Nelson

PEDIATRIC SYMPTOM-BASED DIAGNOSIS

Common Diseases and their Mimics

EDITION

2

Nelson

PEDIATRIC SYMPTOM-BASED DIAGNOSIS

Common Diseases and their Mimics

ROBERT M. KLIEGMAN, MD

Professor of Pediatrics
Nelson Service for Undiagnosed and Rare Diseases
Medical College of Wisconsin
Milwaukee, Wisconsin

HEATHER TOTH, MD

Professor of Pediatrics
Program Director, Internal Medicine-Pediatrics Residency Program
Hospitalist, Departments of Medicine and Pediatrics
Medical College of Wisconsin
Milwaukee, Wisconsin

BRETT J. BORDINI, MD

Associate Professor of Pediatrics
Section of Hospital Medicine
Nelson Service for Undiagnosed and Rare Diseases
Medical College of Wisconsin
Milwaukee, Wisconsin

DONALD BASEL, MD

Professor of Pediatrics
Section Chief, Division of Medical Genetics
Medical College of Wisconsin
Milwaukee, Wisconsin

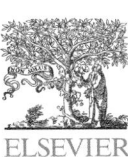

ELSEVIER

Elsevier
1600 John F. Kennedy Blvd.
Ste 1800
Philadelphia, PA 19103-2899

NELSON PEDIATRIC SYMPTOM-BASED DIAGNOSIS, SECOND EDITION ISBN: 978-0-323-76174-1

Notice

Practitioners and researchers must always rely on their own experience and knowledge in evaluating and using any information, methods, compounds or experiments described herein. Because of rapid advances in the medical sciences, in particular, independent verification of diagnoses and drug dosages should be made. To the fullest extent of the law, no responsibility is assumed by Elsevier, authors, editors or contributors for any injury and/or damage to persons or property as a matter of products liability, negligence or otherwise, or from any use or operation of any methods, products, instructions, or ideas contained in the material herein.

Previous edition copyrighted 2018.

International Standard Book Number: 978-0-323-76174-1

Publisher: Sarah Barth
Senior Content Development Specialist: Jennifer Shreiner
Publishing Services Manager: Catherine Jackson
Health Content Management Specialist: Kristine Feeherty
Design Direction: Renee Duenow

Printed in India

Last digit is the print number: 9 8 7 6 5 4 3 2

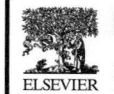

Working together
to grow libraries in
developing countries

www.elsevier.com • www.bookaid.org

This book is dedicated to the residents at Children's Wisconsin.
Their enthusiasm, thirst for knowledge,
and desire to become outstanding pediatricians inspire us.

We further dedicate this textbook to the many patients and their families
who continue to teach us important diagnostic considerations
during their odyssey toward improved health.

CONTRIBUTORS

Omar Ali, MD
Division of Pediatric Endocrinology
Valley Children's Hospital
Madera, California

Louella B. Amos, MD
Associate Professor of Pediatrics
Division of Pulmonary and Sleep
  Medicine
Medical College of Wisconsin
Milwaukee, Wisconsin

Bethany Auble, MD
Assistant Professor of Pediatrics
Medical College of Wisconsin
Milwaukee, Wisconsin

Donald Basel, MD
Professor of Pediatrics
Section Chief, Division of Medical
  Genetics
Medical College of Wisconsin
Milwaukee, Wisconsin

Shannon H. Baumer-Mouradian, MD
Director of Quality Improvement
Assistant Professor of Pediatrics
Medical College of Wisconsin
Milwaukee, Wisconsin

Ashley Beattie, MD
Fellow in Child and Adolescent Psychiatry
Medical University of South Carolina
Charleston, South Carolina

Geetanjali Bora, MD
Fellow in Pediatric Gastroenterology
Medical College of Wisconsin
Milwaukee, Wisconsin

Brett J. Bordini, MD
Associate Professor of Pediatrics
Section of Hospital Medicine
Nelson Service for Undiagnosed and Rare
  Diseases
Medical College of Wisconsin
Milwaukee, Wisconsin

Brian R. Branchford, MD
Assistant Professor of Pediatrics
Division of Pediatric Hematology/Oncology/
  Bone Marrow Transplant
Medical College of Wisconsin
Milwaukee, Wisconsin

Amanda M. Brandow, DO, MS
Associate Professor of Pediatrics
Medical College of Wisconsin
Milwaukee, Wisconsin

Ryan Byrne, MD
Child and Adolescent Psychiatrist
Coastal Empire Community Mental Health
  Center
Beaufort, South Carolina

Gisela G. Chelimsky, MD
Professor of Pediatrics
Medical College of Wisconsin
Division of Pediatric Gastroenterology
Children's Hospital Milwaukee
Milwaukee, Wisconsin

Thomas C. Chelimsky, MD
Professor of Neurology
Medical College of Wisconsin
Milwaukee, Wisconsin

Paula Cody, MD, MPH
Associate Professor of Pediatrics
University of Wisconsin School of Medicine
  and Public Health
Madison, Wisconsin

Gary Cohen, MD, MS
Associate Professor of Pediatrics
Medical College of Wisconsin
Milwaukee, Wisconsin

Deborah M. Costakos, MD, MS
Professor of Ophthalmology
Medical College of Wisconsin
Milwaukee, Wisconsin

Emily M. Densmore, MD, MS
Assistant Professor of Pediatrics
Medical College of Wisconsin
Milwaukee, Wisconsin

John C. Densmore, MD
Professor of Surgery
Medical College of Wisconsin
Milwaukee, Wisconsin

Patricia A. Donohoue, MD
Professor and Section Chief
Pediatric Endocrinology and Diabetes
Medical College of Wisconsin
Milwaukee, Wisconsin

Amy L. Drendel, DO, MS
Professor of Pediatrics
Medical College of Wisconsin
Milwaukee, Wisconsin

Garrett Elsner, MD
Fellow in Child and Adolescent Psychiatry
Medical University of South Carolina
Charleston, South Carolina

Raquel Farias-Moeller, MD
Assistant Professor of Neurology and
  Pediatrics
Medical College of Wisconsin
Milwaukee, Wisconsin

Shayne D. Fehr, MD
Associate Professor of Orthopaedic
  Surgery
Medical College of Wisconsin
Milwaukee, Wisconsin

Susan Feigelman, MD
Professor of Pediatrics
University of Maryland School of
  Medicine
Baltimore, Maryland

Veronica H. Flood, MD
Professor of Pediatrics
Division of Pediatric Hematology/Oncology/
  Bone Marrow Transplant
Medical College of Wisconsin
Milwaukee, Wisconsin

Jessica Francis, MD
Assistant Professor
Director, Residency Program
Department of Obstetrics and
  Gynecology
Medical College of Wisconsin Affiliated
  Hospitals
Milwaukee, Wisconsin

Julia Fritz, MD
Pediatric Gastroenterology
Maine Medical Partners
Portland, Maine

Sandra Gage, MD, PhD
Associate Professor of Pediatrics
University of Arizona College of Medicine -
  Phoenix
Phoenix, Arizona

Bhaskar Gurram, MBBS, MD
Associate Professor of Pediatrics
Division of Pediatric Gastroenterology,
  Hepatology, and Nutrition
University of Texas Southwestern Medical
  Center
Dallas, Texas

Matthew M. Harmelink, MD
Assistant Professor, Section of Child
  Neurology
Department of Neurology
Medical College of Wisconsin
Milwaukee, Wisconsin

Kristen E. Holland, MD
Associate Professor of Dermatology
Medical College of Wisconsin
Milwaukee, Wisconsin

Stephen R. Humphrey, MD
Assistant Professor of Dermatology
Children's Hospital of Wisconsin
Medical College of Wisconsin
Milwaukee, Wisconsin

Anna R. Huppler, MD
Assistant Professor
Pediatrics (Infectious Diseases) and
    Microbiology & Immunology
Medical College of Wisconsin
Milwaukee, Wisconsin

Susan L. Jarosz, DO
Assistant Professor, Pediatric Urology
Baylor College of Medicine
Texas Children's Hospital
Houston, Texas

S. Anne Joseph, MD
Attending Physician
Neurology
Associate Professor of Pediatrics
Northwestern University Feinberg School of
    Medicine
Chicago, Illinois

Alvina R. Kansra, MD
Associate Professor of Pediatrics
Medical College of Wisconsin
Wauwatosa, Wisconsin

Virginia Keane, MD
Mt. Washington Pediatric Hospital
Baltimore, Maryland

Robert M. Kliegman, MD
Professor of Pediatrics
Nelson Service for Undiagnosed and Rare
    Diseases
Medical College of Wisconsin
Milwaukee, Wisconsin

Julie M. Kolinski, MD
Assistant Professor
Department of Pediatrics and Internal
    Medicine
Medical College of Wisconsin
Milwaukee, Wisconsin

Chamindra G. Konersman, MD
Associate Professor of Neurosciences
University of California, San Diego
San Diego, California

Kathleen A. Koth, DO, DFAACAP
Associate Professor of Psychiatry and
    Behavioral Medicine
Medical College of Wisconsin
Milwaukee, Wisconsin

Katja Kovacic, MD
Associate Professor of Pediatrics
Division of Pediatric Gastroenterology
Medical College of Wisconsin
Milwaukee, Wisconsin

**Amornluck Krasaelap,
MD, FAAP**
Assistant Professor of Pediatrics
Children's Mercy Hospital
Kansas City, Missouri

John V. Kryger, MD
Chief of Pediatric Urology
Children's Hospital of Wisconsin
Professor
Department of Urology
Medical College of Wisconsin
Milwaukee, Wisconsin

Sara M. Lauck, MD
Assistant Professor of Pediatrics
Medical College of Wisconsin
Milwaukee, Wisconsin

Tracey H. Liljestrom, MD
Assistant Professor of Medicine and Pediatrics
Medical College of Wisconsin
Milwaukee, Wisconsin

Ahmad Marashly, MD
Assistant Professor
Department of Neurology
University of Washington/Seattle Children's
    Hospital
Seattle, Washington

Seema Menon, MD
Pediatric and Adolescent Gynecology
    Program Director, Children's Hospital of
    Wisconsin
Associate Professor
Obstetrics and Gynecology
Medical College of Wisconsin
Milwaukee, Wisconsin

Adrian Miranda, MD
Professor of Pediatrics
Division of Pediatric Gastroenterology,
    Hepatology, and Nutrition
Medical College of Wisconsin
Milwaukee, Wisconsin

Michelle L. Mitchell, MD
Assistant Professor of Pediatrics
Division of Pediatric Infectious
    Diseases
Medical College of Wisconsin
Milwaukee, Wisconsin

Amy Moskop, MD, MS
Assistant Professor
Pediatric Bone Marrow Transplant and
    Cellular Therapy
Medical College of Wisconsin
Milwaukee, Wisconsin

Michael Muriello, MD
Assistant Professor of Pediatric Genetics
Medical College of Wisconsin
Milwaukee, Wisconsin

James J. Nocton, MD
Professor of Pediatrics
Medical College of Wisconsin
Milwaukee, Wisconsin

Joshua Noe, MD
Associate Professor of Pediatric
    Gastroenterology, Hepatology, and
    Nutrition
Department of Pediatrics
Medical College of Wisconsin
Milwaukee, Wisconsin

Cynthia G. Pan, MD
Professor
Department of Pediatrics
Medical College of Wisconsin
Milwaukee, Wisconsin

Andrew N. Pelech, MD
Professor of Pediatrics
University of California, Davis
Sacramento, California

Brittany Player, DO, MS
Fellow
Section Pediatric Infectious Disease
Medical College of Wisconsin
Milwaukee, Wisconsin

Jacquelyn M. Powers, MD, MS
Assistant Professor of Pediatrics
Baylor College of Medicine
Houston, Texas

Angela L. Rabbitt, DO
Associate Professor of Pediatrics
Medical College of Wisconsin
Milwaukee, Wisconsin

Amanda Rogers, MD
Assistant Professor of Pediatrics
Medical College of Wisconsin
Milwaukee, Wisconsin

John M. Routes, MD
Professor of Pediatrics
Medical College of Wisconsin
Milwaukee, Wisconsin

Mark Simms, MD, MPH
Emeritus Professor of Pediatrics
Medical College of Wisconsin
Milwaukee, Wisconsin

Rajasree Sreedharan, MD
Associate Professor
Pediatrics/Nephrology
Medical College of Wisconsin
Wauwatosa, Wisconsin

Alyssa Stephany, MD, SFHM, FAAP
Associate Professor
University of Kansas School of Medicine
Associate Professor
University of Missouri-Kansas City School
    of Medicine
Children's Mercy Kansas City
Kansas City, Missouri

Julie Talano, MD
Professor of Pediatrics
Pediatric Bone Marrow Transplant and
    Cellular Therapy
Medical College of Wisconsin
Milwaukee, Wisconsin

Grzegorz W. Telega, MD
Associate Professor of Pediatrics
Medical College of Wisconsin
Milwaukee, Wisconsin

Heather Toth, MD
Professor of Pediatrics
Program Director, Internal Medicine-
    Pediatrics Residency Program
Hospitalist, Departments of Medicine and
    Pediatrics
Medical College of Wisconsin
Milwaukee, Wisconsin

Scott K. Van Why, MD
Professor
Department of Pediatrics
Medical College of Wisconsin
Milwaukee, Wisconsin

Sarah Vepraskas, MD
Associate Professor of Pediatrics
Section of Hospital Medicine
Medical College of Wisconsin
Milwaukee, Wisconsin

James W. Verbsky, MD, PhD
Professor of Pediatrics
Medical College of Wisconsin
Milwaukee, Wisconsin

Bernadette Vitola, MD, MPH
Associate Professor of Pediatrics
Pediatric Gastroenterology, Hepatology, and
    Nutrition
Medical College of Wisconsin
Milwaukee, Wisconsin

Kevin D. Walter, MD, FAAP
Associate Professor of Pediatric Orthopedics
    and Pediatric Sports Medicine
Medical College of Wisconsin
Milwaukee, Wisconsin

Michael Weisgerber, MD, MS
Associate Professor of Pediatrics
Section of Hospital Medicine
Program Director, Pediatric Residency
    Program
Program Director, Pediatric-Anesthesia
    Combined Program
Medical College of Wisconsin
Milwaukee, Wisconsin

Peter M. Wolfgram, MD
Associate Professor of Pediatrics
Medical College of Wisconsin
Milwaukee, Wisconsin

Sarah C. Yale, MD
Assistant Professor of Pediatrics
Medical College of Wisconsin
Division of Hospital Medicine
Children's Wisconsin
Milwaukee, Wisconsin

Alicia C. Zolkoske, MD
Assistant Professor of Orthopaedic
    Surgery
Medical College of Wisconsin
Milwaukee, Wisconsin

This book is intended to help the reader begin with a specific chief complaint that may be seen in many different disease entities. It is arranged in chapters that cover specific symptoms mirroring clinical practice. For example, patients do not usually present with a chief complaint of cystic fibrosis; rather, they may present with a cough, respiratory distress, or chronic diarrhea.

With a user-friendly, well-tabulated, illustrated approach, this text will help the reader differentiate between the many disease states causing a common symptom. The inclusion of many original tables and figures will help the reader identify distinguishing features of diseases and work through a diagnostic approach to the symptom. Modified and borrowed figures and tables from other outstanding current sources have been added as well. The combination of these illustrations and tables with diagnostic clues within the text will help provide a quick visual guide to the differential diagnosis of the various diseases under discussion. The diagnostic approach includes standard laboratory and radiologic testing, as well as advanced imaging studies and genetic-based analysis.

In addition, we have incorporated our experience with patients from our **Undiagnosed and Rare Disease Program** and have included uncommon disorders and those diseases that often remain undiagnosed, which may present with common symptoms. Furthermore, we discuss disease mimics or look-alike disorders as well as distinguishing features that may suggest a less common disease presenting with a common symptom.

We appreciate the hard work of our contributing authors. Writing a chapter in this type of format is quite different from writing in the format of a disease-based book. In addition, we thank Sarah Barth, Jennifer Shreiner, and Kristine Feeherty of Elsevier, whose patience and expertise contributed to the publication of this book. We are all also greatly appreciative of Carolyn Redman at the Medical College of Wisconsin Department of Pediatrics, whose editorial assistance and organization have made this new edition a reality. Finally, we are ever grateful for the understanding and patience of Diane Basel, Jessica Bordini, Ryan Festerling, and Sharon Kliegman in supporting this work.

CONTENTS

Nelson

PEDIATRIC SYMPTOM-BASED DIAGNOSIS

Common Diseases and their Mimics

Disease Mimics: An Approach to Undiagnosed Diseases

Brett J. Bordini and Donald Basel

"Getting the right diagnosis is a key aspect of health care, as it provides an explanation of a patient's health problem and informs subsequent health care decisions."
The Institute of Medicine; The National Academies of Sciences, Engineering, and Medicine, 2015

At its core, medicine is committed to identifying, preventing, and treating disease to maintain or restore health. Fundamental to this commitment is **diagnosis**, the process of uncovering the cause of a patient's health-related concerns. Patients rarely present to their physicians with a diagnosis already identified, even with the widespread and increasing availability of health-related information and technology. Rather, patients present with a **symptom**: a subjective physical finding, sensation, or phenomenon that indicates to them that they may no longer be in their baseline state of health. A symptom may be accompanied by a **sign**: an objective finding on physical examination, laboratory investigation, or imaging study that indicates an abnormal deviation from homeostasis. Some signs, like elevated blood pressure, may not be associated with any noticeable symptoms. While not all symptoms or signs denote underlying pathophysiology, their mere presence is often unsettling to the person experiencing them, requiring either reassurance in instances of benign etiologies or a specific diagnosis and management plan in instances of pathology. Diagnosis is the process by which the health care team uncovers the precise explanation for those symptoms and signs so as to inform any subsequent health care–related decisions. The diagnostic process is complex, *iterative, collaborative*, often subject to revision, and fraught with the possibility of *diagnostic error*, yet when properly engaged holds the potential for restoring a patient to health.

DIAGNOSIS: IT ALL STARTS WITH A SYMPTOM

While asymptomatic individuals may have abnormalities detected on screening investigations, most patients enter into the diagnostic process by virtue of symptoms. With the exception of certain pathognomonic findings, such as Koplik spots in measles, presenting features rarely correlate directly and discretely to one individual disease process. It is up to the diagnostician to methodically gather information, categorizing and assigning importance to each historical and physical finding, noting both what is present and what is absent, so that this information can define the patient's **phenotype**, the unique constellation of subjective and objective information indicating the functional health status of the patient, how current physiology differs in ways that may suggest pathology, and the context in which these changes are occurring. Establishing this phenotype is the starting point for developing a structured working **differential diagnosis**, the possible diseases and mechanisms by which the patient's symptoms are produced, which then drives additional investigation. This process is not random but rather has evolved through years of collective experience and analysis into the evidence-based standard of care (Fig. 1.1). Advances in medical science have been accompanied by refinements and improvements in diagnosis, ranging from enhanced understanding of physiology, allowing for more rapid and sophisticated identification of pathology, to the development of diagnostic technologies, such as MRI, molecular genetic assays, or the use of data aggregation and machine learning, allowing for the implementation of artificial intelligence–assisted diagnosis (Fig. 1.2).

DIAGNOSIS AS AN ITERATIVE PROCESS

Diagnosis is an *iterative* process, progressing in a stepwise fashion from an undifferentiated primary medical concern, or chief complaint, to an identified cause of the patient's concerns with an associated management plan. The iterative process often requires one to go back to the beginning and, based on new data from the history, physical exam, imaging, or diagnostic tests, to re-evaluate the original hypothesis. Regardless of the ways in which diagnostic techniques and modalities have advanced over time, the fundamental components of diagnosis remain relatively unchanged and begin with establishing the history of the presenting concern.

History

The goal of obtaining the medical history is to develop a comprehensive yet concise narrative summary of the patient's primary health concern, while placing that concern in the context of the patient's past medical history, determining what social and environmental factors may be contributing to the patient's health, eliciting which health conditions may have a familial tendency, and delineating what other symptoms or signs may be associated with the presenting concern. The scope of history gathering during any patient encounter is highly individualized and depends on both the clinician's experience and the circumstances of the encounter; for example, an annual health supervision visit in an

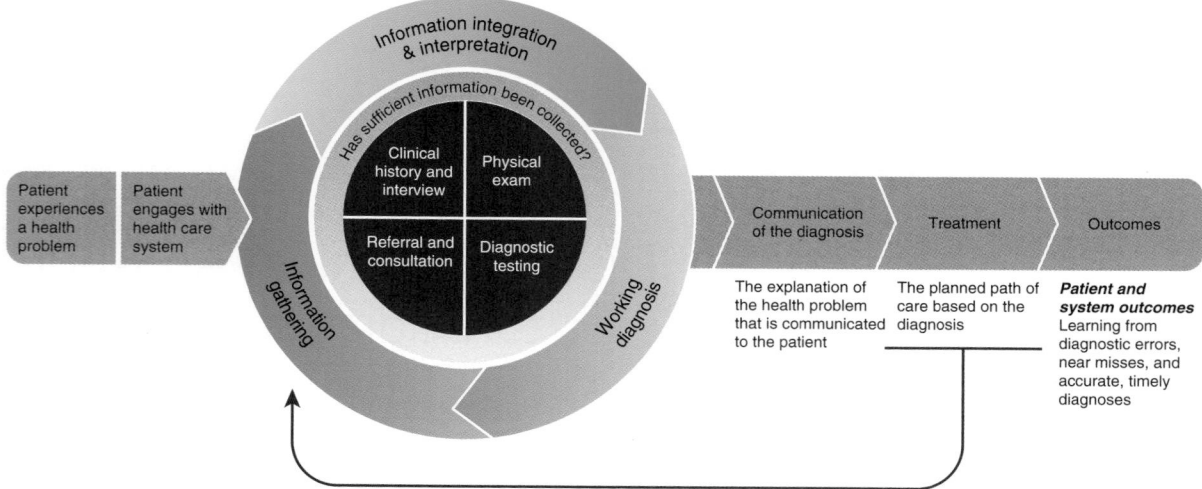

Fig. 1.1 An overview of the diagnostic process. (From Balogh EP, Miller BT, Ball JR, Committee on Diagnostic Error in Health Care; Board on Health Care Services; Institute of Medicine. *Improving Diagnosis in Health Care*. Washington, DC: National Academies Press; December 29, 2015: Fig. 2.1.)

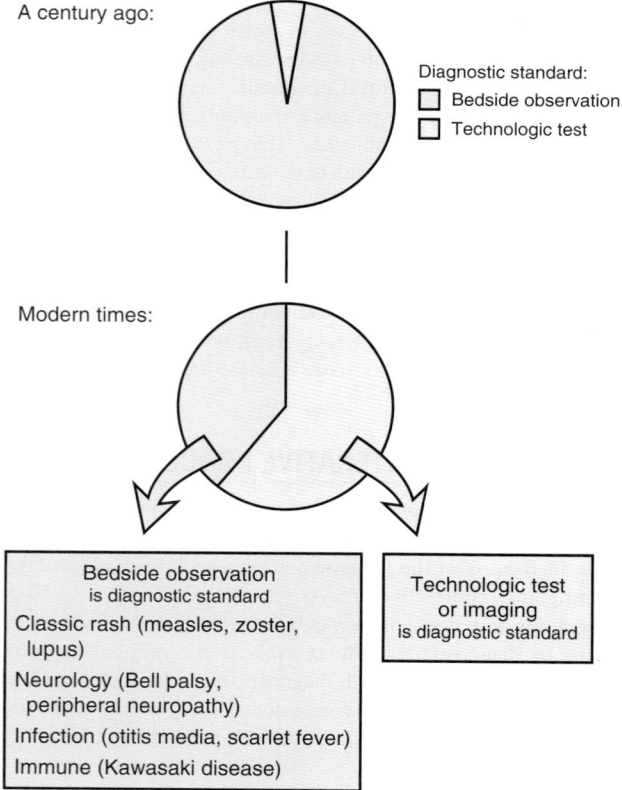

Fig. 1.2 The evolution of the diagnostic evaluation over time and with advances in diagnostic technology. (Modified from McGee S. *Evidence-Based Physical Diagnosis*. 3rd ed. Philadelphia: Elsevier; 2012.)

outpatient clinic and an emergency department visit for acute lateralized weakness would generate vastly different sets of questions.

While matching the pace and scope of history gathering to the acuity of the patient's presentation, the physician should conduct the medical interview in a manner that establishes trust, confidence, and rapport with the patient; creates sufficient space for the patient to tell the story; and focuses on eliciting high-yield information in a timely fashion. To accomplish these aims, a combination of patient-driven, clinician-driven, and evidence-based medical interview techniques are employed. Typically, these interview styles are not implemented in isolation, but rather are blended to nurture conversational flow while allowing for comprehensive information gathering. The patient-centered portions focus on encouraging the patient to express what is most important, while the clinician-centered portions allow the physician to expand, clarify, and refine the history so that it is both comprehensive and specific. Evidence-based elements allow for probing aspects of the history and physical examination with higher-yield questions that help distinguish diagnostic possibilities with a high likelihood from those with a lower likelihood. This discrimination is best accomplished through the use of *key pointer questions*. These questions are often disease or specialty specific and are designed to tease out the nuances of relevant or pertinent information during history taking. When deciding if a suggestive history and physical examination are consistent with Kawasaki disease, a rheumatologist knows to investigate not simply whether the patient does or does not have conjunctivitis, but rather whether conjunctivitis is purulent (exclude), nonpurulent (include), limbic sparing (include), or not (exclude). Such questions leverage high likelihood ratios for crucial aspects of the history and physical examination to allow for more rapid refinement of the differential diagnosis (Fig. 1.3).

In addition to providing crucial information regarding the patient's concerns, the medical history is an interactive process that allows the clinician to establish rapport and hopefully to avoid scenarios in which the patient or family state that the clinician "is a good doctor but never listens to what I say." Building trust, setting expectations, and establishing the primacy of the patient-clinician relationship can be just as crucial as collecting informative data. Listening and being aware of nonverbal cues such as vocal inflection and body language can inform the data collection process as much as directive questioning. In some cases, obtaining that critical piece of information is highly dependent on the tone of the relationship between the two parties.

The medical history, and the quality of data obtained from it, can also be enhanced by the electronic medical record and the ways in which technology has evolved to facilitate good patient care and a good patient experience. *Pre-charting*, or familiarizing oneself with what is already known of the patient's medical history, should be encouraged for any

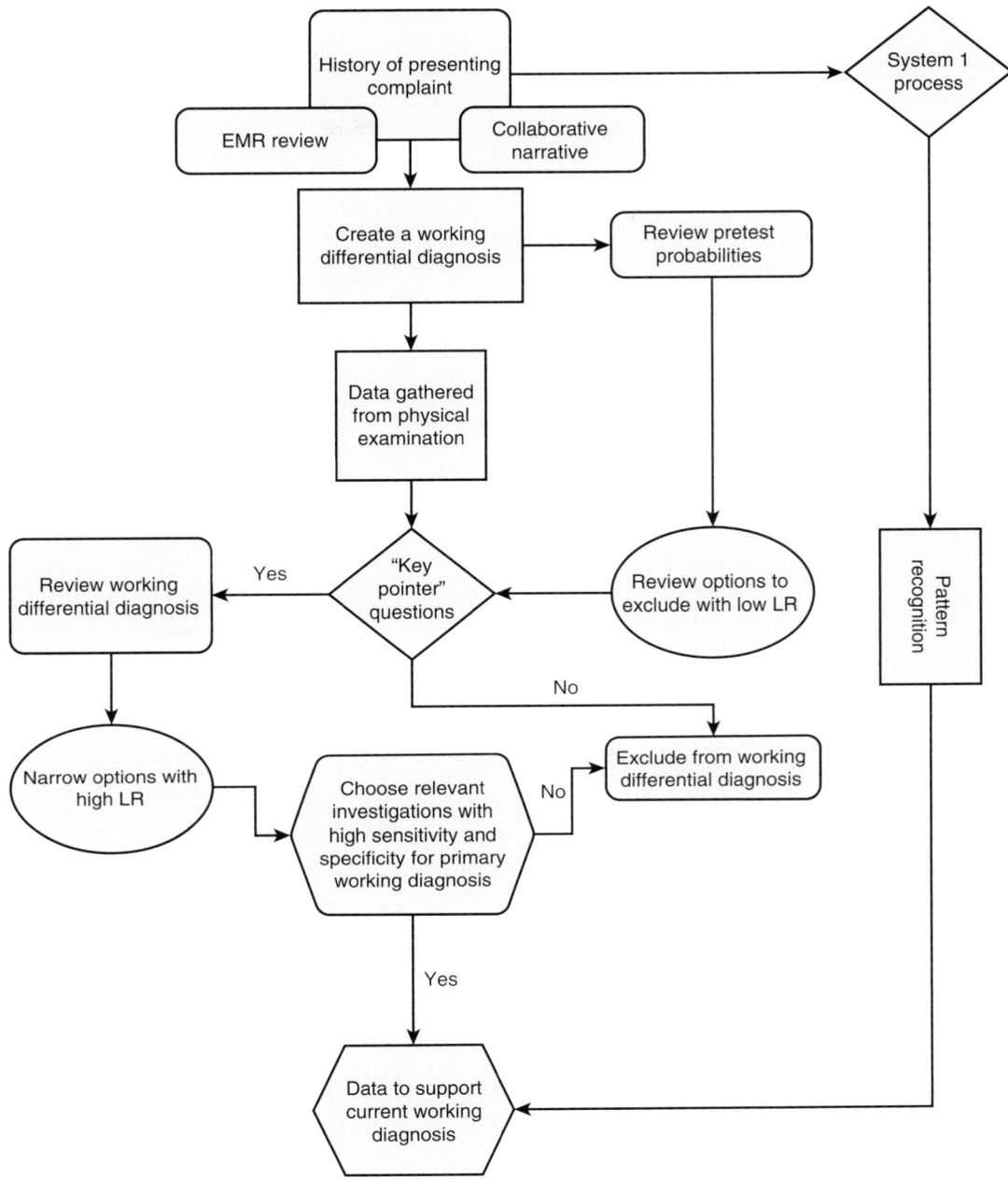

Fig. 1.3 The use of "key pointer" questions in developing a deliberate and analytical diagnosis. EMR, electronic medical record; LR, likelihood ratio.

nonurgent health visit, as a comprehensive chart review can save a significant amount of time during the patient encounter and can create an immediate sense of clinician engagement for the patient, wherein the patient knows that the physician has taken an interest in and has an immediate knowledge of the past history. This preparatory information should always be confirmed though, as diagnostic labels and medical problem lists can sometimes be inaccurate and perpetuate incorrect information about the patient that can increase the risk of diagnostic error.

Physical Examination

While advances in medical technology have changed the degree to which diagnosis is solely reliant on physical examination findings, comprehensive physical examination remains a cornerstone in identifying key phenotypic features that can then be further informed by

applying appropriate technologic testing (see Fig. 1.2). The office visit is a snapshot in time of the person being evaluated, and not all pertinent features are necessarily present for this evaluation: a fever noted at home may resolve or a rash may fade by the time of the appointment; new features may evolve following the medical evaluation. These reported findings, even if not present during the actual physical examination, should still be considered in the diagnostic formulation, given that many diseases and their associated findings are dynamic.

When examining a patient, the traditional dichotomous concept of "positive" and "negative" findings either supporting or negating the possibility of a diagnosis remains important; however, the presence or absence of findings is not weighted equally and requires the application of evidence to determine significance. When evaluating the significance of a finding or result of a test, there are four concepts to consider:

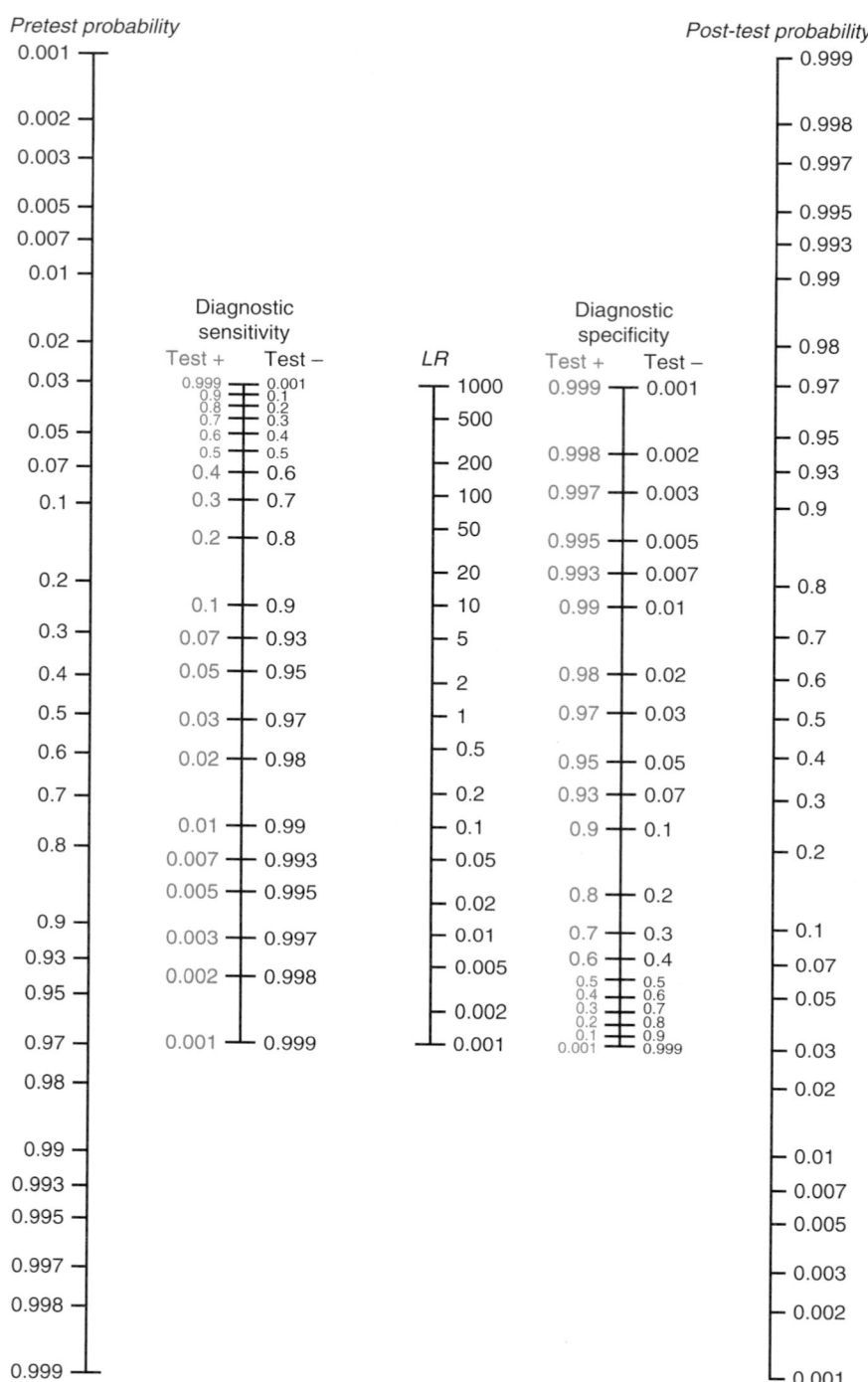

Fig. 1.4 The extended Fagan nomogram for the use of likelihood ratios and pretest probability to determine post-test probability according to Bayes' theorem. LR, likelihood ratio.

pretest probability, sensitivity, specificity, and likelihood ratios (Figs. 1.4 and 1.5).

Pretest Probability

The pretest probability is the general prevalence of the condition within the patient population being evaluated. In this context it is the population risk prior to any bias of the examination or testing.

Sensitivity

Sensitivity refers to the ability of a test to correctly identify the presence of disease in a population of people who are affected by the disease.

Specificity

Specificity refers to the ability of a test to accurately identify the absence of disease through a negative test result.

Likelihood Ratio

Likelihood ratios (LRs) synthesize sensitivity and specificity of examination findings or test results to inform the probability of the presence or absence of disease for the individual patient. The greater the absolute value of the LR, the higher the clinical utility of the test in establishing or excluding a particular disease. Thus, it could be seen as a measure of how "useful" a particular test is in the context of the diagnosis in question. Considered from a diagnostic perspective, it is also a measure of the likelihood of the presence or absence of disease in a patient after the test has been performed (i.e., the post-test probability of a specific diagnosis). The accuracy of an LR is entirely dependent on the quality of data used to generate the LR.

Relying purely on clinical findings, without the aid of additional testing, can on occasion lead the physician to the wrong diagnosis. Fever, cough, rhinorrhea, abdominal pain, headache, tonsillar exudate, and palatal petechiae all have low sensitivity and specificity when considering streptococcal pharyngitis, despite being common findings in patients with streptococcal pharyngitis. The positive predictive value of these signs and symptoms is no more than 50%; other clinical features carry more diagnostic weight: sore throat, tonsillar swelling, anterior cervical adenopathy, and scarlatiniform rash have all been shown to have a significant correlation with culture-positive group A β-hemolytic streptococcal pharyngitis. Therefore, it is important to focus on features with high likelihood ratios when formulating differential diagnoses and testing strategies. When doing so, it may be tempting to aggregate likelihood ratios into clinical reasoning, using the post-test probability of one finding to serve as the pretest probability for the next finding, but when using these tools, each point needs to be considered in isolation and cannot be cascaded to inform one another. In addition, diseases are often complex, and thinking of disease paradigms as either present or absent does not account for the real-life variability in clinical presentation and severity that results from the unique interplay between the patient's individual health status and the dynamic nature of many diseases. It is precisely this interplay that can lead to certain unrelated disorders presenting with similar features (**mimic**), or the same disorder presenting differently in different patients or with changing features over time in the same patient (**chameleon**). An example of considering mimics in the differential diagnosis while looking for distinguishing features is noted in Table 1.1. An example of the same disease with different manifestations acting as chameleons is noted in Table 1.2. At the gene level there are multiple genes producing the Noonan phenotype, while one gene (ADA-2 deficiency) may

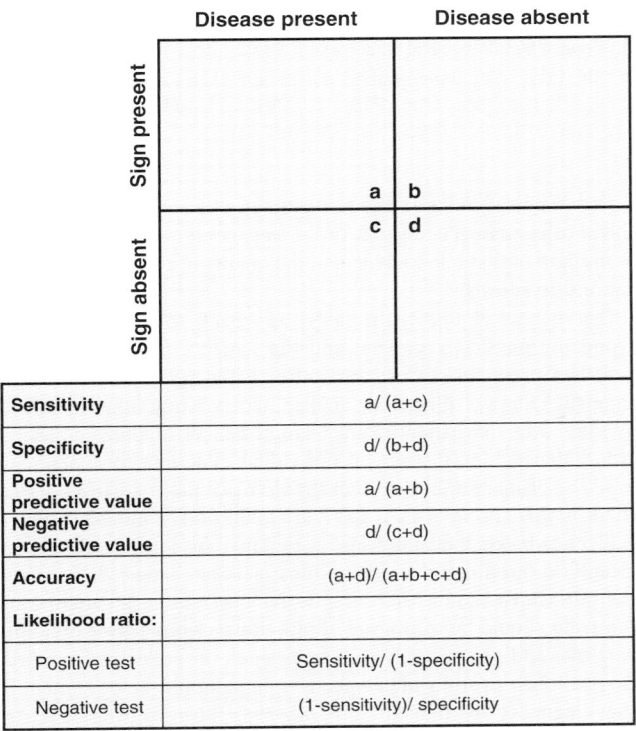

	Disease present	Disease absent
Sign present	a	b
Sign absent	c	d

Sensitivity	a/ (a+c)
Specificity	d/ (b+d)
Positive predictive value	a/ (a+b)
Negative predictive value	d/ (c+d)
Accuracy	(a+d)/ (a+b+c+d)
Likelihood ratio:	
Positive test	Sensitivity/ (1-specificity)
Negative test	(1-sensitivity)/ specificity

Fig. 1.5 Formulas used to calculate sensitivity, specificity, positive predictive value, negative predictive value, accuracy, and likelihood ratios.

TABLE 1.1	MRI Red Flags for the Diagnosis of Children with Acquired Demyelinating Syndromes	
MRI Finding	**Differential Diagnosis**	**Distinguishing Features**
Leptomeningeal enhancement	SVcPACNS Infection Tumor HLH	Leptomeningeal enhancement is not a feature of MS in adults and emerged as a red flag for vasculitic or malignant processes in the pediatric cohort.
Lesion expansion	Tumor Lymphoma PML Sarcoidosis	Increased size of T2 lesions on serial imaging is well recognized in MS, although this should always prompt consideration of malignancy. Increasing size of a white matter–predominant lesion without lesion enhancement in a patient treated with immunosuppressant therapy (or a patient with known HIV) should prompt consideration of PML. PML is a risk for MS patients exposed to more intense immunosuppressive therapies.
Hemorrhage	ANE Stroke Cerebellitis AHLE Large-vessel CNS vasculitis SVcPACNS	Although susceptibility-weighted imaging reveals tiny microfoci of hemosiderin in MS patients, hemorrhage large enough to be visible on conventional MRI sequences is not a feature of ADS or MS and should prompt consideration of disorders in which the cerebral vasculature is specifically involved.

ADS, acquired demyelinating syndrome; AHLE, acute hemorrhagic leukoencephalitis; ANE, acute necrotizing encephalopathy; CNS, central nervous system; HLH, hemophagocytic lymphohistiocytosis; MS, multiple sclerosis; PML, progressive multifocal leukoencephalopathy; SVcPACNS, small-vessel childhood primary angiitis of the central nervous system.
From O'Mahony J, Shroff M, Banwell B. Mimics and rare presentations of pediatric demyelination. *Neuroimag Clin N Am.* 2013;23(2):321–336 (Table 2, p. 323).

TABLE 1.2 Guillain-Barré and Miller Fisher Syndromes and Their Subtypes

Guillain-Barré Syndrome
- Paraparetic variant*
- Pharyngeal-cervical-brachial weakness*

  Acute pharyngeal weakness* †
- Bifacial weakness with paraesthesias*

Miller Fisher Syndrome
- Acute ataxic neuropathy†
- Acute ophthalmoparesis†
- Acute ptosis†
- Acute mydriasis†
- Bickerstaff brainstem encephalitis‡

  Acute ataxic hypersomnolence† ‡

*Localized forms.
†Incomplete forms.
‡Central nervous system form.
From Wakerley BR, Yuki N. Mimics and chameleons in Guillain-Barré and Miller Fischer syndromes. *Pract Neurol.* 2015;15:90–99, Box 1, p. 91.

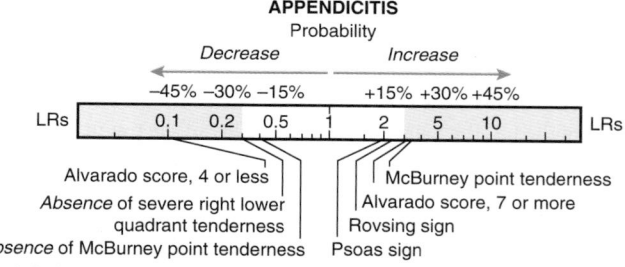

Fig. 1.6 Clinical evidence-based evaluation of the likelihood of appendicitis. LR, likelihood ratio. (From McGee S. *Evidence-Based Physical Diagnosis.* 3rd ed. Philadelphia: Elsevier; 2012.)

produce what appears as unrelated phenotypes (stroke, cytopenias, intestinal lesions). The application of sensitivity, specificity, and LRs thus needs to be judicious, with insight into what is being offered to aid the question at hand. Applied appropriately, these tools offer an established methodology for adjusting disease probability in the context of a specific defined parameter (see Fig. 1.4).

Physical examinations have two paradigms, one in which no additional evidence is required and one that is reliant on advanced testing. Certain presenting disorders remain clinical diagnoses. The diagnosis of otitis media relies on clinical features: the presence of fever along with an erythematous tympanic membrane that has limited mobility on pneumatic otoscopy or a middle ear effusion on visual inspection. Conversely, the definitive diagnosis of a structural malformation in congenital heart disease requires advanced imaging technology such as an echocardiogram to accurately make the diagnosis. When there is a recognized standard-of-care evaluation or investigation that is codependent on the physical findings to achieve a clear clinical diagnosis, this element of the physical examination is considered evidence based. When considering the example of an adolescent biological male presenting to the emergency room with right-sided lower quadrant pain, requesting a pregnancy test is unlikely to yield an informative result as pretest probability is negligible. Rather, applying appropriate clinical reasoning and looking for information to support a more decisive diagnosis may lead to the consideration of appendicitis (Fig. 1.6).

Incorrect application of these diagnostic aids or inaccurate assimilation of phenotypic data forms the basis of diagnostic error. High-quality information, properly synthesized, is important. Diagnostic aids such as artificial intelligence (e.g., machine learning), even when using natural language processing algorithms, require accurate subjective and objective phenotypic data to perform well.

DIAGNOSIS AS A COLLABORATIVE PROCESS AND THE TEAM-BASED APPROACH

The success of any diagnostic endeavor depends on the nature of the relationship forged with the patient, any of the patient's family members or caregivers, and the health care team. The value of any subjective information gathered, whether it be the narrative history of the

primary medical concern, the features and nuances of symptoms, the context of any associated signs, or the impact on daily life, depends on the strength of that relationship and the quality of communication that relationship affords.

The success of this **team-based approach** to diagnosis extends beyond the physician, patient, and the patient's family and caregivers. When presentations are atypical or when patients have endured diagnostic delays or diagnostic errors, incorporating other health care providers into the patient's care team enhances diagnostic accuracy beyond that achieved even by individual experienced expert clinicians. The primary aphorism that should drive the evaluation of every patient is that "none of us is as smart as all of us"; indeed, collective intelligence-based medical decision-making has consistently and significantly outperformed even the most accurate single diagnostician in certain clinical contexts. To the degree possible, each patient evaluation team should be composed of individuals from a wide breadth of disciplines and perspectives so as to broaden the collective knowledge base and solicit a variety of perspectives on pathophysiology and differential diagnoses that may not have otherwise been considered had the patient been evaluated in individual specialty settings. This collaborative and more deliberate approach to diagnosis additionally encourages the generation of multiple diagnostic hypotheses and testing strategies. The end goal and product of this process is the **group phenotype**, in which the evaluation team has collectively—as a *group*—analyzed the patient's primary concerns, physical findings, and objective data into discrete phenotypic phenomena. These phenomena can then be explored further in attempts to uncover hypothesized underlying and unifying pathophysiologic mechanisms that can be investigated with further testing.

Diagnostic Error

Despite the best efforts and intentions of the health care team, the diagnostic process is at risk for error: depending on the clinical setting, diagnostic errors have been identified in up to 15% of patient encounters. Diagnostic error may consist of a missed, delayed, or wrong diagnosis, and the error may be attributable to faults within the structure and function of the health care system, such as the unavailability or inaccuracy of a particular diagnostic modality, or to factors beyond the control of the patient or clinician (e.g., "no fault" error), such as a disease process presenting with such atypical or subtle features as to completely preclude proper diagnosis. Most diagnostic error is attributable to cognitive errors related to **cognitive bias**.

Dual process theory holds that clinicians engaging in medical reasoning typically utilize either a predominantly intuitive approach, termed a **system 1 process**, or a more analytical approach, termed a **system 2 process**. System 1 processes are based in **heuristics**, which rely on pattern recognition and rules of thumb to rapidly sort large amounts of clinical information into an *illness script* that allows for the

TABLE 1.3   Cognitive Biases Related to Heuristic Failure

Bias	Definition
Anchoring	Locking into a diagnosis based on initial presenting features, failing to adjust diagnostic impressions when new information becomes available
Confirmation bias	Looking for and accepting only evidence that confirms a diagnostic impression, rejecting or not seeking contradictory evidence
Diagnostic momentum	Perpetuating a diagnostic label over time, usually by multiple providers both within and across health care systems, despite the label being incomplete or inaccurate
Expertise bias/yin-yang out	Believing that a patient who has already undergone an extensive evaluation will have nothing more to gain from further investigations, despite the possibility that the disease process or diagnostic techniques may have evolved so as to allow for appropriate diagnosis
Overconfidence bias	Believing one knows more than one does, acting on incomplete information or hunches, and prioritizing opinion or authority as opposed to evidence
Premature closure	Accepting the first plausible diagnosis prior to obtaining confirmatory evidence or considering all available evidence; "when the diagnosis is made, thinking stops"
Unpacking principle	Failing to explore primary evidence or data in its entirety and subsequently failing to uncover important facts or findings, such as accepting a biopsy report or imaging study report without reviewing the actual specimen or image

TABLE 1.4   Cognitive Biases Related to Errors of Attribution

Bias	Definition
Affective bias	Allowing emotions to interfere with a diagnosis, either positively or negatively; dislikes of patient types (e.g., "frequent flyers")
Appeal to authority	Deferring to authoritative recommendations from senior, supervising, or "expert" clinicians, independent of the evidentiary support for such recommendations
Ascertainment bias	Maintaining preconceived expectations based on patient or disease stereotypes
Countertransference	Being influenced by positive or negative subjective feelings toward a specific patient
Outcome bias	Minimizing or overemphasizing the significance of a finding or result, often based on subjective feelings about a patient, a desired outcome, or personal confidence in one's own clinical skills; the use of "slightly" to describe abnormal results
Psych-out bias	Maintaining biases about people with presumed mental illness

quick elaboration of a diagnosis. System 2 processes, on the other hand, rely on deliberate counterfactual reasoning and hypothesis generation tailored to individual patient circumstances to arrive at a more robust differential diagnosis. While clinicians predominantly engage system 1 processes and achieve relatively accurate diagnoses for most patients under most circumstances, heuristics can fail when patient presentations are multisystem, atypical, complex, or evolving, instead becoming a form of bias that can result in diagnostic error (Table 1.3). Biases may also be the result of **errors of attribution**, in which perceived characteristics or motivations of patients, family members, or members of the medical evaluation team are given undue weight in the diagnostic formulation. These factors can influence the affective state of the clinician and the integrity of cognition, increasing the likelihood of error. Examples of attribution-related errors are listed in Table 1.4.

Cognitive bias may also be a product of the context in which a diagnostic evaluation takes place. With **context-related biases**, the setting of the diagnostic evaluation influences how clinicians perceive and process the information used in medical decision-making. External factors such as an increased patient volume, higher patient acuity, or staffing shortages, as well as internal factors such as sleep deprivation, stress, and physician burnout, can amplify individual cognitive burden and increase the likelihood of diagnostic error. Independent of cognitive burden, context can introduce bias by causing physicians to consciously or subconsciously de-emphasize relevant information and amplify impertinent information while formulating a diagnosis. Most common among context-related biases is the *framing effect*, in which the manner or setting of a patient's presentation implicitly restricts the breadth of differential diagnoses considered. This framing effect is often more prominent in contexts where patient handoffs occur frequently and diagnostic labels can take on an independent momentum, leaving little opportunity for physicians to challenge their appropriateness, or in specialty care settings, where patient symptoms are more likely to be considered primarily within the scope of that specialty's pathophysiologic mechanisms. Specialty-specific settings may also increase the risk of *availability bias*, in which familiar and more frequently encountered diagnoses are more readily recalled and are given greater weight in the differential diagnosis. When framing effects and availability heuristics are invoked early, they may perpetuate anchoring biases and result in a diagnostic momentum that precludes consideration of alternate diagnoses, producing both erroneous diagnoses and significant delays in proper diagnosis. Further examples of context-related biases are listed in Table 1.5.

The Well-Calibrated Diagnostician

Effective diagnosis extends beyond applying factual recall to the information gathered from a standardized medical history and instead requires the integration of experiential knowledge with individualized information derived from the patient, family, members of the care team, and diagnostic testing to develop diagnostic considerations based on evidence. The general challenge is being able to access information quickly, at the appropriate time, and in a manner that enables seamless patient care. It is not uncommon that clinicians need to engage these more analytical diagnostic approaches while simultaneously focusing on and reacting to tenuous physiology in a critically ill patient. Under circumstances such as these, determining whether the patient warrants a more deliberate, analytical evaluation may be difficult. Confidence

TABLE 1.5   Cognitive Biases Related to Errors of Context

Bias	Definition
Availability bias	Basing decisions on the most recent patient with similar symptoms, preferentially recalling recent and more common diseases
Base-rate neglect	Over- or underestimating the prevalence of a disease, typically overestimating the prevalence of common diseases and underestimating the prevalence of rare diseases
Framing effect	Being influenced by how or by whom a problem is described, or by the setting in which the evaluation takes place
Frequency bias	Believing that common things happen commonly and are usually benign in general practice
Hindsight bias	Reinforcing diagnostic errors once a diagnosis is discovered in spite of these errors; may lead to clinicians overestimating the efficacy of their clinical reasoning and may reinforce ineffective techniques
Posterior probability error	Considering the likelihood of a particular diagnosis in light of a patient's prior or chronic illnesses (new headaches in a patient with a history of migraines may in fact be a tumor)
Representative bias	Basing decisions on an expected typical presentation; not effective for atypical presentations; overemphasis on disease diagnostic criteria or "classic" presentations; "looks like a duck, quacks like a duck"
Sutton's slip	Ignoring alternate explanations for "obvious" diagnoses (Sutton's law is that one should first consider the obvious)
Thinking in silo	Restricting diagnostic considerations to a particular specialty or organ system; each discipline has a set of diseases within its comfort zone, which reduces diagnostic flexibility or team-based communication
Zebra retreat	Lacking conviction to pursue rare disorders even when suggested by evidence

in a proposed or working diagnosis may bias or impede consideration for a more appropriate diagnosis. The degree of concordance between diagnostic confidence and diagnostic accuracy is termed **diagnostic calibration**. Given the magnitude of this challenge, in the context of a busy service, be it the intensive care unit, emergency room, or routine office visit in the middle of a pandemic, a variety of cognitive biases may result in poor diagnostic calibration, as a result of either bias-induced overconfidence or cognitive burden–related complacency, in which a clinician may be aware of the possibility of diagnostic error but underestimates or trivializes its frequency or impact. One mechanism to avoid such diagnostic errors is the **diagnostic timeout**. When the natural history or progression of an illness fails to conform to the original diagnosis, or when new physical examination, laboratory, or imaging findings contradict that diagnosis or suggest alternate diagnoses, the entire diagnostic formulation must be re-evaluated without being anchored to the original and possibly wrong diagnosis (Table 1.6).

These biases may interfere with the ability to recognize when a patient's physiology or response to treatment fails to support the

TABLE 1.6   Diagnostic Timeout

- Identify the clinical issues, dilemmas, or concerns needing a timeout.
- Remove all previous diagnoses and re-examine all labs, imaging, and other information including the history and physical exam.
- Did we consider the risks of heuristic (intuitive) thinking? (See Table 1.3.)
- Do we have biases? (See Tables 1.4 and 1.5.)
- What are the diseases we must not miss?

proposed diagnosis, such as when a child with known asthma does not respond to bronchodilation in the treatment room and aspiration of a foreign body is not considered, or when difficulty ventilating indicates interstitial lung disease or surfactant protein deficiency as opposed to bronchopulmonary dysplasia in a neonate. Revisiting the initial working diagnosis and reassessing when these red flags indicate a parallel diagnosis is an essential part of nurturing the skills required to being a well-calibrated diagnostician.

SUMMARY AND RED FLAGS

Diagnosis most often begins with a symptom and is a complex, iterative, and collaborative process. Despite the incorporation of evidence-based tools, the risk of diagnostic error is always present and most often results from cognitive biases that can lead the clinician to de-emphasize relevant clinical information or overemphasize impertinent findings. The path from symptom to diagnosis is rarely straightforward, and it is improved by building strong relationships with patients, employing a team-based approach whenever possible, and being aware of the cognitive biases that can increase the risk of

diagnostic error. Clinicians should also be aware of and consider rarer disorders that may *mimic* more common diseases, as well as atypical, variable, or slowly evolving presentations of common diseases (*chameleons*). When presentations are complex or confounding, pausing the diagnostic process to engage more deliberate analytical approaches is warranted. One must always consider the complexity of the diagnostic process and emphasize the importance of developing a differential diagnosis that includes common disorders, atypical presentations, imitative mimics, and rare zebras.

BIBLIOGRAPHY

A bibliography is available at ExpertConsult.com.

2

Sore Throat

Sarah C. Yale

Most causes of sore throat are nonbacterial and neither require nor are alleviated by antibacterial therapy (Tables 2.1, 2.2, and 2.3). Accurate diagnosis is essential. Acute streptococcal pharyngitis warrants proper diagnosis and prompt therapy to prevent serious suppurative and nonsuppurative sequelae. Life-threatening complications of oropharyngeal infections, whether caused by streptococci or other pathogens, may manifest initially with poorly differentiated symptoms of mouth pain and pharyngitis and then extend into the parapharyngeal space, cause jugular venous thrombophlebitis, or result in critical airway obstruction (Tables 2.4 and 2.5). Noninfectious causes of sore throat, such as solid tumors, hematologic malignancy, or Kawasaki disease, if not appropriately diagnosed, may similarly carry a high risk of morbidity and even mortality. In most cases, history and physical examination identify the etiology of a sore throat or sufficiently narrow the differential diagnosis so as to direct an evaluation strategy or empiric treatment. **It is important to note that in many of these diseases sore throat is not the defining symptom but part of a systemic illness (e.g., measles, COVID-19, Kawasaki disease).**

VIRAL PHARYNGITIS

Most episodes of pharyngitis are caused by viruses (see Tables 2.2 and 2.3). It is difficult to precisely distinguish between viral and bacterial pharyngitis on clinical grounds, though certain clues may help. Accompanying findings of rhinitis, conjunctivitis, cough, croup, laryngitis, or discrete oropharyngeal ulcerations are common with viral infection but are rare in bacterial pharyngitis (Table 2.6).

Many viruses can produce pharyngitis (see Tables 2.2 and 2.3). Some cause distinct clinical syndromes that are readily diagnosed without laboratory testing (Table 2.7; see also Tables 2.1 and 2.4). In pharyngitis caused by parainfluenza viruses, influenza viruses, rhinoviruses, coronaviruses, and respiratory syncytial viruses, symptoms of coryza and cough often overshadow sore throat, which is generally mild. Parainfluenza viruses are associated with croup and bronchiolitis; minor sore throat and signs of pharyngitis are common at the outset but rapidly resolve. Influenza infection is often associated with high fever, cough, headache, malaise, myalgia, and cervical adenopathy in addition to pharyngitis. In young children, croup or bronchiolitis may develop. When influenza is suspected on clinical and epidemiologic grounds or confirmed by testing (polymerase chain reaction [PCR] is most accurate), specific antiviral therapy is available for treatment of

patients and prophylaxis of family members and other close contacts. In young children, respiratory syncytial virus (RSV) infection is associated with bronchiolitis and, to a lesser degree, pneumonia and croup. In older children, RSV infection is usually indistinguishable from a simple upper respiratory tract infection. Pharyngitis is not a prominent finding of RSV infection in any age group. Infections caused by parainfluenza, influenza, and RSV are often seen in seasonal (winter) epidemics. *Many viral pathogens can be identified using multiplex or targeted PCR testing, but there is rarely reason to test patients in the outpatient setting and infrequent benefit to testing in the inpatient setting, except to confirm and treat influenza.*

Adenoviruses can cause upper and lower respiratory tract disease, ranging from ordinary colds to severe pneumonia and multisystem disease, including hepatitis, myocarditis, and myositis. The incubation period of adenovirus infection is 2–4 days. Upper respiratory tract infection typically produces fever, erythema of the pharynx, and follicular hyperplasia of the tonsils, together with exudate. Enlargement of the cervical lymph nodes occurs frequently. When conjunctivitis occurs in association with adenoviral pharyngitis, the resulting syndrome is called **pharyngoconjunctival fever**. Pharyngitis may last as long as 7 days and does not respond to antibacterials. There are many adenovirus serotypes; adenovirus infections may therefore develop in children more than once. Outbreaks have been associated with swimming pools and contamination in health care workers. If obtained, laboratory studies may reveal a leukocytosis and an elevated ESR.

The **enteroviruses** can cause sore throat. High fever is common, and the throat is mildly erythematous; tonsillar exudate and cervical adenopathy are unusual. Symptoms usually resolve within a few days. Enteroviruses historically were classified as nonpolio enteroviruses, coxsackie A viruses, coxsackie B viruses, and echoviruses, though with increasing recognition of the multitude of enterovirus serotypes they are now numbered consecutively as novel serotypes are identified. Enteroviruses can also cause meningitis, acute flaccid myelitis, myocarditis, rash, and two specific syndromes that involve the oropharynx: herpangina and hand-foot-mouth disease. **Herpangina** is characterized by distinctive discrete, painful, gray-white papulovesicular lesions distributed over the posterior oropharynx (see Table 2.7). The vesicles are 1–2 mm in diameter and are initially surrounded by a halo of erythema before they ulcerate (Fig. 2.1). Fevers are typically present at illness onset, last several days before abating, and may reach 39.5°C or higher. The illness is typically caused by coxsackie A viruses and

TABLE 2.1   Etiology of Sore Throat

Infection

Bacterial (see Tables 2.2 and 2.3)
Viral (see Tables 2.2 and 2.3)
Fungal (see Table 2.3)
Neutropenic mucositis (invasive anaerobic mouth flora)
Tonsillitis
Epiglottitis
Uvulitis
Tracheitis
Peritonsillar abscess (quinsy)
Retropharyngeal abscess (prevertebral space)
Ludwig angina (submandibular space)
Lateral pharyngeal space cellulitis or abscess
Buccal space cellulitis
Suppurative thyroiditis
Lemierre syndrome (septic jugular thrombophlebitis)
Vincent angina (mixed anaerobic bacteria–gingivitis–pharyngitis)

Irritation

Cigarette or electronic cigarette/vaping use
Inhaled irritants; occupational, environmental
Reflux esophagitis
Allergic rhinitis
Chemical toxins (caustic agents including household cleaners, laundry
   detergent pods)
Medications
Paraquat ingestion
Smog, air pollutants
Dry, hot air
Hot foods, liquids
Shouting

Other

Tumor, including Kaposi sarcoma, leukemia
Granulomatosis with polyangiitis (formerly Wegener granulomatosis)
Sarcoidosis
Glossopharyngeal neuralgia
Foreign body
Stylohyoid syndrome
Behçet disease
Kawasaki disease
Posterior pharyngeal trauma—pseudodiverticulum
Pneumomediastinum with air dissection
Hematoma
Systemic lupus erythematosus
Bullous pemphigoid
Syndrome of periodic fever, aphthous stomatitis, pharyngitis, cervical
   adenitis (PFAPA)

TABLE 2.2   Infectious Etiology of Pharyngitis

Definite Causes

Streptococcus pyogenes (group A streptococci)
Corynebacterium diphtheriae
Arcanobacterium haemolyticum
Neisseria gonorrhoeae
Epstein-Barr virus
HIV (primary infection)
Parainfluenza viruses (types 1–4)
Influenza viruses
Rhinoviruses
Enteroviruses
Coronavirus, including SARS-CoV-2
Adenovirus (types 3, 4, 7, 14, 21, others)
Respiratory syncytial virus
Herpes simplex virus (types 1, 2)

Probable or Occasional Causes

Group C streptococci
Group G streptococci
Chlamydia pneumoniae
Chlamydia trachomatis
Mycoplasma pneumoniae
Toxoplasma gondii

SARS-CoV-2, severe acute respiratory syndrome-coronavirus 2.

TABLE 2.3   Additional Potential Pathogens Associated with Sore Throat

Bacteria

Fusobacterium necrophorum (Lemierre syndrome)
Neisseria meningitidis
Yersinia enterocolitica
Tularemia (oropharyngeal)
Yersinia pestis
Bacillus anthracis
Chlamydia psittaci
Secondary syphilis
Mycobacterium tuberculosis
Lyme disease
Corynebacterium ulcerans
Leptospira species
Mycoplasma hominis
Coxiella burnetii

Virus

Cytomegalovirus
Viral hemorrhagic fevers
HIV (primary infection)
Human herpesvirus 6
Measles
Varicella
Rubella

Fungus

Candida species
Histoplasmosis
Cryptococcosis

generally lasts <7 days, but severe pain may impair fluid intake and occasionally necessitates medical support. **Hand-foot-mouth disease** is also caused by enteroviruses, most commonly coxsackievirus A16. Painful vesicles that ulcerate can occur throughout the oropharynx, as opposed to the lesions of herpangina, which tend to be restricted to the posterior oropharynx. Vesicles also develop on the palms and soles and, less often, on the trunk, extremities, or diaper region (Fig. 2.2). Fever is present in most cases, but many children do not appear seriously ill. Illness typically lasts <7 days.

Primary infection caused by **herpes simplex virus (HSV)** (Fig. 2.3) usually produces high fever with acute gingivostomatitis, involving

TABLE 2.4   Distinguishing Features of Parapharyngeal–Upper Respiratory Tract Infections

	Peritonsillar Abscess	Retropharyngeal Abscess (Cellulitis)	Submandibular Space (Ludwig Angina)*	Lateral Pharyngeal Space	Masticator Space*	Epiglottitis	Laryngotracheobronchitis (Croup)	Bacterial Tracheitis	Postanginal Sepsis (Lemierre Syndrome)
Etiology	Group A streptococci, oral anaerobes†	Staphylococcus aureus, oral anaerobes,† group A streptococci, "suppurative adenitis"	Oral anaerobes†	Oral anaerobes†	Oral anaerobes†	Haemophilus influenzae type b (rarely), group A streptococci, Streptococcus pneumoniae, Staphylococcus aureus, and non–type b H. influenzae	Parainfluenza virus; influenza, adenovirus, and respiratory syncytial virus less common	Moraxella catarrhalis, S. aureus, H. influenzae type b or nontypeable	Fusobacterium necrophorum
Age	Teens	Infancy, preteens, occasionally teens	Teens	Teens	Teens	2–5 yr	3 mo–3 yr	3–10 yr	Teens
Manifestations	Initial episode of pharyngitis, followed by sudden worsening of unilateral odynophagia, trismus, hot potato (muffled) voice, drooling, displacement of uvula	Fever, dyspnea, stridor, dysphagia, drooling, stiff neck, cervical pain, adenopathy, swelling of posterior pharyngeal space Descending mediastinitis (rare) Lateral neck radiograph reveals swollen retropharyngeal prevertebral space: infants, >1× width of adjacent vertebral body (>2–7 mm); teens, >1/3× width of vertebral body (>1–7 mm) CT distinguishes cellulitis from abscess	Fever, dysphagia, odynophagia, stiff neck, dyspnea; airway obstruction, swollen tongue and floor of mouth (tender) Muffled voice	Severe pain, fever, trismus, dysphagia, edematous appearing, painful lateral facial (jaw) or neck swelling (induration) May lead to Lemierre syndrome	Pain, prominent trismus, fever Swelling not always evident	Sudden-onset high fever, "toxic" appearance; muffled voice; anxiety; pain, retractions; dysphagia; drooling; stridor; sitting-up, leaning-forward tripod position; cherry-red swollen epiglottis Usually not hoarse or coughing Lateral neck radiograph shows "thumb sign" of swollen epiglottis	Low-grade fever, barking cough, hoarseness, aphonia, stridor; mild retractions; radiograph shows "steeple sign" of subglottic narrowing on anteroposterior neck view	Prior history of croup with sudden onset of respiratory distress, high fever, "toxic" appearance, hoarseness, stridor, barking cough, tripod sitting position; radiograph as per croup plus ragged tracheal air column	Prior pharyngitis with sudden-onset fever, chills, odynophagia, neck pain, septic thrombophlebitis of internal jugular vein with septic emboli (e.g., lungs, joints), bacteremia

*Often odontogenic; check for tooth abscess, caries, tender teeth.
†Peptostreptococcus, Fusobacterium, Bacteroides.

TABLE 2.5   Red Flags Associated with Sore Throat

Toxic appearance
Shock
Fever >2 wk
Duration of sore throat >2 wk
Dysphagia
Trismus
Stridor
Drooling
Dysphonia
Cyanosis
Hemorrhage
Asymmetric tonsillar swelling or asymmetric cervical adenopathy
Respiratory distress (airway obstruction or pneumonia)
Suspicion of parapharyngeal space infection
Suspicion of diphtheria (bull neck, uvula paralysis, thick membrane)
Apnea
Severe, unremitting pain
Tripod sitting position
"Hot potato" or muffled voice
Chest or neck pain
Weight loss
Systemic lymphadenopathy
Pharyngeal pseudomembrane
Marked neck swelling (bull neck)
Uvula paralysis
Travel or exposure to individuals from diphtheria endemic region
HIV behavioral risk

TABLE 2.6   Findings Suggestive of Group A *Streptococcus* and Viral Pharyngitis

Suggestive of Group A *Streptococcus*

Sudden onset
Sore throat
Fever >100.4°F
Headache
Nausea, vomiting, and abdominal pain
Erythema of pharynx and tonsils
Patchy discrete exudates
Tender, enlarged anterior cervical nodes
Patient aged 3–15 yr
Presentation in winter or early spring
History of exposure
Scarlet fever

Suggestive of Viral Etiology

Conjunctivitis
Coryza
Cough
Hoarseness
Diarrhea
Discrete ulcerative lesions
Myalgia
Typical viral rash (measles, etc.)
Posterior cervical or generalized lymphadenopathy
Hepatosplenomegaly
EBV-ampicillin rash

EBV, Epstein-Barr virus.

vesicles throughout the anterior portion of the mouth, including the lips; vesicles eventually ulcerate. There is sparing of the posterior pharynx in herpes gingivostomatitis; the infection usually occurs in young children. High fever is common, pain is intense, and intake of oral fluids is often impaired, which may lead to dehydration and need for medical support. In adolescents, HSV may manifest as poorly differentiated pharyngitis. Approximately 35% of new-onset HSV-positive adolescent patients have herpetic lesions; most teenage patients with HSV pharyngitis cannot be distinguished from patients with other causes of pharyngitis. The classic syndrome of herpetic gingivostomatitis in infants and toddlers lasts up to 2 weeks; data on the course of more benign HSV pharyngitis infections in older children and adolescents are lacking. The differential diagnosis of vesicular-ulcerating oral lesions is noted in Tables 2.7 and 2.8.

Infants and toddlers with **measles** often have prominent oral findings early in the course of the disease. In addition to high fever, cough, coryza, and conjunctivitis, the pharynx may be intensely and diffusely erythematous, without tonsillar enlargement or exudate. **Koplik spots**, the pathognomonic white or blue-white enanthem of measles, appear on the buccal mucosa near the mandibular molars, generally before the typical measles rash develops. Complications of measles include ear infections, pneumonia, and encephalitis. In the United States, widespread measles vaccination virtually eliminated transmission of natural measles infection except among unvaccinated subpopulations (e.g., children younger than 12 months old, families who have refused immunization). Most recent cases are related to unimmunized visitors from countries with endemic measles, although there has been a rise in cases within the United States due to increasing rates of unvaccinated children.

The lesions of **herpangina**, hand-foot-mouth disease, herpes gingivostomatitis, and measles should be distinguished from noninfectious aphthous ulcers, colloquially referred to as canker sores. Aphthous ulcers are typically discrete, 3–5 mm in diameter, round or ovoid, with a peripheral erythematous halo and a white to yellow-white covering exudate. Lesions tend to be painful, though some may be noted only incidentally. An isolated episode of individual or clustered lesions may be related to physical or chemical irritation, a reaction to an allergic or infectious exposure, nutritional deficiency, or immune-mediated inflammation. Individuals with **recurrent aphthous stomatitis** may lack associated features during or between episodes and experience one to several outbreaks per year, a condition known as simple aphthosis. The outbreaks of simple aphthosis tend to start in late childhood or adolescence, last up to 2 weeks, and abate by adulthood. Patients with complex aphthosis tend to have more frequent outbreaks, have more numerous and painful lesions, and occasionally have lesions on the genital mucosa as well. In such circumstances, complex aphthosis must be distinguished from **Behçet disease**, the latter of which is a systemic inflammatory disorder that may include arthritis, neurologic manifestations, and cutaneous lesions, in addition to orogenital mucosal aphthae (see Table 2.6).

An autoinflammatory periodic fever syndrome known as **PFAPA (periodic fever, aphthous stomatitis, pharyngitis, and cervical adenitis)** occurs predictably every 2–8 weeks. The onset of PFAPA is usually before the age of 5 years. In addition to aphthous stomatitis and pharyngitis, PFAPA is characterized by high fever lasting 4–6 days. The diagnosis is clinical and is typically made in patients with a phenotype consistent with PFAPA after excluding cyclic neutropenia, other periodic fever syndromes, infections, malignancy, and the persistence of elevated acute-phase reactants between episodes. Individual episodes resolve spontaneously but may respond to oral prednisone. Cimetidine in PFAPA syndrome is ineffective. As corticosteroids do not prevent future fever cycles, long-term intervention may also

TABLE 2.7 Vesicular-Ulcerating Eruptions of the Mouth and Pharynx

	Gingivostomatitis	Herpangina	Hand-Foot-Mouth Disease	Chickenpox	Systemic Lupus Erythematosus (SLE)	Inflammatory Bowel Disease (IBD)	Aphthous Stomatitis	Behçet Disease	Vincent Stomatitis	Recurrent Scarifying Ulcerative Stomatitis (Sutton Disease)
Etiology	Herpes simplex virus (HSV I)	Coxsackievirus A, B; echovirus or HSV (rarely)	Coxsackievirus A, coxsackievirus B (rarely)	Varicella-zoster virus	Autoimmune	Autoimmune	Unknown	Unknown; vasculitis	Unknown; or anaerobic bacteria	Unknown
Location	Ulcerative vesicles of pharynx, tongue, and palate plus lesions of mucocutaneous (perioral) margin	Anterior fauces (tonsils), soft palate (uvula), less often pharynx	Tongue, buccal mucosa, palate, palms, soles, anterior oral cavity	Tongue, gingiva, buccal mucosa, marked cutaneous lesions; trunk > face	Oral, nasal mucosa; palate, pharynx, buccal mucosa	Lips, tongue, buccal mucosa, oropharynx	As in IBD	Oral (similar to IBD); genital ulcers	Gingiva, ulceration at base of teeth	Tongue; buccal mucosa
Age	<5yr	3–10yr	1yr–teens	Any age	Any age	Any age	Teens and adulthood	Teens, adulthood, occasionally <10yr	Teens; if younger, consider immunodeficiency and blood dyscrasia	Teens
Manifestations	Fever, mouth pain, toxic, fetid breath, drooling, anorexia, cervical lymphadenopathy; cracked, swollen hemorrhagic gums; secondary inoculation possible (fingers, eye, skin); reactivation with long latency (any age)	Fever, sore throat, odynophagia; summer outbreaks; 6–12 lesions (2–4 mm papule) → vesicle → ulceration; headache, myalgia	Painful bilateral vesicles, fever	Fever, pruritic cutaneous vesicles, painful oral lesions	Renal, central nervous system, arthritis, cutaneous, hematologic, other organ involvement; ulcers minimally to moderately painful; may be painless	Multiple recurrences; painful ulcerations 1–2 mm, but may be 5–15 mm; abdominal pain, diarrhea, hematochezia, weight loss	Similar to IBD	Painful ulcerations (heal without scarring); uveitis, arthralgia, arthritis, lower gastrointestinal ulceration (similar to IBD); recurrences; spontaneous remissions	Fever, bleeding gums; gray membrane	Deep, large, painful ulcerations; relapsing; scarring with distortion of mucosa

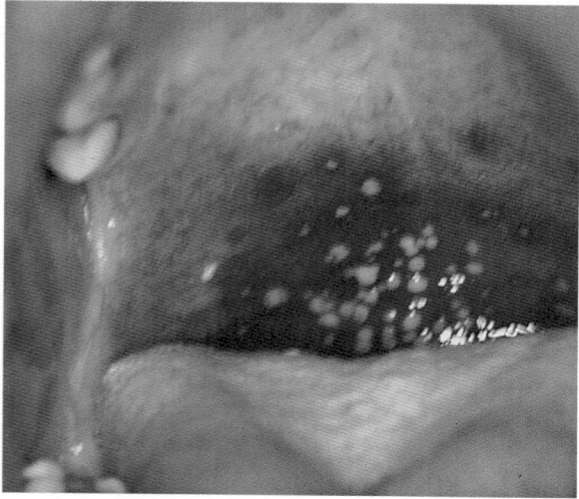

Fig. 2.1 Herpangina with shallow ulcers in the posterior oropharynx. (From Cohen J, Powderly WG. *Infectious Diseases.* 2nd ed. St Louis: Mosby; 2004.)

include tonsillectomy with or without adenoidectomy, although risks of surgical intervention such as anesthetic and postoperative complications must be considered. In most patients PFAPA completely resolves without sequelae before puberty; a few persist into adulthood. Some patients initially diagnosed as having PFAPA actually had a monogenetic recurrent fever syndrome (see Chapter 54).

INFECTIOUS MONONUCLEOSIS

Pathogenesis

Acute exudative pharyngitis commonly occurs with infectious mononucleosis caused by primary infection with the Epstein-Barr virus (EBV). Mononucleosis is a febrile, systemic, self-limited lymphoproliferative disorder that is usually associated with hepatosplenomegaly and generalized lymphadenopathy. Acute pharyngitis may be mild or severe, with erythema, impressive tonsillar exudates, and significant tonsillar hypertrophy that can result in airway obstruction. Regional lymph nodes may be particularly enlarged and slightly tender. Infectious mononucleosis usually occurs in adolescents and young adults; EBV infection is generally milder or subclinical in preadolescent children. In U.S. high school and college students, attack rates are 200–800 per 100,000 per year. EBV is transmitted primarily by saliva.

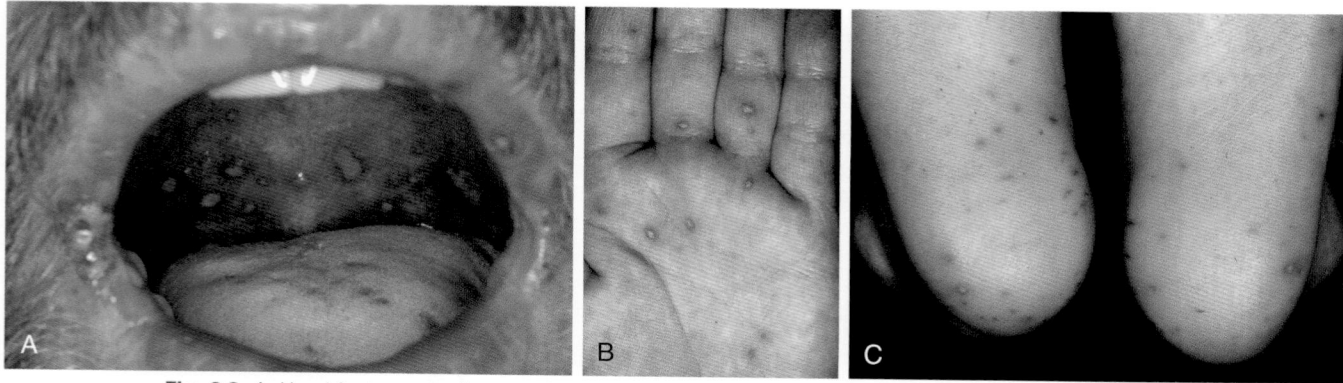

Fig. 2.2 *A,* Hand-foot-mouth disease. Aphthae-like erosions may appear anywhere in the oral cavity. *B,* Hand-foot-mouth disease. Cloudy vesicles with a red halo are highly characteristic of this disease. *C,* Hand-foot-mouth disease. The pale, white, oval vesicles with a red areola are a distinguishing feature of this disease. (From Dinulos JGH. *Habif's Clinical Dermatology.* 7th ed. Philadelphia: Elsevier; 2021, Figs. 14.4, 14.6, and 14.7.)

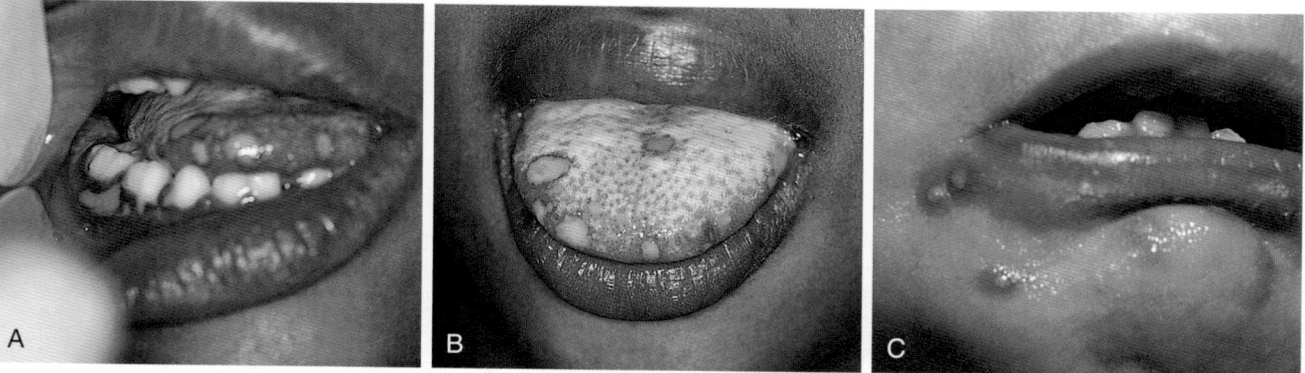

Fig. 2.3 Herpes simplex infections. *A,* Herpetic gingivostomatitis is characterized by discrete mucosal ulcerations and diffuse gingival erythema, edema, and friability in association with fever, dysphagia, and cervical adenopathy. *B,* Numerous yellow ulcerations with thin red halos are seen on the patient's tongue as well. *C,* Thick-walled vesicles on an erythematous base were noted in this child, who showed early findings of intraoral involvement. (From Michaels MG, Williams JV. Infectious diseases. In Zitelli BJ, McIntire SC, Nowalk AJ, eds. *Zitelli and Davis' Atlas of Pediatric Physical Diagnosis.* 7th ed. Philadelphia: Elsevier; 2018, Fig. 13.3.)

TABLE 2.8 Broad Differential Diagnosis of Oral Ulceration

Condition	Comment
Common	
Aphthous ulcers (canker sores)	Painful circumscribed lesions; recurrences
Traumatic ulcers	Accidents, chronic cheek biter, after dental local anesthesia
Hand-foot-mouth disease	Painful; lesions on tongue, anterior oral cavity, hands, and feet
Herpangina	Painful; lesions confined to soft palate and oropharynx
Herpetic gingivostomatitis	Vesicles on mucocutaneous borders; painful, febrile
Recurrent herpes labialis	Vesicles on lips; painful
Other viruses	HIV, varicella, EBV
Chemical burns	Alkali, acid, aspirin; painful
Heat burns	Hot food, electrical
Drugs	NSAIDs, chemotherapy, sulfa drugs, phenytoin, ACE inhibitors, others
Uncommon	
Neutrophil defects	Agranulocytosis, leukemia, cyclic neutropenia; painful
Systemic lupus erythematosus	Recurrent; may be painless or bullous
Behçet syndrome	Resembles aphthous lesions; associated with genital ulcers, uveitis
Necrotizing ulcerative gingivostomatitis	Vincent stomatitis; painful
Syphilis	Chancre or gumma; painless
Oral Crohn disease	Aphthous-like; painful
Histoplasmosis	Lingual
Pneumococcal sepsis or pneumonia	Gingival cystic ulcerations
Pemphigus	May be isolated to the oral cavity
Stevens-Johnson syndrome	May be isolated to or appear initially in the oral cavity
Mycoplasma (MIRM)	Rash may be absent
RIME	Non-mycoplasma infections; lesions similar to MIRM; may be reactive
PFAPA	Unknown etiology recurrent autoinflammatory fever syndrome
Celiac disease	Primary or nutritional deficiencies
Nutritional deficiencies	Vitamin B_{12}, iron, folate

ACE, angiotensin-converting enzyme; EBV, Epstein-Barr virus; MIRM, mycoplasma-induced rash and mucositis; NSAIDs, nonsteroidal antiinflammatory drugs; PFAPA, periodic fever, aphthous stomatitis, pharyngitis, adenitis syndrome; RIME, reactive infectious mucocutaneous eruption.

Clinical Features

After a 2–4-week incubation period, patients with infectious mononucleosis usually experience an abrupt onset of malaise, fatigue, fever, and headache, followed closely by pharyngitis. The tonsils are enlarged with exudates and cervical (often posterior) adenopathy. More generalized adenopathy with hepatosplenomegaly often follows. Fever and pharyngitis typically last 1–3 weeks, and lymphadenopathy and hepatosplenomegaly resolve over 3–6 weeks. Malaise and lethargy can persist for several months and can affect school or work performance.

Diagnosis

The findings of acute exudative pharyngitis together with hepatomegaly, splenomegaly, and generalized lymphadenopathy suggest infectious mononucleosis. Early in the disease and in cases without liver or spleen enlargement, differentiation from other causes of pharyngitis, including streptococcal pharyngitis, is difficult. Indeed, a small number of patients with infectious mononucleosis have a throat culture positive for group A streptococci, though these patients are likely streptococcal carriers. Patients with infectious mononucleosis treated for presumed streptococcal pharyngitis with antibacterials, particularly with ampicillin or amoxicillin, frequently develop a diffuse, erythematous, papular exanthem during the course of therapy that retrospectively suggests infectious mononucleosis due to

EBV. An indistinguishable mononucleosis syndrome can occur with cytomegalovirus, but differentiation is rarely of clinical importance. Acute toxoplasmosis may also present similarly. Serologic evidence of mononucleosis should be sought when splenomegaly or other features are present or if symptoms persist longer than expected. Laboratory studies of diagnostic value include atypical lymphocytosis; these lymphocytes are primarily EBV-specific, cytotoxic T lymphocytes that represent a reactive response to EBV-infected B lymphocytes. A modest elevation of serum aminotransferase levels, reflecting EBV hepatitis, is common. Tests useful for diagnosis include detection of heterophile antibodies that react with bovine erythrocytes (most often detected by the monospot test) and a specific antibody against EBV viral capsid antigen (VCA), early antigen (EA), and nuclear antigen (EBNA). Acute infectious mononucleosis is usually associated with a positive heterophile antibody test result and the presence of antibodies to VCA and EA in a specific pattern; subacute and remote infections produce distinct antibody profiles (Fig. 2.4). In young children, the monospot may be negative.

Primary infection with **HIV** may produce a mononucleosis-like illness with sore throat, fever, lymphadenopathy, rash, myalgia, and hepatosplenomegaly. Early infection may be detected by viral RNA or DNA load because immunoglobulin M (IgM) or immunoglobulin G (IgG) titers may have not yet developed.

BACTERIAL PHARYNGITIS

Group A Streptococcal Infection

In evaluating a patient with sore throat, the primary concern is usually accurate diagnosis and treatment of pharyngitis caused by group A streptococci (GAS), also known as *Streptococcus pyogenes*, which accounts for up to 30% of all episodes of pharyngitis in children in the United States. The sequelae of GAS pharyngitis, especially acute rheumatic fever (ARF) and poststreptococcal glomerulonephritis (PSGN), at one time resulted in considerable morbidity and mortality in the United States and continue to do so in other parts of the world. Prevention of ARF in particular depends on timely diagnosis of streptococcal pharyngitis and prompt antibacterial treatment. Group A streptococci are characterized by the presence of group A carbohydrate in the cell wall, and they are further distinguished by several cell wall protein antigens (M, R, T). These protein antigens, especially the M protein, a virulence factor, are useful for studies of epidemiology and pathogenesis but are not used in clinical care.

Epidemiology

Group A streptococcal pharyngitis is endemic in the United States; epidemics occur sporadically. Episodes peak in the late winter and early spring. Rates of GAS pharyngitis are highest among children aged 5–11 years old. Spread of GAS in classrooms and among family members is common, especially in the presence of crowded living conditions. Transmission occurs primarily by the inhalation of organisms in large droplets or by direct contact with respiratory secretions. Pets do not appear to be a frequent reservoir. Untreated streptococcal pharyngitis is particularly contagious early in the acute illness and for the first 2 weeks after the organism has been acquired. Antibacterial therapy effectively prevents disease transmission: Within 24 hours of institution of therapy with penicillin, it is difficult to isolate GAS from patients with acute streptococcal pharyngitis, and infected children can return to school.

Molecular epidemiology studies of streptococcal pharyngitis have shown that the prevalent M protein types vary among communities and over time. Numerous distinct strains of GAS can circulate simultaneously in a community during the peak season. Molecular genetic studies can establish the specific M protein gene (i.e., *emm* gene); M protein identification is not available or useful for clinical care. Children with streptococcal pharyngitis can serve as a local reservoir for strains that cause invasive disease (e.g., sepsis, streptococcal toxic shock syndrome, cellulitis, necrotizing fasciitis) in the same geographic area and season.

Clinical Features

Acute streptococcal pharyngitis classically presents with the sudden onset of fever and sore throat (see Table 2.6). Headache, malaise, abdominal pain, nausea, and vomiting occur frequently. Cough, rhinorrhea, conjunctivitis, stridor, diarrhea, discrete ulcerated lesions, and hoarseness are distinctly unusual and suggest a viral etiology (see Table 2.6).

Physical examination reveals marked pharyngeal erythema. Petechiae may be noted on the palate but can also occur in viral pharyngitis, especially mononucleosis. Tonsils are enlarged, symmetric, and bright red, with patchy exudates on their surfaces. Anterior cervical lymph nodes are often tender and enlarged.

Combinations of these signs can be used to assist in diagnosis; in particular, tonsillar exudates in association with fever, palatal petechiae, and tender anterior cervical lymphadenopathy strongly suggest infection with GAS. However, other diseases can produce this constellation of findings, including infectious mononucleosis. Some or all

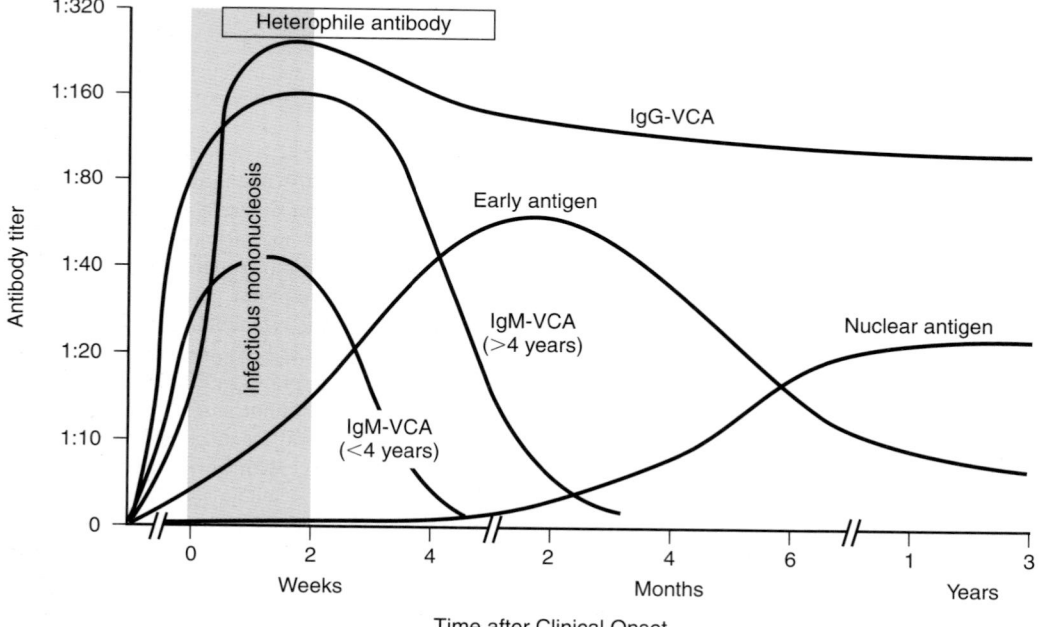

Fig. 2.4 Schematic representation of the evolution of antibodies to various Epstein-Barr virus antigens in patients with infectious mononucleosis. The titers are geometric mean values expressed as reciprocals of the serum dilution. The minimal titer tested for viral capsid antigen (VCA) and early antigen antibodies was 1:10; for Epstein-Barr nuclear antigen, it was 1:2.5. The immunoglobulin M (IgM) response to capsid antigen was divided because of the significant differences noted according to age. IgG, immunoglobulin G. (From Jenson HB, Ench Y, Sumaya CV. Epstein-Barr virus. In: Rose NR, de Macario EC, Folds JD, et al., eds. *Manual of Clinical Laboratory Immunology.* 5th ed. Washington, DC: American Society for Microbiology; 1997:634–643.)

of these classic characteristics may be absent in patients with streptococcal pharyngitis. Symptoms usually resolve within 5 days even in the absence of antibacterial therapy. Younger children can have a syndrome called **streptococcosis**—coryza with crusting below the nares, more generalized adenopathy, and a more chronic course. When rash accompanies the illness, accurate clinical diagnosis is easier. **Scarlet fever**, so-called because of the characteristic fine, diffuse red rash, is essentially pathognomonic for infection with group A streptococci. Scarlet fever is rarely seen in children younger than 3 years old or in adults.

Scarlet Fever

The rash of scarlet fever is caused by infection with a strain of GAS that contains a bacteriophage encoding for production of an erythrogenic (redness-producing) toxin, usually erythrogenic (also called pyrogenic) exotoxin A (designated SPE A). Scarlet fever is simply GAS pharyngitis with a rash and should be explained as such to patients and their families. Although patients with streptococcal toxic shock syndrome are also infected with GAS that produces SPE A, most GAS pharyngeal infections are not associated with development of severe invasive or systemic disease.

The rash of scarlet fever has a texture like sandpaper and blanches with pressure (Figs. 2.5 and 2.6). It usually begins on the face, but after 24 hours, it becomes generalized. The face is red, especially over the cheeks, and the area around the mouth often appears pale in comparison, giving the appearance of circumoral pallor. Accentuation of erythema occurs in flexor skin creases, especially in the antecubital fossae, a finding termed Pastia lines. The papillae of the tongue may be red and swollen, hence the designation "strawberry tongue." The erythema begins to fade within a few days. Desquamation begins within a week

of onset on the face and progresses downward, often resembling that seen after mild sunburn. On occasion, sheetlike desquamation occurs around the free margins of the fingernails; this is usually coarser than the desquamation seen with Kawasaki disease. The differential diagnosis of scarlet fever includes Kawasaki disease, measles, and staphylococcal toxic shock syndrome (Table 2.9).

Diagnosis

Although signs and symptoms may strongly suggest acute streptococcal pharyngitis, laboratory diagnosis is strongly recommended, even for patients with scarlet fever (Fig. 2.5). Scoring systems for diagnosing acute GAS pharyngitis on clinical grounds, such as the McIsaac or Centor criteria, have not proved very satisfactory. Using clinical criteria alone, physicians overestimate the likelihood that patients have streptococcal infection. Historically, the throat culture on blood agar plate was used to diagnose streptococcal pharyngitis, but results were typically not available for 24–48 hours. Rapid antigen detection tests (RADTs) that take <15 minutes can detect the presence of the cell wall group A carbohydrate antigen after acid extraction of organisms obtained by throat swab. These RADTs are highly specific (generally >95%) when compared to throat culture. One recommendation is that two throat swabs be obtained simultaneously from patients with suspected GAS pharyngitis. One swab is used for a rapid test. When the RADT result is positive, it is highly likely that the patient has GAS pharyngitis, and the extra swab can be discarded. When the RADT is negative, GAS may nonetheless be present; thus, the extra swab should be processed for culture. One of the best validated scoring systems for determining pretest probability in children is the McIsaac criteria (fever, cervical adenopathy, tonsillar exudates, no cough, 3–15 years old), but the positive predictive value of the highest McIsaac score is

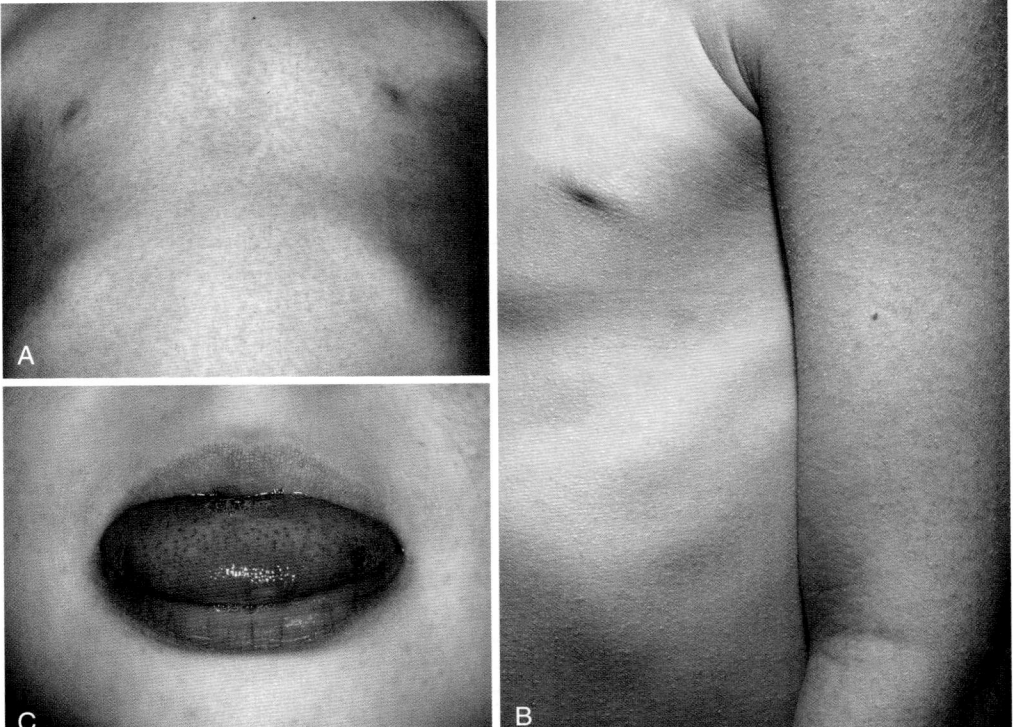

Fig. 2.5 *A,* Scarlet fever. Early eruptive stage on the trunk showing numerous pinpoint red papules. *B,* Fully evolved eruption. Numerous papules giving a sandpaper-like texture to the skin. *C,* Portions of the white coat remain in the center, but the remainder of the tongue is red with engorged papillae ("strawberry tongue"). (From Dinulos JGH. *Habif's Clinical Dermatology.* 7th ed, Philadelphia: Elsevier; 2021, Figs. 14.9, 14.10, and 14.11.)

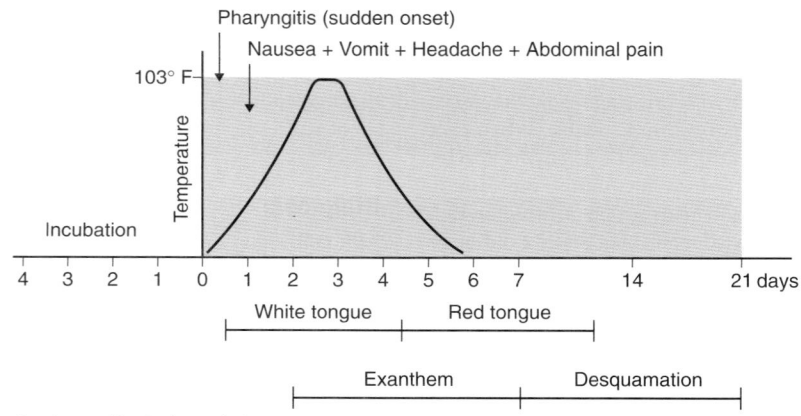

Fig. 2.6 Scarlet fever. Evolution of signs and symptoms. (From Dinulos JGH. *Habif's Clinical Dermatology.* 7th ed. Philadelphia: Elsevier; 2021, Fig. 14.8.)

TABLE 2.9   Differential Diagnosis of Scarlet Fever

	Scarlet Fever	Kawasaki Disease	Measles	Staphylococcal Toxic Shock Syndrome	Staphylococcal Scalded Skin Syndrome
Agent	Group A streptococci	Unknown	Measles virus	*Staphylococcus aureus*	*S. aureus*
Age range	All (peak, 5–15 yr)	Usually <5 yr	<2 yr, 10–20 yr	All (especially >10 yr)	Usually <5 yr
Prodrome	No	No	Fever, coryza, cough, conjunctivitis	Usually no	No
Enanthem	No	Occasionally	Koplik spots	No	Limited
Mouth	Strawberry tongue, exudative pharyngitis, palatal petechiae	Erythema; red, cracked lips; strawberry tongue	Diffusely red, no cracked lips	Usually normal	Erythema
Rash	Fine, red, "sandpaper," membranous desquamation, circumoral pallor, Pastia lines	Variable polymorphic; erythematous face, trunk, and diaper area; tips of fingers and toes desquamate 10–28 days after onset	Maculopapular; progressing from forehead to feet; may desquamate	Diffuse erythroderma; desquamates	Erythema, painful bullous lesions; positive Nikolsky sign; desquamates
Other	Cervical adenitis, gallbladder hydrops, fever	Coronary artery disease; fever >5 days; conjunctival (nonpurulent) injection; tender, swollen hands and feet; cervical adenopathy (size >1.5 cm); thrombocytosis; pyuria (sterile); gallbladder hydrops	"Toxic" appearance; dehydration; encephalitis, pneumonia;	Shock (hypotension, including orthostatic); encephalopathy; diarrhea; headache	Fever, cracked lips; conjunctivitis

only about 60%. In contrast, a score ≤2 is associated with a negative predictive value of about 80%. The presence of viral symptoms such as cough, rhinorrhea, conjunctivitis, laryngitis, stridor, croup, or diarrhea decreases the likelihood that the illness is due to GAS. Patients with a negative RADT result should not be treated before culture verification unless there is a particularly high suspicion of GAS infection (e.g., scarlet fever, peritonsillar abscess, or tonsillar exudates in addition to tender cervical adenopathy, palatal petechiae, fever, and recent exposure to a person with GAS pharyngitis).

Nucleic acid amplification tests (NAATs) for GAS are available for use in hospital and reference laboratories and are supplanting RADTs in many settings. These simplified molecular tests use methods that amplify the DNA of a specific GAS gene. They take <1 hour to perform and are reported to have both sensitivity and specificity ≥99% when compared to standard throat culture and PCR. They can be used as a "stand-alone" test for GAS or as a confirmatory test when the RADT is negative. There are three concerns with these molecular tests: (1) they are so sensitive it is likely they may identify more patients who are carriers than would ordinarily be identified by RADT and/or culture; (2) unless rigorous technique is followed, they may be prone to contamination with exogenous GAS DNA from other swabs, a particular concern in physician offices when performed by staff who are not trained laboratory technologists; and (3) depending on the institution, they can be more expensive than throat culture, and their costs may not be covered by all insurance plans. As NAAT testing becomes more cost efficient the use will likely continue to rise as these assays can provide sensitive and actionable results quicker than a traditional culture.

Testing patients for serologic evidence of an antibody response to extracellular products of GAS is not useful for diagnosing *acute* pharyngitis. Because it generally takes several weeks for antibody levels to rise, streptococcal antibody tests are valid only for determining past infection. Specific antibodies that are often measured in the appropriate

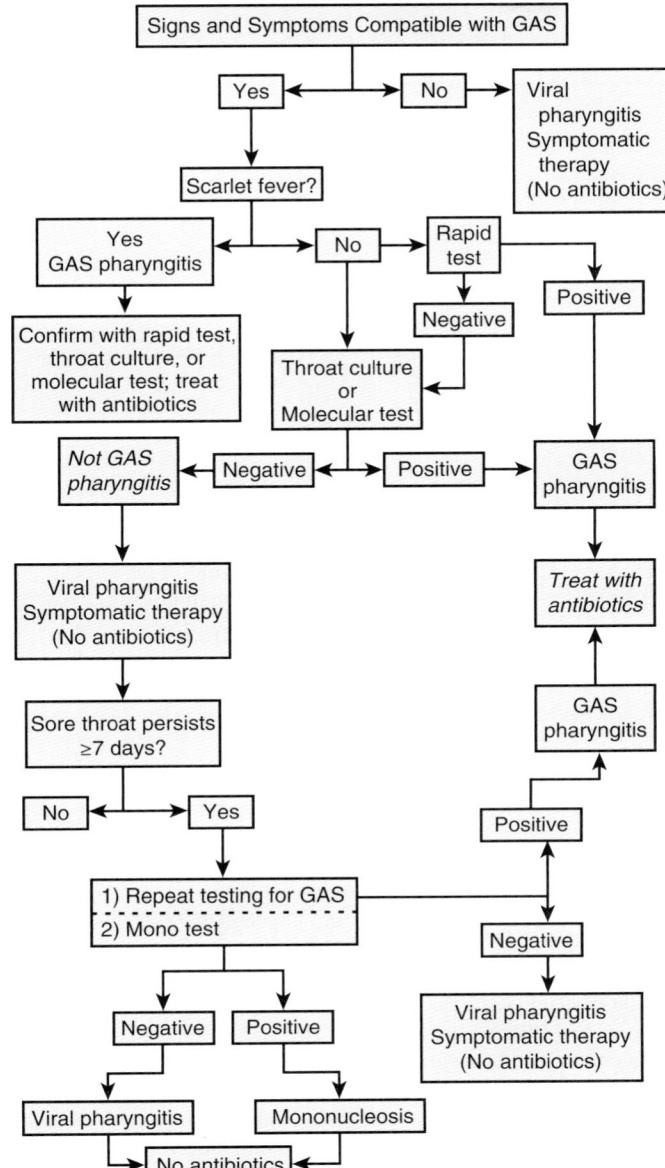

Fig. 2.7 Management of patients with sore throat. GAS, group A streptococci.

clinical setting include antistreptolysin O (ASO), anti–DNase B, and antihyaluronidase (AHT). When antibody testing is desired to evaluate a possible poststreptococcal illness, more than one of these tests should be performed to improve sensitivity.

Treatment

Treatment begun within 9 days of the onset of GAS pharyngitis is effective in preventing ARF. Therapy does not affect the risk of acute poststreptococcal glomerulonephritis. Antibacterial therapy also reduces the incidence of suppurative sequelae of GAS pharyngitis, such as peritonsillar abscess and cervical adenitis. In addition, treatment produces a more rapid resolution of signs and symptoms and terminates contagiousness within 24 hours. For these reasons, antibacterials should be instituted as soon as the diagnosis is supported by laboratory studies.

There are numerous antibiotics available for treating streptococcal pharyngitis (Table 2.10). The drugs of choice are penicillin and amoxicillin. Despite the widespread use of penicillin to treat streptococcal

and other infections for many decades, resistance of GAS to penicillin or any other β-lactam antibiotic has not developed. Amoxicillin has been demonstrated to be effective in eradicating GAS when given by mouth once daily for 10 days.

Patients who are allergic to penicillin can receive a cephalosporin if they have not had an immediate hypersensitivity reaction. Erythromycin or another non–β-lactam antibiotic, such as clarithromycin, azithromycin, or clindamycin, can be used. Resistance of GAS to macrolides has increased dramatically in many areas of the world where erythromycin has been widely used. Macrolide resistance also affects azithromycin and can affect clindamycin.

Suppurative Complications

Antibacterial therapy has greatly reduced the likelihood of developing suppurative complications caused by spread of GAS from the pharynx to adjacent parapharyngeal structures. **Peritonsillar abscess** ("quinsy") manifests with fever, severe throat pain, dysphagia, "hot potato voice," pain referred to the ear, and bulging of the peritonsillar area with asymmetry of the tonsils and sometimes displacement of the uvula to the opposite side (Fig. 2.8; see also Table 2.4). There can be peritonsillar cellulitis without a well-defined abscess cavity. Trismus may be present. When an abscess is found clinically or by an imaging study such as a CT scan, needle aspiration or surgical drainage is indicated. Peritonsillar abscess occurs most commonly in older children and adolescents. Group A streptococcus is recovered from the abscess in ~50%; other organisms include other streptococci and oral anaerobic bacteria.

Retropharyngeal abscess represents extension of an infection from the pharynx or peritonsillar region into the retropharyngeal (prevertebral) space, which is rich in lymphoid structures (Figs. 2.9 and 2.10; see also Table 2.4). Penetrating trauma from a foreign object (e.g., fish bone) may rarely cause this. Children younger than 4 years old are most often affected. Fever, dysphagia, drooling, stridor, extension and limited motion of the neck, and a mass in the posterior pharyngeal wall may be noted. Retropharyngeal abscesses may rarely extend into the posterior mediastinum. The organisms are often polymicrobial and include streptococci, *Staphylococcus aureus*, and anaerobic bacteria. Surgical drainage is often required if frank suppuration has occurred.

Spread of GAS via pharyngeal lymphatic vessels to regional nodes can cause **cervical lymphadenitis**. The markedly swollen and tender anterior cervical nodes that result can suppurate. Otitis media, mastoiditis, and sinusitis also may occur as complications of GAS pharyngitis. Additional parapharyngeal suppurative infections that may mimic streptococcal disease are noted in Table 2.4. Furthermore, any pharyngeal infectious process may produce **torticollis** if there is inflammation that extends to the paraspinal muscles and ligaments, producing pain, spasm, and, on occasion, rotatory subluxation of the cervical spine, a condition termed **Grisel syndrome.** Oropharyngeal torticollis lasts <2 weeks and is not associated with abnormal neurologic signs or pain over the spinous process. Invasive sterile site or bacteremic infections with GAS are unusual sequelae of pharyngitis.

Nonsuppurative Sequelae

Nonsuppurative complications include ARF, PSGN, and possibly reactive arthritis or synovitis. In addition, an association between streptococcal infection and neuropsychiatric disorders such as tic disorder, obsessive-compulsive disorder, and Tourette syndrome has been postulated. This possible association has been called PANDAS (pediatric autoimmune neuropsychiatric disorders associated with streptococci). The terminology has been modified to "pediatric acute-onset neuropsychiatric syndrome" (PANS) or "childhood acute neuropsychiatric syndrome" (CANS), in recognition that the etiologic role of GAS and benefit from antibacterial treatment have been difficult to establish, and it is likely

TABLE 2.10 Recommended Treatment Regimens for Acute Streptococcal Pharyngitis*

	Dose/Route	Duration	Frequency
Standard Treatment			
Amoxicillin	50 mg/kg up to 1,000 mg/oral	10 days	Once daily
Penicillin V	250 mg (weight <27 kg)/oral 500 mg (weight >27 kg) for adolescents and adults/oral	10 days	b.i.d.
Benzathine penicillin G	600,000 U (weight <27 kg)/IM 1.2 million U (weight ≥27 kg)/IM	N/A N/A	Once

	Oral Dose	Duration	Frequency
Treatment for Penicillin-Allergic Patients			
Clarithromycin	15 mg/kg/day up to 500 mg/day	10 days	b.i.d.
Azithromycin[†]	12 mg/kg on day 1 then 6 mg/kg/day on days 2–5	5 days	Once daily
Clindamycin	21 mg/kg/day up to 900 mg/day	10 days	t.i.d.
Cephalosporins[‡]			
Cephalexin	40 mg/kg/day up to 1,000 mg/day	10 days	b.i.d.
Cefadroxil	30 mg/kg/day up to 1,000 mg/day	10 days	Once daily

*Based on Infectious Diseases Society of America 2012 and AAP Red Book recommendations.
[†]Maximum dose for children is 500 mg/day. Adult dosage: 500 mg the first day, 250 mg the subsequent 4 days.
[‡]First-generation cephalosporins (e.g., cephalexin and cefadroxil) are preferred but all cephalosporins are effective. Dosage and frequency vary among agents. Avoid use in patients with history of immediate (anaphylactic) hypersensitivity to penicillin or other β-lactam antibiotics.
b.i.d., two times a day; IM, intramuscular; t.i.d., three times a day.

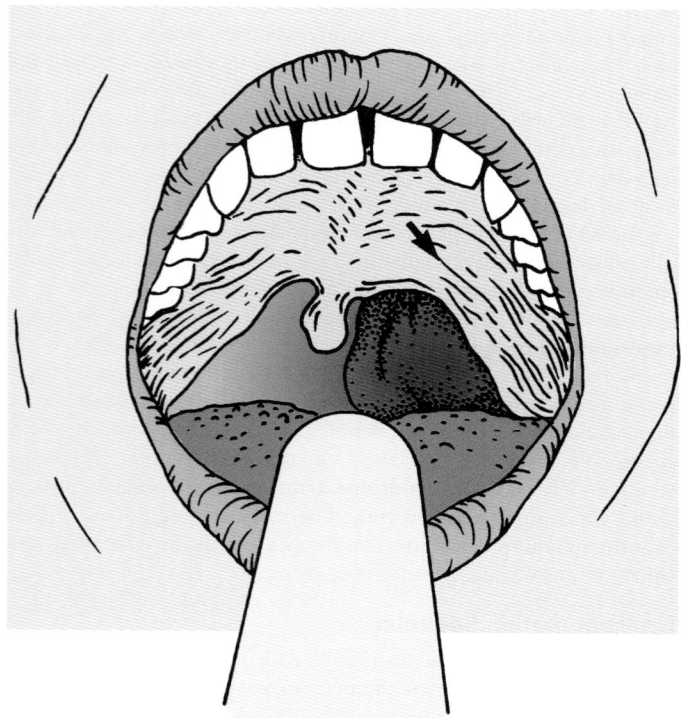

Fig. 2.8 Peritonsillar abscess (quinsy, sore throat). The left tonsil is asymmetrically inflamed and swollen; there is displacement of the uvula to the opposite side. The supratonsillar space *(arrow)* is also swollen; this is the usual site of the surgical incision for drainage. Prominent unilateral cervical adenopathy typically coexists. (From Reilly BM. Sore throat. In: *Practical Strategies in Outpatient Medicine.* 2nd ed. Philadelphia: WB Saunders; 1991.)

that infections other than GAS infection are associated with the development, recurrence, or exacerbation of neuropsychiatric symptoms.

Therapy with an appropriate antibacterial within 9 days of onset of symptoms is highly effective in preventing ARF. Except in certain geographic areas (e.g., Salt Lake City) and populations (e.g., Hasidic Jewish communities), ARF is quite rare in North America. The impressive reduction in ARF prevalence in the United States since the mid-1960s may be related to reductions in the prevalence of so-called "rheumatogenic" GAS M types. The reason for the near disappearance of rheumatogenic types in the United States is unknown. Areas of the world with persistently high rates of ARF have different M types than the United States had in the past and has currently. PSGN is not prevented by treatment of the antecedent streptococcal infection. Pharyngitis caused by one of the "nephritogenic" strains of GAS precedes glomerulonephritis by about 10 days. Unlike ARF, which occurs only after GAS pharyngitis, PSGN also can follow GAS skin infection.

Treatment Failure and Chronic Carriage

Treatment with penicillin cures GAS pharyngitis but does not eradicate GAS from the pharynx in as many as 25% of patients (Fig. 2.11), causing considerable consternation among affected patients and their families. Resistance to penicillin is not the cause of treatment failure. A few such patients are symptomatic and are characterized as having clinical treatment failure. Reinfection with the same strain or a different strain is possible, as is intercurrent viral pharyngitis. Some of these patients may be chronic pharyngeal carriers of GAS who are suffering from a new superimposed viral infection; others may have been nonadherent to therapy. Many patients who continue to have positive tests for GAS despite antimicrobial treatment are asymptomatic and are identified only when follow-up throat swabs are obtained, a practice that is usually unnecessary in North America. Patients who adhered to therapy are at minimal risk for ARF. One explanation for asymptomatic persistence of GAS after treatment is that these patients are chronically colonized with GAS, were initially

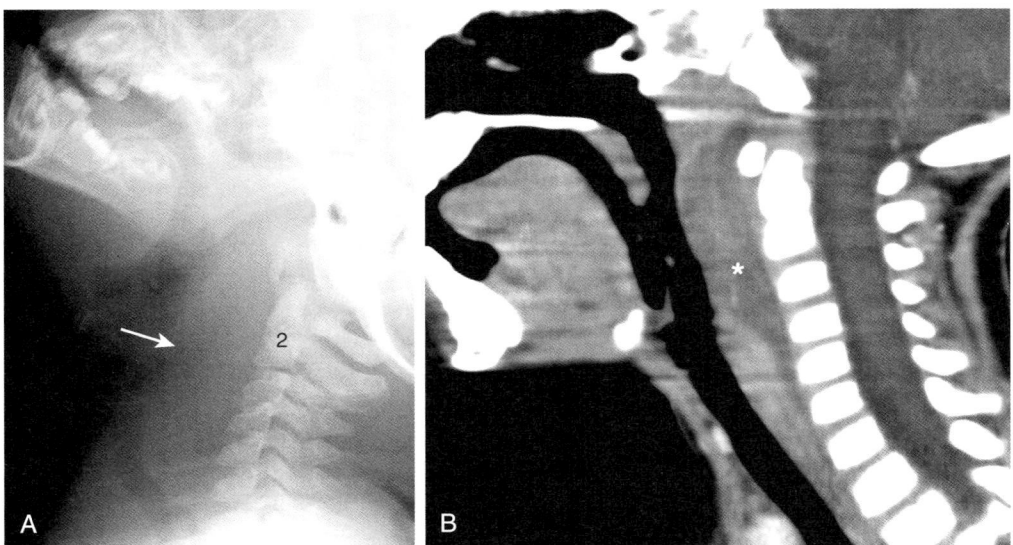

Fig. 2.9 Retropharyngeal abscess in a 3-year-old female with sore throat and fever. *A,* Lateral soft tissue neck radiograph reveals extensive soft tissue swelling displacing the airway anteriorly from the skull base to C6 *(arrow).* *B,* Sagittal reconstructed contrast-enhanced CT confirms thickened, enhancing retropharyngeal soft tissues indicating cellulitis. Region of hypoattenuating fluid is concerning for retropharyngeal abscess *(asterisk).* (From Lowe LH, Smith CJ. Infection and inflammation. In: *Caffey's Pediatric Diagnostic Imaging.* 12th ed. Philadelphia: Elsevier; 2013:138, Fig. 15.4.)

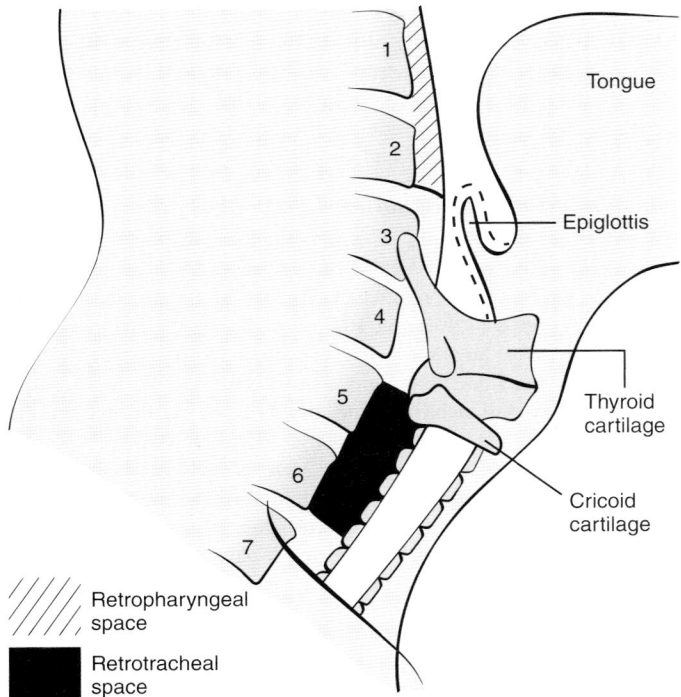

Fig. 2.10 In an adolescent, the retropharyngeal space normally does not exceed 7 mm when measured from the anterior aspect of the C2 vertebral body to the posterior pharynx. In infants the retropharyngeal space is usually less than one width of the adjacent vertebral body. However, during crying, this distance may be three widths of the vertebral body. In addition, under normal circumstances, the retrotracheal space does not exceed 22 mm in adolescents when measured from the anterior aspect of C6 to the trachea. *Dotted lines* depict the "thumbprint" sign, noted on a lateral neck radiograph, made by a swollen epiglottis. (From Reilly BM. Sore throat. In: *Practical Strategies in Outpatient Medicine.* 2nd ed. Philadelphia: WB Saunders; 1991.)

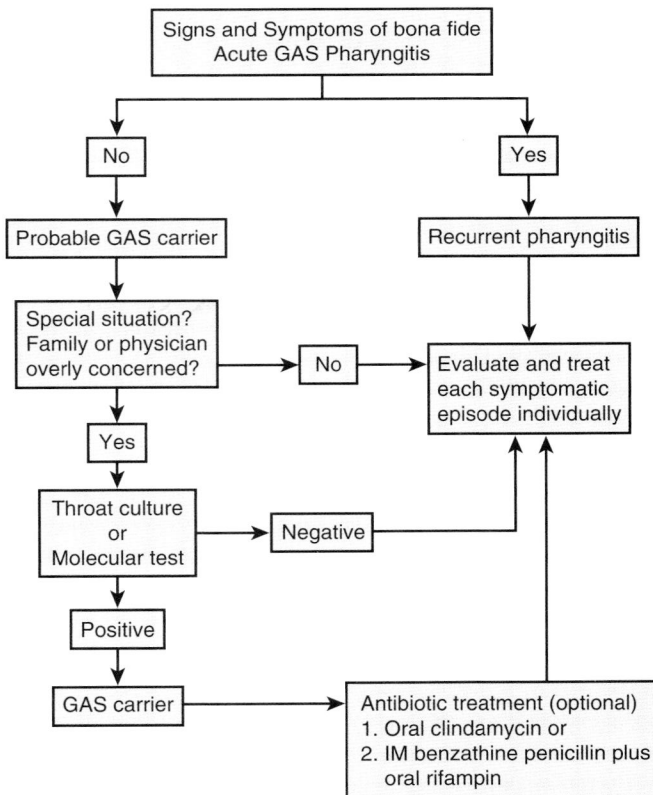

Fig. 2.11 Management of patients with repeated or frequent positive rapid tests or throat cultures. GAS, group A streptococci; IM, intramuscular.

symptomatic because of a viral pharyngitis, and did not truly have acute streptococcal pharyngitis.

Patients who are chronically colonized with GAS are called chronic carriers. Carriers do not appear to be at risk for ARF or for development of suppurative complications, and are rarely sources of spread of GAS in the community. There is no reason to exclude carriers from school. There is no easy way to identify chronic carriers prospectively among patients with symptoms of acute pharyngitis. The pathophysiology of chronic carriage is unknown. As resistance to penicillin is not a factor, many other causes have been hypothesized including nonadherence to antibacterial treatment, tolerance to antibacterials (suppression but lack of killing by antimicrobials), internalization of GAS by epithelial cells, and presence of β-lactamase-producing "co-pathogens," but none has been proven. The clinician should consider the possibility of chronic GAS carriage when a patient or a family member has multiple test-positive episodes of pharyngitis, especially when symptoms are mild or atypical. A culture or other test is usually positive for GAS when the suspected carrier is symptom-free or is receiving antibacterial treatment (intramuscular benzathine penicillin is recommended to eliminate concerns about compliance).

Carriers often receive multiple unsuccessful courses of antibacterial therapy in attempts to eliminate GAS. Physician and patient/family anxiety is common and can develop into "streptophobia." Unproven and ineffective therapies include tonsillectomy, prolonged administration of antibacterials, use of β-lactamase-inhibiting antibacterials, and culture or treatment of pets. Available options for approaching the patient with chronic streptococcal carriage include the following:

1. Evaluate for GAS pharyngitis by throat swab each time the patient has pharyngitis with features that suggest streptococcal pharyngitis. Treat as acute GAS pharyngitis with amoxicillin or penicillin (or an alternative agent) each time a test is positive; this will prevent ARF if the GAS identified has been newly acquired. Avoid testing patients who do not have signs and symptoms suggestive of acute GAS pharyngitis.
2. Treat with one of the regimens effective for terminating chronic carriage.

The first option is simple, as safe as amoxicillin and penicillin, and appropriate for most patients. The second option should be reserved for particularly anxious patients/families; those with a history of ARF or living with someone who had it; or those living or working in nursing homes, chronic care facilities, and hospitals. Two antibacterial treatment regimens have been demonstrated in randomized trials to be effective for eradication of the carrier state:

- Intramuscular benzathine penicillin plus oral rifampin (10 mg/kg/dose up to 300 mg, given twice daily for 4 days beginning on the day of the penicillin injection)
- Oral clindamycin, given for 10 days (20 mg/kg/day up to 450 mg, divided into three equal doses)

Clindamycin is easier to use than intramuscular penicillin plus oral rifampin and may be somewhat more effective. Amoxicillin-clavulanate (40 mg amoxicillin/kg/day up to 2,000 mg amoxicillin/day divided t.i.d. for 10 days) has also been used. Successful eradication of the carrier state makes evaluation of subsequent episodes of pharyngitis much easier, although chronic carriage can recur upon re-exposure to GAS.

Recurrent Acute Pharyngitis

Some patients seem remarkably susceptible to developing GAS pharyngitis. The reasons for frequent *bona fide* acute GAS pharyngitis are obscure. In contrast to chronic carriers, appropriate antibacterial treatment of each episode results in eradication of the organism.

The role of tonsillectomy in the management of patients with multiple episodes of streptococcal pharyngitis is controversial. The presence of tonsils is not necessary for GAS to infect the throat. Fewer episodes of sore throat were reported among patients treated with tonsillectomy (in contrast to patients treated without surgery) during the first 2 years

after operation. Patients had experienced numerous episodes of pharyngitis over several years, and it appears that not all episodes were caused by GAS. By 2 years after tonsillectomy there was no difference between the groups in the frequency of pharyngitis. The postoperative complication rate among tonsillectomy patients was 14%. *Tonsillectomy cannot be recommended for treatment of* recurrent *pharyngitis except in unusual circumstances.* It is preferable to treat most patients with penicillin or amoxicillin whenever symptomatic GAS pharyngitis occurs. Obtaining follow-up throat specimens for lab testing can help distinguish recurrent pharyngitis from chronic carriage but is unnecessary in most instances.

INFECTION WITH STREPTOCOCCI THAT ARE NOT GROUP A (NON-A STREPTOCOCCI)

Certain β-hemolytic streptococci of serogroups other than group A cause acute pharyngitis. Well-documented *epidemics* of food-borne group C and group G streptococcal pharyngitis have been reported in young adults. In these situations, a high percentage of individuals who had ingested the contaminated food promptly developed acute pharyngitis, and throat cultures yielded virtually pure growth of the epidemiologically linked organism. There have been outbreaks of group G streptococcal pharyngitis among children. However, the role of non-A streptococcal organisms as etiologic agents of acute pharyngitis in *endemic* circumstances has been difficult to establish. Group C and group G streptococci may be responsible for acute pharyngitis, particularly in adolescents. However, the exact role of these agents, most of which are carried asymptomatically in the pharynx of some children and young adults, remains to be fully characterized. When they are implicated as agents of acute pharyngitis, group C and G organisms do not appear to necessitate treatment, inasmuch as they cause self-limited infections. ARF is not a sequela to these non-A streptococci infections, but acute glomerulonephritis has been documented in rare cases after epidemic group C and group G streptococcal pharyngitis.

Fusobacterium necrophorum

Fusobacterium necrophorum, an anaerobic gram-negative organism, is increasingly recognized as a cause of pharyngitis in older adolescents and adults aged up to approximately 30 years. Prevalence in studies in Europe is reported to be about 10% in patients with pharyngitis not caused by GAS, but large surveillance studies have not been performed. In a U.S. study of students at a university health clinic, *F. necrophorum* was detected by PCR in 20.5% of patients with pharyngitis and 9.4% of an asymptomatic convenience sample; some had more than one bacterium detected by PCR of throat swabs. Many of the pharyngitis patients with *F. necrophorum* had signs and symptoms indistinguishable from patients with increased likelihood for GAS pharyngitis: About one third had fever, one third had tonsillar exudates, two thirds had anterior cervical adenopathy, and most did not have cough. The symptomatic overlap of *F. necrophorum* and GAS and the presence of asymptomatic carriage could complicate the clinical assessment of sore throat in adolescents, but *F. necrophorum* is difficult to culture from the throat and neither a rapid test nor PCR is available for use in clinical care.

F. necrophorum pharyngitis can be associated with development of septic thrombophlebitis of the internal jugular vein, known as **Lemierre syndrome** (Fig. 2.12). Approximately 80% of cases of Lemierre syndrome are due to this gram-negative rod, but the proportion of patients infected or colonized with *F. necrophorum* who develop pharyngitis and Lemierre syndrome is unknown. Patients present initially with fever, sore throat, exudative pharyngitis, and/or peritonsillar abscess. The symptoms persist, severe neck pain and swelling develop, and the patient appears toxic. Septic shock may ensue along with metastatic complications, especially septic pulmonary emboli. Diagnosis is confirmed by CT or MRI of the neck and isolation of the organism

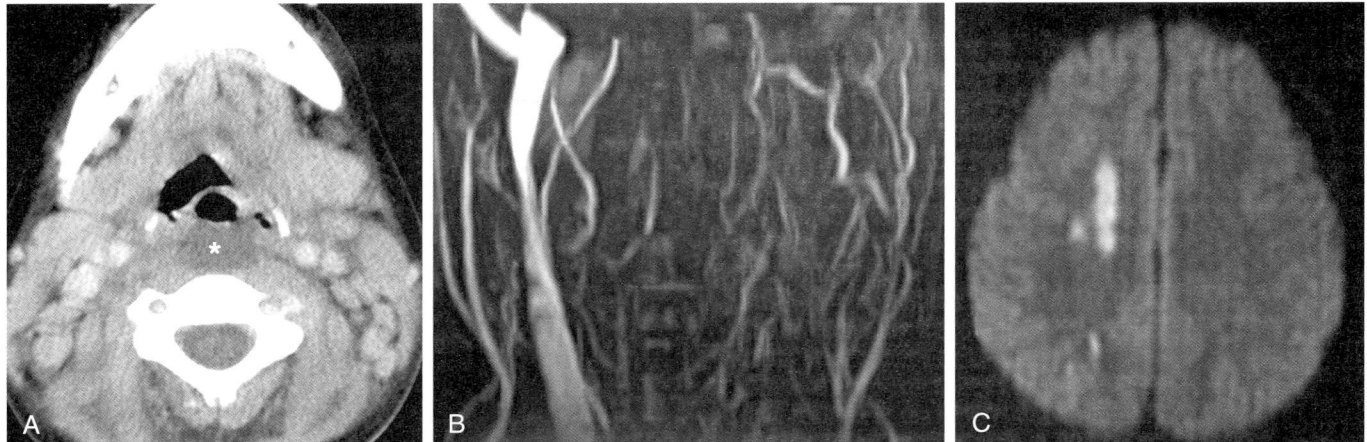

Fig. 2.12 Lemierre syndrome (*Fusobacterium necrophorum* infection) complicated by stroke in a 6-year-old female presenting with fever, difficulty swallowing, and nuchal rigidity. *A,* Axial contrast-enhanced CT image shows low-attenuation retropharyngeal fluid *(asterisk). B,* MRI 2 days later, performed because of acute left arm weakness, confirms lack of left internal jugular vein patency on magnetic resonance venogram. *C,* Diffusion-weighted image of the brain reveals multiple small foci of bright signal infarction secondary to emboli from thrombophlebitis, vasospasm, or both. (From Lowe LH, Smith CJ. Infection and inflammation. In: *Caffey's Pediatric Diagnostic Imaging.* 12th ed. Philadelphia: Elsevier; 2013:137, Fig. 15.2.)

on anaerobic blood culture. *F. necrophorum* is usually sensitive to metronidazole, clindamycin, a carbapenem, and β-lactam in combination with a β-lactamase inhibitor (such as ampicillin-sulbactam). The septic thrombophlebitis of Lemierre syndrome can also be polymicrobial (*Bacteroides, Prevotella*); combination antibacterial therapy may be beneficial. Some patients require surgical debridement and/or incision and drainage. The case-fatality rate may be as high as 9%.

Arcanobacterium Infection

Arcanobacterium haemolyticum is a gram-positive rod that has been reported to cause acute pharyngitis and scarlet fever–like rash, particularly in teenagers and young adults. Detecting this agent requires special methods for culture, and it has not routinely been sought in patients with scarlet fever or pharyngitis. The clinical features of *A. haemolyticum* are indistinguishable from GAS pharyngitis; pharyngeal erythema is present in almost all patients, patchy white to gray exudates in about 70%, cervical adenitis in about 50%, and moderate fever in 40%. Palatal petechiae and strawberry tongue may also occur. The scarlatiniform rash usually spares the face, palms, and soles. The rash is erythematous and blanches; it may be pruritic and demonstrate minimal desquamation. Erythromycin appears to be the treatment of choice.

Epiglottitis and Bacterial Tracheitis

Epiglottitis (or supraglottitis) is a life-threatening infection of the airway proximal to the vocal cords (Fig. 2.13; see also Fig. 2.10). Historically, it was an infection in 1- to 4-year-old children caused by *Haemophilus influenzae* type b. Epiglottitis presents with acute onset of fever and severe sore throat. This disease progresses rapidly to airway compromise. Patients are often drooling and leaning forward with the neck extended. Some patients may have stridor, but a muffled voice is more common. Management depends on establishing a secure airway by intubation and treating with antibacterials. When epiglottitis is suspected, the oropharynx should not be visualized or manipulated except in a controlled environment (e.g., intensive care unit or operating room) by someone with expertise in management of the airway who is prepared to immediately intubate the patient. Vaccination against *H. influenzae* type b has nearly eliminated this disease in childhood; however, epiglottitis caused by GAS, *Streptococcus pneumoniae, S. aureus,* and non–type b *H. influenzae* occurs occasionally.

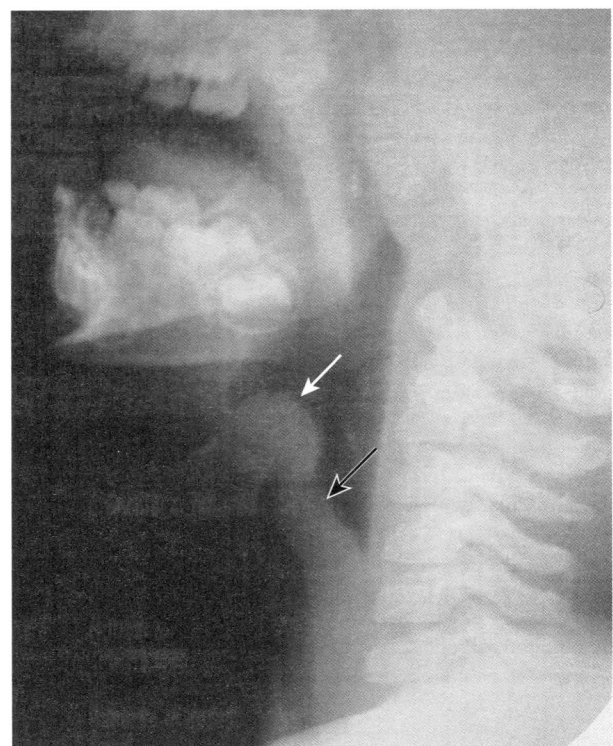

Fig. 2.13 Epiglottis in a 5-year-old boy with respiratory distress and drooling. A lateral soft tissue neck radiograph shows a markedly thickened epiglottis *(white arrow),* which is referred to as the "thumb" sign. The aryepiglottic folds *(black arrow)* also are thickened. (From Laya BF, Lee EY. Upper airway disease. In: *Caffey's Pediatric Diagnostic Imaging.* 12th ed. Philadelphia: Elsevier; 2013:529, Fig. 51.2.)

Bacterial tracheitis (bacterial croup, bacterial laryngotracheitis) is a rare complication of viral croup. *S. aureus* is the most common superinfecting bacterium identified. Patients have a history of prolonged croup symptoms that become dramatically worse with fever and signs of airway obstruction. While sore throat may have been present at the onset of croup, it is not a prominent complaint once bacterial infection of the airway occurs. The clinical appearance of patients with bacterial tracheitis may mimic that of patients with epiglottitis.

DIPHTHERIA

Diphtheria is a very serious disease that is caused by pharyngeal infection by toxigenic strains of *Corynebacterium diphtheriae*. It has become very rare in the United States and other developed countries because of immunization but is endemic in Asia, the Middle East, Eastern Europe, Haiti, and the Dominican Republic. The few diphtheria cases recognized annually in the United States usually occur in unimmunized individuals; the fatality rate is about 5%.

Pathogenesis

The pathogenesis of diphtheria involves nasopharyngeal mucosal colonization by *C. diphtheriae* and toxin elaboration after an incubation period of 1–5 days. Toxin leads to local tissue inflammation and necrosis, producing an adherent grayish membrane made up of fibrin, blood, inflammatory cells, and epithelial cells; toxin is absorbed into the bloodstream. Fragment B of the polypeptide toxin binds particularly well to cardiac, neural, and renal cells, and the smaller fragment A enters cells and interferes with protein synthesis. Toxin fixation by tissues may lead to fatal myocarditis with arrhythmias within 10–14 days and to peripheral neuritis within 3–7 weeks.

Clinical Features

Acute tonsillar and pharyngeal diphtheria is characterized by sore throat, anorexia, malaise, and low-grade fever. The grayish membrane forms within 1–2 days over the tonsils and pharyngeal walls and occasionally extends into the larynx and trachea. Cervical adenopathy varies but may be severe and associated with development of a "bull neck." In mild cases, the membrane sloughs after 7–10 days and the patient recovers. In severe cases, an increasingly toxic appearance can lead to prostration, stupor, coma, and death within 6–10 days. Distinctive features include palatal and uvula paralysis, laryngeal paralysis, ocular palsies, diaphragmatic palsy, and myocarditis. Airway obstruction from membrane formation may complicate the toxigenic manifestations.

Diagnosis

Accurate diagnosis requires isolation of *C. diphtheriae* on culture of material from beneath the membrane, with confirmation of toxin production by the organism isolated. Laboratories must be forewarned that diphtheria is suspected. Other tests are of little value.

GONOCOCCAL PHARYNGITIS

Acute symptomatic pharyngitis caused by *Neisseria gonorrhoeae* occurs occasionally in sexually active individuals from oral-genital contact. In cases involving young children, sexual abuse must be suspected. The infection usually manifests as an ulcerative, exudative tonsillopharyngitis but may be asymptomatic and resolve spontaneously. Gonococcal pharyngitis is more readily transmitted via fellatio than via cunnilingus. Gonorrhea rarely is transmitted from the pharynx to a sexual partner, but pharyngitis can serve as a source for gonococcemia. Diagnosis requires culture on appropriate selective media (e.g., Thayer-Martin medium). NAAT may also detect the organism from pharyngeal and other sites. Examination and testing for other sexually transmitted infections and pregnancy are recommended.

CHLAMYDIAL AND MYCOPLASMAL INFECTIONS

Chlamydia species and *Mycoplasma pneumoniae* may cause pharyngitis, although the frequency of these infections is unclear. *Chlamydia*

trachomatis has been implicated serologically as a cause of pharyngitis in as many as 20% of adults with pharyngitis, but isolation of the organism from the pharynx has proved more difficult. *Chlamydia pneumoniae* has also been identified as a cause of pharyngitis. Because antibodies to this organism show some cross reaction with *C. trachomatis*, it is possible that infections formerly attributed to *C. trachomatis* were really caused by *C. pneumoniae*. Diagnosis of chlamydial pharyngitis is difficult, whether by culture or serologically, and neither method is readily available to the clinician.

M. pneumoniae most likely causes pharyngitis. Serologic (positive mycoplasma IgM) or, less often, culture methods can be used to identify this infectious agent, which was found in 33% of college students with pharyngitis in one study. PCR is diagnostic but there is no need to seek evidence of these organisms routinely in pharyngitis patients in the absence of ongoing research studies of nonstreptococcal pharyngitis. The efficacy of antibacterial treatment for *M. pneumoniae* and chlamydial pharyngitis is not known, but these illnesses appear to be self-limited.

ORAL-PHARYNGEAL FACIAL SPACE PAIN

Facial space infections are usually polymicrobial, are odontogenic in origin, and develop after a periapical tooth abscess spreads through the maxillary or mandibular bone (Figs. 2.14, 2.15, and 2.16 and Table 2.11). In many of these infections there is localized swelling often out of proportion to facial tenderness, erythema, and specific tooth tenderness.

Lateral (buccal side) extension of an infected molar produces marked lateral facial swelling (**buccal space**), while involvement of canines (**canine space**) produces anterior mid-facial edema, which may extend to the periorbital space. Extension to the angle of the jaw (**parotid space**) may be confused with parotitis.

Abscess spread toward the medial-lingual location may irritate muscles of mastication producing trismus, while further extension may produce **lateral pharyngeal space** infection with the risk of involvement of the internal jugular vein and carotid artery as well as producing airway compromise. Other complications may include cavernous sinus thrombosis and brain abscess.

Submandibular and sublingual spread produces **Ludwig angina**, a potentially life-threatening rapidly spreading indurated cellulitis manifest by brawny nonpitting edema, an elevated swollen tongue, pain, trismus, fever, drooling, and a risk for airway compromise (Fig. 2.17).

Dominant bacteria include a combination of anaerobic gram-negative rods and gram-positive cocci plus facultative and

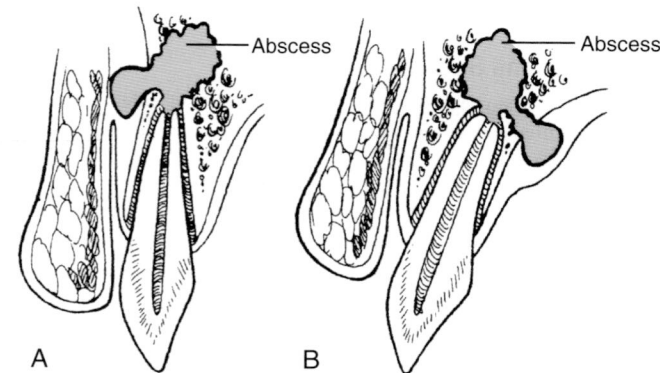

Fig. 2.14 When the infection process is allowed to progress, it erodes through the nearest cortical plate. *A,* Tooth apex is near thin labial bone, so infection erodes onto labial side. *B,* Apex is near palatal side and erodes through that side. (Modified from Christian JM. Odontogenic infections. In: Flint PW, Haughey BH, Lund VJ, et al., eds. *Cummings Otolaryngology Head & Neck Surgery.* 5th ed. Philadelphia: Elsevier; 2010, Fig. 12.1.)

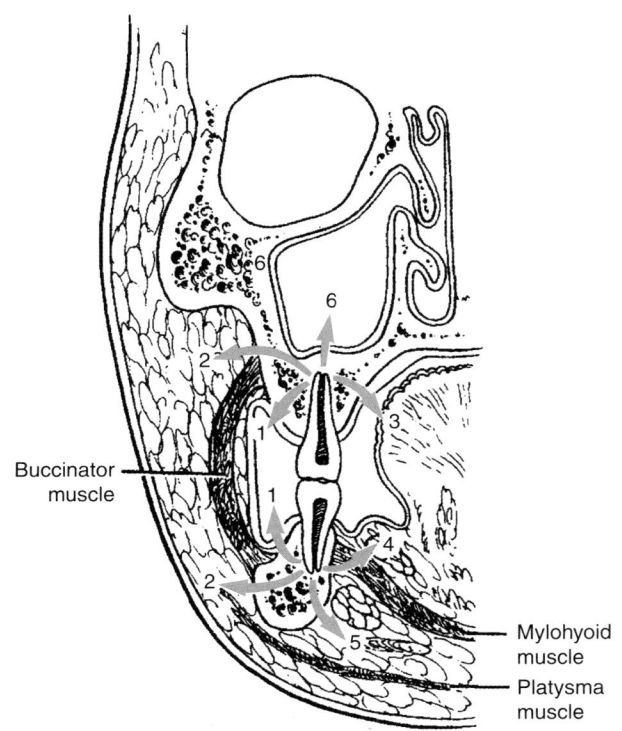

Fig. 2.15 As the infection erodes through the bone, it can express itself in a variety of places, depending on thickness of overlying bone and relationship of muscle attachments to the site of perforation. This illustration notes six possible locations: *1,* vestibule; *2,* buccal space; *3,* palate; *4,* sublingual space; *5,* submandibular space; and *6,* maxillary sinus. (From Christian JM. Odontogenic infections. In Flint PW, Haughey BH, Lund VJ, et al., eds. *Cummings Otolaryngology Head & Neck Surgery.* 5th ed. Philadelphia: Elsevier; 2010, Fig. 12.2.)

TABLE 2.11 Clinical Presentation of Odontogenic Infections by Location

Type of Infection	Clinical Presentation
Dentoalveolar infection	Swelling of the alveolar ridge with periodontal, periapical, and subperiosteal abscess.
Submental space infection	Firm midline swelling beneath the chin. Caused by infection from the mandibular incisors.
Submandibular space infection	Swelling of the submandibular triangle of the neck around the angle of the mandible. Infection is caused by mandibular molar infections. Trismus is typical.
Sublingual space infection	Swelling of the floor of the mouth with possible elevation of the tongue and dysphagia.
Retropharyngeal space infection	Stiff neck, sore throat, dysphagia, raspy voice. These infections are caused by infections of the molars. The retropharyngeal space infection has a high potential to spread to the mediastinum.
Buccal space infection	Swelling of the cheek. Caused by infection of premolar or molar tooth.
Masticator space infection	Swelling on either side of the mandibular ramus. Caused by infection of the mandibular third molar. Trismus is present.
Canine space infection	Swelling of the anterior cheek with loss of the nasolabial fold and possible extension to the infraorbital region.

From Ogle OE. Odontogenic infections. *Dent Clin North Am.* 2017;61(2):235–252 (Table 1, p. 236).

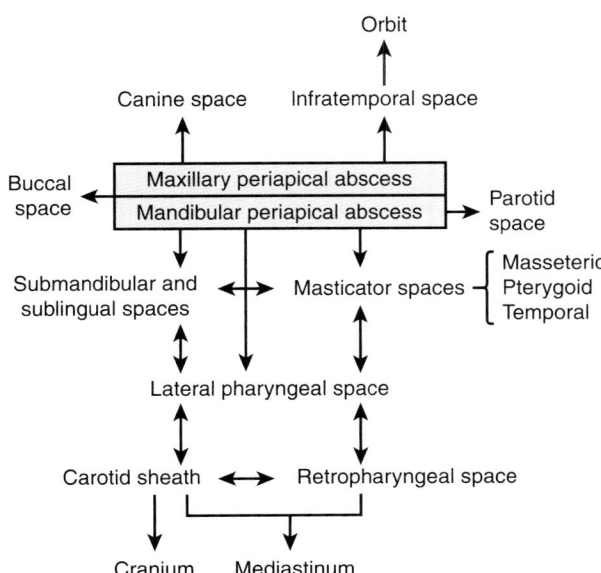

Fig. 2.16 Potential pathways of extension in deep fascial space infections. (From Chow AW. Infections of the oral cavity, neck, and head. In: Bennett JE, Dolin R, Blaser MF, eds. *Mandell, Douglas, and Bennett's Principles and Practices of Infectious Diseases.* 9th ed. Philadelphia: Elsevier; 2020, Fig. 64.6.)

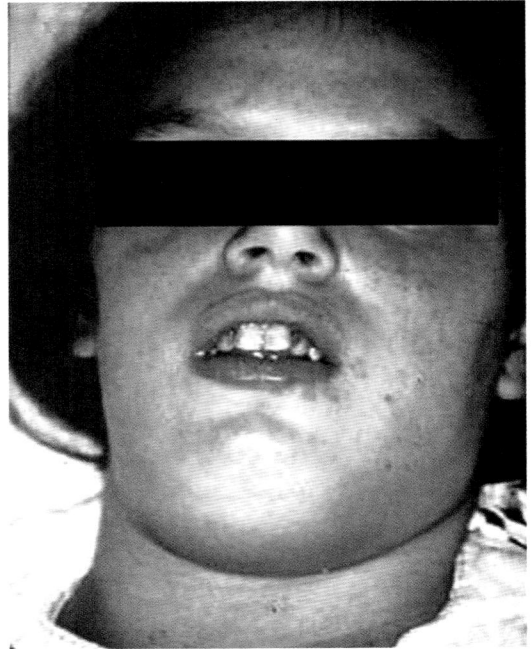

Fig. 2.17 Early appearance of a patient with Ludwig angina with a brawny, boardlike swelling in the submandibular spaces. (From Megran DW, Scheifele DW, Chow AW. Odontogenic infections. *Pediatr Infect Dis.* 1984;3:262; with permission.)

microaerophilic streptococci. Panoramic x-rays and CT imaging help confirm the diagnosis and characterize facial space involvement. Treatment includes involved tooth abscess drainage, root canal or tooth extraction, and surgical debridement of the other infected tissue.

Antibiotic therapy includes clindamycin or ampicillin-sulbactam plus metronidazole. Concerning features include swelling involving the submandibular and submental spaces, swelling in the floor of the mouth, drooling, sitting-up "sniffing" posture, and fever >38.9°C.

SUMMARY AND RED FLAGS

Sore throat is a common pediatric complaint. Most children with acute sore throat have a viral illness. Accurate diagnosis of acute streptococcal pharyngitis is essential because appropriate therapy ensures prevention of serious suppurative and nonsuppurative complications. Life-threatening infectious complications of oropharyngeal infections may manifest with mouth pain, pharyngitis, parapharyngeal space infectious extension, and/or airway obstruction. Other red flags are prolonged fever, prolonged sore throat, drooling, muffled voice, trismus, and severe, unremitting pain (see Table 2.5). Considering noninfectious mimics of pharyngitis with or without oral lesions, such as solid tumors, hematologic malignancy, Kawasaki disease, and other noninfectious inflammatory conditions, is essential prior to instituting therapy.

BIBLIOGRAPHY

A bibliography is available at ExpertConsult.com.

3

Cough

Louella B. Amos

INTRODUCTION

Cough is an important defense mechanism of the lungs and is a common symptom, particularly during winter months. In most patients, it is self-limited. However, cough can be ominous, indicating serious underlying disease, because of accompanying problems (hemoptysis) or because of serious consequences of the cough itself (e.g., syncope and hemorrhage), or cough may present as an uncommon disorder that mimics a common disease.

Pathophysiology

The cough reflex serves to prevent the entry of harmful substances into the tracheobronchial tree and to expel excess secretions and retained material from the tracheobronchial tree. Cough begins with stimulation of cough receptors, located in the upper and lower airways, and in many other sites such as the ear canal, tympanic membrane, sinuses, nose, pericardium, pleura, and diaphragm. Receptors send impulses via vagal, phrenic, glossopharyngeal, or trigeminal nerves to the "cough center," which is in the medulla. Because cough is not only an involuntary reflex activity but also one that can be initiated or suppressed voluntarily, "higher centers" must also be involved in the afferent limb of the responsible pathway. The neural impulses go from the medulla to the appropriate efferent pathways to the larynx, tracheobronchial tree, and expiratory muscles.

The act of coughing (Fig. 3.1) begins with an inspiration, followed by expiration against a closed glottis (compressive phase), resulting in the buildup of intrathoracic pressures (50–300 cm H_2O). These pressures may be transmitted to vascular, cerebrospinal, and intraocular spaces. Finally, the glottis opens, allowing for explosive expiratory airflow (300 m/sec) and expulsion of mucus, particularly from the larger, central airways. The inability to seal the upper airway (e.g., endotracheal tube or tracheostomy) impairs the effectiveness of cough. Respiratory muscle weakness (e.g., muscular dystrophy) impairs both the inspiratory and the compressive phase.

History

The history often provides the most important body of information about a child's cough. A diagnosis can often be discerned with relative certainty from the environmental and exposure history, family history, timeframe, and characterization of the cough.

Demographics

The patient's age (Table 3.1) helps to focus the diagnostic possibilities. Congenital anatomic abnormalities may be symptomatic from birth, whereas toddlers, who may have incomplete neurologic control over swallowing and often put small objects in their mouths, are at risk for foreign body aspiration; adolescents may experiment with smoking traditional cigarettes, e-cigarettes, or vaping. Socioeconomic factors must be considered; a family that cannot afford central heating may use a smoky wood-burning stove; spending time at a daycare center may expose an infant to respiratory viruses; and several adult smokers in a small home expose children to a high concentration of respiratory irritants.

Characteristics of the Cough

The various cough characteristics can help determine the cause of cough. The causes of acute, recurrent, and chronic coughs may be quite different from each other (Fig. 3.2; see also Table 3.1). A cough can be paroxysmal, brassy, productive, weak, volitional, and "throat-clearing," and it may occur at different times of the day (Tables 3.2 and 3.3). The previous response or lack of response to some therapies for recurrent and chronic cough can provide important information (see Table 3.3). Furthermore, some coughs may be caused or worsened by medications (Table 3.4).

Associated Symptoms

A history of accompanying signs or symptoms, whether localized to the respiratory tract (e.g., wheeze, stridor, transient tachypnea of the newborn) or elsewhere (e.g., failure to thrive, frequent malodorous stools) can give important clues (Table 3.5; see also Tables 3.2 and 3.3). It is essential to remember that the daily language of the physician is full of jargon that may be adopted by parents but with a different meaning from that understood by physicians. If a parent says that a child "wheezes" or "croups" or is "short of breath," it is important to find out what the parent means by that term and ask them to mimic the sound or action.

Family and Patient's Medical History

Because many disorders of childhood have genetic or environmental familial components, the family history can provide helpful information:
- Are there older siblings with cystic fibrosis (CF) or asthma?
- Is there a coughing sibling whose kindergarten class has been closed because of pertussis or COVID-19?
- Is there an adolescent or adult with chronic cough (bronchitis) who may have pertussis or tuberculosis?
- Was the child premature, and if so, did they spend a month on the ventilator, and do they now have chronic lung disease (bronchopulmonary dysplasia)?
- Did the toddler choke on a carrot or other food a few months ago?
- Did the child have respiratory syncytial virus (RSV), bronchiolitis, or rhinovirus infection as an infant?
- Did the child receive a bone marrow transplant?
- Is the child fully immunized?
- Did the infant have a tracheoesophageal fistula repaired in the neonatal period?

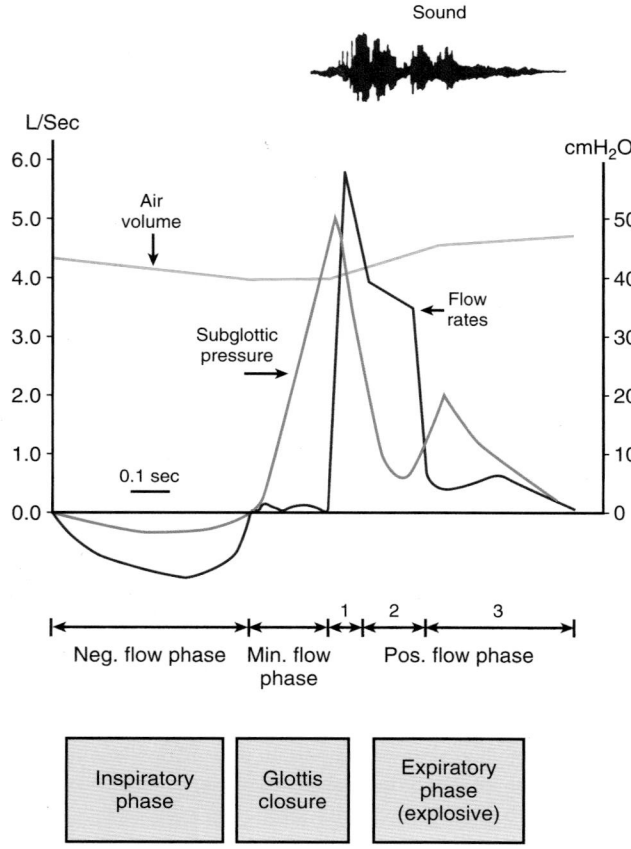

Sound

Fig. 3.1 Cough mechanics, showing changes in expiratory flow rate, air volume, subglottic pressure, and sound recording during cough. (Modified from Yanagihara N et al. The physical parameters of cough: the larynx in a normal single cough. *Acta Otolaryngol.* 1996;61:495–510.)

Physical Examination

Inspection

Initial inspection often reveals the seriousness of an illness:

- Is the child struggling to breathe (dyspnea)?
- Does the child have an anxious look?
- Is the child in respiratory distress?
- Can the child be calmed or engaged in play?
- Are there audible respiratory sounds?
- Is the child's skin blue (representing cyanosis) or ashen?
- Does the child appear wasted, with poor growth that may indicate a chronic illness?

The respiratory rate is often elevated with parenchymal lung disease or extrathoracic airway obstruction. Respiratory rates vary with the age of the child (Fig. 3.3) and with pulmonary infection, airway obstruction, activity, wakefulness and sleep, fever, metabolic acidosis, and anxiety.

Odors may also give helpful clues. Does the examining room or the clothing smell of stale cigarette smoke? Is there a foul odor from a diaper with a fatty stool, which may suggest pancreatic insufficiency and CF? Is the child's breath malodorous, as can be noticed in sinusitis, nasal foreign body, lung abscess, or bronchiectasis?

Fingers. Cyanotic nail beds suggest hypoxemia, poor peripheral circulation, or both. The examiner looks for the presence of **digital clubbing** (Fig. 3.4), which makes asthma or acute pneumonia extremely unlikely. The absence of digital clubbing but a history of severe chronic cough in an older child makes CF unlikely.

TABLE 3.1	**Causes of Cough**		
Age Group	**Acute**	**Recurrent**	**Chronic (>4 wk)**
Infants	Infection[1]*	Asthma[1]	Asthma[1]
	Aspiration[2]	CF[1]	CF[1]
	Foreign body[3]	GER[1]	GER[1]
		Aspiration[2]	Aspiration[2]
		Anatomic abnormality[3]†	Pertussis[2]
			Anatomic abnormality[3]†
		Passive smoking[3]	Passive smoking[3]
Toddlers	Infection[1]	Asthma[1]	Asthma[1]
	Foreign body[2]	CF[1]	CF[1]
	Aspiration[3]	GER[1]	GER[1]
		Aspiration[2]	Aspiration[2]
		Anatomic abnormality[3]	Pertussis[2]
		Passive smoking[3]	Anatomic abnormality[3]
		Protracted bacterial bronchitis[1]	Passive smoking[3]
			Protracted bacterial bronchitis[1]
Children	Infection[1]	Asthma[1]	Asthma[1]
	Foreign body[3]	CF[1]	CF[1]
		GER[1]	GER[2]
		Passive smoking[3]	Pertussis[2]
		Protracted bacterial bronchitis[1]	Mycoplasma[3]
			Habit[3]
			Anatomic abnormality[3]
			Passive smoking[3]
			Protracted bacterial bronchitis[1]
Adolescents	Infection[1]	Asthma[1]	Asthma[1]
	Vaping	CF[1]	CF[1]
		GER[1]	GER[2]
		Aspiration[2]	Smoking[2]
		Anatomic abnormality[3]	Tuberculosis[3]
		Protracted bacterial bronchitis[1]	Habit[2]
			Pertussis[3]
			Aspiration[3]
			Anatomic abnormality[3]
			Tumor[3]
			Protracted bacterial bronchitis[1]

*Infections include upper (pharyngitis, sinusitis, tracheitis, rhinitis, otitis) and lower (pneumonia, abscess, empyema) respiratory tract disease.
†Anatomic abnormality includes tracheobronchomalacia, tracheoesophageal fistula, vascular ring, abnormal position, or take-off of large bronchi.
[1]Common.
[2]Less common.
[3]Much less common.
CF, cystic fibrosis; GER, gastroesophageal reflux.

Chest, abdomen, and spine. The shape of the chest gives information. Is the anteroposterior (AP) diameter increased, which indicates hyperinflation of the lungs from obstruction of small airways (e.g., asthma, bronchiolitis, CF)? Is this diameter small, as can be seen with some restrictive lung diseases with small lung volumes (e.g., muscular dystrophy, spinal muscular atrophy)? The normal infant has a "round" chest configuration, with the AP diameter of the chest about 84% of the transverse (lateral) diameter. With growth, the chest becomes more flattened in the AP dimension, and the AP-to-transverse ratio is between 70% and 75%. Although obstetric calipers can be used

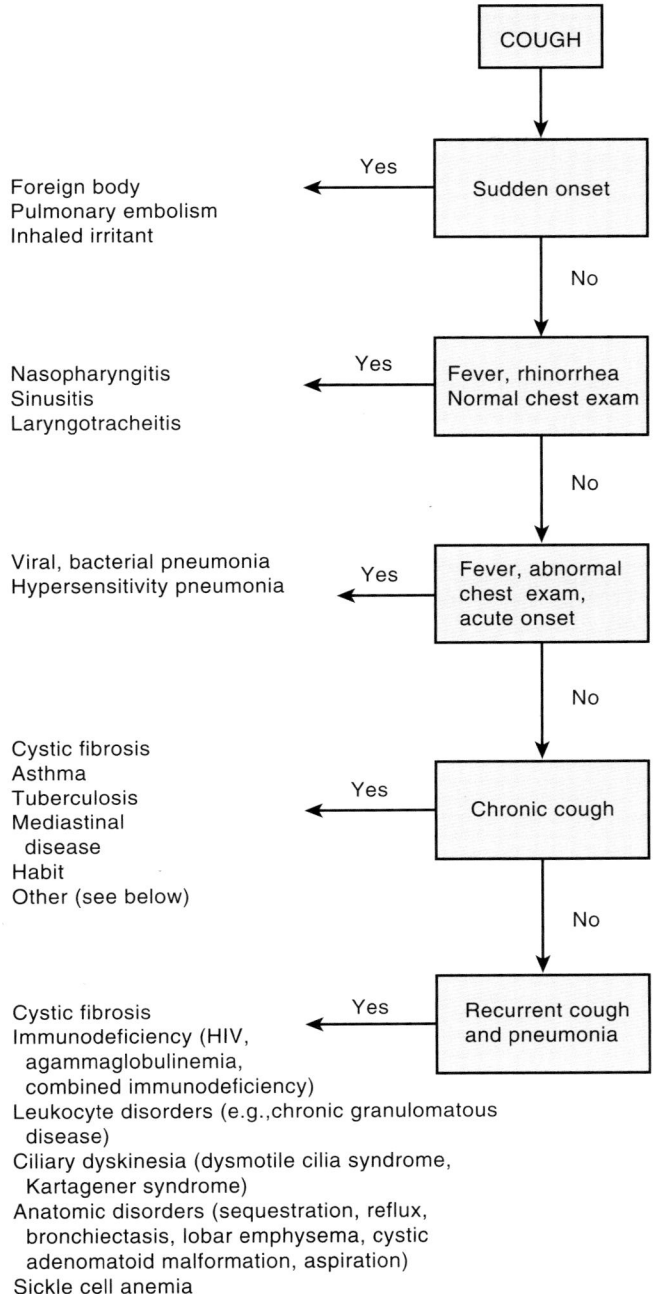

Foreign body
Pulmonary embolism
Inhaled irritant

COUGH → Sudden onset — Yes

Nasopharyngitis
Sinusitis
Laryngotracheitis

Fever, rhinorrhea
Normal chest exam — Yes

Viral, bacterial pneumonia
Hypersensitivity pneumonia

Fever, abnormal
chest exam,
acute onset — Yes

Cystic fibrosis
Asthma
Tuberculosis
Mediastinal
  disease
Habit
Other (see below)

Chronic cough — Yes

Cystic fibrosis
Immunodeficiency (HIV,
  agammaglobulinemia,
  combined immunodeficiency)
Leukocyte disorders (e.g.,chronic granulomatous
  disease)
Ciliary dyskinesia (dysmotile cilia syndrome,
  Kartagener syndrome)
Anatomic disorders (sequestration, reflux,
  bronchiectasis, lobar emphysema, cystic
  adenomatoid malformation, aspiration)
Sickle cell anemia

Recurrent cough
and pneumonia — Yes

Fig. 3.2 Algorithm for differential diagnosis of cough.

TABLE 3.2	**Clinical Clues About Cough**
Characteristic	**Think of**
Staccato, paroxysmal	Pertussis, cystic fibrosis, foreign body, *Chlamydia* species, *Mycoplasma* species, parapertussis
Followed by "whoop"	Pertussis
All day, rarely during sleep, honking	Habit
Barking, brassy	Croup, habit, tracheomalacia, tracheitis, epiglottitis
Staccato	Chlamydia
Hoarseness	Laryngeal involvement (croup, recurrent laryngeal nerve involvement)
Abrupt onset	Foreign body, pulmonary embolism
Follows exercise	Asthma
Accompanies eating, drinking	Aspiration, gastroesophageal reflux, tracheoesophageal fistula
Throat clearing	Postnasal drip
Productive (sputum)	Infection
Sputum casts	Plastic bronchitis
Night cough	Sinusitis, asthma
Seasonal	Allergic rhinitis, asthma
Immunosuppressed patient	Bacterial pneumonia, *Pneumocystis jirovecii*, *Mycobacterium tuberculosis*, *Mycobacterium avium–intracellulare*, cytomegalovirus
Dyspnea	Hypoxia, hypercarbia
Animal exposure	*Chlamydia psittaci* (birds), *Yersinia pestis* (rodents), *Francisella tularensis* (rabbits), Q fever (sheep, cattle), hantavirus (rodents), histoplasmosis (pigeons)
Geographic	Histoplasmosis (Mississippi, Missouri, Ohio River Valley), coccidioidomycosis (Southwest), blastomycosis (North and Midwest)
Workdays with clearing on days off	Occupational exposure

Less easy to notice than intercostal retractions is their bulging out with expiration in a child with expiratory obstruction (asthma). Contraction of the abdominal muscles with expiration is easier to notice and is another indication that a child is working harder than normal to push air out through obstructed airways.

Inspection of the spine may reveal kyphosis or scoliosis. There is a risk of restrictive lung disease if the curvature is severe.

Palpation

Palpating the trachea, particularly in infants, may reveal a shift to one side, which suggests loss of volume of the lung on that side or extrapulmonary gas (pneumothorax) on the other side. Placing one hand on each side of the chest while the patient breathes may enable the examiner to detect asymmetry of chest wall movement, either in timing or in degree of expansion. The former indicates a partial bronchial obstruction, and the latter suggests a smaller lung volume, voluntary guarding, or diminished muscle function on one side. Palpating the abdomen gently during expiration may allow the examiner to feel the contraction of the abdominal muscles in cases of expiratory obstruction. Hyperinflation may push the liver down, making it palpable below the costal margin.

Palpation for tactile fremitus, the transmitted vibrations of the spoken word ("ninety-nine" is the word often used to accentuate these

to give an objective assessment of the AP diameter of the chest, most clinicians rely on their subjective assessment of whether the diameter is increased: does the patient look "barrel-chested"?

Intercostal, subcostal, suprasternal, and supraclavicular retractions (inspiratory sinking in of the soft tissues) indicate increased effort of breathing and reflect both the contraction of the accessory muscles of respiration and the resulting difference between intrapleural and extrathoracic pressure. Retractions occur most commonly with obstructed airways (upper or lower), but they may occur with any condition leading to the use of the accessory muscles. Any retractions other than the mild normal depressions seen between an infant's lower ribs indicate a greater-than-normal work of breathing. Audible end-expiratory "grunting" is suggestive of alveolar fluid from pulmonary, cardiac, or inflammation; it is often associated with severe disease.

TABLE 3.3 Cough: Some Aspects of Differential Diagnosis

Cause	Abrupt Onset	Only When Awake	Yellow Sputum	Responds to Inhaled Bronchodilator (by History)	Responds to Antibiotics (by History)	Responds to Steroids (by History)	Failure to Thrive	Wheeze	Digital Clubbing
Asthma	+	++	++	+++	+	+++	+	+++	–
Cystic fibrosis	+	++	++	+	+++	+	++	++	+++
Infection	+	+	++	–	++	–	+	+	–
Aspiration	+	+	+	+	+	+	++	++	+
Gastroesophageal reflux	+	++	–	–	–	+	++	++	–
Foreign body	+++	+	++	+	++	+	+	++	+
Habit	–	+++	–	–	–	–	–	–	–

+++, very common and suggests the diagnosis; ++, common; +, uncommon; –, almost never and makes examiner question the diagnosis.

TABLE 3.4 Drugs Causing Cough

Drug	Mechanism
Tobacco, marijuana	Direct irritants
β-Adrenergic blockers	Potentiate asthma
ACE inhibitors	↑ Bradykinin (protussive mediator)
Bethanechol	Potentiates asthma
Nitrofurantoin	(?) Via oxygen radicals vs autoimmunity
Antineoplastic agents	Various (including pneumonitis/fibrosis, hypersensitivity, noncardiogenic pulmonary edema)
Sulfasalazine	(?) Causes bronchiolitis obliterans
Penicillamine	(?) Causes bronchiolitis obliterans
Diphenylhydantoin	Hypersensitivity pneumonitis
Aspirin, NSAIDs	Potentiate asthma
Nebulized antibiotics	(?) Direct irritant
Inhaled/nebulized bronchodilators	Increases tracheal/bronchial wall instability in airway malacia; or via reaction to vehicle
Theophylline, caffeine	Indirect, via worsened gastroesophageal reflux (relaxation of lower esophageal sphincter)
Metabisulfite	Induces allergic asthma
Cholinesterase inhibitors	Induce mucus production (bronchorrhea)

ACE, angiotensin-converting enzyme; NSAIDs, nonsteroidal antiinflammatory drugs.

TABLE 3.5 Nonpulmonary History Suggesting Cystic Fibrosis

Maldigestion, malabsorption, steatorrhea (in 80–90%)
Poor weight gain
Family history of cystic fibrosis
Salty taste to skin
Rectal prolapse (up to 20% of patients)
Digital clubbing
Meconium ileus (in 10–15%)
Intestinal atresia
Intestinal obstruction after infancy
Neonatal cholestatic jaundice
Male sterility
Chronic sinusitis

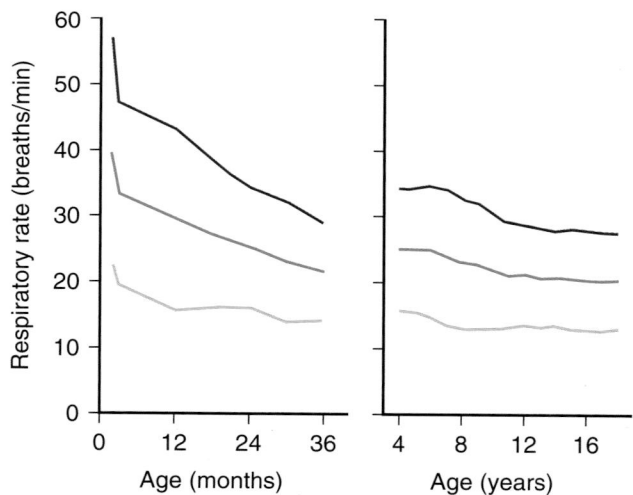

Fig. 3.3 Mean values *(blue line)* ±2 standard deviations *(red and yellow lines)* of the normal respiratory rate at rest (during sleep in children younger than 3 years). There is no significant difference between the genders. (Data from Pasterkamp H. The history and physical examination. In: Chernick V, ed. *Kendig's Disorders of the Respiratory Tract in Children.* 6th ed. Philadelphia: WB Saunders; 1998:88.)

vibrations), helps determine areas of increased parenchymal density and hence increased fremitus (as in pneumonic consolidation) or decreased fremitus (as in pneumothorax or pleural effusion).

Percussion

The percussion determined by the examiner's tapping of one middle finger on the middle finger of the other hand, which is firmly placed over the patient's thorax, may be dull over an area of consolidation or effusion and hyperresonant with air trapping. Percussion can also be used to determine diaphragmatic excursion. The lowest level of resonance at inspiration and expiration determines diaphragmatic motion.

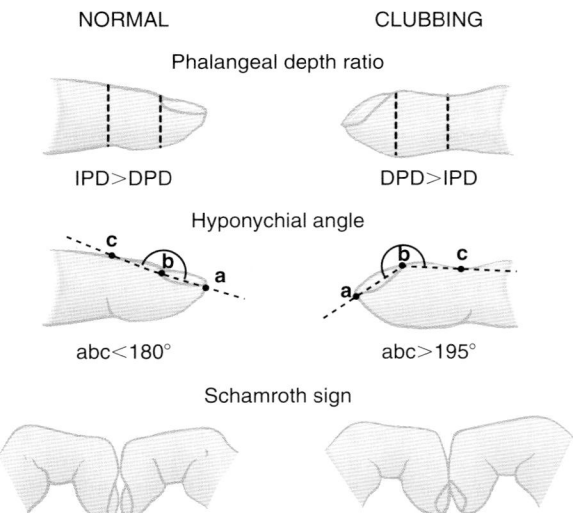

NORMAL   CLUBBING

Phalangeal depth ratio

IPD>DPD   DPD>IPD

Hyponychial angle

abc<180°   abc>195°

Schamroth sign

Fig. 3.4 Measurement of digital clubbing. The ratio of the distal phalangeal depth (DPD) to the interphalangeal depth (IPD), or the phalangeal depth ratio, is normally <1 but increases to >1 with finger clubbing. The DPD/IPD ratio can be measured with calipers or, more accurately, with finger casts. The hyponychial angle is measured from lateral projections of the finger contour on a magnifying screen and is normally <180 degrees but >195 degrees with finger clubbing. Schamroth sign is useful for bedside assessment. The dorsal surfaces of the terminal phalanges of similar fingers are placed together. With clubbing, the normal diamond-shaped aperture or "window" at the bases of the nail beds disappears, and a prominent distal angle forms between the end of the nails. In normal subjects, this angle is minimal or nonexistent. (From Pasterkamp H. The history and physical examination. In: Chernick V, ed. *Kendig's Disorders of the Respiratory Tract in Children*. 6th ed. Philadelphia: WB Saunders; 1998.)

Auscultation

Because lung sounds tend to be higher pitched than heart sounds, the diaphragm of the stethoscope is better suited to pulmonary auscultation than is the bell, whose target is primarily the lower-pitched heart sounds (Table 3.6). The adult-sized stethoscope generally is superior to the smaller pediatric or neonatal diaphragms, even for listening to small chests, because its acoustics are better (Figs. 3.5 and 3.6).

Adventitious sounds come in a few varieties, namely, stridor, crackles, rhonchi, and wheezes. Other sounds should be described in clear, everyday language.

- **Stridor** is a continuous musical sound usually heard on inspiration and is caused by narrowing in the extrathoracic airway, as with croup or laryngomalacia.
- **Crackles** are discontinuous, representing the popping open of air-fluid menisci as the airways dilate with inspiration. Fluid in larger airways causes crackles early in inspiration (congestive heart failure). Crackles that tend to be a bit lower in pitch ("coarse" crackles) than the early, higher-pitched ("fine") crackles are associated with fluid in small airways (pneumonia). Although crackles usually signal the presence of excess airway fluid (pneumonia, pulmonary edema), they may also be produced by the popping open of noninfected fibrotic or atelectatic airways. Fine crackles are not audible at the mouth, whereas coarse crackles may be. Crackles is the preferred term, rather than the previously popular "rales."
- **Rhonchi**, or "large airway sounds," are continuous gurgling or bubbling sounds typically heard during both inhalation and exhalation. These sounds are caused by movement of fluid and secretions in larger airways (in asthma, viral upper respiratory infection [URI]). Rhonchi, unlike other sounds, may clear with coughing.
- **Wheezes** are continuous musical sounds (lasting longer than 200 msec), caused by vibration of narrowed airway walls, as with asthma, and perhaps vibration of material within airway lumens.

TABLE 3.6 Physical Signs of Pulmonary Disease

Disease Process	Mediastinal Deviation	Chest Motion	Fremitus	Percussion	Breath Sounds	Adventitious Sounds	Voice Signs
Consolidation (pneumonia)	No	Reduced over area, splinting	Increased	Dull	Bronchial or reduced	Crackles	Egophony,* whispering pectoriloquy increased†
Bronchospasm	No	Hyperexpansion with limited motion	Normal or decreased	Hyperresonant	Normal to decreased	Wheezes, crackles	Normal to decreased
Atelectasis	Shift toward lesion	Reduced over area	Decreased	Dull	Reduced or absent	None or crackles	None
Pneumothorax	Tension deviates trachea and PMI to opposite side	Reduced over area	None	Resonant, tympanitic	None	None	None
Pleural effusion	Deviation to opposite side	Reduced over area	None	Dull	None	Friction rub; splash, if hemopneumothorax	None

*Egophony is present when *e* sounds like *a*.
†Whispering pectoriloquy produces clearer-sounding whispered words (e.g., "ninety-nine").
Modified from Dantzker D, Tobin M, Whatley R. Respiratory diseases. In: Andreoli TE, Carpenter CJ, Plum F, Smith LH, eds. *Cecil Essentials of Medicine*. Philadelphia: WB Saunders; 1986:126–180.
PMI, point of maximal impulse.

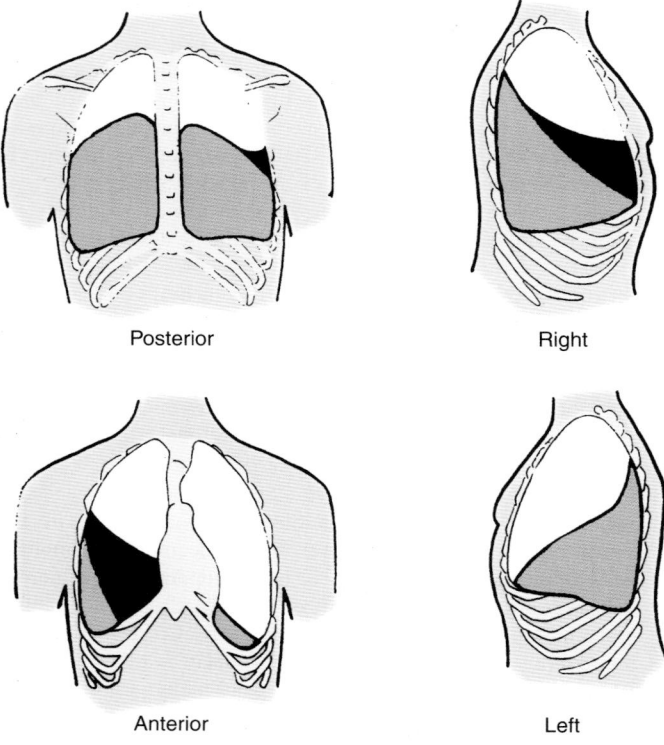

Posterior   Right

Anterior   Left

Fig. 3.5 Projections of the pulmonary lobes on the chest surface. The upper lobes are *white*, the right-middle lobe is *black*, and the lower lobes are *purple*. (From Pasterkamp H. The history and physical examination. In: Chernick V, ed. *Kendig's Disorders of the Respiratory Tract in Children*. 6th ed. Philadelphia: WB Saunders; 1998.)

These sounds are much more commonly heard during expiration than inspiration.

Diagnostic Studies

Radiography

The chest radiograph is often the most useful diagnostic test in the evaluation of the child with cough. Table 3.7 highlights some of the radiographic features of the most common causes of cough in pediatric patients. Radiographic findings are often similar for a number of disorders, and thus these studies may not indicate a definitive diagnosis. Chest radiographs are normal in children with psychogenic (habit) cough and in children with sinusitis or gastroesophageal reflux (GER) as the primary cause of cough. A normal chest radiograph indicates the unlikelihood of pneumonia caused by RSV, influenza, parainfluenza, adenovirus, *Chlamydia* species, or bacteria. Although children with cough resulting from CF, *Mycoplasma* species, tuberculosis, aspiration, a bronchial foreign body, or an anatomic abnormality usually have abnormal chest radiographs, a normal radiograph does not exclude these diagnoses. Hyperinflation of the lungs is commonly seen on chest radiographs of infants with RSV bronchiolitis or *Chlamydia* pneumonia, and a lobar or round (coin lesion) infiltrate is the radiographic hallmark of bacterial pneumonia. Normal sinuses on radiograph or CT scan exclude sinusitis. In some causes of cough, the chest x-ray may be unrevealing; CT angiography is often very helpful in these circumstances, which may include COVID-19, vaping injury, pulmonary embolism, bronchiectasis, granulomatous diseases, and diseases associated with hilar or mediastinal lymphadenopathy.

Hematology/Immunology

The white blood cell (WBC) count may help exclude or include certain entities for a differential diagnosis. For example, a WBC count of 35,000

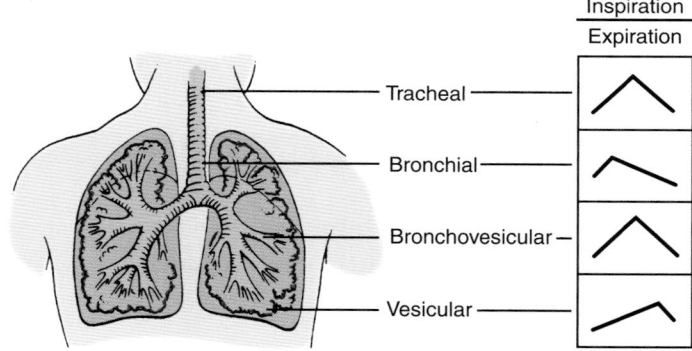

Characteristic	Tracheal	Bronchial	Bronchovesicular	Vesicular
Intensity	Very loud	Loud	Moderate	Soft
Pitch	Very high	High	Moderate	Low
I:E ratio*	1:1	1:3	1:1	3:1
Description	Harsh	Tubular	Rustling, but tubular	Gentle rustling
Normal locations	Extrathoracic trachea	Manubrium	Over mainstem bronchi	Most of peripheral lung

*Ratio of duration of inspiration to expiration.

Fig. 3.6 Characteristics of breath sounds. Tracheal breath sounds are very harsh, loud, and high pitched; they are heard over the extrathoracic portion of the trachea. Bronchial breath sounds are loud and high pitched; normally, they are heard over the lower sternum and sound like air rushing through a tube. The expiratory component is louder and longer than the inspiratory component; a definite pause is heard between the two phases. Bronchovesicular breath sounds are a mixture of bronchial and vesicular sounds. The inspiratory (I) and expiratory (E) components are equal in length. They are usually heard only in the first and second interspaces anteriorly and between the scapulae posteriorly, near the carina and mainstem bronchi. Vesicular breath sounds are soft and low pitched; they are heard over most of the lung fields. The inspiratory component is much longer than the expiratory component; the latter is softer and often inaudible. (From Swartz MH, ed. The chest. In: *Textbook of Physical Diagnosis: History and Examination*. Philadelphia: WB Saunders; 1989.)

TABLE 3.7 Cough: Radiologic and Laboratory Evaluation

	CHEST RADIOGRAPH					Abnormal Sinus Radiograph	COMPLETE BLOOD COUNT				IMMUNOGLOBULINS			+ NP PCR	Other
	Normal	Hyper	Lobar Infil	Diff Infil	Other		↑WBC	↑LY	↑EOS	↑PMN	↑IgG	↑IgM	↑IgE		
Asthma	+	++	−	−	−	+	+	+	++	−	+	+	++		+Bdilator[1]
Cystic fibrosis	+	++	+	+	++	++	++	+	+	++	++	+	+		See Table 3.8
Other infection															
Croup	++	+	+	+	++[2]	−	−	+	+	−				Paraflu +++	
Epiglottitis	++	+	+	+	++[3]	−	+++	+	+	+++	+	+			Direct look
Sinusitis	+++	−	−	−	−	+++	++	−	+	++	++	−	+		
Bronchiolitis	−	+++	+	++	+	−	+	+	+	+				RSV, human metapneumovirus +++	
Pneumonia															
Influenza	−	++	+	++	+	−	++	−	−	+	+	+	−	++	
Paraflu	−	+	+	++	+	−	++	−	−	+	+	+	−	++	
Coronaviruses	−	++	+	++	+	−	++	−	−	+	+	+	−	++	
Adenovirus	−	−	+	++	+	−	++	+	−	++	+	+	−	++	
Pertussis	++	+	−	+	+	−	+	++	++	+	++	+	−	++[4]	
Chlamydia	−	+++	+	+++	+	−	+	+	++	+	+++	+++	−	+++	
Mycoplasma	+	+	+	+	++[5]	+	+	+	++	+	−	++	−	++	+Cold agglutinin
TB	+	−	++	+	++	−	+	+	++	+					+PPD, QuantiFERON
Bacterial	−	+	+++	+	++[5]	−	+++	+	+	+++	++	+	+	+	+Bld cult[6]
Foreign body	−	++[7]	++	−	++[7]	−	++	+	+	++					Bronch
GE reflux	+++	+	−	−	−	+	−	−	−	−	−	−	+	−	Esoph pH[8]
Aspiration	+	+	+	+	++[9]	+	+	−	−	+	−	−	+	−	[10]
Anatomic	+	+	+	−	++[11]	−	+	−	−	+	−	−	−	−	[12]
Habit	+++	−	−	−	−	−	−	−	−	−	−	−	−	−	

[1] Positive response to bronchodilators, either as a home therapeutic trial or in a pulmonary function test in the laboratory.

[2] "Steeple" sign: narrowing of upper tracheal air column.

[3] "Swollen thumb": sign of thickened epiglottis.

[4] Low yield in paroxysmal stage.

[5] Pleural effusion relatively common.

[6] Blood culture positive in 10%; needle aspiration of pleural fluid or lung fluid may yield organism; bacterial antigen in urine. In older infants and children, common pathogens include pneumococci and group A streptococci; Staphylococcus aureus is rare and may be associated with pneumatoceles or empyema.

[7] Localized hyperinflation is common; localized atelectasis is common; inspiratory-expiratory radiographs may show ball-valve obstruction.

[8] Esophageal biopsy specimen shows esophagitis.

[9] Multilobular or multisegmental, dependent lobes.

[10] (?) Lipid-laden macrophages from bronchoscopy or gastric washings; barium swallow or radionuclide study showing aspiration.

[11] Right-sided arch, mass effect on airways, mass identified; MRI.

[12] Bronchoscopy; computed tomography; MRI.

+++, almost always—if not present, must question diagnosis; ++, common; +, less common; −, seldom—if present, must question diagnosis. +Bld cult, blood culture may be positive; Bronch, bronchoscopy can reveal the foreign body; Diff, diffuse or scattered; ↑EOS, increased eosinophil count; Esoph pH, prolonged esophageal pH probe monitoring; GE, gastroesophageal; Hyper, hyperinflated; Ig, immunoglobulin; Infil, infiltrates; ↑LY, increased lymphocyte count; +NP aspirate PCR, nasopharyngeal positive for specific organism; Paraflu, parainfluenza virus; PCR, polymerase chain reaction; ↑PMN, increased polymorphonuclear neutrophil count; PPD, purified protein derivative (TB); RAD, reactive airways disease; RSV, respiratory syncytial virus; TB, tuberculosis; ↑WBC, increased white blood cell count.

with 85% lymphocytes strongly suggests pertussis, but not every child with pertussis presents such a clear hematologic picture. The presence of a high number or large proportions of immature forms of WBCs suggests an acute process, such as a bacterial infection. Immunoglobulins provide supportive evidence for a few diagnoses, such as chlamydial infection, which rarely occurs without elevated serum concentrations of immunoglobulin G (IgG) and immunoglobulin M (IgM).

Bacteriology/Virology

Specific bacteriologic or virologic diagnoses can be made in a number of disorders causing cough, including RSV, influenza, parainfluenza, coronaviruses, adenovirus, enteroviruses, metapneumovirus, *Mycoplasma,* and *Chlamydia* pneumonia. In most cases, the viruses can be rapidly identified with amplification of the viral genome through polymerase chain reaction (PCR). In bacterial pneumonia, the offending organism can be cultured from the blood in a small proportion (10%) of patients. A positive culture provides definitive diagnosis, but a negative culture specimen is not helpful. Throat cultures are seldom helpful (except in CF) in identifying lower respiratory tract bacterial organisms. Sputum cultures and Gram stains may help guide initial empirical therapy in older children with pneumonia or purulent bronchitis, but their ability to identify specific causative organisms with certainty (with the exception of CF) has not been shown clearly.

Infants and young children usually do not expectorate but rather swallow their sputum. Specimens obtained via bronchoscopy may be contaminated by mouth flora, but heavy growth of a single organism from a bronchoalveolar lavage in the presence of polymorphonuclear neutrophils certainly supports the organism's role in disease. If pleural fluid or fluid obtained directly from the lung via needle aspiration is cultured, the same rules apply: Positive cultures and nucleic acid amplification tests are definitive, but negative cultures are not.

Other Tests

A number of specific tests can help to establish diagnoses in a child with cough (see Table 3.7). These include a positive response to bronchodilators in a child with asthma; visualizing the red, swollen epiglottis in epiglottitis (to be done only under very controlled conditions);

the bronchoscopic visualization of the peanut, plastic toy, or other offender in foreign body aspiration; a positive purified protein derivative (PPD) or QuantiFERON assay in tuberculosis; and several studies of the esophagus in GER. Several imaging techniques, such as CT or MRI, can help to delineate various intrathoracic anatomic abnormalities, pulmonary embolism, and bronchiectasis. Multiple tests can be employed to confirm the diagnosis of CF (Table 3.8).

Differential Diagnosis and Treatment

Infection

Infections are the most common cause of acute cough in all age groups and are responsible for some chronic coughs. The age of the patient has a large impact on the frequency of the type of infection.

Infections in infants. Viral upper respiratory infections (common cold); croup (laryngotracheobronchitis); viral bronchiolitis, particularly with RSV or human metapneumovirus; and viral pneumonia are the most frequently encountered respiratory tract infections and hence the most common causes of cough in infancy. Viral illness may predispose to bacterial superinfection (e.g., croup and *Staphylococcus aureus* tracheitis or influenza and *Haemophilus influenzae* or *S. aureus* pneumonia).

Viral upper respiratory infections. Viral URI symptoms and signs usually include nasal congestion and discharge, sore throat, and sneezing. There may be fever, constitutional signs (irritability, myalgias, and headache), or both. Cough is common and may persist for 5–7 days. The mechanism by which URIs cause cough in children is undetermined. In adults, it is generally thought that "postnasal drip"—that is, nasal or sinus secretions draining into the posterior nasopharynx—causes cough and, in fact, may be one of the most frequent causes of cough. Indeed, sinus CT in older patients with URIs often reveals unexpected involvement of the sinus mucosa. Other authorities believe that cough in a child with a URI indicates involvement (inflammation or bronchospasm) of the lower respiratory tract. Over-the-counter cough and cold medications are commonly used. Evidence of efficacy of these medications for children with URI is lacking. Because of the known risk for unintentional overdose from these medications, their use is not recommended in children under age 4 years.

TABLE 3.8	**Laboratory Tests for Cystic Fibrosis**		
Usefulness	**Test**	**Sensitivity**	**Specificity**
Definitive	Sweat chloride test	.99+	.95+
	DNA analysis	.85–.90	.99
Suggestive	Throat or sputum culture* positive for mucoid *Pseudomonas aeruginosa*	.70–.80	.85
	Sinus radiographs		
	Pansinusitis	.95	.90
	Positive IRT newborn screen	.98	.25
Supportive	Fecal elastase		
	Pulmonary function tests:		
	Obstructive pattern, especially small airways and especially if patient is poorly responsive to bronchodilator	.70+	?
	Chest radiograph:		
	Hyperinflation, ± other findings; especially with right upper lobe infiltrate/atelectasis	.70+	?
	Throat or sputum culture*:		
	Positive for *Staphylococcus aureus*	.20	.20
	Positive for *Haemophilus influenzae*	.05–.20	.15

*Throat is usually deep pharyngeal culture.
IRT, immunoreactive trypsinogen.

Common viral pathogens include rhinovirus, RSV, coronaviruses, and parainfluenza viruses. The differential diagnosis includes allergic rhinitis, which often demonstrates clear nasal secretions with eosinophils and pale nasal mucosa, and sinusitis, which presents with mucopurulent nasal secretions containing neutrophils and erythematous mucosa.

Croup (laryngotracheobronchitis). Infectious croup (see Chapter 4) is most common in the first 2 years of life. Its most dramatic components are the barking ("croupy") cough and inspiratory stridor, which appear a few days after the onset of a cold. In most cases, the patient has a low-grade fever, and the disease resolves within a day or two. In severe cases, the child can be extremely ill and is at risk for complete laryngeal obstruction. There may be marked intercostal and suprasternal retractions and cyanosis. *Stridor at rest signifies significant obstruction.* Diminishing stridor in a child who is calm is a good sign, but diminishing stridor in and of itself is not necessarily good: If the child becomes fatigued because of the tremendous work of breathing through an obstructed airway and can no longer breathe effectively, smaller-than-needed tidal volumes make less noise.

It is important to distinguish croup from epiglottitis in the child with harsh, barking cough and inspiratory stridor because the natural histories of the two diseases are quite different (see Table 3.7). Epiglottitis is uncommon but occurs in unimmunized patients (see Chapter 4).

Treatment of mild croup is usually not needed. For decades, pediatricians have recommended putting a child with croup in a steamy bathroom or driving to the office or emergency department with the car windows rolled down. It is likely that these remedies are effective because of the heat exchange properties of the upper airway; air that is cooler or more humid than the airway mucosa will serve to cool the mucosa, thus causing local vasoconstriction and probably decreasing local edema.

In a child who has stridor at rest, evaluation is indicated. Symptomatic, often dramatic relief through decreased laryngeal edema can usually be achieved with aerosolized racemic epinephrine (2.25% solution, 0.25 to 0.5 mL/dose). It is essential to remember that the effects of the epinephrine are transient, lasting only a few hours, although the course of the illness is often longer. The result is that when the racemic epinephrine's effect has worn off, the child's cough and stridor will probably be as bad or even worse than before the aerosol was administered. This is not a "rebound" effect: The symptoms are not worse because of the treatment but, rather, because of the natural progression of the viral illness. Repeating the aerosol will probably again have a beneficial effect. A child who responds favorably to such an aerosol needs to be observed for several hours because further treatment may be needed. A single dose of dexamethasone (0.6 mg/kg orally, intramuscularly, or intravenously, maximum dose 16 mg) reduces the severity and hastens recovery.

Bronchiolitis. Bronchiolitis is a common and potentially serious lower respiratory tract disorder in infants (see Chapter 4). It is caused usually by RSV but on occasion by parainfluenza, influenza, human metapneumovirus, adenovirus, enterovirus, and human rhinovirus. It mostly occurs in the winter months, often in epidemics. RSV bronchiolitis is seen uncommonly in children older than 4 years. Typically, "coldlike" symptoms of rhinorrhea precede the harsh cough, increased respiratory rate, and retractions. Respiratory distress and cyanosis can be severe. The child's temperature is seldom elevated above 38°C.

The chest is hyperinflated, widespread crackles are audible on inspiration, and wheezing marks expiration. The chest radiograph invariably reveals hyperinflation, as depicted by a depressed diaphragm, with an enlarged retrosternal air space in as many as 60% of patients,

peribronchial thickening in approximately 50%, and consolidation and/or atelectasis in 10–25%.

The diagnosis is confirmed with demonstration of RSV by PCR of nasopharyngeal secretions. In most cases, no treatment is needed because the disease does not interfere with the infant's eating or breathing. Apnea is a common complication of RSV bronchiolitis in *neonates* and may necessitate close monitoring. In severe cases, often those in which there is underlying chronic heart, lung, or immunodeficiency disease, RSV can be life threatening. In severe cases, hospital care with supplemental oxygen and intravenous fluids is indicated. Suctioning of secretions is an essential part of the treatment. Many other treatment modalities have been tried for hospitalized infants with bronchiolitis. Aerosolized bronchodilators and systemic glucocorticoids do not seem to alter clinical outcome and are not recommended in most patients. Nebulized saline may reduce the length of hospitalization. Use of a high-flow nasal cannula may reduce the need for more invasive forms of respiratory support in infants with impending respiratory failure.

Viral pneumonia. Viral pneumonia can be similar to bronchiolitis in its manifestation, with cough and tachypnea, after a few days of apparent URI. There can be variable degrees of fever and of overall illness. Infants and children with viral pneumonia may appear relatively well or, particularly with coronavirus, adenovirus, or influenza, may have a rapidly progressive course. Frequent symptoms include poor feeding, cough, cyanosis, fever (some patients may be afebrile), apnea, and rhinorrhea. Frequent signs include tachypnea, retractions, crackles, and cough. Cyanosis is less common.

The most common agents causing viral pneumonia in infancy and childhood are RSV, influenza, and parainfluenza. Adenovirus is less common, but it is important because it can be severe and cause residual lung disease, including bronchiectasis and bronchiolitis obliterans. Adenovirus pneumonia is often accompanied by conjunctivitis and pharyngitis, in addition to leukocytosis and an elevated ESR; the ESR and leukocyte count are usually not elevated in other types of viral pneumonia. Additional viral agents include enteroviruses, human metapneumovirus, and rhinovirus. Radiographs most often reveal diffuse, bilateral peribronchial infiltrates, with a predilection for the perihilar regions, but occasionally lobar infiltrates are present. Pleural effusions are not common. Human coronaviruses account for 5–10% of acute upper respiratory infections in adults; infants with coronaviruses often have coinfections with other respiratory viruses and may not have respiratory symptoms, suggesting that some endemic coronaviruses may have low pathogenicity in healthy infants. Older children and adolescents are at risk for severe pneumonia from severe acute respiratory syndrome-coronavirus 2 (SARS-CoV-2), which causes COVID-19 (see later and Chapter 4). Vaccination is now available for COVID-19.

Treatment is largely supportive, with oxygen and intravenous fluids. Mechanical ventilation may be necessary in a small minority of infants.

Pertussis (whooping cough). Pertussis is a relatively common cause of lower respiratory tract infection in infants, children, adolescents, and adults, especially in those who are underimmunized or not immunized. The causative organism, *Bordetella pertussis*, has a tropism for tracheal and bronchial ciliated epithelial cells; thus, the disease is primarily bronchitis, but spread of the organism to alveoli, or secondary invasion by other bacteria, can cause pneumonia. The disease can occur at any age, from early infancy onward, although its manifestations in young infants and in those who have been partially immunized may be atypical; infants may present with apnea and minimal or no cough.

Most commonly, pertussis has three stages:
- Catarrhal, in which symptoms are indistinguishable from a viral URI

- Paroxysmal, dominated by repeated forceful, paroxysmal coughing spells; spells may be punctuated by an inspiratory "whoop," post-tussive emesis, or both
- Convalescent, in which the intensity and frequency of coughing spells gradually diminish

Each stage typically lasts 1–2 weeks, except the paroxysmal stage, which lasts many weeks. (Pertussis is known as the "100-day cough" in China.) Most children are entirely well between coughing spells, when physical findings are remarkably benign. The paroxysmal cough recurs with subsequent respiratory illnesses for many months after illness. Infants younger than 6 months of age are at highest risk for complications. The majority of infants with pertussis need to be hospitalized.

Diagnosis can be difficult because the definitive result—namely, culturing the organism from nasopharyngeal secretions—requires special culture medium (Bordet-Gengou, which must be prepared fresh for each collection). Culture specimens are much less likely to be positive during the paroxysmal stage than during the catarrhal stage, when the diagnosis is not being considered. PCR assay of an adequate nasopharyngeal (NP) specimen is the most commonly used test because of improved sensitivity and faster turnaround time compared to culture. An elevated WBC count, as high as 20,000–50,000, with lymphocytes predominating is suggestive of pertussis in infants and children but often absent in adolescents. Chest radiographic findings are nonspecific.

Treatment is largely supportive, with oxygen; fluids; and small, frequent feedings for patients who do not tolerate their normal feedings. Treatment with azithromycin decreases infectivity and may ameliorate the course of the disease if given during the catarrhal stage.

Complications include those related to severe coughing (Table 3.9) and those specific to pertussis, such as seizures and encephalopathy. The risk of acquiring pertussis is markedly reduced by immunizations (three primary immunizations and regular booster immunizations). Neither pertussis infection nor immunization produces lifelong immunity.

Chlamydial infection. *Chlamydia trachomatis* can cause pneumonia in young infants following acquisition from the maternal genitourinary tract, particularly those aged 3–12 weeks. Cough, nasal congestion, low-grade or no fever, and tachypnea are common. Conjunctivitis is an important clue to chlamydial disease but is present in only 50% of infants with chlamydial pneumonia at the time of presentation. Affected infants may have a paroxysmal cough similar to that of pertussis, but post-tussive emesis is less common. Crackles are commonly heard on auscultation, but wheezing is much less common than the overinflated appearance of the lungs on radiographs would suggest. The organism may be recovered from the nasopharynx by culture or antigen testing. The CBC may reveal eosinophilia. Chlamydial infection responds to oral erythromycin or azithromycin therapy.

In young infants, the **afebrile pneumonia syndrome** may be caused by *Chlamydia*, *Ureaplasma*, or *Mycoplasma* species; cytomegalovirus; or *Pneumocystis jirovecii*. In this syndrome, cough and *tachypnea* are common. Severe pneumonia may develop in neonates as a result of herpes simplex.

Ureaplasmal infection. *Ureaplasma urealyticum* pneumonia is difficult to diagnose but causes cough in some infants. There are no particularly outstanding features to distinguish this relatively uncommon infection from viral pneumonias.

Bacterial pneumonia. Bacterial pneumonia is less common in infants than is viral pneumonia but can cause severe illness, with cough, respiratory distress, and fever. Chest radiographs are abnormal, and the WBC count is elevated.

Treatment is with antibiotics effective against pneumococci, group A streptococci, and, if illness is severe, *S. aureus*.

Infections in toddlers and children

Viral URIs. In early childhood, as children attend daycare and nursery schools, they are constantly exposed to respiratory viruses to which

TABLE 3.9	Potential Complications of Cough	
Musculoskeletal	Rib fractures
	Vertebral fractures
	Rupture of rectus abdominis muscle
	Asymptomatic elevation of serum creatine phosphokinase
Pulmonary	Chest wall pain*
	Bronchoconstriction
	Pneumomediastinum
	Pneumothorax
	Hemoptysis
	Subcutaneous emphysema
	Irritation of larynx and trachea
Cardiovascular	Rupture of subconjunctival,* nasal,* and anal capillaries or veins
	Bradycardia, heart block
	Transient hypertension
Central nervous system	Cough syncope
	Headache
	Subarachnoid hemorrhage
Gastrointestinal	Hernias (ventral, inguinal)
	Emesis
	Rectal prolapse
	Pneumoperitoneum
Miscellaneous	Anorexia*
	Malnutrition
	Sleep loss*
	Urinary incontinence
	Disruption of surgical wounds
	Vaginal prolapse
	Displacement of intravenous catheters
	Petechiae

*Common.

they have little or no immunity (e.g., RSV, rhinoviruses, adenoviruses, parainfluenza, and enteroviruses). Young children may have as many as six to eight or even more URIs in a year. The remarks concerning colds and cough in infants (see previous discussion) apply to this older age group. The differential diagnosis of rhinorrhea is noted in Table 3.10.

Sinusitis. The sinuses may become the site for viral and subsequent secondary bacterial infection spreading from the nasopharynx (Fig. 3.7). The signs and symptoms are usually localized, including nasal congestion, a feeling of "fullness" or pain in the face (Fig. 3.8), headache, sinus tenderness, day or night cough, and fever. Maxillary toothache, purulent nasal discharge for more than 10 days, and positive transillumination (opacification) are important clues. Sinus radiographs or (more accurate) a CT scan may facilitate the diagnosis of sinusitis by demonstrating opacification of the sinus with mucosal thickening. Sinusitis is thought to be a cause of cough in adults and can probably be listed, with lower certainty, as a cause of cough in children.

Sinusitis is frequently seen in other conditions known to cause cough, especially CF, asthma, primary ciliary dyskinesia, and granulomatosis with polyangiitis with or without eosinophilia. It may be difficult to ascertain whether the cough is a direct result of the sinus infection or the underlying problem (purulent bronchitis in the child with CF or ciliary dyskinesia, exacerbation of asthma). In the first two situations, it may not matter because treatment is the same. In the case of the child with asthma, it is important to treat the asthma with bronchodilating and antiinflammatory agents, as well as to treat the infected sinuses with antibiotics.

TABLE 3.10 Differential Diagnosis of Rhinorrhea

Etiology	Frequency	Duration*	Discharge	Comment
Viral	Common	Acute	Purulent	Polymorphonuclear neutrophils in smear
Allergic	Common	Acute/chronic	Clear	Eosinophils in smear, seasonal
Vasomotor	Common	Chronic	Variable	? Environmental triggers
Sinusitis	Common	Chronic	Purulent	Sinus tenderness
Rhinitis medicamentosa	Common	Chronic	Variable	Medication use
Response to stimuli	Common	Acute	Clear	Odors, exercise, cold air, pollution
Nasal polyps	Uncommon	Chronic	Variable	Consider cystic fibrosis
Granulomatous disease	Uncommon	Chronic	Bloody	Sarcoid, granulomatosis with polyangiitis, midline granuloma
Cerebrospinal fluid fistula	Uncommon	Chronic	Watery	Trauma, encephalocele
Foreign body	Uncommon	Chronic	Purulent	Often malodorous
Tumor	Uncommon	Chronic	Clear to bloody	Angiofibroma, hemangioma, rhabdomyosarcoma, lymphoma, nasopharyngeal carcinoma, neuroblastoma
Choanal atresia, stenosis	Uncommon	Chronic	Clear to purulent	Congenital
Nonallergic eosinophilic rhinitis syndrome	Uncommon	Chronic	Clear	Eosinophils in smear
Septal deviation	Unknown	Chronic	Clear	Congenital, trauma
Drugs	Uncommon	Chronic	Variable	Cocaine, glue and organic solvents, angiotensin-converting enzyme inhibitors, β blockers
Hypothyroidism	Uncommon	Chronic	Clear	
Cluster headache	Uncommon	Intermittent	Clear	Associated tearing, headache
Horner syndrome	Uncommon	Chronic	Clear	Ptosis, miosis, anhidrosis

*Less than 1 week is considered acute.

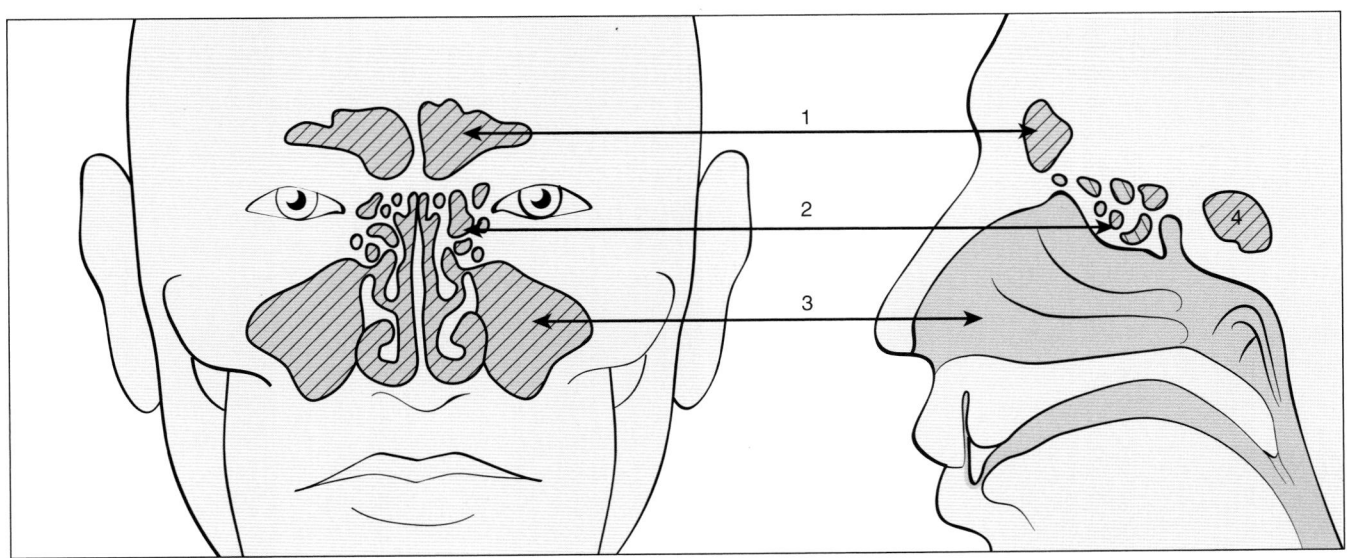

Fig. 3.7 The paranasal sinuses. *1*, Frontal. *2*, Ethmoid. *3*, Maxillary. *4*, Sphenoid. (From Smith RP. Common upper respiratory tract infections. In: Reilly B, ed. *Practical Strategies in Outpatient Medicine*. 2nd ed. Philadelphia: WB Saunders; 1991.)

The treatment of sinusitis involves the use of oral antibiotics active against the common pathogens (i.e., *Streptococcus pneumoniae*, non-typable *H. influenzae*, *Moraxella catarrhalis*, and, in rare cases, anaerobic bacteria or *Streptococcus pyogenes*). Treatment regimens include the use of amoxicillin, amoxicillin-clavulanate, cefuroxime, cefpodoxime, or cefdinir. Amoxicillin is considered the initial agent of choice. Oral (pseudoephedrine, phenylephrine) or topical (phenylephrine, oxymetazoline) decongestants may be of benefit by increasing the patency of the sinus ostia, which permits drainage of the infected and obstructed sinuses. Oral antihistamines may benefit patients with an allergic history. Treatment with antimicrobial agents should continue for at least 7 days after the patient has responded. This may require 14–21 days of therapy. Many patients with presumed sinusitis recover without antibiotic therapy.

Complications of acute sinusitis include orbital cellulitis, abscesses (orbital, cerebral), cranial (frontal) osteomyelitis (Pott puffy tumor), empyema (subdural, epidural), and thrombosis (sagittal or cavernous sinus).

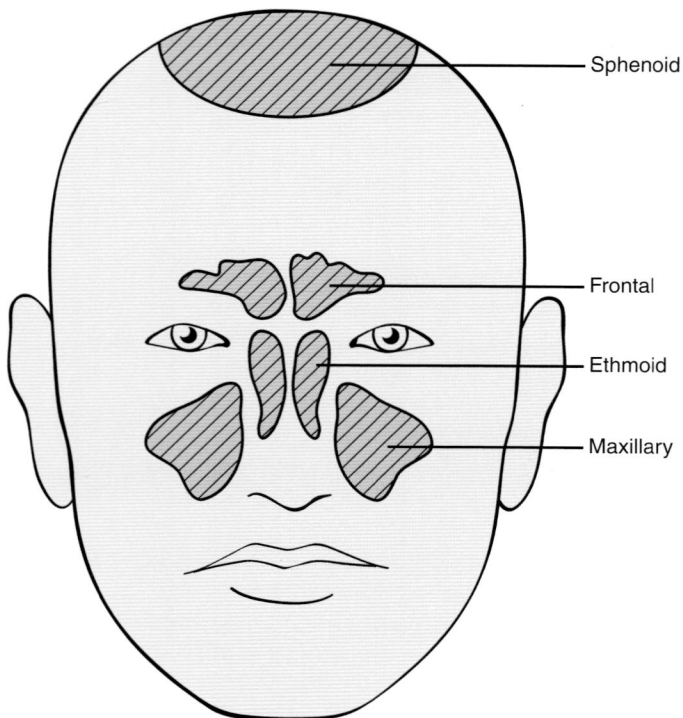

Sphenoid

Frontal

Ethmoid

Maxillary

Fig. 3.8 Typical pain locations in patients with various anatomic sites of acute sinusitis. (From Smith RP. Common upper respiratory tract infections. In: Reilly B, ed. *Practical Strategies in Outpatient Medicine.* 2nd ed. Philadelphia: WB Saunders; 1991.)

Protracted bacterial bronchitis. Protracted bacterial bronchitis (PBB) is a cause of chronic, productive cough in young children. Suggested clinical criteria include a productive cough for at least 4 weeks, no other symptoms, normal spirometry, normal chest x-ray (but may have peribronchial thickening), and possible improvement/resolution after 2 weeks of antibiotics. *H. influenzae, S. pneumoniae,* and *M. catarrhalis* may be the most common pathogens. Treatment of PBB requires an initial 2-week course of an appropriate antibiotic, with the preferred choice being amoxicillin-clavulanate. If cough persists, a more prolonged antibiotic course may be needed (up to 4 weeks). Bronchoscopy with bronchoalveolar lavage may help guide antibiotic treatment, particularly in those with refractory cough despite 4 weeks of antibiotics.

Pneumonia. The features discussed for viral pneumonia in infants are relevant for viral pneumonia in older children. The differentiation of viral or atypical pneumonia from classical bacterial pneumonia is noted in Table 3.11. Adenovirus and influenza pneumonia may present similar to bacterial pneumonia in severity and acuteness and with elevated acute-phase reactants (ESR, CRP, procalcitonin). Etiology clues are noted in Tables 3.12, 3.13, and 3.14. Bacterial pneumonia is more common in toddlers and older children than in infants. The most common pathogen is *S. pneumoniae* (see Table 3.12). Cough may not be as prominent a presenting symptom or sign as tachypnea and grunting. Raised respiratory rates (>50 in infants 2–12 months old, >40 in children 1–5 years old) plus retractions and grunting with or without hypoxemia (oxygen saturation <90%) have a high specificity and sensitivity for pneumonia. Chest pain, abdominal pain, headache, or any combination of these symptoms may occur. Upper lobe pneumonia may produce meningeal signs, and lower lobe involvement may cause abdominal pain and an ileus.

TABLE 3.11   Differentiation of Classical Bacterial Pneumonia from Viral and Atypical Pneumonias*

	Bacterial	Viral/Atypical Bacterial
History	Precedent URI	Headache, malaise, URI, myalgias
Course	Often biphasic illness	Often monophasic
Onset	Sudden	Gradual
Temperature	High fever	Low-grade fever
Rigors	Common	Uncommon
Vital signs	Tachypnea, tachycardia	Usually normal
Pain	Pleuritic	Unusual
Chest examination	Crackles, signs of consolidation	Consolidation unusual
Pleural effusion	Common	Uncommon
Sputum	Productive, purulent, many PMNs, one dominant organism on Gram stain	Scant, no organisms; PMNs or mononuclear cells
ESR	Elevated	Usually normal
CRP	Elevated	Usually normal
Procalcitonin	Elevated	Normal
WBC count	Elevated; left shift	Often normal; predominant lymphocytes
Chest radiography	Lobar consolidation, round infiltrate, parapneumonic effusion; may be "bronchopneumonia"	Diffuse, bilateral, patchy, interstitial or bronchopneumonia; lower lobe involvement common; chest radiograph may look worse than patient's condition
Progression	May be rapid	Rapid if *Legionella* species, hantavirus, SARS, herpesvirus, adenovirus, COVID-19
Diagnosis	Blood, sputum, and pleural fluid specimens for culture; antigen detection possible; BAL if progressive	Viral, chlamydial culture or PCR detection; acute and convalescent titers; BAL if progressive

*Atypical pneumonias include *Chlamydia pneumoniae, Mycoplasma pneumoniae, Legionella* species (*Legionella pneumophila, Legionella micdadei*), Q fever, psittacosis, tularemia.
BAL, bronchoalveolar lavage; CRP, C-reactive protein; PMNs, polymorphonuclear neutrophils; SARS, severe acute respiratory syndrome; URI, upper respiratory tract infection; WBC, white blood cell.

Examination of the chest shows tachypnea but may be otherwise surprisingly normal. In older children, there may be localized dullness to percussion, with crackles or amphoric (bronchial) breath sounds over a consolidated lobe. The chest radiograph may be normal in the first hours of the illness, inasmuch as the radiographic findings often lag behind the clinical manifestations. Nonetheless, both anterior-posterior and lateral views are the main diagnostic tools; lobar consolidation is usual, with or without pleural effusion. In infants, the pattern may be more diffuse and extensive.

Some clinical and radiographic features may be suggestive of the bacterial cause of pneumonia. Children (especially infants) with staphylococcal pneumonia are more likely to have a rapid, overwhelming course. Staphylococcal pneumonia may be accompanied by more extensive radiographic abnormalities, including multilobar consolidation, pneumatocele formation, and extensive pleural (empyema) fluid (Fig. 3.9). The presence of a pleural effusion is not helpful in indicating the specific bacterial diagnosis because other bacterial pneumonias may be accompanied by pleural effusion (Fig. 3.10). Pleural effusions may represent a reactive parapneumonic effusion or an empyema. Pleural fluid may be characterized as transudate, exudate, or empyema (Table 3.15). If the effusion is of sufficient size, as demonstrated by a lateral decubitus radiograph or ultrasonography, a thoracentesis may be indicated to differentiate the nature of the effusion and to identify possible pathogens. For young children who require sedation for thoracentesis and who have an effusion needing drainage, a primary chest tube placement is preferred over thoracentesis due to the risks of multiple procedures with sedation.

Differentiating among the causes of bacterial pneumonia can be done with certainty only with positive cultures from blood, pleural fluid (including PCR testing), or, in rare cases, sputum. Current or previous antibiotic treatment diminishes the yield of such cultures. Bronchoscopy with or without lavage may yield helpful specimens from the progressively ill child or the child who has not responded promptly to empirical antibiotics.

Treatment of uncomplicated presumed bacterial pneumonia is with antibiotics. Ampicillin is the drug of choice for the previously healthy

TABLE 3.12 Causes of Infectious Pneumonia

Bacterial

Common

Streptococcus pneumoniae	See Table 3.11
Group B streptococci	Neonates
Group A streptococci	See Table 3.11
Mycoplasma pneumoniae*	Adolescents; summer-fall epidemics
Chlamydia pneumoniae*	Adolescents (see Table 3.11)
Chlamydia trachomatis	Infants
Mixed anaerobes	Aspiration pneumonia
Gram-negative enteric	Nosocomial pneumonia

Uncommon

Haemophilus influenzae type B	See Table 3.11
Staphylococcus aureus	Pneumatoceles; infants
Moraxella catarrhalis	
Neisseria meningitidis	
Salmonella species	
Francisella tularensis	Animal, tick, fly contact
Nocardia species	Immunosuppressed persons
Chlamydia psittaci*	Bird contact
Yersinia pestis	Plague
Legionella species*	Exposure to contaminated water; nosocomial

Viral

Common

Respiratory syncytial virus	See Table 3.11
Parainfluenza types 1–4	Croup, types 3 and 4 seen in the summer
Influenza A, B	High fever; winter months
Adenovirus 1, 2, 3, 5, 14	Can be severe; occurs all year round
Human metapneumovirus	Similar to RSV
Rhinovirus	Rhinorrhea, wheezing
SARS-CoV-2 (COVID-19)	Pandemic

Uncommon

Enteroviruses	Neonates
Herpes simplex	Neonates
Cytomegalovirus	Infants, immunosuppressed persons
Measles	Rash, coryza, conjunctivitis
Varicella	Adolescents
Hantavirus	Southwestern United States
SARS-CoV-1	Asia

Fungal

Histoplasma capsulatum	Geographic region; bird, bat contact
Cryptococcus neoformans	Bird contact
Aspergillus species	Immunosuppressed
Mucormycosis	Immunosuppressed
Coccidioides immitis	Geographic region
Blastomyces dermatitidis	Geographic region

Rickettsial

Coxiella burnetii*	Q fever, animal (goat, sheep, cattle) exposure
Rickettsia rickettsiae	Tick bite

Mycobacterial

Mycobacterium tuberculosis	See Table 3.16
Mycobacterium avium–intracellulare	Immunosuppressed persons

Parasitic

Pneumocystis jirovecii	Immunosuppressed, steroids
Eosinophilic	Various parasites (e.g., Ascaris, Strongyloides species)

*Atypical pneumonia syndrome (see Table 3.11); atypical in terms of extrapulmonary manifestations, low-grade fever, patchy diffuse infiltrates, poor response to penicillin-type antibiotics, and negative sputum Gram stain.
CoV, coronavirus; SARS, severe acute respiratory syndrome.

TABLE 3.13   Pneumonia: Etiology Suggested by Exposure History

Exposure History	Infectious Agent
Exposure to concurrent illness in school dormitory or household setting	*Neisseria meningitidis,* *Mycoplasma pneumoniae*
Environmental Exposures	
Exposure to contaminated aerosols (e.g., air coolers, hospital water supply)	Legionnaires disease
Exposure to goat hair, raw wool, animal hides	Anthrax
Ingestion of unpasteurized milk	Brucellosis
Exposure to bat droppings (caving) or dust from soil enriched with bird droppings	Histoplasmosis
Exposure to water contaminated with animal urine	Leptospirosis
Exposure to rodent droppings, urine, saliva	Hantavirus
Potential bioterrorism exposure	Anthrax, plague, tularemia
Zoonotic Exposures	
Employment as abattoir worker or veterinarian	Brucellosis
Exposure to cattle, goats, pigs	Anthrax, brucellosis
Exposure to ground squirrels, chipmunks, rabbits, prairie dogs, rats in Africa or southwestern United States	Plague
Hunting or exposure to rabbits, foxes, squirrels	Tularemia
Bites from flies or ticks	Tularemia
Exposure to birds (parrots, budgerigars, cockatoos, pigeons, turkeys)	Psittacosis
Exposure to infected dogs and cats	*Pasteurella multocida,* Q fever (*Coxiella burnetii*)
Exposure to infected goats, cattle, sheep, domestic animals, and their secretions (milk, amniotic fluid, placenta, feces)	Q fever (*C. burnetii*)
Travel Exposures	
Residence in or travel to San Joaquin Valley, Southern California, southwestern Texas, southern Arizona, New Mexico	Coccidioidomycosis
Residence in or travel in Mississippi or Ohio River Valleys, Caribbean, Central America or Africa, South Asia	Histoplasmosis, blastomycosis
Residence in or travel to southern China	SARS, avian influenza
Residence in or travel to Arabian Peninsula	MERS-CoV
Residence in or travel in Southeast Asia	Paragonimiasis, melioidosis
Residence or travel to West Indies, Australia, or Guam	Melioidosis

MERS-CoV, Middle Eastern respiratory syndrome-coronavirus; SARS, severe acute respiratory syndrome.
From Bennett JE, Dolin R, Blaser MJ. *Mandell, Douglas, and Bennett's Principles and Practice of Infectious Diseases.* 9th ed., Vol 1. Elsevier; 2020:894, Table 67.3.

child who requires hospitalization with lobar pneumonia who is fully immunized. If the child is not fully immunized, ceftriaxone is indicated. For the critically ill child, vancomycin and ceftriaxone may be considered for possible drug-resistant *S. pneumoniae* and methicillin-resistant *S. aureus* (MRSA). Many children with pneumonia do well with oral antibiotics and respond within hours to the first dose. Repeated or follow-up chest radiographs may remain abnormal for 4–6 weeks after appropriate treatment and are not indicated for a single episode of uncomplicated pneumonia (i.e., no effusion, no abscess, and good response to treatment).

Mycoplasma pneumoniae is a common cause of pneumonia among school-aged children. The disease often occurs in community outbreaks in the fall. The illness typically begins with extrapulmonary symptoms (i.e., sore throat, myalgias, headache, fever), which then progress to include cough, which can be paroxysmal at times. Patients do not often appear acutely ill, but cough may persist for weeks. There may be no specific abnormalities on the chest examination, although a few crackles may be heard, and about one third of younger patients wheeze.

The radiographic findings in mycoplasma pneumonia can mimic almost any intrathoracic disease; scattered infiltrates with nonspecific "dirty" lung fields, predominantly perihilar or lower lobes, are common, and lobar infiltrates and pleural effusion are occasionally seen. Laboratory data (CBC, ESR, sputum culture) may not be helpful. A rise in anti-mycoplasma IgG over 1–2 weeks may be demonstrated but is seldom helpful in guiding therapy. A positive IgM response may be useful, although it can persist in serum for several months and, consequently, may not indicate current infection. *PCR is the most helpful test.* The cold agglutinin test yields positive results in about 70% of patients with mycoplasma pneumonia, but they are also positive in other conditions, including adenovirus infection. The more severe the illness is, the greater is the frequency of positive cold agglutinins. The diagnosis is often made from the history of an older child who has a lingering coughing illness in the setting of a community outbreak, unresponsive to most (non-erythromycin) antibiotic regimens.

Treatment with azithromycin, clarithromycin, or erythromycin in children younger than 8 years old or tetracycline or doxycycline

TABLE 3.14 Guide to Differential Diagnosis of Pneumonia Based on Radiologic Characteristics

Imaging Characteristics	Possible Pathogens
Chest Radiograph	
Dense segmental or lobar consolidation	More likely bacterial pathogens
Unilateral or bilateral homogenous consolidation	*Streptococcus pneumoniae, Legionella* spp., *Mycoplasma pneumoniae*
Lower lobe	Aspiration-anaerobes, gram-negative rods
Unilobar with air bronchograms	*Chlamydia*
Bulging fissure sign	*Klebsiella* spp.
Bronchopneumonia—result of bronchial inflammation, epithelial ulceration, fibropurulent exudate	*Staphylococcus aureus, Haemophilus influenzae*, fungi
Interstitial infiltrates or interstitial-alveolar infiltrates (diffuse pneumonitis)	More likely viral or *Mycoplasma*
Bilateral with hypoxia out of proportion to imaging abnormalities	*Pneumocystis jirovecii* (PCP)
Patchy, peribronchiolar opacities or ill-defined reticulonodular opacities	Primary viral infection including CMV, HSV, adenovirus *M. pneumoniae*
Diffuse bilateral bronchopneumonia	CMV, HSV, adenovirus
Unilateral or bilateral interstitial basilar infiltrates progressing to severe symmetrical air-space disease	Coronavirus including SARS, MERS
Cavitary Lung Lesions	
Upper lobe	Tuberculosis or nontubercular mycobacteria
Unilateral or lower lobe	Anaerobic lung abscess
Multiple, may be pleural based	Endemic and opportunistic fungi
Cavities that evolve from lobar consolidation and coalescence of latencies	*S. aureus, Pseudomonas aeruginosa, Klebsiella pneumoniae*
Pleural effusion	Large effusions support a bacterial cause
In association with necrosis, pneumatoceles or empyema	*S. aureus, Streptococcus pyogenes, S. pneumoniae*
With multilobular infiltrates	Primary viral especially metapneumovirus, bocavirus
Pneumatoceles	*S. aureus, Klebsiella* spp., *Haemophilus* spp., *S. pneumoniae*
Multiple nodules	Bacteremic spread of *S. aureus* Endemic or opportunistic fungi
Hilar adenopathy	Tuberculous or nontuberculous mycobacteria, endemic fungi
With upper lobe infiltrate	*Mycobacterium tuberculosis*
With homogenous opacities, may cavitate	Coccidioidomycosis
With signs of obstruction	Malignancy with bacterial infection
Computed Tomography	
Ground-glass opacities—localized increase in lung attenuation	*Pneumocystis, Mycoplasma,* fungi, CMV, COVID-19, and other viruses
Tree-in-bud pattern—reflects presence of bronchioles filled with inflammatory material	Bacteria, mycobacteria, fungi, viruses including RSV and parainfluenza virus, and other atypical pathogens
Central density sparing subpleural space	Vaping injury

CMV, cytomegalovirus; HSV, herpes simplex virus; MERS, Middle East respiratory syndrome; PCP, *P. jirovecii* pneumonia; RSV, respiratory syncytial virus; SARS, severe acute respiratory syndrome.
Data from Franquet T. Imaging of pneumonia: trends and algorithms. *Eur Resp J.* 2001;18:196–208; and Franquet T. Imaging of community-acquired pneumonia. *J Thorac Imaging.* 2018;33:282–294.
From Bennett JE, Dolin R, Blaser MJ. *Mandell, Douglas, and Bennett's Principles and Practice of Infectious Diseases.* 9th ed., Vol. 1. Elsevier; 2020:901, Table 67.4.

in children 8 years old or older usually shortens the course of illness. Extrapulmonary complications of mycoplasma infection include aseptic meningitis, transverse myelitis, peripheral neuropathy, erythema multiforme, myocarditis, pericarditis, hemolytic anemia, and bullous otitis media (myringitis). In patients with sickle cell anemia, severe respiratory failure and acute chest syndrome may develop. Infection with *Chlamydia pneumoniae* mimics respiratory disease resulting from *M. pneumoniae*, inasmuch as it occurs in epidemics, is seen in older children, and produces an atypical pneumonia syndrome and pharyngitis.

Tuberculosis. Tuberculosis is uncommon in developed countries; 95% of the disease burden worldwide is in developing countries. Tuberculosis must be considered in the child with chest disease that is not easily explained by other diagnoses, especially if the child lives in or has migrated from an endemic area of the world or has been exposed to an adult with active tuberculosis. Nonetheless, tuberculosis is an infrequent cause of cough in children, even in those with active disease.

The diagnosis is made primarily by skin testing (purified protein derivative [PPD]) or a positive QuantiFERON test; a history of contact with a person who has tuberculosis; and recovery of the organism from

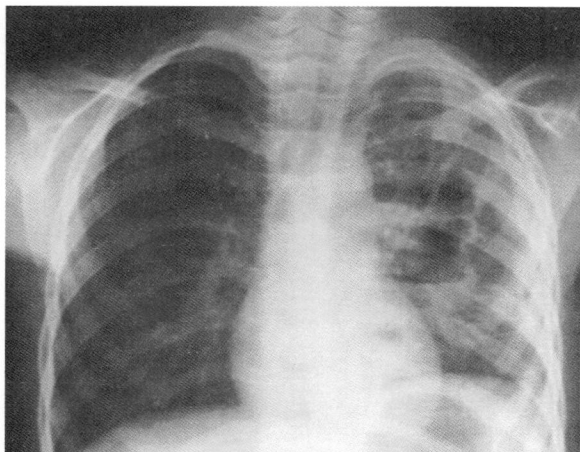

Fig. 3.9 Pneumatocele formation in the left upper lobe of a patient with staphylococcal pneumonia. (From Daly JS, Ellison RT. Acute pneumonia. In: Bennett JE, Dolin R, Blaser MF, eds. *Mandell, Douglas, and Bennett's Principles and Practices of Infectious diseases*. 9th ed. Philadelphia: Elsevier; 2020, Fig. 67.10.)

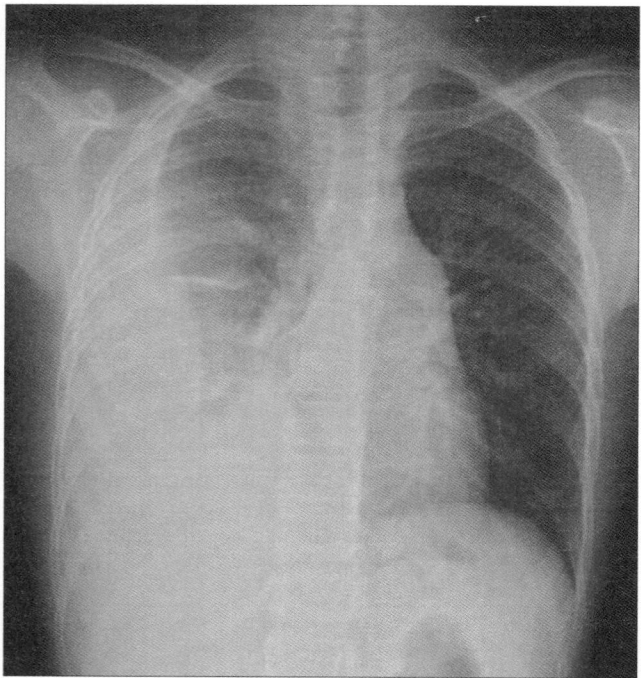

Fig. 3.10 Chest radiograph of large right-sided pleural effusion complicating community-acquired pneumonia. (From de Benedictis FM, Kerem E, Chang AB, et al. Complicated pneumonia in children. *Lancet*. 2020;396:786–798, Fig. 1.)

sputum, bronchoalveolar lavage, pleural fluid or biopsy, or morning gastric aspirates (Table 3.16). The yield from these procedures is relatively low, even from children with active pulmonary tuberculosis.

The patterns of disease in normal hosts include primary pulmonary tuberculosis, with subsequent inactivation usually noted in young children and reactivation of pulmonary disease among adolescents. **Primary pulmonary disease** is often noted as a lower or middle lobe infiltrate during the period of T-lymphocyte reaction to the initial infection. Before resolution, the *Mycobacterium tuberculosis* infection may disseminate to the better-oxygenated upper lobes and

extrathoracic sites, such as bone, or the central nervous system. If the immune response contains the initial infection, the radiographic findings may be indistinguishable from those of any other pneumonic process. In some young patients or those with altered immune function, however, there may be progressive disease, dissemination to **miliary pulmonary disease**, or early reactivation (months to 5 years) at distal sites, which produces tuberculous meningitis or osteomyelitis. **Reactivation** of upper lobe pulmonary disease may produce cavities that are similar to the disease among adults. Cavitary and endobronchial lymph node involvement are highly infectious, in contrast to the much less contagious nature of the hypersensitivity reaction noted in primary pulmonary disease.

Aspiration

Inhaling food, mouth or gastric secretions, or foreign bodies into the tracheobronchial tree causes acute, recurrent, or chronic cough. Interference with normal swallowing disrupts the coordination of swallowing and breathing that prevents aspiration. Structural causes of disordered swallowing include repaired or unrepaired esophageal atresia, strictures, webs, or congenital stenoses. Mediastinal lesions (tumors, lymph nodes), including vascular rings, may compromise the esophageal lumen and esophageal peristalsis, increasing the likelihood of aspiration. Functional disorders include central nervous system dysfunction or immaturity, dysautonomia, achalasia, and diffuse esophageal spasm. Prior neck surgery, including tracheostomy, may alter normal swallowing. Tracheoesophageal fistula and laryngeal clefts are congenital malformations with direct physical connections between the tracheobronchial tree and the upper gastrointestinal tract; thus, oral contents enter the lungs directly.

Making the diagnosis of aspiration as the cause of cough may be difficult. Barium contrast studies during swallowing may help characterize these disorders if barium enters the trachea. Because most patients aspirate sporadically, a normal barium swallow does not rule out aspiration. Radionuclide studies can be helpful if ingested radiolabeled milk or formula is demonstrated over the lung fields at several-hour intervals after the meal. Bronchoscopy and bronchoalveolar lavage that recover large numbers of lipid-laden macrophages suggest that aspiration has taken place; however, the finding is neither sensitive nor specific for aspiration.

Treatment depends largely on the cause of aspiration. Because many patients who aspirate do so because of lack of neurologic control of swallowing and breathing, it is often difficult to prevent. Even gastrostomy feedings cannot prevent aspiration of oral secretions. In extreme cases, tracheostomy with ligation of the proximal trachea has been employed. This not only prevents aspiration but also prevents phonation, and it must be considered only in unusual situations. Aspiration pneumonia is often treated with intravenous ampicillin-sulbactam or clindamycin to cover mouth flora of predominant anaerobes. Additional coverage against gram-negative organisms may be indicated if the aspiration is nosocomial.

Foreign Body

Any child with cough of abrupt onset should be suspected of having inhaled a foreign body into the airway. Toddlers, who by nature put all types of things into their mouths and who have incompletely matured swallowing and airway protective mechanisms, are at high risk. Infants with toddlers or young children in the household who may "feed" the baby are also at risk. In older children, it is usually possible to obtain an accurate history of the aspiration event. These events are described as choking, gagging, and coughing while something (e.g., peanuts, popcorn, small toys, sunflower seeds) is in the mouth. However, in toddlers, ~50% may have no witnessed history of gagging. The child may come

TABLE 3.15 Differentiation of Pleural Fluid

	Transudate	Exudate	Complicated Empyema
Appearance	Clear	Cloudy	Purulent
Cell count	<1,000	>1,000	>5,000
Cell type	Lymphocytes, monocytes	PMNs	PMNs
LDH	<200 U/L	>200 U/L	>1,000 U/L
Pleural/serum LDH ratio	<0.6	>0.6	>0.6
Protein >3 g	Unusual	Common	Common
Pleural/serum protein ratio	<0.5	>0.5	>0.5
Glucose*	Normal	Low	Very low* (<40 mg/dL)
pH*	Normal (7.40–7.60)	7.20–7.40	<7.20
Gram stain	Negative	Usually positive	>85% positive unless patient received prior antibiotics

LDH, lactate dehydrogenase; PMNs, polymorphonuclear neutrophils.
*Low glucose or pH may be seen in malignant effusion, tuberculosis, esophageal rupture, pancreatitis (positive pleural amylase), and rheumatologic diseases (e.g., systemic lupus erythematosus).

TABLE 3.16 Definitions of Positive Tuberculosis (TB) by Mantoux Skin Test (5 TU)

Cutaneous Induration ≥5 mm
- Close exposure to known or suspected active TB
- Chest radiograph consistent with TB (old or active)
- Clinical evidence of TB
- Children receiving immunosuppressive therapy or with immunosuppressive conditions

Cutaneous Induration ≥10 mm
Children at increased risk
- Age <4 yr of age
- *High risk* conditions (chronic renal failure, malnutrition, diabetes mellitus, lymphoma)
Children with likelihood of increased exposure
- Children born in high-prevalence regions of the world
- Children who travel to high-prevalence regions of the world
- Children frequently exposed to adults who are HIV infected, homeless, users of illicit drugs, residents of nursing homes, incarcerated, or institutionalized

Cutaneous Induration ≥15 mm
- All children without any identifiable risk

*BCG vaccination status not relevant.
BCG, bacille Calmette-Guérin; TB, tuberculosis; TU, tuberculin units.
Data from American Academy of Pediatrics. Tuberculosis. In: Kimberlin DW, Brady MT, Jackson MA, et al., eds. *2015 Red Book: Report of the Committee on Infectious Diseases*. 30th ed. Elk Grove Village, IL: American Academy of Pediatrics; 2015:806.

to the physician with cough and wheeze immediately after the event, with a clear history and a straightforward diagnosis. In many children with a tracheobronchial foreign body, however, the initial episode is not recognized; these children may not come to medical attention for days, weeks, or even months. The initial episode may be followed by a relatively symptom-free period lasting days or even weeks, until infection develops behind an obstructed segmental or lobar bronchus. At this point, cough, perhaps with hemoptysis, with or without wheeze, recurs.

On physical examination early after an aspiration episode, there is cough, wheeze, or both, often with asymmetry of auscultatory findings. There may be locally diminished breath sounds. Later, localized wheeze or crackles may be detected. The triad of wheezing, coughing, and decreased breath sounds is present in fewer than 50% of patients. The presence of laryngotracheal foreign bodies often manifests with stridor, retractions, aphonia, cough, and normal radiographs.

Chest radiographs may be normal in 15% of patients with intrathoracic foreign bodies but should be obtained in both inspiration and expiration because in some cases the only abnormality is unilateral or unilobar air trapping, which is occasionally more clearly identified with an expiratory radiograph. In this view, an overdistended lung that had appeared normal on the inspiratory view does not empty, but the normal, unobstructed lung empties normally. This phenomenon causes a shift of the mediastinum toward the emptying lung, away from the side with the obstructing foreign body (Fig. 3.11). In other patients, localized infiltrate or atelectasis may be present behind the obstructing object. In a few patients, it may be possible to identify the foreign body itself; nonetheless, most inhaled food particles are not radiopaque and cannot be seen on radiographs. Aspiration is usually unilateral (80%); 50–60% of the objects are in the right lung (the lobe depends on body position—supine vs standing—but is often the right middle lobe). The definitive diagnostic and therapeutic maneuver is bronchoscopy; either the flexible or rigid bronchoscope enables direct visualization of the object; the rigid instrument also enables its removal.

Gastroesophageal Reflux

GER is a common cause of cough in all age groups (see Chapter 15). The typical patient is an infant in the first 6 months of life who spits up small amounts frequently after feedings. This "regurgitant reflux" most commonly resolves by 1 year of age. However, many toddlers and children continue to have reflux, although it may be "silent" or nonregurgitant (without spitting up).

In most people with GER, it is merely a nuisance or not noticed. In some there are sequelae, and this condition is designated gastroesophageal reflux disease (GERD). One manifestation is cough; the mechanisms for the cough are not fully understood. Aspiration of refluxed material is one mechanism for cough but is probably not very common in neurologically intact children. A major mechanism for GERD with cough is mediated by vagal esophagobronchial reflexes (bronchoconstriction), stimulated by acid in the esophagus. Whether acid in the

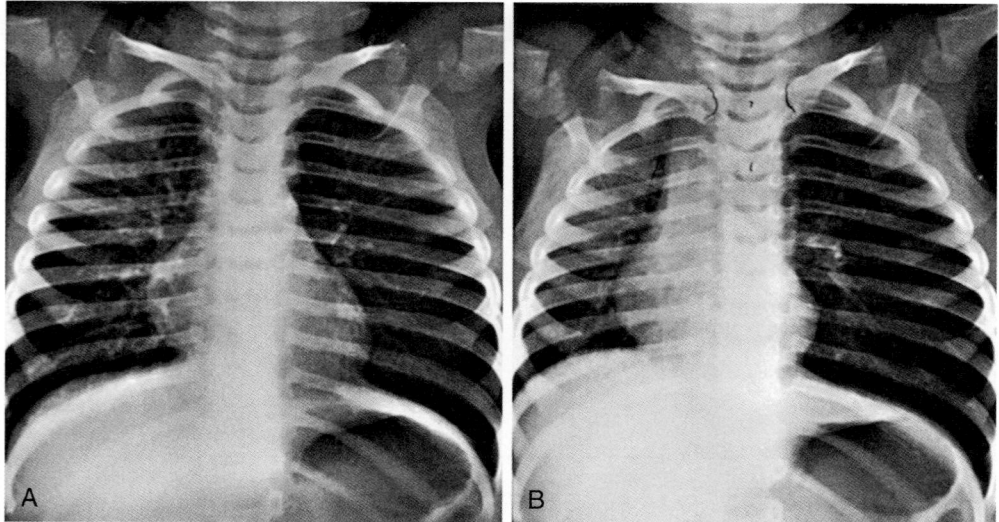

Fig. 3.11 *A,* Normal inspiratory chest radiograph in a toddler with a peanut fragment in the left main bronchus. *B,* Expiratory radiograph of the same child showing the classic air trapping on the involved side. (From Hammer AR, Schroeder JW Jr. Foreign bodies in the airway. In: Kliegman RM, St. Geme JW III, Blum NJ, et al., eds. *Nelson Textbook of Pediatrics.* 21st ed. Philadelphia: Elsevier; 2020, Fig. 411.2.)

esophagus is sufficient stimulus to cause bronchoconstriction by itself or whether it merely heightens bronchial reactivity to other stimuli is not yet clear. Many children with asthma have cough or wheeze that is difficult to control until their concurrent GER is also treated. Many episodes of cough caused by GERD occur in children with asthma that is difficult to control.

The diagnosis of GERD must also be considered in the child with chronic or recurrent cough with no other obvious explanation. The child who coughs after meals or at night, when the supine position may provoke GER, should be evaluated for GER. If GER is confirmed, the next step is a therapeutic trial of antireflux therapy.

Treatment in a child whose cough is related to GER may be accomplished by treating the reflux (see Chapter 15) or by a combination of antireflux and antiasthma treatment. On occasion, the cough may be abolished by stopping all antiasthma medications. In such cases, the cough was a manifestation of bronchospasm with esophageal acidification as the trigger for bronchospasm; the esophageal acidification was caused by the bronchodilator effects on the lower esophageal sphincter.

Asthma

Cough is frequently the sole or most prominent manifestation of asthma; wheezing may be entirely absent. In fact, asthma is almost certainly the most common cause of recurrent and chronic cough in childhood (see Chapter 4). Some of the features that characterize the cough of a child with asthma are listed in Table 3.17. Treatment for asthma manifesting as cough is the same as the treatment for asthma.

Cystic Fibrosis

CF is a common cause of recurrent or chronic cough in infancy and childhood. CF occurs in 1 in 2,000–3,000 live births among White persons, is far less common among African Americans (1 in 15,000), and is rare among Native Americans and Asians. Early diagnosis improves the prognosis for untreated CF; if untreated, many patients die in infancy or early childhood. The median length of survival is in the upper 30s; based on 2018 CF Patient Registry data, the median life expectancy of people with CF who are born between 2014 and 2018 is

TABLE 3.17	**Asthma as a Cause of Cough: History**
Any age (even infants)
Coexistence of allergy increases likelihood, but absence of allergy does not decrease likelihood
Wheeze need not be present
↑ Cough with upper respiratory infections
↑ Cough with (and especially after) exercise
↑ Cough with hard laughing or crying
↑ Cough with exposure to cold
↑ Cough with exposure to cigarette smoke
↑ Nocturnal cough
↑ Exercise-induced dyspnea or cough
Usually a history of dramatic response to inhaled β-agonists

predicted to be 44 years. Of children born in 2018, half are predicted to survive to 47 years or older.

CF is a genetic disorder, inherited as an autosomal recessive trait. The CF gene is on the long arm of chromosome 7; more than 1,900 gene variants have been identified at the CF locus. Of these variants, one (ΔF508, indicating a deletion, Δ, of a single phenylalanine, F, at position 508 of the protein product) is the most common, responsible for 70–75% of all CF chromosomes. The variant affects the gene's protein product, termed cystic fibrosis transmembrane regulator (CFTR), which acts as a chloride channel and affects other aspects of membrane transport of ions and water. Not all the consequences of the defective gene and protein have been determined. In general, however, the defective gene product results in the long-observed clinical manifestations of the disease, including thick, viscid mucus in the tracheobronchial tree, leading to purulent bronchiolitis and bronchitis with subsequent bronchiectasis, pulmonary fibrosis, and respiratory failure; pancreatic duct obstruction, leading to pancreatic insufficiency with steatorrhea and failure to thrive; and abnormally high sweat chloride and sodium concentrations. The airway disease in CF is characterized by infection, inflammation, and endobronchial obstruction. The infection begins with *S. aureus, H. influenzae, Escherichia coli, Klebsiella* species, or

TABLE 3.18 Physical Examination Features of Cystic Fibrosis

General
Low weight for height (>50% of patients)

Head, Eyes, Ears, Nose, and Throat
Nasal polyps (20%)

Chest
Cough
Barrel chest (↑ anteroposterior diameter)
Intercostal, suprasternal retractions
Crackles, especially upper lobes
Wheeze

Abdomen
Hepatomegaly (10%)
Right lower quadrant fecal mass (5–10%)

Extremities
Digital clubbing (80%)

Reproductive Tract
Bilateral atresia or absence of vas deferens (>95% of males)

TABLE 3.19 Causes of Digital Clubbing in Children

Pulmonary
- Cystic fibrosis ++
- Non–cystic fibrosis bronchiectasis +
- Primary ciliary dyskinesia
- Bronchiolitis obliterans
- Interstitial lung diseases
- Empyema
- Lung abscess
- Malignancy
- Tuberculosis
- Pulmonary arteriovenous fistula

Cardiac
- Cyanotic congenital heart disease ++
- Bacterial endocarditis +
- Chronic congestive heart failure

Gastrointestinal
- Crohn disease
- Ulcerative colitis
- Celiac disease +
- Severe gastrointestinal hemorrhage
- Small bowel lymphoma
- Multiple polyposis

Hepatic
- Biliary cirrhosis
- Chronic active hepatitis

Hematologic
- Thalassemia
- Congenital methemoglobinemia

Miscellaneous
- Familial
- Thyroid deficiency
- Thyrotoxicosis
- Chronic pyelonephritis
- Heavy metal poisoning
- Scleroderma
- Lymphoid granulomatosis
- Hodgkin disease
- HIV

++, very common cause of digital clubbing; +, common cause of digital clubbing.

combinations of these organisms but eventually is dominated by non-mucoid or mucoid *Pseudomonas aeruginosa*. Other organisms, such as *Burkholderia cepacia*, *Stenotrophomonas maltophilia*, *Alcaligenes xylosoxidans*, *Aspergillus fumigatus*, or nontuberculous mycobacteria may also appear. In some patients, *B. cepacia* has been associated with rapid deterioration and death, and in others, *Aspergillus* species has caused allergic bronchopulmonary aspergillosis (ABPA). The airway inflammation in all patients with CF appears to be the result of endogenous toxic substances, including elastase, released by neutrophils as they respond to the endobronchial infection and by exogenous enzymes released by the invading organisms.

CF may manifest at birth with meconium ileus (20% of patients), or later, with steatorrhea and failure to thrive despite a voracious appetite, in an apparent effort to make up for the calories that are lost in the stool (see Chapter 12). The most common presenting symptom after the newborn period is cough, which may appear within the first weeks of life or may be delayed for decades. The cough can be dry, productive, or paroxysmal. Cough may respond to antibiotics or perhaps steroids, but it is less likely to improve with bronchodilators (see Tables 3.3 and 3.5). Because CF is a recessive genetic disease, there is often no family history. Furthermore, in atypical cases, patients may not have pancreatic insufficiency (~10% of patients) and thus may not demonstrate steatorrhea and failure to thrive. In addition, malabsorption may not be evident in the neonatal period.

There is no such thing as a child who looks "too good" to have CF; common abnormalities found on physical examination are noted in Table 3.18. One of the most important physical findings is digital clubbing. In most patients with CF, clubbing develops within the first few years of life. Although the list of conditions associated with digital clubbing (Table 3.19) is long, they are less common than CF, or the incidence of digital clubbing with these conditions is low. There is some relationship between the degree of pulmonary disease severity and the degree of digital clubbing. A child who has had years of severe respiratory symptoms without digital clubbing is not likely to have CF.

The diagnosis is confirmed by a positive sweat chloride test or confirming the presence of two CF variants on chromosome 7. The sweat test, if not performed correctly in a laboratory with extensive experience with the technique (as, for example, in an accredited CF center), yields many false-positive and false-negative results. The proper technique is to use quantitative analysis of the concentration of chloride in the sweat produced after pilocarpine iontophoretic stimulation. Chloride concentration ≥60 mmol/L is considered positive, ≤29 mmol/L is negative (normal), and 30–59 mmol/L is intermediate, suggestive of possible CF, and requires further evaluation, including a repeat sweat test and CFTR gene sequencing. Healthy adults have slightly higher sweat chloride concentrations than do children, but the same guidelines hold for positive tests in adults. The non-CF conditions yielding elevated sweat chloride concentrations are listed in Table 3.20. False-negative results of sweat tests can be seen in CF children presenting

TABLE 3.20 Conditions Other Than Cystic Fibrosis with Elevated Sweat Chloride

Adrenal insufficiency (untreated)
Ectodermal dysplasia
Autonomic dysfunction
Hypothyroidism
Malnutrition, including psychosocial dwarfism
Mucopolysaccharidosis
Glycogen storage disease (type I)
Fucosidosis
Hereditary nephrogenic diabetes insipidus
Mauriac syndrome
Pseudohypoaldosteronism
Familial cholestasis
Nephrosis with edema

TABLE 3.21 Indications for Sweat Testing

Pulmonary Indications
- Chronic or recurrent cough
- Chronic or recurrent pneumonia (especially RUL)
- Recurrent bronchiolitis
- Atelectasis
- Hemoptysis
- Staphylococcal pneumonia
- *Pseudomonas aeruginosa* in the respiratory tract (in the absence of such circumstances as tracheostomy or prolonged intubation)
- Mucoid *P. aeruginosa* in the respiratory tract

Gastrointestinal Indications
- Meconium ileus
- Neonatal intestinal obstruction (meconium plug, atresia)
- Steatorrhea, malabsorption
- Failure to thrive
- Hepatic cirrhosis in childhood (including any manifestations such as esophageal varices or portal hypertension)
- Pancreatitis
- Rectal prolapse
- Vitamin K deficiency states (hypoprothrombinemia)

Miscellaneous Indications
- Digital clubbing
- Family history of cystic fibrosis (sibling or cousin)
- Salty taste when kissed; salt crystals on skin after evaporation of sweat
- Heat prostration, especially under seemingly inappropriate circumstances
- Hyponatremic hypochloremic alkalosis in infants
- Nasal polyps
- Pansinusitis
- Aspermia

RUL, right upper lobe.
From Kercsmar CM. The respiratory system. In: Behrman RE, Kliegman RM, eds. *Nelson Essentials of Pediatrics.* 2nd ed. Philadelphia: WB Saunders; 1994:451.

with edema or hypoproteinemia and in samples from children with an inadequate sweat rate. Sweat testing can be performed at any age. Newborns within the first few weeks of life may not produce a large enough volume of sweat to analyze (75 mg minimum), but in those who do (the majority), the results are accurate. Indications for sweat testing are noted in Table 3.21.

In patients for whom sweat testing is difficult (e.g., because of distance from an experienced laboratory, small infants who have not produced enough sweat, patients with extreme dermatitis, or patients with intermediate-range sweat chloride concentrations), CFTR gene sequencing can be useful. Demonstration of two known CF variants confirms the diagnosis. Finding one or no known variant makes the diagnosis less likely but is not exclusive, inasmuch as there are patients with not-yet-characterized variants.

Recovery of mucoid *P. aeruginosa* from respiratory tract secretions is strongly suggestive of CF. Similarly, pansinusitis is nearly universal among CF patients but is quite uncommon in other children. All 50 states are using a neonatal screen for CF. The CF screen assays include measuring serum immunoreactive trypsinogen (IRT) levels, which are elevated in most infants with CF for the first several weeks of life, and DNA analysis for CFTR variants. The main drawback of the IRT assay is that it has relatively poor specificity; as many as 90% of the positive results on the initial screen are false-positive results. If an infant's IRT screen is positive, the test should be repeated, or DNA analysis for the 23 most common CFTR variants should be performed. At 2–3 weeks of age, which is when the IRT is repeated, the false-positive rate has fallen dramatically but is still quite high (25%). Definitive testing with the sweat chloride test needs to be carried out on infants with positive screening results.

Laboratory data that may support the diagnosis of CF include low levels of fecal elastase. This suggests pancreatic insufficiency, which occurs most commonly in CF but can be seen in other diseases. The test is not perfect for confirming CF as some CF patients have sufficient pancreatic function. Pulmonary function test findings with an obstructive pattern, incompletely responsive to bronchodilators, are consistent with CF but, of course, can be seen in other conditions. Conversely, some patients with CF also have asthma and may show a marked response to a bronchodilator. Complications of CF that suggest the diagnosis are noted in Table 3.22.

The treatment of patients with CF requires a comprehensive approach, best performed in, or in conjunction with, an approved CF center. Several studies have shown survival to be significantly better in center-based care than in non–center-based care. CFTR gene modulator therapy aims to increase or improve the function of the abnormal CFTR protein and has shown promising results over the past 5 years.

Anatomic Abnormalities

Table 3.23 lists the main anatomic abnormalities that cause cough.

Vascular rings and slings. Vascular rings and slings are often associated with inspiratory stridor because the abnormal vessels compress central airways, most commonly the trachea (see Chapter 4). The patient may also have difficulty swallowing if the esophagus is compressed.

The diagnosis may be suspected from plain radiographs of the chest, especially those showing tracheal deviation and a right-sided aortic arch. Further support for the diagnosis can be found at bronchoscopy (which shows extrinsic compression of the trachea or a mainstem bronchus), barium esophagram (which shows esophageal compression), or both. The definitive diagnosis is made with CT angiography or magnetic resonance angiography. Treatment is surgical.

Pulmonary sequestration. Pulmonary sequestration is relatively unusual, occurring in 1 in 60,000 children. It occurs most commonly in the left lower lobe and can manifest in several ways (Fig. 3.12; see also Table 3.23). The chest radiograph usually shows a density in the left lower lobe; this density often appears to contain cysts (Fig. 3.13). The feature distinguishing a sequestered lobe from a complicated pneumonia is that the blood supply arises from the systemic circulation and not the pulmonary circulation. Doppler ultrasonography and CT

TABLE 3.22 Complications of Cystic Fibrosis

Pulmonary Complications

- Bronchiectasis, bronchitis, bronchiolitis, pneumonia
- Atelectasis
- Hemoptysis
- Pneumothorax
- Nasal polyps
- Sinusitis
- Bronchospasm
- Cor pulmonale
- Respiratory failure
- Mucoid impaction of the bronchi
- Allergic bronchopulmonary aspergillosis

Gastrointestinal Complications

- Meconium ileus
- Meconium peritonitis
- Distal intestinal obstruction syndrome (meconium ileus equivalent) (non-neonatal obstruction)
- Rectal prolapse
- Intussusception
- Volvulus
- Appendicitis
- Intestinal atresia
- Pancreatitis
- Biliary cirrhosis (portal hypertension: esophageal varices, hypersplenism)
- Neonatal obstructive jaundice
- Hepatic steatosis
- Gastroesophageal reflux
- Cholelithiasis
- Inguinal hernia
- Growth failure
- Vitamin deficiency states (vitamins A, D, E, K)
- Insulin deficiency, symptomatic hyperglycemia, diabetes

Other Complications

- Infertility
- Edema/hypoproteinemia
- Dehydration/heat exhaustion
- Hypertrophic osteoarthropathy/arthritis
- Delayed puberty
- Amyloidosis

From Kercsmar CM. The respiratory system. In: Behrman RE, Kliegman RM, eds. *Nelson Essentials of Pediatrics*. 2nd ed. Philadelphia: WB Saunders; 1994:451.

angiography provide the definitive diagnosis. The treatment is surgical removal.

Congenital pulmonary airway malformation. Congenital pulmonary airway malformations (CPAMs) (formerly known as congenital cystic adenomatoid malformations or CCAMs) are rare. They manifest in infancy with respiratory distress in nearly 50% of cases; the other half may manifest as cough with recurrent infection later in childhood or even adulthood. The chest radiograph reveals multiple cysts, separated by dense areas. Chest CT scans can help make the diagnosis with near certainty. Surgical removal is the treatment of choice, particularly if the lesion is symptomatic.

Congenital lobar emphysema. Congenital lobar emphysema has a prevalence of 1 in 20,000–30,000. It can manifest dramatically with respiratory distress in the neonatal period or later (Fig. 3.14), with cough or wheeze, or as an incidental finding on a chest radiograph. Radiography shows localized overinflation, often dramatic, with compression of adjacent lung tissue and occasionally atelectasis of the contralateral lung because of mediastinal shift away from the involved side. The appearance on chest CT scan is typical, with widely spaced blood vessels (as opposed to congenital cysts, for example, which have no blood vessels within the overinflated area). Bronchoscopy can document patent bronchi and should probably be performed in older children in whom congenital lobar emphysema can be confused with acquired overinflation of a lobe as the result of bronchial obstruction, as with a foreign body. If the disease is symptomatic, treatment is surgical.

Tracheoesophageal fistula. Tracheoesophageal fistula is common, with an incidence of about 1 in 2,500–4,500 live births. Of these fistulas, the large majority (85%) are associated with esophageal atresia; only 3% are the isolated, H-type fistula (a patent esophagus with fistulous tract connecting the esophagus and trachea). A neonate with esophageal atresia experiences respiratory distress, excessive drooling, and choking and gagging with feeding. The H-type fistula causes more subtle signs and may be undiagnosed for months or even years. The child may have only intermittent feeding trouble, especially with liquids. There may be recurrent lower respiratory tract infections.

The diagnosis is not challenging in the infant with esophageal atresia; a nasogastric tube cannot be passed, and swallowed barium outlines the trachea. In the older child with H-type fistula, a barium esophagogram may or may not reveal the fistula. Bronchoscopy and esophagoscopy should permit direct visualization of the fistula; however, the opening may be hidden in mucosal folds.

Treatment is surgical. Many children born with tracheoesophageal fistula have recurrent cough and lower respiratory tract infection for many years, even after successful surgical correction. The cough is characteristically the harsh cough of tracheomalacia, which is present at the site of the fistula. The infections result from several causes, including GER due to impaired esophageal motility, with or without aspiration, and altered mucociliary transport. Treatment involves regular chest physiotherapy and early and aggressive use of antibiotics whenever there is evidence of increased pulmonary symptoms.

Hemangiomas. Hemangiomas may be present within the airway and can cause cough, rarely with hemoptysis. Stridor (if the hemangioma is high in the airway) and respiratory distress (if the hemangioma is large) may also occur. In rare cases, with very large airway hemangiomas, there may even be dysphagia from extrinsic compression. Children with cutaneous hemangiomas in the mandibular or neck region ("beard" distribution) are at risk for an airway hemangioma.

The diagnosis is made with bronchoscopy. These lesions may resolve spontaneously over the first year or so. However, if they cause symptoms, it may not be advisable or possible to wait for them to resolve.

Many airway hemangiomas regress with steroid treatment; however, due to the side effect profile, propranolol is considered the treatment of choice. Asthma is a contraindication for propranolol treatment due to its beta-blocking effect and potential to worsen asthma. Laser ablation may be indicated in some refractory cases that do not respond to first-line treatment. In the case of a large subglottic hemangioma, a tracheostomy is performed and maintained until the mass regresses.

Enlarged lymph nodes. Enlarged mediastinal lymph nodes, such as those resulting from tuberculosis, leukemia, other hematologic malignancies, or other infections, are occasionally a cause of cough in children (Table 3.24; see also Table 3.23). These nodes are usually seen on plain radiographs of the chest. The x-ray study or bronchoscopy may show extrinsic compression of the trachea. Treatment is directed at the underlying cause.

Bronchial stenosis. Occasionally bronchial stenosis, either congenital or acquired, may cause cough. The diagnosis is made with

TABLE 3.23   Anatomic Abnormalities Causing Cough

Condition	Other Symptoms	Diagnostic Evidence	Treatment
Vascular ring/sling	Stridor; dysphagia, emesis	Radiographic: deviated trachea, right-sided arch Barium swallow: esophageal indentation Bronchoscopy: extrinsic compression Chest CT angiography: definitive	Surgical
Pulmonary sequestration	Fever, dyspnea; may be asymptomatic	Radiographic: most commonly in the left lower lobe, usually with cysts Angiography: systemic blood supply	Surgical
Congenital pulmonary airway malformation	Respiratory distress; recurrent infection	Radiographic: multiple cysts alternating with solid areas	Surgical
Congenital lobar emphysema	Respiratory distress; wheeze; may be asymptomatic	Radiographic: localized overinflation, other lobes (even other lung) collapsed Bronchoscopy to rule out foreign body	Surgical (if symptomatic)
Tracheoesophageal fistula or cleft	Gagging, choking with feeds; respiratory distress (especially with esophageal atresia)	Barium esophagram: barium in tracheobronchial tree Bronchoscopy: direct visualization	Surgical
Airway hemangioma	Stridor; wheeze; dysphagia; hemoptysis	Bronchoscopy	Propranolol, steroids; laser; occasionally tracheostomy required
Mediastinal lymph nodes	Stridor	Radiographic: hilar nodes; compressed tracheal air column	Treat cause
Bronchial stenosis	Wheeze; recurrent pneumonia	Bronchoscopy	Balloon dilatation; surgery
Bronchogenic cysts	Wheeze, stridor	Radiographic: hyperinflation of one lung; visible mass (carina, posterior mediastinum) Bronchoscopy: extrinsic compression CT: often definitive	Surgical
Tumors (see Tables 3.24, 3.25)	Cough, wheeze, hemoptysis	CT, MRI	Based on tumor type

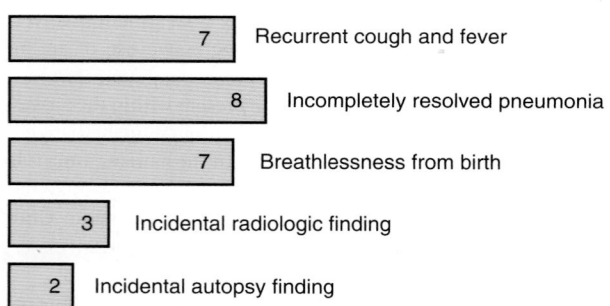

7	Recurrent cough and fever
8	Incompletely resolved pneumonia
7	Breathlessness from birth
3	Incidental radiologic finding
2	Incidental autopsy finding

Fig. 3.12 Different modes of presentation of sequestered lobe and number of children with each problem. (From Phelan PD, Olinsky A, eds. *Respiratory Illness in Children.* Oxford: Wiley-Blackwell; 1994.)

bronchoscopy, after suspicion has been raised by the child having recurrent infiltrates in the same lobe, especially with localized wheeze.

Treatment may be difficult. In some cases, endoscopic balloon dilatation or airway stent placement is successful; in others, surgical resection of stenotic areas may be necessary.

Bronchogenic cysts. Bronchogenic cysts are uncommon, but they can cause cough, wheeze, stridor, or any combination of these. They may also cause recurrent or persistent pneumonia if they block a bronchus sufficiently to interfere with normal drainage of the segment or lobe. Radiography may show localized overinflation if the cyst causes a ball-valve–type obstruction. The cyst itself may or may not be seen on plain radiographs. Bronchoscopy reveals extrinsic compression of the airway. CT studies often definitively show the lesion. Surgical removal is indicated.

Other rare causes of cough. Certain genetic disorders such as hereditary sensory and autonomic neuropathies (HSANs), in the absence of significant autonomic features, may first present with unexplained chronic cough and GER.

Habit (Psychogenic) Cough

On occasion, a school-aged child may develop a cough that lasts for weeks, often after a fairly typical cold. This cough occurs only during wakefulness, never during sleep. In many cases, the cough is harsh and sounds like a foghorn. It can disrupt the classroom, and the child may be asked to leave. The child is otherwise well and may seem unbothered by the spectacle created. There is no response to medications. It seems that this type of cough, previously termed "psychogenic" or "psychogenic cough tic," now called habit cough, has given the child valuable attention. This attention then serves as the sustaining force, and the cough persists beyond the original airway inflammation. In the small minority of cases, there may be deep-seated emotional problems of which the cough is the physical expression.

During the history or physical examination, the child appears completely well and may cough when attention is drawn to the child or when the word "cough" is uttered. The physical examination findings are otherwise completely normal, as are laboratory values. Because this may occur in any child, evidence of mild asthma (history or pulmonary function testing) does not rule out the diagnosis. Once a physician has seen a child with this problem, it is usually possible to make the diagnosis with certainty on entering the examining room or, indeed, from the hallway outside the room.

Treatment can prove more difficult. The child and family should be reassured that the child is well. Suggestion therapy empowers and

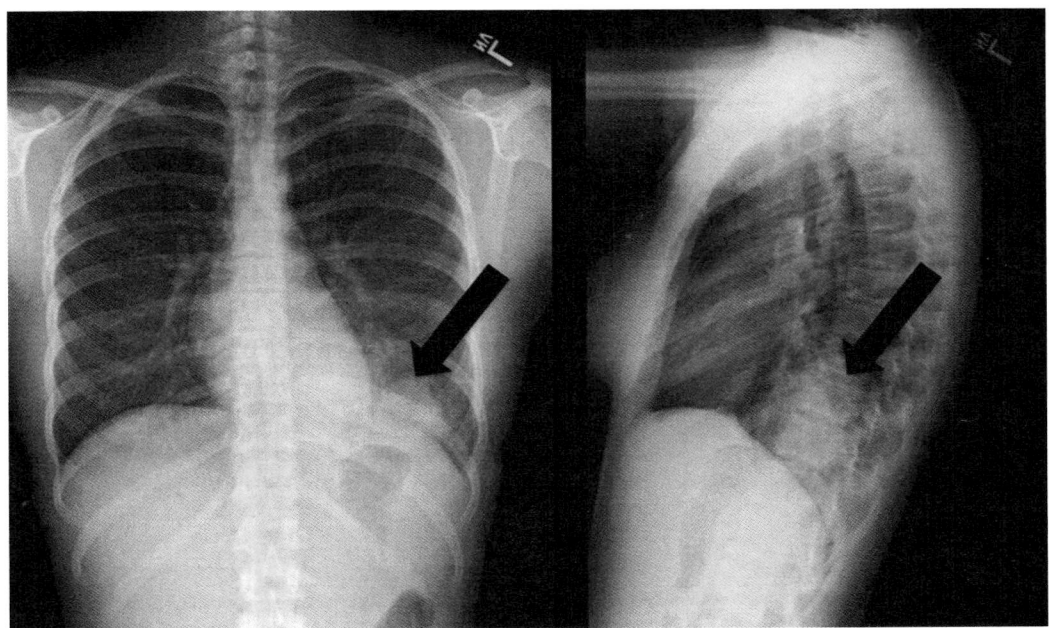

Fig. 3.13 Anterior-posterior and lateral chest radiographs showing a left lower lobe pulmonary sequestration *(bold arrow)* in a 15-year-old girl.

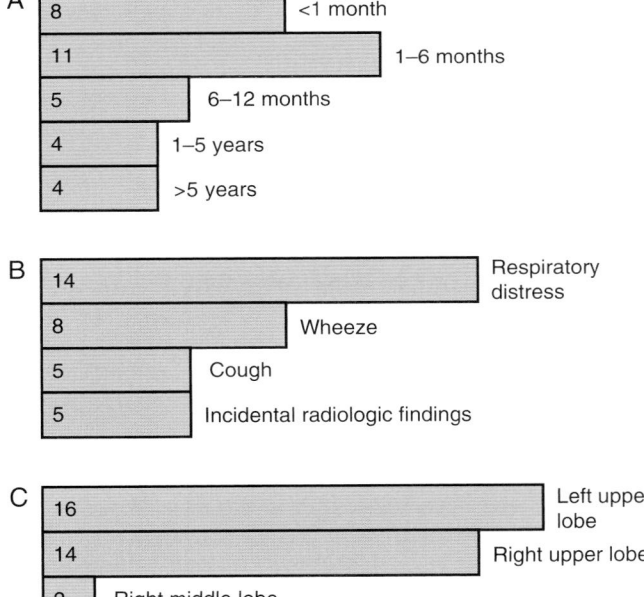

Fig. 3.14 Different modes of presentation of congenital lobar emphysema. *A,* Age at presentation. *B,* Symptoms at presentation. *C,* Involved lobe. Numbers refer to the number of children in each category. (From Phelan PD, Olinsky A, eds. *Respiratory Illness in Children.* Oxford: Wiley-Blackwell; 1994.)

TABLE 3.24	**Intrathoracic Mass Lesions**

Anterior Mediastinum
- Thymus tumor
- T-cell lymphoma
- Teratoma
- Thyroid lesions
- Pericardial cyst
- Hemangioma
- Lymphangioma

Hilar–Middle Mediastinum
- Tuberculosis
- Histoplasmosis
- Coccidiomycosis
- Acute lymphocytic leukemia/lymphoma
- Hodgkin disease
- Sarcoidosis
- Hiatal hernia
- Pericardial cyst
- Bronchogenic or enteric cyst

Posterior Mediastinum
- Neuroblastoma/ganglioneuroma
- Other neural tumors
- Neuroenteric lesions
- Esophageal lesions (duplication)
- Vertebral osteomyelitis
- Diaphragmatic hernia
- Meningocele
- Aortic aneurysm

encourages the patient to suppress the cough for short increments of time. The goal is for them to gradually lengthen the cough-free intervals. Speech therapy may be helpful (Table 3.25).

Other Causes of Cough

Table 3.26 lists several miscellaneous causes of cough in children.

Bronchiectasis. Bronchiectasis is defined as an abnormal dilatation of the subsegmental bronchi and is usually associated with chronic cough and purulent sputum production. It occasionally occurs after severe pneumonias (bacterial or viral); it eventually develops in nearly all patients with CF. Recurrent protracted bacterial bronchitis (over three episodes in 1 year) may be a sign of or a precursor to bronchiectasis. Diagnosis may, on occasion, be made with plain

TABLE 3.25 Speech Therapy Techniques for Treating Habit Cough

Increase abdominal breathing
Reduce muscle tension in neck, chest, and shoulders
Interrupt early cough sensation by swallowing
Substitute gentle cough for hacking cough
Interrupt cough sequence with diaphragm breathing and tightly pursed lips
Increase the patient's awareness of initial sensations that would trigger cough

TABLE 3.26 Miscellaneous Causes of Cough in Children

Postnasal drip	Cerumen impaction
Bronchiectasis	Irritation of external auditory canal
Primary ciliary dyskinesia	Bronchiolitis obliterans
Interstitial lung disease	Follicular bronchiolitis
Heart failure/pulmonary edema	Mediastinal disease (nodes,
Pulmonary hemosiderosis	pneumomediastinum)
Drug induced (see Table 3.4)	Nasal polyps
α_1-Antitrypsin deficiency	Hypersensitivity pneumonitis
Graft-versus-host disease	(extrinsic allergic alveolitis)
Bronchopulmonary dysplasia	Thyroid lesions
Tumor (see Table 3.27)	Subphrenic abscess
Alveolar proteinosis	Sarcoidosis
Tracheomalacia, bronchomalacia	Anaphylaxis
Spasmodic croup	Pulmonary embolism
	Lung contusion

TABLE 3.27 Pulmonary Tumors

Primary Malignant
Bronchial carcinoid*
Mucoepidermoid carcinoma*
Adenoid cystic carcinoma*
Pleuropulmonary blastoma*
Inflammatory myofibroblastic tumor*
Germ cell
Thymoma
Thymolipoma
Bronchogenic carcinoma (squamous cell and bronchioalveolar)
FLIT
NUT midline carcinoma

Primary Benign
Hamartoma
Arteriovenous malformation
Hemangioma
Leiomyoma

Metastatic
Adrenocortical carcinoma
Thyroid carcinoma
Teratoma
Hepatoblastoma
Neuroblastoma
Wilms tumor
Ewing sarcoma
Osteosarcoma
Rhabdomyosarcoma

*Commonest primary lung tumors.
FLIT, fetal lung interstitial tumor; NUT, nuclear protein in testis.

chest radiographs, but high-resolution CT scanning is the diagnostic procedure of choice. Treatment of bronchiectasis consists of airway clearance with chest physiotherapy and postural drainage or high-frequency chest wall oscillation, occasionally bronchodilators and mucolytic agents, and antibiotic therapy during exacerbations. Surgical resection may be indicated in cases that are progressive and localized when medical therapy has failed. The prognosis of bronchiectasis depends on the underlying cause. CF-associated bronchiectasis is a major cause of CF-related morbidity and mortality, whereas non-CF bronchiectasis may remain stable or even regress with therapy.

Primary ciliary dyskinesia. Conditions in which the cilia do not function properly (immotile cilia or ciliary dyskinesia) lead to cough, usually because infection (and bronchiectasis) occurs in the absence of normal mucociliary transport. Diagnosis includes exhaled or nasal low nitric oxide levels, bronchoscopic biopsy, and specific genetic testing. Treatment is similar to that for CF, with regular chest physiotherapy and frequent and aggressive use of antibiotics at the first sign of airways infection, most commonly increased cough.

Interstitial lung disease. Interstitial lung diseases are classified based on those that occur during the neonatal period and those that are not as prevalent in infancy. Interstitial lung diseases that manifest with cough include aspiration (chronic and recurrent) pneumonitis, hypersensitivity pneumonitis, bronchiolitis obliterans, and cryptogenic organizing pneumonia (formerly known as bronchiolitis obliterans organizing pneumonia or BOOP). Lung biopsy may be required for a diagnosis.

Pulmonary hemosiderosis. Pulmonary hemosiderosis is a rare, and often fatal, condition of bleeding into the lung that can manifest with cough. If sputum is produced, it is often frothy and blood-tinged. There may be frank hemoptysis. However, the cough may be nonproductive, or the sputum may be swallowed. Some cases are associated with milk hypersensitivity (**Heiner syndrome**), and others are associated

with collagen vascular disorders. Radiographs usually show diffuse fluffy infiltrates, and there is invariably iron-deficiency anemia. The diagnosis is based on lung biopsy findings.

Primary and metastatic tumors. Tumors causing cough are rare in childhood. Cough usually occurs because of bronchial obstruction, either extrinsic or endobronchial, resulting at times in recurrent obstructive pneumonias (Table 3.27).

Bronchogenic tumors (carcinoid, mucoepidermoid carcinoma [MEC], bronchial adenocarcinoma [BAC], inflammatory myofibroblastic tumor [IMT]) may present with cough, recurrent obstructive pneumonias, wheezing, hemoptysis, and chest pain (Fig. 3.15). Carcinoid is the most common bronchial tumor followed by MEC, BAC, and IMT. Carcinoid tumors rarely manifest vasoactive carcinoid syndrome symptoms (<5%) but may be associated with Cushing syndrome.

Pleuropulmonary blastoma (PPB) usually presents under age 3 years and is often associated with the *DICER1* tumor susceptibility syndrome, an autosomal dominant disease. There are four subtypes: 1, cystic; 2, mixed; 3, solid; and 1r, regressing. Type 1 may be confused with a cystic CPAM. PPB may present with cough, wheezing, pneumonia, or pneumothorax.

The evaluation of a suspected primary or metastatic tumor includes chest x-ray, bronchoscopy, CT angiography, and, to evaluate for metastatic disease, PET-MRI (see Fig. 3.15). Treatment usually requires surgical resection in addition to other tumor-specific therapies.

Tracheomalacia and bronchomalacia. Isolated tracheomalacia or bronchomalacia is uncommon but can cause cough in some children. The cough of tracheomalacia is typically harsh and brassy. Specific treatment is difficult but, fortunately, is seldom needed.

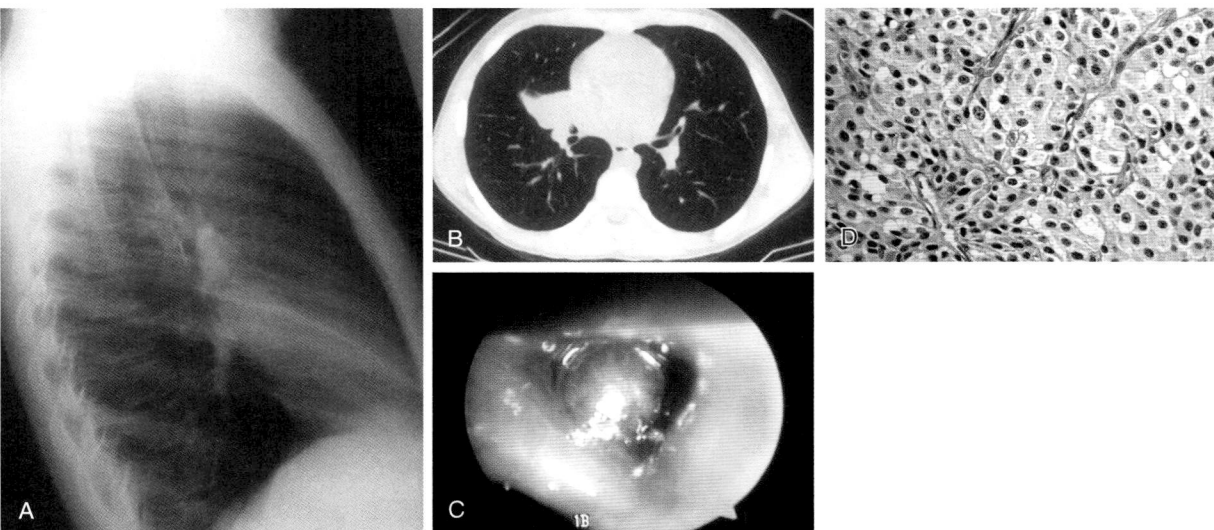

Fig. 3.15 Lateral chest radiograph *(A)* of an 11-year-old boy who presented with intermittent cough. It revealed collapse of the middle lobe, which was confirmed on the CT *(B)*. Subsequent bronchoscopy *(C)* revealed a lesion obstructing the bronchus intermedius, presumed to be a carcinoid tumor, which was confirmed *(D)* on subsequent pathology. (From Weldon CB, Shamberger RC. Pediatric pulmonary tumors: primary and metastatic. *Semin Pediatr Surg.* 2008;17:17–29, Fig. 3.)

Spasmodic croup. Some children, usually preschoolers, may episodically awaken at night with stridor and a harsh, barking cough indistinguishable from that of viral croup. This entity is termed spasmodic croup and is of unclear origin. Viral and allergic causes have been postulated. GER may be the cause in some patients.

Treatment with cool mist or racemic epinephrine is effective in most patients. If GER is the underlying cause, antireflux treatment is beneficial.

Bronchiolitis obliterans. Bronchiolitis obliterans (BO) is very rare except in lung and bone marrow transplant recipients. In other instances, it may arise after adenovirus, measles, or influenza pneumonia; after exposure to certain toxins; or in other rare circumstances. Children may exhibit cough, respiratory distress, and exercise intolerance.

The diagnosis is suggested by the pulmonary function test or radiographic evidence of small airways obstruction; however, these findings are not always present. Not all chest radiographs show overinflated lungs, and not all pulmonary function tests show decreased small airways function.

The definitive diagnosis is histologic via open or transbronchial biopsy. No specific treatment is available. Most children with BO recover but many progress to chronic disability or death.

Hemoptysis

The child who coughs out blood or bloody mucus presents special diagnostic and therapeutic challenges. Although hemoptysis is relatively uncommon in children, particularly among those without CF, many conditions can cause it (Table 3.28). It is important (and not always easy) to distinguish cases in which blood has originated in the tracheobronchial tree (true hemoptysis), the nose (epistaxis), and the gastrointestinal tract (hematemesis). Table 3.29 gives some guidelines to help localize sites of origin of blood that has been reported or suspected as hemoptysis. None of these guidelines is foolproof, partly because blood that has originated in one of these sites might well end up in another before being expelled from the body; for instance, blood from the nose can be swallowed and vomited or aspirated and expectorated.

Infection is among the most common causes of hemoptysis. Lung abscess and tuberculosis need to be considered. Bronchiectasis can readily cause erosion into bronchial vessels, often made tortuous by years of local inflammation, and produce hemoptysis. Other infectious causes are less common and include necrotizing pneumonias and fungal and parasitic lung invasion.

Foreign bodies in the airway can cause hemoptysis by direct irritation, by erosion of airway mucosa, or by secondary infection.

Pulmonary embolus is uncommon in children and adolescents, but it needs to be considered in the differential diagnosis of an adolescent with hemoptysis of unclear origin. Clues to the diagnosis of pulmonary embolus include a positive family history, severe dyspnea, chest pain, hypoxia, a normal chest radiograph, an accentuated second heart sound, an abnormal compression ultrasonographic study of the leg veins, a positive Homans sign, a positive helical CT scan, and a high-probability lung ventilation-perfusion scan.

The diagnosis of several causes of hemoptysis is straightforward. For example, hemoptysis that occurs immediately after a surgical or invasive diagnostic procedure in the chest should suggest an iatrogenic problem. The chest radiograph can help suggest lung abscess, pulmonary sequestration, bronchogenic cyst, or tumor. Chest CT can help with cases of arteriovenous malformations, and additional laboratory values can support the diagnosis of collagen vascular disease. Bronchoscopy can sometimes localize a bleeding site, identify a cause (e.g., a foreign body or endobronchial tumor), or recover an offending bacterial, fungal, or parasitic pathogen. In many instances, bronchoscopy does not help except by excluding some possibilities, because either no blood or blood throughout the tracheobronchial tree is found. Chest CT angiography may help to identify the involved vessel or vessels.

Treatment of hemoptysis depends on the underlying cause. It can be a terrifying symptom to children and their parents, and a calm, reassuring approach is essential. Because hemoptysis is seldom fatal in children, reassurance is usually warranted. Furthermore, hemoptysis most often resolves, and treatment of the bleeding itself is not often needed. What is required is treatment of the underlying cause of the hemoptysis, such as therapy for infection, removal of a foreign body, or control of collagen vascular disease. When death occurs from hemoptysis, it is more likely to be from suffocation than from exsanguination. In cases of massive bleeding, the rigid open-tube bronchoscope may help

TABLE 3.28   Hemoptysis: Differential Diagnosis

Infection	Lung abscess
	Pneumonia*
	Tuberculosis
	Bronchiectasis* (cystic fibrosis, ciliary dyskinesia)
	Necrotizing pneumonia
	Fungus (especially allergic bronchopulmonary aspergillosis or mucormycosis)
	Parasite
	Herpes simplex
Foreign body	Retained
Congenital defect	Heart (various)
	Primary pulmonary hypertension
	Eisenmenger syndrome
	Arteriovenous malformation
	Telangiectasia (Osler-Weber-Rendu)
	Pulmonary sequestration
	Bronchogenic cyst
Autoimmune-inflammatory	Henoch-Schönlein purpura
	Goodpasture syndrome
	Systemic lupus erythematosus
	Sarcoidosis
	Granulomatosis with polyangiitis
Pulmonary hemosiderosis	Idiopathic or with milk allergy (Heiner syndrome)
Trauma	Contusion*
	Fractured trachea, bronchus
Iatrogenic	After surgery
	After transbronchial lung biopsy*
	After diagnostic lung biopsy*
Tumors	Benign (neurogenic, hamartoma, hemangioma, carcinoid)
	Malignant (adenoma, bronchogenic carcinoma)
	Metastatic (Wilms tumor, osteosarcoma, sarcoma)
Pulmonary embolus	Cardiogenic
	Deep vein thrombosis
Other	Factitious
	Endometriosis
	Coagulopathy*
	Congestive heart failure
	After surfactant therapy in neonates
	Kernicterus
	Hyperammonemia
	Intracranial hemorrhage
	Epistaxis*
	Idiopathic

*A common cause of hemoptysis.

TABLE 3.29   Hemoptysis: Differentiating Sites of Origin of Blood

	Pulmonary	Gastrointestinal Tract	Nose
History	Cough, with or without gurgling in lung before episode	Nausea, vomiting, abdominal pain	With or without nosebleed dripping in back of throat
Physical	Cough; localized crackles or decreased breath sounds; digital clubbing	↑ Liver, spleen, epigastric tenderness	Blood in nose

TABLE 3.30   Red Flags for Cough

If associated with severe, acute:
   Hemoptysis
   Dyspnea
   Hypoxemia
   Choking, gagging
If associated with chronic:
   Failure to thrive
   Steatorrhea
   Decreased exercise tolerance
   Digital clubbing
   Cough starting in infancy
   Dyspnea
   Neurodevelopmental delay
Persistence of:
   Cough for 4 wk or more
   Radiographic abnormality, especially if asymmetric
Failure to respond to empirical therapy:
   Antibiotics for presumed infection
   Bronchodilators for presumed bronchospasm

with occlusive substances (embolization). In extremely rare instances, emergency lobectomy may be indicated.

WHEN COUGH ITSELF IS A PROBLEM

Cough itself seldom necessitates specific treatment. Nonetheless, cough is not always completely benign (see Table 3.9). Most complications are uncommon, and most accompany only very severe cough, but some are serious enough to justify treatment of the cough itself.

Cough suppressants include codeine, hydrocodone (two narcotics), or dextromethorphan (a non-narcotic D-isomer of the codeine analog of levorphanol). Such agents should be used only for severe cough that may produce significant complications (see Table 3.9). For most diseases, suppressing the cough offers no advantage. Disadvantages include narcotic addiction and loss of the protective cough reflex with subsequent mucous retention and possible superinfection. Demulcent preparations (sugar-containing, bland soothing agents or honey) temporarily suppress the cough response from pharyngeal sources, and decongestant-antihistamine combinations may reduce postnasal drip. Cough medications should not be used in children under 4 years of age.

suction large amounts of blood while ventilating and keeping unaffected portions of the lung clear of blood. Interventional radiologists treat as well as localize a bleeding site by injecting the offending vessel

■ SUMMARY AND RED FLAGS

Cough is important because it is a symptom and sign of underlying disease that frequently merits treatment. In the acute setting, severe disease, including massive hemoptysis or profound dyspnea or hypoxemia, warrants immediate attention, rapid diagnosis, and rapid management. Certain chronic conditions, including those that suggest CF and those in which symptoms have persisted and interfere with a child's daily activities and quality of life, warrant further evaluation and treatment. Finally, a child whose cough fails to respond to what should have been reasonable treatment should be referred to a pulmonary specialist (Table 3.30).

BIBLIOGRAPHY

A bibliography is available at ExpertConsult.com.

4

Respiratory Distress

Alyssa Stephany

The main function of the respiratory system is to supply oxygen to meet the body's demands and remove excess carbon dioxide. Many processes are involved in ensuring that this occurs, including ventilation (gas delivery to and from the lungs), perfusion (blood supply to the lungs), and diffusion (the exchange of gases along the alveoli). Respiratory distress arises when there is impaired air exchange that leads to decreased ventilation and oxygenation, and can be caused by problems in any of these pathways. It is essential to identify and treat the location and cause of respiratory distress to prevent respiratory failure, which ensues if the respiratory effort is inadequate to provide appropriate tissue oxygenation and maintenance of blood pH.

Respiratory distress occurs for a variety of reasons and with many levels of severity. There are also age-related etiologies (Table 4.1). It can be caused by intrapulmonary pathology (airway, alveolar, interstitium, vascular) or a change in respiratory drive, impaired neuromuscular reserve, or increased ventilatory demand (Table 4.2).

DIAGNOSTIC APPROACH

Signs and symptoms of respiratory distress vary, depending on the severity and cause. The initial approach to a patient includes determining the severity of illness and then determining if immediate treatment is needed by first ensuring that airway, breathing, and circulation are intact. After these steps are completed, further work-up into the cause of respiratory distress may be done. A careful history and physical examination are often sufficient to elucidate the cause of respiratory distress. Not all causes of respiratory distress arise within the respiratory tract. Heart failure, neuromuscular disorders, toxic ingestion, and central nervous system disorders may all manifest with respiratory signs and symptoms. In severe respiratory distress or suspicion of airway obstruction, a feeding trial should not be done as this may increase the risk of aspiration or further respiratory compromise.

HISTORY

An appropriate medical history is important in the child with respiratory distress. The chief complaint provides insight into the nature of the distress (i.e., cough, wheezing, stridor, cyanosis, dyspnea, and/or chest pain). The onset, duration, and chronicity of symptoms should also be obtained. It is important to obtain data regarding any prodrome, exacerbating or ameliorating factors, history of trauma, previous occurrence of similar symptoms, and response to any therapy. Questions should also be directed toward any change in voice or cry, change with positioning, feeding problems, or any choking episodes. The possibility of a foreign body should be raised, although this is often not observed. Past medical history of neonatal events (prematurity), previous endotracheal intubation, recurrent infections, hospitalizations, noisy breathing, and prior gagging or choking episodes may also

provide valuable information. A family history of asthma and allergies, travel, and environmental exposure (i.e., smoking, pets, or irritants) may also uncover etiologic clues. A review of systems with regard to systemic signs and symptoms associated with respiratory disease, such as fever, weight loss, night sweats, or dysphagia, is useful (Table 4.3). Determining whether the respiratory difficulties are acute or chronic or an acute worsening of an underlying chronic respiratory condition is important to address the child's condition.

PHYSICAL EXAMINATION

Pulmonary Physical Examination

The physical examination begins with measurement of vital signs, with attention paid to respiratory rate, pulse oximetry, heart rate, and blood pressure. Tachypnea is often the most prominent manifestation of respiratory distress. A respiratory rate of more than 50 breaths/min in infants 2–12 months of age, 40 breaths/min in children 1–5 years, and 30 breaths/min in children older than 5 years is abnormal. The physical examination should be performed in a warm, well-lit room, preferably with the child in the parent's lap and the child's chest exposed. It is essential to observe the child's general appearance, sense of well-being, degree of dyspnea or cyanosis, and respiratory pattern, including nasal flaring, retractions, and accessory muscle use. **Central cyanosis** (lips, tongue, sublingual tissue as well as hands and feet) is related to both the degree of oxygen desaturation and the hemoglobin level (Table 4.4). Cyanosis is detected when the average amount of deoxygenated hemoglobin is 5 g/dL. Any posture assumed in an effort to minimize the airway difficulties should be determined. The degree and location of retractions should be noted. Retractions may be intercostal, subcostal, or suprasternal, and often signify worsening respiratory distress, particularly in the older child. Infants have a particularly compliant chest wall and are therefore more predisposed to intercostal and sternal retractions; in older children, these features may be less prominent. Nasal flaring and accessory muscle use signify significant respiratory distress; and, as fatigue sets in, head bobbing and/or grunting can be noted, which requires prompt management as this may be a sign of impending respiratory failure. Altered mental status (either agitation or somnolence) may be indicative of severe respiratory distress, hypoxemia, hypercapnia, and impending respiratory failure. Palpation of the chest wall and cervical region may enable the examiner to detect the presence of subcutaneous emphysema indicative of pulmonary air leak. On percussion of the chest and back, a hyperresonant note during percussion of the chest wall indicates hyperinflation, whereas dullness to percussion suggests atelectasis, pulmonary consolidation, or pleural effusion.

Auscultation of the chest should focus on identifying the degree of air exchange and the presence, timing, and symmetry of adventitious breath sounds. Air entry should be evaluated over all discrete

TABLE 4.1   Age-Related Causes of Respiratory Distress

Cause	Full-Term Neonate	Infant-Toddler	Child	Adolescent
COMMON	Meconium aspiration pneumonia	Bronchiolitis	Pneumonia[ǁ]	Pneumonia[#]
	Congenital heart disease	Viral pneumonia[†]	Asthma	Asthma
	Transient tachypnea	Bacterial pneumonia[‡]	Cystic fibrosis	Sickle cell acute chest crisis
	Persistent fetal circulation	Croup (infectious, spasmodic)	Sickle cell acute chest crisis	Tonsillitis
	Congenital pneumonia	Aspiration[§]	Aspiration[§]	Peritonsillar abscess
		Cystic fibrosis	Tonsillitis	Cystic fibrosis
		Laryngomalacia		Panic attack
		Asthma		E-cigarette or vaping associated lung injury (EVALI)
UNCOMMON	Pneumothorax	Congenital anomalies	ARDS	ARDS
	Congenital anomalies*	Epiglottitis	Anaphylaxis	Spontaneous pneumothorax
	Pneumopericardium	Near drowning	Interstitial lung disease[¶]	Pulmonary embolism
	Polycythemia	Pulmonary hemosiderosis	Hemoptysis	Drug induced**
	Vocal cord paralysis	Pulmonary hemorrhage	Retropharyngeal abscess	Interstitial lung disease[¶]
	Pleural effusions	Retropharyngeal abscess	Near drowning	Collagen vascular disease[††]
	Severe anemia	Trauma	Hydrocarbon aspiration	Hypersensitivity pneumonitis[‡‡]
	Pulmonary hypoplasia	Hydrocarbon aspiration	Trauma	Allergic bronchopulmonary aspergillosis
	Surfactant protein deficiency	Smoke inhalation (burn)	Pulmonary fibrosis	Alveolar proteinosis
	Pulmonary lymphangiectasia	Airway hemangioma	Desquamating interstitial pneumonia	Trauma
		Papilloma of vocal cords	Pulmonary alveolar proteinosis	Anaphylaxis
		Bacterial tracheitis	Smoke inhalation (burn)	Smoke inhalation (burn)
		Heart failure	HIV associated[ǁǁ]	Scoliosis
		HIV associated[ǁǁ]	Primary ciliary dyskinesia	Bronchiectasis
		Primary ciliary dyskinesia		Mediastinal mass[§§]
				Hemoptysis
				HIV associated[ǁǁ]

*Congenital anomalies = tracheoesophageal fistula; choanal atresia; tracheal web-stenosis-atresia-cleft; diaphragmatic hernia; eventration of the diaphragm; congenital pulmonary airway malformation (previously called cystic adenomatoid malformation); lobar emphysema; cleft palate–macroglossia (Pierre Robin syndrome); thyroid goiter; pulmonary hypoplasia, including Potter syndrome (renal agenesis, oligohydramnios, pulmonary hypoplasia); lung cysts; chylothorax; pulmonary lymphangiectasia; asphyxiating thoracic dystrophy; vascular rings and slings; arteriovenous malformation; subglottic stenosis.

[†]Viral pneumonia: see Table 4.12 for common causes.

[‡]Pneumonia (infant–toddler): see Table 4.12 for common causes.

[§]Aspiration = gastric fluid or formula aspiration in gastroesophageal reflux, foreign body aspiration.

[ǁ]Pneumonia (child): see Table 4.12 for common causes.

[¶]Interstitial lung disease = idiopathic, rheumatoid, infection (*Pneumocystis carinii*), Langerhans cell histiocytosis, hypereosinophilia syndromes, Goodpasture syndrome, LIP, alveolar proteinosis, familial fibrosis, chronic active hepatitis, inflammatory bowel disease, vasculitis (granulomatosis with polyangiitis with or without eosinophilia, hypersensitivity), graft-versus-host disease, pulmonary venoocclusive disease, sarcoidosis, leukemia, lymphoma, neurofibromatosis, tuberous sclerosis, Gaucher disease, Niemann-Pick disease, Weber-Christian disease, organic dusts (e.g., farmer's lung, humidifier/air-conditioner lung, bird feeder, pancreatic extract, rodent handler, cheese worker), inorganic dusts (pneumoconiosis), irradiation.

[#]Pneumonia (adolescent): see Table 4.12 for common causes.

**Drugs = azathioprine, bleomycin, cyclophosphamide, methotrexate, nitrosoureas, busulfan, nitrofurantoin, penicillin, sulfonamides, erythromycin, isoniazid, hydralazine, phenytoin, carbamazepine, imipramine, naproxen, penicillamine, cromolyn sodium, mineral oil, paraquat, inhaled drugs (cocaine, hydrocarbons), talc, shoe spray.

[††]Collagen vascular disease = rheumatoid arthritis, progressive systemic sclerosis, systemic lupus erythematosus, dermatomyositis, mixed connective tissue disease.

[‡‡]Hypersensitivity pneumonia (also called extrinsic allergic alveolitis): see[¶] above for some specific organic dusts (antigens).

[§§]Mediastinal masses = anterior (teratoma, T-cell lymphoma, thymus, thyroid), middle (lymph nodes–infection–tumor–sarcoidosis, cysts), posterior (neuroenteric cysts–duplication, meningocele, neural tumors–neuroblastoma, ganglioneuroblastoma, neurofibroma, pheochromocytoma), and parenchymal tumors (hamartoma, arteriovenous malformation, carcinoid, adenoma; metastatic–osteogenic sarcoma, Wilms tumor).

[ǁǁ]HIV associated = P. jiroveci, LIP, CMV, *Mycobacterium tuberculosis*, atypical mycobacteria, measles, common bacterial pathogens.

ARDS, acute respiratory distress syndrome; BPD, bronchopulmonary dysplasia; CMV, cytomegalovirus; LIP, lymphocytic interstitial pneumonia; RDS, respiratory distress syndrome; RSV, respiratory syncytial virus.

TABLE 4.2	**Causes of Respiratory Distress**
Extrathoracic	**Intrathoracic**
Nervous System–Metabolic	**Pulmonary**
Intracranial hemorrhage	Airway obstruction
Acidosis	Parenchymal lesions: pneumonia,
Ingestion (aspirin)	hemorrhage, malformation
Ketoacidosis (diabetes)	Air leaks: pneumomediastinum,
Meningitis	pneumothorax
Shock/sepsis	Pleural effusion, empyema
Neuromuscular disease	Acute respiratory distress syndrome
Diaphragmatic paralysis, paresis	Chest wall trauma
Psychologic (anxiety)	Pulmonary embolus
Vocal cord dysfunction	Foreign body (airway or esophagus)
Panic attack	Tumor (cyst, adenoma)
Lesions of Upper Airway	Cystic fibrosis
Malacia	Primary ciliary dyskinesia
Web	**Cardiac**
Cyst	Myocarditis
Hemangioma	Cardiomyopathy
Stenosis (glottic or choanal)	Shunt (left to right)
Papillomatosis	Congestive heart failure
Miscellaneous	Pulmonary edema
Abdominal masses, distention	Pericardial effusion
Ascites	
Anemia	

anatomic locations bilaterally. Homologous segments of each lung should be examined sequentially to compare similar areas. The presence of adventitious sounds should be determined next. The most encountered sounds are wheezing, stridor, crackles, and rhonchi (Table 4.5).

Crackles (previously called "rales") are intermittent, nonmusical low- or higher-pitched, largely inspiratory noises that are produced by the opening (reinflation) of groups of alveoli closed during the previous expiration.

Wheezing is a continuous, high-pitched musical noise, similar to a hiss or whistle.

Rhonchi are continuous sounds that are lower pitched and more rumbling or sonorous, heard more during expiration, and primarily heard over the trachea and bronchi; however, if loud enough they can be heard throughout all lung fields.

Stridor is a high-pitched musical noise generated by turbulent flow of air through the large upper airways.

Other adventitious breath sounds that are described include **pleural rub,** which has a grating quality heard best during inspiration, and **stertor,** a low-pitched, nonmusical noise generated by the vibration of the pharyngeal tissues (nasopharynx, oropharynx, soft palate) due to significant upper respiratory obstruction and subsequent turbulent airflow downstream in the upper airway heard only during inspiration. Determination of the timing (inspiration, expiration, or biphasic) and distribution of the adventitious sounds offers clues as to the site of airway and lung involvement. Wheezing that is continuous and heard equally over both lung fields is associated with diffuse airway narrowing and limitation of airflow, whereas unilateral or very localized wheezing or decreased breath sounds suggest segmental airway obstruction, such as that found with retained foreign body aspiration, mucus plugging, or

atelectasis. Additionally, inspiratory stridor is characteristic of partial airway obstruction at or above the vocal cords, whereas biphasic or expiratory stridor is characteristic of airway obstruction in the subglottic space or trachea (Fig. 4.1).

Other Parts of the Physical Examination

Other elements of the physical examination may have direct bearing on the respiratory system. **Pulsus paradoxus**, the difference between the systolic blood pressure obtained during inspiration and during exhalation, is exaggerated by airway obstruction and pulmonary hyperinflation. As pulmonary overinflation gets worse, pulsus paradoxus values increase and correlate well with the degree of airway obstruction. It is difficult to measure pulsus paradoxus in young children with rapid heart rates. A method that allows a reasonable approximation of the pulsus paradoxus can be obtained by using a sphygmomanometer and noting the difference between the pressure at which the first sporadic faint pulse sounds and the pressure at which all sounds are heard. Values >10 mm Hg are abnormal, and values >20 mm Hg are consistent with severe airway obstruction. Although **digital clubbing** is very rarely seen as a normal and familial variant, its presence in a child with respiratory distress suggests an acute illness superimposed on an underlying chronic respiratory condition. The most common pulmonary causes of digital clubbing in pediatric patients are cystic fibrosis, bronchiectasis, and other destructive pulmonary diseases. Digital clubbing is rarely seen in children with asthma. Other physical findings to observe include mouth breathing and morphologic features suggestive of craniofacial anomalies, such as maxillary hypoplasia, nasal septal deflection, micrognathia, retrognathia, absent nasal airflow (choanal obstructions), platybasia, or macroglossia.

LABORATORY TESTS

The arterial blood gas analysis, obtained while the patient is breathing a known fraction of inspired oxygen (FIO_2), is the "gold standard" for assessing oxygenation, ventilation, and acid-base status. In lieu of an arterial blood gas determination, capillary or venous blood gases may be utilized, but these are less helpful for evaluating oxygenation. Non-invasive measurement of oxygenation by pulse oximetry can provide valuable information. Oximetry measures the degree of hemoglobin saturation with oxygen and should not be confused with partial pressure of oxygen in the blood, as measured by blood gas analysis or estimated by transcutaneous measures. At or near sea level, hemoglobin oxygen saturation lower than 93% indicates that significant hypoxemia may be present, and saturations of 90% or lower are clearly abnormal. A blood gas analysis may be necessary to confirm the presence and degree of hypoxemia, as well as information on acid-base status (pH) and ventilation ($PaCO_2$). Hemoglobin oxygen saturation, measured by pulse oximetry, cannot detect significant hypoxia, but it is relatively accurate at oxygen saturations of 70% or more. Various conditions, such as poor circulation, presence of carboxyhemoglobin or methemoglobin, nail polish, and improper sensor alignment and motion, can result in inaccurate oximetry measures.

IMAGING

Radiography

A plain x-ray of the chest, taken in the posterior-anterior and lateral projections, should be obtained in any patient with respiratory distress in which an etiology has not been determined from the history and physical examination. Important information regarding the presence of parenchymal

TABLE 4.3   Focused History for a Patient with Respiratory Distress

Component	Comments and Examples
Onset, duration, and chronicity	Abrupt onset: suggests upper airway conditions such as foreign body, allergy, anaphylaxis, irritant exposure, or pulmonary embolism Gradual onset: more consistent with process such as infection or heart failure
Alleviating and provoking factors	A child with respiratory distress caused by upper airway obstruction may have some degree of relief by assuming the "sniffing position" to maximize airway patency
Treatment attempted	A child with wheezing secondary to asthma may respond readily to inhaled bronchodilators, but a child with wheezing caused by foreign body aspiration may continue to show symptoms after treatment
Respiratory symptoms	Cold symptoms: may indicate viral upper respiratory infection Cough: "seal-like" or "barky" cough is commonly heard in patients with croup Eliciting descriptions of the difficulty breathing may provide clues to the underlying cause (e.g., supraclavicular or suprasternal retractions point to upper airway obstruction) Color change: Pallor may indicate anemia; cyanosis is indicative of decreased oxygen content in the blood, as seen in some forms of congenital heart disease and in methemoglobinemia Respiratory effort: Poor effort may be seen in patients with underlying muscular dystrophies Change in voice: Whereas muffled or hoarse voice points to upper airway pathology, lower airway disease does not typically change the character of the voice
Systemic or associated symptoms	Fever: Presence suggests an infectious cause Hydration status, including intake and output (urine, emesis, diarrhea, excessive perspiration, or high respiratory rate) Weight loss or failure to gain weight: may indicate systemic process (e.g., inborn error of metabolism) or the severity of respiratory distress is impairing growth (as seen in congestive heart failure) Abdominal pain: may suggest abdominal pathology such as obstruction or appendicitis or may represent referred pain from diaphragmatic irritation (as in basilar pneumonia) Other organ involvement: AKI, myocarditis, rash, cytopenias, thrombosis, shock, emesis, diarrhea, jaundice
Past medical history	Underlying disorders may predispose patients to certain conditions: For example, a patient with sickle cell disease and respiratory distress may be exhibiting signs of acute chest syndrome; a patient with known gastroesophageal reflux and coarse lung findings on examination could have an aspiration pneumonia. History of vaping or smoking
Exposures or environmental factors	For example, a patient involved in a fire may be affected by not only thermal injury to the airways but also systemic toxins such as carbon monoxide and cyanide A patient with allergy and a potential exposure to the allergen could be showing signs of anaphylaxis Exposure to sick contacts
Trauma	History of trauma suggests diagnoses such as pneumothorax, flail chest, cardiac tamponade, or abdominal injury
Immunization status	Children with incomplete or lack of immunization against *Haemophilus influenzae* type B are at increased risk for epiglottitis
Last oral intake	If advanced airway management becomes necessary (e.g., positive-pressure ventilation), the presence of stomach contents may increase the risk of pulmonary aspiration

AKI, acute kidney injury.
From Viteri SD, Sampayo EM. Respiratory distress. In: Florin TA, Ludwig S, eds. *Netter's Pediatrics*. Philadelphia: Elsevier; 2011:17–23.

TABLE 4.4   Cyanosis and Hemoglobin Concentration

| Hemoglobin Concentration (g/dL) | CYANOSIS APPEARS AT* | |
	Oxygen Saturation (%) Below:	Arterial P_{O_2} (mm Hg) Below:
6	60	31
8	70	36
10	76	40
12	80	45
14	83	47
16	85	50
18	87	54
20	88	56

*These figures assume that central cyanosis begins to appear when 2.38 g/dL of deoxygenated hemoglobin accumulates in arterial blood. The corresponding P_{O_2} was obtained from standard hemoglobin dissociation curves for oxygen.
From McGee S. Cyanosis. In: *Evidence-Based Physical Diagnosis*. 3rd ed. Philadelphia: Elsevier; 2012:71.

TABLE 4.5   Classification of Common Lung Sounds

	Acoustic Characteristics	American Thoracic Society Nomenclature	Common Synonyms
Normal	200–600 Hz Decreasing power with increasing Hz	Normal	Vesicular
	75–1,600 Hz Flat until sharp decrease in power (900 Hz)	Bronchial	Bronchial Tracheal
Adventitious		Adventitious	Abnormal
	Discontinuous, interrupted explosive sounds (loud, low in pitch), early inspiratory or expiratory	Coarse crackles	Coarse crackles
	Discontinuous, interrupted explosive sounds (less loud than above and of shorter duration; higher in pitch than coarse crackles or crackles), mid- to late inspiratory	Fine crackles	Fine crackles, crepitation
	Continuous sounds (>250 msec, high pitched; dominant frequency of 400 Hz or more, a hissing sound)	Wheezes	Sibilant rhonchus, high-pitched wheeze
	Continuous sounds (>250 msec, low pitched; dominant frequency <200 Hz, a snoring sound)	Rhonchi	Sonorous rhonchus, low-pitched wheeze

From Davis JL, Murray JF. History and physical examination. In: Broaddus VC, Mason RJ, Ernst JD, et al., eds. *Murray and Nadel's Textbook of Respiratory Medicine.* 6th ed. Philadelphia: Saunders-Elsevier; 2016:263–277.e2.

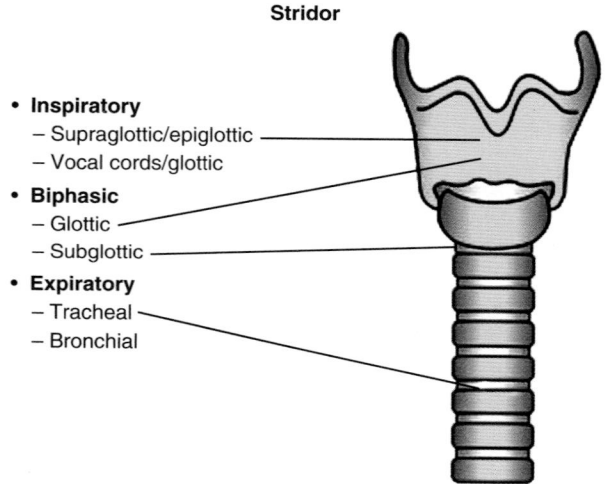

Stridor

- **Inspiratory**
  - Supraglottic/epiglottic
  - Vocal cords/glottic
- **Biphasic**
  - Glottic
  - Subglottic
- **Expiratory**
  - Tracheal
  - Bronchial

Fig. 4.1 Stridor. Inspiratory stridor is characteristic of partial airway obstruction at or above the vocal cords (supraglottic/epiglottic and glottis areas). Biphasic stridor is characteristic at the glottis or subglottic areas, and is typically caused by a fixed obstruction. Expiratory stridor is characteristic of a high tracheal lesion as there is a decrease in airway diameter with expiration. (From Ida JB, Thompson DM. Pediatric stridor. *Otolaryngol Clin North Am.* 2014;47:795–819.)

infiltrates, pleural effusions, airway obstruction, cardiac size, pulmonary vascular markings, extrapulmonary air leaks, and the presence of radiopaque foreign bodies may be obtained from this test. Radiopaque foreign bodies are generally seen easily on a radiograph. If there is a possibility of a radiolucent foreign body, inspiratory and expiratory chest radiographic studies must be performed. Demonstration of unilateral hyperinflation or a mediastinal shift during expiration suggests localized bronchial obstruction, such as a retained foreign body. Lateral decubitus positioning of the patient during the radiographic procedure can reveal a pleural effusion in the lower dependent lung. Ultrasonography of the chest is also useful in detecting pleural fluid and loculations within pleural effusions.

In patients with stridor, anteroposterior and lateral soft tissue radiographic studies of the neck and chest are frequently needed. These should be obtained during inspiration, because the soft tissues of the pharynx may bulge with expiration, causing a false-positive finding of a soft tissue mass that may mimic a retropharyngeal infection.

Computed Tomography

CT of the upper airway and chest can help detect the relationship of the vasculature to the airways (trachea and large central airways); pulmonary parenchymal lesions (infiltrates, abscesses, cysts) or lesions (abscesses, inflammation) in the airway; and central airway caliber. Rapid, fine-cut CT is a technique of high resolution and short duration, which increases its acceptability for pediatric patients. It is the method of choice for noninvasive detection and evaluation of bronchiectasis and interstitial lung disease. In some patients with a normal chest x-ray, the CT will be abnormal. Helical CT is a valuable method of detecting pulmonary embolism. A **PET scan** may be used in combination with a CT scan to evaluate for malignancy or other etiologies.

Magnetic Resonance Imaging

MRI of the pulmonary system may also be useful in elucidating the relationship of the great vessels to the airways and may be superior to CT for this purpose. MRI is less useful for imaging the lung parenchyma. The need for long imaging times often means sedation for young children, and this limits the utility of MRI of the chest for some pediatric patients. Sedatives must be used very carefully, particularly in patients with respiratory distress, and only in monitored situations with the availability of experienced personnel and equipment to provide possible resuscitation.

Fluoroscopy

Fluoroscopic examination of the chest may be useful in determining the cause of respiratory distress. Real-time visualization of the diaphragm can determine whether paralysis or paresis of this major muscle of respiration is contributing to respiratory distress. Asymmetric chest wall motion or unilateral hyperinflation during the respiratory cycle suggests bronchial obstruction, such as that seen with a retained foreign body in the airways. An upper gastrointestinal series is useful to assess for abnormalities of swallowing causing aspiration, presence of tracheoesophageal fistula, or presence of a vascular ring.

TABLE 4.6 Causes of Wheezing in Childhood

ACUTE	CHRONIC OR RECURRENT
Reactive Airways Disease Asthma* Exercise-induced asthma* Hypersensitivity reactions Anaphylaxis	***Reactive Airways Disease (Same as in Acute)*** ***Hypersensitivity Reactions, Allergic Bronchopulmonary*** ***Aspergillosis*** ***Dynamic Airways Collapse*** Bronchomalacia Tracheomalacia* Vocal cord adduction*
Bronchial Edema Infection* (bronchiolitis, ILD, pneumonia) Inhalation of irritant gases or particulates Increased pulmonary venous pressure	***Airway Compression by Mass or Blood Vessel*** Vascular ring/sling Anomalous innominate artery Pulmonary artery dilation (absent pulmonary valve) Bronchial or pulmonary cysts Lymph nodes or tumors
Bronchial Hypersecretion Infection Inhalation of irritant gases or particulates Cholinergic drugs	***Aspiration*** Foreign body Gastroesophageal reflux* Tracheoesophageal fistula (repaired or unrepaired)
Aspiration Foreign body* Aspiration of gastric contents (reflux, H-type TEF)	***Bronchial Hypersecretion or Failure to Clear Secretions*** Bronchitis, bronchiectasis Cystic fibrosis* Primary ciliary dyskinesia Immunodeficiency disorder Vasculitis Lymphangiectasia α_1-Antitrypsin deficiency
E-cigarette- or Vaping-Associated Lung Injury	***Intrinsic Airway Lesions*** Endobronchial tumors Endobronchial granulation tissue Plastic bronchitis syndrome Bronchial or tracheal stenosis Bronchiolitis obliterans Sequelae of bronchopulmonary dysplasia Sarcoidosis
	Congestive Heart Failure/Pulmonary Edema

*Common.

ILD, interstitial lung disease; TEF, tracheoesophageal fistula.

Modified from Kercsmar CM. The respiratory system. In: Behrman RE, Kliegman RM, eds. *Nelson Essentials of Pediatrics.* 2nd ed. Philadelphia: WB Saunders; 1994:445.

Endoscopy

Endoscopy can provide direct visualization of the cause of the airway obstruction and lung lesions; its use involves manipulation of the airway, which should not be undertaken unless the personnel and equipment are present to manage possible worsening airway compromise. Flexible, direct laryngoscopy is widely used to visualize the upper airway without the need for sedation. Rigid bronchoscopy provides visualization of both the upper and lower airways; cardiopulmonary monitoring and intravenous access for sedative administration are required. In cases of significant upper airway obstruction necessitating intervention, or if there is any likelihood of a foreign body, direct laryngoscopy and rigid bronchoscopy in the operating room are the safest procedures that can secure the airway, provide a diagnosis, and accomplish treatment.

CAUSES OF RESPIRATORY DISTRESS

Wheezing

Wheezing is best characterized as a continuous musical sound most often heard on expiration, but it may occur in both phases of respiration. The most common causes of acute wheezing in children are bronchiolitis and asthma. However, it is critical to rule out other causes of wheezing that necessitate different therapy (Table 4.6). Anatomic abnormalities of the airway, such as vascular ring, tracheobronchomalacia, primary ciliary dyskinesia, and foreign body aspiration, may cause airway obstruction and wheezing, especially in infants and young children. Viral infections, notably those of respiratory syncytial virus (RSV), human metapneumovirus, adenovirus, parainfluenza, and influenza, are also common causes of wheezing (bronchiolitis) in

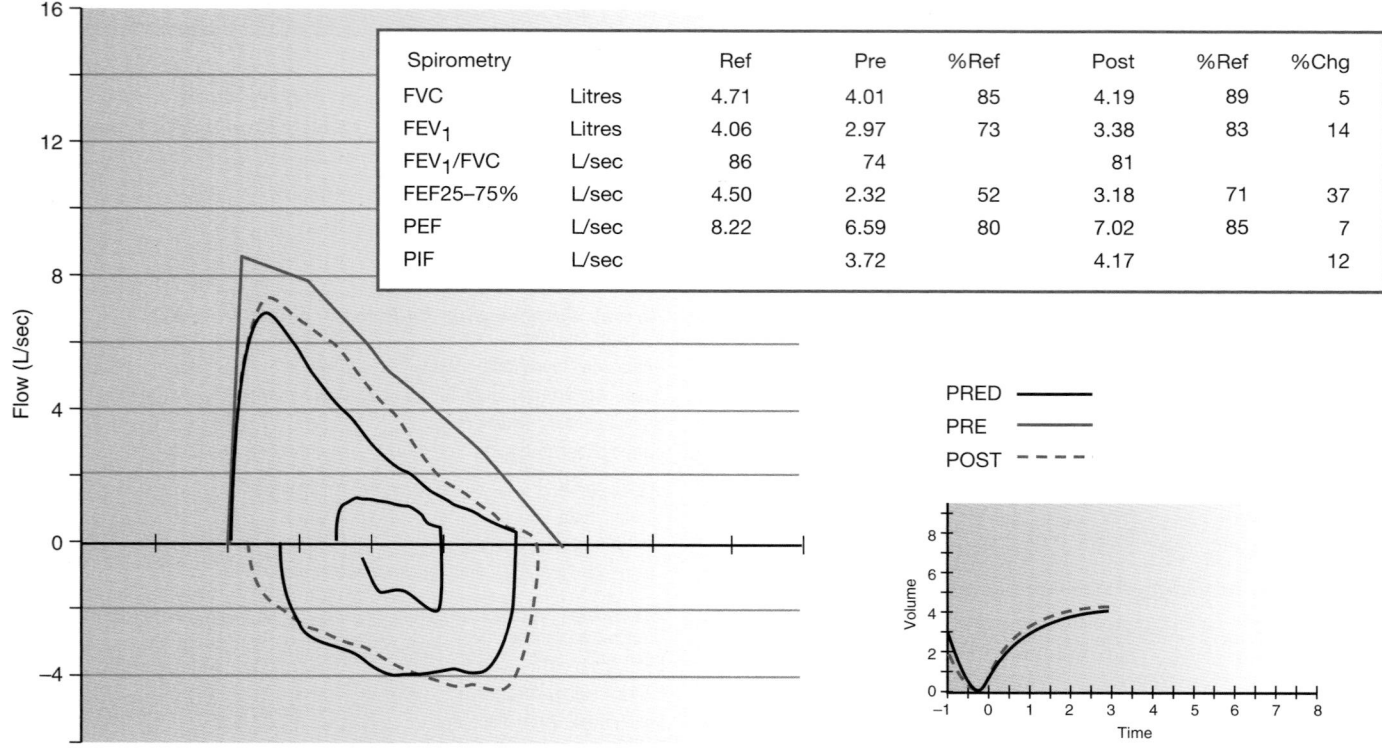

Spirometry		Ref	Pre	%Ref	Post	%Ref	%Chg
FVC	Litres	4.71	4.01	85	4.19	89	5
FEV$_1$	Litres	4.06	2.97	73	3.38	83	14
FEV$_1$/FVC	L/sec	86	74		81		
FEF25–75%	L/sec	4.50	2.32	52	3.18	71	37
PEF	L/sec	8.22	6.59	80	7.02	85	7
PIF	L/sec		3.72		4.17		12

Fig. 4.2 Spirometry demonstrating a scooped flow volume loop seen in obstructive disease in asthma. Following bronchodilator use (PRED, predicted), there is a positive bronchodilator response of >12% in forced expiratory volume in 1 second (FEV$_1$). FEF, forced expiratory flow rate; FVC, forced vital capacity; PEF, peak expiratory flow rate; PIF, peak inspiratory flow rate. (From South M, Isaacs D. *Practical Paediatrics*. 7th ed. Oxford: Churchill Livingstone; 2013.)

infants and young children. Infection with *Mycoplasma* species may produce airway hyperactivity in older children. Other entities to consider are cystic fibrosis, interstitial lung disease, or vocal cord dysfunction. In comparison with asthma, one key distinguishing feature of these diagnoses is that the wheezing does not respond to treatment with bronchodilators.

Asthma

Asthma is defined as airway obstruction that is reversible either spontaneously or with the use of medication. Chronic airway inflammation and bronchial hyperresponsiveness are the likely causes of the airway obstruction. The airways of patients with even mild asthma demonstrate inflammation, manifested as mucosal edema, hypersecretion of mucus, smooth muscle constriction, and inflammatory cell infiltrate. Even when asthma symptoms are not present, airway inflammation may be demonstrated. Furthermore, bronchial hyperresponsiveness, the tendency of airway smooth muscle to constrict in response to a variety of environmental stimuli, is present in virtually all children with asthma and may be exacerbated by airway inflammation. Airway remodeling, the deposition of collagen in the subepithelial basement membrane area, occurs in some but not all asthmatic patients. Fixed airway obstruction is a long-term complication that may occur as a result of airway remodeling.

The diagnosis of asthma is made by a combination of history, physical examination, and spirometry testing. For the child with acute wheezing and respiratory distress, a therapeutic trial of an inhaled β-agonist is the best "diagnostic test" for reversible airway obstruction. Once the acute symptoms have improved, other diagnostic studies can be undertaken. Spirometry, particularly measurement of the forced

expiratory volume in 1 second (FEV$_1$) and mid-maximal forced expiratory flow rates (FEF$_{25-75\%}$), provides a good indication of airflow obstruction in the larger and smaller airways, respectively. If airway obstruction is detected in the resting state, a bronchodilator (typically albuterol) is administered, and spirometry is repeated. An improvement of ≥12% and ≥200 mL in FEV$_1$ above baseline is considered significant and indicative of reversible airway obstruction (Fig. 4.2). If the baseline spirometry is normal, an inhalation challenge test, with either increasing doses of methacholine or hyperventilation of cold, dry air, can provoke a statistically (but usually not clinically) significant decrease in FEV$_1$; a fall in FEV$_1$ of 10% or greater is considered diagnostic of airway hyperresponsiveness and asthma. In children too young to perform spirometry (typically under the age of 5 years), the repeated nature of wheezing episodes and the improvement in symptoms after treatment with antiinflammatory agents and bronchodilators, peripheral blood eosinophilia (>4%), a family history of atopy, and/or a personal history of atopy (eczema, food allergy, or allergic rhinitis) are strongly suggestive of the diagnosis of asthma. Other studies include measurement of total serum immunoglobulin E (IgE) levels. This immunoglobulin is often elevated in individuals with asthma and/or allergy, as well as in those predisposed to asthma.

Patients with acute asthma typically present with shortness of breath, wheezing, cough, and increased work of breathing. Persistent cough may be the most prominent or even sole feature of acute asthma (see Chapter 3). Many asthma episodes are misdiagnosed as bronchitis (which is rare in children). Chest wall retractions and the use of accessory muscles indicate significant airway obstruction. Acute asthma exacerbations that are unresponsive to aggressive bronchodilator administration are termed **status asthmaticus**. The severity of asthma

TABLE 4.7 Severity of Asthma Exacerbations

	Mild	Moderate	Severe	Respiratory Arrest Imminent
Symptoms				
Breathlessness	While walking	While at rest (infant—softer, shorter cry; difficulty feeding)	While at rest (infant—stops feeding)	
	Can lie down	Prefers sitting	Sits upright	
Talks in	Sentences	Phrases	Words	
Alertness	May be agitated	Usually agitated	Usually agitated	Drowsy or confused
Signs				
Respiratory rate	Increased	Increased	Often >30/min	
		Guide to rates of breathing in awake children:		
		Age / Normal rate <2 mo / <60/min 2–12 mo / <50/min 1–5 yr / <40/min 6–8 yr / <30/min		
Use of accessory muscles; suprasternal retractions	Usually not	Commonly	Usually	Paradoxical thoracoabdominal movement
Wheeze	Moderate, often only end expiratory	Loud; throughout exhalation	Usually loud; throughout inhalation and exhalation	Absence of wheeze
Pulse/minute	<100	100–120	>120	Bradycardia
		Guide to normal pulse rates in children:		
		Age / Normal rate 2–12 mo / <160/min 1–2 yr / <120/min 2–8 yr / <110/min		
Pulsus paradoxus	Absent <10 mm Hg	May be present 10–25 mm Hg	Often present >25 mm Hg (adult) 20–40 mm Hg (child)	Absence suggests respiratory muscle fatigue
Functional Assessment				
PEF percent predicted or percent personal best	≥70%	~40–69% or response lasts <2 hr	<40%	<25% Note: PEF testing may not be needed in very severe attacks
Pao₂ (on air)	Normal (test not necessary)	≥60 mm Hg (test not usually necessary)	<60 mm Hg: possible cyanosis	
and/or Pco₂	<42 mm Hg (test not usually necessary)	<42 mm Hg (test not usually necessary)	≥42 mm Hg: possible respiratory failure	
Sao₂ (on air) at sea level	>95% (test not usually necessary)	90–95% (test not usually necessary)	<90%	

Hypercapnia (hypoventilation) develops more readily in young children than in adults and adolescents.

Pao₂, arterial oxygen pressure; Pco₂, partial pressure of carbon dioxide; PEF, peak expiratory flow; Sao₂, oxygen saturation.
From NHLBI/National Asthma Education and Prevention Program, Expert Panel Report 3: Guidelines for the Diagnosis and Management of Asthma. NIH Publication; 2007.

exacerbation may be assessed with the parameters presented in Table 4.7. Common triggers of acute asthma episodes include upper respiratory tract infections, exposure to cold air, exercise, allergens, pollutants, strong odors, and tobacco smoke.

A brief history should be obtained for every child with acute asthma to determine the duration of symptoms, the character of previous episodes (severity, need for hospitalization, and need for intensive care, including mechanical ventilation), antecedent illness, symptoms, exposures, and both chronic and acute use of medications, including dose and time of last administration. History should also focus on identifying risk factors for severe asthma (Table 4.8) and classification of asthma type, which are based on age (Figs. 4.3,

4.4, and 4.5). It is also important to assess the degree of asthma control. The physical examination should focus on respiratory rate, air exchange, degree and localization of wheezing, other adventitious lung sounds, mental status, presence of cyanosis, and degree of fatigue. A chest radiograph should be obtained for all patients with a first episode of wheezing to evaluate for other causes of wheezing if clinically indicated. Patients with recurrent asthma should have a chest radiograph if there is evidence for a foreign body or pneumonia, or concern for a pneumothorax. Chest radiograph findings in asthma are nonspecific, but they usually show symmetric hyperinflation and increased peribronchial thickening. Spirometry has limited efficacy in the emergency management of status asthmaticus.

Although peak expiratory flow rates are often measured, this test is a measure of large airway function only, is effort dependent, and may be unreliable in an anxious, untrained patient. The major value of peak flow measurements in acute asthma is to provide an objective trend indicative of improvement (or lack thereof) in airway caliber if frequent and scheduled treatments are needed.

A CBC is not of use unless other complicating conditions (i.e., bacterial infection, anemia, hemoglobinopathy) are suspected. Serum electrolyte measurements are of little value unless dehydration is suspected. Hypokalemia can be associated with the frequent administration of β-agonists.

Treatment of acute asthma should be instituted in any child with wheezing, dyspnea, cough, and no other immediately discernible cause of the symptoms. Patients with moderate to severe airway obstruction can have significant hypoxemia as a result of ventilation-perfusion mismatch. Consequently, supplemental humidified oxygen should be administered to any child who has significant wheezing, accessory muscle use, or an oxygen saturation of <93%. The mainstay of treatment for an asthma exacerbation is the administration of an inhaled β-adrenergic agonist and systemic corticosteroids. Inhalation of β-agonist by nebulizer or metered-dose inhaler is the route of choice because the onset of action is rapid, sustained, and relatively free of significant side effects even in the most severely affected patients. Anticholinergic agents (ipratropium bromide), when combined with a β-agonist as inhaled treatment, can provide additional bronchodilation. The effect is most marked in children who present to the emergency department with significant airway obstruction. With few exceptions, any patient who presents with wheezing responsive to bronchodilator therapy or any patient requiring hospital admission should receive corticosteroids. In severe respiratory distress, intravenous magnesium or theophylline (or the intravenous formulation aminophylline) may be of benefit. A small percentage of children with acute asthma progress to severe status asthmaticus and respiratory failure. A number of clinical signs and symptoms define respiratory failure in such severely affected patients: a Pao_2 <60 mm in room air or cyanosis in 40% Fio_2, a $Paco_2$ of 40 mm or higher or rising and accompanied by respiratory distress, deterioration in clinical status in spite of aggressive treatment, a change in mental status, and fatigue. Patients meeting any of these criteria should be admitted to an intensive care unit.

TABLE 4.8   Risk Factors for Death from Asthma

Asthma History

Previous severe exacerbation (e.g., intubation or ICU admission for asthma)

Two or more hospitalizations for asthma in the past year

Three or more ED visits for asthma in the past year

Hospitalization or ED visit for asthma in the past month

Using more than two canisters of SABA per month

Difficulty perceiving asthma symptoms or severity of exacerbations by patient, family, and physician

Other risk factors: lack of a written asthma action plan, sensitivity to *Alternaria*

Social History

Low socioeconomic status or inner-city residence

Illicit drug use

Major psychosocial problems

Comorbidities

Cardiovascular disease

Other chronic lung disease

Chronic psychiatric disease

ED, emergency department; ICU, intensive care unit; SABA, short-acting β2-agonist.
From National Heart, Lung and Blood Institute. Expert Panel Report 3 (EPR 3). Guidelines for the Diagnosis and Management of Asthma. Available at: http://www.nhlbi.nih.gov/guidelines/asthma/asthgdln.htm

---

Key: EIB, exercise-induced bronchospasm

Notes

- The stepwise approach is meant to assist, not replace, the clinical decision-making required to meet individual patient needs.

- Level of severity is determined by both impairment and risk. Assess impairment domain by patient's/caregiver's recall of previous 2–4 weeks. Symptom assessment for longer periods should reflect a global assessment such as inquiring whether the patient's asthma is better or worse since the last visit. Assign severity to the most severe category in which any feature occurs.

- At present, there are inadequate data to correspond frequencies of exacerbations with different levels of asthma severity. For treatment purposes, patients who had ≥2 exacerbations requiring oral systemic corticosteroids in the past 6 months, or ≥4 wheezing episodes in the past year, and who have risk factors for persistent asthma may be considered the same as patients who have persistent asthma, even in the absence of impairment levels consistent with persistent asthma.

Components of Severity		Classification of Asthma Severity (0–4 years of age)			
			Persistent		
		Intermittent	Mild	Moderate	Severe
Impairment	Symptoms	≤2 days/week	≥2 days/week but not daily	Daily	Throughout the day
	Nighttime awakenings	0	1–2x/month	3–4x/month	>1x/week
	Short-acting beta2-agonist use for symptom control (not prevention of EIB)	≤2 days/week	>2 days/week but not daily	Daily	Several times per day
	Interference with normal activity	None	Minor limitation	Some limitation	Extremely limited
Risk	Exacerbations requiring oral systemic corticosteroids	0–1/year	≥2 exacerbations in 6 months requiring oral systemic corticosteroids, or ≥4 wheezing episodes/1 year lasting >1 day AND risk factors for persistent asthma		
		Consider severity and interval since last exacerbation. Frequency and severity may fluctuate over time. Exacerbations of any severity may occur in patients in any severity category.			
Recommended Step for Initiating Therapy		Step 1	Step 2	Step 3 and consider short course of oral systemic corticosteroids	
		In 2–6 weeks, depending on severity, evaluate level of asthma control that is achieved. If no clear benefit is observed in 4–6 weeks, consider adjusting therapy or alternative diagnoses.			

Fig. 4.3 Classifying asthma severity ages 0–4. (From NHLBI/National Asthma Education and Prevention Program, Expert Panel Report 3: Guidelines for the Diagnosis and Management of Asthma. NIH Publication; 2007.)

Notes

- The stepwise approach is meant to assist, not replace, the clinical decision-making required to meet individual patient needs.

- Level of severity is determined by both impairment and risk. Assess impairment domain by patient's/caregiver's recall of the previous 2–4 weeks and spirometry. Assign severity to the most severe category in which any feature occurs.

- At present, there are inadequate data to correspond frequencies of exacerbations with different levels of asthma severity. In general, more frequent and intense exacerbations (e.g., requiring urgent, unscheduled care, hospitalization, or ICU admission) indicate greater underlying disease severity. For treatment purposes, patients who had ≥2 exacerbations requiring oral systemic corticosteroids in the past year may be considered the same as patients who have persistent asthma, even in the absence of impairment levels consistent with persistent asthma.

Components of Severity		Classification of Asthma Severity (5–11 years of age)			
		Intermittent	Persistent		
			Mild	Moderate	Severe
Impairment	Symptoms	≤2 days/week	>2 days/week but not daily	Daily	Throughout the day
	Nighttime awakenings	≤2x/month	3–4x/month	>1x/week but nightly	Often 7x/week
	Short-acting beta$_2$-agonist use for symptom control (not prevention of EIB)	≤2 days/week	>2 days/week but not daily	Daily	Several times per day
	Interference with normal activity	None	Minor limitation	Some limitation	Extremely limited
	Lung function	• Normal FEV$_1$ between exacerbations • FEV$_1$ >80% predicted • FEV$_1$/FVC >85%	• FEV$_1$ = >80% predicted • FEV$_1$/FVC >80%	• FEV$_1$ = 60–80% predicted • FEV$_1$/FVC = 75–80%	• FEV$_1$ <60% predicted • FEV$_1$/FVC <75%
Risk	Exacerbations requiring oral systemic corticosteroids	0–1/year (see note)	≥2/year (see note) →		
		← Consider severity and interval since last exacerbation. → Frequency and severity may fluctuate over time for patients in any severity category.			
		Relative annual risk of exacerbations may be related to FEV$_1$.			
Recommended Step for Initiating Therapy		Step 1	Step 2	Step 3, medium-dose ICS option and consider short course of oral systemic corticosteroids	Step 3, medium-dose ICS option, or step 4
		In 2–6 weeks, evaluate level of asthma control that is achieved, and adjust therapy accordingly.			

Fig. 4.4 Classifying asthma severity ages 5–11. (From NHLBI/National Asthma Education and Prevention Program, Expert Panel Report 3: Guidelines for the Diagnosis and Management of Asthma. NIH Publication; 2007.)

Identification and treatment of chronic asthma require careful assessment of the severity of the disease, according to frequency and intensity of symptoms, and subsequent grading into mild, moderate, and severe categories (see Figs. 4.3, 4.4, and 4.5). All patients except those with mild intermittent disease are best managed with chronic administration of an inhaled antiinflammatory agent (corticosteroids) and the intermittent use of an inhaled β-agonist for treatment of acute wheezing episodes. Leukotriene receptor antagonists may be considered as an alternative preventive therapy for mild asthma. Oral corticosteroids are administered for short intervals to control more severe exacerbations. Avoidance of environmental triggers (allergens, tobacco smoke) is also paramount to successful management.

Bronchiolitis

Bronchiolitis is a common, acute viral infection of the distal lower respiratory tract, and is characterized as lower airway obstruction secondary to airway edema, mucus, and cellular debris. Impaired gas exchange can occur as a result of airway obstruction and ventilation-perfusion inequalities. RSV is the most important respiratory pathogen in infants and young children. In addition, it has been identified as the etiologic agent in 5–40% of pneumonias in young children. Other viruses, such as adenovirus, influenza, human metapneumovirus, parainfluenza, and coronavirus, can also cause bronchiolitis. The most severe disease occurs in infants younger than 6 months. By 5 years of age, 95% of all children have serologic evidence of RSV infection. Reinfections are common in older children and adults, because immunity to RSV is short lived and incomplete. In older children and adolescents, infections with RSV are often limited to the upper respiratory tract. In temperate climates, RSV epidemics occur yearly, beginning in midwinter and persisting through early spring.

In infected infants, upper respiratory tract symptoms usually precede the lower respiratory tract involvement by 3–7 days. Low-grade fever, rhinitis, and pharyngitis are common signs in the initial phase of the disease. This then progresses to cough, increased work of breathing, and wheezing (see Chapter 3). Apnea may also occur, particularly in infants younger than 3 months of age. Chest wall retractions and dyspnea are frequently observed, and adventitious sounds (wheezing, crackles) are appreciated on auscultation of the chest. Most children with bronchiolitis demonstrate clinical improvement after 5–7 days, but the duration of illness can be as long as 21 days. *Bacterial superinfection of the lower respiratory tract is rare.* Approximately 30% of infants with bronchiolitis caused by RSV have recurrent episodes of wheezing caused by bronchial hyperactivity and are diagnosed with asthma. This is in part due to persistent inflammation of the distal respiratory tract produced by the viral infection.

The clinical determination of the severity of the lower respiratory tract involvement in infants infected with bronchiolitis can be difficult. Physical findings often associated with respiratory distress, such as tachypnea, intercostal retractions, and wheezing, are not necessarily correlated with the level of hypoxemia. Carbon dioxide retention secondary to alveolar hypoventilation is not a common finding in otherwise previously normal children, but hypercapnia and acute respiratory acidosis can be serious problems in infants with chronic pulmonary disease or congenital heart disease. Chest radiograph findings include a diffuse interstitial pneumonitis and bilateral lung overinflation; alveolar infiltrates or consolidation are present in approximately 20% of children. Infants with congenital heart disease, pulmonary hypertension, prematurity, and young age (younger than 12 weeks) have an increased rate of severe disease and mortality; the course of illness is usually prolonged, and intensive care and mechanical ventilation are frequently needed.

Key: FEV$_1$, forced expiratory volume in 1 second; FVC, forced vital capacity; ICU, intensive care unit

Notes:

- The stepwise approach is meant to assist, not replace, the clinical decision-making required to meet individual patient needs.

- Level of severity is determined by assessment of both impairment and risk. Assess impairment domain by patient's/caregiver's recall of previous 2–4 weeks and spirometry. Assign severity to the most severe category in which any feature occurs.

- At present, there are inadequate data to correspond frequencies of exacerbations with different levels of asthma severity. In general, more frequent and intense exacerbations (e.g., requiring urgent, unscheduled care, hospitalization, or ICU admission) indicate greater underlying disease severity. For treatment purposes, patients who had ≥2 exacerbations requiring oral systemic corticosteroids in the past year may be considered the same as patients who have persistent asthma, even in the absence of impairment levels consistent with persistent asthma.

Components of Severity		Classification of Asthma Severity ≥12 years of age			
		Intermittent	Persistent		
			Mild	Moderate	Severe
Impairment Normal FEV$_1$/FVC: 8–19 yr 85% 20–39 yr 80% 40–59 yr 75% 60–80 yr 70%	Symptoms	≤2 days/week	≥2 days/week but not daily	Daily	Throughout the day
	Nighttime awakenings	≤2x/month	3–4x/month	>1x/week but not nightly	Often 7x/week
	Short-acting beta$_2$-agonist use for symptom control (not prevention of EIB)	≤2 days/week	>2 days/week but not daily, and not more than 1x on any day	Daily	Several times per day
	Interference with normal activity	None	Minor limitation	Some limitation	Extremely limited
	Lung function	• Normal FEV$_1$ between exacerbations • FEV$_1$ >80% predicted • FEV$_1$/FVC normal	• FEV$_1$ >80% predicted • FEV$_1$/FVC normal	• FEV$_1$ >60% but <80% predicted • FEV$_1$/FVC reduced 5%	• FEV$_1$ <60% predicted • FEV$_1$/FVC reduced >5%
Risk	Exacerbations requiring oral systemic corticosteroids	0–1/year (see note)	≥2/year (see note) ⟶		
		Consider severity and interval since last exacerbation. ⟵⟶ Frequency and severity may fluctuate over time for patients in any severity category. Relative annual risk of exacerbations may be related to FEV$_1$.			
Recommended Step for Initiating Treatment		Step 1	Step 2	Step 3	Step 4 or 5 and consider short course of oral systemic corticosteroids
		In 2–6 weeks, evaluate level of asthma control that is achieved, and adjust therapy accordingly.			

Fig. 4.5 Classifying asthma severity ages 12 and older. (From NHLBI/National Asthma Education and Prevention Program, Expert Panel Report 3: Guidelines for the Diagnosis and Management of Asthma. NIH Publication; 2007.)

The diagnosis of bronchiolitis is usually made on clinical grounds. Bronchiolitis is most common in children under 2 years of age and should be suspected in the wheezing child who has current or antecedent upper respiratory tract infection symptoms in the late fall or winter months. The definitive diagnosis of RSV or other viral infection is based on the presence of the viral genome in respiratory secretions. This testing is often not needed if the clinical findings are consistent with bronchiolitis. Polymerase chain reaction (PCR) testing is specific and accurate, and has a short turnaround time in identifying the virus from nasopharyngeal swabs.

Suctioning and supplemental oxygen remain the cornerstone of treatment for bronchiolitis if needed. Unlike asthma, the wheezing accompanying bronchiolitis is often less responsive to bronchodilators. Nonetheless, patients with significant hypoxia and hypercapnia may receive a *trial treatment* with aerosol bronchodilators to determine if this may improve symptoms, which may be continued if infants do show improvement. Infants with bronchiolitis do not respond to treatment with antiinflammatory agents, such as corticosteroids, so these are not recommended. Severely ill patients may require mechanical ventilation; heated, humidified, high-flow nasal cannula oxygen decreases intubation rates and is used in children with severe respiratory distress. Other modalities, such as hypertonic or normal saline aerosols, positive expiratory pressure (PEP) therapy, and chest physiotherapy have shown mixed results but may be of benefit for patients who are hospitalized.

Monthly administration (intramuscularly) of a humanized monoclonal antibody (palivizumab) against RSV can reduce morbidity from bronchiolitis but does not completely prevent infection. Infants at high risk (infants who are premature, those with bronchopulmonary dysplasia or other forms of chronic obstructive pulmonary disease, those with complex congenital heart disease) who are younger than 2 years are most likely to benefit.

Mycoplasma pneumoniae Infections

One of the basic tenets regarding respiratory infections in children is that "bacteria do not make you wheeze." *Mycoplasma pneumoniae* is an exception to that rule and should be considered in an older child who presents with new-onset wheezing. In addition, infections with *M. pneumoniae* can precipitate exacerbations in patients with asthma. Productive or dry coughs secondary to tracheobronchitis are the most common symptoms of *M. pneumoniae* infections. Pulmonary symptoms span from mild viral symptoms to more severe presentations of pneumonia. Other clinical manifestations of *M. pneumoniae* infections include fever/chills, rhinorrhea, and otitis media (see Chapter 5). Extrapulmonary manifestations not only are due to the infection itself but also can be due to immune or vascular complications. Examples of *M. pneumoniae* extrapulmonary findings include hemolytic anemia, rash, mucositis, cardiac disease, polyarthritis, transverse myelitis, rhabdomyolysis, and central nervous system disease. The incidence of *M. pneumoniae* infection peaks between the ages of 5 and 19 years; the organism usually does not produce disease in children younger than age 2. Infections with *M. pneumoniae* tend to be seasonal, occurring most frequently during autumn and early winter.

The findings of *M. pneumoniae* on chest radiographs are variable. In about 5% of patients, the chest radiograph appears normal. A diffuse, bilateral, reticular infiltrate is the classic appearance in about half of patients. However, lobar, alveolar, and interstitial infiltrates have also been described (Fig. 4.6). Enlargement of hilar or peritracheal lymph nodes may also be evident. Pleural effusions (usually small) are found in 14% of patients with *M. pneumoniae*. Atypical pneumonia (diffuse infiltrates with nonlobar pattern; fever, malaise, myalgias) is often caused by *M. pneumoniae* but may also be caused by *Chlamydia pneumoniae*, *Legionella* species, and other

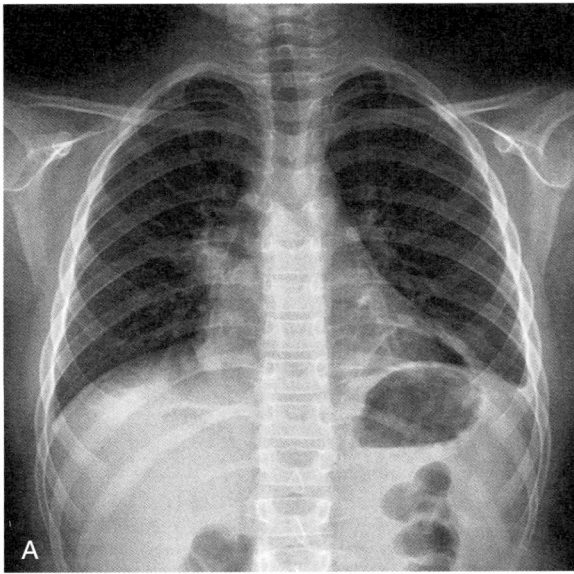

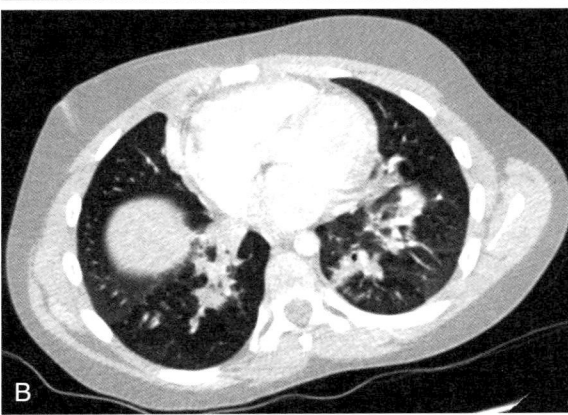

Fig. 4.6 Mycoplasma atypical pneumonia in an 8-year-old girl who presented with fatigue, low-grade fever, and cough. *A,* The chest radiograph shows irregularity of the right hilum and bibasilar infiltration. *B,* Contrast-enhanced CT demonstrates bilateral bronchopneumonia in the lower lobes. A direct fluorescent antibody test from nasopharyngeal aspirate confirmed the diagnosis. (From Coley BD, ed. *Caffey's Pediatric Diagnostic Imaging.* 13th ed. Philadelphia: Elsevier; 2019:519, Fig. 54.16.)

related pathogens. PCR may help to confirm a diagnosis. Many *M. pneumoniae* infections are self-limiting within 7–10 days. When antibiotics are used, treatment is with azithromycin. Doxycycline or fluoroquinolones may also be used in older children, although there is increasing emergence of *M. pneumoniae* resistance to macrolides in some areas of the world.

Vocal Cord Dysfunction

A functional disorder that mimics asthma, vocal cord dysfunction is typically manifested as wheezing, dyspnea, and shortness of breath refractory to treatment with inhaled bronchodilators. Vocal cord dysfunction should be considered in patients with wheezing who present with atypical findings or those who are difficult to treat. The wheezing is produced by adduction of the vocal cords during inspiration and expiration. The resultant high-pitched inspiratory and expiratory noises are transmitted to the chest, although the sounds are best appreciated over the larynx. Despite the patient's apparent dyspnea, gas exchange is usually unaffected. Spirometry

shows variable flattening of the inspiratory flow loop. The diagnosis is established by direct laryngoscopy, which demonstrates paradoxical motion of the vocal cords. Speech therapy is the treatment of choice.

Foreign Body Aspiration

Aspiration of a foreign body into the intrathoracic airways must be considered in the differential diagnosis of a child with the sudden onset of respiratory distress or wheezing. If both main stem bronchi and the trachea are obstructed (typically by larger foreign bodies), the patient may have asphyxia and sudden death; aspiration of foreign bodies in the distal airways often takes a more indolent course. Aspiration of foreign bodies is most common in children between 1 and 4 years of age, particularly in males or in children with neurologic disorders or delayed development. It is rare in children younger than 6 months. The most common objects aspirated by children are small toy parts, coins, marbles, balloons, and food products (e.g., hot dogs, popcorn, seeds, nuts, grapes, carrots, and beans). Endobronchial aspiration of peanuts, raisins, popcorn kernels, or seeds tends to produce more difficulties than other kinds of foreign bodies (metallic or plastic objects) because, in addition to causing physical obstruction of the airway, vegetable matter produces an intense, local inflammatory response secondary to chemical and allergic bronchitis. Larger objects, such as coins, usually lodge in the esophagus. Esophageal foreign bodies can produce significant respiratory symptoms as a result of extrinsic compression of the posterior trachea. This compression can produce respiratory distress, stridor, and wheezing, especially in infants and young children. Dysphagia and vomiting can be late symptoms associated with an esophageal foreign body.

The typical clinical manifestation after the acute event is abrupt respiratory distress, characterized by choking, gagging, cyanosis, and a harsh, paroxysmal cough (see Chapter 3). However, because many aspiration events occur while children are unsupervised, the history of foreign body ingestion or aspiration is frequently not elicited. Chronic cough, dyspnea, hemoptysis, and wheezing may develop. Because the object is most frequently aspirated into the main stem or segmental bronchi (distal airway), the wheezing is typically unilateral. Physical examination may also reveal a decrease in breath sounds on the obstructed side, prolongation of the expiratory phase, and a tracheal shift. In some instances, retained foreign bodies in the airways can produce a persistent pneumonitis, and the chronic inflammatory response can result in bronchiectasis or lung abscess. Retained foreign body should be considered in a child with presumed asthma or pneumonia who is not improving with appropriate treatment.

The diagnosis of foreign body aspiration can be difficult to establish and necessitates a combination of clinical examination, radiographic studies, and ultimately endoscopic visualization. Radiopaque foreign bodies are generally easily visualized by radiographic studies. Radiolucent foreign bodies may become apparent on inspiratory or expiratory chest radiographs, lateral decubitus films, fluoroscopy, or barium swallow studies when an esophageal foreign body could be compressing the posterior tracheal wall (Fig. 4.7). Because an occasional foreign body may not lodge in a bronchus, typical radiologic findings may not be seen. If a foreign body is likely to be present, rigid bronchoscopy for examination of the lower airway and foreign body removal is indicated. Flexible bronchoscopy provides an excellent visualization of the airway and should be reserved for when other diagnoses appear to be much more likely.

Stridor

Stridor, a harsh medium-pitched sound typically heard on inspiration, is caused by turbulent airflow in the upper airway. The phase of

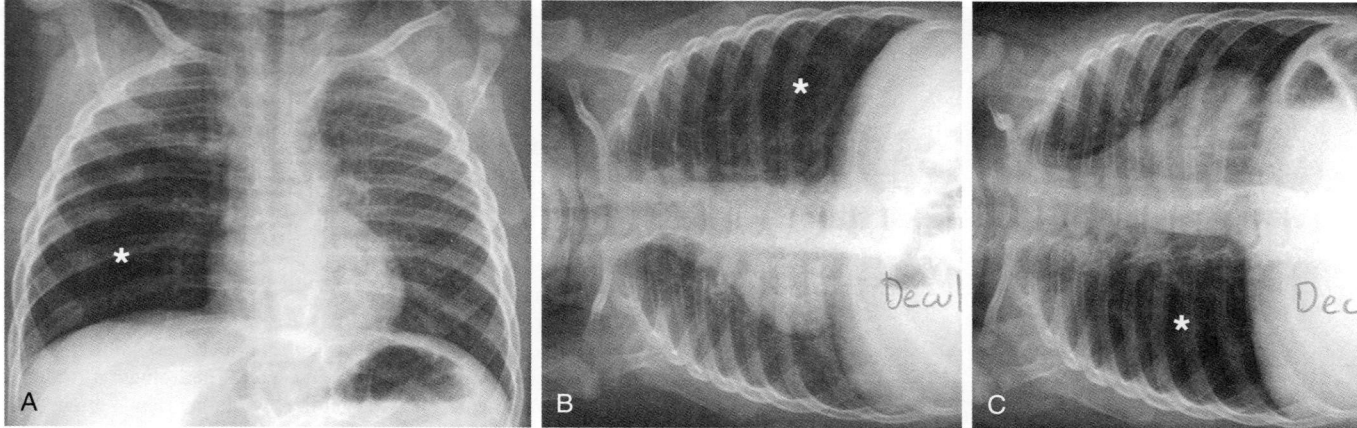

Fig. 4.7 Nonradiopaque foreign body aspiration in a 5-year-old girl who presented with persistent coughing and respiratory distress while eating popcorn. *A,* Frontal chest radiograph obtained at end-inspiration shows mild hyperinflation *(asterisk)* of the right lower lobe. *B,* Frontal chest radiograph obtained at end-inspiration in the left lateral decubitus position demonstrates normal volume loss in the left lung and mild hyperinflation *(asterisk)* of the right lower lobe. *C,* Frontal chest radiograph obtained at end-inspiration in the right lateral decubitus position shows persistent hyperinflation *(asterisk)* of the right lower lobe. (From Coley BD, ed. *Caffey's Pediatric Diagnostic Imaging.* 13th ed. Philadelphia: Elsevier; 2019:490, Fig. 52.7.)

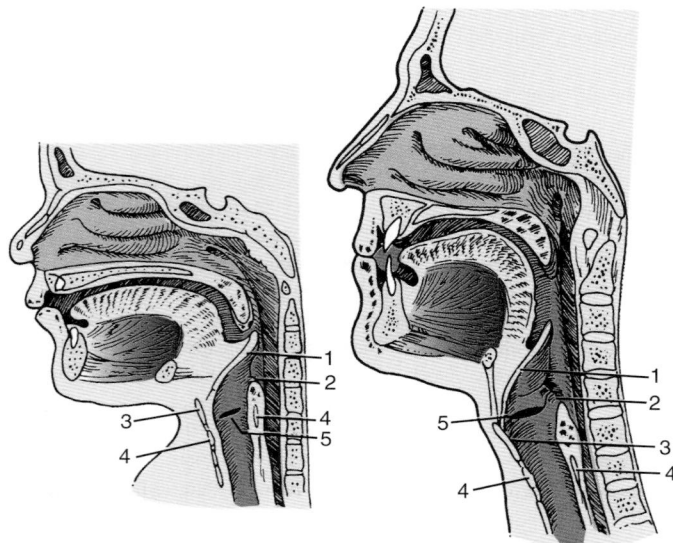

Fig. 4.8 Anatomy of upper airway. Relative comparative anatomy of the larynx in an infant *(left)* and an adult *(right).* Specific landmarks: *1,* epiglottis; *2,* arytenoid cartilages; *3,* thyroid cartilage; *4,* cricoid cartilage; *5,* laryngeal ventricle, the air space below the false vocal cords and above the true vocal cords. Its radiolucency is an excellent landmark on lateral radiograph. The infant larynx is situated relatively high in the cervical region. In addition, the base of the infant's tongue is close to the larynx, and the epiglottis is located near the palate. These anatomic differences partially explain the predominantly obligate nose breathing of the young infant, as well as the relative ease with which upper airway obstructions develop in infants.

respiration in which stridor occurs is helpful in identifying the site of the airway obstruction (see Fig. 4.1). The relative anatomy of the upper airway in an adult versus in an infant is shown in Figure 4.8. The most common cause of stridor of infants and young children is **laryngomalacia**. Congenital anomalies should be suspected in children with recurrent or persistent stridor. Acute inspiratory stridor is most commonly caused by acute inflammation/infection, typically **croup**; however, an acute foreign body aspiration in the upper airway may also cause acute-onset stridor. Epiglottitis is the most serious life-threatening infection in this area and must be identified quickly. A history of prior intubation in a patient with stridor and respiratory distress should raise concern for vocal cord paralysis or subglottic stenosis. An age-related differential diagnosis is noted in Table 4.9. Differentiating features of common disorders are noted in Table 4.10.

Croup

Laryngotracheal bronchitis (croup) is generally a slowly progressive, mild, self-limited viral inflammation of the subglottic larynx occurring in infants and young children. The most common causes are parainfluenza virus types 1 and 3, influenza A, respiratory syncytial virus, and adenovirus. The circumferential cricoid cartilage, which consists of the subglottic airway just below the vocal cords, is the narrowest part of the upper airway in a child (see Fig. 4.8). The inflammation associated with a viral infection in this location causes airway obstruction as edema develops within the confines of the cricoid cartilage. Most patients will develop mild rhinorrhea, cough, and low-grade fever prior to characteristic barky cough and inspiratory stridor (see Chapter 3). The cry or voice may become hoarse. Stridor typically worsens when the patient is upset or active and improves with warm humidified air. Unless the airway obstruction is severe, the child generally has no trouble handling saliva. If a patient develops drooling or rapid progression of respiratory distress, epiglottitis or bacterial tracheitis should be considered. The diagnosis is usually apparent from the history and physical examination. If the diagnosis is not clear, obtaining a lateral neck radiograph is indicated and will show the classic "steeple" sign (Fig. 4.9).

Management varies from outpatient observation with parent education to endotracheal intubation. For mild cases, the patient must be well hydrated; the use of extra humidity is soothing to the airways and helps to keep secretions from being tenacious, so that they are less likely to become obstructive. In more severe cases (stridor at rest, retractions), nebulized epinephrine used as a mucosal vasoconstrictor may provide relief. Usually, patients being treated in this manner are observed in the hospital for a possible "rebound" effect that may occur 2–6 hours after treatment. Parenteral or oral dexamethasone is a safe and effective additional therapy for moderate to severe croup;

TABLE 4.9 Age-Related Differential Diagnosis of Airway Obstruction

Newborn	**Toddler**
Foreign material (meconium, amniotic fluid)	Viral croup (most common etiology in children 3 mo–4 yr of age)
Congenital subglottic stenosis (uncommon)	Bacterial tracheitis (toxic, high fever)
Choanal atresia	Foreign body (sudden cough; airway or esophageal) (see Chapter 3)
Congenital cysts	Spasmodic (recurrent) croup (see Chapter 3)
Micrognathia (Pierre Robin syndrome, Treacher Collins syndrome, DiGeorge syndrome)	Laryngeal papillomatosis
Macroglossia (Beckwith-Wiedemann syndrome, hypothyroidism, Pompe disease, trisomy 21, hemangioma)	Retropharyngeal abscess
Laryngeal web, clefts, atresia	Diphtheria (uncommon)
Laryngospasm (intubation, aspiration, hypocalcemia, transient)	**Infant Older Than 2–3 Yr**
Lingual thyroid	Epiglottitis (epiglottis, aryepiglottic folds)
Vocal cord paralysis (weak cry; unilateral or bilateral, with or without increased intracranial pressure from Arnold-Chiari malformation or other CNS pathology; birth trauma)	Inhalation injury (burns, toxic gas, hydrocarbons)
	Foreign bodies
	Angioedema (family history, cutaneous angioedema)
Tracheal web, stenosis, malacia, atresia	Anaphylaxis (allergic history, wheezing, hypotension)
Pharyngeal collapse (cause of apnea in preterm infant)	Peritonsillar abscess (adolescents)
Tumors*	Ludwig angina
	Diphtheria
Infant	Parapharyngeal abscess
Laryngomalacia (most common cause)	Tumors*
Subglottic stenosis (congenital; acquired after intubation)	Trauma (blunt or penetrating airway injury; tracheal/larynx fracture; chemical burns, e.g., caustic ingestions)
Tumors*	
Tongue tumor (dermoid, teratoma, ectopic thyroid)	
Laryngeal papillomatosis	
Vascular rings	

*Tumors include lymphangiomas, hemangiomas, papillomas, neuroblastoma, lymphoma, rhabdomyosarcoma, and chondrosarcomas.
CNS, central nervous system.
Modified from Kercsmar C. The respiratory system. In: Behrman RE, Kliegman RM, eds. *Nelson Essentials of Pediatrics*. 2nd ed. Philadelphia: WB Saunders; 1994:444.

steroid use has decreased the requirement for endotracheal intubation. Patients with severe croup are usually admitted to the hospital for observation. If intubation is needed, an endotracheal tube one-half to one size smaller than that used for a child with a normal airway of the same age and size is chosen. In atypical cases of recurrent croup or in patients in whom extubation is difficult, an endoscopic evaluation of the airway with laryngoscopy and bronchoscopy is necessary to exclude an underlying anatomic abnormality.

Bacterial Tracheitis

Bacterial tracheitis is a bacterial superinfection of a previous tracheal (croup, influenza virus) viral process and is usually caused by *Staphylococcus aureus*. A variety of other organisms, including *Moraxella catarrhalis*, *Streptococcus pneumoniae*, and non-typable *Haemophilus influenzae*, have also been identified as being occasionally involved. There is generally a virus-like mild phase, followed by a rapid deterioration, during which the patient clinically appears more ill with high fever and respiratory distress. Some patients have a two-phased illness with croup, initial recovery, followed by tracheitis. Neck and chest radiographs often show irregular scalloping of the trachea. Radiopaque densities from inspissated mucus may be seen. Close monitoring and intravenous antibiotic treatment directed toward the likely causative organisms are required. Endotracheal intubation for control of the airway is usually necessary, particularly in younger patients. Extubation is performed on the basis of clinical improvement and a resolution of excessive amounts of purulent secretions. Sometimes the exudate secondary to the tracheitis is thick and can cause airway obstruction similar to that from a foreign body. Antistaphylococcal antibiotic therapy is indicated.

Epiglottitis

Epiglottitis is an acute, rapidly progressive, potentially lethal infection of the epiglottis, aryepiglottic folds, and false vocal cord area. It is an emergency because of the potential for rapid airway obstruction; evaluation and treatment are directed toward establishing an airway while the physician is confirming the diagnosis and treating the infection. In the past, epiglottitis was caused by *H. influenzae* type b in nearly 100% of cases. Since the introduction of the polysaccharide conjugated *H. influenzae* type b vaccine, there has been a dramatic fall in the incidence of acute epiglottitis in the United States. However, in an internationally mobile world, patients who have not been vaccinated may acquire epiglottitis in any country. In addition, other, less common pathogens, such as *S. pneumoniae*, *S. aureus*, and β-hemolytic streptococci, may produce epiglottitis. Unusual presentations will also become more common, with children presenting at a younger age and immunosuppressive diseases being caused by atypical organisms.

Typically, there is an abrupt onset, usually without an obvious prodrome, with rapid progression toward airway compromise. Initially, complaints of sore throat and odynophagia are common. Patients are usually febrile, and drooling is present. The typical presentation is an ill-appearing child sitting forward with their head hyperextended who does not want to lie down (Fig. 4.10). There is a "hot potato" voice and drooling, the mouth is open, and the tongue is protruding. Mild inspiratory stridor and retractions may be present, but these are usually not obvious, because the patient generally takes short, shallow breaths. An intraoral examination is contraindicated because it may predispose to laryngospasm and airway obstruction.

TABLE 4.10 Differential Diagnosis of Upper Airway Obstruction

	Laryngotracheobronchitis (Croup)	Laryngitis	Spasmodic Croup	Epiglottitis	Membranous Croup (Bacterial Tracheitis)	Retropharyngeal Abscess	Foreign Body	Angioedema	Peritonsillar Abscess	Laryngeal Papillomatosis
Age	3 mo–3 yr	5 yr–teens	3 mo–3 yr	2–6 yr	Any age (3–10 yr)	<6 yr	6 mo–5 yr	All ages	>10 yr	3 mo–3 yr
Location	Subglottic	Subglottic	Subglottic	Supraglottic	Trachea	Posterior pharynx	Supraglottic, subglottic, variable	Variable	Oropharynx	Larynx, vocal cords, trachea
Etiology	Parainfluenza, influenza virus, RSV; rarely Mycoplasma, measles, adenovirus	As per croup	Unknown	Haemophilus influenzae type b	Prior croup or influenza virus with secondary bacterial infection by Staphylococcus aureus, Moraxella catarrhalis, H. influenzae	S. aureus, anaerobes	Small objects, vegetable, toys, coins	Congenital C-1 esterase deficiency; acquired anaphylaxis	Group A streptococci, anaerobes	HPV
Prodrome onset	Insidious, URI	As per croup	Sudden onset at night; prior episodes	Rapid, short prodrome	Biphasic illness with sudden deterioration	Insidious to sudden	Sudden	Sudden	Biphasic with sudden worsening	Chronic
Stridor	Yes—biphasic	No	Yes	Yes—soft inspiratory	Yes	No	Yes	Yes	No	Possible
Retractions	Yes	No	Rare	Yes	Yes	Yes	Yes (variable)	Yes	No	No
Voice	Hoarse	Hoarse; whispered	Hoarse	Muffled	Normal or hoarse	Muffled	Complete obstruction—aphonic; other variable	Hoarse, may be normal	"Hot potato," muffled	Hoarse
Position and appearance	Normal	Normal	Normal	Tripod sitting, leaning forward; agitation	Normal	Arching of neck or normal	Normal	Normal; may have facial edema	Normal	Normal
Swallowing (dysphagia)	Normal	Normal	Normal	Drooling	Normal	Drooling	Variable; usually normal	Normal	Drooling, trismus	Normal

TABLE 4.10　Differential Diagnosis of Upper Airway Obstruction—cont'd

	Laryngotracheobronchitis (Croup)	Laryngitis	Spasmodic Croup	Epiglottitis	Membranous Croup (Bacterial Tracheitis)	Retropharyngeal Abscess	Foreign Body	Angioedema	Peritonsillar Abscess	Laryngeal Papillomatosis
Barking cough	Yes	Rare	Yes	No	Yes	No	Variable; brassy if tracheal	Possible	No	Variable
Toxicity	Rare	No	No	Severe	Severe	Severe	No, but dyspnea	No, unless anaphylactic shock or severe anoxia	Dyspnea	None
Fever	<101°F	<101°F	None	>102°F	>102°F	>101°F	None	None	>101°F	None
Radiographic findings	Subglottic narrowing; steeple sign	Normal	Subglottic narrowing	Thumb sign of thickened epiglottis	Ragged irregular tracheal border; as per croup	Thickened retropharyngeal space	Radiopaque object may be seen	As per croup	None needed	May be normal
WBC count	Normal	Normal	Normal	Leukocytosis with left shift	Leukocytosis with left shift	Leukocytosis with left shift	Normal	Normal	Leukocytosis with left shift	Normal
Therapy	Racemic epinephrine: aerosol, systemic steroids, aerosolized steroids, cool mist	None	Cool mist; occasionally as for croup	Endotracheal intubation, ceftriaxone	Vancomycin; ceftriaxone; intubation if needed	Clindamycin; ampicillin-sulbactam (or vancomycin); ceftriaxone; surgical drainage if abscess	Endoscopic removal	Anaphylaxis; epinephrine, IV fluids, steroids; C-1 esterase deficiency; replacement infusion therapy	Penicillin; aspiration	Laser therapy, repeated excision, interferon
Prevention	None	None	None	H. influenzae type b conjugated vaccine	None	None	Avoid small objects; supervision	Avoid allergens; FFP for hereditary angioedema	Treat group A streptococci early	Treat maternal genitourinary lesions; possible cesarean section? HPV vaccine to mother

FFP, fresh-frozen plasma; HPV, human papillomavirus; IV, intravenous; RSV, respiratory syncytial virus; URI, upper respiratory tract infection; WBC, white blood cell.

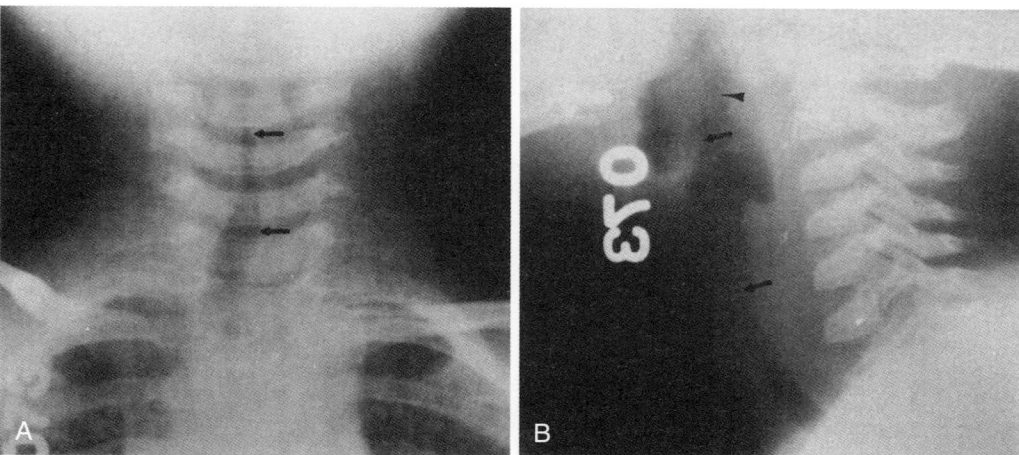

Fig. 4.9 Croup in a 1-year-old child. *A,* Frontal radiograph of the neck shows a tapered reduction of the sub-glottic tracheal caliber from the level of the vocal cords *(upper arrow)* to the normal-caliber trachea below *(lower arrow).* The right mild tracheal deviation is a normal sign resulting from the left aortic arch. *B,* Lateral view shows a normal epiglottis *(upper arrow),* distention of the pharynx, normal palatine tonsils *(arrowhead),* and increased density in the subglottic trachea *(lower arrow).*

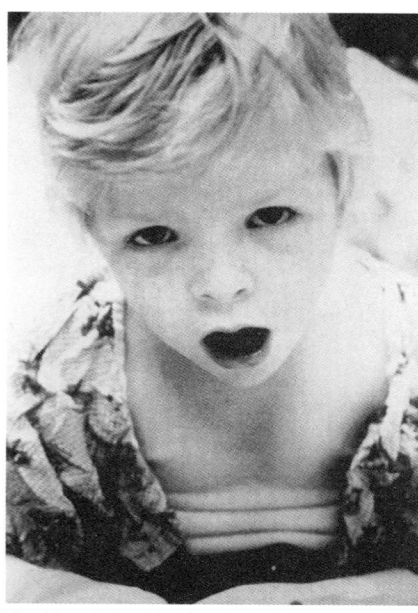

Fig. 4.10 Child with epiglottitis. Characteristic posture in a patient with epiglottitis. The child is leaning forward and drooling, and the neck is hyperextended.

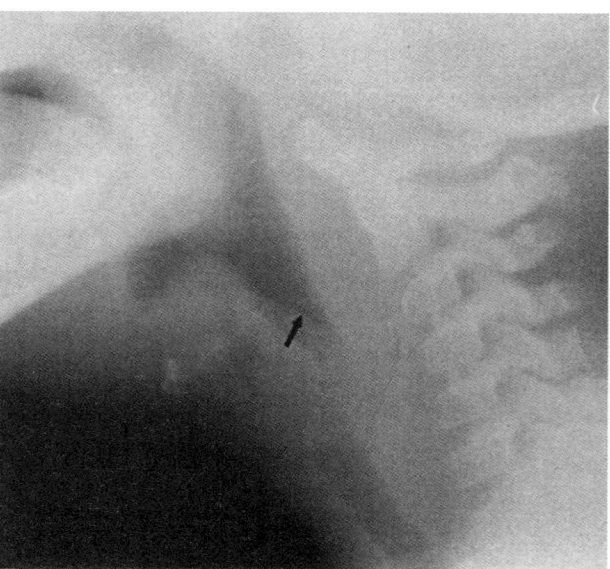

Fig. 4.11 Epiglottitis. The patient is a 3½-year-old child with fever and sudden onset of stridor. Lateral radiograph shows an enlarged epiglottis ("thumbprint" sign) and aryepiglottic folds *(arrow)* and distention of the pharynx.

If there is any question as to the diagnosis, a lateral soft tissue radiograph of the neck can be confirmatory (Fig. 4.11). Someone who has the expertise and equipment to handle sudden airway decompensation in a pediatric patient should accompany the patient to the radiology suite. When a clinical diagnosis of epiglottitis is at all likely, the patient should be taken immediately to the operating room and cared for by experienced pediatric anesthesiology and otolaryngology personnel capable of endotracheal intubation or less often tracheostomy.

Once the airway is secured and the diagnosis confirmed, blood specimens are obtained for culture and treatment is begun with ceftriaxone. Patients usually require 36–48 hours of endotracheal intubation, with observation in the pediatric intensive care unit. If there is a question of safety of extubation, a second laryngoscopy is indicated.

Laryngomalacia

Laryngomalacia is the most common cause of inspiratory stridor and noisy respiration in neonates and infants. It is caused by the inspiratory collapse of the laryngeal cartilages, with prolapse of the epiglottis or arytenoid cartilages into the airway during inspiration. It typically presents with high-pitched inspiratory stridor. Stridor may occur at birth, but the onset is often delayed, occurring at 2–4 weeks of age. The condition is usually self-limited and resolves with time: often by 8–12 months of age but occasionally not until 18–24 months of age. Laryngomalacia should be suspected in infants with recurrent croup, as acute viral infections or agitation can worsen symptoms. Patients often will have associated gastroesophageal reflux disease, and some may have feeding difficulties or failure to thrive. Severe cases may cause apneic events or pulmonary hypertension.

The diagnosis is made on the basis of the clinical presentation (stridor is worse when the patient is supine or during activity, and exacerbations occur with upper respiratory tract infections) and findings on flexible laryngoscopy. Approximately 15–25% of patients with laryngomalacia may have other airway lesions. Therefore a complete airway evaluation with rigid bronchoscopy has been recommended in patients with severe respiratory distress, failure to thrive, or any underlying concern for a concurrent airway lesion, and if the stridor of laryngomalacia does not follow the typical course. Unusually severe cases of laryngomalacia may necessitate operative intervention, such as a supraglottoplasty to trim redundant soft tissue or even a temporary tracheotomy. Laryngomalacia may be accompanied by tracheomalacia, a partial collapse of the tracheal cartilages with respiration. Tracheomalacia may be congenital or secondary to extrinsic compression by vascular rings or tumors. Patients with tracheomalacia manifest with wheezing, cough, stridor, dyspnea, tachypnea, or cyanosis.

Vocal Cord Paralysis

Vocal cord paralysis is a common cause of congenital neonatal laryngeal obstruction, but can also occur in older children. Vocal cord paralysis may be bilateral or unilateral, and it often can cause difficulty feeding, respiratory distress, and a weak cry. In neonates with no surgical history, it is associated with neurologic syndromes, such as the Arnold-Chiari malformation. Traction on the brainstem or increased intracranial pressure and herniation put pressure on the vagus nerve, which is thought to cause the paralysis. It can also be iatrogenic, particularly in neonates with a history of thoracic surgery or difficult birth delivery. Tracheotomy is often necessary to maintain the airway in bilateral vocal cord paralysis, and neurologic and MRI evaluation should be performed to identify any central causes. Vocal cord paralysis also occurs in older children and may be caused by a polyneuropathy (Guillain-Barré syndrome), brainstem encephalitis, neck or thoracic surgery, or compression by local masses.

Vascular Rings

Vascular rings are common and can produce symptoms related to compression of the trachea and/or the esophagus (Table 4.11). Feeding often exacerbates manifestations when the obstructed esophagus acts as an additional extrinsic force on the trachea. Patients present with cough, dysphagia, odynophagia, tachypnea, emesis, noisy breathing, stridor, and/or wheezing. Because they handle oral secretions poorly, they may develop aspiration pneumonia. They also do not tolerate neck flexion. The two most common symptomatic lesions are the right aortic arch with a left ligamentum arteriosus (or patent ductus arteriosus) and the double aortic arch. The diagnosis may be suspected on a chest radiograph by a demonstrated right-sided aortic arch or a narrow displaced trachea. An upper gastrointestinal series demonstrates the indentation of the anterior and/or posterior esophagus, whereas endoscopy demonstrates the pulsatile extrinsic compressing vessels (Fig. 4.12). MRI or echocardiography is usually diagnostic; angiography is not needed to find most of these lesions.

Subglottic Stenosis

Congenital subglottic stenosis occurs when the subglottic space is narrowed, and typically presents in children younger than 3 months with respiratory distress, biphasic or inspiratory stridor, and recurrent croup. *Acquired* subglottic stenosis may develop secondary to endotracheal intubation, particularly if the intubation has been prolonged for several months, if an oversized tube was used, or if multiple intubations were required. Subglottic stenosis should be suspected in any child with these risk factors who does not tolerate extubation because of upper airway obstruction. Laryngoscopy and bronchoscopy are required for evaluation to diagnose subglottic stenosis and also evaluate for other lesions such as subglottic cysts or hemangiomas. Acquired subglottic stenosis is often more severe than the congenital type. In both types of subglottic stenosis, infection and gastroesophageal reflux may exacerbate symptoms and contribute to narrowing of the airway. A cricoid split operation, tracheotomy, or laryngotracheal reconstruction may be needed. Serial dilatations are no longer commonly used because they may continue to injure the cartilage and its overlying mucosa.

Cough

Cough is a common complaint in children (see Chapter 3). The nature of the cough is often helpful in establishing the etiology of respiratory distress. For example, a barky cough is typically associated with viral croup, whereas a more productive cough can be associated with pneumonia. Pneumonia is most commonly caused by bacteria or viruses; however, there are other common noninfectious causes of pneumonia and pneumonitis.

Viral and Bacterial Pneumonia

Pneumonia is defined as acute inflammation of the lung parenchyma, and can be caused by viruses, bacteria, or fungi (see Chapter 3). Clinically, it is often defined as a lower respiratory tract infection, associated with fever, respiratory symptoms, and evidence of lung parenchyma involvement, either by physical examination or chest radiograph findings. *S. pneumoniae* is the most common bacterial pathogen of community-acquired pneumonia; *H. influenzae* and *S. aureus* are less common causes. Viral pathogens are a common cause of pneumonia in young children; it can be difficult to discern which pathogen is causing the clinical symptoms. Atypical pathogens, such as *M. pneumoniae*, are a common cause of pneumonia in school-aged children (Table 4.12). Children with immunodeficiency, sickle cell disease, cystic fibrosis, or HIV may present with more atypical pathogens.

Patients will often begin with an upper respiratory infection with rhinitis and cough (see Chapter 3). They then develop tachypnea and fever and then may develop respiratory distress with subcostal, intercostal, and suprasternal retractions; nasal flaring and use of accessory muscles; and hypoxia. Tachypnea and worsening cough are commonly noted. Patients with lower lobe pneumonias may also present with abdominal pain. Early in the course of illness, crackles, rhonchi, and wheezing are common findings. Later in the course of illness, as lungs consolidate and/or pleural effusions or empyema develops, decreased breath sounds and dullness to percussion may develop. Wheezing is more likely in viral or atypical pneumonia; however, unilateral wheezing may also correlate with a bacterial lobar pneumonia.

Diagnosis is made by chest radiograph, which will show a consolidation, and may show empyema or pleural effusion if present (Fig. 4.13). However, it is important to note that in children with mild lower respiratory tract disease with clinical symptoms consistent with pneumonia, a chest radiograph is not needed to make a diagnosis. Patchy infiltrates are most suggestive of atypical or viral pneumonia. A lobar consolidation or large pleural effusion is likely from a bacterial etiology. Laboratory testing may be helpful in patients with more severe disease, but is not necessary in all patients. Peripheral white blood cell (WBC) count and acute phase reactants are likely elevated, and can be used to follow response to therapy along with clinical response. Blood cultures should be obtained for patients with moderate to severe disease, or who fail to demonstrate improvement after the initiation of antibiotics. Viral or atypical pathogen testing

TABLE 4.11 Vascular Rings

Lesion	Symptoms	Plain Film	Barium Swallow	Bronchoscopy	MRI Echocardiography	Treatment
Double arch	Stridor, respiratory distress Swallowing dysfunction Reflex apnea	AP—wider base of heart Lat.—narrowed trachea displaced forward at C3–C4	Bilateral indentation of esophagus	Bilateral tracheal compression—both pulsatile	Diagnostic	Ligate and divide smaller arch (usually left)
Right arch and ligamentum/ductus	Respiratory distress Swallowing dysfunction	AP—tracheal deviation to left (right arch)	Bilateral indentation of esophagus R > L	Bilateral tracheal compression—R pulsatile	Diagnostic	Ligate ligamentum or ductus
Anomalous innominate	Cough Stridor Reflex apnea	AP—normal Lat.—anterior tracheal compression	Normal	Pulsatile anterior tracheal compression	Unnecessary	Conservative
Aberrant right subclavian	Occasional swallowing dysfunction	Normal	AP—oblique defect upward to right Lat.—small defect on right posterior wall	Usually normal	Diagnostic	Ligate artery
Pulmonary sling	Expiratory stridor Respiratory distress	AP—low L hilum, R emphysema/atelectasis Lat.—anterior bowing of right bronchus and trachea	±Anterior indentation above carina between esophagus and trachea	Tracheal displacement to left Compression of right main bronchus	Diagnostic	Detach and reanastomose to main pulmonary artery in front of trachea

AP, anteroposterior; L, left; Lat., lateral; R, right.
From Kliegman RM, Greenbaum LA, Lye PS. *Practical Strategies in Pediatric Diagnosis and Therapy.* 2nd ed. Philadelphia: Elsevier; 2004:88.

may be helpful as this may decrease the need for additional testing or antibiotic use.

Treatment for bacterial pneumonia is antibiotics directed at the suspected cause of pneumonia and supplemental care (oxygen, intravenous fluids) as indicated based on the patient's clinical presentation. Hospitalization may be required for patients with hypoxia or toxic appearance, moderate to severe respiratory distress, or age younger than 6 months, or if there are concerns about observation or compliance with therapy at home. Those with complicated pneumonia (pleural effusion, empyema, abscess, or extrapulmonary infection) or suspected/documented pathogen with increased virulence are also likely to require hospitalization and further interventions.

Hypersensitivity Pneumonitis

Hypersensitivity pneumonitis, or extrinsic allergic alveolitis, results from the inhalation of organic dust particles. Although numerous causes have been identified, the clinical features of the various types of hypersensitivity pneumonitis are similar and depend on the intensity and frequency of exposure to the allergen; both acute and chronic forms have been described.

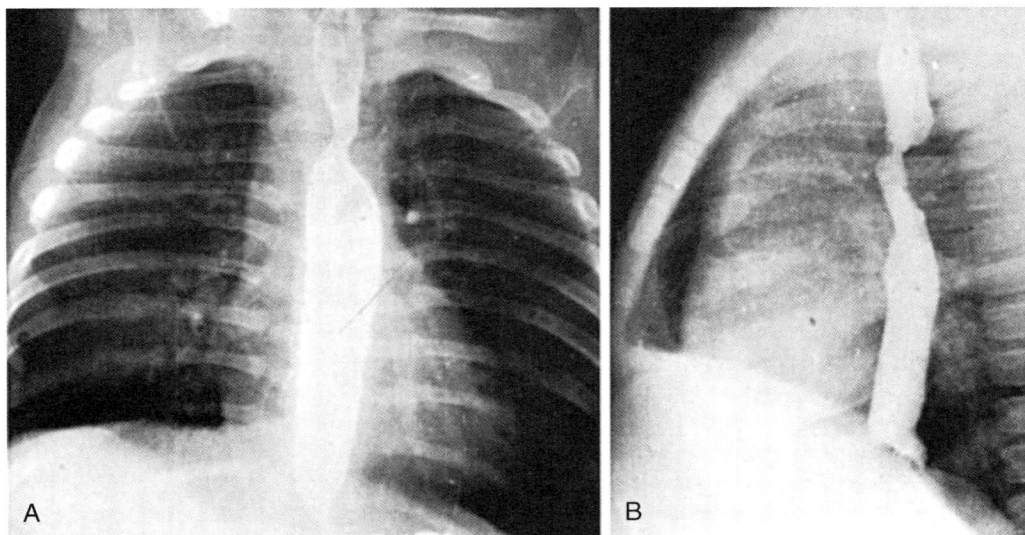

Fig. 4.12 Double aortic arch in an infant aged 5 months. *A,* Anteroposterior view. The barium-filled esophagus is constricted on both sides. *B,* Lateral view. The esophagus is displaced forward. The anterior arch was the smaller and was divided at surgery. (From Bernstein D. Other congenital heart and vascular malformations. In Kliegman RM, St. Geme JW III, Blum NJ, et al., eds. *Nelson Textbook of Pediatrics.* 21st ed. Philadelphia: Elsevier; 2020:2422, Fig. 459.2.)

TABLE 4.12	**Etiologic Agents of Pneumonia Grouped by Age of the Patient**
Age Group	**Frequent Pathogens (in Order of Frequency)**
Neonates (<3 wk)	Group B streptococcus, *Escherichia coli,* other gram-negative bacilli, *Streptococcus pneumoniae, Haemophilus influenzae* (type b,* nontypable), herpes simplex
3 wk–3 mo	Respiratory syncytial virus, other respiratory viruses (rhinoviruses, parainfluenza viruses, influenza viruses, adenovirus, coronavirus), *S. pneumoniae, H. influenzae* (type b,* nontypable); if patient is afebrile, consider *Chlamydia trachomatis*
4 mo–4 yr	Respiratory syncytial virus, other respiratory viruses (rhinoviruses, parainfluenza viruses, influenza viruses, adenovirus, coronavirus), *S. pneumoniae, H. influenzae* (type b,* nontypable), *Mycoplasma pneumoniae,* group A streptococcus
≥5 yr	*M. pneumoniae, S. pneumoniae, Chlamydophila pneumoniae, H. influenzae* (type b,* nontypable), influenza viruses, adenovirus, coronaviruses, other respiratory viruses, *Legionella pneumophila*

* H. influenzae type b is uncommon with routine *H. influenzae* immunization.
From Kelly MS, Sandora TJ. Community acquired pneumonia. In: Kliegman RM, St. Geme JW III, Blum NJ, et al., eds. *Nelson Textbook of Pediatrics.* 21st ed. Philadelphia: Elsevier; 2020.

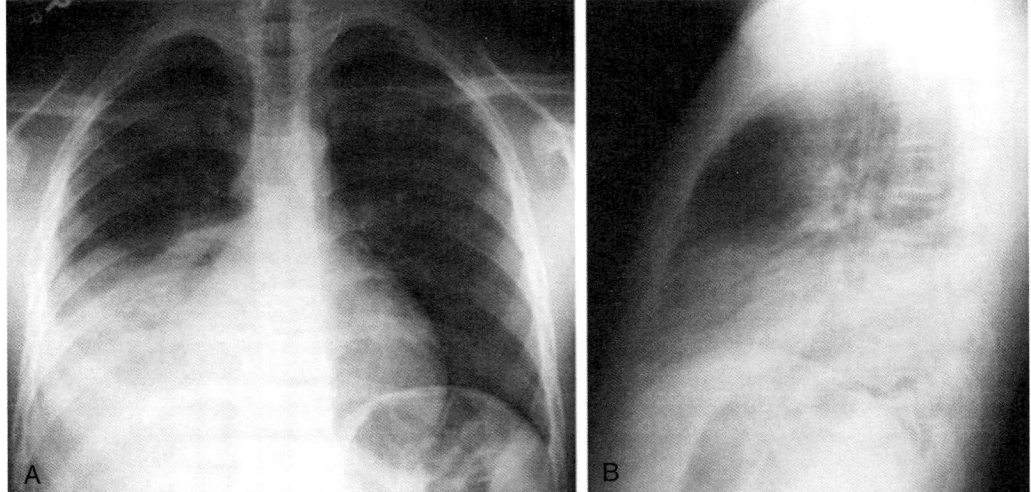

Fig. 4.13 Radiographic findings characteristic of pneumococcal pneumonia in a 14-year-old boy with cough and fever. Posteroanterior *(A)* and lateral *(B)* chest radiographs reveal consolidation in the right lower lobe, strongly suggesting bacterial lobar pneumonia. (From Kelly MS, Sandora TJ. Community acquired pneumonia. In Kliegman RM, St. Geme JW III, Blum NJ, et al., eds. *Nelson Textbook of Pediatrics.* 21st ed. Philadelphia: Elsevier; 2020: Fig. 428.3.)

TABLE 4.13   Classification of Interstitial Lung Disease (Pediatric Diffuse Lung Disease)*

I. Disorders More Prevalent in Infancy	II. Disorders Not Specific to Infancy

A. Diffuse developmental disorders
  1. Acinar dysplasia
  2. Congenital alveolar dysplasia
  3. Alveolar–capillary dysplasia with pulmonary vein misalignment
B. Growth abnormalities
  1. Pulmonary hypoplasia
  2. Chronic neonatal lung disease
C. Prematurity-related chronic lung disease (bronchopulmonary dysplasia)
D. Acquired chronic lung disease in term infants
E. Structural pulmonary changes with chromosomal abnormalities
  1. Trisomy 21
F. Others
  1. Associated with congenital heart disease in chromosomally normal children
G. Specific conditions of undefined etiology
  1. Pulmonary interstitial glycogenosis
  2. Neuroendocrine cell hyperplasia of infancy
H. Surfactant dysfunction mutations and related disorders
  1. *SPFTB* pathologic genetic or gene variants—PAP and variant dominant histologic pattern
  2. *SPFTC* pathologic genetic or gene variants—CPI dominant histologic pattern; also DIP and NSIP
  3. *ABCA3* pathologic genetic or gene variants—PAP variant dominant pattern; also CPI, DIP, NSIP
  4. Others with histology consistent with surfactant dysfunction disorder without a yet recognized genetic disorder
	A. Disorders of the normal host
	  1. Infectious and postinfectious processes
	  2. Disorders related to environmental agents: hypersensitivity pneumonia, toxic inhalation
	  3. Aspiration syndromes
	  4. Eosinophilic pneumonia
	B. Disorders related to systemic disease processes
	  1. Immune-related disorders
	  2. Storage disease
	  3. Sarcoidosis
	  4. Langerhans cell histiocytosis
	  5. Malignant infiltrates
	C. Disorders of the immunocompromised host
	  1. Opportunistic infection
	  2. Disorders related to therapeutic intervention
	  3. Disorders related to transplantation and rejection syndromes
	  4. Diffuse alveolar damage of unknown etiology
	D. Disorders masquerading as interstitial disease
	  1. Arterial hypertensive vasculopathy
	  2. Congestive vasculopathy, including venoocclusive disease
	  3. Lymphatic disorders
	  4. Congestive changes related to cardiac dysfunction
	
	III. Unclassified
	A. Includes end-stage disease, nondiagnostic biopsies, and those with inadequate material

*Many of these entities may present as child interstitial lung disease syndromes.

CPI, chronic pneumonitis of infancy; DIP, desquamative cell interstitial pneumonia; NSIP, nonspecific interstitial pneumonia; PAP, pulmonary alveolar proteinosis.

From Kurland G, Deterding RR, Hagood JS, et al. An official American Thoracic Society clinical practice guideline: classification, evaluation, and management of childhood interstitial lung disease in infancy. *Am J Resp Crit Care Med.* 2013;188:376–394.

In the **acute** form of the disease, the patient typically has fever, rigors, cough, and dyspnea several hours after exposure. The symptoms usually resolve within 24 hours of the onset once the offending material is removed. In the **chronic** or subacute forms of hypersensitivity pneumonitis, the affected individual may have exercise intolerance, anorexia, weight loss, and a productive cough. Diffuse crackles are the prominent finding on physical examination; the patient may be cyanotic if gas exchange is significantly impaired. Digital clubbing is an unusual finding. In acute cases, inflammation of the alveoli and pulmonary interstitium are common reactions, whereas the chronic form can result in interstitial fibrosis and noncaseating granulomas. Chronic hypersensitivity pneumonitis can insidiously lead to respiratory failure and cor pulmonale.

A number of laboratory studies may be helpful in confirming the diagnosis of hypersensitivity pneumonitis. Chest radiograph demonstrates diffuse reticulonodular infiltrate. Pulmonary function studies (spirometry) characteristically show a restrictive defect, and the carbon monoxide diffusion capacity is reduced. During the acute phase of the disease, the patient may have a peripheral leukocytosis and eosinophilia. Serologic studies looking for precipitating immunoglobulin G antibodies to specific antigens are useful in identifying the offending agent. However, these antibodies may be found in asymptomatic individuals exposed to the allergen, and thus their presence is not necessarily correlated with severity of pulmonary disease. Percutaneous or intradermal tests may also be useful, particularly if an avian hypersensitivity pneumonitis is suspected.

Removal of the specific organic dust from the patient's environment is critical to treatment. Mild episodes of hypersensitivity pneumonitis may resolve spontaneously once the offending allergen is eliminated. Severe exacerbations often necessitate treatment with systemic corticosteroids; bronchodilators may be beneficial if the patient is experiencing symptoms of bronchospasm. Hypersensitivity pneumonitis must be differentiated from other causes of interstitial or diffuse lung disease (Table 4.13).

Allergic Bronchopulmonary Aspergillosis

Allergic bronchopulmonary aspergillosis (ABPA) is an immunologic disorder identified in patients with chronic lung disease, in which airway colonization (but not invasive infection) with *Aspergillus fumigatus* causes chronic antigen exposure and increased bronchial hyperactivity. This condition can lead to bronchiectasis, pulmonary fibrosis, and progressive respiratory insufficiency. Hypersensitivity to other fungal species that produces a clinical picture similar to that of ABPA has been reported.

It is important that the diagnosis of ABPA be made and that appropriate therapy with systemic corticosteroids be instituted, because this condition can result in irreversible lung damage. ABPA is characterized by fever, weight loss, wheezing, and productive cough yielding purulent or rust-colored sputum. This condition should be considered in patients with chronic or atypical and progressive or frequently relapsing lung diseases, such as asthma or cystic fibrosis, who have undergone clinical deterioration. In developing countries, it is often misdiagnosed as pulmonary tuberculosis. ABPA is associated with peripheral eosinophilia and markedly elevated serum IgE levels. Although these laboratory findings are not pathognomonic for this condition, the presence of a normal serum IgE makes the diagnosis of active disease unlikely. Affected individuals have evidence of hypersensitivity to *A. fumigatus*, and sputum evaluation may demonstrate *Aspergillus* hyphal elements. Elevated levels of specific IgE and immunoglobulin G antibodies to *A. fumigatus* can be useful in establishing the diagnosis.

The typical chest radiographic findings include increased bronchopulmonary markings, opacification of the affected area, and localized pulmonary consolidation. Linear radiolucencies and parallel markings radiating from the hilum ("tram lines") caused by dilated, thickened bronchi may also be present. Chest CT may demonstrate bronchiectasis, mucoid impaction, and pleuropulmonary fibrosis. The treatment of choice is systemic corticosteroids, administered for weeks to months. Antifungal agents, such as itraconazole, may be effective in preventing exacerbations, but are not helpful in treating acute exacerbations; therefore, these may be a helpful adjunctive therapy.

Other Causes of Respiratory Distress

Aspiration of Oropharyngeal Contents

Central nervous system or neuromuscular disease in infants and children can result in dysfunction of the swallowing mechanism, leading to repeated episodes of pulmonary aspiration. Aspiration is the most common cause of respiratory distress in such children and typically manifests with intractable wheezing, chronic airway inflammation, and recurrent pneumonias.

Video fluoroscopic swallow studies, in which barium mixed with foods of a variety of textures and consistencies are fed to a child under direct visualization and fluoroscopy, can be useful in making the diagnosis and establishing that the child has an abnormal swallowing mechanism. These studies can be helpful with regard to therapy and may determine the appropriate feeding techniques, food consistencies, and feeding volumes that are less likely to cause aspiration in a vulnerable child.

Nasogastric tube or gastrostomy tube feedings may be necessary in children who do not respond to conservative management and who continue to have repeated episodes of aspiration. Nevertheless, the affected child can continue to have periodic aspiration of oropharyngeal secretions despite these interventions. A Nissan fundoplication or jejunostomy tube may be needed to reduce the incidence of gastric aspiration.

Gastroesophageal Reflux

Gastroesophageal reflux can be a primary cause of or an exacerbating factor in wheezing in infants and young children (see Chapter 15). Direct inhalation of stomach contents into the lungs can produce bronchospasm and a chemical pneumonitis. Gastroesophageal reflux with aspiration has also been implicated in cases of bacterial pneumonia, bronchiectasis, obliterative bronchiolitis, and lung abscesses. Tachypnea, wheezing, and cough are the usual clinical findings, typically occurring within 1 hour of the aspiration event. The signs and symptoms of the pneumonitis, however, can be delayed.

Although pulmonary aspiration of gastric contents was once assumed to be the basis of reflux-induced wheezing, reflex bronchoconstriction in response to esophageal acidification can also produce bronchospasm in some patients. Other respiratory symptoms associated with gastroesophageal reflux, such as stridor and obstructive apnea, can manifest as the result of reflex laryngospasm. Gastroesophageal reflux can also complicate and worsen underlying lung diseases, such as asthma or subglottic stenosis, by provoking bronchospasm and potentiating airway or laryngeal inflammation and possibly bronchial hyperactivity.

Pneumothorax

A pneumothorax occurs when air leaks from the alveoli or airways into the pleural space. The most common cause of pneumothorax in children is chest wall trauma. Children with asthma or other underlying chest disease may also develop a pneumothorax. However, spontaneous pneumothorax can occur in otherwise healthy children with no antecedent illness or injury, most commonly adolescent males or young adult men who are tall, thin, and athletic (Fig. 4.14). In patients with an acute pneumothorax with no history of trauma or asthma, the presence of Marfan or Ehlers-Danlos syndromes should be considered. Familial autosomal dominant pneumothorax may be a forme fruste of **Birt-Hogg-Dube syndrome** due to pathologic variants in the *FLCN* gene. Clinical presentation usually includes acute onset of dyspnea and chest or shoulder pain. The physical examination reveals hyperresonance to percussion over the ipsilateral chest, with decreased breath sounds auscultated on the affected side. If the air dissects up through the mediastinum, it may escape into the subcutaneous tissues, producing subcutaneous emphysema. Diagnosis can be confirmed by chest radiograph. Progressive air leak without air escape can lead to a tension pneumothorax. With increasing pressure, there is mediastinal shift, airway compression, and a decrease in cardiac output. Tension pneumothorax can be life-threatening if it is not recognized and treated rapidly. Small, spontaneous pneumothoraces will often resolve with supportive care and supplemental oxygen. The treatment of choice for a pneumothorax of greater than 20% volume is drainage with needle aspiration or with an indwelling chest tube.

Pneumomediastinum

Pneumomediastinum is the presence of air or other gas in the mediastinum and is characterized as either traumatic or spontaneous. Blunt or penetrating trauma to the chest or iatrogenic (i.e., during surgical procedures) can cause a traumatic pneumomediastinum. Spontaneous pneumomediastinum can be either primary, where there is no underlying airway/lung condition that would predispose an individual to an air leak, or secondary, where a predisposition is from an underlying airway/lung condition such as asthma or cystic fibrosis. In general, spontaneous pneumomediastinum is uncommon in pediatrics; however, it should be kept in the differential in children presenting with sudden chest pain or shortness of breath.

Cystic Fibrosis

Cystic fibrosis is a multisystem disorder that involves the eccrine and mucous secretory glands. Inherited as an autosomal recessive trait, cystic fibrosis is the most common life-shortening genetic disease in Caucasian children of northern European ancestry and is an important cause of chronic suppurative lung disease (see Chapter 3). Chronic infection and inflammation lead to the weakening and destruction of the airway wall, which results in bronchiectasis, the abnormal dilatation of the subsegmental airways, and in pulmonary abscesses. The pulmonary deterioration characteristic of cystic fibrosis is rather insidious and is characterized

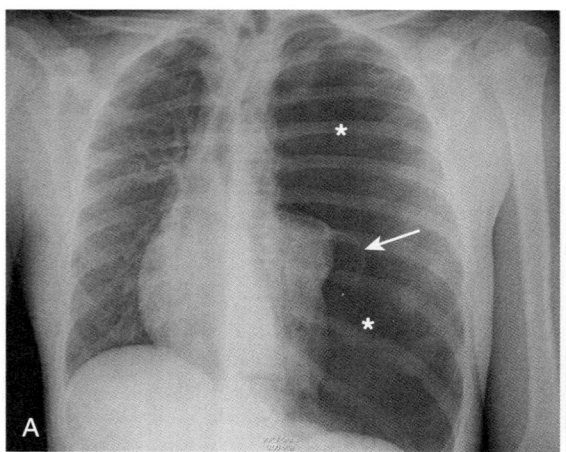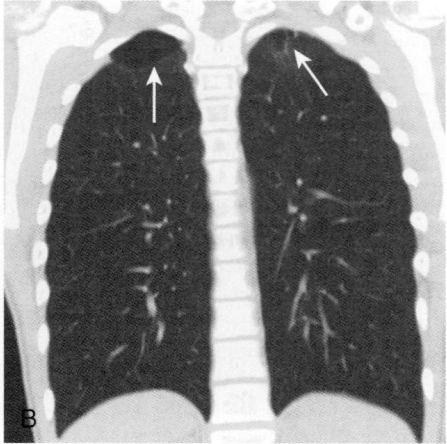

Fig. 4.14 Spontaneous pneumothorax in a tall, thin teenager presenting with tachypnea, tachycardia, and normal blood pressure. *A,* Frontal chest radiograph shows a large pneumothorax occupying the entire left hemithorax *(asterisks),* with a mild cardiomediastinal shift to the right. A bleb is noted along the surface of the collapsed left lung *(arrow). B,* Coronal CT image obtained 1 month after thoracostomy tube removal shows biapical blebs *(arrows),* which are larger on the right. The right apical bleb was not seen on the chest radiographs. (From Coley BD, ed. *Caffey's Pediatric Diagnostic Imaging.* 13th ed. Philadelphia: Elsevier; 2019:585, Fig. 60.6.)

by increasing airway obstruction over a period of years. However, some infants and children with cystic fibrosis can present in acute respiratory distress because of pneumonia, empyema, or pneumothorax.

Primary Ciliary Dyskinesia

Primary ciliary dyskinesia (PCD), another progressive lung disease (ciliopathy), occurs in approximately 1 in 16,000 children and is the result of ultrastructural abnormalities of the cilia (see Chapter 3). The absence of dynein arms (inner and outer) is the most common form of the syndrome, but other structural abnormalities can result in decreased or absent ciliary movement. Acquired ciliary dyskinesia may be caused by a number of different environmental and infectious agents and is usually a temporary condition. The abnormal mucociliary clearance of endobronchial secretions causes a chronic bronchitis. Wheezing is a common clinical manifestation resulting from the obstruction of the airways by mucus. Neonatal tachypnea is the earliest manifestation. Repeated or persistent severe upper respiratory tract infections, usually in the form of chronic pansinusitis or recurrent suppurative otitis media, are typical. Male sterility resulting from the impaired movement of spermatozoa is also present. Although Kartagener initially described several patients with *situs inversus totalis,* chronic sinusitis, and bronchiectasis, dextrocardia is present in only 50% of patients with this syndrome.

Arriving at a diagnosis necessitates a high index of suspicion and warrants pursuit in the child with recurrent wheezing, bronchitis, sinusitis, and otitis media. Findings on chest radiographs are generally nonspecific, and frequently demonstrate areas of pulmonary consolidation. Extensive atelectasis with significant respiratory distress has been described in neonates with this condition. Bronchiectasis is a late sequela of dyskinetic cilia syndrome. Functional assays for mucociliary clearance or examination of nasal or tracheal epithelial cells for ultrastructural ciliary defects with electron microscopy is necessary to establish a diagnosis. Exhaled nitric oxide fraction (FeNO) is very low in PCD. Genetic testing is also available for the ~30 etiologic genes; nonetheless, ~50% have no identifiable pathologic gene variant. Most cases are inherited as autosomal recessives; however, autosomal dominant and X-linked inheritance have been reported.

Hemoptysis

Hemoptysis is the expectoration of blood or blood-tinged sputum and is a rare finding in pediatric patients. First, one must differentiate if the blood is from the airway or an extrapulmonary source. Oral or nasopharyngeal causes as well as hematemesis from the gastrointestinal tract can present similarly. The most common cause of hemoptysis in pediatrics is lower respiratory infections like pneumonia or tracheobronchitis—most of which cases are mild and self-limiting. Foreign body aspiration where the bleeding is caused from mechanical injury to the airway is the second most likely etiology of hemoptysis in children. Other potential etiologies that can lead to severe hemoptysis and respiratory compromise include vascular abnormalities, interstitial or granulomatous lung disease resulting in diffuse alveolar hemorrhage, or pulmonary hemosiderosis (Table 4.14). A CBC to help quantify the amount of blood lost as well as look for thrombocytopenia is important in these cases. Inflammatory markers and coagulation studies can also be useful. A plain chest radiograph is normal in 33–55% of patients, but can be helpful to evaluate for a foreign body or signs of infection. CT scanning with contrast angiography can assist in finding vascular abnormalities. Acute hemorrhage on CT scan will appear as focal consolidation with surrounding ground-glass appearance. Ultimately, bronchoscopy is indicated if a foreign body is suspected, the etiology remains unknown, or respiratory compromise is occurring. Specifically, rigid bronchoscopy allows visualization of the airway as well as potential therapy for the etiology—injection of hemostatic agents, tamponading of a lesion if necessary—while providing a way for mechanical ventilation.

Electronic Cigarette, or Vaping, Product Use–Associated Lung Injury

The use of electronic cigarettes (e-cigarettes), also known as vaping, where a battery-powered device produces aerosol for inhaling, has been associated with respiratory distress. These devices are commonly used for inhaling nicotine and/or tetrahydrocannabinol

(THC). The syndrome is named e-cigarette, or vaping, use–associated lung injury (EVALI). A diagnosis of EVALI should be suspected in any patient with a history of using e-cigarette or vaping products within the prior 3 months presenting with shortness of breath, cough, respiratory distress, myalgias, headaches, or gastrointestinal symptoms like nausea, vomiting, diarrhea, or abdominal pain (Table 4.15). Pulmonary infiltrates are usually noted on chest x-ray but are universally noted on chest CT. The typical CT findings include lower lobe "crazy paving" consisting of ground-glass opacities (GGOs) combined with thickened interlobular septa and subpleural sparing. In addition, there may be ground-glass nodules and consolidation (Figs. 4.15 and 4.16). Although alternative diagnoses need to be excluded, it is important to note that influenza, COVID-19, or other respiratory infections cannot be readily distinguished from EVALI by signs, symptoms, presentation, or imaging. The inhalation injury that has been seen associated with e-cigarettes/vaping includes exacerbation of asthma, hypersensitivity pneumonitis, eosinophilic pneumonia, lipoid pneumonia, and diffuse alveolar hemorrhage. The severity of the illness ranges from minimal or no respiratory support to the need for invasive mechanical ventilation, extracorporeal membrane oxygenation (ECMO), and death. Vitamin E acetate, an additive in some of the THC-containing e-cigarette/vaping products, is strongly linked to EVALI. Systemic glucocorticoids provide patients with clinical improvement. Treating any concurrent or possible other infections, connecting patients with services for cessation of e-cigarette/vaping products, and close follow-up are also necessary. Figure 4.17 shows the clinical algorithm for patients hospitalized with suspected EVALI.

COVID-19

Severe acute respiratory syndrome–associated coronavirus 2 (SARS-CoV-2) produces a broad spectrum of presentations and manifestations within the COVID-19 (coronavirus disease 2019) pandemic. Many pediatric patients are asymptomatic or minimally symptomatic, while others develop various degrees of pulmonary symptoms: *mild-moderate* (mild pneumonia), *severe* (dyspnea, hypoxia, or >50% lung involvement on imaging), and *critical* (respiratory failure, shock, or multiorgan system dysfunction) often in the context of the multisystem inflammatory syndrome in children (MIS-C) (Table 4.16) (see Chapter 53). The case definition for other presentations of COVID-19 is noted in Table 4.17. The presentation may depend on the stage of the illness (Fig. 4.18). Early systemic features include fever, cough, headache, myalgias, and gastrointestinal manifestations (abdominal pain, emesis, and diarrhea). In patients with a pulmonary presentation, COVID-19 pneumonia presents with cough, dyspnea, cyanosis, and fever. Chest x-rays are usually abnormal, and CT imaging demonstrates the "crazy paving" pattern predominantly with bilateral multifocal GGOs or a combination of GGOs with consolidation usually of the lower lobes with a subpleural predominance (Figs. 4.19 and 4.20). The differential diagnosis of COVID-19 pneumonia includes other causes of acute respiratory distress syndrome, pneumocystis or adenovirus pneumonia, EVALI, hypersensitivity pneumonia, granulomatosis with polyangiitis, Lemierre disease, and acute or chronic interstitial lung disease in childhood. The diagnosis is confirmed by nasopharyngeal PCR viral testing (usually in the acute COVID pneumonia syndrome) or by immunoglobulin M and immunoglobulin G antibodies to COVID-19 (usually the later inflammatory MIS-C).

TABLE 4.14 Etiology of Pulmonary Hemorrhage (Hemoptysis)
Focal Hemorrhage
Bronchitis and bronchiectasis (especially cystic fibrosis related)
Infection (acute or chronic), pneumonia, abscess
Tuberculosis
Trauma
Pulmonary arteriovenous malformation (with or without hereditary hemorrhagic telangiectasia)
Foreign body (chronic)
Neoplasm including hemangioma
Pulmonary embolus with or without infarction
Bronchogenic cysts
Diffuse Hemorrhage
Idiopathic of infancy
Congenital heart disease (including pulmonary hypertension, venoocclusive disease, congestive heart failure)
Prematurity
Cow's milk hyperreactivity (Heiner syndrome)
Goodpasture syndrome
Collagen vascular diseases (systemic lupus erythematosus, rheumatoid arthritis)
Henoch-Schönlein purpura and vasculitic disorders
Granulomatous disease (granulomatosis with polyangiitis)
Celiac disease
Coagulopathy (congenital or acquired)
Malignancy
Immunodeficiency
Exogenous toxins, especially inhaled
Hyperammonemia
Pulmonary hypertension
Pulmonary alveolar proteinosis
Idiopathic pulmonary hemosiderosis
Tuberous sclerosis
Lymphangiomyomatosis or lymphangioleiomyomatosis
Physical injury or abuse
Catamenial

From Kliegman RM, St. Geme JW III, Blum NJ, et al., eds. *Nelson Textbook of Pediatrics*. 21st ed. Philadelphia: Elsevier; 2020:2313, Table 436.4.

NONPULMONARY CAUSES OF RESPIRATORY DISTRESS

Cardiac

Cardiac disease is an important and common nonpulmonary cause of respiratory distress. Increased work of breathing and respiratory distress most commonly occur in cardiac diseases caused by large left-to-right shunts, dysfunction of the systemic ventricle, and vascular lesions that obstruct the airway (see Chapter 9). Cardiac failure from any cause is often manifested as respiratory distress. Infants with congenital heart defects that produce a large left-to-right shunt that results in pulmonary vascular engorgement, edema formation, and reduced lung compliance demonstrate tachypnea, dyspnea, and grunting. Wheezing or "cardiac asthma" can occur when there is compression of intrathoracic airways by vascular engorgement and interstitial edema. With most

TABLE 4.15   CDC Surveillance Case Definitions* for Severe Pulmonary Disease Associated with E-cigarette Use (August 30, 2019)

Case Classification	Criteria
Confirmed	Using an e-cigarette ("vaping") or dabbing[†] during the 90 days before symptom onset
	AND
	Pulmonary infiltrate, such as opacities on plain film chest radiograph or ground-glass opacities on chest computed tomography
	AND
	Absence of pulmonary infection on initial work-up: Minimum criteria include negative respiratory viral panel influenza polymerase chain reaction or rapid test if local epidemiology supports testing. All other clinically indicated respiratory infectious disease testing (e.g., urine antigen for *Streptococcus pneumoniae* and *Legionella*, sputum culture if productive cough, bronchoalveolar lavage culture if done, blood culture, HIV-related opportunistic respiratory infections if appropriate) must be negative
	AND
	No evidence in medical record of alternative plausible diagnoses (e.g., cardiac, rheumatologic, or neoplastic process)
Probable	Using an e-cigarette ("vaping") or dabbing[†] in 90 days before symptom onset
	AND
	Pulmonary infiltrate, such as opacities on plain film chest radiograph or ground-glass opacities on chest computed tomography
	AND
	Infection identified via culture or polymerase chain reaction, but clinical team[§] believes this is not the sole cause of the underlying respiratory disease process OR minimum criteria to rule out pulmonary infection not met (testing not performed) and clinical team* believes this is not the sole cause of the underlying respiratory disease process
	AND
	No evidence in medical record of alternative plausible diagnoses (e.g., cardiac, rheumatologic, or neoplastic process)

*These surveillance case definitions are meant for surveillance and not clinical diagnosis; they are subject to change and will be updated as additional information becomes available if needed.
[†]Using an electronic device (e.g., electronic nicotine delivery system [ENDS], electronic cigarette [e-cigarette], vaporizer, vape[s], vape pen, dab pen, or other device) or dabbing to inhale substances (e.g., nicotine, marijuana, tetrahydrocannabinol, tetrahydrocannabinol concentrates, cannabinoids, synthetic cannabinoids, flavorings, or other substances).
[§]Clinical team caring for the patient.
From Schier JG, Meiman JG, Layden J, et al. Severe pulmonary disease associated with electronic-cigarette–product use — interim guidance. *MMWR Morb Mortal Wkly Rep.* 2019;68:787–790. https://doi.org/10.15585/mmwr.mm6836e2external icon

congenital heart defects with left-to-right shunts, an abnormal heart murmur and cardiomegaly are prominent clues to the diagnosis. Acute myocarditis, usually of viral etiology, can manifest with tachypnea, dyspnea, grunting, and diaphoresis. The physical examination reveals tachycardia and decreased heart sounds, and chest radiography shows an enlarged heart. Cardiomyopathy may be congenital, may have a metabolic or toxic cause, may be familial, or may be idiopathic. Other causes of cardiac failure, such as severe hypertension, renal failure, and severe anemia, should also be sought. Systemic ventricular failure caused by obstructing lesions, such as aortic stenosis, coarctation of the aorta, or mitral stenosis, also causes increased pulmonary vascular engorgement and edema, which results in the same symptoms as those for a large left-to-right shunt. Depending on the severity of the left ventricular outflow obstruction, systemic blood flow may be decreased, resulting in poor perfusion and metabolic acidosis. If blood flow into the systemic ventricle from the pulmonary veins or left atrium is decreased or obstructed, as in total anomalous pulmonary venous return or mitral stenosis, then severe pulmonary edema, hypoxemia, and respiratory distress ensue. Many of these lesions manifest early in infancy. Tachypnea, wheezing, cyanosis,

and metabolic acidosis are typical presenting signs. Accurate diagnosis depends on echocardiography; cardiac catheterization may be needed in complex cases.

Neurologic

Children with certain primary neurologic disorders, such as increased intracranial pressure or neuromyopathic weakness, may present in respiratory distress. Common symptoms include irregular respirations, hypoventilation, and hyperventilation. These symptoms, accompanied by an altered mental status, should prompt an evaluation of the central nervous system for problems such as meningitis, cerebritis or encephalitis, intracranial hemorrhage, mass lesion, or toxic ingestion.

Other

Metabolic derangement that results in acidosis can produce tachypnea and possible dyspnea. Common causes of acidosis include diabetic ketoacidosis, sepsis, and ingestions (such as aspirin). The presence of multisystem involvement in addition to respiratory distress should lead to arterial blood gas determination, urinalysis, and possibly a toxicology screen.

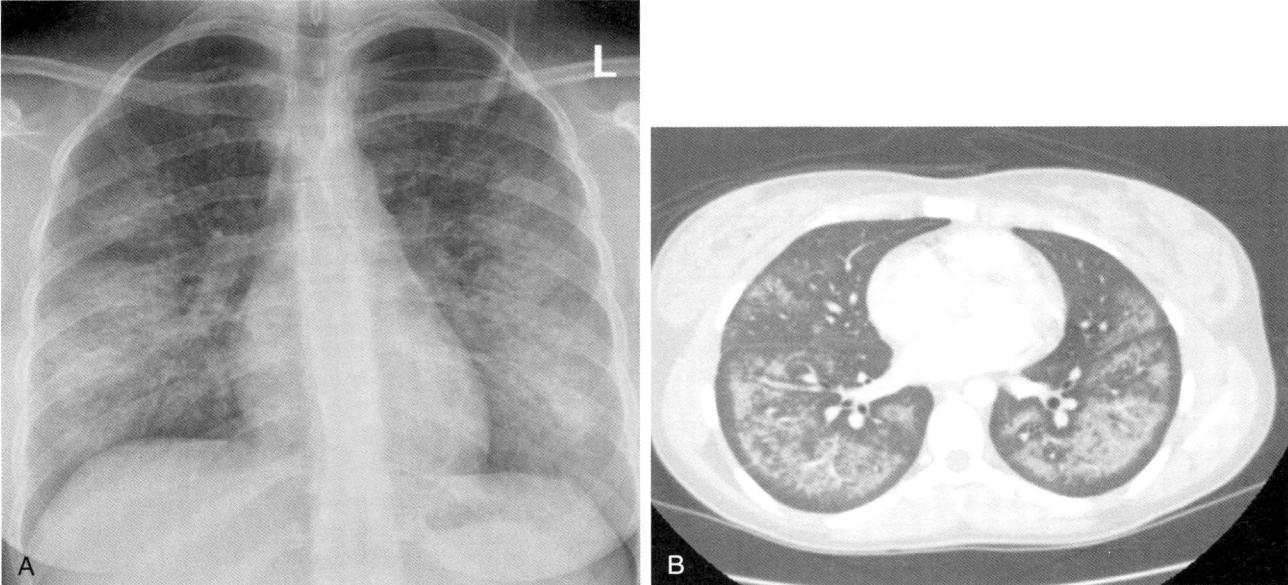

Fig. 4.15 *A,* Chest x-ray of a patient with *E-cigarette or Vaping-product associated lung injury* showing significant bilateral alveolar opacities. *B,* CT scans in axial view showing bilateral ground-glass opacities and dependent consolidations with a subpleural sparing pattern. (From Cherian SV, Kumar A, Estrada-Y-Martin RM. E-Cigarette or Vaping Product-Associated Lung Injury: A Review. *Am J Med.* 2020;133:657–663. Fig. 2.)

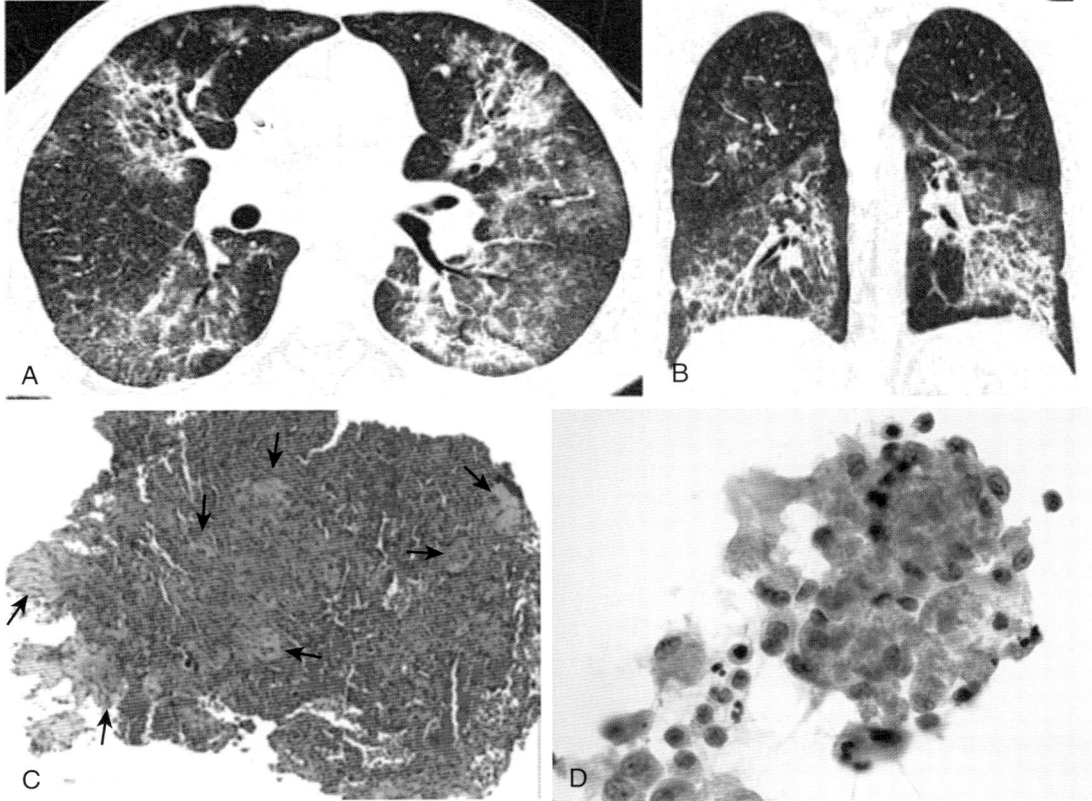

Fig. 4.16 *A–B,* Axial and coronal images of a high-resolution CT chest scan significant for diffuse mid- and lower zone predominant airspace abnormalities comprising ground-glass opacities and consolidation. *C,* Transbronchial biopsy with organizing pneumonia, characterized by numerous airspace plugs of fibromyxoid tissue *(arrows)* (hematoxylin and eosin stain, original magnification ×150). *D,* Scant acute inflammatory cells and associated pulmonary macrophages (Papanicolaou stain, original magnification 60×). (From MacMurdo M, Lin C, Saeedan MB, et al. e-Cigarette or Vaping Product Use-Associated Lung Injury: Clinical, Radiologic, and Pathologic Findings of 15 Cases. *Chest.* 2020;157:e181–e187. Fig. 1 A-D, Case 4.)

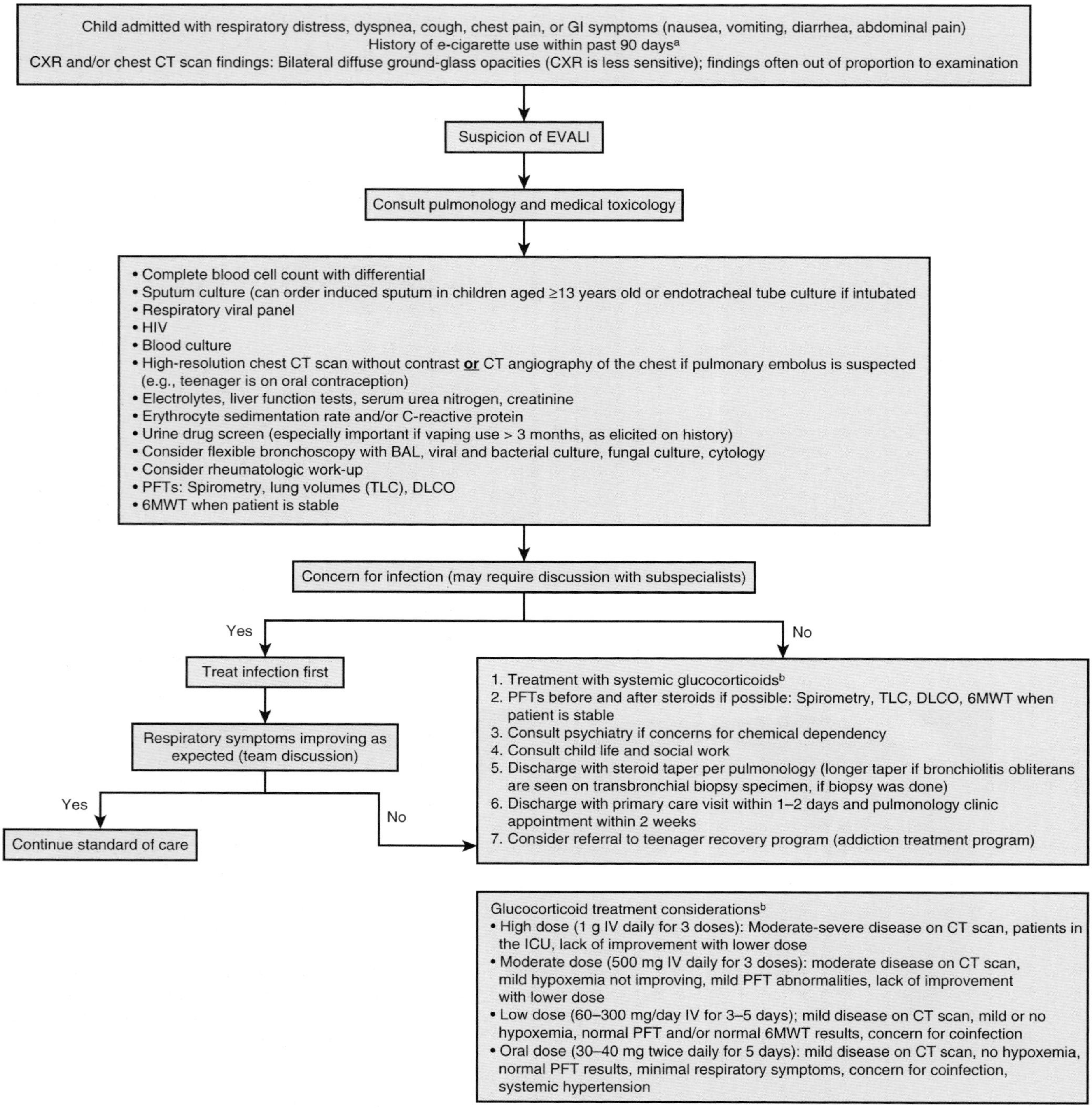

Child admitted with respiratory distress, dyspnea, cough, chest pain, or GI symptoms (nausea, vomiting, diarrhea, abdominal pain)
History of e-cigarette use within past 90 days[a]
CXR and/or chest CT scan findings: Bilateral diffuse ground-glass opacities (CXR is less sensitive); findings often out of proportion to examination

Suspicion of EVALI

Consult pulmonology and medical toxicology

- Complete blood cell count with differential
- Sputum culture (can order induced sputum in children aged ≥13 years old or endotracheal tube culture if intubated
- Respiratory viral panel
- HIV
- Blood culture
- High-resolution chest CT scan without contrast **or** CT angiography of the chest if pulmonary embolus is suspected
  (e.g., teenager is on oral contraception)
- Electrolytes, liver function tests, serum urea nitrogen, creatinine
- Erythrocyte sedimentation rate and/or C-reactive protein
- Urine drug screen (especially important if vaping use > 3 months, as elicited on history)
- Consider flexible bronchoscopy with BAL, viral and bacterial culture, fungal culture, cytology
- Consider rheumatologic work-up
- PFTs: Spirometry, lung volumes (TLC), DLCO
- 6MWT when patient is stable

Concern for infection (may require discussion with subspecialists)

Yes

Treat infection first

No

1. Treatment with systemic glucocorticoids[b]
2. PFTs before and after steroids if possible: Spirometry, TLC, DLCO, 6MWT when patient is stable
3. Consult psychiatry if concerns for chemical dependency
4. Consult child life and social work
5. Discharge with steroid taper per pulmonology (longer taper if bronchiolitis obliterans are seen on transbronchial biopsy specimen, if biopsy was done)
6. Discharge with primary care visit within 1–2 days and pulmonology clinic appointment within 2 weeks
7. Consider referral to teenager recovery program (addiction treatment program)

Respiratory symptoms improving as expected (team discussion)

Yes

No

Continue standard of care

Glucocorticoid treatment considerations[b]
- High dose (1 g IV daily for 3 doses): Moderate-severe disease on CT scan, patients in the ICU, lack of improvement with lower dose
- Moderate dose (500 mg IV daily for 3 doses): moderate disease on CT scan, mild hypoxemia not improving, mild PFT abnormalities, lack of improvement with lower dose
- Low dose (60–300 mg/day IV for 3–5 days); mild disease on CT scan, mild or no hypoxemia, normal PFT and/or normal 6MWT results, concern for coinfection
- Oral dose (30–40 mg twice daily for 5 days): mild disease on CT scan, no hypoxemia, normal PFT results, minimal respiratory symptoms, concern for coinfection, systemic hypertension

Fig. 4.17 Clinical algorithm for pediatric patients hospitalized for suspected electronic cigarette or vaping product use–associated lung injury (EVALI). The algorithm includes U.S. Centers for Disease Control and Prevention (CDC)-based diagnostic criteria, recommended consultations, laboratory work-up and imaging, and recommended treatment and follow-up.[a] May need to speak with peers and family, especially for patients who are intubated. [b]Glucocorticoid dosage considerations. 6MWT, 6-minute walk test; CXR, chest radiography; DLCO, diffusing capacity for carbon monoxide; GI, gastrointestinal; IV, intravenously; PFT, pulmonary function test; TLC, total lung capacity. (From Rao DR, Maple KL, Dettori A, et al. Clinical features of e-cigarette, or vaping, product use-associated lung injury in teenagers. *Pediatrics*. 2020;146[1]:e20194104. https://doi.org/10.1542/peds.2019-4104.)

TABLE 4.16 Case Definition for Multisystem Inflammatory Syndrome in Children (MIS-C)

- An individual aged <21 yr presenting with fever,* laboratory evidence of inflammation,[†] and evidence of clinically severe illness requiring hospitalization, with multisystem (two or more) organ involvement (cardiac, renal, respiratory, hematologic, gastrointestinal, dermatologic, or neurologic); **AND**
- No alternative plausible diagnoses; **AND**
- Positive for current or recent SARS-CoV-2 infection by RT-PCR, serology, or antigen test; or COVID-19 exposure within the 4 wk prior to the onset of symptoms

*Fever >38.0°C for ≥24 hr, or report of subjective fever lasting ≥24 hr.
[†]Including, but not limited to, one or more of the following: an elevated C-reactive protein, erythrocyte sedimentation rate, fibrinogen, procalcitonin, d-dimer, ferritin, lactic acid dehydrogenase, or interleukin 6, elevated neutrophils, reduced lymphocytes, and low albumin.
RT-PCR, reverse transcription polymerase chain reaction.
From Centers for Disease Control and Prevention (https://emergency.cdc.gov/han/2020/han00432.asp).

TABLE 4.17 Clinical Criteria for COVID-19

In the absence of a more likely diagnosis:
- At least two of the following symptoms:
  - Fever (measured or subjective)
  - Chills
  - Rigors
  - Myalgia
  - Headache
  - Sore throat
  - Nausea or vomiting
  - Diarrhea
  - Fatigue
  - Congestion or runny nose

  OR
- Any one of the following symptoms:
  - Cough
  - Shortness of breath
  - Difficulty breathing
  - New olfactory disorder
  - New taste disorder

  OR
- Severe respiratory illness with at least one of the following:
  - Clinical or radiographic evidence of pneumonia
  - Acute respiratory distress syndrome (ARDS)

Laboratory Criteria
Laboratory evidence using a method approved or authorized by the Food and Drug Administration (FDA) or designated authority:

Confirmatory* laboratory evidence:
- Detection of severe acute respiratory syndrome–coronavirus 2 ribonucleic acid (SARS-CoV-2 RNA) in a clinical or an autopsy specimen using a molecular amplification test

Presumptive* laboratory evidence:
- Detection of SARS-CoV-2 by antigen test in a respiratory specimen

Supportive* laboratory evidence:
- Detection of specific antibody in serum, plasma, or whole blood
- Detection of specific antigen by immunocytochemistry in an autopsy specimen

Epidemiologic Linkage
<u>One</u> or more of the following exposures in the prior 14 days:
- Close contact[†] with a confirmed or probable case of COVID-19 disease
- Member of a risk cohort as defined by public health authorities during an outbreak

Criteria to Distinguish a New Case from an Existing Case
A repeat positive test for SARS-CoV-2 RNA using a molecular amplification detection test within 3 mo of the initial report should not be enumerated as a new case for surveillance purposes. To date, there has been minimal evidence of reinfection among persons with a prior confirmed COVID-19 infection and growing evidence that repeat positive RNA tests do not correlate with active infection when viral culture is performed. Similarly, the experience with other coronaviruses is that reinfection is rare within the first year. NOTE: The time period of 3 mo will be extended further when more data become available to show that risk of reinfection remains low within 1 yr of the initial report.

Case Classification
Suspect
- Meets supportive laboratory evidence[‡] with no prior history of being a confirmed or probable case.

Probable
- Meets clinical criteria **AND** epidemiologic linkage with no confirmatory laboratory testing performed for SARS-CoV-2
- Meets presumptive laboratory evidence
- Meets vital records criteria with no confirmatory laboratory evidence for SARS-CoV-2

Confirmed
- Meets confirmatory laboratory evidence

Other Criteria
Vital Records Criteria
- A death certificate that lists COVID-19 disease or SARS-CoV-2 as an underlying cause of death or a significant condition contributing to death.

*The terms confirmatory, presumptive, and supportive are categorical labels used here to standardize case classifications for public health surveillance. The terms should not be used to interpret the utility or validity of any laboratory test methodology.

†Close contact is generally defined as being within 6 feet for at least 15 min. However, it depends on the exposure level and setting; for example, in the setting of an aerosol-generating procedure in health care settings without proper personal protective equipment (PPE), this may be defined as any duration. Data are insufficient to precisely define the duration of exposure that constitutes prolonged exposure and thus a close contact.

‡For suspect cases (positive serology only), jurisdictions may opt to place them in a registry for other epidemiologic analyses or investigate to determine probable or confirmed status.

From Centers for Disease Control and Prevention. Coronavirus disease 2019 (COVID-19): 2020 interim case definition. Approved August 5, 2020. https://wwwn.cdc.gov/nndss/conditions/coronavirus-disease-2019-covid-19/case-definition/2020/08/05/

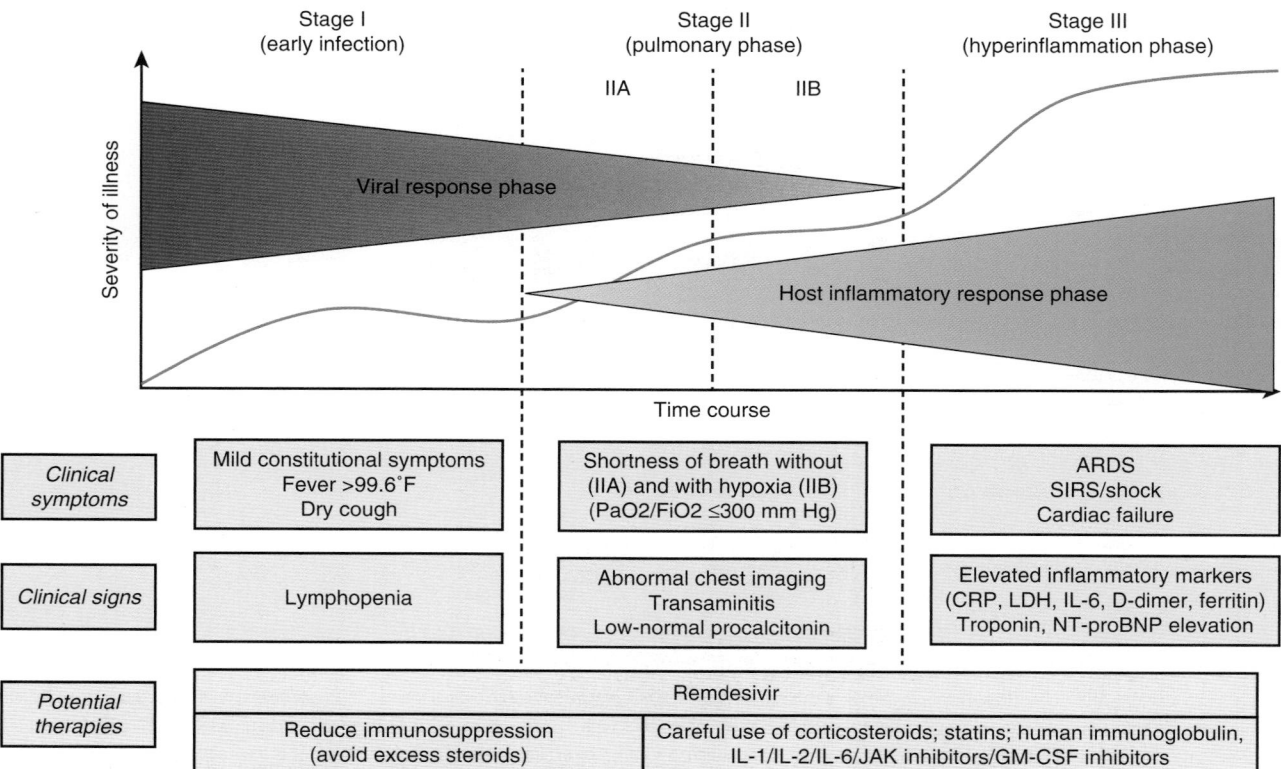

Fig. 4.18 Staging of acute COVID-19 infection. Classification of COVID-19 disease states and potential therapeutic targets. The figure illustrates three escalating phases of COVID-19 disease progression, with associated signs, symptoms, and potential phase-specific therapies. ARDS, acute respiratory distress syndrome; JAK, Janus kinase; LDH, lactate dehydrogenase; NT-proBNP, N-terminal pro B-type natriuretic peptide; SIRS, systemic inflammatory response syndrome; GM-CSF, granulocyte macrophage colony-stimulating factor. (Modified from Siddiqi HK, Mehra MR. COVID-19 illness in native and immunosuppressed states: a clinical-therapeutic staging proposal. *J Heart Lung Transpl.* 2020;39[5]:405–407 [Fig. 1, p. 406].)

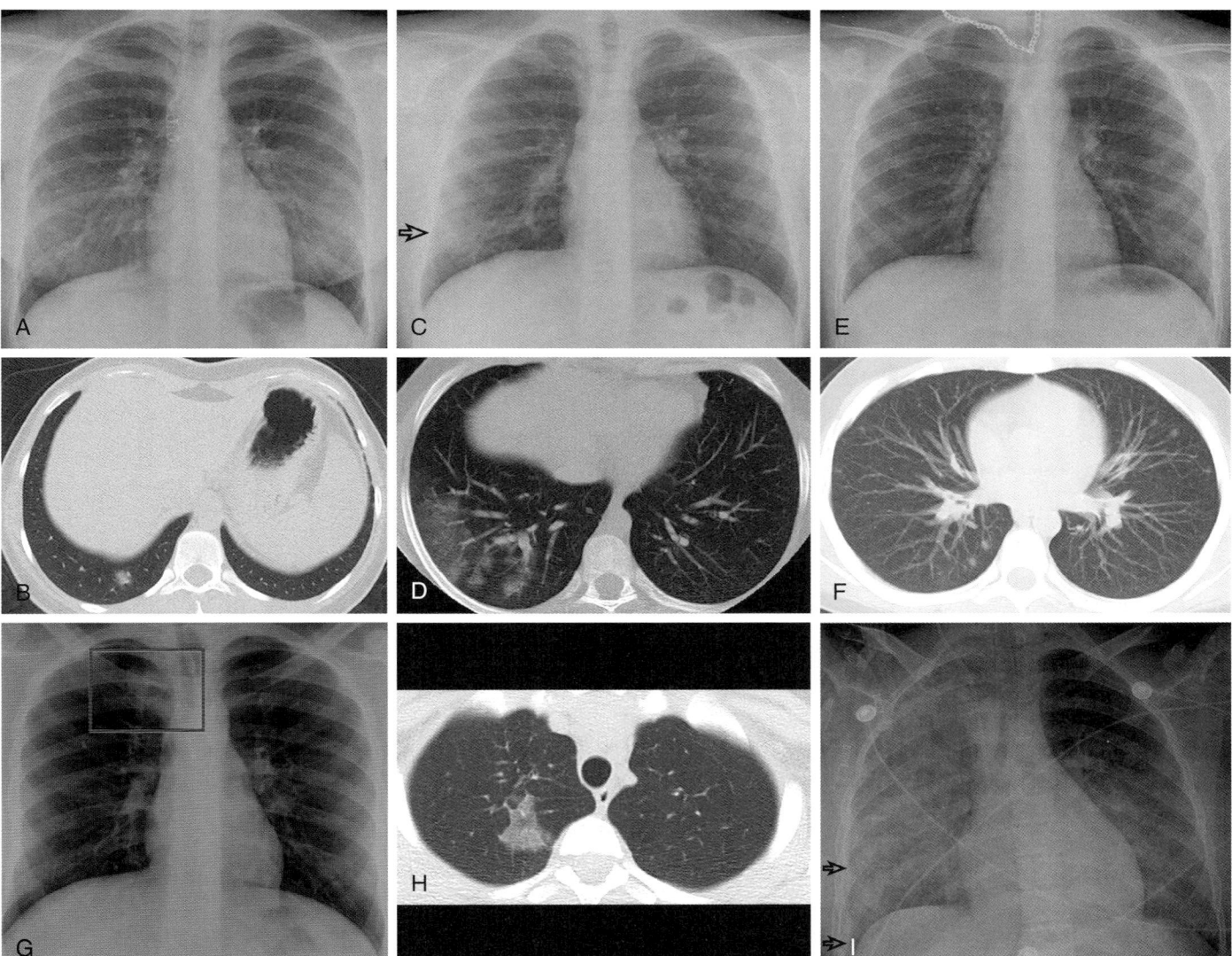

Fig. 4.19 Chest radiography and chest CT findings of children with COVID-19 in conjunction with symptom and time interval between imaging studies. (*A* and *B*) Imaging findings of a 13-year-old female patient with COVID-19. *A,* Posteroanterior chest radiograph of a 13-year-old female patient presented with fever for 2 days. Chest radiography and chest CT images were obtained on the same day. The chest radiography was normal. *B,* Chest CT image in the axial plan revealed a single, peripheral located, ground-glass opacity (GGO) at the posterobasal segment of the right lower lobe. The opacity was obscured with the right liver lobe and diaphragm on chest radiography. (*C* and *D*) Imaging findings of a 10-year-old male patient with COVID-19. *C,* Posteroanterior chest radiograph of a 10-year-old male patient presented with cough and fever for 2 days. Chest radiography and chest CT images were obtained on the same day. The chest radiography revealed peripheral GGO *(arrow)* at the basal segments of the right liver lobe. *D,* Axial section chest CT examination revealed bronchovascular distributed GGOs in a 10-year-old male patient at the periphery of the basal segments of the right lower lobe. (*E* and *F*) Imaging findings of a 13-year-old male patient with COVID-19. *E,* Posteroanterior chest radiograph of a 13-year-old male patient presented with cough and fever for 2 days. Chest radiography and chest CT images were obtained on the same day. The chest radiography was interpreted as normal. *F,* Axial chest CT image of the 13-year-old male patient without contrast demonstrates bilateral, multifocal, peripheral, and perivascular distributed millimetric nodular-shaped GGOs. The opacities were not detected on chest radiography due to the smaller size and lower density. (*G* and *H*) Imaging findings of a 16-year-old female patient with COVID-19. *G,* Posteroanterior chest radiograph of the 16-year-old female patient presented with cough and fever for 3 days. Chest radiography and chest CT images were obtained on the same day. The chest radiography demonstrates paramediastinal GGO at the right upper lobe *(red frame).* *H,* Axial chest CT image of the 16-year-old female patient without contrast demonstrates peripherally distributed GGO at the right upper lobe with an interlobular interstitial thickening. *I,* Anteroposterior chest radiography of an intubated 15-year-old female patient who presented with diarrhea and hypotension on the 4th day of fever demonstrates diffusely distributed GGOs in the right lung in addition to left perihilar and basilar opacities. Right-sided pleural effusion *(arrows)* was also depicted. The patient was diagnosed with multisystem inflammatory syndrome associated with COVID-19, and she was the only patient that resulted in COVID-19–related pediatric death in our clinic. Laboratory examinations revealed lymphopenia (6.64 × 10 9/L), thrombocytopenia (94 × 10 9/L), elevated creatinine (1.24 mg/dL), troponin-T (37.45 pg/mL), PRO-BNP (5578 pg/mL), bilirubin (0.48 mg/dL), alanine transaminase (43.8 (U/L), and C-reactive protein (377 mg/L). (From Bayramoglu Z, Canıpek E, Comert RG, et al. Imaging Features of Pediatric COVID-19 on Chest Radiography and Chest CT: A Retrospective, Single-Center Study. *Acad Radiol.* 2021;28:18–27. Fig. 1.)

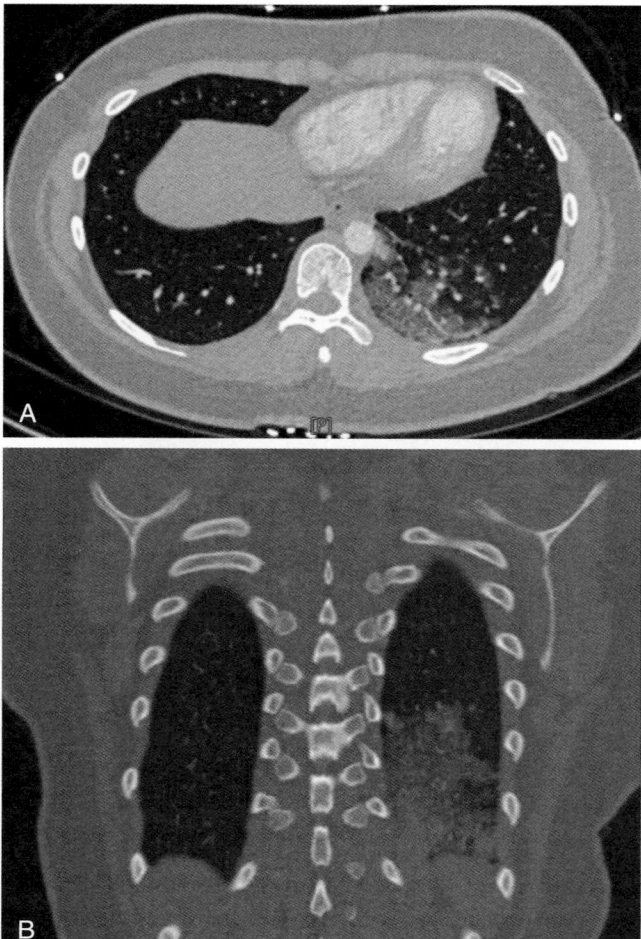

Fig. 4.20 Axial *(A)* and coronal *(B)* contrast enhanced chest CT in a 16-year-old female with cough, fever, and tachycardia, who was COVID-19 positive. The images show geographic ground-glass opacities with septal thickening (crazy paving) in the left lower lobe, with increased density near the diaphragm. (From Romberg EK, Menashe SJ, Kronman MP, et al. Pediatric radiologic manifestations of COVID-19. *Clin Imaging.* 2021;75:165–170. Fig. 6.)

SUMMARY AND RED FLAGS

Respiratory distress may be a result of disorders of the extrathoracic or intrathoracic airways (intrinsic or extrinsic compression-obstruction), alveoli, pulmonary vasculature, pleural spaces, or thorax. The distress may be secondary to pulmonary, cardiovascular, hematologic, or central nervous system diseases. The most important aspect of the evaluation of a child with respiratory distress is observation of the child's breathing pattern and a brief, directed history and physical examination. Laboratory testing, imaging studies and/or endoscopy may be required. Once the cause is identified, treatment should be started quickly to avoid progression to respiratory failure.

Red flags for impending respiratory failure include cyanosis, dyspnea as well as sudden onset of distress (epiglottitis, foreign body aspiration), hemoptysis, severe retractions, lethargy, a sitting up–leaning forward posture, dysphagia, drooling, and aphonia. It is imperative to identify the symptoms of impending respiratory failure (decreased mental status, cyanosis) and not delay treatment with unnecessary clinical or radiologic studies. It is also important not to miss a foreign body, which with time may produce chronic respiratory disease that is often confused with pneumonia or asthma.

Signs of a more chronic process include lack of resolution with normal therapy, chronicity of symptoms, positive family history, digital clubbing, weight loss, and/or failure to thrive. These signs should prompt further work-up and consultation with a pulmonary specialist as needed. Asthma will rarely cause digital clubbing, so its presence should raise concern for another underlying primary lung disease process.

BIBLIOGRAPHY

A bibliography is available at ExpertConsult.com.

5

Earache

Brittany Player

Earache (otalgia) is pain that arises from a pathologic process in the external, middle, or inner ear or that is referred to the ear from another structure. Acute otitis media (AOM) is the most common cause of otalgia in children (Table 5.1). At least 80% of children will experience one or more episodes of AOM in the first 3 years of life. The second most common cause of ear pain is otitis externa, followed by dermatitis and infections of the pinna (Table 5.2). Other causes of otalgia are rare (Table 5.3). A careful examination of the pinna, external auditory canal, and tympanic membrane can identify most causes of ear pain. When the findings are normal, referred pain should be considered (Table 5.4).

HISTORY

Older, verbal children with ear pain are often able to localize and accurately describe their symptoms. Younger children often cannot localize their pain and may present with a variety of nonspecific symptoms, including fever, irritability, emesis, rhinorrhea from an associated upper respiratory tract illness (URI), and ear rubbing or pulling. *Even though ear pulling is associated with ear pain, it is neither specific nor sensitive in the diagnosis of ear disease.* In addition, infants with AOM may occasionally be afebrile and present with various degrees of irritability, such as sleep disturbances and/or eating or drinking inadequately. Ear disease should be considered in infants during the first year of life or in any preschool child with fever, irritability, or a URI.

In taking a history from a child who presents with ear pain, true ear pain must be distinguished from the sensation of fullness and discomfort that children experience when they have an effusion or retracted tympanic membrane secondary to a dysfunctional eustachian tube. The clinician should review the child's history for factors placing the child at risk for infection such as craniofacial abnormalities (e.g., cleft palate), immunodeficiencies, autoimmune disease, diabetes, previous ear infections, placement of tympanostomy tubes, and recent dental procedures, trauma, and air travel. Immunization status should also be reviewed. A careful review of systems should elicit associated fevers, sore throat, reflux symptoms, otorrhea, neurologic symptoms, and symptoms of sinusitis. Children with a middle ear effusion may have decreased hearing acuity.

Acute otitis media presents with abrupt onset of otalgia associated with middle ear fluid, signs and symptoms of inflammation, and local or systemic infection. Risk factors for AOM include a family or personal history of recurrent AOM, trisomy 21, household cigarette smoke exposure, lack of breast-feeding, lower socioeconomic status, males, cleft palate, immunodeficiency, and group daycare attendance or siblings in the household. Children with **otitis externa** ("swimmer's ear") present with either ear pain, purulent otorrhea, or both as well as ear fullness, localized ear pain with mastication, and ear itching. **Relapsing polychondritis** is a rare multisystemic inflammatory disorder that targets cartilaginous structures throughout the body. If the external ears are involved, symptoms may include episodic swelling and redness of the pinnae that is usually bilateral and recurrent. Other cartilaginous structures are often affected, though if findings are unilateral and subtle, the disorder may mimic otitis externa and the diagnosis may remain elusive until symptoms recur. With referred ear pain, such as from tooth decay or teething, there are often additional symptoms associated with the respective head and neck structures (see Table 5.4). Patients with ear pain secondary to maxillary sinusitis may also complain of headaches and purulent rhinorrhea.

PHYSICAL EXAMINATION

In a child presenting with a chief complaint of ear pain, the general examination includes the temperature, the respiratory rate, and a determination of whether the infant or child has a toxic appearance. Then the clinician proceeds with the complete head, eyes, ears, nose, oral cavity, and throat examination and with an appropriately focused physical examination of other pertinent systems.

The examination of the ear begins with the less symptomatic ear. The clinician should inspect the pinna and adjacent tissues for dermatitis, redness, and edema. The mastoid process and the pinna, including its cartilaginous portions, are palpated for any tenderness. Erythema, swelling, and tenderness over the posterior auricular mastoid process suggest **mastoiditis**, whereas localization of these findings to the external auditory canal and the pinna suggests otitis externa. In both conditions, the swelling may be so severe that the pinna is laterally displaced. The opening of the external ear canal is also examined for the presence of discharge or exudate. Manipulating the tragus and pinna causes extreme pain with otitis externa. Most disorders of the external ear can be detected through this examination (see Tables 5.2 and 5.3).

Otoscopy provides an opportunity to indirectly view the middle ear through the tympanic membrane. The middle ear is normally an air-filled cavity that transmits sound from the eardrum to the ossicle and then into the internal ear (Fig. 5.1). Otoscopy begins by properly positioning and, if necessary, gently restraining the patient. Both shoulders and hips need to be stabilized so that the patient cannot roll during the examination. Infants are best examined on an examining table in the prone position, with a parent or an attendant firmly holding the patient's shoulders, thus preventing the patient from moving. Toddlers should sit on a parent's lap, with the examiner sitting in a chair opposite them. The child is held against the parent's chest, with one of the parent's hands and arms holding the child's arms and the other around the child's head so that one ear is exposed. To avoid trauma with movement, the otoscope should be held in the examiner's hand making direct contact with the patient's head, allowing the otoscope to move with the head.

TABLE 5.1   Differential Diagnosis of Painful Middle Ear Disorders

Disorder	Clinical Features
Acute otitis media	Immobile tympanic membrane that may appear bulging, red, and/or opaque
Bullous myringitis	Hemorrhagic or serous bullae on the tympanic membrane; more severe pain than acute otitis media
Mastoiditis	Tenderness and erythema over mastoid with periostitis process; no destruction of bone trabeculae
Acute mastoid osteitis	Destruction of bone trabeculae; tenderness and erythema over mastoid process coupled with outward displacement of pinna
Granulomatosis	Severe necrotizing vasculitis; ulcerative and destructive granulomatous lesions of upper and lower respiratory tract with polyangiitis
Langerhans cell histiocytosis	Pituitary dysfunction, exophthalmos, seborrheic dermatitis, and bone lesions; if bone lesions involve the ear, patient presents with mastoid tenderness and otorrhea

TABLE 5.2   Differential Diagnoses of Painful External Ear and Auditory Canal Disorders

Disorder	Clinical Features
Acute otitis externa	Diffuse redness, swelling, and pain of the canal with greenish to whitish exudate; often very tender pinna
Necrotizing (malignant) otitis externa (± skull base osteomyelitis)	Rapidly progressive, severe swelling and redness of pinna; pinna may be laterally displaced; risk factors include diabetes mellitus, congenital or acquired immunodeficiency, severe neutropenia
Dermatitis	
Eczema	History of atopy, presence of lesions elsewhere; lesions are scaly, red, pruritic, and weeping
Contact	History of cosmetic use or irritant exposure; lesions are scaly, red, pruritic, and weeping
Seborrhea	Scaly, red, papular dermatitis; scalp may have thick, yellow scales
Psoriasis	History or presence of psoriasis elsewhere; erythematous papules that coalesce into thick, white plaques
Cellulitis	Diffuse redness, tenderness, and swelling of the pinna
Furuncles	Red, tender papules in areas with hair follicles (distal third of the ear canal)
Infected periauricular cyst	Discrete, palpable lesions; history of previous swelling at same site; cellulitis may develop, obscuring cystic structure
Insect bites	History of exposure; lesions are red, tender papules
Herpes zoster oticus	Painful, vesicular lesions in the ear canal and tympanic membrane, hearing loss, vestibulitis; with addition of seventh cranial nerve palsy—Ramsay Hunt syndrome
Perichondritis	Inflammation of the cartilage, usually secondary to cellulitis
Relapsing polychondritis	Recurrent episodes, involves other cartilage sites (nose)
Granulomatosis with polyangiitis	Fever, weight loss, respiratory and/or renal manifestations
Tumors including Langerhans cell histiocytosis	Palpable mass, destruction of surrounding structures
Foreign body	Foreign body may cause secondary trauma to the ear canal or become a nidus for an infection of the ear canal
Trauma	Bruising and swelling of external ear; there may be signs of basilar skull fracture (cerebrospinal fluid otorrhea, hemotympanum)

Cerumen (ear wax) is a waxy substance consisting of glandular discharge from cells in the outer external canal mixing with exfoliated epithelial cells. Cerumen can both obscure visualization of the eardrum leading to diagnostic errors and be a cause of otalgia if impaction occurs. To view the eardrum properly, the examiner should remove the wax by irrigating the ear canal gently with lukewarm water, lifting the wax out with a blunt curette, or dissolving the wax by placing 1–2 drops of docusate sodium liquid in the canal for 10–15 minutes. Contraindications for irrigation or use of a cerumenolytic solution are the presence of a tympanostomy tube, a perforated tympanic membrane, or an organic foreign body (e.g., legumes swell in contact with fluids).

During the insertion of the speculum, the clinician should note any redness, edema, tenderness, exudate, furuncles, or vesicles that may be present in the external auditory canal. In some illnesses such as otitis externa, the ear canal may be so edematous that the speculum cannot be inserted, and the eardrum cannot be seen. In addition, in neonates and in some children with craniofacial anomalies such as trisomy 21 or Goldenhar syndrome, the external canal may be so small that it precludes an accurate assessment of the tympanic membrane.

Pneumatic otoscopy allows evaluation of the tympanic membrane's mobility. Because it is more accurate than otoscopy alone in detecting middle ear effusion, pneumatic otoscopy should be part of every ear examination. In performing pneumatic otoscopy, the examiner should select a speculum that fits snugly in the external auditory canal. The examiner then partially depresses the rubber bulb of the pneumatic otoscope and inserts the otoscope into the ear canal (Fig. 5.2). Once the eardrum is seen, the examiner should observe the color, appearance, position, bony landmarks, and mobility of the tympanic membrane (Table 5.5 and Fig. 5.3). If the eardrum is not perforated, the clinician observes its mobility by alternating positive and negative pressure by gently depressing and releasing the bulb of the pneumatic otoscope. Poor mobility of the eardrum may be secondary to middle ear effusion, a perforated tympanic membrane, or lack of an airtight seal (Fig. 5.4).

In neonates and young infants, the eardrum is less perpendicular to the observer, the bony landmarks are less distinct, and the eardrum is less mobile than in older infants and children. Failure to appreciate these normal otoscopic findings may lead to the overdiagnosis of middle ear effusion.

In the first few hours of AOM, the middle ear cavity may not yet be filled with fluid, and the mobility may be normal. By the time the patient is examined, though, the middle ear is usually filled with fluid, and the eardrum is opaque and bulging with decreased mobility (see Fig. 5.4). A reddened eardrum may indicate inflammation of the tympanic membrane (TM), but this physical finding is not specific because crying alone can induce diffuse redness of the eardrum. In addition, differentiation of color is highly variable among observers, which may in part result from the intensity and type of light source used in otoscopy.

TABLE 5.3 Causes of Otalgia and Sources for Referred Pain

Intrinsic	Extrinsic
I. External Ear	**I. Trigeminal Nerve**
External otitis	Dental
Cerumen impaction	Jaw
Foreign body	Temporomandibular joint
Perichondritis	Oral cavity (tongue)
Preauricular cyst or sinus	Infratemporal fossa tumors
Impacted insects	**II. Facial Nerve**
Myringitis	Bell palsy
Trauma	Tumors
Tumor	Herpes zoster
Infection	**III. Glossopharyngeal Nerve**
II. Middle Ear, Eustachian Tube, and Mastoid	Tonsil
Barotrauma	Oropharynx
Middle ear effusion	Nasopharynx
Negative intratympanic pressure (eustachian tube dysfunction)	**IV. Vagus Nerve**
Acute otitis media	Laryngopharynx
Mastoiditis	Esophagus
Gradenigo syndrome (eye pain, otorrhea, cranial nerve VI weakness ± petrositis)	Gastroesophageal reflux
Aditus block	Thyroid
Complication of otitis media	**V. Cervical Nerves**
Tumor	Lymph nodes
Eosinophilic granuloma	Cysts
Granulomatosis with polyangiitis	Cervical spine
	Neck infections
	VI. Miscellaneous
	Migraine
	Neuralgias
	Paranasal sinuses
	Central nervous system
	Drug induced (mesalazine, sulfasalazine)
	Factitious disorder by proxy

From Bluestone CD, Stool SE, Alper CM, et al. *Pediatric Otolaryngology.* 4th ed. Vol 1. Philadelphia: Saunders; 2003:288.

In **otitis media with effusion (OME)**, also known as serous otitis media, the cardinal sign is decreased mobility of the eardrum. The eardrum may be opaque, but not bulging or grossly inflamed (see Fig. 5.5 and Table 5.5). A challenge for the clinician is the child with symptoms consistent with AOM (ear pain) but with the physical findings of OME. In such cases, it is difficult to decide whether there is an acute infection of the middle ear or whether it is OME with an illness at another site causing the symptoms.

When the external ear and tympanic membrane are normal in a child with an earache, the clinician must consider the possibility of referred pain (see Table 5.4). Innervation of the external and middle ear includes pain fibers of the trigeminal, glossopharyngeal, and vagus nerves and, to a lesser extent, the facial nerve and upper cervical nerves. The clinician should examine the neck, parotid gland, thyroid, mouth, tongue, teeth, temporomandibular joint, tonsils, and throat. In children, the cause of referred pain is usually infectious rather than noninfectious (e.g., a tumor).

DIAGNOSTIC TESTS

Bacterial Cultures

Routine cultures of middle or external ear fluid are not required because most infections are self-limited and respond to empiric antimicrobial therapy. In selected instances (e.g., persistent treatment failure, severe pain, an immunocompromised host, a neonate), culture of otorrhea from the external auditory canal or cultures of middle ear fluid by tympanocentesis may guide therapy. In a child with AOM, the offending pathogen is usually also present in the nasopharynx. Unfortunately, nasopharyngeal cultures are not helpful in directing therapy because multiple pathogens are typically isolated, and it is unclear which organism is actually causing the middle ear infection. With the emergence of strains of *Streptococcus pneumoniae* that are resistant to commonly used antibacterials, the incidence of treatment failures may increase. This increasing rate of treatment failure may necessitate a greater reliance on tympanocentesis for culture of middle ear fluid to determine the appropriate antimicrobial agent.

Tympanometry

Tympanometry is an objective, painless method for detecting the presence of middle ear effusion by providing information about tympanic membrane compliance. A soft plastic probe is inserted into the external auditory canal to obtain an airtight seal. The tympanometer measures the flow of sound energy into the middle ear under conditions of changing air pressure. When the air pressure is equal on both sides of an intact eardrum, with the drum in neutral position, the transmission of sound energy through the tympanic membrane is at its maximum. The peak on the tympanogram represents the pressure at which the flow of sound energy is maximal. For example, in a normal air-filled

TABLE 5.4 Causes of Referred Ear Pain

Neck
Cervical lymphadenitis
Infected cervical cysts
Subluxation of the atlantoaxial joint (torticollis and otalgia)

Salivary Glands
Parotitis

Thyroid
Thyroiditis

Teeth and Gums
Dental caries
Dental abscess
Impacted teeth
Gingivitis

Temporomandibular Joint
Temporomandibular disorder
Arthritis, juvenile idiopathic arthritis
Spasm from bruxism or dental malocclusion

Tonsils
Tonsillitis
Peritonsillar abscess
Post-tonsillectomy neuralgia

Pharynx
Pharyngitis

Paranasal Sinuses
Maxillary sinusitis

Other
Herpes zoster (Ramsay Hunt syndrome: postherpetic neuralgia)
Bell palsy
Migraine
Tumors (e.g., of facial nerve)

middle ear cavity, the peak occurs at ambient atmospheric pressure (Fig. 5.6A). With eustachian tube dysfunction (a retracted eardrum but no middle ear effusion), the peak occurs in the negative pressure range on the recording (Fig. 5.6C). With middle ear effusion, the sound energy flowing into the middle ear is reduced, which produces a flat tympanogram (Fig. 5.6B). A flat tympanogram may also result from cerumen, a foreign body, or occlusion of the opening of the probe by the wall of the external auditory canal. In these circumstances, the tympanogram is flat and the estimated volume of the ear canal is lower than anticipated. In a perforated eardrum, the sound energy is readily transmitted through the hole in the drum throughout the entire pressure range, resulting in a flat tympanogram with a higher-than-anticipated ear canal volume.

The use of tympanometry can be limited by patient age and cooperation with testing, cerumen impaction, and the skill of the individual performing the testing. When performed by experts, tympanometry and pneumatic otoscopy have equivalent sensitivity (approximately 90%) and specificity (70–80%). Tympanometry is neither more accurate nor more convenient than is properly performed pneumatic otoscopy. Some tympanometers do not perform well in infants younger than 6 months of age. Tympanometry is advantageous if the clinician is unsure of the otoscopic findings. *Tympanometry can only indicate presence of middle ear effusion but cannot distinguish between AOM and OME.*

Acoustic Reflectometry

Acoustic reflectometers are used to detect middle ear effusion. The device directs sonar-like sound waves of varying frequency toward the tympanic membrane and measures the intensity of reflected sound. This hand-held instrument is similar in size to an otoscope. The tip of the reflectometer is inserted into the ear canal. In contrast to tympanometry, an airtight seal is not required. The frequency of maximal reflected sound depends on the distance of the probe from the eardrum. Middle ear effusion is detected not by the frequency but by the magnitude of maximal reflected sound. When middle ear effusion is present, reflectance is increased in comparison with that in the air-filled middle ear.

Improvements in technology have been made such that reflectometry includes spectral gradient analysis. Reflectometry is easily learned, quick, convenient, and useful in a crying child. It has a lower sensitivity and specificity than properly performed pneumatic otoscopy in detecting middle ear effusion. Because the accuracy of current models decreases in infants younger than 1 year, this technique should not be used in infants younger than 6 months of age. Like tympanometry, reflectometry can reveal only whether middle ear effusion is present and cannot reveal whether the effusion is secondary to AOM or OME. Reflectometry is useful if otoscopic findings are indeterminate.

Diagnostic Imaging

Radiologic techniques are rarely required in the evaluation of external or middle ear disease, but may be useful in the assessment of intratemporal and intracranial complications of otitis media or mastoiditis. Opacification of the normally aerated mastoid air cells is usually seen in AOM because the mastoid air cells communicate with the middle ear space. By definition, this is **acute mastoiditis**; however, this opacification resolves concomitantly with the successful treatment of AOM. In contrast, in *acute mastoid osteitis*, also called acute coalescent mastoiditis, there is destruction of bone trabeculations in the mastoid air cells. CT scan is the preferred imaging modality to aid in this diagnosis. Imaging studies can be useful in evaluating a patient for other intracranial complications of AOM. CT scans of the head can evaluate for suspected cholesteatomas. MRI should be used for diagnosing intracranial mass lesions (e.g., brain abscess) and soft tissue sequelae of infection, while magnetic resonance venography may identify dural sinus thrombosis.

DIFFERENTIAL DIAGNOSIS

Most disorders of the external and middle ear are readily apparent after the examination of the ear (see Tables 5.1 to 5.3). If examination findings are unremarkable, the clinician should consider referred pain (see Table 5.4). Most cases of otitis media are uncomplicated; however, the clinician should be alert to the complications and sequelae of AOM (Table 5.6).

OTITIS EXTERNA

Otitis externa is mainly an inflammation of the external ear canal with or without involvement of the pinna or tympanic membrane, typically secondary to acute bacterial infection. Excessive moisture may cause small abrasions in the protective lipid layer of skin in the external canal, making it vulnerable to infection by normal external

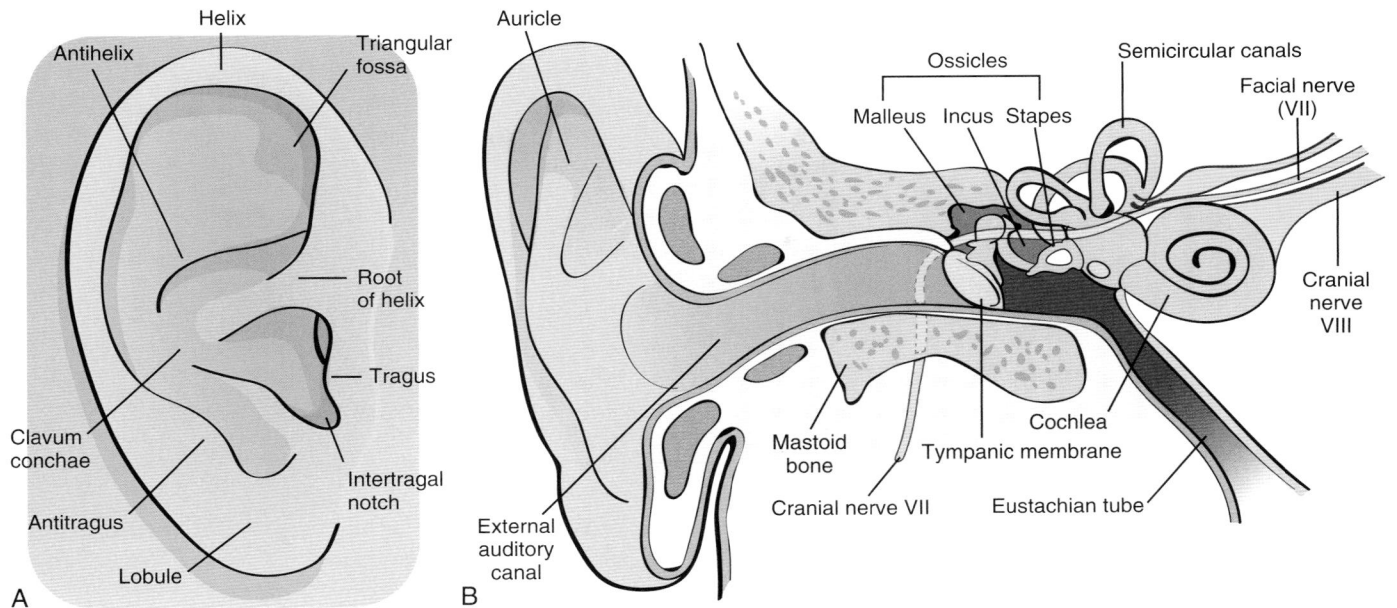

Fig. 5.1 Anatomy of the ear. *A,* A normal external ear (auricle or pinna) is shown, with its various landmarks labeled. It is helpful to refer to such a diagram in assessing congenital anomalies. *B,* This coronal section shows the various structures of the hearing and vestibular apparatus. The three main regions are the external ear, middle ear, and inner ear. The eustachian tube connects the middle ear and the nasopharynx and serves to drain and ventilate the middle ear. (From Yellon R, Chi D. Otolaryngology. In: Zitelli B, ed. *Atlas of Pediatric Physical Diagnosis.* 7th ed. Philadelphia: Elsevier; 2018:869.)

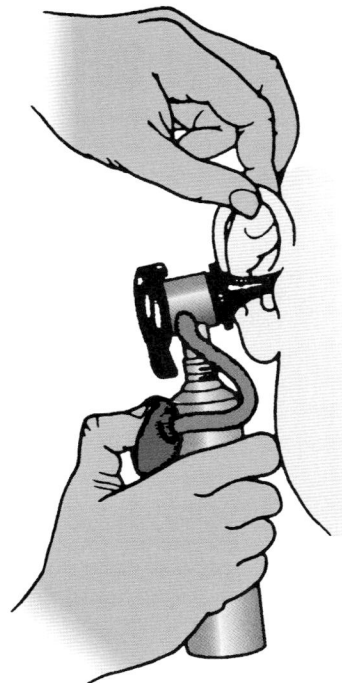

Fig. 5.2 Technique for pneumatic otoscopy. (From Bluestone CD, Klein JO. *Otitis Media in Infants and Children.* 2nd ed. Philadelphia: WB Saunders; 1995:92.)

ear flora or pathogenic bacteria. Dryness or presence of underlying skin conditions (such as eczema) and trauma (including cotton ear swabs) can also predispose the external canal to infection. Less commonly, otorrhea draining from a perforated tympanic membrane secondary to otitis media may cause otitis externa. Cerumen has protective effects by decreasing the pH, thereby inhibiting infection; removal of cerumen alters this pH, leaving the canal vulnerable. Additionally, cerumen impaction can trap water and bacteria in the external canal, leading to infection.

The presenting symptoms are often rapid onset of intense pain (especially with manipulation of the pinna, pressure on the tragus, or jaw movement), erythema, and otorrhea. On physical examination, the ear canal will be red, edematous, and tender. Occasionally, the edema and pain may be so severe as to prevent complete examination of the entire canal and tympanic membrane. Otorrhea may be present in the external canal. While otitis externa can occur at all ages, occurrence peaks between 7 and 12 years of age, with 10% of people having an episode in their lifetime. Otitis externa is rarely bilateral in nature.

Pseudomonas aeruginosa is the predominant organism causing otitis externa and is isolated in up to 60% of microbiologically confirmed cases, but staphylococcal (*Staphylococcus aureus* and coagulase-negative staphylococci) and streptococcal species have been isolated. Gram-negative organisms, such as *Enterobacter, Proteus,* and *Klebsiella* species, and fungal organisms, such as *Candida* and *Aspergillus* species, have also been isolated.

Treatment consists of a topical suspension, commonly ofloxacin or ciprofloxacin combined with hydrocortisone or dexamethasone. The addition of the topical steroid is associated with improvement in pain. Most patients respond within a few days. If there is marked edema of the canal, antibacterials may not reach the site of infection. In this case, the canal should be cleaned with gentle suction, and a cotton wick should be inserted into the auditory canal. Antibacterial suspension is then dripped into the wick, which allows the medication to diffuse farther into the ear canal. In some cases, daily cleaning and replacement of the wick are necessary. If the infection progresses and/or the patient has associated fever and lymphadenitis, the patient may need oral or

Characteristic	Normal Findings	Acute Otitis Media	Otitis Media with Effusion	Comments
Color	Gray to pink	Often red from inflammation; yellow to white from purulent fluid behind tympanic membrane	Usually gray to pink, but may still be yellow or white; not red	Interobserver variation of color is high; redness can occur from crying alone
Appearance	Translucent	Opaque	Translucent or opaque	Opacity is caused by opaque fluid or by scarring of tympanic membrane
Position	Neutral	Fluid under pressure produces bulging of tympanic membrane; bony landmarks may be distorted and the light reflex lost	Not bulging; may be retracted	
Mobility	Tympanic membrane moves freely	Mobility to positive and negative pressure reduced	Mobility to positive and negative pressure reduced	
Other findings		Perforation with otorrhea		

TABLE 5.5   The Tympanic Membrane in Acute Otitis Media and Otitis Media with Effusion

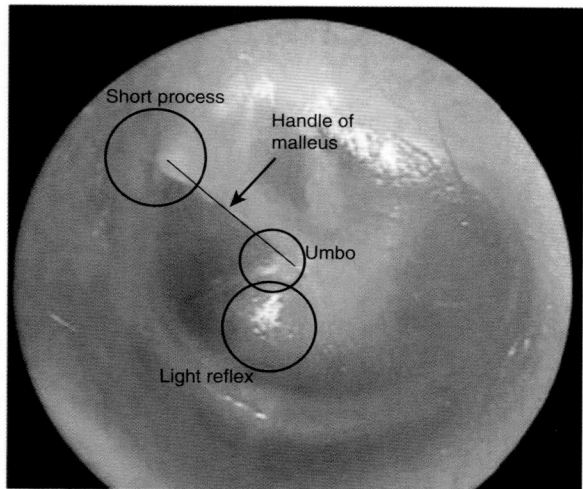

Fig. 5.3 Normal tympanic membrane with normal landmarks identified. (From Cherry JD, Harrison GJ, Kaplan SL, et al., eds. *Feigin and Cherry's Textbook of Pediatric Infectious Diseases.* 8th ed. Philadelphia: Elsevier; 2019:154, Fig. 16.7.)

parenteral antimicrobials and consultation with an otolaryngologist. Prevention should be aimed at keeping the ear canal dry and maintaining healthy skin within the canal.

Chondritis is a potential complication of severe otitis externa and occurs when the infection progresses into the cartilaginous structures of the ear canal. This complication is rare without a history of previous trauma (including ear piercing) or surgery. The most common pathogens are *Pseudomonas* and *S. aureus.* Treatment requires systemic antibacterials, removal of foreign bodies such as earrings, and, if necessary, surgical debridement of tissue.

Furunculosis is an infection of a hair follicle in the outer third of the external ear that can mimic acute external otitis. The causative organism is typically *S. aureus.* Symptoms include a focal area of erythema, swelling, and pain. Draining the abscess and antistaphylococcal antibiotics provide appropriate treatment.

NECROTIZING (MALIGNANT) OTITIS EXTERNA

Necrotizing otitis externa is an extension of infection to the temporal bone and skull base causing extensive tissue destruction (skull base osteomyelitis). The illness may result in chondritis and osteitis of both

the middle and inner ears. This condition is rare in pediatrics, occurring primarily in neutropenic or other immunocompromised patients. In adults, diabetes mellitus is a common predisposing condition, though it is not a common comorbidity in children with diabetes. Presenting symptoms include a markedly swollen and laterally displaced pinna associated with fever, malaise, and persistent, deep-seated otalgia out of proportion to findings on examination. Occasionally, facial nerve paralysis, vertigo, and sensorineural hearing loss may be noted. Diagnosis is supported by radiologic imaging, including CT scan and MRI, which help to characterize the anatomic extent of disease as well as the soft tissue and bone involvement. Aggressive treatment with broad-spectrum parenteral antibiotics is indicated. *P. aeruginosa* is the most commonly isolated pathogen, and coverage should include antibacterials directed against it. Other, less commonly isolated organisms include *Klebsiella* species, *S. aureus, Staphylococcus epididymis,* and *Aspergillus.* Surgical intervention may be necessary to obtain cultures for therapy guidance and provide local tissue debridement.

ACUTE OTITIS MEDIA

Acute otitis media is most commonly a bacterial complication of a preceding or concurrent viral URI, usually occurring several days after the onset of the URI. The viral infection enables pathogenic bacteria in the nasopharynx to ascend through the eustachian tube into the middle ear either by impairing local host defenses or by eustachian tube dysfunction. The bacterial pathogens then cause a secondary infection.

A diagnosis of AOM should be made in children presenting with the following:

- Moderate to severe bulging of the TM or new onset of otorrhea not due to acute otitis externa
- Mild bulging of the TM and recent (<48 hours) onset of significant TM erythema or ear pain (Fig. 5.7; see Table 5.5)

Erythema of the TM is not specific and therefore should be considered a characteristic of AOM only if associated with bulging of the TM.

Microbiology

The leading bacterial pathogens isolated from middle ear fluid in children with AOM are *S. pneumoniae,* nontypable *Haemophilus influenzae,* and *Moraxella catarrhalis. S. aureus* and group A streptococci are uncommon pathogens, though *S. aureus* should be considered in patients with persistent otorrhea after tympanostomy tube placement. In the first month of life (especially the first 2 weeks), gram-negative enteric bacteria (e.g., *Escherichia coli, Klebsiella pneumoniae*) or group B streptococcus may also be isolated. Otitis media associated with an

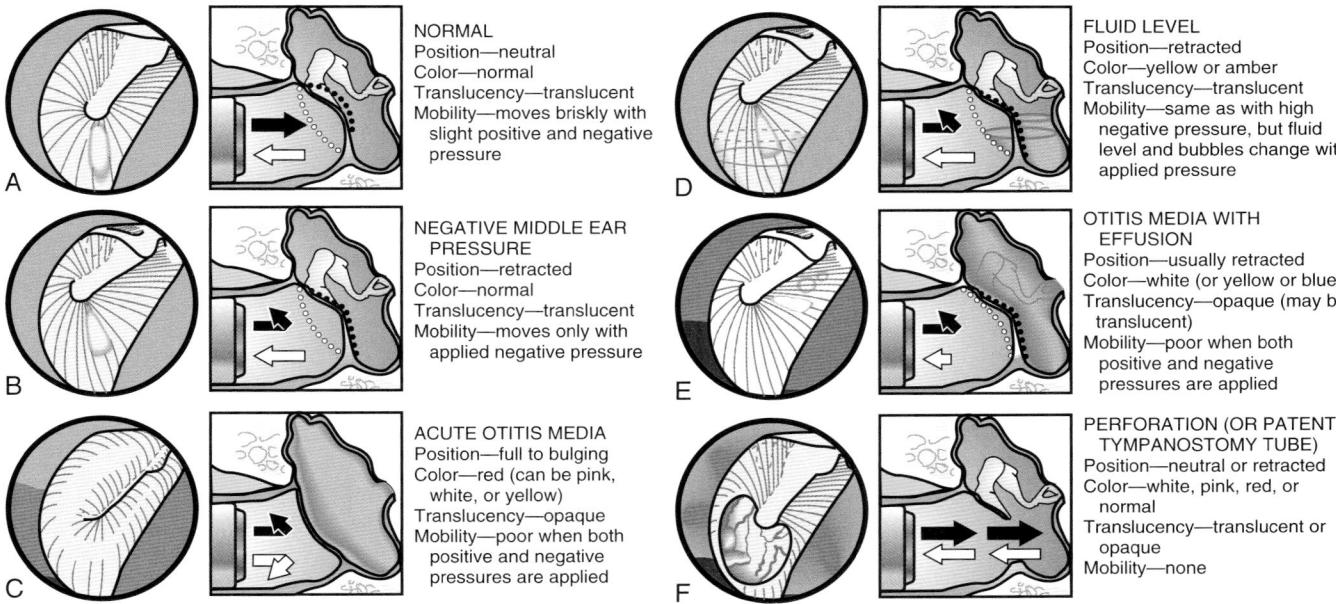

Fig. 5.4 *A–F*, Common conditions of the middle ear, as assessed with the otoscope. (From Bluestone C, Klein J. *Otitis Media in Infants and Children*. 3rd ed. Philadelphia: Saunders; 2001:131.)

NORMAL
Position—neutral
Color—normal
Translucency—translucent
Mobility—moves briskly with slight positive and negative pressure

NEGATIVE MIDDLE EAR PRESSURE
Position—retracted
Color—normal
Translucency—translucent
Mobility—moves only with applied negative pressure

ACUTE OTITIS MEDIA
Position—full to bulging
Color—red (can be pink, white, or yellow)
Translucency—opaque
Mobility—poor when both positive and negative pressures are applied

FLUID LEVEL
Position—retracted
Color—yellow or amber
Translucency—translucent
Mobility—same as with high negative pressure, but fluid level and bubbles change with applied pressure

OTITIS MEDIA WITH EFFUSION
Position—usually retracted
Color—white (or yellow or blue)
Translucency—opaque (may be translucent)
Mobility—poor when both positive and negative pressures are applied

PERFORATION (OR PATENT TYMPANOSTOMY TUBE)
Position—neutral or retracted
Color—white, pink, red, or normal
Translucency—translucent or opaque
Mobility—none

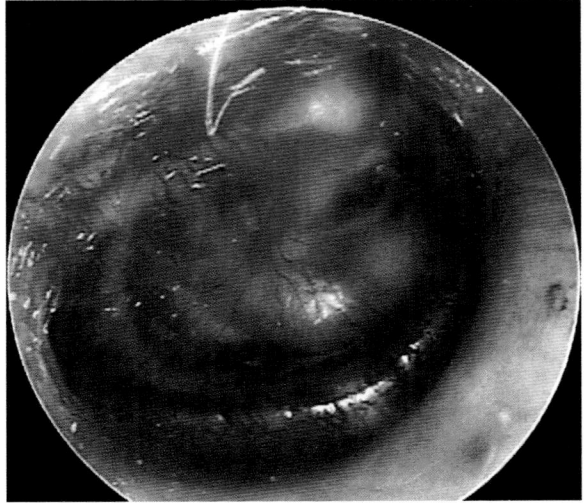

Fig. 5.5 Tympanic membrane in otitis media with effusion. (From Kerschner J, Preciado D. Otitis media. In: Kliegman RM, St. Geme JW III, Blum NJ, et al., eds. *Textbook of Pediatrics*. 21st ed. Philadelphia: Elsevier; 2020:3421.)

erythematous ipsilateral conjunctivitis with purulent exudate is often caused by nontypable *H. influenzae*.

The pneumococcal conjugate vaccine (PCV) 7 was introduced in 2000, covering serotypes 4, 6B, 9V, 14, 18C, 19F, and 23F of *S. pneumoniae*. Widespread use of this vaccine resulted in a 29% reduction in AOM caused by all pneumococcal strains in children prior to 24 months of age. There was also a reduction in tympanostomy tube placement. In the first few years following introduction of PCV7, a shift from *S. pneumoniae* to nontypable *H. influenzae* as the leading pathogen causing AOM was noted. Shortly thereafter, there was a shift to non-PCV7 *S. pneumoniae* isolates as the primary pathogen of AOM, including multiresistant serotype 19A, which was responsible for more cases of AOM and for more severe and invasive infections. Licensing and widespread use of the PCV13 vaccination began in 2010 in the United States, adding coverage for an additional

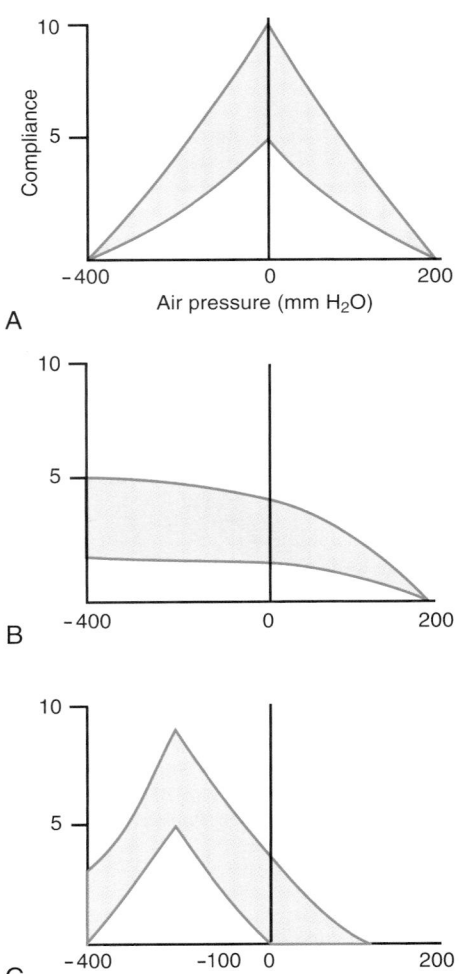

Fig. 5.6 *A*, A normal tympanogram with a peak at atmospheric pressure, indicating an air-filled middle ear with normal (atmospheric) pressure. *B*, A "flat" tympanogram, indicating middle ear effusion. *C*, A tympanogram with a negative peak pressure, indicating eustachian tube obstruction.

TABLE 5.6   Manifestations of the Sequelae and Complications of Otitis Media

Complication	Clinical Features
Acute	
Perforation with otorrhea	Immobile tympanic membrane secondary to visible perforation, exudate in ear canal
Acute mastoiditis with periostitis	Tenderness and erythema over mastoid process, no destruction of bony trabeculae
Acute mastoid osteitis	Destruction of bony trabeculae; tenderness and erythema over mastoid process coupled with outward displacement of pinna
Petrositis	Infection of perilabyrinthine cells; may present with otitis, paralysis of lateral rectus, and ipsilateral orbital or facial pain (Gradenigo syndrome)
Facial nerve palsy	Peripheral cranial nerve VII paralysis
Labyrinthitis	Vertigo, fever, ear pain, nystagmus, hearing loss, tinnitus, nausea and vomiting
Lateral sinus thrombosis	Headache, fever, seizures, altered states of consciousness, septic emboli
Meningitis	Fever, headache, nuchal rigidity, seizures, altered states of consciousness
Extradural empyema	Fever, headache, seizures, altered states of consciousness
Subdural empyema	Fever, headache, seizures, altered states of consciousness
Brain abscess	Fever, headache, seizures, altered states of consciousness, focal neurologic examination
Nonacute	
Chronic perforation	Immobile tympanic membrane secondary to perforation
Otitis media with effusion (OME)	Immobile, opaque tympanic membrane
Adhesive otitis	Irreversible conductive hearing loss secondary to chronic OME
Tympanosclerosis	Thickened white plaques, may cause conductive hearing loss
Chronic suppurative otitis media	Following acute otitis media with perforation, secondary infection with *Staphylococcus aureus*, *Pseudomonas aeruginosa*, or anaerobes develops, causing chronic otorrhea
Cholesteatoma	White, pearl-like destructive tumor with otorrhea arising near or within tympanic membrane; may be secondary to chronic negative middle ear pressure
Otitic hydrocephalus	Increased intracranial pressure secondary to acute otitis media; signs and symptoms include severe headaches, blurred vision, nausea, vomiting, papilledema, diplopia (abducens paralysis)

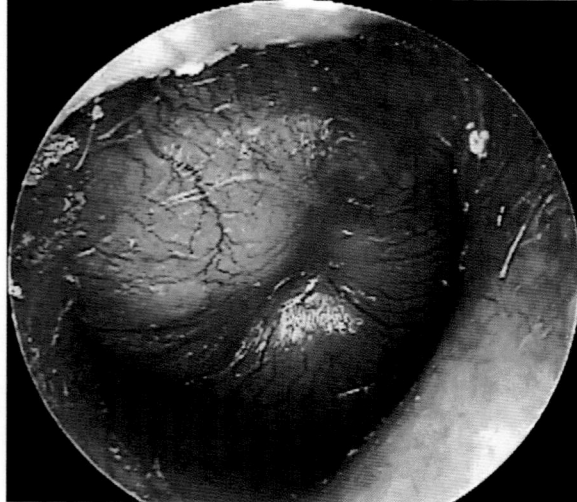

Fig. 5.7 Tympanic membrane in acute otitis media. (From Kerschner J, Preciado D. Otitis media. In: Kliegman RM, St. Geme JW III, Blum NJ, et al., eds. *Nelson Textbook of Pediatrics,* 21st ed. Philadelphia: Elsevier; 2020:3419.)

six serotypes of *S. pneumoniae* (serotypes included in the PCV7 vaccination plus serotypes 1, 3, 5, 6A, 7F, and 19A). Subsequently, there has been emergence of nonvaccine strains of *S. pneumoniae*, though there has been an overall decrease in *S. pneumoniae* as the cause of AOM.

Viruses also have an important etiologic role. It is not clear whether the virus alone or a combination of virus and bacteria are involved in the pathogenesis. Several studies have documented the presence of viruses (in up to 44% of cases, with or without bacteria) in the middle ear fluid of children with otitis media. URIs secondary to respiratory syncytial virus, influenza, and adenovirus have been associated with up to 40% of AOM cases in children attending daycare. To a lesser degree, URIs secondary to parainfluenza, rhinovirus, and enteroviruses have also been associated with AOM. Viruses enhance bacterial adherence and colonization in the nasopharynx, impair local host immune defenses, and cause eustachian tube dysfunction.

Strains of *S. pneumoniae* have emerged with altered penicillin-binding proteins on the bacterial cell wall, which makes them less susceptible to β-lactam drugs such as penicillins and cephalosporins. In addition, because resistance genes are frequently linked, organisms with resistance to β-lactam drugs are more likely to be resistant to sulfa antibacterials and to the macrolide class. Nonetheless, high-dose amoxicillin remains the best oral antibiotic available for drug-resistant *S. pneumoniae*. Approximately 40% of *H. influenzae* strains and nearly all strains of *M. catarrhalis* produce β-lactamase enzymes, which hydrolyze penicillins and some cephalosporins, making them resistant to beta-lactam antibiotics. Use of β-lactamase inhibitors such as clavulanate can overcome this resistance.

Treatment

The goals of treatment in AOM are to relieve discomfort and to prevent infectious complications (Fig. 5.8). Evaluating the treatment of otitis media is complicated by the high rate of spontaneous resolution of the

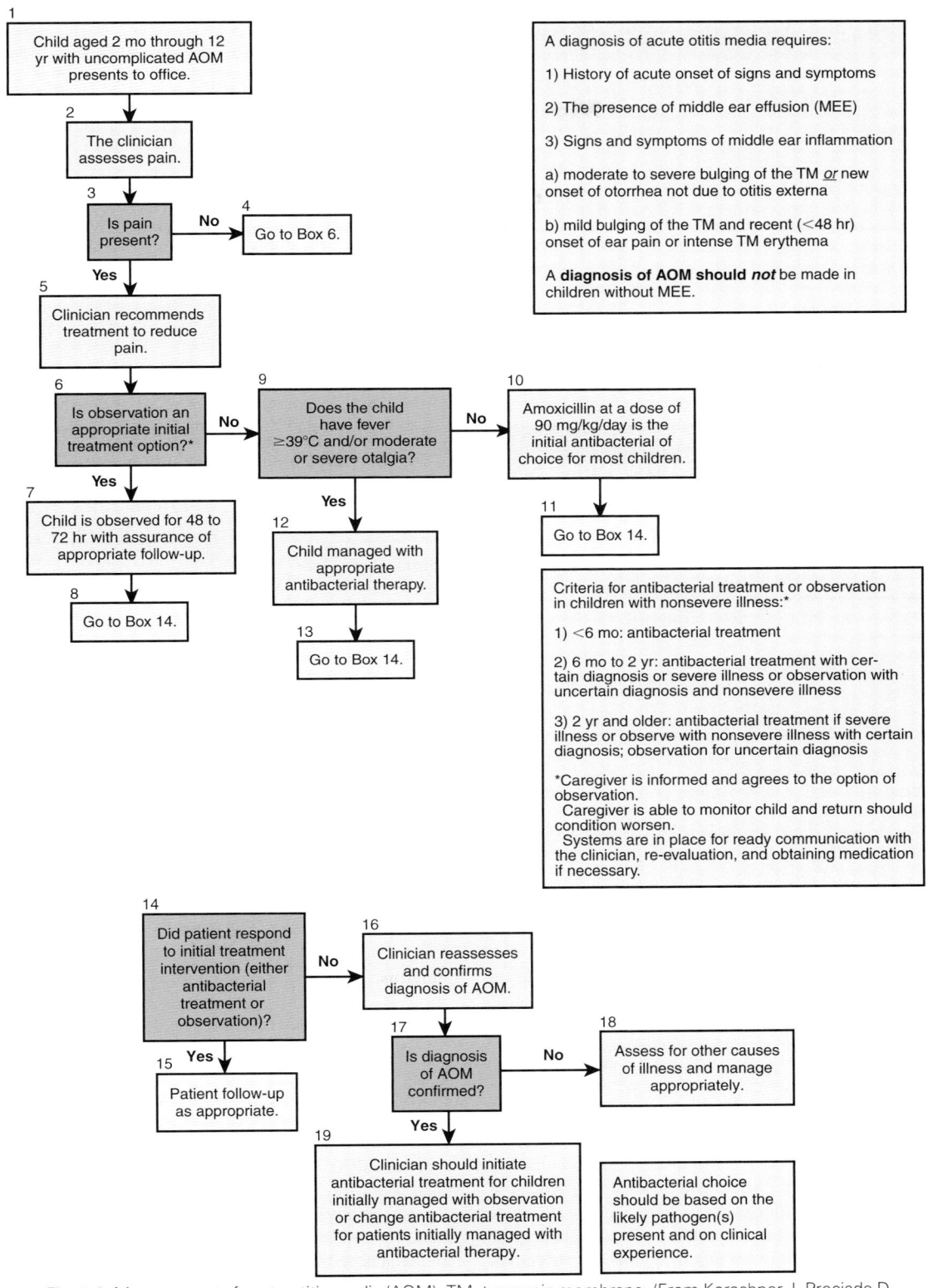

Fig. 5.8 Management of acute otitis media (AOM). TM, tympanic membrane. (From Kerschner J, Preciado D. Otitis media. In: Kliegman R, ed. *Nelson Textbook of Pediatrics*. 21st ed. Philadelphia: Elsevier; 2020:3424.)

infection: In children with AOM, up to 19% with *S. pneumoniae* and 48% with *H. influenzae* cultured on initial tympanocentesis are culture negative within 1 week without antibacterial therapy. Despite *M. catarrhalis* resistance to amoxicillin, approximately 75% of children infected with

that organism demonstrated cure when treated with amoxicillin. The emergence of drug-resistant *S. pneumoniae* strains and concerns about treating a disease with a high rate of spontaneous resolution have led to change in the recommended treatment for otitis media (see Fig. 5.8).

TABLE 5.7   Recommendations for Initial Management for Uncomplicated Acute Otitis Media (AOM)*

Age	Otorrhea with AOM	Unilateral or Bilateral AOM with Severe Symptoms[†]	Bilateral AOM Without Otorrhea	Unilateral AOM Without Otorrhea
6 mo–2 yr	Antibiotic therapy	Antibiotic therapy	Antibiotic therapy	Antibiotic therapy or additional observation
≥2 yr	Antibiotic therapy	Antibiotic therapy	Antibiotic therapy or additional observation	Antibiotic therapy or additional observation[‡]

*Applies only to children with well-documented AOM with high certainty of diagnosis (see Fig. 5.8).

[†]A toxic-appearing child, persistent otalgia more than 48 hr, temperature ≥39°C (102.2°F) in the past 48 hr, or if there is uncertain access to follow-up after the visit.

[‡]This plan of initial management provides an opportunity for shared decision-making with the child's family for those categories appropriate for additional observation. If observation is offered, a mechanism must be in place to ensure follow-up and begin antibiotics if the child worsens or fails to improve within 48–72 hr of AOM onset.

From Lieberthal A, Carroll A, Chonmaitree T, et al. The diagnosis and management of acute otitis media. *Pediatrics.* 2013;131:e976.

TABLE 5.8   Recommended Antibacterials for (Initial or Delayed) Treatment and for Patients Who Have Failed Initial Antibacterial Treatment

INITIAL IMMEDIATE OR DELAYED ANTIBIOTIC TREATMENT		ANTIBIOTIC TREATMENT AFTER 48–72 HR OF FAILURE OF INITIAL ANTIBIOTIC TREATMENT	
Recommended First-Line Treatment	Alternative Treatment (if Penicillin Allergy)	Recommended First-Line Treatment	Alternative Treatment
Amoxicillin (90 mg/kg/day divided b.i.d.) or Amoxicillin-clavulanate (90 mg/kg/day of amoxicillin divided b.i.d.) or Ceftriaxone (50 mg/kg/day IM or IV for 1–3 days)	Cefdinir (14 mg/kg/day once daily or divided b.i.d.) or Cefpodoxime (10 mg/kg/day divided b.i.d.) or Ceftriaxone (50 mg/kg/day IM or IV for 1–3 days)	Amoxicillin-clavulanate (90 mg/kg/day of amoxicillin divided b.i.d.)	Ceftriaxone 50 mg/kg/day daily IM or IV for 1–3 days or Clindamycin (30–40 mg/kg/day in 3 divided doses) *Failure of second antibiotic:* Clindamycin (30–40 mg/kg/day in 3 divided doses) Tympanocentesis* Consultation with otolaryngology[†]

*May be considered in patients in whom response to therapy has been inadequate or when identification of the causative organism and susceptibility profile are necessary.

[†]Consultation with a specialist (i.e., otolaryngology) to perform a tympanocentesis.

b.i.d., twice daily; IM, intramuscular; IV, intravenous.

Adapted from Lieberthal A, Carroll A, Chonmaitree T, et al. The diagnosis and management of acute otitis media. *Pediatrics.* 2014:133:347; Molloy L, Barron S, Khan N, et al. Oral B-lactam antibiotics for pediatric otitis media, rhinosinusitis, and pneumonia. *J Pediatr Health Care.* 2020;34(3):291–300. Kerschner J, Preciado D. Otitis media. In: Kliegman R, ed. *Nelson Textbook of Pediatrics.* 21st ed. Philadelphia: Elsevier; 2020:3418–3431.

Withholding antibacterials in children at low risk for complications may be appropriate under certain circumstances. In the Netherlands, antibacterial therapy is commonly delayed for 48–72 hours following diagnosis to determine whether there is spontaneous resolution. While antibacterial use is lower, rates of acute mastoiditis may be higher, emphasizing the need for close follow-up of patients in whom a watchful waiting approach is employed. There are specific guidelines on the use of watchful waiting and patients for whom its use may be appropriate (Table 5.7). *However, the key to observation prior to antibacterial initiation is close follow-up for assessment of worsening symptoms or spontaneous resolution.* Additionally, adequate analgesia, including acetaminophen and/or ibuprofen, should be provided during the observation period. *While watchful waiting is appropriate for certain populations, the benefits of antibacterial treatment are most clearly seen in children younger than 2 years.*

When an antibacterial is used, efficacy against *S. pneumoniae* is the most important consideration. In addition, the clinician must consider the drug safety, convenience, palatability, and cost. High-dose amoxicillin (90 mg/kg/day given in two divided doses) is the appropriate initial therapy for most cases (Table 5.8). Because otitis media is usually a self-limited illness, the use of broad-spectrum antibacterials for the initial treatment should be discouraged because of high cost, the increased risk of adverse reactions, and the increased likelihood of the development of resistant strains.

The dose of amoxicillin depends on the risk for the presence of drug-resistant pneumococci. Risk factors for drug resistance include age younger than 2 years, daycare attendance, recent antibacterial exposure, and cigarette smoke exposure. In addition, clinicians should consider community resistance patterns. In penicillin-allergic patients, the cross-reactivity between penicillins and cephalosporins is likely lower than previously reported. Cephalosporins are therefore an alternative therapy option in patients without severe and/or recent allergic reaction to penicillins (see Table 5.8). Clindamycin is not effective against *H. influenzae* but may be effective against some penicillin-resistant strains of *S. pneumoniae*. Macrolides (i.e., erythromycin, azithromycin) are minimally effective against *S. pneumoniae* or *H. influenzae* and therefore not appropriate alternatives.

Patients with Persistent Symptoms

After 48–72 hours of antibacterial therapy, most patients are either asymptomatic or improving. Beyond this time period, many patients with ongoing symptoms may have an active viral infection, whereas others may have a persistent inflammatory reaction despite elimination of viable bacteria. Studies are conflicting regarding continued presence of bacteria in the middle ear of persistently symptomatic patients, with some finding ongoing bacterial presence while others report sterile bacterial cultures of middle ear fluid in up to 50% of patients with persistent symptoms. Therefore, in children with mild persistent symptoms, a clinician should consider analgesic-antipyretic medications for relief of symptoms while addressing any issues of drug nonadherence, including palatability and dosing interval. In children with more severe, persistent signs of AOM without otologic improvement, prescribing an alternative antibiotic effective against possible resistant *S. pneumoniae* and β-lactamase–producing *H. influenzae* and *M. catarrhalis* such as amoxicillin-clavulanate (90 mg/kg/day of the amoxicillin component) or 3 days of intramuscular ceftriaxone should be considered (see Table 5.8). With the emergence of *S. pneumoniae* resistance, tympanocentesis with culture of middle ear effusion should be considered for bacteriologic diagnosis and susceptibility testing.

Recurrent Acute Otitis Media

Recurrent otitis media is defined as three episodes of AOM in a 6-month period or four episodes in a 12-month period with at least one episode in the preceding 6 months. Risk factors for recurrent AOM include the following:

- Onset of AOM in the first year of life, especially if the first episode is before the patient is 6 months of age
- Males
- A sibling's history of recurrent AOM
- Cleft palate
- Craniofacial anomalies
- Trisomy 21
- Daycare attendance
- Household cigarette smoke exposure
- HIV infection
- Lack of breast-feeding
- History of atopy/allergies

Children with recurrent otitis media present a particular challenge with regard to treatment options. Long-term, low-dose antibacterial agents have been used as a method of prophylaxis in children with recurrent AOM in attempts to prevent additional episodes. While there is some evidence of decreased episodes of AOM, this benefit only occurred while receiving the prophylactic antibacterial, without benefits after discontinuation of the antibacterial. Other studies have not demonstrated a difference in recurrence of AOM among children with or without prophylactic antibacterials. Given the risks of emergence of antibacterial resistance, side effects of antibacterials, and cost of therapy weighed against the questionable benefits of long-term antibacterial use, *prophylaxis is not recommended.*

The benefits of placing tympanostomy tubes for recurrent AOM or OME include improving hearing, decreasing effusion burden, decreasing episodes of acute otitis media, and improving quality of life for children that suffer from recurrent AOM or chronic effusion. As with any surgical procedure, the benefits must be weighed against the risks, including cost of the procedure and risks of anesthesia. Tympanostomy tubes are eventually extruded from the eardrum by the normal process of epithelial growth. Recurrent episodes of otitis media may then resume. Long-term consequences of tympanostomy tubes include focal atrophy, tympanosclerosis, and chronic perforation at the site of tube insertion.

OTITIS MEDIA WITH EFFUSION

Otitis media with effusion, also known as "glue ear," may occur after an acute episode of otitis media or because of eustachian tube

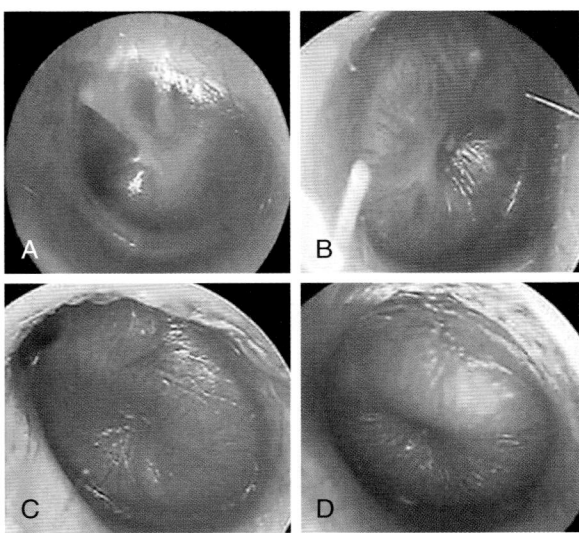

Fig. 5.9 Examples of normal tympanic membrane *(A)* and of mild bulging *(B)*, moderate bulging *(C)*, and severe bulging *(D)* of the tympanic membrane from middle ear effusion. (From Kerschner J, Preciado D. Otitis media. In: Kliegman R, ed. *Nelson Textbook of Pediatrics.* 21st ed. Philadelphia: Elsevier; 2020:3419.)

obstruction resulting from another cause, most commonly URI. OME differs from AOM in that there is middle ear effusion present without signs or symptoms of acute infection (Fig. 5.9). The most common presenting complaint with OME is decreased hearing. Middle ear fluid can persist for weeks after AOM. Two weeks after AOM, approximately 75% of children will have persistent effusion. The percentage drops to 50% at 1 month and 10–25% at 3 months post-AOM. Because most cases of OME resolve without treatment, a period of observation is the most appropriate initial strategy. If effusion persists for 3 months or longer, or if at any time there is concern for language delay, learning difficulties, or significant hearing loss, hearing testing should be performed.

The guideline for affected children between 2 months and 12 years distinguishes between children with OME at risk for speech, language, or learning problems and children not at risk for such problems. The clinician should document laterality, duration, and severity of effusion with pneumatic otoscopy and confirmation of effusion by tympanometry when pneumatic otoscopy is inconclusive. Based on the updated guidelines, use of decongestants, steroids (intranasal or systemic), antihistamines, and/or antibacterial agents are not recommended in the management of persistent OME. Antihistamines, decongestants, and nonsteroidal antiinflammatory agents do not promote the resolution of middle ear effusion and should not be used. With systemic corticosteroids (prednisone), the effusion may resolve initially, but it recurs within a few weeks of steroid discontinuation. Additionally, the side effect profile of systemic steroids precludes its use in children with OME. Although bacteria may be present in some cases, antibacterial therapy has only a minimal effect on the resolution of effusion and does not demonstrate long-term benefit. A period of observation is recommended before surgical intervention is considered.

MASTOIDITIS

Mastoiditis is a potentially serious acute or chronic suppurative complication of otitis media, occurring in approximately 1–4 cases per 100,000 children younger than 2 years old. Life-threatening complications of mastoiditis are related to intracranial extension of the suppurative process. Mastoiditis begins with the development of hyperemia

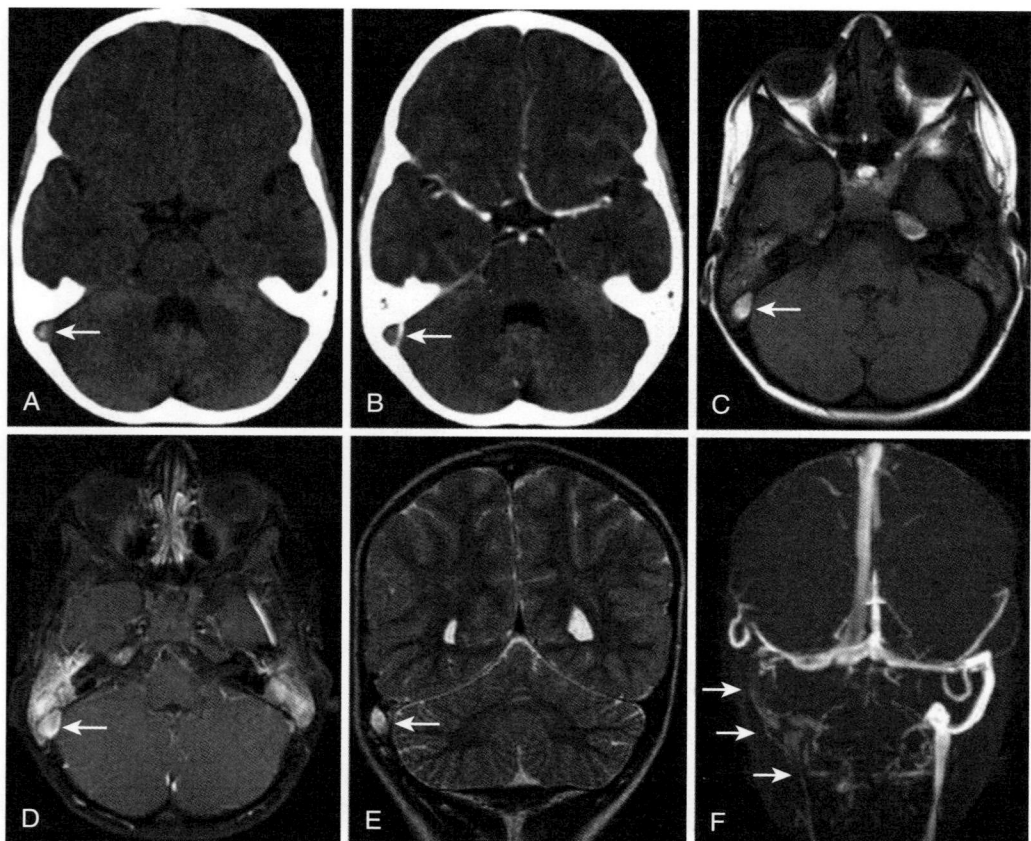

Fig. 5.10 Transverse sinus thrombosis associated with otomastoiditis or middle ear disease. A patient with otitis media, headache, and papilledema. Axial noncontrast *(A)* and contrast-enhanced *(B)* CT of the head through the level of the posterior fossa, axial magnetization transfer T1 precontrast *(C)* and postcontrast *(D)* MRI scans, coronal T2 *(E)* and coronal multiple intensity projection image from a three-dimensional time-of-flight magnetic resonance venogram (MRV) *(F)* were obtained. Note the dense appearance within the right transverse sinus on the noncontrast CT study *(arrow* in *A)*, with corresponding lack of contrast filling on the postcontrast CT study *(arrow* in *B)*. Corresponding T1 shortening is seen in the precontrast MRI *(arrow* in *C)*, with corresponding abnormal signal on the postcontrast images in keeping with clot or slow flow within the region of the right transverse sinus or sigmoid sinus *(arrow* in *D)*. Corresponding T2 prolongation is seen on the coronal T2 image *(arrow* in *E)*. Note the striking asymmetry of flow within the right posterior fossa dural venous system or internal jugular vein on the right on the three-dimensional time-of-flight MRV *(arrows* in *F)*. (From Coley BD, ed. *Caffey's Pediatric Diagnostic Imaging.* 12th ed. Vol 1. Philadelphia: Elsevier; 2013:360.)

and edema of the mastoid process, which then progresses to a suppurative process that may produce demineralization and necrosis of bone, abscess formation, and contiguous spread to intracranial or other head and neck soft tissue areas. Mastoiditis with periosteitis indicates that the infection has spread to the periosteum of the mastoid process and manifests most commonly in children younger than 2 years, although children of any age may be affected. Diagnosis typically relies on history and physical examination findings. Otalgia, posterior ear pain, fever, and otorrhea are frequent symptoms. Posterior auricular tenderness and erythema, anterior-inferior pinna protrusion, loss of the posterior auricular crease, middle ear effusion, a bulging or perforated tympanic membrane, and sagging of the posterior auditory canal wall are observable signs. Acute mastoid osteitis designates further spread of infection causing bony trabeculae destruction. Mastoiditis may result in transverse sinus thrombosis (Fig. 5.10), hearing loss, and labyrinthitis.

Petrositis occurs when the infection spreads medially to the petrous portion of the temporal bone and manifests as eye pain secondary to irritation of the ophthalmic branch of cranial nerve V (Fig. 5.11). **Gradenigo syndrome** is the triad of ipsilateral orbital or facial pain, paralysis of the lateral rectus muscle, and suppurative otitis media. Rarely,

the infection can spread externally to musculature of the neck resulting in a neck abscess **(Bezold abscess)**.

The pathogens responsible for mastoiditis are the same as those of AOM, including *S. pneumoniae* and *H. influenzae*, though *Pseudomonas* and group A streptococci are also causative agents (Table 5.9). A CT scan is usually diagnostic and reveals various stages of mastoiditis, including mastoiditis with periostitis and mastoiditis with osteitis with or without subperiosteal abscess. Treatment is based on the stage and extent of disease. High-dose intravenous antibacterials and myringotomy with or without tympanostomy tube placement are important therapeutic (for drainage) and diagnostic (for culture) procedures. If there is no improvement after 2 days, mastoidectomy may be indicated. Mastoidectomy with myringotomy and tympanostomy tube placement is indicated if a subperiosteal abscess is present.

CHOLESTEATOMA

Cholesteatomas are cystlike growths of the middle ear or mastoid formed by keratinizing squamous epithelial cells (Fig. 5.12) and can be either congenital or acquired. *Congenital* cholesteatomas likely

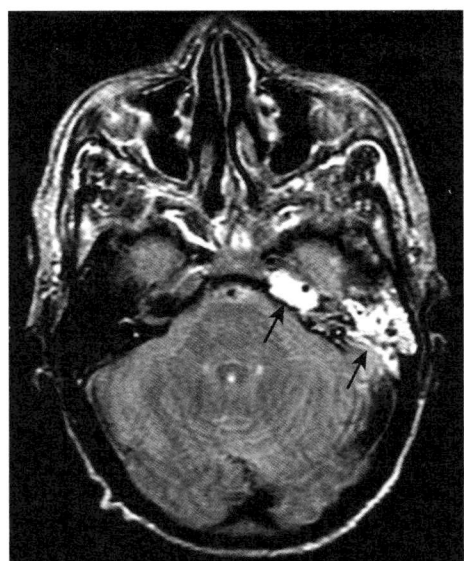

Fig. 5.11 Axial T2-weighted MRI showing left mastoiditis and petrous apicitis *(arrows)* as high signal in mastoid and petrous apex. (From Flint PW, Haughey BH, Lund VJ, et al., eds. *Cummings Otolaryngology Head & Neck Surgery*. 5th ed. Vol. 2. Philadelphia: Elsevier; 2010.)

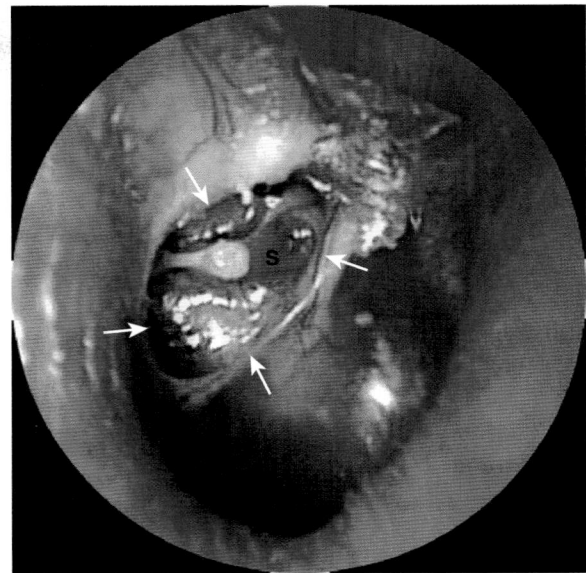

Fig. 5.12 A retraction-pocket cholesteatoma of the posterosuperior quadrant. The incus long process is eroded, which leaves the drum adherent to the stapes head *(S)*. An effusion is present in the middle ear, and squamous debris emanates from the attic. (From Isaacson G. Diagnosis of pediatric cholesteatoma. *Pediatrics*. 2007;120:603–608.)

TABLE 5.9 Etiology of Acute Mastoiditis	
Bacteria	**Frequency**
Streptococcus pneumoniae	10–51%
Streptococcus pyogenes	0–12%
Staphylococcus aureus	2–10%
Pseudomonas aeruginosa	~10%
Haemophilus influenzae	2–3%
No growth	20–40%

From Faria J, Chun R, Kerschner J. Acute mastoiditis. In: Kliegman R, ed. *Nelson Textbook of Pediatrics*. 21st ed. Philadelphia: Elsevier; 2020:3432.

result from epithelial cells implanted during otologic development in utero. *Acquired* cholesteatomas are potential complications from chronic otitis media or secondary to a deep retraction pocket (or invagination) in the tympanic membrane. The condition can also develop after tympanostomy tube placement. Cholesteatomas can cause bony resorption by expansion, often to the mastoid, but occasionally intracranially with potentially life-threatening consequences. This condition should be suspected in children with history of chronic otitis media, persistent otorrhea, and a tympanic membrane with a retraction pocket or perforation with white debris overlying the area. Cholesteatomas commonly present over the superior portion of the tympanic membrane. Urgent otolaryngology consultation should be obtained as delay in treatment can result in intracranial extension, permanent hearing loss, facial nerve injury, and middle and inner ear destruction.

INTRACRANIAL COMPLICATIONS

Meningitis, epidural or subdural empyema, brain abscess, and sigmoid or lateral sinus thrombosis can develop as complications of acute or chronic ear or mastoid infection. If suspected, imaging of the head should be done prior to lumbar puncture to evaluate for hydrocephalus

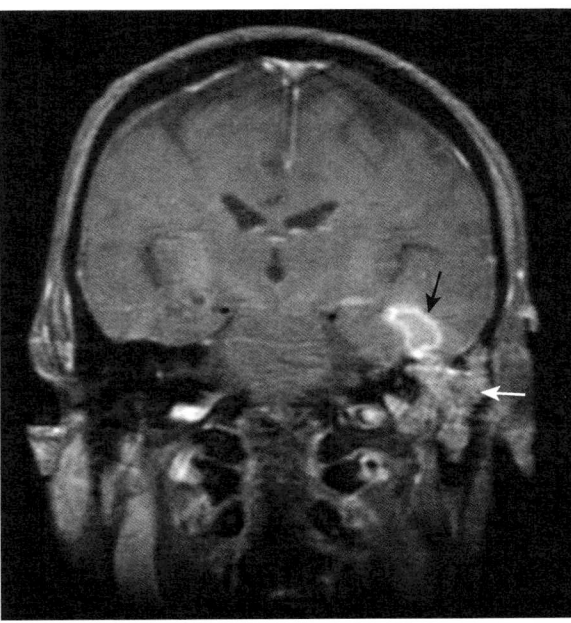

Fig. 5.13 Coronal enhanced T1-weighted MRI of the patient showing enhancing tissue in left mastoid *(white arrow)* and temporal lobe abscess with enhancing capsule *(black arrow)*. (From Flint PW, Haughey BH, Lund VJ, et al., eds. *Cummings Otolaryngology Head & Neck Surgery*. 5th ed. Vol 2. Philadelphia: Elsevier; 2010:1995.)

or mass effect. Meningitis most commonly results from hematogenous spread of the infection and is diagnosed by cerebrospinal fluid (CSF) analysis and culture. Tympanocentesis should be performed for bacterial culture to aid in diagnosis and management choices. Brain abscess can occur from direct extension of acute or chronic otitis media or can develop adjacent to petrositis (Fig. 5.13). Clinical signs and symptoms should lead one to suspect this complication, and diagnosis can be made with CT or MRI. CSF for culture should be obtained to aid in directing therapy; culture may be negative depending on the location and loculation of the abscess. Lateral sinus thrombosis, also known as sigmoid sinus thrombosis, forms when infection from the adjacent mastoid contacts and penetrates the venous wall and forms a thrombus. Embolization of the thrombus can cause distal disease. These intracranial complications require broad-spectrum antibacterials and consultation with otolaryngology and neurosurgery for possible surgical interventions.

SUMMARY AND RED FLAGS

A careful examination of the pinna, external auditory canal, and tympanic membrane can identify most causes of ear pain. If findings are normal, the clinician should consider pain referred from another source (see Table 5.3). Because young children may have trouble localizing their pain, clinicians should be highly suspicious of ear disease in any infant or preschool child with fever, irritability, or URI.

Even though most conditions causing ear pain respond readily to therapy, the clinician must be aware of the following red flags associated with these conditions:

- Laterally displaced pinna (malignant otitis externa, mastoid osteitis)
- Mastoid tenderness (mastoid osteitis)
- Perforated tympanic membrane
- A pearl-like tumor in the tympanic membrane (cholesteatoma)
- Subacute headache, meningismus, and altered mental status (brain abscess, subdural or epidural empyema)

BIBLIOGRAPHY

A bibliography is available at ExpertConsult.com.

6

Apparent Life-Threatening Event/ Brief Resolved Unexplained Event

Amanda Rogers and Sandra Gage

A brief resolved unexplained event (BRUE) is a term used to describe events occurring in infants younger than 1 year of age that are characterized by the observer as "brief" (lasting <1 minute but typically <20–30 seconds) and "resolved" (meaning the patient returned to baseline state of health after the event) and with a reassuring history, physical examination, and vital signs at the time of clinical evaluation by trained medical providers (Table 6.1). A BRUE is diagnosed only when there is no explanation for a qualifying event after conducting an appropriate history and physical examination.

DEFINITION

The term BRUE (pronounced "*brew*") is defined as an event lasting <1 minute in an infant younger than 1 year of age that is associated with at least one of the following: cyanosis or pallor; absent, decreased, or irregular breathing; marked change in muscle tone (hypertonia or hypotonia); and altered level of responsiveness. BRUE occurs in a patient who was asymptomatic prior to the event, at the time of examination is well-appearing and has returned to baseline level of function, and after evaluation has no condition that could explain the event (see Table 6.1). It was introduced as a replacement for the term ALTE (apparent life-threatening event).

The definition of ALTE presented challenges due to the subjectivity and vagueness of the described symptoms. This made it difficult to standardize the care of these patients, due to possible causation by a wide range of disorders. In addition, it relied on the subjective report of the observer rather than on pathophysiology and implied the event was "life-threatening" when it generally was not. The term BRUE serves to remove the "life-threatening" label, more narrowly define the event, and better reflect the transient nature and lack of a clear cause.

In development of the BRUE clinical practice guideline, a systematic review of ALTE literature that allowed for the identification of BRUEs found two subsets of BRUE patients based on their risk for adverse outcomes. Those at **lower risk** are defined as >60 days old, gestational age ≥32 weeks and postconceptual age ≥45 weeks, no prior BRUEs and not occurring in a cluster, event duration <1 minute, no cardiopulmonary resuscitation administered by a trained medical provider, and no concerning historical features or physical exam findings. These patients can likely be managed in the outpatient setting without need for extensive evaluation (Fig. 6.1). Any patient not meeting these criteria are classified as **higher risk** for adverse outcomes.

EPIDEMIOLOGY

Because the term BRUE was introduced in 2016, the incidence of these events is not well known. Prior to the introduction of the term BRUE, the exact incidence of ALTEs was also unclear, due to the subjectivity of the definition and the probability that not all children with ALTE presented for evaluation. Reported figures may have underestimated the true incidence as studies may not have included those cases where the underlying cause was ultimately identified. Various studies estimate the incidence of ALTE to be between 0.46 and 2.46/1,000 live births, accounting for 0.6–1% of all emergency department visits by patients younger than 1 year and 2% of pediatric hospitalizations. Studies attempting to identify BRUE patients among those classified as ALTE found that less than half met the criteria for BRUE. The mortality rates reported to be associated with ALTE vary widely depending on the definition and the population. However, review of these prior studies focused on the outcomes of patients who met the criteria for BRUE did not identify deaths or significant morbidities in that population.

ETIOLOGY

By definition BRUEs are unexplained events with no identifiable underlying cause. It is important for providers presented with a suspected BRUE to consider additional diagnoses that may present similarly. Based on broad symptomatology, the differential diagnosis for BRUEs is large (Table 6.2). Comorbid conditions are frequently identified, but it can be challenging to identify true causation. Thus, caution must be used when implicating a specific diagnosis as the true cause of an event. Prior literature reported that a suspected diagnosis was found in approximately 50% of patients presenting with an ALTE. These diagnoses encompass a wide range of etiologies and systems and should also be considered as alternative etiologies for patients presenting with a BRUE.

The most commonly cited alternative diagnoses include gastroesophageal reflux (GER), seizures, and lower respiratory tract infections. However, numerous less common but potentially dangerous and/or treatable conditions can also present similarly (see Table 6.2). These need to be carefully considered to provide prompt lifesaving or outcome-altering treatment. A thorough and thoughtful history and physical examination are extremely important in the evaluation of a patient with a BRUE, as they provide essential clues to help narrow the differential and perform risk stratification. It is often helpful to consider the differential diagnosis by a systems-based approach, considering both common and rare but concerning diagnoses in each category. Key systems-based historical and physical examination findings may help discriminate among possible etiologies (see Table 6.2).

CLINICAL EVALUATION

History

The most important diagnostic tool in the evaluation of a BRUE is a thorough history elicited from the caretaker who observed the episode. History taking should start with open-ended questions to

TABLE 6.1   BRUE Definition and Factors for Inclusion and Exclusion of BRUE Diagnosis

	Includes	Excludes
Brief	Duration <1 min; typically 20–30 sec	Duration ≥1 min
Resolved	Patient returned to their baseline state of health after the event Normal vital signs Normal appearance	At the time of medical evaluation: 　Fever or recent fever 　Tachypnea, bradypnea, apnea 　Tachycardia or bradycardia 　Hypotension, hypertension, or hemodynamic instability 　Mental status changes, somnolence, lethargy 　Hypotonia or hypertonia 　Vomiting 　Bruising, petechiae, or other signs of injury/trauma 　Abnormal weight, growth, or head circumference 　Noisy breathing (stridor, stertor, wheezing) 　Repeat event(s)
Unexplained	Not explained by an identifiable medical condition	Event consistent with GER, swallow dysfunction, nasal congestion, etc. History or physical examination concerning for child abuse, congenital airway abnormality, etc.
Event Characterization		
Cyanosis or pallor	Central cyanosis: blue or purple coloration of face, gums, trunk Central pallor: pale coloration of face or trunk	Acrocyanosis or perioral cyanosis Rubor
Absent, decreased, or irregular breathing	Central apnea Obstructive apnea Mixed obstructive apnea	Periodic breathing of the newborn Breath-holding spell
Marked change in tone (hyper- or hypotonia)	Hypertonia Hypotonia	Hypertonia associated with crying, choking, or gagging due to GER or feeding problems Tone changes associated with breath-holding spell Tonic eye deviation or nystagmus Tonic-clonic seizure activity Infantile spasms
Altered responsiveness	Loss of consciousness Mental status change Lethargy Somnolence	Loss of consciousness associated with breath-holding spell Postictal phase due to seizure

BRUE, brief resolved unexplained event; GER, gastroesophageal reflux.
From Tieder JS, Bonkowsky JL, Etzel RA, et al. Brief resolved unexplained events (formerly apparent life-threatening events) and evaluation of lower-risk infants. *Pediatrics.* 2016;137(5):e20160590 (Table 1).

obtain the story from the caretaker, followed by specific questions geared at characterizing certain key aspects of the episode. The history should focus on the activities and behaviors preceding the event, characteristics of the episode itself, interventions performed and their effect, and postepisode events and behavior. A comprehensive past medical history, social history, and family history should also be obtained for identifying clues that may aid in narrowing the focus of the investigation. Information essential to a complete history is outlined in Table 6.3. Key historical findings by system can be useful in narrowing the differential (see Table 6.2).

The patient's activities and behaviors immediately preceding the episode are important to consider and may provide clues to the diagnosis. Key associations include those with sleep, feeding, crying, cough, and emesis. The location and position of the child prior to the event should also be noted, such as placement in a car seat, on a soft or firm surface, prone or supine, and with or without surrounding blankets or pillows.

Key characteristics of the actual event include color change, respiratory effort, change in tone or movements, and level of alertness at onset and during the episode. Careful review of these signs and symptoms

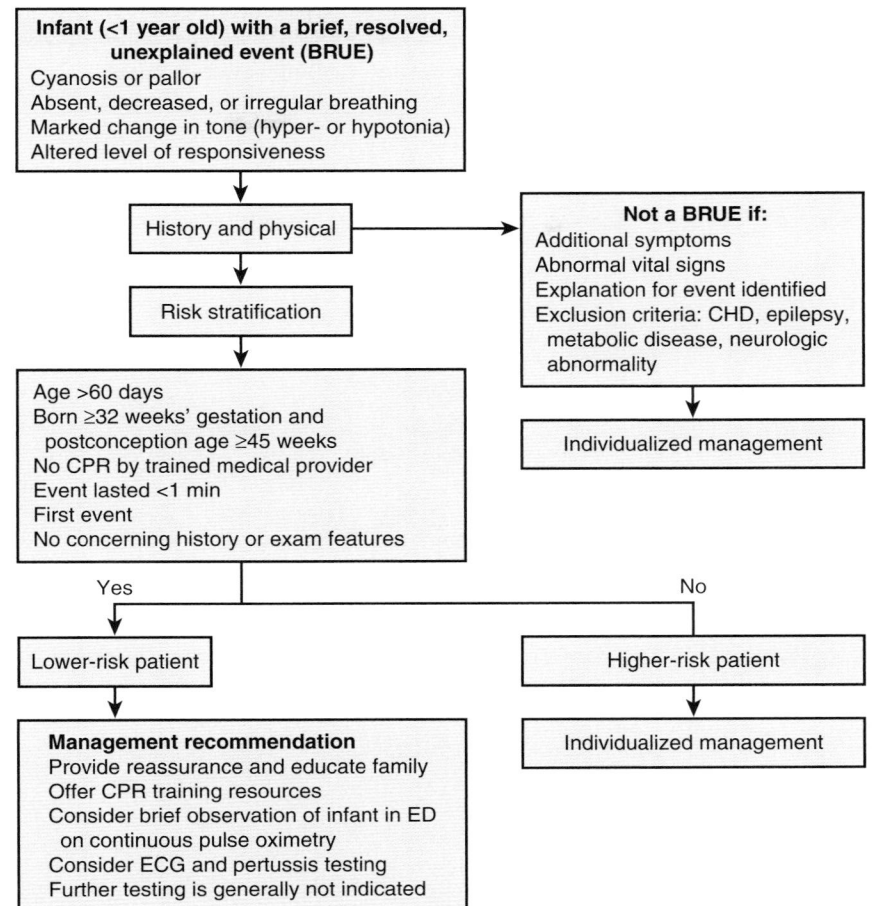

Figure 6.1 Algorithm for diagnosis, risk stratification, and management of a brief resolved unexplained event (BRUE). CHD, congenital heart disease; ECG, electrocardiogram; ED, emergency department. (From The Johns Hopkins Hospital [Baltimore, Maryland], ed. *The Harriet Lane Handbook*. 22nd ed. Philadelphia: Elsevier; 2020.)

aids in the identification and classification of a BRUE, and they are important clues to potential alternative diagnoses.

Color: The specifics of any change in color should be clearly noted, and the hue of the change is significant. Unlike in the term ALTE where any change of color was considered, BRUE more precisely defines concerning color change as episodes of cyanosis or pallor. Episodes of rubor are not consistent with a BRUE, because they are common in healthy infants. The location of the change should also be noted, such as central cyanosis versus peripheral acrocyanosis, as the latter may be consistent with normal changes in perfusion.

Change in breathing: The term BRUE expands the respiratory criteria for ALTE beyond apnea to include absent breathing, diminished breathing, and other breathing irregularities. If apnea is noted, the duration of respiratory cessation aids in the determination of true pathologic apnea. Apnea is defined as cessation in breathing that is prolonged (>20 seconds) or associated with cyanosis, marked pallor or hypotonia, or bradycardia. The degree of respiratory effort noted assists in differentiating central versus obstructive processes. **Central apnea** with no respiratory effort may suggest underlying neurologic, cardiac, metabolic, or infectious causes, while **obstructive processes** include GER, respiratory tract infections, foreign body, suffocation, or airway anatomic anomalies.

Tone: It is important to determine if tone was increased or decreased during or after the event. If abnormal movements were identified, it should be noted if the movements were generalized or localized to a

certain part of the body and the timing. The ability to suppress any abnormal movements should be documented, as this makes conditions such as seizure less likely.

Altered level of responsiveness: Specific note of the level of responsiveness is another criterion under the BRUE definition and is significant to note as it can be associated with episodic but serious cardiac, respiratory, metabolic, or neurologic events.

Of note, if the event was noted to consist primarily of choking or gagging without any of the other features listed earlier, unlike in the former ALTE definition, this would not be included within the current definition of BRUE. Choking and gagging usually indicate easily identifiable common diagnoses such as GER or respiratory infections and therefore are not considered a BRUE.

Additional history should include any interventions performed, by whom, and the effects of the interventions. The need for resuscitation, especially when performed by health care providers, has been associated with more severe and significant underlying etiologies and classifies the event as a higher-risk BRUE. Obtaining a direct history from any emergency personnel who may have been involved with the case is important.

Postepisode behavior should be carefully documented. Level of alertness following the event and time until return to normal behavior are also of particular importance.

Regarding **past medical history**, it is essential to note the birth history including gestational age, any prior similar episodes, preceding

TABLE 6.2   Differential Diagnosis and System-Based Approach to BRUEs

Diagnostic Categories	Common and/or Concerning Causes to Consider	Suggestive Historical Findings	Suggestive Physical Examination Findings	Testing to Consider
Gastrointestinal	GER Intussusception Volvulus Swallowing abnormalities	Coughing, vomiting, choking, gasping Feeding difficulties Recent preceding feed Irritability following feeds Milk in mouth/nose Bilious emesis Pulling legs to chest Bloody/mucousy stool Lethargy following event	Gastric contents in the nose and mouth Abdominal distention Abdominal tenderness	Upper GI to assess for anatomic anomalies Swallow evaluation Abdominal ultrasound or pH probe
Infectious	Upper and lower respiratory tract infection (RSV, pertussis, pneumonia) Bacteremia Meningitis Urinary tract infection	Preceding URI symptoms Multiple events on the day of presentation Sick exposures Foul-smelling urine	Fever/hypothermia Lethargy Ill appearance Coryza Cough Wheeze Tachypnea	NP swab for RSV, pertussis, COVID-19 Chest radiograph CBC and blood culture Cerebrospinal fluid analysis and culture Urinalysis and culture
Neurologic	Seizures Breath-holding spells Congenital central hypoventilation syndrome Neuromuscular disorders Congenital malformations of the brain and brainstem Malignancy Intracranial hemorrhage	Multiple events Loss of consciousness Change in tone Abnormal muscular movements Eye deviation Preceding triggers	Papilledema Abnormal muscular movements Hypertonicity or flaccidity Abnormal reflexes Micro- or macrocephaly Dysmorphic features Ptosis Bulging fontanel	EEG Neuroimaging
Respiratory/ENT	Apnea of prematurity Apnea of infancy Periodic breathing Airway anomaly Aspiration Foreign body Obstructive sleep apnea	Prematurity Foreign body Aspiration Noisy breathing	Wheezing Stridor Crackles Rhonchi Tachypnea	Chest radiograph Neck radiograph Laryngoscopy Bronchoscopy Esophagoscopy Polysomnography
Child maltreatment	Nonaccidental head trauma Smothering Poisoning Factitious syndrome (formerly Munchausen syndrome) by proxy	Multiple events Unexplained vomiting or irritability Recurrent events Historical discrepancies Family history of unexplained death, BRUEs, SIDS, or ALTEs Single witness of event Delay in seeking care	Bruising (especially in a nonmobile child) Ear trauma, hemotympanum Acute abdomen Painful extremities Oral bleeding/trauma Frenulum tears Unexplained irritability Retinal hemorrhages Depressed mental status	Skeletal survey CT of the head Dilated funduscopic examination Toxicology screen
Cardiac	Dysrhythmia (prolonged QT syndrome, Wolff-Parkinson-White syndrome) Cardiomyopathy Congenital heart disease Myocarditis	Abrupt onset Feeding difficulties Failure to thrive Diaphoresis Prematurity	Abnormal heart rate/rhythm Murmur Decreased femoral pulses	Four-extremity blood pressure Pre- and postductal oxygen saturation measurements ECG Echocardiogram Serum electrolytes, calcium, magnesium

Continued

TABLE 6.2	Differential Diagnosis and System-Based Approach to BRUEs—cont'd			
Diagnostic Categories	**Common and/or Concerning Causes to Consider**	**Suggestive Historical Findings**	**Suggestive Physical Examination Findings**	**Testing to Consider**
Metabolic/genetic	Inborn errors of metabolism Electrolyte abnormalities Genetic syndromes including those with craniofacial malformations	Severe initial event Multiple events Event associated with period of stress or fasting Developmental delay Associated anomalies Failure to thrive Severe/frequent illnesses Family history of a BRUE, ALTE, consanguinity, seizure disorder, or SIDS	Dysmorphic features Microcephaly Hepatomegaly	Serum electrolytes; glucose, calcium, and magnesium levels Lactate Ammonia Pyruvate Urine organic and serum amino acids Newborn screen

ALTE, apparent life-threatening event; BRUE, brief resolved unexplained event; ENT, ear, nose, and throat; GER, gastroesophageal reflux; GI, gastrointestinal; NP, nasopharyngeal; RSV, respiratory syncytial virus; SIDS, sudden infant death syndrome; URI, upper respiratory infection.

illnesses, and known medical conditions. Family history should also be obtained with a focus on the presence of BRUEs, ALTEs, sudden infant death syndrome (SIDS), early deaths, and metabolic or neurologic disorders in first- or second-degree family members. Social factors to consider include a full list of caregivers, siblings, and other children in the home; illness exposures; medications in the home; exposure to smoke; or prior Child Protective Services involvement.

Major factors suggestive of risk for future adverse events and/or a serious underlying diagnosis include age, prematurity, multiple events, and the need for CPR by trained medical providers. Prematurity is a frequently noted risk factor for a BRUE/ALTE, perhaps due in part to the preterm infants' immature respiratory centers, arousal mechanisms, and airway reflexes. The risk is increased for infants born at <32 weeks' gestation, and the risk decreases once they reach 45 weeks' postconception age. A history of multiple events raises the concern for serious underlying pathology and progression of future events. With a history of multiple events over days to months, the concern for child maltreatment, seizures, intracranial pathology, and inborn errors of metabolism increases. Multiple events occurring over the course of the day of presentation escalate concern for serious infections and child maltreatment.

Physical Examination

One of the diagnostic challenges of the evaluation of a child with a BRUE is that the patient has returned to their baseline state of health after the event and has a reassuring physical examination and vital signs when evaluated by a trained medical provider. Infants should undergo a complete head-to-toe examination fully unclothed, including vital signs with pulse oximetry, growth parameters with head circumference, and complete ear, nose, throat, cardiac, respiratory, abdominal, neurologic, musculoskeletal, and skin examinations to note any abnormalities or clues to suggest an alternative diagnosis.

Abnormalities noted on the presenting examination may indicate various possible diagnoses and should prompt additional evaluation for the suggested etiology (see Table 6.2). Particular attention should be paid to the child's general appearance for dysmorphic features that might suggest an underlying genetic or metabolic syndrome. Abnormal growth parameters may identify failure to thrive, which can be suggestive of pathologic reflux, cardiac disease, or metabolic disorders. Signs of trauma, including retinal hemorrhages, unexplained bruising, or evidence of oral pharyngeal trauma (torn frenulum), suggestive

of child maltreatment should also be noted. A full neurologic examination may raise concern for an intracranial bleed or mass requiring prompt attention.

Diagnostic Evaluation

A comprehensive history is essential both in performing a risk stratification to determine if the event would be classified as higher or lower risk and in identifying indications of potential alternative diagnoses.

For patients identified as **lower risk**, laboratory studies, imaging studies, and other diagnostic procedures are unlikely to be useful or necessary (see Fig. 6.1). Low-risk patients should not be admitted to the hospital solely for cardiorespiratory monitoring or undergo extensive evaluations. Two evaluations that are recommended for consideration in the lower-risk population include an ECG and pertussis in conjunction with brief monitoring on a continuous pulse oximeter with serial exams. ECGs may be useful in identifying channelopathies, ventricular pre-excitation, cardiomyopathy, or other heart disease. Although the incidence of these is low, the benefit of identifying a patient at risk of sudden cardiac death may outweigh the cost and risk of potential false positives leading to additional evaluation. Pertussis and respiratory syncytial virus (RSV) have been reported to cause BRUE-like events with gasping, color change, and apnea and may not have associated fever or respiratory symptoms particularly when present in young infants.

When evaluating patients presenting with a *higher-risk* BRUE, it is often difficult to determine the degree to which diagnostic work-up is indicated, especially in well-appearing infants with a nonspecific history and physical examination. A potential framework for the approach to evaluation of a higher-risk BRUE suggests consideration of the following: continuous pulse oximetry monitoring for at least 4 hours; consultation with a social worker; a bedside feeding evaluation; ECG; laboratory studies including consideration of a rapid viral respiratory panel and pertussis testing, hematocrit, blood glucose, bicarbonate or venous blood gas, and lactate; consultation with a child abuse expert; head imaging with CT or MRI, and skeletal survey if concerned for child maltreatment; and then additional consultation and evaluation as indicated based on the clinical context. The level of evidence varies for each of these recommendations and the clinical context should be carefully considered when approaching the evaluation of a BRUE. Prior data from the ALTE literature suggests that in approximately 20% of patients the history and physical examination alone yield the cause; in

TABLE 6.3 Important Historical Features in the Evaluation of a Possible BRUE

Prior to Event	
Condition of child	Awake vs asleep
Location of child	Prone vs supine, in crib/car seat, with pillows, blankets
Activity	Feeding, crying
During Event	
Respiratory effort	None, shallow, gasping, increased Duration of respiratory pauses
Color	Pallor, red, cyanotic Peripheral, whole body, circumoral
Tone/movement	Rigid, tonic-clonic, decreased, floppy Focal vs diffuse Ability to suppress movements
Level of consciousness	Alert, interactive, sleepy, nonresponsive
Duration	Time until normal breathing, normal tone, normal behavior Detailed history of caregiver actions during event to aid in defining time course
Associated symptoms	Vomiting, sputum production, blood in mouth/nose, eye rolling
Postevent	
Condition	Back to baseline, sleepy, postictal, crying If altered after event, duration of time until back to baseline
Interventions	
What was performed	Gentle stimulation, blowing in face, mouth-to-mouth, cardiopulmonary resuscitation
Who performed intervention	Medical professional vs caregiver
Response to intervention	Resolution of event vs self-resolving
Duration of intervention	How long was intervention performed
Medical History	
History of present illness	Preceding illnesses, fever, rash, irritability, sick contacts
Past medical history	Prenatal exposures, gestational age, birth trauma Any medical problems, prior medical conditions, prior hospitalizations Developmental delay Medications
Feeding history	Gagging, coughing with feeds, poor weight gain
Family history	Neurologic problems Cardiac arrhythmias Sudden death, childhood deaths, ALTEs, BRUEs Neonatal problems Consanguinity
Social history	Home situation Caregivers Smoke exposure Medications in the home Prior Child Protective Services involvement

ALTE, apparent life-threatening event; BRUE, brief resolved unexplained event.

about 50% of patients, a likely diagnosis is suspected from the history and physical examination and is subsequently confirmed by diagnostic testing. Diagnostic testing alone yields an etiology in approximately 15% of patients. When testing is performed, it is most successful when done in a focused and targeted manner geared toward diagnoses suggested by the history and physical examination, specifically addressing concerning features identified.

DIFFERENTIAL DIAGNOSIS BY SYSTEM

Gastrointestinal

A variety of gastrointestinal (GI) etiologies can mimic a BRUE on presentation, including GER, intussusception, and volvulus.

GER is one of the most commonly cited comorbid conditions in patients presenting with concerning events. Some infants will present with overt symptoms such as coughing, choking, and laryngospasm following regurgitation. Others may present without visible regurgitation but rather with posturing including arching of the back, torsion of the neck, and lifting up of the chin. This phenomenon, known as **Sandifer syndrome**, can be frightening to the observer and is often confused with seizure activity. Historical findings that should raise the index of suspicion for GER include a history of frequent reflux, the event being immediately preceded by a feeding, poor weight gain, irritability following a feed, or gastric contents noted in the infant's nose or mouth during the episode. However, one must be careful when attributing the event to GER. Approximately 50% of all normal infants younger than 3 months of age experience daily regurgitation, and temporal association does not necessarily equate with causation. Although GER may occasionally cause apneic episodes, GER also occurs very commonly in most healthy infants without any sequelae. It is therefore important not to let a history of GER in an infant presenting with a BRUE preclude the consideration of other underlying causes.

Although less common, additional GI pathology can present similar to a BRUE, including conditions such as intussusception or volvulus. Patients who present with these conditions will typically have additional historical and examination findings to suggest their underlying etiology. Patients with **intussusception** can have sudden and severe abdominal pain demonstrated by inconsolable crying and drawing up of the legs to the abdomen. The classic presentation of intussusception is the triad of abdominal pain, a sausage-shaped abdominal mass, and currant-jelly stool. However, this classic triad is frequently not seen at presentation. Some infants present solely with lethargy or altered consciousness. Similarly, infants with **volvulus** can present with sudden-onset abdominal pain accompanied by emesis. Volvulus is a medical emergency, which can lead to bowel necrosis and death. **Oropharyngeal dysphagia** is another consideration. This dysfunctional coordination of the suck, swallow, and breathe mechanism is common when infants are first learning to feed and can be associated with aspiration, laryngeal food penetration, or nasopharyngeal reflux. This etiology should be considered if there are symptoms of choking, gagging, or color change with feeds; prolonged feeds; or pooling of feeds in the mouth.

Obtaining a careful feeding history is critical in the evaluation of potential GI etiologies for patients presenting with a suspected BRUE, but most studies do not support routine testing for GER in these patients. Because there is a high prevalence of GER in infants, it is expected that a high number of these patients will have positive GER testing. When testing is considered, it is important to understand the utility of various modalities. Upper gastrointestinal fluoroscopy is frequently performed. Although this can be useful in identifying underlying anatomic anomalies that can lead to concerning events, it should not be used to delineate GER as the cause for the event. This study frequently demonstrates regurgitation in normal infants, and a positive finding on the study does not necessarily indicate that GER was the cause of the inciting event. Although typically not indicated, if further GER testing is desired, esophageal pH analysis via a pH probe could be considered to help demonstrate a causal link by correlating low pH findings with documented apnea on concurrent cardiorespiratory monitoring (see Chapter 15).

Infectious Disease

Various infectious etiologies can mimic a BRUE on presentation, ranging from common illnesses caused by respiratory viruses to less common but serious infections such as bacteremia and meningitis. A history of multiple events on the day of presentation is often associated with an infectious etiology. Additional historical clues include recent fever, irritability, altered level of arousal, cough, or coryza. Physical examination findings may confirm the suspicion of an infectious etiology, while hypothermia and ill appearance at presentation exclude the event from being characterized as a BRUE and should lead to concern for more serious infectious etiologies. Of note, fever and typical infectious symptoms may be absent in younger infants with immature immunologic and neurologic systems. Prematurity, complicated birth history, or prior antibiotic administration should raise concerns for potential infectious etiologies.

Viral respiratory infections can present with findings similar to that of a BRUE, particularly in young infants. In this population, apnea may be the presenting symptom of viral lower respiratory tract infections, with the telling symptoms of coryza and cough delayed by hours to days. In particular, pertussis and infection caused by RSV are commonly reported conditions associated with apnea in young infants. Suspicion of respiratory infection must remain high, especially during peak respiratory illness periods, or if there is a history of recent exposure. Influenza and coronavirus should also be considered. Neonates with pertussis may present with or develop few other symptoms, so a careful history of potential exposure is essential for early diagnosis. Although uncommon in infants with pertussis, the development of a staccato cough with posttussive emesis, or a classic "whoop," should prompt treatment while awaiting appropriate testing.

Although the incidence of **bacteremia or meningitis** is low in patients presenting with BRUE-like events, the morbidity and mortality of these diagnoses are such that they should always be considered. A history of irritability and/or altered level of arousal may suggest these and other serious infections. Paradoxical irritability (crying when held) suggests soft tissue or bone infection or a fracture. Examination findings of concern include ill appearance, fever, hypothermia, lethargy, nuchal rigidity, and poor peripheral perfusion. Prompt action is required for the evaluation and treatment of these infants.

Urinary tract infections (UTIs) have also been shown to be a potential cause of BRUE-like events. The infection can lead to cardiorespiratory compromise, which can manifest as apnea, color change, altered levels of consciousness, or change in muscle tone. The majority of patients with UTIs significant enough to cause those symptoms will be ill-appearing at presentation. Therefore, most studies indicate that urinalysis and urine culture can be reserved for infants who are febrile, are ill-appearing, or have other clinical symptoms consistent with a UTI.

Neurologic

Neurologic disorders that can present similar to a BRUE include seizure, breath-holding spells, congenital central hypoventilation syndrome (Ondine's curse), metabolic encephalopathies, and brain or brainstem abnormalities.

The most common identifiable neurologic disorder associated with these symptoms is **seizure**, with a rate of up to 25%. Factors that support the diagnosis of seizure include a history of loss of consciousness, poor tone, unresponsiveness, eye deviation, or rhythmic movements that are not able to be suppressed. A history of choking is typically absent in those presenting with seizure. Lack of this historical fact should raise the suspicion for seizure in the differential.

Breath-holding spells have been reported to present to medical attention with a BRUE-like event. These are typically divided into two types: cyanotic and pallid. In cyanotic breath-holding spells, there is usually an emotional trigger such as anger or frustration. The infants cry, then become silent and hold their breath in expiration with subsequent cyanosis. This can then be followed by limpness and possible loss of consciousness. Pallid breath-holding spells are less common and are typically triggered by pain or fright. The child may gasp, then lose consciousness and become pale, diaphoretic, and limp. This can be followed by a period of increased tone and clonic movements. To determine if the event is consistent with a breath-holding spell, it is important to obtain a stepwise history of the event, including any emotional or painful precipitant.

Congenital central hypoventilation syndrome (CCHS) is a rare but important cause of BRUE-like events. This is classically characterized by near-adequate ventilation while awake but significant hypoventilation while asleep. Most patients with CCHS present at ≤1 month of age; however, late-onset central hypoventilation syndrome (LOCHS) may present up to age 10 years. In addition to hypoventilation, there may be associated autonomic dysfunctions or other manifestations (Table 6.4). Infants with no prior history of sleep-related hypoventilation may become apneic after a triggering event such as an upper respiratory tract infection, sedation, or endotracheal intubation. *PHOX2B* gene polyalanine repeat expansion mutations (PARMs) are responsible for ~90% of affected patients in this autosomal dominant disorder. The differential diagnosis of the central hypoventilation seen in CCHS and LOCHS includes Prader Willi syndrome, Chiari I or II malformations, familial dysautonomia, congenital myasthenia, congenital myopathy, mitochondrial defects (Leigh syndrome), and ROHHAD (rapid-onset obesity, hypoventilation, and hypothalamic and autonomic dysfunction). An approach to the evaluation of hypoventilation is noted in Figure 6.2.

Additional rare, but potentially life-threatening, neurologic disorders to consider include brain tumors, neuromuscular disorders, metabolic encephalopathies, and malformations of the brain and brainstem. Examiners should therefore pay particular attention to any focal weakness, cranial nerve abnormalities, or signs of increased intracranial pressure, including papilledema and Cushing triad (bradycardia, respiratory irregularities, and hypertension).

Given the relatively high incidence of seizures in infants presenting with a suspected BRUE, some diagnostic algorithms recommend EEGs as part of the initial investigation. However, at only 15%, the sensitivity of EEGs in diagnosing future epilepsy is poor. Since infants who go on to develop epilepsy will likely have recurrent events, most experts recommend that EEGs be reserved for those patients with recurrent events or history or physical examination findings specifically concerning for seizures. In patients with suspected seizures, evaluation of serum electrolytes may also be beneficial to identify possible derangements including hypo- or hypernatremia, hypocalcemia, or hypoglycemia. If specific electrolyte abnormalities are identified, further work-up should be undertaken to determine underlying pathology.

Neuroimaging may be considered in patients presenting with a BRUE. Current evidence does not support routine neuroimaging for asymptomatic infants with a BRUE-like presentation given the low diagnostic yield, high cost, and sedation or radiation concerns.

TABLE 6.4	**Clinical Manifestations of CCHS**
Organ System	**Clinical Manifestations**
Ophthalmologic	Decreased/absent pupillary light response
	Anisocoria
	Strabismus
	Lack of convergent gaze
	Marcus Gunn jaw winking
Respiratory	Alveolar hypoventilation
	Absent perception of dyspnea
Cardiovascular	Bradycardia
	Prolonged sinus pauses (>3 sec)
	Transient asystole
	Decreased heart rate variability
	Low normal daytime BP
	Orthostatic hypotension
	Nondipping BP circadian pattern
	Decreased BP response to exercise
	Syncope
GI	Hirschsprung disease (20%)
	Constipation
	Esophageal dysmotility
Endocrine	Hyperinsulinism
	Hypoglycemia
	Hyperglycemia
Neurologic	Decreased anxiety
	Decreased pain perception
	Seizures
	Neurocognitive deficits
Skin	Sporadic profuse sweating
Tumors	Neuroblastoma
	Ganglioneuroma
	Ganglioneuroblastoma
Others	Decreased baseline body temperature
	Poor heat tolerance

BP, blood pressure; CCHS, congenital central hypoventilation syndrome; GI, gastrointestinal.
From Bishara J, Keens TG, Perez IA. The genetics of congenital central hypoventilation syndrome: clinical implications. *Appl Clin Genet.* 2018;11:135–144 (Table 1, p. 136).

However, neuroimaging must be considered in the infant with an abnormal neurologic examination, recurrent events, or a clinical concern for seizure, child maltreatment, metabolic encephalopathies, or tumor.

Airway/Pulmonary

Infections of the upper and lower respiratory tract are common causes of BRUE-like events, but other respiratory etiologies have been cited as well. These include apnea of prematurity and infancy, periodic breathing, and airway abnormalities.

The most common cause of apnea in preterm infants is **apnea of prematurity**. It occurs in virtually all infants born at <28 weeks' gestation, and the frequency is indirectly proportional to the gestational age. Apnea of prematurity is thought to be due to immature respiratory control in premature infants and typically presents with either central or mixed (central and obstructive) apnea. Following the perinatal period, it is a diagnosis of exclusion and should be considered only after other etiologies have been ruled out. The apneic events typically begin within the first week of life, and as such, symptom onset after that time should stimulate consideration of other causes. Apnea of prematurity typically resolves by 37–40 weeks' postconceptual age in infants delivered at ≥28 weeks but can persist later in infants delivered prior to 28 weeks.

Apnea of infancy (AOI) refers to apnea that develops in neonates older than 37 weeks' postconception. The etiology is unknown. It is reserved for cases when a cause is not identified and is typically seen as a diagnosis of exclusion.

Periodic breathing is a common entity that is often confused by parents as a BRUE. Periodic breathing is defined as three or more respiratory pauses of >3 seconds' duration within a 20-second portion of the breathing cycle. Sometimes several pauses occur, one after the other, followed by a set of short, rapid respirations before the respiratory rhythm is restored. Importantly, no associated change in color, tone, or heart rate and no prolonged respiratory pauses (>20 seconds) are reported in association with periodic breathing. A clear history of the event is essential in differentiating true apnea from periodic breathing. Video of concerning events can prove very helpful. If determined to be periodic breathing, it is a benign entity and does not require any additional work-up or intervention.

Less common respiratory etiologies to consider include **anatomic airway abnormalities** such as anomalies of the pharynx (adenotonsillar hypertrophy), the larynx (laryngomalacia, edema, subglottic ductal cyst, subglottic stenosis), or the trachea (tracheomalacia, aberrant innominate artery). A history of associated respiratory distress, obstructive apnea, positional symptoms, or noisy breathing, or physical examination findings such as stridor should raise the index of suspicion for these otolaryngologic etiologies. Aspiration can also present with features similar to a BRUE and can be the result of a foreign body, neurologic abnormalities leading to swallowing dysfunction, or anatomic disorders such as cleft palate or tracheoesophageal fistula.

Chest and neck radiographs can be beneficial in assessing for signs of airway abnormalities or radiopaque foreign bodies. If there is high concern for anatomic abnormalities, evaluation by direct laryngoscopy, bronchoscopy, and/or esophagoscopy could be considered. However, in patients who are well-appearing without clinical concern for airway anomalies, the yield for these tests is low. Polysomnography can be useful in differentiating between central versus obstructive processes (see Fig. 6.2). This may be a consideration in patients with prematurity, noisy breathing, or recurrent/severe events when obstruction in suspected.

Child Maltreatment

Child maltreatment should always be considered in infants presenting with BRUE-like symptoms (see Chapter 30). Possible etiologies include head trauma (direct injury or repetitive shaking), smothering, toxic ingestions, and factitious syndrome (formerly Munchausen syndrome) by proxy.

Concerning historical facts include unexplained vomiting or irritability, recurrent events, historical discrepancies (history is confusing, varies among caregivers, changes over the course of the evaluation), or a family history of BRUEs, ALTEs, SIDS, or unexplained death. There is a higher rate of child maltreatment in infants presenting with more severe initial episodes and in those requiring resuscitation.

Any bruising should be noted, especially in a nonambulatory infant. A careful ear, nose, and throat examination should be performed,

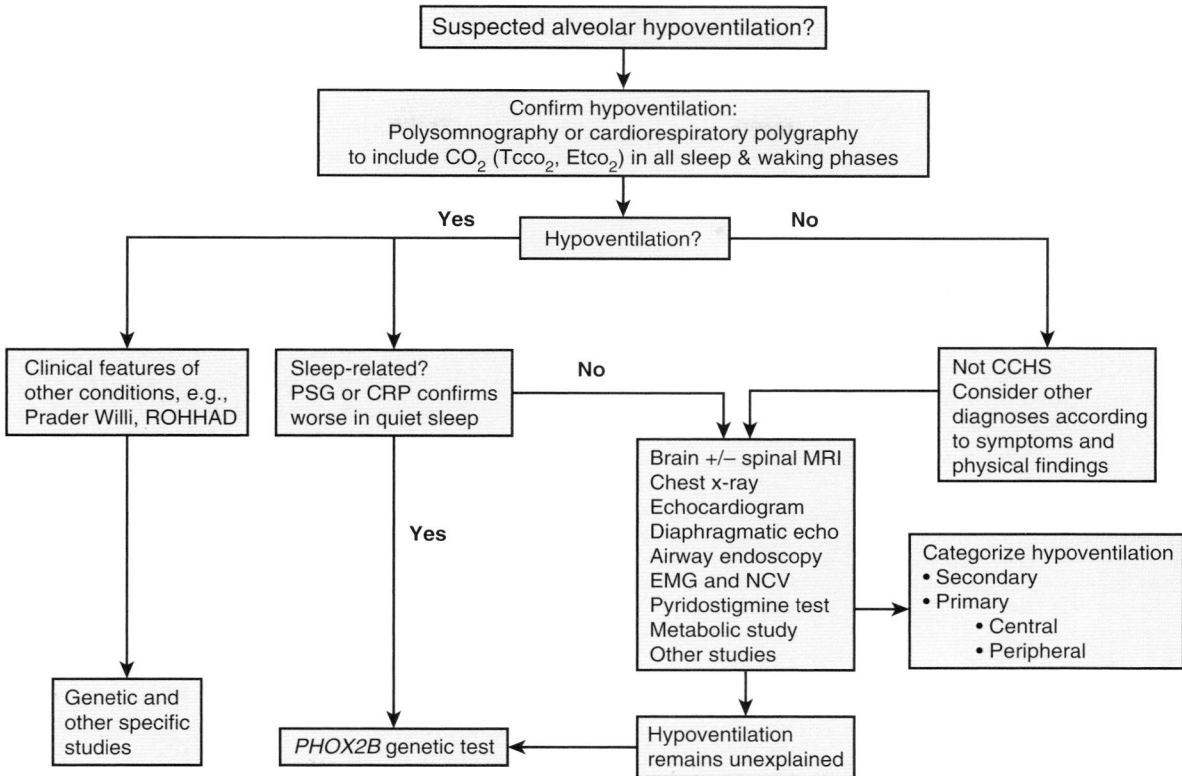

Figure 6.2 Diagnostic algorithm for alveolar hypoventilation. CCHS, congenital central hypoventilation syndrome; CRP, cardiorespiratory polygraphy; EMG, electromyogram; Etco$_2$, end-tidal co$_2$; NCV, nerve conduction velocity; PHOX2B, paired-like homeobox 2B; PSG, polysomnography; ROHHAD, rapid-onset obesity with hypoventilation, hypothalamic dysfunction, and autonomic disregulation; Tcco$_2$, transcutaneous Pco$_2$. (From Trang H, Samuels M, Ceccherini I, et al. Guidelines for diagnosis and management of congenital central hypoventilation syndrome. *Orphanet J Rare Dis.* 2020;15:252 [Fig. 1, p. 3].)

noting any ear bruising, bleeding from the nose or mouth, or frenulum tears. A thorough neurologic examination is also essential, assessing for altered sensorium, fontanel fullness, pupillary abnormalities, or other focal neurologic findings. These findings should all raise suspicion for child maltreatment. However, it is also important to note that infants with child maltreatment may appear well on presentation with no external signs of trauma; the absence of these findings does not rule out maltreatment as the cause for the event.

If there is clinical suspicion for child maltreatment, a skeletal survey, cranial/brain imaging, select laboratory studies, and a dilated funduscopic examination should be considered to assess for supportive findings. Video surveillance while the infant is hospitalized can also be considered in these cases. In addition, if there is concern for possible intentional or unintentional poisoning, a toxicology screen should be considered to identify the presence of medications that could cause the presenting symptoms. However, in patients without historical or physical examination findings concerning for child maltreatment, the evidence does not support the routine use of any of these assessments.

Cardiac

Though relatively rare, with a reported rate of 0–2%, cardiac pathology can lead to BRUE-like events in myriad ways. Children with structurally normal hearts may experience events due to arrhythmias, cardiomyopathy, and myocarditis. Those with structurally abnormal hearts, such as vascular anomalies, cyanotic heart disease, and left-sided

obstruction, may also present with symptoms similar to a BRUE. A history of multiple and/or escalating events over days to weeks, feeding difficulties, diaphoresis, failure to thrive, long QT syndrome, or a positive family history of an ALTE, BRUE, cardiac disease, or sudden unexplained death before the age of 35 years should raise the index of suspicion for cardiac pathology. A complete cardiac examination should be performed, noting abnormalities that might suggest underlying cardiac pathology, such as irregular rhythms, decreased femoral pulses, or murmurs.

Given the low rate of cardiac disease in patients presenting with a BRUE, routine echocardiograms are generally not useful in the initial work-up of these patients. ECGs may be a more useful screening tool, as they are relatively easy to perform and are highly sensitive in identifying cardiac abnormalities. Therefore, ECG could be considered to help exclude cardiac etiologies in patients where this is a clinical concern. However, the examiner should note that there is a high false-positive rate for ECGs in these patients, which could lead to additional unnecessary testing. If arrhythmia is strongly suspected or identified, assessment for electrolyte disturbances, such as hypo- or hyperkalemia, should be undertaken.

Metabolic/Genetic

BRUE-like events can be the initial presentation of various metabolic disorders including organic acidemias, urea cycle disorders, fatty acid oxidation disorders, and mitochondrial disorders. Similarly, this type of event can be the presenting symptom of hypoglycemia and

TABLE 6.5   Red Flags in Infants Presenting with a Suspected BRUE

Age <60 days

Prematurity (gestational age ≤32 wk and postconceptual age ≤45 wk)

Duration >1 min

Cardiopulmonary resuscitation by a trained medical provider

Recurrent events

Concerning historical features

- Inconsistent history/history incompatible with the child's developmental age (concern for child abuse)
- Congenital anomalies, autonomic dysfunction, or known syndromes
- Family history of BRUE, ALTE, SIDS, or unexplained death

Concerning physical exam findings

- Unexplained bruising, torn labial or lingual frenulum, signs of trauma (concern for child abuse)
- Fever or persistent respiratory symptoms (concern for infection)
- Dysmorphic feature
- Abnormal physical examination findings at the time of presentation; no recovery from event

ALTE, apparent life-threatening event; BRUE, brief resolved unexplained event; SIDS, sudden infant death syndrome.

hypocalcemia. Although metabolic entities are rare, they can be progressive and life-threatening and therefore should be considered in the differential for these patients.

Clinical findings that may suggest an inborn error of metabolism include recurrent or severe events, associated developmental delay, failure to thrive, or positive family history of seizure disorders, SIDS, or early infant deaths. Physical findings such as dysmorphic features should also be noted as these could suggest an underlying syndromic etiology. Disorders of the face and upper airway, such as cri du chat and Pierre Robin syndromes, can lead to obstructed respiratory patterns.

Serum chemistries, while not necessarily diagnostic of an inborn error of metabolism, can be helpful in screening patients with potential metabolic abnormalities and should be considered in patients when this is a clinical concern. Serum glucose, bicarbonate, ammonia, lactate, and pyruvic acid levels are useful screening tests in these patients because abnormalities signal the possibility of metabolic disorders requiring additional evaluation. The **newborn metabolic screen** should also be reviewed to ensure no abnormalities were identified. If there is a high index of suspicion, it is prudent to repeat the newborn screen to ensure that the findings remain normal following the introduction of enteral feeds.

SUMMARY AND RED FLAGS

A thorough history and physical examination are paramount in the evaluation of patients with a suspected BRUE. Concerning historical factors and physical examination findings, such as prematurity, age <60 days, multiple events, or requirement for resuscitation, should prompt consideration of further evaluation (Table 6.5).

BIBLIOGRAPHY

A bibliography is available at ExpertConsult.com.

7

Syncope and Dizziness

Gary Cohen

Dizziness is a common but very nonspecific chief complaint about which some elaboration by the patient is generally required for the physician to understand exactly what the patient is experiencing. The description of the sensation is critical in distinguishing whether it is caused by vertigo, disequilibrium, lightheadedness, presyncope, or ataxia (Table 7.1). Although the differential diagnoses of these entities may overlap, there are conditions that are most specific to the individual symptom. All the entities are conditions that may affect children at any age, but older children are more capable of articulating the abnormal sensation they feel. Children younger than 6 years of age may present with nausea, vomiting, ataxia, or syncope.

Syncope is the abrupt transient loss of consciousness and postural tone that results from inadequate cerebral perfusion. There is a rapid and spontaneous recovery. Syncope is a common phenomenon in children and adolescents that is usually benign. Between 30% and 40% of all adolescents and young adults have had one episode of syncope.

Presyncope is the feeling that the person is "about to pass out." The patient feels as if they are going to lose consciousness but does not. The patient may experience lightheadedness, tunnel vision, graying out, and a spectrum of altered consciousness without loss of consciousness. Presyncope may or may not reflect the same pathophysiologic process as true syncope. Presyncope may abort or progress to syncope. The diagnostic approach to presyncope is the same as for syncope.

Dizziness must be considered a change in mental status. It may potentially herald serious underlying central nervous system dysfunction. Dizziness must be better defined to distinguish vertigo from lightheadedness. The principal distinction with *vertigo* is the description of perceived environmental motion: swaying, whirling, or spinning. **Lightheadedness** is frequently associated with psychological stress, including anxiety, hyperventilation, depression, and panic attacks. The history surrounding episodes of lightheadedness is vital for formulating the differential diagnosis.

Disequilibrium refers to "balance problems" without vertigo. The characteristic historical feature is difficulty ambulating. A rare complaint among children, disequilibrium in the young is most often caused by vestibular or cerebellar dysfunction and manifests as ataxia. **Ataxia** is an impairment of coordination, movement, and balance; this impairment is generally associated with dysfunction of the cerebellum or of the sensory and/or motor pathways connecting to the cerebellum. There are transient forms and progressive degenerative conditions that produce ataxia.

SYNCOPE

Syncope is a common phenomenon among children and adolescents. As many as 40% of children experience a syncopal event between the ages of 8 and 18 years. Before age 6 years, syncope is very unusual except in the setting of seizure disorders, breath-holding spells, systemic illnesses, and primary cardiac dysrhythmias. Syncopal episodes cause a large number of health care visits and a number of admissions to hospitals. Neurocardiogenic syncope (vasovagal) is reported as the most common cause followed by cardiogenic syncope. The differential diagnosis of syncope is noted in Tables 7.2 and 7.3; distinguishing features are noted in Tables 7.4 and 7.5.

The pathophysiologic mechanism of syncope follows a common pathway with many inciting stimuli. Cerebral perfusion is compromised by a transient decrease in cardiac output as a result of vasomotor changes, decreasing venous return, primary dysrhythmia, or impairment of cerebral vascular tone. Adolescents with syncope subjected to a head-up tilt-table test reported blurred vision and constriction of visual fields before losing consciousness, as well as nausea, pallor, sweating, and dizziness, which may be accompanied by hypotension (systolic blood pressure <60 mm Hg) or bradycardia (heart rate <40 beats/min) with an occasional junctional rhythm and occasionally asystole. Symptoms are relieved rapidly by returning to the supine position. Several situational factors can exacerbate this response, including warm temperature, a confined space such as being in a crowded room, anxiety or fear, sudden surprise, the sight of blood, and pain such as from needle sticks or shots. Other situational factors include urination, swallowing, coughing, defecation, and hair combing.

This response is caused by an imbalance of parasympathetic and sympathetic tone, which results in peripheral vasodilation, including venodilation, but in no augmentation of venous return, because there is no accompanying increase in large skeletal muscle activity to augment systemic venous return and maintain cardiac filling. Subsequent vagal output results in inappropriate bradycardia and further compromises cardiac output. The child faints and becomes supine, which restores systemic venous return. Awakening is accompanied by increased sympathetic output, which restores the heart rate. The episode tends to be brief but may recur if the patient stands too quickly after the event.

In obtaining the history of a syncopal episode, attention should be paid to the time of day, time of last meal, activities leading up to the event, and associated symptoms such as palpitations, racing heartbeat, chest pain, headache, shortness of breath, nausea, diaphoresis, visual

TABLE 7.1   Syncope and Dizziness

	Vertigo	Presyncope	Disequilibrium	Lightheadedness
Patient complaint	"My head is spinning" "The room is whirling"	"I feel I might pass out" "I feel faint" "I feel like blacking out"	"I feel unsteady" "My balance is off"	"I feel dizzy" "I feel disconnected, drugged"
Associated features	Motion, swaying, spinning, nystagmus	Syncope: loss of postural tone, brief loss of consciousness Situational	Poor balance No vertigo or ataxia	Anxiety, hyperventilation, paresthesias, respiratory alkalosis, panic attacks
Usual cause	Vestibular disorders	Impaired cerebral perfusion	Sensory and/or central neurologic dysfunction	Anxiety and/or depressive disorders
Key differential diagnoses	Peripheral (labyrinthine-cochlear) vs Central neurologic disorder	Neurocardiogenic (vagal) vs Cardiac syncope vs Neuropsychiatric syncope	Sensory deficit vs Central neurologic disease	Anxiety/depression vs Hyperventilation vs Medication effects

TABLE 7.2   Noncardiac Causes of Syncope

- **Reflex vasodepressor syncope**
  - Neurocardiogenic (vasovagal)
  - Emotion (seeing blood)
  - Pain (needle phobia)
- **Miscellaneous situational reflex**
  - Tussive
  - Sneeze
  - Exercise, after exercise
  - Swallowing
  - Stretching
  - Defecation
  - Micturition
  - Hair grooming
  - Valsalva (increased intrathoracic pressure)
  - Trumpet playing
  - Weightlifting
  - Breath-holding spells
- **Systemic illness**
  - Hypoglycemia
  - Anemia
  - Infection
  - Hypovolemia, dehydration
  - Adrenal insufficiency
  - Narcolepsy, cataplexy
  - Pulmonary embolism
  - Pheochromocytoma
  - Carcinoid
  - Mastocytosis
  - Ruptured ectopic pregnancy
- **Central nervous system**

- Seizure (atonic, absence, myoclonic-astatic)
- Stroke, transient ischemic attack
- Subarachnoid hemorrhage
- Myotonic dystrophy
- Kearns-Sayre syndrome
- Friedreich ataxia
- Basilar artery migraine
- Dysautonomia
- Congenital myasthenia gravis
- Syringomyelia
- Arnold Chiari malformation
- **Drug effects**
  - β-Blocking agents
  - Vasodilating agents
  - Opiates
  - Sedatives
  - Drugs prolonging QT interval
  - Diuretics
  - Anticonvulsant agents
  - Antihistamines
  - Antidepressant agents
  - Anxiolytic agents
  - Drugs of abuse
  - Insulin, oral hypoglycemic agents
  - Carbon monoxide
- **Other etiologies**
  - Carotid sinus sensitivity
  - Subclavian steal
  - Panic attack, anxiety
  - Conversion disorder

From Kliegman RM, St. Geme JW III, Blum NJ, et al., eds. *Nelson Textbook of Pediatrics.* 21st ed. Philadelphia: Elsevier; 2020:567, Table 87.1.

changes, and hearing changes. **Cataplexy** may be confused with syncope and is characterized by partial or complete paralysis of skeletal muscles resulting in a rapid progression of weakness of the face and neck followed by the muscles of the trunk and extremities. The patient loses tone and may fall to the floor but remains awake and immobile for 1–2 minutes. The patient usually senses an episode and may sit or lie down. Cataplexy is seen in patients with narcolepsy characterized by daytime sleepiness, hypnagogic hallucinations, or sleep paralysis.

Triggers of cataplexy include intense positive or negative emotions, such as laughing, frustration, fright, surprise, or anger. Details of the syncopal event, such as the patient's position (syncope while supine suggests a cardiac arrhythmia) when symptoms appeared, duration of the episode, and characterization of the patient's appearance during and immediately after the episode, are also important. Almost without exception, by the time the patient presents to the office or emergency room, the physical examination findings are normal. Therefore, the history becomes

TABLE 7.3 Causes of Cardiovascular Syncope: Potentially Fatal if Unrecognized

1. ARRHYTHMIAS
   - A. Bradyarrhythmias
     - a. Sinus node dysfunction (especially in patients with congenital heart defects)
     - b. Atrioventricular block (congenital or acquired, Lyme, Fabry, Chagas diseases)
     - c. Kearns-Sayre syndrome
     - d. Pacemaker malfunction
   - B. Tachyarrhythmias
     - a. Supraventricular
       1. Wolff-Parkinson-White syndrome
       2. Supraventricular tachycardia/atrial arrhythmias (especially in patients with congenital heart defects)
     - b. Ventricular: ventricular tachycardia/torsades/ventricular fibrillation
       1. Channelopathies
          - a. Long QT syndromes
          - b. Catecholaminergic polymorphic ventricular tachycardia
          - c. Brugada syndrome
          - d. Short QT syndrome
       2. Drug induced
       3. Idiopathic
          - a. Ventricular fibrillation
          - b. Ventricular tachycardia from outflow tract
2. STRUCTURAL/FUNCTIONAL HEART DISEASE
   - A. Cardiomyopathy
     - a. Hypertrophic cardiomyopathy
     - b. Dilated cardiomyopathy
     - c. Arrhythmogenic right ventricular dysplasia
     - d. Left ventricular noncompaction
   - B. Coronary anomalies
     - a. Anomalous origin
     - b. Kawasaki disease
     - c. COVID-19
   - C. Valvar aortic mitral or pulmonary stenosis
   - D. Takotsubo disease
   - E. Acute myocarditis
   - F. Congenital heart disease (repaired and unrepaired)
   - G. Pulmonary hypertension, pulmonary embolus
   - H. Aortic dissection (Marfan syndrome)
   - I. Cardiac masses (myxoma, rhabdomyoma, thrombus)
   - J. Eisenmenger syndrome

From MacNeill E, Vashist S. Approach to syncope and altered mental status. *Pediatr Clin N Am.* 2013;60:1083–1106.

TABLE 7.4 Clinical Features Suggesting Specific Causes of Syncope

Diagnostic Consideration

Neurocardiogenic
Symptoms after prolonged motionless standing, sudden unexpected pain, fear, or unpleasant sight, sound, or smell
Syncope in a well-trained athlete after exertion (without heart disease)
Situational syncope during or immediately after micturition, cough, swallowing, or defecation
Syncope with throat or facial pain (glossopharyngeal or trigeminal neuralgia)

Organic Heart Disease (e.g., Coronary Artery Disease, Aortic Stenosis, Primary Arrhythmia, Obstructive Hypertrophic Cardiomyopathy, Pulmonary Hypertension)
Brief sudden loss of consciousness, no prodrome, history of heart disease
Syncope with exertion, while sitting or supine
History of palpitations
Family history of sudden death

Neurologic
Seizures: longer period of being unconscious and confusion for >5 min after regaining consciousness (postictal)
Transient ischemic attack, subclavian steal, basilar migraine: syncope associated with vertigo, dysarthria, diplopia, arm exercise
Migraine: syncope associated with antecedent headaches

Other Vascular
Carotid sinus: syncope with head rotation or pressure on the carotid sinus (as in tumors, shaving, tight collars)
Orthostatic hypotension: syncope immediately on standing
Subclavian steal or aortic dissection: differences in blood pressure or pulse between the two arms

Drug Induced
Patient is taking a medication that may lead to long QT syndrome, orthostasis, or bradycardia

Psychiatric Illness
Frequent syncope, somatic complaints, no heart disease

Modified from Kapoor WN. Syncope. *N Engl J Med.* 2000;343:1856–1862.

the most important piece of information for developing the differential diagnosis, diagnostic evaluation, and management plan.

NEUROCARDIOGENIC SYNCOPE

There are several causes of **neurocardiogenic syncope** (vasovagal); this is the dominant etiology of syncope in children and adolescents. Excessive vagal tone may be primary or secondary to breath holding, cough, deglutition syncope, micturition, defecation, carotid sinus pressure sensitivity, and orthostasis. Neurocardiogenic syncope has been described in association with hair brushing, swallowing, stretching, orthodontic maneuvers, anomalies of the cervical spine, and dental trauma. Many of these episodes may be forms of carotid sinus sensitivity. Cough syncope may be related to prolongation of high intrathoracic pressure that results in decreased venous return and subsequent decreased cardiac output.

The prodromal history is very important in evaluating neurocardiogenic syncope. *Syncope without warning, while the patient is supine, or during exercise implies a primary cardiac cause and a more serious etiology; it is associated with greater morbidity and potential mortality* (see Table 7.3).

Neurocardiogenic syncope is a type of autonomic dysfunction that is also referred to as **vasodepressor syncope**, **vasovagal syncope**, and **reflex syncope**. Presentations include:

1. Primary bradycardia, sometimes to the extreme of sinus arrest or even brief asystole, with subsequent hypotension. This is known as the cardioinhibitory response.
2. Primary vasodepressor response that is characterized by hypotension with the heart rate relatively preserved.
3. Mixed response, the most common response that features *simultaneous* hypotension and bradycardia.

The common pathway producing the heart rate and blood pressure responses and cerebral hypoperfusion is the Bezold-Jarisch reflex (Fig. 7.1). For most children and adolescents, **prodromal warning signs** herald the impending syncopal episode and can, after the first episode, allow the child enough time to prevent fainting by sitting with the head between the knees or by lying supine.

The physiologic mechanisms of neurocardiogenic syncope have been demonstrated with head-up tilt-table testing. **Tilt-table testing** can be performed with or without invasive blood pressure monitoring. The goal is to reproduce the patient's symptoms under close

TABLE 7.5 Comparison of Clinical Features of Syncope and Seizures

Features	Syncope	Seizures
Relation to posture	Common	No
Time of day	Diurnal	Diurnal or nocturnal
Precipitating factors	Emotion, injury, pain, crowds, heat, exercise, fear, dehydration, coughing, micturition	Sleep loss, drug/alcohol withdrawal
Skin color	Pallor	Cyanosis or normal
Diaphoresis	Common	Rare
Aura or premonitory symptoms	Long	Brief
Convulsion	Rare, brief	Common
Other abnormal movements	Minor twitching	Rhythmic jerks
Injury	Rare	Common (with convulsive seizures)
Urinary incontinence	Rare	Common
Tongue biting	No	Can occur with convulsive seizures
Postictal confusion	Rare	Common
Postictal headache	No	Common
Postevent recovery	Seconds to minutes	Often delayed
Focal neurologic signs	No	Occasional
Cardiovascular signs	Common (cardiac syncope)	No
Abnormal findings on EEG	Rare (generalized slowing may occur during the event)	Common

From Bruni J. Episodic impairment of consciousness. In: Daroff RB, Jankovic JM, Mazziotta JC, Pomeroy SL, eds. *Bradley's Neurology in Clinical Practice.* 7th ed. Philadelphia: Elsevier; 2016:9.

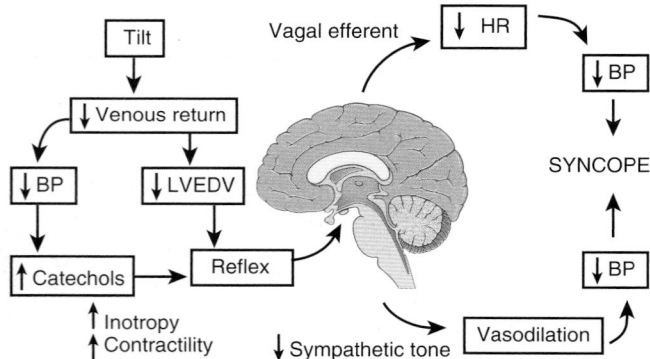

Fig. 7.1 Tilt-table testing: the Bezold-Jarisch reflex. BP, blood pressure; HR, heart rate; LVEDV, left ventricular end-diastolic volume.

monitoring. Various tilt angles and durations have been described, as has the use of isoproterenol as a provocative stimulus.

If the history suggests the diagnosis of neurocardiogenic syncope with normal physical examination findings and a normal ECG, treatment may be empirically started.

An ECG is recommended for all patients with syncope. Even when no longer symptomatic, the ECG may demonstrate characteristic features of Wolff-Parkinson-White syndrome, Brugada syndrome, long and short QT syndromes, hypertrophic cardiomyopathy, arrhythmogenic right ventricular dysplasia, and heart block.

Guidelines for the treatment of neurocardiogenic syncope are found in Table 7.6. The first line of treatment is education and counseling. Most patients will eventually outgrow neurocardiogenic syncope. Patients should maintain hydration and increase dietary salt if there are not any contraindications. Patients should be counseled to avoid situations that precipitate an event and taught to abort an event by lying

down. Physical counterpressure maneuvers are helpful when there is a prodrome (see Table 7.6).

If the patient fails conservative therapies, pharmacologic treatments may be tried. Physicians have used fludrocortisone with increased salt intake, β-adrenergic blockers, and midodrine, which has had promising results.

ORTHOSTATIC SYNCOPE

Conditions that produce **hypotension** (orthostatic or supine) frequently produce syncope or presyncope. Cardiac function and structure are usually normal before the episode; during the predisposing illness, cardiac filling pressures are often reduced because of reduced venous return from hypovolemia or decreased peripheral vascular resistance (peripheral pooling of blood). Dehydration from diarrhea and vomiting, hyperthermia, hyperpyrexia, heat exhaustion, polyuria (diabetes mellitus), or poor intake from anorexia, together with the systemic effects of the primary illness, may produce orthostatic or true hypotension and syncope. In these conditions, dizziness, hypotension, or syncope occurs rapidly when the patient assumes an upright position. Prolonged bed rest, combined with poor fluid intake during an illness, may also result in syncope or presyncope when the child arises to leave the bed. In most of these situations, fluid administration is sufficient to restore intravascular volume and venous return to alleviate postural or supine hypotension.

POSTURAL ORTHOSTATIC TACHYCARDIA SYNDROME

Postural orthostatic tachycardia syndrome (POTS) is characterized by recurrent (often daily) and long-standing symptoms of orthostatic intolerance, exercise intolerance, lightheadedness, fatigue, sweating,

TABLE 7.6 Treatment of Neurocardiogenic Syncope/Vasovagal Syncope (VVS)

RECOMMENDATIONS

Patient education on the diagnosis and prognosis of VVS is recommended.
  In all patents with the common faint or VVS, an explanation of the diagnosis, education targeting awareness of and possible avoidance of triggers (prolonged standing, warm environments, coping with dental and medical settings), and reassurance about the benign nature of the condition should be provided.

Physical counterpressure maneuvers can be useful in patients with VVS who have a sufficiently long prodromal period.
  Patients with a syncope prodrome should be instructed to assume a supine position to prevent a faint and minimize possible injury. In patients with a sufficiently long prodrome, physical counter-maneuvers (leg crossing, limb and/or abdominal contraction, squatting, isometric handgrip, arm tensing) are a core management strategy.

Midodrine is reasonable in patients with recurrent VVS with no history of hypertension, heart failure, or urinary retention.
  Midodrine is a prodrug that is metabolized to desglymidodrine, which is a peripherally active α-agonist used to ameliorate the reduction in peripheral sympathetic neural outflow responsible for venous pooling and vasodepression in VVS.

The usefulness of orthostatic training is uncertain in patients with frequent VVS.
  There are two main methods of orthostatic training. Patients undergo repetitive tilt-table tests in a monitored setting until a negative tilt-table test occurs and then are encouraged to stand quietly against a wall for 30–60 min daily, or patients simply stand quietly against a wall at home for a prolonged period of time daily.

Fludrocortisone might be reasonable for patients with recurrent VVS and inadequate response to salt and fluid intake, unless contraindicated.
  Fludrocortisone has mineral corticoid activity resulting in sodium and water retention and potassium excretion, which results in increased blood volume. Serum potassium level should be monitored because of potential drug-induced hypokalemia. POST II (Prevention of Syncope Trial II) reported a marginally insignificant 31% risk of reduction in adults with moderately frequent VVS, which was significant in patients after 2 wk dose stabilization period.

Encouraging increases in salt and fluid intake may be reasonable in selected patients with VVS, unless contraindicated.
  Evidence for the effectiveness of salt and fluid intake for patients with VVS is limited. Nonetheless, in patients with recurrent VVS and no clear contraindication, such as a history of hypertension, renal disease, heart failure, or cardiac dysfunction, it may be reasonable to encourage ingestion of 2–3 L of fluid per day and a total of 6–9 g (100–150 mmol) of salt per day, or about 1–2 heaping teaspoonfuls. The long-term balance of risks and benefits of a strategy of increasing salt and water intake is unknown.

In selected patients with VVS, it may be reasonable to reduce or withdraw medications that cause hypotension when appropriate.
  A careful examination of the patient's history for medications that may lower blood pressure (hypotensive agents) should be performed. Care should be taken to withdraw or reduce medications only when safe to do so and in conjunction with the prescribing health care provider.

In patients with recurrent VVS, a selective serotonin reuptake inhibitor might be considered.
  Serotonin has central neurophysiologic effects on blood pressure and heart rate and acutely induces syncope during tilt-table testing.

Modified from Shen W-K, et al. 2017 ACC/AHA/HRS guideline for the evaluation and management of patients with syncope: a report of the American College of Cardiology/American Heart (e84-85). Association Task Force on Clinical Practice Guidelines and the Heart Rhythm Society. *Circulation.* 2017;136:e60–e122.

headache, chest tightness, brain fog, palpitations, anxiety, tremor, and presyncope when upright. The syndrome may be secondary to autonomic dysfunction. Symptoms are improved with lying down. Criteria to diagnose POTS include symptoms that have lasted >6 months; heart rate that increases by at least 40 beats/min or a maximum rate of 130 if younger than 18 years or 30 beats/min or a maximum rate of >125 if older than 18 years after assuming a standing from supine position for at least 10 minutes; symptoms worsen with standing and improve with recumbence; and the absence of other overt causes of orthostatic intolerance.

Several different pathophysiologic mechanisms have been described in patients with POTS, including:

1. Peripheral autonomic denervation (neuropathic) leading to reduced venoconstriction and venous pooling with secondary tachycardia
2. Hypovolemia
3. Hyperadrenergic POTS associated with elevated systolic blood pressure and increased norepinephrine levels after standing for 10 minutes
4. Poor exercise tolerance
5. POTS associated with other diseases including autoimmunity

A detailed history of orthostatic intolerance may identify symptoms of headache, fatigue, sleep disorder, weakness, hyperventilation, shaking, sweating, anxiety, dizziness, and presyncope. An evaluation for POTS may include a CBC, glucose, electrolytes, and thyroid function. Cardiac evaluation should include an ECG. A tilt-table test is helpful to demonstrate the effects of orthostatic stress (increased heart rate).

There is no specific treatment for POTS. Medications that may aggravate symptoms of POTS should be avoided, including antihypertensive agents, sedatives, and many other psychiatric medications. Patients should avoid aggravating factors, such as dehydration, extreme heat, and alcohol. Nonpharmacologic treatment includes aerobic exercise, compressive stockings, and increased fluid and salt intake. Pharmacologic treatment should be tailored to the variant the patient exhibits (Table 7.7).

Inappropriate sinus tachycardia (IST) presents with palpitations, fatigue, dizziness, and near syncope. It may be initially confused with POTS. In IST, the heart rate is elevated at rest (>100 beats/min) when supine and increases further with exercise. The mean 24-hour heart rate is >90 beats/min. The differential diagnosis includes hyperthyroidism and pheochromocytoma. Treatment is difficult, but ivabradine with or without metoprolol may be effective.

CARDIAC SYNCOPE/SUDDEN CARDIAC DEATH

A variety of cardiac conditions can result in hypotension and syncope (Tables 7.8, 7.9, and 7.10; see Table 7.3). Dysrhythmias are common and are usually silent between episodes (see Table 7.8). Supraventricular tachycardia, ventricular tachycardia, and heart block are the most common types of dysrhythmia and may be primary or result from medications or illicit drugs. Any form of acquired heart block carries a high mortality rate (Fig. 7.2). A common cause of acquired heart block is Lyme disease. Heart block may necessitate temporary or permanent electronic pacing to maintain cardiac output.

TABLE 7.7 Treatment for Postural Orthostatic Tachycardia Syndrome (POTS)

A regular, structured, and progressive exercise program.

Acute intravenous infusion of up to 2 L of saline if short-term clinical decompensation.

Patients with POTS need a multidisciplinary approach.

The consumption of up to 2–3 L of water and 10–12 g of NaCl daily may be considered.

Fludrocortisone or pyridostigmine.

Treatment with midodrine or low-dose propranolol may be considered.

Those with prominent hyperadrenergic features are treated with clonidine or α-methyldopa.

Drugs that block the norepinephrine reuptake transporter can worsen symptoms in patients with POTS.

Regular intravenous infusions of saline are not recommended in the absence of evidence, and chronic or repeated intravenous cannulation is potentially harmful.

Radiofrequency sinus node modification, surgical correction of a Chiari malformation type I, and balloon dilation or stenting of the jugular vein are not recommended for routine use in patients with POTS and are potentially harmful.

Modified from Sheldon RS, et al. 2015 Heart Rhythm Society expert consensus statement on the diagnosis and treatment of postural tachycardia syndrome, inappropriate sinus tachycardia and vasovagal syncope. *Heart Rhythm.* 2015;12:e44.

TABLE 7.8 Primary Electrical Abnormalities: Features, ECG, and Treatment

Primary Electrical Abnormalities	Features	ECG	Treatment
LQTS: Romano-Ward, Jervell–Lange-Nielsen, acquired	Familial genetic disorder Ion channel variant Presents in torsades de pointes Romano-Ward is MC inherited LQTS Jervell–Lange-Nielsen has congenital deafness	Prolonged QT measured from the onset of the Q wave to the end of the T wave in lead II Varies with HR but >0.44 in men, >0.46 in children and women for HR 50–90 beats/min is prolonged Torsades de pointes can occur Can deteriorate from polymorphic ventricular tachycardia to ventricular fibrillation	β Blocker therapy Recommendations on exercise intensity by a cardiologist ICD if β blockers fail
Brugada syndrome	Inherited autosomal dominant arrhythmogenic syndrome characterized by life-threatening ventricular arrhythmias Genetic variant in *SCN5A* and 13 other genes	ECG abnormalities are from repolarization and depolarization abnormalities Coved-type ST segment elevations in the right precordial leads J wave amplitude ≥2 mm followed by a negative T wave	Placement of ICD
Wolff-Parkinson-White	Owing to one or more re-entrant pathways inducing SVT or atrial fibrillation Up to 14% associated with malignant tachycardias Malignant arrhythmias from short re-entrant pathway repolarization or multiple pathways	Short PR interval Delta waves present	Undergo EPT and ablation
Dilated cardiomyopathy: ventricular tachycardia/fibrillation	Cardiac dilation and systolic dysfunction Inherited or acquired Lamin AC gene variant a common cause of DCM and SCD	Marked LVH Poor R wave progression Left atrial enlargement Right axis deviation	Permanent pacemaker and ICD placement
Catecholamine-exercise: ventricular tachycardia	Ventricular ectopy induced by exercise or emotional stress Variant in gene that encodes Ca-mediated sarcoplasmic fibers Lethal in 30–50% if left untreated	Pre-exercise ECG is usually normal, stress testing recommended ECG with exercise Nonsustained wide ventricular tachycardia	β Blocker therapy Recommendations on exercise intensity by a cardiologist ICD if β blockers fail

DCM, dilated cardiomyopathy; EPT, electrophysiologic testing; HR, heart rate; ICD, implantable cardioverter defibrillator; LQTS, long QT syndrome; LVH, left ventricular hypertrophy; MC, most common; SCD, sudden cardiac death; SVT, supraventricular tachycardia.
From Ellison S. Sudden cardiac death in adolescents. *Prim Care Clin Office Pract.* 2015;42:57–76.

TABLE 7.9 Potential Causes of Sudden Death in Infants, Children, and Adolescents

SIDS and SIDS "Mimics"

SIDS
Long QT syndromes*
Inborn errors of metabolism
Child abuse
Myocarditis
Ductal-dependent congenital heart disease

Corrected or Unoperated Congenital Heart Disease

Aortic stenosis
Tetralogy of Fallot
Transposition of great vessels (postoperative atrial switch)
Mitral valve prolapse
Hypoplastic left-heart syndrome
Eisenmenger syndrome

Coronary Arterial Disease

Anomalous origin*
Anomalous tract (tunneled)
Kawasaki disease
COVID-19
Periarteritis
Arterial dissection
Marfan syndrome (rupture of aorta)
Myocardial infarction

Myocardial Disease

Myocarditis
Hypertrophic cardiomyopathy*
Dilated cardiomyopathy
Arrhythmogenic right ventricular dysplasia
Lyme carditis
Takotsubo syndrome

Conduction System Abnormality/Arrhythmia

Long QT syndromes*
Brugada syndrome
Proarrhythmic drugs
Pre-excitation syndromes
Heart block
Commotio cordis
Idiopathic ventricular fibrillation
Arrhythmogenic right ventricular dysplasia
Catecholaminergic polymorphic ventricular tachycardia
Heart tumor (myxoma, rhabdomyoma)

Miscellaneous

Pulmonary hypertension
Pulmonary embolism
Heat stroke
Cocaine and other stimulant drugs or medications
Anorexia nervosa
Seizures
Electrolyte disturbances

SIDS, sudden infant death syndrome.
*Common.
From Van Hare GF. Sudden death. In: Kliegman RM, Stanton BF, St. Geme JW III, Schor NF, eds. *Nelson Textbook of Pediatrics*. 20th ed. Philadelphia: Elsevier; 2016:2262.

Primary cardiac conduction abnormalities that may result in syncope include Wolff-Parkinson-White syndrome, long QT syndromes, and catecholamine-sensitive ventricular tachycardia. **Wolff-Parkinson-White syndrome** is characterized by a *short PR interval*, pre-excitation seen as a widened QRS duration, and a delta wave on the proximal portion of the QRS. The delta wave represents the presence of accessory electrical tissue from atria to ventricle, with rapid antegrade conduction causing excitation of ventricular tissue before atrioventricular node–His bundle stimulation. If that pathway can conduct in the retrograde manner, a re-entrant circuit is created, causing a narrow QRS complex tachycardia. This greatly shortens the diastolic ventricular filling time and results in diminished left ventricular end-diastolic volume, with subsequently decreased stroke volume and decreased cardiac output. Although the tachycardia is rarely sufficiently fast to result in syncope, some children have profound hypotension and a rapid loss of consciousness. In adults, a similar mechanism results from atrial flutter or fibrillation if the ventricular response rate is fast.

Long QT syndromes are inherited (usually autosomal dominant) or acquired abnormalities in the electrical recovery (repolarization) of the heart (Fig. 7.3). Prolongation of the repolarization phase results in the risk of simultaneous depolarization, the "R-on-T" phenomenon, which causes disorganized ventricular electrical stimulation characterized by **torsades de pointes** (coarse ventricular tachycardia), a potentially lethal dysrhythmia (Fig. 7.4). There may be a family history of sudden cardiac death. Family studies with the same gene variant have demonstrated that affected patients may not always have a long QT interval on ECG as defined for the syndrome, but an increased QT interval may become evident with exercise or during catecholamine infusion. Long QT syndromes may be responsible for some cases of sudden infant death syndrome and drowning. Although additional genetic forms have been described, most gene variants for prolonged QT involve either a potassium or sodium ion channel (see Table 7.10). There is some genotype-phenotype correlation in LQT genes: LQT1 events are frequently associated with stress, exercise, emotion, or swimming; LQT2 events are associated with auditory triggers (alarm clocks); while LQT3 events may be associated with sleep. Long QT syndromes may present as a syncopal episode, seizures, palpitations, or presyncope. Diagnosing long QT syndromes is based on clinical history and ECG findings of a prolonged rate-corrected QT interval. Genetic testing may identify approximately 75% of patients. Acquired prolongation of the QT interval is seen in electrolyte abnormalities (hyperkalemia) and with a variety of medications (Table 7.11). A drug history and toxicology screen may be warranted if there is any question of QT prolongation.

Patients who have undergone **corrective or palliative surgery** for congenital cardiac disease are at risk for both early- and late-onset dysrhythmias that might result in syncope. Sinus node disease (in patients undergoing atrial surgery) may result in tachycardia-bradycardia episodes that can be associated with hypotension. Ventricular dysrhythmias are particularly common after repair of tetralogy of Fallot, double-outlet right ventricle, truncus arteriosus, and pulmonary atresia involving right ventriculotomy with subsequent ventricular scar formation.

Uncorrected structural heart disease is a relatively rare cause of a sudden decrease in cardiac output. However, **hypertrophic cardiomyopathies** can result in obstruction of left ventricular outflow with resultant high transmural pressure and secondary cardiac ischemia, which can be fatal. This type of obstruction is exacerbated by high sympathetic tone, causing increased contractility, and is a frequent mechanism of syncope associated with exercise in competitive athletes. The presence of an outflow tract murmur in the setting of syncope, especially if there is a positive family history, warrants evaluation with *both* electrocardiography and echocardiography. Any condition that impedes left ventricular outflow (valvular aortic stenosis or subaortic stenosis), left ventricular inflow or filling (mitral stenosis or pericardial tamponade), or blood flow through the pulmonary vasculature (primary or secondary pulmonary hypertension) may result in syncope. In almost all cases, characteristic physical findings lead the clinician to the diagnosis. Pulmonary hypertension may be associated with cyanosis, in which case there is cerebral hypoxia resulting from right-to-left

TABLE 7.10 Summary of Heritable Arrhythmia Syndrome Susceptibility Gene

Gene	Locus	Protein
Long QT Syndrome (LQTS)		
Major LQTS Genes		
KCNQ1 (LQT1)	11p15.5	I_{Ks} potassium channel α subunit (KVLQT1, K_v7.1)
KCNH2 (LQT2)	7q35-36	I_{Kr} potassium channel α subunit (HERG, K_v11.1)
SCN5A (LQT3)	3p21-p24	Cardiac sodium channel α subunit (Na_v1.5)
Minor LQTS Genes (listed alphabetically)		
AKAP9	7q21-q22	Yotiao
CACNA1C	12p13.3	Voltage-gated L-type calcium channel (Ca_v1.2)
CALM1	14q32.11	Calmodulin 1
CALM2	2p21	Calmodulin 2
CALM3	19q13.2-q13.3	Calmodulin 3
CAV3	3p25	Caveolin-3
KCNE1	21q22.1	Potassium channel β subunit (MinK)
KCNE2	21q22.1	Potassium channel β subunit (MiRP1)
KCNJ5	11q24.3	Kir3.4 subunit of I_{KACH} channel
SCN4B	11q23.3	Sodium channel β_4 subunit
SNTA1	20q11.2	Syntrophin-α_1
Triadin Knockout (TKO) Syndrome		
TRDN	6q22.31	Cardiac triadin
Andersen-Tawil Syndrome (ATS)		
KCNJ2 (ATS1)	17q23	I_{K1} potassium channel (Kir2.1)
Timothy Syndrome (TS)		
CACNA1C	12p13.3	Voltage-gated L-type calcium channel (Ca_v1.2)
Cardiac-Only Timothy Syndrome (COTS)		
CACNA1C	12p13.3	Voltage-gated L-type calcium channel (Ca_v1.2)
Short QT Syndrome (SQTS)		
KCNH2 (SQT1)	7q35-36	I_{Kr} potassium channel α subunit (HERG, K_v11.1)
KCNQ1 (SQT2)	11p15.5	I_{Ks} potassium channel α subunit (KVLQT1, K_v7.1)
KCNJ2 (SQT3)	17q23	I_{K1} potassium channel (Kir2.1)
CACNA1C (SQT4)	12p13.3	Voltage-gated L-type calcium channel (Ca_v1.2)
CACNB2 (SQT5)	10p12	Voltage-gated L-type calcium channel β_2 subunit
CACN2D1 (SQT6)	7q21-q22	Voltage-gated L-type calcium channel 2 δ_1 subunit
Catecholaminergic Polymorphic Ventricular Tachycardia (CPVT)		
RYR2 (CPVT1)	1q42.1-q43	Ryanodine receptor 2
CASQ2 (CPVT2)	1p13.3	Calsequestrin 2
KCNJ2 (CPVT3)	17q23	I_{K1} potassium channel (Kir2.1)
CALM1	14q32.11	Calmodulin 1
CALM3	19q13.2-q13.3	Calmodulin 3
TRDN	6q22.31	Cardiac triadin
Brugada Syndrome (BrS)		
SCN5A (BrS1)	3p21-p24	Cardiac sodium channel α subunit (Na_v1.5)
Minor BrS Genes (listed alphabetically)		
ABCC9	12p12.1	ATP-binding cassette, subfamily C member 9
CACNA1C	2p13.3	Voltage-gated L-type calcium channel (Ca_v1.2)
CACNA2D1	7q21-q22	Voltage-gated L-type calcium channel 2 δ_1 subunit
CACNB2	10p12	Voltage-gated L-type calcium channel β_2 subunit
FGF12	3q28	Fibroblast growth factor 12
GPD1L	3p22.3	Glycerol-3-phosphate dehydrogenase 1–like
KCND3	1p13.2	Voltage-gated potassium channel (I_{to}) subunit K_v4.3
KCNE3	11q13.4	Potassium channel β_3 subunit (MiRP2)
KCNJ8	12p12.1	Inward rectifier K^+ channel Kir6.1

Continued

TABLE 7.10 Summary of Heritable Arrhythmia Syndrome Susceptibility Gene—cont'd

Gene	Locus	Protein
HEY2	6q	Hes-related family BHLH transcription factor with YRPW motif 2
PKP2	12p11	Plakophilin-2
RANGRF	17p13.1	RAN guanine nucleotide release factor 1
SCN1B	19q13	Sodium channel β_1
SCN2B	11q23	Sodium channel β_2
SCN3B	11q24.1	Sodium channel β_3
SCN10A	3p22.2	Sodium voltage-gated channel α_{10} subunit (Na$_v$1.8)
SLMAP	3p14.3	Sarcolemma-associated protein
Early Repolarization Syndrome (ERS)		
ABCC9	12p12.1	ATP-binding cassette, subfamily C member 9
CACNA1C	2p13.3	Voltage-gated L-type calcium channel (Ca$_v$1.2)
CACNA2D1	7q21-q22	Voltage-gated L-type calcium channel 2 δ_1 subunit
CACNB2	10p12	Voltage-gated L-type calcium channel β_2 subunit
KCNJ8	12p12.1	Inward rectifier K$^+$ channel Kir6.1
SCN5A	3p21-p24	Cardiac sodium channel α subunit (Na$_v$1.5)
SCN10A	3p22.2	Sodium voltage-gated channel α_{10} subunit (Na$_v$1.8)
Idiopathic Ventricular Fibrillation (IVF)		
ANK2	4q25-q27	Ankyrin B
CALM1	14q32.11	Calmodulin 1
DPP6	7q36	Dipeptidyl-peptidase-6
KCNJ8	12p12.1	Inward rectifier K$^+$ channel Kir6.1
RYR2	1q42.1-q43	Ryanodine receptor 2
SCN3B	11q23	Sodium channel β_3 subunit
SCN5A	3p21-p24	Cardiac sodium channel α subunit (Na$_v$1.5)
Progressive Cardiac Conduction Disease/Defect (PCCD)		
SCN5A	3p21-p24	Cardiac sodium channel α subunit (Na$_v$1.5)
TRPM4	19q13.33	Transient receptor potential cation channel, subfamily M, member 4
Sick Sinus Syndrome (SSS)		
ANK2	4q25-q27	Ankyrin B
HCN4	15q24-q25	Hyperpolarization-activated cyclic nucleotide–gated channel 4
MYH6	14q11.2	Myosin, heavy chain 6, cardiac muscle, α
SCN5A	3p21-p24	Cardiac sodium channel α subunit (Na$_v$1.5)
"Ankyrin-B Syndrome"		
ANK2	4q25-q27	Ankyrin B
Familial Atrial Fibrillation (FAF)		
ANK2	4q25-q27	Ankyrin B
GATA4	8p23.1-p22	GATA-binding protein 4
GATA5	20q13.33	GATA-binding protein 5
GJA5	1q21	Connexin 40
KCNA5	12p13	I$_{Kur}$ potassium channel (K$_v$1.5)
KCNE2	21q22.1	Potassium channel β subunit (MiRP1)
KCNH2	7q35-36	I$_{Kr}$ potassium channel α subunit (HERG, K$_v$11.1)
KCNJ2	17q23	I$_{K1}$ potassium channel (Kir2.1)
KCNQ1	11p15.5	I$_{Ks}$ potassium channel α subunit (KVLQT1, K$_v$7.1)
NPPA	1p36	Atrial natriuretic peptide precursor A
NUP155	5p13	Nucleoporin 155 KD
SCN5A	3p21-p24	Cardiac sodium channel α subunit (Na$_v$1.5)

From Tester DJ, Ackerman MJ. Genetics of cardiac arrhythmias. In: Zipes DP, Libby P, Bonow RO, et al., eds. *Braunwald's Heart Disease*. 11th ed. Philadelphia: Elsevier; 2019:605–606, Table 33.1.

shunting, as well as decreased left ventricular output resulting from poor transpulmonary flow and decreased left ventricular filling.

Other rare causes of cardiac syncope are thoracic masses and intracardiac tumors or masses, coronary artery abnormalities, and inflammatory cardiac diseases (myocarditis). Masses or tumors, such as myxomas, fibromas, and rhabdomyomas, tend to produce paroxysmal symptoms, which are often associated with position changes, especially from the recumbent position. **Coronary artery anomalies** are usually not accompanied by signs of ischemia. Rather, the most common manifestation is syncope or sudden cardiac death from compression of the anomalous left main coronary artery as it courses between the pulmonary outflow and the aortic root (Fig. 7.5). This usually occurs in a competitive athlete whose hypertrophied heart responds to catecholamine stimulation during activity and inadvertently compresses the anomalous coronary artery. Inflammatory conditions, such as heart block associated with Lyme disease and ventricular tachycardia associated with myocarditis or pericarditis, predispose to dysrhythmias.

Cardiac syncopal episodes can be accompanied by brief tonic-clonic seizure activity known as **Stokes-Adams syndrome**. The seizure activity appears 10–20 seconds after the onset of asystole and is usually of short duration with no subsequent postictal phase. Many children with cardiac syncope are initially referred to a neurologist.

Sudden cardiac death is discussed with cardiac causes of syncope because cardiac causes of syncope may also produce sudden death (see Table 7.3). Sudden cardiac arrest or death is defined as the abrupt and unexpected loss of heart function. Structural causes include valvular aortic stenosis, coronary artery anomalies, cardiomyopathies, and myocarditis. Cardiac arrhythmias associated with sudden death include Wolff-Parkinson-White syndrome and prolonged QT syndrome. A less common cause is **commotio cordis** resulting from nonpenetrating blunt trauma to the chest. Warning events or symptoms may not always be evident prior to sudden cardiac death; if it presents, patients may complain of episodes of dizziness, lightheadedness, presyncope, syncope, dyspnea, or palpitations. Other relevant history may

include fatigue, unexplained seizure, or chest pain. It is important for the physician to perform a detailed history and physical examination to look for warning signs of cardiovascular disease in the patient *and* family (Table 7.12). Key elements of the physical examination should include measurement of blood pressure and a complete cardiovascular exam with attention to heart rate, rhythm, murmurs, pulses, and features of possible hereditary disorders with recognizable phenotypes such as Marfan syndrome.

Predictors of a cardiac etiology of syncope versus a more benign etiology such as neurocardiogenic syncope include:
1. Syncope associated with activity or while sitting or supine
2. Family history of cardiac disease or sudden/unexplained cardiac death
3. Physical examination consistent with cardiac disease
4. Abnormal ECG
5. Palpitations

NEUROLOGIC CAUSES OF SYNCOPE-LIKE EPISODES

Primary neurologic causes of syncope are more unusual in otherwise healthy children and adolescents than in adults. Seizures must be considered if there is a history of an aural prodrome, focal or generalized tonic-clonic activity, and a prolonged postictal phase of lethargy or confusion (see Tables 7.4 and 7.5). Prolonged postevent lethargy is unusual with more common causes of syncope if the vital signs have returned to normal. Seizures are a common cause of loss of consciousness in the recumbent patient. Seizures are often accompanied by tachycardia and normal or elevated blood pressure. A premonitory aura may herald vertebrobasilar vascular spasm, which appears to occur when syncope is with **basilar type migraines**. There may be a history of unilateral visual changes; the loss of consciousness usually has a somewhat longer onset and duration. The patient frequently complains of headache after regaining consciousness. Basilar type migraine or migraine affecting the vertebrobasilar circulation can cause dizziness, vertigo,

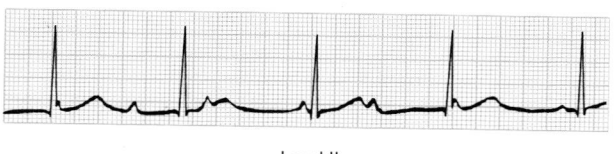

Lead II

Fig. 7.2 Congenital complete atrioventricular (AV) block. The ventricular rate is regular at 53 beats/min. The atrial rate is somewhat variable, from 65 to 95 beats/min, and completely dissociated from the ventricle. The QRS morphology is normal, which is common in congenital complete AV block. (From Van Hare GF. AV block. In: Kliegman RM, Stanton BF, St. Geme JW III, Schor NF, eds. *Nelson Textbook of Pediatrics*. 20th ed. Philadelphia: Elsevier; 2016:2260.)

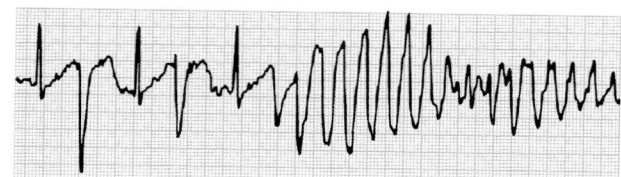

Fig. 7.4 Episode of torsades de pointes in a patient with long QT syndrome. (From Van Hare GF. Sudden death. In: Kliegman RM, Stanton BF, St. Geme JW III, Schor NF, eds. *Nelson Textbook of Pediatrics*. 20th ed. Philadelphia, Elsevier; 2016:2262.)

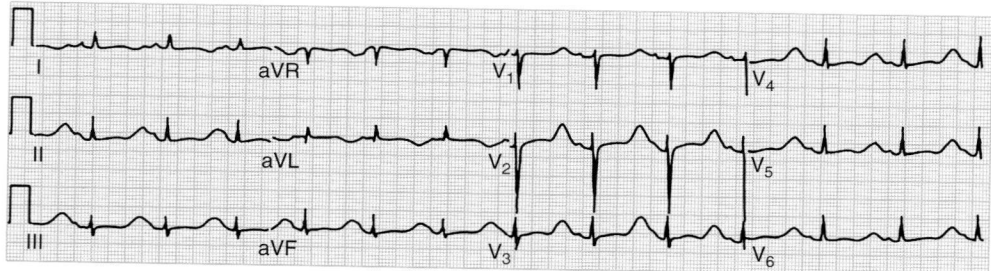

Fig. 7.3 An ECG showing a QT interval of 640 milliseconds in a patient with LQT1 syndrome, with the terminal portion of the T wave merging with the P wave. (From Garan H. Ventricular arrhythmias. In: Goldman L, Schafer AI, eds. *Goldman-Cecil Medicine*. 25th ed. Philadelphia: Elsevier; 2016:373.)

ataxia, confusion, and headache. There is often a positive family history of migraines.

METABOLIC CAUSES OF SYNCOPE

Hypoglycemia should always be included as a cause of syncope, but it is rare in children and adolescents except in patients with insulin-dependent diabetes or inborn errors of glucose, glycogen, fatty acid metabolism, or adrenal insufficiency (see Chapter 57). With hypoglycemia, the patient feels weak, hungry, sweaty, agitated, and confused and eventually experiences altered mental status. Onset is gradual, and the patient remains hemodynamically stable, although tachycardia may be evident. Ingestion of oral hypoglycemic agents may exceed the body's normal glucose homeostasis, resulting in hypoglycemia.

TABLE 7.11 Drugs That Prolong the QT Interval and Produce Torsades de Pointes	
Drugs Commonly Involved	**Other Drugs**
Disopyramide	Amiodarone
Dofetilide	Arsenic trioxide
Ibutilide	Cisapride
Procainamide	Calcium channel blockers: lidoflazine (not marketed in the United States)
Quinidine	
Sotalol	Anti-infective agents: clarithromycin, erythromycin, halofantrine, pentamidine, quinoline-class antibiotics, hydroxychloroquine
Bepridil	
	Antiemetic agents: domperidone, droperidol
	Antipsychotic agents: chlorpromazine, haloperidol, mesoridazine, thioridazine, pimozide
	Methadone

From Roden D. Drug-induced prolongation of the QT interval. *N Engl J Med.* 2004;350:1013–1022.

SYNCOPAL-LIKE EPISODES IN INFANTS AND TODDLERS

Reflex asystolic syncope, also known as "pallid breath-holding spells," is often initiated in a toddler-aged child with a minor stimulus (bump to the head). This is not true breath holding; the child becomes pale, loses tone, and may have asystole and on awakening red color returns to the child's face. This may be an early predictor of vasovagal syncope in an older child.

Cyanotic breath-holding spells are triggered by pain or frustration in a toddler-aged infant. The child experiences a prolonged expiratory apnea and loses tone. Treatment is reassurance and iron supplementation if the serum ferritin level is low.

Infant hyperekplexia manifests with hypertonia, apnea, exaggerated startle response to unexpected stimuli (noise), and poststartle rigidity. Associated gene variants include *GLRA1, SLC6A5, GLRB, GPHN,* and *ARHGEF9* (X-linked). Most are autosomal dominant, but autosomal recessive and X-linked inheritance is possible. Treatment includes clonazepam and placing the patient in a curled-up position during an episode.

Paroxysmal extreme pain disorder may manifest in the neonate and infant and is often triggered by defecation or by changes in temperature, emotional distress, eating spicy foods, or drinking cold fluids in an older child (see Chapter 39). The manifestations include flushing (occasionally Harlequin change), apnea, stiffening, and paroxysmal localized pain (jaw, perianal area). Gene variants in *SCN9A* cause this autosomal dominant disorder. The differential diagnosis includes erythromelalgia and hyperekplexia. Carbamazepine has been one effective medication to manage the neuropathic pain.

PSYCHIATRIC CAUSES OF SYNCOPE

Patients with a history of panic attacks may become syncopal secondary to hyperventilation. The mechanism is not completely understood but may involve the reaction of cerebral blood flow in response to hypocapnia and respiratory alkalosis. Tetany or paresthesias may be present in some patients. The history of the episode is critical, and witnesses are especially helpful. The patient frequently relates a feeling of suffocation, smothering, shortness of breath, or chest tightness. In

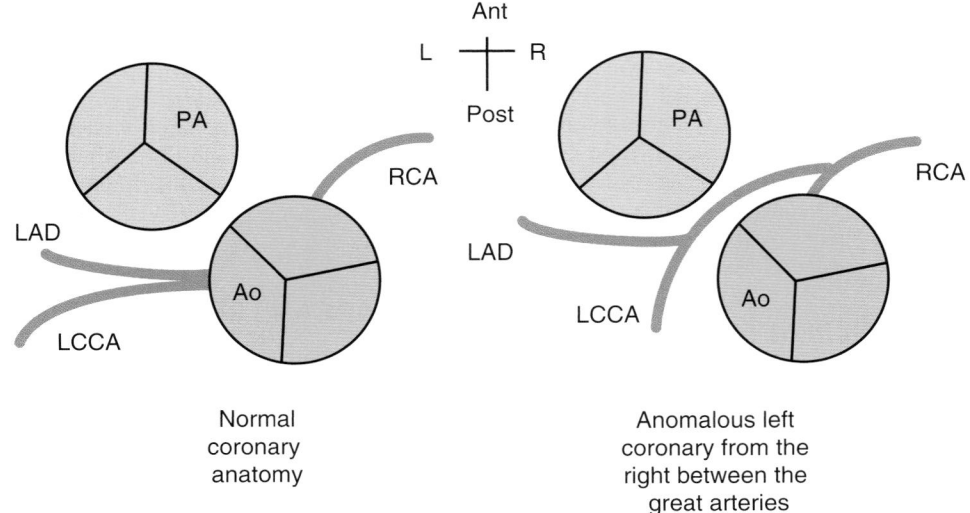

Fig. 7.5 Coronary artery anomalies associated with sudden cardiac death. Ant, anterior; Ao, aorta; L, left; LAD, left anterior descending coronary artery; LCCA, left circumflex coronary artery; PA, pulmonary artery; Post, posterior; R, right; RCA, right coronary artery.

TABLE 7.12 Pediatric Sudden Cardiac Death Risk Assessment*

Patient History Questions:

Tell Me About Any of These in Your Child ... Yes or No

Has your child fainted or passed out during or after exercise, emotion, or startle?

Has your child ever had extreme shortness of breath and/or discomfort, pain, or pressure in their chest during exercise?

Has your child had extreme fatigue associated with exercise (different from other children)?

Has a doctor ever ordered a test for your child's heart?

Has your child ever been diagnosed with an unexplained seizure disorder? Or exercise-induced asthma not well controlled with medication?

Family History Questions:

Tell Me About Any of These in Your Family...

Are there any family members who had a sudden, unexpected, unexplained death before the age of 50 (including sudden infant death syndrome, car crash, drowning, others) or near drowning?

Are there any family members who died suddenly of "heart problems" before the age of 50?

Are there any family members who have had unexplained fainting or seizures?

Are there any relatives with certain conditions, such as:

    Enlarged heart: hypertrophic cardiomyopathy

    Dilated cardiomyopathy

    Heart rhythm problems: long QT syndrome

    Short QT syndrome

    Brugada syndrome

    Catecholaminergic ventricular tachycardia

    Arrhythmogenic right ventricular cardiomyopathy

    Marfan syndrome (aortic rupture)

    Heart attack, age 50 or younger

    Pacemaker or implanted defibrillator

    Deaf at birth (congenital deafness)

Please Explain More About Any "Yes" Answers.

*Ask these questions (or have parents complete for your review) at periodic times during well-child visits (neonatal, preschool, before or during middle school, and before or during high school).

From Campell R, Berger S, Ackerman M, et al. Policy statement pediatric sudden cardiac arrest. *AAP Pediatr.* 2012;e1094–e1102.

retrospect, the patient may also admit to numbness and tingling of the extremities and visual changes. Hyperventilation and hypocapnia may be detected during a tilt-table test by measuring end-tidal CO_2.

A psychiatric cause of syncope (pseudosyncope) is a diagnosis of exclusion. The patient is usually an adolescent and frequently has episodes in the presence of others. The patient is unusually calm in describing the episodes and relates details that may indicate no loss of consciousness. During the episode, there are no associated hemodynamic changes and no pallor, sweating, or respiratory changes. Typically, the patient falls without injury. The key is to define what secondary gain the patient attains through the disorder.

EVALUATION OF THE SYNCOPAL CHILD

History

The history of the event is the critical information for most patients (see Table 7.4). A detailed account of what the patient felt immediately before losing consciousness, what the patient was doing, what the posture or position was, how the patient looked, how long the episode lasted, and associated signs or symptoms direct the diagnostic work-up. A thorough and detailed family history is necessary to

discover risk for sudden death, dysrhythmia, heart disease, seizures, and metabolic disorders. The medication history, including over-the-counter, prescribed, and illicit drugs, as well as any accessible medication of other family members should be gathered.

Physical Examination

Any person who has a syncopal episode should undergo a thorough physical examination, with special attention to the cardiovascular and neurologic systems. The examination should include obtaining vital signs with the patient supine and after standing for 5–10 minutes. Upon careful auscultation, the presence of an outflow tract murmur radiating to the neck, an abnormally loud second heart sound, or the presence of a long decrescendo diastolic murmur at the apex leads to more involved diagnostic testing. A complete neurologic exam should be performed. In most cases, patients with a history of syncope have normal physical findings at the time of the examination.

Diagnostic Tests

Because the child or adolescent who has had a syncopal episode is often evaluated hours or days after the episode, testing serum glucose, electrolytes, or urine toxicology screening is usually of no value. The routine use of blood tests without an indication are of low diagnostic value. *All patients presenting with syncope need an ECG* (Fig. 7.6). The ECG should be inspected for the rhythm, with special attention to nonsinus rhythms and bradycardia. Measurements of the intervals should be performed manually regardless of any preprogrammed measurements printed on the ECG. Abnormalities of the PR, QRS, or QT/corrected QT (QTc) interval imply an underlying conduction abnormality. The P wave, QRS, and T wave amplitudes may indicate chamber enlargement or hypertrophy, each of which carries an increased risk for dysrhythmia. In the patient who also has a history of **palpitations** associated with syncope, long-term cardiac monitoring, with or without a subsequent patient-activated cardiac event recorder monitor, may help capture the cardiac rhythm when the patient is symptomatic. If a heart murmur is appreciated, if there is a family history of sudden death or cardiomyopathy, or if the ECG is at all questionable, a cardiology consultation should be obtained, and two-dimensional, Doppler, and color-flow echocardiography should be performed. If the syncopal event is associated with exercise, echocardiography is critical; if the results are normal, a graded treadmill exercise stress test should be performed with full ECG and blood pressure monitoring. Patients with primary dysrhythmias may require cardiac catheterization and electrophysiologic testing. Patients suspected of having a congenital dysrhythmia syndrome or cardiomyopathy should undergo specific gene panel or exome genetic testing.

Patients exhibiting prolonged loss of consciousness, seizure activity, and a postictal phase of lethargy or confusion should be referred for neurologic consultation and EEG. Without this history, the reported positive yield of EEG is less than 1 in 300 studies. Likewise, neuroimaging studies generally have an exceptionally low yield in the absence of abnormality upon physical examination (see Fig. 7.6).

SUMMARY AND RED FLAGS

Hypotension, both supine and orthostatic, is a major red flag, as are associated palpitations, exertional symptoms, or chest pain (Tables 7.13 and 7.14); participation in gym class or sports must be restricted until a complete diagnostic work-up is completed. Additional red flags include syncope while supine, a positive family history of heart disease or sudden death, prolonged loss of consciousness, prolonged seizures, prolonged postevent neurologic signs, and abrupt onset with no prodrome. Laboratory tests, except for the ECG, which is mandatory,

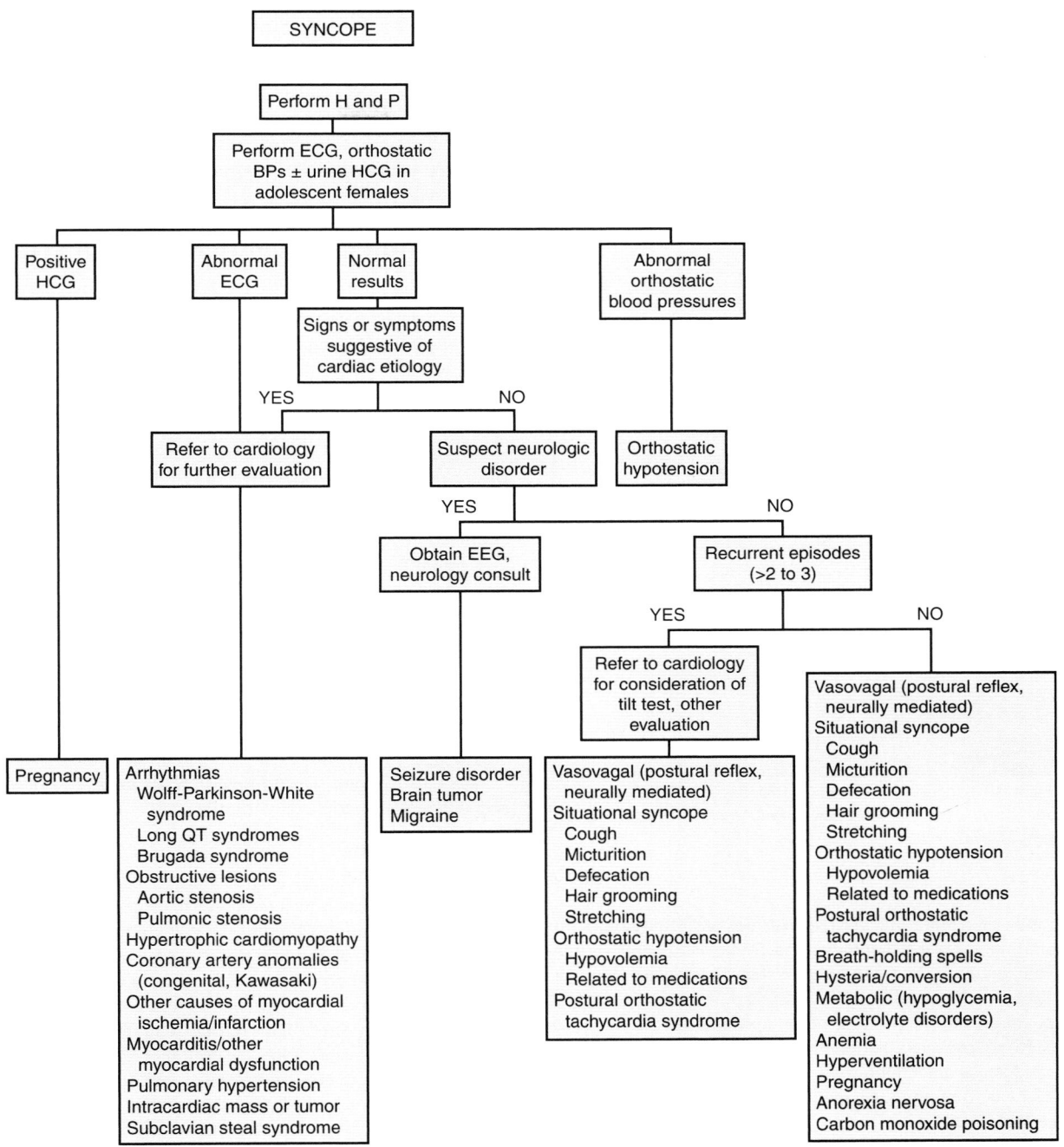

SYNCOPE

Perform H and P

Perform ECG, orthostatic BPs ± urine HCG in adolescent females

Positive HCG

Abnormal ECG

Normal results

Abnormal orthostatic blood pressures

Signs or symptoms suggestive of cardiac etiology

YES — Refer to cardiology for further evaluation

NO — Suspect neurologic disorder

Orthostatic hypotension

YES — Obtain EEG, neurology consult

NO — Recurrent episodes (>2 to 3)

YES — Refer to cardiology for consideration of tilt test, other evaluation

NO — Vasovagal (postural reflex, neurally mediated) / Situational syncope...

Pregnancy

Arrhythmias
  Wolff-Parkinson-White
    syndrome
  Long QT syndromes
  Brugada syndrome
Obstructive lesions
  Aortic stenosis
  Pulmonic stenosis
Hypertrophic cardiomyopathy
Coronary artery anomalies
  (congenital, Kawasaki)
Other causes of myocardial
  ischemia/infarction
Myocarditis/other
  myocardial dysfunction
Pulmonary hypertension
Intracardiac mass or tumor
Subclavian steal syndrome

Seizure disorder
Brain tumor
Migraine

Vasovagal (postural reflex,
  neurally mediated)
Situational syncope
  Cough
  Micturition
  Defecation
  Hair grooming
  Stretching
Orthostatic hypotension
  Hypovolemia
  Related to medications
Postural orthostatic
  tachycardia syndrome

Vasovagal (postural reflex,
  neurally mediated)
Situational syncope
  Cough
  Micturition
  Defecation
  Hair grooming
  Stretching
Orthostatic hypotension
  Hypovolemia
  Related to medications
Postural orthostatic
  tachycardia syndrome
Breath-holding spells
Hysteria/conversion
Metabolic (hypoglycemia,
  electrolyte disorders)
Anemia
Hyperventilation
Pregnancy
Anorexia nervosa
Carbon monoxide poisoning

Fig. 7.6 Syncope algorithm. BP, blood pressure; H, history; HCG, human chorionic gonadotropin; P, physical examination. (From Pomeranz A, Sabnis S, Busey SL, Kliegman RM, eds. *Pediatric Decision-Making Strategies*. Philadelphia: Elsevier; 2016:59.)

are generally of limited value unless guided by pertinent findings in the history and physical examination. The ECG allows screening for Wolff-Parkinson-White syndrome, heart block, and long QT syndrome as well as hypertrophic cardiomyopathies and myocarditis. The most common identifiable etiology in an otherwise healthy child or adolescent is neurocardiogenic syncope, usually a benign and transient condition.

VERTIGO

The characteristic description of vertigo is the illusion of **motion** usually described as the environment spinning or whirling. The perception

of motion may be internal ("My head is [or eyes are] spinning") or external ("The room is spinning or moving"). The sensation is usually rotatory, but it can be linear ("It feels like the swaying of a boat").

Obtaining an accurate description from younger children is difficult. Using terms that the child may understand such as "sliding" or "swinging" may be helpful. The patient's description is critical although potentially vague; further questioning may lead to the rather discrete differential diagnosis of vertigo.

The presence of associated symptoms may help locate the pathology to a central or peripheral cause of vertigo (Tables 7.15, 7.16, and 7.17). Fortunately, peripheral causes of vertigo are more common. Spontaneous rotary vertigo, **nystagmus**, and abnormal head positions are

TABLE 7.13 "Red Flags" in the Evaluation of Patients with Syncope

Syncope with activity or exercise or supine

Syncope not associated with prolonged standing

Syncope precipitated by loud noise or extreme emotion

Absence of presyncope or lightheadedness

Family history of syncope, drowning, sudden death, familial ventricular arrhythmia syndromes, cardiomyopathy

Syncope requiring CPR

Injury with syncope

Anemia

Chest pain

Dyspnea

Palpitations

History of cardiac surgery

History of Kawasaki disease

Implanted pacemaker

Abnormal physical examination

Murmur

Gallop rhythm

Loud and single second heart sound

Systolic click

Increased apical impulse (tachycardia)

Irregular rhythm

Hypo- or hypertension

Clubbing

Cyanosis

From Van Hare GF. Syncope. In: Kliegman RM, Stanton BF, St. Geme JW III, Schor NF, eds. *Nelson Textbook of Pediatrics*. 20th ed. Philadelphia: Elsevier; 2016:515.

symptoms associated more with peripheral causes of vertigo along with nausea, vomiting, sweating, faintness, and fright. Peripheral vertigo results in stimulation of the autonomic nervous system with resultant intense nausea, vomiting, pallor, and diaphoresis. If the vertigo occurs with abrupt changes in the position of the head, peripheral causes of vertigo should be suspected. Peripheral vertigo can be caused by the following: middle ear infections, paroxysmal positional vertigo, labyrinthitis, vestibular neuronitis, Ménière disease (rare in pediatrics), or trauma (see Table 7.16).

Patients suffering from acute ongoing peripheral vertigo appear very ill and very uncomfortable. Because middle ear infection can cause peripheral vertigo, some children seen with otitis media and vomiting may in fact have peripheral vertigo and secondary vomiting.

Benign paroxysmal vertigo of childhood is a common cause of episodes of vertigo in pediatrics. It is thought to be a precursor of future migraines. The episodes may be associated with imbalance and nystagmus. The child will have recurrent brief attacks of vertigo that resolve quickly. There is no associated headache. The episodes improve with age; however, later in life the patient may develop migraine headaches.

A more indolent course, a change in consciousness or behavior, or seizures may indicate a central origin of vertigo (see Table 7.17). Underlying causes of central vestibular dysfunction include acute vascular ischemic or thromboembolic events, acute demyelinating diseases, and pharmacologic vertigo (alcohol, barbiturates, benzodiazepines). More indolent causes of vertigo include tumors of the brainstem or cerebellum, chronic demyelinating diseases, or trauma (see Table 7.17).

Rare syndromes producing vertigo include Cogan syndrome (interstitial keratitis, sensorineural hearing loss, Ménière-like symptoms), Vogt-Koyanagi-Harada syndrome (uveomeningitis, sensorineural hearing loss), Susac syndrome (microangiopathy, stroke, visual loss, sensorineural hearing loss), relapsing polychondritis, and granulomatosis with polyangiitis.

EVALUATION OF THE PATIENT WITH VERTIGO

History

A careful, detailed description of the prodrome and the actual symptoms, including timing, duration, associated symptoms, preceding infections (especially of the upper respiratory tract, such as otitis media or sinusitis), medications, and a history of trauma, must be documented. A past, personal, or family history of vertigo or any other neurologic condition is important.

Physical Examination

Special attention must be paid to the head, ears, eyes, nose, and throat examination. Good visualization of the tympanic membranes and of their mobility is necessary, along with testing both air and bony conduction with a tuning fork (Figs. 7.7 and 7.8). Visualization of the fundi is important. Testing of all the cranial nerves should be performed along with a complete neurologic exam.

The neurologic examination must include an evaluation of the gait, a Romberg test, and an assessment of the visual fields and visual acuity (Fig. 7.9). In most children and adolescents, the physical examination results are normal with only subtle findings when the symptoms are provoked.

The HINTS exam (Head Impulse, Nystagmus, Test of Skew) may help differentiate peripheral vs central causes of vertigo (Table 7.18).

Diagnostic Tests

The history and physical examination results direct the diagnostic work-up and indicate which tests need to be performed. Imaging studies important in the work-up of the vertiginous patient include MRI with visualization of the inner ear, the labyrinthine apparatus, the brainstem, and the cerebellum. If an infectious cause is suspected, it may be useful to perform a lumbar puncture if increased intracranial pressure is not suspected. In the setting of trauma, the simple use of the pneumatic otoscope may allow the examiner to perform a "fistula test," reproducing or worsening the patient's symptoms because of an abnormal communication to the labyrinthine system. If hearing loss is a feature, audiometry and evoked response testing should be considered.

SUMMARY AND RED FLAGS

Vertigo is characterized by the perception of movement, particularly rotational movement, and can be a most distressing and incapacitating phenomenon. The history and examination should allow the examiner to distinguish between peripheral and central vestibular dysfunction.

In children and adolescents, peripheral vertigo is far more common than central vertigo. However, in certain at-risk populations, such as children with sickle cell disease, hemophilia, or congenital heart disease (especially children with right-to-left shunts or mixing lesions) and children receiving anticoagulation therapy, the central causes resulting from hemorrhagic and thromboembolic phenomena must be considered. Chronicity, persistence, vertical nystagmus, and signs of increased intracranial pressure are red flags. Because the diagnosis of vertigo requires that the patient be able to articulate the perception

TABLE 7.14 Summary of Clinical Recommendations for Transient Loss of Consciousness

Topic	Recommendations
Initial assessment	Detailed history, especially from witnesses Full clinical examination 12-lead ECG
Uncomplicated faints	Suggestive features include: 　Posture: occurrence during prolonged standing or previous similar episodes avoided by lying down Provoking factors, such as pain or a medical procedure 　Prodromal symptoms, such as sweating or feeling warm or hot before TLoC 　Further investigation and specialist referral are not needed.
Epilepsy	Suggestive features are a bitten tongue; head turning to one side during TLoC; no memory of abnormal behavior that occurred before, during, or after TLoC; unusual posturing; prolonged limb jerking; confusion after the event; or prodromal déjà vu or jamais vu. If features of epilepsy are present, arrange for early review by an epilepsy specialist. Do not arrange for EEG before neurologic assessment. Note that brief seizure-like activity often occurs during syncope, including uncomplicated faints. Do not suspect epilepsy unless suggestive features are present. Arrange for cardiovascular assessment if the cause of TLoC is unclear.
Urgent specialist referral	Give immediate treatment for clinically urgent problems (such as complete AV block or severe bleeding). Arrange for urgent specialist cardiovascular assessment for patients at risk for a severe adverse event (such as those with long QT interval, cardiac arrhythmia, or structural heart disease).
Further cardiovascular assessment	Focus on specific disorders that may cause TLoC, such as orthostatic hypotension, the carotid sinus syndrome, structural heart disease, or cardiac arrhythmia. Assessment should include repeated history, clinical examination, and 12-lead ECG. For suspected cardiac arrhythmia or unexplained TLoC, use ambulatory ECG for further assessment: 　Very frequent episodes: use 24- to 48-hr Holter monitoring. 　Moderately frequent episodes: use external event monitoring. 　Infrequent episodes: use an implantable event recorder.

AV, atrioventricular; TLoC, transient loss of consciousness.
Modified from Cooper PN, et al. Synopsis of the National Institute for Health and Clinical Excellence Guideline for management of transient loss of consciousness. *Ann Intern Med.* 2011;155:543–549.

TABLE 7.15 Differences Between Peripheral and Central Vestibular Dysfunctions

Symptom/Sign	Peripheral	Central
Severity of vertigo	Marked	Often mild
	Nausea and vomiting common	
Nystagmus	Bilateral	Bilateral or unilateral
	Unidirectional	Bidirectional or unidirectional
	Rotatory/horizontal	May be vertical
	Never vertical	Usually no change with visual fixation
	Fast phase usually opposite to side of lesion	
	Improves with visual fixation	
	Begins within 2–10 sec	Begins immediately
	Fatigues with time	Persistent
	Habituates	Reproducibly repetitive
Direction of environmental spin	Toward fast phase of nystagmus	Variable
Direction of past pointing	Toward slow phase of nystagmus	Variable
Tinnitus/deafness	Often present	Usually absent
Examples	Labyrinthitis	Multiple sclerosis
	Ménière disease	Vertebrobasilar ischemia (see Table 7.17)
	Positional vertigo (see Table 7.16)	

Modified from Reilly BM. *Practical Strategies in Outpatient Medicine.* 2nd ed. Philadelphia: WB Saunders; 1991:191.

TABLE 7.16   Peripheral Vestibulopathy

Syndrome	Usual Presentation	Typical Course	Hearing Loss?	Diagnosis
Benign paroxysmal positional vertigo	Paroxysmal, brief, purely positional vertigo	Often polyphasic illness with gradual improvement but intermittent brief recurrences for weeks/months Does not cause ongoing severe vertigo	No	History Nylen-Bárány maneuvers
Vestibular neuronitis	Acute-onset, severe vertigo, sometimes after viral respiratory infection	Severe ongoing vertigo for many hours or a few days Monophasic illness Resolves spontaneously No hearing loss	No	Clinical history Normal hearing Peripheral nystagmus Rapid (hours–days) resolution without recurrence
Infectious labyrinthitis	Usually, mild vertigo accompanying obvious sinusitis, otitis media, or serous otitis	Resolves over several days with resolution of otitis/sinusitis Very rarely: severe purulent labyrinthitis, mastoiditis, meningitis	No, unless conductive loss due to otitis associated	ENT examination: otitis media? serous otitis? sinusitis?
Toxic vestibulopathy	Vertigo and/or hearing loss associated with use of toxic drugs	Usually dose related and reversible after withdrawal or dose reduction of offending drug	Depends on drug, but sensorineural deafness is common with aminoglycosides, aspirin, loop diuretics, platinum; hearing is usually normal with alcohol and quinidine	Peripheral vertigo with or without hearing loss while/after patient takes vestibulotoxic drugs; most are reversible with discontinuation of drug
Cervicogenic vestibulopathy	Brief positional vertigo, associated with head and neck movements	Usually recurrent, brief, nondebilitating vertigo in patients with cervical spondylosis or other craniovertebral disease (rheumatoid arthritis, Klippel-Feil deformity)	No (but unrelated presbycusis common in this age group)	Typical history Nylen-Bárány maneuvers not consistent with benign positional vertigo Exclude: Vertebrobasilar ischemia Carotid sinus hypersensitivity
Cholesteatoma	Recurrent, often positional vertigo in patients with a history of chronic otitis, TM perforation, mastoiditis	Indolent progression of symptoms	Conductive	Usually visible (at superior border of tympanic membrane) on otoscope examination of ear
Otosclerosis	Progressive hearing loss, sometimes with intermittent vertigo	Indolent progressive hearing loss	Conductive	Family history Audiometry
Post-Traumatic Basilar (temporal bone) fracture	Severe vertigo, often with profound hearing loss immediately after head trauma	Gradual (days–weeks) resolution of vertigo; hearing loss, facial nerve injury often permanent	Often: sensorineural	Radiograph: fracture Hemotympanum? CSF otorrhea? Facial paresis?
Postconcussive	Ongoing, often mild/chronic vertigo after concussion, without fracture	Gradual resolution but often delayed for months–years	No	Persistent/chronic symptoms without evidence of other post-traumatic syndromes
Cupulolithiasis	Classic benign positional vertigo, but after head trauma	Same as for benign positional vertigo	No	Clinical history Nylen-Bárány maneuvers Exclude fistulas
Perilymphatic fistula	Trauma may be remote or indirect (swimming, diving injuries) Usually, positional vertigo, recurrent; or mild persistent vertigo	Post-traumatic vertigo that does not improve over time	Often: mixed or sensorineural	Clinical history Positive fistula test Valsalva maneuver: symptoms worsen?
Whiplash	Positional vertigo, worse with neck extension or turning, after deceleration neck injury	Gradual but slow improvement with resolution of neck symptoms	Usually none	Clinical history Exclude fractures and fistulas
Ossicular disruption	Hearing loss, acute vertigo, following head/facial trauma	Gradual (days) resolution of vertigo; hearing loss persists	Conductive	Clinical history Audiometry Exclude fistulas

CSF, cerebrospinal fluid; ENT, ear–nose–throat; TM, tympanic membrane.
Modified from Reilly BM. *Practical Strategies in Outpatient Medicine.* 2nd ed. Philadelphia: WB Saunders; 1991:196–197.

TABLE 7.17 Central Vertigo

Cause	Clinical Clues	Diagnosis
Vertebrobasilar ischemia	Known (suspected) vascular disease: hypertensive, diabetic Almost always accompanied by brainstem symptoms and signs: diplopia, dysarthria, dysesthesias, motor weakness	TIA: clinical history Stroke: neurologic examination CT scan may be unreliable MRI more sensitive Angiography?
Cerebellar hemorrhage	Hypertensive, anticoagulated, post-traumatic Sudden headache: diplopia, ataxia usually more prominent than vertigo	CT scan
Cerebellopontine angle tumors (acoustic neuroma)	Hearing loss, tinnitus much more prominent than vertigo Mild disequilibrium Early: normal neurologic examination, except sensorineural hearing loss Later: cranial nerves V and VII abnormal; papilledema?	Audiometry: retrocochlear, sensorineural hearing loss CT scan, MRI Internal audiometry canal tomography ENG, ABER
Multiple sclerosis	Optic neuritis Internuclear ophthalmoplegia Spastic paraparesis/incontinence Vertigo first isolated symptom in only 10% of cases	Multiplicity of symptoms and signs dissociated in time and space MRI scanning CSF: oligoclonal bands
Drug toxicity	Alcohol, sedatives, tranquilizers, opiates, anticonvulsants	Discontinue drug
Basilar migraine	Vertigo part of headache syndrome Usually positive family history	Clinical history
Vertiginous (temporal lobe) epilepsy	Vertigo as aura prior to loss of consciousness Very rare	Clinical history Exclude other diagnoses EEG

Cranial neuropathy	Many types, all uncommon:
	  Herpes zoster: external ear/palate skin lesions and cranial nerve VIII symptoms
	  Postinfectious: after viral syndromes: polyneuritis and/or cerebellitis and/or encephalitis
	  Chronic meningitis: syphilis, tuberculosis, sarcoid, carcinomatous
	  Vasculitis: Cogan syndrome, polyangiitis with granulomatosis, temporal arteritis, syphilis
	  Head and neck carcinoma
	  Vascular compression syndromes	

Others: heredofamilial disorders (Friedreich ataxia, spinocerebellar degeneration, olivopontocerebellar degeneration)
Cerebellar degeneration (alcohol, cancer)
Tumor of brainstem, cerebellum
Syrinx cervical cord
Post-traumatic concussion

ABER, auditory brainstem-evoked response; CSF, cerebrospinal fluid; ENG, electronystagmography; TIA, transient ischemic attack.
Modified from Reilly BM. *Practical Strategies in Outpatient Medicine.* 2nd ed. Philadelphia: WB Saunders; 1991:200.

of movement, it is difficult to make this diagnosis in young children; the condition must be carefully distinguished from other movement impairments, especially disequilibrium.

DISEQUILIBRIUM

When a "dizzy" patient describes feeling unsteady on their feet, off balance, or uncoordinated, the patient is describing a disturbance in the body's equilibrium system. The fundamental complaint is difficulty in walking, not from weakness but from a feeling of lack of control.

Walking is a complex activity. The constant integration of visual, vestibular, and proprioceptive afferent information regarding the changing spatial orientation is performed by using all levels of the central nervous system: the cerebral cortex, cerebellum, brainstem, spinal cord, and peripheral neuromuscular system. These spatial data are then utilized by the efferent system, producing both voluntary and involuntary movements and spatial adjustments (Fig. 7.10). Disturbances in any of these pathways can result in difficulty with locomotion.

Disequilibrium, therefore, may result from any perceptual distortion of spatial orientation. Humans depend heavily on visual perception to orient themselves in space. Vestibulocochlear dysfunction can also severely impair a person's ability to ambulate. Peripheral neuropathies affecting proprioceptive function impair the ability of the central nervous system to accurately perceive the position of the limbs with regard to one another and to either the ground or the body. Disorders causing diffuse damage to the integrative mechanism or cortical or cerebellar diseases can impair proprioception as well. Likewise, efferent motor disability produces impairment of locomotion by producing weakness or apraxias (Table 7.19).

The history is critical for patients complaining of dizziness or difficulty ambulating. For children, this includes a detailed developmental history, because the differential diagnosis varies significantly for

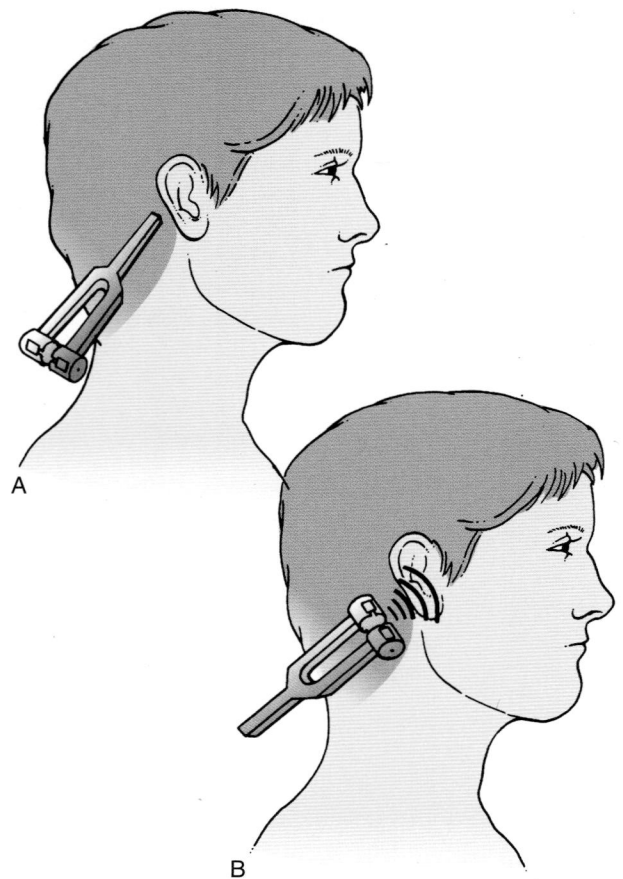

Fig. 7.7 The Rinne test. The tuning fork is first placed on the mastoid process *(A)*. When the sound can no longer be heard, the tuning fork is placed in front of the external auditory meatus *(B)*. Normally, air conduction is better than bone conduction. (From Swartz MH. *Textbook of Physical Diagnosis: History and Examination.* Philadelphia: WB Saunders; 1989:175.)

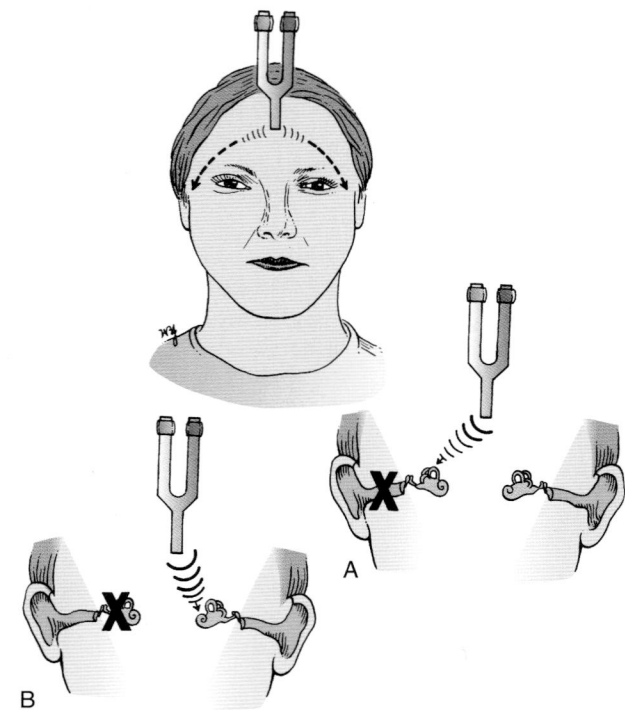

Fig. 7.8 The Weber test. When a vibrating tuning fork is placed on the center of the forehead, the sound is normally heard in the center without lateralization to either side *(top)*. A, In the presence of a conductive hearing loss, the sound is heard on the side of the conductive loss. B, In the presence of a sensorineural loss, the sound is better heard on the opposite (unaffected) side. (From Swartz MH. *Textbook of Physical Diagnosis: History and Examination.* Philadelphia: WB Saunders; 1989:175.)

children who were walking and then stop and for those who do not achieve that milestone. For younger children, it may be very difficult to determine whether refusal or reluctance to walk is related to imbalance, pain, or weakness. Nausea and vomiting are usually associated with vertigo but tend to be rare with disequilibrium. Nausea and vomiting may accompany a viral illness that results in an **acute cerebellar ataxia** and thus may precede the onset of disequilibrium. If nausea is simultaneous with the disequilibrium, drug or alcohol intoxication must be considered. Morning nausea or vomiting can be seen with increased **intracranial pressure**, as in hydrocephalus and posterior fossa tumors. Any history of head trauma, especially in toddlers, and any history of congenital heart disease with the potential for paradoxical embolization, including septic emboli resulting in brain abscess, must be considered.

It is important to distinguish acute intermittent ataxia from more chronic or progressive forms (Tables 7.20 and 7.21). Drugs and **postviral cerebellitis** are common causes of acute sudden-onset ataxia. Varicella-associated postinfectious acute cerebellar ataxia usually comes after the infection, but in rare instances, it may occur before or during chickenpox. Its nature is benign. **Metabolic hereditary disorders** may cause intermittent symptoms provoked by fever, as in maple syrup urine disease, ataxia-telangiectasia, Hartnup disease, Refsum disease, pyruvate decarboxylase deficiency, abetalipoproteinemia, biotinidase deficiency, and some enzyme deficiencies. These must be distinguished from hypothyroidism, demyelinating disorders, muscular dystrophies, and neoplasms of the posterior fossa, brainstem, and spinal cord. **Paraneoplastic effects** of neuroblastoma produce ataxia, opsoclonus, and myoclonus. The Miller Fisher variant of **Guillain-Barre syndrome** produces ataxia, ophthalmoplegia, and areflexia.

Progressive ataxias have a poorer prognosis. Age at onset can be used to distinguish some causes: Posterior fossa tumors and neuroblastoma generally occur within the first decade, Friedreich ataxia and Duchenne muscular dystrophy during the late first to second decades, and multiple sclerosis and diabetic peripheral neuropathy in the second decade.

Observation of the child's gait is an important component of the physical examination. Sufficient room should be found to allow the child to initiate walking, to proceed in a straight line for 10–20 paces, and to turn and return. The normal child, older than 2–3 years, initiates walking without hesitation and steps smoothly with a consistent stride length and height and a narrow base. The arms should swing freely and rhythmically, alternating with the feet, and there should be little sway in the trunk. When the child stops, there should be no hesitation again and no wavering or compensation.

One of the most common gait abnormalities in children is the **wide-based gait.** Careful observation of toddlers at various stages of development familiarizes the observer with the transition from the wide-based, lurching steps of a 12 month old to the smooth, sure, rhythmic stride of children older than 2–3 years. Excessive trunk sway is typical of cerebellar ataxia. Waddling tends to be caused by proximal muscle weakness with a forward-leaning, stiff appearance. It is important to

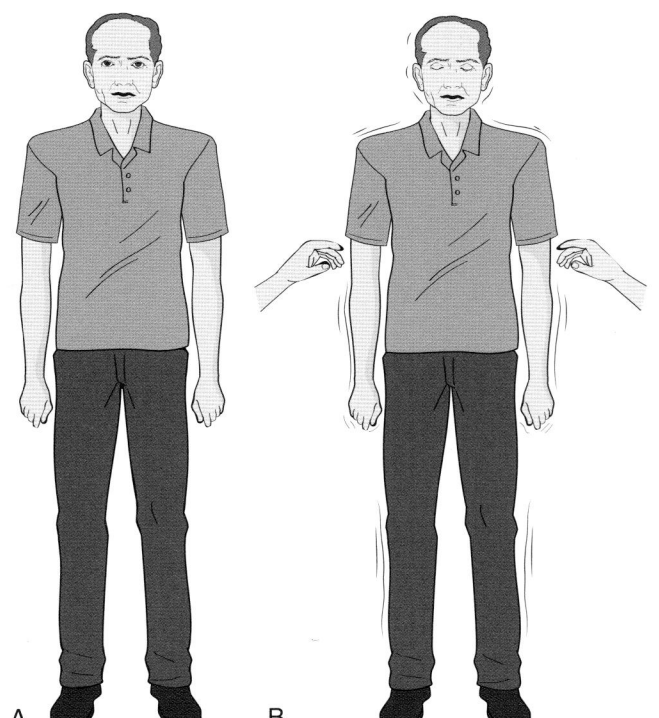

Fig. 7.9 The Romberg test. The patient stands upright, feet together, arms at sides. The examiner should stand next to the patient. The test is performed in two stages: with the patient's eyes open and then with the eyes closed. Even a normal person may experience mild subjective disequilibrium and may "waver" with the eyes closed. Thus, the Romberg test can sometimes stimulate the feeling of disequilibrium. *A,* With the eyes open, the patient can stand unsupported without difficulty. *B,* With the eyes closed, the patient loses their balance. This test result suggests peripheral neuropathy or vestibular dysfunction or both. Cerebellar disease more often results in an inability to maintain posture with the eyes either open or closed. (From Reilly BM. *Practical Strategies in Outpatient Medicine.* 2nd ed. Philadelphia: WB Saunders; 1991:168.)

distinguish an unsteady gait with irregular steps from a limp or a sensory deficit resulting in a high step with a slapping foot plant.

In a toddler, passive and active range of motion exercises should be performed to ensure the observer that there is no joint or muscle pain. Reflexes, including the Babinski sign, should be carefully tested. Testing the sensory system in a toddler, especially proprioception, vibration, and two-point discrimination, can be a challenge. The Romberg test may also be difficult for younger children.

Evaluation of the Patient with Disequilibrium

History

A detailed developmental history, especially for a younger child, is obtained. The family history should also be complete. The examiner should check for prodromal illnesses, especially viral in nature:

Is there any history of trauma?

What is the character of the disability?

Does the child feel unsteady standing, starting to walk, stopping, or turning?

How do the parents characterize the child's gait?

Are there associated symptoms, such as nausea, vomiting, pain, or vertigo?

Does the child take or have access to any medications or drugs?

Is the disequilibrium intermittent or constant?

Are there any other medical conditions?

TABLE 7.18	Interpretation of the HINTS Exam	
HINTS Exam Component	**Peripheral Vertigo**	**Central Vertigo**
Head Impulse Test (HIT)	Loss of eye fixation with head impulse; "positive" or "abnormal"	Intact vestibulo-ocular reflex; "negative" or "normal"
Nystagmus (N)	None or horizontal unidirectional	Vertical, rotatory, or horizontal bidirectional
Test of Skew (TS)	No skew; "negative"	Skew; "positive"

From Quimby AE, Kwok ESH, Lelli D, et al. Usage of the HINTS exam and neuroimaging on the assessment of peripheral vertigo in the emergency department. *J Otolaryngol Head Neck Surg.* 2018;47:54.

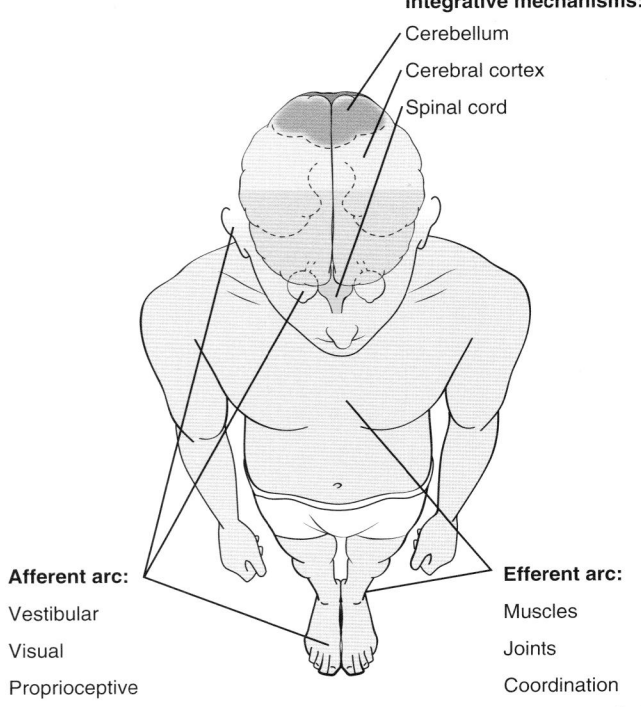

Fig. 7.10 The afferent, integrative, and efferent components of the equilibrium system. (From Reilly BM. *Practical Strategies in Outpatient Medicine.* 2nd ed. Philadelphia: WB Saunders; 1991:166.)

Physical Examination

A thorough general physical examination should precede a very detailed neuromuscular examination. The presence of a goiter, cutaneous lesions of neurofibromatosis, or tuberous sclerosis may point to a diagnosis immediately. The neuromuscular examination should proceed from head to toe in an organized and systematic manner. Muscle tone, bulk, and symmetry of the face, trunk, and extremities are important. Cranial nerves should be examined, as should the sensory system. During the motor examination, the physician should isolate muscle groups and joints by observing the gait more than once before assessing overall function. The Romberg test should be performed in all patients old enough to cooperate, as should the lateralizing cerebellar tests, such as the finger-to-nose and rapid, alternating movements.

TABLE 7.19 Disequilibrium

Cause	Clues	Gait/Romberg Test Result
Most Common		
Multiple sensory deficits	Visual impairment? Hearing/vestibular dysfunction? Neuropathy? Spondylosis/degenerative joint disease? Neuropathy? Weakness?	Timid: slow, short-stepped, apprehensive Remarkably improved with sensory assist (cane, companion) Romberg: normal or sensory
Hyperventilation/anxiety disorders	Young, healthy, anxious patient with *episodic "spells"* of disequilibrium *or* Constant, chronic, elusive disequilibrium with or without obvious medical/psychosocial stress	Usually normal gait Romberg: normal *or* "Nonphysiologic"
Vestibular disorders	*Chronic* unilateral vestibulopathy may cause ongoing disequilibrium: Ménière disease, cholesteatoma, fistula, acoustic neuroma, drug-induced vestibulopathy	Usually normal gait May veer to side of vestibular lesion Romberg: sensory
Drug induced	Central nervous system agents: tranquilizers, barbiturates, sedatives, alcohol, H_2 blockers, β blockers, calcium agents, indomethacin Vestibulotoxic agents: aspirin, loop diuretics, aminoglycosides, quinidine	Timid and/or ataxic gait Romberg: normal or cerebellar Romberg: sensory or normal
Alcoholic	Heavy alcohol abuse may cause cerebellar and/or sensory degeneration Nystagmus uncommon	Ataxic gait Romberg: cerebellar or sensory
Painful ambulation	Arthritis? Claudication? Pain is limiting factor!	Limping? Waddling? Normal gait? Romberg: usually normal
Fear of falling	Normal examination No apraxia or ataxia Rarely, phobic	Timid gait Romberg: often cerebellar but fluctuates, inorganic
Less Common		
Hypothyroidism	Weight gain or poor growth, cold intolerance, hoarseness, fatigue	Usually normal gait Severe: ataxic gait
Hypoglycemia	Episodic	Romberg: usually normal
Apraxia	Usually diffuse cortical dysfunction or frontal lobe disease Usually apraxic in execution of other skilled movements (e.g., combing hair, brushing teeth)	Apraxic gait Romberg: normal
Peripheral disease	Diabetes, alcoholism, pernicious anemia Only very severe (proprioceptive) neuropathy causes gait disorder	Sensory gait: footdrop and/or circus clown Romberg: sensory
Cerebellar disease (nonalcoholic)	See text	Ataxic gait Romberg: cerebellar
Spasticity	Multiple sclerosis, spinal cord tumor/trauma Legs: weak, hyperreflexic, clonus Often bowel/bladder dysfunction	Spastic, scissors gait Romberg: often normal
Normal-pressure hydrocephalus	Urinary incontinence Cognitive impairment Gait disturbance	Ataxic/apraxic
Hemiplegia	Prior cerebrovascular accident Hemiparesis on neurologic examination	Hemiplegic gait Romberg: often normal (if able to perform at all)
Proximal myopathy	Severe bilateral proximal leg weakness: hip disease, muscular dystrophy, myositis, etc.	Waddling gait Romberg: normal
Somatic symptom disorder	Unpredictable, intermittent or bizarre "Secondary gain"	Gait varies: sometimes normal, timid, limping, apraxic Romberg: often cerebellar, but fluctuates, inorganic

CNS, central nervous system; CSF, cerebrospinal fluid.
Modified from Reilly BM. *Practical Strategies in Outpatient Medicine.* 2nd ed. Philadelphia: WB Saunders; 1991:172–173.

TABLE 7.20 Acute or Recurrent Ataxia

Brain tumor
Conversion reaction
Drug ingestion
Encephalitis (brainstem)
Genetic disorders
    Dominant recurrent ataxia
    Episodic ataxia type 1
    Episodic ataxia type 2
    Hartnup disease
    Maple syrup urine disease
    Pyruvate dehydrogenase deficiency
Migraine
    Basilar
    Benign paroxysmal vertigo
Postinfectious/immune
    Acute disseminated encephalomyelitis
    Acute postinfectious cerebellitis (varicella)
    Miller Fisher syndrome
    Multiple sclerosis
    Myoclonic encephalopathy/neuroblastoma
    Pseudoataxia (epileptic)
    Trauma
    Hematoma
    Postconcussion
    Vertebrobasilar occlusion
Vascular disorders
    Cerebellar hemorrhage
    Kawasaki disease

From Augustine E, Mink J. Movement disorders. In: Kliegman R, Stanton B, Schor N, et al, eds. *Nelson Textbook of Pediatrics*. 19th ed. Philadelphia: Elsevier; 2011:2053–2055.

Attention to detail in the history and physical examination findings usually yields a diagnosis.

Diagnostic Tests

Testing for drugs/medications may be the most useful test for children with ataxia. Neuroimaging is indicated for acute ataxia when associated with focal findings on exam, increased intracranial pressure, a history of trauma, or altered mental status. Imaging is indicated for patients with findings concerning for an intracranial mass. Lumbar puncture should be performed for concern of infection or Guillain-Barre syndrome. Metabolic tests and thyroid function tests are indicated by either history or physical findings. When weakness is associated with the disequilibrium, electromyography and nerve conduction studies may be indicated.

SUMMARY AND RED FLAGS

Ataxia can be seen in children at any age; it may portend serious pathologic processes, including posterior fossa tumors, leukodystrophies, metabolic disorders, and familial-hereditary disorders. The history must be obtained carefully, with attention to developmental milestones, family history, specifics of prodromal illnesses, associated symptoms, and a description of the gait. The physical examination must also be detailed and methodical, with special emphasis on the neuromuscular examination. Imaging studies of the central nervous system are usually required, especially for younger children, in whom the possibility of neoplasms is the greatest.

LIGHTHEADEDNESS

Lightheadedness is the most difficult to characterize without using the term "dizzy." The lightheaded patient's description is usually vague

TABLE 7.21 Chronic or Progressive Ataxia

Brain Tumors
Cerebellar astrocytoma
Cerebellar hemangioblastoma (von Hippel–Landau disease)
Ependymoma
Medulloblastoma
Supratentorial tumors

Congenital Malformations
Basilar impression
Cerebellar aplasias
Cerebellar hemisphere aplasia
Dandy-Walker malformation
Vernal aplasia
Chiari malformation

Hereditary Ataxias
Autosomal dominant inheritance
Autosomal recessive inheritance
Abetalipoproteinemia
Ataxia-telangiectasia
Ataxia without oculomotor apraxia
Ataxia with episodic dystonia
Friedreich ataxia
Hartnup disease
Juvenile GM2 gangliosidosis
Juvenile sulfatide lipidoses
Maple syrup urine disease
Marinesco-Sjögren syndrome
Pyruvate dehydrogenase deficiency
Ramsay Hunt syndrome
Refsum disease (HSMN IV)
Respiratory chain disorders

X-Linked Inheritance
Adrenoleukodystrophy
Leber optic neuropathy
With adult-onset dementia
With deafness
With deafness and loss of vision

From Augustine E, Mink J. Movement disorders. In: Kliegman R, Stanton B, Schor N, et al, eds. *Nelson Textbook of Pediatrics*. 19th ed. Philadelphia: Elsevier; 2011:2053–2055.

and nonspecific. The key is to elicit an adequate description from the patient to rule out vertigo, disequilibrium, and presyncope. The differential diagnosis for lightheadedness is then rather short in comparison with the other "dizziness" conditions (Fig. 7.11). It is often difficult to distinguish lightheadedness from presyncope.

In the patient who complains of lightheadedness, voluntary hyperventilation may reproduce the patient's symptoms. Voluntary hyperventilation in normal subjects produces a variety of symptoms (Table 7.22). This test is predictive only if the patient's symptoms are precisely reproduced and all other investigation results are negative.

Lightheadedness that is episodic frequently follows a pattern related to the underlying psychogenic disorder: phobic disorders, posttraumatic stress syndrome, panic attacks, and anxiety disorders. Such situational anxieties, phobias, or panic attacks may occur with or without hyperventilation. Careful history taking is the key to recognizing the pattern. If the history is that of constant lightheadedness, the origin is almost always psychogenic. This is a **somatization** generally of anxiety disorder or depression. The clinician must nonetheless remain cautious with predictable episodes because postural episodes, drug-related episodes, and perimenstrual episodes can follow a pattern and represent physiologic abnormalities that predispose to lightheadedness.

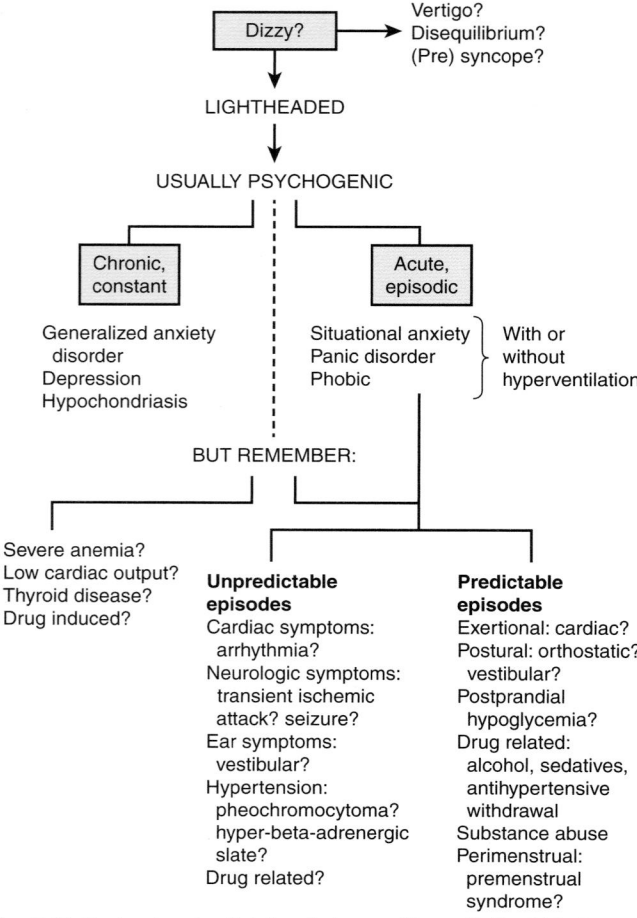

Fig. 7.11 Evaluation for lightheadedness. (From Reilly BM. *Practical Strategies in Outpatient Medicine*. 2nd ed. Philadelphia: WB Saunders; 1991:206.)

If the episodes of lightheadedness are unpredictable, the clinician is advised to consider a broader differential diagnosis. Severe anemia, low cardiac output, thyroid disease, and medications may produce occasional lightheadedness. Of greater concern are episodes of lightheadedness associated with other symptoms, chest pain, seizures, confusion, and visual or auditory changes. Exertional lightheadedness must be pursued to rule out a cardiac dysrhythmia.

If hyperventilation reproduces the patient's symptoms, it is not the diagnosis in and of itself. Hyperventilation is a feature of many psychogenic syndromes and may be acute or chronic. Part of the performance of the hyperventilation should be educating the patient to the feelings and the scenario leading to the hyperventilation reaction. Even young children can then be trained to regulate their breathing to avoid the symptoms. However, this does not address the underlying cause of the hyperventilation reaction; that requires patient, nonjudgmental, longer-term counseling and careful categorization of the underlying disorder. The clinician should not hesitate to consult a psychiatrist to facilitate this process as well as treat the definitive psychogenic disorder.

EVALUATION OF THE PATIENT WITH LIGHTHEADEDNESS

History

The examiner should listen for descriptions suggesting vertigo, disequilibrium, or presyncope and should establish whether there is any

TABLE 7.22	Symptoms Associated with Hyperventilation
General	
Fatigue	
Diffuse weakness	
Insomnia	
Nightmares	
Headache	
"Feel cold"	
Sweats	
Cardiovascular	
Palpitations	
Tachycardia	
Precordial pain	
Raynaud phenomenon	
Respiratory	
Shortness of breath	
Chest pain	
Sighing respirations	
Yawning	
"Can't get deep breath"	
Paroxysmal nocturnal dyspnea	
Unexplained cough	
Dry mouth	
Musculoskeletal	
Muscle spasm	
Tremors	
Twitching	
Tetany	
Neurologic	
Dizziness	
Paresthesias (especially distal)	
Unsteadiness	
Impaired memory and/or concentration	
Slurred speech	
Blurred vision	
Gastrointestinal	
Globus hystericus	
Mouth dryness	
Dysphagia	
Bloating	
Belching/flatulence	
Abdominal pain	
Psychic	
Tension	
Anxiety	
Depression	
Apprehension	

From Reilly BM. *Practical Strategies in Outpatient Medicine*. 2nd ed. Philadelphia: WB Saunders; 1991:208.

pattern to the occurrence of the feeling of lightheadedness. History should include associated symptoms, such as diaphoresis, hyperpnea, pallor or flushing, headache, and chest pain. After the more serious physiologic disorders are ruled out by history, physical examination, or diagnostic testing, psychogenic disorders should be pursued.

Physical Examination

After a thorough general physical examination including examination of the fundi, a full, detailed neurologic examination should be performed. In addition to allowing primary cardiac, endocrine, or neurologic disorders to be ruled out, the examination allows the clinician to gain the confidence of the patient and demonstrates the physician's concern about the patient's complaints.

Diagnostic Tests

Diagnostic testing is directed by the history and physical examination findings. In the setting of lightheadedness, tests are generally done to rule out potentially serious cardiovascular and neurologic conditions.

SUMMARY AND RED FLAGS

Lightheadedness must be distinguished from vertigo, disequilibrium, and presyncope. Frequently, the patient's description of the sensation is vague and uncertain. A pattern of the appearance of the symptoms may suggest an underlying cause. The coexistence of any other symptoms must be carefully sought. Physical findings are generally normal, including the neurologic examination; specific attention is given to cerebellar, vestibular, and sensory function. Voluntary hyperventilation in the supine position frequently reproduces the patient's lightheadedness. Hyperventilation may be acute or chronic and is a symptom itself, rarely a diagnosis.

Treatment must address the underlying psychogenic cause to be successful.

BIBLIOGRAPHY

A bibliography is available at ExpertConsult.com.

8

Chest Pain

Julie M. Kolinski

Chest pain in children is a common complaint; however, it is rarely due to underlying cardiac illness. This underscores the importance of avoiding a false sense of safety in low-risk causes and maintaining vigilance for potential life-threatening etiologies. Chest pain can be the presenting complaint for a child describing chest tightness, burning, pressure, stabbing sensations, palpitations, and/or heartburn. It can be encountered in outpatient, emergency, and urgent care settings. This variability in complaint and care setting can make quickly discerning an etiology difficult, particularly in young children who are not able to verbalize precise symptoms. Chest pain as a symptom affects equal numbers of females and males and children under and over 12 years of age. Diagnostically, children younger than 12 years with chest pain are more likely to have cardiorespiratory etiologies for their pain, whereas adolescents are more likely to have musculoskeletal or psychogenic etiologies.

The general public has been adequately educated on the significant morbidity and mortality that chest pain can imply in adults in the form of cardiac ischemia. Therefore, when children complain of chest pain, it can provide significant anxiety for patients, families, and providers. Due to this anxiety, cardiology consultation is often sought. Only up to 6% of children without known congenital heart disease are found to have a cardiac etiology after evaluation. This number is likely higher than it actually is noted in some studies as only referrals to pediatric cardiology may be analyzed. The challenge for the medical care provider is to distinguish chest pain as a commonly benign pediatric complaint from significant cardiac disease, limit unnecessary evaluation, and provide adequate reassurance for an anxious patient and family.

Due to the rarity of cardiac pathology as the cause for chest pain, it is difficult to develop evidence-based guidelines for evaluation, and the implication of a misdiagnosis of a serious disorder is high. Chest pain caused by noncardiac causes may be the combination of multiple diagnoses, leaving medical providers seeking to "rule out" life-threatening cardiac causes of chest pain. The evaluation, if inconclusive, can leave patients and families without precise answers. Most final diagnoses of noncardiac chest pain represent clinical impressions rather than confirmed diagnoses. Between 20% and 45% of pediatric cases of chest pain are labeled idiopathic. The lack of a defined etiology or the presence of multiple causes for a particular patient can heighten worry, anxiety, and subsequent morbidity, which is reflected in missed days of school, reduced exercise, and psychologic distress. Furthermore, chest pain can become a chronic condition in the pediatric population; up to 45–69% of patients have been noted to have persistent symptoms, with 19% of patients reporting symptoms lasting for more than 3 years.

Overall, if medical providers systematically approach a child's or an adolescent's complaint of chest pain, they can provide thoughtful diagnostic evaluations that not only discover serious cardiac pathology if present but also reassure families when a noncardiac etiology is suspected. Evaluation relies heavily on a thorough history and physical examination with subsequent electrocardiogram and further studies if cardiac etiologies remain on the list of possibilities.

CAUSES OF CHEST PAIN

The most common causes of chest pain in descending frequency include idiopathic, musculoskeletal, psychologic, gastrointestinal, pulmonary, and cardiac diagnoses. A differential diagnosis of pediatric chest pain is listed in Table 8.1. The etiology of chest pain in the absence of cardiac pathology can be multifactorial and can include multiple items on this list.

APPROACH TO THE PATIENT WITH CHEST PAIN

A practical approach to chest pain first requires a detailed history and physical examination. An awareness of indicators (red flags) and prioritization that may suggest serious disease and necessitate immediate treatment are essential (Table 8.2). A deliberate, orderly, and complete approach to the clinical evaluation often calms an anxious child and family.

History

The goal of a thorough history of a patient with chest pain is to determine if the etiology is life threatening, a manifestation of a chronic condition with possible serious complications, a specific acute cause, or multiple acute and/or chronic causes. Although chest pain affects children and adolescents of all ages equally, the age of a child can assist in diagnosis. Adolescents are more likely to have musculoskeletal or psychogenic causes of chest pain, while younger children have more respiratory disorders and vague complaints.

One possible approach includes a stepwise, directed history that includes:
- Description of pain
- Assessment for red-flag symptoms (see Table 8.2), including targeted family history
- Medication review
- Review of known illnesses
- Review of systems including psychosocial evaluation

Eliciting the basics of the chest pain's duration, quality, propensity to radiate, severity, and timing is essential. Details that have been noted to be particularly helpful include duration, aggravating and relieving factors, and associated symptoms. Severe pain that lasts only a few seconds up to 1 or 2 minutes is often from the chest wall, but chest pain that persists longer is more likely to be organic in nature. Aggravating and alleviating factors can include position changes that accompany the pain from pericarditis or onset after eating spicy foods in gastroesophageal reflux. The character and location of the pain in pediatric patients are less helpful in the diagnostic evaluation due to often vague

TABLE 8.1 Differential Diagnosis of Pediatric Chest Pain

Musculoskeletal
Trauma (accidental, abuse)
Exercise, overuse injury (strain)
Costochondritis
Tietze syndrome
Precordial catch syndrome
Slipping rib syndrome
Fibromyalgia
Spinal cord or nerve root compression
Muscle strain (overuse injuries)

Pulmonary
Asthma
Pneumonia
Pleurisy
Cough
Pneumothorax, pneumomediastinum
Pulmonary embolism
Tumor
Foreign body

Psychiatric
Hyperventilation
Anxiety
Panic disorder

Gastrointestinal
Achalasia
Gastroesophageal reflux
Esophageal foreign body including pill esophagitis
Esophageal spasm
Esophageal rupture
Cholecystitis
Subdiaphragmatic abscess
Perihepatitis (Fitz-Hugh–Curtis syndrome)
Peptic ulcer disease
Pancreatitis

Cardiac
Hypertrophic cardiomyopathy
Aortic stenosis
Pulmonary stenosis
Mitral valve prolapse
Dilated cardiomyopathy
Pericarditis
Myocarditis
Endocarditis
Idiopathic ventricular tachycardia
Exercise-induced ventricular tachycardia
Wolff-Parkinson-White syndrome
Aortic dissection
Pulmonary hypertension
Eisenmenger syndrome
Ischemia (anomalous coronary artery, systemic lupus erythematosus, post–heart transplant, Kawasaki disease, sympathomimetic drugs, hypercholesterolemia)

Other
Herpes zoster (cutaneous)
Sickle cell anemia vasoocclusive crisis (rib infarction)
Primary or metastatic cancer
Splenic rupture
Drug related: cigarette smoking, vaping, cocaine use, sympathomimetic use, tetracycline ingestion
Anorexia nervosa
Breast-related disease

TABLE 8.2 Red Flags That Increase the Likelihood of a Cardiac Cause for Chest Pain

Sudden onset of severe pain
Pain radiating to right or left arm or shoulder
Pain occurs with exercise
Described as pressure
Exertional syncope
Pain that awakens the patient from sleep
Palpitations and/or dysrhythmias
Family history of sudden death, young-onset ischemic heart disease, inherited arrhythmias such as long QT syndrome or Brugada syndrome, deep vein thrombosis or pulmonary embolism
Cyanosis
Diaphoresis
Personal past or current history of congenital heart disease
Personal history of connective tissue disease, hypercoagulable or hypercholesterolemic state, systemic lupus erythematosus, Kawasaki disease, sickle cell anemia, Marfan syndrome, cystic fibrosis, Ehlers-Danlos syndrome
Personal history of cocaine, huffing, vaping, and/or amphetamine use

descriptions; nonetheless, medical providers should continue to obtain this information to understand the whole picture. Providers should remember that children often complain of chest pain when the pain is in a different place, such as the epigastrium or flank. Finally, it is important to determine whether the chest pain has had an impact on the child's activity (Table 8.3).

Red-flag symptoms (see Table 8.2) are high-yield, must-know characteristics of a child's or an adolescent's chest pain. Oftentimes, after a patient's complete description of the pain, a medical provider will already know the answers to multiple red-flag symptoms, such as when the pain occurs, if it wakes the patient from sleep, and if it is associated with syncope. A targeted family history includes asking about inherited conditions such as familial hypercholesterolemia, hypertrophic cardiomyopathy, and Marfan syndrome. It also can provide information regarding relatives with adult-onset cardiac illnesses associated with chest pain, such as heart failure or ischemia, which may be providing added anxiety for the family.

Medications that the child may already be taking are important to consider. Some medications have specific links to etiologies of chest pain, such as tetracyclines with erosive esophagitis or oral contraceptives with pulmonary embolism. Other recreational drugs such as cocaine, other sympathomimetic agents (such as amphetamines, synthetic marijuana), and vaping have been associated with chest pain. A child's known underlying illnesses and surrounding medical complaints discovered in a review of systems can complete the clinical picture for medical providers. The presence of joint pain or rash could suggest collagen vascular disease, or the presence of increased drooling could represent an esophageal foreign body.

A full psychosocial review should be performed on each patient to ensure that details of personal stressors and behaviors emerge. It is useful to learn about these aspects of the child's chest pain from the child and the parent/family separately. Make sure to interview the patient alone if the child is older or an adolescent. It is difficult for children to discuss areas of difficulty, such as family relationships, school

difficulties, or concerns about physical development, with family present. It is useful to ask, "What are you concerned that this pain is caused by?" of both the patient and the family. This question frequently gives information about overriding fears and concerns that can help medical providers know how to appropriately reassure the family in the likely event that the chest pain has a benign, noncardiac etiology.

Musculoskeletal

Musculoskeletal chest wall pain is perhaps the most identifiable cause of chest pain due to its association with localized tenderness elicited by specific manipulation of the thorax (Fig. 8.1). Pain can involve the ribs, costochondral junctions (such as in costochondritis), costal cartilages, intercostal muscles, sternum, clavicle, or spine. The pain is often worse with movement, coughing, and inspiration. In considering musculoskeletal etiologies, thoroughly consider any trauma to the chest wall. Both contusion and rib fracture can have exquisite tenderness on palpation and pain on inspiration. Table 8.4 highlights common causes of musculoskeletal chest pain.

In general, chest wall pain can result from the strain of any muscle group present in the chest; however, multiple syndromes have been described in relation to specific patterns of muscular pain (Fig. 8.2). Some of these syndromes include pectoral syndrome (pain in a band across the anterior parasternal chest wall on the right or the left), coracoid syndrome (pain at the site of the pectoralis minor muscle with tenderness at its insertion onto the coracoid process), and xiphoid process syndrome (pain over the xiphoid process).

Psychogenic

Psychogenic causes of chest pain are more common in adolescents than in children under the age of 12. Patients with psychogenic etiologies of chest pain may also have additional physiologic causes of pain; psychologic risk factors can amplify the clinical presentation

TABLE 8.3	Historical Features of Chest Pain That Are Essential to Its Assessment
Duration of pain (how long present but also duration of each episode)
Acuteness of onset
Severity of pain (use scale of 1–10)
Associated symptoms
Precipitating and ameliorating factors
Quality of pain (pleuritic, sharp, dull)
Location of pain
Limitation of activities by pain
Radiation of pain
Time of day that pain occurs
Recent activity, injury, and stresses
Full psychosocial review, including behaviors
Medical history
Family medical history

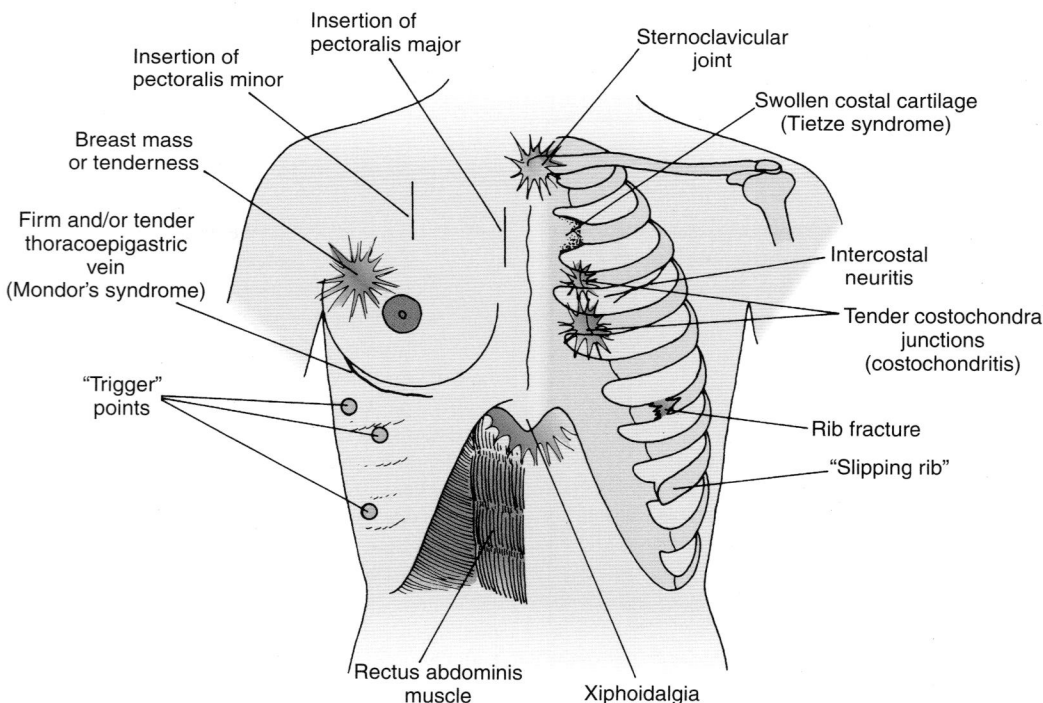

Fig. 8.1 Palpable and/or visible abnormalities of the chest wall that may be found in different chest wall syndromes. In addition, various proximal abdominal causes of chest pain, such as disease of the gallbladder, liver, stomach, pancreas, or subdiaphragmatic space, must be considered. (From Reilly BM. Chest pain. In: *Practical Strategies in Outpatient Medicine.* 2nd ed. Philadelphia: WB Saunders; 1991.)

TABLE 8.4 Manifestations and Causes of Musculoskeletal Chest Pain

Signs and Symptoms	Diagnosis
Aching, localized pain after new or intense exercise or repetitive coughing Can appear up to 2 days later Can have localized swelling or erythema Pain reproduced by range-of-motion testing or palpation	Muscular strain
Sharp, anterior pain over costochondral junctions, often along the sternal border Exacerbated by deep breathing First through fifth ribs are most common and often more than one costochondral junction affected Can be related to growth spurts	Costochondritis (also called costosternal syndrome, parasternal chondrodynia, or anterior chest wall syndrome)
Can be considered a variant of costochondritis Sharp, localized pain at only one costochondral junction Area is swollen, ± warm, erythematous bulbous or fusiform 1–4 cm mass Second or third costochondral junction is most common Age predominance in adolescence and early 20s	Tietze syndrome
Pain and increased mobility due to subluxation of 8th, 9th, or 10th ribs (which are not attached to the sternum), resulting in impingement of superior intercostal nerve Intermittent sharp pain in chest or upper abdomen Brought on by exertion, especially sudden upward and anterior movement ("hooking maneuver"; see Fig. 8.2) Can have popping sensation at onset of pain Caused by trauma or dislocation of these ribs	Slipping rib syndrome (lower rib pain syndrome)
Brief (30 sec–3 min), nonradiating, well-localized, sharp pain in the left parasternal area or cardiac apex ("Texidor twinge") Occurs at rest or with mild activity Exacerbated with inspiration and alleviated by shallow breathing or straightened position Related to poor posture	Precordial catch syndrome
Pain over both anterior chest and back Spasm in muscles innervated by nerve root causes pain No midline spine bony tenderness History of vertigo, headache, pain after prolonged recumbence or straining	Spinal cord or nerve root compression, typically lower cervical or upper thoracic spine
Chronic aching and stiffness Multiple points of tenderness on palpation of muscle with minimal pressure Associated with fatigue and sleep disturbance	Fibromyalgia

of chest pain. Psychologic forms of chest pain are typically recurrent with stressors. Children and adolescents may have a history of anxiety and/or stressful life events that are not easily apparent but can have a large impact on their perception of pain. Many psychologic factors, such as anxiety, depression, and psychosomatic features, often coexist. Patients with psychogenic causes of chest pain are the most likely to have other somatic symptoms, including breathlessness, fatigue, nervousness, near-syncope, and palpitations. These patients also often demonstrate more bodily worries, more limitation of general activity, and more school absences. The most common etiologies of psychogenic chest pain are hyperventilation and underlying psychiatric illness, such as anxiety, depression, or somatoform disorders (conversion or somatization).

Hyperventilation, most often in the setting of a **panic attack**, is characterized by rapid breathing accompanied with dyspnea and anxiety to the degree that systemic symptoms result, such as paresthesias, dizziness/lightheadedness, palpitations, and confusion. This can occur as an acute one-time episode or can represent an underlying panic disorder if recurrent. These symptoms are manifestations of physiologic phenomena caused by hypocapnic respiratory alkalosis, chest muscle strain from use of accessory muscles, tachycardia and arrhythmias, spasm of the diaphragm, and gastric distention caused by aerophagia (Fig. 8.3). Typically, the patient's chest pain complaint due to hyperventilation will include sharp, nonradiating pain over the left precordium. It is the easiest to diagnose when these symptoms arise without exertion. However, it is often difficult to differentiate hyperventilation from asthma as both diagnoses can include dyspnea, chest tightness, cough during exercise, and symptoms characteristic of bronchospasm. Hyperventilation can also occur concurrently with costochondritis or asthma, further complicating diagnosis.

Anxiety, depression, and somatoform disorders can cause episodic chest pain with or without hyperventilation. Within anxiety disorders, chest pain and other symptoms are typically temporally related to stressful situations. Anxiety-related psychogenic chest pain is four times as likely to occur in a patient with a family history of chest pain (often an adult with a history of cardiac ischemia), and the pain is often fleeting and vague in its description.

Gastrointestinal

Esophagitis (reflux, infectious, eosinophilic) and esophageal motility disorders (diffuse esophageal spasm, achalasia) can cause chest pain in both adults and children. Esophagitis (commonly generalized within the term *gastroesophageal reflux*) is characterized by symptoms typical of "heartburn," a substernal burning sensation that is exacerbated by eating or position changes, specifically lying supine. However, heartburn is less common in children than in adults. More commonly, children will have the presence of epigastric tenderness on exam. In fact, epigastric tenderness is one of the best indicators of a gastrointestinal etiology of pain in a child. To manage this diagnosis, first assess if there are triggering factors, such as overeating or spicy foods. Avoidance of

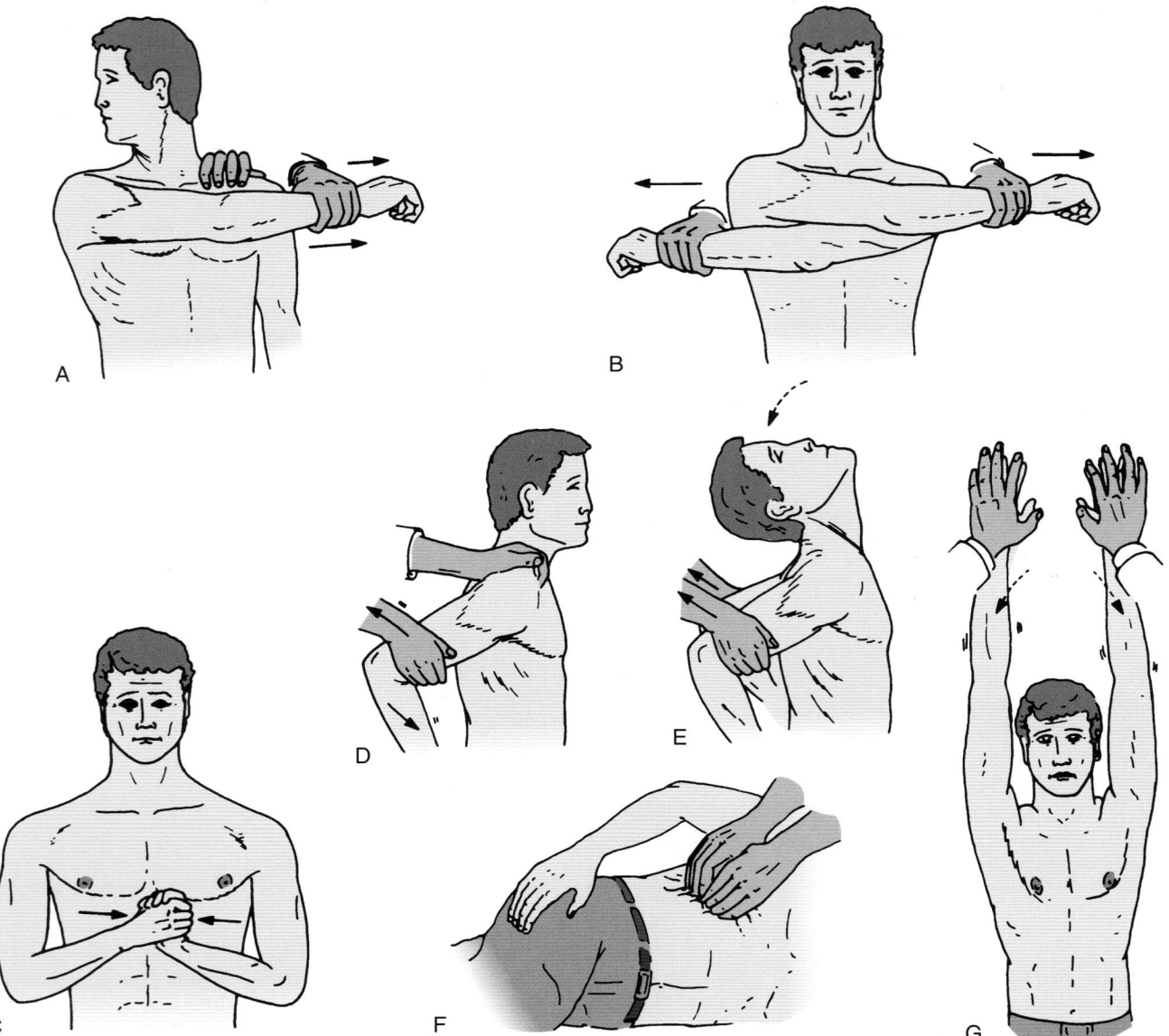

Fig. 8.2 Chest wall maneuvers. *A, B,* The "scissors" maneuver. The patient's arm is adducted across the anterior chest, and the examiner pulls the patient's hand beyond the contralateral shoulder *(A)*. When both arms are tested together, traction is applied to both *(B)*; the patient turns the head to either side, and the arms form a "scissors." Pain originating in the scapula, thoracic spine, pectoral muscles, or ribs and intercostal structures is often precipitated by the scissors maneuver. *C,* The "hedge clipper" maneuver. The pectoralis major muscles are stressed by the patient's pressing the palms forcefully together with the elbows flexed anterior to the chest. The pectoral muscles are thus more clearly defined, and pain is often appreciated within the muscles or at their insertion in the upper parasternal area (see Fig. 8.1). *D,* The "racing dive" maneuver. The pectoralis minor muscles are stressed by forcefully resisting the patient's attempt to throw forward the shoulder and upper arm from an initial position behind (dorsal to) the chest wall. The attempted arm motion is that of flinging the arm and hand forward, as a swim racer would when beginning a racing dive. The examiner resists this forward arm and shoulder motion. *E,* The "crowing rooster" maneuver. The patient hyperextends the neck while the examiner lifts both of the patient's arms backward and superiorly. Pain originating in the cervical spine or anterior chest wall or both is often thus reproduced. *F,* The "hooking" maneuver. With the patient supine, the examiner stands at the patient's side, facing the patient's feet. The examiner then "hooks" their fingers around the lower costal margin of the patient's rib cage and pulls anteriorly (ventrally) and superiorly (cephalad). This maneuver may elicit pain when costochondritis or traumatic rib injuries involve the lower rib cage, when the upper rectus abdominis muscle is torn, or when a "slipping rib" is the problem. *G,* The "high 10" maneuver. The patient raises both hands overhead, elbows extended, and then presses forward with the hands against resistance offered by the examiner. Pain originating in the anterior rib cage, thoracic spine, or pectoral muscles may be elicited here. (*A, B,* and *G* from Reilly BM. Chest pain. In: *Practical Strategies in Outpatient Medicine.* 2nd ed. Philadelphia: WB Saunders; 1991.)

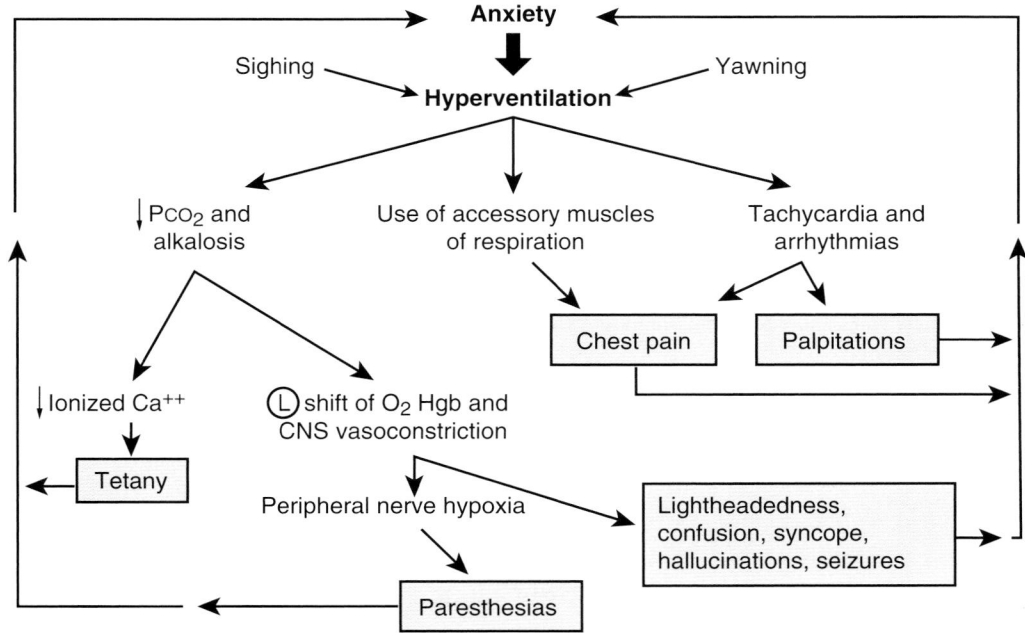

Fig. 8.3 Pathophysiologic mechanisms of hyperventilation. CNS, central nervous system; Hgb, hemoglobin; O_2 Hgb, oxyhemoglobin dissociation curve; P_{CO_2}, carbon dioxide pressure. (From Herman SP, Stickler GB, Lucas AR. Hyperventilation syndrome in children and adolescents: long-term follow-up. *Pediatrics.* 1981;67:183–187.)

these triggers can be adequate treatment to diagnose and treat. If pain persists, a trial of H_2-blocking agents or proton pump inhibitors helps diagnostically and therapeutically in the evaluation of esophagitis.

Motility disorders of the esophagus cause chest pain that lasts from only a few seconds to several hours. The pain is nonexertional but can be exacerbated by bending forward. Achalasia classically causes dysphagia, nocturnal regurgitation, and chest pain. It can occur at any age and the chest pain is variably associated with the diagnosis (19–95% of the time). Eosinophilic esophagitis can cause chest pain secondary to esophageal inflammation, dysmotility, and reflux. Other notable gastrointestinal disorders that also cause chest pain include esophageal foreign body such as pill esophagitis, gastric and duodenal ulcers, cholecystitis, pancreatitis, hepatitis, and infections of the subdiaphragmatic space. Esophageal rupture is a rare cause of chest pain; it has been described in patients with bulimia nervosa or after surgical repair of a tracheoesophageal fistula.

Pulmonary

Pulmonary causes of chest pain are often diagnosed through history and general appearance of the patient (Table 8.5). Some of these causes can require urgent evaluation and treatment. In a patient with sudden, significant chest pain, medical providers should consider acute pneumothorax or acute pulmonary embolism (along with acute pericarditis, myocarditis, or aortic dissection). Underlying history is essential to understand as in a recent trauma or underlying asthma or cystic fibrosis for pneumothorax (which can be spontaneous or secondary to the noted conditions; see Chapter 4). Known obesity, malignancy, prolonged immobilization, or adolescents taking birth control increase risk for pulmonary embolism. Asthma or reactive airway disease is more likely in a patient with audible wheezing and cough. Notably, patients with chest pain from undiagnosed causes after complete evaluation have a greater likelihood than normal control subjects to have abnormal results on methacholine challenges and exercise testing, indicating that reactive airway disease (a typical sign of potential underlying asthma) is a more common etiology of chest pain than providers

TABLE 8.5 Manifestations and Respiratory Causes of Chest Pain

Signs and Symptoms	Diagnosis
Unilateral pain associated with severe dyspnea	Pneumothorax, primary or secondary
Can have radiation to ipsilateral shoulder	
Degree of pain does not correlate to extent of pneumothorax	
Risk factors include tall and thin body habitus, asthma, cystic fibrosis, inhalation of cocaine/marijuana	
Sudden pain, dyspnea, tachycardia ± hypoxia	Pulmonary embolism
Pain is pressure-like or pleuritic	
Can have hemoptysis (rare)	
Risk factors include central venous catheter, trauma, malignancy, immobilization, oral contraceptive use, recent abortion or surgery, hypercoagulable state	
ECG with sinus tachycardia, right heart strain	
Wheeze, ± shortness of breath, ± cough	Asthma, reactive airway disease
Often perceive "tightness" as pain	
If exercise induced, can cause chest pain in absence of wheeze	
Fever, cough ± sputum production	Pneumonia with pleurisy
Midsternal or parasternal pain that can be diffuse	
Pain exacerbated by deep breathing, coughing, straining	

realize. Finally, pneumonia and respiratory infections are the most common causes of chest pain when it presents with fever. Children typically cannot expectorate mucus until at least 8 years of age; therefore, clinical signs of pneumonia can include vomiting and abdominal pain in addition to the more typical symptoms of fever, cough, chest pain, and tachypnea. Vaping-associated lung injury may present with fever, dyspnea, and chest pain (see Chapter 4).

Cardiac

Although cardiac disease is a rare cause of chest pain, there is potential for dangerous morbidity and mortality if left undiagnosed. One of the foremost concerns of families with children who have chest pain is whether or not their child is having a heart attack, although this is extremely uncommon in the pediatric population. Etiologies of chest pain due to cardiac disease include arrhythmias, ischemia, structural abnormalities, and pericardial or myocardial disorders (Tables 8.6, 8.7, and 8.8). Arrhythmias are the most common, whereas patients with myocarditis or myocardial infarction are often the most acutely ill. Heart disease is more commonly found in adolescents than in younger children who complain of chest pain, and adolescents represent the largest group of patients between 1 and 21 years of age who die suddenly of cardiac causes. Perhaps the most important evaluation that should be done in each patient with concern for chest pain secondary to a cardiac etiology is to assess for pediatric sudden cardiac arrest. Four questions that should be asked during this assessment include:

1. Have you ever fainted, passed out, or had a seizure suddenly and without warning, especially during exercise or in response to auditory triggers such as doorbells, alarm clocks, and ringing telephones?
2. Have you ever had exercise-induced chest pain or shortness of breath?
3. Are you related to anyone with sudden, unexplained, and unexpected death before age 50 years?
4. Are you related to anyone who has been diagnosed as having a sudden death–predisposing heart condition such as hypertrophic cardiomyopathy, long QT syndrome, or catecholaminergic polymorphic ventricular tachycardia?

Red-flag symptoms as previously noted are essential to capture in the history (see Table 8.2). Lower-risk findings for cardiac disease include pleuritic, positional, or sharp pain as well as tenderness produced by chest palpation. Children rarely come in complaining of "shortness of breath on exertion" or "palpitations." Instead, children should be asked if they keep up with their same-age peers when participating in activities, if they finish last in races, or whether they must pause in the middle of a flight of stairs. If concerned for palpitations, a provider can ask if a child's heart ever skips a beat or seems to do flip-flops or somersaults in their chest. Even with these questions, a child with palpitations may only be able to describe their symptoms as pain. If red flags are not present but a potentially serious noncardiac etiology of chest pain is suspected, a continued investigation of the pain itself is necessary to make a diagnosis. Supraventricular and ventricular tachyarrhythmias can put adolescents at risk for sudden death.

TABLE 8.6 Causes of Pediatric Anginal Chest Pain

Critical aortic stenosis

Hypertrophic cardiomyopathy

Coronary artery atherosclerosis (hypercholesterolemia)

Anomalous origin of left coronary artery from the pulmonary artery

Acute inflammatory coronary arteritis or aneurysm in context of Kawasaki syndrome, multisystem inflammatory syndrome in children, or vasculitis disorder

Chronic coronary artery stenotic sequalae of acute inflammatory coronary artery diseases

Origin of left coronary artery from right sinus of Valsalva

Ectopic origin from aortic sinus

Coronary artery fistula

Associated with other congenital heart diseases

Cocaine use

Coronary vasospasm

TABLE 8.7 Structural Cardiac Abnormalities That Can Cause Chest Pain

Signs and Symptoms	ECG	Diagnosis
Chest pain with associated dyspnea is brought on by exercise Patient history of syncope, presyncope Seen in adolescence due to rapid growth of left ventricle in puberty Crescendo-decrescendo systolic ejection murmur from outflow tract gradient	Prominent septal Q wave, left ventricular hypertrophy, left axis deviation	Hypertrophic cardiomyopathy
Chest pain is brought on intermittently Patient history of tiring easily, exertional dyspnea ± syncope, cool extremities Signs of right heart failure is a late finding High-pitched, early diastolic decrescendo murmur (pulmonary regurgitation)	Right ventricular hypertrophy	Pulmonary hypertension (primary or secondary to pulmonary stenosis or Eisenmenger complex)
Chest pain is brought on with exercise Patient history of syncope at late stages Harsh crescendo-decrescendo systolic murmur radiating to carotid arteries ± thrill	Left ventricular strain	Aortic stenosis
Chest pain that is vague and nonexertional, but most children are asymptomatic Patient history of postural hypotension, palpitations, or syncope Late to midsystolic click preceding a systolic murmur	Normal, T-wave abnormalities or prominent U waves	Mitral valve prolapse
Chest pain that is acute, present on anterior or posterior chest that can migrate to arms, abdomen, and legs Patient history may include Marfan syndrome, Ehlers-Danlos syndrome, previously healthy weight-lifting athletes High-pitched early diastolic decrescendo murmur (aortic regurgitation)	Normal, can have low QRS voltages	Aortic dissection
Chest pain may be present but unclear due to patient age (for example, symptoms occur at 2–3 mo of age) Patient history of poor feeding, diaphoresis, tachycardia, irritability Signs of heart failure can be present	Anterolateral myocardial infarction pattern with Q waves and ST changes	Anomalous left coronary artery from pulmonary artery

TABLE 8.8 Etiology of Pericarditis and Pericardial Effusion

Idiopathic (Presumed Viral or Autoinflammatory)

Infectious Agents

Bacterial: Group A streptococci, *Staphylococcus aureus*, pneumococci, meningococci,* *Haemophilus influenzae*,* *Salmonella* species, *Mycoplasma pneumoniae*, *Borrelia burgdorferi*, *Mycobacterium tuberculosis*, rickettsiae, tularemia

Viral[†]: Coxsackievirus (group A, B), echovirus, mumps, influenza, Epstein-Barr virus, cytomegalovirus, herpes simplex, herpes zoster, hepatitis B virus, COVID-19, parvovirus

Fungal: *Histoplasma capsulatum*, *Coccidioides immitis*, *Blastomyces dermatitidis*, *Cryptococcus neoformans*, *Candida* species, *Aspergillus* species

Parasitic: *Toxoplasma gondii*, *Entamoeba histolytica*, schistosomes

Collagen Vascular–Inflammatory and Granulomatous Diseases

Rheumatic fever

Systemic lupus erythematosus (idiopathic and drug induced)

Juvenile idiopathic arthritis (JIA)

Kawasaki disease

Scleroderma

Mixed connective tissue disease

Reactive arthritis

Inflammatory bowel disease

Granulomatosis with polyangiitis

Dermatomyositis

Behçet syndrome

Sarcoidosis

Vasculitis

Familial Mediterranean fever

Serum sickness

Stevens-Johnson syndrome

Traumatic

Cardiac contusion (blunt trauma)

Penetrating trauma

Postpericardiotomy syndrome

Radiation

Contiguous Spread

Pleural disease

Pneumonia

Aortic aneurysm (dissecting)

Metabolic

Hypothyroidism

Uremia

Gaucher disease

Fabry disease

Chylopericardium

Neoplastic

Primary

Contiguous (lymphoma)

Metastatic

Infiltrative (leukemia)

Others

Drug reaction

Pancreatitis

Post–myocardial infarction

Thalassemia

Central venous catheter perforation

Heart failure

Hemorrhage (coagulopathy)

Chylous

Biliary-pericardial fistula

*Infectious or immune complex.

[†]Common (viral pericarditis or myopericarditis is probably the most common cause of acute pericarditis in a previously normal host).

Supraventricular tachycardia (SVT), a narrow complex tachycardia, is the most common arrhythmia in children. In children under 12 years, the most common cause of SVT is an accessory atrioventricular pathway, whereas in teenagers, it tends to be atrioventricular node re-entry tachycardia. Patients with pre-excitation or accessory pathways that cause an arrhythmia such as Wolff-Parkinson-White syndrome are at the highest risk for SVT. Alternatively, ventricular tachycardia is a wide complex tachycardia that is often associated with mitral valve prolapse, viral myocarditis, or long QT syndrome. Chest pain caused by an arrhythmia is typically associated with palpitations and/or dyspnea but not necessarily with exercise. The pain is caused by an imbalance of myocardial oxygen supply and demand, subendocardial wall stress, and diminished diastolic coronary perfusion. The pain itself is typically intermittent as most arrhythmias are inherently sporadic in their onset and resolution.

Chest pain that increases during physical exertion or other stress, is relieved by rest, is poorly localized to the substernal area, and possibly radiates to the left arm and/or jaw is likely secondary to a cardiac etiology. This pain is often referred to as anginal and can be secondary to ischemia, although ischemia is not common in children or adolescents. Other conditions that can cause anginal chest pain in children are listed in Table 8.6. Any sign of anginal chest pain should prompt investigation of obstructive, structural cardiac abnormalities and anomalies of the coronary arteries. Associated presyncope, syncope, and/or palpitations

with these symptoms should significantly raise a provider's suspicion for underlying cardiac disease, and a complete physical examination with an ECG is essential initial diagnostic evaluation.

Structural abnormalities lead to chest pain through altered cardiac output, which can lead to syncope or death. Tables 8.7 and 8.9 review the signs, symptoms, and ECG findings of the structural cardiac abnormalities that can cause chest pain.

Acute pericarditis causes substernal chest pain that is sharp, stabbing, and aggravated by deep inspiration, coughing, or straining. Typical pericarditis pain is improved by being in the sitting position, and patients will avoid lying supine. There are many causes of pericarditis and/or pericardial effusion (see Table 8.8). Idiopathic or viral pericarditis has a preceding or accompanying flulike illness with myalgias, arthralgias, and fever. Evaluation for acute pericarditis includes physical examination during which a three-component pericardial rub (atrial systole, ventricular systole, diastolic filling) may be present on auscultation. Of note, this rub may disappear with the development of pericardial effusion. Electrocardiogram findings of acute pericarditis go through a four-stage evolution. Stage 1, the most classic stage for diagnosis (Fig. 8.4), may reveal diffuse PR depressions with upright P waves followed by J-point ST elevations. The ST elevations noted in pericarditis are referred to as J-point elevations due to their upsloping "J" shape. Subsequently, stage 2 shows descent of the J-point elevations followed by stage 3 with T-wave inversions. Stage 4 then shows

TABLE 8.9	**Systolic Murmurs Important in the Diagnosis of Chest Pain**	
Innocent ejection murmur	Loudest left sternal border at base, 1–3 intensity, peaks early in systole; no click, gallop, heave, or diastolic murmur	Diminishes with standing and Valsalva maneuver
Valvular aortic stenosis	*Mild:* Similar to innocent murmur but ejection click is possible *Severe:* Loudest over right second intercostal space, peaks late in systole; delayed carotid upstroke, thrill present; left ventricular heave; audible S$_4$ gallop; aortic insufficiency murmur may also be present	
Hypertrophic cardiomyopathy	Loudest over left second intercostal space, peaks in midsystole; carotid upstroke brisk or bisferiens; no diastolic murmur	Increases with standing or Valsalva maneuver; decreases on squatting
Pulmonic stenosis	*Mild:* Similar to innocent murmur but ejection click is possible *Severe:* Loudest over left second intercostal space; loud, widely split S$_2$; thrill present; right ventricular heave; ejection click at left second intercostal space	
Mitral valve prolapse	Loudest at left sternal border and apex; mid- to late-systolic murmur; click precedes murmur	Increases with standing after squatting and during expiration

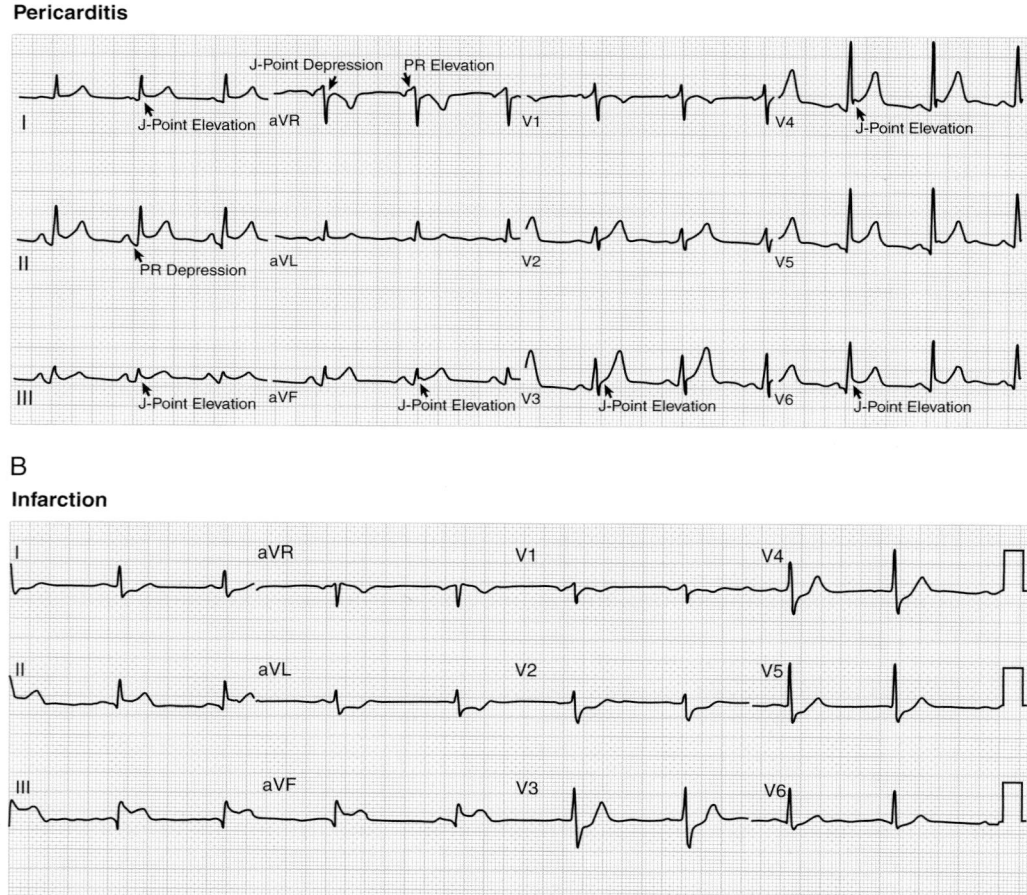

Fig. 8.4 *A,* Acute pericarditis. Note diffuse J-point ST elevations and near-ubiquitous PR segment depressions. *B,* Acute ST elevation myocardial infarction: Note dome-shaped, sometimes referred to as "tombstone-shaped," ST elevations in leads II, III, and aVF with reciprocal ST depressions in leads I, aVL, and V$_1$–V$_5$ consistent with an acute inferior wall myocardial infarction. (*A* from Spodick DH. Acute pericarditis: current concepts and practice. *JAMA.* 2003;289:1150–1153; B from Hwang C, Levis JT. ECG diagnosis: ST-elevation myocardial infarction. *Perm J.* 2014;18:e133.)

restitution back to the child's baseline ECG. These J-point ST elevations are markedly different from ST elevations caused by cardiac ischemia, which are more dome shaped (see Fig. 8.4). A chest x-ray may show an enlarged cardiac silhouette. In pericarditis, perform an echocardiogram to clarify the amount of pericardial fluid present and whether or not there is ventricular dysfunction.

Acute myocarditis often is caused by or follows viral infections. Symptoms of acute myocarditis include lethargy, pallor, low-grade fever, anorexia, chest or abdominal pain, and signs of congestive heart failure. ECG abnormalities tend to be diffuse and nonspecific, and complications of myocarditis include arrhythmias and conduction blocks; chest x-ray may show an enlarged cardiac silhouette. Often, patients can merely have persistent tachycardia. Patients with myocarditis have the propensity to become severely ill and often require inpatient or even intensive care hospitalization.

Other

Other causes of chest pain are diverse and variable. Patients with herpes zoster often experience chest pain *prior* to the typical vesicular rash over a unilateral dermatome. These patients can continue to have burning chest pain for weeks to months. Breast-related causes of chest pain can occur in both males and females. Females may complain of throbbing or burning chest pain caused by fibrocystic disease, fibroadenoma, swelling with menstruation, mastitis, or pregnancy. Gynecomastia in males can lead to unilateral or bilateral chest pain. Substance abuse of tobacco and/or cocaine in addition to other sympathomimetic substances can also cause chest pain. Other medications, such as tetracyclines, iron, or nonsteroidal antiinflammatory agents, can cause pill-induced esophagitis. Foreign bodies in the airways and/or esophagus can be unusual causes of chest discomfort; these diagnoses are typically evident due to other symptoms such as dysphagia, drooling, choking, stridor, or dyspnea. Neoplastic diseases such as mediastinal tumors or lymphomas can also manifest primarily as chest pain.

In addition, certain underlying disease processes have clinical courses that can manifest as chest pain. In patients with sickle cell anemia, chest pain can be secondary to acute chest syndrome and rib or pulmonary infarction. Long-term complications of Kawasaki disease include coronary artery stenosis and coronary artery aneurysm, both of which can present as chest pain. Patients with these cardiac complications of Kawasaki disease often have associated symptoms of fatigue, shortness of breath, and diaphoresis. Patients with Marfan syndrome are at high risk for dissecting aortic aneurysm, as are patients with Turner syndrome, type IV Ehlers-Danlos syndrome, and homocystinuria (Table 8.10). A dissecting aortic aneurysm will often have the history of a sharp, sudden onset of chest pain with radiation to the back. Rheumatic fever is an acquired condition that can present with the major manifestations of carditis, which may include tachycardia out of proportion to degree of fever, mitral regurgitation or aortic regurgitation, and signs of pericarditis or heart failure. Chest pain also can be present before the onset of lower spinal symptoms in ankylosing spondylitis, a disease of the sacroiliac joints with variable involvement in the thoracic and cervical spine. A phenomenon that can occur with any cardiac procedure is postpericardiotomy syndrome, which includes fever, chest pain, and an audible friction rub approximately 1–2 weeks postsurgery.

COVID-19 and Multisystem Inflammatory Syndrome in Children

Chest pain is not a symptom commonly reported with acute COVID-19 syndrome. However, multisystem inflammatory syndrome, characterized by fever, multisystem organ involvement, and laboratory markers of inflammation, has been reported to cause critical illness in >50% of cases. Cardiac involvement is common in children with multisystem inflammatory syndrome in children (MIS-C). Specifically, children with MIS-C should be monitored for shock, cardiac arrhythmias, pericardial effusion, and coronary artery dilation. Evaluation of children with MIS-C should include a cardiac troponin, an N-terminal pro–B-type natriuretic peptide, and inflammatory markers including CRP, ferritin, and D-dimer (see Chapters 4 and 53). All patients with suspected MIS-C should receive an ECG, and if there are abnormalities in biochemical markers, pediatric cardiologists often recommend echocardiogram evaluation to better understand the impact of this newly developing disease. Long-lasting effects of this disease and of acute COVID-19 in the pediatric population are yet to be fully understood.

Physical Examination

A physical examination can often confirm a medical provider's suspicion of a particular diagnosis or diagnoses, especially when it comes to the complaint of chest pain. The cardiovascular assessment of children requires patience, thoroughness, and flexibility to adapt to children who may not desire you to examine them. All physical examinations for the complaint of chest pain should start with observing the child for general states of distress, pain with breathing, and interaction with parents. Vital signs can indicate the presence of pain by revealing signs of tachycardia and tachypnea, and can provide information regarding potential serious medical illness, including fever, hypoxia, or hypotension. Blood pressures should be obtained in all four upper and lower extremities, monitoring closely for a gradient between extremities. All vital signs should be evaluated in the context of reference ranges for a child's age and height.

A helpful physical exam finding is elicitation of chest wall tenderness upon palpation of the thorax, which is pathognomonic for chest wall pain (see Fig. 8.1). Therefore, medical providers are encouraged to palpate over the chest including the ribs, intercostal areas, sternum, xiphoid, manubrium, axilla, clavicles, epigastric area, spinous processes, and paraspinal areas. Chest wall maneuvers can also be performed to better understand what muscle group is causing the pain (see Fig. 8.2).

Palpation of the chest wall should be performed to identify the point of maximal intensity and to determine if there is a cardiac heave or thrill. Palpation of the abdomen should be done for tenderness and organomegaly. Both distal and proximal pulses should be felt for equality and caliber. After palpation, percussion over the thorax should be done. Dullness to percussion can suggest consolidation, effusion, or atelectasis, whereas hyperresonance to percussion can suggest pneumothorax or asthma.

Every medical provider should allow ample time for auscultation of the lungs and heart. Medical providers should follow a constant, systemic procedure for listening to heart sounds (see Table 8.9). Heart sounds include S_1–S_4. S_1 is caused by mitral and tricuspid valve closure, and S_2 is caused by aortic and pulmonary valve closure. The sounds caused by these valves opening are not heard in healthy individuals. Because the left-sided valves close before the right-sided valves, the S_2 heart sound can be physiologically split into the aortic valve and then the pulmonic valve closing during inspiration. S_3 and S_4 are harder to understand and hear. S_3 is a result of the deceleration of blood at the end of early rapid filling of the ventricles. An S_3 is normal in children with hyperdynamic circulations (such as athletes) and thin chest walls (of note, in adults an S_3 is always abnormal). An S_4 is a result of deceleration of blood at the end of late rapid filling of the ventricles. Audible S_4 sounds are always abnormal, no matter what age the patient is. Therefore, a gallop rhythm (third heart sounds) can be normal or abnormal.

Subsequently, medical providers must listen to what occurs between S_1 and S_2. A midsystolic click is often an indicator of the mitral valve

TABLE 8.10 TAA Syndromes and Diseases from a Heritable or Genetic Cause

Gene (Protein)	Syndrome or Disease	Clinical Features
Extracellular Matrix Protein Genes		
FBN1 (fibrillin-1)	Marfan syndrome	Aortic root aneurysm, AD, TAA, MVP, long bone overgrowth, scoliosis, pectus deformities, ectopia lentis, myopia, tall stature, PTX
FBN2 (fibrillin-2)	Congenital contractural arachnodactyly, Beals syndrome	MVP, arachnodactyly, marfanoid habitus, digital contractures, mild aortic dilation
COL3A1 (type 3 procollagen)	Vascular Ehlers-Danlos syndrome	TAA, AAA, arterial rupture, AD, MVP, bowel and uterine rupture, PTX, translucent skin, atrophic scars, small joint hypermobility, easy bruising
EFEMP2 (fibulin-4)	Cutis laxa	TAA, arterial tortuosity, arterial stenosis, hypertelorism, arachnodactyly
MFAP5 (microfibrillar-associated protein 5)	FTAAD, AAT9	TAA, AD
TGF-β Signaling Pathway Genes		
TGFBR1 (TGF-β receptor 1)	Loeys-Dietz syndrome type 1, Furlong syndrome, FTAAD, AAT5	TAA, branch vessel aneurysms, AD, arterial tortuosity, craniosynostosis, hypertelorism, bluish sclera, bifid/broad uvula, translucent skin, visible veins, MVP, clubfoot, easy bruising
TGFBR2 (TGF-β receptor 2)	Loeys-Dietz syndrome type 2, FTAAD, AAT3	TAA, branch vessel aneurysms, AD, arterial tortuosity, craniosynostosis, hypertelorism, bluish sclera, bifid/broad uvula, translucent skin, visible veins, MVP, clubfoot, easy bruising
SMAD3 (SMAD3)	Aneurysm-osteoarthritis syndrome, LDS 3	TAA, branch vessel aneurysms, AD, arterial tortuosity, overlapping phenotype with LDS 1 and 2 and marfanoid features, bifid uvula, premature osteoarthritis, osteoarthritis dissecans
TGFB2 (TGF-β 2 ligand)	FTAAD, LDS 4	TAA, arterial tortuosity, AD, MVP, PDA, overlapping features of MFS and LDS, bifid uvula, hypertelorism
TGFB3 (TGF-β 3 ligand)	Rienhoff syndrome, LDS 5	TAA, AAA, AD, hypertelorism, bifid uvula, overlapping features of MFS and LDS, MVP
SKI (v-SKI sarcoma oncogene homolog)	Shprintzen-Goldberg syndrome (velocardio-facial syndrome)	TAA, marfanoid habitus, craniosynostosis, intellectual disability, skeletal muscle hypotonia
SLC2A10 (glucose transporter 10)	Arterial tortuosity syndrome	Widespread aortic and branch vessel tortuosity, TAA, aortic and arterial dissection, keratoconus, marfanoid habitus, joint contractures
SMAD2 (SMAD2)	FTAAD	TAA, AD, cervicocranial arterial dissection
SMAD4 (SMAD4)	Juvenile polyposis syndrome, HHT, FTAAD	Telangiectasia, AVMs, TAA, AD
Vascular Smooth Muscle Contraction Components or Cytoskeleton Genes		
ACTA2 (α-smooth muscle actin)	FTAAD, AAT6	TAA, AD, BAV, moyamoya disease, premature CAD and CVD, livedo reticularis, iris flocculi
MYH11 (myosin heavy chain-11)	FTAAD, AAT4	TAA, AD, PDA
MYLK (myosin light chain kinase)	FTAAD, AAT7	AD at relatively small aortic size
PRKG1 (protein kinase cGMP dependent)	FTAAD, AAT8	Aortic root aneurysm and AD
MAT2A (MAT IIα)	FTAAD	TAA, AD, BAV
FLNA (filamin A)	EDS with periventricular nodular heterotopia and cardiac valve dysplasia	X-linked, TAA, BAV, MV disease, seizures, joint hypermobility
Bicuspid Aortic Valve–Associated Ascending Aortic Aneurysm		
NOTCH1 (NOTCH1)	BAV with TAA	Aortic stenosis, TAA
TGFBR1, TGFBR2, TGFB2, TGFB3, ACTA2, MAT2A, GATA5, SMAD6, LOX	BAV with TAA	Syndromic and nonsyndromic FTAAD with increased frequency of BAV
XO, Xp	Turner syndrome	BAV, COA, TAA, AD, short stature, lymphedema, webbed neck, premature ovarian failure; affects 1 in 2,500 live-born girls

AAA, abdominal aortic aneurysm; AAT, aortic aneurysm syndrome; AD, aortic dissection; AVM, arteriovenous malformation; BAV, bicuspid aortic valve; CAD, coronary artery disease; COA, coarctation of the aorta; CVD, cerebrovascular disease; EDS, Ehlers-Danlos syndrome; FTAAD, familial thoracic aortic aneurysm and dissection syndrome; HHT, hereditary hemorrhagic telangiectasia; LDS, Loeys-Dietz syndrome; MFS, Marfan syndrome; MV, mitral valve; MVP, mitral valve prolapse; PDA, patent ductus arteriosus; PTX, pneumothorax; TAA, thoracic aortic aneurysm; TGF, transforming growth factor.

From Zipes DP, et al. *Braunwald's Heart Disease – A Textbook of Cardiovascular Medicine*. 11th ed. Vol. 2. Elsevier; 2019:1301, Table 63.1.

TABLE 8.11 Appropriate Use Criteria for Initial Transthoracic Echocardiography in Outpatient Pediatric Cardiology in Children Seen with Chest Pain

Appropriate use of echocardiography	Exertional chest pain
	Nonexertional chest pain with abnormal ECG findings
	Chest pain with a family history of sudden unexplained death or cardiomyopathy
Echocardiography may be appropriate	Chest pain with other symptoms or signs of cardiovascular disease, a benign family history, and normal ECG findings
	Chest pain with a family history of premature coronary artery disease
	Chest pain with recent onset of fever
	Chest pain with recent illicit drug use
Echocardiography is rarely appropriate	Chest pain with no other symptoms or signs of cardiovascular disease, a benign family history, and normal ECG findings
	Nonexertional chest pain with no recent ECG
	Nonexertional chest pain with normal ECG findings
	Reproducible chest pain with palpation or deep inspiration

Adapted from Barbut G, Needleman J. Pediatric chest pain. *Pediatr Rev.* 2020;41(9):469–480.

prolapsing into the left atrium. It can be a single click or series of clicks. Then, the medical provider should listen for heart murmurs. Heart murmurs can provide additional clinical evidence for potential cardiac causes of chest pain. Listening for heart murmurs should be performed with the patient supine, sitting, standing, squatting, and standing after squatting. Many murmurs increase in intensity with decreased ventricular filling or decreased afterload (standing, release of Valsalva, squatting); however, hypertrophic cardiomyopathy's murmur does the opposite. It increases in intensity with the Valsalva maneuver and decreases with squatting. Of note, all diastolic murmurs or murmurs grade 3/6 or higher should be further evaluated with an echocardiogram. The presence of a gallop rhythm or a friction rub can make an immediate cardiac diagnosis. A pericardial friction rub is a scratchy, high-pitched, to-and-fro sound caused by the inflamed pericardial surfaces rubbing together during cardiac motion and that is loudest when the patient is upright and leaning forward. Finally, the patient should be assessed for extremity edema. It is important to stress that if a patient's examination is unrevealing, it is imperative that providers pay close attention to vital signs. Tachypnea, tachycardia, hypoxemia, or hypertension without an obvious cause always warrants further evaluation.

Electrocardiogram

An ECG may be helpful if there is a suggestive history and/or physical examination for potential cardiac disease. In the absence of a suggestive history and physical, the yield of an ECG is considered low as it may be normal in patients with structural heart disease or arrhythmias. Regardless, because of its relatively low cost and noninvasive nature, electrocardiograms should be performed in the evaluation of chest pain if there are any concerns discovered in the history assessment or physical examination. After a medical provider obtains an ECG, there are a few important principles to keep in mind. ECG findings are age specific (e.g., infants have a right ventricular–dominant ECG and T waves are usually inverted), arrhythmias are often not found on routine ECGs, and providers should be careful in using the "machine" read in regard to myocardial infarction, pericarditis, or long QT syndrome (the computer is prone to overdiagnosis).

Further Diagnostic Testing

Cardiac consultation is reasonable for any child with red-flag symptoms, specifically chest pain associated with exertion, syncope with exertion, chest pain with concurrent palpitations, abnormal findings on cardiac examination or ECG, a history of cardiac surgery/intervention, or a high-risk family history. If a patient has chest pain with

concurrent fever or signs of hemodynamic instability, the child should be referred to the emergency department for further evaluation for myocarditis.

When the previous evaluation results in a positive screening result, echocardiogram is the diagnostic test of choice for further assessment. However, referral to a cardiologist is generally more cost-effective than obtaining an echocardiogram without a cardiologist. The decision to do an echocardiogram should be judicious due to the low probability of significant findings (Table 8.11). An echocardiogram should be obtained urgently if there are signs of cardiac tamponade (hypotension, tachycardia, pulsus paradoxus) or poor cardiac output. It is also useful if mitral valve prolapse, valvular heart disease, hypertrophic cardiomyopathy, septal defects, endocarditis, or pericarditis is suspected.

Other diagnostic modalities can include chest radiographs, exercise stress tests, and Holter monitors. A chest radiograph is helpful if there is a clinical finding that needs further investigation, such as a history of trauma or fever. Other than pulmonary disease, a chest radiograph can note cardiomegaly or pneumothorax. Regardless, a chest radiograph in the absence of febrile illness, trauma, or lung findings on physical examination has not been shown to be largely beneficial as the likelihood of finding bone or intrathoracic abnormalities in the absence of these features is low. Exercise stress tests should be reserved for anginal cardiac pain in the setting of other normal testing. Due to the difficulty of determining anginal chest pain in the pediatric population, there has been an increased frequency of exercise stress tests ordered. However, medical providers should remember that in the setting of chest pain with a normal echocardiogram evaluation, an exercise stress test has low yield. A 24-hour Holter monitor or a 30-day loop recorder only should be utilized if an arrhythmia is suspected but the resting ECG is normal. Testing for other underlying abnormalities as the cause of noncardiac chest pain can include pulmonary function testing and/or methacholine challenge testing as well as esophageal manometry testing.

The standardized clinical assessment and management plan (SCAMP) is used to reduce practice variation, optimize resource use, and improve patient care through algorithms. One study showed that utilization of SCAMPs reduced cost by 27.5% in assessing and managing pediatric chest pain. It suggests that the diagnostic approach to chest pain in pediatric patients should use only data gathered from the history and physical in conjunction with ECG to suggest when further testing is indicated. Laboratory testing for biochemical markers of cardiac damage is used extensively in the adult population, primarily to diagnose and assist in management of acute myocardial infarction and in children with MIS-C. The biochemical marker most utilized is the high-sensitivity troponin T. The MB isoenzyme of creatinine kinase is rarely used and only utilized if the troponin T is found to be elevated. Troponin T is a protein present in high concentrations in the myocardium but not in other tissues and is released rapidly after myocardial injury in direct proportion to the extent of injury. Troponin T has a high specificity and a low sensitivity for myocardial injury; therefore, false positives often occur, especially in pediatrics where the prevalence of myocardial ischemia and injury is extremely low. Troponin T levels are elevated in postoperative cardiac surgery patients and in diagnoses of myocarditis. Cutoff values have not been well defined; however, low-level troponin T elevations can signify serious disease in children, as opposed to adults, where these small elevations would be considered insignificant. Additional studies in pediatrics are continually ongoing regarding the potential usefulness of cardiac biochemical markers in diseases with muscle breakdown such as Duchenne muscular dystrophy or in determining subtle cardiac dysfunction after convulsive seizures.

Treatment

Medical providers should refer patients to cardiology specialists if cardiac etiologies are still a concern after thorough history, physical, and necessary ancillary studies such as ECGs. Unfortunately, a precise diagnosis is not made in a high percentage of cases. It is up to the medical provider to carefully deal with uncertainty, not over-test or over-refer, and provide ongoing care that minimizes anxiety. Most importantly, if a noncardiac etiology is the highest consideration, medical providers should thoughtfully provide extensive reassurance that includes a symptomatic treatment approach and a plan for appropriate follow-up. It is of the utmost importance that providers provide this reassurance and follow-up to avoid a chronic course of chest pain with potential disability. Of note, families should be specifically asked about school absenteeism so that recommendations for returning to school can be given. Treatment plans should be tailored to both the most likely diagnosis and the patient's individual concerns. Musculoskeletal chest pain can be treated with heat, antiinflammatory medications, or specific exercises. Psychogenic causes of chest pain are perhaps the hardest to treat, often requiring consultation with behavioral health specialists, counselors, and/or psychologists. Primary care providers can start this treatment by having their patients keep pain diaries to help facilitate follow-up discussions. Gastrointestinal causes of chest pain can be diagnosed and treated with a trial of H_2-blocking agents or proton pump inhibitors in addition to reflux precautionary behaviors such as avoiding foods that worsen the symptoms, not eating close to bedtime, and elevating the head of the bed at night. Pulmonary causes of chest pain require therapies to treat the underlying cause, most frequently reactive airway disease.

Overall, because etiologies of chest pain are so often multifactorial and require ongoing evaluation and treatment, the primary care physician must stay actively involved in the patient's care over time.

BIBLIOGRAPHY

A bibliography is available at ExpertConsult.com.

9

Murmurs

Andrew N. Pelech

A heart murmur is a sign, the audible turbulence of blood flow through the heart or the major vessels; symptoms associated with heart murmurs vary by the underlying cause, as well as the nature and severity of any cardiac lesion producing the murmur. While the majority of heart murmurs are normal or innocent, they must be distinguished from the pathologic murmurs of congenital or acquired cardiac disease. Whereas <1% of the population has significant structural congenital cardiac disease, as much as 85% of the population may have a heart murmur during childhood; causes vary by the age of the patient at presentation (Table 9.1). The causes of congenital heart disease are varied and include genetic disorders, metabolic disorders, teratogens, and syndrome complexes (Table 9.2). The causes of acquired heart diseases in children include rheumatic fever, endocarditis, and cardiac injury caused by systemic illnesses. Whereas the echocardiogram defines the significance of pathologic heart abnormalities, the only way to definitively diagnose an innocent murmur is with a stethoscope.

THE THORAX

Knowing the location of the heart chambers and valves within the thorax helps in the interpretation of the heart sounds (Fig. 9.1). The left atrium is located posteriorly, close to the spine. The right atrium and right ventricle are located anteriorly, immediately beneath the sternum. The outflow tract of the right ventricle, which contains the pulmonary valve, rises to the left of the sternum. The parts of the left side of the heart that are close to the chest wall include the left ventricular apex and the ascending aorta as it passes up to the right of the sternum. In other areas, lung tissue lies between the heart and chest wall, which may diminish or distort the intensity of heart sounds.

ORIGINS OF THE HEART SOUNDS

Normal heart sounds originate from the vibration of heart valves when they close and from heart chambers when they fill rapidly. The amount of pressure that forces valve closure influences the intensity of a heart sound. Other mechanical factors such as valve stiffness, thickness, and excursion have lesser effects on sound intensity.

Cardiac murmurs are the direct result of blood flow turbulence. The amount of turbulence and consequently the intensity of a cardiac murmur are directly proportional to both the pressure difference or gradient across a narrowing or defect and the blood flow or volume moving across the site. In contrast to intensity, the frequency or pitch of a cardiac murmur is proportional to pressure difference or gradient alone.

As sound radiates from its source, sound intensity diminishes with the square of the distance. Consequently, heart sounds should be loudest near the point of origin. However, factors other than distance may influence this relationship. Sound passage through the body is affected by the transmission characteristics of the tissues through which the sound is being transmitted. Fat has a more pronounced dampening effect on higher frequencies than does more dense tissue such as bone. If the difference in tissue density is significant—for example, between the heart and lungs—more sound energy is lost. Only the loudest sounds may be heard when lung tissue is positioned between the heart and chest wall.

THE CARDIAC CYCLE

The timing of events in the cardiac cycle allows for a more thorough understanding of heart sounds and murmurs. The relationship between the normal heart cycle and that of the heart sounds is noted in Figure 9.2.

The cardiac cycle begins with **atrial systole**, the sequential activation and contraction of the two thin-walled upper chambers. Atrial systole is followed by the delayed contraction of the more powerful lower chambers, termed **ventricular systole**. Ventricular systole has three phases:

1. **Isovolumic contraction:** the short period of early contraction when the pressure builds within the ventricle but has yet to rise sufficiently to permit ejection
2. **Ventricular ejection:** when the ventricles eject blood to the body (via the aorta) and to the lungs (via the pulmonary artery)
3. **Isovolumic relaxation:** the period of ventricular relaxation when ejection ceases and pressure falls within the ventricles

During ventricular contraction, the atria relax (**atrial diastole**) and receive venous return from both the body and the lungs. Then, in **ventricular diastole**, the lower chambers relax, allowing initial passive filling of the thick-walled ventricles and emptying of the atria. Later, during the terminal period of ventricular relaxation, the atria contract. This atrial systole augments ventricular filling just before the onset of the next ventricular contraction.

The sequence of contractions generates pressure and blood flow through the heart. The relationship of blood volume, pressure, and flow determines opening and closing of heart valves and generates characteristic heart sounds and murmurs.

CHANGES IN THE CIRCULATION AT BIRTH

The majority of significant structural congenital heart disease is recognizable in the first few weeks of life. The age at recognition or presentation often correlates with the nature of the cardiac anomaly and the urgency with which assessment and treatment are necessary.

In the fetus, oxygen is acquired from the placenta and returns via the umbilical vein and through the ductus venosus to enter the inferior vena cava and right atrium (Fig. 9.3). Preferentially, flow is directed across the foramen ovale to enter the left atrium and, subsequently, the left ventricle. Deoxygenated blood returning from the superior vena cava and upper body segment is preferentially directed by the flap of the eustachian valve to enter the right

TABLE 9.1   **Causes of Heart Murmurs by Age at Presentation**

Neonate*	Infant	Older Child
Transient patency of the ductus arteriosus	Congenital heart disease (L→R shunt or R→L shunt)[†]	Congenital valvular obstruction
Peripheral pulmonic stenosis	Ejection murmurs (normal)	Ejection murmurs (normal)
Cyanotic congenital heart disease	Anemia	Repaired congenital heart disease
Congenital valvular obstruction	Arteriovenous malformation	Anemia
Arteriovenous malformation (CNS, hepatic, pulmonary)	Infective endocarditis	Mitral valve prolapse
Anemia	Kawasaki disease	Venous hum
Asphyxia-related myocardial ischemia (transient TI or MI)	Hunter syndrome	Infective endocarditis
Pulmonary hypertension	Hurler syndrome	Rheumatic fever
	Fabry syndrome	Marfan syndrome
		Prosthetic valves
		Obstructive (hypertrophic) cardiomyopathy (subaortic stenosis)
		Carotid or abdominal bruit
		Tumor (atrial myxoma)
		Thyrotoxicosis
		Systemic lupus erythematosus
		Pericardial friction rub

ASD, atrial septal defect; CNS, central nervous system; L, left; MI, mitral insufficiency; PDA, patent ductus arteriosus; R, right; TI, tricuspid insufficiency; VSD, ventricular septal defect.

*Common causes of congenital heart disease in low birthweight infants include PDA, VSD, tetralogy of Fallot, coarctation of the aorta–interrupted aortic arch, hypoplastic left heart syndrome, heterotaxy, and dextrotransposition of the great arteries, in that order. Common causes of congenital heart disease in term infants include VSD, dextrotransposition of the great arteries, tetralogy of Fallot, coarctation of the aorta, pulmonary stenosis, hypoplastic left heart syndrome, and PDA; other causes represent a smaller percentage.

†The relative percentages of congenital heart lesions are VSD (25–30%); ASD (6–8%); PDA (6–8%); coarctation of aorta (5–7%); tetralogy of Fallot (5–7%); pulmonary valve stenosis (5–7%); aortic valve stenosis (5–7%); dextrotransposition of great arteries (3–5%); and hypoplastic left ventricle, truncus arteriosus, total anomalous venous return, tricuspid atresia, single ventricle, and double-outlet right ventricle representing 1–3% each. Other and more complex lesions (e.g., forms of heterotaxy) together represent 5–10% of all lesions.

ventricle and then, via the ductus arteriosus, to enter the descending aorta to return via the umbilical arteries to the placenta. The pressures within both ventricles are essentially equal, inasmuch as both chambers pump to the systemic circulation. However, in utero, the right ventricle does the majority of the work, pumping 66% of the combined cardiac output. At transition (see Fig. 9.3), with the first breath, pulmonary arterial resistance begins to fall as the lungs begin the process of respiration. Pulmonary venous return to the left atrium closes the flap of the foramen ovale. Through mechanical and chemical mechanisms, the ductus arteriosus begins to close. In the normal full-term infant, this is accomplished by 10–15 hours after birth. Intermittent right-to-left atrial level shunting through the foramen ovale may occur, particularly if pulmonary vascular resistance fails to drop.

The time when congenital heart disease becomes symptomatic is influenced by the specific lesion. Some structural cardiac abnormalities *require* patency of the ductus arteriosus for maintenance of either pulmonary blood flow (e.g., pulmonary atresia) or systemic blood flow (e.g., hypoplastic left heart syndrome). These and other ductus-dependent abnormalities, such as transposition of the great arteries, coarctation of the aorta, or significant outflow obstruction (e.g., critical aortic valve stenosis), manifest in the first few hours or days after birth when the ductus arteriosus begins to close. In the absence of an associated anomaly, hemodynamically significant ventricular septal defects (VSDs) do not manifest before 2–4 weeks after birth. Atrial septal defects (ASDs) are seldom symptomatic in infancy.

NORMAL INTRACARDIAC PRESSURES

In the neonate, after birth and successful transition, resistance to flow in the pulmonary circuit is much lower than in the systemic circuit. As such, the pressures in the right-sided chambers are lower than those in the left-sided chambers. The higher values within the ventricles reflect the pressure during the period of ventricular systole in a normal heart (see Fig. 9.3). Pressure in the great vessels during systole is identical to that in the corresponding ventricles, though this relationship changes if there is outflow obstruction. In ventricular diastole, the semilunar valves (aortic and pulmonary) close. Resistance to blood flow in the vascular bed determines the diastolic pressures in the great arteries. The thin-walled atria generate much lower pressures than do the ventricles, both during the phase of passive atrial filling (**v wave**) and during atrial contraction (**a wave**). Only the mean (m) or average atrial pressure is shown in Figure 9.3. During ventricular relaxation, the diastolic pressures are lower than those in the atria, enabling filling.

PEDIATRIC CARDIOVASCULAR EVALUATION

History

Historical assessment of the pediatric patient referred for evaluation of a cardiac murmur should include questions about the family history, pregnancy (including fetal ultrasonography), and perinatal course, in addition to questions about symptoms of cardiovascular disease. An assessment of exercise or play or feeding capacity should be sought, as should an assessment of growth and development. The presence of congenital abnormalities of other major organ systems is associated with structural cardiac problems in as many as 25% of patients.

Structural heart disease is frequently seen in association with recognizable syndromes (see Table 9.2). Children with clearly definable chromosomal disorders known to be strongly associated with structural cardiac abnormalities, such as trisomy 21 or Turner syndrome, should be referred for further diagnostic evaluation. Family history of sudden unexplained death, rheumatic fever, sudden infant death syndrome, or a structural cardiac abnormality in a first-degree relative may be relevant. Hypertrophic cardiomyopathy in a first-degree relative is associated with

TABLE 9.2   Congenital Malformation Syndromes Associated with Congenital Heart Disease

Syndrome	Features
Chromosomal Disorders	
Trisomy 21 (Down syndrome)	Endocardial cushion defect, VSD, ASD
Trisomy 21p (cat-eye syndrome)	Miscellaneous, total anomalous pulmonary venous return
Trisomy 18	VSD, ASD, PDA, TOF, coarctation of aorta, bicuspid aortic or pulmonary valve
Trisomy 13	VSD, ASD, PDA, coarctation of aorta, bicuspid aortic or pulmonary valve
Trisomy 9	Miscellaneous, VSD
XXXXY	PDA, ASD
Penta X	PDA, VSD
Triploidy	VSD, ASD, PDA
XO (Turner syndrome)	Bicuspid aortic valve, coarctation of aorta
Fragile X	Mitral valve prolapse, aortic root dilatation
Duplication 3q2	Miscellaneous
Deletion 4p (Wolf-Hirschhorn syndrome)	VSD, PDA, aortic stenosis
Deletion 9p	Miscellaneous
Deletion 5p (cri du chat syndrome)	VSD, PDA, ASD, TOF
Deletion 10q	VSD, TOF, conotruncal lesions*
Deletion 13q	VSD
Deletion 18q	VSD
Deletion 1p36	ASD, VSD, PDA, TOF, cardiomyopathy
Deletion/duplication 1q21.1	ASD, VSD, PS
Deletion 7q11.23 (Williams syndrome)	Supravalvular AS, branch PS
Deletion 11q 24-25 (Jacobsen syndrome)	VSD, left-sided lesions
Syndrome Complexes	
CHARGE association (*c*oloboma, *h*eart, *a*tresia choanae, growth *r*etardation, *g*enital, and *e*ar anomalies)	VSD, ASD, PDA, TOF, endocardial cushion defect
DiGeorge syndrome, CATCH 22 (*c*ardiac defects, *a*bnormal facies, *t*hymic aplasia, *c*left palate, *h*ypocalcemia, and deletion 22q11)	Aortic arch anomalies, conotruncal anomalies
Alagille syndrome (arteriohepatic dysplasia)	Peripheral pulmonic stenosis, PS, TOF, abdominal coarctation
VATER association (*v*ertebral, *a*nal, *t*racheo*e*sophageal, *r*adial, and *r*enal anomalies)†	VSD, TOF, ASD, PDA
OAVS (*o*culo-*a*uriculo *v*ertebral *s*pectrum), including Goldenhar syndrome	TOF, VSD
CHILD (*c*ongenital *h*emidysplasia with *i*chthyosiform erythroderma, *l*imb *d*efects)	Miscellaneous
Mulibrey nanism (muscle, liver, brain, eye)	Pericardial thickening, constrictive pericarditis
Asplenia syndrome	Complex cyanotic heart lesions with decreased pulmonary blood flow, transposition of great arteries, anomalous pulmonary venous return, dextrocardia, single ventricle, single atrioventricular valve
Polysplenia syndrome	Acyanotic lesions with increased pulmonary blood flow, azygos continuation of inferior vena cava, partial anomalous pulmonary venous return, dextrocardia, single ventricle, common atrioventricular valve
PHACE syndrome (*p*osterior brain fossa anomalies, facial *h*emangiomas, *a*rterial anomalies, *c*ardiac anomalies and aortic coarctation, *e*ye anomalies)	VSD, PDA, coarctation of aorta, arterial aneurysms
Teratogenic Agents	
Congenital rubella	PDA, peripheral pulmonic stenosis
Fetal hydantoin/phenytoin syndrome	VSD, ASD, coarctation of aorta, PDA
Fetal alcohol syndrome	ASD, VSD, TOF
Fetal valproate effects	Coarctation of aorta, hypoplastic left side of heart, aortic stenosis, pulmonary atresia, VSD
Maternal phenylketonuria	VSD, ASD, PDA, coarctation of aorta
Retinoic acid embryopathy	Conotruncal anomalies

Continued

TABLE 9.2 **Congenital Malformation Syndromes Associated with Congenital Heart Disease—cont'd**

Syndrome	Features
Others	
Apert syndrome	VSD
Autosomal dominant polycystic kidney disease	Mitral valve prolapse
Carpenter syndrome	PDA
Char syndrome	PDA
Conradi syndrome	VSD, PDA
Cornelia de Lange syndrome	VSD, TOF
Crouzon disease	PDA, coarctation of aorta
Cutis laxa	Pulmonary hypertension, pulmonic stenosis
Ellis–van Creveld syndrome	Single atrium, VSD
Holt-Oram syndrome	ASD, VSD, first-degree heart block
Infant of diabetic mother	Hypertrophic cardiomyopathy, VSD, conotruncal anomalies
Kartagener syndrome	Dextrocardia
Laurence-Moon	TOF, VSD
Marfan	Aortic root dissection, mitral valve prolapse
Meckel-Gruber syndrome	ASD, VSD
Noonan syndrome (with or without multiple lentigines)	Pulmonic stenosis, ASD, cardiomyopathy
Pallister-Hall syndrome	Endocardial cushion defect
Pierre Robin sequence	ASD, VSD, PDA, coarctation of aorta
Primary ciliary dyskinesia	Heterotaxy disorders
Rubinstein-Taybi syndrome	PDA, PS, coarctation of aorta, VSD
Scimitar syndrome	Hypoplasia of right lung, anomalous pulmonary venous return to inferior vena cava
Smith-Lemli-Opitz syndrome	VSD, PDA
TAR syndrome (thrombocytopenia and absent radius)	ASD, TOF, VSD
Treacher Collins syndrome	VSD, ASD, PDA

ASD, atrial septal defect; AV, aortic valve; PDA, patent ductus arteriosus; PS, pulmonary stenosis; TOF, tetralogy of Fallot; VSD, ventricular septal defect.
*Conotruncal includes TOF, pulmonary atresia, truncus arteriosus, and transposition of great arteries.
†Also known as VACTERL (vertebral, anal, cardiac, tracheo-esophageal fistula, renal, limb).
Modified from Bernstein D. History and physical examination in cardiac evaluation. In: Kliegman RM, St. Geme JW III, Blum NJ, et al., eds. *Nelson Textbook of Pediatrics.* 21st ed. Philadelphia: Elsevier; 2020:2346–2354.e1, Chapter 449.

a high incidence of inheritance, and this condition is sufficiently subtle that echocardiographic screening is mandatory. Unexplained fever, lethargy, a history of intravenous drug use, or additional symptoms arising after recent dental work should arouse suspicion of possible endocarditis.

Infants born to mothers with diabetes mellitus (type 1 or gestational) have as high as a 30% chance of transient hypertrophic cardiomyopathy and are also at risk for congenital structural abnormalities. Additional maternal risk factors for congenital structural heart disease include acute or chronic maternal illness, vertically transmitted infections, illicit drug use, or the use of certain teratogenic medications.

SYMPTOMS AND SIGNS OF HEART DISEASE

The general health of a child with a suspected cardiac malformation is important to assess. Particularly relevant are the rate of growth and history of past illnesses. Although symptoms of **failure to thrive** are nonspecific, patterns of growth reflect the severity of the disease and effectiveness of treatment (see Chapter 12). In an infant, feeding difficulties are often the first evidence of congestive heart failure. Feeding problems are common manifestations of cardiac disease and may be evidenced as disinterest, excessive fatigue, long feeding duration, diaphoresis, tachypnea, dyspnea, or a change in the pattern of respiration. It is important to obtain an objective measure of caloric intake by quantitating the number and/or volume of feedings. Some index of

exertional tolerance should be sought in all children as an index of cardiovascular fitness and a sign of functional capability. This index should be age relevant and, in an infant, might include assessment of the vigor and duration of feeding and the time period of interactive play. In a toddler, the index might include the ability to keep up with peers, climb stairs, or walk for extended periods. In an older child, a comparison with peer sporting interactions, level of function in physical education, and an index of aerobic ability should be sought.

Tachypnea may occur as a consequence of increased pulmonary blood flow. With increasing pulmonary congestion, particularly obstruction to pulmonary venous drainage, dyspnea is manifested as an anxious look with grunting, flaring of the alae nasi, head bobbing, and intercostal, suprasternal, and subcostal retractions. Respiratory rates and the pattern of breathing should be assessed for a full minute in the quiet infant because rates may vary considerably with activity and feeding (Table 9.3), or even over shorter time periods in a quiet infant. Cardiac asthma or exercise-inducible reactive airway disease may occur as a consequence of passive or active pulmonary congestion (see Chapter 4). Compression of airways by plethoric vessels may contribute to the stasis of secretions and atelectasis, which predisposes to respiratory tract infections.

Cyanosis in association with a cardiac murmur suggests a structural lesion with restriction to pulmonary blood flow (Table 9.4). Cyanosis, or a blue discoloration of the skin and mucous membranes, is a consequence of reduced hemoglobin being present in >5 g/dL of

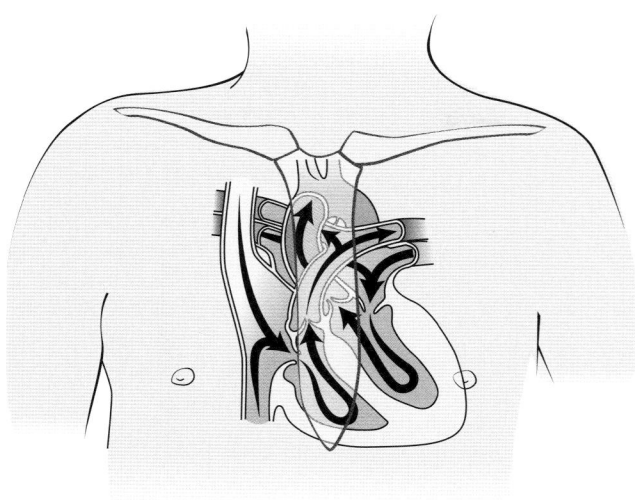

Fig. 9.1 Location of the heart within the thorax. The right atrium and right ventricle lie immediately beneath the sternum. The left atrium lies posteriorly against the spine. The left ventricle extends laterally toward the chest wall, whereas the left ventricular outflow tract extends to the right side of the sternum, going up toward the cardiac base.

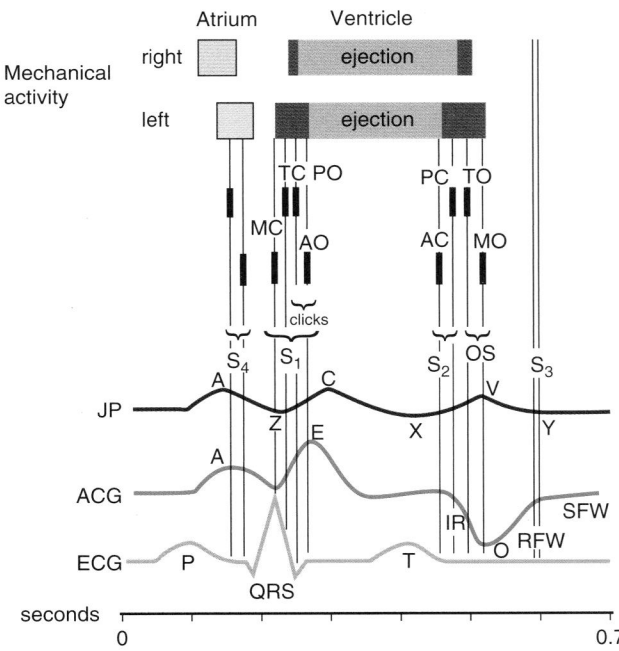

Fig. 9.2 The cardiac cycle. Relationship among electrical and mechanical events, valvular motion, heart sounds (S_1, S_2, S_3, and S_4), the jugular pulse wave (JP), and the apexcardiogram (ACG). AC and AO, aortic component and opening; IR, isovolumic (isochronic) relaxation wave; MC and MO, mitral component and opening; O, opening of mitral valve; OS, opening snap of atrioventricular valves; PC and PO, pulmonic component and opening; RFW, rapid-filling wave; SFW, slow-filling wave; TC and TO, tricuspid component and opening. (From Tilkian AG, Conover MB. *Understanding Heart Sounds and Murmurs: With an Introduction to Lung Sounds.* 3rd ed. Philadelphia: WB Saunders; 1993.)

hemoglobin and is evident in one third of infants with potentially lethal congenital heart disease. Central cyanosis is distinguished from acrocyanosis (peripheral cyanosis) by involvement of the warm mucous membranes, including the tongue and buccal mucosa. Acrocyanosis or peripheral cyanosis is generally confined to the perioral and perinasal regions, extremities, or nail beds and occurs in the child who is cold, vasoconstricted, or at rest. A distinctive feature is that central cyanosis generally worsens with activity and increasing cardiac output, whereas acrocyanosis generally improves or resolves with increased activity.

General Physical Examination
Overall Appearance
Height and weight should be measured and plotted on a growth chart. An assessment of the child's overall growth, appearance, and state of distress serves as a guide to the urgency of further investigation and management. The sick infant often appears anxious, fretful, diaphoretic, pale, or breathless and is seldom consolable. Cyanosis, pallor, digital clubbing, an abnormal pattern of respiration, and possible dysmorphic features may suggest specific structural cardiac anomalies.

Vital Signs
Normal resting heart rates and respiratory rate values for age are presented in Table 9.3. Blood pressure should be measured using an appropriately sized cuff. Every child should have a comparison of upper and lower blood pressures on at least one occasion. The lower limb systolic blood pressure is normally 10 mm Hg higher than the upper limb pressure in older children. On occasion, the subclavian arteries may arise aberrantly beyond the site of ductal ligament insertion. Therefore, both upper limb pressures should be measured and compared with the lower limb pressure. Normal values for blood pressure in children are presented in Figure 9.4.

Respiratory Assessment
Respiratory distress may suggest cardiac disease. In addition to noting the rate, depth, and effort of respiration, the inspection should include observation for evidence of air trapping, increased chest diameter, or the presence of Harrison sulci (horizontal grooves in the anterior chest at the diaphragm insertion site along the sixth and seventh costal cartilages) as an indication of chronic upper airway obstruction. Midfacial hypoplasia with chronic mouth breathing may also suggest upper airway obstructive disease with predisposition to hypercapnia and pulmonary hypertension. Although crackles in the lungs in infants and even young children usually indicate infection, pulmonary edema should also be a consideration.

CARDIOVASCULAR ASSESSMENT
Arterial Examination
Pulses should be assessed for rate, rhythm, volume, and character. The dynamic character of the pulse may provide information about the cardiac output. A clinical index of cardiac output includes the warmth of the digits and measured capillary refill time, obtained by blanching the nail beds or digits and estimating the time to full reperfusion, which is normally <2 seconds. Initially, the radial and brachial pulses should be assessed simultaneously in the upper limb. By palpating the pulse at two sites and altering the pressure applied by the palpating fingers, a more accurate assessment of the rate of rise, volume, and contour may be obtained. Assessment of the femoral pulse requires that the infant be quiet. Palpating parallel to the inguinal crease and allowing the leg to continue to flex is generally more effective than extending the leg. Blood pressures in the arm and leg should be assessed, and the radial and femoral pulses should be palpated simultaneously. Whenever possible, the radial pulse should be brought in close apposition to the femoral pulse to compare for any delay, allowing for a more accurate appreciation of any temporal delay and enabling more accurate detection of the presence of **coarctation of the aorta**. The presence of a palpable femoral pulse is by itself an inadequate screen for coarctation

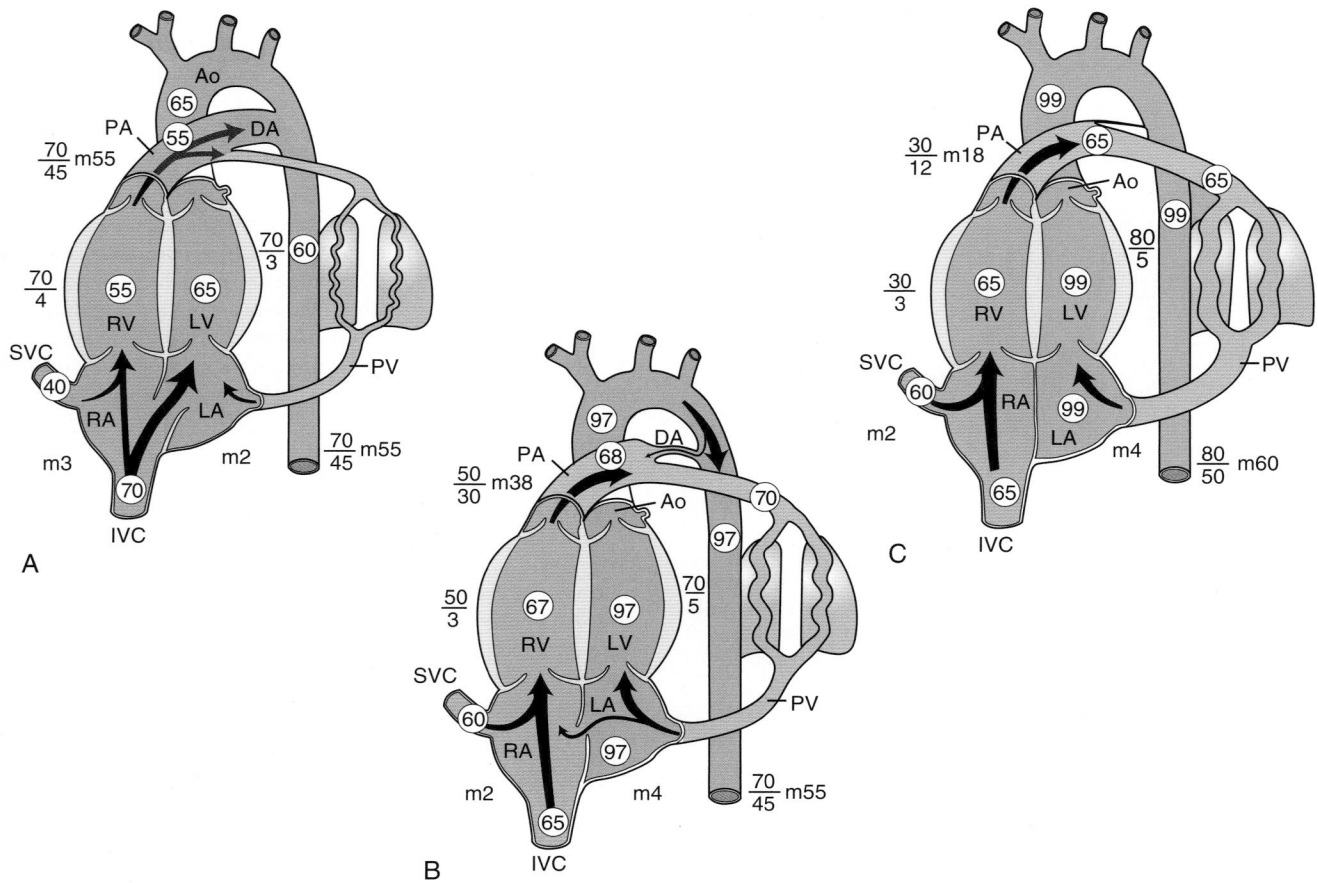

Fig. 9.3 Fetal *(A)*, transitional *(B)*, and neonatal *(C)* circulations. The course of the circulation in the heart and great arteries of the late-gestation fetal lamb, within a few hours of delivery and as a newborn, are presented. The figures in the circles within the chambers and vessels represent percent oxygen saturation. The numbers alongside the chambers and vessels are pressures in mm Hg related to amniotic fluid pressure as zero. Ao, aorta; DA, ductus arteriosus; IVC, inferior vena cava; LA, left atrium; LV, left ventricle; m, mean; PA, pulmonary artery; PV, pulmonary vein; RA, right atrium; RV, right ventricle; SVC, superior vena cava. (Modified from Rudolph AM. Chapters 2 and 3. In: *Congenital Disease of the Heart*. Chicago: Year Book Medical; 1974.)

because a widely patent ductus arteriosus (PDA) or collateral vessels, particularly in the older patient, may provide delayed perfusion. Previous arterial instrumentation, injury, or congenital variability may account for reduction in palpable peripheral pulses.

Venous Examination

In infants and young children, the liver size and character offer more reliable indicators of right atrial pressure and systemic congestion than does the jugular venous pressure. The position, size, and consistency of the liver should be assessed with quiet respiration. The character of the normal liver margin is generally likened to that of the cartilage of the external pinna, and the margin should be sharp and angulated. In the newborn, the liver may be normally palpable at 1.5–2.5 cm below the right costal margin in the midclavicular line. This distance decreases to approximately 1–2 cm by 1 year of age and remains just palpable until school-entrance age. In the presence of congestive heart failure, the liver enlarges and distends downward. The congested liver margin becomes rounded and firm and is often more difficult to feel. An enlarged liver may be tender, and aggressive palpation may cause discomfort and tensing of the abdominal musculature, making accurate assessment difficult. A transverse liver is suggestive of a **heterotaxy syndrome** with abnormal abdominal organ location (i.e., situs abnormalities) and complex congenital heart lesions. The spleen should

always be sought; enlargement suggests endocarditis in the patient with a heart murmur. Splenic enlargement in association with congestive heart failure is unusual (see Chapter 17).

Precordial Examination

Inspection of the chest may suggest the presence of a precordial bulge of long-standing right ventricular volume overload. The examiner's entire palm and hand should be warmed and then fully applied to the patient's chest wall to maximize ability to detect thrills or heaves. Whereas the examiner's fingertips are best utilized to localize an abnormality, the palmar surface of the metacarpals and first phalanges is more sensitive for the detection of low-frequency events. The fingertips should be used to localize the most lateral displacement of the apical impulse. In patients of all ages, the apical impulse should be confined to one intercostal interspace, in which case the impulse would be described as localized; however, if the apical impulse is equally dynamic in two or more interspaces, then it is best described as diffuse. In the neonate, a right ventricular impulse may be felt close to the sternum. Later in life, the same degree of parasternal activity is likely to suggest pulmonary hypertension, right-sided heart volume overload, or right ventricular outflow obstruction. The lateral displacement of the apex, normally located in the midclavicular line, should be compared to existing landmarks. A dynamic or thrusting character to an apical impulse may be detected in association with an

TABLE 9.3 Normal Values of Respiratory and Heart Rates in Infants and Children

	AGE				
	Birth–6 Wk	6 Wk–2 Yr	2–6 Yr	6–10 Yr	Older Than 10 Yr
Respiratory rate	45–60/min	40/min	30/min	25/min	20/min
Heart rate	125 ± 30/min	115 ± 25/min	100 ± 20/min	90 ± 15/min	85 ± 15/min

TABLE 9.4 Categories of Cyanotic Heart Lesions in the Neonate

Group	Heart Size	Pulmonary Blood Flow	Low Cardiac Output	Respiratory Distress	Examples
I	Small	Reduced	No	None	Hypoplastic RV with pulmonary atresia Hypoplastic RV with tricuspid atresia Tetralogy of Fallot (severe)
II	Small or slight cardiomegaly	Increased	No	Moderate	Transposition of great arteries with intact ventricular septum
III	Large	Increased	Yes	Yes	Complicated coarctation of aorta with VSD, hypoplastic LV
IV	Small	Pulmonary venous congestion	Yes	Yes	Obstructed total anomalous pulmonary veins

LV, left ventricle; RV, right ventricle; VSD, ventricular septal defect.
Modified from Gillette PC. The cardiovascular system. In: Behrman RE, Kliegman RM, eds. *Nelson Essentials of Pediatrics*. 2nd ed. Philadelphia: WB Saunders; 1994:503.

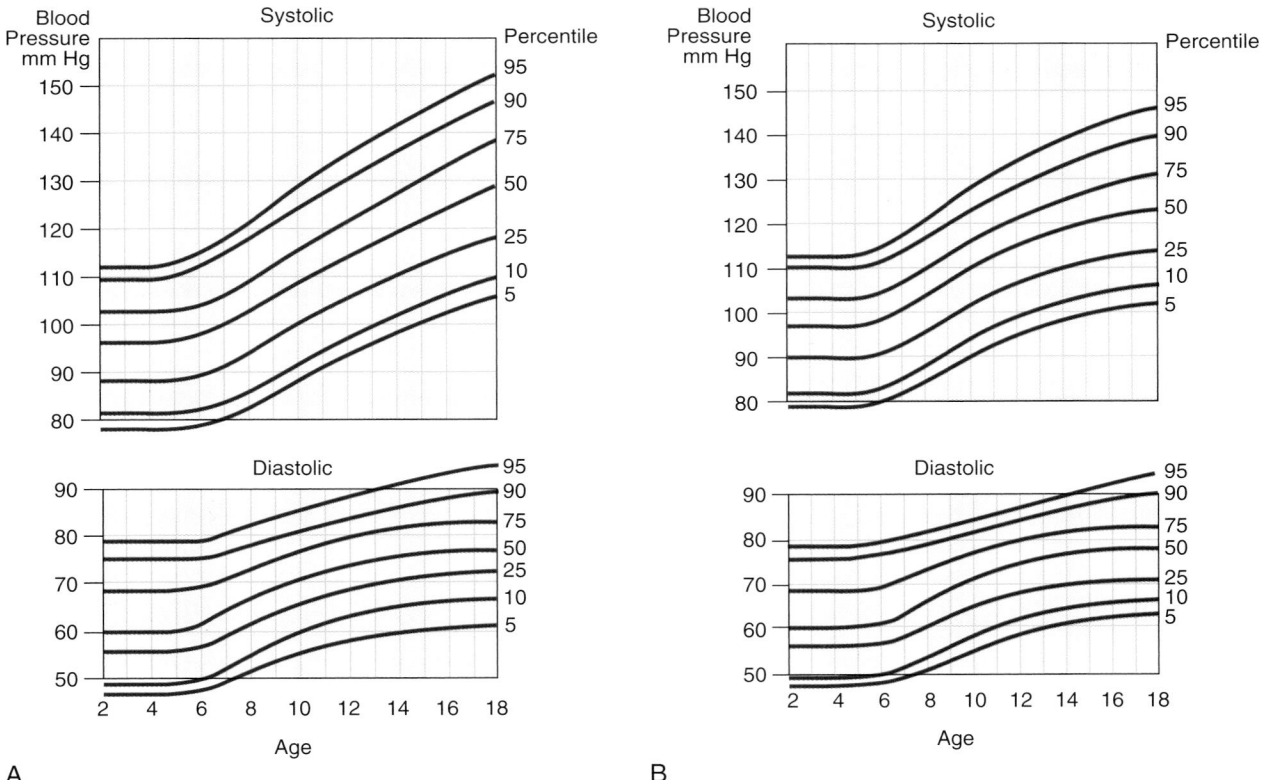

A   B

Fig. 9.4 Normal blood pressure percentiles for boys *(A)* and girls *(B)*, aged 2–18 years. The Korotkoff IV sound is used for diastolic blood pressure. (Modified from the National Heart, Lung, and Blood Institute. Report of the Second Task Force On Blood Pressure Control In Children, 1987. *Pediatrics*. 1987;79:1.)

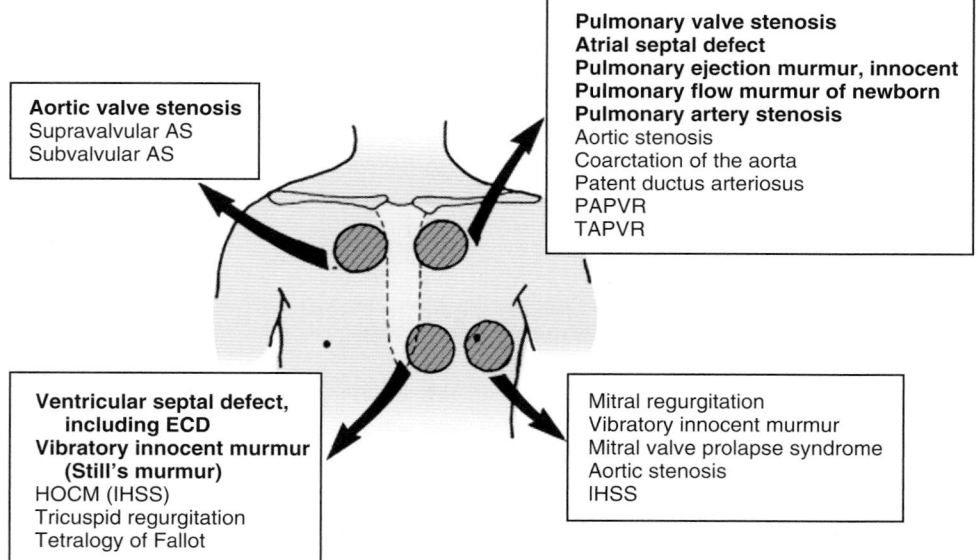

Fig. 9.5 Diagram showing the locations at which certain systolic murmurs are most readily auscultated. Less common conditions are shown in smaller type. AS, aortic stenosis; ECD, endocardial cushion defect; HOCM, hypertrophic obstructive cardiomyopathy; IHSS, idiopathic hypertrophic subaortic stenosis; PAPVR, partial anomalous pulmonary venous return; TAPVR, total anomalous pulmonary venous return. (From Park MK. *Park's Pediatric Cardiology for Practitioners*. 6th ed. Philadelphia: Elsevier; 2014:33, Figure 2-12.)

elevated cardiac output or various forms of obstruction to left ventricular outflow. On occasion, an apical filling impulse, coinciding with an audible S$_3$, may be normally palpable, particularly in the adolescent or athlete with a relative bradycardia and increased stroke volume.

A **thrill** is a palpable murmur and should be sought in the precordial and suprasternal areas. The palmar surface of the examiner's hand is most sensitive in detection of a thrill; however, only the tips of the digits fit in the patient's suprasternal notch. A palpable second heart sound (S$_2$), indicative of a significant level of pulmonary hypertension, may be detected as a sharp or distinctive impulse in the pulmonary outflow.

Auscultation

Thorough auscultation in the cooperative patient may take as long as 5–10 minutes and should include listening in the principal areas of the precordial auscultation (tricuspid, pulmonary, mitral, and aortic) with both the bell and diaphragm of the stethoscope, with the patient in the supine, sitting, and standing positions. These four areas serve as a guide to auscultation of the heart (Fig. 9.5). These are the optimal sites for listening to sounds that arise within the chambers and great vessels:

1. The **tricuspid area** is represented by the fourth and fifth intercostal spaces along the left sternal edge but extends to the right of the sternum as well as downward to the subxiphisternal area.
2. The **pulmonary area** is the second intercostal space along the left sternal border. Murmurs that are best heard in this area may also extend to the left infraclavicular area and often lower, along the left sternal edge to the third intercostal space.
3. The **mitral area** involves the region of the cardiac apex and generally is at the fifth intercostal space in the midclavicular line. This area may also extend medially to the left sternal edge and laterally to the region of the axilla.
4. The **aortic area**, although centered at the second right intercostal space, may extend to the suprasternal area, to the neck, and inferiorly to the third left intercostal space.

The margins of these areas are ill defined, and auscultation should not be limited to these sites and may extend to the axillae, neck, back, or infraclavicular areas.

A step-by-step auscultation—first for heart sounds, subsequently for systolic murmurs, and then separately for diastolic murmurs—is essential. The ability to clearly characterize the S$_2$ is perhaps more crucial than for any other sound; the effects of respiration are important. The components of the S$_2$ in childhood are normally split with inspiration and become single on expiration. A loud pulmonary closure sound should suggest the possibility of pulmonary artery hypertension. The S$_2$ may be widely split and/or fixed in association with right ventricular volume overload or delayed right ventricular conduction. Normal inspiratory splitting of the S$_2$ should be sought and established in all patients. As timing may be difficult in the infant with a rapid respiratory rate, the presence of splitting at any time during the respiratory cycle may be accepted as normal.

The right ventricle is normally just beneath the sternum. This proximity generally makes sounds emanating from the right heart louder and less diffuse. In addition, right heart sounds and murmurs are more influenced by the effects of respiration.

Heart Sounds

Examination should first focus on identifying the normal heart sounds in sequence; subsequent attention should be directed at establishing the effects of inspiration and expiration on the heart sounds. Next, examination should address the presence or absence of additional heart sounds and murmurs. Finally, examination should ascertain any variability that occurs with a change of body position.

First Heart Sound

The first heart sound (S$_1$) (see Fig. 9.2) arises from closure of the atrioventricular (mitral and tricuspid) valves in early isovolumic ventricular contraction and, consequently, is best heard in the mitral and tricuspid valve areas. Mitral valve closure occurs slightly in advance of tricuspid valve closure, and, on rare occasion, near the lower left sternal edge two components (splitting) of the S$_1$ may be heard. There is usually a single first heart sound. The S$_1$ is most easily heard when the heart rate is slow because the interval between the S$_1$ and S$_2$ is shorter than the interval between the S$_2$ and subsequent S$_1$. The intensity of the S$_1$ is influenced by the position of the atrioventricular valve at the onset of ventricular contraction.

Second Heart Sound

Shortly after the onset of ventricular contraction, the semilunar valves (aortic and pulmonary) open and permit ventricular ejection. This opening does not usually generate any sound. The atrioventricular valves remain tightly closed during ventricular ejection. As ventricular ejection nears completion, the pressure begins to fall within the ventricles, and the semilunar valves snap closed. This prevents regurgitation from the aorta and pulmonary artery back into the heart. The closure of the semilunar valves generates the S_2 (see Fig. 9.2). The S_2 usually consists of a louder and earlier aortic valve closure sound (A_2), followed by a later and quieter pulmonary valve closure sound (P_2). Normal physiologic splitting or variability is generally only appreciated in the pulmonary area during or near the end of inspiration. During expiration, the aortic and pulmonary valves close almost synchronously and produce a single or narrowly split S_2. Normal splitting of S_2 is caused by (1) increased right-sided heart filling during inspiration because of increased blood volume returning via the venae cavae and (2) diminished left-sided heart filling because blood is retained within the small blood vessels of the lungs when the thorax expands. During inspiration, when the right ventricle is filled more than the left, it takes slightly longer to empty. This causes the noticeable inspiratory delay in P_2 in relation to A_2. *Splitting of the S_2 during inspiration is a normal finding and should be sought in all patients.*

The aortic and pulmonary pressure in diastole close the semilunar valves. Many forms of congenital or acquired heart disease have an impact on the pulmonary circulation and, consequently, often affect the S_2. Thus, the higher the pulmonary artery diastolic pressure, the more intense and earlier the P_2 is. Pulmonary hypertension in children is suggested when the P_2 is palpable, loud, and narrowly split or cannot be separated from A_2. If the P_2 is audible outside of the pulmonary area, particularly at the apex, then pulmonary hypertension is likely. A single or narrow split S_2 may also be noted in patients with severe pulmonic or aortic valve stenosis, tetralogy of Fallot, truncus arteriosus, pulmonary atresia, hypoplastic left heart syndrome, tricuspid valve atresia, or Eisenmenger syndrome with a VSD. In the presence of moderate to severe pulmonic stenosis, there is low pulmonary artery diastolic pressure. The pulmonary valve closure is therefore delayed and of decreased intensity and is occasionally inaudible.

The S_2 may be widely split and/or fixed in association with right ventricular volume overload or delayed right ventricular conduction.

Third Heart Sound

The third heart sound (S_3) (see Fig. 9.2), which is of very low frequency, occurs about a third of the way into diastole, at the time of the most rapid filling of the ventricles. It is most likely caused by sudden tension of the ventricles, enough to produce sound vibrations within the myocardial wall. Vibrations in the atrioventricular valve itself, as well as in the chordae, may also contribute to the sound. The amplitude of S_3 increases with an increased ventricular filling rate. When heard at the apex, S_3 is considered left ventricular in origin, and when heard at the lower left sternal border, S_3 is likely to be right ventricular in origin. An apical S_3 of soft to moderate intensity is readily heard in most children and young adults. An S_3 in association with tachycardia is termed a **gallop** and may be caused by lesions associated with left or right ventricular diastolic overload or diminished ventricular compliance.

Fourth Heart Sound

The fourth heart sound (S_4) (see Fig. 9.2) is also of low frequency and can be both left-sided and right-sided in origin. It occurs with atrial contraction against a high resistance and is therefore heard just before S_1. It is more difficult to hear than S_3, particularly in children, in whom the PR interval is usually shorter than that in the adult. The S_4 is thought to be caused by a forceful atrial contraction against a poorly compliant left ventricle (e.g., as in diastolic overload). The sound is readily heard in adults with significant chronic hypertension or left ventricular cardiomyopathy and, except for its timing, sounds much like an S_3. In a young baby with total anomalous pulmonary venous return, low pulmonary vascular resistance, and significantly increased right ventricular and pulmonary blood flow, a loud right ventricular S_4 (as well as S_3) may be heard as part of a quadruple rhythm at the lower left sternal border. An intermittent S_4 may be heard in children with complete atrioventricular block. *Whereas an S_3 may be heard in a normal adolescent and can be physiologic, the S_4 only occurs in a pathologic condition.*

Ejection Click

An audible ejection click (see Fig. 9.2) is abnormal and is related to either the hemodynamics associated with a dilated root of the aorta (**aortic ejection click**) or a dilated root of the pulmonary artery (**pulmonary ejection click**) or the effects of a thickened and immobile semilunar valve. The sound is sharp and of very high frequency. The pulmonary ejection click is best heard at the upper left sternal border, whereas the aortic ejection click is usually best heard at the apex. It may also be heard at the upper right sternal border, but if so, it is always louder at the apex or the lower left sternal border. The click arises either from sudden tension of the semilunar valve or from sudden distention with lateral pressure at the root of the aorta or pulmonary artery. The sound is present in aortic or pulmonary valve stenosis. In such cases, the rapid movement of the stenotic valve is suddenly checked. An aortic ejection click may be heard in the presence of a normal aortic valve (as in severe tetralogy of Fallot with a large aortic root); a pulmonary ejection click may be heard with a normal pulmonic valve (as in Eisenmenger syndrome with a large pulmonary root). The aortic ejection click, best heard at the apex, does not vary with respirations. However, the pulmonary ejection click, best heard at the upper left sternal border, is better heard on expiration than inspiration.

An ejection click or a sharp sound present at the upper left sternal border, louder with expiration or heard only on expiration, is characteristic of **pulmonary valve stenosis**. The ejection click follows the period of isovolumic contraction and occurs as a consequence of restricted semilunar pulmonary valve excursion at the onset of ventricular ejection. When the ejection sound occurs at the upper right sternal border or at the apex, a bicuspid or stenotic aortic valve disease is suggested. In contrast to ejection clicks, right-sided cardiac murmurs are accentuated with inspiration. Left-sided heart auscultatory abnormalities vary little with the respiratory cycle.

In the case of the aortic ejection click, the sound is usually well separated from S_1. However, the pulmonary ejection click is usually closer to S_1 than is an aortic click. In some moderate to severe cases, the pulmonary ejection click occurs at the same time as S_1. If one perceives a split S_1, one is most likely hearing an ejection click as the causes of a true split S_1 are very rare.

Opening Snap

The opening snap is present only in rheumatic mitral valve stenosis when the anteromedial leaflet is immobile; is heard early in diastole, usually above the apex; and is of medium frequency. Because the leaflets are fused, the downward movement of the opening valve is suddenly checked, resulting in the opening snap. This sound is often confused with an S_3. The frequency is somewhat higher and the timing is earlier than those of an S_3. The opening snap and the S_3, although similar in timing, can never occur together in the same patient.

Non-Ejection Click

Non-ejection clicks are heard at the apex and occur one third to half of the way between S_1 and S_2. Thus, they are commonly called **mid-systolic clicks**. The sounds are of medium to high frequency. The sound is caused by the sudden tensing of the posterior mitral valve leaflet as it prolapses into the left atrium; in rare cases, there may be multiple mid-systolic clicks. The clicks may be loud, but they may also be soft and easily missed.

CLASSIFICATION OF CARDIAC MURMURS

Heart murmurs are the consequence of turbulent blood flow. Turbulence may arise as a result of
- high flow through abnormal or normal valves
- normal flow through narrow or stenotic valves or vessels
- backward or regurgitant flow through incompetent leaky valves
- flow through congenital or surgical communications
- anemia with high flows and decreased blood viscosity
  Not all cardiac murmurs indicate heart problems.

The clinician should be able to determine and describe the following seven characteristics of heart murmurs:
1. Timing: the relative position within the cardiac cycle relative to S_1 and S_2
2. Intensity or loudness: murmurs are graded as
   - grade I: heard only with intense concentration
   - grade II: faint but heard immediately
   - grade III: easily heard, of intermediate intensity
   - grade IV: easily heard and associated with a thrill (a palpable vibration on the chest wall)
   - grade V: very loud, with a thrill present, and audible with only the edge of the stethoscope on the chest wall
   - grade VI: audible with the stethoscope off the chest wall
3. Location: on the chest wall with regard to
   - area where the sound is loudest (point of maximal intensity)
   - area over which the sound is audible (extent of radiation)
4. Shape: to include the duration (the length of the murmur from beginning to end) and configuration (the dynamic changing nature of the murmur)
5. Pitch: the frequency range of the murmur, generally described as low, medium, or high pitched
6. Quality: aspect that relates to the presence of harmonics and overtones
7. Physiologic effects: of different positions, manipulations, or maneuvers

PEDIATRIC MURMUR EVALUATION

After the neonatal period, an innocent murmur may be detected at some time in the majority of children before school age. The clinical diagnosis of a normal ejection or innocent murmur should only occur in the setting of an otherwise normal history, physical examination, and appearance (Table 9.5 and Fig. 9.6).

Thorough auscultation in the cooperative patient should include listening in the principal areas (tricuspid, pulmonary, mitral, and aortic) of the precordium with both the bell and diaphragm of the stethoscope and with the patient in the supine, sitting, and standing positions.

SYSTOLIC MURMURS

Systolic murmurs begin with or follow the S_1 and end before the S_2 (Fig. 9.7).

Holosystolic murmurs, beginning abruptly with S_1 and continuing at the same intensity to S_2, are graphically shown as a rectangle. This murmur begins during the period of isovolumic contraction and thus occurs when there is a regurgitant atrioventricular valve (tricuspid or mitral) or in association with a VSD.

TABLE 9.5 **Common Innocent Heart Murmurs in Children**		
Type (Timing)	**Description of Murmur**	**Age Group**
Classic vibratory murmur (Still murmur) (systolic)	Maximal at MLSB or between LLSB and apex Grade 2–3/6 in intensity Low-frequency vibratory, "twanging string," groaning, squeaking, or musical	3–6 yr Occasionally in infancy
Pulmonary ejection murmur (systolic)	Maximal at ULSB Early to mid-systolic Grade 1–3/6 in intensity Blowing in quality	8–14 yr
Pulmonary flow murmur of newborn (systolic)	Maximal at ULSB Transmits well to the left and right chest, axilla, and back Grade 1–2/6 in intensity	Premature and full-term newborns Usually disappears by 3–6 mo of age
Venous hum (continuous)	Maximal at right (or left) supraclavicular and infraclavicular areas Grade 1–3/6 in intensity Inaudible in the supine position Intensity changes with rotation of the head and compression of the jugular vein	3–6 yr
Carotid bruit (systolic)	Right supraclavicular area and over the carotids Grade 2–3/6 in intensity Occasional thrill over a carotid	Any age

LLSB, lower left sternal border; MLSB, mid-left sternal border; ULSB, upper left sternal border.
From Park MK. *Park's Pediatric Cardiology for Practitioners*. 6th ed. Philadelphia: Elsevier/Saunders; 2014:36, Table 2-8.

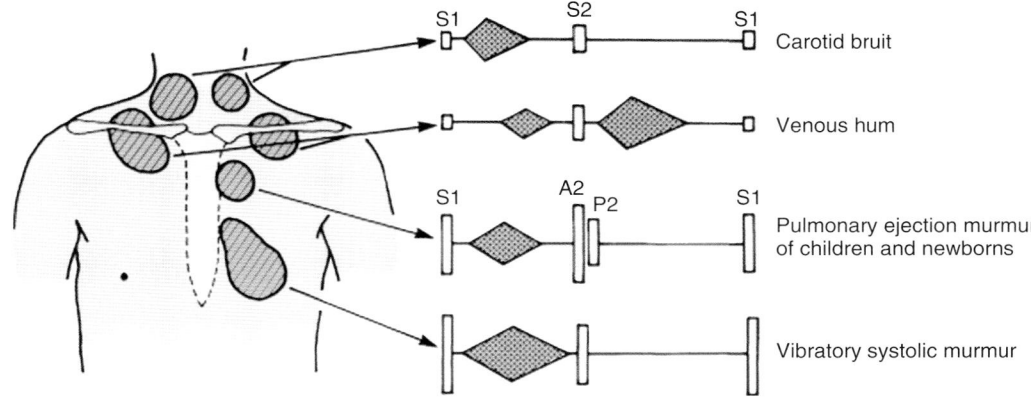

Fig. 9.6 Diagram of innocent heart murmurs in children. (From Park MK. *Park's Pediatric Cardiology for Prac-titioners*. 6th ed. Philadelphia: Elsevier; 2014:37, Figure 2-14.)

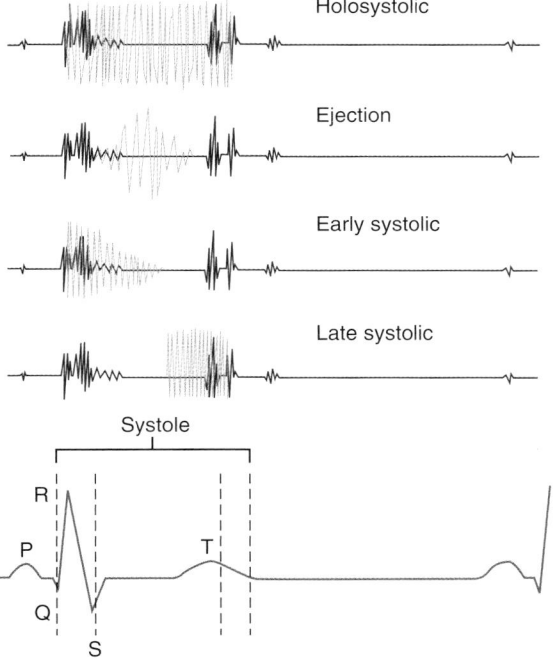

Fig. 9.7 Four classes of systolic heart murmurs. The holosystolic or pansystolic murmur begins abruptly with the first heart sound (S_1) and proceeds at the same intensity to the second heart sound (S_2). The ejection systolic or crescendo-decrescendo murmur begins with the onset of volume ejection from the heart. As the flow increases, the murmur varies both in intensity and frequency and subsequently tapers as the period of ejection ceases, before the S_2. The early systolic murmur begins, as does the holosystolic murmur, abruptly with S_1 but terminates in mid-systole with the cessation of shunt flow. The late systolic murmur begins well after S_1, commencing in mid- to late systole in association with the development of valve insufficiency, and proceeds at this intensity to S_2. (From Pelech AN. The cardiac murmur. *Pediatr Clin North Am*. 1998;45:107–122.)

Ejection murmurs are crescendo-decrescendo or diamond-shaped murmurs that may arise from narrowing of the semilunar valves or outflow tracts. The rising-and-falling nature of the murmur reflects the periods of lower flow at the beginning and near the end of ventricular systole.

Innocent murmurs are almost exclusively ejection systolic in nature (see Table 9.5). They are generally soft, are never associated with a palpable thrill, and are subject to considerable variation with positioning changes.

Early systolic murmurs start abruptly with S_1 but taper and disappear before the S_2 and are exclusively associated with small muscular VSDs.

Mid-systolic to late systolic murmurs begin midway through systole and are often heard in association with the mid-systolic clicks and insufficiency of mitral valve prolapse.

DIASTOLIC MURMURS

Diastole, the period between closure of the semilunar valves (S_2) and subsequent closure of the atrioventricular valves (S_1), is normally silent because of relatively low flow through large valve orifices. Regurgitation of the semilunar valves, stenosis of the atrioventricular valves, or increased flow across the atrioventricular valves all cause turbulence and may produce diastolic heart murmurs (Fig. 9.8).

Early diastolic murmurs are decrescendo in nature and arise from either aortic or pulmonary valve insufficiency (regurgitation).

Mid-diastolic murmurs are diamond shaped and occur because of either (1) increased flow across the normal tricuspid or mitral valve or (2) normal flow across an obstructed or stenotic tricuspid or mitral valve.

Late diastolic or crescendo murmurs are created by stenotic or narrowed atrioventricular valves and occur during atrial contraction.

CONTINUOUS MURMURS

Flow through vessels, channels, or communications beyond the semilunar valves is not confined to either systole or diastole. Thus, there may be turbulent flow throughout some or all of the cardiac cycle (Fig. 9.9). The resulting murmur that extends beyond the S_2 has been classically termed "continuous." The continuous murmur can be heard through part or all of diastole. Continuous murmurs are generally pathologic; the venous hum is an exception.

MURMURS IN CHILDREN WITH NORMAL HEARTS

"Innocent" murmurs occur in the absence of structural or physiologic cardiac disease. Innocent murmurs have been called functional, benign, innocuous, or physiologic but are perhaps best termed normal to accurately convey to parents the favorable impression and outcome that should accompany the diagnosis. After the neonatal period, a normal murmur may be detected in the majority of children at some time before school age.

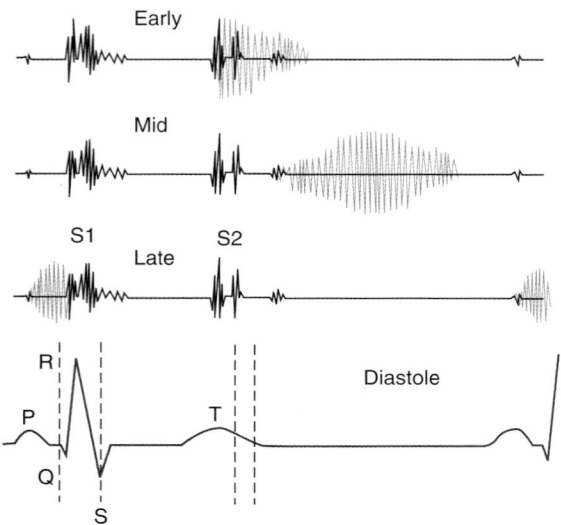

Fig. 9.8 Diastolic murmurs. The early diastolic or decrescendo murmur occurs in association with closure of the semilunar valves (second heart sound) and tapers through part or all of diastole. The mid-diastolic murmur rises and falls in intensity with atrial volume entering the ventricle. The late systolic or crescendo diastolic murmur occurs late in diastole with atrial contraction, before systole, and ascends to the first heart sound. (From Pelech AN. The cardiac murmur. *Pediatr Clin North Am.* 1998;45:107–122.)

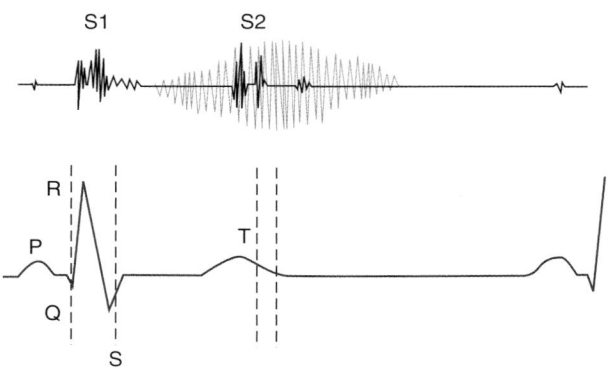

Fig. 9.9 Continuous murmur. The continuous murmur begins in systole and proceeds up to and through the second heart sound, proceeding through part or all of diastole. (From Pelech AN. The cardiac murmur. *Pediatr Clin North Am.* 1998;45:107–122.)

The normal murmurs of childhood are composed of five systolic and two continuous types but are never solely diastolic (see Table 9.5 and Fig. 9.6). The intensity or loudness of the murmur is grade III or less and consequently is never associated with a palpable thrill. The majority of all murmurs, both innocent and organic, are accentuated by fever, anemia, or increased cardiac output.

Vibratory Still Murmur

The most common innocent murmur in children is the vibratory systolic murmur described by Sir George Still. The murmur is typically audible in children between ages 2 and 6 years but may be present as late as adolescence or as early as infancy. The murmur is low to medium in pitch, confined to early systole, generally grade II (range I–III), and heard maximally at the lower left sternal edge and extending to the apex. The murmur is loudest when the patient is in the supine position and often changes in character, pitch, and intensity with upright positioning.

The most characteristic feature of the murmur is its vibratory, musical, harmonious quality described as a "twanging" sound, very like that made by strumming a piece of tense string. The quality of the murmur can thus never be described as "noisy" or "rough." Quite characteristically, the intensity of the murmur diminishes and the pitch changes with upright positioning; it seldom disappears entirely.

The origins of the murmur are obscure and have been ascribed to vibration of the pulmonary valves during systolic ejection, vibrations arising from the shift in blood mass in the dynamically contracting ventricle, physiologic narrowing of the left ventricular outflow tract, and the presence of ventricular false tendons or bridging bands. Phonocardiographic recordings have shown the innocent murmur to arise from either the right ventricular or left ventricular outflow tracts.

Pulmonary Flow Murmur

An innocent pulmonary outflow tract murmur may be heard in children, adolescents, and young adults. The murmur is a crescendo-decrescendo, loudest in early- to mid-peaking ejection systolic murmur confined to the second and third interspaces at the left sternal border. It

is of low intensity (grades II–III) and transmits to the pulmonary area. It is rough and dissonant without the vibratory musical quality of the Still murmur. The murmur is best heard in the supine position and is exaggerated by the presence of a pectus excavatum, a straight back, or kyphoscoliosis, which results in compression or approximation of the right ventricular outflow tract to the chest wall. This murmur may be heard in association with anemia or a thin body build. The murmur is augmented in full exhalation while the patient is supine, rarely resulting in the perception of a palpable thrill, and is diminished by upright positioning and held inspiration.

The murmur of an ASD is attributable to increased flow through the pulmonary outflow tract and may be indistinguishable from the innocent pulmonary flow murmur. However, the hyperdynamic right ventricular impulse, wide splitting of the pulmonary component of the S_2, and presence of a mid-diastolic flow rumble should enable distinction.

The murmur of pulmonary valve stenosis may be distinguished from the innocent pulmonary flow murmur by the frequent presence of a systolic thrill, higher pitch, longer duration, and/or presence of an ejection click. The presence of an ejection click signifies improper opening of a semilunar valve and is usually of pathologic origin. In pulmonary stenosis, the S_2 may be widely split and the P_2, when audible, is of diminished intensity.

Peripheral Pulmonary Arterial Stenosis Murmur

A common murmur heard frequently in newborns and in infants younger than 1 year is the audible turbulence of peripheral branch pulmonary arterial stenosis, angulation, or narrowing. These ejection character murmurs are typically grade I or II, are low to moderate in pitch, begin in early to middle systole, and extend up to and occasionally just after the S_2. These murmurs are most often present in normal newborns but may be associated with viral lower respiratory tract infections and reactive airway disease in older infants. In the fetus, the pulmonary trunk is a relatively dilated, domed structure because it receives the majority of combined cardiac output from the high-pressure right ventricle. Right and left pulmonary artery branches arise from this major trunk as comparatively small lateral branches that receive little intrauterine flow because of high pulmonary artery resistance. When the lungs expand at birth, the relative disparity transiently persists. The branches also arise at comparatively sharp angles from the main pulmonary trunk, accounting for turbulence and a recognized physiologic drop in pressure from the main trunk to the proximal branch pulmonary arteries. In association with a respiratory tract infection, regional vascular reactivity and pulmonary blood flow redistribution may account for the reappearance of the murmur after the neonatal period.

The murmurs are often best heard peripherally in the axillae and back with both regional and temporal variability. Because of the rapid respiratory rate of infants, similar sound frequency composition of breath sounds, and peripheral location of the murmurs, these murmurs are often overlooked. In infancy, they often may be evident in association with a viral respiratory illness. Of importance is that the murmur of peripheral branch stenosis changes with heart rate, increasing in intensity with heart rate slowing as the stroke volume increases and, conversely, diminishing with tachycardia and reduction in stroke volume. Therefore, the murmur becomes louder with slowing of the heart rate and diminishes with tachycardia and increasing cardiac output.

The normal peripheral branch stenosis murmur may be indistinguishable from the peripheral murmur of significant stenosis of the branch pulmonary vessels seen in Williams or rubella syndrome or from accompanying hypoplasia or narrowing of the pulmonary arteries. Murmurs of significant anatomic narrowing may be distinguished by their higher pitch and extension after the S_2 in children after the first few months of life. The pulmonary flow murmur of an ASD may mimic this murmur but is not heard in this age group. Proximal pulmonary valve or right ventricular outflow obstruction may also closely resemble this murmur, but these obstructions are often of louder intensity, possibly associated with an ejection click, and heard maximally lower along the left sternal border.

Supraclavicular or Brachiocephalic Systolic Murmur

A supraclavicular systolic crescendo-decrescendo murmur may be heard in children and young adults. This systolic murmur is audible maximally above the clavicles and radiates to the neck but may be present to a lesser degree on the superior chest. The murmur is low to medium in pitch, of abrupt onset, brief, and maximal in the first half or two thirds of systole. High pitch or extension into diastole is unusual and suggests significant vascular obstruction.

The murmur is present in both supine and sitting positions but varies with hyperextension of the shoulders. The shoulders can be hyperextended with the elbows brought behind the back until the shoulder girdle is taut. When this maneuver is done rapidly, the murmur diminishes or disappears altogether. Supraclavicular systolic murmurs are thought to originate from turbulence within the major brachiocephalic vessels as they arise from the aorta.

Aortic Systolic Murmur or "Athlete's Murmur"

Innocent systolic flow murmurs may arise from the outflow tract in older children and young adults. The murmurs are ejection in character, confined to systole, and audible maximally in the aortic area. In children, these murmurs may arise secondarily to extreme anxiety, anemia, hyperthyroidism, fever, or any condition of increased systemic cardiac output.

In trained athletes, slower heart rates with increased stroke volume may give rise to short crescendo-decrescendo murmurs of low to medium pitch. Physical examination may suggest a relatively displaced thrusting apex and a physiologic S_3.

These murmurs must be distinguished from the systolic murmur of hypertrophic cardiomyopathy obstructions of the left ventricular outflow tract. The presence of a family history for hypertrophic cardiomyopathy or a family history of unexplained death in a young individual, particularly if associated with activity, is suggestive of hypertrophic cardiomyopathy. A systolic murmur that gets louder with performance of the Valsalva maneuver is considered almost diagnostic of hypertrophic cardiomyopathy with systolic anterior motion of the mitral valve. A reduction in venous return results in closer apposition of the septum and mitral valve and dynamic narrowing of the left ventricular outflow tract. In contrast, rapid squatting improves venous return; the left

ventricular chamber size is enlarged, the mitral valve and septum are farther apart, and the murmur of hypertrophic cardiomyopathy gets softer. It is often difficult to be certain of the cause of this type of aortic murmur, and further investigations may be indicated.

Normal Continuous Murmurs

Venous Hum

The most common type of continuous murmur heard in children is the innocent cervical venous hum, which is most audible on the low anterior part of the neck just lateral to the sternocleidomastoid muscle but often extends to the infraclavicular area of the anterior chest wall. The murmur is generally louder on the right than on the left, is louder when the patient is sitting than when lying down, and is accentuated in diastole. Intensity varies from faint to grade III. Patients are occasionally aware of a loud hum. The murmur is quite variable in character, always low pitched, and often described as rumbling, roaring, or whirring.

The venous hum is best accentuated or elicited with the patient in a sitting position and looking away from the examiner. The murmur often resolves or changes in character with lying down and may be eliminated or diminished by gentle compression of the jugular vein or turning the head toward the side of the murmur. The murmur is thought to arise from turbulence at the confluence of flow as the internal jugular and subclavian veins enter the thoracic inlet or perhaps from angulation of the internal jugular vein as it courses over the transverse process of the atlas.

Mammary Arterial Souffle

The mammary arterial souffle occurs most frequently late in pregnancy and in lactating women but may occur in rare cases in adolescence. The term *souffle* refers to a murmur with a blowing quality on auscultation that is typically caused by a vascular structure. The murmur arises in systole but may extend well into diastole, being audible maximally on the anterior chest wall over the breast. There is usually a distinct gap between the S_1 and the origin of the murmur; this gap is thought to relate to the delayed arrival of cardiac stroke volume at the peripheral vasculature. The murmur is generally high pitched and has an unusual superficial character but may vary considerably from day to day. Firm pressure with the stethoscope or digit pressure on the chest wall occasionally abolishes the murmur. The murmur is thought to be arterial in origin, arising from the plethoric vessels of the chest wall. The murmur must be distinguished from the continuous high-pitched murmur of an arteriovenous fistula or a PDA. Characteristically, the mammary arterial souffle varies significantly from day to day, is present in a most distinctive patient population, and resolves with termination of lactation.

MURMURS CAUSED BY COMMON LESIONS WITH LEFT-TO-RIGHT SHUNT

Atrial Septal Defects

The most common form of ASD (Fig. 9.10) is the ostium secundum defect in the floor of the fossa ovalis. Blood flow through an ASD in the low-pressure atria is inaudible. The auscultatory findings in ASD are related to the consequences of increased blood volume that enters the right side of the heart. The right ventricular volume overload is associated with right ventricular overactivity and a right ventricular parasternal tap.

The right atrium and ventricle receive the blood returning from the body plus the blood shunted from left to right through the ASD. This causes a prolongation of right-sided heart emptying. The P_2 of the second heart sound is therefore widely split and fixed (no respiratory variation).

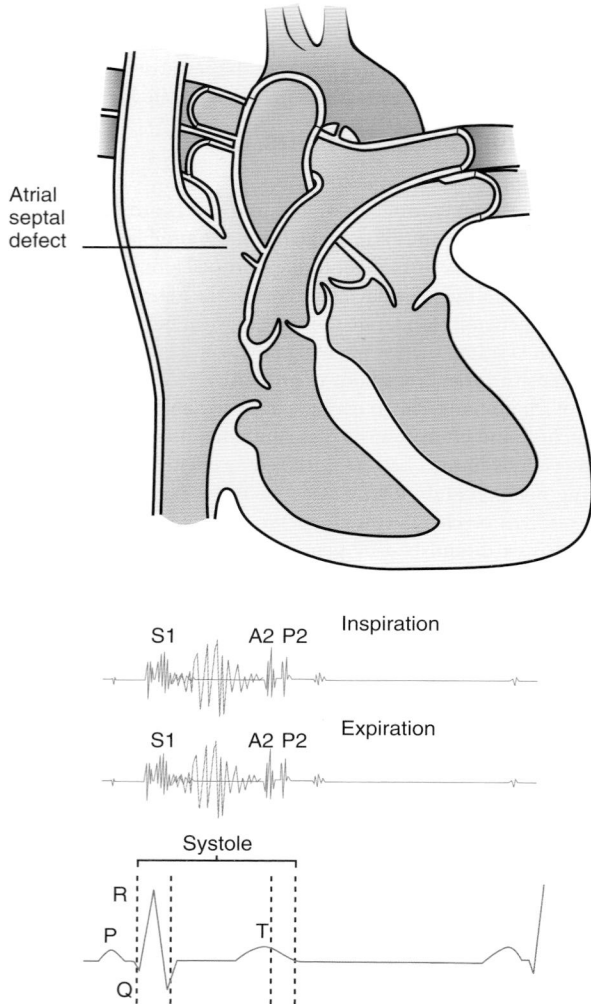

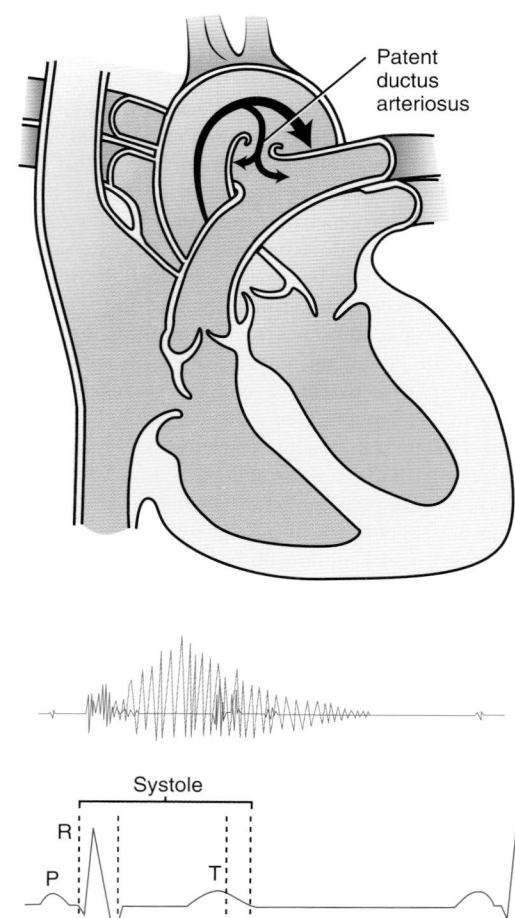

Fig. 9.11 The patent ductus arteriosus consists of residual patency of a fetal communication between the two great arteries. Because the shunt occurs outside the heart, the murmur is continuous and high pitched, provided that the defect is restrictive and the pulmonary artery pressures are low.

Fig. 9.10 Atrial septal defects. The most common type of defect, the secundum atrial septal defect, is shown. Characteristically, in association with a large left-to-right shunt, wide and fixed splitting of the second heart sound occurs. The murmur is that of increased flow through the right ventricular outflow tract. The shunt flow through the defect, which occurs at low pressure, is inaudible.

Two types of murmur may be audible:

1. The typical pulmonary flow murmur is ejection systolic in character, generally of low intensity (grade II or III), and of low pitch. The crescendo-decrescendo murmur begins shortly after the S_1 and ends well before the S_2.
2. In patients with a large atrial shunt, there is typically a well-localized, low-pitched mid-diastolic flow rumble in the tricuspid area because of increased flow across the tricuspid valve.

ASDs may lead to pulmonary hypertension in the second and third decades of life. Treatment is surgical or by device closure during cardiac catheterization.

PATENT DUCTUS ARTERIOSUS

In this condition, the connection between the aorta and pulmonary artery that exists prenatally remains open after birth (Fig. 9.11).

The amount of shunt flow is dependent not only on the size of the ductus communication but also on the differential resistances of the systemic and pulmonary circulations. In some children, the PDA may produce significant left-sided heart volume overload and signs of high-output congestive heart failure.

The peripheral pulses associated with significant diastolic runoff to the pulmonary vascular area are bounding. Palpation may reveal a thrill in systole at the upper left sternal edge when the murmur is grade IV or greater; an abnormal left ventricular impulse; and, if the left-to-right shunt is large, a hyperdynamic, diffuse, and displaced apical impulse. The majority of patients have an asymptomatic murmur.

Premature infants often have persistence of ductal patency after birth. Initially, in the presence of neonatal lung disease and elevated pulmonary vascular resistance, the shunt volume is not large. After the lung disease improves, the presence of a PDA becomes apparent through the detection of a cardiac murmur and bounding pulses. Preterm infants with a PDA may show signs of heart failure, pulmonary edema, a hyperdynamic precordium, and difficulty in weaning from the ventilator. Treatment in preterm infants may include intravenous indomethacin, ibuprofen, acetaminophen, and fluid restriction; if these measures are unsuccessful, surgical ligation or device closure is indicated.

Beyond the neonatal period, the PDA causes a continuous rough murmur, best heard in the pulmonary area. The murmur is generally

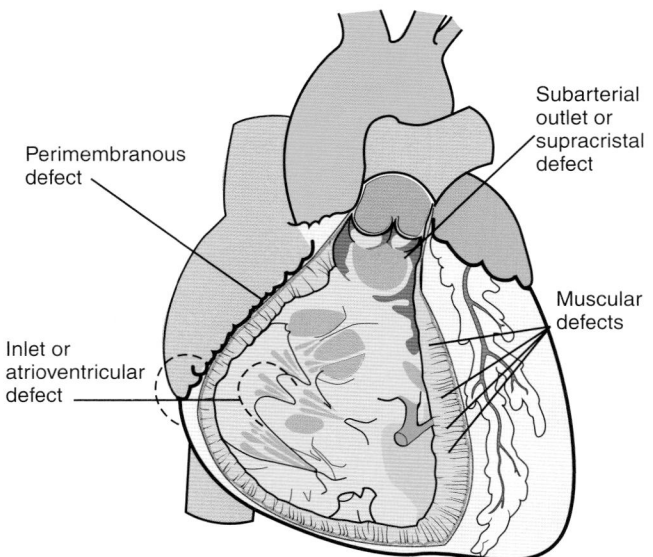

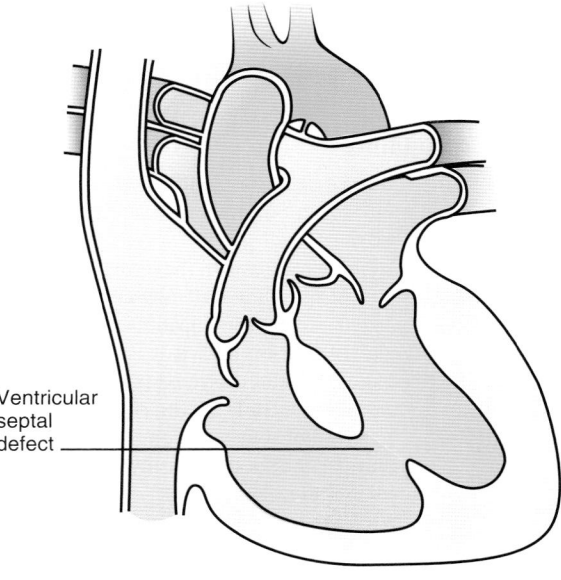

Fig. 9.12 Anatomic types of ventricular septal defects. The four types of defects of the ventricular septum are shown. The most common type is the muscular defect, which commonly occurs in the anterior trabecular area of the septum. The perimembranous (often called membranous) defect occurs in the regions of the pars membranacea, or the embryonic bulboventricular foramina. The subarterial outlet, or supracristal defect, extends to the fibrous ring of the semilunar valves. The inlet or atrioventricular septal defect is that of the atrioventricular canal or embryonic atrioventricularis communis.

high pitched, peaks in late systole, and continues well through the S_2. If the PDA is large, a mid-diastolic flow rumble may be heard at the apex because of relative mitral valve stenosis. Treatment is surgical ligation or device closure during cardiac catheterization.

VENTRICULAR SEPTAL DEFECTS

These common developmental communications between the two ventricles (Fig. 9.12) may be classified as
- perimembranous
- muscular
- atrioventricular or inlet
- subarterial or outlet (supra cristal)
  The acoustic findings depend on five factors:
1. Size
2. Location
3. Shunt or defect flow
4. Pulmonary hypertension
5. Associated anomalies
   All of these factors need to be addressed in the clinical description of a VSD.

The VSD (Fig. 9.13) causes a left-to-right shunt or, in rare cases, a right-to-left shunt, depending on the resistance to the flow of blood leaving the ventricles. The turbulence and thus the intensity of the murmur are directly proportional to the flow and pressure difference between the ventricles.

Size

A moderate-sized VSD that is restrictive (i.e., a pressure difference exists between the ventricles) causes a harsh blowing holosystolic murmur, which is often very loud and frequently associated with a palpable thrill.

The very restrictive or small VSD creates a high-pitched systolic murmur and causes little or no physiologic disturbance. Small

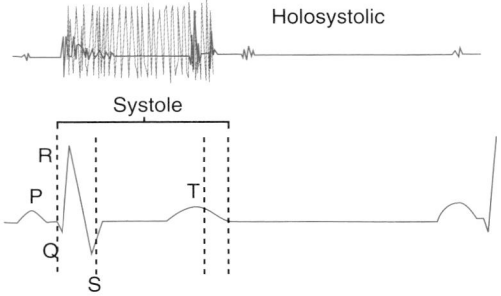

Fig. 9.13 Ventricular septal defects. A ventricular septal defect is a communication between the high-pressure left ventricle and the lower-pressure right ventricle. The shunt flow begins with the onset of ventricular contraction before the period of ejection (isovolumic contraction) and consequently gives rise to a holosystolic murmur that obscures the first and often the second heart sounds. The murmur is high pitched if the defect is restrictive and the right-sided heart pressures are low; however, the murmur may be low pitched or even inaudible if the defect is large or if the pulmonary artery pressures are high, as occurs in the newborn.

muscular defects may close in mid-systole, which then abruptly stops shunt flow and the murmur before S_2.

In an unrestrictive or large VSD, no pressure difference exists between the two ventricles. This results in less turbulence and therefore a reduced intensity of the murmur.

Location

The perimembranous defect is best heard at the left sternal edge in the third left intercostal space. Muscular defects are heard variably from the sternal edge to the apex. Outlet or subarterial defects are best heard higher along the sternum.

Shunt Flow

If the volume of flow through the VSD (shunt flow) is large (i.e., more than 2–3 times normal ventricular outflow), a low-pitched, mid-diastolic flow rumble may be heard in the mitral area. The extra volume of blood returning from the pulmonary circulation to the left side of the heart creates this murmur of "relative" (not true anatomic) mitral valve stenosis.

Pulmonary Hypertension

High pressure in the pulmonary artery limits left-to-right shunt flow and murmur intensity. The pulmonary closure sound is louder and is either narrowly split or single.

Associated Anomalies

Frequently there are anomalies associated with a VSD, such as right- or left-sided heart outflow obstruction or aortic insufficiency. This may affect the character of the murmur.

The VSD murmur begins very early with the onset of left ventricular contraction, which may precede right ventricular contraction because the left ventricle is activated earlier. The murmur commences during the period of isovolumic contraction and, if it is loud (grade III or greater), often obscures the S_1. Blood is ejected from the left ventricle to the right ventricle throughout systole, giving rise to a classical full-length, or "holosystolic," murmur. On occasion, VSD murmurs may not be full length. This may occur characteristically in a small muscular VSD that coapts or closes in mid-systole.

Analysis of the S_2 in a VSD is important and, in conjunction with precordial palpation, enables estimation of the pulmonary artery pressure. The larger the defect, the higher the pulmonary artery pressure and the earlier and louder the P_2. Thus, the physiologic split of S_2 may become very narrow, or the S_2 may even become single, a finding of great concern. In large defects, a balance exists between delayed P_2, caused by large pulmonary blood flow, and early P_2, caused by high pulmonary artery pressure. The wider the split of S_2, the less the concern is, because pulmonary vascular resistance is then likely to be low.

The intensity or loudness of a murmur relates to the combination of both flow and gradient across the defect. Pitch or frequency relates to gradient alone. Thus, very small defects with small left-to-right shunt flow may have a soft, high-pitched murmur. In moderate-sized defects, the murmur is loud, often associated with a palpable thrill. In large defects with no restriction between the right and left ventricles, the murmur is low pitched and less intense as the pulmonary artery and right-sided heart pressures equate with the left-sided heart pressure.

In many children, the VSD spontaneously closes and the murmur becomes softer and softer until it disappears with defect closure. In patients who develop increased pulmonary vascular resistance and a reduction in shunt flow and who are at risk for progressing to **Eisenmenger syndrome** (irreversible pulmonary vascular disease and cyanosis with right-to-left ventricular level shunt), the murmur also becomes quieter. Thus, a diminishing VSD murmur may be evolving into either a good or bad outcome. The treatment of a large VSD currently includes management of heart failure and, most frequently, surgery.

COMPLETE ATRIOVENTRICULAR SEPTAL DEFECTS

There is great variation in the anatomy of atrioventricular septal defects (AVSDs). AVSDs (Fig. 9.14) occur in complete, partial, and intermediate forms. In the complete AVSD, the intracardiac defect extends between both the atria and ventricles. Either the atrial or ventricular extent of the defect may be the primary level of shunt flow; consequently, the defect may manifest primarily as either an ASD or a VSD. Often the defects are large and unrestrictive. In addition, a common accompaniment of AVSD is a cleft in the left-sided atrioventricular valve, which may cause varying degrees of valve insufficiency. Approximately half of the children born with **trisomy 21 (Down syndrome)** have congenital heart disease, the most common abnormality of which is complete AVSD. Maturation of the pulmonary arteries and small muscular arteries is delayed in children with Down syndrome, and elevated pulmonary vascular resistance early in life is common. Therefore, the lesion may be missed early in life because signs of congestive

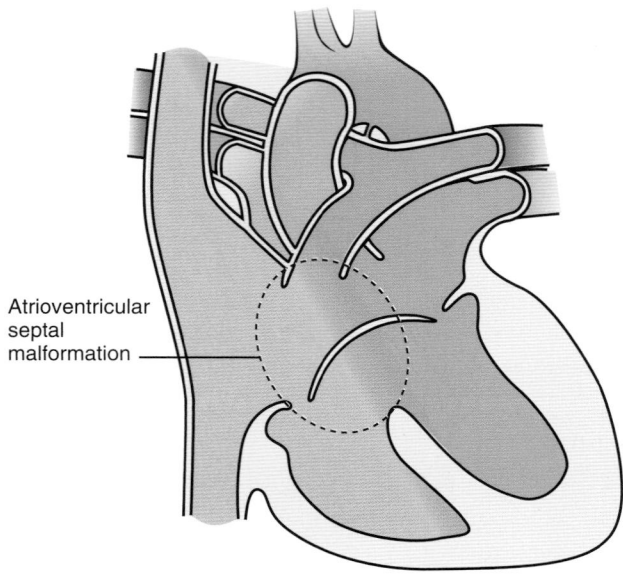

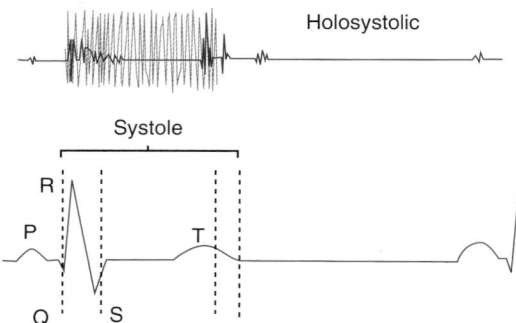

Fig. 9.14 Complete atrioventricular septal malformation. The atrioventricular septal malformations vary markedly from a large atrial component with a restrictive ventricular communication to a large unrestrictive inlet ventricular septal defect. Consequently, their clinical manifestations also vary from that of an atrial septal defect to that of an unrestrictive ventricular septal defect.

heart failure may not occur. It is recommended that all children with Down syndrome undergo echocardiographic evaluation. In patients with complete AVSDs, the electrocardiogram demonstrates an abnormally counterclockwise superior vector due to displacement of the AV node. Intermediate or partial AVSDs are less frequently associated with Down syndrome.

In the partial form of AVSD, absence of the lower part of the interatrial septum, the **ostium primum**, is the major component of the abnormality. In such patients, the manifestation and examination are similar to those described for a secundum type of ASD. Often, mitral regurgitation is present and is apparent as an apical holosystolic murmur that obscures S_1. If the amount of mitral valve insufficiency is large, a mid-diastolic flow rumble of increased filling may be heard.

The manifestation and consequently the clinical signs in patients with AVSD vary considerably, depending on the patient's age, pulmonary vascular resistance, size and level of the defects, amount of valve insufficiency, and ventricular function. Patients with an AVSD often manifest the signs of congestive heart failure early in infancy. Surgical repair provides definitive treatment.

MURMURS CAUSED BY COMMON LESIONS WITH RIGHT-TO-LEFT SHUNT AND CYANOSIS

Tetralogy of Fallot

The tetralogy (Fig. 9.15) has four anatomic features:

1. VSD
2. Pulmonary stenosis
3. Dextroposition or rightward position of the aorta
4. Right ventricular hypertrophy

The functional significance of this anomaly is related to the degree of right ventricular outflow tract obstruction. There is a harsh ejection systolic murmur, heard best in the pulmonary area but also widely transmitted through the chest. The right ventricular outflow obstruction is most frequently a combination of muscular, annular, and valvular narrowing. Consequently, the P_2 is soft, delayed, and often inaudible. The VSD is typically large and unrestrictive. The prominent systolic murmur in tetralogy of Fallot is therefore not caused by the septal defect.

Patients with tetralogy of Fallot may present with moderate to severe degrees of right ventricular outflow obstruction, right-to-left ventricular level shunting, and varying degrees of cyanosis. Alternatively, the outflow obstruction may be mild, providing a predominant left-to-right shunt and causing the "acyanotic" or "pink" form of tetralogy of Fallot. In these patients, the degree of outflow obstruction becomes progressive; bidirectional flow develops and, finally, a dominant right-to-left shunt emerges.

One aspect of tetralogy physiology is the variable degree of desaturation that may occur as a consequence of the reactive nature of the right ventricular outflow obstruction. The sudden development of severe reactive obstruction in response to temperature, fever, illness, dehydration, or intense crying may precipitate a **hypercyanotic** or **tetralogy ("tet") spell**. Either increased infundibular reactivity or decreased systemic vascular resistance is responsible for the diminished pulmonary blood flow. This life-threatening event manifests as profound cyanosis, tachypnea, and dyspnea, progressing to acidosis, unconsciousness, and death. During a spell, the outflow tract murmur disappears with the diminution in pulmonary blood flow.

Tetralogy of Fallot is a consequence of developmental anterior displacement of the conal or outlet septum and failure to adjoin with the muscular trabecular interventricular septum. Because conal tissue is needed for closure of the membranous ventricular septum, the anterior displacement and hypoplasia of the conus results in a VSD, which is characteristically unrestrictive. The aorta extends more to the right, which results in overriding of the aorta.

In cases in which there is a predominant left-to-right shunt, the murmur is a long, loud ejection systolic murmur and may overwhelm and obscure the S_2. The murmur extends up the left sternal border (pulmonary area) and throughout both lung fields. The right ventricle is at systemic pressure, and the pitch of the murmur is quite high. There is a right ventricular parasternal impulse and often a palpable thrill in the pulmonary outflow region.

In cyanotic tetralogy of Fallot, the loudness or intensity of the murmur diminishes as the pulmonary blood flow decreases. The systolic murmur remains high pitched, harsh, and ejection in shape. The S_1 remains loud or normal; the S_2 is single.

In the most severe form of tetralogy, pulmonary atresia with VSD, there is no pulmonary outflow murmur at all. Definitive corrective treatment of tetralogy of Fallot is surgical.

TRICUSPID VALVE ATRESIA

In tricuspid valve atresia (Fig. 9.16), the tricuspid valve does not develop and in its place there may be an imperforate membrane or a thick muscle wedge. The right ventricle is usually very small; the left

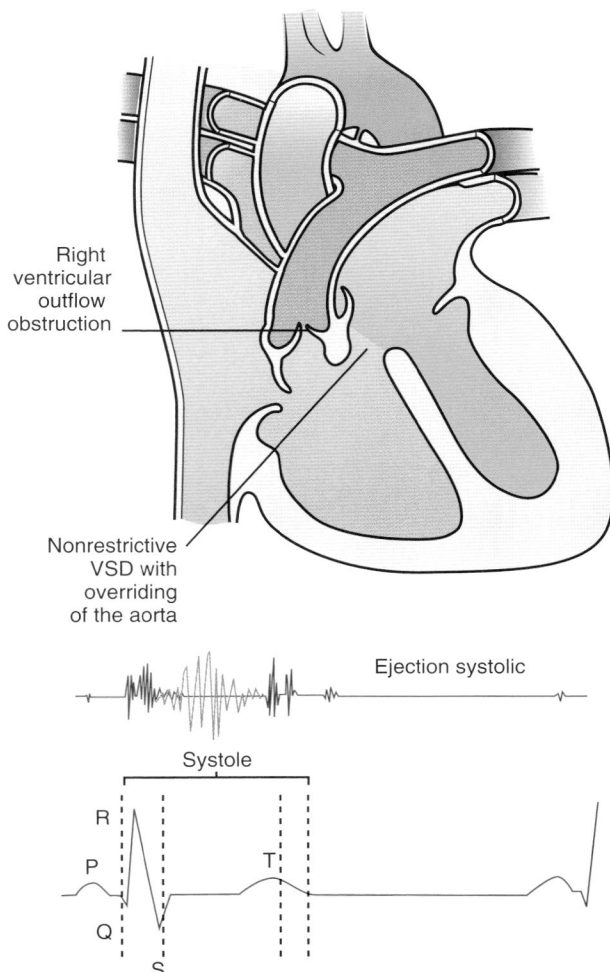

Fig. 9.15 Tetralogy of Fallot. The four anatomic malformations seen in association with tetralogy of Fallot include an unrestrictive perimembranous ventricular septal defect (VSD), overriding of the aorta, right ventricular hypertrophy, and an obstructive right ventricular outflow tract. The cardiac murmur in tetralogy, a harsh loud ejection systolic murmur, arises from the turbulence generated in the right-sided heart outflow. Because the VSD is unrestrictive and the right- and left-sided heart pressures are equal, the VSD generates no sound. The pulmonary closure sound is often soft or inaudible.

ventricle compensates and is large. A dynamic diffuse left ventricular cardiac impulse is palpable. All systemic venous blood returning to the right atrium must pass across at the atrial septal level to enter the left atrium and then the left ventricle. Pulmonary blood flow occurs most often as a consequence of a VSD or, in rare cases, is dependent on the ductus arteriosus. The ECG reveals an abnormally superior left axis. Examination reveals a VSD murmur. The softer and shorter the murmur, the less the pulmonary blood flow is, so that, just as in tetralogy of Fallot, the softer the murmur, the more severe the cyanosis is. If there is enough pulmonary blood flow, both P_2 and A_2 may be heard. Palliative surgery is required.

PULMONARY ATRESIA WITH INTACT VENTRICULAR SEPTUM

There are two forms of pulmonary valve atresia. The first is pulmonary atresia with VSD and generally a long fibrous or muscular outflow atresia, which is the most severe malformation on the spectrum of tetralogy of Fallot. The second form occurs in association with an

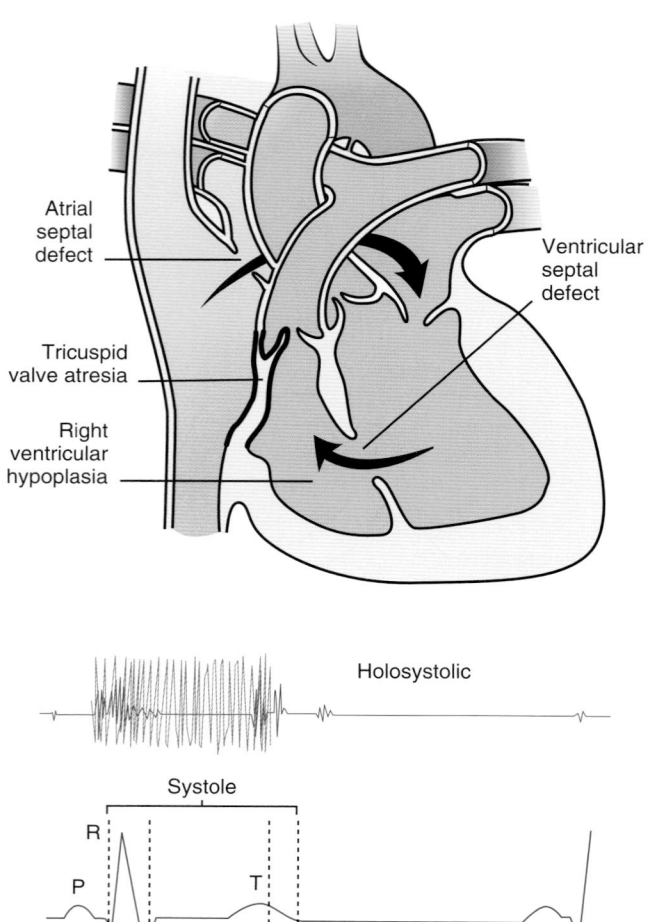

Fig. 9.16 Tricuspid valve atresia. In this condition, the murmur most often detected is a holosystolic murmur of a communicating ventricular septal defect or an ejection systolic murmur related to an obstructing pulmonary outflow.

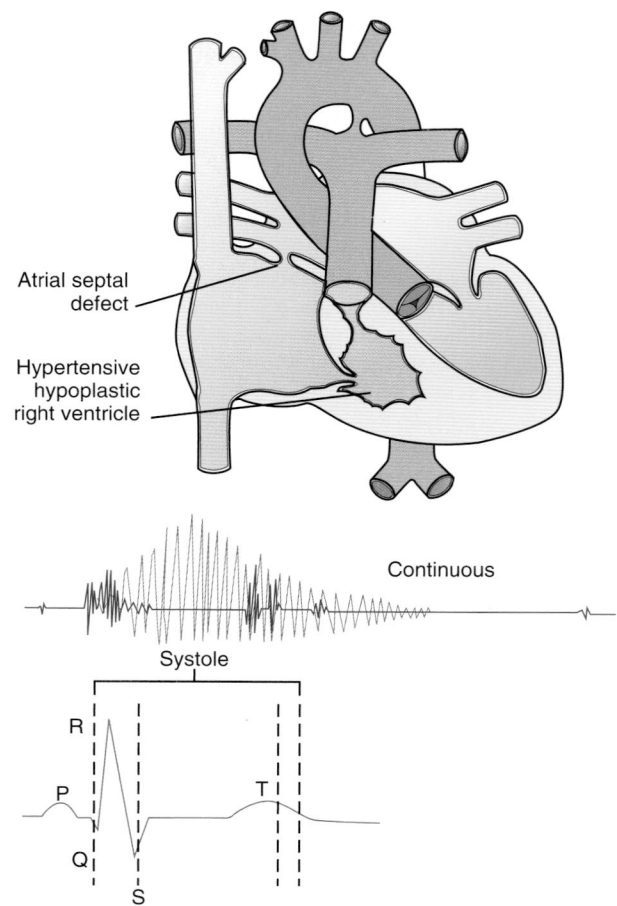

Fig. 9.17 Pulmonary atresia with intact septum. Characteristically, the defect manifests in the cyanotic neonate. Most often, a continuous murmur of a patent ductus arteriosus is audible. Less often, a high-pitched murmur of tricuspid valve insufficiency may be heard.

intact interventricular septum (Fig. 9.17), wherein right-sided heart hypoplasia is usually then present.

The cardiac impulse in a hypoplastic right ventricle with pulmonary atresia may be right ventricular even though the dominant ventricle is the left. In contrast to tricuspid valve atresia, a VSD is not part of this lesion. The source of the pulmonary blood flow in the neonate is a ductus arteriosus with left-to-right shunt. A murmur from this ductus may be audible. There is a single S_2 (aortic closure). On occasion, there is tricuspid valve regurgitation, which may be confused with a VSD murmur. The murmur is high pitched, because the right ventricular pressures are very high. The ECG helps differentiate tricuspid valve and pulmonary atresia. In both disorders, left ventricular hypertrophy is present, but in pulmonary atresia, there is a normal inferior vector. Echocardiography confirms the diagnosis. There is usually profound cyanosis.

Intravenous prostaglandin therapy is required to ensure ductal patency and pulmonary blood flow in the neonatal period. Surgical repair is usually palliative.

TRANSPOSITION OF THE GREAT ARTERIES

In transposition of the great arteries (Fig. 9.18), the aorta arises from the morphologic right ventricle, and the pulmonary artery arises from the morphologic left ventricle. In transposition of the great arteries,

desaturated systemic venous blood returns to the right atrium, passes to the right ventricle, and is returned to the aorta and thus to the systemic circulation. Any oxygenation occurring in this setting is the result of mixing of blood with the pulmonary circulation at the ductal, atrial, or ventricular level.

Transposition of the great arteries with an intact ventricular septum manifests in the neonatal period with profound cyanosis in an infant whose saturations do not improve with oxygen administration the **hyperoxia test**. There is a pronounced right ventricular impulse, and the A_2 is loud because it is anterior. There may be a faint, soft short ejection murmur that is audible along the left sternal border as a result of increased pulmonary blood flow. However, there are often no murmurs. Heart failure is not expected. The P_2 is often not heard.

If there is a VSD, the patient may not present in the neonatal period. The minimal cyanosis may be difficult to detect. Such infants usually become ill at 2–3 weeks of age as a result of congestive heart failure rather than hypoxia. The examination findings are very different, because both ventricles are very hyperdynamic. The heart is large; there is often a palpable thrill and a loud systolic murmur.

Treatment consists of corrective surgical switching of the great vessels.

HYPOPLASTIC LEFT HEART SYNDROME

Hypoplastic left heart syndrome (Fig. 9.19) consists of varying degrees of left-sided heart (mitral valve, left ventricle, aortic valve, or arch)

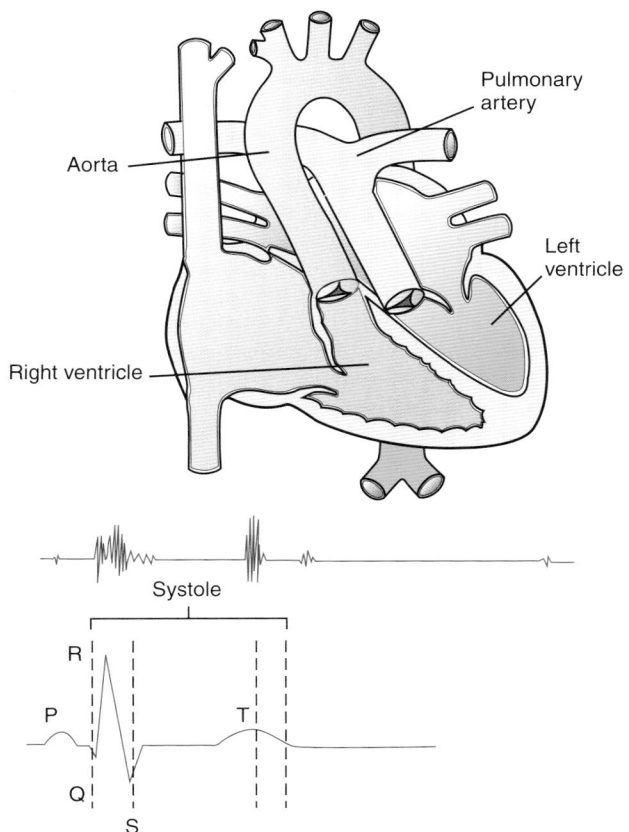

Fig. 9.18 Transposition of the great arteries. The aorta in this condition arises anteriorly, giving rise to a loud, single second heart sound. Many profoundly cyanotic full-term newborns with no audible murmur have transposition of the great arteries.

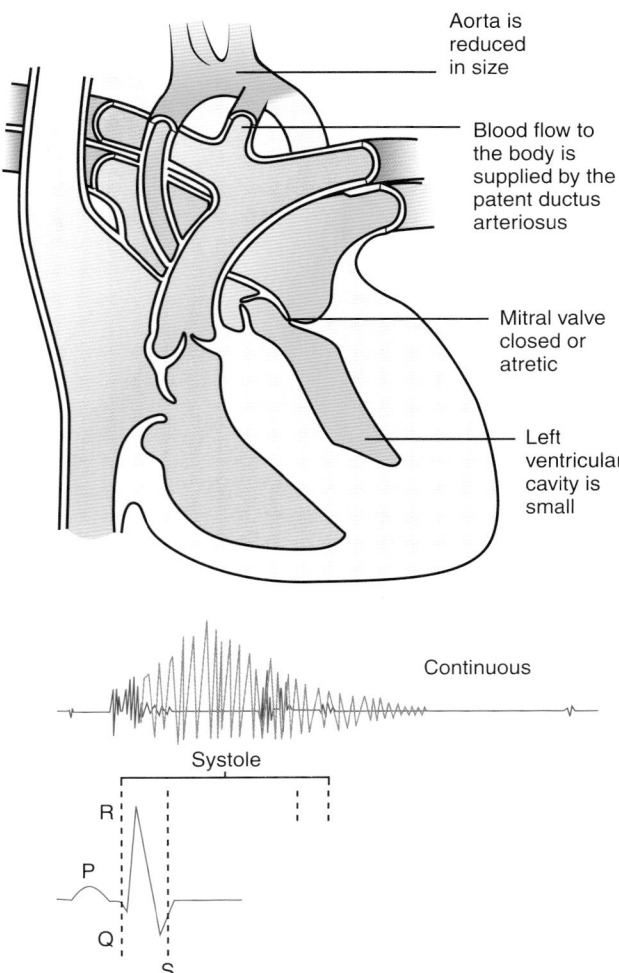

Fig. 9.19 Hypoplastic left heart syndrome. In this condition, the systemic circulation is supplied from the right ventricle via the ductus arteriosus. The continuous murmur of ductal flow that may be heard is generally low pitched as a result of equal pulmonary and aortic pressures.

hypoplasia or atresia such that the left ventricle cannot support the systemic circulation. In the first day or two after birth, the neonate may not be recognized as being ill if the ductus arteriosus remains open and the right ventricular output sustains the systemic output. When the ductus begins to close, perfusion deteriorates, the pulses are diminished, acidosis develops, and death ensues.

The affected infant is often tachypneic, gray, and poorly perfused. There may be considerable pulmonary blood flow and a dynamic right ventricle impulse. An ejection systolic murmur may be audible in the pulmonary area. The heart function may be very poor, and the precordial and auscultatory examination findings may be quiet. A significantly restrictive ASD may cause profound pulmonary venous congestion and poor oxygenation.

After intravenous prostaglandin E_1 has been given, causing opening of the ductus arteriosus, a reasonable systemic output and palpable pulses should return.

Treatment includes the staged Norwood palliative repair to single-ventricle Fontan operation or heart transplantation.

MURMURS CAUSED BY COMMON LESIONS WITH SIMPLE OBSTRUCTION

In areas of obstruction, the gradient or pressure difference across an obstruction relates to the severity of the narrowing, the flow across the narrowing, and the pressure able to be generated (i.e., the cardiac function).

PULMONARY VALVE STENOSIS

The hemodynamic abnormality in pulmonary valve stenosis (Fig. 9.20) is attributable to increased pressure within a right ventricle that is attempting to eject through a narrowed or an obstructed valve. The more severe the stenosis, the higher the intraventricular pressure is until cardiac failure occurs.

This condition is characterized by an ejection systolic murmur, heard best in the pulmonary area. The murmur is diamond-shaped. With increasing valvular obstruction, the murmur becomes louder and higher pitched and peaks later in systole. The P_2 is very helpful because the more severe the pulmonary valve stenosis, the more delayed and less intense the P_2 is.

An ejection click, caused by abrupt arrest of leaflet excursion in early systole, frequently precedes the ejection systolic murmur. The more severe the pulmonary valve stenosis, the earlier and softer the pulmonary ejection click is. In other forms of right ventricular outflow obstruction, such as supravalvular stenosis and subvalvular stenosis, or in the setting of a dysplastic or malformed pulmonary valve, an ejection click is not audible.

In newborns with very severe critical pulmonic stenosis, cyanosis, and low cardiac output, the examination findings may be quite

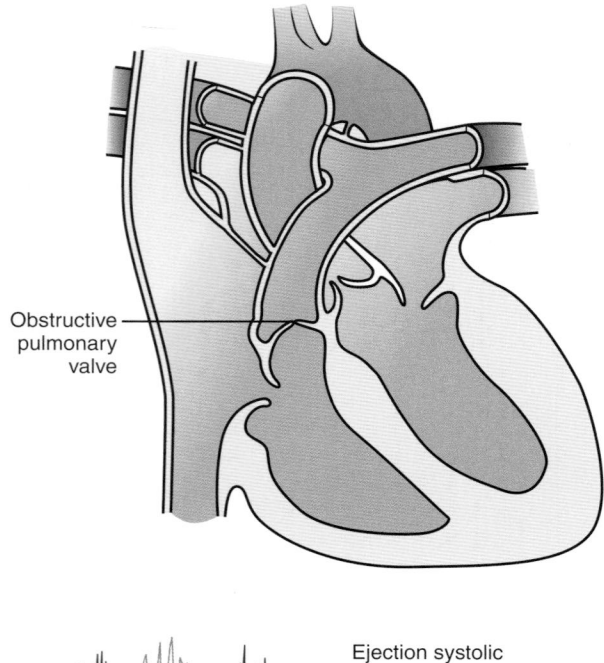

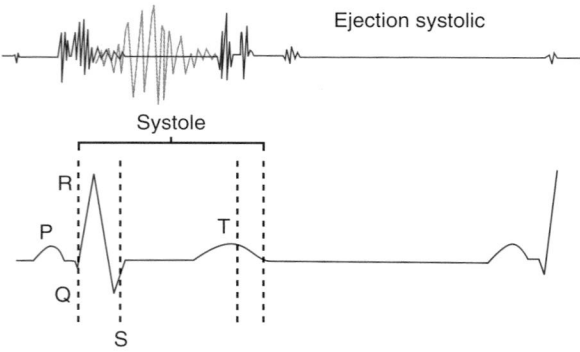

Fig. 9.20 Pulmonary valve stenosis. Pulmonary valve stenosis gives rise to a rough ejection systolic murmur that is most prominent in the pulmonary area and radiates equally to both lung fields. The presence of an ejection click distinguishes valve obstruction from subvalvular or supravalvular stenosis.

different. There may be no pulmonary ejection click, and the murmur may be very short, soft, or both.

Palpation in pulmonic valve stenosis may reveal a palpable thrill in the pulmonary area and an abnormal right ventricular impulse (except in mild cases).

Treatment is transcatheter balloon valve dilatation.

AORTIC VALVE STENOSIS

The hemodynamic impact of aortic valve stenosis (Fig. 9.21) is increased pressure in the left ventricle. The more severe the stenosis, the higher the left ventricular pressure is until heart failure ensues.

The apex beat is of a thrusting character and is not displaced in the absence of left-sided heart failure. Palpation, except in very mild cases, reveals a suprasternal notch thrill and often a carotid systolic thrill. If the murmur is grade IV or greater, a precordial thrill is also palpable at the upper right sternal border (aortic area).

The murmur of aortic stenosis is a rough, harsh, diamond-shaped ejection systolic murmur. It is heard best in the aortic area but often extends into the neck and throughout the precordium.

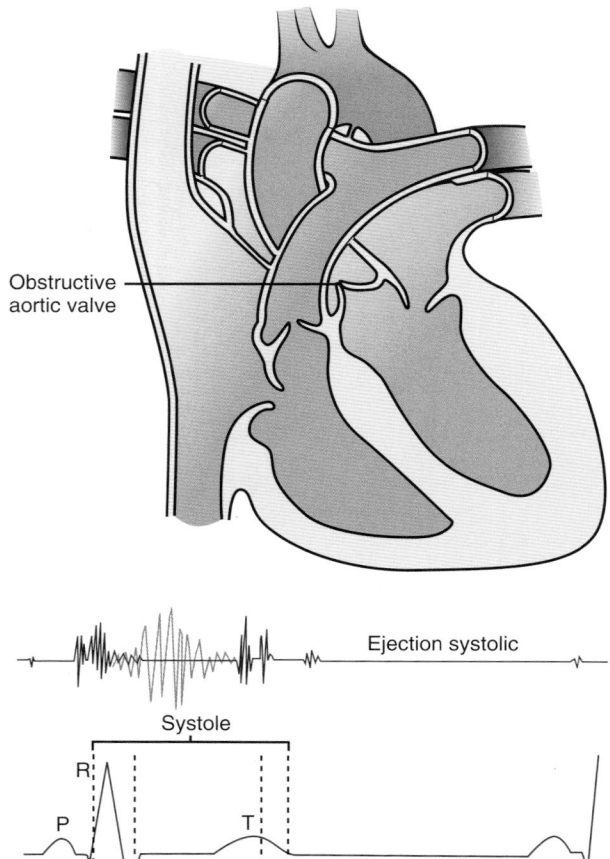

Fig. 9.21 Aortic valve stenosis. The ejection systolic murmur from aortic valve stenosis is audible both at the apex and in the aortic area. The aortic area extends up to the carotid arteries. There is often a palpable thrill in the suprasternal notch. The pitch and peaking of the murmur allow an estimate of the severity of stenosis. Note that a quiet and low-pitched murmur may suggest poor ventricular function and low output.

A soft, short ejection murmur that peaks in systole indicates a mild degree of valve obstruction, whereas a loud, long, and late-peaking murmur, often associated with a palpable thrill, reflects more severe stenosis.

An ejection click often precedes the murmur and is heard best at the apex. The click intensity is inversely proportional to the severity of the valve narrowing. A loud aortic valve **ejection click** is often present in patients with a two-leaflet or bicuspid aortic valve even if there is no valve stenosis.

The splitting of the S_2 is normal. The paradoxical split, occurring when there is a large delay of A_2, is quite rare in children and young adults; it is seen in older people with calcific aortic valve stenosis and a failing left ventricle.

In newborns with severe or critical aortic stenosis and low cardiac output, the examination findings may be very different. There is often no aortic ejection click, and, strikingly, the murmur may be short, soft, or both. Significant heart failure and poor perfusion are present in such neonates.

Two other major types of aortic stenosis exist: subvalvular and supravalvular. Neither has an aortic ejection click. In **supravalvular aortic stenosis** (the major cardiac lesion associated with Williams syndrome), the murmur is usually in the aortic area, whereas in

subvalvular aortic stenosis, the murmur position may extend to the left sternal border or the apex.

The **bicuspid aortic valve** is the most common of all congenital malformations of the heart, found in almost 2% of the general population. The normal aortic valve has three leaflets of equal size. The bicuspid valve has two functional leaflets, one generally larger than the other. The bicuspid aortic valve is often only mildly stenotic or is often unobstructed. The anomaly is recognized from the presence of an aortic ejection click. The ejection click is often mischaracterized as a split S_1, which is a very rare occurrence in children. Asymmetric stresses on the valve leaflets predispose to calcification, dysfunction, and deterioration after many years. The valve is also at risk for the development of infective endocarditis.

Treatment of severe aortic valve stenosis may include surgical or balloon valvotomy and often eventual valve replacement.

COARCTATION OF THE AORTA

Coarctation occurs in association with congenital cardiac anomalies or in isolation. There are fundamentally two forms of coarctation (Fig. 9.22). The more common form has been termed **juxtaductal** or **adult coarctation** and is typically a discrete area of aortic narrowing or indentation of ductal tissue in relationship to the ductus arteriosus or ligamentum. The second type of coarctation has been termed **infantile coarctation** and includes varying degrees of transverse and isthmic aortic arch hypoplasia.

The hemodynamic abnormality caused by a coarctation of the aorta is a high systolic pressure proximal to the area of narrowing, in the ascending aorta, the brachiocephalic vessels, and the left ventricle.

The diagnosis of coarctation of the aorta is made from recognition of systemic hypertension in the right arm and decreased arterial pulsation in the femoral arteries in comparison with that in the brachial arteries. The femoral pulses may be absent, or they may be diminished and delayed. In some cases, the left brachial pulse may be diminished as a result of involvement of the left subclavian artery in the site of narrowing. In rare cases, the right subclavian artery may arise aberrantly below the level of the coarctation, causing the pulse in this arm to be diminished. Therefore, brachial pulses must be felt on both sides and compared with the femoral pulses. The blood pressure must be obtained in both arms as well as in one leg. There is seldom any significant or consistent alteration in the heart sounds unless there is associated aortic valve disease. Up to 40% of patients with juxtaductal coarctation of the aorta have an associated bicuspid aortic valve, usually without stenosis. In these cases, there is an aortic ejection click. More complicated heart lesions, often unrestrictive VSDs or AVSDs, are often seen in association with isthmic arch hypoplasia.

The murmur of coarctation is of the ejection or continuous type, is rarely louder than grade III, starts well after S_1, and may peak late in systole or extend into diastole. The point of maximal cardiac activity is variable and is most often palpable in the fifth or sixth intercostal space, extending out to the axillary line. The murmur of coarctation extends to and is often loudest in the interscapular area posteriorly.

As with aortic stenosis and obstruction of the left heart outflow, the newborn with coarctation may present with signs of low output and heart failure. Prostaglandins have proved useful in this circumstance, alleviating the obstruction by dilating reactive muscle in the aortic wall, which may have extended from the ductus or with opening of the ductus itself, enabling right-to-left ductal flow to the lower body and relieving associated pulmonary hypertension.

Treatment in the neonate is surgical. However, after infancy, aortic coarctation angioplasty with balloon or stent placement may be considered, as may surgery.

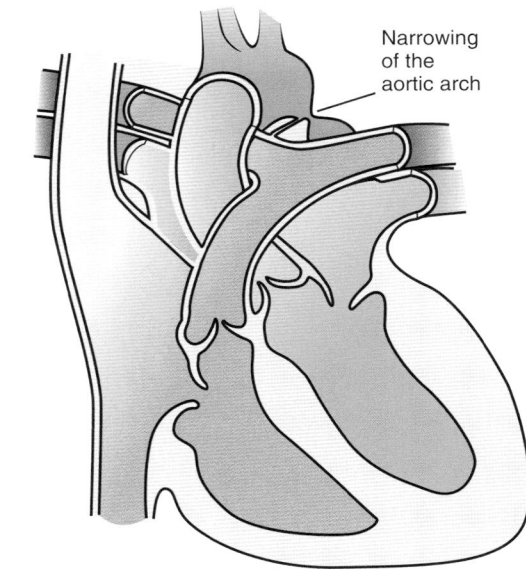

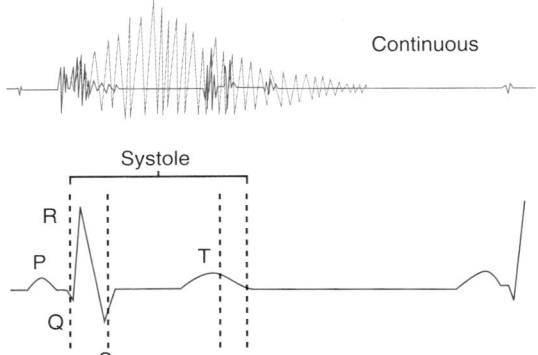

Fig. 9.22 Coarctation of the aorta. The murmur of coarctation is often audible both anteriorly and posteriorly between the scapulae. It is a continuous murmur extending well into diastole.

MITRAL VALVE STENOSIS

Congenital mitral valve stenosis (Fig. 9.23) is uncommon. When it occurs, it is usually in association with additional left-sided heart obstructive abnormalities, particularly coarctation of the aorta, which is termed the **Shone complex**. The most common type of significant mitral stenosis is caused by a **single** or **"parachute" papillary muscle.** In its most severe form, it is part of the hypoplastic left heart syndrome, in which the valve is small, very stenotic, or atretic. In affected patients, cyanosis, heart failure, and poor perfusion are evident within the first few days after birth.

The leaflets in congenital stenosis are very immobile, and there is seldom the accentuation of the S_1 or an opening snap, which is characteristic of acquired or rheumatic mitral valve stenosis.

The murmur of mitral valve stenosis arises from the increased velocity of blood flow across the relatively immobile mitral leaflets during diastolic filling of the left ventricle. This causes a characteristic low-pitched mid-diastolic flow rumble best heard in the mitral area.

Rheumatic mitral valve stenosis is common in many areas of the world but is uncommon in North America. As a consequence of mitral obstruction, the left atrial and pulmonary venous pressures are elevated. Often there is a reflex or secondary elevation of pulmonary

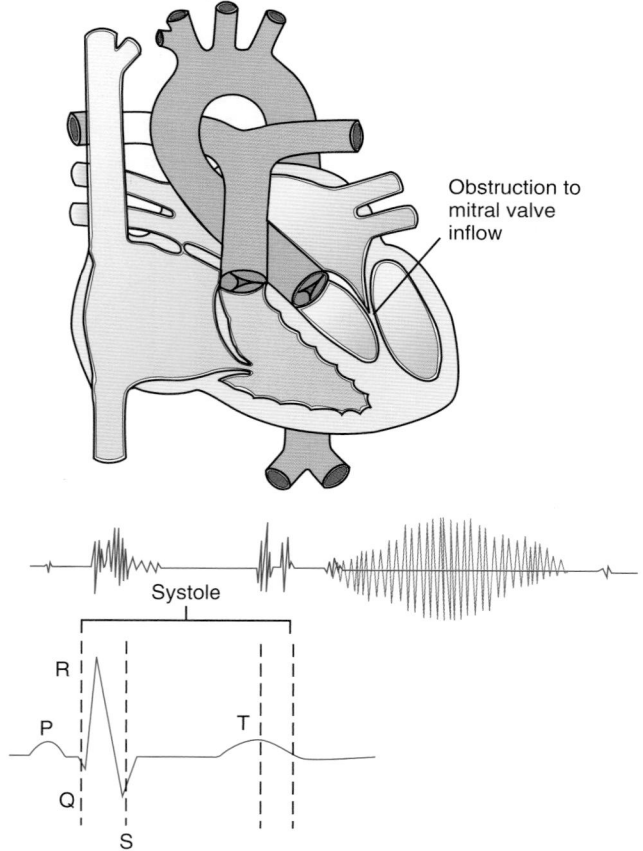

Fig. 9.23 Mitral valve stenosis. The murmur of mitral valve stenosis occurs during the period of passive and active filling of the ventricle as turbulence occurs across the obstructive mitral valve. Pulmonary hypertension often arises as a consequence of the downstream obstruction.

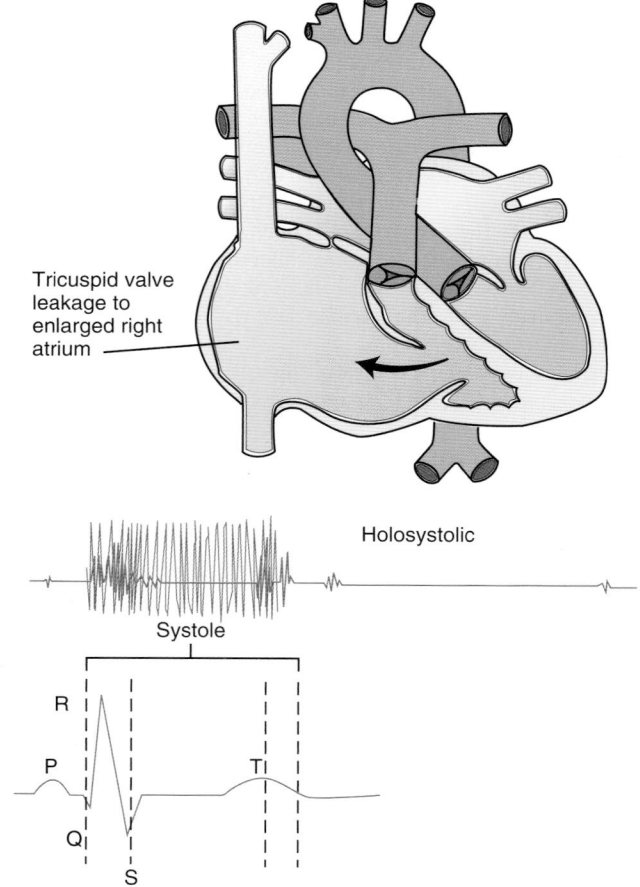

Fig. 9.24 Tricuspid valve insufficiency. The holosystolic murmur of tricuspid valve insufficiency is low pitched in the absence of any pulmonary outflow obstruction, which makes tricuspid valve insufficiency very challenging to hear.

artery pressures caused by constriction and thickening of small muscular pulmonary arteries. The features of pulmonary hypertension, including a prominent right ventricular tap, single loud or palpable S_2, and a high-pitched pulmonary insufficiency, may be apparent.

Excursion of the thickened leaflets often causes an early diastolic high-pitched opening snap before the onset of the murmur. In severe stenosis, strong atrial contraction late in diastole may create a late diastolic crescendo murmur. A loud S_1 is often heard in this condition.

MURMURS CAUSED BY ATRIOVENTRICULAR VALVE AND SEMILUNAR VALVE INSUFFICIENCY

Tricuspid Valve Regurgitation

Tricuspid valve regurgitation (insufficiency) (Fig. 9.24) is uncommon in childhood in the absence of additional abnormalities. It may be a consequence of pulmonary artery hypertension, in which the high-pressure right ventricle contributes to a high-pitched holosystolic murmur at the lower left or lower right sternal border (tricuspid area).

Less often, tricuspid valve insufficiency may occur in association with a displaced and malformed tricuspid valve (**Ebstein anomaly**), in which case the pulmonary arterial and right ventricular pressures are not elevated, and the holosystolic murmur is low pitched. The features of right-sided cardiac murmurs vary much more with the respiratory cycle than do left-sided heart murmurs. There may be signs of right-sided heart failure: an enlarged pulsatile liver and, in the older child, a prominent V wave pulsation in the neck veins.

Mitral Valve Insufficiency

Mitral valve insufficiency (Fig. 9.25) is associated with a diffuse and dynamic apical impulse. If the volume of regurgitant flow is great, a bifid or double apical impulse of a palpable S_3 may be apparent.

The insufficiency jet of blood from the powerful left ventricle to the thin-walled left atrium causes a high-pitched blowing holosystolic murmur that has an abrupt onset. This murmur is heard best with the diaphragm of the stethoscope placed anteriorly in the mitral area. The systolic murmur radiates to the axillae.

The S_1 is usually of normal to increased intensity, but if the valve abnormality is rheumatic in origin, it may be sufficiently deformed that S_1 is quite soft. If the mitral regurgitation is quite significant, an S_3 filling sound is heard, often associated with a mid-diastolic flow rumble of "relative" mitral valve stenosis. Mitral valve insufficiency may be seen as a congenital lesion, in response to dilated annulus secondary to heart failure, during acute rheumatic fever, or as part of the mitral valve prolapse spectrum.

Mitral Valve Prolapse

This common condition of adolescents and young adults manifests as laxity of the mitral valve and results in slippage or displacement of one or both valve leaflets backward into the left atrium during systole (see Fig. 9.25 and Fig. 9.26). Mitral valve prolapse may be isolated or syndromic (Table 9.6). Isolated mitral valve prolapse may be an autosomal

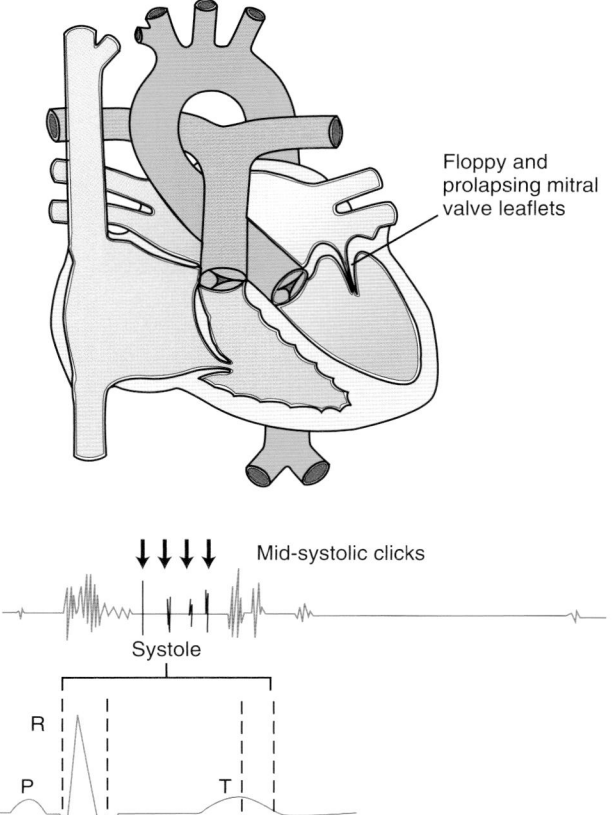

Fig. 9.25 Mitral valve prolapse. The auscultatory examination findings can be very distinctive, with one or more sharp clicks being heard throughout systole. A late systolic high-pitched murmur may arise if mitral valve insufficiency occurs.

dominant disorder with variable penetrance; an X-linked mitral valve prolapse disorder is less common due to pathologic variants in *FLNA*.

The sudden tensing of the mitral valve often causes a *mid-systolic click* or sometimes multiple clicks that can be heard best in the mitral area. The click is frequently followed by a late high-pitched systolic murmur of mitral valve insufficiency. The timing of the click or clicks and the intensity of the murmur often vary with body position. When the patient is sitting up (and even more so during standing), the murmur gets louder or may be heard even when no murmur was heard when the patient was lying down. This is because the left ventricular architecture changes in the upright position. In rare cases, the position change may result in a late systolic murmur becoming full length, although with late accentuation. The ECG often shows unusually anterior and superior T waves with prominent U waves, which suggests papillary muscle dysfunction.

Mitral valve prolapse does not usually progress in childhood, but it may be associated with supraventricular tachycardia, chest pain, and possibly endocarditis or cerebrovascular embolism. Ventricular tachycardia and fibrillation may occur in adults, but sudden cardiac death is very unusual during childhood and adolescence. Thickening of the valve, in addition to prolapse, increases the risk of these complications.

Pulmonary Valve Insufficiency

Pulmonary valve insufficiency (Fig. 9.27) rarely if ever occurs in isolation. Most often, congenital regurgitation of the pulmonic valve occurs in association with a pulmonary outflow obstruction such as in the **absent pulmonary valve syndrome**.

When the pulmonary arterial pressure is low, valve insufficiency is recognized by a very low- to medium-pitched early diastolic murmur that starts with P_2. This is heard best in the pulmonary area and extends for a short distance down the left sternal edge.

The more common types of pulmonary regurgitation are acquired, commonly after surgery for severe pulmonary valve stenosis, as occurs with tetralogy of Fallot, when a pulmonary outflow patch may be placed and the valve leaflets are deficient or absent. Because no P_2 exists, the murmur often appears to start significantly after S_2. Because these patients often have surgically acquired right bundle branch block, the pulmonary valve closure would be well separated from aortic valve closure if the sound could be heard. The diastolic decrescendo murmur begins at that time.

Pulmonary hypertension, particularly when associated with a high pulmonary vascular resistance, is a common cause of secondary pulmonary insufficiency. Often, a pulmonary ejection click may be present because of the dilated pulmonary root. The S_2 is narrowly split or single because the high pulmonary artery diastolic pressure closes the valve early. A diastolic decrescendo murmur then begins with pulmonary valve closure and is high in frequency because the pulmonary artery pressure is high, the so-called **Graham-Steele** murmur.

Aortic Valve Insufficiency

Congenital insufficiency of the aortic valve (Fig. 9.28) is rare and is usually mild and may not be audible. The valve may or may not be bicuspid. There is usually an aortic ejection click that is well separated from S_1, does not vary with respiration, and is usually best heard at the apex. The S_2 split is normal, although the A_2 may be loud and may have a "tambour" quality.

After closure of the aortic valve (A_2), regurgitation of leakage at this site creates the high-pitched, early diastolic decrescendo murmur of aortic insufficiency. This murmur is heard best at the third left or right intercostal space while the patient is sitting. The pulse pressure is normal if the leak is mild.

The most common form of aortic insufficiency is acquired, most often as a consequence of severe **rheumatic carditis**, and can be present in both acute rheumatic fever and chronic rheumatic heart disease. In acute insufficiency, there is usually no aortic ejection click. The left ventricular impulse is abnormal and hyperdynamic, and a wide pulse pressure is present.

A long, low-frequency musical diastolic rumble beginning one third of the time into diastole may occur, especially in the left lateral decubitus position in patients with significant valve insufficiency. This is called the **Austin Flint murmur**. It is believed to be related to regurgitant aortic flow passing across the anterior mitral valve causing fluttering of the leaflet in conjunction with mitral valve inflow.

MISCELLANEOUS CARDIAC ANOMALIES

Pericardial Disease

Many infectious and noninfectious diseases may cause inflammation of the pericardial sac and surrounding structures. The presence of fluid in the pericardial sac may compromise cardiac filling and result in life-threatening impairment of cardiac output, "pericardial tamponade." The auscultatory findings in these cases often include friction rubs.

These variable sounds are high-pitched, superficial, and scratching noises. They occur in synchrony with cardiac movement and can be heard during the early period after myocardial infarction and often frequently are heard after cardiac surgery.

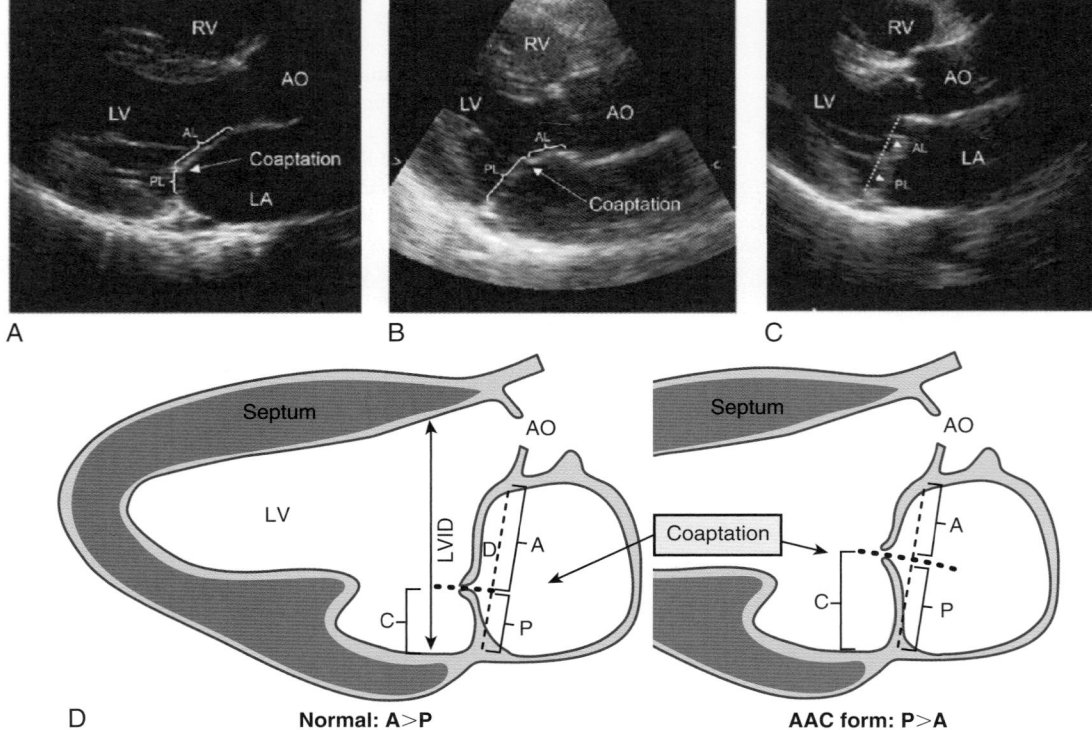

Fig. 9.26 Two-dimensional parasternal long-axis images of posteriorly coapting leaflets (anterior leaflet [AL]; posterior leaflet [PL]) in a normal individual *(A)* vs increased coaptation height and an elongated posterior leaflet in an individual with abnormal anterior coaptation (AAC) features *(B)* and in a patient with bileaflet mitral valve prolapse (MVP) into the left atrium (LA; *C*). Schematics *(D)* showing the projections of anterior (A) and posterior (P) leaflets onto the mitral annular diameter (D). C indicates the coaptation height relative to the annulus and is calculated as P/D or C/LVID, where LVID is left ventricular internal diameter. AO, aorta; LV, left ventricle; RV, right ventricle. (From Delling FN, Vasan RS. Epidemiology and pathophysiology of mitral valve prolapse: new insights into disease progression, genetics, and molecular basis. *Circulation.* 2014;129[21]:2158–2170 [Fig. 4, p. 2165].)

TABLE 9.6	Genetic Anomalies Associated with Mitral Valve Prolapse in Humans	
	Gene or Chromosome	**Defect Localization/Mechanism**
Rare Causal Genetic Defects		
Syndromic MVP		
Trisomies 18, 13, 15	Chr 18, 13, 15	—
Marfan syndrome	*FBN1-TGFβR2-TGFβ2*	ECM/TGFβ pathway
Loeys-Dietz	*TGFβR1-TGFβR2*	TGFβ pathway
Juvenile polyposis syndrome	*SMAD4-BMPR1A*	TGFβ pathway
Aneurysm-osteoarthritis syndrome	*SMAD3*	TGFβ pathway
Ehlers-Danlos syndrome	Collagen types I, III, V, and XI and tenascin	ECM
Osteogenesis imperfecta	Collagen type I	ECM
Williams-Beuren syndrome	Elastin	ECM
Pseudoxanthoma elasticum	*MRP6 (ABCC6)*	ECM
BDCS or FTH syndromes	*SH3PXD2B*	Podosomes/cell migration
Larsen-like syndrome	*B3GAT3*	ECM/glycosaminoglycans
Syndrome with sinus node dysfunction, arrhythmias, LVNC	*HCN4*	Ionic channel/heart development
Nonsyndromic MVP		
Filamin A-MVD	*FLNA*	Mechanotransduction
Myxomatous disease		
MMVP1	Chr 16p	—
MMVP2	*DCHS1*	Cell migration and polarity
MMVP3	Chr 13	—

BDCS, Borrone dermato-cardio-skeletal; Chr, chromosome; ECM, extracellular matrix; FTH, Frank-Ter Haar; GWAS, genome-wide association study; LVNC, left ventricular noncompaction; MVD, mitral valve disease; MVP, mitral valve prolapse; TGF, transforming growth factor.
Modified from Le Tourneau T, Merot J, Rimbert A, et al. Genetics of syndromic and non-syndromic mitral valve prolapse. *Heart.* 2018;104(12):978–984 (Table 1, p. 980).

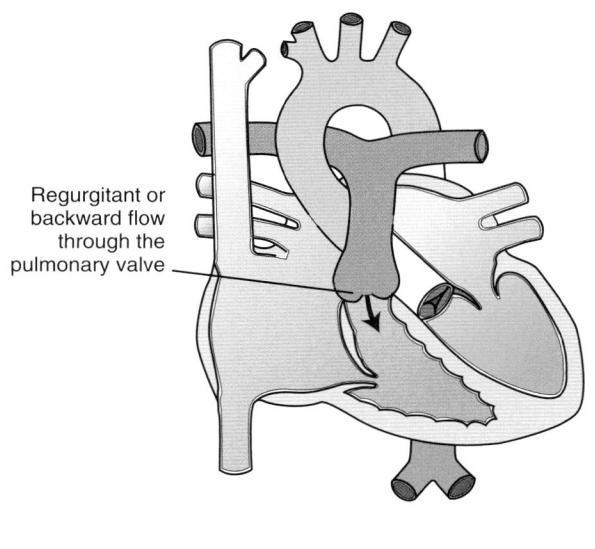

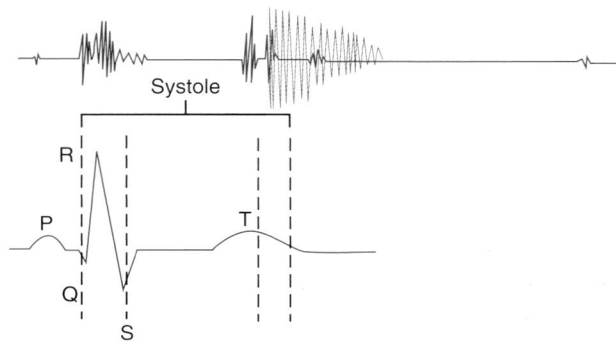

Fig. 9.27 Pulmonary valve insufficiency. A low-pitched early diastolic murmur is heard just after the second heart sound. The murmur characteristically tapers into diastole.

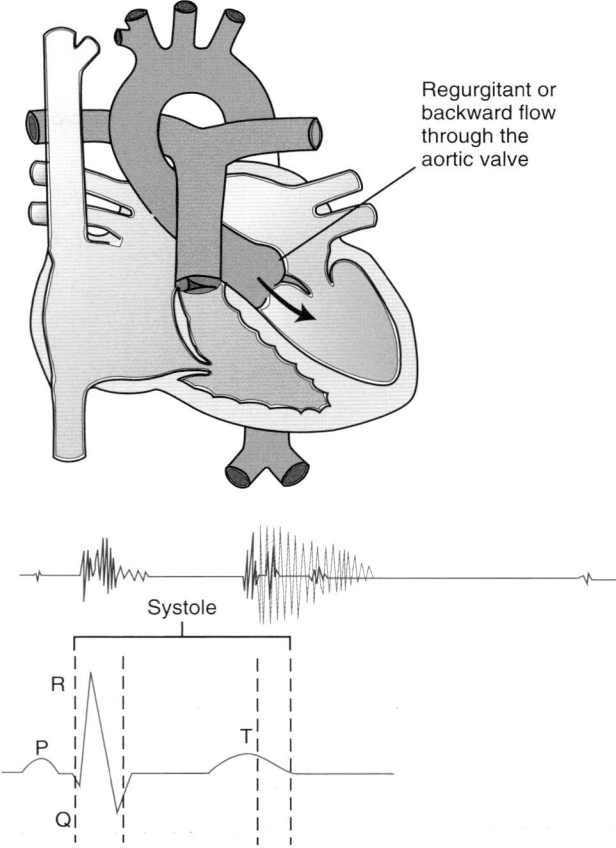

Fig. 9.28 Aortic valve insufficiency. In contrast to the low-pressure murmur of pulmonary valve insufficiency (in the absence of pulmonary hypertension), the murmur of aortic valve insufficiency is high pitched and audible from the aortic area extending to the apex. The peripheral pulses and the intensity and length of the murmur provide clinical quantification of the magnitude of regurgitant flow.

PULMONARY HYPERTENSION

After the neonatal period, pressures in the pulmonary circulation are normally low (approximately 25 mm Hg systolic, or about one fourth of the pressure in the systemic circulation or aorta). Many diseases have profound effects on the pulmonary circulation and can elevate pressures within the pulmonary arteries. These include diseases of the lung parenchyma, pulmonary vasculature, heart, or liver; collagen vascular diseases; and obstruction of the upper airways.

One consistent physical finding detected in pulmonary hypertension is an active right ventricular parasternal tap with a distinctive, sharp, palpable P_2. The P_2 is of increased intensity, and there is a single or narrowly split S_2. There may be no audible murmur; a high-pitched murmur of pulmonary valve insufficiency or a high-pitched systolic murmur of tricuspid valve insufficiency may be present.

Recognition of pulmonary hypertension warrants a diligent search for the underlying cause. If the reason for the elevated pulmonary artery pressure remains unclear, the disorder is referred to as **idiopathic** or **primary pulmonary hypertension**. If an etiology can be found, the disorder is termed **secondary pulmonary hypertension**.

APPROACH TO CONGENITAL HEART DISEASE

Congenital heart disease may produce an asymptomatic murmur, heart failure, cyanosis, cyanosis with heart failure, or severe cardiogenic shock (Fig. 9.29). Malformations associated with profound and fixed cyanosis

without heart failure are usually associated with right-sided obstructive lesions and a right-to-left shunt (e.g., pulmonary atresia, tetralogy of Fallot). Transposition of the great arteries with intact ventricular septum also manifests with profound and fixed hypoxia, with mild tachypnea, and with no heart failure. Malformations associated with cyanosis and heart failure have a large mixing lesion (single ventricle, truncus arteriosus, transposition plus a VSD), in which pulmonary oxygenated venous return mixes with desaturated systemic venous return before ejection to the systemic arterial circulation. In addition, obstructed total anomalous pulmonary veins may produce severe cyanosis, pulmonary venous engorgement, and pulmonary hypertension. Lesions associated with left-sided obstruction (critical aortic stenosis, interrupted aortic arch, hypoplastic left heart syndrome) produce significant cardiogenic shock, poor perfusion, and profound lactic acidosis.

The chest radiograph may provide helpful clues to the cause of the lesion, depending on the paucity (pulmonary atresia) or plethora (obstructed total anomalous pulmonary venous return) of the pulmonary vascular markings; the left- or right-sided (tetralogy of Fallot, truncus arteriosus) position of the aorta; the configuration of the heart (boot-shaped, as in tetralogy of Fallot; egg-shaped, as in transposition of the great arteries; or massive enlargement, as in Ebstein anomaly); or the side of the chest (risk of heart disease is higher with dextrocardia, especially if the stomach bubble is on the left side of the abdomen or if the liver is midline) (Fig. 9.30). The chest radiograph is of some help

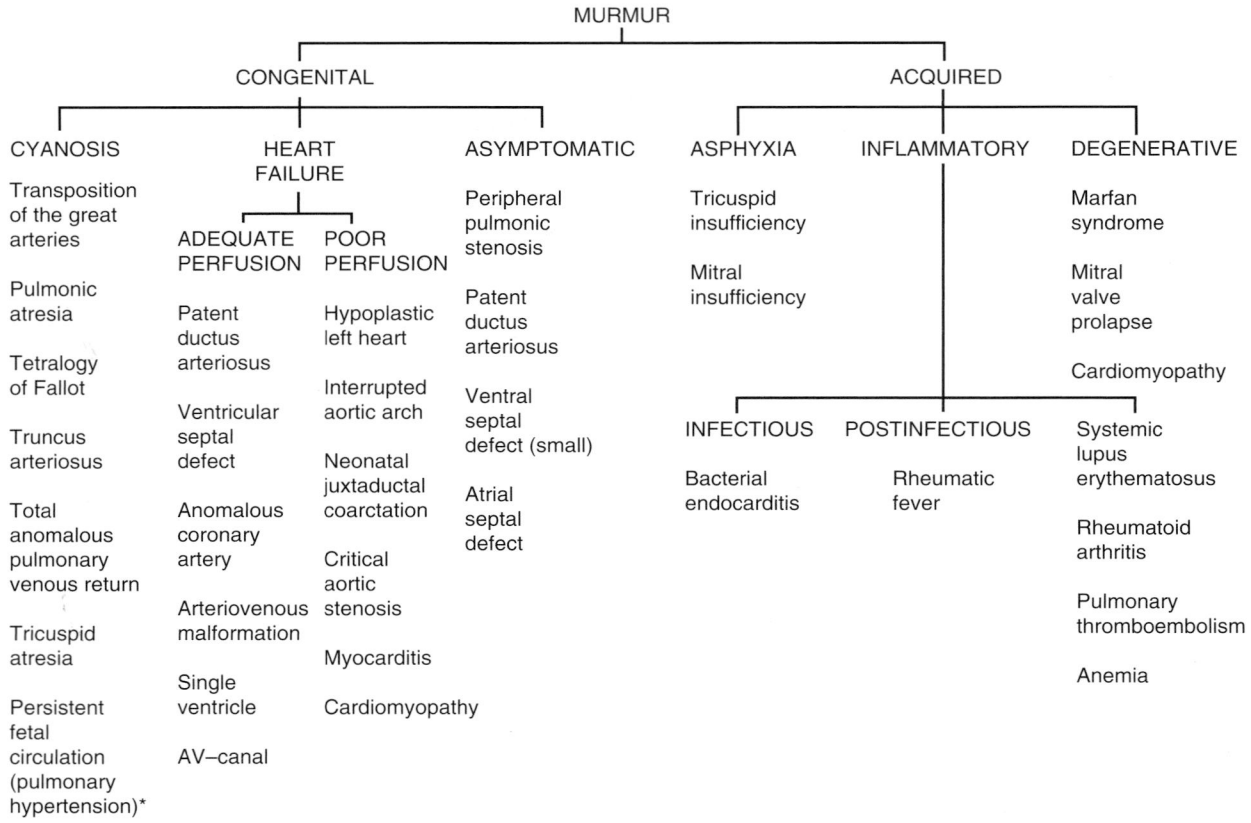

MURMUR

CONGENITAL | ACQUIRED

CYANOSIS

Transposition of the great arteries

Pulmonic atresia

Tetralogy of Fallot

Truncus arteriosus

Total anomalous pulmonary venous return

Tricuspid atresia

Persistent fetal circulation (pulmonary hypertension)*

HEART FAILURE

ADEQUATE PERFUSION

Patent ductus arteriosus

Ventricular septal defect

Anomalous coronary artery

Arteriovenous malformation

Single ventricle

AV–canal

POOR PERFUSION

Hypoplastic left heart

Interrupted aortic arch

Neonatal juxtaductal coarctation

Critical aortic stenosis

Myocarditis

Cardiomyopathy

ASYMPTOMATIC

Peripheral pulmonic stenosis

Patent ductus arteriosus

Ventral septal defect (small)

Atrial septal defect

ASPHYXIA

Tricuspid insufficiency

Mitral insufficiency

INFLAMMATORY

INFECTIOUS

Bacterial endocarditis

POSTINFECTIOUS

Rheumatic fever

DEGENERATIVE

Marfan syndrome

Mitral valve prolapse

Cardiomyopathy

Systemic lupus erythematosus

Rheumatoid arthritis

Pulmonary thromboembolism

Anemia

*Murmur represents tricuspid insufficiency (usually no murmur in persistent fetal circulation).

Fig. 9.29 Algorithmic approach to the child with a heart murmur. AV, atrioventricular.

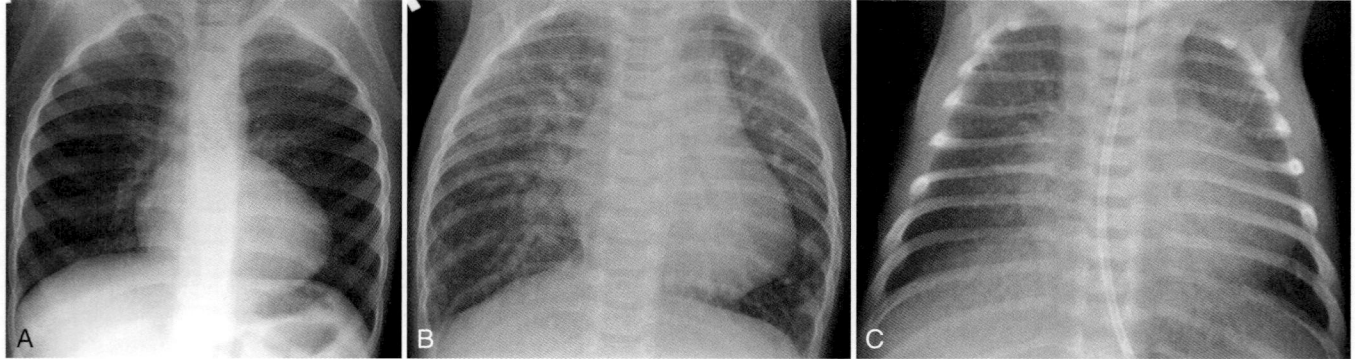

Fig. 9.30 Physiology of congenital heart disease delineated by chest radiography. *A,* Mild cardiomegaly with an upturned cardiac apex, a concave main pulmonary artery segment, and symmetric, severely diminished pulmonary blood flow in a 4-year-old with tetralogy of Fallot/pulmonary atresia. *B,* Moderate cardiomegaly and symmetric, increased pulmonary blood flow in a 3-month-old with a large atrial septal defect and ventricular septal defect. *C,* Moderate cardiomegaly with interstitial edema in an 8-day-old with critical aortic stenosis. (From Frost JL, Krishnamurthy R, Sena L. Cardiac imaging. In: Walters MM, Robertson RL, eds. *Pediatric Radiology: The Requisites.* 4th ed. Philadelphia: Elsevier; 2017:68, Fig. 3.9.)

in distinguishing heart disease from congenital pneumonia, respiratory distress syndrome, pneumothorax, and congenital diaphragmatic hernia.

The ECG in infancy is of help in discriminating atrial and ventricular enlargement or hypertrophy and very helpful when there is an abnormal superior vector (complete atrioventricular canal, tricuspid atresia).

Two-dimensional real-time color Doppler echocardiography is most useful in identifying the anatomy of congenital heart lesions. The echocardiogram enables assessment of the four chambers, the interconnecting valves, the great arteries, the pulmonary venous return, and the anatomic relationships between these structures. Furthermore, color Doppler flow studies can determine the presence, direction, and magnitude of

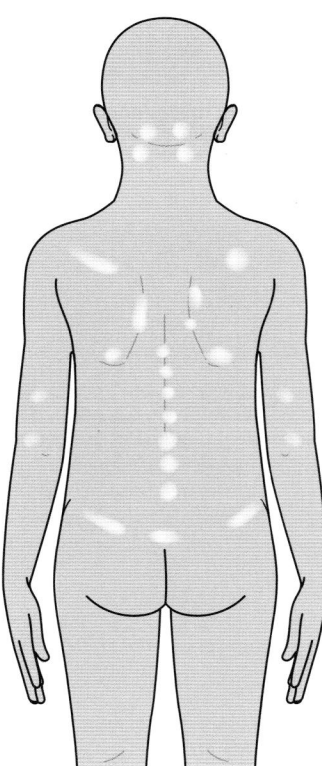

Fig. 9.31 Subcutaneous nodules. (Modified from Shulman ST, Jaggi P. Nonsuppurative poststreptococcal sequelae: rheumatic fever and glomerulonephritis. In: Bennett JE, Dolin R, Blaser MJ, eds. *Mandell, Douglas, and Bennett's Principles and Practices of Infectious Diseases.* 9th ed. Philadelphia: Elsevier; 2020:2466, Fig. 198.3.)

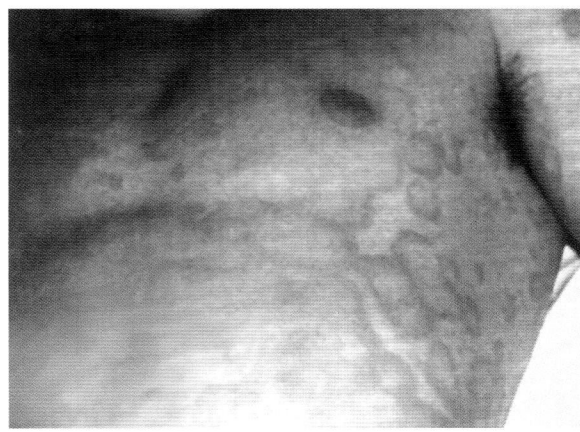

Fig. 9.32 Rash of erythema marginatum in an adolescent boy with acute rheumatic fever showing its characteristic serpiginous and erythematous margins. (From Alsaeid K, Uziel Y, Weiss PF. Reactive arthritis. In: Petty RE, Laxer RM, Lindsley CB, et al., eds. *Textbook of Pediatric Rheumatology.* 8th ed. Philadelphia: Elsevier; 2021, Fig. 46.10.)

right-to-left or left-to-right shunts. Echocardiography has replaced cardiac catheterization for all but the most complex congenital heart lesions.

ACUTE RHEUMATIC FEVER AND RHEUMATIC HEART DISEASE

Rheumatic fever is a postinfectious, immunologically mediated inflammatory disease of the heart, joints, brain, and skin that is caused by group A streptococcus. Migratory polyarthritis is the most common presentation followed by carditis; chorea, subcutaneous nodules (usually with mitral regurgitation) (Fig. 9.31), and erythema marginatum (Fig. 9.32) are much less common. Valvulitis, as manifested by specific and new heart murmurs, is often part of the initial clinical presentation. There are three specific heart murmurs: mitral regurgitation, aortic regurgitation (usually with mitral regurgitation), and the rare Carey-Coombs murmur, a mid-diastolic rumble at the apex. Pericarditis, usually associated with valvulitis, may produce a friction rub. Rheumatic cardiac disease may present with pancarditis (valvulitis, pericarditis, and myocardial involvement). Valvulitis (endocarditis) is the most common cardiac lesion; pericarditis or myocarditis in the absence of valvulitis should suggest another disorder. Recurrent episodes of rheumatic fever create the greatest risk for chronic valve abnormalities.

After the acute rheumatic fever has run its course, any remaining murmurs become part of chronic rheumatic heart disease. If the patient has continued permanent reliable penicillin prophylaxis, the severity of the mitral regurgitation often disappears; this happens less commonly with aortic regurgitation. The development of mitral valve stenosis is

part of the natural history of severe repeated episodes of acute rheumatic fever. Pure aortic stenosis does not develop, although in the presence of long-standing rheumatic heart disease with severe aortic regurgitation, some aortic stenosis may be present. In some very severe cases, tricuspid valve regurgitation has been documented, but it is rare.

The diagnosis of acute rheumatic fever is suggested, although not definitively confirmed, by application of the revised Jones criteria, last edited in 2015 (Table 9.7). In addition, evidence of a group A streptococcal pharyngitis must be present, which may include a positive throat culture, positive streptococcal antigen or antistreptococcal antibody, or history of prior episodes of rheumatic fever. In cases where carditis may be subclinical (no audible murmur), the diagnosis is supported by echocardiographic evidence of subclinical carditis (Table 9.8). The differential diagnosis is limited but in the presence of pericarditis or carditis *and* arthritis may include juvenile idiopathic arthritis and systemic lupus erythematosus (see Chapter 44).

INFECTIVE ENDOCARDITIS

An acute or subacute infection of the cardiac valves produces infective endocarditis. Infection may involve a native, previously normal heart valve; a valve or structure that is altered as the result of congenital heart disease or prior insult; or a prosthetic device (e.g., valve, conduit, patch, graft, shunt, or pacemaker).

Endocarditis may affect congenital heart lesions (most commonly, tetralogy of Fallot, VSD, aortic stenosis, PDA, transposition of the great arteries), valves affected by rheumatic heart disease, and mitral valve prolapse. Endocarditis may develop in congenital heart anomalies in the unoperated and the postoperative states. Furthermore, up to 30% of cases of infective endocarditis occur on previously normal native valves.

Bacterial endocarditis is the result of a bacteremia, which in a normal host is usually transient, asymptomatic, and without sequelae. The presence of a damaged valve, a jet stream–injured endocardium, or a foreign body (e.g., central catheter, graft, shunt, or patch) creates a nidus of infection that permits the bacteria to bind, proliferate, and remain sequestered from normal host defense mechanisms. Transient and predisposing episodes of bacteremia occur during dental procedures that

TABLE 9.7 Guidelines for the Diagnosis of Initial or Recurrent Attack of Rheumatic Fever (Jones Criteria, Updated 2015)

Major Manifestations	Minor Manifestations	Supporting Evidence of Antecedent Group A Streptococcal Infection
Carditis	**Clinical Features**	Positive throat culture or rapid streptococcal antigen test
Polyarthritis	Arthralgia	
Erythema marginatum	Fever	Elevated or increasing streptococcal antibody titer
Subcutaneous nodules		
Chorea	**Laboratory Features**	
	Elevated acute-phase reactants:	
	Erythrocyte sedimentation rate	
	C-reactive protein	
	Prolonged P-R interval	

1. **Initial attack:** two major manifestations, or one major and two minor manifestations, plus evidence of recent GAS infection. **Recurrent attack:** two major, or one major and two minor, or three minor manifestations (the latter only in the moderate/high-risk population), plus evidence of recent GAS infection (see text).
2. **Low-risk population** is defined as ARF incidence <2 per 100,000 school-age children per year, or all-age RHD prevalence of <1 per 1,000 population. **Moderate/high-risk population** is defined as ARF incidence >2 per 100,000 school-age children per year, or all-age RHD prevalence of >1 per 1,000 population.
3. Carditis is now defined as clinical and/or subclinical (echocardiographic valvulitis).
4. Arthritis (major) refers only to polyarthritis in low-risk populations, but also to monoarthritis or polyarthralgia in moderate/high-risk populations.
5. Minor criteria for moderate/high-risk populations only include monoarthralgia (polyarthralgia for low-risk populations), fever of >38°C (>38.5°C in low-risk populations), ESR >30 mm/hr (>60 mm/hr in low-risk populations).

ARF, acute rheumatic fever; GAS, group A streptococci; RHD, rheumatic heart disease.
From Gewitz MH, Baltimore RS, Tani LY, et al. Revision of the Jones criteria for the diagnosis of acute rheumatic fever in the era of Doppler echocardiography: a scientific statement from the American Heart Association. *Circulation*. 2015;131(20):1806–1818.

TABLE 9.8 Echocardiographic Findings in Rheumatic Valvulitis

Pathologic Mitral Regurgitation (All Four Met)	Pathologic Aortic Regurgitation (All Four Met)
1. Seen in at least two views	1. Seen in at least two views
2. Jet length ≥2 cm in at least one view	2. Jet length ≥1 cm in at least one view
3. Peak velocity >3 meters/sec	3. Peak velocity >3 meters/sec
4. Pan-systolic jet in at least one envelope	4. Pan-diastolic jet in at least one envelope

From Shulman ST. Group A streptococcus. In: Kliegman RM, Stanton BF, St. Geme III JW, et al., eds. *Nelson Textbook of Pediatrics*. 20th ed. Philadelphia: Elsevier; 2016.

induce bleeding (even dental cleaning); tonsillectomy or adenoidectomy; intestinal (e.g., endoscopy, gall bladder), urinary (e.g., catheterization, dilatation), prostatic (e.g., cystoscopy), or respiratory surgery; esophageal manipulation (e.g., sclerotherapy, dilatation), incision and drainage of infected tissue; and gynecologic procedures (e.g., vaginal hysterectomy, vaginal delivery).

Bacterial vegetations grow and produce cardiovascular, embolic, or immune complex–mediated signs and symptoms (Table 9.9). Responsible bacteria are noted in Table 9.10; *Staphylococcus aureus*, α-hemolytic oral mucosa–derived streptococci, and enterococci are the dominant pathogens in native normal and unoperated anomalous valves. *Staphylococcus epidermidis* and *S. aureus* are common pathogens in the postoperative patient and in patients with prosthetic devices. Fungal endocarditis is rare and is typically associated with species of *Candida*. Risk factors include indwelling catheters and the use of parenteral nutrition. Risk factors for culture-negative endocarditis and diagnostic strategies are noted in Table 9.11.

The definitive diagnosis of infective endocarditis includes recovery of a microorganism from culture or histologic study of a heart, an embolized vegetation, or an intracardiac abscess (Tables 9.12

and 9.13). Vegetations may be demonstrated by the sensitive technique of transesophageal echocardiography but are usually seen on transthoracic echocardiography in children. In the absence of direct definitive evidence, the following are important diagnostic factors: persistently positive blood cultures with a pathogen compatible with the diagnosis; echocardiographic evidence of an intracardiac mass, vegetations, perivalvular abscess, or new partial dehiscence of a prosthetic valve; and a new valvular murmur (regurgitation or worsening or changing of a pre-existing murmur). Blood cultures are helpful if two or more drawn 12 hours apart are positive or if a majority (e.g., three or four) of separate cultures drawn in 1 hour are positive. More than 85% of first blood cultures are positive; the yield approaches 95% with obtaining a second blood culture. Sufficient blood must be inoculated into the media to detect the low-grade bacteremia of infective endocarditis; excessive blood inoculation may inhibit bacterial growth by continued activity of leukocytes unless the technique involves centrifugation lysis. The cultures should be incubated for more than the routine 72 hours (often 1–2 weeks), and the laboratory should be notified of the possible diagnosis so that laboratory personnel can enrich the media to encourage the growth of fastidious nutrient-dependent organisms.

TABLE 9.9 Frequency of Findings in Pediatric Infective Endocarditis

Symptom	Frequency (%)
Malaise	50–75
Anorexia/weight loss	25–50
Heart failure	25–50
Arthralgia	17–50
Chest pain	0–25
Neurologic symptoms (focal neurologic deficit, aseptic meningitis)	0–25
Gastrointestinal symptoms	0–50

Sign	Frequency (%)
Fever	75–100
Splenomegaly	50–75
Petechiae	21–50
Embolic phenomenon	25–50
New or changed murmur	21–80
Clubbing	0–10
Osler nodes	0–10
Roth spots	0–10
Janeway lesions	0–10
Splinter hemorrhages	0–10
Conjunctival hemorrhages	0–10

Abnormal Laboratory Finding	Frequency (%)
Positive blood culture	75–100
Elevated erythrocyte sedimentation rate	75–100
Anemia	75–90
Presence of rheumatoid factor	25–50
Hematuria	25–50
Low serum complement	5–40

From Levasseur S, Saiman L. Endocarditis and other intravascular infections. In: Long SS, Prober CG, Fischer M, eds. *Principles and Practice of Pediatric Infectious Diseases.* 5th ed. Philadelphia: Elsevier; 2018:264, Table 37.4.

TABLE 9.10 Microbiologic Agents in Pediatric Infective Endocarditis

Common: Native Valve or Other Cardiac Lesions
Viridans group streptococci *(Streptococcus mutans, Streptococcus sanguinis, Streptococcus mitis)*
Staphylococcus aureus
Group D streptococci *(Streptococcus gallolyticus)*
Enterococcus faecalis

Uncommon: Native Valve or Other Cardiac Lesions
Streptococcus pneumoniae
Haemophilus influenzae
Coagulase-negative staphylococci
Abiotrophia defectiva (nutritionally variant streptococcus)
Coxiella burnetii (Q fever)*
Neisseria gonorrhoeae
*Brucella**
*Chlamydia psittaci**
*Chlamydia trachomatis**
*Chlamydia pneumoniae**
*Legionella**
*Bartonella**
*Tropheryma whipplei** (Whipple disease)
HACEK group[†]
*Streptobacillus moniliformis**
Atypical mycobacterium
*Pasteurella multocida**
Campylobacter fetus
Culture negative (6% of cases)

Prosthetic Valve
Staphylococcus epidermidis
S. aureus
Viridans group streptococci
Pseudomonas aeruginosa
Serratia marcescens
Diphtheroids
Legionella species *
HACEK group[†]
Fungi[‡]

*These fastidious bacteria plus some fungi may produce culture-negative endocarditis. Detection may require special media, incubation for more than 7 days, multiplex polymerase chain reaction on blood or valve for 16S rRNA (bacteria) or 18S rRNA (fungi), or serologic tests.
[†]The HACEK group includes *Haemophilus Aggregatibacter* (formerly *Actinobacillus*), *Cardiobacterium, Eikenella,* and *Kingella* species.
[‡]*Candida* species, *Aspergillus* species, *Pseudallescheria boydii, Histoplasma capsulatum.*
From Bernstein D. Infective endocarditis. In: Kliegman RM, Stanton BF, St. Geme III JW, et al., eds. *Nelson Textbook of Pediatrics.* 20th ed. Philadelphia: Elsevier; 2016.

Additional criteria for diagnosing infective endocarditis include fever, predisposing heart lesions and procedures (many patients have undergone no identifiable procedure), vascular phenomena (embolism, Janeway lesions, petechiae, septic pulmonary infarcts, intracranial hemorrhage), immune lesions (glomerulonephritis, Roth spots, Osler nodes) (Fig. 9.33), a suggestive but not definitive echocardiogram, and microbiologic criteria (positive blood culture but not as defined earlier; serologic evidence of active infection).

To prevent infective endocarditis, high-risk patients, procedures, and factors that predispose to bacteremia need to be identified (Table 9.14). Patients needing infective endocarditis prophylaxis include those with intracardiac foreign bodies (prosthetic valve, grafts), prior episodes of infective endocarditis, a heart transplant with abnormal valve function, and certain congenital heart abnormalities including the following: (1) cyanotic congenital heart disease that has not been fully repaired, including children who have had surgical shunts and conduits; (2) a congenital heart defect that has been repaired with prosthetic material or a device for the first 6 months after the repair procedure; and (3) repaired congenital heart disease with residual defects, such as persisting leaks or abnormal flow at or adjacent to a prosthetic patch or prosthetic device.

TABLE 9.11 Causes of Culture-Negative Endocarditis

Organism	Epidemiology and Exposures	Diagnostic Approaches
Aspergillus and other noncandidal fungi	Prosthetic valve	Lysis-centrifugation technique; also culture and histopathologic examination of any emboli
Bartonella spp.	*Bartonella henselae:* exposure to cats or cat fleas *Bartonella quintana:* louse infestation; homelessness, alcohol abuse	Most common cause of culture-negative IE in United States; serologic testing (may cross-react with *Chlamydia* spp.); PCR assay of valve or emboli is best test; lysis-centrifugation technique may be useful
Brucella spp.	Ingestion of unpasteurized milk or dairy products; livestock contact	Blood cultures ultimately become positive in 80% of cases with extended incubation time of 4–6 wk; lysis-centrifugation technique may expedite growth; serologic tests are available
Chlamydia psittaci	Bird exposure	Serologic tests available but exhibit cross-reactivity with *Bartonella*; monoclonal antibody direct stains on tissue may be useful; PCR assay now available
Coxiella burnetii (Q fever)	Global distribution; zoonosis, wide range of mammals	Serologic tests (high titers of antibody to both phase I and phase II antigens); also PCR assay on blood or valve tissue
HACEK spp.	Periodontal disease or preceding dental work	Although traditionally a cause of culture-negative IE, HACEK species are now routinely isolated from most liquid broth continuous monitoring blood culture systems without prolonged incubation times
Legionella spp.	Contaminated water distribution systems; prosthetic valves	Serology available; periodic subcultures onto buffered charcoal yeast extract medium; lysis-centrifugation technique; PCR assay available
Abiotrophia and *Granulicatella* spp.	Slow and indolent course	Supplemented culture media or growth as satellite colonies around *Staphylococcus aureus* streak; antimicrobial susceptibility testing often requires processing specialized microbiology laboratory
Tropheryma whipplei (Whipple disease)	Typical signs and symptoms include diarrhea, weight loss, arthralgias, abdominal pain, lymphadenopathy, central nervous system involvement; IE may be present without systemic symptoms	Histologic examination of valve with periodic acid–Schiff stain; valve cultures may be done using fibroblast cell lines; PCR assay on vegetation material

HACEK, *Haemophilus, Aggregatibacter* (formerly *Actinobacillus*), *Cardiobacterium, Eikenella, Kingella*; IE, infective endocarditis; PCR, polymerase chain reaction.
From Holland TL, Bayer AS, Fowler Jr VG. Endocarditis and intravascular infections. In: Bennett JE, Dolin R, Blaser MJ, eds. *Mandell, Douglas, and Bennett's Principles and Practice of Infectious Diseases.* 9th ed. Philadelphia: Elsevier; 2020:1088, Table 80.6.

TABLE 9.12 Definitions of Major and Minor Criteria Used in the Duke Schema for the Diagnosis of Infective Endocarditis

Major Criteria

1. Positive blood culture for IE
   - Typical microorganism consistent with IE from two separate blood cultures:
     - Viridans streptococci
     - *Streptococcus gallolyticus*
     - HACEK group
     - *Staphylococcus aureus*
     - Community-acquired enterococci (without a primary focus)
   - Microorganism consistent with IE from persistently positive blood cultures if:
     - At least two positive blood cultures sampled more than 12 hr apart
     - All three or a majority of more than four blood cultures
   - Single positive blood culture for *Coxiella burnetii* or IgG antibody titer >1:800
2. Evidence of endocardial involvement by positive echocardiogram for IE, defined as:
   - Oscillating intracardiac mass on valve or supporting structures, in the path of regurgitant jets, or on implanted material
   - Abscess
   - New partial dehiscence of prosthetic valve
   - New valvular regurgitation (worsening or changing of pre-existing murmur not sufficient)

Minor Criteria

1. Predisposing heart condition or intravenous drug abuse
2. Fever: temperature >38°C
3. Vascular phenomena: major arterial emboli, septic pulmonary infarcts, mycotic aneurysm, intracranial hemorrhage, conjunctival hemorrhages, Janeway lesions
4. Immunologic phenomena: glomerulonephritis, Osler nodes, Roth spots, rheumatoid factor
5. Microbiologic evidence: positive blood culture but does not meet major criteria or serologic evidence of active infection with organism consistent with IE

HACEK, *Haemophilus, Aggregatibacter* (formerly *Actinobacillus*), *Cardiobacterium, Eikenella, Kingella*; IE, infective endocarditis; IgG, immunoglobulin G.
Modified from Li JS. Sexton DJ, Mick N, et al. Proposed modifications to the Duke criteria for the diagnosis of infective endocarditis. *Clin Infect Dis.* 2000;30:633–638.
From Levasseue S, Saiman L. Endocarditis and other intravascular infections. In: Long SS, Prober CG, Fischer M, eds. *Principles and Practice of Pediatric Infectious Diseases.* 5th ed. Philadelphia: Elsevier; 2018:266, Box 37.2.

TABLE 9.13 Modified Duke Clinical Criteria for Diagnosis of Infective Endocarditis*

Definite Infective Endocarditis
Pathologic Criteria
- Microorganisms demonstrated by culture or histology in a vegetation, embolized vegetation, or intracardiac abscess
- Pathologic lesions (vegetation or intracardiac abscess) with active endocarditis confirmed by histology

Clinical Criteria
- Two major criteria
- One major and three minor criteria
- Five minor criteria

Possible Infective Endocarditis
- One major criterion and one minor criterion
- Three minor criteria

Rejected
- Firm alternative diagnosis for manifestations of endocarditis
- Resolution of endocarditis manifestations with antibiotic therapy ≤4 days
- No pathologic evidence of infective endocarditis at surgery or autopsy with antibiotic therapy for ≤4 days
- Does not fulfill criteria above

*Any one of the findings listed is taken as evidence.
Modified from Li JS, Sexton DJ, Mick N, et al. Proposed modifications to the Duke criteria for the diagnosis of infective endocarditis. *Clin Infect Dis.* 2000;30:633–638.

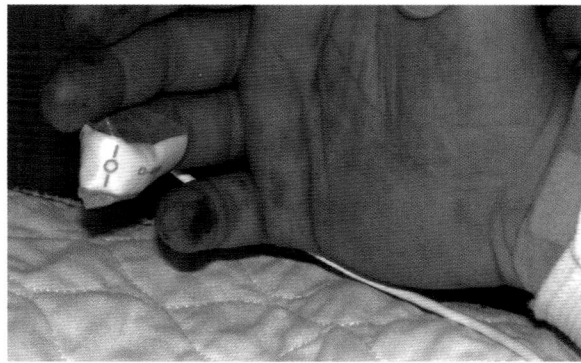

Fig. 9.33 Osler node in infective endocarditis. (From Fowler JR VG, Bayer AS, Baddor LM. Infective endocarditis. In: Goldman L, Schafer AI, eds. *Goldman-Cecil Medicine.* 26th ed. Philadelphia: Elsevier; 2020:420, Fig. 67.2.)

TABLE 9.14 2007 Statement of the American Heart Association (AHA): Cardiac Conditions Associated with the Highest Risk of an Adverse Outcome from Infective Endocarditis for Which Prophylaxis with Dental Procedures Is Reasonable

Prosthetic cardiac valve or prosthetic material used for cardiac valve repair

Previous infective endocarditis

Congenital heart disease (CHD)*

  Unrepaired cyanotic CHD, including palliative shunts and conduits

  Completely repaired CHD with prosthetic material or device, whether placed by surgery or catheter intervention, during the 1–6 mo after the procedure[†]

  Repaired CHD with residual defects at the site or adjacent to the site of a prosthetic patch or prosthetic device (which inhibits endothelialization)

Cardiac transplantation recipients who develop cardiac valvulopathy

*Except for the conditions listed here, antibiotic prophylaxis is no longer recommended by the AHA for any other form of CHD.
[†]Prophylaxis is reasonable because endothelialization of prosthetic material occurs within 6 mo after the procedure.
From Wilson W, Taubert KA, Gewitz M, et al. Prevention of infective endocarditis. Guidelines from the American Heart Association. *Circulation.* 2007;116:1736–1754.

SUMMARY AND RED FLAGS

Murmurs (audible blood flow turbulence) may be caused by cardiac or noncardiac lesions and may be congenital or acquired. Murmurs in the asymptomatic neonate are often transient, as a result of the changing hemodynamics of the transitional circulation between fetal and neonatal life. Most murmurs at all ages are not caused by cardiac disease and are not associated with symptoms or increased risk for disease.

Red flags in the neonatal period include cyanosis or heart failure with or without the presence of other congenital anomalies or syndromes such as trisomy 21. Such syndromes often manifest with multiple congenital anomalies, including those involving the cardiovascular, gastrointestinal, and central nervous systems. In the neonatal period, things not to miss include ductus-dependent lesions, in which systemic blood flow (as in interrupted aortic arch, hypoplastic left heart syndrome) or pulmonary blood flow (as in pulmonary atresia) is through the PDA. Sudden deterioration, cyanosis, or heart failure with increasing metabolic acidosis and a reduction in the murmur suggests closure of the ductus arteriosus. Another condition not to miss is the murmur associated with an arteriovenous malformation, such as the cerebral vein of Galen malformation, which manifests with heart failure and a cranial bruit. Finally, obstructed total anomalous venous return may be confused with persistent fetal circulation or pulmonary infections, and it may be difficult to establish the diagnosis. Total anomalous venous return is associated with fixed, profound cyanosis (Pao_2 <35 mm Hg), severe pulmonary venous congestion, and a small heart radiographically.

Acquired murmurs or symptomatic murmurs that change in quality should suggest acute or recurrent rheumatic fever or infective endocarditis. Systemic symptoms and peripheral signs associated with these disorders are suggestive of the diagnosis. Arthritis (associated with rheumatic fever or endocarditis-induced immune complexes), fever, anemia, leukocytosis, cutaneous manifestations (erythema marginatum and subcutaneous nodules in rheumatic fever; Osler nodes, Janeway lesions, petechiae, and splinter hemorrhages in infective endocarditis), and evidence of prior infection (streptococcal antibodies) or current infection (positive blood cultures or PCR) help identify the nature of the acquired heart disease. Finally, heart murmurs in a normal heart may be caused by hemodynamic factors, such as severe anemia or thyrotoxicosis.

BIBLIOGRAPHY

A bibliography is available at ExpertConsult.com.

10

Shock

Shannon H. Baumer-Mouradian and Amy L. Drendel

WHAT IS SHOCK: PATHOPHYSIOLOGY

Shock is a condition in which inadequate tissue perfusion results in an insufficient delivery of oxygen to meet the body's metabolic needs. Tissue perfusion is dependent on cardiac output. Cardiac output (CO) is determined by the heart rate (HR) and the stroke volume (SV): $CO = HR \times SV$. If either the *heart rate* or the *stroke volume* does not allow for proper tissue perfusion, the patient has shock. Patients are considered in compensated shock if their blood pressure remains in the normal range despite other abnormal vital signs or abnormal tissue perfusion. A child with decompensated shock (abnormal blood pressure) is at high risk for associated morbidity and mortality.

Heart Rate: An increased heart rate is the primary compensatory mechanism that enables children to maintain adequate blood pressure, cardiac output, and tissue perfusion. It is dependent on an intact cardiac conduction system and a responsive autonomic nervous system. There are several conditions whereby heart rate is inadequate, resulting in reduced cardiac output. Newborns and infants have a higher resting heart rate, so their ability to further increase their heart rate to improve cardiac output may be limited. While an adolescent can double their heart rate from 70 to 140, an infant cannot double their heart rate from 150 to 300. A child with an arrythmia will have an ineffectual heart rate that may result in shock. Both atrial and ventricular arrhythmias can cause shock. In children arrhythmias are due to either structural abnormalities or drug intoxication. A child with abnormal sympathetic venous tone that is associated with neurogenic shock will also have an inappropriately low heart rate that results in shock. *A heart rate out of proportion to the degree of fever should suggest septic shock or an arrythmia.*

Stroke Volume: Stroke volume is determined by three elements: preload, cardiac contractility, and afterload. Inadequate stroke volume will result in reduced cardiac output and shock.

Preload is based on the filling volume of the ventricle at the end of diastole. Inadequate preload is most often due to hypovolemia or insufficient circulating volume. *Hypovolemic shock is the most common cause of shock in children.* Hypovolemia may be due to excessive intravascular losses caused by blood loss associated with trauma, or it may be due to excessive fluid losses caused by vomiting and diarrhea or excessive urinary losses associated with diabetes. Young children are at increased risk of having profound volume depletion despite shorter duration of illness. If the circulating volume is not adequate to perfuse the tissues, the patient will show signs of shock.

Cardiac contractility is the inotropic force generated by the ventricles to pump blood. Newborns and infants are known to have stiffer, less compliant myocardium, which limits contractility in this age group. However, compared to adults, inadequate contractility due to an injury to the heart muscle caused by infectious, inflammatory, or familial causes is rare in children. **Cardiac tamponade**, when pressure due to blood or retained fluid within the pericardial sack limits cardiac contractility, may result in **obstructive shock**. Toxins associated with ingestions may inhibit the heart's contractility and lead to shock. Children with septic shock may also have release of toxins that can affect the heart's contractility, resulting in shock. Children with congenital heart disease, particularly left-sided obstructive lesions, may have lesions that result in a pump that does not work properly.

Afterload is the systemic vascular resistance or pressure within the blood vessels that the ventricle must contract against to eject blood to perfuse the body. Sympathetic activation and increased systemic vasoconstriction are compensatory mechanisms for children. This preserves central perfusion by redistributing blood flow to the critical organs. When systemic vascular resistance is low, the patient may be in shock, with increased cardiac output. However, this results in abnormal blood flow and inadequate tissue prefusion that results in signs and symptoms of shock. Loss of vascular resistance is noted in sepsis with the release of toxic chemicals that vasodilate, IgE-medicated release of histamine during anaphylaxis, and a loss of sympathetic venous tone associated with injury to the spinal cord.

Oxygen Delivery: The pediatric patient may also be in shock due to inadequate delivery of oxygen to meet the body's metabolic needs if the oxygen-carrying capacity is limited. Conditions such as severe anemia whereby there is inadequate hemoglobin to deliver oxygen to the tissues or carbon monoxide poisoning and methemoglobinemia in which oxygen cannot be delivered to the tissues can also result in shock.

KEY HISTORICAL ELEMENTS TO AID IN DIAGNOSIS AND ETIOLOGY OF SHOCK

Initial historical elements should focus on evidence of decreased end-organ perfusion. The family should be asked if the child has had a change in behavior or activity. Altered mental status may suggest poor brain perfusion. Hypotonia or weakness may suggest decreased perfusion of the muscles. Reduced urine output is associated with poor perfusion of the kidneys.

Historical elements that are specific to the possible etiology of the shock should also be investigated. A history that quickly evaluates the most common causes of pediatric shock may lead the clinician to the most likely etiology (Figs. 10.1 and 10.2). Query about any recent high or low temperatures or illnesses, particularly if the child is very young or immunocompromised, because this may be associated with untreated or fulminant infection that could lead to septic shock. Ask whether the oral intake of the child has decreased and/or whether the urine and stool output has increased, which may result in hypovolemic shock. Poor oral intake also may be a nonspecific sign of illness in general. Any traumatic mechanism may suggest an injury-related shock. However, for pediatric patients, nonaccidental

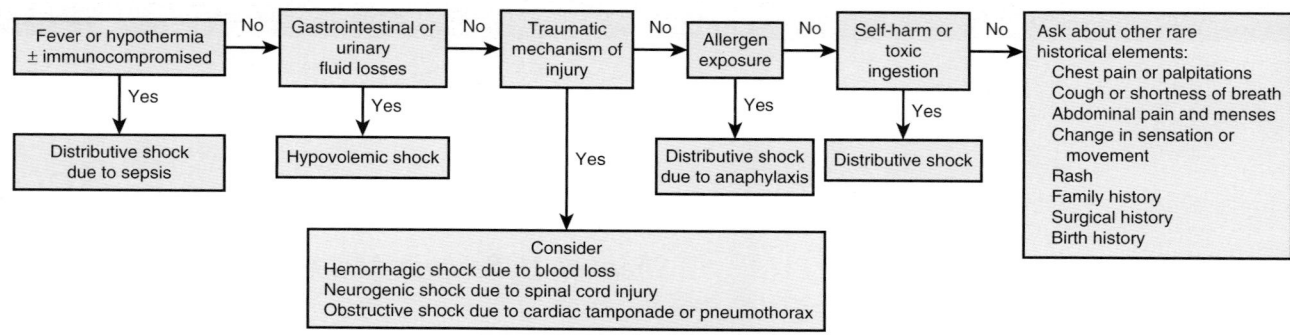

Fig. 10.1 Algorithm for historical elements to determine shock etiology.

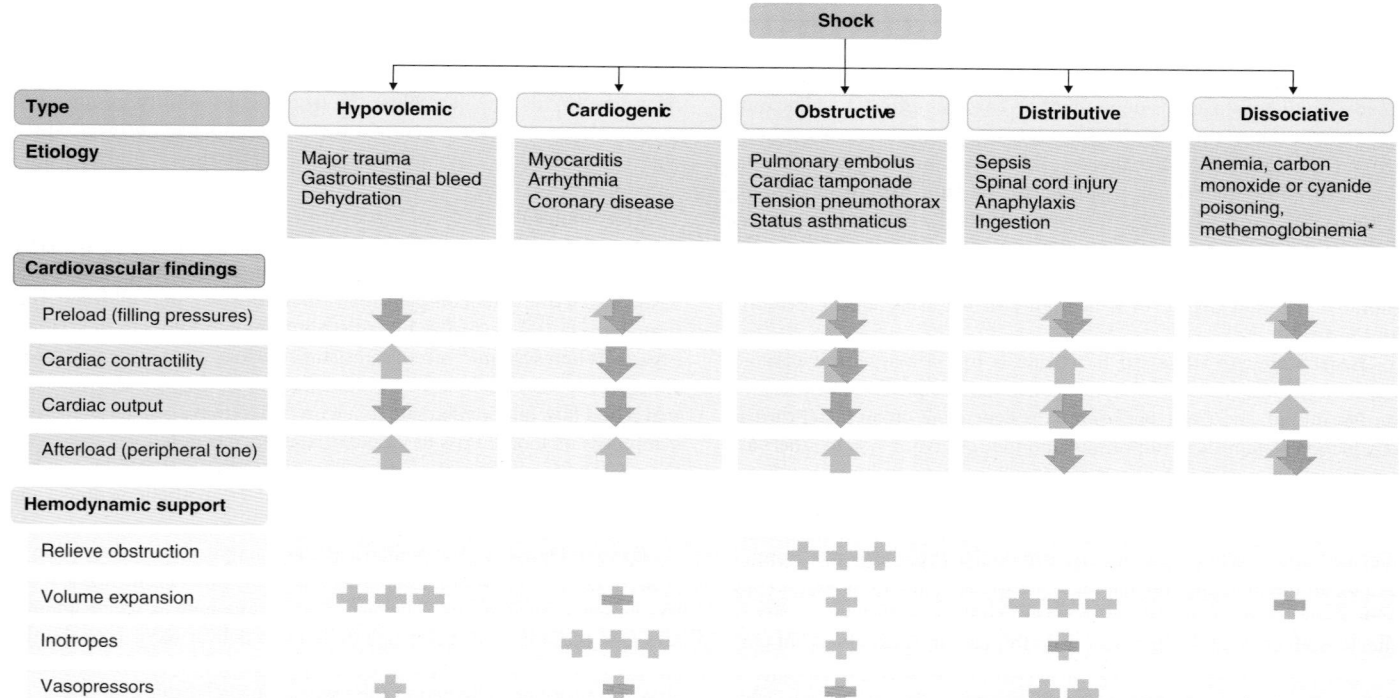

Fig. 10.2 The causes, cardiovascular findings, and hemodynamic support for different types of shock. Under cardiovascular findings, *bidirectional arrows* indicate variation in findings among patients with the particular type. Under hemodynamic support, the number of + *signs* indicates the importance of therapy. A combined + *and* − indicates that the intervention could help some patients but must be used with caution. *Treat specific etiology transfusion or specific antidotes. (Modified from Goldman L, Schafer AI, eds. *Goldman-Cecil Medicine.* 26th ed. Philadelphia: Elsevier; 2020:642, Fig. 98-1.)

trauma must also be considered, and historians may not be forthcoming with accurate details about the mechanism of injury. Allergen exposure with stridor or wheezing may be related to distributive shock due to anaphylaxis. Toxic ingestion may result in distributive shock. Chest pain and palpitations may be associated with arrhythmias or other intrathorax-related etiology. Cough or shortness of breath may suggest pneumonia as a source of septic shock. Abdominal pain should be evaluated in patients with shock related to trauma or infection. Last menstrual period should be obtained to evaluate for pregnancy-related concerns or retained tampon placing the child at risk of toxic shock. Any weakness, numbness, or difficulties with movement should lead the provider to consider neurogenic causes of shock. Rash suggests allergic, immunologic, and infectious etiologies. Suicidal ideation or self-injury suggests a toxic ingestion.

Other important elements to inquire about include a family history evaluating for familial cardiomyopathies or metabolic conditions that may be associated with shock. Surgical history should be queried to evaluate for underlying disorders or recent procedures that may put the patient at risk for infection or blood loss. Birth history may identify congenital malformations that may be associated with shock.

PHYSICAL EXAMINATION TO ASSESS AND MANAGE SHOCK

The initial assessment of a child who may have shock should be focused on "airway, breathing, and circulation," also referred to as the ABCs, to determine if emergent resuscitation is needed. "DE" is included for "disability and exposure" to guide the initial assessment of the patient who may have shock. Shock is a medical emergency that requires timely interventions to improve the patient's conditions as well as aid in coming to a proper diagnosis.

Airway should be assessed to determine if the child is able to protect their airway because inadequate perfusion of the brain may diminish this ability. Asking the child their name is an excellent assessment of their ability to protect their airway and is also the first step in evaluating their mental status. For an infant or nonverbal child, crying or verbalizing may be the best sign of an intact airway.

Breathing assessment should include a determination of whether tachypnea is present to alert the provider to a compensatory response to metabolic acidosis that occurs with shock. Evaluation of breath sounds may tip the provider off to a pneumonia that could be the source of septic shock. Asymmetric breath sounds may be associated with a pleural effusion or a pneumothorax that can cause obstructive shock or with a hemothorax associated with hypovolemic shock. Wheezing may be a sign of anaphylactic shock.

Circulatory assessment is critical to the evaluation of a patient with concerns for shock. The circulatory exam includes auscultation of the chest to determine heart rate and rhythm, palpation of central and peripheral pulses, and assessment of distal cutaneous capillary refill time. Pulses can be assessed *centrally* at the femoral or brachial sites. *Peripheral* pulses can be palpated at the radial or dorsalis pedis sites. Tachycardia is an expected compensatory response. Heart tones should be evaluated for evidence of murmur or muffled heart sounds that are associated with pericardial tamponade. For infants during the first 2 weeks of life, the lack of a murmur that was previously noted can suggest closure of a patent ductus arteriosus that can result in shock for patients with congenital heart disease. Careful evaluation of heart rhythm is important since arrhythmias may be a source of shock. Vasoconstriction results in decreased capillary refill time, reduced pulses, and cool and mottled distal extremities. Sometimes vasodilation may result in *flash capillary refill time*, bounding pulses, and flushed hyperemic skin. These seemingly contradictory findings, both associated with shock, highlight the diagnostic challenge that providers are faced with when evaluating children who may have shock.

Disability assessment provides insights into the mental state of the child. Inability to respond in an age-appropriate manner is a sign of inadequate perfusion of the brain. Typically, infants and children under 2 years do not cooperate with a thorough examination; therefore complete cooperation or sleeping during an exam should be concerning for possible altered mental status. Agitation can also be a sign of decreased brain perfusion; observing the child's interaction with family can aid in determining whether it is fear of the medical examination or a sign of shock.

Exposure identifies any source of active bleeding that could be the source of shock. With full exposure of the patient, the provider will be able to perform a thorough head-to-toe examination. Care must be taken to ensure that the child does not remain completely exposed for long periods of time because children are at an increased risk of hypothermia, particularly in shock states.

Vital signs are particularly critical to assess and monitor in a child with concerns for shock. Elevated heart rate is a common compensatory response in the early phase of shock. Compensatory tachypnea (to metabolic acidosis) can also be noted. Hypotension is a late finding for patients with shock. Healthy children can lose over 30% of their circulating blood volume before the development of hypotension. An oxygen saturation that is abnormal could be a sign of pulmonary pathology associated with shock. Abnormal or difficult-to-obtain

TABLE 10.1 Normal Vital Signs by Age of the Patient

Age	Heart Rate (beats/min)	Blood Pressure (mm Hg)	Respiratory Rate (breaths/min)
Premature	110–170	SBP 55–75, DBP 35–45	40–70
0–3 mo	110–160	SBP 65–85, DBP 45–55	35–55
3–6 mo	110–160	SBP 70–90, DBP 50–65	30–45
6–12 mo	90–160	SBP 80–100, DBP 55–65	22–38
1–3 yr	80–150	SBP 90–105, DBP 55–70	22–30
3–6 yr	70–120	SBP 95–110, DBP 60–75	20–24
6–12 yr	60–110	SBP 100–120, DBP 60–75	16–22
>12 yr	60–100	SBP 110–135, DBP 65–85	12–20

DBP, diastolic blood pressure; SBP, systolic blood pressure.
Adapted from Goldstein B, Giroir B, Randolph A. International Pediatric Sepsis Consensus Conference: definitions for sepsis and organ dysfunction in pediatrics. *Pediatr Crit Care Med.* 2005;6(1):2–8.

oxygen saturation may be due to poor perfusion of the extremity where the probe is placed. For the pediatric patient, normal vital signs change with age, so utilization of an age-appropriate table can help the provider to better identify abnormal vital signs (Table 10.1). For children over 1 year of age, a simple calculation can be relied on by providers to determine the minimum systolic blood pressure: age × 2 + 70. Providers should be vigilant to abnormal vital signs and continuously monitor patients at risk for shock.

In addition to the initial assessment of the ABCs, a head-to-toe physical examination is essential, and an orderly top-to-bottom approach can ensure that nothing on examination is missed (Table 10.2 and Fig. 10.3). Pupillary examination requires the patient to open their eyes, providing insight into their mental alertness. Mucous membrane assessment may show pallor that is associated with blood loss. Dry mucous membranes are associated with hypovolemic shock. A gag reflex will also cue the provider to the patient's level of alertness. Reduced neck mobility can be seen with meningitis and septic shock. Jugular venous distension is associated with cardiac tamponade and pneumothorax, and it may also be seen in cardiogenic shock due to the heart's poor contractility. The abdominal examination should evaluate for bowel sounds and any signs of tenderness or distension. Abdominal pain may be an indication of an intraabdominal infection causing septic shock or intraabdominal bleeding in trauma patients that can result in hypovolemic shock. Careful evaluation for hepatomegaly that is associated with heart failure may be the key to identification of cardiogenic shock. Pelvic stability should be assessed in the trauma patient since pelvic blood loss can be very difficult to identify but can be associated with severe morbidity and mortality. The skin of the extremities should be assessed for evidence of rash that may be associated with infection (purpura) or anaphylaxis (urticaria). Skin tenting can be found with severe hypovolemia and shock. Frequent reassessment of the distal skin perfusion initially evaluated during the circulatory assessment is important during ongoing resuscitation. A femur fracture can result in significant blood loss and shock and thus should be evaluated for in a trauma patient. Neurologic assessment including movement of the extremities on command is a good assessment of mental status. Lack of extremity movement should cue the provider to consider neurogenic shock associated with a spinal cord injury. If there is no movement of the lower extremities and a rectal

TABLE 10.2	**Physical Examination and Selected Laboratory Signs in Shock**
Central nervous system	Acute delirium, restlessness, disorientation, confusion, and coma, which may be secondary to decreased cerebral perfusion pressure (mean arterial pressure minus intracranial pressure). Patients with chronic hypertension or increased intracranial pressure may be symptomatic at normal blood pressures. Cheyne-Stokes respirations may be seen with severe decompensated heart failure. Blindness can be a presenting complaint or complication.
Temperature	Hyperthermia results in excess tissue respiration and greater systemic oxygen delivery requirements. Hypothermia can occur when decreased systemic oxygen delivery or impaired cellular respiration decreases heat generation.
Skin	Cool distal extremities (combined low serum bicarbonate and high arterial lactate levels) aid in identifying patients with hypoperfusion. Pallor, cyanosis, sweating, and decreased capillary refill and pale, dusky, clammy, or mottled extremities indicate systemic hypoperfusion. Dry mucous membranes and decreased skin turgor indicate low vascular volume. Low toe temperature correlates with the severity of shock.
General cardiovascular	Neck vein distention (e.g., heart failure, pulmonary embolus, pericardial tamponade) or flattening (e.g., hypovolemia), tachycardia, and arrhythmias. Decreased coronary perfusion pressures can lead to ischemia, decreased ventricular compliance, and increased left ventricular diastolic pressure. A "mill wheel" heart murmur may be heard with an air embolus.
Heart rate	Usually elevated. However, paradoxical bradycardia can be seen in patients with pre-existing cardiac disease and severe hemorrhage. Heart rate variability is associated with poor outcomes.
Systolic blood pressure	May actually increase slightly when cardiac contractility increases in early shock and then fall as shock advances.
Diastolic blood pressure	Correlates with arteriolar vasoconstriction and may rise early in shock and then fall when cardiovascular compensation fails.
Pulse pressure	Defined as systolic minus diastolic pressure and related to stroke volume and the rigidity of the aorta. Increases early in shock and decreases before systolic pressure decreases.
Pulsus paradoxus	An exaggerated change in systolic blood pressure with respiration (systolic blood pressure declines >10 mm Hg with inspiration) seen in asthma, cardiac tamponade, and air embolus.
Mean arterial blood pressure	Diastolic blood pressure + [pulse pressure/3]
Shock index	Heart rate/systolic blood pressure. Normal = 0.5–0.7. A persistent elevation of the shock index (>1.0) indicates impaired left ventricular function (as a result of blood loss or cardiac depression) and is associated with increased mortality.
Respiratory	Tachypnea, increased minute ventilation, increased dead space, bronchospasm, hypocapnia with progression to respiratory failure, acute lung injury, and adult respiratory distress syndrome.
Abdomen	Low-flow states may result in abdominal pain, ileus, gastrointestinal bleeding, pancreatitis, acalculous cholecystitis, mesenteric ischemia, and shock liver.
Renal	Because the kidney receives 20% of cardiac output, low cardiac output reduces the glomerular filtration rate and redistributes renal blood flow from the renal cortex toward the renal medulla, thereby leading to oliguria. Paradoxical polyuria in early sepsis may be confused with adequate hydration.
Metabolic	Respiratory alkalosis is the first acid-base abnormality, but metabolic acidosis rapidly occurs as shock progresses. Hyperglycemia, hypoglycemia, and hyperkalemia may develop.

From Goldman L, Schafer AI, eds. *Goldman-Cecil Medicine.* 26th ed. Philadelphia: Elsevier, 2020:643, Table 98-1.

examination finds the patient to have a lack of rectal tone, this may also be indicative of a spinal cord injury.

DIAGNOSTIC EVALUATION OF SHOCK

Evaluation should include laboratory tests to detect an etiology and to assess poor end-organ perfusion (Table 10.3). Poor oxygen delivery results in anaerobic metabolism, which produces lactic acid. A CBC can evaluate for hypovolemic shock due to blood loss or dissociative shock due to anemia. If these are likely, a type and cross-match should be performed. Leukocytosis or leukopenia may be found in septic shock. Electrolyte abnormalities may be found in children with hypovolemic shock due to gastroenteritis. Obtaining a glucose level is particularly important because young infants may become hypoglycemic in shock states. Alternatively, hyperglycemia can be seen due to the release of hormones such as catecholamines, corticosteroids, and glucagon. A chest radiograph can evaluate a number of different sources of shock including a pericardial or pleural effusion pneumothorax, pneumonia associated with septic shock, and secondary signs of cardiogenic shock (cardiomegaly, pulmonary edema). An abdominal image can assess for signs of intestinal perforation or obstruction. A bedside focused assessment with sonography in trauma (FAST) abdominal point-of-care ultrasound examination can evaluate for intraabdominal injuries. Consideration of an ECG and, for concerns of cardiogenic shock, an echocardiogram is indicated.

TYPES OF SHOCK

Pediatric shock can be divided into five categories based on the source and subsequent pathophysiology of the shock (Table 10.4 and Fig. 10.2). These include hypovolemic, cardiogenic, distributive, obstructive, and dissociative shock. The most common type of shock is hypovolemic shock, which includes both nonhemorrhagic and hemorrhagic shock. Worldwide, hypovolemic shock due to gastroenteritis is the most common cause of pediatric shock. Children with hypovolemic shock present with a history of either volume loss (vomiting, diarrhea) or both inadequate volume intake and a mechanism of injury suggesting blood loss. Cardiogenic shock can be difficult to diagnose based on history, but careful attention to the cardiac examination can sometimes identify abnormalities suggesting a cardiogenic etiology. Additionally, children with cardiogenic shock do not have improvement in perfusion with large-volume intravenous

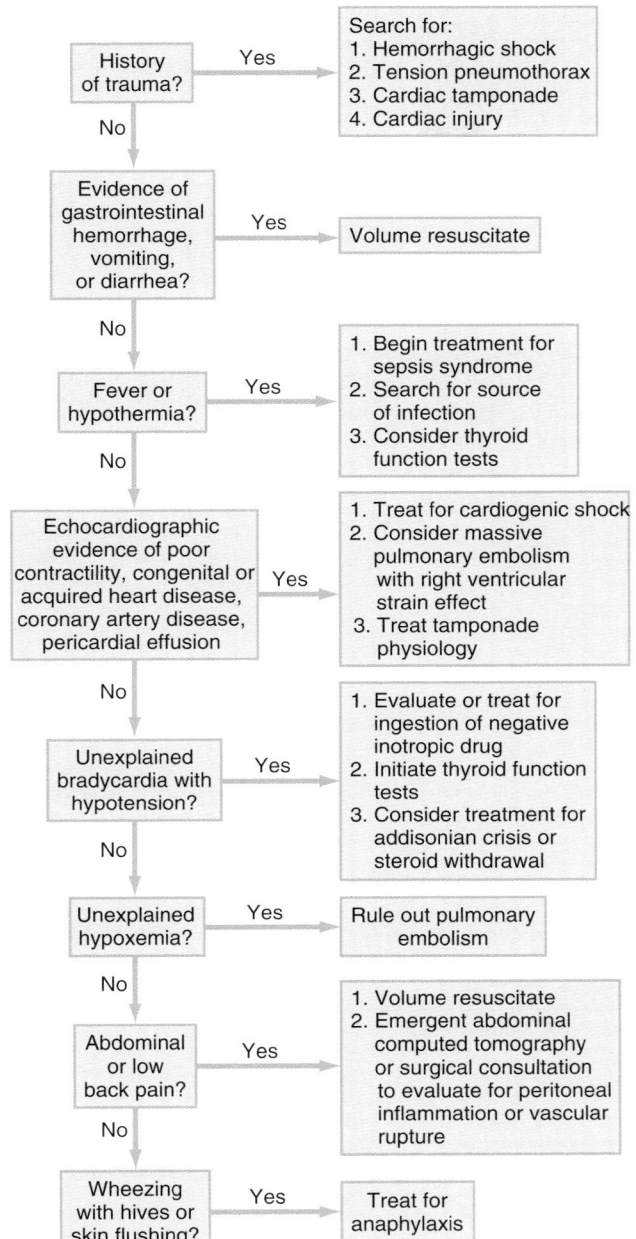

Fig. 10.3 Flow diagram to classify undifferentiated shock. (Modified from Walls R, Hockberger R, Gausche-Hill M. *Rosen's Emergency Medicine: Concepts and Clinical Practice.* 9th ed. Philadelphia: Elsevier; 2018:71, Fig. 6.1.)

TABLE 10.3 Diagnostic Evaluation of Shock for Pediatric Patients
ALL SHOCK ETIOLOGY
Blood sample:
Rapid blood glucose
Blood gas
CBC with differential
Chemistry panel
Blood lactate
Urine sample:
Urinalysis
Imaging:
Chest radiograph, two views
TRAUMATIC ETIOLOGY
Blood sample: type and cross-match and coagulation studies
Point-of-care ultrasound examination of the abdomen
CARDIOLOGY ETIOLOGY
Electrocardiogram
Echocardiogram
SEPSIS ETIOLOGY
Blood sample: inflammatory markers, coagulation studies, and blood culture
Urine and spinal fluid for analysis and culture

PEDIATRIC SEPTIC SHOCK

Septic shock is a leading cause of morbidity and mortality in U.S. children and infants. There are pediatric-specific definitions for systemic inflammatory response syndrome (SIRS), infection, sepsis, severe sepsis, and septic shock (Table 10.5). Pediatric septic shock is defined as a vital sign abnormality with cardiovascular compromise. Pediatric sepsis is defined as the presence of SIRS plus suspected or proven infection. SIRS is defined as abnormal temperature or leukocyte count plus either tachycardia or tachypnea. There are many sepsis mimics that also present as SIRS (Table 10.6).

Early recognition of septic shock and initiation of goal-directed therapy including intravenous fluid boluses, vasopressors, and antibiotics have demonstrated improved pediatric sepsis-associated mortality. Key components of early goal-directed therapy include (1) first-hour fluid resuscitation and inotrope therapy directed to goals of threshold heart rates, normal blood pressure, and capillary refill ≤2 seconds, as well as evaluation after each bolus for fluid overload; (2) first-hour broad-spectrum antibiotics; and (3) goal-directed hemodynamic support (Table 10.7).

FIRST CRITICAL ACTIONS IN THE EVALUATION AND TREATMENT OF SHOCK

The patient should be placed on monitors for continuous evaluation of the heart rate, blood pressure, and oxygenation if there is concern for shock. The overall goal of the treatment of shock is to increase oxygen delivery and decrease oxygen demand. Simply administering oxygen will improve the delivery of oxygen to tissues for nearly all causes of shock. The goal is to eliminate hypoxemia, and placing an oxygen mask with high-flow oxygen requires little technical skill but sometimes is forgotten.

fluid administration. Distributive shock includes septic shock due to infection, shock due to toxins, anaphylactic shock, and neurogenic shock. Septic shock is a common etiology for children, particularly those who are very young or have other chronic diseases that leave them immunosuppressed. Obstructive shock is much less common in children. Dissociative shock is high cardiac output failure due to inadequate oxygen-releasing capacity. Appropriate diagnosis of the type of shock is necessary to choose the correct medical management and can be made based on history and clinical exam findings as well as response to intravenous fluid administration.

TABLE 10.4 Types of Shock

Types of Shock	Pathophysiology	Appearance	Examples	Treatments
Hypovolemic shock*	Decreased cardiac output due to volume depletion → decreased preload	Tachycardia and vasoconstriction maintain adequate circulation up to 30% of circulating volume Narrowed pulse pressure, delayed capillary refill, orthostatic changes, late hypotension, AMS, and decreased UOP	Nonhemorrhagic (vomiting and diarrhea) Hemorrhagic (trauma)	IV fluid bolus Vasopressors Blood replacement
Cardiogenic shock	Decreased cardiac output due to myocardial dysfunction, increased afterload, and/or lack of ventricular filling	Tachycardia, vasoconstriction, cool extremities, narrow pulse pressure, delayed capillary refill, respiratory distress, rales or gallop rhythm, enlarged liver, JVD, cardiomegaly on chest radiograph Significant gradient between upper and lower extremity blood pressures	Cardiomyopathies, infectious myocarditis, and systemic inflammatory process, autoimmune disease, impaired coronary perfusion, cardiopulmonary bypass, acidosis, HIE, and dysrhythmias Infants: ductal dependent lesions, tachydysrhythmias	Judicious IV fluid resuscitation, ionotropic agents to improve contractility, vasodilators to reduce afterload, and management of tachyarrhythmias PGE for infants <2 mo
Distributive shock	Decreased cardiac output and systemic vascular resistance due to peripheral vasodilation → decreased afterload and preload, redistribution of blood flow away from vital organs, and loss of sympathetic outflow	Tachycardic, vasodilated, flushed, warm extremities, wide pulse pressure, bounding pulses, flush capillary refill Anaphylaxis: rash; facial swelling; lip, tongue, or airway swelling; bronchospasm; hypotension Spinal shock: unable to raise HR, hypotension	Septic shock Toxic ingestions Anaphylaxis Spinal cord injuries	IV fluids, vasopressors, antibiotics Specific antidotes Remove triggers, IV fluids, IM epinephrine, antihistamines, vasopressors IV fluids, vasoconstrictors
Obstructive shock	Decreased cardiac output due to increased afterload of the right ventricle from an obstructive process	Tachycardia, delayed capillary refill, cool extremities, narrow pulse pressure, distended neck veins, distant heart tones, asymmetric breath sounds	Tension pneumothorax Pulmonary embolism Cardiac tamponade	Evacuate pneumothorax Anticoagulants Drain pericardial effusion
Dissociative shock	High cardiac output failure due to inadequate oxygen-releasing capacity	Tachycardia, +/- delayed capillary refill, cool extremities, weakened pulse pallor or flushed cheeks	Anemia Carbon monoxide Methemoglobinemia Cyanide	Gradual fluid replacement and blood replacement 5 mL/dL Oxygen, hyperbaric chamber Methylene blue Hydroxocobalamine and cyanide antidote kit (sodium thiosulfate, sodium nitrate, amyl nitrite) plus oxygen.

AMS, altered mental status; HIE, hypoxic ischemic encephalopathies; HR, heart rate; IM, intramuscular; IV, intravenous; JVD, jugular venous distention; PGE, prostaglandin; UOP, urine output.
*Most common.

TABLE 10.5 Definitions for Terminology Used for Septic Shock States

Sepsis	SIRS	Temperature abnormality	Fever >38.5°C or <36°C
		Leukocyte count elevated or depressed for age	
		Plus either	
		HR abnormality	HR >2 SD above normal without external stimulus or bradycardia in child <1 yr old without a source
		RR abnormality	RR >2 SD above normal for age or mechanical ventilation
	Infection		Suspected or proven caused by any pathogen based on exam or laboratory and imaging findings
+ Cardiac Dysfunction	Cardiac dysfunction (Despite >40 mL/kg isotonic fluid in 1 hr)	Hypotension	<5th percental for age
		Need for vasoactive drug	
		Or two of the following:	
		Unexplained metabolic acidosis	Base deficit >5.0 mEq/L
		Increased arterial lactate	>2× the upper limit of normal
		Oliguria	Urine output <0.5 mL/kg/hr
		Prolonged cap refill	>5 sec
		Core-to-peripheral temp gap	>3°C

HR, heart rate; RR, respiratory rate; SIRS, systemic inflammatory response syndrome.

TABLE 10.6 Differential Diagnosis of Systemic Inflammatory Response Syndrome (SIRS)

Infection
- Bacteremia or meningitis (*Streptococcus pneumoniae, Haemophilus influenzae* type b, *Neisseria meningitidis*, group A *Streptococcus, Staphylococcus aureus*)
- Viral illness (influenza, enteroviruses, hemorrhagic fever group, herpes simplex virus, respiratory syncytial virus, cytomegalovirus, Epstein-Barr virus, COVID-19)
- Encephalitis (arboviruses, enteroviruses, herpes simplex virus)
- Rickettsiae (Rocky Mountain spotted fever, *Ehrlichia*, Q fever)
- Syphilis
- Vaccine reaction (pertussis, influenza, measles)
- Toxin-mediated reaction (toxic shock, staphylococcal scalded skin syndrome)

Cardiopulmonary
- Pneumonia (bacteria, virus, mycobacteria, fungi, allergic reaction)
- Pulmonary emboli
- Heart failure
- Arrhythmia
- Pericarditis
- Myocarditis

Metabolic-Endocrine
- Adrenal insufficiency (adrenogenital syndrome, Addison disease, corticosteroid withdrawal)
- Electrolyte disturbances (hypo- or hypernatremia, hypo- or hypercalcemia)
- Diabetes insipidus
- Diabetes mellitus
- Inborn errors of metabolism (organic acidosis, urea cycle, carnitine deficiency, mitochondrial disorders)
- Hypoglycemia

Gastrointestinal
- Gastroenteritis with dehydration
- Volvulus
- Intussusception
- Appendicitis
- Peritonitis (spontaneous, associated with perforation or peritoneal dialysis)
- Necrotizing enterocolitis
- Hepatitis
- Hemorrhage
- Pancreatitis

Hematologic/Immune
- Anemia (sickle cell disease, blood loss, nutritional)
- Methemoglobinemia
- Splenic sequestration crisis
- Leukemia or lymphoma
- Hemophagocytic syndromes
- Cytokine release syndrome s/p CAR-T therapy
- Immune reconstitution syndrome
- Graft versus host disease

Neurologic
- Intoxication (drugs, carbon monoxide, intentional or accidental overdose)
- Intracranial hemorrhage
- Infant botulism
- Trauma (child abuse, accidental)
- Guillain-Barre syndrome
- Myasthenia gravis

Other
- Anaphylaxis (food, drug, insect sting, idiopathic)
- Hemolytic-uremic syndrome
- Kawasaki disease
- Erythema multiforme, toxic epidermal necrolysis
- MIS-C
- Poisoning, iron, cyanide
- Toxic envenomation
- Systemic JIA
- Macrophage activation syndrome
- Idiopathic systemic capillary leak (Clarkson) syndrome

CAR-T, chimeric antigen receptor T-cell; JIA, juvenile idiopathic arthritis; MIS-C, multisystem inflammatory syndrome in children; S/P, status post.

In shock, obtaining rapid vascular access is required to restore circulating volume, obtain blood samples, and administer vasoactive medications and antibiotics if indicated. Ideally vascular access would be obtained in the first 5 minutes after recognition of shock. Although intravenous vascular access protocols can vary, traditionally, after two attempts at peripheral access, alternative methods should be used. Intraosseous access has been shown to be a rapid and effective method to obtain access within 2 minutes with an 80–100% success rate. Optimally, a patient with shock should have two large-bore intravenous lines placed.

Once intravenous access is obtained, administration of intravenous fluids will treat shock, and the patient's response to the fluids administered will also aid in the determination of the etiology of the shock (Table 10.8). Fluid boluses of 20 mL/kg of isotonic crystalloid fluid should be administered as quickly as possible. In neonates or children with pre-existing cardiovascular compromise, a fluid bolus of 10 mL/kg of isotonic fluid may be considered with careful assessment after each bolus, and repeat boluses as needed to treat shock. Monitor for signs of fluid overload, including rales, respiratory distress, or hepatomegaly. Several intravenous fluid infusion strategies exist and vary based on speed of infusion rate, equipment and preparation needed, unique benefits, and limitations.

Rapid identification of reversible causes of shock should be prioritized by clinicians as intravenous access is being obtained. If the patient has a traumatic mechanism of injury, then active bleeding, tension pneumothorax, and cardiac tamponade should be identified and appropriate interventions initiated. If the child is known to have been exposed to an allergen, then treatment of anaphylaxis should be pursued. If the ECG identifies a cardiac arrythmia, then treatment for life-threatening causes should be pursued. If the patient is an infant within the first month of life, a ductal-dependent cardiac lesion may cause shock and initiation of prostaglandins should be considered. If the patient is not responsive to interventions or there is concern for adrenal insufficiency, then systemic corticosteroids should be administered.

TABLE 10.7 Pediatric Sepsis Management Algorithm

Time	Intervention
0 min	Recognize signs of severe sepsis Identify temperature and HR abnormality + either altered mental status, perfusion, other vitals, or high risk for sepsis Provider notification
5 min	Provider/RN assessment ABCDE, mental status Monitor and complete VS Immediate IV access Obtain labs Administer high-flow O_2 Order antibiotics
5–20 min	Rapid-push fluid resuscitation, 20 mL/kg isotonic saline Repeat boluses as needed if no hepatomegaly, rales, or crackles Initiate IV antibiotics Order vasopressors to the bedside **Fluid refractory shock:** initiate vasopressors Cold shock: epinephrine or dopamine if epinephrine not available Warm shock: norepinephrine or dopamine if norepinephrine is not available Notify PICU
20–40 min	Monitor response MS, VS, airway, breathing, perfusion Detailed H&P to identify infection source
40–60 min	Catecholamine-resistant shock Consider hydrocortisone if at risk for absolute adrenal insufficiency Consider additional inotropes, vasopressors, and vasodilators as clinically indicated Goal is normal MAP/CVP, $Scvo_2$ >70%, and CI 3.3–6.0 L/min/m^2 Persistent catecholamine-resistant shock Evaluate for pericardial effusion or pneumothorax Refractory shock ECMO

ABCDE, airway, breathing, circulation, disability, exposure; CI, cardiac index; CVP, central venous pressure; ECMO, extracorporeal membrane oxygenation; H&P, history and physical examination; HR, heart rate; IV, intravenous; MAP, mean arterial pressure; MS, mental status; PICU, pediatric intensive care unit; $Scvo_2$, central venous oxygen saturation; VS, vital signs.

ANAPHYLAXIS

Anaphylaxis is an acute life-threatening allergic reaction that may be initially overlooked as a cause of shock. The presentation is often rapid (usually minutes or hours) following exposure to a triggering agent (Fig. 10.4 and Tables 10.9 and 10.10). The skin and respiratory systems are the most commonly affected sites. The differential diagnosis is noted in Table 10.11. Elevated serum tryptase levels may be present within 5 hours of onset but should not be relied upon to initiate therapy. Treatment relies on epinephrine as the first-line and most important agent (Table 10.12).

TABLE 10.8 Five Categories of Shock According to Primary Treatment of Causes and Problems

PRIMARILY INFUSION OF VOLUME

Hemorrhagic shock
  Traumatic
  Gastrointestinal
  Body cavity
Hypovolemia
  Gastrointestinal losses
  Dehydration from insensible losses
  Third-space sequestration from inflammation

VOLUME INFUSION AND VASOPRESSOR SUPPORT

Septic shock
Anaphylactic shock
Central neurogenic shock
Drug overdose

IMPROVEMENT IN PUMP FUNCTION BY INFUSION OF INOTROPIC SUPPORT OR REVERSAL OF THE CAUSE OF PUMP DYSFUNCTION

Myocardial ischemia
  Coronary artery thrombosis
  Arterial hypotension with hypoxemia
Cardiomyopathy
  Acute myocarditis
  Chronic diseases of heart muscle (ischemic, diabetic, infiltrative,
    endocrinologic, congenital)
Cardiac rhythm disturbances
  Atrial fibrillation with rapid ventricular response
  Ventricular tachycardia
  Supraventricular tachycardia

Septic shock with myocardial failure (hypodynamic shock)
Overdose of negative inotropic drug
  β Blocker
  Calcium channel antagonist
Structural cardiac damage
  Traumatic (e.g., flail mitral valve)
  Ventriculoseptal rupture
  Papillary muscle rupture

IMMEDIATE RELIEF FROM OBSTRUCTION TO CARDIAC OUTPUT

Pulmonary embolism
Cardiac tamponade
Tension pneumothorax
Valvular dysfunction
  Acute thrombosis of prosthetic valve
  Critical aortic stenosis
Congenital heart defects in newborn (e.g., closure of patent ductus
  arteriosus, with critical aortic coarctation)
Critical idiopathic subaortic stenosis (hypertrophic obstructive
  cardiomyopathy)

SPECIFIC ANTIDOTES DUE TO CELLULAR OR MITOCHONDRIAL POISONS

Carbon monoxide
Methemoglobinemia
Hydrogen sulfide
Cyanide

From Walls R, Hockberger R, Gausche-Hill M. *Rosen's Emergency Medicine: Concepts and Clinical Practice.* 9th ed., Vol. 1. Philadelphia: Elsevier; 2018:69, Box 6.1.

Anaphylaxis is likely when any one of the three criteria is fulfilled:

1
Acute onset of an illness (minutes to several hours) with involvement of:

Skin and/or mucosa

Pruritus
Flushing
Hives
Angioedema

And either

Respiratory compromise

Dyspnea
Wheeze-bronchospasm
↓ Peak expiratory flow
Stridor
Hypoxemia

Or

↓ BP or end-organ dysfunction

Collapse
Syncope
Incontinence

2
2 or more of the following that occur rapidly after exposure to a likely allergen for that patient:

Skin and/or mucosa

Pruritus
Flushing
Hives
Angioedema

Respiratory compromise

Dyspnea
Wheeze-bronchospasm
↓ Peak expiratory flow
Stridor
Hypoxemia

↓ BP or end-organ dysfunction

Collapse
Syncope
Incontinence

Persistent GI symptoms

Vomiting
Crampy abdominal pain
Diarrhea

3
After exposure to known allergen for that patient (minutes to several hours):

↓ BP

Fig. 10.4 Visual presentation of anaphylaxis criteria. (From Campbell RL, Li JTC, Nicklas RA, et al. Emergency department diagnosis and treatment of anaphylaxis: a practice parameter. *Ann Allergy Asthma Immunol.* 2014;113:599–608.)

TABLE 10.9 Symptoms and Signs of Anaphylaxis in Infants

Anaphylaxis Symptoms That Infants Cannot Describe	Anaphylaxis Signs That May Be Difficult to Interpret/Unhelpful in Infants (and Why)	Anaphylaxis Signs in Infants
GENERAL		
Feeling of warmth, weakness, anxiety, apprehension, impending doom	Nonspecific behavioral changes such as persistent crying, fussing, irritability, fright	
SKIN/MUCOUS MEMBRANES		
Itching of lips, tongue, palate, uvula, ears, throat, nose, eyes, etc.; mouth tingling or metallic taste	Flushing (may also occur with fever, hyperthermia, or crying spells)	Rapid onset of hives (potentially difficult to discern in infants with acute atopic dermatitis; scratching and excoriations will be absent in young infants); angioedema (face, tongue, oropharynx)
RESPIRATORY SYSTEM		
Nasal congestion, throat tightness, chest tightness, shortness of breath	Hoarseness, dysphonia (common after a crying spell), drooling or increased secretions (common in infants)	Rapid onset of coughing, choking, stridor, wheezing, dyspnea, apnea, cyanosis
GASTROINTESTINAL SYSTEM		
Dysphagia, nausea, abdominal pain/cramping	Spitting up/regurgitation (common after foods), loose stool (normal in infants, especially if breastfed), colicky abdominal pain	Sudden, profuse vomiting
CARDIOVASCULAR SYSTEM		
Feeling faint, presyncope, dizziness, confusion, blurred vision, difficulty in hearing, palpitations	Hypotension (need appropriate-size blood pressure cuff; low systolic blood pressure for children is defined as <70 mm Hg from 1 mo to 1 yr, and less than (70 mm Hg + [2 × age in yr]) from 1 to 2 yr; tachycardia, defined as 120–130 beats/min from 3 mo to 2 yr; loss of bowel and bladder control (ubiquitous in infants)	Weak pulse, arrhythmia, diaphoresis/sweating, collapse/unconsciousness
CENTRAL NERVOUS SYSTEM		
Headache	Drowsiness, somnolence (common in infants after feeds)	Rapid onset of unresponsiveness, lethargy, or hypotonia; seizures

Adopted from Simons FER. Anaphylaxis in infants: can recognition and management be improved? *J Allergy Clin Immunol.* 2007;120:537–540.

TABLE 10.10 Anaphylaxis Triggers in the Community

Allergen Triggers (IgE-Dependent Immunologic Mechanism)*	Other Immune Mechanisms (IgE Independent)
Foods (e.g., peanuts, tree nuts, shellfish, fish, milk, egg, wheat, soy, sesame, meat [galactose-α-1,3-galactose])	IgG mediated (infliximab, high-molecular-weight dextrans)
Food additives (e.g., spices, colorants, vegetable gums, contaminants)	Immune aggregates (IVIG)
Stinging insects: *Hymenoptera* species (e.g., bees, yellow jackets, wasps, hornets, fire ants)	Drugs (aspirin, NSAID, opiates, contrast material, ethylene oxide/dialysis tubing)
Medications (e.g., β-lactam antibiotics, ibuprofen)	Complement activation
Biologic agents (e.g., monoclonal antibodies [infliximab, omalizumab] and allergens [challenge tests, specific immunotherapy])	Physical factors (e.g., exercise,† cold, heat, sunlight/ultraviolet radiation)
Natural rubber latex	Ethanol
Vaccines	Idiopathic*
Inhalants (rare) (e.g., horse or hamster dander, grass pollen)	
Previously unrecognized allergens (foods, venoms, biting-insect saliva, medications, biologic agents)	

IgE, immunoglobulin E; IVIG, intravenous immune globulin; NSAID, nonsteroidal antiinflammatory drug.

*In the pediatric population, some anaphylaxis triggers, such as hormones (progesterone), seminal fluid, and occupational allergens, are uncommon, as is idiopathic anaphylaxis.

†Exercise with or without a co-trigger, such as a food or medication, cold air, or cold water.

Adapted from Leung DYM, Sampson HA, Geha RS, et al. *Pediatric Allergy Principles and Practice*. Philadelphia: Elsevier; 2010:652.

TABLE 10.11 Differential Diagnosis of Anaphylaxis

- Acute generalized urticaria
- Asthma exacerbation
- Pulmonary embolus
- Syncope
- Adverse cutaneous drug reaction
- Anxiety/panic attacks

Flush Syndrome
- Flushing associated with food
  - Alcohol
  - MSG
  - Sulfites
  - Scombroidosis
- Carcinoid tumor
- Perimenopause
- Thyrotoxicosis
- Basophilic leukemia
- Mastocytosis (systemic mastocytosis *and* urticaria pigmentosa)
- Vasointestinal peptide tumors
- Auriculotemporal syndrome (Frey syndrome-gustatory flushing)

Shock Syndromes
- Septic shock
- Hypovolemic shock
- Cardiogenic shock
- Distributive shock

Miscellaneous
- Hypoglycemia
- Acquired and HAE
- ACE inhibitor–associated angioedema
- Red man syndrome (vancomycin)
- Neurologic disorders (seizure, stroke, autonomic epilepsy)
- Vocal cord dysfunction syndrome
- Pheochromocytoma

ACE, angiotensin-converting enzyme; HAE, hereditary angioedema; MSG, monosodium glutamate.

Modified from Walls R, Hockberger R, Gausche-Hill M. *Rosen's Emergency Medicine: Concepts and Clinical Practice*. 9th ed. Philadelphia: Elsevier; 2018:1424, Box 109.6.

TABLE 10.12   Treatment Algorithm for Anaphylaxis

Emergency Measures (Taken Simultaneously)

Remove any triggering agent.

Place patient in supine position.

Begin cardiac monitoring, pulse oximetry, and blood pressure autonomic monitoring.

Begin supplemental oxygen if indicated.

Establish large-bore IV lines (e.g., 16 or 18 gauge).

Establish a patent airway.

Be prepared for endotracheal intubation with or without rapid sequence intubation.

Be prepared to use adjunct airway technique (e.g., awake fiberoptic intubation, surgical airway).

Start rapid infusion of isotonic crystalloid (normal saline):

   Adult: 1,000 mL IV in the first 5 min in the adult (several liters of normal saline may be required)

   Pediatric: 20–30 mL/kg IV increments

Anaphylaxis Treatment Medications

First-Line Agent

Epinephrine is the first-line medication and should be given immediately at the first suspicion of an anaphylactic reaction.

   Adult: 0.3–0.5 mg IM (1:1,000 concentration) in anterolateral thigh every 5–10 min as necessary

   Pediatric: 0.01 mg/kg IM (1:1,000 concentration) in anterolateral thigh every 5–10 min as necessary

Alternatively, epinephrine (EpiPen, 0.3 mL; or EpiPen Jr, 0.15 mL) can be administered into anterolateral thigh.

Second-Line Agents (Should Not Precede the Administration of Epinephrine)

Antihistamines

Diphenhydramine:

   Adult: 50 mg IV or 50 mg oral

   Pediatric: 1 mg/kg IV or oral

Ranitidine*:

   Adult: 50 mg IV (150 mg oral)

   Pediatric 1 mg/kg IV or oral

Aerosolized β-Agonists (if Bronchospasm Is Present)

Adult:

   Albuterol: 2.5 mg, diluted to 3 mL of normal saline; may be given continuously

   Ipratropium: 0.5 mg in 3 mL of normal saline; repeat as necessary

Pediatric:

   Albuterol: 2.5 mg, diluted to 3 mL of normal saline; may be given continuously

   Ipratropium: 0.25 mg in 3 mL of normal saline; repeat as necessary

Glucocorticoids (No Benefit in the Acute Management)

Methylprednisolone:

   Adult: 125–250 mg IV

   Pediatric: 1–2 mg/kg IV

Prednisone/prednisolone:

   Adult: 40–60 mg oral

   Pediatric: 1–2 mg/kg oral

Refractory Hypotension

Consider continuous IV epinephrine drip (dilute 1 mg [1 mL 1:1,000] in 1,000 mL of normal saline or D_5W to yield a concentration of 1 μg/mL)

Adult: 1–10 μg/min IV (titrated to desired effect)

Pediatric: 0.1–1.5 μg/kg/min IV (titrated to desired effect)

Other Vasopressors to Consider

Dopamine: 5–20 μg/kg/min continuous IV infusion (titrated to desired effect)

Norepinephrine: 0.05–0.5 μg/kg/min (titrated to desired effect)

Phenylephrine: 1–5 μg/kg/min (titrated to desired effect)

Vasopressin: 0.01–0.4 units/min (titrated to desired effect)

Patients Receiving β-Blockade

Glucagon: 1–5 mg IV over 5 min, followed by 5–15 μg/min continuous IV infusion

IM, intramuscular; IV, intravenous.

*Alternate drugs include cimetidine or famotidine in appropriate dosages.

From Walls R, Hockberger R, Gausche-Hill M. *Rosen's Emergency Medicine: Concepts and Clinical Practice.* 9th ed, Vol. 2. Philadelphia: Elsevier; 2018:1426, Box 109.7.

■ SUMMARY AND RED FLAGS

Shock is a serious result of many pediatric diseases with distinct patterns (see Fig. 10.2 and Table 10.4). A careful history and physical exam will help identify both predisposing conditions (congenital anomalies, immunosuppression, immune deficiencies) and possible etiologies (gastroenteritis, hemorrhage, fever, rash).

SIRS is a final common pathway for many inflammatory conditions (see Table 10.6); sepsis is a leading cause, although there are serious disorders that "mimic" sepsis.

Red flags of shock/SIRS are noted in Table 10.13 (next page).

TABLE 10.13 Red Flags of Shock/SIRS

General

Recurrent episodes
Culture-negative presumed sepsis
Fluid unresponsive shock
Atypical or unusual rashes
Medical devices: CVL, urinary catheter
Weight loss
Night sweats
Travel to endemic areas
Exposure to infected people
Coagulopathy (DIC)
Salt craving, pigmentation
Weaning chronic steroids

Cardiogenic Concerns

Cardiomegaly
↑ Tachypnea, tachycardia during fluid resuscitation
Pulmonary edema, hypoxia during fluid resuscitation
Elevated troponin
Elevated BNP
Criteria for Kawasaki disease
Criteria for MIS-C
History of palpitations or chest pain

Anaphylaxis Concern

Sudden onset
Urticaria/angioedema
Stridor
Wheezing
Exposure to medication, venoms
Anxiety

Intraabdominal Concern

Tender distended abdomen out of proportion to an ileus or shock
Bile-stained emesis
Hepatic failure
Elevated lipase
Ascites
Hematemesis
Hematochezia

Immune Dysfunction Concern

Asplenia, splenectomy, sickle cell anemia
Cytopenia
Lymphopenia
Splenomegaly
Lymphadenopathy
Recurrent fevers
Elevated acute-phase reactants: CRP, ESR, procalcitonin
Elevated ferritin
High total protein
Criteria for MAS
Criteria for HLH
Abnormal newborn screen

BNP, brain natriuretic peptide; CVL, central venous line; DIC, disseminated intravascular coagulation; HLH, hemophagocytic lymphohistiocytosis; MAS, macrophage activation syndrome; MIS-C, multisystem inflammatory syndrome—children; SIRS, systemic inflammatory response syndrome.

BIBLIOGRAPHY

A bibliography is available at ExpertConsult.com.

Hypertension

Scott K. Van Why and Rajasree Sreedharan

The first step in the evaluation of a child for hypertension is to define whether the child is in fact hypertensive. For children under 13 years of age, the normative data for blood pressure are interpreted based on gender, age, and height because all these are variables that influence blood pressure norms. The current hypertension definition and staging lead to seamless interfacing with the 2017 American Heart Association (AHA) and American College of Cardiology (ACC) adult hypertension guidelines for children over 13 years of age (Table 11.1).

Data on blood pressure tracking from childhood to adulthood demonstrate that higher blood pressure in childhood correlates with hypertension in young adulthood. Autopsy and imaging studies reveal that hypertension is associated with poorer markers of vascular aging, which are known to predict cardiovascular events in adults.

PRESENTATION

Symptoms

Hypertension can be silent or may present with symptoms related to high blood pressure or the primary disease producing the hypertension (e.g., pheochromocytoma, lupus). Chronic hypertension is silent in most cases, but acute hypertension is typically symptomatic. A detailed history and physical examination will help guide the assessment of etiology and urgency for management. Summaries are provided in Tables 11.2 and 11.3. Eliciting symptoms related to acute hypertension that could indicate urgency is critical in the initial assessment and management. Presentations with severe headache, vision changes, chest pain, respiratory distress, abdominal pain, seizure, or acute neurologic changes with elevated blood pressure should be considered emergent in any age group and need immediate attention.

In addition to symptoms secondary to the hypertension, those related to potential etiology should be sought, especially since most hypertension in children is not primary hypertension. Renal causes are high in the differential in all children but vary according to age. Potential causes for each age group (Tables 11.4 and 11.5) help guide the symptoms to be elicited and focus the physical examination. Neonates may present with gross hematuria or an abdominal mass. In later infancy the presentation may be similar to that in neonates, but edema would suggest glomerular pathology. Infants may also present with nonspecific symptoms of poor growth, weight loss, and/or fussiness. Childhood and adolescent acute hypertension may present with symptoms of gross hematuria, edema, rash, joint complaints, respiratory symptoms, or diarrhea depending on the etiology. Urinary symptoms can be a presentation of hypertension in childhood that would suggest a urologic abnormality not previously discovered. In later childhood and adolescence, the risk of recreational drug use increases, so symptoms of lethargy, irritability, anorexia, and poor school performance are relevant. Sleep problems could be related to sleep apnea or illicit drug use. Episodic palpitation or flushing may be symptoms related to

catecholamine-secreting tumors or hyperthyroidism. Some disorders produce transient or intermittent hypertension (Table 11.6).

Physical Examination

Accurate blood pressure measurement is fundamental in identification of hypertension. Manual, auscultatory blood pressure is the most accurate, and the normative data are based on this method of blood pressure measurement. An accurate reading depends on positioning and appropriate cuff size. Sitting relaxed with uncrossed feet on the floor with the back supported and using a cuff with a bladder that covers a minimum of 80% midarm circumference and 40% of arm length are optimal.

In infants and those in whom Korotkoff sounds are not well heard, Doppler can be used to measure blood pressure accurately, but only systolic readings are obtained by that method. An oscillatory method may not be accurate but is useful as a screening tool, if done with a device calibrated for pediatric use. In an emergency setting a manual blood pressure measurement may not be feasible initially. A well-calibrated oscillatory device can be used for initial screening and frequent monitoring, and then validated with auscultatory method at the earliest opportunity.

Blood pressure measurement should be done on the right arm, unless there is known atypical anatomy that can confound that assessment. If blood pressure is found there to be elevated, four extremity readings should be obtained to evaluate for vascular anomalies, in particular aortic coarctation, which might further be suggested by the presence of a heart murmur. Lower extremity blood pressure is typically equal or higher than upper extremity blood pressure. Finding right upper extremity blood pressure >10 mm Hg above that of lower extremity blood pressure is a strong indication of aortic coarctation.

If the initial blood pressure reading is in the elevated blood pressure or stage 1 hypertension range, additional readings should be obtained on different days over days to weeks to confirm the presence of true hypertension. If there is concern that anxiety with clinic visits is affecting blood pressure assessment, 24-hour ambulatory blood pressure monitoring (ABPM) can be used to separate those with sustained hypertension from those with "white coat hypertension." ABPM provides frequent readings in the home setting with diurnal information. The standards used for these readings are different from the casual blood pressure reading guidelines mentioned earlier.

Other pertinent physical examination information is critical in determining the urgency of the situation as well as the etiology. Abnormal fundoscopic findings such as papilledema and retinal hemorrhages and focal neurologic or encephalopathic findings are indicative of acute hypertensive emergency and the need for immediate therapeutic intervention along with prompt evaluation to identify the etiology. The physical findings help lead to both the effects of hypertension and the potential etiology. The presence of a gallop rhythm and rales on

TABLE 11.1	2017 American Heart Association (AHA) and American College of Cardiology (ACC) Adult Hypertension Guidelines for Children over 13 Years of Age	
	For Children Aged 1 to <13 yr	**For Children Aged ≥13 yr**
Normal BP	<90th percentile	<120/<80 mm Hg
Elevated BP	≥90th to <95th percentile or 120/80 mm Hg to <95th percentile (whichever is lower)	120–129/<80 mm Hg
Stage 1 Hypertension	≥95th to <95th percentile + 12 mm Hg or 130–139/80–89 mm Hg (whichever is lower)	130–139/80–89 mm Hg
Stage 2 Hypertension	≥95th percentile + 12 mm Hg or ≥140/90 mm Hg (whichever is lower)	≥140/90 mm Hg

Data extracted from Gidding SS, Whelton PK, Carey RM, et al. Aligning adult and pediatric blood pressure guideline. *Hypertension*. 2019;73:938–943.

TABLE 11.2	History and Physical Exam in the Evaluation of Hypertension
History	*Hypertension-related symptoms:* headache, dizziness, blurry vision, altered mental status, chest pain, palpitations *Etiology-related symptoms:* hematuria, joints, swelling edema, rash, cardiac/respiratory issues, voiding problems *Past history:* prematurity and related issues, intensive care unit stay and related issues, urinary issues including infection *Social history:* include drug and supplement history *Family history:* renal issues or blood pressure problems
Physical exam	• Accurate method for casual measurement 　• Relaxed child in exam room with uncrossed feet on floor and back supported 　• Auscultatory method 　• Appropriate-size cuff 　　• Bladder length 80% of the midarm circumference 　　• Bladder width at least 40% 　• All-extremity blood pressure measurements • Confirm 　• Measure on 3 different days 　• ABPM • Findings in symptomatic hypertension 　• Focal neurologic finding 　• Papilledema 　• Gallop cardiac rhythm on auscultation • Other findings 　• Constitutional: obesity, syndromic features 　• Fundus: retinal hemorrhage, arterial narrowing, papilledema 　• Skin: rash, purpura, café-au-lait 　• Swelling: Edema: periorbital or extremity 　• Cardiac: femoral radial pulse lag, murmur 　• Abdominal mass, bruit • Occasional findings 　• Coloboma 　• Ear tag/pit 　• Webbed neck 　• Genital abnormality

ABPM, ambulatory blood pressure monitoring.

auscultation of the heart and lungs, along with edema, indicates volume overload as the cause of severe symptomatic hypertension, possibly from underlying glomerulonephritis. Edema, rash, and arthritis would suggest hypertension secondary to renal involvement from potential autoimmune disease. Diminished lower extremity pulses with discrepancy between upper and lower extremity blood pressures, along with a heart murmur, point to coarctation of the aorta. Abdominal or flank bruit may be present with renal artery stenosis. Findings of body habitus suggestive of Cushing syndrome, ambiguous genitalia, or features of hyperthyroidism can direct evaluation to endocrine causes. Physical exam findings associated with genetic syndromes that can have hypertension caused by abnormal renal or vascular development include coloboma, lens dislocation, ear tags, brachial cysts, café-au-lait spots, or a webbed neck (see Table 11.3).

ETIOLOGY

Hypertension in children is uncommon and when present is usually from an identifiable cause other than primary essential hypertension. The preponderance of hypertension in adulthood is either primary hypertension, formerly called "essential hypertension," or hypertension secondary to diabetic nephropathy. While the prevalence of primary hypertension is rising in childhood, the cause of hypertension in children and adolescents usually is secondary to an identifiable cause, and is most often from renal disease. Disease processes that cause hypertension in childhood typically manifest at different ages, with the major differences being between infants and older children.

INFANTILE HYPERTENSION

Neonatal

Causes of hypertension identified during infancy can be separated into neonatal forms and those identified later during infancy (see Table 11.4). During the neonatal period causes of elevated blood pressure are typically identified in the context of prenatal fetal imaging, premature birth, or perinatal stress. The principal causes in this age group can be separated between abnormalities in the vasculature or renal architecture. With premature birth, vital signs are routinely monitored, so hypertension is readily identified in this group. In apparently healthy term neonates blood pressure is not routinely assessed after discharge from the nursery, so hypertension is often not identified unless symptoms or signs dictate, such as development of a cardiac murmur, gross hematuria, presentation in extremis from severe hypertension, or palpation of an intraabdominal mass.

The most common cause of hypertension in the neonate is hypertension associated with premature birth. In this context the majority of causes are vascular related, with the preponderance secondary to having had an **umbilical artery catheter (UAC)** for needed vascular access. While rarely identifiable by any imaging study, presumptively these infants sustain a focal thromboembolic insult to a kidney that then drives the elevation in blood pressure. This cause of hypertension tends to improve over time. Often antihypertensive treatment for this cause can be discontinued during later infancy or early childhood. However, hypertension can then recur later in childhood. Less commonly, having had a UAC is associated with being found to have renal

TABLE 11.3 **Findings to Look for on Physical Examination in Patients with Hypertension**

Physical Findings	Potential Relevance	Physical Findings	Potential Relevance
General		**Cardiovascular Signs**	
Pale mucous membranes, edema, growth retardation	Chronic renal disease	Absent of diminished femoral pulses, low leg pressure relative to arm pressure	Aortic coarctation
Elfin facies, poor growth, retardation	Williams syndrome	Heart size, rate, rhythm; murmurs; respiratory difficulty, hepatomegaly	Aortic coarctation, congestive heart failure
Webbing of neck, low hairline, widespread nipples, wide carrying angle	Turner syndrome	Bruits over great vessels	Arteritis or arteriopathy
Moon face, buffalo hump, hirsutism, truncal obesity, striae, acne	Cushing syndrome	Rub	Pericardial effusion secondary to chronic renal disease
Habitus		**Pulmonary Signs**	
Thinness	Pheochromocytoma, renal disease, hyperthyroidism	Pulmonary edema	Congestive heart failure, acute nephritis
Virilization	Congenital adrenal hyperplasia	Picture of bronchopulmonary dysplasia	Bronchopulmonary dysplasia—associated hypertension
Rickets	Chronic renal disease	**Abdomen**	
Skin		Epigastric bruit	Primary renovascular disease or in association with Williams syndrome, neurofibromatosis, fibromuscular dysplasia, or arteritis
Café-au-lait spots, neurofibromas	Neurofibromatosis, pheochromocytoma		
Tubers, "ash-leaf" spots	Tuberous sclerosis		
Rashes	Systemic lupus erythematosus, vasculitis (Henoch-Schönlein purpura), impetigo with acute nephritis	Abdominal masses	Wilms tumor, neuroblastoma, pheochromocytoma, polycystic kidneys, hydronephrosis, dysplastic kidneys
Pallor, evanescent flushing, sweating	Pheochromocytoma	Jaundice	Alagille arteriohepatic dysplasia
Needle tracks	Illicit drug use	**Neurologic Signs**	
Bruises, striae	Cushing syndrome	Neurologic deficits	Chronic or severe acute hypertension with stroke
Acanthosis nigricans	Type 2 diabetes, insulin resistance	Muscle weakness	Hyperaldosteronism, Liddle syndrome (hypokalemic low renin hypertension)
Eyes		**Genitalia**	
Extraocular muscle palsy	Nonspecific, chronic, severe	Ambiguous, virilized	Congenital adrenal hyperplasia (11β- or 17α-hydroxylase deficiencies)
Fundal changes	Nonspecific, chronic, severe		
Proptosis	Hyperthyroidism	**Skeletal**	
Head And Neck		Short metacarpal (4th, 5th) bones, short stature	Autosomal dominant hypertension with brachydactyly (Bilginturan disease)
Goiter	Thyroid disease		
Adenotonsillar hypertrophy	Sleep-disordered breathing		
Webbed neck	Turner syndrome		

From Kliegman RM, St. Geme JW III, Blum NJ, et al, eds. *Nelson Textbook of Pediatrics*. 21st ed. Philadelphia: Elsevier; 2020:2494, Table 472.

artery stenosis later during infancy or early childhood, presumptively acquired from focal injury to the ostium of the renal artery that then progresses to ostial stenosis and subsequent hypertension.

Renal vein thrombosis occurs in infants subjected to perinatal stress or volume depletion but can occur spontaneously in an otherwise healthy infant. The combination of gross hematuria, hypertension, and low platelet count should alert the clinician to this possibility. Doppler study of the renal veins typically identifies a significant thrombus, at times with associated diminished global renal perfusion.

Congenital vascular abnormalities that cause hypertension in the neonate include congenital renal artery stenosis and aortic coarctation. The former is a difficult diagnosis to establish during infancy. Aortic coarctation is readily identified with four-extremity blood pressure measurement and confirmation with echocardiography.

With the routine use of prenatal fetal ultrasound, the majority of renal structural causes of neonatal hypertension are identified prior to birth. These are broadly categorized as **congenital abnormalities of the kidneys and urinary tract (CAKUT)** and include cystic kidney disease and abnormalities of drainage of the urinary tract. While many forms of CAKUT do not cause hypertension, those associated with urinary tract obstruction are more likely to have hypertension as a manifestation. This includes any form of bladder outlet obstruction, such as with neurogenic bladder or urethral valves in males, and ureteral obstruction, most often at the ureteropelvic junction. A multicystic dysplastic kidney on occasion can cause hypertension, but typically hypertension is seen in those associated with ureteral obstruction.

Polycystic kidney disease (PKD) manifested in infancy is rare, but if seen it is almost always associated with severe hypertension. In this context, the kidneys typically are readily palpable on physical exam and found on ultrasound study to be massively enlarged with cysts. The cause may be either autosomal recessive (ARPKD) or infantile-onset autosomal dominant (ADPKD). Imaging, including the finding of associated liver abnormalities in ARPKD, may differentiate between the two diagnoses. However, ARPKD and ADPKD at times may not be able to be differentiated solely on imaging findings or family history. In that instance genetic testing can be helpful, especially for providing a diagnosis of ARPKD.

TABLE 11.4 Causes of Infantile Hypertension

Neonatal
- Vascular
  - Thrombotic/thromboembolic: UAC associated or renal vein thrombosis
  - Aortic coarctation
  - Renal artery stenosis: congenital or acquired
- Congenital urinary tract malformations: obstructive
- Polycystic kidney disease

Later infancy
- Prematurity associated
  - History of thrombotic/thromboembolic renal insult
  - Renal artery stenosis: congenital or acquired
  - Immature kidneys, history of renal insults: AKI, nephrotoxins
  - Bronchopulmonary dysplasia
- Congenital urinary tract malformations: obstructive
- Polycystic kidney disease
- Aortic coarctation
- Tumors: nephroblastoma, neuroblastoma
- Glomerulopathy
  - Congenital infection
  - Congenital/infantile nephrotic syndrome, familial FSGS, Denys-Drash syndrome
  - Atypical HUS

AKI, acute kidney injury; FSGS, focal segmental glomerulosclerosis; HUS, hemolytic uremic syndrome; UAC, umbilical artery catheter.

TABLE 11.5 Causes of Childhood Hypertension

Common Causes
- Primary obesity associated (metabolic syndrome)
- Parenchymal renal disease
  - Acute and chronic glomerulonephritis
    - Postinfectious glomerulonephritis
    - Systemic vasculitis with renal involvement (SLE, HSP, ANCA vasculitis)
    - Primary, idiopathic (IgA nephropathy, FSGS, crescentic glomerulonephritis)
  - Hemolytic uremic syndrome
  - Hereditary cystic kidney disease: PKD, MCKD, nephronophthisis
  - Sickle cell disease
  - Interstitial nephritis
- End-stage kidney disease of unknown etiology
- Congenital urinary tract malformations: obstructive or cystic dysplasia, either isolated or syndromic
- Scarred kidney: congenital Ask-Upmark kidney or acquired from renal injury (e.g., pyelonephritis)
- Drug induced: therapeutic and recreational

Less Common Causes
- Vascular/renal artery stenosis
  - Aortic coarctation
  - Fibromuscular dysplasia
  - Syndromic: Williams syndrome, neurofibromatosis, Turner syndrome, middle aortic syndrome
  - Tumor-associated extrinsic compression: Wilms tumor, neuroblastoma, lymphoma
  - Large-vessel vasculitis: Takayasu, moyamoya, polyarteritis nodosum
  - Trauma-associated perirenal hematoma
- Neoplasia: nephroblastoma (Wilms tumor), neuroblastoma, pheochromocytoma, infiltrative lymphoma
- Persistent or late-onset hypertension from perinatal renal insult, prematurity associated
- Neurologic
  - High intracranial pressure from head trauma, intracranial tumor, or pseudotumor cerebri
  - Secondary to seizure
  - Peripheral neuropathies: Guillain-Barré, poliomyelitis

Rare causes
- Monogenic
  - Liddle syndrome
  - Hyperaldosteronism: familial and glucocorticoid remedial
  - Congenital adrenal hyperplasia
  - Gordon syndrome: pseudohypoaldosteronism
  - Apparent mineralocorticoid excess
  - Mineralocorticoid receptor gain-of-function mutations (Geller syndrome)
- Dysautonomia
- Endocrine
  - Thyroid disease
  - Cushing syndrome
  - Catecholamine-secreting tumors
  - Hypercalcemia: vitamin D intoxication, hyperparathyroidism, malignancy associated

ANCA, antineutrophil cytoplasmic antibody; FSGS, focal segmental glomerulosclerosis; HSP, Henoch-Schönlein purpura; MCKD, multicystic dysplastic kidney; PKD, polycystic kidney disease; SLE, systemic lupus erythematosus.

Later Infancy

Most of the causes of hypertension in the neonatal period may also present during later infancy. However, in the latter context the hypertension is not found incidentally, but rather often is found due to associated symptoms or signs. This is because blood pressure measurement is not commonly performed in otherwise healthy-appearing infants because obtaining a valid blood pressure in an infant is challenging.

Several of the causes of hypertension associated with premature birth may persist or may not manifest until later in infancy. These include intrarenal thrombotic and thromboembolic injury to the kidney that may not have caused hypertension earlier in the neonatal course but present later in infancy. In addition, even without any evident risk factors for a thrombotic or thromboembolic cause, premature birth alone, especially severely premature birth, is associated with early-onset hypertension. The etiology in this scenario is thought to be from the complication of incompletely developed, immature kidneys at birth complicated by events during the early course after birth. Events predisposing to later-onset hypertension include subclinical insults to the kidneys, such as from multiple nephrotoxins and transient hypotensive events, causing occult acute kidney injury. In this setting, bronchopulmonary dysplasia itself is associated with development of hypertension in later infancy.

Congenital vascular and renal architecture abnormalities that cause hypertension may present later in infancy if not found as a neonate. Those caused by CAKUT are found in later infancy either during evaluation for urinary tract infection that can be the presenting feature of CAKUT, from evaluation for symptomatic hypertension, or when blood pressure is measured for an acute illness unrelated to the underlying cause of hypertension. Polycystic kidney disease, especially ARPKD in which progression often manifests as rapidly enlarging kidneys during infancy, may be found by palpation of an abdominal mass. Blood pressure when then measured typically is severely elevated.

TABLE 11.6 Conditions Associated with Transient or Intermittent Hypertension in Children

Renal
Acute postinfectious glomerulonephritis
Henoch-Schönlein purpura with nephritis
Hemolytic uremic syndrome
Acute kidney injury
After renal transplantation (immediately and during episodes of rejection)
Hypervolemia
Pyelonephritis
Renal trauma
Leukemic infiltration of the kidney

Drugs and Poisons
Cocaine
Oral contraceptives
Sympathomimetic agents
Amphetamines
Phencyclidine
Corticosteroids and adrenocorticotropic hormone
Cyclosporine, sirolimus, or tacrolimus treatment after transplantation
Licorice (glycyrrhizic acid)
Lead, mercury, cadmium, thallium
Antihypertensive withdrawal (clonidine, methyldopa, propranolol)
Vitamin D intoxication
Ma-huang

Central and Autonomic Nervous System
Increased intracranial pressure
Guillain-Barré syndrome
Burns
Familial dysautonomia
Stevens-Johnson syndrome
Posterior fossa lesions
Porphyria
Poliomyelitis
Encephalitis
Spinal cord injury (autonomic storm)

Miscellaneous
Preeclampsia
Pain, anxiety
Hypercalcemia
After coarctation repair
White blood cell transfusion
Extracorporeal membrane oxygenation
Closure of abdominal wall defect

Modified from Kliegman RM, St. Geme JW III, Blum NJ, et al., eds. *Nelson Textbook of Pediatrics*. 21st ed. Philadelphia: Elsevier; 2020:2492, Table 472.3.

Rare causes of hypertension in infancy include intraabdominal tumors, found by palpation of a mass or on imaging for gastrointestinal symptoms. The two most likely tumors in this age group are nephroblastoma or neuroblastoma. Both of these tumors may cause hypertension by compromising the renal vasculature. Neuroblastoma also can cause hypertension by obstructing the urinary tract, depending on location and size of the tumor, or by secreting catecholamines.

Rarely, glomerulopathies may manifest in infancy leading to hypertension. These include those secondary to congenital infection such as syphilis and cytomegalovirus (CMV). Congenital or infantile nephrotic syndrome, such as familial focal and segmental glomerulosclerosis (FSGS) or the glomerulopathy of Denys-Drash syndrome, often present with hypertension. Atypical, nondiarrheal, hemolytic uremic syndrome with accompanying glomerulopathy is rare but can present in infancy with anemia and thrombocytopenia, renal insufficiency, and hypertension. The lack of a diarrheal prodrome is a hallmark of the disease.

CHILDHOOD HYPERTENSION

While much of childhood hypertension is discovered during evaluation for an acute illness or symptomatic hypertension, with progression in age hypertension becomes more often found incidentally during examination on a well-child visit. Table 11.5 outlines common and less common causes of hypertension that present during childhood. Several of the diseases that cause hypertension during early or later childhood may be present during infancy but may not progress to cause significant hypertension until later in the course of the disease. Examples of these include hereditary cystic kidney diseases such as PKD, medullary cystic kidney disease, nephronophthisis, or any form of CAKUT with an obstructive lesion. CAKUT that can cause hypertension may become apparent in childhood in those who have been diagnosed with a syndrome that has increased risk of associated urinary tract or renal anomalies. These include Turner syndrome, branchio-oto-renal syndrome, and coloboma-renal syndrome. Renal injury sustained early in life, in the setting of either premature birth, perinatal complications, or early pyelonephritis with associated later development of renal scar, may not result in manifested hypertension until later in childhood.

Common Causes

The younger the child, the more likely it is that there will an *identifiable* cause of elevated blood pressure; thus, secondary hypertension will be found with appropriate investigation. Primary hypertension, then, is a diagnosis of exclusion. Primary hypertension in years past was a rare cause of hypertension in childhood. However, the childhood obesity epidemic that has ensued in the past couple of decades has unmasked primary hypertension earlier in life, and lately brought it into prominence during later childhood and adolescence. When secondary hypertension has been ruled out, primary hypertension is presumed when blood pressure elevation in an older child is not severe, is asymptomatic, is associated with obesity, and there is family history of early-onset primary hypertension.

Acute and symptomatic hypertension in childhood is most likely to be secondary to glomerular disease. **Acute postinfectious glomerulonephritis** is the most common cause of nephritis in childhood, and often may present with symptomatic hypertension when gross hematuria is not the heralding symptom. Patients with systemic vasculitis with renal involvement, including lupus, Henoch-Schönlein purpura, and antineutrophil cytoplasmic autoantibody (ANCA) vasculitis, at presentation and during flares of the disease often have significant hypertension as a prominent feature. **Hemolytic uremic syndrome (HUS)**, both toxigenic and atypical familial forms, routinely have associated hypertension during the episode. The hypertension from HUS may abate after the HUS episode resolves, although it may be persistent and become a long-term sequela requiring chronic treatment.

Patients with **crescentic glomerulonephritis**, whether idiopathic or secondary to other identifiable nephropathy, typically have significant and often severe hypertension at presentation. Primary idiopathic forms of glomerulonephritis such as immunoglobulin A (IgA) nephropathy and focal segmental glomerulosclerosis (FSGS) may be indolent and not have hypertension at presentation. However, if severe

TABLE 11.7 Causes of Renovascular Hypertension in Children

Fibromuscular dysplasia
Syndromic causes
    Neurofibromatosis type 1
    Tuberous sclerosis
    Williams syndrome
    Marfan syndrome
    Other syndromes

Vasculitis
    Takayasu arteritis (disease)
    Polyarteritis nodosa
    Kawasaki disease
    Other systemic vasculitides

Extrinsic compression
    Neuroblastoma
    Wilms tumor
    Other tumors
    Other causes
    Radiation
    Umbilical artery catheterization
    Trauma
    Congenital rubella syndrome
    Transplant renal artery stenosis

From Kliegman RM, St. Geme JW III, Blum NJ, et al., eds. *Nelson Textbook of Pediatrics.* 21st ed. Philadelphia: Elsevier; 2020:2495, Table 472.7.

TABLE 11.8 Features Suggestive of Pheochromocytoma

Hypertension, Persistent or Paroxysmal
Markedly variable blood pressures (± orthostatic hypotension)
Sudden paroxysms (± subsequent hypertension) in relation to:
    Stress: anesthesia, angiography, parturition, exercise
    Pharmacologic provocation: histamine, nicotine, caffeine, β blockers,
      glucocorticoids, tricyclic antidepressants
    Manipulation of tumors: abdominal palpation, urination
Rare patients persistently normotensive
Unusual settings
Childhood, pregnancy, familial
Multiple endocrine adenomas: medullary carcinoma of the thyroid (MEN-2),
    mucosal neuromas (MEN-2B)
Von Hippel–Lindau syndrome
Neurocutaneous lesions: neurofibromatosis

Associated Symptoms
Sudden spells with headache, sweating, palpitations, nervousness, nausea,
    vomiting
Pain in chest or abdomen

Associated Signs
Sweating, tachycardia, arrhythmia, pallor, weight loss

From Zipes DP, et al. *Braunwald's Heart Disease: A Textbook of Cardiovascular Medicine.* 11th ed., Vol. 1. Philadelphia: Elsevier; 2019:925, Table 46.8.

and therapy for the primary process is not effective, hypertension then becomes a nearly uniform feature in these patients.

Early-onset hypertension in patients with sickle cell disease is usually associated with overt **sickle cell nephropathy**, with significant proteinuria and developing renal insufficiency that can become manifest during adolescence. However, even without overt sickle cell nephropathy, this population appears to be prone to earlier-onset hypertension. The predisposition to hypertension in those with sickle cell disease appears to be secondary to endothelial cell dysfunction.

Drug-induced hypertension is common in childhood and adolescence. Usual agents that cause hypertension include several classes of therapeutic medications, illicit drugs, and other agents including supplements (see Table 11.6). The majority of these agents cause hypertension by enhancing vasoconstriction. Any child or adolescent presenting with severe and symptomatic hypertension who does not have evident renal disease on initial testing and is not on a prescribed medication known to cause hypertension should be evaluated for the possibility of drug-induced hypertension.

Less Common Causes

While less common than renal parenchymal causes of hypertension, vascular causes of hypertension should always be considered in a child with significant hypertension (Table 11.7). Often a child with a vascular cause of hypertension presents with asymptomatic and severe hypertension with no evident renal disease based on urinalysis or blood tests. Because the hypertension has been long-standing and gradual, those with aortic coarctation or renal artery stenosis typically present with incidentally found severe hypertension that is asymptomatic. Renal artery stenosis can be idiopathic, such as with fibromuscular dysplasia, or syndromic. Any child who carries a diagnosis of Williams syndrome, Turner syndrome, or neurofibromatosis should be routinely screened for hypertension, since aortic coarctation (Williams and

Turner syndromes) or renal artery stenotic lesions associated with these syndromes are typically asymptomatic and can become manifest as severe hypertension at any time during childhood.

Renal vascular stenosis or compromise can be acquired acutely and in that setting more often presents as symptomatic hypertension. Tumor compression of renal vasculature from Wilms tumor, abdominal neuroblastoma, or lymphoma can cause severe acute hypertension. Large-vessel vasculitis, such as Takayasu arteritis or moyamoya disease, may be occult but then presents with neurologic symptoms and severe hypertension.

Neoplastic disease, separate from those that cause compromise of the major renal vasculature, can directly cause hypertension. Nephroblastoma or lymphoma may cause hypertension by direct infiltration of normal renal parenchyma. Pheochromocytoma and neuroblastoma cause hypertension through elaboration of excessive catecholamines. This may result in severe and symptomatic hypertension at presentation, especially with pheochromocytoma (Table 11.8).

Neurologic injury or disease often has associated elevation in blood pressure. Typically, the elevated blood pressure is acute and transient, not resulting in long-standing hypertension. Increased intracranial pressure from head trauma, intracranial tumor, or idiopathic intracranial hypertension (pseudotumor cerebri) often results in high blood pressure, which if present speaks to the severity of the intracranial pressure and need for acute intervention for the primary problem. Peripheral neuropathies such as from Guillain-Barré syndrome or poliomyelitis commonly have hypertension from autonomic dysfunction in the acute phase of the disease. Hypertension in this setting typically resolves with recovery from the illness, but in some cases can persist.

Blood pressure is often elevated during seizure activity and does not require antihypertensive treatment or specific evaluation if seizure alone is clearly the cause of the elevated blood pressure. However, since hypertensive crisis caused by several underlying diseases, such as acute glomerulonephritis, may present with new-onset seizures, it must always be considered whether the finding of elevated blood pressure is

TABLE 11.9 Clinical Findings in Patients with Mineralocorticoid Excess

Condition	Clinical Presentation
CAH: 11β-hydroxylase deficiency	Early growth spurt initially, then short adult stature; advanced bone age, premature adrenarche, acne, precocious puberty in males, amenorrhea/hirsutism/virilism in females (autosomal recessive)
CAH: 17α-hydroxylase deficiency	Pseudohermaphroditism (male), sexual infantilism (female) (autosomal recessive)
Apparent mineralocorticoid excess	Growth retardation/short stature, nephrocalcinosis (autosomal recessive)
Liddle syndrome	Severe hypertension, hypokalemia, and metabolic alkalosis, muscle weakness (autosomal dominant)
Mineralocorticoid receptor gain-of-function mutation	Early onset of hypertension (before age 20 yr), exacerbated in pregnancy
Glucocorticoid remediable aldosteronism (GRA) (familial aldosteronism type 1)	Early onset of hypertension, presence of family history of mortality or morbidity from early hemorrhagic stroke (autosomal dominant)
Pseudohypoaldosteronism type 2 (Gordon syndrome)	Short stature, hyperkalemic and hyperchloremic metabolic acidosis, borderline blood pressure (autosomal dominant)
Glucocorticoid resistance (children) (Chrousos syndrome)	Ambiguous genitalia, precocious puberty; women may have androgen excess: acne, excessive hair, oligo/anovulation, infertility (familial or sporadic)

CAH, congenital adrenal hyperplasia.

Modified from Kliegman RM, St. Geme JW III, Blum NJ, et al, eds. *Nelson Textbook of Pediatrics.* 21st e. Philadelphia: Elsevier; 2020:2493, Table 472.4.

the cause or effect of the seizure. If hypertension is the effect of the seizure, blood pressure usually returns to normal rapidly after the seizure resolves. However, if blood pressure remains persistently and significantly elevated with resolution of seizure activity, hypertension causing the seizure then becomes much more likely. In that instance treatment of and evaluation for the underlying cause of symptomatic hypertension are imperative.

Rare Causes

While well known to cause elevated blood pressure, endocrine causes of hypertension are rare in childhood (see Table 11.5). Other than catecholamine-secreting tumors, endocrine causes of hypertension do not typically present as hypertension as the principal feature. More often high blood pressure is found when being evaluated for other signs or symptoms attributable to the underlying endocrine disorder. The hypertension resolves when the underlying disorder is discovered and effectively treated. Mineralocorticoid excess from monogenetic etiologies or other causes frequently produces hypertension (Table 11.9).

Monogenic forms of hypertension (see Table 11.5) are exceedingly rare and considered only when renal disease or other identifiable causes of secondary hypertension have been ruled out, and the child does not fit the clinical picture of primary or obesity-associated hypertension. A unifying feature of most monogenic forms of hypertension is that the causative single-gene variant effects enhanced renal sodium resorption, which leads to volume expansion with resultant hypertension. A clue that a monogenic cause of hypertension might be present is that abnormalities in blood potassium may be found because several of the gene variants in this group of disorders affect mineralocorticoid pathways. **Hyperkalemia** and a metabolic acidosis are noted in pseudohypoaldosteronism type 2 (familial hyperkalemic hypertension: **Gordon syndrome**). Gordon syndrome is an autosomal dominant disorder in most patients; the involved genes include *KLHL3*, *CUL3*, *WNK1*, and *WNK4*. **Hypokalemia** is suggestive of **Liddle syndrome** (autosomal dominant; epithelial sodium channel), **Geller syndrome** (autosomal dominant; gain of function in mineralocorticoid receptor), glucocorticoid remedial aldosteronism, and other hyperaldosteronism-like states. In those conditions, hypokalemia is variable and a metabolic alkalosis may also be present.

EVALUATION

In all pediatric patients found to have hypertension, the initial approach is garnering a thorough history and physical examination. Not only does this direct the practitioner to investigations likely to identify the cause, but also it identifies those patients in whom investigation must move quickly. The speed and breadth of needed evaluation are driven by the severity of blood pressure elevation and whether there are associated signs and symptoms that indicate a potentially serious underlying disease or hypertensive crisis.

Secondary hypertension must always be considered in all children who have clearly defined persistent or symptomatic hypertension. Because of the high incidence of specific, identifiable causes of hypertension in the young, even the older child or adolescent who may on initial evaluation seem to fit the picture of primary hypertension requires investigation to rule out more common causes of secondary hypertension. Therefore, in all pediatric patients with clearly defined sustained hypertension, even if mild, focused work-up for an underlying cause is warranted. The younger the child, the more likely it is that an identifiable cause of secondary hypertension is present, to where in infancy nearly all cases have a cause found (Fig. 11.1).

INVESTIGATION OF INFANTILE HYPERTENSION

Most important in neonates/infants is the need for renal imaging. Renal ultrasound *with* Doppler investigation of the major vessels is the primary study recommended in this age group. Cystic kidney disease and CAKUT are readily identified with ultrasound. In addition, the tumors of infancy that can cause hypertension are also typically seen on renal ultrasound.

The Doppler study is primarily performed to rule out thrombus in a major vessel of a kidney, especially in the main renal vein, but also on rare occasion a major renal artery thrombus is found. Doppler study of the renal arteries has low sensitivity for identifying renal artery stenosis (RAS), either acquired or congenital. Thus, if not found by Doppler study, RAS is not ruled out. A clue that there may be underlying unilateral RAS is significant size discrepancy on ultrasound between the kidneys, which otherwise have normal architecture and echogenicity. If other entities are ruled out and RAS is suspected, an angiographic study is required to provide the diagnosis. Direct, invasive angiography to evaluate for RAS carries significant risk in early infancy, so it is typically deferred until late infancy or later, depending on the severity of hypertension and ability to control the hypertension with medication. The first step to evaluate for RAS is noninvasive methods, either CT or magnetic

resonance angiography. As image resolution of the vasculature using either of these methods improves with the age of the infant, the timing of performing the study is commonly determined by a nephrologist in consultation with an imaging specialist, with the same consideration of whether the study is urgent based on the ability to control the infant's hypertension with medication.

While imaging is the primary investigation that reveals the cause of hypertension in infancy, additional studies are indicated at the start of the investigation for hypertension in this group. Urinalysis should be performed on a sample obtained by bag collection, which helps avoid a false-positive result for blood, which often occurs when the sample is collected by catheterization. The lack of blood or protein on the urinalysis effectively rules out a rare congenital or acquired glomerulopathy of infancy. CBC should also be performed as thrombocytopenia may herald an occult major thrombus, such as a renal vein thrombus, or a microangiopathy affecting the kidneys, such as a rare atypical HUS. Finally, renal function should be assessed by measuring blood electrolytes and creatinine levels.

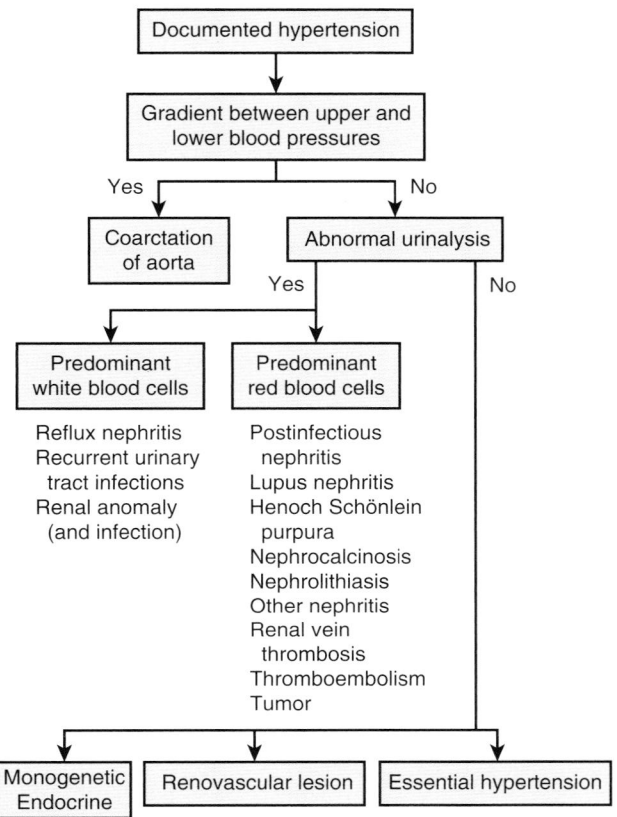

Fig. 11.1 Initial diagnostic algorithm in the evaluation of hypertension. (Modified from Kliegman RM, St. Geme JW III, Blum NJ, et al., eds. *Nelson Textbook of Pediatrics.* 21st ed. Philadelphia: Elsevier; 2020:2493, Fig. 472.1.)

INVESTIGATION OF SYMPTOMATIC CHILDHOOD HYPERTENSION (FIG. 11.2 AND TABLE 11.10)

Children who present with symptomatic hypertension, whether the symptoms be from the hypertension (e.g., headache, visual disturbance, seizure, or other neurologic symptoms) or associated with the underlying disease causing the hypertension (e.g., constitutional symptoms, joint symptoms, skin lesions, gross hematuria, or edema), are likely to have an acute glomerular disease. Initial investigation should be prompt and focus on potential etiologies. Initial testing should include blood and urine tests to screen for acute glomerulopathy. Urinalysis showing blood and/or protein in the urine is indicative of likely underlying glomerular disease. Urine microscopy showing red blood cell (RBC) casts confirm glomerulonephritis, but unfortunately the vast majority of clinical laboratories are unable to identify RBC casts when present, so the lack of RBC casts does not rule out glomerulonephritis (see Chapter 23). A complete metabolic panel may reveal renal insufficiency, with high BUN and creatinine supporting further investigation of renal cause for the hypertension. Low blood albumin on that panel may either indicate nephrotic level of proteinuria or be secondary to

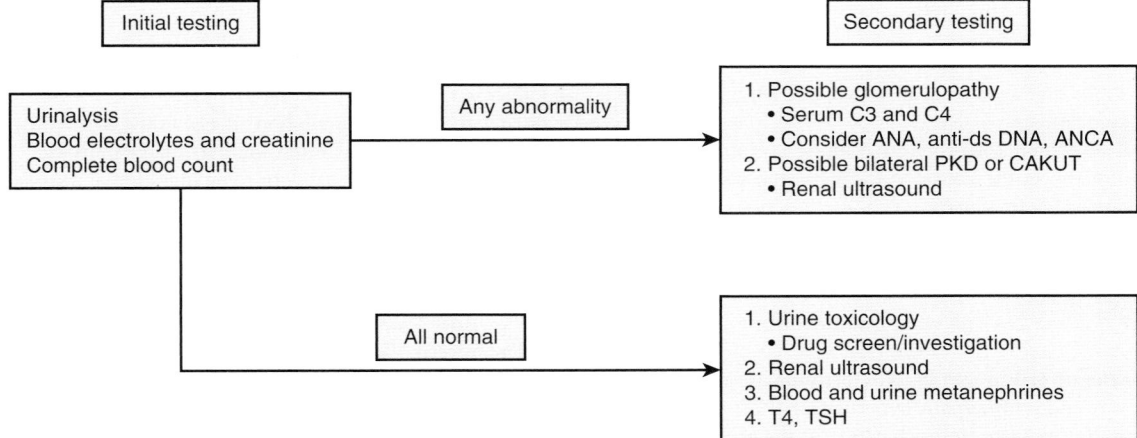

Fig. 11.2 Evaluation of symptomatic hypertension. ANA, antinuclear antibody; ANCA, antineutrophil cytoplasmic antibody; C3 and C4, complement levels; CAKUT, congenital abnormalities of the kidneys and urinary tract; PKD, polycystic kidney disease; T4, thyroxine test; TSH, thyroid-stimulating hormone.

TABLE 11.10   Clinical Evaluation of Confirmed Hypertension

Study or Procedure	Purpose	Target Population
Evaluation for Identifiable Causes		
History, including sleep history, family history, risk factors, diet, and habits such as smoking and drinking alcohol; physical examination	History and physical examination help focus subsequent evaluation	All children with persistent BP ≥90th percentile
Blood urea nitrogen, creatinine, electrolytes, urinalysis, and urine culture	R/O renal disease and chronic pyelonephritis, mineralocorticoid excess states	All children with persistent BP ≥95th percentile
Complete blood count	R/O anemia, consistent with chronic renal disease	All children with signs of chronic kidney disease
Renal ultrasound	R/O renal scar, congenital anomaly, or disparate renal size	All children with signs or symptoms concerning for secondary cause of hypertension
Evaluation for Comorbidity		
Fasting lipid panel, fasting glucose	Identify hyperlipidemia, metabolic abnormalities	Overweight patients with BP at 90th–94th percentile; all patients with BP ≥95th percentile; family history of hypertension or cardiovascular disease; child with chronic renal disease
Drug screen	Identify substances that might cause hypertension	History suggestive of possible contribution by substances or drugs
Polysomnography	Identify sleep-disordered breathing	History of loud, frequent snoring or daytime somnolence
Evaluation for Target-Organ Damage		
Echocardiogram	Identify left ventricular hypertrophy and other indications of cardiac involvement	Patients with comorbid risk factors* and BP 90th–94th percentile; all patients with BP ≥95th percentile
Retinal exam	Identify retinal vascular changes	Patients with comorbid risk factors and BP 90th–94th percentile; all patients with BP ≥95th percentile
Additional Evaluation as Indicated		
Ambulatory blood pressure monitoring	Identify white coat hypertension, abnormal diurnal BP pattern, BP load	All children with persistent BP ≥95th percentile
Renovascular imaging: magnetic resonance or CT angiography	Identify renovascular disease	Young children with stage 1 hypertension and any child or adolescent with stage 2 hypertension
Arteriography: digital subtraction or classic		
Plasma and urine catecholamines: MRI with PET scan	Identify catecholamine-mediated hypertension	Patients with signs and symptoms concerning for pheochromocytoma

BP, blood pressure; R/O, rule out.
*Comorbid risk factors also include diabetes mellitus and kidney disease.
From Kliegman RM, St. Geme JW III, Blum NJ, et al., eds. *Nelson Textbook of Pediatrics.* 21st ed. Philadelphia: Elsevier; 2020:2495, Table 472.6.

inflammation from underlying systemic vasculitis. CBC is also indicated at presentation. Anemia along with low platelet count raises the possibility of HUS but also may indicate hematologic involvement from systemic lupus erythematosus, in which case leukopenia often is an accompanying feature.

If there is clear evidence on the initial blood and urine tests that acute glomerulopathy is the cause of the hypertension, then renal imaging is not needed. In that instance, further investigation with serologic studies to determine the precise cause of the glomerulopathy is indicated. If the pattern does not fit HUS, then additional testing should include C3 and C4 blood complement levels along with antinuclear antibody (ANA) panel and antineutrophil cytoplasmic antibody.

However, if the urinalysis and blood creatinine are normal, other etiologies of severe and symptomatic hypertension must be pursued. If neurologic symptoms are a prominent feature of the presentation and brain imaging is unremarkable, drug ingestion needs to be considered. Urine toxicology screen can rapidly identify common agents that cause symptomatic hypertension, such as cocaine and amphetamines, but is not able to identify a variety of other illicit drugs that can cause severe

hypertension. So, if drug ingestion is suspected and prompt return of the urine toxicology screen is not informative, the urine sample should also be sent for a full drug investigation. The latter testing takes much longer to complete, but if that investigation is not considered and sent during the acute presentation, the window to identify this cause of acute symptomatic hypertension may then be missed.

If acute glomerulopathy or toxic ingestion appears to be ruled out, renal imaging is then indicated, since other forms of parenchymal renal disease may present as severe hypertension at any age and on occasion have associated symptoms. Renal ultrasound in this setting readily identifies congenital urinary tract abnormalities as well as cystic kidney diseases that may present primarily with hypertension, including severe hypertension.

Investigation for Asymptomatic, Less Common, and Rare Causes of Childhood Hypertension (Fig. 11.3 and see Table 11.10)

If the blood creatinine and urinalysis are normal on initial screening and renal ultrasound is normal, an abnormality in blood electrolytes on the chemistry panel may suggest other etiologies for the significant

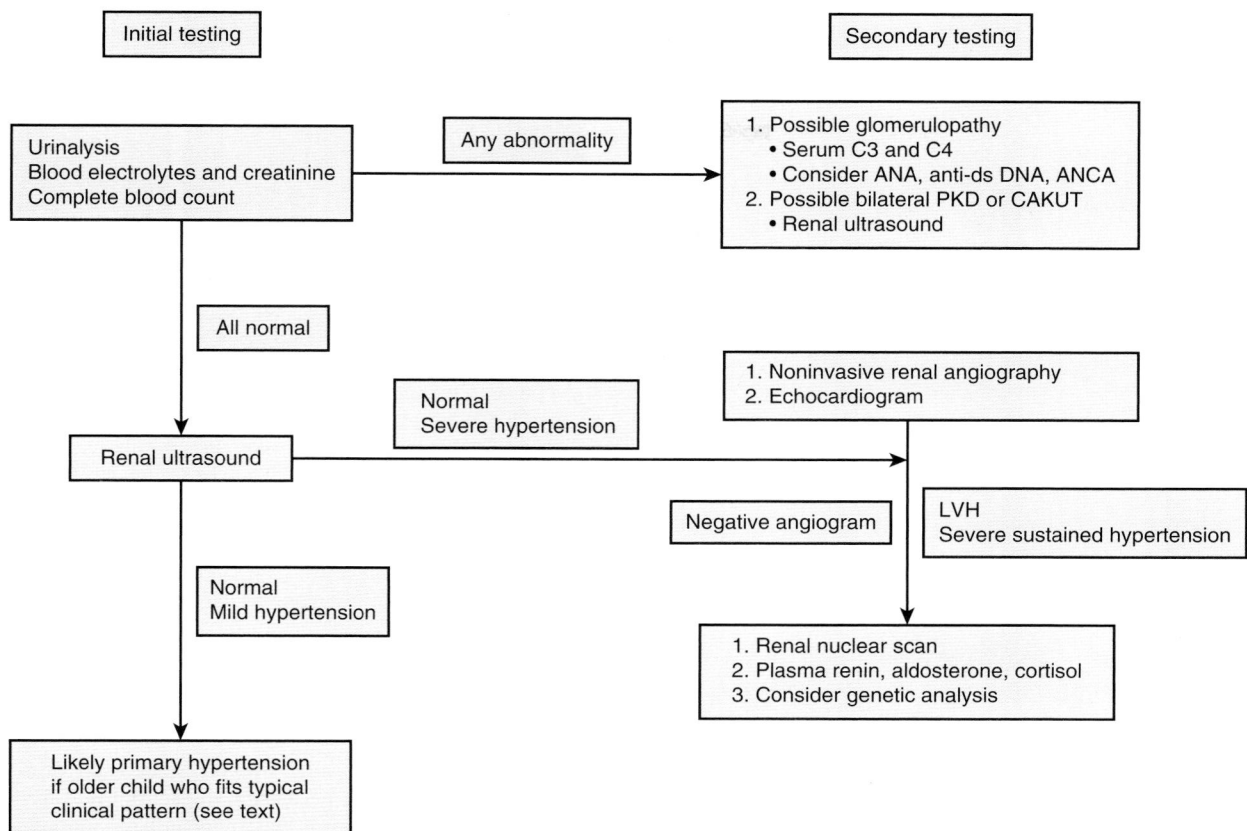

Fig. 11.3 Evaluation of asymptomatic hypertension. ANA, antinuclear antibody; ANCA, antineutrophil cytoplasmic antibody; C3 and C4, complement levels; CAKUT, congenital abnormalities of the kidneys and urinary tract; LVH, left ventricular hypertrophy; PKD, polycystic kidney disease.

hypertension. Low blood potassium is commonly seen when renal artery stenosis is present, as the hypertension is secondary to prominent activation of the renin-angiotensin system. In addition, several of the monogenic causes of hypertension have associated abnormality of blood potassium, especially those with low potassium level from hyperaldosteronism.

If the hypertension is severe at presentation and the more common etiologies of secondary hypertension have been ruled out with the initial investigations as noted earlier, the possibility of an underlying renovascular cause then needs to be explored. Aortic coarctation should always be considered and is simply ruled out on examination using four-extremity blood pressure measurements (see "Physical Examination" section previously). The first step to evaluate for a possible renal artery stenosis is with a noninvasive abdominal CT or magnetic resonance angiogram. If these are negative, an actual angiogram may need to be performed (Fig. 11.4).

Nuclear scans may identify isolated renal vascular or focal parenchymal disease as the cause of hypertension. A radionucleotide renal perfusion scan can identify an area of segmental poor renal perfusion indicative of a scar from a previous renal insult, such as from an episode of pyelonephritis or an occult segmental renal infarction as may occur from thromboembolism or secondary to vasculitis. Unilateral poor global perfusion of a kidney on a captopril renal perfusion scan is indicative of unilateral renal artery stenosis. The need to use a captopril renal scan to identify likely renal artery stenosis has waned as the resolution of the renal vasculature imaging by CT and magnetic

resonance angiograms has improved substantially to provide the diagnosis.

An echocardiogram can serve two roles in the evaluation of a hypertensive patient. First, it has high sensitivity in confirming aortic coarctation in a patient who has strong evidence for coarctation based on the physical examination revealing the typical discrepancy between arm and leg blood pressure values. Second, an echocardiogram can help assess the significance of the hypertension in patients whose blood pressure is difficult to measure consistently, and can also give some sense of duration of hypertension in those who present with symptomatic or severe hypertension. Finding significant left ventricular hypertrophy (LVH) on echocardiogram indicates end-organ effect from hypertension that is not acute, and may have been occult and long-standing. If LVH is present on echocardiogram and initial studies have not found one of the more common causes of hypertension, it then becomes imperative to pursue further diagnostic studies, including those for rare forms of hypertension.

Rare causes of hypertension are pursued as symptoms suggest or if hypertension is significant and otherwise unexplained. Associated symptoms or signs of tachycardia and flushing suggest the possibility of a catecholamine-secreting tumor or thyroid disease. In that scenario, thyroid function tests or blood and urine catecholamine studies reveal the etiology. If an endocrine cause other than thyroid disease is suspected (see Table 11.5) based on clinical presentation or blood electrolyte abnormality on screening studies, blood renin, aldosterone, and cortisol levels are tested. If a pheochromocytoma is suspected

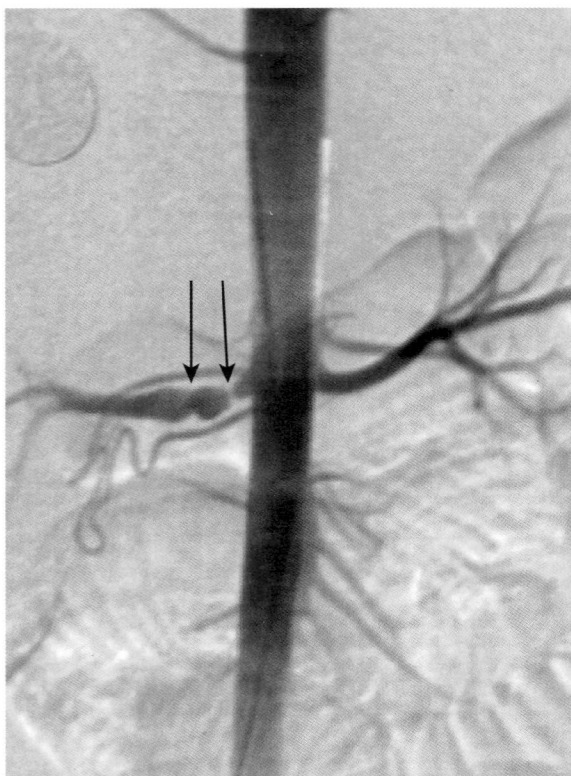

Fig. 11.4 Renal angiogram in 7-year-old boy with hypertension. Right renal artery is visible with a string-of-beads appearance characteristic of fibromuscular dysplasia *(arrows)*. The aorta and left renal artery appear normal. (From Kliegman RM, St. Geme JW III, Blum NJ, et al., eds. *Nelson Textbook of Pediatrics*. 21st ed. Philadelphia: Elsevier; 2020:2496, Fig. 472.2.)

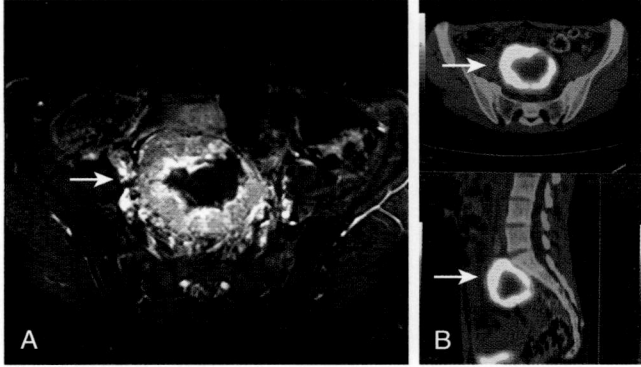

Fig. 11.5 *A,* A 14-year-old girl with paroxysmal hypertension, tachycardia, and biochemical evidence of catecholamine excess with almost exclusively norepinephrine secretion (fractionated 24-hour urinary normetanephrine 15,245 µg/24 hours, n.r. 88–444, and metanephrines <32 µg/24 hours, n.r. 52–341). MRI of the abdomen revealed a 7.5 pelvic mass with high signal intensity on T2 weighted sequences and areas of necrosis. *B,* The mass had increased uptake on ^{18}F-FDG PET/CT (SUVmax 12.4). Histology confirmed paraganglioma, and genetic testing revealed *SDHB* mutation. (Modified from Delivanis DA, Vassiliadi DA, Tsagarakis S. Adrenal imaging in patients with endocrine hypertension. *Endocrinol Metab Clin N Am.* 2019;48:667–680 [Fig. 4, p. 676].)

(see Table 11.8), plasma-free metanephrines are the initial test but followed by a 24-hour urinary metanephrine *and* catecholamine test. Adrenal CT or MRI is the initial imaging study, but CT or MRI combined with PET scanning is the most accurate study for neuroendocrine tumors (Figs. 11.5 and 11.6).

Monogenic forms of hypertension are not usually explored unless the clinical pattern does not fit that of primary hypertension, all other potential identifiable causes are ruled out, or an abnormality on blood electrolytes, especially blood potassium level consistent with a monogenic cause of hypertension, is present. When considering a monogenic form of hypertension, blood renin and aldosterone levels are measured initially, since many of the single-gene variants that cause hypertension impact the aldosterone pathway. All monogenic causes of hypertension have suppressed renin levels (Fig. 11.7). However, the most effective method to make a diagnosis of a monogenic form of hypertension is by genetic sequencing and analysis.

There is no specific test to make the diagnosis of primary hypertension. It is effectively a diagnosis of exclusion made in the context of the typical clinical pattern. It requires ruling out common identifiable causes of hypertension in a child presenting with asymptomatic and mild hypertension. The diagnosis is made, then, when the following pattern is met: the patient is an older child or adolescent, the patient is asymptomatic, the level of hypertension is mild, and there is no evidence of significant end-organ effect (e.g., no LVH on echocardiogram). In addition, there are no abnormalities on the initial screening studies and no history to suggest a renal injury having occurred earlier in the child's life, such as in the perinatal period. There is usually a family history of early-onset hypertension and concomitant significant obesity, bordering on developing associated metabolic syndrome.

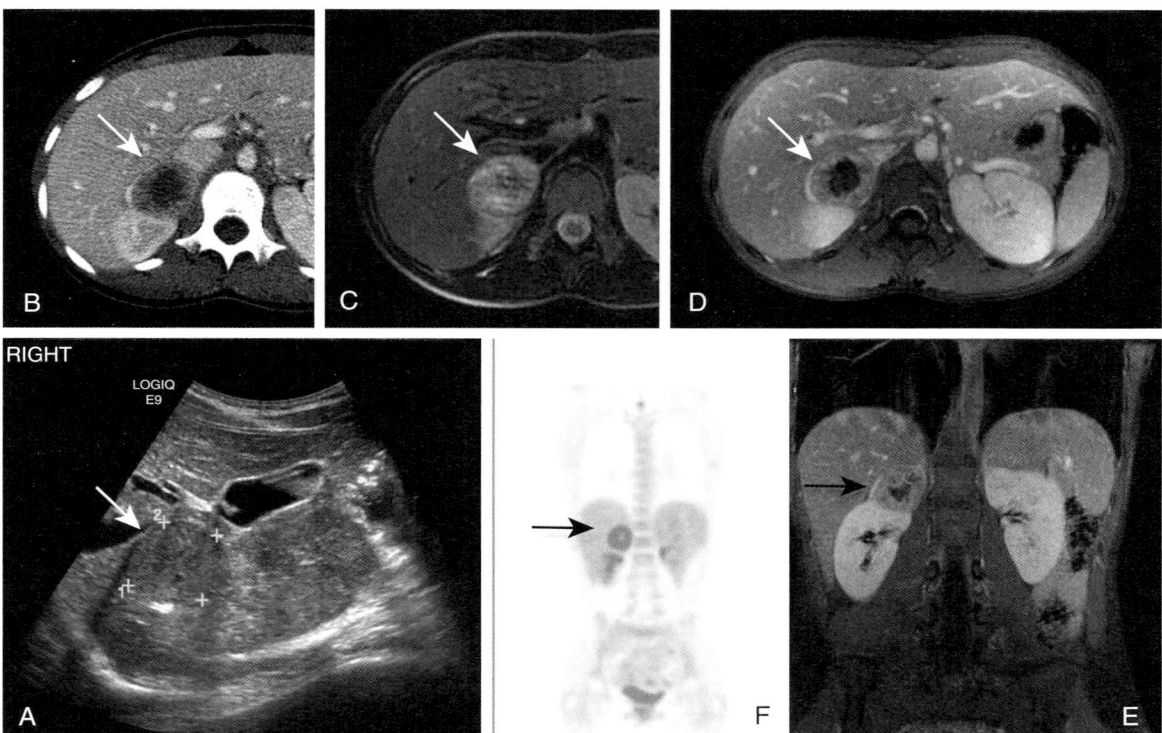

Fig. 11.6 Pheochromocytoma. A young male presented with episodes of hypertension and headaches. *A,* Ultrasound shows a heterogeneously hypoechoic right adrenal mass. *B,* CT shows peripheral thick rind of enhancement and central necrosis. MRI showed high T2 *(C)* signal (light bulb sign) and peripheral enhancement on T1 weighted images *(D). E,* Coronal image shows the right adrenal pheochromocytoma and its relationship with the right kidney. *F,* PET/CT performed for staging showed intense peripheral hypermetabolism (SUVmax of 10.8) and central photopenia (necrosis). No evidence of metastatic disease was seen and the patient underwent surgical resection. (From Bhargava P, Sangster G, Haque K, et al. A multimodality review of adrenal tumors. *Curr Prob Diag Radiol.* 2019;49:605–615 [Fig. 12, p. 611].)

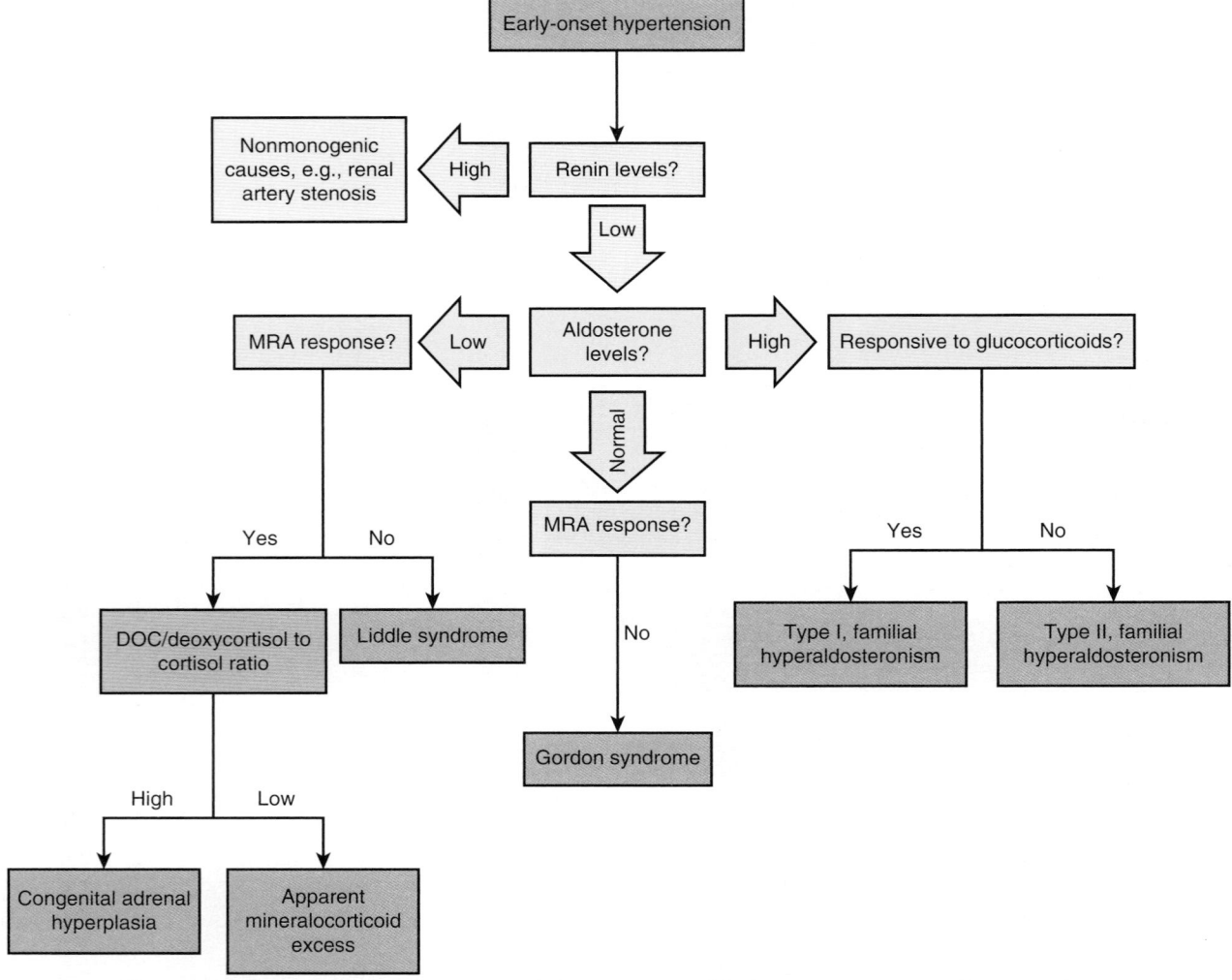

Fig. 11.7 Diagnostic evaluation for monogenic hypertension. DOC, deoxycorticosterone; MRA, mineralocorticoid receptor antagonist. (From Raina R, Krishnappa V, Das A, et al. Overview of monogenic or mendelian forms of hypertension. *Front Pediatr.* 2019;7:263 [Fig. 1].)

RED FLAGS

Symptoms of mental status change, severe headache, and/or blurry vision associated with stage 2 hypertension require urgent evaluation and management. Physical findings of papilledema on fundoscopy, gallop rhythm on cardiac exam, or any neurologic finding also indicates the need for urgent evaluation and management. Associated hematuria and/or generalized edema should be promptly evaluated.

Four-extremity blood pressure with discrepancy between lower and upper extremities or lag in pulse intensity between upper and lower extremities indicates coarctation of the aorta. Symptomatic acute hypertension in later childhood with normal initial testing should raise concern for drug-induced hypertension.

BIBLIOGRAPHY

A bibliography is available at ExpertConsult.com.

12

Failure to Thrive

Susan Feigelman and Virginia Keane

Calories from food provide energy for the body's maintenance functions of repair, regulation, metabolism, replacement of losses, and daily activity. Children have additional caloric requirements because they are growing. Children under the age of 3 years whose caloric needs are not met do not grow according to published norms and are said to have failure to thrive (FTT) or growth faltering. FTT raises serious concerns. It is important to have a systematic, stepwise approach to the diagnosis and management of poor growth in young children and to follow growth over time.

The term **failure to thrive** describes growth failure that accompanies many pathologic as well as psychosocial causes. Differentiation between organic (biomedical) and nonorganic (psychosocial/environmental) is not always useful; children often have a combination of psychosocial and biomedical problems. Children with medical conditions will often have psychosocial issues related to eating and dysfunctional feeding patterns. Children with primarily social or emotional issues around eating may develop medical consequences of undernutrition.

The best diagnostic tool available to the clinician is a comprehensive history, including diet, growth (over time), family and social histories, and a complete review of systems. A thorough physical examination is necessary. Further work-up should be directed by results from this initial evaluation. There is a poor yield from exhaustive laboratory evaluations. Children with either biomedical or psychosocial causes of FTT may or may not gain weight in institutional settings; short-term outcome may not be diagnostic.

NORMAL GROWTH

Newborns typically lose up to 10–12% of their birthweight during the first few days of life and regain this weight by the age of 2 weeks. Subsequently, they gain weight at a steady pace of about 1 ounce per day for the first 2 or 3 months; they gain at half to two thirds that rate for the next 3 months and half to two thirds again for the next 6 months. This results in a doubling of birthweight by the age of 4–6 months and a tripling at about 1 year. Height and head circumference grow at similar well-defined rates. These three growth parameters, along with weight/length, should be plotted on appropriate growth charts and monitored for adherence to standard growth rates. Children grow in a stepwise manner, but on average their growth pattern follows the accepted curves (see Chapter 56). Online tools are available to assist with the determination of growth status (http://peditools.org).

By the age of 3 years, if caloric intake is normal, the child's growth adjusts to their genetic potential. Ultimate height is determined by additional factors, among them rates of bone maturity and pubertal development (see Chapter 56). Considerable energy from ingested food is required to achieve this growth. The energy balance can be described by the following equation, in which E equals energy:

$$E_{IN} = E_{OUT} + E_{growth} + E_{stored}$$

E_{OUT} is the sum of the basal metabolic rate, energy expended in physical activity, and energy needed for food digestion. Children should be in a positive energy balance for growth. Any imbalance in this energy equation (losing or using more calories than are ingested) results in abnormal growth patterns. Weight is usually affected first, followed by height and finally head circumference if the energy imbalance is severe and prolonged in young children.

DEFINITIONS

FTT is a sign, not a diagnosis. FTT is generally used to describe children younger than 2 or 3 years who meet any of the following criteria:
1. Growth under the third percentile on World Health Organization (WHO) weight-for-age growth charts (less than 2 standard deviations [SD] below mean)
2. Weight for height or body mass index (BMI) less than the third percentile
3. Growth patterns that have crossed two major percentiles downward on the weight-for-age charts within 6 months
4. Growth velocity less than normal for age

There are inherent problems with these definitions. Two percent of the normal population is under 2 SD below the mean; those who are growing appropriately per their genetic potential must be differentiated from those with growth problems. The child who has been obese and is now approaching normal weight, crossing major weight percentiles in the process, should not be considered a child with FTT. Some children are naturally slim. The clinician must exercise considerable judgment before raising the concern of poor growth.

Additional terms are used to describe children who are not growing well. A child has **wasting** if the weight for length (or height) is below −2 SD (or −2 z-scores, which is equal to <2nd centile). **Stunting** is defined as a child whose height or length is less than −2 z-scores due to chronic undernutrition. In the third year of life, children are described

TABLE 12.1		Three Major Anthropologic Categories of Failure to Thrive			
	Weight	Length/ Height	Weight/Length or BMI	Head Circumference	Associated Diseases
Type I	Decreased	Decreased/ normal	Decreased	Normal	Malnutrition of organic or nonorganic etiology, usually secondary to intestinal, pancreatic, or liver diseases; systemic illness; or psychosocial factors
Type II	Decreased	Decreased	Increased, decreased, or normal	Normal	Endocrinopathies, bony dystrophy, constitutional or genetic short stature
Type III	Decreased	Decreased	Increased, decreased, or normal	Decreased	Chromosomal (including microdeletions), metabolic disease, intrauterine and perinatal insults, severe malnutrition, congenital syndromes

Modified from Shashidar H, Toila V. Failure to thrive. In: Wyllie R, Hyams JS, Kay M, eds. *Pediatric Gastrointestinal and Liver Disease*. 4th ed. Philadelphia: Elsevier; 2011:137.

as underweight if weight/age is <3% or if BMI is <5%. Short stature or microcephaly alone is not due to nutritional deficiencies (Table 12.1).

INTERPRETATION OF GROWTH CHARTS

The evaluation for any child who is not growing well includes a careful analysis of the growth pattern over time. Measurements of length are the most susceptible to error; standard procedures should be used (see Chapter 56). Possible errors in weight, head circumference, date of birth, or plotting on the growth chart should all be considered. Once the correct data are available, the charts should be examined to answer the following questions:

- Are the measurements of length and weight proportional?
- Has the head grown adequately?
- How severe are the deficits of each measurement, relative to what is expected?
- When did the problem start; what is the progression?
- What environmental factors were present at the start of this process (weaning, introduction of new foods, food insecurity)?

Although weight is usually the most readily available measurement, measurement of length is particularly critical, because it serves as the point of reference for other diagnostic considerations. The best way to obtain accurate length measurements is to use a specially calibrated length board with a fixed headpiece and a movable footpiece. In the absence of such a device, the examiner can use a table or desk with the infant's head pressed against the wall and a firm square box or thick textbook for the sliding footer. Measurements obtained with the infant lying on a mattress and marked with a pen on the sheet are not accurate (see Chapter 56).

The choice of growth curves is important. In the United States, the recommendation is to use the WHO charts from *birth through the second year of life* (http://www.cdc.gov/growthcharts/who_charts.htm) (see Chapter 56). Some children previously classified as FTT will fall into the normal range. Their health status may be poorer than those within normal ranges on both charts. The 2000 age- and gender-specific National Center for Health Statistics growth charts published by the Centers for Disease Control and Prevention combined data across geographic and ethnic populations and are appropriate to use for children *over* 24 months of age.

Conventions (for premature infants) differ in whether to plot age in relation to actual birth date or to use corrected gestational age. Growth charts following children prenatally to infancy are available (see Fenton and Olsen at http://peditools.org). Beyond the equivalent of 40 weeks of gestation, standard charts can be used, keeping in mind that premature infants may not catch up on all parameters for 2 or 3 years.

Because infants with FTT no longer follow their growth curves, the usual convention of expressing growth measurements in relation to

normal percentiles is not always useful; weight/length or BMI z-scores better define and assess the degree of malnutrition. Children with moderate wasting have weight for height below −2 SD of the WHO Child Growth Standards median; severe wasting is defined as weight for height below −3 SD.

It is important to note the following points:

1. Infants and toddlers who are short in proportion to weight should be considered to have primary growth problems, including various endocrine (often growth hormone) and skeletal dysplasias (see Chapter 56) (see Table 12.1).
2. Infants who have had inadequate caloric intake will be abnormally thin. If the problem developed at some time after birth, weight will drop off before changes in length or head circumference.
3. Infants with disproportionately small heads may have primary neurologic or genetic (monogenetic, microdeletion, aneuploidy, syndromic) problems affecting brain growth because head growth is the last to be affected by malnutrition and is not characteristic of primary skeletal growth problems (see Table 12.1). An alternative diagnosis is craniosynostosis, or early closure of skull growth plates.

Several examples of how these patterns may be interpreted are presented in Figures 12.1 to 12.4. Growth charts adjusted for abnormal head size (micro- or macrocephaly) are not available. This factor becomes relatively less important as the child ages, but during infancy it may significantly affect the weight percentile and requires clinical judgment to assess.

Syndrome-specific growth charts have been developed for certain populations (e.g., trisomy 21, skeletal dysplasias). Their use is most appropriate for conditions that affect muscle and bone development (e.g., Russell-Silver syndrome). All other disease-specific charts should be used in conjunction with the WHO charts. Accuracy of some of these charts is suspect.

EPIDEMIOLOGY

FTT is found in all populations but has a higher prevalence among children of low socioeconomic status compared to those in higher socioeconomic groups. FTT accounts for up to 5% of all hospitalizations; up to 10% of children may have FTT at some point in time. Most affected children with nutritional problems present before the age of 3 years.

CLINICAL PRESENTATION

Parents often voice concerns about their young child's weight gain. They may complain that their child is a picky eater or seems not to drink enough formula, or they worry that breast milk supply is inadequate. Very commonly, parents complain that their child is not as big

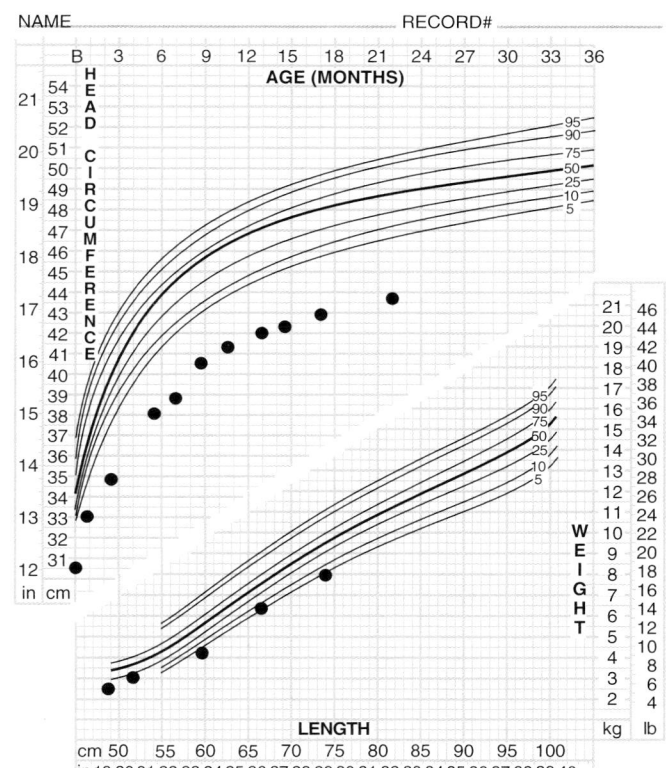

GIRLS: BIRTH TO 36 MONTHS
PHYSICAL GROWTH
NCHS PERCENTILES*

NAME _____ RECORD# _____

GIRLS: BIRTH TO 36 MONTHS
PHYSICAL GROWTH
NCHS PERCENTILES*

NAME _____ RECORD# _____

Fig. 12.1 Growth curve of an infant female with unexplained chronic failure to thrive, which affected weight and head growth more than length, which suggested an organic disorder. Intrauterine growth restriction without postnatal catch-up growth is demonstrated (see Chapter 56). (Modified from National Center for Health Statistics: NCHS growth charts. *Monthly Vital Statistics Report.* 1976;25:76–1120. Rockville, MD: Health Resources Administration, June 1976. Data from The Fels Research Institute, Yellow Springs, Ohio. Copyright 1976, Ross Laboratories.)

as a similar-aged child or a sibling at that age. Many such children are growing normally. Plotting the child's growth and reviewing it with the parents may be reassuring, or it may serve to confirm the parents' concerns. When families raise concerns about growth, regardless of whether a problem exists, the child and the weight have already become a focus of concern for that family. Often parents have already put a great deal of effort into changing the child's eating patterns, leading to intrafamily conflict. In this setting, conversations about the child's growth may carry a high emotional charge.

However, it is often the physician who is first to raise concerns. These suspicions can be confirmed by carefully plotting the growth parameters. The clinician must then prioritize the clinical issues and decide whether the FTT should be addressed immediately or deferred for evaluation and management at another time in the very near future. In rare cases, the growth failure is so severe that immediate hospitalization is indicated for nutritional rehabilitation. In this case, the

evaluation can take place over several days, while therapeutic nutritional interventions are ongoing.

APPROACH TO DETERMINING ETIOLOGY

Clinicians need to have a broad approach to determining etiology of FTT for each child. Many children with FTT, particularly those with chronic diseases, have a mixed pattern of increased needs or losses attributable to organic causes, along with environmental causes leading to calorie deprivation.

There are several growth conditions that result in smaller than normal size that are not due to calorie insufficiency. Infants who are born *symmetrically* small in all growth parameters are believed to have a reduced number of somatic cells in relation to their normal-sized peers as a result of an early intrauterine event. Infants who are *asymmetrically* small for gestational age, with sparing of the head circumference and

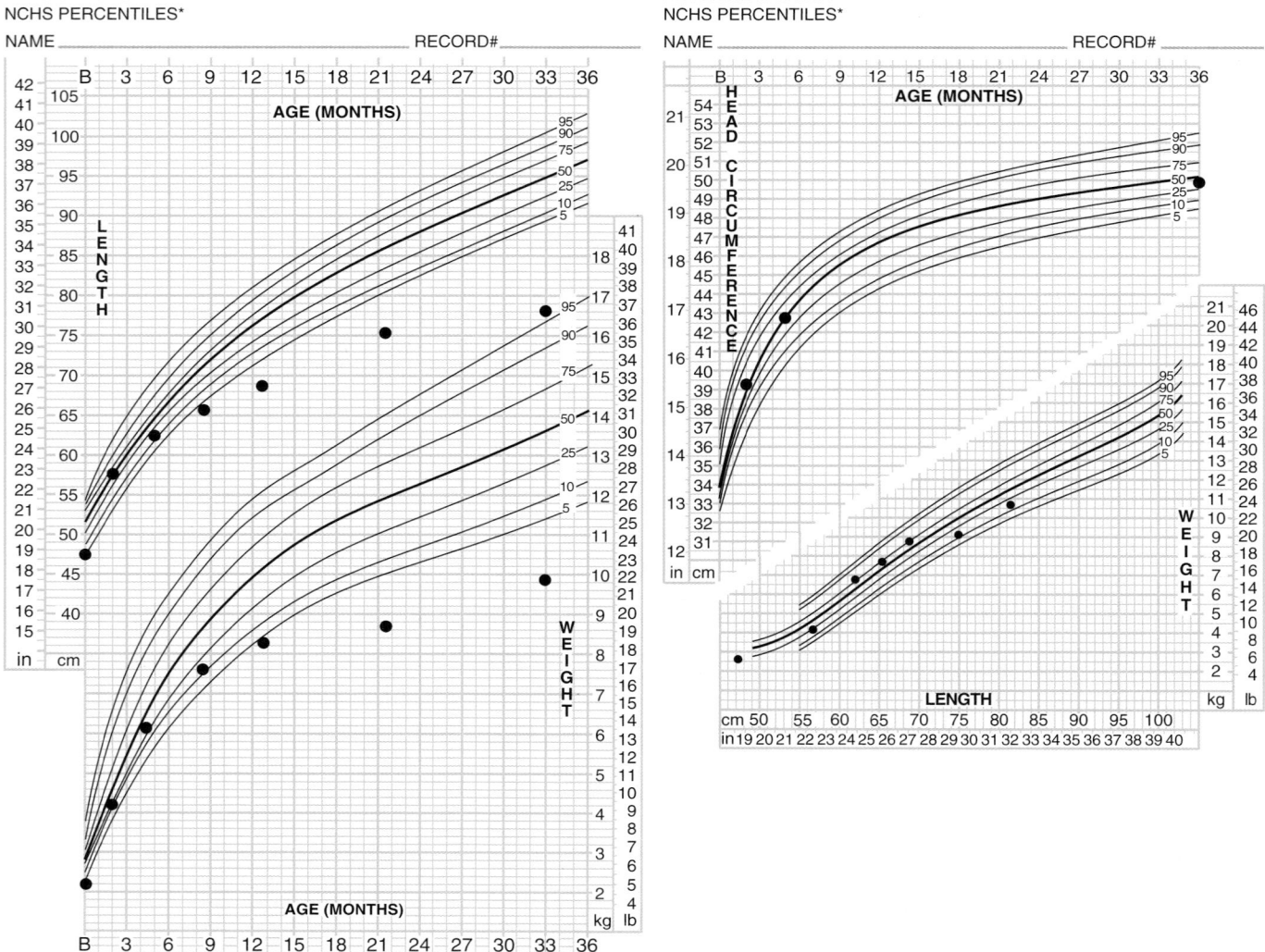

BOYS: BIRTH TO 36 MONTHS
PHYSICAL GROWTH
NCHS PERCENTILES*

NAME _____ RECORD# _____

BOYS: BIRTH TO 36 MONTHS
PHYSICAL GROWTH
NCHS PERCENTILES*

NAME _____ RECORD# _____

Fig. 12.2 Growth curve of an infant male with untreated growth hormone deficiency. Note that weight and length remain proportionate, whereas head growth is less affected. (Modified from National Center for Health Statistics: NCHS growth charts. *Monthly Vital Statistics Report.* 1976;25:76–1120. Rockville, MD: Health Resources Administration, June 1976. Data from The Fels Research Institute, Yellow Springs, Ohio. Copyright 1976, Ross Laboratories.)

possibly length, had a late intrauterine event, such as poor maternal nutrition or placental insufficiency. These infants often eat voraciously and experience catch-up growth early in life. Children with *constitutional growth delay* usually grow normally over the first few years, but weight and height decelerate to near or below the 2nd percentile followed by growth at normal rates along their new curve (see Chapter 56). The symmetric deceleration of height and weight is a clue that the child does not have calorie insufficiency. Children with genetic causes of short stature have short height for age with appropriate low weight (see Table 12.1).

Children with FTT caused by calorie insufficiency typically have decreased weight gain, at first with sparing of height and head circumference (wasting). Long-standing calorie insufficiency results in height deceleration (stunting). Decrease in height or length is the best predictor of chronic malnutrition. Only in the worst, long-standing cases is head growth decreased. This typical pattern suggests calorie insufficiency and informs the clinician of the chronicity of the problem.

There are several approaches to the differential diagnosis. The functional approach determines whether there is a problem with inadequate calorie intake, increased calorie requirement or utilization, or increased calorie loss (Table 12.2). The systems approach focuses on the identification of the organ system(s) responsible for poor growth (Table 12.3).

Another approach is to consider the age at onset, the child's developmental level, and the conditions likely to manifest at that stage of development. The causes of prenatal growth problems include environmental toxins, maternal drug and alcohol use, prenatal infection, congenital syndromes, placental insufficiency, and poor prenatal nutrition. Poor growth immediately after birth can be associated with maternal postpartum depression, bonding and attachment disorders, incorrect formula preparation, failure to establish breast-feeding, and congenital anomalies or metabolic conditions. Difficulty with transition to solid foods results in poor growth from 6 to 12 months. In children older than 9 months, issues of separation and autonomy may result in power

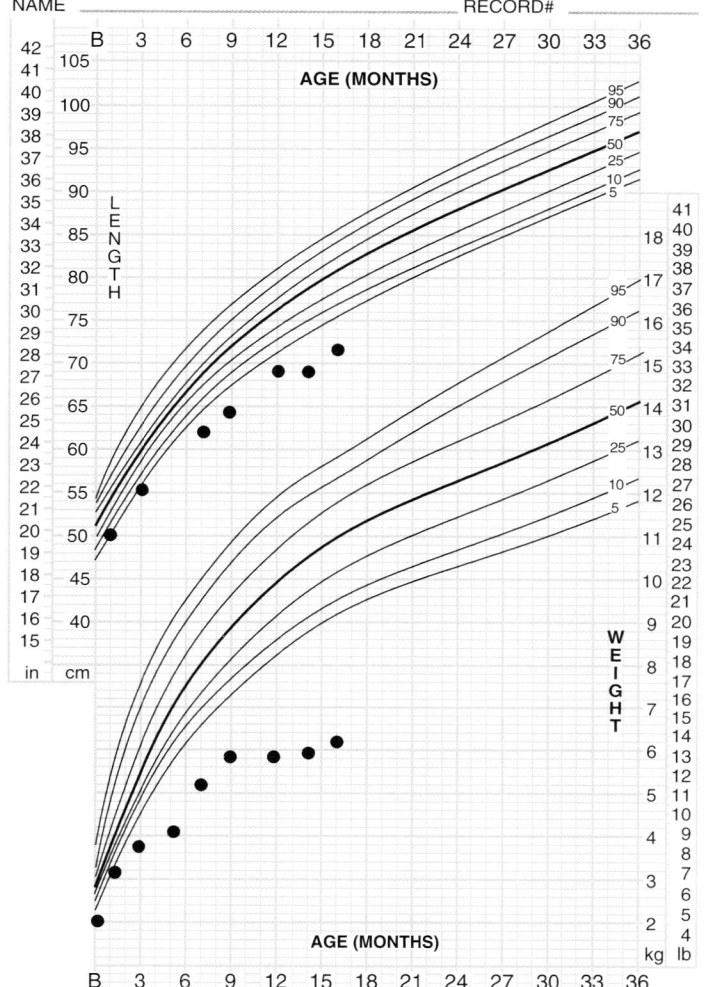

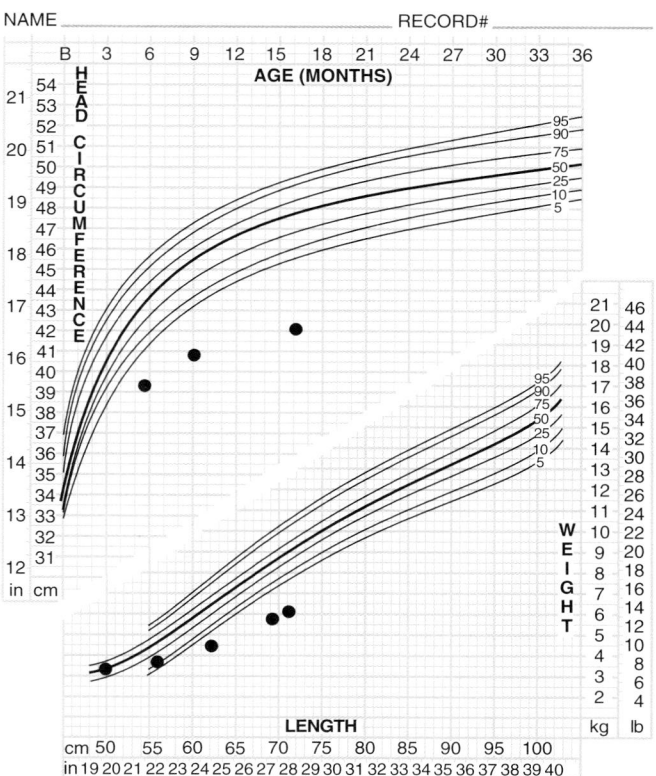

Fig. 12.3 Growth curve of an infant male with severely impaired head growth, poor weight gain, and less impairment of length. Most obvious is the marked microcephaly associated with developmental delay, suggestive of an underlying neurologic disorder. (Modified from National Center for Health Statistics: NCHS growth charts. *Monthly Vital Statistics Report.* 1976:25:76–1120. Rockville, MD: Health Resources Administration, June 1976. Data from The Fels Research Institute, Yellow Springs, Ohio. Copyright 1976, Ross Laboratories.)

struggles over eating, resulting in insufficient intake. For toddlers, poor food choices (empty calories found in juice drinks and snack foods), dysfunctional feeding interaction (restriction of self-feeding or lack of structure around meals), and distraction (chaotic home environment, television and electronic devices) may interfere with adequate food intake.

History

The history is the most important part of the evaluation of the child with FTT and guides the evaluation.

History of the Present Illness

The clinician who first notices poor growth should identify whether the family perceives a problem. What is the family members' perception of the child's food intake? When, if ever, was the problem suspected? What changes have they made to address the problem? Asking these

questions in a nonjudgmental manner will reassure the family that the clinician regards them as partners in the task of improving the child's growth.

A detailed feeding history should start with infant feeding; dietary sources and growth patterns should be chronologically reviewed. Was the child breast- or formula-fed? If breast-fed, were there any problems with milk sufficiency? Did the mother feel emotionally supported in her choice to breast-feed? If the child was formula-fed, what was the formula; how was it mixed; was there ever any reason to change formula? Was feeding a pleasurable or a difficult experience for the parent and child? These questions may give insight into problematic early parent-child interaction.

If the child is beyond infancy, when and how were solid foods introduced? Were there any specific food refusals that might indicate an allergy or intolerance? How did the child accept solids? What are the child's food preferences? When did the child start to self-feed and how

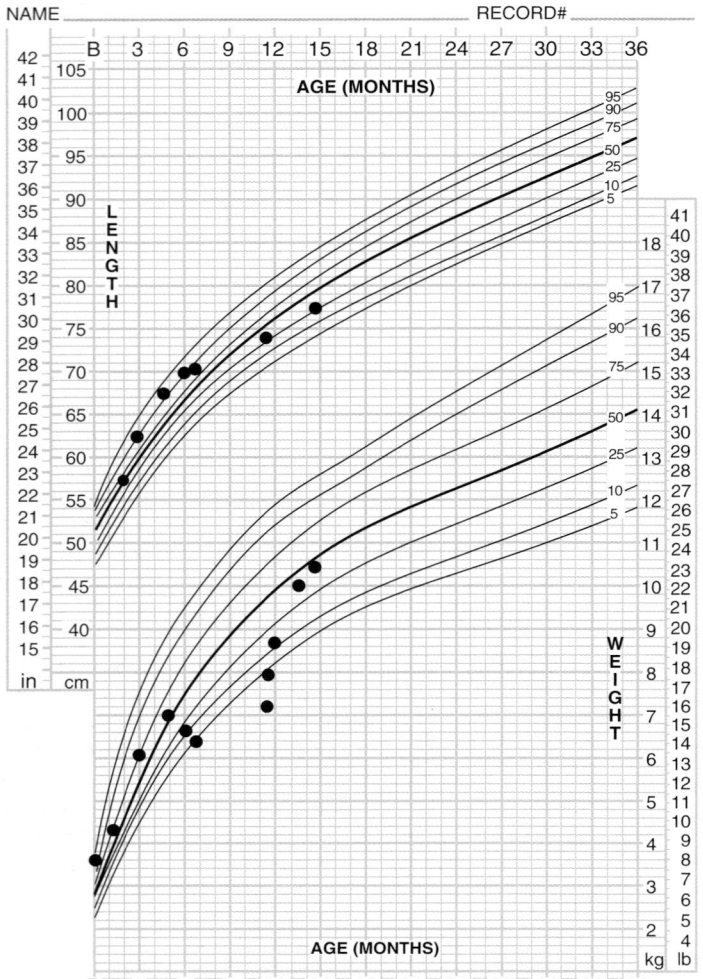

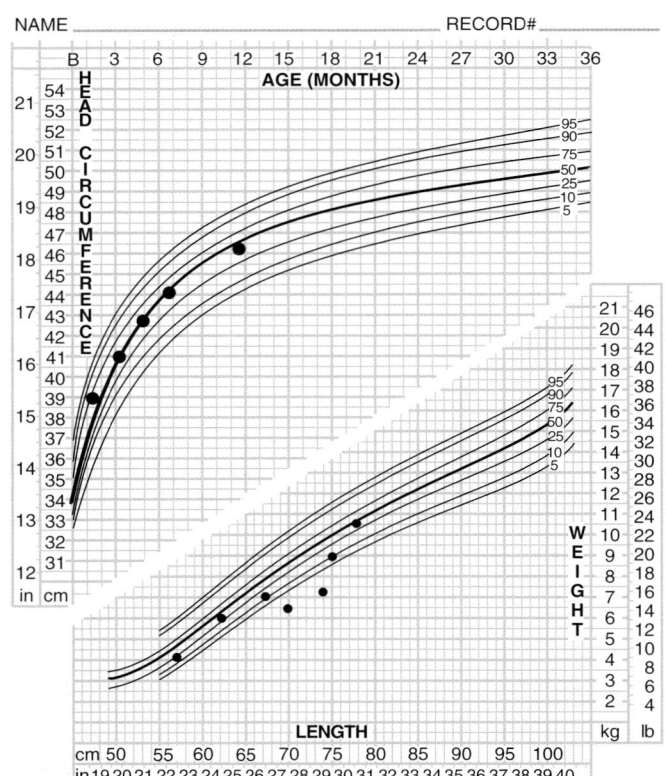

Fig. 12.4 Growth curve of an infant male with acute weight loss and catch-up weight gain. Before the age of 4¹/₂ months, there was normal growth while he was breast-feeding. After a change to an inadequate weaning diet, severe weight loss developed, but less impairment of length occurred. Head size was not affected. An acute episode of diarrhea led to multiple dietary changes that resulted in further weight loss. With a proper diet history, nutritional rehabilitation with a balanced diet resolved this child's problem. This may also be a pattern of a child with celiac disease. (Modified from National Center for Health Statistics: NCHS growth charts. *Monthly Vital Statistics Report.* 1976:25:76–1120. Rockville, MD: Health Resources Administration, June 1976. Data from The Fels Research Institute, Yellow Springs, Ohio. Copyright 1976, Ross Laboratories.)

did the family manage messiness? Where does the child eat? Is there a high chair or booster seat? Are there family meals, or does the child eat alone? What is going on in the immediate environment when the child is eating? Did a traumatic event trigger the eating problem? These questions can reveal dysfunctional eating behaviors that can affect the child's intake.

Questions about unusual eating habits or pica may indicate nutritional deficiencies, such as iron deficiency (Table 12.4). Children with difficult temperaments may have problematic eating behaviors. Are the parents forcing the child to eat?

Does the child have difficulty taking or manipulating food in the mouth? Is there frequent choking on food? Does the child drool? Is there food refusal or aversion suggesting **dysphagia**? If the response

to any of these questions is confirmatory, consider difficulty with oral motor control. This is common among children with neurologic problems.

Obtaining a daily schedule of meals and activities is very helpful. What foods are prepared and offered by other caregivers? Is there a difference in how the child eats when the child is with the parents in comparison to other caretakers?

A careful *dietary* history is imperative. The 24-hour recall is standard, although some authorities question its validity. The clinician asks the parent to remember everything the child ate in the past 24 hours and whether that was a typical day. It is helpful to start with the present and work backward. Alternatively, the parent may keep a 3-day food diary. The diary should be structured so that the type of food, quantity,

TABLE 12.2 Differential Diagnosis by Functional Category

Excessive Calorie Needs

Diabetes mellitus

Cystic fibrosis

Chronic respiratory or cardiovascular disease

Hyperthyroidism

Cerebral palsy/spasticity

Chronic infection or inflammatory diseases

Inadequate Calorie Intake

Family education and mental health: maternal depression/anxiety, psychosis, substance use, lack of parental knowledge of child nutrition needs

Parent-child interaction: parental emotional distance, mealtime distractions (e.g., television), lack of family mealtime, overindulgent or overcontrolling parent, parental inability to read hunger or satiety cues

Poor food choices: allows grazing, excessive juice intake, fad diet, fear of allergies

Child factors: neuromuscular disease, poor oral motor coordination, chronic disease with easy tiring and failure to complete meals, difficult temperament, hyperactivity, inability to display hunger cues

Economic factors: food insecurity, diluting formula, early conversion from formula to cow's milk

Food aversion: impaired swallowing, oropharyngeal or esophageal inflammation, anorexia-causing conditions, psychosocial factors

Increased Calorie Loss/Failure to Incorporate Ingested Calories

Diabetes mellitus

Malabsorption syndromes (celiac disease, lactose intolerance, cystic fibrosis, other causes of pancreatic insufficiency, chronic cholestasis)

Inborn errors of metabolism

Chronic diarrhea (multiple etiologies)

Gastroesophageal reflux and other conditions with chronic vomiting, eosinophilic gastroenteritis

Short gut syndrome

method of preparation, and amount eaten are recorded; beverages should be included. The caregiver should receive prior instruction regarding how to estimate portions and to include only what the child actually eats.

Diet review is a good opportunity to explore parental beliefs about food and the feeding of children (e.g., children must drink water, they need lots of milk, juice is good for them, fat should be restricted to prevent obesity and heart disease). It may be useful to explore parent assumptions about food based on their own experiences or beliefs. The parent who sees the child as vulnerable may be overanxious and rigid about food intake. Cultural norms may dictate certain food choices, which may not provide optimal nutrition. Vegetarian diets may provide insufficient protein, vitamins D and B_{12}, and iron. Parents may substitute goat's milk (deficient in folate) or rice or almond milk (low in protein) for cow's milk–based nutrition.

Medical History

The prenatal and perinatal history begins with the mother's age, general health, and parity. Was this pregnancy planned? What were the parents' reactions to the pregnancy? Did the mother have any emotional problems during or before her pregnancy? What was her alcohol, tobacco, and drug intake during pregnancy? When was prenatal care begun? Were there sufficient visits to monitor the pregnancy? How much weight did she gain? Were there any complications such as sexually transmitted and other infections? Were they hoping for a boy or a girl?

The perinatal history includes problems with labor, method of delivery, gestational age, and the newborn's growth parameters at birth (i.e., appropriate [AGA], small [SGA], or large [LGA] for gestational age). Is this an SGA infant who needs extra calories for catch-up growth or a newborn with intrauterine growth restriction who is small in all growth parameters? Did the baby have any problems in the nursery? A nursery stay of more than 2–3 days following a vaginal birth may indicate a problem with the newborn. Did the baby have feeding problems after birth? Was breast-feeding begun immediately?

The child's medical history should be reviewed for chronic conditions and recurrent, acute conditions, such as recurrent emesis, diarrhea, constipation, neurologic symptoms, or recurrent infections. Hospitalizations, surgical procedures, medications, allergies, and immunization status should be ascertained. Among children hospitalized with FTT, over 40% have an underlying chronic condition and some have two or more chronic conditions. It is essential to document neurodevelopmental progress, because motor or cognitive delays could be associated with neurologic dysfunction that increases calorie requirements and/or decreases feeding efficiency.

Family History

The clinician should ascertain the growth of siblings and other family members. Are there patterns of growth in the family that might result in a child growing slower than expected? What differences or similarities do the parents notice between this child and their other children? What were the growth patterns and ultimate sizes of the parents and grandparents? Document the age at menarche and puberty in parents and siblings. Creating a two-generation genogram that includes the height and weight of each family member may provide clues to the growth potential of the patient. Plotting the mean parental height on the child's height curve will help to predict ultimate stature.

A thorough family history is important. This should include early childhood deaths and any family members with genetic or metabolic conditions. Is there a family history of mental illness that might affect the child or the caretakers? Is there consanguinity?

Social History

Many cases of FTT do not have a primary medical etiology, and thus the social history is vital. Determine the family constellation. What is the relationship of the adults in the household, and how do they get along? Are the parents working, and if so, who cares for the child? Children with FTT come from all socioeconomic groups. Do the parents have nearby food stores as well as adequate storage, refrigeration, and food preparation space? Are there adequate eating facilities and implements? Are there siblings who might eat the child's food? Is the child enrolled in the Women, Infants, and Children (WIC) program? Food insecure families may be eligible for the Supplemental Nutrition Assistance Program (SNAP); both are programs of the U.S. Department of Agriculture. What is the cultural context of food selection and eating behavior?

More difficult social issues must be approached carefully, with a statement to the family that all patients with this problem are asked these routine questions. Families should be screened for substance use that might result in use of food money for tobacco, alcohol, or drugs,

TABLE 12.3   Failure to Thrive: Differential Diagnosis by System

Psychosocial/Behavioral

Inadequate diet because of poverty/food insecurity, errors in food preparation, fad diet, fear of allergy

Poor parenting skills (lack of knowledge of sufficient diet)

Child/parent interaction problems (autonomy struggles, coercive feeding)

Food refusal/aversion/dysphagia

Parental cognitive or mental health problems

Child abuse or neglect

Neurologic

Oral motor dysfunction (dysautonomia, brainstem lesion, cerebral palsy, Chiari malformation, myopathies)

Spasticity

Developmental delay

Increased intracranial pressure

Diencephalic syndrome

Renal

Urinary tract infection

Renal tubular acidosis

Renal failure

Endocrine

Diabetes mellitus

Hypothyroidism/hyperthyroidism

Growth hormone deficiency

Adrenal insufficiency

Genetic/Metabolic/Congenital

Cystic fibrosis

Sickle cell disease

Inborn errors of metabolism (organic acidosis, hyperammonemia, storage diseases)

Fetal alcohol syndrome

Skeletal dysplasias

Chromosomal disorders: aneuploidy, microdeletion/duplication, imprinting

Monogenetic disorders

Multiple congenital anomaly syndromes (VATER, CHARGE)

Gastrointestinal

Pyloric stenosis

Gastroesophageal reflux

Eosinophilic esophagitis

Malrotation

Malabsorption syndromes

Celiac disease

Formula intolerance (lactose, protein)

Pancreatic insufficiency syndromes

Chronic cholestasis

Inflammatory bowel disease

Chronic congenital diarrhea states including IPEX and IPEX-like monogenetic disorders

Pseudo-obstruction

Cardiac

Cyanotic heart lesions

Congestive heart failure

Pulmonary/Respiratory

Severe asthma

Cystic fibrosis; bronchiectasis

Chronic respiratory failure

Bronchopulmonary dysplasia

Adenoid/tonsillar hypertrophy

Obstructive sleep apnea

Miscellaneous

Autoimmune diseases

Autoinflammatory–recurrent fever syndromes

Malignancy

Primary immunodeficiency

Transplantation

Infections

Perinatal infection

Occult/chronic infections

Parasitic infestation

Tuberculosis

HIV

CHARGE, coloboma, heart disease, choanal atresia, retarded growth and retarded development and/or central nervous system anomalies, genital hypoplasia, and ear anomalies and/or deafness; IPEX, immune disregulation polyendocrinopathy enteropathy X-linked; VATER, vertebral defects, imperforate anus, tracheoesophageal fistula, and radial and renal dysplasia.

as well as inadequate child care. Prior involvement of child protection authorities is relevant.

Is the child in group daycare, or has the family traveled to or emigrated from an area where a chronic infection such as a parasite might have been acquired? Although the social history can be the most revealing part of the history, it can be the most difficult to elicit. Often the clinician must establish trust with the family before they can reveal the source of their inability to meet their child's nutritional needs.

Review of Systems

A thorough review of systems can help to reveal organic conditions. A few areas merit special attention to determine sources of calorie loss or increased metabolic demands.

Constitutional: The examiner should ask whether there are any fevers, night sweats, or changes in activity. Assess sleep hygiene, amount of sleep, and whether sleep is disrupted by snoring or awakenings.

Gastrointestinal: Inquire about choking, swallowing, dysphagia, vomiting, spitting up, and rumination. Pocketing food, or retaining food in the mouth, may indicate oral motor dysfunction that impedes adequate intake. Night waking and coughing may indicate reflux. Diarrhea, constipation, abdominal pain, early satiety, distention, and discomfort indicate organic conditions.

Cardiopulmonary: The examiner should ask about coughing, wheezing, shortness of breath, exercise intolerance, and early tiring during feeding.

Renal: Inquire about dysuria, hematuria, increased urinary frequency or volume, secondary enuresis, and urine that seems unusually dilute or concentrated.

Physical Examination

The examination should start with accurate measurements of height or length, weight, and head circumference; these parameters should be plotted on a standard growth curve. Weight for height or BMI (if older than 2 years of age) should also be plotted. Historical events

TABLE 12.4   Characteristics of Mineral Deficiencies

Mineral	Function	Manifestations of Deficiency	Comments	Sources
Iron	Heme-containing macromolecules (e.g., hemoglobin, cytochrome, myoglobin)	Anemia, spoon nails, reduced muscle and mental performance	History of pica, cow's milk, gastrointestinal bleeding, excessive milk in diet	Liver, meat, eggs, grains
Copper	Redox reactions (e.g., cytochrome oxidase)	Hypochromic anemia, neutropenia, osteoporosis, hypotonia, hypoproteinemia, poor growth	Inborn error, Menkes kinky hair syndrome, occipital horn syndrome, long-term TPN	Liver, oysters, meat, nuts, grains, legumes, chocolate
Zinc	Metalloenzymes (e.g., alkaline phosphatase, carbonic anhydrase, DNA polymerase; wound healing)	Acrodermatitis enteropathica; poor growth, acroperioral-perianal rash, alopecia, delayed sexual development, hypogeusia, infection	Protein-calorie malnutrition; weaning; malabsorption syndrome	Meat, grains, cheese, nuts
Selenium	Prevents oxidative damage	Keshan cardiomyopathy in China, poor growth	Endemic areas; long-term TPN	Meat, vegetables
Chromium	Insulin cofactor	Poor weight gain, glucose intolerance, neuropathy	Protein-calorie malnutrition, long-term TPN	Yeast, breads
Fluoride	Strengthens dental enamel	Caries	Supplementation during tooth growth, narrow therapeutic range; fluorosis may cause staining of the teeth	Seafood, supplemented water
Iodine	Thyroxine, triiodothyronine production	Simple endemic goiter Myxedematous cretinism: congenital hypothyroidism Neurologic cretinism: intellectual disability, deafness, spasticity, normal T_4 level at birth	Endemic in New Guinea, the Congo; endemic in Great Lakes area before iodized salt available	Seafood, iodized salt, most food in nonendemic areas

T_4, thyroxine; TPN, total parenteral nutrition.
From Tershakovec AM, Stallings VA. Pediatric nutrition and nutritional disorders. In: Behrman RE, Kliegman RM, eds. *Nelson Essentials of Pediatrics.* 2nd ed. Philadelphia: WB Saunders; 1994:81.

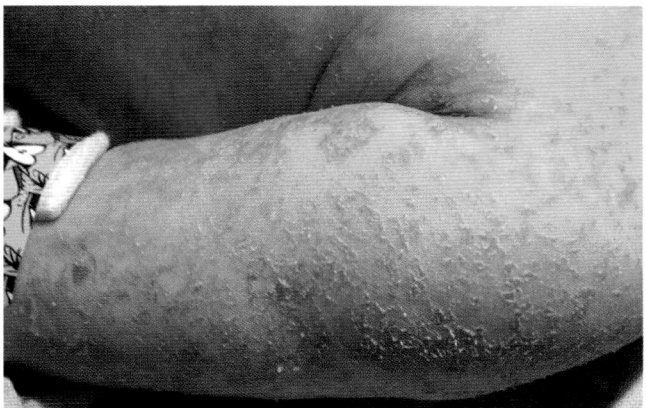

Fig. 12.5 A 14-month-old girl with "flaky paint" dermatitis. (From Katz KA, Mahlberg MH, Honig PJ, et al. Rice nightmare: kwashiorkor in 2 Philadelphia-area infants fed Rice Dream beverage. *J Am Acad Dermatol.* 2005;52[5 Suppl 1]:S69–S72.)

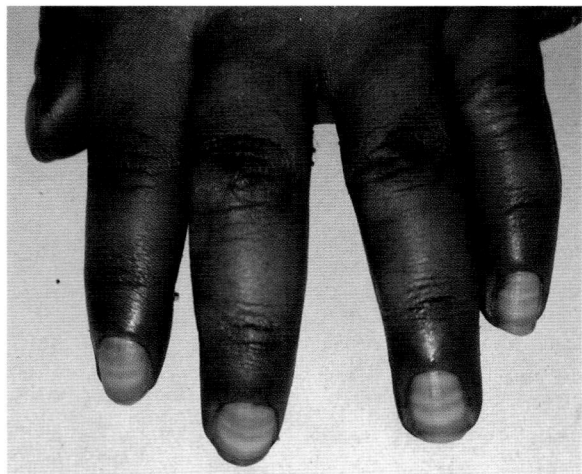

Fig. 12.6 Paired, transverse, homogeneous, and smooth-bordered lines noted in all fingernails, suggestive of Muehrcke lines in an infant fed diluted cow's milk since birth. (From Williams V, Jayashree M. Muehrcke lines in an infant. *J Pediatr.* 2017;189:234.)

should be identified and plotted to discover impact on growth patterns.

As part of a complete physical examination, the following signs should be sought:

General: degree of emaciation, fat distribution and muscle mass, dysmorphic features, vital signs (including blood pressure), hydration status.

Head, eyes, ears, nose, and throat: fontanel size, evidence of chronic ear infections, allergic facies, patency of upper airway, status of teeth

Cardiorespiratory: respiratory effort, lower airway sounds, cardiac sounds, pulses, edema

Gastrointestinal: organomegaly, abdominal distention, rectal fissures or prolapse

Genitourinary: renal masses, Tanner staging

Musculoskeletal: joint swelling, bone deformities

Skin: hydration, bruising or scarring, rashes, hair quality and distribution, nails (Figs. 12.5 and 12.6)

Lymph nodes: local vs generalized (see Chapter 48)

Neurologic: muscle volume, tone (hypo- or hypertonic), strength, coordination, swallowing and drooling, assessment of development and interaction with the examiner

Abnormalities associated with pathologic biomedical conditions should prompt a search for a specific diagnosis (see Table 12.3). On occasion, growth failure as well as other physical findings can

TABLE 12.5   Characteristics of Vitamin Deficiencies

Vitamin	Function	Manifestations of Deficiency	Comments	Sources
Water-Soluble				
Thiamine (B_1)	Coenzyme in ketoacid decarboxylation (e.g., pyruvate → acetyl-CoA transketolase reaction)	Beriberi: polyneuropathy, calf tenderness, heart failure, edema, ophthalmoplegia	Inborn errors of lactate metabolism; boiling milk destroys B_1	Liver, meat, milk, cereals, nuts, legumes
Riboflavin (B_2)	FAD coenzyme in oxidation-reduction reactions	Anorexia, mucositis, anemia, cheilosis, nasolabial seborrhea	Photosensitizer	Milk, cheese, liver, meat, eggs, whole grains, green leafy vegetables
Niacin (B_3)	NAD coenzyme in oxidation-reduction reactions	Pellagra: photosensitivity, dermatitis, dementia, diarrhea, death	Tryptophan is a precursor	Meat, fish, liver, whole grains, green leafy vegetables
Pyridoxine (B_6)	Cofactor in amino acid metabolism	Seizures, hyperacusis, microcytic anemia, nasolabial seborrhea, neuropathy	Dependency state; deficiency secondary to drugs	Meat, liver, whole grains, peanuts, soybeans
Pantothenic acid	CoA in Krebs cycle	None reported	—	Meat, vegetables
Biotin	Cofactor in carboxylase reactions of amino acids	Alopecia, dermatitis, hypotonia, death	Bowel resection, inborn errors of metabolism, and ingestion of raw eggs	Yeast, meats; made by intestinal flora
B_{12}	Coenzyme for 5-methyl-tetrahydrofolate formation; DNA synthesis	Megaloblastic anemia, peripheral neuropathy, posterior lateral column disease, vitiligo, encephalopathy	Vegans; fish tapeworm; transcobalamin or intrinsic factor deficiencies	Meat, fish, cheese, eggs
Folate	DNA synthesis	Megaloblastic anemia	Goat's milk deficient; drug antagonists; heat inactivates	Liver, greens, vegetables, cereals, cheese
Ascorbic acid (C)	Reducing agent; collagen metabolism	Scurvy: irritability, purpura, bleeding gums, periosteal hemorrhage, aching bones	May improve tyrosine metabolism in preterm infants	Citrus fruits, green vegetables; cooking destroys it
Fat-Soluble				
A	Epithelial cell integrity; vision	Night blindness, xerophthalmia, Bitot spots, follicular hyperkeratosis, poor growth	Common with protein-calorie malnutrition; malabsorption	Liver, milk, eggs, green and yellow vegetables, fruits
D	Maintains serum calcium, phosphorus levels	Rickets: reduced bone mineralization, poor growth	Prohormone of 25- and 1,25-vitamin D; malabsorption	Fortified milk, cheese, liver
E	Antioxidant	Hemolysis in preterm infants; areflexia, ataxia, ophthalmoplegia	May benefit patients with G6PD deficiency; malabsorption	Seeds, vegetables, germ oils, green leafy vegetables
K	Post-translation carboxylation of clotting factors II, VII, IX, and X and proteins C and S	Prolonged prothrombin time; hemorrhage; elevated PIVKA	Malabsorption; breast-fed infants, prolonged antibiotic therapy	Liver, green vegetables; made by intestinal flora

CoA, coenzyme A; FAD, flavin adenine dinucleotide; G6PD, glucose-6-phosphate dehydrogenase; NAD, nicotinamide adenine dinucleotide; PIVKA, protein induced in vitamin K absence.
Modified from Tershakovec A, Stallings VA. Pediatric nutrition and nutritional disorders. In: Behrman RE, Kliegman RM, eds. *Nelson Essentials of Pediatrics*. 2nd ed. Philadelphia: WB Saunders; 1994:74.

be associated with specific nutrient deficiencies (Tables 12.4, 12.5, and 12.6).

Laboratory Evaluation

Almost any serious chronic illness may result in FTT; therefore, the examiner must have a broad diagnostic screening approach and simultaneously consider the more likely possibility that nonmedical processes are the cause. In most cases of chronic "organic" illness, there is likely some indication in the history, physical examination, or selected diagnostic screening tests (Table 12.7). In cases where an underlying illness is not detected by these screening tests, the condition may become evident when the infant does not respond to nutritional rehabilitation. If, however, the examiner attempts to pursue every conceivable diagnostic test for organic causes of FTT before implementing vigorous nutritional rehabilitation, the examiner is

likely to run out of time, patience, and resources and come to no conclusion. Some unusual cases may take months or years before a diagnosis can be made.

The choice of the appropriate initial laboratory tests may include several general screening tests to detect treatable conditions. A CBC can reveal clinically inapparent anemia, which, although usually secondary to the poor nutritional state, can sometimes contribute to the poor dietary intake or suggest anemia of chronic disease. A UA and urine culture can reveal evidence of an occult urinary tract infection or renal tubular acidosis. Serum electrolytes with BUN level may detect metabolic conditions. An ESR or CRP may provide evidence of chronic inflammation or infection. The examiner may need to test for celiac disease; poor weight gain may be the only symptom for many years. Other specific tests are directed by the history and physical examination (see Table 12.7). For example, for a child with developmental delay

TABLE 12.6 Clinical Signs of Malnutrition

Site	Signs
Face	Moon face (kwashiorkor), simian facies (marasmus)
Eye	Dry eyes, pale conjunctiva, Bitot spots (vitamin A), periorbital edema
Mouth	Angular stomatitis, cheilitis, glossitis, spongy bleeding gums (vitamin C), parotid enlargement
Teeth	Enamel mottling, delayed eruption
Hair	Dull, sparse, brittle hair; hypopigmentation; flag sign (alternating bands of light and normal color); broomstick eyelashes; alopecia
Skin	Loose and wrinkled (marasmus); shiny and edematous (kwashiorkor); dry, follicular hyperkeratosis; patchy hyper- and hypopigmentation ("crazy paving" or "flaky paint" dermatoses); erosions; poor wound healing
Nails	Koilonychia; thin and soft nail plates, fissures, or ridges
Musculature	Muscle wasting, particularly buttocks and thighs; Chvostek or Trousseau sign (hypocalcemia)
Skeletal	Deformities, usually as a result of calcium, vitamin D, or vitamin C deficiencies
Abdomen	Distended: hepatomegaly with fatty liver; ascites may be present
Cardiovascular	Bradycardia, hypotension, reduced cardiac output, small vessel vasculopathy
Neurologic	Global developmental delay, loss of knee and ankle reflexes, impaired memory
Hematologic	Pallor, petechiae, bleeding diathesis
Behavior	Lethargic, apathetic, irritable on handling

From Kliegman RM, St. Geme JW III, Blum NJ, et al., eds. *Nelson Textbook of Pediatrics*. 21st ed. Philadelphia: Elsevier; 2020:337, Fig. 57.6.

and FTT, a blood lead test, metabolic screening tests, a karyotype or other genetic testing (microarray), imaging of the head, or HIV screening may be necessary, whereas a child with apparent malabsorption is evaluated completely differently (targeting cystic fibrosis, inflammatory bowel disease, celiac disease, or parasitic infection). An endoscopy may be needed to determine eosinophilic infiltration into the gastrointestinal mucosa. If height growth is affected, a bone age may determine if an endocrine evaluation is necessary. Consultation with specialists will be needed in many cases.

OVERALL APPROACH TO MANAGEMENT

The evaluation of a child with FTT should proceed in a stepwise manner (Fig. 12.7). Once the clinician has arrived at a working diagnosis, treatment can be instituted. It is important to develop a therapeutic alliance with family members. Parents whose children are not growing according to expectation may feel guilty or may have a sense of failure. A nonjudgmental approach, avoiding the assignment of blame, is important. Although the clinician can make suggestions, it is the family that must feel empowered to implement the plan.

Providing specific information that can be easily implemented in the family's home environment will be more successful than giving general advice. Suggestions that a parent feed more food to a child may be disregarded, particularly when the family members believe they are already doing their best. Pressuring parents may increase caregiver guilt, frustration, and anxiety if the child does not grow as expected.

Even with the strong suspicion of a biomedical cause, it is reasonable to give specific advice on enhancing calorie intake while further evaluation and treatment are ongoing. If the condition is chronic, the child may need long-term nutritional supplementation. If the condition is acute and treatable, the child needs extra calories for catch-up growth.

Steps to Improve Calorie Intake

Mealtime Behavior

A pleasant, safe setting should be created for mealtime. An infant seat is appropriate for the first several months. Once a child can sustain a sitting position, a high chair is advantageous. The high chair allows the child to feel safe from falling, frees up the child's hands for feeding, and keeps the child confined in one place to focus on the meal. A bib prevents the need for frequent changes of clothing. For an older child, a booster seat is appropriate along with child-sized utensils. Parents who feed an infant or toddler while holding the child in their laps find that the meal is a struggle; this also prevents the child from developing self-feeding skills.

To promote the important social aspect of mealtime, family members should be seated and eat together whenever possible. Use of a small, child-sized table and chair prevents the child from observing and learning from siblings and adults during family meals. Toddlers and older infants are usually interested in the food served to other family members, leading to experimentation with new foods. There should be conversation during the meal, but the child's food intake should not be the focus of the conversation.

Distractions should be minimized during meals. The television and other electronic media should be off. There should not be other commotion in the kitchen. However, for the infant, a small washable toy on the tray or table may help keep attention on the meal.

Parents should understand that experimenting with food is part of the natural curiosity of older infants and toddlers. If the parent is constantly wiping the child and berating the child for getting messy, the child cannot learn that eating can be a fun experience. If a parent has difficulty with messiness, the examiner can suggest spreading newspaper or a plastic sheet under the high chair. Another simple technique is the "two-spoon method"; the child holds a spoon to dip into the food, and the parent has the second spoon, which provides most of the feeding.

Once the child has communicated that the meal is finished, the parent can offer one or two more bites but then should accept that the child is no longer hungry, and the meal should be ended. The duration of the meal for a toddler is typically not more than 15 or 20 minutes. Food should not be brought out until the next scheduled meal or snack.

Beverages

Exclusive breast-feeding is the preferred nutritional source for infants from birth to at least 6 months. Formula-fed infants should be held during a feeding until they are able to sit on their own and hold the bottle. Both breast milk and formula can be fortified for additional calories per ounce. Bottles should never be propped. After 1 year of age, breast milk may continue but formula is changed to cow's milk. Although 1–2% milk is acceptable, whole milk is preferred for underweight toddlers. The volume of formula or whole cow's milk consumed should be about 24 ounces per day. If a child is drinking an excessive

TABLE 12.7 Some Causes of Failure to Thrive and Screening Tests

Cause	Screening Tests
Environmental and Psychosocial*	
Inadequate caloric intake	History; observation in hospital
Emotional deprivation and disruptions	History; observation in hospital
Rumination; chronic diarrhea, gastroesophageal reflux	History; observation in hospital
Anorexia nervosa and bulimia	History; examination
Secondary to impact of organic disease	History and observation
Organic	
Central nervous system abnormalities, infection	Neurodevelopmental assessment; brain MRI
Malabsorption, cystic fibrosis, inflammatory bowel disease, parasites, aganglionic megacolon; liver disease; food intolerance; celiac disease; gastroesophageal reflux, eosinophilic esophagitis	Examination of stools: stool fat and elastase, sweat test, stool ova and parasites; tissue transglutaminase antibodies; liver function tests; barium swallow, ESR, food challenge, esophageal and intestinal biopsy
Partial cleft palate	Physical examination; observation of feeding
Chronic heart failure	Physical examination; chest x-ray; echocardiography
Endocrine disorders	Growth chart; thyroid function tests; bone age, cortisol level, GH testing
Bronchopulmonary dysplasia; bronchiectasis; cystic fibrosis	Physical examination; chest x-ray; tuberculin test, pulmonary function tests, sweat test, newborn screen
Anomalies; infection; renal failure; renal tubular disorder	UA; BUN; ultrasonography; urinary amino acid screen; urine pH
Chromosomal disorders or syndromes; Turner syndrome Skeletal dysplasias	Chromosomal analysis (microarray, exome); identification of peculiar facies or multisystem defects, skeletal radiographs
Other metabolic, syndromic, or inborn errors	Urine and blood amino and organic acids, lactate, mitochondrial DNA, specific gene panels, exome
Tuberculosis, mycotic, congenital, AIDS	Tuberculin skin test or interferon-gamma release assay; appropriate laboratory identification of infectious agent, (antigen, antibody, or PCR)
Juvenile idiopathic arthritis, SLE	Physical examination; ESR; CBC, ANA
DiGeorge syndrome; severe combined immunodeficiency syndrome	History of rash and diarrhea; thymus size; tonsil size; skin tests; CBC, immunoglobulins, lymphocyte cell markers, FISH for DiGeorge syndrome, newborn screen
AIDS or AIDS-related complex	HIV rapid antigen, antibody test
Malignancies (kidney, hematologic, adrenal, brain)	Imaging (CT, ultrasonography) of abdomen, chest; brain CT or MRI, bone marrow
Congenital syndromes caused by alcohol, Dilantin, other drugs, infection	Physical examination; history, TORCH evaluation

*Nonorganic may also be combined with organic.
ANA, antinuclear antibodies; CBC, complete blood cell count; FISH, fluorescent in situ hybridization; GH, growth hormone; PCR, polymerase chain reaction; SLE, systemic lupus erythematosus; TORCH, toxoplasmosis, other, rubella, cytomegalovirus, herpes simplex.
Modified from Barbero GJ. Failure to thrive. In: Behrman RE, ed. *Nelson Textbook of Pediatrics.* 14th ed. Philadelphia: WB Saunders; 1992:215.

amount of formula, review the preparation procedures to ensure that the proper dilution is used.

Children naturally enjoy sweet foods. However, if they are introduced early or used instead of more nutritionally complete foods, children may develop a preference for sweets, especially juices. In particular, toddlers who are allowed to have bottles with sweetened juices throughout the day eat little at mealtime, resulting in undernutrition. In addition, because of limited absorption of dietary sugars, particularly in juices with high fructose-to-glucose ratios (such as apple and pear juice), excessive juice intake may result in bloating, excessive flatulence, abdominal pain, and chronic diarrhea due to carbohydrate malabsorption. Juice should not be introduced until after 12 months of age. When introduced, only 100% fruit juice should be offered in a cup. Intake should be limited to 4 ounces per day for toddlers, 4–6 ounces per day for preschoolers, and 8 ounces per day for older children and adolescents.

Various methods are available to enhance the calorie density of infant dietary beverages for nutritional supplementation. Formulas can be made with less water. Polycose and vegetable oils can be added. Pumped/expressed breast milk can be enhanced with breast milk fortifier (premature infants) or powdered formula (full-term infants).

Food Selection

Complementary foods should be introduced after 4 or 6 months. Infants and young toddlers may have preferences for certain food textures, temperatures, and presentations. These preferences are often short-lived. Normal children may become "picky" eaters in the second and third years of life, generally refusing vegetables and fruits. New foods should routinely be introduced but not forced on the child. With reintroduction (up to 10 times may be required) and modeling, children will try new foods. For some children, food preferences may

PART A

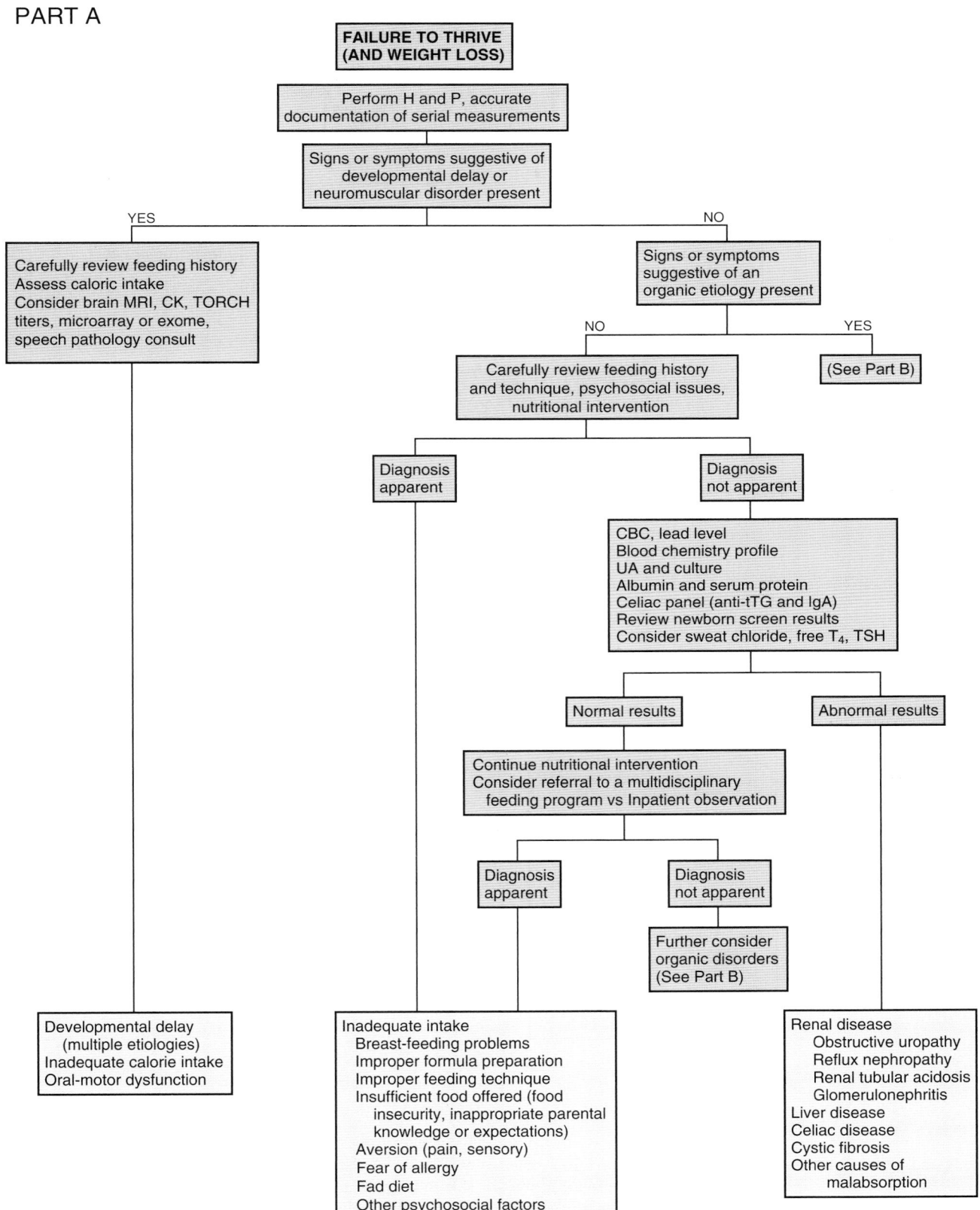

Fig. 12.7 Flow chart for the stepwise evaluation of a child with failure to thrive (and weight loss). anti-tTG, anti–tissue transglutaminase; CK, creatine kinase; ENT, ear, nose, and throat; GER, gastroesophageal reflux; GERD, gastroesophageal reflux disease; H, history; ICP, intracranial pressure; IgA, immunoglobulin A; IgE, immunoglobulin E; O&P, ova and parasites; P, physical examination; PPD, purified protein derivative; T₄, thyroxine; TORCH, toxoplasmosis, other, rubella, cytomegalovirus, herpes simplex; TSH, thyroid-stimulating hormone; UGI, upper gastrointestinal series. (From Pomeranz AJ, Sabnis S, Busey SL, et al., eds. *Pediatric Decision-Making Strategies.* 2nd ed. Philadelphia: Elsevier; 2016.)

PART B

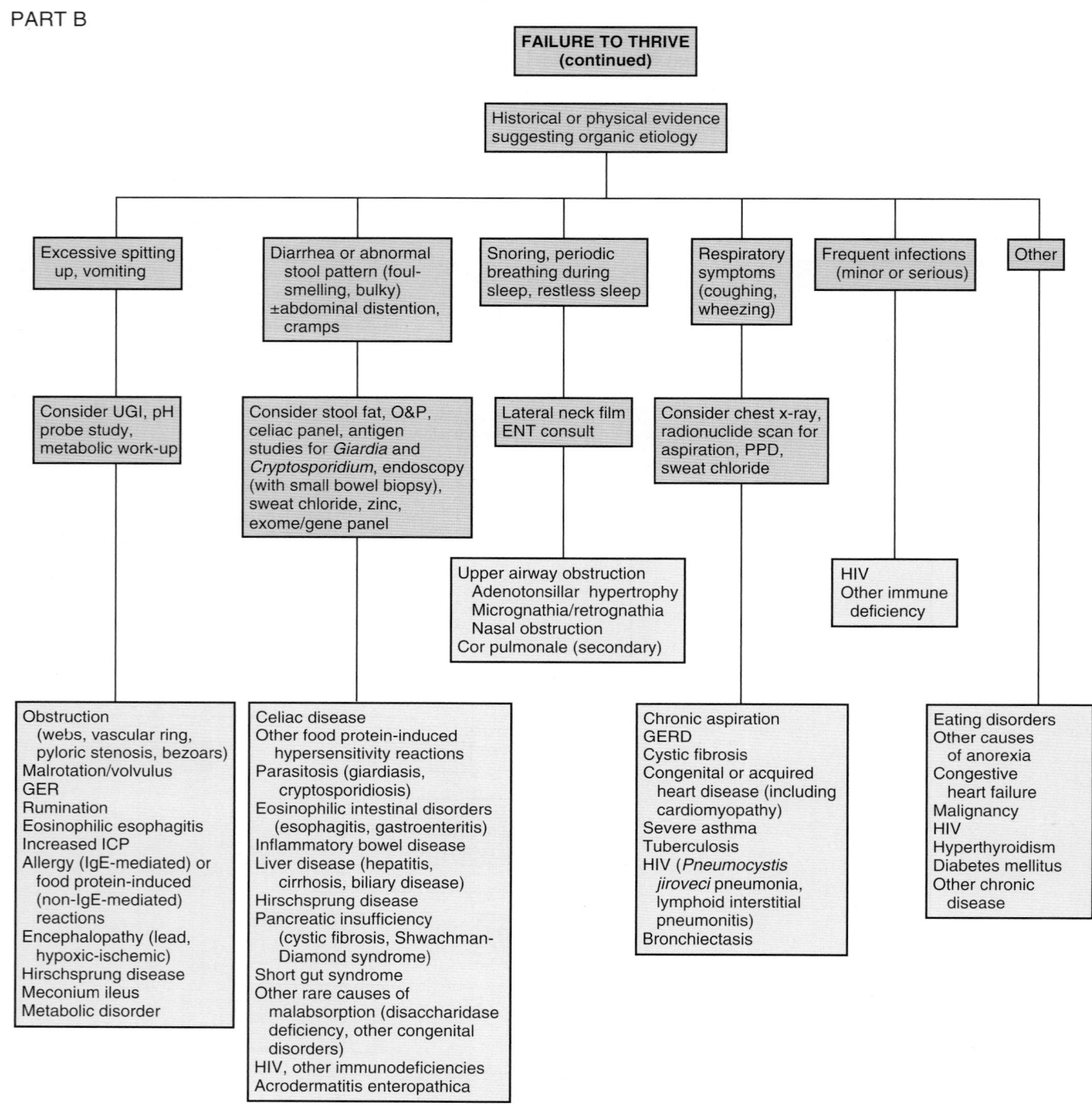

Fig. 12.7, cont'd

be strong and cyclic. For example, a child may go through a cycle in which they request peanut butter and jelly sandwiches for nearly every meal. If a variety of fruits or vegetables are given along with the sandwich, this may be a reasonable compromise. Including older children in food shopping and preparation will increase interest in eating. At mealtime, older toddlers and preschool-aged children may be permitted some flexibility in food selection from two or three choices. Providing choices allows the child to assume some control over the meal. Each choice must be nutritionally sound and acceptable to the parent. Parents should not become bound by social constraints when it comes to foods served at certain meals.

Although it is the caregiver's responsibility to provide appropriate food, it is the child's responsibility to decide on the quantity of food to be eaten. "Force feeding" will convince the child that mealtime is something to be feared. Parents must learn to read a child's cues for hunger and satiety.

TABLE 12.8 Normal Calorie Requirements and Weight Gain by Age

	Calorie Requirement (kcal/kg/day)	Weight Gain* (g/day)
Premature	150	20–40
Full-term to 3 mo	100–120	25–39
3–6 mo		14–20
6–9 mo	90–100	9–13
9–12 mo		7–10
Toddler	75–85	6–9

*Based on WHO growth charts (5% and 95%).

Daily Routines and Snacks

Once children are receiving solid foods, they should be on a regular schedule of meals served at predictable times during the day. This generally means three meals and two or three snacks per day for infants and toddlers. The practice of "grazing"—having food available to the child throughout the day—should not be allowed. Frequent snacking allows the child to be satiated, preventing interest in standard meals and resulting in poor nutrition. Planned snacks afford the opportunity to supplement the child's diet with high-quality foods with good nutritional content. For toddlers and preschool-aged children, beverages should be introduced only after a good portion of the meal has been eaten.

Calculating Caloric Need

To calculate the minimal daily caloric requirements needed for catch-up growth, determine the weight age (age at which current weight would be at 50%) and recommended calories for weight age (Table 12.8). The ideal weight for current height (50% weight for current height) should also be determined. Calories needed for catch-up growth are calculated as:

$$\frac{\text{(kcal/kg for weight age)} \times \text{(ideal weight for height in kilograms)}}{\text{actual weight in kilograms}}$$

Required kcal/kg by age are the following:
0–6 months = 108 kcal/kg
6–12 months = 98 kcal/kg
1–3 years = 102 kcal/kg
4–6 years = 90 kcal/kg

For most children, calories needed for catch-up growth can be easily calculated as:

$$\frac{\text{(120 kcal/kg)} \times \text{(ideal weight for height in kilograms)}}{\text{actual weight in kilograms}}$$

Most infants will achieve catch-up growth on 160–180 kcal/kg/day. Some infants may need considerably more, up to 1.5–2 times the daily requirements for catch-up. Caloric intake can be estimated from the diet history.

NUTRITIONAL SUPPLEMENTATION FOR THE OLDER INFANT AND CHILD

Several products are available for nutritional supplementation. The complete liquid formulations are excellent products; very similar nutritional value can be found in packaged instant-breakfast drinks when mixed with whole milk, at much lower cost. These nutrient-dense beverages should supplement the child's diet, not supplant food.

Many food products (powdered milk, margarine, cheese, wheat germ, peanut butter) can be added to acceptable foods to increase calories. It is easier to increase caloric density than increase the amount of food eaten. Attention should be paid to maximizing protein intake needed for growth.

If a child does not seem to be taking an adequate variety of foods, a supplement of multivitamins with minerals may be indicated. Particularly during periods of rapid catch-up growth, additional vitamins and minerals can be beneficial. Iron and zinc deficiencies may impede normal growth (see Table 12.4). Supplementation of zinc and other trace minerals has been shown to enhance catch-up growth in malnourished children. A trial of an appetite stimulant, such as cyproheptadine, can be effective in some children.

Referral Resources and Other Options
Multidisciplinary Team

Children with FTT have complex medical and psychosocial issues. A multidisciplinary approach is beneficial in complicated cases by relieving the primary medical care provider of the responsibilities of investigating the home situation, reviewing the family's finances and resources, and observation of mealtime. Improvement is most likely when children are referred at younger ages. The team might include a physician, social worker, psychologist, nutritionist, nurse, child life specialist, and home visitor. The team then discusses the case and develops a plan for ongoing management. Children treated by teams have better outcomes than children receiving routine care.

The psychological evaluation may identify children with developmental delays and can assess family stressors and identify strengths and weaknesses in the family. In some families, the child may be the indicator that there is an underlying disturbance, such as depression or marital stress. The psychologist can also offer support and reassurance as the family goes through a difficult period caused by potential long-term nutritional rehabilitation of the child. In addition, the psychologist can help the caregiver understand that improving the feeding situation takes a great effort on the part of the parent as well as the child and that new strategies are required for successful weight gain.

The nutritionist's expertise is essential for a thorough evaluation and follow-up plan. When taking a complete nutritional history, the nutritionist can analyze the nutritional and caloric values of the foods eaten. Alternative meal plans can be developed to maximize calories and nutritional content.

A social worker's contribution to the team is an assessment of the child's environment and factors that may be contributing to the child's poor growth. Areas for investigation include social supports, housing conditions (crowding, space for food storage, proper refrigeration), and food insecurity. Families may need assistance with arranging work leave, rearranging work schedules, transportation, or respite care. Families can be directed to community support services that focus on both social/emotional and material/financial issues. Participation in the WIC and SNAP programs ameliorates food insecurity. If child maltreatment is suspected, the social worker assists with communication with the appropriate social service agency.

When feasible, home observation provides a wealth of information to the clinician about the environment in which the child resides and eats meals. Does the child have an appropriate place in which to eat? Is there a supply of appropriate foods in the home? What are the other environmental factors that may be impeding the child's growth? Studies of home interventions have had mixed success, but young children with the highest risks have improved developmental outcomes with home intervention.

Recording or Direct Observation

Observation or recording of a meal provides an opportunity to assess the child's willingness and ability to participate in the meal, the parenting style, and the interaction between the child and parents. Feeding is most successful when the parent is responsive to the child's cues. Parents who are controlling, overly permissive, or neglectful will find the feeding situation unsuccessful. Parent and child strengths should be pointed out to the parent. Problematic communication, both verbal and nonverbal, should be reviewed. Difficulties that are observed should be discussed and become the basis for further intervention.

Involvement of Social Service Agencies

Clinicians caring for children with FTT often find themselves working in conjunction with other agencies, including *social service agencies*. Children who are refused food or are abused in any way must be reported. It may, however, be difficult to determine what constitutes neglectful care. Families that are disorganized and overwhelmed, have other pressing social issues, or refuse to follow recommendations, resulting in lack of sufficient progress in the child's growth, must be reported to the local agency. This may include parents with cognitive deficits, mental health problems, or substance abuse. It is important for all agencies to work together and articulate a plan, so that the families involved do not receive conflicting instructions and messages.

Behavioral Strategies

In some situations, behavior modification programs are used. These may include strategies to determine specific parameters in the feeding environment that will improve the child's intake. These may include colors, textures, tastes, etc. In more difficult cases, a strict behavior modification program may be used.

Non-Oral Enteral Feeding

For some children, maximizing oral intake may nonetheless provide insufficient calories for catch-up growth. The clinician may consider other forms of enteral feeding. This intervention is needed if, despite all other attempts to maximize oral feeding, the child's growth is falling further below the third percentile or if the child is showing signs of severe malnourishment (e.g., hypoalbuminemia, or low prealbumin levels).

Initially, nasogastric (NG) feeding can be used for night feedings. The child should be encouraged to eat orally during the day. If the need for the NG tube is extended for a longer duration (some authorities use 3 months), then a referral should be made for placement of a percutaneous gastrostomy tube (G-tube). This is used for supplemental nutrition for most children and is not a substitute for oral intake. Children receiving supplemental alimentation should be monitored very closely. Once the weight for height is approaching the 50th percentile, the supplement should be adjusted to prevent obesity. The G-tube is removed when the child can sustain an adequate growth rate with oral intake only.

It is very important that some oral stimulation continue even if the G-tube is the main source of nutrition. If children are denied the chance to develop competence in age-appropriate feeding behaviors, they are likely to develop food aversions. This makes reintroduction of oral intake extremely difficult.

CHILDREN WITH SPECIAL HEALTH CARE NEEDS

This category encompasses a variety of children: children with isolated dysphagia for whom eating represents more work than pleasure, children with sensory issues for whom food tastes and textures can be experienced as adverse, and children who are technology dependent and not able to self-regulate caloric intake.

During the medical assessment, if a child is found to have drooling, coughing, gagging, pocketing of food in the cheek, or retention of food in the mouth, consider oral motor problems. An assessment by a speech therapist or occupational therapist with specific training in oral motor therapy can help reveal specific problems that are amenable to therapy. A modified barium swallow may be recommended to assess the risk of aspiration. Some children with oral motor dysfunction develop food aversion, as if it is not worth the effort to put anything in their mouths. Oral motor therapy or involvement in an intensive feeding program that addresses feeding therapy in a multidisciplinary fashion may be indicated for these children.

Children with **autism** often have sensory issues that cause feeding aversion. Again, oral motor evaluation and therapy may be of help, but the therapy may need to focus on oral desensitization rather than motor skills. These children will sometimes accept only a very limited number of foods, or a single color or texture. The clinician can ensure adequate micronutrient intake with vitamins and other supplements but may need to disguise them in the accepted foods.

Technology-dependent children represent a very different challenge. Here, it is necessary to monitor growth regularly and adjust caloric intake as necessary. Increased activity or work, due perhaps to improved motor skills or decrease in respiratory support, can abruptly increase a child's caloric need and cause weight loss if caloric intake is not increased. In general, increases of 10% are well tolerated and can be adequate to improve growth. This can be done by increasing volume or caloric density depending on the particular patient's clinical situation. Follow-up weight checks in 2–4 weeks can inform the clinician if the increase was adequate or excessive, and additional adjustments can be made. Failure to gain weight appropriately even with additional calories should prompt further evaluation for increased utilization or improper home feeding.

CRITERIA FOR HOSPITALIZATION

Decisions about when to hospitalize a child with FTT are inevitably influenced by practical considerations of the availability and quality of hospital services, cost, and distance from the family's home. The medical issues are whether hospitalization will facilitate further diagnostic steps and whether the affected child is malnourished enough to create a sense of urgency about nutritional rehabilitation. Weight loss resulting in weight for height below −3 SD constitutes severe malnutrition and may require hospitalization. In addition, hospitalization is indicated if there is a concern about **factitious disorder (Munchausen syndrome by proxy)**. In this situation, a parent may be purposefully manipulating the child to produce FTT or other symptoms.

Most children with FTT gain weight in the hospital within 1–2 weeks, but obtaining a weight gain in a short amount of time does not prove that the home environment was the problem. Alternatively, even a 1–2-week hospitalization in a child without an organic cause of the growth failure may not produce a sustainable weight gain. The foreign surroundings and lack of familiar faces might prevent the child from eating appropriately. Parents may not be able to remain with the child in the hospital if they have other small children to attend to at home.

Sufficient time must be anticipated in the hospital for substantial recovery; in severe cases, full recovery requires about 6 weeks. After

TABLE 12.9 Features of Protein-Energy Malnutrition Syndromes in Children

Parameter	Kwashiorkor	Marasmus	Nutritional Dwarfism
Appetite	Poor	Good	Good
Edema	Present	Absent	Absent
Mood	Irritable when picked up, apathetic when alone	Alert	Alert
Weight for age (% expected)	60–80	<60	<60
Weight for height	Normal or decreased	Markedly decreased	Normal

From Feldman M, Friedman LS, Brandt LJ, eds. *Sleisenger and Fordtran's Gastrointestinal and Liver Disease*. 10th ed. Philadelphia: Elsevier; 2016:74, Table 5-17.

initial stabilization and reassurance that the infant is doing well, the child can spend much of this recovery period in a less expensive, non-intensive supervised medical care facility that emphasizes nutritional support and psychosocial stimulation. Creative approaches to well-organized outpatient day programs or frequent home visiting by properly trained health care workers may provide an attractive alternative to hospitalization.

MONITORING

Long-term follow-up with periodic visits is required to ensure that initial weight gains are sustained. At the follow-up visits, the 24-hour diet recall is assessed, or a 3-day diet history is brought by the family. At all visits, the child's growth parameters must be plotted. Dividing weight gained by the number of days since the last measurement provides a mean growth rate. This can be compared with the normal growth rate in children by age group (see Table 12.8). A child in need of catch-up growth should exceed the expected growth rate for normal children. Periodically, the family can be observed or recorded during a feeding session to determine improvement from prior sessions.

LONG-TERM OUTCOMES

Children with early FTT may suffer long-term consequences such as shorter adult height, less schooling, and diminished economic productivity through changes in brain growth and function. However, outcomes may not be as ominous as early studies suggested. Parental self-perceived competence, child adaptability, and adherence to nutritional and behavioral plans have been associated with good outcomes. Among those referred for management, younger child age and multiple child and family risk factors are associated with better weight gain.

Poverty and associated family and environmental problems may exacerbate the negative effects of FTT. Children with FTT who experience neglect are more likely to have poor outcomes. However, children who are diagnosed early and given appropriate treatment and family support services have better recovery than those who are treated later.

Children with a biomedical etiology that can be successfully managed often do well. For those with undetermined causes or persistent FTT, outcomes can be poor. Growth may continue to be delayed. Ultimate stature may be shorter than that predicted from mean parental heights (see Chapter 56).

Of interest is that with long-term follow-up, some children with FTT and rapid nutritional rehabilitation have been observed to develop obesity with long-term consequences of insulin resistance and cardiovascular risk. While rapid catch-up growth may be desirable in some infants, slower weight recovery in other children may have long-term benefits. The factors that lead some children to develop these consequences of overnutrition are not fully understood.

Poor developmental and cognitive outcomes have been found in many children with FTT; however, it is difficult to ascribe outcomes solely to the nutritional deficiencies. Those who were symmetrically small for gestational age and those with microcephaly are particularly at risk for diminished cognitive potential; nutritional enhancement may have minimal effect. Children who are stunted in the first 2 years of life have poor long-term outcomes. Home intervention by child development specialists may lessen the impact of FTT on cognitive skills. Children should be referred for early intervention services as soon as deficits are detected. Better success will be achieved if intervention is started early.

Children with FTT may manifest behavioral problems, even after the nutritional issues appear to be resolved. If the behaviors are particularly difficult to manage, the services of a psychologist or behavior specialist are warranted.

PROTEIN ENERGY MALNUTRITION

Protein energy malnutrition (PEM) is traditionally a disorder of resource-poor countries with multiple risk factors, the major risk being food insecurity. Features are noted in Table 12.9.

There is an increasing awareness of the presence of PEM in developed countries, most often due to parental beliefs that include food elimination diets from fear of food allergies or food protein–induced enterocolitis syndrome (Fig. 12.8). Other risk factors include restrictive diets (autism, eating disorders), cultural remedies to treat feeding intolerance or other illnesses, and food fads. Concerns for cow's milk protein allergy has resulted in food substitutions with low-protein or low-caloric-density foods such as rice milk, nondairy creamers, formula dilution, home remedies of barley or potato juice or fruit purees, and poorly balanced vegan diets.

Hypoalbuminemia and edema are often present with a diffuse erythematous crusting, erosive, and desquamating rash (see Fig. 12.5). The differential diagnosis of the rash includes Langerhans cell histiocytosis, acrodermatitis enteropathica, eczema, and scabies. The differential diagnosis of the edema includes nephrotic syndrome; liver disease; and, because diarrhea is often present in PEM, a protein-losing enteropathy (Table 12.10). Management is noted in Figure 12.8.

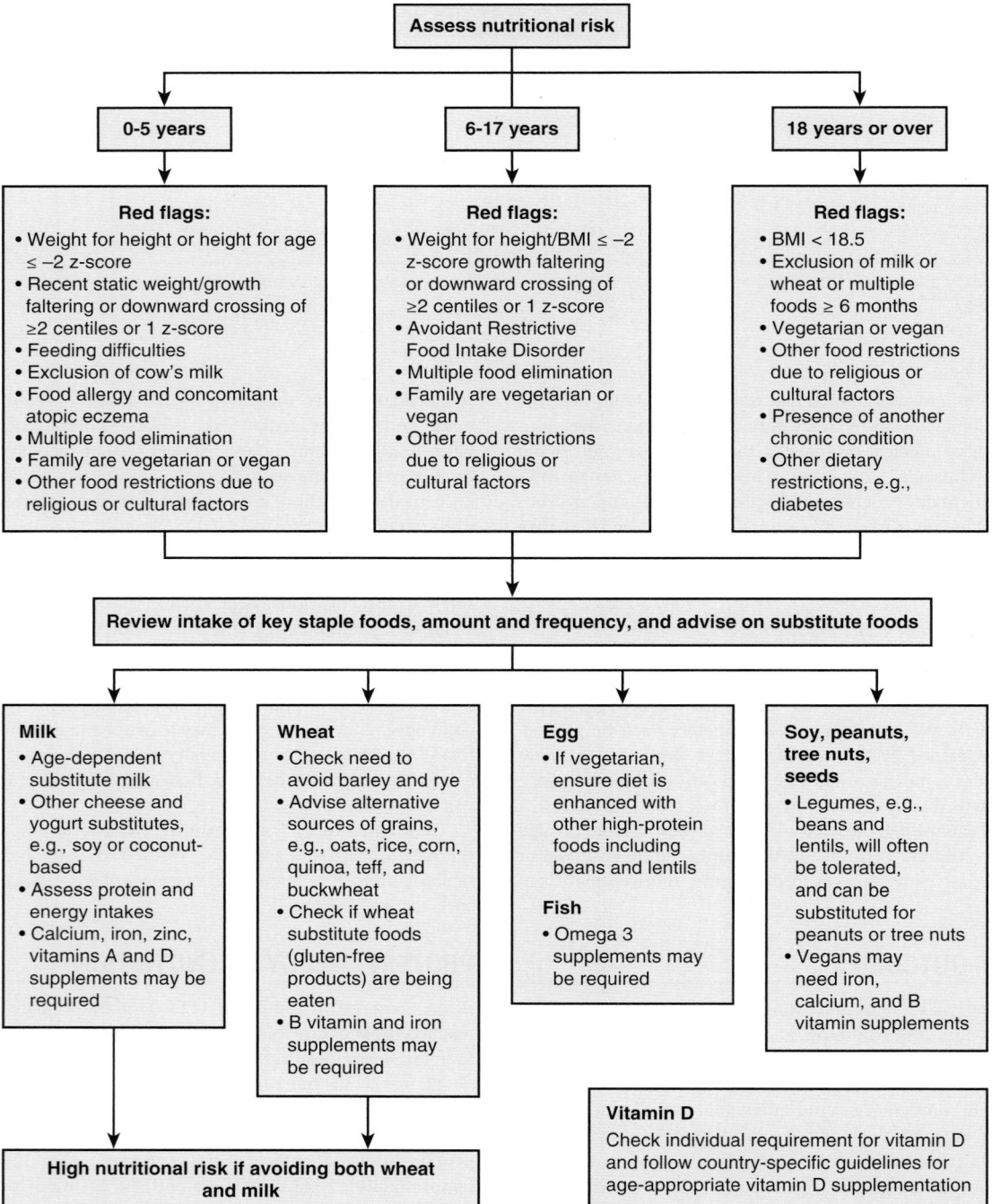

Fig. 12.8 Approach to evaluate risk for adverse elimination diets. BMI, body mass index. (From Skypala IJ, McKenzie R. Nutritional issues in food allergy. *Clin Rev Allergy Immunol.* 2019;57:166–178 [Fig. 1, p. 172].)

TABLE 12.10 Etiology of Protein-Losing Enteropathy

Categories		Agent, Diseases (Gene)
Gastrointestinal infections		CMV, rotavirus, HIV enteropathy
		Salmonella, Shigella, Campylobacter, Clostridium difficile, Helicobacter pylori
		Whipple disease
		Small bowel bacterial overgrowth
		Giardiasis
		Strongyloides stercoralis
		Tuberculosis
Gastrointestinal inflammatory disorders		Menetrier disease
		Eosinophilic gastroenteropathy
		Food (milk, others)-induced enteropathy
		Celiac disease, Crohn disease
		Ulcerative colitis, tropical sprue
		Radiation enteritis
		GVHD, NEC
		Malrotation/volvulus
		Lymphoproliferative disorder (post transplant)
Malignancies		Adenocarcinomas
		Lymphomas
		Kaposi sarcoma
		Neuroblastoma
Vasculitic disorders		Henoch-Schönlein purpura
		Systemic lupus erythematosus
Drugs		NSAID-induced enteropathy
Metabolic/genetic		Congenital disorders of glycosylation (CDG)
		Variants in *DGAT1* gene
		Variants in CD55
		Congenital enterocyte heparan sulfate deficiency (*ALG6*)
		PVLAP-associated diarrhea
		Infantile systemic hyalinosis
Intestinal lymphangiectasia	Congenital/primary IL	Turner, Noonan, Klippel–Trenaunay–Weber
	• Syndromal/genetic/ metabolic	Hennekam (*CCBE1, FAT4*) syndromes
		PLE with skeletal dysplasia (*FGFR3*)
		Generalized lymphatic dysplasia (*PIEZO1*)
	Secondary	
	• Inflammation	Sarcoidosis
	• Radiotherapy	Retroperitoneal fibrosis
	• Neoplastic disorders	Retroperitoneal malignancies, lymphoma
	• Cardiac disorders	Constrictive pericarditis, after Fontan operation, CHF
	• Other	Budd-Chiari syndrome, lymphatic-enteric fistula

CDG, carbohydrate-deficient glycoprotein; CHF, congestive heart failure; CMV, cytomegalovirus; GVHD, graft versus host disease; IL, intestinal lymphangiectasia; NEC, necrotizing enterocolitis, NSAID, nonsteroidal antiinflammatory drug; PLE, protein-losing enteropathy.

▮ SUMMARY AND RED FLAGS

FTT (or growth faltering) is a complex condition encompassing biomedical and psychosocial causes. In the United States, it is most often associated with various psychosocial attributes of the parents, family, or child. The keys to determining the cause are a thorough history and physical examination, including assessment of the growth pattern over time. Red flags include refusal to eat, poor response to feedings, multiple formula or diet changes, unusual parental food beliefs or fear of food allergies, an inappropriately small head size, and abnormal physical signs. Clinicians should be vigilant in identifying chronic disease as well as indicators of child abuse and neglect (see Table 12.3). Recurrent emesis, altered mental status, metabolic acidosis, and hypoglycemia should raise suspicions of an inborn error of metabolism. Microcephaly, seizures, developmental delay or developmental regression, and hypo- or hypertonia should lead to suspicions of a chronic neurologic problem. Identifying and treating the medical and psychosocial causes while enhancing calorie intake can result in better outcomes.

BIBLIOGRAPHY

A bibliography is available at ExpertConsult.com.

13

Abdominal Pain

Adrian Miranda

Acute abdominal pain is usually a self-limiting, benign condition that is commonly caused by gastroenteritis, constipation, or a viral illness. The challenge is to identify children who require immediate evaluation for potentially life-threatening conditions. Chronic abdominal pain is also a common complaint in pediatric practices, as it makes up 2–4% of pediatric visits. At least 20% of children seek attention for chronic abdominal pain by the age of 15 years. Up to 28% of children complain of abdominal pain at least once per week and only 2% seek medical attention. The primary care physician, pediatrician, emergency physician, and surgeon must be able to distinguish serious and potentially life-threatening diseases from more benign problems (Table 13.1). Abdominal pain may be a single acute event (Tables 13.2 and 13.3), a recurring acute problem (as in abdominal migraine), or a chronic problem (Table 13.4). The differential diagnosis is lengthy, differs from that in adults, and varies by age group. Although some disorders occur throughout childhood (constipation, gastroenteritis, lower lobe pneumonia, urinary tract infections), others are more common in a specific age group (see Table 13.2).

PATHOPHYSIOLOGY OF ABDOMINAL PAIN

Abdominal pain results from stimulation of nociceptive receptors and afferent sympathetic stretch receptors. The pain is classified as visceral or parietal (somatic).

Visceral Pain

Visceral pain receptors are located on the serosa surface, in the mesentery, within intestinal muscle, and within mucosa of hollow organs. Pain is initiated when receptors are stimulated by excessive contraction, stretching, tension, or ischemia of the walls of hollow viscera, the capsule of a solid organ (liver, spleen, kidney), or the mesentery. Increased contraction of the smooth muscle of hollow viscera may be caused by infection, toxins (bacterial or chemical agents), ulceration, inflammation, or ischemia. Increased hepatic capsule tension may be secondary to passive congestion (heart failure, pericarditis) or inflammation (hepatitis).

Afferent fibers involved in processing visceral pain are unmyelinated C-fibers that enter the spinal cord bilaterally, resulting in dull, poorly localized pain. Visceral pain is often of gradual onset, and although localization may be imprecise, some general rules may be helpful (Fig. 13.1).

Parietal Pain

Parietal pain arises from direct noxious (usually inflammation) stimulation of the contiguous parietal peritoneum (e.g., right lower quadrant at the McBurney point, appendicitis) or the diaphragm (splenic rupture, subdiaphragmatic abscess). Parietal pain is transmitted through A-delta fibers to specific dorsal root ganglia and thus is usually sharp and more intense. It can usually be exacerbated by movement or cough, is accompanied by tenderness over the site of irritation, and lateralizes to one of four quadrants. Because of the relative localization of the noxious stimulation to the underlying peritoneum and the more anatomically specific and unilateral innervation (peripheral-nonautonomic nerves) of the peritoneum, it is usually easier to identify the precise anatomic location that is producing parietal pain (Fig. 13.2).

ACUTE ABDOMINAL PAIN

The clinician evaluating the child with abdominal pain of acute onset must decide quickly whether the child has a "surgical abdomen" (a serious medical problem necessitating treatment and admission to the hospital) or a process that can be managed on an outpatient basis. Even though surgical diagnoses are fewer than 10% of all causes of abdominal pain in children, they can be life threatening if untreated. Approximately 55% of children evaluated for acute abdominal pain have a specific medical diagnosis; in another 45%, the cause is never defined.

History

Obtaining an accurate history is critical for making an accurate diagnosis but is dependent both on the ability and willingness of the child to communicate and on the skill of the parent or guardian as an observer. The person providing an infant's care is the best source of information about the current illness; the examining physician should try to elicit as much information from the child as possible. Some children give a good account of their illness when they are simply asked to describe it; most children must be asked open-ended, nonleading questions. To determine the presence of anorexia, the physician must ask questions about food intake, the time the food was eaten, and how that behavior compares to the child's normal intake. The answers are often quite different from the responses to the more general questions "Are you hungry?" and "Have you eaten today?"

During the history taking, the child should remain in the parent's arms, at play, or comfortably seated beside the parent, as appropriate for the child's age. While the history is obtained, there is no particular reason that the child should be undressed. The clinician must resist the urge to speed things up by examining the child while taking the history. On occasion, when seeing a seriously ill child, the physician may need to abbreviate the diagnostic process, but taking shortcuts may lead to inaccurate conclusions.

Essential Components of the History

Time of onset of pain. Pain of fewer than 6 hours' duration is accompanied by nonspecific findings, and observation is often needed to determine the nature of the illness. Pain lasting from 6 to 48 hours is more apt to have a cause that warrants medical

TABLE 13.1 Distinguishing Features of Abdominal Pain in Children

Disease	Onset	Location	Referral	Quality	Comments
Functional: irritable bowel syndrome	Recurrent	Periumbilical	None	Dull, crampy, intermittent; duration is variable	Caused by disorder of brain-gut interaction; diarrhea/constipation are symptoms
Gastroenteritis	Acute or gradual	Periumbilical, rectal tenesmus	None	Crampy, dull, intermittent	Emesis, fever, watery diarrhea or dysentery (mucus and blood)
Esophageal reflux	Recurrent, after meals, bedtime	Substernal	Chest	Burning	Sour taste in mouth, Sandifer syndrome
Duodenal ulcer	Recurrent, before meals, at night	Epigastric	Back	Severe burning, gnawing	Relieved by food, milk, antacids; family history
Pancreatitis	Acute	Epigastric/hypogastric	Back	Constant, sharp, boring	Nausea, emesis, marked tenderness
Intestinal obstruction	Acute or gradual	Periumbilical–lower abdomen	Back	Alternating cramping (colic) and painless periods	Distention, obstipation, bilious emesis, increased bowel sounds
Appendicitis	Acute or gradual (1–2 days)	Initially periumbilical or epigastric; later localized to the right lower quadrant	Back or pelvis if retrocecal	Sharp, steady	Nausea, emesis, local tenderness with/without fever; patient is motionless
Meckel diverticulitis (mimics appendicitis)	Recurrent or constant	Generalized diffuse with perforation: periumbilical–lower abdomen	None	Sharp	Hematochezia: painless unless intussusception, diverticulitis, or perforation
Inflammatory bowel disease	Recurrent	Depends on site of involvement		Dull cramping, tenesmus	Weight loss, with/without diarrhea or hematochezia
Intussusception	Acute	Periumbilical–lower abdomen	None	Cramping, with painless periods	Guarded position with knees pulled up, "currant jelly" stools
Disaccharidase deficiency (lactase or sucrase)	Recurrent with ingestion of dairy or sugar	Lower abdomen	None	Cramping	Distention, gaseousness, diarrhea
Eosinophilic esophagitis	Recurrent	Generalized or epigastric	None	Dull or cramping	With or without dysphagia; history of atopy
Celiac disease	Recurrent	Generalized	None	Dull	Constipation, poor weight gain
Anterior cutaneous nerve entrapment (ACNE)	Acute	Right lower abdominal wall		Sharp pain, reproducible with light palpation	Nausea; condition more common in athletes
Abdominal migraine	Acute	Generalized	None	Dull or cramping	Pain causes child to wake up in middle of night; history of similar episodes in the past that resolved abruptly
Urolithiasis	Acute, sudden	Back	Groin	Severe colicky pain	Hematuria; calcification on KUB x-ray study, CT scan
Pyelonephritis	Acute, sudden	Back	None	Dull to sharp	Fever, costochondral tenderness, dysuria, pyuria, urinary frequency
Cholecystitis/cholelithiasis	Acute	Right upper quadrant	Right shoulder, scapula	Severe colicky pain	Hemolysis with/without jaundice

KUB, kidney, ureter, and bladder.

Data from Andreoli TE, Carpenter CJ, Plum F, et al. *Cecil Essentials of Medicine.* Philadelphia: WB Saunders; 1994:326; Behrman R, Kliegman R. *Nelson Essentials of Pediatrics.* 2nd ed. Philadelphia: WB Saunders; 1994:396.

TABLE 13.2 Causes of Acute Abdominal Pain by Age Group

Neonate	**Infant (<2 yr)—cont'd**
Necrotizing enterocolitis*	Gastroenteritis* †
Obstruction*	Intestinal obstruction
Malrotation with volvulus*	Malrotation with volvulus
Idiopathic or drug (indomethacin, steroid)–induced intestinal perforation	Trauma (e.g., abuse)
	Pneumonitis (lower lobe)
Infant (<2 yr)	Hirschsprung disease
Intussusception*	Aerophagia
Incarcerated hernia*	Spontaneous bacterial peritonitis
Urinary tract infection*	Gastroesophageal reflux

Continued

TABLE 13.2   Causes of Acute Abdominal Pain by Age Group—cont'd

Child (2–11 yr)	Adolescent (12–19 yr)
Appendicitis*	Appendicitis*
Gastroenteritis* †	Pelvic inflammatory disease*
Trauma*	Trauma*
Henoch-Schönlein purpura	Anterior cutaneous nerve entrapment syndrome
Abdominal migraine	Tubo-ovarian abscess
Hemolytic uremic syndrome	Perihepatitis (Fitz-Hugh-Curtis syndrome)
Hepatitis	Labor (pregnancy)
Peptic ulcer disease	Hepatitis
Sickle cell anemia: vasoocclusive crisis	Pancreatitis (any cause)
Pancreatitis	Ectopic pregnancy
Pneumonia (lower lobe)	Crohn disease
Abdominal tumors	Ovarian cyst/mittelschmerz*
Pyelonephritis/cystitis	Sickle cell crisis
Testicular torsion	Peptic ulcer disease
Torsed cryptorchid testis	Omental torsion
Incarcerated hernia	Psoas abscess or hemorrhage
Typhlitis	Mesenteric adenitis
Pharyngitis/tonsillitis	Urinary tract infection
Meckel diverticulitis	Muscle strain (exercise, coughing)
Superior mesenteric artery syndrome	DKA
Mesenteric adenitis	Testicular torsion
Spontaneous bacterial peritonitis	Idiopathic*
DKA	
Streptococcal pharyngitis	
Idiopathic*	

*Most commonly seen problem.
†Gastroenteritis indicates intestinal infection with viral, bacterial, protozoal, or parasitic agents. Giardiasis and cryptosporidiosis are particularly common and may produce acute or chronic pain.
DKA, diabetic ketoacidosis.

TABLE 13.3   Sudden Acute Excruciating Abdominal Pain (Within Minutes)

Intestinal Perforation	Luminal Occlusion
Peptic ulcer disease	Urolithiasis
Appendicitis	Cholelithiasis
Diverticula	Strangulated hernia
Vascular Occlusion	**Intraabdominal Hemorrhage**
Midgut volvulus	Ectopic pregnancy
Emboli	Ruptured aortic aneurysm
Endocarditis	Ruptured spleen
Strangulated hernia	
Ovarian torsion	
Testicular torsion	

TABLE 13.4   Causes of Chronic and Recurrent Abdominal Pain by Age Group*

Infant (<2 yr)	Child (2–11 yr)	Adolescent (12–19 yr)
Colic†	Constipation†	Irritable bowel syndrome†
Inguinal hernia	Functional pain†	Psychogenic factors†
Malabsorption‡	Celiac disease	Dysmenorrhea†
Milk allergy	Eosinophilic esophagitis	Mittelschmerz†
Hirschsprung disease	Giardiasis†	Abdominal wall pain
Cystic fibrosis	Peptic ulcer disease	Peptic ulcer disease
Rotational defects	Toxins (lead)	Gallbladder disease
Malformations	Pancreatitis	Pelvic inflammatory disease
Esophagitis	Parasites	Ovarian cysts
	Tumors/masses	Diabetes mellitus
	Diskitis/osteomyelitis	Inflammatory bowel disease
	Abdominal migraine	Malignancy
	Diabetes mellitus	Giardiasis
	Volvulus	Serositis (e.g., SLE, familial
	Intraabdominal abscess§	Mediterranean fever)
	Choledochal cyst	Intraabdominal abscess§
		Hereditary angioedema

*See also Table 13.6.
†Most common diagnoses.
‡Includes lactose and sorbitol (and other fruit juice polyalcohol) intolerance.
§Hepatic, pancreatic, subphrenic, psoas, perinephric, renal, pelvic.
SLE, systemic lupus erythematosus.

intervention, although delays in presentation and diagnosis in children are not unusual. Timing of the progression of symptoms must be detailed.

Location of pain. The location of the pain at its onset and any change in location are very important (Table 13.5; see also Table 13.1). Most intraperitoneal visceral pain is a response to the stimulation of stretch fibers in the bowel wall and is mediated through the spinal nerves. This pain is sensed as a deep, aching periumbilical pain. Pain caused by inflammation of the parietal peritoneum (acute appendicitis) is localized to the area of the inflamed organ or is diffuse if the

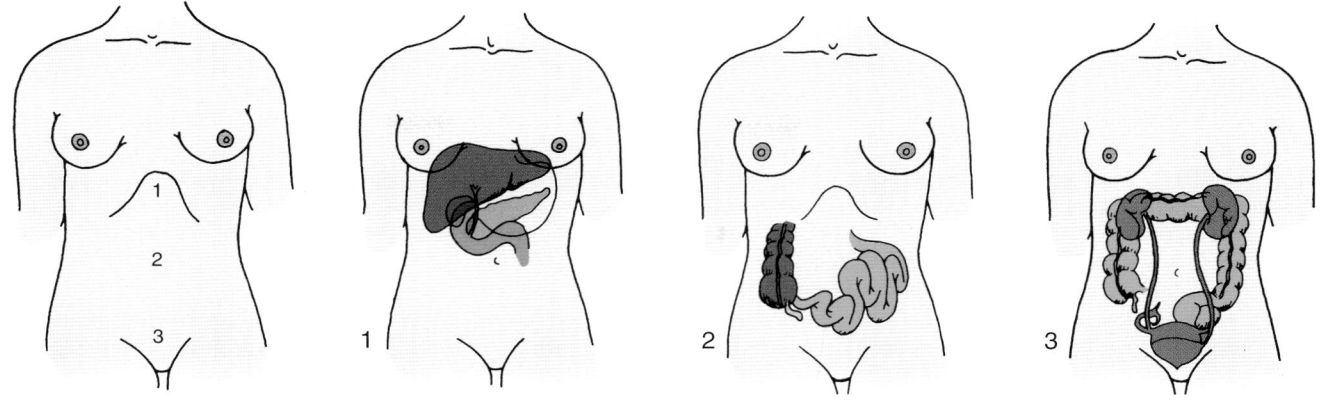

Fig. 13.1 "Visceral" abdominal pain: deep, dull, diffuse. The three general localizations of midline "visceral" abdominal pain are epigastric *(1)*, periumbilical *(2)*, and hypogastric *(3)*. *1*, Epigastric pain usually suggests disease of the thorax, stomach, duodenum, pancreas, liver, or gallbladder. *2*, Periumbilical pain usually implies disease of the small intestine, cecum, or both. *3*, Hypogastric pain usually implicates the large intestine, pelvic organs, or urinary system. (From Reilly BM. Abdominal pain. In: *Practical Strategies in Outpatient Medicine*. 2nd ed. Philadelphia: WB Saunders; 1991:702.)

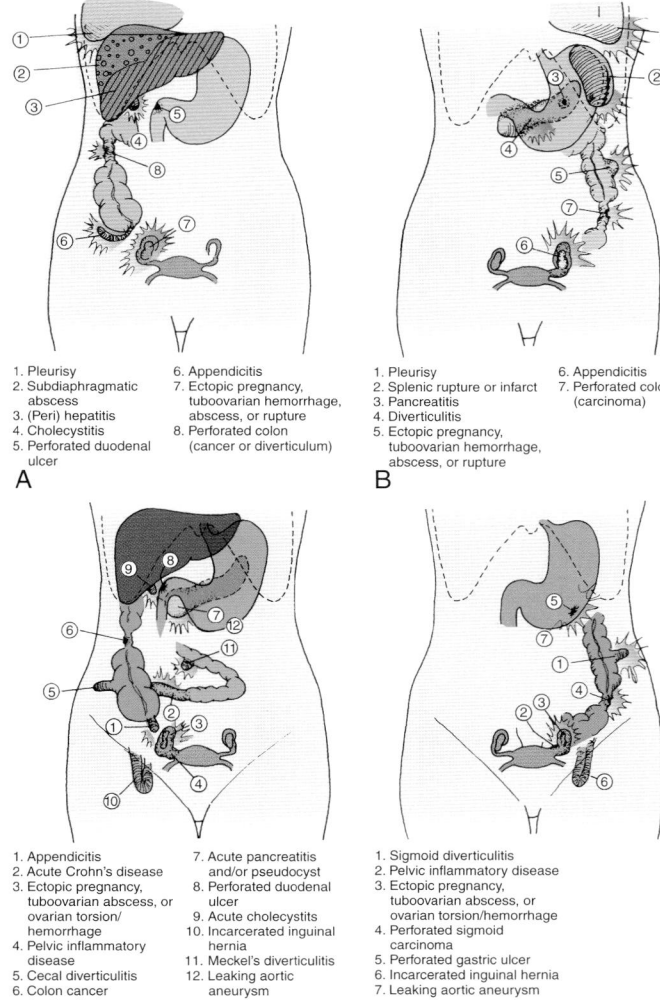

A

1. Pleurisy
2. Subdiaphragmatic abscess
3. (Peri) hepatitis
4. Cholecystitis
5. Perforated duodenal ulcer
6. Appendicitis
7. Ectopic pregnancy, tuboovarian hemorrhage, abscess, or rupture
8. Perforated colon (cancer or diverticulum)

B

1. Pleurisy
2. Splenic rupture or infarct
3. Pancreatitis
4. Diverticulitis
5. Ectopic pregnancy, tuboovarian hemorrhage, abscess, or rupture
6. Appendicitis
7. Perforated colon (carcinoma)

C

1. Appendicitis
2. Acute Crohn's disease
3. Ectopic pregnancy, tuboovarian abscess, or ovarian torsion/ hemorrhage
4. Pelvic inflammatory disease
5. Cecal diverticulitis
6. Colon cancer (perforation)
7. Acute pancreatitis and/or pseudocyst
8. Perforated duodenal ulcer
9. Acute cholecystitis
10. Incarcerated inguinal hernia
11. Meckel's diverticulitis
12. Leaking aortic aneurysm

D

1. Sigmoid diverticulitis
2. Pelvic inflammatory disease
3. Ectopic pregnancy, tuboovarian abscess, or ovarian torsion/hemorrhage
4. Perforated sigmoid carcinoma
5. Perforated gastric ulcer
6. Incarcerated inguinal hernia
7. Leaking aortic aneurysm

Fig. 13.2 Common and uncommon conditions that may cause "parietal" pain and localized peritonitis in the various quadrants of the abdomen. *A*, Right upper quadrant. *B*, Left upper quadrant. *C*, Right lower quadrant. *D*, Left lower quadrant. (From Reilly BM. Abdominal pain. In: *Practical Strategies in Outpatient Medicine*. 2nd ed. Philadelphia: WB Saunders; 1991:703.)

TABLE 13.5 **Localization of Abdominal Pain: Referred or Radiated**	
REFERRED	
Extraabdominal Lesion Pain Referred to Abdomen	**Intraabdominal Extraperitoneal Origin**
Thorax	Pancreas
Spine	Kidney
Hips	Ureters
Pelvis	Great vessels
	Pelvic organs
	Retroperitoneal space
RADIATED	
Origin Is Primary Site with Simultaneously Perceived Pain in a Secondary Site	
Cholecystitis radiates to subscapular area	
Splenic injury radiates to shoulder	
Ureteral colic (stones) radiates to testis, upper leg, or groin	
Pancreatitis radiates to back	

inflammation is extensive and involves more of the peritoneal cavity. Pain resulting from obstruction of an organ is localized to the area of that organ and radiates to the commonly innervated region (e.g., stones in the ureter cause intense flank pain with radiation into the groin). Pain that is migratory or fleeting in location is rarely suggestive of a problem requiring operative intervention. Of note, many young children may point to the umbilicus to localize their pain although the pain may be elsewhere in the abdomen.

Character of pain. The character of the pain is often difficult for the child to describe. Some older children may be able to differentiate cramping, aching, and burning sensations, but most children do not do this well. Children can relate whether the pain comes and goes or is continuous and unrelenting. The character of the pain is usually unknown in the toddler and infant, although the parent can determine whether the discomfort is constant, cramping, or intermittent. If the child intermittently draws the legs up in a flexed position and cries, the clinician can assume that intermittent pain is present.

Child's activity level. The effect of the pain on the child's activities is an important indicator of the severity of the underlying disease, although it is important to note that children with chronic functional abdominal pain may wake up from sleep and may miss favorite activities due to pain and functional disability. Asking whether motion worsens the pain helps differentiate peritoneal irritation or musculoskeletal diseases from more nonspecific problems. The child with acute appendicitis lies motionless, whereas the child with a renal stone, gallstone, gastroenteritis, or pancreatitis may toss and turn and writhe in discomfort. Localized, superficial, tender trigger points in the abdominal wall may suggest abdominal wall (muscle, cutaneous) pain. The localized pain results from entrapment of cutaneous terminal branches of intercostal nerves (7th–12th) penetrating the rectus abdominis muscle and can easily be missed without the proper history or exam.

Gastrointestinal symptoms. The presence or absence of gastrointestinal symptoms may differentiate intestinal problems (acute appendicitis, gastroenteritis, acute cholecystitis) from those arising from other intraabdominal organs (urinary tract infection, ovarian disease, abdominal wall pain).

Anorexia and nausea are difficult symptoms for a small child to describe. Often, if simply asked whether they are hungry, a child will respond in the affirmative. Questions about recent food intake, normal eating habits, the last normal meal, and the current desirability of a favorite food often provide more accurate information about the presence or absence of anorexia and nausea than do direct questions about appetite or nausea.

Vomiting associated with acute pain is usually related to intestinal disease, such as ileus, gastroenteritis, or acute problems of the gastrointestinal tract that warrant surgery (see Chapter 15). However, vomiting may occur as a response to severe nonintestinal pain such as in testicular torsion; this vomiting is usually not recurring and is not a prominent feature. Vomiting that occurs with acute pain in the middle of the night can also be associated with abdominal migraine or cyclic vomiting syndrome, particularly if the history suggests similar episodes in the past that resolved spontaneously. Oftentimes, the child has been misdiagnosed with multiple bouts of acute gastroenteritis that occurred over the course of several weeks or months. Vomiting may also be a sign of increased intracranial pressure, which may or may not be accompanied by associated headache or vital sign changes (bradycardia, hypertension, irregular respirations), a bulging fontanel, an altered level of consciousness, or neurologic findings (third or sixth cranial nerve palsies). Care should be taken to determine whether the pain occurs before or after the onset of the vomiting. With acute surgical lesions (those caused by intestinal obstruction, acute appendicitis, acute cholecystitis), the pain usually occurs before or during the vomiting. If the vomiting occurred before the onset of pain, the clinician should suspect gastroenteritis or another nonspecific problem. The appearance of the vomited material is also important. Feculent or dark-green material suggests intestinal obstruction. Dark brown or frankly bloody material indicates gastritis, prolapse gastropathy, or peptic ulcer disease as the source of pain.

Diarrhea occurs commonly in intestinal diseases of viral, parasitic, or bacterial origin (see Chapter 14). The stool volume is large, and defecation is usually preceded by cramping pain that is alleviated by the passage of the diarrheal stool. Diarrhea may also occur in the presence of acute appendicitis or other pelvic infections (such as those resulting from pelvic inflammatory disease, tubo-ovarian abscess); in these cases, diarrhea is caused by inflammation and irritation of an area of the colon adjacent to an inflammatory mass. The diarrhea in this instance is of small volume and is frequent. It is important to obtain an estimate of the volume and consistency of stool. Diarrhea may also occur in lesions that cause partial obstruction of the bowel, such as strictures, adhesions, and Hirschsprung disease. In this situation, the patient also has some degree of abdominal distention. **Constipation** alone can cause

acute abdominal pain and may also indicate other gastrointestinal dysfunction. Some constipated children present with a picture very similar to that seen in acute appendicitis but have a large amount of stool filling the entire colon. It is therefore important to obtain a good history of not only bowel movement frequency but also consistency (see Chapter 19). The history and exam are sufficient to make the diagnosis of constipation, and imaging is usually not necessary. Once the diagnosis is made, appropriate treatment should start with a proper clean-out followed by maintenance therapy. The clinician should not be fooled by the symptom of tenesmus, where the patient has a feeling of constantly needing to pass stools despite having an empty colon. Tenesmus can be seen in the setting of proctocolitis or inflammatory bowel disease and is often misinterpreted by the patient as constipation.

Associated symptoms. The presence of headache, sore throat, and other generalized aches and pains moves the examiner away from a diagnosis of an acute problem warranting surgery and strongly suggests a viral flulike illness. Asking the child to point to the area of worst pain sometimes results in the child pointing to the head or throat. The examiner must be careful to remember the whole child and not to focus on the abdomen just because that is the area of the presenting complaint. Many systemic diseases directly or indirectly produce abdominal pain and must be considered in the differential diagnosis (Table 13.6).

Family history and personal medical history. Viral gastroenteritis, other viral syndromes, and food poisoning may affect the patient's family or schoolmates; it is important to ask about other family members, classmates, or playmates who have recently had similar symptoms. Certain systemic and inherited diseases, such as sickle cell anemia, diabetes mellitus, celiac disease, spherocytosis, familial Mediterranean fever, and porphyria, are associated with episodes of abdominal pain. A strong family history of migraine headaches in a child with several previous episodes of intense abdominal pain that have resolved, who presents with a new "attack," suggests the possibility of abdominal migraine. The family must be asked about familial diseases and any previous episodes of pain in the child. Previous intraabdominal operations may result in adhesions that can cause pain, intestinal obstruction, or both. A history of previous intraabdominal surgeries suggests the possibility of bowel obstruction. Some specific medical illnesses result in identifiable or predictable causes of abdominal pain (Table 13.7).

Physical Examination

The physical examination begins when the clinician enters the room and observes the child's activity and demeanor while obtaining the history. Does the child appear ill? Is the patient lethargic, rolling about in discomfort, alert but lying very still, or bouncing all over the room? Each of these activities conveys a message. The listless, lethargic child may be in shock, dehydrated, and very ill. The child who is crying out loudly and generally dominating the scene probably does not have a problem that warrants surgery and may have mild pain that is self-resolving. The child who seems only mildly ill but moves with great care, if at all, is assumed to have an inflammatory process until it is proven otherwise.

Physical examination techniques and findings are age dependent. Younger children may have difficulty cooperating because of fear or discomfort. Younger children may be more cooperative if kept on their parent's lap. Older children should be asked to get onto the examination table with as little assistance as possible. If the child does this easily, the probability of an acute intraabdominal inflammatory process is quite low. Outer bulky clothing should be removed to allow good exposure of the abdomen without the child having to feel vulnerable.

TABLE 13.6 Systemic Causes of Acute Abdominal Pain

Metabolic, Hematologic
Acute porphyria
Hereditary angioedema
Sickle cell crisis
Hemolytic transfusion reaction
Leukemia
Acute hemolytic states
Diabetic ketoacidosis
Hemolytic uremic syndrome
Addison disease
Uremia
Electrolyte disturbances
Hyperparathyroidism-hypercalcemia (urolithiasis, pancreatitis)
Hypertriglyceridemia (pancreatitis)
Fabry disease

Musculoskeletal
Arthritis
Spondylodiskitis
Thoracic nerve root dysfunction
Trauma/child abuse
Hernia
Psoas abscess or hemorrhage

Neurologic
Abdominal epilepsy
Abdominal migraine
Brain tumor
Multiple sclerosis
Radiculopathy
Neuropathy
Herpes zoster
Dysautonomia (Riley-Day syndrome)

Drugs, Toxins
Heavy metal poisoning
  Lead
  Arsenic
  Mercury
Mushroom ingestion
Narcotic withdrawal
Black widow spider bite

Infectious, Inflammatory
Acute rheumatic fever
Infectious mononucleosis
Rocky Mountain spotted fever
Measles
Mumps
Pneumonia (lower lobe)
Pericarditis
Pharyngitis
Epididymitis/orchitis
Henoch-Schönlein purpura
Inflammatory bowel disease
Hemolytic uremic syndrome
Systemic lupus erythematosus
Endocarditis
Anaphylaxis
Familial Mediterranean fever and other genetic fever syndromes

Other
Pneumothorax
Pulmonary embolism
Disorder of the brain-gut interaction
Aerophagia

TABLE 13.7 Current or Past Aspects of Medical History That May Suggest Cause of Abdominal Pain

Historical Factor	Cause of Pain
Cystic fibrosis	Pancreatitis, diabetes mellitus, meconium ileus equivalent, appendicitis, intussusception, biliary or urinary stones
Sickle cell anemia	Vasoocclusive crisis, cholelithiasis, hepatitis, hemolytic crisis, renal infarction, splenic sequestration
Diabetes mellitus	Pancreatitis, gastric neuropathy
Cirrhosis, nephrotic syndrome	Primary bacterial peritonitis
SLE, other autoimmune disorders	Vasculitis, pancreatitis, serositis, infarction
Corticosteroids	Gastric ulceration, pancreatitis
NSAID	Ileal perforation, gastric ulceration, renal-papillary necrosis
HIV	Gastroenteritis, hepatitis, pancreatitis, esophagitis, lymphoma
Mononucleosis	Hepatitis, splenic rupture
Henoch-Schönlein purpura	Mucosal hemorrhage, intussusception
Crohn disease	Small bowel stricture, intraabdominal or psoas abscess
Hemolytic uremic syndrome	Colitis
Upper respiratory tract infection	Pneumonia, mesenteric adenitis
Pneumonia	Mesenteric adenitis
Prior surgery	Abscess, adhesions, obstruction, stricture, pancreatitis, ectopic pregnancy
Inborn errors of metabolism, hypertriglyceridemia, hypercalcemia	Pancreatitis
Drugs (valproic acid)	Pancreatitis
Adolescent	Ovarian torsion, sexually transmitted infection, ectopic pregnancy

NSAID, nonsteroidal antiinflammatory drug; SLE, systemic lupus erythematosus.

The examination must be performed in a relaxed, friendly manner with attention fully focused on the child. An accurate examination depends on the child's trust and cooperation. A conversation with the child about family, friends, pets, school, sports, music, or other specific interests of that child diverts attention (distraction) from the examination and increases cooperation. The examiner should never surprise the child and should never lie. The first surprise or untruth, such as the statement "This won't hurt," destroys any trust that has developed.

Vital signs are important as **low-grade fever** (<38.3°C) is seen in early appendicitis but is also common in many other diseases. The absence of fever does not exclude the diagnosis of acute appendicitis or other problems necessitating surgical intervention. Tachycardia may reflect anxiety or may be caused by dehydration, shock, fever, or pain. Tachypnea suggests a metabolic acidosis (shock, diabetes mellitus, or toxic ingestion), an intrapulmonary process, sepsis, or fever. Blood pressure may demonstrate a widened pulse pressure as seen in sepsis. The vital signs must be viewed in context but may be the first clue to a serious illness.

Examination of the head, neck, chest, and extremities may precede the abdominal examination. In children too young to describe the location of the pain, a careful examination of the ears is important, but can be performed at the end of the examination. Streptococcal pharyngitis or mononucleosis is sometimes accompanied by severe abdominal pain. Affected children will present with fever, appear ill, and have tender cervical adenopathy and an obvious tonsillitis, pharyngitis, or both.

Decreased breath sounds and/or rales in a lower-lung lobe may indicate pneumonia. Children with lower lobe bacterial pneumonia may present with severe abdominal pain, high fever, tachypnea, cough, and, on occasion, vomiting. This presentation could mimic that of a child with peritonitis; however, the abdominal findings are not consistent with the diagnosis of an acute intraabdominal process, and examination of the lungs should demonstrate the pneumonia.

The abdominal examination should be performed systematically and with the child as comfortable as possible. Before the examiner actually touches the child's abdomen, they should observe it, looking for distention, inguinal masses, peristaltic waves, and scars from old injuries or surgical incisions. Inguinal and femoral hernias are often overlooked but a common cause of abdominal pain. Next, the child should be asked to indicate with one finger the point of greatest pain. The point may be a vague circle in the area of the umbilicus, but if the child specifies a defined spot, the examiner should avoid that area until the remainder of the abdomen has been palpated.

Gentleness is essential to successful palpation of the abdomen. The examiner must warm both hands and the stethoscope before touching the patient. The stethoscope is an excellent tool for palpation of the abdomen. Auscultation of the chest can simply be extended to the abdomen, with the examiner assuring the child that the stethoscope did not hurt on the chest. The initial examination of the abdomen with the stethoscope should be just for listening, with no pressure exerted, so that no discomfort results.

Bowel sounds are usually nonspecific in most children with abdominal pain; however, in certain processes, they are helpful. High-pitched tinkling sounds or rushes are usually associated with an obstructive process. Bowel sounds in gastroenteritis are ordinarily very active and loud but may be normal. Acute appendicitis is accompanied by normal sounds in the early stages, but bowel sounds disappear with diffuse peritonitis.

Watching the child's reaction to the auscultation may be a valuable clue to areas of true tenderness. As the examiner continues to listen over the entire anterior abdomen, the pressure on the head of the stethoscope increases until the examiner is, in fact, palpating with the stethoscope. This often is a much more reliable method of eliciting true tenderness and guarding than is the palpating hand.

Palpation is begun as far away from the area of pain identified by the child as possible. The examiner's hand should be softly placed flat (in parallel) on the child's abdomen. Directing fingers into the abdomen (perpendicular) as a method of palpation is unnecessary and often frightening. The clinician should watch the child's face, not the abdomen, during the palpation. Some children are extremely stoic, and only the slightest grimace betrays the discomfort they are experiencing. Attention is paid during palpation to the presence of masses. The examiner should focus on finding the location of pain and the presence or absence of guarding or rebound tenderness. **Guarding** refers to the voluntary or involuntary (often referred to as rigidity) contraction of the abdominal musculature. Fear of pain, rather than actual pain elicited by palpation, is the most common cause for voluntary guarding, while involuntary guarding results from reflexive spasms of the abdominal musculature in the setting of peritoneal irritation. A **rigid** or **boardlike** abdomen is the result of involuntary guarding and cannot be overcome by distraction. Voluntary guarding usually starts before the palpation starts and can be overcome by asking the child to take deep breaths, flexing the knees and hips, or by using other distractions appropriate to the child's age and temperament. When encountering tenderness, the examiner should palpate only deeply enough to elicit the complaint of pain and some guarding. There is no need to bring on unnecessary pain by deep palpation.

Rebound pain is an indicator of peritoneal irritation and is elicited during examination of the anterior abdominal wall. It occurs when an inflamed focus within the abdomen is compressed and the pressure is then quickly released, resulting in sudden and sometimes severe pain. The standard method to elicit rebound pain is to palpate deeply, then suddenly remove the palpating hand. *Although this sign aids in the determination of the presence of an intraperitoneal inflammatory process, it is not necessary to cause extra discomfort or stress, particularly in younger children; it is not recommended.* Peritoneal irritation can also be detected by maneuvers such as asking the child to jump or cough or tapping the feet while observing for facial signs of discomfort.

Other areas of inflammation can be detected by maneuvers that move muscles adjacent to the inflammation. A positive **Carnett test** occurs when pain is unchanged or increased when the supine patient tenses the abdominal wall by lifting the head and shoulders off the examining table. Carnett sign is a sensitive tool to discriminate *abdominal wall* pain from visceral pain. The **psoas sign** occurs when elevation and flexion of the leg against the pressure of the examiner's hand (or passive extension of the leg toward the back) causes pain. An inflammatory mass, such as an inflamed appendix, a psoas abscess, or a perinephric abscess, in contact with the psoas muscle is the cause of this pain. Likewise, the **obturator sign** is pain with flexion of the thigh at right angles to the trunk and external rotation of the same leg while the patient is in the supine position. This sign results from contact of an inflammatory mass with the obturator muscle (Fig. 13.3).

The flanks and back must be inspected and palpated. Percussion at the costovertebral angle elicits pain in the presence of renal or perinephric inflammation. Vertebral body and disk disease may be detected by palpitation of the spine. The perineum and genitalia must be inspected and palpated as necessary. External examination of the genitalia in prepubertal girls is adequate. If a more thorough examination or an intravaginal examination is needed in prepubertal girls, it should generally be performed with the patient under anesthesia. In postpubertal girls, a pelvic examination may be valuable, regardless of the patient's sexual activity history.

The need for a **rectal examination** is controversial. If a diagnosis is already obvious, the rectal examination may be deferred. If an imaging study or colonoscopy is planned, a rectal examination may be unnecessary. If constipation is suspected as the cause for pain, rectal

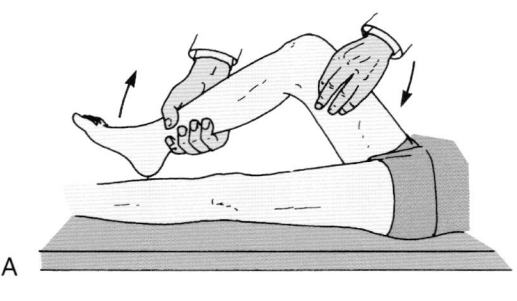

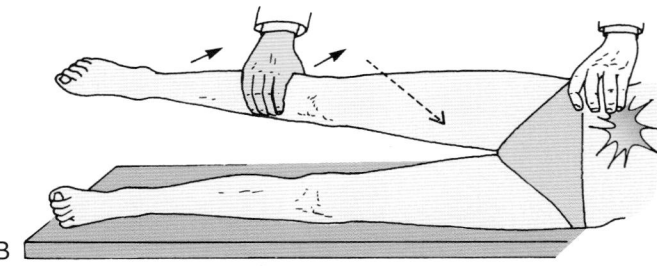

Fig. 13.3 *A,* The obturator sign. Pain occurs when the hip is flexed and rotated. Internal rotation is most likely to cause pain as a result of pelvic or retroperitoneal disease or both. *B,* The psoas sign. The test may be performed passively or actively. The hip is passively extended, thus stretching the psoas muscle *(solid arrow).* The hip is actively flexed usually against resistance, thus tensing the psoas muscle *(dotted arrow).* (From Reilly BM. Abdominal pain. In: *Practical Strategies in Outpatient Medicine.* 2nd ed. Philadelphia: WB Saunders; 1991:714.)

TABLE 13.8   **Red Flags and Clues to an Organic Cause of Abdominal Pain**
Age <4 yr old
Localized pain in nonperiumbilical site
Referred pain
Sudden onset of excruciating pain
Crescendo nature of pain
Sudden worsening of pain
Fever (high fever >39.4°C suggests pneumonia, pyelonephritis, dysentery, cholangitis, more than perforation or abscess)
Jaundice
Distention*
Dysuria
Emesis (especially bilious)
Anorexia
Weight loss
Positive family history (metabolic disorders, peptic ulcer disease)[†]
Change in urine or stool color (blood, acholic) or frequency
Vaginal discharge
Menstrual abnormalities (amenorrhea)
Sexual activity
Delayed sexual development (chronic pain)
Anemia
Elevated erythrocyte sedimentation rate
Elevated stool calprotectin
Specific physical findings (hepatomegaly, splenomegaly, absent bowel sounds, adnexal tenderness, palpable mass, involuntary guarding, focal or diffuse tenderness, positive rectal examination results, perianal disease, joint swelling, rashes)

*Consider 5 Fs: fat, feces, flatus (aerophagia, obstruction), fluid (ascites, hydronephrosis, cysts), fetus (pregnancy or fetal-like abnormal growth [e.g., tumors]).
[†]Family history is also positive for chronic pain syndromes (constipation, irritable bowel, dysmenorrhea, and lactase or sucrase deficiency).

examination should be performed but should be the last part of the physical examination and should be performed only once. The child should be relaxed and should be given an honest explanation of the procedure. The examiner should use plenty of lubricant and should perform the rectal examination very gently. If the child strongly resists, it is pointless to perform a forceful examination. This is when the rectal examination may truly be deferred. Lateralizing pain, masses, and the presence and character of stool in the rectum are assessed. The stool should always be tested for blood except in children with gastrostomy or nasogastric tubes since it will invariably be positive and can be misleading.

Clues to an organic and at times more serious cause of abdominal pain are noted in Table 13.8. Furthermore, peritoneal signs, which suggest a "surgical abdomen," most often caused by peritonitis are noted in Table 13.9. In addition, the presence of shock suggests other serious diseases (see Table 13.9).

Laboratory Evaluation

After a careful history is obtained and thorough physical examination is performed, the diagnosis or a short list of possible diagnoses should be apparent. Laboratory data are supportive in confirming or ruling out suspected disease.

Complete Blood Cell Count

The hemoglobin and hematocrit levels can reveal anemia caused by acute or chronic blood loss (as with ulcers, inflammatory bowel disease, Meckel diverticula) or the anemia of chronic disease (as with systemic lupus erythematosus, inflammatory bowel disease). The white blood cell count indicates the possibility of infection or blood dyscrasias. In uncomplicated acute appendicitis, the white blood cell count ranges from normal values to as high as 16,000. A very high white blood cell count (>18,000/mm³) indicates intestinal gangrene, perforation, peritonitis, or abscess formation, but this count may also be high in acute

bacterial gastroenteritis, streptococcal diseases, pyelonephritis, pelvic inflammatory disease, hemolytic uremic syndrome, and pneumonia.

The differential cell count may also be helpful. In studies of children with acute appendicitis, 95% had neutrophilia, but only half had leukocytosis in the first 24 hours. If the child's history and physical examination findings are highly suggestive of appendicitis, a normal or mildly elevated white blood cell count should not dissuade the clinician from that diagnosis. However, a striking lymphocytosis may suggest gastroenteritis or a systemic illness. Overreliance on the CBC alone can cause delay in reaching the correct diagnosis.

Urinalysis

The UA is an important and useful laboratory test in the evaluation of abdominal pain. The presence of ketones and a high specific gravity suggest poor food intake and dehydration. Large amounts of glucose and ketones in the urine indicate diabetic ketoacidosis. A pregnancy test should be performed on postpubertal girls, regardless of sexual activity history. The presence of both white cells and bacteria indicates a urinary tract infection; either finding alone may not be sufficient for that diagnosis (see Chapter 21). White blood cells may be present in the urine from irritation caused by an inflammatory mass adjacent to the bladder or ureter; hematuria may be seen with nephrolithiasis (see Chapter 23).

TABLE 13.9 Peritoneal Signs of a "Surgical Abdomen"

Severe pain

Patient's eyes anxiously open during examiner's palpation

Patient is motionless

Absent bowel sounds

Extreme tenderness to palpation

Voluntary guarding with gentle palpation

Involuntary guarding: boardlike rigidity

Rebound tenderness (do not intentionally elicit)

Pain with movement or cough

If Shock Is Present, Consider:

Severe pancreatitis

Trauma: intraabdominal hemorrhage

Ruptured spleen (trauma, mononucleosis)

Spontaneous bacterial peritonitis

Intestinal perforation (appendicitis, ulcer, inflammatory bowel disease, *Clostridioides difficile* colitis, penetrating trauma)

Intussusception

Urosepsis

Associated severe gastrointestinal bleeding

Rupture of fallopian tube from ectopic pregnancy

Pulmonary embolism

Aortic dissection

Volvulus

Child abuse

Addisonian crisis (adrenal insufficiency)

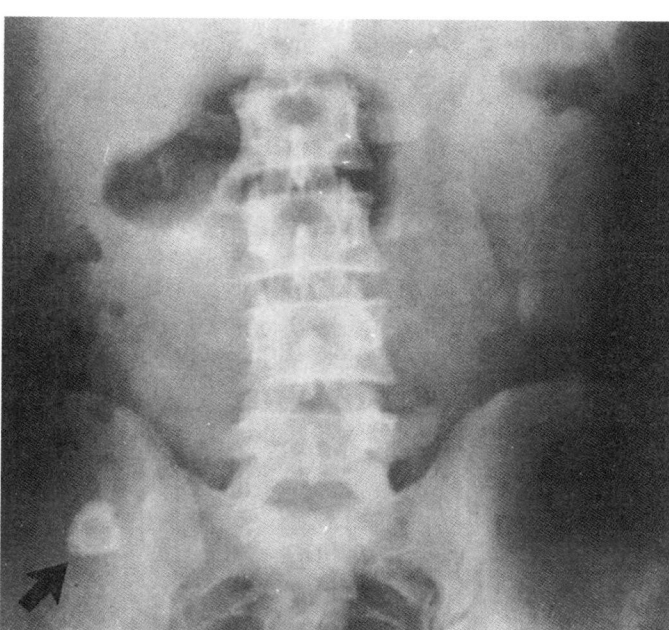

Fig. 13.4 The patient described the gradual onset of anorexia, nausea, and vague periumbilical abdominal pain. Twenty-four hours later, the pain was much more severe in the right lower quadrant, where localized peritoneal signs were apparent. The radiographic film of the abdomen reveals a huge calcified density in the right lower quadrant; it proved to be an appendiceal fecalith at surgery. (From Reilly BM. Abdominal pain. In: *Practical Strategies in Outpatient Medicine.* 2nd ed. Philadelphia: WB Saunders; 1991:16.)

Other Laboratory Tests

Other laboratory tests, such as measurement of serum electrolytes, amylase, and lipase; liver function studies including γ-glutamyl transpeptidase (GGT); inflammatory markers (CRP or sedimentation rate); blood cultures; stool cultures; and viral tests should be ordered on the basis of the differential diagnosis after a thorough history and physical examination are completed.

Imaging Evaluation

Multitudes of imaging studies are available; none should be obtained until the patient has been examined.

Plain Radiography

Plain radiographs, especially kidney-ureter-bladder (KUB) films, with or without upright lateral views of the chest and abdomen, are routinely obtained in most emergency departments as part of the evaluation of acute abdominal pain. The chest film helps assess the presence of a lower lobe pneumonia, which often causes severe abdominal pain, especially in small children. However, early in the disease, the physical examination may be more helpful. Often, if the KUB-abdominal radiographic study includes the lower lobes, the chest radiographic study can be deferred and performed only if the KUB demonstrates lung abnormalities.

Only approximately 10% of abdominal radiographic studies are positive when they are obtained as part of the routine work-up for abdominal pain. Of those that are limited to patients with serious illness, 46% of the results are positive. Plain abdominal radiographs may be helpful to confirm the presence of intestinal obstruction, pneumatosis intestinalis, renal or biliary tract calculi, calcified fecaliths, or intestinal perforation (pneumoperitoneum–free air). These studies detect bowel distention (air-fluid levels on upright views), calcification, free air, and large masses but are not helpful in detecting most other diseases. If free air or intestinal obstruction is suspected, the abdominal films must include a flat and upright or decubitus view of the abdomen to demonstrate the air-fluid interface.

In **acute appendicitis**, a calcified appendicolith (appendiceal fecalith) may be seen (Fig. 13.4). This finding automatically makes the diagnosis of appendiceal dysfunction and confirms the need for appendectomy. The absence of an appendicolith on KUB does not rule out appendicitis. More often, the noncalcified appendicolith may obstruct the appendix; ultrasonographic or CT imaging is necessary to visualize this lesion. If an inflammatory mass lies near the iliopsoas muscle, mild lumbar scoliosis may be present as a result of spasm of the muscle.

Radiographic studies are not always necessary. If the diagnosis is already obvious, specific therapy is indicated. In some situations, other types of imaging studies are more useful, and plain radiographs are not prerequisite.

Ultrasonography

Ultrasonographic examination is ideal for children. It is usually painless, is readily available, emits no radiation, requires no intravenous contrast material, and can be performed without sedation. Unfortunately, it is operator dependent and can be difficult to perform in the setting of extreme pain or lack of cooperation. Lower abdominal **gynecologic pain** in females, especially in adolescent females, can be confused with appendicitis. Pelvic ultrasonography demonstrates pathologic processes of the ovaries and fallopian tubes, the size of the uterus, and the presence of free fluid in the pelvis. An enlarged,

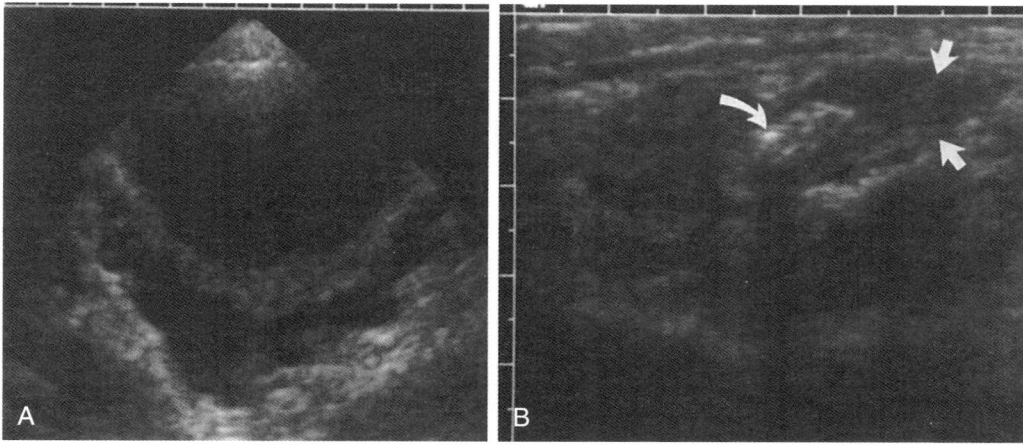

Fig. 13.5 A transverse scan of the pelvis shows free fluid pooling behind the bladder *(A)*. The longitudinal scan of the right lower quadrant *(B)* shows a shadowing appendicolith *(curved arrow)* in a thick-walled appendix, typical of appendicitis. *Straight arrows* outline the appendiceal tip, which looks ready to perforate. Free fluid in the pelvis always increases the suspicion of appendicitis. (From Teele R, Share J. Appendicitis and other causes of intraabdominal inflammation. In: *Ultrasonography of Infants and Children*. Philadelphia: WB Saunders; 1991:349.)

inflamed appendix can also be visualized (Fig. 13.5). Any female with abdominal pain in whom the diagnosis is not obvious should undergo an ultrasonographic examination.

Gallstones, a dilated thick-walled gallbladder, or a dilated common bile duct can be visualized by ultrasonography; all three support the diagnosis of biliary disease. Edema and enlargement of the pancreas are seen in acute pancreatitis. Ultrasonography also details the character of abdominal masses, differentiating cystic from solid masses, and can be helpful in demonstrating free fluid or abscesses. The anatomy of the urinary tract is well defined by ultrasonography; nephromegaly may be seen with pyelonephritis. The choice of ultrasonography versus CT is dependent on the expertise of the regional imaging center. Abdominal ultrasonography is an excellent screening method for detecting intussusception and midgut volvulus. If an ileus or intestinal obstruction is present, interpretation of the ultrasonographic examination becomes difficult because of the multiple air-filled loops of intestine.

Contrast Studies

In some situations, certain bowel lesions are best delineated with a contrast medium placed in the bowel, either in an upper gastrointestinal series or by enema. If a colonic obstruction is suspected, such as in **Hirschsprung disease**, the appropriate contrast material is a barium enema. However, the sensitivity and specificity of contrast enema for detection of Hirschsprung disease are approximately 70% and 83%, respectively. If the suspicion is high for the disease, the patient should be referred for further evaluation with either suction rectal biopsy or anorectal manometry. If the presence of gastrointestinal perforation is possible, regardless of the etiology, a water-soluble agent should be used instead of barium.

Malrotation of the midgut with a volvulus in infants and older children is often seen on ultrasonography but can be diagnosed by an upper gastrointestinal study. In the infant who presents with an acute abdomen and bilious vomiting and in the older child who manifests chronic abdominal pain and intermittent vomiting, the oral barium contrast study is highly reliable to rule out causes of obstruction such as intestinal malrotation with midgut volvulus or other causes for anatomic obstruction (duodenal web, annular pancreas, superior mesenteric artery syndrome).

Intussusception is both diagnosed and treated by means of air or barium enema; however, initial diagnosis is possible with ultrasonogra-

phy. The sudden onset of severe, diffuse pain, along with the suggestion of a soft, nontender mass in the right upper quadrant of the abdomen in a previously well young child, constitutes the classical picture of intussusception. Evidence of blood in the stool is usually a late finding and should not be expected early in the disease process. The plain films may be nonspecific, may show evidence of intestinal obstruction, or may show a mass in the right upper quadrant. A high index of suspicion is all that is needed to justify the air or barium enema study. Sedation with morphine is helpful for comforting the child and for performing a useful study. The air or barium enema often completely reduces the intussusception, eliminating the need for surgical intervention. This study should always be performed in consultation with a surgeon and with the child prepared to go to the operating room in case of failure of reduction or perforation of the colon. Successful hydrostatic reduction of the intussusception is accomplished in 50–75% of cases. Contraindications for reduction enemas include perforation and signs of peritonitis. It should be kept in mind that patients beyond the usual age range (3 months–6 years) for intussusception often have an anatomic lead point (polyp, Meckel diverticulum, lymphoma); successful hydrostatic reduction may not be possible in these situations. In the presence of pneumoperitoneum, peritonitis, or unsuccessful hydrostatic reduction, surgical intervention is indicated. Recurrences occur in 5% of patients treated with reduction enemas.

A mass from appendicitis that is pressing against the cecum or thickening of the cecal wall may be seen on the barium enema study, but ultrasonography and CT scanning with oral contrast media are much more reliable.

Computed Tomography

While ultrasound is an important diagnostic tool in the evaluation of acute abdominal pain in children, abdominal CT scan may also be valuable. Clinicians are reluctant to perform a CT scan due to the risk of radiation, especially in young children who are particularly sensitive to the adverse effects of radiation exposure. CT is very useful in the initial evaluation of abdominal trauma and in the determination of the extent of abdominal masses. Intravenous and gastrointestinal contrast must be used in CT of the abdomen to obtain the most information, especially if inflammatory bowel disease is suspected. CT is usually not helpful in the evaluation of chronic abdominal pain in children,

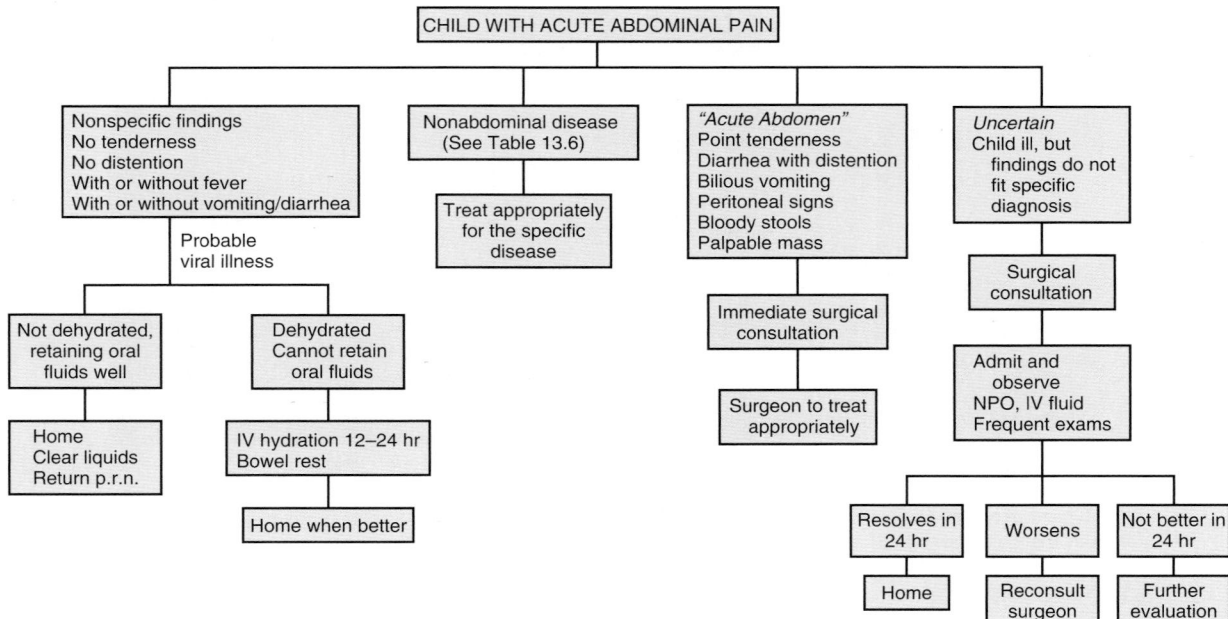

Fig. 13.6 Algorithm for evaluating acute abdominal pain. IV, intravenous; NPO, nil per os (no oral intake); p.r.n., as needed.

and while it may be useful to evaluate a chronic, undefined inflammatory process, MRI has superior accuracy over CT with no radiation risk. MRI is not always easily accessible on an emergency basis and the examination can be time consuming.

Management

The immediate concern in management is the differentiation of serious surgical and medical problems from the more common but less serious causes of acute abdominal pain. A guide to the treatment of the child with acute-onset abdominal pain is noted in Figure 13.6. A mild, nonspecific illness may be treated on an outpatient basis, with follow-up by telephone or in the office. However, the child with abdominal pain who appears ill without a specific diagnosis may warrant evaluation by a pediatric surgeon. If the diagnosis is still not apparent, the child should be admitted for active observation, which includes no oral food or liquid, appropriate intravenous fluids, hourly vital signs, and frequent examinations. If the abdominal examination is difficult because of poor cooperation, or severe pain, analgesia is appropriate. In the case of appendicitis, morphine therapy does not reduce the diagnostic accuracy by an experienced clinician. Analgesics may permit an adequate abdominal examination but do not eliminate the tenderness caused by an inflammatory process. The examination should be repeated every 2–3 hours. About 10% of children admitted for observation go on to show obvious signs of a process warranting surgery in the first few hours. In approximately 50% of the observed children, a specific nonsurgical diagnosis becomes apparent.

SPECIFIC CAUSES OF ACUTE ABDOMINAL PAIN

Appendicitis

Appendicitis is an acute inflammation of the appendix that may be initiated by luminal obstruction by a fecalith, lymphoid hyperplasia (secondary to viral infections), inflammation, or, in rare cases, parasites (pinworm, *Ascaris* species). Obstruction with ongoing distal secretion of mucus causes distention of the appendix, increased luminal pressure, and subsequent arterial obstruction and ischemia. Mucosal ulceration,

fibropurulent serosal exudates, and bacterial infection lead to gangrene from vascular obstruction with subsequent perforation. On occasion, the greater omentum may seal over a ruptured appendix, producing a right lower quadrant mass and periappendiceal abscess.

Appendicitis may be simple (focal inflammation, no serosal exudate), suppurative (obstructed, inflamed, edematous, increased local peritoneal fluid with omental and mesenteric containment, or walled off), gangrenous (similar to suppurative, plus gray-green or red-black areas of gangrene, with or without microperforations, and purulent peritoneal fluid), ruptured (gross perforation, usually on antimesenteric side; peritonitis present), or abscessed (development of pus from rupture into right ileal fossa, lateral to cecum or retrocecal, subcecal, or pelvic). The bacteriologic components of appendicitis include normal intestinal flora, such as enterococci, *Escherichia coli*, *Pseudomonas* species, *Klebsiella* species, and anaerobic bacteria, such as *Clostridium* and *Bacteroides* species.

Appendicitis affects approximately 60,000 children each year in the United States; it primarily affects adolescents and young adults but may develop at any age, even in neonates. The disease is particularly severe in very young children, often because of a delay in diagnosis with subsequent perforation. Appendicitis in young children is difficult to diagnose because of atypical manifestations and the clinician's inability to obtain an accurate history. The thinness of the appendix and the paucity of the omentum in younger children may result in rapid, unimpeded spread of intraabdominal infection after rupture.

Diagnosis

An accurate and early diagnosis is critical for avoiding perforation and peritonitis and for excluding other causes of abdominal pain. Appendicitis usually manifests initially with a gradual onset of periumbilical (occasionally epigastric) pain, which may begin as a dull ache but becomes constant (or, less often, colicky) and of mild to moderate intensity. This is then followed by anorexia, nausea, and sometimes emesis. Emesis preceding the pain is more typical of gastroenteritis. On occasion, an inflamed appendix irritates the colon, producing diarrhea. Furthermore, the appendix may irritate the bladder, causing urinary frequency and dysuria. Pain may transiently stop, but as local peritonitis develops, the pain will continue but shift to the right lower quadrant. The shifting of pain from the periumbilical area to the right lower quadrant area may take 12–36 hours but usually occurs in 2–8 hours and may not yet be evident in an acute onset of <4–6 hours. McBurney point corresponds to the location of the base of the appendix and is found by placing the little finger of one hand in the umbilicus and the thumb on the anterior superior ileal spine. The index finger, if extended perpendicularly to the abdominal wall, identifies McBurney point. Unfortunately, the appendix is not always in its classic position; thus, appendicitis may produce pain in the pelvis, in the retrocecal area (back or flank pain, psoas muscle spasm with limp), or elsewhere (Fig. 13.7). With these locations, the psoas or obturator sign may be positive (see Fig. 13.3).

Patients with unperforated appendicitis may present with a low-grade fever (<38.5°C) and display very characteristic behaviors. They can be anxious while watching where examiners place their hands, be motionless, walk slowly, get on the examining table with difficulty, or exhibit a nondistended but tender abdomen with voluntary guarding, reduced bowel sounds, and point tenderness in any area overlying the appendix. Rectal examination may reveal right-sided or diffuse tenderness and a mass.

Perforation or extensive gangrene should be suspected in the presence of progression for more than 36–48 hours; high fever; diffuse abdominal pain and tenderness; a rigid, boardlike abdomen; leukocytosis; a right lower quadrant mass; and other signs of generalized peritonitis (see Table 13.9).

Laboratory and Radiographic Testing

Ultrasonography has been of benefit in the diagnosis of appendicitis and in excluding other important disease processes (Table 13.10). Helpful ultrasonographic features suggestive of appendicitis include a noncompressible appendix, an inability to visualize the appendix when ruptured, the presence of periappendiceal fluid, or the presence of an appendicolith (Figs. 13.8 and 13.9). Ultrasonography helps define other disease processes, such as mesenteric adenitis (Fig. 13.10) and gynecologic processes. These conditions must be considered in all female patients. Ectopic pregnancy is a particularly serious condition that must not be missed (Fig. 13.11). Gastroenteritis is one of the more common conditions to be considered in the differential diagnosis (Table 13.11).

Treatment

Appendicitis is treated mainly by surgical appendectomy and ligation of the stump by open or more often laparoscopic methods, although there are advantages to medical-only management. If an abscess is present in the right lower quadrant and the patient demonstrates few signs of toxicity, elective nonurgent appendectomy may be delayed to permit preoperative rehydration and broad-spectrum antibiotic therapy. If the appendix is not perforated and no fecalith is present, some centers treat with only broad-spectrum antibiotics. In operative appendicitis, parenteral antibiotics are given before surgery and are continued postoperatively only in the presence of frank contamination, such as gangrenous or perforated appendicitis. The duration of antibiotic therapy is determined by the presence of infectious complications. If the appendix appears normal, other intraabdominal sources of pain should be sought during the surgery.

Complications of appendicitis are uncommon but include sepsis, intraabdominal abscess formation, wound infections, hepatic abscesses, ileus, and peritoneal adhesion formation. There is subsequent risk for intestinal obstruction and tubal infertility in females.

Pancreatitis

Acute pancreatitis is an acute inflammatory condition of the pancreas and recent studies estimate the incidence at approximately 1 in 10,000 children per year. Release and activation of pancreatic digestive enzymes subsequently result in extensive destruction (autodigestion) and necrosis of pancreatic and, if severe, adjacent tissue. Proteolysis, fat necrosis, and hemorrhage are noted in severe or fatal cases of pancreatitis, which is often complicated by

TABLE 13.10 Final Diagnoses in Cases of Clinically Suspected Appendicitis	
Appendicitis	Perforated peptic ulcer
Gastroenteritis	Urinary tract infection
Pelvic inflammatory disease	Meckel diverticulitis
Ovarian cyst: torsion	Pancreatitis
Ectopic pregnancy	Primary peritonitis
Crohn disease	Cholecystitis
Mesenteric adenitis	

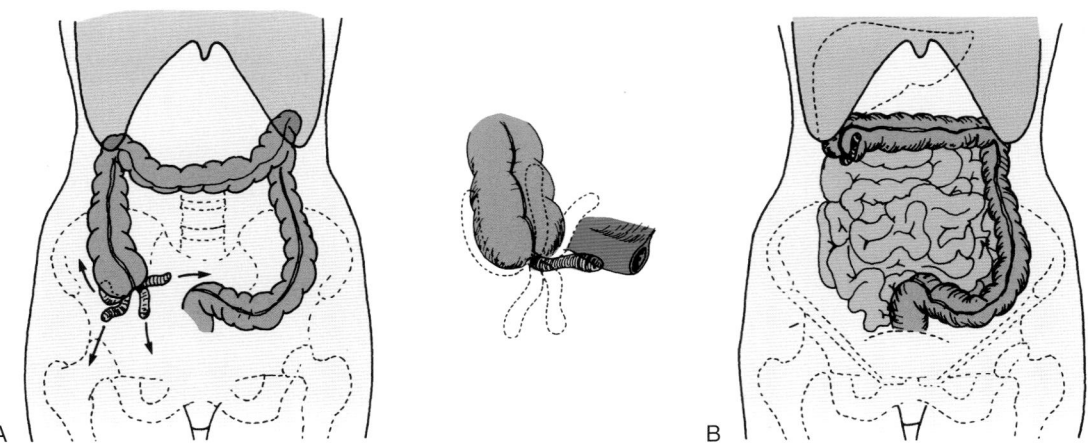

Fig. 13.7 The appendix. *A*, The appendix may be located anteriorly, medially, or retrocecally or in the pelvis. *B*, The location of the appendix depends on the location of the cecum. Because the bowel may be quite mobile in some patients, the appendix may be located in many different sites in the abdomen. In this figure, the appendix is in the right upper quadrant. (From Reilly BM. Abdominal pain. In: *Practical Strategies in Outpatient Medicine*. 2nd ed. Philadelphia: WB Saunders; 1991:728.)

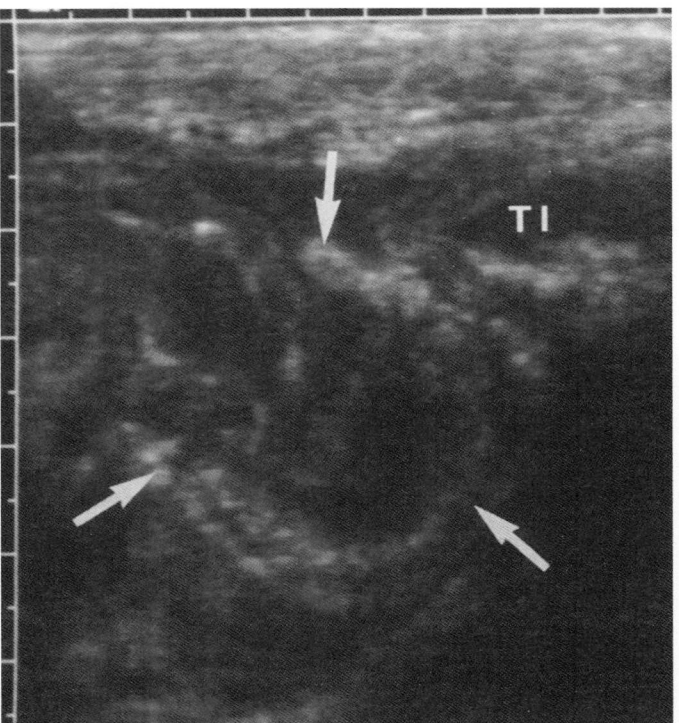

Fig. 13.8 An ultrasound scan of the right lower quadrant in a 6-year-old girl, demonstrating a thick-walled cecum *(arrows)* outlined by echogenic fluid. No appendix was found in spite of careful ultrasonographic searching. During surgery, the patient was found to have a perforated appendix and early periappendiceal abscess. TI, terminal ileum. (From Teele R, Share J. Appendicitis and other causes of intraabdominal inflammation. In: *Ultrasonography of Infants and Children*. Philadelphia: WB Saunders; 1991.)

multiorgan dysfunction syndrome (e.g., hypotension, acute respiratory distress syndrome, acute kidney injury, cardiogenic shock). Pancreatitis is less common in children than in adults, in whom the cause is often alcohol ingestion or gallstones. The etiologic factors in childhood encompass a broad differential diagnosis and often include passage of biliary stones, drugs (valproate), multisystem diseases (hemolytic uremic syndrome, cystic fibrosis), trauma (including child abuse), biliary or pancreatic anatomic anomalies, infections, and metabolic conditions (hypercalcemia, hypertriglyceridemia) (Table 13.12).

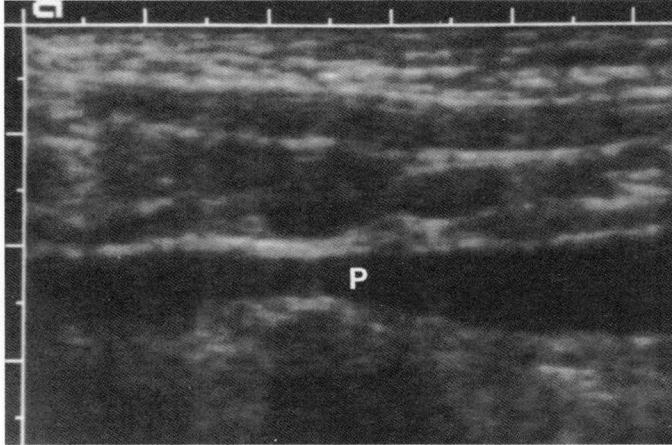

Fig. 13.10 This longitudinal scan of the right lower quadrant shows lymph nodes arranged in a line along the psoas muscle *(P)*. These are nodes enlarged from mesenteric adenitis. The patient did not have appendicitis. (From Teele R, Share J. Appendicitis and other causes of intraabdominal inflammation. In: *Ultrasonography of Infants and Children*. Philadelphia: WB Saunders; 1991.)

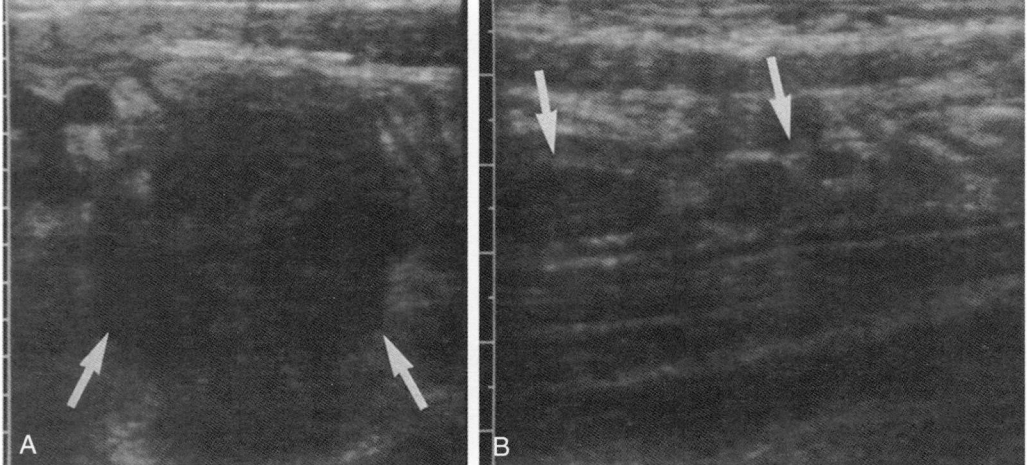

Fig. 13.9 An 11-year-old girl presented with fever, diarrhea, and vomiting. Ten days before admission to the hospital, she was seen by a physician because of abdominal pain. She had been partially treated with antibiotics for a presumed "strep throat" in the interim. When she presented to the hospital, she again had pain in the right lower quadrant, especially when the ultrasound transducer was pressed over the area. *A,* The right lower quadrant abscess *(arrows)* was quickly identified. The appendix could not be visualized. *B,* In scans along the psoas, multiple lymph nodes *(arrows)* were apparent. The child's appendix had ruptured 1 week before admission, but her symptoms had been masked by the antibiotics that she had been given. (From Teele R, Share J. Appendicitis and other causes of intraabdominal inflammation. In: *Ultrasonography of Infants and Children*. Philadelphia: WB Saunders; 1991:348.)

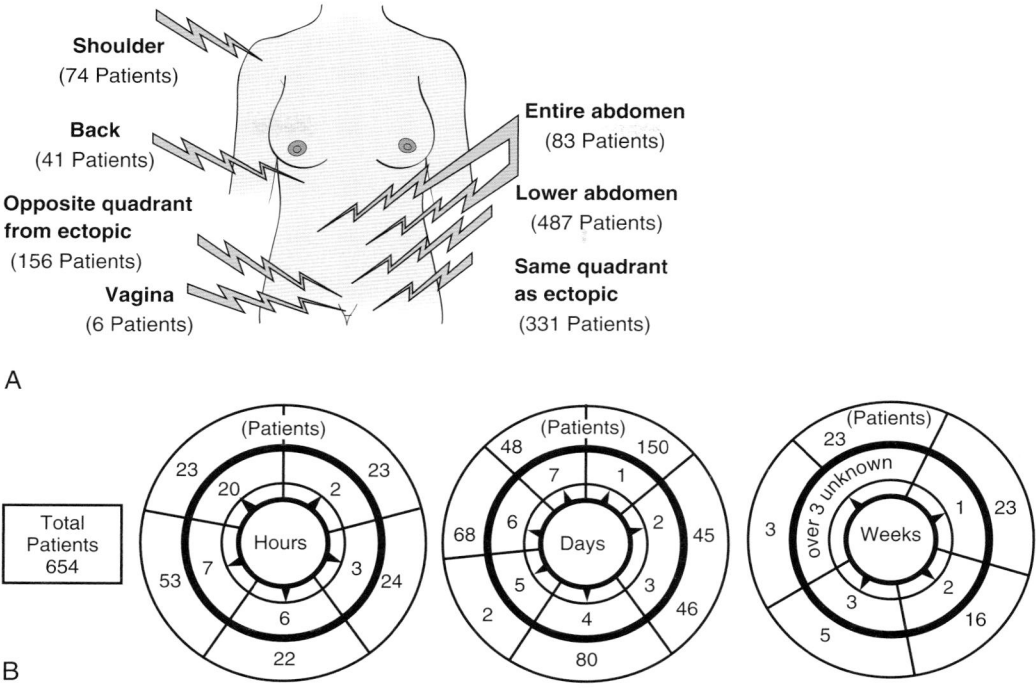

Fig. 13.11 Ectopic pregnancy. *A,* Anatomic location of pain in 654 patients with ectopic pregnancy. *B,* Duration of abdominal pain before the diagnosis of ectopic pregnancy was confirmed among 654 patients. (Modified from Breen JL. A 21-year survey of 654 ectopic pregnancies. *Am J Obstet Gynecol.* 1970;136:1304–1319.)

TABLE 13.11 Comparison of Gastroenteritis and Appendicitis

	Gastroenteritis	Appendicitis
Pain	Diffuse, cramps, intermittent	Periumbilical shifting to RLQ; constant
		Exacerbated by movement, coughing
Vomiting	With or before pain	Follows pain
Diarrhea	Frequent, large volume	Can occur; small volume (from irritation of bowel); may be watery too
Fever	Variable	Low grade, goes up with gangrene or perforation
Course	Intermittently improves	Worsens with time
Systemic symptoms	Variable: headache, malaise, myalgia, arthralgia, sore throat	Rare
Physical examination	General: fussy, restless, frequent motion	Quiet, discomfort with movement
	Abdomen: soft, mild, diffuse tenderness, hyperactive bowel sounds	Abdomen: RLQ tenderness, guarding peritoneal signs, with/without rectal tenderness/mass, absent bowel sounds
Laboratory values	WBC count: variable, may be quite high	WBC count: mild elevation, early left shift; becomes high only with gangrene or perforation
	CRP: variable	CRP: elevated
	Urine: nonspecific	Urine: may have WBCs and/or RBCs if bladder irritated, ketosis if vomiting is prolonged
Imaging studies	Abdominal films: nonspecific ileus	Abdominal films: often nonspecific, with/without fecalith, with/without loss of psoas definition, with/without scoliosis caused by inflammation in RLQ
	Ultrasonography: not indicated	Ultrasonography: enlarged appendix, peritoneal fluid, RLQ abscess, absent appendix, fecalith

RBC, red blood cell; RLQ, right lower quadrant; WBC, white blood cell.

TABLE 13.12   Causes of Acute Pancreatitis in Children

Drugs and Toxins	**Obstructive**
Alcohol	Ascariasis
Acetaminophen	Biliary sludge
Azathioprine	Biliary tract malformation
L-Asparaginase	Cholelithiasis
Cimetidine	Crohn disease
Corticosteroids	Duplication cyst
Didanosine	Pancreatic pseudocyst
Estrogens	Pancreas divisum
Furosemide	Postoperative
Gila monster bite	Sphincter of Oddi dysfunction
6-Mercaptopurine	Tumor
Methyldopa	**Systemic Disease**
Organophosphates	α_1-Antitrypsin deficiency
Pentamidine	Cystic fibrosis
Scorpion bites	Diabetes mellitus
Spider bites	Henoch-Schönlein purpura
Sulfonamides	Hemochromatosis
Tetracycline	Hemolytic uremic syndrome
Thiazides	Hyperlipidemia types I, IV, and V
Valproic acid	Hyperparathyroidism
Hereditary Pancreatitis	Hypothermia
SPINK1	Kawasaki syndrome
CFTR	Systemic lupus erythematosus
Cationic trypsinogen	Malnutrition
Infections	Organic acidemias
Coxsackievirus B	Periarteritis nodosa
Epstein-Barr virus	Peptic ulcer
Hepatitis A, B	Postpancreatic transplantation
HIV	Refeeding after malnutrition
Influenza A	Reye syndrome
Leptospirosis	Uremia
Measles	**Traumatic**
Mumps	Blunt injury
Mycoplasma	Child abuse
Rubella	Post-ERCP
Reye syndrome	Surgical trauma
	Total body cast

CFTR, cystic fibrosis transmembrane conductance receptor; ERCP, endoscopic retrograde cholangiopancreatography; SPINK1, serine protease inhibitor Kazal type 1.
Modified from Behrman RE, ed. *Nelson Textbook of Pediatrics.* 14th ed. Philadelphia: WB Saunders; 1992:999.

Manifestations

Manifestations of acute pancreatitis include intense epigastric abdominal pain that may be described as steady, boring, constant, achelike, knifelike, and exacerbated by recumbency, that radiates to the back, upper abdominal quadrants, or the scapula. Emesis is common, often protracted, and occasionally bilious. Fever is usually low to moderate grade; high fever (>39°C) suggests the presence of a primary infectious process with or without secondary pancreatitis or bacterial superinfection and pancreatic abscess formation. The patient often assumes a hunched-over or knee-chest lateral fetal posture and may manifest epigastric tenderness; bowel sounds may be reduced or absent. Signs of peritonitis suggest more extensive necrosis, as do signs of spreading hemorrhage, such as blue-green discoloration of the flanks (Grey Turner sign) or of the periumbilical region (Cullen sign). Intravascular fluid depletion, cardiogenic shock, hemorrhagic shock, hypocalcemic tetany, or systemic inflammatory response syndrome with multiorgan system failure may ensue. Pain may last for 3–10 days.

The diagnosis of acute pancreatitis in children requires at least two of three of the following be met: (1) abdominal pain compatible with pancreatitis, (2) elevated serum amylase and/or lipase that is three times the upper limit of normal, and (3) imaging consistent with pancreatitis. Initial imaging should start with transabdominal ultrasonography.

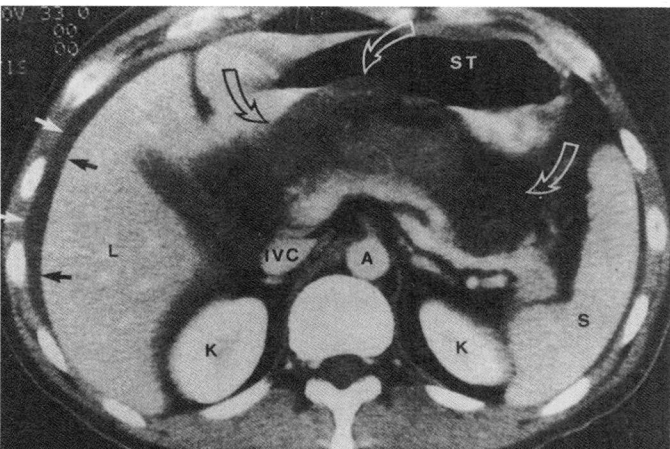

Fig. 13.12 Acute pancreatitis. CT scan through the body of the pancreas demonstrates a halo of decreased attenuation around the pancreas that represents a peripancreatic zone of edema and fluid *(curved arrows)*. Note the pancreatic ascites, most obvious lateral to the liver *(small arrows)*. If intravenous contrast were administered before the CT scan, the inflamed pancreas would appear more dense (whiter). A, aorta; IVC, inferior vena cava; K, kidney; L, liver; PV, portal vein; S, spleen; ST, stomach. (From Freeny P, Lawson T. In: Putman CE, Ravin CE, eds. *Textbook of Diagnostic Imaging.* Philadelphia: WB Saunders; 1988.)

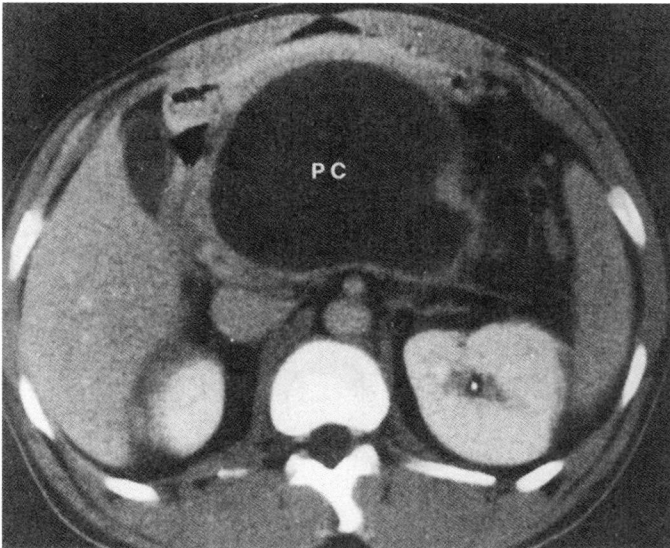

Fig. 13.13 Pseudocyst. Follow-up CT scan (same patient as in Fig. 13.12) 5 months after the episode of acute pancreatitis demonstrates a large pseudocyst *(PC)*. This large pseudocyst will probably not resolve spontaneously and may need drainage. (From Freeny P, Lawson T. In: Putman CE, Ravin CE, eds. *Textbook of Diagnostic Imaging.* Philadelphia: WB Saunders; 1988.)

Ultrasonography and CT scan are helpful in identifying the acutely inflamed pancreas (Fig. 13.12), the degree of necrosis, and the later development of a pancreatic pseudocyst (Fig. 13.13).

Testing for children with a first episode of acute pancreatitis in addition to a CBC, amylase, and lipase should start with liver enzymes (alanine aminotransferase, aspartate aminotransferase, gamma-glutamyl transferase, alkaline phosphatase, bilirubin), triglyceride level, and calcium level. This is based on the most common causes and those for which therapeutic options exist. The differential diagnosis of

TABLE 13.13 Differential Diagnosis of Hyperamylasemia

Pancreatic Pathology
Acute or chronic pancreatitis
Complications of pancreatitis (pseudocyst, ascites, abscess)
Factitious pancreatitis
Complication of ERCP

Salivary Gland Pathology
Parotitis (mumps, *Staphylococcus aureus*, CMV, HIV, EBV)
Sialadenitis (calculus, radiation)
Eating disorders (anorexia nervosa, bulimia)

Intraabdominal Pathology
Biliary tract disease (cholelithiasis)
Peptic ulcer perforation
Peritonitis
Intestinal obstruction
Appendicitis

Systemic Diseases
Metabolic acidosis (diabetes mellitus, shock)
Renal insufficiency, transplantation
Burns
Anorexia-bulimia
Pregnancy
Drugs (morphine)
Head injury
Cardiopulmonary bypass

CMV, cytomegalovirus; EBV, Epstein-Barr virus; ERCP, endoscopic retrograde cholangiopancreatography.
Modified from Kliegman RM, St. Geme JW, eds. *Nelson Textbook of Pediatrics.* 21st ed. Philadelphia: Elsevier; 2020:2076, Table 378.2.

hyperamylasemia is seen in Table 13.13. Adverse prognostic factors in severe acute pancreatitis include the presence of leukocytosis (white blood count >16,000/mm³), hyperglycemia (glucose level >200 mg/dL), a high lactic dehydrogenase level (>350 U/L), and a high aspartate aminotransferase level (>250 U/L) on admission and a decrease in hematocrit value (>10%), an increase in BUN level (>5 mg/dL), a low calcium level (<8 mg/dL), hypoxia (Pao₂ <60 mm Hg), acidosis (base deficit >4 mmol/L), or severe dehydration by 48 hours of hospitalization. The degree of pancreatic necrosis may be determined from the failure of CT scans to depict intravenous contrast parenchymal enhancement; severe pancreatitis is associated with more than 50% necrosis of the gland.

Complications

Complications of pancreatitis include local tissue necrosis with or without superinfection (pancreatic abscess), fistulization (to colon), left-sided pleural effusion, gastrointestinal hemorrhage (ulceration, vascular rupture, splenic rupture), shock, coagulopathy, acute kidney injury, myocardial depression, acute respiratory distress syndrome, hyperglycemia, hypocalcemia, subcutaneous nodules (fat necrosis), hypoalbuminemia, mental changes, and retinopathy.

Management

The management of acute pancreatitis consists of supportive care, such as nasogastric tube decompression for patients with an ileus or severe emesis, administration of intravenous fluids, administration of

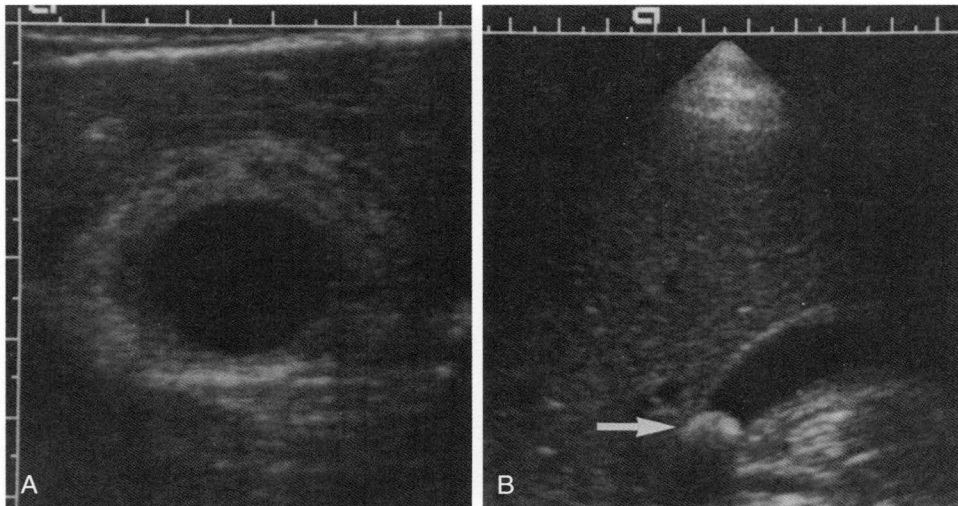

Fig. 13.14 Transverse scan with linear array transducer shows pericolic edema in a teenaged boy, who presented with severe pain in the right upper quadrant from acute cholecystitis *(A)*. A longitudinal scan of the right upper quadrant *(B)* shows a stone *(arrow)* that was thought to be impacted in the neck of the gallbladder because it did not change at all with position. The patient had severe pain with palpation over the gallbladder. (From Teele R, Share J. The liver. In: *Ultrasonography of Infants and Children*. Philadelphia: WB Saunders; 1991.)

narcotics for pain, and therapy for accompanying complications (e.g., shock, adult respiratory distress syndrome, and acute kidney injury). Endoscopic sphincterotomy by endoscopic retrograde cholangiopancreatography (ERCP) is of benefit if gallstones are present, although ERCP has risks that include the induction of pancreatitis.

After initial fluid resuscitation with either normal saline or lactated ringers, maintenance intravenous fluids should be provided at 1.5–2 times with close monitoring of urine output.

In children with mild acute pancreatitis, starting enteral nutrition early (within 48–72 hours of presentation) has been shown to decrease length of stay and decrease risk of organ dysfunction.

There is no role for antibiotics in the management of acute pancreatitis in children, except in the presence of documented infected necrosis, or in children with necrotizing pancreatitis who are not improving or who demonstrate a worsening clinical course.

Cholelithiasis

Gallstones are uncommon in children, but they complicate chronic diseases, such as hemolytic anemia (sickle cell anemia, spherocytosis), cholestatic jaundice in which total parenteral nutrition is given, and other cholestatic diseases. Gallstones may result from prematurity or drug intake (furosemide, ceftriaxone), or they may be idiopathic. Biliary obstruction (stone in cystic or common bile duct) often results in jaundice; sudden onset of severe, sharp right upper quadrant pain; localized deep tenderness in the right upper quadrant (superficial tenderness suggests an associated cholecystitis); and emesis. The pain is episodic and colicky, but often constant and superimposed with waves of more intense pain, and may radiate to the angle of the ipsilateral scapula, back, or other areas of the abdomen or chest. Patients frequently move about to find a comfortable position. There may be associated diaphoresis, pallor, tachycardia, weakness, nausea, and lightheadedness. A round or pear-shaped tender mass may be palpated in the right upper quadrant of the abdomen if the gallbladder is distended. The pain may be diurnal, with increased intensity at night. Many patients with single or multiple gallstones without obstruction are asymptomatic.

Acute cholecystitis is caused by inflammation of the gallbladder wall as a result of duct obstruction (i.e., calculus) or nonobstructing (i.e., acalculous) conditions and is manifested by fever, mild jaundice, severe abdominal pain, emesis, nausea, and leukocytosis. Pain may be similar to that in cholelithiasis and radiates to the right scapula, shoulder, or chest. The Murphy sign is demonstrated by palpating an acutely inflamed gallbladder, which causes the patient to halt respiration and feel the pain. Fever of >39.5°C suggests perforation or gallbladder gangrene, whereas a high direct bilirubin level (>4 mg/dL) suggests a common duct stone. Pain may last for 5–10 days. Passage of stones or microlithiasis (sludge) may also produce acute pancreatitis. Intolerance to fatty foods is, unfortunately, a nonspecific observation.

Diagnosis

The diagnosis is confirmed by ultrasonography that demonstrates acalculous or calculus-induced cholecystitis or acute duct obstruction by a stone (Fig. 13.14).

Treatment

Some treatment of obstructing stones may include endoscopic, open, or laparoscopic cholecystectomy. Some patients may go directly to surgery. However, supportive therapy with proper analgesia and rehydration is of critical importance. Effective pain relief should include nonsteroidal antiinflammatory drugs with an attempt to avoid opioids. Antibiotic therapy should almost always be implemented in the setting of acute cholecystitis, regardless of etiology. Although most cases of acute, acalculous cholecystitis have a viral etiology, antibiotic therapy is often prescribed to prevent further complications and should include coverage against both gram-negative and anaerobic microorganisms.

Peptic Ulcer Disease

Peptic ulceration is becoming recognized in children with increasing frequency (see Chapter 16). Risk factors for peptic ulcer disease include gastritis, a positive family history of ulcer disease, presence of *Helicobacter pylori*, treatment with nonsteroidal antiinflammatory agents and corticosteroids, cigarette smoking, and severe injury (burns, head injury, shock). Manifestations include pain, gastrointestinal bleeding (melena, hematemesis, anemia), emesis, and, in rare cases, perforation. Nocturnal pain, pain relieved by food, and a family history of peptic ulcer disease are often present in older affected children. The pain is often chronic, recurrent, and located in the epigastrium; tenderness may be localized to the epigastric region, but this is an inconsistent finding.

Acute perforation is uncommon in children but is characterized by sudden worsening of pain or a new abrupt onset of excruciating epigastric pain. There is associated pallor, faintness, weakness, syncope, diaphoresis, and a rigid abdomen.

Abdominal Wall Pain

Abdominal pain localized to abdominal muscles, particularly the rectus muscles, may be due to thoracoabdominal nerve entrapment as the anterior branches enter the rectus channel or when the accessory nerves branch within the rectus channel. The nerve, artery, and vein form a neurovascular unit then may be compressed by the fibrous ring or the rectus aponeurosis.

Anterior cutaneous nerve entrapment syndrome (ACNES) may present with acute or chronic pain that is usually unilateral and localized to the lateral aspect of the rectus muscle. The pain may radiate across the abdomen or down the lower abdomen. Traction, increased abdominal pressure, sitting, exercise (sit-ups, crunches, straight leg lifts), or twisting may aggravate the pain. Localizing (point) tenderness is usually present along the lateral aspect of the rectus muscle. Treatment includes local injection of lidocaine or other anesthetic agents and, if not successful, anterior neurectomy.

CHRONIC ABDOMINAL PAIN

Recurrent abdominal pain (RAP) in children remains one of the most challenging common conditions treated by pediatricians. Intermittent severe, episodic pain can be frightening to both families and care providers because it may be an indication of serious disease. It has been reported to occur in 10–15% of children between the ages of 4 and 16 years. In only a small minority of patients with RAP, the symptoms can be explained by discernable organic disease. However, the term *RAP* is a descriptive term and should not be used as a diagnosis. RAP may be caused by several different conditions that include, but are not limited to, celiac disease, inflammatory bowel disease, peptic ulcer, biliary tract disease, pancreatitis, or functional pain. Pain pathways can initially be influenced by the presence of pathology such as inflammation or tissue damage that often persists despite the absence of identifiable pathology.

The term **functional abdominal pain** refers to pain that has no anatomic, histologic, or "organic" etiology. This type of pain is the hallmark of functional abdominal pain disorders (FAPDs) that are subclassified, utilizing Rome IV criteria, into a number of clinically distinct entities, namely irritable bowel syndrome (IBS), functional dyspepsia, abdominal migraine, and functional abdominal pain not otherwise specified (FAP-NOS) (Table 13.14). A common feature among patients with functional gastrointestinal disorders is the heightened sensitivity to experimental pain, also known as **visceral hyperalgesia**. A unifying theory of all functional gastrointestinal disorders is the alteration of the brain-gut axis that can present with clusters of symptoms related to abnormal signals arising from the gastrointestinal tract or abnormal processing of signals in the central nervous system. Without proper explanation of the term *functional*, most families would not understand the condition since the term is very vague and nondescriptive. Thus, FAPDs should be referred to as "disorders of gut-brain interaction" given that their bio-psychosocial etiology involves complex interactions within the gut-brain axis. Symptoms are physiologic and modifiable by sociocultural and psychologic influences. Functional pain can be triggered or influenced by gastrointestinal infections, food, allergies, stress, and physical or sexual abuse. These experiences may have a long-lasting impact on a child and make the child more susceptible to the development of FAPDs by affecting intestinal motility, altered intestinal permeability, or visceral hyperalgesia, which conversely impacts the development of altered or maladaptive coping skills later in life. The *functional* nature of this pain does not mean that the pain is imaginary or that it may not interfere with the child's daily activities. Patients with functional abdominal pain experience real pain and should not be considered to be faking it or not experiencing it at all. Psychosocial factors, along with altered gut physiology, ultimately play an important role in the development of FAPDs including functional abdominal pain, IBS, functional dyspepsia, and abdominal migraine.

The diagnostic Rome criteria for each of these disorders permit clinicians to make a clinical diagnosis with limited diagnostic testing. Applying the criteria in the clinical setting allows the care provider to validate the reality of the symptoms and develop an appropriate physician-patient relationship aimed at improving symptoms and functioning. All too often, the clinician repeatedly performs unnecessary diagnostic tests to rule out pathology. This often leads to dismissal of the patient's concerns or prevents an effective collaboration in the patient's care that promotes a vicious cycle of symptom anxiety and health-seeking behavior. Applying the Rome criteria along with a proper history and physical examination that includes "red flags" is most of the time sufficient to make a clinical diagnosis of an FAPD and to initiate proper treatment (see Table 13.8).

MAKING A DIAGNOSIS OF FUNCTIONAL ABDOMINAL PAIN

The history should be detailed and, in most instances, obtained separately from the parents and the child. A private conversation with each often provides better insight into all factors affecting the child. In addition to covering the historical information already detailed, the clinician should pay attention to factors in the child's environment, family, school, and social interactions that may be sources of undue stress. Care providers often have difficulty making a positive diagnosis of a functional gastrointestinal disorder, particularly since there are no biologic markers. The diagnostic evaluation of a child with abdominal pain begins with a history to distinguish chronic from acute pain and addressing red flags. The revised **Rome IV criteria** for childhood functional abdominal pain are met if the duration of pain exceeds 2 months (episodic or continuous). Children with FAPDs may be subclassified into one of four clinical diagnostic categories that include (1) **functional dyspepsia** (abdominal pain associated with symptoms centered in the upper abdomen), (2) **irritable bowel syndrome** (abdominal pain associated with altered bowel pattern), (3) **functional abdominal pain** not otherwise specified (isolated paroxysmal abdominal pain not otherwise specified), or (4) **abdominal migraine** (paroxysmal intense pain that can be associated with either pallor, headache, photophobia, nausea, or vomiting) (see Table 13.14). The diagnosis of abdominal migraine is sometimes easier to make since symptoms are episodic and occur abruptly after periods of normal well-being. It is not uncommon to get a history of the child waking up in the middle of the night with pain and vomiting and then having complete resolution of symptoms after 1–2 days. The frequent occurrence or change in location of pain or alternating bowel habits in the same patient, however, is not uncommon. Clinicians do not always feel comfortable simply relying on Rome criteria or are unaware that they exist. Functional pain should be considered when abdominal pain persists a month beyond the usual course of an acute illness (i.e., gastroenteritis). Children often present with intermittent, periumbilical pain that usually waxes and wanes and can often experience other comorbid symptoms, including headaches, joint pain, dizziness, pallor, and diaphoresis. Nausea occurs in as many as 50% of children with FAPDs and is a major factor contributing to significant disability.

TABLE 13.14 **Rome IV Diagnostic Criteria for Functional Abdominal Pain Disorders**

Disorder	Diagnostic Criteria
Functional dyspepsia	Must include at least one of the following for at least 4 days per month: • Postprandial fullness • Early satiation • Epigastric pain or burning not associated with defecation Criteria must be fulfilled for at least 2 mo.
Irritable bowel syndrome (IBS)	Must include all of the following: • Abdominal pain at least 4 days per month associated with at least one of the following: related to defecation, a change in stool frequency, or a change in appearance of stool • In children with constipation, pain continues despite resolution of constipation (if pain resolves, the child has functional constipation) Criteria must be fulfilled for at least 2 mo.
Abdominal migraine	Must include all of the following occurring at least twice: • Sudden episodes of intense, acute abdominal pain lasting at least 1 hr • Episodes are separated by weeks to months of mild or no abdominal pain • Typical pattern for each child • Pain is associated with at least two of the following: anorexia, nausea, vomiting, headache, photophobia, or pallor Criteria must be fulfilled for at least 6 mo.
Functional abdominal pain not otherwise specified (FAP-NOS)	Must include all of the following for at least 4 days per month: • Episodic or continuous abdominal pain not solely related to physiologic events (like eating or menses) • Does not meet criteria for other FAPDs Criteria must be fulfilled for at least 2 mo.

FAPDs, functional abdominal pain disorders.
From Wyllie R, Hyams JS, Kay M, eds. *Pediatric Gastrointestinal Liver Disease*. 6th ed. Philadelphia: Elsevier; 2021:57, Table 6.1.

Severity and Location of Pain

Functional pain can vary in intensity, ranging from mild intermittent pain to severe intense pain that disrupts a child's life, family, and school attendance. Excluding organic causes of chronic abdominal pain remains a challenge for pediatricians, particularly given the heterogeneity of FAPD symptoms. Although the location of pain does not always help differentiate between functional and organic causes, periumbilical pain has been shown to be most likely associated with functional pain. Substernal pain should raise the suspicion for an esophageal cause, such as erosive esophagitis from gastroesophageal reflux. Chronic abdominal pain in the presence of dysphagia or history of food impaction should prompt a referral to the specialist to rule out **eosinophilic esophagitis**. In school-age children (9–13 years old) with eosinophilic esophagitis, abdominal pain may be the only presenting symptom, whereas in younger children (4–13 years old), vomiting may be a more common symptom. Epigastric pain can be caused from pathology in the esophagus, stomach, duodenum, and pancreas or from functional dyspepsia. Pain originating from hepatobiliary

structures, including the gallbladder, liver, and head of the pancreas, usually is primarily in the right upper quadrant. Certain conditions must be considered in patients who present with chronic pain in the right lower quadrant and these include chronic appendicitis, abdominal wall pain, and Crohn disease. Identifying certain characteristics or "red flags" that can assist the clinician in detecting organic disease in patients with chronic abdominal pain would be important, since it could limit unnecessary diagnostic testing in those with FAPDs and potentially prevent a delay in the diagnosis of a specific organic disease. Determination of fecal calprotectin is increasingly being utilized as a noninvasive screen for Crohn disease. It is a marker of intestinal mucosal inflammation and appears to be superior to standard serologic testing such as CBC or CRP. A normal calprotectin level in children would minimize the need for colonoscopy in children with chronic abdominal pain.

Approach to Treatment

The first goal is to identify physical and psychologic stress factors that may have an important role in onset, severity, exacerbations, or maintenance of pain. Equally important is to reverse environmental factors that serve as reinforcers of the pain behavior. Parents and the school must work together to support the child. Regular school attendance is extremely important and should be encouraged even in the presence of pain. It is oftentimes helpful for the care provider to communicate directly to school officials to explain the nature of the problem. At home, less attention should be directed toward the symptoms. In the clinic, defining the problem and establishing an effective physician-patient relationship is an important part of therapy. Attention should focus on improvement of daily symptoms and quality of life, as well as the child's return to normal activities. Once the evaluation, including the history, physical examination, and appropriate screening laboratory tests, has been completed and findings are normal, a search for nonorganic sources of pain should not be continued. Instead, the appropriate treatment should be initiated. The child with functional pain may improve once the child and the family understand the nature of the pain and a proper explanation is given by the provider. Knowing that there is no serious organic disease and that the sensations are not imaginary is usually welcome information to the family. However, the conversation about functional abdominal pain should be brought up during the first visit and should not be discussed only after doing extensive testing. The family should understand that testing is only to confirm the absence of other disorders and confirm the possibility of functional pain.

There is a spectrum of functional pain in terms of severity. Some patients have minimal severity and frequency of pain while others have daily, unremitting pain that results in school absences, functional disability, and diminished quality of life. The total number of days missed from school is a good indicator of disability and should always be asked during the visit. For those with mild symptoms not interfering with daily activities, simple treatment strategies such as stool softeners for constipation often provide sufficient relief, such that the child can resume a more normal life. Similarly, dietary manipulation with lactose, sucrose, or fructose avoidance is often an important first step in the child with mild, chronic abdominal pain. **Carbohydrate malabsorption** or intolerance from lactose, sucrose, sorbitol, or high-fructose corn syrup (fruit juices and sodas) may produce pain that responds to dietary elimination of the offending sugar. These simple strategies should not be tried on the child with significant disability and school absences, mainly because they are unlikely to work and time would be lost in trying to get the child back to functioning. The clinician should refrain from talking to patients and family using negative comments such as "You will have to learn to live with this pain." This leads to considerable gloom and hopelessness and will make the condition much more difficult to treat. Sometimes, despite diligent evaluation by the most skilled and patient clinician, symptoms can persist. There are no U.S.

Food and Drug Administration (FDA)–approved drugs for the treatment of chronic abdominal pain in children and there is little evidence of efficacy for most commonly used medications. It is important to consider that the clinician must spend time educating the family regarding the suspected mechanisms and how and why pharmacotherapy may or may not work. In the more severe, disabled patients, patient education should be considered part of a therapeutic program that includes physical reconditioning, exercise, sleep restoration, and, in many cases, thought reprocessing. The FDA has approved IB-Stim, a nonimplantable, percutaneous electrical nerve field stimulation device for the treatment of adolescents with functional abdominal pain associated with IBS. The auricular stimulation targets the brain-gut axis through low-frequency electrical stimulation of auricular cranial nerves and was shown to improve abdominal pain, global symptoms, and functional disability compared to placebo. The novelty of this approach comes at a critical time when the development of nonpharmacologic and nonaddictive therapies to treat chronic pain has become a major priority. Psychologic therapies such as cognitive-behavioral therapy, hypnosis, relaxation, meditation, or biofeedback have been shown to be as effective as, and sometimes better than, pharmacologic therapy. Families should always be educated on the potential modification of the "pain behavior" and potential benefits of lifestyle modifications.

A therapeutic trial with medications should be discussed with the family and should have a well-defined duration and goals. Also, the dose should be adequate to achieve the desired effect. If history and physical examination suggest dyspepsia or epigastric pain without red flags, a trial of acid suppression is very appropriate as an initial step. Similarly, if the history and physical examination suggest constipation as the cause for pain, then the proper therapy with osmotic laxatives or cathartics should be initiated. Pharmacologic therapy, including anticonvulsant or antidepressant agents, has not consistently proven to be effective in children with functional abdominal pain. Such therapy has sometimes been effective in young adults but is not recommended for younger children under 8 years of age. Amitriptyline has been used in small doses and anecdotally has been successful in alleviating functional abdominal pain. It is widely used for chronic pain conditions including migraine headaches, fibromyalgia, and neuropathic pain and is considered to be effective at much lower doses than those used for depression.

Cyproheptadine is an antagonist of serotonin, histamine H_1, and muscarinic receptors. It has been used to treat allergic rhinitis and migraine headaches and anecdotally as an appetite stimulant in children. Antispasmodics such as hyoscyamine or dicyclomine can produce significant anticholinergic side effects including dry mouth, dizziness, and blurred vision. Most antispasmodics should be used as adjuvant therapy for the treatment of chronic abdominal pain and only for episodic pain and not as daily treatment.

Small intestinal bacterial overgrowth may be a cause of chronic abdominal pain. Rifaximin has low systemic absorbance and localized effect on intestinal flora and is approved for diarrhea-predominant IBS in adults. In adolescents with functional pain, bloating, and/or diarrhea, empirical treatment with this antibiotic may be considered. Although short-term treatment appears to be well tolerated in adults, multiple treatments with rifaximin may be needed, which increases the concern for antimicrobial resistance.

The dearth of successful treatment options for chronic abdominal pain often results in patients opting for alternative methods. There appears to be a growing desire among patients and families for a more "natural" approach to therapy. It has been suggested that approximately 35% of adult patients with functional bowel disorders use complementary or alternative medicine despite the perceived lack of efficacy by some clinicians.

If the symptoms are mild and not severe enough to interfere with a child's school or daily activities, using alternative therapies for which there is some scientific evidence of benefit may be a good starting point. These include peppermint oil, melatonin, and STW5 (Iberogast). Concentrated peppermint oil is increasingly being used in the treatment of abdominal pain in children. The menthol component of peppermint oil acts as a calcium channel blocker that causes relaxation of intestinal smooth muscle. Peppermint oil, administered in pH-dependent, enteric-coated capsules, has been shown to reduce abdominal pain severity over placebo in both adults and children. Melatonin is likely to be effective in less severe patients with functional pain with minimal comorbidities and has the added benefit of having a low side effect profile. Iberogast is a mixture of nine herbal plant extracts that is being used as an alternative approach for the treatment of functional dyspepsia and IBS. The exact mechanism of this herbal preparation is not known but several trials have suggested that it is effective in alleviating symptoms of functional dyspepsia and IBS. The combination consists of liquid extracts from chamomile flowers, bitter candytuft, angelica root, caraway fruits, milk thistle, lemon balm leaves, greater celandine, licorice root, and peppermint leaves.

RED FLAGS

Red flags or "alarm signals" are critical to investigate in the history and physical exam of abdominal pain (see Table 13.8). The presence of red flags raises the suspicion of an underlying organic disorder and includes pain localized away from the umbilicus, pain related to menstrual cycle, back pain, multisystem complaints, anorexia, weight loss, evidence of gastrointestinal bleeding (anemia, hematemesis, melena, hematochezia, rectal bleeding, occult bleeding), profuse diarrhea, extraintestinal symptoms (fever, rash, recurrent aphthous ulcers), and a positive family history of inflammatory bowel disease, celiac disease, or peptic ulcers. Anemia, hematochezia, and weight loss in children with chronic abdominal pain are predictive of IBD. Physical findings of linear growth deceleration, localized fullness or mass effect, hepatomegaly, splenomegaly, back or costovertebral angle tenderness, perianal skin tags or fistulas, soiling, or occult blood in stools should be taken seriously and should prevent the diagnosis of a FAPD until further work-up is completed. Biochemical analysis that raises suspicion for organic disorders includes iron deficiency anemia, high sedimentation rate or CRP, hypoalbuminemia, abnormal liver or kidney function tests, or elevated amylase and lipase. A high stool calprotectin level suggests an inflammatory process and should be obtained if there is any suspicion for Crohn disease. In cases in which recurrent vomiting is a significant part of the history, an upper gastrointestinal series should be obtained to rule out gastric outlet disorder, malrotation, or partial small bowel obstruction. An abdominal ultrasound should also be considered to investigate the possibility of gallstones, pseudocyst, ureteropelvic junction obstruction, or a retroperitoneal mass. Contrast CT scans in the evaluation of chronic functional pain is seldom helpful and should not be part of the work-up unless a specific cause is being investigated.

BIBLIOGRAPHY

A bibliography is available at ExpertConsult.com.

14

Diarrhea

Bhaskar Gurram

Diarrhea is the passage of unusually loose or watery stools, typically at least three times in a 24-hour period, and should be considered in a child who is passing stools more frequently than usual with a consistency looser than what is considered normal for that individual. Diarrhea is classified broadly by the duration of symptoms. **Acute diarrhea** is usually a self-limited illness that lasts for 2 weeks or less. **Chronic diarrhea** persists for more than 2 weeks. The etiologies of acute and chronic diarrhea differ by age (Table 14.1).

Diarrhea is further classified by pathophysiology, which typically involves one or more of the following mechanisms: (1) **osmotic diarrhea**, characterized by an increased intraluminal osmotic load leading to passive diffusion of fluid into the gastrointestinal lumen; (2) **secretory diarrhea**, characterized by increased active secretion of fluid into the gastrointestinal lumen beyond the capacity to be reabsorbed; and (3) altered gastrointestinal tract motility. Differentiating osmotic from secretory diarrhea allows for a more directed diagnostic evaluation (Table 14.2). **Osmotic diarrhea** may be related to the malabsorption of carbohydrate, fat, or protein or to the presence of nonabsorbable substances in the gastrointestinal lumen. The characteristics of the stool may provide information that allows for the identification of the malabsorbed substance, particularly for isolated carbohydrate and fat malabsorption (Table 14.3). **Secretory diarrhea** is characterized by an excess of crypt cell fluid and electrolyte secretion that exceeds the absorptive capabilities of the villi and is classified by the presence or absence of normal villi. **Inflammatory diarrhea** of both infectious and noninfectious etiologies usually involves both osmotic and secretory components. Finally, surgical bowel resection may decrease the surface area available for the resorption of both fluid and solutes, leading to both secretory and osmotic diarrhea. The causes of diarrhea based on pathophysiology are presented in Table 14.4.

ACUTE DIARRHEA

History

Acute diarrhea in children is most often infectious (Table 14.5), although it may be secondary to noninfectious inflammatory processes, toxins, or medications. The etiology of acute diarrhea is suggested by both the history and characteristics of the stool (Fig. 14.1 and Table 14.6). Fever or blood in the stool suggests an infectious cause. Watery diarrhea is typical of viral gastroenteritis, as well as some bacterial and parasitic infections. **Dysentery**, characterized by severe diarrhea and the presence of blood and mucus in the stool, suggests bacterial colitis. Vomiting and diarrhea developing within hours of food ingestion suggests exposure to preformed toxins in the food, rather than the acquisition of an enteric pathogen from the food, which is characterized by a predominantly diarrheal illness developing within days of exposure (Fig. 14.2). A recent history of

travel suggests **traveler's diarrhea**, more than 80% of which is caused by bacterial species that are endemic to the area of travel, to which the patient has not been previously exposed. Recent travel may also suggest parasitic or helminthic infection. Exposure to health care settings suggests **nosocomial diarrhea**. Patients with a history of immunodeficiency or malnourishment may be more likely to have an infection with atypical or opportunistic organisms or to have a more protracted and severe course. Hematuria or oliguria may suggest **hemolytic uremic syndrome (HUS)** as a complication of infection with *Escherichia coli* 0157:H7 or *Shigella*. Other extraintestinal manifestations may also provide a clue to the diagnosis (Table 14.7).

Physical Examination

Physical examination should focus on assessing the level of hydration and the need for fluid resuscitation (Table 14.8). The general examination may reveal nonenteric infections that could present with diarrhea, such as otitis media, pneumonia, or sepsis. Abdominal tenderness or masses suggest appendicitis, intussusception, or, less commonly, toxic megacolon. Generalized toxicity or shock may occur with HUS or with sepsis, such as from invasive *Salmonella* or staphylococcal toxic shock syndrome.

Viral Diarrhea

Rotavirus Infection

Rotavirus is the most frequent cause of severe diarrhea in unvaccinated infants and young children. The introduction of an effective vaccine has decreased the incidence, with most infections occurring in unvaccinated children under 3 years of age. In countries with a higher baseline socioeconomic status, it is typically seen in winter months, with prevalence decreasing substantially in summer months. Transmission is by the fecal-oral route and the incubation period ranges from 1 to 3 days. Patients typically present with the acute onset of fever and vomiting followed 1–2 days later by watery diarrhea. Symptoms generally persist for 3–8 days. In moderate to severe cases, dehydration, electrolyte abnormalities, and acidosis may occur. In immunocompromised children, persistent infection and chronic diarrhea can develop, with persistently positive diagnostic assays. Chronic infection is to be differentiated from postinfectious malabsorption seen in some immunocompetent children, in whom the small intestinal mucosa may require 3–8 weeks to recover its absorptive ability. Diagnosis is confirmed by nucleic acid amplification assays, enzyme immunoassay (EIA), immunochromatography, or latex agglutination assay for group A rotavirus antigen detection in the stool.

Norovirus Infection

Norovirus is a single-stranded RNA virus of the *Calciviridae* family and is the leading cause of epidemic outbreaks of acute gastroenteritis, as well as the most common cause of foodborne illness and foodborne

TABLE 14.1   Differential Diagnosis of Acute and Chronic Diarrhea by Age

Infants	Children	Adolescents
ACUTE		
Common	Infectious gastroenteritis	Infectious gastroenteritis
Infectious gastroenteritis	Food poisoning	Food poisoning
Systemic infection	Antibiotic-associated diarrhea	Antibiotic-associated diarrhea
Medication induced (e.g., antibiotics, laxatives)	Food poisoning	Hyperthyroidism
Food protein–induced enterocolitis syndrome (FPIES)	Systemic infection	
Food poisoning		
Overfeeding		
Rare		
Hirschsprung-associated enterocolitis		
Neonatal opioid withdrawal		
CHRONIC		
Disorders of Absorption and Transport of Nutrients and Electrolytes	***Disorders of Absorption and Transport of Nutrients and Electrolytes***	***Disorders of Absorption and Transport of Nutrients and Electrolytes***
Primary lactase deficiency	Lactose intolerance	Lactose intolerance
Secondary (e.g., postinfectious) lactase deficiency	Secondary (e.g., postinfectious) lactase deficiency	Laxative abuse
Congenital sucrose-isomaltase deficiency	Congenital sucrose-isomaltase deficiency	***Disorders of Intestinal Motility***
Trehalase deficiency	Primary bile acid diarrhea	Irritable bowel syndrome
Congenital chloride diarrhea	Familial diarrhea syndrome	Pseudoobstruction and bacterial overgrowth
Congenital sodium diarrhea	***Disorders of Intestinal Motility***	***Infectious Etiologies***
Acrodermatitis enteropathica	Toddler's diarrhea	Giardiasis
Glucose-galactose malabsorption	Irritable bowel syndrome	*Cryptosporidium*
Fanconi-Bickel syndrome	***Infectious Etiologies***	***Neuro-Enteroendocrine Diarrhea***
Lysinuric protein intolerance	Giardiasis	Primary adrenal insufficiency
Chylomicron retention disease	*Cryptosporidium*	***Defects in Intestinal Immune-Related Homeostasis***
Abetalipoproteinemia	***Defects in Enterocyte Structure***	Inflammatory bowel disease
Enterokinase deficiency	Trichohepatoenteric syndrome (syndromic diarrhea)	Celiac disease
Maltase-glucoamylase deficiency	***Neuro-Enteroendocrine Diarrhea***	Eosinophilic gastroenteritis and colitis
Primary bile acid diarrhea	Proprotein convertase 1/3 deficiency	***Pancreatic Insufficiency***
Familial diarrhea syndrome	X-linked lissencephaly	Chronic pancreatitis
Diarrhea-associated *DGAT1* variants	Secretory tumors (e.g., neuroblastoma, VIPoma)	
Defects in Enterocyte Structure	***Defects in Intestinal Immune-Related Homeostasis***	
Congenital tufting enteropathy	Celiac disease	
Microvillus inclusion disease	Inflammatory bowel disease	
Trichohepatoenteric syndrome (syndromic diarrhea)	Eosinophilic gastroenteritis and colitis	
Neuro-Enteroendocrine Diarrhea	Early-onset enteropathy with colitis	
Enteric anendocrinosis	XIAP deficiency	
Mitchell-Riley syndrome	Autoimmune enteropathy	
Proprotein convertase 1/3 deficiency	***Pancreatic Insufficiency***	
X-linked lissencephaly	Cystic fibrosis	
Secretory tumors (e.g., neuroblastoma)	Chronic pancreatitis	
Defects in Intestinal Immune-Related Homeostasis		
Cow's milk or soy milk protein colitis		
Eosinophilic gastroenteritis and colitis		
Early-onset enteropathy with colitis		
IPEX syndrome		
IPEX-like disorders		
XIAP deficiency		
Autoimmune enteropathy		
Other primary immune deficiency disorders (e.g., SCID)		
Pancreatic Insufficiency		
Cystic fibrosis		
Shwachman-Diamond syndrome		
Johansson-Blizzard syndrome		
Pearson syndrome		

DGAT1, diacylglycerol O-acyltransferase 1; IPEX, immune disregulation, polyendocrinopathy, enteropathy, X-linked; SCID, severe combined immunodeficiency; VIP, vasoactive intestinal peptide; XIAP, X-linked inhibitor of apoptosis.

disease outbreaks in the United States. Young children have the highest incidence of infection. Transmission is via the fecal-oral route or through contaminated food or water. Norovirus gastroenteritis typically presents with the abrupt onset of vomiting accompanied by watery diarrhea, abdominal cramps, nausea, and vomiting. Systemic manifestations, including myalgia, fatigue, and headache, may accompany gastrointestinal symptoms. Diagnosis is confirmed by nucleic acid amplification assays that detect viral RNA from the stool. Norovirus can cause persistent infection in immunocompromised patients and is difficult to clear without reconstitution of the immune system.

Bacterial Diarrhea

Most bacterial diarrheal illnesses are foodborne and affect infants and young children more frequently than adults. Bacterial infections of the intestine cause diarrhea via direct invasion of the intestinal mucosa, followed by intraepithelial cell multiplication or invasion of the lamina propria. Cellular invasion may be followed by the production of cytotoxin, which disrupts cell function, and/or the production of enterotoxin, which alters cellular electrolyte and water balance. Bacterial adherence to the mucosal surface may result in flattening of the microvilli and disruption of normal cell functioning. Symptomatic differentiation from viral causes of diarrhea may be difficult, and sequelae or extraintestinal manifestations of infections are varied (see Table 14.7).

Salmonella Infection

Nontyphoidal *Salmonella* organisms are estimated to cause 1 million annual gastrointestinal infections in the United States. The attack rate is highest in infancy; the incidence of symptomatic infections is lower in patients older than 6 years. *Salmonella* infection may cause an asymptomatic intestinal carrier state that is rare in children, enterocolitis with diarrhea, or bacteremia without gastrointestinal manifestations but with subsequent local infections, such as meningitis or osteomyelitis. *Salmonella* infection is usually spread through contaminated water supplies or food (e.g., meat, chicken, eggs, raw milk, and fresh produce). Most infections in the United States are sporadic rather than epidemic. Although an infected food handler may contaminate food sources, farm animals or pets are more often the vector. Cats, turtles, lizards, snakes, and iguanas may also harbor *Salmonella* organisms.

Outbreaks may occur among children in institutional settings; outbreaks in daycare centers are rare.

After a 12- to 72-hour incubation period, gastroenteritis develops and is characterized by the sudden onset of diarrhea, abdominal cramps and tenderness, and fever. The diarrhea is watery, with stools containing polymorphonuclear leukocytes and, on occasion, blood. The peripheral blood white blood cell count is usually normal. Symptoms slowly resolve within 3–5 days, although excretion of the organism may persist for several weeks. The organism is readily isolated from culture of the stool or a rectal swab or may be identified via multiplex PCR assays that detect multiple bacterial, viral, and parasitic enteric pathogens.

Shigella Infection

Most *Shigella* infections in the United States occur in young children aged 1–4 years, with a peak seasonal incidence in late summer and early autumn. It may also be the most common bacterial cause of diarrhea outbreaks in daycare settings. The organism is transmitted via the fecal-oral route, most often by the hands. During a 12- to 72-hour incubation period, patients may develop a nonspecific prodrome characterized by fever, chills, nausea, and vomiting. A predominantly rectosigmoid colitis develops and results in abdominal cramps and watery diarrhea. In more severe infections (**bacillary dysentery**), blood and mucus are passed in small, very frequent stools (see Table 14.6). High fever in young infants may induce febrile seizures, and some patients may develop HUS. Bacterial culture of the stool or a rectal swab, or the use of multiplex PCR assays, allows for differentiating this organism from other pathogens. If positive, antibiotic treatment is usually indicated.

Campylobacter Infection

Many animal species, including poultry, farm animals, and household pets, serve as reservoirs for *Campylobacter jejuni*. Transmission occurs through ingestion of contaminated food, especially undercooked food, and through person-to-person spread via the fecal-oral route. The disease is common in infants and adolescents, and both daycare and college outbreaks have been reported. Asymptomatic carriage is uncommon. *Campylobacter* infection symptoms may range from mild diarrhea to frank dysentery. The organism causes diffuse, invasive enteritis that involves the ileum and colon. Fever, cramping, abdominal pain, and bloody diarrhea are characteristic and may mimic symptoms of acute appendicitis or inflammatory bowel disease (IBD). Fever and diarrhea usually resolve after 5–7 days; prolonged illness or relapse occasionally occurs. *Campylobacter* infection is also known to cause meningitis, abscesses, pancreatitis, and pneumonia. Guillain-Barré syndrome has been reported after *Campylobacter* infection. Identification is via stool or rectal swab bacterial culture or via multiplex PCR assay. If positive, antibiotic treatment is indicated.

Yersinia Infection

Infection with either *Yersinia enterocolitica* or *Yersinia pseudotuberculosis* may cause various clinical syndromes, including gastroenteritis,

TABLE 14.2 Differentiating Osmotic from Secretory Diarrhea

	Osmotic	Secretory
Stool volume	Small (<200 mL/24 hr)	Large (>200 mL/24 hr)
Response to fasting	Diarrhea improves	Diarrhea continues
Stool sodium	<70	>70
Stool osmotic gap*	>50	<50
Stool pH	<5	>6

*Stool osmotic gap = 290 − 2 (stool Na+ + stool K+).

TABLE 14.3 Distinguishing Isolated Carbohydrate from Isolated Fat Malabsorption

	Isolated Carbohydrate Malabsorption	Isolated Fat Malabsorption
Stool character	Loose and watery, non–foul-smelling	Bulky large stool, foul-smelling, oil droplets visible
Perianal rash/skin erosion	Present	Present
Signs of fat-soluble vitamin deficiency	Variable	Present
Stool pH	Acidic (usually <6)	Alkaline
Stool reducing/nonreducing substances	Present	Absent

TABLE 14.4 Differential Diagnosis of Diarrhea by Pathophysiology

Osmotic Diarrhea

1. Carbohydrate malabsorption
   - Lactose intolerance
   - Osmotic laxatives (lactulose, polyethylene glycol 3350)
   - Antacids (magnesium hydroxide)
   - Ingestion of excessive amounts of nonabsorbable sugar or sugar alcohols (sorbitol in chewing gum, diet candy, sucralose)
   - Dietary ingestion of excessive fructose (high-fructose corn syrup, ingestion of high-fructose–containing fruits in excessive amounts)
   - Disaccharidase deficiency (sucrose-isomaltase deficiency, glucose-galactose malabsorption, maltase-glucoamylase deficiency, congenital lactase deficiency, trehalase deficiency)
   - Gastrocolic fistula, jejunoileal bypass, short-bowel syndrome
2. Fat malabsorption
   - Pancreatic insufficiency
   - Defective handling of bile acids (e.g., primary bile acid malabsorption, cholestasis)
   - Defective mucosal lipid handling (e.g., intestinal lymphangiectasia, abetalipoproteinemia, chylomicron retention disease)
3. Protein malabsorption
   - Primary enterokinase deficiency
   - Hartnup disease

Secretory Diarrhea

1. Normal villous architecture
   - Chloride-losing diarrhea (Cl^- – HCO_3^- exchanger defect)
   - Sodium-losing diarrhea (Na^+ – H^+ exchanger defect)
   - Familial diarrhea syndrome (gain-of-function variant of guanylate cyclase 2C)
   - Neurogenin-3 pathogenic variants
2. Villous atrophy
   - Microvillus inclusion disease
   - Tufting enteropathy
   - Acrodermatitis enteropathica
   - Trichohepatoenteric syndrome (phenotypic or syndromic diarrhea)
   - Congenital disorders of glycosylation defects
3. Autoimmune polyglandular syndrome type 1
4. Neuroendocrine tumors

Inflammatory (Combination of Secretory and Osmotic)

1. Infectious
2. Celiac disease
3. Inflammatory bowel disease
4. Autoimmune enteropathy and infantile-onset inflammatory bowel disease
   - Interleukin-10 and interleukin-10 receptor defects
   - Hyperimmunoglobulin D from mevalonate kinase deficiency presenting as severe neonatal colitis
   - IPEX/IPEX-like syndrome
5. Postinfectious enteropathies
6. Eosinophilic gastroenteritis
7. Idiopathic

Decreased Surface Area for Absorption

1. Short-bowel syndrome

IPEX, immune disregulation, polyendocrinopathy, enteropathy, X-linked.

mesenteric adenitis, pseudoappendicitis, and postinfectious reactive arthritis. The organism is present in animals and may be spread to humans by consumption of undercooked meat (especially pork), unpasteurized milk, and other contaminated foods. Person-to-person spread also occurs. Young children are particularly susceptible to

disease, and the frequency of infections increases during the summer months.

The organisms may be identified via multiplex PCR assay or may be cultured from rectal swab or stool specimens, but selective media are required, and the organism may not be identified via culture for several weeks. The microbiology laboratory should be notified if *Yersinia* infection is suspected. Neonates, immunocompromised patients, and patients with bacteremia or extraintestinal infection should receive antibacterial therapy; treatment decreases the duration of fecal excretion and can additionally be considered in immunocompetent patients with moderate to severe symptoms.

Escherichia coli Infection

Although *E. coli* make up the predominant normal flora in the colon, some strains are pathogenic. Diarrhea caused by *E. coli* can be watery, inflammatory, or bloody, depending on the strain involved. These diarrheagenic *E. coli* strains are classified into five major groups on the basis of serogrouping or pathogenic mechanisms: (1) enteropathogenic *E. coli* (EPEC), an important cause of diarrhea in infants; (2) enterotoxigenic *E. coli* (ETEC), a cause of diarrhea in infants and a cause of traveler's diarrhea; (3) enteroinvasive *E. coli*, a cause of watery ETEC-like illness or, less commonly, a dysentery-like illness; (4) enterohemorrhagic *E. coli*, a cause of hemorrhagic colitis and HUS; and (5) enteroaggregative *E. coli*, a cause of persistent diarrhea.

Enteric infections with *E. coli* are acquired via the fecal-oral route. Enterohemorrhagic strains are the only diarrhea-producing *E. coli* strains common in the United States and have been associated with foodborne epidemic outbreaks transmitted in some cases by undercooked meat.

EPEC is a well-established cause of infantile diarrhea, especially in countries with a lower baseline socioeconomic status. Asymptomatic carriage is common. At least two separate mechanisms are responsible for diarrhea: adherence to intestinal epithelial cells leading to villous injury and mucosal inflammation, and production of a toxin similar to that of *Shigella* organisms. Chronic infection resulting in failure to thrive may also occur.

ETEC is the major cause of traveler's diarrhea; occasional nosocomial outbreaks have also occurred in hospitalized infants. At least three different types of *E. coli* enterotoxins (heat-labile, heat-stable toxin A, and heat-stable toxin B) have been identified. Definitive diagnosis requires enterotoxin identification, and this method is not widely available.

Enterohemorrhagic *E. coli* produces a **Shiga-like cytotoxin** and causes diarrhea, hemorrhagic colitis, and, in about 20% of infected persons, **hemolytic uremic syndrome (HUS)**. Both epidemic and sporadic cases have been recognized. Infection is more common in the summer and fall. A particular serotype, *E. coli* 0157:H7, has been linked to the development of HUS in young children. The most common manifestations of enterohemorrhagic *E. coli* infection begin with severe abdominal cramps and watery diarrhea, followed by grossly bloody stools and emesis. Fever is uncommon. Fecal leukocytes are absent or few. Other manifestations include asymptomatic infection and watery diarrhea without progression to hemorrhagic colitis. *E. coli* 0157:H7 is cleared from the stool in 5–12 days. If HUS develops, symptoms become noticeable in the week after the onset of diarrhea and consist of oliguric renal failure, microangiopathic hemolytic anemia, thrombocytopenia, and diarrhea. There is no role for antimicrobial therapy in enterohemorrhagic *E. coli* disease. Antibiotics neither shorten the duration of disease nor prevent progression to HUS; they may predispose to HUS.

Clostridioides difficile Infection

Clostridioides difficile (previously termed *Clostridium difficile*) causes acute and chronic diarrhea in children when the normal colonic flora is disrupted. **Pseudomembranous colitis** is the most severe form of this

TABLE 14.5	**Common Gastrointestinal Pathogens and Their Key Epidemiologic Features**
Organism	**Key Epidemiologic Features**
Viruses	
Adenovirus	Serotypes 40 and 41 among the leading causes of infantile gastroenteritis globally
Astrovirus	Outbreaks in closed populations
Norovirus	Most common cause of medically attended gastroenteritis in United States; winter vomiting illness; environmentally hardy
Rotavirus	Most common global cause of gastroenteritis in young children, particularly in settings without rotavirus vaccination
Sapovirus	Mainly affects infants and toddlers
Bacteria	
Aeromonas spp.	Widely distributed in aquatic environments; may cause diarrhea or extraintestinal infection
Bacillus cereus	Vomiting illness; rare fatal cases with hepatic necrosis; testing for toxin available
Campylobacter jejuni	Associated with poultry; common cause of traveler's diarrhea in Asia; associated with postinfectious arthritis and Guillain-Barré syndrome
Clostridioides difficile	Leading cause of mortality from gastrointestinal infection in United States; community acquired and antibiotic associated
Clostridium botulinum	Vomiting illness due to preformed toxin ingestion; infant botulism due to germination of spores presents with progressive weakness
Enteroaggregative *Escherichia coli*	Persistent diarrhea in young children, associated with malnutrition
Enterohemorrhagic *E. coli* (STEC)	Associated with hemolytic uremic syndrome in children
Enteroinvasive *E. coli*	Associated with dysentery
Enteropathogenic *E. coli*	Acute watery diarrhea
Enterotoxigenic *E. coli*	Most common cause of traveler's diarrhea
Listeria	Associated with raw dairy products; pregnancy complications with systemic illness
Nontyphoidal *Salmonella* spp.	Intestinal carriage can be prolonged
Plesiomonas shigelloides	May cause watery diarrhea, dysentery, or extraintestinal infection
Shigella spp.	Most common global cause of dysentery
Staphylococcus aureus	Vomiting due to preformed staphylococcal enterotoxin ingestion
Vibrio cholerae	Outbreaks of watery diarrhea associated with lack of sanitation and humanitarian crises
Vibrio parahaemolyticus	Associated with shellfish consumption
Yersinia enterocolitica	Zoonosis; able to grow in refrigerated food; associated with postinfectious polyarthritis
Yersinia pseudotuberculosis	Appendicitis-like syndrome
Protozoa	
Cryptosporidium hominis/parvum	Major cause of childhood diarrhea in children in low-income countries; daycare centers
Cyclospora cayetanensis	Opportunistic infection; associated with foodborne outbreaks
Cystoisospora belli	Tropical and subtropical areas; opportunistic infection
Entamoeba histolytica	May cause liver abscess
Giardia lamblia	Associated with drinking from contaminated streams; daycare centers
Microsporidium	Ubiquitous in the environment; opportunistic infection
Parasites	
Anisakis simplex	Vomiting illness after consuming raw fish

STEC, Shiga toxin–producing enterohemorrhagic *E. coli* (original, alternative definition of enterohemorrhagic *E. coli*).
Modified from Bennett JE, Dolin R, Blaser MJ, eds. *Mandell, Douglas, and Bennett's Principles and Practices of Infectious Diseases.* 9th ed. Philadelphia: Elsevier; 2020:1332, Table 96.1.

infection, occurring as a result of a severe inflammatory response to the *C. difficile* toxins. Transmission occurs through person-to-person contact and through environmental contamination via the spores formed by *C. difficile,* which retain viability for up to 1 week on dry surfaces.

The prevalence of carrier status for *C. difficile* in healthy, asymptomatic outpatients is as high as 50% in healthy infants but is usually less than 5% in patients over 5 years of age. *C. difficile* and its toxin have been identified in the feces of healthy infants in concentrations similar to those found in adults with pseudomembranous colitis. The apparent resistance of infants to *C. difficile* and its toxin is related to the developmental absence of the toxin-binding site in the immature intestine. Asymptomatic carriage rates in hospitalized patients may be as high as 20%. Infection is highly associated with recent antibiotic exposure, particularly to broad-spectrum antibiotics, which disrupt the endogenous colonic flora that inhibits the growth of *C. difficile.* Other risk factors for *C. difficile* diarrhea include IBD, cystic fibrosis, use of proton pump inhibitors, indwelling enteral feeding tubes, and immunocompromised status.

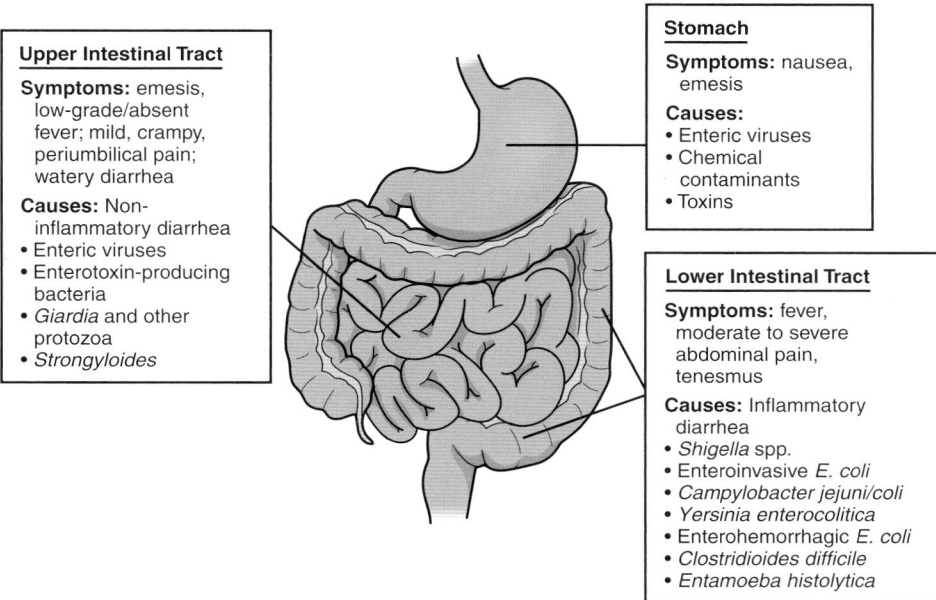

Upper Intestinal Tract

Symptoms: emesis, low-grade/absent fever; mild, crampy, periumbilical pain; watery diarrhea

Causes: Non-inflammatory diarrhea
• Enteric viruses
• Enterotoxin-producing bacteria
• *Giardia* and other protozoa
• *Strongyloides*

Stomach

Symptoms: nausea, emesis

Causes:
• Enteric viruses
• Chemical contaminants
• Toxins

Lower Intestinal Tract

Symptoms: fever, moderate to severe abdominal pain, tenesmus

Causes: Inflammatory diarrhea
• *Shigella* spp.
• Enteroinvasive *E. coli*
• *Campylobacter jejuni/coli*
• *Yersinia enterocolitica*
• Enterohemorrhagic *E. coli*
• *Clostridioides difficile*
• *Entamoeba histolytica*

Fig. 14.1 Localizing gastrointestinal tract signs and symptoms and possible causes of illness. (From Long SS, Prober CG, Fischer M, eds. *Principles and Practice of Pediatric Infectious Diseases.* 5th ed. Philadelphia: Elsevier; 2018:54, Fig. 55.2.)

TABLE 14.6 Clinical Syndromes Associated with Community-Acquired Gastrointestinal Infection

Clinical Syndrome	Signs and Symptoms	Pathogenic Mechanism	Example Pathogens
Acute watery diarrhea*	Loose stools, often with mucus but not blood Occasional vomiting and anorexia Low-grade fever Malaise	Local infection in the gut	Norovirus genogroups I, II, and IV; enteric adenovirus types 40 and 41; rotavirus; enterotoxigenic *Escherichia coli*; enteropathogenic *E. coli*; *Cryptosporidium*; *Clostridium perfringens*; *Bacillus cereus*
Dysentery (acute bloody diarrhea)	Loose stools with gross blood and mucus Fever Abdominal cramps and, in some cases, tenesmus May be clinically toxic	Local invasion of the gut	*Shigella*, enteroinvasive *E. coli*, *Campylobacter jejuni*, *Entamoeba histolytica*, nontyphoidal *Salmonella*, *Yersinia enterocolitica*, *Aeromonas*, *Plesiomonas*, *Clostridioides difficile*
Profuse purging	Copious watery stools resembling "rice water" Low-grade fever Overt signs of dehydration	Toxin mediated	*Vibrio cholerae* O1 and O139, enterotoxigenic *E. coli*
Persistent diarrhea	Similar to acute diarrhea, but symptoms persist for at least 14 days	Local infection in the gut and/or immune compromise of host	*Giardia lamblia*, *Cryptosporidium hominis/parvum*, *Cystoisospora belli*, *Cyclospora cayetanensis*, enteropathogenic *E. coli*, enteroaggregative *E. coli*
Acute vomiting	Sudden onset of nausea and vomiting Little or no diarrhea	Local infection in the gut or intoxication	Norovirus, food poisoning due to *Staphylococcus aureus*, *Bacillus cereus*
Enteric fever	Fever Lymphadenopathy	Local invasion of the gut with systemic spread	*Salmonella enterica* serovar Typhi, *S. enterica* serovar Paratyphi A, B, or C

*Etiologic agents that can cause dysentery can also cause acute watery diarrhea.
From Bennett JE, Dolin R, Blaser MJ, eds. *Mandell, Douglas, and Bennett's Principles and Practices of Infectious Diseases.* 9th ed. Philadelphia: Elsevier; 2020:1335, Table 96.3.

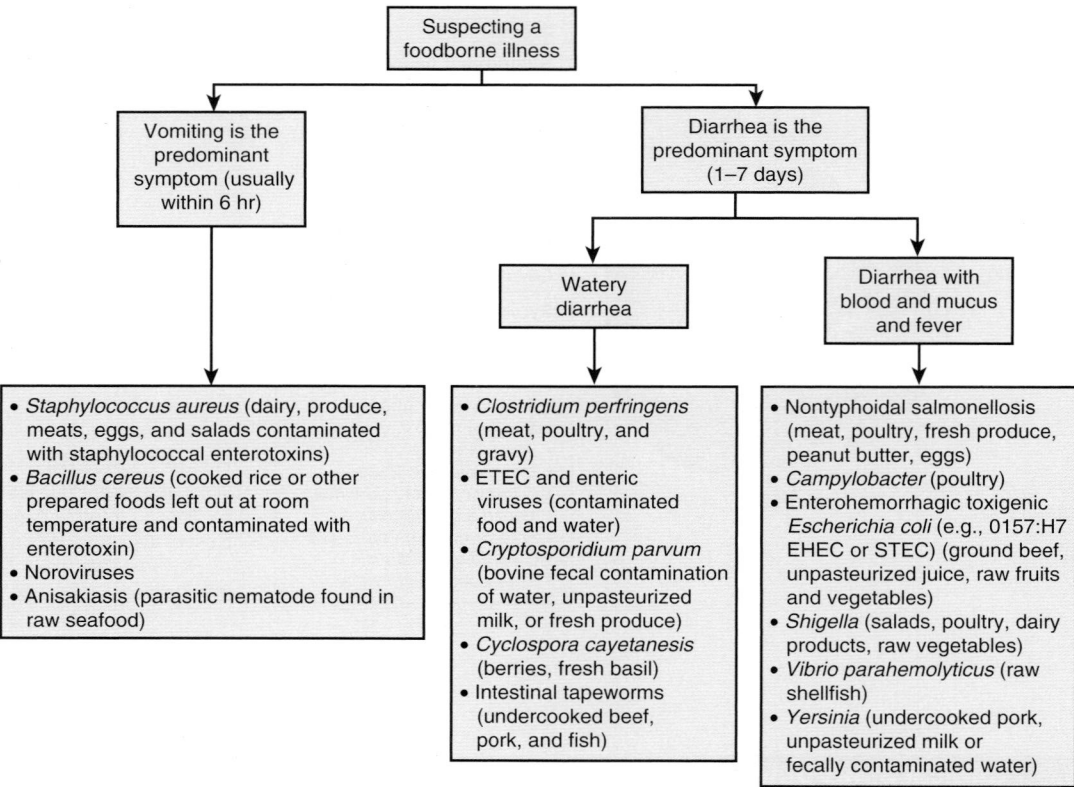

Fig. 14.2 Differentiating causes of foodborne illness. EHEC, enterohemorrhagic *Escherichia coli*; ETEC, enterotoxigenic *E. coli*; STEC, Shiga toxin–producing *E. coli*.

TABLE 14.7   Extraintestinal Manifestations of Enteric Pathogens

Manifestation	Related Enteric Pathogens
Erythema nodosum*	*Yersinia* spp., *Campylobacter* spp., *Salmonella* spp.
Glomerulonephritis*	*Shigella* spp., *Campylobacter* spp., *Yersinia* spp.
Guillain-Barré syndrome*	*Campylobacter* spp.
Hemolytic anemia*	*Campylobacter* spp., *Yersinia* spp.
Hemolytic uremic syndrome*	STEC
Immunoglobulin A nephropathy*	*Campylobacter* spp.
Reactive arthritis*	*Salmonella* spp., *Shigella* spp., *Yersinia* spp., *Campylobacter* spp., *Cryptosporidium* spp.
Postinfectious irritable bowel syndrome	*Campylobacter* spp., *Salmonella* spp., *Shigella* spp., STEC, *Giardia intestinalis*
Meningitis	*Listeria monocytogenes*, *Salmonella* spp. (infants ≤3 mo at high risk)
Intestinal perforation	*Salmonella* spp. (including Typhi), *Shigella* spp., *Campylobacter* spp., *Yersinia* spp.
Encephalopathy, seizure	*Shigella* spp.
Toxic megacolon	*Shigella* spp., *Clostridioides difficile*
Aortitis, osteomyelitis	*Salmonella* spp.

STEC, Shiga toxin–producing *Escherichia coli*.
*Immune-mediated extraintestinal manifestations.
Modified from Long SS, Prober CG, Fischer M, eds. *Principles and Practice of Pediatric Infectious Diseases*. 5th ed. Philadelphia: Elsevier; 2018:54, Table 55.3.

C. difficile infection should be considered in patients in whom diarrhea develops during or within several weeks of antibiotic therapy. Illness associated with this organism varies from a mild, self-limited, nonbloody diarrhea to severe hemorrhagic colitis, protein-losing enteropathy, toxic megacolon, colonic or cecal perforation, peritonitis, sepsis, shock, and death. In rare cases, manifestations of *C. difficile* infection include fever or abdominal pain without diarrhea.

The colitis is caused by potent toxins produced by the organism: **toxin A**, a lethal enterotoxin that causes hemorrhage and fluid secretion in the intestines, and **toxin B**, a cytotoxin detectable by its cytopathic effects in tissue culture. Both toxins play a role in disease pathogenesis, although toxin B may be more important.

Recommendations for diagnosis of *C. difficile* infection are to consider a two-step method to exclude false-positive testing, particularly in the setting of asymptomatic carriage in infants and younger children: nucleic acid amplification testing to identify microbial *toxin genes* and an enzyme immunoassay for *toxins* in stool. Testing is typically performed only on patients with diarrhea who are not concurrently taking laxatives or promotility agents that could otherwise explain the diarrhea; testing may be considered for patients without loose stools if *C. difficile*–induced ileus or toxic megacolon is suspected. Sigmoidoscopy or colonoscopy reveals pseudomembranes in up to 50% of cases, typically in association with more severe disease. Treatment is dependent on the severity of the disease and whether the infection is primary or recurrent. Antibacterials include metronidazole, oral vancomycin, and, in adults, fidaxomicin.

Aeromonas Infection

Aeromonas species are gram-negative bacilli that are found in a variety of freshwater sources and that are capable of causing a wide array

TABLE 14.8 Assessment of Degree of Dehydration

General Appearance	Mild	Moderate	Severe
Infants/young children	Thirsty; alert; restless	Thirsty; restless or listless	Drowsy or lethargic; limp, cold, sweaty, cyanotic
Older children	Thirsty; alert; restless	Thirsty; alert (usually)	Usually conscious (but at reduced level), apprehensive; cold, sweaty, cyanotic extremities; wrinkled skin on fingers/toes; muscle cramps
Signs and Symptoms			
Tachycardia	Absent	Present	Present
Palpable pulses	Present	Present (weak)	Decreased
Blood pressure	Normal	Orthostatic hypotension	Hypotension
Cutaneous perfusion	Normal	Normal	Reduced/mottled
Skin turgor	Normal	Slight reduction	Reduced
Fontanel	Normal	Slightly depressed	Sunken
Mucous membranes	Moist	Dry	Very dry
Tears	Present	Present/absent	Absent
Respirations	Normal	Deep, may be rapid	Deep and rapid
Urine output	Normal	Oliguria	Anuria/severe oliguria

of disease, including a mild, self-limited diarrheal illness in children. Occasionally, *Aeromonas* may cause dysentery or a protracted diarrheal illness. The most common manifestation is a watery, nonbloody, nonmucoid diarrhea seen during the late spring, summer, and early fall. More severe infections may resemble ulcerative colitis, with chronic bloody diarrhea and abdominal pain.

Plesiomonas Infection

Plesiomonas shigelloides is a *Vibrio*-like organism found in soil and warmer (>8°C) fresh or brackish water that is sometimes implicated in childhood diarrhea. It has been linked to consumption of raw shellfish or contaminated water, exposure to reptiles and tropical fish, and travel to endemic areas. The organism is most frequently found in subtropical or tropical climates though has a wide geographic distribution. After an incubation period of 1–2 days, patients typically develop watery diarrhea and vomiting, although some may develop dysentery. Diagnosis is via stool culture. Symptoms may last up to 2 weeks, although the disease is typically self-limited in immunocompetent individuals.

Parasitic Diarrhea

Giardiasis

Giardia intestinalis is a flagellated protozoan that can cause diarrhea, malabsorption, abdominal pain, and weight loss. It spreads through contaminated food and water, as well as through person-to-person contact via the fecal-oral route. The latter mode of transmission is responsible for outbreaks of diarrhea in daycare centers and residential facilities. Infection is often asymptomatic. Symptomatic illness usually develops 1–3 weeks after exposure and may mimic acute gastroenteritis with low-grade or no fever, nausea, vomiting, and watery diarrhea. In some patients, a chronic illness develops, characterized by intermittent, foul-smelling diarrhea, abdominal bloating, nausea, abdominal pain, and weight loss. Up to 40% of patients may develop secondary lactase deficiency following infection. Diagnosis is via EIA or direct fluorescent antibody (DFA) tests, which offer superior sensitivity and specificity compared to microscopy. If microscopy is performed, three separate samples of fresh stool should be examined for cysts or trophozoites, because excretion of the organism is only intermittent. Treatment is typically indicated in the presence of symptoms, to prevent institutional outbreaks, or to prevent spread to immunocompromised individuals.

Entamoeba histolytica Infection

Entamoeba histolytica is acquired in warm climates via the ingestion of cysts in fecally contaminated food or water. Infected individuals are often asymptomatic. Amebic dysentery may occur, but hepatic abscess and other focal infections are uncommon. Because cysts are shed in the stool on an intermittent basis, examination of several fecal specimens may be required for identification. Stool antigen detection assays allow for differentiation between *E. histolytica* and the more prevalent though less pathogenic *E. dispar*, which may also be detected on microscopy. Treatment is indicated to prevent the development of extraintestinal manifestations or spread to other individuals.

Cryptosporidium Infection

This intracellular protozoan causes watery diarrhea in both immunocompetent and immunocompromised hosts and is an important cause of severe diarrhea in individuals infected with HIV. *Cryptosporidium* has also been recognized as an occasional cause of self-limited diarrhea in travelers, as well as in children in daycare centers and persons in residential institutions. The mechanisms by which these organisms cause diarrhea are unknown. Nucleic acid amplification assays and EIA tests are available for diagnosis. Identification via microscopy requires specialized staining techniques that should be requested if *Cryptosporidium* infestation is suspected.

Other Causes of Acute Diarrhea

Parenteral Secondary Diarrhea

Acute diarrhea that accompanies infections outside of the gastrointestinal tract is termed **parenteral diarrhea**. Upper respiratory tract and urinary tract infections may be associated with increased bowel movement frequency or stool water. The mechanism is unclear but may involve alterations in bowel motility, changes in diet, or the effects of antibiotic treatment.

Medications

Various nonlaxative prescription and over-the-counter medications may cause acute diarrhea (Table 14.9). The most implicated agents are antibiotics, acting through mechanisms other than *C. difficile*.

TABLE 14.9 Medications and Substances Associated with Diarrhea in Children

Agent	Mechanism
Stimulant laxatives (e.g., senna, bisacodyl)	Increased intestinal secretion (phenolphthalein, bisacodyl)
Antacids	Osmotic effect (Mg^{2+})
Prokinetic agents	Increased peristalsis (metoclopramide, bethanechol, cisapride)
Measles-mumps-rubella vaccine	Unknown
Thyroid hormone	Increased peristalsis
Chemotherapeutics	Intestinal mucosal injury
Heavy metals	Toxic effect
Organophosphates	Cholinergic effects
Diuretics	Unknown
Digitalis	Unknown
Colchicine	Unknown
Indomethacin	Prostaglandin synthesis inhibition
Theophylline	Increased peristalsis

Food Poisoning (Table 14.10; see Fig. 14.2)

Staphylococcal food poisoning results from ingestion of preformed enterotoxin, produced in contaminated food that has incubated at or above room temperature for a suitable period. Staphylococcal food poisoning is suggested by the sudden onset of vomiting that is followed by explosive diarrhea, usually within 4–6 hours after ingestion of the contaminated food. The illness is self-limited and usually resolves within 12–24 hours. The diagnosis is based on the typical historical presentation. Treatment is supportive; antibiotics are not indicated.

Bacillus cereus, a gram-positive sporulating organism found in soil, is usually associated with contamination of refried rice or vegetables. Two food poisoning syndromes can occur. A *short incubation* period disease (1–6 hours) results from ingestion of preformed toxin and is characterized by nausea, vomiting, and diarrhea, similar to staphylococcal food poisoning. A *long incubation* period disease (8–16 hours) is caused by in vivo production of an enterotoxin and is characterized by abdominal pain, tenesmus, and profuse watery diarrhea. Vomiting is usually absent. Both syndromes resolve spontaneously within 24 hours and are managed with supportive care.

Clostridium perfringens food poisoning has been associated with ingestion of contaminated beef and poultry. The disease results from the production and release of an enterotoxin into the lower bowel 8–24

TABLE 14.10 Foodborne Gastrointestinal Illnesses

Cause	Incubation Period	Clinical Clues	Common Vehicle	Diagnosis
Heavy metals (copper, zinc, cadmium, tin)	Minutes to 2 hr	Metallic taste, diarrhea, prominent vomiting, no fever	Carbonated or acidic beverages in metal containers	Chemical study of implicated beverage
Mushroom poisoning*	Minutes to 2 hr	Altered mental status with visual disturbance (encephalopathy)	Noncommercially obtained mushrooms	Identify mushroom and/or toxic chemical (e.g., muscarine, psilocybin)
Fish/shellfish-related toxins*				
Scombrotoxin poisoning	Minutes to 2 hr	Histamine reaction: flushing, headache, dizziness, burning of throat and mouth	*Scombridae* fish (includes tuna, mackerel, and bonito species), mahi-mahi	Identify fish and/or chemical toxin (ciguatoxin, tetrodotoxin, histamine, etc.)
Paralytic shellfish poisoning	Minutes to 2 hr	Paresthesia, dizziness, sometimes paralysis	Mussels, clams, oysters, scallops contaminated with toxins, typically from dinoflagellate algae species	
Tetrodotoxin poisoning	Minutes to 2 hr	Paresthesia	Various pufferfish and angelfish species. The toxin is produced by symbiotic or infecting bacteria in the fish species	
Ciguatoxin poisoning	2–24 hr	Itching, arthralgia, metallic taste, paresthesia, cramps, visual disturbances, "loose" painful teeth	Barracuda, red snapper, grouper, amberjack	
Norovirus	24–48 hr	Epidemic watery diarrhea	Contaminated ice machines, shellfish, ready-to-eat foods	Nucleic acid amplification assays
Staphylococcal enterotoxins	2–8 hr	Prominent vomiting, no fever, duration <24 hr	Ham, poultry, pastries (cream-filled), mixed salads, egg salad	Identification of preformed toxin or isolation of 10^5 colony-forming units of organism from food
Bacillus cereus				
Emetic form: short incubation	2–8 hr	Prominent vomiting, no fever, duration <48 hr	Fried rice, macaroni and cheese, vegetables, other ready-to-eat foods left at room temperature. Symptoms and rapidity of onset are due to presence of preformed toxin	Identification of preformed toxin or isolation of 10^5 colony-forming units of organism from food

TABLE 14.10 Foodborne Gastrointestinal Illnesses—cont'd

Cause	Incubation Period	Clinical Clues	Common Vehicle	Diagnosis
Diarrheal form: longer incubation	8–14 hr	Abdominal cramps, severe diarrhea, no fever, duration <48 hr	Fried rice, macaroni and cheese, vegetables, other ready-to-eat foods left at room temperature. Symptoms are due to in vivo toxin production	Identification of preformed toxin or isolation of 10^5 colony-forming units of organism from food or stool
Clostridium perfringens	8–14 hr	Abdominal cramps, severe diarrhea, no fever, duration <48 hr	Meat, poultry, gravy	Identification of preformed toxin or isolation of 10^5 colony-forming units of organism from food or stool
Enterotoxigenic *Escherichia coli* (ETEC)	12 hr to several days	Abdominal cramps, watery diarrhea may be prolonged up to 7 days	Incomplete data (rarely reported)	Identification of enterotoxin or isolation of organism from stool
Invasive *E. coli*	12 hr to days	Prolonged febrile diarrhea and/or dysentery	Incomplete data (rarely reported)	Isolation of organism from stool
Vibrio cholerae	12 hr to days	Abdominal cramps, watery diarrhea (rice-water stools). May be prolonged up to 1 wk	Contaminated food and water (very rare in United states)	Isolation of organism from food or stool
Vibrio parahaemolyticus	12 hr to days	Prolonged febrile diarrhea and/or dysentery	Seafood	Stool culture (or food culture)
Shigella species	12 hr to days	Prolonged febrile diarrhea and/or dysentery	Fish, mixed salads	Stool culture (or food culture)
Campylobacter species	12 hr to days	Prolonged febrile diarrhea and/or dysentery	Unpasteurized milk, poultry or meat	Stool culture (or food culture)
Clostridium botulinum	12 hr to days	Diarrhea, constipation Guillain-Barré syndrome	Home-canned foods, fish, honey	Botulinum toxin in food, stool, and serum
Yersinia enterocolitica	Uncertain	Prolonged diarrhea and/or dysentery	Milk, pig intestine	Stool culture

*Potentially dangerous; observation in hospital often required.
Modified from Reilly BM. *Practical Strategies in Outpatient Medicine*. 2nd ed. Philadelphia: WB Saunders; 1991:888.

hours after ingestion of the vegetative form of the organism. Onset is sudden, with abdominal pain and watery diarrhea. Fever and vomiting are absent. Treatment is supportive.

CHRONIC DIARRHEA

The etiology of chronic diarrhea is dependent on the age of the patient (see Table 14.1) and is additionally influenced by socioeconomic factors and the clinical setting. In countries with a lower baseline socioeconomic status, chronic diarrhea may be caused by acute infections, as malnutrition can prolong the course of infectious enterocolitis. The most common etiologies of chronic diarrhea in countries with a higher baseline socioeconomic status are functional intestinal disorders, nutrient malabsorption (e.g., cystic fibrosis), celiac disease, and IBD, but persistent infections of the intestinal tract may also occur. Neonatal or early-infancy-onset chronic diarrhea is often due to monogenic disorders (Tables 14.11 and 14.12).

History

The history should establish the age of onset, as well as the frequency and nature of the stools, including the presence of blood, nighttime stooling, urgency, weight loss, and any associated systemic symptoms. History should also ascertain any recent travel, other sick contacts, or swimming in freshwater sources. A history of recurrent infections, use of intravenous drugs, or other signs, symptoms, or risk factors for immunodeficiency should be documented. Family history should be probed for the presence of gastrointestinal disorders or immunodeficiency.

Physical Examination

Hydration status should be assessed. Growth parameters should be obtained and charted on age-matched growth charts. The physical examination should assess for signs of malnutrition, vitamin and micronutrient deficiency, and dermatologic manifestations of systemic diseases. Jaundice may suggest hemolysis or hepatic dysfunction. Signs of fat-soluble vitamin deficiency include bone deformities in vitamin D deficiency, dry scaly skin and Bitot spots (superficial buildup of keratin in the conjunctivae) in vitamin A deficiency, hyporeflexia or gait abnormalities in vitamin E deficiency, and bruises or bleeding in vitamin K deficiency. Joint examination may reveal arthritis associated with IBD. Abdominal examination may reveal evidence suggestive of neuroendocrine tumors, and perianal examination may reveal evidence of IBD (fistula, skin tags).

Diagnostic Evaluation

The clinician should try to focus the diagnostic evaluation on only those conditions suggested by the history and physical examination. Invasive diagnostic procedures should be limited to those patients whose presentation contains red flags for serious disease (Table 14.13). Laboratory investigation should begin with microbiologic studies for bacteria and parasites in the stool. Acute infection with bacteria, such as *Yersinia*, *E. coli*, and *Salmonella*, may develop into a chronic

TABLE 14.11 Disorders Leading to Early-Onset Chronic Diarrhea

Category	Disorder	Gene(s) Involved	Inheritance	Features
Defects in epithelial nutrient and electrolyte transport	Congenital chloride diarrhea	SLC26A3	AR	• High chloride in stools • Founder effect from Saudi Arabia (Taif region) and Finland • Premature with IUGR • Absence of meconium • Polyhydramnios and dilated loops of bowel on prenatal imaging, abdominal distension after birth • 24% had renal involvement (chronic kidney disease) • Dental carries • Some overlap with Bartter and Gitelman syndrome
	Congenital sodium diarrhea	SLC9A3 GUCY2C	AR AD	• Increased risk of development of IBD • Polyhydramnios and dilated loops of bowel on prenatal imaging • High sodium in stools • Diarrhea may improve with time
	Glucose-galactose malabsorption	SLC5A1	AR	• Treatment requires avoidance of all sugars other than fructose
	Primary bile acid diarrhea	SLC10A2 SLC51B	AR AR	• Associated with cholestasis, increased gamma-glutamyl transferase level, and fat-soluble vitamin deficiency
	Acrodermatitis enteropathica	SLC39A4	AR	• Perioral and extremity lesions, alopecia, and diarrhea • Recurrent infection from immune dysfunction
Defects in epithelial enzymes and metabolism	Congenital lactase deficiency	LCT	AR	• Rare form of inherited diarrhea
	Congenital sucrase-isomaltase deficiency	SI	AR	• Bloating, diarrhea, and rarely associated with failure to thrive • High prevalence in Greenland and Inuit (5%), with 0.2% prevalence in Europeans • Variable phenotype
	Trehalase deficiency	TREH	AR	• Up to 8% of Greenland population • Similar to lactase deficiency
	Enterokinase deficiency	TMPRSS15	AR	• Deficiency of activator of pancreatic enzymes
	DGAT1 deficiency	DGAT1	AR	• Fat-soluble vitamin deficiency • Avoidance of enteral lipids seems to help
	Sieving protein-losing enteropathy	PLVAP	AR	• Protein loss of specific sizes • Syndromic with hydrops, dysmorphic facies, cardiac and renal abnormalities
	Abetalipoproteinemia	MTTP	AR	• Enterocytes show lipid-filled vacuoles
	Hypobetalipoproteinemia	APOB	AR	• Steatorrhea and failure to thrive
	Chylomicron retention disease	SAR1B	AR	• Later noted to have fat-soluble vitamin deficiency and bleeding issues
	Dyskeratosis congenita	DKC1 RTEL1	X AR	• Nail pitting, leukoplakia, and immune defects
	Kabuki syndrome	KMT2D	AD	• Multiple congenital anomalies with varying phenotype
Defects in epithelial trafficking and polarity	Microvillus inclusion disease	MYO5B	AR	• Microvilli seen on electron microscopy are periodic acid–Schiff positive • May be associated with Fanconi syndrome
		STX3	AR	• Rare form. May be associated with neurologic findings
	Tufting enteropathy	EPCAM	AR	• Teardrop-shaped tufts of enterocytes throughout the intestine
	Syndromic sodium-losing diarrhea	SPINT2	AR	• Phenotype similar to tufting enteropathy, but with sodium-losing diarrhea
	Trichohepatoenteric syndrome	TTC37 SKIV2L	AR AR	• Woolly hair, SCID-like phenotype and hepatic defects
	Familial hemophagocytic lymphohistiocytosis type 5	STXBP2	AR	• Recurrence after HSCT, villous blunting
	Multiple intestinal atresia	TTC7A	AR	• Variable phenotype with multiple intestinal atresia, SCID-like phenotype, and enterocolitis

TABLE 14.11 Disorders Leading to Early-Onset Chronic Diarrhea—cont'd

Category	Disorder	Gene(s) Involved	Inheritance	Features
Enteroendocrine cell dysfunction	Enteric anendocrinosis	NEUROG3	AR	• Severe malabsorptive diarrhea, neonatal-onset diabetes mellitus, and normal intestinal biopsies
	Proprotein convertase 1/3 deficiency	PCSK1	AR	• Age-dependent phenotype. Infants have TPN-dependent diarrhea and failure to thrive. Later appear to lose intestinal phenotype and develop multiple endocrine abnormalities
	X-linked lissencephaly with abnormal genitalia	ARX	X	• Seizures, abnormal genitalia, survival between 6 days and 6 yr
	Mitchell-Riley syndrome	RFX6	AR	• Lack of enteroendocrine cells
	Intractable congenital diarrhea in infants	ICR	AR	• Secretory diarrhea caused by a noncoding variant with wide-ranging effects on multiple intestinal genes
Immune disregulation–associated enteropathy	Immune disregulation, polyendocrinopathy, enteropathy X-linked	FOXP3	X	• Polyendocrinopathy
	Common variable immune deficiency (CVID) type 1	ICOS	AR	• Variable presentation. May have dietary-induced diarrhea
	CVID type 8	LRBA	AR	
	ADAM17 deficiency	ADAM17	AR	• Fatal in most patients
	EGFR deficiency	EGFR	AR	• Described in three patients
	CTLA-4	CTLA-4	AD	• Similar to LRBA. May respond to abatacept
	CD55 deficiency	CD55	AR	• Protein-losing enteropathy and thrombosis
	X-linked inhibitor of apoptosis	XIAP	X	• Responsive to HSCT

AD, autosomal dominant; AR, autosomal recessive; EGFR, epidermal growth factor receptor; HSCT, hematopoietic stem cell transplantation; IBD, inflammatory bowel disease; IUGR intrauterine growth restriction; SCID, severe combined immunodeficiency; TPN, total parenteral nutrition; X, X-linked.
From Elkadri AA. Congenital diarrheal syndrome. *Clin Perinatol.* 2020;47:87–104 (Table 2, pp 94–96).

TABLE 14.12 Pancreatic Disorders Leading to Early-Onset Chronic Diarrhea

Cystic fibrosis	AR Pathologic genetic variants involving CFTR. More than 1,300 pathologic genetic variants have been described. Most common is pathologic genetic variant ΔF508	Meconium ileus in neonate Megacolon Chronic diarrhea from pancreatic insufficiency starting from 1 mo of age Failure to thrive Conjugated hyperbilirubinemia	Low stool elastase High sweat chloride (>60 mEq/L) Newborn screening Molecular genetic testing
Shwachman-Diamond syndrome	AR SBDS gene in over 90%	Chronic diarrhea from pancreatic insufficiency Bone marrow failure Skeletal changes Pancreatic lipomatosis on diagnostic imaging (ultrasound or computed tomography)	Clinical features Molecular genetic testing
Johanson-Blizzard syndrome	AR UBR1 gene	Chronic diarrhea from pancreatic insufficiency Dysmorphic features: aplastic alae nasi, extension of the hairline to the forehead with upswept frontal hair, low-set ears, large anterior fontanel, micrognathia, thin lips, microcephaly, aplasia cutis (patchy distribution of hair with areas of alopecia), dental anomalies, poor growth, and anorectal anomalies (mainly imperforate anus)	Clinical features Molecular genetic testing
Pearson syndrome	Sporadic: caused by de novo single, large deletions of mtDNA, which can range from 1,000 to 10,000 nucleotides	Chronic diarrhea from pancreatic insufficiency Sideroblastic anemia, variable neutropenia, thrombocytopenia, and vacuolization of bone marrow precursors Lactic acidosis and liver failure	Clinical features Molecular genetic testing

AR, autosomal recessive; CFTR, cystic fibrosis transmembrane conductance regulator; cGMP, cyclic immunoglobulin; mtDNA, mitochondrial DNA.

TABLE 14.13   Red Flags in the Evaluation of Diarrhea

Presence of blood in stools
Iron-deficiency anemia
Persistent right upper or right lower quadrant abdominal pain
Involuntary weight loss or growth failure
Delayed puberty
Presence of associated symptoms, such as unexplained fever, suggesting inflammatory arthritides or other systemic diseases
Nocturnal fecal urgency or diarrhea
Perirectal/perianal disease
Persistent dysphagia
Edema, hypoalbuminemia
Cutaneous lesions

illness and can be detected by routine stool cultures and multiplex PCR assays. *C. difficile* testing should be performed, especially in the presence of risk factors. Antigen detection and PCR-based assays for *Giardia* and *Cryptosporidium* are more sensitive and specific than routine microscopy-based examinations and are indicated if these infections are suspected.

Except in the setting of neonatal-onset diarrhea and factitious diarrhea, stool electrolytes and osmolality are of limited use. The differentiation of osmotic and secretory diarrhea is typically made by a trial of fasting and determining if there is improvement in the stool output: osmotic diarrhea improves or resolves upon fasting, whereas secretory diarrhea does not. **Stool reducing substances** are positive in the setting of osmotic diarrhea secondary to carbohydrate malabsorption. In patients with osmotic diarrhea and negative reducing substances, it is essential to determine whether steatorrhea is present. If qualitative assays for fecal fat are negative, a more precise indication of steatorrhea may be obtained by quantifying fecal fat and calculating the coefficient of fat absorption, which requires a 72-hour collection of stool. Low fecal elastase suggests pancreatic insufficiency. Elevated levels of **stool α_1-antitrypsin (A1AT)** are suggestive of protein-losing enteropathy (PLE). Elevated **fecal calprotectin** or **fecal lactoferrin** are indicative of intestinal inflammation. The presence of fecal leukocytes or occult blood may indicate mucosal inflammation as well, though neither is sufficiently sensitive nor specific.

Blood tests should include a CBC to evaluate for anemia and thrombocytosis, which may suggest blood loss and inflammation, respectively. In the presence of anemia, red blood cell indices may reveal a microcytosis potentially indicative of iron deficiency or a macrocytosis suggestive of vitamin B_{12} or folate deficiency. A normocytic anemia may be seen in chronic inflammatory diseases. White blood cell count and differential and quantification of immunoglobulins A, G, and M screen for immune deficiency disorders. Elevated ESR and CRP indicate inflammation but are nonspecific. Low albumin could be indicative of an inflammatory process or PLE. Elevated antitissue transglutaminase immunoglobulin A (IgA) antibody is sensitive and specific for celiac disease, but a low total serum IgA level may result in a false-negative test. Levels of the fat-soluble vitamins A, 25-OH vitamin D, vitamin E, and vitamin K (reflected by prothrombin time) may be measured if fat malabsorption is suspected.

The algorithmic approach to evaluating chronic diarrhea is depicted in Figure 14.3*A* and *B* and is enumerated in Table 14.14.

Disorders of Carbohydrate Malabsorption

The brush border epithelium of the small bowel contains enzymes necessary for carbohydrate digestion. These enzymes hydrolyze disaccharides and oligosaccharides into monosaccharides that are then absorbed by transporters on the luminal surface of enterocytes. Carbohydrate malabsorption is secondary to either deficiency of a particular enzyme (e.g., congenital sucrase-isomaltase deficiency) or an abnormality in a transport protein involved with the absorption of monosaccharides (e.g., glucose-galactose malabsorption). The onset of various carbohydrate malabsorption syndromes can vary based on the timing of the introduction of particular carbohydrates (Table 14.15).

Patients with carbohydrate malabsorption disorders present with severe watery diarrhea, which results from osmotic action exerted by the malabsorbed carbohydrate in the intestinal lumen. Colonic bacteria ferment the malabsorbed sugars, which generates a mixture of gases (e.g., hydrogen, methane, and carbon dioxide) and short-chain fatty acids. These gases form the basis of carbohydrate-specific breath hydrogen testing, which is often used in diagnosis. The stools become acidified to a pH of less than 7, which can lead to diaper dermatitis.

Disaccharidase Deficiency

Congenital sucrase-isomaltase deficiency (CSID). CSID is an inherited deficiency of the ability to hydrolyze sucrose, maltose, and starch. Exposure to these substances leads to osmotic diarrhea, pain, bloating, abdominal distension, and, at times, chronic malnutrition and failure to thrive. The sucrase-isomaltase gene is located on chromosome 3 (3q25.2-q26.2) and more than 25 pathogenic variants in the gene have been identified. These variants result in a variety of defects in the structure and function of the enzyme, including isolated deficiencies in sucrase activity or isomaltase activity. This genetic heterogeneity results in phenotypic variability ranging from completely absent to low-residual sucrase activity, and from completely absent to normal isomaltase activity. Because sucrase-isomaltase is responsible for up to 80% of the maltase activity in the brush border, maltase activity is significantly reduced in almost all cases.

The exact prevalence of CSID is unclear, although rates are as high as 10% in the Greenland Inuit population, 7% in Canadians of indigenous ancestry, and about 3% in Alaskans of indigenous ancestry. Estimates of the prevalence of CSID in other North American and European populations generally range from 1 in 500 to 1 in 2,000.

The classic presentation of CSID is severe watery diarrhea, failure to thrive, irritability, and diaper dermatitis in a 9- to 18-month-old infant who has been exposed to sucrose and starch in the form of fruit juices, fruit purees, and starch-laden foods such as crackers and cookies (see Table 14.4). Intrinsic factors that contribute to the severity of presentation during infancy include the shorter length of the colon and a decreased capacity for colonic reabsorption of fluid and electrolytes, more rapid small intestinal transit, a high-carbohydrate diet, and lower levels of amylase prior to 2 years of age. Some patients with milder sucrase deficiency may improve with age as their colonic bacteria develop an increased capacity to ferment residual sucrose and the intestinal tract develops an increased capacity for reabsorption. Patients may be misdiagnosed as having food allergies or irritable bowel syndrome (IBS) or may remain undiagnosed. Symptoms may abate with the restriction of carbohydrate in the diet or with the use of enteral sucrase enzyme supplements.

Diagnosis typically involves endoscopy for histologic examination of small bowel morphology and measurement of disaccharidase levels on biopsy specimens. Diagnosis requires the following:
1. Normal small bowel morphology
2. Absent or markedly reduced sucrase activity
3. Isomaltase activity varying from absent to full activity

4. Reduced maltase activity
5. Normal lactase activity, or in the setting of reduced lactase, a sucrase:lactase ratio of <1.0

Other less invasive methods of diagnosis include sucrose breath hydrogen quantification and differential urinary disaccharide assessment; however, both modalities are associated with high false-positive and false-negative rates. Furthermore, differential urinary disaccharide testing requires a 10-hour urine collection specimen, which is often impractical in infants and younger children.

Maltase-glucoamylase deficiency. Maltase-glucoamylase is a brush border hydrolase that serves as an alternate pathway for starch digestion that complements sucrase-isomaltase activity. Congenital maltase-glucoamylase deficiency is rare, with only several cases described in the literature. Genetically, maltase-glucoamylase shares approximately 59% of its sequence with sucrase-isomaltase, and the enzyme has two catalytic sites that are identical to those of sucrase-isomaltase. Symptoms are similar to those seen in CSID. Diagnosis requires the demonstration of reduced glucoamylase activity in the setting of normal small bowel histology and normal pancreatic amylase activity.

Congenital glucose-galactose malabsorption (CGGM). Congenital glucose-galactose malabsorption results from defective sodium-coupled transport of glucose and galactose into enterocytes. It is a rare autosomal recessive disorder that results from pathogenic variants in the sodium-glucose cotransporter gene *SGLT1* located on chromosome 22q12.3. CGGM presents as a neonatal-onset profuse, watery diarrhea that ceases immediately following the elimination of glucose and galactose sources from the diet. Symptoms recur if the patient is fed formula containing either of these carbohydrates, including polymers such as sucrose and lactose. The disorder may lead to dehydration and electrolyte abnormalities, both of which can become life threatening, and patients may be hypoglycemic. Stool reducing substances are

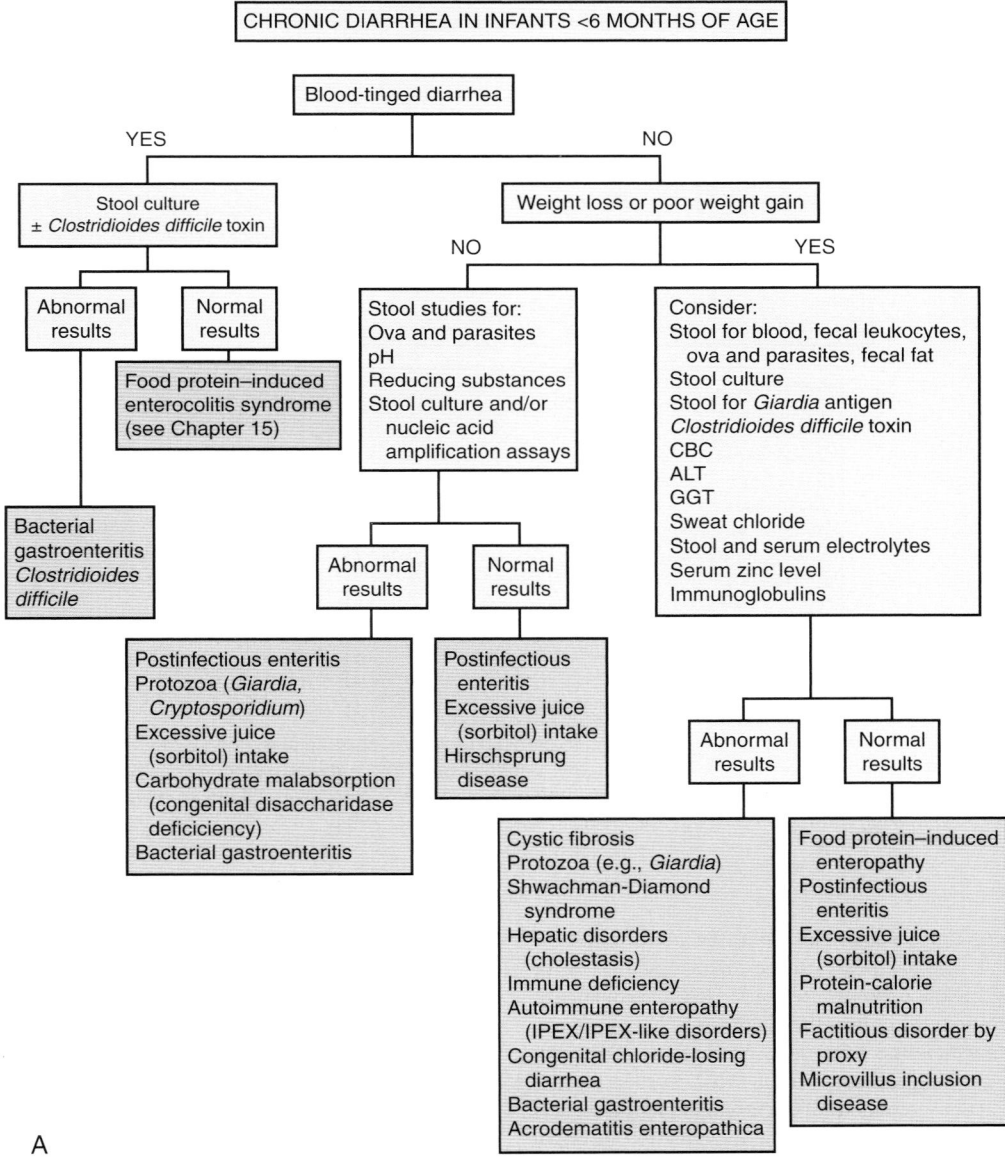

Fig. 14.3 *A,* The algorithmic approach to chronic diarrhea in infants younger than 6 months of age. ALT, alanine aminotransferase; GGT, gamma-glutamyl transferase; IPEX, immune disregulation, polyendocrinopathy, enteropathy, X-linked.

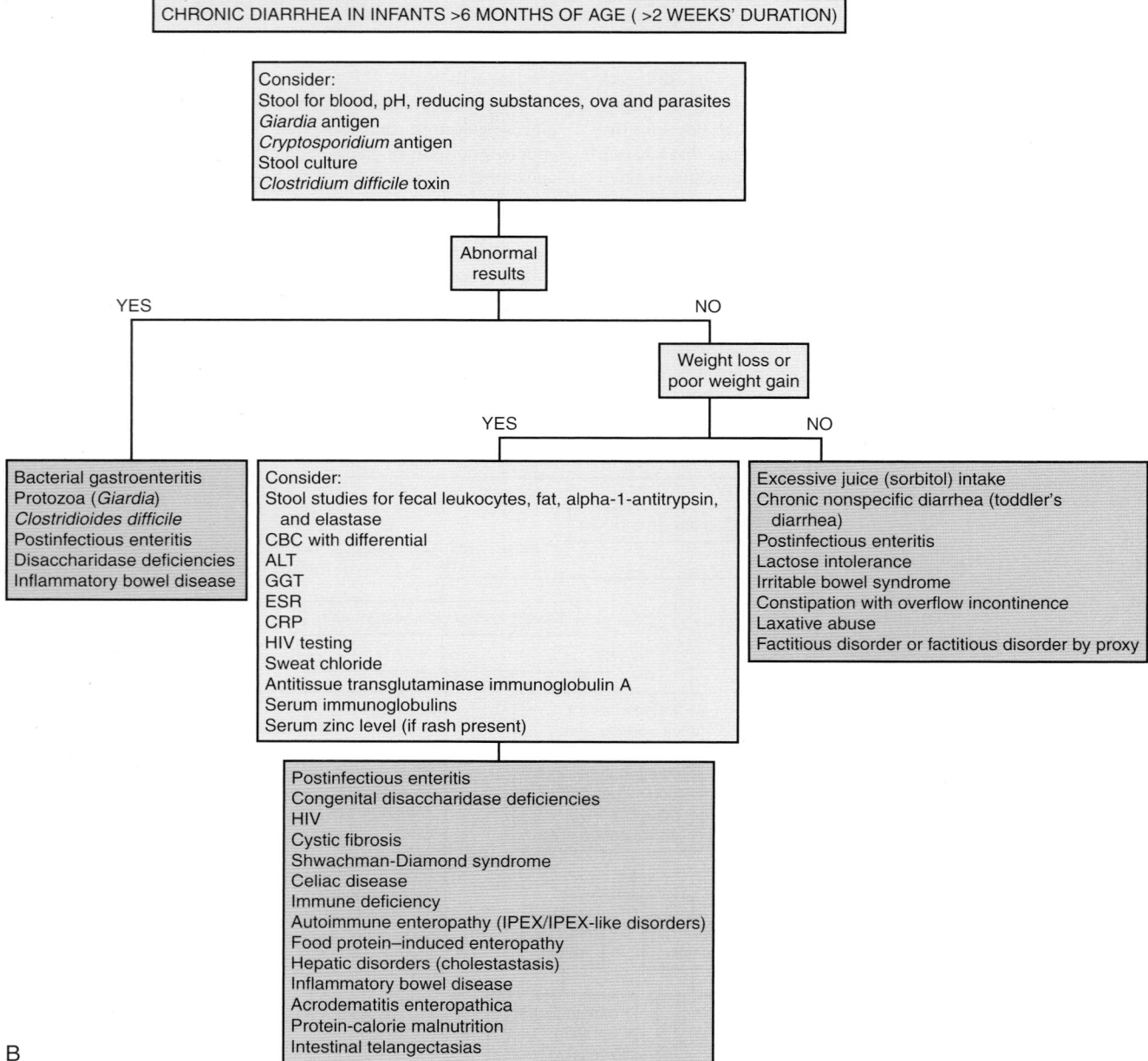

CHRONIC DIARRHEA IN INFANTS >6 MONTHS OF AGE (>2 WEEKS' DURATION)

Consider:
Stool for blood, pH, reducing substances, ova and parasites
Giardia antigen
Cryptosporidium antigen
Stool culture
Clostridium difficile toxin

Abnormal results

YES / NO

Weight loss or poor weight gain

YES / NO

Bacterial gastroenteritis
Protozoa (*Giardia*)
Clostridioides difficile
Postinfectious enteritis
Disaccharidase deficiencies
Inflammatory bowel disease

Consider:
Stool studies for fecal leukocytes, fat, alpha-1-antitrypsin, and elastase
CBC with differential
ALT
GGT
ESR
CRP
HIV testing
Sweat chloride
Antitissue transglutaminase immunoglobulin A
Serum immunoglobulins
Serum zinc level (if rash present)

Excessive juice (sorbitol) intake
Chronic nonspecific diarrhea (toddler's diarrhea)
Postinfectious enteritis
Lactose intolerance
Irritable bowel syndrome
Constipation with overflow incontinence
Laxative abuse
Factitious disorder or factitious disorder by proxy

Postinfectious enteritis
Congenital disaccharidase deficiencies
HIV
Cystic fibrosis
Shwachman-Diamond syndrome
Celiac disease
Immune deficiency
Autoimmune enteropathy (IPEX/IPEX-like disorders)
Food protein–induced enteropathy
Hepatic disorders (cholestasis)
Inflammatory bowel disease
Acrodematitis enteropathica
Protein-calorie malnutrition
Intestinal telangectasias

B

Fig. 14.3, cont'd *B,* The algorithmic approach to chronic diarrhea in children older than 6 months of age. ALT, alanine aminotransferase; GGT, gamma-glutamyl transferase; IPEX, immune disregulation, polyendocrinopathy, enteropathy, X-linked. (Modified from Pomeranz AJ, Sabnis S, Busey SL, Kliegman RM, eds. *Pediatric Decision-Making Strategies.* 2nd ed. Philadelphia: Elsevier; 2016:87–89.)

positive secondary to the presence of glucose in the stools. Intestinal morphology is normal. The diagnosis can be further established by an abnormal glucose breath hydrogen test and *SGLT1* sequencing, although neither is required to confirm the diagnosis.

Congenital lactase deficiency. A rare autosomal recessive disorder leading to very low or complete absence of brush border lactase-phlorizin hydrolase activity, **congenital lactase deficiency** usually presents with diarrhea starting soon after the introduction of breast milk or any lactose-containing formula. Most infants manifest within the first 10 days of life. Unless the disorder is recognized and treated quickly, the condition is life-threatening secondary to dehydration and

electrolyte abnormalities. Small bowel biopsies reveal normal histology but low or completely absent lactase concentrations. A presumptive diagnosis can be made if osmotic diarrhea in a neonate resolves by introducing lactose-free formula.

Primary lactase deficiency (lactose intolerance). Approximately 65% of the world's population has primary lactase deficiency, although prevalence varies by ethnicity. While primary lactase deficiency is nearly universal in Asian and Native American populations and is as high as 80% in Latino, Black, and Ashkenazi Jewish populations, as few as 2% of individuals of northern European ancestry are affected. Age of onset varies by ethnicity as well. Approximately 20% of Latino, Asian,

TABLE 14.14 Diagnostic Studies in the Evaluation of Chronic Diarrhea

Initial Studies

Stool examination for blood, leukocytes, reducing substances, and *Clostridioides difficile* toxin; stool examination for ova and parasites and cultures or nucleic acid amplification testing for infectious pathogens

Complete blood count

Serum electrolytes, blood urea nitrogen, creatinine, calcium, phosphorus, albumin, total protein

Urinalysis and culture

Stool electrolytes

Fecal calprotectin or lactoferrin if inflammatory bowel disease suspected

Second-Phase Studies

Sweat chloride test

Breath analysis

D-Xylose test

Serum carotene, folate, vitamin B_{12}, and iron levels

Fecal α_1-antitrypsin level

Fecal fat studies or coefficient of fat absorption studies

Fatty test meal, Lundh test meal

Third-Phase Studies

Fat-soluble vitamin levels: A, 25-hydroxy D, and E

Contrast radiographic studies: upper gastrointestinal series or barium enema

Small intestinal biopsy for histology and mucosal enzyme determination

Bentiromide excretion test

Specialized Studies

Schilling test

Serum/urine bile acid determination

Endoscopic retrograde pancreatography

Provocative pancreatic secretion testing

Exome sequencing for monogenic disorders

From Wyllie R, Hyams JS, eds. *Pediatric Gastrointestinal Disease*. 2nd ed. Philadelphia: WB Saunders; 1999:283.

TABLE 14.15 Typical Age of Presentation of Carbohydrate Malabsorption Syndromes

Carbohydrate Malabsorption Syndrome	Age of Symptom Onset
Congenital glucose-galactose malabsorption	Neonatal period
Congenital lactase deficiency	
Sucrase-isomaltase deficiency	Weaning age
Glucoamylase deficiency	
Primary lactase deficiency	Uncommon before 2 or 3 yr of age
	Around 5 yr of age in Asian, Latino, and Black populations
	Over 5 yr of age, more typically in adolescence in Caucasians of European descent

and Black children younger than 5 years of age are affected, while White children typically do not develop symptoms of lactose intolerance until after 5 years of age. Children with clinical signs of lactose intolerance at an earlier age than would be typical for their ethnicity may warrant an evaluation for an alternate cause.

Symptoms typically develop insidiously over the course of many years, with most affected individuals experiencing onset of symptoms in late adolescence or adulthood. Within 30 minutes to 2 hours of ingesting lactose, patients develop abdominal cramping and distension, foul-smelling flatulence, nausea, and diarrhea. While the severity of symptoms is directly correlated with the quantity of ingested lactose, each individual exhibits a unique dose threshold beyond which symptoms develop.

Diagnosis is suggested historically. When lactose intolerance is suspected, a trial of a lactose-free diet can aid in confirming the diagnosis. Patients must be sure to eliminate all sources of lactose, including some that may be hidden (Table 14.16). Generally, a 2-week trial of a strict lactose-free diet producing resolution of symptoms, followed by a subsequent reintroduction of dairy foods resulting in recurrence of symptoms, is diagnostic. In subtler cases, hydrogen breath testing is the least invasive and most helpful test to diagnose lactose malabsorption.

Secondary lactase deficiency. Secondary lactase deficiency develops when an inflammatory process, such as a viral gastrointestinal infection, damages the brush border epithelium and leads to the loss of the lactase-containing epithelial cells from the tips of the villi. The immature epithelial cells that replace these are often lactase deficient, leading to lactose malabsorption. Secondary lactase deficiency in most children with acute gastroenteritis is rarely clinically significant. *Most affected children can safely continue breast milk or standard lactose-containing formula without any significant effects, although infants under 3 months of age may develop*

TABLE 14.16 Hidden Sources of Lactose

- Bread and other baked goods
- Waffles, pancakes, biscuits, cookies, and the mixes to make them
- Processed breakfast foods such as doughnuts, frozen waffles and pancakes, toaster pastries, and sweet rolls
- Processed breakfast cereals
- Instant potatoes, soups, and breakfast drinks
- Potato chips, corn chips, and other processed snacks
- Processed meats such as bacon, sausage, hot dogs, and lunch meats
- Margarine
- Salad dressings
- Liquid and powdered milk-based meal replacements
- Protein powders and bars
- Candies
- Nondairy liquid and powdered coffee creamers
- Nondairy whipped toppings
- Certain medications

If a food label includes any of the following words, the product contains lactose:
- Milk
- Lactose
- Whey
- Curds
- Milk by-products
- Dry milk solids
- Nonfat dry milk powder

From National Digestive Diseases Information Clearinghouse. Lactose intolerance. 2015. http://digestive.niddk.nih.gov/ddiseases/pubs/lactoseintolerance.

clinically significant symptoms. Giardiasis, cryptosporidiosis, and other parasites that infect the proximal small intestine often lead to lactose malabsorption from direct injury to the epithelial cells by the parasite. Secondary lactase deficiency with clinical signs of lactose intolerance can be seen in celiac disease, Crohn disease, and immune-related and other enteropathies and should be considered if children with these diagnoses have symptoms of lactose intolerance. Diagnostic evaluation should be directed toward these entities when secondary lactase deficiency is suspected and an infectious etiology is not found.

Severe malnutrition can also produce secondary lactose intolerance via small bowel atrophy. Most infants and children with malabsorption attributable to malnutrition are able to continue to tolerate dietary carbohydrates, including lactose. However, the World Health Organization recommends avoidance of lactose in children with persistent postinfectious diarrhea lasting more than 14 days, if they fail a dietary trial of milk or yogurt. Treatment of secondary lactase deficiency and lactose malabsorption attributable to an underlying condition generally does not require elimination of lactose from the diet but, rather, treatment of the underlying condition.

Trehalase deficiency. Trehalose is an $\alpha(1,1)$-linked glucose dimer that is produced by certain bacteria, fungi, plants, and invertebrates as an energy source and as a method of surviving freezing temperatures or lack of water. Potential dietary sources include mushrooms and processed foods that have trehalose added to improve frozen shelf life. Symptoms are similar to lactose intolerance. Deficiency is rare in most populations though is estimated to affect up to 8% of the indigenous population in Greenland.

Tables 14.11 and 14.12 list additional important causes of chronic neonatal or infantile diarrhea.

Functional Diarrhea (Chronic Nonspecific Diarrhea)

Functional diarrhea, previously termed chronic nonspecific diarrhea or **toddler's diarrhea,** typically affects children between 1 and 3 years of age and is characterized by the passage of several watery and unformed stools each day. Stools are typically relatively well formed in the morning but become looser as the day progresses. The stools often have undigested vegetable matter but lack blood, mucus, or excessive fat. Children with functional diarrhea, if offered an unrestricted and age-appropriate diet, gain weight normally. However, in an attempt to treat the diarrhea, many children are placed on restrictive diets that may lack dairy, fats, and occasionally starches; such restrictions lead to failure to thrive. Rome IV diagnostic criteria specify that all of the following must be present:

1. Daily painless, recurrent passage of four or more large, unformed stools
2. Symptoms lasting more than 4 weeks
3. Onset of symptoms between 6 and 60 months of age
4. No failure to thrive if caloric intake is adequate

Chronic nonspecific diarrhea is thought to be a variant of IBS, and a family history of IBS is common. The pathophysiology may involve abnormal intestinal motility with decreased mouth-to-anus transit time. Excessive fruit juice intake may also contribute to the diarrhea by overwhelming the carbohydrate absorptive ability of the gut. Chronic nonspecific diarrhea is a benign and self-limited condition that usually resolves without intervention by 3–4 years of age. Parents should be reassured and encouraged to place the child on a regular, unrestricted diet to provide adequate calories. The diarrhea often improves with removal of prior dietary restrictions and by limiting fruit juice intake. Some patients may improve with increasing the fat content of the diet (e.g., switching from low-fat milk to whole milk), which can slow gastrointestinal transit time.

Small Intestinal Bacterial Overgrowth

The normal small intestine is colonized with relatively few bacteria, typically $<10^4$ organisms/mL, with lower concentrations in the duodenum and jejunum, and higher concentrations in the ileum. Various conditions such as short bowel syndrome, malnutrition, pseudoobstruction, bowel strictures, and achlorhydria from medications such as proton pump inhibitors may result in overgrowth of aerobic and anaerobic bacteria in the small bowel. Symptoms of abdominal pain, bloating, abdominal distension, and diarrhea arise as bile acids are deconjugated and fatty acids are hydroxylated by bacteria, leading to an osmotic diarrhea. The diagnosis can be made by breath hydrogen testing showing early and late rise in breath hydrogen after ingestion of lactulose. Quantitative jejunal aspirate cultures showing $>10^5$ organisms/mL are suggestive of small intestinal bacterial overgrowth, although established cutoff ranges and specificity are imperfect.

Irritable Bowel Syndrome

IBS is characterized by recurrent abdominal pain and altered bowel habits and typically presents in adolescence. Symptoms include abnormal stool frequency (either four or more stools per day or two or fewer stools per week), abnormal stool form (either loose and watery or lumpy and hard), abnormal passage of stool (e.g., straining, urgency, feeling of incomplete evacuation), the passage of mucus, and bloating or distension. Diagnosis requires that patients have a normal physical examination and growth curve and meet both of the following criteria at least once per week for at least 2 months before diagnosis:

1. Abdominal pain at least 4 days per month associated with one or more of the following:
   a. Pain related to defecation
   b. Change in the frequency of stool
   c. Change in the form or appearance of stool
2. After appropriate evaluation, the symptoms cannot be fully explained by another medical condition

The etiology and pathogenesis of IBS are not well understood. Visceral hypersensitivity has been well documented in children with IBS. Genetic predisposition, early stressful events, and ineffective coping mechanisms are compounding factors. Additional mechanisms may include infection, inflammation, intestinal trauma, allergy, and disordered gut motility.

Celiac Disease

Celiac disease is an immune-mediated systemic disorder elicited by exposure to gluten and related proteins in genetically susceptible individuals. Clinical presentations vary, although the hallmarks of celiac disease include enteropathy and the presence of disease-specific antibodies. Prevalence is as high as 1% in Western nations, with most affected individuals presenting in childhood. A genetic predisposition is suggested by familial aggregation and the high concordance in monozygotic twins, which approaches 100%. A strong association with human leukocyte antigen (HLA)-DQ2.5, and to a lesser degree HLA-DQ8, has been identified. A family or personal history of autoimmune disease and certain genetic conditions confers a higher risk (Table 14.17).

The pathogenesis of celiac disease involves exposure to **gliadin,** a protein component of **wheat gluten,** or structurally related storage proteins (prolamines) found in rye and barley. Altered processing by intraluminal enzymes, changes in intestinal permeability, and activation of the innate immune response precede the development of an adaptive immune response that results in systemic autoimmunity and an inflammatory enteropathy characterized by **villous atrophy,** elongated crypts, and intraepithelial lymphocytosis.

Celiac disease symptoms are protean and reflect its systemic nature. The age of onset is variable, and a high degree of suspicion is needed. Manifestations include recurrent abdominal pain, nausea and vomiting, iron deficiency with or without anemia, short stature, aphthous stomatitis, chronic fatigue, arthritis, raised aminotransferase levels, and reduced bone mineral density (osteopenia). Rare manifestations include ataxia; **dermatitis herpetiformis**, which is a blistering rash with pathognomonic cutaneous IgA deposits; and **celiac crisis**, which is a rare life-threatening syndrome mostly observed in children that is characterized by severe diarrhea, hypoproteinemia, and metabolic and electrolyte imbalances. The classic presentation of a toddler with chronic diarrhea, abdominal distension, and failure to thrive is uncommon. Most patients are identified via serologic screening in the context of a strong family history or other risk factors.

Serologic tests are the cornerstone of screening for celiac disease in patients with risk factors or a suggestive history (Table 14.18). Establishing the diagnosis is dependent on the levels of disease-specific antibodies detected. Total serum IgA should be obtained to exclude IgA deficiency. If total serum IgA is normal and antitissue transglutaminase IgA antibodies are negative, celiac disease is unlikely. Patients with positive antitissue transglutaminase IgA antibodies that are <10 times the upper limit of normal should undergo upper endoscopy with multiple biopsies. If biopsies demonstrate total or partial villous atrophy, elongated crypts, and increased intraepithelial lymphocytes (>25 lymphocytes/100 enterocytes), the diagnosis is confirmed. Patients with positive antitissue transglutaminase IgA antibodies that are ≥10 times the upper limit of normal should have antiendomysial IgA antibodies and HLA testing performed. If the patient is positive for antiendomysial IgA antibodies and is positive for HLA-DQ2 or HLA-DQ8 testing,

the diagnosis is confirmed; if either or both are negative, the patient should undergo biopsy.

Patients with celiac disease experience relief in their symptoms when placed on a strict gluten-free diet. Complications associated with untreated celiac disease include osteoporosis, impaired splenic function, neurologic disorders, infertility or recurrent spontaneous abortion, ulcerative jejunoileitis, and cancer. Enteropathy-associated T-cell lymphoma and adenocarcinoma of the jejunum are rare complications of celiac disease. **Refractory celiac disease** is diagnosed when there are persistent or recurrent malabsorptive symptoms and signs of villous atrophy on biopsy despite strict adherence to a gluten-free diet for more than 12 months. Refractory celiac disease can be classified as **type 1** (characterized by the presence of normal intraepithelial lymphocytes) or **type 2** (characterized by abnormal intraepithelial lymphocytes; clonal intraepithelial lymphocytes lacking surface markers CD3, CD8, and T-cell receptors; or both). Type 2 refractory celiac disease is associated with a higher risk of ulcerative jejunoileitis and lymphoma.

Inflammatory Bowel Disease

IBD is divided broadly into **ulcerative colitis** and **Crohn disease**, idiopathic systemic chronic inflammatory diseases whose primary symptoms are related to relapsing gastrointestinal tract inflammation. Common signs and symptoms include diarrhea, abdominal pain, blood in the stools, and nutritional compromise. Ulcerative colitis consists of mucosal inflammation restricted to the colon, while Crohn disease consists of **transmural inflammation** that affects all layers of the intestinal wall and may involve any portion of the gastrointestinal tract from the mouth to the anus. Ulcerative colitis involves the colon in a continuous fashion, typically starting in the rectum and extending proximally to variable degrees. Crohn disease is characterized by **skip lesions**, in which there are areas of normal-appearing mucosa interspersed with inflammatory lesions.

The prevalence of ulcerative colitis is as high as 246 per 100,000 persons, and the prevalence of Crohn disease is as high as 199 per 100,000 persons. Approximately 25% of all IBD is diagnosed in children and adolescents.

Clinical Presentation

Up to 80% of children with Crohn disease will present with diarrhea. Stool may contain microscopic blood although may not be grossly bloody, especially in the absence of significant left-sided colonic disease. Diarrhea is more common in colonic disease and may be absent altogether in cases of isolated small bowel inflammation. In ulcerative colitis, diarrhea is a more consistent presenting feature, often insidious in its development but eventually progressing to hematochezia. Nocturnal diarrhea with urgency may be a sign of left-sided colonic inflammation in both entities. Gastrointestinal and extraintestinal manifestations otherwise vary between Crohn disease and ulcerative colitis (Table 14.19). Extraintestinal manifestations are present in up to 23% of children at diagnosis, with a higher frequency in those over 6 years of age.

TABLE 14.17 Conditions Whose Presence Confers a Higher Risk of Celiac Disease

Condition	Incidence of Celiac Disease (%)
First-degree relative with celiac disease	2–20
Type 1 diabetes mellitus	3–12
Juvenile idiopathic arthritis	1.5–2.5
Trisomy 21	0.3–5.5
Turner syndrome	6.5
Williams syndrome	9.5
IgA nephropathy	4
IgA deficiency	3
Autoimmune thyroid disease	3
Autoimmune liver disease	13.5

IgA, immunoglobulin A.

TABLE 14.18 Serologic Tests for Celiac Disease

Test	Sensitivity (Percent)	Specificity (Percent)	Comments
Antitissue transglutaminase IgA	>95 (73–100)	>95 (77–100)	Recommended screening test
Antitissue transglutaminase IgG	Widely variable (12.6–99.3)	Widely variable (86.3–100)	Useful in patients with IgA deficiency
Antiendomysial antibody IgA	>90.0 (82.6–100)	98.2 (94.7–100)	Useful in patients with an uncertain diagnosis. Expensive.
Antideamidated gliadin peptide IgG	>90.0 (80.1–98.6)	>90.0 (86.0–96.9)	Useful in patients with IgA deficiency and young children

IgA, immunoglobulin A; IgG, immunoglobulin G.

TABLE 14.19 Clinical Manifestations of Inflammatory Bowel Disease

Manifestation	Comments
Gastrointestinal	
Diarrhea with or without blood	Isolated small bowel Crohn disease may not manifest with diarrhea or grossly bloody stools
Abdominal pain	
Hematochezia	More common in ulcerative colitis
Anorexia, weight loss, and fatigue	More common in Crohn disease
Growth failure and pubertal delay	More common in Crohn disease
Abdominal mass	Only in Crohn disease
Fever and night sweats	More common in Crohn disease
Vomiting and nausea	Seen in both but severe would suggest intestinal obstructive process from Crohn disease
Extraintestinal	
Iritis and uveitis	More common in Crohn disease
Aphthous ulceration	More common in Crohn disease
Erythema nodosum	More common in Crohn disease
Pyoderma gangrenosum	More common in ulcerative colitis
Musculoskeletal • Axial arthropathy and ankylosing spondylitis • Polyarticular arthritis • Pauciarticular arthritis • Osteoporosis	
Liver • Primary sclerosing cholangitis • Autoimmune hepatitis and overlap syndrome • Cholelithiasis	
Autoimmune pancreatitis	
Cardiovascular • Myocarditis • Pericarditis	
Pulmonary Crohn disease	Commonly involves large airways, but parenchymal disease, such as organizing pneumonia, interstitial disease, and necrobiotic nodules, has been described
Renal • Nephritis • Amyloidosis • Urolithiasis (especially oxalate stones)	More common in Crohn disease compared to ulcerative colitis
Hematologic • Iron-deficiency anemia, anemia of chronic disease, vitamin B_{12} deficiency or folate deficiency • Immune thrombocytopenia • Deep vein thrombosis	

TABLE 14.20 Comparison of Crohn Disease and Ulcerative Colitis

Feature	Crohn Disease	Ulcerative Colitis
Malaise, fever, weight loss	Common	Common
Rectal bleeding	Sometimes	Usual
Abdominal mass	Common	Rare
Abdominal pain	Common	Common
Perianal disease	Common	Rare
Ileal involvement	Common	None (backwash ileitis)
Strictures	Common	Unusual
Fistula	Common	Very rare
Skip lesions	Common	Not present
Transmural involvement	Usual	Not present
Crypt abscesses	Variable	Usual
Intestinal granulomas	Common	Rarely present
Risk of cancer*	Increased	Greatly increased
Erythema nodosum	Common	Less common
Mouth ulceration	Common	Rare
Osteopenia at onset	Yes	No
Autoimmune hepatitis	Rare	Yes
Sclerosing cholangitis	Rare	Yes

*Colonic cancer, cholangiocarcinoma, lymphoma in Crohn disease.
From Bishop WP, Ebach DR. Intestinal tract. In: Marcdante KJ, Kliegman RK, eds. *Nelson Essentials of Pediatrics.* 7th ed. Philadelphia: Saunders; 2015:437–444.

Physical examination should establish nutritional status and include an assessment of growth parameters, including the review of previous growth charts. Pubertal status should also be recorded. Oral cavity examination should look for aphthous ulcers that are present in approximately 10% of IBD patients (more commonly in Crohn disease). An eye examination should look for **episcleritis**, painful inflammation of the outer layer of the sclera, and patients with known IBD should be followed by an ophthalmologist to assess for **uveitis** and **keratopathy**. A detailed abdominal examination should document abdominal distension, mass, tenderness, and hyper- or hypoactive bowel sounds. Particular attention should be paid to assessing the perianal region for any abscesses or fistulas. Skin examination should look for **erythema nodosum**, painful raised red lesions about 1–3 cm in diameter typically found on the shins; **pyoderma gangrenosum**, a severe ulcerating rash; and psoriatic lesions. Two clinical features suggest a diagnosis of Crohn disease over ulcerative colitis: the presence of perianal disease and the presence of stricturing and fistulizing disease of the bowel. No other systemic or extraintestinal manifestations reliably suggest one diagnosis over the other (Table 14.20).

Diagnosis

IBD is a clinical diagnosis that integrates history and physical findings with objective data from imaging studies, laboratory evaluation, and endoscopic findings including histopathology. Diagnosis should neither be confirmed nor excluded on any one variable or result: up to 54% of patients with mild ulcerative colitis and 21% of patients with mild Crohn disease have normal hemoglobin, albumin, CRP, and ESR levels at the time of initial diagnosis. Important mimics of IBD include IBS, Behçet disease, infectious enterocolitis (particularly enterovirus and *Yersinia*), and tuberculosis (Tables 14.21 and 14.22). As such, every

TABLE 14.21 Differential Diagnoses of Presenting Symptoms of Crohn Disease

Primary Presenting Symptom	Differential Diagnosis
Right lower quadrant abdominal pain, with or without mass	Appendicitis, infection (e.g., *Campylobacter, Yersinia* species, tuberculosis, or atypical mycobacteria), lymphoma, intussusception, mesenteric adenitis, Meckel diverticulitis, ovarian cyst or ovarian torsion, ectopic pregnancy
Chronic periumbilical or epigastric abdominal pain	Irritable bowel syndrome, constipation, lactose intolerance, peptic ulcer disease, functional dyspepsia
Rectal bleeding, no diarrhea	Fissure, polyp, Meckel diverticulum, solitary rectal ulcer syndrome
Bloody diarrhea	Infection, allergic colitis, hemolytic uremic syndrome, Henoch-Schönlein purpura, ischemic bowel, radiation colitis
Watery diarrhea	Irritable bowel syndrome, lactose intolerance, giardiasis, *Cryptosporidium* infection, sorbitol, laxatives
Perirectal disease	Fissure, hemorrhoid (rare), streptococcal infection, condyloma (rare)
Growth delay	Endocrinopathy
Anorexia, weight loss	Celiac disease, other systemic illnesses, anorexia nervosa
Arthritis	Collagen vascular disease, infection
Liver abnormalities	Chronic hepatitis
Oral ulcers	Celiac disease

TABLE 14.22 Infectious Agents Mimicking Inflammatory Bowel Disease

Agent	Manifestations	Diagnosis	Comments
Bacteria			
Campylobacter jejuni	Acute diarrhea, fever, fecal blood and leukocytes	Culture or nucleic acid amplification assay	Common in adolescents, may relapse
Yersinia enterocolitica	Acute diarrhea that can become chronic, right lower quadrant pain, mesenteric adenitis—pseudoappendicitis, fecal blood and leukocytes Extraintestinal manifestations may mimic Crohn disease	Culture or nucleic acid amplification assay	Common in adolescents as fever of unknown origin, weight loss, abdominal pain
Clostridioides difficile	Onset during or following a course of antibiotics, watery → bloody diarrhea, pseudomembrane on sigmoidoscopy	Cytotoxin assay or nucleic acid amplification assay	May be nosocomial Toxic megacolon possible
Escherichia coli O157:H7	Colitis, fecal blood, abdominal pain	Culture and typing or nucleic acid amplification assay	Hemolytic uremic syndrome possible
Salmonella	Watery → bloody diarrhea, foodborne, fecal leukocytes, fever, pain, cramps	Culture or nucleic acid amplification assay	Usually acute
Shigella	Watery → bloody diarrhea, fecal leukocytes, fever, pain, cramps	Culture or nucleic acid amplification assay	Dysentery symptoms
Edwardsiella tarda	Bloody diarrhea, cramps	Culture	Ulceration on endoscopy
Aeromonas hydrophila	Cramps, diarrhea, fecal blood	Culture	May be chronic May be acquired from contaminated drinking water or swimming in contaminated pools or freshwater sources
Plesiomonas shigelloides	Diarrhea, cramps	Culture	Shellfish source
Tuberculosis	Rarely bovine, now *Mycobacterium tuberculosis* Ileocecal area, fistula formation	Culture, purified protein derivative, biopsy, interferon gamma release assay	Can mimic Crohn disease
Parasites			
Entamoeba histolytica	Acute bloody diarrhea and liver abscess, colic	Trophozoite in stool, colonic mucosal flask ulceration, serologic tests	Travel to endemic area
Giardia lamblia	Foul-smelling, watery diarrhea, cramps, flatulence, weight loss; no colonic involvement	"Owl"-like trophozoite and cysts in stool; rarely duodenal intubation	May be chronic
Opportunistic Organisms in the Setting of Immune Deficiency			
Cryptosporidium	Chronic diarrhea, weight loss	Stool microscopy	Mucosal findings not like inflammatory bowel disease
Isospora belli	Chronic diarrhea, weight loss	Stool microscopy	Tropical location
Cytomegalovirus	Colonic ulceration, pain, bloody diarrhea	Culture, biopsy	More common when on immunosuppressive medications

From Grossman AB, Baldassano RN. Chronic ulcerative colitis. In: Kliegman RM, Stanton BF, St. Geme JW III, et al., eds. *Nelson Textbook of Pediatrics.* 20th ed. Philadelphia: Elsevier; 2016:1823.

patient with a history and examination suggestive of IBD should have stool studies for infectious organisms and special request should be made for *Yersinia* culture if multiplex PCR assays that include *Yersinia* testing are not available. Patients presenting with suggestive symptoms prior to 6 years of age may require an evaluation for an underlying immune disregulation disorder as an additional mimic of IBD (Table 14.23). Stool biomarkers such as calprotectin and lactoferrin should be utilized to exclude noninflammatory causes before considering endoscopic procedures. The suggested diagnostic evaluation of suspected IBD is presented in Table 14.24.

TABLE 14.23 Known Defects Associated with Very Early-Onset Inflammatory Bowel Disease and Associated Extraintestinal Manifestations and Laboratory Findings

Defects	Gene Defect	Extraintestinal Immune, Hematologic, or Somatic Manifestations	Laboratory Findings and Functional Evaluation
IPEX and IPEX-Like Disorders			
IPEX	FOXP3	Autoimmune endocrinopathy, cytopenia, hepatitis and kidney disease, eczema, food allergy, eosinophilia	Decrease in regulatory T-cell number and function Decreased FOXP3 expression
CD25 deficiency	CD25	Autoimmune endocrinopathy, cytopenia, eczema, gingivitis, alopecia universalis, bullous pemphigoid, CMV, EBV disease	Absent CD25 expression
STAT5b deficiency	STAT5B	Autoimmune endocrinopathy, eczema, short stature, interstitial pneumonitis, alopecia universalis, bullous pemphigoid, varicella and herpes zoster infections	Variable immune abnormality Normal to low T, B, and NK cells
STAT1 GOF variant	STAT1	Mucocutaneous candidiasis, short stature, eczema, autoimmune endocrinopathy, sinopulmonary infection, hypertension, aneurysm	Most have normal regulatory T-cell number and FOXP3 expression, abnormal STAT1 phosphorylation studies
STAT3 GOF variant	STAT3	Multisystem autoimmunity, variable short stature, lymphoproliferation	Hypogammaglobulinemia Decreased class-switched memory B cells
LRBA deficiency	LRBA	Multisystem autoimmunity, cytopenia, arthritis, recurrent sinopulmonary infection, granuloma, hypogammaglobulinemia	Hypogammaglobulinemia Decreased class-switched memory B cells
CTLA4 haploinsufficiency	CTLA4	Diarrhea, enteropathy, hypogammaglobulinemia, granulomatous lymphocytic interstitial lung disease, multisystem autoimmunity	Hypogammaglobulinemia Decreased class-switched memory B cells
ADA-2 deficiency	ADA2	Multiorgan disease, vasculopathy, stroke, IBD-like GI illness, autoimmune, autoinflammatory, livedo racemosa	Cytopenias, hypogammaglobulinemia
Defects in IL-10 Signaling			
Defects in IL-10 and IL-10R	IL-10RA IL-10RB IL-10	Perianal fistula, folliculitis, arthritis, abscess, lymphoma	STAT3 phosphorylation by IL-6 and IL-10 studies*
Defects in Neutrophil Function			
CGD	CYBB CYBA NCF1 NCF2 NCF4	Perianal fistula, recurrent cold abscess from catalase-positive organisms,† gastric outlet obstruction	Decreased neutrophil oxidative burst study Elevated IgG
Glycogen storage disease 1b	SLC37A4	Recurrent bacterial infections, hypoglycemic seizures, hepatomegaly	Neutropenia, hypoglycemia, hyperuricemia, hyperlipidemia
Leukocyte adhesion defect	ITGB2	Neutrophilia, recurrent bacterial infections, delayed separation of umbilical cord, poor wound healing	Leukocytosis Absent CD18 expression
Congenital neutropenia	G6PC3	Cutaneous vascular malformation and cardiac defect	Severe neutropenia
Hyperinflammatory Disorders			
XIAP	BIRC4	Perianal fistula, recurrent HLH, EBV, and CMV infections, hypogammaglobinemia	Markedly elevated IL-18 Decreased or absent XIAP protein expression by flow
NLRC4 GOF variant	NLRC4	Recurrent macrophage activation, rash	Markedly elevated IL-18
Mevalonate kinase deficiency	MVK	Recurrent fever, rash, abdominal pain, and emesis	Elevated inflammatory markers Elevated IgD Elevated urine mevalonate

TABLE 14.23 Known Defects Associated with Very Early-Onset Inflammatory Bowel Disease and Its Associated Extraintestinal Manifestations and Laboratory Findings—cont'd

Defects	Gene Defect	Extraintestinal Immune, Hematologic, or Somatic Manifestations	Laboratory Findings and Functional Evaluation
Familial Mediterranean fever	MEFV	Recurrent fever, abdominal pain, arthralgia, peritonitis	Elevated inflammatory markers
Familial HLH type 5	STXBP2	HLH, hypogammaglobinemia, sensorineural hearing loss	Marked elevated ferritin and sIL-2R Decreased CD107a degranulation
Hermansky-Pudlak syndrome	HPS1 HPS4 HPS6	Partial albinism, bleeding tendency, recurrent infection, and immunodeficiency	Decreased CD107a degranulation
Defects in Epithelial Barrier Function			
TTC7A deficiency	TTC7A	Varying degree of intestinal atresia, T-cell immune defect, and recurrent infections	Mild to severe T-cell immune deficiency Hypogammaglobinemia
X-linked ectodermal immunodeficiency (NEMO deficiency)	IKBKG	Varying degree of ectodermal dysplasia, conical teeth, space and brittle hair; recurrent bacterial, viral, and mycobacterial infections	Hypogammaglobinemia Decreased class-switched memory B cells
ADAM17 deficiency	ADAM17	Neonatal inflammatory skin and bowel disease, generalized pustular rash	Normal T-cell and B-cell numbers
Dystrophic epidermolysis bullosa	COL7A1	Blistering disorder primarily affects the hands, feet, knees, and elbows	Unremarkable immune findings
Kindler syndrome	FERMT1	Acral skin blistering, photosensitivity, progressive poikiloderma, and diffuse cutaneous atrophy	Eosinophilia
Isolated or Combined T-Cell and B-Cell Immune Defects			
X-linked agammaglobulinemia	BTK	Recurrent sinopulmonary infection	Absent B cells in peripheral blood Absent plasma cells in tissue Decreased class-switched memory B cells
Common variable immune defect (CVID)		Heterogeneous group of defects with sinopulmonary infections, autoimmunity, lymphoproliferation, and variable T-cell immune defect	Hypogammaglobinemia Variable T-cell lymphopenia
X-linked hyper IgM (CD40L)	CD40L	Sclerosing cholangitis, cryptosporidium diarrhea, and pneumocystis infection	Elevated or normal IgM, neutropenia Absent class-switched memory B cells
Wiskott-Aldrich syndrome	WAS	Eczema, recurrent infection, autoimmunity, vasculitis	Microthrombocytopenia Variable lymphopenia, low IgM Decreased WAS protein
Leaky SCID or Omenn	RAG1, RAG2 IL-7Ra IL-2RG	Generalized erythroderma, hepatosplenomegaly, lymphadenopathy	Eosinophilia T-cell lymphopenia Decreased naïve T cells

CGD, chronic granulomatous disease; CMV, cytomegalovirus; EBV, Epstein-Barr virus; GI, gastrointestinal; GOF, gain of function; HLH, hemophagocytic lymphohistiocytosis; IBD, inflammatory bowel disease; IgD, immunoglobulin D; IgG, immunoglobulin G; IgM, immunoglobulin M; IL, interleukin; IPEX, immune disregulation, polyendocrinopathy, enteropathy, X-linked; NEMO, nuclear factor-kappa B essential modulator; XIAP, X-linked inhibitor of apoptosis.
*STAT3 signaling following IL-6 and IL-10 will only identify IL-10R A and B defects; it will not identify IL-10 deficiency.
†*Staphylococcus aureus, Serratia marcescens, Burkholderia cepacia, Aspergillus,* and *Candida.*
Modified from Chandrakasan S, Venkateswaran S, Kugathasan S. Nonclassic inflammatory bowel disease in young infants. *Pediatr Clin N Am.* 2017;64:139–160 (Table 2, pp. 148–150).

TABLE 14.24 Suggested Evaluation in Suspected Inflammatory Bowel Disease

Test	Common Abnormalities/Comments
Complete blood count with differential	Anemia, especially iron deficiency
Comprehensive metabolic panel	Hypoalbuminemia, elevated liver enzymes, low alkaline phosphatase (likely secondary to associated zinc deficiency)
Erythrocyte sedimentation rate	Elevated in CD > UC
C-reactive protein	Elevated in CD > UC
Stool cultures with *Yersinia*; ova and parasites	Always rule out infectious causes as the likely reason for symptoms
Clostridioides difficile toxin assay or polymerase chain reaction assay	Could be an isolated reason for symptoms or could be a superimposed illness
Fecal occult blood	Positive in vast majority of patients. No need for this test if patient has grossly bloody stools

Continued

TABLE 14.24   **Suggested Evaluation in Suspected Inflammatory Bowel Disease—cont'd**

Test	Common Abnormalities/Comments
Fecal calprotectin (or lactoferrin)	To distinguish inflammatory bowel disease from irritable bowel syndrome prior to considering invasive procedures such as endoscopy
Esophagogastroduodenoscopy and ileocolonoscopy	After ruling out other causes of patient's symptoms
Imaging studies • MRI and MRE • CT abdomen • Abdominal ultrasound	Consider for evaluation of patients presenting with fistulizing or stricturing disease. Also used for evaluation of small bowel after endoscopic procedures
Wireless capsule endoscope	Consider for evaluation of small bowel in very young children in whom MRE is difficult or in situations where conventional endoscope and imaging tools have been nondiagnostic

CD, Crohn disease; MRE, magnetic resonance enterography; UC, ulcerative colitis.

■ SUMMARY AND RED FLAGS

Acute diarrhea is a common childhood illness. For most children, the etiologic agent is of no therapeutic significance. Exceptions are giardiasis, pseudomembranous colitis, dysentery suggestive of *Shigella* infection, amebiasis, or *Campylobacter* infection, all of which necessitate specific treatment. Oftentimes of greater importance are the secondary complications associated with fluid and electrolyte losses and the reduced oral fluid intake, which may result in shock and its systemic complications.

Red flags for acute diarrhea are the manifestations of dehydration (see Table 14.8). Young age (younger than 6 months) is associated with a greater risk of dehydration, as are 10 or more stools a day and frequent emesis and fever (see Table 14.13).

Chronic diarrhea may be benign or may signify a more serious illness associated with malabsorption, inflammation, or congenital defects. Red flags include onset of diarrhea in the neonatal period, weight loss, growth stunting, anorexia, fever, fatty stools, blood in stools, extraintestinal manifestations associated with intestinal disease, history of travel to countries with poor sanitation and water supply, and specific nutritional deficiencies associated with malabsorption.

BIBLIOGRAPHY

A bibliography is available at ExpertConsult.com.

15

Vomiting and Regurgitation

Geetanjali Bora and Katja Kovacic

DEFINITIONS

Vomiting/emesis is a protective reflex in response to a variety of stimuli that results in forceful ejection of stomach contents. The emetic reflex is complex and composed of three sequential events. Initially there is a prodromal phase characterized by nausea and autonomic changes, followed by retching and finally vomiting or forceful expulsion of gastric contents through the oral cavity. These events may occur independent of each other. In some cases, nausea may not progress to vomiting, while vomiting may occur without preceding nausea.

Nausea is defined as a vague, unpleasant epigastric or abdominal sensation that presents in a wavelike pattern and is associated with a feeling of imminent vomiting. Nausea is accompanied by a variety of autonomic changes including increases in salivation, diaphoresis, pupillary dilation, tachycardia, and changes in respiration. The gastrointestinal (GI) motor response during nausea comprises inhibition of spontaneous contractions of the GI tract, relaxation of the proximal stomach, and contraction of the esophageal longitudinal muscle, which pulls the lower esophageal sphincter (LES) and proximal stomach into the thoracic cavity. This is followed by a retrograde peristaltic contraction from the small intestine to the gastric antrum called the retrograde giant contraction, which propels duodenal contents into the stomach.

Retching is defined as strong, involuntary efforts to vomit, which may be seen as preparatory maneuvers to vomiting. These efforts consist of spasmodic contractions of the diaphragm and abdominal wall, resulting in increased abdominal pressure and decreased intrathoracic pressure, facilitating the relaxed LES and dilated proximal stomach to slide further into the thoracic cavity. This enables the free flow of gastric content into the esophagus though this material may be returned to the stomach by secondary (nonswallow) esophageal peristalsis resulting in a to-and-fro movement.

Vomiting (emesis) differs from retching in that gastric content is expelled from the mouth. This is fostered by relaxation of the diaphragm and reversal of intrathoracic pressure from negative to positive, leading to increase of intraluminal pressure in the esophagus. It is accompanied by relaxation of the upper esophageal sphincter and closure of the glottis.

Regurgitation is considered a form of gastroesophageal reflux and should be differentiated from vomiting. It is characterized by nonforceful expulsion of gastric content through the oral cavity, and as such, is caused predominantly by transient LES relaxations. It is generally not accompanied by prodromal symptoms or retching. Although apparently effortless, it may be triggered by contractions of abdominal wall musculature as occurs in rumination syndrome. This propulsion perhaps distinguishes regurgitant from nonregurgitant reflux, which remains in the esophagus.

NEUROANATOMY OF VOMITING

The emetic reflex consists of an afferent limb (receptor and pathway), central integration and control, and an efferent limb (pathway and effector). The diverse afferent pathways may originate within the oropharynx, GI tract, renal system, vestibular system, or central nervous system (e.g., hypothalamus, cortex). These afferent pathways can be triggered by various stimuli including visceral pain and inflammation, toxins, motion, pregnancy, radiation exposure, postoperative states, and unpleasant emotions. Tactile stimulation to the back of the throat can also stimulate emesis. Mechanoreceptors located in the muscularis layer of the GI tract can trigger the emetic reflex in response to passive distension and strong contractions as seen in cases of mechanical obstruction. Chemoreceptors located in the mucosa of the stomach and proximal small bowel can be stimulated by a wide array of chemical irritants and toxins, leading to emesis. Similarly, such receptors can be found in other organ systems such as the pelvic ureteral system, which can induce emesis in response to distension, irritation, and other insults.

The afferent pathways originating from the GI tract are principally mediated via vagal afferent fibers. Vomiting in response to drugs and toxins circulating in the blood is thought to be mediated via the "chemoreceptive trigger zone" in the area postrema located on the dorsal surface of the floor of the fourth ventricle outside the blood-brain barrier. Substances in the blood and cerebrospinal fluid can be detected by chemosensitive receptors in this area. Activation of the afferent limb of the vomiting reflex may also occur through real or apparent motion of the body. This occurs when the brain receives conflicting information about body movement from the visual, vestibular, and proprioceptive systems, referred to as "sensory mismatch." Higher cortical areas (supramedullary) can also induce vomiting in response to central nervous system diseases and emotional stress via cortical afferent nerves.

The afferent pathways terminate centrally in the nucleus tractus solitarius (NTS) and the surrounding reticular area located in the dorsolateral medulla. The NTS is the beginning of the final common pathway by which all emetic pathways are thought to induce vomiting. The NTS signals to the emetic central pattern generator (CPG). Contrary to past beliefs, there is no isolated central "vomiting center" but rather a group of loosely organized neurons scattered throughout the medulla that need to be activated in an appropriate sequence by the CPG to control the bodily functions associated with emesis. In the final step, the stereotypical motor response of vomiting is generated and is mediated by efferent fibers in the vagal, phrenic, and spinal nerves.

NEUROCHEMICAL BASIS OF VOMITING

A wide variety of neurotransmitters and neuropeptides are involved in the vomiting reflex. The chemoreceptor trigger zone (CTZ) in the area postrema contains receptors for dopamine (D_2-receptor), serotonin (5HT-3), histamine (H_1), substance P (neurokinin-1 [NK-1]), acetylcholine (muscarinic), and opioid (μ and δ). These receptors are meant to detect the presence of the associated neurotransmitter in the blood and at a certain level will activate the emetic pathway.

Serotonin receptors (5HT-3) are also found in the vagal afferent fibers of the GI tract, and evidence suggests that chemotherapeutic agents, radiation, and noxious stimuli act directly on these GI tract vagal fibers, inducing the release of serotonin. Substance P and its receptor (NK-1) are widely distributed in the central and peripheral nervous system, and blockade of this receptor prevents emesis due to both central and peripheral stimuli. Animal models have demonstrated that physical and psychological stress can trigger the release of corticotropin-releasing hormone, which acts via the CRF-2 receptor located in the brainstem to induce emesis and mediate gastric stasis.

DATA TO GUIDE THE DIAGNOSIS

History and Demographics

The child's age is an important guide to the diagnostic possibilities (Table 15.1). While most congenital anomalies of the GI tract present in the neonatal period, others such as antropyloric webs, malrotation,

TABLE 15.1 Etiology of Vomiting by Organ System and Age at Presentation

Cause	Neonate (<1 mo)	Infant (1–12 mo)	Child (1–11 yr)	Adolescent (>11 yr)
Non-GI Infections				
Otitis media		+	+	−
Acute or chronic sinusitis	−		+	+
Streptococcal pharyngitis	−		+	+
Pneumonitis		+	+	−
Pyelonephritis	+	+	+	+
Meningitis	+	+	+	+
Sepsis	+	+	+	+
GI Infections				
Gastroenteritis		+	+	+
Infectious colitis		−	+	+
H. pylori gastritis			+	+
Parasitic infection			+	+
Hepatitis		−	+	+
Hepatic abscess		−	+	−
Anatomic Defects				
Esophageal				
Congenital atresia, stricture, webs	+	+	−	−
Tracheoesophageal fistula	+	+	−	
Vascular ring	+	+	+	
Gastric				
Pyloric stenosis	+	+	−	−
Antral webs	+	+	+	−
Bezoars			+	+
Intestinal				
Stenosis and atresia	+	+		
Webs and duplications	+	+	+	−
Imperforate anus	+			
Meconium ileus	+			
Obstructed inguinal hernia	+	+	+	+
Malrotation with volvulus	+	+	+	+
Intussusception		+	+	−
DIOS	+	+	+	+
SMA syndrome			+	+
Duodenal hematoma		−	+	+
Surgical adhesions		+	+	+
Appendicitis			+	+
Mucosal Injuries				
GERD/reflux esophagitis	+	+	+	+
Eosinophilic esophagitis		−	+	+
Gastritis ± H. pylori		−	+	+
Peptic ulcer or duodenitis			+	+

TABLE 15.1 Etiology of Vomiting by Organ System and Age at Presentation—cont'd

Cause	Neonate (<1 mo)	Infant (1–12 mo)	Child (1–11 yr)	Adolescent (>11 yr)
Mucosal Injuries—cont'd				
Eosinophilic gastritis			+	+
Celiac disease	–		+	+
Inflammatory bowel disease	–		+	+
Ménétrier disease			+	+
Chronic granulomatous disease	–		+	–
Nutrient intolerance (dairy, soy)	+	+		
GI Motility Disorders				
Achalasia	–	–	–	+
Gastroparesis			+	+
Paralytic ileus	+	+	+	+
Hirschsprung disease	+	+	–	
Intestinal pseudo-obstruction	+	+	–	–
Pancreaticobiliary				
Cholecystitis	–	–	–	+
Cholelithiasis			–	+
Choledochal cyst	+	+	–	
Pancreatitis			+	+
Gallbladder dyskinesia			–	+
Intestinal Ischemia/Hypoperfusion				
Necrotizing enterocolitis	+	–		
Cardiac defects	+	+	+	–
Mesenteric vessel thrombosis	–	–	+	+
Endocrine				
Adrenal hyperplasia	+	+		
Addison disease	+	+	+	+
Diabetic ketoacidosis			+	+
Pheochromocytoma			–	–
Metabolic Disorders				
Organic acidemia	+	+	–	
Aminoacidemia	+	+	–	
Fatty acid oxidation defects	–	+	+	
Urea cycle defect	+	+	–	
Hereditary fructose intolerance	–	+		
Mitochondriopathies	–	+	+	
Storage disorders	–	+	+	
Acute intermittent porphyria			–	+
Genitourinary Causes				
Ureteropelvic obstruction		+	+	–
Renal stones			+	+
Uremia			+	+
Pregnancy				+
Ovarian torsion			–	+
Neurologic Causes				
Hydrocephalus with shunt malfunction	+	+	+	+
Arnold-Chiari defect		+	+	–
Posterior fossa tumors		–	+	+
Intracranial bleeds	+	+	+	+
Concussions		–	+	+

Continued

TABLE 15.1	Etiology of Vomiting by Organ System and Age at Presentation—cont'd			
Cause	**Neonate (<1 mo)**	**Infant (1–12 mo)**	**Child (1–11 yr)**	**Adolescent (>11 yr)**
Neurologic Causes—cont'd				
Pseudotumor cerebri			+	+
Migraine headaches			+	+
Abdominal migraine			+	+
Vestibular disease (motion sickness)			−	+
Cyclical vomiting syndrome			+	+
Miscellaneous				
Rumination			+	+
Functional vomiting			+	+
Eating disorders				+
Toxic ingestion		−	+	+
Food poisoning		−	+	+
Medication-induced			+	+
Munchausen by proxy (ipecac poisoning)	+		+	

+, typically presents in this age group; − occasionally or rarely present; empty box signifies not present.
DIOS, distal intestinal obstruction syndrome; GERD, gastroesophageal reflux disease; *H. pylori, Helicobacter pylori;* SMA, superior mesenteric artery syndrome.
Modified from Li BUK, Kovacic K. Vomiting and nausea. In: Wyllie R, Hyams JS, Kay M, eds. *Pediatric Gastrointestinal and Liver Disease.* 5th ed. Philadelphia: Elsevier; 2016:88.

and intestinal duplications may be discovered at any age. Other important etiologies of vomiting to consider in the neonatal period are inborn errors of metabolism and sepsis. Older infants presenting with vomiting may have less severe structural or metabolic disorders, or they may have common acquired disorders such as gastroenteritis, mild systemic infections, gastroesophageal reflux, or allergies. Some metabolic disorders first manifest in older infants when novel dietary introductions expose them to provocative foods. Gastroenteritis and other infections are important considerations in these younger patients with relatively naïve immune systems. Toddlers frequently experience repeated episodes of gastroenteritis due to a variety of infectious organisms. Although gastroenteritis may initially present with emesis, there is usually *both* vomiting and diarrhea and, depending on the pathogen, abdominal pain. *Vomiting in the absence of diarrhea should suggest another etiology.* However, this age group also presents with acquired obstructive GI disorders such as intussusception or volvulus or with vomiting caused by ingested poisons.

Throughout childhood and adolescence, a wide variety of acquired disorders become symptomatic, and more subtle congenital malformations may also first become evident at these older ages. Metabolic disorders continue to be an important but infrequent cause of recurrent vomiting throughout childhood. In adolescents, pregnancy, drug ingestion, chronic marijuana use, and eating disorders should be added to the diagnostic considerations.

Temporal Pattern of Vomiting

Vomiting may be acute or recurrent. The recurrent pattern can be categorized as chronic recurrent or cyclic recurrent (Fig. 15.1 and Table 15.2). Differential diagnoses based on temporal pattern of vomiting are extensive (Tables 15.3 and 15.4). Acute vomiting is the most common pattern encountered in the pediatric population due to the frequent nature of infectious triggers. Acute causes of emesis usually present with multiple episodes of emesis per day, lasting for a few days, and may result in dehydration. This can also be encountered in association with acute GI obstructions, food poisoning, or toxin ingestion as well as an acute rise in intracranial pressure as seen with

encephalitis or intracranial space-occupying lesions. The recurrent pattern of vomiting can be chronic, low grade, characterized by one to two episodes of emesis per day. These patients are generally mildly ill and not dehydrated.

About 30% of recurrent emesis manifests with a cyclic pattern as in **cyclic vomiting syndrome (CVS)**. This presents with intermittent episodes of high-frequency vomiting interspersed with periods of normal health. Episodes are often stereotypical and associated with pallor, listlessness, and dehydration. In those with a chronic emesis pattern, the GI causes exceed the non-GI causes by 7:1. The most common etiologies

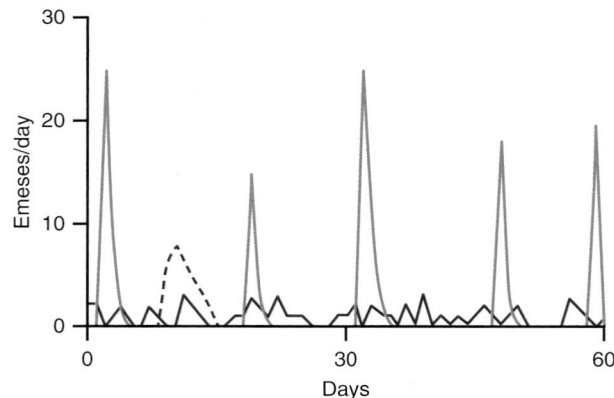

Fig. 15.1 Representation of acute, chronic, and cyclic patterns of vomiting. Three temporal patterns of vomiting are depicted: *acute (dotted purple line), chronic (solid purple line),* and *cyclic (solid blue line).* The number of emeses per day is plotted on the vertical axis over a 2-month period. The *acute* pattern is represented by a single episode of moderate vomiting intensity; the *chronic* pattern by a recurrent low-grade vomiting pattern that occurs on a daily basis; and the *cyclic* pattern by recurrent, discrete episodes of high-intensity vomiting that occur once every several weeks with normal health in between. (From Mokha J. Vomiting and nausea. In: Wyllie R, Hyams JS, Kay M, eds. *Pediatric Gastrointestinal and Liver Disease.* 6th ed. Philadelphia: Elsevier; 2021:72, Fig. 8.2.)

TABLE 15.2   Differentiating Acute, Chronic, and Cyclic Patterns of Vomiting

Clinical Feature	Acute	Chronic Recurrent	Cyclic Recurrent
Epidemiology	Most common	Two thirds of recurrent vomiting cohort	One third of recurrent vomiting cohort
Acuity	Moderate-severe, ± dehydration	Not acutely ill or dehydrated	Severe, dehydrated
Vomiting intensity	Moderate to high	Low, 1–2 emeses/hr at the peak	High, ~6 emeses/hr at peak
Recurrence rate	No	Frequent, >2 episodes/wk	Infrequent, ≤2 episodes/wk
Stereotypy	Unique—*if child has had 3 similar episodes, consider cyclic pattern*	No	Yes
Onset	Variable	Daytime	Early morning
Symptoms	Fever, diarrhea	Abdominal pain, diarrhea	Pallor, lethargy, nausea, abdominal pain
Household contacts affected	Usually	No	No
Family history of migraine headaches		14% positive	82% positive
Causes	Viral infections	Ratio of GI to extra-GI causes 7:1; upper GI tract mucosal injury most common (esophagitis, gastritis)	Ratio of extra-GI to GI causes 5:1; cyclic vomiting syndrome most common (also hydronephrosis, metabolic)

GI, gastrointestinal.
From Li BUK, Kovacic K. Vomiting and nausea. In: Wyllie R, Hyams JS, Kay M, eds. *Pediatric Gastrointestinal and Liver Disease*. 5th ed. Philadelphia: Elsevier; 2016:87.

of chronic emesis include GI mucosal inflammation or defects such as eosinophilic esophagitis, gastritis, peptic ulcer disease, and Crohn disease, but psychobehavioral causes such as rumination and bulimia nervosa should be kept in mind. On the contrary, the diagnostic profile of cyclic vomiting is reversed with a ratio of non-GI causes outnumbering GI causes by 5:1. While CVS is the most common cause of this pattern, an episodic pattern of vomiting can also be a manifestation of renal (e.g., acute hydronephrosis from ureteropelvic obstruction), endocrine (e.g., diabetic ketoacidosis, Addison disease), or metabolic disorders (e.g., mitochondrial, fatty acid oxidation defects).

Characteristics of Vomiting

The contents of the vomitus narrow the diagnostic possibilities. Hematemesis and bilious vomiting, in particular, are approached in a manner very different from that of vomiting without these characteristics and may represent more serious underlying disorders (see Chapter 16). Effortless vomiting is witnessed in reflux and rumination, while more forceful vomiting is often noted with upper GI tract obstruction, CVS, and toxins.

Associated Symptoms

Temporal associations of vomiting with specific time of the day, relation to meals, intake of specific foods, and other inciting events can give important diagnostic clues (see Table 15.4). Of all the causes of early morning emesis, the most worrisome is increased intracranial pressure. More common causes of early morning nausea and vomiting are CVS, dysautonomia, and chronic sinusitis with postnasal drip. *Pregnancy should be ruled out in all sexually active females.* Post-tussive emesis should direct diagnostic attention to the cause of the cough itself. Food vomited many hours after its consumption is suspicious for delayed gastric emptying or gastric outlet obstruction. Episodic vomiting associated with abdominal pain precipitated after consumption of a large quantity of fluids and resolving after diuresis can be a result of intermittent hydronephrosis caused by ureteropelvic junction (UPJ) obstruction.

Associated symptoms (Table 15.5) can be crucial in differentiating serious life-threatening conditions that require urgent intervention from the more benign causes of vomiting. Vomiting with neurologic signs such as headache, altered sensorium, and seizures should alert providers to consider intracranial or metabolic disorders. Abdominal pain is a central symptom associated with vomiting and its character

and location can further help narrow the diagnosis (see Chapter 13). Abdominal pain can be categorized as visceral, parietal, or referred pain. Visceral pain is caused by excessive contraction, distension, inflammation, or ischemia of the walls of hollow viscera (stomach, intestines, bile duct, ureter) or the capsule of solid organs (liver, spleen, kidney). Patients usually have difficulty describing visceral pain. It can be dull, intermittent, vague, or colicky and is poorly localized, often to the midline. Common examples are pain secondary to infectious gastroenteritis, functional abdominal pain disorders, toxic irritation, intestinal obstruction, etc. Parietal pain is sharp, constant, and well localized to the area of the underlying problem. It signifies inflammation of the contiguous peritoneum. It is exacerbated with movement, is associated with localized tenderness on examination, and requires immediate medical attention. Parietal pain is present in conditions such as acute cholecystitis, pancreatitis, appendicitis, and perforation of viscus. Referred pain describes pain perceived in an area remote from the site of the inciting pathologic process. Abdominal pain may therefore be a symptom of disease localized in the thorax, pelvis, or retroperitoneum.

When suspecting a psychosocial cause of vomiting, providers should inquire about anxiety, binge eating, body image, and any recent stressors. Minor head injury can also present as vomiting in children, especially toddlers. There is evidence to suggest that vomiting after a minor head injury may be related to intrinsic patient factors rather than the severity of the injury. Vomiting that is persistent or latent in onset may be more likely to signify head injury. Emesis following a recent history of blunt abdominal trauma should raise the suspicion of a duodenal hematoma.

Medical, Family, and Social History

Previous surgery, hospitalizations, and medications may provide important clues. A family history of fetal or neonatal deaths suggests a genetic or metabolic cause; similar illness in family members or other contacts may suggest infections or common toxic exposures. Psychosocial stressors may be found in adolescents with bulimia, peptic ulcer disease, chronic marijuana use, or intentional self-poisonings.

Physical Examination

Although vomiting is a "gastrointestinal" symptom, it can be a manifestation of disease in multiple systems of the body (see Table 15.5). Vital signs identify fever, which is important in narrowing the

TABLE 15.3 Causes of Vomiting by Temporal Pattern

Category	Acute	Chronic	Cyclic
Infectious	Gastroenteritis* Otitis media* Streptococcal pharyngitis Acute sinusitis Hepatitis Pyelonephritis Meningitis	*Helicobacter pylori** Giardiasis Chronic sinusitis*	Chronic sinusitis*
Gastrointestinal	Inguinal hernia Intussusception Malrotation with volvulus Appendicitis Cholecystitis Pancreatitis Distal intestinal obstruction syndrome	Anatomic obstruction GERD ± esophagitis* Eosinophilic esophagitis* Gastritis* Peptic ulcer or duodenitis* Achalasia SMA syndrome Stricturing Crohn disease Rumination Functional	Malrotation with volvulus Cyclic vomiting syndrome*
Genitourinary	Pyelonephritis UPJ obstruction	Pyelonephritis Pregnancy Uremia	Acute hydronephrosis secondary to UPJ obstruction
Endocrine, metabolic	Diabetic keto-acidosis	Adrenal hyper-plasia	Diabetic ketoacidosis Addison disease MCAD deficiency Partial OTC deficiency MELAS syndrome Acute intermittent porphyria
Neurologic	Concussion Subdural hematoma Encephalitis Migraine	Arnold-Chiari malformation Subtentorial neoplasm	Abdominal migraine* Migraine headaches* Arnold-Chiari malformation Subtentorial neoplasm Metabolic enceph-alopathy
Other	Toxic ingestion Chronic marijuana use: hypereme-sis syndrome Food poisoning	Bulimia Pregnancy	Factitious disorder by proxy (e.g., ipecac poisoning)

*Most common disorders.

GERD, gastroesophageal reflux disease; MCAD, medium-chain acyl-coenzyme A dehydrogenase deficiency; MELAS, mitochondrial myopathy, encephalopathy, lactic acidosis, and strokelike episodes; OTC, ornithine transcarbamylase deficiency; SMA, superior mesenteric artery; UPJ, ureteropelvic junction.
From Li BUK, Kovacic K. Vomiting and nausea. In: Wyllie R, Hyams JS, Kay M, eds. *Pediatric Gastrointestinal and Liver Disease.* 5th ed. Philadelphia: Elsevier; 2016:88.

TABLE 15.4 Temporal Associations of Chronic or Recurrent Vomiting

Temporal Associations	Diagnosis	Other Clues
Time of day: early morning	Increased intracranial pressure Sinusitis with postnasal mucus Pregnancy Uremia	Headache, papilledema Sinus tenderness Secondary amenorrhea
During or after meals		
Any meals	Peptic ulcer disease, reflux	Epigastric pain, heartburn
Specific foods		
Fructose	Hereditary fructose intolerance	Hypoglycemia
Galactose	Galactosemia	Cataracts
High protein	Metabolic inborn error	Hyperammonemia, acidosis
Specific protein		
Cow, soy	Cow's or soy milk intolerance	Stool guaiac positive
Gluten	Gluten-sensitive enteropa-thy (celiac)	Failure to thrive
Various (especially egg, wheat, fish, nuts)	Miscellaneous allergic, eosinophilic gastroen-teropathies	History of asthma, hives, ↑ eosinophils, family history of allergies
After fasting		
Food vomited	Gastric stasis/obstruction	Distention, tympany
Clear vomitus	Metabolic disease	See Table 15.8
Other precipitants		
Cough	Post-tussive	Respiratory disease
Infections	Recurrent gastroenteritis	Fever, diarrhea, sick contacts
Vestibular stimulation	Motion sickness	Nystagmus Vertigo
Hyperhydration	Ureteropelvic junction obstruction ("Dietl crisis")	Spontaneous resolution with normal hydration
Menses	Dysmenorrhea associated Acute intermittent porphyria Pelvic inflammatory disease	Relief with NSAIDs Nonperitonitis pain, distention, tachycardia, constipation Vaginal discharge
Medications, toxins	Local GI irritation: NSAIDs, ingested poison CTZ stimulation: chemotherapeutics, opioids, ipecac Steroid withdrawal: adrenal crisis Drug-induced pancreatitis, hepatitis Drug-precipitated acute intermittent porphyria	Ipecac abuse in anorexia History of L-asparaginase, valproate, isoniazid, etc. Oral contraceptives, sulfa drugs, barbiturates
Episodic/cyclic	See Table 15.3	See Table 15.2

CTZ, chemoreceptor trigger zone; GI, gastrointestinal; NSAIDs, nonste-roidal antiinflammatory drugs.

TABLE 15.5   Associated Symptoms and Signs for Vomiting

Associated Symptom or Sign	Diagnostic Consideration	Associated Symptom or Sign	Diagnostic Consideration
Systemic Manifestations		**Neurologic Symptoms**	
Acute illness, dehydration	Infection, ingestion, cyclic vomiting, possible surgical emergency	Headache	Allergy, chronic sinusitis, migraine, increased intracranial pressure
Chronic malnutrition	Malabsorption syndrome	Postnasal drip, congestion	Allergy, chronic sinusitis
Gastrointestinal Symptoms		Vertigo	Migraine, inner ear disease
Nausea	Absence of nausea can suggest increased intracranial pressure	Seizures	Epilepsy
		Abnormal muscle tone	Cerebral palsy, metabolic disorder, mitochondrial disorder
Substernal	Esophagitis	Abnormal funduscopic exam or bulging fontanel	Increased intracranial pressure, pseudotumor cerebri
Epigastric	Upper GI related (reflux, gastritis, PUD), pancreatitis		
Right upper quadrant	Hepatitis, cholecystitis, pancreatitis, cholelithiasis, biliary colic, right lower pneumonia, right pyelonephritis	**ENT Symptoms**	
		Postnasal drip, congestion	Allergy, chronic sinusitis
Left upper quadrant	PUD, pancreatitis, splenic enlargement, left lower lobe pneumonia, left pyelonephritis	Sore throat, ear pain	Streptococcal pharyngitis, acute otitis media
		Cardiac Symptoms	
Periumbilical	Nonspecific, small bowel obstruction	History of valvular disease	Mesenteric arterial thrombosis/emboli
Right/left flank	UPJ obstruction, renal stones, pyelonephritis, adrenal hemorrhage	Hypotension	Intestinal ischemia, mesenteric arterial thrombosis/emboli
Right lower quadrant	Appendicitis, right tubo-ovarian disease		
Left lower quadrant	Sigmoid related, left tubo-ovarian disease	Hypertension	Porphyria, some variants of cyclic vomiting syndrome
Diarrhea	Gastroenteritis, bacterial colitis	**Renal Symptoms**	
Constipation	Hirschsprung disease, pseudo-obstruction, hypercalcemia, hypokalemia, lead poisoning, porphyria	Dysuria, hematuria, renal hypertension	Pyelonephritis, calculi, hydronephrosis
		Gynecologic Symptoms	
Dysphagia	Eosinophilic esophagitis, achalasia, esophageal stricture	Menstrual irregularity	Pregnancy, ectopic pregnancy
		Vaginal discharge	Pelvic inflammatory disease
Malodorous breath	*H. pylori*	Menses associated	Porphyria, endometriosis, dysmenorrhea
Jaundice	Hepatitis, cholecystitis, hepatobiliary obstruction	**History of Head Trauma**	Concussion, intracranial hemorrhage
Visible peristalsis	Gastric outlet obstruction		
Surgical scars	Surgical adhesions, surgical vagotomy	**History of Abdominal Trauma**	Duodenal hematoma
Succussion splash	Gastric outlet obstruction with gastric distention		
Bowel sounds	Decreased: paralytic ileus; increased: mechanical obstruction	**Family History and Epidemiology**	
		Peptic ulcer disease	Peptic ulcer disease, *H. pylori* gastritis
Severe abdominal tenderness with rebound	Perforated viscera and peritonitis	Migraine headaches	Abdominal migraine, cyclic vomiting syndrome
Abdominal mass	Pyloric stenosis, congenital malformations, Crohn disease, ovarian cyst, pregnancy, abdominal neoplasm	Contaminated water	*Giardia, Cryptosporidium*, other parasites
		Travel	Traveler's (*Escherichia coli*) diarrhea, giardiasis

GI, gastrointestinal; *H. pylori, Helicobacter pylori*; PUD, peptic ulcer disease; UPJ, ureteropelvic junction.

Modified from Li BUK, Kovacic K. Vomiting and nausea. In: Wyllie R, Hyams JS, Kay M, eds. *Pediatric Gastrointestinal and Liver Disease*. 5th ed. Philadelphia: Elsevier; 2016:91.

differential diagnosis. Tachypnea may signify pneumonia or a metabolic acidosis, which is seen with vomiting from inborn errors of metabolism or poisoning. Intense vomiting as seen with infection, toxin ingestion, cyclic vomiting, or a possible surgical emergency can present with signs of severe dehydration or hypovolemic shock. Presence of failure to thrive or chronic malnutrition can be suggestive of malabsorption syndromes or metabolic conditions. A thorough neurologic exam including examination of optic fundi is warranted in all patients. The absence of venous pulsations or sharp optic disc margins may be the only evidence of a brain tumor or other intracranial lesion causing vomiting. When in doubt, a formal ophthalmologic examination is warranted.

Abdominal Examination

Simple observation of operative scars may suggest the possibility of obstruction from intestinal adhesions, and visible distention may represent ascites caused by liver disease or intraluminal distention caused by intestinal obstruction or ileus. The order of the examination is important because auscultation performed after stimulation of intestinal motility by palpation may artifactually change the auscultatory findings. An important distinction in the vomiting child is whether bowel sounds are increased, as in gastroenteritis or in bowel obstructions, or absent, as in ileus caused by peritonitis or in chronic intestinal pseudo-obstruction. Increased bowel sounds resulting from luminal obstruction are often characterized by intermittent "rushes" of high-pitched sounds that are coordinated with episodes of colicky pain. Although seen infrequently, visible peristalsis in infants and a succussion splash in children are indications of a gastric outlet obstruction that is causing gastric distension and retention of fluid. Palpate the abdomen and pelvis for area of tenderness and signs of peritoneal inflammation as they often represent disorders necessitating further imaging and/or surgery. Also palpate for presence of organomegaly and abdominal masses. Hepatosplenomegaly can be found in various metabolic or inflammatory diseases. Abdominal masses can be congenital (e.g., mesenteric cyst) or acquired (e.g., neuroblastoma) and result in bowel obstruction (see Chapter 20). Examine genitalia and hernia sites for ambiguous genitalia, ovarian/testicular torsion, and strangulated hernias. Vague periumbilical pain is quite nonspecific, but the localized, very sharp pain signifying inflammation of the peritoneum requires immediate attention. Initial luminal obstruction may progress to ileus as peritonitis intervenes. Localization of nonperiumbilical pain or tenderness helps a great deal in determining the diseased intraabdominal organ (see Table 15.5).

Rectal Examination

A rectal examination may be helpful in the vomiting child as the presence and consistency of rectal stool may be determined. A large fecal impaction may possibly contribute to vomiting in some young children. Pelvic masses and tenderness identified by rectal exam may represent appendicitis, ovarian torsion, or pelvic inflammatory disease. The stool should always be tested for blood and should be considered for testing for pH, reducing substances, fat, leukocytes, and infectious organisms, depending on the presentation.

Evaluation

The evaluation of a patient with vomiting is usually performed in a primary care or emergency department setting. Initial evaluation is directed at assessment of airway, breathing, and circulation as well as hydration status. Clinically diagnosed dehydration without any laboratory confirmation is usually a sufficient basis to initiate rehydration therapy. Look for the presence of red flag signs (Table 15.6) that suggest more ominous causes of vomiting. If the physical examination reveals signs of acute abdomen (bilious emesis, peritonitis, shock), obtaining abdominal imaging and seeking urgent surgical consultation are

indicated. Presence of brisk hematemesis warrants an urgent gastroenterology consult. Altered mental status suggests toxin ingestion, inborn errors of metabolism, acquired metabolic conditions such as hyperammonemia, diabetic ketoacidosis, and neurologic causes.

Laboratory Data

Well-appearing infants with typical regurgitant reflux usually require no laboratory evaluation, except possibly a GI contrast study if they do not respond readily to conservative therapy (see later discussion). Similarly, a single, brief episode of mild vomiting with no suggestion of dehydration or other complications may necessitate no laboratory studies. Most children with presumed infectious gastroenteritis or colitis do not need to undergo microbiologic stool testing to identify underlying pathogens since these are self-limiting conditions. Other children, those with severe acute vomiting or with chronic or recurrent vomiting, should have screening studies of blood or urine (Table 15.7). Presence of glucose and ketones in urine suggests diabetic ketoacidosis; red blood cells suggest a renal cause (nephritis, Henoch-Schönlein purpura, renal calculi, or trauma); and leukocytes or nitrites suggest a urinary tract infection. Screening blood investigations should include a total blood count, blood sugar, serum electrolytes, blood gases, liver enzymes, lipase, and renal function tests. Elevated leucocyte count suggests presence of infection or inflammation; anemia could be secondary to chronic malabsorption, occult GI losses, or a hemolytic process such as hemolytic uremic syndrome. Typical electrolyte abnormalities

TABLE 15.6 Red Flag Signs in a Child Presenting with Vomiting

- Altered level of consciousness or mental status
- Toxic appearance (shock, sepsis)
- Bilious or bloody vomiting
- Vomiting without diarrhea
- Repeated episodes of emesis with mental status changes
- Developmental delay
- Macro- or microcephaly
- Suspicion of ingestion (toxidromes)
- Signs of trauma/abuse
- Hematochezia or hematemesis
- Abdominal heterotaxia syndromes
- Prior abdominal surgery
- Presence of inconsolable cry or excessive irritability
- Severe dehydration
- Severe malnutrition or failure to thrive
- Bent-over posture, drawing legs up to chest, pained avoidance of unnecessary movement typical of peritonitis
- Silent abdomen
- Tender abdomen

TABLE 15.7 Laboratory Work-Up

Laboratory Test	Possible Significance
CBC	• Anemia: blood loss, chronic malabsorption • Leukocytosis: inflammatory process • Eosinophilia: eosinophilic gastroenteropathy
Electrolytes, glucose, BUN, creatinine	• Metabolic acidosis or alkalosis, hypokalemia: consequence of vomiting • Hyperglycemia: diabetic ketoacidosis • Hypoglycemia: dehydration, metabolic disorder • Azotemia: dehydration
Pancreatic enzymes (amylase, lipase)	• Elevated in pancreatitis
Liver enzymes (ALT, AST, ALP, GGT)	• Elevated in hepatitis, biliary obstruction, metabolic disease
Metabolic work-up (blood gas, ketones, ammonia, lactate, pyruvate, amino acid, organic acid, carnitine, acylcarnitine, porphobilinogen deaminase, toxicology)	• Ketonemia: DKA, dehydration, metabolic diseases • Lactic acidosis: metabolic diseases • Aminoacidemia: e.g., MSUD, tyrosinemia • Organic acidemia: e.g., propionic acidemia, MMA • Hyperammonemia: urea cycle defect, liver failure • Decreased porphobilinogen deaminase: acute intermittent porphyria • Toxicology: ingested poison, drug
Urine (microscopy, culture, β-HCG, reducing substance, ketones, amino acid, organic acid, toxicology, porphobilinogen, δ-ALA)	• Leukocytes: urinary tract infection • Blood: urinary tract infection, renal stones • Ketones: starvation, metabolic disease • Reducing substances: galactosemia • Porphobilinogen, δ-ALA: acute intermittent porphyria

ALA, aminolevulinic acid; ALP, alkaline phosphatase; ALT, alanine aminotransferase; AST, aspartate aminotransferase; β-HCG, β-human chorionic gonadotropin; DKA, diabetic ketoacidosis; GGT, γ-glutamyltransferase; MMA, methylmalonic acidemia; MSUD, maple syrup urine disease.

occur in an infant with projectile vomiting from pyloric stenosis (hypochloremic, hypokalemic metabolic alkalosis) and congenital adrenal hyperplasia or Addison disease (hyperkalemia and hyponatremia). Blood and urine screening for several metabolic disorders are positive only during an actual vomiting episode; therefore, when suspecting a metabolic cause, attempts should be made to obtain specimens at these times, which may increase the diagnostic yield. Metabolic work-up includes acid-base, serum ammonia and lactate, serum and urine carnitine (possible fatty acid oxidation defect), serum amino acids (possible aminoacidemia), urine organic acids (possible organic acidemia), and urine aminolevulinic acid and porphobilinogens (possible acute intermittent porphyria) (Table 15.8).

Radiographic and Procedure Data

If the history and physical examination suggest the possibility of abdominal disease, endoscopic evaluation or abdominal plain films (including a second image such as an upright film) are usually warranted (Table 15.9). Endoscopy is particularly useful in hematemesis,

in suspected peptic ulcer disease, or when tissue is needed for histologic study (e.g., establishing a diagnosis of *Helicobacter pylori* gastritis or of eosinophilic gastroenteropathy). Radiographic testing is useful in most other situations. Further evaluation, such as contrast studies, ultrasonography, CT, or MRI, is tailored to the suspected diagnoses. In some cases, manometric evaluation is prompted by the suggestion of GI motility disorders, such as achalasia and chronic intestinal pseudo-obstruction.

TABLE 15.8 When to Consider Metabolic Work-Up

Nutritional abnormalities	Failure to thrive, anorexia
Dietary provocations	Fructose, galactose, protein, fasting
Neurologic abnormalities	Lethargy, coma Tone ↑ or ↓, developmental delay Seizures
Liver abnormalities	Hepatosplenomegaly Jaundice
Respiratory abnormalities	Apnea Hyperpnea (caused by metabolic acidosis or hyperammonemia)
Odd odors (breath, urine, ear wax)	Cabbage: tyrosinemia Sweaty feet: isovaleric acidemia Musty: phenylketonuria, hepatic coma (fetor hepaticus) Fruity: ketones (many, nonspecific) Maple syrup: maple syrup urine disease Other: 3-methylcrotonyl-CoA carboxylase deficiency Multiple carboxylase deficiency Acyl-CoA dehydrogenase deficiency Putrid: sinusitis Alcohol: alcohol ingestion
Miscellaneous abnormalities	Eye abnormalities (cataracts) Hair abnormalities (fragile) Pigmentation of skin ("tan") and mucosa Adrenal calcifications Ambiguous genitalia Cardiomyopathy Family history of fetal or neonatal deaths; consanguinity
Screening study abnormalities	Metabolic acidosis Hypoglycemia (hyperketonuric or hypoketonuric) Hyperkalemia (with hyponatremia) Hyperammonemia Hypertransaminasemia Anemia, leukocytopenia, thrombocytopenia Urinary non–glucose-reducing substance Urinary Fanconi syndrome

CoA, coenzyme A.

TABLE 15.9 Other Diagnostic Tests

Test	Findings	Possible Significance
Imaging		
Plain abdomen (supine, upright)	Multiple air fluid levels	Bowel obstruction, ileus
	Distended bowel loops	Ileus
	Double bubble	Duodenal atresia
	Calcifications	Biliary, renal stones, appendicitis
	Free air	Intestinal perforation
	Free fluid	Ascites
	Foreign bodies	
	Organomegaly, masses	
Contrast study (barium or Gastrografin)		
1. Upper fluoroscopy	Malrotations, obstructions	
2. Enteroclysis	Distal obstructions	
3. Lower fluoroscopy	Intussusception, obstructions	Therapeutic: intussusception, meconium ileus, DIOS
Ultrasonography	Mass, cyst, abscess, pyloric stenosis; hepatobiliary, pancreatic, urinary, gynecologic lesions	
CT/MRI abdomen	Mass, cyst, inflammatory lesions, hepatobiliary, pancreatic, urinary, gynecologic lesions	
MRI/CT head	CNS lesions	Neurogenic vomiting
Endoscopy		
Upper		
Diagnostic	Obstruction, hemorrhage, *Giardia* or *Helicobacter pylori* infection	
Therapeutic		Hematemesis
Lower		
Diagnostic	Distal obstruction, infection	Obstruction, infection
Therapeutic		Sigmoid volvulus
Manometry		
Esophagus	Failure of sphincter relaxation	Achalasia
	Dysmotility	Esophageal dysmotility
Small bowel	Dysmotility	Pseudo-obstruction
Rectum/colon	Failure of sphincter relaxation	Hirschsprung disease
	Dysmotility	Pseudo-obstruction

CNS, central nervous system; DIOS, distal intestinal obstruction syndrome.

Differential Diagnosis

General Approach

Cardinal symptoms or signs accompanying the vomiting direct the differential diagnosis. When vomiting is a result of intraabdominal disease, it is useful to define whether obstruction, dysmotility, inflammation, or ischemia is the mechanism. Abdominal pain, which frequently accompanies vomiting, can suggest both the type of disorder and the organ involved (see Table 15.5). Symptoms referable to non-GI organ systems direct attention to those systems. For example, accompanying neurologic symptoms may direct attention to central nervous system disorders, metabolic disease, poisonings, or psychobehavioral disease.

Gastrointestinal Obstruction (Table 15.10)

Esophageal Obstruction

Esophageal strictures or obstruction produces dysphagia with welling up or drooling of oropharyngeal secretions or esophageal contents rather than actual vomiting; the material is undigested. Respiratory symptoms from aspiration may be prominent.

Esophageal Atresia

Esophageal atresia is a congenital malformation defined by the discontinuity of the esophagus. Infants present at birth with a prenatal history of polyhydramnios and intolerance of initial feeding. The esophageal atresia is accompanied by a distal tracheoesophageal fistula (TEF) in 85% of cases, by a proximal fistula in a small percentage, and by no fistula in the remainder (Fig. 15.2). Esophageal atresia is associated with other anomalies in 15–50% of patients; cardiac, anorectal, and genitourinary defects are most common. Ten percent of all esophageal atresia patients and 25% of those without a fistula have the VATER or VACTERL (vertebral, anorectal, cardiac, tracheoesophageal, renal, radial, limb) association. As many as 33% of affected infants are premature. Diagnosis can usually be made by plain films after passage of an opaque rubber catheter, which coils in the upper pouch (Fig. 15.3). Treatment is surgical.

Congenital Esophageal Stenosis

Congenital esophageal stenosis is defined as an intrinsic narrowing of the esophagus present at birth. Infants usually tolerate breast-feeding and start to present with vomiting and regurgitation with the introduction of semisolid or solid food. A milder degree of stenosis may not present until later in childhood. Stenoses are categorized into three histopathologic types: tracheobronchial remnants that often contain cartilage, fibromuscular stenoses, and membranous webs. Contrast radiography can diagnose the first two, while endoscopy is needed to diagnose webs. Tracheobronchial rings generally necessitate surgery, membranous webs can be treated with endoscopic dilation, and muscular stenoses may respond to dilation or may necessitate surgery.

Esophageal Strictures

Esophageal strictures (Fig. 15.4) are acquired lesions that can be categorized as inflammatory (secondary to gastroesophageal reflux disease [GERD] and eosinophilic esophagitis), anastomotic (post-TEF repair), or related to corrosive injury (acid, alkali, pills, battery ingestions). The clinical presentation is the same for all these conditions: patients primarily present with dysphagia, recurrent vomiting, or food impaction. The strictures are best demonstrated with contrast radiography; endoscopic biopsies may be important for diagnosis of the etiology. GERD may be treated pharmacologically but may also require an antireflux surgery (fundoplication). Endoscopic dilation of the stricture is performed repeatedly with balloons or semirigid bougies until the strictured site remains patent.

TABLE 15.10	Causes of Gastrointestinal Obstruction
Esophagus	
Congenital	Esophageal atresia (with or without fistula)
	Isolated esophageal stenosis
	Duplication
	Vascular ring
Acquired	Caustic agent esophageal stricture
	Inflammatory stricture: peptic, EOE
	Achalasia
Stomach	
Congenital	Antral webs
Acquired	Pyloric atresia*
	Bezoars/foreign body
	Pyloric stenosis
	Pyloric stricture (ulcer)
	Crohn disease
	Eosinophilic gastroenteropathy
	Prostaglandin-induced pyloric stenosis
	Chronic granulomatous disease
Small Intestine	
Congenital	Intestinal atresia
	Annular pancreas
	Malrotation/volvulus
	Duplications
	Meconium ileus
	Obstructed inguinal hernia
Acquired	Postsurgical adhesions or strictures
	Crohn disease (stricture)
	Intussusception
	Duodenal hematoma (abuse, trauma)
	Meconium ileus equivalent (DIOS)
	Superior mesenteric artery syndrome
Colonw	
Congenital	Meconium plug
	Hirschsprung disease
	Colonic atresia, stenosis
	Rectal stenosis
	Imperforate rectum/anus
	Malrotation/volvulus
	Small left colon syndrome (IDM)
Acquired	Ulcerative colitis (toxic megacolon)†
	Crohn disease (stricture)
	Postsurgical adhesions or strictures

*Often associated with epidermolysis bullosa.
†Produces an ileus.
DIOS, distal intestinal obstruction syndrome; EOE, eosinophilic esophagitis; IDM, infant of diabetic mother.
Modified from Behrman R, Kliegman R. *Nelson Essentials of Pediatrics.* 2nd ed. Philadelphia: WB Saunders; 1994:407.

Miscellaneous Causes

Foreign body ingestion is a common pediatric problem with up to 75% of cases in children age 4 years or younger. Coins are the most commonly ingested foreign body. The esophagus, in particular the upper one third, is a common site for obstruction. Patients may present with drooling, vomiting, cough, and stridor, and if lodged in the esophagus, urgent endoscopic removal is required.

Extrinsic esophageal compression may result from an aberrant subclavian artery, vascular ring, and mediastinal masses (lymphoma,

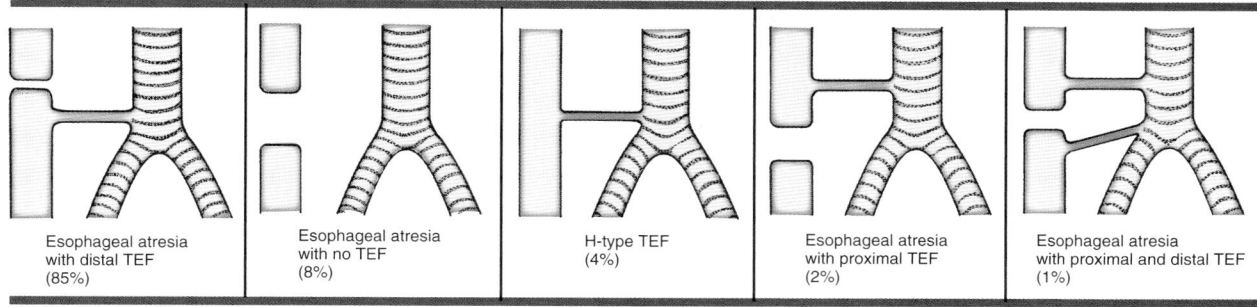

| Esophageal atresia with distal TEF (85%) | Esophageal atresia with no TEF (8%) | H-type TEF (4%) | Esophageal atresia with proximal TEF (2%) | Esophageal atresia with proximal and distal TEF (1%) |

Fig. 15.2 Various types of tracheoesophageal fistulas (TEFs) with relative frequency (%).

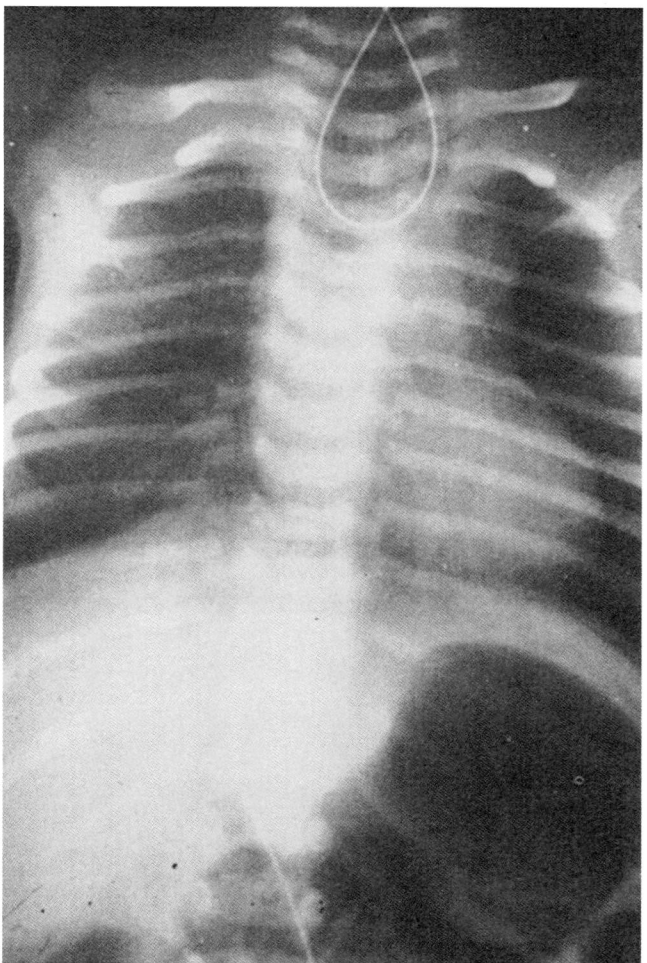

Fig. 15.3 Tracheoesophageal fistula. Coiled radiopaque nasogastric tube in blind upper pouch.

germ cell tumors). Vascular rings occur when the esophagus and trachea are encircled, displaced, or compressed by the aorta or its aberrant branches and can present with stridor, dysphagia, and emesis. It is often an incidental finding on chest x-ray. In symptomatic cases, even after a vascular ring has been detected by plain radiography or esophagography, advanced cross-sectional imaging is recommended for more detailed evaluation.

Gastric Outlet Obstruction

Hypertrophic Pyloric Stenosis

Hypertrophic pyloric stenosis (HPS) is the most common cause of gastric outlet obstruction in infancy with an incidence rate of 1:400 infants. It manifests with nonbilious projectile vomiting beginning at 2–3 weeks of age and increasing during the next month or so, usually in a first-born male child. The vomitus may rarely contain some blood, and propulsive gastric waves can be seen across the abdominal wall. Dehydration, poor weight gain, hypochloremic hypokalemic metabolic alkalosis, and mild jaundice are sometimes evident. A palpable "olive" in the epigastrium (felt best during or after feeding) represents the hypertrophied pyloric muscle. Gastric distention is seen on the plain film, and a contrast study shows the "string sign" of contrast passing through the narrowed pyloric channel. Ultrasound diagnosis is less invasive and demonstrates increase of the pyloric channel length and muscle thickness (Fig. 15.5). Laparoscopic pyloromyotomy is the treatment of choice. Preoperative correction of dehydration and electrolyte imbalance reduces perioperative morbidity. Junctional epidermolysis bullosum is associated with pyloric stenosis.

Other Causes of Gastric Outlet Obstruction

Eosinophilic gastroenteritis can mimic clinical signs and ultrasound appearance of HPS. Clues to diagnosis are eosinophilic infiltrate of endoscopic antral biopsies, peripheral eosinophilia, and an excellent response to treatment with a casein hydrolysate or elemental "hypoallergenic" formula. Prolonged use of prostaglandin infusion in neonates with congenital heart disease may cause transient HPS. The clinical and radiologic features of HPS are relieved after stopping prostaglandin E infusion.

In older children, gastric outlet obstruction may result from chronic peptic ulcer disease, chronic granulomatous disease, gastroduodenal Crohn disease, anatomic abnormalities such as gastric antral web, foreign bodies, and bezoars. Bezoars may be caused by hair, vegetable matter, milk curds, or medications. Contrast radiography, endoscopy, and, in some cases, histopathology is needed to make the diagnosis.

Intestinal Obstruction

The classical clinical tetrad is colicky abdominal pain, nausea and vomiting, abdominal distention, and constipation-to-obstipation. Examination may demonstrate a tympanic abdomen, hyperactive bowel sounds, and signs of dehydration. Severe direct tenderness, involuntary guarding, abdominal rigidity, and rebound tenderness suggest advanced intestinal obstruction, as do marked leukocytosis, neutrophilia, left shift, and lactic acidosis. Obstructions may be categorized by site and type (see Table 15.10). Vomiting is a cardinal sign of intestinal obstruction, being more prominent in high small bowel obstruction than in low small bowel or colon obstruction. With high obstructions, vomiting is not feculent, the onset is often acute, and crampy pain may occur at frequent intervals, while abdominal distention is less prominent. With low obstructions, the vomiting may be feculent and less acute in onset, the interval between cramping is longer, and distention is more notable. Identification of the site of obstruction is aided by the plain film and by other radiographic studies (see Table 15.9). Intraluminal lesions (e.g., tumors, intussusceptions, or extrinsic material such as feces, foreign bodies, bezoars, and

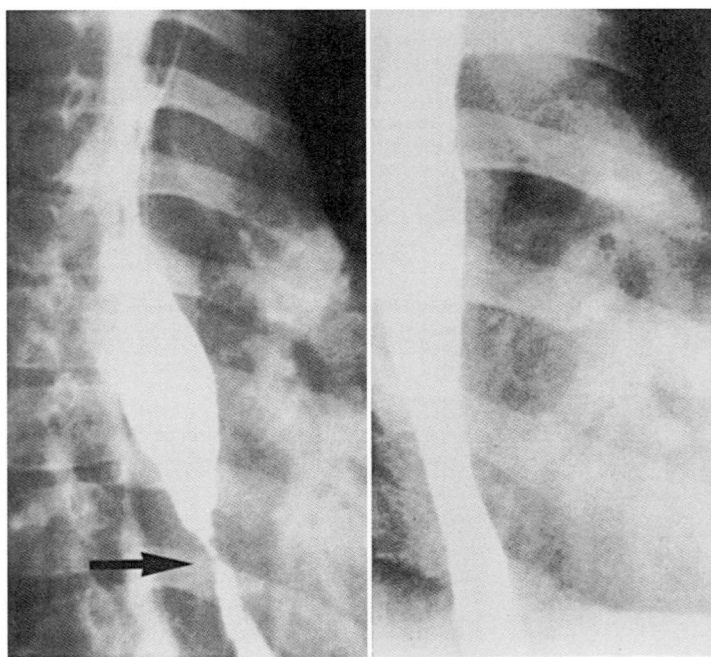

Fig. 15.4 Esophageal stricture. Radiograph of a peptic esophageal stricture *(arrow)* before and after treatment with dilations.

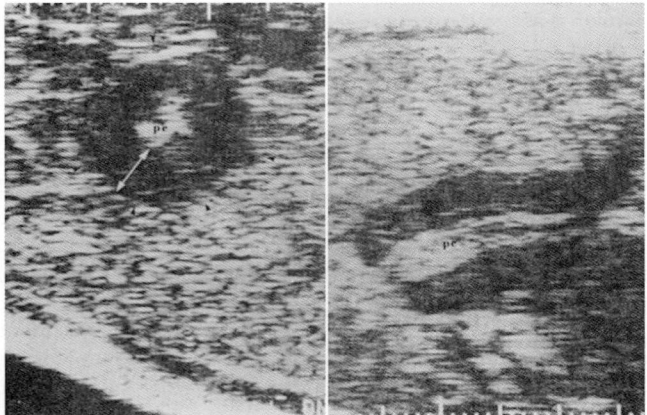

Fig. 15.5 Pyloric stenosis. Cross-sectional *(left)* and transverse *(right)* sonograms of hypertrophic pyloric stenosis, showing increased thickness and length of pyloric muscle. pc, pyloric channel.

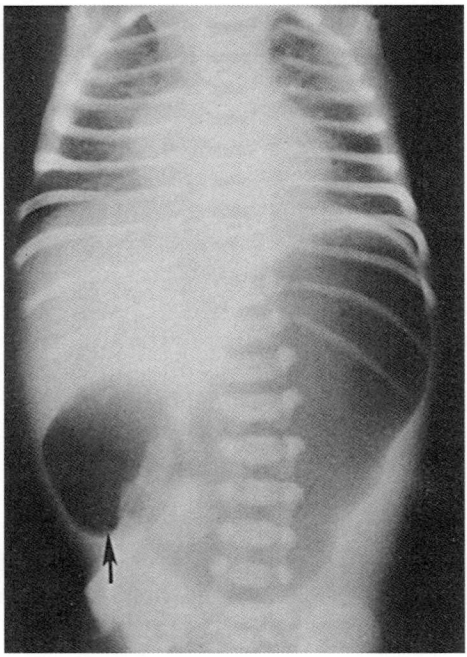

Fig. 15.6 "Double-bubble" sign *(arrow)* in duodenal obstruction.

gallstones) can be differentiated from bowel wall lesions (strictures, stenoses, atresias) and from extraluminal lesions (adhesions, congenital bands, tumors, volvulus) through imaging. Radiographic studies are useful, beginning with the plain film and progressing to ultrasonography or CT. Abdominal CT with oral and intravenous contrast and fluoroscopy with contrast are both sensitive and specific in detecting and characterizing intestinal obstruction. However, the decision to introduce contrast into an intestine that may perforate or be operated on must be made with surgical and radiologic consultation. Often the decision to operate can be made without certain identification of the lesion, and contrast studies are unnecessary.

Infantile bilious vomiting is an important symptom of intestinal obstruction, which often signals a congenital GI anomaly, particularly intestinal obstruction below the ampulla of Vater. Surgical consultation is needed early in these infants because they often require emergency therapy.

Duodenal Atresia, Stenosis, and Web; Annular Pancreas

The juxta-ampullary duodenum is susceptible to a cluster of obstructing congenital anomalies. Infants with complete duodenal obstruction, most commonly atresia, present with bilious vomiting and a radiographic "double-bubble" sign (Fig. 15.6). Associated prematurity (and polyhydramnios) or anomalies, including renal, cardiac, and vertebral defects, occur in approximately 75% of infants; trisomy 21 is seen in about 50%. Double atresias, duplications, and malrotations are frequently seen. Infants with a partial duodenal obstruction caused by a stenosis or web may have such mild symptoms that they do not come to medical attention until regurgitation produces esophagitis or until a foreign body or bezoar is trapped at the obstruction. Treatment is surgical.

Duodenal Hematoma

Blunt abdominal trauma (seatbelt, steering wheel, bicycle handlebar injury; child abuse), or even endoscopic biopsies in the context of a coagulopathy, can produce an obstructing duodenal hematoma. Endoscopy in the setting of stem cell transplantation or other hematopoietic disease may place a patient at greater risk of such hematoma, requiring special consideration of the need for duodenal biopsies in these individuals. Therapy is symptomatic; jejunal feeding that bypasses the obstruction or parenteral nutrition may be required as the problem resolves.

Jejunal Atresia, Ileal Atresia, and Ileal Stenosis

Patients with these congenital lesions present with bilious vomiting and more abdominal distention than those with duodenal lesions. The atresias are readily suspected and diagnosed in the neonatal period. Stenotic lesions may require radiography for diagnosis. Treatment is surgical.

Intestinal Strictures

Strictures produce partial obstruction of the GI tract and may be located anywhere from the esophagus to the anus. They may occur postsurgically (anastomotic), may follow necrotizing enterocolitis, may be caused by penetrating Crohn disease or intestinal graft versus host disease, or may be sequalae of drug-induced ulcers (nonsteroidal antiinflammatory medications or high-dose pancreatic enzymes). Some patients may be treated with endoscopic dilatation, but many require surgical stricturoplasty (opening the bowel longitudinally and closing it transversely) or resection.

Adhesions

Obstructive symptoms in the child with a history of prior abdominal surgery may be caused by adhesive bands.

Duplications

GI tract duplication cysts are rare congenital anomalies and can occur in any portion of the GI tract but are more commonly encountered in the small intestine. These uncommon lesions may cause vomiting by extrinsic obstruction of the intestine or by intussusception. On examination, an abdominal mass may be palpable. Treatment is surgical resection.

Meconium Ileus and Distal Intestinal Obstruction Syndrome

Approximately 20% of infants with cystic fibrosis present in the newborn period with failure to pass meconium, caused by meconium ileus (MI). The sticky, poorly hydrated intestinal mucus plays a role. It can present in two forms: simple or complex MI. In simple MI, viscid meconium physically obstructs the terminal ileum and results in the dilation of the proximal small intestine. In complex MI, the meconium-distended segments of ileum can give rise to complications like prenatal volvulus, ischemic necrosis, or perforation and extrusion of the meconium into the peritoneum. The classic "soap bubble" sign may be seen on abdominal x-ray when meconium mixes with swallowed air (Fig. 15.7).

Simple MI may be treated with hyperosmolar contrast (Gastrografin) enema performed under fluoroscopic guidance. Surgery is required for complex MI or those simple cases resistant to enema. Virtually all infants with MI have cystic fibrosis; the diagnosis should be confirmed by sweat test or DNA analysis.

Older children with cystic fibrosis who stop defecating and have abdominal pain and occasional vomiting are said to have **distal**

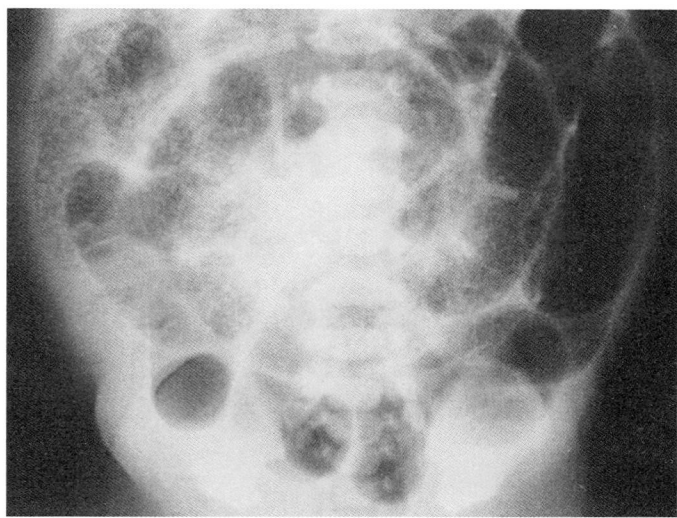

Fig. 15.7 Soap-bubble appearance in meconium ileus.

intestinal obstruction syndrome (DIOS), formerly termed meconium ileus equivalent. Initial treatment consists of rehydration, stool softening laxatives, or intestinal lavage and enemas. If not successful, then Gastrografin, administered orally or as enema often at times mixed with N-acetylcysteine (mucolytic), is nearly always successful. Surgery is rarely required. Close attention to fluid and electrolyte balance is vital in all infants and children treated with a hyperosmolar contrast medium. Avoiding dehydration and optimizing pancreatic enzyme dosage may reduce the chance of further episodes.

Incarcerated Hernia

Whenever vomiting is accompanied by signs of obstruction, sites of potential herniation should be examined for incarceration of a loop of bowel (Fig. 15.8). Inguinal incarceration is most common, but other types of hernias are femoral, obturator, spigelian, umbilical (1 in 1,500 incarcerate), epigastric, mesenteric, and postoperative incisional hernias.

Inguinal hernias are often reduced by gentle, firm, constant pressure that is directed through the scrotum toward the inguinal canal. Sedation and the Trendelenburg position may facilitate reduction.

Malrotation and Volvulus

Volvulus is the twisting of a loop of bowel on the mesentery. Midgut volvulus occurs most often in the context of congenital intestinal malrotation, in which the small intestine is not normally fastened in place. This may only be clinically apparent on upper GI fluoroscopy when the duodenum and distal small bowel are seen to fill with contrast right of midline without crossing to the left upper quadrant (Fig. 15.9). More than half of patients found to have malrotation present symptomatically (the rest of such cases are discovered incidentally), and about half of the symptomatic patients present in the neonatal period with bilious vomiting caused by volvulus. Those presenting later often do not have bilious vomiting; the vomiting may be intermittent for years.

Volvulus is an extremely hazardous obstructing lesion. The luminal obstruction is closed at both ends, which leads to sepsis from rapidly proliferating and translocating bacteria. There is also vascular obstruction caused by the root of the mesentery getting twisted, which quickly produces ischemia of the small intestine. Even if volvulus is diagnosed and repaired promptly, massive intestinal resection may be necessary secondary to underlying necrosis; this produces short bowel syndrome. Because volvulus may be intermittent, it may produce episodic or

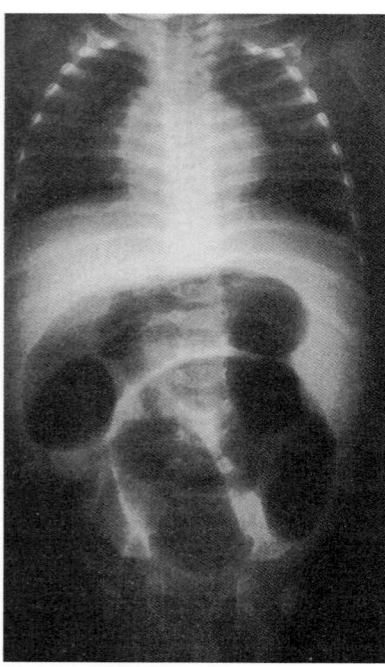

Fig. 15.8 Diffusely dilated bowel loops in intestinal obstruction.

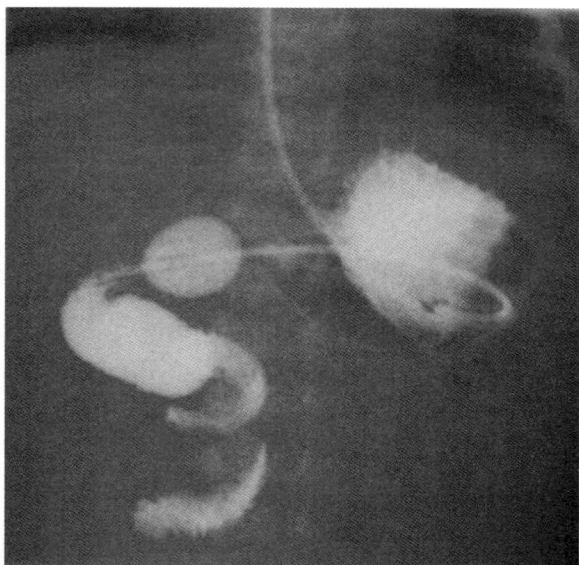

Fig. 15.10 Corkscrew sign: spiral appearance of the distal duodenum and proximal jejunum in the setting of midgut volvulus on contrast studies.

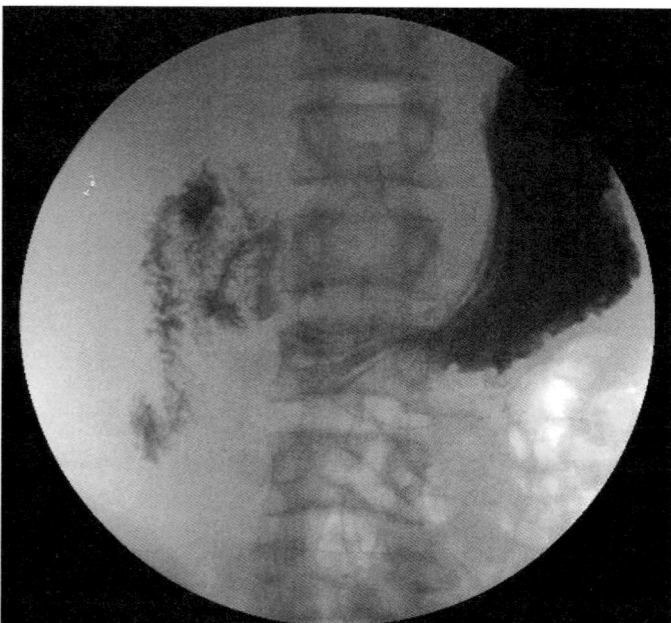

Fig. 15.9 Contrast fluoroscopy (upper gastrointestinal series) demonstrating malrotation. Note the small bowel fills with contrast all to the right of midline and does not cross over the left upper quadrant where the ligament of Treitz would be normally located.

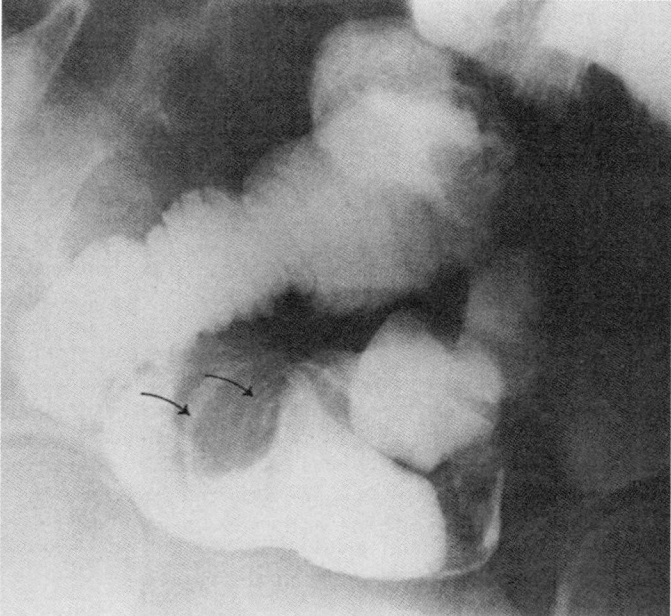

Fig. 15.11 Enteroenteric intussusception *(arrows)*.

chronic intermittent vomiting or nonspecific abdominal pain before a lethal event. Therefore, upper intestinal contrast radiographs should be considered in all patients with intermittent vomiting, and surgery must be performed if a malrotation is found (i.e., if the ligament of Treitz is not to the left of the spine), even if volvulus is not present at the time of the examination. In an infant in whom an ongoing volvulus is suspected, a contrast study may show a "volvulus/corkscrew" pattern (Fig. 15.10). In the sick infant or child in whom volvulus seems likely, surgery without contrast studies may be preferred. Surgery involves correction of any present volvulus, functional positioning of malrotation,

and lysis of potentially obstructing peritoneal (Ladd) bands that cross the abdomen.

Other types of volvulus not associated with malrotation include cecal, sigmoid, and transverse colonic volvulus. They are less common in children and less apt to produce short bowel syndrome, but they too may manifest with vomiting and result in death if untreated. Sigmoid volvulus is sometimes treated nonoperatively via endoscopic release.

Meckel Diverticulum

Meckel diverticulum is a small intestinal diverticulum that represents the fibrous remnant of the omphalomesenteric duct. Although painless GI bleed is the most common presentation, it can present as intestinal obstruction or inflammation (diverticulitis). It may lead to obstructive vomiting by causing intussusception (Fig. 15.11) or intestinal volvulus around the diverticular axis. It can get inflamed, leading to peritonitis (mimics appendicitis or peptic ulcer disease) and sometimes perforation, which can induce vomiting. The "rule of 2s" identifies characteristic findings: diverticula are present in 2% of the population; only 2% are symptomatic; the male:female ratio is 2:1; the diverticula occur within 2 feet of the ileocecal valve and are 2 inches long; there are 2 major types of heterotopic mucosa (gastric and pancreatic); and the condition is confused with 2 diseases (appendicitis and peptic ulcer). Treatment is surgical resection.

Intussusception

The normal function of the intestine is to constrict above and relax below an intraluminal bolus. When such a bolus (a "lead point") is attached to the intestinal wall, the propulsive activity of the intestine produces telescoping of proximal intestine (intussusceptum) into distal intestine (intussuscipiens), causing both luminal obstruction and mesenteric vascular compromise (see Fig. 15.11). Abdominal pain occurs in nearly all children with intussusception, whereas vomiting results in about 65%, and "currant-jelly stools" (from mucosal hemorrhage) occur in fewer than 20%. The pain is severe, crampy, and often contemporaneous with the vomiting. Between cramps, the child may be listless, may sleep, or may even play. Vomiting and bloody stools are more common in younger infants and in those with longer duration of symptoms. An abdominal mass is palpable in about 25% of patients.

The lead point of a symptomatic intussusception is usually ileal, producing intussusception that is ileocecal or ileocolonic. It is probable that prominent ileal lymphoid nodules provide the lead point for most young children presenting with intussusception, 66% of whom are younger than 2 years, with a peak incidence late in the first year of life. Other lead points to be considered are Meckel diverticulum, appendix, enteral duplication cyst, intraluminal polyp, lymphoma, hematoma from trauma, Henoch-Schönlein purpura, or inspissated stool in cystic fibrosis. Transient recurrent small bowel intussusception may also be a feature of celiac disease.

Ultrasound is the diagnostic modality of choice for intussusception in children as it has a high sensitivity and specificity. In stable children without signs of peritonitis, nonoperative reduction is the treatment of choice, preferably with pneumatic (gas) reduction enema. Approximately 10% of patients experience recurrences.

Superior Mesenteric Artery Syndrome

Superior mesenteric artery (SMA) syndrome is caused by extrinsic compression of the duodenum, which is trapped between the SMA anteriorly and the aorta posteriorly as the SMA crosses over the duodenum in the root of the mesentery. The angle at which the SMA comes out from the aorta is normally 25–60 degrees; in people with SMA syndrome, this angle is reduced. Loss of the mesenteric fat pad normally found between these two arteries is the most common cause of reduction in the angle. Most affected individuals have recently undergone significant weight loss (anorexia nervosa, severe burns, neoplastic disease, malabsorptive states). Certain orthopedic surgeries (scoliosis correction) and treatments (hip spica, full body casts) as well as abdominal surgeries (total proctocolectomy and ileal J-pouch anal anastomosis) can also trigger SMA syndrome.

Patients may present both acutely and insidiously, thus making the diagnosis challenging. Adolescents are most often affected with a female:male ratio of 3:2. It should be suspected in a patient with the aforementioned risk factor who presents with early satiety and postprandial abdominal pain, nausea, and bilious emesis. The pain is described as crampy and is relieved by prone or knee-chest positions.

The traditional diagnostic test with barium contrast can be used to visualize the common but nonspecific image showing dilated proximal duodenum with breakup of barium in the distal third of the duodenum. CT and MRA are the most valuable tests for diagnosing SMA syndrome as they are good at evaluating the aortomesenteric angle and provide other anatomic information. Nutritional rehabilitation, preferably by the enteral route via nasojejunal feeds, is the cornerstone of therapy and generally resolves SMA syndrome. The prone position may improve duodenal emptying. Surgery may be needed if there are chronic symptoms despite nutritional rehabilitation.

Constipation, Meconium Plug, and Anal Stenosis

These distal colonic problems produce obstipation primarily, but if they are severe and persistent, vomiting may result. Rectal examination provides the diagnosis. Enemas, laxatives, dietary changes, and behavioral modification are useful in treating constipation, whereas surgery is usually necessary to treat anal atresia or stenosis. Infants with meconium plug syndrome need clinical follow-up to monitor for the presence of coexistent Hirschsprung disease.

Gastrointestinal Dysmotility

Achalasia

Achalasia is an uncommon esophageal dysmotility disorder characterized by emesis of undigested food from the esophagus and history of dysphagia to solids and liquids. Concurrent weight loss is common. The etiology is unknown, but some cases are familial and in other cases it may be part of the triple A syndrome (achalasia, adrenocorticotropic hormone–resistant adrenal insufficiency, alacrima). In endemic areas, Chagas disease should be considered. In addition, achalasia has been associated with trisomy 21, congenital hypoventilation syndrome, and familial dysautonomia. Contrast swallow study or esophagogram and preferably esophageal manometry are needed to confirm diagnosis. The classic finding on manometry is insufficient relaxation of the LES and loss of esophageal peristalsis. Barium swallow demonstrates esophageal dilation, aperistalsis, poor emptying of contrast, and "bird-beak" appearance (Fig. 15.12). Nifedipine, sildenafil, and botulinum toxin have been reported to produce at least temporary clinical benefit in many patients. However, for sustained benefit, first-line therapy is surgical (Heller) myotomy or, in certain cases, pneumatic balloon dilation.

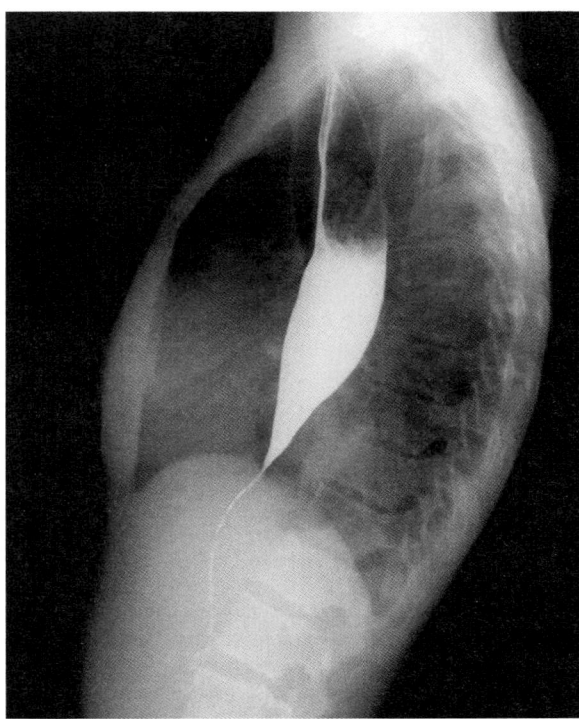

Fig. 15.12 Bird-beak appearance of distal esophagus seen in esophageal achalasia.

Gastroesophageal Reflux

Gastroesophageal reflux (GER) is defined as regurgitation of gastric contents into the esophagus with or without vomiting. GER is of particular importance because (1) it is the most common cause of "vomiting" in infants, (2) physiologic reflux must be distinguished from reflux necessitating evaluation and therapy, and (3) the practitioner must be vigilant to avoid misdiagnosing other infantile vomiting diseases as reflux.

Reflux typically is a benign feature in healthy infants as a result of weak LES tone, which improves and resolves in a predictable manner as a function of growth, development, acquiring upright positions, and introducing some solids in the diet. In these infants, regurgitation will be effortless and will not have associated failure to gain weight, feeding problems, or airway symptoms.

Gastroesophageal reflux disease (GERD) is defined as GER that leads to troublesome symptoms and/or complications (Table 15.11). Reflux may cause failure to gain weight resulting from regurgitation of caloric feedings, odynophagia from esophagitis, or parental reluctance to feed a recurrently spitting infant.

Infants with more problematic regurgitant reflux should undergo upper GI radiography and/or ultrasonography to rule out the possibility of anatomic causes such as malrotation and gastric outlet obstruction such as from hypertrophic pyloric stenosis. Endoscopy with biopsy is warranted in infants with anorexia and irritability who have failed optimal therapies. An older child with atopic history and symptoms of reflux and/or failure of acid suppression therapy needs consideration of endoscopy to rule out alternative causes such as eosinophilic esophagitis. A pH impedance study can be considered if persistent troublesome symptoms correlate with feedings/reflux events. However, such tests should be performed with caution as a significant degree of reflux is physiologic and there is insufficient normative data in infants and children.

Management of regurgitant reflux in infants is outlined in Figure 15.13. First-line therapy includes modifying feed volume and frequency according to age of infant to avoid overfeeding. Thickening of the feeds with 1 tablespoon of dry rice cereal per ounce of formula helps reduce symptoms. Breast-feeding mothers can pump breast milk and add thickeners. Positional therapy and probiotics are not universally recommended because of a lack of data on efficacy. If symptoms persist after the aforementioned measures, a 2–4-week empiric trial of a protein hydrolysate or elemental formula should be attempted for cow's milk protein allergy since there is a high degree of symptom overlap with GERD. Breast-feeding mothers will need to eliminate dairy from their diet. If symptoms do not respond to the aforementioned measures, a referral to a pediatric gastroenterologist is warranted. If timely referral is not possible, a 4–8-week, time-limited trial with an oral H_2-receptor antagonist or proton pump inhibitor (PPI) can be considered in infants. Given increased knowledge of side effects from chronic acid suppression and insufficient randomized controlled data to support its use, empiric acid suppression therapy for infants is not recommended based on expert consensus guidelines. As some benefit is demonstrated in older children with GERD, a short (4–8-week) diagnostic trial of acid suppression therapy can be justified. It is important to avoid long-term use when possible and to initiate a wean if symptoms improve. Refractory GERD is defined as symptoms that do not respond to 4–8 weeks of acid suppression therapy and requires exclusion of alternative diagnoses and evaluation of treatment efficacy.

The rare child who does not improve and develops nutritional, respiratory, or peptic complications from reflux may deserve evaluation for surgical fundoplication if all other therapies fail and excessive reflux is documented by pH impedance study (Fig. 15.14).

TABLE 15.11	**Common Signs and Symptoms of Gastroesophageal Reflux in Infants**
Symptoms	**Signs**
General	**General**
• Discomfort/irritability*	• Dental erosion†
• Failure to thrive	• Anemia
• Feeding refusal	**Gastrointestinal**
• Dystonic neck posturing (Sandifer syndrome)	• Esophagitis
	• Esophageal stricture†
Gastrointestinal	• Barrett esophagus†
• Recurrent regurgitation	**Airway**
• Hematemesis	• Apneic spells
• Dysphagia/odynophagia	• Asthma
Airway	• Recurrent otitis media
• Wheezing	• Recurrent pneumonia with aspiration
• Stridor	
• Cough	
• Hoarseness	

*If excessive irritability and pain is the single manifestation, then it is unlikely to be related to gastroesophageal reflux.
†In older children.
Adapted from Rosen R, Vandenplas Y, Singendonk M, et al. Pediatric Gastroesophageal Reflux Clinical Practice Guidelines: Joint Recommendations of the North American Society for Pediatric Gastroenterology, Hepatology, and Nutrition and the European Society for Pediatric Gastroenterology, Hepatology, and Nutrition. *J Pediatr Gastroenterol Nutr.* 2018;66(3):516–554.

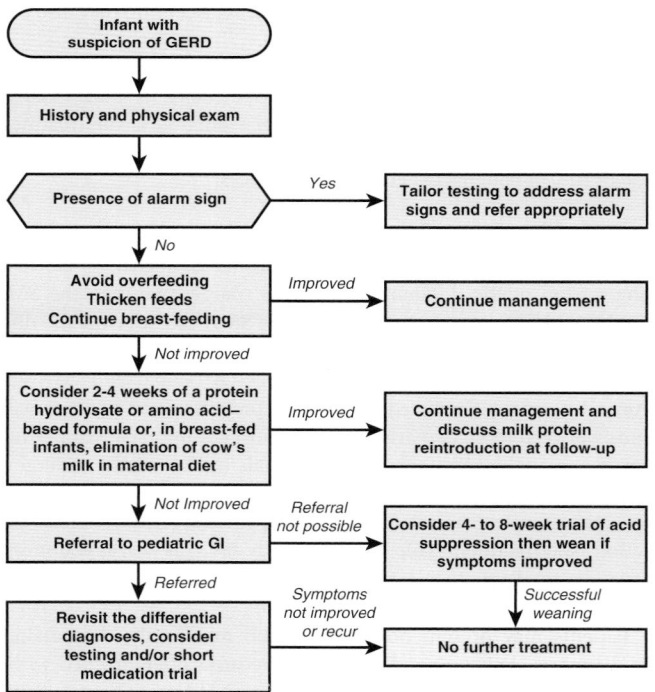

Fig. 15.13 Management of symptomatic infant with gastroesophageal reflux disease (GERD). (Modified from Rosen R, Vandenplas Y, Singendonk M, et al. Pediatric Gastroesophageal Reflux Clinical Practice Guidelines: Joint Recommendations of the North American Society for Pediatric Gastroenterology, Hepatology, and Nutrition and the European Society for Pediatric Gastroenterology, Hepatology, and Nutrition. *J Pediatr Gastroenterol Nutr.* 2018;66[3]:516–554, Fig. 6.)

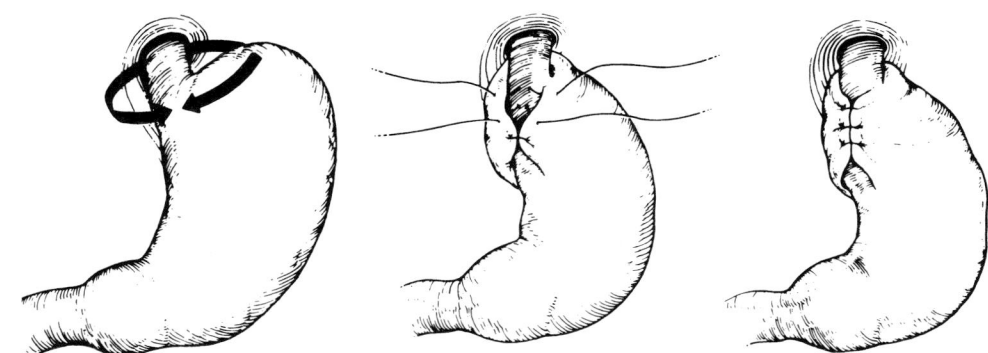

Fig. 15.14 Nissen fundoplication. Fundus is wrapped around the lower esophagus and secured with sutures. This anchors the lower esophageal sphincter below the diaphragm.

Gastroparesis

Gastroparesis is characterized by delayed transit of gastric contents into the duodenum in the absence of mechanical obstruction. It is suggested by the vomiting of food eaten hours earlier and accompanied by abdominal pain and nausea. Diabetic gastroparesis, secondary to autonomic neuropathy and gastric atony, is the classic example of this disorder but is rare in childhood. The etiology in pediatrics is often idiopathic but among the known causes, postinfectious gastroparesis is the most common. Respiratory and GI viruses are implicated, most notably rotavirus, norovirus, cytomegalovirus, Epstein-Barr virus, and varicella. Other etiologies of gastroparesis in children include autonomic nervous system (ANS) disorders, connective tissue (Ehlers-Danlos) or mitochondrial disorders, muscular dystrophies, inflammatory conditions (cow's milk protein allergy, celiac disease), critical illness, and medications (e.g., anticholinergics). Certain anatomic abnormalities (repaired congenital diaphragmatic hernia, intestinal malrotation) are associated with gastroparesis. An upper GI contrast study should be performed to rule out mechanical obstruction. The 4-hour gastric emptying scintigraphy using a radiolabeled solid meal is currently the gold standard for diagnosing gastroparesis. This test needs to be used with caution as there are no pediatric norms to interpret results against.

Pharmacotherapy with prokinetic medications (e.g., erythromycin, metoclopramide) along with dietary modification is the first line of treatment.

Ileus

Paralytic ileus is defined as functional obstruction caused by paralysis of intestinal muscles in response to various stimuli. The common causes of paralytic ileus are postoperative state, following an episode of infectious gastroenteritis, sepsis, peritonitis, or intestinal ischemia. Other causes of paralytic ileus are drugs (narcotics, laxative abuse, anticholinergics), electrolyte disturbances (hypokalemia, hypercalcemia), endocrinopathies (hypothyroidism), status post-chemo- or radiotherapy, or injuries (spinal fractures). Intestinal contents fail to progress, causing abdominal pain and vomiting. Typically, the bowel sounds are decreased or absent; there may be abdominal distention. Signs of ileus may follow signs of intestinal obstruction; in this context, ileus is an ominous sign. Treatment of ileus requires correction of any correctable provocative abnormalities and nasogastric tube decompression until normal peristalsis resumes.

Intestinal Pseudo-obstruction

Chronic pediatric intestinal pseudo-obstruction (PIPO) is a rare disorder defined by either continuous or intermittent symptoms of bowel obstruction in the absence of a lumen-occluding lesion (see Chapter 19). It represents severe GI dysmotility where coordinated peristalsis in the intestinal tract becomes altered or inefficient. Its chronicity sets it apart

from the far more common acute paralytic ileus. PIPO can be categorized into two broad categories: congenital and acquired, which has been further subdivided histologically as myopathic vs neuropathic types.

Most congenital subtypes are sporadic, while family history is present in 20–30%. The myopathic causes (10%) include myositis or muscle fibrosis secondary to collagen vascular disease (e.g., progressive systemic sclerosis), various muscular dystrophies, and familial visceral myopathies. The neuropathic causes (90%) include Hirschsprung disease, Chagas disease, diabetic and other autonomic neuropathies, multiple endocrine neoplasia, and familial visceral neuropathies.

The disorder may involve any part of or the entire luminal GI tract and occasionally (in up to 10% of patients) involves the urinary tract. Common symptoms of PIPO include abdominal pain and distension, nausea, vomiting, and constipation. Symptoms can worsen during acute exacerbations of pseudo-obstruction, which can be triggered by viral or bacterial infections, general anesthesia, psychological stress, and malnutrition. Nearly 65% of the children with PIPO present in infancy, with the very severe cases presenting in the neonatal period. Antenatal ultrasound may show polyhydramnios, megacystis, and distended bowel loops.

To accurately diagnose PIPO, imaging studies and manometry evaluation are generally required. Antroduodenal and colon manometry studies can evaluate the strength and coordination of contractions of the gastric antrum, small bowel, and colon. The main value of manometry testing is to confirm diagnosis/predict prognosis and to help differentiate between myopathic and neuropathic lesions. Histologic evaluation of full-thickness biopsies and genetic testing can aid in diagnosis. **Small intestinal bacterial overgrowth** is a common complication of chronically dilated bowel and is associated with steatorrhea and fat-soluble vitamin and vitamin B_{12} deficiency and can be treated with judicious use of antibiotics. PIPO patients are at increased risk of chronic malnutrition, which is contributed by recurrent vomiting, bacterial overgrowth–induced malabsorption, and intolerance to enteral feeds.

Promotility agents (metoclopramide, erythromycin, pyridostigmine) can be helpful, but pharmacotherapy is often ineffective. Intensive nutritional rehabilitation, via both enteral and parenteral routes, remains the cornerstone of therapy. Children with poor quality of life despite appropriate medical management or those who have developed complications of parenteral nutrition are candidates for intestinal transplantation.

Gastrointestinal Inflammation

Esophagitis

Esophagitis may be associated with vomiting in the setting of eosinophilic esophagitis (EoE), where patients may also experience nausea and/or dysphagia. With regard to reflux disease, esophagitis is secondary to vomiting.

Gastroenteritis

Gastroenteritis is a frequent cause of acute vomiting illness in childhood and frequently associated with diarrhea, abdominal pain, or fever. Rotavirus, especially in infants, is notable for its prominent vomiting, which often precedes the diarrhea. "Food poisoning" also produces vomiting and diarrhea, often caused by bacterially derived toxin. The novel coronavirus COVID-19 has also been associated with gastroenteritis. Microbiologic investigations may be considered in children with underlying chronic conditions or immunodeficiencies (e.g., oncologic diseases, inflammatory bowel disease, etc.), in those with severe symptoms or bloody diarrhea, or in those with prolonged symptoms in whom specific treatment is considered.

Treatment of acute gastroenteritis mandates attention to hydration and supportive care. Oral rehydration is feasible in many children with gastroenteritis, but a common error is to use clear liquids longer than 24 hours; this leaves nutritional needs unmet. Early refeeding in gastroenteritis is most successful when the food is low in fat and lactose and high in complex carbohydrates.

Acid Peptic Disease

Acid peptic disease includes gastritis, gastric ulcer, duodenitis, and duodenal ulcer. In contrast to adults, these disorders frequently cause vomiting in association with abdominal pain in pediatrics. The acidic gastric contents, which normally aid in digestion, become corrosive when there is an increase in acid production or a disruption of protective factors such as a mucous layer, a pH-neutral buffer zone, an epithelial layer, and a rich gastric blood supply. Defined causes for acid peptic disease include infections (*H. pylori* infection being the most well recognized), bile reflux gastritis, medication induced (nonsteroidal antiinflammatory agents, high-dose corticosteroids, etc.), and rare gastrin-secreting tumors (Zollinger-Ellison syndrome). Stress ulcers occur in the context of sepsis, burns, surgery, head trauma, and severe acute illness.

The optimal diagnostic method is endoscopy, with evaluation for *H. pylori* or elevated gastrin in appropriate cases. Acid suppression is the preferred treatment. *H. pylori* infections are treated with evolving regimens of triple antibiotics plus acid suppression drugs; eradication rate is approximately 85% for most treatments. Zollinger-Ellison syndrome is optimally treated by tumor resection and evaluation for related endocrine tumors; PPI treatment is helpful if complete tumor resection is impossible. Complications of acid peptic disease include GI bleeding, intestinal perforation, and gastric outlet obstruction.

Meckel Diverticulitis

In addition to presenting as GI bleeding or obstruction, Meckel diverticula may become inflamed and mimic appendicitis. Treatment is surgical and further information about Meckel diverticulum is discussed previously.

Mesenteric Adenitis

Mesenteric adenitis is often found on CT scans and refers to inflammation of lymph nodes in the mesentery. It is probably caused by viral (adenovirus, measles) or bacterial (*Yersinia enterocolitica*) infection, but the symptoms are similar enough to appendicitis that the diagnosis is usually not made before surgery. Ultrasonography can readily distinguish mesenteric adenitis from appendicitis.

Appendicitis

When vomiting occurs in appendicitis, it follows the periumbilical pain but may precede the localization of the pain to the McBurney point, two thirds of the way between the umbilicus and the right anterior iliac spine. Before perforation, there is only occasional vomiting. After perforation, the fever may be higher; the child lies still with the right hip flexed, and vomiting may be more frequent and feculent. In appendicitis, there is later vomiting, less diarrhea, fewer bowel sounds, and more rectal or rebound tenderness than in gastroenteritis. It is also associated with less diarrhea, less fever, and less leukocytosis than is bacterial enteritis, although *Yersinia*, in particular, has caused right lower quadrant pain closely mimicking appendicitis. Crohn disease is usually more chronic than is appendicitis but sometimes is diagnosed by surgeons at the time of appendectomy based on serosal changes to the bowel.

Inflammatory Bowel Disease

Crohn disease, in particular, may produce vomiting on occasion, particularly when obstructing intestinal strictures develop. Other extraintestinal manifestations of Crohn disease also, in rare cases, produce vomiting.

Allergic Enteropathy, Eosinophilic Gastroenteropathy, and Eosinophilic Esophagitis

Vomiting is a frequent response to ingestion of allergens and may occur as early as the first weeks of life in infants with allergy (non–immunoglobulin E [IgE] or IgE mediated) to cow's milk or soy and in older children as potentially allergenic foods are introduced. There may be associated diarrhea and hematochezia and, in some children, urticaria or other systemic signs of allergy. A strong family history of allergic disorders is suggestive. Laboratory studies may show peripheral blood eosinophilia and positive radioallergosorbent test (serum-specific IgE) to individual foods.

In infants, the simplest diagnostic test is a change to a protein hydrolysate or elemental formula for at least 2 weeks. In breast-fed infants, the mother should start a strict dairy-free diet. If the vomiting (and other symptoms) resolves, it is generally not necessary to rechallenge for diagnosis, but empirical treatment can be continued for several months. Because infants usually outgrow these formula protein intolerances between 10 and 24 months of age, a normal diet can later be introduced as tolerated. Older children with vomiting that represents IgE-mediated food allergy or eosinophilic gastroenteropathy are less likely to outgrow the allergy over time.

IgE-mediated food allergy has a rapid onset of symptoms after exposure to allergic food and reaction can vary from mild to severe, with anaphylaxis being the most severe form. The diagnosis of IgE-mediated food allergy requires a history of classic clinical symptoms and evidence of food-specific IgE by either skin-prick or serum-specific IgE testing. **Eosinophilic GI diseases,** on the other hand, are a group of chronic inflammatory conditions characterized histologically by eosinophilic infiltration of the GI tract and varying degree of villous injury. It is composed of EoE, eosinophilic gastritis, eosinophilic gastroenteritis, or eosinophilic colitis. Diagnosis is made by endoscopy with biopsies. EoE may occur independently of eosinophilic gastroenteropathy and should be kept in mind, particularly with patients manifesting dysphagia or reflux symptoms poorly responsive to standard therapy. At endoscopy, the esophageal mucosa displays a ringed or furrowed appearance with granularity (Fig. 15.15), with pathology specimens confirming a high eosinophil cell count.

If sensitization to particular foods is identified through radioallergosorbent (serum-specific IgE testing) or skin testing, an elimination diet is employed; patients with prohibitive numbers of food allergies may require an amino acid–based diet. Steroids may be necessary for children with negative investigation findings for food allergy or for whom compliance with a restricted diet is problematic.

Similarly, **celiac disease** (i.e., gluten enteropathy) may present with chronic vomiting in association with other GI symptoms, most commonly abdominal pain, bloating, and altered stool habits. Diagnosis is made by serum tissue transglutaminase (TTG) and total IgA level (as IgA-deficient individuals may have a falsely normal TTG) and confirmed by endoscopic duodenal biopsies.

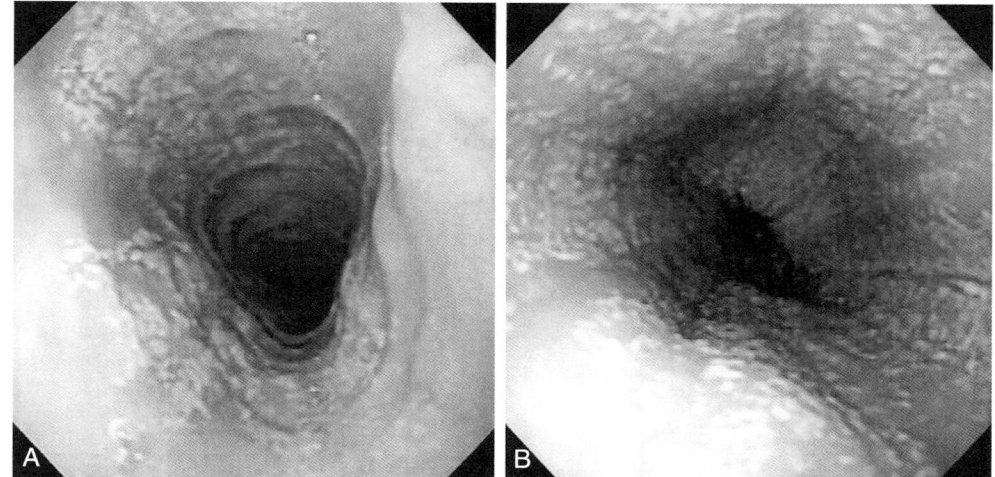

Fig. 15.15 Endoscopic appearance of eosinophilic esophagitis, demonstrating concentric rings in proximal esophagus *(A)* and granularity with mucosal furrowing in distal esophagus *(B)*.

Functional Gastrointestinal Disorders

Functional GI disorders, also known as disorders of gut-brain interaction, are highly prevalent and among the most common conditions referred to GI subspecialists. In the absence of specific biomarkers or tests, functional GI disorders are diagnosed clinically when, after appropriate medical evaluation, symptoms cannot be attributed to another medical condition. They are thought to arise from aberrant gut-brain signaling as a result of complex interplay of various biopsychosocial factors in genetically susceptible individuals. Functional nausea and vomiting disorders form a separate category defined by the Rome IV expert consensus criteria. This category includes CVS, functional nausea and functional vomiting, rumination syndrome, and aerophagia.

Cyclic Vomiting Syndrome

CVS is a chronic, potentially disabling condition marked by a history of three or more bouts of intense, acute nausea and vomiting that may last hours or days, punctuated by entirely symptom-free intervals lasting weeks to months (Table 15.12). Work-up, which may ultimately include endoscopy and imaging studies of the GI tract, urinary tract, and brain, reveals no evidence of significant underlying primary disease. Mean age of presentation is 5 years. CVS has a distinctive pattern of emesis, which is essential for diagnosis (see Fig. 15.15). The vomiting episodes are discrete, recurrent, and relentless as well as stereotypical in each patient as to time of onset (often early morning), duration (hours or days), and symptoms (pallor, listlessness). Four phases are described: the prodromal phase, the emetic phase, the recovery phase, and the interepisodic or asymptomatic phase. The prodromal phase is characterized by nausea, pallor, diaphoresis, fatigue, insomnia, and a sense of impending attack. This is the optimal time to intervene with rescue therapies to prevent progression to the emetic cascade. The emetic phase heralds with emesis that is frequent, is forceful, may contain bile or blood, and is associated with intractable nausea, which is relieved only with deep sleep. Other features include listlessness, pallor, drooling, diarrhea, dizziness, and diaphoresis. About 50% of cases demonstrate photophobia and phonophobia, and a majority are associated with abdominal pain. CVS is associated with poor quality of life with as many as 58% of children with CVS requiring intravenous fluids during episodes and an average of 10 visits to the emergency department annually. An inciting event such as an infection,

TABLE 15.12 Diagnostic Criteria for Cyclic Vomiting Syndrome

At least 5 episodes overall or a minimum of 3 episodes noted in a 6-mo period
Recurrent episodes of vomiting and nausea lasting 1 hr to 10 days and occurring at least 1 wk apart
Stereotypical pattern and symptoms in the individual patient
Vomiting during episodes occurring at least 4 times per hr for at least 1 hr
Returning to baseline health between episodes
Not attributable to another disorder

From Li BUK, Kovacic K. Vomiting and nausea. In: Wyllie R, Hyams JS, Kay M, eds. *Pediatric Gastrointestinal and Liver Disease.* 5th ed. Philadelphia: Elsevier; 2016:98.

emotional excitement, negative stress, or lack of sleep can be identified in 80% of patients.

The pathophysiologic process of CVS remains speculative at this time but, at least in a subset, may overlap with that of migraine disorders. One hypothesis purports that stress-initiated release of corticotropin-releasing hormone leads to cascading production of substances, such as adrenocorticotropic hormone, antidiuretic hormone, histamine, and catecholamines, which in turn mediates the signs and symptoms. Some children may harbor subclinical defects in mitochondrial fatty acid oxidation metabolism or neuronal ion channel function that heighten their susceptibility to attacks when confronted by the increased cellular energy needs created by a physiologic or emotional stressor. A baseline ANS dysfunction is also reported in the literature. Although CVS is well recognized, the provider needs to remain vigilant to other treatable, "look-alike" organic conditions. Reported cases of organic disease mislabeled as "cyclic vomiting" have included intermittent intussusception or volvulus caused by enteric duplication, diverticulum, or malrotation; increased intracranial pressure; toxic or metabolic disease; obstructive uropathy; porphyria; and familial dysautonomia. Medications potentially useful in CVS prophylaxis and in treatment of acute episodes are listed in Table 15.13.

Abdominal Migraine

Abdominal migraine is a periodic syndrome similar to CVS and included in the Rome IV functional abdominal pain disorders category (in addition to functional dyspepsia, irritable bowel syndrome, and functional abdominal pain—not otherwise specified). Abdominal

TABLE 15.13 Treatment of Cyclic Vomiting Syndrome

Rescue and Abortive Pharmacotherapy

Antimigraine	Sumatriptan intranasal 10–20 mg or 3–6 mg SC (>5 yr), 25 mg PO (>17 yr) at onset of symptoms and may repeat once *SE: chest and neck burning, coronary vasospasm, headache*
Antiemetic	Ondansetron 0.2–0.3 mg/kg per dose q4–6h IV/PO/rectal/topical *SE: headache, drowsiness, dry mouth*
	Aprepitant 3-day regimen: 125, 80, 80 mg one q.d. at onset Fosaprepitant 3–4 mg/kg (max 115 mg) IV day 1 followed by 80 mg aprepitant on day 2, 3 *SE: fatigue, dizziness, diarrhea*
Sedatives	Lorazepam 0.05–0.1 mg/kg per dose q6h IV/PO *SE: sedation, respiratory depression*
	Chlorpromazine 0.5–1 mg/kg per dose q6h IV/PO *SE: drowsiness, hypotension, seizures*
	Diphenhydramine 1.25 mg/kg per dose q6h IV/PO *SE: hypotension, sedation, dizziness*
Analgesics	Ketorolac 0.5–1 mg/kg per dose q6h IV/PO *SE: gastrointestinal bleeding, dyspepsia*

Prophylactic Pharmacotherapy

Antimigraine	Amitriptyline, start at 0.2 mg/kg, advance to 1–1.5 mg/kg q.h.s. First choice ≥5 yr old *SE: QT prolongation (monitor EKG), sedation, anticholinergic*
	Propranolol 0.25–1 mg/kg/day divided b.i.d or t.i.d. *SE: hypotension, bradycardia (monitor resting heart rate), fatigue*
	Cyproheptadine 0.25–0.5 mg/kg/day divided b.i.d. or q.h.s. First choice <5 yr old *SE: sedation, weight gain, anticholinergic*
Anticonvulsant	Topiramate titrate to 1.5–2.0 mg/kg/day divided b.i.d. *SE: appetite suppression, cognitive dysfunction, renal stones* Alternative: levetiracetam, valproate, carbamazepine, gabapentin
NK-1 antagonist	Aprepitant 125 mg PO twice weekly (>60 kg); 80 mg (40–60 kg); 40 mg (<40 kg) *SE: fatigue, dizziness, diarrhea*
Mitochondrial supplements	L-carnitine 50–100 mg/kg ≤2 g/day divided b.i.d. *SE: diarrhea, fishy body odor*
	Coenzyme Q10 10 mg/kg/divided b.i.d. ≤600 mg/day
	Riboflavin 10 mg/kg/day divided b.i.d. ≤400 mg/day

b.i.d., twice daily; IV, intravenously; max, maximum; PO, orally; q4–6h, every 4–6 hr; q6h, every 6 hr; q.d., once a day; q.h.s., each bedtime; SC, subcutaneously; SE, side effects; t.i.d., three times daily.

Data from Li BU, Lefevre F, Chelimsky GG, et al. North American Society for Pediatric Gastroenterology, Hepatology, and Nutrition consensus statement on the diagnosis and management of cyclic vomiting syndrome. *J Pediatr Gastroenterol Nutr.* 2008;47:379–393. Sunku B, Li BUK. Cyclic vomiting syndrome. In: Guandalini S, ed. *Textbook of Pediatric Gastroenterology and Nutrition.* London: Taylor and Francis Group; 2004:289 -302; Abell TL, Adams KA, Boles RG, et al. Cyclic vomiting syndrome in adults. *Neurogastroenterol Motil.* 2008;20:269–284; Van Calcar SC, Harding CO, Wolff JA. L-carnitine administration reduces number of episodes in cyclic vomiting syndrome. *Clin Pediatr (Phila).* 2002; 41:171–174; and Li BU. Cyclic vomiting syndrome. *Curr Treat Options Gastroenterol.* 2000; 3:395–402.

migraine is characterized by paroxysmal episodes of intense periumbilical, midline, or diffuse abdominal pain. The episodes are associated with intense nausea, vomiting, anorexia, pallor, headache, or photophobia. A pathophysiologic overlap with CVS and migraine headache is proposed based on similar symptom pattern and response to therapy. When these abdominal symptoms coexist with head pain, a diagnosis of migraine headache is made. Similarly, if the predominant symptom is emesis, CVS is the most accurate diagnostic term. Although there is a high degree of overlap, the predominant and most consistent symptom during episodes defines the illness. Most evolve into typical migraine headaches during preteen years, and by age 18 years, 75% have transitioned their symptoms for migraine headaches. Usually, isolated abdominal migraine attacks occur suddenly, last an hour to days, and, as in CVS, are consistent in character within the same individual. There is usually a family history of migraine, and patients are asymptomatic between attacks. A personal history of car (motion) sickness may be present. Therapy is similar to CVS. Abortive therapy is composed of triptans, while prophylactic antimigraine medications such as propranolol, cyproheptadine, or amitriptyline often help prevent attacks.

Functional Vomiting

Functional vomiting refers to chronic, recurrent vomiting at least once per week that is not self-induced and occurs in the absence of eating disorders, major psychiatric diseases, or other medical diseases. The absence of organic causes illustrates the prominent influence that cortical and psychologic inputs may have in stimulating nausea and vomiting. The proposed features of functional vomiting include chronicity, association with stress, absence of cachexia or anorexia, and commonly relief by hospitalization or higher-level care. An example would be of a child who involuntarily vomits every time before a school test or on Monday mornings due to heightened anxiety but is otherwise well and recovers when the stressor is absent. Although a clear relationship with gastric motor disorders such as gastroparesis has not been established due to lack of diagnostic tests, these conditions may overlap and complicate management. Close evaluation of specific clinical features such as emesis of undigested food and significant postprandial distress as occurs in gastroparesis is essential prior to committing to a diagnosis of functional vomiting.

Rumination Syndrome

Rumination syndrome is characterized by repeated, effortless food regurgitation during or soon after eating (generally within 15 minutes), followed by rechewing, reswallowing, or spitting out the regurgitant. This syndrome can be disabling and lead to medical complications (weight loss, electrolyte imbalance) and, even more so, significant functional limitations and psychosocial stigma (school absenteeism, avoiding social eating). The regurgitation behavior is a habit/reflex that arises as a conditioned response to certain stimuli (e.g., particular foods, environments, activities). It is hypothesized that prior to the act of regurgitation, patients feel a premonitory urge often described as a visceral sensation (e.g., abdominal pressure). To relieve the urge, the patient regurgitates by contracting the abdominal wall muscles. Once the material is brought up, the premonitory urge temporarily subsides, leading to relaxation of abdominal muscles. Other clinical features include general lack of retching and nausea as well as absence of symptoms during sleep. Patients sometimes recognize an inciting event retrospectively (e.g., a respiratory or GI infection, psychosocial stressor, or medical procedure). The disorder tends to cluster more in patients with underlying anxiety, adolescent girls, and children with autism spectrum disorders. In infants and intellectually disabled individuals, rumination can have a positive function of alleviating anxiety and is recognized as a self-soothing mechanism. Treatment may be challenging and focuses on behavioral therapy of unlearning the conditioned rumination behavior. Successful therapy often requires multidisciplinary care in specialized treatment centers.

Functional Dyspepsia

Functional dyspepsia is characterized by chronic postprandial fullness, early satiety, and epigastric pain or burning. Although part of the functional abdominal pain disorders category, postprandial nausea is often severe and patients may have intermittent emesis. The clinical features overlap significantly with those of gastroparesis and these conditions may be difficult to distinguish. However, dyspeptic patients tend to have postprandial emesis in closer temporal association with the meal as opposed to gastroparesis, where emesis is generally delayed.

Gastrointestinal Ischemia and Vascular Insufficiency

Some of the causes of GI ischemia can produce perforation, peritonitis, and death quite rapidly. A high degree of suspicion is useful because the signs are nonspecific.

Vasculitis

Inflammation of the mesenteric vessels is uncommon but may cause GI complaints, including vomiting, abdominal pain, diarrhea, and GI bleeding. Henoch-Schönlein purpura is the most common pediatric vasculitis. Systemic lupus erythematosus, dermatomyositis, polyarteritis nodosa, adenosine deaminase-2 (ADA-2) deficiency, and other hypersensitivity vasculitides are occasional causes. The most diagnostic sign of Henoch-Schönlein purpura is the palpable purpuric rash, typically found on the buttocks, posterior legs, and feet in 97% of patients. However, because the vomiting or hematemesis and the nonspecific abdominal pain (found in nearly 90%) may precede the rash, the diagnosis may initially be obscure. Repeated examination of the skin of a child with persistent vomiting and pain is therefore useful, particularly when the GI symptoms are accompanied by polyarthritis, which occurs in 65% of such patients. Platelet function and coagulation studies are normal; hematuria is often present. Steroids may shorten the abdominal pain by 1 or 2 days, but they might also mask symptoms of accompanying intussusception or perforation.

Mesenteric Ischemia

The mesenteric arteries may be occluded by emboli from a diseased heart or from thrombi formed locally. Nonocclusive ischemia may be caused by poor cardiac output, hypotension, dehydration, or endotoxemia. Mesenteric venous occlusion is very rare. Severe, crampy, diffuse abdominal pain may be accompanied by vomiting, diarrhea, or constipation. If no interventions are taken, the crampy pain becomes continuous and gangrene, peritonitis, and shock set in. Acute mesenteric arterial occlusion may be preceded by chronic symptoms of "abdominal angina," which are episodes of several hours of crampy pain beginning about 20 minutes after meals. Such premonitory symptoms in suggestive settings (heart disease, inherited thrombophilia) should receive serious attention and require mesenteric and celiac angiography and emergency surgery.

Hepatobiliary Disorders

Hepatitis

The presence of acute viral hepatitis is usually suspected in patients who have jaundice, but up to 50% of patients with hepatitis A are anicteric, and even those in whom jaundice develops have a pre-icteric prodrome lasting up to a week. In children with acute hepatitis, therefore, the presenting symptom may be vomiting, another reason for including liver enzymes in the screening evaluation of the ill-appearing vomiting child. The vomiting is often accompanied by fatigue, fever, headache, rhinorrhea, sore throat, and cough.

The findings of serum antigens and antibodies to hepatitis viruses establish the diagnosis. Acute hepatitis with vomiting is treated symptomatically. Management also includes watching for the ominous findings of progressive encephalopathy, ascites, and coagulopathy.

Biliary Colic and Cholecystitis

Biliary obstruction produces vomiting and abdominal pain in children. Biliary colic is visceral pain resulting from transient obstruction of the cystic duct, usually by a gallstone. Biliary colic produces several hours of steady, vaguely localized pain, often in the right upper quadrant; most patients also have vomiting. Episodes of biliary colic commonly recur at unpredictable intervals, from weeks to months. Acute cholecystitis may ensue if the obstruction persists and leads to inflammation of the gallbladder. The pain may localize more clearly to the right upper quadrant and may radiate to the back or shoulder. There may be fever or mild jaundice. Serum alanine aminotransferase, aspartate aminotransferase, γ-glutamyl transpeptidase, alkaline phosphatase, and bilirubin levels may be elevated. In both biliary colic and acute cholecystitis, abdominal films and ultrasonography may disclose stones or gallbladder thickening. Common bile duct stones may produce concurrent elevations of liver enzymes and pancreatic enzymes. Recurrent biliary colic and cholecystitis are managed by cholecystectomy, which can be performed laparoscopically in many children. Endoscopic removal of common bile duct stones is also possible, although it does not prevent recurrence.

Pancreatitis

Pancreatitis is usually associated with epigastric abdominal pain, which may radiate to the back and may have associated emesis. Elevated serum amylase and lipase levels usually confirm the diagnosis.

Gynecologic and Urologic Disorders

Pyelonephritis

High fever, chills, nausea, vomiting, and, less often, diarrhea develop rapidly. There may be symptoms of cystitis with dysuria, frequency, urgency, and suprapubic pain. Costovertebral angle tenderness focuses the diagnosis to the urinary tract. The UA shows pyuria and bacteriuria, and the hemogram shows leukocytosis. Treatment is with antibiotics.

Ureteropelvic Junction Obstruction and Hydronephrosis

Ureteropelvic junction obstruction is the most common congenital anomaly affecting the urinary tract and is often detected on antenatal ultrasound. It is more common in males and 60–90% cases are unilateral. It is caused by intrinsic stenosis of the proximal ureter at the ureteropelvic junction and less commonly by an extrinsic compression (aberrant accessory renal artery).

Congenital cases are usually diagnosed in the first year of life (usually on the basis of a renal hydronephrotic mass or urinary tract infection). About 10–30% of affected older children present with intermittent, acute painful episodes referred to as "Dietl crisis" that are characterized by flank or periumbilical pain, which is frequently accompanied by vomiting. Given the episodic nature, the clinical presentation may mimic CVS.

Typically, symptoms commence in the evening after an increased fluid intake, although the hyperhydration history is often unclear. The child's pain and vomiting usually remit spontaneously in several hours, as dehydration gradually relieves the renal pelvic distention. Superimposed unilateral urinary tract infection may cause additional findings of fever, failure to thrive, and pyuria. Ultrasonography at the time of an episode demonstrates hydronephrosis and provides the diagnosis. Once hydronephrosis is confirmed, diuretic renography (radionuclide scan) is ordered to assess the degree of obstruction as well as the level of renal function. The treatment is surgical.

Renal Colic

Passage of a renal stone usually causes more pain than vomiting. Lateralized colicky pain, hematuria, and confirmatory radiologic studies assist the diagnosis.

Dysmenorrhea, Endometriosis, and Pelvic Inflammatory Disease

These gynecologic disorders manifest with lower abdominal pain but only occasionally with vomiting. Association with menses or vaginal discharge aids the diagnosis. Cervical motion exacerbates the pain in pelvic inflammatory disease.

Ovarian Torsion

Torsion of a normal ovary occasionally occurs in girls of any age, probably caused by laxity of adnexal supports. Repeated attacks of crampy, lower abdominal pain culminate in a final acute episode with severe retching and vomiting, an enlarged ovarian mass, and eventual signs of peritonitis. Leukocytosis may be accompanied by fever. The location of the pain suggests the diagnosis, and the treatment is surgical.

Hyperemesis Gravidarum

Hyperemesis gravidarum is a severe and prolonged form of nausea and vomiting thought to be caused by increased level of circulating β-human chorionic gonadotropin (β-HCG) during early pregnancy. All pubertal adolescent females with symptoms should be tested for pregnancy.

Testicular Torsion

Testicular torsion is a vascular emergency. It is readily diagnosed by the site of pain; surgical treatment is required.

Respiratory Disorders

Sinusitis, Pharyngitis, and Otitis

Sinusitis may induce chronic, unexplained vomiting. The vomiting is more apt to occur in the morning and must be differentiated from serious intracranial processes. It is usually characterized by a cough-vomit cycle. Sinus tenderness and sinus CT scans suggest the diagnosis, and a successful trial of antibiotic therapy confirms it. Less often, pharyngitis or otitis media may manifest acutely with nonspecific vomiting.

Pneumonia

Emesis along with respiratory signs/symptoms may be a manifestation of pneumonia. As pneumonia can also be caused by vomiting secondary to aspiration, it is important to consider the direction of causality in children with pneumonia and vomiting. Aspiration of vomitus is particularly likely to occur in the context of obtundation or other neurologic dysfunction.

Central Nervous System Disorders

Increased Intracranial Pressure

Increased intracranial pressure (ICP) could be secondary to a brain parenchymal lesion (e.g., tumor), vascular malformations, hydrocephalus (e.g., Arnold-Chiari malformation, shunt malfunction), or central nervous system infection or be idiopathic (e.g., pseudotumor cerebri). It presents with headaches, vomiting, diplopia, and irritability. The vomiting is typically described as projectile, not associated with retching, and occurs more commonly upon awakening.

A careful neurologic and ophthalmologic examination may show decreased visual acuity, visual field defects, papilledema, and sixth cranial nerve palsy. General exam should include measurement of blood pressure, occipitofrontal head circumference, and body mass index

(BMI). Relevant radiologic studies (CT or MR scans) should help the examiner make the diagnosis.

Pseudotumor cerebri (meaning "false brain tumor"), also known as idiopathic intracranial hypertension, is the presence of high ICP in the absence of any space-occupying lesion. It is diagnosed by the presence of high opening cerebrospinal fluid (CSF) pressure on lumbar puncture and an otherwise normal CSF analysis and neuroimaging. It is almost always associated with papilledema. Pseudotumor cerebri is more common in obese adolescent females. In most cases, the etiology is unidentifiable, but at times, a secondary cause may be identified. Secondary causes include medication induced (tetracyclines, oral contraceptive pills, chemotherapeutic agents, steroids), endocrine disorders such as hypoparathyroidism, Addison disease, growth hormone therapy, and nutritional disorders such as hypo- or hypervitaminosis A as well as refeeding syndrome. Optic atrophy and visual impairment are the most serious long-term complications. Underlying causes, if identified, should be treated (weight loss, discontinuing medication). Acetazolamide (carbonic anhydrase inhibitor) is an effective medication and works by decreasing CSF production. In some cases, removal of CSF by repeated lumbar puncture may be necessary to reduce ICP and resolve symptoms.

Occlusion or infection of a ventriculoperitoneal shunt may produce vomiting on a neurologic basis, whereas the intraabdominal end of the shunt may provoke intestinal obstruction by volvulus, adhesions, or loculations. These possibilities must be kept in mind for the vomiting patient with a shunt.

Abdominal Epilepsy

Abdominal epilepsy is an uncommon cause of recurrent abdominal pain. It is characterized by paroxysmal episodes of abdominal pain, diverse GI complaints (e.g., nausea, vomiting, diarrhea, bloating), and central nervous system manifestations such as headache, dizziness, confusion, or temporary blindness. Although symptoms overlap strongly with those of abdominal migraines, patients with abdominal epilepsy have definite EEG abnormalities (generally the temporal area) and favorable response to anticonvulsant therapy.

Vestibular Disorders, Motion Sickness

Motion sickness is a common experience. Vestibular disorders produce similar symptoms. Because of the symptoms of nausea, nystagmus, vertigo, and dizziness, the diagnosis is usually obvious. Acute unilateral vestibular neuritis is a common diagnosis in children and occurs in association with respiratory viral infections and is self-limited. Antihistamines and anticholinergics are particularly useful for motion sickness.

Psychobehavioral Disorders

Eating Disorders

Anorexia and bulimia nervosa are eating disorders associated with purging behavior such as self-induced vomiting and laxative abuse. Malnutrition and electrolyte imbalance associated with eating disorders can negatively impact gastric motility and intestinal transit, which in turn can bolster typical symptoms of eating disorders such as loss of appetite, constipation, and bloating and therefore may benefit from prokinetic agents.

Psychiatric Disorders

GI symptoms including recurrent vomiting are not uncommon manifestations of underlying psychiatric disorders including generalized anxiety, depression, bipolar disease, obsessive-compulsive disorder, and post-traumatic stress disorder. A careful history including trauma and abuse screening is essential to help differentiate a psychiatric etiology from anxiety and stress related to an unresolved medical condition.

Munchausen by Proxy

Although rare, providers should remain vigilant to the possibility of Munchausen syndrome by proxy in cases of refractory vomiting along with other nonspecific GI symptoms and absence of findings. This is a mental health disorder in which a caregiver fabricates or causes illness in a child. Given the paucity of diagnostic tests and biomarkers for many functional and motility disorders of the GI tract, GI complaints are among the most common complaints reported in Munchausen by proxy. Red flags include an excessive number of normal investigations and procedures.

Management

Psychiatric and psychology consultation and therapy are often needed for eating disorders, rumination, functional vomiting, and psychiatric causes of recurrent emesis. Principles of behavior modification such as stress reduction techniques, cognitive-behavioral therapy, and hypnotherapy have proven beneficial. Biofeedback techniques such as diaphragmatic breathing have a therapeutic role in rumination syndrome.

Nasogastric or nasojejunal feedings can be used to guarantee nutritional rehabilitation if voluntary oral nutrition is not readily reestablished. Such tube feedings may also provide the child with the incentive to return to oral nutrition. Refeeding syndrome should be monitored for.

Metabolic Disorders

Metabolic diseases that cause vomiting are difficult to diagnose because they are both rare and diverse. Their diagnosis and treatment, however, are crucial because of the potential for severe morbidity and death and their amenability to treatment. They are also important because of their relevance to genetic counseling as most metabolic disorders are hereditary on an autosomal recessive basis. Situations that should prompt consideration of metabolic diseases are listed in Table 15.8. The screening studies (see Table 15.7) should be done while the child is symptomatic.

Poisonings and Drugs

Most ingested poisons, and some absorbed by inhalation, skin contact, or intravenous administration, induce vomiting, which can be seen as a physiologic protection against harmful substances. Symptoms and signs of some of the most common pediatric poisonings along with laboratory findings and treatment are indicated in Table 15.14. Acute known poisonings, either accidental or intentional, are a management rather than diagnostic problem and a Poison Control Center or other toxicology resources are helpful.

Initial diagnostic evaluation can be directed by a careful search of the environment for poisonous items and by toxicology screens on blood, urine, vomitus, and stool; these materials should not be discarded. A few agents, such as lead, cause chronic poisoning, manifested by vomiting, among other symptoms. Since it may be particularly difficult to suspect and treat these poisonings, an index of suspicion of poisoning is important in the chronically vomiting child. **Cannabinoid (marijuana) hyperemesis syndrome** is often seen in a previously well adolescent (no prior history of emesis or CVS), who is a chronic (~ daily) heavy user of marijuana. Nausea and abdominal discomfort may precede the acute onset of emesis characterized by intense and frequent episodes often relieved by taking multiple warm showers. It resembles CVS and many patients have been misdiagnosed with CVS.

Hematemesis

Hematemesis is vomiting of blood, which may be obviously red or have the appearance of coffee grounds (see Chapter 16). The source of bleeding is usually the upper GI tract proximal to the ligament of Treitz. A rapid initial assessment of the actively bleeding child is mandatory and includes checking circulation, airway, and breathing while establishing intravenous access. A quick focused history of bleeding disorders, liver disease, GI diseases, and ingestion of medications, especially nonsteroidal antiinflammatory drugs, or foreign bodies should be taken. On exam the presence of pallor and orthostatic changes could point toward significant blood loss, while presence of jaundice and hepatosplenomegaly suggests chronic liver disease. Endoscopic evaluation and therapy are often needed for children with hematemesis. Important causes of hematemesis are listed in Table 15.15.

Overall, peptic ulcer disease secondary to *H. pylori* is the most common cause of hematemesis in children. Etiologies such as stress gastritis, vascular malformation, and coagulopathies are common in all age groups. In newborns, swallowed maternal blood (uterine, breast milk), trauma secondary to suction of nasogastric tube, and necrotizing enterocolitis need to be considered. In preschool children, peptic ulcer disease, foreign body, and caustic ingestion are important causes, while in older children and adolescents, premalignant lesions such as Barrett esophagus, peptic ulcers, medication-induced gastritis/ulcers, and Mallory-Weiss tear should be considered. Variceal bleeding is uncommon but serious. Gastric vascular malformations are rare, may lead to copious bleeding, and may be difficult to diagnose. Duplications are lined by gastric mucosa in 30% of affected patients. If they are located above the ligament of Treitz, they may cause hematemesis. Obstructive lesions such as pyloric stenosis and antral webs are occasionally associated with hematemesis. The metabolic and toxic (iron, salicylates, theophylline, corrosives, isopropyl alcohol, mushroom poisoning) causes of hematemesis should be kept in mind.

Therapy of hematemesis includes, as needed, correction of any abnormalities of coagulation: stabilization of hemodynamic status and direct attention to the bleeding site by hemostasis endoscopically (e.g., heater probe, injection therapy) or surgically. Reduction of gastric acid secretion pharmacologically is useful in virtually all cases of hematemesis and carries minimal risk.

Other Causes of Vomiting

Chemotherapy

Chemotherapy causes predictable vomiting, which is usually not a diagnostic but a management problem. It may be complicated by anticipatory vomiting. The theories hypothesized for chemotherapy-induced vomiting are direct GI mucosal insult leading to release of serotonin or activation of receptors located in the area postrema by the circulating drug. Factors known to increase the incidence of chemotherapy-induced vomiting include younger age, female gender, emetogenicity of the chemotherapy agent, higher dose, and rate of administration.

The cornerstone of treatment is 5HT-3 and NK-1 receptor antagonists. Steroids, cannabinoids, and anxiolytics may also be beneficial.

Radiation Therapy

Like chemotherapy, radiation therapy may cause acute vomiting. It is thought to be caused by release of various neurotransmitters that activate the emetogenic reflex. Subacutely, diarrhea predominates as a complication of radiation therapy. Months to years later, vomiting may again be a result of radiation therapy, often caused by inflammatory ulcers and strictures. These lesions are difficult to treat without surgery.

Postoperative

The incidence of postoperative nausea and vomiting (PONV) in the pediatric population is as high as 33–82% depending on risk factors. Symptoms are most prominent in the first 24 hours postoperatively but can occur up to 7 days after surgery. Risk factors include age older than

TABLE 15.14   Common Poisoning Agents

Agent	Signs and Symptoms*	Laboratory†	Level	Lavage‡	Charcoal and 70% Sorbitol§	Diuresis, Hemodialysis	Specific Treatment
Ipecac	Acute: diarrhea Chronic: cardiomyopathy, muscle weakness	Abnormal ECG	•	•	•		
Salicylates	Tinnitus Hyperventilation Confusion, seizure, coma	Respiratory alkalosis Non-anion gap metabolic acidosis Uremia Hypoglycemia	•	•	•	•	Fluids Urinary alkalization
Acetaminophen	Early: abdominal pain, anorexia Late: jaundice, confusion, coma	Abnormal LFT Coagulopathy Abnormal KFT	•	•	•		N-acetylcysteine
Iron	Early: abdominal pain, bloody diarrhea Late: seizure, hypotension, shortness of breath, jaundice	Metabolic acidosis Abnormal LFT Coagulopathy	•	•	No		Deferoxamine
Lead	Abdominal pain Constipation Anorexia, fatigue Headache, seizure Learning disability	Microcytic anemia KUB: radiopaque flecks Skeletal x-ray: lead lines	•				BAL-CaEDTA Succimer
Opiates	Pinpoint pupil Respiratory depression Hypotension Ileus	Respiratory acidosis	•				Narcan
Opiate withdrawal	Irritability Dilated pupils Diaphoresis Seizures Abdominal cramps						Methadone Benzodiazepines
Organophosphate	Salivation Lacrimation Diaphoresis Diarrhea Wheezing Hypotension Pupillary constriction Garlic breath	Respiratory acidosis, metabolic acidosis					Supportive Atropine Pralidoxime
Corrosives	Oral pain, ulceration Abdominal pain Respiratory distress	CXR		No	No	No	Supportive Endoscopy
Methanol	Acetone breath Confusion, seizures Decreased vision Abdominal pain	Anion gap metabolic acidosis Abnormal KFT	•		No		Ethanol

TABLE 15.14 Common Poisoning Agents—cont'd

Agent	Signs and Symptoms*	Laboratory†	Level	Lavage‡	Charcoal and 70% Sorbitol§	Diuresis, Hemodialysis	Specific Treatment
Ethanol	Ataxia Confusion, seizures Cyanotic Hypopnea Hypothermia	Hypoglycemia	•	•	No		Dextrose-containing IV fluids, supportive
Ethylene glycol	Confusion, seizures Anuria Dysrhythmias	Non-anion gap metabolic acidosis, abnormal KFT, hypocalcemia				•	Ethanol Calcium gluconate
Digitalis	Confusion Bradydysrhythmias	Hypokalemia Hypomagnesemia Hypercalcemia ECG	•				Digibind (antibody) Antiarrhythmics
Food poisoning	Diarrhea Abdominal pain Suggestive history						Supportive
Seafood poisoning	Paresthesia Respiratory paralysis						Supportive
Mushroom poisoning	Diarrhea Salivation Lacrimation Diaphoresis Wheezing	Respiratory acidosis, metabolic acidosis					Supportive For muscarine-containing mushrooms: atropine Penicillin for *Amanita* mushrooms
Venomous bite	Puncture wound Local swelling, bruising, bleeding, Paresthesia, visual disturbance, coma	Myoglobinuria Low platelets Anemia Coagulopathies					Supportive Antivenom

Black dot (•) indicates recommended.

* Other than nausea and vomiting.

†Other than laboratory suggestive of dehydration secondary to vomiting including ketosis, metabolic acidosis, and azotemia.

‡The utility of emesis/lavage varies with the poison, the amount ingested, and the duration since ingestion. If obtunded, lavage requires endotracheal tube airway protection.

§Avoid charcoal/sorbitol in recent bowel surgery or ileus.

BAL-CaEDTA, 2,3-dimercaptopropanol–edathamil calcium disodium; CXR, chest x-ray; IV, intravenous; LFT, liver function test; KFT, kidney function test; KUB, kidney, ureter, and bladder.

TABLE 15.15   Causes of Hematemesis

Source of Blood	Lesion	Clues Regarding Source
Nasopharynx, respiratory	Epistaxis	Nosebleed history
	Hemoptysis	Cough, other respiratory symptoms
Esophageal	Varices	Copious blood; splenomegaly, chronic liver disease
	Esophagitis, Barrett ulcer	Heartburn
	Foreign body erosion	Foreign body history
	Aortoesophageal fistula	Copious blood; esophageal intubation
	Duplication	
Gastroduodenal	Mallory-Weiss tear	Retching and emesis before hematemesis
	Peptic ulcer disease	History: smoking, alcohol, NSAIDs, *H. pylori* infection, pain in relation to meals
	Gastritis, ulcer	
	Duodenitis, ulcer	
	Stress ulcer	Critically ill patients, extensive burns, increased intracranial pressure.
	Vascular malformation (Dieulafoy ulcer, AVM)	Copious blood, recurrent (may have a negative endoscopy)
	Aortoenteric fistula	"Herald bleed," arterial graft or aneurysm
	Duplication	
	Pyloric stenosis, web	Vomiting containing food from prior meal
	Hemobilia	Trauma, gallstones, pain, jaundice
Coagulopathy (PT ↑, PTT ↓)	Vitamin K deficiency	Newborn, fat malabsorption
	Inherited coagulopathies	Specific factor deficiency
	Acquired coagulopathies	Liver failure
	DIC	Sepsis
	Drugs	History of warfarin, coumadin intake
Thrombocytopenia	Hypersplenism	Splenomegaly (Hct ↓, WBC ↓)
	Chemotherapy	(Hct ↓, WBC ↓)
	DIC	Sepsis
Maternal	Intrapartum	Apt test
	Mastitis, cracked nipples	Maternal history, Apt test
Factitious	Psychologic	Affect, secondary gain
Nonblood	Red or brown food or medicine	Guaiac-negative

AVM, arteriovenous malformation; DIC, disseminated intravascular coagulation; *H. pylori, Helicobacter pylori*; Hct, hematocrit; NSAIDs, nonsteroidal antiinflammatory drugs; PT, prothrombin time; PTT, partial thromboplastin time; WBC, white blood cell count.

3 years; duration of surgery >30 minutes; ear, nose, and throat (ENT) and ocular surgeries (e.g., tonsillectomy, strabismus surgery); inhaled anesthetic agents; higher postoperative pain; use of opioids; prolonged preoperative fasting; dehydrated state; and a family history of PONV. The higher the number of risk factors, the greater the chance of PONV. If the susceptible child is identified from these risk factors, prophylactic therapy is generally effective. Combination therapy with dexamethasone and 5HT-3 antagonists have been found most effective.

Porphyria

Acute intermittent porphyria is an autosomal dominant disorder of episodic abdominal pain (85–95% of patients); 40–90% of patients have associated vomiting. The association of neurologic symptoms such as mental status symptoms (50%), muscle weakness (50%), sensory loss (20%), and convulsions (15%); onset after puberty; and the frequent association with menses or provocative drugs (sulfonamides, phenobarbital) are suggestive. Elevated levels of porphobilinogen and δ-aminolevulinic acid in urine are suggestive, and decreased red blood cell porphobilinogen deaminase is diagnostic.

Familial Mediterranean Fever (Benign Paroxysmal Peritonitis, Periodic Peritonitis, Polyserositis)

Episodic attacks of abdominal pain with rapid development and resolution (within 48 hours) of peritoneal signs (fever, vomiting, absent bowel sounds) occurring in a child of Israeli or North African descent should suggest this autosomal recessive diagnosis. Synovitis, pleuritis, and an erysipelas-like skin lesion are also characteristic. The ESR is raised. Fifty percent of patients have their first attack between 1 and 10 years of age; 90%, by age 20. Definitive genetic testing is available for detection of the familial Mediterranean fever gene.

Dysautonomia

Familial dysautonomia is an autosomal recessive disorder of the sensory and autonomic nervous systems affecting children of Ashkenazi Jewish descent. The gene for familial dysautonomia has been identified, allowing for both prenatal diagnosis and identification of carriers. Associated symptoms include disturbed swallowing, drooling, frequent pneumonias, absence of overflow tearing, erratic temperature control, skin blotching, postural hypotension, relative indifference to pain, corneal anesthesia, breath-holding spells, motor incoordination, spinal curvature, and growth retardation. Glossal fungiform papillae are also absent. The disease is diagnosed with the intradermal histamine test or the conjunctival methacholine (or pilocarpine) test. Management is complex and requires a multidisciplinary team.

Complications of Vomiting

The complications of vomiting are outlined in Table 15.16. Their importance is twofold. First, these complications must be promptly treated, and second, there may be diagnostic implications.

Metabolic Complications

Dehydration results from decreased fluid intake because of anorexia or nausea, as well as from the loss of secretions in the emesis. The electrolyte disturbance can vary depending upon the varying losses of gastric hydrogen chloride (HCl), pancreatic bicarbonate (HCO₃), and GI sodium chloride (NaCl). In high-grade gastric outlet obstruction, prolonged vomiting causes loss of gastric HCl and produces an increase in plasma bicarbonate to compensate for loss of chloride. Potassium and sodium are also lost in the vomitus and are subsequently wasted by the kidneys when they accompany the renal excretion of bicarbonate caused by the alkalosis. This leads to the classically described hypochloremic hypokalemic metabolic alkalosis. In states of marked alkalosis, urine pH is 7 or 8, and urinary sodium and potassium levels are high, despite serum sodium and potassium depletion. Urine chloride, however, remains low, reflecting the nonrenal losses of chloride. Intravenous fluid therapy is often required, and must be designed with an understanding of the sodium and potassium deficits. Preoperative restoration of electrolyte imbalance reduces perioperative morbidity in cases of gastric outlet obstruction.

TABLE 15.16 Complications of Vomiting

Complication	Pathophysiology	History, Physical Examination, and Laboratory Studies
Metabolic	Fluid loss in emesis	Dehydration, metabolic acidosis
	HCl loss in emesis	Alkalosis; hypochloremia
	Na, K loss in emesis	Hyponatremia; hypokalemia
Nutritional	Emesis of calories and nutrients Anorexia	Malnutrition: "failure to thrive"
Mallory-Weiss tear*	Retching → tear at lesser curve of gastroesophageal junction	Forceful emesis → hematemesis
Esophagitis	Chronic vomiting → esophageal acid exposure	Heartburn; hemoccult + stool
Aspiration	Aspiration of vomitus, especially in context of obtundation	Pneumonia; neurologic dysfunction
Shock	Severe fluid loss in emesis and/or accompanying diarrhea	Dehydration, metabolic acidosis
	Severe blood loss in hematemesis	Blood volume depletion

*Occasionally produces blood in the initial vomitus. Invisible radiographically, it is diagnosed endoscopically (if necessary).
HCl, hydrogen chloride; K, potassium; Na, sodium.

TABLE 15.17 Supportive and Nonpharmacologic Therapies for Vomiting Episodes

Disease	Therapy
All	Treat cause: obstruction → operate; allergy → change diet (± steroids); metabolic error → Rx defect; acid peptic disease → H$_2$RAs, PPIs, etc.
Complications	
Dehydration	IV fluids, electrolytes
Hematemesis	Transfuse, correct coagulopathy
Esophagitis	H$_2$RAs, PPIs
Malnutrition	NG or NJ drip feeding useful for many chronic conditions
Meconium ileus	Gastrografin enema
DIOS	Gastrografin enema; balanced colonic lavage solution (e.g., GoLytely)
Intussusception	Barium enema; air reduction enema
Hematemesis	Endoscopic: injection sclerotherapy or banding of esophageal varices; injection therapy, fibrin sealant application, or heater probe electrocautery for selected upper GI tract lesions
Sigmoid volvulus	Colonoscopic decompression
Reflux	Positioning; dietary measures (infants: rice cereal, 1 tbs/oz of formula)
Psychogenic components	Psychotherapy; tricyclic antidepressants; anxiolytics (e.g., diazepam: 0.1 mg/kg/t.i.d.–q.i.d. PO)

DIOS, distal intestinal obstruction syndrome; GI, gastrointestinal; H$_2$RAs, histamine$_2$-receptor antagonists; IV, intravenous; NG, nasogastric; NJ, nasojejunal; PO, orally; PPIs, proton pump inhibitors; q.i.d., four times a day; Rx, prescription; tbs, tablespoon; t.i.d., three times a day.

Nutritional Complications

The nutritional deficits resulting from chronic vomiting and associated anorexia are obvious. No more than a day or two of fluid therapy should take place without attention to nutritional needs. Frequent, small, high-carbohydrate feedings may minimize the stimulation to vomit, but continuous nasogastric or nasojejunal feedings are sometimes needed for cases of chronic vomiting. The presence of metabolic or allergic disease should be considered when the reintroduction of protein leads to relapse of symptoms. In severely malnourished individuals, rapid reinstitution of nutrition can lead to refeeding syndrome, which is characterized by metabolic disturbances such as low phosphate, potassium, and magnesium, which, if severe enough, can be fatal. During refeeding the insulin secretion is triggered in response to increased blood sugar, thus increasing the synthesis of glycogen, protein, and fat. This process requires phosphate, potassium, and magnesium, the stores of which are already low and get quickly depleted, leading to cardiac, pulmonary, and neurologic complications. Gradual introduction of calories and close monitoring of blood chemistry are therefore necessary during the early refeeding period.

Mallory-Weiss Tear

This linear mucosal laceration in the juxtaesophageal gastric mucosa usually occurs after prolonged forceful retching or vomiting. Invisible radiographically, it is diagnosed endoscopically (if necessary). Mallory-Weiss tears usually necessitate no treatment and supportive care.

Peptic Esophagitis

Esophagitis, similar to that resulting from gastroesophageal reflux, may result from chronic vomiting from many causes. Diagnosed

endoscopically or histologically, it should be treated. The treatment of esophagitis usually includes H$_2$-receptor antagonists or PPIs; prokinetic agents may also be needed.

Therapy

Therapy of vomiting starts with treatment of the cause, treatment of complications, and treatment of behavioral aspects that may perpetuate the vomiting. General supportive and more specific pharmacologic approaches to therapy are outlined in Tables 15.17 and 15.18. The physician should be very careful about treating the vomiting symptom without diagnosing and treating its cause. In several situations, diagnostic procedures, such as Gastrografin enema for fecal obstructions in cystic fibrosis, barium enema for intussusception, and endoscopy with sclerotherapy for variceal hematemesis, are also therapeutic. As noted, many causes of vomiting involve psychologic and higher cortical influences. In these cases, psychobehavioral and multidisciplinary approaches are often essential to successful management. Such therapies are focused on returning the disabled child to proper functioning and school attendance while eliminating secondary gain for vomiting and reducing surrounding anxiety. Cognitive-behavioral and psychologic therapies may be helpful in isolation or with concurrent pharmacotherapy.

Antiemetic Drugs

In situations of persistent vomiting, antiemetic drugs are useful to reduce the metabolic and nutritional consequences and interrupt vicious circles in which psychogenic factors may also participate. Since multiple neurotransmitters and chemoreceptors are involved in emetic

TABLE 15.18 Pharmacologic Therapies for Vomiting

Drug Class/Generic	Dosages	Mechanism	Side Effects	Indications
5HT-3 Receptor* Antagonist				
• Ondansetron	0.15 mg/kg q6–8h IV/PO	Action at CTZ and vagal afferents in gut	Headache, QT prolongation	Chemotherapy induced, postoperative, CVS
• Granisetron	10 µg/kg IV q6h			
Substituted* Benzamides				
• Cisapride	0.2–0.3 mg/kg t.i.d.–q.i.d. PO	5HT-4 Rcp agonist in gut	Diarrhea, abdominal pain, headache	GER, gastroparesis
• Metoclopramide	0.1 mg/kg up to q.i.d. IM/IV/PO	D2 Rcp antagonist at CTZ, 5HT-4 agonist in gut	Extrapyramidal reactions	GER, gastroparesis, chemotherapy induced
Antihistamines[†]				
• Diphenhydramine	1.25 mg/kg q6h PO/IV	Vestibular suppression, anti-Ach effect, and H1 Rcp antagonist	Sedation, anticholinergic side effects	Motion sickness, CVS, chemotherapy induced
• Hydroxyzine	0.5 mg/kg q6h PO			
Phenothiazines[‡]				
• Promethazine	0.25–0.5 mg/kg q4–6h PR/IM	D2 receptor antagonist at CTZ, H1 Rcp antagonist	Anticholinergic, extrapyramidal side effects	Chemotherapy induced, CVS
• Prochlorperazine	>10 kg: 0.1 mg/kg q6–8h PO/PR, max 10 mg/dose			
Anticholinergic[†]				
• Scopolamine		Vestibular suppression, anti-Ach effect on CNS	Sedation, anticholinergic side effect	Prophylaxis of motion sickness
NK-1 Receptor Antagonists[§]				
• Aprepitant	3-day regimen: 125, 80, 80 mg	NK-1 Rcp antagonist in CTZ	Fatigue, dizziness, diarrhea	Chemotherapy induced, CVS
• Fosaprepitant	1 q.d. PO/IV			
Benzodiazepines[†]				
• Lorazepam	0.05–0.1 mg/kg/dose IV	Enhanced central GABAergic inhibition inducing anxiolysis, sedation	Sedation, respiratory depression	Chemotherapy induced, CVS adjunct
• Diazepam	0.1–0.3 mg/kg IV Max: <0.6 mg/kg/24 h			
Cannabinoids[‡]				
• Dronabinol	>12 yr: 5 mg/m^2/dose q4–6h PO	Unknown	Disorientation, vertigo, hallucinations	Chemotherapy
Corticosteroids[‡]				
• Dexamethasone	Initial dose: 5–10 mg/m^2 IV, max 20 mg, then 5 mg/m^2 q12h	Unknown	Hyperglycemia, mood lability, gastritis	Adrenal suppression, chemotherapy induced

*High antiemetic activity.
[†]Minimal antiemetic activity.
[‡]Mild to moderate antiemetic activity.
[§]Moderate to high antiemetic activity.
Ach, acetylcholine; b.i.d., twice daily; CTZ, chemoreceptor trigger zone; CVS, cyclical vomiting syndrome; GER, gastroesophageal reflux; IM, intramuscularly; IV, intravenously; max, maximum; PO, orally; q4–6h, every 4–6 hr; q6h, every 6 hr; q6–8h, every 6–8 hr; q.i.d., four times daily; Rcp, receptor; t.i.d., three times daily.
Modified from Li BUK, Kovacic K. Vomiting and nausea. In: Wyllie R, Hyams JS, Kay M, eds. *Pediatric Gastrointestinal and Liver Disease.* 5th ed. Philadelphia: Elsevier; 2016:91.

pathways, most antiemetics can be broadly classified based on their mechanism of action as follows:

Serotonin receptor antagonists: Ondansetron and granisetron are the most used drugs in this category and are available as both intravenous and oral preparations. They act by blocking serotonin 5HT-3 receptors at both peripheral and central levels. Side effects include possible QTc prolongation.

Dopamine receptor antagonists: Dopamine receptor antagonists antagonize the D_2-receptor in the area postrema. Metoclopramide,

prochlorperazine, and promethazine are common drugs in this class. Metoclopramide promotes foregut motility by other mechanisms, while the latter two have additional anticholinergic and antihistamine effects. Extrapyramidal symptoms (tardive dyskinesia, dystonia) are possible serious side effects. Domperidone is a peripheral D_2-receptor antagonist and has antiemetic and promotility effects as well.

Anticholinergics: Scopolamine is an anticholinergic that antagonizes the muscarinic receptor and is predominantly used to prevent motion sickness. Common side effects include dry mouth, drowsiness, and vision changes.

Antihistamines: Antihistamines act on the H_1- and H_2-receptors and the most common reported side effect is drowsiness. Examples are promethazine and diphenhydramine.

NK-1 antagonists: NK-1 antagonists are inhibitors for the NK-1 receptor, which prevents binding of substance P (a known emetogen). Aprepitant (orally) and fosaprepitant (intravenously) are the commonly used drugs in this category. NK-1 antagonists were initially developed for treatment of chemotherapy-induced emesis but have also proven beneficial in other etiologies such as CVS. Side effects are uncommon but may include headache, dizziness, and hypersensitivity reactions.

Anxiolytics: Benzodiazepines are commonly used and particularly helpful in anxiety-induced emesis and when sedative effects are needed as for acute/abortive therapy of CVS episodes.

Cannabinoids: Cannabinoids are controversial antiemetics given the possibility of psychedelic and addictive effects with long-term use. At this time, use is limited to chemotherapy-induced nausea, vomiting, and anorexia.

Corticosteroids: Corticosteroids have limited use in chemotherapy- and irradiation-induced nausea and vomiting and cases of adrenal crisis. The mechanism of action as an antiemetic is not clear.

Promotility agents: Erythromycin acts on the motilin receptors located in the gastric smooth muscle, enhancing gastric motility. Cisapride, a 5HT-4-receptor agonist, also facilitates gastric motility, but due to its arrhythmogenic potential it is only available in the United States via restricted, compassionate care protocols.

In some settings, the diverse sites of action account for the useful additive effects of these drugs. Optimal therapy for vomiting caused by chemotherapy, for example, may include several agents to provide blockade of the multiple receptor types. Serotonin and dopamine receptor antagonists are the most widely used general antiemetic agents.

Although treatment for many functional GI and motility causes of emesis is often empiric, disease-specific therapies and guidelines are available for certain syndromes. For example, treatment for CVS can be divided into lifestyle modification, abortive or rescue therapy to prevent progression from the prodromal to emetic phase, supportive therapy during episodes, and prophylactic daily therapy to prevent future episodes (see Table 15.13). Lifestyle changes include adequate fluid intake, frequent calorie intake, and regimented sleep along with stress reduction.

Supportive therapy includes dextrose 10% containing intravenous fluids to diminish catabolism, less stimulating environment, and a combination of antiemetics and sedatives/anxiolytics to attenuate symptoms. Many of these agents can also help abort an early episode.

SUMMARY AND RED FLAGS

Vomiting and regurgitation are commonly encountered in pediatrics and can signify underlying problems with a wide array of body systems. Although acute vomiting most commonly results from self-resolving infectious illnesses, the medical provider needs to carefully evaluate for red flags that may herald serious emergencies and surgical conditions.

When emesis becomes chronic, the specific temporal pattern and associated signs and symptoms should direct further diagnostic work-up. Although therapy is often empiric, treatment trials should be tailored to the underlying cause and the individual patient. Red flags are noted in Table 15.6.

BIBLIOGRAPHY

A bibliography is available at ExpertConsult.com.

16

Gastrointestinal Bleeding

Julia Fritz, Amornluck Krasaelap, and Bernadette Vitola

Gastrointestinal (GI) bleeding in children can range from small amounts of blood in the stool, associated with milk protein allergy or anal fissure, to life-threatening hemorrhage, associated with portal hypertension or peptic ulcer disease. Severe bleeding is a true medical emergency and necessitates prompt diagnostic attention and appropriate management since overall mortality of children hospitalized in the United States with GI bleeding is approximately 2%. *Hemodynamic stabilization of the patient with severe bleeding should always precede diagnostic studies.* An accurate history and thorough physical examination usually allow the physician to categorize the problem as mild or severe and to direct evaluation at the appropriate pace.

DEFINITIONS

Children with GI bleeding generally present with hematemesis, hematochezia, or melena, although the clinical manifestation can be as subtle as evidence of occult blood loss. An **upper GI bleed** is bleeding from the esophagus, stomach, or duodenum. Upper sources account for the majority of GI bleeds in children. If the site of bleeding is distal to the ligament of Treitz, it is a **lower GI bleed**. Blood passed per rectum can originate from either an upper or lower GI source. Occult bleeding may occur from disorders at numerous sites.

Hematemesis

Vomited blood can be either red or the color of coffee grounds. Hematemesis is most commonly associated with an upper GI bleed, although swallowed blood produces the same clinical picture. Bright red hematemesis suggests active bleeding that has not had prolonged contact with gastric secretions. When gastric secretions interact with the blood, the blood will darken in color as the iron oxidizes and leads to dark red or "coffee ground" emesis.

Hematochezia and Melena

The presence of hematochezia (bright red blood) is generally associated with colonic bleeding, although it may result from a brisk upper bleed. Maroon stools from the rectum are generally associated with a lower GI bleed. The presence of melena—passage of black, tarry stools—generally results from significant blood loss proximal to the ileocecal valve, with up to 90% originating proximal to the ligament of Treitz. The color results from bacterial breakdown of the hemoglobin. *Up to 10–15% of upper GI bleeds present with melena in the absence of hematemesis.* These patients are more likely to have a clinically significant bleed.

Occult Gastrointestinal Bleeding

In contrast to overt GI bleeding as in hematemesis, hematochezia, or melena, occult GI bleeding is a positive fecal blood test when there is no visible blood loss.

Mimics of Gastrointestinal Bleeding

Hemoptysis may occasionally be mistaken for hematemesis. Melena may be confused with menstrual bleeding. In addition, certain medications, supplements (such as iron), foods, and dyes may turn stool or emesis red or maroon color, mimicking blood. A thorough history including respiratory symptoms, menstrual history, medications, and diet history is important.

APPROACH TO GASTROINTESTINAL BLEEDING

The first step is to determine whether the problem is actually GI bleeding. Many substances and non-GI sources may simulate GI bleeding (Table 16.1). Occult blood testing consists of guaiac-based tests from the stool or emesis (gastric occult blood), which measure heme, and fecal immunochemical tests (FITs), which measure the globin portion of human hemoglobin. Recommendations for guaiac-based testing from manufacturers are to avoid red meat, citrus fruits and juices,

TABLE 16.1 Mimics of Gastrointestinal Bleeding

Foodstuffs:
- Beets
- Blueberries
- Food coloring
- Gelatin
- Licorice
- Punch
- Red candy
- Spinach
- Tomato skins
- Watermelon

Medications:
- Phenytoin
- Bismuth
- Iron supplementation
- Rifampin
- Diazepam
- Cefdinir
- Phenolphthalein

Bleeding from other locations:
- Epistaxis
- Hemoptysis
- Menses
- Recent dental work or tonsillectomy

Swallowed maternal blood in breast-fed or newborn infant
Munchausen (factitious disorder) syndrome by proxy
Factitious disorder

supplemental vitamin C in excess of 250 mg/day for 3 days prior to testing, and antacids for at least 60 minutes prior to testing. Nonsteroidal antiinflammatory drugs (NSAIDs) should be avoided for 1 week prior to testing and aspirin exposure should be minimized; however, it is uncertain whether these products affect the reliability of the test. In addition, although iron preparations may blacken stools, they do not lead to false-positive results. Female patients should be told not to collect test samples for 3 days after or during a menstrual period. To avoid potential false-positive or false-negative results, stool should be collected from diapers or from disposable collection devices rather than directly from toilet water. Finally, an alkali denaturation test, also known as the Apt-Downey or Apt test, should be performed when a breast-fed infant vomits bright red blood or passes red bloody stools to distinguish whether it is maternal or fetal hemoglobin.

Once GI bleeding is confirmed, the evaluation, differential diagnosis, and therapeutic interventions will depend on the age of the patient, severity of bleeding, and whether the bleed is coming from the upper or the lower GI tract (Tables 16.2, 16.3, 16.4, and 16.5). A nasogastric (NG) tube may be placed in the appropriate patient when the source of bleeding is not clear. Bloody aspirate from the stomach is confirmation of upper GI bleeding. The tube may then be used to lavage the stomach with warm saline. If aspirated saline clears after repeated lavage, the bleeding has likely stopped or is from a different source.

HEMATEMESIS AND MELENA: UPPER GASTROINTESTINAL BLEED

History

Neonates who did not receive prophylactic vitamin K are at risk for hemorrhagic disease of the newborn (see Chapter 51) and additional perinatal factors may place them at risk for sepsis or other stress that could lead to gastritis. Infants who require intensive care may have trauma from an NG tube, and infants with neonatal umbilical vein catheterization or neonatal omphalitis are at risk for portal vein

TABLE 16.2 Differential Diagnosis for Upper Gastrointestinal Bleeding

Infants	Ill-appearing	Stress ulcer
		Hemorrhagic gastritis
		Sepsis with DIC
		Vitamin K deficiency
		Infection—CMV, herpes, parasites, fungal
	Well-appearing	Trauma
		Milk protein sensitivity
		Mallory-Weiss tear
		Prolapse gastropathy
		Reflux esophagitis
		Reactive gastritis
		Anatomic anomalies (duplication)*
		Vascular anomalies (hemangioma/vascular malformation)*
Children	Ill-appearing	Esophageal varices
		Stress ulcer
		Sepsis with DIC
		Hemobilia
	Well-appearing	Esophagitis including pill ulceration (alendronate, tetracycline, quinidine, potassium chloride, aspirin, NSAIDs)
		Reflux esophagitis
		Gastritis
		• NSAIDs
		• *Helicobacter pylori*
		Ulcer from foreign body
		Mallory-Weiss tear
		Prolapse gastropathy
		Vascular malformation*
		• Dieulafoy lesion (artery that protrudes through mucosa)
		Anatomic anomalies (duplication)*
		Infection—CMV, herpes, parasites, fungal

CMV, cytomegalovirus; DIC, disseminated intravascular coagulation; NSAIDs, nonsteroidal antiinflammatory drugs.
*Patient is usually well-appearing but may deteriorate due to high rate of bleeding.

TABLE 16.3 Differential Diagnosis for Lower Gastrointestinal Bleeding

Infants	Ill-appearing	Infectious—*Salmonella*, *Shigella*, *Escherichia coli* O157:H7, *Campylobacter* species, *Yersinia* species, *Entamoeba histolytica*, CMV
		Ischemia—volvulus or necrotizing enterocolitis
		Sepsis with DIC
		Vitamin K deficiency
		Hirschsprung enterocolitis
		Intussusception
	Well-appearing	Trauma
		Anal fissure
		Milk protein sensitivity/eosinophilic proctocolitis
		Lymphonodular hyperplasia
		Vascular anomalies (hemangioma/vascular malformation)*
		Anatomic anomalies
Children	Ill-appearing	Infectious—above plus *Clostridium difficile*
		Intussusception
		Meckel diverticulum
		Inflammatory bowel disease
		Ischemia
		Typhlitis
		Henoch-Schönlein purpura
		Trauma
	Well-appearing	Anal fissure
		Milk and other protein sensitivity
		Juvenile polyp
		Medication
		• NSAIDs
		• Mycophenolate
		Lymphonodular hyperplasia
		Hemorrhoid (in chronic liver disease)
		Vascular anomalies (hemangioma/vascular malformation)*
		Anatomic anomalies

CMV, cytomegalovirus; DIC, disseminated intravascular coagulation; NSAIDs, nonsteroidal antiinflammatory drugs.
*Patient is usually well-appearing but may deteriorate due to high rate of bleeding.

TABLE 16.4 Causes of Occult Gastrointestinal Bleeding

Inflammatory Causes

Peptic esophagitis

Crohn disease

Ulcerative colitis

Mild enterocolitis

Celiac disease

Eosinophilic gastroenteritis

Meckel diverticulum

Solitary rectal ulcer

Vascular Causes

Angiodysplasia and vascular ectasias

Gastroesophageal varices

Congestive gastropathy

Hemangiomas

Drugs

Nonsteroidal antiinflammatory drugs

Extragastrointestinal Causes

Hemoptysis

Epistaxis

Oropharyngeal bleeding

Infectious Causes

Hookworm

Strongyloidiasis

Ascariasis

Tuberculosis enterocolitis

Amebiasis

Tumors and Neoplastic Causes

Polyps

Lymphoma

Leiomyoma

Lipoma

Carcinoma

Artificial Causes

Hematuria

Menstrual bleeding

Nonspecific test positivity

Miscellaneous Causes

Long-distance running

Coagulopathies

Factitious

Modified from Ahlquist DA. Approach to the patient with occult gastrointestinal bleeding. In: Yamada T, ed. *Textbook of Gastroenterology.* Philadelphia: JB Lippincott; 1991:620.

TABLE 16.5 Rare/Atypical Causes of Gastrointestinal Bleeding in Children

Hematemesis/Melena

- Hemobilia—nontraumatic
- Spontaneous intramural hematoma
- Burkitt lymphoma
- Collagenous gastritis/duodenitis
- Superior mesenteric artery aneurysm
- Ectopic pancreas
- Hemosuccus pancreaticus
- Gastric volvulus
- Ectopic varices
- Aortoesophageal fistula
- Gastrointestinal stromal tumor (GIST)

Hematochezia

- Eosinophilic colitis
- Cytomegalovirus colitis (non–inflammatory bowel disease)
- Granulomatous colitis (non–Crohn disease)
- Sarcoidosis
- Abdominal tuberculosis
- Chronic granulomatous disease
- Hermansky-Pudlak syndrome
- Ileal GIST
- Intestinal Behçet disease
- Langerhans cell histiocytosis
- IPEX (immune disregulation, polyendocrinopathy, enteropathy)
- Wiskott-Aldrich syndrome
- Juvenile hyaline fibromatosis
- Spontaneous intramural hematoma
- Ectopic varices

From Wyllie R, Hyams JS, Kay M, eds. *Pediatric Gastrointestinal and Liver Disease.* 5th ed. Philadelphia: Elsevier; 2016:153, Box 13-11.

Information regarding chronic pulmonary disease, renal disease, bleeding disorders such as hemophilia, platelet dysfunction or von Willebrand disease, and liver disease, including a history of jaundice, should be obtained in all children. Patients with cystic fibrosis are at risk not only for the development of esophageal varices caused by biliary cirrhosis but also for coagulopathies from vitamin K deficiency. They may also have hemoptysis, which can be misinterpreted as hematemesis. In patients with renal disease, uremia will cause platelet dysfunction, which may manifest as a GI bleed. The family history should address the presence of bleeding disorders, peptic ulcer disease, and possible *Helicobacter pylori* exposure. Other genetic disorders may be elicited in the family history such as VMCM (venous malformations, multiple cutaneous and mucosal, OMIM 600195), hereditary hemorrhagic telangiectasia, Peutz-Jeghers syndrome, and blue rubber bleb nevus syndrome that cause variable GI bleeding.

Physical Examination

Immediate attention must be given to signs of hypovolemia, anemia, or shock. An orthostatic change, such as a pulse rate increase of 20 beats/min or a drop in systolic blood pressure of more than 10 mm Hg when the patient changes from supine to standing, is a sensitive index of significant volume depletion. Blood pressure may remain normal up to the point of circulatory collapse in children and a normal blood pressure should not be reassuring in the setting of other signs of hypovolemia such as tachycardia or delayed capillary refill.

In addition to close attention to changes in vital signs, a physical exam with emphasis on potential sources of bleeding is essential (Table 16.6). The oropharynx and nasal canals should be examined for lesions

thrombosis and resultant later onset of esophageal varices. In older children, a recent history of vomiting, regurgitation, or abdominal pain suggests a mucosal lesion. Forceful, repeated vomiting may result in a Mallory-Weiss tear or prolapse gastropathy. Reactive gastritis can be due to medications such as NSAIDs as well as alcohol or ingestion of caustic substances. Providers must ask about recent bleeding such as epistaxis or dental procedures, which could lead to hematemesis without a GI source of bleeding.

TABLE 16.6 Pertinent Physical Findings in Gastrointestinal Bleeding

Exam Finding	Associated Disorder
Splenomegaly Caput medusae	Portal hypertension and esophageal varices
Palmar erythema Spider angioma Jaundice Ascites	Liver disease
Hemangioma	Hemangioma in gastrointestinal tract
Port-wine stain	Vascular malformation in gastrointestinal tract
Palpable purpura	Henoch-Schönlein purpura or other vasculitis
Hyperpigmented lesions of the oral or anal mucosa	Peutz-Jeghers syndrome (gastrointestinal polyps)
Lip, oral mucosal telangiectasias	Hereditary hemorrhagic telangiectasia
Oral ulcers Perianal fistula Perianal skin tag Erythema nodosum Pyoderma gangrenosum	Inflammatory bowel disease

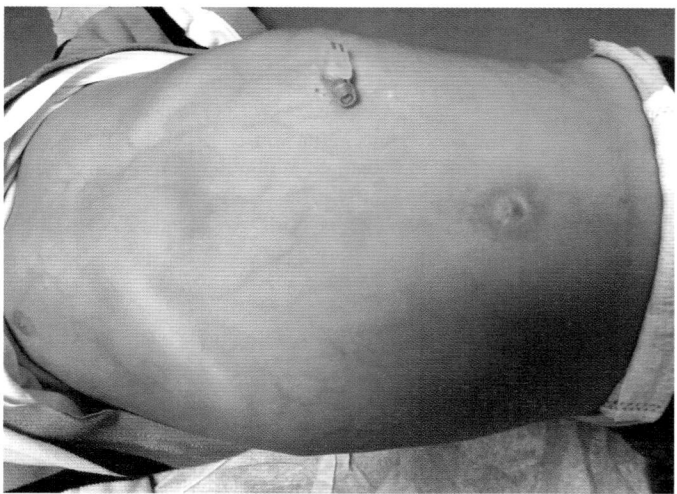

Fig. 16.1 Prominent venous pattern on the abdomen.

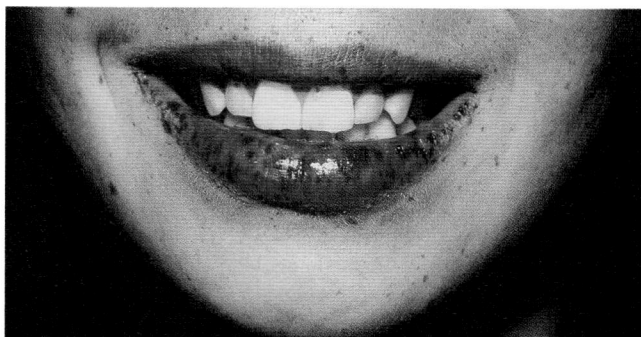

Fig. 16.2 Peutz-Jeghers syndrome. This smiling, 12-year-old girl developed progressive lentigines on her face, particularly her lips, in early childhood. She also has involvement of the extremities, trunk, and mucous membranes. (From Cohen BA, ed. *Pediatric Dermatology*. 4th ed. Philadelphia: Saunders; 2013:152, Fig. 6.6.)

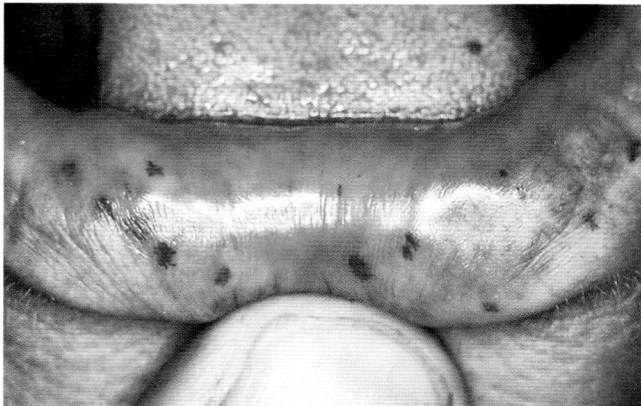

Fig. 16.3 Hereditary hemorrhagic telangiectasia. Telangiectasias are found on the lips, oral mucosa, nasal mucosa, skin, and conjunctiva. Epistaxis is the most common manifestation of the disease. Blood transfusions may be required. (From Dinulos GHJ. *Habif's Clinical Dermatology*. 7th ed. Philadelphia: Elsevier; 2021:925, Fig. 23.42.)

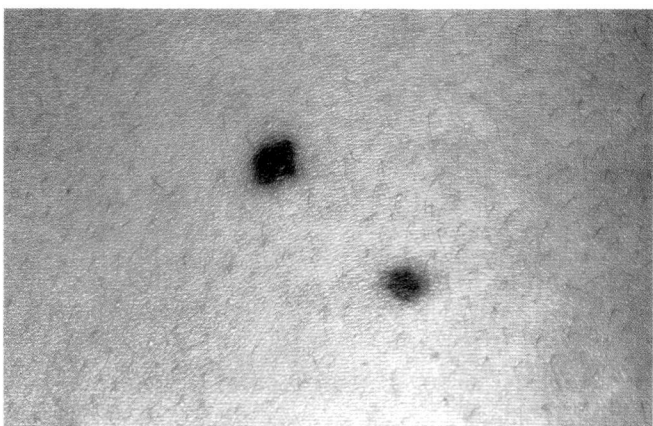

Fig. 16.4 Blue rubber bleb nevus syndrome. A 16-year-old girl was evaluated for multiple 3 mm–1 cm blue nodules on the skin. She had a history of similar lesions in the gastrointestinal tract, which were discovered during surgery for small bowel obstruction from intussusception. (From Cohen BA, ed. *Pediatric Dermatology*. 4th ed. Philadelphia: Saunders; 2013:51, Fig. 2.70.)

as the cause of bleeding. Palpation to evaluate organomegaly should begin at the iliac crests so as not to miss a hugely enlarged liver or spleen. A prominent venous pattern on the abdomen (Fig. 16.1), splenomegaly, and ascites may suggest portal hypertension. Tenderness and guarding indicate a significant inflammatory process.

In addition to assessing for pallor, cutaneous lesions may help determine the underlying cause of bleeding. Petechiae can indicate disseminated intravascular coagulation, hypersplenism, or another bleeding abnormality. Hyperpigmented lesions of the oral or anal mucosa may indicate Peutz-Jeghers disease (Fig. 16.2). Cutaneous telangiectasia and hemangiomas may indicate such diseases as Osler-Weber-Rendu syndrome (a.k.a. hereditary hemorrhagic telangiectasia) (Fig. 16.3) and ataxia-telangiectasia, or they may simply suggest a predisposition for vascular malformations. However, only about 2% of individuals with cutaneous vascular lesions will also have GI involvement. Blue cutaneous nodules suggest blue rubber bleb nevus syndrome (Fig. 16.4). Palmar erythema, spider angioma, or jaundice suggests underlying liver

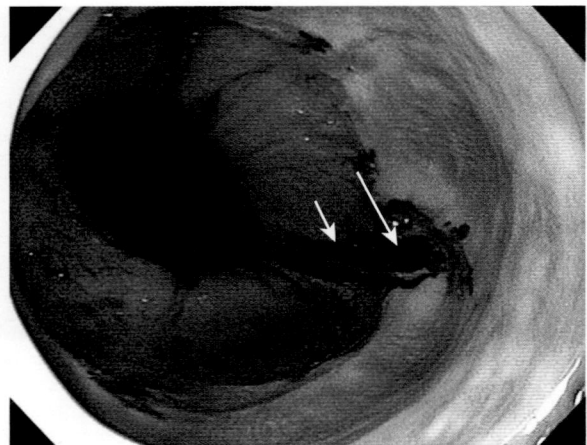

Fig. 16.5 Endoscopic appearance of a Mallory-Weiss tear with mild oozing. Note that the tear starts at the gastroesophageal junction *(long arrow)* and extends distally into the hiatal hernia *(short arrow)*. (From Feldman M, Friedman LS, Brandt LJ, eds. *Sleisenger and Fordtran's Gastrointestinal and Liver Disease.* 11th ed. Philadelphia: Elsevier; 2021, Fig. 20-14.)

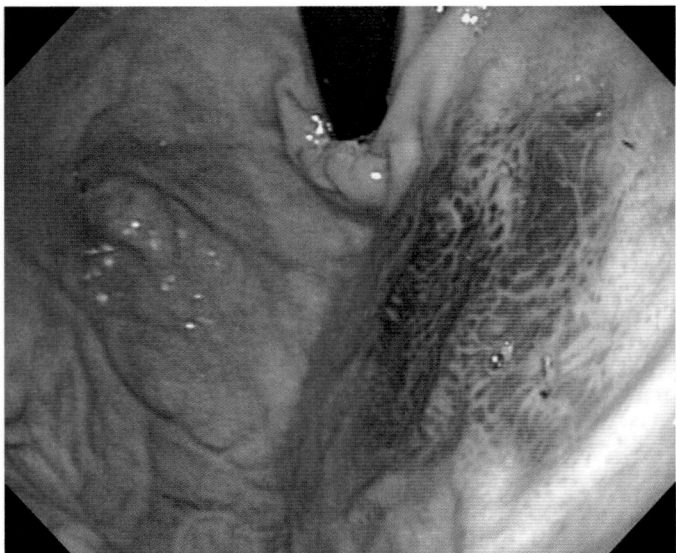

Fig. 16.6 Endoscopic view of fundus showing area of prolapse gastropathy.

disease. Scleral icterus may be subtle but can be the first sign of liver disease and may be more easily appreciated than jaundice in darker-skinned individuals.

Differential Diagnosis

In infants, esophagitis, gastritis, and ulcers are the most common causes of upper GI bleeding. Esophagitis may be associated with dysphagia, irritability, and arching with feeds (see Chapter 15). Milk protein sensitivity should be considered as well, although it more often presents with blood in stool. Trauma or infection (such as cytomegalovirus, herpes simplex, parasites, or fungal) can cause mucosal irritation presenting as hematemesis. Anatomic abnormalities including duplication cysts or vascular abnormalities may also lead to hematemesis or melena in infants.

In older children, mucosal lesions remain common causes of bleeding. Mallory-Weiss tears are associated with repeated forceful vomiting from a variety of causes (e.g., acute gastroenteritis) (Fig. 16.5). The forcefulness of the vomiting causes a tear in the distal esophagus at the level of the lower esophageal sphincter. The history is generally one of frequent nonbloody vomiting that then becomes hematemesis. Prolapse gastropathy, caused by prolapse of gastric mucosa into the distal esophagus, can similarly occur after forceful vomiting and lead to hematemesis (Fig. 16.6). Reactive gastritis secondary to medication (NSAIDs) or infection (*H. pylori*) is also a common cause of upper GI bleeding. Children with known or unknown liver disease can develop esophageal varices that may lead to large-volume hematemesis and melena (or hematochezia if bleeding is brisk). Ulcers, although rare, can also lead to significant blood loss and may be related to *H. pylori* infection, stress such as surgery or burns, and foreign body ingestion, specifically button batteries, which can lead to significant bleeding.

HEMATOCHEZIA: LOWER GASTROINTESTINAL BLEED

History

Chronicity of bleeding is essential to ascertain because infectious colitis may cause acute bloody diarrhea, while inflammatory bowel disease generally presents with a more prolonged history (see Chapter 14). Presence or absence of pain can also help distinguish between causes of

bleeding. Severe, acute abdominal pain is often present in patients with vascular compromise, such as in intussusception, midgut volvulus, and bowel ischemia (e.g., Henoch-Schönlein purpura), while painless rectal bleeding suggests a Meckel diverticulum, polyp, or angiodysplasia. Growth failure is suggestive of inflammatory bowel disease, specifically Crohn disease; constipation points to the possibility of an anal fissure (see Chapter 19) or Hirschsprung disease with enterocolitis. Information regarding travel (either by the patient or by visitors), sick contacts, daycare exposure, camping, and antibiotic exposure may reveal potential infectious causes. Family history of polyps or colon cancer is important given the inherited polyposis syndromes, as is a family history of inflammatory bowel disease.

Physical Examination

Physical exam in any patient with GI bleeding must begin with assessment of hemodynamic status. In addition to a general exam, for patients with hematochezia, a rectal exam is important to evaluate for fissures as well as skin tags and fistulas, which may be seen in Crohn disease (Fig. 16.7). Local intense tenderness, fever, and erythema of the perianal area may suggest group A β-hemolytic streptococcus infection. Infants and toddlers may have a palpable right lower quadrant abdominal mass, which suggests intussusception. Skin examination may show purpura, which, although not always present initially, is seen in Henoch-Schönlein purpura; it may also be seen in hemolytic uremic syndrome. Erythema nodosum or pyoderma gangrenosum is present in approximately 3% of children with inflammatory bowel disease and may correlate with disease severity.

Differential Diagnosis

Anal fissures are probably the most frequent cause of streaks of bright red blood mixed with stool. The bleeding may be associated with hard bowel movements but may occur from straining with normal bowel movements. There is also an association with group A streptococcal perianal cellulitis and bleeding. Anal fissure may be a manifestation of milk protein allergy with resultant perianal inflammation and subsequent constipation to avoid painful defecation. More often, a milk protein allergy will present with specks of blood within the stool. There may be a history of increasing frequency and amount of blood and mucus in the stool. The infant may exhibit cramping with bowel movements

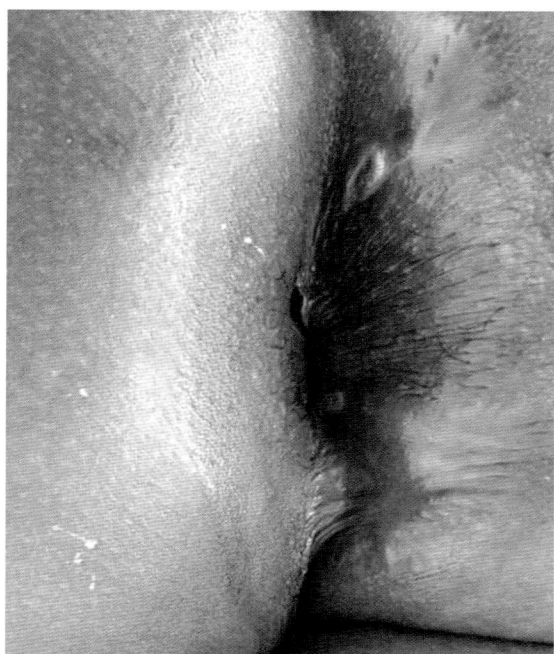

Fig. 16.7 Skin tags and fistulas as in Crohn disease.

and vomiting may be part of the presentation. Often there is a family history of food allergies. Milk protein allergy can be seen in infants fed cow's milk– or soy protein–based formulas, as well as in breast-fed infants. Ischemic bowel disease, including necrotizing enterocolitis and volvulus, may lead to rectal bleeding and an acutely ill, sick-appearing neonate or infant. Risk factors for necrotizing enterocolitis include prematurity, cardiac surgery, polycythemia, chronic diarrhea, and GI malformations.

Infectious colitis is common in both infants and children and causes frequent, often watery, bloody bowel movements (see Chapter 14). There may be cramping pain before and during the bowel movement as a result of the colitis. Common pathogens include *Salmonella* and *Shigella* organisms, especially with dysentery type stools, but *Escherichia coli* O157:H7, *Campylobacter* species, *Yersinia* species, and *Entamoeba histolytica* should also be considered. *Clostridium difficile* is a common cause of hematochezia in older children but is also found in healthy infants without causing disease due to lack of toxin receptors in the immature colon.

For young children, intussusception and Meckel diverticulum are common causes of hematochezia. The hallmark of intussusception is the presence of "currant jelly" stools associated with colicky abdominal pain, lethargy, or irritability. Meckel diverticulum occurs in 1–3% of the population and manifests by the age of 2 years in about 50% of patients. Bleeding results from mucosal ulceration secondary to secretion of gastric acid or pepsin from ectopic gastric or pancreatic tissue, respectively, in the tip of the diverticulum. It is usually brisk and painless with blood ranging from dark red to bright red.

Juvenile polyps also present with painless rectal bleeding but are uncommon in children under 1 year of age with peak incidence between ages 5 and 7 years. They are more common in males and non-Caucasian people. Most juvenile polyps occur in the distal colon and may cause bleeding from autoamputation as they outgrow their blood supply. Juvenile polyps can be classified to juvenile polyposis syndrome (JPS) based on the number (five or more), distribution, and family history. Polyps are generally benign but some may suggest an inherited disorder, such as Peutz-Jeghers disease or adenomatous polyps in familial adenomatous polyposis (FAP). Affected individuals with FAP

are at significant risk for the development of colonic carcinoma and require repeated colonoscopies and, eventually, prophylactic colectomy and ileoanal pouch procedures.

In older children, inflammatory bowel disease becomes a more common cause of hematochezia. The rectal bleeding varies from occult to frank blood in the bowel movements. Blood is present in 100% of cases of ulcerative colitis but in only 30–50% of cases of Crohn disease. Inflammatory bowel disease is generally accompanied by fever, weight loss, and rectal bleeding (see Chapter 14).

Henoch-Schönlein purpura is an IgA vasculitic syndrome that can cause bloody stools. It is often accompanied by cramping abdominal pain, purpuric rash (palpable purpura), joint swelling, scalp edema (infants and toddlers), and, occasionally, nephritis (see Chapter 22).

OCCULT GASTROINTESTINAL BLEEDING

Occult gastrointestinal bleeding (OGIB) is defined as bleeding that is unknown to the patient. This condition most often presents as iron-deficiency anemia or positive occult blood during evaluation for abdominal pain, vomiting, diarrhea, or weight loss. Normal fecal blood loss ranges from 0.5 to 1.5 mL/day. In occult bleeding, a patient can lose up to 100 mL/day and the stool can still appear grossly normal.

History

While the history of iron-deficiency anemia might be the only clinical clue to diagnose OGIB, it should always be in the differential diagnosis of chronic iron-deficiency anemia. Due to a very low degree of bleeding, symptoms are minimal and typically related to iron-deficiency anemia including irritability, anorexia, and lethargy.

Physical Examination

In contrast to overt GI bleeding, changes in hemodynamic status or vital signs are unlikely. Pallor is usually seen at palmar creases, nail beds, and conjunctivae. Other physical examinations to determine the underlying cause of bleeding are similar to those for upper and lower GI bleeding.

Differential Diagnosis

OGIB in children can be caused by any lesion in the GI tract, particularly in the upper GI tract and small intestine. The causes of OGIB are similar to those of overt bleeding discussed previously.

Angiodysplasia/Angioectasia

These abnormal vascular lesions are dilated, tortuous mucosal small blood vessels of unknown etiology that can produce occult (occasionally acute) upper or lower intestinal blood loss (~50% are in the small bowel) (Fig. 16.8). They are more common in older adults but may produce recurrent and chronic intestinal bleeding in children, particularly those with hereditary hemorrhagic telangiectasia, von Willebrand disease, aortic stenosis, and end-stage renal disease, although they are often independent of an underlying disorder. They may be isolated or multiple. Other vascular etiologies of intestinal blood loss are noted in Table 16.7.

DIAGNOSTIC EVALUATIONS

Laboratory Evaluation

Initial laboratory evaluation should include a CBC with differential and platelet count, coagulation profile, and a comprehensive metabolic profile with total and direct bilirubin (Table 16.8). Patients with clinical signs of significant blood loss should have a blood typing with cross match sent. Occult blood testing can be performed on stool or emesis to confirm presence of blood. In patients with lower GI bleeding, stool

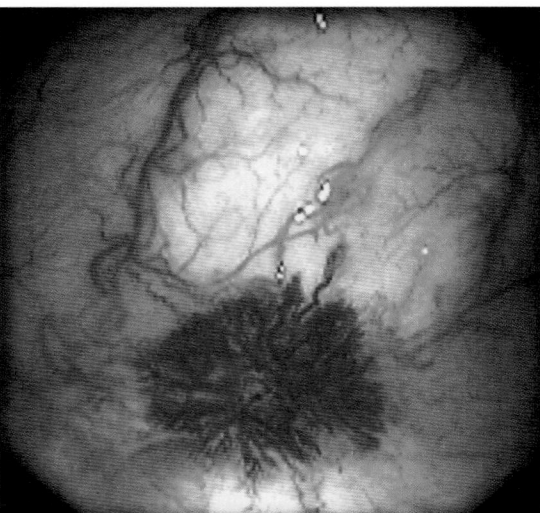

Fig. 16.8 Endoscopic image of an angioectasia (AE) in the ascending colon. This AE has a typical coral reef–like pattern of small vessels distorting the mucosa and submucosa. A tortuous submucosal vein, which is the earliest stage in the development of AE, is probably present among the linear vessels intersecting the ectasia but cannot be distinguished. (From Feldman M, Friedman LS, Brandt LJ, eds. *Sleisenger and Fordtran's Gastrointestinal and Liver Disease*. 11th ed. Philadelphia: Elsevier; 2021, Fig. 38-1.)

should be sent for analysis of infectious causes. UA may be useful in patients with hematochezia with suspicion for hemolytic uremic syndrome. Iron studies should also be tested to evaluate for iron deficiency secondary to bleeding.

Imaging

Radiographs

Abdominal radiographs should be obtained in all infants with acute hematochezia to look for pneumoperitoneum, pneumatosis intestinalis, or hepatic portal vein gas suggesting necrotizing enterocolitis. Flat plate films may also identify intussusception, volvulus, abdominal masses, or foreign bodies (Fig. 16.9). Upper GI contrast studies can discern anatomic lesions, such as strictures, stenosis, atresias, malrotation, large ulcerations, and masses. Small bowel follow-through examination allows evaluation of the small bowel from the ligament of Treitz to the ileocecal valve. Areas of ulceration, mucosal thickening, and narrowing may be appreciated. An air or water-soluble enema should be performed in infants and children in whom there is a concern of distal intestinal obstruction, such as intussusception (see Chapter 13). In cases of intussusception, the enema not only aids in diagnosis but also may be therapeutic. Crohn disease and ulcerative colitis may be suggested by results of this test, but endoscopy is necessary for histologic confirmation of these diagnoses.

Abdominal Ultrasound

An ultrasound may be useful in patients with suspected liver disease to evaluate for portal hypertension. It may also be used in potential cases of intussusception or suspected large vascular malformations (Fig. 16.10).

Computed Tomography

CT scans may be useful in evaluating possible anatomic anomalies and may reveal signs of inflammation related to infectious or inflammatory colitis. CT enterography can localize an *active* lower GI bleed. Given the radiation exposure, the value of a CT over other diagnostic modalities must be considered.

TABLE 16.7 **Vascular Lesions of the GI Tract**
Primary Vascular Lesions
Aneurysms of the aorta and its branches
Angioectasia (angiodysplasia, vascular ectasia)
Arteriovenous malformation
Blue rubber bleb nevus
Capillary phlebectasia
Dieulafoy lesion
Glomus tumor
Hemangioma
Hemangiomatosis
Hemangioendothelioma
Hemangiopericytoma
Hemangiosarcoma
Hemorrhoids
Kaposi sarcoma
Diseases and Syndromes with Vascular Lesions
Blue rubber bleb nevus syndrome
Ehlers-Danlos syndrome
Hereditary hemorrhagic telangiectasia (Osler-Weber-Rendu disease)
Klippel-Trenaunay or Parkes Weber syndrome
Kohlmeier-Degos syndrome
Marfan syndrome
Pseudoxanthoma elasticum
PSS (scleroderma, CREST)
Scurvy
Turner syndrome
von Willebrand disease
Systemic Disorders Associated with Vascular Lesions
Portal hypertension
Congestive gastropathy and colopathy
GAVE (watermelon stomach)
Spider telangiectasias
Varices
Renal failure
GI telangiectasias
Vasculitis (e.g., polyarteritis nodosa)
Iatrogenic lesions
Radiation telangiectasia

CREST, calcinosis, Raynaud phenomenon, esophageal dysmotility, sclerodactyly, telangiectasia; GAVE, gastric antral vascular ectasia; GI, gastrointestinal; PSS, progressive systemic sclerosis.
From Feldman M, Friedman LS, Brandt LJ, eds. *Sleisenger and Fordtran's Gastrointestinal and Liver Disease*. 11th ed. Philadelphia: Elsevier; 2021:618, Box 37-1.

Magnetic Resonance Enterography

Magnetic resonance enterography (MRE) can be useful in cases of occult bleeding or in suspected and known inflammatory bowel disease to evaluate for areas of inflammation in the small bowel that may be causing blood loss. Patients must be awake and able to stay still through the prolonged study, which limits its utility in younger patients.

Angiography

Angiography may help identify the source of bleeding but is only sensitive for an active bleed at a rate of at least 0.5 mL/min. The diagnostic efficacy can be improved with provocative measures by using anticoagulants, vasodilators, and fibrinolytic agents to prolong, augment, or reactivate the bleeding. The safety of provoking bleeding in the patient must be considered. The classic angiographic finding that confirms active bleeding is extravasation of contrast material such as in a Meckel diverticulum or the presence of vascular malformations of the bowel, which may be acquired or congenital. Therapeutic angiography can also be used to control GI bleeding.

TABLE 16.8 Laboratory Findings Suggestive of a Diagnosis

Lab Finding	Significance
Hgb/HCT	Normal hemoglobin or hematocrit does not rule out significant bleed as it may take time to equilibrate
Low MCV	Chronic blood loss
Low platelets	HUS, hypersplenism (secondary to portal hypertension), ITP, DIC
High platelets	Chronic blood loss, inflammation, IBD
Elevated prothrombin time	Liver disease, coagulation disorder, DIC
Elevated BUN/normal Cr	UGI bleed more likely
Elevated BUN/elevated Cr	HUS or HSP
Decreased albumin	IBD or liver disease
Elevated ESR/CRP	IBD
Elevated AST/ALT	Liver disease
Elevated bilirubin	Liver disease
Fecal calprotectin	IBD, infectious enteritis
Eosinophilia	Parasitic infestation

ALT, alanine aminotransferase; AST, aspartate aminotransferase; Cr, creatinine; DIC, disseminated intravascular coagulation; Hgb/HCT, hemoglobin/hematocrit; HSP, Henoch-Schönlein purpura; HUS, hemolytic uremic syndrome; IBD, inflammatory bowel disease; ITP, immune thrombocytopenic purpura; MCV, mean corpuscular volume; UGI, upper gastrointestinal.

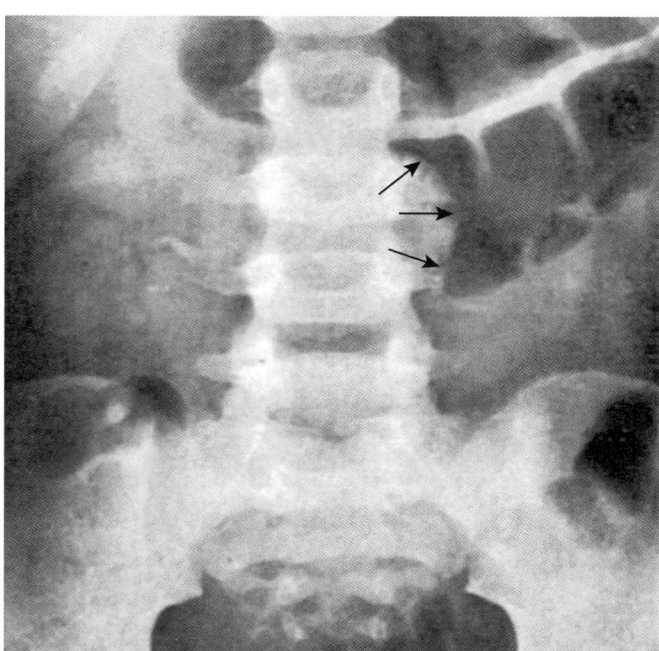

Fig. 16.9 Flat plate film demonstrating intussusception *(arrows)*.

Nuclear Imaging

Nuclear medicine may determine the site of bleeding with minimal complications; it is associated with minimal radiation exposure and requires minimal sedation. Technetium 99m (99mTc) pertechnetate is rapidly taken up by gastric mucosa, and it is useful in identifying sites of bleeding secondary to ectopic gastric mucosa. Gastric mucosa is found in 90% of bleeding Meckel diverticula, and in these patients the Meckel scan has a sensitivity of 94% and a specificity of 97% in the pediatric population (Fig. 16.11). False-negative results have been reported frequently because of insufficient gastric tissue mass, downstream washout of isotope, impaired blood supply, or suboptimal techniques. Positive identification may be improved by the administration of ranitidine to prevent excretion of pertechnetate from gastric tissue.

Bleeding scans are performed by intravenously injecting technetium sulfur colloid. The agent is distributed quickly and is rapidly taken up by the reticuloendothelial system. It can detect a rate of bleeding of 0.1 mL/min. However, because the technetium is taken up by the reticuloendothelial system, this may hinder the search for bleeding sites behind the liver or spleen. Finally, the clearance is very rapid, with a half-life of 2 minutes, which means that bleeding has to be occurring at the time of the scan.

The 99mTc pertechnetate–labeled red blood cell scan is a sensitive and accurate test for the localization of active bleeding. In cases of intermittent bleeding, a single injection of labeled cells allows repeated scans for up to 24 hours. It can detect as little blood as 0.5 mL/min.

Procedural Evaluations

Upper Endoscopy or Esophagogastroduodenoscopy

Esophagogastroduodenoscopy (EGD) is the procedure of choice in identifying the site of upper GI bleeding. EGD can also allow direct

intervention at the bleeding site, as in the case of esophageal varices or a visible vessel in an ulcer crater. Endoscopic visualization of the stomach and duodenum should be performed even if the bleeding is thought to originate from esophageal varices. Of patients with proven esophageal varices, 50% may manifest bleeding from gastritis or peptic ulcer disease rather than the varices. Endoscopy, however, should not be performed until the patient is as hemodynamically stable as possible. Gastric lavage may be useful prior to upper endoscopy to remove any blood present in the stomach to allow for better views as well as to determine whether there is still active bleeding. Erythromycin can be given prior to endoscopy to accelerate gastric emptying and removal of blood from the stomach.

Lower Endoscopy

Lower GI tract bleeding can also be evaluated endoscopically. Procedures frequently used in children include proctosigmoidoscopy and flexible colonoscopy. With the patient under appropriate sedation, lower GI endoscopy allows for full exploration of the colon; identifies the presence of multiple lesions; allows for therapeutic intervention to bleeding lesions through electrocoagulation, laser therapy, or thermocoagulation; and allows for removal of bleeding lesions, such as polyps. Colonoscopy is indicated when there is melena or severe bleeding with no evidence of upper GI lesions, when stools are guaiac positive over a long time, and when examination of the terminal ileum is indicated to determine whether inflammatory bowel disease is present. One disadvantage is that large amounts of luminal blood obscure visualization of a lesion. Before lower GI colonoscopy, intestinal lavage with oral administration of polyethylene glycol should be used to remove as much of the luminal blood and stool as possible.

Small Bowel Enteroscopy

Small bowel enteroscopy refers to endoscopic examination of the small intestine, extending into the jejunum and/or ileum. Enteroscopy can be useful in the evaluation of occult bleeding. While its diagnostic yield

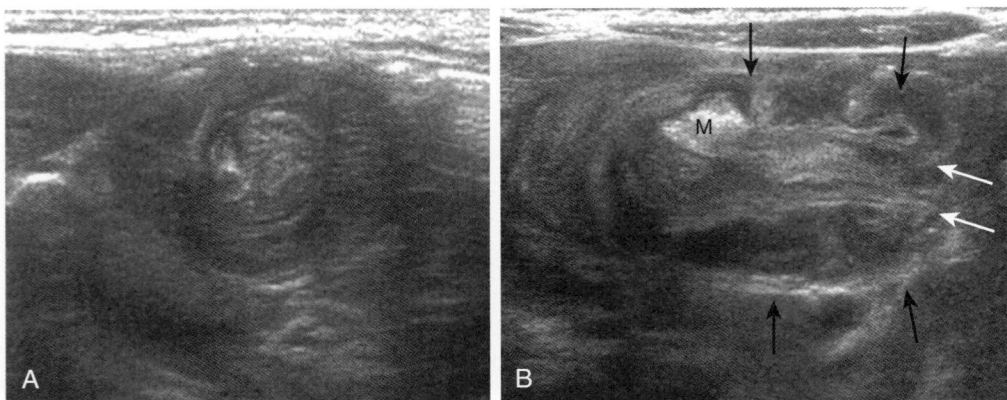

Fig. 16.10 Abdominal ultrasound illustrating intussusception. *A,* Transverse plane shows target-like appearance of bowel. *B,* Longitudinal plane shows inner bowel loops *(white arrows)* telescoping through outer bowel loops *(black arrows).* Edema of affected bowel causes hyperechoic mucosa *(M).*

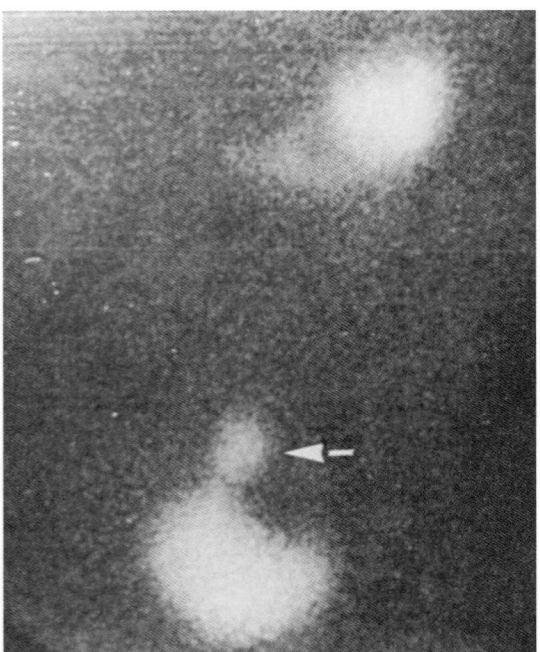

Fig. 16.11 Positive Meckel scan. *Arrow* indicates abnormal area of increased uptake in lower abdomen above bladder, consistent with gastric mucosa containing Meckel diverticulum.

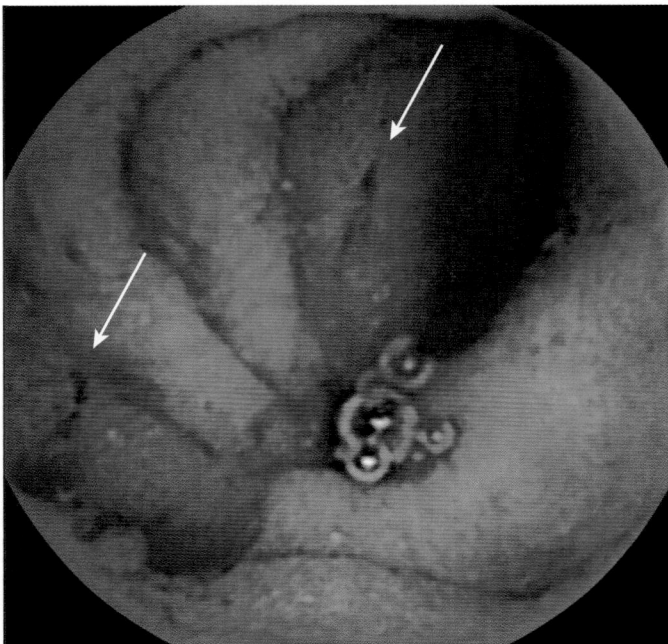

Fig. 16.12 Capsule endoscopy image revealing jejunal bleeding *(arrows)* from a vascular malformation in a patient who presented with anemia refractory to iron supplementation.

varies by study, it allows for direct intervention if the source of bleeding is found. In addition, it has been employed intraoperatively to help identify lesions and guide surgical intervention.

Capsule Endoscopy

Wireless camera capsule endoscopy may be useful in patients with occult or apparent bleeding when other work-up, including an upper and lower endoscopy, has been negative. The patient swallows or has the capsule placed endoscopically and images are taken as the capsule passes through the small and large intestines, which can identify vascular malformations and other sources of bleeding (Fig. 16.12). The main risk is capsule retention and so children must be of a certain size and be evaluated for possible stricture prior to the study.

Treatment

Resuscitation

The severity of bleeding determines the general guidelines for treatment. For severe bleeding, initial management re-establishes and maintains the intravascular volume. Subsequently, the site of blood loss must be determined and attempts made to stop the hemorrhage. Severe anemia also necessitates packed red blood cell transfusions after the intravascular volume deficit is corrected (Table 16.9).

Although parents tend to overestimate the amount of blood lost by their child, a major error in the management of GI bleeding is underestimating blood loss. The hematocrit may remain unchanged initially, despite significant blood loss, and therefore is not a good indicator of significant bleeding. If orthostatic blood

TABLE 16.9 Initial Management of Patients with Hypovolemia Secondary to Gastrointestinal Hemorrhage

1. Establish adequate intravenous (IV) access by placing two IV catheters.
   - Recommended catheter size:
     - Infant: 20 gauge
     - Child: 18 gauge
     - Adolescent: 16 gauge
2. Rapidly infuse saline or lactated Ringer solution; use smaller boluses and frequent monitoring in patients with suspected varices to avoid rapid increase in venous pressure and worsening of variceal bleed.
3. Carefully monitor pulse, blood pressure, and central venous pressure to avoid fluid overload.
4. Monitor urine output, skin perfusion, and orthostatic changes in pulse and blood pressure for early recognition of shock.
5. Transfuse with packed red blood cells to return oxygen-carrying capacity to normal.
6. Carefully record all fluids transfused, and estimate and record all recognized fluids lost.

Modified from Olson AD, Hillemeier AC. Gastrointestinal hemorrhage. In: Wyllie R, Hyams JS, eds. *Pediatric Gastrointestinal Disease*. Philadelphia: WB Saunders; 1993:253.

pressure changes or tachycardia is present, the initial goal of treatment should be to hemodynamically stabilize the patient, maintain the intravascular volume, and provide adequate oxygen delivery to the tissues. A second potential error is the failure to establish adequate intravenous (IV) access. The largest possible IV catheter must be rapidly placed in a child with active bleeding. Blood loss should be replaced immediately with a crystalloid solution, such as normal saline or lactated Ringer solution. Initially, a fluid push of 20 mL/kg should be given, although resuscitation should be performed cautiously in patients who may have portal hypertension as overly aggressive resuscitation raises the venous pressure and could worsen bleeding from varices. In these patients, small, repeated fluid boluses with close monitoring are preferred to large-volume boluses. If blood loss continues and the patient appears to be at risk for hypovolemic shock, infusion of normal saline or colloid solutions (5% albumin) can be continued until blood is available. Plasma is indicated if coagulation factors are depleted. Once bleeding has stopped, transfusions of packed red blood cells should continue, to slowly raise the hematocrit to 30% (10 g/dL hemoglobin) (for patients with variceal bleeding the goal is instead hemoglobin of 8–9 g/dL). If continued blood loss necessitates multiple transfusions, fresh frozen plasma and calcium should be given to replace coagulation factors and correct the hypocalcemia caused by the citrate in blood products. The platelet count in such patients must be monitored because thrombocytopenia may develop.

If an NG tube is inserted, the tube size is determined by the child's age and size. A 12 French tube is used in infants and preschool children; a 14 or 16 French tube is appropriate for children of elementary school age or older. Gastric lavage should be undertaken with room temperature normal saline. The color of the gastric lavage fluid gives the physician an indication of the rate of bleeding. Lavage returns that are bright red indicate significant ongoing bleeding; pink-tinged or brown flecks in the solution indicate less significant or minimal bleeding.

Maintaining a gastric pH of more than 4 is considered standard therapy for upper GI mucosal bleeding. This can be accomplished with either H_2-receptor antagonists or proton pump inhibitors.

Vasoactive Agents

In patients with suspected variceal bleeding, a continuous infusion of octreotide may be started. This agent reduces splanchnic blood flow with minimal disturbance to other organs. It is safer than vasopressin but has not been shown to have benefit in nonvariceal bleeding. Customarily, a bolus of octreotide (1–2 µg/kg) is given over 5–10 minutes, and this is followed by a continuous infusion of 1 µg/kg/hr, although higher doses may be required. The infusion may help control the bleeding until definitive therapy (banding or sclerotherapy) is performed. After endoscopic intervention, octreotide infusions may be weaned slowly (every 12 hours) with close monitoring of the patient to ensure varices do not rebleed. See Table 16.10 for additional pharmacotherapy.

Endoscopic Modalities

Most patients with GI bleeding will undergo upper and/or lower endoscopy for definitive diagnosis and treatment. The aim of therapeutic endoscopy is to stop bleeding and prevent rebleeding. Endoscopy should be performed when the patient has been stabilized, and preferably within 24 hours of bleeding presentation. For patients with mucosal lesions, such as ulcers or bleeding polyps, there are multiple therapeutic interventions available. Injection therapy with diluted epinephrine and sclerosants, ablative therapy (contact methods such as thermocoagulation heater probe and electrocoagulation; noncontact methods such as argon plasma coagulation), mechanical therapy (such as with hemoclips and band ligation), and hemostatic powder spray can be used to stop active bleeding. Vascular lesions may also be treated endoscopically. For patients with colitis, colonoscopy is used primarily to confirm diagnosis and extent of disease.

Variceal banding is the preferred method for treating bleeding esophageal varices (Fig. 16.13*A* and *B*). Ideally, the banding takes place after good control of acute bleeding, affording the endoscopist an unobstructed view of the varices. Side effects of this therapy are minimal, and the procedure is repeated weekly to monthly until the varices are obliterated. Sclerotherapy is also effective in controlling the acute bleeding from esophageal varices and may be performed weekly to monthly until the varices resolve. In young children whose upper esophageal sphincter is too small for the endoscopic banding device to pass, sclerotherapy may be the only option. Complications include esophageal ulceration and esophageal stricture. A number of sclerosing agents (e.g., ethanolamine, sodium morrhuate, ethanol, tetradecyl sulfate) are efficacious in treating varices. Empiric broad-spectrum antibiotics are also typically administered in patients with liver disease causing variceal bleeding due to a high association of infection with bleeding.

Interventional Radiology

Selective embolization during angiography can be used to treat vascular malformations and to control bleeding from ulcers. The rate of complications from angiography is 2%, whether the procedure is diagnostic or therapeutic. In patients with intrahepatic portal hypertension with bleeding from GI sites inaccessible to sclerotherapy or banding, coiling of varices or transjugular intrahepatic portosystemic shunting may be beneficial.

Surgical Intervention

Surgical intervention is a definitive treatment for many of the anatomic anomalies causing GI bleeding and may be performed in conjunction with endoscopy to identify the lesion. Despite effective nonoperative therapeutic interventions, traditional operations such as suture ligation, lesion or organ excision, vagotomy, portosystemic anastomosis, and devascularization procedures continue to be helpful in many instances.

TABLE 16.10   Pharmacotherapy in Pediatric Gastrointestinal Bleeding*

Medication	Dosage
Proton Pump Inhibitor†—Acid Reducer	
Pantoprazole†	*IV:* ≥2 yr: 0.8 or 1.6 mg/kg once daily (max dose: 80 mg/dose) *Oral:* ≤5 yr: 1.2 mg/kg/day once daily >5 yr: 20 (<40 kg) or 40 mg once daily (>40 kg)
Esomeprazole†	*IV:* <1 yr: 0.5 mg/kg once daily >1 yr: <55 kg: 10 mg once daily >55 kg: 20 mg once daily *Oral:* 3–5 kg: 2.5 mg once daily 5–7.5 kg: 5 mg once daily 7.5–20 kg: 10 mg once daily ≥20 kg: 10–20 mg once daily
Omeprazole†	*Oral:* 5 kg to <10 kg: 5 mg once daily 10–20 kg: 10 mg once daily ≥20 kg: 20 mg once daily (max 40 mg/day)
Lansoprazole†	*Oral:* Infants 1–2 mg/kg/day ≤30 kg: 15 mg once daily >30 kg: 30 mg once daily
H₂-Receptor Antagonist—Acid Reducer (Alternative If IV PPI is Not Available)	
Ranitidine‡	*IV:* ≤16 yr: 2–4 mg/kg/day divided every 6–8 hr (max dose: 50 mg/dose) >16 yr: 50 mg every 6–8 hr

Medication	Dosage
	Oral: ≤16 yr: 4–8 mg/kg/day divided twice daily (max dose: 300 mg/day) >16 yr: 150 mg twice daily
Famotidine	*IV* 0.25 mg/kg/dose every 12 hr (max dose: 20 mg/dose) *Oral:* ≤16 yr: 0.5 mg/kg/day nightly or divided twice daily (max dose: 40 mg/day) >16 yr: 40 mg/day nightly or divided twice daily (max dose: 40 mg/day)
Vasoactive Agent—Somatostatin Analog, Selectively Decreases Splanchnic Blood Flow	
Octreotide	*IV:* 1–2 µg/kg initial bolus followed by 1–2 µg/kg/hr continuous infusion (doses up to 4 µg/kg/hr have been used) Following endoscopic intervention may taper dose by 50% every 12 hr and discontinue when dose is 25% of initial dose
Mucosal Coating Agent—Coats Mucosal Injury, Binds Bile Acids to Prevent Further Injury, Inhibits Pepsin in the Presence of Acid	
Sucralfate§	*Oral:* 40–80 mg/kg/day divided every 6 hr (max dose: 1,000 mg/dose)

*Dosages listed are from *Pediatric Lexi-Comp* online formulary and do not apply to infants aged <3 mo. Evidence-based dosing of these medications is not well established.

†Proton pump inhibitors (PPIs) should not be administered in infants aged <1 yr without endoscopic evidence of acid-induced disease.

‡Ranitidine has been withdrawn from the US market.

§Use in conjunction with PPI may limit efficacy.

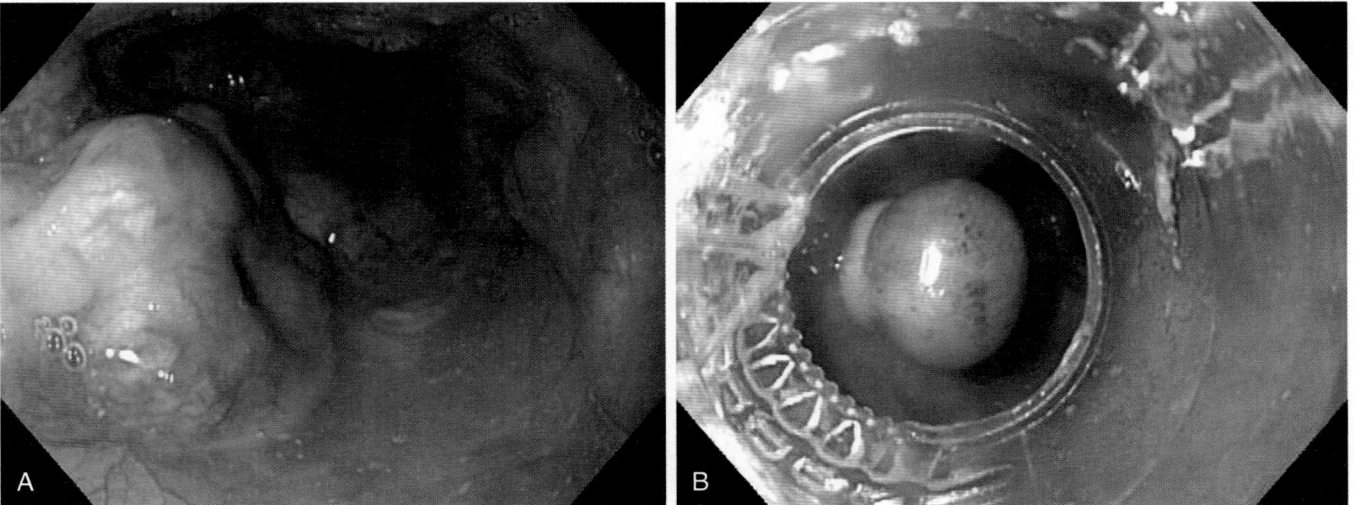

Fig. 16.13 Variceal banding is the preferred method for treating esophageal varices. *A,* Grade 3 esophageal varices in patient with cirrhosis. *B,* View of varices after band application.

SUMMARY AND RED FLAGS

GI bleeding may occur anywhere along the GI tract and can range from occult blood loss to massive hemorrhage. Approach to GI bleeding begins with ensuring hemodynamic stability of the patient while obtaining a thorough history and physical exam to help determine upper versus lower sources of bleeding. Iron-deficiency anemia in a male or premenstrual female should raise the suspicion of occult blood loss. Red flags include hemodynamic instability that necessitates immediate attention. Laboratory, radiologic, endoscopic, and surgical evaluation are used for confirmation of diagnosis and potential treatment.

BIBLIOGRAPHY

A bibliography is available at ExpertConsult.com.

17

Hepatomegaly

Grzegorz W. Telega

Hepatomegaly can occur as a feature of primary liver disease or as a result of systemic disorders such as congenital anomalies, inborn errors of metabolism, and perinatal or postnatal infections (Tables 17.1 and 17.2). Common symptoms of hepatic dysfunction, such as fatigue, fever of unknown origin, pruritus, failure to thrive, confusion, change in mental status, and/or diarrhea, are nonspecific. Hepatomegaly and jaundice are frequently the findings that lead to an evaluation for liver disease. Causes of hepatomegaly associated with jaundice are discussed in Chapter 18.

ASSESSMENT OF THE LIVER

An accurate assessment of liver size is an important initial step. Considerable patience may be necessary to obtain the required information. The patient should lie down in a supine position with the knees flexed. The abdominal muscles should be relaxed as much as possible. The provider should become familiar with the sensation of pressure over the abdominal wall in the lower abdomen in order to detect the difference palpating while transitioning over the liver edge. The examiner should also be sure that the lower border of a massively enlarged liver is not missed by failure to palpate below the umbilicus. The lower edge of the liver should be determined by palpation just lateral to the right rectus muscle. Careful palpation of the liver edge along the lower border is important as enlargement of the liver can be asymmetrical in chronic cirrhosis, such as in Budd-Chiari syndrome and with liver tumors.

The lower edge of the liver is usually palpable in normal subjects with deep inspiration when it moves downward 1–3 cm. In the newborn, the liver edge may be palpable 2–3 cm below the right costal margin, but that distance is usually less than 2 cm by 4–6 months of age. In older children, the liver edge is usually not more than 1 cm below the right costal margin except on deep inspiration. The liver may be normally palpable in the midline several centimeters below the xiphoid.

Palpation should always be combined with percussion of the upper and lower boundaries of the liver. The upper edge of the liver is determined through percussion passing downward from the nipple line. The examiner may also define the lower edge through light percussion, moving upward from the umbilicus toward the costal margin. The anterior span of the liver is the difference between the highest and lowest points of hepatic dullness in the right midclavicular line.

In the scratch test, the stethoscope is placed over the right lower costal area. The examiner then scratches the skin of the abdomen and uses auscultation to detect the lower liver edge by using the difference in sound transmission over solid liver and hollow intestine.

It is important to remember that physical examination has limitations. It may be difficult to detect the borders of the liver in patients with morbid obesity, ascites, pleural effusion, or extensive surgical scars, or resisting exam. Physical examination determines only the external borders of the liver and does not truly measure liver volume. A downward, tonguelike projection of the right lobe—the Riedel lobe—is a normal anatomic variant that is more commonly found in girls. It is a common error to express liver size and to define hepatomegaly on the basis of only the liver edge felt below the right costal margin. The liver may be displaced downward in patients with pulmonary disease, particularly with hyperaeration of the lungs. It may be difficult in some cases to distinguish masses arising from the right kidney or adrenal gland from an enlarged liver.

Liver size changes with age in proportion to the body size (Table 17.3). At birth, the liver constitutes approximately 4% of body weight and normally occupies a larger portion of the abdominal cavity than it does later in life. Liver weight increases twofold by the end of the first year of life, triples by the age of 3 years, and is increased sixfold by the age of 9 years. In the adult, liver weight is approximately 12 times that in the neonate.

The consistency and surface of the liver should be noted, including whether the liver edge is sharp or rounded and whether the liver surface is soft, hard, or irregular. The liver edge is normally soft, fairly sharp, and nontender. Livers enlarged because of congestive heart failure or because of acute infiltration by inflammatory cells or tumor are firm, have a somewhat rounded edge, and have smooth surfaces. In cirrhosis, the liver is hard and may have an irregular surface and edge. Tenderness generally suggests an acute process, as rapid distention of the liver capsule causes pain.

Hepatomegaly may resolve rapidly when congestive heart failure is controlled, biliary obstruction is relieved, diabetes is better controlled, or massive liver cell necrosis leads to collapse of the liver tissue.

History and Physical Examination

Once the presence of hepatomegaly is established, the provider should focus on the aspects of the history and physical examination that will direct the diagnostic evaluation (Tables 17.4 and 17.5). Review of systems should focus on growth, achievement of developmental milestones, changes in mental status, vomiting, diarrhea, fevers, pruritus, easy bruising, bleeding, urine output, and abdominal distention. Obtaining a detailed family and travel history is important, as many conditions leading to hepatomegaly are genetic in nature or are a result of infections. The possibility of intentional or accidental drug intake along with herbal or over-the-counter supplements should always be entertained. On physical examination, it is important to determine the presence or absence of jaundice, splenomegaly, ascites, change in mental status, tremors, neurologic abnormalities, fever, signs of malnutrition, prominent vascular patterns on the anterior abdominal wall (caput medusae, spider angiomas), arterial hypertension, hypotension, bruising, petechiae, hemangiomas, pallor, obesity, renal enlargement, masses outside of the liver, lymphadenopathy, muscle weakness, cyanosis, heart murmurs, tachypnea, tachycardia, abnormal eye exam (cataracts, Kayser-Fleischer ring), bone and joint abnormalities, and dysmorphic features. A pelvic exam in sexually active females may detect signs of a sexually transmitted infection, which can lead to perihepatitis (formerly Fitz-Hugh–Curtis) syndrome.

TABLE 17.1 Causes of Hepatomegaly in Infants and Children

Infection and Inflammation

Viral hepatitis (hepatitis A, B, C, D, E; EBV; adenovirus, echovirus, TORCH)

Autoimmune hepatitis

Sepsis

Perinatal infections

Allograft rejection

Graft versus host disease

Systemic lupus erythematosus

Juvenile idiopathic arthritis

Primary sclerosing cholangitis

Systemic granulomatous disorders with hepatic involvement

Sarcoid

Tuberculosis

Hepatic abscess (bacterial and parasitic)

Parasitic infection

Visceral larva migrans

Schistosomiasis

Leishmoniasis

Malaria

Liver flukes

Kupffer cell hyperplasia

Macrophage activation syndrome

Gestational alloimmune liver disease

Biliary Obstruction

Biliary atresia

Choledochal cysts

Stricture of common bile duct

Primary sclerosing cholangitis

Infiltration

Extramedullary hematopoiesis

Erythroblastosis fetalis

Thalassemias

Metastatic tumors

Neuroblastoma

Wilms tumor

Leukemia

Lymphoma

Hemophagocytic lymphohistiocytosis (HLH)

Langerhans cell histiocytosis

Storage/Metabolic Disease

α_1-Antitrypsin deficiency

Wilson disease

Infants of diabetic mothers

Glycogen storage disease

Galactosemia

Tyrosinemia

Cystic fibrosis

Gaucher disease

Niemann-Pick disease

Gangliosidoses

Hereditary fructose intolerance

Mitochondrial hepatic disorders including DNA depletion syndrome

Mucopolysaccharidoses

Amyloidosis

Hepatic porphyrias

Expansion of Extracellular Matrix

Cirrhosis

Fibrocystic disease (congenital hepatic fibrosis)

Steatosis

Malnutrition

Nonalcoholic steatohepatitis (obesity)

Cystic fibrosis

Parenteral nutrition

Diabetes mellitus

Hereditary fructose intolerance

Galactosemia

Wolman disease

Cholesterol ester storage disease

Mitochondrial hepatopathies

β-Oxidation defects

Medication toxicity (tetracycline, valproic acid)

Hepatic Malignancy/Tumor (see Table 17.2)

Primary or metastatic

Vascular Congestion

Congestive heart failure

Budd-Chiari syndrome

Venoocclusive disease (VOD): radiation, high-dose chemotherapy, stem cell transplant, bush tea, pyrrolizidine alkaloids, familial VOD with immunodeficiency

Cystic Disease

Fibrocystic disease

Autosomal dominant polycystic kidney disease

Congenital hepatic fibrosis

Caroli syndrome

Isolated polycystic liver disease

EBV, Epstein-Barr virus; TORCH, toxoplasmosis, other infections, rubella, cytomegalovirus, herpes simplex virus.

TABLE 17.2 Hepatic Tumor Characteristics

	Clinical Findings	Age	Radiology Findings	Laboratory Findings	Biopsy Findings	Therapy	Prognosis
Hepatic hemangioma (focal, multifocal, and diffuse)	Screening for cutaneous lesions, mass, or hemodynamic effects	Generally, under 1 yr of age, up to 3 yr of age	Focal, multifocal, or diffuse vascular tumor; larger mass with necrosis, hemorrhage, and/or calcifications	Decreased T_3, T_4; normal AFP	Capillary-like vascular proliferation lined by plump endothelial cells. No significant cytologic atypia, GLUT-1 positive in multifocal and diffuse	Observation, surgery, corticosteroids or propranolol	Favorable, most involute, those with cardiac failure and hypothyroidism often require treatment
Focal nodular hyperplasia	Bleeding, torsion, hepatic mass	Adolescents 10–18 yr, post-chemotherapy for other malignancy	Well-demarcated mass with central scar	Normal AFP	Central scar with portal tracts and bile ductal proliferation, often damaged or abnormal vessel associated with scar, maplike pattern of glutamine synthetase staining	Observation, surgery	Favorable
Hepatic adenoma	Hepatic mass, often found incidentally	Adolescent late teens	Well-demarcated mass, heterogeneous appearance, intratumoral hemorrhage is common	Normal AFP	Usually solitary mass consisting of benign hepatocytes with isolated (unpaired) arteries, serum amyloid–associated protein positive	Observation, surgery	Favorable, chance of hemorrhage
Mesenchymal hamartoma	Liver mass, more often right lobe	Within the first 2 yr	Cystic mass in right lobe (75%)	Normal to slightly elevated AFP	Cystic tumor with a mixture of loose edematous/myxoid tissue with entrapped bile ducts and hepatocytes	Surgery	Favorable. Local recurrence without complete resection, small number associated with undifferentiated embryonal sarcoma (UES)
Hepatoblastoma	Liver mass, often with weight loss and hematologic paraneoplastic syndromes	70% by age 2 and 90% by age 5	Solid and nodular but can show cystic degeneration/hemorrhage or necrosis. Some with calcifications	Elevated AFP in 90% of cases	Various morphology either pure epithelial or mixed epithelial and mesenchymal components; often with necrosis and hemorrhage	Chemotherapy and surgery	Quite variable based on risk factors (staging, histology, and AFP level)
Hepatocellular carcinoma	Liver mass	In endemic HBV areas can be under 10 yr, most cases after 10 yr of age; HCV as risk factor	Can be solitary or multifocal solid lesions often with necrosis and hemorrhage. Fibrolamellar variant with central scar	Elevated AFP in two-thirds of cases	Various pattern and subtypes, loss of portal tracts, loss of reticulin network, mild to marked cellular atypia	Surgery, transarterial chemoembolization (TACE), chemotherapy	Unfavorable. Overall 5-yr survival ~24%. Better prognosis in fibrolamellar variant ~80%
Biliary tract rhabdomyosarcoma	Obstructive jaundice	Under 5 yr of age	Hilar mass with dilated biliary tree	Obstructive cholestasis, normal to slightly elevated AFP	One of two subtypes with intrabiliary growth and projections with myxoid stroma with cambium layer	Chemotherapy, radiation therapy, and surgery	Favorable. Event-free survival of 60–90%
Undifferentiated embryonal sarcoma	Liver mass, more often right lobe	5–10 yr of age	Solid and cystic areas, more often in the right lobe	Normal to slightly elevated AFP	Variable mesenchymal components with large cystic and myxoid areas with hemorrhage and necrosis	Chemotherapy and surgery	Historically, unfavorable, but recent studies suggest improved outcomes

AFP, α-fetoprotein; HBV, hepatitis B virus; HCV, hepatitis C virus; T_3, triiodothyronine; T_4, thyroxine.
From Wyllie R, Hyams JS, Kay M, eds. *Pediatric Gastrointestinal and Liver Disease.* 6th ed. Philadelphia: Elsevier; 2021:727, Table 66.3.

TABLE 17.3 Normal Liver Span in Infants and Children

Age	Span (cm)
Preterm infant	4–5
Full-term infant	5–6.5
1–5 yr	6–7
5–10 yr	7–9
10–16 yr	8–10

TABLE 17.4 Historical Features in the Diagnostic Evaluation of Hepatomegaly or Hepatosplenomegaly

Symptom	Diagnosis
Failure to thrive	Glycogen storage disease (infancy) types I, III, IV, IX, X Hereditary fructose intolerance Organic acidemias Wolman disease Cystic fibrosis Hemophagocytic lymphohistiocytosis Cholestatic liver disease
Fever	Acute and chronic hepatitis Systemic illness Hepatic abscess Hemophagocytic lymphohistiocytosis Viral infection
Diarrhea	Wolman disease Cholestatic liver disease
Peculiar odor	Organic acidemias Hepatic failure
Neurologic/psychiatric symptoms in older child	Wilson disease Porphyria Hyperammonemia (urea cycle disorders, organic acidemias) Drug intoxication/toxicity Hypoglycemia (glycogen storage disease, organic acidemias, β-oxidation defects)

Pathophysiology

The pathophysiologic mechanisms underlying the enlargement of the liver are complex and heterogeneous. Hepatomegaly may reflect proliferation or enlargement or malfunction of one or more component structures of the liver, including liver parenchyma (hepatocytes), bile ducts (cholangiocytes, cysts), the reticuloendothelial system (Kupffer cells), interstitial tissue (stellate cells, collagen), blood (including hematopoietic cells), and blood vessels (endothelial cells). The liver also increases in size as a result of hepatic tumors, benign cysts, and infiltration of inflammatory or malignant cells.

The liver is particularly susceptible to injury not only from drugs and other exogenous toxins but also from endotoxins that arise after the activation of inflammatory cells and the production of cytokines. Inborn errors of metabolism can be responsible for disturbances of liver structure and function and can produce hepatomegaly. The liver can be enlarged because of storage of glycogen, lipid, or glycolipids within the hepatocyte. In glycogen storage disease, the cytoplasm of enlarged hepatocytes is filled with dense pools of glycogen particles that displace other organelles. Steatosis is a frequent finding in diabetic or obese patients and is characterized via ultrasound showing large lipid

inclusions, which may almost entirely fill the cytoplasm of hepatocytes. In lysosomal storage disorders such as Gaucher disease and Niemann-Pick disease, there is marked involvement of Kupffer cells with lysosomal inclusions characteristic of each disorder. Inclusions may also be present within hepatocytes; they contribute to hepatomegaly.

In many cases of biliary obstruction, such as biliary atresia, there may be significant hepatic enlargement, related in part to fibrosis and portal tract edema. As part of the liver's response to biliary obstruction, there may also be marked proliferation of small bile ductules that contribute to liver mass. Other conditions in which this could occur include choledochal cysts and common bile duct strictures.

The liver is the largest reticuloendothelial organ, and Kupffer cells, which are intensely phagocytic cells that line the sinusoids, constitute 15% of all the cells in the liver. In septicemia, hepatitis, and several other inflammatory conditions, hepatomegaly may result from proliferation and hyperplasia of Kupffer cells. Kupffer cells also contribute to hepatomegaly in lysosomal storage disorders.

Resident stellate cells produce collagen, leading to fibrosis and eventually cirrhosis in response to injury of the liver from numerous causes, including infection, drug toxicity, and biliary obstruction. Hepatocellular injury activates stellate cells leading to the production of collagen and fibrosis. Fibrosis is a long-standing process, which may evolve over time leading to complete disruption of hepatic architecture and cirrhosis. Although an end-stage cirrhotic liver is usually small, it may be enlarged during the early stages of evolution. Congenital hepatic fibrosis is an inherited malformation of the liver characterized by the presence of broad bands of fibrous tissue and numerous distorted bile ducts and vascular structures. All of these abnormal components contribute to marked enlargement and hardening of the liver.

About 15% of the liver is occupied by sinusoidal and vascular structures. The liver is capable of rapid and massive enlargement in association with increased venous pressure. Distention of hepatic sinusoids can be present in congestive heart failure, constrictive pericarditis, or obstruction of hepatic venous outflow resulting from thrombosis or endothelial damage from drug toxicity (venoocclusive disease).

Since the liver serves as a secondary site of hematopoiesis, hepatomegaly can be caused by extramedullary hematopoiesis, particularly in young infants. Extramedullary hematopoiesis can be the result of chronic inflammation, hemolysis, hemophagocytic lymphohistiocytosis (HLH), or bone marrow failure.

Hepatomegaly can occur as a result of cellular infiltration by inflammatory cells. Lymphocytic infiltrate is present in various forms of acute and chronic viral hepatitis, or in autoimmune hepatitis. Plasma cells are a prominent part of the infiltrate in autoimmune disease. Macrophages may be seen, particularly in reaction to liver cell necrosis. The increase in liver size resulting from cellular infiltration may be balanced by loss of liver cell mass from liver cell necrosis or apoptosis.

Cellular infiltration of the liver may also occur in malignant disorders such as leukemia. A number of intraabdominal malignancies such as neuroblastoma may metastasize to the liver, producing hepatomegaly.

A variety of space-occupying lesions can lead to hepatomegaly. Cysts, either isolated or communicating with the biliary tract; tumors intrinsic to the liver; and hepatic abscesses can all be associated with hepatomegaly. Each must be differentiated by clinical features and defined more precisely by imaging studies.

EVALUATION OF THE CHILD WITH HEPATOMEGALY

Laboratory Studies

Laboratory assessment of liver function is essential (Table 17.6). Because of the large functional reserve of the liver, hepatomegaly may be the only clinical indication of liver disease. The onset of symptoms such as jaundice and bleeding may be delayed long after laboratory

TABLE 17.5   Physical Signs in the Differential Diagnosis of Hepatomegaly

Sign	Differential Diagnosis	Sign	Differential Diagnosis
Asymmetric hepatomegaly	Tumor, cyst, abscess	Neurodegeneration	Mucopolysaccharidoses (types IH, II, III)
Abdominal mass	Congenital hepatic fibrosis/polycystic kidneys		Gaucher disease types II and III
	Extrahepatic tumors (neuroblastoma, Wilms tumor)		GM_2 gangliosidosis
	Choledochal cysts		Niemann-Pick disease types A, B, C
	Adenoma		Glycoproteinoses
	Hepatoblastoma		Mucolipidoses
	Hepatocellular carcinoma		Disorders of protein glycosylation
Hepatic bruit	Hemangioendothelioma		Peroxisomal disorders (Zellweger syndrome)
Splenomegaly	Congenital infection		Mitochondrial disorders
	Systemic infection (viral, bacterial, fungal)	Hypotonia	Glycogen storage disease type II
	Cirrhosis		Peroxisomal disorders (Zellweger syndrome)
	Portal hypertension		Mitochondrial disorders
	Lysosomal storage disease		Mucolipidoses
	Lymphoma	Malnutrition	Cystic fibrosis
Cutaneous hemangioma or telangiectasia	Hemangioendothelioma		Steatosis
	Hereditary hemorrhagic telangiectasia	Virilization	Hepatoblastoma
	Cirrhosis (vascular spiders)		Nonalcoholic fatty liver
Coarse/dysmorphic facial features	Mucopolysaccharidosis	Eye findings	
	GM_1 gangliosidosis	Cataracts	Galactosemia
	Glycoproteinoses (sialidosis, mucolipidosis II)	Kayser-Fleischer rings	Wilson disease
	Disorders of protein glycosylation	Telangiectasias	Hereditary hemorrhagic telangiectasia
	Glycogen storage disease type I	Iritis	Primary sclerosing cholangitis
	Alagille syndrome	Chorioretinitis	Congenital or acquired infections
	Zellweger syndrome	Cherry red spot	Lysosomal storage diseases
Episodic acute encephalopathy/coma	Disorders of fatty acid β-oxidation		GM_2 gangliosidosis
	Hyperammonemia (urea cycle disorders, organic acidemias)		Niemann-Pick disease type B
	Mitochondrial disorders	Posterior embryotoxon	Alagille syndrome
	Some urea cycle disorders (arginosuccinate lyase deficiency)	Liver tenderness	Acute hepatitis (viral, toxic, autoimmune)
	Drug toxicity		Congestion (heart failure, hepatic vein obstruction)
Skeletal deformities	Sialidosis (dysostosis multiplex)		Trauma (subcapsular hematoma, fracture, laceration)
	Mucopolysaccharidoses (dysostosis multiplex)		Abscess (hepatic, subphrenic)
	Gaucher disease (marrow infiltration, deformities, fractures)		Cholangitis
	Mucolipidosis II (restricted joint mobility)		Perihepatitis
Skin findings			
Papular acrodermatitis	Hepatitis B		
Eczematoid rash	Histiocytosis		

evidence of disturbed liver function is evident. Patients with progressive liver disease, such as chronic viral hepatitis, Wilson disease, or α_1-antitrypsin deficiency, may be asymptomatic for years or even decades. The pattern of liver test abnormalities may be helpful in suggesting whether the patient's liver disease is primarily hepatocellular or biliary in nature. Laboratory studies, particularly when followed sequentially, may provide information about the synthetic, exocrine, metabolic (glucose, amino acids, lipids, detoxification), and endocrine (hyperaldosteronemia, vitamin D activation) liver function. Laboratory data provide input into several prognostic models used in assessment of the mortality risk and in evaluation for liver transplant.

All patients with hepatomegaly should have a complete metabolic panel (sodium, potassium, chloride, bicarbonate, creatinine, BUN, aspartate aminotransferase [AST], serum alanine aminotransferase [ALT], albumin, glucose, lactate dehydrogenase [LDH], alkaline phosphatase, total bilirubin, total protein), fractionated bilirubin (conjugated and unconjugated bilirubin), CBC, UA, prothrombin time (PT), partial thromboplastin time (PTT), and fibrinogen.

D-dimers should also be tested in patients with suspected sepsis or thrombosis.

Hepatocellular Injury

Serum ALT and AST are indicators of hepatocellular injury. The aminotransferases may be elevated as a result of hepatocyte necrosis induced by a number of infectious, inflammatory, or metabolic disorders or by drug toxicity. ALT is present in much lower concentration in most tissues other than the liver. AST is less specific, as it is present not only in the liver but also in muscle and the brain. Some patients with a systemic viral illness such as influenza may have acute rhabdomyolysis, which leads to a very marked increase in serum AST. Hemolysis may also lead to an elevation of this enzyme. Although in most cases of liver disease there is some elevation of aminotransferase values, significant liver disease (hepatic steatosis, hepatitis C infection, congenital hepatic fibrosis, and many metabolic disorders) may be present even when these test results are normal. Aminotransferases do not necessarily reflect liver function and may have little correlation with the specific diagnosis or prognosis.

TABLE 17.6 Helpful Laboratory Abnormalities in the Evaluation of Hepatomegaly

Vacuolated white blood cells in peripheral smear	Wolman disease GM$_1$ gangliosidosis
Neutropenia	Glycogen storage disease type I Organic acidurias Shwachman-Diamond syndrome Hemophagocytic lymphohistiocytosis Sepsis Leukemia Neuroblastoma Portal hypertension (hypersplenism)
Hemolytic anemia	Wilson disease Autoimmune hepatitis Hemoglobinopathy (with extramedullary hematopoiesis)
Hypophosphatemia	Glycogen storage disease type I Hereditary fructose intolerance
Hypertriglyceridemia	Glycogen storage disease type I Hemophagocytic lymphohistiocytosis Nonalcoholic fatty liver
Elevated creatinine	Disorders of fatty acid β-oxidation Reye syndrome Congenital hepatic fibrosis/autosomal recessive polycystic kidney disease
Renal tubular dysfunction	Tyrosinemia Glycogen storage disease type I Hereditary fructose intolerance Wilson disease Galactosemia

Biliary Injury

Alkaline phosphatase and γ-glutamyltransferase (GGT) are expressed in the bile ducts. Their elevation can occur in both intrahepatic and extrahepatic cholestasis. Alkaline phosphatase is found in bile ducts and also in several other tissues, including bone, small intestine, placenta, and kidney. Because children have a significant proportion of serum alkaline phosphatase activity originating from bone, this test may be of less value in the assessment of pediatric liver disease. Even minor bone trauma or vitamin D deficiency can lead to elevation of alkaline phosphatase. The tissue origin of alkaline phosphatase can be determined by fractionation of alkaline phosphatase isoenzymes. The normal newborn may have very high levels of GGT, up to 10 times the upper limit of normal for adults. Values of GGT for premature babies may be higher than those for term infants during the first weeks after birth. In comparison with other standard serum assays, GGT may be the most sensitive indicator of biliary disease, but it does not determine a specific diagnosis. The highest levels of GGT are usually found in biliary obstruction. GGT levels may be paradoxically normal or low in progressive familial intrahepatic cholestasis types 1 and 2 and in some inborn errors of bile acid metabolism.

Exocrine Function

Disposal of bilirubin requires conjugation with glucuronic acid in the hepatocyte, excretion across the canalicular membrane, and unobstructed passage through the biliary tree. As a result, the serum concentration of conjugated bilirubin represents a test of exocrine liver function. Despite the diagnostic value of conjugated bilirubin, it is important to remember that the pathophysiologic consequences of cholestasis are more directly related to bile acid excretion. Insufficient bile acid concentration in the intestinal lumen leads to fat malabsorption, fat-soluble vitamin deficiencies, and steatorrhea. Analysis of serum bile acid levels, vitamin A, 25-hydroxy vitamin D, vitamin E, PT/international normalized ratio (INR), and measurement of fecal fat may further define the extent of exocrine dysfunction (see Chapter 18).

Synthetic Function

Albumin is the principal serum protein synthesized by the liver and has a half-life in serum of approximately 20 days. A decrease in serum albumin concentration may result from decreased production by the liver. Serum albumin may also be low because of loss into the urine or the gastrointestinal tract.

The liver plays a central role in the production of coagulation factors. The PT and PTT are easily available tests of liver synthetic capacity once vitamin K deficiency has been excluded. All the clotting factors except factor VIII are exclusively made by the hepatocytes. The half-life of several clotting factors is short (factor VII has a half-life of 3–5 hours), and so the PT rapidly reflects changes in hepatic synthetic function and serves as a prognostic indicator in patients with fulminant hepatic failure. Caution should be used in interpreting a prolonged PT or PTT in the setting of sepsis as disseminated intravascular coagulation may cause abnormalities.

Metabolic Function

Many tissues can break down glycogen or produce glucose-6-phosphate via the gluconeogenesis pathway for local energy production inside the cell. The liver is the only organ that can release glucose into circulation. Hypoglycemia may be a feature of hepatic failure, glycogen storage diseases, mitochondrial diseases, fatty acid β-oxidation defects, pyruvate metabolism defects, Krebs cycle and gluconeogenesis defects, organic acidurias, or hereditary fructose intolerance. Blood glucose level determination is essential in the evaluation of hepatomegaly, particularly in patients with alterations of mental status. In most conditions, hypoglycemia is associated with ketosis and lactic acidosis. Hypoglycemia in the absence of or with low levels of ketones in the urine strongly suggests a fatty acid β-oxidation defect or a mitochondrial disorder. Blood gas (and anion gap), serum amino and urinary organic acids, lactate, pyruvate, acylcarnitines, acylglycines, cortisol, insulin, thyroid function, and adrenocorticotropic hormone (ACTH) as well as the ratios of total and esterified to free serum carnitine concentrations should be determined in follow-up studies.

The urea cycle is a series of enzymatic reactions converting highly toxic ammonia into less toxic urea. Ammonia is a ubiquitous byproduct of amino acid metabolism. The urea cycle takes place exclusively in the liver. In liver disease, impairment of the urea cycle can be caused by destruction of hepatocytes, metabolic block at the level of the urea cycle, organic acid catabolism defects, or mitochondrial electron transport defects. Shunting of portal blood in cirrhosis or in congenital portosystemic shunts permits large amounts of ammonia and other toxins to bypass the liver and reach the systemic circulation directly.

Hepatomegaly with an acute change in mental status should raise the possibility of a serious metabolic condition. Since both hypoglycemia and hyperammonemia can lead to severe and irreversible brain damage, correction of these abnormalities should be considered an emergency.

The liver is the main site of biosynthesis and processing of cholesterol, lipids, and lipoproteins. Liver disease may profoundly affect serum lipid and lipoprotein concentrations. In cholestatic liver disease there may be extreme elevations of free cholesterol and phospholipids. These abnormalities are accompanied by the presence of an abnormal low-density lipoprotein fraction called lipoprotein X. In end-stage liver disease and acute liver failure, serum cholesterol may be low.

Enzymatic analysis of cultured lymphocytes or hepatic tissue may aid in the diagnosis. Genetic diagnosis is possible in many of these disorders.

Extrahepatic Involvement

High levels of unconjugated bilirubin suggest the possibility of a concurrent hemolytic disorder or may reflect inborn errors of conjugation (see Chapter 18).

Neutropenia can be associated with splenomegaly/hypersplenism from portal hypertension, glycogen storage disease type Ib, Shwachman-Diamond syndrome, HLH, sepsis, leukemia, and neuroblastoma.

Renal involvement can be reflected by elevated creatinine, inability to concentrate urine, or Fanconi syndrome. This could raise suspicion for autosomal recessive polycystic kidney disease, tyrosinemia, glycogen storage disease type Ib, Wilson disease, hereditary fructose intolerance, or galactosemia.

Imaging Studies

Ultrasonography is the most useful initial imaging modality. It can assess gallbladder size, detect gallstones and sludge in the bile ducts and gallbladder, demonstrate ascites, and define cystic or obstructive dilatation of the biliary tree. Extrahepatic anomalies may also be detected. Mass lesions in the liver, including tumors, cysts, abscesses, vascular malformations, and hematomas, can be defined. Abnormal echogenicity may suggest diffuse parenchymal liver disease including fatty infiltration or fibrosis. Doppler studies may be used to differentiate between vascular and nonvascular structures and potential thrombi. Portal venous flow may be decreased or reversed, which suggests portal hypertension.

A plain film of the abdomen is *not* the study of choice for evaluation of hepatomegaly. If performed, it may support the diagnosis of hepatomegaly if seen. Air may be noted within the portal venous system, a late finding in bowel infarction and necrosis, intraabdominal sepsis, or complicated inflammatory bowel disease. Air may also be present within the biliary tree, especially in patients who have undergone recent biliary tract surgery or who have an enterobiliary fistula. Coarse calcifications may be found in hepatoblastoma and laminated calcifications in hepatocellular carcinoma. Subacute abscesses and echinococcal cysts may also contain calcium and be seen on a plain film.

CT with contrast provides useful information in differentiation of liver masses. CT angiograms and/or venograms are useful in defining the anatomy of vascular anomalies. Disadvantages of CT scans are the frequent need for sedation, potential renal toxicity of contrast, and risks from ionizing radiation.

MRI provides additional information about liver anatomy, particularly in differentiation of liver tumors. Magnetic resonance angiography (MRA) may be of value in assessing the vascularity of masses within the liver. Magnetic resonance cholangiography is commonly used to assess the biliary tract with visualization of details previously possible only with transhepatic or endoscopic retrograde cholangiography.

Hepatic scintigraphy can be useful for assessing the liver parenchyma and biliary tree. The most frequently performed study is hepatobiliary scintigraphy performed with a technetium 99m (^{99m}Tc)–labeled iminodiacetic acid derivative. Biliary imaging with this technique provides information about patency of the biliary tract and gallbladder. ^{99m}Tc–sulfur colloid scanning may be used in assessing a patient with a mass. ^{99m}Tc–sulfur colloid accumulates in Kupffer cells. Most malignant tumors, hemangiomas, abscesses, and cysts lack Kupffer cells and appear as "cold" spots on these scans. In contrast, a nodule taking up the isotope suggests a benign lesion containing Kupffer cells, such as a regenerative nodule of cirrhosis, fatty change, or focal nodular hyperplasia.

Liver Biopsy

Percutaneous, transjugular, or open-liver biopsy is one of the most important diagnostic tests in evaluating a child with hepatomegaly. Liver biopsy is used to establish a diagnosis and score severity of disease in chronic viral hepatitis, drug-induced liver disease, autoimmune hepatitis, and various metabolic disorders. Abnormal material in hepatocytes or Kupffer cells and viral inclusions suggest storage disorders. Electron microscopy and immunohistochemical methods may aid in identification and localization of these abnormalities. Liver tissue may also be frozen for later biochemical or molecular analysis.

SPECIFIC ISSUES IN THE DIAGNOSIS AND TREATMENT OF HEPATOMEGALY

The clinical challenge in the evaluation of hepatomegaly is that there is a very broad differential with many relatively rare conditions. Tables 17.5 and 17.6 list some of the physical signs and laboratory abnormalities that may be associated with hepatomegaly. Table 17.7 lists a stepwise approach for devising the differential diagnosis and directing the investigation. The first goal is to identify potentially life-threatening conditions, to focus on emergency measures to manage immediate threats to life, and to prevent irreversible end-organ damage. The second goal is to identify potentially treatable disorders requiring timely interventions. Ultimately, the clinician should focus on other chronic conditions to establish proper diagnosis and prognosis. Some disorders may be corrected by liver transplantation; such patients should be promptly referred to a transplant center for evaluation.

Hepatomegaly in the Infant

Hepatomegaly in the neonate is commonly associated with liver dysfunction and jaundice (see Chapter 18). In infants, jaundice is a frequent presenting feature of liver disease rather than a later manifestation of advanced liver disease, as in the older child or adult. The majority of infants with cholestatic liver disease manifest the disease during the first month of life.

Changes in mental status, such as irritability or lethargy, poor feeding, and vomiting, are frequent symptoms in metabolic disorders. Urea cycle defects lead to hyperammonemia and acute encephalopathy associated with astrocyte swelling without axonal damage. Patients present with a change in mental status or ataxia. Severe or prolonged hyperammonemia ultimately leads to progressive irreversible brain damage characterized by cortical and brainstem gliosis and neuronal atrophy. Symptomatology of galactosemia and tyrosinemia depends on the presence of nutritional substrates; thus irritability, lethargy, hepatomegaly, ascites, edema, and coagulopathy may manifest soon after feedings are initiated and evolve over the first weeks of life.

A profound impairment of hepatic synthetic function, often in excess of that expected for the degree of cholestasis, may be an early indication of metabolic liver disease. Hepatic failure may be present in mitochondrial disorders, including both mitochondrial DNA variants and mitochondrial DNA depletion syndromes. In addition to the liver, other organs (brain, heart, skeletal muscle) may be involved. Affected patients often have lactic acidosis, hypoglycemia, hypertriglyceridemia, and an abnormal acylcarnitine profile.

Gestational alloimmune liver disease (GALD, formerly neonatal hemochromatosis) may manifest with hepatic failure at birth. Patients with GALD benefit from early treatment with plasmapheresis and intravenous immunoglobulin (IVIG) but may require liver transplantation if there is no resolution of synthetic liver failure. Diagnosis of GALD bears significance for future pregnancies. GALD will develop in up to 80% of infants of mothers with a previous child diagnosed with this condition. GALD is caused by maternal alloantibodies crossing the

TABLE 17.7   Evaluation of Patients with Hepatomegaly

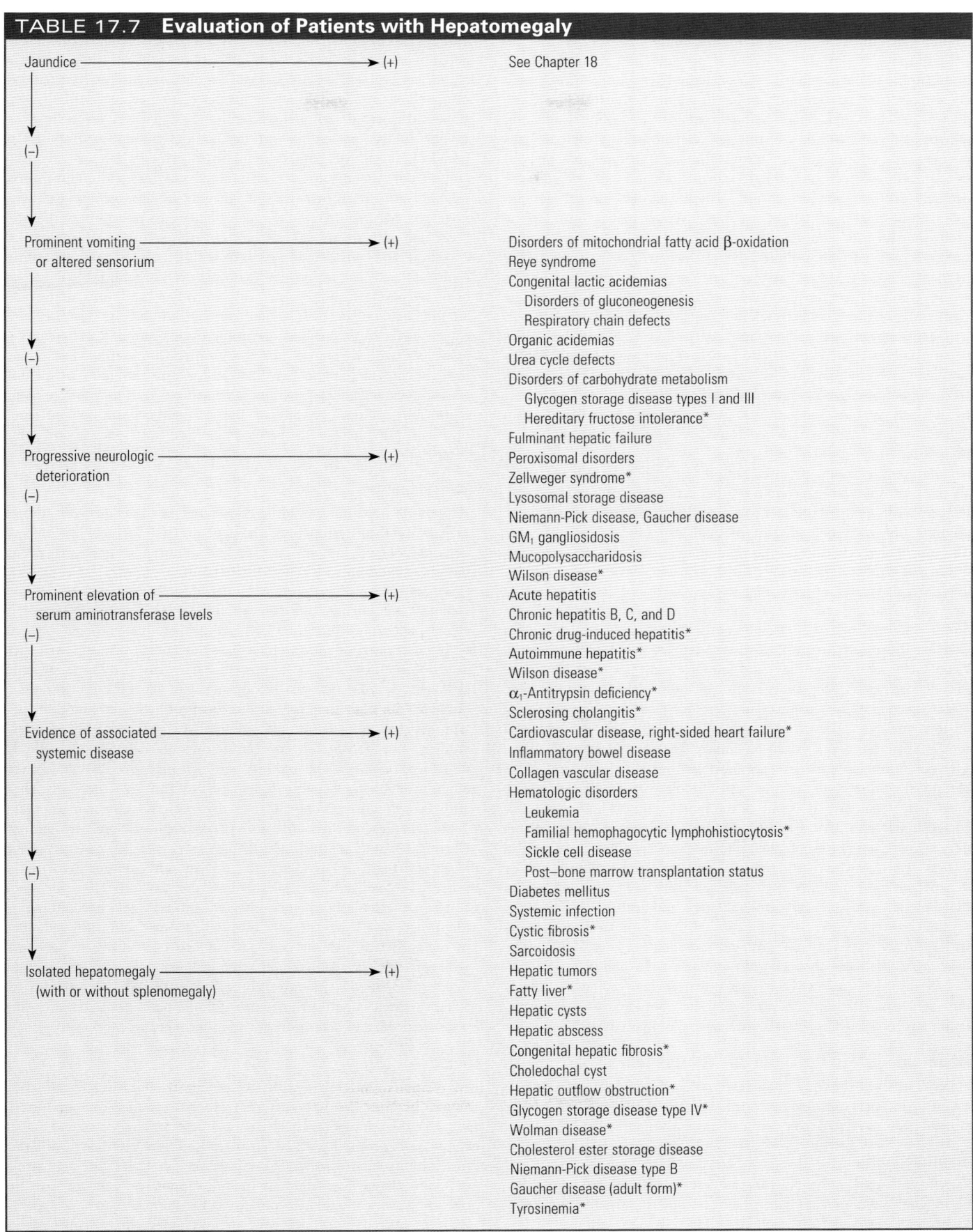

Jaundice ──────────────────────→ (+) See Chapter 18

│
↓
(−)
│
↓

Prominent vomiting ──────────────→ (+)
or altered sensorium

│
↓
(−)
│
↓

Progressive neurologic ──────────→ (+)
deterioration
(−)
│
↓

Prominent elevation of ──────────→ (+)
serum aminotransferase levels
(−)
│
↓

Evidence of associated ──────────→ (+)
systemic disease

│
↓
(−)
│
↓

Isolated hepatomegaly ───────────→ (+)
(with or without splenomegaly)

Disorders of mitochondrial fatty acid β-oxidation
Reye syndrome
Congenital lactic acidemias
   Disorders of gluconeogenesis
   Respiratory chain defects
Organic acidemias
Urea cycle defects
Disorders of carbohydrate metabolism
   Glycogen storage disease types I and III
   Hereditary fructose intolerance*
Fulminant hepatic failure
Peroxisomal disorders
Zellweger syndrome*
Lysosomal storage disease
Niemann-Pick disease, Gaucher disease
GM_1 gangliosidosis
Mucopolysaccharidosis
Wilson disease*
Acute hepatitis
Chronic hepatitis B, C, and D
Chronic drug-induced hepatitis*
Autoimmune hepatitis*
Wilson disease*
α_1-Antitrypsin deficiency*
Sclerosing cholangitis*
Cardiovascular disease, right-sided heart failure*
Inflammatory bowel disease
Collagen vascular disease
Hematologic disorders
   Leukemia
   Familial hemophagocytic lymphohistiocytosis*
   Sickle cell disease
   Post–bone marrow transplantation status
Diabetes mellitus
Systemic infection
Cystic fibrosis*
Sarcoidosis
Hepatic tumors
Fatty liver*
Hepatic cysts
Hepatic abscess
Congenital hepatic fibrosis*
Choledochal cyst
Hepatic outflow obstruction*
Glycogen storage disease type IV*
Wolman disease*
Cholesterol ester storage disease
Niemann-Pick disease type B
Gaucher disease (adult form)*
Tyrosinemia*

*Disease that may result in cirrhosis.

placenta and damaging the liver; the severity of injury can be alleviated by prenatal administration of IVIG to the mother.

A number of clinical features may provide clues about the cause of hepatomegaly in newborns. An enlarged liver with a firm or hard consistency is more commonly found in infants with extrahepatic bile duct obstruction or neonatal hemochromatosis. Congenital infection may be associated with low birthweight, hepatomegaly, microcephaly, purpura, and chorioretinitis. Dysmorphic facial features may be seen in association with chromosomal abnormalities and with Alagille syndrome. Congenital malformations, including cardiac anomalies, polysplenia, intestinal malrotation, and situs inversus, may be found in the syndromic form of biliary atresia. Abnormal lateralization syndromes can be associated with a midline liver, which may be palpable in the hypogastrium. The spleen may also be enlarged with infection or as a result of portal hypertension. Hepatomegaly, as well as a mass in the right upper quadrant, may be felt in infants with a choledochal cyst.

Infants may present with hepatomegaly, cholestasis, and sometimes hepatic failure related to infection such as cytomegalovirus, herpes simplex virus, enteroviruses, echovirus, coxsackievirus, or parvovirus B19. Hepatomegaly and cholestasis can also be associated with bacterial sepsis, syphilis, tuberculosis, and toxoplasmosis. α_1-Antitrypsin deficiency can also present as hepatomegaly associated with cholestasis in infants.

Infants with **storage diseases** can present with isolated hepatomegaly or hepatosplenomegaly and few other symptoms in the early stages. Hepatomegaly is a feature of these disorders because of a pathologic accumulation of undegraded or partially degraded macromolecules. The mucopolysaccharidoses, the lipid storage diseases, the mucolipidoses, and glycoprotein storage disease are examples of these disorders. The clinical features of lysosomal storage diseases are determined by where the deficient enzyme is expressed and the rate of accumulation of the abnormal material. Hepatomegaly in the neonate can occur in Gaucher disease, Niemann-Pick disease type A, and Wolman disease. Neonatal hepatosplenomegaly and jaundice may occur in Niemann-Pick disease type C. Progressive neurologic dysfunction may occur later. Hepatosplenomegaly accompanied by coarse facial features and skeletal abnormalities is present in infants with the GM_2 gangliosidoses and mucopolysaccharidoses. Based on clinical features and manifestations, specific enzymatic activities may be determined in peripheral white blood cell culture or in cultured skin fibroblasts to establish a precise diagnosis. Hepatomegaly is one of the most common findings in glycogen storage disorders. A common feature of **glycogen storage disorders** is inefficient release of glucose from glycogen stores; this can lead to hypoglycemia when fasting. Since brain energy metabolism heavily depends on the availability of glucose, severe hypoglycemia can lead to metabolic strokes, irreversible brain damage, and death.

Enzyme replacement therapies are available for treating patients with Gaucher disease type I, glycogen storage disease type II (Pompe disease), and mucopolysaccharidoses types I, II, and VI. Glycogen storage disorders can also be managed with dietary therapy maintaining euglycemia. Although of limited efficacy, bone marrow transplantation has been used in patients with several of these disorders.

Hepatomegaly in the Child and Adolescent

Hepatomegaly in the child or adolescent may be an isolated finding on a routine physical examination or may be associated with many other clinical features related to systemic disease or impaired liver function.

Steatohepatitis

Fatty liver disease in the child and adolescent is associated with childhood obesity. An increase in serum ALT value is found in 6% of overweight children and 10% of obese children. A large number of U.S. adolescents may have fatty infiltration of the liver (**nonalcoholic steatohepatitis or nonalcoholic fatty liver disease**). Nonalcoholic steatohepatitis should be suspected in any obese child with hepatomegaly and/or abnormal liver test results. Many of these children have features of metabolic syndrome, such as insulin resistance, arterial hypertension, and elevated serum cholesterol and triglyceride levels. In overweight children presenting with hepatomegaly and liver dysfunction, nonalcoholic steatohepatitis should be the primary diagnostic consideration, but other disorders, such as autoimmune hepatitis and chronic viral hepatitis, must be ruled out. Imaging studies, including ultrasonography, MRI, and CT, may suggest altered composition of the liver consistent with steatosis. Liver biopsy is the definitive diagnostic test and should be considered in patients with persistently abnormal aminotransferases. The purpose of the biopsy is to establish the diagnosis of nonalcoholic steatohepatitis, rule out other conditions, and evaluate the degree of steatosis, inflammation, and fibrosis. Steatohepatitis can progress to cirrhosis and chronic liver failure. Steatohepatitis is associated with increased mortality from cardiovascular disease and liver cancer. Obese patients with steatohepatitis should be enrolled in a weight management program. Medications such as vitamin E and metformin could be considered. Bariatric surgery can be considered in select individuals with nonalcoholic fatty liver disease and other comorbidities.

Viral Hepatitis

Acute viral hepatitis should be considered in the child with hepatomegaly and liver dysfunction. The patient may be acutely ill with sudden onset of fever, anorexia, nausea, and vomiting. Jaundice may occur, but many children with acute viral hepatitis are anicteric. On physical examination, varying degrees of tender hepatomegaly may be defined. Hepatitis is confirmed by an elevation in serum aminotransferase levels. Hepatitis may be caused by hepatotropic viruses (hepatitis A, B, C, D, or E) or by other viral infections that can involve the liver, such as cytomegalovirus (CMV), Epstein-Barr virus (EBV), adenovirus, enterovirus, and echovirus. Serodiagnosis of all of these infections is possible. The evaluation for various forms of hepatitis should include anti–hepatitis A virus immunoglobulin M (IgM), hepatitis B surface antigen, anti–hepatitis B core antibody, anti–hepatitis C antibody, CMV IgM or CMV PCR, and EBV serologic profile or EBV PCR. Therapy is available for hepatitis B, hepatitis C, and CMV hepatitis. Hepatitis B or C has the potential to evolve to cirrhosis over many years. Table 17.8 presents the main causes of chronic liver disease in children. Chronic hepatitis B infection is defined by persistently elevated serum levels of hepatitis B DNA. Hepatitis C is an indolent infection with the potential to evolve to cirrhosis over several decades. However, some children, particularly when co-infected with HIV, may have more rapidly progressive liver disease. Chronic hepatitis C infection is defined by the persistent presence of hepatitis C RNA in serum. As new antiviral agents are available, eradication of hepatitis C is possible in the majority of patients. The novel coronavirus COVID-19 has been associated with elevated liver enzymes, although additional research and time are needed to determine any long-term health effects.

Toxins

All patients presenting with hepatomegaly and liver dysfunction should be questioned about recent exposure to medications, including over-the-counter and herbal supplements or environmental toxins. Acute and chronic hepatitis can be caused by a number of different medications such as isoniazid and methyldopa. Treatment of drug- or toxin-related liver injury is mainly supportive. Contact with the offending agent should be avoided. Corticosteroids may have a role in immune-related injury, as may occur with phenytoin. N-acetylcysteine

TABLE 17.8 Causes of Chronic Liver Disease in Children

Autoimmune hepatitis
    Type 1 (anti–smooth muscle antibody, antinuclear antibody positive)
    Type 2 (anti–liver-kidney microsomal antibody)
α_1-Antitrypsin deficiency
Wilson disease
Primary sclerosing cholangitis (overlap syndrome with autoimmune hepatitis)
Viral hepatitis
    Hepatitis B
    Hepatitis C
    Hepatitis D
Drugs

therapy, by stimulating glutathione synthesis, is effective in preventing hepatotoxicity when administered within 16 hours after an overdose of acetaminophen and appears to improve survival in patients with severe liver injury even 36 hours after toxin ingestion. Liver injury in most cases is completely reversible when the hepatotoxic drug is withdrawn. With continued use of certain drugs, such as methotrexate or amiodarone, the effects of hepatotoxicity may proceed insidiously to cirrhosis.

α_1-Antitrypsin Deficiency

Children and adolescents with α_1-antitrypsin deficiency may present with manifestations of chronic liver disease or cirrhosis with evidence of portal hypertension. Liver biopsy may show a chronic hepatitis with varying degrees of fibrosis. The diagnosis is established by determination of the α_1-antitrypsin phenotype (phenotypes ZZ and SZ cause liver disease) and may be confirmed by liver biopsy. Periportal hepatocytes demonstrate periodic acid–Schiff–positive diastase-resistant intracytoplasmic globules. Immunocytochemical studies confirm that this material is the abnormal α_1-antitrypsin. It is important to manage the complications of cirrhosis, cholestasis, and portal hypertension. Patients with α_1-antitrypsin deficiency are at increased risk of hepatocellular carcinoma. Liver transplantation is curative, though the majority of the patients with α_1-antitrypsin deficiency do not require liver transplantation.

Wilson Disease

Wilson disease is a metabolic disorder that may manifest with hepatic disease in childhood, ranging from asymptomatic hepatomegaly (with or without splenomegaly) to subacute or chronic hepatitis or fulminant hepatic failure. Initial manifestations of Wilson disease may include portal hypertension, ascites, edema, and esophageal hemorrhage. Wilson disease can also present with extrahepatic symptoms, such as hemolytic anemia, movement disorders, or mood disorders. Wilson disease is due to variants in a copper-transporting P-type adenosine triphosphatase, which leads to a failure of biliary copper excretion and a progressive accumulation of copper in the liver and other organs. Lipid peroxidation, particularly of mitochondrial membranes, results from copper overload leading to the functional alterations in the liver and the brain. A low serum ceruloplasmin level suggests the diagnosis of Wilson disease. Serum copper levels may also be elevated, and urinary copper excretion is high, often up to 1,000 μg or more per day. The diagnosis is confirmed with a quantitative determination of copper in a liver biopsy specimen. Treatment of Wilson disease involves chelation and urinary excretion of the excess copper. The most frequently employed agents are penicillamine and trientine. In response to chelation therapy, urinary copper excretion increases markedly, and this is associated with

a gradual clinical improvement. Liver transplantation may be required for treatment of fulminant Wilson disease or in patients with decompensated cirrhosis.

Autoimmune Liver Disease

Several forms of autoimmune liver disease may also manifest with hepatomegaly during childhood and adolescence. Autoimmune hepatitis is defined as a continuing inflammatory process manifested by elevated aminotransferases, immunoglobulin G, and autoantibodies (antinuclear antibodies, smooth muscle, actin, microsomal antibodies). The severity at presentation is highly variable, ranging from laboratory abnormalities to cirrhosis and hepatic failure. In 25–30% of patients with autoimmune hepatitis, particularly children, the illness may have acute onset; however, in most patients, the onset is insidious with few nonspecific symptoms. The patient may be asymptomatic or have fatigue, malaise, behavioral changes, anorexia, and amenorrhea. Months or even years may pass before a liver problem is recognized with onset of jaundice or bleeding. Autoimmune hepatitis is frequently associated with other autoimmune disorders, including arthritis, vasculitis, nephritis, thyroiditis, celiac disease, inflammatory bowel disease, and Coombs-positive anemia.

Laboratory studies in autoimmune hepatitis reveal a moderate elevation, usually <1,000 IU/L, of serum aminotransferases. Serum bilirubin levels can be mildly elevated but can also be normal. Serum alkaline phosphatase activity is normal or only slightly increased. A diagnosis of autoimmune hepatitis may initially be suggested by marked elevation of serum gamma globulin levels. Characteristic patterns of serum autoantibodies may be present. Type 1 autoimmune hepatitis is associated with antiactin (smooth muscle) and antinuclear antibodies, and type 2 with microsomal antibodies. In type 1 autoimmune hepatitis, most patients present between 10 and 20 years of age. Type 2 usually affects children between the ages of 2 and 14 years. Liver biopsy is useful in confirming the diagnosis and assessing the degree of liver damage. Cirrhosis may be present at the time of diagnosis.

Immunosuppressive medications are necessary to treat autoimmune hepatitis. Corticosteroid therapy, in combination with azathioprine, improves the clinical, biochemical, and histologic features in most patients and prolongs transplant-free survival in most patients with severe disease.

Primary Sclerosing Cholangitis

Primary sclerosing cholangitis is an autoimmune disorder with the focus of injury being the biliary tract. The disorder may be difficult to distinguish from autoimmune hepatitis, and some patients have an overlap syndrome with features of both disorders. Hepatomegaly is frequently present. Patients may be asymptomatic or have jaundice, pruritus, or abdominal pain. Although serum aminotransferase levels are elevated, there is more striking elevation of serum alkaline phosphatase and GGT activities. **Inflammatory bowel disease** occurs in 50–75% of patients and may manifest at any time in the course of the liver disease. Magnetic resonance cholangiography reveals beading and irregularity of the intrahepatic and extrahepatic bile ducts. There is no definitive treatment. The course of the disorder is slowly progressive and eventually necessitates liver transplantation.

AIDS

Hepatobiliary manifestations are common in patients with AIDS. Hepatomegaly may be present, caused by a heterogeneous group of issues that includes viral hepatitis, opportunistic infections, medication-induced hepatic injury, malnutrition, peliosis hepatis, AIDS cholangiopathy, and neoplasms. Pathologic features that are most typical of pediatric AIDS include giant cell transformation and diffuse

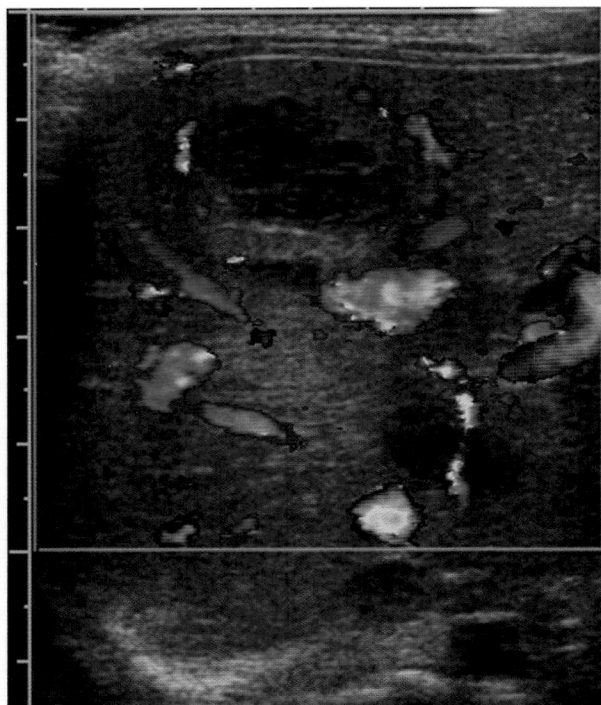

Fig. 17.1 *Escherichia coli* abscess in a 3-week-old with sepsis. A transverse color Doppler ultrasound image through the right hepatic lobe shows a complex, septated cystic lesion with intense peripheral vascularity and no blood flow centrally. (From Walters MM, Robertson RL, eds. *Pediatric Radiology: The Requisites.* 4th ed. Philadelphia: Elsevier; 2017:124, Fig. 5.11.)

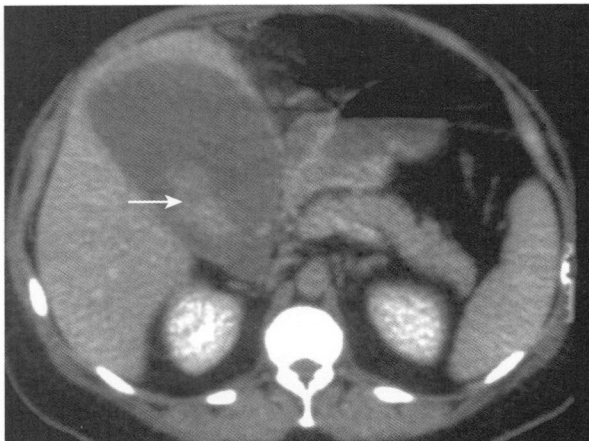

Fig. 17.2 Amebic abscess. Axial contrast-enhanced CT image shows a large, exophytic low-attenuation cyst with hyperdense central debris *(arrow)*. (From Coley BD, ed. *Caffey's Pediatric Diagnostic Imaging.* 13th ed. Philadelphia: Elsevier; 2019:835, Fig. 90.8.)

parenchymal lymphoplasmacytic infiltrates, the latter being associated with lymphoid interstitial pneumonitis.

Other Infections

Hepatosplenomegaly and anicteric hepatitis have been reported with cat-scratch disease, typhoid, brucellosis, tularemia, syphilis, Lyme disease, leptospirosis, Rocky Mountain spotted fever, Q fever, tuberculosis, and actinomycosis.

Perihepatitis Syndrome

Perihepatitis (formerly Fitz-Hugh–Curtis) syndrome is associated with acute salpingitis. Symptoms and signs include acute onset of severe right upper quadrant abdominal pain, friction rub over the anterior liver surface, and physical signs of pelvic inflammatory disease on pelvic examination (see Chapter 21).

Hepatic Abscess

A pyogenic, fungal, or parasitic hepatic abscess is an unusual infection in children. Common clinical findings are fever, abdominal pain, and hepatomegaly, with or without tenderness.

Pyogenic abscesses occur most frequently in infants who have had sepsis or umbilical infections (Fig. 17.1). Cases in older children are usually associated with underlying host-defense defects, particularly HIV, chronic granulomatous disease, and leukemia, or with occurrence of previous blunt trauma to the liver. Pyogenic abscess may follow an episode of appendicitis. Liver abscess may also occur in previously healthy children. *Staphylococcus aureus* and enteric and anaerobic bacteria are common etiologic agents. Liver function test results are commonly normal. Ultrasonography or CT scan confirms the presence and number of lesions. Echogenic debris or gas may be seen.

Amebiasis occurs in clusters in the southern United States, with person-to-person transmission in association with poor sanitation and crowding. Amebic abscess follows portal invasion by the parasite (Fig. 17.2). The diagnosis is established by demonstrating a positive result on enzyme-linked immunosorbent assay for antibody to *Entamoeba histolytica* or by finding trophozoites or cysts in the stool. Toxocariasis and echococcosis are caused by abortive infection of the liver in humans with the natural parasite of dogs or cats (Fig. 17.3). The diagnosis is confirmed by specific serologic profiles.

Endocrine Disorders

Hepatomegaly and mild elevations of aminotransferase levels and bilirubin are common in hypothyroidism and are occasionally observed in hyperthyroidism. An enlarged liver is often found in patients with poorly controlled diabetes mellitus, mainly as a result of excessive glycogen deposition. An extreme, rare case of this process is represented by **Mauriac syndrome**, which is characterized by dwarfism, obesity, moon facies, hypercholesterolemia, and marked hepatomegaly. Patients with acromegaly can also have mild to severe hepatomegaly as part of a generalized visceromegaly associated with the disease.

Liver Tumors

Liver tumors are the third most common solid abdominal tumors, after neuroblastoma and Wilms tumor (see Chapter 20, Table 17.2). Hepatic metastatic disease can also occur with many childhood neoplasms, most frequently neuroblastoma, leukemia, and lymphoma (Fig. 17.4). The primary tumor location is usually known.

Benign liver tumors account for 33% of cases of primary hepatic tumors. Benign liver tumors include hemangioendotheliomas, mesenchymal hamartomas, focal nodular hyperplasia (Fig. 17.5), and adenomas. Malignant tumors include hepatoblastoma (Fig. 17.6), hepatocellular carcinoma, and undifferentiated embryonal cell sarcoma. Of all hepatic neoplasms, hepatoblastoma, hepatocellular carcinoma, and infantile hemangioendothelioma are the three most common, accounting for 65% of cases. Most hepatic tumors are asymptomatic or may manifest with abdominal distention, abdominal pain, weight loss, vomiting, or diarrhea. Any hepatic mass can present with acute abdominal pain caused by hemorrhage into the tumor or peritoneal cavity.

Hemangioendotheliomas are the most common benign hepatic tumors. Nearly 95% of all hemangioendotheliomas manifest in the first year of life. Congestive heart failure due to hyperdynamic circulation may be present in 10–15% of cases. In addition to the liver, hemangiomas may be present in the skin, lungs, lymph nodes, pancreas, retroperitoneum, intestine, or bone and be seen with hepatic hemangioendotheliomas. Liver ultrasound shows a hyperechogenic mass frequently associated with increased vascular flow on Doppler evaluation. MRI or CT with intravenous contrast can be useful to further define the mass if sonographic evaluation is not conclusive.

Mesenchymal hamartomas, which consist of multiple cysts filled with serous fluid separated by myxomatous stroma, have no capsule. Of mesenchymal hamartomas, 70% manifest in the first 2 years of life. Hepatic adenoma is a rare benign tumor of the liver. Oral contraceptives, diabetes mellitus, glycogen storage disease, portosystemic shunts, and androgen therapy increase the risk of adenoma.

Focal nodular hyperplasia (FNH) is caused by nodular regeneration of the liver around a focal scar of the liver parenchyma. FNH is seen predominantly in females and may occur at all ages. FNH is more common in patients who have congenital portosystemic shunts (Abernethy anomaly).

The majority of patients with **hepatoblastoma** present before 2 years of age and 90% by the age of 4. **Hepatocellular carcinoma** and, less commonly, undifferentiated embryonal sarcoma occur primarily in older children. Tyrosinemia, ataxia-telangiectasia, glycogen storage disease type I, chronic hepatitis B or hepatitis C, α_1-antitrypsin deficiency, autoimmune hepatitis, and cholestatic

cirrhosis are associated with higher risk of hepatocellular carcinoma. Serial screening with periodic liver sonograms is indicated for patients with these diseases. If nodules are identified, the nature of the mass can be clarified with CT with contrast (triphasic CT) or MRI with contrast.

Serum α-fetoprotein (AFP) is the useful marker of malignant liver tumors; 80–90% of hepatoblastomas and 60–90% of hepatocellular carcinomas are positive. The serum AFP level is normal in mesenchymal hamartoma, focal nodular hyperplasia, and adenoma. The diagnosis of liver tumors is confirmed by needle biopsy, usually with ultrasound or CT guidance.

Hepatic Cysts

The origin of solitary cysts is unknown. They are probably the sequelae of focal intrahepatic hemorrhage. **Peliosis hepatis**, characterized by multiple blood-filled spaces of varying sizes within the liver parenchyma, can be a complication of long-term treatment with anabolic steroids. Hepatomegaly, often with tenderness, may be present before any evidence of liver biochemical abnormality is evident.

Choledochal cysts are defined as congenital dilation or outpouching of large bile ducts. Though the majority of choledochal cysts are

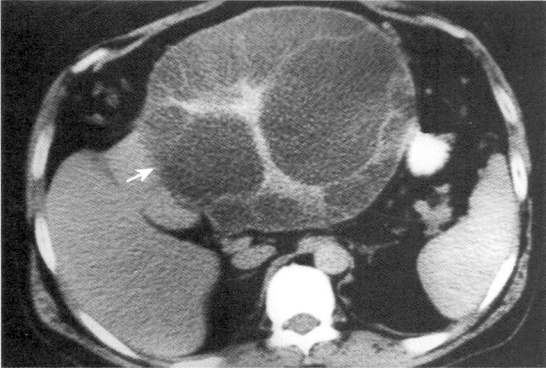

Fig. 17.3 An axial computed tomography image shows a liver abscess (arrow) in a child with *Echinococcus* infection. A large, complex cystic lesion is seen, with multiple daughter cysts noted. (From Walters MM, Robertson RL, eds. *Pediatric Radiology: The Requisites.* 4th ed. Philadelphia: Elsevier; 2017:125, Fig. 5.14.)

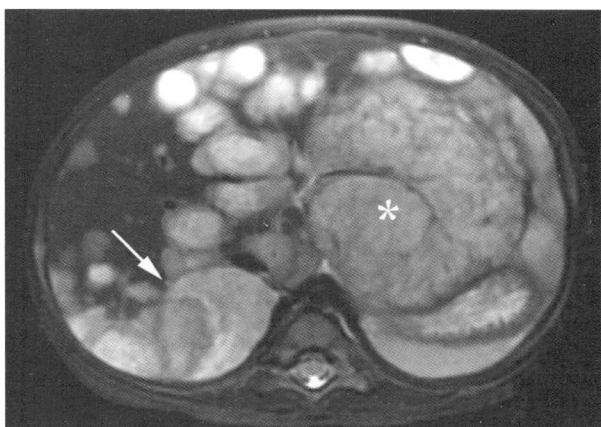

Fig. 17.4 Metastatic neuroblastoma in a 6-week-old infant with hepatomegaly. An axial T2-weighted image with fat saturation through the upper abdomen shows multiple T2 bright metastatic hepatic nodules, with a large metastatic lesion in the left hepatic lobe (asterisk). A right adrenal primary tumor is shown (arrow). (From Walters MM, Robertson RL, eds. *Pediatric Radiology: The Requisites.* 4th ed. Philadelphia: Elsevier; 2017:130, Fig. 5.21.)

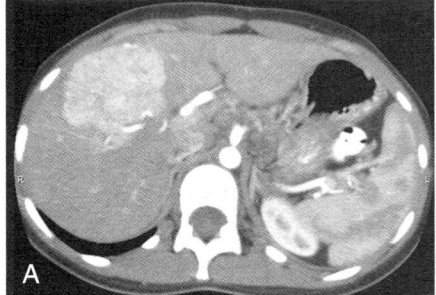 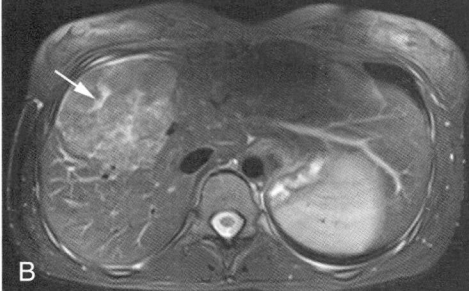 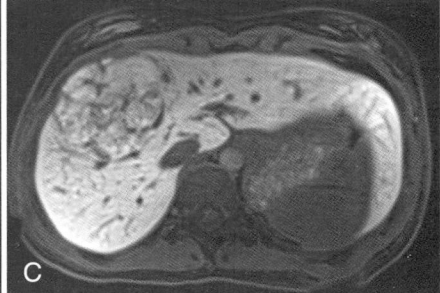

Fig. 17.5 Focal nodular hyperplasia incidentally found in a 15-year-old girl. *A,* An axial contrast-enhanced CT image shows a lobulated, heterogeneously enhancing mass. *B,* An axial T2-weighted MRI with fat saturation shows a heterogeneously hyperintense mass with a hyperintense central scar (arrow). *C,* An axial T1-weighted MRI with fat saturation obtained 20 minutes after the intravenous injection of gadoxetic acid disodium shows accumulation of contrast in hepatocytes within the lesion. (From Walters MM, Robertson RL, eds. *Pediatric Radiology: The Requisites.* 4th ed. Philadelphia: Elsevier; 2017:128, Fig. 5.18.)

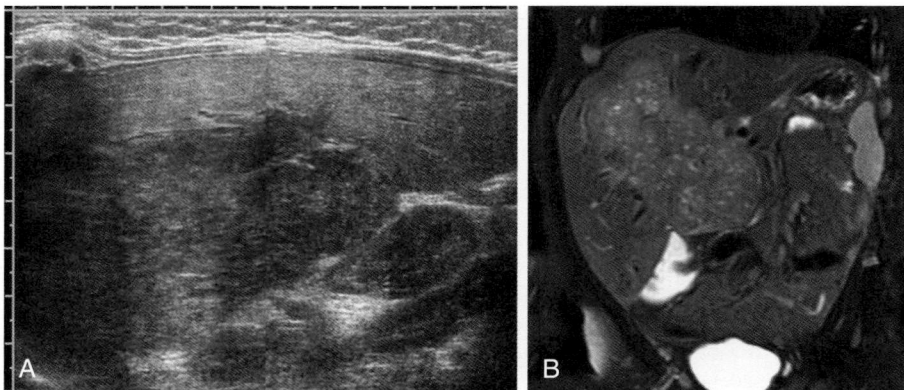

Fig. 17.6 Hepatoblastoma in a 5-month-old infant with an abdominal mass. *A,* A composite sagittal ultrasound image of the right hepatic lobe shows a complex, heterogeneously hypoechoic solid mass compressing surrounding liver parenchyma. *B,* A coronal T2-weighted MRI with fat saturation shows a heterogeneous, hyperintense mass extending into the porta hepatis and causing intrahepatic biliary ductal dilatation. (From Walters MM, Robertson RL, eds. *Pediatric Radiology: The Requisites.* 4th ed. Philadelphia: Elsevier; 2017:129, Fig. 5.19.)

diagnosed in the first year of life, later presentation is possible. Choledochal cysts are associated with an increased risk of ascending cholangitis and cholangiocarcinoma; thus, they should be surgically removed.

Congenital hepatic fibrosis is almost universally associated with autosomal recessive polycystic kidney disease (ARPKD). Approximately 40% of patients with congenital hepatic fibrosis have involvement of large bile ducts, which can be visualized by magnetic resonance cholangiogram as multiple cystic dilations of the intrahepatic bile ducts (Caroli disease). **Caroli disease** is associated with an increased risk of ascending cholangitis and sepsis, particularly in patients who underwent kidney transplantation for ARPKD. Recurrent cholangitis in patients with ARPKD can be an indication for combined liver/kidney transplantation.

Hepatic Venous Outflow Obstruction

Hepatic venous outflow obstruction is classified into three categories by the level of obstruction. Obstruction can occur at the level of hepatic venules (sinusoidal obstruction syndrome: venoocclusive disease), hepatic veins (Budd-Chiari syndrome), or suprahepatic vena cava. Hepatic venous outflow obstruction manifests with acute ascites and tender hepatomegaly. Abdominal pain, distention, and splenic enlargement may be prominent. Elevation of the aminotransferases or serum bilirubin level is present in the acute stage.

The pathologic hallmark of **venoocclusive disease (VOD)** is occlusion of central and sublobular hepatic veins by intimal edema and fibrosis. The illness classically follows ingestion of plants that contain a toxic pyrrolizidine alkaloid, which can be present in bush teas and herbal medicines. Venoocclusive disease may also occur as a hepatic response to irradiation and induction for bone marrow transplantation. A familial autosomal recessive form of venoocclusive disease associated with immunodeficiency usually presents at or before 1 year of life. Immunodeficiency is manifest by combined hypogammaglobulinemia and T-cell defects; identifying *SP11O* pathologic gene variants establishes the diagnosis.

The clinical diagnosis of VOD is based on either the McDonald (modified Seattle) or Jones (Baltimore) criteria. The McDonald criteria require the presence of two features from hepatomegaly with right upper quadrant pain, total bilirubin of 34.2 μmol/L or more (normal range <20 μmol/L), and ascites or unexplained weight gain >2% of baseline. The Jones criteria require a total bilirubin of 34.2 μmol/L or more and presence of at least two of the following: hepatomegaly, ascites, and weight gain >5% of baseline.

Budd-Chiari syndrome develops in a variety of conditions that predispose to thrombosis, including intake of oral contraceptives, pregnancy, trauma, tumor invasion, cirrhosis, inflammatory bowel disease, collagen vascular disease, protein C deficiency, sickle cell anemia, polycythemia vera, paroxysmal nocturnal hemoglobinuria, and lymphoproliferative disorders. Membranous obstruction of the suprahepatic vena cava is the most common cause of suprahepatic outflow obstruction. However, thrombosis of the suprahepatic vena cava can occur in any condition that may precipitate Budd-Chiari syndrome. Diagnostic evaluation begins with pulsed Doppler sonography of the hepatic vessels. CT angiogram can further define the anatomy of the outflow obstruction. Liver biopsy in hepatic outflow obstruction reveals a characteristic pattern of sinusoidal dilatation with centrilobular congestion. Cirrhosis is a poor prognostic sign.

■ SUMMARY AND RED FLAGS

Hepatomegaly that is persistent suggests a chronic illness, which with time may produce serious morbidity or mortality, despite an initial well appearance of the patient. It is important to determine whether the hepatomegaly is a result of a specific liver disease or whether it is part of a generalized systemic illness. Red flags include signs of acute hepatic failure (coma, hemorrhage), developmental delay, failure to thrive, and those noted in Table 17.9.

TABLE 17.9	Red Flags Suggesting Serious Liver Disease in a Patient with Hepatomegaly
History	**Physical Examination—cont'd**
History of prolonged hyperbilirubinemia in infancy	Digital clubbing
History of neurologic or psychiatric disease	Palmar erythema
Previous blood transfusion, intravenous drug use	Spider angiomata
Past history of hepatitis	Arthritis
Delayed puberty	Papular acrodermatitis
Gastrointestinal bleeding	Kayser-Fleischer rings
Family history of chronic liver or kidney disease	Encephalopathy
Physical Examination	Asterixis
Hard or nodular liver	**Laboratory Test Results**
Splenomegaly	Prolonged prothrombin time
Ascites	Hypoglycemia
Prominent abdominal venous pattern	Hyperammonemia
Growth retardation	Decreased serum albumin
Muscle wasting	

BIBLIOGRAPHY

A bibliography is available at ExpertConsult.com.

18

Jaundice

Grzegorz W. Telega

Jaundice, the yellow discoloration of skin and sclerae, results when the serum level of bilirubin, a pigmented compound, is elevated. Jaundice is not evident until the total serum bilirubin is at least 2–2.5 mg/dL in children out of the neonatal period.

Bilirubin is formed from the degradation of heme-containing compounds, particularly hemoglobin (Fig. 18.1). Microsomal heme oxygenase, located principally in the reticuloendothelial system, catabolizes heme to biliverdin, which is then reduced to bilirubin by biliverdin reductase. This unconjugated bilirubin (UCB) is lipophilic and cannot be easily eliminated via the kidney because of its insolubility in water. It can easily cross cell membranes and the blood-brain barrier. UCB is transported bound primarily to albumin. A receptor on the hepatocyte surface facilitates bilirubin uptake. Bilirubin is then conjugated with glucuronic acid by bilirubin uridine diphosphate glucuronosyltransferase (UDPGT). UDPGT can be induced by a variety of drugs (e.g., narcotics, anticonvulsants, and oral contraceptives) and by bilirubin itself. Enzyme activity is decreased by restriction of calorie and protein intake.

Conjugated bilirubin (CB) is a polar, water-soluble compound. It is excreted from the hepatocyte to the canaliculi, through the biliary tree, and into the duodenum. Once CB reaches the colon, bacterial hydrolysis converts CB to urobilinogen. A small amount of urobilinogen is reabsorbed and returned to the liver via enterohepatic circulation or excreted by the kidneys. The remainder is converted to stercobilin and excreted in feces. In neonates, β-glucuronidase in the intestinal lumen hydrolyzes CB to UCB, which is then reabsorbed and returned to the liver via the enterohepatic circulation.

Hyperbilirubinemia can result from alteration of any step in this process. Hyperbilirubinemia can be classified as conjugated (direct) or unconjugated (indirect), depending on the concentration of CB in the serum. Conjugated and unconjugated are more accurate terms, because "direct" and "indirect" refer to the van den Bergh reaction, historically used for measuring bilirubin. In this assay, the unconjugated fraction is determined by subtracting the direct fraction from the total and, therefore, is an indirect measurement. The direct fraction includes both conjugated bilirubin and Δ-bilirubin, an albumin-bound fraction. Conjugated hyperbilirubinemia exists when more than 20% of the total bilirubin or more than 2 mg/dL is conjugated. If neither criterion is met, the hyperbilirubinemia is classified as unconjugated.

Unconjugated hyperbilirubinemia can be caused by any process that results in increased production, decreased delivery to the liver, decreased hepatic uptake, decreased conjugation, or increased enterohepatic circulation of bilirubin. The primary concern in patients with high levels of unconjugated bilirubin is kernicterus, resulting from the neurotoxicity of UCB across the blood-brain barrier mostly in the basal ganglia, pons, or cerebellum. This is a concern primarily in neonates.

Conjugated hyperbilirubinemia can occur due to hepatocellular dysfunction, biliary obstruction, and abnormal excretion of bile acids or bilirubin.

DIAGNOSTIC STRATEGIES

The causes of jaundice in the neonate and older infant are not the same as the causes of jaundice in the older child or adolescent (Figs. 18.2 and 18.3). The approach to the problem varies with age.

Bilirubin

In any patient with jaundice, the total serum bilirubin should be fractionated, as the differential diagnosis of unconjugated hyperbilirubinemia is distinct from that of conjugated hyperbilirubinemia (see Figs. 18.2 and 18.3). On occasion, hemolysis interferes with some assays and may result in a falsely elevated conjugated fraction. This can be problematic with specimens obtained by heelstick or fingerstick. If the clinical picture is consistent with unconjugated hyperbilirubinemia, the assay should be repeated with a venous sample.

Aminotransferases

Aspartate aminotransferase (AST) and alanine aminotransferase (ALT) are frequently used as markers of hepatocellular injury. AST is expressed in mitochondria of the liver and cytosol of red blood cells and muscles; thus, it is not specific for liver injury. Since ALT is less abundant outside of the liver, an increased ALT level is more suggestive of liver disease. Levels of both are markedly elevated (>5- to 10-fold normal) with hepatocellular injury caused by hepatitis, hepatotoxicity, ischemia, and genetic or metabolic liver disorders. Elevation of AST in excess of ALT suggests an extrahepatic source of injury. With acute biliary obstruction, there are initial sharp increases in ALT and AST levels and a rapid decline in 12–72 hours as obstruction is relieved. In chronic cholestasis, aminotransferases are usually only mildly elevated. With hepatocellular injury, ALT and AST levels tend to remain more significantly elevated longer. In acute liver failure a rapid decline in ALT and AST levels with worsening coagulopathy is a poor prognostic factor.

It is important to remember that aminotransferases reflect cell injury, not liver function. *There is no correlation between the severity of the liver dysfunction and the degree of elevation of ALT and AST levels.* Temporal trends in serum aminotransferase levels are useful in monitoring disease activity in chronic viral and autoimmune hepatitis.

Alkaline Phosphatase

Alkaline phosphatase is an enzyme found in bile ducts, bone, intestine, placenta, and tumors. Elevations in the serum alkaline phosphatase level occur with hepatobiliary disease but also normal growth, healing fractures, vitamin D deficiency, bone disease, pregnancy, and malignancy. Fractionation of the alkaline phosphatase isoenzymes can help to determine its site of origin. A mild increase can be seen transiently in normal individuals. In the evaluation of conjugated hyperbilirubinemia, an alkaline phosphatase level of >3 times normal indicates cholestasis; a milder elevation is more consistent with hepatocellular disease.

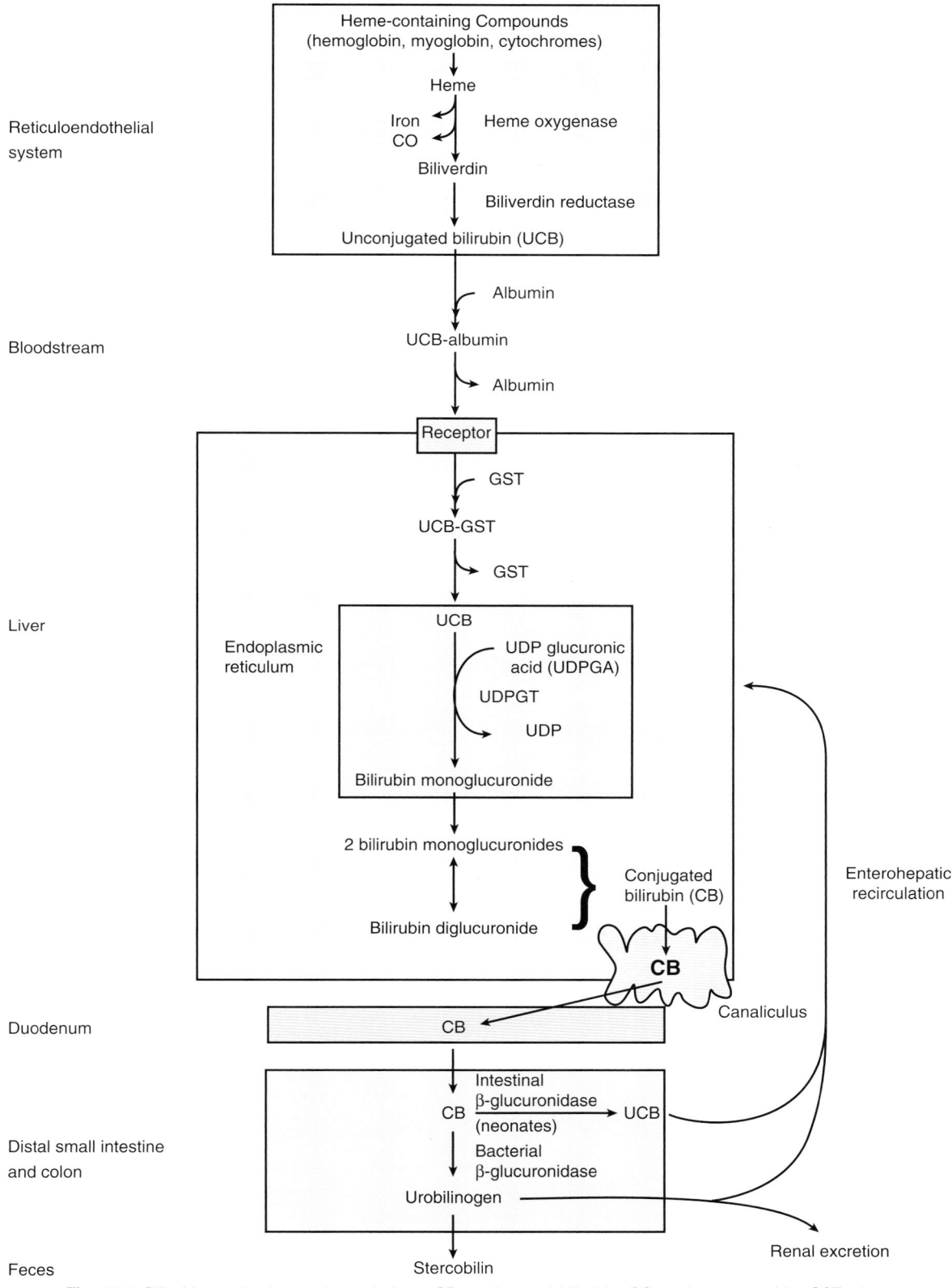

Fig. 18.1 Bilirubin production and metabolism. CB, conjugated bilirubin; CO, carbon monoxide; GST, gluta-thione S-transferase B; UCB, unconjugated bilirubin; UDP, uridine diphosphate; UDPGA, uridine diphosphate glucuronic acid; UDPGT, uridine diphosphate glucuronosyltransferase. (Modified from Gourley GR. Jaundice. In: Wyllie R, Hyams JS, eds. *Pediatric Gastrointestinal Disease: Pathophysiology, Diagnosis, Management.* 2nd ed. Philadelphia: WB Saunders; 1999:89.)

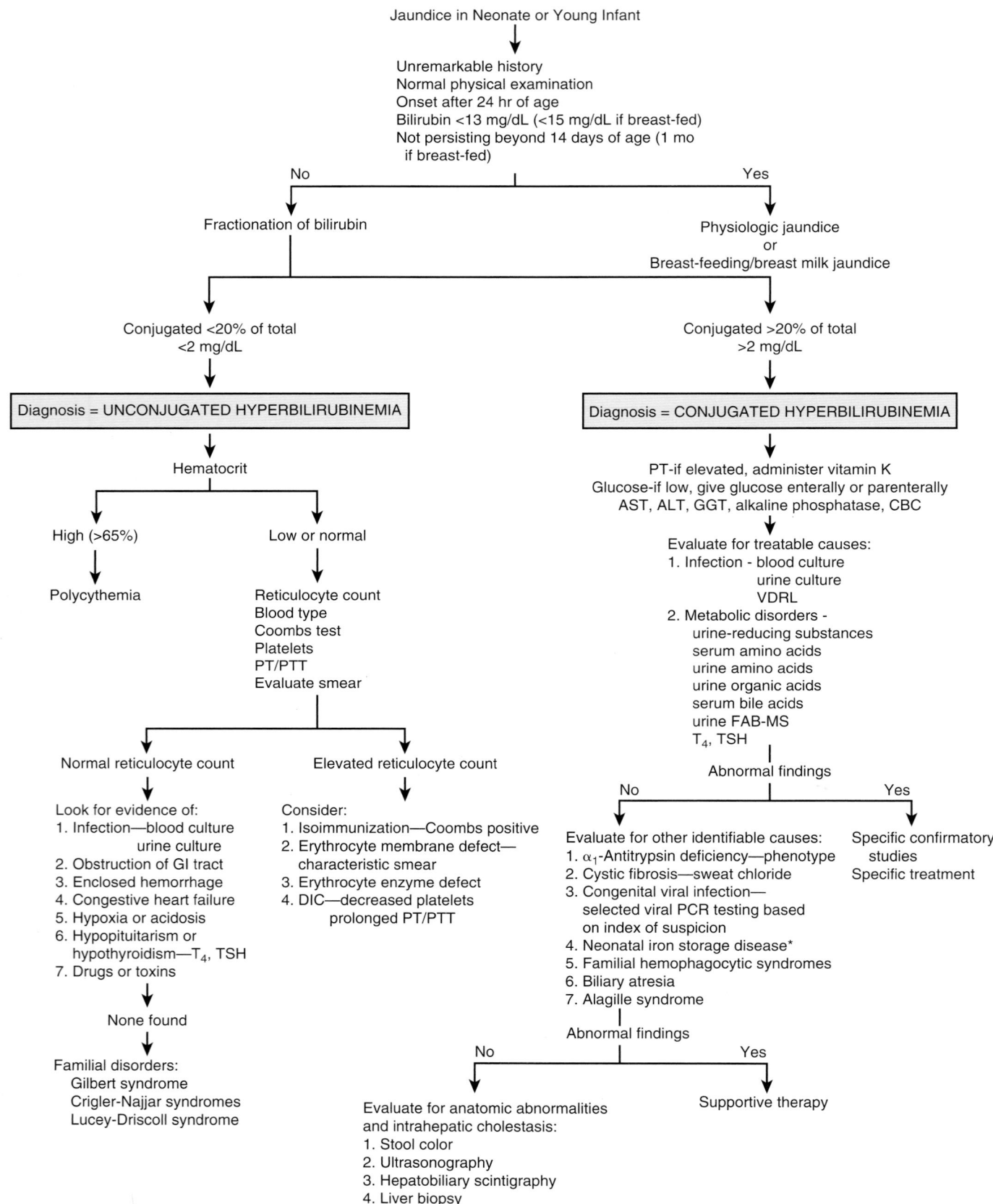

Fig. 18.2 Diagnostic approach to the neonate or infant with hyperbilirubinemia. *Also called congenital alloimmune hepatitis or neonatal hemochromatosis. ALT, alanine aminotransferase; AST, aspartate aminotransferase; DIC, disseminated intravascular coagulation; FAB-MS, fast atom bombardment mass spectrometry; GGT, γ-glutamyltransferase; GI, gastrointestinal; PT, prothrombin time; PTT, partial thromboplastin time; T_4, thyroxine; TSH, thyroid-stimulating hormone; VDRL, Venereal Disease Research Laboratory.

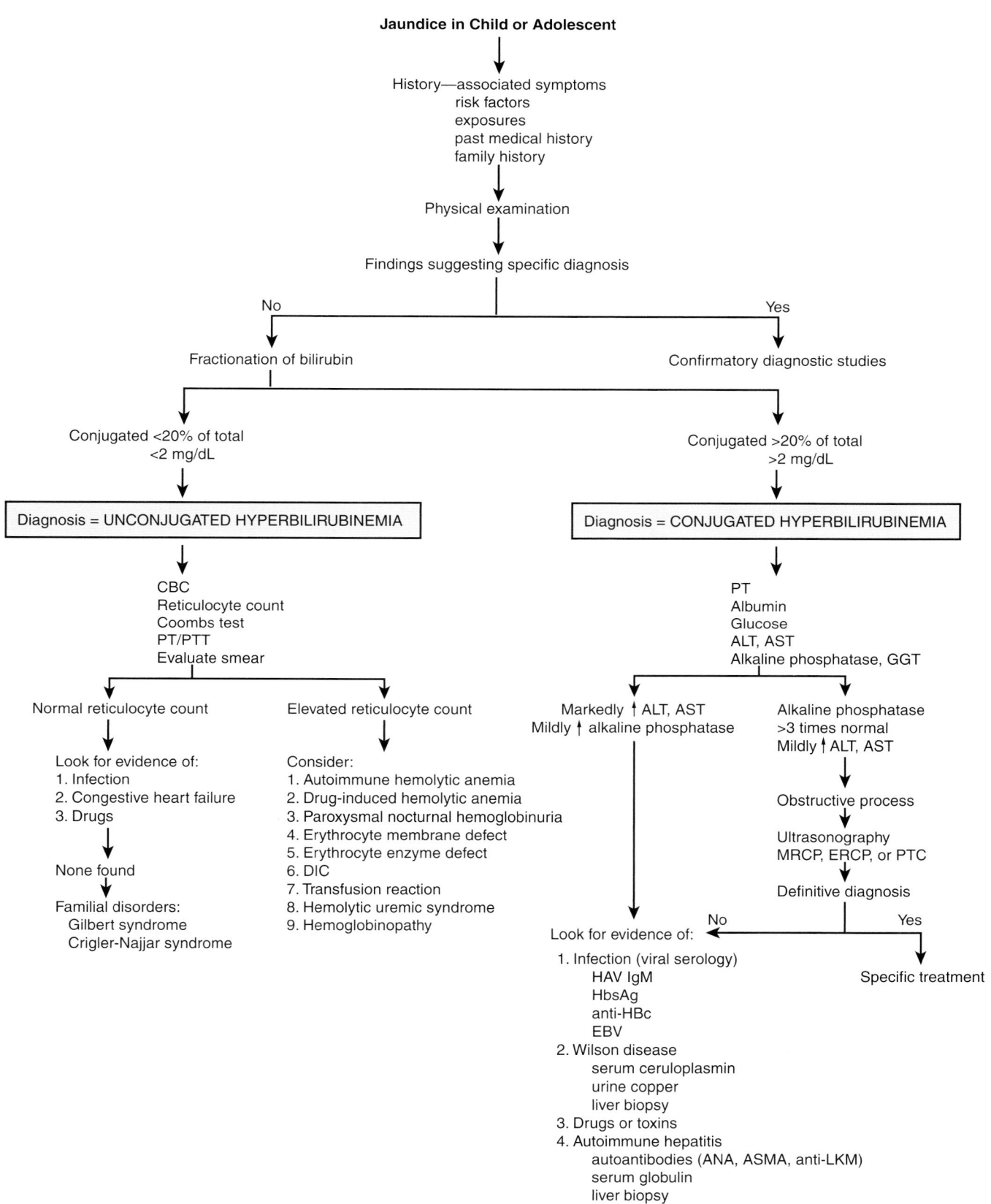

Fig. 18.3 Diagnostic approach to the child or adolescent with hyperbilirubinemia. ALT, alanine aminotransferase; ANA, antinuclear antibody; ASMA, anti–smooth muscle antibody; AST, aspartate transaminase; DIC, disseminated intravascular coagulation; EBV, Epstein-Barr virus; ERCP, endoscopic retrograde cholangiopancreatography; GGT, γ-glutamyltransferase; HAV, hepatitis A virus; HBc, hepatitis B core; HBsAg, hepatitis B surface antigen; IgM, immunoglobulin M; LKM, liver-kidney microsomal; MRCP, magnetic resonance cholangiopancreatography; PT, prothrombin time; PTC, percutaneous transhepatic cholangiography; PTT, partial thromboplastin time.

γ-Glutamyltransferase

The γ-glutamyltransferase (GGT) level is more specific for biliary tract disease than are ALT and AST levels. GGT elevations are inducible by alcohol and certain drugs, including phenytoin and phenobarbital. GGT is found in a variety of tissues and can be elevated in chronic pulmonary disease, renal failure, and diabetes mellitus. The GGT concentration is most helpful in confirming that an elevated alkaline phosphatase level is a result of liver disease rather than bone disease and in differentiating familial cholestatic syndromes.

Bile Acids

Serum bile acids are a very sensitive measure of cholestatic disease. Bile acid levels may be elevated before an increase in bilirubin. Levels are generally very high in primary cholestasis and biliary obstruction but only mildly increased (more than twice normal) in hepatocellular disease. Bile acids should be measured while fasting.

Albumin

Albumin is produced in the liver, and levels can reflect hepatic synthetic function. Serum albumin levels can be useful in monitoring progression of chronic liver disease and in discriminating an acute illness from a previously unrecognized chronic disorder. Hypoalbuminemia can also be secondary to nephrotic syndrome or a protein-losing enteropathy. Due to a long half-life (20 days), albumin is of limited use in assessing synthetic dysfunction in acute liver failure.

Prothrombin Time

Prothrombin time (PT) is the best marker of hepatic synthetic function, as most clotting factors are produced in the liver. It is important not only to measure the PT but also to document the response to parenteral administration of vitamin K because vitamin K deficiency may be an alternative explanation of the elevation of the PT. With severe hepatocellular injury, there is little improvement in the PT. Disseminated intravascular coagulation and thrombosis of a major blood vessel should not be overlooked as the cause of a prolonged PT.

Ultrasonography

Ultrasound studies are useful, noninvasive, relatively inexpensive diagnostic tools for the evaluation of liver disease. Ultrasonography provides information on the size and consistency of the liver and spleen and anatomic abnormalities of the biliary tree, gallstones, and hepatic masses such as cysts, tumors, or abscesses. Dilated intrahepatic ducts may indicate extrahepatic obstruction; however, the absence of dilation on ultrasonography cannot exclude obstruction, and further studies are required for definitive diagnosis. The utility of ultrasonography is limited in obese patients and in patients with excessive bowel gas. Doppler ultrasonography also demonstrates dynamic flow in hepatic blood vessels and the portal vein; it can identify vascular anomalies of the liver and suggest presence of portal hypertension. Ultrasound elastography can provide an indirect measure of liver fibrosis.

Scintigraphy

Hepatobiliary scintigraphy can aid in the diagnosis of biliary atresia. In a healthy individual, hepatic uptake and excretion of the radionuclide via the biliary system are prompt. When there is an injury to the hepatocyte, the uptake of radionuclide by the liver is diminished; however, the tracer should eventually be visualized in the intestinal tract. With obstructive processes, such as biliary atresia, uptake should be relatively normal unless the problem has been present long enough to have caused hepatocellular injury; however, there is no excretion into the intestinal tract. Administration of phenobarbital (5 mg/kg/day) for 5 days before the study may increase bile flow and thus can increase the

diagnostic accuracy. Unfortunately, a significant percentage of patients with intrahepatic cholestasis and neonatal hepatitis do not demonstrate biliary excretion, and further evaluation is needed; thus, final diagnosis is delayed. In patients with high level of suspicion for biliary atresia (acholic stools, high GGT), liver biopsy and percutaneous cholangiogram provide a faster and more direct way to reach the diagnosis.

Computed Tomography

CT is useful for identifying mass lesions within the liver and when there are technical problems with ultrasonography. CT with contrast can be used to define the nature of liver tumors. CT angiography can define the anatomy of portal and hepatic circulation. CT has limited value in the evaluation of biliary anatomy.

Magnetic Resonance

Magnetic resonance (MR) studies provide valuable information regarding the anatomy of the liver. Since many imaging protocols can be used depending on the purpose of the study, contacting a radiologist prior to ordering the study is recommended. Cost and frequent need for sedation make MR evaluation the tool for secondary evaluation after screening imaging with ultrasound leaves diagnostic questions. MRI can demonstrate storage of heavy metals, such as iron in neonatal iron storage disease. MR with contrast can define the nature of liver tumors. MR angiography is useful in studying the vascular system, including the vascular supply of tumors. MR cholangiopancreatography (MRCP) visualizes abnormalities of the intrahepatic and extrahepatic biliary tree and is also quite useful in evaluating the pancreatic duct system. At this point resolution of MRCP is inadequate to diagnose biliary atresia. Unlike endoscopic retrograde cholangiopancreatography (ERCP) or percutaneous transhepatic cholangiography (PTC), MRCP is noninvasive.

Endoscopic Retrograde Cholangiopancreatography

ERCP is performed for the evaluation of biliary anatomy in situations when endoscopic intervention is likely. Unlike MRCP, ERCP is both diagnostic and potentially therapeutic for common duct stones and for strictures. Complications of the procedure include cholangitis and pancreatitis. ERCP is recommended for evaluation of the biliary tree when therapeutic intervention is likely.

Percutaneous Transhepatic Cholangiography

PTC can be used as an alternative to ERCP as a diagnostic and therapeutic tool in evaluating the biliary tree. Under ultrasound guidance, a needle is passed through the liver and into the biliary tree, and contrast material is injected. If obstruction is identified, biliary drainage, if required, can be performed at the same time. PTC is contraindicated if there are marked ascites or irreversible coagulopathy. The complications of PTC include bleeding, pneumothorax, infection, and bile leakage.

Liver Biopsy

Percutaneous liver biopsy is often necessary to determine the cause of conjugated hyperbilirubinemia. In some instances, a specific pattern of injury, such as paucity of bile ducts or bile duct proliferation, may be evident. In other cases, specific markers of disease may be identified (the distinctive inclusions in α_1-antitrypsin deficiency) or measured (metabolic enzyme activity). Ultrasound-guided biopsy is useful when a specific lesion needs to be evaluated or if there is abnormal anatomy of the liver. An open biopsy may be necessary when a large sample of tissue is needed or when there are contraindications to the percutaneous approach, such as ascites or severe coagulopathy. Transjugular liver biopsy can reduce the risk of bleeding in patients with coagulopathy. The complications of liver biopsy are the same as those for PTC.

JAUNDICE IN THE NEONATE AND INFANT

History

Evaluation of the infant with jaundice starts with a thorough history, including age at onset and duration of jaundice (see Fig. 18.2). In the neonate, the causes of jaundice range from a benign, self-limited process associated with immaturity of bilirubin excretion (physiologic jaundice) to life-threatening biliary atresia or metabolic disorders (galactosemia, fructosemia, tyrosinemia). In older infants, there are fewer benign explanations for jaundice. For example, physiologic jaundice generally resolves by 1–2 weeks of age, and jaundice associated with breast milk usually resolves by the time the infant is 1 month old.

Acholic stools usually indicate obstruction of the biliary tree; however, nonpigmented stools can be seen with severe hepatocellular injury. The clinician should document the presence or absence of acholic stool in every infant evaluated for jaundice. The center of the stool should be examined because the outside may be lightly pigmented from sloughed jaundiced cells of the intestinal tract. Delayed passage of meconium may be secondary to cystic fibrosis or Hirschsprung disease. Delayed passage of stools, by itself, can lead to increased enterohepatic circulation of bilirubin.

Clues to the diagnosis of hyperbilirubinemia are often found in the prenatal and perinatal history (Table 18.1). Maternal infections that can be transmitted to the fetus or neonate, such as syphilis, toxoplasmosis, cytomegalovirus (CMV), hepatitis B, enterovirus, herpes simplex, and HIV, are rare causes of cholestatic liver disease in the neonate. Prenatal growth pattern should be carefully evaluated. Perinatal infections such as CMV, rubella, and toxoplasmosis can present with intrauterine growth restriction. Premature infants are prone to higher bilirubin levels and more prolonged hyperbilirubinemia; they are also more likely to have risk factors for hyperbilirubinemia such as delayed enteral feedings, require parenteral nutrition, and have perinatal insults with hypoxia and acidosis.

Delay of feeding can contribute to both conjugated and unconjugated hyperbilirubinemia; this effect is usually transient and should not be overinterpreted. Breast-feeding is associated with higher levels of unconjugated bilirubin and a longer duration of jaundice than in formula-feeding. Even when diagnosis of breast milk jaundice is likely, conjugated bilirubin should be checked because it provides an easy screening tool for liver disorders, including biliary atresia. Galactosemia does not manifest in the infant who receives a lactose-free formula. Hereditary fructose intolerance is not clinically apparent until the infant ingests fluids or solids containing fructose or sucrose. Infants with metabolic disorders often present with a history of vomiting, lethargy, and poor feeding. Vomiting may also be a symptom of intestinal obstruction including malrotation/volvulus.

The family history can often provide direction to the evaluation, particularly with some of the less common hereditary disorders. This can include most of the metabolic disorders, hemolytic diseases, and disorders associated with intrahepatic cholestasis (Tables 18.2 and 18.3). Diseases that lead to severe liver dysfunction resulting in neonatal hepatic failure have some characteristic features (Table 18.4).

Physical Examination

With increasing levels of bilirubin, neonatal icterus becomes more extensive, spreading in a cephalopedal direction. **Pallor** may indicate hemolytic disease. **Petechiae** alert the clinician to thrombocytopenia, possible sepsis, congenital infections, or severe hemolytic disease.

Dysmorphic face can be present in Zellweger syndrome or Alagille syndrome (see Table 18.1). The characteristic facies of Alagille syndrome may not be recognizable until later in childhood. Microcephaly that accompanies jaundice is associated with congenital viral infections.

An **ophthalmologic examination** can demonstrate a variety of abnormalities. Cataracts are seen in galactosemia and rubella.

TABLE 18.1 Diagnostic Clues in the Evaluation of Infants with Jaundice

Symptom	Possible Diagnosis
Prenatal/Perinatal Findings	
Polyhydramnios	Intestinal atresia
In utero growth restriction	Cytomegalovirus; rubella; toxoplasmosis
Vomiting/poor feeding	Metabolic disorders
Delayed passage of meconium	Cystic fibrosis; Hirschsprung disease
Constipation, hypotonia, hypothermia	Hypothyroidism
Maternal preeclampsia	HELLP: fatty acid oxidation disorders
Microphallus	Hypopituitarism associated with SOD
Intrahepatic cholestasis of pregnancy	PFIC type 2 and 3
Repeated affected neonates	Alloimmune hepatitis
Characteristic Facies	
Narrow cranium, prominent forehead, hypertelorism, epicanthal folds, large fontanel	Zellweger syndrome
Triangular face with broad forehead, hypertelorism, deep-set eyes, long nose, pointed mandible	Alagille syndrome
Microcephaly	Congenital viral infections
Ophthalmologic Findings	
Cataracts	Galactosemia; rubella
Chorioretinitis	Congenital infections
Nystagmus with hypoplasia of optic nerve	Hypopituitarism with SOD
Posterior embryotoxon	Alagille syndrome
Perinatal Infections	
Syphilis	Syphilis
Toxoplasmosis	Toxoplasmosis
Cytomegalovirus	Cytomegalovirus
Hepatitis B	Hepatitis B
Herpes simplex	Herpes simplex
Enterovirus	Enterovirus
HIV	HIV infection
Renal Disease	
RTA	Tyrosinemia
RTA	Galactosemia
Congenital hepatic fibrosis	ARPKD
Alagille syndrome	Alagille syndrome
Arthrogryposis	RTA–cholestasis syndrome
Fibrocystic disease	Congenital hepatic fibrosis

ARPKD, autosomal recessive polycystic kidney disease; HELLP, hemolysis, elevated liver enzymes, low platelets; PFIC, progressive familial intrahepatic cholestasis; RTA, renal tubular acidosis; SOD, septo-optic dysplasia.

Chorioretinitis accompanies congenital infections (toxoplasmosis, syphilis, rubella, CMV, herpes simplex virus). Nystagmus with hypoplasia of the optic nerve suggests hypopituitarism associated with septo-optic dysplasia. Posterior embryotoxon is found in Alagille syndrome.

A **heart murmur** may be caused by an underlying congenital heart disease, which may be associated with Alagille syndrome, one of the trisomies, and syndromic forms of biliary atresia

TABLE 18.2 Differential Diagnosis of Unconjugated Hyperbilirubinemia in Neonates and Infants

Physiologic Jaundice	**Infection**
Breast-Feeding/Breast Milk Jaundice	**Intestinal Obstruction**
Polycythemia	Pyloric stenosis
Diabetic mother	Intestinal atresia
Fetal transfusion (maternal, twin)	Hirschsprung disease
Intrauterine hypoxemia	Cystic fibrosis
Delayed cord clamping	**Enclosed Hematoma (Cephalohematoma, Ecchymoses)**
Congenital adrenal hyperplasia	**Congestive Heart Failure**
Neonatal thyrotoxicosis	**Hypoxia**
Hemolysis	**Acidosis**
Isoimmune	**Hypothyroidism or Hypopituitarism**
Rh incompatibility	**Drugs/Toxins**
ABO incompatibility	Maternal oxytocin
Other (M, S, Kidd, Kell, Duffy)	Vitamin K
Erythrocyte membrane defects	Antibiotics
Hereditary spherocytosis	Phenol disinfectants
Hereditary elliptocytosis	Herbs
Infantile pyknocytosis	**Familial Disorders of Bilirubin Metabolism**
Erythrocyte enzyme defects	Gilbert syndrome
Glucose-6-phosphate dehydrogenase	Crigler-Najjar syndrome types I and II
Pyruvate kinase	Lucey-Driscoll syndrome
Hexokinase	
Other	
Hemoglobinopathy	
Thalassemia	
Sepsis	
Hemangioma	
Congenital erythropoietic porphyria	
Familial TTP (*ADAM TS13*)	

TTP, thrombotic thrombocytopenic purpura.

Modified from Balistreri WF. Liver disease in infancy and childhood. In: Schiff ER, Sorrell MF, Maddrey WC, eds. *Schiff's Diseases of the Liver*. 8th ed. Philadelphia: Lippincott-Raven; 1999:1364.

(polysplenia syndrome). Heart disease that results in hepatic ischemia or congestion can be a cause of conjugated or unconjugated hyperbilirubinemia.

Hepatomegaly, splenomegaly, and ascites may be caused by both hepatic and nonhepatic etiologies, but they always require evaluation as they are not associated with physiologic or breast milk jaundice.

Microphallus can be associated with septo-optic dysplasia and hypopituitarism.

Differential Diagnosis

When a neonate has jaundice, a thorough history, including the obstetric history, and physical examination should provide most of the information necessary to determine whether the condition represents physiologic jaundice (see Fig. 18.2). A total and fractionated bilirubin measurement should be performed if there is any question about the diagnosis of physiologic jaundice.

Physiologic and Breast Milk Jaundice

In neonates, increased bilirubin production is caused by the normally increased neonatal red blood cell mass and the decreased life span of the red blood cells (80 vs 120 days). Albumin binding is decreased because of lower albumin concentrations and diminished binding capacity, which results in decreased transport of UCB to the liver with increased deposition in tissues. Uptake of bilirubin by the hepatocytes during the first weeks of life is defective. Low levels of glutathione S-transferase B decrease intracellular binding, which may impede the transport of UCB to the endoplasmic reticulum. Conjugation is impaired by decreased activity of UDPGT. Secretion into the canaliculi is impaired. There is increased enterohepatic circulation of unconjugated bilirubin as a result of increased activity of β-glucuronidase in the intestinal lumen and as a result of intestinal bacterial flora with lower capacity for urobilinogen formation (see Fig. 18.1).

These features contribute in varying degrees to **physiologic jaundice**, characterized by a peak bilirubin level of <13 mg/dL on postnatal days 3–5, a decrease to normal by 2 weeks of age, and a conjugated fraction of <20%. In premature, breast-fed infants, infants of diabetic mothers, and Asian and Native American infants, the peak is higher and lasts longer. Conjugated bilirubin should be checked if there is any question of the nature of jaundice.

Breast-feeding has been associated with an increased incidence of unconjugated hyperbilirubinemia outside the expected range (>13 mg/dL). Jaundice of this level may occur in 10–25% of breast-fed infants, in contrast to 4–7% of formula-fed infants. It can occur within the first 5 days of life and is referred to as "early" or "breast-feeding" jaundice. Breast-feeding jaundice is seen in infants who are not feeding adequately and may be dehydrated or malnourished. In a second group of breast-fed infants, the jaundice develops slowly, occurring after the first

TABLE 18.3 Mechanistic Classification of the Etiologies of Neonatal Cholestasis

Impaired bile flow
  Extrahepatic ducts
    Biliary atresia
    Choledochal cyst
    Spontaneous bile duct perforation
    Choledocholithiasis, biliary sludge
    Duct compression (may also be intrahepatic), e.g., hepatoblastoma, neuroblastoma, rhabdomyosarcoma, neonatal leukemia, systemic juvenile xanthogranuloma, Langerhans cell histiocytosis
    Bile duct stenosis
  Intrahepatic duct obstruction/formation
    Alagille syndrome
    "Nonsyndromic paucity of interlobular bile ducts," e.g., Williams syndrome
    Cystic fibrosis
    Ductal plate malformations: congenital hepatic fibrosis; ARPKD; Caroli disease; Ivemark, Jeune, Joubert, Bardet-Biedl syndromes
    Neonatal sclerosing cholangitis
  Canalicular membrane transporters
    PFIC type 1, BRIC, Nielsen syndrome (familial Greenland cholestasis)
    PFIC type 2
    PFIC type 3
    Neonatal Dubin-Johnson syndrome
    Villin functional defect
    Overload of excretory mechanism capacity: ABO blood group incompatibility with hemolysis
  Hepatocyte tight junctions
    Neonatal ichthyosis–sclerosing cholangitis syndrome–claudin-1 protein
    Familial hypercholanemia due to TJP2 (zonulin-2) deficiency
  Hepatocyte dysfunction
  Bile acid synthesis
    First-degree: BASD
    3-Oxo-Δ4-steroid 5β-reductase deficiency
    3β-Hydroxy-Δ5-C27-steroid dehydrogenase/isomerase deficiency
    Oxysterol 7α-hydroxylase deficiency
    Familial hypercholanemia due to BAAT deficiency
    Second-degree: organelle dysfunction
    Smith-Lemli-Opitz syndrome (cholesterol formation)
    Peroxisomal disorders: Zellweger, infantile Refsum, neonatal ALD
  Infectious
    Bacterial: sepsis (endotoxemia, e.g., UTI, gastroenteritis)
    Listeria
    Syphilis
    TB
  Viral: herpes viruses: CMV, HSV, HHV-6
    Parvovirus B19
    Hepatitis A, B, C
    Enterovirus: coxsackieviruses, echoviruses, "numbered" enteroviruses
    Adenovirus
    Rubella
    HIV
    Paramyxovirus
  Protozoal
    Toxoplasmosis
  Toxic
    Parenteral nutrition–associated liver disease
    Fetal alcohol syndrome
    Drugs: maternal amphetamines, anticonvulsants; infant antifungals

Endocrine
  Panhypopituitarism
  Hypothyroidism, cortisol deficiency
  McCune-Albright syndrome
  Donohue syndrome (leprechaunism)
Metabolic
  α_1-Antitrypsin deficiency
  Carbohydrate disorders
  Galactosemia
  Fructosemia (hereditary fructose intolerance)
  Glycogen storage disease type IV (Andersen disease)
  Amino acid disorders
  Tyrosinemia type I
  Lipid disorders
  Niemann-Pick disease type C
  Gaucher disease
  Cerebrotendinous xanthomatosis
  Farber disease
  β-Oxidation defects: short- and long-chain acyl-CoA dehydrogenase deficiencies
  Lysosomal storage disorders
  Niemann-Pick disease, type C
  Gaucher disease
  Farber disease
  Mucopolysaccharidosis VI (Maroteaux-Lamy syndrome)
  Mucolipidosis II (I-cell disease)
  Urea cycle defects
  Citrin deficiency (formerly type II citrullinemia)
  Mitochondrial respiratory chain disorders
  Growth retardation, amino aciduria, cholestasis, iron overload, lactic acidosis, and early death (GRACILE)
Immune mediated:
  Gestational alloimmune liver disease
  Neonatal lupus erythematosus
  Autoimmune hemolytic anemia with giant cell hepatitis
  Hemophagocytic lymphohistiocytosis
Other:
  Hypoxic/ischemic/vascular
  Shock/hypoperfusion/hypoxia
  Budd-Chiari syndrome
  Cardiac insufficiency (congenital heart disease, arrhythmia)
  Multiple hemangiomata
  Sinusoidal obstruction syndrome
  ARC syndrome (arthrogryposis–renal tubular dysfunction–cholestasis; defective vacuolar protein sorting)
  Chromosomal: trisomy 18, 21
  Congenital disorders of glycosylation
  Hardikar syndrome
  Lymphedema cholestasis syndrome (Aagenaes syndrome)
  Kabuki syndrome
  North American Indian childhood cirrhosis (defective cirhin protein–unknown function)
  Pseudo-TORCH syndrome
  "Idiopathic neonatal hepatitis"

ALD, adrenoleukodystrophy; ARC, arthrogryposis-renal-cholestasis; ARPKD, autosomal recessive polycystic kidney disease; BAAT, bile acid coenzyme A: amino acid N-acyltransferase; BASD, bile acid synthetic defects; BRIC, benign recurrent intrahepatic cholestasis; CMV, cytomegalovirus; HHV-6, human herpesvirus type 6; HIV, human immunodeficiency virus; HSV, herpes simplex virus; PFIC, progressive familial intrahepatic cholestasis; TORCH, toxoplasmosis, other (syphilis, varicella-zoster, parvovirus B19), rubella, cytomegalovirus, and herpes infections; UTI, urinary tract infection.
From Wyllie R, Hyams JS, Kay M, eds. *Pediatric Gastrointestinal and Liver Disease*. 6th ed. Philadelphia: Elsevier; 2021:745, Table 68.1.

TABLE 18.4   Typical Laboratory Findings in Neonatal Liver Failure

	GALD	HLH	Mitochondrial	Viral	Ischemic
Transaminase levels (IU/L)	Normal/mild increase <100	Moderate/significant increase (>1,000)	Moderate increase (100–500)	Significant increase (>1,000)	Significant increase (>1,000–6,000)
INR	Significant increase	Moderate/significant increase	Moderate/significant increase	Moderate/significant increase	Moderate/significant increase
Ferritin level (ng/mL)	800–7,000	Significant increase (>20,000)	Variable	Significant increase (>20,000)	Variable depending on underlying cause of ischemia
Triglyceride levels	Normal	Increased	Normal	Normal	Normal
Hypoglycemia	Yes	Often	Yes	Often	Variable
Lactic acidosis	Normal	Normal	Increased	Normal unless shock	Often
α-Fetoprotein level (for age)	Increased	Normal	Normal/increased	Normal	Normal
Cholestasis	Progressive after birth	Moderate/significant	Moderate	None/mild at presentation	Mild/moderate

GALD, gestational alloimmune liver disease; HLH, hemophagocytic lymphohistiocytosis.
Data from Sundaram SS, Alonso EM, Narkewicz MR, et al. Characterization and outcomes of young infants with acute liver failure. *J Pediatr.* 2011;159:813–818; Taylor SA, Whitington PF. Neonatal acute liver failure. *Liver Transpl.* 2016;22:677–685; Bitar R, Thwaites R, Davison S, et al. Liver failure in early infancy: aetiology, presentation, and outcome. *J Pediatr Gastroenterol Nutr.* 2017;64:70–75; Fellman V, Kotarsky H. Mitochondrial hepatopathies in the newborn period. *Semin Fetal Neonatal Med.* 2011;16:222–228.

week of life, and peaks between the second and third weeks of life at 10–20 mg/dL. This is referred to as "late" or "breast milk" jaundice. The precise cause of increased bilirubin levels in this latter setting has not been established; alternative theories include inhibition of glucuronosyltransferase activity and increased enterohepatic circulation of UCB. Kernicterus appears to be very rare but has been reported in association with breast-feeding. No treatment is necessary for physiologic jaundice. Practices that support breast-feeding, such as rooming-in on the maternity ward and frequent feedings, decrease the risk for breast-feeding jaundice. If the bilirubin exceeds 20 mg/dL in the breast-fed infant, discontinuing breast-feeding for 24 hours and supplementing with formula feeds results in a decreased bilirubin level. Phototherapy or rarely exchange transfusion may also be needed. Diagnosis of breast milk jaundice should include a blood test for conjugated bilirubin and can be diagnosed only with appropriate clinical history in the absence of conjugated hyperbilirubinemia.

If there are any **red flags** or uncertainty about the diagnosis (Table 18.5), or if treatment is being considered, the hyperbilirubinemia should be investigated further. Any abnormality identified by history, physical examination, or laboratory findings is a matter of concern.

Unconjugated Hyperbilirubinemia

The differential diagnosis of unconjugated hyperbilirubinemia in the neonate and infant is presented in Table 18.2. Unless abnormalities in the history and physical examination direct the evaluation more specifically, hematologic evaluation, which may identify causes of increased bilirubin production, should be performed. This includes a CBC with examination of the smear, a reticulocyte count, a direct Coombs test, and blood typing (mother and infant).

Polycythemia. Neonatal polycythemia, defined as a hematocrit >65% by venipuncture, can be caused by maternal diabetes, twin-twin transfusion, intrauterine hypoxemia, endocrine disorders, and delayed cord clamping (see Table 18.2). Polycythemia results in increased bilirubin production because of the increased red blood cell mass.

Hemolytic disorders. Reticulocytosis, unconjugated hyperbilirubinemia, and an increased nucleated red blood cell count, with either a low or normal hematocrit, suggest hemolysis. This can result from isoimmunization; erythrocyte membrane, hemoglobin, or enzyme defects; or sepsis with disseminated intravascular coagulation. Some causes of isoimmunization have low reticulocyte counts because the antibody binds to these precursor cells. Rarer causes of hemolysis include hemangiomas and congenital erythropoietic porphyria.

Isoimmune hemolytic disease. In this group of disorders, maternal antibodies (immunoglobulin G) to the infant's erythrocytes cross the placenta, resulting in red blood cell destruction. The administration of anti-D gamma globulin (Rh$_O$[D] immune globulin [RhoGAM]) after delivery to women who are Rh-negative has reduced the incidence of Rh sensitization and erythroblastosis fetalis. If a woman has been sensitized, the fetus can be monitored with serial amniocenteses. If necessary, intrauterine transfusion can then be performed to prevent the sequelae of severe hemolysis, which include fetal and neonatal anemia, edema, hepatosplenomegaly, and circulatory collapse or stillbirth of an infant with hydrops fetalis. If the problem has not been recognized prenatally, the infant with Rh incompatibility presents with pallor, hepatosplenomegaly, and rapidly developing jaundice.

The diagnosis is confirmed by demonstrating that the infant is Rh-positive, that the direct Coombs test result is positive, and that maternal antibody is coating the infant's red blood cells. These test results are modified with in utero transfusions with Rh-negative cells. Depending on the degree of hemolysis, postnatal phototherapy and/or exchange transfusion may be required.

ABO blood type incompatibility causes a less severe form of isoimmune hemolytic disease with a less rapid development of jaundice. It is more common in infants with blood type A or B who are born to mothers with blood type O. Hemolysis develops in 50% of sensitized infants; of these infants, 50% have a bilirubin level >10 mg/dL. In addition to showing anemia, reticulocytosis, and spherocytes on the smear, the direct Coombs test result is weakly positive, and the indirect Coombs test result is positive. In rare cases, other minor blood group antibodies can also cause hemolysis.

Erythrocyte membrane defects. Red blood cell membrane defects are relatively uncommon causes of unconjugated hyperbilirubinemia. There is often a family history of hemolysis, transfusions, cholecystectomy for bilirubin stones, or splenectomy. Hemolysis results from fragility of the red blood cell membrane. When the defect

TABLE 18.5 Red Flags in the Evaluation of Infants with Jaundice

Onset
<24 hr of age
>2 wk of age

Bilirubin

Conjugated
>20% of total or >2 mg/dL

Total
>13 mg/dL formula-fed
>14–15 mg/dL breast-fed

Course
Increases by >5 mg/dL/day
Persists beyond 14 days of age

Prenatal History
Maternal infection
Maternal diabetes mellitus
Maternal drug use
Polyhydramnios
Intrauterine growth restriction

Delivery
Prematurity
Perinatal asphyxia
Small for gestational age

Feeding
Delayed enteral feeding
Vomiting
Poor feeding
Associated with change in formula

Stools
Acholic
Delayed passage of meconium

Family History
Jaundice
Anemia
Liver disease
Splenectomy
Cholecystectomy

Physical Examination
Ill-appearing
Pallor
Petechiae
Hematoma or ecchymoses
Chromosomal stigmata
Abnormal facies
Microcephaly
Cataracts
Chorioretinitis
Nystagmus
Optic nerve hypoplasia
Posterior embryotoxon
Heart murmur
Hepatosplenomegaly (or isolated hepatomegaly or splenomegaly)
Ascites
Acholic stools
Dark urine
Microphallus
Encephalopathy—seizures, lethargy, coma

is present in infancy, there are anemia, jaundice, and splenomegaly, and the smear is often characteristic (e.g., spherocytosis or elliptocytosis). Spherocytes are also seen with ABO incompatibility. All membrane defects yield negative results of the Coombs tests.

Erythrocyte enzyme defects (see Chapter 49). Glucose-6-phosphate dehydrogenase (G6PD) deficiency is common. Jaundice is seen more frequently in persons with a Mediterranean or Far Eastern ancestry who have a complete absence of the enzyme. In these individuals, hemolysis can occur without a precipitant. In African-American patients, the disease is generally less severe, and hemolysis is rare without exposure to a drug, a toxin, or an infection that causes an oxidant stress. G6PD deficiency can manifest as neonatal jaundice on day 2 or 3 after birth; alternatively, it may not manifest until later in childhood, when jaundice is associated with an acute hemolytic crisis. The diagnosis of G6PD deficiency is confirmed by documenting deficiency of the enzyme in red blood cells.

Numerous deficiencies of enzymes in the glycolytic pathway have been identified. Pyruvate kinase deficiency is the most common of these rare disorders. Most of these disorders are thought to have an autosomal recessive mode of transmission and have been identified in only a small number of individuals. They all result in hemolysis. The time of manifestation depends on the degree of hemolysis.

Other considerations. If the hematocrit is normal and there is no evidence of hemolysis or a consumptive process, other explanations for unconjugated hyperbilirubinemia should be sought. Blood and urine cultures rarely identify infectious etiologic agents if the patient is otherwise clinically normal. Vomiting, abdominal distention, and delayed passage of meconium suggest obstruction of the gastrointestinal tract and should be further investigated by imaging. Clinical examination should also identify cephalohematoma, ecchymoses, heart failure, hypoxia, and acidosis. Thyroxine and thyroid-stimulating hormone levels should be obtained or checked from the state neonatal screening program to look for evidence of hypothyroidism or hypopituitarism.

Drugs, administered to either mother or neonate, and toxins should be identified by careful record review. Examples include oxytocin, excess vitamin K in premature infants, some antibiotics, and phenol disinfectants used in nurseries. Use of herbal remedies should also be investigated.

In the evaluation process, it is important to remember that the division of causes into hemolytic and nonhemolytic is an arbitrary one. Drugs, infection, and G6PD deficiency can contribute to both hemolytic and nonhemolytic neonatal jaundice. In addition, the cause of jaundice can be multifactorial.

Familial disorders of bilirubin metabolism

Gilbert syndrome. Gilbert syndrome is a benign condition that occurs in up to 8% of the population. A familial incidence is reported in 15–40% of cases. Gilbert syndrome is a heterogeneous group of disorders that have in common at least a 50% decrease in UDPGT activity as a result of a defect in the gene responsible for this enzyme. In 20–30% of individuals with Gilbert syndrome, there is also a decrease in hepatocyte bilirubin uptake. Affected individuals are generally asymptomatic and may not present with jaundice until the second or third decade of life. Gilbert syndrome may be responsible for some cases of neonatal jaundice. Mild jaundice with a bilirubin level up to 7 mg/dL can occur transiently with fatigue, exercise, fasting, febrile illness, and alcohol ingestion in older patients. Except for showing an increased indirect bilirubin level, all laboratory studies are normal. The diagnosis is generally a clinical one but can be confirmed by documenting a twofold to threefold rise in unconjugated bilirubin during a 24-hour fast.

Crigler-Najjar syndrome. Crigler-Najjar syndrome types I and II (also known as Arias syndrome) are rare autosomal recessive conditions caused by variants (different alleles from those of Gilbert syndrome) in the gene coding for UDPGT. Crigler-Najjar syndrome type I is characterized by marked hyperbilirubinemia (20–40 mg/dL) in the neonatal period in an otherwise healthy infant. Among untreated infants, kernicterus is universal, and affected individuals usually die with severe neurologic problems. Because UDPGT is undetectable, there is no conjugated bilirubin in the bile or serum, and the bile is colorless. There is no decrease in serum UCB levels during phenobarbital administration. The only therapies are exchange transfusion, intensive phototherapy, and liver transplantation.

The onset of Crigler-Najjar syndrome type II is usually at birth, although it can be in late childhood. There is <5% of the normal UDPGT activity. Bile contains bilirubin monoglucuronides. Bilirubin levels, generally 8–25 mg/dL, respond to phenobarbital administration with a significant decrease. Neurologic disease is rare.

Lucey-Driscoll syndrome. Lucey-Driscoll syndrome is a transient familial neonatal hyperbilirubinemia that appears in the first few days of life and resolves by 2–3 weeks of age. This results from inhibition of UDPGT by a substance that has been found in both maternal and infant serum. The bilirubin level can rise to >60 mg/dL in untreated infants, resulting in severe neurotoxicity. The condition is treated with exchange transfusion.

Therapy. Treatment of unconjugated hyperbilirubinemia depends on the degree of elevation of bilirubin. Considerable controversy exists over which level is toxic and when treatment should be initiated. Because it is lipid soluble, unconjugated bilirubin can diffuse into the central nervous system, which results in neurologic toxicity. Most authorities agree that kernicterus does not occur below a bilirubin level of 20–30 mg/dL in the healthy, full-term infant without evidence of hemolysis. Kernicterus may occur at lower bilirubin levels in premature or sick neonates.

Treatment options include phototherapy and exchange transfusion. Phototherapy produces a reduction of bilirubin by 1–2 mg/dL in 4–6 hours by causing the photoisomerization and photodegradation of unconjugated bilirubin to more water-soluble forms that are more readily excreted in bile and urine. Potential complications include retinal damage, diarrhea, and dehydration. Phototherapy is begun at levels below that for exchange transfusion (~5 mg/dL less) or during preparations for an exchange transfusion.

Exchange transfusion with blood cross-matched against that of the mother is indicated for severe hyperbilirubinemia. This decision must be based not only on the bilirubin level but also, as important, on the infant's age and clinical condition. In full- or near-term infants (>2,000 g in weight) with evidence of hemolysis, exchange transfusion is indicated if the serum unconjugated bilirubin level is higher than 25–30 mg/dL or if the bilirubin level does not rapidly respond to phototherapy. Signs of kernicterus (i.e., a high-pitched cry, gaze paralysis, fever, lethargy, and opisthotonic posture) warrant exchange transfusion, no matter what the bilirubin level.

Neonatal conjugated hyperbilirubinemia. Conjugated hyperbilirubinemia in the neonate and infant has an extensive differential

TABLE 18.6 **Conditions Not to Miss in Infants with Conjugated Hyperbilirubinemia**
Priorities
Hypoprothrombinemia
Hypoglycemia
Extrahepatic biliary atresia
Infections
Sepsis
Urinary tract infection
Syphilis
Toxoplasmosis
Herpes simplex virus
Endocrine Disorders
Hypopituitarism
Hypothyroidism
Metabolic Disorders
Galactosemia
Hereditary fructose intolerance (fructosemia)
Tyrosinemia
Mitochondrial hepatocerebral subtypes
Other
Neonatal hemochromatosis
Bile acid abnormalities
Choledochal cyst
Intestinal obstruction
Familial hemophagocytic syndromes
Heart disease
Toxins

diagnosis (see Table 18.3). It is important to first evaluate the infant for potentially treatable problems (Table 18.6) and institute specific therapy that prevents significant morbidity and may be life-saving. Figure 18.2 outlines a diagnostic approach when the clinical presentation has not suggested a likely diagnosis.

Common to all of these conditions is the potential for coagulopathy. If the PT is prolonged, the infant should be treated with intravenous vitamin K to avoid spontaneous hemorrhage, particularly intracranial. Depending on the degree of hepatocellular damage, vitamin K may not correct the PT. This mandates prompt evaluation for the underlying cause of neonatal liver failure or extrahepatic causes of coagulopathy. Interpretation of PT should be based on neonatal norms, as normal PT is higher in newborns, particularly in premature newborns versus older infants. Even with a normal PT at the outset, infants with conjugated hyperbilirubinemia should be on oral fat-soluble vitamin supplementation until their cholestasis resolves.

Hypoglycemia is another danger that is associated with diseases that cause severe hepatic dysfunction but also with metabolic disorders as well as with hypopituitarism. The infant may be relatively asymptomatic despite significant hypoglycemia. The serum glucose level can be measured before a feeding. If hypoglycemia is present, the infant should receive frequent feedings, continuous feedings, or intravenous dextrose infusions. Glucose level should always be the part of the evaluation of conjugated hyperbilirubinemia.

Hyperammonemia can be present in severe liver dysfunction and metabolic liver disorders. Ammonia should be checked on infants with lethargy or with a change in mental status.

Serum levels of aminotransferases, GGT, and alkaline phosphatase, in addition to a CBC, should be included in the initial evaluation.

Obstructive/anatomic abnormalities, idiopathic cholestasis, and idiopathic neonatal hepatitis

Biliary atresia. Untreated biliary atresia is universally lethal, and only prompt diagnosis and surgical treatment can prevent mortality. Biliary atresia accounts for approximately 30% of cases of neonatal cholestasis seen at major referral centers. It occurs in 1 in 8,000–15,000 live births. It is the result of a progressive inflammatory process leading to obliteration of the lumen of the extrahepatic ducts. It is the leading indication for liver transplantation in the pediatric population. Infants are less often icteric from birth and more often develop jaundice at 2–6 weeks of age. Infants are usually full term and initially appear healthy except for jaundice, dark urine, and acholic stools. The family history usually is negative for liver disease. There appear to be two forms of biliary atresia:

1. In the "embryonic" or "fetal form," which occurs in 15–30% of cases, there is no jaundice-free period. There are often associated other anatomic defects, including cardiac defects, polysplenia, malrotation, and abdominal heterotaxia.
2. In the "perinatal form," there may be a jaundice-free interval after resolution of the normal physiologic jaundice, and there are no associated anomalies.

At the time of presentation, infants with biliary atresia may have an enlarged, firm liver. Pruritus, splenomegaly, and ascites can develop later with advanced disease. The work-up should be performed expeditiously; it is important to identify biliary atresia early because the success of surgical establishment of drainage is correlated with early age at surgery. Surgery performed before the infant is 2 months old carries an approximately 80% rate of success in terms of obtaining some bile flow. This rate decreases to about 20% for surgery performed in patients older than 3 months. Diagnostic work-up includes evaluation of other identifiable causes of neonatal cholestasis including CMV or syphilis infection, α_1-antitrypsin deficiency, hypothyroidism, and other anatomic abnormalities of the biliary tree. Combination of conjugated hyperbilirubinemia, acholic stools, and elevated GGT should trigger prompt evaluation for biliary atresia. An ultrasound study helps exclude other treatable anatomic abnormalities, such as a choledochal cyst. The gallbladder is usually absent or collapsed in infants with biliary atresia. It is strongly recommended that noninvasive work-up is completed by 1 month of age and the infant is referred to a pediatric tertiary center if biliary atresia cannot be ruled out.

Liver biopsy and percutaneous cholangiogram should follow if no alternative cause of jaundice is identified. Characteristic findings on liver biopsy are periportal edema and fibrosis, bile duct proliferation, and bile duct plugs. Some centers utilize hepatobiliary scintigraphy, which demonstrates uptake of the tracer but no excretion into the duodenum if biliary atresia is present. However, this study can lead to delay in diagnosis (requires pretreatment with phenobarbital) and can be inconclusive in hepatic dysfunction due to poor uptake of the tracer.

The diagnosis is confirmed by intraoperative cholangiography at the time of surgery. The surgical procedure, a portoenterostomy, was initially described by Kasai. The porta hepatis is transected, and a loop of intestine is brought up to drain the bile ducts. Those in whom bile drainage is not established require early liver transplantation. In the majority of patients, surgery is palliative, allowing time before liver transplantation is needed; overall and post-transplant mortality are significantly reduced with a timely Kasai procedure.

The important, potentially life-threatening complication of the Kasai procedure is **bacterial ascending cholangitis**. Febrile patients with biliary atresia need to be promptly evaluated for causes of fever. If no alternative source of fever is identified, they should be evaluated for cholangitis.

Most of the patients with biliary atresia remain cholestatic despite the Kasai procedure; thus, they require supplementation with medium-chain triglyceride (MCT) oil (or MCT-enriched formulas) and fat-soluble vitamins. Pruritus can be managed with rifampin or naltrexone. Portal hypertension with splenomegaly, esophageal varices, and ascites can develop over time in many patients with biliary atresia. Due to significant risk of complications and frequent need for liver transplant, patients with biliary atresia should be followed in centers with pediatric transplant/hepatology expertise.

Alagille syndrome. Alagille syndrome is characterized by the abnormal development of multiple organs related to defective JAG-1/NOTCH-2 signaling. Alagille syndrome has an autosomal dominant transmission with highly variable expression. Often other family members are recognized as being affected when an infant is brought to medical attention. There is a high proportion of sporadic cases (up to 70%) with de novo variants in the *JAG-1* gene responsible for this syndrome. Variants of the NOTCH-2 receptor can result in a similar clinical picture, though they are less common than *JAG-1* variants.

The most important clinical feature is a marked reduction in the number of interlobular bile ducts. Jaundice may have its onset in the neonatal period or may not appear until later in childhood. The diagnosis is confirmed by liver biopsy. Symptoms of cholestasis often improve over time.

Additionally, patients with Alagille syndrome can have unusual facies (a triangular face with broad forehead, widely spaced and deep-set eyes, a long nose, and a pointed mandible), vertebral arch defects (butterfly vertebrae, hemivertebrae, decreased interpedicular distance), posterior embryotoxon (ocular), and cardiac anomalies (ranging from peripheral pulmonic stenosis to complex congenital heart disease) (Fig. 18.4). There is a 20–25% rate of mortality from serious cardiac or liver disease. Renal anomalies, pancreatic insufficiency, and growth retardation are present in some patients (Table 18.7). Cerebral vascular anomalies are the main reason for increased mortality later in life. Screening with MR angiography is recommended in school age. By the age of 4–6 months, pruritus develops and can be severe. Pruritus can be managed with rifampin or naltrexone. Xanthomas appear in association with a markedly elevated cholesterol level.

There is a nonsyndromic form of bile duct paucity with cholestasis caused by bile duct paucity but not associated with clinical or genetic variants characteristic of Alagille syndrome. The prognosis for this form is less favorable.

Choledochal cysts. Manifestations include conjugated hyperbilirubinemia with jaundice, vomiting, acholic stools, and hepatomegaly in the neonate. Alternatively, choledochal cysts can manifest with jaundice, abdominal pain, and a right upper quadrant mass in the older child. There are five main anatomic types of cystic dilatations of the extrahepatic or intrahepatic bile ducts (Fig. 18.5). The diagnosis is made by ultrasound studies and confirmed by MR cholangiography or intraoperative cholangiography. Treatment involves surgical excision. Cholangitis may occur postoperatively. If the cyst is not fully excised, cholangiocarcinoma can develop in the residual cyst tissue.

Treatable infections

Bacterial infection. An infant may, in rare cases, appear clinically well, with jaundice as the only sign of a bacterial infection. Blood and urine cultures should be obtained in infants with unexplained conjugated hyperbilirubinemia. Infection is less likely to be missed in the symptomatic infant who presents with poor feeding, lethargy, vomiting, temperature instability, apnea, bradycardia, or shock. *Escherichia coli* is the most common organism identified in either sepsis or urinary tract infection (often with bacteremia) when jaundice is present. The hyperbilirubinemia may be caused by endotoxin-mediated

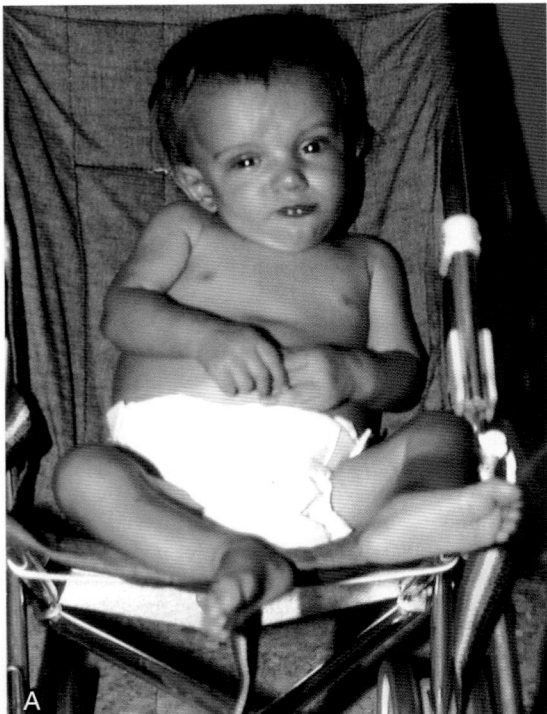

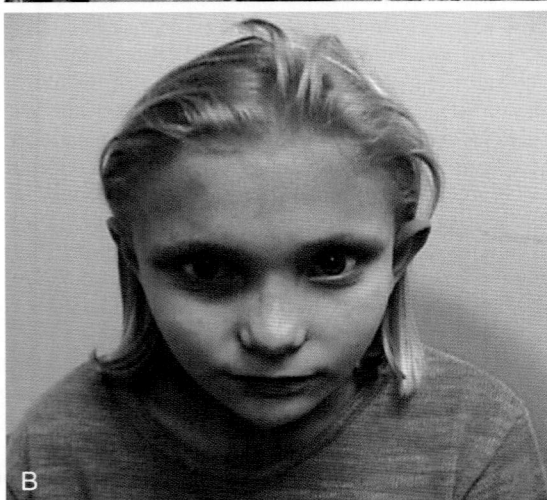

Fig. 18.4 Alagille syndrome. *A,* A 1½-year-old with broad forehead and prominent chin. *B,* Note the deep-set eyes; broad forehead; long, straight nose with flattened tip; and prominent chin. (*A,* From Jones KL, Jones MC, Del Campo M. *Smith's Recognizable Patterns of Human Malformation.* 7th ed. Philadelphia: Elsevier; 2013:760, Fig. 1 A and B; *B,* Courtesy Dr. Ian Krantz, University of Pennsylvania.)

TABLE 18.7 Extrahepatic Manifestations of Alagille Syndrome

Cardiac
Peripheral pulmonary stenosis
Tetralogy of Fallot
Ventricular septal defect
Atrial septal defect
Aortic coarctation
Pulmonary atresia

Skeletal
Short stature
Butterfly vertebrae
Fused vertebrae
Rib anomalies
Spina bifida occulta
Thin cortical bones

Ocular
Posterior embryotoxon
Axenfeld anomaly
Optic disc drusen
Shallow anterior chamber
Microcornea

Vascular
Renal artery stenosis
Intracranial bleeding
Central nervous system malformations

Other
Renal developmental abnormalities
Renal tubulopathies
Pancreatic exocrine and endocrine insufficiency
High-pitched voice
Microcolon
Growth restriction

From Mieli-Vergani G, Hadzic N. Biliary atresia and neonatal disorders of the bile ducts. In: Wyllie R, Hyams JS, Kay M, eds. *Pediatric Gastrointestinal and Liver Disease.* 4th ed. Philadelphia: Elsevier/Saunders; 2011:749.

canalicular dysfunction. Less often, other gram-negative bacilli or *Listeria*, *Staphylococcus*, or *Streptococcus* species may be identified as the causative agent. Although sepsis accounts for only a small percent of the cases of neonatal cholestasis, it is easily diagnosed and treated.

Herpes simplex. Herpes simplex causes a severe neonatal infection that usually manifests at 7–14 days of age with lethargy, poor feeding, a vesicular rash (in 60–70% of patients), jaundice, hepatomegaly, temperature instability, encephalitis, and coagulopathy. The diagnosis is made by identification of the virus in skin lesions through direct fluorescent antibody staining or PCR of herpes simplex DNA in blood or cerebrospinal fluid. Treatment is with intravenous acyclovir. Among infants with disseminated infection, the mortality rate is 15–35%.

Enteroviruses. Maternal infection at the time of delivery may result in severe enteroviral disease in the infant within 1–7 days of birth. Manifestations are similar to that of herpes simplex virus except a macular rash. Severe hepatitis, carditis, or encephalitis or a sepsis picture may develop. Diagnosis is made through PCR or viral culture. Treatment strategies include intravenous immunoglobulin (IVIG) and pleconaril.

Coronavirus (COVID-19). Infection with COVID-19 has been associated with liver dysfunction, although additional studies are needed to understand the severity and long-term effects of this new virus.

Cytomegalovirus infection. CMV infection is common, but 90% of affected infants are asymptomatic at birth. In the severely affected infant with vertical transmission, CMV can manifest within the first 24 hours after birth with intrauterine growth restriction, conjugated hyperbilirubinemia, hemolytic anemia, thrombocytopenic purpura, and hepatosplenomegaly. Often an infant with low birthweight presents with microcephaly, periventricular calcifications, and chorioretinitis. The diagnosis can be made by obtaining urine and saliva specimens for CMV DNA.

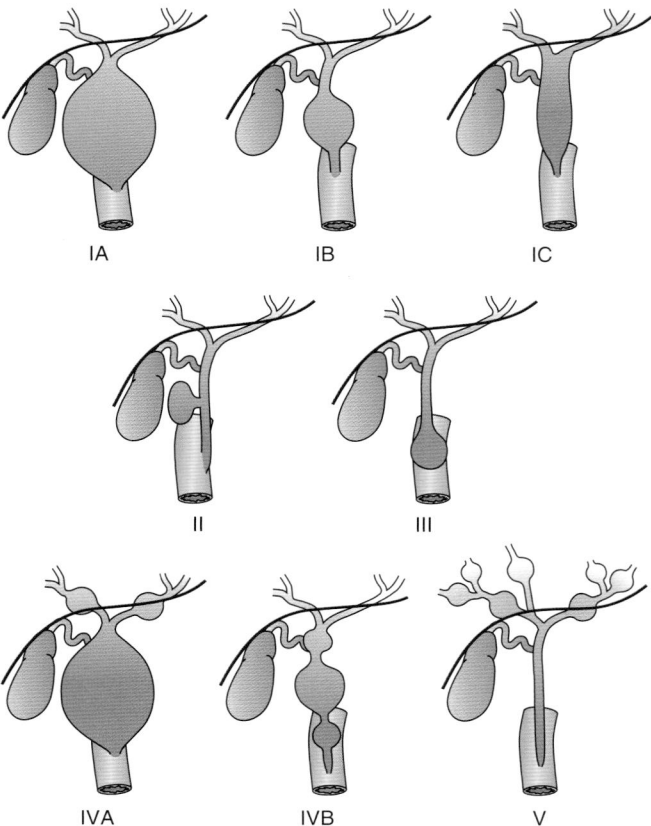

Fig. 18.5 Todani classification of choledochal cysts based on cholangiographic morphology. Types *IA* and *IB* involve cystic dilatation of the common duct, with *IB* limited to the area below the insertion of the cystic duct; *IC* is cylindrical dilatation of the duct. Type *II* is a saccular diverticulum from the common bile duct. Type *III* is a choledochocele at the ampulla of Vater. Types *IVA* and *IVB* are multiple cystic dilatations of both the intra- and extrahepatic ducts and extrahepatic biliary tree only, respectively. Type *V* is equivalent to Caroli disease with numerous intrahepatic cystic dilatations throughout the biliary tree and liver. (From Kim OH, Chung HJ, Choi BG. Imaging of the choledochal cyst. *Radiographics*. 1995;15:69–88.)

Treatment includes the use of ganciclovir and possibly CMV immunoglobulin. The liver disease resolves in most patients, but neurologic sequelae are common. Postnatal acquisition from CMV-positive blood transfusion may produce a sepsis syndrome and hepatitis.

The findings of CMV in a cholestatic infant without other features of congenital CMV infection should not stop the search for other causes of cholestasis, particularly biliary atresia.

Hepatitis B. Hepatitis B infection manifests with jaundice in fewer than 5% of perinatal infections. Perinatal transmission is high when mothers are chronic carriers who are seropositive for hepatitis B e antigen (HBeAg) or when they acquire acute infection in the last trimester. Most infants are asymptomatic, but there is a high incidence of subsequent chronic infection. Perinatal infection can be prevented with hepatitis B immune globulin and vaccination. It is important to identify mothers who are seropositive for hepatitis B surface antigen (HBsAg); identification requires universal screening.

Syphilis. Congenital syphilis remains a problem despite maternal screening. With severe infection, the infant has fever, a diffuse macular-papular rash, hepatosplenomegaly, edema, anemia, and periostitis, in addition to jaundice. Nontreponemal serologic tests (Venereal Disease Research Laboratory) may be routinely performed on cord blood. If the result is positive, the diagnosis should be confirmed on serum from the

infant. Confirmation requires a positive specific test for syphilis such as the immunoglobulin M (IgM) or immunoglobulin G fluorescent treponemal antibody. Treatment is with intravenous penicillin for 10–14 days.

Toxoplasmosis. If toxoplasmosis is suspected on clinical grounds, IgM titers should be obtained, or the placenta should be examined histologically. Most infected infants are asymptomatic. Infants with severe congenital infection may have hydrocephaly or microcephaly, intracranial calcifications, chorioretinitis, aseptic meningitis, jaundice, purpura, and hepatomegaly. Postnatal treatment consists of pyrimethamine and sulfadiazine; folinic acid is added to prevent folate deficiency.

Treatable metabolic disorders. Many metabolic disorders are part of the universal newborn screening program in developed countries. The clinician needs to be aware of which disorders are and which are not screened for in a particular country or state. Even in the presence of universal neonatal screening for metabolic disorders, the test may be falsely negative, particularly if the newborn was tested too early, was premature, or underwent transfusions before the test was performed. In countries with robust neonatal screening programs, repeating the newborn screen may be an easy and cost-effective first step in evaluation for possible metabolic disease. Other useful screening modalities include urine-reducing substances (galactosemia), serum amino acids, ammonia level, urine organic acids, quantitative serum bile acids, qualitative analysis of urinary bile acids by fast atom bombardment mass spectrometry (FAB-MS), the thyroxine level, and the thyroid-stimulating hormone level, succinyl-acetone (tyrosinemia), triglycerides, lactate, pyruvate, and acyl carnitines (mitochondrial disorders).

Galactosemia. Galactosemia, a life-threatening disorder, can easily be detected. It is an autosomal recessive disorder with deficiency of galactose-1-phosphate uridyltransferase, which is required for conversion of galactose to glucose. As a result, galactose-1-phosphate accumulates; this compound is thought to be hepatotoxic. Once lactose (glucose-galactose) is introduced into the infant's diet, vomiting, diarrhea, jaundice, hepatomegaly, and cataracts develop. Affected infants often present with *E. coli* sepsis in the first weeks of life.

Laboratory evaluation may demonstrate elevations of aminotransferase levels, a prolonged PT, hemolytic anemia, and aminoaciduria. The urine yields positive findings for reducing substances (galactose) if the infant is receiving a lactose-containing formula or breast milk. The diagnosis can be confirmed by documenting deficiency of the enzyme in erythrocytes or leukocytes. Transfusions may cause false-negative results. Treatment consists of eliminating galactose from the diet.

Hereditary fructose intolerance (fructosemia) is an uncommon disorder; it can manifest with hepatic failure in an infant exposed to fructose or sucrose in formula, juice, fruit, or medications. A thorough diet history in relation to the onset of jaundice is often the key to this diagnosis. Prompt removal of fructose, sucrose, and sorbitol from the diet is essential.

Tyrosinemia is diagnosed from serum amino acid levels and urine organic acid levels. Elevated urinary succinylacetone is pathognomonic. Treatment involves the dietary restriction of phenylalanine, methionine, and tyrosine and the use of 2-(2-nitro-4-trifluoromethylbenzoyl)-1, 3-cyclohexanedione to prevent the formation of toxic metabolites. Liver transplantation may still be required.

Disorders of bile acid metabolism typically are suggested by conjugated hyperbilirubinemia with low or normal GGT and low or normal total bile acid levels. They can be detected by bile acid FAB-MS analysis of urine. Treatment of some forms of bile acid synthetic disorder is possible with oral cholic acid supplementation.

Fatty acid oxidation defects often present with hypoketotic hypoglycemia, hepatomegaly, variable hyperammonemia, and cholestasis (Table 18.8).

TABLE 18.8   Individual Fatty Acid Oxidation Defects

Defect	Clinical Phenotype	Other Features	Metabolic Abnormalities	Diagnosis Confirmation
Carnitine transporter deficiency	H, C, M		Low free carnitine	EM
Carnitine palmitoyl transferase 1	H, R, M	RTA	High free carnitine	EM
Carnitine/acyl carnitine translocase	H, C, M	Early death	C16 and 18 species	EM
Carnitine palmitoyl transferase 2	H, C, M	RTA	C16 and 18	493C>T
Very long-chain acyl-CoA dehydrogenase	H, C, R, M		C14, 16, and 18	
Medium-chain acyl-CoA dehydrogenase	H, C, R, M		C8 DCA	985A>G in 90% symptomatic cases
Long-chain 3-hydroxyacyl-CoA dehydrogenase/mitochondrial trifunctional protein	H, C, M	Retinopathy, neuropathy	C16 and 18 species DCA	1528G>C
Short-chain 3-hydroxyacyl-CoA dehydrogenase	H	Hyperinsulinism	C4-OH urinary ethylmalonic acid	EM
Multiple acyl-CoA dehydrogenase	H, C, M	Congenital malformations, renal cysts, RTA	C6, 8, 10, and 12 urinary ethylmalonic, glutaric, and adipic acids; DCA	EM

C, acylcarnitine species; C, cardiomyopathy or arrhythmia; DCA, dicarboxylic aciduria; EM, enzyme measurement in cultured fibroblast; H, acute hepatic presentation; M, myopathic presentation; R, rhabdomyolysis; RTA, renal tubular acidosis.
From Wyllie R, Hyams JS, Kay M, eds. *Pediatric Gastrointestinal and Liver Disease*. 6th ed. Philadelphia: Elsevier; 2021:787, Table 71.1.

TABLE 18.9   "Pathognomonic" Presentations of Mitochondrial Disorders with Prominent Hepatic Involvement

Clinical Features	Disorder	Gene(s)
Liver failure and seizures	Alpers-Huttenlocher syndrome	POLG (PEO1, FARS2)
Liver failure and rotatory nystagmus ± developmental stasis/regression and elevated plasma tyrosine	Hepatocerebral MDDS	DGUOK
Liver failure and peripheral neuropathy	Hepatocerebral MDDS	MPV17
Liver disease with sensorimotor neuropathy, corneal anaesthesia/scarring, and acral mutilation	Navajo neurohepatopathy	MPV17
Liver failure, Leigh-like encephalopathy, SNHL, and methylmalonic aciduria	Hepatocerebral MDDS (succinyl-CoA ligase deficiency)	SUCLG1
Liver failure with spontaneous recovery	"Benign reversible" mitochondrial hepatopathy	TRMU
Liver failure and renal tubulopathy	Complex III deficiency	BCS1L
Cholestasis with iron overload, intrauterine growth restriction, amino aciduria, lactic acidosis, and early death	GRACILE syndrome	BCS1L
Liver disease with SNHL, Leigh-like encephalopathy, and 3-methylglutaconic aciduria	MEGDEL syndrome	SERAC1

GRACILE, growth restriction, amino aciduria, cholestasis, iron overload, lactic acidosis, early death; MDDS, mitochondrial DNA depletion syndrome; MEGDEL, 3-methylglutaconic aciduria, deafness, encephalopathy, Leigh like; mtDNA, mitochondrial DNA; SNHL, sensorineural hearing loss.
Modified from Rahman S. Gastrointestinal and hepatic manifestations of mitochondrial disorders. *J Inherit Metab Dis.* 2013;36:659–673.

Mitochondrial disorders with a hepatocerebral phenotype often present in infancy with liver dysfunction, hepatomegaly, and liver failure or cirrhosis (Table 18.9).

Other identifiable infectious and metabolic causes of cholestasis

α_1-**Antitrypsin deficiency.** An α_1-antitrypsin protein immunoelectrophoresis can detect an α_1-antitrypsin deficiency, which is the most common inherited cause of neonatal cholestasis. Deficiency occurs in 1 in 1,600–2,000 live births. α_1-Antitrypsin is a protease inhibitor that is synthesized in the liver and inactivates neutrophil proteases. The normal α_1-antitrypsin phenotype, MM, is found in 80–90% of the population. There are numerous allelic variants. Liver disease is associated with the ZZ phenotype and sporadically with other variants. The exact mechanism of liver injury is unclear, and there is variability in expression so that clinically significant liver disease develops in only 10–15% of individuals with the ZZ phenotype. There is also great variability in manifestation. Commonly, the disorder manifests in early infancy with prolonged conjugated hyperbilirubinemia, failure to thrive, acholic stools, hepatomegaly, and less commonly ascites. In some patients it manifests later in childhood or even adulthood. Manifestations in older individuals include jaundice, hepatosplenomegaly, ascites, portal hypertension with varices, chronic hepatitis, cryptogenic cirrhosis, or, rarely, hepatocellular carcinoma. The diagnosis is established by serum phenotyping (ZZ). Treatment is supportive. Some individuals do very well with minimal liver dysfunction. Others have progressive liver disease, requiring transplantation. α_1-Antitrypsin deficiency can enhance hepatotoxicity of hepatotoxic drugs. All individuals with α_1-antitrypsin deficiency should be aware of the potential for lung disease when they are older.

TABLE 18.10   Progressive Familial Intrahepatic Cholestasis

	PFIC 1	PFIC 2	PFIC 3
Transmission	Autosomal recessive	Autosomal recessive	Autosomal recessive
Chromosome	18q21-22	2q24	7q21
Gene	ATP8B1/F1C1	ABCB11/BSEP	ABCB4/MDR3
Protein	FIC1	BSEP	MDR3
Location	Hepatocyte, colon, intestine, pancreas; on apical membranes	Hepatocyte canalicular membrane	Hepatocyte canalicular membrane
Function	ATP-dependent aminophospholipid flippase; unknown effects on intracellular signaling	ATP-dependent bile acid transport	ATP-dependent phosphatidylcholine translocation
Phenotype	Progressive cholestasis, diarrhea, steatorrhea, growth failure, severe pruritus	Rapidly progressive cholestatic giant cell hepatitis, growth failure, pruritus	Later-onset cholestasis, portal hypertension, minimal pruritus, intraductal and gallbladder lithiasis
Histology	Initial bland cholestatic; coarse, granular canalicular bile on EM	Neonatal giant cell hepatitis, amorphous canalicular bile on EM	Proliferation of bile ductules, periportal fibrosis, eventually biliary cirrhosis
Biochemical features	Normal serum GGT; high serum, low biliary bile acid concentrations	Normal serum GGT; high serum, low biliary bile acid concentrations	Elevated serum GGT; low to absent biliary PC; absent serum LPX; normal biliary bile acid concentrations
Treatment	Biliary diversion, ileal exclusion, liver transplantation, but post-OLT diarrhea, steatorrhea, fatty liver	Biliary diversion, liver transplantation	UDCA if residual PC secretion; liver transplantation

ATP, adenosine triphosphate; BSEP, bile salt export pump; EM, electron microscopy; GGT, γ-glutamyltransferase; LPX, lipoprotein X; OLT, orthotopic liver transplantation; PC, phosphatidylcholine; PFIC, progressive familial intrahepatic cholestasis; UDCA, ursodeoxycholic acid.
From Suchy FJ, Sokol RJ, Balistreri WF, eds. *Liver Disease in Children*. 3rd ed. New York: Cambridge University Press; 2007.

Cystic fibrosis. As many as one third of infants with cystic fibrosis may have evidence of liver involvement, frequently cholestasis. The incidence is increased among infants with meconium ileus. The diagnosis can be confirmed with a sweat chloride test or by detecting the abnormal gene. Although the cholestasis resolves, the infant with cystic fibrosis can develop problems including focal biliary cirrhosis, multilobular cirrhosis, fatty liver, obstruction of the common duct, cholelithiasis, sclerosing cholangitis, and, rarely, cholangiocarcinoma.

Hypothyroidism and hypopituitarism. Jaundice can be a manifestation of both hypothyroidism and hypopituitarism. Hypopituitarism may manifest with hypoglycemia, microphallus, and signs of hypothyroidism in addition to jaundice. Wandering nystagmus is present when hypopituitarism is associated with septo-optic dysplasia. Treatment of the underlying endocrinopathy leads to resolution of the liver disease.

Progressive familial intrahepatic cholestasis. Progressive familial intrahepatic cholestasis (PFIC) is a group of disorders related to defective transport of bile acids (Table 18.10). PFIC is clinically suggested by the presence of cholestasis in the absence of physical damage to the bile ducts. GGT is normal except in PFIC type 3. The molecular defects for three PFIC types involve molecules expressed on the canalicular membrane of the hepatocyte. All types of PFIC are inherited in an autosomal recessive manner. PFIC results in progressive cholestasis and pruritus, leading to cirrhosis and end-stage liver disease. PFIC type 1 has low or normal serum GGT and high serum concentrations of bile acids. The defect of the *FIC-1* gene, which encodes a P-type adenosine triphosphatase (ATP8B1), is involved in phospholipid translocation in the enterocytes and canalicular membrane of the hepatocyte. In addition to cholestasis, patients have chronic secretory diarrhea. PFIC type 1 can also be associated with sensorineural hearing loss and pancreatitis.

Patients with PFIC type 2 also exhibit cholestasis, normal serum GGT, and high levels of serum bile acids. A PFIC type 2 disorder is caused by defective function of the bile salt export pump (BSEP) protein, encoded by the *ABCB11* gene. Since BSEP is expressed only in hepatocytes, symptoms are limited to cholestatic liver disease.

Patients with PFIC type 3 have high serum GGT and cholesterol levels. They demonstrate symptoms later in life and reach end-stage liver disease at a later age. PFIC type 3 is caused by a defect in the *ABCB4* gene, which encodes a phospholipid transporter (MDR3) in the canalicular membrane and results in low biliary phospholipid levels.

Except in cases necessitating liver transplantation, chronic biliary diversion and ursodeoxycholic acid therapy may reduce pruritus and improve liver function. In **benign recurrent intrahepatic cholestasis (BRIC)**, homozygous or compound heterozygous variants of respective genes (*ATP8B1, ABCB11, ABCB4*) develop a milder form of cholestatic liver disease, which generally does not progress to end-stage liver disease. In patients with BRIC jaundice, pruritus or fat malabsorption symptoms can be triggered by pregnancy, toxins, and medications.

Idiopathic neonatal hepatitis. Idiopathic neonatal hepatitis is a descriptive term rather than a specific disease entity. The diagnosis is made by exclusion of other causes of cholestasis, particularly biliary atresia. The infant with neonatal hepatitis is more likely to be premature or small for gestational age. Acholic stools are uncommon but can occur when the hepatitis is severe. In 5–15% of cases, there is a familial incidence. Hepatobiliary scintigraphy demonstrates delayed uptake, but there is usually excretion into the duodenum unless the hepatitis is severe. In this case, intraoperative cholangiography may be required. Biopsy findings include panlobular disarray indicative of severe hepatocellular disease, inflammatory infiltrate in the portal areas, focal hepatocellular necrosis, multinucleated giant cells, and increased extramedullary hematopoiesis.

Treatment is supportive. The outcome is variable and is better for infants with sporadic (nonfamilial) cases; of such infants, approximately 60% recover, 10% have chronic liver disease, and 30% die without liver transplantation. The percentages for recovery and death are reversed (30% and 60%, respectively) in familial cases.

Treatment of cholestasis. Some interventions are essential for all infants with cholestasis. Malabsorption of fats and fat-soluble vitamins occurs as a result of a decreased concentration of bile salts in the intestinal lumen. Affected infants should be given a formula containing

MCTs, which are more easily digested and absorbed in the absence of bile acids. Even with MCT supplementation, many patients will require caloric intake in excess of 150 kcal/kg/day to maintain growth. Due to organomegaly and ascites, weight alone may overestimate nutritional status. Proper monitoring of growth requires a routine anthropometric evaluation of skinfold and mid-arm circumference. Some affected infants require supplemental tube feedings. Supplemental vitamins A, D, E, and K are given to prevent symptoms of vitamin deficiency visual problems, rickets, neuropathy, and coagulopathy, respectively. Fat-soluble vitamin levels need to be monitored. Pruritus is often severe and is not readily treatable. Several medications have been tried, including ursodeoxycholic acid, antihistamines, cholestyramine, rifampin, and naltrexone. Ursodeoxycholic acid is beneficial in some infants with cholestasis, and helps to improve bile excretion, thus reducing serum bile acid levels. Biliary diversion has been effective in some cases. Ascites can be managed with sodium restriction, albumin infusions, and diuretics.

JAUNDICE IN THE CHILD AND ADOLESCENT

History

Chronic fatigue, though nonspecific, is a common symptom of liver disease and should trigger at least a basic evaluation including amino-transferases even in the absence of overt jaundice. Myalgias, nausea, vomiting, and fever are often seen in patients with viral hepatitis or autoimmune hepatitis. **Acute biliary obstruction** is signaled by right upper quadrant pain, vomiting, fever, and acholic stools in addition to jaundice. Neurologic and psychiatric symptoms may be among the manifestations of Wilson disease. Autoimmune hepatitis may or may not be accompanied by manifestations of other autoimmune disorders.

The child's age at the onset of symptoms may be helpful. Wilson disease commonly manifests in school-aged children and adolescents. Similarly, autoimmune hepatitis is most prevalent in school-aged children and adolescents with female predominance. A thorough history should include past and present use of prescription, over-the-counter (e.g., acetaminophen, herbal supplements), and street drugs. Many medications have been associated with hepatobiliary damage; others, with hemolysis. Intravenous drug use is a risk factor for viral hepatitis and HIV. Adolescents in particular should be asked about alcohol use.

Symptoms of cholestasis such as jaundice, dark urine, steatorrhea, symptoms of fat-soluble vitamin deficiency, failure to thrive, and pruritus should be explored in detail.

Information about exposure to viral hepatitis, either by travel to an endemic area or during an outbreak, should be pursued. There is a high transmission rate in daycare centers.

The patient's medical history should be reviewed because some chronic illnesses are associated with specific hepatobiliary complications. These should include AIDS, cystic fibrosis, heart disease, renal disease, hemolytic disorders, autoimmune disorders, celiac disease, and inflammatory bowel disease.

A family history of inheritable disorders, such as Wilson disease, autosomal recessive polycystic kidney disease, Alagille syndrome, or spherocytosis, is informative. Less specific but still useful clues are a history of autoimmune disorders, jaundice, anemia, cholecystectomy, or splenectomy in other family members.

Physical Examination

Some patients present with previously unidentified chronic liver disease. The clinician should focus on signs of portal hypertension: spider angiomas, palmar erythema, dilated abdominal veins, ascites, and splenomegaly with a small liver. Cutaneous excoriation as evidence of pruritus, xanthomas, and jaundice support cholestasis. Clubbing of

TABLE 18.11   Differential Diagnosis of Unconjugated Hyperbilirubinemia in Childhood and Adolescence

Increased Bilirubin Production

Autoimmune hemolytic anemia
   Idiopathic
   Secondary
      Infection (viral, mycoplasma)
      Diseases with autoantibody production
      Immunodeficiency
      Malignancy

Drug-induced hemolytic anemia

Paroxysmal nocturnal hemoglobinuria

Erythrocyte membrane defects
   Hereditary spherocytosis
   Hereditary elliptocytosis

Erythrocyte enzyme defects
   Glucose-6-phosphate dehydrogenase
   Pyruvate kinase
   Hexokinase
   Other

Hemoglobinopathy
   Sickle cell disease
   Thalassemia

Hemolytic uremic syndrome

Thrombotic thrombocytopenia purpura

Sepsis with disseminated intravascular coagulation

Reabsorption of hematoma

Transfusion reaction

Decreased Uptake, Storage, or Metabolism

Congestive heart failure

Sepsis

Acidosis

Gilbert syndrome

Crigler-Najjar syndrome type II

Prolonged fasting

Drugs

Portacaval shunt

digits may suggest hepatopulmonary syndrome. A large, tender liver is suggestive of acute viral hepatitis or congestive heart failure. A small liver may be found in patients with severe hepatitis or cirrhosis. A tender gallbladder is indicative of choledocholithiasis or cholecystitis. Abnormal neurologic findings, including tremor, fine motor incoordination, clumsy gait, and choleriform movements, suggest Wilson disease. A slit-lamp examination should be included to look for the Kayser-Fleischer rings (a brownish discoloration at the periphery of the cornea) of Wilson disease.

Differential Diagnosis

Unconjugated Hyperbilirubinemia

Most causes of unconjugated hyperbilirubinemia in the child and adolescent are secondary to hemolysis (Table 18.11) (see Chapter 49). A CBC with evaluation of the smear, reticulocyte count, and Coombs test can differentiate hemolytic from nonhemolytic disorders.

Erythrocyte membrane defects (spherocytosis) and enzyme defects (pyruvate kinase deficiency, G6PD) may not be apparent until childhood or adolescence. Acquired autoimmune hemolytic anemia is characterized by pallor, abdominal pain, fever, and dark urine in addition to jaundice. Laboratory studies document anemia and reticulocytosis. The direct Coombs test result can be positive in autoimmune hemolytic anemia. Hemolytic anemia can be associated with infection, immunodeficiency, malignancy, hemolytic uremic syndrome, or autoimmune disorders, such as systemic lupus erythematosus, rheumatoid arthritis, thyroid disorders, and autoimmune hepatitis.

Unconjugated hyperbilirubinemia can be caused by congestive heart failure and infection. In such circumstances extrahepatic symptoms, cardiac failure, or sepsis dominate the picture. If no other explanation is found, Gilbert syndrome or Crigler-Najjar syndrome type II should be considered.

Conjugated Hyperbilirubinemia

In the child with conjugated hyperbilirubinemia, the PT, albumin, glucose, AST, ALT, GGT, and alkaline phosphatase levels should be measured. Albumin and PT reflect hepatocyte synthetic function. Hypoglycemia is another marker of severity of hepatocellular damage. This is important in considering how quickly the evaluation should proceed or how closely the patient should be monitored. Patients with coagulopathy, hyperammonemia, encephalopathy, or hypoglycemia should be admitted to the hospital and observed very closely. PT should be repeated after a dose of parenteral vitamin K to differentiate synthetic liver failure from a vitamin K deficiency. Hypoglycemia should be corrected with frequent meals or intravenous dextrose.

Obstruction. The relative elevation of AST/ALT and alkaline phosphatase levels in the context of the clinical picture determines the likelihood of an obstructive cause. Although obstructions occur less commonly in children than in adults, it is important not to miss correctable causes of obstruction that, if left untreated, can cause hepatocellular damage. These patients usually have markedly elevated alkaline phosphatase and minimally elevated AST and ALT levels. They should be evaluated promptly with ultrasonography and possibly with MRCP, ERCP, or PTC. The possible causes of obstruction are listed in Table 18.12.

Gallstones. Gallstones are particularly common in children with hemolytic disorders, such as sickle cell disease, thalassemia, erythrocyte membrane defects, erythrocyte enzyme defects, and autoimmune hemolytic anemia. The mean age at presentation is 12 years. Gallstones are also associated with anatomic abnormalities of the biliary tract, cystic fibrosis, ileal dysfunction, obesity, parenteral nutrition, sepsis, prematurity, and pregnancy. Stones may be found incidentally on abdominal radiographs or ultrasound studies in asymptomatic individuals. Alternatively, gallstones may manifest with symptoms of biliary colic: nausea, vomiting, right upper quadrant or nonspecific abdominal pain, and jaundice. Ultrasonography is a very sensitive diagnostic test. Treatment for symptomatic patients is cholecystectomy. ERCP can be used to remove common bile duct stones.

Primary sclerosing cholangitis. Primary sclerosing cholangitis (PSC) is characterized by focal dilatation and stenosis of the intrahepatic or extrahepatic bile ducts with surrounding fibrosis resulting from an inflammatory process. It can manifest from early childhood through adulthood. In adults, it is frequently associated with inflammatory bowel disease, especially ulcerative colitis. PSC may precede the onset of inflammatory bowel disease by many years. It can occur in the absence of any underlying condition. The onset may be insidious with fatigue and pruritus being the only symptoms. Steatorrhea, weight loss, and symptoms of fat-soluble deficiency can be present in some

patients. Abdominal pain, fever, and jaundice may signify ascending cholangitis with bacterial infection complicating PSC. Diagnostic evaluation includes ultrasound studies, which may show dilated ducts. MR cholangiography can provide a detailed anatomy of the biliary tree and is more sensitive than an ultrasound. ERCP and PTC do not provide an advantage in diagnosing PSC but are useful, minimally invasive procedures that can be performed if the dominant stricture is identified and biliary obstruction can be improved by dilation and/or stent placement. PTC can progress to cirrhosis with ultimate liver failure. Cholangiocarcinoma complicates PTC in 10–15% of adults. No medical therapy has been shown to improve outcomes in PSC; thus, treatment is supportive, focused on management of cholestasis. Liver transplantation is available as curative intervention once disease progresses to end-stage liver disease.

Multiple **biliary strictures** have also been found in association with Langerhans cell histiocytosis, congenital hepatic fibrosis, and autosomal recessive polycystic kidney disease; following ischemic/hypoxic injury; and in immunodeficiency states.

Overlap syndrome with features of both sclerosing cholangitis and autoimmune hepatitis and autoimmune cholangitis with inflammation focused on small bile ducts has been described as variants of the disease. In those conditions, response to immunosuppressive therapy is better than in PSC but worse than in autoimmune hepatitis.

Infection. Infections are a common cause of jaundice in the child and adolescent. The most important step is to evaluate patients for synthetic liver failure and for signs of chronicity (portal hypertension, growth failure, risk factors for blood-borne or sexually transmitted disorders). Patients with synthetic liver failure should be referred for urgent evaluation by the liver transplant center.

Diagnostic work-up should focus on potentially treatable disorders (CMV, hepatitis B and C) and disorders preventable for contacts (hepatitis A). Screening for common community-acquired disorders such as EBV, adenovirus, or enterovirus is optional. In the absence of an identifiable viral agent, idiopathic acute hepatitis can be diagnosed only after the complete resolution of abnormal bilirubin and aminotransferases is documented. If abnormalities persist, a work-up for chronic liver diseases should be initiated.

Hepatitis A. Hepatitis A virus (HAV) infection is usually anicteric or asymptomatic in children younger than 5 years of age. However, in almost 66% of infected patients between 5 and 17 years of age, a symptomatic illness with jaundice develops. Two to 7 days before the onset of jaundice, there is a flulike illness with symptoms that can include malaise, headache, myalgias, anorexia, vomiting, diarrhea, right upper quadrant pain, and fever. Some children present with cough and coryza. The urine becomes dark, and jaundice and pale or acholic stools develop. Aminotransferase levels are 10–100 times normal. The diagnosis is confirmed by an HAV IgM study. Children generally recover within 2 weeks. Rarely fulminant hepatitis develops from HAV infection. Small percentages of patients develop either a relapsing or protracted cholestatic illness lasting up to 8 months. There is no carrier state or chronic illness.

HAV is an enterovirus of the picornavirus group. Transmission is by the fecal-oral route, which may include contaminated water and food, especially shellfish. The greatest fecal excretion is before the onset of jaundice when the disease has not yet been recognized (Fig. 18.6). Transmission rates are high in daycare centers and institutions with developmentally delayed children. The incubation period is 15–40 days. After exposure, infection can be prevented in 85–90% of cases by giving intramuscular immunoglobulin to contacts within 2 weeks of exposure. Hepatitis A vaccine is available for long-term prophylaxis.

Hepatitis B. Hepatitis B virus (HBV) is a DNA virus that is transmitted through blood products, shared needles, and sexual

TABLE 18.12   Differential Diagnosis of Conjugated Hyperbilirubinemia in Childhood and Adolescence

Autoimmune Hepatitis

Anatomic/Obstructive

Gallstones

Primary sclerosing cholangitis

Choledochal cyst

Bile duct stenosis

Anomalies of the choledocho-pancreatico-duodenal junction

Pancreatitis

Caroli disease

Congenital hepatic fibrosis

Tumor

    Hepatic

    Biliary

    Pancreatic

    Duodenal

Infection

Non-A–Non-E hepatitis

Hepatitis A

Hepatitis B

Hepatitis C

Hepatitis D

Hepatitis E

Epstein-Barr virus

Cytomegalovirus

Human herpesvirus 6

Coronavirus (COVID-19)

Herpes simplex virus

Varicella-zoster virus

Enteroviruses

Measles

Parvovirus

Human immunodeficiency virus

Leptospirosis

Sepsis/shock

Liver abscess

Metabolic Disorders

Wilson disease

Cystic fibrosis

Cholesterol ester storage disease

Alpers syndrome

α_1-Antitrypsin deficiency

Navajo neurohepatopathy

Fatty acid oxidation disorders

Drug or Toxin

Drugs*

Chlorpromazine

Hormones (estrogens, androgens)

Antibiotics (amoxicillin-clavulanate, dicloxacillin, erythromycin, sulfonamides, tetracycline)

Anticonvulsants (carbamazepine, phenytoin, valproate)

Acetaminophen

Alcohol

Halothane

Isoniazid

Antineoplastics

Toxins

Amanita phalloides (mushroom)

Insecticides

Carbon tetrachloride

Phosphorus

Herbal teas

Total Parenteral Nutrition

Intrahepatic Cholestasis

Benign recurrent intrahepatic cholestasis

Progressive familial intrahepatic cholestasis type 3

Miscellaneous

Dubin-Johnson syndrome

Rotor syndrome

Budd-Chiari syndrome

Hepatic venoocclusive disease

Systemic lupus erythematosus

Indian childhood cirrhosis (ICC) and ICC-like disorders

Cardiovascular

Ischemia

Congestive heart failure

Cardiomyopathy

Oncologic

Leukemia

Langerhans cell histiocytosis

Lymphoma

Graft versus host disease

Sickle cell disease with intrahepatic sickling

Hemophagocytic lymphohistiocytosis

Heat stroke

*Many other drugs have been implicated in the etiology of conjugated hyperbilirubinemia; these are the most commonly cited.

contact; vertically during childbirth; and from occupational exposure. Infection in the newborn can be prevented by administration of hepatitis B immunoglobulin within 12 hours of birth and a series of three hepatitis B vaccinations. HBV infection is diagnosed mostly in children from countries with high prevalence of hepatitis B and no effective immunization or perinatal screening program. In developed countries, hepatitis B should be suspected in children born from mothers with pre-existing hepatitis B or mothers with no prenatal care. Hepatitis B risk factors in adolescents include intravenous drug use and unprotected sex. The majority of children with hepatitis B are asymptomatic; few develop symptoms of acute or chronic hepatitis. Extrahepatic symptoms of arthritis, polyarteritis, urticaria, and nephritis from circulating immune complexes can be present. HBsAg is the first antigenic marker to appear; it disappears after 1–3 months

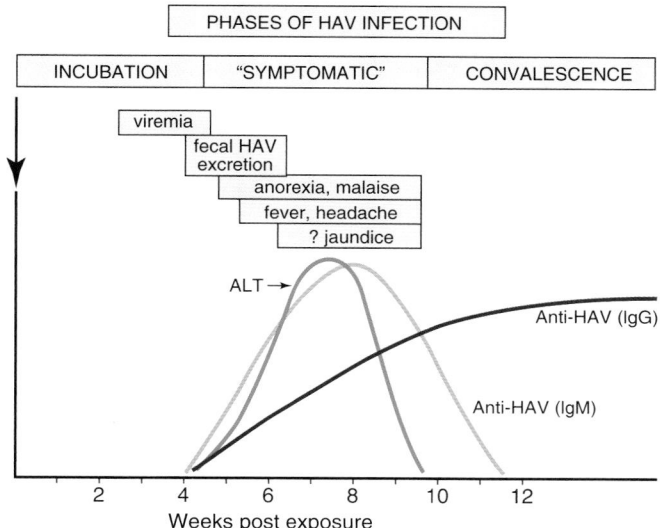

Fig. 18.6 Typical course of hepatitis A virus (HAV) infection. ALT, alanine aminotransferase; IgG, immunoglobulin G; IgM, immunoglobulin M. (From Balistreri WF. Viral hepatitis. *Pediatr Clin North Am.* 1988;35:640.)

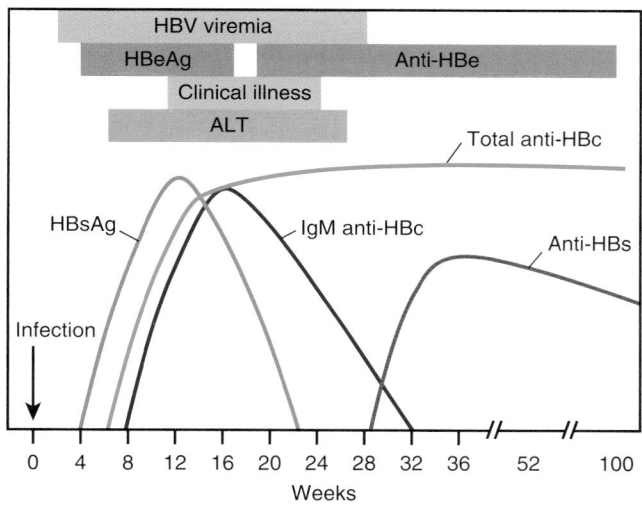

Fig. 18.7 Clinical, virologic, and serologic course of acute hepatitis B virus (HBV) infection. ALT, alanine aminotransferase; HBc, hepatitis B core; HBe, hepatitis B envelope; HBeAg, hepatitis B e antigen; HBs, hepatitis B surface; HBsAg, hepatitis B surface antigen; IgM, immunoglobulin M. (From Bennett JE, Dolin R, Blaser MJ, eds. *Mandell, Douglas, and Bennett's Principles and Practices of Infectious Diseases.* 9th ed. Philadelphia: Elsevier; 2020:1552, Fig. 117.2.)

if HBV resolves (Fig. 18.7). Hepatitis B surface antibody (anti-HBs) is a protective antibody that develops after immunization or resolution of infection. In patients whose infections resolve, there is a window of 2–6 weeks between the disappearance of HBsAg and the appearance of anti-HBs. During this window, anti-HBc or HBV DNA may be the only evidence of infection with HBV. HBeAg correlates with viral replication. HBV DNA is a measure of viral replication. Screening for infection is made with HBsAg and anti-HBc. Although acute HBV infection is rarely a severe illness, fulminant hepatic failure develops in up to 1% of patients. Chronic infection, defined as the persistence of HBsAg for at least 6 months, occurs in 90% of infected neonates, 25–50% of infected children younger than 5 years, and 5–10% of

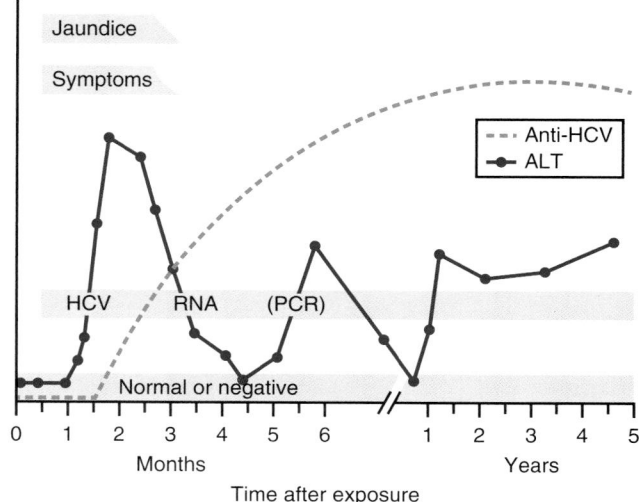

Fig. 18.8 Typical clinical, virologic, and serologic course of chronic hepatitis C virus (HCV). ALT, alanine aminotransferase; PCR, polymerase chain reaction; RNA, ribonucleic acid. (From Hoofnagle JH. Chronic hepatitis. In: Goldman L, Ausiello D, eds. *Cecil Medicine.* 23rd ed. Philadelphia: Saunders; 2008.)

infected adults. Children with chronic active hepatitis B can be treated with antiviral agents.

Hepatitis C. Acute hepatitis C virus (HCV) infection is often mild and usually subclinical. Jaundice is unusual. Chronic infection develops in 40–60% of affected children, in contrast with up to 80% of infected adults, and can progress to cirrhosis (Fig. 18.8). Screening for hepatitis uses anti-HCV antibodies, and infection is confirmed via PCR for HCV RNA. Transmission may be parenteral due to intravenous drug use or exposure to blood, or sexual or vertical transmission is also possible. Elimination of hepatitis C is possible with directly acting antiviral agents. The treatment regimen is selected based on hepatitis C genotype. Highly effective antiviral therapies are available and can lead to complete eradication of hepatitis C virus in the majority of patients with hepatitis C.

Hepatitis D. Hepatitis D virus (HDV) infection can occur only in the presence of HBV as either a co-infection or a superinfection. Its route of transmission is parenteral. As with HBV, it can become chronic. The diagnosis is confirmed by the presence of HDV antibody.

Hepatitis E. Hepatitis E virus (HEV) infection is similar to HAV in its manifestation and mode of transmission. It is a self-limited illness with no chronic state. However, fulminant hepatitis may occur in up to 20% of cases. Serologic diagnosis can be made by finding antibodies to HEV.

Epstein-Barr virus. Epstein-Barr virus infection can mimic HAV, HBV, or HCV infection. Often there is an exudative pharyngitis and lymphadenopathy. Fatal hepatic necrosis can occur. This is rare, but it is of particular concern in the immunocompromised host. The diagnosis is confirmed by elevation of Epstein-Barr virus PCR.

Cytomegalovirus hepatitis can be symptomatic particularly in infants. Hepatitis is usually self-limited. Ganciclovir can be used as treatment in severe cases.

Other viruses. Other viruses including herpes simplex, human herpesvirus 6, parvovirus B19, coronavirus COVID-19, and norovirus can also cause hepatitis, particularly in the immunosuppressed patient.

Wilson disease. Wilson disease is an autosomal recessive disorder of copper metabolism. As a result of ATP7B variant, copper cannot be excreted and it accumulates in the liver, which causes hepatic steatosis and necrosis. Copper is then released into the circulation

TABLE 18.13 Classification of Autoimmune Hepatitis

Variable	Type 1 Autoimmune Hepatitis	Type 2 Autoimmune Hepatitis
Characteristic autoantibodies	Antinuclear antibody* Smooth-muscle antibody* Antiactin antibody[†] Autoantibodies against soluble liver antigen and liver-pancreas antigen[‡] Atypical perinuclear antineutrophil cytoplasmic antibody	Antibody against liver-kidney microsome type 1* Antibody against liver cytosol type 1* Antibody against liver-kidney microsomal type 3
Geographic variation	Worldwide	Worldwide; rare in North America
Age at presentation	Any age	Predominantly childhood and young adulthood
Gender of patients	Female in ~75% of cases	Female in ~95% of cases
Association with other autoimmune diseases	Common	Common[§]
Clinical severity	Broad range, variable	Generally severe
Histopathologic features at presentation	Broad range, mild disease to cirrhosis	Generally advanced
Treatment failure	Infrequent	Frequent
Relapse after drug withdrawal	Variable	Common
Need for long-term maintenance	Variable	~100%

*The conventional method of detection is immunofluorescence.
[†]Tests for this antibody are rarely available in commercial laboratories.
[‡]This antibody is detected by an enzyme-linked immunosorbent assay.
[§]Autoimmune polyendocrinopathy–candidiasis–ectodermal dystrophy is seen only in patients with type 2 disease.
From Krawitt EL. Autoimmune hepatitis. *N Engl J Med.* 2006;354:54–66.

and is ultimately deposited in the central nervous system, kidneys, and cornea. The hepatic manifestation predominates in childhood; a neuropsychiatric manifestation becomes more common later, in adolescence and adulthood. The liver involvement may manifest as acute hepatitis, fulminant hepatic failure, chronic hepatitis, cirrhosis, or asymptomatic elevation of serum aminotransferases. Neurologic symptoms such as dysarthria, clumsiness, tremor, and mood disorders may or may not be present. In the kidney, the result is tubular dysfunction; in the cornea, the result is Kayser-Fleischer rings. Hemolysis can be present as a result of copper toxicity. The diagnosis is supported by documenting a low serum ceruloplasmin level, high urinary copper excretion, and increased hepatic copper concentrations on liver biopsy. D-Penicillamine or trientine to chelate copper can successfully treat Wilson disease. Dietary restriction of copper can aid treatment. Wilson disease requires lifelong therapy. Wilson disease is a potentially lethal treatable disorder that should be promptly diagnosed. Patients presenting with synthetic liver failure should be promptly referred for liver transplant evaluation.

Drugs and toxins. Numerous drugs and toxins are associated with hepatic injury (see Table 18.12) and should be considered in the evaluation of jaundice. The reaction can be idiosyncratic or dose related. In the latter case, this may be associated with either accidental or purposeful overdose. The manifestation can be that of acute hepatitis, fulminant hepatic failure, or cholestatic disease, depending on the drug.

Autoimmune hepatitis. Autoimmune hepatitis (AIH) is a common cause of chronic liver injury (Table 18.13). The most frequent course is insidious with fatigue as a dominant symptom. Autoimmune hepatitis can present acutely with malaise, anorexia, nausea, vomiting, and jaundice. Autoimmune disorders such as arthritis, thyroiditis, vasculitis, nephritis, hemolytic anemia, or diabetes mellitus are often associated with AIH. AIH may be associated with inflammatory bowel disease. Laboratory studies demonstrate elevated aminotransferase levels, mild hyperbilirubinemia, and hypergammaglobulinemia. Antinuclear antibody, actin, or anti–smooth muscle antibody is present in type 1 AIH, whereas anti–liver-kidney microsomal antibody is found in type 2 AIH (see Table 18.13).

Liver biopsy is required for diagnosis. Characteristic findings are plasma cells and an inflammatory infiltrate expanding the portal area and moderate to severe piecemeal necrosis. Treatment consists of steroids and azathioprine.

■ SUMMARY AND RED FLAGS

When evaluating a patient with jaundice, it is important to determine whether the condition represents a hepatobiliary problem, a hematologic disorder, or a systemic illness. If there is conjugated hyperbilirubinemia, it is essential to evaluate for severe dysfunction, as manifest by prolonged PT, hyperammonemia, encephalopathy, and/or hypoglycemia. Coagulopathy, encephalopathy, or hypoglycemia can signify severe hepatic failure, which mandates early intervention.

BIBLIOGRAPHY

A bibliography is available at ExpertConsult.com.

19

Constipation

Joshua Noe

Constipation is defined symptomatically as the *infrequent* passage of *hard* stools, straining while passing a stool, or pain associated with the passage of a hard stool. The range of normal defecation patterns in children is widely variable, though in general, formula-fed infants may have four to five stools per day in the first weeks of life, while breast-fed infants usually pass softer and more frequent stools. Stool frequency in both gradually decreases to one to two per day by 1 year of age. Most children aged 1–4 years have one or two daily bowel movements, with a range of three daily bowel movements to one bowel movement every other day.

Constipation is classified broadly either as functional or as secondary to underlying conditions, such as anatomic abnormalities, metabolic disorders, neurologic dysfunction, or medication effects (Table 19.1). Most childhood constipation is functional. The Rome IV Criteria for Functional Gastrointestinal Disorders defines **functional constipation** in two age groups as noted in Tables 19.2 and 19.3.

Changes in diet, such as formula changes or the addition of solid foods, may lead to transient constipation in infants, with up to 40% of constipation starting during this time period. Minor illnesses, including infectious diarrhea, can subsequently result in episodic constipation as well. More long-standing constipation is often secondary to inadequate intake of dietary fiber, fluid, or both. The evaluation of constipation involves first determining whether the change in the frequency or consistency of stools is secondary to functional constipation or is related to an underlying organic disorder. This determination is based on identifying historical features and examination findings that suggest an underlying disorder and prompt further investigation.

PHYSIOLOGY OF NORMAL DEFECATION AND CONSTIPATION

Fecal continence and physiologic defecation are dependent on the **anal inhibitory reflex**, which is in turn dependent on the proper structure and function of the internal and external anal sphincters and the pelvic floor. The **internal anal sphincter** is an involuntary muscle that is contracted at rest. When a bolus of stool distends the rectum, the internal anal sphincter relaxes. This process generally results in the child sensing the need to defecate. The **external anal sphincter** and the **puborectalis muscle** of the pelvic floor, under voluntary control, contract upon rectal distention, respectively closing the anus and decreasing the rectoanal angle, thus allowing the child to hold stool until it is socially convenient to defecate. Voluntary relaxation of the puborectalis muscle and the external anal sphincter straightens the anorectal angle and allows the child to stool. In situations where there is **encopresis** secondary to **overflow incontinence**, the child typically consciously withholds stool by refusing to relax the external anal sphincter in the setting of a relaxed internal anal sphincter. Over time, the child is not able to keep the external anal sphincter fully contracted and stool leaks out of the anal canal. The presence of overflow incontinence is an important indicator that the anal inhibitory reflex is likely intact, as patients with anatomic or neurologic abnormalities of the distal colon and internal anal sphincter, including Hirschsprung disease, are unable to reflexively relax the internal anal sphincter to allow for the passage of stool.

Patients with chronic constipation have abnormal anorectal manometry. The most consistent abnormality is blunted rectal sensation, rendering the patient unable to sense stool in the rectum. Other findings include incomplete relaxation of the internal anal sphincter and paradoxical contraction of the external sphincter during attempted defecation. Patients who have paradoxical anal contraction, also known as functional dyssynergia, are less likely to respond to routine medical therapy or may be more likely to have recurrent constipation if treatment is withdrawn unless the paradoxical contraction is addressed.

DATA COLLECTION AND ASSESSMENT

History

Functional constipation may be distinguished from secondary causes of constipation by assessing the age of symptom onset, the stool consistency, and the presence of associated signs or symptoms.

The age at symptom onset differentiates disease processes that are congenital versus those that are acquired. Failure to pass meconium in the first 48 hours of life suggests a diagnosis of **Hirschsprung disease**, though up to 50% of patients with Hirschsprung disease will pass meconium prior to this. Constipation in the first month of life or a history of constipation since infancy suggests organic causes, including and in addition to Hirschsprung disease (Table 19.4). The onset of symptoms beyond infancy suggests acquired organic constipation or functional constipation.

Stool consistency in constipation can differ by etiology. Functional constipation tends to produce painful, large, bulky stools, whereas constipation secondary to Hirschsprung disease or other organic etiologies tends to produce harder, pebble-like, or ribbon-like stools. Stool consistency may be objectively rated via use of the **Bristol stool scale** (Fig. 19.1) and can be used to follow response to therapy.

The assessment of associated signs and symptoms should include evaluating for a history of blood in the stool, as well as for the presence of urinary symptoms. Bright red blood on the surface of the stool suggests an anal fissure indicative of straining, which is seen in approximately 25% of patients with constipation. Blood mixed in the stool suggests a more remote source, and thus less likely an anal fissure. **Urinary symptoms** may take the form of either retention or incontinence. Retention may be secondary to congenital or acquired abnormalities in the neurologic regulation of bladder voiding and may be associated with similar abnormalities in the regulation of defecation. **Megacystic megaureter intestinal hypoperistalsis syndrome** is often detected in utero or after birth with massive bladder distention and failure to pass

TABLE 19.1 Causes of Constipation in Infants and Children

Functional
Faulty diet (poor fiber intake, excessive cow's milk, inadequate nutrition)
Inadequate fluid intake
Situational
Depression
Familial-constitutional

Anatomic
Anterior anal displacement
Ectopic anus
Anal stenosis
Malrotation
Colonic anomalies (rectocele, duplications)
Stricture (postsurgical, sequelae of inflammatory disorders including necrotizing enterocolitis)
Painful anorectal lesions (fissures, dermatitis, abscess)
Abnormal abdominal musculature (prune belly, gastroschisis)
Intestinal neoplasm, extraintestinal pelvic mass (teratoma)

Endocrine
Hypothyroidism
Panhypopituitarism
Hypoparathyroidism
Diabetes mellitus
Diabetes insipidus (via dehydration)

Genetic/Metabolic
Hypercalcemia
Metal intoxication (lead, arsenic, mercury)
Dehydration
Cystic fibrosis: DIOS
Hypokalemia
Acute intermittent porphyria
Blue diaper syndrome
Hereditary coproporphyria
Rubinstein-Taybi syndrome
Williams syndrome (hypercalcemia)

Infectious
Typhoid
Infant botulism
Chagas disease

Intrinsic Intestinal Neuronal or Myopathic Disorders
Hirschsprung disease
Intestinal neuronal dysplasia
Hypoganglionosis
Intestinal ganglioneuromatosis
Pediatric intestinal pseudoobstruction (neuropathic or myopathic; primary or secondary)
Megacystis megaureter intestinal hypoperistalsis syndrome
Intestinal sphincter achalasia

Neurologic/Spinal Cord Lesions
Spina bifida and spina bifida occulta
Tethered cord
Spinal cord tumors
Traumatic lesions
Myotonic dystrophy
Cerebral palsy
Muscular dystrophy

Psychologic
Anorexia nervosa
Depression

Medications/Toxins
Anticonvulsants
Antacids (aluminum and calcium)
Iron
Lead
Barium
Opioids (codeine, diphenoxylate–atropine sulfate [Lomotil], loperamide [Imodium])
Antidepressants
Anticholinergics
Phenothiazines
Phenytoin
Methylphenidate
Pancreatic enzymes (fibrosing colonopathy)
Vitamin D intoxication
Vincristine
Calcium channel blockers
Bismuth
Clonidine
Antihistamines
Diuretics

Other
Milk protein–induced anal inflammation and fissure formation
Celiac disease
Collagen vascular disease (SLE, mixed connective tissue disease, scleroderma, dermatomyositis)
Amyloidosis

DIOS, distal intestinal obstruction syndrome; SLE, systemic lupus erythematosus.

TABLE 19.2 Functional Constipation: Infant/Toddler

Diagnostic criteria Must include 1 mo of **at least two** of the following in infants up to 4 yr of age:
1. Two or fewer defecations per week
2. History of excessive stool retention
3. History of painful or hard bowel movements
4. Presence of a large fecal mass in the rectum
5. History of large-diameter stools
In toilet-trained children, the following additional criteria may be used:
6. At least one episode/wk of incontinence after the acquisition of toileting skills
7. History of large-diameter stools that may obstruct the toilet

TABLE 19.3 Functional Constipation: Child/Adolescent

Diagnostic criteria Must include **two or more** of the following at least once a week for a minimum of 1 mo with insufficient criteria for diagnosis of IBS:
1. Two or fewer defecations in the toilet per week in a child with a developmental age of at least 4 yr
2. At least one episode of fecal incontinence per week
3. History of retentive posturing or excessive volitional stool retention
4. History of painful or hard bowel movements
5. Presence of a large fecal mass in the rectum
6. History of large-diameter stools that can obstruct the toilet
After appropriate evaluation, the symptoms cannot be fully explained by another medical condition.

IBS, irritable bowel syndrome.

TABLE 19.4 Causes of Constipation During the Neonatal Period

Meconium plug (rule out cystic fibrosis)
Meconium ileus (rule out cystic fibrosis)
Hirschsprung disease
Pediatric intestinal pseudoobstruction
Anteriorly displaced anus
Ectopic anus
Anal stenosis
Imperforate anus
Spina bifida
Hypothyroidism
Hypercalcemia
Neuronal intestinal dysplasia types A and B
Megacystis megaureter intestinal hypoperistalsis syndrome
Medications (opioids, paralytic agents, magnesium)

meconium. In some patients, it is an autosomal dominant disorder due to variants in the *ACTG2* gene. Patients with primary chronic intestinal pseudoobstruction may also have bladder distention.

Alternately, retention may be secondary to urinary tract outflow obstruction caused by a large stool burden. Incontinence may be due to a large stool mass distending the rectum and placing pressure on the posterior bladder wall or may indicate overflow incontinence in the setting of a neurogenic bladder.

Abdominal pain is common in constipated patients; when present, it is often mild, nonspecific, and periumbilical. Older children may describe discomfort in the lower abdomen and a history of pain relief after passing stool. Appetite is often diminished. A diary recorded over a period of several days to weeks noting the passage of stools, the timing of meals, and the onset of abdominal pain can aid in the diagnosis of constipation and in monitoring therapy. The personal medical history and the family history may reveal illnesses and conditions associated with constipation (Table 19.5; see Table 19.1).

The child's behavior during defecation should be noted. A history of straining, as an index of difficulty in defecation, can be misinterpreted by parents, who often view a child's efforts to withhold stool as efforts to pass a bowel movement. Parents often describe a toddler who hides in a corner, with stiffened straight legs, or who may lean into the wall or hold onto a table while "straining." More often, these actions represent attempts at withholding stool. The young child, having become constipated, passes a painful stool, which, if large, may be associated with an anal fissure. If a fissure is present, a small amount of blood is usually passed with the stool and may create additional worry if noticed by the child. The child associates the passage of stools with pain and tries to prevent further painful episodes by withholding fecal matter. This behavior results in the formation of even larger, harder stools, which are painful to pass, thus establishing a link between pain and defecation that perpetuates the cycle. Children with stool retention may go 3–5 days without defecating. Enuresis and encopresis may occur in this setting. Fecal incontinence is one of the most common presentations of functional constipation and can be misinterpreted by the parent as diarrhea by virtue of constant smearing of stool in the gluteal cleft.

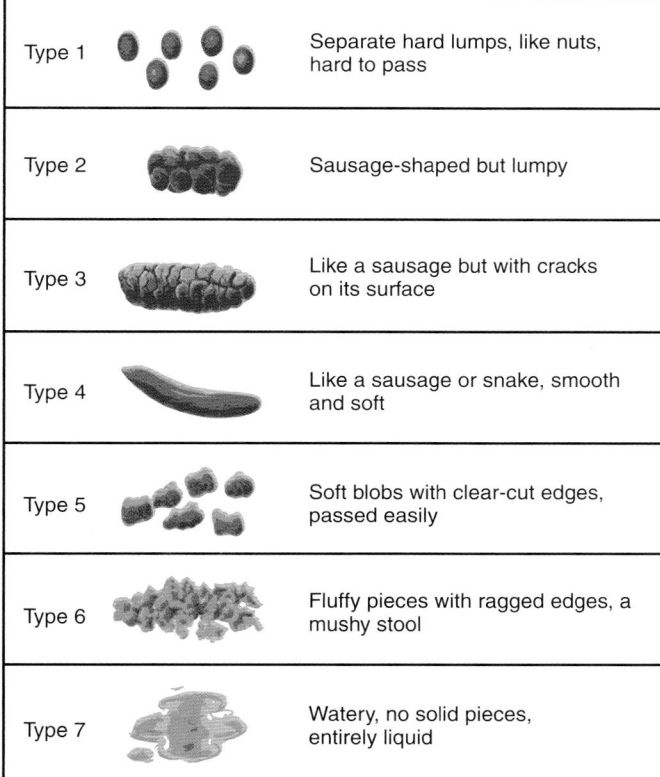

Type 1	Separate hard lumps, like nuts, hard to pass
Type 2	Sausage-shaped but lumpy
Type 3	Like a sausage but with cracks on its surface
Type 4	Like a sausage or snake, smooth and soft
Type 5	Soft blobs with clear-cut edges, passed easily
Type 6	Fluffy pieces with ragged edges, a mushy stool
Type 7	Watery, no solid pieces, entirely liquid

Fig. 19.1 The Bristol stool chart allows for qualitative comparisons of stool consistency in the setting of both constipation and diarrhea.

Physical Examination

Abnormal growth patterns should alert the physician to the possibility of underlying organic disease, such as hypothyroidism or celiac disease (see Table 19.5). Abdominal examination is usually benign; there may be some mild tenderness in the left lower quadrant on palpation of a segment of bowel that is full of stool. Stool may be palpable through the abdominal wall in the sigmoid and descending colon. On occasion, a large, firm fecal mass extends from the symphysis pubis to the umbilicus, which may mimic findings of an abdominal malignancy.

The spine and sacral area should be examined closely. A tuft of hair, a dimple, or a palpable defect or mass in this area should prompt consideration of **spina bifida occulta** or a **tethered spinal cord**. Sensory and motor function should be assessed. A normal **anal wink**, as elicited by gentle stroking of the perianal skin with a sharp object, such as a wooden tongue blade or the corner of a small package of lubricant, gives evidence of intact lumbosacral innervation. A normal **cremasteric reflex** in males also gives evidence of intact lumbosacral innervation. The cremaster muscle, innervated by the genitofemoral nerve of the lumbar plexus, typically contracts when the observer brushes a finger along the upper surface of the inner thigh, resulting in withdrawal superiorly of the ipsilateral testis.

TABLE 19.5 Historical and Physical Findings Suggestive of Organic Etiologies of Constipation	
Symptoms or History	**Physical Findings**
Acute Signs	Severe abdominal distension
Delayed passage of meconium (after 48 hr of life)	Pelvic mass (e.g., sacral teratoma)
Fever, vomiting, or diarrhea	Lumbosacral dimple, hair tuft or lipoma, or deviation of the gluteal cleft
Rectal bleeding (unless attributable to an anal fissure)	Anal scars
Severe abdominal distension	Anteriorly displaced anus
Bilious emesis	Patulous anus (i.e., low resting sphincter tone)
Chronic Signs	Perianal fistula
Constipation present from birth or early infancy	High anal canal tone with empty rectum
Ribbon stools (very narrow in diameter)	Explosive expulsion of stool after digital examination of the rectum
Urinary incontinence or bladder disease	Absent anal wink
Weight loss or poor weight gain	Absent cremasteric reflex
Delayed growth (e.g., decreasing height percentiles)	Decreased lower extremity tone or strength
Extraintestinal symptoms (especially neurologic deficits)	Abnormal lower extremity deep tendon reflex: absence of delay in relaxation
Congenital anomalies or syndrome associated with Hirschsprung disease (e.g.,	phase
Down syndrome, congenital central hypoventilation syndrome, neuroblastoma)	Abnormal thyroid gland
Family history of Hirschsprung disease	Extreme fear during the anal inspection

Modified from Tabbers MM, DiLorenzo C, Berger MY, et al. Evaluation and treatment of functional constipation in infants and children: evidence-based recommendations from ESPGHAN and NASPGHAN. *J Pediatr Gastroenterol Nutr.* 2014;58(2):258.

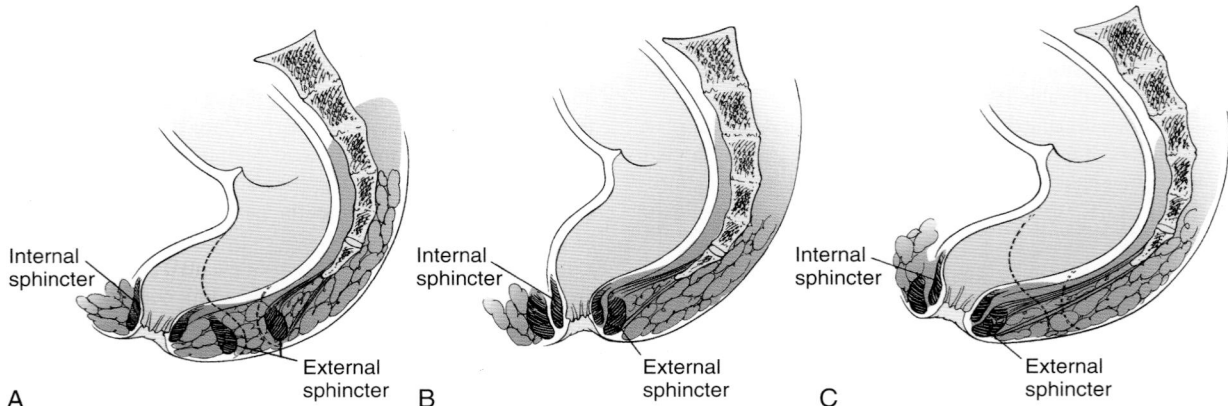

Fig. 19.2 *A,* Anterior ectopic anus. *B,* Normal anal anatomy. *C,* Anterior anal displacement.

The perianal area should be examined for evidence of fissures suggestive of the passage of large, hard stools. The examination is facilitated if an assistant gently spreads the patient's buttocks apart while the examiner illuminates the area. Soiling in the undergarments may indicate fecal impaction with overflow incontinence. The location of the anus in relation to the other perineal structures should be determined to assess for anatomic or structural anomalies, such as **anterior displacement of the anus** (Fig. 19.2). The anus is typically situated in the center of the slightly hyperpigmented skin surrounding the anal sphincter. An anteriorly displaced anus is indicated by an abnormal **anal position index (API)**, which is defined as the ratio of the distance between the anus and the posterior aspect of the genitals (the fourchette in females and scrotum in males) to the distance between the coccyx and the posterior genitals (Fig. 19.3). Measurements may be obtained using calipers or by placing clear plastic tape adjacent to the landmarks and marking with a pen, and then subsequently measuring the distance on the tape. The normal API for females is 0.45 ± 0.15, and for males it is 0.54 ± 0.14.

Digital examination is indicated in the evaluation of infantile constipation, if the cause or degree of constipation is unclear, or if there are signs of organic disease. The examiner should note the patency and tone of the anus. High tone and an empty rectal vault may suggest Hirschsprung disease. If the aganglionic segment is short enough, withdrawal of the finger might result in an explosive release of stool as the finger acts as a dilator to reach the dilated, ganglion-containing segment. Conversely, a dilated rectal vault with a large stool impaction is more suggestive of functional constipation with withholding behavior. In a cooperative patient, the examiner can ask the patient to bear down against their finger as if attempting to push out stool, which should result in relaxation of the anal canal. Patients who have paradoxical contraction of their anal canal upon this request may have **functional dyssynergia**, a condition in which the patient's pelvic floor fails to relax upon attempted defecation.

Diagnostic Evaluation

Routine laboratory evaluation is usually not helpful in the evaluation of constipation, though is indicated if an organic etiology is suspected on the basis of the history or physical examination. Endocrinologic disturbances, such as hypothyroidism, can be associated with constipation. If **celiac disease** (see Chapter 14) is a consideration, serum anti–tissue transglutaminase immunoglobulin A (IgA) antibody levels should be assessed. A total IgA level should be performed concomitantly to exclude IgA deficiency confounding interpretation. If the patient does have IgA deficiency, anti–tissue transglutaminase IgG levels or esophagogastroduodenoscopy with duodenal biopsies can be performed.

Plain films of the abdomen are rarely necessary, although if obtained may demonstrate stool in the large bowel. While this information is occasionally useful in the case of a child with complaints of diarrhea whose symptoms are due to fecal impaction and overflow of liquid stools, a digital rectal exam similarly can supply the information needed. In addition, there is poor correlation between stool burden on abdominal radiography and symptoms of constipation. However, abdominal radiography may be a useful initial study in the evaluation of suspected obstruction or pseudoobstruction, identifying possible transition zones and/or air-fluid levels. Suspected Hirschsprung disease is evaluated radiographically via a liquid contrast enema in children over 1 month of age in whom a transition zone is expected to have developed; in neonates, rectal suction biopsy is the test of choice (Fig. 19.4). A contrast study in neonates may be useful to detect a meconium plug, microcolon, meconium ileus, or congenital anomalies (ileal atresia, colonic duplication).

Neurologic symptoms, lower extremity or midline defects of the lower back or gluteal cleft, or examination findings suggestive of occult spinal dysraphism or tethered cord should be investigated with MRI of the spine and/or brain. MRI can be used if a disorder involving the lumbosacral spine is abnormal. Children with lower extremity and midline defects involving the lower back or gluteal cleft should have this imaging considered. Concerns for intestinal dysmotility may be evaluated with a **colonic transit study**, in which the patient swallows either a capsule of radiopaque circular markers once on day 1 or different-shaped markers on 3 consecutive days and undergoes serial abdominal radiographs to determine the distribution of the markers. After 3 days and by some protocols again after 7 days, any markers that have not yet been evacuated in the stool should be located in the rectum. The presence of markers more proximally in the gastrointestinal tract suggests enteric nervous system or neuromuscular pathology (e.g., pediatric intestinal pseudoobstruction).

A rectal motility evaluation may be helpful in the diagnosis and management of chronic constipation. **Anorectal manometry** can be used to evaluate the integrity of the muscles and the innervation of the defecatory mechanism. Determining the sensory threshold provides valuable diagnostic information: patients who cannot detect a balloon filled with 120 mL of air usually have encopresis. Hirschsprung disease is unlikely if reflexive relaxation of the internal anal sphincter occurs in the presence of rectal distention. Manometry and **electromyography** document the paradoxical contraction of the external anal sphincter on attempted defecation seen in functional dyssynergia. Anorectal manometry can also be used as a therapeutic modality in biofeedback therapy in patients with constipation and encopresis and in patients with paradoxical external anal sphincter contraction. **Total colonic**

Fourchette-
coccygeal
distance
Fourchette-
anal distance
Scroto-
coccygeal
distance
Scroto-
anal distance

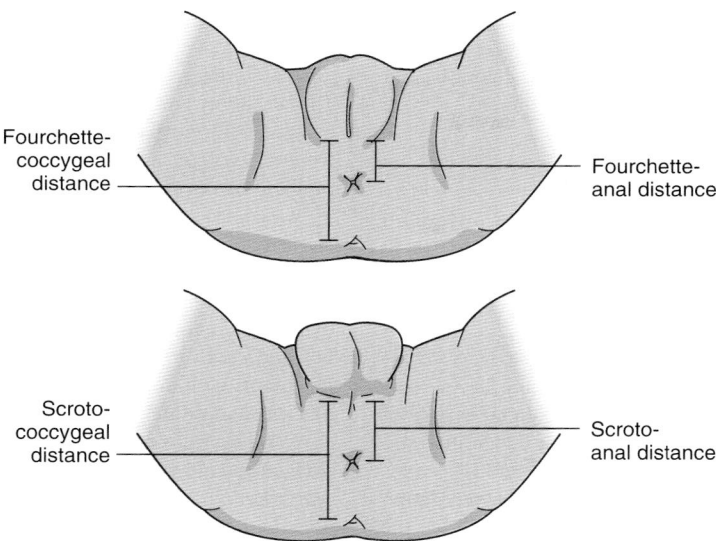

Fig. 19.3 Measuring the anal position index (API) in females and males. The API is defined as the ratio of the distance between the anus and the posterior aspect of the genitals (the fourchette in females and scrotum in males) to the distance between the coccyx and the posterior genitals. (From Alemrajabi M, Moradi M, Jahangiri F, et al. Anal position index; can it predict pelvic organ disorders in adults? *J Coloproctol.* 2019;39[3]:237–241.)

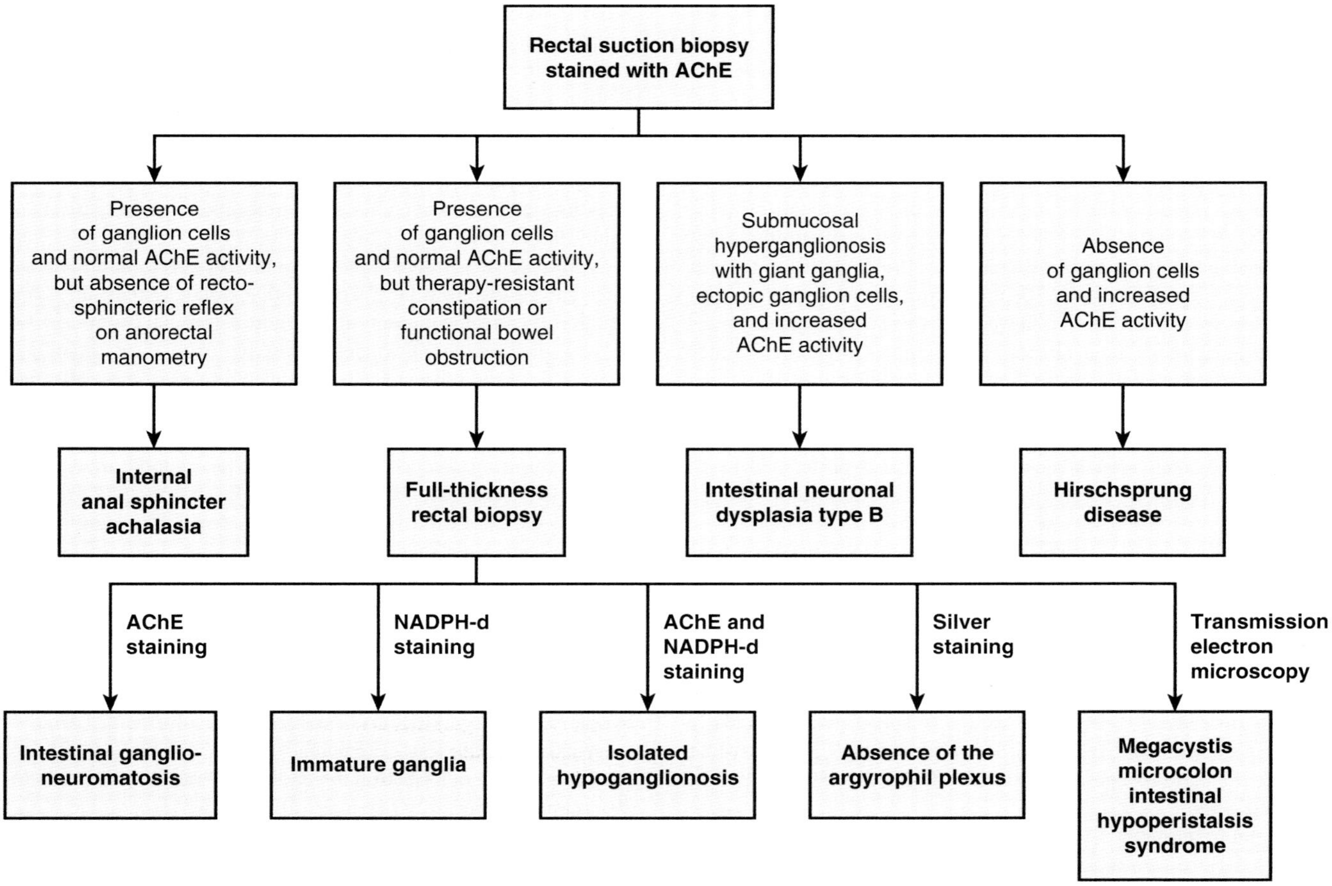

Rectal suction biopsy stained with AChE
Presence of ganglion cells and normal AChE activity, but absence of recto-sphincteric reflex on anorectal manometry
Presence of ganglion cells and normal AChE activity, but therapy-resistant constipation or functional bowel obstruction
Submucosal hyperganglionosis with giant ganglia, ectopic ganglion cells, and increased AChE activity
Absence of ganglion cells and increased AChE activity
Internal anal sphincter achalasia
Full-thickness rectal biopsy
Intestinal neuronal dysplasia type B
Hirschsprung disease
AChE staining
NADPH-d staining
AChE and NADPH-d staining
Silver staining
Transmission electron microscopy
Intestinal ganglio-neuromatosis
Immature ganglia
Isolated hypoganglionosis
Absence of the argyrophil plexus
Megacystis microcolon intestinal hypoperistalsis syndrome

Fig. 19.4 Diagnostic algorithm for investigating chronic constipation and functional bowel obstruction in newborn infants and young children. AChE, acetylcholinesterase; NADPH-d, nicotinamide adenine dinucleotide phosphate diaphorase.

motility is performed by placing a catheter in the colon to monitor pressures from the rectum to the cecum. Motility tracings reveal information about the function of the colon that is useful in diagnosis and treatment, particularly if surgical options need to be explored.

DIFFERENTIAL DIAGNOSIS

The algorithmic approach to evaluating delayed passage of meconium in neonates is presented in Figure 19.4. An algorithmic approach to evaluating pediatric constipation is presented in Figure 19.5.

Hirschsprung Disease

Congenital aganglionic megacolon, or Hirschsprung disease, is a common cause of neonatal intestinal obstruction, occurring in approximately 1:5,000 to 1:15,000 live births, with a male-to-female ratio of about 4:1. The disease is rare in premature births, may be familial, and is associated with trisomy 21, Waardenburg syndrome, multiple endocrine neoplasia type 2A syndrome, congenital central hypoventilation syndrome, and piebaldism. The absence of ganglion cells in both the Meissner (submucosal) plexus and the Auerbach (myenteric) plexus results in an inability of the involved segment of bowel to relax in response to distention from the presence of stool. In the newborn, passage of meconium is often delayed beyond 48 hours after birth. Most affected patients are diagnosed during infancy: 50% are diagnosed in the first months of life, 75% by 3 months, and 80% by the end of the first year. Diagnosis may be delayed into childhood and, in rare cases, into adolescence or even adulthood in some patients with ultra-short-segment disease. These patients complain of constipation; manifestations usually start in infancy. Differentiating Hirschsprung disease from functional constipation may be challenging in older patients or in those with short-segment disease (Table 19.6). Conditions that may mimic Hirschsprung disease include other abnormalities of intestinal innervation such as chronic pediatric intestinal pseudoobstruction and hyperganglionosis (see Table 19.1 and Fig. 19.4).

The lesion begins at the internal anal sphincter and extends continuously into the rectum or the rectosigmoid colon in up to 80% of cases. In 10% of cases, there is total colonic aganglionosis; in another 10%, there is variable involvement of the small intestine in addition to total colonic disease. Delayed passage of meconium is the most common manifestation in the neonate, followed by lower intestinal obstruction (distention, bile-stained emesis), obstipation (no stools), failure to thrive, or, in rare cases, intestinal perforation. Meconium plug syndrome, in which a thick, inspissated cast of meconium obstructs the colonic lumen, may be an initial presentation. In addition, if stool is passed immediately after a rectal examination is performed in an obstipated or constipated patient, Hirschsprung disease should be suspected.

A plain abdominal film occasionally reveals distention of the normally innervated bowel proximal to the affected segment. The most useful radiographic test, though, is a liquid contrast enema, which may demonstrate a small-caliber rectum with a transition in the rectosigmoid to the dilated, obstructed, normal proximal colon. Patients undergoing contrast enema should not undergo preparatory bowel evacuation procedures, which decrease test specificity, particularly in short-segment disease. A delayed lateral radiograph performed 24 hours after the contrast enema aids in identifying a transition zone in the sigmoid colon.

Anorectal manometry is a valuable diagnostic procedure if radiographic procedures are unrevealing. Normal internal anal sphincter relaxation with transient rectal distention rules out Hirschsprung disease. Paradoxical contraction of the internal anal sphincter suggests an absence of ganglion cells and is most common in Hirschsprung disease, though absence of relaxation has also been noted in premature infants, in neonates with infection or sepsis, and in thyroid aplasia; normal function is seen after appropriate therapy for these conditions. The sensitivity and specificity of anorectal manometry vary somewhat by age (children vs infants vs neonates), with a sensitivity that ranges from 0.79 to 0.90, a specificity ranging from 0.97 to 1.00, and a positive predictive value of 0.94–1.00.

A *definitive* diagnosis of Hirschsprung disease requires histologic confirmation of the absence of ganglion cells; such confirmation may be accomplished by a simple submucosal suction biopsy, which may be performed in the physician's office. Suction biopsy excludes the diagnosis if ganglion cells are present. However, there may be a 10% false-negative rate. A full-thickness rectal biopsy procedure is reserved for infants with bowel obstruction and for older children with abnormal rectal motilities and inconclusive suction biopsies.

Complications of undiagnosed Hirschsprung disease include **acute toxic megacolon** or infectious enterocolitis, most frequently caused by *Staphylococcus aureus* or *Clostridioides difficile*. Therapy for these complications includes correcting electrolyte abnormalities (oftentimes hypokalemia), broad-spectrum parenteral antibiotics, bowel rest, rectal tube placement, and, if needed, emergency cecostomy or colectomy. Treatment for Hirschsprung disease is surgical resection of the affected segment of bowel and various strategies for an ileal or colonic rectal pull-through procedure.

Pediatric Intestinal Pseudoobstruction

Chronic intestinal pseudoobstruction is characterized by symptoms of intestinal obstruction without an identifiable lumen-occluding lesion. Pediatric-onset disease differs from adult-onset disease in etiology, symptom onset, phenotypic features, and natural history, and is considered a distinct entity termed **pediatric intestinal pseudoobstruction (PIPO)** (Table 19.7). A variety of primary and secondary etiologies can produce the underlying pathophysiology of PIPO, which may consist of an intestinal **neuropathy,** an intestinal smooth muscle **myopathy**, an intestinal **mesenchymopathy** in which there is dysfunction of the interstitial cells of Cajal (ICC)**,** or a combination of these mechanisms (Table 19.8).

Symptoms vary according to the pathophysiology and the extent to which the gastrointestinal tract and other organ systems are involved, though most affected patients experience abdominal distention, vomiting, and constipation. The majority present during the neonatal period; at onset these symptoms may be nonspecific and mimic colic, feeding intolerance, or other more routine causes of neonatal constipation; up to 80% of patients will present by 1 year of age. The abdominal distention, vomiting, and constipation may be episodic or exacerbated by intercurrent illnesses, surgical procedures, psychologic stressors, or enteral feeds. Over time, intestinal stasis may result in **small intestinal bacterial overgrowth** with resultant worsening abdominal distention and pain, and malabsorption; malnutrition may produce additional manifestations, including growth failure and the sequelae of micronutrient deficiencies. Certain etiologies are more likely to have associated features that may suggest PIPO as the underlying cause of abdominal symptoms; patients with an underlying intestinal smooth muscle myopathy are more likely to have bladder involvement. Earlier onset (<1 year)–associated intestinal malrotation, enteral feeding intolerance, and parenteral nutrition dependence are additional predictors of poor outcome; mortality risk is approximately 20%.

Congenital PIPO may be sporadic or inherited; manifestations differ according to the underlying genetic abnormality (Table 19.9), though variable expressivity and penetrance have been noted within families with the same genetic abnormality as well. One congenital form, **megacystis-microcolon-intestinal hypoperistalsis syndrome,**

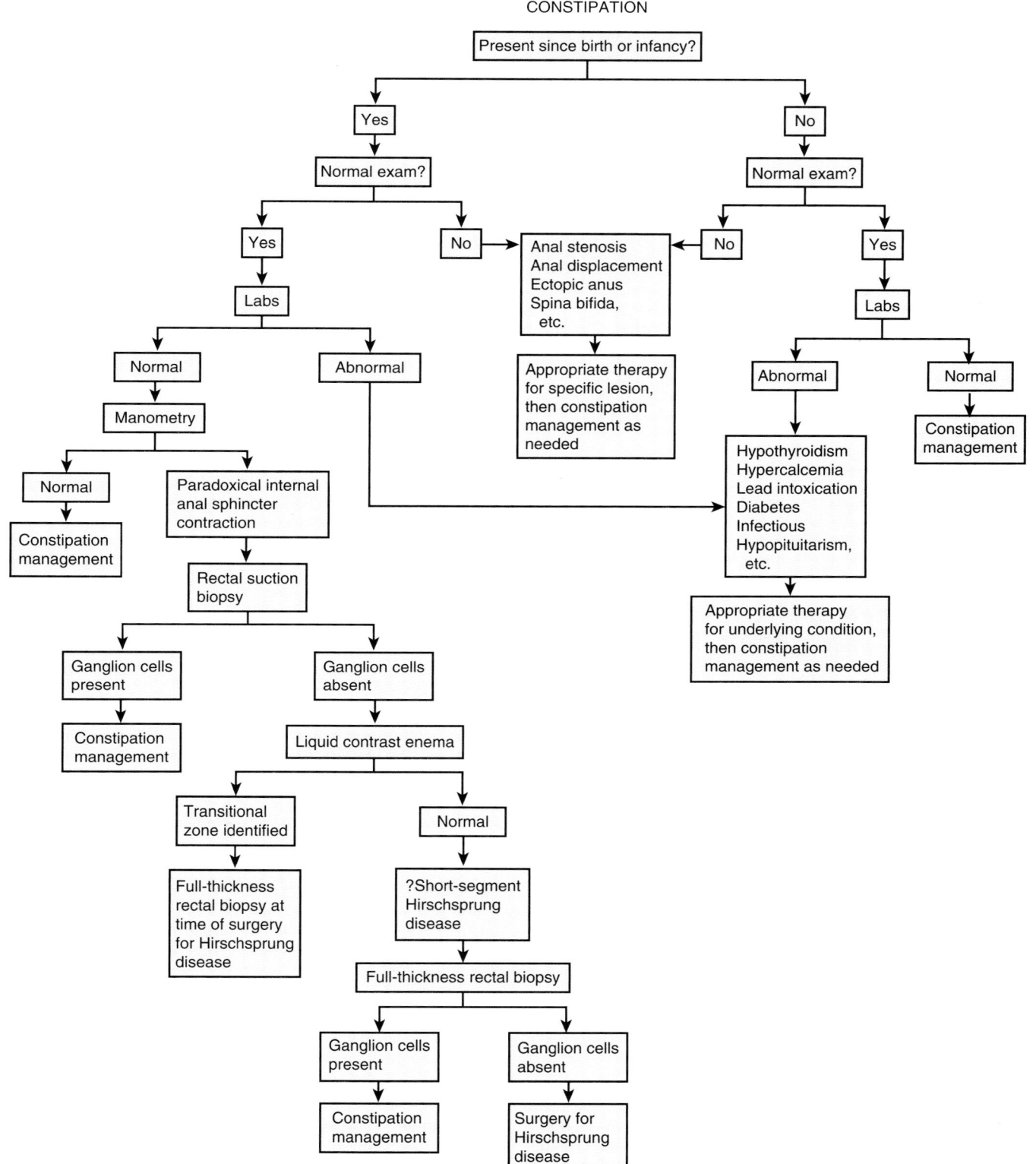

Fig. 19.5 Algorithmic approach to the diagnosis of constipation.

can be suspected antenatally via the demonstration of an enlarged bladder and/or an abnormally narrow colon on fetal ultrasound, with gastrointestinal symptoms developing shortly after birth. The bladder remains enlarged and difficult to empty, contributing to abdominal distension and often requiring catheterization. **Mitochondrial**

neurogastrointestinal encephalopathy (MNGIE) is characterized by ptosis, ophthalmoplegia, peripheral neuropathy, and white matter abnormalities, in addition to pseudoobstruction. Other genetic forms have characteristic phenotypic features that suggest the specific diagnosis (see Table 19.9) and the potential need for either targeted

TABLE 19.6 **Distinguishing Hirschsprung Disease from Functional (Acquired) Constipation**

	Functional Constipation	Hirschsprung Disease*
History		
Gender of patient	Male	Male
Onset of constipation	After 2 yr of age	At birth
Prevalence	1–3% of males	1:5,000–1:15,000
Encopresis	Common	Very rare
Forced bowel training	Usual	None
Stool size	Very large	Small, ribbon-like
Enterocolitis	None	Possible
Abdominal pain	Common	Rare except with obstruction, toxic megacolon, or enterocolitis
Failure to thrive	Uncommon	Common
Examination		
Abdominal distention	Variable	Common
Poor growth	Rare	Common
Anal tone	Patulous	Tight
Rectal examination	Stool in ampulla	Ampulla empty
Malnutrition	Absent	Possible
Laboratory		
Contrast enema	Massive amounts of stool, no transition zone	Transition zone, delayed evacuation (>24 hr)
Rectal biopsy	Normal	No ganglion cells; ↑ acetylcholinesterase staining
Anorectal manometry	Distention of the rectum causes relaxation of the internal sphincter	No sphincter relaxation

*Note that ultrashort-segment Hirschsprung disease may have clinical features of functional (acquired) megacolon (e.g., constipation).
Modified from Behrman RE, ed. *Nelson Textbook of Pediatrics.* 16th ed. Philadelphia: Saunders; 2000:1140.

pseudoobstruction gene panel testing or genome or exome sequencing with copy number variant analysis. Secondary causes of PIPO are diverse, though can be categorized according to pathophysiology or associated disease (see Table 19.8).

The diagnosis should be suspected in patients presenting with symptoms of obstruction in whom anatomic luminal obstruction and malrotation have been excluded. Abdominal radiography may show dilated loops of bowel or multiple air-fluid levels. Luminal contrast studies can help exclude malrotation or obstruction; water-soluble contrast is preferred, as retained barium in the setting of delayed intestinal transit may form a bezoar. CT or MRI may be considered in patients unable to tolerate enteral contrast or in instances where extraluminal pathology is being considered as well. Laboratory evaluation should be directed at excluding secondary causes (see Table 19.8), particularly since therapy for those diseases that are amenable to treatment may reverse the symptoms of PIPO; the evaluation should include a CBC, comprehensive metabolic profile, inflammatory markers, and thyroid and cortisol studies. If history of phenotypic features is suggestive, then additional

studies may include hemoglobin-A1c; anti–tissue transglutaminase IgA and total IgA; antinuclear antibody; anti-double-stranded DNA; anti-Scl-70 antibodies; aldolase and creatine phosphokinase; urine catecholamines; anti-Hu and type 1 anti-neuronal nuclear antibodies; urinary porphyrins; serology for Chagas disease, Epstein-Barr virus (EBV), cytomegalovirus (CMV), JC virus, herpes simplex virus (HSV), and rotavirus; thymidine phosphorylase activity; serum lactic acid; and toxicology screens as indicated based on exposure history.

Manometry can identify the extent of gastrointestinal tract involvement and help distinguish between myopathic and neuropathic etiologies; it may be challenging if disease is more restricted to the small intestine. Normal manometry and the absence of dilated bowel loops on plain radiography suggest alternate diagnoses. Histologic studies can provide more conclusive evidence of pathophysiology and guide prognostication and therapy. Full-thickness biopsies of the gastric antrum, small intestine, and colon should be obtained. Laparoscopic techniques decrease the risk of adhesions, disease exacerbation, or other complications. Neuropathic disease is characterized by loss or inflammatory infiltration of neurons, myopathic disease by smooth muscle atrophy and fibrosis, and mesenchymopathic disease by reduced, absent, or disrupted ICC networks, whereas mixed disease will demonstrate features of all three mechanisms.

Treatment is directed at correcting any underlying conditions resulting in secondary PIPO and at optimizing nutrition and quality of life while minimizing intraabdominal interventions that can exacerbate symptoms or result in adhesions, infection, or other complications. Some patients may tolerate eating orally with the use of pro-motility agents. Others with disease affecting primarily the proximal gastrointestinal tract may be able to tolerate gastric or jejunal feeds via enteral feeding tubes. Most patients will be unable to meet their nutritional requirements via enteral feeds alone and often require some degree of parenteral nutrition support. In these patients, central line complications or infections can be an additional source of morbidity or mortality.

Anterior Anal Displacement

There are two forms of displacement of the anus (see Fig. 19.2). In **anterior ectopic anus**, the anal canal and the internal anal sphincter are displaced anteriorly in the perineum as a unit and are separated from the external anal sphincter, which remains posterior in its usual position. On physical examination, it may be possible to elicit an external sphincter anal wink in the usual location, posterior to the opening of the anal canal. Rectal examination often reveals a sharp posterior angulation in the anal canal. In **anterior anal displacement**, the entire normal anal unit is located in the anterior perineum. Both entities are found more commonly in females. Symptoms of constipation often begin in the neonatal period and are related to the difficulty in expelling stool through a canal that is angled anteriorly. If the displacement is severe enough to cause symptoms, surgical correction may be necessary to relocate the anus and relieve the obstruction.

Anal Stenosis

The diagnosis of **anal stenosis** may be delayed beyond the neonatal period, especially if the degree of stenosis is not severe. Any portion of the anal canal or the entire canal may be involved. The diagnosis can be made by digital examination or by endoscopy. Constipation is caused by fecal retention secondary to outlet obstruction. Treatment is by dilatation or anorectal myectomy.

Imperforate Anus

Imperforate anus is usually diagnosed in the neonatal nursery. Passage of meconium is delayed or is noted to take place through an abnormal

TABLE 19.7 Common and Distinctive Features of Pediatric Intestinal Pseudoobstruction

Etiology	Majority of cases appear to be congenital (up to 80%) and primary; secondary forms rare (<10%)
Disease subtype	Neuropathies more common (~70%) with myopathic forms seen in ~30%
Symptom onset	In utero, from birth, or early infancy (65–80% of patients by 12 mo of age)
Clinical features	• Recurrent or continuous episodes of intestinal pseudoobstruction with symptoms present from birth/early life • Pain infrequently seen (approximately 30%) • Urologic involvement common (36–100%) • Intestinal malrotation in about 30% of cases • High risk of colonic and small bowel volvulus
Natural history	• Poor outcome predicted by myopathic forms of PIPO; urinary involvement; concurrent intestinal malrotation; and inability to tolerate enteral feeds • Risk of mortality in approximately 20% of cases
Diagnostic approach	• Diagnosis relies on clinical picture and radiology together with specialized tests (e.g., intestinal manometry, histopathology) • Dilated bowel loops with fluid levels commonly absent (~40%) in patients presenting in the neonatal period • Histopathology yield high and used to inform management, for example, use of parenteral nutrition in intestinal myopathies and prokinetics in intestinal neuropathies • Apart from specific indications little yield from investigating for secondary PIPO • Need to differentiate from feeding problems and fabricated or induced illness
Nutritional therapy	Significant (~80%) require parenteral nutrition to maintain normal growth and development; specialized feeds (e.g., hydrolyzed protein feeds) and feeding routes (e.g., jejunal) used to promote enteral feed tolerance
Pharmacologic therapy	Minimal evidence from well-designed trials; most medication use is based on anecdotal evidence, case reports, or adult literature
Surgical therapy	Venting ostomies very commonly used to decompress and reduce pseudoobstructive events; surgery as a "bridge" to transplantation may be indicated in highly elected cases

PIPO, pediatric intestinal pseudoobstruction.

From Mousa H, Hyman PE, Cocjin J, et al. Long-term outcome of congenital intestinal pseudoobstruction. *Dig Dis Sci.* 2002;47:2298–2305; Faure C, Goulet O, Ategbo S, et al. Chronic intestinal pseudoobstruction syndrome: clinical analysis, outcome, and prognosis in 105 children. French-Speaking Group of Pediatric Gastroenterology. *Dig Dis Sci.* 1999;44:953–959; Hanks JB, Meyers WC, Andersen DK, et al. Chronic primary intestinal pseudo-obstruction. *Surgery.* 1981;89:175–182; Mann SD, Debinski HS, Kamm MA. Clinical characteristics of chronic idiopathic intestinal pseudo-obstruction in adults. *Gut.* 1997;41:675–681; Pitt HA, Mann LL, Berquist WE, et al. Chronic intestinal pseudo-obstruction. Management with total parenteral nutrition and a venting enterostomy. *Arch Surg.* 1985;120:614–618; Stanghellini V, Camilleri M, Malagelada JR. Chronic idiopathic intestinal pseudo-obstruction: clinical and intestinal manometric findings. *Gut.* 1987;28:5–12; Stanghellini V, Cogliandro RF, De Giorgio R, et al. Natural history of chronic idiopathic intestinal pseudo-obstruction in adults: a single center study. *Clin Gastroenterol Hepatol.* 2005;3:449–458; Vargas JH, Sachs P, Ament ME. Chronic intestinal pseudo-obstruction syndrome in pediatrics. Results of a national survey by members of the North American Society of Pediatric Gastroenterology and Nutrition. *J Pediatr Gastroenterol Nutr.* 1988;7:323–332; Howard L, Ashley C. Management of complications in patients receiving home parenteral nutrition. *Gastroenterology.* 2003;124:1651–1661.

TABLE 19.8 Classification of Pediatric Intestinal Pseudoobstruction (PIPO)

Primary PIPO
- Sporadic or familial forms of myopathy and/or neuropathy and/or mesenchymopathy (abnormal ICC development) that relate to disordered development, degeneration, or inflammation. Inflammatory (including autoimmune) conditions include lymphocytic and eosinophilic ganglionitis and/or leiomyositis
- Mitochondrial neurogastrointestinal encephalomyopathy (MNGIE) and other mitochondrial diseases
- Neuropathy associated with multiple endocrine neoplasia type 2B
- Hirschsprung disease (e.g., total intestinal aganglionosis)*

Secondary PIPO
- Conditions affecting GI smooth muscle:
  - Rheumatologic conditions (dermatomyositis/polymyositis, scleroderma, systematic lupus erythematosus, Ehlers-Danlos syndrome)
  - Other (Duchenne muscular dystrophy, myotonic dystrophy, amyloidosis, ceroidosis/brown bowel syndrome)
- Pathologies affecting the enteric nervous system (familial dysautonomia; primary dysfunction of the autonomic nervous system; neurofibromatosis; diabetic neuropathy; fetal alcohol syndrome; postviral-related inflammatory neuropathy, e.g., cytomegalovirus, Epstein-Barr virus, varicella zoster virus, JC virus)
- Endocrinologic disorders (hypothyroidism, diabetes, hypoparathyroidism, pheochromocytoma)
- Metabolic conditions (uremia, porphyria, electrolyte imbalances, e.g., potassium, magnesium, calcium)
- Gastroschisis
- Neuropathy following neonatal necrotizing enterocolitis
- Other (celiac disease; eosinophilic gastroenteritis; Crohn disease; radiation injury; Chagas disease; Kawasaki disease; angioedema; drugs, e.g., opioids, anthraquinone laxatives, calcium channel blockers, antidepressants; antineoplastic agents, e.g., vinca alkaloids; paraneoplastic CIPO; major trauma/surgery; chromosome abnormalities)

Idiopathic (i.e., where forms of primary or secondary PIPO classified as above do not, as yet, have a defined etiopathogenesis)

CIPO, chronic intestinal pseudoobstruction; GI, gastrointestinal.
*Needs to be excluded in all cases of PIPO.

From Thapar N, Saliakellis E, Benninga MA, et al. Paediatric intestinal pseudo-obstruction: evidence and consensus-based recommendations from an ESPGHAN-led expert group. *J Pediatr Gastroenterol Nutr.* 2018;66(6):991–1019 (Table 3, p. 999).

TABLE 19.9   Primary Disorders Associated with Chronic Intestinal Pseudoobstruction and Identified Genes

Gene	Syndrome	Function	Inheritance	Phenotype	Age of onset
SOX10	Type IV Waardenburg syndrome	Encodes a transcription factor essential for the development of enteric neurons	Autosomal dominant	Peripheral neuropathy with hypomyelination, sensorineural deafness, and pseudoobstruction	Neonatal period
POLG (DNA-polymerase gamma)	Congenital myopathy and gastrointestinal pseudoobstruction	Encodes for the catalytic subunit of the mitochondrial DNA	Autosomal recessive	Associated with mitochondrial depletion and deletions. Severe hypotonia and generalized muscle weakness, severe abdominal distension, and hypoactive bowel	Neonatal period
FLNA (filamin A)	Chronic idiopathic intestinal pseudoobstruction (CIIPX)	Encodes large cytoskeletal proteins	X-linked recessive	Abnormal filamin A leads to cytoskeletal abnormalities and potentially disrupts entericneuron structure and function. Seizures and progressive abdominal distension and obstruction	Neonatal period
L1CAM (L1 cell adhesion molecule)	Hydrocephalus with stenosis of the aqueduct of Sylvius (HSAS) and congenital idiopathic intestinal pseudoobstruction	Encodes a transmembrane glycoprotein involved in neurite outgrowth and neuronal migration	Autosomal recessive	Defect in the differentiation of the interstitial cells of Cajal leading to progressive distension and intermittent episodes of obstruction	Neonatal period
ACTG2 (enteric smooth muscle actin–gamma 2)	Familial visceral myopathy; megacystis–microcolon–intestinal hypoperistalsis syndrome	Encodes enteric smooth muscle actin	Autosomal dominant, sporadic	Altered ACTG2 protein in the muscularis propria leads to impaired contractility	Neonatal to third decade in life
MYH11 (myosin heavy chain 11)	Megacystis–microcolon–intestinal hypoperistalsis syndrome	Encodes myosin light chain	Autosomal recessive	Abnormal MYH11 in smooth muscle myosin leads to impaired contractility	Neonatal to third decade in life
MYLK (myosin light chain kinase)	Megacystis–microcolon–intestinal hypoperistalsis syndrome	Encodes a kinase required for myosin activation and subsequent interaction with actin filaments	Autosomal recessive	Abnormal MYLK leads to impaired smooth muscle cell contraction	Neonatal to third decade in life
LMOD1 (leiomodin 1)	Megacystis–microcolon–intestinal hypoperistalsis syndrome	Encodes visceral smooth muscle cells	Sporadic	Abnormal LMOD1 leads to impaired intestinal smooth muscle contractility	Neonatal to third decade in life
MYL9 (myosin regulatory light chain 9)	Megacystis–microcolon–intestinal hypoperistalsis syndrome	Encodes a regulatory myosin light chain	Autosomal recessive	Abnormal MYL9 leads to impaired intestinal smooth muscle contractility	Neonatal to third decade in life
RET proto-oncogene (receptor tyrosine kinase)	MEN2B	Expressed in the neural crest cells of the enteric ganglia and encodes a member of the receptor tyrosine kinase family of transmembrane receptors	Autosomal dominant	Gain-of-function variant associated with intestinal ganglioneuromas leading to increased cell number in the myenteric plexus and dysmotility	Infancy to third decade of life
TYMP (thymidine phosphorylase)	Mitochondrial neurogastrointestinal encephalomyopathy (MNGIE)	A nucleoside that maintains adequate thymidine in mitochondria	Autosomal recessive	Accumulation of thymidine in mitochondrial DNA leads to impaired function. Multisystem mitochondrial disease with progressive gastrointestinal dysmotility	Infancy to third decade of life

TABLE 19.9 Primary Disorders Associated with Chronic Intestinal Pseudoobstruction and Identified Genes—cont'd

Gene	Syndrome	Function	Inheritance	Phenotype	Age of onset
RAD21	Mungan syndrome	Part of a cohesion complex that controls pairing and unpairing in cell replication. Plays an important role in epithelial and neuronal survival and APOB regulation in the gastrointestinal tract	Autosomal recessive	Pseudoobstruction, megaduodenum, long-segment Barrett esophagus, and cardiac abnormalities	First to second decade of life
SGOL1	Chronic atrial and intestinal dysrhythmia (CAID)	Component of the cohesion pathway	Autosomal recessive	Accelerated cell cycle progression and enhanced activation of TGF-β signaling leading to changes in both the enteric nervous system and smooth muscle	First to fourth decade of life

APOB, apolipoprotein B; MEN2B, multiple endocrine neoplasia type 2B; TGF-β, transforming growth factor-β.
From Gamboa HE, Sood M. Pediatric intestinal pseudo-obstruction in the era of genetic sequencing. *Curr Gastroenterol Rep.* 2019;21:70. https://doi.org/10.1007/s11894-019-0737-y

location as a result of the presence of a fistula (e.g., rectovaginal, rectovesicular, or rectoperineal). Treatment is surgical; the actual procedure depends on the level and the extent of the defect.

Spina Bifida and Spina Bifida Occulta

Defecation disturbances, most frequently constipation, are common in patients with spina bifida and spina bifida occulta, especially if the defect involves the lumbosacral spine. The spinal and nerve root defects result in poor functioning of the terminal bowel. Voluntary external sphincter control and rectoanal sensation are most often diminished or absent, and the degree of difficulty with defecation is related to the degree and the extent of the injury.

Most patients can achieve an acceptable level of continence via an individualized bowel regimen. Dietary fiber, stool softeners, suppositories, and enema continence catheters are treatment options. Biofeedback and pudendal nerve stimulation are successful in some patients. In most patients, a combination of treatment modalities allows social continence to be achieved and dramatically improves the patient's quality of life. Treatment of patients with spinal or nerve injury, or dysfunction from other causes, is similar.

Endocrine and Metabolic Diseases

The appropriate laboratory tests should be performed to rule out the various metabolic and endocrinologic conditions that may manifest with constipation (see Table 19.1). Frequent among these conditions is hypothyroidism, though hypothyroidism manifesting solely with neonatal constipation is rare. Rather, it should be suspected in any infant presenting with constipation, a history of prolonged neonatal jaundice, and other suggestive findings, such as poor feeding or an enlarged fontanelle size.

Neurologic Disease

Children with neurologic disease may have constipation for many reasons, including poor intestinal motility, lack of dietary fiber, and poor awareness of rectal vault distention with stool retention. Any illness affecting the spinal cord or sacral nerves, degenerative muscle diseases, cerebral palsy, and demyelinating diseases can result in constipation.

Medication-Related Constipation

A complete medication and environmental exposure history may reveal substances that can cause constipation (see Table 19.1).

ENCOPRESIS

Idiopathic or functional constipation is much more common than Hirschsprung disease. Long-standing constipation, including functional constipation, leads to **encopresis**, the deposition of stools in the undergarments or other unorthodox locations that persists or occurs beyond the age that is considered culturally appropriate for achieving continence. In some cultures, delayed bowel training up to the age of 6 years is normal. It is generally accepted in the United States that healthy children should be bowel trained by the age of 4 years.

Encopresis is related to the chronic withholding of stool. As the fecal mass accumulates, it causes rectal distention, increases rectal compliance, and eventually results in blunted or absent sensitivity of the rectum to the presence of liquid stool passing around a firm fecal mass. Children with encopresis usually pass small stools and do not completely empty the rectum. Periodically, they pass huge stools, which may block the toilet. It is important to specifically question the patient or parents regarding these massive stools because this information is frequently not volunteered.

Encopresis has been incorrectly considered a symptom or manifestation of psychiatric illness. It was thought that the patient retained stools either consciously or subconsciously as a way to rebel against, please, or anger caretakers. Although encopresis may be seen in association with emotional and behavioral problems, it is usually the result of painful defecation followed by a pattern of stool withholding, leading to chronic constipation, overflow encopresis, and possibly poor relations with peers as a result of fecal soiling. In the few patients in whom encopresis is truly a manifestation of psychiatric disease, there is often no stool retention, and the prognosis for fecal continence with therapy is poor.

Idiopathic constipation with or without encopresis may compress the bladder by a dilated rectum, thus causing stasis and urinary tract infections.

SUMMARY AND RED FLAGS

Constipation is a common concern in infants and young children. A detailed history of bowel patterns identifies many children with normal bowel movements whose parents need reassurance. The majority of patients who do have constipation have functional constipation. The history should include a review of all medications and a search for an associated chronic disease, such as a metabolic or neurologic disease. This complete history, combined with a careful physical examination, including the spine and sacral area, the location of the anus, and a digital rectal examination, should alert the physician to the need for further evaluation. Red flags include onset in the neonatal period, growth failure, prolonged jaundice in the neonatal period, and symptoms of obstruction. Distinguishing features associated with Hirschsprung disease are listed in Table 19.6. Pediatric intestinal pseudoobstruction may initially present with nonspecific symptoms but has a significant risk of morbidity and mortality.

BIBLIOGRAPHY

A bibliography is available at ExpertConsult.com.

20

Abdominal Masses

John C. Densmore and Emily M. Densmore

An abdominal mass or abdominal fullness in a child usually becomes apparent when it enlarges enough to be visualized during bathing or palpable on physical examination. Masses may arise from intraperitoneal, retroperitoneal, or abdominal wall locations and emanate from both solid and hollow viscera (Figs. 20.1 and 20.2). An abdominal mass may prove life threatening (e.g., malignant neoplasm, splenic sequestration crisis in sickle cell disease), arise from congenital malformation or disorganized development (e.g., mesenteric cyst, enteric duplication), or be benign or correctable nonoperatively (e.g., fecaloma, splenomegaly associated with infectious mononucleosis). Hepatomegaly and splenomegaly often indicate systemic illnesses such as infection, hemolysis, storage disease, or malignancy (see Chapter 17). A child with an abdominal mass requires a prompt and thorough work-up with testing guided by history, physical examination findings, age, and gender. Early surgical referral may assist in this work-up following a directed screening approach.

DIAGNOSTIC STRATEGIES

Clinical History

A child's age, gender, and thorough clinical history help to identify the most likely disease category (Tables 20.1 and 20.2). The duration and character of associated symptoms are important for narrowing the differential diagnosis (e.g., fatigue, fever, appetite changes, vomiting, stooling history, weight loss, night sweating, character and frequency of pain, hematuria, flushing, palpitations, lower extremity swelling, lymph nodal prominence, and jaundice). A history of abdominal trauma should be elicited, as solid organ injuries may result in hematoma, seroma, persistent pseudocyst, or arteriovenous malformation. Infectious disease may have sequelae of cyst, lymphadenopathy, or intraabdominal abscess. Some systemic diseases (e.g., glycogen storage, hereditary spherocytosis), genetic syndromes (e.g., Beckwith-Wiedemann, Peutz-Jeghers, von Hippel-Lindau, familial adenomatous polyposis, hereditary pheochromocytoma, *PTEN* hamartoma tumor), and anomalies (aniridia with Wilms tumor, isolated hemihypertrophy with neuroblastoma and Wilms tumor, Hirschsprung with neuroblastoma) are associated with intraabdominal tumors. A family history is pertinent as is a menstrual and sexual history, particularly in adolescent females. Prenatal imaging frequently identifies congenital malformations and neoplasms, requiring postnatal imaging and surgical assessment.

Physical Examination

A complete physical exam should be performed in children with abdominal masses. Attention should be paid to the general condition (fever, pallor, petechiae, cachexia) of the child and to signs of metastatic disease. Enlarged lymph nodes and their locations should be noted, the skin inspected, and the lungs and heart auscultated. Extremities should be evaluated for evidence of swelling, venous phlegmasia, or evidence of embolic disease to bone, muscle, or skin. Genitourinary exam should make note of any inappropriate virilization, testicular changes, and hymenal patency in the case of a female with a low pelvic mass. In addition, a neurologic examination may reveal signs of central or peripheral nervous system involvement. The eyes should be carefully inspected for periorbital ecchymosis, proptosis, squint, opsoclonus-myoclonus syndrome, heterochromia of the iris, Horner syndrome, and scleral icterus. The patient's blood pressure must be determined and may be elevated in patients with Wilms tumor, neuroblastoma, or pheochromocytoma.

To successfully perform abdominal palpation in a child, the clinician must approach the patient calmly and gently, as the most reliable exams are completed in cooperative and relaxed children. Enlarged organs may be missed in a struggling child who does not lie quietly. When cooperation proves difficult in an infant, the examining hand should be placed and remain static on the abdomen and the exam completed between cries or as the child calms in the parent's arms. Creative play is sometimes necessary, with the use of pacifiers or bottles to distract the child from the exam. Re-examination after voiding or defecating elucidates contributions of constipation and urinary retention in the child's presentation.

The abdominal quadrants should be examined systematically (Table 20.3; see Figs. 20.1 and 20.2). With the patient in the supine position, the symmetry of the abdomen should be inspected, and any visible masses or the presence of ascites should be noted. A very enlarged spleen is frequently visible, with fullness of the left side of the abdomen. The presence of tense fluid-filled hernias or prominent periumbilical veins as sequelae of portal hypertension should be noted. The mass should be localized, and its size, shape, texture, mobility, tenderness, and relation to midline noted. The umbilical position is a useful marker of abdominal asymmetry.

Signs of peritoneal inflammation must be sought (see Chapter 13). Dull visceral pain conducted by slow C nerve fibers may be reported for inflammatory processes in the vascular distributions of the celiac, superior mesenteric, and inferior mesenteric arteries and referred to the epigastrium, umbilical region, or hypogastrium, respectively. When the inflamed process contacts the peritoneum, peritoneal fast A nerve fibers allow discrete localization of sharp pain to the abdominal wall. Ultrasound is often a very useful adjunct in the evaluation of an abdominal mass and is often available at the bedside.

Approximately half of abdominal masses in older children are caused by enlargement of the liver or spleen, or both. The liver is normally palpated in the right upper quadrant and epigastrium extending 1–2 cm below the costal margin. The inferior hepatic margin may be palpated in a thin child, is usually nontender, and moves with respiration. Detection of liver edge by auscultation using skin scratches has been proven unreliable and has been supplanted by the use of readily available ultrasound. Hepatomegaly is discussed in detail in Chapter 17. The spleen is located

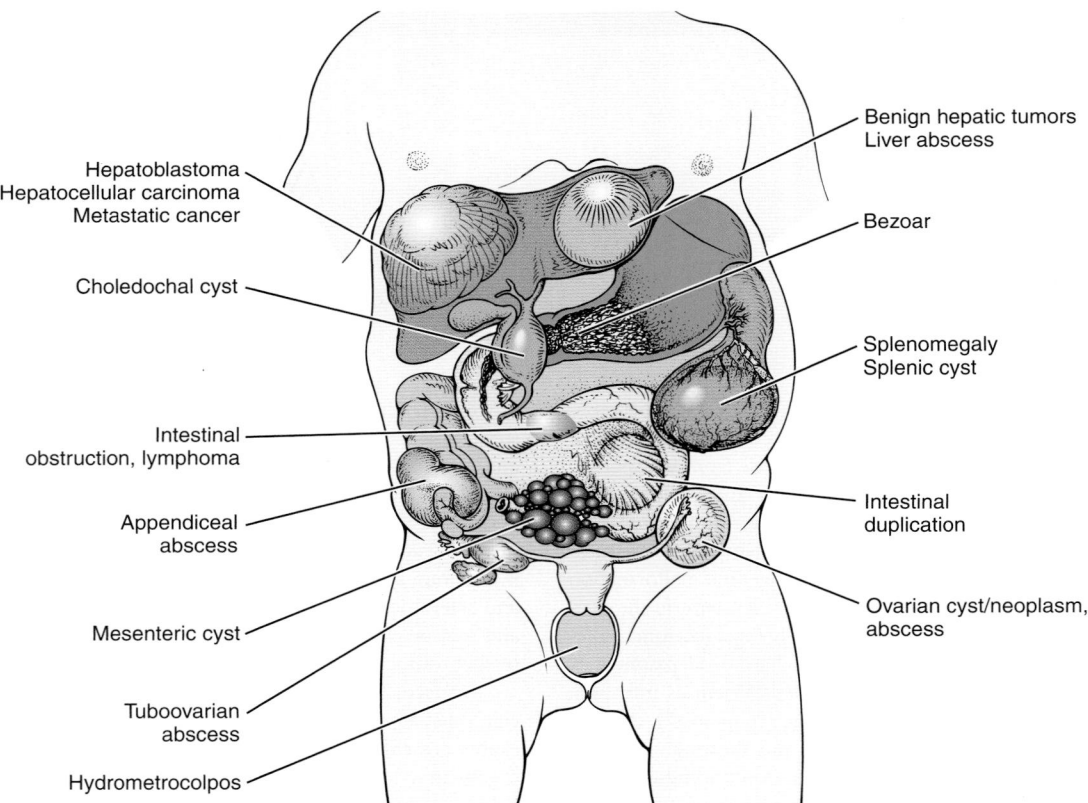

Fig. 20.1 Location of select intraabdominal tumors and masses.

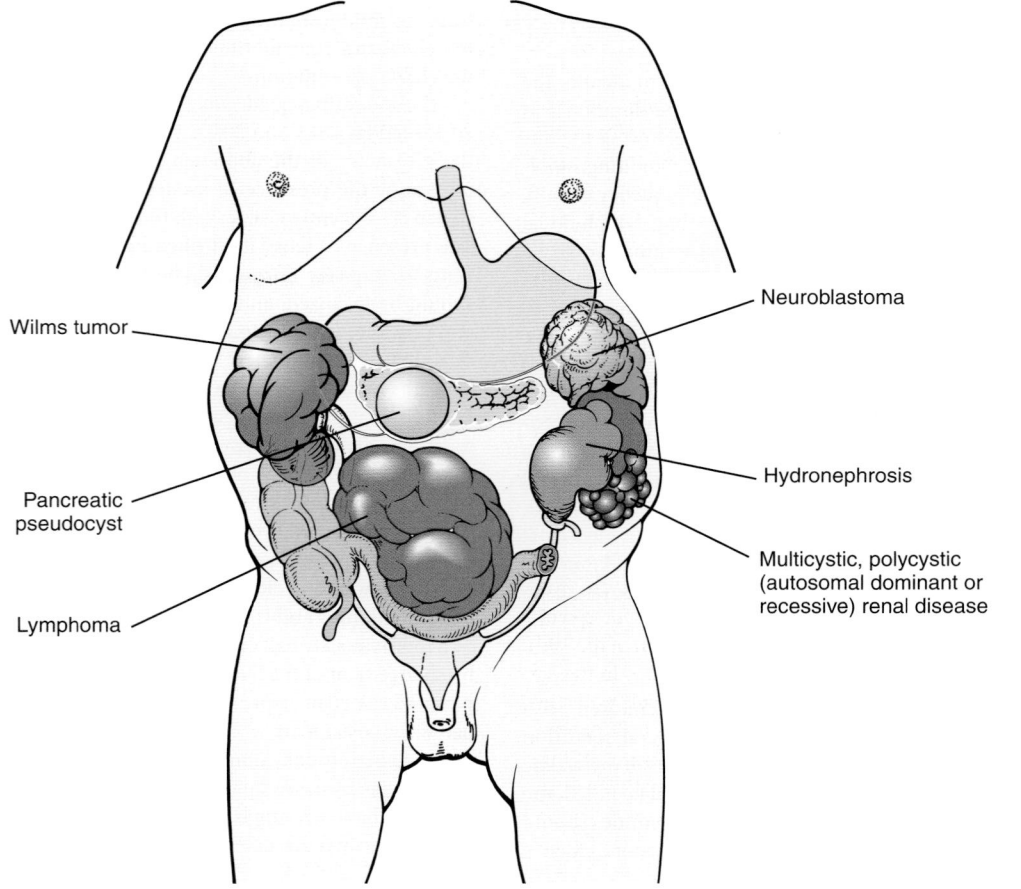

Fig. 20.2 Location of select retroperitoneal tumors and masses.

TABLE 20.1 Stepwise Evaluation of an Abdominal Mass

Clinical History
Age and gender
General symptoms
Pain
Gastrointestinal symptoms
Urogenital symptoms
Pulmonary symptoms
Family history
Sexual history
Weight loss
Travel

Physical Examination
General condition
Lymph nodes
Associated physical findings
Cachexia

Abdominal Palpation
Quadrant of the abdomen
Organ most likely to be affected
Characteristics (soft or hard, mobile or nonmobile, crosses midline, moves with respiration, tender)

Ultrasonography
Location
Solid or cystic

Depending on the Clinical Suspicion, Evaluation Can Be Continued with One or More of the Following:
Laboratory studies: CBC, urinalysis, tumor markers
Imaging studies: plain radiography of chest and abdomen, contrast radiography of the gastrointestinal tract, CT, MRI, angiography, PET scan

TABLE 20.2 Age-Related Etiology of Abdominal Masses

Age	Benign	Malignant
Neonate (0–1 mo)	Congenital hydronephrosis Cystic or dysplastic kidney disease Intestinal duplication Mesenteric/omental cyst Neurogenic bladder Ovarian cyst Renal vein thrombosis Choledochal cyst Mesoblastic nephroma Meconium ileus Hematoma (adrenal, hepatic, splenic)	Neuroblastoma
Infant (0–1 yr)	Intestinal duplication Mesenteric/omental cyst Ovarian cyst Hydronephrosis Mesoblastic nephroma Cystic-dysplastic kidney Liver hamartomas Hepatic cavernous hemangioma Liver hemangioendothelioma Teratoma Lymphatic malformation Intussusception Hepatosplenomegaly Choledochal cyst Megacolon Urachal cyst	Neuroblastoma Hepatoblastoma Wilms tumor (rare) Teratoma
Child	Mesenteric/omental cyst Choledochal cyst Appendiceal abscess Lymphatic malformation	Neuroblastoma (2–10 yr) Hepatoblastoma Wilms tumor Leukemia Lymphoma
Adolescent	Bezoar Hematocolpos Hydrometrocolpos Pregnancy Inflammatory bowel disease Retroperitoneal hematoma (hemophilia) Castleman disease Mesenteric fibromatosis (dermoid)	Neuroblastoma (11–16 yr) Adrenal cortical carcinoma Hepatocellular carcinoma Ovarian or testicular neoplasm Lymphoma Rhabdomyosarcoma Inflammatory myofibroblastic tumor Desmoplastic small round cell tumor

in the left upper quadrant and is nonpalpable in most healthy children. To locate an enlarged spleen, the examiner must begin palpation in the patient's left iliac fossa (to avoid missing a grossly enlarged spleen or liver with extension of the left hepatic lobe into the splenic area in the left upper quadrant); the examiner's right hand should move toward the patient's left upper quadrant to find the spleen's lower pole or medial border. The examiner's left hand is placed in the patient's left flank, and gentle displacement of the thoracic cage toward the examiner's right hand often displaces the spleen forward enough to make it appreciable. The spleen has a rounded tip and should move downward with inspiration and is more superficial than a renal mass. It is equally important for the examiner to palpate the spleen as it is for the spleen to "touch" the examiner during its descent with inspiration. Overaggressive palpation may push the spleen away, whereas gentle or light palpation permits the examiner to feel the spleen's edge passively. Because the extent to which the spleen extends below the costal margin depends heavily on the patient's position, the extent of the spleen below the costal margin should be measured with the patient in the supine position. Measurement from the left costal margin to the lower pole of the spleen defines the splenic axis. Ordinarily, the long axis of the spleen is along the length of the 10th rib. As it enlarges, it extends medially and downward. Masses in the left upper quadrant, especially left renal masses, may be difficult to distinguish from an enlarged spleen. In general, a splenic notch, if present, helps identify the mass as a spleen, but nodular masses, such as Wilms tumors of the kidney, neuroblastomas, and retroperitoneal teratomas, may masquerade as splenomegaly. Many enlarged spleens are not palpable on physical examination because of their relationship to other organs

and the thoracic cage. Hyperinflation of the lungs (as occurs in asthma, bronchiolitis, and ipsilateral pneumothorax) may make a normal-sized liver or spleen palpable.

Flank masses are the next most frequent, particularly in newborn to toddler-aged children. Renal masses extend caudally, are fixed with respiration, and cause abdominal asymmetry. Lower abdominal masses are most commonly caused by constipation or urinary retention. These may be functional or secondary to neurogenic dysfunction. A perforated appendix with resulting abscess formation may create a tender right lower quadrant mass. Ovarian or uterine tumors often

TABLE 20.3 Location and Nature of Abdominal Masses

Organ	Congenital	Benign	Malignant	Acquired
Liver and biliary tract	Hemangioma Choledochal cyst	Hemangioendothelioma Hamartoma	Hepatoblastoma Lymphoma Leukemia Hepatocellular carcinoma	Abscess Hematoma Parasitic disease Hydrops of the gallbladder
Spleen		Cyst	Sarcoma	Splenomegaly (e.g., mononucleosis)
Kidney	Hydronephrosis Cystic disease Duplication		Wilms tumor	Hematoma
Adrenal gland	Neuroblastoma	Pheochromocytoma	Neuroblastoma Pheochromocytoma	Hematoma
Stomach	Duplication Teratoma	Leiomyoma Inflammatory pseudotumor	Leiomyosarcoma Adenocarcinoma	Bezoar
Intestines	Duplication Megacolon	Lymphangioma Hemangioma	Carcinoma Lymphoma	Appendiceal abscess Intussusception Obstipation
Mesentery		Mesenteric/omental cyst		Inflammatory bowel disease Parasitic disease Tuberculosis
Pancreas		Cyst	Carcinoma	Pseudocyst
Uterus	Hydrometrocolpos	Myoma	Rhabdomyosarcoma	Pregnancy
Ovaries	Cyst Teratoma	Cyst Cystic teratoma Cystic adenoma Granulosa cell tumor	Yolk sac tumor Embryonal carcinoma Dysgerminoma Choriocarcinoma	Tuboovarian abscess
Bladder	Urachal cyst Posterior urethral valve	Inflammatory pseudotumor	Rhabdomyosarcoma	Urinary retention
Retroperitoneum	Presacral teratoma Anterior myelomeningocele	Ganglioneuroma	Neuroblastoma	Psoas abscess Aortic aneurysm
Abdominal wall	Hernia Omphalocele Gastroschisis	Hemangioma	Rhabdomyosarcoma	Hematoma Rectus sheath hematoma Abscess

grow undetected in the pelvis until large enough to exit the pelvis as a large palpable abdominal mass.

Laboratory and Imaging Studies

Screening laboratory data, including CBC with differential and cell morphology, measurements of serum electrolytes, urinalysis, urine pregnancy test when appropriate, and inflammatory markers, are broadly applicable. Liver function tests, serum amylase, tumor marker levels (Table 20.4), and renal function tests are often important initial objective data points.

Plain abdominal radiographs may reveal tumor calcifications, organomegaly, excess fecal load, and mass effect upon intestines. Views in at least two different positions should be obtained to appreciate ascites or intestinal obstruction. As a screening modality, ultrasonography is a highly efficient, low-cost, and widely available test. It is noninvasive, is nonirradiating, and can give detailed information on the location, vascularity, and nature of the mass and adjacent structures (Fig. 20.3). The most widely used defining imaging technique is CT (Fig. 20.4), followed by MRI. These modalities often provide radiologic diagnosis, are invaluable for surgical planning, and are unhampered by bowel gas, a common limitation of ultrasound. MRI or CT when combined with functional PET scanning can define primary, metastatic, and recurrent disease (Figs. 20.5 and 20.6).

TABLE 20.4 Tumor Markers

Tumor	Tumor Markers
Neuroblastoma	Urinary catecholamines LDH Ferritin Neuron-specific enolase
Wilms tumor	Erythropoietin
Hepatoblastoma, pancreatoblastoma, yolk sac tumors	α-Fetoprotein (AFP, AFP-L3), PIVKA
Germ cell tumors	β-hCG, α-fetoprotein, LDH
Pheochromocytoma, paraganglioma	Plasma metanephrine, normetanephrine

hCG, human chorionic gonadotropin; LDH, lactate dehydrogenase; PIVKA, protein induced by vitamin K absence.

SPLENOMEGALY

Unlike many other abdominal masses, splenomegaly is usually secondary to a systemic process; it can be caused by diseases that result in hyperplasia of the lymphoid and reticuloendothelial systems (infections, inflammatory disorders), infiltrative disorders (Gaucher disease,

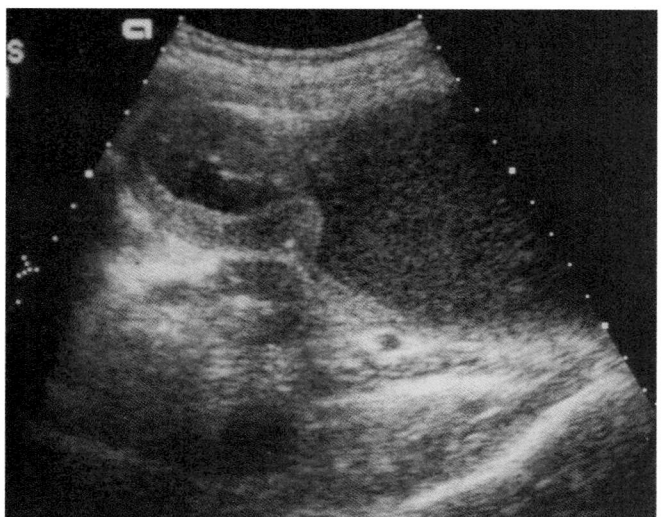

Fig. 20.3 An ultrasonic longitudinal view of the pelvis reveals hydrometrocolpos. The uterus and cervix are readily seen superior to the large collection of fluid in the vagina located at the right of the image.

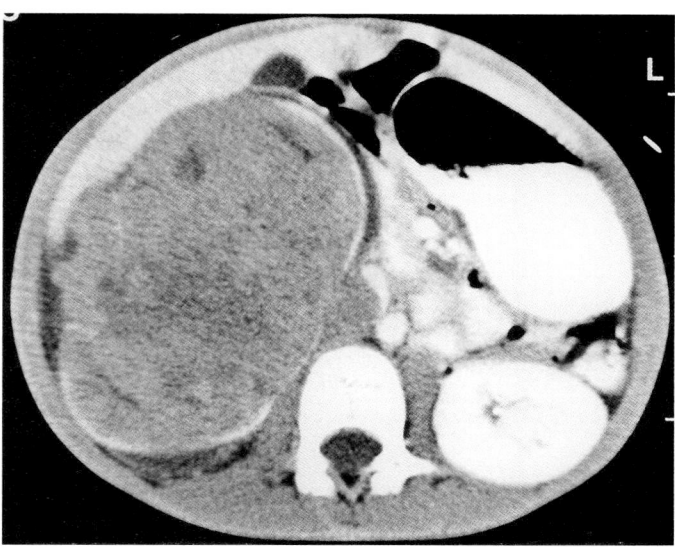

Fig. 20.4 CT revealing a large Wilms tumor replacing the right kidney. Notice that the renal cortex, enhanced by contrast medium, is splayed out around the mass. This characteristic helps differentiate Wilms tumor from neuroblastoma, which would displace a normal-appearing kidney.

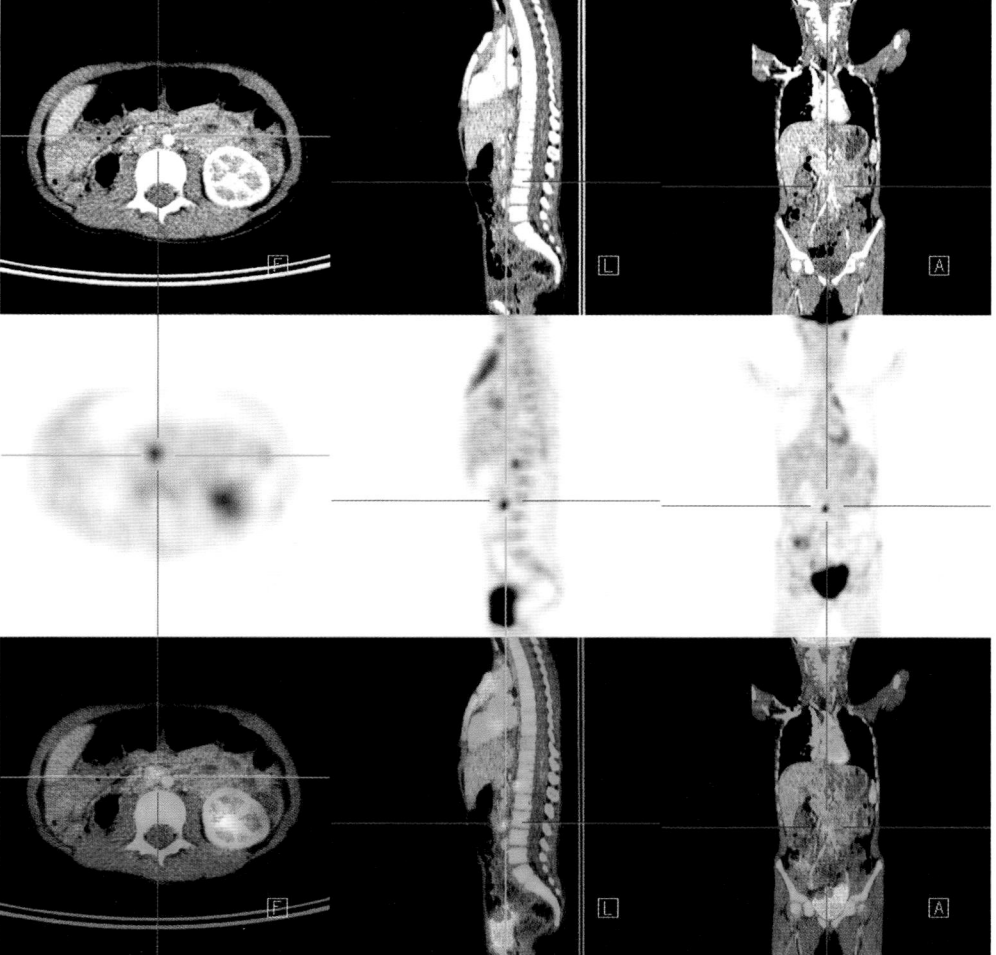

Fig. 20.5 Recurrent anaplastic Wilms tumor with multiple sites of ^{18}F-fluorodeoxyglucose (FDG)-avid disease. Standard CT scan *(top)*. PET scan *(middle)*. PET/CT scan *(bottom)*. (From Murphy JJ, Tawfeeq M, Chang B, et al. Early experience with PET/CT scan in the evaluation of pediatric abdominal neoplasms. *J Pediatr Surg.* 2008;43:2186–2192 [Fig. 2, p. 2188].)

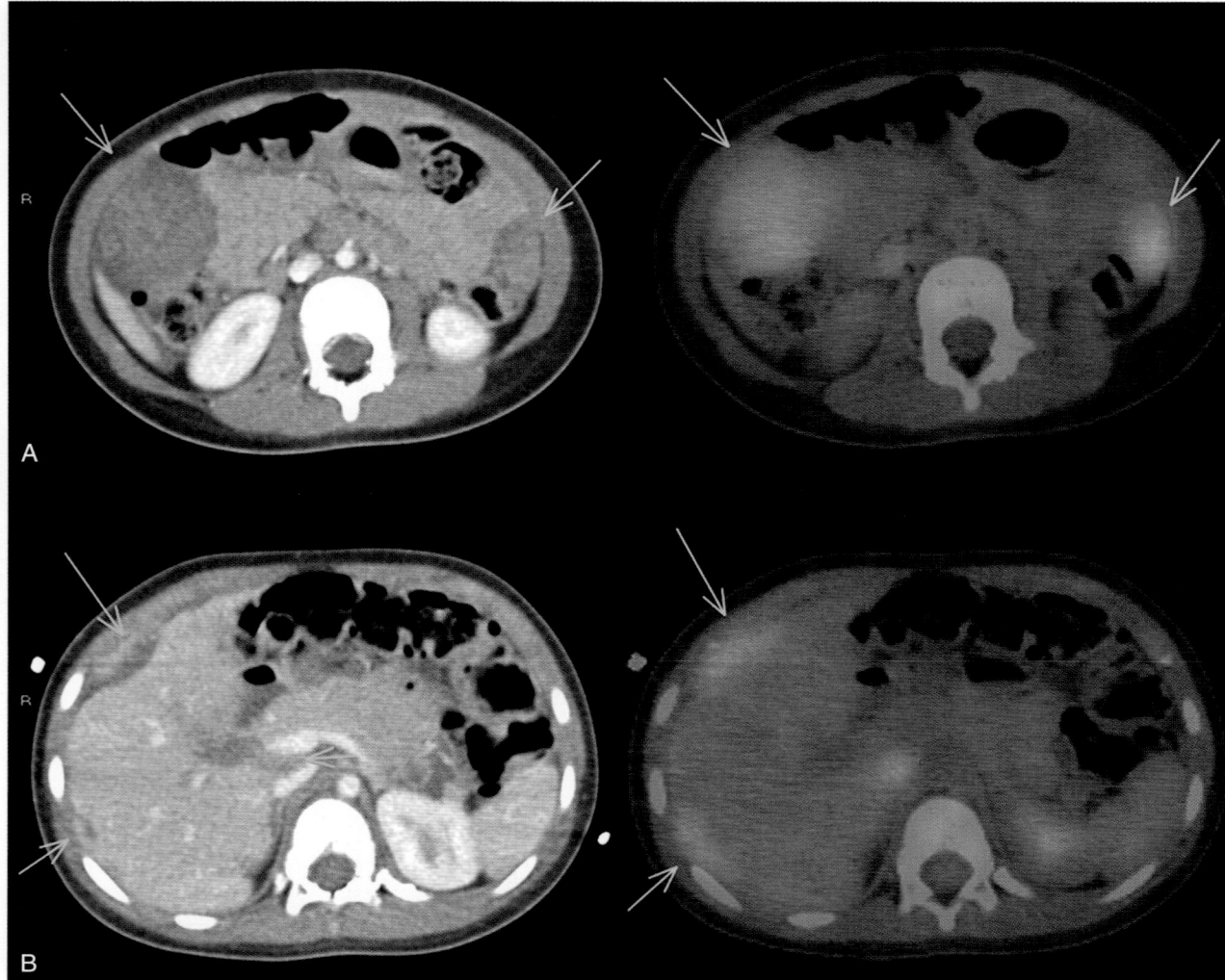

Fig. 20.6 CT (*A*) and PET/CT (*B*) of the abdomen and pelvis, showing multiple FDG-avid peritoneal masses throughout the abdominal cavity. (From Kruger E, Obasaju P, Dunn E, et al. Desmoplastic small round cell tumor presenting as an inguinal mass in a 2-year old boy. *J Pediatr Surg Case Rep.* 2020;58:101479. Fig. 2.)

leukemia, lymphoma, histiocytosis, hemophagocytic lymphohistiocytosis), hematologic disorders (thalassemia, hereditary spherocytosis), and conditions that cause distention of the sinusoids whenever there is increased pressure in the portal or splenic veins (portal hypertension) (Table 20.5). In addition, palpable spleens in children and adolescents are not always indicative of disease. A palpable spleen (≤2 cm below the left costal margin) is a normal finding in a child younger than 3 years and may be a normal finding in an older child. Up to 15% of full-term neonates, 10% of children, and 3% of college freshmen have palpable spleens unassociated with an increase in lymphoreticular malignancy and with equivalent health. However, a spleen that is palpable >2 cm below the left costal margin should be evaluated further. Masses that may be mistaken for splenomegaly include the left lobe of the liver, a left upper quadrant tumor such as Wilms or neuroblastoma, a spleen that is displaced by obstructive lung disease such as asthma or bronchiolitis, or a gastric bezoar. Painful splenomegaly generally follows stretching of the splenic capsule with rapid enlargement of the spleen. Malfixed "wandering" spleens may undergo torsion, presenting the upper pole to the abdominal wall as a prominent painful abdominal mass. Splenic enlargement that is noted not in the context of an acute illness (i.e., it is noted incidentally, for instance, on a well-child examination or checkup) is more likely to be caused from a chronic process such as a storage disease

than splenomegaly that is noted in the context of an acute illness. Acute onset of splenomegaly is most characteristic of an acute infection or a rapidly progressive malignancy (acute leukemia, lymphoma). Chronic splenomegaly (present for ≥1 month) is much more likely to represent a chronic process, such as storage diseases, congestive processes (portal hypertension, congestive heart failure), hemolysis, chronic infection, or inflammation. Massive splenomegaly (a spleen that crosses the midline or reaches the pelvis) indicates leukemia, lymphoma or other lymphoproliferative syndromes (post-transplant, familial hemophagocytic lymphohistiocytosis), hemoglobinopathy, Langerhans cell histiocytosis, visceral leishmaniasis, or a storage disease.

History

Birth and medical history, including transplacentally acquired infections, especially congenital syphilis, are often associated with splenic enlargement. History of a neonatal umbilical venous catheter, perhaps accompanied by occult portal venous injury or thrombosis, may progressively obstruct the extrahepatic portal vein, leading to congestive splenomegaly. Recurrent infections suggest immunodeficiency. Liver disease may lead to portal hypertension, which may in turn lead to splenomegaly. Congestive heart failure and associated congenital cardiac malformations have an increased risk of abdominal heterotaxia

TABLE 20.5   Differential Diagnosis of Splenomegaly by Pathophysiology

ANATOMIC LESIONS

Cysts, pseudocysts

Hamartomas

Polysplenia syndrome

Hemangiomas and lymphangiomas

Hematoma or rupture (traumatic)

Peliosis

HYPERPLASIA CAUSED BY HEMATOLOGIC DISORDERS

Acute and Chronic Hemolysis*

Hemoglobinopathies (sickle cell disease in infancy with or without
  sequestration crisis and side variants, thalassemia major, unstable
  hemoglobins)

Erythrocyte membrane disorders (hereditary spherocytosis, elliptocytosis,
  pyropoikilocytosis)

Erythrocyte enzyme deficiencies (severe G6PD deficiency, pyruvate kinase
  deficiency)

Immune hemolysis (autoimmune and isoimmune hemolysis)

Paroxysmal nocturnal hemoglobinuria

Chronic Iron Deficiency

Extramedullar Hematopoiesis

Myeloproliferative diseases: CML, juvenile CML, myelofibrosis with myeloid
  metaplasia, polycythemia vera

Osteopetrosis

Patients receiving granulocyte and granulocyte-macrophage colony-stimulating
  factors

INFECTIONS†

Bacterial

Acute sepsis: *Salmonella typhi, Streptococcus pneumonia, Haemophilus
  influenzae* type b, *Staphylococcus aureus*

Chronic infections: infective endocarditis, chronic meningococcemia,
  brucellosis, tularemia, cat-scratch disease

Local infections: splenic abscess (*S. aureus,* streptococci, less often *Salmonella*
  spp., polymicrobial infection), pyogenic liver abscess (anaerobic bacteria,
  gram-negative enteric bacteria), cholangitis

Viral*

Acute viral infections

Congenital CMV, herpes simplex, rubella

Hepatitides A, B, and C; CMV

EBV

Viral hemophagocytic syndromes: CMV, EBV, HHV-6

HIV

Spirochetal

Syphilis, especially congenital syphilis

Leptospirosis

Rickettsial

Rocky Mountain spotted fever

Q fever

Typhus

Fungal/Mycobacterial

Miliary tuberculosis

Disseminated histoplasmosis

South American blastomycosis

Systemic candidiasis (in immunosuppressed patients)

Parasitic

Malaria

Toxoplasmosis, especially congenital

Toxocara canis, Toxocara cati (visceral larva migrans)

Leishmaniasis (kala-azar)

Schistosomiasis (hepatic-portal involvement)

Trypanosomiasis

Fascioliasis

Babesiosis

IMMUNOLOGIC AND INFLAMMATORY PROCESSES*

Systemic lupus erythematosus

Juvenile idiopathic arthritis

Mixed connective tissue disease

Systemic vasculitis

Serum sickness

Drug hypersensitivity, especially to phenytoin

Graft versus host disease

Sjögren syndrome

Cryoglobulinemia

Amyloidosis

Sarcoidosis

Autoimmune lymphoproliferative syndrome

Post-transplant lymphoproliferative disease

Large granular lymphocytosis and neutropenia

Histiocytosis syndromes

Hemophagocytic syndromes (nonviral, familial)

MALIGNANCIES

Primary: leukemia (acute, chronic), lymphoma, angiosarcoma, Hodgkin disease,
  mastocytosis

Metastatic

STORAGE DISEASES

Lipidosis (Gaucher disease, Niemann-Pick disease, infantile GM1
  gangliosidosis)

Mucopolysaccharidoses (Hurler, Hunter-type)

Mucolipidosis (I-cell disease, sialidosis, multiple sulfatase deficiency,
  fucosidosis)

Defects in carbohydrate metabolism: galactosemia, fructose intolerance,
  glycogen storage disease IV

Sea-blue histiocyte syndrome

Tangier disease

Wolman disease

Hyperchylomicronemia type 1, IV

CONGESTIVE DISEASE*

Heart failure

Intrahepatic cirrhosis *or* fibrosis

Extrahepatic portal (thrombosis), splenic, and hepatic vein obstruction
  (thrombosis, Budd-Chiari syndrome)

*Common.

†Chronic or recurrent infection suggests underlying immunodeficiency.

CML, chronic myelogenous leukemia; CMV, cytomegalovirus; EBV, Epstein-Barr virus; G6PD, glucose-6-phosphate dehydrogenase; HHV-6, human herpesvirus 6.

From Kliegman RM, St. Geme JW III, Blum NJ, et al., eds. *Nelson Textbook of Pediatrics.* 21st ed. Philadelphia: Elsevier; 2020:2620, Table 513.1.

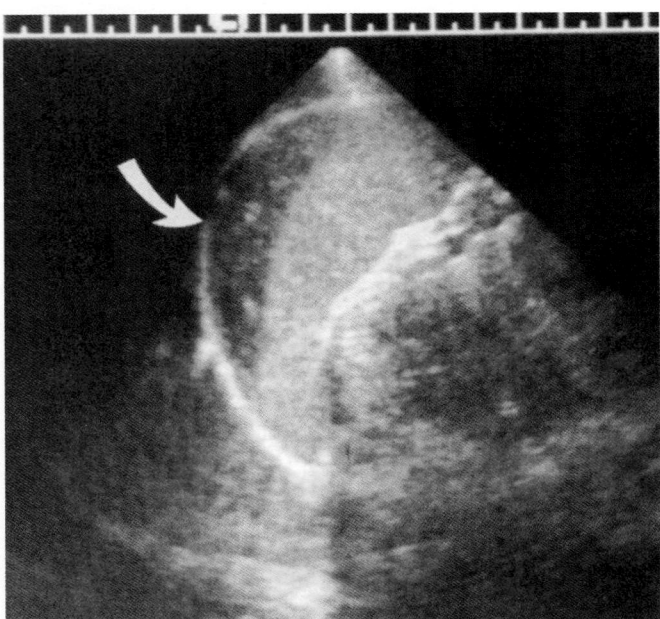

Fig. 20.7 The subcapsular splenic hematoma *(arrow)* in a 15-year-old boy who had been in a motor vehicle crash was best seen on coronal scans through the left intercostal spaces.

with splenic malformation and splenomegaly. Abdominal trauma may acutely produce a splenic hematoma (Fig. 20.7) or may be followed by development of a chronic splenic pseudocyst.

A family history of anemia, transfusions, early biliary stones, cholecystectomy, and splenectomy may indicate hemolytic anemia. Identification of Mediterranean (thalassemia, glucose-6-phosphate dehydrogenase [G6PD] deficiency), African (sickle cell disease, G6PD deficiency), southern Asian (thalassemia, G6PD deficiency), or Ashkenazi Jewish (storage disease) ancestry in patients with splenomegaly is helpful in identifying an inherited process.

Social and behavioral issues of parents, children, and adolescents heavily affect certain risks and exposures. Sexual encounters and intravenous and illicit drug exposure may expose patients to hepatitis, cytomegalovirus, and HIV. Sexual abuse may place even young children at risk; it may be difficult to elicit an accurate history.

A review of systems in a patient with splenomegaly should elucidate related conditions. Systemic symptoms, such as fever or weight loss, are seen in many disorders that manifest splenomegaly, particularly infections, malignancies, and inflammatory or granulomatous processes, such as hemophagocytic lymphohistiocytosis (HLH) and sarcoidosis. When fever is acute in onset, infection is most likely. Chronic fever, often gradual in onset and not associated with chills, is more likely to be caused by inflammatory processes (systemic lupus erythematosus [SLE], juvenile idiopathic arthritis [JIA], sarcoidosis, Langerhans cell histiocytosis) or tumors (lymphomas, especially Hodgkin disease, or leukemia). Exposure to infectious agents or a travel history that might result in exposure to infectious agents unusual for the patient's community (malaria, leishmaniasis, schistosomiasis, trypanosomiasis for U.S. citizens with a travel history to an endemic country) should be determined. Pallor suggests anemia (hemolysis, bone marrow infiltration, hypersplenism); purpura and petechiae suggest thrombocytopenia (bone marrow failure, autoimmune disorder, hypersplenism, bone marrow infiltration); and jaundice and conjunctival icterus suggest hemolytic anemia, liver dysfunction, or both. Rashes caused by a variety of acute and chronic infections and inflammatory diseases

(SLE, JIA, infective endocarditis, HLH) and hemangiomata that are part of a systemic process involving the spleen may provide clues to splenic disease. Dyspnea, cough, orthopnea, and fatigue suggest respiratory disease (Langerhans cell histiocytosis or sarcoidosis), anemia, congestive heart failure, or malignancy (Hodgkin disease). Diarrhea caused by *Salmonella* infection or inflammatory bowel disease may be accompanied by splenic enlargement. Abdominal pain accompanied by splenomegaly may be attributable to acute splenic capsule distention or caused by coincident gallstones, hepatitis, or trauma. Joint pain resulting from SLE, JIA, and other autoimmune inflammatory diseases may be associated with splenomegaly. Bone pain is a feature of bone marrow infiltrative processes, particularly leukemia or neuroblastoma or storage disease (Gaucher disease). Poor vision in an infant with splenomegaly suggests osteopetrosis (with deafness) or uveitis-iritis (sarcoidosis, JIA). Loss of developmental milestones occurs with storage diseases. Splenomegaly may accompany neurologic paraneoplastic syndromes (such as myasthenia gravis) secondary to lymphoma or lymphoproliferative syndromes.

Physical Examination

Nutritional status and growth parameters provide clues to disorders that affect the patient's metabolic state and tissue oxygenation. Malnutrition (as evidenced by such problems as weight loss and failure to thrive) in a child with splenomegaly suggests malignancy, chronic hemolysis, immunodeficiency or chronic infection, a metabolic disorder, or liver disease. Pallor, petechiae, purpura, jaundice, hemangiomata, septic emboli to the skin, infiltrative lesions (leukemia cutis, solid tumors), seborrhea, or eczema (as occurs in Langerhans cell histiocytosis and immunodeficiency) should be noted. Cherry-red retinal spots or cloudy corneas suggest storage diseases. Conjunctival pallor, scleral icterus, fundal hemorrhages, evidence of sinus infection or otitis media, condition of gingivae, and evidence of salivary gland enlargement should be noted. The clinician should look for signs of heart failure or new or changing murmurs, which suggest valvular or other structural heart disease or endocarditis. Any respiratory distress, rales, rhonchi, or suggestion of pneumonia or asthma should be noted. Abdominal distention, prominent veins on the abdomen, hepatomegaly, fluid wave, tenderness, or rebound should be noted, as should specific characteristics and size of the spleen itself. A hard or nodular spleen suggests malignancy or chronic hemolysis. A tender spleen suggests either acute enlargement or infection, or both. A spleen that is more than 5 cm below the left costal margin is usually not transient and represents significant disease. Arthritis, splinter hemorrhages, and poor bone growth (as occurs in storage diseases and osteopetrosis) should be noted. Size, texture, mobility, tenderness, and distribution of lymph nodes should be noted. Enlarged (>1 cm), firm, fixed lymph nodes are suggestive of lymphoma or leukemia. Tender enlarged lymph nodes are suggestive of more common infections. Developmental delay suggests chronic infection, immunodeficiency, or storage diseases.

Approach to the Child with Splenomegaly

The most common cause of splenomegaly in childhood is viral infection, which should induce only moderate splenomegaly (<5 cm below the left costal margin) that is transient, lasting <4–6 weeks. Other common causes include autoimmune disorders and destruction of abnormal blood cells (such as brisk hemolysis). The approach to the child with splenomegaly is affected by several key factors, each of which indicates the probability of significant disease necessitating diagnosis and intervention (Fig. 20.8A and B).

Laboratory Investigation

Table 20.6 summarizes key diagnostic laboratory investigations.

TABLE 20.6 Summary of Laboratory Investigations for Suspected Diagnosis with Splenomegaly

Suspected Diagnosis	Tests to Be Performed
Hemolysis	CBC, reticulocyte count, blood smear, serum bilirubin measurement, Coombs test, osmotic fragility study, RBC enzyme assays, hemoglobin electrophoresis
Infection	CBC, differential, blood cultures, viral studies (EBV, CMV, HIV), toxoplasmosis, Bartonella titers, TB test, malaria blood smear, PCR testing and/or blood smear for babesiosis, CRP, procalcitonin
Liver disease	Liver function tests, albumin measurement, prothrombin time, α_1-antitrypsin, serum copper, ceruloplasmin
Portal hypertension	Liver function tests; albumin measurement; prothrombin time; ultrasonography/CT of portal veins, liver, and spleen
Immunologic and inflammatory disease	ESR, CRP, C3, C4, antinuclear antibody, rheumatoid factor measurements; ferritin, urinalysis; BUN, serum creatinine, and immunoglobulin measurements
Infiltrative disease	CT, enzyme assay for Gaucher disease, tests as indicated for other storage diseases
Malignancy	CBC with differential, peripheral smear, CXR, uric acid, LDH, CT, bone marrow aspiration
Genetic syndrome	Molecular DNA testing or whole exome sequencing

CMV, cytomegalovirus; CXR, chest x-ray; EBV, Epstein-Barr virus; LDH, lactate dehydrogenase; PCR, polymerase chain reaction; RBC, red blood cell; TB, tuberculosis.

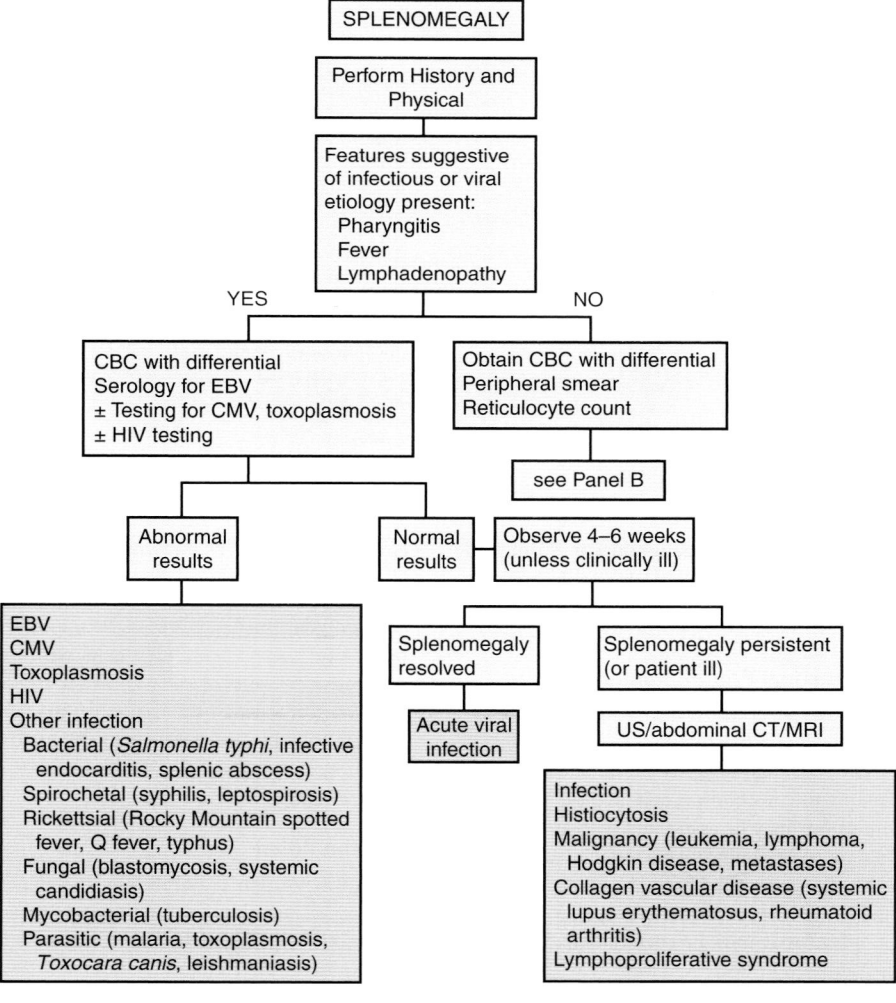

A

Fig. 20.8 *A and B,* Approach to the child with splenomegaly. CMV, cytomegalovirus; CXR, chest x-ray; EBV, Epstein-Barr virus; G6PD, glucose-6-phosphate dehydrogenase; MAS, macrophage activation syndrome; RBC, red blood cell; US, ultrasonography. (Adapted from Pomeranz A, Sabnis S, Busey S, et al. *Splenomegaly: Pediatric Decision-Making Strategies.* 2nd ed. Philadelphia: Elsevier; 2016:106–109.)

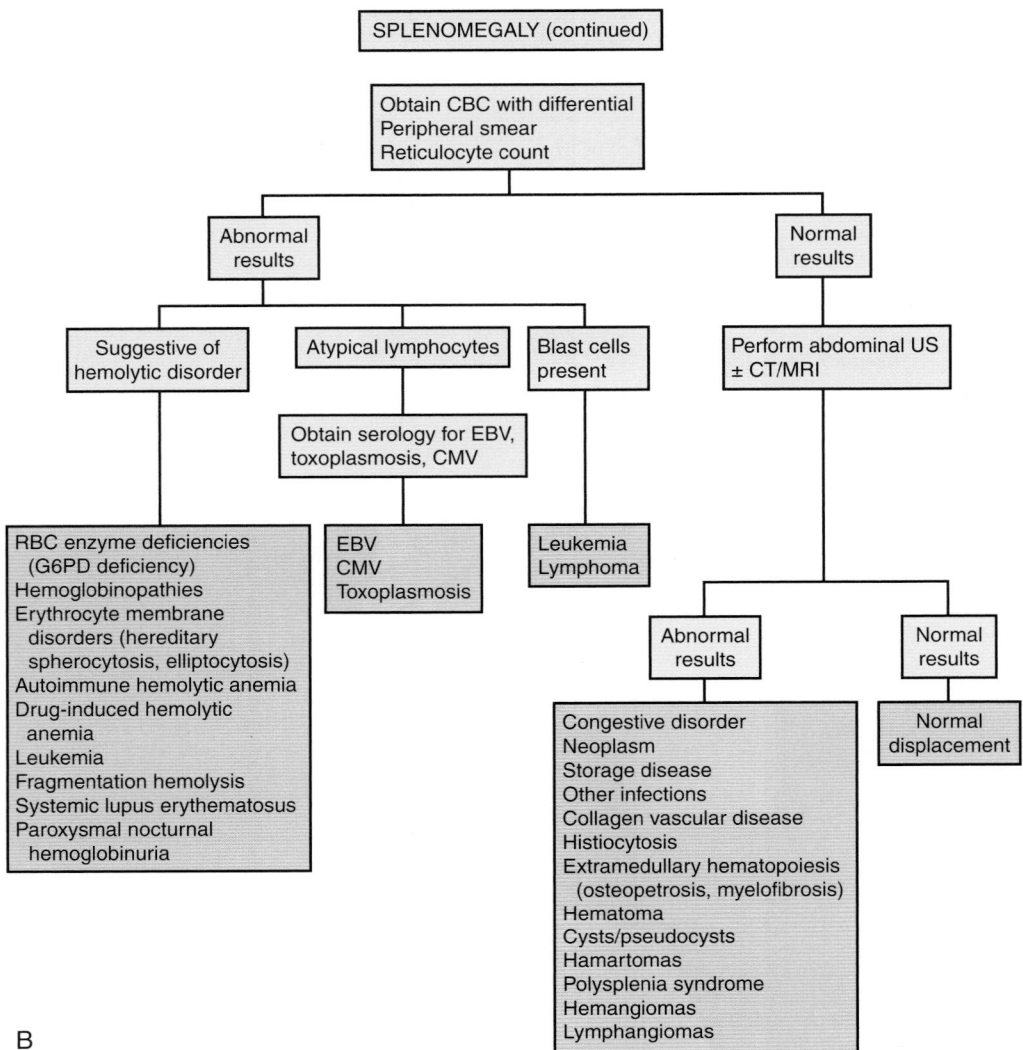

B

Fig. 20.8, cont'd

Complete Blood Cell Count

A CBC is the first test indicated in all patients with undiagnosed spleno-megaly. This count provides extensive information about hematologic, infectious, and inflammatory processes; the result may also be abnormal in patients with hypersplenism caused by portal hypertension.

Leukocyte Count, Differential, and Procalcitonin

A white blood cell (WBC) count above or below the normal range for age, the neutrophil count, the lymphocyte count, and the presence of abnormal cells (atypical lymphocytes, blasts) should be noted. Viral infection is the most common cause of splenomegaly in children, and atypical lymphocy-tosis may be a clue. Viral infections may be associated with an increased (early) or decreased WBC count. Most significant bacterial infections pro-duce neutrophilia and reactive changes in the neutrophils. Infections with intracellular bacteria or some viruses may produce neutropenia. Addition-ally, an elevated procalcitonin level may indicate bacterial infection. Leu-kemia can manifest with an increased or decreased total WBC count. The presence of blasts is confirmatory, but they are not always present.

Hemoglobin, Erythrocyte Morphology, and Reticulocyte Count

Hemolytic anemia may be unsuspected without examination of the blood smear and the reticulocyte count (see Chapters 49 and 50).

Malarial parasites may be seen on the blood smear but may be missed unless a thick preparation is examined. Clues found on the blood smear include spherocytes (present in hereditary spherocytosis and hemolytic anemias); elliptocytes (present in hereditary elliptocyto-sis); polychromasia, poikilocytes, and fragmented cells (present in hemolytic anemias); sickled cells with target cells, spherocytes, and nucleated red blood cells (present in sickle cell anemia and vari-ants); and microcytosis, hypochromia (present in thalassemias), and Howell-Jolly bodies (present in splenic dysfunction). Hypersplenism (pooling or sequestration of blood cells in an enlarged spleen) may cause anemia.

Platelet Count

Thrombocytopenia (<150,000 platelets/mm³) may be caused by decreased platelet production or increased platelet destruction. Production is diminished in conditions characterized by bone mar-row infiltration (leukemia, neuroblastoma). Increased destruction accompanies immunologic processes, drug reactions, HLH, and viral infections. Thrombocytosis (>400,000 platelets/mm³) often accom-panies iron-deficiency or acute infection as an acute-phase reac-tant. Sequestration of platelets within an enlarged spleen may cause thrombocytopenia.

Pancytopenia

Pancytopenia implies bone marrow dysfunction, bone marrow infiltration, or portal hypertension with hypersplenic destruction of all the formed elements of the blood (see Chapter 50). A bone marrow aspiration and biopsy should be performed in any child with splenomegaly and pancytopenia. Tests of liver function, including prothrombin time and albumin, are indicated.

Viral Antibody Titers

Viral antibody titers for Epstein-Barr virus (EBV) and cytomegalovirus should be obtained when a mononucleosis syndrome is present, especially when splenomegaly persists. Heterophile antibody tests are rapid and have a sensitivity of 85% for EBV in older children and adolescents but are not sensitive in children younger than 4 years. Specific serologic testing for EBV is useful in these younger children. The results of these tests rarely affect management but may permit a presumptive diagnosis of a self-limited process to be made, and they may preclude more invasive tests such as imaging and/or bone marrow examination. Toxoplasmosis should also be considered. Primary infection with HIV frequently causes splenomegaly. Acute infection with HIV may not be noted on screening labs, and therefore additional testing may be required.

Erythrocyte Sedimentation Rate and C-Reactive Protein

Elevation of the ESR is nonspecific but suggests infection, especially bacterial, mycobacterial, or fungal infection, or an inflammatory process, such as JIA, HLH, or SLE. The ESR may be normal despite significant inflammation, for example, when there is severe anemia or hypofibrinogenemia. The CRP level may be elevated when the ESR is normal.

Liver Function Tests

Liver function tests are indicated if splenomegaly is significant (>2 cm) or persists longer than 1 month. Portal hypertension is often asymptomatic until hepatic fibrosis is far advanced. Liver synthetic function (albumin, prothrombin time, fibrinogen), direct bilirubin levels, and transaminase levels should be assessed.

Immunologic Evaluation

Immunologic evaluation is needed when autoimmune disorders (JIA, SLE) or immunodeficiency disorders (inherited or acquired) are suspected. This assessment includes measurements of antinuclear antibody titer, immunoglobulin levels, and immunoglobulin subclass levels; tests of neutrophil function; and measurements of T-cell subclasses. Repeated infections stimulate the immune system and may cause splenomegaly.

Cultures

Bacterial, fungal, and other cultures may be necessary and are dictated by the suspected infection.

Genetic Testing

Splenomegaly is a feature in many genetic conditions. A search for splenomegaly on the Online Mendelian Inheritance in Man (OMIM) website returns 205 clinical syndromes for which the molecular basis is known. After a thorough work-up does not reveal a cause for splenomegaly, molecular testing including whole exome sequencing (WES) may be appropriate, especially if there are dysmorphisms, developmental delay, or multiple organ system involvement.

Bone Marrow Examination

Bone marrow examination is appropriate for diagnosing infiltrative processes (acute leukemia and other malignancies), HLH, and some infections that may be difficult to diagnose from other tissues

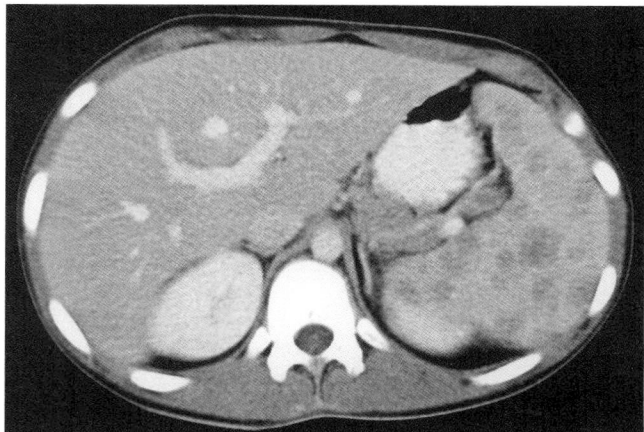

Fig. 20.9 Abdominal CT scan of a 15-year-old with fever, weight loss, and orthopnea. The diagnosis was Hodgkin disease. The spleen shows hypoechoic lesions, typical of lymphoma.

(disseminated histoplasmosis, miliary tuberculosis, bacterial endocarditis, and other chronic infections, especially in immunocompromised patients). While lysosomal storage disorders (Gaucher disease, Niemann-Pick disease, Tay-Sachs disease) may be identified through bone marrow examination in patients for whom malignancy is initially suspected, enzyme and genetic testing are preferred over bone marrow biopsy for the diagnosis of these conditions.

Imaging

Chest radiography is simple and may reveal hilar adenopathy or a mediastinal mass when malignancy is suspected. Imaging of the spleen has several roles but should be performed selectively. It is useful for the confirmation of splenic size, assessment of splenic architecture, and evaluation of other organs involved in the differential diagnosis. It can be useful in determining whether there are other abdominal masses that suggest widespread involvement by tumor, and if there is silent portal hypertension.

The choice of imaging depends on the questions to be asked. Ultrasonography has been the preferred method of imaging as it does not require radiation and is used to assess size and perfusion and to visualize cysts and other lesions. Guidelines are available for the upper limit of normal splenic length (measured as the greatest longitudinal distance between the dome of the spleen and the tip). Doppler flow ultrasonography can detect portal hypertension.

CT of the spleen can define focal lesions (Fig. 20.9) and nonfocal enlargement, as well as evaluate the splenic and portal veins and the vasculature of the spleen. Less common in children than in adults, splenic cysts and pseudocysts may manifest with palpable spleens (Fig. 20.10). Both CT and ultrasonography identify such cysts well, and they also image the pancreas. Pancreatitis is a common cause of splenic cysts. Subcapsular hematoma can also be visualized by ultrasonography. Splenic lacerations are seen well on CT (Fig. 20.11). Persistent splenomegaly after systemic infections may be caused by splenic abscesses, which are visualized with ultrasonography (Fig. 20.12). CT is an alternative imaging procedure for each of these problems.

SPLENECTOMY

Surgery plays an important role in the management of splenomegaly due to congenital hemolytic anemias. Laparoscopic splenectomy procedures have been demonstrated to significantly decrease sequestration events in both hereditary spherocytosis and sickle cell disease. Partial

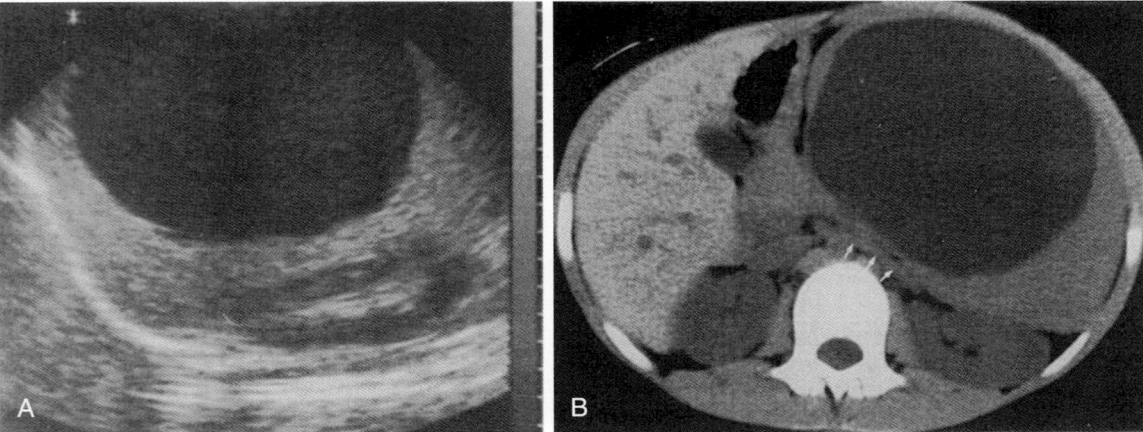

Fig. 20.10 The large epidermoid cyst of the spleen in a boy, shown on ultrasonography *(A)*, is shown by CT scan *(B)* to compress the left renal vein *(arrows)*. The boy presented with varicocele.

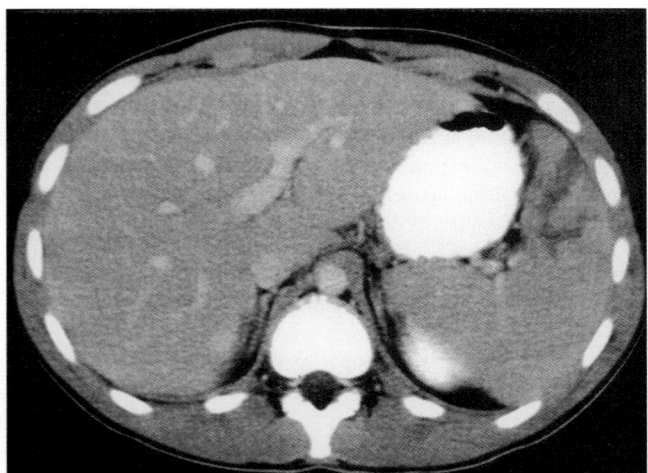

Fig. 20.11 Splenic laceration that resulted from trauma in a 15-year-old boy.

splenectomy outcomes are durable in 5-year follow-up with only a 4.8% failure rate according to the congenital hemolytic anemia registry. The use of partial splenectomy may be helpful in hereditary spherocytosis where total splenectomy has been associated with pulmonary artery hypertension, thrombosis, and overwhelming postsplenectomy sepsis. Pediatric surgeons initiated nonoperative approaches for the management of splenic lacerations resulting from trauma. The American Association for the Surgery of Trauma grading scales for splenic injury have been employed to prospectively follow outcomes in stable pediatric trauma patients. Patients with grade I–II lacerations are confined to bed for 24 hours, and those with grade III–V lacerations are confined to bed for 48 hours with restriction of activity for grade plus 2 weeks postinjury. Even for the highest grades of injury, the need for splenectomy due to hemorrhage and clinical deterioration is <5%.

NEUROBLASTOMA

Neuroblastoma is the most common extracranial solid malignancy in childhood. It accounts for 10% of all childhood tumors and 15% of pediatric cancer deaths. The incidence of neuroblastoma is approximately 10.2 per million U.S. children under age 15 and is more common in males than in females (1.2:1). The tumor affects primarily children younger than 8 years, and more than 50% occur in children older than 2 years of age. Pathologic genetic or gene variant of neural crest cells giving rise to the primitive sympathetic innervation leads to tumor formation. Seventy-five percent of the tumors are abdominal, and 65% of these originate in the adrenal medulla or lumbar sympathetic ganglia. The biology of neuroblastoma is exceptionally heterogeneous as mature lesions, particularly in neonates, may regress spontaneously or mature into more benign forms of ganglioneuroblastoma or ganglioma. Unpredictably, other lesions may degenerate despite intensive chemotherapy. As a derivative of sympathetic ganglia, this tumor produces catecholamines (90%) and expresses surface disialoganglioside 2 (GD2). These features are exploited via MIBG scans and GD2 epitope-directed immunotherapy. Multiple genetic associations have been made including alterations in MYCN and anaplastic lymphoma receptor tyrosine kinase (ALK) variants. MYCN amplification has important prognostic consideration and can lead to postsurgical upstaging and alteration in chemotherapy. Gain-of-function variants in ALK have provided therapeutic targets with ALK inhibitors, including sorafenib. Both staging and multimodal therapy of neuroblastoma are rapidly changing landscapes as interventions become more targeted with the additional aim of decreasing secondary malignancy. Presurgical staging has coalesced competing staging systems into the International Neuroblastoma Risk Group staging system (INRGSS). Isolated lesions <3.1 cm (solid) or 5 cm (cystic) are observed in infants under 6 months of age, and low-risk lesions in older children may be amenable to surgical resection alone.

Toddlers present with progressive abdominal distention or abdominal discomfort. The mass is retroperitoneal and tends to encase rather than displace vessels and viscera. Catecholamine production by the tumor occasionally results in flushing, sweating, and irritability. Vasoactive intestinal polypeptide, also produced by the tumor, may cause secretory diarrhea. A variety of neurologic symptoms (opsoclonus-myoclonus) may also be seen, as may weight loss and anorexia. Most patients have metastases at the time of diagnosis, mainly to regional and distant lymph nodes, bone marrow and bone cortex, the orbit, the liver, and occasionally the lungs. Signs and symptoms related to metastases include bone pain, proptosis, and skin lesions.

Diagnostic studies must define relative anatomy and size of the tumor and determine regional invasion, metastatic disease, function, and ultimately histologic features. In 90% of patients, high levels of catecholamines and their detectable metabolites (homovanillic and vanillylmandelic acid) are found in spot urine samples. Twenty-four-hour urine collections show no additional sensitivity. Ferritin remains

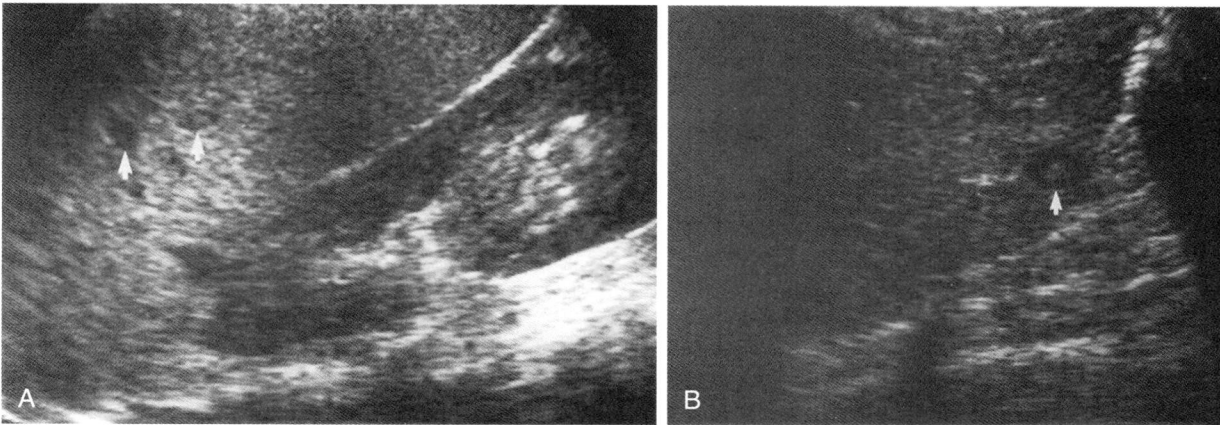

Fig. 20.12 A 10-year-old girl had been treated for acute myelogenous leukemia. She had taken multiple antibiotics for recurrent infections. Unremitting fevers then developed. Candidiasis was strongly suspected, and ultrasonography was requested. Two weeks after the clinical suspicion of candidiasis was raised, obvious focal defects *(arrows)* could be seen within the spleen *(A)* and liver *(B)*.

a useful serum marker, while neuron-specific enolase is more relevant in tumor biopsy immunohistochemistry. A CBC may show anemia. In 50% of cases, a plain radiograph shows finely stippled tumor calcifications and displacement of gas-filled bowel loops. Ultrasonography confirms its solid nature and position in relation to the kidney. CT or MRI should be completed with arterial and venous phase contrast prior to biopsy or resection (Fig. 20.13). Axial imaging may reveal any intraspinal extension of the tumor or its metastases. Bone marrow metastases are detected by bone marrow aspiration. PET scans identify sites of recurrent or residual metastatic lesions. MIBG uptake is useful to study pretherapy to assess the role of MIBG-based therapy (I-131) as part of the multimodal plan.

Surgical resection is the primary treatment of localized neuroblastoma. Two exceptions to this rule exist—neonates with stage MS disease (primary lesion, cutaneous, hepatic, and/or bone marrow metastases) and infants up to 1 year of age with stage L1 small adrenal or periadrenal tumors. In these cases careful observation may be employed with intervention for disease progression. Adjuvant chemotherapy and radiotherapy are employed postoperatively, depending on the stage of the disease. For initially unresectable tumors, a diagnostic open biopsy is preferred to needle biopsy, and preferably retroperitoneally. Bone marrow aspiration findings, necessary for staging, may demonstrate classic small, round blue cells forming rosettes. For large encasing tumors surrounding major vasculature, neoadjuvant chemotherapy may be employed following biopsy and prior to resection. This strategy has been shown to improve resectability, the goal being to achieve >90% tumor volume reduction at resection. In high-risk neuroblastoma, at least four cycles of high-dose chemotherapy precede resection, followed by postoperative radiation therapy, autologous stem cell rescue, and continued chemotherapy. The use of differentiating agents, such as retinoic acid, is indicated in high-risk disease. Interleukin 2 (IL-2), granulocyte macrophage colony-stimulating factor (GM-CSF), and anti-GD2 therapy are also used in high-risk protocols. Staging is based on the regional extension of the tumor, the level of metastatic disease, and the degree of resection. The outcome of the patient is determined primarily by the child's age, tumor stage, histologic classification, and MYCN amplification. Hyperploid DNA is associated with a lower stage and better prognosis (contrary to most other tumors). Overall 5-year neuroblastoma survival is 81% (>95% low risk, >90% intermediate risk, and >40% high risk), a striking shift considering that this tumor was uniformly fatal 30 years ago.

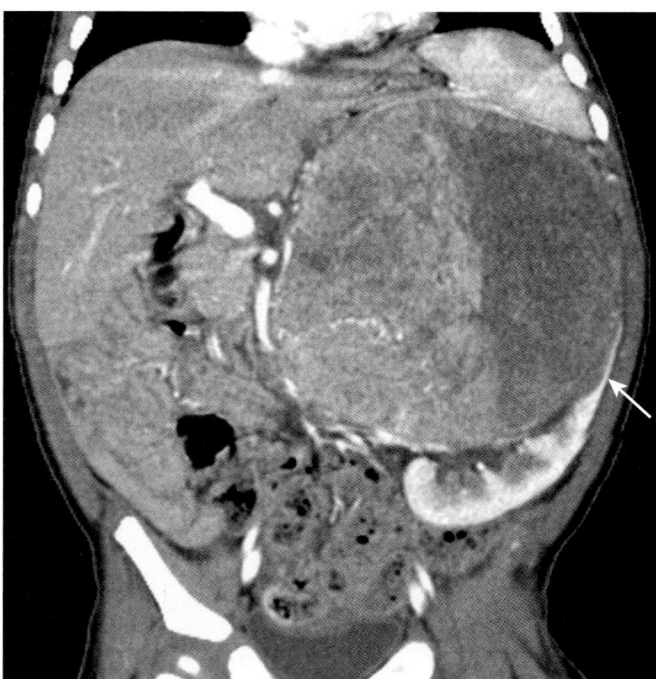

Fig. 20.13 Left adrenal neuroblastoma in a 9-month-old girl. Coronal contrast-enhanced CT image shows a large heterogeneous retroperitoneal mass invading the left kidney. The left kidney is displaced caudally and laterally with suggestion of a partial "claw sign" *(arrow)*, which may lead to the erroneous interpretation that the mass is arising from the left kidney. (From Navarro OM, Daneman A. Acquired conditions. In: Colley BD, ed. *Caffey's Pediatric Diagnostic Imaging.* 13th ed. Philadelphia: Elsevier; 2019:1175, Fig. 122.8.)

RENAL MASSES

The most common causes of a renal mass in neonates and infants are congenital (bilateral or unilateral) hydronephrosis and congenital multicystic-dysplastic kidney (often unilateral). In older infants and toddlers, Wilms tumor (nephroblastoma) emerges as the leading cause. Ultrasonography immediately reveals whether the mass is solid or cystic, thus directing further investigation. An ectopic or horseshoe midline kidney may also be palpable.

Congenital Hydronephrosis

Hydronephrosis secondary to ureteropelvic obstruction due to aberrant renal artery or adhesion may result in a flank mass discovered in the neonatal period or in later childhood. It is more common in males and on the left side. The most common presenting symptom in infants is an abdominal mass or urinary tract infection. In older children, distention of the renal pelvis may cause intermittent pain, and hematuria may occur following minor abdominal trauma.

The diagnosis is confirmed with ultrasonography. A voiding cystourethrogram excludes ureterovesical reflux and posterior urethral valves (in males). Diuretic renal scintigraphy is useful to demonstrate degree of obstruction and relative renal function. Treatment consists of pyeloplasty with resection of the obstruction.

Prenatally diagnosed dilated renal pelvis occurs in 1% of pregnancies and rarely requires fetal intervention (Fig. 20.14). Postnatally, these infants will spontaneously resolve in over 90% of cases. Higher rates of intervention are required in infants with bilateral involvement, advanced grades of calyceal dilatation with parenchymal thinning (Society of Fetal Urology [SFU] grade III/IV), high-grade reflux, and bladder wall thickening. Males with bilateral hydronephrosis should undergo urologic evaluation for presence of obstructing posterior urethral valves.

Cystic Abnormalities of the Kidney

A unilateral multicystic-dysplastic kidney (MCDK) usually manifests as a flank mass in the newborn. Ultrasonography demonstrates a cystic kidney with absence of renal parenchyma and decreased function and readily allows for evaluation of the contralateral kidney. MCDK is differentiated from advanced hydronephrosis by lack of continuity between parenchymal cysts and the collecting system. Treatment rarely consists of surgical excision as the majority of lesions slowly involute and are not associated with increased risk of malignancy. Earlier reports combined cystic Wilms tumor with MCKD, now realized to be discretely different lesions. MCKD requiring resection includes those resulting in continued growth and rarely uncontrolled hypertension or pain. Voiding cystourethrogram (VCUG) is rarely indicated, as MCKD is associated with a very low rate of ureteral reflux.

In the more serious case of autosomal recessive infantile polycystic disease (1/20,000 live births), both kidneys are affected. The kidneys are filled with thousands of small cysts derived from the collecting tubules. The clinical manifestation varies, depending on the degree of renal failure. Unfortunately, 30% of newborns die with pulmonary failure and almost 50% of patients experience severe renal insufficiency before the age of 15 years. The neonatal form is fatal without dialysis and then renal transplantation. Abdominal ultrasonography discloses the cystic nature of the condition, and diuretic renal scintigraphy shows symmetrically diminished function. Following peritoneal dialysis, renal transplantation is the definitive management.

Wilms Tumor (Nephroblastoma)

Wilms tumor (WT) is an embryonal renal neoplasm, one of the most common childhood abdominal malignancies. The estimated incidence is close to 1 in 15,000 live births, with a male-to-female ratio of 0.9:1. The mean age at diagnosis is 3.5 years, and at least 90% of the patients present before the age of 8 years. Between 4% and 10% of children have bilateral disease with a mean age of 2.5 years. Associated conditions include aniridia, hemihypertrophy, genitourinary anomalies, and Beckwith-Wiedemann syndrome. WT arises in precursor lesions called nephrogenic rests, which may be intra- or extralobar and usually spontaneously regress. The tumor suppressor gene *WT1* (11p13) and the transcription factor *WT2* (11p15) are associated with Wilms pathogenesis. Germline variants in these genes induce Wilms-associated syndromes (Denys-Drash, Wilms tumor–aniridia–genitourinary malformation–mental retardation), which are rare. Loss of heterozygosity at 1p and 16q is associated with higher relapse rates, upstages lesions, and is more resistant to current chemotherapy. Microscopic hematuria is present in about 30% of patients. In rare cases, obstruction of the left renal vein may induce a left-sided varicocele via the gonadal vein. Other less common symptoms or signs include anemia, polycythemia, weight loss, hypertension, or frank hematuria.

In infants and toddlers, the most useful imaging modality is a CT scan of the abdomen with arterial and venous phase contrast due to the speed of the study and high resolution afforded for surgical planning (Fig. 20.15). The location, size, and resectability of the tumor; presence of local

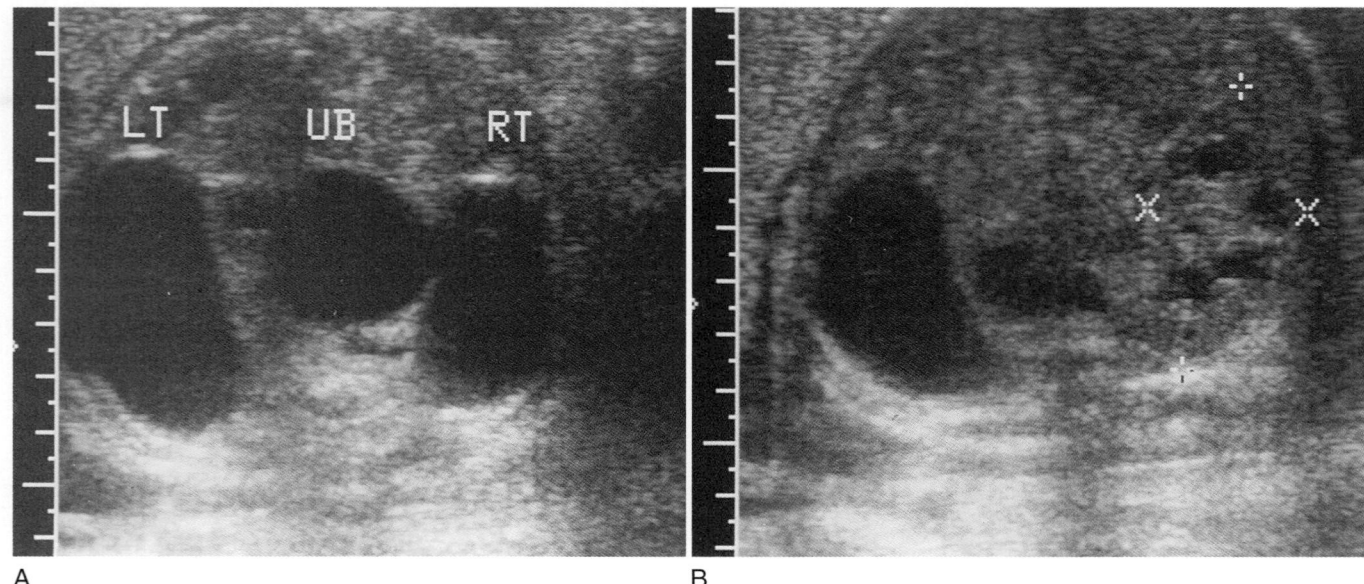

A   B

Fig. 20.14 Fetal ultrasonography showing bilateral hydronephrosis. *A,* The urinary bladder (UB) is seen between the two dilated renal pelvises (LT and RT). *B,* The renal cortex is seen on the right side of the same fetus, between the two Xs.

tumor invasion; and infiltration of the renal vein and inferior vena cava are assessed. Metastatic or bilateral disease must be ruled out. Differentiation of WT from neuroblastoma on axial imaging is based on whether the renal pelvis is splayed by an intrinsic renal mass or simply displaced by a suprarenal mass. In WT, lung metastases from the renal vein and inferior vena cava infiltration may be present, whereas bone metastases are rare; these features distinguish it from neuroblastoma. In some cases, however, the overwhelming size of the tumor may make differentiation between WT and neuroblastoma challenging. A chest CT scan should be completed.

Treatment includes a transabdominal nephrectomy with early ligation of the renal vein to avoid tumor mobilization. Chemotherapy and radiotherapy are added postoperatively, depending on the stage and histologic features of the tumor. For very large or complex tumors, especially those with extension of the tumor into the renal vein, inferior vena cava, and right atrium, preoperative chemotherapy has been employed in selected patients following tumor biopsy. In cases of bilateral disease, partial resection with nephron-sparing surgery is employed. For children with excessive loss of functional renal parenchyma, transplantation is an option.

Tumor staging is based on radiographic evaluation (metastatic disease) and intraoperative findings (tumor size, extrarenal extension of the tumor, tumor spillage, status of local lymph nodes). The stage determines the prognosis and treatment of the disease. Survival depends on the prognostic factors, cytogenetics, the histologic features of the tumor, and the age of the patient. Younger patients have a better prognosis. Most children have either stage I or stage II disease (regional extension of the tumor but complete surgical removal), and most cases of WT have favorable histologic features. Overall, the 5-year survival rate for favorable histology tumors exceeds 90%, with steadily decreasing chemotherapeutic toxicity and radiation exposure called for in evolving treatment protocols. This adjustment in therapy is a model for other cancer types, the result of an ongoing collaboration between the National Wilms Tumor Study (NWTS) Group in the United States and the Societe International D'oncologie Pediatrique (SIOP) group in Europe. Similarly, the amount of cross-sectional imaging used for post-treatment surveillance is steadily decreasing to keep ionizing radiation exposure "as low as reasonably achievable" (ALARA). The late complications of therapy for WT include the development of acute myelogenous leukemia, short stature, and congestive heart failure.

LIVER TUMORS

Hepatomegaly or a hepatic mass may be caused by infection (hepatitis, abscess, cyst), storage disease, extramedullary hematopoiesis, and benign or malignant lesions. Primary liver tumors are uncommon in

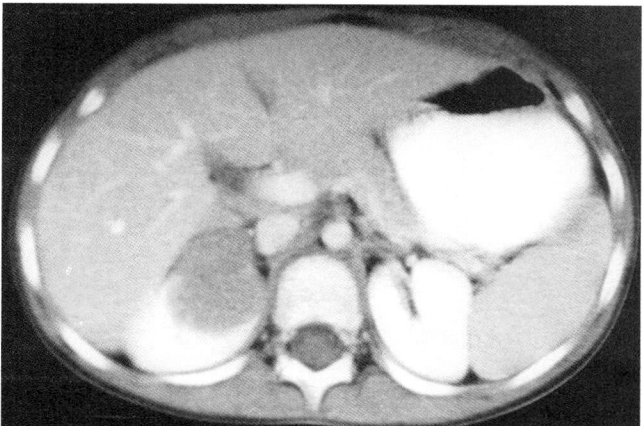

Fig. 20.15 An exophytic Wilms tumor noted incidentally on a CT obtained for trauma.

children, but when they occur, 66% are malignant. Hepatoblastomas predominate, followed by hepatocellular carcinoma, mesenchymoma, and rarely sarcoma.

Hepatic abscesses are caused by pathogens such as *Staphylococcus aureus*, anaerobic bacteria, or *Escherichia coli*. Chronic granulomatous disease, appendicitis, or immunocompromised state may predispose a child to this complication. Amebic infection of the liver caused by *Entamoeba histolytica* and parasite infestation with *Echinococcus* species may also lead to abscess formation in tropical climates. Abscesses are treated with appropriate antibiotics and percutaneous drainage, only rarely requiring surgical intervention.

Benign tumors can be of either mesenchymal or epithelial origin. Mesenchymal tumors include disorders such as hamartomas, cavernous hemangiomas, and infantile hemangioendotheliomas in young children. These conditions manifest as asymptomatic abdominal masses. Hemangiomas, particularly diffuse ones, may be difficult to resect and should be managed nonoperatively unless complications develop. Hamartomas, which usually manifest in the first year of life, should be resected. Epithelial lesions include focal nodular hyperplasia, hepatic adenoma, and nonparasitic solitary or multiple cysts.

The initial radiographic evaluation for liver masses should include plain abdominal radiography to detect calcifications and the mass effect, and ultrasonography to determine the origin, size, and echogenicity of the tumor. In addition, an abdominal CT or MRI scan can be obtained to define the exact localization and extent of the tumor (Fig. 20.16). MRI is more capable of discerning hamartomatous versus malignant lesions than CT scan, especially using EOVIST, a gadolinium agent preferentially taken up by hepatocytes. Angiography is often

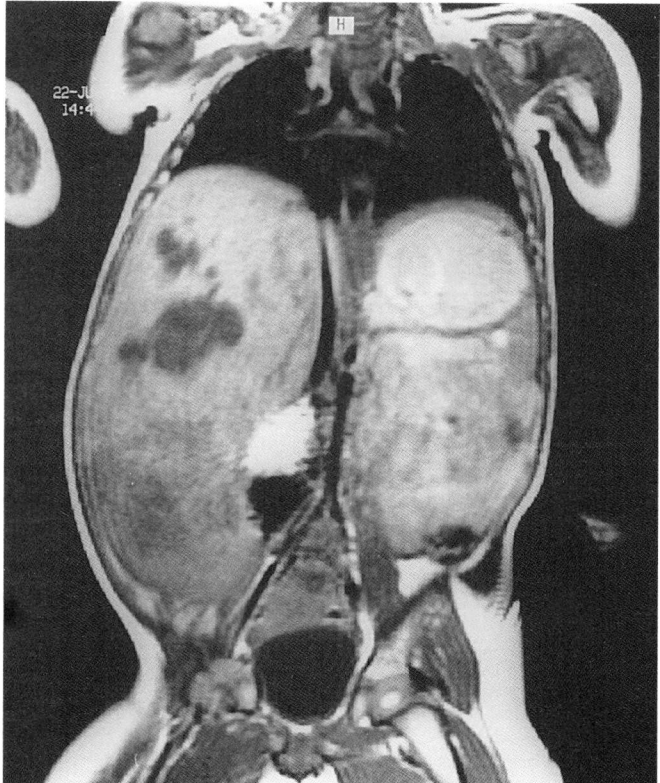

Fig. 20.16 MRI showing a liver hamartoma in a 13-month-old boy. Note the excellent visualization of the blood vessels. The child presented with abdominal distention, poor appetite, and decreased activity. The liver was nontender and was palpated 15 cm below the costal margin. Operative resection was successful.

useful for determining resectability. Chest radiography or CT is used to determine the presence of pulmonary metastases.

Hepatoblastoma

Hepatoblastoma is the most common primary liver tumor in children under 3 years of age affecting 1.5 per 1 million live births, and it is twice as common in males as in females. Premature birth and very low birthweight are associated with increased risk. The most common presentation is a child with a palpable abdominal mass, occasionally associated with anemia, nausea, vomiting, weight loss, or abdominal pain. An unusual manifestation is precocious puberty resulting from tumor secretion of human chorionic gonadotropin. Elevated levels of serum α-fetoprotein are seen in about 90% of cases, and this feature is helpful in the post-therapy monitoring of disease activity. Ultrasonography, MRI, or CT (Fig. 20.17) may be used to image the lesion and assign a PRETEXT (PRETreatment EXTent of Disease) stage. Designed by the International Childhood Liver Tumor Strategy Group (SIOPEL), PRETEXT classifies tumors into four risk groups based upon the number of contiguous uninvolved liver segments as well as metastatic, portal venous, or systemic venous invasion (Fig. 20.18). The goal is to accurately predict resectable lesions and plan for transplantation when appropriate without the complications associated with attempted resection in all cases, as surgical resection of hepatoblastoma is the mainstay of therapy. Core needle biopsy and neoadjuvant chemotherapy are undertaken in unresectable lesions, and axial imaging is repeated. Hepatic transplantation may be undertaken when lesions remain unresectable in the absence of metastatic disease. While PRETEXT I lesions portend a 100% 5-year survival, PRETEXT IV lesions confer 63% 5-year event-free survival with resection and platin-based therapy. Early consultation and use of liver transplantation is the current most effective therapy for advanced stage lesions. Pretreatment variables associated with survival are the extent of the tumor, histologic classification, and the presence of metastases.

Hepatocellular Carcinoma

Hepatocellular carcinoma, more common in adults, usually occurs in an already diseased liver, such as that found after hepatitis B or C virus infection, tyrosinemia, galactosemia, biliary atresia, or cirrhosis. It is

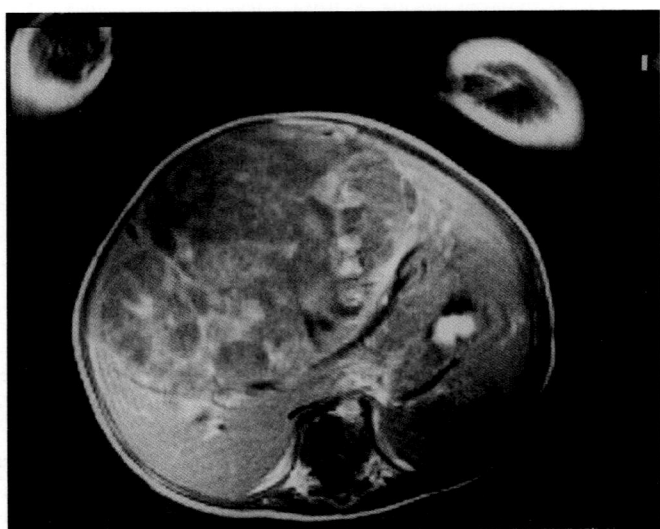

Fig. 20.17 CT of a hepatoblastoma in an 8-month-old girl. The child presented with hepatomegaly, increased abdominal girth, weight loss, and lethargy. The voluminous tumor occupies a large part of the upper abdominal cavity.

PRETEXT (*PRETreatment EXTent of disease*)

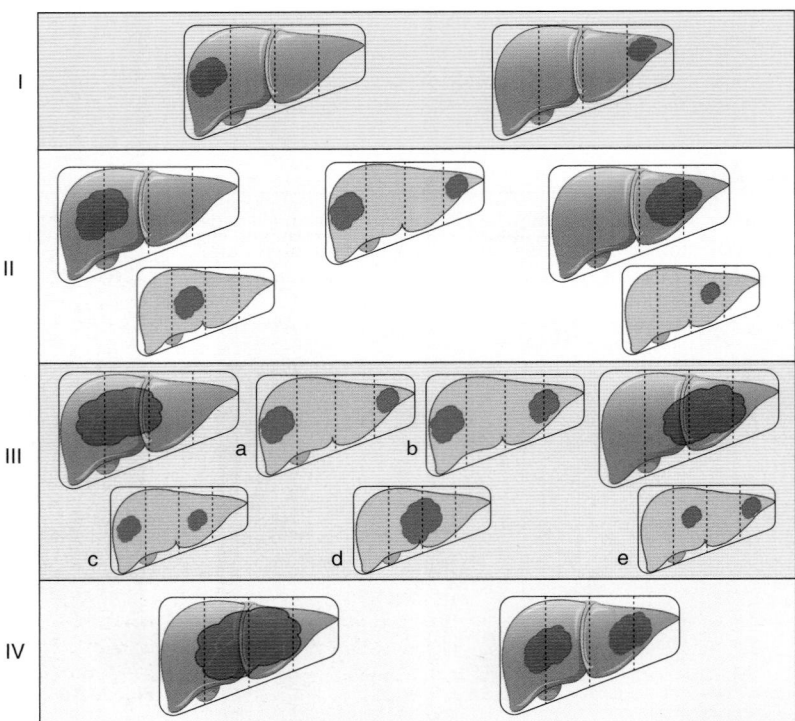

PRETEXT
= Extent of tumor at diagnosis

POSTTEXT
= Extent of tumor after
  neoadjuvant chemotherapy

I ... 3 contiguous sections tumor free
II ... 2 contiguous sections tumor free
III ... 1 contiguous section tumor free
IV ... no contiguous sections tumor free

In addition, any group may have:
V ... ingrowth vena cava, all 3 hepatic veins
P ... ingrowth portal vein, portal bifurcation
E ... extrahepatic
C ... caudate
M ... metastasis

Fig. 20.18 PRETEXT classification of hepatic tumors. Staging considers number of uninvolved contiguous liver segments. (From Meyers R, Aronson D, Zimmermann A. Malignant liver tumors. In: Coran A, ed. *Pediatric Surgery*. 7th ed. Philadelphia: Saunders; 2012:463–482.)

rare in younger children and has a peak incidence between the ages of 10 and 15 years. The tumor manifests as a painful abdominal mass; in more than 65% of patients, it is unresectable. In these cases and in the absence of metastatic disease, liver transplantation should be considered. The diagnostic evaluation, staging, and treatment of hepatocellular carcinoma are similar to those of hepatoblastoma. Tyrosine kinase inhibitors such as sorafenib have emerged as significant treatment adjuncts in the pediatric patient population.

CONGENITAL DILATATION OF THE BILE DUCTS

Any congenital cystic dilatation of the bile ducts is commonly called choledochal cyst. There are several anatomic varieties of this condition, and the cause remains unknown. The most common choledochal cyst is seen when the common bile duct is grossly dilated (Todani type I, Fig. 20.19). However, the size varies, and the child may remain asymptomatic for many years. About 20% of patients present with the classic triad of jaundice, pain, and a right upper quadrant abdominal mass. Obstructive jaundice may result from coincident gallstones, manifesting in pruritus, dark urine, and acholic stools.

Ultrasonography reveals the location, size, and nature of the cyst. If there is any doubt about its origin, magnetic resonance cholangiopancreatography (MRCP) or liver-phase CT scan (Fig. 20.20) may be used to outline the biliary tract and help differentiate it from other lesions such as duodenal duplication. Treatment consists of resection of the cyst and drainage of the hepatic duct into an intestinal segment (Fig. 20.21). Incomplete resection of at least the mucosa of the affected portion of the biliary tree predisposes the patient to the development of cholangiocarcinoma, which is a 20–30% lifetime risk in this population.

INTESTINAL AND PANCREATIC MASSES

Appendiceal Phlegmon and Abscess

Either delayed manifestation (walled off by mesentery) or delayed diagnosis of acute appendicitis may enable the development of a right lower quadrant mass after perforation as the inflamed tissues amalgamate into a phlegmon. Further maturation of this process may lead to an abscess. Diagnosis is often facilitated by the history, which can differentiate from many other causes of abdominal mass by the recent (days to weeks) history of fever associated with abdominal pain and nausea. Antibiotic therapy may mask the diagnosis of appendicitis. Ultrasound is the preferred primary diagnostic modality and may be used in many cases to guide percutaneous drainage (Fig. 20.22). Interval appendectomy in an uninflamed field may be performed safely 6–8 weeks later and is particularly useful in patients without obstructive symptoms. This approach is not appropriate either for suspected uncomplicated acute appendicitis with an appendicolith or for diffuse peritonitis.

Intussusception

Intussusception occurs when peristalsis of a lead point attached to the intestinal wall results in telescoping of proximal intestine into distal intestine causing luminal obstruction. Abdominal pain, vomiting, "currant-jelly stools," and lethargy are common. Two thirds of patients are younger than 2 years of age; the peak incidence is late in the first year of life. Ileocolic intussusception is usually caused by benign ileal lymphoid hyperplasia, whereas ileoileal intussusception or intussusception in an older child should raise concern for a pathologic lead point. An abdominal mass may be palpated in 25% of patients as a "sausage" in the upper abdomen. Ultrasound may be obtained if the

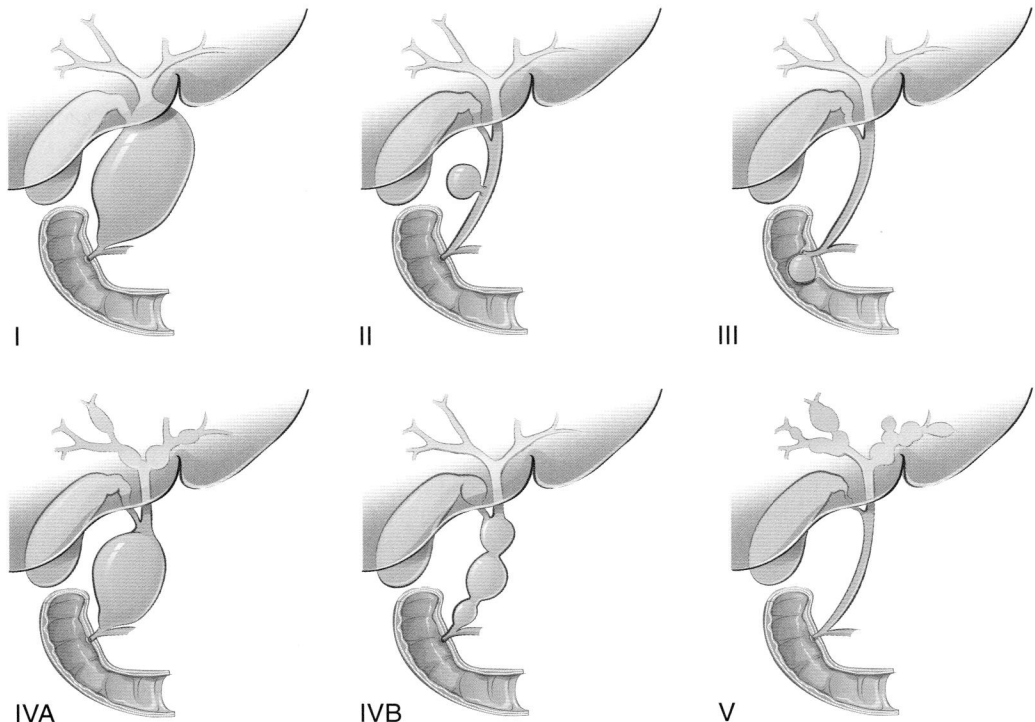

I   II   III

IVA   IVB   V

Fig. 20.19 Todani classification of choledochal cysts. (From Michaelis S, Kalache K. Biliary anomalies. In: Copel J, ed. *Obstetric Imaging*. 1st ed. Philadelphia: Saunders; 2012:114–120; redrawn from Callen PW. *Ultrasonography in Obstetrics and Gynaecology*. 5th ed. Philadelphia: Saunders; 2008.)

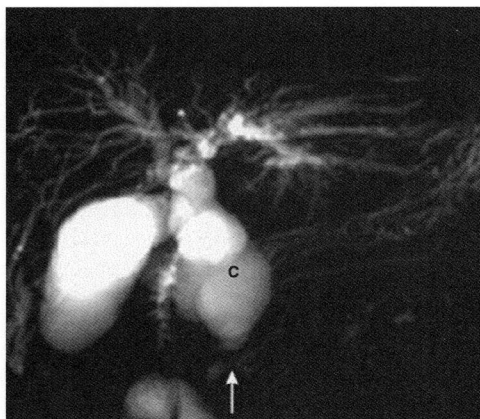

Fig. 20.20 Magnetic resonance cholangiopancreatography demonstrating a pediatric Todani type I choledochal cyst *(C)* and common bile duct–pancreatic duct junction *(arrow).* (From Lim J, Kim K, Choi D. Biliary tract and gallbladder. In: Haaga J, Dogra V, Forsting M, et al., eds. *CT and MRI of the Whole Body.* 5th ed. Philadelphia: Mosby; 2009:1373–1453.)

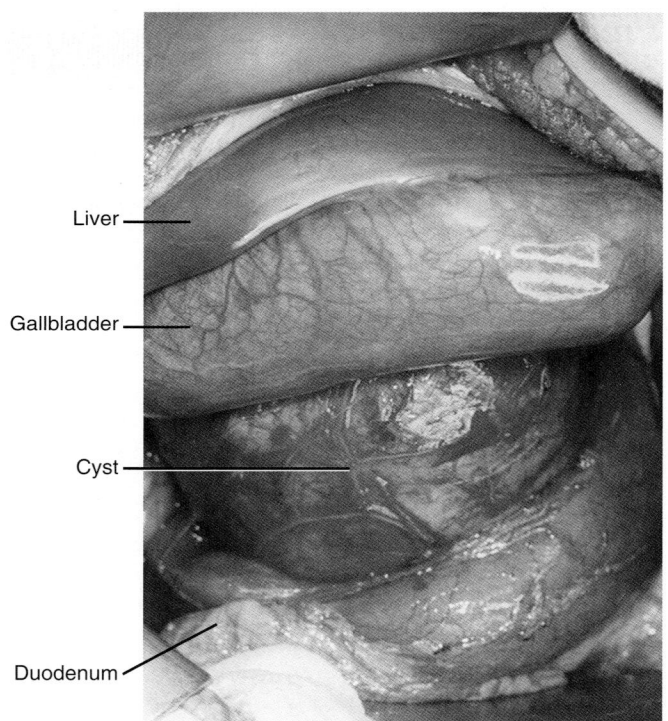

Liver

Gallbladder

Cyst

Duodenum

Fig. 20.21 Operative photograph of a choledochal cyst between the gallbladder and the duodenum, displacing both.

diagnosis is uncertain, but radiologic reduction enemas are diagnostic and therapeutic (see Chapter 13).

Bezoar

Children with psychiatric illness or developmental delay may eat their own hair (trichotillomania) or other indigestible material (e.g., persimmon peel). Most of these patients are females, usually in their teens. A trichobezoar (hair) or a phytobezoar (vegetable matter) forms in the stomach and causes partial gastric outlet obstruction. Gastric bezoars may massively distend the stomach and extend into the small intestine. If hair manages to pass the stomach, it collects in the duodenum and

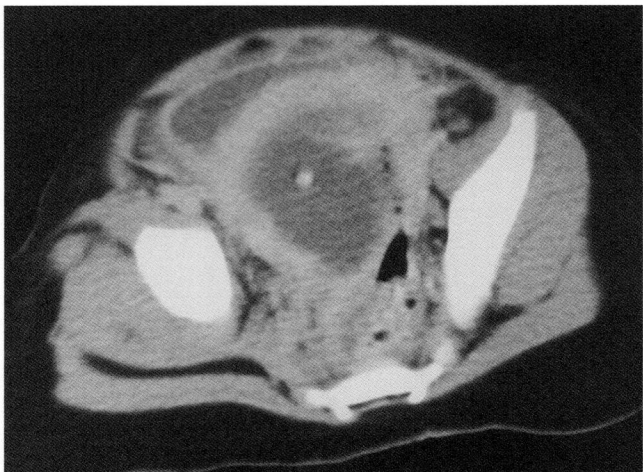

Fig. 20.22 A large appendiceal abscess with a calcified fecalith. The abscess was drained percutaneously and treated with antibiotics. Interval appendectomy was performed 8 weeks later.

causes biliary tract obstruction; if it collects in the ileum, it may lead to intestinal obstruction.

The clinical picture is characterized by poor appetite, vague abdominal discomfort, and intolerance to solid foods. Physical examination reveals loss of hair on the scalp and a movable mass in the epigastrium. Abdominal radiographs will show gastric outlet or intestinal obstruction. Axial imaging subsequently demonstrates the size and location. The bezoar may be removed endoscopically, but operative removal is most frequently required. Bacterial counts within a bezoar are extremely high, and operative removal is associated with a high rate of postoperative infection despite use of perioperative antibiotics and intraoperative wound protectors.

Intestinal Duplications

Duplications of the gastrointestinal tract occur anywhere from the esophagus to the anus and are either cystic or tubular. The more common cystic duplications are lined with endothelium and are enclosed in a muscular wall common with the adjacent intestinal segment. Tubular duplications are located on the mesenteric side of the bowel and are either blind or in communication with the bowel. The lining is usually that of the adjacent intestine but may be heterotopic, such as gastric mucosa in a duplication of the small bowel.

Duplications are often detected prenatally. When discovered, they should be resected after birth as volvulus has been seen as early as 2 postnatal weeks. In older children, the manifestations depend on the size and location of the malformation. Many intraabdominal duplications manifest as an asymptomatic, palpable mass but may also cause pain, intestinal obstruction, hemorrhage, or volvulus. Ultrasonography differentiates the cystic nature of duplications from solid tumors and also demonstrates the intimate association between the duplication and the bowel wall. Treatment consists of resection of the duplication alone or, more commonly, along with the portion of intestine from which the duplication arose, depending on the anatomic location and amount of shared wall and blood supply (Fig. 20.23).

Neoplasms of the Gastrointestinal Tract

Neoplasms of the gastrointestinal tract of children are rare. The symptoms are often nonspecific, and diagnosis tends to be delayed. A gastric teratoma may appear as an epigastric mass, while gastric leiomyomas manifest with bleeding. Gastrointestinal stromal tumors most commonly arise in the small intestine, can cause intussusception or

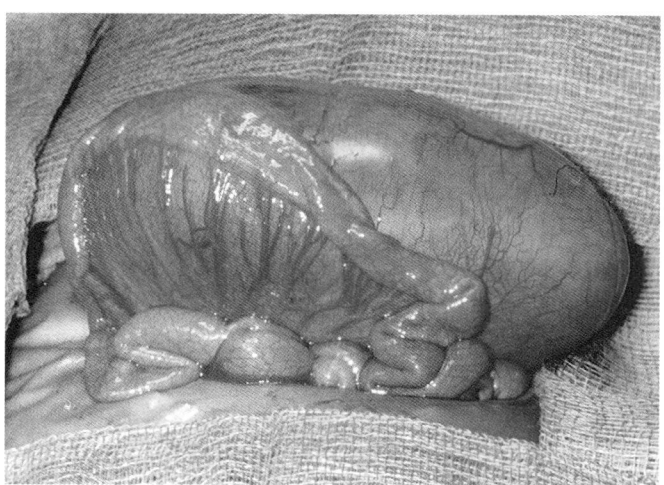

Fig. 20.23 Operative photograph of the typical appearance of an intestinal duplication.

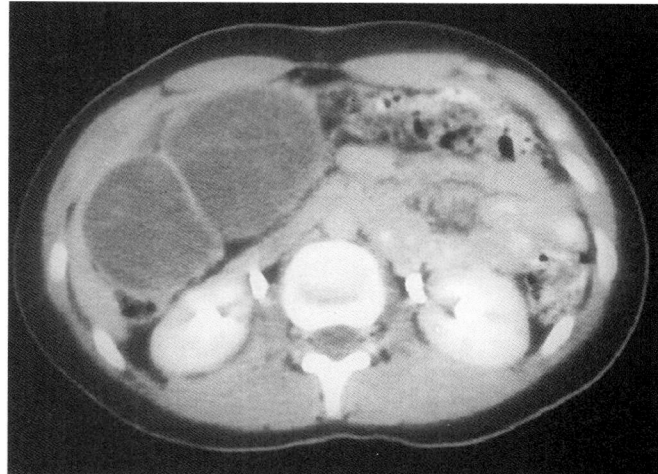

Fig. 20.24 CT scan of the abdomen in an 11-year-old male, showing a mesenteric cyst in the transverse mesocolon.

volvulus, and are highly sensitive to imatinib, a tyrosine kinase inhibitor. Non-Hodgkin lymphoma is the most common malignant tumor of the small intestine and may act as a lead point for intussusception. Other malignant tumors of the small intestine include angiosarcoma and carcinoid tumor. These conditions also occur in the large intestine. Carcinoid tumors are most commonly found in the appendix, where they can cause obstruction and may lead to appendicitis. The colon is the most common site for the rare adenocarcinoma of the gastrointestinal tract in children. Colon adenocarcinoma in children is usually nonsyndromic, mucinous in nature (80%), and often at an advanced stage upon discovery. Benign neoplasms of the small and large intestine include hemangiomas, lymphangiomas, leiomyomas, and polyps. Neoplasms of the intestine require resection for diagnosis and treatment.

Mesenteric, Omental, and Retroperitoneal Cysts

Benign cysts located in the omentum or mesentery can be simple or multilocular and contain clear serous fluid. They arise from a developmental abnormality of the lymphatic system that results in lymphatic obstruction. Most of these cysts are diagnosed during the first 5 years of life. They may be asymptomatic for years or manifest with a distended abdomen, abdominal mass, intestinal obstruction, volvulus, or abdominal pain. The abdomen is usually nontender with a mobile mass. In contrast to ascites, the flanks do not bulge when a child with an abdominal cyst is in the supine position.

A plain abdominal radiograph shows intestinal gas displaced forward in the case of a mesenteric cyst and backward in the case of an omental cyst. Small amounts of calcification may be seen in the wall of the cyst. Ultrasonography, MRI, or CT further elucidates the nature, size, and location of the cyst (Fig. 20.24). An ovarian, pancreatic, or choledochal cyst or an intestinal duplication may be difficult to differentiate from a mesenteric or omental cyst. Cerebrospinal fluid from a **ventriculoperitoneal shunt** or lumbar drain fails to be resorbed because of scarring of the peritoneum, leading to a "CSFoma" (Fig. 20.25), which also may be mistaken for a mesenteric or omental cyst. Treatment of these lesions consists of surgical marsupialization or extirpation, occasionally requiring segmental small bowel resection. Retroperitoneal lymphatic malformations are amenable to percutaneous sclerotherapy with good results.

Rare solid lesions include inflammatory myofibroblastic tumor, Castleman disease, mesenteric fibromatosis, desmoplastic small round cell tumors (Fig. 20.6), or rhabdomyosarcoma.

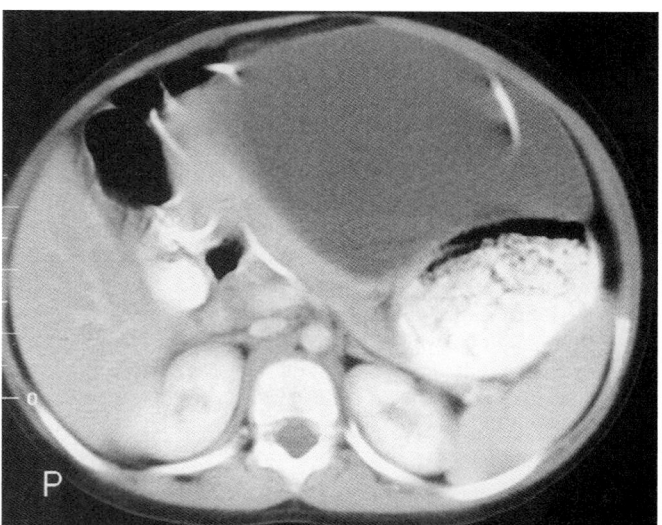

Fig. 20.25 A large fluid collection associated with a ventriculoperitoneal shunt ("CSFoma").

Pancreatic Pseudocyst and Neoplasms

Pancreatic tumors are rare in children and are cystic or solid, benign or malignant. Young children and infants may have pancreatoblastoma. Functional neoplasms arise from the islet cells, and the clinical manifestation is not of an abdominal mass but rather is characterized by the effects of the endocrine substances secreted by the tumor (e.g., hypoglycemia caused by insulinoma). Tumors arising from the acinar or ductal parts of the pancreas are nonfunctional and usually manifest as an abdominal mass. They may be benign (cystadenoma) or malignant (adenocarcinoma). Embryonic pluripotent cells may give rise to solid pseudopapillary tumors, accounting for <5% of all pediatric pancreatic masses. Metastases are common in pancreatic neoplasms given the frequent delay in diagnosis. Diagnosis is aided by ultrasonography, endoscopy, CT, or MRI and, in cases of suspected endocrine tumors, by measurements of active hormones. Both benign and malignant tumors should be surgically resected. Malignant non–multiple endocrine neoplasia pancreatic tumors in children are rare and include Ewing sarcoma family tumors, VIPoma, acinar cell carcinoma, and solid pseudopapillary tumor.

A pancreatic pseudocyst lacks epithelial lining and is the result of pancreatitis or pancreatic blunt trauma. Often, there is a symptom-free interval of several weeks or months between the trauma and the appearance of symptoms. The cause of pancreatic pseudocyst in the absence of trauma should prompt investigation of causes of recurrent pancreatitis including pancreas divisum and variants in *PRSS1* and *SPINK1* genes, allowing inappropriate release of pancreatic trypsin. Typical signs and symptoms are nausea, abdominal pain, and an epigastric mass. Ultrasonography and axial imaging locate the cyst and identify any displacement of the bowel. The cysts usually resolve spontaneously; however, if they do not, they should be drained percutaneously or into the gastrointestinal tract.

OVARIAN TUMORS

Ovarian tumors are common abdominal masses in females leading to 25 per 100,000 children's hospital admissions. They must be considered in any female with lower abdominal pain, an abdominal mass, or precocious puberty. They manifest at any age from birth to adulthood but occur slightly more frequently in children at an average of 13 years of age. The risk of malignancy increases with age. Cystic tumors are more common than solid tumors, and the majority of masses are benign. An ovarian lesion may also be the presenting manifestation of other metastatic diseases, such as neuroblastoma or rhabdomyosarcoma. Malignant gonadal tumors (dysgerminoma, gonadoblastoma) may be seen in females with gonadal dysgenesis and males with cryptorchidism. Other causes of adnexal mass include hydrosalpinx, pregnancy, and imperforate hymen leading to hydrocolpos or hydrometrocolpos.

Diagnosis is made by ultrasonography, which provides information on the size, consistency, location, perfusion, and wall characteristics of the tumor. Abdominal radiography may reveal calcifications. CT can locate local or distant metastases. Endocrinopathies are present in 5–10% of children with ovarian tumors, so consideration of the anterior pituitary–adrenal–gonadal axis is warranted. Levels of tumor markers, such as α-fetoprotein and β-human chorionic gonadotropin

(β-hCG), are uniformly helpful. CA-125 and inhibin A should be considered, especially in children older than 3 years of age, in solid masses >8 cm, with inappropriate virilization, or with other concerns for operative findings consistent with epithelial cancer. Germ cell tumors occur in the setting of a normal karyotype.

A simple cyst may appear in a neonate as a mobile abdominal mass or may even be detected incidentally by ultrasonography. Small cysts (generally <6 cm) can be monitored with ultrasonography and should spontaneously disappear. Larger cysts should be excised, because they can undergo torsion. The symptoms of ovarian torsion in an older child simulate those of appendicitis or ectopic pregnancy (see Fig. 20.26).

All other tumors of the ovaries should be excised, whether benign (cystic teratoma, cystic adenoma, granulosa cell tumor) or malignant (endodermal sinus tumor, yolk sac tumor, embryonal carcinoma, malignant teratoma, adenocarcinoma, dysgerminoma, choriocarcinoma). Great care should be taken to spare as much of the adnexa as possible to preserve future fertility. Unilateral salpingectomy with ovarian preservation is required in the case of symptomatic hydrosalpinx. Depending on the histologic appearance and stage, most malignant lesions should be treated postoperatively with chemotherapy. Survival depends on the nature of the lesion; however, with the exception of highly malignant tumors such as endodermal sinus tumors and embryonal carcinoma, the prognosis is good.

SOFT TISSUE SARCOMA

Soft tissue sarcomas arise from mesenchymal cells and are generally rare tumors. Rhabdomyosarcoma (RMS) arises from striated muscle and accounts for 4% of pediatric tumors, while nonrhabdomyosarcomatous soft tissue sarcoma (NRSTS) is much more heterogeneous and adds an additional 3% of incidence. RMS is the most common pelvic malignancy in children under 3 years of age. In this location, tumors may grow undetected until large enough to palpate. Treatment is surgical resection with sentinel node biopsy and a chemotherapeutic backbone strengthened by mTOR and tubulin inhibitors, with the addition of radiation therapy if the tumor is large and/or incompletely

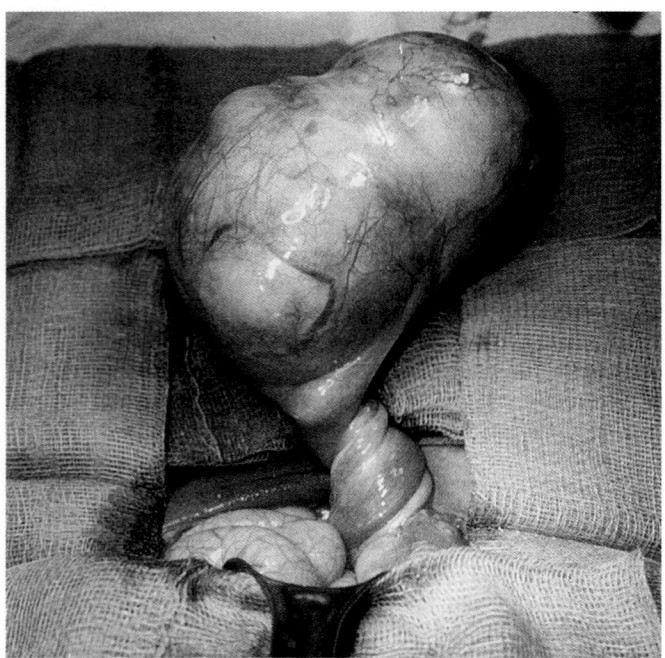

Fig. 20.26 Torsion of an ovarian teratoma in a 5-year-old female. The child presented with acute abdominal pain and a movable mass. A preoperative radiograph showed calcified material in the mass.

TABLE 20.7 **Red Flags**
1. Lower Abdominal Mass in Females
May be an indication of pregnancy, imperforate hymen, torsion of ovarian tumor, tuboovarian abscess
2. Appendiceal Abscess
Can often appear as a small bowel obstruction in younger children, in whom the diagnosis is often missed
3. Nonmobile Mass
Is suggestive of malignancy
4. Skeletal Pain or Pathologic Fracture
Is suggestive of metastatic disease (neuroblastoma) or lymphoma
5. Sudden Increase in Size of Clothing
May represent a mass or ascites
6. Left-Sided Varicocele
May be a consequence of a left-sided Wilms tumor
7. Systemic Signs of Weight Loss, Fever, Night Sweats, Anorexia, Petechiae, Anemia
Should trigger concern for malignancy, inflammatory bowel disease, autoimmune disorders, hemophagocytic lymphohistiocytosis, or atypical infections

resected. Currently 5-year survival for all cases exceeds 70% and is greatly affected by age, group, histology, size, and site of involvement.

NRSTS may arise in multiple areas within the abdomen and pelvis. The most effective therapy is surgical resection, especially for tumors <5 cm, as chemotherapeutic response is less effective than in RMS. Patients with incomplete resection benefit from radiation and proton beam therapy for local control. Tyrosine kinase inhibitors have a select role in treating some tumor subtypes (e.g., desmoid).

SUMMARY AND RED FLAGS

Although the discovery of an abdominal mass in a child is of great concern, the prognoses of most congenital masses are excellent. Splenomegaly is often a manifestation of acute and benign common viral infections in children. Red flags for splenomegaly include chronicity, a positive family or travel history, pancytopenia, and signs of disease in addition to splenomegaly (weight loss, pallor, jaundice, fever, malaise, petechiae). Additional red flags for abdominal masses are listed in Table 20.7. With modern diagnostic techniques and advanced multimodal therapy, the prognoses for malignant tumors continue to improve.

BIBLIOGRAPHY

A bibliography is available at ExpertConsult.com.

21

Dysuria

Paula Cody

Dysuria is defined as painful urination and can be related to uncomfortable contraction of the muscles of the bladder or when urine comes into contact with the inflamed genitourinary mucosa. The differential diagnoses for a patient presenting with dysuria are extensive (Table 21.1) and can be due to infectious or noninfectious causes. The cause of dysuria varies based on age of the child or adolescent; therefore, specific elements of the patient history, potential causes, and diagnostic evaluation will vary with age (Fig. 21.1). With every patient, the provider must elicit a history of signs and symptoms outside the genitourinary tract, including fever, weight loss, generalized rash, involvement of other mucosa, and joint pain or swelling. Physical examination for every patient should include temperature, blood pressure, inspection of the genitals for skin lesions or discharge, abdominal palpation, pelvic examination when indicated, and neurologic examination in children with voiding dysfunction to exclude spinal cord pathology. It is important to also consider less common etiologies of dysuria such as genetic disorders including hyperoxaluria and acute intermittent porphyria.

NEONATES

Neonates and infants cannot complain of dysuria; however, urinary tract infections (UTIs) are prevalent in this age group and a major source of morbidity. In this age group, it is difficult to distinguish between upper UTI (pyelonephritis) and lower UTI (cystitis) based on signs and symptoms alone. Unlike UTIs in older children, neonatal UTIs are more common in male neonates compared to females. In neonates, UTIs are associated with bacteremia and/or congenital abnormalities of the kidney and urinary tract. In term infants, infections tend to be community acquired and present in the 2nd to 3rd week after birth. UTIs can be caused by either hematogenous spread or an ascending infection. In preterm infants, infections are more likely to be hospital acquired.

The symptoms suggestive of a UTI in the neonate are the same as those for **suspected sepsis**; therefore, major presenting symptoms include fever, poor feeding, weight loss, lethargy, and vomiting (see Chapter 52). Neonates may also present with jaundice or abdominal distention. A maternal urinary infection at or near term may increase the risk for neonatal pyelonephritis. A mother whose vaginal culture is positive for group B streptococci or who presents with fever, prolonged rupture of the amniotic membranes (>18 hours), uterine tenderness, or preterm labor is at an increased risk for delivering a premature

baby with pyelonephritis as part of the neonatal sepsis syndrome. Family history is also important. There is a high genetic component to the presence of **vesicoureteral reflux (VUR)**; the siblings of children with known VUR also have a significant risk of reflux, with or without infection. Children with a UTI and VUR are at increased risk of pyelonephritis and renal scarring. However, the screening for VUR in an asymptomatic sibling of an index case of VUR is controversial; a voiding cystourethrogram (VCUG) is recommended if there is evidence of renal scarring on ultrasound or if there is a history of UTI in the sibling who has not been tested. Given that the value of identifying and treating VUR is unproven in the absence of a UTI, an observational approach without screening for VUR may be taken for siblings of children with VUR, with prompt treatment of any acute UTI and subsequent evaluation for VUR.

Physical examination of a neonate suspected of having a UTI should include the palpation of the abdomen to identify hydronephrosis, obstructive lesions, or cystic kidneys. Urine culture should be obtained by suprapubic or bladder catheterization, as bag collection has a high rate of contamination with perineal flora. Because of the associated risk of bacteremia, blood cultures and cerebrospinal fluid (CSF) cultures should be obtained in all neonates in whom UTI is suspected. Initial empirical therapy should be started after collection of urine, blood, and CSF cultures. The empirical therapy should provide broad coverage against probable uropathogens and is initially administered parenterally, as the risk of urosepsis is higher in neonates than in other age groups. Common empirical therapy includes ampicillin in addition to either gentamicin or a third-generation cephalosporin. Therapy is then tailored according to the specific uropathogen identified on culture and the antimicrobial sensitivity.

Ultrasound is the first-line imaging method in neonates after the first UTI. The main purpose of diagnostic imaging is the detection of risk factors, such as anomalies of the kidney and urinary tract or VUR, as well as any renal damage acquired from the infection. Clinical practice guidelines do not recommend DMSA (dimercaptosuccinic acid) scans as part of routine evaluation of infants with their first febrile UTI because the findings rarely affect acute clinical management.

CHILDREN 2–24 MONTHS OF AGE

Like neonates, young children 2–24 months of age cannot report dysuria. Nonetheless, UTIs are common (see Chapter 52). The main

TABLE 21.1 Causes of Dysuria

Infectious causes	Urinary tract infection (cystitis, pyelonephritis)
	Urethritis
	Herpes simplex virus infections
	Varicella infections
	Epstein-Barr virus infections
	Hemorrhagic cystitis (adenovirus)
	Prostatitis
	Vaginitis*
	Renal tuberculosis
	Urinary schistosomiasis
	Sexually transmitted infections
Urinary tract abnormalities (congenital and acquired)	Urinary calculi
	Urethral stricture
	Meatal stenosis
	Prostate enlargement
	Malignancy
	Urethral diverticulum
	Bladder diverticulum
	Idiopathic hypercalciuria
	Bladder outlet obstruction
	Urethral prolapse
Genital tract abnormalities	Sexually transmitted infections
	Vaginitis
	Prostatitis
	Endometritis
	Endometriosis
	Labial adhesions
	Phimosis
	Paraphimosis
	Balanitis
	Foreign body
	Vulva, vaginal ulcerations
Medications and irritants	Primary irritant dermatitis
	Chemical irritants (soaps, detergents, bubble baths, feminine hygiene products, spermicides)
	NSAIDs
	Anticholinergics (amitriptyline, imipramine, and antihistamines)
	Anti-infectives (isoniazid, sulfonamides)
	Chemotherapy-related hemorrhagic cystitis (cyclophosphamide)
Other	Trauma
	Stevens-Johnson syndrome/toxic epidermal necrolysis
	Behçet syndrome
	Inflammatory bowel disease
	Toxic shock syndrome
	Reactive arthritis (in conjunction with urethritis, conjunctivitis)
	Neurologic conditions that impact bladder emptying
	Pinworms
	Lichen sclerosus
	Appendicitis (if inflamed appendix or periappendiceal abscess lies low in iliac fossa)
	Tumor (bladder, kidney, uterus, vagina)
	Foreign body (urethral, vaginal)
	Perianal group A streptococcus

NSAIDs, nonsteroidal antiinflammatory drugs.

*Vaginitis; chemical, nonspecific bacterial, *Candida albicans*, *Trichomonas vaginalis*, herpes simplex, gonorrhea, group A streptococcus, gram-negative organisms.

risk factor for febrile infant males is whether or not they are circumcised; other individual risk factors for UTI in males include temperature >39°C, fever for at least 24 hours, and absence of another source of infection. Individual risk factors for UTI in infant females include age younger than 12 months, temperature of at least 39°C, fever for at least 2 days, and absence of another source of infection (Table 21.2).

The method of collecting urine for testing is dependent on the risk factors of the child. Culture of a urine specimen from a bag attached to the perineal area has a high false-positive rate; this method of urine collection is not suitable for diagnosing UTI. However, a culture of a urine specimen from a sterile bag that shows no growth is strong evidence that UTI is absent; if growth of a single uropathogen is present, it may represent a UTI. Nonetheless, one approach provides several recommendations in testing and treatment of UTIs in febrile infants (Fig. 21.2):

- If a febrile infant (2–24 months) with no apparent source for fever *requires* antibacterial therapy, a urine specimen should be obtained via suprapubic aspiration or catheterization for both culture and UA prior to the initiation of antibacterials.

If immediate empiric antibiotic therapy is not indicated:

- Clinician should obtain urine sample for UA and culture through catheterization or suprapubic aspiration.

or

- Clinician can obtain a clean-void bagged urine sample. If UA results suggest UTI, then an additional urine specimen for culture should be obtained via catheterization or suprapubic aspiration and empiric treatment initiated.

Diagnosing a UTI in young children generally requires both a positive UA (for white cells and/or bacteria) and >50,000 CFU/mL of a single urinary pathogen on urine culture from a suprapubic or catheterized urine specimen. A combination of a positive urine nitrite test plus positive leukocyte esterase plus white blood cells ≥10/mm^3 or ≥5 per high-power field is highly suggestive of a UTI. Some labs also report the microscopic presence of bacteria. Nitrite testing may be negative with high urine flow rates and frequent bladder emptying (bacteria need ~4 hours to produce nitrites); leukocyte esterase may be negative with certain bacteria or localized infections (abscess). Negative leukocytes, nitrites, and leukocyte esterase in the presence of bacteria suggest **asymptomatic bacteriuria,** which requires no treatment.

Sterile pyuria (leukocytes with no bacterial growth) may be seen in a partially treated UTI, renal or perinephric abscess, infection proximal to an obstruction (duplication), nephronia, interstitial nephritis, renal tuberculosis, Kawasaki disease, MIS-C (multisystem inflammatory syndrome in children), adenovirus or JC viruses, endocarditis, sexually transmitted infections (STIs), schistosomiasis, prostatitis, appendicitis, epididymitis, or lupus.

The usual choices for empirical antibacterial therapy include a third-generation cephalosporin, amoxicillin plus clavulanic acid, or trimethoprim-sulfamethoxazole. The clinician should base choice of antibacterial on local antimicrobial sensitivity patterns if available and should adjust according to sensitivity results of the isolated uropathogen. Most well-appearing infants can be treated orally. Fever persisting after 48 hours of appropriate antibiotic therapy raises the suspicion of a complicated UTI (obstructive uropathy, abscess, nephronia).

The rationale for imaging infants with UTI is to identify abnormalities of the genitourinary tract. Renal and bladder ultrasound is the first-line imaging modality to identify anatomic abnormalities. VCUG to detect VUR should not be performed after the first febrile UTI. It is indicated if the ultrasound reveals hydronephrosis, renal

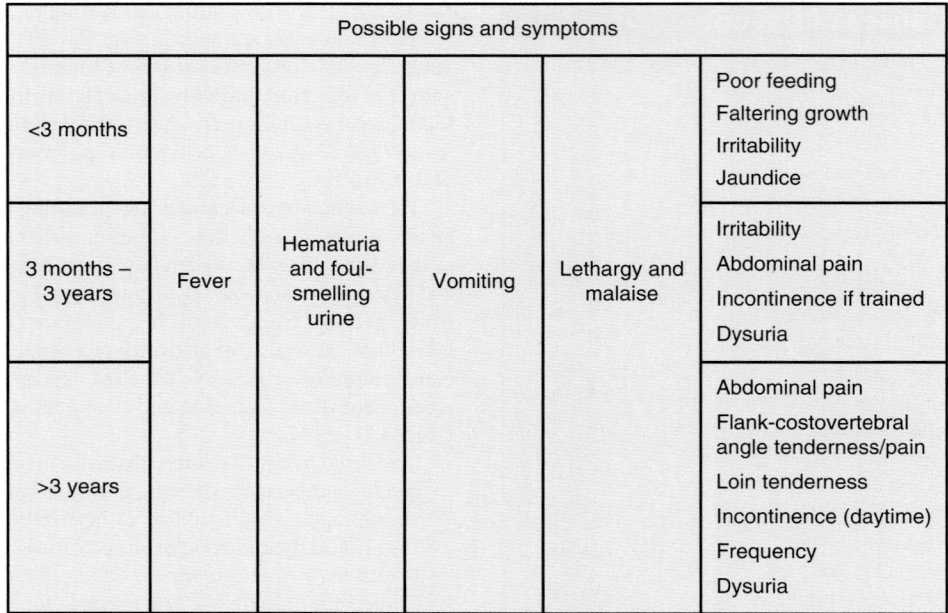

Fig. 21.1 Possible signs and symptoms in children with a urinary tract infection. (Modified from Prajapati H. Urinary tract infections in children. *Pediatr Child Health*. 2018;28[7]:318–323 [Table 2, p. 319].)

TABLE 21.2 Risk Factors for UTI

Past History

Age 2–24 months

Uncircumcised males <2 yr old

Genitourinary anomalies (obstructive uropathies)

Neurogenic bladder (spinal dysraphism, spinal cord injury, megacystic disorders)

Dysfunctional voiding

Constipation

Poor perineal hygiene

History of prior UTI

Current Illness

Males ≤1 yr

Females ≤2 yr and sexually active adolescents

Fever without a focus ≥48 hr

Fever ≥39°C

Foul-smelling urine

Urine positive for nitrites

Urine positive for leukocyte esterase

Pyuria ≥10/mm³ WBC or ≥5 WBC/HPF

Bacteria on microscopy

HPF, high-power microscopic field; UTI, urinary tract infection; WBC, white blood cell.

scarring, or other findings that suggest high-grade VUR or obstructive uropathy.

PRESCHOOL CHILDREN

A young child may or may not be able to verbalize dysuria; they may show signs of urethral irritation including delayed toilet training (especially during the day), secondary enuresis, dribbling, and frequent squatting. Due to the large variability in the time of achievement of daytime dryness (15 months–4 years), delayed toilet training may be an unreliable sign of dysuria; **primary diurnal enuresis** should be evaluated if the child is older than 48 months of age. Nocturnal enuresis is rarely a sign of UTI, but urine cultures should probably be obtained in children who do not stay dry at night by 5 years of age. A more significant symptom in young children is the *acute onset* of daytime enuresis after a period of continence.

UTIs are the most common cause of dysuria in preschool children. It may be difficult to distinguish between pyelonephritis and cystitis in these young children. Both urine and stool withholding have a role in causing UTIs in young children. Bowel/bladder dysfunction is associated with large residual urine volumes after voiding and increased UTI risk, and thus the treatment of constipation leads to a reduction in UTIs. Females are at increased risk of UTI due to the ease with which pathogens can migrate from the gastrointestinal tract to the periurethral area and urethra, and ultimately ascend to the bladder. Improper toileting habits can further increase the risk of UTI. Uncircumcised males, patients with neurogenic bladders (spina bifida), patients with indwelling catheters, and patients with renal or bladder anomalies (e.g., cysts, obstructed hydronephrosis, double collecting systems, ectopic ureter, horseshoe kidney, posterior urethral valves, VUR) are at increased risk for UTI.

Children who are toilet-trained can give a clean-void urine sample. Those who are not toilet-trained can give a urine specimen from a sterile bag attached to the perineal area, although this has a high false-positive rate.

Preschool children may also have irritant urethritis due to bubble baths, perfumed soaps, or detergents.

SCHOOL-AGED/PREPUBERTAL CHILDREN

Dysuria in school-aged children can be due to infectious and noninfectious causes (see Table 21.1). Most children with a UTI present with dysuria, frequency, or fever. It is worthwhile to ask about any urine color change, which suggests the presence of hematuria. The child should be questioned about the frequency, character, and size of their bowel movements. **Constipation** may predispose the school-aged

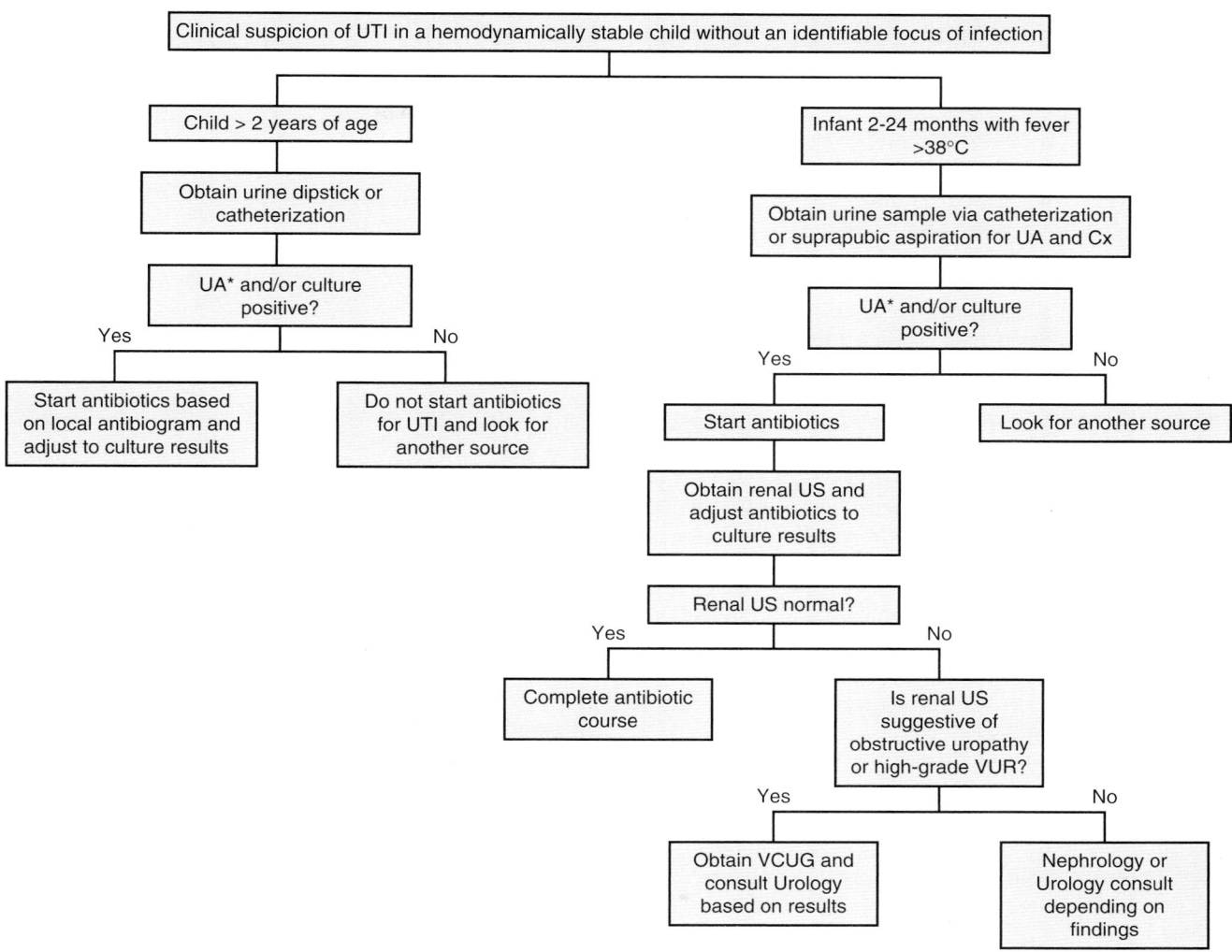

Fig. 21.2 Algorithm for diagnosis and management of UTI in infants and young children. *UA positive for leukocyte esterase, leukocytes, nitrites, or bacteria. Cx, culture; US, ultrasonography; UTI, urinary tract infection; VCUG, voiding cystourethrogram; VUR, vesicoureteral reflux.

child to a UTI; stool softeners, such as mineral oil or fiber, may be indicated. Pyelonephritis can be clinically distinguished from cystitis by presence of systemic features (fever, vomiting) and signs (flank pain, costovertebral angle tenderness).

A careful inspection of the genitals is important in the diagnosis of the cause of dysuria. Males may have nonspecific bacterial infection of the glans penis (**balanitis**); uncircumcised boys can have infection of both the glans and the prepuce (**balanoposthitis**). Both of these are usually accompanied by painful swelling and inflammation. Irritants can cause a nonspecific urethritis in males, with dysuria being the main symptom.

Prepubertal females can have dysuria as the presenting symptom of **vaginitis**, along with other symptoms including vaginal discharge. In prepubertal females, the vulvar mucosa is thin and susceptible to inflammation from chemicals and mechanical irritation. Because the labia are not well developed, the vulvar mucosa is not anatomically shielded and is thus vulnerable to irritation. Vaginitis in prepubertal females can be nonspecific, due to irritants (soaps, detergents), or may be due to the presence of a foreign body (Table 21.3). Whereas vulvovaginal candidiasis is common in postpubertal females, the vaginal environment in prepubertal females is not typically conducive to *Candida* species growth, unless they have an immunodeficiency or recent antibacterial use. In the majority of cases, vulvovaginitis in prepubertal females is a mixed, nonspecific

bacterial infection secondary to contamination by urine and feces. The responsible bacteria are usually normal flora (Table 21.4). Bloody vaginal discharge in young females may be caused by *Shigella* species or group A streptococcal infections, a foreign body (e.g., toilet paper), neoplasm (such as rhabdomyosarcoma), or trauma. Most cases of prepubertal nonspecific vaginitis can be managed with hygiene; some vulvovaginitis may require a course of antibacterial agents or topical estrogen vaginal cream (Table 21.5).

Several **vulvar skin disorders** can be confused with vulvovaginitis and present with dysuria due to contact of urine with inflamed mucosa. **Lichen sclerosus** manifests as white patches on the glabrous skin that are thinned and atrophic and are easily traumatized with resultant bullae (which may be blood-filled) in the vulvar region. **Seborrheic dermatitis** may manifest with inflammation and secondary infection of the intertriginous areas; the face and scalp may be involved as well. Labial or vulvar agglutination may be noted and can be secondary to previous vulvovaginitis of unestrogenized epithelia.

Urethritis caused by herpes simplex virus may occur in both males and females of this age group from autoinoculation from herpes stomatitis; however, presence of genital ulcers should always elicit questioning about sexual activity and/or assault.

Other etiologic factors that may lead to urethritis and resultant dysuria include infection (fungi, pinworms, scabies), irritation (soap,

TABLE 21.3 Causes of Noninfectious Vulvovaginitis and Dysuria

Condition	Historical Cues
Poor hygiene	Infrequent bathing, handwashing, and clothing changes; soiled underwear, toilet independence
Poor perineal aeration	Tight clothing, nylon underwear, tights, leotards; wet bathing suits, hot tubs, obesity
Frictional trauma	Tight clothing, sports, sand from sandbox or beach, obesity, excessive masturbation or sexual abuse
Chemical irritants	Bubble baths, harsh or perfumed soaps or detergents, powders, perfumed and/or dyed toilet paper, ammonia, perfumed and/or dyed sanitary products; douches and feminine hygiene products
Contact dermatitis	Topical creams or ointments, exposure to poison ivy
Vaginal foreign bodies	Wiping habits, excessive masturbation or self-exploration, sexual abuse
Parasites, insect bites, infestations	Home environment, pets, sandboxes, travel, camping, exposure to woods or beach
Medications	Topical steroid or hormone creams, antibiotics, chemotherapy
Generalized skin disorders	History of pruritus, chronic skin lesions, prior diagnosis
Anatomic anomalies	Vesicovaginal or rectovaginal fistula, ectopic ureter, spina bifida, cloacal anomalies, urogenital anomalies
Genetic disorders	Hyperoxaluria, acute intermittent porphyria
Neoplasms	Discharge, bleeding, bulging abdomen, change in bowel or bladder function, premature puberty
Systemic illness (Stevens-Johnson syndrome, Crohn disease, toxic shock syndrome)	Tampon use, systemic evidence of inflammatory bowel disease including rash, oral ulcers, failure to gain weight or height, abdominal pain

Modified from Succato GS, Murray PJ. Pediatric and adolescent gynecology. In: Zitelli BJ, Davis HW, eds. *Atlas of Pediatric Physical Diagnosis*. 7th ed. Philadelphia: Mosby Elsevier; 2018:658–690.

shampoo, detergent, bubble bath), systemic illness (Stevens-Johnson syndrome), and trauma (abuse, play, tight clothing, masturbation).

ADOLESCENTS

There are many causes for dysuria in an adolescent. A detailed sexual history is mandatory (Table 21.6). Greater than 38% of high school students have engaged in sexual intercourse, with an increase to 56% among 12th graders. Over 3% initiated sexual intercourse before 13 years of age, and 27% had a sexual encounter within the previous 3 months. Adolescents are likely to have multiple sexual partners over relatively short periods of time, fail to recognize the symptoms of STIs, and use condoms inconsistently. It is critical that the provider perform a thorough history in a nonjudgmental and nonthreatening manner. Interviewing the adolescent in the room alone (i.e., without a parent present) for at least a portion of the visit is the standard of care for all adolescent health care visits. The terms of a confidential visit should be explained to the adolescent and parent; all information disclosed by the adolescent remains confidential (within the confines of the state's confidentiality laws) unless they reveal a risk of rendering harm to themselves or others, such as with suicidal or homicidal ideation. Ask the adolescent about sexual partners, including anatomy and gender identity, since one's gender identity may not match the sexual anatomy

TABLE 21.4 Normal Vaginal Flora

- Aerobic
  - Gram-positive rods
    - Diphtheroids
    - Lactobacilli
  - Gram-positive cocci
    - *Staphylococcus aureus*
    - *Staphylococcus epidermidis*
    - *Streptococcus* species
      - α-Hemolytic
      - β-Hemolytic
      - Nonhemolytic
      - Group D
  - Gram-negative rods
    - *Escherichia coli*
    - *Klebsiella* and *Enterobacter* species
    - *Proteus* species
    - *Pseudomonas* species
- Anaerobic species
  - *Bacteroides* species
  - *Clostridium* species
  - *Eubacterium* species
  - *Fusobacterium* species

Modified from Larsen B, Monif GRG. Understanding the bacterial flora of the female genital tract. *Clin Infect Dis*. 2001;32(4):e69–e77.

TABLE 21.5 Treatment of Nonspecific Vulvovaginitis in Young Females

- Toilet hygiene
  - Urinate with knees apart
  - Wipe in an anterior-to-posterior direction with supervision
  - Scent- and dye-free wipes may be useful
- Clothing
  - Choose white cotton underpants, may need to change underpants midday if urinary dribbling
  - Wear loose-fitting clothing
  - Change out of wet swimsuits immediately
- Bathing
  - Take sitz baths in clear water up to 4 times a day
  - Wash gently with unperfumed soap
  - Do not use bubble bath or wash hair in bath
  - Rinse perineum with clear water, dry gently with towel
- Management of inflammation and pruritis
  - Premarin vaginal cream topically twice daily for 10–14 days
  - Hydroxyzine, 0.5 mg/kg/dose orally 4 times daily as needed
  - Diphenhydramine, 1.25 mg/kg/dose orally 4 times daily as needed

and can lead to inaccurate assumptions about types of sexual activity. Questions about victimization, trafficking, and abuse are part of the sexual history, regardless of age or gender.

Urinary tract infections (UTIs) are much more common in adolescent females than adolescent males. Risk factors for recurrent UTIs in females include frequency of sexual intercourse (higher frequency leads to higher risk), maternal history of recurrent UTI, a new sexual partner in the past year, and spermicide use in the past year. Common pathogens in this age group include *Escherichia coli*, *Proteus* species, *Klebsiella* species, *Staphylococcus saprophyticus*, and enterococcus. Although often recommended by clinicians, no evidence supports the thought that postcoital urination leads to a reduction in the frequency of UTIs.

One of the most common causes of dysuria in adolescent males and females is **sexually transmitted infections (STIs)** (Table 21.7).

TABLE 21.6 Approach to Clinical Evaluation of Sexually Transmitted Infections: Sexual History

Age at coitarche
Gender identity and anatomy of sexual partners
Date of most recent sexual encounter
Duration of relationship with current partner
Numbers of current, recent (within past 3–6 mo), and lifetime partners
Condom usage (overall consistency)
Contraceptive usage
Vaginal intercourse
Oral intercourse
Anal intercourse
Dyspareunia
Involuntary sexual encounters (abuse, rape)
Partner's sexually transmitted infection symptoms and relevant sexual history (i.e., other sex partners)

TABLE 21.7 Sexually Transmitted Infection Syndromes in Adolescents and Young Adults

Sexually Transmitted Infection Syndrome	Primary Organisms	Other Causal Organisms
Genitourinary Syndromes		
Discharge and dysuria	Chlamydia trachomatis Neisseria gonorrhoeae Trichomonas vaginalis Mycoplasma genitalium	Ureaplasma urealyticum Mycoplasma hominis Herpes simplex virus 1, 2
Proctitis, proctocolitis, and enteritis	Chlamydia trachomatis Neisseria gonorrhoeae Treponema pallidum Herpes simplex virus 1, 2	Campylobacter species Entamoeba histolytica Giardia lamblia Salmonella species Shigella species Cytomegalovirus
Genital ulcer and lymphadenopathy	Herpes simplex virus 1, 2 Treponema pallidum	Calymmatobacterium granulomatis Haemophilus ducreyi Chlamydia trachomatis lymphogranuloma venereum
Pelvic pain (e.g., pelvic inflammatory disease)	Chlamydia trachomatis Neisseria gonorrhoeae Mycoplasma genitalium	Mycoplasma hominis Mixed aerobic and anaerobic bacteria
Scrotal pain (e.g., epididymitis)	Chlamydia trachomatis Neisseria gonorrhoeae	Mycoplasma genitalium Ureaplasma urealyticum
Pharyngeal Syndromes		
Infections of pharyngeal mucosa	Neisseria gonorrhoeae Herpes simplex virus 1, 2	Treponema pallidum Human papillomaviruses
Dermatologic Syndromes		
Genital warts	Human papillomaviruses	—
Molluscum contagiosum	Molluscum contagiosum virus	—
Rash, alopecia	Treponema pallidum	—
Arthritis and dermatitis syndrome	Neisseria gonorrhoeae Chlamydia trachomatis	—
Jaundice, hepatitis	Hepatitis A, B, C viruses	—
Scabies	Sarcoptes scabiei	—
Pubic lice	Phthirus pubis	—

From Long SS, Prober CG, Fischer M, eds. *Principles and Practice of Pediatric Infectious Diseases.* 5th ed. Philadelphia: Elsevier; 2018:350, Table 49-1.

Adolescents represent an age group at high risk for acquisition and transmission of STIs. Although many STIs are asymptomatic and are diagnosed by screening asymptomatic sexually active individuals, STIs can present with dysuria, vaginal discharge, penile discharge, and genital lesions (Table 21.8). The most likely time for this to happen is within 1 month of beginning a relationship with a new sexual partner. Diagnostic testing is highlighted in Table 21.9.

Chlamydial genital infection is the most frequently reported bacterial STI. Infections with *Chlamydia trachomatis* may be asymptomatic or may present with dysuria, discharge, intermenstrual bleeding, or dyspareunia. *C. trachomatis* has also been associated with Fitz-Hugh–Curtis syndrome (perihepatitis) and reactive arthritis. *C. trachomatis* infection may lead to pelvic inflammatory disease (PID), ectopic pregnancy, and infertility. *C. trachomatis* urogenital infection can be detected in women by testing urine or collecting swab specimens from the endocervix or vagina; in men, the diagnosis can be made through urine or urethral swab. Nucleic acid amplification tests (NAATs) are the most sensitive methods for detecting *C. trachomatis.* Treatment of infection improves symptoms, decreases the risk of sequelae, and prevents sexual transmission of the disease (Table 21.10).

Gonorrhea, caused by *Neisseria gonorrhoeae*, is the second most frequently reported bacterial STI. Infections with *N. gonorrhoeae* may be asymptomatic or may present with dysuria, discharge, intermenstrual bleeding, or dyspareunia. *N. gonorrhoeae* infection may lead to PID; late complications include ectopic pregnancy and infertility. *N. gonorrhoeae* urogenital infection can be detected in women by testing urine or collecting swab specimens from the endocervix or vagina; in men, the diagnosis can be made through urine or urethral swab. NAATs are the most sensitive methods for detecting *N. gonorrhoeae.* Treatment of infection improves symptoms, decreases risk of sequelae, and prevents sexual transmission of the disease (see Table 21.10). Treatment of gonorrhea is complicated by the ability of *N. gonorrhoeae* to develop resistance to antibacterials.

Trichomoniasis, caused by *Trichomonas vaginalis*, may be asymptomatic or may present with dysuria, frothy yellow-green vaginal discharge, genital pruritus, or intermenstrual bleeding. Diagnosis of *T. vaginalis* is usually assessed by microscopy of vaginal or urethral secretions; however, there are more sensitive methods of detection, including a specific culture, a nucleic acid probe, and an immunochromatographic capillary flow dipstick. See Table 21.10 for treatment recommendations.

Primary herpes simplex virus (HSV) infection can cause genital ulcers and dysuria, as well as other conditions, including nongenital lesions, cervicitis, urethritis, cystitis, proctitis, and pharyngitis. Systemic complications, such as hepatitis, pneumonia, thrombocytopenia, and monoarticular arthritis, may rarely occur. HSV-infected patients can present with a primary infection, which can be asymptomatic; a first clinical episode, which may not necessarily occur during the primary infection; or a recurrent episode. Usually, the first clinical episodes are more painful and prolonged than are subsequent ones. Recurrent episodes occur less frequently with a genital HSV-1 infection and with intervals between episodes becoming longer, as compared to HSV-2. Treatment for initial and recurrent outbreaks of HSV is listed in Table 21.10.

Vaginitis due to various causes can cause dysuria in adolescent females. Vulvovaginal candidiasis, bacterial vaginosis, and trichomoniasis are common causes of vulvovaginitis in adolescents. Other causes are local chemical or allergic irritants, bacterial infections caused by *Streptococcus* or *Staphylococcus* species, trauma, and secondary infections from foreign bodies. Rare causes of vaginitis and subsequent

TABLE 21.8   Diagnostic Characteristics of Genital Lesions

Syndrome	Appearance	Number of Lesions	Pain	Adenopathy	Occurrence in the United States
Herpes	Vesicles and superficial ulcers on erythematous base (1–2 mm)	Multiple	Often	Bilateral; inguinal; firm; movable; tender	Frequent
Syphilis	Papule and superficial or deep ulcer (5–15 mm)	Single	No	Bilateral; inguinal; firm; movable; nontender	Uncommon
Lymphogranuloma venereum	Ulcer (2–10 mm), resolves quickly	Single	Yes	Unilateral; inguinal; fluctuant; may suppurate; tender	Uncommon
Human papillomavirus	Anogenital exophytic warts; may resemble cauliflower or be papular with projections	Single or multiple	No	None	Frequent
Lice or nits	Tiny (≤1 mm) insects or eggs adherent to hair shaft; excoriations	Multiple	No but pruritic	None	Common
Chancroid	Deep, purulent ulcers (2–20 mm)	Multiple	Yes	Unilateral; inguinal; fluctuant; may suppurate; tender	Rare
Non–sexually acquired genital ulceration (common causes: Epstein-Barr virus, cytomegalovirus, *Mycoplasma*)	Varied—can be shallow or deep, may be necrotic, often in kissing pattern on labia	Single or multiple	Yes	Based on underlying condition	Uncommon

TABLE 21.9   Tests Used to Determine the Cause of Sexually Transmitted Infection Syndromes in Adolescents and Young Adults

STI Syndrome	Office Tests Available	Preferred Laboratory Tests
Genitourinary Syndromes		
Discharge and dysuria	Females: microscopic wet prep vaginal secretions, pH paper, whiff test, KOH; LET; rapid tests for GC, CT, TV, BV, and HIV; UPT Males: Gram stain smear of urethral discharge looking for ≥5 WBCs per oil immersion field and intracellular gram-negative diplococci; LET; microscopic examination of first-void spun urine sediment with ≥10 WBCs per high-power field; rapid tests for GC, CT, and HIV	Females, males: NAATs for GC, CT, and TV; HIV test
Proctitis, proctocolitis, and enteritis	Females, males: Gram stain smear of anorectal exudate; rapid test for HIV Females: UPT	NAATs for GC and CT; see HSV and syphilis under genital ulcer; cultures for other gram-negative pathogens and amoeba; HIV test
Genital ulcer and lymphadenopathy	Females, males: darkfield examination for syphilis; rapid test for HIV Females: UPT	Cultures for HSV-1 and HSV-2 or PCR for HSV; serology for type-specific glycoprotein G to discern HSV-1 or HSV-2 RPR or VDRL and confirmatory tests for syphilis if positive or treponemal EIA or CIA chemiluminescence immunoassays and confirmatory nontreponemal test (RPR or VDRL) if positive NAATs for CT; PCR genotyping or serology for LGV (complement fixation or microimmunofluorescence) Gram stain and culture for chancroid; staining for Donovan bodies on tissue biopsy; HIV test
Pelvic pain (e.g., pelvic inflammatory disease)	Microscopic wet prep vaginal secretions, pH paper, whiff test, KOH; LET; rapid tests for GC, CT, TV, BV, and HIV; UPT	NAATs for GC, CT, and TV; HIV test
Scrotal pain (e.g., epididymitis)	Gram stain smear of urethral discharge looking for ≥5 WBCs per oil immersion field and intracellular gram-negative diplococci; LET; microscopic examination of first-void spun urine sediment with ≥10 WBCs per high-power field on first-void urine; rapid tests for GC, CT, and HIV	NAATs for GC and CT; HIV test
Pharyngeal Syndromes		
Infections of pharyngeal mucosa	Rapid strep test	NAATs or culture for GC and CT; culture or PCR for HSV-1 and HSV-2, serology for type-specific glycoprotein G to discern HSV-1 and HSV-2; RPR or VDRL and confirmatory tests if positive; HIV test

TABLE 21.9 Tests Used to Determine the Cause of Sexually Transmitted Infection Syndromes in Adolescents and Young Adults—cont'd

STI Syndrome	Office Tests Available	Preferred Laboratory Tests
Dermatologic Syndromes		
Genital warts	Characteristic lesions	—
Molluscum contagiosum	Characteristic lesions	Wright or Giemsa staining for intracytoplasmic inclusions
Rash, alopecia	—	RPR or VDRL and confirmatory tests if positive
Arthritis, dermatitis	Males: Gram stain smear urethral discharge looking for ≥5 WBCs per oil immersion field and intracellular gram-negative diplococci; LET Females: Microscopic wet prep vaginal secretions for WBCs; LET; rapid tests for GC, CT; and UPT	Females, males: NAATs or culture for GC and CT from rectum or pharynx Females: NAATs of vaginal swab Males: NAATs of first-void urine
Jaundice, hepatitis	—	Appropriate laboratory tests for hepatitis
Scabies	Microscopic examination of skin and hair	—
Pubic lice	Identification of eggs, nymphs, and lice with naked eye or microscopy	—

BV, bacterial vaginosis; CIA, chemiluminescence immunoassay; CT, *Chlamydia trachomatis*; EIA, enzyme immunoassay; GC, *Neisseria gonorrhoeae*; HSV-1, herpes simplex type 1; HSV-2, herpes simplex type 2; KOH, potassium hydroxide; LET, leukocyte esterase test of urine; LGV, lymphogranuloma venereum; NAATs, nucleic acid amplification tests; PCR, polymerase chain reaction; RPR, rapid plasma reagin; STI, sexually transmitted infection; TV, *Trichomonas vaginalis*; UPT, urine pregnancy test; VDRL, Venereal Disease Research Laboratory; WBCs, white blood cells.
From Long SS, Prober CG, Fischer M, eds. *Principles and Practice of Pediatric Infectious Diseases*. 5th ed. Philadelphia: Elsevier; 2018:351, Table 49-2.

TABLE 21.10 Recommended Treatments of Selected Sexually Transmitted Infections

Pathogen	Recommended Regimen
Chlamydia trachomatis	Azithromycin, 1 g orally in a single dose or Doxycycline, 100 mg orally twice a day for 7 days
Neisseria gonorrhoeae	Ceftriaxone 500 mg (patient weight <300 lb) or 1 g (>300 lb) intramuscularly in a single dose
Trichomonas vaginalis	Metronidazole, 2 g orally in a single dose or Tinidazole, 2 g orally in a single dose
Herpes simplex virus First clinical genital episode	Acyclovir, 400 mg orally 3 times a day for 7–10 days or Acyclovir, 200 mg orally 5 times a day for 7–10 days or Famciclovir, 250 mg orally 3 times a day for 7–10 days or Valacyclovir, 1 g orally twice a day for 7–10 days
Herpes simplex virus Episodic therapy for recurrent genital episodes	Acyclovir, 400 mg orally 3 times a day for 5 days or Acyclovir, 800 mg 3 times a day for 2 days or Acyclovir, 800 mg orally twice a day for 5 days or Famciclovir, 125 mg orally twice a day for 5 days or Valacyclovir, 500 mg orally twice a day for 3 days or Valacyclovir, 1 g orally once a day for 5 days

Modified from Centers for Disease Control and Prevention. Sexually transmitted diseases treatment guidelines 2015. *MMWR*. 2015;64(3):1–135. See full document for alternative treatments and specific treatments in pregnancy and treatment for children younger than 8 yr old.

dysuria include ulcerating conditions of the mucous membranes, such as toxic shock syndrome and Stevens-Johnson syndrome. Epstein-Barr virus, cytomegalovirus, *Mycoplasma pneumoniae*, and other systemic infections can cause non–sexually acquired genital ulcerations. Noninfectious causes of genital ulcers that can be confused with infection include inflammatory bowel disease and Behçet syndrome. Inflammatory bowel disease usually manifests with intestinal symptoms, deeper ulcers, and a longer duration of ulcerative lesions. Behçet syndrome may manifest with lesions of other mucous membranes as well as ocular, central nervous system, and joint manifestations. If the clinical diagnosis is not definitive, viral culture of the lesions is recommended.

Males with dysuria may also have penile pain or dysuria as a result of phimosis, paraphimosis, balanitis, urethral trauma, epididymitis, or meatal stenosis. **Phimosis** is a scarring or narrowing of the preputial opening and manifests as failure to retract the foreskin. The foreskin is normally difficult to retract in neonates, but by 3 years of age, it is easily retracted. **Paraphimosis**, an emergent cause of dysuria and penile pain, is an incarceration of the prepuce behind the glans. Edema, pain, and swelling are present. Balanitis is an infection of the prepuce caused by *Streptococcus* species, *Candida* species, mixed flora, or *Trichomonas* species; it may be recurrent and warrants circumcision.

Evaluation for dysuria in the adolescent female should include a clean-catch (midstream) urine for dipstick, microscopic exam, and culture. The presence of leukocytes on UA may indicate vaginitis due to STIs (*N. gonorrhoeae*, *C. trachomatis*, herpes, *T. vaginalis*). To check for gonorrhea or *Chlamydia*, a first-stream urine or a swab of the vagina or cervix should be obtained. Depending on sexual activity, the pharynx and rectum should also be tested to check for infections in those locations. Any lesions suggestive of HSV should be cultured or tested by polymerase chain reaction (PCR). The evaluation of any vaginal discharge includes description of the vaginal discharge, measurement of vaginal pH, saline preparation, performance of a whiff test, and microscopic examination (Table 21.11 and Figs. 21.3, 21.4, and 21.5). Thick, adherent cottage cheese–like discharge is suggestive of candidiasis; other physical examination findings include erythema, edema, and excoriation of the vagina. Thin, homogeneous, gray-white, foul-smelling discharge is suggestive of bacterial vaginosis (BV). Purulent, profuse, irritating,

TABLE 21.11   Differences in Characteristics Between Bacterial Vaginosis, Trichomoniasis, and Vulvovaginal Candidiasis

Clinical Elements		Normal	Bacterial Vaginosis	Trichomoniasis	Vaginal Candidiasis
Symptoms	Vaginal odor	–	+	+/–	–
	Vaginal discharge	Clear-white	Thin, gray, homogeneous	Green-yellow	White, curdlike
	Vulvar irritation	–	+/–	+	+
	Dyspareunia	–	–	+	–
Signs	Vulvar erythema	–	–	+/–	+/–
	Bubbles in vaginal fluid	–	+	+/–	–
	Strawberry cervix	–	–	+/–	–
Microscopy	**Saline Wet Mount**				
	Clue cells	–	+	–	–
	Motile protozoa	–	–	+	–
	KOH Test				
	Pseudohyphae	–	–	–	+
	Whiff test	–	+	+/–	–
	pH	3.8–4.2	>4.5	>4.5	<4.5

KOH, potassium hydroxide.
Modified from Centers for Disease Control and Prevention. Sexually transmitted diseases treatment guidelines 2015. *MMWR*. 2015;64(3):1–135.

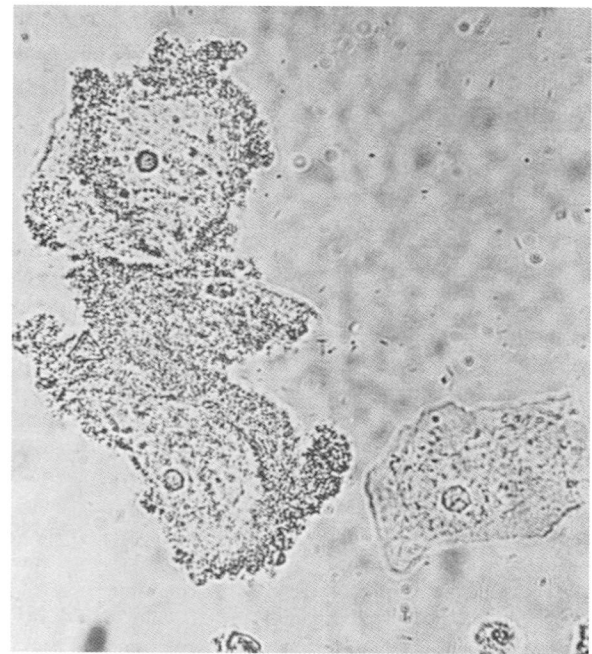

Fig. 21.3 Bacteria are clinging to the sides of a vaginal epithelial cell ("clue cell"). (From Huffman JW. Genitourinary infections. In: Feigen RD, Cherry JD, eds. *Textbook of Pediatric Infectious Diseases*. 2nd ed. Philadelphia: WB Saunders; 1992:570.)

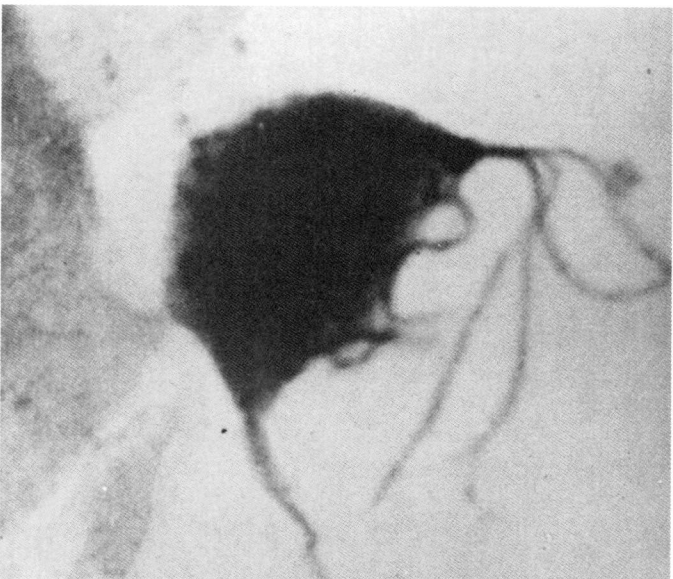

Fig. 21.4 *Trichomonas vaginalis* identified in wet smears of the vaginal discharge. (From Huffman JW. Genitourinary infections. In: Feigen RD, Cherry JD, eds. *Textbook of Pediatric Infectious Diseases*. 2nd ed. Philadelphia: WB Saunders; 1992:568.)

frothy green-yellow discharge often accompanies trichomoniasis. The Amsel criteria for diagnosis and treatment of bacterial vaginosis are listed in Tables 21.12 and 21.13, respectively.

The provider should perform a pelvic examination to exclude **pelvic inflammatory disease (PID)** in all sexually active adolescent females when vaginal discharge and/or pelvic pain are reported (Table 21.14). PID is an acute infection of the upper female genital tract (endometriosis, salpingitis, tubo-ovarian abscess, pelvic peritonitis). Features that suggest PID (vs lower tract infection) include cervical motion tenderness, uterine or adnexal tenderness, temperature >101°F, cervical

mucopurulent discharge or friability, abundant white blood cells on saline prep of vaginal fluid, elevated erythrocyte sedimentation rate and C-reactive protein levels, and a documented cervical infection with *N. gonorrhea* or *C. trachomatis*. Table 21.15 lists differential diagnoses for PID, and Table 21.16 details the recommended treatment regimens for PID. Pregnancy testing is indicated when an adolescent female presents with dysuria or any symptoms of an STI; the test results may influence the treatment plan. *Another important consideration in sexually active adolescents is screening for HIV.*

The Centers for Disease Control and Prevention recommend gonorrhea and *Chlamydia* testing of all males who meet the diagnostic criteria for urethritis. NAATs, the most sensitive gonorrhea and *Chlamydia* diagnostic test, can be performed on a single urine or urethral

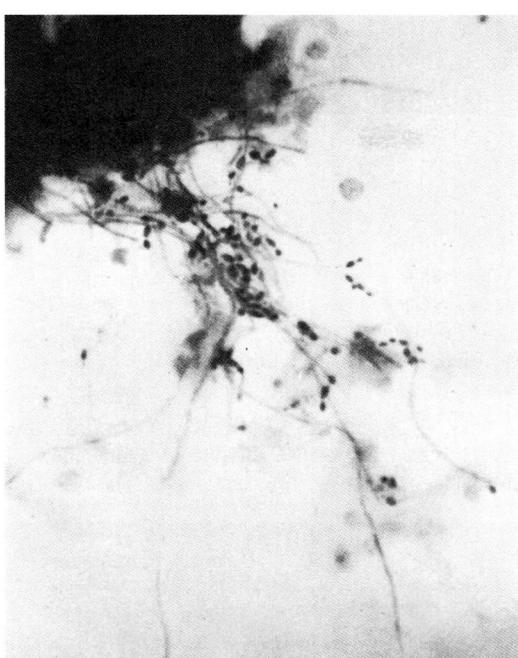

Fig. 21.5 Hyphae of *Candida albicans* on a wet smear of vaginal discharge. (From Huffman JW. Genitourinary infections. In: Feigen RD, Cherry JD, eds. *Textbook of Pediatric Infectious Diseases*. 2nd ed. Philadelphia, WB Saunders; 1992:564.)

TABLE 21.12 Amsel Criteria for the Diagnosis of Bacterial Vaginosis

3 of the following 4 Amsel criteria are considered necessary to diagnose BV:
1. Vaginal discharge: thin, homogeneous, white, uniformly adherent
2. Vaginal pH >4.5
3. Positive result of whiff test: fishy odor after mixing discharge with 10% KOH
4. >20% clue cells on microscopic examination: bacteria-coated squamous epithelial cells, where both the periphery (cell membrane) and cytoplasm have a granular, irregular, "moth-eaten" appearance

KOH, potassium hydroxide.
Modified from Amsel R, Totten PA, Spiegel CA, et al. Nonspecific vaginitis. Diagnostic criteria and microbial and epidemiologic associations. *Am J Med*. 1983;74:14–22.

TABLE 21.13 Treatment Regimens for Bacterial Vaginosis

Nonpregnant Females

Metronidazole, 500 mg orally twice daily for 7 days
or
Metronidazole gel, 0.75%, 1 full applicator (5 g) intravaginally once a day for 5 days
or
Clindamycin cream, 2%, 1 full applicator (5 g) intravaginally once a day for 7 days

Pregnant Females

Metronidazole, 250 mg orally 3 times daily for 7 days
or
Metronidazole 500 mg orally twice daily for 7 days

Modified from Centers for Disease Control and Prevention. Sexually transmitted diseases treatment guidelines 2015. *MMWR*. 2015;64(3):1–135.

TABLE 21.14 Diagnostic Criteria for Pelvic Inflammatory Disease

Minimum Criteria

Uterine or adnexal tenderness (unilateral or bilateral)
or
Cervical motion tenderness

Additional Criteria to Increase Specificity of Minimum Criteria

Abnormal cervical or vaginal mucopurulent discharge
Presence of WBCs on saline microscopy of vaginal secretions
Oral temperature >38.3°C (101°F)
Elevated erythrocyte sedimentation rate or C-reactive protein
Laboratory evidence of *Neisseria gonorrhoeae* or *Chlamydia trachomatis* at cervix

WBCs, white blood cells.
Modified from Centers for Disease Control and Prevention. Sexually transmitted diseases treatment guidelines 2015. *MMWR*. 2015;64(3):1–135.

TABLE 21.15 Differential Diagnosis for Pelvic Inflammatory Disease

Ectopic pregnancy
Ovarian cyst (with or without ovarian torsion)
Acute appendicitis
Endometriosis
Pyelonephritis
Septic or incomplete abortion
Pelvic thrombophlebitis
Functional pain
Psoas-pelvic muscle abscess
Mesenteric adenitis
Pelvic adhesions
Pelvic bone osteomyelitis
Chronic intestinal disease (e.g., inflammatory bowel disease)

TABLE 21.16 Treatment Regimens for Pelvic Inflammatory Disease

Parenteral Regimens (One of the Following)

Cefotetan, 2 g IV q12h, or cefoxitin, 2 g IV q6h, both **plus** doxycycline, 100 mg IV or PO q12h *or*
Ceftriaxone 1 g IV q24h **plus** doxycycline 100 mg PO or IV q12h **plus** metronidazole 500 mg PO or IV q12 hr
Parenteral therapy may be discontinued 24 hr after clinical improvement and continue doxycycline, 100 mg PO twice daily, **and** metronidazole 500 mg twice daily for 14 days of total therapy
For tubo-ovarian abscess, addition of either metronidazole, 500 mg PO twice daily, or clindamycin, 450 mg PO 4 times daily, to oral doxycycline provides better coverage against anaerobes

Outpatient Regimens (One of the Following)

Ceftriaxone, 500 mg IM in a single dose, or cefoxitin, 2 g IM, with probenecid, 1 g PO in a single dose once, or other parenteral 3rd-generation cephalosporin (e.g., ceftizoxime) **plus** doxycycline, 100 mg PO twice daily for 14 days, with metronidazole, 500 mg PO twice daily for 14 days

IM, intramuscularly; IV, intravenously; PO, per os (orally); q6h, every 6 hr; q8h, every 8 hr; q12h, every 12 hr.
Modified from Centers for Disease Control and Prevention. Sexually transmitted diseases treatment guidelines 2015. *MMWR*. 2015;64(3):1–135.

TABLE 21.17 Treatment Regimens for Epididymitis

One of the following:
For epididymitis most likely caused by gonococcal or chlamydial infection:
    Ceftriaxone, 500 mg intramuscularly in a single dose, **plus** doxycycline, 100 mg orally twice daily for 10 days
For epididymitis most likely caused by enteric organism, or for patients who are allergic to cephalosporins and/or tetracyclines:
    Levofloxacin, 500 mg orally once daily for 10 days*†

*Fluoroquinolones have not been recommended for persons younger than 18 yr because they damage articular cartilage in juvenile animal models. Among children treated with fluoroquinolones, no joint damage attributable to therapy has been observed. Quinolones should not be used to treat possible gonorrhea infections acquired in Asia or the Pacific, including Hawaii, or California.
†In men who practice insertive anal sex and are not allergic to ceftriaxone, add ceftriaxone 500 mg IM × 1 dose.
Modified from Centers for Disease Control and Prevention. Sexually transmitted diseases treatment guidelines 2015. *MMWR*. 2015;64(3):1–135.

TABLE 21.18 Common Pitfalls in the Correct Diagnosis of Dysuria

Neonates/Infants

Assume that significant bacteriuria in a bagged urine specimen is a true UTI, and treat before a confirmatory culture is obtained
Fail to obtain a urine culture in a neonate older than 3 days and miss obstructive uropathy with a secondary infection

Toddlers and School-Aged Children

Trust a urine culture from a bagged urine specimen
Accept a laboratory report of "no significant growth" on urine, without knowing that the laboratory reports only >100,000 CFU/mL as "significant"
Fail to label urine as a "catheterized specimen," so that the laboratory can plate 0.1 mL as well as 0.01 mL

Adolescents

Fail to ask about sexual history suggestive of vaginitis, such as a new sexual partner and condom or other birth control device use
Treat pyuria as a UTI in a sample contaminated with vaginal leukocytes

CFU, colony-forming unit; UTI, urinary tract infection.

TABLE 21.19 Red Flags for Referral to a Pediatric Urologist or Nephrologist After a Urinary Tract Infection

- Poor urine stream in males (posterior urethral valves)
- Constant wetting not from urethra (ectopic ureter or patent urachus)
- Dilating VUR (grade III, IV, or V)
- Renal scarring detected on sonography or a DMSA scan obtained >6 mo after the UTI
- Urinary obstruction seen on a sonogram
- Voiding dysfunction (enuresis, frequency, "curtsy" to stop voiding)
- Breakthrough UTI in the child with VUR receiving prophylaxis
- Elevated serum creatinine level
- Hypertension
- Antenatal hydronephrosis that is confirmed after day 3 after birth

DMSA, dimercaptosuccinic acid; UTI, urinary tract infection; VUR, vesicoureteral reflux.

TABLE 21.20 Red Flags and Things Not to Miss: Sexually Transmitted Infections

Diagnosis of More Than One Sexually Transmitted Infection in the Same Patient

- If patient is diagnosed with syphilis, gonorrhea, or HIV
- If patient reports engaging in unprotected sex with multiple partners
- If patient is immunocompromised
- If patient has a history of sexually transmitted infections

Abdominal Pain in an Adolescent Girl

- Pelvic inflammatory disease
- Tubo-ovarian abscess
- Ectopic pregnancy
- Appendicitis
- Ovarian cyst (rupture or torsion)

Fever, Rash, Malaise, Arthralgia

- Disseminated gonococcemia
- Reactive arthritis
- HIV infection

Rape

Pregnancy

Treatment of Partners

Asymptomatic Cervicitis

specimen. Any lesion suspicious for HSV should be cultured. Table 21.8 lists the treatments for selected STIs. Epididymitis, typically presenting as unilateral testicular pain, is most frequently caused by *C. trachomatis* or *N. gonorrhoeae* or a sexually transmitted enteric organism such as *E. coli* and *Pseudomonas* species. On examination, a hydrocele may be present. Treatment of epididymitis is listed in Table 21.17.

SUMMARY AND RED FLAGS

Dysuria in prepubertal children is usually a symptom of a UTI but may also be due to other infectious or noninfectious causes of urethritis and vaginitis. The differential diagnosis expands greatly in adolescents, in whom an STI may be the cause. Table 21.18 demonstrates common pitfalls in the appropriate evaluation of dysuria in children and adolescents. Red flags are noted in Tables 21.19 and 21.20.

Because children younger than 2 years cannot often verbalize a specific complaint of dysuria, the diagnosis of a UTI is more challenging in children this age. Awareness of specific risk factors for UTI (uncircumcised status in boys, height of fever, and lack of other cause for fever on examination) especially in the first year of life will lead to the evaluation of those at highest risk and avoid unnecessary testing in those at low risk. Combining the results of the UA with an appropriately obtained urine culture allows for expeditious treatment and confirmation of the particular pathogen when the culture results are available.

BIBLIOGRAPHY

A bibliography is available at ExpertConsult.com.

22

Proteinuria

Rajasree Sreedharan

Proteinuria can be detected by various means, and the most common is the dipstick test, a calorimetric assay that spots only albumin and not low-molecular-weight proteins. In addition, false-positive dipstick assessment can be seen with highly concentrated urine, alkaline urine, the presence of contrast media, vaginal secretions, or semen. False negatives are less common but can be seen with very dilute urine. Though 24-hour urine collection is the gold standard to quantify the proteinuria, spot urine protein-to-creatinine ratio can be used for initial confirmation after a positive screen with dipstick or to trend proteinuria (Table 22.1). A ratio <0.2 protein mg/creatinine mg is considered normal in children older than 2 years of age and a ratio <0.5 mg/mg is considered normal in younger children between 6 months and 2 years of age. In timed collection, protein excretion >240 mg/m^2 in 24 hours in children younger than 6 months of age and >150 mg/m^2 in older children is considered abnormal, and over 40 mg/m^2/hr (>3 g/1.73 m^2/day) is considered nephrotic range. Qualitative analysis of protein in urine by immunonephelometry or electrophoresis helps distinguish glomerular from tubular proteinuria.

Proteinuria in children can be transient, orthostatic, or persistent. Transient and orthostatic proteinuria are benign conditions and require no treatment. Several factors including fever, stress, hypovolemia, exercise, and seizures can lead to transient proteinuria (Table 22.2). **Orthostatic proteinuria** is defined as increased protein in urine only when upright. In this condition, absence of proteinuria when horizontal and resting can be confirmed by documenting absence of protein in a first morning void. Split day/night urine collection is the gold standard to diagnose orthostatic proteinuria, which is a common benign cause of proteinuria, especially in adolescents. Persistent proteinuria requires meticulous evaluation to rule out renal pathology.

Evaluation of proteinuria begins with a detailed history and physical examination. Pertinent histories that help distinguish pathologic from benign proteinuria include history of respiratory symptoms concurrent with or preceding the proteinuria, presence of red urine, edema, positive family history of kidney disease, or hearing loss. Findings of edema and hypertension suggest pathologic proteinuria. Repeating urine dipstick in asymptomatic children with a negative history can eliminate unnecessary further testing for transient proteinuria. If still positive, spot urine protein-to-creatinine ratio can help confirm the presence of proteinuria. If confirmed, a first morning void protein-to-creatinine ratio can then identify orthostatic proteinuria. Once the benign conditions are ruled out in asymptomatic children, further testing is similar to that of symptomatic children and these children should be referred to nephrologists. This more detailed evaluation begins with 24-hour urine collection where possible, complete urinalysis, and sediment evaluation looking for glomerular or other parenchymal pathology that could be causing the proteinuria (Fig. 22.1). Positive leukocyte esterase, nitrite, and presence of pyuria or bacteriuria suggest a urinary tract infection. If not resolved with treatment of infection, proteinuria will need further evaluation. Low molecular proteins, such as β2-microglobulin, α1-microglobulin, lysozyme, and retinol-binding protein, are found in **tubular proteinuria** as is seen in Fanconi syndrome or Dent disease. Red blood cell (RBC) casts are pathognomonic of **glomerulonephritis**. Serum chemistry including creatinine, BUN, electrolytes, albumin, and cholesterol will also help separate proteinuria secondary to glomerulonephritis or nephrotic syndrome. Lupus antibody studies, streptococcal infection, and complement C3 and C4 levels along with viral studies can help delineate the various causes of glomerulonephritis and nephrotic syndrome. Renal ultrasound should be considered to rule out any gross parenchymal etiology for the proteinuria, such as dysplastic kidney and cystic kidney disease. Renal biopsy may be indicated if there is evidence for worsening of proteinuria, hypoalbuminemia, deteriorating renal function, or a poor response to the initial therapy.

Differential diagnoses for proteinuria are extensive, as described in Table 22.2. The initial evaluation of a patient with proteinuria is presented in Table 22.3. Indications for a referral to a pediatric nephrologist are described in Table 22.4. If there is obvious edema with proteinuria, the diagnostic evaluation noted in Table 22.3 advances directly to the second phase and, if necessary, to the third phase.

The combination of proteinuria, hypoalbuminemia, edema, and hyperlipidemia are the defining features of nephrotic syndrome. Nephrotic syndrome may be a result of many primary etiologic factors, with varying renal pathologic processes and long-term consequences. Proteinuria that causes edema is always clinically significant, although not all edema is secondary to proteinuria (Table 22.5). All children with nephrotic syndrome invariably have "nephrotic range" proteinuria, necessitating detailed evaluation, and most require treatment. In rare cases, a child with asymptomatic proteinuria has nephrotic-range proteinuria. If there is concomitant hypoalbuminemia and hyperlipidemia, the work-up proceeds as if the child presented with nephrotic syndrome, despite the absence of edema. Even without hypoalbuminemia and hyperlipidemia, nephrotic-range proteinuria is less likely to be benign than is less marked asymptomatic proteinuria.

NEPHROTIC SYNDROME IN YOUNG CHILDREN
Differential Diagnosis

Three diseases constitute all cases of isolated nephrotic syndrome: minimal change disease (the most common), focal segmental sclerosis (also called focal glomerular sclerosis), and membranous glomerulopathy. These classifications are based on pathologic findings. Thus, these presentations could be primary or secondary due to other causes. In addition, nephrotic syndrome can be present along with glomerulonephritis (GN), such as postinfectious GN, immunoglobulin A (IgA) GN, or membranoproliferative GN. Systemic diseases also cause childhood nephrotic syndrome, accounting for 10% of cases. The three foremost

TABLE 22.1	Quantification of Proteinuria in Children		
Method	**Indications**	**Normal Range**	**Comments**
Dipstick testing	Routine screening for proteinuria performed in the office	Negative or trace in a concentrated urine specimen (specific gravity: ≥1.020) Test interpretation: 1+ ~30 mg/dL 2+ ~100 mg/dL 3+ ~300 mg/dL	False-positive test can occur if urine is very alkaline (pH >8.0) or very concentrated (specific gravity: >1.025), when there is pus, vaginal secretions, or semen present
24-hr urine for protein and creatinine*excretion	Quantitation of proteinuria (as well as creatinine clearances)	<150 mg/m²/24 hr	More accurate than spot urine analysis; inconvenient for patient; the creatinine content should be measured to determine whether the specimen is truly a 24-hr collection. The amount of creatinine in a 24-hr specimen can be estimated as follows: females, 15–20 mg/kg; males, 20–25 mg/kg
Spot urine for protein/creatinine ratio—preferably on first morning urine specimen	Semiquantitative assessment of proteinuria	<0.2 mg protein/mg creatinine in children older than 2 yr old <0.5 mg protein/mg creatinine in those 6–24 mo old	Simplest method to quantitate proteinuria; less accurate than measuring 24-hr proteinuria
Microalbuminuria	Assess risk of progressive glomerulopathy in patients with diabetes mellitus	<30 mg urine albumin per gram of creatinine on first morning urine	Therapy should be intensified in diabetics with microalbuminuria

Modified from Flores FX. Clinical evaluation of the child with proteinuria. In: Kliegman FM, St. Geme J, eds. *Nelson Textbook of Pediatrics*. 21st ed. Elsevier; 2020:2749–2750.e1.

considerations include systemic lupus erythematosus (SLE), IgA vasculitis (Henoch-Schönlein purpura), and hemolytic uremic syndrome. These diseases have extrarenal manifestations in addition to the proteinuria and must be considered in any child who presents with systemic illness and significant proteinuria. Hereditary forms of nephrotic syndrome are a genetically heterogeneous group of disorders representing a spectrum of hereditary renal diseases (Table 22.6 and Fig. 22.2). Over 45 recessive or dominant genes have been associated with steroid-resistant nephrotic syndrome (SRNS)/hereditary nephrotic syndrome in humans (Table 22.7). Several of the more common disorders along with other causes of nephrotic syndrome are noted in Tables 22.8 and 22.9. Causes of congenital nephrotic syndrome (in infants 3 months of age or younger) are noted in Table 22.10.

MINIMAL CHANGE DISEASE

Most cases of nephrotic syndrome in children are caused by minimal change nephrotic syndrome, defined as normal histologic features of the kidney by light microscopy and immune stains. Preschool-aged children constitute the age group in which minimal change nephrotic syndrome is most common. Patients often present with asymptomatic edema, which may manifest as swollen or puffy eyes upon awakening in the morning; increasing abdominal girth (increased waist or belt size) from ascites; pedal or leg edema, which causes difficulty in putting on their regular-sized shoes, especially after being upright during the daytime; or swelling in other sites, such as the scrotum, penis, vulva, and scalp. Tense edema or ascites is occasionally painful.

Minimal change nephrotic syndrome is slightly more common in males than in females. The hallmark of this disease is total clearing of the proteinuria with oral prednisone therapy. A common misconception is that neither hematuria nor hypertension is present in children with minimal change disease. Microscopic hematuria and hypertension are present in up to 20% of children who have minimal change disease. The BUN or serum creatinine level may also be elevated in up to 30% of the cases, usually from prerenal causes. Serum complement

studies are normal. Older age, hematuria, hypertension, and azotemia may occur with minimal change nephrotic syndrome, but the combination suggests another disease.

Diagnosis

Studies that would help confirm that a patient with nephrotic syndrome has minimal change disease include urinalysis; serum chemistry including BUN, creatinine, albumin, and cholesterol levels; and complements and lupus antibody titers.

The urinalysis would be expected to show 3+ to 4+ protein, which is correlated with a urine concentration of 300–2,000 mg/dL. The urine may also occasionally yield positive results for blood. Microscopic examination of the urine sediment often shows oval fat bodies and/or refractile granular casts, which are seen when there is significant lipiduria. Red blood cells might also be present, but it is unusual to see red blood cell casts. Their presence would suggest a diagnosis of glomerulonephritis (see Chapter 23).

The complement C3 and C4 levels are normal in minimal change disease and are depressed in some other causes of nephritis (see Chapter 23). The serum cholesterol values are elevated in minimal change nephrotic syndrome and are usually >250 mg/dL; levels in the range of 500–600 mg/dL may occur. The serum albumin concentration is invariably <2.5 and often <2.0 g/dL. A renal biopsy is not immediately indicated because most patients (>90%) with minimal change disease respond to prednisone, a response that is considered diagnostic.

Treatment

With a presumptive diagnosis of minimal change nephrotic syndrome, it is recommended that patients be placed on a therapeutic course of prednisone, 60 mg/m²/day or 2 mg/kg/day, up to a maximum of 60 mg for 4–6 weeks, followed by a dose of 40 mg/m² or 1.5 mg/kg (maximum 40 mg) given every other day for another 6 weeks. In most patients, there is total resolution of proteinuria within 10–21 days of initiating therapy. Patients who do not respond to prednisone therapy should be considered candidates for a renal biopsy to guide further therapy.

TABLE 22.2 Causes of Proteinuria

Transient Proteinuria
Fever
Exercise
Dehydration
Cold exposure
Congestive heart failure
Seizure
Stress

Orthostatic (Postural) Proteinuria

Glomerular Diseases Characterized by Isolated Proteinuria
Idiopathic (minimal change) nephrotic syndrome
Focal segmental glomerulosclerosis
Mesangial proliferative glomerulonephritis
Membranous nephropathy
Membranoproliferative glomerulonephritis
Amyloidosis
Diabetic nephropathy
Sickle cell nephropathy

Glomerular Diseases with Proteinuria as a Prominent Feature
Acute postinfectious glomerulonephritis (e.g., streptococcal, endocarditis, hepatitis B or C virus, and HIV)
Immunoglobulin A nephropathy
Henoch-Schönlein purpura nephritis
Lupus nephritis
Serum sickness
Alport syndrome
Vasculitic disorders
Reflux nephropathy

Tubular Diseases
Cystinosis
Wilson disease
Lowe syndrome
Dent disease (X-linked recessive nephrolithiasis)
Galactosemia
Tubulointerstitial nephritis
Acute tubular necrosis
Renal dysplasia
Polycystic kidney disease
Reflux nephropathy
Drugs (e.g., penicillamine, lithium, NSAID)
Heavy metals (e.g., lead, gold, mercury)

NSAID, nonsteroidal antiinflammatory drug.
From Pais P, Avner ED. Fixed proteinuria. In: Kliegman RM, Stanton BF, St. Geme JW III, eds. *Nelson Textbook of Pediatrics.* 20th ed. Philadelphia: Elsevier; 2016:2520, Table 526.1.

Total clearing of proteinuria in response to prednisone is an excellent prognostic sign. Very few patients progress to renal failure, although many patients (~80%) who initially respond to prednisone therapy with total clearing of proteinuria may have relapses and require intermittent prednisone therapy for many years. Approximately 18% of patients treated with prednisone for minimal change nephrotic syndrome respond to therapy and never experience a relapse.

Patients with **recurrent nephrotic syndrome** are subgrouped into those who experience frequent and infrequent relapses. A patient with infrequent relapse has fewer than two relapses in any 6-month period; a person with frequent relapse has two or more relapses within

6 months. Prednisone should be reinitiated at a dose of 60 mg/m^2/day or 2 mg/kg/day until a maximum of 60 mg/day and continued until the urine test results are negative for protein for 3 consecutive days. After that, alternate-day prednisone is given at a dose of 40 mg/m^2 or 1.5 mg/kg (maximum 40 mg) in the morning for another 4 weeks and then discontinued altogether. Relapses are frequent during the influenza virus seasons; any minor upper respiratory infection may trigger a relapse of nephrotic syndrome. Patients who suffer infrequent relapses may be treated with prednisone alone.

Patients with frequently relapsing nephrotic syndrome may be steroid dependent and require constant daily prednisone therapy to maintain a remission. Because constant daily prednisone has significant untoward side effects (growth failure, cushingoid facies, osteoporosis, cataracts, opportunistic infections, hypertension, and glucose intolerance), other therapies need to be considered. A renal biopsy is recommended prior to initiating alternative agents to confirm the diagnosis of minimal change nephrotic syndrome. Treatment strategies with corticosteroid-sparing agents for patients with frequent relapse who develop steroid-related adverse effects include alkylating agents, cyclophosphamide or chlorambucil, and more recently rituximab.

Complications of Nephrotic Syndrome

Even in patients with the frequent relapse variant of minimal change disease, the incidence of renal failure is only 1%. The reported mortality rate remains higher, at approximately 5%.

Infection

The major cause of death in nephrotic syndrome is overwhelming infection, usually secondary to **spontaneous bacterial peritonitis**, which develops in as many as 10% of patients with nephrotic syndrome at some point in the course of illness. Such infection is most frequent in patients who are edematous with significant ascites. Peritoneal fluid interferes with macrophage function, whereas ascitic fluid may dilute local complement or immunoglobulin levels, altering host defense mechanisms in the peritoneum.

The most common pathogen is *Streptococcus pneumoniae. Escherichia coli* and *Staphylococcus aureus* are other etiologic agents that may cause spontaneous peritonitis in patients with minimal change disease. With the use of appropriate antibiotics, mortality from peritonitis is ~10%. Any child with nephrotic syndrome in relapse with evidence of ascites needs to be evaluated quickly if either abdominal pain or fever develops. A blood specimen and paracentesis (e.g., Gram stain, culture, neutrophil count, measurement of glucose and protein levels) should be obtained, and the patient should be started on intravenous cefotaxime and an aminoglycoside or ceftriaxone alone without further delay. The neutrophil count in spontaneous bacterial peritonitis is usually ≥250 cells/mm^3.

Thrombosis

A second serious complication of nephrotic syndrome is spontaneous thrombosis, pulmonary embolus, or both. The blood of patients with nephrotic syndrome is hypercoagulable, and there is an increased incidence of thrombotic phenomena in these children. Children can have arterial thrombosis, as well as venous thrombosis with resultant pulmonary emboli. The renal vein and dural sinus veins are other possible sites of thrombosis. Use of injectable and oral antithrombolytic agents, in addition to heparin, have allowed for more effective treatment of thrombotic complications.

Hyperlipidemia

Hyperlipidemia is treated by some authorities with statins to lower the serum cholesterol levels and theoretically reduce vascular pathologic processes.

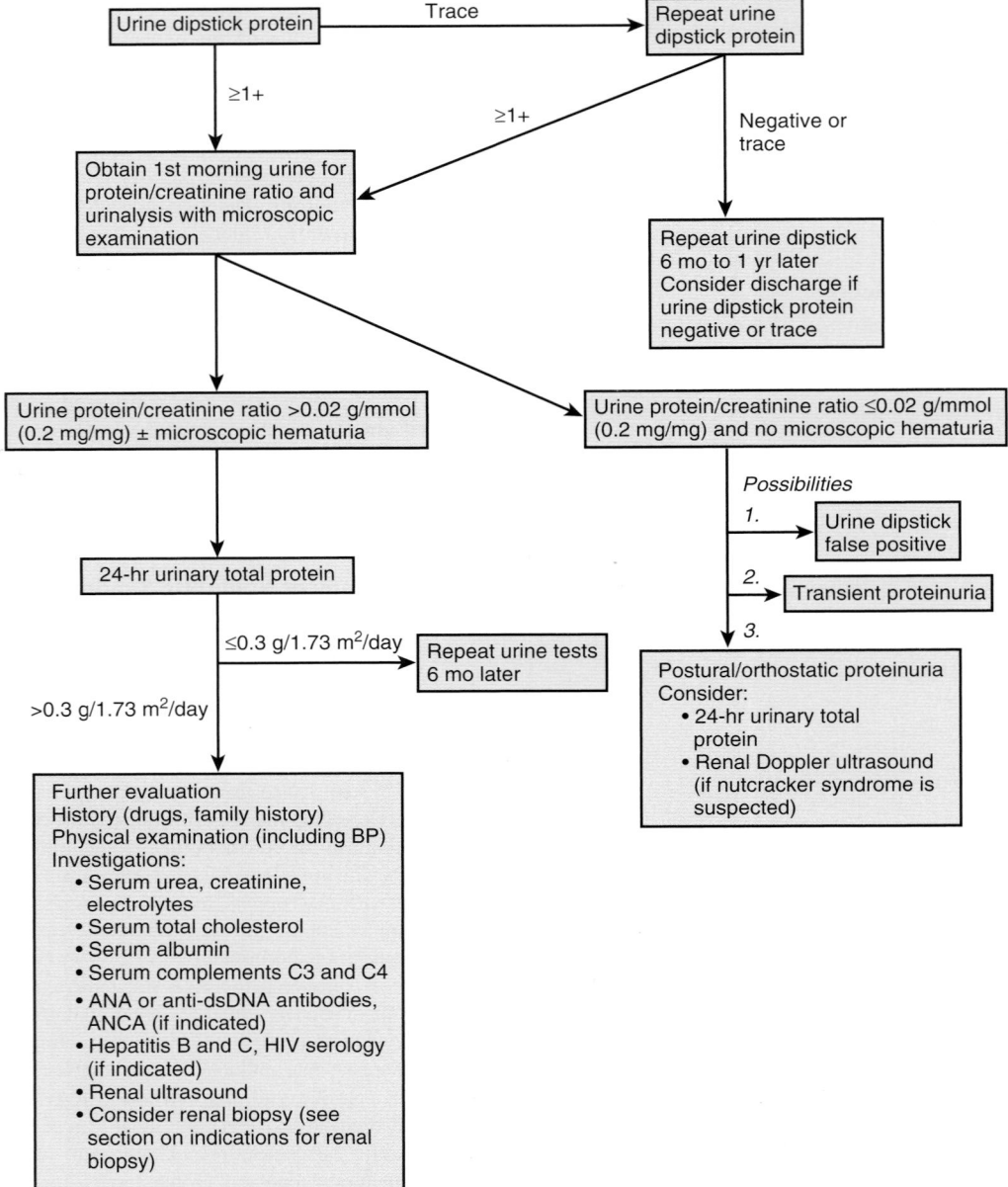

Fig. 22.1 Algorithm for investigating proteinuria. ANA, antinuclear antibody; ANCA, antinuclear cytoplasmic antibody; anti-dsDNA, anti–double-stranded DNA; BP, blood pressure. (From Yap HK, Lau PYW. Hematuria and proteinuria. In: Geary DF, Scharfer F, eds. *Comprehensive Pediatric Nephrology.* Philadelphia: Elsevier; 2008:190.)

OTHER FORMS OF NEPHROTIC SYNDROME

Focal Segmental Sclerosis

Diagnosis

Clinical criteria do not always allow clinicians to differentiate minimal change disease from focal segmental sclerosis before completion of a course of prednisone therapy. Inability to clear proteinuria completely during prednisone therapy may be the first indication of focal segmental sclerosis. Patients who respond to prednisone initially with clearing of proteinuria but do not respond to a course of steroids in a subsequent relapse should also be considered to have focal segmental sclerosis. Such patients represent about 7% of those who have an initial response to prednisone therapy. A patient who does not respond to prednisone with total clearing of proteinuria should undergo renal biopsy.

Focal segmental sclerosis may be primary (idiopathic) or secondary to severe obesity, reflux nephropathy, sickle cell nephropathy, reduced renal mass (single kidney), opiate or analgesic abuse, chronic bacteremia (endocarditis), renal transplant rejection, or nephropathy resulting from HIV infection. Genetic variants in several genes result in focal segmental glomerulosclerosis. The genetic basis of these hereditary focal segmental glomerulosclerotic disorders is genetically heterogeneous. Nine hereditary subtypes have been described. *FSGS1:ACTN4; FSGS2:TRPC6; FSGS3:CD2AP; FSGS4:APOL1; FSGS5:INF2; FSGS6:MYO1E; FSGS7:PAX2; FSGS8:ANLN;* and *FSGS9:CRB2.* Many of these genes code for

TABLE 22.3 Work-up of a Child with Proteinuria

Pediatrician's Work-up: Phase I
Early morning urinalysis to include examination of the sediment
Ambulatory and recumbent urinalyses for dipstick protein testing

Pediatrician's Work-up: Phase II
Blood electrolytes, BUN, creatinine, serum proteins, cholesterol
Timed 12 hr urine collections, recumbent and ambulatory
Renal ultrasonography

Pediatric Nephrologist's Work-up: Phase III
Complement, ANA, viral studies, genetic studies
Renal biopsy
Management of established renal disease

ANA, antinuclear antibody.
Modified from Norman ME. An office approach to hematuria and proteinuria. *Pediatr Clin North Am.* 1987;34:545–562.

TABLE 22.4 When to Refer the Child with Proteinuria to a Nephrologist

Persistent nonorthostatic proteinuria
A family history of glomerulonephritis, chronic renal failure, or kidney transplantation
Systemic complaints such as fever, arthritis or arthralgias, and rash
Hypertension, edema, cutaneous vasculitis, or purpura
Coexistent hematuria with or without cellular casts in the spun sediment
Elevated blood urea nitrogen and creatinine levels or unexplained electrolyte abnormalities
Increased parental anxiety

Modified from Norman ME. An office approach to hematuria and proteinuria. *Pediatr Clin North Am.* 1987;34:545–561, Table 24.9.

TABLE 22.5 Causes of Edema

Kidney Diseases
Acute glomerulonephritis
Nephrotic syndrome
Acute renal failure
Chronic renal failure

Heart Failure

Liver Failure

Nutritional and Gastrointestinal Disorders
Protein-calorie malnutrition
Protein-losing enteropathy
Nutritional edema (especially on refeeding)
Iron deficiency anemia associated

Endocrine Disorders
Hypothyroidism
Mineralocorticoid excess

Miscellaneous
Hydrops fetalis
Venocaval obstruction
Capillary leak syndrome (systemic inflammatory response syndrome)
Turner syndrome (lymphedema)
Allergic reaction (periorbital edema)

proteins that are involved in the structure and function of the podocyte foot process (see Table 22.7).

Treatment

Results of treatment of focal segmental sclerosis have been poor. Patients have severe and unremitting proteinuria despite treatment with prednisone, chlorambucil, or cyclophosphamide. The long-term outcome has been poor; 33% are in renal failure ~10 years after diagnosis, and nearly 100% are in renal failure 20 years after diagnosis. The incidence of focal segmental sclerosis appears to be increasing, possibly related to obesity and genetic predisposition.

Patients with focal segmental sclerosis present two difficult problems. First, renal function may be maintained reasonably well for years, but massive proteinuria persists. Hence, patients are often edematous for months or years, and stigmata of protein malnutrition may develop as a result of large protein losses. Symptomatic therapy with a low-sodium diet and judicious use of diuretics is sometimes effective. Dietary manipulation of protein intake is ineffective; increasing dietary protein intake is accompanied by a concomitant increase in urinary protein excretion. There is no evidence that protein restriction either modifies serum proteins or prevents progression to renal insufficiency.

The second problem occurs when affected patients progress to end-stage renal failure. Recurrence of the disease in transplanted kidneys occurs in 25–30% of recipients. Therefore, many patients undergo a long period of dialysis before receiving a kidney transplant in an effort to diminish the frequency of recurrent disease.

Some patients respond to calcineurin inhibitors, cyclosporine, or tacrolimus, with total clearing of their proteinuria. There may be no progression to renal insufficiency. It is unknown what percentage of patients with focal segmental sclerosis respond to cyclosporine; it is estimated that 25–60% have an initial response.

Membranous Nephropathy

Membranous nephropathy is a pathologic diagnosis made following renal biopsy and may be primary or secondary to other diseases (e.g., hepatitis, SLE, or malignancy) or toxins and drugs such as nonsteroidal antiinflammatory drugs, gold, mercury, bismuth, silver, D-penicillamine, trimethadione, probenecid, and captopril. All the secondary causes must be considered and should be addressed and treated before the condition is considered primary. Antibodies against the phospholipase A_2 receptor (PLA_2R) in the serum or a renal biopsy by immune staining have been identified in 70% of patients with primary or idiopathic membranous nephropathy. Circulating antibodies against thrombospondin type-1 domain-containing 7A (THSD7A) are found in another 5–10% of the remaining patients with primary membranous nephropathy. The changes in the antibody titers correspond to remission or relapse of proteinuria and can be used to monitor the disease.

Treatment

Addressing the triggers of secondary membranous nephropathy in itself may result in resolution of proteinuria in the majority of cases. Membranous nephropathy secondary to SLE is more difficult to treat. In addition, the increased incidence of spontaneous resolution of the proteinuria makes selecting the patients who should be treated very complicated. Close monitoring of primary membranous nephropathy to determine the need for treatment is recommended for 6 months prior to initiating treatment. Sodium restriction, diuretics, and angiotensin-converting enzyme (ACE) inhibitors can be used for control of proteinuria and symptoms. In patients with no decrease of proteinuria, or with

TABLE 22.6   Genetic Heterogeneity of Primary Nephrotic Syndrome and Syndromic Disorders Associated with Nephrotic Syndrome

Location	Phenotype	Inheritance	OMIM	Gene/Locus
Primarily Renal				
1q23.3	Nephrotic syndrome, type 22	AR	619155	NOS1AP
1q25.2	Nephrotic syndrome, type 2	AR	600995	PDCN
1q42.13	Nephrotic syndrome, type 18	AR	618177	NUP133
3p21.31	Nephrotic syndrome, type 5, with or without ocular abnormalities	AR	614199	LAMB2
7q21.11	Nephrotic syndrome, type 15	AR	617609	MAGI2
7q33	Nephrotic syndrome, type 13	AR	616893	NUP205
10q22.1	Nephrotic syndrome, type 14	AR	617575	SGPL1
10q23.33	Nephrotic syndrome, type 3	AR	610725	PLCE1
11p13	Nephrotic syndrome, type 4	AD	256370	WT1
11p11.2	Nephrotic syndrome, type 19	AR	618178	NUP160
12p12.3	Nephrotic syndrome, type 6	AR	614196	PTPRO
12q14.1	Nephrotic syndrome, type 21	AR	618594	AVIL
12q15	Nephrotic syndrome, type 11	AR	616730	NUP107
16p13.13	Nephrotic syndrome, type 10	AR	615861	EMP2
16q13	Nephrotic syndrome, type 12	AR	616892	NUP93
17q22	Nephrotic syndrome, type 7	AR	615008	DGKE
17q22	Hemolytic uremic syndrome, atypical, susceptibility to, 7	AR	615008	DGKE
17q25.1	Nephrotic syndrome, type 17	AR	618176	NUP85
17q25.3	Nephrotic syndrome, type 8	AR	615244	ARHGDIA
19p13.2	Nephrotic syndrome, type 16	AR	617783	KANK2
19q13.12	Nephrotic syndrome, type 1	AR	256300	NPHS1
19q13.2	Nephrotic syndrome, type 9	AR	615573	COQ8B
Xq22.3	Nephrotic syndrome, type 20	XL	301028	TBC1D8B
19q13.2	Glomerulosclerosis, focal segmental, 1	AD	603278	ACTN4
11q22.1	Glomerulosclerosis, focal segmental, 2	AD	603965	TRPC6
6p12.3	Glomerulosclerosis, focal segmental, 3	CD2AP-AD	607832	CD2AP
14q32.33	Glomerulosclerosis, focal segmental, 5	INF2-AD	613237	INF2
15q22.2	Glomerulosclerosis, focal segmental, 6	AR	614131	MYO1E
10q24.31	Glomerulosclerosis, focal segmental, 7	AD	616002	PAX2
2q35	Glomerulopathy with fibronectin deposits 2	AD	601894	FN1
7p14.2	Focal segmental glomerulosclerosis 8	AD	616032	ANLN
9q33.3	Focal segmental glomerulosclerosis 10	AR	256020	LMX1B
1q32	Glomerulopathy with fibronectin deposits 1	AD	137950	GFND1
2q35	Glomerulopathy with fibronectin deposits 2	AD	601894	FN1
Systemic Disorders				
1p33-p31.1	Forsythe-Wakeling syndrome	AR	613606	
17q21.33	Interstitial lung disease, nephrotic syndrome, and epidermolysis bullosa, congenital	AR	614748	ITGA3
3p21.31	Pierson syndrome	AR	609049	LAMB2
15q25.2	Galloway-Mowat syndrome 1	AR	251300	WDR73
Xq28	Galloway-Mowat syndrome 2, X-linked	XLR	301006	LAGE3
14q11.2	Galloway-Mowat syndrome 3	AR	617729	OSGEP
20q13.12	Galloway-Mowat syndrome 4	AR	617730	TP53RK
2p13.1	Galloway-Mowat syndrome 5	AR	617731	TPRKB
21q22.3	Galloway-Mowat syndrome 6	AR	618347	WDR4
12q15	Galloway-Mowat syndrome 7	AR	618348	NUP107
1q42.13	Galloway-Mowat syndrome 8	AR	618349	NUP133

TABLE 22.6 Genetic Heterogeneity of Primary Nephrotic Syndrome and Syndromic Disorders Associated with Nephrotic Syndrome—cont'd

Location	Phenotype	Inheritance	OMIM	Gene/Locus
16p13.3	Congenital disorder of glycosylation, type Ik	AR	608540	ALG1
11p13	Denys-Drash syndrome	AD, SMu	194080	WT1
2q11.2	Autoimmune disease, multisystem, infantile onset, 2	AR	617006	ZAP70
4q21.1	Epilepsy, progressive myoclonic 4, with or without renal failure	AR	254900	SCARB2
2q35	Schimke immunoosseous dysplasia	AR	242900	SMARCAL1
10q24.32	Immunodeficiency, common variable, 10	AD	615577	NFKB2
9q33.2	Amyloidosis, Finnish type	AD	105120	GSN
16p13.2	Congenital disorder of glycosylation, type Ia	AR	212065	PMM2
11p13	Frasier syndrome	AD, SMu	136680	WT1
2q33.1	Autoimmune lymphoproliferative syndrome, type II	AD	603909	CASP10
1p31.3	Autoinflammation, immune disregulation, and eosinophilia	AD	618999	JAK1
Xp11.23	Congenital disorder of glycosylation, type IIm	SMo, XLD	300896	SLC35A2
4q31.3	Amyloidosis, familial visceral	AD	105200	FGA
11q23.3	Amyloidosis, 3 or more types	AD	105200	APOA1
12q15	Amyloidosis, renal	AD	105200	LYZ
15q21.1	Amyloidosis, familial visceral	AD	105200	B2M
2q24.2	Aicardi-Goutieres syndrome 7	AD	615846	IFIH1
3p21.1	Autoimmune lymphoproliferative syndrome, type III	AR	615559	PRKCD
6q13	Sialic acid storage disorder, infantile	AR	269920	SLC17A5
2q36.3	Alport syndrome 2, autosomal recessive	AR	203780	COL4A4
2q36.3	Alport syndrome 2, autosomal recessive	AR	203780	COL4A3
9q33.3	Nail-patella syndrome	AD	161200	LMX1B
Xq22.3	Alport syndrome 1, X-linked	XLD	301050	COL4A5
16p13.3	Familial Mediterranean fever, AR	AR	249100	MEFV
19p13.3	C3 deficiency	AR	613779	C3
12q24.31	Mucopolysaccharidosis-plus syndrome	AR	617303	VPS33A
10p13	Omenn syndrome	AR	603554	DCLRE1C
11p12	Omenn syndrome	AR	603554	RAG1
11p12	Omenn syndrome	AR	603554	RAG2
11p15.5	Nephropathy with pretibial epidermolysis bullosa and deafness	AR	609057	CD151
22q12.3	End-stage renal disease, nondiabetic, susceptibility to		612551	APOL1
22q12.3	Glomerulosclerosis, focal segmental, 4, susceptibility to		612551	APOL1
9q33.3	Ventriculomegaly with cystic kidney disease	AR	219730	CRB2
1q44	Muckle-Wells syndrome	AD	191900	NLRP3
12q13.3	Pseudo-TORCH syndrome 3	AR	618886	STAT2
Xq13.3	Intellectual disability, X-linked 98	XLD	300912	NEXMIF
15q26.1	Arthrogryposis, renal dysfunction, and cholestasis 1	AR	208085	VPS33B
11p15.4	Immunodeficiency 10	AR	612783	STIM1
14q32.32	Imerslund-Grasbeck syndrome 2	AR	618882	AMN
10p14	Hypoparathyroidism, sensorineural deafness, and renal dysplasia	AD	146255	GATA3
12q24.11	Hyper-IgD syndrome	AR	260920	MVK
Xp11.23	Immunodisregulation, polyendocrinopathy, and enteropathy, X-linked	XLR	304790	FOXP3
Xq26.2-q26.3	Lesch-Nyhan syndrome	XLR	300322	HPRT1
12q23.2	Microcephaly 24, primary, autosomal recessive	AR	618179	NUP37

Continued

TABLE 22.6   Genetic Heterogeneity of Primary Nephrotic Syndrome and Syndromic Disorders Associated with Nephrotic Syndrome—cont'd

Location	Phenotype	Inheritance	OMIM	Gene/Locus
1q21	Nephropathy-hypertension	AD	161900	
15q22.31	Melorheostosis, isolated, somatic mosaic		155950	MAP2K1
7q11.23	Cutis laxa, autosomal dominant	AD	123700	ELN
2p21	Cystinuria	AD, AR	220100	SLC3A1
19q13.11	Cystinuria	AD, AR	220100	SLC7A9

AD, autosomal dominant; AR, autosomal recessive; SMo, somatic mosaicism; SMu, somatic mutation; TORCH, toxoplasmosis, other infections, rubella, cytomegalovirus, herpes simplex virus; XL, X-linked; XLD, X-linked dominant; XLR, X-linked recessive.

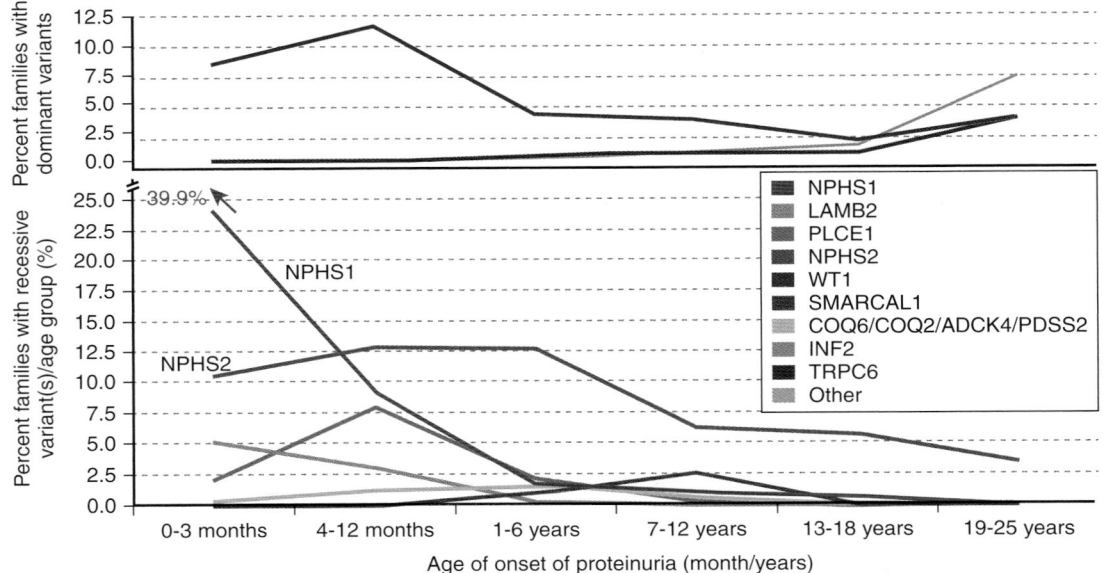

Fig. 22.2 Relative distribution of steroid-resistant nephrotic syndrome (SRNS)-causing genes by their age of onset. Percentages of families in an international cohort with SRNS that manifested at 25 years of age and resulted from variants in monogenic genes are interconnected by lines between age groups and shown in different colors for each causative gene (*lower panel* for recessive genes, *upper panel* for dominant genes). *NPHS1* variants *(red)*, *LAMB2 (orange)*, and *PLCE1 (dark blue)* have early age of onset and are rarely found in patients older than 6 years. The dominant genes *INF2 (light blue)* and *TRPC6 (brown)* manifest in early adulthood, and *WT1 (black)* shows a biphasic distribution with a first peak at 4–12 months and a second peak for age of onset beyond 18 years *(upper panel)*. These findings are compatible with the notion that variants in recessive disease genes are found more frequently in early-onset disease, whereas variants in dominant genes more frequently cause adult-onset disease. (Modified from Sadowski CE, Lovric S, Ashraf S, et al. A single-gene cause in 29.5% of cases of steroid-resistant nephrotic syndrome. *J Am Soc Nephrol.* 2015;26:1279–1289.)

severe, life-threatening symptoms related to the nephrotic syndrome, immunosuppression with steroids and cyclophosphamide can be tried.

NEPHROTIC SYNDROME IN INFANTS YOUNGER THAN 1 YEAR

Nephrotic syndrome that manifests very early in life is a much more serious entity, and the prognosis is guarded (see Table 22.9). The outlook is poorest in younger infants (younger than 6 months of age) and improves as the age at presentation approaches 1 year. Minimal change disease is rarely seen in infants younger than 6 months of age. It is more common in infants who present at 6–8 months. By 1 year, it is the most common cause of nephrotic syndrome.

The conditions that result in nephrotic syndrome in infants differ markedly from those seen in older children. Secondary causes are more prominent and need to be considered, particularly in newborns or very young infants. It is especially important to test for syphilis because the

early institution of penicillin therapy may lead to the resolution of the renal disease and may mitigate the involvement of other organ systems as well. Congenital toxoplasmosis is also treatable with the combination of steroids and pyrimethamine–sulfadiazine–folinic acid. Other congenital infections offer less opportunity for treatment to influence the outcome; extrarenal manifestations of these infections are much more serious than kidney disease.

Primary renal disease–causing nephrotic syndrome in early infancy is most often caused by either congenital nephrotic syndrome or diffuse mesangial sclerosis. In both diseases, the prognosis for survival is poor unless aggressive supportive therapy and kidney transplantation are undertaken.

Congenital Nephrotic Syndrome

Congenital nephrotic syndrome is an autosomal recessive disorder resulting from variants in the gene encoding the protein, nephrin, and other genes (see Table 22.10 and Fig. 22.2). Infants with

TABLE 22.7 Genetic Causes of Nephrotic Syndrome Categorized According to the Location of Abnormal Proteins in Podocytes

Gene	Protein	Inheritance	Locus	Phenotypes
Slit Diaphragm and Adaptor Proteins				
NPHS1	Nephrin	AR	19q13.1	CNS, SRNS (NPHS1)
NPHS2	Podocin	AR	1q25–q31	CNS, SRNS (NPHS2)
PLCE1	Phospholipase C, ε1	AR	10q23	DMS, SRNS (NPHS3)
CD2AP	CD2-associated protein	AD/AR	6p12.3	SRNS (FSGS3)
FAT1	FAT1	AR	4q35.2	NS, ciliopathy
Cytoskeleton Components				
ACTN4	α-Actinin-4	AD	19q13	Late-onset SRNS (FSGS1)
INF2	Inverted formin-2	AD		SRNS (FSGS5), Charcot-Marie-Tooth disease with glomerulopathy
MYH9	Myosin, heavy chain 9	AD	22q12.3–13.1	Macrothrombocytopenia with sensorineural deafness, Epstein syndrome, Sebastian syndrome, Fechtner syndrome
MYO1E	Myosin IE	AR	15q22.2	Childhood-onset SRNS (FSGS6)
ARHGDIA	Rho GDP-dissociation inhibitor (GDI) a1	AR	17q25.3	Childhood-onset SRNS (NPHS8), seizures, cortical blindness
ARHGAP24	Arhgap24 (RhoGAP)	AD	4q22.1	Adolescent-onset FSGS
ANLN	Anillin	AD	7p14.2	FSGS8
GBM and Basal Membrane Proteins and Related Components				
LAMB2	Laminin subunit β2	AR	3p21	Pierson syndrome DMS, FSGS (NPHS5)
ITGB4	Integrin-β4	AR	17q25.1	Epidermolysis bullosa, anecdotic cases presenting with NS and FSGS
ITGA3	Integrin-β3	AR		Epidermolysis bullosa, interstitial lung disease, SRNS/FSGS
CD151	Tetraspanin	AR	11p15.5	Epidermolysis bullosa, sensorineural deafness, ESRD
EXT1	Glycosyltransferase	AR	8q24.11	SRNS
COL4A3,4	Collagen (IV) α3/α4	AD/AR	2q36–q37	Alport syndrome, FSGS
COL4A5	Collagen (IV) α5	XD	Xq22.3	Alport syndrome, FSGS
Apical Membrane Proteins				
TRPC6	Transient receptor potential channel 6	AD	11q21–q22	SRNS (FSGS2)
EMP2	Epithelial membrane protein 2	AD	16p13.2	Childhood SRNS/SSNS (MCD) (NPHS10)
Nuclear Proteins				
WT1	Wilms tumor protein	AD/AR	11p13	SRNS (NPHS4), Denys-Drash syndrome, Frasier syndrome, WAGR syndrome
LMX1B	LIM homeobox transcription factor 1-β	AD	9q34.1	Nail-patella syndrome, NS
SMARCAL1	HepA-related protein	AR	2q35	Schimke immunoosseous dysplasia
PAX2	Paired box gene 2	AD	10q24.3–q25.1	Adult-onset FSGS (FSGS7), renal coloboma syndrome
MAFB	A transcription factor	AD	20q11.2–q13.1	Carpotarsal osteolysis progressive ESRD
LMNA	Lamins A and C	XD	1q22	Familial partial lipodystrophy, FSGS
NXF5	Nuclear RNA export factor 5	XR	Xq21	SRNS/FSGS cardiac conduction disorder
GATA3	GATA binding protein 3	AD	10p14	HDR syndrome (hypoparathyroidism, sensorineural deafness, renal abnormalities)
NUP93	Nucleoporin 93kD	N/A	16q13	SRNS
NUP107	Nucleoporin 107kD	N/A	12q15	Early-childhood-onset SRNS/FSGS
Mitochondrial Proteins				
COQ2	4-Hydroxybenzoate polyprenyl-transferase	AR	4q21–q22	Early-onset SRNS, CoQ10 deficiency

Continued

TABLE 22.7   Genetic Causes of Nephrotic Syndrome Categorized According to the Location of Abnormal Proteins in Podocytes—cont'd

Gene	Protein	Inheritance	Locus	Phenotypes
COQ6	Ubiquinone biosynthesis monooxygenase COQ6	AR	14q24.3	NS with sensorineural deafness, CoQ10 deficiency
PDSS2	Decaprenyl-diphosphate synthase subunit 2	AR	6q21	Leigh syndrome, CoQ10 deficiency, FSGS
MTTL1	Mitochondrially encoded tRNA leucine 1 (UUA/G)	Maternal	mtDNA	Mitochondrial diabetes, deafness with FSGS, MELAS syndrome
ADCK4	aarF domain containing kinase 4	AR	19q13.1	Childhood-onset SRNS (NPHS9), CoQ10 deficiency
Lysosomal Proteins				
SCARB2	Scavenger receptor class B, member 2 (LIMP II)	AR	4q13–q21	Action myoclonus-renal failure syndrome, lysosomal storage disease
NEU1	Sialidase 1			
	N-Acetyl-α-neuraminidase	AR	6p21.33	Nephrosialidosis, SRNS
Other Intracellular Proteins				
APOL1	Apolipoprotein L1	AR	22q12.3	FSGS in African-Americans (FSGS4)
PTPRO	Tyrosine phosphatase receptor-type O (GLEPP1)	AR	12p12.3	SRNS (NPHS6)
CRB2	Crumbs homolog 2	AR	9q33.3	Early-onset familial SRNS (FSGS9)
DGKE	Diacylglycerol kinase-ε	AR	17q22	Atypical hemolytic uremic syndrome, membranoproliferative lesions (NPHS7)
ZMPSTE24	Zinc metalloproteinase	AR	1q34	Mandibuloacral dysplasia, FSGS
PMM2	Phosphomannomutase 2	AR	16p13.2	CDG syndrome, FSGS
ALG1	β1,4 Mannosyltransferase	AR	16p13.3	CDG syndrome, congenital NS
CUBN	Cubilin	AR	10p13	Childhood-onset SRNS megaloblastic anemia
TTC21B	IFT139 (a component of intraflagellar transport-A)	AR	2q24.3	Nephronophthisis (NPHP12), FSGS
WDR73	WD repeat domain 73	AR	15q25.2	Galloway-Mowat syndrome, SRNS/FSGS

ACTN4, actinin-alpha 4; ADCK4, AarF domain containing kinase 4; AD, autosomal dominant; ALG1, asparagine-linked glycosylation protein 1; ANLN, anillin; APOL1, apolipoprotein L1; AR, autosomal recessive; ARHGAP24, Rho GTPase-activating protein 24; ARHGDIA, Rho GDP dissociation inhibitor (GDI) alpha; CD2AP, CD2-associated protein; CDG syndrome, congenital disorders of glycosylation; CNS, congenital nephrotic syndrome; COQ2, coenzyme Q2 4-hydroxybenzoate polyprenyltransferase; COQ6, coenzyme Q6 monooxygenase; CoQ10, coenzyme Q10; CRB2, Crumbs family member 2; DGKE, diacylglycerol kinase epsilon; DMS, diffuse mesangial sclerosis; EMP2, epithelial membrane protein 2; ESRD, end-stage renal disease; EXT1, exostosin 1; FSGS, focal segmental glomerulosclerosis; GBM, glomerular basement membrane; GLEPP-1, glomerular epithelial cell protein 1; HDR syndrome, hypoparathyroidism, sensorineural deafness, and renal abnormalities; ITGA3, integrin alpha 3; ITGB4, integrin beta 4; INF2, inverted formin, FH2 and WH2 domain containing; LAMB2, laminin beta 2; LIMP2, lysosome membrane protein 2; LMX1B, LIM homeobox transcription factor 1 beta; MAFB, v-maf avian musculoaponeurotic fibrosarcoma oncogene homolog B; MELAS syndrome, mitochondrial encephalomyopathy, lactic acidosis, and strokelike episodes; MTTL1, mitochondrially encoded tRNA leucine 1 (UUA/G); MYH9, myosin heavy chain 9, nonmuscle; MYO1E, *Homo sapiens* myosin IE; N/A, not available; NPHS1, nephrin; NPHS2, podocin; NS, nephrotic syndrome; NUP93, Nucleoporin 93 kD; NUP107, Nucleoporin 107 kD; PDSS2, prenyl (solanesyl) diphosphate synthase, subunit 2; PLCE1, phospholipase C, epsilon 1; PTPRO, protein tyrosine phosphatase receptor type O; SCARB2, scavenger receptor class B, member 2; SMARCAL, SWI/SNF-related, matrix associated, actin-dependent regulator of chromatin, subfamily a-like 1; SRNS, steroid-resistant nephrotic syndrome; TRPC6, transient receptor potential cation channel, subfamily C, member 6; TTC21B, tetratricopeptide repeat domain 21B; WAGR syndrome, Wilms tumor, aniridia, genitourinary anomalies, and mental retardation syndrome; WDR73, WD repeat domain 73; WT1, Wilms tumor 1.
From Tae-Sun Ha, MD. Genetics of hereditary nephrotic syndrome: a clinical review. *Korean J Pediatr.* 2017;60(3):55–63.

congenital nephrotic syndrome are often premature, with a low birthweight, placentomegaly, increased amniotic fluid α-fetoprotein levels, and hypogammaglobinemia (decreased immunoglobulin G levels).

Ascites and edema, caused by massive proteinuria, are usually present in affected infants during the first few weeks after birth. Patients do not respond to steroids or cytotoxic therapy. Infections and thrombosis are the two major complications; they cause considerable morbidity and mortality. Because of the massive proteinuria, patients fail to thrive; they require nasogastric feeding with a high-calorie, high-protein formula. Nephrectomy and peritoneal dialysis are often necessary to control protein losses and allow for adequate growth and control of uremia so that the infant can reach a size and nutritional state sufficient for renal transplantation.

Diffuse Mesangial Sclerosis

Diffuse mesangial sclerosis is the other diagnostic entity seen in infants. This disease is similar to congenital nephrotic syndrome, but it often results in less severe protein losses. Patients are often full term and of a normal birthweight. The amniotic fluid α-fetoprotein is normal, and the onset of edema (1 week–33 months) is later than in congenital nephrotic

TABLE 22.8 Causes of Childhood Nephrotic Syndrome

Idiopathic Nephrotic Syndrome
Minimal change disease
Focal segmental glomerulosclerosis
Membranous nephropathy
Glomerulonephritis associated with nephrotic syndrome—membranoproliferative glomerulonephritis, crescentic glomerulonephritis, immunoglobulin A nephropathy

Genetic Disorders Associated with Proteinuria or Nephrotic Syndrome
Over 100 genetic syndromic disorders are associated with proteinuria; the more common disorders are listed below (see Tables 22.6, 22.7, and 22.10)

Nephrotic Syndrome (Typical)
Finnish-type congenital nephrotic syndrome (absence of nephrin)
Focal segmental glomerulosclerosis (variants in nephrin, podocin, *MYO1E*, α-actinin-4, TRPC6)
Diffuse mesangial sclerosis (variants in laminin β_2 chain)
Denys-Drash syndrome (variants in WT1 transcription factor)
Congenital nephrotic syndrome with lung and skin involvement (integrin α_3 variant)
Mitochondrial disorders (rare association, steroid resistance, MELAS)

Proteinuria with or Without Nephrotic Syndrome
Nail-patella syndrome (variant in LMX1B transcription factor)
Alport syndrome (variant in collagen 4 biosynthesis genes)

Multisystem Syndromes with or Without Nephrotic Syndrome
Galloway-Mowat syndrome
Charcot-Marie-Tooth disease
Jeune syndrome
Cockayne syndrome
Bardet-Biedl syndrome

Metabolic Disorders with or Without Nephrotic Syndrome
Alagille syndrome
α_1-Antitrypsin deficiency
Fabry disease
Glutaric acidemia
Glycogen storage disease
Hurler syndrome
Partial lipodystrophy
Mitochondrial cytopathies
Sickle cell disease

Secondary Causes of Nephrotic Syndrome
Infections
Endocarditis
Hepatitis B, C
HIV-1
Infectious mononucleosis
Malaria
Syphilis (congenital and secondary)
Toxoplasmosis
Schistosomiasis
Filariasis

Drugs
Captopril
Penicillamine
Gold
Nonsteroidal antiinflammatory drugs
Pamidronate
Interferon
Mercury
Heroin
Lithium

Immunologic or Allergic Disorders
Vasculitis syndromes
Castleman disease
Kimura disease
Bee sting
Food allergens
Serum sickness

Associated with Malignant Disease
Lymphoma
Leukemia
Solid tumors

Glomerular Hyperfiltration
Oligomeganephronia
Morbid obesity
Adaptation to nephron reduction

Modified from Eddy AA, Symons JM. Nephrotic syndrome in childhood. *Lancet.* 2003;362:629–638; from Pais P, Avner ED. Fixed proteinuria. In: Kliegman RM, Stanton BF, St. Geme JW III, eds. *Nelson Textbook of Pediatrics.* 20th ed. Philadelphia: Elsevier; 2016:2522, Table 527.1.

syndrome (birth–3 months). The patients have hypertension, hematuria, and renal insufficiency at presentation. When diffuse mesangial sclerosis is seen in association with a female phenotype, chromosome typing is recommended to look for patients with Drash syndrome (XY gonadal dysgenesis, nephropathy, and Wilms tumor). When this syndrome is present, bilateral nephrectomy and gonadectomy are recommended because the potential for malignancy is very high.

Treatment is similar to patients with congenital nephrotic syndrome and eventually requires renal transplantation. The major goal is to help these infants achieve the growth and good nutrition necessary for successful renal transplantation. Nephrotic syndrome occasionally occurs after transplantation for congenital nephrotic syndrome, probably secondarily to an autoimmune reaction to nephrin.

ASYMPTOMATIC PROTEINURIA DISORDERS

Many patients have proteinuria, but there is no edema, the blood pressure is normal, and serum protein levels are normal. The extent of the work-up must be tailored to the seriousness of the problem. Whether an evaluation should be performed depends on whether the proteinuria is both persistent and nonorthostatic (Fig. 22.3). A *child younger than 7 or 8 years of age* who has persistent isolated proteinuria, normal blood pressure, renal function, and total protein and serum albumin levels should be observed carefully with repeated urinalyses every 3–6 months and parents counseled with regard to swelling and/or ascites, which may develop in association with influenza or an upper respiratory infection. If there is evidence of overt nephrotic syndrome with

TABLE 22.9 Causes of Nephrotic Syndrome in Infants Younger Than 1 Year

Secondary Causes

Infections

Syphilis
Cytomegalovirus
Toxoplasmosis
Rubella
Hepatitis B
HIV
Malaria
Toxins
Mercury

Other

Systemic lupus erythematosus
Syndromes with associated renal disease
Nail-patella syndrome
Lowe syndrome
Nephropathy associated with congenital brain malformation
Denys-Drash syndrome: Wilms tumor
Hemolytic uremic syndrome

Primary Causes

Congenital nephrotic syndrome (see Table 22.10)
Diffuse mesangial sclerosis
Minimal change disease
Focal segmental sclerosis
Membranous nephropathy

From Kliegman RM, Greenbaum LA, Lye PS. *Practical Strategies in Pediatric Diagnosis and Therapy.* 2nd ed. Philadelphia: Saunders; 2004:418.

TABLE 22.10 The Etiology of Congenital (3 Months of Age or Younger) Nephrotic Syndrome (CNS)

Primary CNS

Nephrin gene variants (*NPHS1*, Finnish type of CNS [CNF])
Podocin gene variants (*NPHS2*)
WT1 gene variants (Denys-Drash, isolated CNS)
LamB2 gene variants (Pierson syndrome, isolated CNS)
PLCE1 gene variants
LMX1B variants (nail-patella syndrome)
LamB3 gene variants (Herlitz junctional epidermolysis bullosa)
Mitochondrial myopathies
CNS with or without brain and other malformations (no gene defect identified as yet)

Secondary CNS

Congenital syphilis
Toxoplasmosis, malaria
Cytomegalovirus, rubella, hepatitis B, HIV
Maternal systemic lupus erythematosus
Neonatal autoantibodies against neutral endopeptidase
Maternal steroid–chlorpheniramine treatment

From Jalanko H. Congenital nephrotic syndrome. *Pediatr Nephrol.* 2009;24:2121–2128 (Table 1, p. 2122).

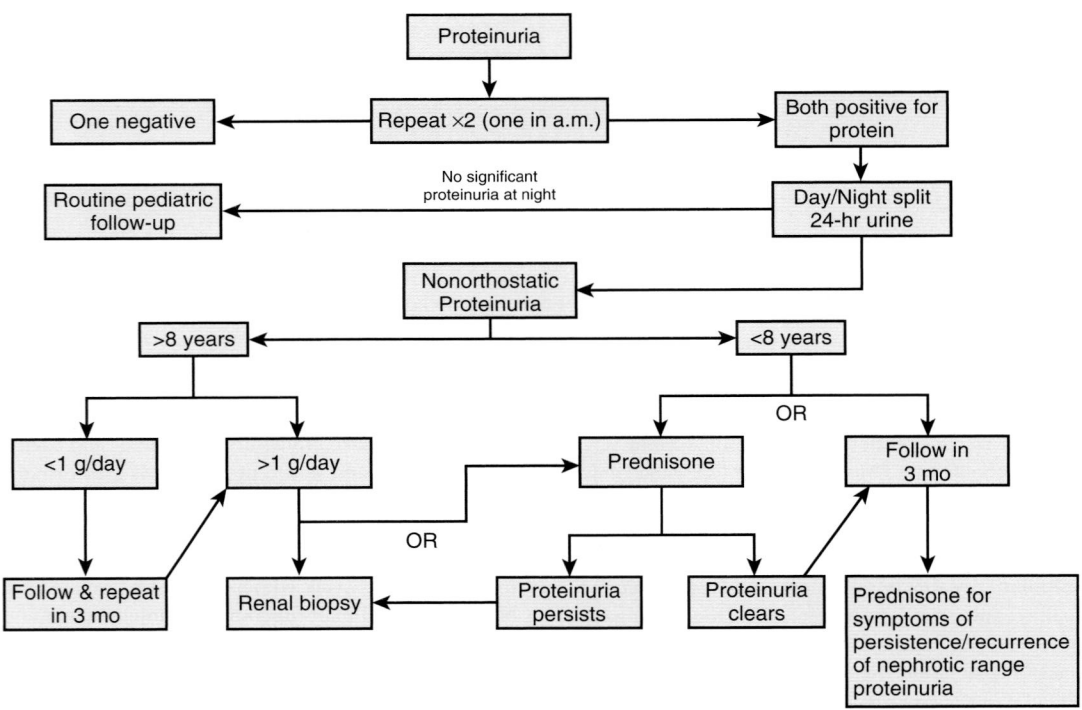

Fig. 22.3 Algorithm for age-based management of proteinuria.

edema, a decrease in serum albumin, and an increase in serum cholesterol, a trial of daily prednisone therapy is indicated. It is good practice to give the pneumococcal vaccine to patients who have persistent proteinuria but no evidence of edema or nephrotic syndrome, because of the risk of pneumococcal peritonitis if nephrotic syndrome develops. If the patient has a more serious lesion, symptoms will develop, at which time evaluation and therapy may be undertaken.

In a *patient older than 8 or 9 years*, once the presence of persistent and nonorthostatic proteinuria is established, the next step is to quantify the amount of protein in a 24-hour specimen. If urinary protein excretion is >1 g/day, a renal biopsy may be considered. Alternatively, these patients can also be treated with steroids and the response assessed. If proteinuria does not clear after 6–8 weeks of therapy, renal biopsy is then indicated. The choice of 1 g/day of proteinuria is arbitrary; nephrotic syndrome is defined as 40 mg/m^2/hr. Hence, an average 8-year-old patient who weighs 30 kg and has surface area 1 m^2 nephrotic syndrome by this definition is at a level of 960 mg/day. Renal biopsy should be considered at lower range if there are additional features suggestive of glomerulonephritis. This guideline helps avoid a biopsy for the patient with minimal proteinuria because isolated proteinuria is an unlikely possibility with membranoproliferative glomerulonephritis (MPGN) or SLE. However, the incidence of focal segmental sclerosis is much higher in adolescents than in younger children. With the possibility of treatment with cyclosporine and/or ACE inhibitors preventing future renal failure, aggressive evaluation is warranted to identify patients who might benefit from these therapies.

Low molecular protein, such as β2-microglobulin, α1-microglobulin, lysozyme, and retinol-binding protein, can be seen in urine in tubular disorders, such as Fanconi syndrome or Dent disease. If associated with acidosis, hypokalemia, and hypophosphatemia, Fanconi syndrome should be considered. In males, if proteinuria is associated with hypercalciuria and nephrocalcinosis, Dent disease, an X-linked proximal tubulopathy that eventually leads to end-stage renal disease, should be considered, and the urine should be tested for β2-microglobulin. Genetic testing can confirm the diagnosis.

The presence of protein in the urine increases the risk of renal insufficiency, regardless of its cause. This has led to therapies that reduce proteinuria, thereby decreasing the risk of a progressive loss of renal function. The traffic of protein across the glomerular capillary membrane appears to stimulate a cascade of inflammatory events that cause interstitial fibrosis. ACE inhibitors result in efferent arteriolar vasodilatation, leading to a decrease in intraglomerular pressure, which in turn leads to a decreased transport of protein across the glomerular filter. Patients who are treated with ACE inhibitors are less likely to increase their level of proteinuria and are less likely to lose their renal function than are patients who are not treated with these agents. This was first apparent in the treatment of diabetic nephropathy, but there is evidence that ACE inhibitors offer advantages to patients with other nephropathies as well. Angiotensin II blockers offer another avenue for accomplishing a decrease in intraglomerular pressures, and these also decrease proteinuria when used alone or in conjunction with an ACE inhibitor. ACE inhibitors and angiotensin II blockers may be useful for patients with proteinuria either as a first step or as adjunctive therapy for those who fail to respond to other medications.

SUMMARY AND RED FLAGS

Asymptomatic proteinuria may be associated with nonspecific febrile benign illnesses, postural mechanisms, and glomerular or tubular dysfunction. Significant proteinuria with edema suggests nephrotic syndrome, which in most children suggests minimal change nephrotic syndrome. An age younger than 1 year or older than 10 years plus significant hematuria, azotemia, and hypertension are red flags that suggest a cause of nephrosis other than the more benign minimal change disease. Additional red flags include a poor response to prednisone therapy and signs of multiple organ system involvement by a primary systemic disease, such as SLE. Fever and abdominal pain in a patient with nephrotic syndrome should suggest spontaneous primary bacterial peritonitis. Severe headache and respiratory distress in a patient with nephrotic syndrome should raise concerns for thrombosis or pulmonary embolus.

BIBLIOGRAPHY

A bibliography is available at ExpertConsult.com.

23

Hematuria

Scott K. Van Why and Cynthia G. Pan

Hematuria is a common issue faced by primary physicians who care for children. While it can cause great anxiety in the patient and family when it presents as gross hematuria, rarely does hematuria alone herald a serious illness during childhood. Indeed, despite thorough evaluation, no cause can be found in a large percentage of children who have hematuria. Nearly 40% of children who present with gross hematuria and 80% of patients with persistent, isolated microscopic hematuria have no identifiable cause despite a thorough investigation. This raises the question of how much investigation should be performed on a child who presents with hematuria, particularly if it is *isolated* microscopic hematuria, because the evaluation can be costly and at times invasive.

How extensive an evaluation is appropriate depends much on the context. Those children who present with gross hematuria or microscopic hematuria with associated signs or symptoms deserve a thorough evaluation. These two groups contain those more likely to have an identifiable cause and include the subset that has an acute or potentially serious illness that can progress to significant morbidity or sequelae if not identified and treated. Associated symptoms and signs that indicate the need for prompt evaluation include other urinary or systemic symptoms that led to testing the urine for blood, and findings of hypertension, edema, poor growth, fever, or other systemic signs at presentation.

The more difficult question is how much testing is required of an apparently healthy child discovered to have isolated microscopic hematuria on routine screening urinalysis. Thorough testing of such a child with no symptoms, a normal physical examination, and no significant family history of kidney disease rarely identifies a cause of hematuria. A screening urinalysis in children, with the potential attendant costly and usually uninformative additional investigation, is not recommended for early school-aged children. It is reasonable to screen children who have a significant family history of kidney disease, particularly if there is a family history of hereditary nephritis.

GROSS HEMATURIA

Gross hematuria, defined as blood in the urine visible to the naked eye, is a dramatic symptom that is usually brought to medical attention, unless an older child with the symptom is too frightened to bring it to the attention of the parents. Carefully defining the appearance of the urine can be the first and a major clue to the origin of the blood. Hematuria emanating from a nonglomerular, lower urinary tract source can present as frankly bloody urine varying in color from dark red, cherry, or pink-tinged urine. On occasion, lower tract hematuria can result in passing blood clots. Seeing blood in the urine only on initiation or at termination of voiding is an additional clue that the source is from the lower tract. Blood seen at the urethral meatus or only on initiation of voiding suggests a urethral source. In contrast, hematuria originating from a glomerular source more often presents with description of other color changes in the urine, such as brown-, cola-, tea-, or, on occasion, even green-colored urine.

The first step when presented with this symptom is to perform a urinalysis. If no hemoglobin is found on macroscopic urinalysis, then causes of urine discoloration other than hematuria need to be considered (Table 23.1). One common presentation that can be particularly frightening to a parent is finding a pink or red-tinged wet diaper, thought to be blood in the urine. This most often is from a simple benign entity commonly called **red diaper syndrome**, caused by precipitation of urate crystals in the diaper. A macroscopic urinalysis negative for heme indicates this to be the most likely cause, and in an otherwise healthy infant, no further investigation is warranted.

If red blood cells (RBCs) are found in the urine of a child with a history suggestive of gross hematuria, then evaluation for potential causes is needed (Tables 23.2 and 23.3 and Fig. 23.1). The first step is a thorough history and physical examination.

History

Development of pain with the onset of hematuria usually indicates a lower urinary tract source. Irritative symptoms, such as dysuria, urgency, or frequency, can be seen in bleeding from the bladder from a variety of causes. Although not a typical feature of urinary tract infection (UTI), the most common identifiable cause of gross hematuria is a UTI and is usually accompanied by significant dysuria or abdominal pain, and sometimes fever. Severe and episodic or colicky flank or abdominal pain should raise suspicion for urolithiasis, which may have accompanying dysuria as the stone is being passed. Urinary tract obstruction, such as posterior urethral valves in males or ureteropelvic junction obstruction in either gender, may remain occult until infection or trauma causes hematuria. In the former, the only preceding symptoms may be a male who voids only infrequently, commonly strains to void, or has ongoing urinary incontinence beyond the toddler years. Bleeding from renal tumors is an uncommon cause of gross hematuria in children but should be considered particularly in the setting of associated abdominal pain, a palpable mass, or passing of blood clots.

Gross hematuria due to glomerular disease is rarely accompanied by significant pain, though some may report mild abdominal pain or flank discomfort. An exception is immunoglobulin A (IgA) vasculitis (Henoch-Schönlein purpura [HSP]), a common pediatric systemic vasculitis, which can have variable, including severe, gastrointestinal disease. Clues to underlying glomerular disease may be a recent history of pharyngitis, streptococcal skin infection, or other febrile illnesses, indicating possible acute postinfectious glomerulonephritis. Patients with glomerulonephritis or renal insufficiency may report shortness of breath, edema, or weight gain from fluid retention. They may also have a headache or visual changes secondary to severe hypertension. Abdominal pain, diarrhea, hematochezia, rash, and arthralgias are symptoms indicative of a systemic vasculitis, such as IgA vasculitis

(HSP). Recurrent, painless gross hematuria is often seen in young patients with IgA nephropathy in association with concurrent respiratory illness. Recurrent fever, weight loss, alopecia, mouth ulcers, chest pain, fatigue, and arthritis suggest systemic lupus erythematosus (SLE). Hemoptysis or cough is seen in pulmonary-renal syndromes caused by antineutrophil cytoplasmic antibody (ANCA)-associated disease, and on occasion in lupus and HSP.

The patient's **medical history** may be most informative. Stressed neonates from birth asphyxia, infection, or volume depletion can develop renal vein thrombus that presents as gross hematuria. Patients with African ancestry should be queried for personal or family history

of sickle cell hemoglobinopathy since gross hematuria from renal papillary necrosis can occur in those with sickle cell disease as well as in children with simple sickle cell trait. Medication history can uncover a cause of gross hematuria from drug-induced interstitial nephritis, seen with several antibiotics, anticonvulsants, or nonsteroidal antiinflammatory drugs; the latter can also cause papillary necrosis. Cyclophosphamide can cause a severe hemorrhagic cystitis, which usually has concomitant prominent bladder symptoms.

A history of frequent or severe bleeding from other sites, such as heavy menses, prolonged nosebleeds, hemarthroses, or significant bleeding associated with surgical procedures, suggests an undiagnosed bleeding disorder. Exposure history to tuberculosis should be obtained, as well as a travel history, as parasitic infections such as schistosomiasis of the bladder, uncommon in Western societies, is common in other parts of the world. Questions specific to other potential sources of blood in the urine include those directed at a foreign body from self-instrumentation of the urethra, trauma, sexual abuse, and menstruation. Extreme sports activities such as running a marathon or long-distance cycling can cause gross hematuria.

Review of the **family history** is important to uncover hereditary nephritis, hereditary cystic kidney disease, or potential benign familial hematuria. A family history of kidney disease leading to end-stage renal failure, especially if in men in multiple generations and if not clearly due to diabetes mellitus, would suggest Alport syndrome, the most common cause of hereditary nephritis. **Alport syndrome** is predominantly an X-linked recessive disorder that may cause gross hematuria in childhood, although more often it is microscopic. When gross hematuria occurs in Alport syndrome, it is often triggered by any infectious process such as a common cold. The gross hematuria then subsequently clears, but microscopic hematuria is a persistent finding. The early clinical features of hereditary nephritis can be exactly the same as benign familial hematuria but then evolve to develop other features. Early in the course of the disease, there is no associated proteinuria, but that feature develops later, often in childhood as the nephropathy progresses. Hearing loss is a common but variable feature of Alport syndrome that tends to run in affected families. Female family members who are carriers usually have persistent and isolated hematuria that does not progress, but on occasion may develop progressive nephritis.

Benign familial hematuria and familial thin basement membrane nephropathy are also responsible for both microhematuria and gross hematuria. The primary difference in family history that separates benign familial hematuria from progressive hereditary nephritis is that

TABLE 23.1 Urine Discoloration from Sources Other Than Hematuria

Pink, Red, Cola-Colored, Burgundy

Disease Associated

Hemoglobinuria*	Porphyrinuria
Myoglobinuria*	

Associated with Drug or Food Ingestion

Aminopyrine	Nitrofurantoin
Anthocyanin	Phenazopyridine
Azo dyes	Phenolphthalein
Beets	Pyridium
Blackberries	Red food coloring
Chloroquine	Rifampin
Deferoxamine mesylate	Rhodamine B
Iron sorbitol	Rhubarb
Methyldopa	Sulfasalazine
	Urates

Dark Brown, Black

Disease Associated

Alkaptonuria	Methemoglobinemia
Homogentisic aciduria	Tyrosinosis
Melanin	Bile pigments

Associated with Food or Drug Ingestion

Alanine	Resorcinol
Cascara	Thymol

*Heme tests positive.

TABLE 23.2 Laboratory Testing in Suspected Glomerulonephritis*

Symptoms	Suspected Glomerulonephritis	Laboratory
History of preceding pharyngitis, URI, or impetigo	Acute postinfectious GN	C3, C4 complement (low C3, normal C4)
Arthralgia, purpura, pedal edema, abdominal pain, hematochezia	IgA vasculitis (Henoch-Schönlein purpura)	Skin biopsy
Arthritis, rash, fever, oral ulcers, weight loss, alopecia, weakness, central nervous system symptoms, other systemic symptoms	Systemic lupus erythematosus	C3, C4 (both low) ANA, anti-dsDNA (both high)
Family history of renal failure, hearing loss, hematuria	Familial nephritis—Alport syndrome	Audiogram, slit-lamp exam, genetic testing
Recurrent, painless gross hematuria	IgA nephropathy	None (kidney biopsy)
Hemoptysis, cough, fevers	Goodpasture syndrome	Anti-GBM Ab
Rash, sinus disease, hemoptysis, systemic symptoms	ANCA-associated vasculitis	ANCA

*All patients: serum creatinine, electrolytes, CBC, random urine protein:creatinine ratio, 24-hr urine collection for protein.
Ab, antibody; ANA, antinuclear antibody; ANCA, antineutrophil cytoplasmic antibody; anti-dsDNA, anti–double-stranded DNA antibody; anti-GBM, anti–glomerular basement membrane antibody; GN, glomerulonephritis; IgA, immunoglobulin A; URI, upper respiratory infection.

TABLE 23.3 Causes of Gross Hematuria in Children

GLOMERULAR

Primary
Acute postinfectious glomerulonephritis
IgA nephropathy*
Mesangial proliferative glomerulonephritis
Membranoproliferative glomerulonephritis
Familial nephritis (Alport syndrome)
Benign familial hematuria—thin basement membrane disease
Rapidly progressive glomerulonephritis

Systemic
IgA vasculitis (Henoch-Schönlein purpura)
Systemic lupus erythematosus
Hemolytic uremic syndrome
ANCA-associated vasculitis
Goodpasture disease (rare in childhood)
Bacterial endocarditis

INTERSTITIAL DISEASE

Pyelonephritis
Acute interstitial nephritis
Polycystic kidney disease (autosomal dominant)

VASCULAR

Trauma
Sickle cell disease and trait
Renal artery/vein thrombosis
Arteriovenous malformation
Nutcracker syndrome
Sports- and exercise-induced hematuria
Hemangioma/hamartoma

NEOPLASTIC

Wilms tumor
Renal cell carcinoma
Uroepithelial tumors
Rhabdoid tumors
Congenital mesoblastic nephroma
Angiomyolipoma

URINARY TRACT

Cystitis
  Bacterial
  Viral (adenovirus)
  Parasitic (schistosomiasis)
  Tuberculosis
  Cyclophosphamide
Urethritis
Urolithiasis
Idiopathic hypercalciuria without urolithiasis
Trauma
Hydronephrosis, severe
Foreign body

BLEEDING DISORDERS

Hemophilia A or B
Platelet disorder
Thrombocytopenia
Coagulopathy, congenital or acquired

*Common cause of asymptomatic gross hematuria.
ANCA, antineutrophil cytoplasmic antibody; IgA, immunoglobulin A.

members of sequential generations of the family with benign familial hematuria, either male or female, have persistent isolated hematuria that never progresses to significant renal disease. The genetics of benign familial hematuria due to thin basement membrane nephropathy has been defined and includes gene variants that are identical to those seen in some patients with autosomal recessive forms of progressive hereditary nephritis. Patients with thin basement membrane nephropathy, or benign familial hematuria, may be carriers of genes that cause autosomal recessive Alport syndrome.

Patients with **autosomal dominant polycystic kidney disease (ADPKD)** may present initially with gross hematuria from spontaneous bleeding into the macrocysts. Because the course of ADPKD can vary widely from one generation to the next, with some members having very mild disease with minimal clinical features until late adulthood, the family history of the disease may not be apparent on presentation. Early onset of hypertension, during youth or young adulthood in a parent of an affected child, may be the only clue to a family member being affected by ADPKD.

Gross hematuria is a presenting complaint in 15% of children with **urolithiasis**. Kidney stone disease can be familial, and in some cases related to specific genes, as in X-linked recessive nephrolithiasis (Dent disease) or primary hyperoxaluria. Therefore, family history of early-onset nephrolithiasis, especially in siblings, should be sought in children presenting with gross hematuria and symptoms or imaging that indicate kidney stone disease as the cause. A family history of a bleeding disorder such as hemophilia or platelet disorders should be sought.

Physical Examination

The initial focus of the physical examination should be for evidence of systemic disease for which the hematuria is one manifestation, and for potential sequelae of renal disease. Accurate measurement and attention to blood pressure, recognizing age differences in blood pressure, is critical. **Hypertension** may be the sole feature on physical examination that indicates underlying acute glomerulonephritis, or chronic kidney disease from several causes. The finding of **edema** in this context is highly suggestive of underlying renal parenchymal disease, either acute or chronic, with likely accompanying renal insufficiency. **Poor growth** or failure to thrive may indicate chronic renal disease. Pallor, fever, rashes, or musculoskeletal findings suggest systemic vasculitis with renal involvement from diseases such as HSP, SLE, or, less often, ANCA-associated disease. Examination of the abdomen may reveal abdominal or flank masses that could be tumors, cystic kidneys, or urinary obstruction. The most common renal tumor in childhood, typically seen in young children (ages 1–4 years), is Wilms tumor, though other types occur. Hydronephrosis or enlarged cystic kidneys may be palpable. Suprapubic tenderness may indicate bladder infection, stone, or other less common causes of bladder pathology as the source of blood. The genitalia should be inspected for blood at the urethral meatus that suggests a urethral source, tears or lacerations due to abuse or accidents such as from straddle injuries, or to look for a foreign body.

Evaluation

Laboratory Tests

Macroscopic and microscopic examination of the urine is the first essential step in laboratory evaluation. If no heme is found on macroscopic examination, then other causes of urine discoloration need to be considered (see Table 23.1 and Fig. 23.1). If the urine is heme positive on macroscopic examination but no red cells are found on microscopic examination of the urine sediment, then myoglobinuria or hemoglobinuria need to be considered as the possible source, since **rhabdomyolysis**

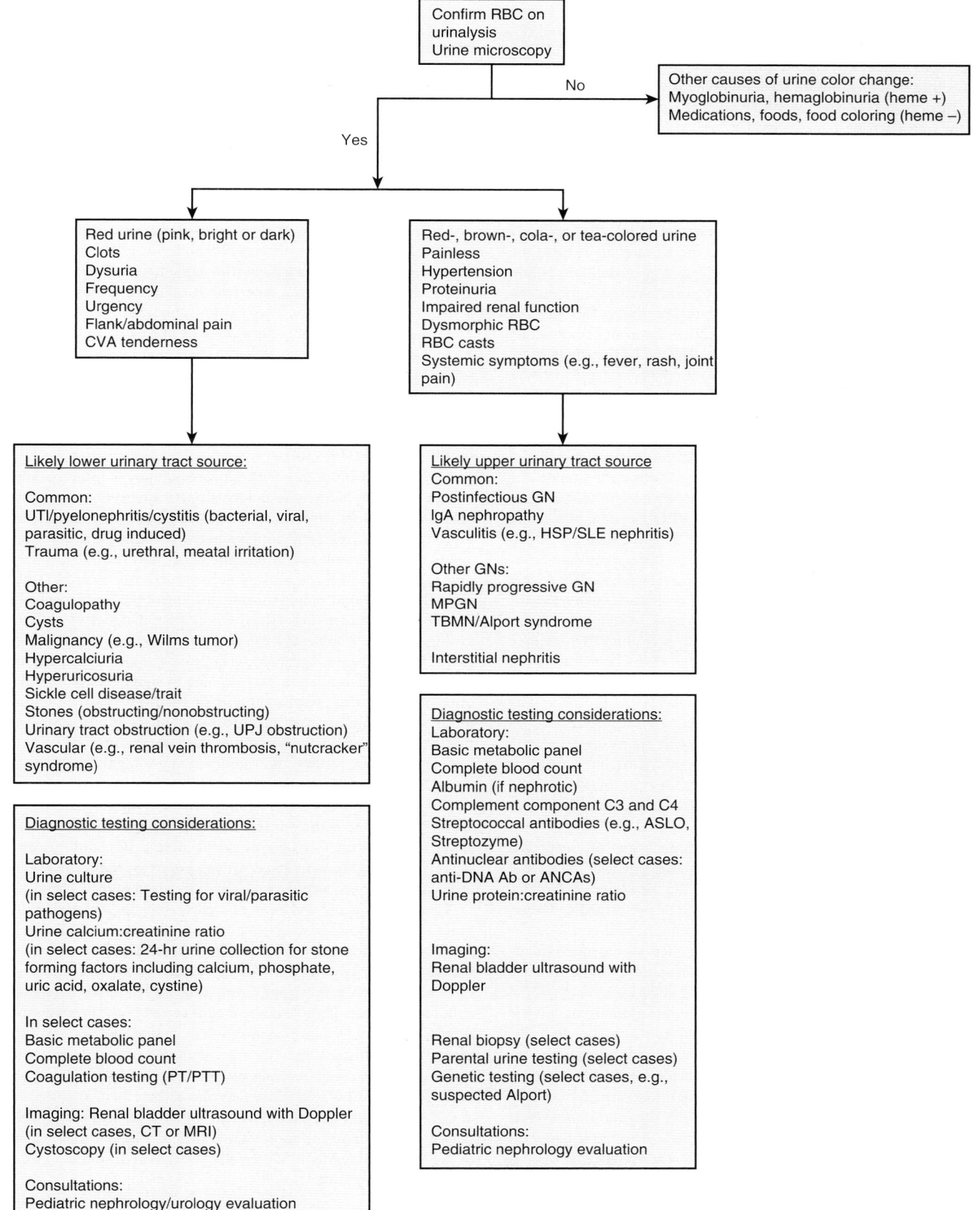

Fig. 23.1 Gross hematuria work-up. Abs, antibodies; ANCAs, antineutrophil cytoplasmic antibodies; CVA, cerebrovascular accident; GN, glomerulonephritis; HSP/SLE, Henoch-Schönlein purpura/systemic lupus erythematosus; IgA, immunoglobulin A; MPGN, membranoproliferative glomerulonephritis; PT/PTT, prothrombin time/partial thromboplastin time; RBC, red blood cell; TBMN, thin basement membrane disease; UPJ, ureteropelvic junction; UTI, urinary tract infection. (From Brown DD, Reidy KJ. Approach to the child with hematuria. *Pediatr Clin N Am.* 2019;66:15–30 [Fig. 2, p. 18].)

and **acute hemolysis** are both potential life-threatening diseases that require immediate attention. If urine is heme positive but no red cells are seen and there is no evidence for rhabdomyolysis or acute hemolytic disease, then other reasons for the findings need to be considered. Urine test strips can on occasion be falsely positive for blood if the urine is infected with peroxidase-producing bacteria. More likely is that red cells were present but lysed in urine that either was very dilute or was held for an extended time before microscopic examination was performed. Finding red cell casts in a resuspended pellet of spun urine (centrifuged 3–5 minutes at 1,500–2,000 rpm) under high-power field is a clear indication that the source of hematuria is glomerular. While the specificity of this finding in localizing the source to the glomerulus is high, the sensitivity of finding red cell casts in the hands of clinical labs is low. When red cell casts have been found in the urine sediment by experienced nephrologists, clinical laboratory reports of finding RBC casts in the urine of the same patients is very low. Unless the urine is thoroughly examined by an experienced clinician, the lack of RBC casts in a lab report does not lower the chance the patient might have a glomerular source of the hematuria. Another finding on microscopic examination of the urine sediment that suggests a glomerular source is the presence of a significant number of dysmorphic red cells (see Fig. 23.1). This finding requires careful inspection of erythrocyte morphology and is best done with a phase-contrast microscope. Clinical labs do not report the number of dysmorphic red cells present, in part because differentiating dysmorphic RBCs from simple crenated RBCs (a result of osmotic shrinkage of RBCs) takes an experienced eye. Keeping these caveats in mind, if an experienced clinician finds RBC casts or a significant number of dysmorphic RBCs in a patient with hematuria, subsequent testing can be focused on identifying potential glomerular causes of hematuria, avoiding unnecessary, costly, or potentially invasive imaging procedures.

An additional feature of urinalysis that may help guide to the source of the red cells is the presence of proteinuria. Gross hematuria from lower tract bleeding can result in urine positive for protein, particularly if any lysis of urinary red cells occurs, but usually is <2+ proteinuria by dipstick reading. *Anything >2+ proteinuria should raise suspicion of glomerular disease, especially if the hematuria is only microscopic.* Bacteria and significant pyuria suggest pyelonephritis or cystitis, but pyuria can also be a feature of acute suppurative glomerulonephritis. Quantification of the gross hematuria using a "urocrit," with a result >1%, can indicate lower tract bleeding.

All patients with suspected glomerulonephritis or suspected chronic kidney disease should have prompt assessment of their renal function with a serum creatinine and a CBC. Serologic studies for immune-mediated glomerulonephritis should be performed including complement levels (C3, C4), antinuclear antibody, and anti–double-stranded DNA antibody. ANCA and anti–glomerular basement membrane antibody titers should also be obtained if vasculitis or pulmonary renal syndromes are suspected (see Table 23.2 and Fig. 23.1).

The diagnosis of most cases of postinfectious glomerulonephritis can be made clinically. The diagnosis of HSP is also made clinically, but skin biopsy of purpuric lesions demonstrating vasculitis with predominantly IgA deposits can be supportive evidence. A kidney biopsy is often needed to define other forms of glomerulonephritis, especially primary, idiopathic glomerulopathies (Fig. 23.2). In addition, even if the diagnosis of vasculitis (Fig. 23.3 and Table 23.4) is made based on clinical and serologic criteria, staging of the severity of renal disease with renal pathology, such as in SLE, HSP, or ANCA-positive disease, is important for guiding therapy. High levels of proteinuria are often an indication to obtain a kidney biopsy to provide a diagnosis or stage the severity of the lesion in several forms of glomerulonephritis. The degree of proteinuria can be assessed with a 24-hour urine collection or with a spot urine protein:creatinine ratio (see Chapter 22).

A urine culture is indicated in patients with any bladder symptoms, fever, flank pain, or abdominal pain. Gross hematuria can also be seen with nonbacterial infections such as tuberculosis, adenovirus, or schistosomiasis. In immunocompromised patients, BK polyomavirus can cause prominent cystitis.

Idiopathic hypercalciuria can be a cause of gross hematuria. It is characterized by excessive urinary calcium excretion in the absence of hypercalcemia or other known causes of hypercalciuria (Table 23.5). The hematuria is thought to be secondary to calcium oxalate and phosphate crystals adhering to urothelium. The risk of developing kidney stones is not known. Although often asymptomatic, hypercalciuria is also implicated in causing urinary symptoms including abdominal and flank pain. Therefore, in a patient who has any such symptom concomitant with gross hematuria, especially if UTI and anatomic causes of hematuria are ruled out, urinary calcium should be measured.

Hypercalciuria is defined by a 24-hour urine for calcium excretion >4 mg/kg/day. A spot urine calcium:creatinine ratio of >0.22 is considered abnormal in the older child and adolescent, but normal values may be significantly higher in younger children, especially those younger than 7 years of age.

Imaging and Cystoscopy

Renal imaging with noninvasive ultrasonography is recommended in all cases of gross hematuria, unless strong evidence for glomerulonephritis is found on clinical grounds as detailed earlier. Ultrasound is excellent in children to investigate potential urologic and congenital abnormalities, as well as certain genetic diseases including polycystic kidney disease and those causing nephrocalcinosis, such as Dent disease. The ultrasound should include imaging of the bladder, which can identify rare bladder tumors, as well as find evidence of obstructive urologic disease. Ultrasound can also provide some evidence for renal parenchymal disease. Enlarged, echogenic kidneys with poor corticomedullary differentiation may be seen in significant glomerular or interstitial nephritis. Nephrolithiasis or calcinosis may be found on ultrasound, as well as hydronephrosis secondary to urinary obstruction from lower tract kidney stones. Urolithiasis may be missed on ultrasound; if the history and examination are highly suggestive of a stone as the source of the hematuria, a CT scan is then necessary.

CT imaging is most useful to identify kidney stones (using the helical technique) and is the primary indication to perform this study. CT also provides detailed images of the bladder, pelvis, and retroperitoneum when looking for masses. Angiogram of the kidney may be necessary to identify an arteriovenous malformation of the kidney.

Cystograms generally have no major role in the evaluation of gross hematuria unless there is ultrasound evidence of bladder outlet obstruction from unrecognized urethral valves, or an unusual mass such as a urothelial tumor, rhabdomyosarcoma, or fibromatous polyp. Cystoscopy is rarely indicated in the usual evaluation of hematuria in children. However, if passing blood clots is part of the presentation, or if renal and bladder ultrasound shows a bladder mass or an obstructive lesion, cystoscopy may then be definitive in diagnosing bladder and ureteral sources of bleeding and provides an opportunity to obtain tissue for diagnosis. Cystoscopy may also be helpful to look for unilateral bleeding from one ureter, which can be seen with renal papillary necrosis, or more uncommon lesions such as vascular malformations or polyps of the bladder or ureter, all of which can be difficult to define by radiologic methods.

MICROSCOPIC HEMATURIA

While thorough evaluation of gross hematuria is always warranted, how far to proceed with the evaluation of microscopic hematuria can

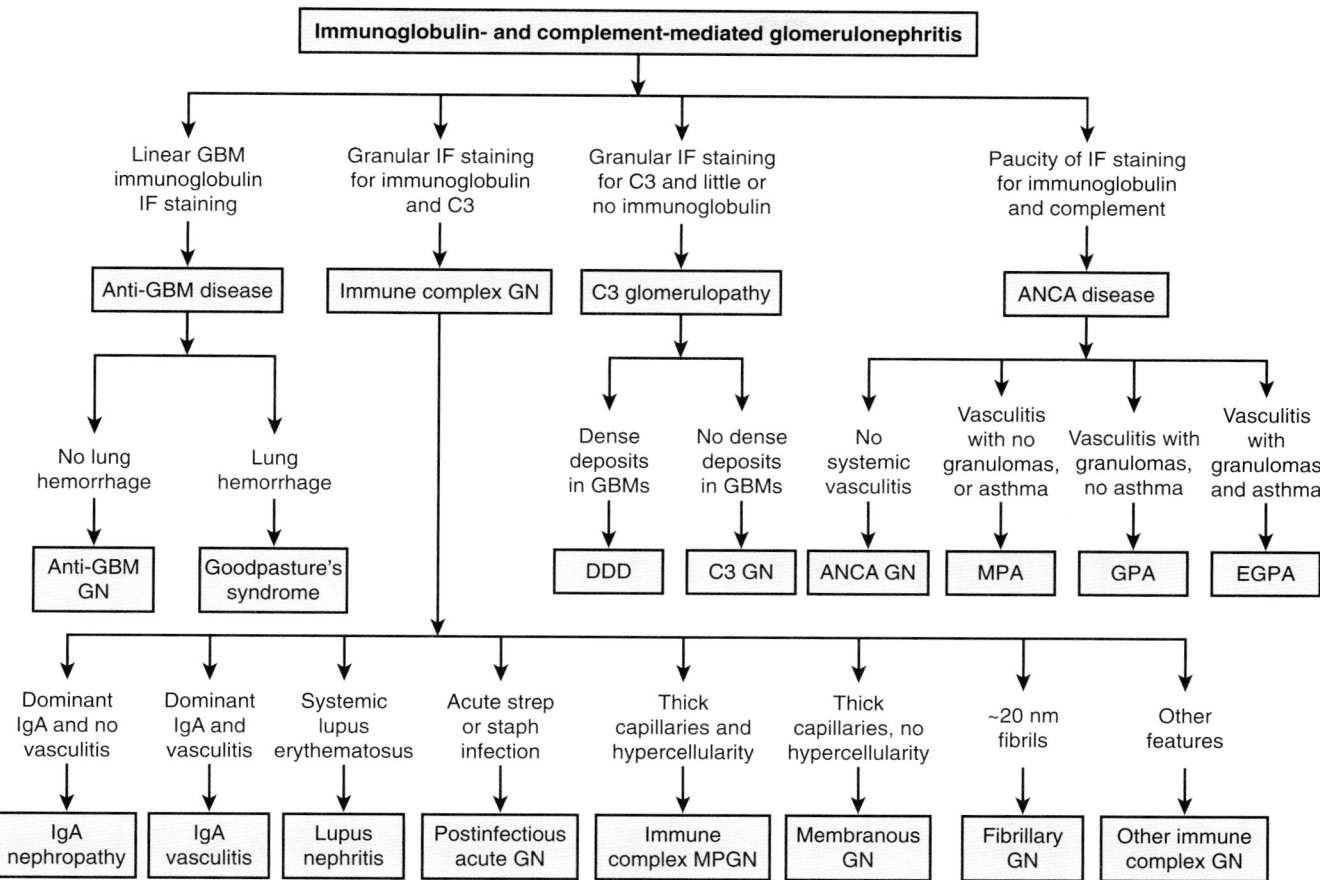

Fig. 23.2 Algorithm for the diagnostic classification of glomerulonephritis that is known or suspected of being mediated by antibodies and complement. Note that the integration of light microscopy, immunofluorescence (IF) microscopy, electron microscopy, laboratory data, and clinical manifestations is required to diagnose glomerulonephritis (GN) precisely. ANCA, antineutrophil cytoplasmic autoantibody; DDD, dense deposit disease; EGPA, eosinophilic granulomatosis with polyangiitis; GBM, glomerular basement membrane; GPA, granulomatosis with polyangiitis; MPA, microscopic polyangiitis. (From Yu ASL, Chertow GM, Luyckx VA, et al., eds. *Brenner & Rector's The Kidney.* 11th ed. Philadelphia: Elsevier; 2020:1072, Fig. 31.35.)

be a difficult question. Much depends on the context in which the microscopic hematuria was identified. Thorough evaluation of microscopic hematuria identified on a screening urinalysis at a well-child visit rarely reveals an etiology. One exception is when there is a **family history** of renal disease known or suggestive to be from hereditary nephritis. In that context, particularly if in a pattern indicative of Alport disease where there can be associated hearing loss, performing a screening urinalysis to determine whether a child may be affected is reasonable. The lack of any hematuria in an older child effectively rules out that child having hereditary nephritis. If microscopic hematuria is found, additional noninvasive study can help define whether a child has Alport disease, including audiometry to evaluate for subclinical high-frequency hearing deficit and examination by an ophthalmologist who can identify retinal or lens abnormalities that are characteristic of Alport disease. If no hearing or ophthalmologic abnormalities are found, and if proteinuria accompanies microscopic hematuria in a child from a family affected by hereditary nephritis, further investigation may include collagen IV gene sequencing or kidney biopsy.

When microscopic hematuria is found on urinalysis performed because of symptoms or signs, further evaluation is then indicated. If the presentation was with urinary symptoms or abdominal or flank pain, urine culture and imaging of the urinary tract, first with ultrasound to include the bladder, is the first step. If those tests are

not revealing, and particularly if abdominal or flank pain is colicky, abdominal CT scan with kidney stone protocol is then indicated. If imaging studies are normal and urine culture is negative, evaluation for idiopathic hypercalciuria may then be pursued.

Abnormalities on physical examination that led to a urinalysis being performed should drive further evaluation for underlying intrinsic kidney disease. Specifically, if hypertension, edema, or failure to thrive triggered the urinalysis, blood tests to assess kidney function and CBC should be performed. If acute glomerulonephritis is suspected because of prodromal illness, hypertension, or edema, blood complement C3 and C4 levels should also be measured. If other symptoms or signs suggest possible systemic vasculitis, testing for lupus or ANCA-associated disease should then be considered. If the patient has had poor growth suggesting a chronic process, or supportive evidence for acute nephritis is lacking, renal ultrasound may identify small kidneys indicating a chronic nephropathy, obstructive nephropathy, or cystic kidney disease as the etiology.

MORE COMMON CAUSES OF HEMATURIA

Postinfectious Glomerulonephritis

Gross hematuria appearing 5 days to 4 weeks after a febrile illness suggests a diagnosis of acute postinfectious glomerulonephritis (PIGN),

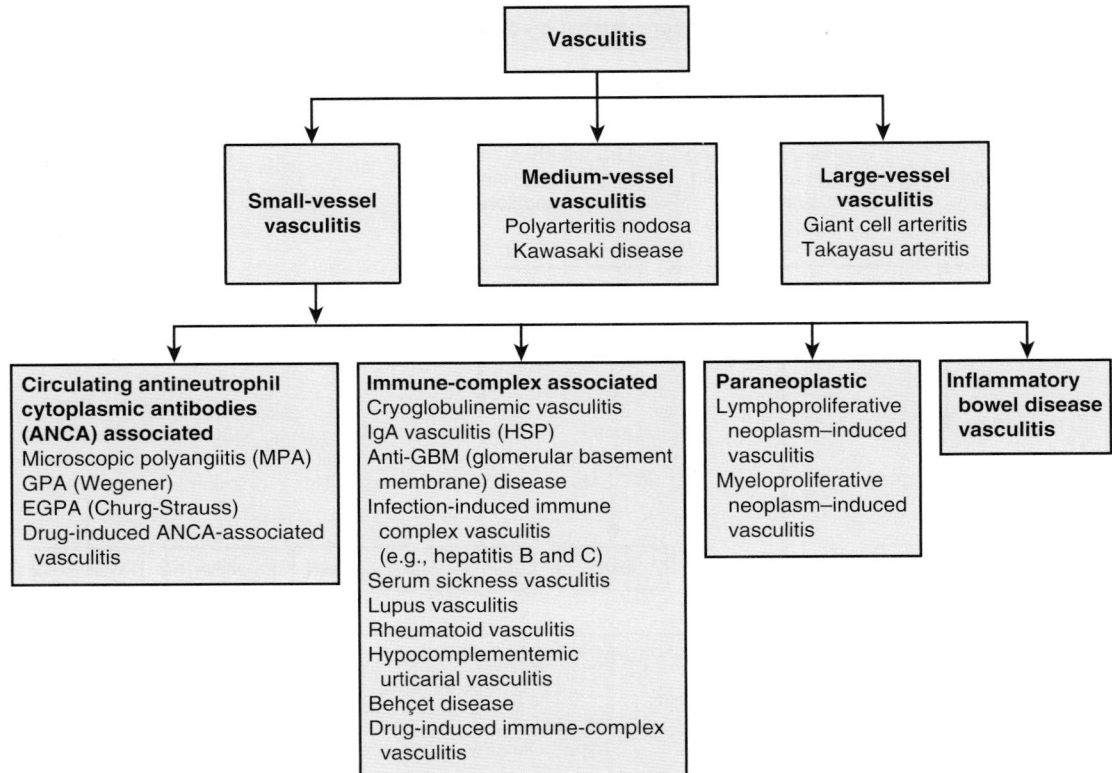

Fig. 23.3 Major categories of noninfectious vasculitis. Not included are vasculitides that are known to be caused by direct invasion of vessel walls by infectious pathogens, such as rickettsial vasculitis and neisserial vasculitis. EGPA, eosinophilic granulomatous polyangiitis; GPA, granulomatous polyangiitis; HSP, Henoch-Schönlein purpura; IgA, immunoglobulin A. (From Feehally J, Floege J, Tonelli M, et al., eds. *Comprehensive Clinical Nephrology.* 6th ed. Philadelphia: Elsevier; 2019:292, Fig. 25.2.)

TABLE 23.4	**Organ System Involvement in Small-Vessel Vasculitis**				
	FREQUENCY OF INVOLVEMENT (%)				
Organ System	**Microscopic Polyangiitis**	**GPA (Wegener)**	**EGPA (Churg-Strauss)**	**IgA Vasculitis (HSP)**	**Cryoglobulinemic Vasculitis**
Kidney	90	80	20	50	55
Skin/cutaneous	40	40	40	90	90
Lungs	50	90	90	<5	<5
Ear, nose, throat	35	90	70	<5	<5
Musculoskeletal	60	60	50	75	70
Neurologic	30	50	40	10	40
Gastrointestinal	50	50	40	60	30

EGPA, eosinophilic granulomatosis with polyangiitis; GPA, granulomatosis with polyangiitis; HSP, Henoch-Schönlein purpura; IgA, immunoglobulin A. From Feehally J, Floege J, Tonelli M, et al., eds. *Comprehensive Clinical Nephrology.* 6th ed. Philadelphia: Elsevier; 2019:294, Table 25.2.

the most common form of acute nephritis in childhood. The typical child with PIGN is school age. The classical findings are hematuria, oliguria, edema, some level of renal insufficiency, and hypertension. It is not uncommon for PIGN to be asymptomatic, and hypertension may not be a feature at initial presentation. The child with suspected PIGN requires close follow-up including monitoring for the development of hypertension, since severe symptomatic hypertension is a common sequela of acute PIGN.

PIGN is a self-limited disease that in the vast majority of cases resolves without the development of chronic kidney disease or established hypertension. Microscopic hematuria is present in virtually all cases; gross hematuria is present in about 30%. The urine is commonly described as smoky or tea- or cola-colored. The gross hematuria usually disappears in 3–5 days; proteinuria disappears in several weeks, and microscopic hematuria resolves in months to 1 year. Group A streptococcal (GAS) infection is the most well-defined cause, described in up to 80% of patients with PIGN, with the triggering infection being either pharyngeal or impetiginous. Other infectious agents have also been implicated in causing PIGN, including several other bacteria and viruses.

The criteria for diagnosis of PIGN relies on defining the clinical picture, supported by finding glomerular hematuria (red cell casts or many

TABLE 23.5 Causes of Hypercalciuria

Physiologic Stimuli to Calcium Excretion
Sodium excretion
Acidosis
Hypophosphatemia

Increased Filtered Load
Hypercalcemia (hyperparathyroidism, dietary, vitamin D excess)
Excess calcium administration

Impaired Renal Tubular Reabsorption of Calcium
Loop diuretics
Selective tubular defects
Bartter syndrome
Hereditary hypophosphatemic rickets with hypercalciuria
Syndrome of hypercalciuria, normocalcemia, growth retardation, polyuria, and proteinuria (Dent disease)
Renal tubular acidosis
Fanconi syndrome

Idiopathic Hypercalciuria
Absorptive
Renal leak

Hypercalciuria of Unknown Cause
Medullary sponge kidney
Diabetes mellitus
Syndrome associated with total parenteral nutrition

From Milliner DS, Stickler GB. Hypercalcemia, hypercalciuria, and renal disease. In: Edelmann CM, ed. *Pediatric Kidney Disease*. 2nd ed. Boston: Little, Brown; 1992:1661–1687.

dysmorphic RBCs) in the urine sediment by an experienced examiner, and a simple serologic pattern. Practitioners will commonly perform serologic testing for streptococcal infection, an old habit that is not typically informative. Serology positive for antistreptococcal antibodies at presentation is neither necessary nor sufficient to confirm, nor does the absence of such antibodies rule out, the diagnosis of PIGN. Evidence of recent streptococcal infection can be helpful and may be provided by positive culture for GAS in the correct time frame preceding onset of nephritis. Most important is testing C3 serum complement level at presentation. In nearly all cases of PIGN, C3 level is low at presentation, then returns to normal by 6–12 weeks after presentation, as the nephritis spontaneously resolves. If the serum C3 level does not return to normal, other causes of nephritis need to be considered, including lupus nephritis, membranoproliferative glomerulonephritis (MPGN), or C3 nephropathy. The complement pattern in active lupus nephritis often is a low C4 along with the low C3 level. In MPGN or C3 nephropathy, C4 is usually normal with persistently low C3. If C3 level is normal at presentation of glomerulonephritis, other etiologies need to be considered, including several idiopathic forms that may only be diagnosed by kidney biopsy (see Tables 23.2 and 23.3).

Therapy for PIGN is symptomatic, with particular attention to hypertension. Early treatment of the streptococcal infection does not prevent development of nephritis. The acute complications from PIGN are principally from hypertension and may include seizures, hypertensive encephalopathy, and heart failure. The prognosis of PIGN is excellent. Mortality is low at ~0.5%. While some level of renal insufficiency is typical, fulminant renal failure is uncommon. Complete recovery occurs in over 95% of patients, with an occasional patient developing rapidly progressive, crescentic glomerulonephritis or indolent chronic glomerulonephritis that progresses to end-stage kidney disease.

Recurrent hematuria and proteinuria can occur in patients who have a nonspecific upper respiratory tract illness within several months following the episode of PIGN, but it is unusual for the other features of acute nephritis (hypertension and renal insufficiency) to recur.

Immunoglobulin A Nephropathy

Recurrent episodes of painless gross hematuria are a common presentation of childhood IgA nephropathy. This form of glomerulonephritis is common in both children and adults, with the mean age of presentation in children being 9–10 years. Episodes of gross hematuria are triggered by upper respiratory illnesses, but in contrast to PIGN where the illness precedes onset of hematuria, in IgA nephropathy the illness is concurrent with onset of gross hematuria. Serum complement is normal. Serum IgA levels have been found to be elevated in only 8–16% of affected children so are not helpful in the diagnosis. Confirmation of the diagnosis is possible only by renal biopsy demonstrating immune deposits of primarily IgA in glomeruli, principally in the mesangium. A wide range of histologic glomerulopathy can be found in IgA nephropathy, ranging from mild mesangial proliferation to crescentic, rapidly progressive glomerulonephritis. Most cases of IgA nephropathy have a benign pattern, with recurrent episodes of gross hematuria during illnesses, followed by complete resolution of gross hematuria within days. Between episodes, the urine may be free of blood or may show persistent microscopic hematuria but lack of proteinuria. This benign pattern commonly does not progress nor require treatment. However, the disease is quite variable between patients, with some developing acute nephritic symptoms, acute renal failure, nephrotic syndrome, or progression to end-stage kidney disease in up to 10% of affected children. Other disorders are also associated with IgA nephropathy (Table 23.6). No specific therapy exists for IgA nephropathy, but an extended course of steroid therapy can be beneficial for patients with more severe forms of IgA nephropathy, including those with acute nephritic syndrome or nephrotic-range proteinuria.

Hereditary Nephritis

A family history of renal disease with progression to renal failure, restricted to male members of the family on the maternal side, suggests a diagnosis of Alport syndrome, a predominantly X-linked recessive nephropathy (Table 23.7). Affected patients uniformly have some level of hematuria beginning at an early age, even in infancy. The majority of affected children develop hematuria in the school-age years. Initially the hematuria is an isolated finding, but as the disease progresses proteinuria develops. Often there is accompanying development of progressive deafness. Female members of the family who carry the gene usually have isolated microscopic and sometimes periodic macroscopic hematuria that does not progress to the other features of the syndrome. However, occasionally such individuals can develop progressive disease similar to male family members. The disease is caused by a pathogenic variant in the *COL4A5* gene on the X chromosome that codes for type IV collagen found in normal glomerular basement membranes; genetic testing can help confirm the diagnosis. Renal biopsy provides a definitive diagnosis, which shows characteristic electron microscopic appearance of attenuation, disruption, and lamellation of the glomerular basement membrane. However, these findings may not occur until a later age when the nephropathy has progressed. Early findings may simply be thin glomerular basement membranes, which can be confused with the more benign entity, thin basement membrane nephropathy. No specific therapy exists, but treatment with an angiotensin-converting enzyme (ACE) inhibitor early in the course of the disease after proteinuria develops can slow the progression of the nephropathy.

There is also an autosomal recessive variant of hereditary nephritis that has been associated with variants in genes that code for other

TABLE 23.6　Diseases Reported in Association with IgA Nephropathy: Common, Reported, and Rare

Disease Group	Common	Reported	Rare
Rheumatic and autoimmune disease	Ankylosing spondylitis Rheumatoid arthritis Reiter syndrome Uveitis	Behçet syndrome* Takayasu arteritis† Myasthenia gravis	Sicca syndrome
Gastrointestinal disease	Celiac disease	Ulcerative colitis	Crohn disease Whipple disease
Hepatic disease	Alcoholic liver disease Nonalcoholic cirrhosis Schistosomal liver disease		
Lung disease	Sarcoid		Pulmonary hemosiderosis
Skin disease	Dermatitis herpetiformis		
Malignancy		IgA monoclonal gammopathy	Bronchial carcinoma Renal carcinoma Laryngeal carcinoma Mycosis fungoides Sézary syndrome
Infection	HIV, hepatitis B (in endemic areas)	Brucellosis	Leprosy
Miscellaneous		Wiskott-Aldrich syndrome‡	

*Behçet syndrome: systemic vasculitis typified by orogenital ulceration and chronic uveitis.
†Takayasu arteritis: systemic vasculitis involving the aorta and its major branches, most often found in young women.
‡Wiskott-Aldrich syndrome: X-linked disorder in which increased serum IgA is associated with the triad of recurrent pyogenic infection, eczema, and thrombocytopenia.
Rare associations have been made in one or two reported cases only. In a disease as common as immunoglobulin A (IgA) nephropathy, it is therefore uncertain whether these are truly related.
From Feehally J, Floege J, Tonelli M, et al., eds. *Comprehensive Clinical Nephrology.* 6th ed. Philadelphia: Elsevier; 2019:272, Fig. 23.1.

TABLE 23.7　Genetic and Possibly Genetic Glomerular Diseases Initially Presenting with Isolated Hematuria

Disease/Syndrome	Zygosity	Gene	End-Stage Renal Disease Estimated Lifetime Risk
X-linked Alport (male)	Hemizygous	COL4A5	>90%
X-linked Alport (female)	Heterozygous	COL4A5	15%
AR Alport	Homozygous	COL4A3/COL4A4	>90%
AR Alport	Heterozygous	COL4A3/COL4A4	10%
AD TBMN	Heterozygous	COL4A3/COL4A4	14%
HANAC	Heterozygous	COL4A1	n/d
Epstein/Fechtner	Heterozygous	MYH9	30%
CFHR5 nephropathy (male)	Heterozygous	CFHR5	80%
CFHR5 nephropathy (female)	Heterozygous	CFHR5	20%
IgA nephropathy (hematuria only)	—	—	Very low within 20 yr of diagnosis

AD, autosomal dominant; AR, autosomal recessive; HANAC, hereditary angiopathy, nephropathy, aneurysms, and muscle cramps; IgA, immunoglobulin A; n/d, not described; TBMN, thin basement membrane nephropathy;
Modified from Gale DP. How benign is hematuria? Using genetics to predict prognosis. *Pediatr Nephrol.* 2013;28:1183–1193 (Table 1, p. 1184).

chains of collagen found in the glomerular basement membrane. Progression of the nephropathy is similar to that of patients with the classical form of Alport disease. Individuals who carry a disease-causing variant in only one of these autosomal recessive genes may have simple, benign, thin basement membrane nephropathy that does not progress.

Some patients with a more common form of familial hematuria demonstrate persistent microscopic and recurrent gross hematuria *without* development of significant proteinuria or deterioration of renal function. This is called **thin basement membrane nephropathy (benign familial hematuria)** (see Table 23.7). Evidence of this cause of hematuria can be obtained when urinalyses are performed on other family members, finding isolated microscopic hematuria in other members of the family. Renal biopsy demonstrates normal light and immunofluorescent microscopic findings. Electron micrographs show uniformly thin basement membranes. It appears to be an autosomal dominant disorder; it is often associated with heterozygous variants of collagen genes (*COL4A3, COL4A4, COL4A5*) that are associated with autosomal recessive hereditary nephritis. This raises the possibility that benign familial hematuria is the hypomorphic state of progressive hereditary nephritis. Indeed, some patients develop abnormal renal function during adolescence and adulthood.

Polycystic Kidney Disease

Autosomal dominant polycystic kidney disease (ADPKD) is a common disorder that mainly affects adults, but development of cysts may well begin in childhood, and in rare cases renal cysts may be present at birth. Usually, the cysts are asymptomatic in childhood unless there is early and substantial cystic disease. Gross hematuria may be the first manifestation of this disorder and occurs in 50% of patients. It may occur spontaneously or be brought on by minimal trauma. The usual manifestations of the disease in adults (hematuria, hypertension, abdominal mass, and uremia) are seldom seen in children. Furthermore, adults tend to have associated problems not commonly seen in affected children, including acute and chronic pain (60%), UTI, and nephrolithiasis (20%). With the widespread use of ultrasonography and CT for routine evaluation of acute abdominal pain, it is more common to detect early evidence of the disease as an incidental finding, sometimes presenting as a single renal cyst during childhood. Diagnosis requires finding multiple bilateral renal cysts. Because the primary gene that causes ADPKD lies near the gene that causes tuberous sclerosis, the two diseases occasionally coexist as a contiguous gene deletion syndrome. Renal involvement in patients with tuberous sclerosis may be isolated to renal angiomyolipomas or may also manifest polycystic kidney disease as well, either of which can be a source of gross hematuria.

In contrast to ADPKD, **autosomal recessive polycystic kidney disease (ARPKD)** typically has early onset and evidence of renal disease is often found on prenatal ultrasound. If not discovered in the perinatal period, it may present later in infancy or early childhood as an abdominal mass with hypertension. Typically, the kidneys are significantly enlarged and have a cystic appearance different from ADPKD. However, it is not always possible to distinguish early-onset ADPKD from ARPKD on radiologic grounds.

Nephrolithiasis can occur at any age and may cause the symptoms of renal colic, manifested as intense, episodic flank pain that often radiates to the groin. In young infants, nephrolithiasis and thus renal colic is rare, and may manifest as generalized irritability or abdominal pain. Gross hematuria has been reported in ~25% of patients with nephrolithiasis. The physical examination may be unrevealing; the urinalysis may contain crystals in addition to RBCs. A high-resolution CT scan is the best study to confirm the presence of a stone. Children with nephrolithiasis should have an evaluation for a metabolic cause of their kidney stones. This begins with a 24-hour urine collection for calcium, urate, citrate, oxalate, cystine, and creatinine. The determination of creatinine excretion is important to ensure that an adequate collection has been obtained (a minimum of 10–15 mg/kg/24 hr, depending on age and body habitus of the child). If an abnormality is found, specific therapy may prevent or delay subsequent complications, which can include frequently recurring stones and acute or chronic renal failure.

Hypercalciuria (defined as urinary calcium levels >4 mg/kg/day) is the most common metabolic abnormality found in children with nephrolithiasis. Furthermore, hypercalciuria without an overt stone can manifest as gross hematuria with abdominal or flank pain. Hypercalciuria can be idiopathic or secondary to another disease, such as renal tubular acidosis. Therapy depends on the cause of the hypercalciuria or the specific type of stone.

Urinary tract infection is the most common identifiable cause of gross hematuria, with as many as 25% of children presenting with gross hematuria having a documented symptomatic UTI. Urine culture is essential for a diagnosis of UTI and should be performed in all children with gross hematuria, especially if any urinary symptoms accompany.

UNCOMMON CAUSES OF HEMATURIA IN CHILDHOOD

Coagulation abnormalities and hemoglobinopathies are rarely found in patients with gross hematuria. **Sickle cell disease** is the most likely cause in this category, and gross hematuria is one of the few manifestations of the carrier state that may develop in those with sickle cell trait. A combination of low oxygen tension, reduced blood flow, low pH, and high osmolality in the renal medulla makes a hostile environment that induces sickling and sludging of erythrocytes there. This results in areas of infarction and hemorrhage and can progress to renal papillary necrosis. While the gross hematuria often is asymptomatic, if papillary necrosis ensues or hemorrhage from the renal medulla is substantial with passage of clots, acquired ureteral obstruction can cause significant associated flank or abdominal pain. Therapy is hydration and rest.

Renal vascular thrombosis, particularly renal vein thrombosis, may present with isolated gross hematuria. Two groups of children are at highest risk for this problem. The first group is sick neonates. Renal vascular thrombosis in this group can originate from events associated with perinatal stress that cause hypotension and decreased perfusion to the kidney, umbilical vascular catheters, trauma, hypercoagulable states, dehydration, or disseminated intravascular coagulation. Infants of diabetic mothers are more prone to renal vein thrombosis, possibly because of polycythemia or other associated perinatal stress. The thrombosis in the neonate can be in the renal artery but most often is in the renal vein. Along with gross hematuria, accompanying clinical features may include a palpable enlarged kidney on the affected side, hypertension, and thrombocytopenia. The second group of children who are susceptible to renal vascular thrombosis are those with **nephrotic syndrome**, with the well-described associated hypercoagulable state (see Chapter 22). The diagnosis of renal vein thrombosis can be suspected from the patient's history and can be confirmed with a Doppler flow study of the renal vasculature. Several treatment approaches have been advocated. In many cases, careful attention to hydration and hemodynamic status in the neonate, or administration of albumin in the patient with nephrotic syndrome, stabilizes the patient with no further progression of the thrombus. With large thrombi that propagate to the vena cava or affect both kidneys, anticoagulation is considered. Renal vein thrombi, even with isolated supportive care, often resolve without late renal sequelae. However, late sequelae of hypertension and renal atrophy can occur. The less common renal artery thrombi more often result in significant renal injury and atrophy.

Renal and bladder **tumors** are rare causes of gross hematuria in children. Wilms tumor, the most common pediatric renal malignancy, usually manifests as a flank or abdominal mass but on occasion can present with gross hematuria. Renal carcinoma is exceedingly rare in childhood but can occur in older children and also may present as gross hematuria. Each of these tumors can be readily detected radiographically through ultrasonography or CT, which is why imaging of the urinary tract to include the bladder is an important part of the evaluation of all children with gross hematuria unless the source of the blood has clearly been defined to be of glomerular origin. Benign polyps in the urinary tract are a rare cause of hematuria and are usually small. They may not be found by imaging and thus may require cystoscopy and ureteroscopy to discover.

Cyclophosphamide treatment can cause **hemorrhagic cystitis**, which can have accompanying severe bladder symptoms and hemorrhage. This results from prolonged contact of the toxic metabolites of cyclophosphamide with the bladder epithelium. Prevention is primarily with increased hydration to ensure high urine flow, and the use of mesna in patients receiving high-dose cyclophosphamide, a drug that prevents bladder mucosa toxicity from the metabolites.

High-intensity or long-duration **physical exertion** (marathons) can cause gross hematuria. Its pathophysiology is not known, but several mechanisms proposed include bladder or kidney trauma, hemolysis, dehydration, peroxidation of red cells, and renal ischemia.

Bleeding from **arteriovenous malformations** of the kidney, ureter, or bladder can manifest as asymptomatic gross hematuria, which often appears bright red. The blood can be localized to the bladder, one kidney, or ureter with cystoscopy. Endoscopic laser treatment can eliminate the source of bleeding. When bleeding from a vascular malformation is severe and not amenable to laser treatment, angiography and surgery are considered.

Nutcracker syndrome occurs when the left renal vein is compressed between the superior mesenteric artery and aorta, causing a rise in pressure and development of collateral veins with varicosities in the renal pelvis, ureter, and gonadal vein. It presents with left flank pain, hematuria, and occasionally a varicocele in males. Diagnosis can be difficult, but Doppler studies of the left renal vein, magnetic resonance angiography, and CT may identify this entity.

Symptoms of urethritis with gross hematuria and a negative urine culture in boys suggest urethrorrhagia or idiopathic urethritis. The most common complaint is blood-stained underwear. Ultrasound including the bladder should be performed to rule out other lesions discussed earlier. Cystoscopy does not show a treatable lesion and may be contraindicated because of the possibility of producing a stricture. Low-dose, long-term antibiotic treatment may help in some cases. Alternately, exploring for symptoms of dysfunctional elimination syndrome and treating with bowel and bladder regimens may resolve the problem. The condition appears to be benign and self-limited, so reassurance is the best approach.

Infections that are unusual in Western societies but more common in other parts of the world can present with gross hematuria. *Schistosoma haematobium* causes bladder lesions, containing eggs and a surrounding granuloma that may hemorrhage. Urinary symptoms of suprapubic pain, dysuria, or urgency are common. Chronic inflammation of the ureters may result in urinary obstruction. Diagnosis is made by biopsy of lesions found in the liver, rectum, or bladder, or by the detection of characteristic eggs in feces or urine.

Mycobacterium tuberculosis infection can involve the kidneys, resulting in formation of tuberculomas that may cavitate, rupture, and disseminate the bacterium throughout the urinary tract. Tuberculosis of the genitourinary tract most often occurs in young adults and is characterized by tubercles at the ureteral orifices.

Adenovirus is a common respiratory infection in children, which can cause a hemorrhagic cystitis. This complication occurs most often in immunocompromised patients but on occasion can also affect normal, healthy children.

▮ RED FLAGS

Blood visible in the urine commonly raises great concern in a child and the parents, and sometimes in the physician, but rarely heralds a serious disease. Parents frequently are concerned that hematuria is a manifestation of a malignancy, so this should be addressed initially with reassurance that it is very rare for the cause of hematuria in a child to be a tumor. The history of recent or current illness and the family history, as well as associated signs or symptoms, can usually direct the appropriate evaluation. The focus of testing initially should be on confirming the presence of hematuria, ruling out urinary infection with culture, assessing renal function with blood tests, and exploring urinary tract anatomy with ultrasound. Invasive studies, such as cystoscopy or renal biopsy, are rarely indicated.

Features of the evaluation that require prompt attention include absence of RBCs in the urine (which raises the concern for possible hemoglobinuria or myoglobinuria), hypertension, azotemia, pain, weight loss, fevers, or a palpable mass. The presence of significant proteinuria suggests glomerular disease, which would require further evaluation by a nephrologist for consideration of renal biopsy.

BIBLIOGRAPHY

A bibliography is available at ExpertConsult.com.

24

Acute and Chronic Scrotal Swelling

John V. Kryger and Susan L. Jarosz

The most serious causes of acute scrotal swelling are testicular torsion and incarcerated inguinal hernia, both of which necessitate immediate surgical correction. Consequently, a prompt, careful approach to a painful or inflamed scrotum is essential. The differential diagnosis of scrotal swelling is extensive and varies depending on the age of the patient (Tables 24.1 and 24.2). The most common causes include testicular torsion, torsion of the appendix testis, and epididymitis.

SCROTAL AND INGUINAL ANATOMY

Inguinal Region

The inguinal canal runs obliquely between the external and internal inguinal rings. The anterior wall of the canal is formed by the external oblique aponeurosis; the posterior wall is formed by the inguinal ligament and conjoined tendon. The oblique direction of the inguinal canal allows for the posterior and anterior walls to coapt with increases in intraabdominal pressure.

Testis Descent

The testes develop in the lumbar region of the abdominal cavity between the peritoneum and the transversalis fascia at approximately 7 weeks of gestation. By the eighth week of gestation, the gubernaculum extends from the caudal end of the epididymis through the inguinal canal to insert on the internal wall of the scrotum. The processus vaginalis, a finger-like outpouching of the peritoneum, extends adjacent to the gubernaculum to form the inguinal canal. As the processus vaginalis descends into the scrotum, it carries extensions of the abdominal wall layers.

The testis normally descends through the inguinal canal into the scrotum before birth. As the testis and spermatic cord descend through the inguinal canal, they are covered by the three concentric layers of the anterior abdominal fascia (Fig. 24.1). When the testis reaches the scrotum, the testis and surrounding layers of fascia and tunica vaginalis fuse to the dartos of the scrotum. The processus vaginalis is initially patent, leaving a connection between the scrotum and the peritoneal cavity. Normally, the processus vaginalis obliterates, leaving a residual tunica vaginalis surrounding the testis. Typically, the tunica vaginalis contains 1–2 mL of clear fluid.

Scrotum

The scrotum has two separate compartments, each containing a testis, epididymis, and distal spermatic cord. It comprises multiple layers that are continuous with the superficial layers of the anterior abdominal wall. The external location of the scrotum results in the temperature of the testes being 2–3°F below the core body temperature, which allows for normal spermatogenesis.

Testis

The testes are the male reproductive organs and are suspended in the tunica vaginalis of the scrotum by the spermatic cords. The epididymis,

attached to the testis posteriorly, consists of the caput (upper pole), corpus (body), and cauda (tail) (Fig. 24.2). The vas deferens can be palpated as a narrow, firm, tubular structure in the spermatic cord. The epididymis is responsible for sperm maturation and storage. Each testis relies on three arteries for its blood supply: the testicular artery, the cremasteric artery, and the deferential artery. Each enters the scrotum through the spermatic cord. The testicle receives both sympathetic and parasympathetic innervation. These autonomic nerves carry impulses that, with testicular stimulation, produce symptoms of deep visceral pain and nausea.

DIAGNOSTIC STRATEGIES

History

In evaluating acute or chronic scrotal swelling, the following historical elements should be established:

1. **Onset of pain**: Testicular torsion has a very sudden onset and can be precipitated by activity or can occur at rest or during sleep. Epididymitis or torsion of the appendix testis or other testicular appendage often has a more insidious onset over the course of days, with progressive pain and swelling.
2. **Duration of pain**: Episodic pain lasting seconds and abating is rarely pathologic, whereas severe pain, persistent pain, or episodes lasting more than 1 hour raise concern.
3. **Associated/radiation of pain**: If there is radiation of pain from the flank, then renal or ureteral pathologic processes, such as an obstructing ureteral calculus, should be considered. Inguinal discomfort may suggest hernia or other inguinal pathology.

Although sometimes nonspecific, associated manifestations are also important:

1. **General systemic**: Fever, chills, or rigors suggest an infectious cause.
2. **Abdominal signs/symptoms**: Nausea, vomiting, and abdominal or inguinal pain are common but nonspecific. They may indicate an intestinal process.
3. **Urologic signs/symptoms**: Dysuria, urinary frequency, hematuria, or penile discharge suggests an infectious process such as urinary tract infection, urethritis, or epididymitis.
4. **Unusual rashes**: Henoch-Schönlein purpura may result in vasculitis of the spermatic cord with associated scrotal pain and swelling.

In addition, a thorough medical history is imperative and should include the following:

1. History of urinary tract infections or renal calculi.
2. Prior sexual activity, which would raise the possibility of a sexually transmitted infection.
3. History of any surgical procedures on the groin, scrotum, or abdomen. Often an orchiopexy performed for an undescended testis

TABLE 24.1 Differential Diagnosis of Scrotal Enlargement/Swelling in Young and Adolescent Males

Painful	Painless*
Testicular torsion	Hydrocele
Torsion of testicular appendage (less common after adolescence)	Inguinal hernia (reducible)
	Varicocele
Epididymoorchitis	Spermatocele (postpubertal males)
Trauma: testicular rupture, hematocele	Testicular tumor (see Table 24.5)
	ALL
Inguinal hernia (incarcerated)	Paratesticular tumor
Mumps orchitis	Idiopathic scrotal edema
Vasculitis	Henoch-Schönlein purpura

*Occasionally associated with discomfort.
ALL, acute lymphoblastic leukemia.

TABLE 24.2 Differential Diagnosis of Scrotal Swelling in Newborns

Hydrocele	Scrotal hematoma
Inguinal hernia (reducible)	Testicular tumor
Inguinal hernia (incarcerated)*	Meconium peritonitis
Testicular torsion*	Epididymitis*

*May be associated with scrotal inflammation.

places the testis in a dartos pouch, which would make testicular torsion unlikely in the future.

4. History of any previous episodes of testicular pain. Previous episodes of intermittent or severe pain in the same testis may be secondary to intermittent torsion of the testis.
5. Lower urinary tract pathologic processes, such as posterior urethral valves, neuropathic bladder, or urethral stricture (e.g., after trauma or hypospadias repair), may predispose to urinary tract infection, which could cause bacterial epididymitis.

Physical Examination

Examination of the scrotal contents should be performed in any male patient presenting with abdominal, inguinal, or scrotal pain. Essential components include inspection, palpation, and transillumination of any masses.

Pubertal development. In prepubertal males, torsion of the appendix testis is more common than testicular torsion (Table 24.3). Conversely, in the postpubertal male, testicular torsion and epididymitis (if the patient is sexually active) are more common.

Scars in the inguinal region. Scars may imply previous surgery for hernia, hydrocele, undescended testis, or varicocele.

Scrotal skin changes and fixation. Erythema suggests an underlying inflammatory process but is nonspecific. Duskiness or fixation of the skin over the testis is suggestive of testicular necrosis.

Testis position within the scrotum. A testis positioned high in the scrotum is suggestive of testicular torsion. The spermatic cord

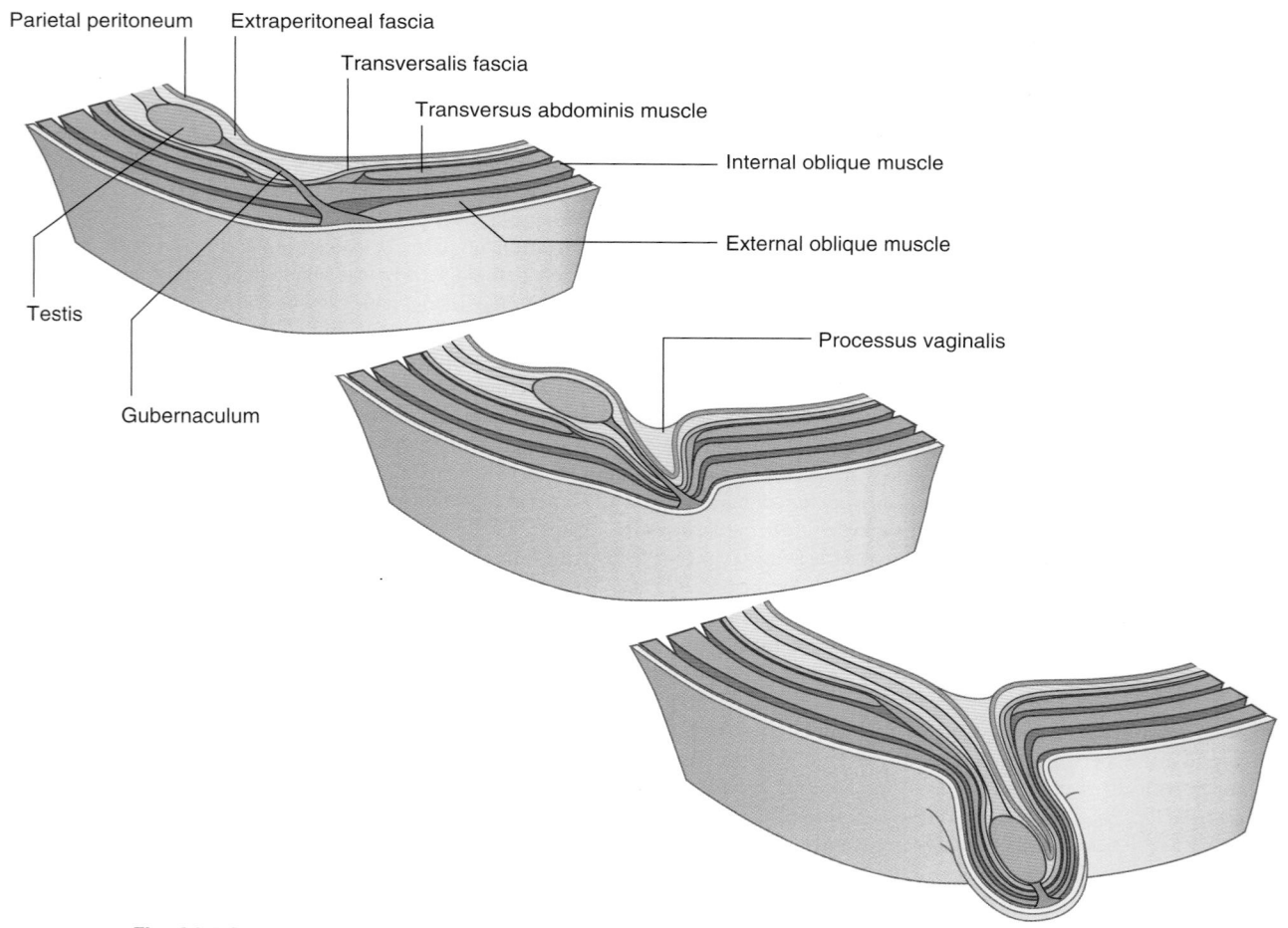

Fig. 24.1 Descent of the testis from week 7 (postfertilization) to birth. As the testis and spermatic cord descend through the inguinal canal, they are covered by the three concentric layers of the anterior abdominal fascia. (From Drake RL, Vogl AW, Mitchell AWM, eds. *Gray's Anatomy for Students.* 3rd ed. Philadelphia: Churchill Livingstone; 2015:253–420.)

shortens as it twists. The affected testis should be compared with the contralateral testis with respect to size, consistency, and tenderness. Accurate localization of pain to the testis, epididymis, or both is important.

Cremasteric reflex. Stimulated by gently scratching the ipsilateral medial thigh, reflexive cremaster muscle contraction causes the scrotum to retract. The presence of a symmetric cremasteric reflex makes testicular torsion less likely. An absent cremasteric reflex is nonspecific. Sometimes with anxiety, the testis of a child will retract high into the inguinal canal. An important maneuver to relax the cremaster muscle is to examine the patient in a seated position with the legs crossed.

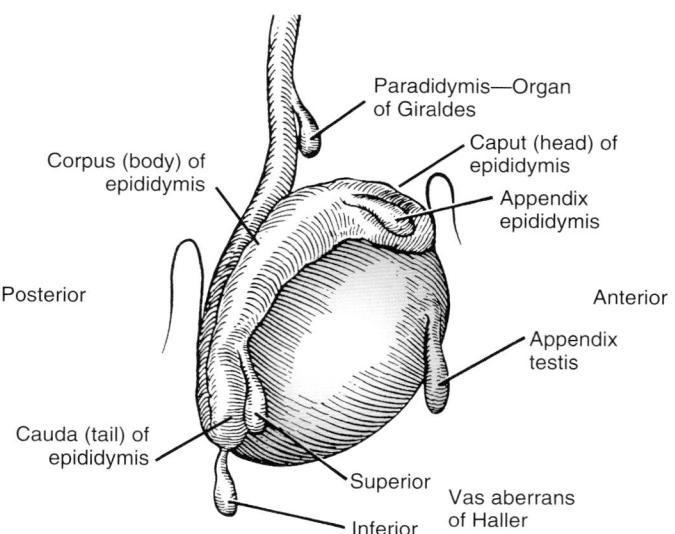

Fig. 24.2 Lateral view of the testis showing the posterior location of epididymis and appendix testes. The appendix testis is present in almost all males, the appendix epididymis is present in approximately 50% of males, and the other appendages are rarely present. (From Kelalis PP, King LR, Belman AB, eds. *Clinical Pediatric Urology.* 2nd ed. Philadelphia: WB Saunders; 1985.)

Laboratory Data

Basic laboratory evaluation of acute and chronic testicular swelling includes UA, urine culture, and tests for *Chlamydia* and gonorrhea if the patient is sexually active.

Imaging Studies

Imaging studies are often helpful in determining the cause of acute and chronic testicular or scrotal swelling. They should not be substituted for a thorough history and careful physical examination performed by a surgical specialist. The conditions necessitating immediate surgical treatment include testicular torsion, incarcerated inguinal hernia, and testicular rupture secondary to trauma; testicular tumor mandates urgent surgical attention. If the history and physical examination strongly support the diagnosis of testicular torsion, then prompt surgical exploration is recommended, without confirmation by an imaging study. If the history or physical findings are equivocal for testicular torsion, or if an alternate diagnosis requires investigation, **color Doppler ultrasonography** should be obtained (Fig. 24.3). Sonography provides a relatively accurate image of the testis and epididymis, and color Doppler imaging assesses blood flow. It is performed by examining the uninvolved testis first and adjusting the color flow settings to detect normal flow. The affected testis is then examined for decreased or absent flow in comparison with the normal testis. Color flow Doppler imaging distinguishes between the increased collateral blood flow within the scrotal skin and the decreased blood flow to the testis in patients with testicular torsion. The sensitivity of Doppler ultrasonography for detecting testicular torsion ranges from 69% to 100%, and specificity ranges from 77% to 100%. Sonography can also help determine if a scrotal hematoma represents a testicular rupture. Color flow Doppler imaging accurately demonstrates increased flow resulting from torsion of the appendix testis or epididymitis but is usually unable to distinguish these two entities. It also cannot distinguish viral from bacterial epididymitis. If a tumor is present, sonography can demonstrate whether the mass arises from the testis or paratesticular structures. It can also distinguish the presence of a hydrocele, cyst, tumor, or varicocele. The test is quick, easy to perform, and noninvasive. There are several important limitations of color Doppler imaging:

TABLE 24.3	Differentiation of Acute Painful Scrotal Swelling in Childhood		
	Testicular Torsion	**Epididymoorchitis**	**Torsion of the Appendix Testis**
Age	Usually perinatal and 12–18 yr, but any age possible	Usually adolescence, but any age possible	2–12 yr
Symptoms and signs	Abrupt onset; may have previous similar episodes	Gradual onset	Gradual onset
Pain	Localized to the testis and may radiate to groin and lower abdomen	Localization to epididymis; may involve entire testis after 24 hr	Localization to upper pole of testis; may involve entire testis after 24 hr
Fever	Rare	Common	Rare
Vomiting	Common	Rare	Rare
Dysuria	Rare	Common	Rare
Physical examination	Testis may be high riding, swollen, exquisitely tender; scrotal erythema may be present; cremasteric reflex absent	Testis and epididymis are firm, tender, swollen; scrotal erythema may be present; cremasteric reflex present	Testis is normal or enlarged; firm mass may be seen or felt at upper pole, distinct from epididymis; scrotal erythema may be present; cremasteric reflex present
Pyuria, urinary infection	Rare	Possible, particularly in bacterial epididymitis	Rare
Blood flow (color Doppler study)	Diminished or absent	Increased	Normal or increased

1. If the duration of torsion is brief and if the torsional rotation is incomplete, there may be venous congestion without impairment of arterial blood flow; color Doppler imaging may demonstrate normal or decreased blood flow.
2. In the prepubertal testis, blood flow may be difficult to demonstrate, even when the testes are normal, and absence of flow may be misinterpreted for testicular torsion.
3. The color Doppler aspect of the study is user dependent.

DIFFERENTIAL DIAGNOSIS

(Table 24.4; see also Table 24.3)

Testicular Torsion

Testicular torsion is a surgical emergency because prolonged periods without blood flow lead to progressive ischemic changes within the testis. The likelihood of testicular survival depends on the duration and severity of torsion. Consequently, testicular survival depends on accurate diagnosis and timely emergency management.

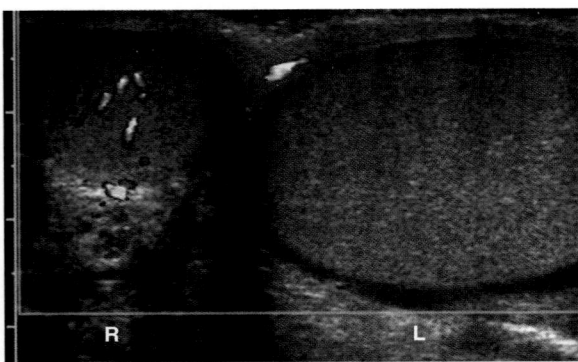

Fig. 24.3 Testicular torsion and axis change. A color Doppler ultrasound in the transverse plane shows color flow in the right testicle. The right testicle *(R)* is oval to circular because it has been evaluated in the transverse plane. The left testicle *(L)* is elongated as if it is in the longitudinal plane. This axis change is the ultrasound equivalent of the worrisome clinical finding suggestive of torsion when accompanied by a history of sudden pain. Lack of color Doppler flow in the left testicle confirms a left testicular torsion. (From Coley BD, ed. *Caffey's Pediatric Diagnostic Imaging*. 13th ed. Philadelphia: Elsevier; 2019: Fig. 126.13.)

The incidence of spermatic cord torsion is 1 in 4,000 among male patients younger than 25 years. The peak ages for testicular torsion are in the neonatal period, as well as from the ages of 12 to 18 years. The pathogenesis of torsion and the presentation in these two age groups are different.

In testicular torsion, the testis and spermatic cord rotate or twist within the tunica vaginalis (termed "intravaginal" torsion), resulting in obstruction of venous drainage, followed by compromise of arterial flow and subsequent infarction (Fig. 24.4). In many instances of torsion occurring beyond the neonatal period, a preexisting anatomic abnormality termed the **bell clapper deformity** increases the likelihood of the testis rotating on the spermatic cord. The "bell clapper" refers to a redundant tunica vaginalis that inserts higher along the spermatic cord, allowing the testis to rotate freely within, and lie more transversely in the scrotum (Fig. 24.5). The deformity is common, present unilaterally in 17% and bilaterally in 40% of males.

TABLE 24.4	Causes of Acute Scrotal Pain
Common	**Uncommon**
Testicular torsion	Granulomatous orchitis*
Torsion of testicular appendage	Drug-induced epididymitis (amiodarone)*
Epididymitis (gonorrheal and/or chlamydial infection in sexually active adolescents)*	Behçet disease
Trauma*	Sarcoidosis
Scrotal edema (Henoch-Schönlein purpura)	Polyarteritis nodosa*
Pain referred to scrotum (nephrolithiasis, ureteropelvic junction obstruction, appendicitis, spinal cord tumor, IgA nephropathy)	Epididymitis (tuberculosis, brucellosis, actinomycosis, leprosy, *Salmonella* infection, fungal infection, parasitic infestation, *Nocardia* infection)
Less Common	Orchitis (rickettsial, *Nocardia* infections, toxoplasmosis, cytomegalovirus, COVID-19)
Orchitis (mumps, varicella, coxsackievirus, dengue)*	Testicular pyocele
Abscess	Fournier gangrene
Infarction	
Malignancy: primary testicular neoplasm (e.g., seminoma), germ cell (usually painless mass)	
Leukemia: primary or relapse (usually painless swelling)*	

*Bilateral involvement possible.
IgA, immunoglobulin A.

The likelihood of irreversible testicular damage depends on the severity and duration of torsion. If the torsion results in complete ischemia, the testis may become necrotic within 6–12 hours; however, if testicular torsion is incomplete, there may be continued arterial perfusion for 24–48 hours. Because the viability of the testis cannot reliably be gauged based on the perceived duration of torsion, immediate surgical exploration should always be considered.

Patients with testicular torsion typically experience the sudden onset of severe testicular pain and swelling. The event is often incorrectly attributed to minor trauma or exercise, but pain may also occur independent of activity or suddenly awaken the patient from sleep. The pain is usually localized to the affected hemiscrotum, and patients may also report inguinal or abdominal pain. Associated symptoms may include nausea and vomiting. Up to half of patients describe previous episodes of severe scrotal pain that resolved spontaneously. Dysuria and other voiding symptoms are absent.

On examination, the scrotum is erythematous and edematous, and the testis is enlarged and extremely tender (Fig. 24.6). If the patient has been experiencing severe pain for more than 24 hours, there may be too much inflammation to delineate the scrotal contents. The cremasteric reflex is usually always absent, although this is not a perfectly reliable sign. The testis may be high in the scrotum with a transverse lie. UA results are negative. If testicular torsion has been present for more than 48 hours, the scrotum is typically severely enlarged, erythematous, and edematous, and the testis is an enlarged and indurated mass. Color Doppler imaging typically reveals hyperemia in the scrotal wall and absent testicular blood flow.

In most cases, the diagnosis of testicular torsion can be made from the history and physical examination. If torsion is the likely diagnosis, scrotal exploration should proceed immediately and should not be delayed awaiting confirmatory imaging. If the diagnosis is uncertain, imaging should be obtained. Color Doppler ultrasonography typically demonstrates absent blood flow.

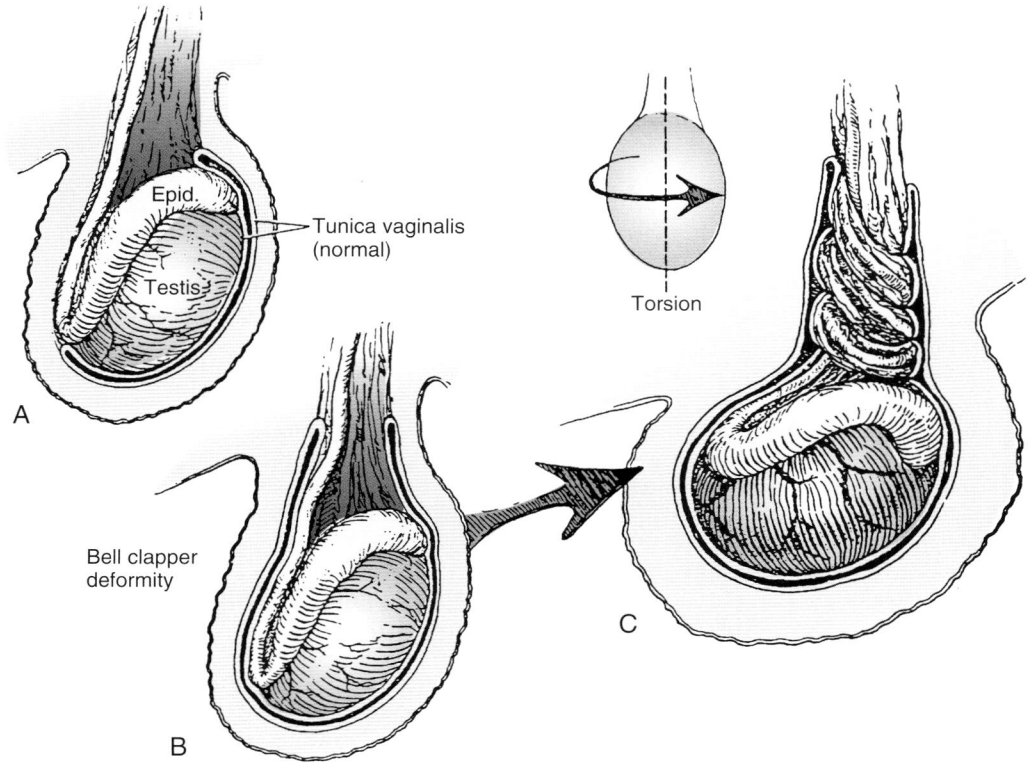

Fig. 24.4 *A* to *C,* Mechanism of testicular torsion associated with the bell clapper deformity. Epid, epididymis. (From Fleisher GR, Ludwig S. *Textbook of Pediatric Emergency Medicine.* 3rd ed. Baltimore: Williams & Wilkins; 1993.)

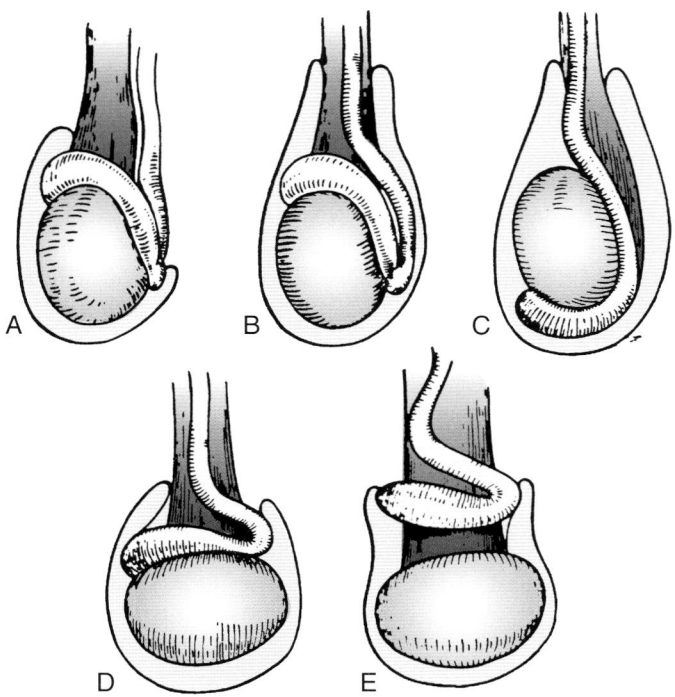

Fig. 24.5 Anomalies of suspension associated with intravaginal testicular torsion. *A,* Normal. *B,* Envelopment by the tunica vaginalis. *C,* Inversion of the epididymis. *D* and *E,* Horizontal lie. Bell clapper deformity is shown in *B* through *E.* (From Kelalis PP, King LR, Belman AB, eds. *Clinical Pediatric Urology.* 2nd ed. Philadelphia: WB Saunders; 1985.)

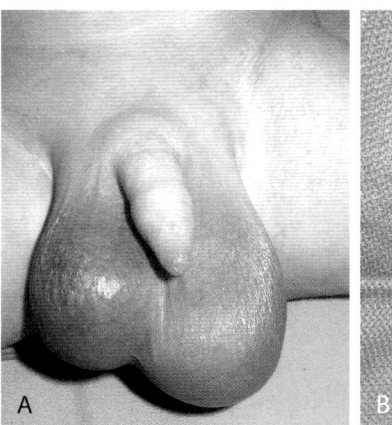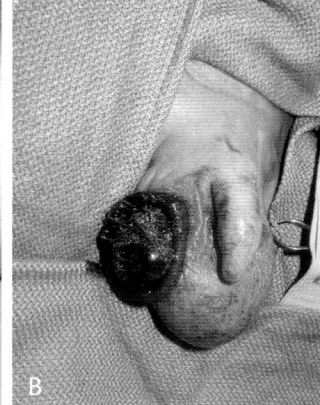

Fig. 24.6 *A* and *B,* Right testicular torsion in a newborn. The right hemiscrotum is darker, and the testis was indurated and enlarged. (From Kliegman RM, St. Geme JW III, Blum NJ, et al., eds. *Nelson Textbook of Pediatrics.* 21st ed. Philadelphia: Elsevier; 2020:2831, Fig. 560.5.)

Some patients present with a history of severe testicular pain that resolved in the emergency room or on the way to the hospital. In these cases, **intermittent torsion** should be suspected. While immediate scrotal orchiopexy is not mandated under these circumstances, surgical fixation should still be considered, as the recurrence rate is high. Furthermore, some patients may fail to seek prompt medical evaluation in the event of recurrence because of fear of surgery or wishful thinking that the torsion will spontaneously resolve again.

Surgical management of testicular torsion consists of exploration, detorsion, and evaluation of testicular viability. An infarcted testicle is removed. If the testis is viable, orchiopexy is performed, in which the viable testis is fixed to the dartos layer of the scrotal wall with nonabsorbable sutures. Contralateral scrotal orchiopexy is also performed given the significant risk of contralateral torsion. If torsion is detected and treated within 4 hours of the onset of symptoms, the salvage rate approaches 100%; at 8–12 hours, it falls to 20%; and after 24 hours, infarction is likely.

Testicular torsion also occurs in the fetus and neonate. In these cases, torsion results from incomplete attachment of the gubernaculum and tunica vaginalis to the scrotal wall. The entire testis, epididymis, and tunica vaginalis twist in a process termed **extravaginal testicular torsion**. If torsion occurs prenatally, the testis is typically large and firm. The ipsilateral hemiscrotum may be ecchymotic if torsion occurred shortly prior to birth, although if torsion occurred more remotely, ecchymoses may have resolved by the time of delivery. Prenatal torsion always results in a nonviable testis. Postnatal extravaginal testicular torsion can occur up to 46 weeks' corrected gestational age. Affected neonates typically have sudden onset of irritability with progressive enlargement of the testis, with associated scrotal erythema. Color Doppler ultrasonography in the neonate is fairly reliable in distinguishing testicular torsion from scrotal hematoma and testicular tumor. Although testicular salvage in neonates with in utero torsion is highly unlikely, urgent exploration is recommended to confirm the diagnosis and to perform a contralateral scrotal orchiopexy to protect the solitary remaining testis, which is also at risk for torsion. If there is a possibility that torsion occurred after birth, there is a chance of saving the testis, and immediate exploration is warranted.

TORSION OF THE APPENDIX TESTIS

The appendix testis, a vestigial remnant of the müllerian duct system, is attached to the upper pole of the testis and is present in approximately 90% of males. The appendix epididymis, a remnant of the wolffian ducts, is present in about 10% of males. When these appendages are long and pedunculated, they tend to twist at their base, resulting in ischemia and eventual infarction (Fig. 24.7). This type of torsion is most common between 2 and 12 years of age and is uncommon in adolescents. Torsion of the appendix testis results in progressive pain and inflammation of the epididymis and scrotum.

The onset of pain and swelling is typically gradual. Affected males often adopt a wide-based gait but otherwise appear comfortable. Constitutional symptoms are usually less severe than with testicular torsion but may include nausea, vomiting, and pain referred to the lower abdomen. Physical examination reveals an erythematous and edematous scrotum. Palpation of the testis may reveal a 3- to 5-mm tender

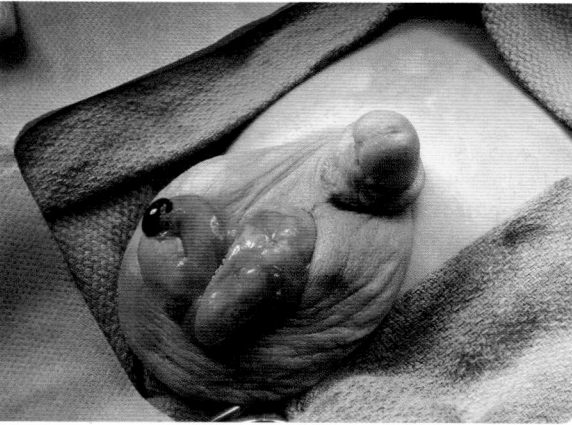

Fig. 24.7 Torsed appendix epididymis.

indurated mass on the upper pole. The torsed appendix testis may be visible through the scrotal skin; this finding is termed the **blue dot sign** and is present in approximately 20% of cases. As the duration of torsion increases, differentiation from testicular torsion becomes increasingly difficult as reactive inflammation of the testis and epididymis worsens. A clinical diagnosis of torsion of the appendix testis should not be made unless the appendix testis is palpated or visualized.

The natural history of torsion of the appendix testis is for the inflammation to resolve gradually after infarction of the appendage. In general, the process is complete within 10 days from the onset of symptoms. Scrotal exploration and excision of the torsed appendage is unnecessary unless there is uncertainty regarding the diagnosis and testicular torsion is possible. If the diagnosis of torsion of the appendix testis is highly likely, color Doppler ultrasonography is optional for confirmation. Management includes strict rest for 2–3 days and nonsteroidal antiinflammatory medications to reduce inflammation and pain. Vigorous activity such as sports should be restricted for at least 7 days, as activity may worsen and prolong pain and swelling. The patient should be instructed to seek prompt medical evaluation if pain does worsen, as such worsening may be indicative of testicular torsion.

EPIDIDYMITIS, EPIDIDYMOORCHITIS, AND ORCHITIS

The inflammation of **epididymitis** may be caused by an infectious process or may be secondary to trauma, torsion of the appendix testis, or sterile reflux of urine down the vas deferens. Pain and swelling are typically insidious in onset. Patients may have associated dysuria, urgency, frequency, and urethral discharge, and some may report transient episodes of inguinal pain that preceded the onset of testicular symptoms and that were secondary to spermatic cord inflammation. The epididymis is tender, enlarged, indurated, and situated posterior to the testis; in **epididymoorchitis**, inflammation progresses to involve the testis, which also becomes enlarged and tender. A reactive hydrocele may be present, obscuring testicular examination. The cremasteric reflex is typically preserved. Isolated **orchitis** is less common, particularly in prepubertal males, though it may be seen in postpubertal males with mumps virus infection.

Bacterial epididymitis usually results from urethral infection passing retrograde through the vas deferens to the epididymis (Fig. 24.8). In prepubertal males, bacterial epididymitis is most frequently secondary to a structural abnormality of the lower genitourinary tract, such as ectopic ureter, ectopic vas deferens, or urethral stricture, or may be secondary to dysfunctional voiding. UA typically demonstrates pyuria, bacteriuria, or both, and bacterial culture of the urine may isolate the causative organism, usually a gram-negative coliform. Given the association with underlying urogenital abnormalities, further evaluation should include renal ultrasonography and voiding cystourethrography. In postpubertal males without underlying genitourinary abnormalities, bacterial epididymitis is most frequently caused by sexually transmitted infection, typically *Chlamydia trachomatis*, although *Neisseria gonorrhoeae* and *Ureaplasma urealyticum* may be causative as well. Additional causes of bacterial epididymitis include extension of urinary tract infection or infection with *Mycoplasma pneumoniae* or mycobacteria. UA and bacterial culture of the urine should be obtained, as should nucleic acid amplification tests for *C. trachomatis* and *N. gonorrhoeae* from urine or urethral swab specimens. Patients whose epididymitis is related to a sexually transmitted infection should further be tested for syphilis and HIV.

Viral epididymitis may be difficult to distinguish from noninfectious inflammatory causes of epididymitis. Enteroviruses and adenoviruses are typically implicated, either as a primary infection or as a postinfectious sequela. The inflammation of **orchitis** most commonly represents an extension of epididymitis; however, isolated orchitis may be seen in males with **mumps infection**. This manifestation is rare in prepubertal males, though it may complicate infection in up to 35% of postpubertal males. The onset of orchitis usually occurs within 1 week of the onset of mumps parotitis and is more frequently unilateral. Diagnosis may be clinical, although given the markedly decreased incidence of mumps following the introduction of an effective vaccine and the possibility of alternate infectious etiologies, confirmatory testing may be obtained. Patients with parotitis may provide buccal swabs or saliva samples for nucleic acid amplification testing. Mumps-specific immunoglobulin M (IgM) antibody testing or acute and convalescent serum immunoglobulin G (IgG) antibody titer quantification may confirm the diagnosis. Up to a third of patients with mumps orchitis develop testicular atrophy and subfertility, although true infertility is rare, even with bilateral testicular involvement.

Noninfectious etiologies of epididymitis include torsion of the appendix testis, trauma, and medication exposure, particularly to amiodarone. Scrotal ultrasonography shows epididymal swelling and hyperemia consistent with epididymitis. Urinalysis and urine culture reveal no evidence of bacterial urinary tract infection.

TRAUMA AND HEMATOCELE

Blunt scrotal trauma can result in a spectrum of injuries ranging from testicular contusion to testicular rupture (Fig. 24.9). Testicular injuries usually result from a fall, kick, or direct blow from a blunt object that compresses the testis up against the pubic bone. A detailed history of the nature of the injury aids in recognizing the likelihood of serious testicular injury. With disruption of the tunica albuginea (capsule) of the testis, there is such significant painful scrotal swelling that the testis cannot be palpated. Often there is associated erythema or ecchymosis of the scrotal wall. In cases of suspected testicular injury, other diagnoses such as torsion and epididymitis should be considered. Scrotal ultrasonography should be performed to assess the integrity of the testis and to assess for torsion. UA should be performed to assess for bacterial epididymitis.

VARICOCELE

A **varicocele** is an abnormal dilation of the veins of the pampiniform plexus in the scrotum. Varicoceles are rare under 10 years of age; approximately 10% of adolescent males and 15% of adult males have a varicocele. The increased prevalence among adolescents and adults is secondary to the increased testicular blood flow that occurs with puberty. More than 95% of varicoceles are left-sided, likely secondary to the higher venous pressure of the left internal spermatic vein and the absence of a venous valve at the insertion of the left internal spermatic vein into the renal vein. If a varicocele is detected on the right side or in a male younger than 10 years old, abdominal ultrasonography is indicated to ascertain whether an abdominal tumor is present.

A varicocele manifests as a painless, paratesticular mass often described as a "bag of worms" (Fig. 24.10). On occasion, patients describe a chronic, dull ache in or adjacent to the testis. Physical examination in both the supine and the upright positions, with and without the Valsalva

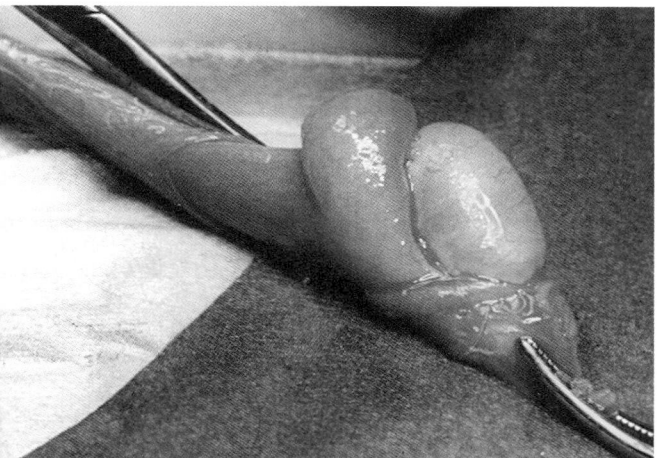

Fig. 24.8 Epididymitis in a 6-year-old male. Note the reactive orchitis as well as the significant enlargement of the epididymis.

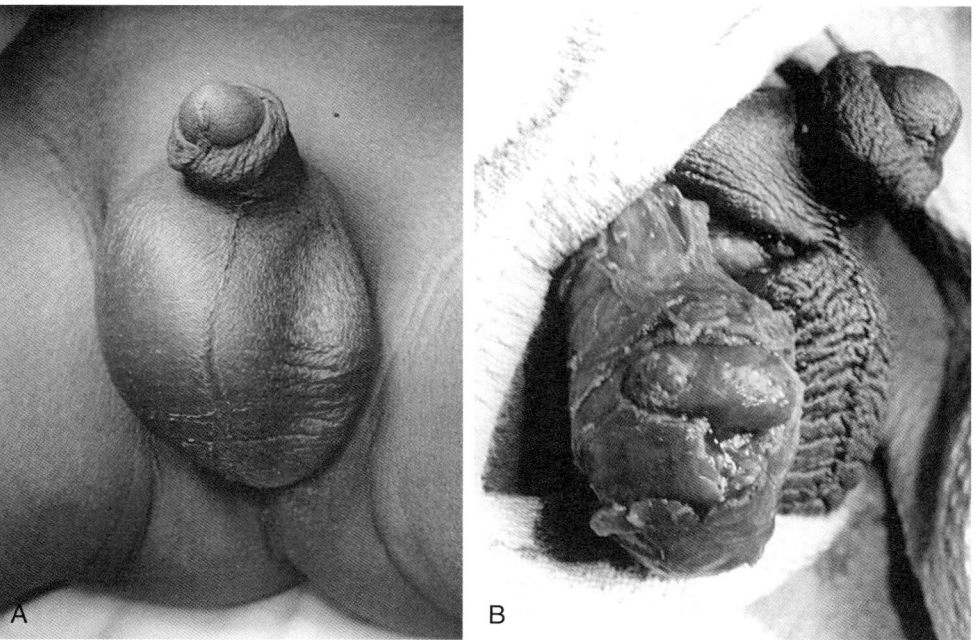

Fig. 24.9 *A*, Appearance in an 8-year-old male kicked in the scrotum while performing karate with his brother. Note right scrotal swelling. An ultrasound study showed scrotal hematoma and a ruptured testis. *B*, Scrotal exploration shows a nonviable testis. Orchiectomy was performed.

maneuver, facilitates the diagnosis. Typically, the varicocele is decompressed while supine and is more prominent when standing. Measuring the volume of both testicles is important to document size discrepancies, as approximately one third of affected males have associated volume loss. Calipers, an orchiometer, or ultrasonography may be used.

Appropriate and timely diagnosis is essential, as an untreated varicocele may lead to degeneration of germinal centers, interstitial fibrosis, and impaired spermatogenesis and testosterone production. Up to 15% of adult males with a varicocele are infertile. The goal in treatment of a varicocele is preservation and restoration of spermatogenesis. Because the majority of testicular volume is composed of seminiferous tubules, if the left testis is significantly smaller than the right, the clinician may presume that the varicocele has affected testicular growth. Typically, after varicocelectomy in an adolescent, the testis shows catch-up growth. Surgical management does not guarantee paternity as an adult.

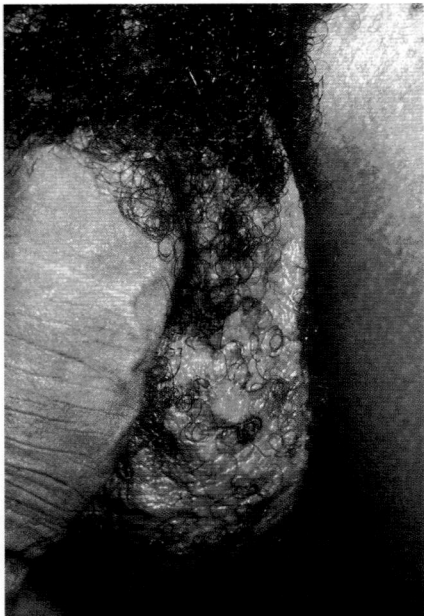

Fig. 24.10 Left varicocele in an adolescent male. (From Kliegman RM, St. Geme JW III, Blum NJ, et al., eds. *Nelson Textbook of Pediatrics.* 21st ed. Philadelphia: Elsevier; 2020:2832, Fig. 560.7.)

INGUINAL HERNIA

Hernias and hydroceles result from incomplete obliteration of the processus vaginalis. Indirect inguinal hernias result from a patent processus vaginalis that allows bowel or omentum to pass through the internal inguinal ring (Fig. 24.11). Patients usually present with inguinal swelling, scrotal swelling, or both. While swelling should reduce with gentle pressure, a hernia that cannot be reduced is called an **incarcerated hernia** and is a surgical emergency, as the vascular supply of the herniated bowel may become compromised (Fig. 24.12). Physical signs of incarceration include inguinal or scrotal erythema, pain, signs of bowel obstruction, and inability to reduce the hernia. Infants with an incarcerated hernia have a 10% incidence of ipsilateral testicular infarction secondary to increased pressure on the spermatic cord.

If an incarcerated hernia is suspected, the child is hospitalized and sedated, and manual reduction of the hernia is attempted. Most

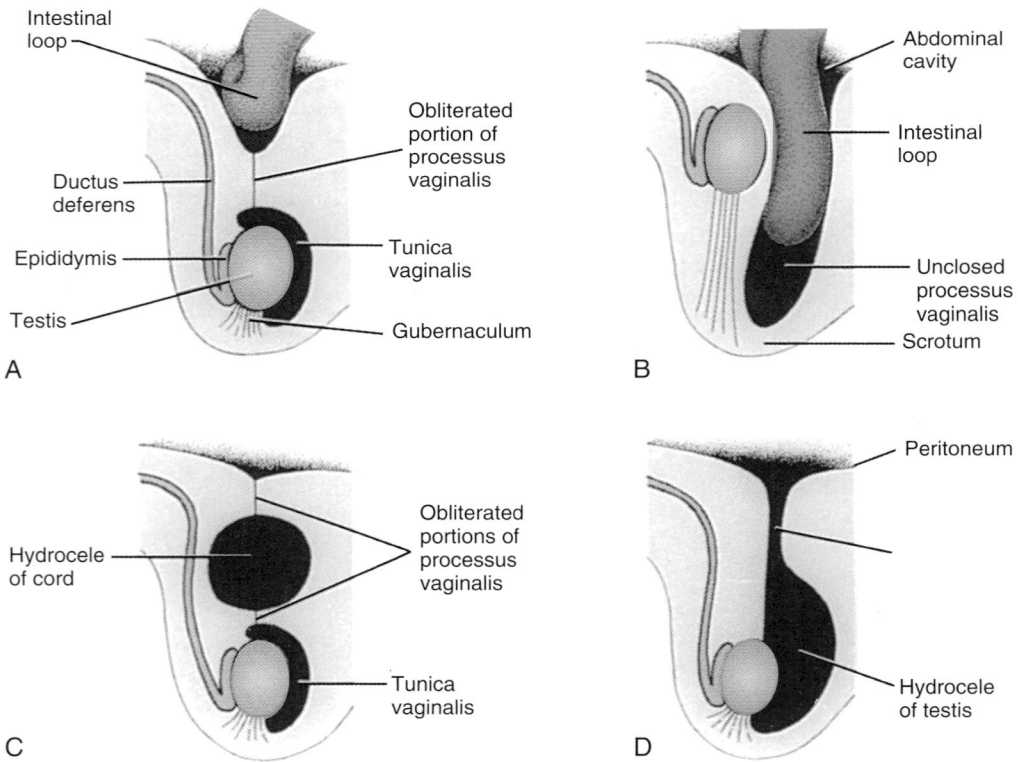

Fig. 24.11 Diagrams of sagittal sections of the inguinal region. *A,* Incomplete indirect inguinal hernia, resulting from persistence of the proximal processus vaginalis. *B,* Indirect inguinal hernia into the scrotum, resulting from persistence of the entire processus vaginalis. Note the presence of an undescended testicle, which is a commonly associated malformation. *C,* Hydrocele of the cord, derived from an unobliterated portion of the processus vaginalis. *D,* Communicating hydrocele, resulting from peritoneal fluid passing through a patent processus vaginalis. (From Moore KL. *Clinically Oriented Anatomy.* 2nd ed. Baltimore: Williams & Wilkins; 1993:299.)

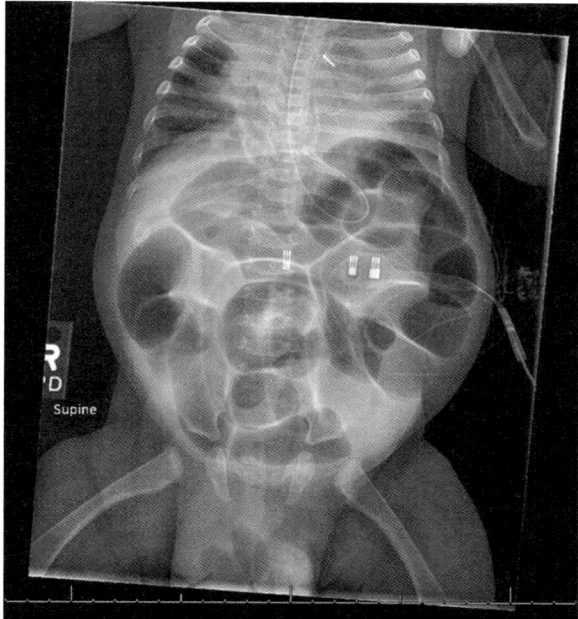

Fig. 24.12 Incarcerated inguinal hernia. Kidney, ureter, and bladder study demonstrating abdominal bowel loops and bowel gas in the scrotum.

incarcerated hernias can be reduced successfully and should be repaired promptly. Children with an easily reducible hernia should also undergo herniorrhaphy within a reasonable time to reduce the possibility of incarceration.

HYDROCELE

A **hydrocele** is an accumulation of fluid within the tunica vaginalis. Communicating hydroceles, defined by a patent processus vaginalis, are present in approximately 2% of newborn males, are more common in preterm infants, and tend to persist (see Fig. 24.11). The diameter of the patent processus vaginalis is much smaller than that seen with a hernia, allowing only peritoneal fluid to pass into the scrotum. Typically, affected males have painless scrotal swelling that progresses over the course of the day and resolves while sleeping or otherwise recumbent, as fluid returns to the peritoneal cavity. Noncommunicating hydroceles are characterized by the presence of an unobliterated portion of the processus vaginalis (see Fig. 24.11) and may be acquired following an inflammatory condition within the scrotum, such as testicular torsion, torsion of the appendix testis, epididymitis, or testicular tumor.

Physical examination reveals a smooth and nontender scrotal mass that is clear upon transillumination (Fig. 24.13). Because hydroceles can be associated with testicular neoplasms in postpubertal males, testicular examination should be performed. If the size of the hydrocele precludes adequate testicular examination, scrotal ultrasonography is advised. Most communicating hydroceles resolve by 1 year of age and can be managed expectantly; however, large and tense masses may be difficult to distinguish from hernias and may require ultrasonography. Large hydroceles or hydroceles persisting beyond the age of 2 years rarely regress spontaneously and may predispose to inguinal hernia.

A severe form of the hydrocele is the **abdominoscrotal hydrocele**, in which the hydrocele sac is tense with fluid and extends from the scrotum proximally through the inguinal canal into the abdominal cavity (Fig. 24.14). On examination, these hydroceles are palpable in the inguinal canal, and an abdominal mass is often present. These hydroceles do not resolve and may cause extrinsic testicular compression. Early repair is recommended.

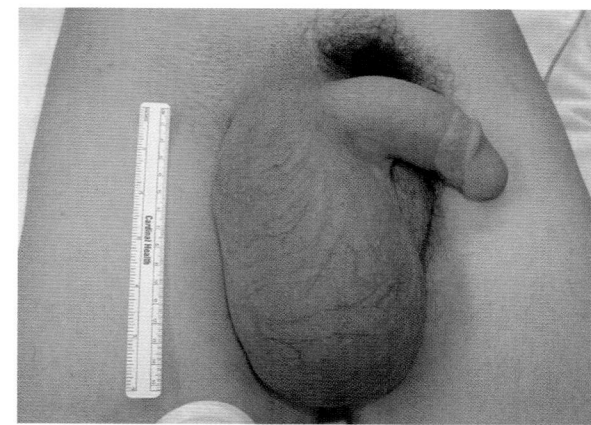

Fig. 24.13 Large hydrocele in a teenage male.

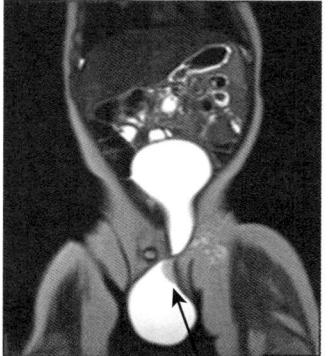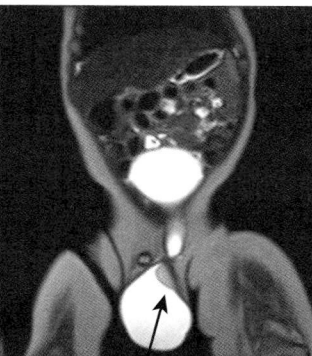

Note: the fusiform shaped testis in the hydrocele

Fig. 24.14 Abdominoscrotal hydrocele.

TESTICULAR TUMORS

Although testicular and paratesticular tumors are uncommon, testicular cancer is the most common solid malignancy in postpubertal males between the ages of 15 and 35 years, with a bimodal age distribution reflecting this age range, and another peak in the first 2 years of life. Most testicular cancers are germ cell tumors, representing approximately 95% of testicular cancers, while the remaining 5% are stromal tumors derived from Leydig, Sertoli, and granulosa cells (Table 24.5). Risk factors for testicular tumors include a history of cryptorchidism, a prior history of testicular cancer in the contralateral testicle, and a family history of testicular cancer. Gonadoblastoma is a complication of phenotypic males with disorders of sexual development (see Chapter 26).

Most patients with testicular tumors present with an incidentally noted nontender, hard mass that fails to transilluminate on examination. Pain is uncommon, although some patients may present with pain secondary to hemorrhage or infarction within the mass. Up to 15% of testicular tumors are associated with a noncommunicating hydrocele, prompting affected patients to seek medical evaluation. Stromal tumors may elaborate hormones that can lead to precocious pseudopuberty, gynecomastia, galactorrhea, or other endocrinologic manifestations.

Scrotal ultrasonography should be performed to confirm the finding of a testicular mass and may help delineate the type of testicular tumor (Fig. 24.15). Serum tumor markers, such as α-fetoprotein and β-human chorionic gonadotropin, should be evaluated before surgical intervention. Partial orchiectomy is typically performed for prepubertal testis tumors with negative α-fetoprotein; radical orchiectomy is

TABLE 24.5 **World Health Organization Classification of Germ Cell Tumors: Male**

Germ Cell Tumors	Sex Cord/Gonadal Stromal Tumors
Intratubular germ cell neoplasia, unclassified	***Pure Forms***
Other types	Leydig cell tumor
Tumors of One Histologic Type	Malignant Leydig cell tumor
Seminoma	Sertoli cell tumor
Seminoma with syncytiotrophoblastic cells	Sertoli cell tumor lipid-rich variant
Spermatocytic seminoma	Sclerosing Sertoli cell tumor
Spermatocytic seminoma with sarcoma	Large cell calcifying Sertoli cell tumor
Embryonal carcinoma	Malignant Sertoli cell tumor
Yolk sac tumor	Granulosa cell tumor
Trophoblastic tumors	Adult type granulosa cell tumor
Choriocarcinoma	Juvenile type granulosa cell tumor
Trophoblastic neoplasms other than choriocarcinoma	Tumors of the thecoma/fibroma group
Monophasic choriocarcinoma	Thecoma
Placental site trophoblastic tumor	Fibroma
Teratoma	Sex cord/gonadal stromal tumor, incompletely differentiated
Dermoid cyst	Sex cord/gonadal stromal tumor, mixed forms
Monodermal teratoma	Malignant sex cord/gonadal stromal tumor
Teratoma with somatic type malignancies	Tumors containing both germ cell and sex cord/gonadal stromal elements
Tumors of More Than One Histologic Type	Gonadoblastoma
Mixed embryonal carcinoma and teratoma	Germ cell–sex cord/gonadal stromal tumor, unclassified
Mixed teratoma and seminoma	
Choriocarcinoma and teratoma/embryonal carcinoma	
Others	

From Orkin SH, Nathan DG, Ginsburg D, et al. *Nathan and Oski's Hematology and Oncology of Infancy and Childhood.* 8th ed., Vol 2. Philadelphia: Elsevier; 2015:2059, Box 63-1.

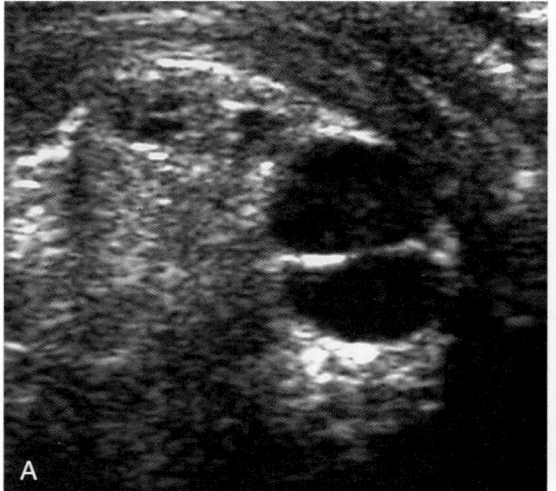
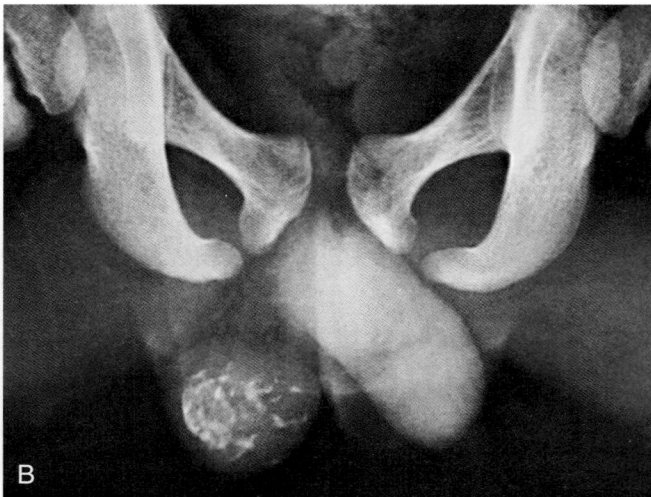

Fig. 24.15 Testicular teratoma. *A,* Transverse grayscale sonogram of the right testicle shows a complex testicular mass with debris-filled cystic foci and surrounding hyperechogenicity. *B,* A coned radiograph of the lower pelvis identifies a calcified right testicular lesion. (From Coley BD, ed. *Caffey's Pediatric Diagnostic Imaging.* 13th ed. Philadelphia: Elsevier; 2019:1198, Fig. 125.21. Courtesy Dr. Leslie E. Grissom.)

performed for postpubertal testis tumors and prepubertal testis tumors with elevated α-fetoprotein, given their higher metastatic potential. After radical orchiectomy, abdominal and chest CT is obtained to evaluate the most common sites of metastatic disease, the retroperitoneum, and lungs.

Leukemia and lymphoma are the most common secondary malignancies to affect the testis. These tumors can present bilaterally, and, because the blood-testis barrier protects the intratesticular cells, the testis may be the site of residual tumor in children after chemotherapy.

Paratesticular structures can give rise to various benign tumors, such as lipomas, leiomyomas, hemangiomas, and fibromas. Malignant paratesticular tumors are rare; rhabdomyosarcoma is the most common malignant paratesticular tumor.

MECONIUM PERITONITIS

Antenatal peritonitis may result from intestinal perforation. Although the intestinal perforation may heal, the intraabdominal meconium may track down the patent processus vaginalis into the scrotum, resulting in the formation of an inflammatory mass. This condition can manifest as bilateral neonatal hydroceles, which eventually regress into firm, nodular masses involving either or both testicles. Scrotal sonography demonstrates multiple areas of echogenic foci suggestive of calcification. In addition, a plain film of the scrotum shows calcification.

SCROTAL WALL SWELLING

Henoch-Schönlein Purpura (Immunoglobulin A Vasculitis)

Henoch-Schönlein purpura is a systemic vasculitis of unknown etiology that involves the skin, gastrointestinal tract, joints, and kidneys. Most affected patients are younger than 7 years. Genitourinary manifestations may include glomerulonephritis (see Chapter 23), ureteritis, renal pelvic bleeding, and acute swelling of the scrotum and spermatic cord. Scrotal wall and testicular involvement has been reported in up to a third of affected patients.

Palpable purpura (the characteristic skin finding in Henoch-Schönlein purpura) often begins in the lower extremities and buttock region. Later, the rash may spread to the scrotum; on occasion, the rash may begin on the scrotum. If scrotal swelling and pain precede the development of the characteristic rash, the presentation may be difficult to distinguish from testicular torsion. However, as these conditions may coexist, if there is any uncertainty regarding the diagnosis, color Doppler ultrasonography should be performed.

Acute Idiopathic Scrotal Wall Edema

Acute idiopathic scrotal wall edema is an uncommon entity that accounts for up to 5% of acute scrotal swelling. The average patient is between 4 and 7 years of age and typically presents with the sudden onset of unilateral or bilateral scrotal wall edema and mild tenderness. The overlying skin is erythematous, and the edema may extend anteriorly onto the abdominal wall or posteriorly into the perineum. The testicles are easily palpable, normal in size, and nontender. The origin of this syndrome is unknown, but allergic causes have been implicated. Most cases spontaneously resolve within 48–72 hours.

Idiopathic Fat Necrosis

Idiopathic fat necrosis is an uncommon cause of acute painful swelling of the scrotum, secondary to necrosis of the intrascrotal fat that is present in prepubertal males. Examination of the underlying testis may be hampered by inflammation within the scrotal wall. The etiology is unknown but may be related to trauma with physical activity. Ultrasonography demonstrates hyperechoic intrascrotal masses with posterior shadowing and a hyperechoic striated scrotal wall with normal-appearing testes and epididymis. Treatment is supportive.

Fournier Gangrene

Fournier gangrene of the scrotum usually affects adults but rarely can afflict infants and children. In children, it occurs primarily as a result of genital insect bites, as a complication of circumcision, or from extension of perianal skin abscesses. Other predisposing factors include diabetes mellitus, trauma, instrumentation, urethral stricture, and inguinal or perineal surgery. Symptoms of this life-threatening infection include acute scrotal swelling with tenderness, erythema, skin necrosis, and systemic manifestations of fever, chills, and septicemia. The most common organisms identified include *Staphylococcus aureus*, *Bacteroides fragilis*, *Escherichia coli*, *Clostridium perfringens*, and streptococcal species. Despite aggressive treatment, mortality rates approach 50%.

REFERRED PAIN

Pain in the scrotum without inflammatory signs or abnormalities on physical examination may be referred pain. Sensory innervation to the scrotum includes the genitofemoral and ilioinguinal nerves. Most common causes include distal ureteral stones and constipation.

▮ RED FLAGS

- An approach to scrotal swelling and pain is noted in Figure 24.16.
- Testicular torsion is a surgical emergency and acute scrotal pain should be evaluated promptly. Physical examination findings suggesting testicular torsion include marked tenderness, high-riding testis, and absent cremasteric reflex.
- Partial or intermittent torsion can present with persistent arterial blood flow on ultrasonography.
- A varicocele before puberty or on the right side is a red flag; abdominal ultrasonography is indicated.

BIBLIOGRAPHY

A bibliography is available at ExpertConsult.com

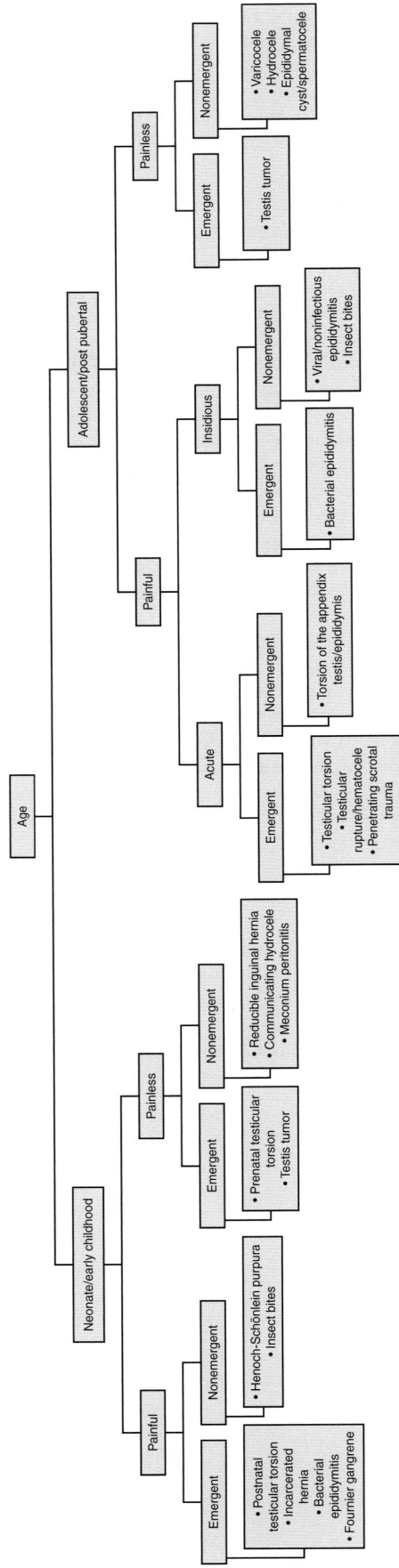

Fig. 24.16 Scrotal swelling algorithm.

25

Menstrual Problems and Vaginal Bleeding

Jessica Francis and Seema Menon

PREPUBERTAL VAGINAL BLEEDING

The source of abnormal vaginal bleeding during prepubertal childhood is much more likely to be the vulva or vagina rather than the uterus. There are unique characteristics making history and physical examination effective in narrowing the diagnostic possibilities as seen in Table 25.1. Collecting information regarding recent trauma, medication exposure, rashes or irritation of the external genitalia, abdominal pain, chronic cough, constipation, and malodorous discharge is essential in making a diagnosis efficiently. A sensitive assessment regarding the possibility of sexual assault should be made, and an age-appropriate physical examination should be conducted noting the presence or absence of other pubertal signs, abnormalities of the vulva or urethra, vaginal discharge, and abdominal or vaginal masses.

Vaginal bleeding presenting within the first several days of life is most commonly due to estrogen withdrawal. Maternal estrogen enters fetal circulation stimulating proliferation of the endometrium. External genitalia examination typically reveals estrogenization, with thickened vulvar mucosa and leukorrhea. Several days after delivery, serum estrogen levels fall significantly, leading to a reduction of blood supply to the endometrium, and the lining sheds as ischemia develops. If vaginal bleeding occurs within the first few days of life with a normal physical examination, a work-up is not needed provided the bleeding spontaneously resolves.

The presence of a **vaginal foreign body** is another common cause of vaginal bleeding in early childhood. This bleeding is often described as persistent, light in quantity, brown colored, and malodorous. The physical examination is unremarkable other than the possible presence of a vaginal malodor. The most common foreign body found in the vagina is toilet paper, although many other solid objects have been reported. Depending on the age and cooperation of the patient, lateral and downward traction of the labia majora may allow direct visualization of the foreign body. Toilet paper can be retrieved in the office by gently irrigating the vagina with water using a small, flexible pediatric feeding tube. In cases where an optimal pelvic examination is not possible, a vaginoscopy under sedation should be performed. One technique is to place an 8 French Foley catheter in the vagina. A 5-mm laparoscope is simultaneously placed in the vagina. Saline is then flushed into the vagina using the Foley catheter while the labia majora are manually held together. The vagina is then distended allowing for complete visualization of the vaginal cavity including the cervix and any foreign body present. Simply removing the foreign body will adequately treat the symptoms; no antibiotic therapy is needed. A vaginal foreign body should not automatically trigger a full sexual assault evaluation; this investigation should be conducted if there is indication by history, or if suspicious scarring of the posterior fourchette is noted.

Prepubertal **vaginal infection** may present with bleeding and discharge. Unlike vaginal foreign body, the bleeding is typically red in color and not malodorous. Vaginal infection is also associated with complaints of external genital irritation. Mucosal erythema on physical examination is notable, particularly when the pathogen is group A β-hemolytic streptococcus. The diagnosis is confirmed with culture of the vaginal canal. A specimen for culture can be collected using the gentle irrigation technique described previously if vaginal swab placement is not possible. In addition to group A β-hemolytic streptococcus, other pathogens that are commonly identified include *Haemophilus influenzae*, *Escherichia coli*, *Shigella*, and *Salmonella* species, with the latter two being particularly associated with vaginal bleeding. A recent history of an upper respiratory infection should raise suspicion of this diagnosis as the majority of vaginal infections arise from autoinoculation. Notably, *Candida* infections of the vagina are uncommon in this population.

Vulvar dermatoses can also present with vaginal bleeding and significant irritation or pain of the external genitalia. In this case, the bleeding is minimal, often caused by trauma from scratching. While vulvar dermatosis in the prepubertal population is relatively uncommon, **atopic dermatitis**, **lichen sclerosus**, and **psoriasis** are the most commonly described conditions (Figs. 25.1 and 25.2). Atopic dermatitis will only occur in regions in contact with the allergen. Suspicion for the latter two conditions should be raised if extragenital skin findings are noted, or if a positive family history is elicited. The typical appearance of lichen sclerosus is white parchment paper–like appearance in an hourglass distribution. Obliteration of the labia minora and clitoris can occur with long-standing disease. Pinpoint bruising can also occur. While this is not the most common presentation, it is worth noting as it can be concerning for trauma. The treatment involves short courses of high-potency topical steroids and usually resolves as serum estrogen levels rise with maturation. Psoriasis typically appears as an erythematous plaque or papule marked by fissures, erosions, or scales. Treatment includes topical steroids, fluorinated ointments, emollients, and newer immunomodulators. In both cases, biopsy is needed to confirm the diagnosis; however, if clinical suspicion is high and symptoms are severe, empiric treatment prior to biopsy is reasonable. Other vulvar lesions that can produce bleeding include hemangiomas and genital warts.

Urethral prolapse is another cause of prepubertal vaginal bleeding associated with a classic physical examination finding (Fig. 25.3). It is seen more commonly in young females. The only complaint is bleeding; there is no coexisting pain or irritation. The limited estrogen levels in childhood leave the urethra vulnerable to prolapse, especially in the setting of frequent Valsalva maneuvers from chronic cough or constipation. On physical examination, the urethra appears prominent, erythematous, and tubular "doughnut shaped," protruding well beyond the urethral meatus. Topical estrogen therapy for 1–2 weeks is typically effective in resolving this condition. Rarely, urethral necrosis or urinary retention can occur. In these cases, topical estradiol therapy may still be effective, but surgical resection may be needed for treatment.

TABLE 25.1 Causes of Prepubertal Bleeding

	Pain or Irritation	Associated Characteristics	Family History
Estrogen withdrawal	No	First week of life (neonates)	No
Foreign body	No	Malodorous	No
Vaginal infection	Yes	Recent upper respiratory infection	No
Vulvar dermatoses	Yes	Vulvar discoloration or lesion Extragenital skin findings	Yes
Urethral prolapse	No	Chronic cough or constipation Red, beefy, protuberant urethra	No
Straddle injury	Yes	Provoking injury Visible laceration	No
Precocious puberty*	No	Cyclic pattern of bleeding Secondary sexual characteristics present	Yes
Vaginal malignancy	Possible	Visible mass	No
Isolated functional ovarian cysts	No	None	No

*McCune-Albright syndrome, central precocious puberty, juvenile granulosa cell tumor, severe hypothyroidism.

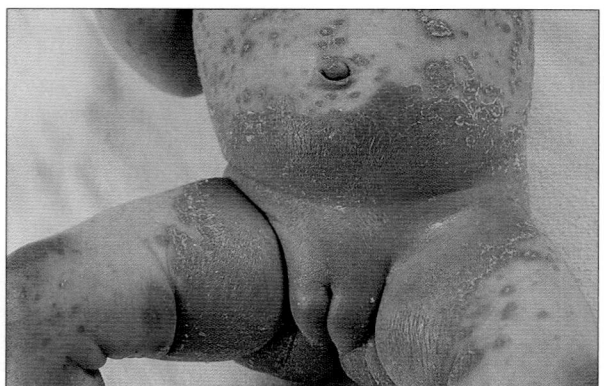

Fig. 25.1 Psoriasis: typical diaper involvement. (From Eichenfield LF, Frieden IJ, Esterly NB, eds. *Textbook of Neonatal Dermatology*. 2nd ed. Philadelphia: Saunders; 2008, Fig. 15.12.)

While the vast majority of lesions of the external genitalia causing prepubertal bleeding are benign, malignancy has been reported. **Sarcoma botryoides**, a variant of rhabdomyosarcoma, is the most common vaginal tumor in childhood. The classic description of this tumor is a protruding vaginal mass with grapelike vesicles. Other malignant tumors of the lower genital tract that have been reported include mesenchymal tumors, neural ectodermal tumors in the Ewing family, and mixed müllerian tumors. Any abnormal-appearing vaginal mass should raise concern for malignancy and should prompt a referral to an appropriate specialist for evaluation.

Bleeding secondary to a **perineal injury** presents acutely with pain and is associated with a clear provoking event unlike the other causes of childhood vaginal bleeding. Straddle injuries are the most common childhood injury to the genitalia and can lead to a bleeding laceration. This injury is caused by a nonpenetrating blunt force to the perineum when the legs are apart. Classic activities associated with straddle injuries include bike riding, playing on a seesaw, and gymnastics. Water-jet injuries related to falls during water sports can also be a mechanism for vaginal laceration and hemorrhage. An examination must be done to determine whether the laceration requires primary closure with suture. Conscious sedation or examination under anesthesia is appropriate for straddle injury evaluations as pain may prohibit a thorough evaluation. If the history does not substantiate the injury, a sensitive interview

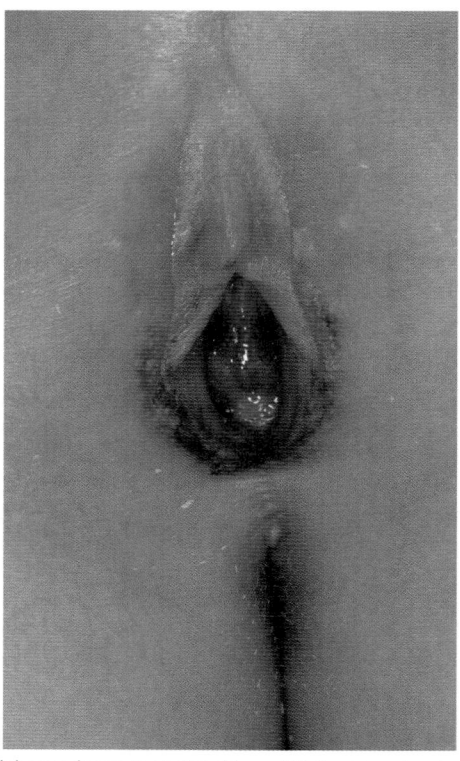

Fig. 25.2 Lichen sclerosus et atrophicus. Whitening, atrophy, inflammation, and purpura of the labia. (From Paller AS, Mancini AJ, eds. *Hurwitz Clinical Pediatric Dermatology*. 5th ed. Philadelphia: Elsevier; 2016:535, Fig. 22.51.)

should be conducted prior to the examination. Co-examination with the sexual assault team is important should there be any suspicion.

Prepubertal vaginal bleeding presenting with breast development and growth acceleration should raise concern for **precocious puberty** (see Chapter 55). Conventional thinking defines pubertal changes before age 8 years as precocious. However, this is debated as hallmarks of puberty have been appearing earlier over the past century and differ by race in the United States. Important historical cues that are helpful in making a diagnosis include symptoms or known central nervous system (CNS) abnormalities, symptoms of hypothyroidism, family

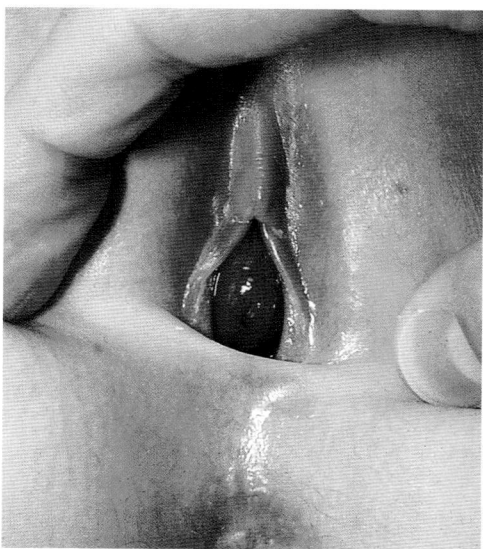

Fig. 25.3 Urethral prolapse. This is a chronic case in which the initial hemorrhagic nature of the acute prolapse has resolved with observation, leaving a protuberant, edematous urethra. (From Zitelli BJ, McIntire SC, Nowalk AJ, eds. *Zitelli and Davis' Atlas of Pediatric Physical Diagnosis.* 7th ed. Philadelphia: Elsevier; 2018:558, Fig. 15.43.)

history of early puberty, Peutz-Jeghers or McCune-Albright syndrome, or neurofibromatosis type 1. Height, Tanner staging of the breasts and pubic hair, and external genital changes consistent with estrogen exposure, such as elongation of the labia minora and thickening of vulvar mucosa, should be specifically evaluated during physical examination. Café-au-lait spots, presence of an abdominal mass, and thyroid gland abnormalities should also be assessed. Radiographic imaging to determine the bone age of the left wrist can identify elevated serum estrogen levels and is a good initial screening test. Laboratory evaluation confirming precocious puberty includes elevated serum estradiol, androgen panel, and gonadotropins. Imaging may also be needed in some clinical scenarios.

Early elevated serum estrogen most commonly occurs because of maturation of the hypothalamic-pituitary-ovarian (HPO) axis, termed gonadotropin-releasing hormone (GnRH)–dependent precocious puberty. In this condition, the pathology is simply the early timing of maturation. Administration of a GnRH analog is effective in temporarily stopping anterior pituitary production of gonadotropins, ultimately preventing sex hormone production from the ovary. The purpose of halting early puberty is to avoid age-inappropriate social contact, and to preserve height, which is particularly effective when treating patients 6 years of age or younger. Rarely, GnRH pulsatile release is stimulated by CNS abnormalities such as infection, tumors, hydrocephaly, meningomyelocele, neonatal encephalopathy, or cranial radiation. Type 1 neurofibromatosis and tuberous sclerosis are also associated with

GnRH-dependent precocious puberty. Imaging of the CNS should be aggressively pursued if there is suspicion of a CNS lesion, if pubertal progression is rapid, or if the child is under age 6.

GnRH-independent precocious puberty is a much less common cause of precious puberty. In this condition, the hypothalamus is not driving ovarian sex steroid hormone production. Conditions such as malignant granulosa cell tumors of the ovary, benign functional ovarian cysts, or tumors of the pituitary or adrenal gland are responsible for the elevated serum estrogens. McCune-Albright syndrome, Peutz-Jeghers syndrome, and hypothyroidism are associated with GnRH-independent precocious puberty as well.

GnRH-dependent and -independent precocious puberty are associated with different history and physical examination cues (Table 25.2). A GnRH stimulation test is effective in differentiating these two processes. A rise in gonadotropins after exogenous administration of GnRH suggests that the HPO axis is active, confirming GnRH-dependent precocious puberty.

ABNORMAL BLEEDING IN ADOLESCENCE

Establishment of the menstrual cycle is a major hallmark of adolescence. The menstrual cycle serves as a marker of health, so much so that it has been heralded as a "vital sign" during adolescence. Irregular menstrual bleeding may simply be related to the maturation of the complex physiologic process leading to puberty. In other cases, irregular menstrual bleeding may be a symptom of a significant medical condition (Table 25.3). A basic understanding of the menstrual cycle is helpful when trying to understand the many causes of abnormal bleeding.

REVIEW OF THE MENSTRUAL CYCLE

Complex interaction between the hypothalamus, pituitary, ovary, and uterus leads to ovulatory menstrual cycles (Fig. 25.4). The hypothalamus releases pulses of GnRH into a portal system to the pituitary gland. The anterior pituitary is stimulated to release the gonadotropins, follicle-stimulating hormone (FSH) and luteinizing hormone (LH), when exposed to GnRH pulses. LH acts on the theca cells of the ovary leading to androgen production; these hormones are aromatized to estrogens in the granulosa cells of the ovary under the influence of FSH. This drives development of the dominant follicle.

Interaction between the anterior pituitary and ovary is complex in that it is bidirectional. Gonadotropin release is stimulated by GnRH and modulated by ovarian hormones, both the sex steroid hormones and the peptide hormones, activin and inhibin. In the first half of the cycle, the dominant follicle grows in size leading to increased estradiol production. A positive feedback relationship is seen between the ovary and the anterior pituitary, with higher levels of estradiol stimulating gonadotropin release. This ultimately leads to the LH surge, triggering ovulation.

TABLE 25.2	Comparison of GnRH-Dependent and GnRH-Independent Precocious Puberty	
	GnRH-Dependent Precocious Puberty	**GnRH-Independent Precocious Puberty**
Prevalence	More common	Less common
Family history of early puberty	Positive	Negative
Unique characteristics	History or symptoms of CNS lesions, tumors, or infections	Symptoms of hypothyroidism, café-au-lait lesions, known Peutz-Jeghers syndrome
GnRH stimulation test	Positive	Negative

CNS, central nervous system; GnRH, gonadotropin-releasing hormone.

TABLE 25.3 Causes of Abnormal Bleeding in Adolescents

	Cycle Length	Intermenstrual Bleeding	Heavy Menses	Unique Characteristics	Family History
Coagulopathy	Prolonged	No	Yes	Bruising Epistaxis Gingival bleeding	Yes
HPO axis immaturity	Variable	No	Variable	None	No
PCOS	Variable	No	Variable	Acne Hirsutism Central obesity	Yes
Endometrial causes	Prolonged	Yes	No	Unprotected sexual activity Vaginal discharge Fever Cervical motion tenderness Uterine tenderness	No
Contraceptive break-through	Prolonged	Yes	No	Progesterone-only contraceptive use Improper use of hormonal contraception	No
Adenomyosis	Prolonged	No	Yes	Symmetrically enlarged uterus	Possible
Leiomyoma	Prolonged	No	Yes	Asymmetrically enlarged uterus	Yes
Polyp	Prolonged	Yes	No	None	No

HPO, hypothalamic-pituitary-ovary; PCOS, polycystic ovary syndrome.

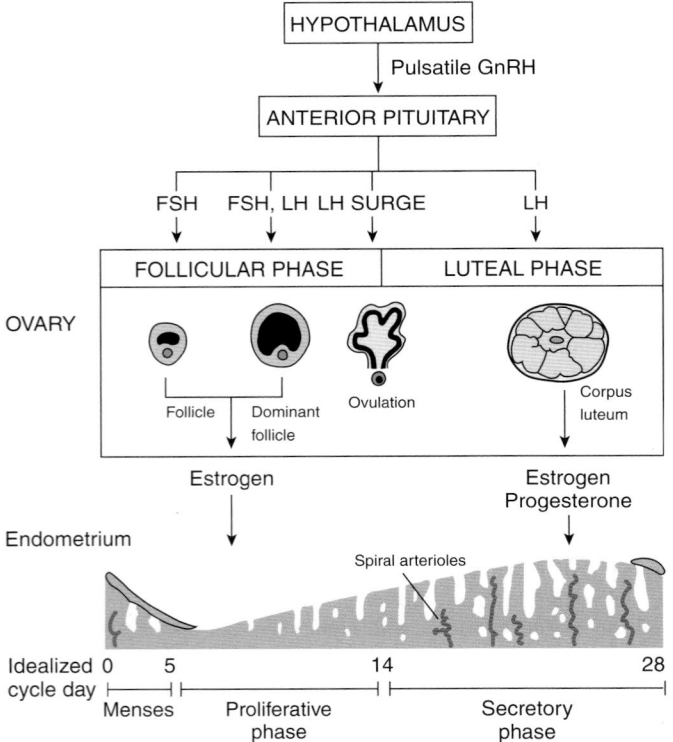

Fig. 25.4 Hypothalamic-pituitary-ovarian endometrial axis: changes over time. FSH, follicle-stimulating hormone; GnRH, gonadotropin-releasing hormone; LH, luteinizing hormone.

Postovulation, the dominant follicle transforms into a progesterone-secreting corpus luteum. During this phase of the cycle, estradiol inhibits gonadotropin release, preventing the development of another dominant follicle. The corpus luteum sustains progesterone secretion for 14 days; beyond this point, continued progesterone secretion is dependent on β-human chorionic gonadotropin (β-hCG) signaling

from a pregnancy. If no pregnancy occurs, the corpus luteum regresses, and progesterone levels drop.

The endometrium is a mucosal surface lining the uterine cavity. Its thickness and composition are under the influence of estradiol and progesterone. During the preovulatory estradiol-dominant phase, termed the *proliferative phase*, the endometrium rapidly grows. The endometrial lining undergoes glandular differentiation to optimize implantation during the postovulatory progesterone-dominant phase, termed the *secretory phase*. If no pregnancy occurs, the spiral arterioles supplying the endometrium undergo spasm secondary to waning estradiol and progesterone levels. The endometrium becomes ischemic and sheds, producing menstrual bleeding. The amount of menstrual blood directly correlates with the thickness of the endometrium, the activity of the coagulation cascade directing the clotting of the vessels, and the re-exposure to estrogen with the start of the new cycle. Any abnormality in these processes can lead to an abnormal bleeding pattern.

Normal parameters of the menstrual cycle should be understood to correctly identify abnormal patterns of bleeding. The cycle interval describes the number of days between the first day of one period and the first day of the next period. A normal cycle *interval* in adolescents is between 21 and 45 days. The cycle *length* describes the number of days menstrual bleeding lasts. A normal cycle length is conventionally described as less than 7 days. The amount of bleeding is much harder to quantify. Greater than 80 mL of menstrual blood loss during a cycle is considered pathologically heavy, with the average blood loss being 30 mL. The clinical impracticality of obtaining this information is obvious. Menstrual blood flow requiring soaked pad changes every 1–2 hours is conventionally considered to be pathologically heavy.

Information regarding the start of menarche, cycle interval, cycle length, bleeding between menses, and questions detailing the quantity of blood flow is essential in the assessment of abnormal bleeding. The acronym **PALM-COEIN** has been devised to categorize the multiple causes of abnormal uterine bleeding (Table 25.4). The conditions falling under the PALM group describe structural abnormalities and are much less common in the adolescent population than the nonstructural conditions falling under the COEIN group.

TABLE 25.4	**Classification System for Abnormal Bleeding**
PALM	**COIEN**
Polyp	Coagulopathy
Adenomyosis	Ovulation dysfunction
Leiomyoma	Iatrogenic causes
Malignancy	Endometrial causes
	Not otherwise specified

PREGNANCY

Pregnancy evaluation is an important early step in the assessment of abnormal bleeding in the adolescent. Bleeding in pregnancy, particularly in the first trimester, is common and can occur with a normal or an abnormal intrauterine pregnancy or an ectopic pregnancy. Pregnancy-associated bleeding can be light or heavy; similarly, it may be painless or associated with uterine cramping. A thorough history is helpful in understanding the heaviness of the current bleeding episode, determining the date of the last normal menstrual cycle, and assessing sexual and contraceptive activity. Physical examination can be helpful if the patient is beyond the first trimester as the uterus may be palpable on abdominal examination. A pelvic examination to assess the size of the uterus is helpful in the first trimester but may not be appropriate for all adolescent patients. If a pregnancy is diagnosed by urine β-hCG testing, the viability of the pregnancy may be determined with ultrasound or serial β-hCG measurements 48 hours apart early in pregnancy. The threshold minimum rise expected depends on the starting β-hCG level: at least 33% if the level is >3,000 mIU/mL to 49% if the level is <1,500 mIU/mL. Dropping or plateauing levels in early pregnancy are typically diagnostic of an abnormal intrauterine or ectopic pregnancy. Early assessment is essential due to the morbidity associated with a delayed diagnosis of an abnormal pregnancy.

COAGULOPATHY

The prevalence of bleeding dyscrasias in the general population is estimated to be 1–2%. Among adolescents with heavy menstrual bleeding the prevalence is approximately 20%. Bleeding dyscrasias, particularly platelet dysfunction and thrombocytopenia, are associated with heavy and prolonged menstrual bleeding. In the adolescent population, menstrual cycles consistently lasting more than 7 days with a gushing sensation or requiring soaked pad changes more frequently than every 2 hours, documented anemia, family history of bleeding disorder or tooth extraction, and delivery or miscarriage associated with excessive bleeding should raise concern for a bleeding dyscrasia. Capturing information related to the cycle length, saturation of pads and frequency of change, frequency of menstrual blood leakage onto clothing, and number of school days or social activities missed is effective in assessing heavy bleeding in the adolescent. Additionally, patients who report easy bruising, gingival bleeding, or frequent epistaxis should raise suspicion for a platelet function defect. A reasonable basic approach to testing involves evaluating the platelet count, prothrombin time/international normalized ratio and partial thromboplastin time, and von Willebrand disease panel. Hematology referral is advisable in patients with severe, heavy, and prolonged bleeding and for those patients whose bleeding is not controlled with standard hormone therapy. Although not as common as platelet function disorders, coagulation factor deficiencies may also present with heavy uterine bleeding during adolescence.

OVULATORY DYSFUNCTION

The complex feedback relationship between estrogen and the anterior pituitary is the last part of the menstrual cycle to mature. Before positive feedback is established, FSH may actually decrease with rising estrogen levels. This stunts dominant follicle development and ovulation does not occur. Without ovulation, the corpus luteum does not develop; consequently, progesterone secretion from the ovary is limited. The endometrial lining is unstable without progesterone influence, leading to an abnormal bleeding pattern. This scenario is often termed *immaturity of the HPO axis*. The associated **anovulatory bleeding** pattern can present as frequent, absent, or heavy uterine bleeding. The abnormal bleeding associated with HPO immaturity is typically seen within the first 3 years of menarche. While this is the most common cause of irregular bleeding in early adolescence, other causes should be considered because immaturity of the HPO axis is a diagnosis of exclusion.

Polycystic ovary syndrome (PCOS) is a complex endocrinopathy that is likely the result of a heterogeneous combination of influences including genetics, the intra- and extrauterine environment, insulin resistance, steroid hormone metabolism, and other metabolic abnormalities. The presenting clinical pattern can include hyperandrogenemia causing hirsutism and acne; infrequent or absent ovulation leading to amenorrhea, oligomenorrhea, and subfertility; polycystic ovaries on ultrasound; and eventual development of metabolic syndrome (obesity, type 2 diabetes, hypertension). The bleeding pattern most commonly associated with PCOS is infrequent or absent menses, although prolonged and heavy bleeding may occur. Diagnosis of PCOS typically relies on a variable presentation of three key features: hyperandrogenism, oligomenorrhea, and polycystic-appearing ovaries (Table 25.5). However, the hormonal changes and physical symptoms associated with PCOS overlap greatly with early adolescence, making the evaluation particularly difficult in this age group. PCOS diagnosis during adolescence is less focused on ovarian ultrasonography as polycystic-appearing ovaries are present in up to 40% of adolescents. Laboratory evaluation of androgen levels can also be problematic as assays vary in sensitivity and normative levels are not perfectly established. Anti–müllerian hormone elevation has also been associated with PCOS, but again, a normative level is not clear. The diagnostic work-up of PCOS also involves the exclusion of mimicking causes such as late-onset (nonclassic) congenital adrenal hyperplasia, androgen-secreting tumors, and Cushing disease. Normal early adolescence should also be considered as a mimicking condition. Therefore, considering this diagnosis within the 2 years of menarche should be done with caution, and only in the case of obvious pathology. Given the association of PCOS with future morbidity, close monitoring and re-evaluation should be considered for adolescents with persistent PCOS symptomatology.

Thyroid dysfunction can lead to an abnormal uterine bleeding pattern by disrupting ovulation. Similar to PCOS, the bleeding pattern most commonly associated with thyroid dysfunction is absent or infrequent menses, but heavy, prolonged bleeding can develop. In this case, severe hypothyroidism leads to significantly elevated levels of thyroid-stimulating hormone. This hormone, also from the anterior pituitary, has FSH-like activity and stimulates the stromal cells of the ovary to produce high levels of estrogen. The disregulated production of estrogen leads to a thickened endometrial lining that eventually outgrows its blood supply, leading to ischemia and shedding. Bleeding is heavy and prolonged because this shedding is asynchronous, and the volume of endometrium is high.

Ovulatory dysfunction often presents as absent menses or amenorrhea. The **amenorrhea presentation** has an extremely wide range of diagnostic possibilities, some of which are associated with significant

TABLE 25.5 Diagnostic Criteria for PCOS

1990 NIH Guidelines

Patient satisfies both criteria:

(1) Clinical or biochemical hyperandrogenism

(2) Oligomenorrhea or oligo-ovulation

Other causes of hyperandrogenism and anovulatory subfertility should be excluded.

2003 ESHRE/ASRM or Rotterdam Guidelines

Patient satisfies two of three criteria:

(1) Oligomenorrhea or oligo-ovulation

(2) Clinical or biochemical hyperandrogenism

(3) Polycystic ovaries on ultrasound

Other causes of hyperandrogenism and anovulatory subfertility should be excluded.

2006 AES Guidelines

Patient satisfies both criteria:

(1) Hyperandrogenism: hirsutism or biochemical hyperandrogenism

(2) Ovarian dysfunction: oligo-anovulation or polycystic ovaries

Other causes of hyperandrogenism and anovulatory subfertility should be excluded.

AES, Androgen Excess Society; ASRM, American Society for Reproductive Medicine; ESHRE, European Society for Human Reproduction and Embryology; NIH, National Institutes of Health; PCOS, polycystic ovary syndrome.
From Rao P, Bhide P. Controversies in the diagnosis of polycystic ovary syndrome. *Ther Adv Reprod Health*. 2020;14:1–11 (Table 1, p. 2).

morbidity and even mortality if not recognized. Significant anatomic abnormalities, male karyotype, tumor of the anterior pituitary gland, significant malnutrition, and premature ovarian insufficiency illustrate the complexity of diagnostic possibilities (Table 25.6).

The first step in accurate diagnosis is determining when amenorrhea is actually pathologic. A work-up for absent menses should be done for adolescents who show no signs of secondary sexual maturation by age 13 or no menses with other sexual characteristics by age 15, or if more than 3 months pass between menstrual cycles. Amenorrhea evaluation can begin at age 14 if hirsutism is noted or low caloric intake is suspected. Starting with a thorough history to identify any risk factors such as known renal anomalies, childhood exposure to chemotherapy or radiation, exercise and nutrition imbalance, galactorrhea, or family history of early menopause is important. A physical examination, including assessment of height, body mass index, acne and hirsutism, Tanner staging of breast and pubic hair development, and confirmation of a patent vagina if appropriate can help to further narrow the diagnostic possibilities. Ultrasound evaluation is a reasonable early test if the patient is not amenable to an examination, particularly if there is high risk of an anatomic abnormality. Laboratory assessment should include a pregnancy test and serum thyroid-stimulating hormone, FSH, and prolactin.

If the thyroid or pregnancy testing is abnormal, the diagnosis is clear. If the prolactin level is elevated and there is no evidence of hypothyroidism, MRI of the anterior pituitary is warranted. Over 50% of the time, an elevated prolactin level is secondary to an anterior pituitary tumor. Other CNS lesions that irritate the pituitary stalk are also associated with elevated prolactin levels. A thorough medication review should also be conducted in the case of hyperprolactinemia as this is a common side effect of antipsychotic medications that competitively bind to dopamine receptors, effectively lowering dopamine activity, leading to an elevation of prolactin secondary to the inhibitory relationship between dopamine and prolactin.

An elevated FSH is associated with complex diagnoses such as premature ovarian insufficiency and gonadal dysgenesis. Immediate karyotype evaluation should be performed with the intent of making an early diagnosis of **Turner syndrome** or **gonadal dysgenesis** involving an XY karyotype. Both of these conditions may be associated with morbidity if early treatment is not initiated. XY karyotype is associated

TABLE 25.6 Characteristics of the Causes of Amenorrhea

	FSH	Karyotype	Family History	Classic Unique Findings
Turner syndrome	Elevated	45,X	Fragile X syndrome for mosaic Turner syndrome	Short stature Webbed neck Lymphedema of hands and feet Low neck hairline
XY gonadal dysgenesis	Elevated	46,XY	No	No secondary sexual development
Hypothalamic amenorrhea	Low or normal	46,XX	No	Low body mass index Poor dentition
Imperforate hymen	Normal	46,XX	No	Pain Bulging hymen
PCOS	Normal	46,XX	Yes	Acne Hirsutism Central obesity
Müllerian anomalies	Normal	46,XX	Possible	Normal breast development Blind vaginal pouch
AIS	Normal	46,XY	No	Normal breast development Scant or no body hair Blind vaginal pouch
Premature ovarian insufficiency	Elevated	46,XX	Yes	Variable presence of secondary sexual characteristics
Kallmann syndrome	Low or normal	46,XX	Yes	Inability to smell Absent secondary sexual characteristics

AIS, androgen insensitivity syndrome; FSH, follicle-stimulating hormone; PCOS, polycystic ovary syndrome.

with malignancy requiring gonadectomy; Turner syndrome is associated with left-sided cardiac abnormalities (bicuspid aortic valve, coarctation of aorta) in 50% of patients. Certainly, emotional support with both individual and family therapy, and referral to a support group, should be considered in patients with elevated FSH as natural fertility is compromised and to support any gender identity concerns that might be raised.

In many cases of amenorrhea, the hormone evaluation and physical examination will be largely normal. Functional hypothalamic amenorrhea, most likely caused by immaturity of the HPO axis, is a diagnosis of exclusion and presents with either normal or low FSH levels. Identification of excessive stress related to either the social environment or a medical condition, sports or exercise activity not supported with sufficient calories, physical examination findings confirming poor nutrition based on low body mass index percentile, or poor dentition from frequent vomiting is important to identify. Amenorrhea with anosmia is suspicious for Kallmann syndrome, which is associated with GnRH deficiency. In the case of functional hypothalamic amenorrhea, MRI of the CNS should be considered when the history interview does not produce any suspicion for stress or nutrition abnormalities, and particularly when symptoms such as nausea, headaches, and vision changes are present.

ENDOMETRIAL CAUSES

Infection and inflammation of the endometrium can lead to an abnormal uterine bleeding pattern. The bleeding pattern can range from light, intermenstrual bleeding to prolonged menstrual bleeding. Infection of the upper genital tract, pelvic inflammatory disease (PID), is a common diagnosis in adolescents and is directly linked to the high prevalence of gonorrhea and chlamydia infections in this population. Treating gonorrhea and chlamydia infections of the lower genital tract has been shown to reduce the risk of PID, which has clinical implications much more severe than abnormal bleeding. Testing for gonorrhea and chlamydia infections is recommended at least annually in sexually active women 25 years of age or younger, regardless of symptoms. Nucleic acid amplification test (NAAT) is the most sensitive and clinically useful as testing can be done on urine specimens and vaginal swabs as well as endocervical specimens. An infectious source of bleeding should be considered when evaluating a sexually active teenager.

IATROGENIC CAUSES

The most common group of medications that lead to abnormal uterine bleeding prescribed to adolescents is hormonal contraceptives. Iatrogenic bleeding is typically described as prolonged or intermenstrual and is rarely heavy, and it is often referred to as **breakthrough bleeding**. Combination contraceptives (pills, transvaginal ring, and transdermal patch) are designed to provide 21 days of hormones for the purpose of blocking ovulation and 7 days of placebo triggering the endometrium to shed, leading to a menstrual cycle. If pills are missed, or if the transdermal patch or ring is left in place longer than prescribed or removed too early, endometrial bleeding will be triggered. In some cases, breakthrough bleeding may occur even if the contraceptive method is being used correctly. Some follicular development has been described particularly with the very low-dosage ethinyl estradiol contraceptive pills. While this is not associated with lower contraceptive efficacy, it may be associated with more ovarian cyst development and irregular bleeding. All progestin-only contraceptive methods are associated with breakthrough bleeding. The majority of women using progesterone-only contraception report abnormal bleeding patterns after 1 year of use; however, the longer these methods are used, the more acceptable the bleeding pattern becomes. The actual mechanism causing breakthrough bleeding when using progesterone-only contraception is not clear; endometrial evaluation shows abnormal, enlarged, thin-walled fragile blood vessels. Both the progestin-releasing and the nonhormonal intrauterine device (IUD) can be associated with an abnormal bleeding pattern after initial insertion. This abnormal bleeding pattern typically improves over time. The majority of hormonal IUD users ultimately experience a decrease in monthly menstrual bleeding, while the majority of nonhormonal IUD users report no change from their preinsertion menstrual pattern after 1 year of use.

Abnormal bleeding in adolescents can be associated with non-hormonal medications as well. Anticoagulation medications can lead to a heavy and prolonged bleeding pattern, especially when supratherapeutic anticoagulation occurs. In some cases, the bleeding associated with anticoagulation is quite heavy and requires acute, aggressive therapy to prevent significant anemia. A strategy to avoid heavy menstrual bleeding from anticoagulation is to start a safe hormonal contraceptive method associated with reducing menstrual blood loss.

NOT YET CLASSIFIED

Persistent abnormal bleeding sometimes requires multiple evaluations over time to identify the cause. In many cases, the initial evaluation, even when complete, may not identify the abnormality. PCOS is a good example of a condition that evolves over time and sometimes requires multiple evaluations to confirm. If the bleeding pattern is causing anemia or significant quality-of-life disruption, treatment should not be withheld simply because a clear diagnosis has not been established.

STRUCTURAL CAUSES: PALM

The structural causes of abnormal bleeding are much less common in the adolescent population. Gynecologic malignancy and hyperplasia in adolescence are rare conditions. In the case of the rare vaginal or cervical malignancy, the abnormal bleeding is typically prolonged or intermenstrual; endometrial malignancies and uterine sarcomas, also exceedingly rare, typically present with heavier bleeding. **Ovarian germ cell** tumors are the most common gynecologic malignancy during adolescence, most commonly presenting in the 15- to 19-year age group. Abnormal uterine bleeding is not a common presenting symptom of germ cell tumors. However, malignant stromal cell tumors of the ovary, specifically juvenile granulosa cell tumors, classically present with heavy and prolonged uterine bleeding. Ultrasound evaluation should be immediately performed if an adolescent presents with abnormal uterine bleeding and an abdominal mass.

In addition to malignancy, ultrasound evaluation is effective in diagnosing leiomyomas (fibroids) and polyps. Both represent a benign overgrowth of uterine tissue and, again, are extremely uncommon in the adolescent population. A **leiomyoma** is a smooth muscle tumor of the myometrium that loses growth regulation and often presents with heavy and prolonged uterine bleeding. A **polyp** is typically an overgrowth of the endometrium or the endocervix and classically presents as intermenstrual bleeding. This structural abnormality is not well reported in the adolescent population. **Adenomyosis** is another abnormality where islands of endometrial tissue are embedded in the myometrium of the uterus. While this condition is rare in the adolescent population, it typically presents with heavy and prolonged bleeding, similar to a leiomyoma. Adenomyosis is also a benign condition, but unlike leiomyoma, the sensitivity of ultrasound diagnosis is low; MRI is more sensitive and reliable for diagnosis.

CONGENITAL ANOMALIES

Müllerian anomalies are another important structural cause of abnormal bleeding. The müllerian ducts, embryonically called the paramesonephric ducts, appear 37 days postfertilization and undergo a process of differentiation, migration, fusion, and canalization to become the fallopian tubes, uterus, cervix, and upper vagina. Müllerian anomalies result from abnormalities in differentiation (agenesis), fusion (uterine didelphys, vaginal septum), and canalization (uterine septum). Absent menstrual bleeding is the most common abnormal bleeding pattern associated with müllerian anomalies, although most anomalies, such as bicornuate, didelphys, and septate uterus, do not result in abnormal bleeding. Anomalies presenting with amenorrhea are associated with an absence of the vagina, uterus, and/or cervix or a complete obstruction such as a transverse vaginal septum.

Anomalies involving a transverse vaginal septum are actually quite rare and may present with prolonged irregular bleeding as well as with amenorrhea. If spontaneous perforation of the vaginal septum occurs, a prolonged, irregular bleeding pattern is produced. Similarly, an obstructed hemivagina that spontaneously ruptures may lead to a similar bleeding pattern. This müllerian anomaly describes uterine didelphys and bicollis with a partial vaginal septum obstructing the outflow of one of the müllerian tracts. A pelvic ultrasound is a good first step when evaluating for a suspected upper genital tract abnormality. MRI is the best imaging modality for confirmation.

A simple external genital examination should always be done during the evaluation of amenorrhea as imperforate hymen, a structural anomaly much more common than müllerian anomalies, is easily diagnosed by inspection. An imperforate hymen is the complete obstruction by the hymenal membrane at the level of the vaginal introitus preventing the passage of menstrual bleeding. Pain is a key complaint. Diagnosis by examination is reliable as the hymenal tissue is often bulging from the pressure resulting from the hematocolpos. In this case, a simple surgical procedure to remove the redundant hymen can be done to achieve normal anatomy. If a patient presents with a bulge at the introitus, pain, and regular menses, you should be suspicious of obstructed hemivagina and can confirm this diagnosis by attempting to pass a lubricated Q-tip into the vaginal canal. Diagnosis of müllerian anomaly warrants imaging of kidneys, as renal anomaly or agenesis is common in these patients.

Mayer-Rokitansky-Küster-Hauser (MRKH) syndrome and androgen insensitivity syndrome (AIS) are two other diagnostic possibilities that present with absent vagina and amenorrhea. In both of these conditions, the müllerian structures are absent and both external genitalia and breast development are consistent with a female phenotype. Karyotype and testosterone level differentiate the two disorders, as MRKH individuals are 46,XX with serum testosterone in the female range, whereas AIS individuals are 46,XY with testosterone levels in the male range. In AIS, the absent androgen activity leads to female external genitalia development and limited body hair, as well as no wolffian structure development. Peripheral conversion of androgens to estrogens leads to estrogenization, specifically breast development, during puberty. The gonads are at risk for malignancy and removal after achievement of adult height is recommended. After gonadectomy, estrogen replacement is needed until natural age of menopause is reached for optimal health. AIS is significantly less common than MRKH (2–5/100,000 vs 4/1,500) and is associated with an X-linked recessive inheritance pattern, whereas MRKH appears to be more sporadic. Of note, individuals with gonadal dysgenesis and a Y chromosome present with amenorrhea and female external genitalia, but unlike AIS breast development

TABLE 25.7	**Contraindications to Estrogen Therapy**
Poorly controlled hypertension, or coexisting vascular disease
Current/history of ischemic heart disease
Liver dysfunction: severe cirrhosis, adenoma, hepatocellular carcinoma
History of venous thromboembolism/known thrombophilia
Complicated valvular heart disease
Migraine with aura
Active cancer or within 6 mo of treatment
<6 mo since diagnosis of peripartum cardiomyopathy
Diabetes with vascular complication
Major surgery with prolonged immobilization
Moderate to severe impairment of cardiac function
Solid organ transplant complicated by graft failure, rejection, cardiac allograft vasculopathy

is minimal and testosterone levels are low. As previously mentioned, gonadectomy should not be delayed in these individuals as the risk of malignancy is higher than in AIS.

TREATMENT

Progestins alone, or in combination with estradiol, are the most effective medical therapy to treat abnormal bleeding in adolescents. Hormones should be considered first-line therapy even when managing adolescents with bleeding dyscrasias or structural abnormalities such as adenomyosis or leiomyomas. When given cyclically, especially in the combination contraceptive formulation, bleeding becomes regular and light. If progestin-only therapy is given continuously, menstrual bleeding may be suppressed, although breakthrough bleeding, as described previously, can occur.

Selecting the best method for abnormal bleeding management should first focus on safety considerations, particularly if an estrogen-containing treatment is selected. Contraindications to estrogen therapy are listed in Table 25.7. Teenagers that smoke should be counseled to quit smoking. After a determination of safety is made, a detailed discussion should be held to determine any potential compliance concerns as improper use of hormone therapy can lead to irregular bleeding and ultimately treatment failure.

Antifibrinolytics, specifically tranexamic acid, are effective nonhormonal medications that can be considered for those adolescents who are not comfortable taking hormonal medications or who have significant contraindications or side effects to hormone therapy. These medications can also be used adjunctively with hormone therapy if bleeding control is suboptimal, but the risk for venous thromboembolism should be discussed with the patient. A platelet transfusion, factor replacement, desmopressin, intravenous immune globulin, or oral corticosteroids may be appropriate adjunctive therapy depending on the etiology. Hormone therapy is effective in controlling bleeding secondary to all of these conditions and should be concurrently administered. In the rare case of a malignancy, polyp, or resectable partial anatomic blockage, surgical management is required.

If abnormal uterine bleeding is profound, producing significant anemia, hormonal therapy remains the mainstay of medical treatment, but with different dosing regimens (Table 25.8). Both estrogens and progestins alone or in combination are effective. High-dose progestin therapy leads to endometrial atrophy. High-dose estradiol therapy is effective by inducing endometrial vascular vasospasm, regenerating denuded epithelium, and increasing clotting factors. Both intravenous and oral high-dose estradiol preparations are available and the

TABLE 25.8 Hormone Treatment Regimens for Acute Heavy Bleeding

IV Estrogen	Combination Oral Contraceptives	Oral Progesterone
Conjugated estrogen 25 mg every 4–6 hr	30–50 μg of ethinyl estradiol–containing tablets every 4–8 hr Taper dosage over several days when bleeding subsides	Medroxyprogesterone 10–20 mg orally b.i.d. to t.i.d. or Norethindrone 5–10 mg orally b.i.d.

b.i.d., two times a day; IV, intravenous; t.i.d., three times a day.

intravenous route may be preferable in patients who are unable to tolerate oral medication secondary to nausea. Regardless of which high-dose hormone regimen is used, once cessation of bleeding has been achieved, transitioning to a progestin-dominant therapy is imperative. If this is not done, sudden stoppage of the high dosage of hormone therapy will lead to withdrawal bleeding. Specific factor replacement, particularly factor VII replacement, may also be effective in controlling profound heavy bleeding, regardless of the cause.

GnRH agonist therapy is another option to acutely control heavy uterine bleeding. The mechanism of action involves decreased expression of GnRH receptors of the anterior pituitary secondary to receptor saturation, which leads to decreasing sex hormone production from the ovaries. This medication should be used with caution as a flare in bleeding may initially occur. Traditional dosing involves an intramuscular injection of either 11.25 mg given at 3-month intervals or monthly dosing of 3.75 mg. GnRH agonist therapy is limited to 12 months of use secondary to the significant lowering of bone mineral density as a result of decreased circulating ovarian estrogens. Vasomotor symptoms are also a common side effect of decreased estrogens; treatment with low-dose progestins or estradiol is typically effective in relieving symptoms.

Management of acute bleeding may require surgical therapy in addition to medical therapy. Placement of a Foley balloon into the endometrium filled with 30 mL of saline can effectively tamponade the bleeding endometrium and reduce the blood supply to the uterus by partially compressing the uterine arteries. The balloon is deflated gradually over 12–24 hours while hormone therapy is ongoing. A dilation and curettage is often performed with Foley balloon placement. This procedure leads to endometrial thinning and can be effective in controlling heavy bleeding on its own, particularly if imaging suggests the presence of a clot in the endometrial cavity. Importantly, in cases of bleeding related to a dyscrasia, the sharp dilation and curettage procedure can increase blood loss. The final two surgical options, uterine artery embolization and hysterectomy, impair fertility and should be reserved as a last resort in life-threatening situations.

MENSTRUAL PAIN IN ADOLESCENTS

Dysmenorrhea, defined as pain during the menstrual cycle, is the most common reason adolescent patients seek gynecologic care. Pain is most commonly in the pelvis secondary to uterine cramping but can also be reported in the back and upper thighs. Sixty to 70% of adolescents report pain during menses, and 15% report significant quality-of-life dysfunction leading to a disruption of normal activities. Dysmenorrhea is associated with ovulatory cycles; therefore, this symptom typically presents in the later adolescent years. Dysmenorrhea, unlike chronic pelvic pain, presents with cyclic pain beginning within 48 hours of the

first day of the menstrual cycle and resolves by menstrual cycle day 2 or 3. Primary dysmenorrhea is significantly more common in adolescents. In this condition, high levels of prostaglandin E_2 and $F_{2\alpha}$, produced by the endometrium, cause painful uterine cramping. Secondary dysmenorrhea is the result of an anatomic abnormality causing uterine cramping. About 10% of adolescents with menstrual pain have secondary dysmenorrhea.

If the physical examination is normal and there are no factors in the medical history raising suspicion for an anatomic abnormality, empirical treatment without laboratory or radiologic evaluation is a reasonable approach. Nonsteroidal antiinflammatory drugs (NSAIDs) are effective therapy as prostaglandin production is directly reduced. This therapy is most effective when started 24–48 hours prior to the onset of pain. Contraceptive agents that block ovulation and limit the growth of the endometrial lining lead to a decrease in prostaglandin production and therefore are also effective in treating dysmenorrhea. Although NSAIDs are traditionally considered first-line therapy for primary dysmenorrhea, starting a contraceptive agent without an NSAID trial is acceptable given the inherent administration difficulty associated with proper NSAID use. Warm baths, heating pads, and exercise may be helpful adjunctive therapies. Nontraditional therapies such as vitamin E, magnesium supplementation, acupuncture, transcutaneous electrical nerve stimulation, and dietary supplements are not well studied.

If menses are reported to be painful, and if there is some persistence of pain between cycles, or if empirical therapy for primary dysmenorrhea is unsuccessful after 3–6 months of treatment, a diagnosis of secondary dysmenorrhea should be considered. Uterine leiomyomas, adenomyosis, and outflow tract abnormalities that block the egress of menstrual blood can cause significant pain during menses and discomfort between menstrual cycles. The most common cause of **secondary dysmenorrhea** during adolescence is **endometriosis.** The prevalence of endometriosis in the adolescent population has not been established, but 60% of adult women with endometriosis report symptoms prior to age 20, and approximately 66% of adolescents undergoing laparoscopy for pain are found to have endometriosis. Confirmation of endometriosis is challenging as no blood test or imaging study is diagnostic. Laparoscopic surgical evaluation of the pelvis can be helpful, but the lesions are often subtle and heterogeneous in appearance and consequently can be missed. The hormonal therapies effective in treating primary dysmenorrhea are also effective in the treatment of secondary dysmenorrhea, with the exception of outflow tract obstruction abnormalities, which always require surgical management. The levonorgestrel IUD has been particularly effective in controlling symptoms of endometriosis and leiomyomas.

While dysmenorrhea is a common premenstrual symptom, it is a different entity than **premenstrual syndrome (PMS)**. The basic diagnostic strategy for PMS involves confirming the presence of at least one somatic complaint (breast tenderness, abdominal bloating, headache, or swelling of extremities) and one affective complaint (depression, angry outbursts, irritability, anxiety, confusion, or social withdrawal) during the 5 days preceding menses for three consecutive menstrual cycles. The symptoms must be resolved by the fourth day of the menses and should not recur until at least 13 days have passed from cycle day 1 of the last menses. For diagnostic purposes, these symptoms should also negatively impact social or school participation.

Premenstrual dysphoric disorder (PMDD) is often grouped with PMS, but the diagnostic criteria differ. The American Psychiatric Association requires at least five of the following symptoms: marked depressed mood, marked anxiety, marked emotional lability, persistent and marked anger, decreased interest in usual activities, difficulty concentrating, lethargy, marked change in appetite, sleep disturbance, loss of control sensation, and physical symptoms of breast tenderness, swelling, headaches, joint pain, muscle pain, bloating, or weight gain. For diagnosis, the symptoms must interfere with activities and relationships, and the symptoms cannot be an exacerbation of a mood or personality disorder. These criteria must be confirmed by daily prospective ratings over two consecutive cycles. The pathophysiology of PMS and PMDD has been linked to the fluctuation of ovarian sex steroid hormones after ovulation. While no difference in hormonal levels have been confirmed in women with PMS/PMDD compared to those that do not have these conditions, there may be a different serotonin activity or γ-aminobutyric receptor activity response to the hormone fluctuations during the luteal phase.

Treatment options include hormonal suppression of ovulation to prevent the luteal phase fluctuation of hormones. Hormonal agents containing the fourth-generation progestin drospirenone have been effective in controlling affective and somatic symptoms. The possible small increased risk of venous thromboembolic events associated with this particular progestin preparation warrants a careful risk-benefit analysis. NSAIDs and spironolactone have been shown to be helpful in the alleviation of the physical symptoms. Selective serotonin reuptake inhibitors (SSRIs) are a first-line treatment option in adult women with severe PMS and PMDD as improvement in both somatic and affective symptoms has been documented. However, the efficacy of these medications in adolescents with PMS/PMDD is unclear, and the association of these medications with increased suicidality has blunted widespread use. Nonpharmacologic therapies that have been utilized include exercise; stress management; heat therapy; cognitive-behavioral therapy; education about the syndrome; supplementation with calcium, magnesium, vitamin B_6, and vitamin E; and chasteberry, ginkgo biloba, and St. John's wort herbal remedies. Data supporting these therapies are promising but limited for conclusions of efficacy. Red flags include a mass, extragenital bleeding, anemia, a positive family history, and the possibility of an abnormal pregnancy.

SUMMARY AND RED FLAGS

Menstrual concerns and abnormal bleeding are common complaints in childhood and adolescence with a wide range of diagnostic possibilities. A thorough history and physical examination help to quickly identify the more likely underlying causes, narrowing the laboratory and imaging evaluation that may be needed to efficiently make an accurate diagnosis. Red flags in the evaluation of vaginal bleeding include prolonged bleeding, nongynecologic bleeding, headache, visual disturbances, galactorrhea, abnormal or pelvic mass, anemia, or fevers. For the vast majority of adolescents presenting with menstrual concerns, treatment can be initiated with limited evaluation secondary to the likelihood of the underlying cause being a benign, transient process. Abnormal bleeding in childhood typically warrants more of a diagnostic work-up, although most often the underlying cause is also benign.

BIBLIOGRAPHY

A bibliography is available at ExpertConsult.com.

26

Disorders of Sex Development

Patricia A. Donohoue

The term *disorders of sex development (DSD)* replaces the former terms *intersex* and *hermaphroditism* (Table 26.1). The most common presenting symptom of DSD is **atypical (ambiguous) genitalia** at birth. Other presenting signs and symptoms include lack of some or all aspects of pubertal development, postnatal virilization of a phenotypic female, or infertility. The classification of DSD is based on broad categories related to blood sex chromosome composition and gonadal structure. These categories include 46,XX DSD, 46,XY DSD, ovotesticular DSD, and sex chromosome DSD (Table 26.2).

The terms *atypical* or *ambiguous genitalia,* in a broad sense, refer to any case in which the external genitalia do not appear completely male or completely female. Although there are standards for genital size dimensions, variations in size of these structures do not always constitute ambiguity.

Development of the external genitalia begins with the potential to be either male or female (Fig. 26.1 and Table 26.3). Virilization of a female, the most common form of DSD, results in varying phenotypes (Fig. 26.2) that develop from the basic bipotential genital appearances of the embryo (see Fig. 26.1). Degrees of virilization at birth are often classified using the **Prader stages** (Fig. 26.3).

OVERVIEW OF SEX DIFFERENTIATION

In typical differentiation from the sexually undifferentiated early fetus, the final phenotype of the external and internal genitalia is consistent with a normal sex chromosome complement (either XX or XY). The process of sex differentiation and development follows a consistent timeline (Fig. 26.4). A 46,XX complement of chromosomes as well as genetic factors, including DAX1, the signaling molecule WNT-4, CTNNB1, and R-spondin 1, are among the many factors needed for the development of normal ovaries and müllerian (paramesonephric) ducts (uterus, fallopian tubes, and upper vagina). Development of the male phenotype requires the product of a Y chromosome gene called *SRY* (Sex-determining Region on the Y chromosome), which, in concert with products of other genes such as *SOX9, SF1, WT1,* and *FGF9,* directs the undifferentiated gonad to become a testis. SRY acts as a transcriptional regulator to increase cellular proliferation, attract interstitial cells from adjacent mesonephros into the genital ridge, and stimulate testicular Sertoli cell differentiation. Sertoli cells act as an organizer of steroidogenic and germ cell lines and produce antimüllerian hormone that causes the female (paramesonephric) duct system to regress. Aberrant genetic recombinations may result in X chromosomes carrying *SRY,* resulting in XX males (46,XX testicular DSD), or Y chromosomes that have lost *SRY,* resulting in XY females (46,XY DSD due to gonadal dysgenesis). Epigenetic causes of abnormal sex differentiation have been shown in plants, invertebrates, and vertebrates and will likely be shown to contribute to human DSD as well.

Antimüllerian hormone (AMH) from the ipsilateral fetal testis causes the müllerian (paramesonephric) ducts to regress. In its absence, they persist as the uterus, fallopian tubes, cervix, and upper vagina. By about 8 weeks of gestation, the Leydig cells of the testis begin to produce testosterone. During this critical period of male differentiation, testosterone secretion is stimulated by placental human chorionic gonadotropin (hCG), which peaks at 8–12 weeks. In the latter half of pregnancy, lower levels of testosterone are maintained by luteinizing hormone (LH) secreted by the fetal pituitary. **Testosterone** produced locally initiates development of the ipsilateral wolffian (mesonephric) duct into the epididymis, vas deferens, and seminal vesicle. Development of the external genitalia also requires **dihydrotestosterone (DHT)**, the more active metabolite of testosterone. DHT is produced largely from circulating testosterone and is necessary for fusion of the genital folds to form the penis and scrotum. DHT is also produced via an alternative biosynthetic pathway from androstanediol, and this pathway must also be intact for normal and complete prenatal virilization to occur. A functional **androgen receptor**, produced by an X-linked gene, is required for testosterone and DHT to produce the androgen effects.

In the XX fetus with normal long and short arms of the X chromosomes, the bipotential gonad develops into an ovary by about the 10th–11th week. This occurs only in the absence of *SRY,* testosterone, and AMH and requires a normal gene in the DSS (Dosage Sensitive Sex reversal) locus of DAX1 (DSS Adrenal hypoplasia congenital region on X, also known as NROB1), WNT-4, and R-spondin 1. A female external phenotype will develop even in the absence of fetal gonads. Unlike development of the male external phenotype, which requires androgen production and its action, estrogen is unnecessary for normal female prenatal sex differentiation. This is demonstrated by 46,XX patients who lack estrogen due to a deficiency of aromatase, the enzyme required for conversion of androgen to estrogen. Development of the ovary was once thought to be a passive process in the absence of SRY. Although the morphologic changes in the developing ovary are less marked than in the testis, there are a number of sequentially expressed genes and pathways that are required for complete ovarian development as well as maintenance of ovarian integrity postnatally. One of these genes is R-spondin 1, which, if variants result in abnormal function, can result in testicular or ovotesticular development in 46,XX individuals. Once developed, the ovary requires FAX12 to preserve its differentiation and stability.

Several genes important to the pathoetiology of DSD are listed in Table 26.4.

OVERVIEW OF GONADAL FUNCTION

Testes

Levels of placental hCG peak at 8–12 weeks of gestation, and in males hCG stimulates the fetal Leydig cells to secrete testosterone, the main hormonal product of the testis. In the classical androgen biosynthetic

TABLE 26.1 Revised Nomenclature

Previous	Currently Accepted
Intersex	Disorders of sex development (DSD)
Male pseudohermaphrodite	46,XY DSD
Undervirilization of an XY male	46,XY DSD
Undermasculinization of an XY male	46,XY DSD
46,XY intersex	46,XY DSD
Female pseudohermaphrodite	46,XX DSD
Overvirilization of an XX female	46,XX DSD
Masculinization of an XX female	46,XX DSD
46,XX intersex	46,XX DSD
True hermaphrodite	Ovotesticular DSD
Gonadal intersex	Ovotesticular DSD
XX male or XX sex reversal	46,XX testicular DSD
XY sex reversal	46,XY complete gonadal dysgenesis

From Lee PA, Houk CP, Ahmed SF, et al. Consensus statement on management of intersex disorders. *Pediatrics.* 2006;118:e488–e500.

pathway (Fig. 26.5), testosterone is then converted by the enzyme 5α-reductase to its more potent metabolite, DHT. This early period is critical for virilization of the XY fetus including fusion of the midline to form the scrotum and extension of the urethral meatus to distal penile opening (see Fig. 26.1). Defects in this process lead to various deviations from typical male development. After virilization, fetal levels of testosterone decrease but are maintained at lower levels in the latter half of pregnancy by LH secreted by the fetal pituitary. This LH-mediated testosterone secretion is required for continued penile growth and, to some degree, for testicular descent.

As part of the normal transition from intrauterine to extrauterine life, perhaps related to the sudden withdrawal of maternal and placental hormones, newborns and young infants experience a transient surge of gonadotropins and sex steroids. This is the so-called *minipuberty.*

In males, LH and testosterone peak at 1–2 months of age and then decline to reach prepubertal levels by 4–6 months of age. Follicle-stimulating hormone (FSH), along with inhibin B, peaks at 3 months and declines to prepubertal levels by 9 and 15 months, respectively. The LH rise is more dominant than that of FSH.

The neonatal surge may be important for postnatal maturation of the gonads, for stabilization of male external genitalia, and perhaps

TABLE 26.2 Etiologic Classification of Disorders of Sex Development

46,XX Disorders of Sex Development (DSD)

Androgen Exposure

Fetal/Fetoplacental Source

Congenital adrenal hyperplasia
  21-Hydroxylase (CYP21A2) deficiency
  11β-Hydroxylase (CYP11B1) deficiency
  3β-Hydroxysteroid dehydrogenase II (HSD3B2) deficiency
Cytochrome P450 oxidoreductase (POR)
Aromatase (CYP19) deficiency
Glucocorticoid receptor gene pathogenic variant

Maternal Source

Virilizing ovarian tumor
Virilizing adrenal tumor
Androgenic drugs

Disorders of Ovarian Development

XX gonadal dysgenesis

Testicular DSD

Undetermined Origin/Associated with Genitourinary and Gastrointestinal Tract Defects

Cloacal exstrophy

MURCS association

Mayer-Rokitansky-Küster-Hauser syndrome

46,XY DSD

Defects in Testicular Development

WT-1 defects
  Denys-Drash syndrome
  Frasier syndrome
  WAGR syndrome

Campomelic syndrome and SOX9 pathogenic variant

SF1 pathogenic variant

Variants in SRY gene (XY pure gonadal dysgenesis, Swyer syndrome)

XY gonadal agenesis (embryonic testicular regression syndrome)

Deficiency of Testicular Hormone Production

Leydig cell aplasia/hypoplasia
  Variants in luteinizing hormone receptor

Congenital adrenal hyperplasia
  Lipoid adrenal hyperplasia (CYP11A1) deficiency; pathogenic variant in StAR (steroidogenic acute regulatory protein)
  3β-Hydroxysteroid dehydrogenase type II (HSD3B2) deficiency
  17-Hydroxylase/17,20-lyase (CYP17A1) deficiency

17β-Hydroxysteroid dehydrogenase (17β-HSD) or 17-ketosteroid reductase deficiency

Smith-Lemli-Opitz syndrome (defect in conversion of 7-dehydrocholesterol to cholesterol [DHCR7])

Persistent Müllerian Duct Syndrome Due to Antimüllerian Hormone Gene Variants, or Receptor Defects for Antimüllerian Hormone

Defect in Androgen Action

Dihydrotestosterone (DHT) deficiency
  5α-Reductase II (SDR5A2) pathogenic variants
  3α-Reductase (AKR1C2/AKR1C4) pathogenic variants

Androgen receptor defects
  Complete androgen insensitivity syndrome (CAIS)
  Partial androgen insensitivity syndrome (PAIS)

Undetermined Causes, Including Those Associated with Other Congenital Defects

Ovotesticular DSD
XX
XY
XX/XY chimeras

Sex Chromosome DSD
45,X (Turner syndrome and variants)
47,XXY (Klinefelter syndrome and variants)
45,X/46,XY (mixed gonadal dysgenesis, sometimes a cause of ovotesticular DSD)
46,XX/46,XY (chimeric, sometimes a cause of ovotesticular DSD)

From Lee PA, Houk CP, Ahmed SF, et al. Consensus statement on management of intersex disorders. *Pediatrics.* 2006;118:e488–e500.

Sexual appearance of fetus at second to third month of pregnancy

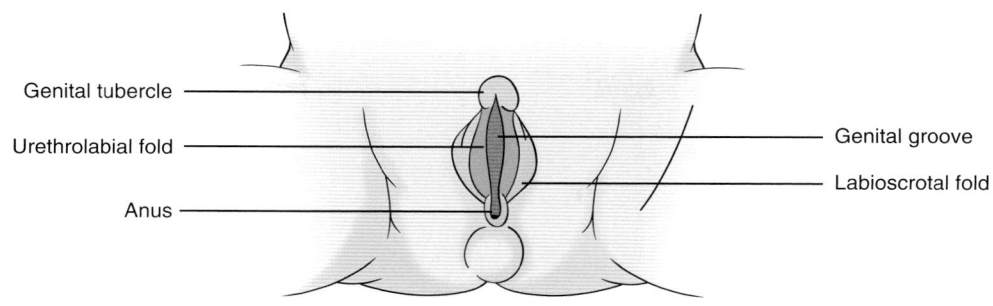

Sexual appearance of fetus at third to fourth month of pregnancy

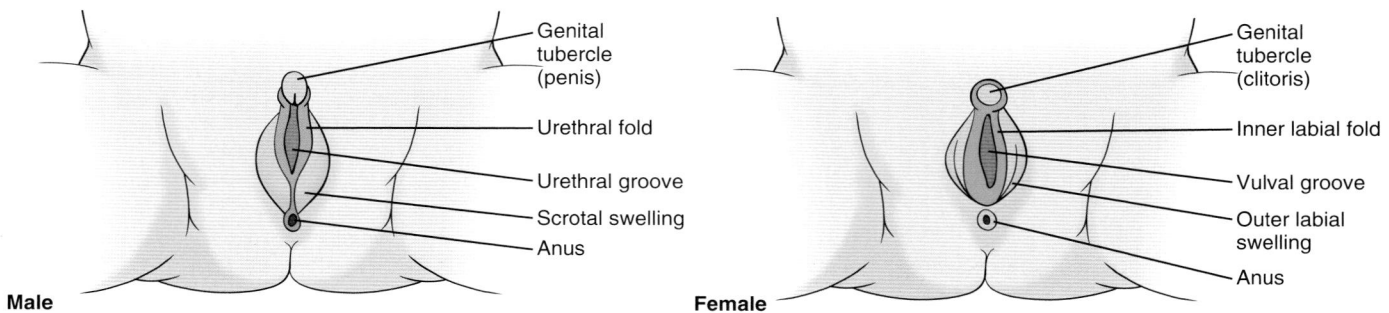

Sexual appearance of fetus at time of birth

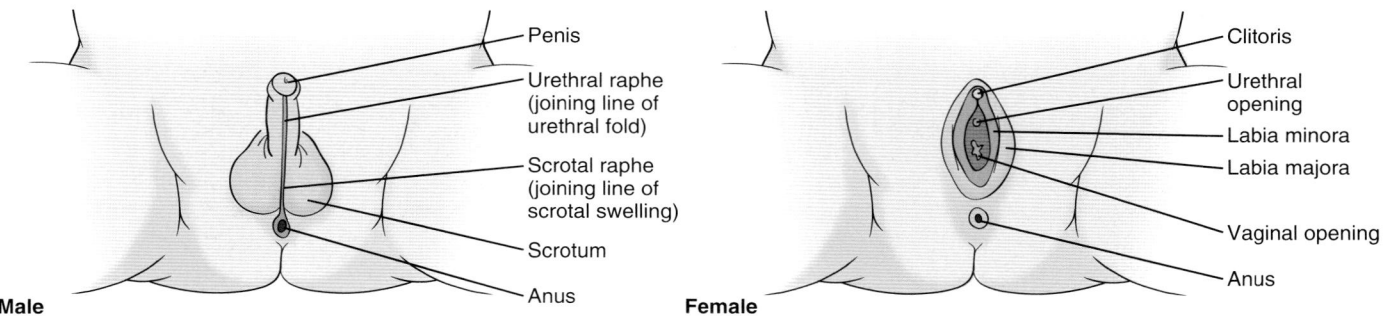

Fig. 26.1 Schematic illustration of differentiation of normal male and female genitalia during embryogenesis. (From Zitelli BJ, Davis HW. *Atlas of Pediatric Physical Diagnosis.* 4th ed. St Louis: Mosby; 2002:328.)

TABLE 26.3 Embryologic Origins of Female and Male Reproductive Structures		
Precursor	**Female**	**Male**
Undifferentiated bipotential gonad	Ovary	Testis
Internal ducts		
Wolffian (mesonephric)	Involution	Epididymis, vas deferens, seminal vesicles
Müllerian (paramesonephric)	Fallopian tubes, uterus, cervix, upper vagina	Involution, prostatic utricle
Urogenital sinus	Lower vagina, urethra	Urethra
External genitalia		
Genital tubercle	Clitoris	Penile corpora cavernosa
Labioscrotal folds	Labia majora	Scrotum
Labiourethral folds	Labia minora	Penile urethra

also for gender identity and sexual behaviors. The postnatal surge in LH and testosterone is absent or blunted in infants with hypopituitarism, cryptorchidism, and complete androgen insensitivity syndrome (CAIS). The development of nocturnal pulsatile secretion of LH marks the advent of puberty.

AMH, inhibin, and activin are members of the transforming growth factor-β (TGF-β) superfamily of growth factors. AMH is the earliest secreted product of the Sertoli cells of the fetal testis. The AMH receptor is expressed in Sertoli cells. In the female it is present in fetal müllerian duct cells and in granulosa cells (fetal and postnatal). During sex differentiation in males, AMH causes involution of the müllerian ducts. AMH is secreted in males by Sertoli cells during both fetal and postnatal life. In females, it is secreted by ovarian granulosa cells from 36 weeks of gestation to menopause, but at lower levels. The serum concentration of AMH in males is highest at birth, whereas in females it is highest at puberty. After puberty, both sexes have similar serum concentrations of AMH. Its role in postnatal life is not yet fully characterized.

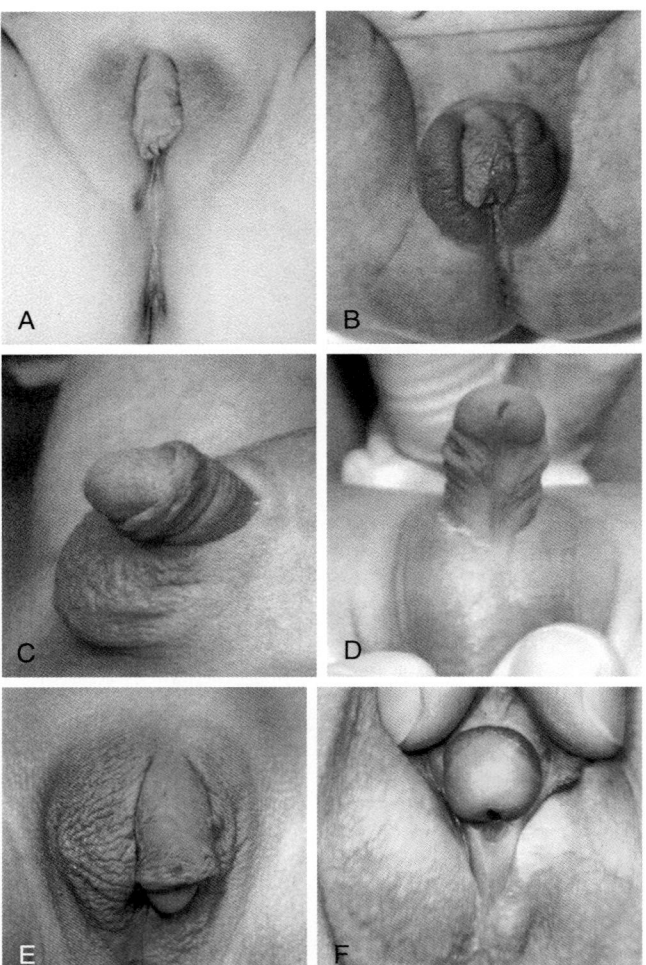

Fig. 26.2 Virilization of external genitalia in 46,XX congenital adrenal hyperplasia (21-hydroxylase deficiency *A–D*). *A,* There is a mild to moderate degree of virilization, with primarily clitoral hypertrophy and significant fusion of the labia. *B,* Virilization is moderate, with clitoromegaly, labial fusion, and rugation of labial folds. *C, D,* Complete masculinization is evident. *E, F,* Asymmetric external genitals with left unilateral descended testis *(E),* penoscrotal hypospadias, and chordee *(F).* Asymmetric external genital development or gonadal descent would be characteristic of mixed gonadal dysgenesis or ovotesticular disorder of sexual development *(E, F).* (From Gleason CA, Juul SE, eds. *Avery's Diseases of the Newborn.* 10th ed. Philadelphia: Elsevier; 2018:1371, Figs. 97.6 and 97.7.)

Inhibin is another glycoprotein hormone secreted by testicular Sertoli cells and ovarian granulosa and theca cells. Inhibin A consists of an α subunit disulfide linked to the β-A subunit, whereas inhibin B consists of the same α subunit linked to the β-B subunit. Activins are dimers of the B subunits, either homodimers (BA/BA, BB/BB) or heterodimers (BA/BB). Inhibins selectively inhibit, whereas activins stimulate pituitary FSH secretion. Inhibin A is absent in males and is present mostly in the luteal phase in women. Inhibin B is the principal form of inhibin in males, and in females during the follicular phase. *Inhibin B is useful as a marker of Sertoli cell function in males.* FSH stimulates inhibin B secretion in females and males, but only in males is there also evidence for gonadotropin-independent regulation. In males with delayed puberty, inhibin B may be a useful screening test to differentiate between constitutional delay of puberty and hypogonadotropic hypogonadism (HH). In HH the serum inhibin B level has been shown to be very low to undetectable.

Like inhibin and activin, follistatin (a single-chain glycosylated protein) is produced by gonads and other tissues such as the hypothalamus, kidney, adrenal gland, and placenta. Follistatin inhibits FSH secretion principally by binding activins, thereby blocking the effects of activins at the level of both the ovary and pituitary.

Many additional peptides act as mediators of the development and function of the testis. They include neurohormones such as growth hormone–releasing hormone, gonadotropin-releasing hormone, corticotropin-releasing hormone, oxytocin, arginine vasopressin, somatostatin, substance P, and neuropeptide Y; growth factors such as insulin-like growth factors (IGFs) and IGF-binding proteins, TGF-β, and fibroblast, platelet-derived, and nerve growth factors; vasoactive peptides; and immune-derived cytokines such as tumor necrosis factor and interleukins IL-1, IL-2, IL-4, and IL-6.

Testicular development is marked by major maturational changes at puberty (see Chapter 55). Clinical patterns of pubertal changes vary widely. In 95% of boys, enlargement of the genitals, which is typically the first sign of puberty, begins between 9.5 and 13.5 years, reaching maturity at 13–17 years. In a minority of normal boys, puberty begins after 15 years of age. In some boys, pubertal development is completed in less than 2 years, but in others it may take longer than 4.5 years. Pubertal development and the adolescent growth spurt occur at an older age in boys than in girls.

The median age of sperm production (spermarche) is 14 years. This event occurs in mid-puberty as judged by pubic hair, testis size, evidence of growth spurt, and testosterone levels. Nighttime levels of FSH are in the adult male range at the time of spermarche; the first conscious ejaculation occurs at about the same time.

Ovaries

In the normal female, the undifferentiated gonad can be identified histologically as an ovary by 10–11 weeks of gestation (see Fig. 26.4), after the upregulation of R-spondin 1. Oocytes are present from the 4th month of gestation and reach a peak of 7 million by 5 months of gestation. For normal maintenance, oocytes need granulosa cells to form primordial follicles. Functional FSH (but not LH) receptors are present in oocytes of primary follicles during follicular development. Two normal X chromosomes are needed for maintenance of oocytes. In contrast to somatic cells, in which only one X chromosome is active, both Xs are active in germ cells. At birth, the ovaries contain about 1 million active follicles, which decrease to 0.5 million by menarche. Thereafter, they decrease at a rate of 1,000/month, and at an even higher rate after the age of 35 years.

The hormones of the fetal ovary are provided mostly by the fetoplacental unit. As in males, peak gonadotropin secretion occurs in fetal life and then again at 2–3 months of life, with the lowest levels at about 6 years of age. In contrast to males, the FSH surge predominates over LH in females. FSH peaks around 3–6 months of age, declines by 12 months, but remains detectable for 24 months. Under LH influence, estradiol peaks at 2–6 months of age. The inhibin B response is variable, peaking at between 2 and 12 months and remaining above prepubertal levels until 24 months. In both infancy and childhood, gonadotropin levels are higher in females than in males.

The most important estrogens produced by the ovary are estradiol-17β (E2) and estrone (E1); estriol is a metabolic product of both, and all three estrogens may be found in the urine of mature females. Estrogens arise from androgens produced by the adrenal glands, the ovaries, or the testes (see Fig. 26.5). This conversion explains why in certain types of 46,XY DSD, feminization occurs at puberty. In HSD17B3 deficiency (see later), for example, the enzymatic block results in markedly

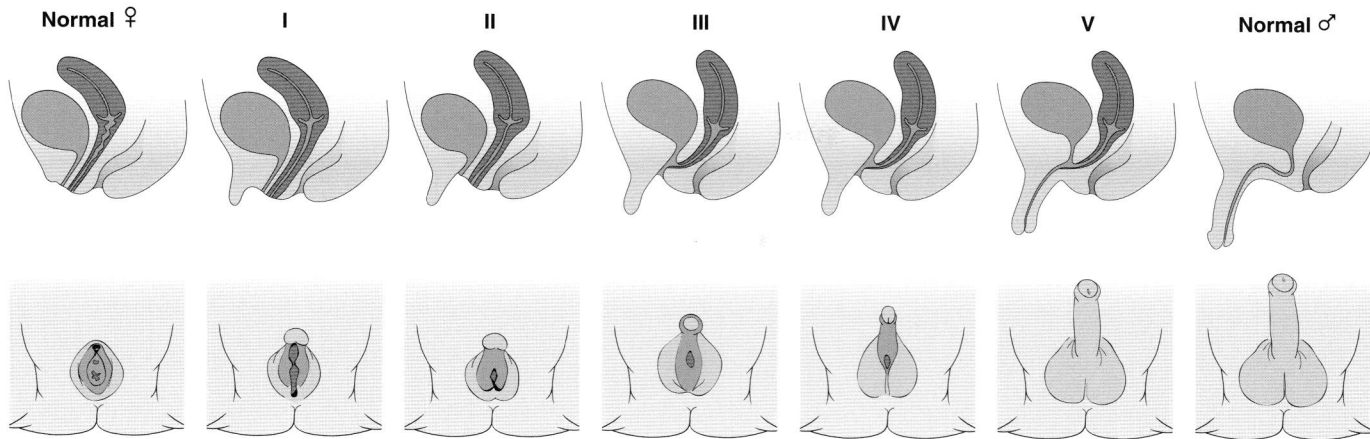

Fig. 26.3 Method of staging the degree of virilization of the external genitalia of females as proposed by Prader (1958). In type I, the only abnormality is a slight enlargement of the clitoris. In type V, there is a markedly enlarged phallus with a penile urethra. (Redrawn from Prader A. Vollkommen männliche äussere gentialentwicklung und salzverlustsyndrom bei madchen mit kongenitalem adrenogenitalem syndrom. *Helv Paediat Acta.* 1958;13:5.)

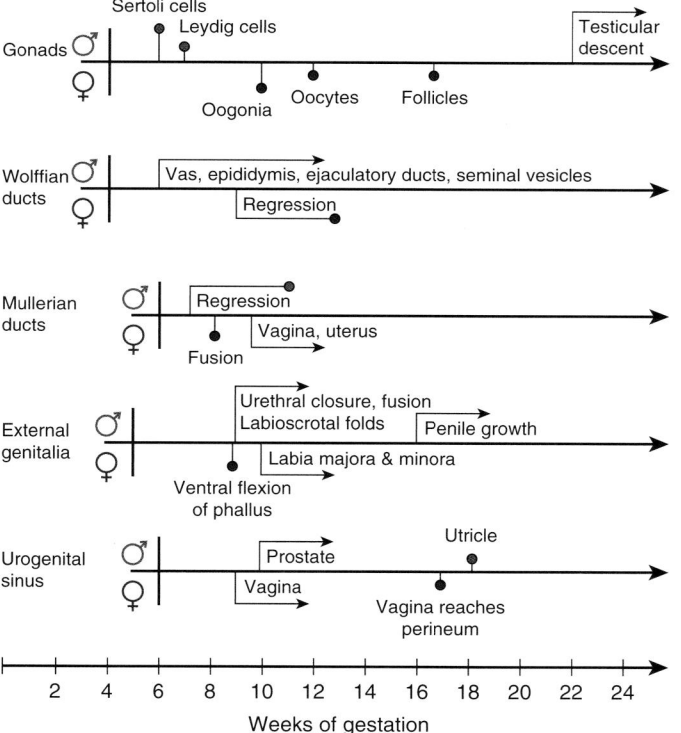

Fig. 26.4 Timing of development of external and internal genitalia. The *solid dot* shows the age at onset of the various developmental changes. Male differentiation is shown above each line, with female differentiation below. (From White PC, Speiser PW. Congenital adrenal hyperplasia due to 21-hydroxylase deficiency. *Endocr Rev.* 2000;21:245–291.)

increased secretion of androstenedione, which is converted in the peripheral tissues to estradiol and estrone. These estrogens, in addition to those directly secreted by the testis, result in breast development. Estradiol produced from testosterone in CAIS causes complete feminization in these XY individuals.

Plasma levels of estradiol increase slowly but steadily with advancing sexual maturation and correlate well with clinical progression of pubertal development, skeletal age, and rising levels of FSH. Levels of LH do not rise measurably until secondary sexual characteristics are present. Estrogens, like androgens, inhibit secretion of both LH and FSH (negative feedback). In females, estrogens also provoke the surge of LH secretion that occurs in the mid-menstrual cycle and results in ovulation. The capacity for this positive feedback is another maturational milestone of puberty.

The average age at menarche in White American girls is about 12.5–13 years, but the range of "normal" is wide, and 1–2% of normal girls have not menstruated by 16 years of age (see Chapter 55). The age at onset of pubertal signs is about 2 years before menarche. This age varies, with some studies suggesting earlier ages than previously thought, especially in the U.S. African-American population. Menarche generally correlates closely with skeletal age. Maturation and closure of the epiphyses is partially estrogen dependent, as demonstrated by a very tall 28-year-old normally masculinized male with continued growth due to incomplete closure of the epiphyses, who proved to have complete estrogen insensitivity due to an estrogen-receptor defect.

DIAGNOSTIC APPROACH TO THE PATIENT WITH ATYPICAL OR AMBIGUOUS GENITALIA

Infants with ambiguous or atypical genitalia should be evaluated and treated at a center with multidisciplinary experience in DSD. The appearance of the external genitalia is rarely diagnostic of a particular disorder, and thus does not often allow distinction among the various forms of DSD. Some clues are noted in Table 26.5. The most common causes of 46,XX DSD are virilizing forms of **congenital adrenal hyperplasia (CAH)**. It is important to note that in 46,XY DSD, the specific diagnosis is not found in up to 50% of cases. At one experienced center, the six most common diagnoses accounted for 50% of the cases. These included virilizing CAH (14%), androgen insensitivity syndrome (10%), mixed gonadal dysgenesis (8%), clitoral/labial anomalies (7%), hypogonadotropic hypogonadism (6%), and 46,XY small-for-gestational age males with hypospadias (6%). The etiology in cases of 46,XY DSD without a known diagnosis can be further delineated using exome sequencing technologies.

The difficulty of establishing a diagnosis in 46,XY DSD and the resulting lack of specific management emphasizes the need for thorough diagnostic evaluations (Fig. 26.6). These include biochemical

TABLE 26.4 Genes Associated with in Disorders of Sex Development

Gene	Protein	OMIM #	Locus	Inheritance	Gonad	Müllerian Structures	External Genitalia	Associated Features/Variant Phenotypes
46,XY DSD								
Disorders of Gonadal (Testicular) Development: Single-Gene Disorders								
WT1	TF	607102	11p13	AD	Testicular dysgenesis	±	Female or ambiguous	Wilms tumor, renal abnormalities, gonadal tumors (WAGR, Denys-Drash, and Frasier syndromes)
SF1 (NR5A1)	Nuclear receptor TF	184757	9q33	AD/AR	Testicular dysgenesis	±	Female or ambiguous	More severe phenotypes include primary adrenal failure; milder phenotypes have isolated partial gonadal dysgenesis; mothers who carry SF1 pathogenic variant have premature ovarian insufficiency
SRY	TF	480000	Yp11.3	Y	Testicular dysgenesis or ovotestis	±	Female or ambiguous	
SOX9	TF	608160	17q24-25	AD	Testicular dysgenesis or ovotestis	±	Female or ambiguous	Campomelic dysplasia (17q24 rearrangements; milder phenotype than point pathogenic variants)
DHH	Signaling molecule	605423	12q13.1	AR	Testicular dysgenesis	+	Female	The severe phenotype of one patient included minifascicular neuropathy; other patients have isolated gonadal dysgenesis
ATRX	Helicase (?chromatin remodeling)	300032	Xq13.3	X	Testicular dysgenesis	–	Female, ambiguous, or male	α Thalassemia, developmental delay
ARX	TF	300382	Xp21.13	X	Testicular dysgenesis	–	Ambiguous	X-linked lissencephaly, epilepsy, temperature instability
MAP3K1		613762	5q11.2	AD	Dysgenetic testes	Streak ovaries, uterus can be normal	Female or ambiguous male (rare)	Sparse axillary and pubic hair, gonadoblastoma
Disorders of Gonadal (Testicular) Development: Chromosomal Changes Involving Key Candidate Genes								
DMRT1 DMRT2	TF	602424	9p24.3	Monosomic deletion	Testicular dysgenesis	±	Female or ambiguous	Developmental delay; Rib/vertebral malformations
DAX1 (NR0B1)	Nuclear receptor TF	300018	Xp21.3	dupXp21	Testicular dysgenesis or ovary	±	Female or ambiguous	
WNT4	Signaling molecule	603490	1p35	dup1p35	Testicular dysgenesis	+	Ambiguous	Developmental delay
DMRT3 OAS3	Regulate ESR1 expression	603351	9p24.3 12q24	Digenic with DMRT3 and OAS3	Testicular dysgenesis		Female or ambiguous	
Disorders in Hormone Synthesis or Action								
LHGCR	G-protein receptor	152790	2p21	AR	Testis	–	Female, ambiguous, or micropenis	Leydig cell hypoplasia
DHCR7	Enzyme	602858	11q12-13	AR	Testis	–	Variable	Smith-Lemli-Opitz syndrome: coarse facies, 2nd–3rd toe syndactyly, failure to thrive, developmental delay, cardiac and visceral abnormalities
StAR	Mitochondrial membrane protein	600617	8p11.2	AR	Testis	–	Female	Congenital lipoid adrenal hyperplasia (primary adrenal failure), pubertal failure
CYP11A1	Enzyme	118485	15q23-24	AR	Testis	–	Female or ambiguous	Congenital adrenal hyperplasia (primary adrenal failure), pubertal failure
HSD3B2	Enzyme	201810	1p13.1	AR	Testis	–	Ambiguous	CAH, primary adrenal failure, partial androgenization due to ↑ DHEA

TABLE 26.4 Genes Associated with in Disorders of Sex Development—cont'd

Gene	Protein	OMIM #	Locus	Inheritance	Gonad	Müllerian Structures	External Genitalia	Associated Features/Variant Phenotypes
CYP17	Enzyme	202110	10q24.3	AR	Testis	–	Female ambiguous or micropenis	CAH, hypertension due to ↑ corticosterone and 11-deoxycorticosterone (except in isolated 17,20-lyase deficiency)
POR (P450 oxidoreductase)	CYP enzyme electron donor	124015	7q11.2	AR	Testis	–	Male or ambiguous	Mixed features of 21-hydroxylase deficiency, 17α-hydroxylase/17,20-lyase deficiency, and aromatase deficiency; sometimes associated with Antley-Bixler skeletal dysplasia
HSD17B3	Enzyme	605573	9q22	AR	Testis	–	Female or ambiguous	Partial androgenization at puberty, ↑ androstenedione:testosterone ratio
SRD5A2	Enzyme	607306	2p23	AR	Testis	–	Ambiguous or micropenis	Partial androgenization at puberty, ↑ testosterone:DHT ratio
AKR1C4	Enzyme	600451	10p15.1	Unclear	Testis	–	Ambiguous or micropenis	DHT deficiency in patients once thought to have 17,20-lyase deficiency; dose effect with AKR1C2 pathogenic variant is possible
AKR1C2	Enzyme	600450	10p15.1	Unclear	Testis	–	Ambiguous or micropenis	DHT deficiency in patients once thought to have 17,20-lyase deficiency; dose effect with AKR1C2 pathogenic variant is possible
AMH	Signaling molecule	600957	19p13.3-13.2	AR	Testis	+	Normal male	Persistent müllerian duct syndrome; male
AMH receptor	Serine–threonine kinase transmembrane receptor	600956	12q13	AR	Testis	–	Normal male	External genitalia, bilateral cryptorchidism
Androgen receptor	Nuclear receptor TF	313700	Xq12	X	Testis	–	Female, ambiguous, micropenis, or normal male	Phenotypic spectrum from complete androgen insensitivity syndrome (female external genitalia) and partial androgen insensitivity (ambiguous) to normal male genitalia/infertility

46,XX DSD

Disorders of Gonadal (Ovarian) Development

Gene	Protein	OMIM #	Locus	Inheritance	Gonad	Müllerian Structures	External Genitalia	Associated Features/Variant Phenotypes
SRY	TF	480000	Yp11.3	Translocation	Testis or ovotestis	–	Male or ambiguous	
SOX9	TF	608160	17q24	dup17q24	ND	–	Male or ambiguous	
R-spondin 1	TF	610644	1p34.3	AR	Ovotestis	+/–	Male or ambiguous	Palmoplantar hyperkeratosis and certain malignancies

Androgen Excess

Gene	Protein	OMIM #	Locus	Inheritance	Gonad	Müllerian Structures	External Genitalia	Associated Features/Variant Phenotypes
HSD3B2	Enzyme	201810	1p13	AR	Ovary	+	Clitoromegaly	CAH, primary adrenal failure, partial androgenization due to ↑ DHEA
CYP21A2	Enzyme	201910	6p21-23	AR	Ovary	+	Ambiguous	CAH, phenotypic spectrum from severe salt-losing forms associated with adrenal failure to simple virilizing forms with compensated adrenal function, ↑ 17-hydroxyprogesterone
CYP11B1	Enzyme	20210	8q21-22	AR	Ovary	+	Ambiguous	CAH, hypertension due to ↑ 11-deoxycortisol and 11-deoxycorticosterone
POR (P450 oxidoreductase)	CYP enzyme electron donor	124015	7q11.2	AR	Ovary	+	Ambiguous	Mixed features of 21-hydroxylase deficiency, 17α-hydroxylase/17,20-lyase deficiency, and aromatase deficiency; associated with Antley-Bixler skeletal dysplasia
CYP19	Enzyme	107910	15q21	AR	Ovary	+	Ambiguous	Maternal virilization during pregnancy, absent breast development at puberty, except in partial cases
Glucocorticoid receptor	Nuclear receptor TF	138040	5q31	AR	Ovary	+	Ambiguous	↑ ACTH, 17-hydroxyprogesterone and cortisol; failure of dexamethasone suppression (patient heterozygous for a pathogenic variant in CYP21)

ACTH, adrenocorticotropic hormone; AD, autosomal dominant (often de novo pathogenic variant); AR, autosomal recessive; CAH, congenital adrenal hyperplasia; DHEA, dehydroepiandrosterone; DHT, dihydrotestosterone; DSD, disorders of sex development; ND, not determined; OMIM #, Online Mendelian Inheritance in Man number; TF, transcription factor; WAGR, Wilms, aniridia, genital anomalies, and retardation; X, X-chromosomal; Y, Y-chromosomal; Y-chromosome.

Data from Lee PA, Houk CP, Ahmed SF, et al. International Consensus Conference on Intersex organized by the Lawson Wilkins Pediatric Endocrine Society and the European Society for Paediatric Endocrinology. Consensus statement on management of intersex disorders. Pediatrics. 2006;118:e488–e500; Baxter RM, Arboleda VA, Lee H, et al. Exome sequencing for the diagnosis of 46,XY disorders of sex development. J Clin Endocrinol Metab. 2015;100:e333–e344.

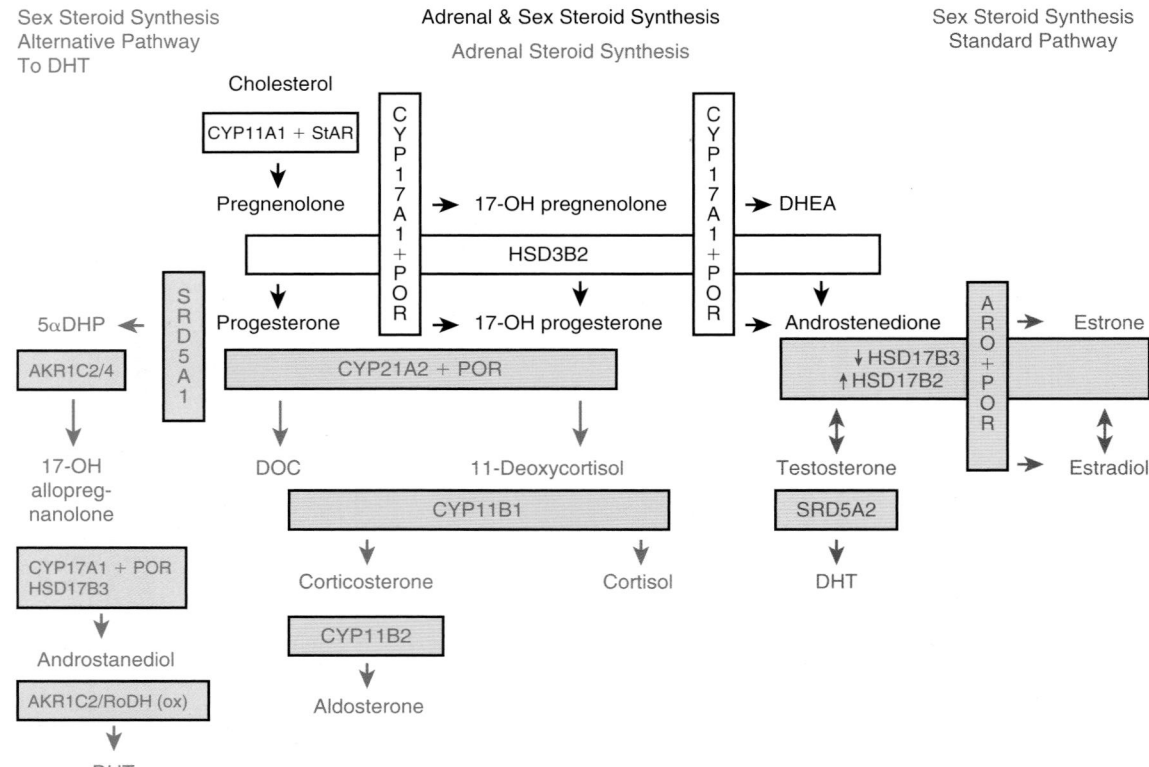

Fig. 26.5 Steroidogenic pathways. CYP11A1: cholesterol side chain cleavage. Enzyme activities include 20-hydroxylase, 22-hydroxylase, and 20,22-lyase; CYP17A1: activities include 17α-hydroxylase and 17,20-lyase; HSD3B2: activities include 3β-hydroxysteroid dehydrogenase type II and D5D4-isomerase; CYP21A2: activity is 21-hydroxylase; CYP11B1: activity is 11β-hydroxylase; CYP11B2: activities include 18-hydroxylase (CMOI) and 18-dehydrogenase (CMOII); SRD5A1: activity is 5α-reductase type I; SRD5A2: activity is 5α-reductase type II; HSD17B2: activity is 17β-hydroxysteroid dehydrogenase type II; HSD17B3: activity is 17β-hydroxysteroid dehydrogenase type III; AKR1C2/4 *(blue)*: activities are 3α-reductase types I and III; AKR1C2/RoDH (ox): activities are 3α-reductase and 3-hydroxyepimerase. ARO, aromatase; DHEA, dehydroepiandrosterone; DHT, dihydrotestosterone; 5αDHP, 5α-dihydroprogesterone; DOC, deoxycorticosterone; POR, P450 oxidoreductase. (Data from Kim MS, Donohoue PA. Adrenal disorders. In: Kappy MS, Allen DB, Geffner ME, eds. *Pediatric Practice Endocrinology*. 2nd ed. New York: McGraw-Hill; 2014; and Flück CE, et al. Why boys will be boys: two pathways of fetal testicular androgen biosynthesis are needed for male sexual differentiation. *Am J Hum Genet*. 2011;89:201–218.)

characterization of possible steroidogenic enzymatic defects, imaging studies to characterize internal genitalia, and determination of genetic sex as well as other genetic studies as determined by each individual patient with atypical genitalia. The parents need counseling about the potentially complex nature of the baby's condition, and guidance as to how to deal with the curiosity of their well-meaning friends and family members. The evaluation and management should be carried out by a multidisciplinary team of experts that include practitioners in pediatric endocrinology, pediatric surgery/urology, pediatric radiology, newborn medicine/neonatology, genetics, and psychology. *On occasion, the sex of rearing will need to be uncommitted until the diagnostic evaluation is completed.* Once the sex of rearing has been agreed on by the family and team, treatment can be organized. Genetic counseling should be offered as part of routine work-up.

After a complete history and physical exam, the common diagnostic approach includes multiple steps that are usually performed at the same time rather than waiting for results of one test prior to performing another, in order to expedite the diagnosis. At many centers, the initial evaluation may include a broad genetic screening panel that simultaneously examines for multiple potential disease-associated genetic variants. Careful attention to the presence of physical features other than the genitalia is crucial to determine if a diagnosis of a particular multisystem syndrome is possible (Table 26.6 and Fig. 26.7). A summary of many features of commonly encountered causes of DSD is provided in Table 26.7.

Diagnostic tests include the following:
1. Blood karyotype, with rapid determination of sex chromosomes (in many centers this is available within 24–48 hours) (see Fig. 26.7).
2. Other blood tests (see Table 26.6)
   a. Screen for congenital adrenal hyperplasia: cortisol biosynthetic precursors and adrenal androgens, particularly serum levels of 17-hydroxyprogesterone and androstenedione for 21-hydroxylase deficiency, the most common form. In the United States, all 50 states have a newborn screen for 21-hydroxylase deficiency.
   b. Screen for androgen biosynthetic defects with serum levels of androgens and their precursors.
   c. Assess for gonadal responsiveness to gonadotropin to screen for testicular gonadal tissue: measure serum levels of testosterone and dihydrotestosterone before and after intramuscular injections of hCG.

TABLE 26.5	Association of Genital Abnormalities
Abnormal Characteristics	**Examples of Associated Disorders**
Male-Appearing Genitalia	
Micropenis	Growth hormone or luteinizing hormone deficiency
	Testosterone deficiency (in 2nd and 3rd trimesters)
	Partial androgen insensitivity
	Syndrome: idiopathic
Hypospadias (more severe)	Disorders of gonadal development 46,XX DSD
	Ovotesticular DSD
	46,XX or 46,XX DSD
	Syndrome: idiopathic
Impalpable gonads	Anorchia
	Persistent müllerian duct syndrome
	46,XX DSD with 21- or 11β-hydroxylase deficiency cryptorchidism
Small gonads	47,XXY, 46,XX DSD
	Dysgenetic or rudimentary testes
Inguinal mass (uterus or tube)	Persistent müllerian duct syndrome, dysgenetic testes
Female-Appearing Genitalia	
Clitoromegaly	XX with 21- or 11β-hydroxylase or 3β-hydroxy dehydrogenase deficiency
	Other 46,XX DSD
	Gonadal dysgenesis, dysgenetic testes, ovotesticular DSD
	46,XY DSD
	Tumor infiltration of clitoris
	Syndrome: idiopathic
Posterior labial fusion	As for clitoromegaly
Palpable gonad(s)	Gonadal dysgenesis, dysgenetic testes, ovotesticular DSD
	46,XY DSD
Inguinal hernia or mass	As for palpable gonad(s)

DSD, disorders of sex development.

From Martin RJ, Fanaroff AA, Walsh MC, eds. *Fanaroff's & Martins's Neonatal-Perinatal Medicine.* 11th ed. Philadelphia: Elsevier; 2020:1674, Table 89.3.

d. Molecular genetic analyses for SRY (sex-determining region of the Y chromosome), other Y-specific loci, and, when appropriate, broad screening for other known single-gene defects associated with DSD (see Table 26.4).
e. Gonadotropin levels (LH and FSH).
f. AMH and inhibin B levels.
3. The internal anatomy of patients with ambiguous genitalia can be defined with one or more of the following studies:
a. Pelvic ultrasound; renal and adrenal ultrasound.
b. Pelvic MRI.
c. Genitourethrograms.
d. Endoscopic examination of the genitourinary tract.
e. Exploratory laparoscopy to locate and characterize/biopsy the gonads.

BASIC APPROACHES TO THE DIAGNOSIS AND MANAGEMENT OF DISORDERS OF SEX DEVELOPMENT

In the neonate, the presence of atypical genitalia requires immediate attention to determine the etiology and then, if necessary, decide on the sex of rearing. In some cases, DSD is associated with other abnormalities that adversely impact the child's health, particularly the salt-losing forms of CAH, adrenal insufficiency related to SF1 defects, and renal abnormalities associated with WT-1 defects.

The family of the infant needs to be informed of the child's condition as early, completely, compassionately, and honestly as possible. Caution must be used to avoid feelings of guilt, shame, and confusion. Guidance needs to be provided to alleviate both short-term and long-term concerns and to allow the child to grow up in a completely supportive environment. The initial care is best provided by a team of professionals who remain focused foremost on the needs of the child. Management of the potential emotional and psychologic effects that these disorders can generate in the child and the family is of paramount importance and requires the involvement of physicians, psychologists, and other health care professionals with sensitivity, training, and experience in this field.

While awaiting the results of blood tests, imaging with pelvic ultrasonography and/or MRI is used to determine the presence of a uterus and ovaries. Presence of a uterus and absence of external palpable gonads often suggest a virilized XX female. A search for the source of virilization includes studies of adrenal hormones to rule out varieties of CAH, and studies of androgens and estrogens may be necessary to rule out aromatase deficiency. Virilized XX females with CAH are generally (but not always) reared as females even when the genitalia are Prader stage 4 or 5 (see Fig. 26.3).

The absence of a uterus, with or without palpable external gonads, may indicate an undervirilized XY male. Measurements of blood levels of gonadotropins, testosterone, AMH, and DHT are necessary to determine whether testicular production of androgen is present and is normal. Undervirilized males who are totally feminized may be reared as females. Certain significantly undervirilized infants, such as those with 5α-reductase deficiency, may be reared as males because these children virilize normally at puberty. Sixty percent of individuals with 5α-reductase deficiency assigned as female in infancy will identify as males as adults. An infant with a comparable degree of undervirilization resulting from an androgen receptor defect, such as androgen insensitivity syndrome (AIS), may be successfully reared as a female, depending on androgen responsiveness.

In some mammals, the female exposed to androgens prenatally or in early postnatal life exhibits nontraditional sexual behavior in adult life. Most, but not all, females who have undergone fetal masculinization from CAH have female sexual identity, although during childhood they may appear to prefer male typical play activities over female typical play activities.

In the past it was thought that surgical treatment of ambiguous genitalia to create a female appearance, particularly when a vagina was present, was more successful than construction of male genitalia. Considerable controversy has developed regarding these decisions. Sexual functioning is to a large extent more dependent on neurohormonal and behavioral factors than the physical appearance and functional capacity of the genitalia. Similarly, controversy exists regarding the timing of the performance of invasive and definitive procedures, such as surgery. Whenever possible, without endangering the physical or psychologic health of the child, an expert multidisciplinary team should consider deferring elective surgical procedures and gonadectomies until the child can participate in the informed consent for the procedure.

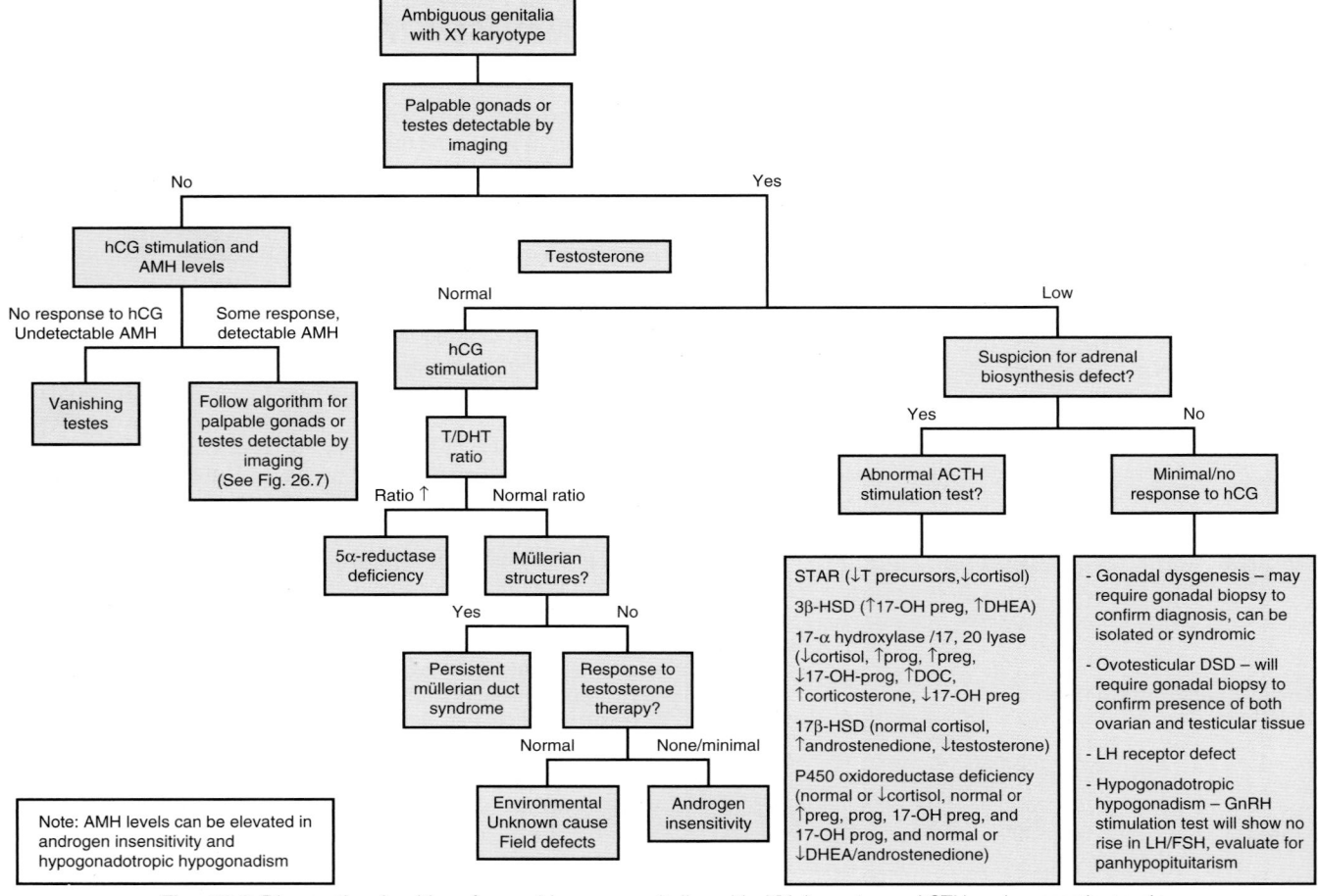

Fig. 26.6 Diagnostic algorithm for ambiguous genitalia with XY karyotype. ACTH, adrenocorticotropic hormone; AMH, antimüllerian hormone; DHEA, dehydroepiandrosterone; DHT, dihydrotestosterone; DOC; deoxycorticosterone; DSD, disorder of sex development; FSH, follicle-stimulating hormone; GnRH, gonadotropin-releasing hormone; hCG, human chorionic gonadotropin; HSD, hydroxysteroid dehydrogenase; LH, luteinizing hormone; preg, pregnenolone; prog, progesterone; STaR, steroidogenic acute regulatory protein; T, testosterone. (From McCann-Crosby B, Sutton R. Disorders of sexual development. *Clin Perinatol.* 2015;42[2]:395–412 [Fig. 3, p. 400].)

For all patients with DSD who have Y-chromosome material and intraabdominal gonads, gonadectomy is generally recommended due to the risk of gonadal tumors developing with increasing age, many of which are malignant. The risk is highest in children with gonadal dysgenesis, partial androgen insensitivity, or Frasier or Denys-Drash syndrome.

The pediatrician, pediatric endocrinologist, and psychologist, along with the appropriate additional specialists, should provide ongoing compassionate, supportive care to the patient and the patient's family throughout childhood, adolescence, and adulthood. Active support groups are available for families and patients with many of the conditions discussed.

SPECIFIC TYPES OF DISORDERS OF SEX DEVELOPMENT

46,XX Disorders of Sex Development

In 46,XX DSD, the sex chromosomes are XX, but the external genitalia are virilized. If the gonads are ovaries, there is no significant AMH production. Thus the uterus, fallopian tubes, cervix, and upper vagina will develop. The varieties and causes of this condition are relatively few. Most cases result from exposure of the female fetus to excessive *exogenous* or *endogenous* androgens during early intrauterine life (see Figs. 26.2 and 26.4 and Table 26.2). The changes consist principally of virilization of the external genitalia (clitoral hypertrophy and labio-scrotal fusion).

Androgen Exposure/Fetoplacental Source

Congenital adrenal hyperplasia. CAH is the most common cause of genital ambiguity and of 46,XX DSD. CAH is caused by an enzymatic defect in the biosynthesis of cortisol. This results in compensatory adrenocorticotropic hormone (ACTH) excess, which stimulates hyperplasia of the adrenal cortex in an attempt to normalize cortisol secretion. There is overproduction of adrenal androgen precursors in the forms of CAH that cause genital ambiguity in 46,XX infants. Females with 21-hydroxylase and 11-hydroxylase deficiency are the most highly virilized (see Fig. 26.2). Minimal virilization also occurs with the type II 3β-hydroxysteroid dehydrogenase (HSD3B2) defect (see Fig. 26.5 for enzymatic pathways). The androgen precursors are converted in extra-adrenal tissues into testosterone and DHT, the potent androgens that bind to the androgen receptor (AR). The treatment for all forms of CAH is cortisol replacement therapy, which reduces ACTH secretion and reverses the androgen excess.

TABLE 26.6 Potential Investigations for Disorders of Sex Development

Approach	Test	Uses
Genetics	FISH* (X- and Y-specific probes)	Rapid analysis of sex chromosome complement on cells
	qfPCR*	Rapid analysis of sex chromosome signal in DNA
	Karyotype*	Analysis of sex chromosomes and autosomes in cells with ability to look for mosaicism by screening multiple cells, as well as detection of major deletions, duplications, and balanced translocations
	Array CGH or SNP microarray*	Analysis of chromosome signal across the genome, with ability to detect smaller copy number variants but not balanced translocations, using DNA
	Multiple ligation probe-dependent amplification	Analysis of the loss or gain of specific exons or whole genes on a predefined panel of probes, such as for DSD genes, using DNA
	Single-gene analysis	Sanger sequencing and analysis of individual genes that are highly likely to be the cause of DSD based on incidence and clinical and biochemical features (e.g., *CYP21A2*)
	Targeted panel sequencing	Analysis of large numbers of known DSD-causing genes using high-throughput sequencing of DNA
	Whole exome sequencing	Analysis of all the coding exons in the DNA, which may show changes in known, putative, or novel DSD-associated genes, using high-throughput sequencing
Endocrine	Routine serum biochemistry*; urinalysis*	May reveal a salt-losing crisis or associated renal disorder (e.g., WT1)
	17-Hydroxyprogesterone,* 11-deoxycortisol, 17-hydroxypregnenolone	May help to diagnose CAH or reveal a specific block in an adrenal pathway relevant to DSD
	Renin, ACTH	May show a salt-losing state or primary adrenal insufficiency
	Testosterone,* androstenedione, DHT	Indicates the degree of androgen production and ratios of androgens in the basal state or following hCG stimulation and may help to diagnose a block in androgen production consistent with a specific diagnosis (e.g., 17β-hydroxysteroid dehydrogenase or 5α-reductase deficiencies); can also reveal androgen production in ovotesticular DSD
	Gonadotropins	May indicate an underlying block in steroidogenesis or androgen insensitivity (LH), or impaired Sertoli cell function (FSH)
	AMH, inhibin B	Can be useful markers of testicular integrity: AMH is detectable throughout childhood and is reduced in testicular dysgenesis or absent if streak gonads or anorchia occur; AMH may be high in AIS or reduced androgen production due to steroidogenic defects; AMH may help to reveal the presence of testicular tissue in 46,XX ovotesticular DSD
	Urinary steroids by GC–MS	Can be used to diagnose specific steroidogenic defects in the newborn period (e.g., 21-hydroxylase deficiency, 11β-hydroxylase deficiency, 3β-hydroxysteroid dehydrogenase deficiency, P450 oxidoreductase deficiency, 17α-hydroxylase deficiency); can reveal 5α-reductase deficiency only after 3–6 mo of life
	Dynamic tests: ACTH stimulation	Used to assess the adrenal gland stress response (quantitative) and can be coupled with measurement of steroid metabolites or poststimulation urine steroid analysis to study ratios of metabolites (diagnostic)
	hCG stimulation	Used in short (3 days) or prolonged (3 wk) formats to assess androgen production (quantitative) and androgen biosynthesis pathways (diagnostic); can also be used to assess for the presence of testicular tissue (e.g., anorchia, ovotestis), although AMH is now more often used initially
	FSH stimulation test	Rarely used to investigate the presence of ovarian tissue by measuring inhibin A and estradiol response
Imaging	Abdominopelvic and renal ultrasound*	Can reveal the size, position, and structure of gonads (especially testes); the presence of müllerian structures; and associated changes (such as renal size or anomalies)
	MRI	Sometimes used to assess internal structures, especially in adolescence
	Cystourethroscopy, sinogram	Can reveal the structure of the bladder, vagina, and common channel
Surgical	Laparoscopy	Can reveal internal structures by direct visualization, such as gonads and müllerian structures
	Gonadal biopsies	Can be used to determine the nature of gonads, especially if testicular dysgenesis or ovotestes are suspected

*Indicates first-line investigations for which results are available within days. For images of G-banded karyotypes and FISH analysis, see Fig. 26.6.
ACTH, adrenocorticotropic hormone; AIS, androgen insensitivity syndrome; AMH, antimüllerian hormone; CAH, congenital adrenal hyperplasia; CGH, comparative genomic hybridization; DHT, dihydrotestosterone; DSD, disorders of sex development; FISH, fluorescent in situ hybridization; FSH, follicle-stimulating hormone; GC–MS, gas chromatography–mass spectrometry; hCG, human chorionic gonadotropin; LH, luteinizing hormone; qfPCR, quantitative fluorescent polymerase chain reaction; SNP, single-nucleotide polymorphism.
From Achermann JC, Hughes IA. Pediatric disorders of sex development. In: Melmed S, Polonsky KS, Larsen PR, et al., eds. *Williams Textbook of Endocrinology*. 13th ed. Philadelphia: Elsevier; 2016:949.

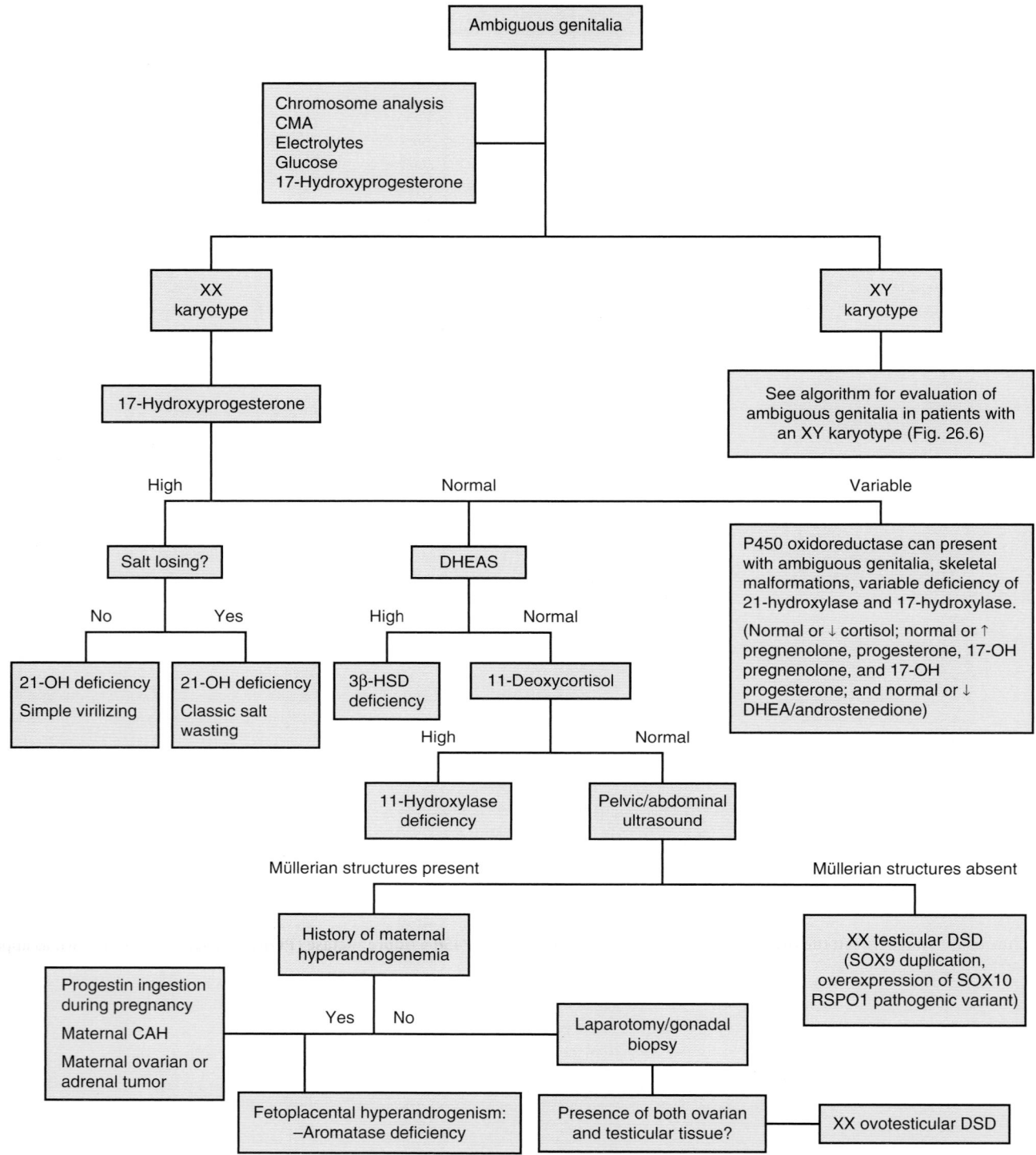

Fig. 26.7 Diagnostic algorithm for patients with ambiguous genitalia. CAH, congenital adrenal hyperplasia; CMA, chromosomal microarray; DHEA, dehydroepiandrosterone; DHEAS, dehydroepiandrosterone sulfate; DSD, disorders of sexual development; HSD, hydroxysteroid dehydrogenase. (From McCann-Crosby B, Sutton R. Disorders of sexual development. *Clin Perinatol.* 2015;42[2]:395–412 [Fig. 2, p. 399].)

Mineralocorticoid replacement may be needed in 21-hydroxylase and HSD3B2 deficiency. The surgical treatment of virilized genitalia in affected females is usually recommended during infancy. However, this remains a controversial topic.

CAH due to 21-hydroxylase deficiency (variants in the *CYP21A2* gene) is one of the most common inherited diseases associated with

DSD. It accounts for more than 95% of cases of adrenal steroidogenic defects and is estimated to occur in about 1 in 14,000 live births. In some genetically isolated populations such as Yupik Eskimos, the incidence is much higher. CYP21A2 deficiency usually presents as one of two clinical syndromes in neonates or very young infants, both of which are associated with glucocorticoid deficiency. If not diagnosed

TABLE 26.7 Atypical/Ambiguous Genitalia: Features Associated with the Most Common Diagnoses

	21-OH Deficiency	Testicular Dysgenesis with Y Chromosome	Ovo-Testicular DSD	Partial Androgen Insensitivity	Dihydrotestosterone (DHT) Deficiency	Block in Testosterone (T) Synthesis
Clinical Feature						
Palpable gonad(s)	–	+/–	+/–	+	+/–	+
Uterus present[†]	+	+	Usually	–	–	–
Increased skin pigmentation	+/–	–	–	–	–	–
Sick baby	+/–	–	–	–	–	+/–
Dysmorphic features	–	+/–	–	–	–	–
Diagnostic Test Results						
Serum 17-OHP	Elevated	Normal	Normal	Normal	Normal	Normal
Electrolytes	Possibly abnormal	Normal	Normal	Normal	Normal	Possibly abnormal
Karyotype	46,XX	45,X/46,XY or others	46,XX	46,XY	46,XY	46,XY
Testosterone response to hCG	NA	Positive	Normal or reduced	Positive	Positive	Reduced or absent
Gonadal biopsy	NA	Dysgenic gonad	Ovotestis	Normal testis with +/– Leydig cell hyperplasia	Normal testis	Normal testis
				DNA screening for AR[‡] or post-receptor pathogenic variants positive in many cases	Elevated T:DHT ratio	Levels of testosterone precursors elevated Testosterone level low

[†]As determined by ultrasound or rectal examination.
[‡]Androgen receptor.
17-OHP, 17-hydroxyprogesterone; 21-OH, 21-hydroxylase; hCG, human chorionic gonadotropin; NA, not applicable.

in the first few weeks, the **salt-wasting form** is associated with dehydration, hyponatremia, hyperkalemia, acidosis, and hypotension with elevated plasma renin activity (PRA) due to mineralocorticoid deficiency. Symptoms of this renal salt loss include lethargy, vomiting, and poor feeding. Adrenal androgen excess results in ambiguous genitalia in affected females. The simple virilizing form also causes prenatal virilization in females but without postnatal salt wasting. In some infants, the distinction between the two forms is not clear due to early detection by newborn screening. Female patients with salt-losing CAH tend to have more virilization than do non–salt-losing female patients. Masculinization may be so intense that the urethral meatus is at the tip of the enlarged clitoris, giving the appearance of a normal penis (see Fig. 26.2). The patient may therefore appear to be a male with bilateral cryptorchidism. Affected males have normal genitalia. **Late-onset forms** of CYP21A2 deficiency present with early pubarche in both sexes, or with hirsutism and menstrual irregularities in older females. These late-onset forms are not causes of DSD.

CAH due to 11β-hydroxylase deficiency (pathogenic variants in the *CYP11B1* gene) is the second most common cause of CAH, and accounts for <5% of CAH cases. As with other causes of CAH, cortisol synthesis is reduced; however, there is excessive mineralocorticoid (deoxycorticosterone [DOC]) secretion accompanying adrenal androgen overproduction. As a result, patients become hypertensive after infancy because of increased sodium retention.

CAH due to 3β-hydroxysteroid dehydrogenase type II deficiency (pathogenic variants in the *HSD3B2* gene) is a rare form of CAH in which synthesis of all steroid hormones is impaired (see Fig. 26.5). Thus, there are deficiencies of glucocorticoids, mineralocorticoids, and potent androgens. Most patients present as neonates or in early infancy. Clinical manifestations are because of both cortisol and aldosterone deficiency as seen in 21-hydroxylase deficiency, including feeding difficulties, vomiting, volume depletion, and subsequent hyponatremia, hyperkalemia, and high PRA. Affected females have mild virilization (an indirect effect of oversecretion of dehydroepiandrosterone [DHEA]). This form of CAH may also cause 46,XY DSD.

P450 oxidoreductase (POR) deficiency is also known as apparent combined CYP21A2 and CYP17A1 deficiency. The underlying defect is a pathogenic variant in the *POR* gene that encodes cytochrome P450 oxidoreductase, a mitochondrial cofactor that transfers electrons to CYP21A2 and CYP17A1 during steroidogenesis. This results in a partial deficiency of the enzymes 21-hydroxylase and 17-hydroxylase. Affected females are born with ambiguous genitalia, suggesting intrauterine androgen excess; however, as opposed to classic CAH, after birth serum androgen concentrations are low, and virilization does not progress. Males may have undervirilization. Mothers may have virilization during pregnancy with an affected fetus. Bone malformations affecting primarily the head and limbs (**Antley-Bixler syndrome**) may be seen in both boys and girls with POR deficiency.

Aromatase deficiency. In 46,XX females, the rare condition of aromatase deficiency during fetal life leads to 46,XX DSD and results in hypergonadotropic hypogonadism at puberty because of ovarian failure to synthesize estrogen from androgen. Examples of this condition include two 46,XX infants who had enlargement of the clitoris and posterior labial fusion at birth. In one instance, maternal serum and urinary levels of estrogen were very low and serum levels of androgens were high. Cord serum levels of estrogen were also extremely low, and those of androgen were elevated. The second case also had virilization of unknown cause since birth, but the aromatase deficiency was not diagnosed until 14 years of age, when she had further virilization and failed to go into female puberty. At that time, she had elevated levels of gonadotropins and androgens but low estrogen levels, and ultrasonography revealed large ovarian cysts bilaterally. Two siblings with aromatase deficiency have also been described. The 28-year-old XX proband was 177.6 cm tall (+2.5 SD) after having received estrogen replacement therapy. Her 24-year-old brother was 204 cm tall (+3.7 SD) and had a delayed bone age of only 14 years due to failure of epiphyseal fusion, which is estrogen mediated.

Cortisol resistance due to glucocorticoid receptor gene pathogenic variants. A 9-year-old female with 46,XX DSD and a history of ambiguous genitalia, thought to be due to 21-hydroxylase deficiency CAH, had elevated cortisol levels both at baseline and after dexamethasone, along with hypertension and hypokalemia, suggestive of the diagnosis of generalized glucocorticoid resistance. A novel homozygous pathogenic variant in exon 5 of the glucocorticoid receptor was demonstrated. Subsequently, additional families with this condition have been identified. Virilization occurs due to excess ACTH stimulation of adrenal steroid production, as the glucocorticoid receptor defect is also present in the pituitary gland, which senses inadequate cortisol effect to provide negative feedback.

Androgen Exposure: Maternal Source

Virilizing maternal tumors. Rarely, a female fetus can be virilized by a maternal androgen-producing tumor. In a minority of cases, the lesion is a benign adrenal adenoma, but the majority are ovarian tumors, particularly androblastomas, luteomas, and Krukenberg tumors. Maternal virilization may be manifested by enlargement of the clitoris, acne, deepening of the voice, decreased lactation, hirsutism, and elevated levels of androgens. In the infant, there is enlargement of the clitoris of varying degrees, often with labial fusion if the tumor produced excess androgen during the 1st trimester. Mothers of children with unexplained 46,XX DSD should undergo physical examination and measurements of their own levels of plasma testosterone, dehydroepiandrosterone sulfate (DHEAS), and androstenedione.

Administration of androgenic drugs to women during pregnancy. Testosterone and 17-methyltestosterone have been reported to cause 46,XX DSD in some instances. The greatest number of cases has resulted from the use of certain progestational compounds for the treatment of threatened abortion. These progestins have been replaced by nonvirilizing ones.

Disorders of Ovarian Development

46,XX testicular DSD. In this condition, also called XX male, the gonads are testicular, and virilization is typically incomplete. Infertility and/or gonadal failure may develop after childhood. Many cases are due to translocation of SRY sequences onto one of the X chromosomes, often paired with duplication of SOX9. The appropriate sex of rearing may be difficult to determine.

46,XX gonadal dysgenesis. These females typically present at puberty with lack of breast development and hypergonadotropic hypogonadism. Normal müllerian structures are present, but ovaries are absent or streaks. They do not have atypical genitalia.

Undetermined/unknown. Rarely, 46,XX DSD can be associated with other congenital anomalies, especially those of the genitourinary or gastroenteric tract, and are thus multifactorial in origin. These include cloacal exstrophy and MURCS association (müllerian hypoplasia, renal agenesis, and cervicothoracic somite abnormalities). Isolated deficiency of müllerian development is known as **Mayer-Rokitansky-Küster-Hauser syndrome**.

46,XY Disorders of Sex Development

In 46,XY DSD, the genotype is XY, and the external genitalia are either not completely virilized, ambiguous (atypical), or completely female. When gonads are found, they typically contain testicular elements; their development ranges from rudimentary to normal. Because the process of normal virilization in the fetus is so complex, it is not surprising that there are many varieties and causes of 46,XY DSD. *The etiology of 46,XY DSD is not identified in up to 50% of cases; however, with advances in rapid and robust genetic testing panels, the proportion of undiagnosed cases is declining.*

Defects in Testicular Development

The first step in male differentiation is development of the bipotential gonad into a testis. In the XY fetus, if there is a deletion of the short arm of the Y chromosome or pathogenic variant of the *SRY* gene, male gonadal differentiation does not occur. The phenotype is female; müllerian (paramesonephric) ducts are well developed because of the absence of AMH, and gonads consist of undifferentiated streaks. By contrast, even extreme deletions of the long arm of the Y chromosome (Yq−) have been found in normally developed males, most of whom have short stature and azoospermia. This indicates that the long arm of the Y chromosome normally has genes that prevent these manifestations. In many syndromes in which the testes fail to differentiate, Y chromosomes appear morphologically normal on karyotyping.

Wilms tumor suppressor gene (WT1) pathogenic variants: Denys-Drash, Frasier, and WAGR syndromes. The constellation of nephropathy with atypical genitalia and bilateral Wilms tumor typifies Denys-Drash syndrome. Müllerian ducts are often present, indicating deficiency of multiple fetal testicular functions. Affected patients with a 46,XX karyotype have normal external genitalia. There is onset of proteinuria in infancy that progresses to nephrotic syndrome and end-stage renal failure by 3 years of age, with focal or diffuse mesangial sclerosis being the most consistent histopathologic finding. Wilms tumor usually develops in children younger than 2 years of age and is frequently bilateral. Gonadoblastomas have also been reported.

A variety of variants of *WT1* have been found in **Denys-Drash syndrome**. *WT1* functions as a tumor suppressor gene and a transcription factor, and is expressed in the genital ridge and fetal gonads. One report found a zinc finger domain variant in the *WT1* alleles of a patient with no genitourinary abnormalities, suggesting that some cases of sporadic Wilms tumor may carry the *WT1* variant. Different pathogenic variants of the *WT1* gene, heterozygous variants at intron 9, have been described in **Frasier syndrome**, a condition of nonspecific focal and segmental glomerulosclerosis, 46,XY gonadal dysgenesis, and frequent gonadoblastoma, but without Wilms tumor.

WAGR syndrome is a contiguous gene deletion syndrome causing **W**ilms tumor, **A**niridia, **G**enitourinary malformations, and intellectual disability (**R**etardation). These children have a deletion of one copy of chromosome 11p13, which may be visible on karyotype analysis. The deleted region encompasses the aniridia gene (*PAX6*) and *WT1*. Only the 46,XY males have genital abnormalities, ranging from cryptorchidism to severe undervirilization. Gonadoblastomas have developed in the dysgenic gonads. Wilms tumor usually occurs by 2 years of age. Some cases also had unexplained obesity, raising the question of an obesity-associated gene in this region of chromosome 11 and naming the syndrome **WAGRO**.

Campomelic dysplasia. This form of short-limbed skeletal dysplasia is characterized by anterior bowing of the femur and tibia; small, bladeless scapulae; small thoracic cavities and 11 pairs of ribs; along with malformations of other organs. It is usually lethal in early infancy. About 75% of reported 46,XY patients exhibit a completely female phenotype with the external and internal genitalia both being female. Some 46,XY patients have atypical genitalia. The gonads appear to be ovaries but histologically may contain elements of both ovaries and testes.

The gene responsible for the condition is *SOX9* (SRY-related HMG-box gene). This gene is structurally related to *SRY* and also directly regulates type II collagen gene (*COL2A1*) development. There is phenotypic variability in that the same pathogenic variants may result in different gonadal phenotypes. Gonadoblastoma was reported in a patient with this condition. The inheritance is autosomal dominant.

Steroidogenic Factor 1 *(SF1)*

Adrenal insufficiency and 46,XY DSD have been described in patients with pathogenic variants of the *SF1* gene. In some patients, *SF1* variants occur without causing adrenal insufficiency. In a number of these families, if the mother shares the same *SF1* variant, she experiences premature ovarian insufficiency.

Other Known Genetic Causes of 46,XY DSD

46,XY DSD has been described in patients with other single-gene pathogenic variants, as well as deletions of parts of autosomal loci on chromosomes 2q, 9p, and 10q. A disorder with digenic inheritance involving coexistence of pathogenic variants in both *DMRT3* and *OAS3* has been described in a Taiwanese kindred. Examples of a number of these genetic conditions are shown in Table 26.4. The use of exome sequencing of targeted genes has enhanced the detection of specific genetic defects in patients with 46,XY DSD.

XY pure gonadal dysgenesis (Swyer syndrome). The designation *pure* distinguishes this condition from forms of gonadal dysgenesis that are of chromosomal origin and associated with somatic anomalies such as 45,X Turner syndrome and 47,XXY Klinefelter syndrome. Affected patients have normal stature as adults and a completely female phenotype at birth, including vagina, uterus, and fallopian tubes. At pubertal age, breast development and menarche fail to occur, and hypergonadotropic hypogonadism is present. None of the other phenotypic features associated with 45,X are present. Familial cases suggest an X-linked or a sex-limited dominant autosomal transmission. Most of the patients with a known genetic cause have had pathogenic variants of the *SRY* gene. The gonads consist of almost totally undifferentiated streaks despite the presence of a cytogenetically normal Y chromosome. The primitive gonad cannot accomplish any testicular function, including suppression of müllerian ducts. There may be hilar cells in the gonad capable of producing some androgens; accordingly, some virilization, such as clitoral enlargement, may occur at the age of puberty. The streak gonads may undergo neoplastic changes, such as **gonadoblastomas** and **dysgerminomas**, and should be removed as soon as the diagnosis is established, regardless of the age of the patient.

XY gonadal agenesis syndrome (embryonic testicular regression syndrome). In this rare syndrome, the external genitalia are slightly atypical but more nearly female. Hypoplasia of the labia; some degree of labioscrotal fusion; a small, clitoris-like phallus; and a perineal urethral opening are present. No uterus, no gonadal tissue, and usually no vagina can be found. At the age of puberty, no sexual development occurs and gonadotropin levels are elevated. Most children have been reared as females. In several patients with XY gonadal agenesis in whom no gonads could be found on exploration, significant rises in testosterone followed stimulation with hCG, indicating Leydig cell function somewhere. Siblings with the disorder are known.

It is presumed that testicular tissue was active long enough during fetal life for AMH to inhibit development of müllerian ducts but not long enough for testosterone production to result in virilization. Testicular degeneration seems to occur between the 8th and the 12th fetal week. Regression of the testes before the 8th week of gestation results in Swyer syndrome; between the 14th and the 20th week of gestation, it results in the rudimentary testis syndrome; and after the 20th week, it results in anorchia with otherwise normal external genitalia.

In **bilateral anorchia**, sometimes referred to as *vanishing testes syndrome*, testes are absent, but the male phenotype is complete; it is presumed that fetal testicular function was active during the critical period of genital differentiation but that sometime later it was damaged. Bilateral anorchia in identical twins and unilateral anorchia in identical twins and in siblings suggest a genetic predisposition. Coexistence of anorchia and the gonadal agenesis syndrome in a sibship is evidence for a relationship between the disorders.

Deficiency of Testicular Hormone Production

Genetic defects have been delineated in the enzymatic steps required for the synthesis of testosterone by the fetal testicular Leydig cells, and a defect in Leydig cell differentiation has also been described. These defects produce 46,XY males with incomplete masculinization. Because levels of testosterone are normally low before puberty except during the period of *minipuberty* at 1–2 months of age, an hCG stimulation test may be needed in children to assess the ability of the testes to synthesize testosterone.

Leydig cell aplasia. Patients with aplasia or hypoplasia of the Leydig cells usually have a female phenotype, but there may be mild virilization. Testes, epididymis, and vas deferens are present; the uterus and fallopian tubes are absent due to normal production of müllerian-inhibiting substance. There are no secondary sexual changes at puberty, but pubic hair may be normal. Plasma levels of testosterone are low and do increase with hCG stimulation; LH levels are elevated. The Leydig cells of the testes are absent or markedly deficient. The defect may involve a lack of receptors for LH. In children, hCG stimulation is necessary to differentiate the condition from the androgen insensitivity syndromes (AISs), as older children with AIS have low testosterone levels when prepubertal. There is male-limited autosomal recessive inheritance. The human LH receptor is a member of the G protein–coupled superfamily of receptors that contains seven transmembrane domains. Several inactivating pathogenic variants of the LH receptor have been described in males with hypogonadism suspected of having Leydig cell hypoplasia or aplasia.

Congenital adrenal hyperplasia. **CAH due to lipoid adrenal hyperplasia:** This is the most severe form of congenital adrenal hyperplasia, and it derives its name from the appearance of the enlarged adrenal glands resulting from accumulation of cholesterol and cholesterol esters. The rate-limiting process in steroidogenesis is the transport of free cholesterol through the cytosol to the inner mitochondrial membrane, where the P450 side-chain cleavage enzyme (CYP11A1) acts. Cholesterol transport into mitochondria is mediated by the steroidogenic acute regulatory protein (StAR) (see Fig. 26.5). Most patients with lipoid CAH have genetic variants of StAR. A minority have variants in CYP11A1.

All serum steroid levels are low or undetectable, and ACTH and PRA levels are very elevated. The phenotype is female in both genetic females and males. Genetic males have no müllerian structures because the testes can produce normal AMH but no steroid hormones. These children present with acute adrenal crisis and salt wasting in infancy. Most patients are 46,XY. In 46,XX patients with StAR defects, ovarian steroidogenesis can occur at puberty, as ovarian estrogen production does not require StAR. These 46,XX patients do not have DSD. All patients have a lifelong requirement for glucocorticoid and mineralocorticoid replacement therapy. Some patients will need estrogen replacement therapy, such as all 46,XX individuals with CYP11A1 pathogenic variants, as well as all 46,XY lipoid CAH patients. Intraabdominal testes should be removed due to the risk of future malignancy.

CAH due to 3β-hydroxysteroid dehydrogenase type II (HSD3B2) deficiency. 46,XY infants with this form of CAH have various degrees of hypospadias, with or without bifid scrotum and cryptorchidism and, rarely, a complete female phenotype. Affected infants usually develop salt-losing manifestations shortly after birth due to an inability to synthesize biologically potent steroid hormones (see Fig. 26.5). Incomplete defects, occasionally seen in infants without salt loss and in boys with premature pubarche, as well as late-onset nonclassic forms have been reported, but these forms do not cause DSD. As described earlier, patients with HSD3B2 deficiency have pathogenic variants involving the gene encoding type II 3β-hydroxysteroid enzyme, resulting in impairment of steroidogenesis in the adrenals and gonads. The impairment may be unequal between adrenals and gonads. Normal pubertal changes in some boys could be explained by the normally present type I 3β-hydroxysteroid dehydrogenase present in many peripheral tissues. Infertility is frequent. There is no correlation between degree of salt wasting and degree of phenotypic abnormality. Replacement therapy with adrenal steroids is required from infancy on, and with sex steroids at puberty. In 46,XY patients with intraabdominal testes who are being raised as females, gonadectomy is recommended.

CAH due to deficiency of 17-hydroxylase/17,20-lyase. A single enzyme (CYP17A1) encoded by a single gene has both 17-hydroxylase and 17,20-lyase activities in adrenal and gonadal tissues (see Fig. 26.5). Genetic males with CYP17A1 deficiency usually have a complete female phenotype or, less often, various degrees of undervirilization, from labioscrotal fusion to perineal hypospadias and cryptorchidism. Pubertal development fails to occur in both genetic sexes.

In the classic disorder, there is decreased synthesis of cortisol by the adrenals and of sex steroids by the adrenals and gonads. Levels of the mineralocorticoid DOC and corticosterone are markedly increased and lead to the hypertension and hypokalemia characteristic of this form of 46,XY DSD. Although levels of cortisol are low, the elevated ACTH and corticosterone levels prevent symptomatic cortisol deficiency. The renin-aldosterone axis is suppressed because of the strong mineralocorticoid effect of elevated DOC. Virilization does not occur at puberty; levels of testosterone are low, and those of gonadotropins are increased. Because fetal production of AMH is normal, no müllerian duct remnants are present. In 46,XY phenotypic females, removal of intraabdominal testes and replacement therapy with hydrocortisone and estrogenic sex steroids are indicated.

CYP17A1 deficiency has autosomal recessive inheritance. Affected 46,XX females are usually not detected until young adult life, when they fail to experience normal pubertal changes and are found to have hypertension and hypokalemia. This condition should be suspected in patients presenting with primary amenorrhea and hypertension whose chromosomal complement is either 46,XX or 46,XY.

Deficiency of 17-ketosteroid reductase. This enzyme, also called 17β-hydroxysteroid dehydrogenase (17β-HSD), catalyzes the final step in testosterone biosynthesis. It is necessary to convert androstenedione to testosterone and also DHEA to androstenediol, and estrone to estradiol (see Fig. 26.5). Enzymatic defects in the fetal testis give rise to males with complete or near-complete female phenotype in 46,XY patients. Müllerian ducts are absent, and a shallow vagina is present. The diagnosis is based on the ratio of androstenedione to testosterone; in prepubertal children a hCG stimulation test may be necessary to make the diagnosis.

The inheritance is autosomal recessive. At least four different types of 17β-HSD are recognized, each encoded by different genes on different chromosomes. Type III (HSD17B3) is the enzyme defect that is especially common in a highly inbred Arab population in Gaza. The gene for the disorder is expressed only in the testes, where it converts androstenedione to testosterone. Most patients are diagnosed at puberty because of virilization and the failure to menstruate. Testosterone levels at puberty may approach normal, presumably as a result of peripheral conversion of androstenedione to testosterone. Some patients spontaneously adopt a male gender role at puberty.

Type I 17β-HSD converts estrone to estradiol and is found in the placenta, ovary, testis, liver, prostate, adipose tissue, and endometrium. Type II, whose gene is on chromosome 16q24, reverses the reactions of types I and III (convert testosterone to androstenedione and estrone to estradiol, respectively). Type IV is similar in action to type II. A late-onset form of 17β-HSD deficiency presents as gynecomastia in young adult males.

Persistent müllerian duct syndrome. In this disorder, there is persistence of müllerian duct derivatives in otherwise completely virilized males. Cases have been reported in siblings and identical twins. Cryptorchidism is present in 80% of affected males; during surgery for this or inguinal hernia, the condition is uncovered when a fallopian tube and uterus are found. The degree of müllerian development is variable and may be asymmetric. Testicular function is normal in most, but testicular degeneration has been reported. Some affected males acquire testicular tumors after puberty. In a study of 38 families, 16 families had defects in the *AMH* gene. They had low blood AMH levels. In 16 families with high AMH levels, the defect was in the *AMH* type II receptor gene, with 10 of 16 having identical deletions.

Treatment consists of removal of as many of the müllerian structures as possible without causing damage to the testis, epididymis, or vas deferens.

Smith-Lemli-Opitz syndrome. Smith-Lemli-Opitz syndrome is an autosomal recessive disorder caused by variants in the sterol Δ7-reductase gene. This prevents normal androgen synthesis. It is characterized by prenatal and postnatal growth retardation, microcephaly, ptosis, anteverted nares, broad alveolar ridges, syndactyly of the second to third toes, and severe intellectual disability. Its incidence is 1/20,000–1/60,000; 70% are male. 46,XY patients usually have genital ambiguity or completely female external genitalia. Müllerian duct derivatives are usually absent. Affected 46,XX patients have normal genitalia. Patients with Smith-Lemli-Opitz syndrome may also develop adrenal insufficiency due to inability to produce sufficient steroid hormones.

Defects in Androgen Action

In the following group of disorders, fetal synthesis of testosterone is normal and defective virilization results from inherited abnormalities in androgen action.

Dihydrotestosterone deficiency. Deficiency of steroid 5α-reductase type II (SRD5A2): SRD5A2 deficiency prevents the conversion of testosterone to DHT in androgen target tissues. Decreased production of DHT in utero results in marked ambiguity of external genitalia of affected 46,XY infants because of the absolute requirement for DHT in completion of prenatal virilization. Biosynthesis and peripheral actions of testosterone are normal.

The phenotype commonly associated with this condition in boys consists of a small phallus, bifid scrotum, urogenital sinus with perineal hypospadias, and blind vaginal pouch (Fig. 26.8). Testes are in the inguinal canals or labioscrotal folds and are normal histologically. There are no müllerian structures. Wolffian (mesonephric) structures (i.e., the vas deferens, epididymis, and seminal vesicles) are present. Most affected patients have been assigned the female sex of rearing. At puberty, virilization occurs; the phallus enlarges, the testes descend and grow normally, and spermatogenesis occurs, as DHT is *not* required for normal virilization at puberty. There is no gynecomastia. Beard growth is scanty, acne is absent, the prostate is small, and recession of the temporal hairline fails to occur. The prenatal virilization of the

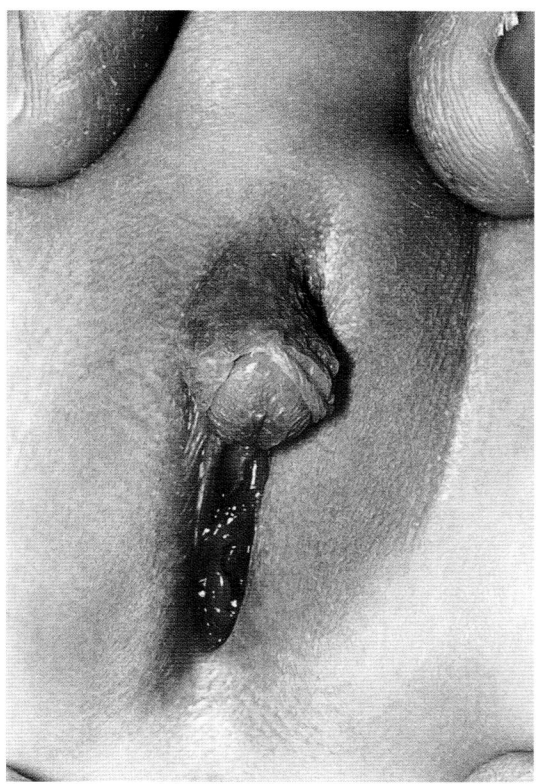

Fig. 26.8 5α-Reductase deficiency. (From Wales JKH, Wit JM, Rogol AD. *Pediatric Endocrinology and Growth.* 2nd ed. Philadelphia: Elsevier; 2003:165.)

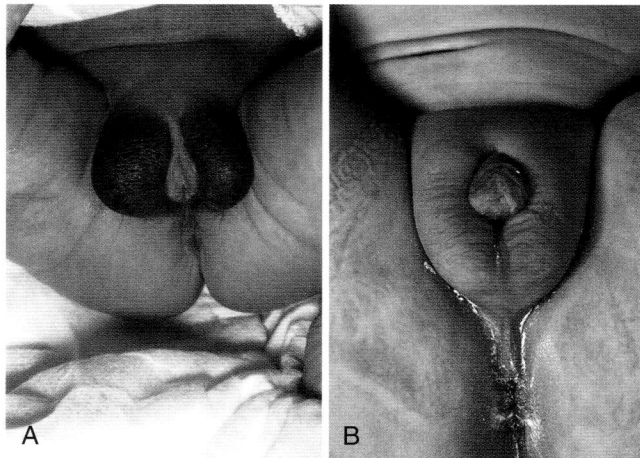

Fig. 26.9 *A,* Partial androgen insensitivity with descended testes in bifid labioscrotal folds. *B,* Less severe partial androgen insensitivity with severe hypospadias and maldescent of testes. (From Wales JKH, Wit JM, Rogol AD. *Pediatric Endocrinology and Growth.* 2nd ed. Philadelphia: Elsevier; 2003:165.)

wolffian ducts is caused by the action of locally produced testosterone itself, although masculinization of the urogenital sinus and external genitals depends on the action of DHT during the critical period of fetal masculinization. Growth of facial hair and of the prostate postnatally also appears to be DHT dependent.

Several different gene defects of SRD5A2 have been identified in patients from throughout the world. Familial clusters have been reported from the Dominican Republic, Turkey, Papua New Guinea, Brazil, Mexico, and the Middle East. There is no reliable correlation between genotype and phenotype.

The disorder is inherited as an autosomal recessive trait but expression is limited to males. Normal homozygous females with normal fertility indicate that in females DHT has no significant role in sex differentiation or in ovarian function later in life. The clinical diagnosis should be made as early as possible in infancy. It is important to distinguish this from partial androgen insensitivity syndrome (PAIS), as patients with PAIS are far less sensitive to androgen treatment than are patients with SRD5A2 deficiency. The biochemical diagnosis of SRD5A2 deficiency is based on finding normal serum testosterone levels and normal or low DHT levels with markedly increased basal and especially hCG-stimulated testosterone:DHT ratios (>17).

It is important to note that most but not all children with SRD5A2 deficiency reared as females in childhood have changed to identify as male around the time of puberty. It appears that exposures to testosterone in utero, early postnatally, and at puberty have variable contributions to the formation of their male gender identity. Much more needs to be learned about the influences of hormones such as androgens as well as the influences of cultural, social, psychologic, genetic, and other biologic factors in gender identity and behavior. Infants with

this condition should be reared as boys whenever practical. Treatment of male infants with DHT results in phallic enlargement. DHT is not commercially available in the United States but can be obtained from European suppliers.

Deficiency of 3α-reductase (AKRC): Another cause of DHT deficiency is a block in an alternative pathway of DHT synthesis (see Fig. 26.5). Patients previously thought to have 46,XY DSD due to isolated deficiency of the 17,20-lyase activity of CYP17A1 have subsequently been characterized as having variants in the *AKR1C2* gene (3α-reductase type III) or both the *AKR1C2* and *AKR1C4* (3α-reductase type IV) genes. These findings show that both the classical and alternative pathways to DHT production must be intact for normal prenatal virilization.

Androgen receptor defects: androgen insensitivity syndromes. The AISs are the **most common** forms of 46,XY DSD, occurring with an estimated frequency of 1/20,000 genetic males. This group of heterogeneous X-linked recessive disorders can result from 1 of more than 150 different variants described in the androgen receptor gene, located on Xq11-12: single point variants resulting in amino acid substitutions or premature stop codons, frameshift and premature terminations, gene deletions, and splice site variants. Post-receptor defects have also been described.

The clinical spectrum seen in patients with AIS, all of whom have a 46,XY chromosomal complement, range from phenotypic females (complete AIS or CAIS) to males with various forms of atypical genitalia and undervirilization (partial AIS or PAIS, as well as clinical syndromes such as Reifenstein syndrome) (Fig. 26.9) to phenotypically normal-appearing males with infertility. In addition to normal 46,XY chromosomes, the presence of testes and normal or elevated testosterone and LH levels are common to all such patients.

In CAIS, an extreme form of failure of virilization, genetic males appear female at birth and are invariably reared accordingly as their condition often goes undetected until childhood or adolescence. The external genitalia are female. The vagina ends blindly in a pouch, and the uterus is absent due to the normal production and effect of AMH by the testes. In about one third of patients, unilateral or bilateral fallopian tube remnants are found. The testes are usually intraabdominal but may descend into the inguinal canal; they consist largely of seminiferous tubules. At puberty, there is normal development of breasts, and the habitus is female, but menstruation does not occur and sexual hair is absent. Adult heights of these women are commensurate with those of normal males despite profound congenital deficiency of androgenic effects.

The testes of affected adult patients produce normal to elevated male levels of testosterone that are converted to normal levels of DHT. Failure of normal male external genitalia differentiation during fetal life reflects a defective response to androgens including DHT starting very early in gestation.

Prepubertal females with this disorder are often detected when inguinal masses prove to be testes or when a testis is unexpectedly found during inguinal herniorrhaphy. *About 1–2% of females with an inguinal hernia prove to have this disorder.* In infants, elevated LH levels should suggest the diagnosis. In older girls and adults, amenorrhea is the usual presenting symptom. In prepubertal children, the condition must be differentiated from other types of 46,XY undervirilized males in which there is complete feminization. These include 46,XY gonadal dysgenesis (Swyer syndrome), true agonadism, Leydig cell aplasia including LH receptor defects, and 17-ketosteroid reductase deficiency; all these conditions, unlike complete AIS, are characterized by low levels of testosterone as neonates and during adult life and by failure to respond to hCG during the prepubertal years. Although patients with complete AIS have unambiguously female external genitals at birth, those with partial AIS have a wide variety of phenotypic presentations ranging from perineoscrotal hypospadias, bifid scrotum, and cryptorchidism to extreme undervirilization appearing as clitoromegaly and labial fusion. Some forms of partial AIS have been known as specific syndromes. Patients with Reifenstein syndrome have incomplete virilization characterized by hypogonadism, severe hypospadias, and gynecomastia (Fig. 26.10). Gilbert-Dreyfus and Lubs are additional syndromes classified as partial AIS. In all cases, abnormalities in the androgen receptor gene or post-receptor defects have been identified.

The diagnosis of patients with partial AIS may be particularly difficult in infancy. The postnatal surge in testosterone and LH is diminished in those with CAIS but not in those with PAIS. In some, especially those sufficiently virilized in infancy, the diagnosis is not suspected until puberty when there is inadequate virilization with lack of facial hair or voice change and the appearance of unusually prominent gynecomastia. Azoospermia and infertility are common. Increasingly, androgen receptor defects are being recognized in adults who have a small phallus and testes and infertility. A single amino acid substitution in the androgen receptor was reported in a large Chinese family in whom some affected members were fertile while others had gynecomastia and/or hypospadias.

In children or young women with CAIS, the historical recommendation has been that testes should be removed prior to adult life, or as soon as they are discovered. *In one third of patients, malignant tumors, usually seminomas, develop by 50 years of age.* Several teenage females have acquired seminomas. Replacement therapy with estrogens is indicated at the age of puberty if the gonads were removed prior to this age. Some patients prefer to retain their gonads until after puberty has completed in order to mimic a more natural pubertal progression based on their own body's timing of gonadotropins.

Normal breasts develop in affected girls who have not had their testes removed by the age of puberty. In these individuals, production of estradiol results from aromatase activity on testicular testosterone. The absence of androgenic activity also contributes to the feminization of these women.

The psychosexual and surgical management of patients with PAIS is extremely complex and depends in large part on the presenting phenotype. Osteopenia is recognized as a late feature of AIS.

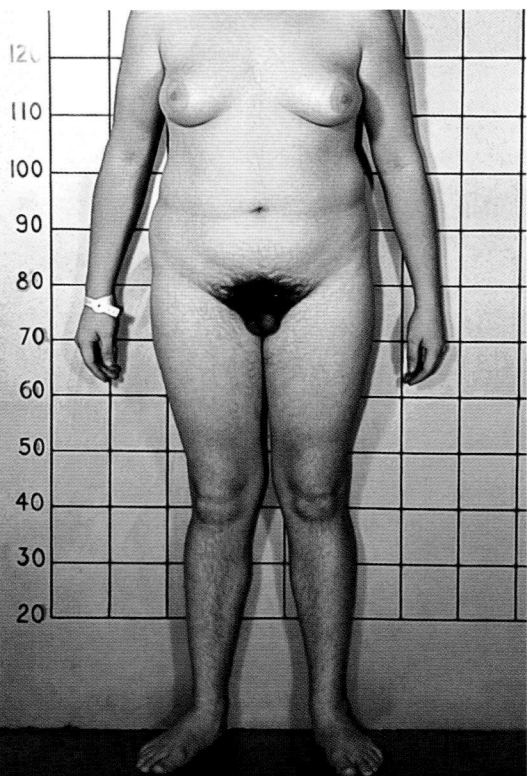

Fig. 26.10 Partial androgen insensitivity syndrome at adolescence, male sex of rearing. Note gynecomastia from peripheral aromatase conversion of testosterone to estradiol. Abundant pubic hair implies only partial resistance. (From Wales JKH, Wit JM, Rogol AD. *Pediatric Endocrinology and Growth.* 2nd ed. Philadelphia: Elsevier; 2003:165.)

Molecular analyses have suggested that phenotype may depend in part on somatic mosaicism of the androgen receptor gene. This was based on the case of a 46,XY patient who had a premature stop codon in exon 1 of the androgen receptor gene but who also had evidence of virilization (pubic hair and clitoral enlargement) explained by the discovery of the wild-type alleles on careful examination of the sequencing data. The presence of mosaicism shifts the phenotype to a higher degree of virilization than expected from the genotype of the mutant allele alone. Genetic counseling is thus challenging in families with androgen receptor gene variants. In addition to lack of genotype-phenotype correlations, there is a high rate (27%) of de novo pathogenic variants in families.

The degree of sex hormone–binding globulin reduction after exogenous androgen administration (stanozolol) has been shown to correlate with the severity of the receptor defect and may become a useful clinical tool. Successful therapy with supplemental androgens has been reported in patients with PAIS and various pathogenic variants of the androgen receptor in the DNA-binding domain and the ligand-binding domain.

Affected androgen receptors are also reported in patients with spinal and bulbar muscular atrophy in whom clinical manifestations including testicular atrophy, infertility, gynecomastia, and elevated LH, FSH, and estradiol levels usually manifest between the 3rd and 5th decades of life. Androgen receptor pathogenic variants have also been described in patients with prostate cancer.

Undetermined Causes of 46,XY Disorders of Sex Development

Other 46,XY undervirilized males display great variability of the external and internal genitalia and various degrees of phallic and müllerian development. Testes may be histologically normal or rudimentary, or there may only be one testis. Other complex genetic syndromes, many resulting from single-gene variants, are associated with varying degrees of ambiguity of the genitalia, particularly in the male. These entities must be identified on the basis of the associated extragenital malformations. Examples include **bladder exstrophy** and **Eagle-Barrett syndrome** (formerly known as prune-belly syndrome). Another such complex syndrome is termed ATRX or X-linked α thalassemia with intellectual disability and genital abnormalities.

Ovotesticular Disorders of Sex Development

In ovotesticular DSD, both ovarian and testicular tissues are present, either in the same or in opposite gonads. Affected patients have ambiguous genitalia, varying from normal female with only slight enlargement of the clitoris to almost normal male external genitalia.

About 70% of all patients have a 46,XX karyotype. Ninety-seven percent of affected patients of African descent are 46,XX. Fewer than 10% of persons with ovotesticular DSD are 46,XY. About 20% have 46,XX/46,XY mosaicism. Half of these are derived from more than one zygote and are chimeras (chi 46,XX/46,XY). The presence of both paternal and maternal alleles for some blood groups are demonstrated. An ovotesticular DSD chimera, 46,XX/46,XY, was reported as resulting from embryo amalgamation after in vitro fertilization. Each embryo was derived from an independent, separately fertilized ovum.

Examination of 46,XX ovotesticular DSD patients with Y-specific probes has detected fewer than 10% with a portion of the Y chromosome including the *SRY* gene. Ovotesticular DSD is usually sporadic, but a number of siblings have been reported. The cause of most cases of ovotesticular DSD is unknown.

The most frequently encountered gonad in ovotesticular DSD is an ovotestis, which may be bilateral. If unilateral, the contralateral gonad is usually an ovary but may be a testis. The ovarian tissue is often normal, but the testicular tissue is usually dysgenic. The presence and function of testicular tissue can be determined by measuring basal and hCG-stimulated testosterone levels as well as AMH levels. Patients who are highly virilized and have had adequate testicular function with no uterus are usually reared as males. If a uterus exists, virilization is often mild and testicular function minimal; assignment of female sex may be indicated. Selective removal of gonadal tissue inconsistent with sex of rearing may be possible; however, it should be noted that microscopic remnants of the undesired gonad may be present and become hormonally active during puberty. In a few families, 46,XY ovotesticular DSD subjects and 46,XX males have been described in the same sibship.

Defects in the ovarian developmental protein R-spondin 1, encoded by the *RSPO1* gene, have also been described in 46,XX ovotesticular DSD.

Pregnancies with living offspring have been reported in 46,XX ovotesticular DSD individuals reared as females, but very few males with ovotesticular DSD have fathered children. About 5% of patients will develop gonadoblastomas, dysgerminomas, or seminomas.

Sex Chromosome Disorders of Sex Development

Some ambiguity of the genitalia is associated with a wide variety of chromosomal aberrations (see Table 26.2), which must always be considered in the differential diagnosis, the most common being the 45,X/46,XY syndrome. It may be necessary to karyotype several tissues to establish mosaicism. The phenotype in 45,X/46,XY individuals may vary from completely female to completely male, and it is reported that there are probably a large number of patients who are never detected and are raised as normal males.

Other conditions included in the broad category of sex chromosome DSD include 45,X Turner syndrome and 47,XXY Klinefelter syndrome, due to their associated gonadal failure. However, patients with these conditions have normal external genitalia at birth.

▌ RED FLAGS

Danger signs include manifestations of adrenal insufficiency, in addition to a male phenotype without a palpable testis in the scrotum, hyperpigmentation (increased ACTH production), and hypertension. Although normal at birth, male patients with CAH may experience an adrenal crisis once circulating placental-maternal steroid hormones are catabolized and excreted. This phenomenon often occurs between the 3rd and 10th days of life. The initial diagnosis in the male with salt-losing CAH may be sepsis, pyloric stenosis, meningitis, or other more common neonatal conditions.

BIBLIOGRAPHY

A bibliography is available at ExpertConsult.com.

27

Intellectual Developmental Disorders (Developmental Delay)

Mark Simms

DEFINITIONS

Intellectual disability (ID) has replaced the older term mental retardation (MR), reflecting a more enlightened and progressive attitude toward individuals with disabilities, both physical and cognitive. ID is characterized by significant limitations in intellectual functioning and in adaptive behavior that begin before age 18 years and are expressed in conceptual, social, and practical adaptive skills. The impairments of ID extend beyond what is measured on a standardized test of intelligence and must take into account the context of an individual's typical environment and their cultural and linguistic backgrounds. Adaptive functioning includes three broad domains: conceptual, social, and practical. The **conceptual domain** involves academic competence, the acquisition of practical knowledge, and judgment in novel situations. The **social domain** involves awareness of others' thoughts and feelings, empathy, friendships, and social judgment. The **practical domain** involves the ability to manage one's own affairs, including school and work responsibilities, money management, and recreation (Table 27.1). Although ID is a lifelong condition, it is recognized that "with appropriate personalized supports over a sustained period, the life functioning of the person with intellectual disability generally will improve." In a long-term study comparing ID and non-ID siblings, those with mild ID (intelligence quotient [IQ] between 64 and 75) were just as likely to find stable employment, to have similar total family incomes, to have stable marriages, and to raise children as their siblings. However, they reported higher rates of psychologic distress and lower rates of participation in formal organizations. Table 27.2 provides descriptions of typical adult functioning in individuals with varying degrees of ID.

The term **developmental disability** includes a diverse group of lifelong physical and mental impairments that negatively affect an individual's ability to function as well as their peers. These conditions begin during childhood (before 22 years of age) and interfere with mobility, acquisition of self-care ability, communication skills, social skills, general learning ability, and independent living. The specific types of conditions and categories of disabilities vary widely. The National Institute for Child Health and Development (NICHD) includes the following conditions: neurologic disorders: cerebral palsy, muscular dystrophy, epilepsy, genetic syndromes, autism, and degenerative disorders; sensory disorders: blindness and deafness; metabolic disorders: phenylketonuria (PKU); and cognitive disorders: intellectual impairment, learning disabilities, and attention-deficit/hyperactivity disorder (ADHD). Developmental disabilities may be isolated, as in a child with impaired vision, or

may be multiple, as in a child with delays in motor, cognitive, language, and social functioning. There may be considerable overlap in specific disorders in terms of the affected functions (Fig. 27.1). In young children, developmental delays may result from a wide range of causes, including early environmental understimulation, chronic physical illness, neuromuscular disorders, central nervous system (CNS) abnormalities, and genetic syndromes (Tables 27.3 and 27.4). Some etiologies are fully or partly amenable to early educational and medical interventions, while others may lead to permanent intellectual impairment or progressive deterioration of functioning. Therefore, until a young child has had the benefit of early intervention services and has matured to the point where formal cognitive, language, and adaptive measures are stable and predictive of future functioning, the descriptive term **global developmental delay** (GDD) is preferred.

EPIDEMIOLOGY

Intellectual Disability

The overall prevalence of ID varies from 1% to 3%, depending on the criteria used and the age of the individual at the time of evaluation. Standardized tests of intelligence have a mean of 100 and standard deviation of 15 points. Statistically, 2.5% of individuals should have an IQ score below 2 standard deviations (70 points) and fit the cognitive criterion for ID. However, because the standard error of measurement is approximately 5 points, extending the IQ score upward to 75 points would almost double the prevalence of ID. This might be countered by secondary criteria involving deficits in adaptive behaviors, since many children with IQ scores in the mildly low range (55–70) will not qualify for a diagnosis of ID because they have adequate adaptive functioning. Many studies have documented a higher rate of mild ID in economically disadvantaged children that stems from a few highly significant sociodemographic risk factors.

Developmental Disability

Developmental disabilities affect approximately one in six children in the United States (16.9%). The prevalence rates vary by specific condition: ADHD (9.54%), learning disability (7.86%), autism (2.49%), and ID (1.17%) are the most common, while epilepsy, deafness, cerebral palsy, and blindness each affect <1%. Males have more than twice the prevalence of any developmental disability, and children insured by Medicaid have a prevalence of disability that is approximately 1½ times greater than those with private insurance. The overall prevalence of disability increased by 9.5% between 2009–2011 and 2015–2017, mostly due to a 122.3% increase in autism (from 1.12% to 2.49%). In addition, the prevalence of ID increased 25.8% (from 0.93% to 1.17%).

Table 27.3 lists the prevalences of selected conditions.

DIAGNOSIS

Identification of a specific cause for delayed development in a child is important and may provide insight into prognosis, recurrence risk, therapies, counseling, and linkage with a supportive group. Identification of the child's functional abilities, strengths and weaknesses, overall physical health, and environmental factors is critical for optimizing the child's health, development, and functioning. In addition, the origin of developmental disability is not apparent in many children, or there may be multiple possible causal factors or multiple disabilities present. For example, 23% of children with developmental disabilities have two disabilities, and 6% have three or more. Even if a specific diagnosis cannot be made,

early identification of developmental delay can lead to a program of early intervention or remediation that may improve the child's ultimate functioning. To identify those disorders that are amenable to intervention, an international consortium has developed both a web-based tool and a mobile application (app) to assist practitioners in the evaluation and management of children with ID (http://www.treatable-id.org/).

IDENTIFICATION

Children who experience significant complications in the perinatal period or who are born with obvious congenital anomalies are at risk for developmental disabilities. In addition, newborn screening programs may identify children with rare but significant problems who require early treatments and interventions. Children with no apparent risk factors or obvious physical or neurologic symptoms may be identified through a process of surveillance and screening during routine child health care visits.

Developmental Risk Factors

Young children's development may be adversely affected by biologic and/or sociocultural risk factors (Table 27.5). Many risk factors can be graded according to severity (e.g., degree of prematurity, intracranial hemorrhage, intrauterine growth restriction), but it is often the cumulative effect of multiple factors that ultimately determines a child's developmental outcome, even when one or more "severe" risks are present. It has been shown that low 5-minute Apgar scores, in the absence of other symptoms of neonatal encephalopathy, may correlate poorly with long-term neurologic dysfunction. Sociocultural risks also can have profound effects on development and may interact with biologic

TABLE 27.1   Diagnosis of Intellectual Disability

Diagnostic Criteria

All Three Criteria Must Be Met

A. Deficits in intellectual function, such as reasoning, problem solving, planning, abstract thinking, judgment, academic learning, and learning from experience, confirmed by both clinical assessment and individualized standardized testing.

B. Deficits in adaptive functioning that result in failure to meet developmental and sociocultural standards for personal independence and social responsibility. Without ongoing support, the adaptive deficits limit functioning in one or more activities of daily life, such as communication, social participation, and independent living, across multiple environments, such as home, school, work, and community.

C. Onset of intellectual and adaptive deficits during the developmental period.

Assumptions

1. Assessments performed on the child are sensitive to differences in culture, language, communication, and behavior.
2. The demands and constraints of the child's environment (home, neighborhood, school) must be considered.
3. Even children with limitations have strengths that should be considered.

Data from American Psychiatric Association. *Diagnostic and Statistical Manual of Mental Disorders (DSM-V)*. 5th ed. Arlington, VA: American Psychiatric Association; 2013.

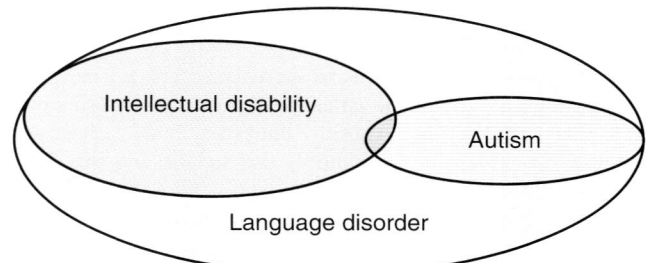

Fig. 27.1 Relationship of autism, language disorders, and intellectual disability. (Modified from Simms MD, Schum RL. Preschool children who have atypical patterns of development. *Pediatr Rev*. 2000;21:147–158.)

TABLE 27.2   Severity of Intellectual Disability and Adult Age Functioning

Level	Mental Age as an Adult*	Adult Adaptation
Mild	9–11 yr	Reads at fourth- to fifth-grade level; simple multiplication/division; writes simple letters, lists; completes job applications; basic independent job skills (arrive on time, stay at task, interact with coworkers); uses public transportation, may qualify for driver's license; keeps house, cooks using recipes
Moderate	6–8 yr	Sight-word reading; copies information, e.g., address from card to job application; matches written number to number of items; recognizes time on clock; communicates; some independence in self-care; housekeeping with supervision or cue cards; meal preparation, can follow picture recipe cards; job skills learned with much repetition; uses public transportation with some supervision
Severe	3–5 yr	Needs continuous support and supervision; may communicate wants and needs, sometimes with augmentative communication techniques
Profound	<3 yr	Limitations of self-care, continence, communication, and mobility; may need complete custodial or nursing care

*International Statistical Classification of Diseases and Related Health Problems. 10th revision. World Health Organization; 2010.
From Schum RL. Grand Rounds Presentation at Children's Hospital of Wisconsin; 2003.

TABLE 27.3   Prevalence of Select Conditions Associated with Developmental Delay

Condition	Prevalence/100,000	Comments
Cerebral palsy	250–270	Represents many causes
Significant hearing loss	150	In neonatal period
Down syndrome	98–125	Prevalence at birth
Fragile X syndrome	117	Predominantly in boys
Meningomyelocele	60–100	Prevalence at birth
Klinefelter syndrome	100	15% have intelligence quotient (IQ) <80
Fetal alcohol syndrome	60–800	Present at birth
Congenital HIV infection	5–50	Preventable with maternal and neonatal therapy
Blindness	41–88	Syndromic, genetic, prematurity risks
Infantile hydrocephalus	64	Prevalence at birth
Neurofibromatosis	33	5% have intellectual disability
Trisomy 18	30	Prevalence at birth
Trisomy 13	20	Prevalence at birth
Turner syndrome	20	IQ may be normal
Prader-Willi syndrome	13–20	In childhood
Galactosemia	14	In infancy
Phenylketonuria	6–12	In infancy
Anophthalmia	6	Consider other anomalies
Rett syndrome	4–5	In females 2–18 yr of age
Histidinemia	3	At birth
Acrocephalosyndactylia (Apert syndrome)	1–2	Present at birth

risk factors to create a greater effect than any single factor alone (so-called "double jeopardy").

Developmental Protective Factors

During the process of developmental surveillance, the clinician should identify and acknowledge the influence of protective and supportive factors that may contribute to positive outcomes. Barring catastrophic circumstances, child-rearing conditions that support and enrich early development may compensate for biologic deficits. Sociocultural factors, such as small family size, higher level of parental education, and fewer changes in residence, have a more powerful positive effect than many biologic risks and seem to be important predictors of developmental functioning beyond infancy. The brains of infants and young children are remarkably resilient and normal cognitive and language outcomes are often seen, even in the face of perinatal stroke or similar focal brain injuries. Neural plasticity also extends to situations of extreme environmental deprivation, providing interventions occur early enough. In addition, preschool early intervention programs that are designed to mitigate the factors that place children at risk for poor outcomes have been shown to have significant short- and long-term educational, behavioral, and economic benefits.

SCREENING FOR SPECIFIC ABNORMALITIES

Deficits in vision, hearing, and language can have devastating effects on development; early intervention to ameliorate these problems can improve outcomes. *All children should be screened on a regular basis for these conditions.*

Visual Deficits

Children at high risk for development of deficits in vision (see Chapter 43) include those with strabismus (especially after 4 months of age), hydrocephalus, congenital infection, neonatal encephalopathy, congenital anomaly of the CNS, prematurity with exposure to oxygen, and

TABLE 27.4   Identification of Cause in Children with Significant Intellectual Disability

Cause	Examples	% of Total
Chromosomal disorder	Trisomies 21, 18, 13 Deletions 1p36, 4p, 5p, 11p, 12q, 17p Microdeletions Klinefelter, 47,XXX, and Turner syndromes	~20
Genetic syndrome	Fragile X, Prader-Willi, Angelman, and Rett syndromes	~20
Nonsyndromic autosomal mutations	Variations in copy number; de novo mutations in *SYNGAP1, GRIK2, TUSC3,* oligosaccharyl transferase, and others	~10
Developmental brain abnormality	Hydrocephalus ± meningomyelocele; schizencephaly, lissencephaly	~8
Inborn errors of metabolism or neurodegenerative disorder	Phenylketonuria, Tay-Sachs disease, various storage diseases	~7
Congenital infections	HIV, toxoplasmosis, rubella, cytomegalovirus, syphilis, herpes simplex, Zika virus	~3
Familial intellectual disability	Environment, syndromic, or genetic	~5
Perinatal causes	Hypoxic-ischemic encephalopathy, meningitis, intraventricular hemorrhage, periventricular leukomalacia, fetal alcohol syndrome	4
Postnatal causes	Trauma (abuse), meningitis, hypothyroidism	~4
Unknown		20

From Kliegman RM, St. Geme J. *Nelson Textbook of Pediatrics.* 21st ed. Vol 1. Philadelphia: Elsevier; 2020:284, Table 53.1.

TABLE 27.5   Risk Factors for Developmental Disabilities

Biologic	Sociocultural
Male	Low parental education
Maternal age above 30 yr old	Maternal depression
Multiple pregnancies	Maternal substance abuse
High birth order	Low socioeconomic status
Preterm birth	Lack of prenatal care
Low birthweight (<750 g)	Inadequate environmental stimulation
Intrauterine growth restriction	
Small head circumference	
Brain malformations	
Holoprosencephaly	
Schizencephaly	
Lissencephaly	
Neonatal complications	
Neonatal encephalopathy	
Intracranial hemorrhage	
Symptomatic hypoglycemia	
Severe hyperbilirubinemia	
Congenital infections	
Acquired central nervous system infections	
Iron and iodine deficiencies	
Brain injury	
Malnutrition	

TABLE 27.6   Risk Indicators Associated with Permanent Congenital, Delayed-Onset, and/or Progressive Hearing Loss in Children

1. Caregiver concern* regarding hearing, speech, language, or developmental delay
2. Family history* of permanent childhood hearing loss
3. Neonatal intensive care stay of >5 days or any of the following, regardless of length of stay: ECMO,* assisted ventilation, exposure to ototoxic medications (gentamicin and tobramycin) or loop diuretics (furosemide/Lasix), and hyperbilirubinemia that requires exchange transfusion
4. In utero infections such as CMV,* herpes, rubella, syphilis, Zika virus, and toxoplasmosis
5. Craniofacial anomalies, including those that involve the pinna, ear canal, ear tags, ear pits, and temporal bone anomalies
6. Physical findings, such as a white forelock, that are associated with a syndrome known to include sensorineural or permanent conductive hearing loss
7. Syndromes associated with hearing loss or progressive or late-onset hearing loss,* such as neurofibromatosis, osteopetrosis, and Usher syndromes; other frequently identified syndromes include Waardenburg, Alport, Pendred, and Jervell and Lange-Nielsen
8. Neurodegenerative disorders* such as Hunter syndrome or sensory motor neuropathies such as Friedreich ataxia and Charcot-Marie-Tooth syndrome
9. Culture-positive postnatal infections associated with sensorineural hearing loss,* including confirmed bacterial and viral (especially herpes viruses and varicella) meningitis
10. Head trauma, especially basal skull/temporal bone fracture* that requires hospitalization
11. Chemotherapy*
12. Recurrent or persistent otitis media for at least 3 mo

CMV, cytomegalovirus; ECMO, extracorporeal membrane oxygenation.
*Risk indicators that are of greater concern for delayed-onset hearing loss.
From American Academy of Pediatrics, Joint Committee on Infant Hearing. *Pediatrics.* 2007;120(4):898–921.

family history of a childhood onset of visual impairment. All neonates should routinely undergo an evaluation of their fundi for the presence of a red reflex, which can be obscured by cataract or tumor, as well as inspection of the globe, which may be enlarged by congenital glaucoma. Infants with nystagmus who do not follow (tract) visually by 3 months of age, who have dissociation between visual behavior and motor behavior, or whose parents express concern about their vision should undergo a formal ophthalmologic evaluation.

Preschool children should undergo periodic evaluations of extraocular movements to rule out strabismus and amblyopia; the evaluation should include visual inspection of the child's eyes, the Hirschberg light test, and the cover-uncover test. As early in the child's development as possible, specific tests of monocular and binocular vision such as Allen cards (3–5 years), the Snellen chart (>5 years), or the Titmus test (>4 years) should be performed.

Loss of Hearing

Early detection of hearing loss is critical for optimizing the language development of these children. Universal newborn hearing screening programs (UNHSPs) can detect infants born with moderate, severe, or profound bilateral hearing impairment. Although the prevalence of congenital deafness is low in the general population (1–3/1,000 infants), it is higher in infants who require neonatal intensive care services (2–4/100 infants). More than half of babies with permanent congenital hearing impairment do not have prospectively identifiable risk factors and would be missed without UNHSPs. They would not receive hearing intervention within the first 6 months of life, a period that is critical for speech, language, and later learning development. Hearing loss can be acquired during infancy or childhood from infection (cytomegalovirus [CMV], meningitis), trauma (particularly basal skull and temporal bone fractures), ototoxic drugs (aminoglycosides, furosemide), or damaging noise levels. A number

of **genetic syndromes** are associated with deafness (Waardenburg, Alport, Pendred, and Jervell and Lange-Nielsen), and progressive or late-onset hearing loss can occur in neurofibromatosis, Usher syndromes, Hunter syndrome, Friedreich ataxia, or Charcot-Marie-Tooth syndrome (Table 27.6). Children with one or more "risk factors" should have hearing screening again at 24–30 months, even if they passed the newborn screening test. In addition, parental concern about hearing loss has a sensitivity of approximately 44%. If parents express concern about their child's ability to hear and if the child has had recurrent episodes of otitis media, mastoiditis, or one of the perinatal or familial risk factors, a formal audiometric screening should be performed. Table 27.7 lists the latest acceptable age ("limit ages") for the appearance of skills related to hearing; absence of these milestones may indicate a disorder of hearing. *Deaf infants may smile, coo, and babble; however, their vocalizations usually cease after 8 months of age.*

Speech and Language Disorders

Disorders of speech and language development, prevalent in 3–20% of preschool children, are the most common reason for referral to early intervention programs and are correlated with subsequent learning problems. Speech refers to the mechanics of oral communication (sound production); language includes the understanding, processing, and production of communication (words). Speech problems may include articulation (pronunciation) deficits (phonologic or apraxic speech disorders), fluency disorders (stuttering), or unusual voice quality. Language delays may be confined to expression with normal receptive abilities or may involve both expressive and receptive abilities. Language delays may be a feature of GDD/ID, autism spectrum disorders (ASDs), or hearing impairment, or may be the result of an isolated disorder (specific language impairment).

Children with speech and language delays often experience emotional and social adjustment difficulties related to their inability to communicate effectively with parents and peers. In general, children with normal comprehension of language and normal nonverbal cognitive abilities have an excellent prognosis, while those with receptive delays are at risk for language-based learning disabilities (reading comprehension and writing disorders) (Table 27.8).

TABLE 27.7 Latest Acceptable Age for Skills Related to Hearing*

Age (mo)[†]	Activity
3	Not startling to loud sounds
6	Not smiling to voice; not vocalizing
9	Does not localize speech or other sounds
12	Not babbling multiple sounds and syllables
18	No words
24	<50% of speech understandable

*A child who does not demonstrate the activity by the stated age should have formal audiometry performed.
[†]Corrected for gestational age.
Modified from the Arizona Speech, Language, Hearing Association.

TABLE 27.8 Speech-Language Screening for Pediatricians

Refer for a Speech-Language Evaluation If:

At Age	Receptive	Expressive
15 mo	Does not look/point at 5–10 objects/people named by a parent	Not using three words
18 mo	Does not follow simple directions ("Get your shoes")	Not using Mama, Dada, or other names
24 mo	Does not point to pictures or body parts when they are named	Not using 25 words
30 mo	Does not verbally respond or nod/shake head to questions	Not using unique two-word phrases, including noun-verb combinations
36 mo	Does not understand prepositions or action words; does not follow two-step directions	Vocabulary <200 words; does not ask for things by name; echolalia to questions; regression of language after acquiring two-word phrases

From Schum RL. Language screening in the pediatric office setting. *Pediatr Clin North Am.* 2007;54:425–436.

Prenatal and Newborn Screening Programs

Prenatal Screening

Prenatal screening has undergone significant changes with the advent of next-generation sequencing (NGS) technologies. The traditional screening takes the form of biochemical and ultrasound tests, which may detect fetuses at high risk for chromosome anomalies and neural tube defects. In the first trimester (11–14 weeks' gestation), measurement of maternal serum levels of human chorionic gonadotropin (hCG) and pregnancy-associated plasma protein A (PAPP-A) and a sonogram measurement of the fluid underneath the skin along the back of the fetus's neck (nuchal translucency) may identify Down syndrome, trisomy 13, or trisomy 18. In the second trimester (15–22 weeks' gestation), a quad screen (α-fetoprotein, hCG, estriol, and inhibin A levels) may identify Down syndrome and neural tube defects (spina bifida, encephalocele). An abnormal result on these screenings is typically followed by high-resolution ultrasonography, chorionic villus sampling or amniocentesis, genetic testing (chromosome analysis or microarray), and genetic counseling. NGS technologies allow for noninvasive prenatal screening (NIPS) on maternal blood samples, also called *cell-free* fetal DNA prenatal screening. These technologies identify possible chromosomal and microdeletion disorders through maternal blood screening. If an abnormality is detected, a confirmatory test is still required through more invasive techniques such as amniocentesis. In addition, prenatal genetic carrier screening can be performed for a large number of disorders; at present, these are the only standard of care for individuals at high risk for certain genetic conditions (e.g., Tay-Sachs).

Newborn Screening

Uniform newborn screening is highly successful in identifying children with rare but serious conditions who can benefit from early intervention. All 50 states, U.S. territories, and the U.S. military routinely test for inborn errors of metabolism (IEMs), congenital hypothyroidism, congenital adrenal hyperplasia, severe T-cell immunodeficiency (SCID), cystic fibrosis, and hemoglobinopathies. Test samples should be collected between 24 and 48 hours of age, but results may be influenced by a variety of maternal and infant factors. Tests for congenital adrenal hyperplasia are sensitive to the weight of the infant and the use of steroids. Screening for hypothyroidism (thyroid-stimulating hormone [TSH]) may be falsely low in premature or low birthweight infants. The use of antibiotics and total parenteral nutrition (TPN) may interfere with interpretation of newborn metabolic screening tests. While all states screen for a "core panel" of 29 conditions, they vary in testing for other conditions. An additional 26 conditions have been recommended for inclusion in the U.S. Health and Human Services Recommended Uniform Screening Panel. Normal newborn screening test results do not eliminate the possibility that a clinically symptomatic child could have one of the disorders in the state's panel.

IDENTIFICATION OF CHILDREN WITH DEVELOPMENTAL DISABILITIES IN PRIMARY HEALTH CARE SETTINGS

Not all developmentally disabling conditions can be identified at or shortly after birth through newborn screening programs. Many disorders may not manifest until children are preschool or school age, and some infrequent disorders cause regression or deterioration of function beginning at different ages (Table 27.9). Therefore, identification of children with developmental disabilities is a continuous process that should take place throughout childhood.

TABLE 27.9 Common Presentations of Intellectual Disability by Age

Age	Area of Concern
Newborn	Dysmorphic syndromes (multiple congenital anomalies), microcephaly Major organ system dysfunction (e.g., feeding, breathing)
Early infancy (2–4 mo)	Failure to interact with the environment Concerns about vision and hearing impairments
Later infancy (6–18 mo)	Gross motor delay
Toddlers (2–3 yr)	Language delays or difficulties
Preschool (3–5 yr)	Language difficulties or delays Behavior difficulties, including play Delays in fine motor skills: cutting, coloring, drawing
School age (>5 yr)	Academic underachievement Behavior difficulties (e.g., attention, anxiety, mood, conduct)

From Kliegman RM, St. Geme J. *Nelson Textbook of Pediatrics.* 21st ed. Vol 1. Philadelphia: Elsevier; 2020:287, Table 53.4.

Parents, caretakers, or teachers who have concerns about the child's behavior or failure to meet age-appropriate developmental expectations often identify children with developmental disabilities. Multiple studies have found parental concern to identify correctly 74–80% of preschool-age children (0–6 years old) with cognitive delays, speech and language delays, and learning disabilities. Conversely, the absence of parental concern correctly identified 70–80% of children without a significant disability. Thus, reliance on parental concern alone as a means of identification matches acceptable standards for more formal developmental screening tests. However, sole reliance on parental concerns will miss a substantial number of children with developmental concerns, especially those with more subtle disabilities, for a variety of reasons. Parents may be unaware of their child's delays, they may lack the confidence to raise their concerns to the health care provider, or the provider may dismiss these concerns and not pursue further investigation. Children without obvious physical impairments may not be identified until they enter a formal school program. Complicating matters further, children with developmental disabilities may experience significant behavioral or emotional difficulties that "mask" (or distract from) their underlying developmental difficulties.

Developmental Screening

Developmental screening involves the routine application of a brief standardized tool when there is no obvious concern. Physicians often rely on their own clinical judgment, which detects fewer than 30% of children with significant developmental disabilities, or on informal and nonstandardized lists of developmental milestones. A more practical and widely accepted alternative is the use of parent-completed developmental questionnaires, such as the Ages and Stages Questionnaire (ASQ) or the Parents' Evaluations of Developmental Status (PEDS) that can be scored by nonphysician staff and interpreted by the health care provider.

Developmental Surveillance

Developmental surveillance is a "flexible, continuous process whereby knowledgeable professionals perform skilled observations of children throughout all encounters during child health care." The goal of developmental surveillance is to identify children who may benefit from further diagnostic evaluations and early intervention services. To be effective, surveillance requires clinicians to be knowledgeable about child development and to recognize both variations of and deviations from normal patterns. Identification of children in need of further evaluation is believed to be improved by incorporating into the process developmental risk factors based on the child's medical history and family history, as well as social and environmental circumstances. Additionally, clinicians are encouraged to include the observations and impressions of preschool teachers, public health nurses, and other professionals involved in the child's care.

A combination of both developmental surveillance at every well-child visit and standardized developmental screening at the 9-, 18-, and 30-month visits is recommended (Fig. 27.2). At any point in this process, children who elicit concern about their development should be referred for further diagnostic evaluations and for early intervention and educational programs.

COMPREHENSIVE DEVELOPMENTAL ASSESSMENT

Children identified with developmental delays should receive a comprehensive, multidisciplinary evaluation including assessments of neurodevelopmental, cognitive, and communication functioning. These assessments should focus both on the child's strengths and functional abilities and on weaknesses and disabilities. Based on the findings from these evaluations, further subspecialty consultations (e.g., neurology, genetics, physical medicine and rehabilitation, ophthalmology, occupational and physical therapy, speech therapy) can be arranged, and a plan for specific laboratory investigations developed. The goals of the evaluations are to identify a specific etiologic diagnosis, prognosis, recurrence risk, and interventions to promote the child's optimal development. Parents may also benefit from associating with a disease-specific support group.

Neurodevelopmental Pediatric Assessment

History

Pediatric evaluation of a child with GDD or ID consists of a complete history and physical examination. Schedule the evaluation as a separate visit with sufficient uninterrupted time (at least 45–60 minutes) to focus on issues related to the child's behavior and development. Unless the child's and family's histories are well known to the provider, parents can be asked to complete detailed history questionnaires and developmental and behavioral rating scales, and to provide any additional information from outside sources (e.g., prior medical records, consultation reports, educational evaluations) prior to this visit that will contribute to assembling a complete record of the child's care. Previsit preparation may help parents to refresh their memory regarding their child's development and to focus their questions and concerns during the evaluation.

Many disabilities have their origin in the prenatal period, so the pregnancy and birth history are reviewed carefully for possible developmental risk factors (Table 27.10). Difficulty in conception or history of recurrent pregnancy loss may suggest the presence of an inherited chromosome anomaly. Maternal illnesses (toxoplasmosis, other [syphilis, varicella-zoster, Zika virus, parvovirus B19], rubella, CMV, and herpes [TORCH] infections; HIV infection) preceding or continuing through pregnancy or exposure to potentially harmful or teratogenic substances (tobacco, alcohol, illicit drugs, radiation exposure, or medications) should be noted. Other pregnancy complications such as intrauterine growth restriction (which may reflect chronic placental insufficiency, uterine anatomic abnormality, or fetal genetic anomaly); bleeding (especially in the third trimester), which can be caused by placenta previa, placental abruption, or hemolysis, elevated liver enzymes, and low platelets (HELLP) syndrome; hypertension (especially leading to eclampsia); complications of maternal diabetes; or limited prenatal care may be associated with poor fetal outcomes. In the perinatal period, signs of fetal distress during labor (heart rate and movement abnormalities associated

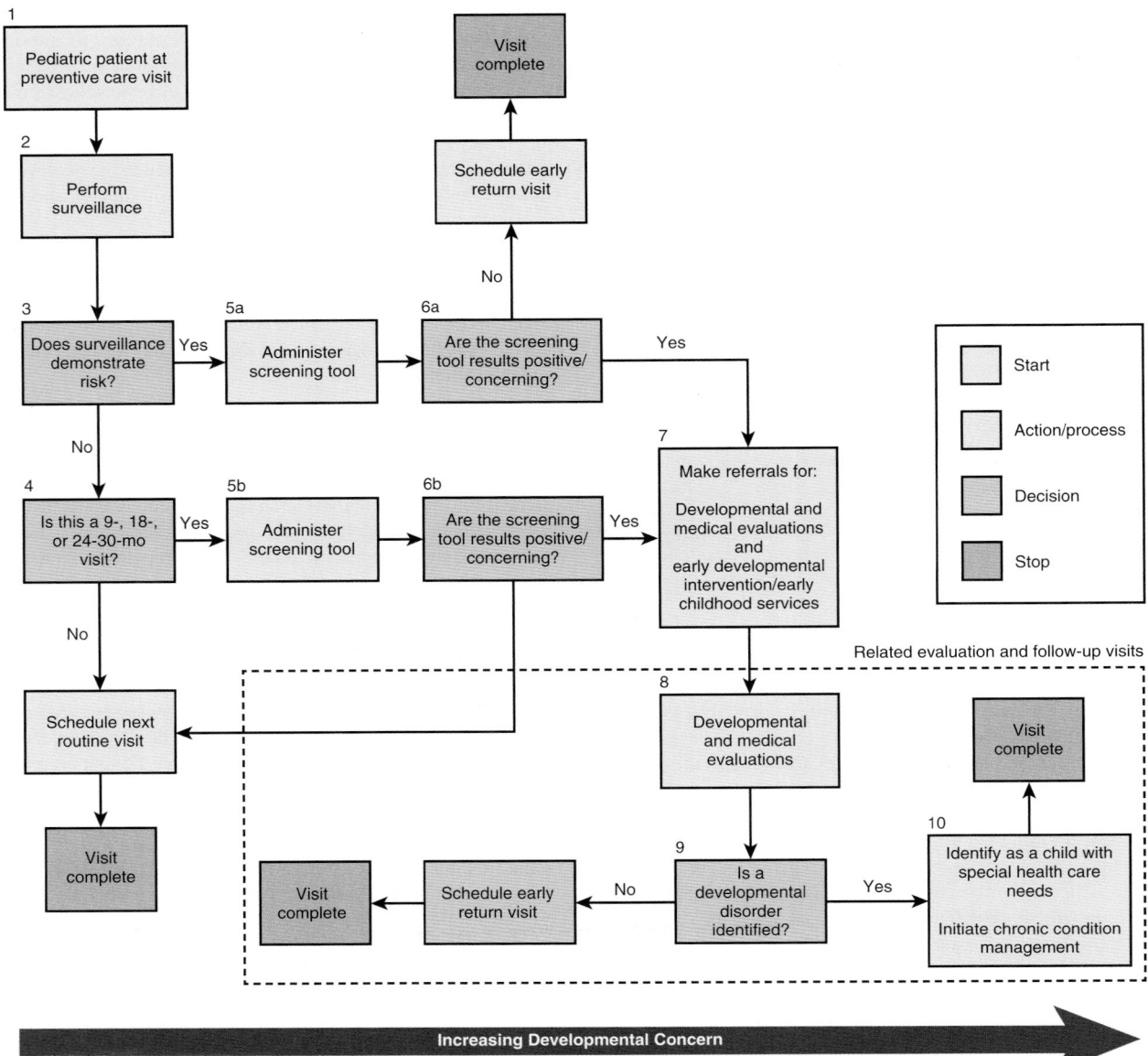

Fig. 27.2 Developmental surveillance and screening algorithm within a pediatric preventive care visit. Numbers refer to steps in the algorithm. (From Council on Children with Disabilities, et al. Identifying infants and young children with developmental disorders in the medical home: an algorithm for developmental surveillance and screening. *Pediatrics*. 2006;118:407.)

with uterine contractions), low Apgar scores, neonatal seizures, or the need for extensive neonatal resuscitation may be the result of acute fetal CNS injury or pre-existing congenital abnormalities that first manifest at the time of birth. The method of delivery and the reason(s) for non-vaginal delivery may reflect on fetal status at the time of birth. Neonatal physical measurements (weight, length, and head circumference) when compared with gestational age are helpful in determining whether the child experienced intrauterine growth restriction. Severe medical complications in the neonatal period such as the presence of neonatal encephalopathy syndrome including seizures and multiorgan compromise, intraventricular hemorrhage, neonatal infections, prolonged requirement for mechanical ventilation, need for extracorporeal membrane oxygenation (ECMO), the presence of complex cardiac anomalies, and necrotizing enterocolitis may be associated with increased risk of developmental disabilities (Table 27.11). Conversely, an infant who did not require care in a neonatal intensive care unit (NICU) or prolonged

stay in the hospital following birth likely experienced no significant perinatal developmental risk factors. When available, reviewing medical records from the neonatal period may be helpful in clarifying what transpired at the time of the infant's birth.

The social and economic circumstances of the family may reveal factors that place the infant at risk for developmental disabilities. The clinician should ask about the highest educational levels achieved by both parents, marital status or stability of the parents' relationship, parental mental health concerns, history of "high-risk behaviors" (illicit drug use), housing status, and presence of a parental support system (close friends and extended family members) to help with care of the infant.

The first weeks and months of life are a "transition period" for both the infant and the family. Children with developmental disabilities may begin to manifest symptoms in this period with difficulties nursing, excessive colic, poor weight gain, onset of seizures, or delayed achievement of motor milestones. Review of prior growth records may help differentiate

TABLE 27.10 Information to Obtain About a Child with Suspected Developmental Disabilities

Item	Possible Significance
Parental Concerns	Parents are quite accurate in identifying developmental problems
Current Levels of Developmental Functioning	Used to monitor child's progress
Temperament	May interact with disability or be confused with developmental delay
Prenatal History	
Alcohol ingestion	Fetal alcohol syndrome; an index of caretaking risk
Illegal drug, toxin, medication exposure	Developmental toxin (e.g., phenytoin); may be an index of caretaking risk
Radiation exposure	Damage to the CNS
Nutrition	Inadequate fetal nutrition
Prenatal care	Index of the social situation
Injuries, hyperthermia	Damage to the CNS
Smoking	Possible CNS damage
Maternal PKU	Maternal PKU effect
Maternal infections	Toxoplasmosis, rubella, CMV, HIV, herpesvirus infections, Zika virus
Perinatal History	
Gestational age, birthweight	Biologic risk from prematurity and small for gestational age
Labor and delivery	Hypoxia or index of abnormal prenatal development
Apgar scores	Hypoxia, cardiovascular impairment
Specific perinatal adverse events; see Table 27.11	Increased risk for CNS damage
Neonatal History	
Illness: seizures, respiratory distress, hyperbilirubinemia, metabolic disorder; see also Table 27.11	Increased risk for CNS damage
Malformations	May represent syndrome associated with developmental delay
Family History	
Consanguinity	Autosomal recessive condition more likely
Mental functioning	Increased hereditary and environmental risks
Illnesses (e.g., metabolic disease)	Hereditary illness associated with developmental delay
Family member died young or unexpectedly	May suggest inborn errors of metabolism or storage disease
Family member requires special education	Hereditary causes of developmental delay
Social History	
Resources available (e.g., financial, social support)	Necessary to maximize child's potential
Educational levels of parents	Family may need help to provide stimulation
Mental health problems	May exacerbate child's conditions
High-risk behaviors (illicit drug use, sexual promiscuity)	Increased risk for congenital infection; index of caretaking risk
Other stressors (e.g., marital discord)	May exacerbate child's conditions or compromise care
Other History	
Sex of the child	Important for X-linked conditions
Developmental milestones	Index of developmental delay, regression may indicate a progressive condition
Head injury	Even moderate trauma may be associated with developmental delay or learning disabilities
Serious infections (e.g., meningitis)	May be associated with developmental delay
Toxic exposure (e.g., lead)	May be associated with developmental delay
Physical growth	May indicate malnutrition; obesity, growth failure caused by genetic disorder
Recurrent otitis media	Associated with hearing loss and abnormal speech development
Visual and auditory functioning	Sensitive index of impairments in vision and hearing
Nutrition	Malnutrition during infancy may lead to delayed development
Chronic conditions such as renal or cyanotic cardiac	May be associated with delayed development

CMV, cytomegalovirus; CNS, central nervous system; PKU, phenylketonuria.

TABLE 27.11   Findings That May Be Used to Identify Neonates at Increased Risk for Developmental Delay

Item	Comment
Apgar scores	<3 at 5 min or <5 at 10 min, and HIE
Abnormal EEG	
Neonatal seizures	Hypoglycemia, hypoxia, intracranial hemorrhage, or infection confer high risk
Intracranial	Grade III or higher; PVL hemorrhage
Hydrocephalus	Especially with other anomalies, thin cortical mantle, or parenchymal lesions
Central nervous system	Seen on CT scan or ultrasonography system anomalies
Prematurity	<32 wk
Small for gestational age	<3rd percentile (intrauterine growth restriction)
Dysmorphic	Three or more minor or one or more major features
Chromosomal	Trisomies, fragile X, XO anomaly
Ventilation required	Longer than 2 wk
Small head	<3rd percentile circumference
Meningitis/encephalitis	Bacterial (group B streptococci, *Escherichia coli*) Viral (herpes simplex)
Hypoglycemia	Symptomatic
Congenital infection	Cytomegalovirus, toxoplasmosis, syphilis, rubella, herpes simplex, varicella-zoster, HIV
Hyperbilirubinemia	Requiring exchange transfusions
Associated medical problems	Such as retinopathy of prematurity, heart disease, bronchopulmonary dysplasia, necrotizing enterocolitis

HIE, hypoxic-ischemic encephalopathy; PVL, periventricular leukomalacia.

between a congenital or acquired disorder. A history of recurrent illness, family/social or environmental stress, trauma (especially to the CNS), or epilepsy may be associated with poor development. *True regression, the loss of previously acquired skills, should be distinguished from failure of development* (see Chapter 28). Newly emerging skills may fluctuate until they are firmly established. In cases of true regression, multiple areas of functioning are affected and do not re-emerge over time.

Ages of achievement of common milestones in motor, language, cognitive, and social development should be reviewed. Parents of infants and toddlers may have more accurate recollections of their child's milestones than parents of older children. In some cases, parents may recall comparing their child's milestones to another child's (sibling, relative, neighbor) or may only recall their child's "major" milestones, such as ages at which the child began walking independently, waving "bye-bye," using first words, or talking in sentences.

A three-generation family pedigree should be reviewed to identify other individuals with conditions similar to the child's, developmental/learning disabilities, or early deaths. Consanguinity may increase the risk of a recessive disorder. A family's ethnic ancestry may suggest potential etiology, since a number of conditions occur at increased frequency among certain ethnic groups (e.g., Tay-Sachs disease among Ashkenazi Jews).

Social and environmental factors such as parental physical or mental illness (including substance abuse), death of a close family member, divorce, domestic abuse, parental incarceration, multiple changes

of dwelling, placement in foster care, or having a sibling with a serious chronic illness may have significant adverse effects on a child's development.

It is important to know whether the child has received any type of educational or therapeutic interventions and the impact those programs have had on the child's behavior and development.

For young children, a description of their play interests, self-help skills, and social interactions with parents, peers, and caretakers/teachers may provide valuable information about the child's level of overall development. A review of common activities of daily living (ADLs), including dressing, eating, toileting, and motor skills, often provides insight about the integrity of the child's cognitive, communication, and neuromotor development. School experiences, academic readiness skills, educational achievement, and behavior patterns at home and school often reflect the cognitive and language development of school-age children and adolescents.

Physical Examination

The physical examination should begin with observations of the general appearance of the child, including overall state of health, visual and auditory responsiveness to the surroundings, and interactions with parents. When the child is at rest, subtle abnormalities of body proportions and movement patterns may be observed. Careful attention should also be paid to physical measurements (length/height, weight, *and head circumference*) with values plotted on standard reference curves. Both poor growth and excessive growth may be associated with metabolic disorders or genetic syndromes. Head circumference measurements may be abnormal (greater or less than 2 standard deviations from the mean) or disproportionate for body size (head circumference should correlate with length/height of the child). Although large or small head size may be associated with significant pathology, a benign form of familial micro- and macrocephaly may be ruled out if one or both parents share the same trait. **Dysmorphic features** may suggest a recognizable pattern of deformation or malformation (Table 27.12) (see Chapter 29). If the child has an unusual appearance, biologic family members should be examined either directly or from photographs to determine any resemblance. Additionally, examining serial photographs of a child at different ages can help to identify "coarsening" of facial features due to a storage disease (mucopolysaccharidosis). Abnormalities of skin pigmentation may suggest the presence of a neurocutaneous disorder (phakomatosis) associated with developmental disability (neurofibromatosis, tuberous sclerosis, Sturge-Weber syndrome) (see Chapter 60). A Wood's lamp examination may be helpful if a depigmented lesion is identified (ash-leaf spots in tuberous sclerosis). Measurements of facial features, such as inner canthal distance, palpebral fissure length, auricular size and position, and development of the philtrum and upper lip, may be associated with structural anomalies of craniofacial development caused by genetic or teratogenic exposure (fetal alcohol syndrome). The oral structures should be examined for the presence of cleft palate (velocardiofacial syndrome, Stickler syndrome), macroglossia (Beckwith-Wiedemann syndrome), or recessed jaw (Pierre-Robin sequence). Anomalies of the neck may indicate vertebral abnormalities (Klippel-Feil syndrome) or genetic disorders (Turner syndrome, Noonan syndrome, Down syndrome). Cardiac anomalies are associated with a large number of syndromes. The abdominal exam may reveal evidence of an enlarged liver (associated with glycogen storage diseases, sphingolipidoses, or mucopolysaccharidoses). Examination of the back should include the "forward bend test" for scoliosis, and the presence of dimpling or a hirsute area in the lower spine that could represent an occult form of spinal dysraphism (tethered cord or other spinal cord anomaly). Anomalies of the extremities (limb proportions, hands, feet, and nails) are associated

TABLE 27.12 **Physical Examination of a Child with Suspected Developmental Disabilities**

Item	Possible Significance
General appearance	May indicate significant delay in development or obvious syndrome
Stature	
Short stature	Malnutrition; many genetic syndromes are associated with short stature (e.g., Turner, Noonan)
Obesity	Prader-Willi syndrome
Large stature	Sotos syndrome
Head	
Macrocephaly	Alexander syndrome, Canavan disease, Sotos syndrome, gangliosidosis, hydrocephalus, mucopolysaccharidosis, subdural effusion
Microcephaly	Virtually any condition that can restrict brain growth (e.g., malnutrition, Angelman syndrome, Cornelia de Lange syndrome, fetal alcohol effects)
Face	
Coarse, triangular, round, or flat face; hypotelorism or hypertelorism; slanted or short palpebral fissure; unusual nose, maxilla, and mandible	Specific measurements may provide clues to inherited, metabolic, or other diseases such as fetal alcohol syndrome, cri du chat (5p–) syndrome, or Williams syndrome
Eyes	
Prominent	Crouzon, Seckel, and fragile X syndromes
Cataract	Galactosemia, Lowe syndrome, prenatal rubella, hypothyroidism
Cherry-red spot in macula	Gangliosidosis (GM$_1$), metachromatic leukodystrophy, mucolipidosis, Tay-Sachs disease, Niemann-Pick disease, Farber lipogranulomatosis, sialidosis type III
Chorioretinitis	Congenital infection with cytomegalovirus, toxoplasmosis, Zika virus, or rubella
Corneal cloudiness	Mucopolysaccharidosis types I and II, Lowe syndrome, congenital syphilis
Ears	
Low-set or malformed pinnae	Trisomies such as Down syndrome, Rubinstein-Taybi syndrome, CHARGE syndrome, cerebro-oculofacioskeletal syndrome, fetal phenytoin effects
Hearing	Loss of acuity in mucopolysaccharidosis; hyperacusis in many encephalopathies
Heart	
Structural anomaly or hypertrophy	CHARGE syndrome, velocardiofacial syndrome, glycogenosis type II, fetal alcohol effects, mucopolysaccharidosis type I; chromosomal anomalies such as Down syndrome; maternal PKU; chronic cyanosis may impair cognitive development

Item	Possible Significance
Liver	
Hepatomegaly	Fructose intolerance, galactosemia, glycogenosis types I–IV, mucopolysaccharidosis types I and II, Niemann-Pick disease, Tay-Sachs disease, Zellweger syndrome, Gaucher disease, ceroid lipofuscinosis, gangliosidosis
Genitalia	
Macro-orchidism	Fragile X syndrome
Hypogenitalism	Prader-Willi, Klinefelter, and CHARGE syndromes
Extremities	
Hands, feet; dermatoglyphics, creases	May indicate a specific entity such as Rubinstein-Taybi syndrome or may be associated with chromosomal anomaly
Joint contractures	Signs of muscle imbalance around the joints; e.g., with meningomyelocele, cerebral palsy, arthrogryposis, muscular dystrophy; also occurs with cartilaginous problems such as mucopolysaccharidosis
Skin	
Café-au-lait spots	Neurofibromatosis, tuberous sclerosis, chromosomal aneuploidy, ataxia-telangiectasia, multiple endocrine neoplasia type 2b Fanconi anemia, Gaucher disease Syndromes: basal cell nevus, McCune-Albright, Silver-Russell, Bloom, Chediak-Higashi, Hunter, Bannayan-Riley-Ruvalcaba, Maffucci
Seborrheic or eczematoid rash	PKU, histiocytosis
Hemangiomas and telangiectasia	Sturge-Weber syndrome, Bloom syndrome, ataxia-telangiectasia
Hypopigmented macules, streaks, adenoma sebaceum	Tuberous sclerosis, hypomelanosis of Ito
Hair	
Hirsutism	De Lange syndrome, mucopolysaccharidosis, fetal phenytoin effects, cerebro-oculofacioskeletal syndrome, trisomy 18, Wiedemann-Steiner syndrome (hypertrichosis cubiti)
Neurologic	
Asymmetry of strength and tone	Focal lesion, hemiplegic cerebral palsy
Hypotonia	Prader-Willi, Down, and Angelman syndromes; gangliosidosis; early cerebral palsy; muscle disorders (dystrophy or myopathy)
Hypertonia	Neurodegenerative conditions involving white matter, cerebral palsy, trisomy 18
Ataxia	Ataxia-telangiectasia, metachromatic leukodystrophy, Angelman syndrome

CHARGE, coloboma, heart defects, atresia choanae, retarded growth, genital anomalies, ear anomalies (deafness); PKU, phenylketonuria.
From Kliegman RM, St. Geme J. *Nelson Textbook of Pediatrics.* 21st ed. Vol 1. Philadelphia: Elsevier; 2020:285, Table 53.2.

TABLE 27.13 Examples of Minor Anomalies and Associated Syndromes*,†

Head	Flat occiput: Down syndrome, Zellweger syndrome; prominent occiput: trisomy 18 Delayed closure of sutures: hypothyroidism, hydrocephalus Craniosynostosis: Crouzon syndrome, Pfeiffer syndrome Delayed fontanel closure: hypothyroidism, Down syndrome, hydrocephalus, skeletal dysplasias	Teeth	Anodontia: ectodermal dysplasia Notched incisors: congenital syphilis Late dental eruption: Hunter syndrome, hypothyroidism Talon cusps: Rubinstein-Taybi syndrome Wide-spaced teeth: de Lange syndrome, Angelman syndrome
Face	Midface hypoplasia: fetal alcohol syndrome, Down syndrome Triangular facies: Russell-Silver syndrome, Turner syndrome Coarse facies: mucopolysaccharidoses, Sotos syndrome Prominent nose and chin: fragile X syndrome Flat facies: Apert syndrome, Stickler syndrome Round facies: Prader-Willi syndrome	Hair	Hirsutism: Hurler syndrome Low hairline: Klippel-Feil sequence, Turner syndrome Sparse hair: Menkes disease, argininosuccinic acidemia Abnormal hair whorls/posterior whorl: chromosomal aneuploidy (e.g., Down syndrome) Abnormal eyebrow patterning: Cornelia de Lange syndrome
Eyes	Hypertelorism: fetal hydantoin syndrome, Waardenburg syndrome Hypotelorism: holoprosencephaly sequence, maternal phenylketonuria effect Inner canthal folds/Brushfield spots: Down syndrome; slanted palpebral fissures: trisomies Prominent eyes: Apert syndrome, Beckwith-Wiedemann syndrome Lisch nodules: neurofibromatosis Blue sclera: osteogenesis imperfecta, Turner syndrome, hereditary connective tissue disorders	Neck	Webbed neck/low posterior hairline: Turner syndrome, Noonan syndrome
		Chest	Shield-shaped chest: Turner syndrome
		Genitalia	Macro-orchidism: fragile X syndrome Hypogonadism: Prader-Willi syndrome
Ears	Large pinnae/simple helices: fragile X syndrome Malformed pinnae/atretic canal: Treacher Collins syndrome, CHARGE syndrome Low-set ears: Treacher Collins syndrome, trisomies, multiple disorders	Extremities	Short limbs: achondroplasia, rhizomelic chondrodysplasia Small hands: Prader-Willi syndrome Clinodactyly: trisomies, including Down syndrome Polydactyly: trisomy 13, ciliopathies Broad thumb: Rubinstein-Taybi syndrome Syndactyly: de Lange syndrome Transverse palmar crease: Down syndrome Joint laxity: Down syndrome, fragile X syndrome, Ehlers-Danlos syndrome Phocomelia: de Lange syndrome
Nose	Anteverted nares/synophrys: de Lange syndrome; broad nasal bridge: fetal drug effects, fragile X syndrome Low nasal bridge: achondroplasia, Down syndrome Prominent nose: Coffin-Lowry syndrome, Smith-Lemli-Opitz syndrome	Spine	Sacral dimple/hairy patch: spina bifida
		Skin	Hypopigmented macules/adenoma sebaceum: tuberous sclerosis Café-au-lait spots and neurofibromas: neurofibromatosis Linear depigmented nevi: hypomelanosis of Ito Facial port-wine hemangioma: Sturge-Weber syndrome Nail hypoplasia or dysplasia: fetal alcohol syndrome, trisomies
Mouth	Long philtrum/thin vermilion border: fetal alcohol effects Cleft lip and palate: isolated or part of a syndrome Micrognathia: Pierre-Robin sequence, trisomies, Stickler syndrome Macroglossia: hypothyroidism, Beckwith-Wiedemann syndrome		

*Increased incidence of minor anomalies has been reported in cerebral palsy, intellectual disability, learning disabilities, and autism.
†The presence of three or more minor anomalies implies a greater chance that the child has a major anomaly and a diagnosis of a specific syndrome.
CHARGE, coloboma, heart defects, atresia choanae, retarded growth, genital anomalies, ear anomalies (deafness).
Modified from Levy SE, Hyman SL. Pediatric assessment of the child with developmental delay. *Pediatr Clin North Am.* 1993;40:465–477.

with a wide range of birth defects and syndromes. The presence of multiple malformations may be an important key to identifying a specific developmental disorder or syndrome. Although minor physical anomalies may be associated with developmental delay, most children with minor anomalies develop normally (Table 27.13).

The neuromotor examination should include observation of muscle bulk and presence or absence of muscle atrophy associated with myopathy. The assessment of cranial nerves includes evaluation for visual responsiveness, pupillary reactivity, presence of red reflexes, fullness of eye movements, and evidence of strabismus. Ptosis, asymmetry of facial expression, or abnormal tongue movement (deviation or fasciculation) suggests muscle weakness or partial paralysis. Muscle strength may be assessed by observing the child move about and manipulate objects. In the first year of life, motor milestones include the ability to sit independently, crawl, cruise, and walk. By 18 months, children should be able to squat and recover. The **Gowers maneuver** is helpful in assessing strength of the quadriceps muscles (see Chapter 35). Decreased muscle tone may be reflected in poor posture or hypermobile joints. Decreased stretch reflex responsiveness may be due to lower motor neuron disease or myopathy. In infants, the persistence

of primitive reflexes or the absence of protective postural reflexes is suggestive of neuromotor dysfunction. In older children, the presence of increased stretch reflexes, clonus, and positive Babinski reflexes are signs of upper motor neuron dysfunction associated with spasticity. Normal gait requires intact and coordinated motor and sensory ability. Unsteady gait or tremor may be a sign of muscle weakness or abnormal cerebellar function or basal ganglia disease. Asymmetry of gait may reflect hemiplegia. Observing the child reaching for objects, extending the arms outstretched, or performing the finger-to-nose test may reveal tremors or difficulty with eye-hand coordination.

FORMAL NEURODEVELOPMENTAL ASSESSMENTS

Psychologic Evaluation

Evaluation by a child psychologist can provide an assessment of a child's strengths and weaknesses across a broad range of cognitive areas. For infants and young children, global measures of development are the most valuable, since the structure of intelligence develops from relatively "general" and homogeneous ability to more complex and differentiated functions over time. Few tasks on measures used for preschool children reflect "pure" abilities in any particular skill. Rather, tasks for infants reflect the child's ability to utilize a combination of cognitive, language, and motor skills to respond. However, tests vary in their ability to separate these component functions. The Bayley Scales of Infant and Toddler Development-3rd Edition (Bayley III) is a widely used tool for assessing children 0–42 months of age. There are several normed measures of verbal and nonverbal abilities that can be used with children older than 2 years of age. Many factors can contribute to the child's performance. Observing how the child responds to a task can be as informative as the accuracy of the response. It is generally recognized that intelligence testing prior to age 6 years is not highly predictive of test results at older ages, but the evaluation provides a measure of the child's abilities at that point in time. In addition, a psychologist is able to observe the child's behavior, attention span, organizational skills, persistence, and frustration tolerance during the evaluation. These informal observations may help to determine the presence or absence of emotional or behavioral problems that stem from, or coexist with, the child's developmental disabilities.

Results of psychologic tests are not indicative of specific etiologies (genetic or acquired biologic conditions) and cannot determine whether a child has suffered a "brain injury," even in the context of a potentially traumatic event. Serial cognitive measures, particularly when there is premorbid information that has changed over time, may suggest the effects of trauma or a progressive disease process.

Speech-Language and Oral Motor Evaluation

The ability to understand and communicate with others has a very strong influence on a child's emotional, behavioral, and social functioning. Communication abilities may or may not reflect the child's intellectual ability. A speech-language pathologist can evaluate a wide range of communication and oral motor skills in children. Even prior to the use of words, infants display "preverbal" communication abilities (gestures) and may recognize a number of spoken words. Older children may suffer from delays in understanding of language (language disorders) or from disorders of speech sound production (apraxia, dysarthria). Many children with neurologic disabilities have oral motor coordination disorders (dysphagia) that interfere with chewing and swallowing and place them at risk for poor weight gain and/or pulmonary aspiration. Drooling management is also a problem for many children with oral motor coordination delays. While it is more common for receptive language ability to exceed expressive language ability, children with Williams syndrome and with spina bifida/hydrocephalus may display conversational skills that exceed their cognitive deficits ("cocktail conversation"). In both conditions, "basic" language abilities (vocabulary and grammar) are relatively well developed, while "higher-level" language functions (semantic knowledge and pragmatic aspects of communication) are deficient.

DIAGNOSTIC STRATEGY

Once a comprehensive profile of the child's strengths and weaknesses has been identified through neurodevelopmental, psychologic, and speech-language evaluations, the next step is to establish a developmental diagnosis.

Cognitive, language, and motor abilities typically develop in a coordinated fashion. Discrepancies in development between different areas of function may point to a specific area of concern or suggest possible clinical diagnoses (Table 27.14). Many disorders can be identified by their characteristic pattern of development over time (e.g., infantile hypotonia evolving into hyperphagia and obesity in Prader-Willi syndrome, regression/microcephaly/hand-wringing behavior in Rett syndrome). In general, motor milestones do not correlate well with intellectual ability, since most children with ID walk at a normal age. Language abilities, when well developed, are usually an excellent indicator of intellectual function. Problem-solving skills (referred to as "adaptive" or "visual-motor" skills) often correlate with nonverbal cognitive abilities. Finally, psychosocial milestones often reflect language ability. A child with delays in all areas likely has a cognitive deficit, while a child whose communication skills are at variance with nonverbal cognitive abilities likely has a language disorder.

Delays isolated to a single, specific area such as expressive language are more likely to be transient than are generalized delays. If the child's development has regressed, a progressive encephalopathy may be present (see Chapter 28).

Genetic Considerations

More than 800 genes have been implicated in GDD/ID as well as more than 1,000 additional "candidate" genes. Of these, more than 400 are autosomal recessive, 180 are autosomal dominant, and 140 are X-linked. Many genes are associated with "syndromic" GDD/ID (i.e., cases in which abnormalities are identified on examination such as micro- or macrocephaly, dysmorphic features, congenital anomalies, failure to thrive, short stature, abnormal neurologic examination, seizures, structural brain abnormalities, sensory deficits [vision or hearing]). Variability of clinical features is the rule, rather than the exception, for most syndromes that cause GDD/ID. Of the more than 200 genes that have been associated with "nonsyndromic" GDD/ID, at least 30 are also associated with syndromic GDD/ID and at least 60 are also associated with other neurologic (i.e., epilepsy) or neuropsychiatric (i.e., autism, schizophrenia) disorders.

A distinction should be made between a clinical diagnosis that is based on descriptions and measurements of various functional abilities and an etiologic diagnosis that attributes the problem(s) to a specific cause. For most developmental disabilities, a specific etiology cannot be established with absolute certainty. Clinical diagnoses such as cerebral palsy or ID can result from multiple etiologies, and, conversely, the same etiology can manifest in a variety of ways. As medical diagnostic

TABLE 27.14	Differential Diagnosis of Atypical Patterns of Development				
	Intellectual Disability	**Developmental Language Disorder**	**Specific Language Impairment**	**Autism Spectrum Disorder**	**Social Pragmatic Communication Disorder**
Cognitive ability	Delayed	Normal/delayed	Normal	Normal/delayed	Normal
Language ability	Delayed	Disordered	Disordered	Disordered	Normal
Social ability	Normal	Normal	Normal	Abnormal	Abnormal
Family history	Negative	Speech/language	Speech/language	Affective disorder	Social deficits

Modified from Simms MD, Schum RL. Preschool children who have atypical patterns of development. *Pediatr Rev.* 2000;21:147–158.

technologies have improved, the number of individuals for whom an etiologic diagnosis can be established has increased. Even when a specific *etiologic* diagnosis cannot be determined, an accurate *clinical* diagnosis is often helpful in designing treatment recommendations because most treatments are based on an educational-developmental model and are successful for a range of underlying etiologies.

Although most parents will pursue further evaluations when they are concerned about their child's development, not all are willing or able to have their child undergo medical diagnostic testing procedures when they are very young. Instead, parents typically want to know what they can do to help their child "catch up" with their peers. This concept is often reinforced by referring to the problem as a developmental "delay." Unless there are signs of regression or failure to thrive that would make diagnostic testing urgent, "watchful waiting" while the child enters a program of interventions is an accepted strategy. If, despite these measures, developmental concerns persist, families may be more willing to obtain further diagnostic testing. It is often helpful to share with parents that the probability of establishing a medical diagnosis with current technology is 30–40%, unless specific syndromes or disorders are suspected from the history and physical examination. While in most situations a specific diagnosis will not result in a cure for the underlying disorder, if a specific etiology can be established, it may result in effective treatments and preventive measures for other medical concerns associated with the diagnosis. Medical treatment for the circadian rhythm dysfunction associated with Smith-Magenis syndrome can be very successful in improving sleep patterns and daytime behaviors. In addition, children can be monitored on an expectant basis for complications that occur frequently with specific disorders (Wilms tumor in Beckwith-Wiedemann syndrome).

LABORATORY TESTING

When a specific diagnosis is suspected based on the history and physical examination, a "targeted" approach to confirm that condition (single-gene tests, specific metabolic studies, neuroimaging) is warranted (Tables 27.15 and 27.16). If no clinical diagnosis is suspected, current guidelines for comprehensive evaluation recommend a "tiered approach" (Fig. 27.3).

Genetic Tests

The first-tier test for all children with "nonspecific" GDD/ID is a chromosomal microarray (CMA). If a specific diagnosis is not established by CMA, referral for consultation with a geneticist should also be arranged.

NGS with broad screening panels within a group of phenotypes (e.g., X-Linked Intellectual Disability [XLID] panel) and whole exome sequencing (WES) are transforming the diagnostic process for children with disabilities. While the diagnostic yield of CMA in unexplained ID is 10–15%, diagnosis in approximately 36% of affected children with GDD/ID can be achieved with WES. The diagnostic rate is higher for syndromic GDD/ID and lower for isolated ASD (see Fig. 27.3). Some genomic sequencing (exome/genome) labs are able to report large chromosomal deletions and duplications (if they span multiple exons), complementing CMA testing.

There are disease-causing variants that are not detected by WES or CMA. Karyotype will detect balanced translocations if there is no loss or gain of chromosomal material. Fragile X repeat expansions are not covered on either technology. The yield of testing for fragile X is low unless there are typical clinical features (long face with large ears, prominent forehead and prominent jaw; hypotonia, joint laxity) or a suggestive family history (X-linked intellectual disability with anticipation, premature ovarian failure, or adult-onset neurologic disease). Whole genome sequencing is an emerging option for cases unsolved by WES and increases the diagnostic rate by up to 10% by detecting variants missed by both WES and CMA (small deletions/duplications, intronic and intergenic single nucleotide variants, structural variants, and some repeat expansions). There is always the possibility of finding *variants of uncertain significance* that have not yet been associated with GDD/ID or that may not cause any medical problems. In this case, it may be necessary to test both parents to determine if the variant was inherited or de novo. If the variant is de novo in the child, it is more likely to be significant. If the same variant is found in an unaffected parent, it is more challenging to interpret the significance of the variant. There are numerous examples of unaffected parent carriers with chromosomal deletions (reduced penetrance) and wide variability in phenotypic expression within affected families who have the same variant (variable expressivity). Including parents in WES (*Trio sequencing*)

TABLE 27.15 Chromosomal Abnormalities in Which Developmental Delay Is a Major Feature

Condition	Incidence	Comments
Trisomy 21	1/700	Down syndrome
Fragile X syndrome	1/800	Macro-orchidism, hyperactivity, autistic-like behavior
47,XXY (Klinefelter syndrome)	1/1,000	Small testes, problems in language skills
47,XXX	1/1,000	Females with learning and language problems may have 48,XXXX
45,X (Turner syndrome)	1/2,000	Females with short stature, broad neck, gonadal dysgenesis; visuospatial deficits common
Prader-Willi syndrome (abnormality of contiguous genes on chromosome 15; inherited from deletions of paternal chromosomes—monoparental disomy)	1/5,000	Hypotonia in infancy, obesity, short stature, mild intellectual disability
Angelman syndrome (chromosome anomaly similar to that in Prader-Willi syndrome; inherited from maternal deletion in chromosome 15—monoparental disomy)	Unknown	Ataxia, prognathism, absence of speech, severe intellectual disability, inappropriate laughter
Trisomy 18	1/8,000	Multiple congenital anomalies, severe developmental delay
Trisomy 13	1/20,000	Multiple congenital anomalies, severe developmental delay
5p– (cri du chat syndrome)	1/100,000	High-pitched cry, small stature, speech and language delays
4p– (Wolf-Hirschhorn syndrome)	1/100,000	Midline deficiencies, profound intellectual disability, seizures
11p– (Wilms tumor, aniridia)	1/100,000	Ambiguous genitalia, aniridia, cataracts
17p– (Miller-Dieker syndrome)	1/100,000	Lissencephaly, microcephaly, seizures, cryptorchidism

TABLE 27.16 Suggested Evaluation of the Child with Intellectual Disability/Global Developmental Delay

Test	Comments
In-depth history	Includes pre-, peri-, and postnatal events (including seizures); developmental attainments; and three-generation pedigree in family history
Physical examination	Particular attention to minor or subtle abnormalities; neurologic examination for focality and skull abnormalities Behavioral phenotype
Vision and hearing evaluation	Essential to detect and treat; can mask as developmental delay
Gene microarray analysis	A 7.8% yield overall (10% in syndromic and 6.5% in nonsyndromic intellectual disability) Better resolution than karyotype. May identify up to twice as many abnormalities as karyotyping. Excellent in detecting de novo microdeletions or microduplications
Karyotype	Yield: 4% in global developmental delay/intellectual disability Best for inversions and balanced insertions, reciprocal translocations, and polyploidy
Fragile X screen	Combined yield: 2% Preselection on clinical grounds can increase yield to 7.6%
X-linked candidate intellectual disability genes	May explain up to 10% of intellectual disability Yield may be as high as 42% if there is a definite family history and as high as 17% from a possibly linked kindred
Exomic gene sequencing	Detects inherited and de novo point mutations, especially in nonsyndromic severe intellectual disability
Neuroimaging	MRI preferred. Positives increased by abnormalities of skull contour or microcephaly and macrocephaly, or focal neurologic examination. Overall, has a higher yield than CT Identification of specific etiologies is rare. Most conditions that are found do not alter the treatment plan. Need to weigh risk of sedation against possible yield
Thyroid (T_4, TSH)	Near 0% in settings with a universal newborn screening program
Serum lead	If there are identifiable risk factors for excessive environmental lead exposure
Metabolic testing	Yield: 0.2–4.6% based on clinical indicators and tests performed Urine organic acids, plasma amino acids, ammonia, lactate, and a capillary blood gas. Focused testing based on clinical findings is warranted Tandem mass spectrometry newborn screening has allowed for identification of many disorders in the perinatal period and has decreased yield in older children. Other disorders have emerged; e.g., congenital disorders of glycosylation and disorders of creatine synthesis and transport
MECP2 for Rett syndrome	1.5% of females with severe intellectual disability 0.5% of males
EEG	May be deferred in absence of history of seizures
Repeated history and physical examination	Can give time for maturation of physical and behavioral phenotype. New technology may be available for evaluation

MECP2, methyl CpG-binding protein 2; T_4, thyroxine; TSH, thyroid-stimulating hormone.
Modified from Michelson DJ, Shevell MI, Sherr EH, et al. Evidence report: genetic and metabolic testing on children with global developmental delay: report of the Quality Standards Subcommittee of The American Academy of Neurology and The Practice Committee of Child Neurology. *Neurology.* 2011;77:1629–1635; Curry CJ, Stevenson RE, Aughton D, et al. Evaluation of mental retardation: recommendations of a consensus conference: American College of Medical Genetics. *Am J Med Genet.* 1997;12:72:468–477; Shapiro BK, Batshaw ML. Mental retardation. In: Burg FD, Ingelfinger JR, Polin RA, et al., eds. *Gellis and Kagan's Current Pediatric Therapy.* 18th ed. Philadelphia: Saunders; 2005, used with permission; and Shevell M, Ashwal S, Donley D, et al. Practice parameter: evaluation of the child with global developmental delay. *Neurology.* 2003;60:367–380.

is preferred and improves diagnostic outcomes, increasing yield and decreasing variants of uncertain significance. No patient who remains undiagnosed after genomic sequencing should be lost to follow-up because WES/whole genome sequencing data can be reanalyzed every 1–2 years until a diagnosis is made.

Metabolic Tests

Inborn errors of metabolism may present with progressive neurologic impairment (see Chapter 28). There is, however, great variability, and consideration for broad metabolic screening should always be considered if a causative etiology for ID/GDD remains unresolved. The current standard for static encephalopathy includes screening plasma amino acids, serum acylcarnitines, and urine organic acids. There are certain specific clinical presentations that

should raise the question for treatable metabolic disorders (such as language impairment in the context of seizures associated with creatine transport disorders).

Neuroimaging

Ultrasonography

An ultrasound study of the head performed before the anterior fontanel closes can provide a general anatomic picture of the brain, including a view of the posterior fossa. This technique is insensitive to lesions involving the subdural space, and its success depends more on the skill of the interpreter than that of the other imaging studies. It does not expose the child to radiation, nor is sedation required in most instances. Its primary uses include identifying and monitoring

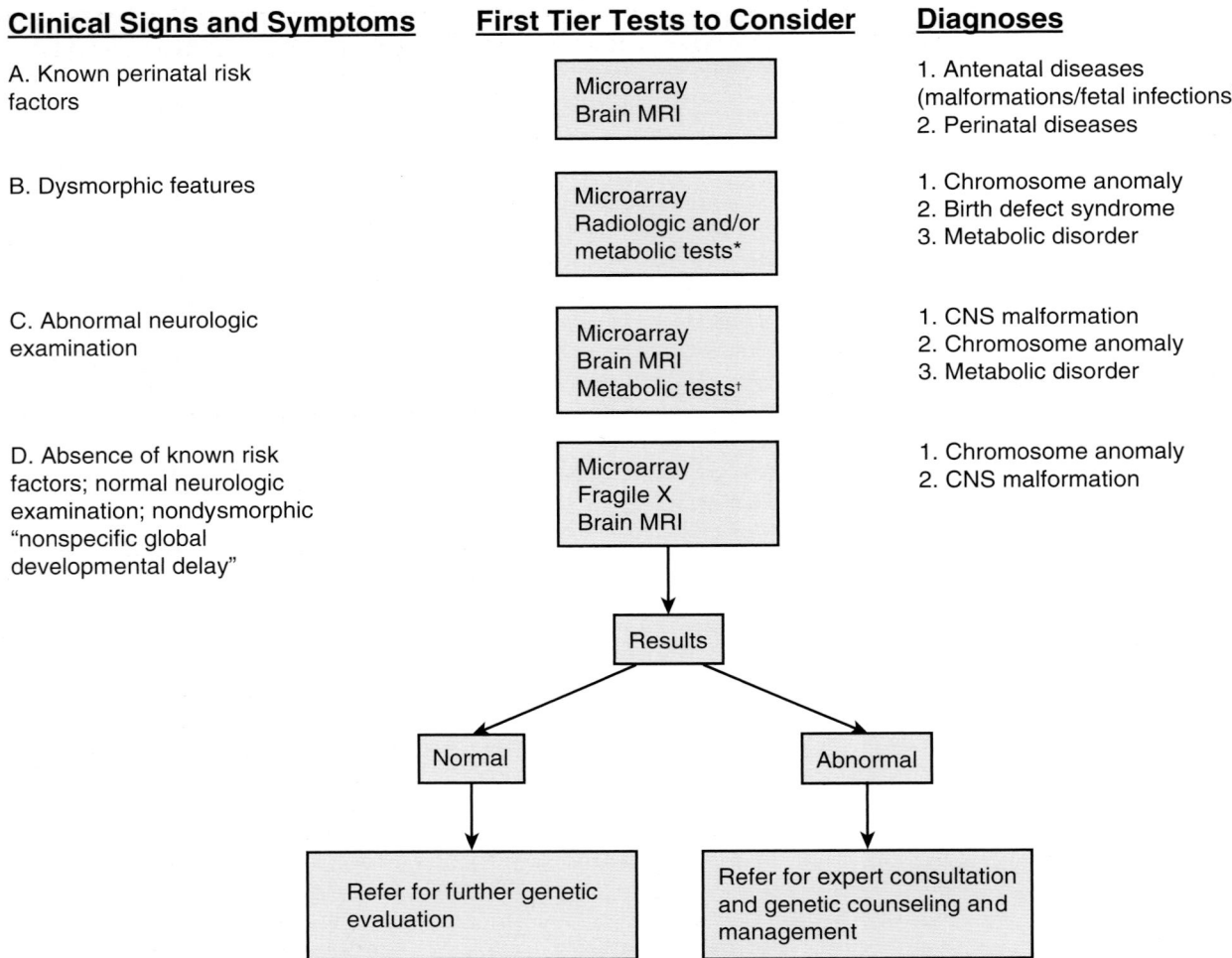

Fig. 27.3 Evaluation of infants with developmental delay without regression. *Mucopolysaccharide screening. †Urine organic acids; plasma amino acids; acylcarnitine profile. CNS, central nervous system.

intraventricular hemorrhage and hydrocephalus; these functions are useful, especially in the preterm infant.

Computed Tomography Scans

CT provides more detail than ultrasonography, including details of bone structures and the subdural space. Using contrast material will further delineate structures such as tumors or differentiate white from gray matter. However, CT exposes the child to radiation, and most young children require sedation to undergo this procedure.

Magnetic Resonance Imaging

MRI provides the greatest detail of the nonbone aspects of the CNS. The scanning time is longer than for CT, and most young children require sedation. The contrast material used, gadolinium, is generally safer than the contrast agents used for CT. MRI is superior to CT in the evaluation of the posterior fossa. MRI is used for imaging the spinal cord. MRI can differentiate abnormalities of gray and white matter, as well as deep and cortical gray matter lesions. Special techniques include magnetic resonance angiography, which can identify blood flow, and cerebrospinal fluid flow imaging, which can identify flow in conditions such as Chiari malformation. Magnetic resonance spectroscopy identifies metabolites in the brain such as lactate, N-acetylaspartate, and choline. Conditions such as phenylketonuria, maple syrup urine disease, and Canavan disease have distinctive patterns on spectroscopy.

Indications for Various Imaging Modalities

Many studies have identified abnormalities in the brains of children with developmental delay on MRI that were not evident on CT. These abnormalities include delayed myelination, focal lesions, and hypoplastic white matter. In approximately 33% of children with developmental delay, the MRI is abnormal. This increases if the child has microcephaly or associated neurologic findings such as focal motor deficits, seizures, or a pattern of regression/degeneration. Neuroimaging in children with GDD may reveal evidence of cerebral injury, brain malformation, or markers of cerebral dysgenesis. Injury may be due to hypoxic-ischemic encephalopathy ("watershed" or deep gray matter lesions in term infants and periventricular leukomalacia common in premature infants) or signs of intrauterine infection. Malformations may result from disorders of ventral induction (holoprosencephaly, agenesis of the corpus callosum, septo-optic dysplasia), migrational abnormalities (lissencephaly, schizencephaly, pachygyria, polymicrogyria, band heterotopias), and aberrant white matter development (demyelinating/dysmyelinating syndromes). At times, neuroimaging may provide information about the possible timing of the event (whether injury or dysgenesis). Serial imaging studies may help to distinguish a static from a progressive course and aid in prognosis. However, in many instances, abnormal findings may not be sufficient for determining the specific underlying cause of the disability. Furthermore, there may be

TABLE 27.17 Types of Abnormalities Identified by Neuroimaging

- Malformations of cortical development:
  - Midline defects: holoprosencephaly; callosal agenesis; cerebellar hypoplasia
  - Migration defects: lissencephaly; bands; schizencephaly; pachygyria/microgyria
  - Hydrocephalus, hemimegalencephaly
  - Neurocutaneous syndromes: tuberous sclerosis; neurofibromatosis
  - Trauma: hypoxic-ischemic encephalopathy; stroke
- Metabolic and neurodegenerative disorders:
  - Cortical gray matter: lysosomal enzyme defects (lipidoses: GM_1 gangliosidosis, neuronal ceroid lipofuscinosis) and mucolipidoses
  - Corpus striatum (caudate and putamen): mitochondrial disorders, organic acidopathies, aminoacidopathies, Wilson disease, juvenile Huntington disease
  - Globus pallidus: Hallervorden-Spatz disease, methylmalonic acidemia, hyperbilirubinemia
  - White matter (leukoencephalopathies): peroxisomal disorders (adrenoleukodystrophies), lysosomal leukodystrophies (metachromatic, globoid cell); other white matter diseases (Pelizaeus-Merzbacher, Canavan, Alexander, Cockayne, Aicardi Goutières syndrome)
  - Congenital infection: cytomegalovirus; HIV; toxoplasmosis
- Neoplastic disorders

a very weak correlation between neuroimaging findings and the child's clinical picture. As an unintended consequence, neuroimaging studies may reveal incidental findings that are unrelated to the child's developmental delay, for example, nonspecific findings such as mild ventriculomegaly and enlargement of the subarachnoid spaces, or patchy areas of white matter gliosis of uncertain origin (Table 27.17). In many instances, these are benign variations of normal or clinically insignificant anomalies. In some cases, these findings may require consultation with a pediatric neurosurgeon, but it is important to avoid unnecessary additional tests or interventions whenever possible.

Other Tests

Most neurometabolic disorders can be identified through serum, plasma, and urine tests in conjunction with neuroradiologic investigations. However, other tests can be helpful for identifying specific diseases. Analysis of cerebrospinal fluid for elevated protein levels may help in the diagnosis of a disease affecting white matter; the presence of measles antibody can help identify subacute sclerosing panencephalitis. On occasion, cerebrospinal fluid evaluation of lactate, pyruvate, and amino acids may be helpful. Peripheral nerve conduction tests and electromyography may help confirm that the condition is associated with peripheral neuropathy. Diminished deep tendon reflexes and prolonged nerve conduction times are noted in Krabbe disease, Refsum disease, metachromatic and adrenal leukodystrophy, and infantile neuroaxonal dystrophy (see Chapter 35).

Skin and muscle biopsies may identify conditions in which abnormal material is stored in cells, such as neuronal ceroid lipofuscinosis. Brainstem auditory evoked response is useful as an evaluation of hearing in infants and is used to evaluate brainstem functioning. Visual evoked response can be useful in determining the integrity of the visual pathways; however, it cannot determine visual acuity.

Discussing a Developmental Diagnosis with Parents

When a specific developmental diagnosis is established, it should be shared with the family in an objective but sensitive manner. Facts about the condition and prognostic information should be presented with an explanation of the margin of uncertainty around any disorder. Each child is unique; therefore, making a prognosis for an individual child solely based on data is risky. When appropriate, parents should be reassured that they did not do anything to cause the child's disease, since feelings of guilt in this situation are universal. All parents want some measure of hope and assurance that they will have help from competent professionals who will care for their child.

When the child is an infant or toddler, a frank discussion about the child's profile of developmental strengths and weaknesses relating skills to a "developmental age" may help parents to align their expectations to the child's functional abilities. All parents want to help their child grow and develop to their potential, and the clinician should make a plan for follow-up to evaluate the child's progress. For children under age 3 years, follow-up in 6 months will provide a time frame in which significant change can be observed. For older children, yearly intervals are appropriate.

SPECIFIC CONDITIONS

Cerebral Palsy

Cerebral palsy (CP) is the leading cause of motor disability in children. CP is a clinical diagnosis characterized by significant impairment of movement and posture that begins in infancy or early childhood. Worldwide, CP affects 1–5 in every 1,000 live births. The cause is often brain dysgenesis or injury (prenatal or perinatal from hypoxic-ischemic encephalopathy, intraventricular hemorrhage, or periventricular leukomalacia). There is an inverse relationship between birthweight and CP, ranging from 51–73/1,000 in very low birthweight (<1,500 g) neonatal survivors to 1–2/1,000 in normal birthweight (>2,500 g) infants. The effects of improvements in neonatal intensive care have both increased the survival of low birthweight and premature infants and have decreased the incidence of CP among survivors. However, more than half of children diagnosed with CP were born at term or near term, and there has not been a decrease in CP prevalence over time. In a large population-based study in Western Australia, approximately 76% of children with CP were born at term after an uncomplicated perinatal course without evidence of neonatal encephalopathy. One study identified clinically significant copy number variants in 31% of children with no obvious etiology (so-called "cryptogenic" CP). Thus, the etiology of CP appears to be multifactorial with a largely prenatal onset including genetic, environmental, inflammatory, and infectious influences on fetal development.

Although the underlying pathology is nonprogressive, the clinical manifestations may change over time. An infant with CP may initially present as hypotonic but then develop spasticity, and functional disability may increase if joint contractures or scoliosis develops. CP is associated with a wide range of other disabilities, including sensory impairment (hearing and vision), dysphagia, epilepsy, and ID (40–65%).

Some IEMs present with features of CP ("CP mimics") and are amenable to treatment that can improve the neurologic outcome. A number of symptoms should raise the "index of suspicion" that an IEM may be responsible for the clinical picture of CP (Tables 27.18 and 27.19 and Fig. 27.4).

Important "mimics" include pediatric-onset hereditary spastic paraplegia syndromes (Table 27.20) and dopa-responsive (Segawa disease) and other monoamine-related dystonias (Fig. 27.5).

Autism Spectrum Disorder

(See Chapter 32.)

Fragile X Syndrome

Fragile X (FRAXA) syndrome is the most commonly diagnosed genetic cause of ID in males. It affects 1 in 4,000 males and 1 in 8,000

TABLE 27.18   Clinical Features That Should Prompt Evaluation for Genetic and Metabolic Conditions in a Patient Presenting with Symptoms of Cerebral Palsy

Absent history of any perinatal risk factor for brain injury

Family history of sibling with similar neurologic symptoms

Motor symptom onset after an initial period of normal development

Developmental regression

Progressive neurologic symptoms

Paroxysmal motor symptoms or marked fluctuation of motor symptoms

Clinical exacerbation in the setting of a catabolic state (e.g., febrile illness)

Isolated generalized hypotonia

Prominent ataxia

Signs of peripheral neuromuscular disease (reduced or absent reflexes, sensory loss)

Eye movement abnormalities (e.g., oculogyria, oculomotor apraxia, or paroxysmal saccadic eye-head movements)

From Pearson TS, Pons R, Ghaoui R, et al. Genetics of cerebral palsy. From Pearson TS, Pons R, Ghaoui R, et al. Genetic mimics of cerebral palsy. *Mov Disord.* 2019;34:625–636 (Table 1, p. 628).

TABLE 27.19   Brain MRI Findings Suggestive of Selected Genetic CP Mimics

Finding	Selected Conditions
Hypomyelination	*PLP1*-related dysmyelinating disorders H-ABC (*TUBB4A* mutation) AGS (may also have basal ganglia and WM calcification) GM$_1$ gangliosidosis
Demyelination	Krabbe disease Metachromatic leukodystrophy
Thin corpus callosum	HSP (i.e., SPG4, SPG11, SPG15, and others)
Globus pallidus lesions	T$_2$-hypointense: NBIA (SN also involved in BPAN, MPAN), fucosidosis T$_2$-hyperintense: MMA, PDH deficiency, creatine deficiency syndromes
Focal atrophy or hypoplasia	Glutaric aciduria type 1 (frontotemporal), H-ABC (cerebellum ± putamen), Joubert syndrome (cerebellum)

AGS, Aicardi-Goutières syndrome; BPAN, β-propeller protein-associated neurodegeneration; CP, cerebral palsy; H-ABC, hypomyelination with atrophy of the basal ganglia and cerebellum; HSP, hereditary spastic paraplegia; MMA, methylmalonic aciduria; MPAN, mitochondrial membrane protein-associated neurodegeneration; NBIA, neurodegeneration with brain iron accumulation; PDH, pyruvate dehydrogenase; WM, white matter.

From Pearson TS, Pons R, Ghaoui R, et al. Genetic mimics of cerebral palsy. *Mov Disord.* 2019;34:625–636 (Table 2, p. 628).

females. FRAXA syndrome is found in all racial and ethnic groups. The disorder is the result of an inheritable unstable DNA in the *FMR1* gene of the X chromosome. Normal individuals may have fewer than 40 triplet repeats. Females with between 55 and 200 repeats are said to have *FMR1* premutation, since the number of repeats is likely to expand in cells that become eggs. Males with >200 repeats are clinically symptomatic and will likely have a moderate degree of ID. In addition, speech and language delays, attention difficulty, anxiety disorder, and autism are associated with FRAXA syndrome. Full-mutation females may have a mild degree of ID. Because characteristic physical symptoms of FRAXA are difficult to identify in infants and young children, routine molecular testing for the *FMR1* gene may identify 2–6% of males and 2–4% of females with nonspecific ID. In older children and adults, characteristic physical features and a distinct "behavioral phenotype" may suggest a diagnosis of FRAXA syndrome (Table 27.21).

Inborn Errors of Metabolism and Storage Diseases

IEMs may manifest in variable ways but should always be considered in the differential diagnosis if there is an atypical progression or lack of response to proven interventions (see Chapter 28).

Congenital Infections

Bacteria, parasites, or viruses acquired before, during, or after birth may cause CNS infection and injury. The diagnosis is based on the clinical manifestations (Table 27.22) and polymerase chain reaction (PCR), culture, or serologic evidence of infection (Table 27.23).

Postnatal Infections

CNS infection during infancy or childhood may cause encephalitis or meningoencephalitis with resultant ID. Bacterial (pneumococcus, *Mycobacterium tuberculosis*, meningococcus) and viral (herpes simplex type 1 or 2, eastern or western equine encephalitis virus, West Nile virus, St. Louis encephalitis virus, HIV; in rare cases, mumps, enteroviruses, or California encephalitis virus) cases occur in infancy and early childhood and variably have neurodevelopmental sequelae. Secondary problems caused by the infection such as hearing or visual loss must also be considered. Late sequelae or prior viral infection such

as measles or rubella panencephalitis may appear 10–20 years after the initial CNS disease and manifest as dementia, poor school performance, and progressive encephalopathy.

TREATMENT

The treatment of a child with a developmental or intellectual disability includes routine health maintenance, treatment of the underlying condition (if possible), treatment of associated conditions (such as hyperactivity, seizures, or drooling), relief of symptoms, anticipatory guidance to prevent secondary conditions, and environmental, educational, and family support. The overriding goal is to optimize the functional status and prognosis of the child.

Health maintenance for children with developmental disabilities should be the same as that provided for all children, including immunizations, regular monitoring of physical growth and development, and screening for conditions such as anemia, tuberculosis, and lead intoxication. Use of standardized growth charts will reflect the child's individual pattern over time. Specific growth charts are available for some conditions, including Down syndrome, Prader-Willi syndrome, and FRAXA syndrome. Nutritional recommendations are available for children with CP.

Very few conditions that lead to developmental delay can be "cured." However, medical treatment of associated conditions can help reduce pain and discomfort. For example, many children with CP have drooling and spasticity. Drooling can be controlled by the use of glycopyrrolate, scopolamine patch, or surgery to the salivary glands. Spasticity can be managed with oral baclofen, periodic injections of botulinum toxin, tizanidine, or dorsal root rhizotomy. Behavioral or psychiatric problems may benefit from counseling, support, or psychopharmacologic medications. These medications can be used

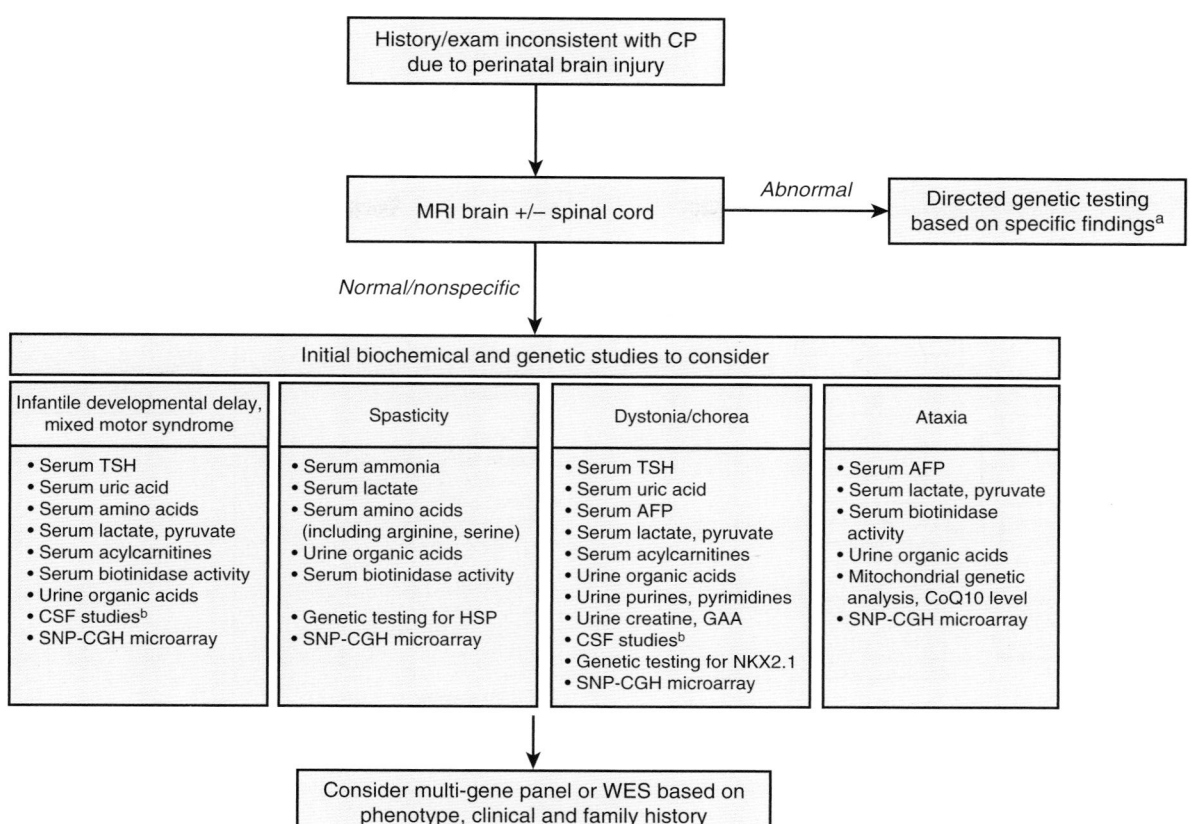

Fig. 27.4 General diagnostic approach to the patient with an infantile-onset, apparently nonprogressive motor disorder. Studies are grouped by predominant clinical presentation; it may be appropriate to consider investigations from more than one group depending on the specific clinical context. [a]See examples in Table 27.19. [b]CSF studies: glucose (+serum glucose), lactate, pyruvate, neurotransmitter metabolites (biogenic amines + γ-aminobutyric acid), pterins, 5-methyltetrahydrofolate. AFP, α-fetoprotein; CP, cerebral palsy; CSF, cerebrospinal fluid; GAA, guanidinoacetate; HSP, hereditary spastic paraplegia; SNP-CGH, single-nucleotide polymorphism-comparative genomic hybridization; TSH, thyroid-stimulating hormone. (From Pearson TS, Pons R, Ghaoui R, et al. Genetic mimics of cerebral palsy. *Mov Disord.* 2019;34:625–636 [Fig. 1, p. 627].)

TABLE 27.20 Clinical and Neuroimaging Findings in Hereditary Spastic Paraplegias (HSPs) with Pediatric Onset*

HSP Form	HSP Type	Inheritance	Gene	Childhood Onset	Disease Characteristics[†]	Neuroimaging Findings (Brain)
Pure	SPG3A	Aut. dom	*ATL1*	+++	None	Normal
Pure	SPG4	Aut. dom	*SPAST*	++	None	Leukoencephalopathy, thin corpus callosum
Pure	SPG6	Aut. dom	*N1PA1*	+	None	Normal
Pure	SPG10	Aut. dom	*KIFSA*	+++	Neuropathy	Normal
Pure	SPG12	Aut. dom	*RTN2*	+++	None	Normal
Pure	SPG31	Aut. dom	*REEP1*	++	None	Normal
Complicated	SPG1	X-linked	*L1CAM*	+++	Intellectual disability, adducted thumb	Thin corpus callosum
Complicated	SPG2	X-linked	*PLP1*	++	Intellectual disability, epilepsy	Normal
Complicated	SPG7	Aut. rec	*SPG7*	+	Optic atrophy, neuropathy, cerebellar ataxia	Cerebellar atrophy
Complicated	SPG11	Aut. rec	*KI AA 1840*	+++	Intellectual disability, neuropathy	Leukoencephalopathy, thin corpus callosum
Complicated	SPG15	Aut. rec	*ZFYVE26*	+++	Intellectual disability, retinopathy, cerebellar ataxia	Leukoencephalopathy, thin corpus callosum
Complicated	SPG17	Aut. rec	*BSCL2*	+	Neuropathy	Normal

*Onset before 18 yr of age.

[†]Other than the classic HSP symptoms, including spastic paraparesis, atrophy of the distal lower extremities, and neurogenic bladder dysfunction.

Aut. dom, autosomal dominant; Aut. rec, autosomal recessive; +, occasional; ++, common; +++, characteristic.

From Lee RW, Poretti A, Cohen JS, et al. A diagnostic approach for cerebral palsy in the genomic era. *Neurol Med.* 2014;16:821–844 (Table 5, p. 832); and Kliegman RM, St. Geme J. *Nelson Textbook of Pediatrics.* 21st ed. Vol 2. Philadelphia: Elsevier; 2020:3171, Table 616.2.

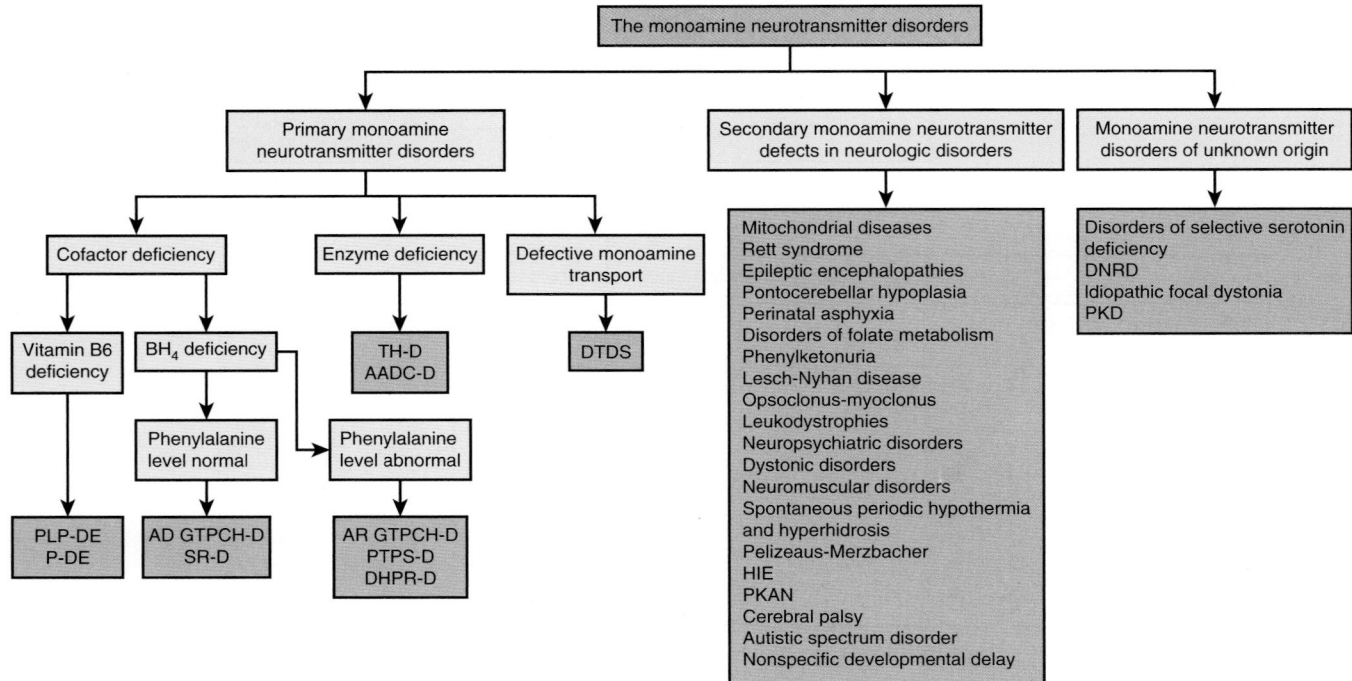

Fig. 27.5 Classification of the monoamine neurotransmitter disorders. AADC-D, aromatic L-amino acid decarboxylase deficiency; AD GTPCH-D, autosomal dominant GTP cyclohydrolase 1 deficiency; AR GTPCH-D, autosomal recessive GTP cyclohydrolase 1 deficiency; BH$_4$, tetrahydrobiopterin; DHPR-D, dihydropteridine reductase deficiency; DNRD, dopa-nonresponsive dystonia; DTDS, dopamine transporter deficiency syndrome; HIE, hypoxic ischemic encephalopathy; P-DE, pyridoxine-dependent epilepsy; PKAN, pantothenate kinase-associated neurodegeneration; PKD, paroxysmal kinesigenic dyskinesia; PLP-DE, pyridoxal-phosphate–dependent epilepsy; PTPS-D, 6-pyruvoyltetrahydropterin synthase deficiency; SR-D, sepiapterin reductase deficiency; TH-D, tyrosine hydroxylase deficiency. (From Kurian MA, Gissen P, Smith M, et al. The monoamine neurotransmitter disorders: an expanding range of neurological syndromes. *Lancet Neurol.* 2011;10:721–731, Fig. 1.)

TABLE 27.21 Scoring System for Screening Individuals for Fragile X Syndrome*

Category	Score	Criteria
Family history	2	Intellectual disability in sibling, maternal uncle, aunt, nephew, niece, first cousin
	1	Any other affected relative
	0	No family history of retardation
Personality	2	Shyness, lack of eye contact followed by friendliness, verbosity, and echolalia
	1	Some of these characteristics
	0	No characteristic
Ears	2	Large and protruding
	1	Large, not protruding
	0	Other
Face	2	Long jaw, high and wide forehead
	1	Only one finding
	0	No findings
Body habitus	2	Slim, tall, rounded shoulders, hyperextensible fingers, lack of body hair, **or** obese with female fat distribution, striae, soft skin, lack of body hair (in males)
	2	Slim **or** obese (females)
	1	Only some features
	0	No features

*A score of 5 or greater has a sensitivity of 0.88 and specificity of 0.98 in comparison with chromosome analysis.

to reduce arousal symptoms and to improve affect, perceptual functioning, cognitive processing, communication, and behavior (Table 27.24). Attention must be paid to the use of medications in specific conditions. Valproic acid is more likely to cause hepatotoxicity in GM$_2$ gangliosidosis, spinocerebellar degeneration, Friedreich ataxia, Lafora body disease, Alpers disease, and myoclonic epilepsy with ragged red fibers. Parents and capable children should be informed about the medication prescribed, including side effects. Some written guidelines for parents and youth are available for psychopharmacologic medications.

Anticipatory guidance for parents of children with developmental disabilities involves the same categories used in all children but may be modified because of the unique features of the child's condition. For example, parents of children with CP should be aware of the possibility that their child may be at risk for poor weight gain and aspiration pneumonia because of oral motor dysphagia; strabismus, spinal scoliosis, and deformities (contractures) of the foot, knee, and hip because of muscle spasticity; osteoporosis; decubitus ulcers; epilepsy; and learning difficulties.

Although there are many different causes, children with developmental disabilities and their families share many common characteristics, including chronicity of the condition (with no cure in most instances); inability to participate in peer activities; parental feelings of guilt and loss of the "ideal" child; increased expense to care for a disabled child; lost economic opportunities (such as the inability of a parent to return to work because they must care for the child at home); need for personal care (because the child cannot be left alone or with a sitter); confusing systems of health care, insurance coverage, and governmental agencies and rules; and social isolation.

TABLE 27.22 Maternal Infections Affecting the Fetus or Newborn

Infection	Mode(s) of Transmission	Neonatal Outcome
Bacteria		
Group B streptococcus	Ascending cervical	Sepsis, pneumonia
Escherichia coli	Ascending cervical	Sepsis, pneumonia
Listeria monocytogenes	Transplacental	Sepsis, pneumonia
Mycoplasma hominis	Ascending cervical	Pneumonia
Chlamydia trachomatis	Vaginal passage	Conjunctivitis, pneumonia
Syphilis	Transplacental, vaginal passage	Congenital syphilis
Neisseria gonorrhoeae	Vaginal passage	Ophthalmia (conjunctivitis), sepsis, meningitis
Mycobacterium tuberculosis	Transplacental	Prematurity, fetal demise, congenital tuberculosis
Virus		
Rubella	Transplacental	Congenital rubella
Cytomegalovirus	Transplacental, breast milk (rare)	Congenital cytomegalovirus or asymptomatic
HIV	Transplacental, vaginal passage, breast milk	Congenital or acquired immunodeficiency syndrome
Hepatitis B	Vaginal passage, transplacental, breast milk	Neonatal hepatitis, chronic hepatitis B surface antigen carrier state
Hepatitis C	Transplacental and vaginal passage	Rarely neonatal hepatitis. –5% chronic carrier state possible
Herpes simplex type 2 or 1	Intrapartum exposure	Neonatal herpes simplex virus Neonatal encephalitis, disseminated viremia, or cutaneous infection
Varicella-zoster	Transplacental: Early Late	Congenital anomalies Neonatal varicella
Parvovirus	Transplacental	Fetal anemia, hydrops
Coxsackievirus B	Fecal-oral	Myocarditis, meningitis, hepatitis
Rubeola	Transplacental	Abortion, fetal measles
West Nile	Transplacental (rare) Possible perinatal	Uncertain, possible rash, encephalitis
Zika	Transplacental	Congenital microcephaly, intracranial calcifications, brain abnormalities, retinal lesions
Chikungunya	Transplacental (rare), perinatal	Neonatal encephalitis
Dengue	Transplacental, perinatal	Neonatal sepsis-like symptoms
Parasites		
Toxoplasmosis	Transplacental	Congenital toxoplasmosis
Malaria	Transplacental	Abortion, prematurity, intrauterine growth restriction
Fungi		
Candida	Ascending, cervical	Sepsis, pneumonia, rash

From Kliegman RM, St. Geme J. *Nelson Textbook of Pediatrics.* 21st ed. Vol 1. Philadelphia: Elsevier; 2020:879, Table 114.3.

Environmental support may be needed and may take the form of family therapy, financial counseling, and referral to a disease-oriented volunteer support group or in a "Big Brothers/Big Sisters" program. Formal support includes early intervention for children from birth to 3 years of age, preschool intervention through the school district for children 3–5 years of age, and special education services provided under the Individuals with Disabilities Education Act (IDEA) and Section 504 of the Rehabilitation Act for school-age children. Families may also need assistance in transitioning their adolescent child from school to a work or independent living situation. At each stage in the child's life, the clinician should review the services the child is receiving and determine whether the family might benefit from additional support. The mnemonic "MD's DD BASICS" provides a list of content areas for review at each visit (Table 27.25). Checklists to monitor the care of children

with specific problems such as Down syndrome are also available (Table 27.26).

PITFALLS AND HAZARDS IN DEVELOPMENTAL DIAGNOSIS

The identification of "risk factors" does not imply a specific etiology or diagnosis. It is important to avoid a logical fallacy (post hoc attribution) and not base a diagnosis on a specific cause unless there is positive evidence to confirm that cause. A history of a low 5-minute Apgar score with no other symptoms of neonatal encephalopathy is not likely to be the cause of a child's subsequent developmental disability.

Dysmorphic and physically disabled children are often assumed to have GDD/ID, and, conversely, children with normal facial appearance and motor skills may not be identified early as having

TABLE 27.23   Laboratory Tests in the Diagnosis of Specific Perinatal Infections

Infectious Agent	Acceptable Specimen(s) from Infant Unless Otherwise Indicated	Laboratory Test
Chlamydia trachomatis	Conjunctiva, nasopharyngeal swab, tracheal aspirate	Culture using special transport media Nucleic acid amplification tests (NAATs) are not U.S. Food and Drug Administration approved for specimens from neonates*
Genital mycoplasmas (*Mycoplasma hominis, M. genitalium, Ureaplasma urealyticum*)	Tracheal aspirate, blood, or cerebrospinal fluid (CSF)	Culture using special transport media Real-time polymerase chain reactions (PCRs)
Neisseria gonorrhoeae	Conjunctiva, blood, CSF, or synovial fluid	Finding gram-negative intracellular diplococci on Gram stain is suggestive Culture on special media establishes the diagnosis
Syphilis (*Treponema pallidum*)	Serum (mother) Serum CSF	Rapid plasma reagin (RPR), and, if reactive, a specific treponemal test† RPR Venereal Disease Research Laboratories (VDRL)
Cytomegalovirus (CMV)	Urine, saliva, blood, or CSF	PCR for detection of CMV DNA Obtain within 2–4 wk of birth
Enteroviruses	Blood, nasopharyngeal swab, throat swab, conjunctival swab, tracheal aspirate, urine, stool, rectal swab, or CSF	PCR Cell culture (sensitivity depends on serotype and cell lines used)
Hepatitis B	Serum (mother) Serum	Hepatitis B surface antigen (HBsAg) If mother's HBsAg is positive, at age 9 mo, test the infant for HBsAg and hepatitis B surface antibody
Herpes simplex viruses 1 and 2	Conjunctiva, skin vesicle scraping, whole blood, or mouth vesicles CSF "Surface cultures" (mouth, nasopharynx, conjunctiva, and anus)	PCR or cell culture PCR PCR or cell culture
HIV	Serum (mother) Whole blood	Fourth-generation HIV antigen/antibody test HIV DNA PCR
Candida species	Blood, skin biopsy, or CSF	Culture
Zika virus	Blood, urine, CSF	NAAT and serum immunoglobulin M (IgM) NAAT may be falsely negative Immunoglobulin G (IgG) antibodies may reflect maternal exposure Antibodies may cross-react with other flaviviruses

*Published evaluations of NAATs for these indications are limited, but sensitivity and specificity are expected to be at least as high as those for culture.
†Treponemal tests include the *T. pallidum* particle agglutination (TP-PA) test, *T. pallidum* enzyme immunoassay (TP-EIA), *T. pallidum* chemiluminescent assay (TP-CIA), and fluorescent treponemal antibody absorption (FTA-ABS) test.
From Kliegman RM, St. Geme J. *Nelson Textbook of Pediatrics.* 21st ed. Vol 1. Philadelphia: Elsevier; 2020:1012, Table 131.6.

TABLE 27.24   Psychopharmacologic Agents That May Be Useful in the Treatment of Children with Developmental Disabilities

Medication	Possible Indications
Carbamazepine	Mania, bipolar disorder, impulsivity, aggression, seizures, trigeminal neuralgia
Clomipramine	Obsessive-compulsive disorder, depression
Clonazepam	Mania, bipolar disorder, seizure
Clonidine, guanfacine	Manic episodes, attention-deficit/hyperactivity disorder, aggression
Sertraline, other SSRIs, risperidone, olanzapine, aripiprazole	Obsessive-compulsive disorder, depression, anxiety Aggressive, self-injurious behavior
Methylphenidate	Attention-deficit/hyperactivity disorder: dextroamphetamine Aggression, impulsivity
Valproic acid	Bipolar disorder, especially rapidly cycling

SSRIs, selective serotonin reuptake inhibitors.

GDD/ID. Cognitive development is usually unaffected in a number of striking dysmorphic syndromes (e.g., Treacher Collins syndrome, achondroplasia).

Children with physical disabilities, language disorders, ADHD, or anxiety disorder may be misdiagnosed as having an intellectual disorder unless appropriate measures are used to account for these comorbid conditions. A child with mild cerebral palsy may score low on tasks that require motor responses. In this situation, a motor-free cognitive test should be used to judge intellectual ability. Similarly, a child with low language abilities may show a wide discrepancy between subnormal verbal scores and average nonverbal scores, making a "composite IQ" score invalid. Alternatively, a nonverbal test of cognitive ability can be used. Evaluation of children with behavioral and/or emotional challenges should include appropriate accommodations, such as frequent breaks during testing or extending testing over several sessions, to ensure that the results reflect the child's innate ability and not the impact of other, extraneous, factors.

Identifying a child as being "at risk" for developmental delay may alter the family's perceptions, making the child vulnerable. This might lead to constraints on the child's experiences and diminished expectations of

TABLE 27.25 Providing Primary Care to Children with Developmental Disabilities Using the Mnemonic "MD'S DD BASICS"

MD'S DD BASICS	Things to Check	Potential Consultant(s)
Motor	Ambulation, seating, position, spine	Orthopedist, physiatrist, PT, OT
Diet	Weight, fat stores, diet, feeding problems	Nutritionist/dietitian, speech pathologist, OT
Seizures	Seizure record; drug levels and side effects	Neurologist
Dermatology	Skin breakdown	Nursing, plastic surgeon
Dentistry	Teeth, gums	Dentist
Behavior	Aggression, self-injury, sleep, pica, interfering behavior	Psychologist, psychiatrist
Advocacy	Finances, family support, program aid	Social worker
Sensory	Vision, hearing	Ophthalmologist, audiologist
Infections	Immunizations, environment, lungs, urine	Infection control nurse
Constipation	Stools, gastroesophageal reflux	Gastroenterologist
Sexuality	Menses, sexual activity, masturbation, contraception, prevention of sexually transmitted diseases	Gynecologist, habilitation program

OT, occupational therapist; PT, physical therapist.
Modified from Sulkes S. MD's DD BASICS: identifying common problems and preventing secondary disabilities. *Pediatr Ann*. 1995;24:245–254.

TABLE 27.26 Medical Checklist for a Child with Down Syndrome

Age	Condition	Monitoring
Birth to 2 mo	Etiology, recurrence risk	Chromosome analysis and genetic counseling
	Hypothyroidism	TSH, T_3, and T_4
	Congenital heart defect	Pediatric cardiology evaluation, including echocardiography
	Family stress	Referral to Down Syndrome Association
2–12 mo	Refractive errors, cataracts	Pediatric ophthalmologic evaluation
	Hearing loss; recurrent otitis media	Auditory brainstem evoked response
	Delayed development	Formal developmental evaluations
1–12 yr	Delayed development	Enrollment in early intervention program
	Hypothyroidism	Annual TSH
	Hearing loss	Auditory testing: annually between 1 and 3 yr and every 2 yr between 3 and 13 yr
	Refractive error	Ophthalmologic examination every 2 yr
	Atlantoaxial instability	Cervical spine roentgenography at 2 and 12 yr
	Routine care	Dental examination at 2 yr, then every 6 mo (prophylaxis for subacute bacterial endocarditis, if indicated)
12–18 yr	Hypothyroidism	TSH annually
	Decreased hearing	Auditory testing every 2 yr
	Refractive error	Ophthalmologic examination every 2 yr
	Mitral valve prolapse	Echocardiography

T_3, triiodothyronine; T_4, thyroxine; TSH, thyroid-stimulating hormone.

performance. When a child is born with a single risk factor, such as prematurity, the parents may be afraid to place demands on the child, creating a vicious cycle of "learned helplessness" and immature behaviors.

Parents of children who are informed that their child is not normal often grieve for their "lost" (typically developing) child. This process of grieving involves stages that include denial, sadness, anger, and guilt. One parent may be experiencing persistent anger while another is still sad or depressed. This difference in stages may make communication between them exceedingly difficult. Grieving may occur at times other than the initial diagnosis, for example, on the first day of kindergarten. These feelings may be expressed in nonfunctional ways, such as denial that leads to unending shopping for professionals who will "cure" the child or anger that is expressed at the clinician, thereby thwarting efforts at building a trusting and supportive relationship. However, many authorities believe that these emotions are essential steps that allow the parents to release the old dreams and secure new ones. The goal of the therapeutic clinician is to accept the parents at whatever stage they are in and to help them understand the normalcy of the stages.

▉ SUMMARY AND RED FLAGS

Developmental disabilities are common. Identifying children with developmental delay involves both specific attention to children with biologic and/or sociocultural risks and routine developmental surveillance and screening during well-child visits. All children with suspected developmental delay should receive a formal multidisciplinary assessment that includes a systematic diagnostic approach with a "tiered" strategy for laboratory and neuroimaging evaluations. Developmental regression, vomiting, seizures, or lethargy suggests the presence of a potentially life-threatening metabolic disorder. Parents need to understand that it is not always possible to identify a single defined disease process responsible for their child's developmental disability. Even if a specific etiology is not found, comprehensive clinical assessments can identify the child's profile of strengths and weaknesses. Children with developmental disabilities will require meticulous monitoring over time and coordination of care to optimize their functional status. All children with developmental disabilities will benefit from early intervention, therapeutic, and special education services to help maximize their developmental potential and to promote independence and personal autonomy.

Red flags include developmental regression (see Chapter 28), dysmorphology, developmental delay associated with vomiting or lethargy (consider IEMs), failure to thrive, seizures, and recognition of a treatable cause of delay or CP (http://www.treatable-id.org/).

BIBLIOGRAPHY

A bibliography is available at ExpertConsult.com.

28

Neurocognitive and Developmental Regression

Michael Muriello

The etiology of intellectual developmental disabilities includes a wide spectrum of disorders that may present at different periods of development (infantile, juvenile, adult) and with different trajectories (Fig. 28.1). Some are static encephalopathies (cerebral palsy, hypoxic-ischemic encephalopathy), while others are progressive, resulting in intellectual, neurologic, and/or developmental regression (Table 28.1).

Dominant etiologic categories include:
- Storage diseases including leukoencephalopathies
- Inborn errors of metabolism including mitochondrial disorders
- Genetic and idiopathic epilepsy encephalopathies
- Cerebrovascular diseases
- Trauma

Progressive neurocognitive regression is an uncommon but important presentation to recognize, diagnose, and potentially treat. The cardinal feature is usually first stagnation and then loss of developmental milestones in young children or loss of abilities, especially cognitive, in older children. The deficits can be slow or rapidly progressive and may or may not be accompanied by other neurologic signs and symptoms. Early recognition and treatment, when possible, may prevent permanent neurologic deficits. Distinguishing delayed development from arrested development or loss of skills can be challenging, especially on first presentation when there are insufficient data to predict the overall trajectory. The recognition of subtle features depends on both parental reporting and careful developmental screening by primary care providers. Overt symptomatology or rapid decline is unlikely to go unnoticed and requires urgent evaluation in all cases. The differential diagnosis of neurodegenerative conditions is broad and includes genetic, neurologic, infectious, immunologic, endocrine, traumatic, and idiopathic conditions. Initial referral to multiple specialists may be needed.

DIAGNOSTIC APPROACH

Distinguishing delayed development from arrested development can be challenging, especially on first presentation when there are insufficient data to predict the overall trajectory. Normal development can include brief, transient plateaus or minor losses of skills that occur prior to a significant leap forward in overall development or during concurrent illness. In such cases careful observation and close follow-up will be reassuring. There are certain key elements to consider when taking a history or examining a patient that may trigger deeper exploration for the possibility of regression or intellectual disability (ID) (Tables 28.2 and 28.3). Careful neurocognitive assessment is essential when there are subtle or ill-defined but concerning losses of skills or arrest of development. Referral for neuropsychologic evaluation is essential to correctly establish the specific areas of weakness or change and establish a baseline for the developmental diagnosis.

Developmental regression should be considered as a separate diagnostic entity, unique from global developmental delay (GDD) or ID (see Chapter 27) even though there are overlapping conditions. Identifying true regression, rather than failure of development, may be challenging and require close follow-up over a period of time. Once regression is identified, evaluation is warranted.

If the arrest in development is more abrupt, global, or associated with other neurologic signs and symptoms, urgent evaluation is indicated. This may include referral to neurology and/or medical genetics, both basic labs (comprehensive metabolic panel, thyroid studies, blood counts) and specific laboratory studies based on accompanying symptoms, brain MRI, and EEG (Table 28.4 and Figs. 28.2 and 28.3). A specific subset of metabolic disorders can present with regression and various treatment options are available; it is thus important to recognize and diagnose these potentially treatable disorders (Tables 28.5 and 28.6). An exception to this rule is the loss of social and communication skills that precedes a diagnosis of autism in ~30% of cases. Neuropsychologic evaluation is required to determine whether the regression is part of the autistic spectrum (see Chapter 32).

More than 300 neurodegenerative disorders have been described including genetic, neurologic, infectious, immunologic, endocrine, traumatic, and idiopathic conditions; additional classification based on progression and age is noted in Table 28.7 and in Figure 28.2. Neurodegenerative disorders are often categorized as involving white matter, gray matter, basal ganglia, or the entire central nervous system. **White matter diseases** (e.g., adrenoleukodystrophy) affect long tracts and manifest with loss of motor skills, spasticity, disturbed gait, areflexia (if peripheral nerve is also involved), or ataxia, whereas **gray matter diseases** (e.g., ceroid lipofuscinoses) manifest with seizures and abnormalities of cognition, vision, and hearing. Many disorders commonly classified as "white matter" or "gray matter" manifest with a mixed picture of signs and symptoms. Diseases that involve primarily the **basal ganglia** (deep gray matter), such as Huntington disease, manifest with cognitive deterioration, behavioral changes, rigidity, dystonia, ataxia, dysarthria, seizures, and incoordination. When these diseases progress, neurologic signs and symptoms may become more widespread and less specific.

Progressive disorders may be the result of metabolic or storage diseases or due to a genetic syndrome (Rett syndrome). In contrast, static encephalopathies are usually the result of structural abnormalities due to abnormal development or trauma (see Tables 28.6 and 28.7).

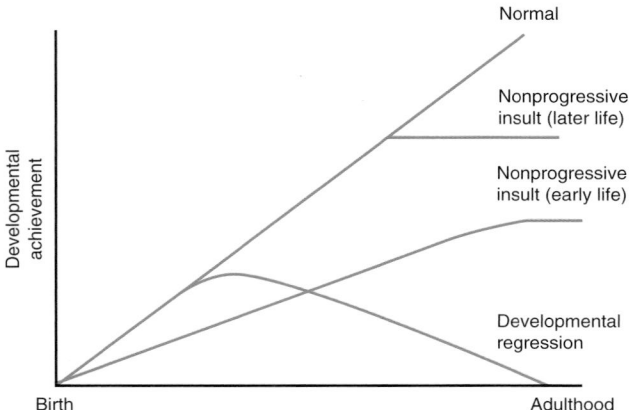

Fig. 28.1 Potential developmental trajectories. (From Holland J, Brown R. Developmental regression: assessment and investigation. *Paediatr Child Health.* 2017;27[6]:253–259 [Fig. 1, p. 253].)

TABLE 28.1   Criteria for Regression

Any child who fulfills **all** the following three criteria:
- Progressive deterioration for more than 3 mo **with**
- Loss of already attained intellectual/developmental abilities **and**
- Development of abnormal neurologic signs

Excluding: static intellectual loss, e.g., after encephalitis, head injury, or near drowning

Including:
- Children who meet the case definition even if specific neurologic diagnoses have been made
- Metabolic disorders leading to neurologic deterioration
- Seizure syndromes (epileptic, encephalopathies) if associated with progressive deterioration
- Pre-existing developmental delay with acute deterioration

Modified from Holland J, Brown R. Developmental regression: assessment and investigation. *Paediatr Child Health.* 2017;27(6):253–259 (Box 1, p. 254).

GENETIC EVALUATION

The genetic considerations for ID are detailed in Chapter 27. Next-generation sequencing (NGS) technology provides broad screening panels within a group of phenotypes (e.g., X-Linked Intellectual Disability [XLID] panel). Genomic sequencing (whole exome sequencing [WES] and whole genome sequencing [WGS]) is transforming the diagnostic process for children with neurodegenerative disorders. Consideration for genome or exome sequencing as a ***first-line*** approach in the presence of neurologic regression is becoming the standard of care. If there is progressive neurodevelopmental regression, exome/genome sequencing should be considered early in the diagnostic evaluation because many treatable disorders have improved outcomes with earlier initiation of therapy (i.e., mucopolysaccharidoses, Krabbe disease). This is especially true for young patients or more rapidly progressive neurodegenerative disease processes. Rapid genome/exome sequencing can provide results in as little as 5–10 days but is typically reserved for the intensive care setting.

TABLE 28.2   Elements in History That Are Red Flags for Regression

General
- Age at presentation: certain disorders present within specific age ranges
- Trigger: some disorders manifest more symptoms during intercurrent illness
- Nature of progression of symptoms (slow, sharp, or stepwise decline)
- Other neurologic symptoms (movement disorders, gait disturbances, behavioral changes, ataxia, seizures, signs of increased intracranial pressure)
- Seizures, if present: type, nature, frequency, and response to treatment
- Endocrine disorders: adrenal dysfunction in peroxisomal disorders (Zellweger)

Developmental History
- Milestones: rate achieved, change in progression

Family Health History
- Family history of neurodegenerative disorders
- Consanguinity
- Ancestry (e.g., Tay-Sachs in Jewish and Amish communities)

Metabolic Tests

Inborn errors of metabolism (IEMs) should be suspected in children with acute or episodic neurologic abnormalities in whom there is unexplained altered mental status, vomiting, an unusual smell to the urine or body odor, metabolic acidosis, elevated lactate, hypoglycemia, or renal stones. IEMs may manifest as episodic acute encephalopathy (from an organic acidemia or hyperammonemia) or as a chronic progressive encephalopathy (with associated cardiomyopathy, spasticity, hyperreflexia, or liver dysfunction), often as a result of mitochondrial disorders or storage diseases (Tables 28.8 and 29.9). Routine neonatal screening for metabolic disorders may identify infants with IEMs that are associated with GDD. However, not all children with IEMs manifest soon after birth, and normal results do not eliminate the possibility that an IEM is present. Targeted biochemical lab testing can be performed when a specific disease is considered (7-dehydrocholesterol for Smith-Lemli-Opitz syndrome, very-long-chain fatty acids for peroxisomal disorders, thyroxine [T_4]/thyroid-stimulating hormone [TSH] for hypothyroidism, creatinine kinase for Duchenne muscular dystrophy, glycosaminoglycans and oligosaccharides for lysosomal storage disorders such as Hunter or Hurler disease) (see Fig. 28.3). In general, few IEMs result in GDD/ID in the absence of other neurologic symptoms (see Table 28.8). To date, 89 IEMs (and more, other disorders) have been identified that are amenable to treatment of the underlying defect and/or pathogenetic mechanism (Table 28.10). Of these, 54 (60%) can be identified by blood (plasma amino acids, homocysteine, copper, ceruloplasmin) and urine (creatine metabolites, glycosaminoglycans, oligosaccharides, organic acids, and pyrimidines) tests. The remaining 35 (40%) are identified by specific tests and molecular analysis. A digital app (TIDE BC) is freely available (http://www.treatable-id.org) and provides an information portal about these diseases and their treatments. Although the yield from metabolic studies in "nonsyndromic" GDD/ID is relatively low (0.2–2.5%), IEMs are amenable to treatment, so metabolic testing should be considered in all cases of unexplained GDD/ID.

TABLE 28.3 Elements on Physical Examination That Are Red Flags for Regression

Head Circumference
- Macrocephaly (white matter disorders, hydrocephalus): especially if crossing centiles
- Microcephaly (gray matter disorders)

Dysmorphic Features
- Coarse facial features in mucopolysaccharidosis
- Tall forehead, depressed nasal bridge, micrognathia in peroxisomal biogenesis disorders

Ophthalmology
- Ptosis (mitochondrial disorders, myasthenia syndromes, Menkes syndrome)
- Retinal degeneration (gray matter disease)
- Optic atrophy (white matter disease)
- Cherry-red spots ($GM_{1/2}$ [Tay-Sachs] gangliosidosis, Krabbe leukodystrophy, metachromatic leukodystrophy)

Neurology
- Long tract signs in raised intracranial pressure
- Abnormal tone (spasticity, dystonia, hypotonia)
- Movement disorder (ataxia, chorea)

Skin
- Café-au-lait spots in neurofibromatosis, Chediak-Higashi syndrome, Gaucher disease, Hunter syndrome
- Hypopigmented macules and Shagreen patch in tuberous sclerosis
- Abnormal "kinky" hair in Menkes syndrome
- Severe, intractable eczema in biotinidase deficiency

Visceromegaly
- Hepatosplenomegaly is a frequent manifestation of a number of storage disorders

Other
- Skeletal manifestations: dysostosis multiplex in lysosomal disorders, stippling in peroxisomal disorders
- Cardiac valvular disease in lysosomal storage disorders

TABLE 28.4 Tiered Approach to Evaluating Regression*

Blood
Genetic testing: genomic approach—exome/genome or large gene panel on exome backbone if more targeted
Full blood count, urea and electrolytes, liver function test, bone profile, thyroid function test, ESR, ammonia, lactate, uric acid
Very long-chain fatty acids
Biotin
Copper and ceruloplasmin
Amino acids
Free carnitine and acylcarnitine profile
Lysosomal enzyme assay in leukocytes
Vitamin B_{12} and E levels
Heavy metals: lead, mercury

Cerebrospinal Fluid
Amino acids (with plasma amino acids simultaneously)
Lactate and pyruvate
Glucose (with plasma levels simultaneously)
Neurotransmitters and neuroinflammatory markers (N-methyl-D-aspartate receptor antibodies)

Urine
Organic acids
Glycosaminoglycans and oligosaccharides through mass spectrometry

BRAIN MRI with consideration for targeted spectroscopy

TISSUE BIOPSY and analysis as indicated
Muscle for mitochondrial testing
Liver for assessment of copper, iron, or electron microscopy

*This evaluation is often coincident with the evaluation for intellectual disability (see Chapter 27).

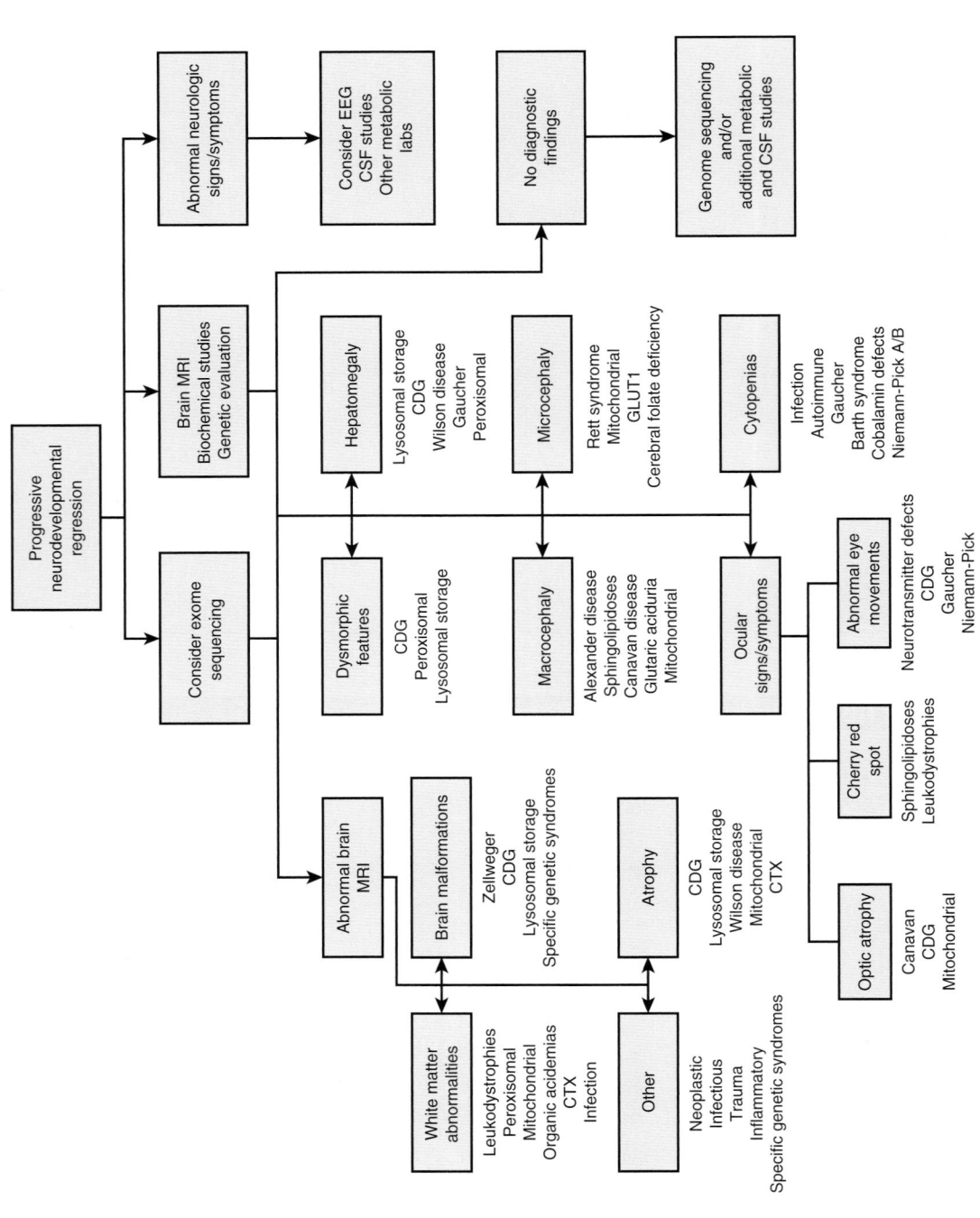

Fig. 28.2 Evaluation of children with progressive cognitive, developmental, and neurologic deterioration. CDG, congenital disorders of glycosylation; CSF, cerebrospinal fluid; CTX, cerebrotendinous xanthomatosis. (Modified from Fenichel GM. *Clinical Pediatric Neurology: A Signs and Symptoms Approach.* 2nd ed. Philadelphia: WB Saunders; 1993:138.)

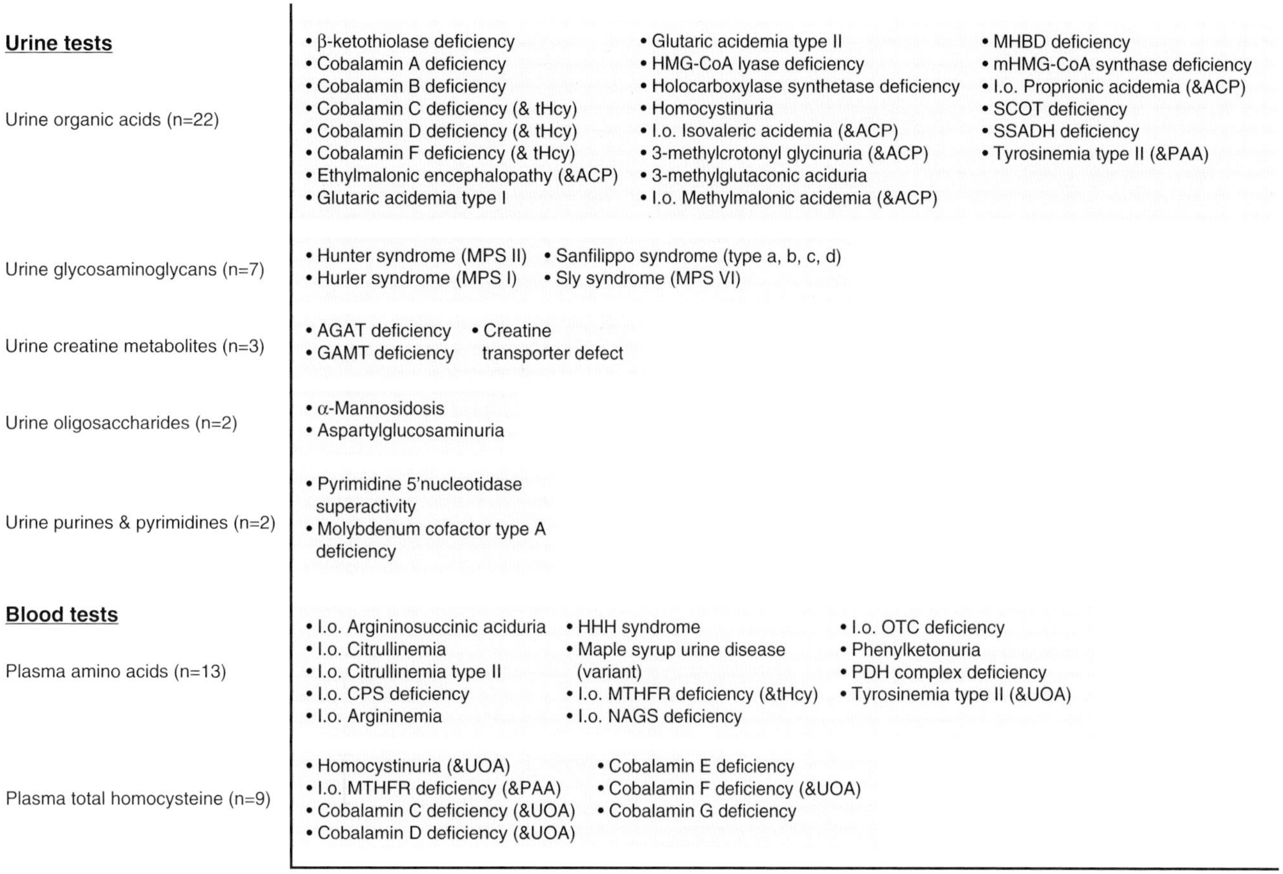

Urine tests

Urine organic acids (n=22)

- β-ketothiolase deficiency
- Cobalamin A deficiency
- Cobalamin B deficiency
- Cobalamin C deficiency (& tHcy)
- Cobalamin D deficiency (& tHcy)
- Cobalamin F deficiency (& tHcy)
- Ethylmalonic encephalopathy (&ACP)
- Glutaric acidemia type I

- Glutaric acidemia type II
- HMG-CoA lyase deficiency
- Holocarboxylase synthetase deficiency
- Homocystinuria
- I.o. Isovaleric acidemia (&ACP)
- 3-methylcrotonyl glycinuria (&ACP)
- 3-methylglutaconic aciduria
- I.o. Methylmalonic acidemia (&ACP)

- MHBD deficiency
- mHMG-CoA synthase deficiency
- I.o. Proprionic acidemia (&ACP)
- SCOT deficiency
- SSADH deficiency
- Tyrosinemia type II (&PAA)

Urine glycosaminoglycans (n=7)

- Hunter syndrome (MPS II)
- Hurler syndrome (MPS I)

- Sanfilippo syndrome (type a, b, c, d)
- Sly syndrome (MPS VI)

Urine creatine metabolites (n=3)

- AGAT deficiency
- GAMT deficiency

- Creatine transporter defect

Urine oligosaccharides (n=2)

- α-Mannosidosis
- Aspartylglucosaminuria

Urine purines & pyrimidines (n=2)

- Pyrimidine 5'nucleotidase superactivity
- Molybdenum cofactor type A deficiency

Blood tests

Plasma amino acids (n=13)

- I.o. Argininosuccinic aciduria
- I.o. Citrullinemia
- I.o. Citrullinemia type II
- I.o. CPS deficiency
- I.o. Argininemia

- HHH syndrome
- Maple syrup urine disease (variant)
- I.o. MTHFR deficiency (&tHcy)
- I.o. NAGS deficiency

- I.o. OTC deficiency
- Phenylketonuria
- PDH complex deficiency
- Tyrosinemia type II (&UOA)

Plasma total homocysteine (n=9)

- Homocystinuria (&UOA)
- I.o. MTHFR deficiency (&PAA)
- Cobalamin C deficiency (&UOA)
- Cobalamin D deficiency (&UOA)

- Cobalamin E deficiency
- Cobalamin F deficiency (&UOA)
- Cobalamin G deficiency

Fig. 28.3 Bar graph depicting the yield of "metabolic screening tests." For the mucopolysaccharidoses, enzyme activity should be measured as a next step: Hurler (iduronidase); Hunter syndrome (iduronate-2-sulfatase); Sanfilippo syndrome (IIIa = heparan-N-sulfatase, IIIc = acetyl CoA glucosamine N-acetyl transferase, IIId = N-acetyl-glucosamine-6-sulfatase); Sly syndrome (β-glucuronidase). ACP, plasma acylcarnitine profile; HHH, hyperornithinemia-hyperammonemia-homocitrullinuria; MPS, mucopolysaccharidosis; PAA, plasma amino acids; tHcy, total homocysteine; UOA, urine organic acids. (From van Karnebeek CDM, Stockler S. Treatable inborn errors of metabolism causing intellectual disability: a systematic literature review. *Mol Genetic Metab.* 2012;105:368-381 [Fig. 1, p. 374].)

TABLE 28.5   Select "Intrinsic" Conditions Associated with Developmental Regression

Age at Onset (yr)	Conditions	Comments
<2, with hepatomegaly (see Chapter 17)	Fructose intolerance	Vomiting, hypoglycemia, poor feeding, failure to thrive (when given fructose)
	Galactosemia	Lethargy, hypotonia, icterus, cataract, hypoglycemia (when given lactose)
	Glycogenosis (glycogen storage disease) types I–IV	Hypoglycemia, cardiomegaly (type II)
	Mucopolysaccharidosis types I and II	Coarse facies, stiff joints
	Niemann-Pick disease, infantile type	Gray matter disease, failure to thrive
	Tay-Sachs disease	Seizures, cherry-red macula, edema, coarse facies
	Zellweger (cerebrohepatorenal) syndrome	Hypotonia, high forehead, flat facies
	Gaucher disease type II	Extensor posturing, irritability
	Carbohydrate-deficient glycoprotein syndromes	Dysmyelination, cerebellar hypoplasia
<2, without hepatomegaly	Krabbe disease	Irritability, extensor posturing, optic atrophy, and blindness
	Rett syndrome	Females with deceleration of head growth, loss of hand skills, hand wringing, impaired language skills, gait apraxia
	Maple syrup urine disease	Poor feeding, tremors, myoclonus, opisthotonos
	Phenylketonuria	Light pigmentation, eczema, seizures
	Menkes kinky hair disease	Hypertonia, irritability, seizures, abnormal hair
	Subacute necrotizing encephalopathy of Leigh	White matter disease
	Cerebro-oculofacioskeletal syndrome (of Pena and Shokeir)	Reduced white matter, failure to thrive
	Canavan disease	White matter disease
	Pelizaeus-Merzbacher disease	White matter disease
2–5	Niemann-Pick disease types III and IV	Hepatosplenomegaly, gait difficulty
	Wilson disease	Liver disease, Kayser-Fleischer ring; deterioration of cognition is late
	Gangliosidosis type II	Gray matter disease
	Ceroid lipofuscinosis	Gray matter disease
	Mitochondrial encephalopathies (e.g., myoclonic epilepsy with ragged red fibers [MERRF])	Gray matter disease
	Ataxia-telangiectasia	Basal ganglia disease
	Huntington disease (chorea)	Basal ganglia disease
	Hallervorden-Spatz syndrome	Basal ganglia disease
	Metachromatic leukodystrophy	White matter disease
	Adrenoleukodystrophy	White matter disease, behavior problems, deteriorating school performance, quadriparesis
5–15	Adrenoleukodystrophy	Same as for adrenoleukodystrophy in 2–5 yr olds
	Multiple sclerosis	White matter disease
	Neuronal ceroid lipofuscinosis, juvenile and adult (Spielmeyer-Vogt and Kufs disease)	Gray matter disease
	Schilder disease	White matter disease, focal neurologic symptoms
	Refsum disease	Peripheral neuropathy, ataxia, retinitis pigmentosa
	Sialidosis type II, juvenile form	Cherry-red macula, myoclonus, ataxia, coarse facies
	Subacute sclerosing panencephalitis	Diffuse encephalopathy, myoclonus; may occur years after measles

TABLE 28.6 Select "Extrinsic" Conditions Associated with Developmental Regression

Neoplasms and their therapy	Vitamin B_{12} and E deficiencies
Leukemia	Hypothyroidism
Tumors	Chronic lead poisoning
Langerhans cell histiocytosis	Adrenocortical insufficiency
Hemophagocytic lymphohistiocytosis	Autoimmune encephalitis (e.g., N-methyl-D-aspartate receptor [NMDAR] encephalitis)
Increased intracranial pressure	
Hydrocephalus, including ventricular shunt malfunctions	Collagen vascular disease (e.g., systemic lupus erythematosus)
Subdural hematoma or effusion	"Pseudo" regression
Infections	• Child abuse
Encephalitis, including HIV infection, toxoplasmosis	• Behavioral disorders
Meningitis	• Bullying
Endocrine disorders	• Medication, recreational drug effects

TABLE 28.7 Causes of Developmental Regression

Onset Before Age 2 yr

AIDS

Encephalopathy*

Autism Spectrum Disorder

Disorders of Amino Acid Metabolism
Guanidinoacetate methyltransferase deficiency*
Homocystinuria
Maple syrup urine disease (intermediate and thiamine response forms)*
Phenylketonuria
Hyperammonemic disorders

Disorders of Lysosomal Enzymes
Ganglioside storage disorders
 • GM_1 gangliosidosis
 • GM_2 gangliosidosis (Tay-Sachs disease, Sandhoff disease)
Gaucher disease type II (glucosylceramide lipidosis)*
Globoid cell leukodystrophy (Krabbe disease)
Glycoprotein degradation disorders
I-cell disease
 • Mucopolysaccharidoses*
 • Type I (Hurler syndrome)*
 • Type III (Sanfilippo disease)
Niemann-Pick disease type A (sphingomyelin lipidosis)
Sulfatase deficiency disorders
 • Metachromatic leukodystrophy (sulfatide lipidoses)
 • Multiple sulfatase deficiency

Carbohydrate-Deficient Glycoprotein Syndromes

Hypothyroidism*

Mitochondrial Disorders
Alexander disease
Mitochondrial myopathy, encephalopathy, lactic acidosis, stroke
Progressive infantile poliodystrophy (Alpers disease)
Subacute necrotizing encephalomyelopathy (Leigh disease)
Trichopoliodystrophy (Menkes disease)

Neurocutaneous Syndromes
Chediak-Higashi syndrome
Neurofibromatosis*
Tuberous sclerosis*

Other Disorders of Gray Matter
Infantile ceroid lipofuscinosis (Santavuori-Haltia disease)
Infantile neuroaxonal dystrophy
Lesch-Nyhan disease*
Progressive neuronal degeneration with liver disease
Infantile spasms (West, Lennox-Gastaut)
Epileptic encephalopathies (monogenetic, idiopathic)
Rett syndrome
Aicardi-Goutieres syndrome

Other Disorders of White Matter
Aspartoacylase deficiency (Canavan disease)
Galactosemia: transferase deficiency*
Neonatal adrenoleukodystrophy
Pelizaeus-Merzbacher disease
Progressive cavitating leukoencephalopathy

Progressive Hydrocephalus*

Continued

TABLE 28.7 Causes of Developmental Regression—cont'd

Onset After Age 2 yr	Other Disorders of Gray Matter—cont'd
Disorders of Lysosomal Enzymes Gaucher disease type III (glucosylceramide lipidosis) Globoid cell leukodystrophy (late-onset Krabbe disease) Glycoprotein degradation disorders Aspartylglycosaminuria Mannosidosis type II GM$_2$ gangliosidosis (juvenile Tay-Sachs disease) Metachromatic leukodystrophy (late-onset sulfatide lipidoses) Mucopolysaccharidoses types II and VII Niemann-Pick type C (sphingomyelin lipidosis)	Huntington disease Biotin-thiamine-responsive basal ganglia disease Mitochondrial disorders • Late-onset poliodystrophy • Mitochondrial neurogastrointestinal encephalomyopathy (MNGIE) • Myoclonic epilepsy and ragged-red fibers Progressive neuronal degeneration with liver disease Xeroderma pigmentosum Wilson disease Neurodegeneration with brain iron accumulation (NBIA) Pantothenate kinase neurodegeneration
Infectious Disease AIDS encephalopathy* Congenital syphilis* Subacute sclerosing panencephalitis	**Other Disorders of White Matter** Adrenoleukodystrophy Alexander disease Cerebrotendinous xanthomatosis Progressive cavitating leukoencephalopathy Epileptic aphasia • Landau-Kleffner syndrome Febrile infection-related epilepsy syndrome (FIRES)
Other Disorders of Gray Matter Ceroid lipofuscinosis • Juvenile • Late infantile (Bielschowsky-Jansky disease)	

*The most common conditions and the ones with disease-modifying treatments.
Modified from Pina-Garza JE. *Fenichel's Clinical Pediatric Neurology: A Signs and Symptoms Approach*. 7th ed. Philadelphia: Saunders; 2013.

TABLE 28.8 Features Suggestive of Inherited Neurometabolic Disorders

Encephalopathy	Systemic Features
Intellectual disability	Urinary odor
Developmental regression	Intrauterine growth restriction
Cerebral palsy	Failure to thrive
Spastic diplegia	Poor sucking
Spastic quadriplegia	Vomiting repeatedly
Depressed sensorium	Weak cry
Lethargy	Cardiomyopathy
Irritability	Hepatomegaly
Stupor	Fatty liver
Coma	Fibrosis/cirrhosis
Dementia	Hepatosplenomegaly
Hypotonia	Renal tubular acidosis
Seizures	Susceptibility to infections
Myoclonus	Bone marrow depression
Infantile spasms	Neutropenia
Extrapyramidal symptoms	Thrombocytopenia
Dystonia	Pancytopenia
Opisthotonos	Seborrhea
Choreoathetosis	Alopecia
Microcephaly	Abnormal hair
Macrocephaly	Pili torti
Speech problems	Trichorrhexis nodosa
Eye-related problems	
Abnormal movements	
Apraxia	
Cherry-red spot	
Nystagmus	
Optic atrophy	
Tapetoretinal degeneration (hereditary)	

Modified from Chaves-Carballo E. Detection of inherited neurometabolic disorders. A practical clinical approach. *Pediatr Clin North Am*. 1992;39:801–820.

TABLE 28.9 Key Features in Select Metabolic Disorders

- **Sphingolipidoses** (Tay-Sachs disease, Niemann-Pick disease, GM$_1$ gangliosidosis) are associated with a cherry-red retinal spot, hepato- and/or splenomegaly, intellectual disability (ID), dystonia, and seizures.
- **Glycoprotein degradation disorders** (e.g., mannosidosis, fucosidosis) may variably manifest with coarse facies, ID, hepatosplenomegaly, and vacuolated lymphocytes.
- **Mucopolysaccharidoses** (e.g., the Hurler, Hunter, and Sanfilippo syndromes) may manifest with coarse facies, ID, hepatosplenomegaly, dysostosis multiplex, and corneal clouding.
- **Neuronal ceroid lipofuscinosis** may manifest with ID, vision loss, ataxia, and myoclonic seizures.
- **Peroxisomal disorders** (Zellweger syndrome, X-linked adrenoleukodystrophy, Refsum disease) variably manifest with ID, encephalopathy, seizures, blindness, dysmorphic features, deafness, and adrenal insufficiency in males (X-ALD).

TABLE 28.10   Conditions in Which Early Treatment May Significantly Improve the Course of the Disease

Condition	Treatment
Galactosemia	Lactose-free diet
Fructosemia	Fructose-free diet
Phenylketonuria	Phenylalanine-free diet
Maternal phenylketonuria	Phenylalanine-free diet during pregnancy
Maple syrup urine disease	Diet restricted in branched-chain amino acids + dialysis or exchange transfusion
Hypoglycemia from any cause	Prevent hypoglycemia and/or provide glucose
Lead intoxication	Separate child from source of lead; chelation therapy
Hypothyroidism	Thyroid replacement
Recurrent otitis media	Antibiotic prophylaxis, pressure-equalizing tubes
Malnutrition	Adequate nutrition
Increased intracranial pressure (e.g., hydrocephalus, neoplasm)	Shunt ventricles or cystic structure
Congenital HIV infection	Prenatal/postnatal treatment with AZT (zidovudine)
Congenital toxoplasmosis	Prenatal treatment with spiramycin, pyrimethamine, and sulfonamide
Dopa-responsive dystonia	Responds to levodopa; may be misdiagnosed as cerebral palsy
Biotinidase deficiency	Oral biotin
Biotin-thiamine-responsive basal ganglia disease	Biotin, thiamine
Wilson disease	Copper chelation; liver transplant
Cerebral folate disorder	Folinic acid
Creatine disorders	Creatine monohydrate
Vitamin B_{12} deficiency	Vitamin B_{12}
Cerebral glucose transporter defect	Ketogenic diet
Metachromatic leukodystrophy	BMT
Niemann-Pick disease	BMT, liver transplantation, implanted amniotic epithelial cells
Adrenoleukodystrophy	BMT
Glycogen storage disease type IV	Liver transplantation
Menkes disease	Parenteral copper histidinate
Lesch-Nyhan syndrome	Allopurinol + bone marrow transplantation
Krabbe disease	BMT
α-Mannosidosis	ERT: velmanase alfa
Aspartylglucosaminuria	BMT
Gaucher disease type III	ERT: Ceredase; SRT: Cerdelga; PCT: Mucosolvan
Hunter syndrome (MPS II)	ERT: Elaprase
Hurler syndrome (MPS I)	ERT: Aldurazyme
Sanfilippo syndrome A (MPS IIIa)	SRT: Genistein
Sanfilippo syndrome B (MPS IIIb)	SRT: Genistein
Sanfilippo syndrome C (MPS IIIc)	SRT: Genistein
Sanfilippo syndrome D (MPS IIId)	SRT: Genistein
Sly syndrome (MPS VII)	ERT: Mepsevii
Neuronal ceroid lipofuscinosis type II	ERT: Brineura

BMT, bone marrow transplant; ERT, enzyme replacement therapy; MPS, mucopolysaccharidosis; PCT, pharmacologic chaperone therapy; SRT, substrate reduction therapy.

SUMMARY AND RED FLAGS

Developmental regression is important to differentiate from ID as it implies an active or ongoing process resulting in neurologic degeneration. Red flags for potentially life-threatening metabolic disorders include vomiting, intractable seizures, unexplained lethargy, or altered mental status. Tables 28.2 and 28.3 provide further clues for the treating provider. Recognition of treatable disorders allows for timely intervention and will impact long-term outcomes (http://www.treatable-id.org).

BIBLIOGRAPHY

A bibliography is available at ExpertConsult.com.

29

Dysmorphology

Donald Basel

With advancing genomic technology, disorders previously identified to be unique phenotypes are now recognized as sharing common pathways or developmental mechanisms. The clinical diagnostic paradigm is evolving to a "genomic" first approach and is less reliant on the detailed phenotype to select single-gene tests to reach a diagnosis. Technology has also introduced machine learning in the form of facial recognition linked to diagnostic databases to facilitate syndromic diagnosis. Dysmorphology is not losing its relevance. It remains a key component of an evaluation to identify and characterize the dysmorphic phenotype, which can help to inform or interpret the outcome of genomic testing and resolve indeterminate variants.

Dysmorphology evolved as a subset of clinical genetics that focused on standardizing the descriptive terminology used to define deviations from normal structural development in the context of syndromic disorders. These traits were termed *birth defects* and result from malformations, deformations, or disruptions, which generally have a significant and obvious effect on appearance (Table 29.1 and Fig. 29.1). The incidence of congenital birth anomalies is common, with estimates that up to 15% of newborns have one minor anomaly. If more than one anomaly is present, the likelihood of an underlying major malformation is up to fivefold that of the general population. If there are three or more minor anomalies, the risk of a major anomaly is 20–30%. A careful and detailed evaluation is thus necessary if multiple minor anomalies are present. Minor anomalies are typically not of medical importance and are more of a cosmetic nature; a common example would be an accessory nipple. Additional examples are provided in Table 29.2; major malformations, conversely, are of clinical importance and more frequently impact the health care management of an affected individual (Table 29.3). To identify the abnormal state, one has to be familiar with normal developmental stages, the timing of specific organ development, and developmental vulnerable periods (Fig. 29.2). The dysmorphic physical examination is directed to overcome some of the clinical challenges of identifying and describing birth defects by providing a framework in which to differentiate normal human variable morphology from the abnormal in the context of a specific diagnosis.

An international initiative to standardize the nosology used in clinical dysmorphology has been adapted to the Internet as an online resource supported by the National Human Genome Research Institute (NHGRI): https://elementsofmorphology.nih.gov/. These terms in themselves are of no clinical utility (aside from communicating the appropriate malformation to other providers) but, when used with available database tools, can be a powerful adjunct to determining the final diagnosis. Examples of these terms are noted in Table 29.4. The importance of reaching a diagnosis is to provide insight into the nature of the condition, enable appropriate counseling of recurrence risk, guide the necessary management recommendations, and provide the family with an overall framework of the natural history and prognosis of the disorder.

DIAGNOSTIC APPROACHES

Often the geneticist-dysmorphologist is asked to view a child with the expectation that the total picture will lead to an instant identification of a syndrome or condition. Instant identification happens more frequently with the common or better-known conditions, but most often, making a diagnosis is more challenging with complex disorders. The diagnostic process frequently relies on additional technologic tools in combination with review of literature.

Human Variation

Human variation is the norm. A common-sense argument can be made for variation by pointing out the ability of people to recognize and differentiate thousands of individuals whom they have met; computer programs for facial recognition are based on this premise. Nonetheless, humans differ little from one another at their DNA level; variation is currently estimated at approximately 0.1% or 1 base of DNA/1,000 bases, which equates to roughly 6 coding variants/gene.

The advent of molecular and biochemical diagnostic methods for identifying genes and gene products has begun to ease the burden on the geneticist by providing diagnostic and confirmatory tests for syndrome identification. Sequencing of the Human Genome clarified many prior preconceived notions regarding human genetics. Prior to the completion of the project, it was estimated that humans had approximately 100,000 genes, whereas this number is closer to 23,000 genes. Of these genes, less than half have been associated with human disease and many have no clear function assigned to them at this time. This gene coding portion of the genome only accounts for approximately 1% of the total genomic code, which consists of roughly 3 billion nucleotides. DNA analysis when available may provide the genotype and confirm the diagnosis, but it cannot unerringly define the phenotype.

There is still much to learn about our genetic code and how genes are expressed and regulated; even if we could perform genomic sequencing on every patient, there would be a number of patients in whom the molecular diagnosis remained elusive. One meta-analysis of the outcomes of genomic sequencing applied to children presenting with both syndromic and nonsyndromic intellectual disability supported a mean diagnostic rate of 36% with the range extending from 15% through 80%.

There are common genetic pathways that relate genes within a pathway to common groups of disorders. This has provided an

TABLE 29.1 Mechanisms, Terminology, and Definition of Dysmorphology

Terminology	Definition	Example
Malformation sequence	Single, local tissue morphogenesis abnormality that produces a chain of subsequent defects	DiGeorge sequence of primary 4th brachial arch and 3rd and 4th pharyngeal pouch defects that lead to aplasia or hypoplasia of the thymus and parathyroid glands, aortic arch anomalies, and micrognathia
Deformation sequence	Mechanical (uterine) forces that alter structure of intrinsically normal tissue	Oligohydramnios produces deformations by in utero compression of limbs (dislocated hips, equinovarus foot deformity), crumpled ears, dislocated nose, or small thorax
Disruption sequence	In utero tissue destruction after a period of normal morphogenesis	Amnionic membrane rupture sequence, leading to amputation of fingers/toes, tissue fibrosis, and destructive tissue bands
Dysplasia sequence	Poor organization of cells into tissues or organs	Neurocutaneous melanosis sequence with poor migration of melanocyte precursor cells from the neural crest to the periphery, manifesting as melanocytic hamartomas of skin, meninges, and so forth
Malformation syndrome	Appearance of multiple malformations in unrelated tissues without an understandable unifying cause; with enhanced genetic investigation, a single etiology may become identified	Trisomy 21 Teratogens

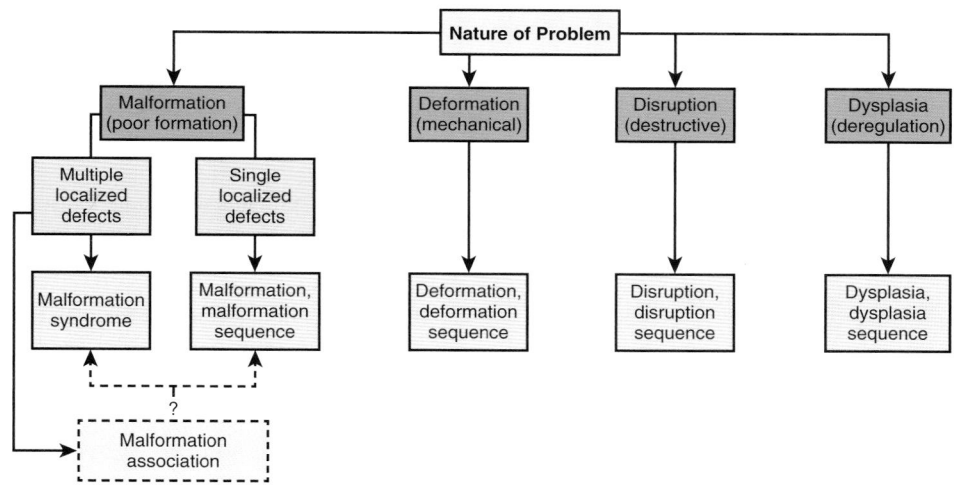

Fig. 29.1 Most patients with multiple structural defects will fall into one of these categories (e.g., malformation, deformation, disruption, or dysplasia). The prognosis, management, and recurrence-risk counseling may vary considerably among these categories. (From Jones KL, Jones MC, Del Campo M, eds. *Smith's Recognizable Patterns of Human Malformation.* 7th ed. Philadelphia: Elsevier; 2013:3.)

explanation to clinicians why seemingly disparate disorders share certain disease associations but remain clinically distinct. An example of this is the **RASopathies** (Fig. 29.3), in which *germline* pathogenic variants in *KRAS* can result in the classic Noonan phenotype or cardiofaciocutaneous syndrome. There is genetic heterogeneity in this group of disorders that share several overlapping features. In addition, *somatic* mosaicism for genes in this pathway has been identified to cause several capillary/vascular malformation disorders and *KRAS* is a frequently identified somatic variant in cancer/tumor tissue. Another example is the allelic disorders involving the *TRPV4* gene, which include brachyolmia type 3, digital arthropathy–brachydactyly, hereditary motor and sensory neuropathy type IIc, metatropic dysplasia, parastremmatic dwarfism, scapuloperoneal spinal muscular atrophy, spondyloepiphyseal dysplasia Maroteaux type, spinal muscular atrophy, and spondylometaphyseal

dysplasia Kozlowski type. The wide phenotypic variability ranging from primary skeletal dysplasias to isolated neuromuscular disease speaks to the complexities of gene regulation and tissue-specific expression. Another example is seen in the sonic hedgehog pathway (Fig. 29.4).

In addition to the primary gene code, there are tertiary elements that can be *imprinted*, in which gene expression is controlled by parent of origin, or can even be affected by the environment, the concept of **epigenetic** control. Further variability exists in genomic **copy number variations**, some of which are considered normal variants, while others result in recognizable microdeletion or microduplication disorders such as velocardiofacial syndrome (VCFS) and Smith–Magenis syndrome.

Not all congenital malformations or birth defects are primarily genetic. Teratogenic exposure, vascular events, and extrinsic factors,

TABLE 29.2 Minor Anomalies and Phenotype Variants

Craniofacial
- Large fontanel
- Flat or low nasal bridge
- Saddle nose, upturned nose
- Micrognathia
- Cutis aplasia of scalp

Eye
- Palpebral fissures
  - Telecanthus
  - Slanting of palpebral fissures
- Hypertelorism
- Brushfield spots

Ear
- Lack of helical fold
- Posteriorly rotated pinna
- Preauricular tags with or without auricular skin tags
- Small pinna
- Auricular (preauricular) pit or sinus
- Folding of helix
- Darwinian tubercle
- Crushed (crinkled) ear
- Asymmetric ear sizes
- Low-set ears

Skin
- Dimpling over bones
- Capillary hemangioma (face, posterior neck)
- Dermal melanosis (African-Americans, Asians)*
- Sacral dimple

- Pigmented nevi
- Redundant skin
- Cutis marmorata

Hand
- Simian creases
- Bridged upper palmar creases
- Clinodactyly of 5th digit
- Hyperextensibility of thumbs
- Single flexion crease of 5th digit (hypoplasia of middle phalanx)
- Partial cutaneous syndactyly
- Polydactyly
- Short, broad thumb
- Narrow, hyperconvex nails
- Hypoplastic nails
- Camptodactyly
- Shortened 4th digit

Foot
- Partial syndactyly of 2nd and 3rd toes
- Asymmetric toe length
- Clinodactyly of 2nd toe
- Overlapping toes
- Nail hypoplasia
- Wide gap between hallux and 2nd toe
- Deep plantar crease between hallux and 2nd toe

Others
- Mild calcaneovalgus
- Hydrocele
- Shawl scrotum
- Hypospadias
- Hypoplasia of labia majora

*Congenital dermal melanocytosis.

TABLE 29.3 Major Anomalies

Neurologic
- Severe hydrocephalus
- Lissencephaly
- Schizencephaly
- Megalencephaly
- Neural tube defect
  - Spina bifida
  - Meningomyelocele
  - Encephalocele

Cardiovascular
- Various congenital heart malformations
- Cardiomyopathy
- Severe arrhythmia

Genitourinary
- Ambiguous genitalia
- Kidney malformations
- Urachal defects

Craniofacial
- Craniosynostosis
- Facial cleft
- Cleft lip and palate
- Structural eye defects
  - Coloboma
  - Aniridia
- Structural ear defects
  - Microtia
  - Aplasia of the auditory canal

Limb
- Amelia
- Split hand/split foot malformation
- Significant syndactyly requiring surgery

Respiratory
- Congenital pulmonary airway malformation (CPAM)
- Tracheoesophageal fistula

Abdominal Wall
- Gastroschisis
- Omphalocele

such as amniotic bands, all have the potential to result in deviations from normal morphologic development (Fig. 29.5).

TERATOLOGY

Teratogens are agents that affect normal development and can give rise to congenital anomalies. It is not uncommon for the parents of a child born with birth defects to attribute the cause to themselves, looking for answers in events preceding or during the pregnancy. They frequently question benign infections and routine medication; it is important to address these concerns because guilt can impair the critical bonding between parent and child. Teratogens are usually considered chemical agents, such as thalidomide or alcohol. However, perinatal infections with cytomegalovirus would fall into this broad category, as would significant radiation exposure. The minority of fetuses exposed to potential teratogens show effects, even if exposed at the same time with the same dose of the agent (e.g., alcohol, 30%; thalidomide, 20%; hydantoins, 10%; warfarin, 8%; lithium, 7%; and diazepam, 1%).

The exact determinants why some fetuses are affected are poorly understood. It is estimated that approximately 10% of birth defects are caused by recognizable teratogens and up to 40% remain without an identifiable cause.

Embryologic timing is one of the critical elements that define the final outcome. There are broadly three periods identified in fetal development (see Fig. 29.2):

Implantation: Period of fertilization through gastrulation and formation of the embryonic plate (first 2 weeks after fertilization). Significant interference with development during this time usually results in loss of conceptus.

Embryonic: This is the period of primary tissue differentiation, and thus, the period at greatest risk for major malformations (weeks 3–8).

Fetal: At this time, primary organogenesis is complete, but growth and neuronal migration proceed. The central nervous system (CNS) is at risk and many of the minor birth defects arise during this time (9 weeks through birth).

Some teratogens may have delayed effects, and these do not result in an overt congenital malformation; diethylstilbestrol (DES) exposure in a female fetus can predispose to vaginal clear cell carcinoma in puberty.

Embryogenesis

The developmental timing of the event that results in the final phenotype is one of the critical determinants of the phenotypic outcome. The timing is important because multiple developmental processes are occurring at the same time and thus a number of malformations present concomitantly as a result of interference with everything developing at the same embryonic time; radial ray defects may be seen with cardiac septal defects as in Holt–Oram syndrome. The common embryologic origin of various elements can give rise to overlapping disorders with

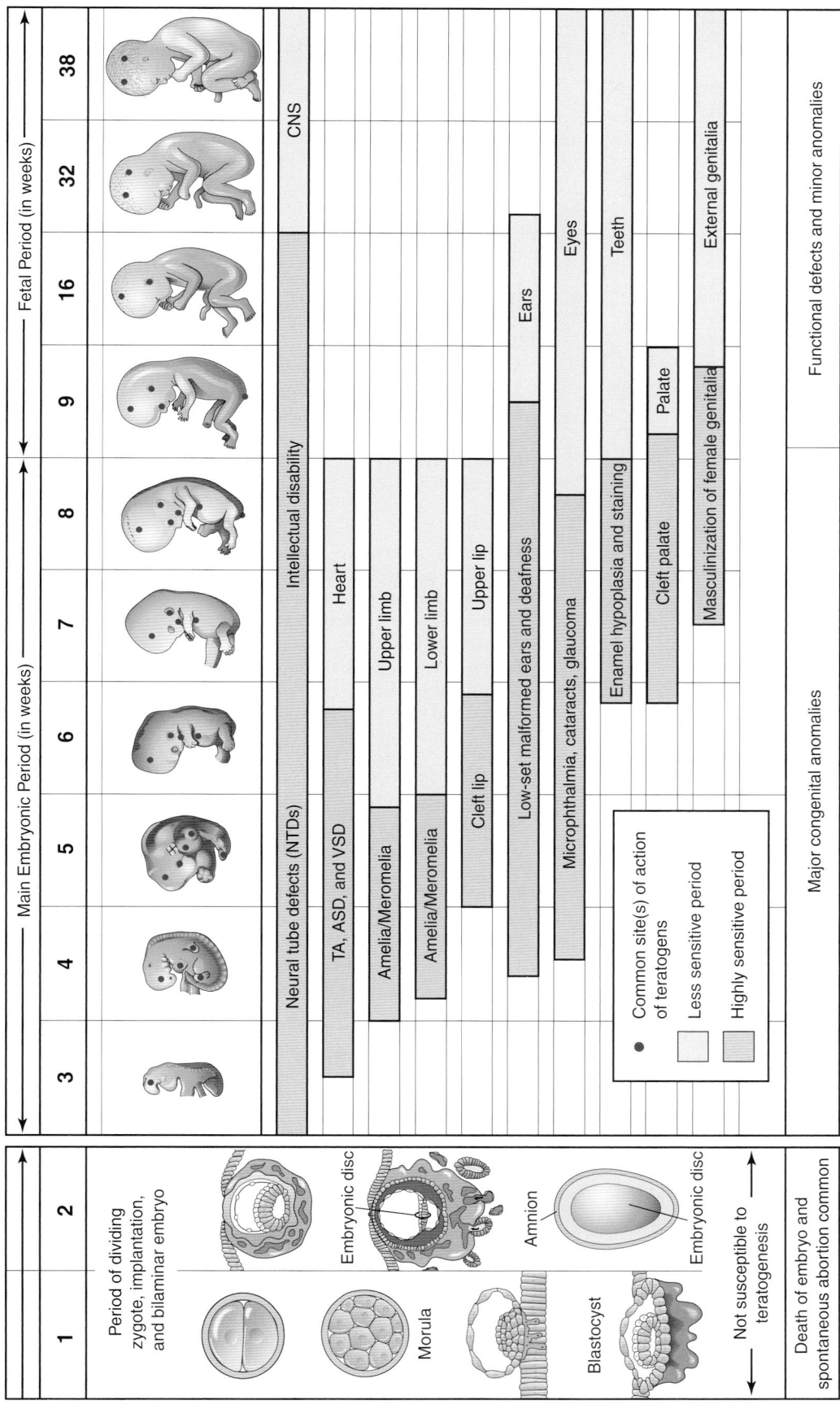

Fig. 29.2 Critical periods in human prenatal development. During the first 2 weeks of development, the embryo is usually not susceptible to teratogens; a teratogen damages all or most of the cells, resulting in death of the cells, allowing the conceptus to recover and the embryo to develop without birth defects. During highly sensitive periods (mauve), major birth defects may be produced (e.g., amelia, absence of limbs, neural tube defects, spina bifida cystica). During stages that are less sensitive to teratogens (green), minor defects may be induced (e.g., hypoplastic thumbs). ASD, atrial septal defect; CNS, central nervous system; TA, truncus arteriosus; VSD, ventricular septal defect. (From Moore KL, Persaud TVN, et al. *The Developing Human.* 10th ed. Philadelphia: Elsevier; 2016.)

TABLE 29.4 Glossary of Selected Terms Used in Dysmorphology

Terms Pertaining to the Face and Head

Brachycephaly: A condition in which head shape is shortened from front to back along the sagittal plane; the skull is rounder than normal

Canthus: The lateral or medial angle of the eye formed by the junction of the upper and lower lids

Columella: The fleshy tissue of the nose that separates the nostrils

Glabella: Bony midline prominence of the brows

Nasal alae: The lateral flaring of the nostrils

Nasolabial fold: Groove that extends from the margin of the nasal alae to the lateral aspects of the lips

Ocular hypertelorism: Increased distance between the pupils of the 2 eyes

Palpebral fissure: The shape of the eyes based on the outline of the eyelids

Philtrum: The vertical groove in the midline of the face between the nose and upper lip

Plagiocephaly: A condition in which head shape is asymmetric in the sagittal or coronal planes; can result from asymmetry in suture closure or from asymmetry of brain growth

Scaphocephaly: A condition in which the head is elongated from front to back in the sagittal plane; most normal skulls are scaphocephalic

Synophrys: Eyebrows that meet in the midline

Telecanthus: A wide space between the medial canthi

Terms Pertaining to the Extremities

Brachydactyly: A condition of having short digits

Camptodactyly: A condition in which a digit is bent or fixed in the direction of flexion (a "trigger finger"–type appearance)

Clinodactyly: A condition in which a digit is crooked and curves toward or away from adjacent digits

Hypoplastic nail: An unusually small nail on a digit

-melia: A suffix meaning "limb" (e.g., amelia—missing limb; brachymelia— short limb)

Polydactyly: The condition of having 6 or more digits on an extremity

Syndactyly: The condition of having 2 or more digits at least partially fused (can involve any degree of fusion, from webbing of skin to full bony fusion of adjacent digit)

From Behrman RE, Kliegman RM. *Nelson Essentials of Pediatrics.* 4th ed. Philadelphia: Saunders; 2002:149.

shared elements: branchial arch developmental field defects in VCFS or disorders caused by abnormal neural crest cell migration. Critical embryologic events can give rise to disorders due to failure of a specific embryologic process: Neural tube defects arise because of abnormal neural tube fusion/closure.

BIRTH DEFECTS

It is estimated that approximately 15% of newborns have one minor anomaly, 0.8% have two minor anomalies, and 0.5% have three. The more minor anomalies that are present, the greater is the probability that an underlying syndrome or a major organ anomaly is also present. Statistically, this equates to a fivefold risk if two minor anomalies are present and a 20–30% probability that there is a major anomaly (congenital heart disease, renal, CNS, limb) if three minor anomalies are present. Approximately 50% of major anomalies involve the head and neck region. The Centers for Disease Control and Prevention statistics

for the United States assert that a baby is born with a birth defect every 4.5 minutes; in 2010, birth defects accounted for about one in five infant deaths in the United States. Examples and potential etiologies are noted in Table 29.5.

Persons in the same family or ethnic group may superficially resemble one another; any attempt at identifying a condition as an abnormality should include inspection of close relatives. *Unusual morphologic findings in a child who resembles their parents does not exclude a dysmorphic condition.* The parents might have variation in expression of the disorder, or there could be additional features that are distinct that need to be separated from the common familial morphology.

CLINICAL CLASSIFICATION

Single-System Defects

- Most common of all birth defects
- Isolated to a single organ system
- Clinically similar to organ malformations seen in syndromes due to common pathways and same-organ end-point
- Examples: isolated cleft lip/palate; congenital heart disease; distal limb anomalies

Association

- Statistically ascertained nonrandom co-occurrences of multiple anomalies in which a single underlying cause is not identifiable. Usually, a diagnosis of exclusion
- Creates an awareness to evaluate for associated anomalies
- <1% risk for recurrence
- Example: VATER/VACTERL (vertebral, anal atresia, cardiac, tracheoesophageal fistula, renal anomalies, limb malformations—typically radial ray) (Figs. 29.6 and 29.7)

Sequence

- A cascade of effects from a single localized abnormality in early morphogenesis that results in multiple congenital anomalies
- Example: Potter sequence secondary to renal agenesis and severe oligohydramnios (Figs. 29.8 and 29.9)

Syndrome

- The presence of multiple structural/functional defects due to a single cause
- Example: Down syndrome caused by trisomy for chromosome 21 (Fig. 29.10) or other trisomies (Fig. 29.11 and Tables 29.6, 29.7, and 29.8)

Complex

- Denotes a malformation arising from the effects of an event affecting a single developmental field in the embryo. Typically relates to aberrant vasculature or vascular events
- Example: sacral agenesis, Poland anomaly

DYSMORPHIC EVALUATION

The first step toward a dysmorphic evaluation is an index of suspicion. In a neonate with birth defects, this is often a logical step, but in a child with failure to thrive or short stature, someone has to initiate a more detailed evaluation for a syndromic entity, or it will be delayed. It is not uncommon for a young female to be diagnosed with monosomy X (Turner syndrome) when she fails to enter puberty.

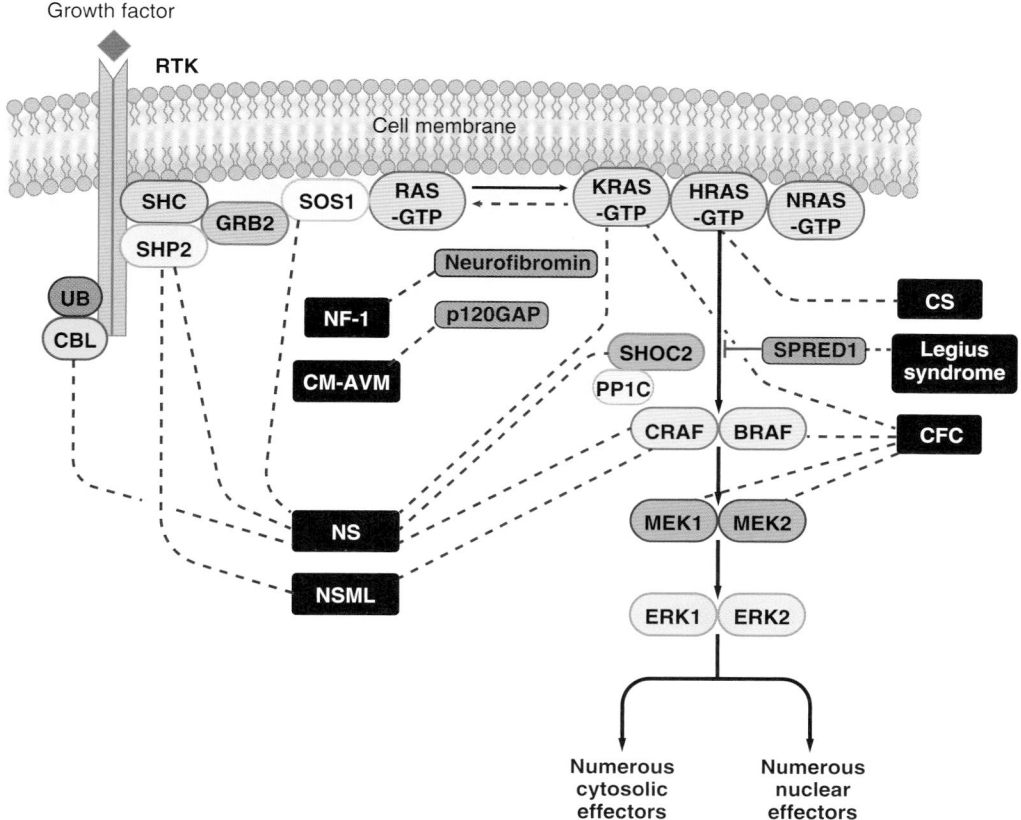

Fig. 29.3 The RAS/MAPK signal transduction pathway. The MAPK signaling pathway of protein kinases is critically involved in cellular proliferation, differentiation, motility, apoptosis, and senescence. The RASopathies are medical genetic syndromes caused by pathogenic variants in genes that encode components or regulators of the RAS/MAPK pathway (indicated by *dashed lines*). These disorders include neurofibromatosis type 1 (NF1), Noonan syndrome (NS), Noonan syndrome with multiple lentigines (NSML), capillary malformation–arteriovenous malformation syndrome (CM-AVM), Costello syndrome (CS), cardiofaciocutaneous syndrome (CFC), and Legius syndrome. RAS/MAPK, RAS protein family/mitogen-activated protein kinase. (From Rauen KA. The RASopathies. *Annu Rev Genomics Hum Genet.* 2013;14:355–369.)

Components of Dysmorphic Evaluation

Detailed History

- A family health history (three-generation pedigree analysis) (Figs. 29.12 and 29.13) (about 5% of children have a biologic father who is not the reported partner)
- Pregnancy history with detail to exposures (teratogens) and general health (gestational diabetes)
- Birth history and neonatal status
- Participation in state newborn screening
- General growth and developmental history; *regression is very important to document*
- Complete medical history, including details of the minutiae of symptom presentation and progression

Some sensitivity surrounding the history taking should be exercised as it is common for a parent to perceive responsibility for the outcomes. Most birth defects occur sporadically without a family history. Autosomal recessive disorders typically happen in one or more siblings without a family history; many autosomal dominant conditions occur as new pathogenic variants. Sex-linked conditions may have no prior family occurrence or an occurrence identified in a remote relative such as the maternal grandmother's brother.

Family health history. It is customary to start with the siblings of the patient (**the proband**), proceed to the parents and the parents' siblings and their children, and then consider the four grandparents and their siblings. This approach is more helpful than the generic question "Does anyone in the family have anything like this?" Many parents may be unaware of neonatal deaths in older relatives (the proband's grandparents or uncles and aunts). Most people are unfamiliar with the term *consanguinity,* but the examiner can ask whether there are ancestors in common or inquire about the place of origin and the size of the community from which the families derive. Maiden names of women should always be noted. Self-identified, remote ancestry may help identify a fruitful area to investigate because certain conditions may be more common in certain ethnic population groups. Consanguinity refers to couples who have ancestors in common within two or three generations, whereas group identity is not consanguinity.

Pregnancy and birth history. Maternal health and concurrent illness with treatment is a critical part of the evaluation. Details of participation in prenatal screening programs and prenatal evaluations can help resolve uncertainties that arise during the evaluation. On occasion, a discrepancy is discovered between an ultrasound report and a neonatal clinical finding: for example, a "normal" cerebellum reported at 17 weeks of gestation and absence of the cerebellum at term. Before concluding that some process happened between 17 and 40 weeks of gestation, it is important to review the actual studies done at 17 weeks. This type of investigation can help pinpoint the timing of in utero problems or can eliminate erroneous hypotheses if the

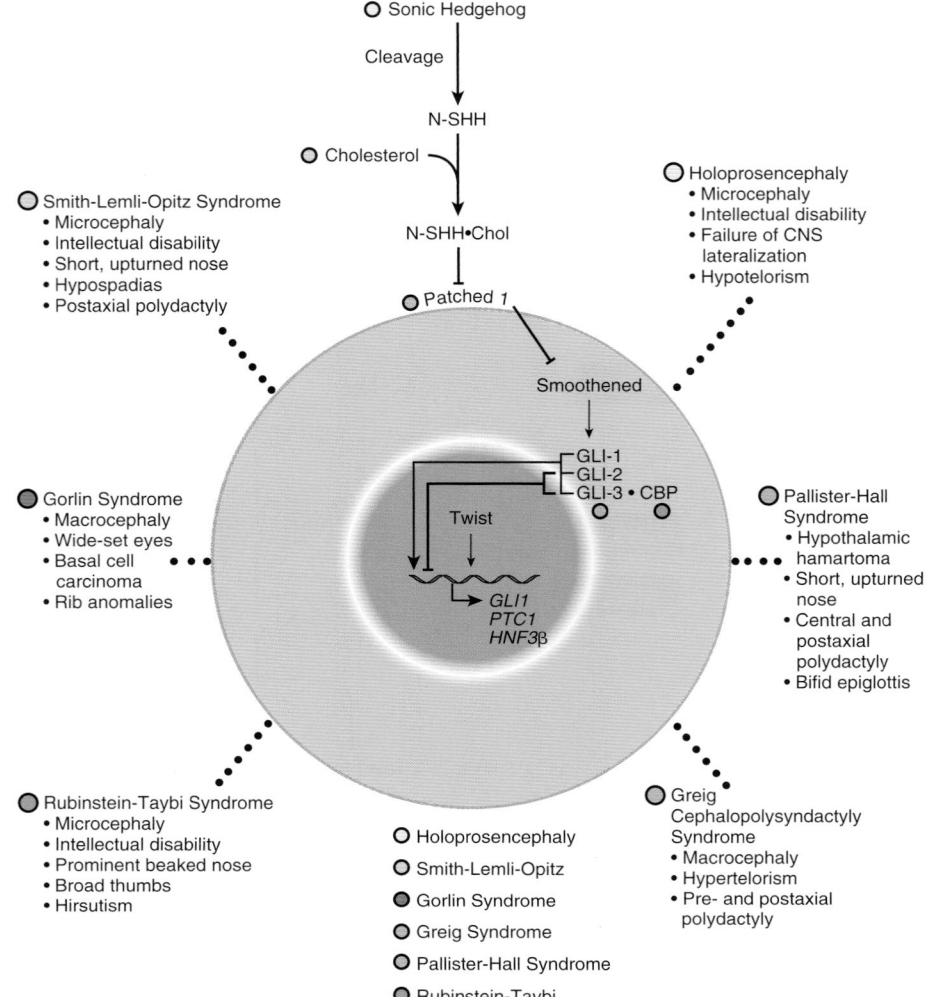

Fig. 29.4 Deleterious sequence variants in genes that function together in a developmental pathway typically have overlapping clinical manifestations. Several components of the sonic hedgehog (SHH) pathway have been identified and their relationships elucidated (see text for further details). Pathogenic variants in several members of this pathway result in phenotypes with facial dysmorphism, as seen in holoprosencephaly, Smith-Lemli-Opitz syndrome, Gorlin syndrome, Greig cephalopolysyndactyly syndrome, Pallister-Hall syndrome, and Rubinstein-Taybi syndrome. CNS, central nervous system. (From Kliegman RM, St. Geme JW III, Blum NJ, et al, eds. *Nelson Textbook of Pediatrics.* 21st ed. Philadelphia: Elsevier; 2020:989, Fig. 128.2.)

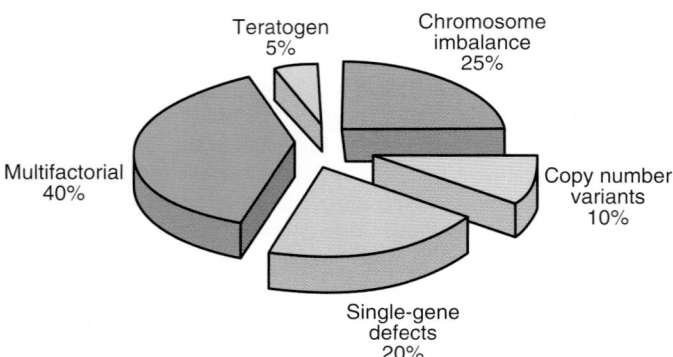

Fig. 29.5 Causes of congenital malformation. (From Nussbaum RL, et al. *Thompson and Thompson Genetics in Medicine.* 8th ed. Philadelphia: Elsevier; 2016.)

study of the fetus at 17 weeks was incomplete or inconclusive. Viral and other infectious illnesses and rashes are germane to note, as are times of exposure during the pregnancy. Parvovirus B19, rubella virus, cytomegalovirus, *Toxoplasma* species, herpes simplex virus, varicella virus, Zika virus, and *Treponema pallidum* (syphilis) are microorganisms that can be teratogenic or affect organ function. Fetal exposure to these organisms at a vulnerable time can be critical; conversely, exposures after formation of an organ are not expected to have a morphologic effect on the organ. Perinatal anoxia is often blamed for infants' problems, but infants with a syndrome or genetic condition may be predisposed to perinatal problems, including fetal distress or neonatal adaptive difficulties.

Developmental history. A developmental history establishes the pattern for acquisition of developmental milestones. A screening tool such as the Denver Developmental Assessment Test can assist in the evaluation of younger children. It is important to establish whether

TABLE 29.5 Causes of Congenital Malformations

Monogenic (7.5% of Serious Anomalies)
X-linked hydrocephalus
Achondroplasia
Ectodermal dysplasia
Apert disease
Treacher Collins syndrome

Chromosomal (6% of Serious Anomalies)
Trisomies 21, 18, 13
XO, XXY
Deletions 4p–, 5p–, 7q–, 13q–, 18p–, 18q–, 22q–
Prader–Willi syndrome (50% have partial deletion of chromosome 15)

Maternal Infection (2% of Serious Anomalies)
Intrauterine infections (e.g., herpes simplex, CMV, varicella-zoster, rubella, and toxoplasmosis)
Zika virus

Maternal Illness (3.5% of Serious Anomalies)
Diabetes mellitus
Phenylketonuria
Hyperthermia

Uterine Environment (% Unknown)
Deformation
Uterine pressure, oligohydramnios: clubfoot, torticollis, congenital hip dislocation, pulmonary hypoplasia, 7th nerve palsy

Disruption
Amniotic bands, congenital amputations, gastroschisis, porencephaly, intestinal atresia

Twinning
Conjoined twins, intestinal atresia, porencephaly

Environmental Agents (% Unknown)
Polychlorinated biphenyls
Herbicides
Mercury
Alcohol

Medications (% Unknown)
Thalidomide
Diethylstilbestrol
Phenytoin
Warfarin
Cytotoxic drugs
Isotretinoin (vitamin A)
D-Penicillamine
Valproic acid

Unknown Etiologies
Polygenetic
Anencephaly/spina bifida
Cleft lip/palate
Pyloric stenosis
Congenital heart disease

Imprinting of Genes
Prader–Willi syndrome
Beckwith–Wiedemann syndrome

Sporadic Syndrome Complexes (Anomalads)
CHARGE syndrome
VATER syndrome
Pierre Robin syndrome
Prune-belly syndrome

Nutritional
Low folic acid–neural tube defects

CHARGE, coloboma, heart defects, atresia choanae, retarded growth, genital anomalies, ear anomalies (deafness); CMV, cytomegalovirus; VATER, vertebral defects, anal atresia, tracheoesophageal fistula with esophageal atresia, and radial and renal anomalies.
From Behrman RE, Kliegman RM. *Nelson Essentials of Pediatrics.* 4th ed. Philadelphia: Saunders; 2002:148.

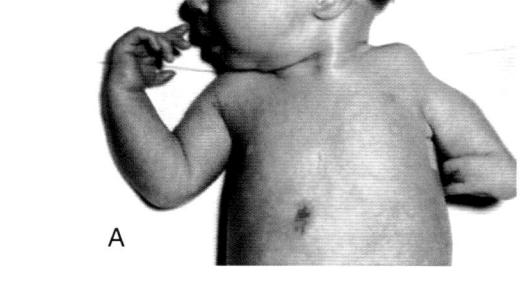

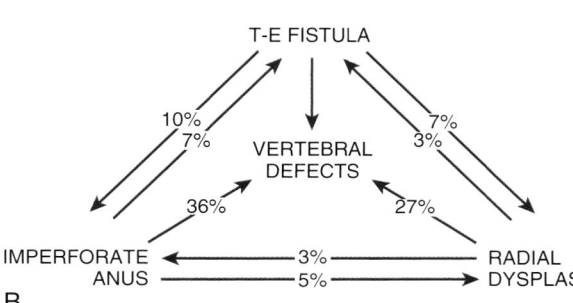

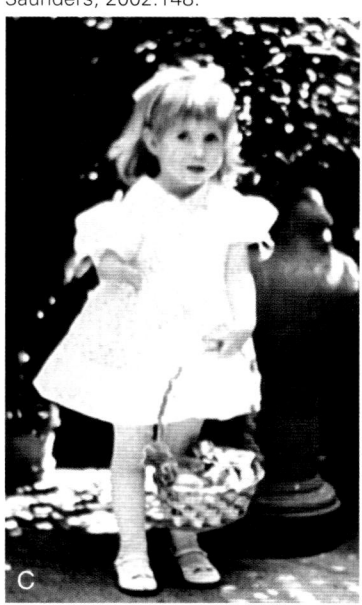

Fig. 29.6 VATER association as initially set forth. *A,* Young infant with vertebral anomalies, anal atresia, esophageal atresia with tracheoesophageal fistula, radial aplasia on the left, and thumb hypoplasia on the right. *B,* Relative frequencies of some of the other VATER association defects when the patient is ascertained by virtue of having one of the defects. *C,* Same patient at 2 years of age, with normal intelligence. T-E, tracheoesophageal. (From Jones KL, Jones MC, Del Campo M, eds. *Smith's Recognizable Patterns of Human Malformation.* 7th ed. Philadelphia: Elsevier; 2013:852.)

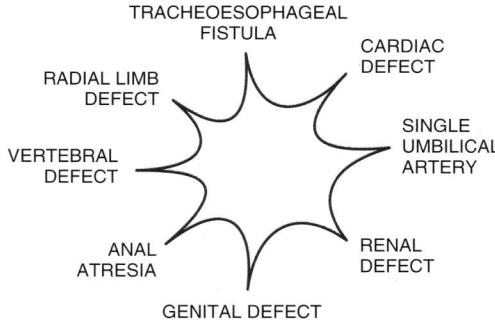

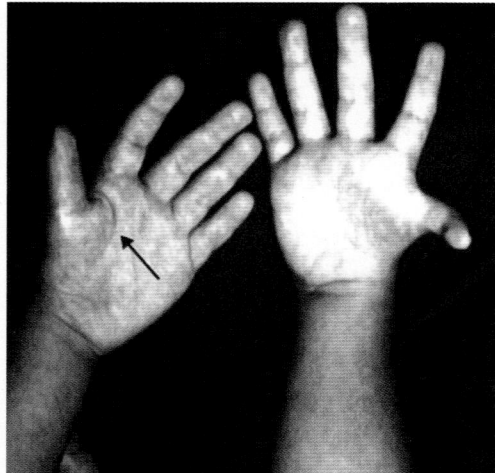

Fig. 29.7 *Top,* Expanded VACTERL association of defects. *Bottom,* Note the relatively severe thumb *(radial)* defect of the right hand and the much more subtle "radial" defect of the left hand *(arrow).* The *arrow* depicts a hypoplastic thenar eminence and crease. (From Jones KL, Jones MC, Del Campo M, eds. *Smith's Recognizable Patterns of Human Malformation.* 7th ed. Philadelphia: Elsevier; 2013:853.)

a child is making progress, remaining static, or showing signs of **developmental regression** (see Chapter 28) by losing landmarks of development. The last possibility is the most ominous for prognosis and warrants aggressive evaluation for diagnosis and possible treatment.

Prior medical concerns including all evaluations and investigations to date should be reviewed. It is often necessary to delay the initial consult so that past medical records can be made available for thorough review.

Examination

The details of morphology are documented in much more detail than is ordinarily the case in a general physical examination. Diagnosis is often based on the language used in the description. Even if a diagnosis is not clear, the description is the starting point of the evaluation. It is helpful to have an anatomic outline for assessing morphology in an orderly and systematic manner.

There are few opportunities to follow a predetermined flow for the examination in most young children, but it is important to maintain a level of structure to the data collection process so as not to overlook a critical finding. It is also good practice to obtain photographs of the face with frontal and side profiles for later reflection and utilization of newer facial recognition tools. When documenting your findings, aim to use standardized terminology in alignment with Human Phenotype Ontology (HPO) as this will aid in the diagnostic analysis and

if machine learning tools with natural language processing are ever applied to the medical record for diagnostic purposes.

Initial Inspection

General observation of the patient is important. The office visit is a small snapshot in the life of the person being evaluated. Subtle movements, behaviors, and social interactions may be key to the underlying diagnosis. Children with Williams syndrome are exceptionally sociable with verbose language skills and frequently have a coarse character to their voice, whereas on the opposing end, children with autism may not permit you to perform a complete physical examination and the greatest opportunity to evaluate movements and physical traits is while you are initially interviewing the parents or caregivers.

Anthropometrics

The Centers for Disease Control and Prevention has published growth curves for children and adolescents that are based upon a heterogeneous U.S. population more representative of various ethnic and ancestral groups than were previous charts. There are separate curves for height, weight, head circumference, and stature for males and females aged 0–36 months, and there are corresponding curves for males and females aged 2–18 years, in addition to curves for body mass index, but without curves for head circumference. There are also references for anthropometric measurements of various body parts from the fetus to adult age. If a child's measurements are discrepant from the norms—that is, *over the 97th percentile* or *under the 3rd percentile*—it is possible to transpose the actual measurement up or down to the 50th percentile on the same line to determine the height age or weight age equivalent. Height can be plotted versus weight on the stature curve to determine whether these parameters are proportional. Thus, a child can be identified as small or tall for age and appropriate or inappropriate in weight (either too heavy or too thin) for height. A child with short stature and proportionate weight has proportionate short stature. Head growth is an important factor in assessing brain growth as well as skull growth and suture closure. Abnormally small head size (**microcephaly**) and abnormally large head size (**macrocephaly**) are considered in proportion to stature with consideration for chronologic age. A child 7 years of age but with a height age of 4 years and proportionate weight and head circumference does not truly have microcephaly but proportionate growth failure. Standardized tables exist in various reference resources for several ethnic groups that allow for assessment across racial barriers. Additionally, standardized charts exist for known syndromes so that normal growth can be appropriately evaluated in a child with a known diagnosis.

A helpful diagnostic assessment for children of discrepant size is the **bone age**, determined by radiograph of the left hand and wrist, according to the standards of Gruleich and Pyle, but occasionally, for infants, by radiograph of the hemiskeleton.

The data collection should include the following highlights with more detail completed as needed.

Head and Neck

- Hair: distribution, texture, pigmentation, low posterior hairline (Fig. 29.14)
- Skull: shape, fontanel
- Neck: mobility, adenopathy, thyroid, embryonic remnants (branchial arch)

Face

- Forms the largest and most important aspect of the dysmorphic evaluation

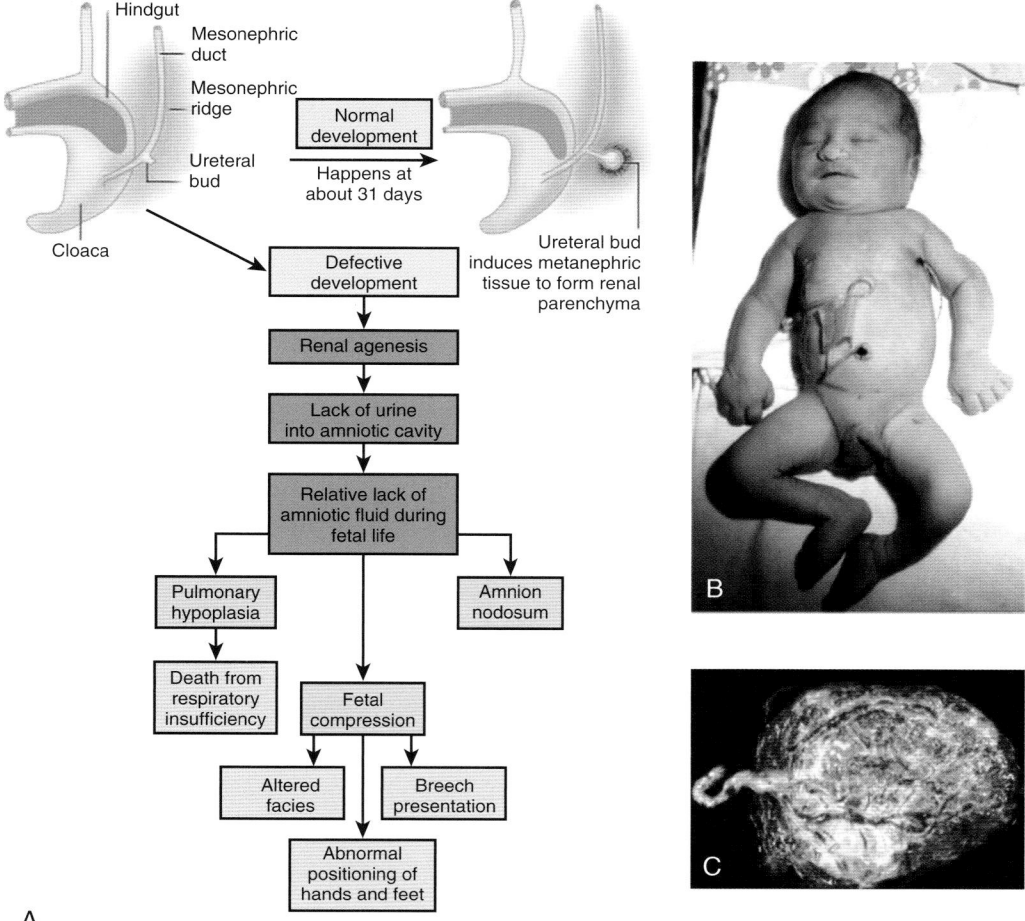

Fig. 29.8 *A–C,* The consequences of renal agenesis. Note the multiple deformational defects in *B,* and the amnion nodosum (brown-yellow granules from vernix that have been ribbed into defects of the amniotic surface) in *C.* (From Jones KL, Jones MC, Del Campo M, eds. *Smith's Recognizable Patterns of Human Malformation.* 7th ed. Philadelphia: Elsevier; 2013:821.)

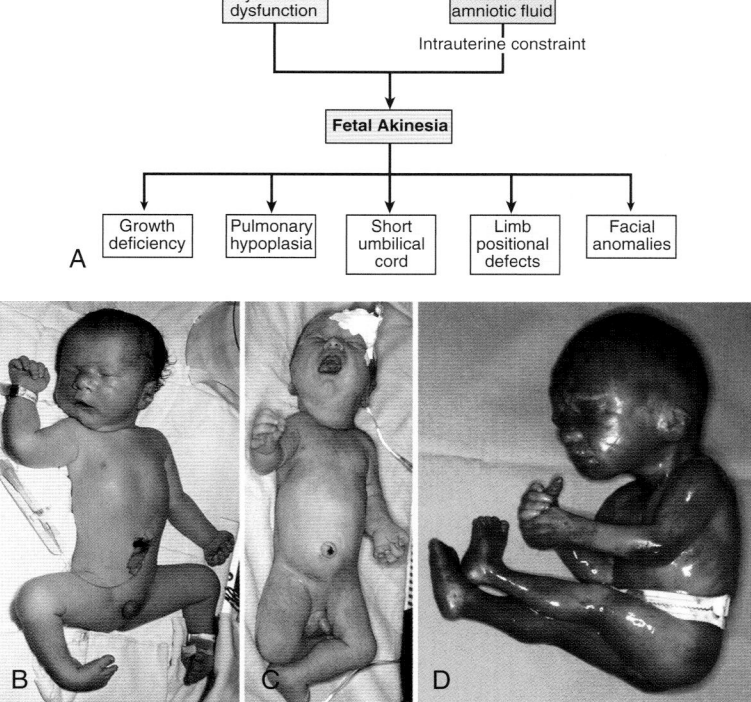

Fig. 29.9 *A,* This diagram demonstrates the etiologically heterogeneous phenotype that results from fetal akinesia. *B,* This infant was born with myotonic dystrophy to a mother with the same condition. He had multiple joint contractures with thin bones and respiratory insufficiency. *C,* This infant was immobilized in a transverse lie after amnion rupture at 26 weeks. *D,* This fetus had bilateral renal agenesis resulting in oligohydramnios. (From Graham JL. *Smith's Recognizable Patterns of Human Malformation.* 3rd ed. Philadelphia: Elsevier; 2007:287. Fig. 47-2.)

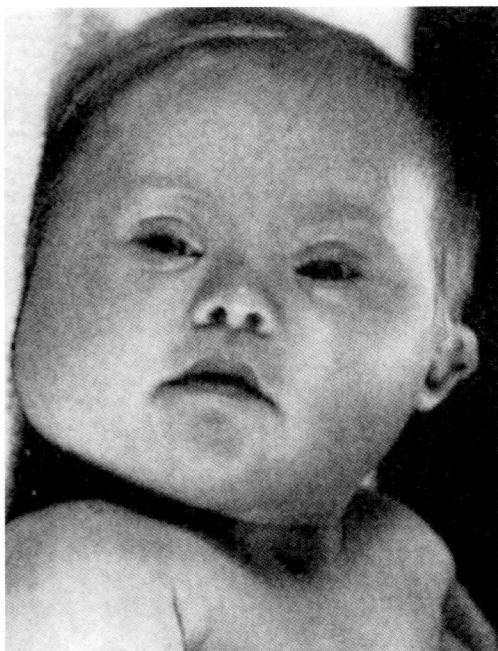

Fig. 29.10 Facial appearance of a child with Down syndrome. (From Wiedemann HR, Kunze J, Dibbern H. *Atlas of Clinical Syndromes: A Visual Guide to Diagnosis.* 3rd ed. St. Louis: Mosby; 1989.)

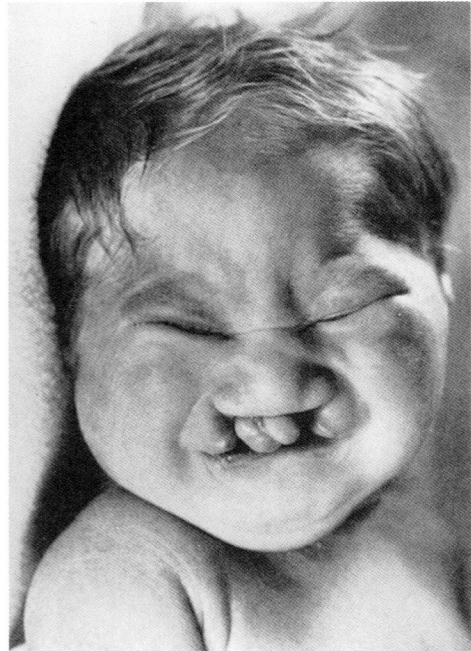

Fig. 29.11 Facial appearance of a child with trisomy 13. (From Wiedemann HR, Kunze J, Dibbern H. *Atlas of Clinical Syndromes: A Visual Guide to Diagnosis.* 3rd ed. St. Louis: Mosby; 1989.)

General "Rules"

- 1/3s = forehead-nasion:nasion-subnasale:subnasale-chin = 1:1:1
- Perpendicular from pupils should meet corners of mouth
- Inner canthal distance should allow space for an additional eye (on MRI space between globes should allow an additional globe)

TABLE 29.6	Clinical Findings That May Be Present with Trisomy 21*
Stature smaller than that of peer age group	Lax joints, including laxity of the atlantoaxial articulation (the latter predisposing the patient to C1–C2 dislocation)
Developmental delays	
Congenital heart disease (e.g., endocardial cushion defect and ventricular septal defect)	Short, broad hands, feet, and digits; single palmar crease, clinodactyly
Structural abnormalities of the bowel (e.g., tracheoesophageal atresia, duodenal atresia, annular pancreas, duodenal web, and Hirschsprung disease)	Exaggerated space between 1st and 2nd toes
	Velvety, loosely adhering mottled skin (cutis marmorata) in infancy; coarse, dry skin in adolescence
Central hypotonia	
Brachycephaly	
Delayed closure of fontanels	Statistically increased risk for leukemia, Alzheimer disease, hypothyroidism
Small midface, hypoplastic frontal sinuses, myopia, and small (short) ears	

*An individual may exhibit any combination of these findings. There is no correlation between the number of physical findings and eventual level of mental performance. The increased risk for leukemia is significant, but probably not >1% for any individual. Alzheimer disease is relatively common in persons with trisomy 21 who die in middle adult life, but its frequency in all adults with Down syndrome is not known.
From Behrman RE, Kliegman RM. *Nelson Essentials of Pediatrics.* 4th ed. Philadelphia: Saunders; 2002:142.

- Top of ear should align with eyebrow/line through pupils should align with root of outer helix
- Forehead: slope, breadth, height, prominence
- Eyebrows: thickness/fullness, arch
- Eye: distance (hyper- or hypotelorism), color, pupil shape, presence of epicanthus or telecanthus, alignment (up- or down-slanting)
- Ears: overall shape/architecture, position, rotation, pits, creases, hearing
- Nose: root, bridge, tip, columella, nasolabial fold, alae nasi, philtrum
- Mouth: lip thickness and shape, lip pits, mucosal lesions, dental alignment, dentition, palate, uvula
- Chest: shape, pectus, nipples, breathing
- Abdomen: organomegaly, masses, hernia
- Genitalia: structure, size, Tanner stage, anus, and perineum
- Musculoskeletal: spine alignment, joint mobility (see Chapter 47), proportions, finger length, palmar surfaces, nail health
- Neurologic evaluation: complete including development, behavior and modified mini-mental examination, and observation for unique movements or behaviors

If a child has an unusual appearance and the differences do not seem to be familial variations as judged by observing the parents, it is necessary to describe how the child appears different. When the variation is a discontinuous variable—that is, a birth defect (e.g., there is an extra digit on the ulnar side of each hand; there is a cleft of the lip on the left that extends into the left nostril, and there is a notch in the gum behind the cleft)—the task is easier. Such birth defects may be considered major abnormalities. The subtle malformations are often minor abnormalities, but both major and minor findings are relevant to diagnosis. Some conditions may be obvious on inspection alone, especially to an experienced observer. Typical manifestations of Down syndrome (Figs. 29.15 and 29.16; see also Tables 29.6 and 29.7 and Fig. 29.10),

TABLE 29.7 Ultrasonographic and Pathologic Findings of Trisomic Conditions

Abnormality	Trisomy 21	Trisomy 18	Trisomy 13
IUGR	+	++	++
CNS abnormalities	–	+	++
Holoprosencephaly	–	–	++
Mild ventricular dilatation	+	+	+
Agenesis of the corpus callosum	–	+	+
Dandy–Walker variant	–	++	+
Spina bifida, NTD	–	++	+
Face	–	+	++
Cyclopia	–	–	++
Cleft lip or palate	–	+	++
Microphthalmia	–	++	+
Duodenal atresia	++	–	–
Esophageal atresia	+	++	–
Cardiac defects	+	++	++
Echogenic intracardiac foci	+	–	++
Diaphragmatic hernia	–	++	+
Cystic hygroma	+	+	+
Hydrops	+	+	+
Omphalocele	–	+	+
Echogenic bowel	++	+	+
Short femur or humerus	+	++	–
Radial aplasia or limb reduction	–	++	+
Clenched hands or wrists	–	++	+
Polydactyly	–	–	++
Club feet or rocker-bottom feet	–	++	++
Renal abnormalities	+	+	++
Choroid plexus cysts	+?	++	–
Single umbilical artery	–	++	++

CNS, central nervous system; IUGR, intrauterine growth restriction; NTD, neural tube defect.
From Nyberg DA, Souter VL. Sonographic markers of fetal aneuploidy. *Clin Perinatol.* 2002;27:762.

TABLE 29.8 Findings That May Be Present in Trisomy 13 and Trisomy 18

	Trisomy 13	Trisomy 18
Head and face	Scalp defects (e.g., cutis aplasia)	Small and premature appearance
	Microphthalmia, corneal abnormalities	Tight palpebral fissures
	Cleft lip and palate in 60–80% of cases	Narrow nose and hypoplastic nasal alae
	Microcephaly	Narrow bifrontal diameter
	Microphthalmia	Prominent occiput
	Sloping forehead	Micrognathia
	Holoprosencephaly (arhinencephaly)	Cleft lip or palate
	Capillary hemangiomas	Microcephaly
	Deafness	
Chest	Congenital heart disease (e.g., VSD, PDA, and ASD) in 80% of cases	Congenital heart disease (e.g., VSD, PDA, and ASD)
	Thin posterior ribs (missing ribs)	Short sternum, small nipples
Extremities	Overlapping of fingers and toes (clinodactyly)	Limited hip abduction
	Polydactyly	Clinodactyly and overlapping fingers; index over 3rd, 5th over 4th; closed fist
	Hypoplastic nails, hyperconvex nails	
		Rocker-bottom feet
		Hypoplastic nails
General	Severe developmental delays and prenatal and postnatal growth retardation	Severe developmental delays and prenatal and postnatal growth retardation
	Renal abnormalities	Premature birth, polyhydramnios
	Nuclear projections in neutrophils	Inguinal or abdominal hernias
	Only 5% live >6 mo	Only 5% live >1 yr

ASD, atrial septal defect; PDA, patent ductus arteriosus; VSD, ventricular septal defect.
From Behrman RE, Kliegman RM. *Nelson Essentials of Pediatrics.* 4th ed. Philadelphia: Saunders; 2002:142.

trisomy 13 or 18 (Figs. 29.17 and 29.18; see also Table 29.8 and Fig. 29.10), severe manifestations of Cornelia de Lange syndrome, and those of Williams syndrome may represent a quick diagnosis; however, even these classical syndromes may manifest in atypical and subtle ways, and careful assessment is necessary to identify them. The expectation that, with enough experience, a physician, even a geneticist or a dysmorphologist, can unerringly identify every case of a common syndrome (even one so common and well known as trisomy 21) is not true. Human diversity is so great that even the most experienced clinicians are glad for confirmatory tests. Most cases of trisomy 21 can be identified by inspection, but there is not the same degree of certainty about every dysmorphic patient.

ASSEMBLING THE DATA

After the history and examination are complete, the abnormal findings are listed. In general, the order is in a sequence ranked by

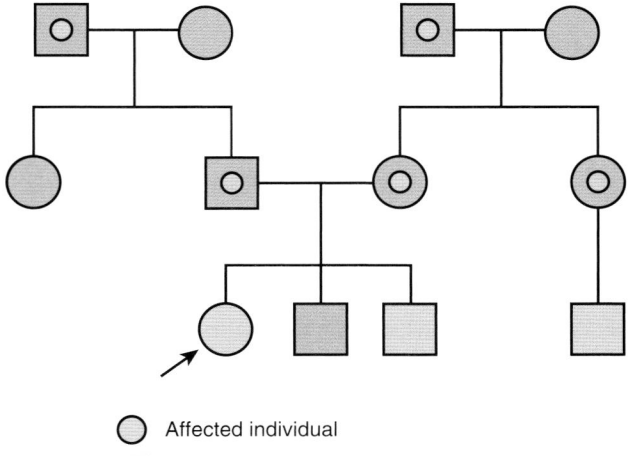

Affected individual

Carrier (heterozygote)

Fig. 29.12 Pedigree showing affected individuals and carriers. (From Marcdante KJ, Kliegman RM. *Nelson Essentials of Pediatrics.* 7th ed. Philadelphia: Elsevier; 2015:147, Fig. 47-1.)

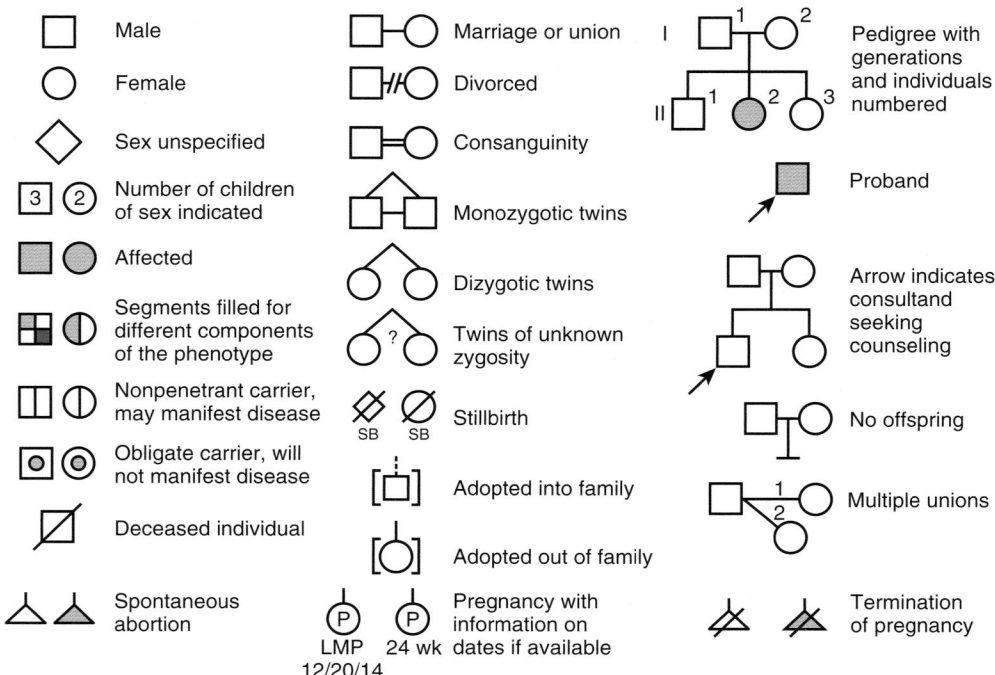

Fig. 29.13 Symbols commonly used in pedigree charts. Although there is no uniform system of pedigree notation, the symbols used here are according to recent recommendations made by professionals in the field of genetic counseling. (From Nussbaum RL, McInnes RR, Willard HF, eds. *Thompson and Thompson Genetics in Medicine.* 8th ed. Philadelphia: Elsevier; 2016:109.)

perceived importance. In determining the order, the clinician may consider the magnitude of the deviation, but uniqueness is important in differentiating conditions. Subtleties can be significant; for example, **inverted nipples** (common in carbohydrate-deficient glycoprotein syndrome) or **redundant umbilical skin** (in company with abnormal anterior chamber of the eye and abnormally shaped teeth in Rieger syndrome) can be very helpful in identifying a condition.

The description of history and morphology becomes the working diagnosis. Even if the clinician cannot find a match in the standard references concerning the syndrome identification, a descriptive diagnosis is invaluable for providing the constellation of findings that delineate the problems.

MINIMAL DIAGNOSTIC CRITERIA

The key phenotypic elements of a syndrome, which unquestionably identify it and differentiate it from all other similar conditions, have been termed the *minimal diagnostic criteria.* In the absence of a definitive laboratory test, establishing the diagnostic criteria is a logical and ideal goal for achieving uniformity of diagnosis.

Unfortunately, minimal diagnostic criteria are difficult to decide upon and are enumerated for only a few conditions. Reasonably successful efforts for identifying diagnostic criteria for two relatively common conditions, **neurofibromatosis type 1 (NF1)** (Table 29.9) and **Marfan syndrome** (Table 29.10), have been achieved and updated through consensus conferences. The molecular abnormalities for each condition have been identified, but the absence of a molecular result does not exclude the diagnosis, and in the case of Marfan syndrome, the molecular finding itself is not sufficient for a diagnosis.

In NF1, a family history that includes an affected parent is a major help (and major criterion) for diagnosis. When there is no positive family history, an index case requires additional criteria. The criteria are quite specific and include easily documented findings. However, criteria do not include learning disabilities, intellectual disability, scoliosis, short stature, asymmetric limb growth, endocrine and neuroendocrine tumors, hypertension, or epilepsy, any of which may be present in NF1. These conditions are germane but not unique to NF1.

The concept of minimal diagnostic criteria is laudable but difficult to achieve. When available, the minimal diagnostic criterion is the confirmatory laboratory test; however, the confirmatory laboratory test does not necessarily define the parameters of the phenotype of the syndrome as is noted in the example of Marfan syndrome and *FBN1* gene variants.

TOOLS TO ASSIST THE DIAGNOSTIC ODYSSEY

Reference books on syndromology, human malformations, and deformations are excellent resources for assistance with diagnosis; however, most illustrations in texts focus on individuals with the most exaggerated findings to illustrate the condition. Birth defects are discrete (discontinuous) variables, but human features occur in a continuum. Diagnosis becomes a process of identifying the variables by a systematic evaluation of the entire individual.

Technology has eliminated some of the art forms once in common practice (e.g., dermatoglyphics or the analysis of finger and palm ridge patterns).

Syndrome recognition is usually performed with genetic and morphometric technologies that may blur the margins between various syndromes and enable syndrome recognition through the application of various computational tools. These methods include facial

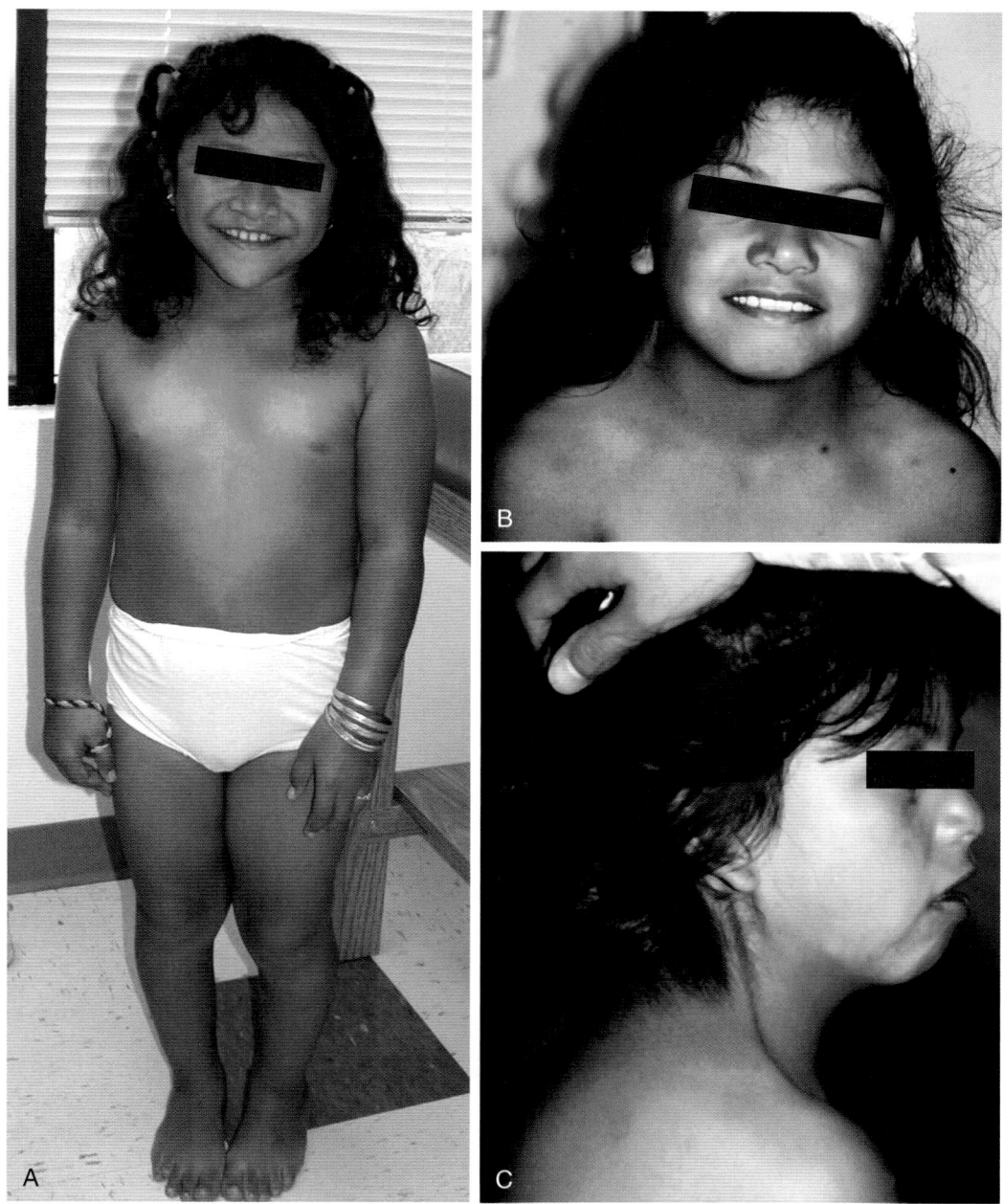

Fig. 29.14 Turner syndrome. *A–C,* Note prominent ears, loose folds of skin in posterior neck with low hairline, and broad chest with widely spaced nipples. (Courtesy Dr. Lynne M. Bird, Children's Hospital, San Diego; From Jones KL, Jones MC, Del Campo M, eds. *Smith's Recognizable Patterns of Human Malformation.* 7th ed. Philadelphia: Elsevier; 2013:81.)

recognition software for syndromic identification (Fig. 29.19). These tools are not diagnostic but offer rank-listed possibilities for diagnostic consideration. Such methods extract features from training images and perform classification of images, often identifying features such as image texture that would not have been identified by human diagnosticians. One of the more widely implemented tools is the free resource Face2Gene®, which, in addition to the facial computational analysis, enables adjunct HPO terminology to be entered to further refine the phenotype. The machine learning aspect of these tools ensures that, over time, their accuracy will improve. The knowledge base is continually expanded through "crowdsourcing" the expertise of recognized experts who continue to train the system by entering molecularly confirmed diagnoses.

The advent of broad molecular diagnostic tests has eliminated the original quest for a clinical diagnosis, which would then serve to focus targeted single-gene testing. Copy number variations (CNVs or microdeletion/duplication disorders) still represent 10–15% of all syndromic disorders presenting for diagnosis, which has established chromosome microarrays as the first-line standard of care in the evaluation of a child with multiple congenital anomalies, developmental delays, or autism spectrum behaviors (Table 29.11). This is supported by the American College of Medical Genetics as well as the U.S. Food and Drug Administration (FDA). Common chromosomal deletion and duplication disorders can be identified in this way (Table 29.12). Current technologies offer the capability of sequencing over 2,000 genes known to cause both syndromic and nonsyndromic

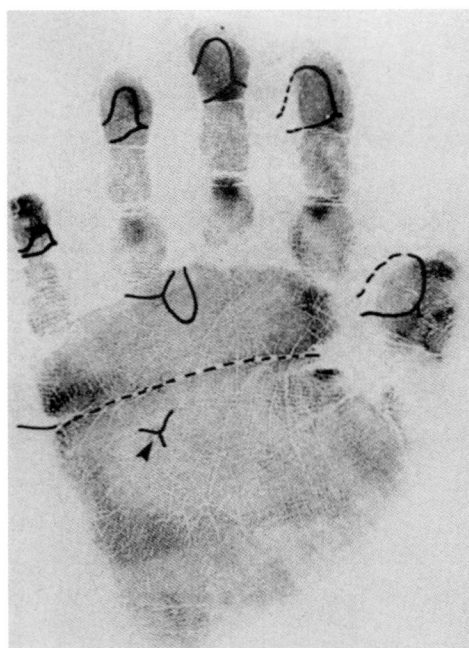

Fig. 29.15 Characteristic dermal patterns of the palm of a child with Down syndrome: a single flexion crease (simian crease), axial triradius *(arrowhead)* in distal position, a pattern area on the palm between the 3rd and 4th digits, and ulnar loops on all 10 digits. (From Nussbaum RL, McInnes RR, Willard HF. *Thompson and Thompson Genetics in Medicine.* 6th ed. Philadelphia: Saunders; 2001:160.)

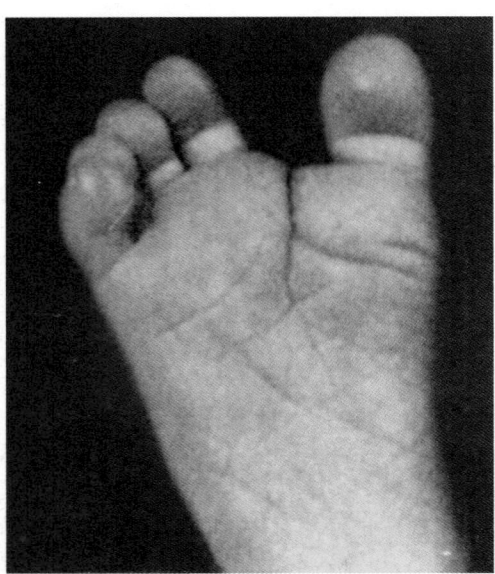

Fig. 29.16 "Prehensile" foot in a 1-month-old child. (From Wiedemann HR, Kunze J, Dibbern H. *Atlas of Clinical Syndromes: A Visual Guide to Diagnosis.* 3rd ed. St. Louis: Mosby; 1989.)

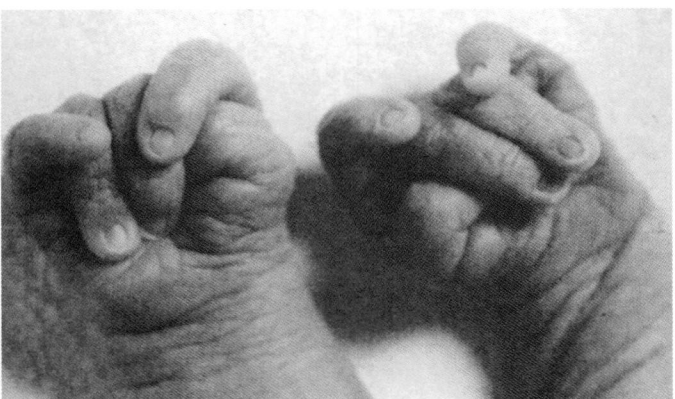

Fig. 29.17 Trisomy 18: Overlapping finger and hypoplastic nails. (From Wiedemann HR, Kunze J, Dibbern H. *Atlas of Clinical Syndromes: A Visual Guide to Diagnosis.* 3rd ed. St. Louis: Mosby; 1989.)

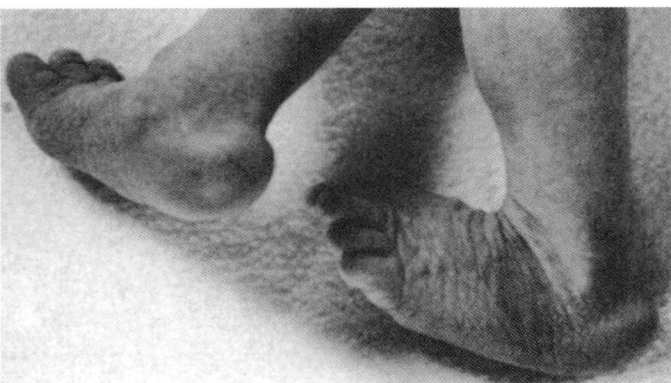

Fig. 29.18 Trisomy 18: Rocker-bottom feet (protruding calcanei). (From Wiedemann HR, Kunze J, Dibbern H. *Atlas of Clinical Syndromes: A Visual Guide to Diagnosis.* 3rd ed. St. Louis: Mosby; 1989.)

TABLE 29.9 **Diagnostic Criteria for Neurofibromatosis Type 1***
1. Family history (an affected parent)
2. 6 or more café-au-lait spots
>0.5 cm in prepubertal children
>1.5 cm in postpubertal children
3. 1 or more plexiform neurofibromas
4. 2 or more neurofibromas
5. Freckling of the armpits or in skinfolds
6. 2 or more Lisch modules of the iris
7. Optic glioma
8. Osseous dysplasia of the sphenoid bone and/or long bones

*There must be positive findings in 2 or more categories.
From National Institutes of Health Consensus Developmental Conference. Neurofibromatosis conference statement. *Arch Neurol.* 1988;45:575.

intellectual disability or autism and in addition can use complex algorithms to assess CNVs, which is typically less expensive than running a microarray. *There is a strong rationale for a exome- or genome-first approach because these technologies can provide comprehensive sequencing with CNV analysis at minimal additional burden to health care expenditure.*

Utilization of specific genetic databases such as POSSUM (Pictures of Standard Syndromes and Undiagnosed Malformations) or LMD (London Medical Databases) relies on cross-referencing the presence of specific dysmorphologic features to create differential diagnoses. Another diagnostic support tool that includes genetic disorders but expands the differential diagnosis to include all pediatric onset conditions is SimulConsult (https://simulconsult.com/). These resources, however, require an annual subscription and are curated by affiliated academic programs. Free resources that use the standardized ontologic nosology include OMIM (Online Mendelian

TABLE 29.10 Revised Ghent Criteria for the Diagnosis of Marfan Syndrome

The revised criteria place more emphasis on aortic root dilatation/dissection and ectopia lentis

I: In the **absence of family history**: MFS DX if:

(1) Aortic root dilated/dissected (Z ≥2) AND EL*

(2) Aortic root dilated/dissected (Z ≥2) AND FBN1

(3) Aortic root dilated/dissected (Z ≥2) AND Syst (≥7 points)*

(4) Ectopia lentis with normal aortic root AND FBN1 pathogenic variant associated with aortic root dilated/dissected

II: In the **presence of family history**: MFS DX if:

(5) EL AND FH of MFS

(6) Systemic feature score (≥7 points) AND FH of MFS*

(7) Ao (Z ≥2 above 20 yr old, ≥3 below 20 yr) + FH of MFS*

*Caveat: without discriminating features of Shprintzen–Goldberg syndrome, LDS, or vEDS **AND** after TGFBR1/2, collagen biochemistry, COL3A1 testing if indicated *(Other conditions/genes will emerge with time.)*

Scoring of systemic features: Max total: 20 points; score ≥7 points indicates systemic involvement

- Wrist AND thumb sign **[3]** (wrist OR thumb sign **[1]**)
- Pectus carinatum deformity **[2]** (pectus excavatum or chest asymmetry **[1]**)
- Hindfoot deformity **[2]** (plain pes planus **[1]**)
- Pneumothorax **[2]**
- Dural ectasia **[2]** *(sensitive, but not specific; not considered equal to lens dislocation or aortic root enlargement)*
- Protrusio acetabuli **[2] AP pelvis:** medial protrusion of the acetabulum at least 3 mm beyond the ilioischial line
- ↓ US/LS** **AND** ↑ arm span/height (>1.05) AND no severe scoliosis **[1]**
- Scoliosis (≥2 degrees) or thoracolumbar kyphosis **[1]**
- Reduced elbow extension **[1]** 170 degrees or less upon full extension
- Facial features (3/5) **[1]** (dolichocephaly, enophthalmos, down-slanting palpebral fissures, malar hypoplasia, retrognathia)
- Skin striae **[1]** *(abnormal position or excessive)*
- Myopia >3 diopters **[1]**
- Mitral valve prolapse (all types) **[1]**

US/LS** (normal upper to lower segment ratios)

White adults, 0.85; Black adults, <0.78

Children 0–5 yo <1; 6–7 yo <0.95; 8–9 yo <0.9

Major Differential Diagnoses

Ectopia lentis syndrome: EL with or without Syst AND with an FBN1 not known with Ao or no FBN1

MASS phenotype: Ao (Z <2) AND Syst (≥5 with at least 1 skeletal feature) without EL

Mitral valve prolapse syndrome: MVP AND Ao (Z <2) AND Syst (<5) without EL

Differential expanded, conditions with:

aortic aneurysms: LDS, bicuspid aortic valve, familial thoracic aortic aneurysm, vEDS, arterial tortuosity

ectopia lentis: ectopia lentis syndrome, Weill–Marchesani syndrome, homocystinuria

Stickler syndrome systemic features: Shprintzen–Goldberg syndrome, CCA, LDS, MASS phenotype and MVPS

Ao, aortic root dilatation/dissection; AP, anteroposterior; CCA, congenital contractural arachnodactyly; DX, diagnosis; EDS, Ehlers-Danlos syndrome; EL, ectopia lentis; FH, family history; LDS, Loeys-Dietz syndrome; LS, lower segment; MASS, Mitral valve, myopia, Aorta, Skin, and Skeletal features; MFS, Marfan syndrome; MVPS, mitral valve prolapse syndrome; Syst, systemic feature score; US, upper segment; vEDS, vascular type of Ehlers-Danlos syndrome; yo, years old.

From Loeys BL, Dietz HC, Braverman AC, et al. The revised Ghent nosology for the Marfan syndrome. *J Med Genet.* 2010;47:476–485.

Inheritance in Man; http://www.omim.org/) and Phenomizer (http://compbio.charite.de/phenomizer/), which similarly allow the end user to generate lists of potential diagnoses.

Genetic Testing

The catalog of available genetic tests has greatly expanded, and as large-scale sequencing becomes more accessible and affordable, genomic analysis is becoming the standard of care. The primary limitation of this testing is our ability to interpret all the variation and to connect relevance of this variation to the clinical phenotype being evaluated. It thus remains important to collect and identify crucial/significant phenotypic data elements that assist in the interpretation of the tests ordered. Broad panels encompassing common phenotypes are available for complex heterogeneic disorders such as epilepsy or cardiomyopathy. To assist in the identification of laboratories offering specific testing, a few reference websites have been established offering global laboratory listings; two of these resources include https://www.ncbi.nlm.nih.gov/gtr/ and https://app.concertgenetics.com/. Given the variability of the testing methodology and the genes included in various panel tests, it is important for the ordering practitioner to understand not only which genes are included but also what technology is being utilized so as to truly appreciate the negative predictive value in relation to the disorder within the differential diagnosis. For example, some tests do not offer copy number evaluation, and if the disorder you have near the top of your differential is most commonly caused by a deletion of a gene, then the test being ordered may provide a false-negative result (i.e., miss the diagnosis).

Testing itself should be judiciously selected to confirm a diagnosis or gather more information to enable a diagnosis to be formulated (see Chapter 1: Evidence-Based Technologic Testing). Before any laboratory or imaging testing is done, the examiner should address the question "Does the description correlate with a described condition or syndrome?" Often, the working diagnosis is the succinct and relevant description of the child, which amounts to a list of findings arranged in order of importance or significance from the perspective of the examiner.

A further advance in molecular understanding is the identification of metabolic disorders that are associated with intellectual disability but have proven treatments. The publication *The Treatable Intellectual Disability* (https://www.treatable-id.org) presents a digital tool to enhance diagnosis and care for rare diseases and impacted the initial testing recommendations for children with intellectual disability, and recommendations for initial evaluations as listed in Tables 29.13 and 29.14 have become more broadly implemented. Thus, metabolic screening for disorders that would not have been detected through national newborn screening programs is routinely used in the evaluation of children with intellectual disability. The development of *metabolomic analysis* has additionally improved the ability for diagnosing rare metabolic disorders in individuals presenting with multisystem complex phenotypes and has become routine in the evaluation of undiagnosed and rare disorders. Metabolomic analysis refers to the cross-correlation of multiple analytes in several samples (serum, urine, and/or cerebrospinal fluid) aided by machine learning tools that have metabolic signatures for numerous diseases.

Diagnostic imaging is invaluable in assessing CNS malformations, cardiac structure and function, skeletal deformity, and abdominal organs. The rapid advances in imaging technology and resolution are additionally enabling functional studies as well as real-time metabolic analysis with spectroscopy when using MRI to study the brain.

Bone age testing is indicated with short stature, growth delay, or large stature. Complete skeletal surveys are one of the only ways to help delineate skeletal dysplasias but require expert interpretation.

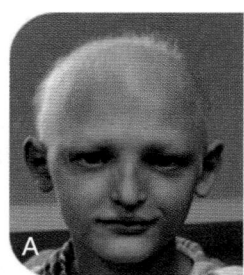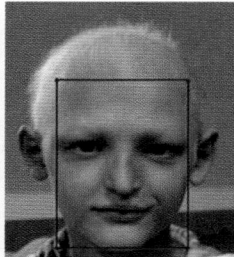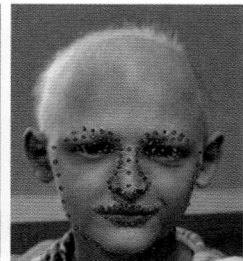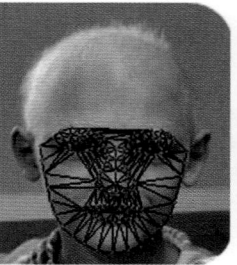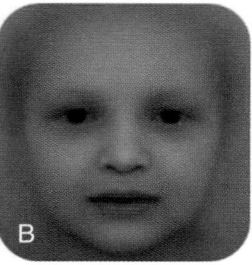

Fig. 29.19 Image analysis process of the automated facial recognition technology. *A,* A face is detected in the frontal image and anatomic points are automatically identified. The face is divided into multiple regions, whose appearance is analyzed. *B,* Last, a mask depicting the characteristic appearance of each syndrome is created. (From Basel D. Dysmorphology in a genomic era. *Clin Perinatol.* 2020;47:15–23 [Fig. 5, p. 21].)

TABLE 29.11 Common Microdeletion and Duplication Syndromes and Frequency of Occurrence

Condition; Genomic Location	Incidence	Major Phenotypic Features
16p11.2 duplication	1/1,900	Normal to DD, ASD, ADHD, microcephaly, psychiatric conditions
16p11.2 deletion	1/2,300	ID/DD, ASD, ADHD, macrocephaly, psychiatric conditions
16p13.11 deletion	1/2,300	ID/DD, seizures, schizophrenia
1q21.1 duplication	1/3,300	Normal to motor skill and articulation difficulty, ID/DD, ASD, ADHD, scoliosis, abnormal gait, macrocephaly, short stature, psychiatric conditions (schizophrenia, anxiety, depression), CHD (especially tetralogy of Fallot)
22q11.2 duplication	1/4,000	Normal to ID/DD, growth retardation, hypotonia
1p36 deletion syndrome	1/5,000	ID/DD, hypotonia, seizures, structural brain abnormalities, CHD, vision and hearing issues, skeletal anomalies, characteristic facies
Charcot–Marie–Tooth type 1A; 17p12 duplication	1/5,000–1/10,000	Slowly progressive neuropathy causing distal muscle weakness and atrophy, sensory loss, and slow nerve conduction velocity first noticeable in the 1st or 2nd decade
X-linked ichthyosis; Xp22.31 deletion	1/6,000	ID/DD, ichthyosis, Kallmann syndrome, short stature, ocular albinism
7q11.23 duplication	1/7,500	DD, normal to ID, speech problems, hypotonia, problems with movement and walking, behavioral abnormalities, seizures, aortic enlargement
17q12 deletion	1/14,500	Kidney/urinary abnormalities, diabetes, ID/DD, ASD, psychiatric conditions
Sotos syndrome; 5q35 deletion	1/15,000	ID/DD, overgrowth, characteristic facies
Cri-du-chat; 5p15 deletion	1/15,000–1/50,000	High-pitched cry, microcephaly, hypotonia, characteristic facies, ID/DD, CHD
Koolen de Vries; 17q21 deletion	1/16,000	ID/DD, sociable personality, hypotonia, seizures, distinct facial features, CHD, kidney anomalies, foot deformities
Potocki–Lupski syndrome; 17p11.2 duplication	1/20,000	ID/DD, ASD, hypotonia, CHD

ADHD, attention-deficit/hyperactivity disorder; ASD, autism spectrum disorder; CHD, congenital heart defect; DD, developmental delay; ID, intellectual disability.

Modified from Norton ME, Kuller JA, Dugoff L, eds. *Perinatal Genetics.* Elsevier; 2019:129, Table 12.2.

TABLE 29.12 Examples of Some Chromosomal Deletion Syndromes for Which There Is a Commercially Available DNA Probe for Fluorescent In Situ Hybridization Analysis

Condition	Brief Description	Probe
Williams syndrome	Proportionate short stature, mild–moderate to severe intellectual disability, cocktail patter for conversation, stellate pattern of iris pigmentation, supravalvular aortic stenosis, recessed nasal bridge, and wide mouth with full lips	7q11
WAGR syndrome	Wilms tumor, aniridia, growth delay, intellectual disability, and genitourinary anomalies	11p13
Prader–Willi syndrome Angelman syndrome	Distinct syndromes with common or overlapping areas of deletion; phenotype depends on gender of the parent of origin of the deletion *Prader–Willi syndrome:* hypotonia in infancy, short stature, obesity, mild–moderate and occasionally severe intellectual disability, small hands and feet (caused by paternal deletion of 15q11-13 or maternal uniparental disomy for chromosome 15) *Angelman syndrome:* severe intellectual disability, absence of speech, ataxia, tremulous movements, large mouth, frequent drooling (caused by maternal deletion of chromosome 15q11-13 or paternal uniparental disomy)	15q11
Smith–Magenis syndrome	Brachycephaly, prognathism, self-destructive behavior, wrist biting, pulling out nails, head banging, indifference to pain, severe intellectual disability, hyperactivity, social behavior problems	17p11.2
Miller–Dieker syndrome	Microcephaly, narrow temples, hypotonia/hypertonia, abnormal posturing, seizures, severe to profound intellectual disability, poor growth, lissencephaly and other brain abnormalities on CT or MRI	17p13
Velocardiofacial (VCF) syndrome (overlaps with DiGeorge syndrome)	*VCF:* cleft palate, congenital heart disease, learning and/or behavior problems, long face, prominent nose, limb hypotonia, slender hands with tapering fingers *DiGeorge syndrome:* T-cell deficiency, immunoglobulin deficiency	22q11

WAGR, Wilms tumor, aniridia, genitourinary anomalies, and mental retardation.

TABLE 29.13 Genetics and Biochemical Developmental Delay Evaluation

Tier One	Acylcarnitine profile
	Amino acids (plasma)
	Ammonia
	Urine organic acids
	Ceruloplasmin
	Copper (blood)—if abnormal repeat with 24-hr urine
	DNA microarray
	Homocysteine (blood)
	Lactic acid and pyruvic acid (blood) to determine lactate:pyruvate ratio in mitochondrial disorders
Tier Two	Mucopolysaccharides screen
	Congenital disorders of carbohydrate glycosylation
	Chromosome Fragile X
	Prader–Willi and Angelman (methylation testing)
	Creatine/guanidinoacetate (blood)
	Creatine/guanidinoacetate (urine)
	Purine pyrimidine panel (urine)
	Very long chain fatty acids (blood)

TABLE 29.14 Genetic Testing in Congenital Heart Disease

Patient Features	What to Order
CHD with features suggestive of trisomy 21 or 45X	Karyotype
CHD with features of trisomy 13 or 18	STAT chromosome FISH 21/18/13
Conotruncal congenital heart lesion • Interrupted aortic arch • Pulmonary atresia with ventricular septal defect • Tetralogy of Fallot • Truncus arteriosus • Malaligned ventricular septal defect and/or features typical of 22q11.2 deletion syndrome	DNA microarray
Heterotaxy	DNA microarray Next-generation sequencing heterotaxy panel
CHD with or without dysmorphic features/multiple anomalies	DNA microarray

CHD, congenital heart disease; FISH, fluorescent in situ hybridization.

Specialized laboratory testing is reserved to aid specific diagnostic investigation (e.g., muscle biopsy, fibroblast culture for enzyme analysis, electron microscopy of arterial walls or blood buffy coat). These specialized tests are performed by a small number of laboratories to aid the diagnosis of rare disorders and should ideally be left to the expert physician.

BIBLIOGRAPHY

A bibliography is available at ExpertConsult.com.

30

The Irritable Infant

Angela L. Rabbitt

An irritable infant is a challenge to the caregiver and medical provider and is a common presenting complaint in early infancy. An irritable infant is defined here as a patient younger than 1 year of age who, according to the caregiver, cries excessively or is excessively fussy without a specific defined time period. In addition, this chapter also addresses issues of an irritable toddler (~2–3 years of age). There are many causes, but most irritable infants do not have significant underlying pathologic processes. However, there are serious entities that must not be missed (Table 30.1).

Medical providers should also recognize the profound anxiety and stress that infant crying may place on families and other caregivers. Although excessive crying generally resolves with time, the family's beliefs about the cause of the crying can have a lasting effect on the way they interact with the child and their beliefs about the infant's health. Caregivers who perceived their infant's crying as excessive or inconsolable described higher rates of depression, strained family relationships, and guilt about their inability to calm the infant. Excessive crying may even trigger thoughts of harming the infant and is reported as a common trigger for child physical abuse. Additionally, infants with early cry-fuss problems in combination with family dysfunction are at higher risk for ongoing behavioral problems, highlighting the need for early identification and intervention in this population. Therefore, the provider's response when evaluating an irritable infant should be focused on diagnosing potentially treatable medical conditions including rare disorders and on addressing the caregiver's understanding and response to the crying.

DIAGNOSTIC APPROACH

Less than 5–10% of infants who present for medical care due to excessive crying will have a serious underlying etiology. However, a thorough medical evaluation including a detailed history and physical examination is needed to identify the minority of infants with treatable issues, and in healthy infants a thorough evaluation may reassure caregivers. The initial evaluation should focus on ruling out potentially emergent conditions (Fig. 30.1). The physical examination should include a complete examination of all body systems with the clothing removed. Table 30.2 lists elements of the history and physical examination suggestive of emergent and common diagnoses that may present with a chief complaint of crying. The history should be comprehensive, given the wide array of possible diagnoses to consider. The history should include questions about the characteristics of the cry (the time of day, duration, whether it is associated with feeds) and any changes to the infant's typical crying pattern. Infants with a sudden increase in the frequency and duration of inconsolable crying compared to their normal crying pattern are more likely to have an underlying medical condition. Clinicians should also ask caregivers why they think the infant is crying to specifically address any fears about the infant's health.

In most cases, the history and/or physical examination will suggest the diagnosis, which can be confirmed with the judicious use of laboratory and imaging studies. However, providers should be aware of potentially serious diagnoses that may present with vague symptoms of fussiness and few other signs or symptoms on physical examination, including neurologic conditions and certain fractures. In very young infants, the neurologic exam is a poor screening tool to detect subtle neuropathology, and intracranial injury may not be accompanied by external evidence of trauma. In cases of physical abuse, an accurate history of injury may be concealed or unknown to the presenting caregiver, and the child may present for medical care after the symptoms of acute injury have resolved. In addition to questions about recent symptoms, medical providers assessing crying complaints should ask about any remote history of bruising or other injury. A history of previous neurologic symptoms, such as episodes of unexplained seizures, apnea, altered mental status, developmental delay, or periods of extreme lethargy, may suggest an occult head injury or other nontraumatic neuropathology. Consider head imaging and a skeletal survey in infants with a history of neurologic symptoms or prior injury.

Growth parameters, including head circumference, should be obtained. Increasing head circumference percentile may point to increased intracranial pressure in infants with otherwise vague symptoms. Though conditions such as constipation, gastroenteritis, and gastroesophageal reflux are most often benign, poor growth or developmental delay may indicate more severe disease or that another medical condition is causing the symptoms.

A urinary tract infection (UTI) may also present with vague symptoms of irritability in infants. A UTI is one of the few conditions in which laboratory or imaging may lead to a diagnosis in the absence of a suggestive clinical picture. Some suggest that a urinalysis and culture should be a standard screening test in infants who present with crying.

When the history and physical examination do not suggest a diagnosis, additional laboratory or radiographic evaluation may be needed. In particular, if the infant is ill-appearing, has evidence of poor growth or developmental delay, or is persistently inconsolable beyond the initial assessment, laboratory and radiographic studies should be done (Table 30.3). Patients may need to be monitored in the hospital until a diagnosis can be established. Some tests to consider include:

- A CBC with differential, ESR, and/or CRP measurement (for infection or inflammation, anemia)
- Analysis of cerebrospinal fluid (for meningitis or encephalitis)
- Blood culture
- Serum pH and complete metabolic panel, amylase, and lipase (for electrolyte abnormalities, metabolic diseases, abdominal trauma)
- UA and culture (for trauma or infection)
- Stool guaiac (for intussusception, gastroenteritis, cow's milk allergy)
- A skeletal survey (for trauma)

TABLE 30.1 Differential Diagnosis in the Irritable Infant

Emergent/Urgent Diagnoses	Nonemergent/Urgent Diagnoses
Eyes, Ears, Nose, Throat	
Choanal atresia	Otitis externa
Corneal abrasion	Teething
Foreign body	Stomatitis
Glaucoma	
Otitis media	
Respiratory	
Airway obstruction (croup, foreign body)	Upper respiratory tract infection
Lower respiratory tract infection (pneumonia, bronchiolitis)	
Cardiovascular	
Congestive heart failure	
Supraventricular tachycardia	
Anomalous coronary artery	
Myocarditis	
Kawasaki disease	
Gastrointestinal System	
Incarcerated hernia	Constipation
Gastrointestinal obstruction (intussusception, volvulus, pyloric stenosis, Hirschsprung disease)	Uncomplicated gastroenteritis
	Anal fissure
Abdominal trauma	Gastroesophageal reflux
Peritonitis (appendicitis, spontaneous)	Inappropriate feeding volume or technique
	Milk or soy protein allergy
Genitourinary System	
Testicular torsion	
Ovarian torsion	
Urinary tract infection	
Orchitis	
Balanitis	
Epididymitis	
Musculoskeletal System	
Osteomyelitis	Minor, soft tissue injury
Diskitis	
Septic arthritis	
Fractures	
Radial head subluxation	
Leukemia, neuroblastoma	
Skin	
Cellulitis	Impetigo
Tourniquet syndrome (digit, genitalia)	Dermatitis
	Insect bites
	Minor injury
Central Nervous System	
Encephalitis	
Meningitis	
Increased intracranial pressure (trauma, hydrocephalus, intracranial hemorrhage)	
Intracranial mass	
Miscellaneous	
Drug ingestion	Vaccine reaction
Neonatal abstinence syndrome	Poor caregiver-infant interaction
Inborn error of metabolism	Normal crying
Sepsis	
Sickle cell crisis	
Physical abuse	
Familial pain syndromes	

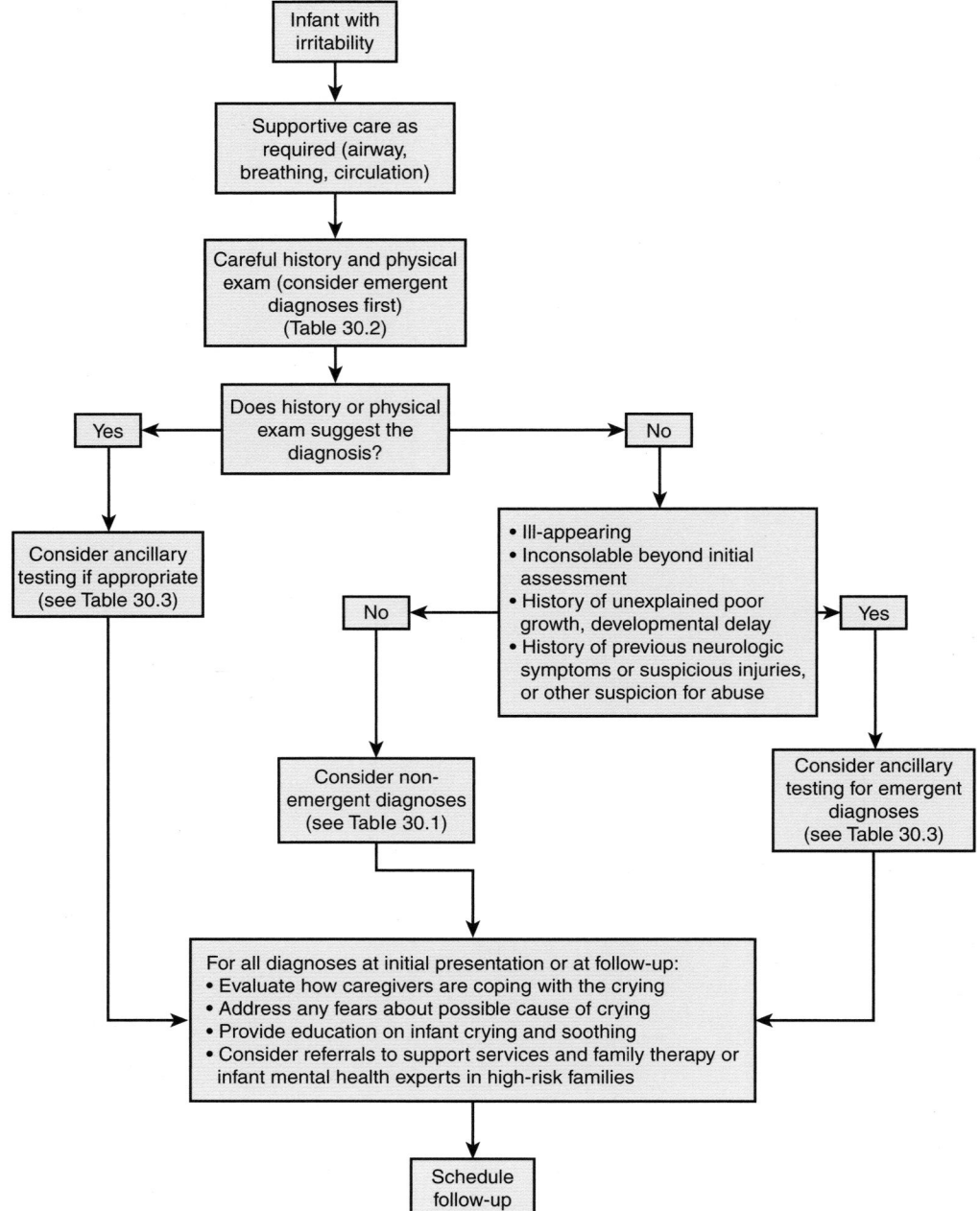

Fig. 30.1 Initial approach to the irritable infant.

- CT scan or MRI of the head (for intracranial hemorrhage, mass, or hydrocephalus)
- Comprehensive urine drug screen (for ingestion)

In the **consolable infant** without history or physical examination findings suggestive of a serious condition, nonemergent causes of crying are more likely (see Table 30.1). The most likely diagnosis in infants younger than 4 months of age is above-average crying in a normal infant. However, because a definitive diagnosis has not been established, infants should receive a follow-up evaluation within 24 hours to ensure that a more serious illness was not missed and to address any additional concerns or questions about the crying. This element is especially critical if the clinician has any doubt concerning the establishment of the correct diagnosis.

Paradoxical irritability occurs when a parent attempts to console a crying infant but in the process of holding or cuddling the child, there is an exacerbation of crying. This should suggest that a painful site has been touched or moved and is seen in septic arthritis, osteomyelitis, meningitis, or a fracture.

ADDRESSING CAREGIVERS' RESPONSE TO CRYING

The distress, frustration, and anxiety that persistent or inconsolable crying may cause caregivers should be recognized and acknowledged with empathy, regardless of the cause. After addressing any urgent medical needs, caregivers should be educated about the normal pattern of infant crying and methods to soothe the infant.

TABLE 30.2 Clinical Presentation of Selected Diagnoses in Infants Presenting with Crying

Review of Systems	Possible Physical Exam Findings	Diagnoses to Consider
Eyes, Ears, Nose, Throat		
• Pain or irritation of one eye • Chronic or intermittent tearing	• Photophobia • Tearing • Foreign body seen on lid inversion • Corneal enlargement or clouding • Ocular enlargement • Optic nerve cupping	• Foreign body • Corneal abrasion • Glaucoma
• Difficulty breathing and cyanosis during feeds; symptoms improve with crying	• Inability to pass a nasogastric tube • Decreased air movement through nares	• Choanal atresia
• Otorrhea • Fever • Ear tugging • Decreased appetite	• Bulging or immobile tympanic membrane • Abnormal color or perforated tympanic membrane • Otorrhea	• Otitis media • Otitis externa
• Excessive drooling • Decreased appetite	• Inflamed gums • Tooth eruption • Erythema over frenulum • Sores or ulcerations	• Teething • Lacerated frenulum • Herpetic stomatitis
Respiratory		
• Trouble breathing, cough, congestion	• Abnormal breath sounds • Respiratory distress	• Airway obstruction (foreign body, croup) • Pneumonia • Bronchiolitis • Chest trauma
Cardiovascular		
• Tachypnea and diaphoresis with feeds • Trouble breathing • Easy fatigability • Pallor, cyanosis	• Tachycardia • Respiratory distress • Poor perfusion • Abnormal heart sounds • Abnormal breath sounds • Hepatomegaly • Cardiomegaly	• Congestive heart failure • Supraventricular tachycardia • Anomalous coronary artery • Myocarditis
Gastrointestinal System		
• Constipation (hard stools, less than two per week)	• Nonspecific exam • Stool mass in left lower quadrant • Anal fissure	• Constipation
• Delayed passage of meconium, poor growth, vomiting	• Abdominal distention • Tight anal canal with empty ampulla	• Hirschsprung disease
• Vomiting • Poor feeding with or without poor weight gain • Crying associated with feeds • Diarrhea	• Nonspecific exam • Hematochezia • Atopic dermatitis	• Milk and/or soy protein allergy • Gastroesophageal reflux disease • Gastroenteritis
• Sudden-onset intermittent pain • Vomiting • Lethargy • Poor feeding • Hematochezia	• Abdominal distention • Abdominal tenderness, guarding • Abdominal or pelvic mass	• Intestinal obstruction (volvulus, intussusception) • Peritonitis
• History of injury • No history or history of prior suspicious injury in abusive trauma	• With or without evidence of injury on exam • Nonspecific abdominal exam	• Abdominal trauma
• Forceful vomiting • Hungry between episodes of emesis	• Dehydrated • Palpable pyloric sphincter	• Pyloric stenosis

Continued

TABLE 30.2 Clinical Presentation of Selected Diagnoses in Infants Presenting with Crying—cont'd

Review of Systems	Possible Physical Exam Findings	Diagnoses to Consider
• Improper formula volume or mixing • Frustration with feeds • Poor latch • Feeding aversion • Poor growth • Vomiting • Excess gas	• Nonspecific exam	• Inappropriate feeding volume or technique
Genitourinary System • Testicular swelling	• Testicular swelling, tenderness	• Testicular torsion • Orchitis • Epididymitis
• Previous urinary tract infection	• Suprapubic tenderness • Fever • Nonspecific exam	• Urinary tract infection
Musculoskeletal System • Decreased movement of an extremity • Increased crying with movement	• Swelling, tenderness, warmth, erythema, pain or crepitus with palpation or movement • Fever • Pseudoparalysis	• Fractures • Soft tissue injury • Osteomyelitis • Septic arthritis • Diskitis • Malignancy
Skin • Rash • Purulent drainage • Itching	• Swelling, tenderness, warmth, erythema, rash	• Infection • Dermatitis • Insect bites
• Swollen appendage	• Well-demarcated line separating normal tissue from a distal dusky edematous appendage • Ligature deeply imbedded in a groove covered by edematous tissue	• Tourniquet syndrome
• Sudden onset of irritability • History of injury • No history of injury, history of prior suspicious injury in abusive trauma	• Bruising, laceration, burns	• Abusive or nonabusive trauma
• Hernia	• Dusky or nonreducible umbilical or inguinal bulge	• Incarcerated hernia
Central Nervous System • Lethargy • Vomiting • Seizures • With or without fever • May present with subtle nonspecific symptoms	• Abnormal neurologic exam • Ill-appearing • Fever • Papilledema • Enlarged head circumference • Bulging fontanel	• Meningitis • Encephalitis • Increased intracranial pressure (hydrocephalus, intracranial hemorrhage) • Intracranial mass
• No history, or history of prior suspicious injury • Prior history of symptoms of increased intracranial pressure	• Nonspecific exam • Retinal hemorrhages (present in 85% of patients with abusive head trauma) • With or without other injuries	• Abusive or nonabusive head trauma
Miscellaneous • Medication administration • Illicit drug use by caregivers • Seizures	• Nonspecific exam • Altered mental status • Tachycardia • Respiratory or cardiac compromise • Seizures	• Drug ingestion

Continued

TABLE 30.2 **Clinical Presentation of Selected Diagnoses in Infants Presenting with Crying—cont'd**

Review of Systems	Possible Physical Exam Findings	Diagnoses to Consider
• Maternal drug use during pregnancy • Poor feeding • Vomiting • Sneezing, hiccups, diarrhea • Poor sleep • Tremors • Seizures	• Nonspecific exam	• Neonatal abstinence syndrome
• Vomiting • Poor growth • Developmental delay or regression • Seizures	• Dehydration and shock • Organomegaly • Abnormal neurologic exam • Jaundice • Dysmorphic features • Abnormal odor • Tachypnea	• Inborn error of metabolism
• Lethargy • With or without fever • Seizures	• Ill-appearing • Cardiorespiratory compromise	• Sepsis
• Infant or family history of sickle cell disease • Trouble breathing	• Respiratory distress • Splenomegaly • Swelling and tenderness of the hands and feet	• Sickle cell crisis
• Recent immunizations	• Nonspecific exam	• Vaccine reaction
• Dysfunctional or chaotic home environment • Significant caregiver stress	• Nonspecific exam	• Poor infant-caregiver interaction
• Content between crying bouts • Feeding well • Normal growth and development	• Nonspecific exam	• Normal infant crying

Normal infant crying progressively increases after 2 weeks and peaks in the 2nd month of life, then gradually decreases by the 4th or 5th month. It generally peaks in the late afternoon and evening within the first 6 months of life. At times it may be unrelated to the needs of the infant. Therefore, even in healthy infants some episodes of fussiness will not be soothed with typical caregiver attempts to soothe, such as feeding, cuddling, carrying, and diapering, and may occur for up to 4–5 hours per day. This pattern of crying is consistent among normal infants regardless of caretaking styles, cultural groups, and socioeconomic status, and has been demonstrated even in some nonhuman mammalian species. The pattern may reflect a developmental stage characterized by infants' increased reactivity to their environment and an immature ability to self-regulate. Though this crying pattern seems to be universal, the frequency and duration of crying varies significantly between infants. This variation is due to several factors, including infant temperament, the caregivers' response to crying, and likely other unidentified factors.

Caregivers should be reassured that physical contact in the form of carrying and feeding on demand within the first months of life will not spoil the infant. Responding promptly to crying in very young infants before it becomes inconsolable may reduce the amount of crying over the long term by creating a more secure attachment between the infant and caregiver. Room sharing, with the infant's crib or bassinet in the caregiver's bedroom, may also decrease infant crying in the first 3 months of life. Conversely, in infants older than 3–4 months of age a consistent daily routine of feeding and sleeping and reasonable delays in caregiver responses to crying may encourage infants to develop autonomous settling and improve infants' ability to self-regulate.

Soothing techniques (swaddling, pacifier use, rocking the baby in a calm environment, or providing some background noise or vibration) are inconsistently effective in studies assessing their efficacy to reduce infant crying. However, these techniques cost nothing and are not associated with adverse effects. It is reasonable to recommend these techniques as an initial response to infant crying.

Despite caregivers' best efforts, there will be times even healthy infants may not be soothed. The caregivers' inability to soothe the infant is often their primary source of negative feelings such as frustration, anger, or guilt, creating a loss of confidence in parenting skills and feelings of resentment toward the infant. Infants then respond to caregiver anxiety with increased crying. Caregivers may be reassured by information that bouts of fussing do not necessarily indicate illness or pain but may simply reflect the infant's inability to regulate the crying once it has started. Medical providers can also reassure caregivers that most infant cry-fuss problems are transient and not necessarily predictive of ongoing behavior problems in childhood. In a prospective, community-based study of outcomes in infants with sleep and cry-fuss problems, only 5% of mothers reported persistent problems at age 2 years.

The clinician must be aware that parental distress from prolonged, unexplained crying can lead to the use of ineffective, inappropriate, or even dangerous remedies. Fennel extract may show promise as a way to decrease crying, although additional study of this treatment and possible negative effects is needed. If herbal teas containing fennel replace infant formula, they may lead to malnutrition and electrolyte abnormalities. Treatments that have been shown to have no significant or reproducible effect in treating crying are acupuncture, reflexology,

TABLE 30.3   Initial Ancillary Testing or Referrals to Consider for Specific Diagnoses

Potential Diagnoses	Ancillary Testing or Consultations to Consider
Eyes, Ears, Nose, Throat	
Corneal abrasion or foreign body	Fluorescein stain
Glaucoma	Ophthalmology consult
Foreign body	Radiographs and/or ENT consult
Respiratory	
Pneumonia or bronchiolitis	Chest radiography, pulse oximetry, nasopharyngeal viral testing
Airway obstruction (croup, foreign body)	Chest and/or neck radiography, pulse oximetry, ENT consult for bronchoscopy
Cardiovascular	
Congestive heart failure	Chest radiography, pulse oximetry, electrocardiogram, echocardiography, CBC, CMP, BNP, troponin, Cardiology consult
Supraventricular tachycardia	
Anomalous coronary artery	
Myocarditis	
Gastrointestinal System	
Incarcerated hernia	Ultrasonography with Doppler, Surgical consult
Gastrointestinal obstruction (intussusception, volvulus, pyloric stenosis, Hirschsprung disease), peritonitis, abdominal trauma	CBC, CMP, amylase, lipase, abdominal and pelvic radiography, abdominal ultrasound, upper gastrointestinal contrast study, abdominal and pelvic CT, air contrast enema for intussusception, Surgical consult
Milk and/or soy protein allergy	Hemoccult testing
Genitourinary System	
Testicular torsion	Ultrasonography with Doppler, Surgical consult
Ovarian torsion	Pelvic ultrasonography or CT, Surgical consult
Urinary tract infection	UA with culture, CBC, blood culture
Musculoskeletal System	
Osteomyelitis	CBC, ESR, CRP, blood culture, radiography, MRI, Orthopedics and Infectious Disease consult
Septic arthritis	
Fractures	Skeletal survey
Diskitis	ESR, spine radiographs, spine MRI
Leukemia, metastatic neuroblastoma	CBC, bone marrow, abdominal imaging
Skin	
Cellulitis, infection	CBC, wound culture
Central Nervous System	
Encephalitis	Lumbar puncture, head CT or MRI, CBC, blood culture, EEG
Meningitis	
Increased intracranial pressure (abusive or nonabusive trauma, hydrocephalus, intracranial hemorrhage), neoplasm	Head CT or MRI
Miscellaneous	
Drug ingestion	Comprehensive urine drug screen (with confirmatory testing)
Neonatal abstinence syndrome	Urine or meconium drug screen
Inborn error of metabolism	CBC with differential, ABG, CMP, serum ammonia, serum uric acid, LDH, blood glucose, aldolase, creatine kinase, UA, urine reducing substances, serum amino acids, urine organic acids, serum acylcarnitine profile, lactate, Genetics consult
Sepsis	CBC, LP, UA, urine and blood culture
Sickle cell crisis	CBC, reticulocyte count, chest radiography, pulse oximetry
Physical abuse	Injury surveillance: Skeletal survey; head CT or MRI in infants <6 mo of age or current or prior symptoms of head injury; AST, ALT, amylase, lipase; comprehensive urine drug investigation screen with confirmatory testing, Child Protection Team consult

ABG, arterial blood gas; ALT, alanine aminotransferase; AST, aspartate aminotransferase; BMP, basic metabolic panel; BNP, brain natriuretic peptide; CMP, comprehensive metabolic panel; EEG, electroencephalogram; ENT, Otolaryngologist; LDH, lactate dehydrogenase; LP, lumbar puncture; UA, urinalysis.

TABLE 30.4	Location of Cutaneous Injuries
Locations That May Raise Concern for Abuse	**Common Locations of Accidental Injury in Mobile Infants**
Any bruising in a precruising infant	Nose
Upper arms	Shins
Soft parts of the trunk	Bony prominences of the trunk
Ears	Occiput
Soft parts of the face	Forehead
Neck	Chin
Genitals	
Buttocks	
Hands and feet	

soy formula, simethicone, gripe water, glucose, sucrose, dimethicone, fiber-enriched formula, and the introduction of lactase enzyme into the infant's milk. Treatment with anticholinergic drugs (dicyclomine hydrochloride, dicycloverine, and cimetropium bromide) was effective in reducing infant crying but is associated with unacceptable side effects. In addition, several reports have been published of hospitalization or death in infants treated for excessive crying with sedating medications such as dextromethorphan and diphenhydramine, dimenhydrinate, and opiates. Clinicians should counsel caregivers about the dangers of using these medications in young infants.

Given the stress that crying can place on a family and the fact that all families will inevitably be faced with the challenge of a fussy infant, this education should be a routine part of each well-child evaluation in the 1st year of life. It should not only be given to the caregiver who presents with the child for medical care, but also to all adults who will be caring for the child.

More intensive educational and behavior modification interventions directed toward families with persistently fussy infants have shown promise to reduce crying, improve parent-child relationships, and positively influence behavioral development in infants. Successful programs generally assess and address caregiver needs, sources of vulnerability, and infant health. They also provide respite and educate families about infant crying, soothing, and ongoing emotional care. In addition, multidisciplinary approaches may include family therapy or referrals to perinatal and infant mental health experts who can support caregiver-infant interactions.

SPECIFIC DIAGNOSES

Child Maltreatment

Caregiver perceptions of prolonged or inconsolable crying place the infant at risk of abuse; caregivers may smother, slap, or shake their baby in response to crying. Crying is a common stimulus for abusive head trauma, and the abuse is often repeated because the head injury stops the crying.

Any injury in a noncruising infant raises concern for abusive trauma and should prompt an evaluation for additional injuries. In older infants and children who can independently ambulate, most accidental bruising occurs over bony prominences on the anterior surface of the body. Bruising to the ears, neck, genitals, and buttocks is unusual in nonabused children (Table 30.4). Abusive bruises tend to be larger, often clustered, and associated with other cutaneous injury. Patterned injuries and any significant, unexplained, or poorly explained injury also may suggest abuse (Figs. 30.2, 30.3, and 30.4). The purpose of additional testing when infants present with suspicious findings is injury surveillance and identification of medical conditions that may

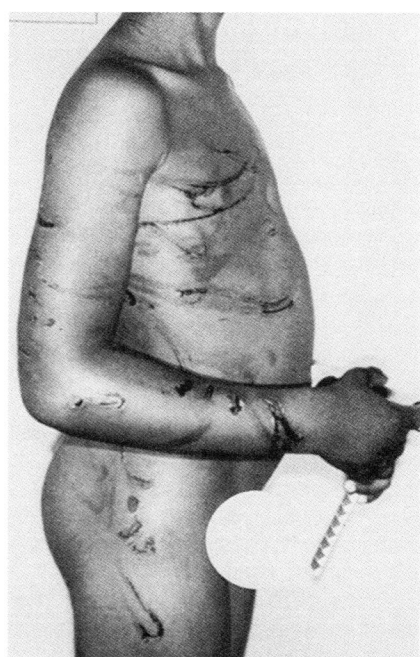

Fig. 30.2 Lash marks from an electric cord. Such marks are distinctive. The deep lacerations, which are looped if the cord is looped, result in deep tissue damage, and there is the potential for keloid formation on healing. (From Johnson CF. Inflicted injury versus accidental injury. *Pediatr Clin North Am.* 1990;37:791–815.)

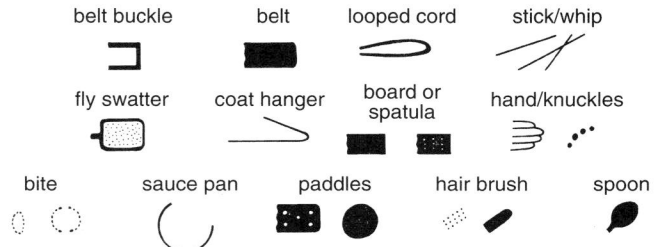

Fig. 30.3 Marks from objects. (From Johnson CF. Inflicted injury versus accidental injury. *Pediatr Clin North Am.* 1990;37:791–815.)

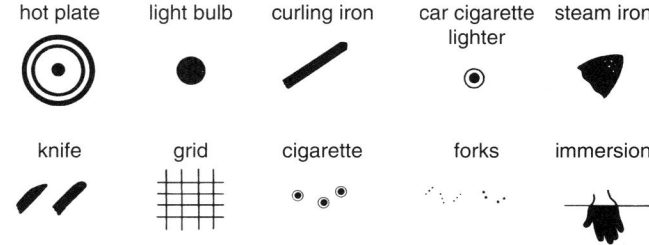

Fig. 30.4 Marks from burns. (From Johnson CF. Inflicted injury versus accidental injury. *Pediatr Clin North Am.* 1990;37:791–815.)

mimic abusive trauma. The absence of additional injury does not rule out abuse. Even in isolation, the presence of a suspicious injury places the infant at risk for more severe ongoing abuse. In infants who were ultimately diagnosed with physical abuse, almost 30% of the infants had a history of previous, more minor suspicious injuries. Medical providers were reportedly aware of these injuries in 40% of cases but did not recognize them as concerning (Table 30.5). If there are doubts about whether an injury should be considered suspicious or what tests are indicated, providers should consult a child abuse specialist.

TABLE 30.5 Pitfalls in Child Abuse Evaluation: 12 Costly Errors

1. A desire to not make the diagnosis
2. Failure to assemble past information on medical conditions and medical encounters
3. Too great a reliance on the information developed by others
4. Transference-countertransference with custodial parent (formation of alliances or development of hostilities)
5. Overinterpretation or underinterpretation of signs and symptoms
6. Overinterpretation or underinterpretation of physical findings
7. Failure to know about conditions mistaken for sexual abuse
8. Faulty laboratory techniques resulting in either false-positive or false-negative reports
9. Use of techniques easily challenged in court
10. Impatience about arriving at a diagnostic conclusion
11. Failure to understand normative data with regard to psychosexual development
12. Failure to prepare adequately for court appearances

TABLE 30.6 Skeletal Injuries from Child Abuse

High-Specificity Findings
- Classic metaphyseal lesions
- Posterior rib fracture
- Scapular fracture
- Sternal fracture
- Spinous process fracture
- First rib fracture

Moderate-Specificity Findings
- Multiple fractures
- Fractures of differing age
- Spine fracture
- Complex skull fracture
- Physeal fractures of the long bones
- Digital fractures

Low-Specificity Findings
- Diaphyseal fractures of the long bones
- Simple skull fractures
- Clavicle fracture
- Subperiosteal new bone formation

From Coley BD, ed. *Caffey's Pediatric Diagnostic Imaging*. 13th ed. Philadelphia: Elsevier; 2019:1455, Box 143.2; modified from Kleinman PK. *Diagnostic Imaging of Child Abuse*. 2nd ed. St. Louis, MO: Mosby; 1998.

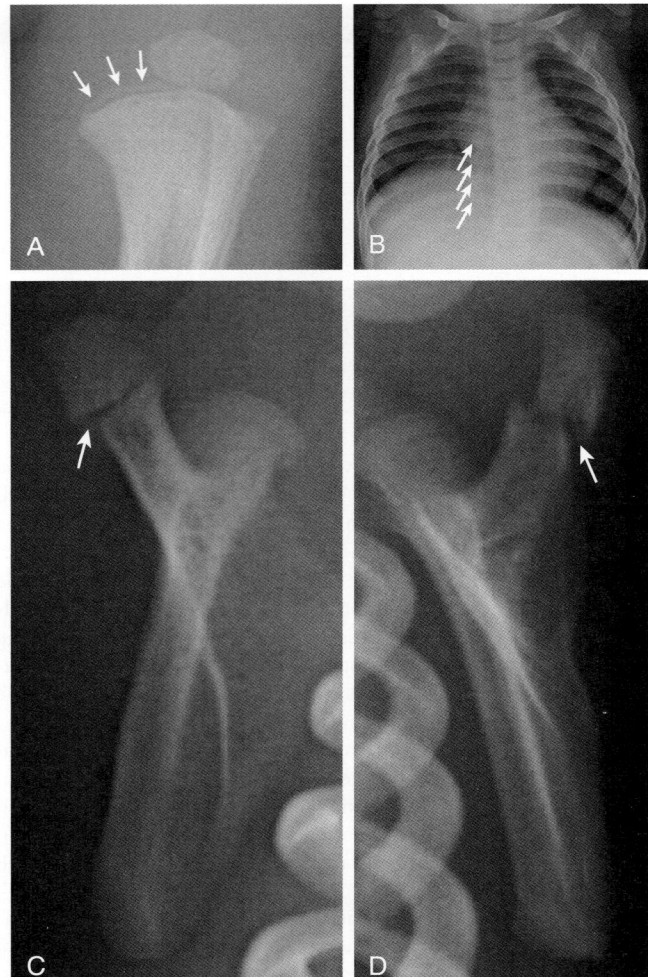

Fig. 30.5 Child abuse. *A*, Radiograph of the proximal lower leg in a 23-day-old infant with fussiness and suspected lower extremity pain reveals a classic metaphyseal lesion of the proximal tibia with a bucket-handle configuration *(arrows)*. *B*, Chest radiograph in a 12-month-old boy presenting with constipation reveals multiple consecutive rib fractures, seen posteriorly near the costovertebral junctions *(arrows)*. Fractures are healing, with callous formation evident. The patient had several additional rib head fractures better profiled on other views obtained as part of a complete skeletal survey. *C, D*, Radiographic views of the bilateral scapulae reveal minimally displaced fractures of the acromion processes *(arrows)* in an infant with multiple fractures of different ages on skeletal survey. (From Walters MM, Ronertson RL, eds. *Pediatric Radiology: The Requisites*. 4th ed. Philadelphia: Elsevier; 2017:2599, Fig. 7.123.)

An evaluation for suspected child abuse may need to include imaging studies (Table 30.6 and Fig. 30.5) as well as an eye exam by an experienced ophthalmologist looking for traumatic retinal hemorrhage. Retinal hemorrhages may occur in a significant number of normal neonates after birth; over 75% resolve by 10 days of life, while all resolve by 2 months. Retinal hemorrhages atypical for a neonate or after 1–2 months suggest child abuse (Fig. 30.6).

Medical providers are in a unique position to identify infants at risk for maltreatment when they present for medical care, and to provide education and resources to high-risk families. In infants hospitalized for abusive head trauma, the majority of victims' caregivers sought medical care for excessive crying prior to the abuse. Multiple phone calls and visits to the pediatrician for excessive crying is a warning sign that it is causing significant distress in the family. Ask caregivers how the crying is affecting the family and address any feelings of guilt or frustration. Clinicians can also ask how caregivers typically respond to the crying. All families who present with a fussy infant should be encouraged to seek support and periodic relief from the infant's care. Instruct the caregivers to safely place the infant in a crib or other safe location and walk away for a short time if they feel frustrated and at risk of harming the infant.

Infantile Colic

The definition of infantile colic varies within the medical literature. The most commonly used definition is derived from Wessel's Criteria, where crying occurs for at least 3 hours a day, at least 3 days a week,

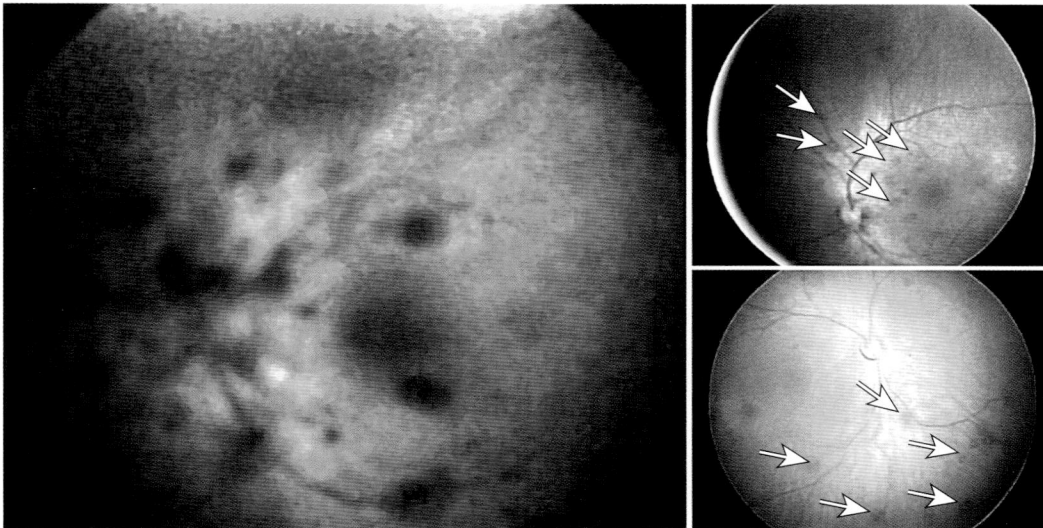

Fig. 30.6 Retinal hemorrhages. *Arrows* point to hemorrhages of various sizes. (From Kliegman RM, St. Geme JW III, Blum NJ, et al., eds. *Nelson Textbook of Pediatrics.* 21st ed. Philadelphia: Elsevier; 2020:104, Fig. 16.9.)

for at least 3 weeks in an otherwise healthy infant. Crying from colic generally occurs in the evenings, usually starts between 3 and 21 days of age, peaks at ~6 weeks, and subsides by 3–4 months of age. During crying bouts, parents describe that colicky infants often flex their legs over the abdomen or may arch their backs with a "pained" look on their face. However, many of these criteria, including the appearance of pain, are also common features of normal infant crying. It is not clear whether the appearance of pain in these infants is due to a true organic etiology or related to caregivers' anxiety about the duration and unsoothable nature of the cry.

The definition of colic for clinical purposes has shifted to remove strict criteria regarding the duration and characteristics of crying in colic. The 2016 Rome IV Criteria for Functional Gastrointestinal Disorders in Infants and Toddlers support a diagnosis of colic in an infant who (1) is younger than 5 months of age when the symptoms start and stop; (2) experiences prolonged periods of infant crying, fussing, or irritability reported to occur without obvious cause, which cannot be prevented or resolved by caregivers; and (3) has no evidence of infant failure to thrive, fever, or illness.

A single clear cause of colic remains elusive. Some suggest that the crying from colic is a response to pain from gastrointestinal (GI) dysfunction, such as milk protein or lactose intolerance, gastroesophageal reflux disease, abnormal peristalsis, excessive gas, or altered GI microbiota. However, objective testing for these disorders has not revealed significant differences between colicky and noncolicky infants, and treatments for most have been inconsistently effective. Systematic reviews of complementary and alternative treatments of infant crying have found moderately strong evidence that some probiotics may reduce crying in breast-fed infants, supporting a possible connection between altered GI microbiota and crying in some cases.

Many theorize that colic symptoms are not caused by a single condition, but rather are a common end-point for multiple processes, including infant temperament and caregivers' responses to the crying. In this view, the term "colic" is used to describe a constellation of common symptoms rather than an underlying disease. Because of the significant overlap in the pattern and characteristics of crying in infants diagnosed with colic and normal infants, colic may represent a point further along a continuum of normal infant behavior. This perspective suggests that, in healthy infants, the clinical focus should be shifted

from attempting to diagnose and treat a particular medical condition to providing education and support to caregivers. From a practical standpoint, the clinician should follow the same method of evaluation that would be initiated for any crying infant regardless of whether the crying meets the definition of colic. The duration and frequency of crying in this population can be particularly distressing for caregivers, and education on soothing and coping with the crying should be emphasized.

Feeding and Gastrointestinal Dysfunction

A subset of otherwise healthy infants who present with excessive crying will have some form of GI dysfunction. A history of crying that is associated with vomiting or hematochezia or is temporally related to feeds may increase the likelihood. Common causes include constipation, gastroesophageal reflux disease (GERD), eosinophilic esophagitis, excessive gas, and cow's and/or soy milk protein allergy or intolerance. Congenital lactose intolerance is rare, but infants may develop transient intolerance from inflammation of the intestinal villi due to gastroenteritis or a milk protein allergy. In infants with hematochezia, a milk protein allergy is most likely. However, in less clear-cut cases, improper feeding volume or technique can cause symptoms that may be misdiagnosed as GERD or a milk protein allergy. Formula changes and pharmacologic interventions may not be without undesirable consequences, including premature cessation of breast-feeding or the development of parental anxiety concerning the possibility of an intrinsic abnormality in their infant.

When GI dysfunction is suspected, and after potentially serious medical conditions are ruled out, clinicians should first evaluate feeding volume and technique. Over- or underfeeding may contribute to infant irritability. Using a slow-flow nipple can cause excessive air intake in a very vigorous feeder. Appropriate burping, feeding the infant in an upright position, using a formula thickener, and using bottles with collapsible bags may also help reduce fussing from excessive intestinal gas or GERD. Poor attachment, latch, and oral motor dysfunction may contribute to feeding problems, fussing, and even infant aversion to feedings. Consider consultation with a lactation specialist in breast-feeding infants.

Unfortunately, no specific laboratory test exists for diagnosing protein allergy in relation to excessive infant crying, and the symptoms of

GERD are often nonspecific. In fact, inflammation of the GI tract from cow's milk protein allergy may be the cause of the vomiting and symptoms of pain in up to 40% of infants diagnosed with GERD. Clinicians should inquire about a past medical or family history of atopy, which may increase the likelihood of a cow's milk protein allergy. Guidelines caution against empiric treatment with acid-reducing medications to diagnose GERD in young infants with nonspecific symptoms due to potential side effects with the overuse of these medications, and because their efficacy in decreasing crying is low. There is evidence that a trial of an extensively hydrolyzed or amino acid–based formula, or a milk- and egg-free diet in breast-feeding mothers, may decrease crying compared to controls in otherwise healthy infants with suspected GI dysfunction. The introduction of soy formula may not resolve symptoms because a significant number of infants with milk protein allergies are also allergic to soy protein. There is also evidence that probiotics may be beneficial to reduce low-grade intestinal inflammation and crying in some infants, especially breast-fed infants and those with symptoms of GERD or constipation. When potentially serious medical conditions have been excluded, and the infant's feeding volume and technique are appropriate, it is reasonable to try these interventions. Changes should be implemented one at a time and continued for at least 2 weeks to evaluate the effects of each change. If a 2–4 week trial of hydrolyzed or amino acid–based formula is beneficial, a cow's milk–based formula challenge should be planned to confirm the diagnosis of cow's milk allergy. In infants with persistent symptoms and suspicion of GERD, clinicians can consider a trial of a proton pump inhibitor and/or referral to a gastroenterologist.

Teething

Many complaints, ranging from fever to irritability, have been ascribed to teething. The most common symptoms associated with teething are irritability, excessive drooling, and loss of appetite. Some studies do support the belief that teething is associated with low-grade fever and diarrhea, but this finding is not consistent. No symptom or cluster of symptoms can reliably exclude other medical conditions; therefore, teething should be considered a diagnosis of exclusion.

Management consists of allowing the infant to bite on any appropriate hard object, such as a teething ring. Objects that are small or may break into pieces such as teething biscuits or frozen foods are not recommended due to the risk of choking. Chilling the object in the refrigerator may reduce gum inflammation and pain. However, plastic teething rings should not be frozen or boiled unless directed by the manufacturer. Extreme temperatures may damage plastic teething rings and cause fluid to leak, and frozen rings may injure gums. An oral systemic analgesic such as acetaminophen may provide additional relief, but topical anesthetic agents are not recommended due to potential serious side effects (methemoglobinemia) with the overuse of these medications.

Drug Reactions

Some therapeutic medications and illicit drugs may cause infant irritability when directly ingested or when transferred to the infant through breast milk. Substances associated with irritability include cocaine, amphetamines, opiates (from withdrawal), fluoxetine, theophylline, clemastine, and caffeine. Pseudoephedrine use in breast-feeding mothers may be associated with infant irritability, but this finding is not consistent among studies. However, when directly ingested by infants, pseudoephedrine can cause irritability as well as other more serious and life-threatening complications. In the evaluation of the irritable infant, a careful infant and maternal drug history are important to obtain along with a comprehensive urine drug screen if indicated.

In the neonate, irritability may also be a symptom of drug withdrawal or the continued effects of in utero exposure. Drugs associated with **neonatal abstinence syndrome (NAS)** include benzodiazepines, methamphetamine, heroin, methadone, buprenorphine, and other prescription opioid analgesics. Some antidepressants and anxiolytics have been found to potentiate withdrawal in infants as well. Manifestations include irritability, jitteriness, sneezing and congestion, emesis, seizures, poor feeding, hiccups, diarrhea, sleeplessness, hyperactivity, and tremors. Caregivers often describe the crying as high-pitched and inconsolable. NAS usually begins in the 1st week of life and may last for up to a month, depending on the type of substance used. This initial phase may be followed by a relapsing course that includes ongoing irritability and may last for several months. Newborns exposed to cocaine may display similar symptoms of irritability soon after birth, but these likely represent continued effects of the drug rather than withdrawal symptoms.

Mild cases of NAS are often treated with behavioral management such as reducing stimulation, swaddling, demand feeding, and other calming techniques. Pharmacotherapy is required when supportive therapy fails, or if more serious side effects such as seizures and dehydration develop. Education on coping with infant crying and methods to soothe the infant, as well as close monitoring of the home environment, are particularly important in this population due to the challenges of caring for an infant with irritability from NAS and to the lack of caregiver resources and coping skills often associated with maternal drug use.

Monogenetic Pain Syndromes

Heterozygous gain-of-function pathologic gene variants involving various channelopathies may result in an autosomal dominant form of familial painful peripheral neuropathy. Of interest, loss-of-function gene variants in the same gene may be associated with hereditary insensitivity to pain syndromes (Table 30.7).

Familial episodic pain syndrome type 1 (FEPS) is an autosomal dominant disorder due to pathologic variants in the *TRPA1* gene. The onset is during infancy and is characterized by arm and chest pain, tachycardia, and diaphoresis, which is triggered by cold, hunger (fasting), or physical stress (exertion). Episodes last ~1–2 hours. **FEPS type 2** is seen predominantly in adults. **FEPS type 3** is an autosomal dominant disorder due to pathologic variants in the *SCN11A* gene, producing a small-fiber painful neuropathy seen predominantly in adults. Infants may present with recurrent episodes of crying due to limb and distal joint pain. Fatigue, intercurrent illnesses, and weather changes are common triggers.

Paroxysmal extreme pain disorder (PEPD) (aka familial rectal pain syndrome) is an autosomal dominant, painful neuropathy due to pathologic gain-of-function variants in the *SCN9A* gene. Pain may begin after birth and is often stimulated by defecation or perineal irritation (wiping, rectal thermometer). Jaw pain may be initiated by cold fluids, spicy foods, and emotions; ocular pain may be caused by cold wind. The pain is severe, paroxysmal, and associated with harlequin color change, lacrimation, rhinorrhea, and tonic stiffening episodes, which may be confused with seizures, syncope, or hyperekplexia. The painful episodes last seconds to a few minutes. Treatment is difficult and has included carbamazepine, mexiletine, topical lidocaine, and stool softeners.

Inherited erythromelalgia (aka primary erythermalgia) (IEM) is due to pathologic gain-of-function genetic variants in *SCN9A* and is characterized by recurrent episodes of bilateral burning pain, erythema, and swelling primarily of the feet but also the hands. Over time, the face and ears may be involved; the pain may become constant. It is more common during childhood, but episodes may begin in infancy. Triggers include a warm environment or prolonged standing. Treatment includes cooling with a fan or ice; the latter may

TABLE 30.7   Clinical Features of Human Disorders Caused by Mutations in Ion-Channel Genes That Lead to Altered Pain Perception and Are Inherited in a Mendelian Manner

	Mutated Gene (Protein)	Type and Effect of Mutation	Main Phenotype	Additional Features
Inherited erythromelalgia	SCN9A (Na$_v$1.7)	Heterozygous, activating	Onset by age 20 yr; episodic pain triggered by warmth; feet affected more frequently than hands	Erythema of feet
Paroxysmal extreme pain disorder	SCN9A (Na$_v$1.7)	Heterozygous, activating	Onset at birth; episodic pain; sacral region is affected most frequently, face is affected more often than the limbs; physical triggers include defecation	Erythema of the sacrum; tonic attacks
Small-fiber neuropathy	SCN9A (Na$_v$1.7)	Heterozygous, activating	Onset at any age but more common in early adulthood; persistent burning pain; feet affected more frequently than hands	Could be autonomic features
Small-fiber neuropathy	SCN10A (Na$_v$1.8)	Heterozygous, activating	Persistent burning pain	Could be autonomic features
Familial episodic pain syndrome type I	TRPA1 (TRPA1)	Heterozygous, activating	Onset at birth or in infancy; episodic chest or arm pain; triggers are hunger and cold	—
Familial episodic pain syndrome type III	SCN11A (Na$_v$1.9)	Heterozygous, activating	Onset in 1st decade; episodic hand and foot pain; triggers are intercurrent illness or exercise	—

Na$_v$, sodium ion channel.
Modified from Bennett DLH, Woods CG. Painful and painless channelopathies. *Lancet Neurol.* 2014;13:587–599 (Table 1, p. 590).

produce cold injury if used too often. Medical therapy is similar to PEPD. The differential diagnosis includes Fabry disease (may initially present in infancy with painful feet and hands) and secondary autoimmune causes of erythromelalgia.

Pathologic genetic variants in *SCN2A* cause benign familial infantile seizures, febrile seizures plus syndrome, and intractable epilepsy of infancy. A gain-of-function genetic variant is associated with neonatal seizures, episodic ataxia, myoclonus, and pain.

STING-associated vasculopathy infantile onset (SAVI) is a severe autosomal dominant autoinflammatory disorder due to a pathologic gain-of-function variant in *TMEM173*, which encodes the STING protein (stimulator of interferon genes). Interferon-driven inflammation (**interferonopathy**) results in painful ulcerating lesions (digits, face, nose, ears) that become eschars and necrotic. Associated features include interstitial lung disease, livedo reticularis, Raynaud phenomenon, and elevated ESR and CRP. The differential diagnosis includes juvenile idiopathic arthritis, granulomatosis with polyangiitis, and other infant-onset autoinflammatory diseases (see Chapter 54).

Aicardi-Goutières syndrome is an autosomal recessive (occasionally autosomal dominant), systemic autoinflammatory interferonopathy that presents in infancy with irritability and progresses to dystonia, seizures, developmental delay, and progressive microcephaly. Some patients may develop systemic lupus erythematosus (SLE)-like symptoms as well as cold-induced chilblains. **Familial chilblain lupus** is another interferonopathy with early childhood onset of acral lesions (fingers, toes, nose, cheeks, ears). This disorder is a monogenetic form of cutaneous lupus with autosomal dominant inheritance (*TREX1*, *SAMHD1*, *STING* gene variants)

SUMMARY AND RED FLAGS

Although at times a simple diagnosis is easily established, the infant with excessive irritability often presents a significant challenge. Establishment of the likely diagnosis, combined with exclusion of significant pathophysiologic processes (see Table 30.1) and rare causes, is a prerequisite to the formulation of an appropriate management plan. Through a logical and stepwise approach, the clinician can usually establish the cause and develop a treatment plan. When the clinician cannot determine the underlying cause, close follow-up monitoring should result in optimal patient care.

Red flags include inconsolability, paradoxical irritability, abnormal level of consciousness, abnormal vital signs, evidence of trauma or anemia, prior suspicious injuries, abdominal tenderness or distention, eye tearing, photophobia or conjunctival irritation, and abnormalities of growth including increasing head circumference percentile. Consolability by being held by the caregiver is often reassuring. In contrast, paradoxical crying or irritability when being held suggests that the holding process aggravates a painful process such as a fracture, osteomyelitis, or meningitis.

In all cases, clinicians should evaluate the level of distress that the crying is causing caregivers and should provide education and support. Families with a history of maltreatment, mental illness or drug use in caregivers, caregivers with limited social support, or those who frequently seek medical care or report significant distress and frustration from the crying are at a higher risk for adverse outcomes. When these risk factors are identified, a multidisciplinary approach involving education and resources for the caregivers, medical care for the infant, and family therapy or referrals to perinatal and infant mental health experts can improve caregiver-infant interactions and long-term outcomes for the child.

BIBLIOGRAPHY

A bibliography is available at ExpertConsult.com.

31

Emotional and Behavioral Symptoms

Ryan Byrne, Garrett Elsner, and Ashley Beattie

The history is the most important tool for identifying a psychiatric disorder. The initial focus in conducting the history is to establish rapport and to ensure the child's safety. Safety should always be assessed and should include risk of suicide, homicide, and abuse (physical, sexual, emotional, and neglect). The history should then focus on delineating the specific behaviors of concern, on identifying any stressors that may be precipitating the behavior (Table 31.1), and on recognizing any associated symptoms that may differentiate which disorder or disorders are causing the behavior (Table 31.2). In addition to primary psychiatric diagnoses, the clinician should focus on possible medical causes of the behaviors in question, including medication side effects, substance misuse, and medical illnesses (Tables 31.3 and 31.4). Comorbidity is common in children with psychiatric illnesses, and as such, the clinician should consider whether a combination of medical *and* psychiatric diagnoses may be producing the patient's symptoms.

Information should be obtained from multiple sources whenever possible. This can include any adults who have spent significant time with the child, such as parents, other family members, guardians, and teachers. The child should be interviewed separately so as to provide a better chance of obtaining their perspective of the presenting symptoms. The patient may also be more comfortable disclosing a history of abuse or destructive behaviors, such as substance misuse, self-harm, or high-risk sexual activity, during an individual interview. Because some psychiatric disorders demonstrate a strong genetic predisposition, a detailed psychiatric family history should be obtained. Psychiatric illness in family members may be undiagnosed; the clinician should inquire about the presence of symptoms in addition to formal diagnoses in the family.

The following validated principles should guide history taking, particularly when discussing sensitive topics such as substance use, sexual abuse, and suicidal ideation or intent:

1. **Behavioral analysis**: The clinician should break down complex patterns of behavior into discrete incidents and focus on concrete details chronologically. Doing so allows the clinician to objectively establish the sequence of behaviors behind sensitive events, particularly when the patient's subjective responses to the events may influence recall or reporting.
2. **Shame attenuation**: The clinician should assume a stance of unconditional positive regard so as to minimize the influence of guilt or shame while discussing taboo subjects.
3. **Gentle assumption**: By framing questions based on the assumption that a behavior exists, the clinician may overcome patient hesitation to acknowledge the presence of that behavior (e.g., "How often do you have suicidal thoughts?").
4. **Symptom amplification**: By assuming a high frequency of the behavior and inquiring in a concrete manner (e.g., "How many days a week do you drink? 5–6?"), the clinician may make the patient feel more at ease by acknowledging the existence of a particular behavior, particularly if a patient is troubled by the frequency of the behavior.
5. **Denial of the specific:** By asking specific questions, the clinician may elicit more accurate information by prompting recollection of particular behaviors that may otherwise be denied when asked in general terms. Asking the patient whether they have ever used marijuana may be more likely to elicit a positive response than asking the patient whether they have ever used illegal drugs.
6. **Normalization:** By simply describing common patterns of symptoms or behaviors, the clinician may help the patient feel more at ease by endorsing the presence of similar patterns in their behaviors.

The history allows the clinician to define patterns of behavior that suggest a differential diagnosis. The *Diagnostic and Statistical Manual of Mental Disorders,* Fifth Edition (DSM-5), contains descriptive diagnostic criteria based on the presence or absence of various symptoms and aids the clinician in assigning a specific diagnosis to these behavior patterns and symptom clusters. Terms frequently used in the diagnosis of psychotic illnesses are noted in Table 31.5. The persistence, frequency, and severity of behaviors should be used to distinguish a behavior that is symptomatic from a behavior that is within normal limits. When a behavior does not meet a clinical threshold, it can be just as important for the provider to reassure a family and provide support during a difficult time of normal development. A classic example would be a 2 year old expressing their autonomy or a teenager struggling to establish their individual identity.

CONDITIONS CHARACTERIZED BY ABNORMAL BEHAVIORS

Disruptive behaviors are broadly categorized by whether they affect the patient or others, then further classified by whether there is associated difficulty in regulating emotions or behaviors (see Table 31.2).

Behaviors That Primarily Affect the Patient

Attention-Deficit/Hyperactivity Disorder

The cardinal features of attention-deficit/hyperactivity disorder (ADHD) are hyperactivity, distractibility, and impulsivity. Manifestations of these symptoms must be present in more than one setting (school *and* home) and must interfere with functioning or development. Prevalence increases with the child's age and is approximately 9–15% in school-aged children. ADHD is more frequent in males than in females with a ratio of about 2:1 for the predominantly inattentive type and 4:1 for the predominantly hyperactive type. Females may be underdiagnosed as they are more likely to present with the inattention symptoms as compared to the hyperactivity symptoms that tend to be more disruptive and more likely to reach the threshold for seeking care. The DSM-5 specifies that there must be a persistent pattern of inattention and/or hyperactivity–impulsivity with six or more symptoms in either category lasting at least 6 months. Adolescents 17 years of age or older require only five symptoms; however, symptoms should be present prior to 12 years of age.

Inattention

1. Lack of attention to detail or inaccurate work
2. Difficulty sustaining attention
3. Failure to listen when spoken to directly
4. Lack of follow-through
5. Disorganization
6. Avoidance of activities requiring sustained attention
7. Frequent loss of items
8. Easy distraction by extraneous stimuli
9. Forgetfulness

Hyperactivity/Impulsivity

1. Frequent fidgeting or squirming
2. Frequent need to walk around
3. Restlessness or need to run around/climb
4. Difficulty engaging in quiet activities
5. Acting "on the go," restlessness, or difficulty of caregivers to keep up with
6. Talking excessively
7. Frequently interrupting
8. Difficulty waiting turn
9. Intrusiveness

The chronicity of the **hyperactivity** in this disorder may be subtle. Although children with ADHD tend to move around more than other children, the hyperactivity may be of concern only in certain situations in which the child is expected to be quiet (e.g., in school or places of worship). Some children with ADHD can sit and be attentive in quiet and relaxed situations, whereas a noisy and active setting, such as an unstructured classroom, precipitates inappropriate behavior. When these children become older, they often become less overtly hyperactive. An adolescent may mostly feel restless without acting upon that feeling in a disruptive manner. This restlessness may contribute significantly to academic underachievement. Despite intentions for diligent studying, the restlessness may cause the affected teenager to feel the need to walk around, distracting from studying.

Impulsivity significantly contributes to morbidity. The impulsivity applies not only to actions but also to emotions. An impulsive child whose emotions change quickly is at risk for physically aggressive behaviors, such as hitting or biting. In school-aged children, the impulsive aggression is often manifested as explosive behavior. Because of their explosive behavior, inability to wait their turn in a game, and difficulty regulating emotions when interacting with teachers, these children have great difficulty with both peer and teacher relations. Impulsivity can also be potentially life threatening because the child may act before considering the consequences. Impulsivity may manifest as *risk-taking behaviors* in both children (e.g., running into the street after a ball without checking for traffic) and adolescents (high-risk sexual activity or substance misuse).

Hyperactivity and impulsivity in children are often readily apparent to adults; however, the manifestations of **inattention and distractibility** are often not as overt. In young children, inattentive behavior can consist of shifting from one activity to another and having difficulty finishing tasks. The parents may incorrectly consider these actions to represent lack of motivation. In adolescence, inattentive behavior may result in poor school performance. These children may forget to do homework or may need excessively long periods to complete assignments because of their inability to focus on their work. They may be mislabeled as being lazy.

The challenge in diagnosing ADHD lies in defining when specific behaviors are abnormal, particularly when those behaviors may not be apparent in all situations or contexts. The clinician should not rely solely on observations obtained in the clinic setting, but should instead gather information from multiple sources, including parents, teachers, daycare workers, and even a direct classroom observation from a trained health care professional. Being in the clinic can be overstimulating or

TABLE 31.1 Common Precipitants of Psychiatric Symptoms

| Substance misuse |
| Stress |
| Death or illness of family or friend |
| Interpersonal conflict, including bullying |
| Rejection or abandonment |
| Significant change in routine |
| Homelessness |

TABLE 31.3 The MIDAS Mnemonic for Screening for Medical Illness

| M: Do you take any **M**edications? |
| I: Do you have any medical **I**llnesses? |
| D: Do you have a primary care **D**octor? |
| A: Have you ever had any **A**llergies, reactions, or side effects? |
| S: Have you ever had any **S**urgery? |

From Carlat DJ. *The Psychiatric Interview*. 3rd ed. Philadelphia: Lippincott Williams & Wilkins; 2011.

TABLE 31.2 Disruptive Behavior Disorders

Symptom	Intermittent Explosive Disorder	Disruptive Mood Dysregulation Disorder	Oppositional Defiant Disorder	Conduct Disorder
Aggressive outbursts	+	+	+	+
Property destruction or physically assaultive	+	+	+	+
Persistently irritable	−	+	+/−	−
Purposefully defiant	−	−	+	+
Vindictive	−	−	+	+
Argues with authority	−	−	+	+
Stealing	−	−	−	+
Use of a weapon or fire setting	−	−	−	+
Run away from home/truancy	−	−	−	+

A "+" indicates symptoms are seen in the disorder. A "−" indicates symptoms are not seen in the disorder.

TABLE 31.4   Medical (Secondary) and Psychiatric (Primary) Causes of Psychosis and/or Depression

Category	Disorders	Category	Disorders
Psychiatric	Schizophrenia Schizoaffective Schizophreniform Brief psychotic Major depression Bipolar Postpartum	Demyelinating, dysmyelinating	Multiple sclerosis Acute disseminated encephalomyelitis Adrenoleukodystrophy Metachromatic leukodystrophy
Head trauma	Traumatic brain injury Subdural hematoma	Inherited metabolic	Wilson disease Posterior horn syndrome Tay-Sachs disease (adult onset) Neuronal ceroid lipofuscinosis Niemann-Pick disease type C Acute intermittent porphyria Mitochondrial encephalopathy, lactic acidosis, and stroke-like episodes (MELAS) Mitochondrial neurogastrointestinal encephalopathy (MNGIE) Cerebrotendinous xanthomatosis Homocystinuria Ornithine transcarbamylase deficiency Phenylketonuria
Infectious	Viral infections/encephalitides (HIV infection/encephalopathy, herpes encephalitis, cytomegalovirus. Epstein-Barr virus, COVID-19) Lyme disease Cerebral malaria Endocarditis Neurosyphilis Whipple disease		
Inflammatory	Autoimmune encephalitis: NMDAR, limbic, others Systemic lupus erythematosus Sjögren syndrome Hashimoto encephalopathy (steroid-responsive encephalopathy associated with autoimmune thyroiditis [SREAT]) Sydenham chorea Sarcoidosis Celiac disease	Syndromes	Williams Prader-Willi Marfan Fragile X Deletion 22q11.2 Rapid-onset obesity with hypothalamic dysfunction, hypoventilation, autonomic dysregulation (ROHHAD) Klinefelter
Neoplastic	Primary or secondary cerebral neoplasm Paraneoplastic encephalitis: ovarian teratoma-associated autoimmune encephalitis Systemic neoplasm Pheochromocytoma	Epilepsy	Ictal Interictal Postictal Postepilepsy surgery Lafora progressive myoclonic epilepsy Complex partial (temporal lobe)
Endocrine or acquired metabolic	Hepatic encephalopathy Uremic encephalopathy Hypo/hyperparathyroidism Hypo/hyperthyroidism Addison disease Cushing disease Vitamin deficiency: vitamin B_{12}, folate, niacin, vitamin C, thiamine Gastric bypass–associated nutritional deficiencies Hypoglycemia Hyponatremia	Substance induced (medications)	Analgesics Acyclovir Androgens (anabolic steroids) Antiarrhythmics Anticonvulsants Anticholinergics Antihypertensives Antineoplastic agents β-Blocking agents Cefepime Clarithromycin Cyclosporine Dextromethorphan Dopamine agonists Ketamine Fluoroquinolones Metronidazole Sulfamethoxazole-trimethoprim Oral contraceptives Sedatives/hypnotics Selective serotonin reuptake inhibitors (SSRIs) (serotonin syndrome) Steroids
Vascular	Cerebral autosomal dominant arteriopathy with subcortical infarcts and leukoencephalopathy (CADASIL) Other vasculitis syndromes Stroke		
Degenerative	Idiopathic basal ganglia calcifications, Fahr disease Neuroacanthocytosis Neurodegeneration with brain iron accumulation (NBIA) Tuberous sclerosis Huntington disease Corticobasal ganglionic degeneration Multisystem atrophy, striatonigral degeneration, olivopontocerebellar atrophy		

TABLE 31.4   Medical (Secondary) and Psychiatric (Primary) Causes of Psychosis and/or Depression—cont'd

Category	Disorders	Category	Disorders
Substance induced	Alcohol Amphetamines Cocaine LSD Marijuana and synthetic cannabinoids Methylenedioxymethamphetamine (MDMA, Ecstasy) Phencyclidine Mescaline Psilocybins (mushrooms)	Toxins	Heavy metals: lead, mercury, arsenic Carbon monoxide Inhalants Organophosphates St. John's Wort
Drug withdrawal syndromes	Alcohol Barbiturates Benzodiazepines Amphetamines SSRIs	Other	Normal-pressure hydrocephalus Ionizing radiation Decompression sickness Narcolepsy

anxiety provoking for the child. The classroom teacher represents an excellent resource for determining whether the patient's level of activity and degree of impulsivity are abnormal. Standardized behavioral checklists (such as the Vanderbilt Rating Scale) filled out by the parents and teachers quantify the degree of abnormal behaviors with regard to an age-specific reference population.

Before establishing a diagnosis of ADHD, the clinician must rule out other psychiatric and medical causes of the patient's symptoms. With respect to psychiatric conditions, the differential diagnosis of ADHD includes learning disorders, oppositional behavior, mood disorders, anxiety disorders, and substance abuse. *Because of the high association of learning disorders with ADHD, the evaluation should include an assessment for learning problems.*

With respect to medical conditions, the differential diagnosis of ADHD includes iron deficiency, lead toxicity, thyroid disorders, seizures, hearing loss, and substance misuse. Screening for symptoms of sleep disturbances or sleep apnea is essential because chronically ineffective or inefficient sleep can produce symptoms of inattention and hyperactivity.

Tic Disorders

Tics are motor movements or vocalizations that are sudden, rapid, recurrent, nonrhythmic, and involuntary. Tics often become worse during stress but may improve during activities requiring moderate physical or mental activity. Tics need to be differentiated from other abnormal movements, such as chorea, athetosis, dystonia, myoclonus, and hemiballismus (Chapter 40). These other movements may be associated with an underlying neurologic condition or may be medication induced. Tics are common with 5–24% of school-aged children having a history of tics. Most do not require treatment and do not progress to a more serious tic disorder. **Simple motor tics** are defined as repetitive movements of single muscle groups. They may consist of eye blinking, neck jerking, or shoulder shrugging. **Complex motor tics** are repetitive movements of several muscle groups in coordination, such as repetitive grooming behaviors, deep knee bends, or smelling of objects. **Simple vocal tics** are defined as nonverbal noises, such as throat clearing or grunting sounds, whereas **complex vocal tics** are intelligible words. Complex vocal tics may rarely manifest as **coprolalia**, the repetitive, stereotyped vocalization of obscenities.

The DSM-5 categorizes tic disorders as follows:
1. **Provisional tic disorder:** motor and/or vocal tics lasting less than a year
2. **Chronic motor or vocal tic disorder:** either motor or vocal tics lasting longer than a year
3. **Tourette disorder:** both multiple motor and one or more vocal tics lasting longer than a year

The incidence of Tourette disorder is 4–5/10,000. In some families, this illness is inherited as an autosomal dominant condition, with 70% penetrance in females and near-complete penetrance in males. Because of this difference in penetrance, Tourette disorder is 1.5–3 times more common in males than in females. The median age at presentation is 7 years, though some children may present as early as 2 years. While coprolalia is popularly thought to be a common feature of Tourette disorder, fewer than 10% of affected patients have this form of complex vocal tics.

The DSM-5 criteria for Tourette disorder are as follows:
1. Multiple motor and one or more vocal tics must be present, although not necessarily concurrently, lasting longer than a year with no tic-free intervals longer than 3 months
2. Symptom onset before age 18 years
3. No medical cause for the tics

Tics may lead to the patient being socially ostracized. Children with chronic tic disorders frequently have other psychologic conditions, such as ADHD or obsessive-compulsive disorder (OCD), which may lead to further difficulties in peer interactions and frequent frustration of teachers and family members. Such stressors can worsen the tics, which can further compound the problem.

Behaviors That Affect Others

Disruptive Mood Dysregulation Disorder

While the predominant characteristic of disruptive mood dysregulation disorder (DMDD) is chronic, persistent, and severe irritability, it is often the behavioral issues that prompt presentation to a clinician. DMDD often manifests as irritable, depressed mood and temper tantrums with a low frustration tolerance. The DSM-5 requires the following for diagnosis:
1. Severe recurrent temper outbursts that manifest with verbal or behavioral aggression out of proportion to the situation in intensity or duration

---

TABLE 31.5 Psychiatric Terms

Abulia is the state of reduced impulse to act and think associated with indifference about consequences of action.

Affect is the examiner's observation of the patient's emotional state. Frequently used descriptive terms include the following:

    Constricted affect is reduced range and intensity of expression.

    Blunted affect is further reduced. Usually, there is little facial expression and a voice that is monotone and lacking normal prosody.

    Flat describes severely blunted affect in which there is no affective expression.

    Inappropriate affect is an incongruous expression of emotion or behavior relative to the content of a conversation or social norms.

    Labile affect exhibits abrupt and sudden changes in both type and intensity of emotion.

Anxiety is the feeling of apprehension caused by anticipation of danger that may be internal or external.

Apathy is dulled emotional tone associated with detachment or indifference.

Comportment refers to self-regulation of behavior through complex mental processes that include insight, judgment, self-awareness, empathy, and social adaptation.

Compulsion is the uncontrollable impulse to perform an act repetitively.

Confusion is the inability to maintain a coherent stream of thought owing to impaired attention and vigilance. Secondary deficits in language, memory, and visual spatial skills are common.

Delusion is a false, unshakable conviction or judgment that is out of keeping with reality and with socially shared beliefs of the individual's background and culture. It cannot be corrected with reasoning.

Depression is a sustained psychopathologic feeling of sadness often accompanied by a variety of associated symptoms, particularly anxiety, agitation, feelings of worthlessness, suicidal ideation, abulia, psychomotor retardation, and various somatic symptoms and physiologic dysfunctions and complaints that cause significant distress and impairment in social functioning.

Hallucination is a false sensory perception not associated with real external stimuli.

Mood is the emotional state experienced and described by the patient and observed by others.

Obsession is the pathologic persistence of an irresistible thought or feeling that cannot be eliminated from consciousness by logical effort. It is associated with anxiety and rumination.

Paranoia is a descriptive term designating either morbid-dominant ideas or delusions of self-reference concerning one or more of several themes, most commonly persecution, love, hate, envy, jealousy, honor, litigation, grandeur, and the supernatural.

Prosody is the melodic patterns of intonation in language that convey shades of meaning.

Psychosis is the inability or impaired ability to distinguish reality from hallucinations and/or delusions.

Russell sign is calluses on the knuckles or back of the hand due to repeated self-induced vomiting over long periods of time.

Thought process and content. Common descriptive terms include the following:

    Circumstantial thought follows a circuitous route to the answer. There may be many superfluous details, but the patient eventually reaches the answer.

    Linear thought demonstrates goal-directed associations and is easy to follow.

    Loose associations are thoughts that have no logical or meaningful connection with ensuing thoughts.

    Tangential thoughts are initially clearly linked to a current thought but fail to maintain goal-directed associations; the patient never arrives at the desired point or goal.

    Clang associations describe speech in which the sounds of words are similar but not the meanings. The words have no logical connection to each other.

    Flight of ideas describes a rapid stream of thoughts that tend to be related to each other.

    Magical thinking describes the belief that thoughts, words, or actions have power to influence events in ways other than through reality-based mechanisms.

    Thought blocking is characterized by abrupt interruptions in speech during conversation before an idea or thought is finished. After a pause, the individual indicates no recall of what was being said or what was going to be said.

From Perez DL, Murray ED, Price BH. Depression and psychosis in neurological practice. In: Daroff RB, Jankovic J, Mazziotta JC, Pomeroy SL, eds. *Bradley's Neurology in Clinical Practice.* 7th ed. Philadelphia: Elsevier; 2015.

---

2. Behavior is inconsistent with developmental level
3. Behavior occurs on average 3 or more times per week
4. The mood between outbursts is persistently irritable or angry
5. Symptoms present for 12 or more months
6. Symptoms present in at least two settings
7. Age of onset of symptoms must be before age 10 years, but diagnosis should not be made before age 6 years or after age 18 years

The overall prevalence of DMDD among children and adolescents is as high as 5%. Rates are higher in males and school-aged children than in females and adolescents. DMDD can cause significant difficulties with school performance and family/peer relationships. Many children with DMDD will also meet criteria for ADHD, mood disorders, or anxiety disorders. The diagnosis of DMDD should be distinguished from bipolar disorder, which must have distinct episodes of mania or hypomania (Table 31.6). The age of the patient can also help differentiate DMDD and bipolar disorders because bipolar disorders rarely present prior to adolescence. Individuals who meet criteria for

DMDD and oppositional defiant disorder (ODD) should only be given the diagnosis of DMDD.

Intermittent Explosive Disorder

Intermittent explosive disorder (IED) is an impulse control disorder where the child will have significant recurrent behavioral outbursts that are seen as out of proportion to the situation. The outbursts can be violent but are not premeditated. The outbursts can cause significant distress to both the patient and family. IED does not have the persistently angry or irritable mood in between outbursts that is present in DMDD. The DSM-5 requires the following for diagnosis:

1. Recurrent behavioral outbursts representing failure to control aggressive impulses
2. Verbal or physical aggression toward property, animals, or other individuals occurring on average twice weekly for 3 months or three behavioral outbursts involving destruction of property and/or physical assault within a 12-month period

TABLE 31.6 Diagnostic Features of Primary Psychiatric Disorders

The following conditions require clinically significant distress or impairment in social or occupational functioning:

- **Schizophrenia** is a disorder that lasts for at least 6 mo and includes at least 1 mo of active symptoms (two or more of the following: delusions, hallucinations, disorganized speech, grossly disorganized or catatonic behavior, or negative symptoms).
- **Schizoaffective disorder** is a disorder in which a mood episode and the active symptoms of schizophrenia occur together and were preceded or are followed by at least 2 wk of delusions or hallucinations without prominent mood symptoms.
- **Major depressive disorder** is characterized by one or more major depressive episodes (at least 2 wk of depressed mood or loss of interest accompanied by at least four additional symptoms of depression). Additional symptoms of depression may include significant weight changes, sleep dysfunction, psychomotor agitation or retardation, fatigue or loss of energy, feelings of worthlessness or guilt, diminished concentration, and suicidal ideation or thoughts of death.
- A **manic episode** is defined by an abnormally and persistently elevated, expansive, or irritable mood persisting for at least 1 wk (or less if hospitalization is required). At least three of the following symptoms must be present if the mood is elevated or expansive (four symptoms are required if the mood is irritable): inflated self-esteem or grandiosity, decreased need for sleep, pressured speech, flight of ideas, distractibility, increased goal-directed activities or psychomotor agitation, and excessive involvement in pleasurable activities with a high potential for painful consequences. Psychotic features may be present.
- **Bipolar I disorder** is characterized by the presence of both manic and major depressive episodes or manic episodes alone.
- **Bipolar II disorder** is characterized by the presence of major depressive episodes alternating with episodes of hypomania.
- **Hypomania** is characterized by an abnormally and persistently elevated, expansive, or irritable mood persisting for at least 4 days. Other criteria required for diagnosis are identical to that of a manic episode except that the symptoms are not so severe as to cause marked impairment in social or occupational functioning, hospitalization is not required, and no psychotic symptoms are present.

From Perez DL, Murray ED, Price BH. Depression and psychosis in neurological practice. In: Daroff RB, Jankovic J, Mazziotta JC, Pomeroy SL, eds. *Bradley's Neurology in Clinical Practice.* 7th ed. Philadelphia: Elsevier; 2015.

3. Aggression grossly out of proportion to trigger
4. Outbursts are not premeditated
5. Chronological age is at least 6 years (or equivalent development level)
6. The outbursts cause marked distress in the individual or impairment in interpersonal functioning

The diagnosis of IED can be made in addition to ADHD, conduct disorder, oppositional defiant disorder, or autism spectrum disorder. It cannot be made with a diagnosis of DMDD. It is important to rule out other potential causes for the outbursts including bipolar disorder, substance use disorders, and traumatic brain injury.

Substance Use Disorder

Substance use can lead to a wide range of disturbances in mood and behavior. The disturbance can occur during both the period of intoxication *and* the period of withdrawal. The hallmark of a substance use disorder is the continued use of a substance despite it causing ongoing negative cognitive, behavioral, and physiologic symptoms. The other hallmark of substance use disorder is the significance of the negative behaviors, such as verbal or physical aggression, defiance, lying, or stealing. Sometimes these behaviors will reach the point of violating the rights of family and friends.

Oppositional Defiant Disorder

The characteristic feature of ODD is a persistent pattern of both defiant behavior and an angry/irritable mood, argumentative/defiant behavior, or vindictiveness. Affected individuals exhibit at least four of the following behaviors in a consistent manner over a 6-month period:

1. Frequently losing temper
2. Often arguing with authority figures
3. Defying rules
4. Deliberately annoying adults
5. Blaming others for their actions
6. Becoming easily annoyed by others
7. Being angry
8. Being vindictive

ODD should not be diagnosed if the patient meets the DSM-5 criteria for conduct disorder or if the symptoms occur in the context of a mood, an anxiety, or a psychotic disorder, in which children exhibit oppositional behavior as a reaction to their illness.

Prevalence ranges from 1% to 11%, depending on the population. In prepubertal children, it occurs more frequently in males; however, in adolescents, its incidence is equal in both sexes. Most children present before 8 years of age. Affected preschool-aged children sometimes exhibit increased motor activity, difficulty being comforted, and overreacting to situations. Affected school-aged children have low self-esteem and a low tolerance for frustration. The disorder commonly occurs in families with a history of mood or psychotic disorders—particularly maternal depression—and with chronic disruptive behaviors, such as ADHD or conduct disorder.

Children with this disorder are at marked risk for other psychiatric disorders, such as ADHD. In addition, these patients may be at increased risk for conduct disorder, antisocial personality disorder as adults, substance abuse, major depressive disorder, and suicide.

Conduct Disorder

A child has conduct disorder if they have repetitively violated the rights of others and of society. Children with this diagnosis have performed three or more of the following behaviors within the past year and with at least one occurring in the previous 6 months:

1. Aggression toward people or animals, such as intimidation, initiation of fights, use of weapons, cruelty to people, cruelty to animals, rape, confrontational theft, or mugging
2. Destruction of property, such as arson or vandalism
3. Deceitfulness or theft, such as breaking into houses or cars or stealing items of nontrivial value
4. Serious violation of rules, such as curfew violation, running away, or truancy before the age of 13 years (for running away to qualify as a symptom, it must occur twice, or once if it was lengthy, and must not be an attempt to escape sexual or physical abuse)

Conduct disorder is classified as **childhood onset** if symptoms occur before 10 years of age and **adolescent onset** if symptoms occur at or after 10 years of age. It may have the qualifier of "limited prosocial emotions" such as lack of remorse or guilt, callous lack of empathy, unconcerned about performance, and shallow affect. It is further subdivided by severity of offense: mild (e.g., truancy), moderate (e.g., vandalism, nonconfrontational theft), and severe (e.g., rape,

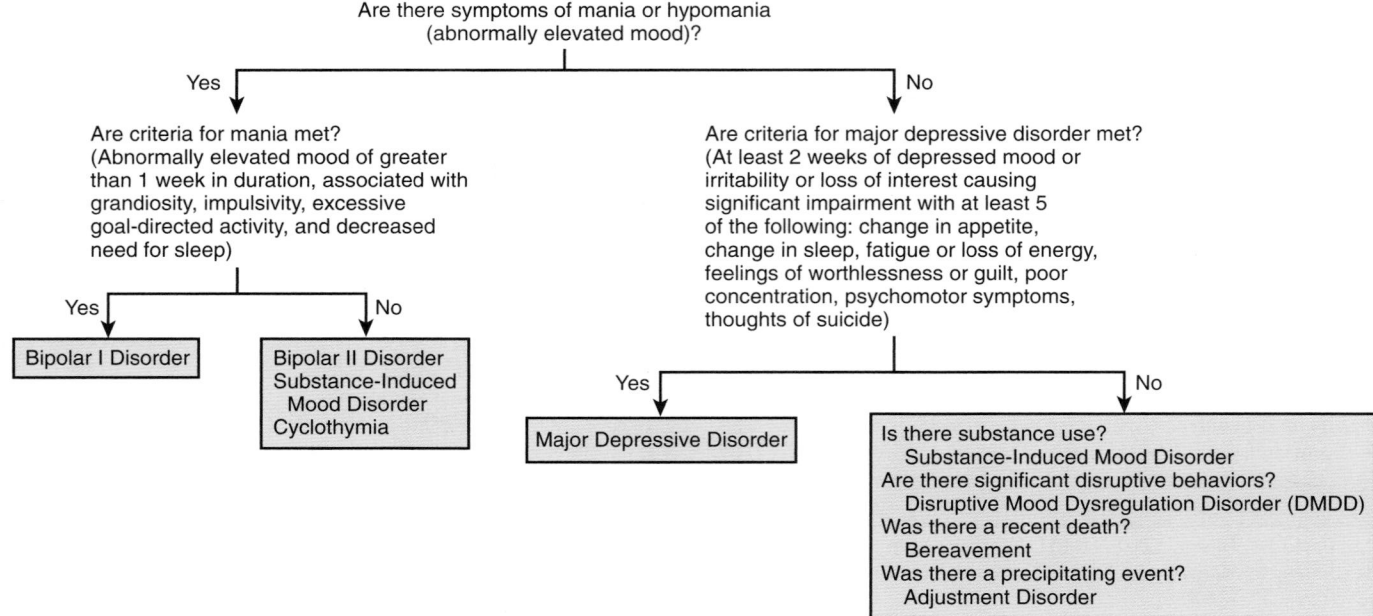

Fig. 31.1 Evaluation of mood disorders.

confrontational theft). The prevalence of conduct disorder is higher in males than in females. Children initially present with lying, initiating fights, and truancy; as they get older, they progress to more violent acts. Males are more likely to exhibit acts of violence, such as fighting and stealing, than are females, who are more likely to exhibit truancy, runaway behavior, and high-risk sexual activity. Half of these children may develop **antisocial personality disorder**, which is a severe conduct disorder of adulthood that is usually associated with criminal activity. The earlier the onset of conduct disorder, the greater the risk of developing antisocial personality disorder as an adult. These children also have a high frequency of depression, suicidal ideation, personality disorders, anxiety disorders, ADHD, and substance abuse.

CONDITIONS CHARACTERIZED BY DISRUPTION IN MOOD

Mood disorders are divided into those characterized by a depressed mood and those characterized by extremes of mood lability. When assessing mood disturbances, it is essential to screen for symptoms suggestive of bipolar illness as these patients have a risk of becoming manic when treated with antidepressants (Fig. 31.1). The evaluation of any patient with a disruption in mood should include an assessment of the risk of suicide.

Conditions Characterized by Depressed Mood

Depressive disorders that may present in childhood include DMDD, major depressive disorder, premenstrual dysphoric disorder, persistent depressive disorder (i.e., dysthymia), substance/medication-induced depressive disorder, adjustment disorder with depressed mood, and depressive disorder related to another medical condition.

Major Depressive Disorder

Major depressive disorder is associated with serious risks of suicide, significant social isolation, and academic impairment (see Table 31.6). Presentations may be subtle. While children and adolescents can present with classic sad or depressed mood, they may also present with irritability. Patients may also present with somatic complaints, psychosis,

or both. The psychotic symptoms are typically *mood-congruent* auditory hallucinations and delusions of guilt, medical illnesses, or deserving punishment. DSM-5 criteria for major depressive disorder consist of at least a 2-week period of a depressed mood—or irritability in some children—or loss of interest in pleasurable activities, resulting in significant impairment. During this period, the patient has to have at least five of the following symptoms:

1. Depressed mood or irritability in some children
2. Loss of interest or pleasure
3. Loss of appetite or overeating
4. Insomnia or hypersomnia
5. Fatigue or loss of energy
6. Feelings of worthlessness or guilt
7. Poor concentration or indecisiveness
8. Suicidal ideation or thoughts of death
9. Psychomotor agitation or retardation

These symptoms should not be secondary to bereavement, medical conditions, substance abuse, or bipolar disorders. Emotional reaction to adverse stressors is a normal part of life. The clinician must decide whether the reaction to the stressor is normal, an adjustment disorder, or major depression.

The occurrence of major depressive disorders in adolescence is as high as 5%, with a cumulative prevalence in adolescence of 12% in females and 7% in males. There is also a threefold increase in major depression in children who have a parent with depression. The differential diagnosis of major depression encompasses various medical disorders, including neurologic disorders, endocrine disorders such as hypothyroidism or hyperparathyroidism, side effects from medications such as H₂-blockers or isotretinoin, and substance abuse or use (see Table 31.4). Numerous psychiatric conditions are comorbid with major depression. Among these are ODD, conduct disorder, ADHD, anxiety disorders, eating disorders, and substance abuse.

Major depressive disorder can manifest at any age; most patients present in early adulthood. Children usually present with somatic complaints, social withdrawal, and irritability, whereas adolescents often present with psychomotor retardation, thoughts of guilt and worthlessness, and excessive sleep. Approximately 15% of children with major depression eventually develop bipolar disorders. Fifty percent of children with major depression have multiple episodes, frequently associated with significant stressors. Approximately 25% of patients with certain chronic medical conditions such as cancer or diabetes develop a major depressive episode during the course of the illness. The main difficulty in diagnosing major depression is that the gravity of the depressive mood is often not always apparent to the parent and the clinician. Children and adolescents suffering from depression often have a broader range of affect compared with adults, who often appear more sullen. Given that children and adolescents often present with irritability or mean-spiritedness, the parents and/or clinician may attribute this behavior to typical adolescent behavior. These children do not always appear sad and the clinician should have a high index of suspicion of major depression in any child who presents with sullenness and irritability. Guidelines for evaluating such a patient are as follows:

1. Assess suicidal ideation and ensure the patient's safety.
2. Obtain collateral information from other sources to determine the child's functioning and symptoms.
3. Obtain a thorough family history for symptoms and formal diagnoses of mood disorders.
4. Rule out bipolar disorders by assessing for symptoms of mania or hypomania.
5. Investigate primary or comorbid conditions, such as substance abuse.
6. Consider the role of life stressors in relationship to the symptoms.

Premenstrual Dysphoric Disorder

Both physical and mood symptoms can occur prior to a female's menstrual cycle. When the symptoms are severe, they may constitute premenstrual dysphoric disorder, the primary features of which are mood lability, irritability, dysphoria, and anxiety that appear recurrently during the premenstrual phase of a female's cycle and then resolve around the onset of menses. Delusions or hallucinations have been described but are rare. The 12-month prevalence is as high as 6% of menstruating women. Onset can be any time after menarche. Factors such as stress, a history of trauma, and seasonal changes can contribute. The DSM-5 states that the following criteria must be met:

1. In the majority of cycles, at least four of the following symptoms: marked affective lability (mood swings, increased sensitivity to rejection), irritability or anger, increased interpersonal conflicts, depressed mood, feelings of hopelessness or self-deprecating thoughts, anxiety, or tension
2. At least one of the following: decreased interest in activities, difficulty concentrating, lack of energy, change in appetite, change in sleep, sense of being out of control, physical symptoms of breast tenderness, joint pain, bloating, or weight gain
3. Symptoms present during the majority of cycles over the year prior

The severity of symptoms is similar to that in other psychiatric disorders, such as major depression or generalized anxiety disorder, though the duration of symptoms is shorter. Nonetheless, symptoms do need to be severe and cause marked impairment in functioning to satisfy diagnostic criteria. To confirm the diagnosis, daily prospective symptom ratings are required for at least two cycles.

Substance-Induced Mood Disorders

Substance-*induced* disorders are distinct from substance *use* disorders. Whereas the latter refer to the negative consequences of substance use over time, the substance-induced disorders refer to the immediate effects of substance use—**intoxication** and **withdrawal**—and to the **substance-induced mental disorders**, which include psychotic disorders, anxiety disorders, depressive disorders, bipolar and related disorders, obsessive-compulsive and related disorders, sleep disorders,

sexual dysfunction, delirium, and neurocognitive disorders. The hallmark of substance-induced mental disorders is that the symptoms of the disorder are attributable to the ingestion or chronic use of the substance and were not present prior to substance use. While symptoms may abate as the pharmacologic activity of the substance abates, repeated use may lead to chronic changes in neurophysiology, and as such, behavioral effects may persist even when the substance is no longer used.

The substances specified in the DSM-5 include alcohol, caffeine, cannabis (also synthetic cannabinoids), hallucinogens (including phencyclidine and others), inhalants, opioids, sedatives/hypnotics/anxiolytics, stimulants, tobacco, and "other." Defining the symptom complex associated with each individual substance is out of the purview of this text; however, the possibility of substance use/abuse as a cause for behavioral and mood disruption is critical for all physicians to recognize. The patient interview should include time to speak with the patient individually, without a parent or other caregiver present, so as to establish rapport, to incorporate the techniques of normalizing and remaining nonjudgmental, and to encourage a patient to discuss their substance use.

Adjustment Disorder

Adjustment disorder is an excessive or maladaptive response to a stressor, and diagnosis is contingent upon the recognition of a particular stressor. Typical stressors for children and adolescents include separations, painful injuries, illness, hospitalization or surgery, parental divorce, change of residency, academic failure, and conflict with peers. The DSM-5 criteria for adjustment disorder are as follows:

1. The symptoms develop within 3 months of the stressor.
2. Significant social and/or academic impairment results.
3. The symptoms do not meet criteria for mood or anxiety disorder.
4. The symptoms do not represent bereavement.
5. The symptoms abate 6 months after termination of the stressor.

This disorder is further classified by the patient's symptoms, such as **depressed mood**, **anxiety**, and/or **conduct disorder**. Affected patients may be at increased risk for suicide, particularly if social and/or academic impairment are severe. If the stressor is an illness or its treatment, the morbidity of the medical condition may increase as a consequence of noncompliance. The differential diagnosis of adjustment disorder is a mood or anxiety disorder, a disruptive behavior disorder, or post-traumatic stress disorder (PTSD).

Conditions Characterized by Extremes of Mood Lability

The **bipolar disorders** include bipolar I disorder, bipolar II disorder, and cyclothymic disorder. All are characterized by the presence of either mania or hypomania. **Mania** manifests acutely, leads to significant functional impairments, and is characterized by racing thoughts, distractibility, delusions of grandeur, and other disturbances in thinking. Problematic behaviors during a manic episode include recklessness (e.g., excessive participation in social activities, high-risk sexual activity, spending sprees, extreme gambling), agitation, decreased sleep, and excessive talkativeness. A **manic episode** is defined as an abnormally elevated, euphoric, expansive, or irritable mood for at least 1 week unless treated. This mood disturbance is associated with at least three of the following symptoms or four if the mood is irritable:

1. Grandiosity
2. Decreased need for sleep
3. Talkativeness
4. Racing thoughts
5. Distractibility
6. Excessive goal-directed activity or psychomotor agitation
7. Reckless pursuit of pleasure

TABLE 31.7 Columbia Suicide Severity Rating Scale–Screener

1. Have you wished you were dead or wished you could go to sleep and not wake up?
2. Have you actually had any thoughts about killing yourself?
   If Yes to 2, answer questions 3, 4, 5, and 6. If No to 2, go directly to question 6.
3. Have you thought about how you might do this?
4. Have you had any intention of acting on these thoughts of killing yourself, as opposed to you having the thoughts but you definitely would not act on them?
5. Have you started to work out or worked out the details of how to kill yourself? Do you intend to carry out this plan?
6. Have you done anything, started to do anything, or prepared to do anything to end your life?

   Response Protocol to Screening, based on last item answered YES.
   Item 1 – Mental Health Referral at discharge
   Item 2 – Mental Health Referral at discharge
   Item 3 – Care Team Consultation (Psychiatric Nurse) and Patient Safety Monitor/Procedures
   Item 4 – Psychiatric Consultation and Patient Safety Monitor/Procedures
   Item 5 – Psychiatric Consultation and Patient Safety Monitor/Procedures
   Item 6 – If over a year ago, Mental Health Referral at discharge
   If between 1 wk and 1 yr ago, Care Team Consultation (Psychiatric Nurse) and Patient Safety Monitor
   If 1 wk ago or less, Psychiatric Consultation and Patient Safety Monitor

From Posner K. *Columbia-Suicide Severity Rating Scale: Screener/Recent–Self-Report.* http://www.cssrs.columbia.edu/scales_practice_cssrs.html.

The symptoms of a **hypomanic episode** are the same, though are present for a shorter duration (i.e., 4 days or fewer), are not associated with psychotic symptoms of delusions or hallucinations, and are not severe enough to cause major social or academic dysfunction. Up to 10% of patients with hypomania will eventually develop mania.

Bipolar I disorder is characterized by the presence of manic episodes. Patients may also have prior or subsequent episodes of hypomania or major depression, though these are not required. **Bipolar II disorder** is characterized by the presence of at least one major depressive episode and hypomania. **Cyclothymic disorder** is a chronic, cyclic illness of hypomania and depressive symptoms without episodes of major depression.

Comorbid psychiatric conditions include eating disorders, ADHD, conduct disorders, panic disorders, social phobias, adjustment disorders, substance use disorders, and substance-induced disorders. The lifetime prevalence of bipolar I disorder is as high as 1.6%, and that of bipolar II disorder is 0.5%. Approximately 15% of adolescents with recurrent major depression eventually develop bipolar illnesses.

The differential diagnosis of the bipolar disorders includes schizophrenia and medical conditions that cause changes in mental status, particularly thyroid disorders, Cushing disease, and multiple sclerosis (see Table 31.4). Substance-induced mood disorders must also be considered, particularly those associated with cocaine, tricyclic antidepressants, and selective serotonin reuptake inhibitors. The clinician should obtain a detailed family history as bipolar disorder frequently runs in families. Because the condition is often undiagnosed in parents, the questions should be directed toward the presence of the symptoms for bipolar disorders. The following principles should guide the evaluation of patients with symptoms of depression or mania:

1. Recognize the symptoms of mania and hypomania.
2. Remember that depressed patients often have bipolar disorders.
3. Obtain a thorough family history to look for symptoms of mood disorders.
4. Consider bipolar illnesses in patients with any disruptive disorder that does not respond to treatment.
5. Assess for drug and/or alcohol use as substances may induce bipolar disorder, and substance use is frequently a comorbid condition.

Borderline personality disorder is a chronic personality disorder characterized by intense mood lability, impulsivity, identity disturbances, and unstable relationships. The diagnosis may be challenging in adolescents whose appropriate psychologic development includes the forging of identity and personality traits; however, since borderline personality disorder is associated with significant morbidity and potential mortality, it should be considered in the differential diagnosis of a patient presenting with significant mood or behavioral issues. Diagnosis requires five or more of the following:

1. Significant efforts to avoid real or imagined abandonment
2. Unstable and intense relationships with extremes of idolization and devaluation
3. Marked identity disturbances with unstable sense of self
4. Significant impulsivity in at least two areas that are potentially self-damaging: spending, sexual activity, substance abuse, reckless driving, or binge eating
5. Recurrent suicidal or self-mutilating behavior
6. Intense dysphoria, irritability, or anxiety
7. Chronic feelings of emptiness
8. Inappropriate anger
9. Transient, stress-related paranoia or dissociation

Both genetic and psychosocial factors are believed to be causative. Risk factors for borderline personality disorder include a history of abuse, neglect, or early parental loss. The median population prevalence is approximately 6% in primary care settings and is as high as 10% in outpatient mental health clinics. Females are more frequently diagnosed than males, at a ratio of 3:1.

Addressing Suicidal Thoughts and Attempts

Suicide is the second leading cause of death in adolescents, and assessing the risk of suicide is a critical component in the evaluation of any child or teen. Although depression is an important risk factor for suicide, only half of adolescents who attempt suicide have clinically diagnosable depression. In those without depression, strong predictors of suicide are impulsivity and low frustration tolerance. The approach to evaluating suicidality is complicated and includes a stepwise process of probing first for latent thoughts of suicidality (Table 31.7), then for active suicidal intent. Key to this process is assessing whether the child is considering acting on thoughts of death or suicide. To assess risk, the interviewer should focus on the **risk factors for completed suicide**, which include the following:

1. Male gender
2. Adolescence

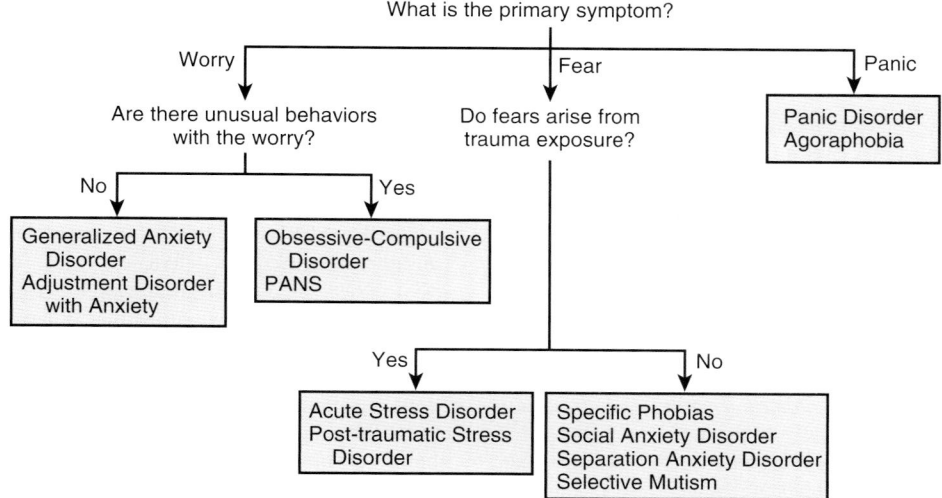

Fig. 31.2 Evaluation of worry, fear, and panic. PANS, pediatric acute onset neuropsychiatric disorder.

3. Formation of a conscious plan
4. Presence of available means (e.g., medications, firearms)
5. Depression
6. Hopelessness
7. Impulsivity
8. Low frustration tolerance
9. Use of intoxicants
10. Sexual identity conflicts
11. Recent death of family member or friend, or significant breakup
12. Previous suicide attempts

Once a patient's thoughts of suicide have escalated to suicide threats, plans, or attempts, this constitutes a medical emergency and the patient should be immediately referred to an experienced mental health professional or emergency department, and psychiatric hospitalization should strongly be considered.

CONDITIONS CHARACTERIZED BY WORRY, FEAR, AND PANIC

These conditions include diagnoses in the broad categories of anxiety disorders, trauma- and stressor-related disorders, and obsessive-compulsive disorder. In childhood, these diagnoses are often comorbid and may include portions of other related disorders. A child with PTSD may experience panic attacks or a child with social anxiety may also have some generalized worries.

Conditions Characterized by Worry

Worries are primarily internal ruminations about the potential to experience negative outcomes from typically benign, everyday events. While often accompanied by somatic symptoms, such as stomach upset and headache, the hallmark of these disorders is the persistence of worry across one or more areas of a child's life. Conditions characterized by worry are categorized by whether they are associated with unusual behaviors (Fig. 31.2).

Worry Without Unusual Behaviors

Generalized anxiety disorder is characterized by excessive worry and concern over many issues. Chronic generalized anxiety may lead to symptoms of depression or somatic complaints, including abdominal pain, nausea, appetite loss, and headaches. DSM-5 criteria are as follows:

1. Excessive anxiety and worry about various issues for more than 6 months
2. Difficulty controlling the worry
3. Anxiety and worry are associated with three of the following:
   a. Restlessness
   b. Being easily fatigued
   c. Difficulty concentrating
   d. Irritability
   e. Muscle tension
   f. Sleep disturbance
4. Anxiety, worry, or physical symptoms cause significant distress or impairment

The lifetime prevalence of generalized anxiety disorder is approximately 5%, with most cases initially presenting during childhood or adolescence. The disorder is chronic and worsens during periods of stress. Comorbid diagnoses include mood disorders, other anxiety disorders, and substance use disorders.

Adjustment disorder with anxiety. The hallmark of adjustment disorders is an excessive or maladaptive response to a stressor that is out of proportion to that stressor. In **adjustment disorder with anxiety**, the maladaptive response manifests as excessive worry. It can occur in both children and adolescents. Stressors that children and adolescents may encounter include social separations, parental divorce, illness, injury, moving, academic failure, and peer conflict. The stressor should not represent a perceived threat to the life of oneself or a loved one, which would suggest PTSD. DSM-5 diagnostic criteria are as follows:

1. Symptoms develop within 3 months of the stressor
2. Significant impairment results
3. The symptoms do not meet criteria for an alternative anxiety disorder
4. The symptoms do not represent bereavement
5. The symptoms abate 6 months after termination of the stress

Worry with Unusual Behaviors

Obsessive-compulsive disorder (OCD) is characterized by obsessive worries that are briefly relieved by compensatory compulsive behaviors. **Obsessions** are recurrent and persistent thoughts, urges, or images that the individual attempts to ignore or suppress. Common obsessions include fear of contamination or illness, guilt regarding sexual thoughts, images of violent or horrific scenes, and urges to injure oneself or others. **Compulsions** are repetitive and excessive acts the patient performs to reduce the anxiety elicited by obsessions. Compulsions may include actions, such as repetitive handwashing or checking locks, or mental acts, such as repeating certain words or counting internally. Some patients need to perform a particular action a specific number of times to satisfy the compulsion. To meet criteria for OCD, the compulsive actions must take over an hour a day or interfere with the patient's day-to-day life.

Lifetime prevalence of OCD is approximately 2.5%. While females are more frequently affected in general, males have a higher prevalence during childhood. Children generally present with vague anxiety symptoms or poor concentration before clear obsessions and compulsions are seen. In children, OCD is highly comorbid with tic disorders and ADHD. Other comorbidities include depression, anxiety disorders, and eating disorders.

Pediatric Acute Onset Neuropsychiatric Disorder. *Pediatric acute onset neuropsychiatric disorder (PANS)* is the term proposed for a group of neuropsychiatric disorders (particularly OCD, tic disorder, and Tourette disorder) with an *acute onset*, triggered by an immune or infectious process. The most common subtypes are pediatric autoimmune neuropsychiatric disorders associated with *Streptococcus pyogenes*, for which a possible relationship with group A streptococcal (GAS) infections has been hypothesized. It has been proposed that this subset of patients with obsessive-compulsive and tic disorders may produce autoimmune antibodies in response to a GAS infection that cross-react with brain tissue similar to the autoimmune response believed to be responsible for the manifestations of Sydenham chorea. Until carefully designed and well-controlled studies have established a causal relationship between neurobehavioral abnormalities and GAS infections, routine diagnostic laboratory testing for GAS and antistreptococcal antibodies, long-term antistreptococcal prophylaxis, or immunoregulatory therapy (e.g., intravenous immunoglobulin, plasma exchange) to treat exacerbations of this disorder is not routinely recommended. The newer, broader diagnosis of PANS follows the suggestion that a broad spectrum of infectious agents may have the ability to trigger exacerbations in children with these neurobehavioral disorders.

Conditions Characterized by Fear

Fear is an intense emotion centered on a belief that something is dangerous, emotionally harmful, or painful. Fears may be spontaneous or may arise from previous traumatic experiences. While all people experience fear as an emotion, in these disorders it causes significant functional impairment.

Fears Arising Spontaneously

Specific phobias. The hallmark of a specific phobia is intense fear upon exposure to a particular stimulus or situation or, occasionally, upon thinking about or visualizing the stimulus. The fear is out of proportion to the actual danger. The fear response in children typically manifests as clinging, crying, having a tantrum, or "freezing." Common specific phobias include animals, heights, enclosed places, exposure to blood, or venipuncture. Specific phobias peak in childhood and early adulthood. Diagnostic criteria of a specific phobia are as follows:
1. Intense fear is caused by a particular stimulus.
2. The object or situation almost always provokes immediate fear or anxiety.
3. Stimuli are avoided or endured with great distress.
4. The fear is out of proportion to the actual danger.
5. The fear persists 6 months or longer.

Social anxiety disorder (social phobia). Social anxiety disorder is a specific phobia in which the stimulus is either a social or performance task. Diagnostic criteria include the following:

1. Marked fear about one or more social situations
2. Individual fears that they will act in a way that will be negatively evaluated
3. Social situations almost always provoke fear or anxiety
4. Social situations are avoided
5. Fear is out of proportion to the actual threat posed by the social situation
6. Fear or anxiety persists 6 months or longer

Social phobia most often begins in adolescence and is one and a half times more frequent in females compared to males. Children with social anxiety often refuse group play, stay close to familiar adults, and appear excessively timid in unfamiliar situations. Children may report somatic complaints, such as headaches or stomachaches, which abate when the child is allowed to remain home and away from social situations, including school. School avoidance due to severe social anxiety can be a significant problem for children and adolescents. Social phobia may be comorbid with panic disorder, other anxiety disorders, mood disorders, and substance abuse.

Separation anxiety disorder. The core fear in separation anxiety disorder is separation from a specific attachment figure or figures. Fear of separation is normal in infants and children aged 6–30 months but should be considered abnormal if increasing or not declining beyond this age range. Diagnosis requires the presence of symptoms for greater than 4 weeks. At least three of the following symptoms must be present:
1. Distress with separation
2. Worry about losing loved ones
3. Worry about an event causing separation
4. Refusal to go away from home
5. Reluctance to be alone
6. Refusal to fall asleep alone
7. Repeated nightmares of separation
8. Somatic complaints when separation occurs or is anticipated

The prevalence of separation anxiety disorder is as high as 5%, with onset typically in early childhood. Patients with separation anxiety disorder often display their worries as demands or behavioral outbursts, which may cause significant family conflict. Comorbid conditions include major depressive disorder and panic disorder with agoraphobia.

Selective mutism. Patients with selective mutism have a persistent failure to speak in specific, but not all, situations. Children with selective mutism are often shy in public but controlling at home in order to maintain proximity to parents. Diagnostic criteria include the following:
1. Consistent failure to speak in specific social situations
2. Failure to speak interferes with achievement or social communication
3. Duration of at least 1 month
4. Failure to speak is not due to lack of knowledge of the spoken language
5. Disturbance is not better explained by a communication or other psychiatric disorder

The differential diagnosis includes communication disorders, autism spectrum disorders, and social anxiety disorder. Selective mutism may be a more severe form of social anxiety disorder.

Fears Arising from Traumatic Events

A **traumatic event** is defined as an exposure to actual or threatened death, serious injury, or sexual violence. Responses to traumatic events include hyperarousal, avoidance of circumstances reminiscent of the event, or re-experiencing the event via nightmares, intrusive thoughts of the event, or flashbacks. **Acute stress disorder** and **PTSD** are characterized by severe and persistent trauma responses that lead to impaired function. Symptoms are divided into four clusters: intrusion, avoidance, negative alteration in cognition and mood, and marked alterations in arousal and activity. **Acute stress disorder** is the persistence of at least 9 of the 14 defined symptoms, regardless of symptom cluster designation, for 3 days to 1 month after exposure to a traumatic event. In contrast to acute stress disorder, **PTSD** must include symptoms from each of the separate symptom clusters. Exposure to the traumatic event includes directly experiencing the event, witnessing the event, learning the event occurred to a family member or close friend (caregiver for children under 6), or experiencing repeated or extreme exposure to details of a traumatic event.

1. Intrusion symptoms
   a. Distressing memories of the event
   b. Dreams in which content or effect of the dream is related to the event (in children, does not need to be related to event)
   c. Dissociative reactions in which the individual feels the event is recurring (flashbacks) (in children, may be re-enactment in play)
   d. Psychologic distress at exposure to reminders of the event
   e. Marked physiologic reactions to reminders of the event
2. Avoidance
   a. Avoidance or efforts to avoid distressing memories (children may avoid places or physical reminders)
   b. Avoidance of external reminders (children may avoid people, conversations, or interpersonal relationships)
3. Negative alterations in cognition and mood
   a. Inability to remember an important aspect of the traumatic event (not a criterion for a child under 6 years of age)
   b. Persistent and exaggerated negative beliefs (not a criterion for a child under 6 years of age)
   c. Persistent, distorted thoughts about cause or consequences of trauma (not a criterion for a child under 6 years of age)
   d. Persistent negative emotional state (fear, guilt, sadness, shame)
   e. Decreased interest in activities (constriction of play in children)
   f. Feelings of detachment (socially withdrawn behavior in children)
   g. Persistent inability to experience positive emotions (express positive emotions in children)
4. Alterations in arousal
   a. Irritable behavior and angry outbursts (with little provocation)
   b. Reckless or self-destructive behaviors (not a criterion in a child under 6 years of age)
   c. Hypervigilance
   d. Exaggerated startle response
   e. Problems with concentration
   f. Sleep disturbance

While as many as 30% of children will have some symptoms of acute stress disorder following a trauma, only 10% will meet diagnostic criteria. The significance of acute stress disorder in predicting eventual development of PTSD remains unclear.

Comorbid diagnoses include panic disorder, social phobia, substance abuse, OCD, somatic symptom disorder, and major depressive disorder. In addition to PTSD, childhood trauma and other significant stressors, together known as **adverse childhood experiences,** have been found to predispose children to future chronic medical and mental health conditions. These medical conditions include ischemic heart disease, cancer, chronic lung disease, skeletal fracture, and liver disease.

Conditions Characterized by Panic

Panic Disorder

Panic attacks may be a component of many psychiatric disorders. While panic disorder is characterized by recurrent and unexpected panic attacks, the hallmark of panic disorder is persistent concern over having additional attacks, worry about the consequences of an attack, or a significant change in behavior related to the attacks. **Panic attacks** occur suddenly, peak within 10 minutes, often resolve without intervention, and consist of at least four of the following symptoms:

1. Palpitations or tachycardia
2. Diaphoresis
3. Trembling or shaking
4. Shortness of breath or sensation of smothering
5. Feelings of choking
6. Chest pain
7. Nausea or abdominal discomfort
8. Dizziness or feeling faint
9. Chills or heat sensation
10. Paresthesias
11. Derealization (feelings of unreality) or depersonalization
12. Fear of losing control or "going crazy"
13. Fear of dying

The 1-year prevalence rate of panic disorder is as high as 3.5%. The age of onset is bimodal, with the largest peak occurring in adolescence and a smaller one in the mid-30s. Panic disorder in prepubertal children is rare.

Patients with panic disorder have a high degree of comorbid conditions. Over half of patients may have major depressive disorder. There is a high frequency of other anxiety disorders, such as social phobia, OCD, and generalized anxiety disorder. Patients with panic disorder are also at great risk for substance abuse, as a consequence of self-medicating. Panic attacks may be inappropriately diagnosed as cardiac, pulmonary, or neurologic emergencies.

Agoraphobia

Agoraphobia is characterized by intense anxiety over developing a panic attack or other incapacitating or embarrassing symptoms in a place from which the person cannot escape or in which help may not be available. Diagnosis requires that the anxiety manifest in at least two of the following situations:

1. Riding public transportation
2. Being in open spaces
3. Being in enclosed spaces
4. Standing in line or in a crowd
5. Being outside of the home alone

The anxiety is present nearly every time an individual is exposed to the situation they fear and may also develop when the child knows that they may be placed in one of these situations. While agoraphobia does present in childhood, the peak of onset is late adolescence and early adulthood. It is seen in about 1.7% of adolescents. Females are affected twice as frequently as males. Agoraphobia is typically preceded by panic disorder, phobias, and separation anxiety disorder. Other comorbidities, such as depression and substance use disorder, often follow the presentation of agoraphobia.

CONDITIONS CHARACTERIZED BY MENTAL STATUS ABNORMALITIES

The evaluation of mental status changes (Fig. 31.3) involves first determining whether the abnormality is limited—such as hallucinations unaccompanied by changes in cognition or consciousness—or pervasive (see also Chapter 41). The abnormality should then be classified by whether it is episodic or persistent. Finally, the mental status change should be classified as either acute or chronic. An example of a limited, episodic, acute change in mental status is the development of hallucinations secondary to acute anxiety. In contrast, autism represents a pervasive, persistent, and chronic alteration in mental status.

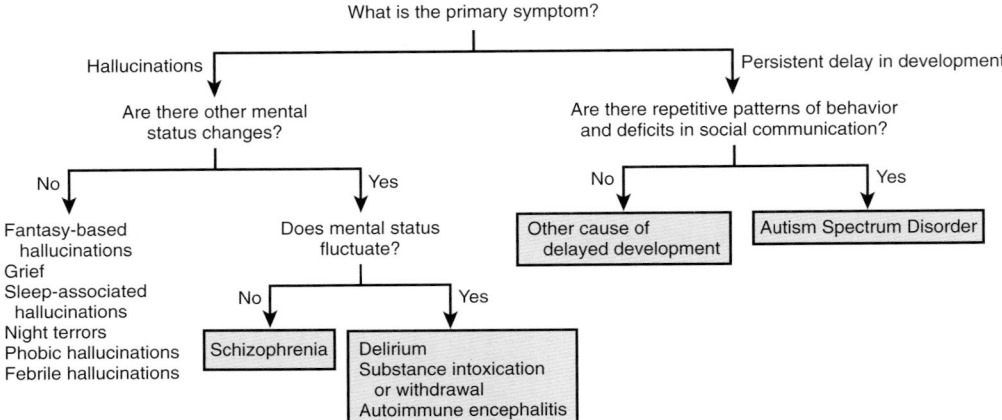

Fig. 31.3 Evaluation of abnormal mental status findings.

Psychosis is an important consideration in any patient with mental status abnormalities. Psychosis has key features including **delusions** (fixed irrational implausible beliefs that may be persecutory, referential, grandiose, erotomanic, nihilistic), **hallucinations, disorganized thinking/speech** (loose associations, tangential, incoherent), **abnormal motor behavior/catatonia,** and **negative symptoms** (diminished emotions, avolition, alogia, anhedonia, asociality). Psychosis, often associated with schizophrenia, has a much broader differential diagnosis (see Table 31.4), which must include drug use and the multiple causes of autoimmune encephalitis (Table 31.8). Clues or red flags for secondary causes of psychosis are noted in Table 31.9.

Catatonia is also often associated with schizophrenia and may be noted more often in patients with secondary causes of psychosis (see Table 31.9). Disorders associated with catatonia include autoimmune encephalitis (particularly N-methyl-D-aspartate receptor related), systemic lupus erythematosus, viral encephalitis, autoimmune thyroid disorders, autism, and demyelinating diseases. Catatonia is characterized by the features in Table 31.10. The diagnosis is suggested by the presence of two or more of these symptoms lasting ≥1 hour. Catatonia may coexist with delirium.

Conditions Characterized by Hallucinations

Hallucinations—the apparent perception of something that does not exist in reality—may be an indication of a medical condition, poor visual or auditory function, the ingestion of a substance, or a psychiatric illness (see Fig. 31.3). The vast majority of hallucinations in preadolescent children do not ultimately represent a serious psychiatric or medical illness. Hallucinations occur in as many as 5% of normal children.

The first step in evaluating hallucinations is to assess the patient's mental status. Most children with hallucinations have an otherwise normal mental status. If the primary alteration in mental status is confusion, medical **delirium** should be considered (see Chapter 41). The presence of **delusions**—beliefs that are maintained despite being objectively contraindicated by reality—should prompt consideration of psychosis, schizophrenia, or mood disorders. Most hallucinations associated with delirium are visual, whereas those observed in psychoses are typically auditory. Auditory hallucinations may be perceived as chatter or as a voice that chastises the child. Culture can often shape the content of hallucinations and whether the sensory experiences are considered worrisome or abnormal by the patient and family. Children with an otherwise normal mental status may hallucinate in the context of fantasy, grief, sleep, acute phobia, and fever.

Fantasy-Based Hallucinations

To define a subjective perceptual experience as hallucinatory, the person experiencing the phenomenon has to be able to distinguish imagination from reality. As they develop, children gradually learn that imagination and reality are two separate entities. Children under 3 years of age confuse reality with imagination. By 4 years of age, children understand the concept of "pretend," and by 7 years of age, they understand imagination but act as though the fantasy is still real. They may still describe having an imaginary friend. By 8 years of age, most children are reliably able to distinguish inner thoughts from voices. Some children are involved in more fantasy than are their peers and may engage in fantasy for entertainment or comfort. On occasion, they may get carried away by their fantasies and become quite fearful. Most of these children proceed to healthy psychologic adjustment. Children who have intellectual disability or other developmental delays may, appropriately, have imaginary friends or voices into adolescence.

Grief-Induced Hallucinations

The grieving process following the death of a loved one may include visual hallucinations of the deceased. These hallucinations can also be auditory, in which the child hears the voice of the deceased speaking to the child. The child's and the family's reaction to these hallucinations is dependent on their cultural and religious beliefs. Some families may perceive these events as a supernatural or a religious experience. Although these experiences may be frightening to some young children, many find reassurance or comfort.

Hallucinations Associated with Sleep

Dreamlike hallucinations can occur during various stages of sleep. Some may be considered bizarre by the patient and may include partial preservation of consciousness. **Hypnagogic hallucinations** occur during sleep onset and **hypnopompic hallucinations** occur during awakening. The overall prevalence of hypnagogic hallucinations is as high as 37%; that of hypnopompic hallucinations is as high as 12.5%. Patients with insomnia or excessive daytime sleepiness may be more likely to experience sleep-related hallucinations. As many as 30% of patients with **narcolepsy** experience both hypnagogic and hypnopompic hallucinations. These hallucinations can also occur as part of PTSD, in which case they often take the form of a flashback or re-experiencing of the traumatic event. **Night terrors** may resemble hallucinations, though are a distinct entity of non–rapid eye movement sleep arousal. The DSM-5 defines **sleep terror disorder** as recurrent episodes of night terrors. During episodes, the child appears to arouse from sleep and cries or screams inconsolably, may speak unintelligibly, and exhibits

TABLE 31.8 Antigenic Targets in Autoimmune Encephalitis with Associated Psychiatric Features

Commonly Targeted Antigens	Antigen Description or Epitope	Main Encephalopathy Syndrome and Psychiatric Features	Other Associated Neurologic Disorders	Main Psychiatric Features
NMDAR	Ligand-gated ion channel	Encephalopathy (frequently extralimbic manifestation)	Post–herpes simplex encephalitis relapse with chorea; pediatric dyskinetic encephalitis lethargica; idiopathic epilepsy; immunotherapy-responsive dementia	Anxiety, agitation, bizarre behavior, catatonia, delusional or paranoid thoughts, and visual or auditory hallucinations; also movement disorder, seizures, autonomic instability
LGI1	VGKC-associated and AMPAR-associated secreted molecule	Limbic encephalitis with or without faciobrachial dystonic seizures; prominent hyponatremia	Morvan syndrome, neuromyotonia, epilepsy, REM sleep behavior disorder; rarely isolated movement disorder (parkinsonism, dystonia, chorea)	Confusion, hallucinations, depression
CASPR2	VGKC-associated adhesion molecule	Morvan syndrome: peripheral nerve hyperexcitability, autonomic instability, encephalopathy	Limbic encephalitis, neuromyotonia, epilepsy; rarely isolated movement disorder (chorea, myoclonus)	Confusion, hallucinations, agitation, delusions
AMPAR	Ligand-gated ion channel	Limbic encephalitis	NA	Personality change, psychosis, apathy, agitation, confabulation
GABA$_A$R	Ligand-gated ion channel	Limbic encephalitis with refractory seizures	Varied presentations	Confusion, anxiety, affective changes (including depression), hallucinations, catatonia
GABA$_B$R	Ligand-gated ion channel	Limbic encephalitis with refractory status epilepticus	Opsoclonus-myoclonus; cerebellar ataxia; PERM	Psychosis, agitation, catatonia
Hu	Intracellular RNA-binding protein	Limbic encephalitis or limbic encephalomyelitis occurring with small cell lung cancer	Painful sensory neuropathy; cerebellar ataxia	Confusion, depression, less commonly hallucinations
Ma2	Intracellular protein involved in mRNA processing or biogenesis	Limbic encephalitis occurring with testicular germ cell tumors; REM sleep disorder is common; frequent short-term memory problems	Visual dysfunction, gait disturbance, hypokinesia	Confusion and anxiety, including obsessions and compulsions
D2R	Metabotropic receptor	So-called basal ganglia encephalitis with prominent movement disorder (i.e., dystonia, parkinsonism, chorea, tics)	Sydenham chorea, PANDAS	Agitation, depression, psychosis, emotional lability
DPPX	Auxiliary subunit of Kv4.2 potassium channels	Limbic encephalitis with enteropathy	PERM	Amnesia, delirium, psychosis, depression
MGluR5	Metabotropic glutamate receptor	So-called Ophelia syndrome: limbic encephalitis in association with Hodgkin lymphoma	Paraneoplastic limbic encephalitis without lymphoma, or nonparaneoplastic limbic encephalitis; immunotherapy-responsive prosopagnosia	Depression, anxiety, delusions, visual and auditory hallucinations, personality change, anterograde amnesia
GFAP	Intracellular (cytosolic) glial intermediate filament protein	Corticosteroid-responsive meningoencephalitis or encephalitis, with or without myelitis; presents with subacute onset of memory loss and confusion	NA	Occurred in 29% in one study but not described in detail; psychosis and behavioral changes reported

AK5, adenylate kinase 5; AMPAR, α-amino-3-hydroxy-5-methyl-4-isoxazolepropionic acid receptor; CASPR2, contactin-associated protein-like 2; D2R, dopamine receptor D2; DPPX, dipeptidyl-peptidase-like protein-6; GABA$_A$R, γ-aminobutyric acid type A receptor; GABA$_B$R, γ-aminobutyric acid type B receptor; GFAP, glial fibrillary acidic protein; LGI1, leucine-rich glioma-inactivated 1; MGluR5, metabotropic glutamate receptor 5; NA, not applicable; NMDAR, N-methyl-D-aspartate receptor; PANDAS, pediatric autoimmune neuropsychiatric disorders associated with streptococcal infections; PERM, progressive encephalomyelitis with rigidity and myoclonus; REM, rapid eye movement; VGKC, voltage-gated potassium channel.

Modified from Pollak TA, Lennox BR, Muller S, et al. Autoimmune psychosis: an international consensus on an approach to the diagnosis and management of psychosis of suspected autoimmune origin. *Lancet Psychiatry*. 2020;7(1):93–108.

TABLE 31.9 Red Flags and Features Suggesting Secondary Etiologies of Psychosis

Atypical Features
- Normal prior to event
- Very early (≤13 yr) age of onset
- Acute or subacute onset (days, ≤1 mo)
- Catatonia
- Dyskinesias
- Isolated misidentification delusion (Capgras syndrome)
- Depressed level of consciousness
- Cognitive and recent memory decline
- Poor orientation
- Intractability despite adequate therapy
- Rapidly progressive and/or fluctuating (polymorphic) symptoms
- Multimodel hallucinations: visual, auditory, olfactory, gustatory

History
- Infectious prodrome
- New or worsening headache
- Paresthesias
- Past, current substance misuse
- Recent onset incontinence
- Anorexia/weight loss
- Risk factors for cerebrovascular disease or central nervous system infections
- Malignancy
- Immunocompromised status
- Head trauma
- Seizures
- Hepatobiliary disorders
- Systemic lupus erythematosus/other autoimmune diseases
- Biological relatives with similar medical complaints

Physical Examination
- Autonomic hyperactivity: tachycardia, hypertension, mydriasis, sleep disturbance
- Incoordination, or gait difficulty
- Toxidrome
- Abnormal neurologic exam: upper and lower motor neuron focal findings
- Movement disorder

Diagnostic Abnormalities
- Abnormal electroencephalogram (extreme delta brush, diffuse slowing)
- Abnormal cerebrospinal fluid (pleocytosis: greater than five lymphocytes)
- Positive urine toxicology
- Screening laboratory tests including N-methyl-D-aspartate receptor and other antibodies
- Abnormal neuroimaging studies (unilateral or bilateral hippocampal/medial temporal lobe hyperdensities: limbic encephalitis)
- Hyponatremia

intense fear and autonomic arousal (e.g., tachycardia, sweating). On awakening, the child has no memory of the event. Episodes of night terrors last from 1 to 10 minutes. Night terrors occur during stage 4 sleep and not during rapid eye movement sleep and tend to occur in the first half of the night. Over 30% of 18-month-old toddlers will experience a night terror, with the prevalence decreasing to 2.2% by adulthood. **Seizures**, especially of the temporal and frontal lobes, can produce fear and complex behavior patterns resembling night terrors, and should be considered in the differential diagnosis of night terrors.

Phobic Hallucinations

Acute phobic hallucinations occur in preschool-aged children and consist of episodes of hallucinations coupled with terror. These hallucinations last from 10 to 60 minutes and may occur any time of the day but mostly at night. During episodes, the child may become very frightened, state that bugs are crawling over them and attempt to remove them, cry, or hide. Because of the acute change in mental status, this condition must be differentiated from the medical and psychotic causes of hallucinations, such as delirium. The cause of acute phobic hallucinations is unknown. Phobic hallucinations are most frequently seen in children with a personal or family history of anxiety. Symptoms usually last 1–3 days and diminish over 1–2 weeks.

Febrile Hallucinations

Preschool-aged children may hallucinate during high fevers. The hallucinations are temporary and are not associated with future psychiatric disorders. The phenomenon may represent a mild form of delirium and typically requires only reassurance for management, as well as evaluation for the source of fever. Persistent hallucinations, impaired consciousness, and changes in cognition, such as not recognizing parents or difficulty completing previously accomplished tasks, suggest frank delirium and require further evaluation.

Schizophrenia

Schizophrenia is a disorder of chronic, persistent psychosis (loss of reality testing) that often presents in adolescence or young adulthood. Symptoms are divided into four domains: positive symptoms, negative symptoms, cognitive symptoms, and mood symptoms. **Positive symptoms** consist of psychotic symptoms (such as hallucinations), delusions (fixed false beliefs), and disorganized speech and behavior (loose associations). **Negative symptoms** consist of social withdrawal, flattening of affect, alogia (i.e., speaking in brief sentences), abulia, apathy, and avolition (i.e., lack of desire to do anything) (see Table 31.5). The flat affect may consist of a reduction in body language, lack of eye contact, and emotional unresponsiveness (see Table 31.5). **Cognitive symptoms** are characterized by deficits in executive function and an inability to appreciate and react appropriately to social cues. **Mood symptoms** often consist of depression though may also consist of context-inappropriate cheerfulness or sadness. The symptoms may fluctuate over time, and as such, schizophrenia is divided into two phases: prodromal and active. Diagnostic criteria for schizophrenia specify two or more of the following **characteristic symptoms:**

1. Delusions
2. Hallucinations
3. Disorganized speech
4. Grossly disorganized or catatonic behavior
5. Negative symptoms, such as flat affect

At least one symptom must be delusions, hallucinations, or disorganized speech and the symptoms must appear in the context of significant social and educational dysfunction. There must also be continuous indications of the disturbance for at least 6 months, with at least 1 month of active-phase symptoms. Medical causes and mood disorders need to be excluded (see Table 31.4). *Orientation and memory are usually intact in schizophrenia.*

During the **prodromal phase**, the patient exhibits progressive **negative symptoms**; these include social withdrawal, flattened affect, or eccentric behaviors. During this period, the patient may also have unusual beliefs that are not of the magnitude of true delusions or hallucinations. The patient may have magical thinking or may perceive that someone is talking to them, but no words are hallucinated.

During the **active phase** of schizophrenia, the patient has at least two characteristic symptoms for more than 1 month, unless the

TABLE 31.10 Catatonia

Excitement: Extreme hyperactivity; constant motor unrest, which is apparently nonpurposeful

Immobility/stupor: Extreme hypoactivity, immobility; minimally responsive to stimuli

Mutism: Verbally unresponsive or minimally responsive

Staring: Fixed gaze, little or no visual scanning of environment, decreased blinking

Posturing/catalepsy: Maintains posture(s), including mundane (e.g., sitting or standing for hours without reacting)

Grimacing: Maintenance of odd facial expressions

Echopraxia/echolalia: Mimics of examiner's movements/speech

Stereotypy: Repetitive, non-goal-directed motor activity (e.g., finger-play; repeatedly touching, patting, or rubbing self)

Mannerisms: Odd, purposeful movements (hopping or walking tiptoe, saluting passersby, exaggerated caricatures of mundane movements)

Verbigeration: Repetition of phrases or sentences

Rigidity: Maintenance of a rigid posture despite efforts to be moved

Negativism: Apparently motiveless resistance to instructions or to attempts to move/examine the patient; contrary behavior does the opposite of the instruction

Waxy flexibility: During reposturing of the patient, offers initial resistance before allowing themselves to be repositioned (similar to that of bending a warm candle)

Withdrawal: Refusal to eat, drink, or make eye contact

Impulsivity: Suddenly engaging in inappropriate behavior (e.g., runs down the hallway, starts screaming, or takes off clothes) without provocation; afterward, cannot explain

Automatic obedience: Exaggerated cooperation with examiner's request, or repeated movements that are requested once

Passive obedience (*mitgehen*): Raising arm in response to light pressure of finger, despite instructions to the contrary

Negativism (*gegenhalten*): Resistance to passive movement that is proportional to strength of the stimulus; response seems automatic rather than willful

Ambitendency: Appears stuck in indecisive, hesitant motor movements

Grasp reflex: Striking the patient's open palm with two extended fingers of the examiner's hand results in automatic closure of the patient's hand

Perseveration: Repeatedly returns to the same topic or persists with the same movements

Combativeness: Belligerence or aggression, usually in an undirected manner, without explanation

Autonomic abnormality: Abnormality of body temperature (fever), blood pressure, pulse rate, respiratory rate, inappropriate sweating

From Dhossche DM, Wachtel LE. Catatonia is hidden in plain sight among different pediatric disorders: a review article. *Pediatr Neurol.* 2010;43:307–315.

symptoms have been shortened by treatment. The most common **delusions** in this disorder are persecutory (e.g., the patient is being spied on) and referential (e.g., external events or comments are directed toward the patient). Other less common delusions may be somatic (e.g., internal organs are replaced by others), religious, or grandiose in nature. Hallucinations are most commonly auditory but may emanate from any sensory modality.

The **disorganized speech** may be incomprehensible, and the patient may be unable to organize a logical conversation. The behavior problems consist of inappropriate dress, disheveled appearance, unprovoked aggression, and **catatonia**, decreased responsiveness to the environment (see Table 31.10). If symptoms have not been present for 6 months, the provisional diagnosis of **schizophreniform disorder** is applied. Approximately 65% of patients with schizophreniform disorder have symptoms that last longer than 6 months and are reclassified as having schizophrenia.

Schizophrenia is exceedingly rare and is often a misdiagnosis prior to 13 years of age. If diagnosed prior to this age, it is labeled as **childhood-onset** or **very early-onset schizophrenia**. *Furthermore, onset prior to age 13 requires a careful evaluation to look for atypical features and to exclude medical causes of psychosis, especially drug ingestion and autoimmune encephalitis* (see Tables 31.8 and 31.9). Prevalence is approximately 2.5/100,000 in children under 13 years of age and 0.5% in adolescents. The differential diagnosis of schizophrenia consists of other causes of psychosis (especially autoimmune encephalitis), delirium, dementia, mood disorder, pervasive developmental disorders, and substance ingestion (see Tables 31.4 and 31.9). The prognosis of schizophrenia is guarded, with significant morbidity and mortality. The risk of suicide is high early in the illness. The disorder is chronic and is associated with exacerbations and remissions. Even with optimal therapy, patients with schizophrenia may have significant social deficits, poor initiative, and abnormal thought processes.

Conditions Characterized by Fluctuating Mental Status

Delirium

Delirium is characterized by deficits in cognition and consciousness that develop over a short time (see Chapter 41). Diagnostic criteria include the following:

1. Disturbance in awareness and attention (i.e., reduced ability to direct, focus, sustain, and shift attention)
2. Change in cognition (e.g., memory deficit, disorientation, language disturbance, perceptual disturbance) that is not better accounted for by a pre-existing, established, or evolving dementia
3. Disturbance develops over a short period of time and tends to fluctuate over time
4. There is evidence of a medical, substance-induced, or toxin-induced cause

Children with delirium may misinterpret auditory or visual stimuli or may have actual hallucinations. The hallucinations of delirium are different from those seen in psychosis in that they are more often visual and acute in onset, whereas those resulting from psychoses are usually auditory and are subacute or chronic.

Besides altered sensorium, patients often have decreased sleep or reversal of the sleep/wake cycle and may exhibit psychomotor agitation or retardation. Delirium is indicative of global cerebral dysfunction. Because causes of delirium are potentially life threatening, an expedient and comprehensive medical evaluation is needed.

Substance Intoxication

Intoxication is defined as clinically significant behavioral or psychologic changes following the use of a substance (Table 31.11). The most common signs of intoxication are changes in perception, wakefulness, attention, thinking, judgment, coordination, and interpersonal

TABLE 31.11   Potential Behavioral and Cognitive Manifestations of Substance Abuse

Depression
Panic attacks
Anxiety
Hallucinations
Delusions
Paranoia
Mania
Depersonalization
Disinhibition

Impulsivity
Cognitive deficits:
    Attention
    Calculation
    Executive tasks
    Memory
Fatigue
Sedation

From Perez DL, Murray ED, Price BH. Depression and psychosis in neurological practice. In: Daroff RB, Jankovic J, Mazziotta JC, Pomeroy SL, eds. *Bradley's Neurology in Clinical Practice*. 7th ed. Philadelphia: Elsevier; 2015.

behavior. Physical findings suggest particular classes of medications and cluster into recognizable patterns of signs and symptoms termed **toxidromes** (Table 31.12). If the suspected cause of altered mental status in a patient is substance intoxication, urine and blood toxicology testing should be performed.

Patients who present with substance intoxication should be evaluated for whether the ingestion represented an attempt at self-harm or suicide. Some substance intoxications will require medical hospitalization, if severe. Patients being treated for psychiatric illnesses may be at risk of two particular toxidromes related to their medical therapy, **serotonin syndrome** and **neuroleptic malignant syndrome**.

Serotonin Syndrome

The triad of cognitive-behavioral changes, autonomic instability, and neuromuscular signs and symptoms are characteristic of the central serotonin syndrome. Patients frequently manifest behavior alterations that include confusion, disorientation, agitation, and irritability. Coma, anxiety, seizures, hallucinations, and hypomania are less common.

Central serotonin syndrome results from excessive central nervous system serotonin activity from dietary supplements or the use of substances that modify central nervous system serotonin levels. Most commonly, these agents are selective serotonin reuptake inhibitors or other substances that inhibit serotonin reuptake, including tricyclic antidepressants, meperidine, dextromethorphan, and

TABLE 31.12   Clinically Relevant Toxidromes

Toxidrome	Clinical Findings	Example Agents
Cholinergic	Diarrhea, fecal incontinence, enuresis, miosis, tachycardia followed by bradycardia, lacrimation, sialorrhea, sweating, muscle fasciculations followed by weakness and/or paralysis, altered mental status	Organophosphate and carbamate insecticides *Amanita muscaria* Nicotine
Anticholinergic	Agitated delirium, flushing, decreased sweating, tachycardia, mydriasis, urinary retention, decreased peristalsis, hyperthermia	Atropine Benztropine Scopolamine Diphenhydramine
Sympathomimetic	Mydriasis, hyperthermia, seizures, hyperactivity, hypertension, tachycardia, diaphoresis, delusions, piloerection	Cocaine Methamphetamine MDMA
Sympatholytic	Miosis, hypotension, bradycardia or reflex tachycardia, CNS depression	Clonidine Methyldopa Oxymetazoline
Opioid	Miosis, CNS depression, respiratory depression or apnea, may have hypotension	Heroin Morphine Fentanyl Oxycodone
Serotonin syndrome	Mental status changes, autonomic hyperactivity, neuromuscular abnormalities, akathisia, tremor, clonus, muscle hypertonicity, hyperthermia	Sertraline Fluoxetine Citalopram Linezolid Trazodone Meperidine Tramadol
Neuroleptic malignant syndrome	Fever, "lead pipe" muscular rigidity, altered mental status, autonomic dysfunction (in setting of recent treatment with neuroleptics)	Haloperidol Chlorpromazine Promethazine Prochlorperazine Ziprasidone Quetiapine

CNS, central nervous system; MDMA, methylenedioxymethamphetamine.
From Skolnik AB, Wilcox SR. General toxicology and toxidromes. In: *Critical Care Secrets*. 5th ed. St. Louis: Mosby; 2013:545–551.

TABLE 31.13 Diagnostic Features of Malingering and Factitious Disorders

	Malingering	Factitious Disorder (Previously Known as Munchausen)	Factitious Disorder Imposed on Another
Primary gain	+/− (primary goal with malingering is external reward rather than sick role)	Goal is to receive medical care/interventions	Parent produces symptoms in child to receive medical care/obtain sick role for child
Secondary gain	+ Economic gain or avoidance of responsibilities	−	−
Age of onset	More common in adults	More common in adults; can start in adolescence/childhood	Adults in a caretaker role
Things to look out for	Misuse of resources/fraudulent behaviors	Avoidance of unnecessary procedures/treatments, especially more invasive procedures; monitor for signs of "doctor shopping"	Concerns for child maltreatment and abuse; safety concerns for children and families

A "+" indicates symptoms are seen in the disorder. A "-" indicates symptoms are not seen in the disorder.

3,4-methylenedioxymethamphetamine (MDMA). Other substances, such as amphetamines, cocaine, and levodopa, increase synaptic serotonin release, while others, such as lithium and lysergic acid diethylamide, are serotonin agonists. Monoamine oxidase inhibitors inhibit serotonin degradation.

Autonomic features of serotonin syndrome include hyperthermia, diaphoresis, and tachycardia. Hypertension, mydriasis, and tachypnea are less common. Neuromuscular features include myoclonus, hyperreflexia, tremor, restlessness, hyperactivity, and ataxia. **Neuroleptic malignant syndrome** is included in the differential diagnosis and is distinguished by neurologic exam since neuroleptic malignant syndrome presents with hyporeflexia and lead-pipe muscular rigidity (Chapter 38).

Neuroleptic Malignant Syndrome

The hallmark of neuroleptic malignant syndrome is severe generalized rigidity, fever, and altered mental status consisting of delirium or stupor. Other findings include diaphoresis, significant creatine kinase elevation, autonomic instability, urinary incontinence, tachypnea, and pallor. While rare, as many as 0.02% of individuals treated with antipsychotics are affected and fatality rates are as high as 20% if the condition is not recognized and managed appropriately. Differentiation from serotonin syndrome is based on medication review, and the presence of significant rigidity, which serotonin syndrome lacks.

CONDITIONS CHARACTERIZED BY PHYSICAL FINDINGS OR COMPLAINTS

Parents may present to the primary care provider with unexplained physical complaints on behalf of the child. These complaints may be inconsistent with the results of the medical evaluation and may fail to respond to any medical therapy. These unexplained physical complaints may be the manner in which a patient copes with a stressor. The patient may not be aware of the stressor, nor may the patient realize that these symptoms emanate from their effort to cope with the problem. The clinician should empathize with the patient, validate the presence of the symptoms, then state which potentially serious medical conditions are reasonably felt to be unlikely based on the patient's history, examination, and diagnostic evaluation. The clinician should highlight the notion that stress can produce or worsen symptoms and should recommend that the possibility of stress be evaluated while the clinician continues to monitor the patient for other medical illnesses. Key to the evaluation is determining whether the symptoms are more concerning primarily to the parent or to the child.

Conditions Characterized by Parental Concerns (Table 31.13)

Parental Worry

Parents may worry excessively about their child's health because of a preceding life-threatening event or illness, because of mistrust of the medical profession, or as an expression of their own fear of having a serious condition themselves. These parents do not invent the child's symptoms but instead experience an exaggerated worry about symptoms. The evaluation of a parent's excessive concern over the child's health may be further subdivided into specific concerns versus general medical worries.

Specific medical concerns are often related to prior life-threatening events or illnesses, or previous negative experiences with the health care system. Reassurance after an appropriate and thorough medical evaluation may reduce parental anxiety. When the parent reveals the past incident that led to distrust of the reassurances of doctors, the clinician may be able to reduce the parent's worry through open discussion on the differences between past and current events.

If the parents report that they worry about everything, the clinician should determine whether this is a recent development or a chronic concern. Parents with an acute onset of general medical worries about their children may suffer from a recent stressor or may have anxiety, depression, or OCD. Reassurance alone may be insufficient under these circumstances and the parents' generalized worries may not improve until their own symptoms improve. In such a case, providing parents with resources for their own mental health treatment may be needed.

Factitious Disorder Imposed on Another (Formerly Munchausen Syndrome by Proxy) (see also Chapter 30)

This disorder is a condition in which the patient either feigns or produces symptoms or physical findings in their child to fulfill an underlying need to assume the caregiver role for a sick child. There is no external reward for these symptoms, in contrast to **malingering**, in which the symptoms result in either economic gain or avoidance of responsibilities.

Red flags include unexplained and prolonged illnesses, incongruous symptoms and signs, ineffective medical treatments, and prior episodes of sudden infant death syndrome. The offending caregiver may not seem worried about the child's medical condition. Some caregivers may form an unusually close relationship with the medical staff; however, there are many exceptions, in which the caregiver is instead neglectful, disruptive, and argumentative.

When this entity is suspected, the first step in evaluation is to ensure the child's safety, which may require hospitalization on a medical ward.

TABLE 31.14   **Diagnostic Features of Conditions Characterized by Patient's Physical Complaints**

	Illness Anxiety Disorder	Somatic Symptom Disorder	Conversion Disorder
Presenting complaint	Primary concern is the development of a serious illness—does not require specific symptoms	Primary concern is a specific symptom; generally presents with a more specific physical complaint	Presents with new-onset neurologic or physical symptom; patient may or may not be concerned about this new symptom
Medical correlation to complaint	Generally present with more vague complaints than a specific symptom; not usually explained by medical work-up	Patient can have a medical explanation for their symptom; however, the worry about the seriousness of the symptom is disproportionate or excessive	Physical and neurologic findings do not correlate with patient's presentation
Course of disease	Often associated with other anxiety disorders; can be chronic	Chronic; rarely remits	Generally acute onset; can recur with same or different presenting symptom(s)

With safety assured, the next step is to develop a definitive investigative plan with a multidisciplinary team consisting of mental health professionals, physicians, social services, child abuse specialists, and the legal system. This plan will be most successful when combined with thorough and timely documentation of findings and concerns.

Conditions Characterized by the Patient's Physical Complaints

Psychologic and social stressors may result in the development of physical symptoms. These symptoms seem real to the child and cause a great deal of distress. Extreme manifestations of these concerns include the somatic symptom disorders (Table 31.14).

Illness Anxiety Disorder (Hypochondriasis)

In illness anxiety disorder, the child either fears that they have a serious illness or focuses on minor discomforts with a worry that they may have a life-threatening illness. The hallmark is not the physical symptom itself but the anxiety over what the symptom represents. Illness anxiety disorder is often associated with other anxiety and depressive disorders; consequently, these patients may appear sad, irritable, or fatigued and should be screened for suicidal ideation or intent, as well as evidence of other comorbid psychiatric disorders.

Somatic Symptom Disorder

Somatic symptom disorder requires the presence of a physical symptom that is distressing. That symptom must then lead to one of the following three behaviors:
1. Disproportionate and persistent thoughts about the seriousness of one's symptoms
2. Persistently high level of anxiety about health or the symptom
3. Excessive time and energy devoted to the health concern

In addition, the patient must have at least one symptom for 6 months. This is separate from illness anxiety disorder as the patient's complaints are focused on the symptom, not anxiety about developing a life-threatening illness. It is important to note that, in contrast to conversion disorder, the symptom does not have to be medically unexplainable.

Associated comorbid conditions are major depressive disorder, panic disorder, substance abuse, borderline personality disorder, and antisocial personality disorder. This is a chronic condition that rarely remits. The psychiatric differential diagnosis is extensive and includes major depression, schizophrenia with somatic delusions, panic disorders (in which symptoms occur only during an attack), generalized anxiety disorder, and factitious disorder.

Factitious Disorder

Factitious disorder consists of a patient inducing symptoms or signs to assume the role of being sick and to receive care. There is no secondary gain, such as escaping responsibilities or receiving money, as is found with malingering. The onset of this disorder usually occurs in early adulthood; it can also occur in childhood. Patients are at risk for substance use disorders (secondary to using agents to induce symptoms) as well as for complications from associated diagnostic evaluations and unnecessary surgical procedures. On confrontation, they may either change their symptoms or try to seek medical care elsewhere.

Conversion Disorder (Functional Neurologic Symptom Disorder)

The diagnosis of conversion disorder is based on the presence of one or more symptoms of altered voluntary motor or sensory function. Symptoms may take the form of weakness, paresthesias, vision changes, or paroxysmal episodes of erratic movements that may be mistaken for seizure activity. The history, physical examination, and neurologic diagnostic evaluation, including the use of long-term video electroencephalogram monitoring in the case of paroxysmal movements, demonstrate incompatibility between the symptom and any medical condition. Unlike somatic symptom disorder, in which patients have excessive thoughts, feelings, or behaviors associated with the voluntary motor or sensory function, conversion disorder is an unconscious phenomenon.

Onset is usually in late adolescence or early adulthood. A typical episode is acute, follows a recent stressor, and is of relatively short duration, typically <4 weeks. The symptoms may solve a psychologic conflict. For example, complaints of blindness may prevent a patient from being witness to traumatic events in their environment. Common childhood stressors associated with conversion disorders are grief, bullying, and abuse. Major depressive disorder and anxiety disorders are associated with conversion disorders.

Conditions Characterized by Changes in Eating

The disorders combined under eating disorders (Table 31.15) are most often thought of as leading to weight loss. However, these disorders may be better conceptualized by their pattern of eating than weight changes that may result.

Conditions Characterized by Decreased Eating

Anorexia Nervosa

Anorexia nervosa is an eating disorder in which the patient restricts caloric intake due to a significant fear of gaining weight and distorted body image. There are two subtypes, **restricting type** and **binge-eating/purging type**. Diagnostic criteria are as follows:
1. Restriction of energy intake leading to a significantly low body weight
2. Intense fear of gaining weight or becoming fat

3. Distorted perception of body size, undue influence of body weight or shape on self-evaluation, or lack of recognition of severity of low body weight

Patients with anorexia nervosa will often go to great lengths to hide their intent and symptoms, oftentimes by wearing baggy clothes, by explaining that excessive and vigorous exercise is required for sports participation, by rationalizing food restriction as health consciousness, by complaining that allergies ruin the taste and smell of food, or by concealing purging behaviors, such as induced vomiting or diarrhea. Because of frequent concealment, the detection of these behaviors is challenging.

The prevalence of anorexia nervosa is as high as 1%; almost 90% of cases occur in females. Although this condition is associated with higher socioeconomic status, it can occur in persons from a variety of socioeconomic backgrounds and in all ethnic groups.

Besides weight loss, patients with anorexia nervosa may develop symptoms of depression or may withdraw socially secondary to the physiology of starvation. Actual loss of appetite is rare, though patients with anorexia have been found to have higher levels of leptin, which suppresses appetite. Patients with anorexia may develop obsessive-compulsive behavior regarding food, such as collecting recipes or hoarding food. These patients may also have inflexible thinking or feel the need to control their environment.

Anorexia nervosa may affect every organ system, and presenting symptoms and signs are secondary to malnutrition and purging. The symptoms of **malnutrition** are fatigue, depression, and amenorrhea. The physical findings of malnutrition are bradycardia, hypothermia, hypotension, emaciation, hair loss, yellow skin, and lanugo. If the patient controls caloric intake through **purging** via vomiting, findings may include hypertrophic salivary glands, dental erosions secondary to gastric acid irritation, and abrasions or calluses on the dorsum of the hand secondary to manual induction of vomiting (**Russell sign**). The metabolic abnormalities related to starvation and purging consist of leukopenia, anemia, hyperamylasemia from parotid gland irritation, vomiting-related metabolic alkalosis or laxative-associated metabolic acidosis, thyroid abnormalities, hypomagnesemia, hypocalcemia, hypozincemia, and electrolyte abnormalities resulting from diuretic abuse and dehydration. These patients also have regression of the hypothalamic-pituitary-gonadal axis, which results in low estrogen levels in girls and low testosterone levels in boys.

In evaluating an adolescent with unexplained weight loss, the examiner must rule out the medical causes of cachexia such as malignancy, malabsorption (celiac disease), or inflammatory bowel disease. Interview data that support a diagnosis of anorexia nervosa are a restrictive dietary history, distorted perception of body shape, and rationalization of the causative behaviors. Once the medical causes for weight loss have been ruled out, the examiner must consider the psychiatric differential diagnosis for anorexia nervosa and its associated comorbid conditions. These conditions are major depressive disorder, the abuse of stimulants, OCD, social phobia, body dysmorphic disorder, and bulimia nervosa. If the patient has symptoms of depression that fail to resolve with the correction of malnutrition, the clinician should also consider the diagnosis of major depressive disorder.

Anorexia nervosa is associated with both life-threatening psychologic conditions (i.e., suicide) and medical conditions (e.g., electrolyte abnormalities, cardiac failure, starvation). The lifelong rate of mortality secondary to anorexia nervosa in patients who require hospitalization is more than 10%. Some of the possible medical complications are osteoporosis resulting from hypocalcemia with low serum estrogen levels, cardiomyopathy, anemia, sepsis resulting from malnutrition-induced immunodeficiency, arrhythmias resulting from electrolyte abnormalities, and superior mesenteric artery syndrome. **Superior mesenteric artery syndrome**, which is characterized by postprandial vomiting and

pain secondary to intermittent gastric outlet obstruction, is more common in anorexia nervosa as profound weight loss is believed to result in the loss of the intraabdominal fat pad between the duodenum and superior mesenteric artery.

Avoidant/Restrictive Food Intake Disorder

The hallmark of avoidant/restrictive food intake disorder (ARFID) is avoidance or restriction of food intake in infancy or early childhood that is not related to a disturbance in the way in which one's body weight or shape is experienced. The restriction in eating must be associated with one or more of the following:
1. Significant weight loss
2. Significant nutritional deficiency
3. Dependence on enteral feeding tubes or supplements
4. Marked interference with psychosocial functioning

Two common reasons that patients develop ARFID are an aversion to the sensory characteristics of food and a conditioned negative response to eating. Examples of sensory aversions include extreme sensitivity to appearance, color, smell, texture, or taste of food. It is separate from "picky eating" in that the restriction leads to one of the aforementioned outcomes. A conditioned negative response to eating could result from an episode of choking, trauma to or traumatic investigations of the throat or upper gastrointestinal tract, or repeated vomiting. Risk factors for ARFID include anxiety disorders, autism spectrum disorder, OCD, ADHD, familial anxiety, gastroesophageal reflux disease, vomiting, and other gastrointestinal conditions.

Conditions Characterized by Binge Eating

Bulimia Nervosa

Diagnostic criteria for bulimia nervosa are as follows:
1. Recurrent episodes of **binge eating** (eating more than what most individuals would eat in a discrete period and a sense of lack of control over eating)
2. Recurrent inappropriate **purging** (compensatory behaviors for controlling weight gain, such as induced vomiting, laxative misuse, diuretic misuse, prolonged fasting, or excessive exercise)
3. Binge eating and compensatory measures occur at least once a week for 3 months
4. Self-evaluation is unduly influenced by body shape and weight
5. Does not occur within anorexia nervosa

Bulimia nervosa is twice as common as anorexia nervosa and has a later onset, typically in late adolescence. Unlike anorexia nervosa, there is not significant food restriction or low body weight. Like anorexia nervosa, it is more common in females (90%) and can occur in any socioeconomic background. Almost 90% of patients control their weight gain by purging. Other methods for controlling weight are excessive exercise and fasting before binge eating.

Comorbid psychologic conditions are common in bulimia nervosa and include mood disorders, personality disorders, anxiety disorders, and substance use. Approximately 30% of patients who use medications to control weight also have substance use disorders, typically of alcohol or stimulants. In contrast to anorexia nervosa, significant medical complications occur less commonly in bulimia nervosa. If present, comorbid medical conditions of bulimia nervosa are associated with vomiting or medication abuse. These conditions are esophagitis and gastritis, cardiomyopathy (particularly if syrup of ipecac is used to induce vomiting), hypokalemia and nephrolithiasis from diuretic abuse, metabolic alkalosis from vomiting and metabolic acidosis from laxative abuse, and increased amylase levels.

Concealment of symptoms coupled with the lack of cachexia makes bulimia nervosa difficult to detect. Some patients may present to the

TABLE 31.15 Diagnostic Guidelines for Eating Disorders

	Anorexia Nervosa, Restricting Type	Anorexia Nervosa, Binge/Purge Type	Bulimia Nervosa	Binge-Eating Disorder
BMI/weight	Underweight Mild: BMI ≥17 kg/m^2 Moderate: BMI 16–16.99 kg/m^2 Severe: 15–15.99 kg/m^2 Extreme: BMI <15 kg/m^2	Underweight Mild: BMI ≥17 kg/m^2 Moderate: BMI 16–16.99 kg/m^2 Severe: 15–15.99 kg/m^2 Extreme: BMI <15 kg/m^2	May be normal weight or overweight	May be normal weight or overweight/obese
Restricting behaviors	+	+	−	−
Purging behaviors (including excessive exercise, use of laxatives, vomiting)	−	+ Must have recurrent binge-eating or purging behaviors in the last 3 mo	+ Must occur at least one time per week for 3 mo	−
Episodes of binge eating	−	+ Must have recurrent binge-eating or purging behaviors in the last 3 mo	+ Must occur at least one time per week for 3 mo	+ Must occur at least one time per week for 3 mo
Potential medical complications	Hypotension, bradycardia, hypothermia, fatigue, dizziness, leukopenia, anemia, thyroid abnormalities, amenorrhea, electrolyte abnormalities (hyponatremia, hypocalcemia, hypophosphatemia, hypoglycemia, etc.)	Hypotension, bradycardia, hypothermia, fatigue, dizziness, leukopenia, anemia, thyroid abnormalities, amenorrhea, electrolyte abnormalities (can have abnormalities consistent with malnutrition and/or purging behaviors)	Esophagitis, gastritis, cardiomyopathy (especially w/ use of ipecac), electrolyte abnormalities including hypokalemia and nephrolithiasis from diuretic abuse, metabolic alkalosis from vomiting, metabolic acidosis from laxative abuse, and increased amylase levels.	Obesity, metabolic abnormalities
Notable physical findings	Signs of malnutrition: emaciation, hair loss, yellow skin, and lanugo	Signs of malnutrition: emaciation, hair loss, yellow skin, and lanugo If engaging in recurrent vomiting can also have dental erosion, parotid hypertrophy, Russell sign, and pharyngeal irritation	Suggestive of recurrent vomiting: dental erosion, parotid hypertrophy, Russell sign, and pharyngeal irritation	

BMI, body mass index.
A "+" indicates symptoms are seen in the disorder. A "−" indicates symptoms are not seen in the disorder.

clinician because of a parent's detection of binge eating and purging. Physical findings that suggest recurrent vomiting are dental erosion, parotid hypertrophy, callus abrasions on the dorsum of the hand known as **Russell sign**, and pharyngeal irritation.

Binge-Eating Disorder

Binge-eating disorder consists of recurrent binge-eating episodes without compensatory behaviors to prevent weight gain. Patients with binge-eating disorder may be of normal weight or overweight. DSM-5 criteria are as follows:

1. Recurrent episodes of binge eating (eating more than what most individuals would eat in a discrete period and a sense of lack of control over eating)
2. Binge-eating episodes are associated with three of the following:
   a. Eating much more rapidly than normal
   b. Eating until feeling uncomfortably full
   c. Eating large amounts of food when not hungry
   d. Eating alone because of embarrassment by how much one is eating
   e. Feeling disgusted, depressed, or guilty afterward
3. Marked distress regarding binge eating is present
4. Binge eating occurs, on average, at least once a week for 3 months

Binge-eating disorder is distinct from obesity as most individuals with obesity do not engage in recurrent binge-eating episodes. At this time, there are limited data regarding the prevalence of binge-eating disorder in youths. In adults, it is roughly twice as common in females.

SUMMARY AND RED FLAGS

Suicide is the second leading cause of death in adolescents. Identifying suicidal ideation and intent is crucial in the evaluation of patients presenting with changes in mood or behavior. Changes in mood or behavior carry a significant burden for patients, their family members, and society as a whole. Many psychiatric illnesses have comorbid psychiatric and medical conditions that require thoughtful and deliberate assessment, and many psychiatric symptoms may be secondary to an underlying medical condition. Red flags include risk-taking behavior, violence, poor school performance, poor attention to personal appearance and hygiene, deteriorating social interaction, reduced appetite, weight loss, reduced or excessive sleeping, delusions, and hallucinations (see Table 31.9).

BIBLIOGRAPHY

A bibliography is available at ExpertConsult.com.

32

Autistic-like Behaviors

Kathleen A. Koth

Autism spectrum disorder (ASD) is a neurobiologic disorder with onset in early childhood; it is characterized by impaired social communication and interaction accompanied by restricted and repetitive behaviors.

With definitions that vary dependent on agencies, schools, and clinicians, there is often confusion surrounding the diagnosis of ASD. This is the term used for all children who were, in previous editions of the *Diagnostic and Statistical Manual of Mental Disorders* (DSM), divided into autism, Asperger syndrome, and pervasive developmental disorder not otherwise specified. The reliability and validity of the separation of these diagnoses were shown to be directly correlated to the diagnosing facility and not a distinct set of diagnostic criteria or biomarkers, and, therefore, the diagnoses were collated under the umbrella of autism spectrum disorder (DSM-5).

Several criteria must be met to enable the diagnosis of ASD beyond difficulties in socialization (Tables 32.1 and 32.2). It should be noted that although these features must be present early in the developmental period, there is no age cutoff for making a diagnosis.

DIAGNOSTIC CRITERIA

The diagnostic criteria in the DSM-5 focus on symptoms in two primary domains. A thorough history of previous behaviors that meet criteria is sufficient for being present early in development. As with all symptoms in the DSM-5, these behaviors must cause significant impairment to be a disorder. Finally, the symptoms cannot be better explained by intellectual disability (intellectual developmental disorder) or global developmental delay (see Table 32.1E) or other disorders (Table 32.3).

There are several modifiers and levels that help clinicians better communicate about the abilities and deficits of an individual with ASD. The modifiers include those for accompanying intellectual impairment, accompanying language impairment, if the diagnosis is associated with a known medical or genetic condition, and if it is associated with another neurodevelopmental, mental, or behavioral disorder. There is also a modifier if catatonia is present. The level system adds a way to indicate how much support an individual needs, from level 1, where minimal support is required and an untrained observer may not quickly notice they have ASD, to level 3, where very substantial support is required due to their symptoms (Table 32.4). Common clinical features are noted in Table 32.5.

MEDICAL WORK-UP

A thorough physical examination can help to guide next steps. Children with ASD frequently react adversely to the focused attention of an examination, and, as a result, indirect techniques such as observation and examination by an experienced clinician are required. A dysmorphology evaluation (see Chapter 29) can aid with identifying comorbid syndromes and guide genetic testing. Facial asymmetry, multiple hair whorls, and prominent forehead have been described as occurring more often in patients with autism. There are reports of rapid head growth in the 1st year of life in some individuals. Specific organ system malformations in individuals with ASD behaviors should raise the suspicion of a **congenital malformation syndrome** associated with autistic-like behavior (Table 32.6).

During the initial physical work-up, it is important to rule out other major medical concerns that can mimic autism (see Table 32.3). A *formal hearing screen* is essential; relying on newborn hearing screening or screening undertaken at school is not sufficient when considering autism. Due to the child's difficulty in participating in the test, it is important to test in a manner that does not involve child response, even if they are older. If a vision screening has not been performed adequately, this should also be included. A Woods lamp examination of the skin should be conducted to rule out neurocutaneous disorders such as tuberous sclerosis and neurofibromatosis type 1.

Screening and Diagnosis for Autism Spectrum Disorder

All children should be screened for autism at the 18- and 24-month well-child visits. There are screening checklists that parents can complete prior to the visit, which are then reviewed by the physician. The Modified Checklist for Autism in Toddlers, Revised (M-CHAT-R) (https://m-chat.org/en-us/page/take-m-chat-test/online) is one of the most widely used at ages 18–30 months. It is free, electronic for easy scoring, and available in many languages. The Social Communication Questionnaire is available for children ages 4 years and older with a mental age above 2 years and contains 40 yes-or-no questions for parents with a simple cutoff score. These and other screening tools are not diagnostic but are meant to screen for parental concerns that could lead to a work-up for ASD.

Autism spectrum disorder is a clinical diagnosis that can be made by qualified clinicians familiar with the diagnostic criteria, nuances of diagnosis, and experience in the field. However, there is an important role for neuropsychologic testing in unclear cases and this is often required for the child to obtain services. The **gold standard test is the Autism Diagnostic Observation Schedule (ADOS),** which is available for individuals 12 months of age through adulthood and requires about an hour to administer. The person administering the exam must have special training and certification in the ADOS. The test has good specificity and sensitivity in laboratory settings but has been met with some criticism in community settings. The Autism Diagnostic Inventory–Revised (ADI-R) can be used with those children who have a mental age of 2 years and older, requires a few hours, and is given by a trained administrator to the caregiver. Its biggest limitation is that it does not include any observation or interaction with the child. The Childhood Autism Rating Scale–2 (CARS-2) is a 10-minute observation tool used by trained neuropsychologists and psychologic testers to observe the child and uses an unscored parent questionnaire.

TABLE 32.1 DSM-5 Diagnostic Criteria for Autism Spectrum Disorder

A.	Persistent deficits in social communication and social interaction across multiple contexts, as manifested by the following, currently or by history:
	1. Deficits in social-emotional reciprocity.
	2. Deficits in nonverbal communicative behaviors used for social interaction.
	3. Deficits in developing, maintaining, and understanding relationships.
B.	Restricted, repetitive patterns of behavior, interests, or activities, as manifested by at least two of the following, currently or by history:
	1. Stereotyped or repetitive motor movements, use of objects, or speech.
	2. Insistence on sameness, inflexible adherence to routines, or ritualized patterns of verbal or nonverbal behavior.
	3. Highly restricted, fixated interests that are abnormal in intensity or focus.
	4. Hyper- or hyporeactivity to sensory input or unusual interest in sensory aspects of the environment.
C.	Symptoms must be present in the early developmental period (may not become fully manifest until social demands exceed limited capacities, or may be masked by learned strategies in later life).
D.	Symptoms cause clinically significant impairment in social, occupational, or other important areas of current functioning.
E.	These disturbances are not better explained by intellectual disability (intellectual developmental disorder) or global developmental delay.

From the *Diagnostic and Statistical Manual of Mental Disorders*. 5th ed. American Psychiatric Association; 2013:50–51.

TABLE 32.2 Associated Features of Autism Not in DSM-5 Criteria

Atypical language development and abilities
Age <6 yr: frequently disordered and delayed in comprehension; two thirds have difficulty with expressive phonology and grammar
Age ≥6 yr: disordered pragmatics, semantics, and morphology, with relatively intact articulation and syntax (i.e., early difficulties are resolved)
Motor abnormalities: motor delay; hypotonia; catatonia; deficits in coordination, movement preparation and planning, praxis, gait, and balance

Adapted from Lai MC, Lombardo MV, Baron-Cohen S. Autism. *Lancet* 2014;383:896–910.

· A neuropsychologic examination of a child with developmental delays or suspected ASD should go beyond testing for autism to determine the child's cognition and adaptive functioning, which is of utmost importance in determining what types of support they need. If the patient is able to participate, intelligence testing is available for verbal and nonverbal children and adults of all ages. This helps screen for **intellectual disability** but also examines what areas of intelligence are strengths and weaknesses for the child and will be used as building blocks for targeted interventions. Adaptive functioning testing, such as the Vineland Adaptive Behavior Scales, can help to identify how the child is functioning overall, which may be the most helpful part of the diagnosis to use in intervention. *Often individuals with autism are not functioning where expected for chronological or*

TABLE 32.3 Conditions Commonly Misdiagnosed as Autism Spectrum Disorder

Primary communication disorder
• Specific language impairment
• Social (pragmatic) communication disorder
Anxiety disorder
• Selective mutism
Reactive attachment disorder
• Post-institutional autistic syndrome
Cognitive impairment
Visual impairment
Hearing impairment
Normal behavioral variations

From Simms MD. When autistic behavior suggests a disease other than classic autism. *Pediatr Clin N Am.* 2017;64(1):127–138 (Box 1, p. 128).

even cognitive age. Very intelligent individuals with ASD can struggle with toilet training, food preparation, and other activities of daily living. Neuropsychologic assessment is also useful in planning school and home interventions.

Common Mimics and Co-occurring Neurodevelopmental Disorders

There are many cognitive and communication difficulties that can appear to be ASD (see Table 32.3). These can also be *co-occurring* with ASD and further complicate the overall picture (Table 32.7).

Communication disorders are difficult to recognize and require careful observation and standardized testing. Communication disorders often do not become apparent until the expectations of the environment exceed the individual's abilities. For severe disorders this could be very early in life, whereas for a mild disorder it could be several years into school when a problem is identified.

Receptive language disorder is a communication disorder where the process of receiving and comprehending language is abnormal. **Expressive language disorder** is difficulty with the production of vocal, gestural, and verbal signals. They do not have to be impaired together because these correlate with separate regions of the brain. Having either one, or both, presents significant challenges. These may present when children have difficulties in school that seem different from attention-deficit/hyperactivity disorder (ADHD) or learning disabilities.

In **receptive language disorders**, individuals have difficulty processing verbal input. They may appear as though they have not been listening. In conversation, it is frequently interpreted that they do not understand what others were saying. When disciplined through verbal command, they appear disobedient and repeat the behaviors. Yet when expressive language is preserved, they can converse, express themselves, and give others direction without apparent concern. This often causes difficulty in school and can have educators and parents blaming the child for not listening or paying attention. They can appear socially awkward or not able to fully participate in peer interactions when understanding is difficult.

When **expressive language disorder** is present, the individual has a difficult time expressing themselves but can understand completely what is being said to them. This can lead to frustration in the child who cannot express questions well to the teacher, cannot explain how they complete a task, or cannot give a presentation to the class. These

TABLE 32.4 DSM-5 Severity Levels for Autism Spectrum Disorder

Severity Level	Social Communication	Restricted, Repetitive Behaviors
Level 3 "Requiring very substantial support"	Severe deficits in verbal and nonverbal social communication skills cause severe impairments in functioning, very limited initiation of social interactions, and minimal response to social overtures from others For example, a person with few words of intelligible speech who rarely initiates interaction and, when they do, they make unusual approaches to meet needs only and respond to only very direct social approaches.	Inflexibility of behavior, extreme difficulty coping with change, or other restricted/repetitive behaviors markedly interfere with functioning in all spheres. Great distress/difficulty changing focus or action.
Level 2 "Requiring substantial support"	Marked deficits in verbal and nonverbal social communication skills; social impairments apparent even with supports in place; limited initiation of social interactions; and reduced or abnormal responses to social overtures from others. For example, a person who speaks simple sentences, whose interaction is limited to narrow special interests, and who has markedly odd nonverbal communication.	Inflexibility of behavior, difficulty coping with change, or other restricted/repetitive behaviors appear frequently enough to be obvious to the casual observer and interfere with functioning in a variety of contexts. Distress and/or difficulty changing focus or action.
Level 1 "Requiring support"	Without supports in place, deficits in social communication cause noticeable impairments. Difficulty initiating social interactions, and clear examples of atypical or unsuccessful responses to social overtures of others. May appear to have decreased interest in social interactions. For example, a person who is able to speak in full sentences and engages in communication but whose to-and-fro conversation with others fails, and whose attempts to make friends are odd and typically unsuccessful.	Inflexibility of behavior causes significant interference with functioning in one or more contexts. Difficulty switching between activities. Problems of organization and planning hamper independence.

From the *Diagnostic and Statistical Manual of Mental Disorders.* 5th ed. American Psychiatric Association; 2013:52.

issues can make the child appear socially awkward as well and lead to embarrassment and social isolation. Not being able to express yourself verbally can also extend to explaining emotions and desires. Behavioral issues can result from the frustration and inability to express those to others.

Pragmatic language disorder is a very narrow spectrum disorder for those individuals who have difficulty in the social rules of verbal and nonverbal communication without any of the other symptoms of ASD such as repetitive behaviors, narrow ranges of interest, or insistence on routines. This diagnosis may apply when social difficulties cannot be better explained by intellectual developmental disorder (IDD) or inattention. Although many children with **ADHD** have deficits in nonverbal communication, this is not considered pragmatic language disorder because the cause is not being able to attend long enough to observe details of others' behavior.

The association of ASD and IDD is often difficult to separate. Approximately 50% or half of people with ASD have IDD. The communication difficulties that many children with ASD have can make formal cognitive assessment challenging, but more so it can make the results inaccurate. How a person with ASD performs on an IQ test may be more representative of their level of function to participate than their actual cognitive ability. In nonautistic individuals IQ test subsets are usually within a narrow range, but in autism they can be scattered over a wide range, indicating strength in some areas and weakness in others. No IQ pattern has been identified to be diagnostic in ASD. Since the diagnosis of IDD no longer requires an IQ score for severity, overall functional cognition can be used in assessment, but participation and effort are required for accurate results. *It is important not to assume overall cognitive strength or functional ability from a single skill.* While completing calculus in their sophomore year of high school, an individual may struggle with reading comprehension on a grade school level, be unable to complete their daily hygiene without direct support, not know what money is, or be unable to prepare food.

IDD is not just cognitive intelligence but also function or adaptive reasoning. The changes in the DSM-5 well articulate the conceptual, social, and practical domains that are affected in IDD. An individual with IDD may socialize more appropriately for their cognitive age than their chronological age. If one is to consider a diagnosis of ASD in addition to IDD, the socialization must be different from that expected for the developmental age with the inclusion of stereotyped or repetitive behaviors, restricted areas of interest, inflexibility of routines, and unusual sensory input that are not expected with that developmental age. This is even more difficult in those with severe and profound IDD who already have very limited social understanding, self-stimulating behaviors, and stereotypies. The diagnosis of ASD should only be added if the symptoms of ASD are above and beyond what can be seen in this population.

The addition of the IDD diagnosis to ASD can be very difficult when the autism symptoms are impairing daily functioning and participation in standardized testing. The use of alternate communication tools and applied behavior analysis (ABA) therapy can help to identify cognitive strengths and functioning that are limited in their expression by autism.

GENETIC TESTING AND DIAGNOSIS

There is a wide spectrum of disorders that have autistic-like behavior (Tables 32.6, 32.8, and 32.9 and Fig. 32.1). There is no definitive monogenetic etiology for most patients with classic ASD; rather, ASD represents diverse pathoetiologic pathways, which overlap in a similar behavioral phenotype. It remains the current recommendation that all children with a developmental disorder such as ASD or IDD undergo genetic testing if a cause of the disorder is not otherwise known. One in five children with a neurodevelopmental disability has an identifiable genetic risk factor and that number is increasing rapidly with the application of advanced genetic diagnostic tools. The importance of reaching a unifying diagnosis can impact numerous areas including screening for comorbidities, helping families understand and accept the diagnosis and natural history, and making important reproductive decisions in addition to the potential development of specific therapy.

TABLE 32.5 Signs and Symptoms of Possible Autism in Preschool Children (or Equivalent Mental Age)

SOCIAL INTERACTION AND RECIPROCAL COMMUNICATION BEHAVIORS

Spoken Language

Language delay (in babbling or using words, e.g., using <10 words by age 2 yr)

Regression in or loss of use of speech

Spoken language (if present) may include unusual features, such as vocalizations that are not speechlike; odd or flat intonation; frequent repetition of set words and phrases (echolalia), use of subjective pronouns, such as you, she, or he, to refer to self after 3 yrs

Reduced and/or infrequent use of language for communication (e.g., use of single words, although able to speak in sentences)

Responding to Others

Absent or delayed response to name being called, despite normal hearing

Reduced or absent responsive social smiling

Reduced or absent responsiveness to other people's facial expressions or feelings

Unusually negative response to the requests of others ("demand avoidance" behavior)

Rejection of cuddles initiated by parent or caregiver, although the child may initiate cuddles

Interacting with Others

Reduced or absent awareness of personal space, or unusually intolerant of people entering their personal space

Reduced or absent social interest in others, including children of own age—may reject others; if interested in others, child may approach others inappropriately, seeming to be aggressive or disruptive

Reduced or absent imitation of others' actions

Reduced or absent initiation of social play with others; plays alone

Reduced or absent enjoyment of situations that most children like (e.g., birthday parties)

Reduced or absent sharing of enjoyment

Eye Contact, Pointing, and Other Gestures

Reduced or absent use of gestures and facial expressions to communicate (although may place an adult's hand on objects)

Reduced and poorly integrated gestures, facial expressions, body orientation, eye contact (looking at people's eyes when speaking), and speech used in social communication

Reduced or absent social use of eye contact (assuming adequate vision)

Reduced or absent "joint attention" (when one person alerts another to something by means of gazing, finger pointing, or other verbal or nonverbal indication for the purpose of sharing interest); this would be evident in the child from lack of:
Gaze switching
Following a point (looking where the other person points to—may look at hand)
Pointing at or showing objects to share interest

Ideas and Imagination

Reduced or absent imagination and variety of pretend play

Unusual or Restricted Interests and/or Rigid and Repetitive Behaviors

Repetitive "stereotypic" movements such as hand flapping, body rocking while standing, spinning, and finger flicking

Repetitive or stereotyped play (e.g., opening and closing doors)

Overfocused or unusual interests

Excessive insistence on following own agenda

Extremes of emotional reactivity to change or new situations; insistence on things being "the same"

Overreaction or underreaction to sensory stimuli, such as textures, sounds, or smells

Excessive reaction to the taste, smell, texture, or appearance of food, or having extreme food fads

Adapted from Baird G, Douglas HR, Murphy MS. Recognizing and diagnosing autism in children and young people: summary of NICE guidance. *BMJ.* 2011;343:d6360 (Box 1, p. 901).

As individuals with specific genetic diagnoses increase, parent support groups allow for sharing of common experience that can help families manage and cope, especially for their neurotypical siblings.

The current standard of care supports genetic testing in the form of a chromosomal microarray for all individuals with IDD or an ASD diagnosis. Fragile X testing should be considered if there is a family history of IDD, premature ovarian failure, or fragile X–associated tremor/ataxia syndrome (FXTAS) in an elderly male relative. With the advance of next-generation sequencing technologies, large IDD/ASD gene panels are available that screen hundreds to thousands of genes simultaneously. These gene panels are curated by the laboratories and are updated frequently based on published gene associations. It is important to be familiar with what test is being offered or to work with a genetic professional when ordering such testing. The current literature supports using exome sequencing as standard of care for first-tier testing, but this test has variable insurance coverage.

The diagnostic testing algorithm detailed in Figure 32.2 provides a comprehensive approach for diagnostic consideration. For patients with seizures see Figure 32.3. Although epilepsy is more common in children with ASD (onset in infancy or adolescence), there are epilepsy syndromes that have autistic-like behaviors (see Table 32.9).

GENETIC DISORDERS THAT CO-OCCUR WITH AUTISM SPECTRUM DISORDER

Fragile X Syndrome

Fragile X syndrome is the leading identifiable monogenetic cause of ASD. IDD is observed in about 85% of males and 20–30% of females with fragile X syndrome; ASD is seen in 30–43% of males and 16–20% of females. Cognitive deficits are seen in executive functioning, working memory, short-term memory, and processing. Hyperarousal to sensory stimuli of all types is common. Individuals with fragile X syndrome have an increased risk of psychiatric co-occurring illnesses such as ADHD and anxiety.

The physical manifestations can be very subtle in the young child showing midface hypoplasia with sunken eyes, large-cupped ears, arched palate, and macro-orchidism. Medical features

TABLE 32.6 Syndromes with Autistic-Like Behaviors

Chromosome Deletions	IDD *CDKL5* (Rett-Like) Regression, Others
1q21	2q37 monosomy
7q11.28	Angelman
16p11.2	Bardet-Biedl
17q12	Cardiofaciocutaneous
2q23.1 (*MBD5* mutations)	CHARGE association
12q24.3	Cohen
Cri-du-chat (5p15.2-p15.33)	Congenital rubella
22q deletion syndrome	Cornelia de Lange
Jacobsen (11q23.2)	Costello
Phelan-McDermid (*SHANK3* mutations; 22q13)	*FOXG1* mutations
Pitt-Hopkins (18q21.2)	Fragile X
	Hypomelanosis of Ito
Chromosome Duplications	Joubert
15q11.1-q13.3	Kleefstra (*EHMT1* mutations)
7q11.23	Lujan-Fryns
18q12.2	Moebius sequence
16p11.2	Muscle-eye brain disease
1q21.1	Myotonic dystrophy
22q11.2	Neurofibromatosis
Potocki-Lupski (17p11.2)	Nonsyndromic intellectual disability due to *SYNGAP1* mutations
Epilepsy Encephalopathies, Epilepsy	Noonan
Cortical dysplasia focal epilepsy	Oculoauriculovertebral spectrum (including Goldenhar)
SCN1A-related syndromes (Dravet, Lennox Gastaut, others)	Partial monosomy 1p36
Early myoclonic encephalopathies (Ohtahara: *STXBP1, ARX, SIK1*)	Partial tetrasomy 15
SCN2A-related syndromes (West, others)	Prader-Willi
SLC6A1 myotonic-atonic epilepsy	PTEN mutations
HCN1-related epilepsies	Rett complex (female >> male)
CDKL5	Ring chromosome 14
SCN8A	*SETD1B* mutations
PCDH19	Sex chromosome aneuploidies
SCL35A2-related disorders	Smith-Lemli-Opitz
Epilepsy-aphasia spectrum (Landau-Kleffner; *GRIN2A*; continuous spike wave during low-wave sleep)	Smith-Magenis
	Sotos
Juvenile myoclonic epilepsy (*RING2*)	Timothy
	Trisomy 21
	Tuberous sclerosis
	WAGR
	Wiedemann-Steiner (*KMT2A* mutations)
	Williams

CHARGE, coloboma, heart, choanal atresia, retardation, genital, ear anomalies; IDD, intellectual developmental disability; WAGR, Wilms tumor, aniridia, genitourinary anomalies, mental retardation.

commonly include mitral valve prolapse, seizures, migraines, neuropathy, otitis media, strabismus, joint laxity, ataxia, fibromyalgia, and gastrointestinal (GI) problems. Sleep disturbances are common and can be accompanied by sleep apnea and restless leg syndrome; affected individuals have difficulty with sleep latency and maintaining sleep.

MECP2-Related Neurodevelopmental Disorders

Pathogenic variants in *MECP2* cause a spectrum of disorders that include Rett syndrome, PPM-X syndrome, MECP2 duplication syndrome, and *MECP2*-related severe neonatal encephalopathy. Rett syndrome affects females and classically presents with a history of normal psychomotor development for the first 6–18 months of life. Development then stagnates for a period before rapid regression

in motor and language skills before long-term stability is reached. During the period of regression, stereotypic hand movements replace purposeful hand movements and are accompanied by behavioral issues with screaming and inconsolable crying. There can be panic-like attacks as well as bruxism and episodic apnea and/or hyperpnea, which make caring for an affected child difficult for parents. Autistic-like features can be present although rarely meeting the diagnostic criteria.

PTEN Hamartoma Syndrome

Rare autosomal dominant disorders of the PTEN pathway include Bannayan-Riley-Ruvalcaba syndrome (BRRS), Proteus and Proteus-like syndromes, and Cowden syndrome. The presentation within each of these clinical subtypes differs. Patients with BRRS have facial

TABLE 32.7 Common Co-occurring Conditions in Autism Spectrum Disorder (ASD)

Comorbidity	Individuals with Autism Affected	Comments
Developmental Disorders		
Intellectual disability	~45%	Prevalence estimate is affected by the diagnostic boundary and definition of intelligence (e.g., whether verbal ability is used as a criterion).
		In individuals, discrepant performance between subtests is common.
Language disorders	Variable	In the DSM-IV, language delay was a defining feature of autism (autistic disorder), but is no longer included in the DSM-5.
		An autism-specific language profile (separate from language disorders) exists, but with substantial interindividual variability.
Attention-deficit/ hyperactivity disorder	28–44%	In the DSM-IV, not diagnosed when occurring in individuals with autism, but no longer so in the DSM-5.
Tic disorders	14–38%	Approximately 6–5% have Tourette syndrome.
Motor abnormality	≤79%	See Table 32.2.
General Medical Disorders		
Epilepsy	8–35%	Increased frequency in individuals with intellectual disability or genetic syndromes.
		Two peaks of onset: early childhood and adolescence.
		Increases risk of poor outcome.
Gastrointestinal problems	9–70%	Common symptoms include chronic constipation, abdominal pain, chronic diarrhea, and gastroesophageal reflux.
		Associated disorders include gastritis, esophagus, gastroesophageal reflux disease, inflammatory bowel disease, celiac disease, Crohn disease, and colitis.
Immune dysregulation	≤38%	Associated with allergic and autoimmune disorders.
Genetic disorders	10–20%	Collectively called syndromic autism.
		Examples include fragile X syndrome (21–50% of individuals affected have autism). Rett syndrome (most have autistic features but with profiles different from idiopathic autism), tuberous sclerosis complex (24–60%), Down syndrome (5–39%), phenylketonuria (5–20%).
		CHARGE syndrome* (15–50%), Angelman syndrome (50–81%), Timothy syndrome (60–70%), and Joubert syndrome (-40%).
Sleep disorders	50–60%	Insomnia is the most common.
Psychiatric Disorders		
Anxiety	42–56%	Common across all age groups.
		Most common are social anxiety disorder (13–29% of individuals with autism) and generalized anxiety disorder (13–22%).
		High-functioning individuals are more susceptible (or symptoms are more detectable).
Depression	12–70%	Common in adults, less common in children.
		High-functioning adults who are less socially impaired are more susceptible (or symptoms are more detectable).
Obsessive-compulsive disorder (OCD)	7–24%	Shares the repetitive behavior domain with autism that could cut across nosologic categories.
		Important to distinguish between repetitive behaviors that do not involve intrusive, anxiety-causing thoughts or obsessions (part of autism) and those that do (and are part of OCD).
Psychotic disorders	12–17%	Mainly in adults.
		Most commonly recurrent hallucinosis.
		High frequency of autism-like features (even a diagnosis of ASD) preceding adult-onset (52%) and childhood-onset schizophrenia (30–50%).
Substance use disorders	≤16%	Potentially because individual is using substances as self-medication to relieve anxiety.
Oppositional defiant disorder	16–28%	Oppositional behaviors could be a manifestation of anxiety, resistance to change, stubborn belief in the correctness of own point of view, difficulty seeing another's point of view, poor awareness of the effect of own behavior on others, or no interest in social compliance.
Eating disorders	4–5%	Could be a misdiagnosis of autism, particularly in females, because both involve rigid behavior, inflexible cognition, self-focus, and focus on details.

TABLE 32.7   Common Co-occurring Conditions in Autism Spectrum Disorder (ASD)—cont'd

Comorbidity	Individuals with Autism Affected	Comments
Personality Disorders[†]		
Paranoid personality disorder	0–19%	Could be secondary to difficulty understanding others' intentions and negative interpersonal experiences.
Schizoid personality disorder	21–26%	Partly overlapping diagnostic criteria.
Schizotypal personality disorder	2–13%	Some overlapping criteria, especially those shared with schizoid personality disorder.
Borderline personality disorder	0–9%	Could have similarity in behaviors (e.g., difficulties in interpersonal relationships, misattributing hostile intentions, problems with affect regulation), which requires careful differential diagnosis. Could be a misdiagnosis of autism, particularly in females.
Obsessive compulsive personality disorder	19–22%	Partly overlapping diagnostic criteria.
Avoidant personality disorder	13–25%	Could be secondary to repeated failure in social experiences.
Behavioral Disorders		
Aggressive behaviors	≤68%	Often directed toward caregivers rather than noncaregivers. Could be a result of empathy difficulties, anxiety, sensory overload, disruption of routines, and difficulties with communication.
Self-injurious behaviors	≤50%	Associated with impulsivity and hyperactivity, negative affect, and lower levels of ability and speech. Could signal frustration in individuals with reduced communication, as well as anxiety, sensory overload, or disruption of routines. Could also become a repetitive habit. Could cause tissue damage and need for restraint.
Pica	~36%	More likely in individuals with intellectual disability. Could be a result of a lack of social conformity to cultural categories of what is deemed edible, or sensory exploration, or both.
Suicidal ideation or attempt	11–14%	Risks increase with concurrent depression and behavioral problems, and after being teased or bullied.

*Coloboma of the eye, heart defects; atresia of the choanae; retardation of growth or development, or both; genital or urinary abnormalities, or both; and ear abnormalities and deafness.
[†]Particularly in high-functioning adults.
DSM-IV, *Diagnostic and Statistical Manual of Mental Disorders*, 4th edition; DSM-5, *Diagnostic and Statistical Manual of Mental Disorders*, 5th edition.
Adapted from Lai MC, Lombardo MV, Baron-Cohen S. Autism. *Lancet*. 2014;383:896–910.

TABLE 32.8   Inborn Errors of Metabolism with Autistic-like Behavior

Adenylosuccinate lyase deficiency
Biotinidase deficiency
Cerebral folate deficiency
Ceroid lipofuscinosis (infantile)
Cystathionine β-synthase deficiency
Dihydropyrimidinase deficiency
Disorders of creatine transport or metabolism
Homocystinuria
Lesch-Nyhan syndrome
Mitochondrial disorders
Mucopolysaccharidosis
Phenylketonuria (untreated)
Sanfilippo syndrome
Succinic semialdehyde dehydrogenase deficiency
Urea cycle disorders

dysmorphic features that include a broad, flat forehead; thick eyebrows; full cheeks; long philtrum; and pointed jaw in addition to macrocephaly. Skin manifestations include papillomatous papules and café-au-lait spots; hyperpigmented macules are common on the glans of the penis.

In BRRS, the diagnosis is frequently made in infancy or childhood due to the significant intellectual disability and/or ASD seen in 25–55% of cases. Cowden syndrome is an adult-onset tumor predisposition syndrome, and Proteus syndrome is characterized by somatic overgrowth of the affected areas.

22q11.2 Deletion Syndrome

22q11.2 microdeletion syndrome has a broad array of phenotypic presentations that have many names including DiGeorge syndrome, velocardiofacial syndrome, Shprintzen syndrome, and conotruncal anomaly facial syndrome. This syndrome can be detected both early and later in life. Early presentations include congenital heart defects, cleft palate, hearing loss, immune dysfunction, and hypocalcemia.

The presence of cognitive impairment is common, but higher rates of ADHD and anxiety are also seen. Despite the presence of

TABLE 32.9   Single Gene and Genomic Copy Number Regions Commonly Associated with Autism and Epilepsy

Gene or Genomic Region	Associated Syndrome	Key Features
15q11-q13	Chromosome 15q11-q13 duplication syndrome	Autism, intellectual disability, ataxia seizures, developmental delays, and behavioral problems Note: Deletion of this region is associated with Angelman syndrome/Prader-Willi syndrome
Chromosome 21	Down syndrome	Distinct facial dysmorphisms, intellectual disability, congenital anomalies, and medical comorbidities
22q13.3/SHANK3	Phelan-McDermid syndrome	Neonatal hypotonia, global developmental delay, absent or severely delayed speech, autistic behavior, and minor dysmorphic features
FMR1	Fragile X syndrome	Moderate to severe intellectual disability, macro-orchidism, and distinct facial features (long face, large ears, and prominent jaw)
TSC1/2	Tuberous sclerosis	Multisystem disorder characterized by hamartomas (brain, heart, lungs, kidneys, and skin)
PTEN	PTEN-related disorders	Hamartoma syndromes and malignancies (breast, thyroid, and endometrial) Macrocephaly and ASD have been reported in children with PTEN mutations
MECP2	MECP2-related disorders	Severe neurodevelopmental disorder characterized by arrest of development between 6 and 18 mo of age, regression of skills, loss of speech, stereotypic hand movements, microcephaly, seizures, and intellectual disability
CDKL5	CDKL5-related disorders	X-linked dominant condition characterized by early onset of seizures, severe global developmental delay, and postnatal microcephaly Other features include subtle dysmorphic facial features, sleep disturbances, gastrointestinal problems, stereotypic hand movements, and intellectual disability
FOXG1	FOXG1-related disorders	Severe neurodevelopmental disorder with features of classic Rett syndrome but earlier onset in the first months of life
MEF2C	MEF2C-related disorders	Severe neurodevelopmental disorder characterized by intellectual disability, epilepsy, and stereotypic movements
CASK	CASK-related disorders	Characterized by a distinct malformation phenotype in females involving postnatal microcephaly and pontine and cerebellar hypoplasia, developmental delay, growth retardation, and eye abnormalities
SCN2A	SCN2A-related disorders	Autosomal dominant seizure disorder characterized by infantile onset or refractory seizures

From Lee BH, Smith T, Paciorkowski AR. Autism disorder and epilepsy: disorders with a shared biology. *Epilepsy Behav.* 2015;47:191–201 (Table 1, p. 193).

social-emotional reciprocity and nonverbal communication, this disorder is rarely characterized by repetitive behaviors or restricted interests, leading few patients to meet the ASD diagnosis.

22q11.2 Duplication Syndrome

The reciprocal duplication of the 22q11.2 deletion syndrome results in a disorder with more notable gross motor delays, although affected children struggle with abstract thinking and social abilities, which becomes more notable as school demands progress in the third or fourth grade. Receptive language is stronger than expressive; verbal memory is stronger than visuospatial memory.

These individuals can be described as shy or withdrawn, emotionally liable, hyperactive, and impulsive. They can move from task to task quickly but are less able to adapt to changes in routine or the environment. Social deficits are often seen including the lack of social-emotional reciprocity. They do not often have the repetitive behaviors and rigidity to fulfill the threshold for diagnosis of ASD. In one study 84% of cases had at least one psychiatric disorder, but only 18% met strict criteria for ASD.

Tuberous Sclerosis

This is an autosomal dominant disorder that results from pathogenic variants in either the *TSC1* or *TSC2* gene. The prevalence is estimated to be 1/6,000–9,000 people. Affected infants can be identified prenatally by the presence of cardiac rhabdomyomas as early as 22 weeks of gestation. Infants can present with infantile spasms, or during an

evaluation for ASD. Most commonly it is identified postnatally with cardiac rhabdomyomas, with hypopigmented macules on the skin, or after the development of seizures. MRI will reveal subependymal nodules and cortical tubers.

IDD can be present, the severity of which is often associated with the age of seizure onset and their severity. Psychiatric comorbidity is significant, with 30–50% having ADHD, 30–60% with depression or anxiety disorders, and 25–50% with ASD.

Timothy Syndrome

Timothy syndrome is a neurodevelopmental disorder that is associated with long QT syndrome. It is caused by pathogenic variants in the *CACNA1C* gene, which encodes a calcium channel. The gene variant allows calcium to enter cells abnormally, which causes a prolonged QT interval that increases the risk of arrhythmias and sudden cardiac death. Physical examination can demonstrate low-set ears, lower nasal bridge, small upper jaw, and widely spaced teeth. Cutaneous syndactyly webbed fingers and toes are commonly found. Seizures, stroke, and blindness can also be found. Developmental delays, including ASD, are common.

Phelan-McDermid Syndrome

Contiguous gene deletion of the 22q13 region that includes *SHANK3* or pathogenic variants in *SHANK3* results in Phelan-McDermid syndrome. *SHANK3*, which encodes for a scaffolding protein in the postsynaptic glutamatergic synapse, plays a critical role in synaptic function. While it

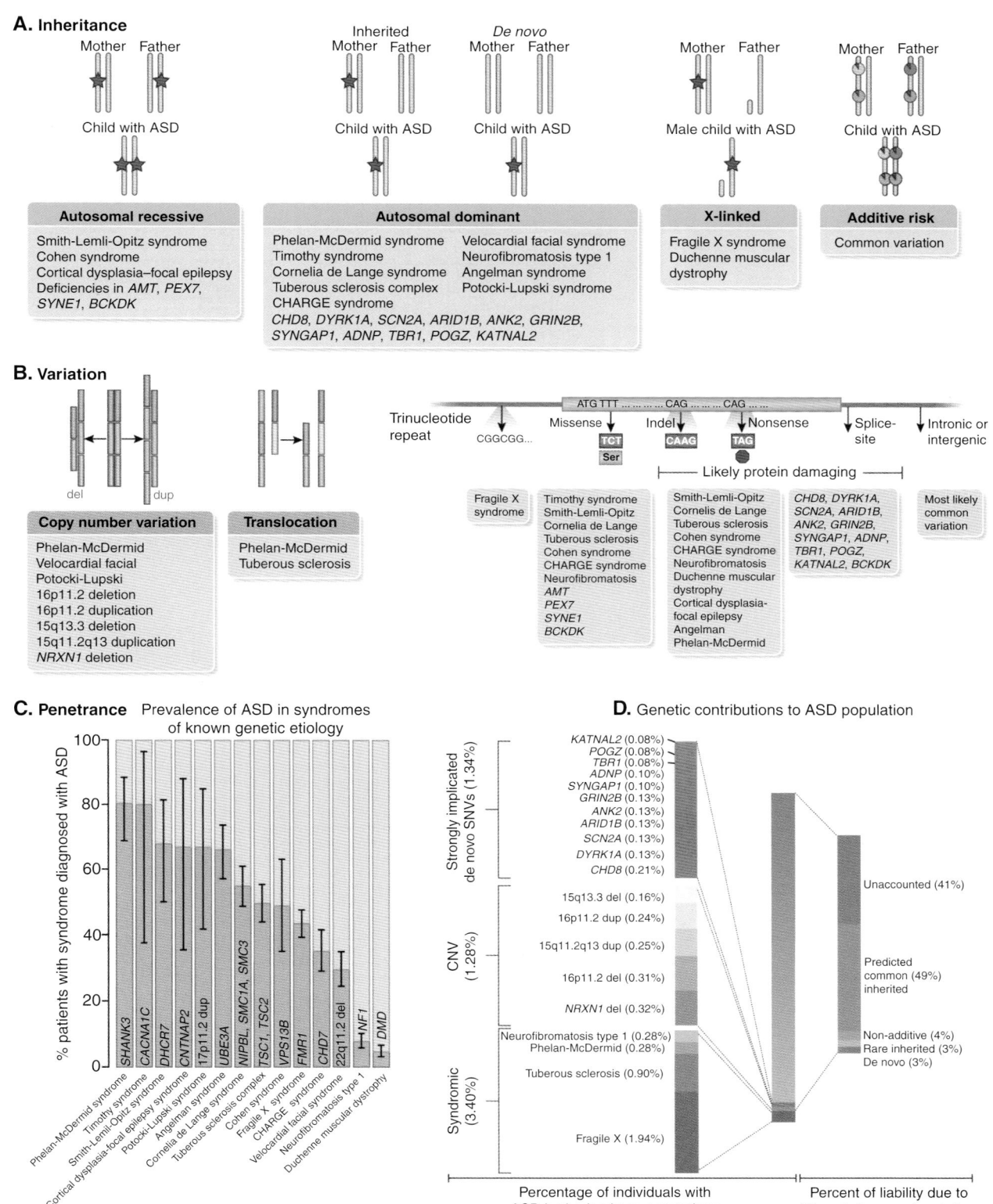

Fig. 32.1 Genetic architecture of autism spectrum disorder (ASD). *A*, The inheritance patterns of syndromes with known genetic etiology and high incidence of autism, as well as that of genes recently identified to be associated with autism. The *red stars* indicate a causal allele and the *red pie charts* indicate a small proportion of risk. Most dominant disorders show de novo inheritance. Autosomal recessive, autosomal dominant, and X-linked inheritance patterns best fit a major gene model, whereas a polygenic model is best represented by additive risk. *B*, The types of genetic variation *(left and middle)* and the developmental disorders *(right)* associated with autism. Genes that have been associated with ASD are also indicated. *C*, The penetrance of known syndromic mutations summarized from multiple studies. Ninety-five percent binomial proportion confidence intervals, based on Wilson's score interval, are shown. *D*, The percentage of individuals with ASD harboring known mutations, as well as the percentage of liability from different classes of mutations. The percentage variance in liability measures the contribution of a particular variant or class of variants relative to the population variance in a theoretical variable called liability. Liability is a continuous and normally distributed latent variable that represents each individual's risk (both genetic and environmental) for developing a disease. Notably, percentage variance in liability is directly dependent on the frequency of the variant and the effect size of the variant, and it is inversely dependent on the frequency of the disease in the population. CNV, copy number variation. (From de la Torre-Ubieta L, Won H, Stein J, et al. Advancing the understanding of autism disease mechanisms through genetics. *Nat Med.* 2016;22[4]:345–361 [Fig. 1, p. 346].)

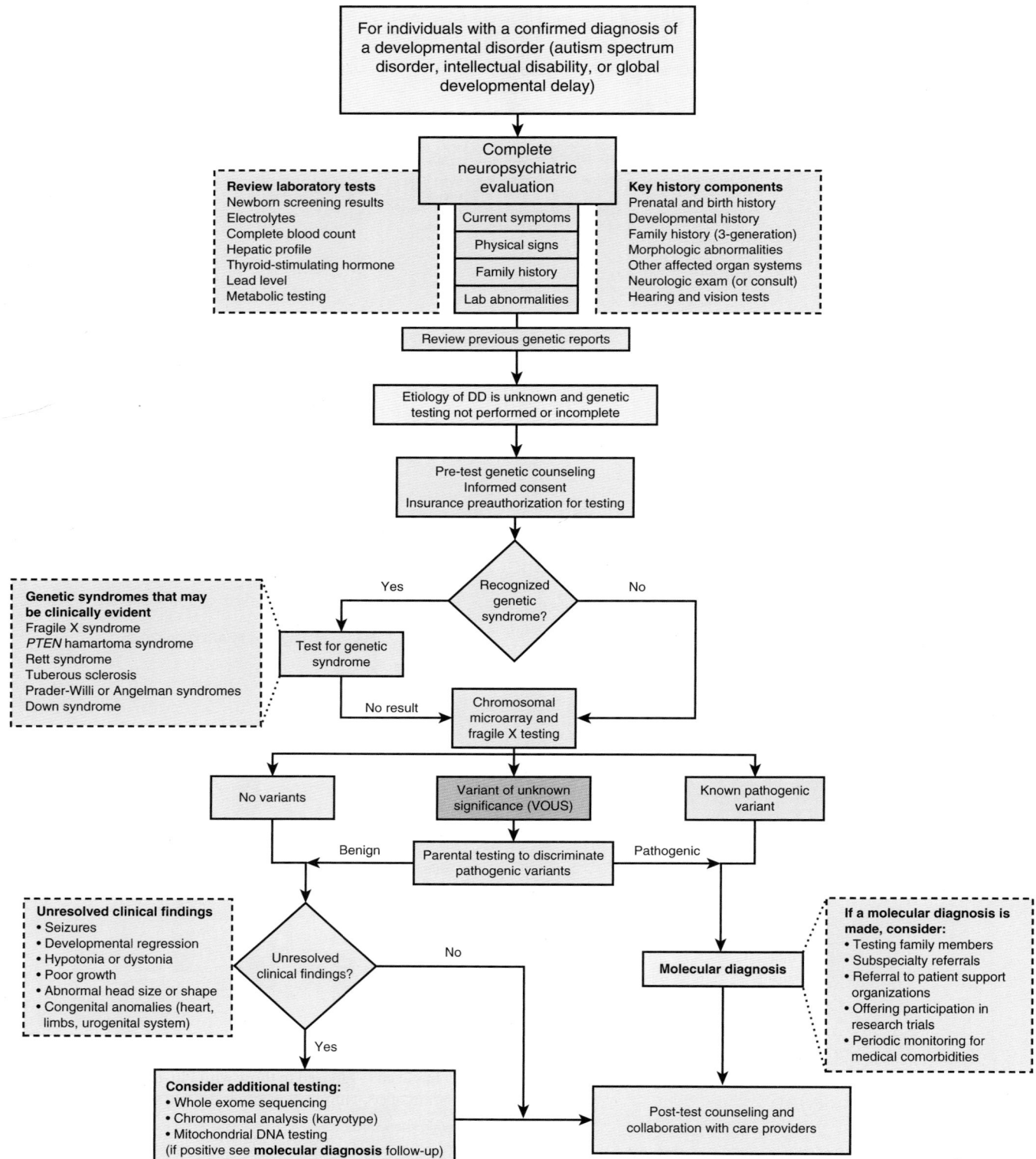

Fig. 32.2 Diagnostic genetic testing algorithm for youth with developmental disorders. JAACAP-D-17-00189. DD, development disorder. (From Muhle R, Reed H, Vo L, et al. Clinical diagnostic genetic testing for individuals with developmental disorders. *J Am Acad Child Adolesc Psychiatry.* 2017;56[11]:910–913.)

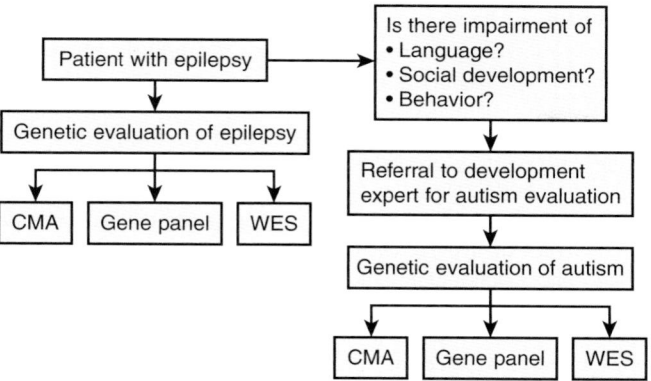

Fig. 32.3 Suggested workflow for evaluation of patients with epilepsy who may be at risk for autism. A patient with epilepsy should be screened for impairment in language, social development, and/or behavior. If warranted, the patient should be referred to a trained expert in autism diagnosis. If a diagnosis of autism is confirmed, or if significant other developmental concerns exist (i.e., intellectual disability), genetic evaluation is appropriate. The clinical genetic evaluation for autism and epilepsy may have overlap and may be tailored by recognition of conditions where autism and epilepsy overlap. Current clinical genetic evaluation includes sequential chromosomal microarray (CMA), autism and epilepsy next-generation sequencing gene panels, and, if necessary, whole exome sequencing (WES). (Modified from Lee BH, Smith T, Paciorkowski AR. Autism disorder and epilepsy: disorders with a shared biology. *Epilepsy Behav.* 2015;47:191–201.)

accounts for a relatively small number of cases of ASD and IDD, the severity of the phenotype increases with the size of the affected region. While 20% of the cases are de novo, parents can carry a balanced chromosomal translocation, increasing the recurrence risk in additional offspring.

Most individuals have at least one visible dysmorphic feature including dolichocephaly, long eyelashes, pointed chin, prominent or dysplastic ears, bulbous nose, and full lips in addition to hypoplastic or dysplastic nails and large, fleshy hands. Hypotonia is often present and can present early in the form of feeding abnormalities and posture. Gait is almost uniformly affected and can range from nonambulatory to having issues with gait, toe walking, and broad-based ataxia. Coordination and motor planning issues are also seen in most cases. An increased risk of scoliosis is present.

Medical comorbidities are common. GI issues are most common and include gastroesophageal reflux disease (GERD), constipation, and diarrhea. Recurrent ear and upper respiratory infections can be linked to immune system abnormalities as well as allergies and asthma. There is an increased incidence of seizures. MRI data have included an increase in brain abnormalities including the corpus callosum, arachnoid cyst, ventriculomegaly, and dysmyelination. There can be significantly delayed or absent speech. Behavioral difficulties are often found but have not been well categorized.

There is an increased incidence of ASD in individuals with Phelan-McDermid syndrome, along with IDD.

Cortical Dysplasia–Focal Epilepsy Syndrome

CNTNAP2 variants can be seen clinically with ASD, focal epilepsy, language regression, and IDD. It can also be associated with Gilles de la Tourette syndrome, ADHD, and schizophrenia.

15q11-13 Deletion or Duplication Maternal/Paternal

The loss or gain of genetic material from 15q11.2-13 has been seen frequently in the context of an ASD diagnosis. Portions of this region are additionally imprinted, and clinically unique syndromes are manifest dependent on whether the loss of material is maternal or paternal.

Angelman syndrome is a result of this alteration in the *maternally* inherited allele. Most individuals with Angelman syndrome have severe IDD are nonverbal, and usually plateau in development between 18 and 24 months. If they do have speech, it is usual phrase speech and receptive language skills are better than expressive. They are happy to engage with others and seek social attention in a developmentally appropriate manner but can have repetitive and restrictive behavior as seen in many with severe IDD. Body movements and mannerisms, such as hand flapping, are very common.

Prader-Willi syndrome is the result of alteration in the *paternally* inherited allele. Individuals have mild to moderate IDD. Social deficits are often reported in individuals with Prader-Willi but often not to the severity of those with ASD. They can have some repetitive and restrictive behaviors, be insistent on routines, arrange objects, and have repetitive speech.

Potocki-Lupski Syndrome

The duplication of 17p11.2 is known as Potocki-Lupski syndrome. Younger children are usually identified due to hypotonia, poor feeding with failure to thrive, sleep-disorder breathing, and cardiovascular anomalies. Older children can have developmental delays and cognitive impairment. For those individuals who have speech it can be marked with precision, referring to themselves in the third person, having running commentaries, or echolalia.

Behavioral issues are seen in most patients including those with attention, hyperactivity, anxiety, somatization, and withdrawal. ASD can be seen in these individuals with motor mannerisms, repetitive behaviors, social aspects of withdrawal, poor eye contact, and difficulty with transitions.

Ring Chromosome 14 Syndrome R(14) Syndrome (OMIM #616606)

This is a rare genetic syndrome for which prevalence and incidence are not known. Moderate to severe IDD is persistent in affected individuals. The level of impairment is largely due to the time of onset of epilepsy and its severity. Language is one of the most affected features. Behaviorally, hyperactivity and stereotypies are often noted. There are reports of ASD being present with the need to adhere to routines as well as being hyper- or hyporeactive to stimuli.

Pitt-Hopkins Syndrome

Pitt-Hopkins syndrome is a neurodevelopmental disorder caused by deletions of the *TCF4* gene located on 18q21.2. Physical signs include abnormal facies and hand abnormalities as well as gross motor deficits. Individuals usually have very limited speech and severe IDD. Many children with this deletion have significant behavioral outbursts with hair pulling, tantrums, inappropriate laughing, and throwing, banging, and kicking objects. There can be self-injurious behaviors or hitting, pinching, and pushing.

ASD has been diagnosed in those with Pitt-Hopkins syndrome. The combination of communication issues driving social interaction issues as well as repetitive behaviors can be present.

METABOLIC DISORDERS THAT PRESENT WITH AUTISTIC-LIKE FEATURES

In addition to genetic syndromes, metabolic disorders can present with autistic-like behaviors (see Table 32.8).

Metabolic disorders remain an important consideration in the differential diagnosis for children presenting with features of autism. Referral to a specialist center for additional testing is recommended as many of these disorders require expert knowledge to ensure that the appropriate testing is requested.

Regression

Loss of developmental milestones may occur in 10–20% of children with ASD often at ~18–24 months. Some children without obvious earlier signs of ASD may show developmental regression by ~3–4 years of age, a condition previously named **childhood disintegrative disorder**; this disorder has been incorporated into the general designation of ASD. In addition, regression may rarely be seen in adolescents with ASD and may be associated with catatonia or seizures.

The cause of regression is often not known; possible etiologies, particularly in those with profound and rapid-onset regression, should include epilepsy syndromes, genetic syndromes (tuberous sclerosis, Rett), neurodegenerative storage diseases (lipid, leukodystrophies), lead poisoning (pica is common in ASD), hypothyroidism, new onset seizures, catatonia, and autoimmune or subacute sclerosing panencephalitis (see Chapter 28).

Catatonia

Catatonia is a serious disorder seen in many neuropsychiatric diseases including ASD. Catatonia usually presents acutely often at the onset of puberty and demonstrates symptoms within motor, speech, and behavioral domains (autism shut down syndrome). Symptoms include stupor, catalepsy, waxy flexibility, mutism, negativism, posturing, mannerisms, stereotypy, agitation, grimacing, echolalia, and echopraxia (diagnostic criteria require 3 of 12 symptoms). Motor manifestations may be hypo- or hyperactivity; self-injurious behaviors may also be present. Behavioral manifestations also include regression, obsessive-compulsive behaviors, withdrawal or depression, sensory sensitivity (light, touch, movement, taste), and a delusional belief that friends or family have been replaced by a double (Capgras syndrome). Treatment includes benzodiazepines and, in refractory patients, electroconvulsive therapy (ECT).

■ SUMMARY AND RED FLAGS

While "unknown" continues to be the current answer for the etiology in the majority of individuals with ASD, it is important for clinicians to be aware of the comorbid disorders and disorders that masquerade as ASD to ensure accurate clinical diagnoses and appropriate utilization of resources for optimal wellness of this population. Red flags or clues to another diagnosis are noted in Table 32.10.

TABLE 32.10   Red Flags
Single or multiple congenital anomalies
Dysmorphic features
Macro- or microcephaly
Epilepsy encephalopathy syndromes
New-onset seizures
Regression
Neurocutaneous lesions
Family history of genetic disease
Catatonia

BIBLIOGRAPHY

A bibliography is available at ExpertConsult.com.

33

Chronic Pain

Gisela G. Chelimsky and Thomas C. Chelimsky

CHRONIC PAIN

Chronic pain is often defined as recurrent or persistent pain lasting ≥3 months. The child may have a definable medical condition but often does not have a specific disease diagnosis or identifiable etiology for the pain other than the pain symptoms (often called chronic primary pain or central pain syndrome), and the central pain syndrome is often associated with other overlapping pain conditions. Chronic primary pain is associated with functional and emotional disabilities but is independent of identifiable biologic or psychologic contributors. The central nature of the pain may occur when the central nervous system's response to pain is hypersensitive. Simple touch that should not be painful is perceived as pain (**allodynia**), or minor noxious stimuli produce an exaggerated pain perception (hyperalgesia). This pain amplification and hypersensitivity to pain create a cascade of events resulting in localized (migraine, low back, jaw) or generalized pain perception. In most patients, the pain is constant but may be intermittent and manifest in a broad spectrum of severity and characterizations (burning, stabbing, dull, paresthesias, sharp). Comorbidities are common and include fatigue, sleep impairment, poor concentration, and disturbances in affect.

Chronic Overlapping Pain Condition

Many pain conditions tend to co-aggregate, coexist, or overlap. Approximately 20% of adults in the United States who report chronic generalized pain will also report having pain in the face or jaw, back, or neck, as well as headache. The National Institutes of Health designated 10 conditions that often co-occur with chronic pain as part of the **chronic overlapping pain conditions (COPCs)**. These conditions include temporomandibular joint (TMJ) disorder, myalgic encephalomyelitis/chronic fatigue syndrome (CFS), fibromyalgia (FM), irritable bowel syndrome (IBS), vulvodynia, painful bladder syndrome/interstitial cystitis (PBS/IC), headaches and migraines, chronic lower back syndrome, and endometriosis. The prevalence of COPCs in adults is ~4-44 million persons. Fifteen percent of the adult population will report neck pain and migraine or severe headache and almost 29% report back pain. Interestingly, when assessing the other comorbid pain conditions, it is important to understand that they will depend on which is the index symptom that is being evaluated. Furthermore, although the cardinal symptom of COPC is pain, other nonpainful symptoms coexist with the COPC such as fatigue, anxiety, depression, sleep disorders, difficulty concentrating, and reduced ability to perform physical activities.

Comorbid Conditions

The term *chronic overlapping pain conditions* implies that these are associated with and comorbid with one another. The concept of comorbidity implies a second condition that either was present or develops during the course of a subject's disease that was a primary initial *index* disorder. In contrast, *multimorbidity* describes the occurrence of two or more conditions without assigning one condition as the index disease. Understanding the pathophysiology of a disorder can be aided by grasping the chronology of disorder development after the index disease. A patient with depression who develops FM should be distinguished from a patient with FM who then develops depression. This distinction is important particularly given traditional beliefs that a psychiatric condition predisposes to a chronic pain condition; however, the evidence does not support this concept. Depression and chronic pain do coexist in 30-50% of patients but may also occur without the other syndrome being present. More than 50% of subjects may have either depression without chronic pain or chronic pain without depression. But in subjects with both conditions, depression and chronic pain have an adverse effect on the other disorder. An antecedent change in either pain or depression predicts subsequent worsening of the other symptom. Depression itself does not cause chronic pain.

A common chronic pain location in adults is the low back, followed in decreasing order by the shoulder, neck or throat, head, hips, abdominal pain, chest/lungs, face/gums, and genital or pelvic pain. Among diagnosed pain conditions, such as FM or migraines, ~60% of adult patients will report multiple pain conditions. The average number of other pain conditions co-occurring with a specific diagnosis varies; cluster headaches, FM, chronic pelvic pain, migraine headaches, and chronic lower back pain have the most other pain conditions. The number of pain conditions and sites involved are predictors of emotional distress. Pain severity itself is not consistently a predictor of depressive or anxiety symptoms. In addition, the number of comorbid disorders is higher with a prior history of post-traumatic stress disorder (PTSD).

Pathophysiology

The pathophysiologic factors for individuals who develop a COPC include certain predispositions such as genetic or epigenetic factors and early-life pain, stress, or traumatic experiences. Later specific environmental changes such as psychologic or physical trauma, infection, or injury may trigger the development of COPC. Patients with COPC have a disordered pain amplification state that is either central or peripherally mediated. A biopsychosocial model may explain the development of and response to a COPC. Most pain syndromes are thought to depend on a neurobiologic mechanism that includes central hyperalgesia, pain amplification, and psychosocial factors that feed back to further amplify pain (Fig. 33.1). These factors include anxiety, depression, history of trauma, current or past stress, previous pain experience, and attitudes and beliefs about pain. In addition, the patient's fear of a significant undiagnosed problem, catastrophizing behaviors or beliefs, loss of control and self-efficacy, and fear avoidance all contribute. Coping strategies play a critical role in managing challenges that the person views as difficult or impossible to deal with based on self-perception and pain beliefs. These strategies require an active effort to overcome thoughts and behaviors that reinforce negative pain beliefs. The pain beliefs constitute the core factor that modulates how the patient will respond to a pain exacerbation ("I am disabled from the pain"; "I will never get back to normal"). **Catastrophizing** reflects the cognitive bias of a negative pain belief, with the expectation that pain will produce a bad outcome in any setting. It contains the three components of *rumination* ("I can't get my mind off the pain"), *amplification* ("My pain is always getting worse"), and *hopelessness* ("Nothing will help my pain"); catastrophizing is associated with a more difficult pain experience, decreased physical and psychosocial function, and more disability.

Pain beliefs are independently associated with physical disability and depression. Poor coping is associated with physical disability, and catastrophizing is associated with depression. It is important to note

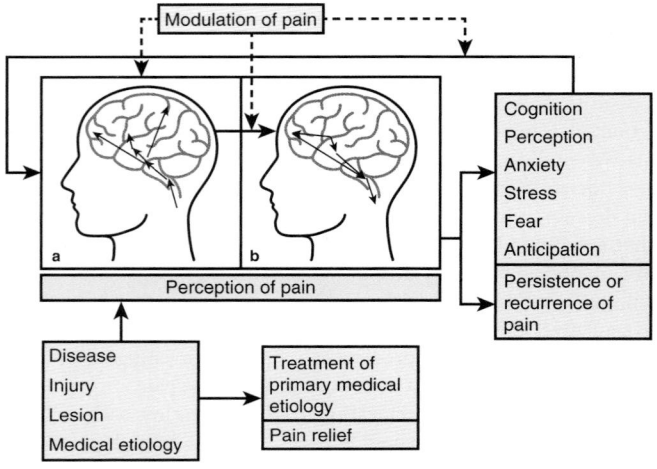

^a Ascending afferent nociceptive pathways for pain perception
^b Descending pain modulatory pathways

Fig. 33.1 Analytic framework or logic model: a possible analytic framework for the effect of the intervention to modulate pain. (From WHO Guideline for the Management of Chronic Pain in Children, https://www.who.int/publications/m/item/guideline-for-the-management-of-chronic-pain-in-children.)

that coping style can be trained and has a major role in the belief system. *Passive* coping strategies reinforce the negative pain construct and learned passivity of the chronic pain syndrome ("When my pain gets bad, I take a pill"), whereas *active* coping strategies constitute an excellent long-term strategy toward chronic pain recovery ("When my pain gets bad, I relax my low back muscles through this exercise"). Pain may also lead to depressed mood probably through fatigue and decreased functionality. Fatigue also contributes to decreased activity and function, worse pain, and poor sleep. Poor sleep, which may be related to pain, in turn leads to decreased pain threshold and more fatigue.

Epidemiology

The prevalence of chronic pain between adult males and females is similar. In adolescents with chronic pain ~30% had both headache and stomachache, ~12% had backache and headache, and ~35% had all three pains (headache, stomachache, and backache), demonstrating the prevalence of these disorders in teens with chronic pain and their overlap. The prevalence of FM in pediatrics is ~6–12% and is associated with generalized aches in >90%, headaches in ~75%, sleep complaints in 70%, reports of joint swelling in 24%, fatigue in 20%, abdominal pain in 17%, and joint hypermobility in 14% (Fig. 33.2). Functional abdominal pain has a high prevalence in pediatrics (2–30%) and is often associated with other chronic pain disorders such as headaches and pain in the extremities, back, and neck.

Management

When evaluating a patient with chronic pain, a careful family and personal history and then a detailed physical exam must occur. Identifying red flags (Table 33.1) should lead to a diagnostic evaluation to uncover their cause. Even when such red flags are not present, the disorders presented in Table 33.2 should always be considered as possible underlying contributors to a chronic pain syndrome.

The practitioner needs to recognize that pain has two critical components: (1) nociception, or sensory pain, the input, and (2) suffering pain, the emotional component. When the patient can distinguish the two components (although the patient may not be able to modify the sensory aspect), they can often learn to modify the emotional response through *active* coping strategies. The approach to the management of chronic pain needs to include an interdisciplinary team. The team typically includes a practitioner who manages medications, a physical

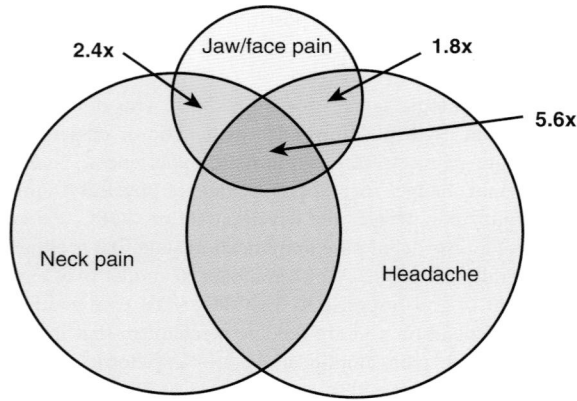

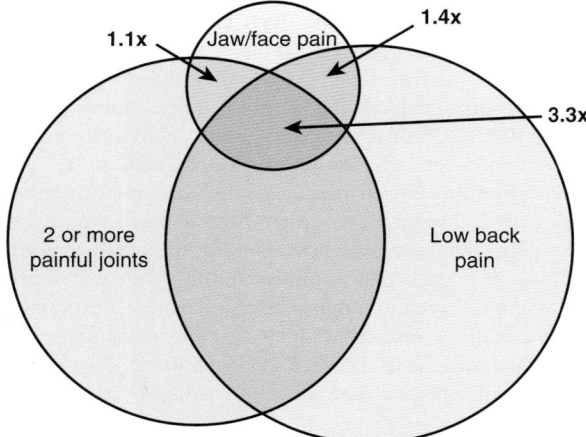

Fig. 33.2 Venn diagram depicting overlap of jaw/face pain and other painful conditions, U.S., adults. Patients with neck pain or headache have about twice the risk of associated jaw/face pain. The association of back pain or joint pain with jaw/face pain was less robust. In both diagrams, the combination of two pain syndromes greatly increased the risk of jaw/face pain (5.6x and 3.3x). (From Maixner W, Fillingham RB, Williams DA, et al. Overlapping chronic pain conditions: implications for diagnosis and classification. *J Pain.* 2016;17[Suppl]:T93–T107 [Fig. 2, p. T96].)

therapist who modifies the motor patterns and behaviors associated with pain, and a psychologist who helps to defuse the negative cognitive set and reduce catastrophizing. Together these specialists set goals to address the easy-to-manage issues based on the patient's goals and motivation. When treating pediatric chronic pain, the practitioner also needs to understand the role parents and patients play in accepting the medical treatment. The factors involved in that decision include the specific pain beliefs and the readiness to take ownership of the disease and engage in the treatment. Chronic pain needs to be understood as a disorder of the brain that requires brain retraining, using the concept of the biopsychosocial model, which includes the social, psychologic, biologic, and behavioral factors that contribute to the manifestation of both health and disease. This model helps the patient move from a pure sensory understanding of pain to a broader understanding that includes the emotional, motor, and stress factors responsible for suffering.

Regardless of whether organic causes are identified that contribute to the chronic pain syndrome, the critical role of the practitioner is *to believe* the patient. Patients with COPC usually have been told that their pain is in their head, that they have school avoidance, that everything is anxiety driven, and to go back to school and stop complaining. To make any progress, a foundation of trust must be built upon the practitioner *listening to* and *validating* the complaints. The history should include enough of a review of systems to understand the extent of the COPC comorbid disorders. The history should also include sleep complaints and fatigue, as well as anxiety, depression, and history of PTSD.

It is useful to ask the patient to keep a diary of their pain and what exacerbates the pain. Often, the patients will report that the pain is exacerbated by stress, bad news, or school activities, or on Sunday night.

The practitioner also needs to elicit the feelings of **catastrophizing**. The clues to catastrophizing may be some variation of the following statements: (1) "I will never get better"; (2) "With this pain, I will never be able to play basketball again"; (3) " I am so tired that I will never be able to get up and start rehab"; and (4) "I will never be able to go to college."

Parents may also express feelings of catastrophizing, which may sound like "We've been to so many doctors without any clear answer they feel hopeless that they will never get better."

Fear avoidance is another factor that interferes with improvement. This can be expressed by the child or by the parent. The child may report that they cannot exercise because of the pain, or the parent may express similar feelings that the abdominal pain is so severe the child cannot start physical therapy.

Readiness for change, measured in pediatrics by the Pain Stages of Change Questionnaire for Adolescents (PSOCQ-A) and for the parents (PSOCQ-P), helps the practitioner understand where the patient and family stand in relation to taking ownership of the disease. These questionnaires have 30 items rated on a 5-point scale. Based on the results, the parents and adolescents can be in the precontemplation, contemplation, and action/maintenance stages (Fig. 33.3). Greater catastrophizing in the parents is correlated with precontemplation. In adolescents, higher catastrophizing is inversely correlated with action and maintenance. The perception that "pain always means a part of the body is damaged" is associated with precontemplation. In contrast, "pain is affected by feeling and emotions" is inversely correlated with

TABLE 33.1 Red Flags

Focal neurologic findings
Abnormal or asymmetric deep tendon reflexes
Papilledema
Age <5 yr
Morning joint stiffness
Pain awakens from sleep
Anemia
Persistent emesis
Chronic diarrhea
Fever, night sweats
Failure to thrive or new weight loss
Bowel, bladder dysfunction
Muscle wasting
Localized pain particularly in distribution of a cranial or peripheral nerve
Positive family history of pain syndromes or chronic medical disorders

TABLE 33.2 Disorders to Consider

Channelopathies
Erythromelalgia: primary (associated with the *SCN9A* gene) or secondary
Paroxysmal extreme pain disorder (*SCN9A* gene)
Small-fiber neuropathy (*SCN9A, SCN10A* genes)
Familial episodic pain syndrome (*SCN11A, TRPA1* genes)

Connective Tissue Disorders
Ehlers-Danlos
Marfan

Immune/Autoimmune
Systemic lupus erythematosus
Sarcoidosis
Juvenile idiopathic arthritis
Sjögren syndrome
Familial Mediterranean fever and other autoinflammatory recurrent fever syndromes
Hereditary angioedema
Chronic recurrent multifocal osteomyelitis
Mononeuritis multiplex associated with vasculitis

Metabolic/Nutrition
Fabry disease
Gaucher disease
Porphyria
Mitochondrial neuropathies
Vitamin deficiency (thiamine, B_{12}, C, D)
X-linked adrenoleukodystrophy

Other
Guillain-Barré syndrome
Multiple sclerosis
Toxic: lead, arsenic, chemotherapy
HIV
Familial amyloid neuropathy
Complex regional pain syndrome types 1 and 2
Sickle cell anemia
Thalamic stroke
Primary, metastatic, or recurrent malignancy (acute lymphocytic leukemia, neuroblastoma)
Neurofibromatosis
Radiculopathy
Nerve entrapment syndromes
  1. Peroneal
  2. Suprascapular
  3. Anterior, posterior hip
  4. Anterior cutaneous nerve (abdominal)

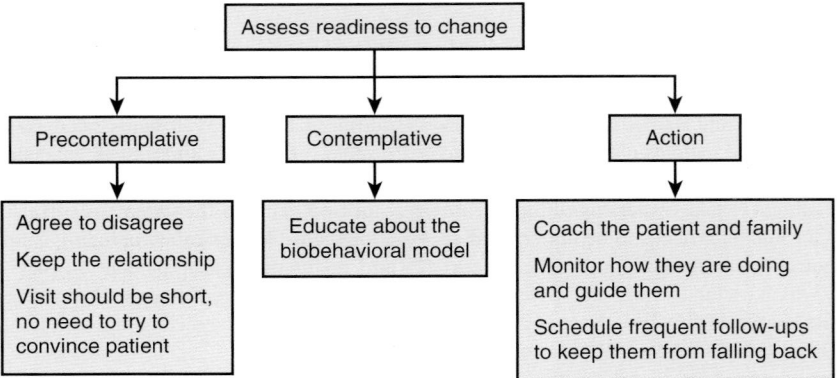

Fig. 33.3 Approach the practitioner should take in each stage of readiness to change.

precontemplation. The **stages of change** are described as follows: (1) *Precontemplation*: The patient and/or parent feel that they have little responsibility for the pain management or control and are not interested in behavioral changes. They feel it is the practitioner's role to manage the pain, therefore still thinking in the biopharmacologic model; they employ a passive coping strategy, which will further amplify the neurobiologic mechanism behind the chronic pain syndrome. (2) *Contemplation*: The patient and/or the parents start realizing that they have some personal responsibility for the pain management/control, and they are considering the biobehavioral role and need to implement behavioral changes. They are still of two minds, one that is resisting and one that is considering the need for behavioral change; their phrases typically include the conjunction "but": "Yes I know I should exercise, but I just don't think I will tolerate it." (3) *Action*: The patient and/or parent are ready to start making behavioral changes.

Knowing in what stage the patient and the parents are determines how the practitioner will manage the patient. If the adolescent or the parents are in the precontemplative stage, the visit should be short, agree to disagree, and build the trust relationship with the patient. Pushing the patient to adopt the biobehavioral model will accomplish nothing or, worse, push them away. With the patient who is a contemplator, educate them about the biobehavioral model and let them think about it, and with the patient who is ready for action, the role of the practitioner is to coach them, monitor how they are doing, guide them, and schedule frequent follow-ups to keep them from falling back.

Therapeutic Approach

The pharmacologic strategy should be viewed as temporary tools (windows of opportunity with lower pain) to help patients start exercising (activation) and advance other behavioral changes through cognitive-behavioral therapy (CBT). The efficacy of pharmacotherapy for the management of chronic pain is limited with a short-lived role. Emphasis should be toward treatments centered on the biopsychosocial or biobehavioral model. Therapy may reduce the perception of pain and enhance positive coping responses, but in general the patient may always have some degree of pain.

Exercise: Often patients have the erroneous concept that exercise will worsen their condition (a common and highly limiting pain belief). Exercise may produce some muscle soreness that resolves over several weeks. The data on improved pain (rather than function or well-being) with exercise are more controversial, with some studies showing improvement and others not, particularly in the shorter term. More importantly, exercise does not worsen pain in the long term, and critically, it improves patient function, leading to greater activation, the definitive treatment of the chronic pain syndrome. Physical activity often improves the psychological well-being of the subjects, leading to less fatigue and depression. When looking at FM in adults,

moderate aerobic exercise or tai-chi is helpful. Tai-chi may produce more improvement in pain than aerobic exercise, probably due to the added mind-body therapeutic effect. When comparing resistance training and aerobic activity, both groups have improvement, but the group that performs aerobic activity has a greater reduction in pain. Water or land aerobic exercises offer similar improvement. Sleep may not necessarily improve with exercise.

Given that hypermobile Ehlers-Danlos syndrome (h-EDS) often is comorbid with FM and other COPCs, it is important to discuss exercise in patients with h-EDS. Children with muscular-skeletal symptoms with h-EDS often complain of pain and have decreased maximal exercise capacity. This is thought to be related to **deconditioning**. Often patients with h-EDS fear movement or activity (fear-avoidance), which leads to increased pain, decreased quality of life, and increased fatigue. Physical therapy improves the pain and quality of life in children with h-EDS and pain; physical therapy is recommended in this setting.

The effectiveness of CBT is often explained by the "neuromatrix theory" of Melzack suggesting that sensory, emotional, and cognitive inputs affect the brain's homeostasis, producing a prolonged stress response with high and continuous cortisol secretion, setting the stage for the development of a chronic pain syndrome. CBT identifies maladaptive thoughts and beliefs and hidden fears and then *reframes* the thinking process to adapt behaviors that will increase function and activation. CBT sessions are aimed at problem solving, goal setting mainly related to doing activities that produce pleasure, exercising and pacing, and some relaxation techniques that the patient can apply at home. An important part of CBT is the assignment of patient homework to practice the new skills and report back.

Patients may be reluctant to see a psychologist because of prior invalidating experiences with practitioners whose message was received as the dismissal "everything is in your head." To avoid this resistance, it is suggested to describe the current biobehavioral model of pain to the patient along with the emotional and sensory components of pain. Patients usually accept this model, and with an appropriate interview and asking what exacerbates their pain and symptoms, they realize that stress is a component and agree to do CBT. Furthermore, the concept of CBT should be introduced early in the relationship to set the foundation for the biobehavioral model. The psychologists should not be introduced late in the relationship when "nothing was found," making the patient feel rejected and dismissed. Rather, the behaviorist is viewed as an active and key member of the team who provides a skillset critical to the recovery process. It should be emphasized that the referral is for the purpose of acquiring a new skillset, and not for any psychiatric diagnosis.

Pharmacologic Management: Opioids *should never* be used in chronic pain syndromes. Prescription of daily opioids, use of extended-release opioids, and combination of opioids with benzodiazepines increase the risk of opioid overdose. Furthermore, every increase in opioid dosage is associated with an 18% increased chance of the pediatric patient overdosing. This risk persists even 6 months after stopping the prescribed opioid medication.

Acceptable pharmacologic interventions include acetaminophen, antidepressants such as amitriptyline or citalopram, antiepileptics such as gabapentin or pregabalin, and serotonin antagonists like pizotifen. One systematic review of the pediatric data did not show convincing evidence that any of these medications was superior to placebo in the very few randomized controlled trial studies in pediatrics. The data available in pediatrics are very limited. In contrast, there is a large body of literature for adult chronic pain. The problem in the pediatric literature is not only the scarcity of publications but also the very low doses of medications used to assess whether tricyclics (amitriptyline), citalopram, and gabapentin were efficacious. Amitriptyline dosage ranged from 10 to 30 mg/day, citalopram from 10 to 20 mg/day, and gabapentin 300 mg t.i.d. Similar data were found with pregabalin (75–450 mg/day) vs placebo in the management of FM, although in this study the doses of pregabalin were higher. When looking at nonsteroidal antiinflammatory drugs, the only reliable studies were done comparing them to other medications. There was no difference in pain improvement between naproxen and meloxicam, celecoxib, or rofecoxib.

In clinical practice when treating adolescents, start with amitriptyline 10 mg at bedtime after checking an ECG for QTc and increase the dosage by 10 mg every 3–4 days to about 1 mg/kg/day if needed. The ECG should be monitored when getting to about 1 mg/kg/day; blood levels can also be monitored. Often if the patient is a rapid metabolizer, doses may need to be increased further while monitoring blood levels and the ECG for prolonged QTc. Similarly, one may use higher doses of gabapentin, sometimes of up to 900 mg t.i.d. Due to fatigue, sometimes we only increase the bedtime dose to 600 or 900 mg.

SUMMARY AND RED FLAGS

COPC is common in pediatrics. The pathophysiology is not well understood, but there is a clear understanding that the chronic pain in COPC is not playing the protective role that it does in acute pain, but rather reinforcing the learned passive role of the patient and reinforcing the neurobiologic basis of the pain syndrome. As a treating physician, it is critical to determine the stage of readiness to change (precontemplative, contemplative, or action) for both the patient and the family, which will dictate the management approach and decrease the time spent in visits when patients or families are not ready to accept the biobehavioral approach. Knowing that the biopharmacologic approach has shown little benefit, practitioners should emphasize gradually increasing activity, exercise, and referral to behavioral health for CBT, with medications playing primarily an adjuvant role when there is need for a "window of opportunity" to pass beyond a physical or behavioral barrier. Red flags (Table 33.1) and disorders not to miss (Table 33.2) are noted in the respective tables.

BIBLIOGRAPHY

A bibliography is available at ExpertConsult.com.

34

Headaches

Sara M. Lauck and Sandra Gage

Headaches are classified as primary or secondary. **Primary headaches** are benign, are not caused by underlying disease or structural problems, and include migraines, tension-type headaches (TTHs), and the trigeminal autonomic cephalgias (TACs). Migraines and TTHs are the most common primary headaches in children and can have less distinct features in children than they do in adults (Table 34.1). While primary headaches may cause significant pain and disability, they are not intrinsically dangerous. **Secondary headaches** are caused by an underlying disease, such as infection, tumor, intracranial hemorrhage, or a vascular disorder, and may indicate an innocuous etiology or portend a serious illness. Most headaches in children are primary headaches or harmless secondary headaches. History and physical examination guide the diagnosis of primary headache disorders, assess the degree of headache-related disability, and reveal information that may prompt evaluation for secondary headaches. Each subsequent visit allows for assessment of the response to therapy and consideration of secondary headaches, the causes of which may confer significant morbidity and in rare cases may be life threatening.

HISTORY

The specific headache diagnosis is determined by the headache phenotype, which is defined in terms of laterality, location (Figs. 34.1, 34.2, and 34.3), timing, frequency, duration, quality, severity, associated symptoms, and alleviating and aggravating factors. In most cases, a single phenotypic headache is present. If the patient has more than one type of headache, the clinician must obtain a specific history for each type. Ideally, the history should be obtained from the child, parent, and any other caregivers, including teachers. Even a young child should be given the opportunity to describe the symptoms experienced with each headache episode and may use drawings to do this.

The laterality and location of the pain should be established (see Figs. 34.1, 34.2, and 34.3). If the pain is unilateral, it should be noted whether the pain is always on one side or if the side varies. The location may be restricted or more widely distributed; if the location varies from one episode to another, this should be noted as well. Unusual locations in pediatrics may include the occipital region. This location should raise index of suspicion for intracranial pathology if there are abnormal neurologic findings or the headache does not meet criteria for a primary headache disorder.

The timing, frequency, and duration of headaches should be described, as the temporal patterns of headaches are useful in creating a differential diagnosis, identifying the need for work-up, and classifying the type of headache. The temporal categories of headache include acute, acute recurrent, chronic nonprogressive, and chronic progressive (Table 34.2).

The severity of a headache does not necessarily correlate with the seriousness of its etiology. Pain caused by brain tumors may initially be mild, whereas the pain of TTHs may be excruciating. Pain is subjective and may be influenced by age, culture, duration, and previous encounters with medical care, leading some patients to unintentionally minimize or exaggerate their pain; as such, pain alone should not be used to narrow the differential diagnosis. An exception to this principle is the **thunderclap headache**, in which the onset of pain is sudden, reaches maximum severity within seconds, and is often described by patients as the worst headache they have ever had. Such headaches may indicate subarachnoid hemorrhage, arterial dissection, or venous sinus thrombosis, among other causes (Table 34.3). Numerical scales, or visual scales for younger children, are helpful for quantifying pain and determining the efficacy of treatment. In older patients, descriptive phrases, such as *mild, moderate, severe,* and *excruciating,* may suffice.

Associated symptoms such as hemiparesis, ataxia, visual loss, diplopia, scotomata, vertigo, seizure-like activity, confusion, mood or behavioral changes, autonomic symptoms, and hemisensory occurrences may suggest neurologic dysfunction or a migraine-related aura. Any history of fevers, syncope, nausea, vomiting, and appetite changes should also be ascertained. Special note should be made if the pain awakens the patient from sleep, is present upon awakening in the morning, or worsens when recumbent; these findings may indicate increased intracranial pressure. Events associated with the onset or aggravation of headaches, such as trauma, intake of particular foods, or physical exertion, may provide insight into the etiology of headaches, as well as potential triggers to avoid.

Alleviation via rest or positional changes should be noted, as should the response of the headaches to medications. A thorough medication history is essential for diagnosing analgesic overuse headaches and headaches caused by medication side effects. The use of over-the-counter medication and prescription medications, including medications that have not been prescribed for the patient, should be delineated, as well as the use of any supplements or traditional remedies. Both primary and secondary headaches may respond to medications and such a response is not diagnostic of any specific headache disorder. For example, relief of an acute headache by triptans is not

TABLE 34.1 Differential Diagnosis of Headache

Headache Type	Genetics	Epidemiology	Characteristic Features	Length	Accompanying Symptoms
Migraine headache	Complex genetics but usually a family history	More frequent in women	Unilateral, bilateral; throbbing; moderate to severe; worsens with activity	Hours to days	Photophobia, phonophobia, nausea and/or vomiting
Tension-type headache	Usually a family history	Equal frequency in men and women	Tight bandlike pain; bilateral; pain may be mild to moderate; improves with activity	Hours to days	No nausea or vomiting; small amount of light or sound sensitivity, but not both
Cluster headache	May have a family history	More frequent in men	Unilateral severe pain in the face	Minutes to hours	Ipsilateral ptosis, miosis, rhinorrhea, eyelid edema, tearing
Paroxysmal hemicrania	Usually no family history	More frequent in women	Unilateral pain in the face	Minutes	Ipsilateral ptosis, miosis, rhinorrhea, eyelid edema, tearing; responds to indomethacin
Short unilateral headache with conjunctival injection, tearing	No family history	More frequent in men	Unilateral eye pain; orbit pain	Typically 4 min or less	Conjunctival injection, tearing
Hemicrania continua	No family history	More frequent in women	Unilateral continuous headache with episodic stabbing pains	Continuous	Ipsilateral ptosis, miosis, rhinorrhea, eyelid edema, tearing

From Digre KB. Headaches and other head pain. In: Goldman L, Schafer AI, eds. *Goldman-Cecil Medicine.* 25th ed. Philadelphia: Elsevier; 2016, Table 398-2.

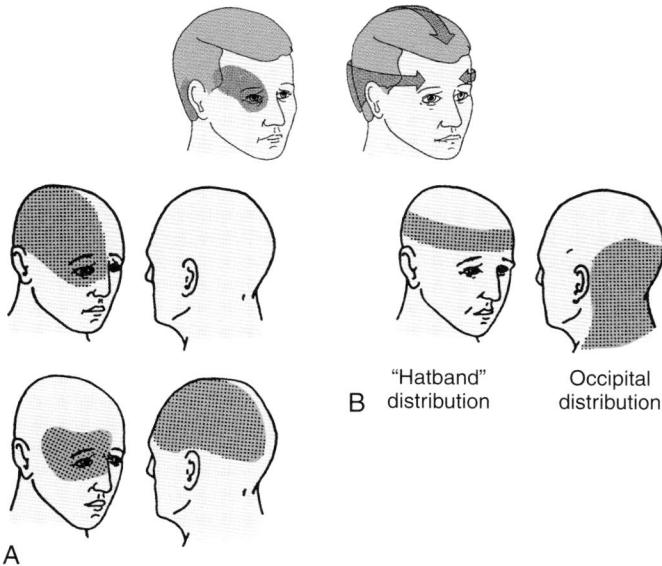

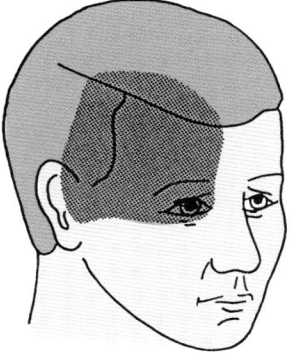

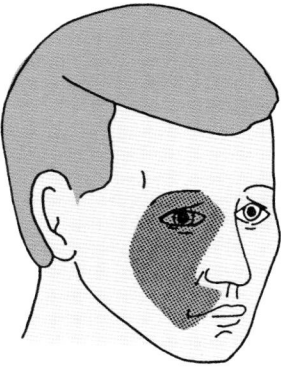

Fig. 34.1 Common location of migraine *(A)* and tension *(B)* headaches. Of note, some tension headaches may be unilateral, while migraines may occur in the same distribution (including bilateral) as tension headaches. (From Reilly BM. *Practical Strategies in Outpatient Medicine.* 2nd ed. Philadelphia: WB Saunders; 1991.)

"Hatband" distribution

Occipital distribution

Ocular disease
Frontal sinusitis
Temporomandibular syndrome
Temporal arteritis
Tension headache
Migraine
Cluster

Ocular disease
Maxillary sinusitis
Dental infection
Allergic/vasomotor rhinitis
Nasopharyngeal tumor
Trigeminal neuralgia
Migraine
Cluster

Fig. 34.2 Periorbital headache. (From Reilly BM. *Practical Strategies in Outpatient Medicine.* 2nd ed. Philadelphia: WB Saunders; 1991.)

diagnostic of migraine, as triptans may also be effective for other causes of headache.

In patients with recurring headaches, the history may be clarified by keeping a **headache diary**, which can additionally determine headache patterns, identify triggers, aid diagnosis, and assess the efficacy of therapy (Table 34.4). A headache diary may also assist in determining the degree of disability caused by the headache. Disability evaluation may be augmented by school attendance and performance records. Headaches that improve with the onset of the summer school holiday may suggest that a child is struggling academically or is being bullied at school. In younger children, where detailed personal descriptions of pain may be more difficult to

obtain and record in a diary, videos of the headache episodes may aid diagnosis.

The past medical history may reveal a risk for potentially serious causes of secondary headaches that require prompt evaluation, such as sickle cell disease, thyroid disorders, parathyroid dysfunction, malignancy, hypercoagulability, hypertension, immunodeficiency, congenital heart disease, autoimmune disorders, and arteriovenous malformations. Allergic rhinitis and other atopic disorders are also associated with headaches. Infantile colic, benign paroxysmal torticollis, cyclic vomiting syndrome, and benign paroxysmal vertigo are considered **episodic syndromes that may be associated with migraine** and may *precede* the development of typical migraine symptoms later in life. In females, a menstrual history should be obtained, including details of the cycle and the timing of headaches with respect to the menstrual cycle. A history of secondary

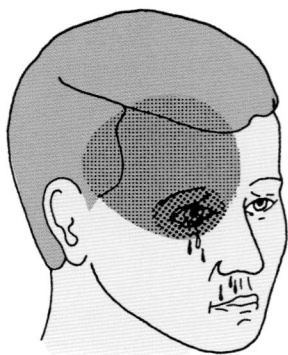

Periorbital or **frontotemporal** location is usual

Tears and **nasal stuffiness,** often unilateral, accompany the headache

Duration is usually brief (1 hour)

Fig. 34.3 Cluster headache. (From Reilly BM. *Practical Strategies in Outpatient Medicine.* 2nd ed. Philadelphia: WB Saunders; 1991.)

TABLE 34.3   Main and Rare Causes of Thunderclap Headache

Main Causes	Rare Causes
Vascular Disorders	
Subarachnoid hemorrhage	Pituitary apoplexy, arteritis, angiitis
Intracerebral hemorrhage	Unruptured vascular malformation,
Cerebral venous thrombosis	aneurysm
Spontaneous intracranial	Arterial hypertension
hypotension	Cerebral segmental vasoconstriction
Cervical artery dissection	
Nonvascular Disorders	
	Greater occipital neuralgia
	Intermittent hydrocephalus by colloid cyst
Infections	
Meningitis, encephalitis	Erve virus (European Nairovirus)
	Sinusitis
Primary Headache Disorders	
Migraine	Cluster headache
Primary thunderclap headache	Tension headache, new daily persistent
Primary exertional headache	headache
Primary cough headache	

From Linn FHH. Primary thunderclap headache. In: Aminoff MJ, ed. *Handbook of Clinical Neurology.* Vol. 97. New York: Elsevier; 2010:473–481.

TABLE 34.2   Four Temporal Patterns of Childhood Headache

Acute: Single episode of pain without a history of such episodes. The "first and worst" headache raises concerns for aneurysmal subarachnoid hemorrhage in adults but is commonly due to *febrile illness* related to upper respiratory tract infection in children. Regardless, more ominous causes of acute headache (hemorrhage, meningitis, tumor) must be considered.

Acute recurrent: Pattern of attacks of pain separated by symptom-free intervals. Primary headache syndromes, such as *migraine or tension-type* headache, usually cause this pattern. Recurrent headaches are occasionally due to specific epilepsy syndromes (benign occipital epilepsy), substance abuse, or recurrent trauma.

Chronic progressive: Implies a gradually increasing frequency and severity of headache. The pathologic correlate is *increasing ICP.* Causes of this pattern include pseudotumor cerebri, brain tumor, hydrocephalus, chronic meningitis, brain abscess, and subdural collections.

Chronic nonprogressive or chronic daily: Pattern of frequent or constant headache. Chronic daily headache generally is defined as >3-mo history of >15 headaches/mo, with headaches lasting >4 hr. Affected patients have normal neurologic examinations; psychologic factors and anxiety about possible underlying organic causes are common.

From Huang Schiller J, Shellhaas RA. Headache and migraine. In: Marcdante KJ, Kliegman RM, eds. *Nelson Essentials of Pediatrics.* 8th ed. Philadelphia: Elsevier; 2019:686.

TABLE 34.4   The Headache Diary for Recurring Headaches*

Date
Time of onset
Time of resolution
Maximum level of pain (mild, moderate, or severe *or* according to a visual or numerical pain scale)
Triggers:
    Sleep
    Foods†
    Activities
    Medications
Modifiers:
    Response to position changes or Valsalva maneuver
    Medications used (dose, response)
    Other modifiers
Additional symptoms

*If more than one type of headache exists, the types should be defined and labeled, and separate data should be recorded for each type.
†Foods are believed to be less associated with triggering migraines than previously.

---

amenorrhea could suggest pituitary or other central nervous system neoplasms.

The family history should be probed for any genetic predisposition to migraines, aneurysms, other vascular malformations, early-onset strokes, or brain neoplasms. A negative family history for primary headaches should cause the clinician to be more cautious in assigning the diagnosis of a primary headache disorder. Social history should investigate for psychosocial factors that may influence or be influenced by headaches, such as school performance, the relationships between family members, recent changes in social structure, and substance abuse in the patient or the family. The provider should also screen for indications of neglect or abuse. Detailed psychologic evaluation with screening for symptoms of depression and anxiety may be indicated.

Some historical components are classic features of primary headaches, while others are concerning for secondary headaches

TABLE 34.5 History-Related Red Flags for Secondary Headaches

Quality:
  "Thunderclap" rapid-onset headache or the "worst headache of my life"
  Recent worsening in severity or frequency
  Change in quality
  New-onset symptoms consistent with cluster headache
Location:
  Unilateral without alteration of sides
  Chronic or recurrent occipital headache
Timing:
  Awakens from sleep
  Occurs in morning or causes morning vomiting
  Acute or chronic progressive pattern
Positional or activity-related variations:
  Worsened in the recumbent position or when bending over
  Headache experienced or worsened with cough or the Valsalva maneuver
Associated neurologic history:
  Neurologic dysfunction other than typical aura
  Altered sensorium during headache
  Sensory deficits or changes in vision, gait, or coordination
  Other focal neurologic deficits
  Seizures or syncope
  Decreased visual acuity
  Mental status changes (e.g., confusion or disorientation)
  Regression in fine or gross motor developmental skills
  Decline in cognition or school performance
  Change in mood, behavior, or personality
Associated general history:
  Vomiting without nausea and morning/fasting nausea or vomiting
  Polyuria or polydipsia
  Preschool or younger age
  History of head trauma
  Neck pain
  Medical comorbidities
  History of ventriculoperitoneal shunt
  Certain medications
  Signs of systemic or localized head/neck infection
  Negative family history of primary headache disorders

TABLE 34.6 Physical Examination Red Flags for Secondary Headaches

Abnormal vital signs:
  Hypertension
  Growth failure
  Increased head circumference or bulging fontanel
  Fever
Meningeal signs with or without fever
Evidence of cranial trauma
Cranial bruit
Frontal bony tenderness
Macrocephaly
Abnormal ophthalmologic findings:
  Papilledema
  Abnormal ocular movements
  Squinting
  Pathologic pupillary response
  Visual field defects
Abnormal neurologic findings:
  Impaired mental status
  Cranial nerve palsy
  Ataxia
  Abnormal gait
  Abnormal coordination
  Abnormal reflexes
  Asymmetric motor or sensory examination
  Hemiparesis
  Developmental regression
Precocious, delayed, or arrested puberty
Skin findings:
  Café-au-lait or ash leaf macules
  Petechiae or purpura
  Facial hemangioma
  Malar rash

(Table 34.5). Throughout the history, the clinician should constantly assess for warning signs of serious and sometimes life-threatening causes of secondary headache. The identification of any of these red-flag symptoms should cause concern and lead promptly to further investigation.

PHYSICAL EXAMINATION

Abnormalities in the examination may provide clues to the underlying etiology of secondary headaches, and red flags may identify specific diagnoses of concern (Table 34.6). Vital signs assessment may reveal elevated blood pressure, which may be the cause of headache, signal increased intracranial pressure, or herald an underlying renal abnormality. Fever may be a sign of an infectious or inflammatory process. Growth parameters, including height, weight, body mass index, and head circumference, should be obtained. Poor weight gain may indicate an underlying chronic illness associated with headaches, such as celiac disease, respiratory disorders, neurofibromatosis type 1, or neglect. Obesity should alert the clinician to assess for symptoms of obstructive sleep apnea or idiopathic intracranial

hypertension (IIH). Enlarged head circumference associated with signs of headache or other evidence of increased intracranial pressure warrants alarm.

The general examination starts with assessment of mental status and overall level of distress. The head and neck examination should assess specifically for nasal congestion, sinus tenderness, and signs of allergic rhinitis, such as boggy nasal turbinates. Frontal bone tenderness could be an early sign of Pott puffy tumor, a complication of frontal sinusitis. Tenderness over the mandibular condyle in children with dental malocclusion, or jaw crepitus in patients with arthritis, may indicate temporomandibular joint dysfunction as a cause of headache. Thorough lymphatic, respiratory, cardiac, and abdominal examinations should also be completed. Genitourinary examination should include pubertal stage, as headaches may be associated with endocrine disorders. Skin should be evaluated for petechiae, atopic or vasculitis findings, and lesions associated with neurocutaneous syndromes such as neurofibromatosis or tuberous sclerosis. Signs of trauma should be noted. Neurologic examination should be detailed and include assessments of mental status, cranial nerves, auditory function, sensation, motor strength, reflexes, gait, coordination, and speech. Whenever possible, a thorough ophthalmologic examination should be undertaken, including visual acuity testing and a funduscopic evaluation for papilledema (Fig. 34.4). In a young child, much of the neurologic examination is completed through observation or engaging the child in play to elicit

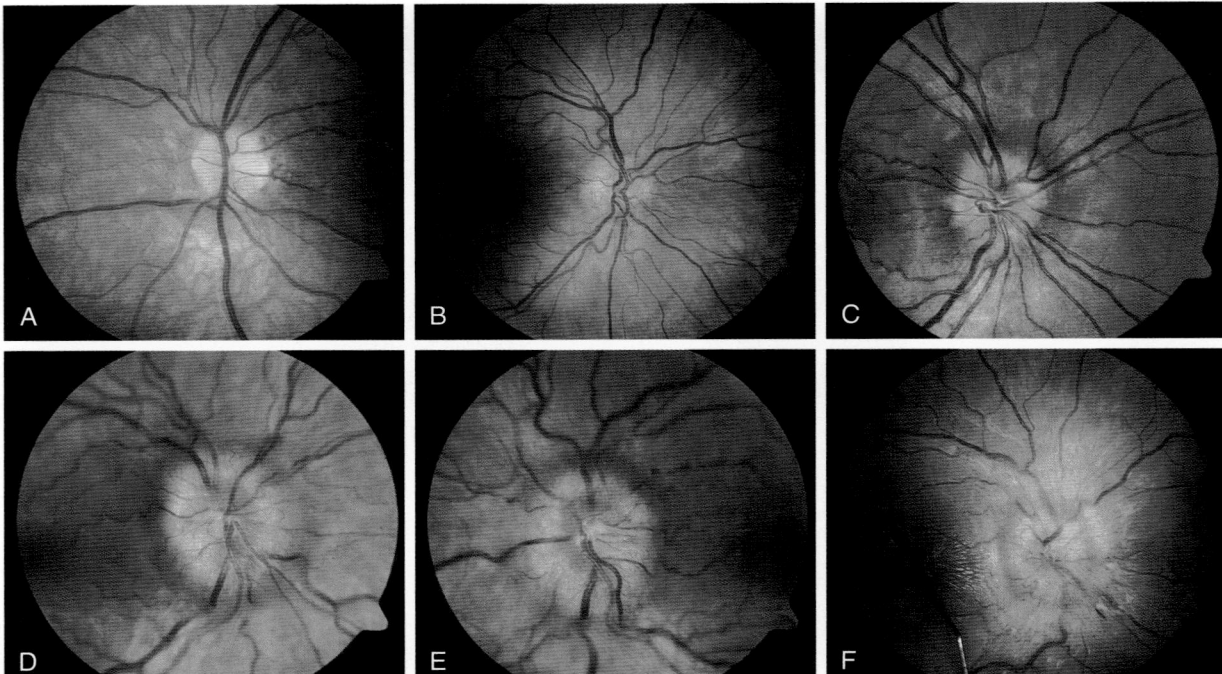

Fig. 34.4 Stages of papilledema (Frisen scale). *A,* Stage 0: normal optic disc. *B,* Stage 1: very early papilledema with obscuration of the nasal border of the disc only, without elevation of the disc borders. *C,* Stage 2: early papilledema showing obscuration of all borders, elevation of the nasal border, and a complete peripapillary halo. *D,* Stage 3: moderate papilledema with elevation of all borders, increased diameter of the optic nerve head, obscuration of vessels at the disc margin, and a peripapillary halo with finger-like extensions. *E,* Stage 4: marked papilledema characterized by elevation of the entire nerve head and total obscuration of a segment of a major blood vessel on the disc. *F,* Stage 5: severe papilledema with obscuration of all vessels and obliteration of the optic cup. Note also the nerve fiber layer hemorrhages and macular exudate. (*A–C* courtesy Dr. Deborah Friedman; *D–F* courtesy Flaum Eye Institute, University of Rochester.)

findings. A complete ophthalmologic evaluation may be limited by lack of cooperation or comprehension. If the clinician is unable to complete or interpret the neurologic and ophthalmologic assessments, the support of a neurologist and an ophthalmologist may be required. If the results of examination suggest a structural brain lesion or increased intracranial pressure, neuroimaging is warranted (Table 34.7). However, many causes of headache, including some serious diseases early in their course, do not present with abnormal findings on physical examination or have fluctuating abnormal findings (Table 34.8). A single normal physical examination does not exclude pathology; thus, periodic reassessments are essential if headache persists.

NEUROIMAGING

Most children do not require neuroimaging for headaches, and it is rarely indicated in children with recurrent headaches and a normal neurologic and ophthalmologic exam. Neuroimaging should be considered when the headache history or symptomatic progression is incompatible with a primary headache disorder or if there is no family history of primary headache disorder. Furthermore, neuroimaging in the assessment of headaches in children is indicated when the following features are present: abnormal neurologic exam or historical findings; new onset of afebrile seizures or alteration in seizure type or frequency; new severe headache; change in frequency or severity of headaches; headache consistent with increased intracranial pressure; association of headache with cough or bending over; concerning past medical history components, including trauma or presence of a ventriculoperitoneal shunt; and age younger than 6 years (Table 34.9). In specific cases, neuroimaging may be considered when there is history of a brain tumor in the family, fear by the patient or the parents of underlying pathology, or inability to obtain an accurate physical examination due to lack of patient cooperation.

MRI and CT are the neuroimaging modalities to consider (Table 34.10). CT remains the most sensitive and rapid method for detecting acute intracranial bleeding and is preferred in emergency situations or when MRI is contraindicated or unavailable. *MRI is otherwise the preferred imaging modality,* offering superior visualization of soft tissue contrast and gray-to-white matter differentiation without exposing the patient to the ionizing radiation associated with CT scanning. While gadolinium contrast for MRI is considered safe, it is not usually necessary. An MRI contrast study should be considered when there is concern for infection or if the noncontrast study is abnormal. MRI may involve the need for sedation, particularly in younger children. Normal neuroimaging and a single normal neurologic examination should not give complete reassurance. Follow-up assessment of ongoing symptoms or for changes in the physical examination remains necessary.

LABORATORY INVESTIGATIONS

Routine blood work is not indicated when history suggests a primary headache disorder and physical and neurologic examinations are normal. Findings in the history, physical examination, or neuroimaging that dictate directed laboratory evaluation are listed in Table 34.11.

TABLE 34.7 Headache Disorders Associated with Neurologic Signs

Headache	Pain Profile	Neurologic Sign
Complicated migraine	AR	Hemiparesis, aphasia, paresthesia, hemianopia
Migraine with brainstem aura	AR	Dysarthria, vertigo, tinnitus, hypoacusis, diplopia, ataxia, decreased level of consciousness
Acute confusional migraine	AR	Alteration in migraine sensorium, stupor, agitation, fugue state
Vasculitis	CP, AR	Seizure, changes in sensorium
Brain neoplasm or mass	CP	Papilledema, focal deficit
Hydrocephalus	CP, AR	Papilledema, bilateral sixth nerve palsies, increased motor tone, impaired upward gaze and Parinaud syndrome
Idiopathic intracranial hypertension	CP	Papilledema, constricted visual fields, enlarged blind spot
Subarachnoid hemorrhage, ruptured aneurysm	A	Changes in sensorium, focal neurologic signs, meningismus
Subdural or epidural hemorrhage	CP	Focal neurologic signs, papilledema, changes in sensorium
Sagittal sinus thrombosis	A	Papilledema, focal neurologic deficits, changes in sensorium, seizures
Meningitis, encephalitis	A	Focal neurologic deficits, changes in sensorium, seizures
Optic neuritis	A	Papillitis, decreased visual acuity, afferent pupillary defect

A, acute; AR, acute recurrent; CP, chronic progressive.

TABLE 34.8 Headache Disorders with No Neurologic Signs

Headache Disorder	Pain Profile
Tension-type headache	CN, AR
Migraine without aura	AR, CN
Cluster headache	AR
Hypertension, uncomplicated	AR, CN
Fever	A
Anoxia	A
Medication overuse	CN
Caffeine withdrawal	A, AR
Early hydrocephalus or brain mass	CP
Cough headache, uncomplicated	AR
Meningitis, uncomplicated	A
Sinusitis, dental or pharyngeal abscess	AR
Temporomandibular joint syndrome	CN
Postconcussive syndrome	CN
Conversion disorder	CN

A, acute; AR, acute recurrent; CN, chronic nonprogressive; CP, chronic progressive.

TABLE 34.9 Reasons to Obtain Neuroimaging in a Child with Headache

Abnormal neurologic findings on examination including papilledema
History of abnormal or focal neurologic symptoms
New onset of afebrile seizures or alteration in seizure type or frequency
Recent onset of severe headache
New headache or change in pattern/severity of previously stable headache
Symptoms concerning for increased intracranial pressure such as headache:
- Occurring in the morning
- Worse in recumbent position
- Waking the child from sleep
- Associated with morning vomiting

Cough headache or headache when bending over
Atypical auras with presumed migraine headache
Headache consistent with trigeminal autonomic cephalgia
Recent or remote trauma
Medical comorbidities such as ventriculoperitoneal shunt
Young age (less than 6 yr) or inability to describe headache
Incompatibility of headache with primary headache disorder
Lack of family history of primary headache disorder

TABLE 34.10 Neuroimaging Modalities

Advantages of MRI

Most vascular malformations are detected
Accurate detection of tumors in temporal lobes and posterior fossa, and small tumors that obstruct CSF flow (e.g., quadrigeminal plate and third ventricular)
Paranasal sinuses usually included in the examination without special request
More sensitive for detecting transependymal CSF in cases of borderline hydrocephalus
Diagnostic for Chiari malformations
Magnetic resonance angiography can detect many aneurysms
Magnetic resonance venography can detect cortical vein and dural sinus thrombosis

Advantages of CT

Can rapidly diagnose intracranial bleed
Shorter imaging time, important in evaluating critically ill patients
May be used in patients with pacemakers, metal implants (surgical clips), and cosmetic tattoos (MRI may turn off pacemakers and dislodge the clips; tattoos distort the image)
Less expensive and easier access than MRI

CSF, cerebrospinal fluid.

CLASSIFICATION OF HEADACHES

Headaches are classified broadly as primary or secondary. The acuity or chronicity of the headache helps to guide the development of the differential diagnosis (Fig. 34.5).

Primary Headaches

There are three categories of primary headaches: TTH, migraine headache, and the TACs. TTH and migraine are the most common headache types in children and adolescents.

Tension-Type Headaches

TTHs are common in pediatrics with a broad prevalence range reported. These headaches have a typical pattern. Patients awaken

TABLE 34.11　Potentially Useful Tests and Studies in Children with Headaches

Laboratory Test	Possible Cause of Headache
CBC	Infection (elevated white blood cell count); bleeding diathesis (thrombocytopenia); anemia
CSF examination with opening pressure	Infection, vasculitis, pseudotumor cerebri, subarachnoid hemorrhage after CT is normal
Toxicology assays	Substance abuse, possible toxin exposure, carbon monoxide
Hypercoagulation panel	Unexplained venous sinus thrombosis
ESR, ANA, ANCA	Vasculitis
Genetic tests	Familial hemiplegic migraine, MELAS, CADASIL, CARASIL
EEG	Seizure disorder
Electrolytes, ECG, UA	Hypertension, renal disease
VP shunt radiographic series	Malfunctioning VP shunt
Blood glucose	Hypoglycemia or hyperglycemia
Serum calcium	Hyperparathyroidism

ANA, antinuclear antibody; ANCA, antineutrophil cytoplasmic antibodies; CADASIL, cerebral autosomal dominant arteriopathy with subcortical infarcts and leukoencephalopathy; CARASIL, cerebral autosomal recessive arteriopathy with subcortical infarcts and leukoencephalopathy; CSF, cerebrospinal fluid; MELAS, mitochondrial encephalomyopathy, lactic acidosis, and strokelike episodes; VP, ventriculoperitoneal.

feeling well, with pain beginning gradually and escalating throughout the day. Pain is constant, squeezing, nonpulsatile, and located in a band extending from the front of the head, across the temples, and toward the occiput or neck. Photophobia and phonophobia may accompany these headaches but are not a constant feature; patients with TTH typically do not experience both photophobia and phonophobia in the context of a single episode. Unlike migraine headaches, routine physical activity does not tend to influence the severity of the headache. In patients with long-standing pain, the headaches may assume characteristics of migraines; indeed, TTHs often accompany other headache disorders.

TTHs are classified by the International Classification of Headache Disorders-3 (ICHD-3) as either episodic or chronic. Both episodic and chronic TTHs are further classified as having associated pericranial tenderness or as lacking such tenderness. This tenderness is typically present between headaches and increases during episodes. **Episodic tension-type headache** (acute recurrent) is categorized as either infrequent or frequent. Infrequent episodic TTH is defined as 10 or more episodes total, occurring less than once per month on average. Frequent episodic TTH is defined as 10 or more episodes total, occurring on 1–14 days per month on average for over 3 months. Individual episodes of either may last from 30 minutes to as long as a week and have at least two of the following features: (1) bilateral location, (2) pressing or tightening (non-pulsating) quality, (3) mild or moderate intensity, and (4) not aggravated by routine physical activity such as walking or climbing stairs. Nausea or vomiting must be absent; if present, migraine should be considered. Either photophobia or phonophobia may be present; if both are present simultaneously, migraine should be considered. **Chronic tension-type headaches** are defined as headaches occurring at least 15 days a month for over 3 months, with features otherwise similar to episodic TTHs.

Psychosocial history may uncover the cause of the headache. Adjustment disorders and depression may be either the underlying causes or

reactions to chronic pain. Sleep disturbances, school absences, and chronic analgesic use are common. In some highly motivated and successful children, the headaches may be a reaction to the stress associated with achievement. In this instance, school attendance is usually perfect, and the patient continues to achieve in all realms. However, some patients with chronic TTH may lack a contributory psychosocial history, and the severe subtypes of TTH are now thought to have a neurobiologic foundation.

Patients with TTHs have normal neurologic and physical findings, except for possible tenderness along the affected muscles. These muscles often feel tight, and palpation may trigger the pain. Laboratory tests are not required in the evaluation of TTHs.

Migraine Headaches

The diagnosis of migraine headache is typically based on the historical description of episodes. Migraine and migraine variants occur in early childhood but with an unknown prevalence, as diagnostic criteria for migraine are often insufficient in young children and infants (Table 34.12). Several features distinguish migraine in children from adult migraine. In children, the headaches are shorter, ranging from 2 to 72 hours, and pain tends to be frontotemporal rather than unilateral. Vomiting and abdominal pain are more common in children than in adults, and while photophobia and phonophobia may be present in children, they may need to be deduced by behavior changes rather than by child report. Thus, 5- to 10-year-old children may present with bilateral frontal headaches and associated abdominal pain, nausea, vomiting, photophobia, phonophobia, and a desire to sleep. Unilateral temporal headache location develops in late adolescence, with onset of aura typically in middle school. A family history of migraines is common, with reports of up to 90% of pediatric patients having a first- or second-degree relative with recurrent headaches.

The prevalence of migraine headaches increases with age throughout childhood and is higher in females following the onset of puberty. While the diagnosis of migraine is typically made later in childhood, a careful retrospective history of infancy and early childhood events may reveal early episodic symptoms consistent with migraine, including pallor, vomiting, fussiness, and sleepiness occurring outside the context of concurrent illnesses. Furthermore, benign paroxysmal torticollis, cyclic vomiting syndrome, and benign paroxysmal vertigo are episodic syndromes that may be associated with the diagnosis of migraines later in life.

Certain exposures trigger migraine attacks in susceptible patients. Precipitants include hunger, dehydration, heat or weather changes, exertion, sleep deprivation or irregularity, substance exposures or withdrawal, and psychologic triggers. Food triggers are now thought to be less common than previously believed. In postmenarchal females, migraines may cluster around particular phases of the menstrual cycle.

Migraines are categorized based on the presence or absence of an associated aura. Migraine without aura is the most common migraine phenotype in pediatric patients.

Migraine without aura. Criteria assist in the diagnosis of **migraine without aura** and are based on the number and duration of episodes, as well as symptoms and associated findings (Table 34.13). Children may have shorter-duration headaches. The pain onset is typically gradual and is dull and constant. At times, though, the pain of an episode may be sudden and severe, prompting concern for a thunderclap headache. More typically, pain increases in severity over the course of an individual episode and becomes throbbing. As the headache proceeds, the pain may generalize to the entire cranium. Intense nausea often accompanies migraines, with occasional vomiting. Skin pallor is a common finding. Nasal congestion and tearing may be present. Because most patients are sensitive to motion, light, and noise during

A   HEADACHE

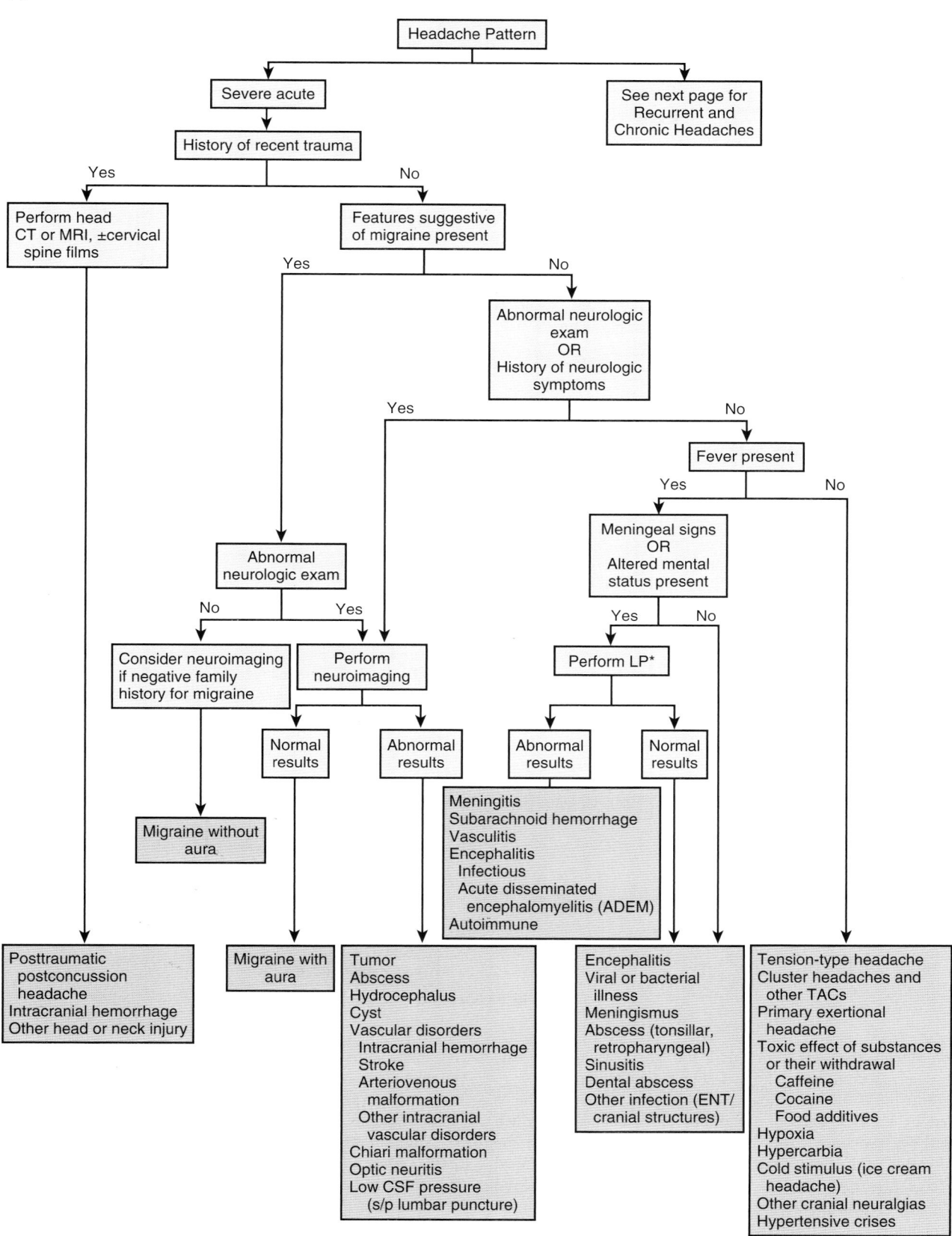

Fig. 34.5 *A–B,* Decision-making algorithm in the assessment of headache. The temporal pattern of the headache must be clarified. Each pattern (acute, acute recurrent, chronic progressive, chronic nonprogressive) has its own differential diagnosis. *Delay LP if signs of increased intracranial pressure but treat and image first. CNS, central nervous system; CSF, cerebrospinal fluid; ENT, ear, nose, and throat; LP; lumbar puncture; s/p, status post; TAC, trigeminal autonomic cephalgia. (From Pomeranz AJ, Sabnis S, Busey SL, et al. *Pediatric Decision-Making Strategies.* 2nd ed. Philadelphia: Elsevier; 2016:185–186.)

Continued

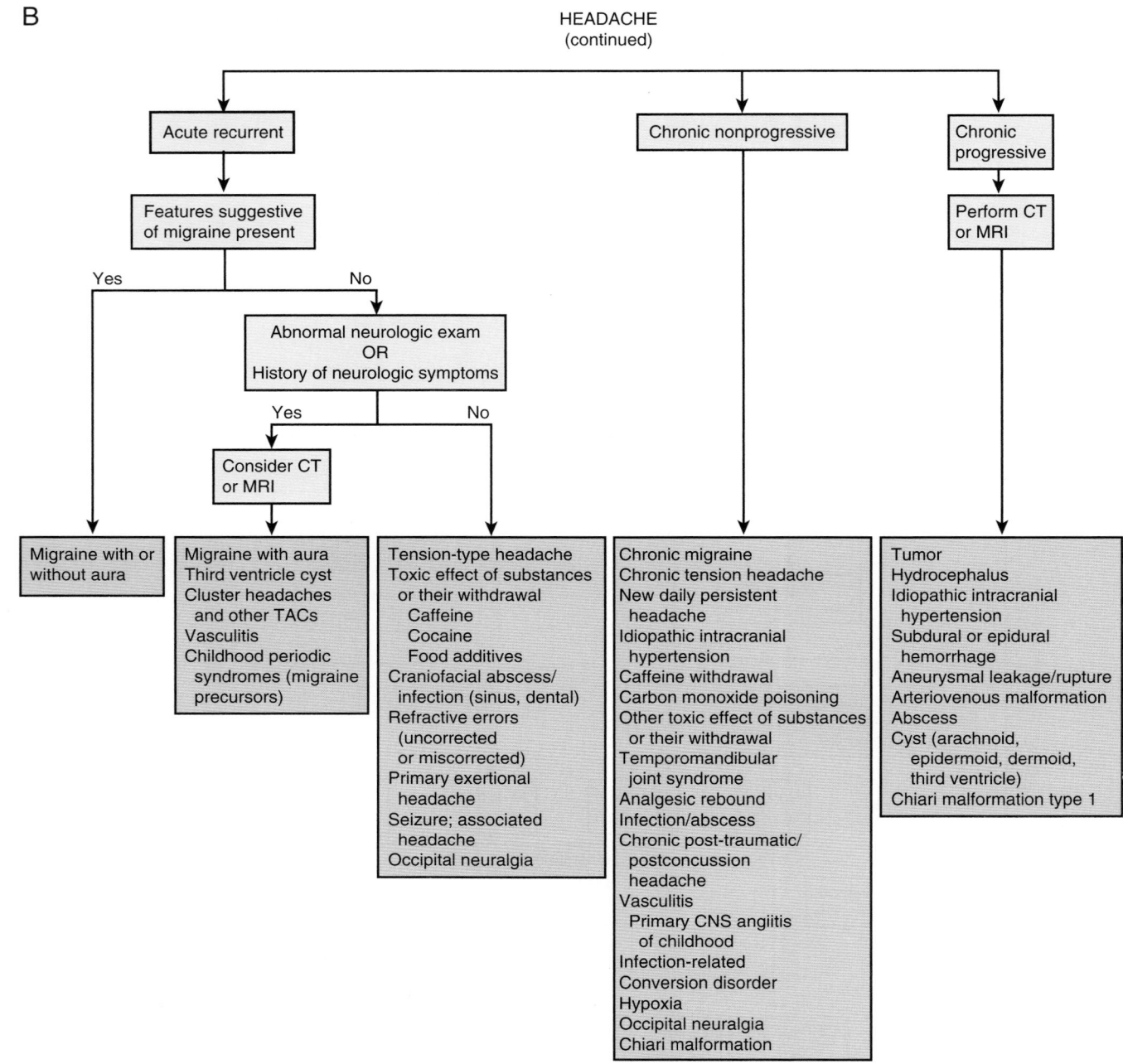

Fig. 34.5, cont'd

a migraine attack, they search for a dark and quiet place to sleep. The patient usually awakens within hours feeling fatigued but pain free.

Migraine with aura. In migraine with aura, the headache is preceded by sensory signs or symptoms termed an **aura,** which is caused by vasoconstriction and diminished blood flow to the affected region of the brain (Table 34.14). In **migraine with typical aura** (Table 34.15), the aura is visual and may consist of blurred vision, spreading scintillating scotomata, flashing lights, zigzag lines, and hemianopia. These features typically last less than 60 minutes. Less classic visual disturbances may occur in children. Sensory auras are less common than visual auras and may consist of numbness or tingling.

Aura should not be confused with a **prodrome,** which may include anxiety, fatigue, hunger, thirst, nausea or depression. A prodrome may

last many hours before a migraine, while an aura usually lasts less than 60 minutes.

Further types of migraine with aura are classified by the specific aura symptoms.

Migraine with brainstem aura (Table 34.16), previously known as *basilar artery migraine,* has aura limited to brainstem symptoms such as dysarthria and ataxia. In some patients, the headache may be a minor component of the syndrome. Visual changes may also occur and may include vivid visual images. Vertigo and tinnitus are less common symptoms. Diplopia, vertigo, and vomiting should prompt evaluation for a posterior fossa abnormality, such as a mass or a vascular malformation.

Hemiplegic migraine has an aura that consists of motor weakness and visual, sensory, and/or speech/language symptoms that are fully reversible. Both familial and sporadic forms have been described. The familial

TABLE 34.12 Migraine Variants

Migraine with or without aura
Acephalic migraine (aura without headache)
Familial (*CACNA1A, ATP1A, SCN1A*) or sporadic hemiplegic migraine
Basilar migraine (ataxia, deafness, tinnitus, vertigo, syncope)
Acute confusional migraine
Vestibular migraine
Paroxysmal torticollis (infants)*
Benign paroxysmal vertigo (infants)*
Transient global amnesia
Abdominal migraine
Retinal (monocular vision loss)
Migralepsy (migraine triggered by seizures)
Cluster migraine
Icepick headache
Migraine strokes

*Episodic syndrome that may be associated with migraine.

TABLE 34.13 Migraine Without Aura

A. At least five attacks fulfilling criteria B–D
B. Headache attacks lasting 4–72 hr (untreated or unsuccessfully treated)
C. Headache has at least two of the following four characteristics:
  1. Unilateral location
  2. Pulsating quality
  3. Moderate or severe pain intensity
  4. Aggravation by or causing avoidance of routine physical activity (e.g., walking or climbing stairs)
D. During headache at least one of the following:
  1. Nausea and/or vomiting
  2. Photophobia and phonophobia
E. Not better accounted for by another ICHD-3 diagnosis

ICHD-3, International Classification of Headache Disorders-3.
Arnold M, Headache Classification Committee of the International Headache Society (IHS). The international classification of headache disorders, 3e. *Cephalalgia.* 2018;38(1):19.

TABLE 34.14 Migraine Auras

Visual
Blurred vision
Zig-zag lines
Scotoma (field deficits)
Scintillations
Black dots
Kaleidoscope
Micropsia, macropsia
Metamorphopsia (Alice in Wonderland)

Basilar
Dysarthria
Vertigo
Tinnitus
Hearing loss
Diplopia
Bilateral vision symptoms
Ataxia
Depressed level of consciousness
Bilateral paresthesias

Other
Cheiro-oral syndrome*
Attention loss (poor concentration)
Confusion
Amnesia
Agitation
Aphasia (expressive, receptive)

*Migrating paresthesia: hand to arm to face to lips to tongue.

TABLE 34.15 Migraine with Typical Aura

A. At least two attacks fulfilling criteria B and C
B. Aura consisting of visual, sensory, and/or speech/language symptoms, each fully reversible, but no motor, brainstem, or retinal symptoms
C. At least three of the following six characteristics:
  1. At least one aura symptom spreads gradually over 5 or more min
  2. Two or more aura symptoms occur in succession
  3. Each individual aura symptom lasts 5–60 min
  4. At least one aura symptom is unilateral
  5. At least one aura symptom is positive (e.g., scintillations or paresthesia)
  6. The aura is accompanied, or followed within 60 min, by headache
D. Not better accounted for by another ICHD-3 diagnosis

ICHD-3, International Classification of Headache Disorders-3.
Arnold M, Headache Classification Committee of the International Headache Society (IHS). The international classification of headache disorders, 3e. *Cephalalgia.* 2018;38(1):20–21.

hemiplegic migraine is an autosomal dominant disorder with genetic variants described in three separate genes: *CACNA1A, ATP1A2,* and *SCN1A.*

Retinal migraine involves monocular visual disturbances that are fully reversible. This migraine subtype is extremely rare, and other causes of the vision disturbance should be investigated prior to designating this diagnosis (see Chapter 43).

The **episodic syndromes that may be associated with migraines,** previously termed **childhood periodic syndromes,** are a group of potentially related symptoms that occur with increased frequency in children with migraine. The hallmark of these symptoms is the recurrent episodic nature of the events. These include gastrointestinal-related symptoms (recurrent gastrointestinal disturbance, cyclic vomiting syndrome, and abdominal migraine), benign paroxysmal vertigo, and benign paroxysmal torticollis.

Acute confusional migraine and **Alice in Wonderland syndrome** are headache conditions that occur primarily in children. Acute confusional migraine, which can be triggered by minor head trauma or have no precipitating event, usually converts to typical migraine with age. Episodes consist of alteration in consciousness, which may include lethargy, agitation, and dysphagia. Attacks last a few hours, with the child eventually falling asleep. The child awakens without memory of the incident. Alice in Wonderland syndrome is characterized by perceptual disturbances in which the sense of proportion or distance, particularly with respect to the body, is distorted. While in adults this syndrome is associated with

migraine episodes, Epstein-Barr virus infection seems to be the most common trigger in children. Migraine mimics are noted in Table 34.17.

Complications of migraine. **Status migrainosus** is defined as a migraine headache that lasts over 72 hours with debilitating pain or associated symptoms. Diagnosis is based on a propensity for previous prolonged migraine attacks. Some patients have an aura that lasts longer than 1 week, termed **persistent aura without infarction.** Conversely, when an aura symptom persists for greater than an hour and neuroimaging demonstrates associated ischemic infarction, **migrainous infarction** is diagnosed. Patients can also have migraine aura-triggered seizures that occur during or within 1 hour of a migraine with aura.

TABLE 34.16   Migraine with Brainstem Aura

A. At least two attacks fulfilling criteria B and C
B. Aura consisting of visual, sensory, and/or speech/language symptoms, each fully reversible, but no motor or retinal symptoms
C. At least three of the following six characteristics:
  1. At least one aura symptom spreads gradually over 5 or more min
  2. Two or more aura symptoms occur in succession
  3. Each individual aura symptom lasts 5–60 min
  4. At least one aura symptom is unilateral
  5. At least one aura symptom is positive (e.g., scintillations or paresthesia)
  6. The aura is accompanied, or followed within 60 min, by headache
D. Aura with at least two of the following fully reversible brainstem symptoms:
  1. Dysarthria (must be distinguished from aphasia)
  2. Vertigo (must be distinguished from dizziness)
  3. Tinnitus
  4. Hypoacusis
  5. Diplopia
  6. Ataxia not attributable to sensory deficit
  7. Decreased level of consciousness (GCS ≤13)
    a. Not better accounted for by another ICHD-3 diagnosis

ICHD-3, International Classification of Headache Disorders-3.
Arnold M, Headache Classification Committee of the International Headache Society (IHS). The international classification of headache disorders, 3e. *Cephalalgia*. 2018;38(1):20–22.

TABLE 34.17   Migraine Mimics and Secondary Migraine

Trigeminal autonomic cephalgias (TACs)
Cluster headache
Hemicrania continua
Short-lasting unilateral neuralgiform headache attacks with or without conjunctival tearing (injection) (SUNCT/SUNA)
Ophthalmoplegic (CN III, IV, VI) migraine
Arterial dissection
Vasculitis/vasculopathies
  Giant cell arteritis
  Moyamoya
  Cerebral autosomal dominant arteriopathy with subcortical infarcts and leukoencephalopathy (CADASIL) *(NOTCH 3)*
  Cerebral autosomal recessive arteriopathy with subcortical infarcts and leukoencephalopathy (CARASIL) *(HTRA1)*
  SLE
  Granulomatosis with polyangiitis
  Primary CNS vasculitis
  Reversible cerebral vasoconstriction syndrome (RCVS)
  Antiphospholipid antibody syndrome
MELAS
Idiopathic intracranial hypertension (pseudotumor cerebri)
Occipital epilepsy
Sudden vision loss
Transient ischemic attack
Acute glaucoma
Sinusitis with intracranial extension
Epilepsy with aura
Transient headache and neurologic deficits with CSF lymphocytosis (HaNDL)
Alternating hemiplegia of childhood *(ATP1A3)*
Fabry disease

CN, cranial nerve; CNS, central nervous system; CSF, cerebrospinal fluid; MELAS, mitochondrial encephalomyopathy with lactic acidosis and strokelike episodes; SLE, systemic lupus erythematosus.

TABLE 34.18   Cluster Headache

A. At least five attacks fulfilling criteria B–D
B. Severe or very severe unilateral orbital, supraorbital, and/or temporal pain lasting 15–180 min (when untreated)*
C. Either or both of the following:
  1. At least one of the following symptoms or signs, ipsilateral to the headache:
    a. Conjunctival injection and/or lacrimation
    b. Nasal congestion and/or rhinorrhea
    c. Eyelid edema
    d. Forehead and facial sweating
    e. Miosis and/or ptosis
  2. A sense of restlessness or agitation
D. Occurring with a frequency between one every other day and eight per day†
E. Not better accounted for by another ICHD-3 diagnosis

*During part, but less than half, of the active time course of cluster headache, attacks may be less severe and/or of shorter or longer duration.
†During part, but less than half, of the active time course of cluster headache, attacks may be less frequent.
ICHD-3, International Classification of Headache Disorders-3.
Arnold M, Headache Classification Committee of the International Headache Society (IHS). The international classification of headache disorders, 3e. *Cephalalgia*. 2018;38(1):41–42.

Trigeminal Autonomic Cephalgias

Trigeminal autonomic cephalgia is rare in children under 7 years of age but has been reported in a child as young as 3 months. Onset typically occurs during adolescence or adulthood. Cluster headaches and paroxysmal hemicranias are types of TAC (see Table 34.1).

Cluster headache. **Cluster headaches** are characterized by episodes of pain interspersed between long periods of remission (Table 34.18). Prevalence in childhood is estimated to be between 0.03% and 0.1%; the disorder is more common in males. Pain is unilateral and localized to the orbital, supraorbital, and/or temporal region. The pain begins suddenly and rapidly increases to an excruciating level. Cluster headaches may be as short as 15 minutes or may last as long as 3 hours; episodes tend to be shorter and less frequent in children. Associated findings include ipsilateral conjunctival injection and/or lacrimation, nasal symptoms, eyelid edema, sweating, miosis, and/or ptosis. Children may have less prominent autonomic features than adults and are most likely to experience lacrimation, conjunctival injection, and nasal discharge. A patient may find it impossible to rest and become agitated and restless during an attack, which is in contrast to migraines, during which the patient becomes quiet and withdraws to a dark, cool room for sleep. However, restlessness may not be as severe or characterizable in children, so observation of behavior is very important.

Cluster headache is categorized as either episodic or chronic. Episodic cluster headaches occur in a series that may last for a week to months, separated by remission periods of months to years, whereas chronic cluster headaches are defined as occurring for at least 1 year without such a remission period or with remission periods that last <3 months. Cluster headaches are more common in individuals who smoke tobacco.

Paroxysmal Hemicrania

Paroxysmal hemicrania is characterized by shorter cluster headache–like attacks, lasting 2–30 minutes, though they can be longer in children. Although the disorder usually begins in adulthood, chronic paroxysmal hemicrania may affect older children and adolescents. Patients have at least five attacks a day, and the pain may awaken the patient from sleep. Children can have facial pallor instead of flushing. This headache typically responds dramatically to indomethacin therapy. Relief of symptoms occurs within a few days of beginning the medication. Other nonsteroidal antiinflammatory drugs (NSAIDs) are of no benefit. Because the symptoms of chronic paroxysmal hemicrania are similar to those of vascular malformations of the brain, a neuroimaging study should be performed to rule out malformation before the diagnosis of chronic paroxysmal hemicrania is made.

Secondary Headaches

Headache Associated with Trauma

Acute headache. If a child presents with a headache after trauma and has abnormal neurologic signs or symptoms, noncontrast CT of the head should be obtained emergently to assess for subarachnoid, subdural, or epidural intracranial bleed. Cervical spine radiographs should be obtained if cervical injury is suspected. If the child has focal neurologic deficits indicating possible vascular injury, MRI is indicated, potentially with magnetic resonance (MR) angiography.

Persistent headache. Headaches may occur as part of the postconcussive or post-traumatic syndrome. The headache is generally constant and may have qualities of both chronic tension-type and migraine headaches. For example, some patients may have nausea, vomiting, and visual auras. Other features of this syndrome are fatigue, dizziness, vertigo, poor memory, decreased reaction times, and inability to concentrate. The neurologic findings are usually normal. Symptoms begin within a week of the head injury and may persist for years. About 70% of patients recover within a year, but 15% are still symptomatic after 3 years. Post-traumatic headache is considered acute if duration is <3 months and chronic if >3 months. The pathophysiology of this syndrome is unknown. Postconcussive syndrome is more common in persons with a history of psychologic or psychosomatic illness. A neuroimaging study may be necessary to exclude the rare possibility of a chronic subdural hematoma. Trauma may also lead to the development of primary headaches such as migraines.

Headaches Associated with Vascular Disorders

Acute ischemic stroke (see Chapter 37). Headache is a feature of up to 30% of acute ischemic strokes. More commonly experienced symptoms are focal neurologic deficits such as weakness of the limbs and face or speech abnormalities; as such, every child presenting with a focal neurologic deficit must undergo evaluation for stroke. CT imaging can show mature acute ischemic stroke; however, cerebral diffusion-weighted MRI is needed to identify early and small infarcts. MR angiography can diagnose vascular occlusion and suggest possible arteriopathy. The headache in acute ischemic stroke is typically of moderate intensity and otherwise lacks consistent features, though may occasionally present as a thunderclap headache. Similar headaches may also accompany transient ischemic attacks.

Aneurysms and arteriovenous malformations. Arterial aneurysms may be congenital (berry) or caused by an infectious process (mycotic). Rupture of an arterial aneurysm is rare in children. The rupture produces an excruciating headache, known as a thunderclap headache. Patients will often describe the pain as the worst headache of their lives. The pain is acute in onset and associated with nuchal rigidity, emesis, and changes in sensorium. The neurologic examination findings may be nonfocal. Noncontrast CT or MRI and an MR angiogram of the head (*neck if arterial dissection is suspected*) are indicated. CT scan reveals blood in the cisterns and meninges in 85% of cases. If the CT scan shows no pathologic process, a lumbar puncture (LP) is necessary in all patients thought to have a ruptured aneurysm. The spinal fluid in a ruptured aneurysm is bloody, xanthochromic, or both. In half of the cases, patients report having previous headaches before having the headache associated with the rupture. These earlier headaches may be caused by leakage of

blood from the aneurysm. If the clinician suspects a leaking or ruptured aneurysm, rapid neurologic and neurosurgical care are mandatory. Arteriovenous malformations may produce similar manifestations.

Venous thrombosis. Cerebral sinovenous thrombosis can present with progressive headache. Additional signs and symptoms can include papilledema, sixth cranial nerve palsy with associated diplopia, focal deficits, seizures, lethargy, and confusion. Prothrombotic states, certain systemic diseases, and head and neck infections (such as meningitis and mastoiditis) and disorders are risk factors for development of cerebral sinus venous thrombosis. Contrast CT venography or MRI venography should be obtained to assess for filling defects, with MRI offering better assessment of parenchyma.

Vascular dissection. Vascular dissection may present with a headache that precedes ischemic symptom development by hours to days. These headaches are typically persistent, nonthrobbing, and unilateral but may be throbbing, thunderclap, and steadily worsening. Infection, coughing, vomiting, and connective tissue disorders such as Ehlers-Danlos disease are risk factors. MRI with angiography of the head and neck is required for diagnosis.

Vasculitis. Vasculitis is an important cause of headaches in adults; in children, headache is rarely the only presenting manifestation of this disorder and is instead a less frequent associated finding. Because of the increased risk of systemic hypertension in patients with vasculitis, it is important to include a blood pressure measurement as part of the complete history and physical examination. When systemic lupus erythematosus and mixed connective tissue disorders affect the central nervous system, children may present with seizures and mental status changes. These symptoms may occur with or without headaches.

Genetic disorders. Patients with **mitochondrial encephalomyopathy, lactic acidosis, and strokelike episodes (MELAS)** may have recurrent migraine episodes and/or acute headache with associated neurologic deficits and/or seizures. MELAS is characterized by strokelike episodes, most commonly in the posterior temporal, parietal, and occipital lobes, as well as lactic acidosis, ragged red fibers on muscle biopsy, and at least two of the following: seizures, dementia, recurrent migraine headache, and vomiting. MELAS is associated with myopathy, short stature, hearing deficits, ophthalmologic problems, learning disabilities, hemiparesis, cardiac problems, and diabetes. Molecular genetic testing is available to identify pathogenic variants in mitochondrial genes associated with the disorder: Over 80% of confirmed cases are related to pathogenic variants in *MT-TL1*; another 10% of confirmed cases are related to pathogenic variants in *MT-ND5*; pathogenic variants in over a dozen additional mitochondrial genes can cause the syndrome as well. Migraines are also common in a variety of other mitochondrial disorders.

Cerebral autosomal dominant arteriopathy with subcortical infarcts and leukoencephalopathy (CADASIL) is a mitochondrial disorder that may present with headaches. Most patients develop symptoms in late adolescence or adulthood, though earlier onset is possible and the disorder should be considered in children with subcortical infarcts, migraines, and multifocal T2/fluid-attenuated inversion recovery (FLAIR) hyperintensities in the deep white matter. CADASIL is inherited in an autosomal dominant fashion and may lead to early stroke or dementia; a suggestive family history should increase suspicion. Pathogenic variants in *NOTCH3* are diagnostic; molecular genetic testing is available. **Cerebral autosomal recessive arteriopathy with subcortical infarcts and leukoencephalopathy (CARASIL)** is due to pathologic variants in *HTRA1*. Associated features include alopecia and spondylosis.

Headaches Associated with Nonvascular Intracranial Disorders

Secondary headaches may be due to a variety of nonvascular intracranial pathology, including increased cerebrospinal fluid (CSF) pressure, decreased CSF pressure, intracranial masses, Chiari type I malformations, and seizures.

Disorders associated with increased CSF pressure. Idiopathic intracranial hypertension (IIH), formally called pseudotumor cerebri, is most commonly seen in obese postmenarchal females, but can occur in prepubertal children. IIH is defined as a new or significantly worsening headache, with associated elevated cerebrospinal fluid opening pressure (>250 mm H_2O or in obese children >280 mm H_2O), that does not meet criteria for another headache diagnosis and has no identifiable cause. Pain is typically worse when recumbent and improves to a degree when upright or standing. The associated headache either develops or worsens with the IIH or leads to its diagnosis and is associated with pulsatile tinnitus and/or papilledema.

Secondary intracranial hypertension may be caused by medication or a variety of medical conditions, including obstructive, toxic, metabolic, infectious, or hormonal causes. History and physical examination will guide whether neuroimaging is indicated (see Table 34.9) and whether evaluation for nonobstructive secondary causes is indicated (Table 34.19). If papilledema is present, neuroimaging should be obtained prior to lumbar puncture to evaluate for other causes of intracranial hypertension, such as a tumor or hydrocephalus. MRI with venography should also be considered in patients who are at risk for venous thrombosis or in those whose presentation does not fit the typical idiopathic intracranial hypertension profile (e.g., males, prepubertal children, and nonobese females), in order to assess for dural sinus thrombosis. In IIH, MRI can show empty sella turcica, distention of the perioptic subarachnoid space, flattening of the posterior sclerae, protrusion of the optic nerve papillae into the vitreous, and transverse cerebral venous sinus stenosis.

All patients with IIH should be monitored closely with special attention to ocular findings, as they are at risk for development of permanent visual impairment secondary to the development of optic atrophy.

TABLE 34.19 Secondary Intracranial Hypertension Without an Obstructive Lesion on MRI	
Hematologic Disorders	**Nutritional Disorders**
Wiskott-Aldrich syndrome	Hypovitaminosis A
Iron-deficiency anemia	Vitamin A intoxication
Aplastic anemia	Hyperalimentation in malnourished patient
Sickle cell disease	Vitamin D–dependent rickets
Polycythemia	
Bone marrow transplantation and associated treatments	**Connective Tissue Disorders**
Prothrombotic states	Antiphospholipid antibody syndrome
Fanconi anemia	Systemic lupus erythematosus
	Behçet disease
Infections	
Acute sinusitis	**Endocrine Disorders**
Otitis media (lateral sinus thrombosis)	Polycystic ovarian syndrome
Mastoiditis	Hypothyroidism
Tonsillitis	Hypoparathyroidism/hyperparathyroidism
Measles	Congenital adrenal hyperplasia
Roseola	Addison disease
Varicella, recurrent varicella-zoster virus infection	Recombinant growth hormone
Lyme disease	
HIV or associated treatment complications	**Other Conditions**
	Dural sinus thrombosis
Drug-Related	Obesity (in pubertal patients)
Tetracyclines	Superior vena cava syndrome
Sulfonamides	Sleep apnea
Nalidixic acid	Guillain-Barré syndrome
Fluoroquinolones	Crohn disease
Corticosteroid therapy and withdrawal	Ulcerative colitis
Nitrofurantoin	Turner syndrome
Cytarabine	Galactosemia
Cyclosporine	Atrial septal defect repair
Phenytoin	Möbius syndrome
Mesalamine	Sarcoidosis
Isotretinoin	
Amiodarone	
Oral contraceptive pills/implants	
Renal Disorders	
Nephrotic syndrome	
Chronic renal insufficiency	
Post–renal transplantation	
Peritoneal dialysis	

From Parker A. Idiopathic intracranial hypertension (pseudotumor cerebri). In: Kliegman RM, St. Geme JW III, Blum NJ, et al., eds. *Nelson Textbook of Pediatrics.* 21st ed. Philadelphia: Elsevier; 2020:3237.

Hydrocephalus usually causes a generalized headache. Slowly developing hydrocephalus initially causes mild pain, whereas rapidly developing hydrocephalus causes severe pain. Most patients with hydrocephalus have morning headaches that lessen after they arise, though pain may also be constant. Physical examination reveals signs of increased intracranial pressure, such as papilledema or tenderness of the neck. Papilledema is usually absent in children with an open fontanel. Macrocephaly is present in young children with unfused cranial sutures and in those with long-standing hydrocephalus. Other signs of hydrocephalus are a bulging fontanel and widened cranial sutures. The head growth chart is especially important in the evaluation of children with hydrocephalus. Head growth is abnormal if the plot of sequential head circumferences crosses percentile lines.

Cough headaches are intermittent headaches caused by transient increases in intracranial pressure resulting from activities that elevate intrathoracic pressure, such as exertion, coughing, or bending. The pain is maximum and severe at the onset of the activity and then resolves in seconds. Patients are usually asymptomatic between events. Cough headaches, which are much shorter than exercise-induced vascular headaches, may be caused by both benign and life-threatening conditions. Structural causes of cough headache include brain tumors, cysts, and Chiari malformations. The results of the physical examination are usually normal, even when structural lesions cause this syndrome. In children, subtentorial tumors account for more than 50% of space-occupying lesions; cough headaches are a cause for concern and warrant an MRI.

Disorders associated with decreased CSF pressure. **Intracranial hypotension** may occur from a tear in the dura caused by trauma, surgery, or lumbar puncture. The etiology of the headache is due to traction on the dura and vessels at the base of the brain. The headache associated with intracranial hypotension typically improves while the patient is recumbent and worsens upon sitting or standing.

The most common cause of a headache from intracranial hypotension is a persistent CSF leak following lumbar puncture. Risk factors for post–lumbar puncture headache include the use of large-bore spinal needles and multiple attempts at obtaining CSF. Patients describe a severe headache within seconds after assuming an upright position. The headache disappears soon after the patient lies down. Other causes of low-pressure headaches include CSF leaks from fractures or tumors at the base of the skull.

Intracranial masses. **Brain neoplasms** are the second most common type of childhood malignancy, though the overall incidence is low. As such, tumor is an infrequent cause of headache in children. The mechanisms by which tumors produce headaches include hydrocephalus from obstruction of CSF flow or direct traction on dural or vascular structures. Headaches caused by hydrocephalus may develop rapidly, whereas traction on dural or vascular structures from tumor growth causes a slow and progressive headache. At the time of presentation, most patients with tumors or hydrocephalus have chronic and progressive headaches, with a history of increasing frequency and severity of pain over time.

Headache secondary to a tumor may or may not be localized to the tumor site. Patients with posterior fossa tumors usually have occipital pain, but if hydrocephalus is also present, the pain may be generalized. Headache secondary to tumor typically demonstrates a slow increase in the severity and frequency of painful episodes; initially, pain may be mild, and over-the-counter analgesics provide adequate pain relief. However, it is important to note that many patients with brain tumors have no particular pattern to their headaches. Patients with brain tumors near the optic chiasm may have visual disturbances, galactorrhea, or other endocrine abnormalities. Diplopia may be present if the third or sixth cranial nerve is compressed; ptosis may also be present.

Other historical features concerning for intracranial neoplasm include changes in school performance, reported motor or balance disturbances, personality or behavior changes, or seizures.

Physical examination often reveals abnormal findings, including papilledema and neurologic deficits. Focal neurologic findings may include eye movement abnormalities, anisocoria, facial weakness, ptosis, swallowing difficulties, hemiparesis, sensory deficits, cranial nerve deficits, altered mental status, and ataxia. Papilledema may be absent in children with posterior fossa tumors (with or without hydrocephalus) or in children with open fontanels. Nonlateralizing signs include increased motor tone as well as third and sixth nerve palsies. Increased motor tone may not be a constant finding and may manifest as transient shivering.

Parinaud syndrome is the triad of upward-gaze paresis, poor pupillary reaction to light, and retraction nystagmus on convergence, and is seen in patients with hydrocephalus or tumors in the pineal region. The presence of Parinaud syndrome always warrants neuroimaging.

Increased intracranial pressure secondary to hydrocephalus and/or a brain tumor should be suspected in any child with chronic progressive headaches, abnormal neurologic examination findings, nuchal rigidity, or abnormal head growth. Patients with these signs and symptoms should undergo neuroimaging (see Table 34.9).

Intracranial cysts are classified as arachnoid, epidermoid, or dermoid. Slow-growing cysts often produce headache patterns similar to those of neoplasms. Epidermoid and dermoid cysts may have sinus tracts that communicate with the skin. Rarely, cysts may rupture and result in increased intracranial pressure and resultant headache. If these cysts become infected, their clinical manifestations resemble that of a brain abscess.

A **colloid cyst of the third ventricle** is a potentially life-threatening cause of headache. With changes in position, this cyst functions as a ball valve and intermittently impedes the flow of CSF. This obstruction causes transient increases in intracranial pressure. During some episodes of obstruction, the patient may be asymptomatic. At other times, symptoms may be severe and include debilitating thunderclap headaches, neurologic posturing, coma, and even death. The intracranial pressure returns to normal when position is changed or when the increased CSF pressure overcomes the obstruction. Physical findings are normal between events. MRI confirms diagnosis. Treatment consists of CSF diversion or removal of the cyst.

Chiari I malformations. **Chiari I malformation** may present with headaches (often occipital and neck) that worsen with cough and Valsalva maneuvers, and may be associated with radicular extremity pain. Patients presenting with this pattern of findings require neuroimaging.

Headaches associated with epileptic seizures. Headache may be a preictal phenomenon in patients with focal epilepsy syndromes or a consequence of an epileptic seizure. Postictal headaches tend to remit within hours of the cessation of seizure activity but may last as long as 72 hours. Headache occurring as an ictal phenomenon in partial seizures remits with, or soon after, the cessation of seizure activity.

Headaches Related to Substances

Medication-overuse headaches. A thorough medication history is essential, as many analgesics may be associated with overuse headaches. All classes of headache medications can paradoxically cause headaches that may be worse on waking and exacerbated by activity. Acetaminophen, nonsteroidal antiinflammatory drugs, triptans, ergot alkaloids, and opiates can be culprits. The diagnostic criteria for medication-overuse headaches include the following: (1) headache occurring on 15 days per month in a patient with a pre-existing headache disorder and (2) regular overuse of the medication taken for acute and/or symptomatic treatment of headache for >3 months. Stopping the medication improves the symptoms.

Caffeine withdrawal headaches. The threshold for withdrawal for each person is variable, but when caffeine is ingested in sufficient quantities for prolonged periods, sudden withdrawal may lead to vascular headaches. In the most common scenario, consumption occurs on weekdays, and because of schedule differences, the caffeinated beverage is not consumed on the weekend. This syndrome is easily diagnosed by history or using a headache diary.

Other substance exposure headaches. **Carbon monoxide poisoning** should be suspected in any child with chronic headaches, as even mild exposure may cause headache and nausea. The diagnosis is difficult to confirm with an arterial hemoglobin carbon monoxide (HbCO) level because the half-life of HbCO in room air is only 4 hours. Hence, the level may be normal only a few hours after exposure. One way of diagnosing and treating this condition is by removing the cause of the exposure. Example sources of carbon monoxide exposure include heavy urban traffic in which the patient is a car passenger, methylene dichloride paint strippers, kerosene space heaters, a gasoline engine running in an attached garage, cigarette smoking, and faulty home furnaces. Typically, co-inhabitants have similar symptoms. Patients exposed to carbon monoxide may have behavioral and neurologic findings days to months later.

Other substance exposures may also lead to headaches. Ingestion of alcohol may lead to headache either during or after consumption. Use of cocaine causes headaches through various mechanisms, including hypertension, vasoconstriction, hypersensitivity vasculitis, and subarachnoid hemorrhage. Elevations in serum lead levels may cause headache (lead encephalopathy).

Headaches Associated with Infections

Infectious causes of headache are common and are typically benign, with the most common etiology being a viral upper respiratory tract infection. However, serious and life-threatening infections may present with headache.

Meningitis and **meningoencephalitis** may present with a headache that is acute in onset and generalized. Fever, nuchal rigidity, alteration in sensorium, and abnormal neurologic findings may be present as well. Children presenting with this constellation of findings require an emergent lumbar puncture with cell counts and differential, glucose and protein quantification with a simultaneous determination of serum glucose, Gram stain, bacterial culture, and any indicated viral studies based on history, physical findings, or local epidemiology.

The child with a **brain abscess** may present with progressive neurologic dysfunction and may deteriorate quickly. Brain abscess should be considered in any child with a right-to-left cardiac shunt, chronic mucosal surface infections (sinus, otitis, dental), endocarditis, and a recent onset of persistent, chronic headaches. These patients may present with focal neurologic findings and signs of increased intracranial pressure rather than fever and nuchal rigidity. Neuroimaging should be considered prior to lumbar puncture, due to risk of herniation with space-occupying lesions.

Headache may accompany infections of the eye and orbit. The signs and symptoms of **periorbital cellulitis** are periorbital redness and tenderness, whereas in **orbital cellulitis**, the patient may also have chemosis, proptosis, ophthalmoplegia, painful extraocular movements, and change in visual acuity. Inflammation of the eye and orbit usually causes localized pain.

The headache associated with **sinusitis** may be acute or chronic. When the frontal or maxillary sinuses are involved, pain is frontal or orbital in location. When the ethmoid or sphenoid sinuses are infected, the headache may be frontal or occipital. Signs and symptoms of sinusitis include purulent rhinorrhea, halitosis, cough, tenderness to palpation over the sinuses

or teeth, and fever. A prior history of allergic rhinitis or sinusitis may be present. The diagnosis of acute bacterial sinusitis in pediatric patients may be made if symptoms of nasal discharge or daytime cough persist without improvement for more than 10 days, clinical course worsens or new symptoms develop after initial symptoms improve, or symptoms are severe at onset with fever of or above 39°C and purulent nasal discharge for at least 3 days. Imaging studies are not required to confirm a diagnosis of sinusitis. However, contrast CT of the head, sinuses, and orbits should be obtained if there are signs of orbital cellulitis, altered mental status, or severe headache associated with sinusitis.

Dental abscesses may produce headaches that are aching or stabbing, and may occur as a complication of dental caries, tooth extractions, or root canal procedures. Physical examination may be normal or may reveal gingival swelling, redness, purulence, or pain. Palpating each tooth individually with a tongue blade may reveal the specific source of pain.

Headaches and/or Facial Pain Related to Dysfunction of Extracranial Structures (Table 34.20)

Asthenopia or eye strain may be a cause of headache and mild, dull, aching discomfort of the eyes. Because it is due to muscle strain that occurs while trying to correct visual acuity, it is not present on awakening and worsens with prolonged visual duties. Referral to an ophthalmologist should be made if asthenopia is suspected. Physical examination is otherwise normal. Abnormal extraocular movements should prompt neuroimaging to evaluate for possible intracranial lesions.

A **corneal abrasion** should be suspected in the irritable infant and in the patient with excruciating eye pain. Diagnosis is made by fluorescein examination of the cornea. Corneal irritation, keratoconjunctivitis sicca, and recurrent erosion syndrome may present with recurrent eye pain that must be differentiated from cluster headaches.

Optic neuritis (inflammation of the optic nerve) often causes ipsilateral retro-orbital pain. Optic neuritis may occur as a single entity, or it may be part of the manifestation of multiple sclerosis. This disorder is rare in children but is more common in adolescents. The ophthalmologic examination reveals papillitis, an afferent pupillary defect, and decreased visual acuity. Often, the findings are normal except for decreased visual acuity. A neuroimaging study should be performed to fully evaluate the orbit and optic nerve and to evaluate for the presence of other demyelinating lesions more consistent with multiple sclerosis.

Malocclusion of the temporomandibular joint (TMJ) may cause chronic headaches. The pain is localized to the side of the affected joint. Some patients report constant pain, whereas others have pain only with jaw movement. An identifying "click" occurs when the patient opens the mouth. Full depression of the mandible may be limited in range. Not every person with a click has TMJ syndrome, and not everyone with TMJ syndrome has headaches. Gum chewing may exacerbate the pain associated with TMJ syndrome. In patients without TMJ syndrome, gum chewing may cause headaches through overuse of the temporalis muscles. Patients with symptomatic TMJ syndrome often find relief with the use of an occlusal splint worn during sleep.

Disorders Affecting Homeostasis

Headaches triggered by **fasting** may occur in individuals with or without primary headache disorders. Children may fast due to dieting or irregular schedules; skipping breakfast before school is associated with increased headache frequency in adolescents. These headaches may occur within 1 hour but generally take 12 hours to develop. A thorough diet history reveals prolonged fasting as the etiology of the headache.

Anoxia and **hypoxia** (<70 mm Hg) may produce headaches through dilatation of cerebral arteries, which in turn causes an increase in cerebral blood flow. Headaches are typically bifrontal, throbbing,

TABLE 34.20 Chronic Facial Pain: Differential Diagnosis

Orbital Pain	Nasal/Cheek Pain
Ocular disease	Sinusitis
Migraine	Facial cellulitis
Cluster headache	Neoplasm (nasopharynx, sinus)
Sinusitis	Vasomotor rhinitis
Orbital cellulitis	Allergic rhinitis
Tolosa-Hunt syndrome	Trigeminal neuralgia
Intracranial aneurysm	Midline granuloma
Cavernous sinus disease (mass, aneurysm)	Granulomatosis with polyangiitis
Giant cell arteritis	TMJ syndrome
Neoplasm	Dental disease
Graves disease	Postherpetic neuralgia
Neoplasm, frontal lobe	Atypical odontalgia
Trigeminal neuralgia	Cluster headache
Postherpetic neuralgia	
Zoster	**Poorly Localized/Vague**
	Sinus disease
Ear/Periauricular Pain	TMJ syndrome
Chronic external otitis	Depression
Relapsing polychondritis	Conversion reaction
Cholesteatoma	Neoplasm
TMJ syndrome	Muscle contraction
Migraine	
Carotidynia	**Dental/Jaw Pain**
Glossopharyngeal neuralgia	Toothache
Thyroiditis	TMJ syndrome
Muscle contraction	Sinusitis
Carotid aneurysm	Neoplasm
Cervical spine disease	Trigeminal neuralgia
Neoplasm	Parotid disease
Zoster	Atypical odontalgia
	Postherpetic neuralgia

TMJ, temporomandibular joint.
Modified from Reilly BM. *Practical Strategies in Outpatient Medicine.* 2nd ed. Philadelphia: WB Saunders; 1991:106.

and worse with exertion, straining, or supine positioning. In children with illnesses that predispose them to hypoxia (chronic lung disease, obstructive sleep apnea), treatment should be directed at alleviating the source of the hypoxia. High altitudes may also lead to an acute hypoxic state. Hypercapnia (levels >50 mm Hg) may also cause throbbing headaches. For nocturnal or morning headaches, in addition to neuroimaging, polysomnography should be considered to assess for obstructive sleep apnea.

Systemic hypertension, both acute and chronic, may be associated with headaches. The pain is related to altered regulation of cerebral blood flow. Acute hypertension typically occurs in a child with underlying renal disease due to poststreptococcal glomerulonephritis, renal failure, or collagen vascular disease. Although hypertension is an uncommon cause of headaches in children, the diagnosis of hypertension is straightforward, and treatment of the hypertension alleviates the headaches. Headaches may be part of **malignant hypertension syndrome**, in which retinal exudates and microscopic hematuria are usually present. Severe hypertension may also cause intracerebral hemorrhage.

Psychologic Factors

There is a high rate of comorbid psychiatric diagnoses in children with primary headaches, of which anxiety and depression are the most common. Primary headaches are more commonly seen in children with a

history of psychiatric disorders. Anxiety and mood disorders are also comorbidities associated with TTHs, especially when chronic, and psychosocial stress may trigger these headaches. Consequently, screening for mental health symptoms and psychosocial stressors should occur in conjunction with the medical history. History should also aim to determine child coping skills, family relationships, and parental reactions to pain.

Conversion disorder may manifest as headaches. Headaches associated with conversion disorder are very difficult to diagnose and treat appropriately. The frequency and severity of these headaches increase without lasting relief from any pharmacologic or physical therapy. Some patients appear as if they are in pain, whereas others look perfectly normal despite claiming to be in considerable pain. Secondary TTH pain may occur, which further complicates the diagnosis. The neurologic findings in conversion disorder are normal.

The two goals in approaching conversion disorder headaches are (1) to convince the family that there is no physical cause for these headaches and (2) to uncover the origin of the conversion disorder. The physician with a pre-established rapport with the family is clearly at an advantage in convincing the family that no physical cause exists for the headaches. The origins of a conversion disorder are difficult to uncover and require the finesse of an experienced therapist. Psychologic intervention is essential, not only to identify the source of the problem but also to offer appropriate counseling.

SUMMARY AND RED FLAGS

Headaches are a common cause of morbidity and health care utilization in children. Most children who present with headaches will have a benign secondary headache or the primary headache disorders of TTH or migraine. However, the clinician must always consider conditions associated with significant morbidity or mortality in the evaluation of each patient with a headache. A thorough history and physical examination are the best tools to aid in determining which patients have a serious and life-threatening cause for their headaches. Certain symptoms and signs should be considered red flags and prompt further evaluation (see Tables 34.5 and 34.6). Blood pressure and fundoscopic exams are essential. Indications for neuroimaging are shown in Table 34.9. In the evaluation of the patient with headache, a single normal neurologic examination or one normal neuroimaging study should not provide complete reassurance. If headache persists, children require continued follow-up and ongoing comprehensive assessments, including detailed general physical and neurologic examinations. Maintenance of a headache diary for patients with frequent or chronic headaches may be invaluable in determining the diagnosis and assessing the response to therapy. Assessment of headaches requires a strong patient-physician relationship to provide continued review of associated symptoms, ongoing assessments, appropriate evaluation, consideration of psychosocial factors, and reassurance when indicated.

BIBLIOGRAPHY

A bibliography is available at ExpertConsult.com.

35

Hypotonia and Weakness

Chamindra G. Konersman

MUSCLE WEAKNESS AND HYPOTONIA

As a symptom, hypotonia may be overt in its presentation, with the manifestations of low muscle tone apparent to family and the medical team alike. Other times, hypotonia may be insidious, subtly presenting to an examiner during a medical evaluation and only rising to the awareness of family when delays or regressions in milestones are pointed out in the process of obtaining a history. **Hypotonia** is defined as decreased resistance to passive movement of a muscle through its range of motion, while **weakness** consists of decreased maximal force of active muscle contraction. Depending on the underlying cause, hypotonia may be associated with either weakness or normal muscle strength; similarly, muscle weakness may be associated with hypotonia, hypertonia, or no apparent change in muscle tone. Hypotonia affects children of all ages and may be congenital or acquired, acute or chronic, progressive or static, isolated or part of a complex clinical situation (Table 35.1). An analytical approach to children with hypotonia requires historical information, clinical observations, and detailed general physical and comprehensive neurologic examinations to localize the source of hypotonia to a specific lesion (Fig. 35.1). This neuraxial localization is then combined with laboratory, imaging, and genetic studies as indicated to arrive at a diagnosis (Tables 35.2 and 35.3).

The generation of normal muscle tone requires the integrity of the entire central and peripheral nervous systems, from the cerebral cortex to cortical white matter pathways, basal ganglia, cerebellum, brainstem, spinal cord, peripheral nerve, neuromuscular junction (NMJ), and muscle. Diseases that affect the function of the nervous system at any of these levels may result in abnormal muscle tone (see Tables 35.2 and 35.3). The primary structure responsible for regulating muscle tone is the **muscle spindle**, a sensory apparatus within the muscle that detects stretching of muscle fibers and that, in response, sends impulses to the spinal cord via sensory afferent pathways. These sensory afferent fibers bifurcate in the spinal cord, with one branch synapsing directly onto anterior horn α motor neurons, producing contraction in the agonist muscle that underwent stretching, while the other branch synapses onto an inhibitory interneuron, inactivating the antagonist muscle. When engaged by stretching of the muscle, this pathway is referred to as the **stretch reflex**, which works to oppose changes in muscle length (Fig. 35.2). Additional inputs to the muscle include excitatory input traveling via α motor neurons that end at the NMJ to produce voluntary contraction, as well as γ motor neurons that end at the muscle spindle, providing inhibitory input to the muscle spindle, setting the level of resting muscle tone. This lower motor neuron pathway of α motor neurons and γ motor neurons is closely monitored and influenced by descending central pathways from the cerebral cortex, basal ganglia, brainstem, and cerebellum. These descending pathways constitute the upper motor neuron pathways that influence resting muscle tone.

Associated symptoms and physical findings in hypotonia vary depending on whether the hypotonia is caused by lesions of the central nervous system (CNS), as opposed to the peripheral nervous system (PNS) (Table 35.4). An estimated 80–90% of infantile hypotonia is central in origin, with the remaining 10–20% being peripheral. Most cases of acute *lateralized* body weakness result from abnormalities of the blood supply to a portion of the CNS. **Stroke** serves as a term to denote the sudden onset of symptoms attributable to such an interruption of cerebral or spinal perfusion and is discussed in Chapter 37.

EVALUATING HYPOTONIA

The systematic evaluation of muscle tone consists first of making the following clinical observations:
- Characterization of spontaneous posture
- Response to postural changes
- Extent of joint mobility
- Response to flapping of distal extremities

Muscle tone is divided into postural and phasic. **Postural tone** is the steady contraction of muscles in uniform resistance to passive movement. Antigravity resistance is an example of postural tone. **Phasic tone** is the catch experienced when an extremity is rapidly flexed or extended across a joint. The method of evaluating muscle tone and strength depends on the age of the patient.

HYPOTONIC INFANT

Clinical Evaluation

In an infant, historical information must include a complete obstetric history, including the amount and quality of fetal movements, amniotic fluid volume, and intrauterine growth restriction, as well as accurate data about perinatal events, diet, toxic exposures, and family history. The muscle strength, passive tone, joint extensibility, and postural reflexes, including responses to traction, axillary suspension, and ventral suspension of the hypotonic infant, should be compared to those of the normal infant (Fig. 35.3).

Muscle Strength

Muscle strength (Table 35.5) cannot be measured directly in infants, but numerous clinical clues allow the careful observer to identify weakness. The most important of these clues is the spontaneous posture. The weak infant has diminished or no spontaneous movement, often in striking contrast to the usual vigorous and plentiful movements of the infant with normal strength. The lower extremities are abducted and the lateral surfaces of the thighs lie against the examination table in a classic "frog leg" position, whereas the upper extremities lie extended alongside the body or flexed in a flaccid position beside the head (Figs. 35.4 and 35.5A). With marked weakness, there are no movements that overcome

TABLE 35.1   Causes of Hypotonia and Weakness

Systemic	Connective Tissue	Cerebral	Spinal Cord	Anterior Horn Cell	Peripheral Nerve	Neuromuscular Junction	Muscle
Common							
Sepsis	Stickler syndrome	Hypoxic-ischemic brain injury	Myelodysplasia	Spinal muscular atrophy	Postinfectious polyneuropathy (Guillain-Barré syndrome)	Botulism	Duchenne muscular dystrophy
Heart failure	Marfan syndrome	Intracranial hemorrhage	Spinal cord tumor			Infantile myasthenia	Becker muscular dystrophy
Acidosis	Achondroplasia	Brain malformation*	Epidural abscess		Toxic neuropathies (isoniazid, vincristine, platinum-based antineoplastic medications, nitrofurantoin)	Transient acquired neonatal myasthenia	Myotonic dystrophy
Hypoxia		Intrauterine infection	Transverse myelitis				Dermatomyositis
Renal failure		Postnatal brain injury	Acute flaccid myelitis				
Hypoglycemia			Trauma (transection or compression)				
Trisomy 21			Syringomyelia				
Prader-Willi syndrome							
Fragile X syndrome							
Hypothyroidism							
Other chromosomal disorders							
Maternal-fetal drug effects							
Uncommon							
Disorders of amino acid metabolism	Ehlers-Danlos syndrome	Progressive encephalopathies	Neonatal spinal cord transection	Möbius syndrome	Chronic inflammatory demyelinating polyneuropathy	Toxic (organophosphate poisoning, aminoglycosides, magnesium)	Pompe disease
Urea cycle disorders	Osteogenesis imperfecta	Mitochondrial disease	Hypoxic-ischemic myelopathy		Charcot-Marie-Tooth disease	Postneuromuscular blocking agents (vecuronium)	
Peroxisomal disorders	Velocardiofacial syndrome		Arteriovenous malformation		Hereditary sensory and autonomic neuropathies		
Scurvy							
Rickets							
Sotos syndrome							
Angelman syndrome							
Rett syndrome							
Smith-Lemli-Opitz syndrome							
Rare							
Lowe syndrome		Miller-Dieker syndrome		Poliomyelitis	Refsum disease	Congenital myasthenic syndromes	Other muscular dystrophies
Zellweger syndrome		Congenital muscular dystrophy		Incontinentia pigmenti	Giant axonal neuropathy		Congenital myopathies
Neonatal adrenoleukodystrophy		Metachromatic leukodystrophy		Fazio-Londe disease	Metachromatic leukodystrophy		Metabolic myopathies
Mucolipidosis type IV		Krabbe disease		Brown-Vialetto-Van Laere syndrome	Krabbe disease		Mitochondrial myopathies
Tay-Sachs disease				Juvenile amyotrophic lateral sclerosis			
Gangliosidosis							
Mannosidosis							
Infantile neuroaxonal dystrophy							

*Examples of brain malformations include agenesis of the corpus callosum, lissencephaly, Joubert syndrome, and Dandy-Walker malformations.

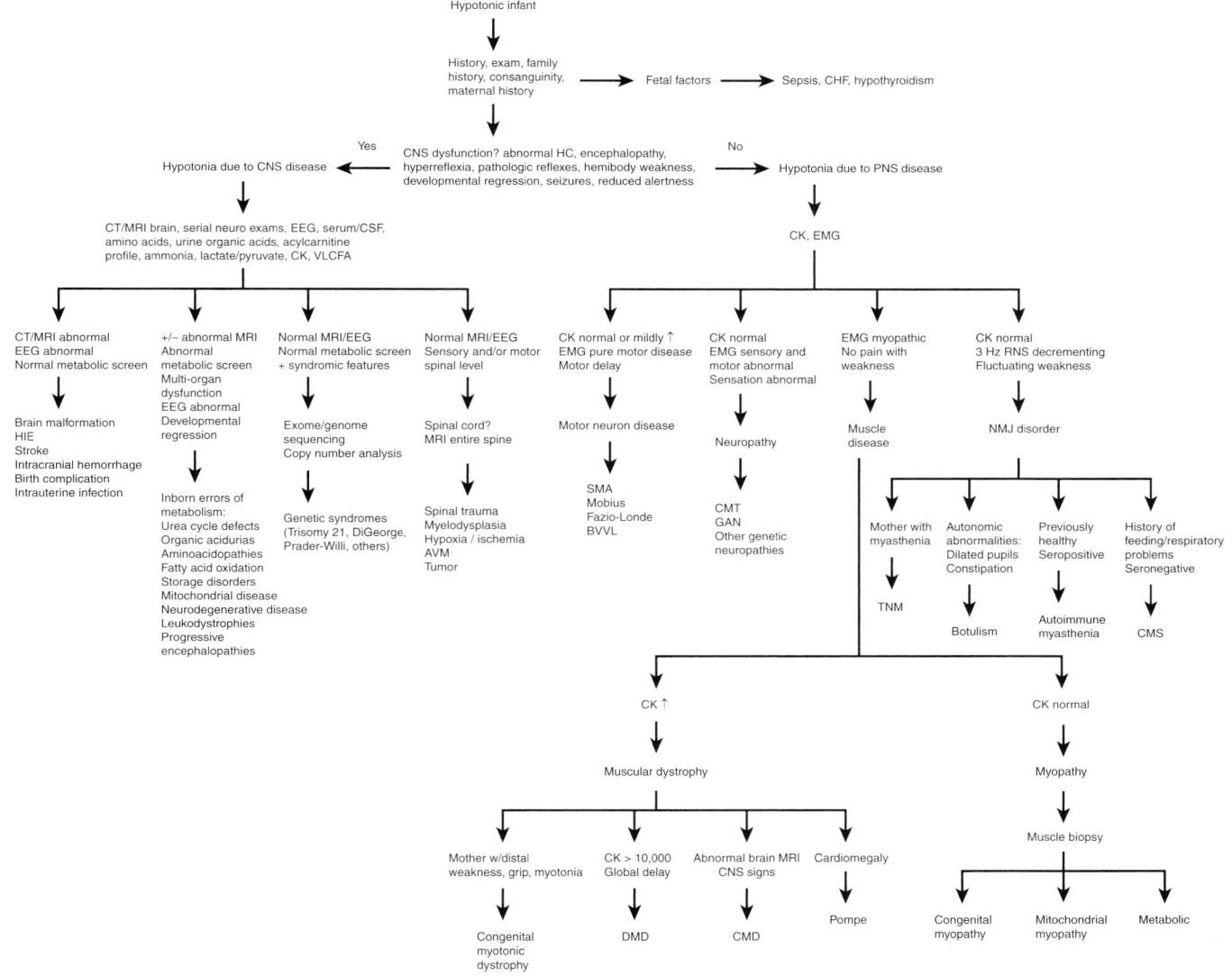

Fig. 35.1 Diagnostic approach to the hypotonic infant. AVM, arteriovenous malformation; BVVL, Brown–Vialetto–Van Laere syndrome; CHF, congestive heart failure; CK, creatine kinase; CMD, congenital muscular dystrophy; CMS, congenital myasthenic syndrome; CMT, Charcot-Marie-Tooth disease; CNS, central nervous system; CSF, cerebrospinal fluid; DMD, Duchenne muscular dystrophy; EMG, electromyography with nerve conduction; GAN, giant axonal neuropathy; HC, head circumference; HIE, hypoxic-ischemic encephalopathy; NMJ, neuromuscular junction; PNS, peripheral nervous system; RNS, repetitive nerve stimulation; SMA, spinal muscular atrophy; TNM, transient neonatal myasthenia; VLCFA, very long-chain fatty acids.

the pull of gravity. The immobility of the weak infant results in flattening of the occipital bone, which is often associated with occipital hair loss. When placed in a sitting posture, the infant droops forward, the shoulders sink, the head falls forward, and the arms hang limply.

Passive Tone

Passive tone can be assessed by evaluating the resistance to movement of the limbs through their range of motion. Evaluation of the shoulders, elbows, wrists, hips, knees, and ankles is especially helpful. In hypotonic infants, the examiner senses a looseness of the limbs as the limbs are moved. In addition, grasping the midportion of the infant's limb and passively flapping the extremity allows the examiner to evaluate the degree of limpness of the distal extremity. In the hypotonic infant, the hands and feet wave limply; in the normal infant, the ankle and wrist are maintained fairly rigidly in line with the rest of the extremity.

Even in normal infants, there is a wide variation of muscle tone. Passive muscle tone varies and is particularly diminished after feeding and before sleep. There is profound hypotonia in all infants during sleep. Premature infants, even those without neurologic injury, have diminished tone relative to term infants, due to incomplete myelination of corticospinal and subcorticospinal tracts. Tone can also be affected by the position of the head. The infant whose head is turned to one side may manifest an **asymmetric tonic neck response**, with increased extensor tone on the side of the body to which the head is turned and increased flexor tone on the contralateral side, resulting in a "fencer's posture" (Fig. 35.6). This asymmetry of tone may be elicited even in the child who does not exhibit the typical fencer's posture. Therefore, examination of an infant should always be conducted while the infant's head is at the midline; the same is true for eliciting muscle stretch reflexes. Hypotonia can also be a secondary finding in a variety

TABLE 35.2   Differentiating the Causes of Infantile Hypotonia

Localization	Cause	History and Exam Findings	Investigation to Aid in Diagnosis
Brain	HIE Intracerebral hemorrhage	Prematurity, difficult delivery	Brain MRI
	Brain malformations	Cranial nerve abnormalities, Babinski sign, gradual development of hypertonia (especially axial), respiratory or feeding difficulties, global delay, micro-macrocephaly	Cerebral ultrasound Brain MRI
	Intrauterine infection	Fever, altered mental status	Microbial cultures/evaluations, CSF evaluation
	Postnatal birth injury	Seizures, focal neurologic deficits	Brain MRI, EEG
	Progressive encephalopathies (leukodystrophies, progressive myoclonic epilepsies, Lennox-Gastaut syndrome, infantile spasms)	Seizures, developmental regression, ataxia, focal neurologic deficits, visual loss	Brain MRI, EEG, EMG/NCS (useful in adrenoleukodystrophy, Krabbe disease, and metachromatic leukodystrophy), specific genetic testing
	Mitochondrial disease	Seizures, focal neurologic deficits, global delay, visual loss, hyper- or hyporeflexia	Brain MRI, lactate, pyruvate, creatine kinase, GDF-15, muscle biopsy, mitochondrial DNA sequencing and deletion/duplication analysis on muscle or affected tissue, EMG/NCS
Brainstem	Joubert syndrome Pontocerebellar hypoplasia Cobblestone malformations	Multiple cranial nerve abnormalities, breathing and feeding difficulties, possible intellectual delay, nystagmus, possible hyperreflexia, ataxia	Brain MRI (molar tooth sign in Joubert syndrome), genetic panels for specific disorders
Spinal cord	Myelodysplasia Spinal cord tumor Syringomyelia Hypoxia-ischemia Trauma AVM	Spinal level on exam, weakness below a defined spinal level, absent reflexes (acutely) or hyperreflexia (chronically) below the level, may have Babinski sign, history of trauma	Brain MRI, complete spinal MRI
Motor neuron	Spinal muscular atrophy	Absence of antigravity movements, tongue fasciculations, absent reflexes to hyporeflexia, normal cognition, breathing/feeding difficulties; weakness in legs more than arms in SMA types II–III	*SMN1* genetic analysis
	Poliomyelitis	Neck stiffness, muscle spasms, areflexia, asymmetric flaccid paralysis of a limb, respiratory distress, muscle atrophy, normal sensation	Isolation of poliovirus from stool, confirmation using RT-PCR, acute and convalescent serology showing fourfold increase in titer, EMG/NCS showing pure motor neuronopathy
	Incontinentia pigmenti	Skin blistering, verrucous skin lesions, hyperpigmented streaks, pale/hairless atrophic linear streaks that respect Blaschko lines, dental abnormalities, intellectual delay	DNA analysis, EMG/NCS showing pure motor neuronopathy
	Fazio-Londe disease Brown–Vialetto–Van Laere syndrome (BVVL)	Optic atrophy, nystagmus, bulbar palsy, facial weakness, hearing loss (BVVL only), tongue fasciculations, ptosis, respiratory compromise, muscle weakness	DNA analysis
Nerve	Guillain-Barré syndrome (GBS) Chronic inflammatory demyelinating polyneuropathy (CIDP)	Sensory ataxia with walking difficulties, rapidly (GBS) or slowly (CIDP) progressive weakness, absent reflexes or hyporeflexia, autonomic dysfunction, antecedent gastrointestinal or respiratory illness in GBS	EMG/NCS with absent or prolonged F-waves, prolonged distal latencies, conduction block, demyelinating nerve conduction velocities, CSF showing cytoalbuminologic dissociation, MRI with edematous enhancing nerve roots
	Toxic neuropathies	History and temporal correlation with exposure to a neurotoxic drug, distal then proximal muscle weakness, absent reflexes or hyporeflexia, sensory ataxia with walking difficulties	EMG/NCS showing mixed axonal/demyelinating features, plasma drug levels
	Charcot-Marie-Tooth disease	Family history of similar disease, pes cavus and hammer toe foot deformities, ataxic gait, foot drop, absent reflexes or hyporeflexia	EMG/NCS to determine if axonal or demyelinating subtypes, DNA analysis
	Hereditary sensory and autonomic neuropathies	Sensory loss in a stocking/glove distribution, chronic skin ulceration and poor wound healing, distal muscle weakness with foot deformity, absent reflexes or hyporeflexia, variable anhidrosis	EMG/NCS showing normal or mildly abnormal motor responses and abnormal sensory responses, nerve biopsy showing reduced myelinated and unmyelinated fibers, DNA analysis

TABLE 35.2 Differentiating the Causes of Infantile Hypotonia—cont'd

Localization	Cause	History and Exam Findings	Investigation to Aid in Diagnosis
Nerve—cont'd	Refsum disease	Autosomal recessive inheritance, stocking/glove distribution of sensory and motor weakness, anosmia, hearing loss, ataxia, ichthyosis, short metacarpals and metatarsals, cardiac arrhythmia, and cardiomyopathy	Elevated plasma phytanic acid concentration, DNA analysis
	Giant axonal neuropathy	Stocking/glove distribution of sensory loss and motor weakness, cerebellar ataxia, absent reflexes or hyporeflexia, kinky hair (tightly curled), nystagmus, dysarthria, pyramidal tract signs, optic neuropathy, seizures	Brain MRI with white matter abnormalities, axonal sensorimotor polyneuropathy on EMG/NCS, nerve biopsy showing giant axons (axonal swelling) and disorganized neurofilaments, DNA analysis
	Metachromatic leukodystrophy Krabbe disease Adrenoleukodystrophy	Developmental regression, absent reflexes or hyporeflexia, Babinski signs	EMG/NCS showing demyelinating neuropathy, brain MRI showing white matter disease, DNA analysis
Neuromuscular junction	Botulism	Sudden poor feeding, constipation, weak cry, gradual muscle weakness, dilated poorly reactive pupils, exposure to soil/dust with bacterium or honey consumption	Presence of toxin in stool/serum, culture bacterium from stool, EMG/NCS showing low-amplitude motor responses or decrement on repetitive nerve stimulation in a weak muscle
	Transient acquired neonatal myasthenia	Ptosis, feeding and respiratory difficulties, aspiration, mother with signs or symptoms of autoimmune myasthenia	Maternal history of myasthenia, EMG/NCS showing decrement on repetitive nerve stimulation in a weak muscle, good response to acetylcholinesterase inhibitors
	Infantile (autoimmune) myasthenia	Ptosis, episodic weakness, recurrent feeding and respiratory difficulties, easy fatigability	EMG/NCS showing decrement on repetitive nerve stimulation in a weak muscle, good response to acetylcholinesterase inhibitors, antiacetylcholine receptor antibody serology
	Congenital myasthenic syndrome	Ptosis, episodic weakness, recurrent feeding and respiratory difficulties, easy fatigability	EMG/NCS showing decrement on repetitive nerve stimulation in a weak muscle, DNA analysis, negative antiacetylcholine receptor antibody serology
Muscle	Duchenne/Becker muscular dystrophy	X-linked pattern of inheritance, enlarged calves, proximal muscle weakness with a Gower maneuver	Markedly elevated CK, DNA analysis
	Congenital myotonic dystrophy	Autosomal dominant pattern of inheritance, frog-leg position, open down-turned mouth, minimal antigravity movements in infants, distal > proximal weakness in children, impaired relaxation of grip, dysarthria, myopathic facies with temporal wasting	Test mother (then father) for clinical myotonia or electrical myotonic discharges, EMG/NCS with myopathy in newborn period and myotonic discharges in older children, normal to mildly elevated CK, *DPMK* gene CTG repeat analysis
	Pompe disease	Absence of antigravity movements, severe cardiomegaly, feeding/respiratory difficulties, hepatomegaly	GAA enzyme activity in dried blood spot, lymphocytes or fibroblasts, *GAA* gene analysis
	Congenital muscular dystrophy	Family history, proximal > distal muscle weakness, feeding and respiratory difficulties, early-onset contractures in specific subtypes, keloids/hyperkeratosis pilaris in specific subtypes, CNS dysfunction in specific subtypes	Brain MRI, mild to markedly elevated CK, muscle biopsy showing dystrophic changes, muscle MRI, EMG/NCS to assess for demyelinating neuropathy component and myopathy, DNA analysis
	Congenital myopathies	Family history, proximal > distal muscle weakness, feeding and respiratory difficulties, ptosis and ophthalmoparesis in specific subtypes	Normal to mildly elevated CK, muscle biopsy showing specific changes (nemaline rods, cores, centrally placed nuclei), DNA analysis
	Metabolic myopathies	Family history, proximal muscle weakness, history of rhabdomyolysis or myoglobinuria, second-wind phenomenon in some subtypes	Normal to markedly elevated CK, EMG/NCS usually myopathic, metabolic evaluation (lactate, pyruvate, acylcarnitine profile, plasma amino acids, urine organic acids), muscle biopsy, DNA analysis
	Mitochondrial myopathies	Maternal inheritance pattern, proximal > distal weakness, ptosis, ophthalmoparesis, short stature, variable cardiac and CNS involvement, recurrent rhabdomyolysis	Normal to moderately elevated CK, abnormal GDF-15, EMG/NCS showing myopathy and variable neuropathy, muscle biopsy with ragged red fibers, mitochondrial DNA analysis

AVM, arteriovenous malformation; CK, creatine kinase; CNS, central nervous system; CSF, cerebrospinal fluid; CTG, cytosine-thymine-guanine; EMG/NCS, electromyography/nerve conduction study; GAA, acid α-glucosidase; GDF-15, growth differentiation factor-15; HIE, hypoxic-ischemic encephalopathy; RT-PCR, reverse transcription polymerase chain reaction; SMA, spinal motor atrophy.

Modified from Sparks SE. Neonatal hypotonia. *Clin Perinatol.* 2015;42:363–371.

TABLE 35.3 Localization of Symptoms on Neural Axis

| | UPPER MOTOR UNIT | | LOWER MOTOR UNIT | | | |
	Brain	Spinal Cord	Alpha Motor Neuron*	Peripheral Nerve	Neuromuscular Junction	Muscle
Level of consciousness	↓	Normal	Normal	Normal	Normal	Normal
Strength	Mild to moderate ↓	Mild to moderate ↓	Marked ↓	Marked ↓	Marked ↓	Marked ↓
Tone	Spastic (hypotonia at onset possible)	↓ Acutely; ↑	↓, flaccid	↓	↓	↓
Deep tendon reflexes	Normal to ↑	↓ Acutely; ↑	↓ to absent	↓ to absent (lost early)	Normal	Normal to ↓ to absent
Babinski	Present	Present usually	Absent	Absent	Absent	Absent
Fasciculations	Absent	Absent	Present	Rarely	Absent	Absent
Atrophy	Mild to moderate	Mild to moderate	Present	Present	Absent	Present pseudohypertrophy
Sensation	Normal	Absent below level of lesion	Normal	Abnormal in defined peripheral nerve distribution or glove/stocking	Normal	Normal
Creatine kinase level	Normal	Normal	Normal to moderately elevated (several 1,000s IU/L)	Normal or mildly elevated (100s IU/L)	Normal	Normal to severely elevated
Overall pattern	Hemibody deficits	Spinal level present	Proximal weakness in SMA; asymmetric weakness in other diseases	Distal, length-dependent usually, defined nerve territory	Symmetric, painless weakness of tonically active muscles	Proximal > distal weakness
Other	Seizures Developmental delay Regression Cortical signs (e.g., language)	Radicular back pain, bowel/bladder dysfunction			Fluctuating diurnal variation Fatigability	Myalgia, Gower sign

SMA, spinal muscular atrophy.

*Originate in anterior horn cells.

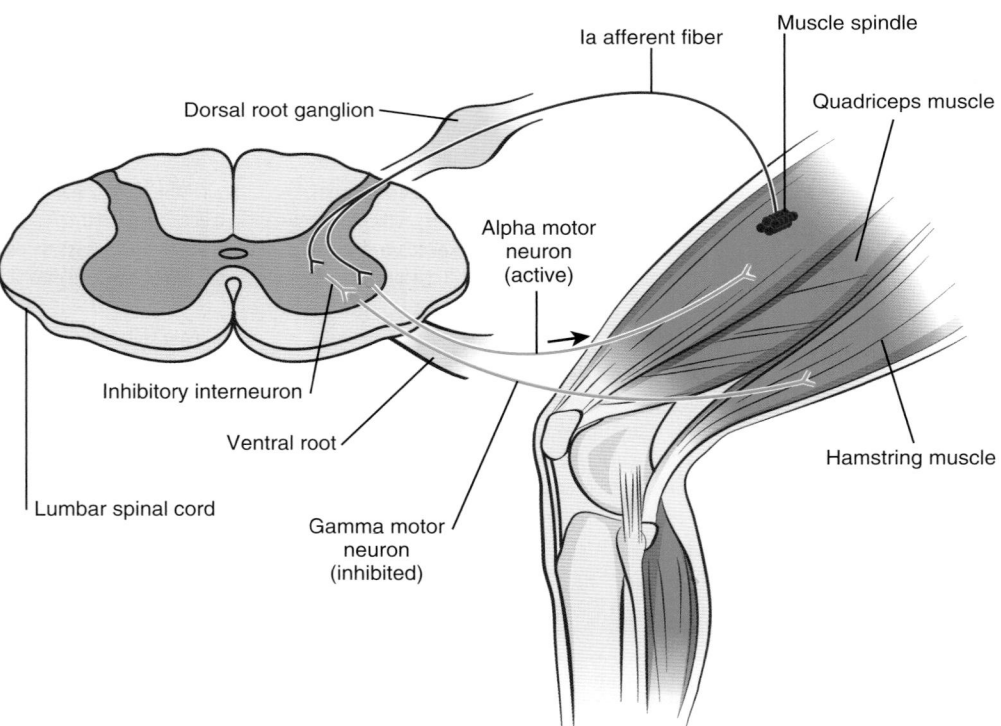

Fig. 35.2 Lower motor neuron pathway influencing resting muscle tone. Stretching of the quadriceps muscle (agonist) will result in relaxation or inhibition of the hamstring muscle (antagonist).

TABLE 35.4   Exam and Historical Findings to Distinguish Central from Peripheral Hypotonia

Finding	Central	Peripheral
Seizures	Present	Absent
Altered mental status	Present	Absent
Delayed cognitive milestones	Present	Absent
Deep tendon reflexes	Normal or increased	Absent or decreased usually
Babinski sign	Present	Absent
Infantile reflexes	Persistent	Not persistent
Pull-to-sit	Minor head lag	Marked head lag
Tongue fasciculations without other cranial nerve deficits	Unlikely	Very likely
Ophthalmoparesis	Present in brainstem disease	Present in some myopathic diseases
Ptosis	Present in some brainstem diseases	Present in some myopathic and neuromuscular junction diseases
Weakness	Mild to moderate	Severe
Antigravity movements	Present	Absent usually
Arthrogryposis	Less common	More common
Muscle atrophy	None to mild	Moderate to severe

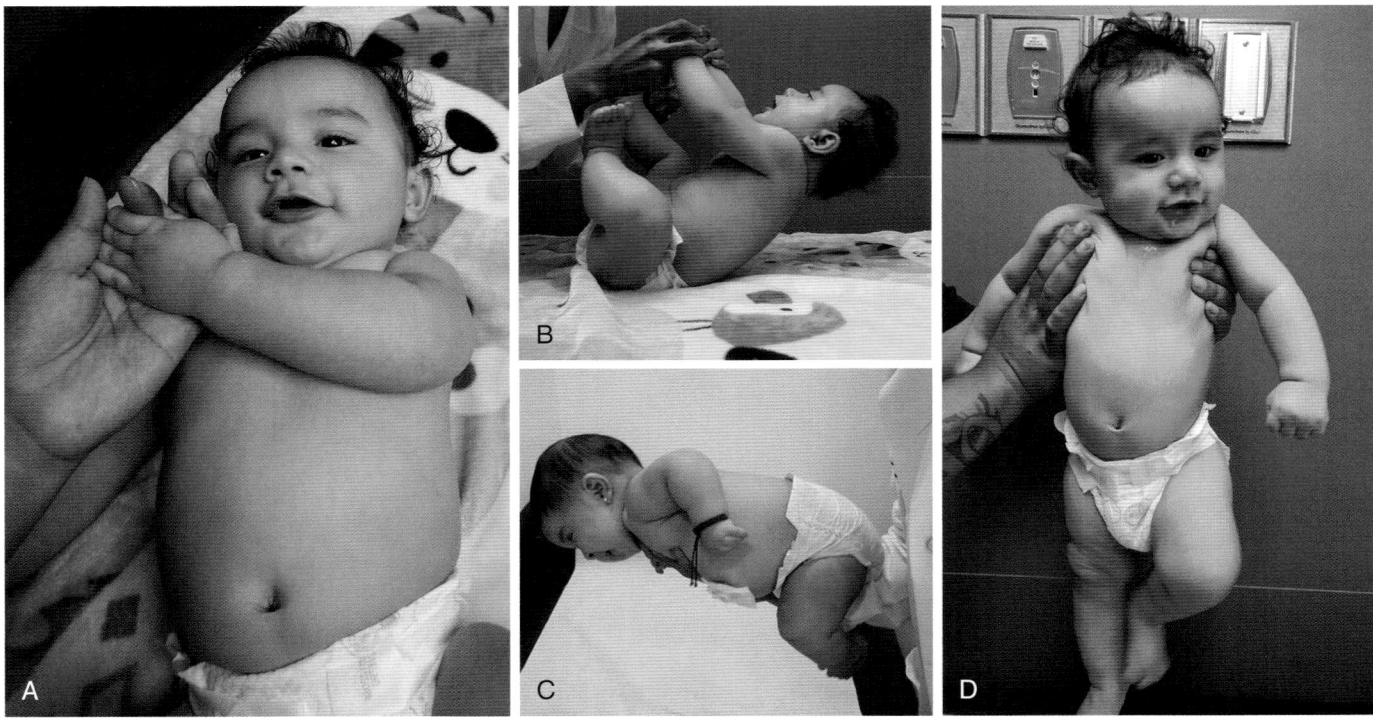

Fig. 35.3 Normal postural responses in a 5-month-old infant showing that the elbow does not extend beyond the midline on joint extensibility testing *(A)*, the head and body in the same plane (no head lag) on pull-to-sit with resistance resulting in flexed elbows and knees *(B)*, and lack of a slip-through with resistance against the examiner's hands, good maintenance of head control, and extension of the head and legs with the steppage reflex *(D)*. An infant with hypoxic-ischemic encephalopathy who was initially hypotonic at the time of delivery was noted to be hypertonic at 8 months with a normal ventral suspension response as evidenced by the ability to keep the head above horizontal *(C)*.

of systemic conditions, such as heart failure, sepsis, acidosis, or failure to thrive (see Table 35.1).

Joint Extensibility

The extent to which the joints may be extensible provides an indirect clue to the presence of hypotonia. Examination of mobility at the elbows, wrists, hips, and knees is helpful. The hypotonic infant may assume unusual postures in the presence of joint hyperextensibility. The **scarf sign** is a useful sign of hyperextensibility in the young infant. With the infant in a semireclining position, the hand is pulled across the chest toward the opposite shoulder and the position of the elbow is noted (see Fig. 35.3A). If the elbow passes the midline, there is hypotonia.

Postural Reflexes

Traction response (pull-to-sit). The traction response is the most useful and most sensitive of the postural reflexes in infants. With the infant lying supine, the infant's hands are grasped, and the infant is pulled up to a sitting position. Once the sitting posture is attained, the head is held erect in the midline. During the maneuver, the examiner notes the infant's attempt to counter the traction by flexion of the arms (see Fig. 35.3B).

In an infant younger than 3 months, the **plantar grasp** should also be evident when grasping the infant's hands to assess the traction response. In addition, there should be flexion at the elbow, knee, and

TABLE 35.5	**Grading Muscle Strength**

0: No contraction
1: Minimal visual or palpable contraction only
2: Moves in horizontal plane but not against gravity
3: Moves against gravity but not against resistance
4: Moves against gravity and minimal resistance
5: Moves against gravity and full resistance

ankle in response to the maneuver. The degree to which the head and neck pull up along with the trunk depends on the child's age.

In infants younger than 33 weeks' gestation, there is no traction response. From 33 weeks to term, the infant has head lag but responds to the traction maneuver by flexing the neck flexors in an attempt to lift the head. The full-term infant exhibits a traction response with minimal head lag, and when the sitting posture is attained, the head may be held erect momentarily and then falls forward.

By age 3 months, there should be no head lag, and the head should be aligned with the plane of the back as the child is pulled to sitting. The absence of flexion of the limbs in response to the examiner's pull and the presence of head lag inappropriate for age suggest hypotonia (see Figs. 35.4D and 35.5C).

Axillary suspension. The response to axillary suspension allows assessment of generalized and shoulder girdle tone. The infant is held under the arms, lifted, and suspended from the axillae without the thorax being grasped. In infants with normal tone and strength, the shoulder girdle muscles exert enough strength to allow the infant to be suspended without slipping through the examiner's grasp. In addition, the infant's head is held midline and the legs are held with some flexion at the hips, knees, and ankles (see Fig. 35.3D). The hypotonic infant droops with legs extended and head falling forward, and the absence of resistance of the muscles of the shoulder girdle allows the infant to slip through the grasp of the examiner as the baby's arms fling upward (see Fig. 35.5B).

Ventral suspension. The response to ventral suspension allows assessment of tone of the trunk, neck, and extremities. The examiner holds the infant, who is lying prone. The infant is supported only by the examiner's hand on the abdomen. A normal infant holds the head erect and the back straight and holds the extremities with some flexion at the elbows, hips, knees, and ankles (see Fig. 35.3C). A full-term neonate makes intermittent attempts to hold the head straight, maintains the back straight, and can flex the limbs. The hypotonic infant droops in the examiner's palm, as if in the shape of an inverted "U," with the head and legs dangling limply (see Fig. 35.4C).

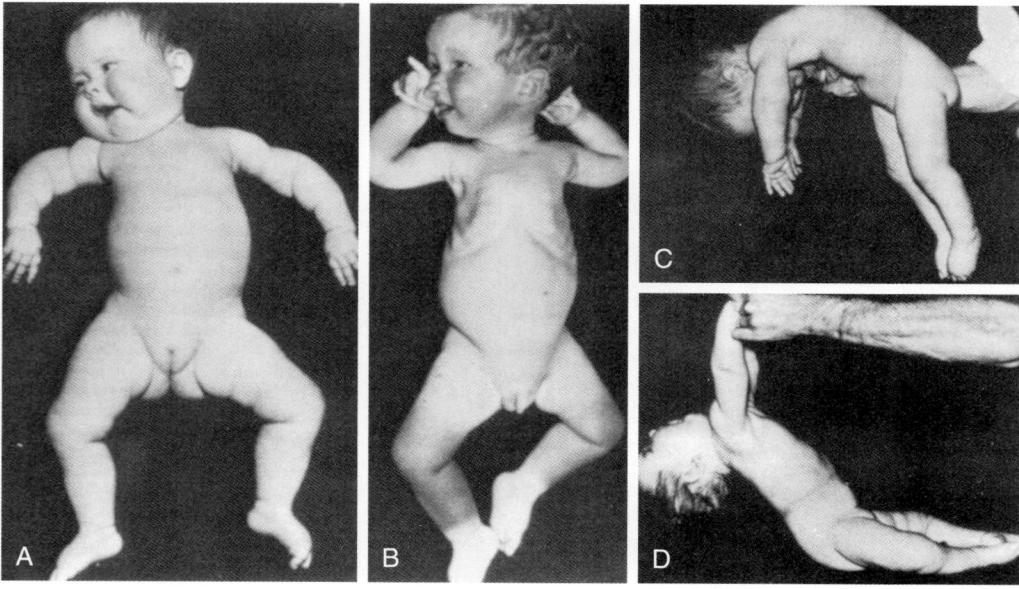

Fig. 35.4 Spinal muscular atrophy I: characteristic postures. *A,* A 6-week-old infant with severe weakness and hypotonia from birth. Note the frog-leg posture of the lower limbs and internal rotation ("jug-handle") at the shoulders. *B,* A 1-year-old infant with frog-leg posture, external rotation at shoulders, intercostal recession, and normal facial expressions. A 6-week-old infant with marked weakness of the limbs and trunk giving the characteristic inverted "U" appearance on ventral suspension *(C)* and pull-to-sit *(D).* (Modified from Volpe JJ, ed. *Neurology of the Newborn.* 5th ed. Philadelphia: Saunders; 2008:770–771.)

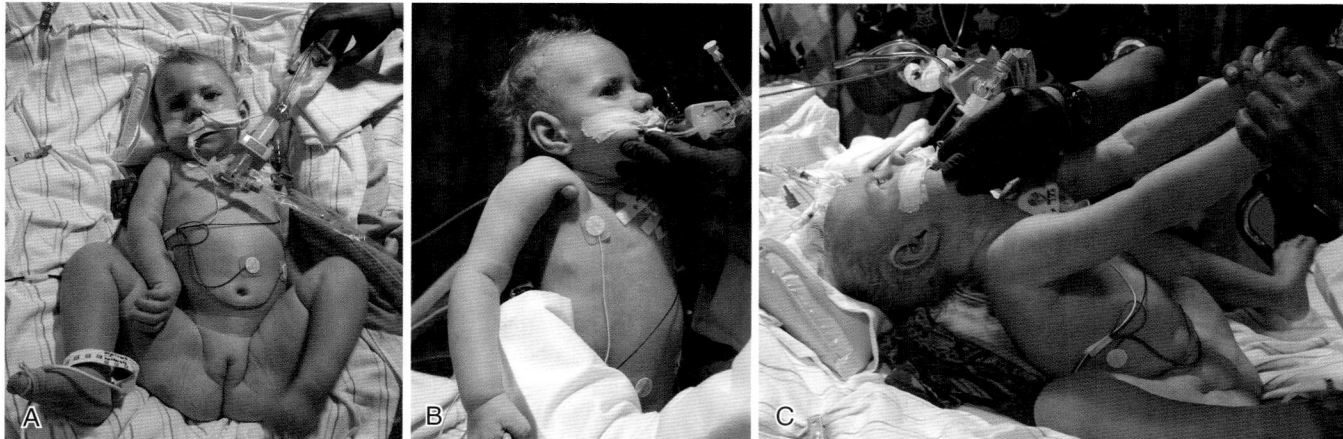

Fig. 35.5 An 18-month-old infant, with an undiagnosed pure motor neuron disorder with severe axial more than appendicular weakness, delays in motor milestones, and respiratory insufficiency, has internal rotation of upper arm and frog-leg position *(A)*, a slip-through appearance on axillary suspension *(B)*, and a prominent head lag on pull-to-sit traction testing *(C)*.

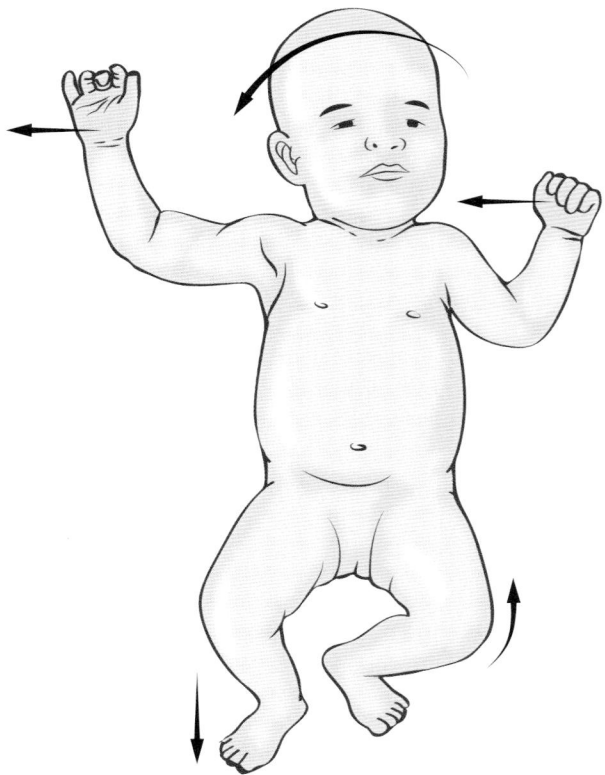

Fig. 35.6 Asymmetric tonic neck reflex. Normally present from birth to 2 months. Turning head to one side when supine elicits extension of arm and leg ipsilateral to side that head is turned and flexion of opposite arm and leg. Persistence beyond 2 months might suggest abnormal development of contralateral motor cortex.

WEAK CHILD

Clinical Evaluation

Posture and Strength

Observation of the child's spontaneous posture may suggest the presence of weakness. Muscle strength can be observed as the child performs functional tasks, including moving from a supine to a seated position, arising to stand from a sitting or lying position, standing on one leg independently, hopping, walking, running, and climbing stairs. The **wheelbarrow**

maneuver, in which the pelvis and lower extremities are supported by the examiner while the child propels themselves forward on the floor using only the arms, can be used to functionally assess strength in the upper extremities. In the child older than 5 years, manual muscle testing can be performed if the child is cooperative (see Table 35.5). The examiner evaluates each muscle group independently, comparing the child's muscle strength in resistance to the examiner's strength. Although a child's strength is not expected to be equal to an adult, the child is given full strength scores if the degree of strength exhibited is substantial for age. The child with muscle weakness has difficulty performing motor tasks and may exhibit unusual postures (e.g., lordosis) or toe walking, and on manual muscle testing may be easily overcome by the examiner's strength.

Passive Tone

Passive muscle tone is more consistent during the waking hours in the child than in the infant. The major joints should be moved through their range of motion and the extent of resistance noted. Flapping the distal extremities provides a useful clue. Briskly lifting the lower extremity at the knee while the patient lies supine is another useful test of muscle tone. In the normal child, the foot briefly drags along the examination table and then rises with the leg. In the hypertonic child, the leg remains extended stiffly at the knee. In the hypotonic child, the lower leg hangs limply and the foot drags as the knee is raised.

Joint Extensibility

The hypotonic child demonstrates hyperextensibility of joints, especially at the elbows, wrists, knees, and ankles. Examination of the small muscles of the fingers across distal joints may also be helpful (Fig. 35.7).

DIAGNOSTIC APPROACH TO THE HYPOTONIC INFANT

The diagnosis of a particular neurologic disorder depends on the location of the lesion (i.e., which part of the nervous system is impaired or abnormal), the patient's age, and whether the condition is progressive or static (see Tables 35.1 to 35.3).

A careful perinatal history is obtained to identify possible features suggestive of perinatal **hypoxic-ischemic brain injury**. The infant who has neurologic dysfunction attributable to perinatal asphyxia typically has a history of an acute encephalopathy during the neonatal period (e.g., disturbance of consciousness, poor feeding, seizures, autonomic dysfunction).

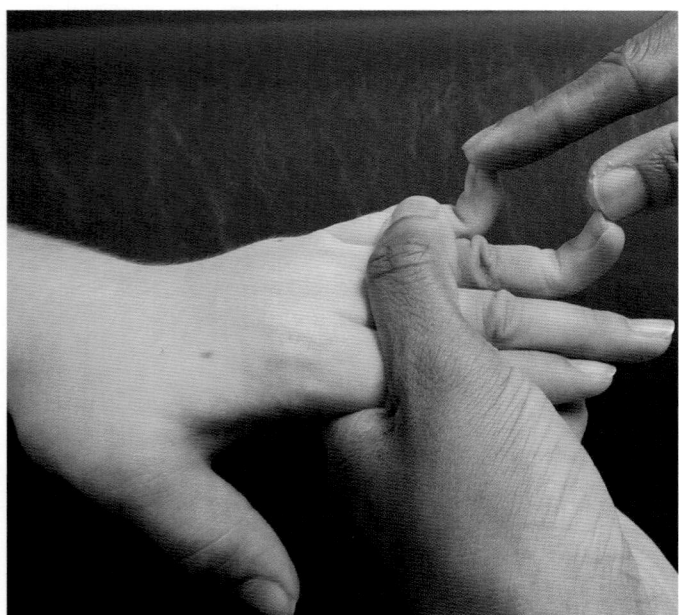

Fig. 35.7 Hyperlaxity at the distal interphalangeal joints in a 9-year-old girl with a congenital myopathy.

A CT study or MRI of the head is helpful to identify evidence of brain malformation, intrauterine infection, hypoxic brain injury, intracranial hemorrhage, or hydrocephalus. If the history suggests seizures, an EEG should be obtained.

An **ophthalmologic evaluation** may detect evidence of ocular malformation (cataracts, microphthalmia, optic hypoplasia), evidence of intrauterine infection (chorioretinitis), or retinal/macular abnormality (retinitis pigmentosa, cherry-red spot) (see Chapter 43).

In some cases, requesting a hearing evaluation or brainstem auditory evoked response may be appropriate. A lumbar puncture is necessary if acute or chronic (intrauterine) meningitis is suspected.

Fig. 35.1 summarizes the diagnostic approach to the hypotonic infant. After a thorough history and detailed general and neurologic examinations, the first priority is to determine if there are signs and symptoms of CNS dysfunction because the majority of hypotonia in infants is central in origin (see Table 35.4). Extraneural involvement such as the presence of multiorgan dysfunction, bone marrow suppression, organomegaly, or heart failure accompanying hypotonia is highly suggestive of a systemic disease, such as a storage disorder or an inborn error of metabolism. Particular attention should be given to family history, perinatal maternal illnesses and exposures, delivery complications, and the possibility of consanguinity. Signs and symptoms of CNS involvement in an infant include abnormal head circumference (either micro- or macrocephaly), reduced levels of alertness (i.e., encephalopathy), seizures, respiratory and feeding difficulties, hypotonia and later hypertonia, hemibody weakness, hyperreflexia, developmental cognitive regression, and pathologic reflexes such as persistence of the Babinski sign in an older infant or child. The hypotonic infant's exam findings may change with age, even on the order of weeks to months. Many hypotonic neonates initially thought to have PNS dysfunction eventually develop hypertonia, hyperreflexia, and pathologic Babinski signs over time, indicative of CNS dysfunction; therefore, serial thorough neurologic exams are essential until confirmatory testing yields a firm diagnosis or until a clinical diagnosis is made with reasonable confidence. An MRI of the head is obtained to detect any anatomic abnormalities or other causative lesions. If CNS dysfunction is present, initial recommended testing includes EEG (which may show seizures or cortical slowing) and a complete metabolic screen—serum amino acids (aminoacidopathies, urea cycle disorders, some organic acidurias), urine organic acids (organic acidurias), ammonia (urea cycle disorders, organic acidurias), acylcarnitine profile (organic acidurias, fatty acid oxidation disorders, riboflavin transporter defect), serum and cerebrospinal fluid (CSF) lactate and pyruvate (mitochondrial disease), serum growth differentiation factor-15 (GDF-15) levels (mitochondrial disease), very long-chain fatty acids (peroxisomal disorders), and lysosomal enzyme panel (lysosomal storage disease), since some conditions are treatable and prompt initiation of therapy may halt or slow progression of disease.

An abnormal brain MRI and EEG with a normal metabolic screen suggests a possible static cause such as brain malformation, hypoxic-ischemic encephalopathy (HIE)/stroke, maternal or fetal infection, or a birth complication. **Developmental regression** is highly suggestive of inborn errors of metabolism, storage disorders, mitochondrial diseases, or neurodegenerative diseases (see Table 35.1 under "systemic" and "cerebral" for specific disorders) (see Chapter 28). Regression coupled with an abnormal metabolic screen may suggest urea cycle defects, organic acidurias, aminoacidopathies, fatty acid oxidation defects, lysosomal and peroxisomal disorders, mitochondrial disease, or certain neurodegenerative disorders and should prompt immediate referral to a metabolic specialist for rapid diagnosis and possible treatment. Many of the treatable metabolic disorders are diagnosed early in the United States via newborn screening programs.

In the setting of persistent hypotonia with normal MRI, EEG, and metabolic screening, syndromic genetic causes should be considered. Common congenital considerations such as Prader-Willi syndrome, spinal muscular atrophy, and myotonic dystrophy type 1 may lack other overt phenotypic features beyond reduced tone and require specific genetic testing to detect the underlying pathogenic genetic abnormalities, which may not be detected on exome or genome sequencing. In the case of Prader-Willi syndrome, DNA methylation testing detects >99% of affected individuals, whereas sequence analysis detects <1%. For patients not identified prenatally or on newborn screening, deletion/duplication analysis of the *SMN1* gene detects >95% of patients with spinal muscular atrophy, whereas sequence analysis typically detects <5%. Targeted analysis of *DMPK* is required to identify pathologic expansion of a CTG trinucleotide repeat leading to myotonic dystrophy type 1. If these targeted analyses are negative in patients with a high suspicion of a genetic disorder, exome sequencing with copy number variant analysis should be pursued to detect other genetic etiologies of hypotonia. Detailed phenotyping is essential in interpreting the results of genetic sequencing. Some syndromes, such as trisomy 21 or 22q11.2 deletion syndrome, have characteristic features that may allow for presumptive clinical diagnosis while awaiting confirmatory genetic testing. For other disorders, dysmorphic facial features to note in infancy include low-set ears, large/small ears, hyper- or hypotelorism, epicanthal folds, asymmetric crying facies, short or webbed neck, cleft lip/palate, and maxillary or mandibular hypoplasia (see Chapter 29). Body dysmorphisms in infancy include abnormal limb length, palmar crease, club feet, polydactyly/syndactyly, genitourinary abnormalities, spinal abnormalities, and ophthalmologic abnormalities. These phenotypic findings may provide additional context for the interpretation of sequence or copy number variants of uncertain significance.

If a careful neurologic exam demonstrates a sensory or motor level, such as strong arms and flaccid legs with a pathologic Babinski sign and lower extremity hyperreflexia, then spinal cord pathology is suspected. MRI of the entire spine (with and without gadolinium) typically captures anatomic abnormalities as well as intra- and extramedullary spinal abnormalities.

If hypotonia persists and MRI of the brain and spine, EEG, metabolic screening, and preliminary genetic syndrome screens are negative, then motor neuron, nerve, muscle, or NMJ diseases should be considered (see Tables 35.1 and 35.3).

Profound and persistent hypotonia in the setting of normal intellectual function is the typical pattern for the majority of PNS diseases, and the physical examination does not tend to evolve as much during infancy as it does in CNS disease. In addition, hyporeflexia and absence of a pathologic Babinski sign are the norm with a few exceptions, such as in congenital muscular dystrophy. The most useful initial tests for these patients are a creatine kinase (CK), thyroid-stimulating hormone (TSH), and electromyography with nerve conduction study (EMG/NCS, or simply EMG). In motor neuron disease, CK is typically normal but occasionally might be slightly elevated, while the EMG shows a pure motor neuropathy (see Table 35.2). When obtaining EMG, at least one sensory and motor nerve conduction assessment should be done in an upper and lower extremity and needle EMG should be performed on at least one proximal and one distal muscle. If ptosis, ophthalmoparesis, episodic weakness, or feeding/breathing difficulties are present clinically, then doing a 3-Hz repetitive nerve stimulation (RNS) on an affected muscle may be informative to assess for fatigability suggestive of NMJ disorders. Needle EMG in newborns can be difficult to interpret; waiting for the child to be at least 2 months old might yield more meaningful results. In the meantime, other avenues of testing, such as muscle biopsy and genetic testing, should be pursued as appropriate.

Nerve disorders demonstrate involvement of both sensory and motor nerves either in an axonal or demyelinating pattern on EMG; CK is normal. Muscle diseases have a myopathic EMG, typically with normal sensory nerve conductions. An elevated CK is a hallmark of muscular dystrophies due to the continual degeneration and regeneration of muscle fibers, whereas myopathies typically have a normal CK. Duchenne muscular dystrophy is the prototypical muscular dystrophy with a markedly elevated CK >10,000 U/L in an infant. A parental history of distal weakness with grip myotonia suggests **congenital myotonic dystrophy**. The congenital muscular dystrophies have variable brain MRI findings ranging from normal to lissencephaly, with clinical findings of intellectual delay and seizures. Pompe disease is characterized by concomitant cardiomegaly, feeding difficulties, and failure to thrive. When EMG suggests a myopathy and the CK is normal, then a muscle biopsy can help distinguish between congenital myopathy, mitochondrial disorders, and metabolic myopathies.

If the 3-Hz RNS shows significant decrement and CK is normal, then an NMJ disorder is likely. Clinically, NMJ disorders appear similar to each other with fluctuating ptosis, ophthalmoparesis, feeding and respiratory difficulties, limb and trunk weakness, and poor head control, but key differences help narrow the differential diagnosis. If the mother is known to have autoimmune myasthenia, then a hypotonic infant may have transplacental-derived **transient neonatal myasthenia.** If the hypotonic infant has autonomic dysfunction such as dilated pupils or constipation, then botulism must be considered. If the infant was previously healthy and then rapidly developed symptoms that localize to the NMJ, autoimmune myasthenia is possible, and antibodies should be tested. A child with a history of persistent feeding and respiratory difficulties since birth, worsened by illness or suddenly without an identified cause, should prompt evaluation for congenital myasthenic syndromes, which are a heterogeneous group of genetic disorders.

Arthrogryposis multiplex congenita, the finding of multiple joint contractures affecting two or more body areas and present at birth, can be caused by lesions anywhere in the neural axis including the CNS and PNS, connective tissue and joint disorders, and maternal and fetal factors (Table 35.6). In an infant with arthrogryposis, determining if the cause is central or peripheral or neither is often crucial to making a diagnosis.

TABLE 35.6 Major Causes of Arthrogryposis Multiplex Congenita

Site of Major Pathologic Findings	Disorder
Cerebrum, brainstem, cerebellum	• Microcephaly • Cortical migrational disorders: lissencephaly-pachygyria (e.g., Zellweger syndrome), polymicrogyria, agenesis of the corpus callosum, schizencephaly • Pontocerebellar hypoplasia (type 1) • Dentato-olivary dysplasia • Cytomegalovirus infection • Leptomeningeal angiomatosis • Encephaloclastic processes: porencephalies, hydranencephaly, multicystic encephalomalacia • Hydrocephalus
Spinal cord	• Cervical spinal atrophy • Lumbosacral meningomyelocele • Sacral agenesis
Motor neuron	• Spinal muscular atrophy type 1 • Spinal muscular atrophy with respiratory distress type 1
Peripheral nerve	• Charcot-Marie-Tooth disease
Neuromuscular junction	• Congenital myasthenic syndromes • Maternal autoimmune myasthenia (rare)
Muscle	• Congenital myotonic dystrophy • Congenital muscular dystrophies • Congenital myopathies (nemaline myopathy, myotubular myopathy, core myopathy) • Distal arthrogryposis syndromes (types 1–10)
Intrauterine/maternal factors	• Amyoplasia (vascular compromise to fetus or placenta during embryogenesis) • Lack of space: multiple pregnancies, uterine abnormality (bicornuate uterus, uterine fibroid) • Fetal alcohol syndrome with contractures • Intrauterine tumors • Amniotic fluid leakage • Disruption (bands) • Maternal illnesses: infections, untreated SLE, metabolic imbalances • Maternal medications (curare, muscle relaxants) • Maternal injuries in the first trimester
Joint and connective tissue abnormalities	• Chondrodysplasia • Congenital contractural arachnodactyly • Marfan syndrome

SLE, systemic lupus erythematosus.
Modified from Volpe JJ, ed. *Neurology of the Newborn.* 5th ed. Philadelphia: Saunders; 2008:760.

the cause is central or peripheral or neither is often crucial to making a diagnosis.

Diagnostic Approach to the Child with Weakness

The diagnostic approach to the weak child is very similar to the hypotonic infant, with emphasis placed on identifying systemic disorders first and then determining if signs and symptoms localize to the CNS or PNS. Fig. 35.8 outlines an algorithm for determining the cause of weakness in a child.

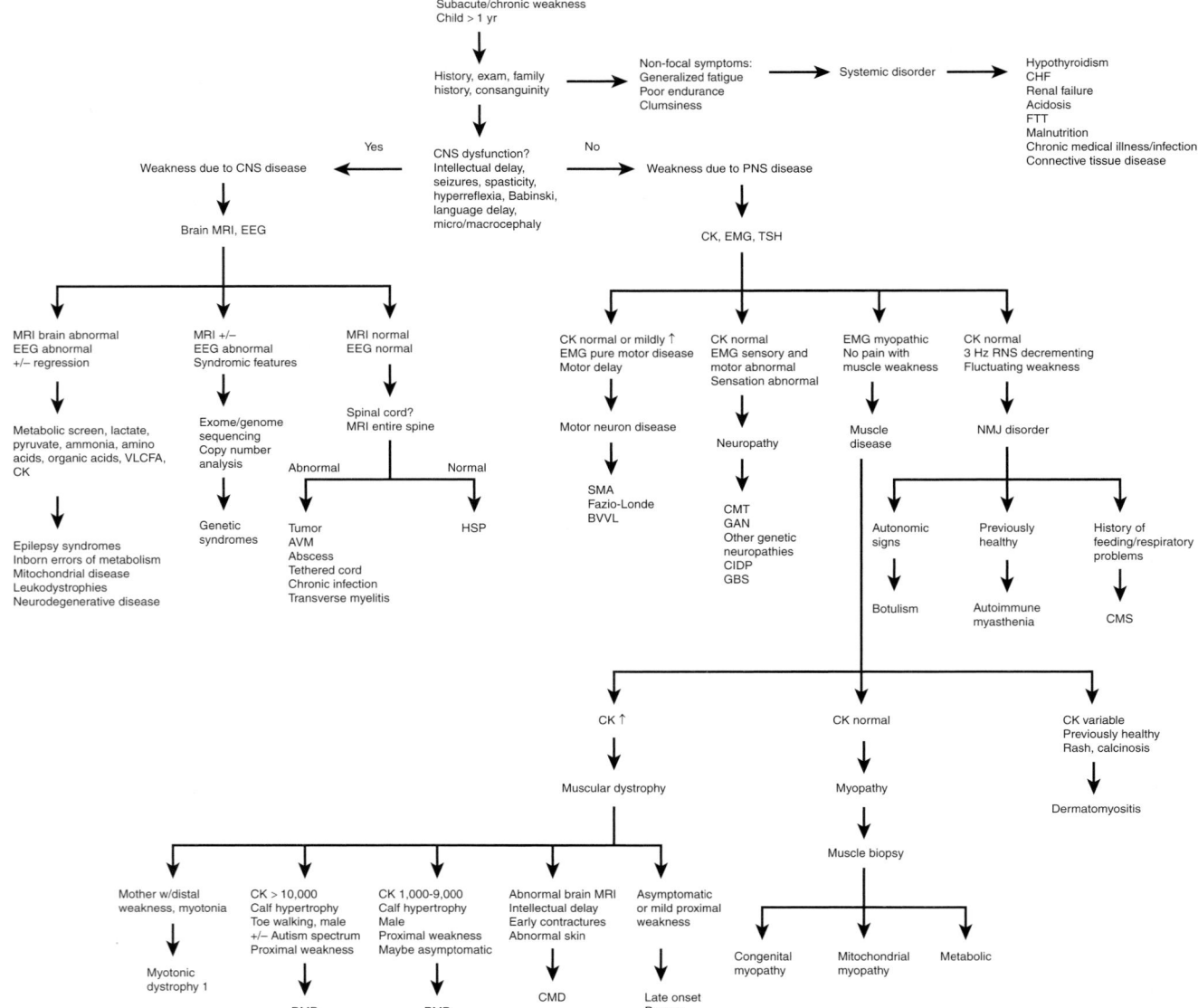

Fig. 35.8 Diagnostic approach to the child with weakness. AVM, arteriovenous malformation; BMD, Becker muscular dystrophy; BVVL, Brown–Vialetto–Van Laere syndrome; CHF, congestive heart failure; CIDP, chronic inflammatory demyelinating polyneuropathy; CK, creatine kinase; CMD, congenital muscular dystrophy; CMS, congenital myasthenic syndrome; CMT, Charcot-Marie-Tooth disease; CNS, central nervous system; DMD, Duchenne muscular dystrophy; EMG, electromyography with nerve conduction; FTT, failure to thrive; GAN, giant axonal neuropathy; GBS, Guillain-Barré syndrome; HSP, hereditary spastic paraplegia; NMJ, neuro-muscular junction; PNS, peripheral nervous system; RNS, repetitive nerve stimulation; SMA, spinal muscular atrophy; TSH, thyroid-stimulating hormone; VLCFA, very long-chain fatty acids.

Disorders of the cerebral cortex commonly cause axial hypotonia but appendicular hypertonia in children. Some progressive neurologic disorders affect both the brain and peripheral nerves (metachromatic dystrophy, Krabbe disease, adrenoleukodystrophies, and some mito-chondrial disorders). Other progressive disorders may affect both brain and muscle (Duchenne muscular dystrophy, myotonic dystrophy, dystroglycanopathies, and some mitochondrial disorders).

Sometimes disturbance of function at one site conveys a predilec-tion for injury to another site in the nervous system, making neuraxial localization more challenging. For instance, children with congenital muscle weakness (e.g., congenital myopathy) are likely to have had severe respiratory impairment at birth that results in secondary anoxic injury to the brain. Because hypotonia itself is nonspecific with regard to localizing the site of nervous system dysfunction, the evaluation of the child with hypotonia must begin with a search for clues that might identify the location of the abnormality.

Is the Problem a Systemic Disorder?

Systemic disorders are a common cause of generalized hypotonia in toddlers and children (see Table 35.1). Hypotonia is commonly seen in association with sepsis and other infections, heart failure, failure to thrive, hypercalcemia, renal failure, hypothyroidism, acidosis, hypoxia, hyperammonemia, hypoglycemia, rickets, scurvy, amino and organic acid disorders, severe malnutrition, and other chronic disorders. This

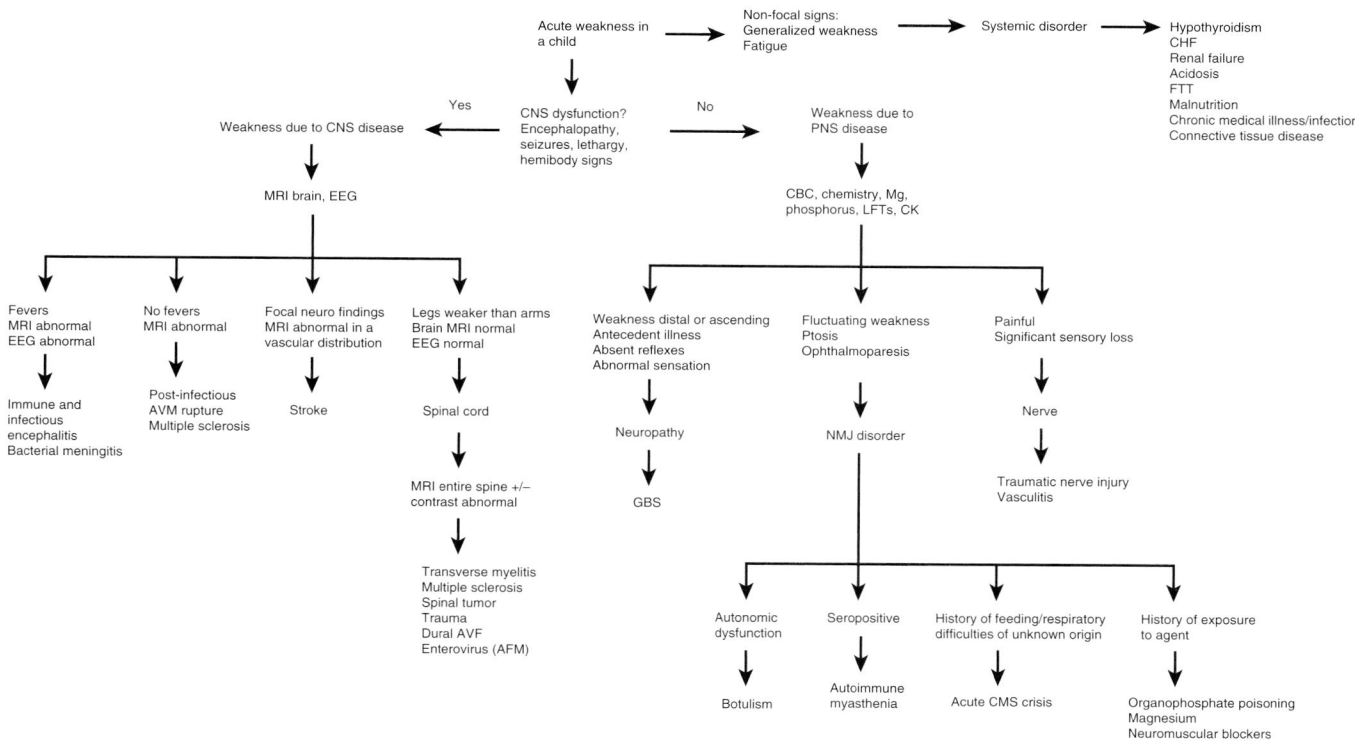

Fig. 35.9 Diagnostic approach to the child with acute weakness. *AFM,* acute flaccid myelitis; *AVF,* arteriovenous fistula; *AVM,* arteriovenous malformation; *CHF,* congestive heart failure; *CK,* creatine kinase; *CMS,* congenital myasthenic syndrome; *CNS,* central nervous system; *FTT,* failure to thrive; *GBS,* Guillain-Barré syndrome; *LFTs,* liver function tests; *NMJ,* neuromuscular junction; *PNS,* peripheral nervous system.

observation warrants a careful search for a systemic or metabolic abnormality in children with hypotonia, particularly (but not exclusively) when the onset of hypotonia is acute (Fig. 35.9).

Frequently overlooked causes of hypotonia are those that are not traditionally considered neurologic disorders, though may mimic neurologic disorders. **Connective tissue disorders** often produce a phenotype similar to those of neurologic causes of hypotonia in infancy and early childhood, with associated delay of developmental milestones. Connective tissue disorders are distinguished by joint hyperextensibility disproportionate to the extent of weakness and by the absence of other neurologic abnormalities or microcephaly (velocardiofacial syndrome, achondroplasia, Marfan syndrome, Ehlers-Danlos syndrome). In several congenital disorders, hypotonia is a regular feature as a result of a combination of abnormalities of neurologic, muscle, and connective tissue function, including Sotos syndrome, Prader-Willi syndrome, Angelman syndrome, Noonan syndrome, Rett syndrome, and Smith-Lemli-Opitz syndrome.

Diagnostic Considerations

Any child with hypotonia and weakness should be evaluated for a systemic disorder. Laboratory evaluation, such as electrolyte measurements, renal function tests, thyroid function tests, and acid-base balance assessment, should be considered. Laboratory evaluation should also be considered for uncommon metabolic disorders in children with chronic hypotonia, especially those with other neurologic findings and those with recurrent bouts of lethargy, episodic severe hypotonia, vomiting, or acidosis. Appropriate metabolic screening tests include plasma and urine amino acid quantification, urine organic acid quantification, and measurements of blood ammonia, blood lactate, pyruvate, and GDF-15.

Genetic analysis should be performed for any hypotonic child who additionally demonstrates microcephaly, growth retardation, congenital malformations, dysmorphism, global developmental delay, or features of specific genetic disorders. If characteristic neurologic or dysmorphic features are present, specific disorders, such as Rett syndrome, Angelman syndrome, Prader-Willi syndrome, Noonan syndrome, Sotos syndrome, and fragile X syndrome, must be considered.

Common Disorders

Trisomy 21. The child with trisomy 21 generally has recognizable features, including microcephaly, up-slanted palpebral fissures, epicanthal folds, flat nasal bridge, protuberant tongue, excess posterior nuchal skin, and single palmar creases (see Chapter 29). Hypotonia and associated weakness are nearly universal findings. As the child grows, the muscle strength generally improves, but the hypotonia persists. The diagnosis is established by genetic analysis showing trisomy 21.

Prader-Willi syndrome. Prader-Willi syndrome manifests in early infancy with marked hypotonia and virtually no other identifiable symptoms, though cryptorchidism in males and features of hypogonadism in both males and females may be apparent. As the child grows, the phenotypic features become more apparent, including microbrachycephaly, almond-shaped palpebrae, short stature, and small hands and feet. At 3–6 years of age, the child develops a disorder of appetite that results in ravenous food-seeking behaviors, impaired satiety, and eventual marked obesity if access to food is not regulated. Weakness associated with the disorder is most prominent in the neonate and older infant and gradually lessens, whereas the hypotonia persists.

DNA methylation analysis is the only technique that accounts for paternal deletion, maternal uniparental disomy, and imprinting defects and identifies >99% of affected patients. Up to 75% of affected children have a deletion of chromosome 15q11-q13 of paternal origin, and 20–25% have maternal disomy. Because the clinical findings are non-specific during the early months, such testing should be performed in any neonate or infant with hypotonia of unknown cause.

Uncommon Disorders

Metabolic disorders. Metabolic disorders that are associated with hypotonia include the following (see Table 35.1):

- Aminoacidopathies, organic acidurias, urea cycle defects, fatty acid oxidation defects
- Lowe syndrome
- Peroxisomal disorders (Refsum syndrome, adrenoleukodystrophy, Zellweger syndrome)
- Acyl coenzyme A dehydrogenase deficiencies
- Storage disorders (mannosidosis, Krabbe disease, sialuria, mucolipidosis type IV, Tay-Sachs disease)

Genetic neurologic disorders. Neurologic disorders associated with hypotonia are often recognizable by unusual neurologic features that include the following:

- **Angelman syndrome**: global developmental delay, wide-based ataxic gait with arms flexed at elbows and hands flapping ("happy puppet"), little or no language, inappropriate laughter, and seizures. A characteristic dysmorphic feature includes a wide mouth with increased space between teeth. DNA methylation analysis reveals that up to 80% have abnormal methylation in the maternally inherited 15q11.2-q13 locus, the same chromosome that is affected in Prader-Willi syndrome.
- **Rett syndrome**: developmental regression characterized by partial or complete loss of previously attained fine motor abilities, language and gait dysfunction, autism, characteristic hand-wringing movements, mostly in females, though affected males present with severe neonatal-onset encephalopathy that is progressive and typically fatal in infancy or early toddlerhood. Genetic sequencing of the *MECP2* gene demonstrates heterozygous pathogenic variants in females and a hemizygous pathogenic variant in liveborn males.

Congenital malformation syndromes. Congenital malformation syndromes are recognizable by their characteristic features:

- **Sotos syndrome**: prominent forehead with dolichocephaly; macrosomia; down-slanted palpebrae; long, narrow face; intellectual delay; mild ventriculomegaly.
- **Noonan syndrome**: short stature, down-slanted palpebrae, low-set posteriorly rotated ears, hypertelorism, congenital heart disease, pectus deformities, webbed/short neck, ptosis, intellectual disability in some. Diagnosis is based on clinical features combined with a comprehensive genetic panel or genomic sequencing demonstrating a disease-causing pathogenic variant.
- **Lowe syndrome**: congenital cataracts, aminoaciduria, metabolic acidosis, hypotonia, global developmental delay, seizures in some, behavioral abnormalities (obsessive-compulsiveness or self-stimulation). Pathogenic variants in the *OCRL* gene are responsible for this syndrome.

Connective tissue disorders. Connective tissue disorders associated with hypotonia, and particularly with joint hyperextensibility, can also generally be recognized by their associated symptoms:

- **Stickler syndrome**: Pierre Robin sequence (micrognathia, cleft palate, glossoptosis), flattened facies, myopia
- **Velocardiofacial syndrome**: congenital heart disease, micrognathia, hypocalcemia, T-cell disorders, cleft palate
- **Achondroplasia**: disproportionate short stature, risk of brainstem compression
- **Ehlers-Danlos syndrome**: skin bruising and scarring, skin hyperelasticity, smooth skin, joint hypermobility

- **Marfan syndrome**: tall stature; long, thin arms and fingers; ectopic lens; blue sclera; aortic dissection; mitral valve prolapse
- **Osteogenesis imperfecta**: frequent fractures, either atraumatic or associated with minimal trauma

Although many of these disorders may result in delayed motor milestones due to the hypotonia or skeletal abnormalities, and a subsequent evaluation for presumed weakness, their underlying condition does not cause primary pathology affecting the neural axis.

Is the Problem in the Cerebrum or Cerebellum?

Diagnostic Considerations

Several clues suggest that hypotonia is caused by an abnormality of cerebral function. The presence of associated symptoms attributable to dysfunction of the cerebral cortex is the most useful and may include the following:

- Acute impairment of consciousness
- Acute or chronic impairment of cognitive abilities (mental status examination or poor school grades, respectively)
- Seizures
- Developmental regression

Delayed language and social development are typical of chronic disorders. The presence of microcephaly or macrocephaly is also an important clue. Brisk reflexes, clonus, an asymmetric tonic neck response, and pathologic Babinski signs suggest possible cerebral cortical dysfunction. The presence of dysmorphism or of congenital malformations suggests the possibility of an underlying cerebral malformation. Congenital ocular malformations (e.g., microphthalmia or optic hypoplasia) are frequently associated with congenital brain malformation as well.

Hypertonia mixed with signs of hypotonia strongly suggests a cerebral origin. Cerebral palsy is often characterized by hypotonia in infancy with later development of spasticity. In some children with cerebral dysfunction, the coexistence of hypotonia and hypertonia is persistent. Thus, an infant with hypotonia of the neck and trunk musculature who also exhibits scissoring of the lower extremities or persistent fisting of the hands (i.e., typical signs of hypertonia) can be presumed to have cerebral dysfunction.

Signs of cerebellar dysfunction (e.g., ataxia, nystagmus, titubation, dysmetria, and impairment of coordination) are often useful diagnostic clues. The cerebellum helps maintain normal muscle tone and diseases of the cerebellum typically are associated with some degree of hypotonia.

Common Disorders

Hypoxic-ischemic encephalopathy. Brain injury resulting from asphyxia, hypoxia, or ischemia is an important cause of neonatal neurologic morbidity. Tissue oxygen deficiency is presumed to underlie the neurologic injury caused by hypoxic-ischemic insults. An oxygen deficit may be incurred by either hypoxemia or ischemia. **Hypoxemia** is defined as diminished oxygen content of blood, while **ischemia** is characterized by reduced blood perfusion in a particular tissue bed. Hypoxemia and ischemia often occur simultaneously or in sequence. Ischemia is likely to be the more significant contributor of these two insults.

Asphyxia denotes an impairment in gas exchange, which results not only in a deficit of oxygen in blood but also in an excess of carbon dioxide with resultant acidosis. Furthermore, sustained asphyxia usually results in hypotension and ischemia, which is consistent with the likely predominant importance of ischemia as the final common pathway to brain injury. Asphyxia is the most common clinical insult resulting in brain injury during the perinatal period.

Evidence of hypoxic-ischemic injury to the neonatal nervous system is reflected by a constellation of signs noticed early after birth. The asphyxiating event or events may occur at any point in the antepartum, intrapartum, or postpartum periods. It is estimated that insults sustained by the fetus during the antepartum period, such as maternal cardiac arrest or hemorrhage leading to transplacental and fetal hypotension, account for approximately 20% of cases of HIE. Intrapartum events, such as placental abruption, uterine rupture, and traumatic delivery, may account for 35% of cases of HIE. In an additional 35% of infants displaying signs of HIE, markers of intrapartum fetal distress and antepartum risk, such as maternal diabetes, intrauterine growth restriction, or maternal infection, are found. Postpartum difficulties, such as cardiovascular compromise, persistent fetal circulation, and recurrent apnea, account for approximately 10% of HIE cases. Postpartum difficulties are found more commonly in premature than in full-term infants. Therefore, for at least 35% of cases of neonatal HIE, difficulties of the intrapartum period alone do not explain the encephalopathy.

Recognition of neonatal HIE requires careful observation and examination of the newborn in the context of a detailed history of pregnancy, labor, and delivery. Newborns who have sustained hypoxic-ischemic insults severe enough to cause permanent neurologic injury usually demonstrate abnormalities on neurologic examination. A combination of low Apgar scores, fetal acidosis or distress, and abnormal neurologic examination findings help define HIE. Nonetheless, if the hypoxic-ischemic damage has occurred well in advance of parturition, it may be asymptomatic in the neonate.

Mild HIE (stage 1) may be characterized by hyperalertness or by mild depression of the level of consciousness, which may be accompanied by uninhibited Moro and brisk deep tendon reflexes, signs of sympathetic activity (dilated pupils), and a normal or only slightly abnormal EEG. Typically, these symptoms last less than 24 hours. **Moderate HIE (stage 2)** may be marked by obtundation, hypotonia, diminished spontaneous movements, and seizures. Infants with **severe HIE (stage 3)** are ill for more than 24 hours and are comatose. These infants are also markedly hypotonic and display bulbar and autonomic dysfunction. The EEG is abnormal and may demonstrate a burst-suppression pattern or seizures, or may be isoelectric.

Neonates with moderate or severe HIE may show variation in the level of consciousness during the first days after birth. Initially, depression of the level of alertness may appear to improve after the first 12–24 hours after birth. However, specific signs of improving alertness such as visual fixation or following are lacking. In addition, other persistent or progressive neurologic deficits, as well as functional deterioration of other extraneural systems, are inconsistent with a true improvement in neurologic state. Coma may persist, supervene, or even progress to brain death by 72 hours of life. If the infant survives 72 hours without losing all cerebral function, a variable amount of improvement may be observed.

Diffuse hypotonia accompanied by a lack of movement constitutes the most frequently observed motor deficit found early in the course of neonatal HIE. By the end of the first day, patterns of weakness that reflect the distribution of cerebral injury from a generalized hypoxic-ischemic insult may emerge. Affected full-term infants may demonstrate quadriparesis with predominant proximal limb weakness. This pattern of weakness derives from ischemia in the watershed or parasagittal region of the brain, which corresponds to the border zones of circulation between the anterior and the middle cerebral arteries and the middle and the posterior cerebral arteries. Affected premature infants may have weakness primarily in the lower extremities because of perinatal ischemic injury of motor fibers serving the legs. These fibers lie dorsal and lateral to the external angles of the lateral ventricles. Focal

ischemia (stroke) may result in focal deficits reflective of the vascular territory in which the injury has occurred. These patterns are relatively subtle. As many as 70% of infants with moderate or severe HIE experience seizures by the end of the first day of life.

There is a direct relationship between motor and cognitive deficits at 1 year of age and the severity of acidosis observed at birth in asphyxiated and symptomatic neonates. The extent of these sequelae is dependent not only on the occurrence of asphyxia but also on its duration. The three stages of HIE also correlate with outcome at 1 year of age. Those neonates with mild (stage 1) HIE or those who demonstrate moderate (stage 2) HIE for <5 days usually develop normally. Persistence of moderate encephalopathy or appearance of severe (stage 3) HIE is associated with seizures and motor and cognitive delay during follow-up. Children with mild HIE as neonates tend to be free of deficits in motor and cognitive functioning or school performance. Greater impairment of performance in each of these developmental spheres is found among children who exhibited moderate or severe neonatal HIE.

The likelihood of long-term neurologic sequelae after HIE is higher in neonates who have seizures. The EEG may provide valuable prognostic information after the occurrence of seizure. Interictal background abnormalities, such as a burst-suppression pattern, persistently low voltage, and electrocerebral inactivity, are highly correlated with poor outcome. Conversely, infants with normal EEGs or those revealing only maturational delay have much more favorable prognoses. Long-term outcomes in moderate and severe HIE include cerebral palsy, hearing loss, visual impairment, poor memory and attention, hyperactivity, irritability, increased support requirements, lower standardized test scores, autism, and psychosis.

Neuroimaging is useful in determining prognosis. Head ultrasonography findings of severe periventricular intraparenchymal echodensities followed by evidence of tissue injury (cyst formation) are correlated with later motor and cognitive deficits in premature infants. MRI performed early in the neonatal course of hypoxic-ischemic brain injury provides useful prognostic information. Most infants with MRI evidence of basal ganglia hemorrhage, periventricular leukomalacia, or multicystic encephalomalacia after asphyxia ultimately demonstrate neurodevelopmental abnormalities. Diffusion-weighted imaging (DWI) reveals evidence of neonatal brain injury earlier than T1- and T2-weighted pulse sequences. Indeed, DWI reveals focal injury when standard MRI and CT are normal (Fig. 35.10).

Advances in neonatal neurocritical care, including the use of therapeutic hypothermia and aggressive seizure management, have improved long-term outcomes in moderate and severe HIE, including children with sustained normal neurodevelopmental trajectories.

Brain malformations. Brain malformation can arise as a result of a chromosomal disorder, as a component of a multiple malformation syndrome, or as an isolated abnormality. When associated with a chromosomal disorder or multiple malformation syndromes, the other associated features are the primary clues to diagnosis. In isolated brain malformation, the primary features include cognitive and motor developmental impairment and, in most cases, microcephaly. The MRI scan can detect abnormalities of development of the hemispheric structures (e.g., agenesis of the corpus callosum, holoprosencephaly), abnormalities of cortical cellular migration (e.g., lissencephaly, pachygyria), and cerebral heterotopias as well as brainstem and cerebellar malformations (e.g., Joubert syndrome).

Uncommon Disorders

Progressive encephalopathies of infancy. Progressive encephalopathies of infancy account for a small number of children with persistent hypotonia (see Chapters 27 and 28). These disorders are recognizable by a progressive deterioration of neurologic function and by diagnostically

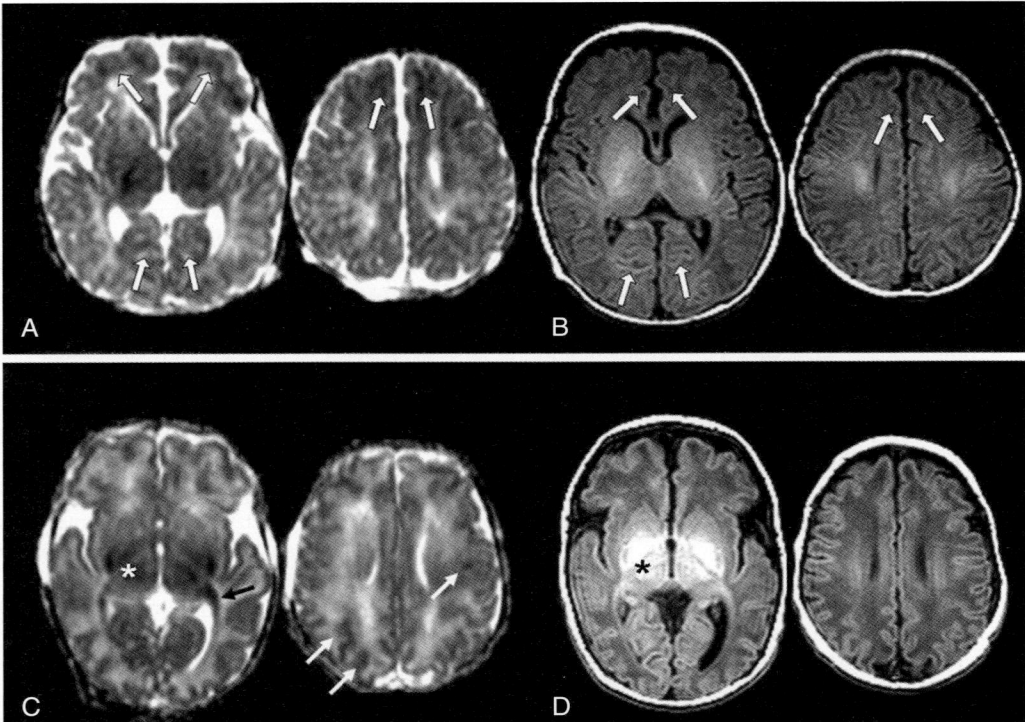

Fig. 35.10 Predominant patterns of brain injury in newborns with hypoxic-ischemic brain injury. These apparent diffusion coefficient maps (*A* and *C*) performed on day 3 of life and T1-weighted images (*B* and *D*) performed on day 10 of life are typical of the two major predominant patterns of brain injury seen in term newborns with hypoxic-ischemic encephalopathy. *A*, In the "watershed" pattern, areas of restricted diffusion are seen in the parasagittal regions *(arrows)*. *B*, One week later, very subtle hyperintensities can be seen in the same areas on the T1-weighted images *(arrows)*. *C*, In the "basal nuclei" predominant pattern, the areas that show restricted diffusion are the thalami and basal ganglia *(white star)* bilaterally. In this example, part of the optic radiation is also affected *(black arrow)*. *D*, On day 10, the injury in the thalami and basal ganglia *(black star)* appears as T1 hyperintensities bilaterally.

specific clues. The infant's development is normal for some time and then plateaus; this plateau is followed by developmental regression with loss of previously acquired skills. Hypotonia is a feature of many of these disorders, at least at some point during the course of the illness. Some disorders feature hypotonia as the result of the combination of CNS injury and an associated polyneuropathy (Krabbe disease and metachromatic leukodystrophy). Progressive disorders that may be associated with hypotonia include neonatal adrenoleukodystrophy, mannosidosis, fucosidosis, Gaucher disease types 2 and 3, GM₁ gangliosidosis, infantile neuroaxonal dystrophy, infantile Refsum disease, Krabbe disease, metachromatic leukodystrophy, mucolipidosis type IV, and Tay-Sachs disease. The diagnosis of these disorders is based on recognition of clinically suggestive clues and on results of specialized biochemical and molecular genetic testing. If such a disorder is suspected, the infant should be referred to appropriate genetic and neurologic specialists.

Mitochondrial diseases. Mitochondrial diseases often affect both the brain and muscle and clinically manifest as hypotonia, likely as a combination of both cerebral dysfunction and myopathy (Tables 35.7 and 35.8). The diagnosis is based on recognition of clinical symptoms, presence of lactic acidosis, an elevation in serum levels of GDF-15, the presence of ragged red fibers on muscle histologic examination, and mitochondrial abnormalities identifiable on a muscle electron microscopic examination (Fig. 35.11). The diagnosis of many mitochondrial diseases is suggested by elevated GDF-15 levels and is made possible by specific mitochondrial DNA testing or analysis of

nuclear genes responsible for mitochondrial structure and function. Not all mitochondrial disorders have an identifiable responsible gene variant or an abnormal muscle biopsy. Other inborn errors of metabolism may produce hypotonia by central mechanisms (organic acidurias, hyperammonemia) or by interfering with muscle metabolism.

Brain malformation syndromes. **Miller-Dieker syndrome** is characterized by severe **lissencephaly** ("smooth brain" with agyria), severe developmental impairment, hypotonia early in life, and hypertonia with age. Facial changes include bitemporal hollowing, upturned nares, thin vermilion border, and small jaw. Microdeletions of 17p13.3 affecting the *PAFAH1B1* and *YWHAE* genes cause 80% of de novo cases, whereas the remaining 20% are inherited from a parent with a balanced chromosomal rearrangement.

Dystroglycanopathies (previously known as **muscle-eye-brain disease**) are a category of congenital muscular dystrophies with eye abnormalities and an assortment of brain malformations including cobblestone lissencephaly type II, focal pachygyria, polymicrogyria, pontocerebellar hypoplasia, and occipital encephalocele. These diseases are characterized by hypotonia in infancy due to a concomitant muscular dystrophy and CNS disease and variable degrees of intellectual disability. **Walker-Warburg syndrome** is the most severe form of dystroglycanopathy, usually resulting with early demise. The list of genes associated with dystroglycanopathy includes *POMT1*, *POMT2*, *POMGnT1*, *POMGnT2*, *FKTN*, *FKRP*, *LARGE*, *ISPD*, *GTDC2*, *B3GALNT2*, *B3GNT1*, *B4GAT1*, *TMEM5*, *POMK*, *DPM1*, *DPM2*, *DPM3*, *DOLK*, *GMPPB*, *RXYLT1*, and *DAG1*.

TABLE 35.7 Clinical Spectrum of Mitochondrial Disease

Nervous System
- Hypotonia
- Failure to thrive
- Motor regression
- Stroke (nonvascular)
- Dementia
- Episodic encephalopathy (elevated cerebrospinal fluid lactate)
- Intellectual disability
- Neuropathy (axonal, demyelinating, or sensory ganglionopathy)
- Ophthalmoparesis (slowly progressive)
- Ptosis (slowly progressive; little diurnal variation; asymmetric at onset)
- Optic atrophy
- Retinitis pigmentosa (perimacular; vision usually spared)
- Ataxia
- Central apnea
- Epilepsy (focal or multifocal myoclonus; status epilepticus; triggered by sodium valproate)
- Migraines
- Sensorineural hearing loss (asymmetric; young onset; partial recovery possible)

Heart
- Cardiomyopathy
- Conduction block or arrhythmia

Skeletal Muscle
- Myopathy (proximal, symmetric weakness; myalgia)
- Exercise intolerance
- Episodic rhabdomyolysis

Other
- Lactic acidosis
- Recurrent bowel obstruction (pseudoobstruction)
- Short stature
- Diabetes (young onset; nonobese)

Modified from Amato A, Russell J. *Neuromuscular Disorders.* 1st ed. New York: McGraw-Hill; 2008; Liang C, Ahmad K, Sue CM. The broadening spectrum of mitochondrial disease: shifts in the diagnostic paradigm. *Biochim Biophys Acta.* 2014;1840:1360–1367.

Is the Problem in the Spinal Cord?

Diagnostic Considerations

Depending on the location of the lesion, spinal cord dysfunction can produce a spectrum of motor findings, from spastic weakness of all four extremities to flaccid paraparesis of the lower extremities (Table 35.9). Different etiologies manifest as specific spinal cord syndromes, many of which are characterized by increased tone (Table 35.10). However, particularly after acute injury to the spinal cord and in some chronic disorders of the spinal cord, hypotonia may be the prominent motor sign. The typical associated findings of hyperreflexia, clonus, Babinski signs, and sensory loss with a sensory level are important clues, as is the disparity between the weakness and sensory impairment of the extremities in contrast to the normal strength and function of the head and neck.

Spinal cord injury resulting from birth trauma is a frequently overlooked cause of hypotonia in the newborn. A history of a lengthy or difficult (e.g., breech or vertex) delivery should suggest spinal cord injury, and care should be taken not to falsely attribute motor dysfunction in these infants to anoxic brain injury; however, many neonates with spinal cord injuries also have anoxic encephalopathy because of the traumatic nature of the delivery, potentially obscuring consideration of spinal cord injury in infants with more prominent signs of brain anoxia. The extent to which the hypotonia of neonatal hypoxic-ischemic injury is caused by hypoxic injury to the spinal cord has not yet been fully elucidated. Any child with suspected spinal cord injury should undergo MRI. Radiographically, the bones of the cervical spine are normal, but MRI demonstrates the cord lesion. As acute neurosurgical intervention is often required, birth-related spinal cord injury should always be considered in hypotonic neonates with prolonged or difficult deliveries. Additional categories of spinal cord disease are outlined in Table 35.11.

Common Disorders

Meningomyelocele. Meningomyelocele is a congenital malformation of the spine, spinal cord, and overlying meninges that affects up to 0.2% of liveborn infants, with some degree of geographic variation in incidence. The spinal defect may be antenatally diagnosed or is obvious at birth, except in milder abnormalities that are covered by skin. The degree to which the lower extremities are hypotonic and flaccid depends on the location of the spinal defect. The presence of a Chiari malformation and associated hydrocephalus must be discerned in every affected patient. Antenatal diagnosis and fetal surgical correction are possible. Maternal screening reveals elevated serum α-fetoprotein, and fetal ultrasound can further delineate the extent of the defect.

Transverse myelitis. Transverse myelitis is a common cause of acute hypotonia and weakness that manifests over hours or several days. The localization is suggested by an identifiable motor-sensory level and by impairment of bowel and bladder function. Reflexes are characteristically depressed at the onset of the disease and then become exaggerated with clonus and Babinski signs. The diagnosis is via MRI and CSF analysis; signal intensity of the involved cord segment is abnormal on MRI, and mild pleocytosis and elevated CSF protein levels are present. Myelitis may occur as part of acute disseminated encephalomyelitis (ADEM), multiple sclerosis (MS), neuromyelitis optica spectrum disorder (NMOSD), or an autoimmune rheumatic disease such as systemic lupus erythematosus (SLE), Sjögren syndrome, or sarcoidosis. CSF assays that demonstrate immunologic activity unique to the intrathecal space, such as oligoclonal bands or an elevated immunoglobulin G (IgG) synthesis index, are clues to disorders such as ADEM, MS, and NMOSD; specific antibody testing of the serum and CSF can provide specific diagnosis. If myelitis is accompanied by severe limb weakness, indicative of motor neuron damage, then a diagnosis of West Nile virus (WNV) or enterovirus-causing acute flaccid myelitis (AFM) needs to be entertained via rapid imaging and microbiologic and serologic assays of the blood and CSF assessing for specific organisms. WNV classically causes a concomitant encephalopathy, unlike AFM. Clinical features of AFM are noted in Table 35.12 and distinguishing features in Table 35.13. Imaging of AFM is noted in Fig. 35.12.

Tethered cord syndrome. Pathologically, tethered cord syndrome (TCS) occurs when the lumbosacral spinal cord is fixed to the sacrum due to a thickened filum terminale, dermal sinus, or lipoma resulting in downward traction as the vertebrae elongate with vertical growth. Physiologically, this traction results in reduced blood flow and ischemia to the cord and cauda equina, causing Wallerian degeneration. In infants and neonates, evidence of spina bifida occulta may be evident externally due to various cutaneous findings such as lipomas, a hair tuft, nevi, hemangiomas, and dermal sinuses (Fig. 35.13). Typical presenting signs and symptoms are anorectal malformation, lower

TABLE 35.8 Select Mitochondrial Disorders with Hypotonia Classified by Clinical Phenotype and Genotype

Clinical Phenotype	Common Clinical Features	Associated Genetic Changes	Mode of Inheritance
MELAS syndrome (mitochondrial encephalopathy, lactic acidosis, and strokelike episodes)	Cardinal—strokelike episodes, intermittent encephalopathy, T2/FLAIR abnormalities on brain MRI that do not respect vascular territory, lactic acidosis Other—hearing loss, diabetes, short stature, gastrointestinal issues	tRNA point mutations: • m.3243A>G in tRNA^{Leu} (~80% of cases) • m.3217T>C in tRNA^{Leu} (~7.5% of cases) • m.13513G>A encoding NADH-ubiquinone (<15% of cases) • m.3252A>G in tRNA^{Leu} (<5% of cases) • Multiple other mtDNA point mutations	Maternal
MERRF syndrome (myoclonic epilepsy with ragged red fibers)	Cardinal—myoclonus, proximal weakness, generalized epilepsy, ataxia Other—multiple lipomatosis, hearing loss, cognitive impairment, neuropathy	tRNA point mutations: • m.8344A>G in tRNA^{Lys} (>80% of cases) • m.8356T>C in tRNA^{Lys} • m.8363G>A in tRNA^{Lys} • m.8361G>A in tRNA^{Lys} • Multiple other mtDNA point mutations	Maternal
KSS (Kearns-Sayre syndrome)	Cardinal—multisystemic disease with progressive external ophthalmoplegia, pigmentary retinopathy, cardiomyopathy before age 20yr Other—short stature, proximal muscle weakness, hearing loss, dementia, ataxia, multiple endocrinopathies (diabetes, hypothyroidism, hypoparathyroidism, hypogonadism	Single large mtDNA deletion (1.1–10 kb) • m.8470_13446del4977 (deletion of 4977 base pairs; most common) • Multiple other mtDNA deletions	Sporadic
CPEO (chronic progressive external ophthalmoplegia)	Cardinal—skeletal muscle disorder with ptosis, ophthalmoparesis, +/− proximal muscle weakness	Single large mtDNA deletion (1.1–10kb) • m.3243A>G in tRNA^{Leu} (most common; same as MELAS) • Multiple other mtDNA point mutations • Multiple mtDNA deletions caused by pathologic variants in the following nuclear genes: *SLC25A4* encoding ANT1, *C10orf2* encoding twinkle, *POLG* encoding mtDNA polymerase, *POLG2*, *OPA1*	Sporadic Maternal Autosomal dominant
Leigh syndrome (subacute necrotizing encephalomyelopathy)	Hypotonia, spasticity, movement disorders (chorea), cerebellar ataxia, neuropathy, bilateral basal ganglia lesions, seizures, lactic acidosis, psychomotor retardation/regression especially with illness between 3 and 12 mo of age Hypertrophic cardiomyopathy	mtDNA pathologic variants: • m.8993T>G or m.8993T>C in *MT-ATP6* (~10% of cases) • Multiple other mtDNA point mutations • m.8470_13446del4977 (deletion of 4977 base pairs; also seen in KSS) Nuclear gene variants resulting in respiratory chain complex deficiencies: • Complex I: *NDUFS1, NDUFS2, NDUFS3, NDUFS4, NDUFS7, NDUFS8, NDUFV1, NDUFV2, NDUFA2, NDUFA9, NDUFA10, NDUFA12, NDUFAF2, NDUFAF4, NDUFAF5, NDUFAF6, NDUFAF8, FOXRED1, NUBPL, TIMMDC1* • Complex II: *SDHA, SDHAF1* • Complex III: *BCS1L, UQCRQ, TTC19* • Complex IV: *SURF1, COX8A, COX10, COX15, SCO2, NDUFA4, PET100, PET117, LRPPRC, TACO1* • Complex V: *ATP5MD*; additional nuclear genes involved in mitochondrial DNA maintenance (e.g., *POLG*), mitochondrial gene expression, cofactor biosynthesis, and other aspects of mitochondrial structure and function have also been associated with Leigh syndrome.	Maternal Sporadic Autosomal recessive

NARP (neurogenic muscle weakness, ataxia, retinitis pigmentosa)	Proximal neurogenic muscle weakness, sensory neuropathy, seizures, ataxia, pigmentary retinopathy, learning difficulties, dementia with onset usually in childhood	• m.8993T>G or m.8993T>C in *MT-ATP6* (50% of cases)	Maternal
Mitochondrial DNA maintenance defects (formerly categorized as mitochondrial DNA depletion syndromes and deletion syndromes)	• **Encephalohepatopathy phenotype:** developmental delay, seizures, hepatic dysfunction and failure, hearing impairment, hypotonia, hypoglycemia, lactic acidosis • **Encephalomyopathy phenotype:** early-onset developmental delay, seizures, hypotonia, hearing impairment, optic atrophy, ophthalmoplegia, ptosis, ataxia • **Encephaloneuropathy phenotype:** hypotonia, vision impairment, hearing impairment, epilepsy, optic atrophy • **MNGIE (mitochondrial neurogastrointestinal encephalopathy):** symmetric distal weakness, demyelinating peripheral neuropathy, paresthesia, ptosis, ophthalmoparesis or ophthalmoplegia, asymptomatic leukoencephalopathy, progressive gastrointestinal dysmotility, hypotonia, proximal muscle weakness, axial weakness, respiratory insufficiency, marked clinical variability with death in infancy to early adulthood due to respiratory insufficiency • **Myopathy:** hypotonia, ptosis, ophthalmoplegia, cataracts, hypertrophic cardiomyopathy • **Ophthalmoplegia:** ptosis, ophthalmoplegia, generalized weakness with easy fatigability, bulbar dysfunction, ataxia • **Optic atrophy:** vision impairment, optic nerve pallor, peripheral neuropathy, muscle weakness • **Neuropathy:** peripheral sensory and motor neuropathy	• **Encephalohepatopathy:** *DGUOK, MPV17, POLG, TFAM, TWNK* • **Encephalomyopathy:** *ABAT, FBXL4, OPA1, POLG, RNASEH1, RRM2B, SUCLA2, SUCLG1* • **Encephaloneuropathy:** *OPA1, POLG, TWNK* • **MNGIE:** *TYMP, POLG, RRM2B* • **Myopathy:** *AGK, DGUOK, DNA2, MGME1, POLG2, SLC25A4, TK2* • **Ophthalmoplegia:** *POLG, RRM2B, SLC25A4, TK2, TWNK* • **Optic atrophy:** *OPA1, MFN2* • **Neuropathy:** *MFN2*	Varied

FLAIR, fluid-attenuated inversion recovery; mtDNA, mitochondrial DNA; NADH, nicotinamide adenine dinucleotide, reduced form; tRNA, transfer RNA.

Data from DiMauro S, Hirano M. MERRF. 2003 June 3. In: *GeneReviews [Internet].* Seattle: University of Washington; 2003; DiMauro S, Hirano M. MELAS. 2001 February 27. In: *GeneReviews [Internet].* Seattle: University of Washington; 2001; Thorburn DR, Rahman S. Mitochondrial DNA-Associated Leigh Syndrome and NARP. 2003 October 30. In: *GeneReviews [Internet].* Seattle: University of Washington; 2003; Liang C, Ahmad K, Sue CM. The broadening spectrum of mitochondrial disease: shifts in the diagnostic paradigm. *Biochim Biophys Acta.* 2014;1840:1360–1367. El-Hattab AW, Craigen WJ, Wong LJC, et al. Mitochondrial DNA maintenance defects overview. 2018 Mar 8. In: Adam MP, Ardinger HH, Pagon RA, et al (eds). *GeneReviews [Internet].* Seattle: University of Washington; 1993–2021.

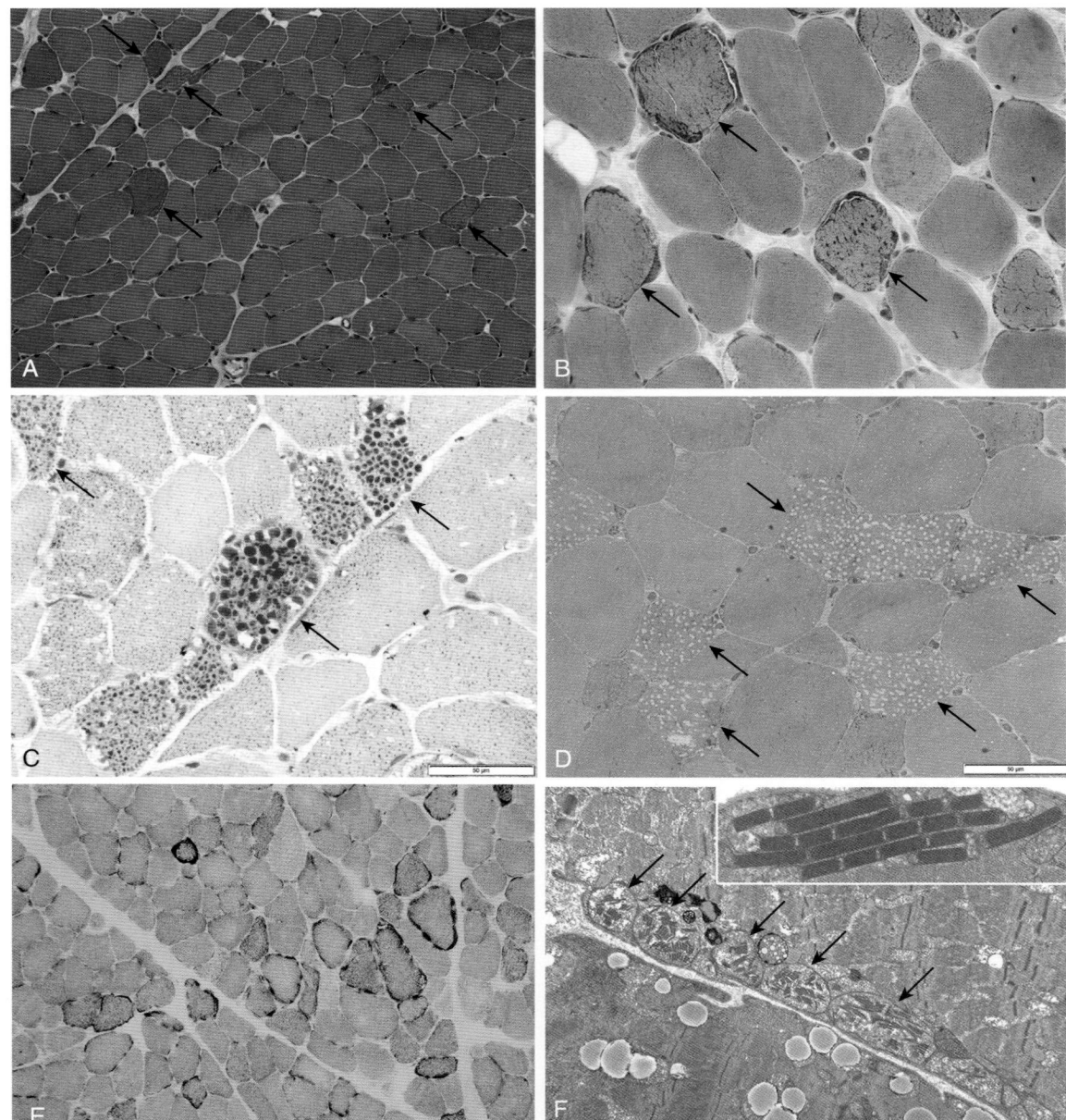

Fig. 35.11 Pathologic changes seen in mitochondrial myopathy. Hematoxylin and eosin stain *(A)* demonstrating increased fiber size variation and subsarcolemmal basophilic deposits *(arrows)* correlating with ragged red fibers *(arrows)* on Gomori trichrome *(B)*, oil red O *(C)*, and toluidine *(D)* staining showing increased lipid deposition in the fibers *(arrows)* indicative of marked mitochondrial dysfunction due to defects in β-oxidation. *E,* Cytochrome c oxidase (COX) (brown stain) with succinate dehydrogenase (SDH) counterstain (blue stain) showing many COX-negative fibers (blue staining fibers) indicative of mitochondrial dysfunction since the COX enzyme is partly encoded within mitochondrial DNA. *F,* Electron microscopy showing classic paracrystalline "parking lot" inclusions within the mitochondria located immediately underneath the sarcolemma that correlate highly with mitochondrial dysfunction *(arrows;* inset with higher magnification) and increased lipid deposition *(ars). (A,* Courtesy Michael Lawlor, MD, PhD, Medical College of Wisconsin, Milwaukee, WI; *C, D,* and *F,* courtesy Karra Jones, MD, PhD, UC San Diego, San Diego, CA; *B, E,* courtesy Chamindra Konersman, MD, Medical College of Wisconsin, Milwaukee, WI.)

extremity deformities or early-onset scoliosis, and urinary dribbling, typically diagnosed on urodynamic studies.

Toddlers and adolescents with TCS usually do not have any cutaneous stigmata but develop slowly progressive gait dysfunction, spasticity, difficulties running, foot deformities, and spastic bladder that is more noticeable after a growth spurt. Examination demonstrates upper motor neuron dysfunction with hyperreflexia and Babinski signs.

Some patients also have variable involvement of the cauda equina as evidenced by a flaccid bladder and atrophy of the lower extremities and relatively reduced reflexes. Diagnosis is confirmed by MRI of the spine showing a low-lying conus below the L1/L2 interspace, usually in association with a thickened filum or lipoma. Neurosurgical decompression can improve gait and bowel and bladder function and prevent further progression of foot deformity.

Hereditary spastic paraplegia. Hereditary spastic paraplegia (HSP) is a large group of genetically and phenotypically heterogenous disorders, with over 70 genetic subtypes, with the common feature of slowly progressive spasticity, hyperreflexia, and Babinski signs. Inheritance patterns include autosomal dominant, recessive, and X-linked recessive. The majority of pathogenic variants in HSP localize to proteins composing the upper motor neuron or oligodendrocyte (Fig. 35.14). In addition to pure spastic forms, patients may have varying degrees of motor and/or sensory neuropathy, cognitive dysfunction, urinary dysfunction, or optic neuropathy, resulting in complex phenotypes. Although most are adult onset, a handful are early onset, ranging from infancy to teenage years. MRI of the spine must be performed to exclude anatomical causes, and is normal in the vast majority of cases. Diagnosis is confirmed via molecular genetic testing. A mimic of cerebral palsy, HSP should be suspected if an infant with isolated spasticity and a presumed diagnosis of cerebral palsy appears to be worsening.

Uncommon Disorders

An **epidural spinal abscess** may manifest in a manner similar to transverse myelitis, except with more back pain, neck pain, fevers, and local tenderness. **Spinal cord tumor**, either primary or metastatic, usually manifests with subacute onset of spastic weakness of the extremities though rarely can manifest as hypotonia (see Table 35.10). Rapid diagnosis with MRI is essential so that medical or neurosurgical intervention can be promptly initiated in an attempt to preserve cord function.

Is the Problem in the Motor Unit?

Diagnostic Considerations

The motor unit is composed of the anterior horn cell (motor neuron), nerve, NMJ, and muscle fibers. Disorders that affect the motor unit produce a common clinical picture characterized by preservation of cognitive function and alertness, absence of seizures, characteristically diminished or absent muscle stretch reflexes, and hypotonia. **Muscle atrophy** is frequently associated with motor unit disorders, but it can also occur in chronic upper motor neuronal causes of hypotonia.

It is not always easy to determine which component of the motor unit is abnormal (anterior horn cell/motor neuron, nerve, NMJ, or muscle), but the following guidelines are useful:

- Fasciculations: motor neuron
- Distal-to-proximal pattern of weakness: nerve > muscle
- Distal-to-proximal pattern of sensory loss: nerve
- Proximal weakness: muscle
- Cramps: motor neuron, muscle, nerve
- Prominent pain: nerve
- Fluctuating weakness: NMJ
- Fluctuating droopy eyelids (ptosis): NMJ
- Painless double vision: NMJ

TABLE 35.9 Motor Involvement in Spinal Cord Lesions

Affected Cord Segment	Motor Involvement
C1–C4	Paralysis of neck, diaphragm, intercostal muscles, and all four extremities
C5	Spastic paralysis of trunk, arms, and legs; partial shoulder control
C6–C7	Spastic paralysis of trunk and legs; upper arm control; partial lower arm control
C8	Spastic paralysis of trunk and legs; hand weakness only
T1–T10	Spastic paralysis of trunk and legs
T11–T12	Spastic paralysis of legs
L1–S1	Flaccid paralysis of legs
S2–S5	Flaccid paralysis of lower legs; bowel, bladder, and sexual function affected

From Swartz MH. *Textbook of Physical Diagnosis: History and Examination.* 2nd ed. Philadelphia: WB Saunders; 1994:496; modified from Fenichel GM. *Clinical Pediatric Neurology: A Signs and Symptoms Approach.* 2nd ed. Philadelphia: WB Saunders; 1993:262.

TABLE 35.10 Spinal Cord Syndromes

Site	Mechanism	Manifestation
Complete—upper cord (above T10)	Space-occupying lesion Trauma	Flaccid symmetric weakness, paralysis, loss of sensation below lesion, areflexia (in spinal shock), reflexes return and are ↑ after recovery from spinal shock, distended bladder, positive Babinski sign, positive Beevor sign*
Conus medullaris (T10–L2)	Space-occupying lesion Trauma	Symmetric weakness, paralysis, ↑ knee deep tendon reflexes, ↑ ankle deep tendon reflexes, positive Babinski sign, spastic bladder and sphincter disturbance
Cauda equina (below L2)	Space-occupying lesion Tethered cord Trauma (rare)	Asymmetric weakness, loss of lower extremity deep tendon reflexes, sensory saddle perineum sensory loss, no Babinski sign, distended atonic bladder with urinary retention and overflow incontinence and decreased rectal tone
Anterior cord	Flexion-rotation force from anterior dislocation or compression fracture of vertebral body (+/– ischemia of anterior spinal artery)	Weakness and reduced pain and temperature sensation
Central cord	Hyperextension injury; tumor, hemorrhage, syringomyelia	Flaccid weakness of arms (lower motor neuron lesion) with strong and spastic lower extremities (upper motor neuron lesion); sacral sensation with bowel and bladder partially affected
Posterior cord	Hyperextension (fractures of posterior vertebra)	Significant ataxia (loss of proprioception); strength and pain and temperature sensations may be spared or less affected
Brown-Séquard syndrome	Laceration (stabs), lateral space-occupying lesions: hemisection	Strength, position, and vibration sensations are affected on the side of the lesion; pain and temperature sensation are affected on the contralateral side

*Beevor sign: superior displacement of umbilicus during attempts to lift shoulders off an examining table, seen in paraplegia.

TABLE 35.11   Spinal Paraplegia

Congenital Malformations
1. Arachnoid cyst
2. Arteriovenous malformations
3. Atlantoaxial dislocation
4. Caudal regression syndrome
5. Dysraphic states
   a. Chiari malformations
   b. Meningomyelocele
   c. Tethered spinal cord
6. Syringomyelia

Familial Spastic Paraplegia
1. Autosomal dominant
2. Autosomal recessive
3. X-linked recessive

Infections—Inflammatory
1. Spondylodiskitis
2. Epidural abscess
3. Herpes-zoster myelitis
4. Polyradiculoneuropathy
5. Tuberculous osteomyelitis
6. Acute flaccid myelitis

Infarction
1. Arterial infarction
2. Dural arteriovenous malformation

Transverse Myelitis
1. Neuromyelitis optica
2. Encephalomyelitis
3. Idiopathic

Trauma
1. Concussion
2. Epidural hematoma
3. Fracture-dislocation
4. Neonatal cord trauma

Tumors
1. Astrocytoma
2. Ependymoma
3. Neuroblastoma
4. Other

Modified from Piña-Garza. *Fenichel's Clinical Pediatric Neurology: A Signs and Symptoms Approach.* 7th ed. Philadelphia: Saunders; 2013.

TABLE 35.12   Clinical Presentation of Acute Flaccid Myelitis

	Estimated Frequency
Age <21 yr	80–90%
Prodromal fever or viral illness	85–95%
Neurologic onset to nadir <10 days	100%
Headache or neck stiffness at onset	12–60%
Asymmetric onset of weakness	65–95%
Limb weakness	85–95%
Upper limb weakness	60–85%
Flaccidity or hyporeflexia of affected limbs	95–100%
Neck, face, extraocular, or bulbar weakness	20–60%
Trunk weakness	30–70%
Requirement for mechanical ventilation	10–40%
Bladder or bowel dysfunction	5–40%
Nonspecific sensory symptoms (e.g., paresthesia)	10–20%
Cardiovascular autonomic dysfunction	<10%
CSF pleocytosis (with testing <5 days after onset)	85–95%
Gray matter–predominant spinal cord lesion(s) on MRI	95–100%
Brainstem lesion(s) on MRI	35–45%
Cerebral deep gray matter lesion(s) on MRI	<5%

CSF, cerebrospinal fluid.
From Murphy OC, Messacar K, Benson L, et al. Acute flaccid myelitis: cause, diagnosis, and management. *Lancet.* 2021;397:334–344 (Table 1, p. 336).

movements. Tongue protrusion tends to exaggerate normal quivering movements, and as such, examining the tongue in its neutral position is typically preferred. Muscle enzymes are usually normal but are occasionally elevated, and NCSs are usually normal (Table 35.14). The electromyogram may demonstrate fibrillations and large motor unit potentials that are reduced in number.

Common disorders. Spinal muscular atrophy (SMA) is characterized by degeneration of anterior horn cells in the spinal cord and brainstem nuclei, leading to progressive loss of motor function. The disorder is inherited in an autosomal recessive fashion and is most often related to homozygous deletions in exon 7 of the *SMN1* (survival motor neuron) gene, though less frequently is caused by a combination of a deletion in one copy of the gene and pathogenic sequence variants in the other. There is a wide spectrum of phenotypes with respect to age of onset, disease manifestations, severity, and prognosis; these phenotypes have been organized into clinical subtypes (Table 35.15). No correlation exists between the type of pathogenic change in *SMN1* and the clinical subtype; however, a related gene, *SMN2*, can occasionally produce functional survival motor neuron gene product, and is considered disease-modifying in a dose-dependent fashion. SMA type I is the prototype for the spinal muscular atrophies. Manifestations begin early in life and even occasionally in the prenatal period (e.g., decreased fetal movements, congenital contractures, polyhydramnios caused by poor in utero swallowing, poor respiratory effort at birth). Neonates and young infants experience progressive weakness and hypotonia, which result in poor head and body control and a flaccid, motionless, extended posture with alert facies (see Fig. 35.4). Fasciculations may be noted in the tongue, over muscles with little subcutaneous fat, and as a fine tremor of the outstretched fingers. Bilateral paralysis of the diaphragm with difficulties breathing and poor feeding are the

- Stridor: motor neuron/nerve/NMJ/muscle
- Foot deformity: motor neuron/nerve/muscle

On examination, the distribution of weakness, the presence or absence and quality of reflexes, and the presence of tongue fasciculations should be assessed. CK, TSH, and EMG should be obtained, and if an acute infectious polyradiculoneuritis is suspected, a lumbar puncture for CSF analysis is performed.

Is the Problem in the Motor Neuron/Anterior Horn Cell?

Diagnostic considerations. **Motor neuron disease** is suggested by hypotonia, weakness, absence of reflexes, and fasciculations. Muscle fasciculations are difficult to appreciate in infants because of the presence of subcutaneous fat. Fasciculations might be seen on the tongue, but they must be distinguished from normal quivering

TABLE 35.13 Differentiating Acute Flaccid Myelitis from Clinical Mimics

	Acute Flaccid Myelitis	Guillain-Barré Syndrome	Acute Transverse Myelitis (Demyelinating or Idiopathic)	Spontaneous Spinal Cord Infarction
Prodromal illness	+++	+++	+/–	–
Temporal evolution	Hours to days	Days to weeks	Days to weeks	Minutes to hours
Pattern of weakness	Asymmetric, arms > legs	Symmetric, ascending	Variable	Symmetric, severe
Facial/bulbar weakness	++	++	+/–	+/–
Respiratory failure	++	++	+/–	+/–
Numbness/paresthesia	+/–	+++ (except AMAN)	+++	+
Sensory level	–	–	++	++
Encephalopathy	–	–	+/– (e.g., ADEM)	–
Bowel/bladder dysfunction	+/–	+/–	++	+++
Possible associated symptoms or syndromes	Headache, neck pain/stiffness, neuropathic pain	Neuropathic pain	Optic neuritis, encephalitis, seizures	Severe back/limb pain at onset
MRI spinal cord	Ill-defined gray matter–predominant lesion, +/– nerve root enhancement	Normal cord, +/– nerve root enhancement	Variable, but usually a well-defined enhancing white > gray matter lesion	No-enhancing anterior cord or gray matter lesion
CSF	Mild–moderate pleocytosis	Elevated protein	Mild–moderate pleocytosis	Sometimes elevated protein or mild pleocytosis
Microbiologic tests	Nasopharyngeal, rectal swabs and CSF for enteroviruses including polio and live polio vaccine virus if indicated. West Nile virus titers	Stool sample: bacterial culture, viral RT-PCR panel; respiratory sample: viral RT-PCR panel; serum: *Campylobacter jejuni* and *Mycoplasma pneumoniae* IgM/IgG; other organisms according to region and season	If indicated based on clinical presentation	Not usually indicated
Other useful tests	+/– EMG/NCS	EMG/NCS; serum: antiganglioside antibodies	Serum: MOG-IgG, aquaporin-4-IgG; CSF: oligoclonal bands	Angiography

AMAN, acute motor axonal neuropathy subtype; ADEM, acute disseminated encephalomyelitis; CSF, cerebrospinal fluid; EMG/NCS, electromyography and nerve conduction studies; MOG, myelin oligodendrocyte glycoprotein.
Modified from Murphy OC, Messacar K, Benson L, et al. Acute flaccid myelitis: cause, diagnosis, and management. *Lancet.* 2021;397:334–344 (Table 2, p. 337).

commonly noted symptoms that bring patients with later disease onset to medical attention.

The majority (95%) of affected individuals have homozygous deletions in exon 7 of *SMN1*; the remainder are compound heterozygotes for a deletion coupled with a pathogenic sequence variant in *SMN1*. Both prenatal testing for at-risk individuals and newborn screening are available. In symptomatic individuals, diagnosis is established by targeted analysis of *SMN1* to determine copy number of exon 7: If two intact copies are found, then alternate diagnoses are explored; if no copies are found, the diagnosis is established; if one copy is found, then sequence analysis is performed to assess for a pathogenic variant in that copy that would then establish the diagnosis. In patients with an established diagnosis, *SMN2* copy number analysis is performed to help prognosticate, since more copies of the *SMN2* gene confer a milder phenotype (see Table 35.15; Fig. 35.15). Timely diagnosis is of paramount importance, as gene therapies can improve survival and motor development in certain affected individuals.

Rare disorders. **Juvenile amyotrophic lateral sclerosis (JALS)** is a rare disorder caused by degeneration of both upper and lower motor neurons and is characterized by mild to moderate muscle atrophy, mostly in the legs and hands, beginning typically around 6 years of age and leading to loss of ambulation in early to mid-adolescence. Additional features include facial muscle spasticity with dysarthria and uncontrolled laughter, as well as a spastic gait. Despite the presence of

facial and bulbar symptoms, atrophy and fasciculation of the tongue are absent. Some patients may have bladder dysfunction and sensory disturbances as well. EMG shows a denervation pattern with normal nerve conduction velocity. Pathogenic variants in *ALS2, SIGMAR1, SPG11,* and *SETX* are associated with various subtypes of JALS, with varying modes of inheritance.

Is the Problem in the Nerve?

Diagnostic considerations. Neuropathies are characterized by hypotonia, weakness, and diminished or absent reflexes. Neuropathies may be primarily motor or sensory, and the child's symptoms may be either acute or chronic weakness or discomfort caused by paresthesia and dysesthesia. The pattern of weakness in most neuropathies is in a **distal-to-proximal gradient** with foot deformity and atrophy resulting in pes cavus and hammer toe deformities. **Pes planus** may be a common feature in a neuropathy during infancy or early childhood due to low tone, with high-arched feet developing only as the patient ages. In chronic sensory neuropathies (with insensitivity to pain), the child may sustain injuries (e.g., burns or even fractures) that are unnoticed. Autonomic symptoms associated with some neuropathies include orthostatic hypotension, gastrointestinal dysmotility, and abnormalities of sweating. In general, the reflexes in neuropathies are diminished disproportionately to the extent of muscle weakness; that is, the reflexes may be markedly reduced or absent, whereas the muscle

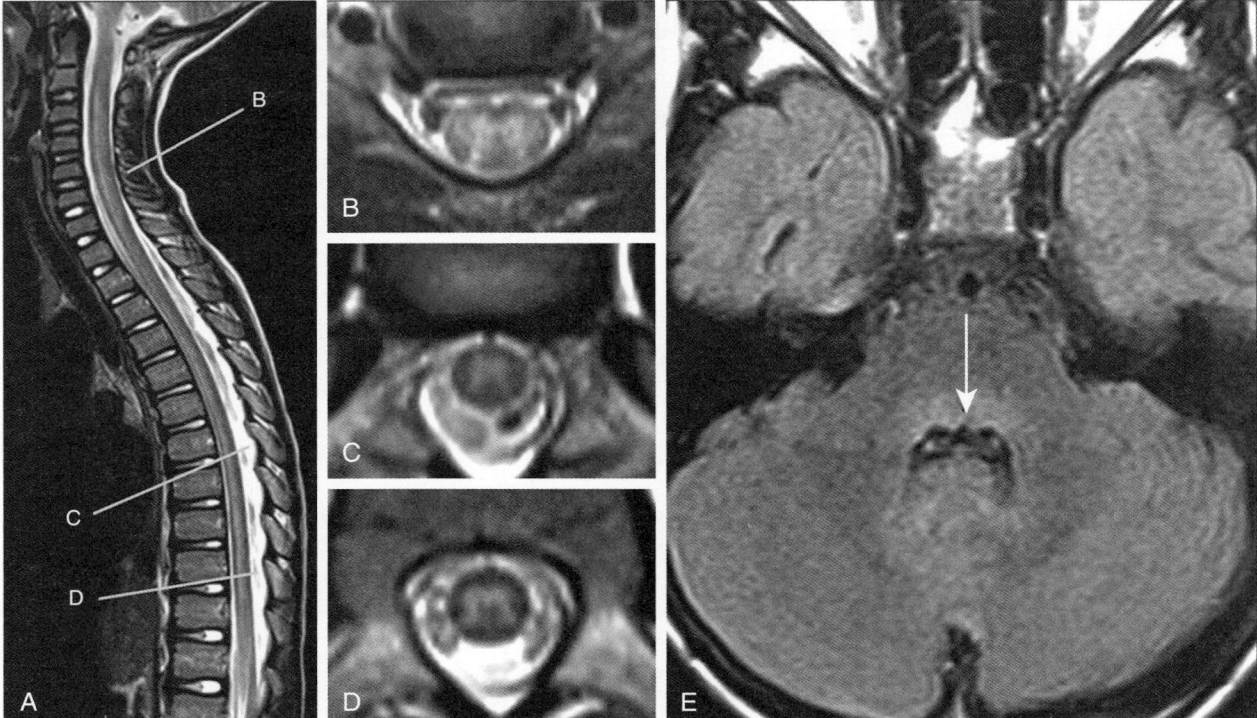

Fig. 35.12 Typical MRI findings in the acute phase of acute flaccid myelitis (AFM). Spinal MRIs are shown of an 8-year-old child with AFM, acquired 24 hours after onset of neurologic symptoms. *A*, Sagittal T2 image showing an ill-defined longitudinally extensive central/anterior spinal cord lesion. *B*, Axial T2 image from C5–C6 shows hyperintensity of the entire gray matter of the spinal cord, with associated edema and some surrounding white matter hyperintensity. *C*, Axial T2 image from T7 shows asymmetric hyperintensity of the gray matter (right more than left). *D*, Axial T2 image from T10 shows hyperintensity of the entire gray matter. *E*, Axial fluid-attenuated inversion recovery (FLAIR) image at the level of the middle cerebellar peduncle demonstrates hyperintensity of the dorsal pons *(arrow)*. (From Murphy OC, Messacar K, Benson L, et al. Acute flaccid myelitis: cause, diagnosis, and management. *Lancet.* 2021;397:334–344 [Fig. 1, p. 338].)

strength is only mildly diminished. NCSs and EMGs demonstrate slowing of nerve conduction velocities and features that suggest either primary axonal involvement (fibrillations, normal or mildly slow nerve conduction velocity) or demyelination (marked slowing of nerve conduction velocity) (see Table 35.14). The differential diagnosis for neuropathy based on category can be remembered by the mnemonic "CHANCE-IT" (Table 35.16). Neuropathies with onset in infancy based on the most salient feature are described in Table 35.17; genetic pediatric-onset neuropathies are noted in Table 35.18.

Common disorders

Guillain-Barré syndrome. Guillain-Barré syndrome (GBS) is an acute inflammatory demyelinating polyneuropathy (AIDP) that is often associated with an antecedent upper respiratory tract infection or an illness with diarrhea, especially those caused by *Campylobacter*. The disorder can occur in childhood or adolescence, though is rare in infancy and is characterized by ascending motor weakness and areflexia. The weakness is usually symmetric, ascends and progresses over time (usually 1–2 weeks), and may cause serious respiratory compromise by producing weakness of the respiratory muscles, often necessitating hospitalization and frequent assessments of respiratory function (e.g., negative inspiratory forces and vital capacity) in affected patients. Children complain of difficulty walking, rising from the floor, and climbing stairs, and become irritable and noticeably clumsier, fall frequently, and may refuse to bear weight. More commonly than adults, children present with acute-onset ataxia with multiple falls and poor balance stemming from sensory disturbance with milder weakness. Children often have more paresthesia and discomfort

than adults, with neck, back, leg, and buttock pain in at least 50% of cases, presumably mimicking a radiculopathy due to nerve root inflammation. In addition to an abnormal nerve conduction velocity, the CSF protein level is usually elevated out of proportion to the white cell count (**cytoalbuminologic dissociation**) after the first week of illness, indicative of an inflammatory process occurring within the CSF space. Postgadolinium enhancement of edematous nerve roots and peripheral nerves as seen on MRI in the cervical and lumbosacral regions is found in ~95% of children with GBS and is highly suggestive, although not specific, for the disease.

Classic AIDP is not commonly associated with an antiganglioside antibody (Table 35.19). The triad of **ophthalmoplegia, areflexia, and ataxia** without overt weakness characterizes **Miller Fisher syndrome (MFS)**, a variant of GBS. This variant is associated with the GQ1b IgG antiganglioside antibody. A severe pure motor variant of GBS called acute motor axonal neuropathy (AMAN) is associated with profound weakness, severe disability, and protracted need for rehabilitation and is associated with GM_1 antiganglioside antibodies. The poorer prognosis and slow recovery of AMAN are related to axonal damage and the slow regeneration of axons at 1 mm/day (~1 inch per month). **Autonomic nervous system** involvement may produce hypotension or hypertension and bradyarrhythmias or tachyarrhythmias. Therefore, due to the risk of respiratory and autonomic dysfunction, all patients suspected of having GBS or its variants should be monitored in the intensive care unit or other setting capable of providing cardiac monitoring, frequent respiratory monitoring, and high-frequency nursing care. The differential diagnosis is noted in Tables 35.12 and 35.16.

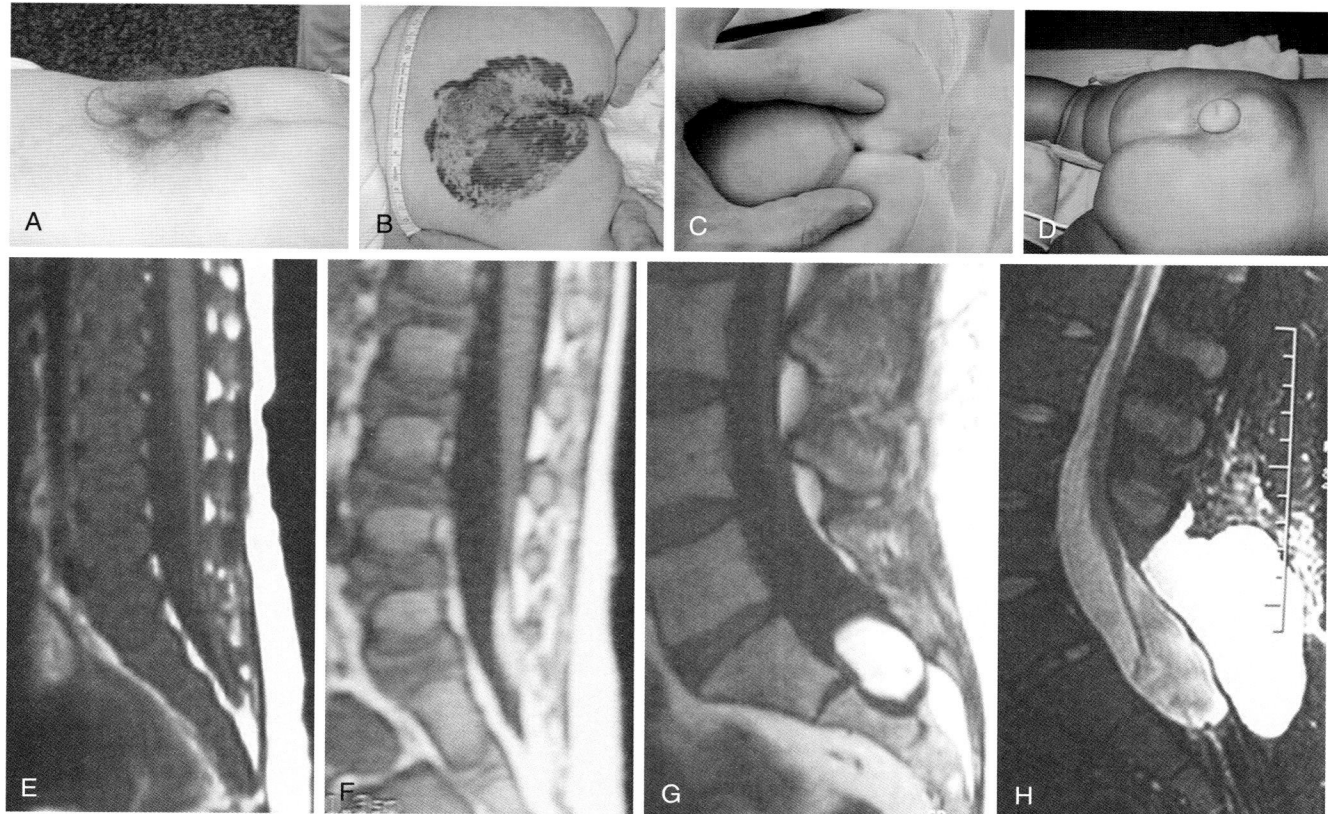

Fig. 35.13 Cutaneous signs of spina bifida and MRI of spine demonstrating various forms of tethered cord syndrome. *A,* Hair tuft. *B,* Hemangioma. *C,* Lipomatous mass with dermal sinus tract. *D,* Skin appendage. MRI showing low-lying conus *(E),* fatty filum terminale *(F),* lumbosacral lipoma *(G),* and lipomyelomeningocele *(H).* (Modified from Lew SM, Kothbauer KF. Tethered cord syndrome: an updated review. *Pediatr Neurosurg.* 2007;43[3]:236–248.)

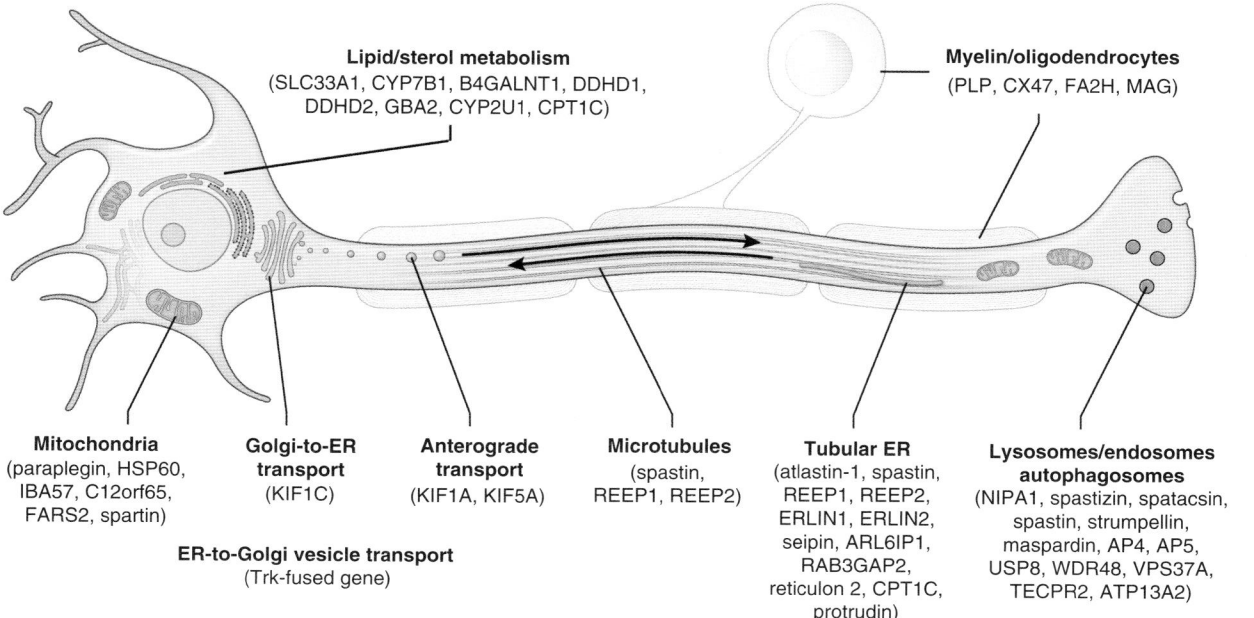

Fig. 35.14 Location of pathologically altered proteins seen in hereditary spastic paraplegia on upper motor neuron with oligodendrocyte demonstrating common pathogenic theme for entire group. (Modified from Blackstone C. Cellular pathways of hereditary spastic paraplegia. *Annu Rev Neurosci.* 2012;35:25–47, Fig. 2.)

TABLE 35.14   Typical Electrophysiologic Features of Nerve and Muscle Diseases

	Motor Nerve Conductions	Sensory Nerve Conductions	F Response	H Reflex	Needle Electromyography
Myopathy (dystrophic, inflammatory)	Normal	Normal	Normal	Normal	• Spontaneous activity: fibrillation potentials and positive sharp waves (muscle membrane irritability) • Volitional activity: small-amplitude myopathic units
Myopathic (mitochondrial, congenital myopathy)	Normal	Normal	Normal	Normal	• Spontaneous activity: usually none • Volitional activity: small-amplitude, short-duration units with rapid recruitment
Axonal neuropathy	• ↓ Amplitude • Normal or mildly slow conduction velocities	↓ Amplitude	Normal	Normal	• Spontaneous activity: fibrillation potentials and positive sharp waves (muscle membrane irritability) especially in distal muscles • Volitional activity: large-amplitude, long-duration units with reduced recruitment
Demyelinating neuropathy	• Markedly slow conduction velocities • Prolonged latencies • ↓ or normal amplitude	• Prolonged latencies • ↓ Amplitude or no response	Delayed or absent	Delayed or absent	• Spontaneous activity: usually none • Volitional activity: large-amplitude, long-duration units with reduced recruitment
Radiculopathy	Normal or ↓ amplitude	Normal	Delayed or absent	Delayed or absent if S1 is involved	• Spontaneous activity: fibrillation potentials and positive sharp waves (muscle membrane irritability); fasciculations • Volitional activity: large-amplitude, long-duration units with reduced recruitment
Motor neuron disease	Normal or ↓ amplitude	Normal	Normal	Normal	• Spontaneous activity: fibrillation potentials and positive sharp waves (muscle membrane irritability); fasciculations • Volitional activity: large-amplitude, long-duration units with reduced recruitment

TABLE 35.15   Spinal Muscular Atrophy (SMA): Clinical and Genetic Characteristics

Phenotype	Age of Onset	Natural Age of Death	Highest Motor Milestones	Other Findings	*SMN2* Copy Number
SMA 0	Prenatal	2–6 mo	None achieved	• Arthrogryposis • Facial diplegia • Decreased fetal movements • Polyhydramnios • Breech presentation • Respiratory failure in early infancy	1
SMA I	<6 mo	Usually ≤2 yr, but may survive longer	Sitting with support	• Prominent tongue fasciculations • Mild joint contractures • Facial weakness • Poor suck and swallow • Small bell-shaped chest • Paradoxical breathing	1–2
SMA II	6–18 mo	70% alive at age 25 yr	Independent sitting when placed	• Legs more affected than arms, with failure to sit alone by 9–12 mo and stand by 1 yr • Postural hand/finger tremor • Lose ability to sit independently by mid-teens	2–3
SMA III	>12 mo	Normal	Independent ambulation	• Legs more affected than arms, manifesting as difficulty walking • Distal then proximal contractures	≥3
SMA IV	Second or third decade	Normal	Walking during adulthood	• May lose ambulation with time	≥4

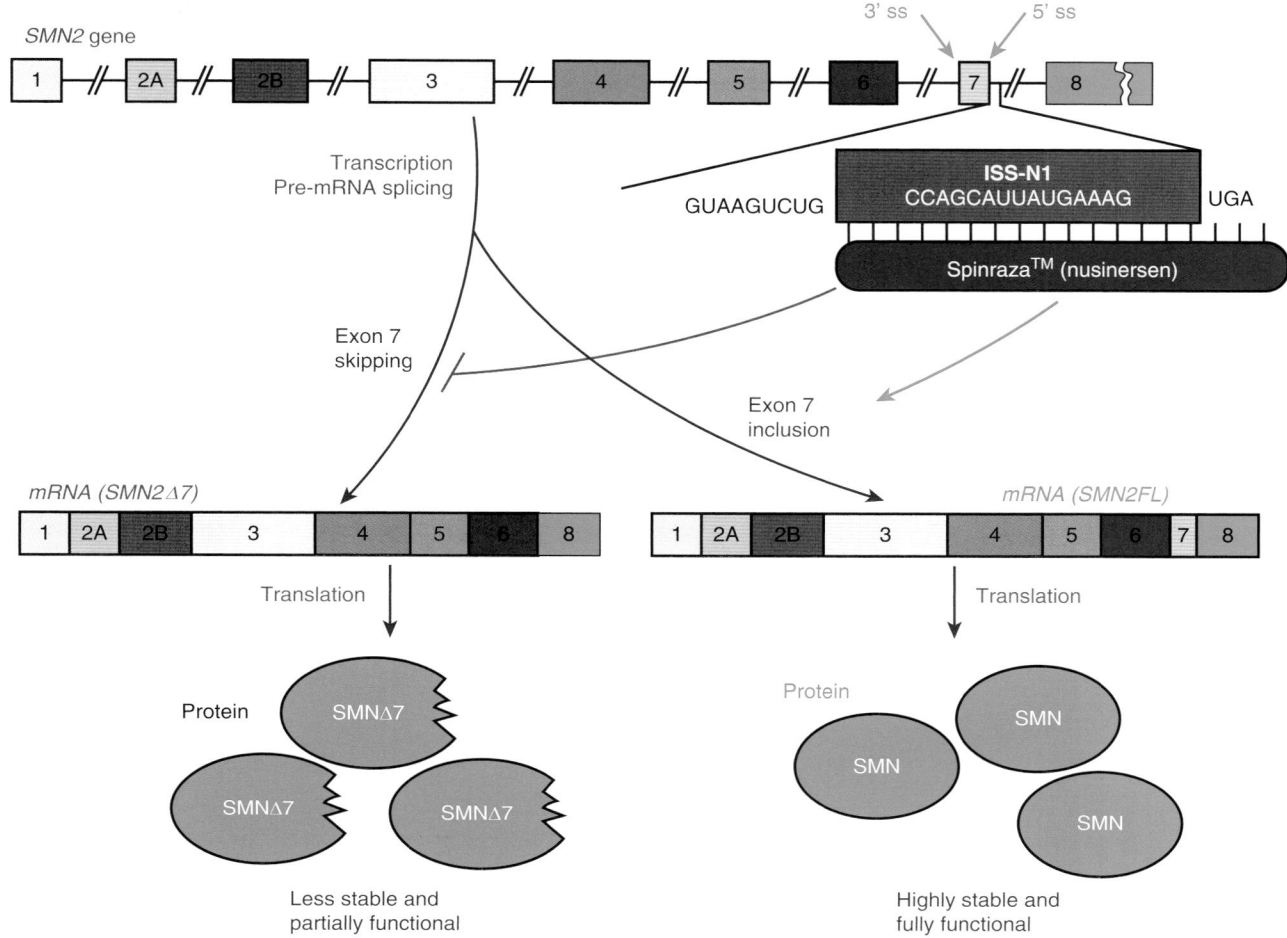

Fig. 35.15 Genetics of spinal muscular atrophy (SMA) and mechanism of action for nusinersen. Patients with SMA typically have homozygous deletions of *SMN1* and a variable number of *SMN2* copies. *SMN2* exons are represented by *colored boxes*, whereas introns are shown as *broken lines*. Normally, SMN2 pre-mRNA splicing results in exon 7-included (SMN2FL, SMN2 full length) 10% of the time and exon 7-skipped (SMN2Δ7) transcripts 90% of the time, translation of which leads to production of the full-length functional SMN protein and a truncated, less stable isoform, respectively. The intronic sequence immediately downstream of exon 7 is shown with the critical splicing region, ISS-N1, highlighted in the *red box*. Nusinersen *(blue box)* binds and blocks the ISS-N1 region to include exon 7 in the final transcript, resulting in full-length SMN2 transcript. Positions to which nusinersen anneals are indicated. (Modified from Singh NN, Howell MD, Androphy EJ, Singh RN. How the discovery of ISS-N1 led to the first medical therapy for spinal muscular atrophy. *Gene Ther.* 2017;24[9]:520–526.)

Intravenous immunoglobulin (IVIG) is the treatment of choice for all variants of GBS; plasma exchange is equally efficacious, though IVIG is typically the preferred method due to ease of administration. Both modalities allow faster recovery and shorten hospital stay. Prognosis in children is more favorable than adults, with shorter duration of illness and more complete recovery. In children, approximately 60% lose ambulation and 20% require ventilation during their illness, which reaches its nadir within 2 weeks of onset, but few have significant disability by 4 months postillness.

Charcot-Marie-Tooth hereditary neuropathy. Charcot-Marie-Tooth disease (CMT) refers to a group of slowly progressive hereditary motor and sensory neuropathies. The disorders are genetically and phenotypically heterogeneous though share certain characteristic features, primarily a slowly progressive distal motor neuropathy of the extremities with varying degrees of sensory neuropathy. Various classification schemata have been adopted historically, principal among these a system based on the mechanism of neuropathy and mode of inheritance, though

with evolving understanding of the underlying genetic mechanisms and associated genes, classification according to underlying genetic abnormality has become more conventional. Over 90% of CMT cases are caused by pathogenic variants in the following four genes, all of which can lead to presentation in infancy or childhood: peripheral myelin protein 22 (*PMP22*), mitofusin 2 (*MFN2*), myelin protein zero (*MPZ*), and gap junction protein beta 1 (*GJB1*) (Table 35.20). Most CMT cases are autosomal dominant, while the remainder are X-linked dominant and autosomal recessive. CMT has considerable clinical variability from mild to severe phenotypes between patients and even within siblings (Fig. 35.16). Infants and children with CMT manifest with hypotonia. The classic CMT phenotype has slowly progressive weakness out of proportion to pain or sensory disturbance, with onset in adulthood presenting with foot drop, hearing loss, frequent falls, and difficulties running, walking long distances, climbing stairs, and walking in the dark. In comparison, childhood-onset CMT exhibits moderate to severe motor delays, moderate to severe foot deformities with pes cavus and hammer

TABLE 35.16   Mnemonic for Neuropathy: CHANCE-IT

Collagen Vascular Diseases	Hereditary	Autoimmune	Nutrition	Cancer	Endocrine	Infectious	Toxin or Trauma
Polyarteritis nodosa	CMT	GBS	Vitamin deficiencies (B_1, B_2, B_6, B_{12}, E), hypokalemia	Lambert-Eaton	Diabetes mellitus	*Campylobacter* (GBS)	Tick toxin
SLE	HSAN	Immunizations			Hypothyroidism	Diphtheria	INH
Vasculitis	Metabolic (porphyria)	Chronic inflammatory demye-linating polyneuropathy			Acromegaly (entrapment)	Lyme	DDI
Angiitis	Refsum disease					Leprosy	DDC
Granulomatous (sarcoidosis)	Leukodystrophies (e.g., Krabbe disease, adrenoleukodystrophy, metachromatic)					HIV	Organophosphates
Granulomatosis with polyangiitis						Herpes-zoster	Lead
ADA-2 deficiency	Amyloid (familial)					Rabies	Mercury
Henoch-Schönlein purpura	Congenital abetalipopro-teinemia						Thallium
Mononeuritis multiplex	Fabry disease						Arsenic
	Tangier disease						Vincristine
	Tyrosinemia						Uremia
							Nitrofurantoin
							Chloramphenicol
							Acrylamide
							Cyanide
							N-Hexane
							Glue sniffing
							Buckthorn toxin
							Puffer fish toxin
							Snake bite
							Carbon monoxide
							Entrapment
							Obstetric trauma

ADA, adenosine deaminase; CMT, Charcot-Marie-Tooth disease; DDC, dideoxycytidine; DDI, dideoxyinosine; GBS, Guillain-Barré syndrome; HSAN, hereditary sensory-autonomic neuropathy; INH, isoniazid; SLE, systemic lupus erythematosus.

TABLE 35.17   Neuropathies with Onset in Infancy

Salient Clinical Feature	Clinical Phenotype	Gene	Mode of Inheritance
Axonal Neuropathies			
Pes cavus with foot drop	CMT2E	*NEFL*	AD, AR
Optic atrophy	CMT2A	*MFN2*	AD, AR
	CMT4A	*GDAP1*	AR
	IOSCA	*C10orf2*	AR
	Infantile neuroaxonal dystrophy	*PLA2G6*	AR
Ophthalmoparesis	Mitochondrial disorders	*SCO2*	AR
		C10orf2	
		TK2	
Skeletal abnormalities	CMT2C, SPSMA, congenital dSMA	*TRPV4*	AD
Arthrogryposis	Congenital dSMA	*TRPV4*	AD
	SMARD1	*IGHMBP2*	AR
	X-linked SMA	*UBE1*	X-linked
	Pontocerebellar hypoplasia type 1	*EXOSC3, VRK1, TSEN54, RARS2*	AR
	SMA with congenital fractures	Unknown	Unknown, presumed AR
Congenital fractures	X-linked SMA	*UBE1*	X-linked
	SMA with congenital fractures	Unknown	Unknown, presumed AR
Vocal cord paresis	CMT2A	*MFN2*	AD, AR
	CMT2C, SPSMA, congenital dSMA	*TRPV4*	AD
	CMT4A	*GDAP1*	AR
	BVVL/Fazio-Londe disease	*SLC52A3*	AR
Early infantile respiratory failure	SMA1	*SMN1*	AR
	SMARD1	*IGHMBP2*	AR
	X-linked SMA	*UBE1*	X-linked
	Pontocerebellar hypoplasia type 1	*EXOSC3, VRK1, TSEN54, RARS2*	AR
	SMA with congenital fractures	Unknown	Unknown, presumed AR
	Lethal neonatal AR axonal sensorimotor polyneuropathy	Unknown	AR
	Congenital axonal neuropathy with encephalopathy	Unknown	Unknown, presumed AR
Predominant motor involvement	Congenital dSMA, SPSMA	*TRPV4*	AD
	SMA1	*SMN1*	AR
	X-linked SMA	*UBE1*	X-linked
	Pontocerebellar hypoplasia type 1	*EXOSC3, VRK1, TSEN54, RARS2*	AR
	SMA with congenital fractures	Unknown	Unknown, presumed AR
	Mitochondrial disorders	*SCO2, TK2*	AR
Kinky hair hepatopathy	Giant axonal neuropathy	*GAN*	AR
	Mitochondrial disorders	*DGUOK*	AR
		C10orf2	
	MTP/LCHAD deficiency	*HADHA/HADHB*	AR
Cardiomyopathy	Mitochondrial disorders	*SCO2*	AR
		TK2	AR
		DGUOK	AR
	MTP/LCHAD deficiency	*HADHA/HADHB*	AR

Continued

TABLE 35.17 Neuropathies with Onset in Infancy—cont'd

Salient Clinical Feature	Clinical Phenotype	Gene	Mode of Inheritance
Axonal Neuropathies—cont'd			
CNS involvement	Pontocerebellar hypoplasia type 1	*EXOSC3, VRK1, TSEN54, RARS2*	AR
	Giant axonal neuropathy	*GAN*	AR
	Infantile neuroaxonal dystrophy	*PLA2G6*	AR
	HMSN/ACC	*KCC3*	AR
	IOSCA	*C10orf2*	AR
	CMTX1	*GJB1*	X-linked
	Mitochondrial disorders	*SCO2*	AR
		TK2	AR
		DGUOK	AR
	Adrenoleukodystrophy	*ABCD1*	X-linked
Developmental regression	Adrenoleukodystrophy	*ABCD1*	X-linked
Dysautonomia, chronic skin ulceration	HSAN III (Riley-Day syndrome)	*IKBKAP*	AR
Demyelinating Neuropathies			
Acute sensory ataxia, walking difficulties in a previously well child	GBS		
Slowly progressive weakness, ataxia in a previously well child; responsive to steroids	CIDP		
Developmental regression	MLD	*ARSA*	AR
	Krabbe disease	*GALC*	AR
Irritable, stiff, crying infant; occasional unexplained fevers	Krabbe disease	*GALC*	AR
Pes cavus with foot drop, marked difficulties walking	CMT1A	*PMP22* point mutations or duplication	De novo (AD), AR
	CMT1B	*MPZ*	De novo (AD)
	CMT1F	*NEFL*	AD, AR
	CMT4C	*SH3TC2*	AR
	CMT4E	*EGR2*	AR, AD
	CMT4F	*PRX*	AR
	CMT4H	*FGD4*	AR
Early respiratory insufficiency	CMT1A	*PMP22* point mutations or duplication	De novo (AD), AR
	CMT1B	*MPZ*	De novo (AD)
	CMT4C	*SH3TC2*	AR
	CMT4E	*EGR2*	AR, AD
Severe scoliosis requiring surgery in infancy	CMT1B	*MPZ*	De novo (AD)
	CMT4C	*SH3TC2*	AR
Facial weakness	CMT4B1	*MTMR2*	AR
	CMT4B2	*SBF2*	AR
	CMT4C	*SH3TC2*	AR
Sensorineural hearing loss	CMT1A	*PMP22* point mutations or duplication	De novo (AD), AR
	CMT4C	*SH3TC2*	AR
	CMT4F	*PRX*	AR
Congenital nystagmus	CMT1B	*MPZ*	De novo (AD)
	CMT4C	*SH3TC2*	AR

AD, autosomal dominant; AR, autosomal recessive; BVVL, Brown–Vialetto–Van Laere syndrome; CMT, Charcot-Marie-Tooth disease; CIDP, chronic inflammatory demyelinating polyneuropathy; CNS, central nervous system; dSMA, distal spinal muscular atrophy; GBS, Guillain-Barré syndrome; HMSN/ACC, hereditary motor and sensory neuropathy with agenesis of the corpus callosum; HSAN, hereditary sensory and autonomic neuropathy; IOSCA, infantile-onset spinocerebellar ataxia; MLD, metachromatic leukodystrophy; MTP/LCHAD, mitochondrial trifunctional protein/long-chain 3-hydroxyacyl-CoA dehydrogenase; SMA, spinal muscular atrophy; SMARD, spinal muscular atrophy with respiratory distress type 1; SPSMA, scapuloperoneal spinal muscular atrophy.

TABLE 35.18 Genetic Disorders Associated with Pediatric-Onset Neuropathy: Clinical Features, Diagnostic Findings, and Molecular Genetics

Disorder	Age of Onset	Neuromuscular Findings	Systemic Findings	Diagnostic Evaluation	Course	Inheritance	Molecular Genetics
Monogenic Neuropathy Disorders							
Hereditary motor-sensory neuropathies (also referred to as Charcot-Marie-Tooth [CMT] hereditary neuropathies)	Typically childhood or adolescence, though infantile hypotonia and developmental delays possible	• Chronic, progressive motor and sensory polyneuropathy • Wasting and weakness of distal extremities • Distal sensory loss • Decreased or absent tendon reflexes • Skeletal deformities (e.g., pes cavus, hammer toes) • Hearing loss, dysphagia (*MPZ* pathologic variants)	• Acrocyanosis • Optic atrophy (*MFN2* pathologic variants) • Vocal cord and respiratory involvement (CMT2c subtype) • Early-onset glaucoma (*MTMR13* pathologic variants) • Vocal cord paresis (*GDAP1* pathologic variants)	• EMG/NCV: axonal or demyelinating sensorimotor polyneuropathy, depending on subtype • MRI: nerve roots on spinal MRI may show the "onion bulb" sign, with T2 hyperintensity and bulbous tapering from the root to the nerve fiber • CSF: elevated protein possible • Blood: neutropenia (*DNM2* pathologic variants) • Other: sural nerve biopsy no longer routinely performed but may show onion bulb formation	Chronic, progressive	Autosomal dominant, autosomal recessive, or X-linked, depending on subtype	Numerous genes are implicated in the pathogenesis of CMT. CMT1 accounts for up to 50% of all cases, and the most common form of CMT1, CMT1a, is caused by duplications in the *PMP22* gene. Duplications have also been identified in subtypes of CMT4. Deletions are implicated in subtypes of CMT2, CMT4, and CMTX. Pathogenic variants detected by sequence analysis will detect most other subtypes
Hereditary sensory and autonomic neuropathies (HSAN)	Early childhood to late adulthood. Symptoms of HSAN4 begin in infancy	• Severe, progressive peripheral sensory loss. Profound and early insensitivity to pain in HSAN4 • Severe, shooting pain in the extremities early in disease • Distal then proximal muscle weakness and atrophy. Strength may be preserved in HSAN5 • Decreased or absent tendon reflexes • Skeletal deformities (e.g., pes cavus) • Dysautonomic crises with gastrointestinal and bladder symptoms, hypotension, temperature and sweating disregulation (HSAN3, also known as familial dysautonomia or Riley-Day syndrome)	• Skin ulcerations and bone necrosis in affected extremities with possible spontaneous amputation • Fractures, infections, and unwitnessed injuries in the extremities secondary to decreased sensation (HSAN2, HSAN4) • Small stature, smooth tongue, cognitive delays, glomerulosclerosis (HSAN3) • Self-mutilating behaviors (HSAN4)	• EMG/NCV: axonal sensorimotor polyneuropathy with chronic denervation changes. Typically normal in HSAN5 • MRI: brain atrophy possible in HSAN3 • Urine: decreased vanillylmandelic acid excretion (HSAN3) • Other: sural nerve biopsy no longer routinely performed but may show loss of myelinated axons without demyelination; abnormal histamine and methacholine challenge responses (HSAN3)	Chronic, progressive	Autosomal dominant, autosomal recessive depending on subtype	Numerous genes are implicated in the pathogenesis of HSAN. Subtypes of HSAN1 are associated with pathologic variants in the *SPTLC1* and *SPTLC2* genes, as well as other genes. Subtypes of HSAN2 are caused by pathologic variants in *WNK1, FAM134B,* and other genes. HSAN3 is caused by pathologic variants in *IKBKAP*. HSAN4 is caused by pathologic variants in *NTRK1*

Continued

TABLE 35.18   Genetic Disorders Associated with Pediatric-Onset Neuropathy: Clinical Features, Diagnostic Findings, and Molecular Genetics—cont'd

Disorder	Age of Onset	Neuromuscular Findings	Systemic Findings	Diagnostic Evaluation	Course	Inheritance	Molecular Genetics
Monogenic Neuropathy Disorders—cont'd							
Hereditary neuralgic amyotrophy	Second or third decade (median: 28 yr)	• Sudden-onset severe pain in the arms or shoulders • Unilateral or bilateral brachial plexopathy developing within weeks of pain onset • Motor > sensory symptoms • Absent or diminished tendon reflexes in affected limbs • Paresthesia and hypoesthesia in affected limb • Atrophy of the upper extremity • Autonomic symptoms possible, primarily vasomotor changes	• Precipitants: infection, immunization, surgery, childbirth, overuse of affected limb, cold exposure • Variable findings: bifid uvula, cleft palate, short stature, partial syndactyly, ocular hypotelorism	• EMG/NCV: chronic denervation changes • MRI: evidence of myelopathy or inflammatory plexopathy possible • CSF: elevated protein possible • Blood: elevated transaminases possible early in attacks • Other: sural nerve biopsy is rarely performed but may show reduction in number of myelinated fibers	Relapsing-remitting/episodic. Persistent and cumulative deficits possible	Autosomal dominant	*SEPT9*: Up to 55% of affected patients have an abnormality in the *SEPT9* gene identified either by sequencing or deletion/duplication analysis
Hereditary neuropathy with liability to pressure palsies (HNPP)	Second or third decade (range: 2–70 yr; mean: 37 yr)	• Acute-onset sensory and motor mononeuropathy in areas of compression (in decreasing order of frequency: peroneal nerve causing foot drop, ulnar nerve at the elbow, median nerve at the wrist causing carpal tunnel syndrome, brachial plexus and radial nerve) • Paresthesia in affected distribution • Reduced or absent tendon reflexes • Mild polyneuropathy (focal weakness, atrophy, or sensory loss) possible • Mild to moderate pes cavus deformity	• None reported	• EMG/NCV: bilateral slowing of distal sensory and motor nerve conduction velocities at the carpal tunnel and at least one additional abnormal finding for motor conduction in one peroneal nerve; abnormal conduction across entrapment sites is supportive • MRI: asymptomatic white matter lesions on brain MRI possible, decreased brain white matter volume possible • Other: sural nerve biopsy shows tomaculous changes though is not specific	• Recurrent acute attacks • Attacks last days to months • Full recovery in approximately 50% of episodes • Incomplete recovery with mild residual deficits is common • Severe disability is rare	Autosomal dominant	*PMP22*: contiguous gene deletion of chromosome 17p11.2 in 80% of affected probands; pathogenic variant in 20% of affected probands
Riboflavin transporter Brown–Vialetto–Van Laere syndrome	Early childhood	• Chronic progressive motor and sensory neuropathy • Ataxia • Bulbar weakness • Sensorineural deafness • Upper extremity weakness > lower extremity	• Optic atrophy • Respiratory insufficiency	• Abnormal acylcarnitine panel • EMC/NC axonal sensory neuropathy	• Chronic, progressive, unless treated with high-dose riboflavin	Autosomal recessive	*SLC52A2* and *SLC52A3* Encoding riboflavin transporters

Mitochondrial Neuropathy Disorders—cont'd

Disorder	Age of Onset	Clinical Features	Diagnostic Testing	Course	Inheritance	Gene
Mitochondrial neurogastrointestinal encephalopathy (MNGIE) disease	Between the first and fifth decades (60% of affected individuals present before age 20 yr)	• Mixed demyelinating > axonal sensorimotor neuropathy • Paresthesia in a stocking-glove distribution • Symmetric distal muscle weakness • Unilateral or bilateral foot drop • Ptosis • External ophthalmoplegia • Asymptomatic leukoencephalopathy • Severe gastrointestinal dysmotility and malabsorption • Cachexia	• EMG/NCV: decreased motor and sensory nerve conduction velocities, prolonged F-wave latency, partial conduction block • MRI: diffuse white matter abnormalities on T2 or FLAIR series • CSF: elevated protein possible • Blood: markedly reduced levels of thymidine phosphorylase enzyme activity, elevated plasma thymidine and deoxyuridine; lactic academia and hyperalaninemia possible • Urine: increased deoxyuridine and thymidine • Other: evidence of mitochondrial dysfunction in affected tissues	Chronic, progressive, degenerative	Autosomal recessive	*TYMP*: pathogenic variants on sequence analysis
Neurogenic muscle weakness, ataxia, and retinitis pigmentosa (NARP)	Early childhood	• Proximal muscle weakness • Sensory or sensorimotor axonal polyneuropathy that can be clinically unapparent with episodic worsening in the setting of viral illnesses • Cerebellar ataxia • Seizures • Learning difficulties • Variable retinitis pigmentosa • Short stature • Cardiac conduction defects	• EMG/NCV: axonal sensory or sensorimotor polyneuropathy • MRI: cerebral and cerebellar atrophy • CSF: elevated lactate • Blood: elevated lactate; elevated alanine concentrations on plasma amino acid analysis • Urine: lactic aciduria • Other: isolated defects of mitochondrial complex I or IV enzymes	Chronic, progressive, degenerative	Mitochondrial	*MT-ATP6*: pathogenic variants in *MT-ATP6* are identified in approximately 50% of affected individuals
Ataxia neuropathy spectrum (*POLG*-related disorders)	Infancy to adulthood	• Sensory ataxia • Cerebellar ataxia • Sensorimotor polyneuropathy • Most affected individuals have encephalopathy and seizures • Variable ophthalmoplegia and dysarthria • Gastrointestinal dysmotility reported with some pathologic variants • Liver disease: elevated transaminases, mild liver synthetic dysfunction, or even liver failure possible	• EMG/NCV: axonal sensory, motor, or mixed polyneuropathy • MRI: hyperintense lesions in the thalami, cerebellar white matter, and inferior olivary nuclei on T2-weighted imaging • CSF: elevated protein possible • Blood: elevated transaminases, mild liver synthetic dysfunction, or even liver failure possible • Other: functional assays may show respiratory chain defects	Chronic, progressive	Autosomal recessive	*POLG*, which encodes DNA polymerase gamma, the only DNA polymerase found in mitochondria

Continued

TABLE 35.18 Genetic Disorders Associated with Pediatric-Onset Neuropathy: Clinical Features, Diagnostic Findings, and Molecular Genetics—cont'd

Disorder	Age of Onset	Neuromuscular Findings	Systemic Findings	Diagnostic Evaluation	Course	Inheritance	Molecular Genetics
Metabolic and Other Neuropathy Disorders—cont'd							
Refsum disease	Infancy to adulthood	• Asymmetric, waxing-waning though chronically progressive sensory and motor polyneuropathy • Distal weakness and paresthesia with muscular atrophy • Late-onset cerebellar ataxia • Sensorineural hearing loss	• Anosmia • Early-onset retinitis pigmentosa • Ichthyosis • Congenitally short metacarpals and metatarsals in ~35% of individuals • Cardiac arrhythmias and cardiomyopathy	• EMG/NCV: primarily demyelinating polyneuropathy with secondary axonal degeneration • MRI: progressive symmetric signal change in the corticospinal tracts, cerebellar dentate nuclei, and corpus callosum • CSF: elevated protein possible • Blood: elevated plasma phytanic acid concentration (typically >200 µmol/L; normal <10 µmol/L) • Other: deficiency of phytanoyl-CoA hydroxylase or PTS2 receptor If molecular genetic testing is negative or ambiguous in patients with elevated plasma phytanic acid levels and a consistent phenotype, enzyme analysis of phytanoyl-CoA hydroxylase should be performed	Chronic, progressive	Autosomal recessive	• >90% of identified affected individuals have pathogenic variants or deletions/duplications in *PHYH*, which encodes phytanoyl-CoA hydroxylase • <10% of identified affected individuals have pathogenic variants or deletions/duplications in *PEX7*, which encodes the PTS2 receptor
Krabbe disease (globoid cell leukodystrophy)	Infantile form presents prior to 6 mo. Late-onset forms present between 6 mo and adulthood	• Infantile form presents with irritability, stiffness, seizures, and developmental delays or regression. A subset of patients present with isolated peripheral neuropathy with absent tendon reflexes and weakness prior to appearance of other symptoms. Affected patients then develop spasticity and severe developmental regression that progresses to decerebrate posturing and blindness • Late-onset forms may present with distal weakness and paresthesia. Hypertonicity and developmental regression follow but may vary in severity	• Sterile pyrexias in infantile form • Fist clenching	• EMG/NCV: slow motor conduction velocities • MRI: diffuse severe demyelination • CSF: elevated protein possible • Blood: decreased (0–5% of normal) galactocerebrosidase enzyme activity • Other: EEG with diffuse slowing of background rhythm	Infantile form is severe and rapidly progressive, with death prior to 2 yr. Late-onset forms are chronic, progressive, and variable in severity	Autosomal recessive	*GALC* pathogenic variants and deletions

Metabolic and Other Neuropathy Disorders—cont'd

Disorder	Age of onset	Clinical features	Associated features	Diagnostic findings	Course	Inheritance	Gene
Acute intermittent porphyria	Adolescence to young adulthood	• Episodic neurovisceral attacks: sudden-onset severe abdominal pain, muscular weakness, autonomic changes (tachycardia, hypertension), mental status changes, possible seizures and hyponatremia • Progressive peripheral neuropathy, primarily motor, that can progress in an ascending fashion to include respiratory insufficiency or failure	• Hypertension • Chronic kidney disease • Risk of hepatocellular carcinoma • Attack triggers: numerous medications, alcohol intake, fluctuations in reproductive hormones, fasting, stress	• EMG: axonal motor neuropathy • MRI: findings consistent with posterior reversible encephalopathy syndrome possible • Urine: increased concentration of porphobilinogen during attacks • Biochemical confirmation via urine with specific quantitative assay necessary for diagnosis due to asymptomatic heterozygotes	Recurrent attacks of variable length and recovery (days to months)	Autosomal dominant	*HMBS*: encodes hydroxymethylbilane synthase. Pathogenic variants and deletions/duplications, with variable penetrance
Myofibrillar myopathies	Infancy through adulthood	• Proximal and distal muscle weakness (proximal > distal in up to a third of affected individuals, distal > proximal in up to a third of affected individuals) • Peripheral neuropathy with weakness and paresthesia	• Cardiomyopathy in up to 30% of affected individuals • Muscle aches and cramps • Restrictive lung disease	• EMG/NCV: fibrillation potentials, positive sharp waves, and other signs of electrical irritability. Mixed myopathic and neurogenic features • MRI: muscle inflammation possible • Blood: mild elevations in serum creatine kinase • Other: muscle histology with abnormal trichrome staining, decreased oxidative enzyme activity, and intense congophilia; muscle immunohistochemistry with ectopic expression of various proteins; muscle electron microscopy with myofibrillar degeneration commencing at the Z-disk	Chronic, progressive, resulting in severe disability or death	Autosomal dominant, with the exception of X-linked *FHL1* pathologic variant and autosomal recessive *CRYAB* pathologic variants	Sequence variants in the following genes have been identified. Deletions or duplications have not been reported: • *DES* • *CRYAB* • *MYOT* • *LDB3* • *FLNC* • *BAG3* • *FHL1* • *DNAJB6*
CD59 deficiency	Infancy through young adulthood	• Recurrent immune-mediated polyneuropathy following febrile illnesses • Risk for strokes	• Coombs-negative hemolysis during episodes	• EMG/NCV: demyelinating, axonal, or mixed polyneuropathy • MRI: spinal root enhancement • CSF: increased protein during episodes • Blood: elevated CRP during episodes	Relapsing, chronic, progressive. Individual episodes respond to immunomodulatory therapy	Autosomal recessive	*CD59*: pathogenic variant CYS89TYR in the *CD59* gene on chromosome 11p13

CSF, cerebrospinal fluid; EMG, electromyogram; FLAIR, fluid-attenuated inversion recovery; NCV, nerve conduction velocity.
Modified from Bordini BJ, Monrad P. Differentiating familial neuropathies from Guillain-Barré syndrome. *Pediatr Clin North Am.* 2017;64(1):231–252 (Table 2, pp. 241–248).

TABLE 35.19   Class and Variant Forms of Guillain-Barré Syndrome (GBS) in Pediatrics: Clinical Features That Distinguish from Acute Inflammatory Demyelinating Polyradiculoneuropathy and Key Diagnostic Features, Including Antiganglioside Antibody Profiles

Variant	Clinical Features	Diagnostic Features
Classic GBS		
AIDP	Acute-onset ascending weakness Frequent falls Refusal to walk, run, climb Numbness, tingling, pain May involve respiration, swallowing, facial muscles, autonomic nervous system	EMG/NCV CSF protein elevation, no pleocytosis MRI bright spinal nerve roots
Ophthalmoplegia-Ataxia-Areflexia Constellation		
Miller Fisher syndrome	Ophthalmoplegia, ataxia out of proportion to sensory loss, absent weakness Clumsiness, dysesthesia, numbness	EMG/NCV studies showing axonopathy, although some patients may have demyelinating features, also with reduced or absent sensory nerve action potentials; antibodies isolated include anti-GT_{1a}, GQ_{1b}, GD_{1b}
Bickerstaff brainstem encephalitis	Considered a subtype of Miller Fisher syndrome; includes ophthalmoplegia, ataxia, encephalopathy, and hyperreflexia	EMG/NCV studies similar to Miller Fisher; MRI findings variable but may include hyperintense foci in the brainstem on T2-weighted imaging, thalamic or cerebellar lesions possible; antibodies isolated include anti-GT_{1a}, GQ_{1b}, GD_{1b}
Plegia/Paresis with or Without Sensory and Autonomic Symptoms Constellation		
Paraparetic GBS	Weakness and paresthesia restricted to the lower extremities	EMG/NCV studies similar to AIDP
Facial diplegia and distal limb paresthesia	Similar to AIDP but with bifacial weakness; rare in children but may present in adolescents No ophthalmoplegia	EMG/NCV studies similar to AIDP; antibodies isolated include anti-GM_2; association with cytomegalovirus infection
Polyneuritis cranialis	Multiple bilateral cranial nerve palsies (often sparing the optic nerve); severe peripheral sensory loss	MRI showing enhancement of cranial nerves; antibodies isolated include anti-GQ_1, GT_1
Pharyngeal-cervical-brachial weakness	Swallowing dysfunction; weakness of oropharyngeal, neck, and shoulder muscles	EMG/NCV studies showing axonopathy; antibodies isolated include anti-GT_{1a}, GQ_{1b}, GD_{1a}
Acute motor axonal neuropathy	Absence of sensory or autonomic symptoms; rapid progression of ascending symmetric weakness; higher likelihood of respiratory failure Ascending weakness may involve respiration, swallowing, or facial muscles	EMG/NCV studies showing motor axonopathy without demyelinating features; antibodies isolated include anti-GM_1, GM_{1b}, GD_{1a}, GalNac-GD_{1a}; strong association with *Campylobacter jejuni* infection
Acute motor-sensory axonal neuropathy	Absence of autonomic symptoms; prolonged course with possible muscle wasting; rare in children	EMG/NCV studies showing motor and sensory axonopathy without demyelinating features; antibodies isolated include anti-GM_1, GM_{1b}, GD_{1a}; strong association with *C. jejuni* infection
Pure sensory GBS	Significant sensory ataxia with absent reflexes and minor motor involvement	EMG/NCV studies with demyelinating features; antibodies isolated include anti-GD_{1b}

AIDP, acute inflammatory demyelinating polyradiculoneuropathy; CSF, cerebrospinal fluid; EMG, electromyogram; GBS, Guillain-Barré syndrome; NCV, nerve conduction velocity.
Modified from Bordini BJ, Monrad P. Differentiating familial neuropathies from Guillain-Barré syndrome. *Pediatr Clin North Am.* 2017;64(1):231–252 (Table 1, pp. 237–238).

toes, claw-hand deformities, respiratory insufficiency, and early-onset scoliosis that may need surgical correction. Nerve biopsy shows onion-bulb formation and axons without evidence of myelination. A severe infancy or childhood-onset phenotype is associated with pathogenic variants in the following genes: *MPZ, EGR2, PMP22, PRX, NEFL, MFN2,* and *GDAP1.*

Uncommon disorders

Chronic inflammatory demyelinating polyneuropathy. Chronic inflammatory demyelinating polyneuropathy (CIDP) is a chronic immune-mediated neuropathy with a childhood incidence of <1 in 200,000. CIDP is more common in childhood and is unlikely to occur

in neonates or infants. Unlike GBS/AIDP, there is no antecedent illness. Immune-mediated targeting of myelin in the motor and sensory neurons is the mechanism of disease.

This neuropathy is characterized by progressive proximal weakness with the nadir reached within 2 months of onset. Symptoms initially manifest in the legs and can progress to the arms and face and then involve swallowing or breathing function. Complete absence of reflexes is typically seen. Diagnosis is conferred when EMG demonstrates multiple segments of motor nerves with conduction velocities in the demyelinating range, with abnormal or absent sensory nerve conductions in the setting of a consistent clinical history. CSF shows

TABLE 35.20 Classification of HMSN or Charcot-Marie-Tooth (CMT) Disease

Type	Gene or Cytogenetic Location	Age of Onset	Evocative Phenotypes
Autosomal Dominant CMT1 (AD-CMT1)			
CMT1A	PMP22 (duplication)	All ages	Classic form. Hypertrophy of nerves
HNPP	PMP22 (deletion)	2–64 yr	Recurrent entrapment neuropathies. Multifocal neuropathies
CMT1B	MPZ	First to second decade	Clinically more severe than CMT1A
CMT1C	LITAF	Childhood	Abnormal gait. Occasional nerve hypertrophy. Rarely deafness
CMT1D	EGR2	First decade	DSS/CHN. Possible cranial nerve involvement. Scoliosis
CMT1E	PMP22	Childhood	Associated with deafness
CMT1F	NEFL	1–13 yr	CMT1 with early onset. Severe disease
CMT "plus"	FBLN5	Fourth to fifth decade	Skin hyperelasticity. Age-related macular degeneration
Autosomal Dominant CMT2 (AD-CMT2)			
CMT2A	MFN2	6 mo–50 yr	Prominent distal weakness. Late proximal weakness. Optic atrophy. CNS involvement
CMT2B	RAB7	Second decade	Severe sensory loss. Foot ulcers. Arthropathy and amputations
CMT2C	TRPV4	Birth to 60 yr	Younger more severe. Motor predominance. Vocal cord, diaphragm, respiratory involvement/dHMN
CMT2D	GARS	16–30 yr	Distal upper limb predominance dHMN
CMT2E	NEFL	First to fifth decade	Hearing loss. Hyperkeratosis
CMT2F	HSPB1	Adult	Classic/dHMN
CMT2G	12q12-q13.2	Second decade	Classic
CMT2I	MPZ	Late	Classic
CMT2J	MPZ	Late	Deafness and pupillary abnormalities
CMT2K	GDAP1	Variable	Vocal paralysis and pyramidal features
CMT2L	HSPB8	15–33 yr	Classic/dHMN
CMT2M	DNM2	First to second decade	Tremor
CMT2N	AARS	15–50 yr	Classic
CMT2O	DYNC1H1	Early childhood	Sometimes learning difficulties
CMT2P	LRSAM1	27–40 yr	Mild. Sometimes asymmetry
CMT2Q	DHTKD1	13–25 yr	Classic CMT
HMSN-P	TFG	17–55 yr	Proximal involvement. Tremor. Diabetes mellitus
CMT2	HARS	Late onset	Sensory predominant
CMT2	MARS	Late onset	Motor-sensory
CMT2	MT-ATP6	First to second decade	Motor predominant. Pyramidal signs
Dominant and Recessive X-Linked CMT			
CMTX1	GJB1	First to second decade	Classic. Occasional deafness
CMTX4	AIFM1	Early childhood	Intellectual disability. Deafness
CMTX5	PRPS1	Childhood	Mild–moderate neuropathy. Deafness. Late optic atrophy
CMTX6	PDK3	Childhood	Classic CMT
Dominant Intermediate CMT			
DI-CMTA	10q24.1-q25.1	7–72 yr	Classic CMT
DI-CMTB (CMT2M)	DNM2	First to second decade	Classic CMT with neutropenia and early-onset cataract
DI-CMTC	YARS	7–59 yr	Classic CMT
DI-CMTD	MPZ	30–50 yr	Sensory loss and weakness. Deafness/pupil disorders
DI-CMTE	INF2	5–28 yr	Glomerulosclerosis and proteinuria
DI-CMTF	GNB4	5–45 yr	Classic CMT

Continued

TABLE 35.20   **Classification of HMSN or Charcot-Marie-Tooth (CMT) Disease—cont'd**

Type	Gene or Cytogenetic Location	Age of Onset	Evocative Phenotypes
Autosomal Recessive CMT1 AR-CMT1 (CMT4)			
AR-CMT1A	GDAP1	<2 yr	Severe and progressive. Vocal cord and diaphragm paralysis in some cases
AR-CMT1B1	MTMR2	3 yr	Severe CMT1. Facial/bulbar weakness. Scoliosis
AR-CMT1B2	MTMR13 (SBF2)	4–13 yr	Severe CMT1. Glaucoma. Kyphoscoliosis
AR-CMT1B3	MTMR5 (SBF1)	5–11 yr	Pes planus. Scoliosis
AR-CMT1C	SH3TC2	Early onset first to second decade	Severe to moderate CMT1. Scoliosis. Deafness
AR-CMT1D	NDRG1	<10 yr	Severe CMT1. Deafness. Tongue atrophy
AR-CMT1E	EGR2	Birth	Congenital hypotonia. Respiratory failure. Arthrogryposis
AR-CMT1F	PRX	Birth to first decade	CMT1. Prominent sensory involvement
AR-CMT1G (HMSN-Russe)	HK1	8–16 yr	Severe to moderate CMT1
AR-CMT1H	FGD4	<2 yr	Delayed milestones. Scoliosis. Severe course
AR-CMT1J	FIG4	Congenital, childhood, or adult	Severe disorder. Similarities to motor neuron disease
AR-CMT1	SURF1	Childhood	Severe. Associated to cerebellar ataxia, brain MRI abnormalities, and lactic acidosis
Autosomal Recessive CMT2 AR-CMT2 (CMT2)			
AR-CMT2A (CMT2B1)	LMNA	Second decade	Severe course. Distal and proximal weakness
AR-CMT2B (CMT2B2)	MED25	28–42 yr	Classic CMT2
AR-CMT2C (CMT2B5)	NEFL	First decade	Severe form
AR-CMT2F/dHMN	HSPB1	Variable	Sometimes proximal leg weakness
AR-CMT2H	GDAP1	First decade	Pyramidal involvement. Vocal cord involvement
AR-CMT2K (rarely AD)	GDAP1	Early-onset form	Severe form. Vocal cord paralysis. Skeletal deformities. Milder dominant form
AR-CMT2P	LRSAM1	Third to fourth decade	Cramps. Erectile dysfunction
(HMSN VI)	MFN2	Early onset	Optic atrophy
ARAN-NM	HINT1	First decade	Neuromyotonia
GAN	GAN	Childhood	Severe axonal neuropathy with early-onset CNS involvement. Milder form CMT-like

AD, autosomal dominant; AR, autosomal recessive; CHN, congenital hypermyelinating neuropathy; CNS, central nervous system; HMSM, hereditary motor and sensory neuropathy; HNPP, hereditary neuropathy with liability to pressure palsies.
From Tazir M, Hamadouche T, Nouioua S, et al. Hereditary motor and sensory neuropathies or Charcot-Marie-Tooth diseases: an update. *J Neurol Sci.* 2014;347:14–22 (Table 2, pp. 16–17).

cytoalbuminologic dissociation, similar to GBS. When the diagnosis is under consideration, infectious and neoplastic etiologies must be excluded.

Unlike GBS, this syndrome requires prolonged, typically lifelong, treatment with immunosuppressants. Good functional recovery is possible with adequate early immunosuppression, with the goal being to maintain the patient on a single steroid-sparing drug long term.

Is It a Problem at the Neuromuscular Junction?

Diagnostic considerations. NMJ disorders are characterized by hypotonia and weakness with preserved reflexes, *except in the case of botulism*, in which reflexes may be diminished or even absent. The hypotonia and weakness in NMJ disorders are characterized by *fatigability* and *diurnal fluctuations*, with symptoms typically worsening over the course of the day, as well as acute exacerbations, sometimes in conjunction with identifiable triggers such as stress

or a febrile illness. Weakness may be generalized or concentrated primarily in proximal muscle groups. Commonly affected are the small muscles of the eyes that are continually contracting when awake, such as the levator palpebrae superioris, resulting in ptosis, as well as the extraocular muscles, resulting in ophthalmoparesis, producing the symptom of diplopia (Fig. 35.17). Diagnostic investigations that help localize hypotonia and weakness to the NMJ include EMG of an affected muscle, which demonstrates a decrementing response to 3-Hz RNS (Fig. 35.18 and Table 35.21), though if the disease is severe and has resulted in static weakness, the needle EMG may be normal or appear myopathic. Motor and sensory nerve conduction velocities are normal, as is the CK, helping suggest against nerve or muscle involvement, respectively. NMJ disorders are difficult to distinguish from each other on clinical grounds. All patients with NMJ disorders should undergo testing for the presence of acetylcholine receptor and muscle-specific kinase antibodies, as positive antibodies are

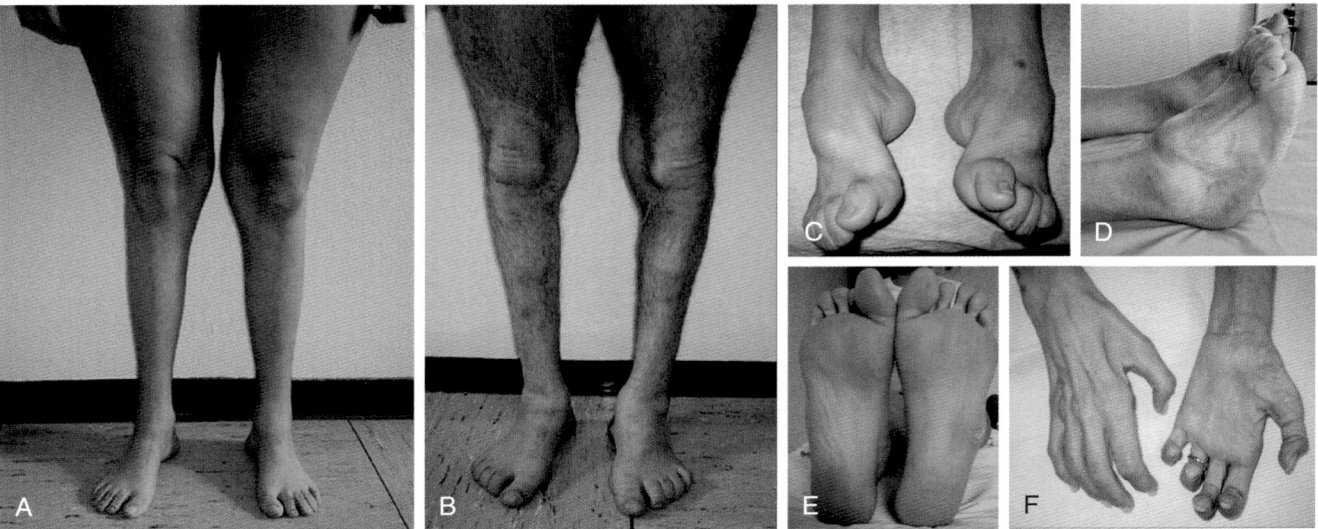

Fig. 35.16 Patients with Charcot-Marie-Tooth disease. *(A-B)* Muscle wasting of the legs and the lower third of the thigh. *(C-E)* Foot deformities of different severities, with high arches, hammer toes, and callosities. *(F)* Severe atrophy of intrinsic hand muscles (*main en griffe* ["claw hand"]). (From Pareyson D, Marchesi C. Diagnosis, natural history, and management of Charcot-Marie-Tooth disease. *Lancet Neurol.* 2009;8[7]:654–667 [Fig. 1, p. 655].)

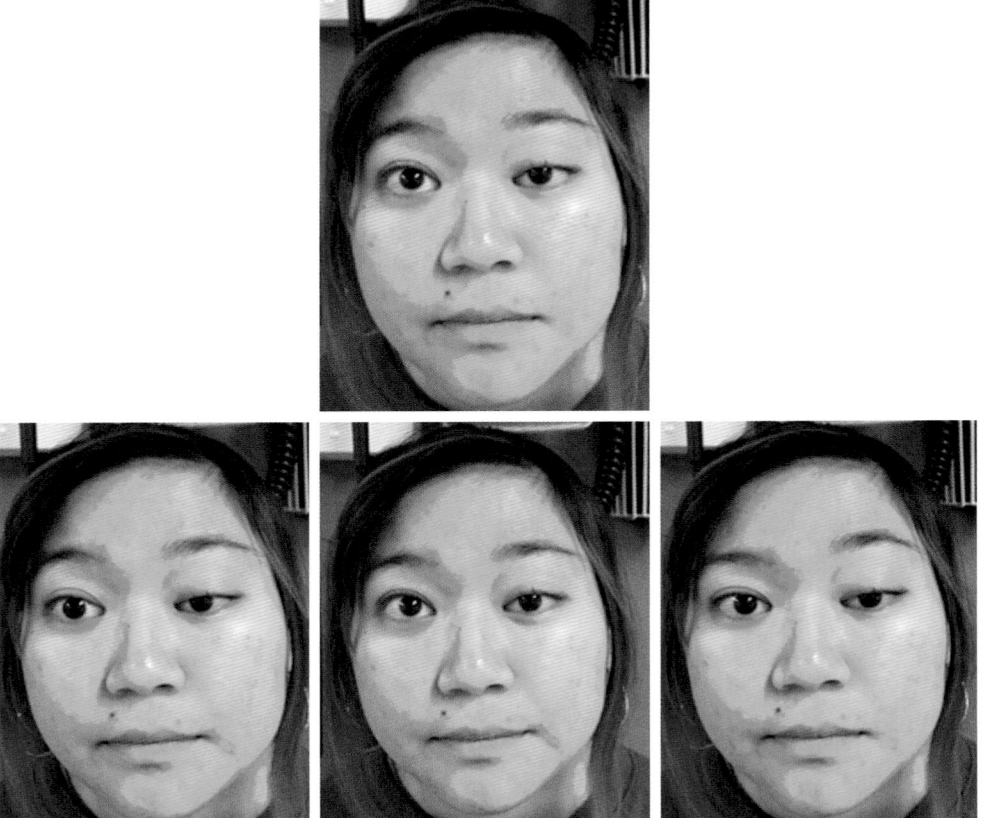

Fig. 35.17 Left ptosis and ophthalmoparesis in nearly all directions of gaze in a 17-year-old female adolescent with acetylcholine receptor antibody–positive generalized myasthenia diagnosed at 12 years of age. Left ptosis is evident on primary gaze *(center)*, with near-complete ophthalmoparesis on up gaze *(top)*, right gaze *(left)*, and left gaze *(right)* with relatively preserved down gaze *(bottom)*. (Photographs courtesy Dr. Chamindra Konersman, used with permission.)

diagnostic of autoimmune myasthenia and provide indication for immunomodulating therapy. Negative antibody status does not preclude autoimmune myasthenia, however.

Common disorders

Autoimmune myasthenia gravis. Up to 15% of all autoimmune myasthenia is pediatric onset. Symptoms include acute diplopia, ptosis, respiratory distress, and feeding difficulties in a previously

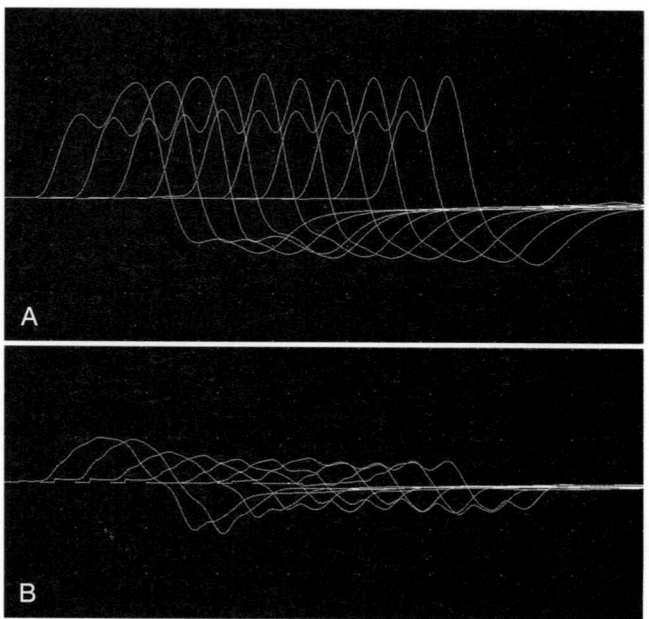

Fig. 35.18 Repetitive nerve stimulation (RNS) at a rate of 3 Hz in a 15-year-old female adolescent with ptosis and generalized weakness diagnosed with seropositive myasthenia. RNS of a clinically strong muscle, the abductor digiti minimi, shows no decremental response (A); however, when performed on a clinically weak muscle, the trapezius, a decremental response of 44% between the first and fifth responses (B) is seen.

healthy infant or child, with symptoms that tend to worsen or be more pronounced later in the day (see Fig. 35.17). Infants may also have stridor. Onset can occur in infancy through adolescence; neonatal presentation is rare. Categorizing each patient into either *generalized* or *ocular* myasthenia is clinically helpful, as the generalized form can be associated with respiratory or swallowing compromise, is potentially life-threatening, and requires hospitalization. Up to 35% of pediatric cases are categorized as ocular at onset, though a proportion of these progress to generalized disease within 2 years of symptom onset; frequent surveillance and reassessment are required.

Autoimmune myasthenia is caused by antibodies directed against specific antigens within the NMJ. The most common antibody is the acetylcholine receptor (AChR) antibody, which mediates disease by binding acetylcholine receptors at the postsynaptic membrane and inducing complement activation, which results in destruction of the receptor, distortion of the membrane, and interference with binding sites on remaining receptors. The AChR antibodies are present in approximately 75% of generalized pediatric myasthenia cases and 40% of ocular cases, similar to adult rates. The next most common auto-antibody is the muscle-specific kinase (MuSK) antibody, occurring in approximately 10% of pediatric myasthenia cases, again similar to adult rates. The prevalence of other more recently identified antibodies, such as the lipoprotein receptor-related membrane protein 4 (LRP-4), is yet to be determined. The presence of either AChR or MuSK antibodies in a patient with symptoms of myasthenia is diagnostic and obviates the need for further diagnostic studies. Seronegative patients should undergo 3-Hz RNS in a clinically weak muscle. A decrementing response confirms that disease is localized to the NMJ and provides evidence for a presumptive diagnosis of myasthenia. RNS has largely replaced edrophonium (Tensilon) testing due to its superior sensitivity and specificity, as well as the relative impracticality of Tensilon testing due to need for cardiac monitoring. Patients who are initially seronegative should be retested at the time of any exacerbations, as approximately 40% of initially seronegative patients become seropositive within 2 years. Childhood autoimmune myasthenia has a higher remission rate than adults; remission is associated with conversion to antibody-negative status. Distinguishing between autoimmune and

TABLE 35.21	Differentiating Between Types of Neuromuscular Junction Disorders			
	Botulism	**Autoimmune Myasthenia**	**Transient Neonatal Myasthenia**	**Congenital Myasthenic Syndrome**
Sudden onset in a previously healthy infant	+	+	−	+/− usually present at birth
Generalized hypotonia and weakness	+	+	+	+
Facial weakness, ptosis	+	+	+	+
Dilated, poorly reactive pupils	+	−	−	− (rare exception)
Constipation	+	−	−	−
Response to anticholinesterases	−	+	+	+/−
3 Hz (low frequency) RNS	Decremental response	Decremental response	Decremental response	Decremental response
High-frequency RNS	Incremental response in mild cases	Decremental response	Decremental response	Decremental response
Family history	−	+/−	+	+/−

*Congenital myasthenia includes congenital myasthenic syndromes, infantile (autoimmune) myasthenia, and transient acquired neonatal myasthenia.
+, present; −, absent; +/−, variable; RNS, repetitive nerve stimulation.
Modified from Volpe JJ, ed. *Neurology of the Newborn.* 5th ed. Philadelphia: Saunders; 2008:791.

genetic forms of myasthenia can be challenging in children, though responsiveness to immunosuppression strongly suggests autoimmune myasthenia.

Evaluation for **thymic hyperplasia or thymoma** via CT of the chest is necessary in all autoimmune myasthenia. Children are rarely found to have thymomas, but thymectomy is recommended in pediatric seropositive myasthenia, especially if response to medical therapy is poor. Unlike adults, thymectomy may prevent progression from ocular to the generalized form and may be beneficial in ocular myasthenia. Thymectomy is not recommended for adult ocular myasthenia. A thymectomy does not preclude the need for medical therapy but affords better disease control and reduced doses of immunosuppression. Symptomatic treatment includes long-acting cholinesterase inhibitors such as pyridostigmine; however, very few patients have complete and sustained resolution of symptoms solely on this drug. Most ocular and nearly all generalized myasthenia patients require early and sufficient disease-modifying treatment with immunosuppressants such as oral prednisone, which has been beneficial in controlling symptoms, reducing permanent weakness, and decreasing progression from ocular to generalized forms. Prednisone is harmful long term; therefore, all patients who respond to steroids should be offered steroid-sparing immunosuppression with azathioprine as the first-line agent for maintenance therapy. Rituximab can also be considered for long-term disease control. IVIG is only recommended for maintenance therapy if a patient cannot tolerate steroids and is added to the regimen if high-dose steroids yield suboptimal disease control.

Acute crises can be life-threatening and should be treated with prompt hospitalization, respiratory support as needed, and either IVIG or plasma exchange for disease control. Good functional recovery is possible with adequate immunosuppression and the goal is to maintain the patient on a single steroid-sparing drug long term.

Botulism. **Infantile botulism** is caused by the ingestion of *Clostridium botulinum* organisms that germinate in the infant's gastrointestinal tract and release botulinum neurotoxin into the bloodstream. The toxin, composed of a heavy and light chain, prevents the release of acetylcholine at motor and autonomic NMJs through a series of steps (Fig. 35.19). Reduced acetylcholine release into the synaptic cleft results in flaccid paralysis of skeletal muscle, flaccid paralysis of smooth muscles of the gut, and autonomic ganglia dysfunction. Symptoms evolve over the course of several days and include constipation, followed then by lethargy, reduced spontaneous movement, hypotonia, and poor feeding. Subsequently, head drop develops, as do ptosis, a weak cry and smile, and mydriasis, as well as a descending paralysis that can compromise respiratory function. Reflexes are often preserved though can be diminished or even absent. Decreased physiologic variability in heart rate can occur in severe cases.

Infantile botulism affects neonates from younger than 1 week of age to 1 year, with 95% of cases occurring in infants younger than 6 months old. The sources of *C. botulinum* include honey, corn syrup, soil, and dust. The immaturity of the gut microbiome in infants is presumed to increase their susceptibility to colonization by *C. botulinum*. Exposure to soil from active construction, whether via a parent who works in construction or via proximity to a construction site, has also been proposed as a means of contracting the disease.

Diagnosis is made by detecting toxin in stool using a neutralizing bioassay. Serum studies for botulinum toxin are unreliable. EMG can help exclude mimics and demonstrates low-amplitude motor conductions at baseline, with an increase of >40% above baseline following exercise or tetanic stimulation at 30–50 Hz.

Prompt diagnosis allows for rapid treatment with intravenous botulism immunoglobulin, allowing for significantly reduced durations of hospital stay and lower durations of mechanical ventilation, enteral feeding tube requirement, or need for parenteral nutrition. Recovery takes

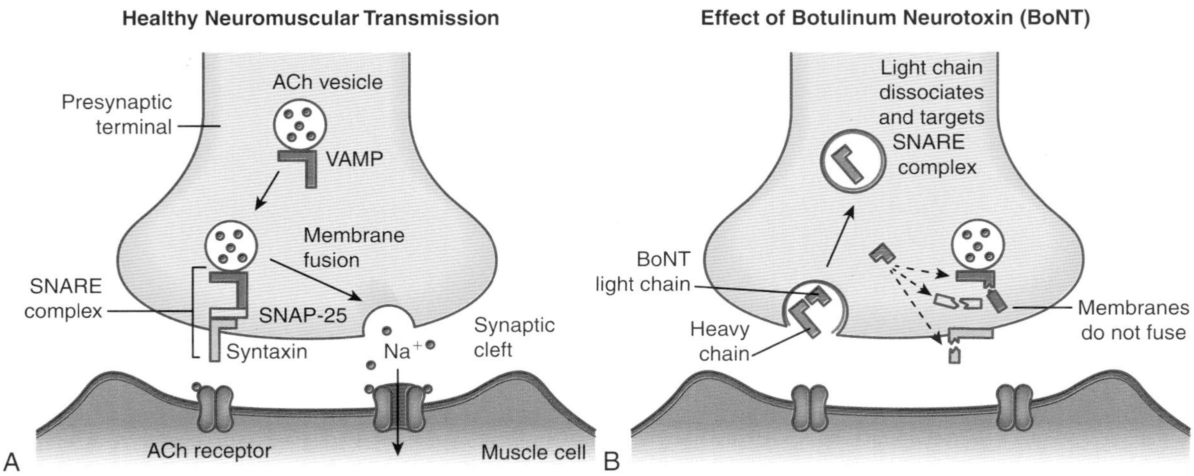

Fig. 35.19 Neuromuscular transmission in botulism compared to normal. *A*, Healthy neuromuscular transmission. Acetylcholine (ACh)-containing vesicles bind to the presynaptic terminal membrane via formation of the soluble N-ethylmaleimide-sensitive factor attachment protein receptors (SNARE) complex, leading to membrane fusion and release of ACh into the synaptic cleft. ACh molecules then bind to receptors on the muscle cell, allowing influx of sodium and muscle contraction. *B*, Effect of botulinum neurotoxin (BoNT). BoNT binds receptors on the presynaptic terminal and is endocytosed. The light chain is dissociated from the heavy chain and translocates into the cytoplasm, where it cleaves specific SNARE proteins according to BoNT subtype. Subtypes A, C, and E target SNAP-25; subtypes B, D, F, and G target vesicle-associated membrane protein (VAMP); and subtype C further targets syntaxin. (From Rosow LK, Strober JB. Infant botulism: review and clinical update. *Pediatr Neurol.* 2015;52[5]:487–492.)

weeks to months, with the diaphragm recovering faster than peripheral muscles. Prognosis is generally excellent if there are no complications.

Food-borne botulism develops after ingestion of preformed toxin in poorly canned foods. Affected children have nausea and vomiting with dilated pupils, diplopia, dysphagia, dysarthria, dry mouth, and hypotonia. Wound botulism is uncommon.

Uncommon disorders

Transient neonatal myasthenia. Transient neonatal myasthenia (TNM) is caused by transplacental transfer of maternal antibodies, even if the mother is seronegative, and occurs in up to 30% of neonates born to mothers with autoimmune myasthenia. The neonate will likely be seropositive for maternal autoantibody. Affected patients usually demonstrate generalized hypotonia, weak cry, respiratory distress, ophthalmoparesis, and difficulty feeding a few hours after birth. Notably, affected neonates are alert with normally reactive pupils.

Treatment is supportive and most infants recover completely within 4–6 weeks. Some require respiratory support until symptoms resolve. Anticholinesterase inhibitor therapy with neostigmine may be needed for a few days to a few weeks. Plasma exchange may also be required for severe cases. Clearance of antibody from the infant's serum correlates with resolution of symptoms. No long-term treatment is necessary.

Rare cases of arthrogryposis multiplex congenita have been described in TNM due to early transplacental transfer of maternal AChR antibodies binding fetal acetylcholine receptors, resulting in reduced fetal movements and development of contractures.

Congenital myasthenic syndrome. Congenital myasthenic syndrome (CMS) is a rare set of genetic disorders stemming from pathogenic variants in over a dozen different genes causing either defective release of acetylcholine (presynaptic), lack of acetylcholinesterase or abnormal clustering of acetylcholine receptors (synaptic), or abnormal acetylcholine receptor response (postsynaptic) (Fig. 35.20).

Clinically, all CMSs are seronegative for AChR and MuSK antibodies and can manifest with ophthalmoparesis, ptosis, and feeding and respiratory difficulties, making them indistinguishable from the autoimmune myasthenia (Fig. 35.21). Lack of a response to immunomodulatory therapy is suggestive, while genetic confirmation of disease is necessary for definitive diagnosis. Treatment with acetylcholinesterase inhibitors needs to be tailored based on the nature of the genetic defect, since a subset of patients will respond with worsening weakness to pyridostigmine.

Is It a Problem in the Muscle?

Diagnostic considerations. The muscle diseases are broadly categorized into muscular dystrophies or myopathies based on clinical and pathologic features. **Muscular dystrophies**, or dystrophinopathies, are a group of relentlessly progressive disorders characterized by ongoing muscle degeneration and regeneration, elevated CK, and a dystrophic pattern on muscle biopsy light microscopy that consists of rounded large and small fibers, many degenerating and regenerating fibers, internal nuclei, and prominent fibrosis between fibers, indicative of scarring. The dystrophic pattern is uniform for all dystrophinopathies, and specialized staining is necessary to distinguish between different types of muscular dystrophy (Fig. 35.22). Variable involvement of other organs, such as the heart, can occur in muscular dystrophies, though a thoughtful approach to assessing for involvement of other organ systems is advised. Notably, concomitant elevations in aspartate aminotransferase (AST) and alanine aminotransferase (ALT) will occur whenever CK is markedly elevated, since AST/ALT are not enzymes specific to the liver and are also found in muscle. Recognition of this laboratory abnormality pattern may prevent an unnecessary liver biopsy or other investigations, as disease restricted to the muscle will lack other markers of hepatic dysfunction, such as elevations in

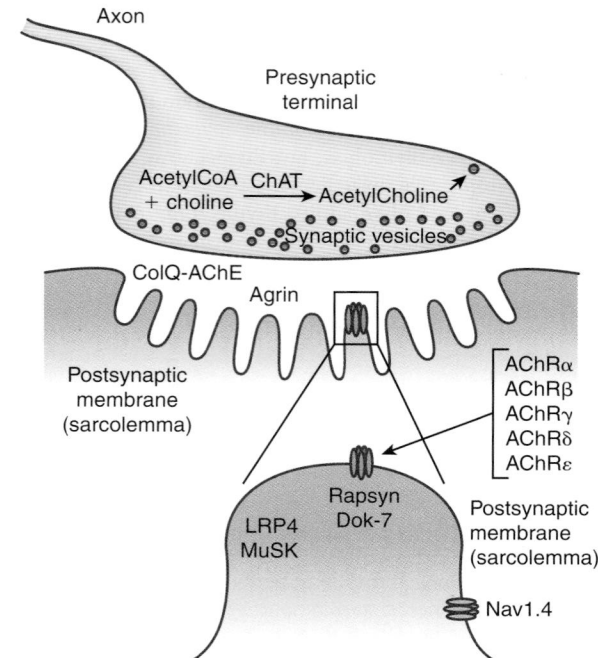

Fig. 35.20 Congenital myasthenic syndrome classified by location of defective protein. (From Shieh PB, Oh SJ. Congenital myasthenic syndromes. *Neurol Clin.* 2018;36[2]:367–378.)

alkaline phosphatase, gamma glutamyl transferase and bilirubin, or coagulation abnormalities.

A **myopathy**, on the other hand, has a structural or functional abnormality in the myofiber resulting from pathogenic genetic variants. Generally, myopathies are less progressive than dystrophinopathies but have the potential to be similarly disabling. Most importantly, myopathies lack the characteristic scarring and muscle turnover on muscle biopsy and instead exhibit unusual features such as cores, rods, vacuoles, or centrally placed nuclei. Due to the lack of increased muscle turnover relative to dystrophinopathies, CK is typically normal. Variable involvement of other organs can occur with myopathies as well.

A stepwise evaluation generally consists of first obtaining a CK to distinguish between muscular dystrophies and myopathies. Lactate, pyruvate, thyroid studies, and a muscle biopsy to differentiate between muscular dystrophy, myopathy, metabolic myopathy, inflammatory myopathy, and mitochondrial disease are subsequent steps in diagnosing a muscle disease. Based on the results of these initial investigations, further genetic and metabolic studies may be necessary for a definitive diagnosis. Metabolic disorders that affect muscle are outlined in Table 35.22.

Common disorders

Duchenne and Becker muscular dystrophy. Duchenne and Becker muscular dystrophy (DMD and BMD) are X-linked disorders caused by pathogenic variants in the *DMD* gene, which encodes dystrophin. The majority of pathogenic changes consist of deletions of one or more exons within the gene, while sequence variants account for the remainder. While DMD is characterized by the absence of dystrophin in muscle, BMD has a partially functional protein product. The difference between the two phenotypes is based on the nature of the underlying genetic abnormality. Typically, copy number or sequence variants causing DMD are "out-of-frame," resulting in a premature termination of translation and subsequent degradation of the protein product, while variants that cause BMD are "in-frame," producing a partly functional, albeit truncated, protein. As an X-linked disorder, biological males are affected far more frequently than females, who are typically carriers though may rarely manifest partial or even complete symptoms.

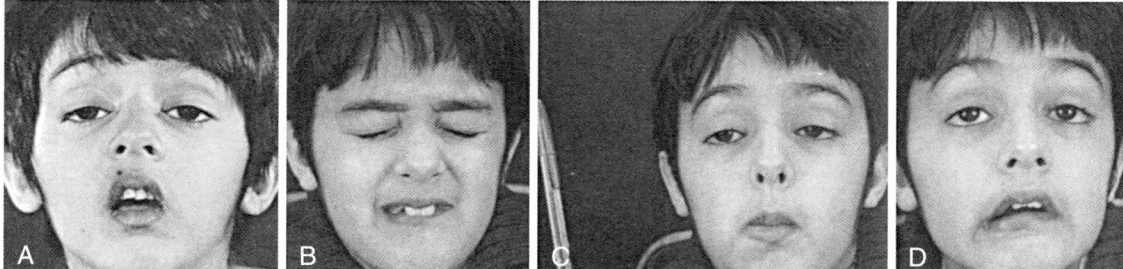

Fig. 35.21 Congenital myasthenic syndrome. This child was referred at 4 years of age with a history of swallowing difficulty. By 2 years, his walking had not progressed further, and he was unable to run or climb stairs. His parents had also noted some ptosis in the first year. On examination, he had obvious ptosis, limited ocular movement, associated weakness of facial movement, an expressionless face, open mouth, and an inability to close the eyes tightly *(A)*. There was general hypotonia with joint laxity. The child got up from the floor with a Gower sign and could not stand on one leg or run. A diagnosis of myasthenia was confirmed by demonstrating a response decrement to repeated ulnar nerve stimulation. A definite improvement in the ptosis and his ability to get up from the floor was noted after intravenous edrophonium chloride (Tensilon). He was treated with pyridostigmine and showed a definite improvement, but with time, he needed an increased dosage and frequency. His performance improved after each dose and tended to wane as the next dose became due. He still had a Gower sign on rising from the floor, marked ptosis, external ophthalmoplegia, and facial weakness *(B–D)*. A history of consanguinity suggested a possible diagnosis of autosomal recessive infantile (congenital) myasthenia. (From Dubowitz V. *Muscle Disorders in Childhood.* 2nd ed. London: WB Saunders; 1995:414.)

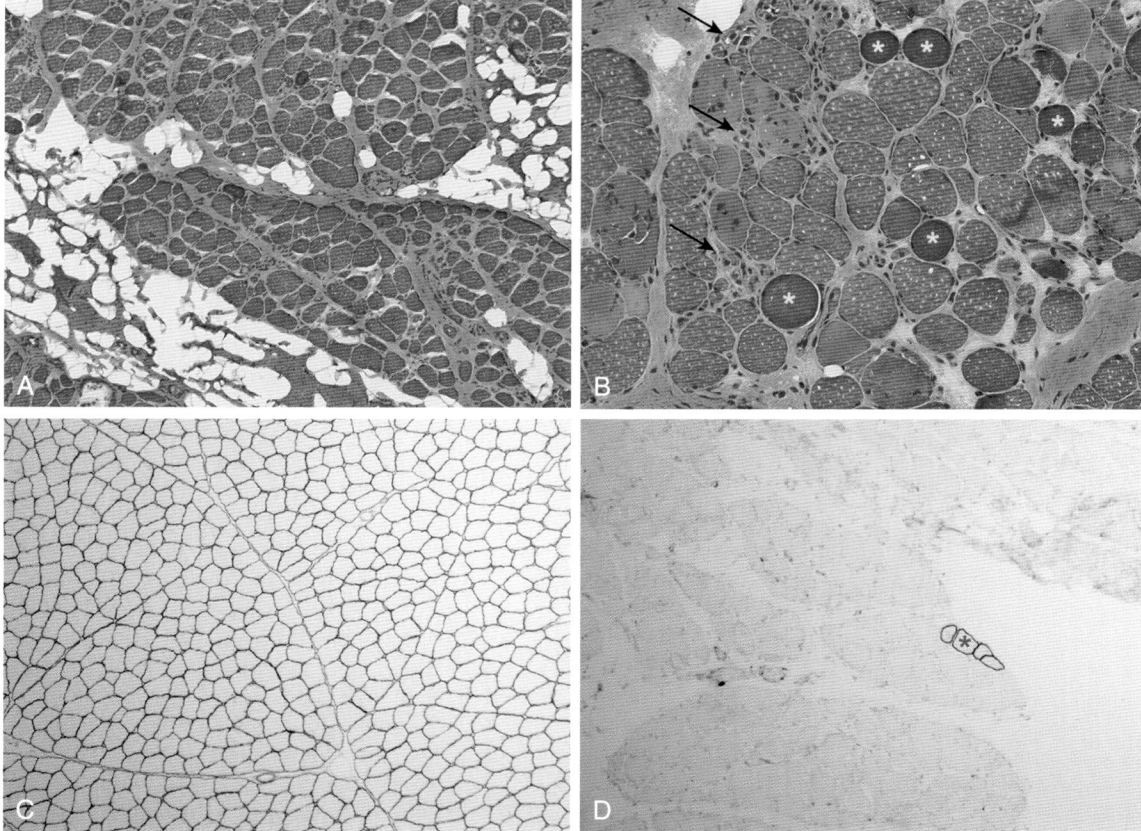

Fig. 35.22 Muscle biopsy in Duchenne muscular dystrophy (DMD) showing prominent dystrophic changes consisting of fiber size variation, thick endomysial (around each myofiber) and perimysial connective tissue, increased internal nucleation, and fatty replacement of muscle tissue on hematoxylin and eosin (H&E) *(A)*. Higher magnification on H&E *(B)* shows mild inflammation consisting of myophagocytes consuming degenerating muscle fibers *(arrows)* and hypercontracted fibers *(yellow asterisks)*. Dystrophin immunohistochemistry demonstrates the normal staining pattern outlining the sarcolemma *(C)* in normal muscle, whereas the absence of staining in nearly all the fibers is seen in a DMD patient *(D)*. A few fibers within the muscle, called "revertant fibers," may have their reading frame spontaneously restored, thus enabling them to express dystrophin *(red asterisk)*. (Courtesy Michael Lawlor, MD, PhD, Medical College of Wisconsin, Milwaukee, WI.)

TABLE 35.22 **Metabolic Diseases That Affect Muscle**

Name(s)	Enzyme Deficiency	Clinical Features	Diagnostic Testing
Glycogen storage disease type II (Pompe disease)	α-1,4-Glucosidase (GAA enzyme)	• Infantile-onset Pompe—poor feeding, motor delay and hypotonia with weakness, respiratory difficulties, cardiac issues (short P-R interval with wide QRS complex, cardiomegaly, LV outflow obstruction, cardiomyopathy) • Late-onset Pompe—limb-girdle pattern of weakness, respiratory insufficiency without clinical heart disease • GAA enzyme replacement therapy available	• Measure acid α-glucosidase (GAA) enzyme activity on dried blood spot to screen • Confirm via *GAA* gene sequencing demonstrating biallelic pathogenic variants for definitive diagnosis • Baseline elevated CK (~10× normal) in infantile-onset form; baseline CK may be normal in adult-onset form • Muscle biopsy may show vacuoles (lysosomes) and glycogen accumulation with positively staining PAS; 20–30% of patients with adult-onset form may not show specific changes on biopsy
Glycogen storage disease type IIIa (Debrancher deficiency, Cori disease, Forbes disease)	Amylo-1,6-glucosidase	• Ketotic hypoglycemia, hepatomegaly, hyperlipidemia, elevated liver enzymes, cardiomyopathy in childhood, limb-girdle pattern of weakness in 20s–30s	• Baseline elevated CK (2–20× normal) • Triglycerides, cholesterol, and liver enzymes are elevated • *AGL* gene sequencing demonstrating biallelic pathogenic variants for definitive diagnosis
Glycogen storage disease type IV (Brancher deficiency, Andersen disease)	Glycogen branching enzyme (GBE)	• Fatal perinatal neuromuscular subtype—fetal akinesia, polyhydramnios, fetal hydrops • Congenital neuromuscular subtype—hypotonic newborn, respiratory distress, dilated cardiomyopathy, death in infancy • Childhood neuromuscular subtype—chronic progressive myopathy, dilated cardiomyopathy	• Demonstrate deficiency of GBE in the liver, muscle, or skin fibroblasts • *GBE1* gene sequencing demonstrating biallelic pathogenic variants for definitive diagnosis
Glycogen storage disease type V (McArdle disease)	Myophosphorylase	• Exercise-induced muscle cramps and pain, especially early in exercise, that improve with rest or lower intensity ("second-wind phenomenon") • Recurrent myoglobinuria +/– rhabdomyolysis	• Baseline elevated CK (>5× normal) • *PYGM* gene sequencing demonstrating biallelic pathogenic variants for definitive diagnosis • Quantitative or qualitative (stain) on muscle biopsy shows virtual absence of enzyme activity • Subsarcolemmal glycogen accumulation on muscle biopsy on LM (either PAS positive or vacuoles on H&E) and EM
Glycogen storage disease type VII (Tarui disease)	Phosphofructokinase	• Classical form—muscle aching, cramping, exercise intolerance, myoglobinuria, nausea/vomiting after intense exercise, starting in childhood; hemolytic anemia • Late-onset form—cramps, myalgia, mild proximal weakness in adulthood • Infantile form—hypotonia, arthrogryposis, intellectual disability, fatal in infancy	• Baseline elevated CK • *PFK* gene sequencing demonstrating biallelic pathogenic variants for definitive diagnosis
Glycogen storage disease VIII (phosphorylase kinase [PhK] deficiency)	Phosphorylase b kinase	• Exercise intolerance, cramps, myoglobinuria, progressive muscle weakness in childhood to adulthood • Hepatomegaly, growth retardation, fasting ketosis and hypoglycemia	• Baseline elevated CK • PhK enzyme activity reduced in muscle • *PHKA1* gene sequencing and/or *PHKB* gene sequencing demonstrating biallelic pathogenic variants for definitive diagnosis
	Phosphorylase a1 kinase	• Same as above but X-linked and very rare	
Glycogen storage disease IX (phosphoglycerate kinase deficiency)	Phosphoglycerate kinase	• Myopathic form—muscle weakness, pain, cramping, especially with exercise with myoglobinuria +/– rhabdomyolysis	• Baseline mildly elevated CK • *PGK1* gene sequencing demonstrating biallelic pathogenic variants for definitive diagnosis
Glycogen storage disease X (phosphoglycerate mutase deficiency)	Phosphoglycerate mutase	• Strenuous exercise intolerance, cramps, myoglobinuria	• Baseline mildly elevated CK • *PGAM2* gene sequencing demonstrating biallelic pathogenic variants for definitive diagnosis
Glycogen storage disease XI (lactate dehydrogenase deficiency)	Lactate dehydrogenase	• Exercise intolerance, cramping, recurrent myoglobinuria	• Normal CK between attacks • *LDHA* gene sequencing demonstrating biallelic pathogenic variants for definitive diagnosis

TABLE 35.22	**Metabolic Diseases That Affect Muscle—cont'd**		
Name(s)	Enzyme Deficiency	Clinical Features	Diagnostic Testing
Systemic primary carnitine deficiency	Solute carrier family 22 (sodium-dependent carnitine transporter)	• Childhood myopathic form—hypotonia, dilated cardiomyopathy that could result in death, proximal muscle weakness in early childhood (2–4 yr) • Adult form—fatigability	• Baseline CK elevated • Reduced plasma carnitine levels • Increased lipid deposition on muscle biopsy • *SLC22A5* gene sequencing demonstrating biallelic pathogenic variants for definitive diagnosis
Carnitine palmitoyltransfer-ase II deficiency	Carnitine palmitoyl-transferase II (CPT II)	• Myopathic form—recurrent myalgia and myoglobinuria after prolonged exercise, cold, or fasting; weakness during attacks; onset from childhood to adulthood • Severe infantile form—liver failure, cardio-myopathy, seizures, hypoketotic hypoglyce-mia, myopathy before 1 yr of age (rare)	• Normal CK between attacks • CPT II gene sequencing demonstrating biallelic patho-genic variants for definitive diagnosis • Muscle biopsy can be normal

CK, creatine kinase; EM, electron microscopy; H&E, hematoxylin and eosin; LM, light microscopy; LV, left ventricular; PAS, periodic acid–Schiff.

The diagnoses of DMD and BMD are suspected from the history (including the family history), physical examination findings, and an elevated serum CK (often 10,000–30,000 IU/L). Genetic testing via *DMD* deletion/duplication with reflexive sequencing analysis confirms the diagnosis. Although muscle biopsy is no longer necessary in DMD, it may still be useful in certain cases of BMD (see Fig. 35.22).

Rarely, infants with DMD may present with failure to thrive and global developmental delay. Some affected individuals have mild delays in their motor or cognitive milestones, but most have normal early milestones and do not come to clinical attention until 2–5 years of age when they are noted to be slower in walking or running, rising from the floor, or climbing stairs compared to their peers. Early in the dis-ease, there is usually *calf pseudohypertrophy* because of a proliferation of fat and collagen and even some small degree of muscle hypertrophy. The classic maneuver employed to rise from the floor is a **Gower sign**, indicative of proximal hip extensor weakness, and is typically seen by 7 years of age (Fig. 35.23). The characteristic phenotype of toe-walking with a waddling Trendelenburg gait, hyperlordosis, and enlarged calves is usually seen by 5–6 years of age. However, atrophy of all muscles occurs with age. Language and cognitive abnormalities are seen in many patients with a high incidence of autism and attention-deficit/hyperactivity disorder.

With time, proximal muscle weakness makes ambulation difficult, necessitating assistive devices such as wheelchairs. With the standard use of steroids, the age of wheelchair dependence ranges between 9 and 14 years. Respiratory muscle failure develops by late adolescence. The pulmonary insufficiency may be aggravated by thoracic kyphoscolio-sis. Nocturnal bilevel ventilation with progression to daytime use to treat hypercapnia due to advancing restrictive lung disease has been instrumental in prolonging life expectancy. Most patients develop **cardiomyopathy** starting in adolescence; screening with serial echo-cardiograms or cardiac MRI begins at 10 years of age. Most affected patients die by 25–35 years of age.

Oral corticosteroids slow progression of disease by improving mus-cle strength, which results in prolonged time to loss of ambulation, less scoliosis, preservation of respiratory function, and possible reduction in cardiac fibrosis. Despite these benefits, the side effects of long-term steroids serve as a deterrent to initiation. More novel therapies include the use of a synthetic antisense oligonucleotide, eteplirsen, that can allow for the restoration of the reading frame and production of a shortened but functional dystrophin protein that can lead to modest delays in disease progression. This medication is only beneficial for

DMD patients with a specific though common pathogenic change in exon 51 that disturbs the reading frame, which is approximately 14% of all DMD cases. Future therapies for DMD are centered on gene replacement with a shortened functional version of the *DMD* gene called *microdystrophin*.

Becker muscular dystrophy has marked clinical heterogeneity with a variable age of onset ranging from childhood to adulthood. Affected patients also have calf pseudohypertrophy, eventually exhibit a Gower maneuver, and have variable degrees of proximal muscle weakness. Other phenotypes in BMD include isolated quadriceps weakness, childhood cramps–myalgia syndrome, exercise-induced myoglobin-uria, and, rarely, asymptomatic elevated CK levels. Childhood-onset weakness typically results in loss of ambulation in the third or fourth decade. Cognition is usually normal but cardiomyopathy occurs fre-quently in this population and rarely may be the heralding symptom. Corticosteroids are not beneficial in most cases of BMD.

Myotonic dystrophy type 1. Myotonic dystrophy type 1 is a common muscle disorder of childhood that is distinct in that it causes primarily a distal distribution of muscle weakness and is associated with *myotonia*, a phenomenon characterized by persistent muscular contraction with apparent delay in relaxation of muscles. A child with myotonia has difficulty letting go of a doorknob or releasing a ball after gripping it tightly. Myotonia usually is present by 10 years of age, but significant distal muscle weakness is not usually evident until the end of the second decade. In **congenital myotonic dystrophy**, the newborn infant has severe generalized hypotonia and weakness, often with swallowing and sucking difficulty, facial diplegia, a down-turned tented mouth, moderate to severe intellectual disability, and congenital joint contractures (e.g., talipes equinovarus, arthrogrypo-sis) (Fig. 35.24). Usually there is a history of polyhydramnios and reduced fetal movements in utero (Table 35.23). If these features are present at birth, then assessing for distal weakness and myotonia in the mother, followed by the father, may aid in the diagnosis.

Myotonic dystrophy type 1 is a slowly progressive disorder with multisystem involvement, including the development of cataracts, premature male-pattern baldness, facial muscle atrophy resulting in a "hatchet face" appearance, cervical kyphosis, cardiac arrhythmias, diabetes, pilomatrixomata, increased risk of thyroid cancer, thy-roid dysfunction, gastrointestinal dysmotility, and testicular atrophy. EMG in children reveals a characteristic myotonic discharge (termed "dive bomber"), but EMG in the neonatal period may not show this characteristic finding. Genetic testing demonstrating a pathologic

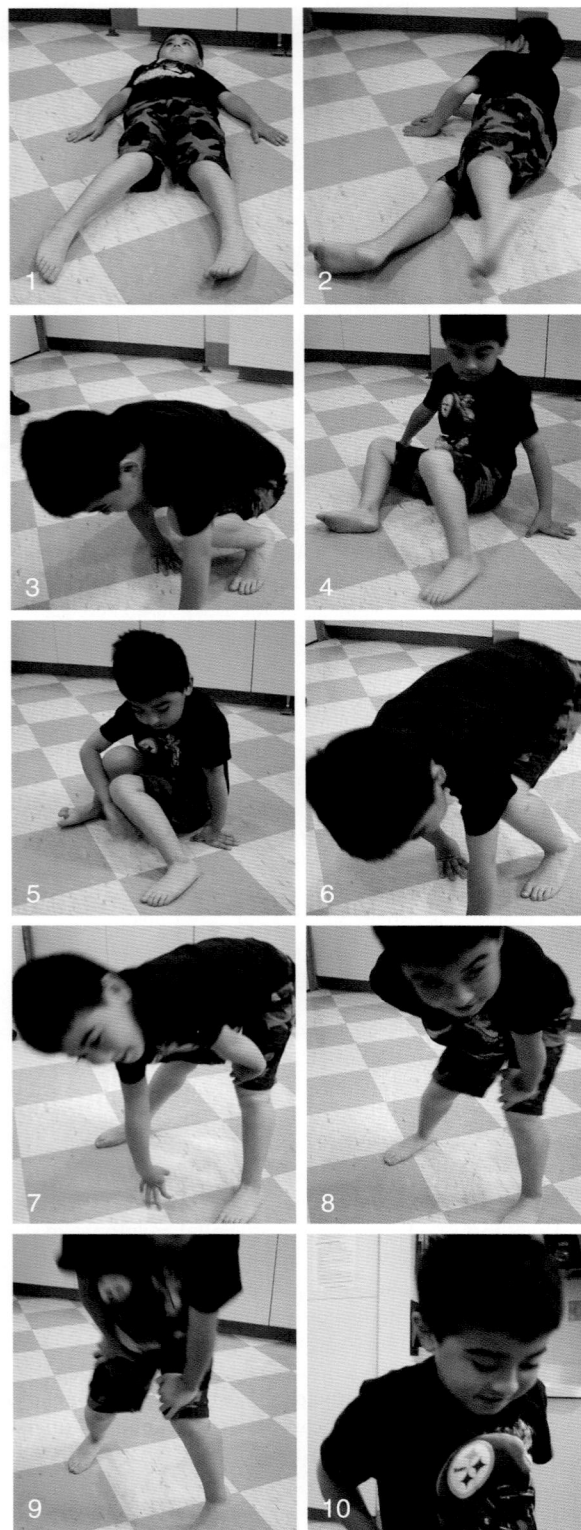

Fig. 35.23 The Gower maneuver in a 7-year-old male child with Duchenne muscular dystrophy: the sequence of postures used in getting up from the ground. *1,* Lying prone. *2–4,* Getting onto the hands and knees. *5–6,* Legs and arms extended and legs brought as close as possible to the arms. *7,* Hand placed on the knee. *8,* Both hands on the knees, knees extended. *9,* Hands moving alternately up the thighs, "climbing up himself." *10,* Erect posture.

cytosine-thymine-guanine (CTG) trinucleotide repeat expansion in the *DMPK* gene of chromosome 19q13.3 establishes the diagnosis. This abnormality, inherited in an autosomal dominant manner, will demonstrate genetic anticipation, resulting in earlier and more severe disease every generation.

Surveillance by a cardiologist for cardiac arrhythmia with timely placement of a pacemaker and implantable cardioverter defibrillator in these patients can prevent significant morbidity and mortality.

Juvenile dermatomyositis. Juvenile dermatomyositis (JDM) is a childhood- to adolescent-onset, systemic autoimmune disease caused by inflammation of small vessels of various organs including muscle, skin, and other major organs. Clinically, JDM presents with subacute-onset proximal muscle weakness and a characteristic heliotrope rash, Gottron papules, and cutaneous calcinosis. Involvement of the lung is a major cause of death in JDM and there is an association with malignancy. CK may be mildly elevated or normal. Autoantibodies are found in more than 60% of children, with each patient being seropositive for a single antibody. Each antibody likely has a specific phenotype and associated prognosis. Anti-tRNA synthetase and anti-MDA5 autoantibodies are associated with interstitial lung disease, anti-NXP-2 autoantibodies are associated with calcinosis, while anti-Mi2 is associated with "classic" JDM. Fundamentally, end-organ tissue is damaged by humoral and cell-mediated immune mechanisms including antibody-mediated destruction, complement activation, neutrophil activation, and small-vessel infarction resulting in necrosis.

Muscle biopsy remains essential for the diagnosis and demonstrates extensive myopathic changes with variability in muscle fiber size, perimysial and perivascular lymphocytic inflammation, membrane attack complex (MAC) deposition on microvasculature, muscle infarction with necrosis, and pathognomonic perifascicular atrophy—smaller muscle fibers on the edge of the fascicle compared to the center (Fig. 35.25).

Uncommon disorders

Pompe disease. Pompe disease, also known as acid maltase deficiency or glycogen storage disease type II, is a severe metabolic disease due to acid α-glucosidase (GAA) enzyme deficiency, resulting in impaired lysosomal glycogen breakdown. Accumulation of glycogen in lysosomes results in rupture and eventual myofibrillar breakdown.

Pompe disease is classified by age of onset, rate of progression, severity, and organ system involvement. The spectrum of disease is related to the level of enzyme activity, with severe early-onset infantile cases having little (<1%) to no enzyme function and late-onset disease having up to 30% enzyme function. Infantile-onset Pompe disease (IOPD) presents before 1 year with a rapidly progressive hypertrophic cardiomyopathy, left ventricular outflow tract obstruction, hypotonia, proximal muscle weakness, respiratory distress requiring ventilatory support, and feeding difficulties. Marked motor developmental delay, macroglossia, and normal intellect are typical. Patients typically die from respiratory failure. Late-onset Pompe disease (LOPD) refers to any infant who presents prior to 12 months of age without cardiomyopathy, or presentation after 12 months of age with or without cardiomyopathy, and can range from having mild proximal weakness and preserved ambulation though significant restrictive lung disease, to asymptomatic elevated CK found on routine blood testing. Patients with LOPD do not have severe cardiomyopathy.

Treatment with exogenously administered enzyme replacement therapy (ERT) has changed the course of IOPD and is the standard of care to treat Pompe disease, resulting in improved cardiac function, reduced risk of death, and decreased risk of invasive ventilation in the first few years of life, though most patients still remain at risk of

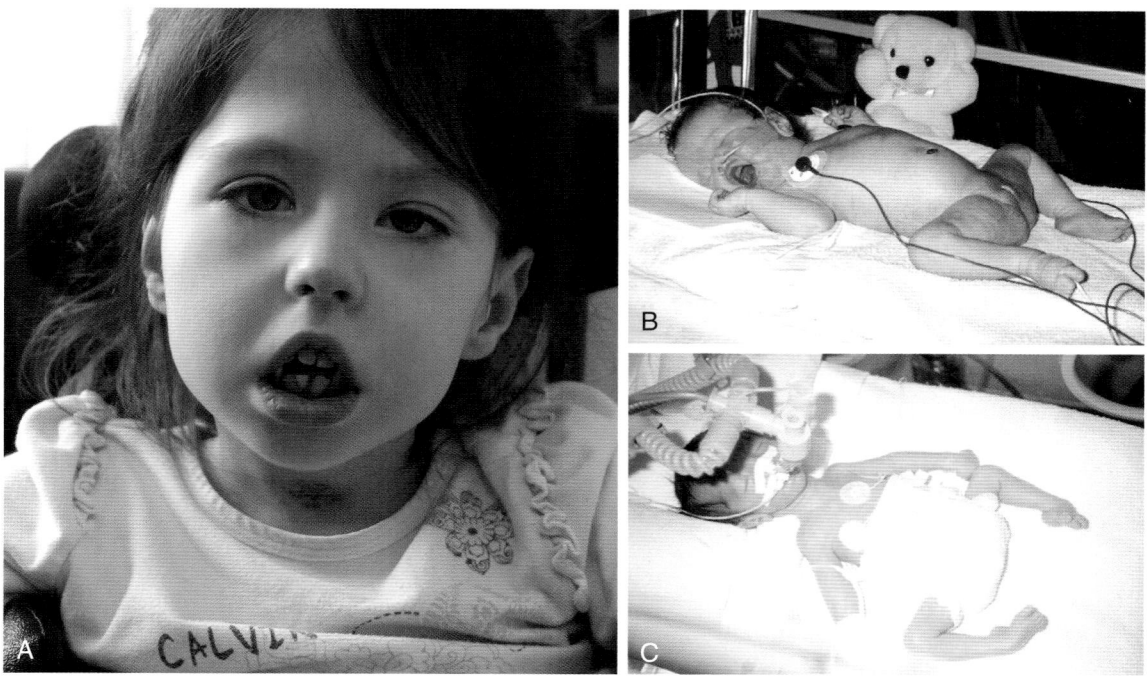

Fig. 35.24 *A,* A 6-year-old with congenital myotonic dystrophy with 1975 cytosine-thymine-guanine (CTG) repeats in the *DMPK* gene showing the characteristic elongated facies, left ptosis, and an open, down-turned (tented) mouth with dental malocclusion. The tracheostomy scar is evidence of the severe respiratory distress requiring intubation at time of birth. *B,* Neonate with congenital myotonic dystrophy also with an open, down-turned mouth and frog-leg position of lower extremities. *C,* A neonate with congenital myotonic dystrophy with severe respiratory distress and arthrogryposis. (*B,* From Johnston H. The floppy weak infant revisited. *Brain Dev.* 2003;25:155–158; *C,* from Echenne B, Bassez G. Congenital and infantile myotonic dystrophy. *Handb Clin Neurol.* 2013;113:1387–1393.)

TABLE 35.23 Clinical Features of Congenital Myotonic Dystrophy

Clinical Feature	% of Cases Exhibiting Feature
Hypotonia	100
Muscle atrophy	100
Transmission via mother	100
Intellectual disability in survivors	100
Facial diplegia	100
Feeding difficulties	92
Respiratory distress	88
Hyporeflexia or areflexia	87
Arthrogryposis	82
Polyhydramnios	80
Reduced fetal movements	68
Edema	54
Premature birth (<36 wk)	52
Elevated right hemidiaphragm	49
Neonatal mortality	41
Infant death in siblings	28

From Volpe JJ, ed. *Neurology of the Newborn.* 5th ed. Philadelphia: Saunders; 2008:802.

requiring invasive ventilation and losing the ability to ambulate as they age. In patients with LOPD, ERT stabilizes but does not improve motor and respiratory function.

Congenital myopathies. Congenital myopathies are genetically and clinically heterogeneous (Table 35.24). These myopathies have characteristic muscle biopsy findings that narrow the differential diagnosis and guide targeted genetic evaluation. Distinguishing features on muscle biopsy include the presence of cores, nemaline rods, central nuclei, or congenital fiber type disproportion (CFTD) (Fig. 35.26). Cores are areas devoid of oxidative enzyme activity, best seen on oxidative stains such as nicotinamide adenine dinucleotide or ATPase. Nemaline rods are red, purple, or blue inclusions best seen on Gomori trichrome stain and vary per fiber, by fiber type, and in their distribution within the myofiber. Centrally placed nuclei are usually large in relation to the myofiber, present in a disproportionate number of fibers, and may be centrally placed along the length of the fiber. CFTD refers to the relative atrophy of type 1 fibers by 35–40% compared to type 2 fibers in the absence of other structural changes such as rods, cores, and central nucleation.

Although onset of weakness is usually at birth, symptoms can develop at any age. A wide range of severity is possible for each subtype, even within the same family. If manifesting in infancy, patients have diffuse weakness, congenital hip dysplasia, and breathing and swallowing dysfunction, with delays in motor milestone development and variable levels of facial involvement. If manifesting in childhood or adolescence, then proximal muscle weakness with a Gower maneuver

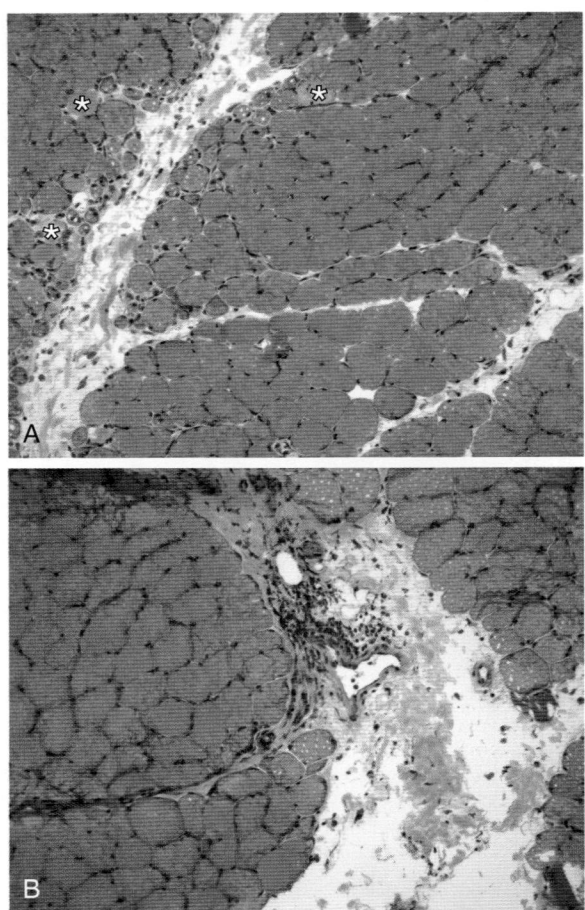

Fig. 35.25 Characteristic histopathologic findings on muscle biopsy in a 15-year-old female adolescent with juvenile dermatomyositis (JDM). *A,* Pathognomonic finding of perifascicular atrophy showing smaller regenerating (purple, basophilic) fibers along the edges of the center and left fascicles compared to the normal-appearing pink fibers in the center of the fascicles. Isolated pale staining necrotic fibers are seen *(asterisks). B,* Perivascular inflammation with many lymphocytes surrounding small vessels. (Images courtesy of Dr. Denise Malicki, University of California, San Diego, and Rady Children's Hospital.)

TABLE 35.24	**Specific Congenital Myopathies: Distinguishing Clinical Features**	
Subcategory	**Distinguishing Clinical Features**	**Associated Genes**
Central core disease	• Facial weakness mostly with *RYR1* • Ophthalmoparesis and ptosis with *RYR1* • High incidence of malignant hyperthermia with *RYR1* • Severe axial/respiratory weakness out of proportion to limb weakness with *SEPN1* • Prominent early fixed kyphoscoliosis with *RYR1* • Rigid spine in older childhood with *SEPN1* • High incidence of club feet, pes cavus, foot drop, and distal hand/foot muscle atrophy with *RYR1*	*RYR1, SEPN1, TTN, MYH7, CCDC78*
Nemaline myopathy	• Prominent facial weakness • Severe bulbar weakness, feeding difficulties, and respiratory compromise in neonatal period or early infancy in some	*ACTA1, NEB, TPM3, TPM2, TNNT1, CFL2, KBTBD13, KLHL40, KLHL41, LMOD3*
Centronuclear myopathy	• Prominent facial weakness • Prominent ophthalmoparesis and ptosis (in infancy) • Prominent bilateral ptosis • Severe bulbar weakness, feeding difficulties, and respiratory compromise in neonatal period or early infancy • Infant that is long for age with elongated hands/feet • High incidence of neonatal/infantile death with *MTM1* • High incidence of club feet, pes cavus, foot drop, and distal hand/foot muscle atrophy with *DMN2*	*MTM1* (causes myotubular myopathy), *DNM2, BIN1, RYR1*
Congenital fiber type disproportion	• Severe axial/respiratory weakness out of proportion to limb with *SEPN1* • Rigid spine in older childhood with *SEPN1*	*TPM3, RYR1, TPM2, SEPN1, ACTA1*

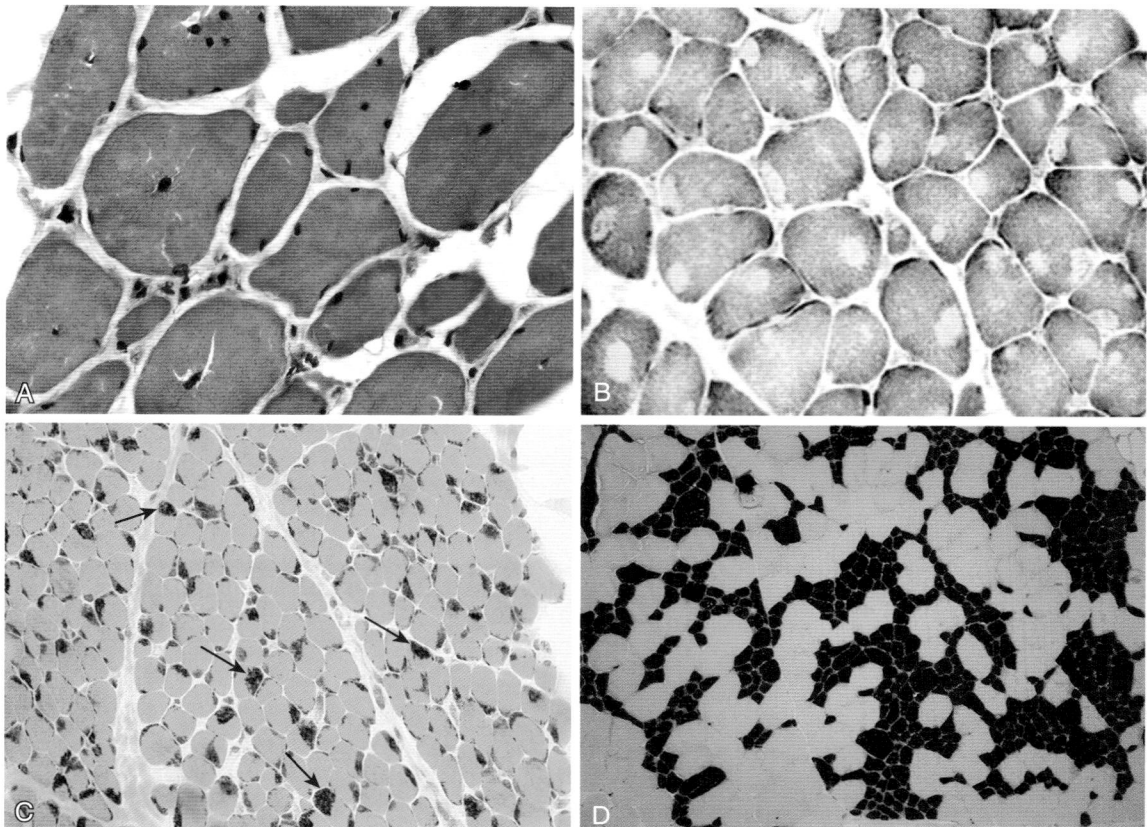

Fig. 35.26 Pathologic changes seen on muscle biopsy in congenital myopathies. Centronuclear myopathy is characterized by a centrally placed nucleus *(A)* seen in a disproportionate number of myofibers on the background of fiber size variability shown here on hematoxylin and eosin (H&E) staining. Core myopathy has well-demarcated centrally or eccentrically placed cores, best visualized on oxidative stains such as succinate dehydrogenase (SDH) *(B)*. Nemaline rods are purple-blue staining rods (few are labeled by *arrows*) best visualized on Gomori trichrome located in a subsarcolemmal position *(C)*. Congenital fiber-type disproportion showing small, dark-staining type 1 fibers (average diameter, 20–40 µm) on ATPase at pH 4.3 relative to the larger, pale-staining type 2 fibers (average diameter, 80–100 µm) *(D)*. *(A*, Courtesy Karra Jones, MD, PhD, University of California, San Diego, San Diego, CA; *B*, from North KN, Wang CH, Clarke N, et al. Approach to the diagnosis of congenital myopathies. *Neuromuscular Disord.* 2014;24:97–116, with permission; *C*, courtesy Michael Lawlor, MD, PhD, Medical College of Wisconsin, Milwaukee, WI; *D*, courtesy Chamindra Konersman, MD, Medical College of Wisconsin, Milwaukee, WI.)

and variable degrees of mobility, restrictive lung disease, scoliosis, rigid spine, thin body habitus, and pectus deformities are typical; intellect is normal. Nemaline rod myopathy has a distinctive facial weakness characteristic by elongated facies and an open mouth that is due to weakness of jaw closure muscles, a phenotype referred to as "myopathic" facies (Fig. 35.27). The centronuclear myopathies characteristically cause ptosis and ophthalmoparesis. One subtype, myotubular myopathy due to pathogenic variants in *MTM1*, is particularly severe, presenting in the neonate with difficulties swallowing and breathing, often requiring enteral feeding tube placement and mechanical ventilation in early infancy. Pathogenic variants in *RYR1* can lead to malignant hyperthermia with exposure to halothane-derived anesthetic agents.

Congenital muscular dystrophies. The congenital muscular dystrophies (CMDs) are another group of clinically and genetically heterogeneous disorders (Table 35.25). These disorders are also typically congenital onset, though symptoms may start later in life. CMDs have elevated CK levels with nonspecific dystrophic changes on muscle biopsy. Inheritance pattern is variable.

Weakness is typically proximal and axial more than appendicular and results in restrictive lung disease, rigid spine, contractures, and variable ability to ambulate. Some CMDs, such as *FKRP*-related CMD, can cause cardiomyopathy. Collagen VI–related dystrophies have characteristic early-onset contractures with skin findings; infantile-onset patients typically never achieve ambulation. *LAMA2*-related dystrophies also result in early-onset proximal contractures and white matter abnormalities on brain MRI. The dystroglycanopathies cause varying degrees of CNS involvement, ranging from severe intellectual disability due to lissencephaly to normal cognition. Salient features of CMDs are highlighted in Table 35.23. The phenotypic spectrum of CMDs are shown in Fig. 35.28.

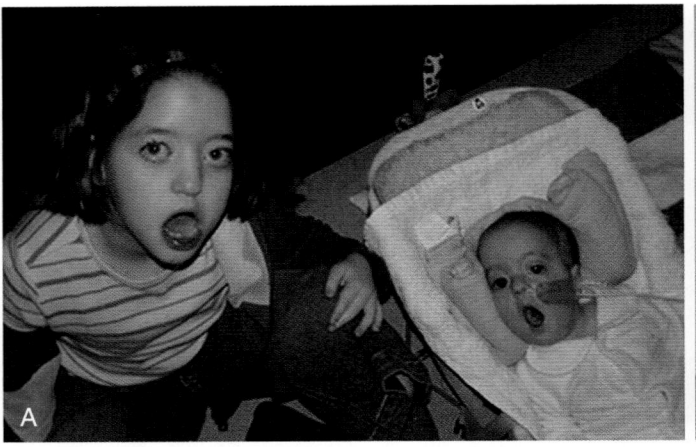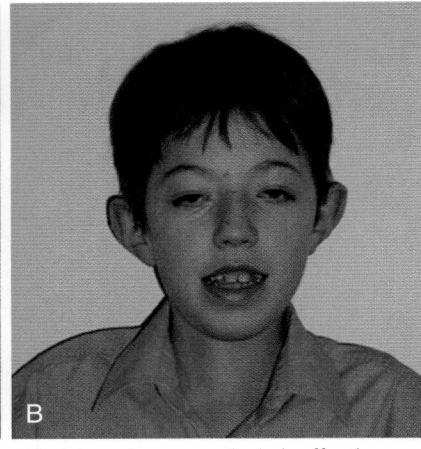

Fig. 35.27 Facial involvement in congenital myopathies. *A,* Pronounced facial weakness, particularly affecting the lower face and mouth resulting in craniofacial dysmorphism ("myopathic facies") in sisters aged 6 years and 3 months with autosomal recessive nemaline myopathy (likely due to nebulin). *B,* Ptosis and ophthalmoplegia in a patient with *DNM2*-related centronuclear myopathy at age 9 years. (From North KN, Wang CH, Clarke N, et al. Approach to the diagnosis of congenital myopathies. *Neuromusc Disord.* 2014;24[2]:97–116.)

TABLE 35.25	Specific Congenital Muscular Dystrophies: Distinguishing Clinical Features	
Subcategory	**Distinguishing Clinical Features**	**Associated Genes**
Collagen VI–related dystrophies	• Proximal muscle weakness in childhood • Severe hypotonia and diffuse weakness in infancy • Infantile onset typically never achieves ambulation • Early-onset proximal contractures diffusely • Distal joint hyperlaxity • Hyperkeratosis pilaris on skin (legs and arms) • Keloids • Atrophic, wide scars • Scoliosis (early) • Very thin body habitus • Severe restrictive lung disease early requiring bilevel ventilation • Normal intellect • CK usually elevated (100–several 1,000 U/L)	*COL6A1, COL6A2, COL6A3*
LAMA2-related dystrophies	• Proximal muscle weakness in childhood • Severe hypotonia and diffuse weakness in infancy • Infantile onset typically never achieves ambulation • Early-onset proximal contractures diffusely • Brain MRI demonstrates white matter disease (clinically not significant) • Some develop seizures • Very thin body habitus • Severe restrictive lung disease early requiring bilevel ventilation • Nerve conductions demonstrate slowing • Normal intellect • CK usually 1,000s	*LAMA2*
Dystroglycan-related disorders (dystroglycanopathies, previously known as muscle-eye-brain disease)	• Mild to severe proximal muscle weakness and hypotonia in infancy • Varying degrees of CNS involvement • Brain MRI may be abnormal—lissencephaly, pachygyria, cerebellar hypoplasia, or dysplasia • *FKRP* and *FKTN* may cause a cardiomyopathy, if late onset • Varying degree of eye involvement—severe myopia, retinal hypoplasia • Intellectual delay ranging from normal to severe disability	*POMT1, POMT2, POMGnT1, POMGnT2, FKTN, FKRP, LARGE, ISPD, GTDC2, B3GALNT2, B3GNT1, B4GAT1, TMEM5, POMK, DPM1, DPM2, DPM3, DOLK, GMPPB, RXYLT1,* and *DAG1*
Myofibrillar myopathy	• Distal and proximal muscle weakness developing in adolescence or early adulthood • Respiratory muscle weakness often necessitating noninvasive or invasive ventilatory support • Rigid spine • Possible sensory neuropathy	*BAG3, CRYAB, DES, FLNC, KY, LDB3, MYOT, PYROXD1*
Selenon-related myopathy	• Severe axial weakness • Early-onset scoliosis • Early-onset restrictive lung disease requiring bilevel noninvasive ventilation, prior to loss of ambulation (characteristic) • Normal intellect	*SEPN1*

TABLE 35.25 Specific Congenital Muscular Dystrophies: Distinguishing Clinical Features—cont'd

Subcategory	Distinguishing Clinical Features	Associated Genes
LMNA-related dystrophy	• Severe hypotonia and diffuse weakness in infancy • Proximal muscle weakness in childhood • Prominent head drop in infancy (dropped-head syndrome); may achieve ambulation despite head drop • At risk of cardiac arrhythmia • Early diffuse contractures • Severe restrictive lung disease requiring bilevel ventilation	*LMNA*

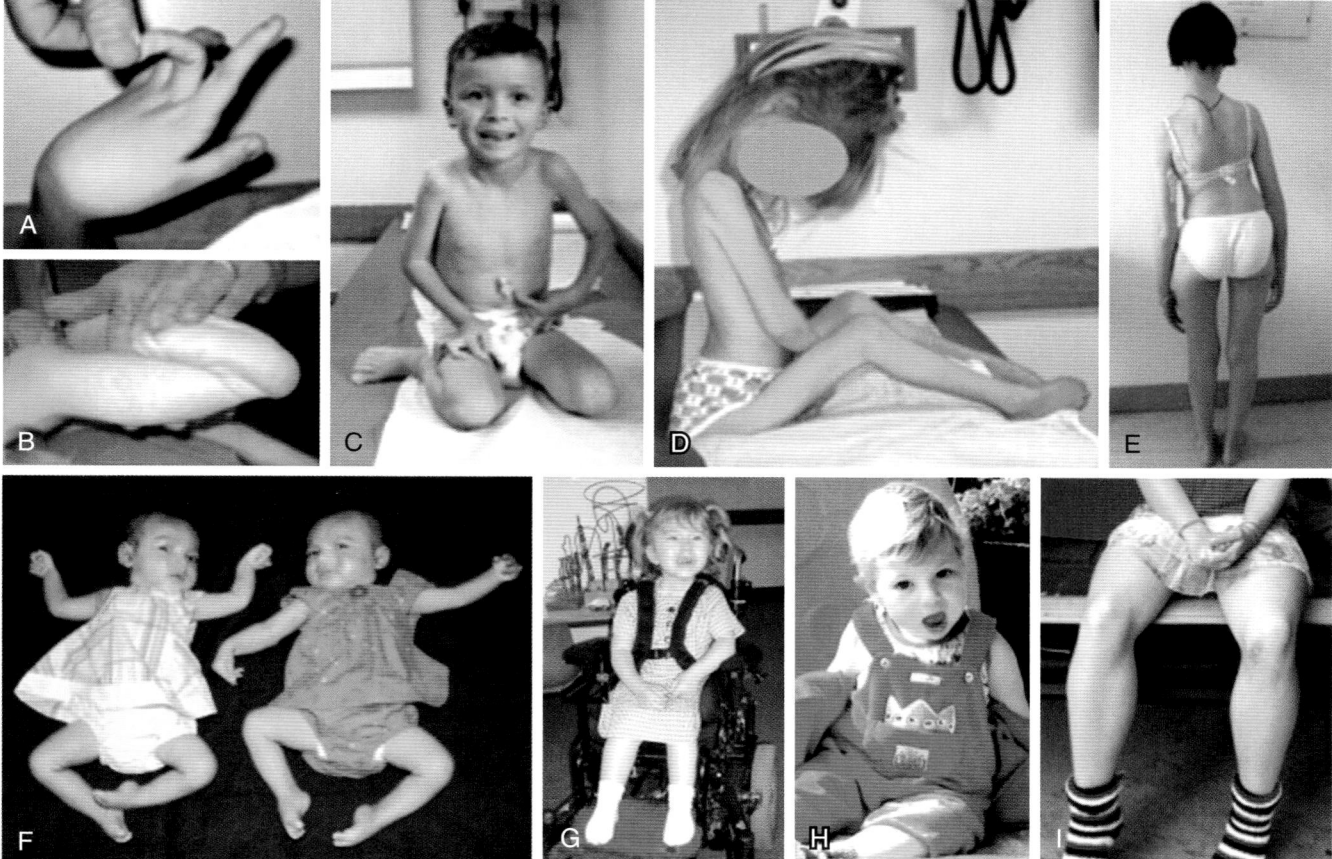

Fig. 35.28 Phenotypic spectrum of congenital muscular dystrophy. *A,* Hand of a patient with collagen VI–related dystrophy. Note the significant hyperlaxity even in the most distal interphalangeal joints. *B,* Foot of an infant with collagen VI–related dystrophy. Note the ability to dorsiflex the foot back to the shin, the soft palmar skin, the pes planus (loss of arch), and the prominent calcaneus. *C,* Patient with collagen VI–related dystrophy. Note flexible fingers and round face with facial erythema. He also has contractures in the elbows and knees. *D,* Patient with *LMNA*-related dystrophy. Note the dropped head, hyperlordosis, and adducted foot indicative of peroneal weakness, and overall thinness. *E,* Patient with selenon-related myopathy. Note atrophy of inner thigh muscles and lateral deviation of spine (status after surgical rod placement). *F,* Twins with *LAMA2*-related dystrophy. Note hypotonic posture with splayed legs ("frog-leg" posture), weak arms, flexed fingers, and foot contractures. *G,* Patient with *LAMA2*-related dystrophy. Note facial weakness and foot contracture. She has no antigravity strength in the upper extremity. *H,* Patient with dystroglycan-related dystrophy (*POMT1*). Note weak sitting posture and hypotonic lower face with open mouth characteristic of congenital myopathic disorders. *I,* Same patient with dystroglycan-related dystrophy (*POMT1*) at an older age. Note calf and quadriceps hypertrophy and mild forearm hypertrophy. (Modified from Bönnemann CG, Wang CH, Quijano-Roy S, et al. Diagnostic approach to the congenital muscular dystrophies. *Neuromuscul Disord.* 2014;24[4]:289–311.)

SUMMARY AND RED FLAGS

Hypotonia and weakness may be manifestations of lesions throughout the neuromuscular axis; the primary responsibility of the clinician is to determine from where along this axis low tone and weakness are originating. History can help differentiate congenital from acquired causes and suggest a mode of inheritance or route of exposure to an inciting trigger. Associated findings, such as seizures, encephalopathy, multisystem organ dysfunction, sensory levels, paresthesia, fatigability, and elevated CK, provide additional clues in localization. Once this initial evaluation has suggested or established a particular station along the neuromuscular axis, more in-depth investigations can provide definitive diagnosis. Major **red flags** include diffuse encephalopathy, seizures, metabolic crisis, and signs of respiratory weakness, though some patients may be too weak to manifest clinically apparent external signs of respiratory distress despite impending respiratory failure. Prompt identification of an etiology allows for initiation of appropriate supportive measures, prognostication, and, in some instances, introduction of targeted therapies.

BIBLIOGRAPHY

A bibliography is available at ExpertConsult.com.

36

Rhabdomyolysis

Matthew M. Harmelink

RHABDOMYOLYSIS

Rhabdomyolysis is an acute muscle injury resulting in myocyte cell death with subsequent release of toxic intracellular compounds producing muscle and systemic symptoms. This differs from **hyperCKemia,** in which there is elevated creatine kinase in the serum secondary to dysfunction of the myocyte sarcolemma. These diagnoses represent a broad category of disease processes with a large differential diagnosis. The difficulty lies in differentiating between the two processes given that the treatment of the former may include hospital admission while the latter often only requires supportive care.

Diagnosis

The surrogate biomarker for rhabdomyolysis, **creatine kinase (CK),** is a poor substitute because it is not possible to differentiate, based upon this value, between rhabdomyolysis and hyperCKemia. The generally accepted **definition of rhabdomyolysis** includes an elevation of CK either >1,000 IU/L or greater than five times the upper limit of normal in a clinical context of acute muscle weakness, myalgia, and muscle swelling (Fig. 36.1).

There are exceptions; focal rhabdomyolysis may result in lower CK levels with the same underlying pathologic processes. Additionally, levels above the limit of 1,000 I/U can be found in patients with acute denervating diseases, in patients with hyperCKemia from intense exercise, and in patients with non-muscle-related diseases. A diagnosis of rhabdomyolysis should not be considered in patients without acute clinical symptoms and acute CK changes from the baseline value. Levels over 5,000 I/U are rarely found in acute or chronic non-muscle-related diseases.

In addition to muscle damage and pain, toxins released into the circulation from the myocyte damage can lead to systemic problems including cardiac arrythmias, encephalopathy, and, most commonly, acute kidney injury.

HyperCKemia

HyperCKemia is diagnosed when the serum elevation of CK is beyond the upper limits for age, gender, race, and muscle mass but in the absence of associated symptoms. Given the sensitive CK fluctuations with exercise, the assessment of hyperCKemia needs to be taken into consideration with the patient's hydration status, previous activity, and timing from any possible inciting event. CK typically begins to increase 24 hours after the onset of a muscle injury or stress, peaks at around 24–36 hours, and, in a monophasic illness, starts to decline. The normal half-life of CK, in a patient without renal failure, is between 24 and 48 hours (Fig. 36.2).

Careful consideration of laboratory norms for CK is essential in interpreting elevated levels during an acute event because normal values correlate to overall muscle bulk, race, and gender. Additionally, frequent exercise in athletes can lead to persistently elevated CK (350–500 IU/L) during training. Obtaining a baseline CK level after a period of rest is required. *There is no risk of renal damage in hyperCKemia given that there is no myoglobin released into the circulation.*

Myoglobinuria

Myoglobinuria is the presence of elevated myoglobin levels in the urine. Myoglobin is a chemical compound that carries oxygen in the myocyte. Upon damage to the cell membrane, it can be released into the blood at higher levels than typically seen. When levels are >0.5–1.5 mg/L, it saturates the serum haptoglobin and α_2-immunoglobulin and the excess is filtered by the glomerulus. Myoglobin sequesters fluid, leading to hypovolemia and renal vasoconstriction. It can release the free iron, which may damage the renal tubules, or it may react directly with the lipid membrane of the kidney, resulting in damage to the proximal tubules.

While there are direct laboratory detection methods, the time to obtain results is not rapid enough to use this value to direct treatment; urine heme when not in the presence of red blood cells is frequently used as a surrogate marker to indicate myoglobinuria in the appropriate acute setting and when clinically suspected. *In this situation, the urine red blood cell (RBC) count should be checked to determine if the heme +++ results in myoglobin or hematuria.* Measuring myoglobin levels remains a valuable differentiator between rhabdomyolysis and hyperCKemia. Normal urine myoglobin levels are <10 mg/dL (and 100 mg/dL in blood); elevated levels indicate rhabdomyolysis.

The typical red- or tea-colored urine described in rhabdomyolysis is not always noted and requires a urine myoglobin concentration >100 mg/dL. In a patient who has been fluid resuscitated, the urinary dilution can mask both the visible and laboratory detection of myoglobinuria. It is important to collect samples during the acute phase of presentation or when fluids are weaned because the urine can then become positive.

Myositis

Myositis is an inflammatory process in the muscle not related to underlying chronic apoptotic muscle disease. In patients with myositis, there is an underlying immune or rheumatologic process resulting in inflammatory cells causing muscle damage, which involves the myocyte membrane. This is in contrast with primary (genetic) muscle diseases in which there can be signs of inflammation secondary to the apoptotic process of cell death. In some cases, such as dysferlinopathies, these can be mistaken for an inflammatory myopathy on the biopsy. However, in isolated myositis, there is not the same release of other biomarkers from the myocytes into the serum as seen in acute rhabdomyolysis. Additionally, other than infectious myositis, most of these disease processes are subacute to chronic in nature with only rare presentations as acute rhabdomyolysis.

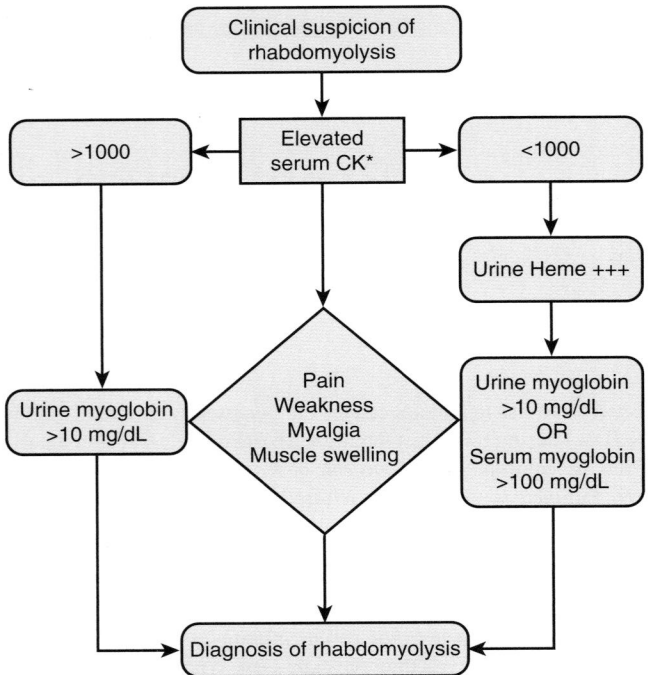

Fig. 36.1 Simplified diagnostic algorithm for rhabdomyolysis. *Some definitions of rhabdomyolysis include CK >5x the normal range for the lab.

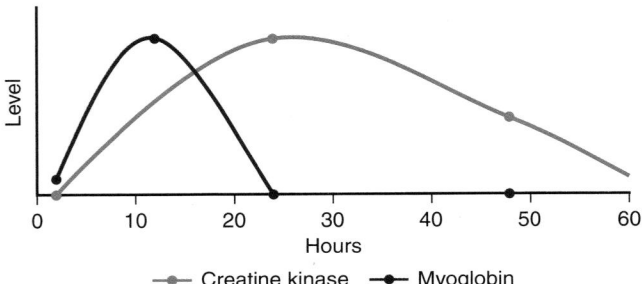

Fig. 36.2 Timing of myoglobin and creatine kinase elevations.

Clinical Presentation

History

The first part of the history of a patient with possible rhabdomyolysis is the history of the acute episode, while the second part is to evaluate for an underlying etiology. The acute history will help differentiate the potential for rhabdomyolysis from other causes of pain and weakness (Table 36.1); once diagnosed, the etiology of the rhabdomyolysis needs to be evaluated.

A child with rhabdomyolysis may present with a variety of symptoms. Most patients present with muscle pain. The remaining 20% do not present with overt signs of muscle disease. Dark urine (myoglobinuria) may be reported in ~5% of patients; an even smaller number develop acute renal failure.

Patients with focal muscle swelling may develop a **compartment syndrome** resulting in local neurovascular features and may develop more systemic disease such as acute kidney injury or encephalopathy with associated seizures, somnolence, and/or other cognitive changes. Cardiac arrythmias may also be present.

Given the half-life and timing of the typical peak for both myoglobin and CK, the timing of the disease onset is important. Patients presenting early in their course may not have an elevation of their CK, whereas patients who have milder symptoms or do not present during

the acute episode may have normal or near-normal lab results. Symptoms of previous episodes for which the patient did not seek clinical care can suggest an underlying etiology; any signs of possible muscle disease including features of muscle dysfunction (weakness, cramps, pain) at baseline as well as during different types of activity (anaerobic vs aerobic and concentric vs eccentric exercise) as well as family history and inciting events or risk factors can be helpful in differentiating these diseases (Fig. 36.3).

Because of the phenotypic variation between some of the underlying genetic disorders that can predispose a patient to rhabdomyolysis, evaluation for diagnostic or subtle symptoms should be considered (Table 36.2; see Fig. 36.3).

Physical Examination

The physical examination must assess and track the degree of muscle injury, evaluate for signs of an underlying etiology, and diagnose secondary complications of rhabdomyolysis. An in-depth neuromuscular exam is warranted with objective tracking of manual muscle testing (MMT)-scored muscle strength (Table 36.3). This helps localize the injury but also assesses for pain-limited features as compared to true muscle weakness. Sequential tracking of muscle symptoms helps determine the disease progression and should be a guiding tool for treatment and hospital discharge.

Acutely in rhabdomyolysis, muscle weakness should not be used to determine an etiologic diagnosis because the ability to differentiate between *baseline* weakness and *current* symptoms can be difficult; historical features are often more helpful. Examples of functional questions to ask can be the ability to go up and down stairs (which have different predominant muscle groups), the ability to be active in sporting activities, and any previous history of muscle cramping, aches, or signs of myalgias. Atrophy or pseudohypertrophy, which suggests a chronic process, can be helpful during the acute phase to evaluate for underlying causes.

Diagnostic Evaluation

Patients are typically diagnosed with rhabdomyolysis based upon serum CK, which is used as a marker for muscle breakdown (see Fig. 36.1). However, very focal rhabdomyolysis can result in CK levels that are not as elevated.

A two-tiered acute approach for patients with possible rhabdomyolysis is recommended given that most pediatric patients have either exertional or infectious etiologies (Tables 36.4 and 36.5). This allows a thoughtful approach to the patient in which etiologic studies may not change management. There is no strong evidence for biochemical or gene sequencing in a patient with a first episode of rhabdomyolysis and no family history of muscle disease.

Muscle Biopsy

While histopathology can be diagnostic of a known (often genetic or immunologic) etiology, the yield of a biopsy *during* an acute episode is very low. This is because the acutely damaged muscle has a similar end-stage appearance due to the diffuse injury, which often masks the more subtle features of the underlying cause. In almost all cases, a muscle biopsy, if needed, should be deferred for at least 3 months after the resolution of the last acute episode to ensure the highest yield.

The muscles selected should be those known to be affected, ideally with a manual muscle strength score between 3–4+ out of 5, and not those with diffuse atrophy. The most common muscle studies are the hamstring muscles, or the vastus lateralis, followed occasionally by the biceps and gastrocnemius. Genetic testing and biochemical analysis are frequently pursued prior to obtaining a muscle sample because they are less invasive and less expensive.

TABLE 36.1 Differential Causes of Acute Muscle Weakness and Pain

Disease	Typical Weakness Pattern	Pain Pattern	Other Symptoms
Rhabdomyolysis	Diffuse or muscles used with exertion, often larger muscles are preferred	Same as muscle pain	Dark or red urine Elevated CK
Guillain-Barré syndrome	Ascending weakness	Neuropathic pain (typically distal)	May have areflexia, autonomic symptoms
Myasthenia gravis	Proximal weakness with/without ocular or bulbar symptoms, often fatigable	No pain	Pupillary-sparing fatigable weakness
Botulism	Descending weakness that involves pupils	No pain	Often GI symptoms
Myalgia	In area of pain	Often muscle or joint pains, large muscles preferred	Often in association with other disease, CK is often normal
Psychogenic	May have non-neurologic pattern of weakness, weakness that varies based upon how it is examined, give-way weakness	Pain and weakness are not always congruent in a physiologic distribution	May have other features of a psychogenic illness Normal CK during an acute episode is not rhabdomyolysis
Nonrheumatologic connective tissue disease (e.g., Ehlers-Danlos syndrome)	Often no overt weakness	Pain is often after activity but more joint related than muscle	Normal CK during an acute episode May have a history of fatigue with endurance activity but normal strength

CK, creatine kinase; GI, gastrointestinal.

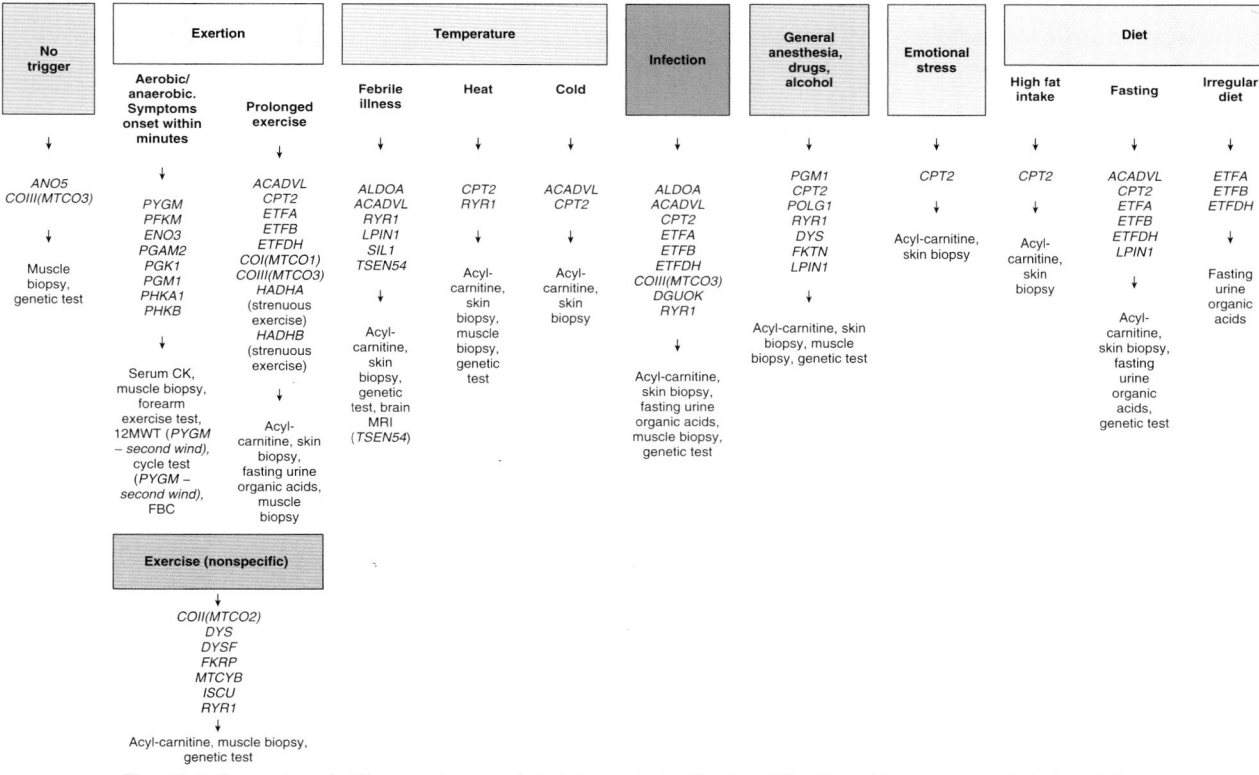

Fig. 36.3 Examples of different triggers of rhabdomyolysis. The identification of triggers may help in guiding genetic testing and may also aid in the interpretation of variants of uncertain significance identified on next-generation sequencing in patients presenting with RM. 12MWT, 12-minute walk test; CK, creatine kinase; FBC, full blood count. (From Scalco RS, Gardiner AR, Pitceathly RDS, et al. Rhabdomyolysis: a genetic perspective. *Orphanet J Rare Dis.* 2015;10:51, Fig. 2.)

TABLE 36.2 Genetic Disorders Associated with Rhabdomyolysis

Gene	OMIM	Cytogenetic Location	Inheritance	Disorder
Muscle Structure and Function				
ATP2A1	601003	16p11.2	AR	Brody myopathy
DMD	300376	Xp21.2	XLR	Dystrophin-associated muscular dystrophy: Becker type
AMPD1	600467	1p13.2	AR	Myopathy due to myoadenylate deaminase deficiency
SCN4A	168300	17q23.3	AD	Paramyotonia congenita
ISCU	255125	12q23.3	AR	Myopathy with lactic acidosis
CAV3	123320	3p25.3	AD	Familial hyperCKemia
CASQ1	114250	1q23.2	AD	Myopathy, vacuolar, with CASQ1 aggregates
Mitochondria/Energy Metabolism				
HADHA HADHB	600467	2p23.3	AR	Mitochondrial trifunctional protein deficiency (MTPD)
MCKAT	602199	Not known	AR	Mitochondrial medium-chain 3-ketoacyl-coenzyme A thiolase (MCKAT) deficiency
CPT2	600467	1p32.3	AR	CPT II deficiency, myopathic, stress induced
ACADVL	600467	17p13.1	AR	VLCAD deficiency
PYGM	600467	11q13.1	AR	McArdle disease, or glycogen storage disease type V (GSD5)
PGAM2	261670	7p13	AR	Glycogen storage disease type X
LDHA	612933	11p15.1	AR	Glycogen storage disease type XI
ALDOA	611881	16p11.2	AR	Glycogen storage disease type XII
SLC25A20	212138	3p21.31	AR	Carnitine-acylcarnitine translocase deficiency
POLG	600467	15q26.1	AD	Autosomal dominant progressive external ophthalmoplegia (adPEO) with mitochondrial DNA (mtDNA) deletions-1 (PEOA1) is caused by variants in the nuclear-encoded DNA polymerase-gamma gene
DGUOK	617070	2p13.1	AR	Progressive external ophthalmoplegia with mitochondrial DNA deletions, autosomal recessive 4
MRM2	600467	7p22.3	AR	Mitochondrial DNA depletion syndrome 17
ATP5F1D	618120	19p13.3	AR	Mitochondrial complex V (ATP synthase) deficiency
FDX2	600467	19p13.2	AR	Mitochondrial myopathy with or without optic atrophy and reversible leukoencephalopathy (MEOAL)
MRPS14	618378	1q25.1	AR	Combined oxidative phosphorylation deficiency 38
TSFM	600467	12q14.1	AR	Combined oxidative phosphorylation deficiency-3 (COXPD3)
Metabolic				
SLC25A42	600467	19p13.11	AR	Metabolic crises with variable encephalomyopathic features and neurologic regression (MECREN)
PGK1	600467	Xq21.1	XLR	Phosphoglycerate kinase-1 deficiency
Other				
CACNA1S MHS4 MHS6 MHS3 MHS2 RYR1	600467 601887 610888 154276 154275 145600	1q32.1 3q13.1 5p 7q21 17q11.2 19q13.2	AD	Malignant hyperthermia susceptibility (multiple types including King-Denborough syndrome)
CACNA1S	188580	1q32.1	AD	Thyrotoxic periodic paralysis associated with malignant hyperthermia allele
CTDP1	600467	18q23	AR	Congenital cataracts, facial dysmorphism, and neuropathy
PGM1	600467	1p31.3	AR	Congenital disorder of glycosylation, type It (CDG1T)
XK	300842	Xp21.1	XL	McLeod syndrome with or without chronic granulomatous disease
CYP2C8	601129	10q23.33	Risk allele	Statin-induced rhabdomyolysis cytochrome P450-drug metabolism, altered, CYP2C8-related
TRAPPC2L	618331	16q24.3	AR	Progressive encephalopathy with episodic rhabdomyolysis (PEERB)
TANGO2	616878	22q11.21	AR	Metabolic encephalomyopathic crises, recurrent, with rhabdomyolysis, cardiac arrhythmias, and neurodegeneration (MECRCN)
SLC16A1	245340	1p13.2	AD	Erythrocyte lactate transporter defect
QARS1	615760	3p21.31	AR	Microcephaly, progressive, seizures, and cerebral and cerebellar atrophy (MSCCA)
LPIN1	268200	2p25.1	AR	Myoglobinuria, acute recurrent, autosomal recessive
HRAS	218040	11p15.5	AD	Costello syndrome/congenital myopathy with excess of muscle spindles
SIL1	248800	5q31.2	AR	Marinesco-Sjögren syndrome

AD, autosomal dominant; AR, autosomal recessive; ATP, adenosine triphosphate; CPT II, carnitine palmitoyl transferase II; VLCAD, very long-chain acyl-CoA dehydrogenase; XLR, X-linked recessive.

TABLE 36.3   Manual Muscle Testing Grading

	Kendall and Kendall	AMA Impairment Rating Guide
Grade 0	No muscle contraction	No muscle contraction
Grade 1	Muscle contraction palpable or seen, but no motion	Muscle contraction palpable or seen, but no motion
Grade 2	Motion of the part with gravity reduced	Motion of the part with gravity reduced
Grade 3	Muscle can hold the part in test position against the resistance of gravity but cannot hold if even slight pressure is added	Muscle can hold the part in the test position against gravity alone
Grade 4	Muscle holds test position against some pressure but breaks away	Patient can move the part through the full active range of motion against some resistance
Grade 5	Muscle holds test position against full pressure	Patient can move the part through the full active range of motion against full resistance

AMA, American Medical Association.
Adapted from Conable KM, Rosner AL. A narrative review of manual muscle testing and implications for muscle testing research. *J Chiropr Med.* 2011;10(3):157–165.

TABLE 36.4   Initial Studies for During Active Episode of Presumed Rhabdomyolysis

First Tier	Second Tier
CBC	Infectious evaluation
CMP	ECG if indicated by electrolytes
CK	Metabolic studies (described in text) if suspected disease on initial presentation
UA, micro and macro	
Urine drug screen	

CK, creatine kinase; CMP, comprehensive metabolic panel.

Treatment

During an acute episode of rhabdomyolysis, the mainstay of treatment is use of sufficient fluids to help diurese the serum electrolytes, chemicals, and toxins. In theory, by ensuring excretion of these chemicals, the nonmuscle complications can be avoided. In adults, the recommendations are to give a fluid bolus followed by starting the patient on 1.5–2 times greater than maintenance fluids. No evidence-based guidelines exist for children; some recommend the titrating of fluids to maintain a urine output 3–4 times normal, or 3–4 mL/kg/hour in a child. Another method is to titrate the fluids to maintain a physiologic creatine kinase half-life, which, in theory, would ensure an appropriate urine output. This method addresses the patient's physiology (Fig. 36.4).

Before discharge the patient must demonstrate appropriate oral intake with continued CK clearance and no myoglobin in the urine. Patients must also have improved and tolerable symptoms but are not expected to have fully resolved their pain or mild weakness. Nonetheless, with underlying myocyte injury, mild pain, weakness, and some limited endurance are expected to last for weeks to months after resolution of the acute event.

Renal Injury Risk

A serious complication of rhabdomyolysis is the potential risk for renal injury. Fortunately, the risk remains relatively low (~5–10% in children). While some evidence suggests that patients with rhabdomyolysis and a CK <5,000 IU/dL are at lower risk of renal involvement, this may reflect patients with hyperCKemia and not rhabdomyolysis. In one study, no patients with initial urinary heme (myoglobin) dipstick results of <2+ developed acute renal failure, compared with ~18% of patients with urinary heme (myoglobin) dipstick results of ≥2+. The

TABLE 36.5   Infectious Causes of Rhabdomyolysis

Viruses
Influenza A or B
Cytomegalovirus
Epstein-Barr virus
HIV: acute retroviral syndrome
Human herpesvirus 6
Respiratory syncytial virus
Coxsackieviruses
Enterovirus
Adenovirus
Echovirus
Cytomegalovirus
Herpes simplex virus
Varicella-zoster virus
West Nile virus
Dengue virus

Bacteria
Group A β-hemolytic streptococci
Legionella species
Salmonella
Salmonella species
Francisella species
Streptococcus pneumoniae
Staphylococcus aureus
Enterococcus
Pseudomonas aeruginosa
Neisseria meningitidis
Haemophilus influenzae
Coxiella burnetii
Leptospira species
Mycoplasma species
Escherichia coli
Rocky Mountain spotted fever

Other
Malaria
Fungal infections
Anaplasmosis
Trichinosis

General Management Guidelines for Pediatric Inpatient Rhabdomyolysis Without Renal Complications

1. **Patient presents clinically with rhabdomyolysis signs and symptoms**
   a. Collect: Basic metabolic panel, creatine kinase, urinalysis
2. **Initiate fluids**
   a. Initiate IV fluids (NS) at rate of 1.5x maintenance
      OR
   b. If there is concern or known metabolic disease, start D10 NS at 1.5x maintenance or as per genetics/metabolic rescue plan based upon glucose infusion rate.
3. **Initial lab evaluation**
   a. Basic metabolic panel
      i. POSITIVE by RIFLE criteria → patient is developing ARF → not eligible for protocol
      ii. NEGATIVE by RIFLE criteria → patient not in renal failure. Repeat Q12.
   b. Urinalysis
      i. POSITIVE myoglobin: Repeat UA Q12 until negative for myoglobin.
      ii. NEGATIVE myoglobin: Do not draw any more UAs. Continue on 1.5x MIVF as above, and monitor CK values per below.
   c. Creatine kinase
      i. POSITIVE: Repeat Q12 hours
      ii. NEGATIVE: Patient is not in rhabdomyolysis, discontinue protocol.
4. **Q12 lab evaluation**
   a. Basic metabolic panel: Repeat as in step 3
   b. Urinalysis: Repeat as in step 3
   c. Creatine kinase
      i. If $T_{1/2}$ <36 hours, decrease IV plus PO fluid rate by 0.5x. Continue to repeat Q12 until patient achieves discharge criteria (as noted in step 5)
      ii. If $T_{1/2}$ >36 hours, increase IV plus PO fluid rate by 0.5x. Continue to repeat Q12 until patient achieves discharge criteria (as noted in step 5)
5. **Eligibility for discharge; repeat step 4 until:**
   a. Patient maintains 1x maintenance fluids orally
   b. CK $T_{1/2}$ is <24 hours
   c. Urinalysis is negative for myoglobin
   d. Patient exhibits little to no signs or symptoms of clinical rhabdomyolysis.

Fig. 36.4 Treatment algorithm for patients with rhabdomyolysis. ARF, acute renal failure; CK, creatine kinase; IV, intravenous; MIVF, maintenance intravenous fluids; NS, normal saline; PO, by mouth; RIFLE, risk, injury, failure, loss of kidney function, and end-stage kidney disease; $T_{1/2}$, half-life.

degree of elevation of the CK does not accurately correlate with the risk of rhabdomyolysis in pediatric patients.

Compartment Syndrome

Compartment syndrome is another serious complication because the swelling can result in vascular and neurologic compression and secondary ischemic injury. Frequent evaluations of distal perfusion and peripheral neurologic findings are warranted until the patient is convalescing. Neurovascular evaluations of the distal extremities are warranted every 2–4 hours during the early phases of injury. Signs of compartment syndrome include pain out of proportion to the examination as well as that induced by manual passive limb movement. Consultation with an orthopedic or general surgeon is warranted to help evaluate the need for a fasciotomy to relieve the pressure.

HOSPITAL FOLLOW-UP

Following discharge, follow-up is recommended for all patients with rhabdomyolysis. For those patients who have an identified etiology, follow-up with their specialist is warranted to help with recovery as well as direct any possible activity level and/or treatment changes.

For patients without a known diagnosis, referral to a neuromuscular specialist or neurologist with an interest and expertise in muscle diseases is warranted. Even though the most common cause of rhabdomyolysis is exertional or infectious, exercise or periods of high energy demand as seen in infection can also induce a patient with an underlying disease to have rhabdomyolysis (see Fig. 36.3). If there is concern for an underlying genetic or metabolic disorder, referral to a geneticist can be helpful to further direct additional genetic and/or metabolic studies. This type of testing would not typically be undertaken during an acute episode of rhabdomyolysis unless a suspicious history is presented and clear etiology is suspected. Obtaining a baseline CK is warranted in every patient 2–3 months after discharge when they have had 48 hours of no exercise (to prevent minimal elevations from activity) to help differentiate between diseases in patients warranting further evaluation or to help screen for muscular dystrophies.

DISEASES

There are many genetic and acquired causes of rhabdomyolysis. Additionally, there are potentially genetic polymorphisms that could predispose certain patients to developing rhabdomyolysis but not significant enough to be defined as a current disease. This is important for those patients with recurrent episodes but no clear genetic cause (see Table 36.2).

Exercise-Induced

Exercise is often the inciting event that causes rhabdomyolysis for patients over the age of 2 years. The type of exercise is often important: prolonged aerobic vs strenuous anaerobic (see Fig. 36.3).

History

In exercise-induced rhabdomyolysis, there is typically a monophasic episode of rhabdomyolysis with a preceding history of a rapid increase in the level of physical activity from the normal baseline. The presence of red or dark urine a few hours following the activity in association with muscle soreness, localized swelling, and pain, which may last several days, is typical. It is not uncommon to discover a history of similar episodes prior to this presentation without seeking care. In the recurrent episodes, concern should be raised for an underlying etiology and additional testing will be guided by the history and physical findings (see Fig. 36.3, Tables 36.2 and 36.6).

Physical Examination

The physical examination may establish a possible underlying etiology as well as assess for emergent complications such as compartment syndrome. The evaluation of strength may be limited by pain and weakness from the muscle damage in the acute setting, and thus the exam should be used to evaluate for possible chronic changes, monitor for progression of the disease process, and ensure there are no systemic or neurovascular complications. In cases where the injury was induced by intense focal activity, such as weight lifting, the areas of involvement may be isolated.

The presence of atrophy, pseudohypertrophy, dysmorphic features, and/or unusual weakness (such as scapular winging, which would be unusual in rhabdomyolysis) suggests an underlying disease.

TABLE 36.6 Inherited Neuromuscular Disorders Associated with Episodes of Rhabdomyolysis*

Gene	Disease Name	Baseline Creatine Kinase Levels	Pattern of Inheritance	Trigger for Rhabdomyolysis
Disorders of Glycogen Metabolism				
PYGM	Glycogen storage disease type V, McArdle disease	High	AR	Aerobic and anaerobic exercise, symptom onset within minutes
PFKM	Glycogen storage disease type VII, Tarui disease	High	AR	Aerobic and anaerobic exercise, symptom onset within minutes
ALDOA	Glycogen storage disease type XII	Normal Mild elevation, high	AR	Febrile illness, infection
ENO3	Glycogen storage disease type XIII	Normal High	AR	Aerobic and anaerobic exercise, symptom onset within minutes
PGAM2	Glycogen storage disease type X	High	AR	Aerobic and anaerobic exercise, symptom onset within minutes
PGK1	Phosphoglycerate kinase 1 deficiency	Normal High	X-linked	Aerobic and anaerobic exercise, symptom onset within minutes
PGM1	Glycogen storage disease type XIV	High	AR	Aerobic and anaerobic exercise, symptom onset within minutes, general anesthesia
PHKA1 PHKB	Glycogen storage disease type IX	?	X-linked AR	Aerobic and anaerobic exercise, symptom onset within minutes
Disorders of Fatty Acid Metabolism				
ACADVL	Deficiency of very long-chain acyl-CoA dehydrogenase	Normal High	AR	Fasting, prolonged exercise, cold, infections, fever
CPT2	Carnitine palmitoyl-transferase deficiency	Normal	AR	Prolonged exercise, fasting, fever, infection, high fat intake, cold exposure, heat, emotional stress, drugs
ETFA ETFB ETFDH	Glutaric aciduria type II Multiple acyl-coenzyme A dehydrogenase deficiency	Normal Mildly to moderately elevated	AR	Physical exercise, fasting, irregular diet or infection
Mitochondrial Disorders				
COI (MTCO1)	Mitochondrial disorder	Normal	Maternal inheritance	Prolonged or repetitive exercise
COII (MTCO2)	Mitochondrial disorder	Normal	Maternal inheritance	Exercise
COIII (MTCO3)	Mitochondrial disorder	Normal	Maternal inheritance	Prolonged exercise, viral illness, unknown cause
DGUOK	Mitochondrial disorder	?	AR	Viral illness
FDX1L	Mitochondrial disorder	Normal High	AR	?After exercise
HADHA HADHB	Mitochondrial trifunctional protein deficiency	Normal	AR	Strenuous physical activity
ISCU	Iron–sulfur cluster deficiency myopathy (mitochondrial disorder)	?	AR	Exercise
MTCYB	Mitochondrial disorder	Normal	?Sporadic pathogenic variants	Exercise
POLG1	One case report of rhabdomyolysis in association with propofol infusion syndrome		AD, AR	Propofol infusion syndrome
Disorders of Intramuscular Calcium Release and Excitation–Contraction Coupling				
RYR1	Malignant hyperthermia susceptibility, exertional rhabdomyolysis, congenital myopathy	Normal or mildly to moderately elevated (usually <1,000 IU/L)	AD, AR	Heat, infection, alcohol, drugs, anesthetic (malignant hyperthermia susceptibility), and exercise
Muscular Dystrophies				
ANO5	Anoctaminopathy-5	High	AR	Unprovoked; no trigger has been identified
DMD	Duchenne muscular dystrophy, Becker muscular dystrophy	High	X-linked	Exercise, anesthetic drugs
DYSF	Limb-girdle muscular dystrophy 2B, Miyoshi myopathy	High	AR	Exercise

Continued

TABLE 36.6   Inherited Neuromuscular Disorders Associated with Episodes of Rhabdomyolysis—cont'd

Gene	Disease Name	Baseline Creatine Kinase Levels	Pattern of Inheritance	Trigger for Rhabdomyolysis
FKTN	Fukuyama congenital muscular dystrophy	High	AR	One case following the use of halothane and succinylcholine
FKRP	Limb-girdle muscular dystrophy 2I	High	AR	Exercise
Miscellaneous				
LPIN1	Phosphatidic acid phosphatase deficiency	Normal, high	AR	Febrile illness, anesthesia, and fasting
SIL1	Marinesco-Sjögren syndrome	Normal, high	AR	Febrile infection
TSEN54	Pontocerebellar hypoplasia type 2	Normal, high	AR	Hyperthermia
TANGO2	Encephalocardiomyopathy	High	AR	Encephalocardiomyopathy crisis

*The table summarizes genes, disease names, baseline serum creatine kinase levels (between acute episodes of rhabdomyolysis), patterns of inheritance, and triggers for rhabdomyolysis. Genes commonly associated with rhabdomyolysis episodes are indicated in bold.
AD, autosomal dominant; AR, autosomal recessive.
From Scalco RS, Gardiner AR, Pitceathly RDS, et al. Rhabdomyolysis: a genetic perspective. *Orphanet J Rare Dis.* 2015;10:51, Table 1.

Diagnostic Evaluation

Once a diagnosis of rhabdomyolysis is established (see Fig. 36.1 and Table 36.4), further evaluation is assessed based on individual clinical findings. For all patients with a clear history of a single episode of isolated exertional rhabdomyolysis, no additional evaluation is recommended. For those with recurrent exertional rhabdomyolysis, the evaluation should be directed for an underlying disease (see Table 36.6 and Fig. 36.3). A baseline CK is warranted, but if no other concerning features exist, further evaluation is not warranted following an isolated event.

Treatment

After the acute episode, it is important to develop an appropriate exercise program. Initially, for 3–4 weeks, strenuous exercise is not recommended because the myofibers remain damaged. However, a slow return to activity, after resolution of any soreness or weakness on exam, can help the child recover.

Hospital Follow-Up

For patients who are following up from presumed exercise-induced rhabdomyolysis, a repeat history of signs and symptoms of an underlying cause is warranted. Additionally, reviewing their baseline CK is important because elevations in CK would prompt the clinician to look for another cause.

INFECTIOUS

Infection is the most common cause of rhabdomyolysis in children under the age of 2 years. While there are a large variety of infections, viral infections, particularly influenza and enteroviruses, are the most common etiologies (see Table 36.5). Any infection producing shock or hypoxia may also be associated with high CK levels.

In infectious rhabdomyolysis, the patient often presents with other symptoms indicative of their disease (fever, myalgias, rash). In some patients with infections and myalgias, consideration of obtaining a CK is warranted. However, for patients in the ambulatory setting who are not limited in their activities, in whom the myalgias are mild, and who have no urine color changes, given the low risk of rhabdomyolysis, this may not be necessary. Viral myositis does not always lead to rhabdomyolysis. Although there is direct virus infection in the muscle for an otherwise healthy patient, the CK level is not as high as in rhabdomyolysis, and myoglobinuria is not expected.

In rare cases, there have been reports of asymptomatic patients who present with rhabdomyolysis with no infectious symptoms. This is an issue in the COVID-19 pandemic where asymptomatic but infected patients are common, thus making the rhabdomyolysis more likely an association than causative.

Viral rhabdomyolysis may have a longer time to convalescence than other monophasic causes (e.g., exercise-induced rhabdomyolysis) given that the infection's duration is greater than that of an exertional trigger. However, treatment remains the same with the goal to avoid renal complications by increasing excretion of the by-products.

TRAUMA

Traumatic rhabdomyolysis includes crush, blast, or electrical injuries, ischemia, and/or prolonged immobility.

There should be a documented history of trauma and/or prolonged immobility. Crush injuries are more likely to be a cause of rhabdomyolysis than other injuries; the injury may be focal rather than a more diffuse process.

DRUG/TOXIN

History

Drug-induced rhabdomyolysis can present in a variety of manners. In the setting of recreational drug use, other signs of drug use can be clues. However, the list of potential causes is extensive, and each may have other associated symptoms (*toxidromes*) (Table 36.7). Opiates, drugs with sympathomimetic properties, and drugs associated with intense (raving) exertion are among the common agents producing rhabdomyolysis.

Evaluation of drug ingestions, intentional or not, and prescription medications or over-the-counter remedies as well as herbal supplements or toxins is warranted for any patient with rhabdomyolysis (Tables 36.7 and 36.8).

Diagnostic Evaluation

For patients presenting without an identifiable etiology for rhabdomyolysis, a drug screen is warranted.

TABLE 36.7 Drugs with Known Associations with Rhabdomyolysis

Recreational/Misused Drugs	Others
Cocaine	Amiodarone
Heroin	Arsenic trioxide
Ethanol	Emetine
Amphetamines	ε-Aminocaproic acid (Amicar)
LSD	Lamotrigine
Phencyclidine	Nicotinic acid
Mushrooms	Vasopressin (from ischemia)
Ecstasy	Zidovudine
	Hemlock
Neuroleptic/Antipsychotic	Acetaminophen
Succinylcholine	Baclofen
Propofol	Caffeine
Valproic acid (in patients with CPT II)	Chloral hydrate
Fenfluramine	Colchicine fibric acid derivatives (bezafibrate, clofibrate, fenofibrate, gemfibrozil)
Lithium	Quinine
Haloperidol	Corticosteroids
Fluphenazine	Statins (atorvastatin, fluvastatin, lovastatin, pravastatin, rosuvastatin, simvastatin, cerivastatin)
Perphenazine	
Chlorpromazine	Theophylline
Cyclic antidepressants	Benzodiazepines
Selective serotonin reuptake inhibitors	Antihistamines
	Phenylpropanolamine
Antibiotics	Ephedra
Fluoroquinolones	Proton pump inhibitors
Pyrazinamide	Ritodrine
Trimethoprim/sulfonamide	Vincristine
Amphotericin B	Salicylates
Itraconazole	
Daptomycin	
Isoniazid	
Pentamidine	

Treatment

Treatment is based upon the exposure. While symptomatic management is available for some toxins and drugs, in most cases these will not affect the rhabdomyolysis. When possible, removal of the exposure is warranted.

Autoimmune

Autoimmune diseases are not common causes of rhabdomyolysis but more so of subacute or chronic elevations of CK. Autoimmune myositis is associated with elevated CK. The progression correlates better to a slow decline of strength, often in proximal muscles. In addition, the patients may have the heliotrope rash as well as telangiectasias, photosensitivity, and/or extensor joint violaceous or red rashes (Gottron papules). Because these can be vasculitic diseases, often there are nailbed capillary changes. The best known of the pediatric autoimmune myositides is **dermatomyositis**; other subtypes exist including lupus myositis and idiopathic inflammatory myopathies.

Patients often have a *proximal* weakness but are less likely to have pain in the muscles. Additionally, atrophy can be indicative of a more chronic process. Other signs of autoimmune disease such as rash, joint pain, and/or systemic disease can be indicative of a more generalized systemic process.

TABLE 36.8 Toxins with Known Associations with Rhabdomyolysis

Buffalo and burbot fish
Birds who eat hemlock: hemlock herbs from quail eggs
Kidney beans
Snake venom (coral, cobra, viper, rattlesnake)
Insect (hornet, African bee, honey bee, and others)
Tricholoma equestre (mushroom)
Carbon monoxide (CO)
Spider venom
Heavy metals
Pesticides
Cyanide
Toluene

The evaluation for autoimmune myositis differs from other causes of rhabdomyolysis in that the *muscle biopsy is often a key component.* Given the process is subacute to chronic, the typical nonspecific muscle breakdown seen in rhabdomyolysis that would contraindicate the biopsy is not present. The addition of rheumatologic studies such as an antinuclear antibody (ANA) as well as muscle-specific antibodies can be helpful in determining the etiology (Table 36.9).

TABLE 36.9 **Myositis-Specific and Myositis-Associated Autoantibodies**

Type of Autoantibodies	Myositis-Specific Antibodies (MSAs)	Myositis-Associated Antibodies (MAAs)	Other Autoantibodies Often Found in Myositis
Autoantibody specificities	Classic MSAs: Jo-1, PL-7, PL-12, EJ, OJ, Mi-2, SRP	PM-Scl, Ku, U1RNP, U1/U2RNP, U3RNP	Ro52, Ro60, Su/Ago2
	New antibodies that can be considered MSAs: KS, TIF1γ/α, TIF1β, MJ/NXP-2, MDA5/CADM-140, SAE	—	—
Association with SARDs	PM/DM, PM/DM overlap syndrome	PM/DM, PM/DM overlap syndrome, SSc, SLE	Various SARDs
Detection in non-PM/DM	Uncommon (anti-ARS can be in overlap syndrome and idiopathic ILD)	Not uncommon	Often
Association with myopathy when found in non-PM/DM	Yes	Yes	No or not established
Prevalence in general population	Almost none	PM-Scl, Ku, U1/U2RNP—almost none; U1RNP, ~0.1%	Relatively common (0.5–1%)

DM, dermatomyositis; ILD, interstitial lung disease; PM, polymyositis; SARDs, systemic autoimmune rheumatic diseases; SLE, systemic lupus erythematosus; SSc, scleroderma, systemic sclerosis.
From Satoh M, Tanaka S, Ceribelli A, et al. A comprehensive overview on myositis-specific antibodies: new and old biomarkers in idiopathic inflammatory myopathy. *Clin Rev Allergy Immunol.* 2017;52(1):1–19 (Table 1, p. 2).

Treatment

The treatment of autoimmune myositis includes immunosuppressing and/or immunomodulating agents. Corticosteroids are initiated before transitioning the patient to steroid-sparing agents, often azathioprine, methotrexate, or mycophenolate mofetil, depending upon the disease process.

MUSCLE DISEASE

The muscle diseases include the muscular dystrophies and myopathies. In the **muscular dystrophies**, the pathology is associated with dysfunction in the genes that are part of the scaffolding of the muscle membrane and connecting to the surrounding extracellular matrix. The **myopathies** are often due to dysfunction in a component of the contractile apparatus. The dystrophies often have hyperCKemia at baseline, whereas the myopathies do not. However, there are many diseases in these categories with possible overlap and differentiation can be difficult.

The risk of **malignant hyperthermia** is not ubiquitous in all muscle disease, but, unless a specific variant analysis is determined, it is safest to use malignant hyperthermia precautions for any anesthesia in a known or suspected patient with muscle disease.

Dystrophinopathy

Dystrophin is an X-linked gene that links the internal contractile apparatus of the myofiber to the sarcolemma, where it connects with other structural proteins that eventually anchor the cell to the extracellular matrix. A defect in this protein results in a progressive muscle disease. There is a large phenotypic variation in which the mildest males with the disease with the slowest progression are able to ambulate into their adult years, while the more severely affected males will lose the ability to walk by age 10–12 years and die in their late teens to early 20s without treatment. Differentiation of this disease is between Becker muscular dystrophy for those males who continue to walk after the age of 12 years and Duchenne muscular dystrophy for those who lose the ability to walk prior to 12 years of age; ~30% of males will have some cognitive deficits. Females may also present with milder symptoms that range from mild cardiac disease in adult years to rarely female children with similar features to the male counterpart.

Patients with dystrophinopathy have baseline hyperCKemia (sometimes up to 40,000 IU/L); they are also at risk for rhabdomyolysis. Rhabdomyolysis may be confused with myalgias and an increase in their already high CK due to muscle activity; dark urine suggests rhabdomyolysis.

Patients rarely present with rhabdomyolysis as an initial manifestation after exercise. In the patient with an undiagnosed but possible muscle disease, a family history is very important because 65% of cases of dystrophinopathy are inherited. For males, this is often from asymptomatic mothers, but there may be a distant family history of a young male who died of a muscle disease in the family.

In a patient presenting with rhabdomyolysis who has, or is suspected of having, a dystrophinopathy, the males often have calf pseudohypertrophy from fatty infiltrates. While during an acute episode of rhabdomyolysis it may be difficult to differentiate baseline weakness from weakness from the rhabdomyolysis, the patients often present with proximal muscle weakness between the ages of 3 and 5 years.

The diagnostic evaluation of a patient with rhabdomyolysis and possible underlying dystrophinopathy begins with a *baseline* CK as an outpatient because all male patients with dystrophinopathy have hyperCKemia at baseline. While other muscular dystrophies can also cause hyperCKemia, dystrophinopathies have the highest incidence in young males. In young females, symptomatic carriers of dystrophinopathies at a young age are less common than some of the other muscle diseases such as the dysferlinopathies or other limb-girdle muscular dystrophies. The use of genetic muscle disease panel testing after the result of an elevated baseline CK can offer rapid diagnostic testing.

Other Muscular Dystrophies

Other muscular dystrophies can also present with rhabdomyolysis. In these cases, the specific gene and genetic change can direct the phenotype further (see Tables 36.2 and 36.6 and Fig. 36.3). The pattern of muscle weakness, age of onset, and progression can vary between many of these diseases and may be used to better phenotype the patients. In some patients, rhabdomyolysis may be the presenting event; these disorders include fukutin-related protein muscular dystrophy, anoctaminopathy, dysferlinopathy, caveolinopathy, and calpainopathy. Exercise or a febrile illness may be precipitating events.

MYOPATHIES

RYR1 and Malignant Hyperthermia

RYR1-related myopathy has a broad phenotypic presentation. In the mildest cases, variants in this gene present only with malignant hyperthermia when given an inciting anesthetic; other patients can present with severe respiratory and muscle weakness as a newborn infant. However, at baseline there is often no hyperCKemia.

In patients with *RYR1*-myopathy-associated rhabdomyolysis with **malignant hyperthermia**, lactic acidosis and hyperthermia are often found; this may not be the case in exertional rhabdomyolysis. Malignant hyperthermia is associated with volatile anesthetics and depolarizing agents.

For patients with *exertional RYR1* rhabdomyolysis, the features are similar to those with exercise-induced rhabdomyolysis; in addition, there may be features of an underlying muscle disease such as ptosis, proximal muscle weakness, and/or difficulty keeping up with their peers. Recurrent symptoms congruent with possible rhabdomyolysis or myalgias are also possible clues in patients with otherwise normal baseline examinations.

A family history of weakness, malignant hyperthermia, or exertional myalgias is also helpful in making this diagnosis.

For patients with malignant hyperthermia–related muscle disease, immediate consideration for a broad muscle disease genetic panel can be helpful. *RYR1* is a large gene with a high degree of commonly occurring variants. This complicates the interpretation of variants identified through gene sequencing, and it is important to provide the family with the most current information regarding a variant identified through testing.

The treatment of malignant hyperthermia differs somewhat from that of typical rhabdomyolysis because there are continued concerns about intense muscle contractions perpetuating the disease; the *RYR1* gene is involved with calcium influx and, thus, avoiding continued depolarization is needed. The first step is to avoid the inciting agent. Dantrolene is beneficial with or without cooling. Avoiding β blockers as well as calcium and calcium antagonists is recommended to help stop perpetuate the mechanism of injury.

GLYCOGEN METABOLISM/MCARDLE DISEASE

There are a variety of glycogen storage diseases associated with rhabdomyolysis, with the best-known being McArdle disease, also known as myophosphorylase deficiency (see Fig. 36.3 and Tables 36.2 and 36.6).

Patients with McArdle disease often describe intolerance to brief intense exercise but do better with moderate exercise; they will describe cramping and muscle swelling. After the patient develops acute myalgias, they will be able to have further activity (the "second-wind phenomenon") if they take a brief rest. However, this is not found in every patient. Weakness in childhood is not common and is mild, if present.

The baseline CK is often elevated above baseline even when at rest. The electromyogram and nerve conduction studies can have myopathic features in some, but not all, patients. Genetic testing is the standard of care in diagnosing this disease.

Carnitine Palmitoyl Transferase II Deficiency

Carnitine palmitoyl transferase II (CPT II) deficiency is an autosomal recessive disease that presents in various forms. The **myopathic** form will have little to no symptoms prior to the onset of rhabdomyolysis. Patients may have some mild myalgias with activity but will often present in an acute decompensation from exercise, cold, fasting, valproate usage, or anesthesia. The **infantile** form is more severe and is a hepato-cardio-muscular systemic disorder presenting with hepatomegaly, hypoglycemia, hypotonia, cardiomyopathy, and seizures.

Patients with CPT II disease have normal CK levels at rest. This is a disease of recurrence presenting with episodes of rhabdomyolysis and a history of myalgias or cramping. Analysis of serum acylcarnitines and total free carnitine is warranted; there is a high ratio of palmitoylcarnitine (C16:0) + oleoylcarnitine (C18:1))/acetylcarnitine (C2) with normal serum carnitine.

Systemic Disease

This category includes hypokalemic as well as thyroid storming or hypothyroidism-associated rhabdomyolysis. Given that thyroid-associated rhabdomyolysis is very rare, unless other features are suggestive, it is not warranted to screen every patient who presents with rhabdomyolysis without other features.

Mitochondrial and Fatty Acid Oxidation Defects

Mitochondrial diseases may have chronic symptoms including other neurologic features, cardiac disease, and weakness (see Tables 36.2 and 36.6). Given the potential heterogeneous presentations of primary mitochondrial diseases, a broad array of multisystem symptoms should be considered as variations in presentation are significant.

The diagnostic evaluation often begins with biochemical testing and in the acute stage this is warranted. In these patients, sending serum lactic acid, pyruvic acid, ammonia, very long-chain fatty acids, an acylcarnitine profile, total and free carnitine, and urine organic acids is appropriate in the acute phase.

Presumed Isolated HyperCKemia

Elevated CK levels in an otherwise asymptomatic patient may be an incidental finding (idiopathic) or an early preclinical manifestation of a muscle disease. These latter disorders include muscular dystrophy (especially female carriers), other mitochondrial myopathies, myoadenylate deaminase deficiency, caveolinopathies, desmin-related myopathies, and inflammatory myositis. Strenuous exercise within 7 days of testing may also produce elevated CK levels.

■ SUMMARY AND RED FLAGS

Rhabdomyolysis is a pathologic process that is the end result from either structural or energy depletion of myocytes. The treatment focuses on protecting the kidneys and other organs from secondary damage from the released intracellular substances into the serum by use of appropriate hydration as well as glucose in patients with suspected metabolic disease.

While most causes of rhabdomyolysis are due to exercise or infection, being aware of signs that may indicate an underlying disease is important and this would warrant treatment. Often, the use of a baseline (at rest and postevent) CK can help differentiate between groups of muscle diseases and help direct further evaluation. Recurrent episodes, a personal or family history (cramping, prolonged postexercise muscle soreness), decompensation or death during surgery (anesthesia), calf pseudohypertrophy, muscle wasting, being unable to keep up with peers, hepatic–cardiac–central nervous system dysfunction, and persistent elevations of CK after recovery strongly suggest an underlying genetic etiology.

BIBLIOGRAPHY

A bibliography is available at ExpertConsult.com.

37

Stroke

Raquel Farias-Moeller

Stroke is a sudden focal neurologic syndrome caused by an abrupt and critical interruption of the normal metabolic function of the central nervous system (CNS), typically due to ischemia or hemorrhage. Depending on where in the CNS this interruption occurs, the symptoms of stroke can be striking, such as acute lateralized weakness, though at times are subtle, mimicking other and sometimes more benign neurologic processes or producing clinically asymptomatic lesions that are discovered only on imaging studies or detailed neuropsychological evaluation. Despite this variability in presentation, stroke is a serious medical emergency and is among the 10 most common causes of death in childhood; prompt recognition and management are essential, as effective interventions that can minimize the sequelae of stroke are time dependent and some must be initiated within hours of symptom onset. The sequelae are not trivial: In addition to lasting lateralized weakness (paralysis, paresis), other symptoms such as learning disabilities, disturbances of language, visual deficits, and seizures may persist throughout adulthood. Physicians should recognize both common and rare disorders that can predispose to stroke to counsel patients and their families on the risk and recognition of stroke and to institute available prophylactic measures to minimize that risk. Additionally, clinicians should be aware of phenomena that can mimic the symptoms of stroke to avoid unnecessary investigations or interventions.

DEFINITIONS

Stroke is a sudden focal neurologic syndrome caused by cerebrovascular disease, which refers to any abnormality of the brain resulting from a pathologic process of the blood vessels, such as occlusion of the lumen by an embolus or thrombus, rupture of a vessel wall or alteration in vessel wall permeability, increased viscosity, vessel inflammatory disorders, or other changes in the quality of blood flow through the cerebral vessels. Brain injury from stroke occurs in one of two general forms:

Ischemia consists of inadequate brain perfusion with consequent lack of oxygen or other blood-delivered substances necessary for normal metabolic function.

Hemorrhage occurs when blood is released into the extravascular cranial space, producing focal brain injury from irritation and pressure exerted by the space-occupying mass of blood.

Rarely *metabolic stroke* due to mitochondrial disorders, hypoglycemia, or organic acidemias may produce stroke in the absence of ischemia or hemorrhage.

Arterial ischemic stroke (AIS) typically occurs via one of three mechanisms: embolism, thrombosis, or global cerebral hypoperfusion. Ischemic brain injury may rarely be secondary to metabolic derangements or arterial vasospasm. Figures 37.1 through 37.4 demonstrate the arterial vascular supply to the brain.

Embolic stroke occurs when material formed within a vessel outside the brain travels to and lodges in a blood vessel supplying the brain, blocking cerebral perfusion. Emboli originate most commonly in the heart, arising from a thrombus on a cardiac chamber wall or from a vegetation on valve leaflets. Artery-to-artery emboli are composed of clot or platelet aggregates that originate in vessels proximal to the brain that ultimately travel to and occlude flow in vessels critical for cerebral perfusion. Systemic vein-to-cerebral artery emboli (i.e., paradoxical emboli) are possible in the presence of the right-to-left shunts of cyanotic congenital heart disease or a patent foramen ovale.

Thrombosis denotes vascular occlusion caused by a localized process within a blood vessel or vessels. Although atherosclerosis underlies most thrombotic processes affecting adults, it is not common in children. Localized luminal clot formation in cerebral vessels occurs in polycythemia or in a hypercoagulable state. Alternatively, anatomic abnormalities may lead to clot formation or mechanical obstruction as is found in fibromuscular dysplasia, arteritis (vasculitis), or arterial dissection.

Global cerebral hypoperfusion due to systemic hypotension or cardiac pump failure (resulting from congenital heart disease or its surgical repair) can result in cerebral ischemic injury. With diminished cerebral perfusion, brain injury is more diffuse than the more focal injuries characteristic of thrombotic and embolic cerebral events.

Metabolic stroke occurs when a physiologic stressor produces metabolic demands that exceed the ability to provide sufficient metabolic substrate to the brain, provoking an energy failure state that results in an acute neurologic deficit. Common stressors include prolonged fasting with hypoglycemia, intercurrent illness, or seizures. Patients with certain inborn errors of metabolism or mitochondrial disorders are more susceptible to metabolic decompensation and therefore metabolic stroke.

Vasospasm, a contraction of the wall of intracranial arteries causing luminal narrowing, is most often seen after subarachnoid hemorrhage but may also occur in the setting of CNS infections. Narrowed vessels are unable to perfuse areas of the brain sufficiently and cerebral ischemia may occur.

Intracranial hemorrhage arises in one of two patterns:

Subarachnoid hemorrhage (SAH) occurs when blood flows out of the intracranial vascular bed onto the surface of the brain to mix with cerebrospinal fluid in the subarachnoid space. The most common source of such intracranial bleeding in early childhood is an **arteriovenous malformation (AVM).** Ruptured **intracranial aneurysms** also cause SAH, especially in older children (Table 37.1).

Intraparenchymal hemorrhage denotes bleeding into the parenchyma of the brain. The severity and spectrum of deficits caused by intraparenchymal hemorrhage are determined by the extent and location of bleeding in the brain (Table 37.2).

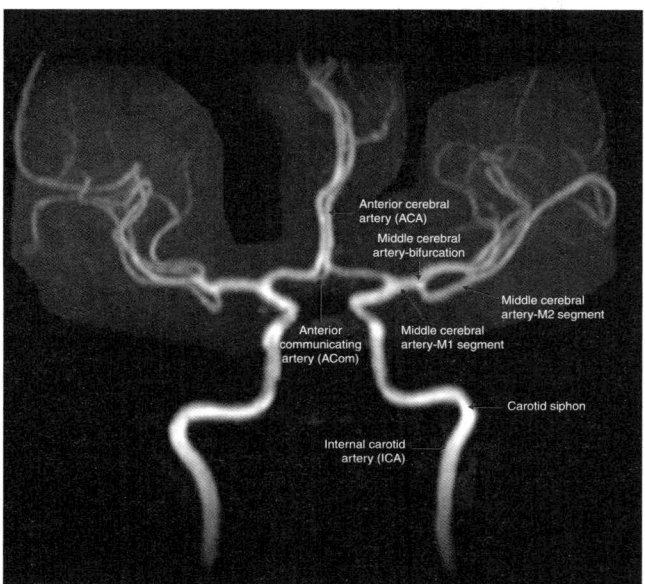

Fig. 37.1 Magnetic resonance angiogram of the intracranial portion of the internal carotid artery and its main branches. (From Goldstein LB. Approach to cerebrovascular diseases. In: Goldman L, Schafer AI, eds. *Goldman-Cecil Medicine.* 26th ed. Philadelphia: Elsevier; 2020:2388, Fig. 378-2.)

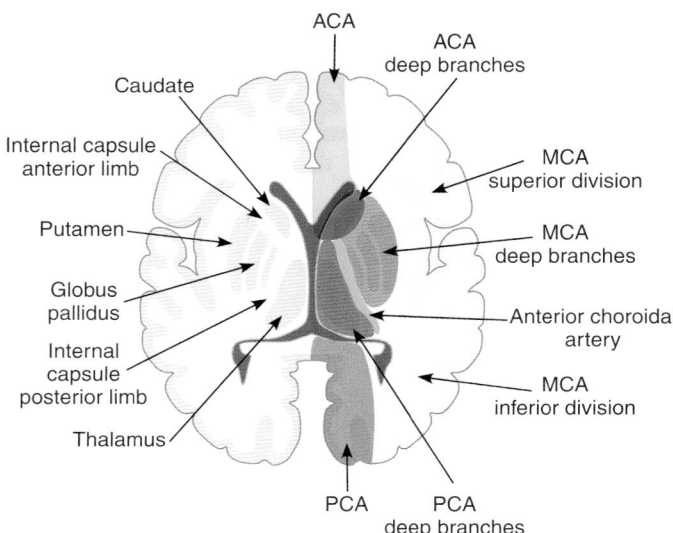

Fig. 37.3 Anatomic distribution of blood flow from major intracranial vessels in the cerebral hemispheres. ACA, anterior cerebral artery; MCA, middle cerebral artery; PCA, posterior cerebral artery. (From Lemkuil BP, Drummond JC, Patel PM. Central nervous system physiology: cerebrovascular. In: Hemmings HC Jr, Egan TD, eds. *Pharmacology and Physiology for Anesthesia.* 2nd ed. Philadelphia: Elsevier; 2019:175, Fig. 9.2A.)

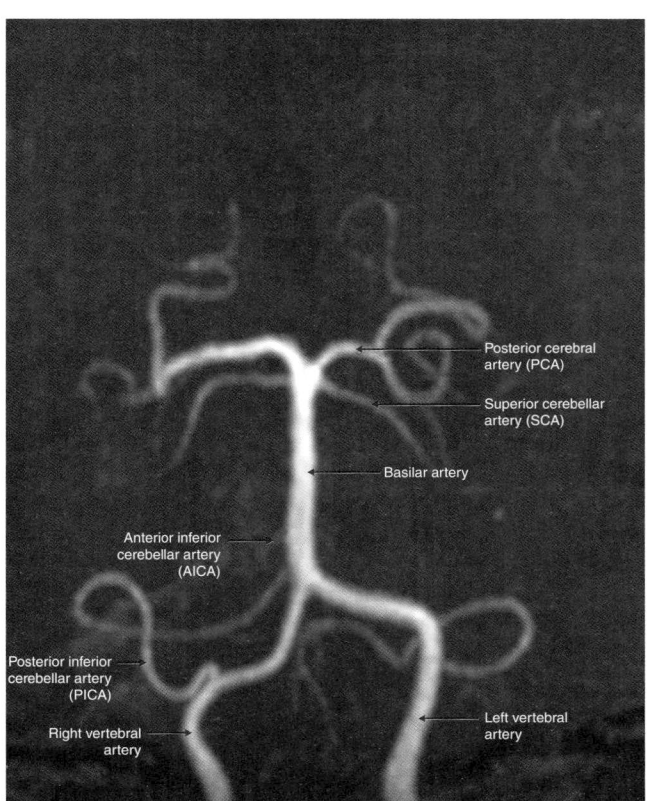

Fig. 37.2 Magnetic resonance angiogram of the intracranial portion of the vertebrobasilar system. (From Goldstein LB. Approach to cerebrovascular diseases. In: Goldman L, Schafer AI, eds. *Goldman-Cecil Medicine.* 26th ed. Philadelphia: Elsevier; 2020:2389, Fig. 378-3.)

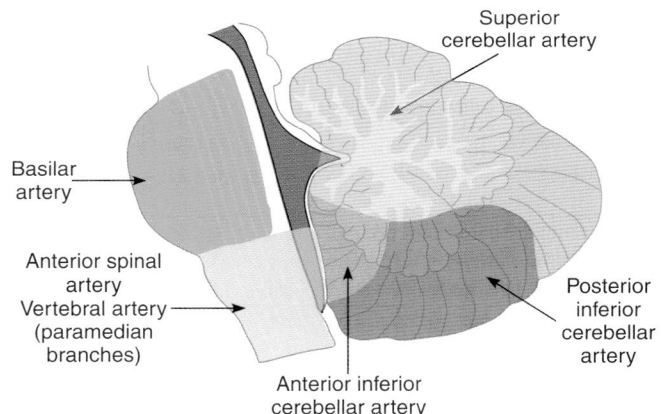

Fig. 37.4 Anatomic distribution of blood flow from major intracranial vessels in the cerebral hemispheres and infratentorial structures. (From Lemkuil BP, Drummond JC, Patel PM. Central nervous system physiology: cerebrovascular. In: Hemmings HC Jr, Egan TD, eds. *Pharmacology and Physiology for Anesthesia.* 2nd ed. Philadelphia: Elsevier; 2019:175, Fig. 9.2B.)

Venous stroke occurs when there is occlusion of the dural venous sinuses (Table 37.3). Thrombosis may occur in cerebral veins that conduct deoxygenated blood from the brain parenchyma to the dural sinus system (Fig. 37.5). These sinuses—the sagittal, straight, transverse, cavernous, and petrous—then convey the blood to the jugular veins. Occlusion of flow anywhere in these venous conduits leads to local underdrainage, which may lead to ischemia and even hemorrhage.

THE SYMPTOMS OF STROKE

The primary symptom of a stroke is a sudden **neurologic deficit**, a localized interruption of the functions for which the compromised area of brain tissue is responsible. The location, or *focality*, of the resultant

TABLE 37.1	Causes of Spontaneous Subarachnoid Hemorrhage in Young Adults	
Cerebral aneurysm rupture	Autoimmune disorders	
Perimesencephalic hemorrhage	Systemic lupus erythematosus	
Vascular malformation rupture (arteriovenous malformation, arteriovenous fistula, cavernous malformations)	Polyarteritis nodosa	
Other	Henoch-Schönlein purpura	
Congenital disorders	Poststreptococcal glomerulonephritis	
Coarctation of the aorta	Kawasaki disease	
Pseudoxanthoma elasticum	Other systemic diseases	
Menkes kinky hair syndrome	Heat stroke	
Sturge-Weber syndrome	Conn syndrome	
Tuberous sclerosis complex	Thyrotoxicosis	
Neurofibromatosis 1 (von Recklinghausen disease)	Wolman disease	
Hereditary hemorrhagic telangiectasia (Rendu-Osler disease)	Spinal endometriosis	
Ehlers-Danlos syndrome	Neoplasms	
Klinefelter syndrome	Gliomas	
Autosomal dominant polycystic kidney disease	Meningiomas	
Systemic vascular disease	Acoustic neuromas	
Hypertension	Choroid plexus papillomas	
Cerebral embolism	Pituitary adenomas	
Moyamoya disease	Pineocytomas	
Cerebral venous occlusive disease	Chordomas	
Eclampsia	Subependymomas	
Hematologic disorders	Metastatic carcinoma	
Hemophilia	Intraspinal neoplasms	
Aplastic anemia	Drugs	
Sickle cell anemia	Amphetamines	
Leukemias	Cocaine	
Thrombocytopenic purpura	Ephedrine	
Anticoagulant therapy	Monoamine oxidase inhibitors	
Thrombolytic therapy	Oral contraceptive pills	
Infectious diseases	Phencyclidine	
Infective endocarditis	Alcohol	
Tuberculous meningitis	Miscellaneous	
Luetic meningoencephalitis	α-Galactosidase deficiency	
Fungal central nervous system infections	α_1-Antitrypsin deficiency	
Infectious mononucleosis	Cystic fibrosis	
Tick-borne relapsing fever	Klippel-Trénaunay-Weber syndrome	
	Parry-Romberg syndrome	
	3-M syndrome	

From Biller J. *Stroke in Children and Young Adults*. 2nd ed. Philadelphia: Saunders; 2009:290, Table 15-1.

deficit depends on the laterality and whether the event occurred in the cortex, the subcortical areas, the cerebellum, or the brainstem, as well as the pathways that were interrupted (Table 37.4). The duration of the neurologic deficit may vary. Focal neurologic deficits in stroke are usually chronic and static, though with intense rehabilitation, some degree of recovery is expected. **Stroke recrudescence**, in which a pre-existing stroke-induced deficit can temporarily worsen during an acute stressor, can occur as well. Finally, although alterations of blood flow often result in permanent deficits, some cause only temporary ones: **transient ischemic attacks (TIAs)** are brief episodes of focal, nonepileptic neurologic deficit attributable to interruption of cerebral perfusion; the onset is abrupt, and, by definition, symptoms last less than 24 hours with complete recovery afterward; most TIAs last only a few minutes.

The degree to which a neurologic deficit is symptomatic is influenced not only by the location of the lesion but also by the age and developmental status of the patient. Neonates and infants often present with vague symptoms that may mimic a variety of conditions, such as lethargy, apnea, or feeding intolerance. Older children and adolescents present similarly to adults, with distinct focal neurologic deficits; however, more globally diffuse presentations can occur and do so more commonly than in adults, and must be distinguished from mimicking conditions such as migraine headache or acute disseminated encephalomyelitis. When symptoms are diffuse or there is a depressed level of consciousness, detailed neurologic examination may uncover subtle focal deficits that increase the suspicion of stroke. Examination may also allow the clinician to determine when symptoms are attributable to CNS-based pathology other than stroke, to pathophysiology outside the CNS, or to a psychogenic cause.

Stroke symptoms, such as weakness or sensory deficits, may present in isolation, but a combination of deficits is common. Similar symptoms may be attributable to strokes affecting different brain territories. Diagnostic delays in pediatric stroke can be related to the lack of awareness among families and medical staff members as to the risk and presentation of pediatric stroke, as well as higher incidence of **stroke mimics**, conditions that present similarly to stroke despite being due to a different etiology. These mimics vary in severity and morbidity

TABLE 37.2 Causes of Spontaneous Intracerebral Hemorrhage in Young Adults

Vascular malformations
    AVMs
    Capillary telangiectasias
    Cavernous malformations
    Developmental venous anomalies
Aneurysms
    Saccular
    Infective
    Traumatic
    Neoplastic
Arterial hypertension
    Secondary
    Primary
Bleeding diatheses
    Leukemia
    Thrombocytopenia
    Disseminated intravascular coagulation
    Polycythemia
    Hyperviscosity syndromes
    Hemophilia
    Hypoprothrombinemia
    Afibrinogenemia
    Selective factor deficiencies
    von Willebrand disease
    Sickle cell anemia
    Antiplatelet therapy
    Anticoagulant therapy
    Thrombolytic therapy
Icelandic form of CAA
Arteritis/arteriopathies
    Infectious vasculitides
    Multisystem vasculitides
    Isolated CNS angiitis
    Moyamoya disease
    HANAC syndrome
Drug related
    Amphetamines
    Cocaine
    Phenylpropanolamine
    Pentazocine-pyribenzamine
    Phencyclidine
    Heroin
    Monoamine oxidase inhibitor
    Other drugs
Intracranial tumors
    Primary malignant or benign
    Metastatic
Cerebral venous occlusive disease
Miscellaneous
    Post–carotid endarterectomy
    Post–selective neurosurgical procedures
    Post–spinal anesthesia
    Postmyelography
    Cold related
    Post–painful dental procedures
    Protracted migraine
    Methanol intoxication

AVM, arteriovenous malformation; CAA, cerebral amyloid angiopathy; CNS, central nervous system; HANAC, hereditary angiopathy with nephropathy, aneurysms, muscle cramps.
From Biller J. *Stroke in Children and Young Adults*. 2nd ed. Philadelphia: Saunders; 2009:263, Table 14-1.

and are often more prevalent in children than in adults. Stroke mimics vary by stroke symptom and differ in etiology according to age (Table 37.5). The following sections describe the most common symptoms with which children with stroke can present.

Weakness

Children with stroke most often present with unilateral weakness secondary to injury of the **corticospinal tract**, which originates in the motor cortex in the precentral gyrus and sends motor information to the spinal cord. **Hemiparesis** manifests as unilateral weakness and **hemiplegia** as unilateral paralysis, or complete loss of strength. The motor cortex is organized by the region of the body it controls (Fig. 37.6). The localization and severity of weakness, as well as the type (flaccid or spastic), depend on the location of the stroke and the timing of examination.

Localization and Severity of Weakness

The upper motor neurons of the corticospinal tracts originate in the cerebral cortex, decussate (i.e., cross sides) in the brainstem, and terminate on lower motor neurons and interneurons in the spinal cord (Fig. 37.7). Due to this crossing, lesions above the decussation cause contralateral motor deficits. In cortical strokes affecting upper motor neurons, the location of the injury determines which body parts are weak, as well as the degree of weakness. Given the large topographic distribution of the motor cortex and different vascular territories that supply it, a substantially large stroke in the motor cortex may cause weakness in only a relatively small area of the body. In contrast, a very small stroke in the internal capsule may cause complete hemiplegia, due to the compact nature of the corticospinal tract in this area. If a stroke in the brainstem causes unilateral weakness, it is typically accompanied by other signs of brainstem dysfunction.

The severity of unilateral weakness may vary from severe hemiplegia to subtle hemiparesis. On examination, hemiparesis may be accompanied by **pronator drift,** slowing of **rapid alternating movements,** or decreased **arm swing** during gait. Pronator drift is assessed by asking the patient to extend the arms at the shoulder while keeping the elbows straight with the palms facing up in a supinated position, as if carrying a tray. The patient is then asked to close the eyes and maintain the arms in this position. In pronator drift, the affected arm will slowly drift down and the hand may pronate. Assessing rapid alternating movements involves asking the patient to perform a series of repetitive movements as quickly though dexterously as possible. Movements include alternating supination and pronation of the forearm to tap the plantar and palmar surfaces of the hands against the thighs, touching each of the fingers to the thumb in succession in a repeating fashion, or tapping the floor by repeatedly flexing and extending the ankles. The weak limb will perform these movements with decreased speed and dexterity in comparison to the unaffected limb. **Decreased arm swing** can be observed when the patient is asked to ambulate; the affected arm does not swing as much as the unaffected arm.

Characterization of Weakness: Flaccid or Spastic

Tone is the resistance of muscle to stretch; the maintenance of normal tone requires intact central and peripheral nervous systems (see Chapter 35). Acutely following a stroke, weakness is usually flaccid, or hypotonic. For infants and young children, the flaccid weakness manifests symptomatically as decreased or absent spontaneous movement of the affected limbs, while passive movements of the affected limbs are met with little to no resistance. Such deficits in older children and adolescents are noticeable to both the patient and observers alike, and muscle group testing can further localize specific areas of weakness.

TABLE 37.3 Causes of Cerebral Venous Thrombosis

Idiopathic	Drugs—cont'd
Prothrombotic state	ε-Aminocaproic acid
Protein C or S deficiency	Cisplatin and etoposide
Antithrombin deficiency	Medroxyprogesterone
Factor V Leiden variant	Heparin (heparin-induced thrombocytopenia)
Activated protein C resistance	Immunoglobulin G (intravenous immunoglobulin)
Prothrombin G20210A variant	Infections
Variants in thrombomodulin	Herpes zoster virus
Platelet glycoprotein IIIa (β_3) variant	Myeloidosis
Heparin cofactor II deficiency	Mucormycosis
Variants in plasminogen gene	Aspergillosis
MTHFR C677 variant	Pneumococcal meningitis
Dysfibrinogenemia	Syphilis
Elevated plasminogen activator inhibitor	HIV
Tissue plasminogen activator deficiency	Otitis media
Increased factors VIII, IX, X; von Willebrand factor	Mastoiditis
Variants in tissue factor pathway inhibitor	Sinusitis
Sickle cell disease and trait	Peritonsillar abscess
Reactive thrombocytosis and essential thrombocythemia	Endotoxemia
Pregnancy and puerperium	Trichinosis
Postoperative state	Sepsis
Antiphospholipid antibody syndrome	Vasculitides
Hyperhomocysteinemia	Behçet disease
Homocystinuria	Sarcoidosis
Cancer	Polyangiitis with granulomatosis
Inflammatory bowel diseases	Systemic lupus erythematosus
Dehydration	Polyarteritis nodosa
Congestive heart failure	Trauma
Paroxysmal nocturnal hemoglobinuria	Head trauma
Marasmus	Neurosurgical procedures
Iron-deficiency anemia	Strangulation
Nephrotic syndrome	Intravenous catheters
Thrombocytopenia	Cardiac pacemakers
Essential thrombocythemia	Others
Disseminated intravascular coagulation	Osteopetrosis
Thrombotic microangiopathies	Malignant atrophic papulosis (Kohlmeier-Degos disease)
Polycythemia vera and secondary polycythemia	Chronic lung disease
Hyperlipidemia	Diabetes mellitus
Familial histidine-rich glycoprotein deficiency	Budd-Chiari syndrome
Drugs	Arteriovenous malformation
Asparaginase	Sturge-Weber syndrome
Estrogen and oral contraceptives	Cerebral arterial occlusions
Androgen	Neoplasm (meningioma, metastasis, glomus tumors)

From Biller J. *Stroke in Children and Young Adults*. 2nd ed. Philadelphia: Saunders; 2009:237, Table 12-3.

With time, patients with weakness from stroke typically develop increased tone, or spasticity, as well as clonus in the affected limbs. **Spasticity** generally involves antigravity muscles, primarily the arm flexors and leg extensors. As a result, the arms become flexed and pronated, while the legs become extended and adducted, with plantar flexion of the foot and inversion of the ankle. If the hand is affected, **cortical thumbing,** consisting of adduction and flexion of the thumb, may occur. Testing for spasticity involves moving the relaxed affected extremity several times through its range of motion and assessing for freedom of movement. The extremity is then suddenly stretched through that range of motion at a higher velocity, at which point, if there is spasticity, tone will notably increase and the limb will "catch," a finding referred to as the *clasp-knife response.*

In addition to developing spasticity, patients with stroke affecting the corticospinal tracts develop brisk and hyperactive deep tendon reflexes due to the interruption of descending inhibitory upper motor

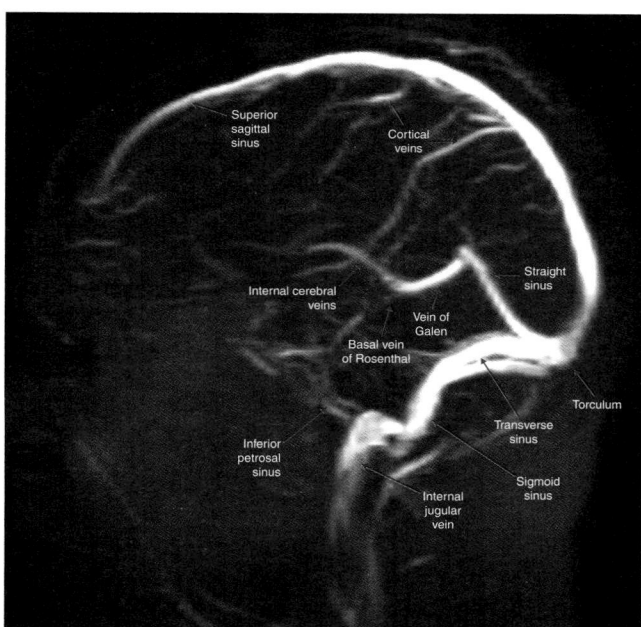

Fig. 37.5 Parasagittal magnetic resonance venogram showing venous structures. (From Goldstein LB. Approach to cerebrovascular diseases. In: Goldman L, Schafer AI, eds. *Goldman-Cecil Medicine.* 26th ed. Philadelphia: Elsevier; 2020:2393, Fig. 378-10.)

TABLE 37.4 Clinical Manifestations of Ischemic Cerebrovascular Disease	
Occluded Artery	**Typical Major Clinical Manifestations***
Internal carotid artery	Ipsilateral visual loss Ipsilateral middle cerebral artery syndrome
Anterior choroidal artery	Contralateral hemiparesis Contralateral sensory impairment Contralateral visual field defect
Anterior cerebral artery	Contralateral leg > arm paresis Contralateral leg > arm sensory deficit
Middle cerebral artery	Contralateral hemiparesis affecting face and arm > leg Contralateral sensory deficit affecting face and arm > leg Contralateral visual field defect Aphasia (dominant hemisphere) Contralateral hemispatial neglect (nondominant or dominant hemisphere)
Posterior cerebral artery	Contralateral homonymous hemianopia (or homonymous superior or inferior quadrantanopia) Contralateral sensory deficits (thalamic involvement)
Basilar artery tip	Bilateral central visual loss Confusion
Basilar artery	Ipsilateral cranial nerve deficit Contralateral hemiparesis Contralateral sensory impairment affecting arm and/or leg Coordination deficit
Vertebral artery, posterior inferior cerebellar artery	Ipsilateral sensory impairment over the face Dysphagia Ipsilateral Horner syndrome Ataxia
Superior cerebellar artery	Gait ataxia Ipsilateral limb ataxia Variable contralateral limb weakness

*Note: Not all may be present.
From Goldman L, Schafer AI, eds. *Goldman-Cecil Medicine.* 26th ed. Philadelphia: Elsevier; 2020:2397, Table 379-2.

neuron pathways and increased activity of the γ neuron reflex loop (see Chapter 35). Hyperactive reflexes are often accompanied by pathologic **clonus,** consisting of repetitive, rhythmic muscle contractions in response to tendon percussion or stretch of that muscle. Healthy neonates may have several beats of physiologic clonus; clonus in older infants or in children, adolescents, or adults is generally considered pathologic. Greater than 10 beats upon elicitation is considered sustained clonus and is indicative of more severe hypertonia. Pathologic **spread of reflexes,** in which antagonist or nearby adjacent muscle groups contract along with the muscle whose stretch reflex is being tested, is an additional sign of hypertonia. Other specific **pathologic reflexes** may be present if the relevant portion of the corticospinal tract is affected. Plantarflexion of the great toe is the physiologic response to stroking the foot in an arc from the heel, along the lateral aspect of the plantar surface, and across the ball of the foot to the great toe. Patients with an upper motor neuron lesion affecting control of the leg and foot will demonstrate the **Babinski response,** in which the great toe dorsiflexes rather than plantarflexes. The **Hoffmann sign** is elicited when the examiner flicks the fingernail of the patient's middle finger rapidly downward; if present, the index finger and the thumb involuntarily flex.

Sensory Deficits

The somatosensory cortex, located in the postcentral gyrus in the parietal lobe, posterior to the motor cortex, interprets sensory information from the periphery. The sensory cortex is organized topographically in a manner similar to the organization of the motor cortex (see Fig. 37.6) and shares the same vascular supply (see Figs. 37.1 and 37.3). Sensory information being received in the somatosensory cortex must first travel through ascending tracts in the spinal cord: the spinothalamic tracts and the dorsal columns (see Fig. 37.7); the former decussate within the spinal cord near their point of origin, whereas the latter cross the midline in the medulla. Each pathway conveys different sensory modalities and both ascend through the brainstem, arriving at the ventral posterior lateral nucleus of the

thalamus. Symptoms vary by where in these pathways stroke occurs. Given the shared blood supply to the motor and sensory cortices, cortical strokes tend to produce combined motor and sensory symptoms. Cortical strokes also tend to interrupt not just primary sensory information, but also the meaningful interpretation of sensory information. In contrast to strokes within the sensory cortex, strokes affecting pathways as they traverse the thalamus and other relays may produce isolated sensory deficits affecting just primary sensory modalities. The sensory tracts may also suffer infarction at the level of the brainstem, in which case cranial neuropathies or brainstem syndromes may ensue.

The most common sensory deficit following a stroke is a loss of sensation, or **hypoesthesia,** which may range from partial to complete numbness. Lesions of the somatosensory cortex may involve more complex sensory deficits like **agraphesthesia,** which refers to the loss of directional orientation across the surface of the skin, and

TABLE 37.5	**Distinguishing Clinical and Imaging Features of Stroke Mimics**	
Disorder	**Clinical Distinction from Stroke**	**Imaging Distinction from Stroke**
Migraine	Evolving or "marching" symptoms, short duration, complete resolution, headache, personal or family history of migraine	Typically normal Migrainous infarction is extremely rare
Seizure*	Positive symptoms, Todd paralysis is postseizure and time limited	Normal or may identify source of seizures (e.g., malformation, old injury)
Infection	Fever, encephalopathy, gradual onset, meningismus	Normal or signs of encephalitis/cerebritis, which are typically diffuse and bilateral. Arterial ischemic stroke and cerebral sinovenous thrombosis can occur in bacterial meningitis
Demyelination	Gradual onset, multifocal symptoms, encephalopathy Accompanying optic neuritis or transverse myelitis	Multifocal lesions, characteristic appearance (e.g., patchy in acute disseminated encephalomyelitis, ovoid in multiple sclerosis), typical locations (e.g., pericallosal in multiple sclerosis), less likely to show restricted diffusion
Hypoglycemia	Risk factor (e.g., insulin therapy), related to meals, additional systemic symptoms	Bilateral, symmetric May see restricted diffusion Posterior dominant pattern
Hypertensive encephalopathy (posterior reversible leukoencephalopathy syndrome)	Documented hypertension, bilateral visual symptoms, encephalopathy	Posterior dominant, bilateral, patchy lesions involving gray and white matter; usually no restricted diffusion
Inborn errors of metabolism	Pre-existing delays/regression, multisystem disease, abnormal biochemical profiles	May have restricted diffusion lesions but bilateral, symmetric, not conforming to established vascular territories. Magnetic resonance spectroscopy changes (e.g., high lactate in mitochondrial myopathy, encephalopathy, lactic acidosis, and strokelike episodes)
Vestibulopathy	Symptoms limited to vertigo, imbalance (i.e., no weakness); gradual onset	Normal
Acute cerebellar ataxia	Sudden-onset bilaterally symmetric ataxia; postviral	Normal
Channelopathy	Syndromic cluster of symptoms not localizing to single lesion; gradual onset, progressive evolution	Normal
Alternating hemiplegia	History of contralateral events Choreoathetosis/dystonia	Normal
Functional neurologic disorders	Recent psychosocial stressors Failure of signs and symptoms to localize to a specific lesion within the neural axis Presence of inconsistent examination findings Positive Hoover sign (when being evaluated for supposed lower extremity weakness, the patient with a functional disorder will exert downward pressure at the heel of the unaffected limb if the examiner holds the heel while asking the patient to raise the affected leg off the bed)	Normal

*Seizures, however, can also herald the onset of true stroke.

which on examination manifests as the inability to recognize a number or letter drawn on the skin. **Extinction to simultaneous stimulation** refers to the inability to recognize a sensory stimulus on the affected side when that stimulus is presented bilaterally at the same time, despite being able to recognize the stimulus on the affected side when it is presented in isolation. A patient may detect light brushing of the skin of the cheek on the affected side when presented in isolation though fail to detect brushing of the cheek on the affected side when both cheeks are brushed simultaneously. In the subacute and chronic stages of stroke a child may have lingering hypoesthesia, but also may have altered sensation, or **dysesthesia**. The ability of children to recognize and describe sensory deficits is dependent on developmental status. Children may use terms like "pins and needles," "burning," "bubbles," or just "pain" to describe dysesthesia. In thalamic strokes that affect the sensory relay nuclei, dysesthesia may provoke severe pain: **Thalamic pain syndrome** (or **Dejerine-Roussy syndrome**) is characterized by a profound hemi-body sensory loss that is eventually replaced by pain, paresthesia, and hyperalgesia of the hemibody contralateral to the stroke.

Language Deficits

Children with acute stroke may present with a sudden language deficit, the nature of which is determined by the location of the stroke. Broca's area, in the inferior frontal gyrus, is mainly responsible for speech

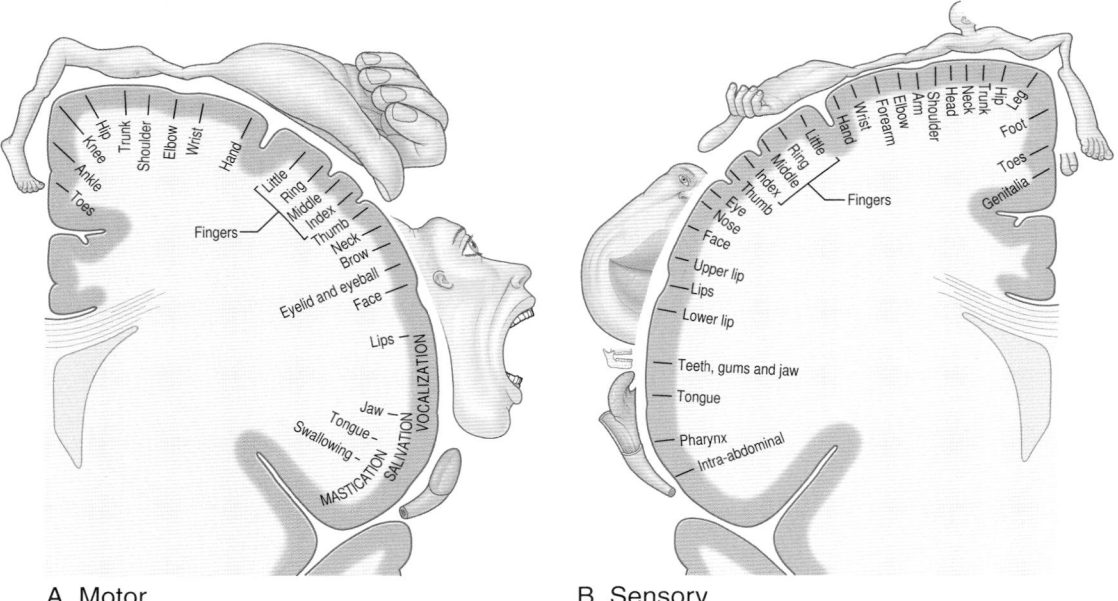

A Motor   **B** Sensory

Fig. 37.6 The topographic organization of the primary somatic sensory *(A)* and motor *(B)* areas of the cortex. The relative size of each body area represented within the homunculus is indicative of the amount of cortical tissue dedicated to processing sensory *(A)* or motor *(B)* information for that body area. (From Huether SE, McCance KL, Brashers VL. *Understanding Pathophysiology.* 7th ed. Philadelphia: Elsevier; 2020, Fig. 14.9.)

production. Wernicke's area, located in the junction of the superior temporal gyrus and the parietal cortex adjacent to auditory regions, is responsible for speech recognition. In most individuals these language areas are located in the *left* hemisphere. Lesions in and around Broca's and Wernicke's areas, or in the white matter tracts connecting these areas, lead to speech disturbances, or **aphasias**.

Types of Aphasias

The examination of a patient with suspected aphasia must consider age and developmental stage, as the evaluation requires pre-existent language production and comprehension, as well as the ability to follow commands, such as the repetition of words. Aphasias can be broadly divided into **expressive** (nonfluent) and **receptive** (fluent) and can be further categorized based on the ability to repeat words or phrases (Table 37.6).

The prototypical expressive aphasia is **Broca aphasia**, the evaluation of which typically reveals a frustrated patient who is able to comprehend language while being unable to speak or repeat phrases. In the most severe form, the patient is mute, whereas in the milder forms the patient may produce speech with frequent paraphasic errors (e.g., responding "pan" when asked to name a pen). An additional expressive aphasia is **transcortical motor aphasia**, in which a patient retains the ability to comprehend and repeat speech but is unable to produce spontaneous speech.

The prototypical receptive aphasia is **Wernicke aphasia**, in which comprehension of language is impaired but prosody or fluency of speech is preserved. The content of speech is often nonsensical and the words are often malformed; however, since the patient cannot understand their own nonsensical speech, frustration or concern with the deficit is absent. With pure Wernicke aphasia repetition is impaired. An additional expressive aphasia in which repetition is preserved is **transcortical sensory aphasia**.

Additional aphasia syndromes include **global aphasia**, in which both production and comprehension are impaired; **mixed transcortical** aphasia, in which both receptive and expressive language are impaired but the repetition of words is preserved; and **conduction aphasia**, in which the comprehension and production of speech are preserved but the repetition of words is impaired.

Visual Deficits

Visual deficits vary depending on the location and extent of stroke; determining the nature and degree of a visual disturbance can aid in localization and assist in visual therapies (Fig. 37.8). The **optic nerves** carry visual information from the nasal and temporal visual fields of each eye. Within the **optic chiasm**, fibers from the nasal visual field of each eye decussate and join with fibers from the temporal visual field, which do not cross the midline, forming the **optic tracts**, such that the left visual fields from both eyes are registered by the right hemisphere, and the right visual fields from both eyes by the left hemisphere. The optic tracts pass from the chiasm to the left and right **lateral geniculate nuclei** of the thalami. From the lateral geniculate nucleus, information travels though superior and inferior **optic radiations**: The superior radiations travel through the parietal lobes and contain information of the inferior visual fields, while the inferior radiations travel through the temporal lobes and carry information of the superior visual fields, with both arriving at the **visual cortex** within the corresponding **occipital lobes**. Fibers specifically serving central vision come together tightly and synapse at the innermost folding of the **calcarine gyrus** in the occipital lobe.

The vascular supply to these areas is varied. The lateral geniculate nucleus is supplied by the anterior choroidal artery, a branch of the internal carotid artery. The superior optic radiation is supplied by a branch of the middle cerebral artery, while the inferior optic radiation is supplied by the middle and posterior cerebral arteries. Lesions in the calcarine gyrus have dual blood supply from the posterior cerebral artery and posterior branches of the middle cerebral artery; an ischemic lesion of one vascular territory often results in a contralateral hemianopia with sparing of the macular or central vision. The occipital cortex itself is in the territory of the posterior cerebral artery.

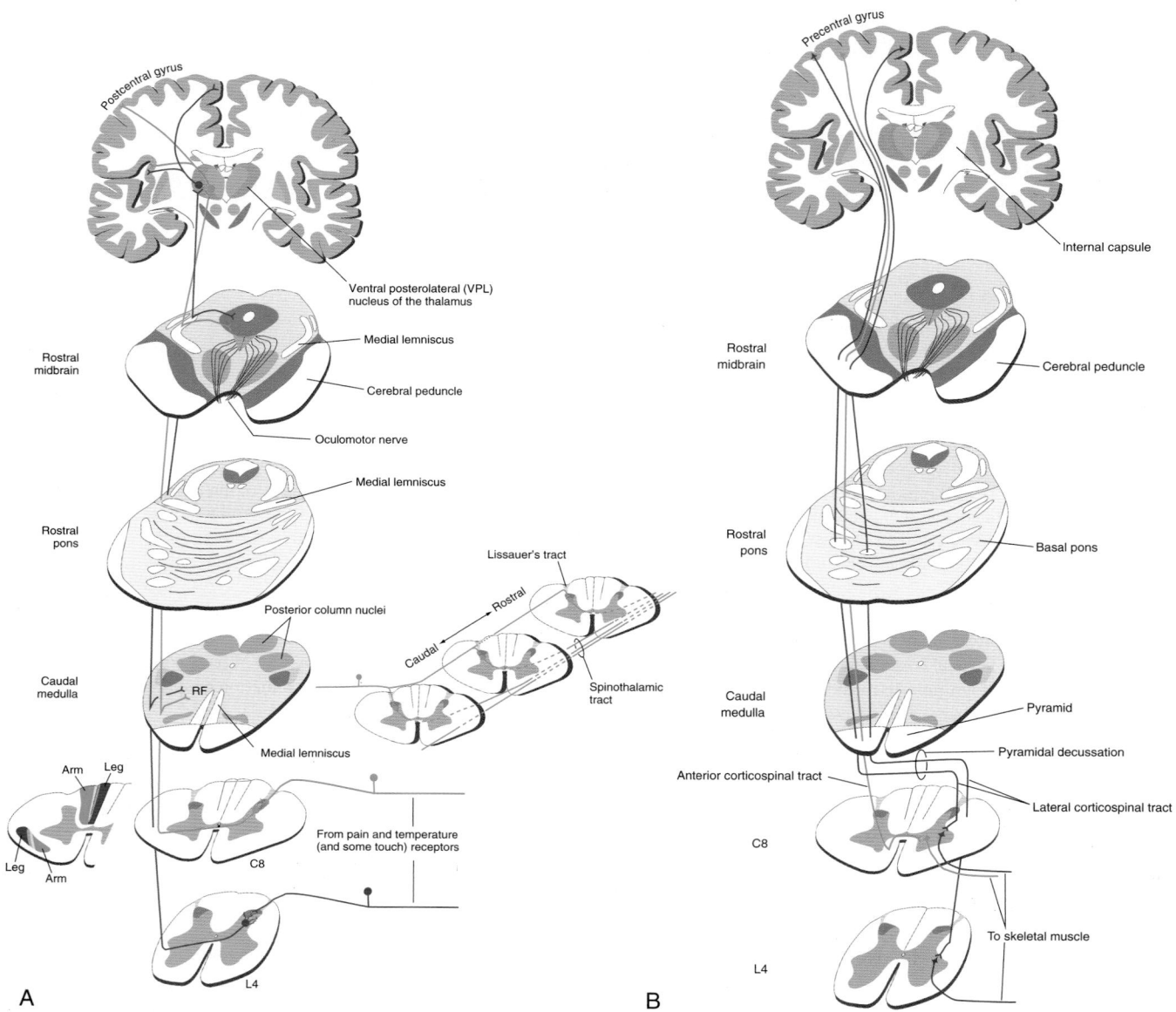

Fig. 37.7 *A,* Corticospinal tracts. Fibers from the precentral gyrus and other nearby cortical areas descend through the cerebral peduncles, pons, and medullary pyramids; most cross in the pyramidal decussation to form the lateral corticospinal tract. Those that do not cross in the pyramidal decussation form the anterior corticospinal tract; most of these fibers cross in the anterior white commissure before ending in the spinal gray matter. Most corticospinal fibers do not synapse directly on motor neurons; they are drawn that way here for simplicity. *B,* Spinothalamic tract. Pain, temperature, and some touch and pressure afferents end in the posterior horn. Second- or higher-order fibers cross the midline, form the spinothalamic tract, and ascend to the ventral posterolateral (VPL) nucleus of the thalamus (and also to other thalamic nuclei not shown). Thalamic cells then project to the somatosensory cortex of the postcentral gyrus, to the insula, and to other cortical areas (also not shown). Along their course through the brainstem, spinothalamic fibers give off many collaterals to the reticular formation (RF). The inset to the left shows the lamination of fibers in the posterior columns and the spinothalamic tract in a leg–lower trunk–upper trunk–arm sequence. The inset to the right shows the longitudinal formation of the spinothalamic tract. Primary afferents ascend several segments in Lissauer's tract before all of their branches terminate; fibers crossing to join the spinothalamic tract do so with a rostral inclination. As a result, a cordotomy incision at any given level will spare most of the information entering the contralateral side of the spinal cord at that level, and to be effective, the incision must be made several segments rostral to the highest dermatomal level of pain. (*A* and *B,* From Vanderah TW, Gould DJ. *Nolte's The Human Brain.* 8th ed. Philadelphia: Elsevier; 2021, Figs. 10-22 and 10-24.)

Ischemic lesions of the visual pathway may involve the retina or optic nerve, though the latter is rare in children, with demyelinating disease being a more common etiology of optic nerve lesions in children and adolescents. Lesions in the retina or optic nerve affect one eye and can result in **scotoma** (i.e., a blind spot), central blurry vision, or, if severe, monocular blindness; pupillary response is often affected, resulting in a **relative afferent pupillary defect,** in which shining a light on the affected eye results in decreased pupillary constriction relative to shining a light in the unaffected eye. Strokes affecting the optic chiasm result in **bitemporal hemianopias**, in which vision loss affects the right and left temporal visual fields, though this finding is less frequently due to stroke and is more commonly due to perichiasmatic masses such as pituitary or sellar masses, craniopharyngiomas, or aneurysms. Retrochiasmatic lesions are associated with **contralateral hemianopias** (visual field defect corresponding to the opposite visual field) or **quadrantanopias** depending on whether the optic tracts, radiations, or occipital lobes are involved (see Fig. 37.8).

Lesions within visual processing centers in the occipital and parietal lobes may produce disorders of visual cognition. Visual information from the occipital lobe is transmitted superiorly to the parietal lobe for spatial processing ("where" pathways) and inferiorly to the temporal lobe for identification ("what" pathways). The left inferior identification pathways are specialized for visual word processing; lesions in the

TABLE 37.6 Aphasia Types and Distinguishing Features			
Aphasia Type	Fluency	Comprehension	Repetition
Broca	Absent	Present	Absent
Transcortical motor	Absent	Present	Present
Wernicke	Present	Absent	Absent
Transcortical sensory	Present	Absent	Present
Mixed transcortical	Absent	Absent	Present
Conduction	Present	Present	Absent
Global	Absent	Absent	Absent

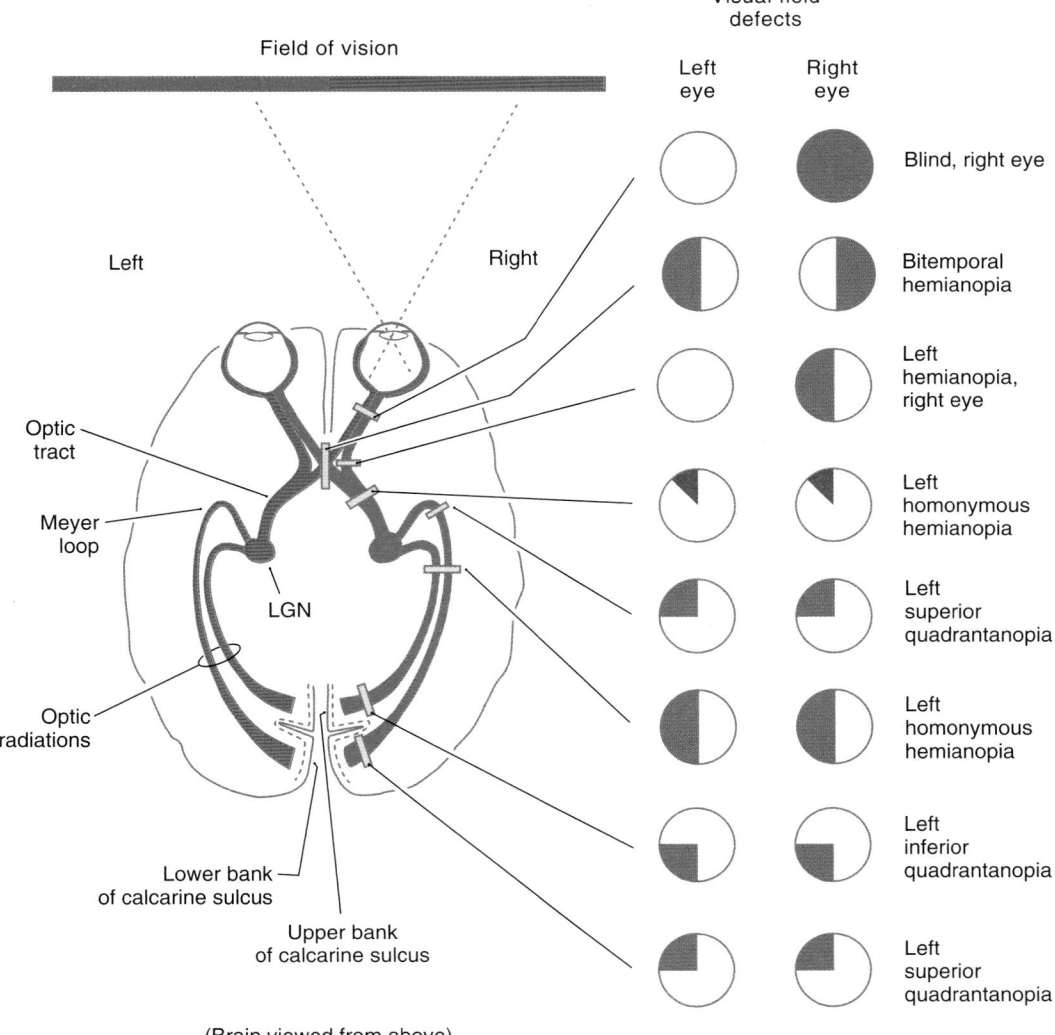

Fig. 37.8 Visual field defects produced by lesions as different places in the visual pathway. Regions of normal vision are indicated in *white*; regions of loss of vision are indicated in *black*. LGN, lateral geniculate nucleus. (From Corbett JJ, Chen J. The visual system. In: Haines DE, Mihailoff GA, eds. *Fundamental Neuroscience for Basic and Clinical Applications*. 5th ed. Philadelphia: Elsevier; 2018:299, Fig. 20.16.)

left inferior temporal occipital region result in **alexia**, the inability to read. The right identification pathways are specialized for processing faces; lesions in the right inferior temporal or occipital regions may lead to an inability to recognize faces, or **prosopagnosia**. When ischemic lesions to the visual pathways occur bilaterally, several syndromes may occur. **Balint syndrome** is characterized by **optic ataxia** (i.e., difficulty using visual attention to guide extremity movements), **ocular apraxia** (i.e., inability to use visual attention to guide ocular movements), and **simultanagnosia** (i.e., inability to visually survey a scene), and is caused by lesions of the bilateral parietal-occipital junctions due to medial cerebral artery-posterior cerebral artery watershed strokes. On examination, a patient with Balint syndrome manifests optic ataxia by misdirecting the finger to the target on finger-to-nose testing. With ocular apraxia, the patient is unable to track the examiner's finger with the eyes when directed but is able to move the eyes to commands such as "look left" or "look right." When assessing for simultanagnosia, the patient may be shown a drawing of one large letter or number composed of smaller versions of a different letter or number. The patient may only see the small letters or numbers, but not the larger letter or number they create.

When a stroke in the bilateral occipital cortex occurs (e.g., from bilateral posterior cerebral artery stroke), **cortical blindness** may occur. With cortical blindness, the pupillary light responses are preserved, but the brain cannot decode visual information. The patient may be clearly visually impaired, stumble with objects or not blink to threat, or even deny the blindness and confabulate what is being seen. The confabulation in the setting of cortical blindness is referred to as **Anton syndrome**. Children who have cortical blindness from a remote stroke may have wandering eyes or roving eye motions, which must be distinguished from the roving eye movements seen in septo-optic dysplasia or the rapid, multidirectional eye movements, *opsoclonus*, seen in opsoclonus-myoclonus-ataxia syndrome. The former is distinguished from cortical blindness by the presence of optic nerve hypoplasia and multiple pituitary deficiencies, whereas the latter is distinguished by the rapid and darting nature of the eye movements, irregular myoclonic jerks, and ataxia, as well as an association with tumors such as neuroblastoma as part of a paraneoplastic syndrome, or as a postinfectious sequela of certain viral or bacterial infections.

Coordination, Precision, and Gait Disorders

Cerebellar strokes may present with acute changes in the quality of movements consisting of incoordination (**ataxia**), loss of precision (**dysmetria**), difficulty with rapid alternating movements (**dysdiadochokinesia**), or gait disorders. Articulation of words (**dysarthria**) is also associated with cerebellar strokes and should be distinguished from aphasia. Infants and younger children may present with an inability to sit unsupported or reach for objects with the precision observed by caregivers prestroke. The older and cooperative child may be examined via the finger-to-nose and heel-to-shin tests: Patients with dysmetria and ataxia will lack coordination and precision, missing and oscillating around the target when using the affected limb. With dysarthria, comprehension and expression should be intact, though it may be difficult to understand the words being spoken. Cerebellar lesions may result in difficulty maintaining a standing position with the feet close together; gait is wide based and unsteady. Ataxia, dysmetria, and dysdiadochokinesia are ipsilateral to the cerebellar hemisphere that has suffered ischemia. If these deficits are bilateral and acute, alternative diagnoses like intoxication or inflammatory, infectious, or postinfectious pathologies must be considered, including acute cerebellar ataxia, cerebellitis, or hemophagocytic lymphohistiocytosis.

Children who present with cerebellar stroke may have significant headache and vomiting due to hydrocephalus from pressure in the posterior fossa crowding the fourth ventricle. More severe cases may result in obtundation from increased intracranial pressure. The blood supply to the cerebellum is via the vertebrobasilar system through the superior cerebellar arteries, the anterior inferior cerebellar arteries, and the posterior inferior cerebellar arteries. These vessels also supply the brainstem; cerebellar stroke is often accompanied by signs and symptoms of brainstem dysfunction.

Brainstem Syndromes

The brainstem contains many critical gray and white matter structures, such as the corticospinal tracts, the dorsal columns and spinothalamic tracts, cranial nerve nuclei, connections with the cerebellum, the reticular activating system, and ascending neurotransmitter-specific projection pathways. The vascular supply of the brainstem corresponds to its three levels, with the midbrain supplied by the superior cerebellar arteries (with the exception of the superior midbrain that is supplied by the posterior cerebral arteries), the pons supplied by the anterior inferior cerebellar arteries, and the medulla supplied by the posterior inferior cerebellar arteries. These three arteries arise from the vertebrobasilar system. Given the dense organization of these structures and the nature of their blood supply, symptoms of brainstem stroke are varied and localization is often challenging. Presenting symptoms, such as nausea or vertigo, are often vague and may mimic migraine, benign positional paroxysmal vertigo, seizure, or other sometimes less emergent diagnoses, leading to diagnostic delays and significant morbidity and mortality.

Table 37.7 describes classic **brainstem syndromes**. The hallmark of a brainstem stroke is **crossed paresis**, which consists of facial weakness ipsilateral to the stroke with contralateral limb hemiparesis. This pattern of findings is due to the notion that all cranial nerves, with the exception of cranial nerve IV, project ipsilaterally and the corticospinal tracts do not cross the midline until the cervicomedullary junction, rostral to the brainstem. Depending on whether a brainstem lesion is located more medially or dorsolaterally determines the nature of symptoms: medial brainstem strokes are primarily motor, whereas dorsolateral brainstem strokes are predominantly sensory. Dorsolateral brainstem strokes may also affect the cerebellar peduncles, leading to deficits in coordination and movement precision. Ventral pontine stroke from a basilar artery thrombosis or embolism may present with **locked-in syndrome**, in which the patient is awake and conscious but unable to move or communicate except for blinking and vertical eye movements. Locked-in syndrome must be distinguished from coma by determining the level of consciousness.

Seizures

Seizures are a common presenting symptom in pediatric stroke, occurring in the majority of neonates and ~30% of older children. Children who have had a stroke are also at risk for developing epilepsy, sometimes years after a stroke; in some cases, seizures may be refractory to treatment and may lead to adverse neurodevelopmental outcomes.

While seizures in neonatal AIS are common, symptoms can be subtle. Pauses in breathing or even true apneic spells may not be noticed if not accompanied by cyanosis or unless continuous cardiorespiratory monitoring is in place; myoclonic activity may be confused for benign neonatal movements. Electroencephalogram can assist in determining whether a particular event of concern is seizure-related. Perinatal stroke is a risk factor for **infantile spasms**, a rare and potentially devastating epileptic syndrome characterized by developmental delays, a specific electroencephalographic pattern termed *hypsarrhythmia*, and frequent seizures. The seizures—*epileptic spasms*—consist of an abrupt,

TABLE 37.7 Common Brainstem Syndromes, Cardinal Symptoms, Anatomic Localization, and Vascular Supply

Syndrome	Signs/Symptoms	Localization	Vascular Supply
Weber (superior alternating hemiplegia)	Ipsilateral CN III palsy, contralateral hemiparesis (including the lower face)	Medial midbrain/cerebral peduncle	Deep penetrating artery from posterior cerebral artery
Benedikt (paramedian midbrain)	Ipsilateral CN III palsy, contralateral involuntary movements	Ventral midbrain involving the red nucleus	Deep penetrating artery from posterior cerebral artery or paramedian penetrating branches of basilar artery
Nothnagel	Ipsilateral CN III palsy, contralateral dysmetria and limb ataxia	Superior cerebellar peduncle	Deep penetrating artery from posterior cerebral artery
Foville (inferior medial pontine)	Ipsilateral CN VI and VII (upper and lower facial weakness) with or without contralateral hemiparesis	Caudal pontine tegmentum involving the facial colliculus	Pontine perforator branches off the basilar artery
One and a half	Ipsilateral CN VI palsy, bilateral internuclear ophthalmoplegia	Paramedian pons involving the paramedian pontine reticular formation and medial longitudinal fasciculi	Paramedian pontine perforators off the basilar artery
Wallenberg (lateral medullary)	Ipsilateral facial and contralateral body hypoalgesia and thermoanesthesia, ipsilateral palatal weakness, dysphagia, dysarthria, nystagmus, vertigo, nausea/vomiting, ipsilateral Horner syndrome, skew deviation singultus	Lateral medulla	Posterior inferior cerebellar artery
Dejerine (medial medullary)	Ipsilateral tongue weakness and contralateral hemiparesis with or without contralateral loss of proprioception and vibratory sense	Medial medulla	Vertebral artery or anterior spinal artery

CN, cranial nerve.

Data from Eckerle BJ, Southerland AM. Bedside evaluation of the acute stroke patient. In: Barrett KM, Meschia JF, eds. *Stroke. Neurology in Practice*. Hoboken, NJ: Wiley-Blackwell; 2013:1Y15.

brief contraction followed by a more sustained but less intense tonic contraction lasting no more than several seconds. The spasms involve the muscles of the neck, trunk, and extremities. Spasms may be flexor, extensor, or mixed and occur in clusters typically after waking from sleep. Infantile spasms are considered a relative neurologic emergency, as treatment must be initiated soon after diagnosis to mitigate neurocognitive deterioration. Infantile spasms typically present months after stroke and are thought to be due to maladaptive changes in regulatory GABAergic pathways of brain development.

Disorders of Consciousness

Pediatric stroke may present with diffuse neurologic features such as alteration in consciousness or coma. Disorders of consciousness may arise from bilateral cerebral hemispheric, bi-thalamic, or brainstem infarctions; however, disordered consciousness may also be due to increased intracranial pressure from a large unilateral infarction leading to herniation and brainstem compression, in which case the **Cushing triad** of hypertension, bradycardia, and abnormal respiration may indicate the need for emergent intervention. Lastly, disordered consciousness may be secondary to prolonged seizures or the effects of medications given to control seizures.

STROKE SYNDROMES BY AGE

The risk factors and etiologies of stroke are diverse, are highly age dependent, and differ based on whether the stroke is ischemic or hemorrhagic, venous or arterial. The evaluation and management of stroke differ depending on the age of the patient and the clinical setting.

Despite these differences, the evaluation of a suspected acute stroke must be done emergently and should include verification of history, vital signs, comprehensive physical examination including detailed neurologic examination, laboratory studies, and neuroimaging. Establishing the *time at which the child was last seen normal* is crucial, as interventions aimed at reperfusing ischemic brain tissue are highly time-dependent. For children over the age of 2 years, examination should include the Pediatric National Institutes of Health (NIH) Stroke Scale (Table 37.8).

Acute laboratory studies should be tailored according to age and often include CBCs, electrolytes, basic chemistry, glucose, prothrombin time, international normalized ratio, partial thromboplastin time, and toxicology screen. These essential screening laboratories aid in detecting stroke mimics such as severe hypoglycemia or toxic ingestion and laboratory derangements that must be urgently addressed, as well as limitations to administer hyperacute therapies for stroke such as thrombolytics in select patients. Once the patient has been stabilized, neuroimaging usually occurs.

Imaging modality depends on acuity, age, and clinical status. In neonates, open fontanels and decreased bone mineralization allow for head ultrasonography to quickly evaluate for intraparenchymal or intraventricular hemorrhage. Outside the neonatal period, or when children present to the emergency department from home, noncontrast CT of the head (CTOH) is often performed first as it is widely available and fast, does not require sedation, is sensitive for acute hemorrhage, and may be used to rule out alternative diagnoses. In ischemic stroke, a noncontrast CTOH may be normal early after symptom onset or show findings of ischemia, which manifest as subtle hypodense areas. With time these hypodensities

TABLE 37.8   Pediatric NIH Stroke Scale: Instructions

1a. Level of Consciousness (LOC): For children age 2 yr and up, the investigator must choose a response, even if a full evaluation is prevented by such obstacles as an endotracheal tube, language barrier, or orotracheal trauma/bandages. A 3 is scored only if the patient makes no movement (other than reflexive posturing) in response to noxious stimulation. *For infants age 4 mo up to age 2 yr, multiply the score for this item by 3, and omit scoring items 1b and 1c.*

1b. LOC Questions: The patient is asked the month and their age. The answer must be correct; there is no partial credit for being close. Aphasic and stuporous patients who do not comprehend the questions will score 2. Patients unable to speak because of endotracheal intubation, orotracheal trauma, severe dysarthria from any cause, language barrier, or any other problem not secondary to aphasia are given a 1. It is important that only the initial answer be graded and that the examiner not "help" the patient with verbal or nonverbal cues.

   Modified for children, age 2 yr and up. A familiar family member must be present for this item: Ask the child, "How old are you?" or "How many years old are you?" for question number 1. Give credit if the child states the correct age or shows the correct number of fingers for their age. For the second question, ask the child, "Where is XX?", with XX referring to the name of the parent or other familiar family member present. Use the name for that person that the child typically uses (e.g., "mommy"). Give credit if the child correctly points to or gazes purposefully in the direction of the family member. Omit this item for infants age 4 mo up to age 2 yr. See comment under item 1a.

**1c. LOC Commands: The patient is asked to open and close the eyes (for children older than age 2 yr, this command to open and close the eyes is suitable *and can be scored as for adults)* and then to grip and release the nonparetic hand. *For children older than age 2 yr, substitute the command to grip the hand with the command "show me your nose" or "touch your nose."* Substitute another one-step command if the hands cannot be used. Credit is given if an unequivocal attempt is made but not completed due to weakness. If the patient does not respond to command, the task should be demonstrated to them (pantomime) and score the result (i.e., follows no, one, or two commands). Patients with trauma, amputation, or other physical impediments should be given suitable one-step commands. Only the first attempt is scored. *Omit this item for infants age 4 mo up to age 2 yr. See comment under item 1a.*

2. Best Gaze: Only horizontal eye movements will be tested. Voluntary or reflexive (oculocephalic) eye movements will be scored, but caloric testing is not done. If the patient has a conjugate deviation of the eyes that can be overcome by voluntary or reflexive activity, the score will be 1. If the patient has an isolated peripheral nerve paresis (CN III, IV, or VI), score a 1. Gaze is testable in all aphasic patients. Patients with ocular trauma, bandages, pre-existing blindness, or other disorder of visual acuity or fields should be tested with reflexive movements and a choice made by the investigator. Establishing eye contact and then moving about the patient from side to side will occasionally clarify the presence of a partial gaze palsy.

3. Visual: Visual fields (upper and lower quadrants) are tested by confrontation, using finger counting (for children older than 6 yr) or visual threat *(for children age 4 mo to 6 yr)* as appropriate. Patient must be encouraged, but if they look at the side of the moving fingers appropriately, this can be scored as normal. If there is unilateral blindness or enucleation, visual fields in the remaining eye are scored. Score 1 only if a clear-cut asymmetry, including quadrantanopia, is found. If patient is blind from any cause, score 3. Double simultaneous stimulation is performed at this point. If there is extinction, patient receives a 1 and the results are used to answer question 11.

4. Facial Palsy: Ask or use pantomime to encourage the patient to show teeth or raise eyebrows and close eyes. Score symmetry of grimace in response to noxious stimuli in the poorly responsive or noncomprehending patient. If facial trauma/bandages, orotracheal tube, tape, or other physical barrier obscures the face, these should be removed to the extent possible.

5 and 6. Motor Arm and Leg: The limb is placed in the appropriate position: extend the arms (palms down) 90 degrees (if sitting) or 45 degrees (if supine) and the legs 30 degrees (always tested supine). Drift is scored if the arm falls before 10 sec or the leg before 5 sec. *For children too immature to follow precise directions or uncooperative for any reason, power in each limb should be graded by observation of spontaneous or elicited movement according to the same two grading scheme, excluding the time limits.* The aphasic patient is encouraged using urgency in the voice and pantomime but not noxious stimulation. Each limb is tested in turn, beginning with the nonparetic arm. Only in the case of amputation or joint fusion at the shoulder or hip, **or immobilization by an IV board,** may the score be 9, and the examiner must clearly write the explanation for scoring as a 9.

7. Limb Ataxia: This item is aimed at finding evidence of a unilateral cerebellar lesion. Test with eyes open. In case of visual defect, ensure testing is done in intact visual field. The finger-nose-finger and heel-shin tests are performed on both sides, and ataxia is scored only if present out of proportion to weakness. *In children, substitute this task with reaching for a toy for the upper extremity, and kicking a toy or the examiner's hand, in children too young (under 5 yr) or otherwise uncooperative for the standard exam item.* Ataxia is absent in the patient who cannot understand or is paralyzed. Only in the case of amputation or joint fusion may the item be scored 9, and the examiner must clearly write the explanation for not scoring. In case of blindness, test by touching nose from extended arm position.

8. Sensory: Sensation or grimace to pin prick when tested, or withdrawal from noxious stimulus in the obtunded or aphasic patient. *For children too young or otherwise uncooperative for reporting gradations of sensory loss, observe for any behavioral response to pin prick, and score it according to the same scoring scheme as a "normal," "mildly diminished," or "severely diminished" response.* Only sensory loss attributed to stroke is scored as abnormal and the examiner should test as many body areas (arms [not hands], legs, trunk, face) as needed to accurately check for hemisensory loss. A score of 2, "severe or total," should only be given when a severe or total loss of sensation can be clearly demonstrated. Stuporous and aphasic patients will therefore probably score 1 or 0. The patient with brainstem stroke who has bilateral loss of sensation is scored 2. If the patient does not respond and is quadriplegic, score 2. Patients in a coma (item 1a = 3) are arbitrarily given a 2 on this item.

9. Best Language: A great deal of information about comprehension will be obtained during the preceding sections of the examination. *For children age 6 yr and up with normal language development before onset of stroke: The patient is asked to describe what is happening, to name the items on the naming sheet, and to read from the list of sentences.* Comprehension is judged from responses here as well as to all of the commands in the preceding general neurologic exam. If visual loss interferes with the tests, ask the patient to identify objects placed in the hand, repeat, and produce speech. The intubated patient should be asked to write. The patient in a coma (question 1a = 3) will arbitrarily score 3 on this item. The examiner must choose a score in the patient with stupor or limited cooperation, but a score of 3 should be used only if the patient is mute and follows no one-step commands. *For children age 2–6 yr (or older children with premorbid language disability), score this item based on observations of language comprehension and speech during the preceding examination. For infants age 4 mo to 2 yr, score for auditory alerting and orienting responses.*

10. Dysarthria: If the patient is thought to be normal, an adequate sample of speech must be obtained by asking the patient to read or repeat words from the list. If the patient has severe aphasia, the clarity of articulation of spontaneous speech can be rated. Only if the patient is intubated or has another physical barrier to producing speech may the item be scored 9, and the examiner must clearly write an explanation for not scoring. Do not tell the patient why they are being tested.

11. Extinction and Inattention (Formerly Neglect): For children age 2 yr and up: Sufficient information to identify neglect may be obtained during the prior testing. If the patient has a severe visual loss preventing visual double simultaneous stimulation, and the cutaneous stimuli are normal, the score is normal. If the patient has aphasia but does appear to attend to both sides, the score is normal. The presence of visual spatial neglect or anosognosia may also be taken as evidence of abnormality. Since the abnormality is scored only if present, the item is never untestable. **For children age 4 mo to 2 yr, score as a 1 if there is either a sensory or motor deficit; score as a 2 if there are both sensory and motor deficits on the general neurologic examination.**

CN, cranial nerve; NIH, National Institutes of Health.

Adapted from Ichord RN, Bastian R, Abraham L, et al. Interrater reliability of the Pediatric National Institutes of Health Stroke Scale (PedNIHSS) in a multicenter study. *Stroke.* 2011;42:613–617.

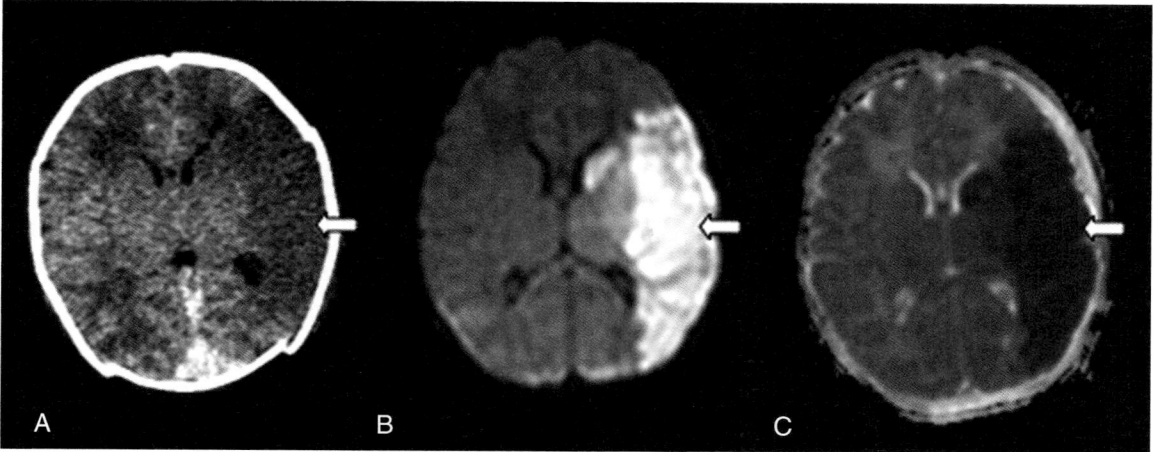

Fig. 37.9 Acute arterial ischemic stroke. CT and MRI demonstrate an arterial ischemic stroke in a 1-day-old term infant who presented with a right focal seizure. *A,* An axial CT image reveals hypodensity *(white arrow)* in the left middle cerebral artery (MCA) territory consistent with acute infarction. *B,* Axial MRI diffusion-weighted trace image of the same patient reveals a clearly demarcated area of infarct as a region of hyperintensity *(white arrow)* in the left MCA territory. *C,* Apparent diffusion coefficient map reveals region of signal hypointensity and restricted diffusion *(white arrow)* to match area of signal hyperintensity observed in *(B).* (With permission from Lehman LL, Rivkin MJ. Perinatal arterial ischemic stroke: presentation, risk factors, evaluation and outcome. *Pediatric Neurol.* 2014;51:760–768, Fig. 2.)

TABLE 37.9	Stroke Appearance According to Timing of Acquisition of MRI				
Timing	**DWI**	**ADC**	**T1**	**T2**	**FLAIR**
Hyperacute, 0–6 hr	Hyperintense	Hypointense			
Acute, 6–24 hr	Hyperintense	Hypointense	Hypointense	Hyperintense	Hyperintense
Subacute, 1–7 days	Hyperintense	Isointense	Hypointense	Hyperintense	Hyperintense
Chronic, >1 mo	Variable	Hyperintense	Hypointense	Hyperintense	Variable

ADC, apparent diffusion coefficient; DWI, diffusion-weighted imaging; FLAIR, fluid-attenuated inversion recovery.
From Tong E, Hou Q, Fiebach J, et al. The role of imaging in acute ischemic stroke. *Neurosurg Focus.* 2014;36:E3.

become more evident. Conversely, CTOH is very sensitive for hemorrhage, which is manifested by hyperintensity in the location of the bleeding. *Brain MRI that includes diffusion-weighted imaging (DWI) and apparent diffusion coefficient (ADC) sequences is more sensitive for the diagnosis of ischemic stroke.* Figure 37.9 demonstrates characteristic CT and MRI changes in acute ischemic stroke, while Table 37.9 describes the typical findings in stroke on MRI based on the timing of imaging. Often imaging of the intracranial and cervical vessels may be necessary and can be done with magnetic resonance angiography (MRA), computed tomography angiography (CTA), or a conventional angiography, depending on the circumstances of the patient. Pediatric stroke algorithms are useful in determining the most appropriate imaging of patients with stroke according to symptoms and availability of imaging modality (Fig. 37.10).

The outcome of stroke varies considerably by age, risk factors, etiology, and management. In general, up to 10% of affected children die, and more than half of the survivors incur a functional or cognitive neurologic deficit. Predictors of poor outcome are not well understood; establishing long-term rehabilitative care, decreasing recurrence risk, and screening for chronic complications of stroke, such as epilepsy and intellectual disability, can improve outcomes.

PERINATAL STROKE

Perinatal stroke is a diverse group of cerebrovascular injuries occurring between 20 weeks of fetal life and 28 days of postnatal life. Strokes affecting early brain development are estimated to have an incidence as high as 1 in 1,600. The consequences of these injuries include cerebral palsy, epilepsy, and cognitive and behavioral challenges. Presentation may be acute or remote, strokes may be due to arterial or venous processes, and injury may be ischemic or hemorrhagic.

Perinatal stroke can be divided broadly into neonatal stroke and presumed perinatal stroke based on the timing of presentation. Neonatal stroke presents acutely and symptomatically during the neonatal period—often within the first week of life—and consists of neonatal AIS, neonatal hemorrhagic stroke, and cerebral sinovenous thrombosis (CSVT). Presumed perinatal stroke presents remotely outside of the neonatal period, may be symptomatic or incidentally identified on neuroimaging, and consists of presumed perinatal AIS, presumed perinatal hemorrhagic stroke, and periventricular venous infarction. Stroke diagnosed in the fetus through the use of fetal imaging or on neuropathologic examination of stillborn children is referred to as in utero stroke and in survivors typically presents as presumed perinatal stroke.

Neonatal Stroke

Stroke is surprisingly common in the neonatal period. The incidence of neonatal AIS is as high as 1 in 2,200 live births, similar to the incidence of large-artery AIS in adults and more than 10 times greater than the incidence of AIS in children; the incidence in neonates born before 34 weeks' gestation is higher than that in term neonates. Neonatal

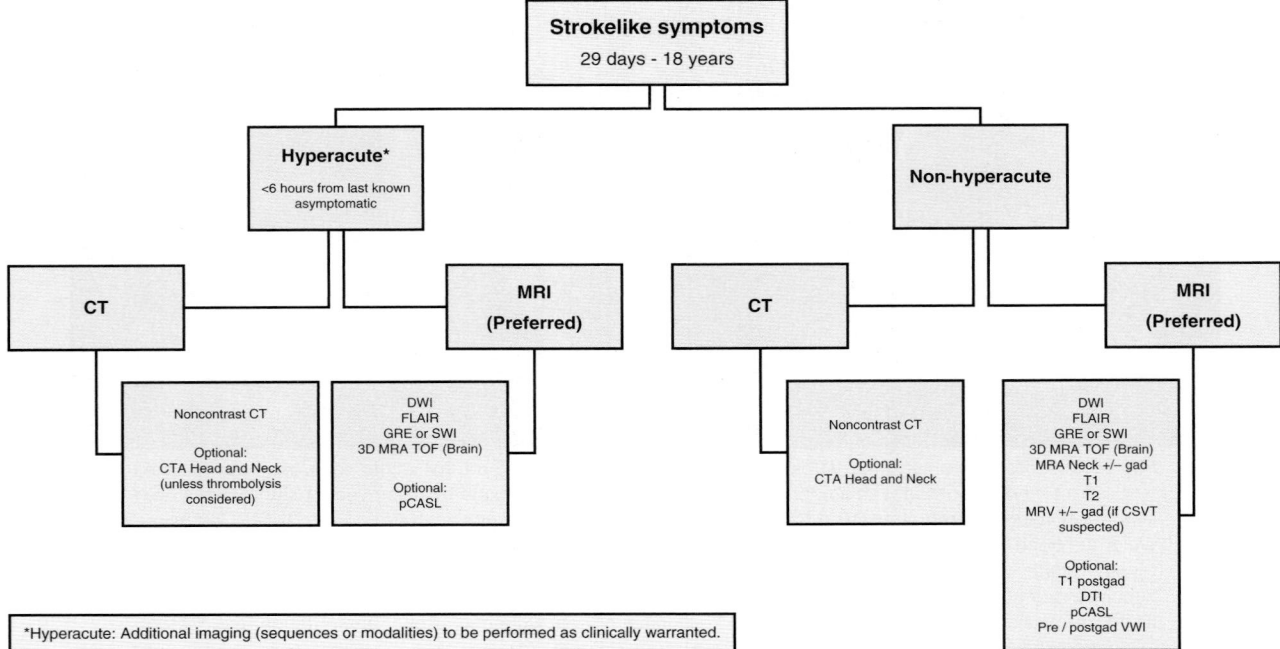

Fig. 37.10 Algorithm demonstrating proposed imaging modalities according to symptomatology and modality of image. CSVT, cerebral sinovenous thrombosis; CT, computed tomography (of the head); CTA, computed tomographic angiography; DTI, diffusion tensor imaging; DWI, diffusion-weighted imaging; FLAIR, fluid-attenuated inversion recovery; gad, gadolinium; GRE, gradient echo; MRA, magnetic resonance angiography; MRI, magnetic resonance imaging (of the brain); pCASL, pseudo-continuous arterial spin labeling; SWI, susceptibility-weighted imaging; TOF, time of flight; VWI, vessel wall imaging. (From Mirsky DM, Beslow LA, Amlie-Lefond C, et al. Pathways for neuroimaging of childhood stroke. *Pediatr Neurol.* 2017;69:11–23, Fig. 5.)

hemorrhagic stroke is less common, affecting approximately 1 in 9,500 live births; neonatal CSVT is even less common.

Clinical Presentation and Mimics

Neonatal AIS is the most common type of perinatal stroke, and focal motor seizures are the most frequent presenting symptom, occurring in up to 90% of affected term newborns. Other presenting symptoms include encephalopathy in ~66% of affected neonates, feeding difficulties, apnea, and tone abnormalities. Lateralized findings, most typically motor weakness or decreased tone, may be present, though their absence does not exclude cerebral infarction. Furthermore, diminished extremity movement on the side of a focal seizure may represent postictal paralysis rather than paresis from upper motor neuron injury caused by cerebral infarction. Preterm neonates with AIS are commonly asymptomatic and may be incidentally diagnosed on routine screening cerebral ultrasound. Preterm infants with AIS most frequently present with respiratory difficulties, though seizures, feeding difficulty, and abnormal tone may occur as well. Presenting features for neonates with AIS are summarized in Table 37.10. Neonates with hemorrhagic stroke and with CSVT present similarly, with a combination of encephalopathy, seizures, feeding and respiratory difficulties, and focal neurologic deficits. Neonates with hemorrhagic stroke may also have a bulging fontanelle or widening of the cranial suture lines.

Seizures are the most common presentation of neonatal stroke, and are also the most common stroke mimic. Neonatal seizures may occur in the setting of hypoxic ischemic encephalopathy (HIE), cerebral malformations, meningitis, sepsis, acute metabolic derangements, inborn errors of metabolism, kernicterus, neonatal abstinence syndrome, and

TABLE 37.10 Symptoms Associated with Perinatal Arterial Ischemic Strokes (AIS)

Symptom	% of Cases
Neonatal AIS in Term Infants	
Seizures (usually focal motor)	69–90
Hemiparesis	~30
Impaired level of consciousness	39
Abnormal tone	38–46
Respiratory difficulties	26
Feeding difficulties	24
Neonatal AIS in Preterm Infants	
Respiratory distress or apnea	83
Seizures	30
Abnormal feeding	26
Abnormal tone	22
Presumed Perinatal AIS	
Early hand preference (<2 yr of age)	81–86
Hand fisting	
Seizures	14–15
Gaze preference	5

From Lehman LL, Rivkin MJ. Perinatal arterial ischemic stroke: presentation, risk factors, evaluation, and outcome. *Pediatr Neurol.* 2014;51:760–768.

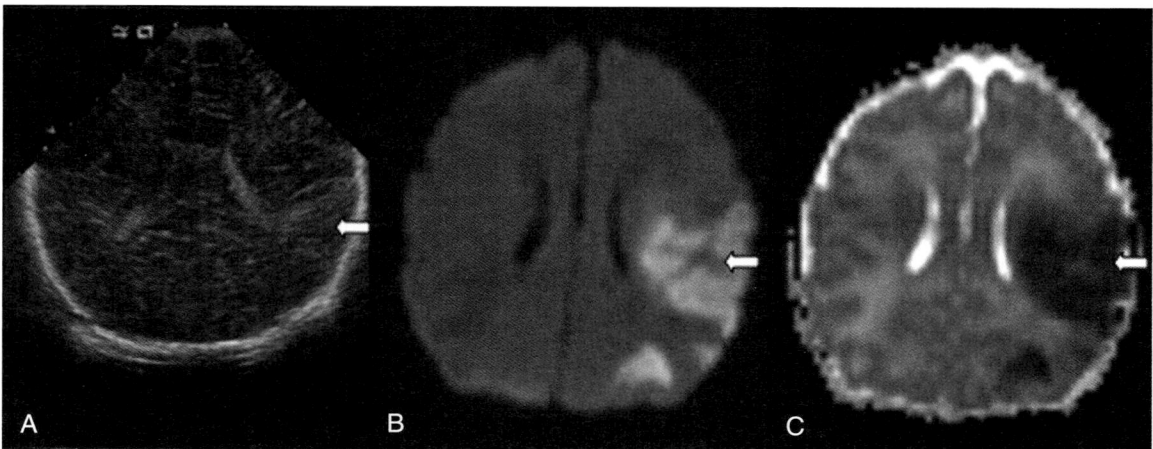

Fig. 37.11 Neonatal arterial ischemic stroke. Ultrasound (US) and MRI of neonatal arterial ischemic stroke in a 1-day-old term infant who presented with a right focal seizure. *A,* US reveals hyperechogenicity in the left cerebral hemisphere (indicated by *white arrow*), concerning for ischemic injury. *B,* Axial MRI diffusion-weighted trace image of the same patient reveals well-defined hyperintensity (indicated by *white arrow*) in the left middle cerebral artery (MCA) territory. *C,* Apparent diffusion coefficient map of the matching slice observed in *(B)* reveals corresponding hypointensity (indicated by *white arrow*) in the left MCA territory. (From Lehman LL, Rivkin MJ. Perinatal arterial ischemic stroke: presentation, risk factors, evaluation, and outcome. *Pediatr Neurol.* 2014;51:760–768, Fig. 1.)

TABLE 37.11	Location of Arterial Strokes in Perinatal Arterial Ischemic Stroke Based on Gestational Age	
Gestational Age	**Location of Arterial Stroke**	**% of Cases**
Full-term neonate	Cortical branch strokes	59
Preterm neonate (overall)	Lenticulostriate (overall)	39
<28–32 wk of gestation	Lenticulostriate	
32–36 wk of gestation	Cortical branch infarcts	

genetic epilepsy syndromes. The timing of seizures, as well as associated findings, can assist in distinguishing etiology: Neonates with seizures secondary to stroke typically have seizure onset after 24 hours of life, have focal motor activity, and remain lucid interictally. In contrast, neonates with HIE typically have seizures within the first 12 hours of life, have an associated antenatal event such as fetal distress or perinatal asphyxia, and have encephalopathy of varying degrees. Neonates with meningitis or sepsis often have associated temperature and hemodynamic instability and may have metabolic derangements and acid-base disturbances. Neonates with inborn errors of metabolism often have hypoglycemia and acid-base disturbances, can have hyperammonemia depending on the metabolic disorder, and may have progressive encephalopathy.

Risk Factors of Neonatal Stroke

For neonatal AIS, the low recurrence rate of <2% suggests the pathophysiology is related to a process unique to the perinatal state. The left hemisphere is the most commonly involved area, with exclusive involvement of the middle cerebral artery territory in up to 90% of perinatal AIS strokes (Fig. 37.11), though the location of stroke varies based on gestational age (Table 37.11). Risk factors for neonatal AIS can be broadly categorized as maternal, fetal, and placental (Table 37.12). Placentally derived emboli may lodge in cerebral vessels.

Congenital heart defects involving right-to-left shunts through septal defects increase the risk of embolic stroke. Congenital defects of coagulation (factor VIII, protein C, protein S, antithrombin III deficiency, and others) or sepsis-induced disseminated intravascular coagulation may also result in neonatal embolic stroke. Fetal head trauma during labor and delivery that results in endothelial damage to cerebral vessels occasionally leads to thrombosis and resultant focal ischemia of the brain. Polycythemia and hypotension can each lead to intravascular stasis and abnormalities in flow, resulting in cerebrovascular thrombosis in neonates. Meningitis and encephalitis cause diffuse or localized thrombosis as a result of vascular inflammation, leading to hemostasis and thrombosis. Lastly, specific neonatal cardiac conditions requiring extracorporeal membrane oxygenation (ECMO) may predispose the neonate to AIS. Many have an unknown etiology.

Neonatal hemorrhagic stroke or **intraparenchymal hemorrhage** (IPH), in the absence of intraventricular hemorrhage (IVH), occurs most commonly in full-term infants. Hemorrhage into the parenchyma of the cerebral hemispheres can be caused by head trauma, vascular malformation (Fig. 37.12), coagulopathy, thrombocytopenia, tumor, or infarction. A common cause of prenatal, intrapartum, and postnatal hemorrhage is alloimmune thrombocytopenia, caused by acquired antiplatelet antibodies when a mother becomes sensitized to paternal antigens on fetal platelets. Maternal immune thrombocytopenia may also affect the fetus, producing thrombocytopenia in utero; however, the incidence of neonatal cerebral hemorrhage is much lower in immune thrombocytopenia than in alloimmune thrombocytopenia. **Vitamin K–deficient bleeding** should be considered as a cause of intracranial hemorrhage for breast-fed full-term neonates or for neonates who were not administered parenteral vitamin K shortly after birth. In the absence of recognized coagulation or anatomic abnormalities, cerebral hemispheric IPH may also be due to hemorrhagic conversion of a previous infarction.

In premature infants, IPH most often occurs in conjunction with severe IVH (Fig. 37.13). Hemorrhage from the friable, unsupported germinal matrix leads to accumulation of intraventricular blood, and

TABLE 37.12 Risk Factors for Perinatal Arterial Ischemic Stroke (AIS)

Type of Risk Factor	Risk Factors
Term Infants with Neonatal AIS	
Maternal	Thrombophilia
	Infertility
	Prolonged rupture of membranes
	Preeclampsia or gestational hypertension
	Smoking
	Intrauterine growth restriction
	Infection
	Maternal fever during delivery
	Smoking
Fetal	Thrombophilia (MTHFR variant, FVL, prothrombin gene variant, protein C/S deficiency)
	Congenital heart disease
	Arteriopathy
	Twin-twin transfusion syndrome
	Hypoglycemia
	Perinatal asphyxia
	Infection (sepsis/meningitis)
	Need for resuscitation
	Apgar score of <7 at 5 min
Placental	Chorioamnionitis
	Placental infarcts
	Distal villous immaturity
	Placenta weighing <10th percentile
Preterm Infants with Neonatal AIS	
Maternal	Infection
	Gestational bleeding
	Maternal smoking
	Maternal drug use
Fetal	Twin-twin transfusion syndrome
	Twin demise
	Abnormal fetal heart rate
	Hypoglycemia
	Thrombophilia (MTHFR variant, FVL)
Presumed Perinatal AIS	
Maternal	Preeclampsia
	Infection
	Gestational bleeding
	Gestational diabetes
	Thrombophilia
Fetal	Congenital heart disease

MTHFR, methylenetetrahydrofolate reductase deficiency; FVL, factor V Leiden deficiency.
Modified from Lehman LL, Rivkin MJ. Perinatal arterial ischemic stroke: presentation, risk factors, evaluation, and outcome. *Pediatr Neurol.* 2014;51:760–768.

often ventricular distention. These events, in turn, cause impairment of blood flow in the medullary veins located in the periventricular white matter, preventing blood drainage into the greater cerebral venous system. Eventually, the periventricular venous congestion leads to ischemia and a resultant venous infarction. If there continues to be difficulty with cerebrospinal fluid production and reabsorption dynamics, the infant may develop posthemorrhagic hydrocephalus and in some instances may need cerebrospinal fluid diversion procedures.

Risk factors for **neonatal CSVT** include thrombophilia, infection, dehydration, polycythemia, congenital heart disease, and ECMO (Table 37.13). The lesions associated with cerebral venous thrombosis include thrombosis in the deep or superficial veins, venous infarction, and hemorrhage (Fig. 37.14). The hemorrhage that typically accompanies CSVT is a result of the increased venous and capillary hydrostatic pressure due to the presence of the clot causing extravasation of fluid and red blood cells.

Evaluation and Management

Imaging. The evaluation of the neonate with suspected stroke requires neuroimaging. Head ultrasonography is typically readily available and is a reliable bedside tool that is often performed initially, as ultrasonography can rapidly detect areas of increased echogenicity in the cerebral cortex that correspond with hemorrhage. In especially severe cases of ischemia, increased echogenicity of injured subcortical structures such as the thalamus and basal ganglia can also be appreciated. Ischemic cortical injury involving the territory of the middle cerebral artery (frontal and parietal lobe regions surrounding the central sulcus) is better revealed by ultrasonography than are other vascular territories. The principal advantages of cranial ultrasonography are its easy portability to the patient's bedside and lack of radiation exposure to the infant; however, reliability is highly operator dependent. CT is usually not recommended due to the radiation exposure as well as the low sensitivity for neonatal AIS in the acute phase. However, CT is sensitive for detecting hemorrhagic stroke and other forms of extra-axial hemorrhagic processes.

MRI is the imaging modality of choice to confirm the diagnosis of neonatal stroke. DWI sequences on MRI can identify areas of recent infarct within hours of onset, earlier than conventional T1- and T2-weighted images. Subsequent images can show chronic changes such as cerebral atrophy, paucity of white matter, delayed myelination, and ventriculomegaly. MRI can be complemented with MRA of the cerebral and neck arteries to assess for arterial occlusion, dissection, anatomic abnormalities, or other lesions. If there is concern for neonatal CSVT, magnetic resonance venography (MRV) should be performed to detect a thrombus or absent flow in the intracranial venous system.

Laboratory Testing. Laboratory testing for the wide variety of etiologic factors underlying stroke should be conducted according to the presentation and symptoms. Investigations should include screening for infection, liver dysfunction, coagulopathy, prothrombotic states, inborn errors of metabolism, urea cycle disorders, and mitochondrial abnormalities. Placenta may be submitted for pathologic examination.

Management

Treatment for neonatal stroke is largely supportive. Neuroprotective approaches are employed to maintain homeostasis in oxygen, temperature, hydration, glucose, and hemodynamics. Electroencephalogram should be performed to screen for interictal abnormalities and subclinical seizures. Seizures are often self-limited though if persistent may be controlled with antiseizure medicines. With recurrence rates of neonatal AIS being low, the use of antithrombotic medications is not recommended unless there is a persistent source of embolism or a severe thrombophilia is documented. In neonatal CSVT, anticoagulation may be considered on a case-by-case basis, especially if there is thrombus propagation on serial imaging. For neonates with hemorrhagic stroke, investigation and correction

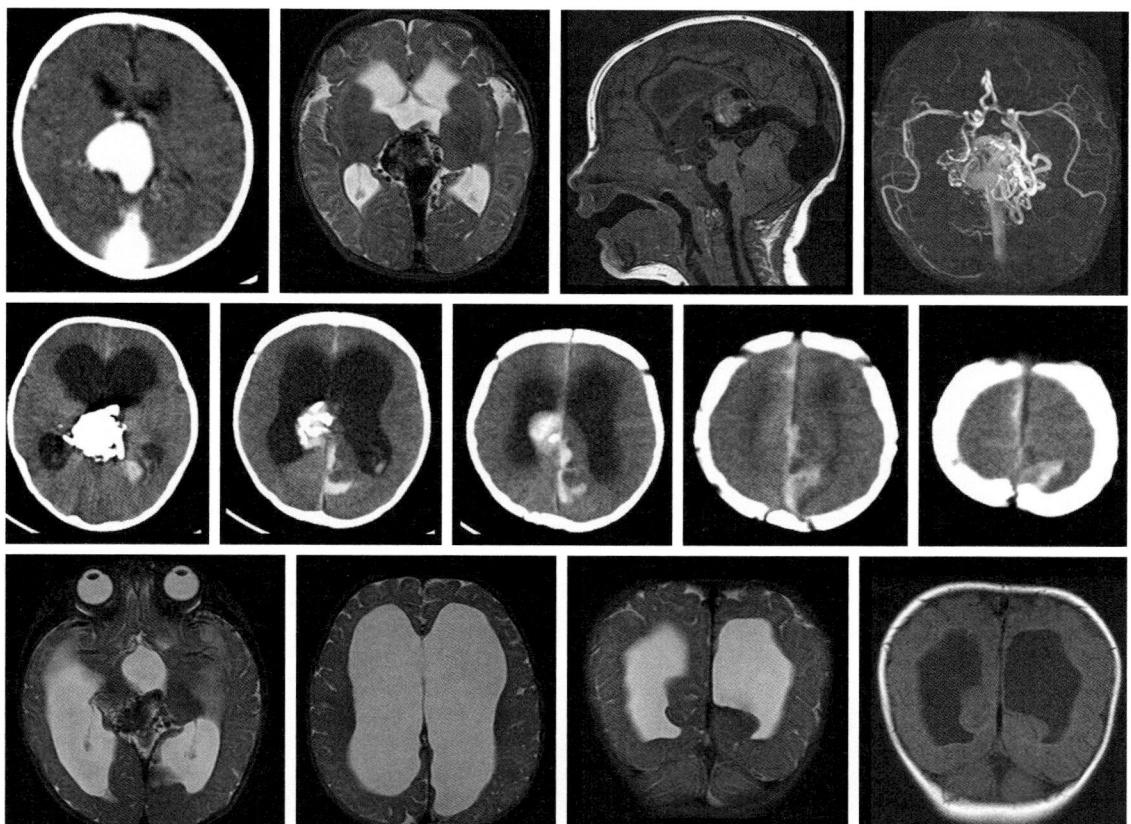

Fig. 37.12 Neonatal vein of Galen malformation and intraventricular hemorrhage. A 5-day-old female born at 38 weeks was noted to be drowsy with poor feeding. She had signs of cardiac failure. A CT scan *(top left)* demonstrates vein of Galen aneurysmal malformation, which was partly treated by transarterial glue embolization without complication but with significant residual arteriovenous shunting (MR images, *top row*). Following a second embolization procedure, there was acute clinical deterioration with signs of raised intracranial pressure *(middle row)*. CT shows acute intraventricular hemorrhage and hydrocephalus, and a left parieto-occipital lobe low-density lesion (*middle*, images 1–3) with adjacent subarachnoid and subdural hematoma (*middle*, images 4 and 5). Some linear hyperdensity was believed to be due to thrombus within the persistent falcine sinus (*middle*, images 4 and 5). Follow-up imaging shows maturation of the focal left parieto-occipital lesion in keeping with an infarct *(bottom row)*, which is probably venous in origin. (From Gunny RS, Lin D. Imaging of pediatric stroke. *Magn Reson Imaging Clin North Am.* 2012;20:1–33, Fig. 18.)

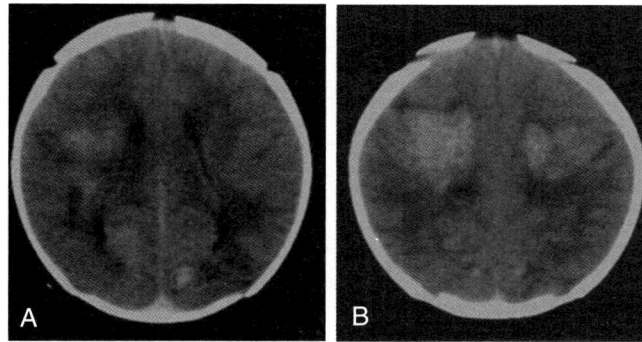

Fig. 37.13 Neonatal intraventricular and intraparenchymal hemorrhages. A term baby delivered by cesarean section for thick meconium and late decelerations, Apgar scores of 1, 6, and 8 (at 1, 5, and 10 minutes), presented with neonatal seizures on the first day of life. *A* and *B*, Axial head CT images show bilateral frontal, parietal, and scattered occipital hemorrhages in the periventricular and subcortical white matter, the largest in the frontal centrum semiovale. (From Gunny RS, Lin D. Imaging of perinatal stroke. *Magn Reson Imaging Clin North Am.* 2012;20:1–33, Fig. 22.)

of bleeding diatheses are crucial. Ruptured vascular lesions may require prompt surgical correction. Acute decompressive craniectomy or hematoma evacuation is rarely performed though may be required. Regardless of the type of stroke or timing, neonates should be referred to rehabilitation therapies and be screened routinely for developmental delays and learning disabilities, especially in the school-age years.

Outcomes

The mortality rate for neonatal AIS is low at 0.16 per 100,000 live births. Stroke recurrence occurs in about 2% of neonates, most of whom have thrombophilia, congenital heart disease, or an arteriopathy. Chronic motor deficits occur in up to 60% of neonates with AIS; infarction in the basal ganglia or posterior limb of the internal capsule in term neonates correlates with long-term hemiparesis. Other long-term sequelae in neonatal AIS include language delays and behavioral disorders such as attention deficit or hyperactivity. Almost half of neonates with AIS develop epilepsy as a result of their stroke.

Developmental outcome in full-term infants with hemorrhagic stroke depends on the location, extent, and underlying cause.

TABLE 37.13	**Risk Factors for Neonatal Cerebral Sinovenous Thrombosis**	
Type of Risk Factor	**Risk Factors (Estimated % of Cases)**
Maternal	Preeclampsia
	Diabetes
Fetal/neonatal	Acute neonatal illness (61–84%)
	Dehydration
	Infection
	Meningitis
	Congenital heart disease
	Thrombophilia (same as in arterial; 15–20%)
	ECMO
	Complicated delivery
	Polycythemia
	Dehydration

ECMO, extracorporeal membrane oxygenation.

Posthemorrhagic hydrocephalus is predictive of abnormal outcomes, including motor impairment and cognitive delay. Epilepsy develops in up to 15% of affected patients. In premature infants, the simultaneous occurrence of IVH with IPH carries high risk for major motor deficits and marked cognitive impairment.

Outcomes of CSVT are difficult to discern due to the high incidence of hemorrhagic complications and their attendant mortality rate, which approaches 20%. Factors associated with a higher risk of adverse outcome include the presence of infarcts, bilateral cerebral involvement, and neurologic comorbidities. Neonates with cerebral venous thrombosis and thalamic hemorrhage are at risk for development of late-onset epilepsy with electrographic status epilepticus of slow wave sleep, which may be associated with cognitive and behavioral sequelae.

Presumed Perinatal Stroke

The prevalence of presumed perinatal stroke is difficult to establish given the large number of minimally symptomatic children or those with delayed presentations, but it is estimated to be around 40 per 100,000.

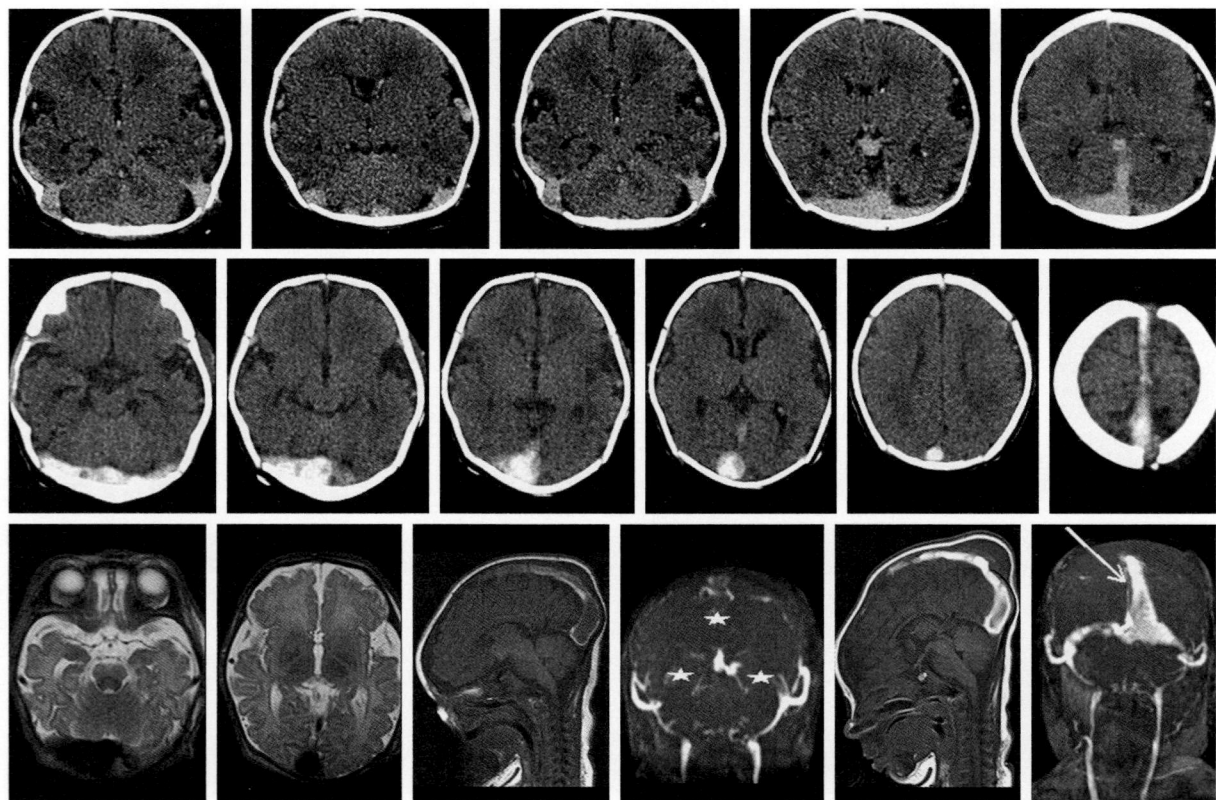

Fig. 37.14 Neonatal cerebral sinovenous thrombosis. A term male neonate was hypotonic at birth with poor respiratory effort requiring resuscitation. Initial CT *(top row)* on day 2 of life shows diffuse brain edema with expanded and hyperdense transverse and sagittal sinuses, torcula, and internal cerebral veins as well as the cerebral cortical veins. CT performed on day 9 *(middle row)* shows resolution of the cerebral edema and increased density of the thrombus within the transverse sinus, torcula, and superior sagittal sinus. MRI on day 9 *(bottom left,* images 1–4) shows mild diffuse cerebral atrophy but no focal venous infarcts, with a persistent thrombus and no flow on the magnetic resonance venography *(stars).* Follow-up MRI on day 15 *(bottom right,* images 5 and 6) shows the evolution of thrombus signal intensity to methemoglobin. Note the effect of T1 shortening within the thrombosed sagittal and transverse sinuses and torcula, mimicking flow within the sinuses *(arrow).* (From Gunny RS, Lin D. Imaging of perinatal stroke. *Magn Reson Imaging Clin North Am.* 2012;20:1–33, Fig. 10.)

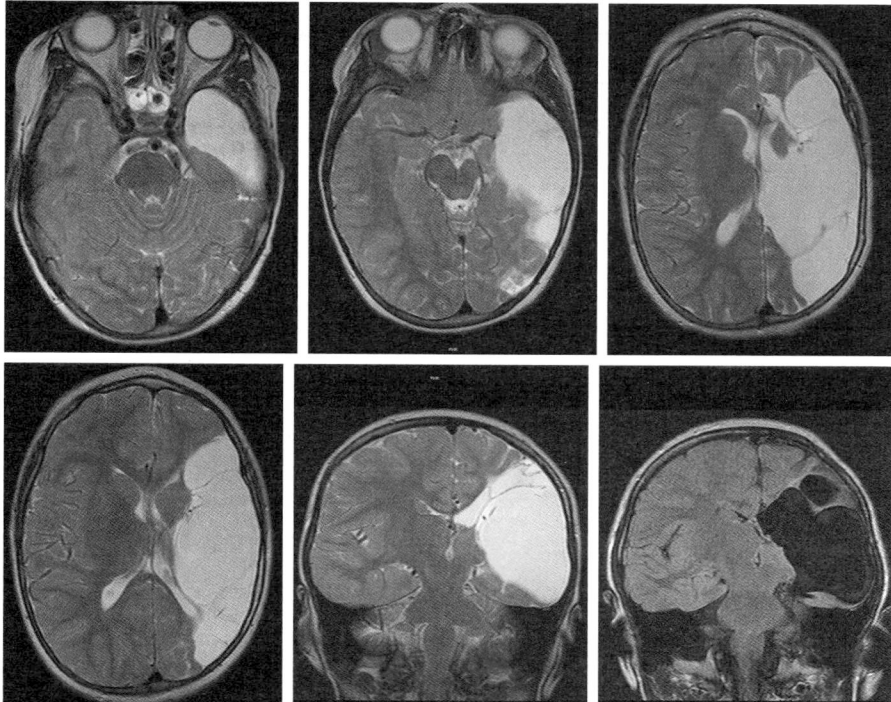

Fig. 37.15 Presumed perinatal arterial ischemic stroke (AIS). MRI of a 5-year-old girl with long-standing right hemiplegia and intractable epilepsy secondary to a left-sided infarct. Note the large area of cystic cavitation in the left temporal (*top left* and *middle* images), frontal (*top right* image), and parietal lobes (*top right* and *bottom left* images) in the extended left middle cerebral artery territory (with some additional anterior choroidal involvement, and atrophy of the left thalamus; *bottom left* image). The left hemicranium is smaller, and there is some expansion of the left calvarial diploic space. There is three-site involvement of the basal ganglia, superficial cortex, and posterior limb of the internal capsule (*bottom row* images). There is imaging evidence of Wallerian degeneration with atrophy, and signal hyperintensity suggestive of gliosis in the ventral midbrain and pons (*bottom middle* and *right* images). (From Gunny RS, Lin D. Imaging of perinatal stroke. *Magn Reson Imaging Clin North Am.* 2012;20:1–33, Fig. 5.)

The risk factors for presumed perinatal stroke are similar to those for neonatal stroke.

Clinical Presentation and Mimics

One of the most frequent presentations of presumed perinatal stroke is **early hand preference** with asymmetric reaching. In patients with early hand preference, neurologic examination may reveal a varied spectrum of impairment, from subtle decrease in hand dexterity to clear paresis with spasticity in the affected limb. Periventricular venous infarctions are more likely associated with lower extremity impairment, whereas presumed perinatal AIS is more likely associated with upper extremity weakness. Mimics of stroke-related early hand preference include brain malformations and brachial plexus injury.

Presumed perinatal stroke frequently presents as symptomatic localization-related epilepsy. Seizure semiology is variable, ranging from focal seizures without alterations in consciousness to generalized seizures with or without focal onset. Seizures may be subtle and in some instances may consist only of electrographic status epilepticus of slow wave sleep, which may present with developmental delays or regression. On some occasions, patients may present with infantile spasms.

Evaluation, Management, and Outcome

MRI of the brain is the imaging modality of choice for presumed perinatal stroke, as MRI establishes the location, extent, and severity of the stroke and can identify other lesions, such as gray matter heterotopia or other brain malformations that may produce similar symptoms. Patients with presumed perinatal AIS may have a porencephalic cyst, an area of cystic encephalomalacia in the location of a brain insult that usually involves the cortex and subcortical structures. In cases of perinatal periventricular infarction, MRI may demonstrate periventricular tissue loss, gliosis, and hemosiderin deposition, which may lead to variable degrees of ventricle deformation and corpus callosum tissue loss (Fig. 37.15).

Given the high rate of symptomatic epilepsy in presumed perinatal stroke, especially in presumed perinatal AIS, assessing for the possibility of seizures, including obtaining an EEG when the history is concerning, is essential. Interictal abnormalities such as spikes or sharp waves may be seen and represent a sign of hyperexcitability and consequent risk for seizures. There may be areas of focal slowing or lower-amplitude waveforms that correspond to areas of focal cerebral dysfunction. These focal abnormalities typically correspond to the location of the stroke; however, there may be additional diffuse findings such as generalized slowing of the background brain wave rhythm, which represents an encephalopathic state. There may also be generalized, multifocal spikes or sharp waves, which may signify the development of an epileptic encephalopathy. If present, seizures may be controlled with antiepileptic medications.

Once the diagnosis of presumed perinatal stroke has been made, early-intervention rehabilitation therapies must be initiated. Patients should be screened for cognitive impairment and learning disabilities even if not manifesting these complaints; deficits may include

TABLE 37.14   Symptoms of Strokes in Children Based on Etiology

Symptoms/Signs	ARTERIAL ISCHEMIC STROKES %	HEMORRHAGIC STROKES %	CEREBRAL VENOUS THROMBOSIS* Symptoms/Signs	%
Hemiparesis	70–80	35	Headache	75
Facial weakness	40–60	35	Altered consciousness	55
Speech disturbance	30–40	10	Focal deficits	40–50
Visual changes	5–15	20	Seizures	25
Limb ataxia	20–25	5		
Focal numbness	20	<5		
Vomiting	10–20	55		
Headache	25–45	75		
Decreased level of consciousness	20–40	50		
Seizures	15–30	20		
Vertigo	10	NDA		
Diplopia	3	NDA		
Papilledema	1	NDA		
No lateralizing symptoms	35	65		
No neurologic signs	10	60		
GCS ≥14	85	60		
GCS 9–13	15	20		
GCS ≤8	0	20		

*Ichord RN, Benedict SL, Chan AK, et al. Paediatric cerebral sinovenous thrombosis: findings of the International Paediatric Stroke Study. *Arch Dis Child*. 2015;100:174–179.

GCS, Glasgow Coma Scale; NDA, no data available.

Data pooled from Mallick AA, Ganesan V, Kirkham FJ, et al. Childhood arterial ischaemic stroke incidence, presenting features, and risk factors: a prospective population-based study. *Lancet Neurol*. 2014;13:35–43; Yock-Corrales A, Mackay MT, Mosley I, et al. Acute childhood arterial ischemic and hemorrhagic stroke in the emergency department. *Ann Emerg Med*. 2011;58:156–163; Wintermark M, Hills NK, deVeber GA, et al. Arteriopathy diagnosis in childhood arterial ischemic stroke: results of the vascular effects of infection in pediatric stroke study. *Stroke*. 2014;45:3597–3605; Lynch J, Hirtz DG, DeVeber G, et al. Report of the National Institute of Neurological Disorders and Stroke Workshop on Perinatal and Childhood Stroke. *Pediatrics*. 2002;109:116–123.

visuospatial, executive, and attention difficulties and may require comprehensive neuropsychological evaluation to identify.

STROKE IN CHILDREN

Stroke in older infants and children is best categorized in three different groups: AIS, intracranial hemorrhage, and venous stroke. For all three groups the clinical presentation is similar, but the risk factors, evaluation, management, and outcomes vary significantly. The incidence of stroke in children declines after the neonatal stage and remains low until mid-adolescence. Biological males have a 1.25 times higher relative risk of stroke when compared to biological females, even adjusting for trauma.

Children with stroke are more likely to present similarly to adults, with focal neurologic deficits; children are more likely to experience delays in recognition and diagnostic evaluation. Diagnostic delays are multifactorial in etiology, though contributing factors include low index of suspicion for pediatric stroke as well as the higher prevalence of stroke mimics in children. Prompt recognition is essential, as children may be candidates for hyperacute therapies such as thrombolysis or thrombectomy in cases of AIS, anticoagulation in cases of venous stroke, or neuroprotective care protocols regardless of etiology.

Presenting symptoms are largely dependent on the type of stroke and the brain region affected (Table 37.14). Possible mimics also vary depending on the nature of the stroke; for patients who present with acute unilateral weakness, common differential diagnoses include postictal hemiparesis (Todd paralysis), brain tumor, hemiplegic migraine, trauma, CNS infection, and conversion disorder. Postictal hemiparesis is typically preceded by clinical seizure activity, though occasionally the seizure activity may be clinically inapparent or the hemiparesis may have onset during the seizure itself. As opposed to the persistent unilateral weakness associated with stroke, postictal hemiparesis is typically transient. Patients who present with hemiplegic migraine generally have associated headache and oftentimes a family history of migraine. Acute hemiparesis with migraine is believed to reflect the involvement of the cerebral circulation derived from the carotid artery. When the vertebrobasilar circulation is involved in migraine, symptoms such as ataxia, cortical blindness, and cranial nerve dysfunction may occur as well.

Rarer mimics include CNS inflammatory conditions such as acute disseminated encephalomyelitis, which is characterized by a coincident encephalopathy, acute flaccid myelitis, alternating hemiplegia of childhood, hypertensive encephalopathy, and strokelike migraine attacks after radiation therapy (**SMART**) syndrome. Thorough clinical examination, history taking, and neuroimaging can discriminate between these conditions and stroke (see Table 37.5). For patients who present with other focal neurologic deficits or alteration in awareness, appropriate differential diagnoses must be considered according to clinical context.

Ischemic Stroke in Children

Risk Factors and Etiology

Ischemic stroke in children is associated with diverse risk factors (Table 37.15); however, despite thorough evaluation, up to one third of childhood AIS is classified as idiopathic. The Childhood AIS Standardized Classification and Diagnostic Evaluation (CASCADE) criteria are used to classify stroke presentation and distribution, offering excellent interrater reliability and consistency when describing pediatric stroke (Fig. 37.16).

Arteriopathies. Arteriopathies are cerebrovascular conditions associated with vessel wall abnormalities and may be unilateral or bilateral, be focal or diffuse, affect small vessels or large, be transient or progressive, and affect different areas within the cerebral vessels. Arteriopathies may be isolated conditions or part of a systemic illness.

Moyamoya arteriopathy is characterized by endothelial proliferation, fibrosis, and intimal thickening within the terminal portion of the internal carotid arteries, leading to progressive narrowing and occlusion. Resultant proliferation of collateral vessels from the basilar skull circulation creates an intricate latticework of compensatory blood flow that has a characteristic appearance: moyamoya means "hazy" or "puff of smoke" and reflects findings seen on conventional angiography (Fig. 37.17). Children usually present with acute hemiplegia as a result of uncompensated occlusion of the internal carotid artery. Because the anatomic abnormality is often bilateral, the hemiplegia may alternate. *Primary or idiopathic* moyamoya demonstrates a genetic predisposition (*ACTA2, GUCY1A3, RNF213* genes) and occurs in the absence of associated conditions, whereas the designation *moyamoya syndrome* is given when the progressive distal internal carotid artery occlusion is secondary to a primary disorder such as sickle cell disease, neurofibromatosis, trisomy 21, tuberculous meningitis, or fibromuscular dysplasia.

Sickle cell disease arteriopathy is a significant source of morbidity in patients with sickle cell disease. By the age of 20 years, approximately 11% of children with sickle cell disease will have had a symptomatic stroke; up to 40% have silent cerebral infarcts in which no overt symptoms occur but changes are seen on brain imaging. Children with sickle cell disease who have silent infarctions may demonstrate school dysfunction or headache as the only manifestation of neurologic involvement of the disease. Stroke recurrences are common.

The arteriopathy often involves the internal carotid or middle cerebral arteries, and in some cases moyamoya syndrome or intracranial hemorrhage can develop. Stroke may occur within the context of a sickle cell vaso-occlusive crisis or may be an isolated event, and typically occurs in watershed distributions between two cerebrovascular territories, affecting both the gray and white matter of the cortex. The proposed pathophysiologic mechanisms consist of both sickling-related occlusion and progressive stenosis in cerebral vessels. Sickled red blood cells (RBCs) flowing through arteries and capillaries activate endothelial proliferation in large vessels, ultimately leading to stenosis. Angiography demonstrates large-vessel vasculopathy in the internal carotid arteries and middle cerebral arteries; microscopic examination reveals endothelial proliferation, disruption of the elastic lamina, and microthrombi. Additional contributing factors include increased RBC adhesion, endothelial activation, inflammation, and coagulation dysregulation. Children with sickle cell disease may also have SAH, though the risk is less than that of infarction, occurring in fewer than 2%. The clinical findings of SAH differ from those of infarction in patients with sickle cell disease. Severe headache, vomiting, and alteration in mental state characterize SAH in children with sickle cell disease. Meningeal signs and focal neurologic deficits may be found on examination.

Transient cerebral arteriopathy consists of focal stenosis or segmental narrowing of the vessel wall that typically affects large vessels in the anterior circulation and fluctuates on serial angiographic studies. Strokes in transient cerebral arteriopathy usually involve the basal ganglia. Pathophysiology is undetermined; association with certain viral infections such as varicella and herpes has been proposed. **Connective tissue disorders** such as Marfan, Ehlers-Danlos, and Loeys-Dietz syndromes may have associated arteriopathies that can result in ischemic stroke; patients with these disorders are also at risk of stroke via **arterial dissection**. Arterial dissections may also occur in otherwise healthy children in the setting of major mechanical injuries such as whiplash and penetrating injuries, or even with minor trauma like neck manipulation, physical effort, or contact sports. Arteriopathies are also seen in rarer **genetic disorders** such as adenosine deaminase 2 deficiency; pathogenic variants in *NOTCH3* and *ACTA2* have been implicated in pediatric stroke.

Cardiac Disease. **Congenital heart disease** is a significant risk factor for childhood stroke. The strokes are typically embolic; children with single-ventricle physiology face the greatest risk, but other cardiac conditions such as arrhythmias, cardiomyopathy, or endocarditis are also associated with stroke. Cardiac defects involving right-to-left shunts allow emboli originating in peripheral venous circulation to bypass their filtration and removal by the pulmonary vascular bed. Emboli entering the heart via venous return may be shunted to the peripheral arterial circulation only to lodge in the cerebrovascular tree.

Patent foramen ovale contributes significantly to stroke in children. Echocardiographic evaluation of patients who have had stroke reveals patent foramen ovale or evidence of right-to-left shunting in many. Transesophageal echocardiography with agitated saline assessing for evidence of direct right-to-left flow is an essential component of the evaluation of children with embolic stroke.

Valvular defects can cause stroke as well. Mitral valve prolapse may result in small emboli being dislodged from the abnormal valve leaflets and has been estimated to underlie up to 30% of strokes in patients younger than 30 years. **Rheumatic valvular disease** of the mitral or aortic valves, once a common cause of embolic stroke, has become an infrequent cause of childhood stroke due to improved diagnosis and treatment of group A streptococcal disease. Infectious vegetations of the mitral and aortic valves in **bacterial endocarditis** pose a considerable risk for embolic stroke, regardless of whether the valve is native, prosthetic, rheumatic, or congenitally abnormal, as these vegetations may dislodge and travel distally to occlude cerebral arteries or seed the adventitia of a cerebral vessel and induce thrombosis or the development of a mycotic aneurysm. The most common organisms found are streptococci and staphylococci. Mycotic aneurysms may lie dormant for some time before their rupture leads to SAH or IPH and resultant neurologic signs.

Left atrial myxoma, atrial fibrillation, nonbacterial valvular lesions, and polycythemia in uncorrected cyanotic heart disease may also be associated with stroke.

Another important risk factor of stroke in children with severe cardiac disease is the utilization of ventricular assist devices or venoarterial ECMO. As blood is circulated with the assistance of these devices, fibrin deposits may be introduced into the arterial circulation and may propagate to the cerebrovascular tree. To prevent thrombosis, patients using these devices are usually administered systemic anticoagulation, which may increase the risk of intracranial hemorrhage.

Prothrombotic Conditions. Several disorders of coagulation can render patients at risk for embolic or thrombotic stroke (see Table 37.15). Adverse consequences of **antiphospholipid antibodies**

TABLE 37.15 Risk Factors and Causes of Stroke in Children

Arteriopathies
Focal or transient cerebral arteriopathy
Craniocervical arterial dissection
Fibromuscular dysplasia
Moyamoya disease or syndrome
Sickle cell arteriopathy
Primary CNS angiitis
HANAC syndrome
Genetic variants (see text and Table 37.17)

Cardiovascular Disease

Congenital
Aortic stenosis
Mitral stenosis
Ventricular septal defects
Patent ductus arteriosus
Patent foramen ovale
PHACE syndrome

Acquired
Endocarditis
Kawasaki disease
Cardiomyopathy
Atrial myxoma
Arrhythmia
Rheumatic heart disease
Prosthetic heart valve
Catheterization/surgery
ECMO

Hematologic Abnormalities
Hemoglobinopathies
Polycythemia
Leukemia/lymphoma
Thrombocytopenia including TTP
Disorders of coagulation
    Protein C deficiency
    Protein S deficiency
    Antithrombin III deficiency
    Factor V (Leiden) resistance to activated protein C
    Lupus anticoagulant
    Oral hormonal contraception
    Pregnancy and the postpartum state
    Disseminated intravascular coagulation
    Paroxysmal nocturnal hemoglobinuria
    Inflammatory bowel disease
    Protein-losing enteropathy
    Nephrotic syndrome
    L-Asparaginase
    Prothrombin G20210A variant
    MTHFR deficiency
    Lipoprotein(a) elevation
    Antiphospholipid antibody syndrome
    PNH

Systemic Disorders
Meningitis
    Viral
    Bacterial
    Tuberculous
Systemic infection
    Viremia
    Bacteremia
    Local head and neck infections, including Lemierre syndrome
    Postinfectious (including varicella and other viruses)
Drug-induced inflammation and vasoconstriction
    Amphetamine
    Cocaine
    Ergot alkaloids
Autoimmune disease
    Systemic lupus erythematosus
    Juvenile idiopathic arthritis
    Takayasu arteritis
    Mixed connective tissue disease
    Polyarteritis nodosa
    Primary CNS vasculitis
Trisomy 21

Metabolic Diseases
Hyperhomocysteinemia/homocystinuria/elevated homocysteine levels
Fabry disease
Pseudoxanthoma elasticum
Sulfite oxidase deficiency

Mitochondrial Disorders
MELAS
Leigh syndrome

Intracerebral Vascular Processes
Ruptured aneurysm
Arteriovenous malformation
Migraine headache
Post–subarachnoid hemorrhage vasospasm
Hereditary hemorrhagic telangiectasia
Sturge-Weber syndrome
Carotid or vertebral artery dissection
Neurofibromatosis type 1
CADASIL
CARASIL

Trauma and Other External Causes
Nonaccidental trauma
Head and neck trauma
Oral trauma
Placental embolism
Neck hyperextension (carotid dissection)
Lollipop stroke (pharyngeal trauma)

CADASIL, cerebral autosomal dominant arteriopathy with subcortical infarcts and leukoencephalopathy; CARASIL, cerebral autosomal recessive arteriopathy with subcortical infarcts and leukoencephalopathy; CNS, central nervous system; ECMO, extracorporeal membrane oxygenation; HANAC, hereditary angiopathy with nephropathy aneurysms, muscle cramps; MELAS, mitochondrial encephalomyopathy, lactic acidosis, strokelike episodes; MTHFR, methylenetetrahydrofolate reductase; PHACE, posterior fossa brain malformations, hemangiomas of the face, neck, and scalp, arterial anomalies, coarctation of the aorta and cardiac anomalies, and eye defects; PNA, paroxysmal nocturnal hemoglobinuria; TTP, thrombotic thrombocytopenic purpura.

have been identified in all age groups. Antiphospholipid antibodies, including **lupus anticoagulant**, are polyclonal antibodies found in serum that bind to both neutral and negatively charged phospholipids. Lupus anticoagulant and **anticardiolipin antibodies**

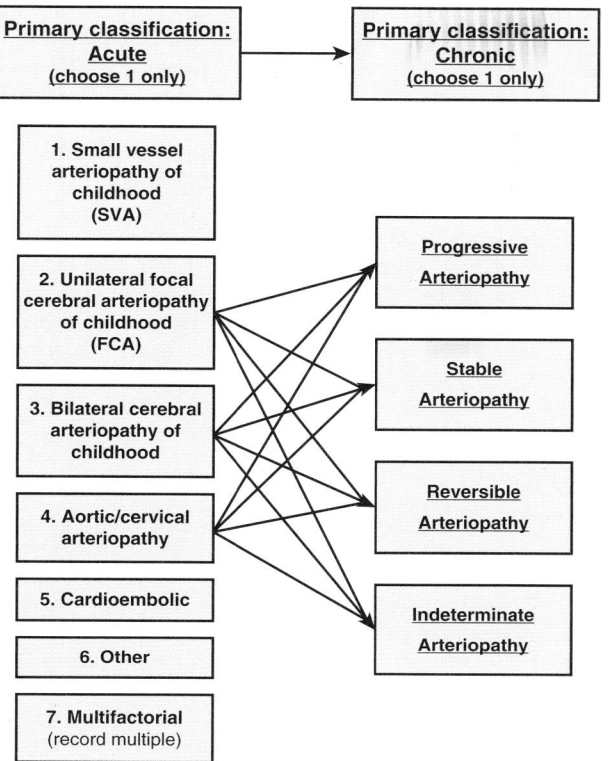

Fig. 37.16 Childhood AIS Standardized Classification and Diagnostic Evaluation (CASCADE) system for classification of childhood arterial ischemic stroke. (From Bernard TJ, Manco-Johnson MJ, Lo W, et al. Towards a consensus-based classification of childhood arterial ischemic stroke. *Stroke.* 2012;43[2]:371–377.)

were first associated with thrombotic or embolic cerebrovascular events in patients with systemic lupus erythematosus (SLE). The antibody prolongs the partial thromboplastin time (PTT) in vitro but acts as a procoagulant in vivo. A common finding associated with coagulation testing among children with AIS is the presence of anticardiolipin antibody. The presence of these antibodies in a patient who concurrently smokes cigarettes, has positive antinuclear antibodies, or suffers from hyperlipidemia may impart a higher risk for stroke than if the patient carries the antibody alone. The antibody's presence is indicated by a prolonged PTT and a falsely positive serum Venereal Disease Research Laboratory (VDRL) result. Although cerebral infarction and TIAs constitute the most frequently observed neurologic manifestations related to the presence of these antibodies, migraine headache, seizures, and monocular visual disturbances are also associated.

Absence of specific serum proteins that act as inhibitors of coagulation may lead to stroke. Two of these proteins, **protein S** and **protein C**, have been associated with thrombotic or embolic cerebrovascular disease. Protein C and its cofactor protein S act as anticoagulants and synergistically attenuate coagulation by deactivating the activated forms of factors V and VIII. Absence of (or resistance to) either of these proteins disrupts the balance of coagulation toward increased spontaneous clotting and can result in stroke. In addition, **antithrombin III** opposes the action of the activated forms of factors II, IX, X, XI, and XII through the irreversible formation of inactivating complexes with these factors. Deficiencies of proteins S and C as well as of antithrombin III may cause arterial thrombotic or embolic stroke or venous infarction. Although their deficiencies are often congenital, they may be acquired through liver disease or nephrotic syndrome. Factor V Leiden, prothrombin 20210A, and lipoprotein A are also important factors that may contribute to the pathogenesis of AIS. A screening hematologic battery of tests, including prothrombin time, PTT, and specific immunologic and functional testing for the proteins suspected of being deficient, is essential for diagnosis.

Paroxysmal nocturnal hemoglobinuria (PNH) and **thrombotic thrombocytopenic purpura (TTP)** predispose to stroke.

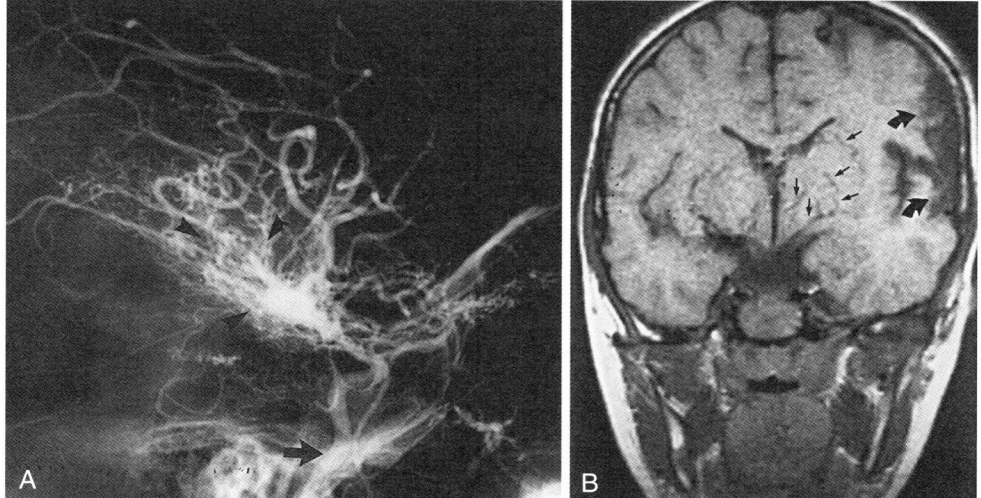

Fig. 37.17 Sudden onset of right hemiparesis in a 6-year-old boy. *A,* Cerebral angiogram shows the left internal carotid artery *(arrow)* leading to a highly arborized, telangiectatic network of vessels *(arrowheads)* characteristic for moyamoya disease. The typical middle cerebral artery vascular tree is absent. *B,* Cranial coronal MRI scan shows region of low signal in the middle cerebral artery territory and denotes infarction *(curved arrows).* Flow voids in the basal ganglia *(straight arrows)* are radiographic manifestations of the basilar collateral circulation typical of this vascular anomaly.

TABLE 37.16 **Autoimmune Disorders Associated with Central Nervous System (CNS) Involvement**

Disorder	CNS Manifestations
Systemic lupus erythematosus	Migraine headache, seizures, stroke, cerebellar dysfunction, transverse myelopathy, aseptic meningitis, psychosis
Mixed connective tissue disease	Seizures, stroke, cerebellar dysfunction, trigeminal neuropathy
Polyarteritis nodosa	Migraine headache, stroke, subarachnoid hemorrhage, seizures
Granulomatosis with polyangiitis	Migraine headache, subarachnoid hemorrhage, stroke
Takayasu arteritis	Seizure, stroke
Henoch-Schönlein purpura	Headache, stroke, seizures, chorea
Primary CNS vasculitis	Headache, stroke, seizure

Autoimmune Conditions. Autoimmune disorders are uncommon causes of stroke in children (Table 37.16). Symptoms of abrupt onset with accompanying deficits referable to the CNS have long been associated with **systemic lupus erythematosus**. A CNS vasculitis had been presumed to underlie the CNS manifestations of SLE; however, an autopsy study of patients who suffered from SLE revealed a virtual absence of cerebrovascular inflammation. Rather, small areas of infarction relate to proliferative changes in cerebral arterioles that lead to luminal occlusion. Large areas of infarction are more probably related to lupus anticoagulant–derived thromboembolism or to embolism from the sterile cardiac valve leaflet vegetations associated with SLE (Libman-Sacks endocarditis). Additional causes of CNS illness include thrombocytopenic hemorrhage, steroid-induced pseudotumor or psychosis, and CNS infection.

True **cerebral arterial vasculitis** may be an isolated disease or seen in association with recognizable systemic autoimmune disorders. Isolated angiitis of the CNS may affect small, medium-sized, or large vessels. Multiple regions of infarction are often found on MRI. Neuropathologic evidence of polymorphonuclear leukocyte or monocyte infiltration leading to intimal proliferation and vessel wall necrosis is found. The inflammation affects blood flow and predisposes to thrombosis.

Stroke may occur in the course of **polyarteritis nodosa**. Involvement of the CNS is found in up to 40% of such patients. **Granulomatosis with polyangiitis,** a necrotizing vasculitis of the upper pulmonary system, rarely affects the CNS; stroke is uncommon. When the CNS is affected, extension of sinus or nasal inflammation into the basilar skull frequently has occurred. **Takayasu arteritis**, involving the aorta and its principal branches, has been associated with thrombotic stroke. Inflammation-induced luminal constriction leading to thrombosis is thought to cause cerebral ischemia in children. **Necrotizing arteritis** with inflammatory infiltrate has been found in both meningeal and cerebral vessels of children suffering from Henoch-Schönlein purpura. Both fixed and transient deficits may occur in this disorder.

Metabolic and Genetic Disorders. There are rare metabolic and genetic conditions associated with stroke (Table 37.17). **Homocystinuria**, a disorder of homocysteine metabolism, can cause thrombotic stroke in children. Abnormal homocysteine metabolism results from one of three inheritable enzymatic defects.

The most striking phenotype results from deficiency of cystathionine synthetase, the enzyme that facilitates the catabolism of homocysteine to cystathionine leading to accumulation of homocysteine. Children affected by this autosomal recessive disorder have marfanoid habitus, global developmental delay, lens dislocation, and thromboembolism. Thromboemboli may travel to cerebrovascular beds, causing stroke. Hyperhomocysteinemia injures the vascular endothelium. The denuded vessel wall then becomes a site for thrombosis. The resulting thrombus may remain at its site of origin or it may embolize to a distal locus. Therefore, stroke may have thrombotic or embolic characteristics. Both arterial and venous infarctions may result. Some patients without homocystinuria but with elevated serum homocysteine levels may be at risk for stroke.

Sulfite oxidase deficiency, another autosomal recessive disorder, results in the accumulation of serum sulfite. The associated phenotype may result from deficiency of either the enzyme or its associated and essential pterin-containing molybdenum cofactor. Intellectual disability, seizures, lens displacement, and acute hemiplegia result. The mechanism of the strokelike episodes has not been fully elucidated. It is possible that ischemic mechanisms are not involved and that direct metabolic neurotoxicity accounts for the sudden onset of deficits resembling those of stroke. Sulfites and S-sulfocysteine accumulate in urine.

Fabry disease, a rare X-linked lipid storage disease attributable to ceramide trihexosidase deficiency, results in accumulation of the sphingolipid trihexoside in the kidneys, vascular endothelium, and corneas. Symptoms become apparent in childhood or adolescence. Angiokeratomas and painful paresthesia often constitute the first symptoms. Renal failure follows. Endothelial accumulation of sphingolipid in vessel walls leads to cerebrovascular occlusion that results in stroke. Recurrent stroke is common.

The manifestations of **mitochondrial disorders** include recurrent and sometimes catastrophic stroke. The syndrome of **mitochondrial encephalomyopathy, lactic acidosis, and strokelike episodes (MELAS)** manifests in childhood and results from a pathogenic variant in mitochondrial DNA. The most common biochemical finding is a deficiency of complex I of the electron transport chain. An elevated serum or cerebrospinal fluid lactate level serves as its biochemical signature, and molecular confirmation of the diagnosis can be secured from blood. Although some features of MELAS are shared with other mitochondrial syndromes, hemiparesis of abrupt onset is fairly specific for this syndrome. An excruciating headache resembling migraine may precede the strokelike episodes. Seizures and sensorineural hearing loss are almost always present at some point in the course of the illness. Neuropathologic study of brains from patients with MELAS has shown cystic cavities and necrosis of cortex with relative sparing of white matter.

Other metabolic disorders have been associated with stroke in childhood. Urea cycle defects, especially ornithine transcarbamylase deficiency manifesting in girls, can cause stroke. Deficiency of arginase, another important enzyme of the urea cycle, has been observed in association with hemiparesis and diparesis of subacute onset. Finally, familial lipoprotein disorders, especially those featuring a dearth of high-density lipoprotein or an abundance of triglycerides, have been associated with stroke in children. In most cases, a family history of hyperlipidemia is found.

Evaluation and Management

Table 37.18 describes the paraclinical assessment of stroke in children. The evaluation of stroke should be focused on determining the etiology as management depends largely on it. Stroke evaluation urgency depends on the acuteness of the presentation. For any patient with

TABLE 37.17 Genetic Associations with Thrombotic, Hemorrhagic, or Vascular Stroke

Lipid and Other Disorders with Atherosclerosis

Hereditary dyslipoproteinemias

    Familial hypercholesterolemia

    Familial hypertriglyceridemia

    Hyperlipoproteinemia (types III and IV)

    Familial hypoalphalipoproteinemia

    Tangier disease

    Progeria (de Lange, Deckel, Bloom, Cockayne syndromes)

Arteriopathy, Angiopathy, Vasculitis

Ehlers-Danlos (type IV) syndrome

Pseudoxanthoma elasticum

Menkes syndrome

Marfan syndrome

Rendu-Osler-Weber syndrome (hereditary hemorrhagic telangiectasia)

Sturge-Weber syndrome

Neurofibromatosis 1

Tuberous sclerosis complex

Polycystic kidney disease (autosomal dominant type 1, 2)

Fibromuscular dysplasia

von Hippel–Lindau syndrome

Bannayan-Zonana syndrome

Moyamoya disease (*ACTA2, GUCY1A3, RNF2B,* unknown)

Fabry disease

CARASIL (*HTRA1*)

CADASIL (*NOTCH3*)

RVCL (*TREX-1*)

DADA2 (*CECR1*)

COL4A1/A2 angiopathies including:

    Hereditary angiopathy nephropathy and cramps (HANAC), and

    Autosomal dominant porencephaly with infantile hemiplegia (POREN1)

FOXC1/PITX2: Digenetic inheritance

CARASAL (*CTSA*)

HCHWA-Dutch type

HCHWA-Icelandic type

FAP

ADA2 deficiency

ACTA2 gene variant

Hematologic Disorders

Antithrombin deficiency

Protein C and S deficiency

Thrombomodulin deficiency

Activated protein C resistance

Factor V Leiden variant

Prothrombin G20210A variant

Sickle cell disease

Hematologic Disorders—cont'd

Factor V, VII, VIII, IX, X, XI, XII, XIII deficiency

Hemoglobinopathies (hemoglobin C or S disorders)

Prekallikrein deficiency

C_2 deficiency

β-thalassemia

Disorders of fibrinogen

    Afibrinogenemia

    Hypofibrinogenemia

    Dysfibrinogenemia

Elevated thrombin-activatable fibrinolysis inhibitor

Elevated factor VIII

Elevated factor IX

Elevated factor XI

Disorders of the fibrinolytic system

    Hypoplasminogenemia

    Tissue plasminogen activator defects

MTHFR gene variant

Heparin cofactor II deficiency

Hereditary platelet defects

Cardiac Disorders

Familial atrial myxomas

Rhabdomyomas (tuberous sclerosis)

Mitral valve prolapse

Cardiac papillary fibroelastoma

Hereditary cardiac conduction disorders

Hereditary cardiomyopathies

Inborn Errors of Metabolism

Mitochondrial abnormalities

    MELAS

    Leigh disease

Organic acidemia

    Methylmalonic acidemia

    Propionic acidemia

    Isovaleric acidemia

Homocystinuria

Glutaric aciduria type II

Sulfite oxidase deficiency

11β-hydroxylase deficiency, 11β-ketoreductase deficiency, 17α-hydroxylase deficiency

3-Methylcrotonyl-CoA carboxylase 3-hydroxy-3-methylglutaryl-CoA lyase deficiency

Other Disorders

CCM1 (*KRIT1*)

CCM2 (*CCM2*)

CCM3 (*PDCD10*)

ADPKD, autosomal dominant polycystic kidney disease; CADASIL, cerebral autosomal dominant arteriopathy with subcortical infarcts and leukoencephalopathy; CARASAL, cathepsin A–related arteriopathy with strokes and leukoencephalopathy; CARASIL, cerebral autosomal recessive arteriopathy with subcortical infarcts and leukoencephalopathy; CCM, cerebral cavernous malformation; DADA2, deficiency of adenosine deaminase 2; FAP, familial amyloid polyneuropathy; HCHWA, hereditary cerebral hemorrhage with amyloidosis; MELAS, mitochondrial encephalopathy, lactic acidosis, and strokelike episodes; RVCL, retinal vasculopathy with deficiency of adenosine deaminase 2.

TABLE 37.18 Radiologic, Laboratory, and Cardiovascular Assessment of Stroke in Children

Radiologic Assessment	**Metabolic Disturbances**
Rapid Detection of Intracranial Blood	Serum electrolytes, glucose
Cranial CT	Serum and urine toxicology screen
Cranial MRI (also detects extravascular blood but is not as rapidly obtained as cranial CT images)	Serum amino acids*
	Urine organic acids*
	Acylcarnitine profile*
Detection of Brain Parenchymal Changes Related to Stroke	GDF-15*
Cranial MRI, including diffusion-weighted imaging	Serum/CSF lactate and pyruvate*
Cranial CT (reveals changes later in course than MRI)	
	Disturbance of Hemoglobin
Detection of Abnormal Vascular Structure	Hemoglobin concentration
Percutaneous cerebral angiogram (provides the most complete and accurate demonstration of extracranial and intracranial vasculature)	Hemoglobin electrophoresis
Cranial MRA	**Inflammatory Disturbances**
	ESR
Laboratory Assessment	ANA
	CSF studies: glucose, protein, cell counts, special stains, cultures
Disturbance of RBC, WBC, or Platelet Number	Serum triglycerides
Hematocrit	Serum cholesterol; if high, obtain fasting HDL
Platelet count	Gene panel or whole exome
WBC count with differential	
	Cardiovascular Assessment
Disturbance of Coagulation	ECG
PT, PTT	Standard and transesophageal echocardiogram
Antithrombin III level	
Protein C level, protein S level; resistance to protein C assay	
Lupus anticoagulant detection, anticardiolipin antibody, antiphospholipid antibody	
MTHFR gene variant, prothrombin 20210A gene variant analysis	

*Consider if marked or persistent abnormalities in glucose homeostasis or acid-base balance.

ANA, antinuclear antibodies; CSF, cerebrospinal fluid; GDF-15, growth differentiation factor-15; HDL, high-density lipoproteins; MRA, magnetic resonance angiography; MTHFR, methylenetetrahydrofolate reductase; PT, prothrombin time; PTT, partial thromboplastin time; RBC, red blood cell; WBC, white blood cell.

acute neurologic deficit in which stroke is suspected, urgent neuroimaging must follow, as well as laboratory data, pertinent history, and directed examination. Patients should be screened for complications of stroke, which include seizures, cerebral edema, hemorrhagic conversion, and stroke recurrence. Neuropsychological testing and rehabilitation strategies must be instituted.

Hyperacute therapies like thrombolysis and thrombectomy, which are directed at revascularizing the brain and preserving the ischemic penumbra, or area of viable tissue around the periphery of an infarct, have revolutionized the care of adolescents and adults with stroke. The evidentiary support for the use of these therapies in pediatrics is insufficient, largely because of the difficulty of studying hyperacute therapies in pediatric stroke. Neuroprotective measures, which include permissive hypertension and reduction of metabolic demand, remain the mainstay of treatment in most pediatric stroke cases.

Strategies to prevent primary stroke or stroke recurrence vary depending on the specific etiology. Patients with sickle cell disease related to hemoglobin SS or hemoglobin S-β^0-thalassemia genotypes are at the highest risk for stroke, compared to other sickle cell disease genotypes, and should be screened on a recurring basis for stroke risk beginning in early childhood. These assessments consist of determining the mean flow velocity in the large intracranial vessels via transcranial Doppler ultrasonography; higher velocities are suggestive of vasculopathy and may portend a higher stroke risk. Those at increased risk should be considered for chronic transfusion therapy to maintain

a lower percentage of hemoglobin S; those unable to tolerate chronic transfusion may be considered for hydroxyurea therapy. These patients should also have at least one MRI during the school-aged years to screen for silent cerebral infarcts. Those who have sustained strokes should also be offered chronic transfusion therapy; alternative therapies include hydroxyurea or even hematopoietic stem cell transplantation, depending on disease severity, recurrence risk, and tolerance of chronic transfusion.

Anticoagulation is commonly used in cardioembolic stroke when the risk for further embolism propagation is present; if due to an abnormal heart rhythm, rate control is established either medically or via ablation procedures. Strokes due to moyamoya disease and syndrome may be prevented by revascularization through indirect and/or direct bypass surgery. In some cases of arteriopathy, antithrombotic therapies may be considered. Treatment of infectious endocarditis consists of parenteral anti-infectives and, if needed, valve replacement or repair. Lastly, in select cases, closure of a patent foramen ovale may be performed to decrease the risk of subsequent stroke.

Outcome

In-hospital mortality from pediatric stroke is approximately 3%. Almost half of children with AIS have neurologic deficits, with the majority having hemiparesis. Cognitive impairments, as well as impairments of higher cortical and executive functioning, such as working memory, processing speed, visual-spatial and visual-constructional

TABLE 37.19 Prevalence of the Causes of Hemorrhagic Stroke in Children	
Etiology	% of Cases
Vascular malformations	54
AVM	30
Cavernous hemangioma	12
Aneurysm	10
Venous malformation	0.5
SAH	2
Medical etiologies	9
Brain tumors	2.5
Trauma/dissection	1
Undetermined	33

AVM, arteriovenous malformations; SAH, subarachnoid hemorrhage.

skills, inhibitory control, and problem solving, may also occur and should be evaluated by neuropsychological testing, so as to allow for identification of specific deficits and the formulation of customized rehabilitation and school accommodation plans. Up to 30% of patients with childhood AIS receive some form of special education in the classroom, and up to 60% have emotional or behavioral difficulties.

Hemorrhagic Stroke in Children

Hemorrhagic stroke may occur from disordered coagulation, thrombocytopenia, vascular lesions, or conversion of ischemic or venous stroke (Table 37.19). Symptoms are similar to ischemic stroke though may also include signs of increased intracranial pressure or even impending cerebral herniation. Evaluation and management depend on etiology. If hemorrhagic stroke is suspected, emergent noncontrast CTOH should be obtained. Any coagulopathy or thrombocytopenia should be promptly corrected. If there is concern for a vascular lesion, such as arterial dissection or an aneurysm, CTA or conventional angiography should be performed; if such a lesion is present, consultation with neurovascular specialists can determine the need for and urgency of intervention. Occasionally patients with large intracranial bleeding must undergo surgical evacuation of a hematoma to control intracranial hypertension and prevent mass effect from damaging adjacent brain structures. In the case of hemorrhagic transformation of an ischemic or venous stroke, neuroprotection must be maximized with normalization of physiologic parameters, control of hypertension, and reduction of brain metabolism. Outcome largely depends on the volume of hemorrhage and the degree of brain injury.

Coagulopathies

Coagulopathies like hemophilia (A and B) are X-linked disorders that may result in intracranial bleeding. Bleeding may occur in either intraparenchymal or subarachnoid locations. Hemophilia A arises from factor VIII deficiency. Patients with this disorder may experience intracranial bleeding in association with head trauma. Spontaneous intracranial bleeding not associated with head trauma also occurs. The risk of spontaneous bleeding rises with the severity of factor VIII deficiency. Hemophilia B derives from a deficiency of factor IX. Intracranial bleeding is seen less frequently among these patients than among patients with hemophilia A, though hemophilia B is encountered much less frequently than hemophilia A, and this difference may account for the less frequent observation of intracranial bleeding. Clinical symptoms depend on the intracranial location of the hemorrhage. If the bleeding occurs in the subarachnoid space, symptoms of severe headache, nuchal rigidity, and meningismus are found. Mental status is frequently altered. If bleeding occurs within brain parenchyma, focal features, including hemiparesis, may be found.

Thrombocytopenia

Severe thrombocytopenia rarely leads to cerebral hemorrhage, especially if the cause is idiopathic (immune) thrombocytopenic purpura. Thrombocytopenia caused by bone marrow failure (e.g., drug-induced suppression, aplastic anemia, malignancy) and TTP pose a greater risk. Significant risk of intracranial hemorrhage is thought not to occur until the platelet count is $<20,000/\text{mm}^3$. Small petechial hemorrhages into white matter are thought to be more common than are large parenchymal hemorrhages. Causes of thrombocytopenia include idiopathic immune thrombocytopenic purpura, TTP, hemolytic uremic syndrome, infection, and malignancy (replacement of bone marrow or drug-induced suppression). The features of these underlying disorders tend to determine the symptomatic presentation beyond intracranial hemorrhage and can assist in establishing the cause (see Chapter 51).

Vascular Malformations

Vascular malformations may predispose children to hemorrhagic stroke. Arteriovenous malformation (AVM) of the brain is the most common cause of intracranial hemorrhage in preadolescent children. The malformation represents a developmental anomaly that manifests with hemorrhage much more frequently in children than in adults; biological males are affected more frequently than biological females. The AVM consists of dilated vascular channels, some of which reveal the highly muscularized walls of arterioles. Gliotic neural tissue resides in and among the vascular branches of the malformation. The most frequent presenting events associated with AVM in children are seizures and hemorrhage. Most AVMs reside in the cerebral hemispheres; 10% arise in the posterior fossa.

The clinical features of AVM hemorrhage consist of those found in IPH. Focal features depend on the area of the brain in which the bleeding has occurred. A higher mortality rate has been observed in children than in adults harboring hemorrhagic AVMs. The risk of hemorrhage from an unruptured AVM is approximately 3% per year. MRI allows for better identification and localization of the malformation (Fig. 37.18).

Intracranial aneurysms constitute the most common cause of intracranial bleeding in all patients younger than 20 years and are more frequent in biological males. The most common site of aneurysmal bleeding in children is along the intracranial portion of the internal carotid artery. The vertebral and basilar arteries are other common sites of intracranial aneurysm in children. In addition, intracranial aneurysms discovered in children tend to be larger than those found in adults. Although most aneurysms constitute vascular developmental anomalies, other causes exist, including mycotic aneurysms associated with bacterial endocarditis (Fig. 37.19), as well as acquired cerebral artery aneurysms in children infected with HIV. Intracranial aneurysms are found with increased frequency among patients suffering from polycystic renal disease, those with aortic coarctation, and those with Ehlers-Danlos syndrome.

Affected patients are usually studied with angiography after aneurysmal bleeding. Patients should be closely observed for development of hydrocephalus and increased intracranial pressure. Aneurysmal bleeding resulting in significant SAH can precipitate cerebral **vasospasm**. Vasospasm, in turn, can cause a secondary cerebral infarction. Vasospasm occurs most commonly 7–10 days after the aneurysmal bleeding.

The syndrome of **posterior fossa brain malformations; *h*emangiomas of the face, neck, and scalp; *a*rterial anomalies; *c*oarctation of the aorta and cardiac anomalies; and *e*ye defects (PHACE)** is a

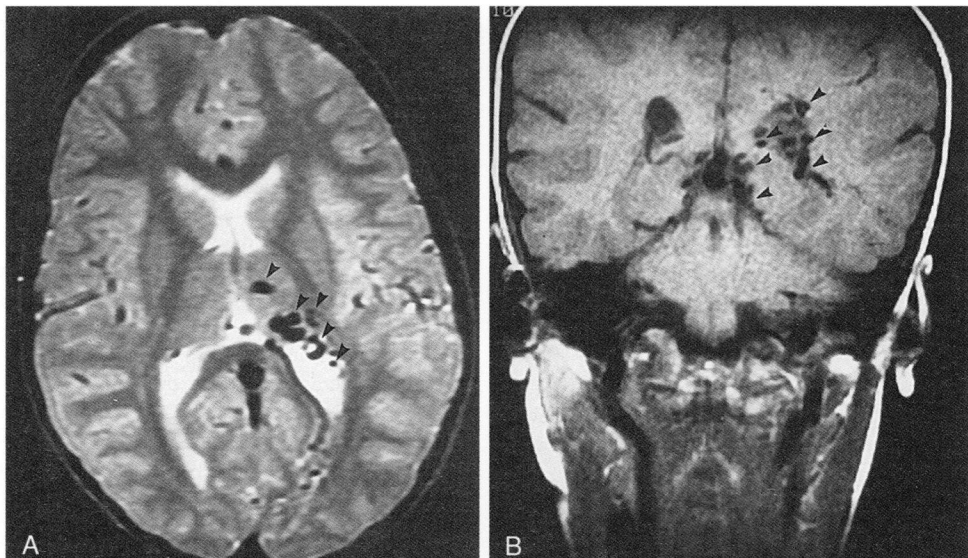

Fig. 37.18 Cranial MRI scan of a 6-year-old girl with recurrent headache. *A,* Axial view demonstrates flow voids deep in the left hemisphere near the lateral ventricle *(arrowheads),* consistent with arteriovenous malformation. *B,* Coronal view through parietal lobes also demonstrates numerous flow voids *(arrowheads)* indicative of arteriovenous malformation.

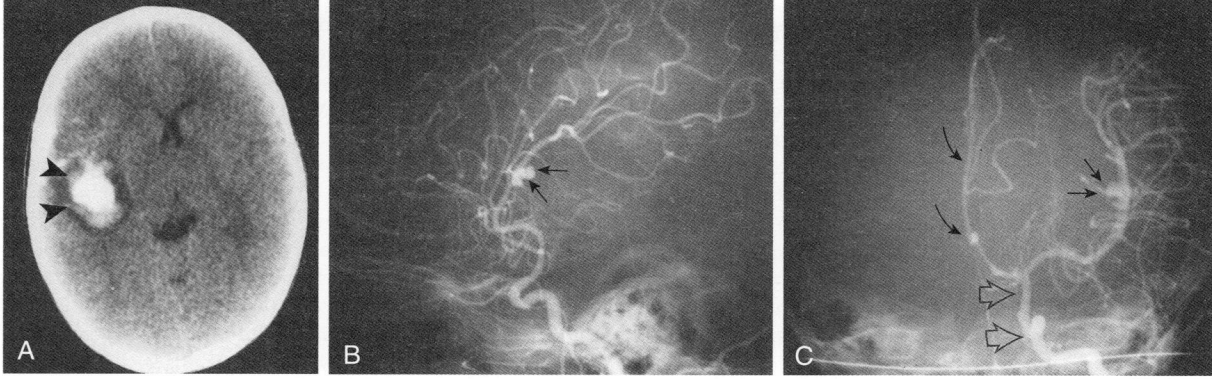

Fig. 37.19 Mycotic cerebral aneurysm hemorrhage. *A,* A cranial CT scan reveals a hyperdense area in the left temporal lobe *(arrowheads)* representing intraparenchymal hemorrhage. *B,* Cerebral angiography in a lateral view shows a lobulated structural abnormality representing the mycotic aneurysm, most probably residing in the middle cerebral artery tree *(arrows).* *C,* An anteroposterior angiographic view confirms the location of the aneurysm in the middle cerebral artery *(straight arrows)* located laterally rather than in the more medial anterior cerebral artery *(curved arrows).* The internal carotid artery *(open arrows)* gives rise to both the anterior and the middle cerebral arteries.

constellation of disorders. CNS malformations affect the posterior fossa and include Dandy-Walker malformation, arachnoid cysts, cerebellar hypoplasia, and enlarged cisterna magna. Vascular anomalies include brachiocephalic artery and aortic arch anomalies (e.g., coarctation of aorta), cerebrovascular arterial hypoplasia, aneurysms, stenosis and aberrancies, and progressive occlusive arterial disease leading to stroke.

Venous Stroke in Children

Venous stroke occurs when a thrombus obstructs the cerebral venous circulation and leads to an increase in the hydrostatic pressure of the veins and capillaries proximal to the thrombus. Redistribution of blood flow through the venous system allows for some degree of compensation, but if the hydrostatic pressure overcomes this compensatory capacity,

venous stroke may occur. The annual incidence of CSVT in children is estimated at seven cases per million and more often the superficial sinuses are involved. The clinical manifestations depend on the area of the brain that has been injured; prior to stroke, antecedent symptoms include headache or blurry vision from papilledema. Due to changes in pressure dissipation and the blood-brain barrier, venous strokes may turn into hemorrhagic strokes. Venous system thrombi may also obstruct cerebrospinal flow and thus cause intracranial hypertension.

Risk Factors

The etiology for CSVT in children is often multifactorial. The most common risk factor for CSVT is head and neck infections such as otitis media, mastoiditis, sinusitis, or Lemierre syndrome (see Chapter 48). Other risk factors include systemic illnesses such as liver disease, nephrotic syndrome, SLE, malignancy, head trauma, or neurosurgery. Rarely, CSVT occurs as a complication of iron-deficiency anemia, β-thalassemia, and sickle cell disease. Thrombophilia plays an unclear role in pediatric CSVT. The association of factor V Leiden and pro-thrombin G20210A polymorphisms appear to have a weaker role in pediatric CSVT than in adult CSVT. Conversely, dehydration is a bigger risk factor for CSVT in children than it is in adults. Often several risk factors are present.

Evaluation and Management

Emergent neuroimaging with a CT scan and corresponding CT venogram or a brain MRI with a corresponding magnetic resonance venogram should be obtained in instances of suspected CSVT. Once venous stroke has been diagnosed, concomitant abnormalities, such as dehydration or infection, must be corrected. High-quality evidence for the role of anticoagulation in children with CSVT is lacking though may be considered, as may endovascular treatment for patients with severe presentations and rapidly deteriorating neurologic function despite anticoagulation. Children should undergo evaluation for CSVT etiology, which should include prothrombotic assessment. If initiated, the duration of anticoagulation is usually 3–6 months for children, but if there is an inherent prothrombotic risk it may be continued for longer.

Outcome

Mortality for children with CSVT is as high as 10%; recanalization rates approach 70%. Recurrence rate in children is as high as 20%. Functional outcomes vary depending on the region of the brain that has suffered infarction. A peculiar characteristic of venous stroke is that vasogenic edema may occur to a different magnitude than does cytotoxic edema; as such, brain tissue damage may be less severe and deficits may be reversible at higher rates than in arterial stroke. Successful recanalization decreases the risk of chronic headache and intracranial hypertension.

STROKE IN ADOLESCENTS

The causes of adolescent stroke include those discussed for preadolescent children though also include causes typically seen in adults as well as other entities not commonly encountered in neonates or preadolescent children. Determination of stroke mechanism—embolic, thrombotic, or hemorrhagic—and whether it is arterial or venous remains important. The management of adolescent stroke depends on etiology; for example, adolescents with cardioembolic strokes may benefit from hyperacute therapies like tissue plasminogen activator and/or thrombectomy.

Fibromuscular Dysplasia

Fibromuscular dysplasia involves arteries throughout the body. First described in renal arteries, the pathologic features of fibromuscular dysplasia have been found in carotid, vertebral, and intracranial arteries. Fibromuscular dysplasia involves irregularly spaced focal zones of fibrous and muscular hyperplasia of the media, disruption of the elastic lamina, and eventration of the media. The constricted regions of vascular fibrosis alternate with regions of luminal dilation to create the characteristic beaded appearance on angiography. Fibromuscular dysplasia is more common in primary school-aged biological females and has been found in adolescents. Findings vary by the site of dysplasia: If the carotid arteries are involved, a bruit may be heard on auscultation; if the renal arteries are affected, hypertension may be present. Neurologic symptoms signifying cerebrovascular involvement most commonly consist of TIAs and mild strokes.

Oral Contraception, Pregnancy, and the Puerperium

Oral hormonal contraceptives have been associated with a slight increase in stroke risk in young women; comorbid procoagulant disorders, migraine headache history, and tobacco use increase this risk further. Pregnancy and the postpartum period are states of hypercoagulability and increased venous stasis, both of which can result in CSVT and subsequent venous stroke. Excessive maternal blood loss during or shortly after delivery can result in hypoperfusion of the pituitary gland with resultant hypopituitarism, a condition termed **Sheehan syndrome**. Finally, though rare, peripartum cardiomyopathy, postpartum cerebral angiopathy, amniotic fluid embolism, and hypertensive disorders of pregnancy may place patients at risk for strokes.

Illicit Substance Use

Several illicit substances such as cocaine, ecstasy, and lysergic acid diethylamide have been associated with stroke. **Cocaine** has been associated with both ischemic and hemorrhagic stroke. The probability of hemorrhagic stroke is higher in cocaine users with occult intracranial aneurysms or AVMs. Irrespective of the method of cocaine administration, SAH may occur, as cocaine produces tachycardia, hypertension, and vasoconstriction. The resultant sudden rise in systemic blood pressure is thought to precipitate SAH. Ischemic lesions have also been found, though intracranial hemorrhage appears to occur more commonly than ischemic infarction. **Amphetamines** can also induce vasospasm, cardiac arrhythmias, and cardiomyopathy and accelerate atherosclerosis. Drugs injected intravenously place adolescents at risk for embolism or endocarditis.

Modifiable Risk Factors

Adolescents and young adults with traditional cerebrovascular disease risk factors (hypertension, diabetes, smoking, obesity, hyperlipidemia) are at risk for stroke.

CAUSES OF STROKE UNRELATED TO AGE

Pharyngeal Infection

Pharyngeal infections have been associated with stroke caused by thrombotic occlusion of the carotid arteries in their cervical course. In childhood, stroke resulting from carotid occlusion more commonly occurs in the intracranial segment of the carotid artery. Infections of the cervical region such as tonsillitis, pharyngitis, cervical lymphadenitis, necrotizing fasciitis, and Lemierre syndrome (see Chapter 48) have been found in children experiencing acute hemiplegia. In these instances, angiography has shown occlusion of the internal carotid artery located in its cervical segment. Neuroimaging has demonstrated ischemic infarction of the cortical region served by the middle cerebral artery, which arises from the carotid circulation. It is speculated that the soft tissue infection leads to an inflammatory arteritis. Vessel wall inflammation and direct pressure on the artery then lead to intravascular thrombosis and occlusion. Neurologic symptoms are noted in a patient with evidence of infection: fever, lethargy, sore throat or neck, difficulty swallowing, or cervical lymphadenopathy.

Head and Neck Trauma

Head and neck trauma is an important cause of stroke in children. Neurologic symptoms may be delayed more than 24 hours in their appearance in relation to the time of the inciting trauma. Stroke caused by carotid artery injury has been well documented. Most often, these cerebrovascular events occur after head and neck trauma sustained in motor vehicle accidents, bicycle accidents, fights, or falls. Hemiparesis is a common symptom at presentation if the cause resides in the carotid artery. Carotid angiography reveals internal carotid artery occlusion.

The site of occlusion most often exists at the level of the carotid bifurcation. Pathologically, an intimal tear is found with attendant thrombus blocking the arterial lumen. In some cases, arterial dissection is found.

Vertebral artery injury from trauma may cause stroke in children. Traction injuries of the neck appear to cause vertebral artery injury. The vertebral artery is most vulnerable to traumatic injury at its atlantoaxial portion. The resultant strokes occur in the vertebrobasilar portion of the cerebral circulation. Symptoms are referrable to the structures receiving blood from this system: brainstem, cerebellum, occipital lobes, and temporal lobes. Clinical symptoms of vertebrobasilar stroke include difficulty swallowing, ataxia, facial weakness, tinnitus, vertigo, anisocoria, extraocular movement palsies, dysmetria, cortical blindness, and mental status changes. Because both the long sensory and the motor tracts course through the brainstem, symptoms of general sensorimotor impairment may be found. Vertebral artery injury in children has been reported in the setting of athletic endeavor or automobile accidents. The resultant vertebrobasilar strokes are caused by thrombosis or vertebral artery dissection.

Migraine Headache

Stroke may occur in the setting of migraine headache. The occurrence of focal motor deficits during a migraine headache denotes complicated migraine (see Chapter 34). Acute hemiparesis has been documented during these episodes and is believed to reflect the involvement of the cerebral circulation derived from the carotid artery. Symptoms such as ataxia, cortical blindness, and cranial nerve dysfunction are correlated with vertebrobasilar circulation involvement. Focal symptoms may be fixed or may occur as TIAs.

Angiographic studies on patients with focal deficits consistent with stroke in the setting of migraine headache reveal vasoconstriction of vessels in either the vertebrobasilar or the carotid circulations. The anatomic position of the constricted vessels correlated with the location of the observed deficits. Ischemia provoked by vasoconstriction during prolonged migraine has been hypothesized as the mechanism of stroke in these patients.

■ SUMMARY AND RED FLAGS

Acute hemiplegia most frequently represents stroke. Mimics of stroke should be considered, though if clinical suspicion of stroke remains, urgent neuroimaging must be performed to further categorize the type of stroke, as acute management largely depends on this categorization. Following stabilization and the initiation of neuroprotective strategies, contributing factors should be determined so as to discern the risk of recurrence and to initiate any indicated prophylactic measures. Stroke complications include seizures, hemorrhagic transformation of ischemic and venous stroke, intracranial hypertension, and long-lasting functional and cognitive deficits. Rehabilitation referrals, including neuropsychological evaluation, should be initiated promptly.

The evaluation of remote stroke is similar though does not necessarily require the same degree of urgency: obtaining neuroimaging, assessing the type of stroke, discerning risk factors and etiology when able to while aiming to prevent stroke recurrence, preventing and treating complications, and optimizing maximal potential for recovery through rehabilitation strategies.

Red flags include status epilepticus, signs of increased intracranial pressure, coma, severe acute (worst ever) headache, nuchal rigidity, extracranial sites of bleeding, fever, and a family or personal history of disorders predisposing to stroke.

BIBLIOGRAPHY

A bibliography is available at ExpertConsult.com.

38

Hypertonicity

Ahmad Marashly

DEFINITIONS

Tone is defined as *resistance to passive stretch* while a patient is attempting to maintain a relaxed state of muscle activity. Tone can be divided into **postural tone,** which represents the steady flexion or extension of a joint caused by the uniform resistance of muscle to passive movement, and **phasic tone,** which represents the catch when an extremity is rapidly flexed or extended. **Hypertonia** describes unusually elevated tone, typically the result of an upper motor neuron disease. Hypertonia itself has three different clinical subtypes that may exist individually or in combination (Table 38.1):

Spasticity: hypertonia in which one or both of the following signs are present: (1) resistance to externally imposed movement increases with increasing speed of stretch and varies with the direction of joint movement, and/or (2) resistance to externally imposed movement rises rapidly above a threshold speed or joint angle.

Dystonia: movement disorder in which involuntary, sustained, or intermittent muscle contractions cause twisting and repetitive movements, abnormal posture, or both. The muscle contractions are the hypertonic component.

Rigidity: hypertonia in which all of the following are true: (1) the resistance to externally imposed joint movement is present at very low speeds of movement, does not depend on imposed speed, and does not exhibit a speed or angle threshold; (2) simultaneous co-contraction of agonists and antagonists may occur, and this is reflected in an immediate resistance to a reversal of the direction of movement about a joint; (3) the limb does not tend to return toward a particular fixed posture or extreme joint angle; and (4) voluntary activity in distant muscle groups does not lead to involuntary movements about the rigid joints, although rigidity may worsen.

The term **motor syndrome** is an alternative term inclusive of the different types of clinical hypertonia as well as other neurologic deficits. A motor syndrome caused by an injury before the age of 2 years is often labeled cerebral palsy (CP), whereas motor syndromes caused by injuries sustained after that age are described by terminology typically related to the etiology.

CP (see Chapter 27) and dystonia syndromes (see Chapter 40) are the two most common etiologies of hypertonia in children.

HISTORY

Elements of the history that should be collected include:
- Onset of increased tone
- Preceding illnesses, traumas, surgeries, or any events prior to the onset of increased tone
- Course of hypertonia including worsening, improvement, or no changes over time since the onset
- Limbs or body parts affected including the part most prominently affected
- Any times of the day when hypertonia is most or least noticeable
- Abnormal posture or movements
- Abnormal gait
- Worsening and alleviating factors
- History of brain or spinal cord injuries
- Drug or toxin exposure
- Pregnancy and birth
- Other medical or surgical conditions
- Family history of any neuromuscular disorders
- Environmental or medical allergies

Physical Examination

A general physical examination includes head and neck, cardiopulmonary, abdominal, skin, and genital examinations. Findings on any of these areas may indicate a syndromic or genetic pathology. Additionally, abnormalities in these systems may have implications on treatment options for hypertonicity.

The neurologic examination includes the following components:

Mental state: This is age dependent and can range from observing the patient interacting with their environment and people around them in the first few years of life to formal mental state testing in the older cooperative child.

Cranial nerves examination includes pupillary reflexes, external eye movements, facial sensation, face symmetry, hearing, tongue and uvula on the midline, neck movements, and shoulder shrug.

A **fundoscopic** examination should be performed whenever possible. Abnormal findings in the retina can be signs of a genetic or systemic pathology or an intracranial pathology leading to increased intracranial pressure.

The **motor** examination is the main tool to assess a patient with hypertonia. Components of the motor exam include:

Strength: The ability to examine strength is also dependent on the patient's age and cooperation and ranges from observing the child moving their limbs against gravity and the examiner's resistance to the more detailed exam of different muscle groups in the child who is able to follow commands. Strength is typically graded as follows: 0: no contraction or movement; 1: muscle contraction but no movement; 2: movement at the level of the bed but not against gravity; 3: movement against gravity but not against resistance; 4: some movement against resistance but not at the expected full level for age; and 5: normal movements against resistance.

Muscle bulk is assessed by inspection and palpation to detect any subtle muscle wasting, fasciculations, or hypertrophy.

Tone: It is important to take a thorough look at the whole musculoskeletal system in a child presenting with increased tone, including the parts that are reportedly unaffected. This allows

TABLE 38.1   Clinical Findings of the Different Hypertonia Subtypes

Clinical Finding	Spasticity	Dystonia	Rigidity
Change in resistance with increasing speed of passive movement	Increases	No effect	No effect
Change in resistance with rapid reversal of direction	Delayed	Immediate	Immediate
Fixed posture	Only in severe cases	Yes	No
Effect of voluntary activity on pattern of activated muscles	Minimal	Yes	Minimal
Effect of behavioral task and emotional state pattern of activated muscles	Minimal	Yes	Minimal

TABLE 38.2   Comparison of Ashworth and Tardieu Hypertonia Scales

	Ashworth Scale	Tardieu Scale
0	No increased tone	No resistance
1	Slight increase in muscle tone, manifested by a catch and release or by minimal resistance at the end of the range of motion when the affected part is moved in flexion or extension	Slight resistance
2	More marked increase in muscle tone through most of the range of motion, but affected part(s) easily moved	Catch followed by a release
3	Considerable increase in muscle tone, passive movement difficult	Fatigable clonus (<10 sec)
4	Affected part(s) rigid in flexion or extension	Infatigable clonus (>10 sec)

for comparison and detection of any unreported abnormalities by history. Inspection will look for size of the muscles, abnormal posture, and abnormal movements.

The child should be relaxed as much as possible and the body part examined supported against gravity. The head should be maintained in the midline to avoid contributions to tone from the tonic neck reflex. The following steps are then performed:

1. Palpate muscles to look for contraction at rest.
2. Measure resistance to movement of the affected joint with the child supine, seated, and standing.
3. Measure passive range of motion at very slow (3 seconds to complete the movement), intermediate (0.5 second to complete the movement), and fast (as rapidly as possible) speeds. Note the resistance at the onset of movement, the presence or absence of a "catch" occurring at some time after the onset of movement, and the joint angle at which the catch occurs.
4. Perform sudden reversal in the direction of movement at slow, intermediate, and fast speeds, and note the presence or absence of increased resistance immediately on reversal (suggesting co-contraction) or at some time after (suggesting a spastic catch), as well as any velocity dependence.
5. Ask the child to move the same joint on the contralateral side and observe for involuntary movement, and then test for a change in resistance to slow, passive movement. Instruct the child to move a distant and unrelated joint (e.g., by opening and closing one fist) on the contralateral side and then the ipsilateral side and observe for involuntary movement or a change in resistance to passive movement.

Reflexes: The main reflexes examined are the biceps, triceps, brachioradials, ankles, and knees.

Gait: When applicable, gait can aid in the determination of the different deficit patterns related to weakness, hypertonia, or movement disorders affecting the lower limbs.

Different scaling systems have been developed to measure hypertonia including the Ashworth, modified Ashworth, and pendulum tests. These tests do not distinguish between the different clinical types of hypertonia but do measure severity. The Tardieu Scale compares the occurrence of a catch at low and high speeds and is effective in measuring the velocity-dependent component of hypertonia (Table 38.2). Other scales are designed to specifically measure dystonia and rigidity such as the Barry-Albright Dystonia Scale. The Hypertonia Assessment Tool (HAT) is a 7-item scaling system designed to assess all three different types of hypertonia for each extremity and has been shown to have good reliability, validity, and inter-rater agreement in identifying

spasticity and the absence of rigidity, and moderate findings for identifying dystonia (Table 38.3).

Etiology

Hypertonia is a result of a pathology to the upper motor neuron pathways in the cortex, basal ganglia, thalamus, cerebellum, brainstem, central white matter, or spinal cord. Hypertonia is not considered to be a sign of a peripheral nerve or muscle pathology.

Hypertonia is a component of many motor disorders. Clinically, motor disorders are often divided into pyramidal and extrapyramidal groups. However, it is increasingly recognized that the pyramidal and extrapyramidal motor systems are highly interconnected and a clear distinction is not always possible; rather, pathology affecting both systems usually exists in the same patient.

Pyramidal motor disorders result from injury to the cortical projections to the brainstem (corticobulbar) and spinal cord (corticospinal) at any point along their tract resulting in a combination of weakness and increased tendon reflexes.

Extrapyramidal motor disorders result from injury to the basal ganglia, cerebellum, or nonprimary motor cortical areas resulting in abnormal motor control without weakness or changes in tendon reflexes.

The coexistence of pyramidal and extrapyramidal signs can make determination of contributions of these systems complex because different clinical types of hypertonia (spasticity, dystonia, and rigidity) often coexist in the same patient to variable degrees.

Furthermore, the ongoing growth, maturation, and prominent plasticity of the central nervous system in children add to the complexity of motor syndromes, which can lead a static injury to the central nervous system to manifest with a dynamically changing clinical picture.

CEREBRAL PALSY

The most common disorder manifesting primarily with hypertonia in children is CP, resulting from an injury to the developing brain before the age of 2 years.

The different subtypes of spastic CP reflect the different variables involved in determining the clinical picture including age, location, and type of injury (Table 38.4).

The overall prevalence of CP is ~2 per 1,000 live births, with much higher prevalence in preterm compared with term infants and decreasing gestational age (GA) and birthweight (BW).

TABLE 38.3 Hypertonia Assessment Tool (HAT) with a Description of the Administration Procedure for Each Item

Items (in Order of Administration)	Type of Hypertonia	Administration of Item	Scoring (Fill Each Box with 0 [Negative] or 1 [Positive])
Increased involuntary movements or postures of the designated limb with tactile stimulus of a distant body part	Dystonia	With the child at rest, observe involuntary movements of the designated limb as you gently rub a distant body part such as the shin or forearm	Dystonia is present if more involuntary movements or postures are observed in the designated limb with the tactile stimulus
Increased involuntary movements or postures with purposeful movement of a distant body part	Dystonia	Observe movements of the designated limb as the child carries out purposeful movements*	Dystonia is present if more involuntary movements or postures are observed in the designated limb with purposeful movement
Velocity-dependent resistance to stretch	Spasticity	Move the limb as described below[†] and assess for a change in muscle resistance between the slow and the fast stretch	Spasticity is present if there is an increase in resistance between the fast stretch compared with the slow stretch
Presence of spastic catch	Spasticity	Note the presence of a rapid rise (spastic catch) in resistance at a particular joint angle when moving the limb as described during the fast stretch[†]	Spasticity is present if a spastic catch is noted
Equal resistance to passive stretch during bidirectional movement of a joint	Rigidity	Assess this item during the fast stretch of the muscle[†]	Rigidity is present if the resistance felt is equal with movement in both directions
Increased tone with movement of a distant body part	Dystonia	Perform two additional fast stretches.[†] During the second stretch ask the child to do a purposeful movement* and assess for an increase in tone	Dystonia is present if greater tone is noticed when child is carrying out the purposeful movements
Maintenance of limb position after passive movement	Rigidity	For the arm, note the original position of the elbow; move the elbow by 45 degrees into either flexion or extension and observe if the elbow returns to its original position. For the leg, note the original position of the ankle; move the ankle into 45-degree further dorsiflexion or plantarflexion and observe if the ankle returns to its original position	Rigidity is present if the limb remains in the final position of stretch rather than returning (partially or fully) to the limb's original position

Before administering the HAT, the child should be supine on the examining table. The child should be as comfortable as possible by having appropriate caregivers present, a roll placed under the knees, a comfortable room temperature, and unrestrictive clothing. Complete all items for the involved extremity being examined before moving on to the next involved extremity.

*Based on the child's ability, ask the child to carry out two of the following for a 10-second period: (1) count to 10 slowly; (2) open and close one hand (into a fist) repeatedly (choose the hand that is not being examined); (3) open and close eyes (tight blinking) repeatedly; (4) reach for an object placed at least 1 foot away; and (5) visually track a brightly colored object (e.g., red-tipped pen) or light source (e.g., flashlight).

[†]Support the limb against gravity. Move the joints of the limb through the child's full range starting with the joint in full flexion or adduction, moving to full extension or abduction, and then returning to flexion or adduction, twice slowly and twice as quickly as possible. Upper extremity: shoulder adduction and abduction—begin with shoulder in full adduction; elbow flexion and extension—begin with elbow in full flexion; forearm pronation and supination—begin with forearm in full pronation; wrist flexion and extension—begin with wrist in full flexion. Lower extremity: hip adduction and abduction—begin with hip in full adduction; knee flexion and extension—begin with knee flexed with the hip in 90-degree flexion; ankle dorsiflexion and plantarflexion—begin with ankle in full plantarflexion.

From Jethwa A, Mink J, Macarthus C, et al. Development of the hypertonia assessment tool (HAT): a discriminative tool for hypertonia in children. *Dev Med Child Neurol.* 2010,52:e83–e87 (Appendix I, p. e87).

Although infants born preterm are at higher risk of developing CP, most CP cases are in infants born after 36 weeks' GA. Of the overall CP cases, ~25% are very preterm (GA <32 weeks), ~10–20% moderately preterm or late preterm (GA 32–36 weeks), and ~60% term (GA >36 weeks).

An approach to neonatal hypertonia is noted in Figure 38.1.

There are a number of genetic and metabolic disorders that present with clinical features of CP (Tables 38.5 and 38.6). Hereditary spastic paraplegia is discussed in Chapter 27.

Testing

The diagnostic approach to evaluating a child with hypertonia includes excluding the disorders in Tables 38.5 and 38.6 and the approach noted in Figures 38.1 and 38.2.

Management

Management of hypertonia depends on the clinical type and is typically a combination of physical, medical, and surgical interventions delivered through a multidisciplinary team of pediatricians, neurologists, physical medicine and rehab specialists, and orthopedic surgeons. Goals and extent of management also differ based on the pathology, functionality, and other comorbidities as not all cases of hypertonia need to be treated. In general, the following principles are observed when formulating a plan for treatment:

1. Distinguish type of clinical hypertonia and how it influences function.
2. For intramuscular injections, identify muscles to be injected. Not all spastic muscles need to be treated, because some patients rely on their hypertonia to maintain certain functions.

TABLE 38.4	**Clinical Features of Spastic Cerebral Palsy (CP) Subtypes**			
CP Subtype	**Location of Hypertonia**	**Common Causes and Location of Injury**	**Age Group**	**Clinical Features**
Spastic diplegic	Both lower limbs and upper limbs relatively or completely preserved	Periventricular leukomalacia Deep white matter	Preterm infants	Hypotonia of the lower limbs for the first 6 mo of life Spasticity evolves by 6 mo of age Flexion, adduction, and internal rotation of the hips with contractures of the hip flexors and hamstring muscles and to a lesser extent knees and elbows Reduced limb length and muscle bulk in lower extremities
Spastic hemiplegic	Hemibody including upper and lower limbs	Neonatal stroke, congenital malformations Cerebral cortex	Term infants of normal birthweight	Weakened and abnormal posturing on one body side Early hand dominance During first 1–2 yr, movement and tone on the affected side typically decrease before tone and tendon reflexes abnormally increase The arm is typically more affected than the leg Typical posture appears by 2 yr of age Arm is adducted at the shoulder and flexed at the elbow, the forearm is pronated, and the wrist and fingers are flexed with the hand closed Hip is partially flexed and adducted, and the knee and ankle are flexed; the foot may remain in the equinovarus or calcaneovalgus position Independent walking usually occurs at the appropriate age or is only slightly delayed
Spastic quadriplegic	All limbs affected	Congenital infections, congenital malformations, ischemic hypoxic encephalopathy Diffuse, cortical, and white matter injury	Most commonly term SGA infants, but can also occur in preterm infants	Moderate or severe psychomotor delay All limbs are affected Poor head control Early spasticity by 2–3 mo of age Adduction of the thighs results in typical scissoring of the legs By 9–10 mo of age, unable to flex the legs with poor truncal balance Upper limbs equally or more involved than lower limbs Severe comorbidities including feeding difficulties, chronic respiratory insufficiency, and epilepsy are common

SGA, small for gestational age.

3. Outcome of treatment depends on clear communication of goals of treatment between the clinician and the patient/family.
4. Regular assessment and evaluation are needed as the clinical picture and effect of treatment may change over time requiring adjusting the treatment regimen, especially in growing children with ever-changing functionality levels and demands.
5. Physical and occupational therapies are the main modality of management for children with hypertonia.

HEREDITARY HYPEREKPLEXIA

Hyperekplexia (HPX), also known as stiff baby syndrome or startle disease, is an inherited disorder (Table 38.7) due to dysfunction of the glycinergic neuronal receptor (see also Chapter 40). HPX manifests with exaggerated startle responses to various stimuli (visual, auditory, and most often tactile) leading to myoclonic jerks and stiffness. Onset is often in neonates, but ambulatory children may fall if an episode occurs while sitting or standing. *Consciousness is retained.* The head retraction reflex is elicited by gently tapping the nose, glabella, lip, or chin. In addition to the exaggerated startle reflexes, patients may present with generalized stiffness after birth or following a startle response. The stiffness

resolves during sleep. Patients have normal development and a normal EEG and MRI. The differential diagnosis of other disorders manifesting with an abnormal startle response is noted in Table 38.8.

STIFF PERSON SYNDROME

Stiff person syndrome (SPS) is most commonly reported in adults as an autoimmune or paraneoplastic disorder that manifests with sensitivity to external stimuli, progressive truncal muscle (paraspinal) rigidity, and muscle spasms.

Variants of adult SPS include:
- SPS associated with myoclonus
- SPS associated with epilepsy and dystonia
- SPS with neuro-ophthalmologic findings
- SPS with progressive rigidity and encephalomyelitis
- SPS cerebellar variant

In children, the disorder is usually associated with immunoglobulin G (IgG) anti–glutamic acid decarboxylase antibodies or anti–glycine receptor antibodies and other coexisting autoimmune diseases including diabetes mellitus, Graves disease, autoimmune thyroiditis, vitiligo, and celiac disease.

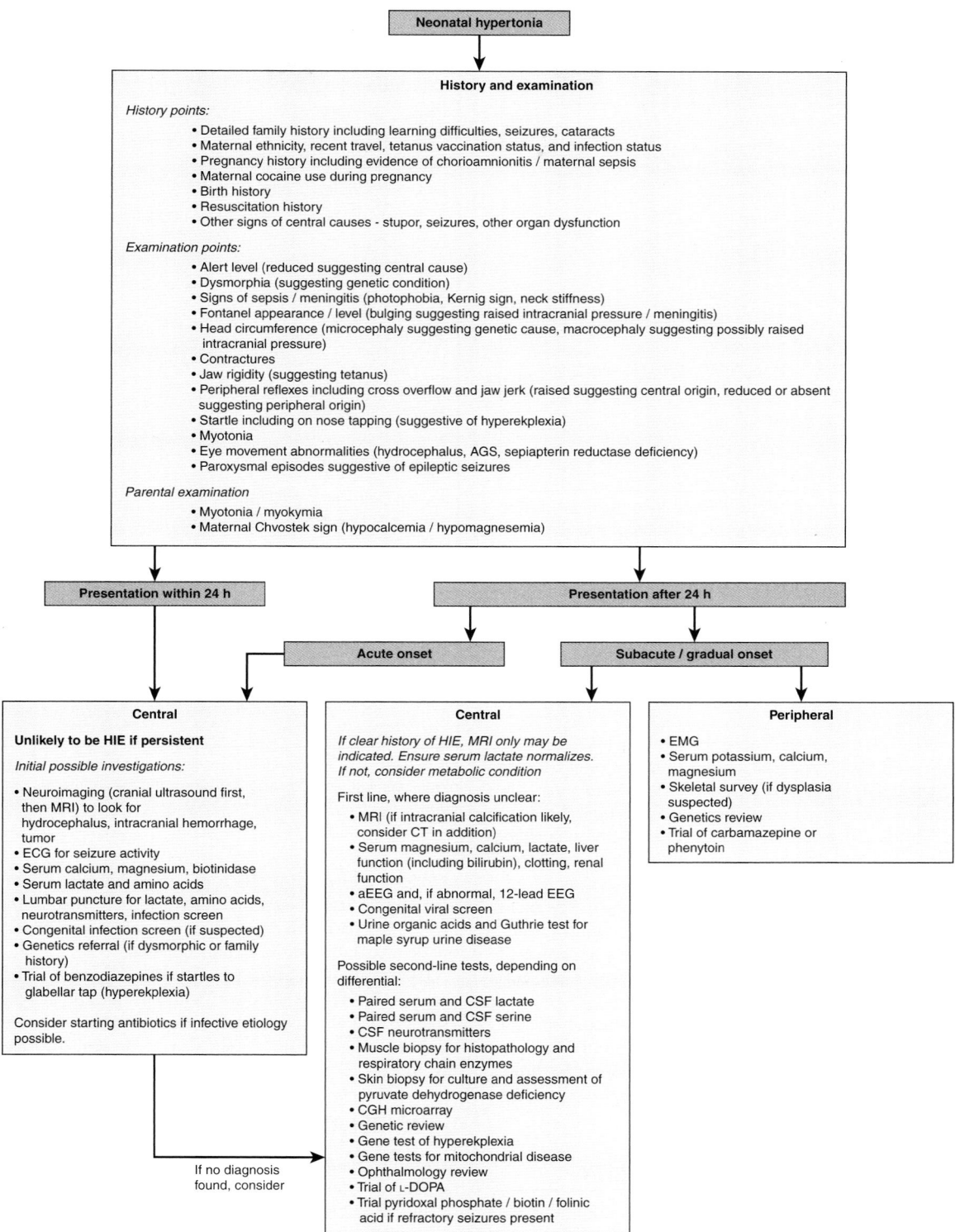

Fig. 38.1 A suggested algorithm for the investigation of neonatal hypertonia. AGS, Aicardi-Goutières syndrome; aEEG, amplitude integrated EEG; CGH, comparative genomic hybridization; CSF, cerebrospinal fluid; EMG, electromyography; HIE, hypoxic-ischemic encephalopathy. (From Hart AR, Sharma R, Rittey CD, et al. Neonatal hypertonia – a diagnostic challenge. *Dev Med Child.* 2015;57:600–610 [Fig. 2, p. 608].)

Presenting manifestations include gait disturbances due to lower extremity stiffness or spasms, lumbar lordosis from paraspinal muscle involvement, and an exaggerated startle response precipitated by anxiety-provoking activities. The classic SPS phenotype is the most prevalent type; variants noted in adults may also occur in children. The differential diagnosis includes hyperekplexia, dystonias, progressive encephalomyelitis with rigidity and myoclonus (PERM), and hereditary spastic paraplegia.

TABLE 38.5   Brain MRI Findings Suggestive of Selected Genetic Cerebral Palsy Mimics

Finding	Selected Conditions
Hypomyelination	*PLP1*-related dysmyelinating disorders H-ABC (*TUBB4A* variant) AGS (may also have basal ganglia and WM calcification) GM1 gangliosidosis
Demyelination	Krabbe disease Metachromatic leukodystrophy
Thin corpus callosum	HSP (i.e., SPG4, SPG11, SPG15, and others)
Globus pallidus lesions	T2 hypointense: NBIA (SN also involved in BPAN, MPAN), fucosidosis T2 hyperintense: MMA, PDH deficiency, creatine deficiency syndromes
Focal atrophy or hypoplasia	Glutaric aciduria type 1 (frontotemporal) H-ABC (cerebellum ± putamen) Joubert syndrome (cerebellum)

AGS, Aicardi-Goutières syndrome; BPAN, β-propeller protein-associated neurodegeneration; H-ABC, hypomyelination with atrophy of the basal ganglia and cerebellum; HSP, hereditary spastic paraplegia; MMA, methylmalonic aciduria; MPAN, mitochondrial membrane protein-associated neurodegeneration; NBIA, neurodegeneration with brain iron accumulation; PDH, pyruvate dehydrogenase; WM, white matter.
Adapted from Pearson TS, Pons R, Ghaoui R, et al. Genetic mimics of cerebral palsy. *Mov Disord.* 2019;34(5):625–636.

TABLE 38.6   Differential Diagnoses in Spastic Paraplegia

Childhood Onset
Diplegic cerebral palsy
Structural (Chiari malformation, atlantoaxial subluxation)
Hereditary spastic paraplegia
Leukodystrophy (e.g., Krabbe)
Metabolic (arginase deficiency, abetalipoproteinemia)
Levodopa-responsive dystonia
Infection (myelitis)
Multiple sclerosis

Adolescent Onset
Cervical spine degenerative disease
Multiple sclerosis
Motor neuron disease
Neoplasm (primary/secondary spinal tumor, parasagittal meningioma)
Infection (myelitis)
Dural arteriovenous malformation
Chiari malformation
Adrenoleukodystrophy
Hereditary spastic paraplegia
Spinocerebellar ataxias
Vitamin deficiency (B$_{12}$ and E)
Lathyrism
Levodopa-responsive dystonia
Infection (syphilis, human T-cell leukemia virus 1, HIV)
Copper deficiency

From Salinas S, Proukakis C, Crosby A, et al. Hereditary spastic paraplegia: clinical features and pathogenetic mechanisms. *Lancet Neurol.* 2008;7:1127–1138 (Panel, p. 1128).

TETANUS

Tetanus is caused by toxin produced by the spore-forming bacteria *Clostridium tetani* and develops after a cutaneous wound in older children or in neonates secondary to umbilical cord infection. Puncture wounds are a high risk and include nails, splinters, intramuscular injections, body piercing, tattoos, and bites (insect, animal, human). Burns, dental abscesses, and compound fractures are additional risks for tetanus. In some patients, the source of tetanus is unknown. The incubation period is ~3–21 days. Risk factors other than wounds include unimmunized status, intravenous drug users, immunosuppressed patients, or neonates born to unimmunized mothers with septic cutting or contamination of the umbilical cord.

Manifestations include risus sardonicus, painful muscle spasms, opisthotonic posturing, and trismus (Tables 38.9 and 38.10). Complications include vocal cord paralysis, autonomic storming, fractures, hernias, and aspiration pneumonia. The differential diagnosis includes strychnine poisoning and dystonic drug reactions.

MYOGENIC ETIOLOGIES OF HYPERTONICITY

Myotonia congenita is either an autosomal dominant (Thomsen disease) or autosomal recessive (Becker disease) disorder and is characterized by generalized stiffness (myotonia, delayed relaxations) after muscle contractions (Table 38.11). Pathologic variants in the chloride channel gene (*CLCN1*) are responsible for both forms of myotonia congenita. Both forms are associated with muscle hypertrophy (legs); myotonia can be demonstrated with hand contraction or eye closure. Transient muscle weakness occurs during exercise but with repeated efforts muscle strength returns to normal (warm-up phenomenon).

Paramyotonic congenita (PMC) presents with myotonia affecting the facial muscles and those of the neck and hands, although all skeletal muscles are involved. PMC is due to pathologic variants in *SCN4A*. Myotonia is exacerbated by exercise and cold exposure. Paradoxical myotonia occurs with repeated muscle contraction because PMC does not demonstrate a warm-up phenomenon.

Hyperkalemic period paralysis is an autosomal dominant disorder (*SCN4A*) and manifests with episodes of weakness or paralysis but may also demonstrate muscle stiffness between attacks of weakness. Hypertonicity may also be present but may instead be myotonia.

DRUG-RELATED HYPERTONICITY

Serotonin syndrome is characterized by mental status changes (agitation, confusion, hypomania, coma), autonomic hyperactivity (tachycardia, labile blood pressure, diaphoresis, diarrhea), and neuromuscular dysfunction (myoclonus, hyperreflexia, clonus, rigidity, tremor, shivering, mydriasis) following exposure to an inciting drug (Tables 38.12 and 38.13).

A simplified diagnostic approach requires any of the following:
- Tremor and hyperreflexia
- Spontaneous clonus
- Muscle rigidity, temperature >38°C, and either ocular clonus or inducible clonus
- Ocular clonus and either agitation or diaphoresis
- Inducible clonus and either agitation or diaphoresis

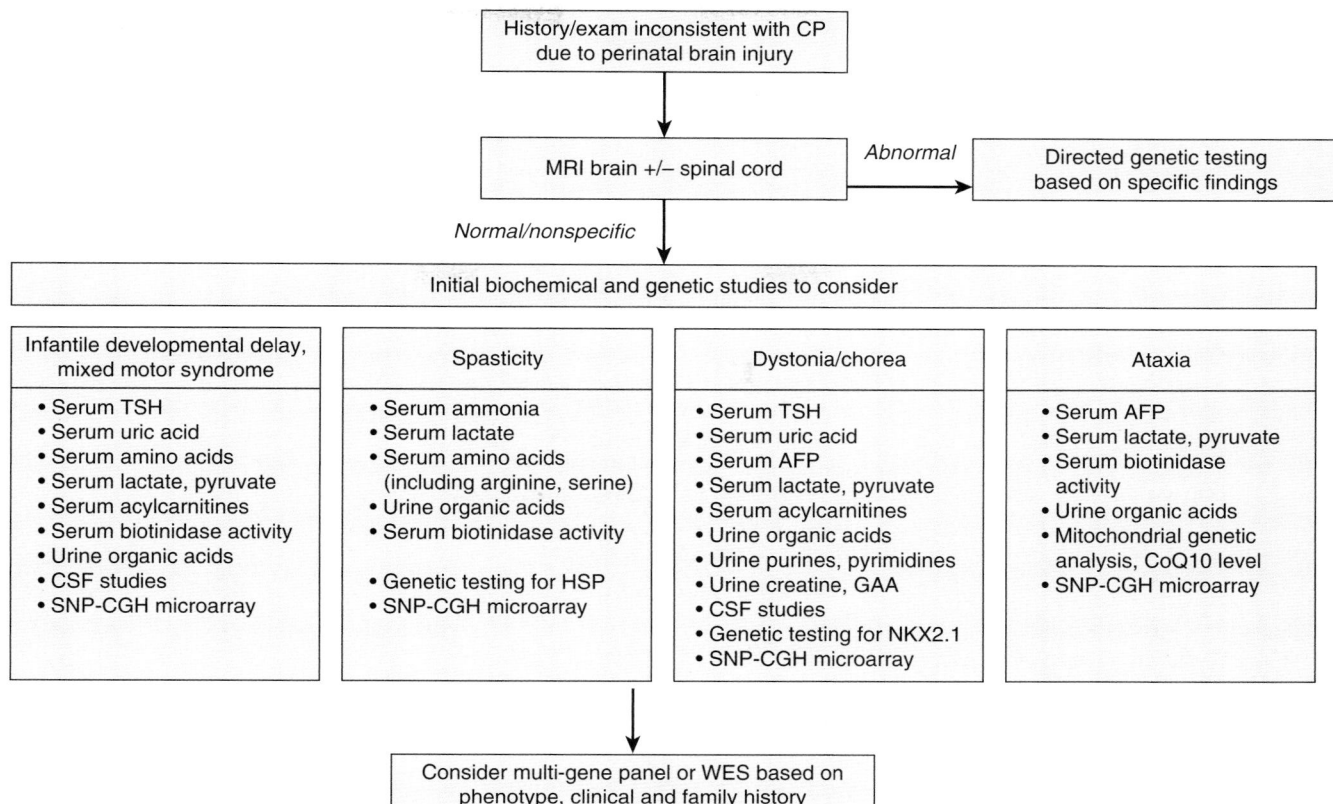

Fig. 38.2 General diagnostic approach to the patient with an infantile-onset, apparently nonprogressive motor disorder. Studies are grouped by predominant clinical presentation; it may be appropriate to consider investigations from more than one group depending on the specific clinical context. CSF studies: glucose (+serum glucose), lactate, pyruvate, neurotransmitter metabolites (biogenic amines + γ-aminobutyric acid [GABA]), pterins, 5-methyltetrahydrofolate. AFP, α-fetoprotein; CP, cerebral palsy; CGH, comparative genomic hybridization; CSF, cerebrospinal fluid; GAA, α-glucosidase; HSP, hereditary spastic paraplegia; SNP, single nucleotide protein; TSH, thyroid-stimulating hormone; WES, whole-exome sequencing. (From Pearson TS, Pons R, Ghaoi R, et al. Genetic mimics of cerebral palsy. *Mov Disord.* 2019;34[5]:625–634 [Fig. 1, p. 627].)

TABLE 38.7 *GLRA1, GLRB,* and *SLC6A5*-Related Hereditary Hyperekplexia (HPX): Modes of Inheritance and Methods of Variant Detection

			PROPORTION OF PROBANDS WITH A PATHOGENIC VARIANT DETECTABLE BY METHOD[†]	
Gene	**Proportion of HPX Attributed to Variant of Gene**	**MOI***	**Sequence Analysis[‡]**	**Gene-Targeted Deletion/ Duplication Analysis[§]**
GLRA1	61–63%	AD and AR	~95%	See footnote[‖]
GLRB	12–14%	AD and AR	11/12	1/12
SLC6A5	25%	AR (rarely AD)	24/24	None reported

AD, autosomal dominant; AR, autosomal recessive; MOI, mode of inheritance; PCR, polymerase chain reaction.

*~85% were AR and ~15% were AD.

[†]Additional affected individuals have been reported, many as case studies. For additional reported variants, see the Human Genome Mutation Database.

[‡]Sequence analysis detects variants that are benign, likely benign, of uncertain significance, likely pathogenic, or pathogenic. Variants may include small intragenic deletions/insertions and missense, nonsense, and splice site variants; typically, exon or whole-gene deletions/duplications are not detected.

[§]Gene-targeted deletion/duplication analysis detects intragenic deletions or duplications. Methods used may include quantitative PCR, long-range PCR, multiplex ligation-dependent probe amplification (MLPA), and a gene-targeted microarray designed to detect single-exon deletions or duplications.

[‖]Deletion of exons 1–7 is common in the Turkish population. Deletion of exons 1–6 and of 4–7 have also been reported.

From Balint B, Thomas R. Hereditary hyperekplexia overview 2007 Jul 21 (Updated 2019 Dec 19). In: Adan MP, Ardinger HH, Pagon RA, et al., eds. *GeneReviews* [Internet]. Seattle: University of Washington; 1993–2021, Table 2.

TABLE 38.8 **Complex Genetic Neurodevelopmental Disorders with an Excessive Startle Response**

Gene	Disorder	MOI	Distinguishing Clinical Features	Reference*
ARHGEF9	Early-infantile epileptic encephalopathy 8	XL	• Severe ID • Epilepsy (often intractable focal seizures or febrile seizures) • Dysmorphic features	OMIM 300607
ASNS	Asparagine synthetase deficiency	AR	• Profound DD and progressive encephalopathy • Microcephaly • Hypotonia followed by spastic quadriplegia • Seizures	Asparagine synthetase deficiency
CACNA1A	Early-infantile epileptic encephalopathy 42	AD	• Epileptic encephalopathy with myoclonic epilepsy • Myoclonic seizures provoked by tactile stimuli and spontaneous and reflex seizures to noise and touch	OMIM 617106
CLPB	CLPB deficiency (3-methylglutaconic aciduria)	AR	• Congenital or infantile cataracts • Neutropenia • Other neurologic signs: hypotonia, spasticity, ataxia, dystonia, epilepsy, or ID	CLPB deficiency
CRLF1	Crisponi syndrome	AR	• Dysmorphic features, camptodactyly • Facial and bulbar weakness	Cold-induced sweating syndrome including Crisponi syndrome
CTNNB1	CTNNB1-related syndrome	AD	• Hyperekplexia is rare in this entity (single case report) • Later onset of hyperekplexia (not congenital but in childhood) and atypical pattern (no generalized stiffness induced by startle) • No congenital stiffness • Progressive neurologic involvement with additional signs (ID, ataxia, spasticity) • Microcephaly	Winczewska-Wiktor et al. (2016)
GPHN	Molybdenum cofactor deficiency, complementation group C	AR	• Intractable seizures • Severe psychomotor retardation • Hypotonia combined w/hyperreflexia • Usually lethal in infancy	OMIM 615501
HEXA	Tay-Sachs disease	AR	• DD or regression • Visual impairment • Epilepsy • Later: macrocephaly, decerebrate posturing, dysphagia, progression to unresponsive vegetative state	Hexosaminidase A deficiency
RPS6KA3	Coffin-Lowry syndrome	XL	• ID • Facial dysmorphism, tapering digits, and skeletal deformity • Besides hyperekplexia, there may be other types of stimulus-induced drop attacks (e.g., cataplexy-like episodes)	Coffin-Lowry syndrome
SCN8A	Early-infantile epileptic encephalopathy 13	AD	Epileptic encephalopathy with DD and ID	*SCN8A*-related epilepsy with encephalopathy
SLC6A9	GLYT1 encephalopathy	AR	• Hypotonia > hypertonicity • Arthrogryposis • Respiratory failure • Dysmorphic features • Encephalopathy	GLYT1 encephalopathy
SUOX	Isolated sulfite oxidase deficiency	AR	• Progressive epileptic encephalopathy • Other neurologic features: opisthotonus, spastic quadriplegia, pyramidal signs • Microcephaly, dysmorphic features	Isolated sulfite oxidase deficiency
TRAK1	Early-infantile epileptic encephalopathy 68	AR	• Hypotonia • Progressive epileptic encephalopathy	OMIM 618201
TSEN54	Pontocerebellar hypoplasia type 2	AR	• Generalized clonus ("jitteriness") • Delayed developmental (motor and cognitive) milestones • Other neurologic signs: spasticity, chorea, visual impairment, epilepsy	*TSEN54*-related pontocerebellar hypoplasia

AD, autosomal dominant; AR, autosomal recessive; DD, developmental delay; ID, intellectual disability; MOI, mode of inheritance; XL, X-linked.

*OMIM phenotype entry or citation is provided if a related *GeneReview* is not available.

From Balint B, Thomas R. Hereditary hyperekplexia overview 2007 Jul 21 (Updated 2019 Dec 19). In: Adan MP, Ardinger HH, Pagon RA, et al., eds. *GeneReviews* [Internet]. Seattle: University of Washington; 1993–2021.

TABLE 38.9 Presenting Features on Admission to Hospital for Non-neonatal Tetanus

- Trismus (93–98%)
- Generalized muscle tension (94–95%)
- Muscle stiffness (96%)
- Dysphagia (83%)
- Dyspnea (7%)
- Muscle spasms (46–80%)
- Body temperature >38.4°C (76%)
- Pulse ≥120 beats/min (34%)

From Yen LM, Thwaites CL. Tetanus. *Lancet*. 2019;393:1657–1666 (Panel 3, p. 1661).

Malignant hyperthermia (MH) occurs rapidly after exposure to an inhaled anesthetic agent or succinylcholine and is characterized by tachypnea, tachycardia, lactic acidosis, muscle rigidity, rhabdomyolysis, and fever. The earliest sign of MH is a rapid rise of end-tidal CO_2. Susceptibility to MH is associated with autosomal dominant pathologic variants on *RYR1*; *CACNA1S* is an uncommon but reported gene. MH has also been reported in patients with scoliosis and various congenital muscle disorders.

Neuroleptic malignant syndrome is similar to MH and follows the administration of neuroleptic antipsychotic agents; fever, muscle rigidity, rhabdomyolysis, autonomic dysfunction, and neutral states changes are also present.

OPISTHOTONUS

Opisthotonus manifests with acute or chronic spastic arching of the neck and back due to tonic contraction of the extensor muscles of the neck, back, and legs. The hyperextension can resemble decerebrate posturing. There are many etiologies that may also be age related (Table 38.14).

TABLE 38.10 Classification of Tetanus Severity

Grade 1: Mild
- Mild to moderate trismus
- Generalized spasticity
- No respiratory compromise
- No spasms
- Little or no dysphagia

Grade 2: Moderate
- Moderate trismus
- Marked rigidity
- Mild to moderate but short spasms
- Moderate respiratory compromise with an increased respiratory rate (>30 breaths/min)
- Mild dysphagia

Grade 3: Severe
- Severe trismus
- Generalized spasticity
- Reflex prolonged spasms
- Increased respiratory rate (>40 breaths/min)
- Apneic spells
- Severe dysphagia
- Tachycardia (>120 beats/min)

Grade 4: Very Severe
- Clinical features of grade 3 tetanus
- Violent autonomic disturbances involving the cardiovascular system
- Severe hypertension and tachycardia alternating with relative hypotension and bradycardia (either of which might be persistent)

From Yen LM, Thwaites CL. Tetanus. *Lancet*. 2019;393:1657–1666 (Panel 2, p. 1660).

TABLE 38.11 Chloride Channel Myotonias

Clinical Features	Autosomal Dominant Myotonia Congenita of Thomsen	Autosomal Recessive Generalized Myotonia of Becker
Inheritance	Dominant	Recessive
Gene defect	Chromosome 7; variant in skeletal muscle chloride channel	Chromosome 7; variant in skeletal muscle chloride channel
Age of onset	Infancy to early childhood	Late childhood, occasionally starts earlier or begins in teens
Myopathy	Muscle hypertrophy frequent; no myopathy, although variants uncommonly develop weakness	Occasional muscle wasting and weakness can occur late; hypertrophy of muscles frequently occurs in legs
Myotonia	Generalized stiffness, especially after rest; improves with exercise; prominent myotonia of eye closure, but not paradoxical myotonia	Generalized stiffness, especially after rest; transient weakness is prominent after complete relaxation for several minutes; myotonia occurs in eyes; no paradoxical myotonia
Provocative stimuli	Prolonged rest or maintenance of the posture	Prolonged rest or maintenance of the same posture
Therapy for symptoms	Exercise; antimyotonia therapy (e.g., mexiletine); Achilles tendon stretching helps prevent need for heel cord–lengthening surgery	Exercise; especially avoiding prolonged rest; antimyotonia therapy (e.g., mexiletine); transient weakness does not improve after mexiletine

From Swaiman KF, Ashwal A, Ferriero DM, et al., eds. *Swaiman's Pediatric Neurology*. 6th ed. Philadelphia: Elsevier; 2018:1151, Table 151-3.

TABLE 38.12 Classes of Medications That Produce Serotonin Syndrome in Psychiatric Patients

Selective serotonin reuptake inhibitors
Monoamine oxidase inhibitors
Atypical antipsychotics
Heterocyclic antidepressants
Trazodone
Dual-uptake inhibitors
Psychostimulants
Buspirone
Mood stabilizers
Analgesics
Antiemetics
Cough suppressants
Dietary supplements

From Goldman L, Schafer AI, eds. *Goldman-Cecil Medicine.* 26th ed. Philadelphia: Elsevier; 2020:2594, Table 406-5.

TABLE 38.13 Signs and Symptoms of Serotonin Syndrome (Review of 100 Cases)

Sign/Symptom	Frequency (%)	Sign/Symptom	Frequency (%)
Cognitive-Behavioral Symptoms	51	**Neuromuscular**	
		Myoclonus	58
Confusion/disorientation	34	Hyperreflexia	52
Agitation/irritability	29	Muscle rigidity	51
Coma/unresponsiveness	15	Restlessness/hyperactivity	48
Anxiety	14	Tremor	43
Euphoria/hypomania	13	Ataxia/incoordination	40
Headache	13	Clonus	23
Drowsiness	12	Babinski sign (bilateral)	16
Seizures	11	Nystagmus	15
Insomnia	6	Trismus	7
Hallucinations (visual and auditory)	5	Teeth chattering	6
		Opisthotonos	6
Autonomic Nervous System		Paresthesias	6
Hyperthermia	45		
Diaphoresis	45		
Sinus tachycardia	36		
Hypertension	35		
Dilated pupils	28		
Tachypnea	26		
Nausea	23		
Unreactive pupils	20		
Flushing	16		
Hypotension	15		
Diarrhea	8		
Ventricular tachycardia	6		
Cyanosis	5		
Abdominal cramps	4		
Salivation	4		

From Shannon MW, Borron SW, Burns MJ, eds. *Haddad and Winchester's Clinical Management of Poisoning and Drug Overdose.* 4th ed. Philadelphia: Elsevier; 2007:571, Table 29-3.

TABLE 38.14 Etiologies of Opisthotonus

Infections
Tetanus

Meningitis

Metabolic
Gaucher disease

Krabbe disease

Kernicterus

Neurodegeneration with brain iron accumulation

Glutaric aciduria

Maple syrup urine disease

Dopa-responsive dystonia

Toxin/Drug
Strychnine

Phenothiazines

Haloperidol

Cyanide

Metoclopramide

Infant alcohol withdrawal

Anatomic
Arnold-Chiari malformation

Brain tumor

Brain hemorrhage

Hydrocephalus

Traumatic brain injury

Dandy-Walker malformations

Other
Cerebral palsy

Stiff person syndrome

Conversion disorder

Anoxic injury

RED FLAGS

In the pediatric population, hypertonia is typically thought of in the context of static, nonprogressive diseases caused by an early one-time insult in life. With this concept in mind, any clinical features that suggest a *progressive* process should be considered as red flags and prompt further work-up for rare yet potentially serious pathologies (see Chapter 28).

Such red flags include developmental regression or loss of already acquired milestones; evolving/worsening focal deficits such as weakness, spasticity, vision, or hearing; marked cranial nerve involvement; extraneurologic system involvement (hepatic or kidney disease, progressive skin rashes); and family history of progressive neurologic diseases.

Some progressive causes of hypertonia in children include childhood-onset Parkinson disease, Wilson disease, leukodystrophies, demyelinating diseases (Alexander disease, Canavan disease, Krabbe disease), mitochondrial disorders, and neuronal ceroid lipofuscinosis.

BIBLIOGRAPHY

A bibliography is available at ExpertConsult.com.

39

Paroxysmal Disorders

Donald Basel

Paroxysmal disorders can be broadly classified into epileptiform and nonepileptic events. The nonepileptic episodes are often referred to by the generic term *spells*. They may mimic epileptic seizures but are not associated with the typical rhythmic EEG patterns characteristic of seizures (Table 39.1; see Chapters 7 and 40). These spells can be a manifestation of myriad etiologies leading to transient loss of consciousness and can be neurologic, cardiovascular, endocrine, psychologic, or gastrointestinal in origin. Most paroxysmal neurologic symptoms can be effectively evaluated, diagnosed, and managed by following a systematic approach. A detailed history will often be sufficient to make the diagnosis or to significantly narrow the diagnostic differential. A few well-selected tests will then allow the correct diagnosis to be made and subsequently enable the appropriate treatment of the child. The principal aim in the assessment is to establish signs of serious or emergent neurologic disease, and second, to form a differential diagnosis to guide further investigations and treatment (Fig. 39.1).

HISTORY

A careful description of the event or events from beginning to end, including re-enactments or videos by the parents of any unclear physical symptoms, is critical.

Pertinent questions include:

- Was this the first such event, or have there been multiple events?
- Is there a single or multiple episodes within the event?
- What was the child doing at the time of each spell—were they awake, asleep, playing, or sitting quietly?
- If they were asleep, how long had they been asleep, or what time of day or night did the spell occur?
- If abnormal tone or movements were involved, was the child rigid or limp, and which limbs were involved? Were the movements rhythmic and synchronous, or were they alternating, migratory, or stop-start?
- If the child was unresponsive or had alteration of awareness, what did the parents do to ascertain their level of responsiveness? Did the parents try touching them to regain their attention, or merely call their name?
- How long did the event last, and how did the child behave afterward?
- Did the child describe any symptoms prior to the onset of the actual event, or was there any abnormal behavior that the parents witnessed prior to the event?
- Were there any signs or symptoms of illness associated with the spell? Were any fevers documented?
- Has there been any behavioral, developmental, or academic regression since the start of the events?
- Is the child developmentally normal? If not, has the child's development always been abnormal, or was there a regression at some point?

- Were there any problems during pregnancy or the delivery?
- Has the child ever had a significant head injury or central nervous system (CNS) infection?
- Is there any family history of similar events, or any other neurologic disorders?

Parents frequently record videos of these spells on their mobile devices, which are ideal for reviewing the episode firsthand.

PHYSICAL EXAMINATION

The physician should compare vital signs, including blood pressure and head circumference, to previous measurements if possible. Elevated blood pressure can be indicative of pain, anxiety, increased intracranial pressure, or hypertensive encephalopathy. Hypotension may suggest syncopal events or sepsis. Dramatic increases in head circumference in infants may indicate intracranial pathology.

A general physical examination, including the cardiopulmonary and abdominal examinations, should be performed; abnormalities may indicate a non-neurologic cause for spells. **Dysmorphic** features or **cutaneous** findings can provide clues toward an underlying syndromic diagnosis.

An **ophthalmologic** examination can be as simple as obtaining a red reflex and observation of eye movements in young children. Eye movements may be observed by having the patient track a moving object or toy; abnormalities such as deviation, nystagmus, or new-onset limitations in range of motion may indicate a structural cause for the spells such as hydrocephalus or a mass lesion. In cooperative older children, the physician should attempt a funduscopic examination. **Papilledema** is a clue to increased intracranial pressure but is only readily appreciable after 2–3 weeks of increased intracranial pressure; it will not be present with acute disturbances leading to increased intracranial pressure.

The child will provide important information about their **mental status** and **developmental status** through simple conversation. Conversations about toys, school, or family members in the room can provide information about orientation, aphasia, dysarthria, and fund of knowledge for age. If there are any questions about whether any facial asymmetry is new-onset, parents may be able to provide old photographs; most people have some degree of facial asymmetry at baseline that may only be noticed after a frightening event causes the parents to observe the child more closely.

Muscle strength can be ascertained by manual testing in a cooperative older child or observing natural play or strength of resistance to examination in a younger child. If a child can easily perform age-appropriate actions such as crawling, walking, running, climbing, or grabbing for objects, and strongly resists examination, they are likely to have grossly normal strength in their major muscle groups. **Tone** can be checked by passively moving the patient's limbs or suspending

TABLE 39.1	Comparison of Generalized Seizures and Some Disorders That Can Mimic Them			
Condition	**Precipitants (May Not Apply to All Patients)**	**Prodrome**	**Ictal Symptoms**	**Postictal Symptoms**
Generalized seizures	Sleep deprivation, television, video games, visual patterns, and photic stimulation	Rarely irritability or nonspecific behavioral changes	Usually 2–3 min Consciousness might be preserved if atonic or, in some, tonic seizures Synchronous bilateral movements Tongue biting	Delayed recovery with postictal depression, incontinence (may be ictal also)
Syncope: vasovagal	Fatigue, emotional stress, dehydration, vomiting, choking, swallowing	Blurring of vision, tinnitus, dizziness, nausea, sweating, crying in breath-holding spells	Loss of consciousness for seconds, pallor, and rarely reflex anoxic seizures	Rapid recovery with no postictal depression
Syncope with reflex anoxic seizures	Minor bump to head, upsetting surprises			
Syncope: trigeminal vagal	Cold water on face			
Syncope: orthostatic	Standing up, bathing, awakening			
Hyperekplexia	Auditory and tactile stimuli	None	Tonic stiffening, cyanosis if severe, nonfatigable nose-tap–induced startles	Depending on severity, may have postictal depression
Cardiac	Exercise	None	Loss of consciousness, often only for a few seconds, pallor	Rarely
Psychogenic	Suggestion, stress	None	Eyes closed, with active opposition to attempts to open them Asynchronous flailing limb movements that vary between attacks Motor activity stops and starts during a spell Weeping and crying No injury May respond to suggestion during "loss of consciousness" Usually longer than 2–3 min	No postictal depression

Adapted from Obeid M, Mikati MA. Expanding spectrum of paroxysmal events in children: potential mimickers of epilepsy. *Pediatr Neurol.* 2007;37(5):309–316.

an infant in your hands to check if they start to slide through your grip. Low tone (hypotonia) can also be detected by observing gait or observing how the child sits; "W"-sitting (sitting with knees together and heels outside of their hips) may be another clue. Low strength (weakness) should be distinguished from hypotonia or ataxia; an example of normal strength but low tone might be an infant with motor delays and head lag who vigorously opposes examination; a child with normal strength but ataxia might vigorously oppose examination but cannot accurately reach to push away the examiner.

A normal physical examination (including vital signs and mental status) does not rule out the presence of a neurologic disorder but generally indicates a disorder that does not require immediate intervention and that more time can be spent carefully evaluating all diagnostic possibilities. In children with baseline neurologic abnormalities, such as children with cerebral palsy, knowledge of their baseline physical examination, abilities, and behavior is critical in deciding how urgently they need to be evaluated further. Parents can be very helpful in determining a child's baseline behavior in this case.

RED FLAGS

After obtaining a history of the events, the presence of "red flags" in the history or examination should strongly prompt referral to the emergency room:

Increased Intracranial Pressure or Large Intracranial Mass

- Hypertension and bradycardia
- Third or sixth nerve palsy; anisocoria, ptosis, diplopia
- Forced-seeming and persistent downward deviation of both eyes (tonic downward gaze deviation)
- Papilledema
- Severe vomiting that is exquisitely positional (i.e., strongly provoked by the transition from lying to sitting)
- Engorged scalp veins
- Bulging fontanel or split cranial sutures in an infant
- Presence of a ventriculoperitoneal shunt (VP shunt) with any of the aforementioned symptoms should prompt concern about shunt malfunction

Ongoing Status Epilepticus

- Waxing and waning responsiveness after a convulsive seizure has ended, particularly with periods of complete unresponsiveness
- Persistent eye deviation after a convulsive seizure has ended
- Persistent tachycardia after a convulsive seizure has ended
- Persistent confusion or delirium, even if the child is able to speak and walk

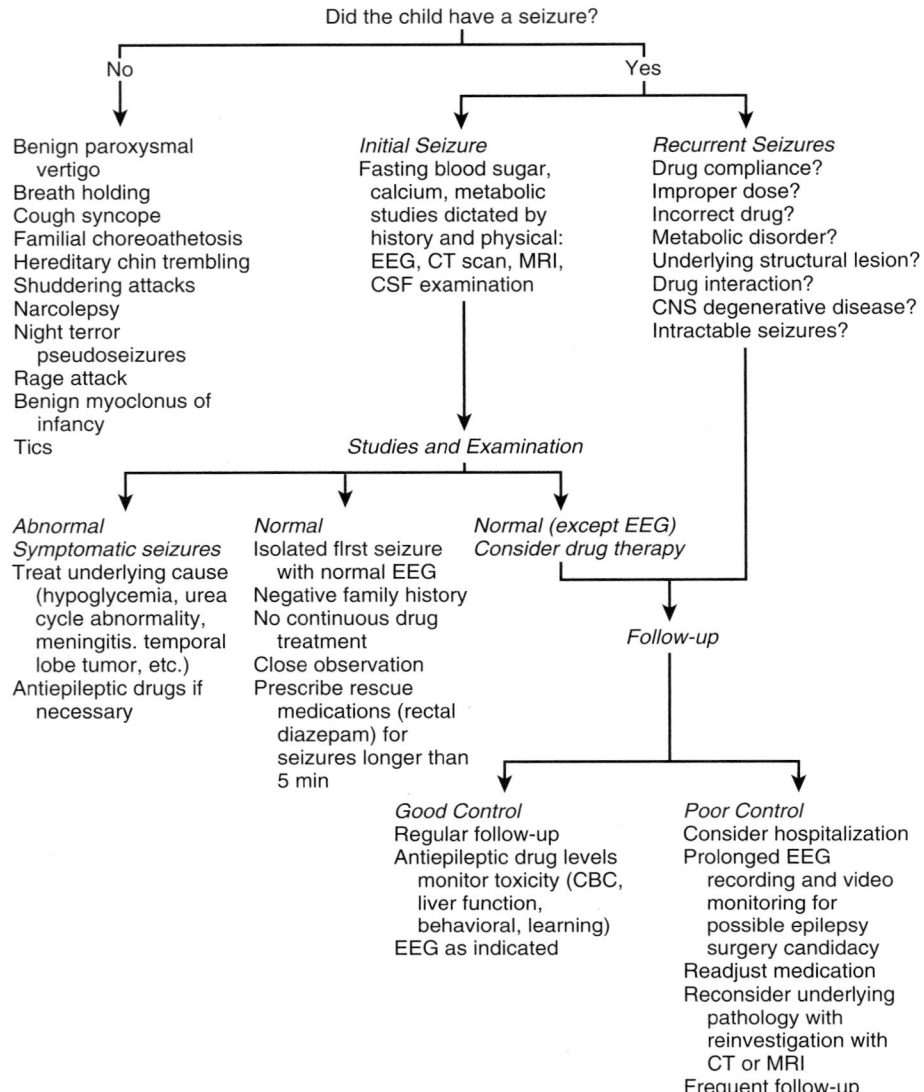

Did the child have a seizure?

No → Benign paroxysmal
vertigo
Breath holding
Cough syncope
Familial choreoathetosis
Hereditary chin trembling
Shuddering attacks
Narcolepsy
Night terror
pseudoseizures
Rage attack
Benign myoclonus of
infancy
Tics

Yes →

Initial Seizure
Fasting blood sugar,
calcium, metabolic
studies dictated by
history and physical:
EEG, CT scan, MRI,
CSF examination

Recurrent Seizures
Drug compliance?
Improper dose?
Incorrect drug?
Metabolic disorder?
Underlying structural lesion?
Drug interaction?
CNS degenerative disease?
Intractable seizures?

Studies and Examination

Abnormal
Symptomatic seizures
Treat underlying cause
(hypoglycemia, urea
cycle abnormality,
meningitis. temporal
lobe tumor, etc.)
Antiepileptic drugs if
necessary

Normal
Isolated flrst seizure
with normal EEG
Negative family history
No continuous drug
treatment
Close observation
Prescribe rescue
medications (rectal
diazepam) for
seizures longer than
5 min

Normal (except EEG)
Consider drug therapy

Follow-up

Good Control
Regular follow-up
Antiepileptic drug levels
monitor toxicity (CBC,
liver function,
behavioral, learning)
EEG as indicated

Poor Control
Consider hospitalization
Prolonged EEG
recording and video
monitoring for
possible epilepsy
surgery candidacy
Readjust medication
Reconsider underlying
pathology with
reinvestigation with
CT or MRI
Frequent follow-up

Fig. 39.1 Approach to the child with a suspected convulsive disorder. CNS, central nervous system; CSF, cerebrospinal fluid.

Stroke or Complicated Migraine

- Focal weakness or numbness, particularly if accompanied by slurred speech or confusion (if the spell is remote and the patient has returned to a normal baseline, suggest expedited referral to a neurologist)

Meningitis

- Fever
- Nuchal rigidity
- Positive Kernig or Brudzinski signs
- Bulging fontanel

The following **red flags** should prompt an urgent or even emergent referral to a pediatric neurologist, including direct communication with a neurologist for proper triaging:

- Infantile spasms
- Clusters of abdominal "crunches" or "startles," particularly when the child is falling asleep or waking up from sleep
- Developmental plateau or regression
- Loss of visual attentiveness

Any developmental regression in infants or toddlers that has been present for more than 1 month (or sooner, for dramatic or progressive regressions) is concerning; change in handedness after 4–5 years of age is also a red flag (see Chapter 28).

PAROXYSMAL SPELLS OF ALTERED BEHAVIOR OR MOVEMENT

Paroxysmal neurologic symptoms can have neurologic, psychiatric, pulmonary, cardiovascular, or gastrointestinal causes (see Table 39.1). For this reason, during the investigation of a paroxysmal event, generic terms such as *spells, convulsions,* or *altered mental status* are more appropriate to use rather than *seizures,* which implies a very specific etiology and may falsely eliminate diagnostic possibilities. Witnesses may use terms such as *grand mal, petit mal,* or even *generalized tonic-clonic* (GTC) to describe events; these descriptors should not be taken at face value or thought to only describe epileptic seizures.

EPILEPTIC SEIZURES

An epileptic seizure is a paroxysmal alteration in behavior, motor function, and/or autonomic function occurring in association with excessive synchronous neuronal activity in the CNS. Seizures may be considered *provoked* or *unprovoked*, referring to whether they were precipitated by an acute cause such as illness, concussion, metabolic disorder, or toxic ingestion. The term *symptomatic* refers to whether the seizures represent a symptom of a known chronic disorder, such as a structural, genetic, or metabolic abnormality. *Epilepsy* is a disorder in which there are *recurrent* unprovoked epileptic seizures; Figure 39.2 outlines the contextual framework when evaluating seizure disorders and Figure 39.3 provides the classification structure. Table 39.2 provides a glossary of terms frequently encountered when considering seizure disorders.

Epileptic seizures must be clearly distinguished from non-neurologic paroxysmal disorders caused by psychiatric, cardiovascular, pulmonary, or gastrointestinal causes. There are also paroxysmal disorders that are neurologic but nonepileptic in nature, such as tics, dystonias, stereotypies, or other movement disorders. The correct diagnosis is critical to avoid unnecessary testing, interventions, and medication trials. However, multiple types of events, both epileptic and

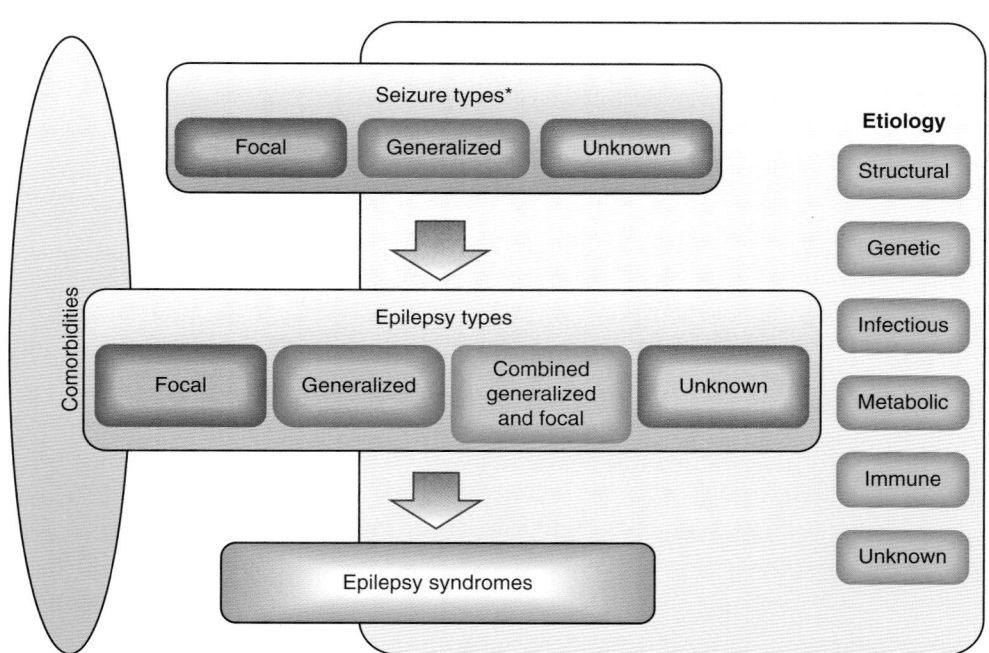

Fig. 39.2 The International League Against Epilepsy (ILAE) 2017 Classification of the Epilepsies. *Denotes onset of seizure. (From Jankovic J, Mazziotta JC, Pomeroy SL, Newman NJ, eds. *Bradley's Neurology in Clinical Practice.* 8th ed. Philadelphia: Elsevier; 2022:1625, Fig. 100.6.)

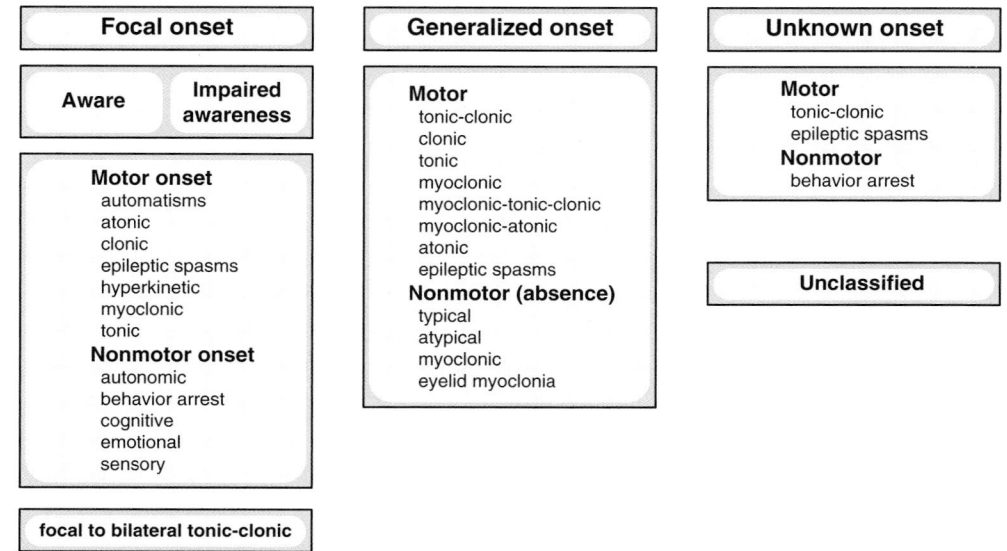

Fig. 39.3 The 2017 International League Against Epilepsy (ILAE) operational classification of seizure types. (Modified from Jankovic J, Mazziotta JC, Pomeroy SL, Newman NJ, eds. *Bradley's Neurology in Clinical Practice.* 8th ed. Philadelphia: Elsevier; 2022:1619, Fig. 100.3.)

TABLE 39.2 Terminology Used in Describing Paroxysmal Episodes

Word	Definition
Absence, typical	A sudden onset, interruption of ongoing activities, a blank stare, possibly a brief upward deviation of the eyes. Usually, the patient will be unresponsive when spoken to. Duration is a few seconds to half a minute with very rapid recovery. Although not always available, an EEG would show generalized epileptiform discharges during the event. An absence seizure is a seizure of generalized onset. The word is not synonymous with a blank stare, which also can be encountered with focal onset seizures
Absence, atypical	An absence seizure with changes in tone that are more pronounced than in typical absence or the onset and/or cessation is not abrupt, often associated with slow, irregular, generalized spike-wave activity
Atonic	Sudden loss or diminution of muscle tone without apparent preceding myoclonic or tonic event lasting ~1–2 sec, involving head, trunk, jaw, or limb musculature
Automatism	A more or less coordinated motor activity usually occurring when cognition is impaired and for which the subject is usually (but not always) amnesic afterward. This often resembles a voluntary movement and may consist of an inappropriate continuation of preictal motor activity
Autonomic seizure	A distinct alteration of autonomic nervous system function involving cardiovascular, pupillary, gastrointestinal, sudomotor, vasomotor, and thermoregulatory functions
Aura	A subjective ictal phenomenon that, in a given patient, may precede an observable seizure
Awareness	Knowledge of self or environment
Behavior arrest	Arrest (pause) of activities, freezing, immobilization, as in behavior arrest seizure
Bilateral	Both left and right sides, although manifestations of bilateral seizures may be symmetric or asymmetric
Clonic	Jerking, either symmetric or asymmetric, that is regularly repetitive and involves the same muscle groups
Cognitive	Pertaining to thinking and higher cortical functions, such as language, spatial perception, memory, and praxis. The previous term for similar usage as a seizure type was psychic
Consciousness	A state of mind with both subjective and objective aspects, comprising a sense of self as a unique entity, awareness, responsiveness, and memory
Dacrystic	Bursts of crying, which may or may not be associated with sadness
Dystonic	Sustained contractions of both agonist and antagonist muscles producing athetoid or twisting movements, which may produce abnormal postures
Emotional seizures	Seizures presenting with an emotion or the appearance of having an emotion as an early prominent feature, such as fear, spontaneous joy or euphoria, laughing (gelastic), or crying (dacrystic)
Epileptic spasms	A sudden flexion, extension, or mixed extension-flexion of predominantly proximal and truncal muscles that is usually more sustained than a myoclonic movement but not as sustained as a tonic seizure. Limited forms may occur: grimacing, head nodding, or subtle eye movements. Epileptic spasms frequently occur in clusters. Infantile spasms are the best-known form, but spasms can occur at all ages
Epilepsy	A disease of the brain defined by any of the following conditions: (1) at least two unprovoked (or reflex) seizures occurring >24 hr apart; (2) one unprovoked (or reflex) seizure and a probability of further seizures similar to the general recurrence risk (at least 60%) after two unprovoked seizures, occurring over the next 10 yr; (3) diagnosis of an epilepsy syndrome. Epilepsy is considered to be resolved for individuals who had an age-dependent epilepsy syndrome but are now past the applicable age or those who have remained seizure free for the last 10 years, with no antiseizure medicines for the last 5 yr
Eyelid myoclonia	Jerking of the eyelids at frequencies of at least 3 per second, commonly with upward eye deviation, usually lasting <10 sec, often precipitated by eye closure. There may or may not be associated brief loss of awareness
Fencer's posture seizure	A focal motor seizure type with extension of one arm and flexion at the contralateral elbow and wrist, giving an imitation of swordplay with a foil. This has also been called a supplementary motor area seizure
Figure-of-4 seizure	Upper limbs with extension of the arm (usually contralateral to the epileptogenic zone) with elbow flexion of the other arm, forming a figure-of-4
Focal	Originating within networks limited to one hemisphere. They may be discretely localized or more widely distributed. Focal seizures may originate in subcortical structures
Focal onset bilateral tonic-clonic seizure	A seizure type with focal onset, with awareness or impaired awareness, either motor or nonmotor, progressing to bilateral tonic-clonic activity. The prior term was seizure with partial onset with secondary generalization
Gelastic	Bursts of laughter or giggling, usually without an appropriate affective tone
Generalized	Originating at some point within, and rapidly engaging, bilaterally distributed networks
Generalized tonic-clonic	Bilateral symmetric or sometimes asymmetric tonic contraction and then bilateral clonic contraction of somatic muscles, usually associated with autonomic phenomena and loss of awareness. These seizures engage networks in both hemispheres at the start of the seizure
Hallucination	A creation of composite perceptions without corresponding external stimuli involving visual, auditory, somatosensory, olfactory, and/or gustatory phenomena. Example: "hearing" and "seeing" people talking

TABLE 39.2	Terminology Used in Describing Paroxysmal Episodes—cont'd
Word	**Definition**
Immobility	Activity arrest
Impaired awareness (impairment of consciousness)	Impaired or lost awareness is a feature of focal impaired awareness seizures, previously called complex partial seizures
Jacksonian seizure	Traditional term indicating spread of clonic movements through contiguous body parts unilaterally
Motor	Involves musculature in any form. The motor event could consist of an increase (positive) or decrease (negative) in muscle contraction to produce a movement
Myoclonic	Sudden, brief (<100 msec) involuntary single or multiple contractions of muscles or muscle groups of variable topography (axial, proximal limb, distal). Myoclonus is less regularly repetitive and less sustained than is clonus
Myoclonic-atonic	A generalized seizure type with a myoclonic jerk leading to an atonic motor component. This type was previously called myoclonic-astatic
Myoclonic-tonic-clonic	One or a few jerks of limbs bilaterally, followed by a tonic-clonic seizure. The initial jerks can be considered to be either a brief period of clonus or myoclonus. Seizures with this characteristic are common in juvenile myoclonic epilepsy
Nonmotor	Focal or generalized seizure types in which motor activity is not prominent
Propagation	Spread of seizure activity from one place in the brain to another, or engaging of additional brain networks
Responsiveness	Ability to appropriately react by movement or speech when presented with a stimulus
Seizure	A transient occurrence of signs and/or symptoms due to abnormal excessive or synchronous neuronal activity in the brain
Sensory seizure	A perceptual experience not caused by appropriate stimuli in the external world
Tonic	A sustained increase in muscle contraction lasting a few seconds to minutes
Tonic-clonic	A sequence consisting of a tonic followed by a clonic phase
Unclassified	Referring to a seizure type that cannot be described by the ILAE 2017 classification either because of inadequate information or unusual clinical features. If the seizure is unclassified because the type of onset is unknown, a limited classification may still derive from observed features
Unresponsive	Not able to react appropriately by movement or speech when presented with stimulation
Versive	A sustained, forced conjugate ocular, cephalic, and/or truncal rotation or lateral deviation from the midline

ILAE, International League Against Epilepsy.
Adapted from Fisher FS, Cross JH, D'Souza C, et al. Instruction manual for the ILAE 2017 operational classification of seizure types. *Epilepsia.* 2017;58(4):531–542 (Table 2, p. 538).

nonepileptic, may occur in the same patient, necessitating that each spell be properly characterized.

EPIDEMIOLOGY AND CAUSES OF SEIZURES AND EPILEPSY

If febrile seizures are included, approximately 3.5% of children experience some kind of seizure by the age of 15 years; most seizures occur before the age of 3 years. Most children who present with a seizure do not have or will not develop epilepsy. Many children presenting with a seizure have febrile convulsions, which are a provoked, age-dependent paroxysmal neurologic condition; 13% of children with seizures have acute symptomatic seizures other than febrile convulsions; and 8% have single, unprovoked seizures of unknown cause. The incidence of acute symptomatic seizures is highest in the first year of life; the most common causes of these predominantly neonatal seizures are genetic, infection, and metabolic disorders. After age 4 years, head trauma is the most common cause of acute symptomatic seizures, and infection is the next most common.

The incidence of epilepsy among children younger than 15 years is 45–85/100,000 in developed countries. It is highest in younger children; in those younger than 1 year, it is ~100/100,000. The prevalence of active epilepsy in patients taking antiepileptic drugs (AEDs) is between 4.3 and 9.3/1,000, or about 0.5–1% of the population. Traditionally, ~60% of children with epilepsy have no identifiable etiologic factors for the disease; next-generation gene sequencing technology has moved the estimated underlying genetic etiology to approximately 40%. Of those children in whom a cause is identified, population-based studies report the following presumed causes: infection in 5%, head trauma in 3%, and miscellaneous causes (tumors, malformations of cortical development, vascular malformations, and cerebral infarction) in 2%. Epilepsy is found in association with other long-standing neurodevelopmental abnormalities in 13% of children.

GENETICS

It is estimated that a genetic etiology underlies epilepsy in approximately 40% of individuals. There are certain patterns and ages of onset that might guide specific genetic consideration (Tables 39.3 and 39.4), but given the wide genetic and phenotypic heterogeneity, it is more practical to do gene sequencing broadly as opposed to trying to narrow down the genetic sequencing unless there is a very clear diagnostic consideration such as Angelman or Rett syndrome. Neonatal-onset seizures require both a metabolic (Table 39.5) and a genomic approach to the diagnostic evaluation because there are several epileptic encephalopathic syndromes that could be treatable and genetic testing generally has a 2–3-month turnaround for results. If rapid genome sequencing is an option, this would supplant the need for metabolic testing as the results of genomic sequencing will be available within a short enough period of time to allow for timely implementation of treatment. Molybdenum cofactor deficiency is a rare example that has a lifesaving orphan drug treatment that needs to be initiated as early as possible to prevent irreversible cystic encephalopathy. Table 39.6 outlines several of the recognizable syndromic genetic disorders as defined by the underlying pathoetiology.

TABLE 39.3 Clinical Conditions for Targeted Gene Sequencing

Targeted Gene Sequencing	Clinical Condition	Advantage of Testing
SCN1A	Dravet syndrome. Consider testing for recurrent episodes of febrile status epilepticus, intractable tonic-clonic seizures during the first year of life, epileptic encephalopathy attributed to vaccination, and adults with a history consistent with Dravet syndrome	Avoidance of sodium channel blockers, aggressive seizure management, justification of stiripentol, bromides, etc.
PCDH19	Females presenting with multiple clusters of brief febrile seizures and developmental delay or regression, particularly if there is a family history consistent with paternal transmission	Prognosis and potential forthcoming treatment options
SLC2A1	Onset of absence seizures at younger than 4 yr old, particularly if there is a family history of paroxysmal exercise-induced dyskinesia	Initiation of a ketogenic diet
POLG	Prior to starting valproic acid in patients with drug-resistant seizures and developmental delay or regression	Avoidance of potentially fatal liver failure starting as early as 2 mo after initiation of valproic acid therapy
HLA-B*1502	Prior to starting carbamazepine, oxcarbazepine, phenytoin, and lamotrigine in patients of Asian descent	Avoidance of a potentially fatal reaction (Stevens-Johnson syndrome/toxic epidermal necrolysis)

Modified from Ream MA, Patel AD. Obtaining genetic testing in pediatric epilepsy. *Epilepsia*. 2015;56:1505–1514.

TABLE 39.4 Identified Genes for Epilepsy Syndromes*†

Epilepsy Type	Gene	Protein
Infantile Onset		
Benign familial neonatal seizures	KCNQ2	Potassium voltage-gated channel
	KCNQ3	Potassium voltage-gated channel
Benign familial neonatal infantile seizures	SCN2A	Sodium channel protein type 2α
Early familial neonatal infantile seizures	SCN2A	Sodium channel protein type 2α
Early infantile epileptic encephalopathy (EIEE)	CDKL5 (EIEE2)	Cyclin-dependent kinase-like 5
	ARX (EIEE1)	Aristaless-related homeobox
	TSC1	Hamartin
	TSC2	Tuberin
	SCN1A (EIEE6)	Sodium channel protein type 1α
	PCDH19 (EIEE9)	Protocadherin-19
	KCNQ2 (EIEE7)	Potassium voltage-gated channel
	STXBP1 (EIEE4)	Syntaxin binding protein 1
	SLC2A1	Solute carrier family 2, facilitated glucose transporter member 1
	ALDH7A1	α-Aminoadipic semialdehyde dehydrogenase (antiquitin)
	POLG	DNA polymerase subunit γ1
	SCN2A (EIEE11)	Sodium channel protein type 2α
	PLCβ1 (EIEE12)	Phospholipase C β1
	ATP6AP2	Renin receptor
	SPTAN1 (EIEE5)	α₂-Spectrin
	SLC25A22 (EIEE3)	Mitochondrial glutamate carrier 1
	PNPO	Pyridoxine-5′-phosphate oxidase
Generalized epilepsy with febrile seizures plus (early onset)	SCN1A	Sodium channel protein type 1α
	SCN1B	Sodium channel protein type 1β
	GABRG2	γ-Aminobutyric acid receptor subunit γ2
	SCN2A	Sodium channel protein type 2α
Childhood Onset		
Childhood-onset epileptic encephalopathies	SCN1A	Sodium channel protein type 1α
	PCDH19	Protocadherin-19
	SLC2A1	Solute carrier family 2, facilitated GTM1
	POLG	DNA polymerase subunit γ1
	SCN2A	Sodium channel protein type 2α

TABLE 39.4 Identified Genes for Epilepsy Syndromes*†—cont'd

Epilepsy Type	Gene	Protein
Childhood Onset—cont'd		
Early-onset absence seizures, refractory epilepsy of multiple types, at times with movement disorder	GLUT-1 deficiency syndrome, SLC2A1 gene	Solute carrier family 2, facilitated GTM1
Generalized epilepsy with febrile seizure plus	SCN1A	Sodium channel protein type 1α
	SCN1B	Sodium channel protein type 1β
	GABRG2	γ-Aminobutyric acid receptor subunit γ2
	SCN2A	Sodium channel protein type 1α
Juvenile myoclonic epilepsy (more commonly presents in adolescence)	EFHC1	EF-hand domain-containing protein 1
	CACNB4	Voltage-dependent L-type calcium channel
	GABRA1	γ-Aminobutyric acid receptor subunit α1
Progressive myoclonic epilepsy (different forms present from infancy through adulthood)	EPM2A	Laforin
	NHLRC1	NHL repeat-containing protein 1 (malin)
	CSTB	Cystatin-B
	PRICKLE1	Prickle-like protein 1
	PPT1, TPP1, CLN3, CLN5, CLN6, CLN8, CTSD, DNAJC5, MFSD8	Multiple proteins causing neuronal ceroid lipofuscinosis
Autosomal dominant nocturnal frontal lobe epilepsies (presents in childhood through adulthood)	CHRNA4	Neuronal acetylcholine receptor α4
	CHRNB2	Neuronal acetylcholine receptor β2
	CHRNA2	Neuronal acetylcholine receptor α2
Adolescent Onset		
Juvenile myoclonic epilepsy (JME)	See Childhood-Onset JME	
Progressive myoclonic epilepsy (PME)	See Childhood-Onset PME	
Autosomal dominant nocturnal frontal lobe epilepsies (AD-NFLE)	See Childhood-Onset AD-NFLE	
Autosomal dominant lateral temporal lobe epilepsy (usually presents in adulthood)	LGI1	Leucine-rich glioma-inactivated protein 1

*Note that the same gene (different variants) often appears as causing different epilepsy syndromes.
†Most of these genes can be tested for through commercially available targeted single-gene sequencing or through commercially available gene panels or through exome sequencing (http://www.ncbi.nlm.nih.gov/sites/GeneTests/review?db=genetests).

In some circumstances, unique clinical phenotypes can guide the initial clinical differential diagnosis. Severe **metabolic acidosis** resulting in shock and requiring intubation and ventilation is seen in metabolic epileptic encephalopathic syndromes such as nonketotic hyperglycinemia, pyridoxine-5′-phosphate oxidase deficiency, molybdenum cofactor deficiency, pyridoxine-dependent epilepsy, and Leigh syndrome. Table 39.7 provides an overview of the clinical associations of metabolic disorders associated with epilepsy. The characteristic **syndactyly** of the second and third toes is seen in steroid metabolism disorders, Smith-Lemli-Opitz syndrome in particular, which additionally has associated genitourinary tract abnormalities. Skin **exanthems** are highly suggestive of biotinidase deficiency. Atypical coarse or thin hair and wormian bones are seen in copper disorders such as Menkes syndrome. **Cardiomyopathy** is characteristic of mitochondrial disorders including Barth syndrome and fatty acid oxidation disorders and is also seen in RASopathies and cobalamin C deficiency. **Atypical fat distribution** and a prominent suprapubic fat pad are seen in congenital disorders of glycosylation. The circumstances in which genetic testing is offered varies widely between centers. Gene panels are offered by several laboratories and do not all include the same genes. It is thus important to understand the benefits and limitations of the test requested. Exome sequencing should not be considered "end of the line" or "last resort," as the window of opportunity for targeted intervention may pass while more conventional options are investigated.

This is particularly relevant in new-onset intractable or refractory seizures. In addition, there are several cases with digenic seizure disorders or rare metabolic disorders that will not be easily detected through more routine analysis but benefit from early targeted intervention to reduce morbidity and improve overall quality of life. The consensus for evaluating patients with suspected congenital disorders of glycosylation, mitochondrial disorders, or otherwise complex atypical disorders is to utilize exome sequencing as a first-line diagnostic test, with yields of up to 30% in these circumstances.

SEIZURE CLASSIFICATION AND TERMINOLOGY

Seizures are characterized according to their clinical semiology and presumptive etiology (see Figs. 39.2 and 39.3). Seizures can be difficult to classify and identify without a careful description of their onset, unfolding, and aftermath. Multiple seizure types may have the same brief general description, such as "twitching" or "staring." Without further details as to duration, additional symptoms, and postictal behavior, they may be incorrectly classified as to type, even if they are accurately determined to be seizures. This is clinically relevant because improper classification can lead to inappropriate treatment; for example, some antiepileptic medications for focal seizures will exacerbate generalized seizures. Table 39.8 aligns some of the older terminology with the newer classification.

TABLE 39.5 Inborn Errors of Metabolism (IEMs) Identified by Each of the Tier 1 Diagnostic Tests

Source	Diagnostic Test	Related IEM	Source	Diagnostic Test	Related IEM
BLOOD	Comprehensive metabolic panel	Glucose (low in FAODs and HIHA)	**BLOOD—cont'd**		Isolated sulfite oxidase deficiency (low Cys, high Tau)
		Anion gap (elevated in organic acidemias)		Plasma acylcarnitines	FAODs
		Liver transaminases (elevated in CDGs and mitochondrial depletion syndromes)			Organic acidemias
					Ethylmalonic encephalopathy
		Alkaline phosphatase (low in hypophosphatasia, elevated in GPI biosynthesis defects)		Copper and ceruloplasmin	Menkes disease (low)
	Blood gases	Organic acidemias (low pH)			Wilson disease (low)
		Urea cycle disorders (high pH)		Plasma total homocysteine	Cobalamin C disease (high)
	Ammonia	Urea cycle disorders			MTHFR deficiency (high)
		Organic acidemias			Molybdenum cofactor deficiency (low)
		HIHA			Isolated sulfite oxidase deficiency (low)
		HHH syndrome	**URINE**	Urinalysis	Organic acidemias (elevated ketones)
		Lysinuric protein intolerance			MSUD (elevated ketones)
		Pyruvate carboxylase deficiency		Urine AASA	PDE
	Creatine kinase	FAODs			Molybdenum cofactor deficiency
		Dystroglycanopathy type-CDG			Isolated sulfite oxidase deficiency
	Uric acid	Molybdenum cofactor deficiency (low)		Urine purines and pyrimidines	Adenylosuccinate lyase deficiency (high succinyladenosine)
	Lactate/pyruvate	PDH deficiency			Molybdenum cofactor deficiency (high xanthine and hypoxanthine)
		Pyruvate carboxylase deficiency		Creatine metabolites	AGAT deficiency (low GAA and creatine)
		Biotinidase deficiency			GAMT deficiency (high GAA, low creatine)
		Mitochondrial respiratory chain defects			Creatine transporter deficiency (high creatine)
		Lipoic acid synthesis defects		Urine organic acids	PNPO deficiency (vanillactate)
	Plasma amino acids	Urea cycle defects (elevated Glu)			Organic acidurias
		MSUD (elevated branched-chain amino acids)			OTC deficiency (orotic acid)
		Tetrahydrobiopterin deficiencies (elevated Phe)			Cobalamin C deficiency (MMA)
		Lactic acidemias (elevated Ala)			Biotinidase deficiency and holocarboxylase synthetase deficiency (3-hydroxypropionic acid, 3-hydroxyisovaleric acid, 3-methylcrotonylglycine, methylcitrate)
		Pyruvate carboxylase deficiency (elevated Cit, Pro, and Lys; low Glu)			Fumarate hydratase deficiency (fumarate)
		PNPO deficiency (high Gly and Thr)			SSADH deficiency (4-hydroxybutyric acid)
		PDE (high Gly and Thr)			Ethylmalonic encephalopathy (EMA)
		Nonketotic hyperglycinemia (elevated Gly)			Mitochondrial short-chain enoyl-CoA hydratase 1 deficiency (methacryloylglycine, 3-hydroxyisobutyric acid, S-2-carboxypropyl-cysteine, and S-2-carboxypropylcysteamine)
		Hyperprolinemia type 2 (elevated Pro)			
		Lipoic acid synthesis disorders (elevated Gly)			
		Serine biosynthesis disorders (low Ser)			
		Glutamine synthetase deficiency (low Gln)			
		Asparagine synthetase deficiency (low Asn)			
		GABA transaminase (elevated GABA, elevated β-Ala)			
		Mitochondrial glutamate transporter deficiency (elevated Pro)			
		Molybdenum cofactor deficiency (low Cys, high Tau)			

AASA, α-aminoadipic semialdehyde; AGAT, arginine:glycine amidinotransferase; CDG, congenital disorders of glycosylation; EMA, ethylmalonic acid; FAODs, fatty acid oxidation disorders; GAA, guanidinoacetate; GABA, γ-aminobutyric acid; GAMT, guanidinoacetate methyltransferase; GPI, glycosylphosphatidylinositol; HHH, hyperornithinemia-hyperammonemia-homocitrullinuria; HIHA, hyperinsulinism-hyperammonemia syndrome; MMA, methylmalonic acidemia; MSUD, maple syrup urine disease; MTHFR, methylenetetrahydrofolate reductase; OTC, ornithine transcarbamylase; PDE, pyridoxine-dependent epilepsy; PDH, pyruvate dehydrogenase; PNPO, pyridox(am)ine 5'-phosphate oxidase; SSADH, succinic semialdehyde dehydrogenase.

From van Karnebeek CDM, Sayson B, Lee JJY, et al. Metabolic evaluation of epilepsy: a diagnostic algorithm with focus on treatable conditions. *Front Neurol.* 2018;9:Article 1016 (Table 3). https://doi.org/10.3389/fneur.2018.01016.

TABLE 39.6   Epilepsy Genes and Phenotypes Catalogued in Online Mendelian Inheritance in Man (OMIM) Since 2016

Gene	Phenotype	OMIM
Chromatin Remodeling		
ACTL6B	Epileptic encephalopathy, early infantile, 76	618470
SMARCC2	Coffin-Siris syndrome 8	618362
STAG2	Neurodevelopmental disorder, X-linked, with craniofacial abnormalities	301022
Intracellular Signaling		
CSF1R	Brain abnormalities, neurodegeneration, and dysosteosclerosis	618476
YWHAZ	Popov-Chang syndrome	618428
CHP1	Spastic ataxia 9, autosomal recessive	618438
Ion Channels and Neurotransmitter Receptors		
CACNA1E	Epileptic encephalopathy, early infantile, 69	618285
GABRG2	Epileptic encephalopathy, early infantile, 74	618396
CACNA2D2	Cerebellar atrophy with seizures and variable developmental delay	618501
HCN1	Generalized epilepsy with febrile seizures plus, type 10	618482
CACNA1B	Neurodevelopmental disorder with seizures and nonepileptic hyperkinetic movements	618497
KCNK4	Facial dysmorphism, hypertrichosis, epilepsy, intellectual/developmental delay, and gingival overgrowth syndrome	618381
SLC25A42	Metabolic crises, recurrent, with variable encephalomyopathic features and neurologic regression	618416
ATP1A1	Hypomagnesemia, seizures, and intellectual disability	618314
SLC28A1	Uridine-cytidineuria	618477
SCN8A	Myoclonus, familial, 2	618364
SLC9A7	Intellectual developmental disorder, X-linked 108	301024
Metabolism		
GLS	Epileptic encephalopathy, early infantile, 71	618328
PARS2	Epileptic encephalopathy, early infantile, 75	618437
RNF13	Epileptic encephalopathy, early infantile, 73	618379
FCSK	Congenital disorder of glycosylation with defective fucosylation 2	618324
PPP3CA	Arthrogryposis, cleft palate, craniosynostosis, and impaired intellectual development	618265
PPP2CA	Neurodevelopmental disorder and language delay with or without structural brain abnormalities	618354
MTHFS	Neurodevelopmental disorder with microcephaly, epilepsy, and hypomyelination	618367
P4HTM	Hypotonia, hyperventilation, impaired intellectual development, dysautonomia, epilepsy, and eye abnormalities	618493
DHPS	Neurodevelopmental disorder with seizures and speech and walking impairment	618480
MAST1	Mega-corpus-callosum syndrome with cerebellar hypoplasia and cortical malformations	618273
DEGS1	Leukodystrophy, hypomyelinating, 18	618404
MYORG	Basal ganglia calcification, idiopathic, 7, autosomal recessive	618317
ALKBH8	Intellectual developmental disorder, autosomal recessive 71	618504
NAXD	Encephalopathy, progressive, early onset, with brain edema and/or leukoencephalopathy, 2	618321
KDM6B	Neurodevelopmental disorder with coarse facies and mild distal skeletal abnormalities	618505
HS6ST2	Paganini-Miozzo syndrome	301025
TRMT1	Intellectual developmental disorder, autosomal recessive 68	618302
COLGALT1	Brain small vessel disease 3	618360
IREB2	Neurodegeneration, early onset, with choreoathetoid movements and microcytic anemia	618451
PIGB	Epileptic encephalopathy, early infantile, 80	618580
Mitochondrial Metabolism		
MICOS13	Combined oxidative phosphorylation deficiency 37	618329
GFM2	Combined oxidative phosphorylation deficiency 39	618397
Neuronal Development		
NFASC	Neurodevelopmental disorder with central and peripheral motor dysfunction	618356
NHLRC2	Fibrosis, neurodegeneration, and cerebral angiomatosis	618278

Continued

TABLE 39.6 **Epilepsy Genes and Phenotypes Catalogued in Online Mendelian Inheritance in Man (OMIM) Since 2016—cont'd**

Gene	Phenotype	OMIM
Nucleoplasmic Transport		
NUP133	Galloway-Mowat syndrome 8	618349
NUP214	Susceptibility to acute infection-induced encephalopathy 9	618426
Regulation of Cell Morphology and Motility		
BICD2	Spinal muscular atrophy, lower extremity predominant, 2b, prenatal onset, autosomal dominant	618291
DOCK3	Neurodevelopmental disorder with impaired intellectual development, hypotonia, and ataxia	618292
PHACTR1	Epileptic encephalopathy, early infantile, 70	618298
MACF1	Lissencephaly 9 with complex brainstem malformation	618325
DYNC1I2	Neurodevelopmental disorder with microcephaly and structural brain anomalies	618492
Synaptic Vesicle Cycle		
NEUROD2	Epileptic encephalopathy, early infantile, 72	618374
MAPK8IP3	Neurodevelopmental disorder with or without variable brain abnormalities	618443
Transcriptional Regulation		
ATN1	Congenital hypotonia, epilepsy, developmental delay, and digital anomalies	618494
RORB	Susceptibility to idiopathic generalized epilepsy 15	618357
ZNF142	Neurodevelopmental disorder with impaired speech and hyperkinetic movements	618425
RSRC1	Intellectual developmental disorder, autosomal recessive 70	618402
TCF20	Developmental delay with variable intellectual impairment and behavioral abnormalities	618430
EIF3F	Intellectual developmental disorder, autosomal recessive 67	618295
ZBTB11	Intellectual developmental disorder, autosomal recessive 69	618383
CNOT1	Holoprosencephaly 12 with or without pancreatic agenesis	618500
NFIB	Macrocephaly, acquired, with impaired intellectual development	618286
SOX4	Coffin-Siris syndrome 10	618506
TRRAP	Developmental delay with or without dysmorphic facies and autism	618454
Transmembrane Protein		
TMEM94	Intellectual developmental disorder with cardiac defects and dysmorphic facies	618316
Structural Protein		
COL3A1	Polymicrogyria with or without vascular-type Ehlers-Danlos syndrome	618343
Nuclear DNA Polymerase		
POLE	Intrauterine growth retardation, metaphyseal dysplasia, adrenal hypoplasia congenita, genital anomalies, and immunodeficiency	618336
Multiple Functions		
WDR4	Microcephaly, growth deficiency, seizures, and brain malformations	618346
Intracellular Trafficking		
TRAPPC2L	Encephalopathy, progressive, early onset, with episodic rhabdomyolysis	618331

From Hebbar M, Mefford HC. Recent advances in epilepsy genomics and genetic testing. *F1000Res.* 2020;9(F1000 Faculty Rev):185; last updated Mar 12 2020 (Table 1). https://www.ncbi.nlm.nih.gov/pmc/articles/PMC7076331/pdf/f1000research-9-23530.pdf.

Clonic movements are rhythmic, nonsuppressible, position-independent jerking movements (low frequency, high amplitude) caused by involvement of the motor cortex. They can be unilateral or bilateral and can start with one body part and spread. If bilateral, they are synchronous and do not alternate from one side to the other in a bicycling fashion. This should be distinguished from **clonus**, which is rhythmic twitching of a limb, generally the foot, caused by hyperreflexia and lack of descending cortical inhibition due to CNS injury such as is seen in cerebral palsy or stroke. This is generally provoked by movement, excitement, and positioning and can be suppressed or halted by gently repositioning the affected limb. There is no alteration of alertness with clonus. In newborns, **jitteriness** (high frequency, low amplitude) may also be mistaken for clonic seizure activity; this tends to be stimulus-provoked and suppressible.

The term **tonic** refers to a change in tone as a manifestation of seizure activity, which clinically presents as stiffening or arching. This can occur as the only manifestation of a seizure (tonic seizure) or may be

TABLE 39.7 Summary of Clinical, Laboratory, EEG, and Neuroimaging Findings of Metabolic Epilepsy

IEM	Neurologic	Non-neurologic	Laboratory	EEG	Brain MRI	Brain MRS
Urea cycle disorders	Encephalopathy	Liver disease (sometimes)	Hyperammonemia Respiratory alkalosis Increased glutamine	Slow background	Cortical and subcortical edema BG T2 hyperintensity with thalamic sparing Scalloped ribbon of DWI restriction at insular gray-white matter interface	Prominent Glx peak
Organic acidemias	Encephalopathy Choreoathetosis	Cytopenias Pancreatitis Cardiomyopathy (PA) Renal disease (MMA)	Hyperammonemia High anion gap metabolic acidosis Ketotic hyperglycinemia	Slow background Burst-suppression possible	Diffuse swelling neonatally; delayed myelination and globi pallidi lesions later	Decreased Glx peak (PA)
Disorders of biotin metabolism	Encephalopathy	Erythroderma or ichthyosis	Hyperammonemia High anion gap metabolic acidosis Lactic acidosis Ketosis	Burst-suppression	Intraventricular hemorrhage Subependymal cysts	Lactate peak
MSUD	Encephalopathy Opisthotonos Bicycling/fencing movements	Sweet ("maple syrup") smell	Ketosis Hypernatremia Increased BCAAs and BCKAs	Comblike rhythm	Increased signal and cytotoxic edema myelinated structures, vasogenic edema of unmyelinated tracts	BCAA/BCKA peak (0.9 ppm)
Fatty acid oxidation defects	Encephalopathy ("Reye syndrome")	Lipid storage myopathy Liver disease Renal cysts (GA2)	Hypoketotic hypoglycemia	Slow background	T2 hyperintensities in periventricular and subcortical WM (GA2)	Lipid peak (0.9 and 1.3 ppm)
Primary lactic acidosis	Encephalopathy Infantile Parkinsonism (PC deficiency)	Dysmorphic features (PDH deficiency)	Lactic acidosis	Slow background, multifocal spikes	T2 hyperintensities and DWI restriction of dorsal brainstem, cerebral peduncles, corticospinal tracts; subependymal cysts	Lactate peak
Glycine encephalopathy	Seizures	None	High CSF glycine and CSF/plasma glycine ratio	Burst-suppression	Dysgenesis of the CC T2 hyperintensities and DWI restriction of myelinated tracts	Glycine peak (3.55 ppm)
Molybdenum cofactor/sulfite oxidase deficiency	Seizures Hyperekplexia	None	Elevated S-sulfocysteine; low cysteine, high taurine Increased AASA and pipecolic acid	Burst-suppression	Diffuse swelling followed by cystic changes	S-sulfocysteine peak (3.61 ppm); taurine peak (3.24 and 3.42 ppm)
Disorders of GABA metabolism	Seizures Hypersomnolence Choreoathetosis	Overgrowth (GABAT)	Elevated urine 4-hydroxybutyric acid (SSADH); elevated GABA, β-alanine, and homocarnosine (GABAT)	Slow background, multifocal spikes, burst-suppression	T2 hyperintensities of globi pallidi, dentate and subthalamic nucleus (SSADH)	GABA peak (2.2–2.4 ppm; GABAT)
PDE	Seizures	None	Increased AASA and pipecolic acid	Slow background, multifocal spikes, burst-suppression	Usually normal; can have dysgenetic CC	Decreased NAA peak (over time)
Serine biosynthesis disorders	Microcephaly Seizures	Ichthyosis Ectropion, eclabion (Neu-Laxova)	Low serine in plasma and CSF	Multifocal spikes; hypsarrhythmia	Hypomyelination	Decreased NAA peak; increased choline peak
Lysosomal storage disorders	Neurodegeneration	Hydrops fetalis Dermal melanosis Ichthyosis (Gaucher type 2)	Decrease in specific enzyme activity Vacuolated lymphocytes (CLN3 disease)	Fast central spikes (Tay-Sachs); vertex sharp waves (sialidosis)	Hypomyelination (GM1 and GM2 gangliosidosis, fucosidosis, Salla disease) Subdural fluid collections (NCLs)	Broad peak centered around 3.7 ppm

Continued

TABLE 39.7 **Summary of Clinical, Laboratory, EEG, and Neuroimaging Findings of Metabolic Epilepsy—cont'd**

IEM	Neurologic	Non-neurologic	Laboratory	EEG	Brain MRI	Brain MRS
Peroxisomal disorders	Hypotonia Seizures	Cholestasis; renal cysts; epiphyseal stippling Dysmorphic features	Elevated VLCFA, phytanic acid, bile acid intermediates, pipecolic acid, low plasmalogens	Multifocal spikes; hypsarrhythmia	Perisylvian polymicrogyria and pachygyria; hypomyelination; subependymal cysts	Lipid peak (0.9 and 1.3 ppm)
Congenital disorders of glycosylation	Hypotonia Seizures	Inverted nipples Abnormal fat pads	Elevated transaminases; coagulopathy; endocrine abnormalities	Multifocal epileptic discharges	Pontocerebellar hypoplasia	Decreased NAA peak
Disorders of copper metabolism	Seizures	Pili torti Cutis laxa Bladder diverticula Metaphyseal lesions Wormian bones	Low serum copper and ceruloplasmin; high urine copper	Burst-suppression	Arterial tortuosity Subdural collections	Decreased NAA peak
GLUT1 deficiency	Seizures Abnormal eye movements	Hemolytic anemia, pseudohyperkalemia, cataracts (specific variants)	Low CSF glucose and lactate; low CSF/serum glucose ratio	Variable depending on type of seizure	Normal	Normal

AASA, α-aminoadipic semialdehyde; BCAAs, branched-chain amino acids; BCKAs, branched-chain ketoacids; BG, basal ganglia; CC, corpus callosum; CSF, cerebrospinal fluid; DWI, diffusion-weighted imaging; GA2, glutaric aciduria type 2; GABA, γ-aminobutyric acid; GABAT, GABA transaminase; Glx, glutamine/glutamate; IEM, inborn error of metabolism; MMA, methylmalonic acidemia; MRS, magnetic resonance spectroscopy; MSUD, maple syrup urine disease; NAA, N-acetylaspartate; NCLs, neuronal ceroid lipofuscinosis; PA, propionic acidemia; PC, pyruvate carboxylase; PDE, pyridoxine-dependent epilepsy; PDH, pyruvate dehydrogenase; SSADH, succinic semialdehyde dehydrogenase deficiency; VLCFA, very long-chain fatty acids; WM, white matter.
From van Karnebeek CDM, Sayson B, Lee JJY, et al. Metabolic evaluation of epilepsy: a diagnostic algorithm with focus on treatable conditions. *Front Neurol.* 2018;9:Article 1016 (Table 2). https://doi.org/10.3389/fneur.2018.01016.

followed by clonic jerking, which is the generalized tonic-clonic seizure (GTC or grand mal). **Atonic** seizures refer to seizures where a sudden, brief loss of tone in the neck or entire body causes a head nod or fall to the ground. This type of seizure must be distinguished from falls due to complete loss of consciousness or those due to tonic stiffening of the entire body. With atonic seizures, the loss of tone is sudden but brief, and the patient is quickly responsive afterward.

Automatisms are semipurposeful movements that usually occur with impairment of consciousness either during or after a seizure and can be very useful for identifying a spell as a seizure. They may be a perseveration of an activity in progress at ictal onset, such as turning pages of a book, or novel semipurposeful movements arising during the seizure. These novel movements are most often a mixture of masticatory, oral, and lingual movements (lip smacking or grimacing) and simple fragmentary limb movements, such as fidgeting with a held object or pulling at clothing. In infants, orofacial automatisms are more likely than complex gestures and must be distinguished from the normal behavior of infants. Automatisms can be seen both in focal seizures, specifically those of temporal lobe onset, and in some generalized seizures, specifically absence epilepsy, so they are not specific to a broad category of seizure.

Impairment of consciousness, defined as an alteration in awareness of external stimuli, may be combined with a complete loss or impairment of responsiveness to external stimuli. Assessment of consciousness during seizures is often difficult, particularly in young children. It is possible to be unresponsive because of an inability to speak or articulate clearly (aphasia, apraxia, or paralysis). It is also possible to be responsive to external stimuli but to have altered awareness, often demonstrated by complete amnesia for events immediately

before, during, or after the seizure, which implies that memory was not acquired during the seizure because of ongoing neuronal dysfunction. It is possible to have complex motor behaviors without loss of complete awareness or amnesia; frontal lobe seizures commonly have this presentation and must be carefully distinguished from nonepileptic events. Both focal and generalized seizures can be associated with impairment of consciousness; the term **dyscognitive** is used to describe this symptom (see Table 39.2).

Seizure etiology was previously divided into *idiopathic, cryptogenic,* and *symptomatic*. There were also separate categories for infantile spasms and neonatal seizures. The terms *genetic, structural, metabolic,* and *unknown* are currently used to characterize presumptive etiologies (Table 39.9).

FOCAL SEIZURES

Localization-Related Seizures, Partial Seizures

Focal seizures are seizures in which the first clinical and EEG changes indicate initial activation of a system of neurons limited to part of one cerebral hemisphere. The clinical symptoms and signs of focal seizures reflect the functional anatomy of the region of the brain undergoing the abnormal neuronal discharge.

When consciousness is impaired, this was historically known as a **complex** partial seizure; if there is no apparent loss of consciousness, this was known as a **simple** partial seizure. These terms have been replaced by the more descriptive terms **focal seizure with impairment of consciousness** or **focal dyscognitive seizure** in the case of complex partial seizures, and **focal seizure without impairment of consciousness** for simple partial seizures (see Table 39.8).

TABLE 39.8 Mapping of Old to New Seizure Classifying Terms

Old Term for Seizure	New Term for Seizure [Choice] (Optional)	Old Term for Seizure	New Term for Seizure [Choice] (Optional)
Absence	**(Generalized) absence**	Infantile spasms	**[Focal/generalized/unknown] onset epileptic spasms**
Absence, atypical	(Generalized) absence, atypical	Jacksonian	Focal aware motor (Jacksonian)
Absence, typical	(Generalized) absence, typical	Limbic	Focal impaired awareness
Akinetic	Focal behavior arrest, generalized absence	Major motor	Generalized tonic-clonic, focal-onset bilateral tonic-clonic
Astatic	[Focal/generalized] atonic		
Atonic	**[Focal/generalized] atonic**	Minor motor	Focal motor, generalized myoclonic
Aura	Focal aware	**Myoclonic**	**[Focal/generalized] myoclonic**
Clonic	[Focal/generalized] clonic	Neocortical*	Focal aware or focal impaired awareness
Complex partial	**Focal impaired awareness**	Occipital lobe*	Focal
Convulsion	[Focal/generalized] motor [tonic-clonic, tonic, clonic], focal to bilateral tonic-clonic	Parietal lobe*	Focal
		Partial	Focal
Dacrystic	Focal [aware or impaired awareness] emotional (dacrystic)	**Petit mal**	**Absence**
Dialeptic	Focal impaired awareness	**Psychomotor**	**Focal impaired awareness**
Drop attack	[Focal/generalized] atonic, [focal/generalized] tonic	Rolandic	Focal aware motor, focal to bilateral tonic-clonic
Fencer's posture (asymmetric tonic)	Focal [aware or impaired awareness] motor tonic	Salaam	[Focal/generalized/unknown onset] epileptic spasms
		Secondarily generalized tonic-clonic	Focal to bilateral tonic-clonic
Figure-of-4	Focal [aware or impaired awareness] motor tonic	**Simple partial**	**Focal aware**
Freeze	Focal [aware or impaired awareness] behavior arrest	Supplementary motor	Focal motor tonic
		Sylvian	Focal motor
Frontal lobe*	Focal	**Temporal lobe***	**Focal aware/impaired awareness**
Gelastic	Focal [aware or impaired awareness] emotional (gelastic)	**Tonic**	**[Focal/generalized] tonic**
Grand mal	**Generalized tonic-clonic, focal to bilateral tonic-clonic, unknown-onset tonic-clonic**	**Tonic-clonic**	**[Generalized/unknown] onset tonic-clonic, focal to bilateral tonic-clonic**
Gustatory	Focal [aware or impaired awareness] sensory (gustatory)	Uncinate	Focal [aware impaired awareness] sensory (olfactory)

Note that there is not a one-to-one correspondence, reflecting reorganization as well as renaming.
The most important terms are set in bold.
*Anatomic classification may still be useful for some purposes, for example, in evaluation for epilepsy surgery.
From Fisher FS, Cross JH, D'Souza C, et al. Instruction manual for the ILAE 2017 operational classification of seizure types. *Epilepsia*. 2017;58(4):531–542 (Table 3, p. 540).

An **aura** is the portion of a seizure that is experienced before any loss of consciousness. Some auras can be difficult for a patient to describe; asking them if they know a seizure will happen before it happens, even if they cannot articulate precisely what they are experiencing, is one way to approach the topic. Examples of auras include an epigastric rising sensation; nausea; visual, auditory, or olfactory hallucinations; or limbic symptoms such as fear or a sensation of déjà vu. An aura may be suspected in very young children if there is a change in behavior before seizures, such as interrupting an activity to seek out parents or complaining of abdominal pain. The presence of an aura is traditionally thought to be indicative of a focal seizure without impairment of consciousness, as it implies focal cortical dysfunction, but some studies have reported that up to 64% of patients with documented idiopathic generalized epilepsy experience some form of aura, possibly due to asymmetric propagation of the discharges through the thalamocortical networks.

Nonepileptic events such as **migraines** or **syncope** may also have a prodrome, further highlighting the value of a comprehensive history in distinguishing types of events.

The progressive symptoms of some seizures after the initial aura reflect the spread of the abnormal electrical discharge beyond the region of onset, which is why a detailed history is critical for evaluating paroxysmal spells and determining the likelihood that they represent seizure activity.

Focal seizures can have motor and/or sensory components, depending on which areas of what is termed *eloquent cortex* become involved in the seizure. However, the seizure may originate in a portion of the cortex that does not produce obvious physical symptoms (termed the *silent* or *noneloquent cortex*), and physical signs of the seizure only develop if the seizure discharge spreads to involve eloquent cortex. Seizures with clear electrical abnormalities but minimal or absent physical symptoms are commonly referred to as *electrographic seizures* or *subclinical seizures*. Subclinical electrographic seizures, particularly during sleep, can be associated with deterioration in development, behavior, attention, and learning.

Focal motor seizures produce rhythmic jerking (clonic) movements of the limb or limbs *contralateral* to the primary motor cortex involved. Other focal motor seizures include involuntary turning of the head and eyes in one direction (version), vocalization, and speech arrest. There may be tonic stiffening and extension of the arm ipsilateral to the seizure onset.

Involvement of the sensory cortex produces simple *somatosensory* experiences such as paresthesia or numbness, often with a dysesthetic quality, and visual, auditory, olfactory, or gustatory phenomena. Some

TABLE 39.9   Suggested Scheme for an Etiologic Classification of Epilepsy

Main Category	Subcategory	Examples*
Idiopathic epilepsy	Pure epilepsies due to single-gene disorders	Benign familial neonatal convulsions; autosomal dominant nocturnal frontal lobe epilepsy; generalized epilepsy with febrile seizures plus; severe myoclonic epilepsy of childhood; benign adult familial myoclonic epilepsy
	Pure epilepsies with complex inheritance	Idiopathic generalized epilepsy (and its subtypes); benign partial epilepsies of childhood
Symptomatic epilepsy Predominantly genetic or developmental causation	Childhood epilepsy syndromes	West syndrome; Lennox-Gastaut syndrome
	Progressive myoclonic epilepsies	Unverricht-Lundborg disease; dentato-rubro-pallido-luysian atrophy; Lafora body disease; mitochondrial cytopathy; sialidosis; neuronal ceroid lipofuscinosis; myoclonus renal failure syndrome
	Neurocutaneous syndromes	Tuberous sclerosis; neurofibromatosis; Sturge-Weber syndrome
	Other neurologic single-gene disorders	Angelman syndrome; lysosomal disorders; neuroacanthocytosis; organic acidurias and peroxisomal disorders; porphyria; pyridoxine-dependent epilepsy; Rett syndrome; urea cycle disorders; Wilson disease; disorders of cobalamin and folate metabolism
	Disorders of chromosomes	Down syndrome; fragile X syndrome; 4p– syndrome; isodicentric chromosome 15; ring chromosome 20
	Developmental anomalies of the cerebral structure	Hemimegalencephaly; focal cortical dysplasia; agyria-pachygyria-band spectrum; agenesis of the corpus callosum; polymicrogyria; schizencephaly; periventricular nodular heterotopia; microcephaly; arachnoid cyst
Predominantly acquired causation	Hippocampal sclerosis	Hippocampal sclerosis
	Perinatal and infantile causes	Neonatal seizures; postneonatal seizures; cerebral palsy
	Cerebral trauma	Open head injury; closed head injury; neurosurgery; epilepsy after epilepsy surgery; nonaccidental head injury in infants
	Cerebral tumor	Glioma; ganglioglioma and hamartoma; DNET; hypothalamic hamartoma; meningioma; secondary tumors
	Cerebral infection	Viral meningitis and encephalitis; bacterial meningitis and abscess; malaria; neurocysticercosis; tuberculosis; HIV
	Cerebrovascular disorders	Cerebral hemorrhage; cerebral infarction; degenerative vascular disease; arteriovenous malformation; cavernous hemangioma
	Cerebral immunologic disorders	Rasmussen encephalitis; SLE and collagen vascular disorders; inflammatory and immunologic disorders
	Degenerative and other neurologic conditions	Alzheimer disease and other dementing disorders; multiple sclerosis and demyelinating disorders; hydrocephalus and porencephaly
Provoked epilepsy	Provoking factors	Fever; menstrual cycle and catamenial epilepsy; sleep-wake cycle; metabolic and endocrine-induced seizures; drug-induced seizures; alcohol- and toxin-induced seizures
	Reflex epilepsies	Photosensitive epilepsies; startle-induced epilepsies; reading epilepsy; auditory-induced epilepsy; eating epilepsy; hot water epilepsy
Cryptogenic epilepsies†		

*These examples are not comprehensive, and in every category there are other causes.
†By definition, the causes of the cryptogenic epilepsies are "unknown." However, these are an important category, accounting for at least 40% of epilepsies encountered in adult practice and a lesser proportion in pediatric practice.
DNET, dysembryoplastic neuroepithelial tumor; SLE, systemic lupus erythematosus.
From Shorvon SD. The etiologic classification of epilepsy. *Epilepsia.* 2011;52:1052–1057.

of these sensory phenomena can be quite complex, including structured visual hallucinations, sensations of depersonalization, and affective symptoms such as anxiety or fear. Epileptic phenomena are a rare cause for such phenomena, and a broad differential diagnosis should be considered for paroxysmal spells where the primary symptoms are sensory or affective.

As the seizure continues to spread, both cerebral hemispheres may become engaged, and there is generalized clonic jerking of the body that closely resembles a GTC seizure. These secondarily generalized seizures may be mistaken for a generalized seizure if the onset is not witnessed. Occasionally after a seizure, there is persistent focal weakness or hemiparesis known as **Todd palsy**, which is strongly suggestive of a contralateral focal onset to the seizure.

Generalized Seizures

Generalized seizures are defined as seizures in which the first clinical changes indicate initial involvement of both hemispheres. Motor involvement, if present, is bilateral, as are the initial EEG changes.

Consciousness is impaired in most generalized seizures, but not in all; for instance, brief myoclonic seizures and some atonic seizures may not be associated with any impairment of consciousness.

Absence (petit mal) seizures begin with sudden interruption of activity and staring; they are usually brief and end abruptly without postictal confusion. Simple absence seizures consist of only motionlessness and a blank stare lasting for several seconds, with immediate postictal reanimation. Lip-smacking, fumbling or searching hand movements, or convulsive swallowing can appear during longer seizures, or preictal activities may be continued in a slow, automatic manner. Paroxysmal alterations in autonomic function may also accompany absence seizures, including pupillary dilation, pallor, flushing, sweating, salivation, piloerection, or a combination of these. Absence seizures that are more typically accompanied by eyelid fluttering, facial twitching, or myoclonic jerks of the trunk or extremities are referred to as *complicated* absence seizures. Atypical absence seizures are described as absence seizures with a less abrupt beginning and end, with more pronounced changes in muscle tone, and of longer duration. Distinctions should be made between the clinical features of absence seizures, focal dyscognitive seizures, and episodic daydreaming (Table 39.10). Staring spells that are prolonged beyond 15–20 seconds are less likely to represent absence seizures due to incorrect duration. Staring spells in infants and toddlers are also unlikely to represent absence seizures due to incorrect age of onset. Early-onset generalized epilepsy is associated with rare genetic syndromes. Children with prolonged staring spells, particularly starting at a young age, are at higher risk of partial-onset seizures or behavioral spells.

Tonic-clonic seizures are perhaps the most dramatic of the epileptic seizures. The **tonic phase** begins with sudden sustained contraction of facial, axial, and limb muscle groups, and there may be an initial involuntary stridorous cry or a moan secondary to contraction of the diaphragm and chest muscles against a partially closed glottis (the *ictal cry*). The tonic contraction is maintained for seconds to 10s of seconds, during which time the child falls if standing, is apneic and may become cyanotic, may bite the sides of their tongue, and may pass urine. The **clonic phase** of the seizure begins when the tonic contraction is repeatedly interrupted by momentary relaxation of the muscular contraction. This gives the appearance of generalized jerking as the contraction resumes after each relaxation. At the end of the clonic phase, the body relaxes, and the patient is unconscious with deep respiration. If roused, the patient is confused, may complain of muscle soreness, and usually wishes to sleep.

Myoclonic seizures are sudden, brief, shocklike contractions of muscles. They may involve the whole body or a portion of the axial musculature such as the face and trunk, or they may be limited to the limbs. They can be isolated or repetitive, irregular or rhythmic. Myoclonic seizures arise from the cortex and are associated with a distinct EEG pattern. Some forms of myoclonus are of brainstem or spinal origin; those occurring without other seizure types are not regarded as epileptic myoclonus but thought of as *movement disorders*.

Generalized tonic seizures begin in the same way as tonic-clonic seizures; a massive, generalized contraction produces any combination of facial grimacing, neck and trunk flexion or extension, abduction or elevation of the arms, and flexion of the hips. Subtle tonic seizures may produce only facial grimacing and slight neck and trunk flexion. Tonic seizures may be accompanied by pronounced autonomic activity with diaphoresis, flushing, pallor, and tachycardia, even when the muscular contraction is slight.

Atonic seizures are characterized by a sudden decrease or loss of postural muscle tone. The extent of muscle involvement may vary; an atonic seizure may be limited to a sudden head drop with slack jaw or may result in a fall because of loss of axial and limb muscle tone. The falls are referred to as *drop attacks*, and because they are unexpected and sudden in onset, they often result in injury.

DIAGNOSTIC EVALUATION OF A SEIZURE DISORDER

Electroencephalographic Studies

The incidence of EEG epileptiform activity in normal children without a history of seizures is very low (<2%); such findings are associated with a strong family history of genetic epilepsy. The incidence of recurrent epileptic seizures in patients with focal EEG spikes is 83%. In a child with suspected seizures, the finding of focal or generalized epileptiform activity on the EEG supports a diagnosis of epilepsy, whereas multiple negative EEG studies capturing both wakefulness *and* sleep argue against such a diagnosis and should prompt the physician to consider alternative diagnoses and to attempt to record the episodes.

There are two basic types of EEGs: *conventional* and *amplitude-integrated*. A conventional EEG utilizes 19 or more electrodes distributed symmetrically over both hemispheres and along the midline. A routine outpatient EEG is run for at least 20 minutes, and more often 40–60 minutes. A prolonged EEG, or long-term monitoring, is run for over 24 hours, and can even be performed for over a week at a time. This type of prolonged study can be performed on an ambulatory basis at home or as an inpatient in an epilepsy monitoring unit. Amplitude-integrated EEG, by contrast, utilizes only two or four EEG electrodes and is primarily used in neonatal intensive care units.

An EEG should always attempt to capture sleep, and most will include hyperventilation and photic stimulation, all of which potentially activate epileptiform discharges, increasing the diagnostic yield. Hyperventilation produces absence seizures in about 80% of children with childhood

TABLE 39.10 Differential Diagnosis of Episodic Unresponsiveness Without Convulsions

Clinical	Absence Seizures	Focal Dyscognitive Seizures	Staring, Inattention
Frequency	Multiple daily	Rarely more than one to two per day	Daily, situation dependent: e.g., may occur only at school
Duration	Often <10 sec, rarely >30 sec	Average duration >60 sec, rarely <10 sec	Seconds to minutes
Aura	Not present	May be present	Not present
Abrupt interruption of child's activity	Yes: e.g., speech arrest midsentence; pause while eating, playing, or fighting	Yes	Activities such as play or eating are not abruptly interrupted, no sudden onset
Eyelid flutter	Common, often with upward eye movement	Uncommon, but may be present	No
Myoclonic jerks	Common	Uncommon	Not present
Automatisms	Occur in longer absences, usually mild	Frequent and often prominent	No
Responsiveness	Unresponsive	Unresponsive	Responds to touch
Postictal impairment	None	Postictal confusion and malaise is typical; drowsiness may also occur	No
EEG	Generalized 3-Hz spike-and-wave complexes	Regional epileptic discharges (most often frontal or temporal)	Normal
MRI	Normal	Focal structural lesions not uncommon (e.g., tumor)	Normal
First-line medication	Valproate, ethosuximide	Carbamazepine, phenytoin, valproate	None

absence epilepsy. Intermittent photic stimulation produces generalized epileptic discharges in several of the generalized epileptic syndromes, but photosensitivity is overall rare in epilepsy. Recording during wakefulness and sleep performed after sleep deprivation may have the highest yield. Overnight recording in the hospital provides for prolonged sampling of the interictal EEG in wakefulness and spontaneous sleep. For any patient with refractory seizures or an uncertain diagnosis, the use of video and EEG monitoring is usually helpful in clarifying the diagnosis. Defining the exact seizure type may lead to modification of drug treatment or consideration of epilepsy surgery, or a nonepileptic paroxysmal disorder may be discovered.

A single normal EEG does not definitively exclude a seizure disorder, particularly in people with infrequent seizures or seizures in specific contexts, such as illness or sleep.

Neuroimaging Studies

MRI is superior to CT for the evaluation of epilepsy. Any patient with a history or examination suspicious for focal-onset epilepsy should have MRI of the brain unless the syndrome is clearly that of benign focal epilepsy of childhood with centrotemporal spikes. MRI may also reveal an abnormality in patients with symptomatic generalized epilepsy. Functional neuroimaging is important in the assessment of candidates for surgical resection in patients with intractable seizures (Fig. 39.4).

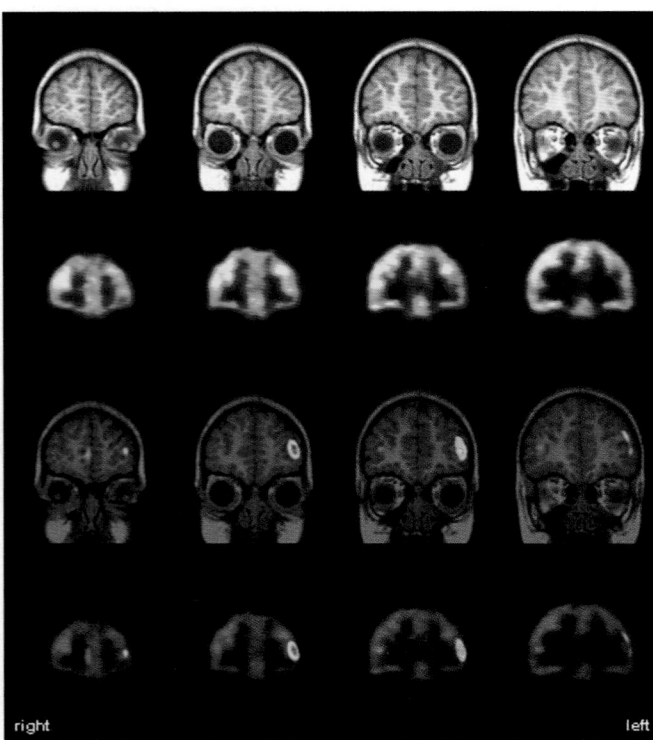

Fig. 39.4 Fluorodeoxyglucose F 18 ([18F]FDG) PET and ictal [99mTc] ethyl cysteinate dimer ([99mTc]ECD) single photon emission computed tomography (SPECT) in left frontal lobe epilepsy. This patient's MRI scan *(top row)* was normal, whereas [18F]FDG PET showed extensive left frontal hypometabolism *(second row)*. Additional ictal and interictal [99mTc] ECD SPECT scans were performed for accurate localization of seizure onset. Result of a SPECT subtraction analysis (ictal-interictal; blood flow increases above a threshold of 15%, maximum 40%) was overlaid onto the MRI and [18F]FDG PET scan *(third and fourth rows,* respectively), clearly depicting the zone of seizure onset within the functional deficit zone given by [18F]FDG PET. (From Jankovic J, Mazziotta JC, Pomeroy SL, Newman NJ, eds. *Bradley's Neurology in Clinical Practice.* 8th ed. Philadelphia: Elsevier; 2022:593, Fig. 42.18.)

When available, a 3.0 Tesla MRI of the brain with specific protocols dedicated to epilepsy evaluation (e.g., proper alignment of the imaging axis with the hippocampi) is preferred. It is important to note that generalized seizures associated with status epilepticus may also produce nonspecific and reversible findings on MRI (Fig. 39.5).

Evaluation of the First Seizure

There is no clinical sign or diagnostic investigation that determines with certainty whether a child presenting with a first seizure has epilepsy or has had an isolated seizure. The assessment of patients with a first seizure must include a search for etiologic agents and features that may indicate the risk of recurrence. Factors to be considered include the circumstances of the seizure, the health of the child in the time before the seizure, the recent sleep patterns, the possibility of abuse or trauma, and the chance of ingestion of prescription or street drugs or syndromes such as the neurocutaneous disorders (Table 39.11).

The recurrence risk after a first unprovoked seizure, usually defined as a seizure or flurry of seizures within 24 hours in patients older than 1 month, is ~40–50%.

The most important predictor of recurrence appears to be the existence of an underlying neurologic disorder. The existence of intellectual disability or cerebral palsy is a common antecedent to epilepsy, as is a history of significant head injury. An EEG with generalized or focal epileptiform discharges or with focal or generalized slowing is also predictive of recurrence. Focal seizures are more likely to be associated with recurrence, although patients with such seizures are also more likely to have an existing neurologic deficit or an abnormal EEG. The duration of the first seizure or a presentation in status epilepticus is not associated with a higher incidence of recurrence. A family history of epilepsy is not a predictor of recurrence. Earlier age at onset, particularly before the age of 12 months, has been associated with a higher risk of recurrent seizures.

Most authorities believe that the majority of patients with a first seizure should not be treated unless the risk of recurrence is judged to be significantly higher than average. An abnormal neurologic examination, an abnormal MRI of the brain, and abnormal EEG all increase the risk of recurrence; the greater the number of risk factors, the more likely an AED may be initiated after a first known seizure, although some neurologists will still elect to wait for a second confirmed seizure. In adults or adolescents, the issues of driving and employment may influence the decision to treat a first seizure, but in otherwise healthy and developmentally normal children, there is almost no indication for chronic AED treatment in response to a single seizure. Activities such as bathing, driving, and swimming must be carefully supervised.

The decision to begin AED therapy is usually made after a patient has had two or more seizures in a short interval of time (6–12 months). Treatment with AEDs lowers the recurrence rate by about 50% (Fig. 39.6).

STATUS EPILEPTICUS

Status epilepticus *is a medical emergency* where epileptic seizures are prolonged or occur in rapid succession without recovery between the seizures. There are two general categories of status epilepticus: convulsive and nonconvulsive ("subclinical") status epilepticus. **Convulsive status epilepticus** may involve repetitive or prolonged GTC, myoclonic, or tonic seizures. **Nonconvulsive status epilepticus** may involve repeated or continuous absence seizures or focal dyscognitive seizures with an altered state of consciousness lasting hours or even days.

A common duration of a seizure defined as status epilepticus is 30 minutes or longer, but seizures continuing for more than 5–10 minutes warrant immediate attention, as they are statistically likely to progress to status epilepticus. The tonic-clonic phase of generalized seizures

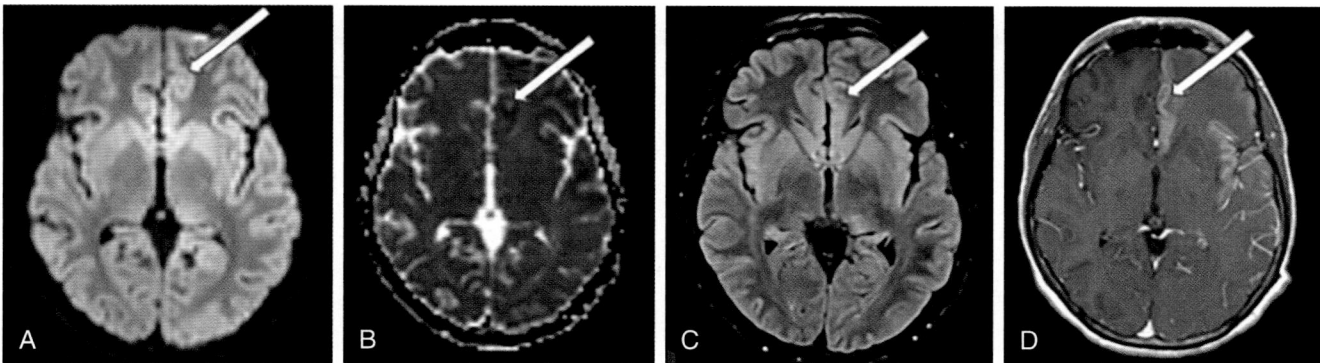

Fig. 39.5 Common MRI findings due to status epilepticus. Diffusion-weighted imaging (DWI) *(A)* sequence reveals increased intensity in the left insular and frontal cortices *(white arrows)* with corresponding decreased apparent diffusion coefficient *(B)*. There are similar regions of increased intensity on fluid-attenuated inversion recovery imaging *(C)* and contrast enhancement *(D)* implying a component of vasogenic edema. These changes resolved on repeat MRI 1 week later. (From Guerriero RM, Gaillard WD. Imaging modalities to diagnose and localize status epilepticus. *Seizure Eur J Epilepsy.* 2019;68:46–51 [Fig. 1, p. 48].)

usually lasts <2 minutes; such seizures lasting ≥5 minutes usually evolve into status epilepticus. One third of children presenting with status epilepticus have no history of epilepsy, another third have a history of chronic epilepsy, and an acute illness or injury has caused status epilepticus in another third. One of the most common precipitants of status epilepticus in people with a known history of epilepsy is abrupt *discontinuation* of a daily AED.

Status epilepticus has a significant acute mortality rate, partly because of the underlying cause of the seizures; intracranial infections (meningitis, encephalitis), poisoning, acute metabolic disorders, and head injuries are some of the most common causes.

The goals of the emergency management of status epilepticus are as follows:

1. Maintain normal cardiorespiratory function and cerebral oxygenation.
2. Stop clinical and electrical seizure activity and prevent its recurrence.
3. Identify precipitating factors.
4. Correct any metabolic disturbances (hypoglycemia, hyponatremia) and prevent systemic complications such as cardiovascular collapse, cardiac arrhythmia, pneumonia, and renal failure.

Table 39.12 sets out a plan of initial assessment and management of convulsive status epilepticus. Lorazepam and diazepam are rapidly acting anticonvulsants when given intravenously but must be combined with a primary AED, as their duration of action is short. Side effects include sedation, depressed respiration, decreased ability to protect the airway, and hypotension.

Phenytoin, fosphenytoin, phenobarbital, or valproic acid could be used in conjunction with the benzodiazepines in providing longer-lasting anticonvulsive action.

Phenytoin is less commonly used. It has a rare but serious complication called *purple glove syndrome,* which occurs in 1.7–5.9% of intravenous administrations; within 2 hours of administration, there is pain, bluish discoloration, and swelling of the affected limb. Treatment involves discontinuation of the phenytoin and elevation and icing of the affected limb; compartment syndrome is a potential complication.

Fosphenytoin, a prodrug of phenytoin, can be administered either intravascularly or intramuscularly. Fosphenytoin has a maximum infusion rate of 150 mg PE/min; when it is infused faster, hypotension and arrhythmias may occur.

Valproate can be given intravenously and may be the appropriate therapy for patients with known idiopathic and symptomatic generalized epilepsies. It is also generally appropriate for children with a known static cerebral injury presenting with status epilepticus as their first seizure, such as a child with a history of neonatal hypoxic-ischemic encephalopathy who presents at age 4 in status epilepticus. It is contraindicated in children with known or suspected mitochondrial disease, multisystemic disease of unknown etiology, or known hepatic disease, or in children under the age of 2 years.

Nonconvulsive status epilepticus may arise when frequent focal dyscognitive seizures or absence seizures occur. In both settings, discrete seizures may not be identifiable; instead, the child may present with confusion, clouded consciousness, and partial responsiveness or a stuporous state, all of which can last hours or even days. It should be treated urgently as soon as it is identified, especially if focal dyscognitive status is suspected, in which case treatment should follow that outlined for convulsive status epilepticus. In absence status epilepticus, intravenous benzodiazepines are usually effective but should be used in conjunction with intravenous valproate or oral ethosuximide.

CLASSIFICATION OF EPILEPSIES AND EPILEPTIC SYNDROMES

The clinician should attempt to determine whether the seizure disorder is focal or generalized, and then whether there is evidence of underlying brain dysfunction. Both the focal and generalized epilepsies in otherwise developmentally normal children respond favorably to treatment, and there is a good chance of long-term remission. Structural epilepsies may benefit from surgical intervention. Genetic and metabolic epilepsies respond less predictably to treatment, and the chance of remission is less certain.

Identification of one of the epileptic encephalopathies of infancy and childhood has grave prognostic significance (Table 39.13). These epilepsies vary in the seizure types and EEG features but have certain features in common: specific age at onset and expression, intractable seizures, cognitive dysfunction, arrest in development, conspicuous interictal epileptic discharges on the EEG, and a poor response to treatment.

Neonatal Period

The paroxysmal disorders seen in the neonatal period (birth to 8 weeks) are presented in Table 39.14.

TABLE 39.11 Neurocutaneous Syndromes

Clinical Syndromes and Findings	Investigations
Sturge-Weber Syndrome	
Facial hemangioma, "port-wine stain" upper face, division of cranial nerve V; bilateral in 30%, absent in 5%, associated truncal and limb hemangiomas in 45%	CT scan: calcification, MRI scan with gadolinium
Intracranial leptomeningeal angiomatosis	EEG: attenuation of background rhythms, epileptiform discharges
Epilepsy in 70–90%, usually before 2 yr and before hemiparesis, intractable in 35%	
Intellectual disability in 50–60%	
Hemiparesis in 30%, often with hemisensory deficit and hemianopia	
Tuberous Sclerosis	
Diagnostic Criteria*	
Any One of the Following:	
Facial angiofibroma (adenoma sebaceum, nasolabial folds, and nose becomes more prominent with age) or periungual fibromas	Physical examination
Cortical tubers, subependymal nodule, giant cell astrocytoma	MRI examination: T1 and T2 sequences with gadolinium
Multiple retinal hamartomas (usually asymptomatic) or multiple renal angiomyolipomas (usually asymptomatic, may manifest as hematuria, hypertension, or renal failure)	Funduscopic examination and renal ultrasonography, abdominal CT scan
Or Any Two of the Following:	
Infantile spasms (seizures in 90%, most commonly generalized; infantile spasms and myoclonus)	History and physical, EEG; focal or generalized abnormalities
Hypomelanotic papules (ash leaf spots; in 80–90%, 1–2 cm oval or leaf-shaped)	Wood lamp examination in darkened room
Single retinal hamartoma	Funduscopic examination
Subependymal or cortical calcification on CT scan	CT scan of the brain
Single renal angiomyolipomas or cysts	Renal ultrasonography or abdominal CT scan
Cardiac rhabdomyomas (single or multiple; may obstruct outflow, cause arrhythmias, or cause conduction defects)	Echocardiography, ECG
First-degree relative with tuberous sclerosis (autosomal dominant disorder, 80% of cases represent new variants)	Examination of parents; echocardiography, MRI scans
Also Associated:	
Intellectual disability in 50–66%	
Shagreen patches; hamartomatous skin lesion in lumbosacral region in 50%	
Pulmonary involvement, fibrosis	Chest radiograph
Skeletal abnormalities	Hand, feet (cystic), long bone (sclerotic) radiographic changes
Epidermal Nevus Syndrome	
Hamartomatous lesions; subclassified according to most predominant histologic and clinical features (e.g., linear nevus sebaceus, see below)	Careful examination of the scalp, skin folds, and conjunctiva; funduscopic examination
Sporadic, affects both sexes equally; CNS abnormalities are common with epidermal nevus syndrome, including seizures (25% of patients), intellectual disability, and neoplasia; also, skeletal abnormalities, including kyphoscoliosis and hemiatrophy	Spine and limb radiographs, as appropriate
Linear nevus sebaceus; hairless verrucous yellow-orange or hyperpigmented plaques on the face and scalp	
Epilepsy in 76%	
Intellectual disability in 60%	
Associated neuronal migration disorders	MRI scan of the brain
Malignant transformation of a skin lesion	
Other Neurocutaneous Syndromes Associated with Seizures	
Neurofibromatosis; cutaneous lesions include café-au-lait spots, axillary freckling, neural tumors; seizure types include generalized tonic-clonic, partial complex, and partial simple-motor	MRI scan of the brain
Incontinentia pigmenti; involvement includes linear papular-vesicular cutaneous lesions at birth, later pigmentation, ocular and dental anomalies; female-to-male ratio >20:1 (boys may die in utero); seizure types include neonatal onset and later generalized tonic-clonic	Skin biopsy; ophthalmology examination
Hypomelanosis of Ito (incontinentia pigmenti achromians)	

*See http://www.tsalliance.org/healthcare-professionals/diagnosis/.
CNS, central nervous system.

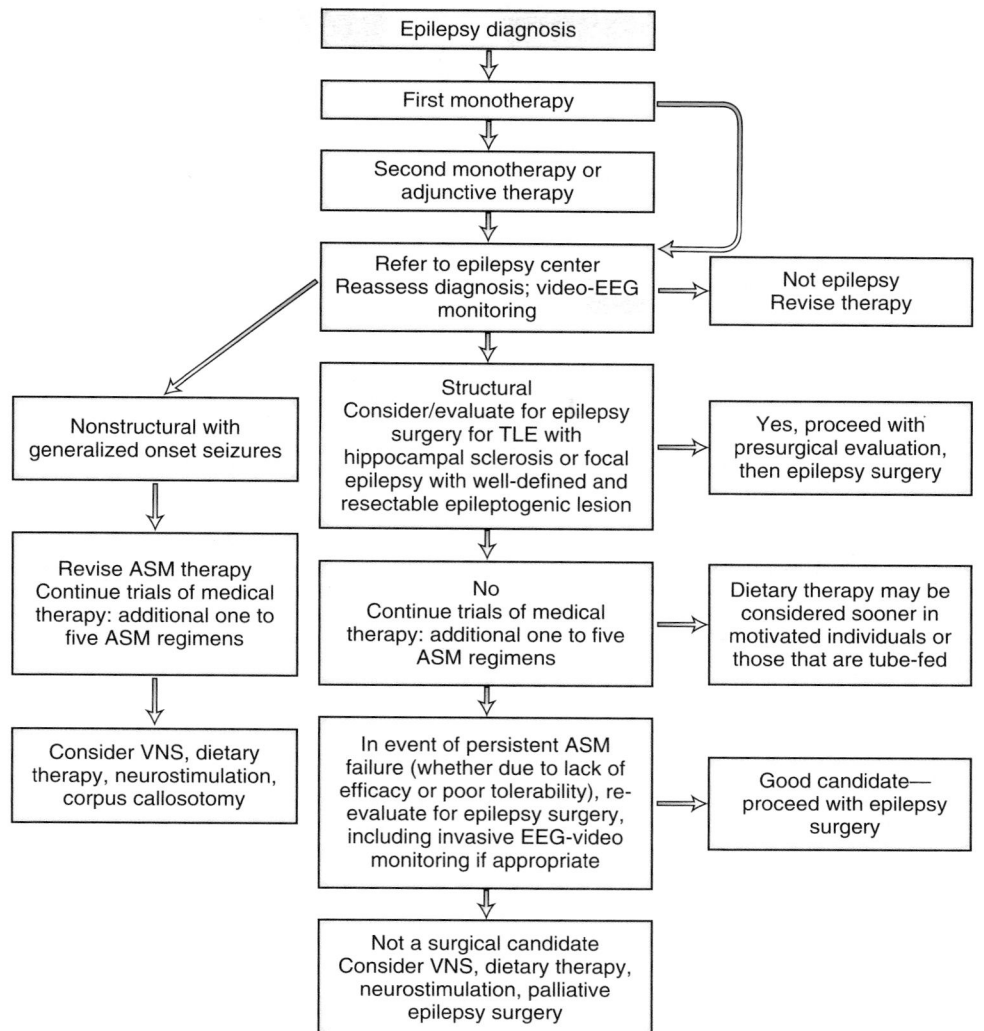

Fig. 39.6 Additional steps assume that seizures are not controlled despite adequate trial of well-tolerated medication. AED, antiepileptic drug; ASM, antiseizure medication; TLE, temporal lobe epilepsy; VNS, vagus nerve stimulation. (From Jankovic J, Mazziotta JC, Pomeroy SL, Newman NJ, eds. *Bradley's Neurology in Clinical Practice.* 8th ed. Philadelphia: Elsevier; 2022:1649, Fig. 100.19.)

Paroxysmal Nonepileptic Disorders

Jitteriness. Jitteriness or tremulousness is a common movement disorder of neonates. It can be confused with seizures, especially if superimposed on normal tonic postural reflexes. Jitteriness, characterized by rhythmic alternating movements of all extremities with equal velocity in flexion and extension, only occasionally has a true synchronized clonic appearance. Jitteriness is not accompanied by eye deviation or staring, is stimulus sensitive, and can usually be stopped by gentle passive flexion of the moving limb.

Jitteriness in the newborn can be associated with hypoxic-ischemic encephalopathy, hypoglycemia, hypocalcemia, and drug withdrawal; if any of these causative factors are identified, there may also be a higher risk of epileptic seizures. In otherwise healthy infants, jitteriness seems to be a benign movement disorder, resolving by 10–14 months of age.

Benign Neonatal Sleep Myoclonus

Myoclonic jerks may appear during sleep in some healthy neonates. It has been reported within hours of birth and may disappear over the next few months or persist into childhood. The jerks can be bilateral and synchronous or asymmetric; they may migrate between muscle groups during an episode. They are repetitive but do not disturb sleep. These jerks have been described in all stages of sleep but are most prominent in quiet sleep; they are not confined to sleep onset. Features distinguishing this phenomenon from epilepsy are its presence exclusively during sleep with disappearance on awakening, normal EEGs, and normal psychomotor development.

Acute Symptomatic Seizures and Occasional Seizures

Most neonatal seizures are acute symptomatic seizures, and the number of children who continue to have seizures after the neonatal period is relatively small. Neonatal seizures have been classified according to the clinical features as subtle, tonic, clonic, and myoclonic. However, not all of these clinical seizure types have consistent ictal EEG patterns. The classification of neonatal seizures reflects the variable, poorly organized, and often subtle clinical expression of epileptic seizures at this age. Typical GTC or absence seizures are not seen at this age, perhaps because of the limited capacity of the neonatal brain for interhemispheric synchrony. Patterns include the following:

- Clinical seizures *consistently* associated with an EEG seizure pattern:
  - *Clonic seizures* with focal or multifocal jerking of the face or extremities fit this category, as do focal tonic seizures with focal

TABLE 39.12   Management of Convulsive Status Epilepticus

Priority	Examination and Laboratory Investigations	Management
On arrival	Airway patency and respiratory rate, inspect pharynx, chest auscultation, BP, pulse, temperature; level of consciousness; response to command, pain; serum Na, K, glucose, creatinine, Ca, Mg; CBC, liver function studies, AED levels; serum and urine toxins screen; arterial blood gases, chest radiograph	Airway protection; suction pharynx and give supplemental oxygen Rectal antipyretic to lower temperature if elevated, IV access and administer: 25% glucose IV, 2–4 mL/kg, and lorazepam* IV, 0.1 mg/kg (to a maximum of 8 mg) as a bolus and fosphenytoin IV, 20 mg/kg at 150 mg/min with ECG monitoring and collection of serum level after loading dose *If immediate IV access is not possible, give diazepam 0.3–0.5 mg/kg rectally and fosphenytoin IM and arrange for central line or intraosseous access
After initial treatment	Neck stiffness, funduscopy, signs of trauma, rashes, symmetry of motor function and reflexes	If patient is febrile: appropriate cultures, other studies depending on age and other symptoms If any suspicion of head injury: obtain urgent CT scan
If seizures continue	Patient's level of consciousness becomes depressed with lorazepam and PB, and an EEG is necessary to assess adequacy of therapy	Arrange ICU bed and consider intubation; give further bolus of lorazepam 0.05–0.1 mg/kg, and push PHT serum level above 30 mg/L with further loading dose (~10 mg/kg) In an ICU setting, if seizures continue with PHT levels of 30–40 mg/L, then add PB 20 mg/kg IV loading over 15–30 min Continued clinical or electrical seizures may necessitate induction of pentobarbital therapy: loading dose of 5–15 mg/kg, followed by IV infusion of 1–3 mg/kg/hr titrated by EEG monitoring to achieve burst-suppression pattern; maintain for 24–48 hr and review Elective intubation and ventilation, arterial line, BP monitoring
After stabilization or in tandem with escalating therapy	LP; if acute febrile illness with papilledema or focal neurologic signs, then CT/MRI first	If LP is delayed and intracranial infection is suspected, then cover with antibiotic and antiviral therapy

*Give lorazepam if actively convulsing; this may not be required in patients with serial seizures who can be quickly loaded with fosphenytoin.

AED, antiepileptic drug; BP, blood pressure; Ca, calcium; ICU, intensive care unit; IM, intramuscularly; IV, intravenously; K, potassium; LP, lumbar puncture; Na, sodium; Mg, magnesium; PB, phenobarbital; PHT, phenytoin.

TABLE 39.13   Cryptogenic and Symptomatic Epileptic Encephalopathies

Neonates and Infants

Early infantile epileptic encephalopathy (Ohtahara syndrome)
Early infantile myoclonic epilepsy
Migratory partial seizures of infancy
West syndrome (infantile spasms)
Severe myoclonic epilepsy of infants (Dravet syndrome)
Epilepsy restricted to females with cognitive impairment
Atypical Rett syndrome with early epilepsy
Epilepsy in association with inherited disorders of metabolism (see Table 39.7)
    Lysosomal storage disorders
    Urea cycle disorders
    Aminoacidurias

Children and Adolescents

Lennox-Gastaut syndrome
Myoclonic-astatic epilepsy
Atypical benign partial epilepsy
Acquired epileptic aphasia (Landau-Kleffner syndrome)
Continuous spike-and-wave patterns in slow-wave sleep
Epilepsy in association with inherited disorders of metabolism
Mitochondrial encephalomyopathies
Progressive myoclonus epilepsies
Epilepsy in association with systemic disorders involving the central nervous system
Systemic lupus erythematosus, other vasculitides

TABLE 39.14   Paroxysmal Disorders of the Neonatal Period

Paroxysmal Nonepileptiform Disorders

Jitteriness
Benign neonatal sleep myoclonus

Acute Symptomatic Seizures and Occasional Seizures

Hypoxic-ischemic encephalopathy
Intraventricular hemorrhage
Acute metabolic disorders*
Sepsis-meningitis

Epileptic Syndromes

Benign idiopathic neonatal convulsions
Familial
Nonfamilial
Ohtahara (see EIEE) (see Table 39.18)
Symptomatic focal epilepsy
Brain tumor
Malformations of cortical development
Inherited metabolic disease; mitochondrial disorders
Early-onset generalized epileptic syndromes with encephalopathy
Early myoclonic encephalopathy
Early infantile epileptic encephalopathy (EIEE)

*Hypoglycemia, hypocalcemia, hypomagnesemia, hyponatremia, hypernatremia, hyperammonemia.

tonic posturing of a limb or asymmetric posturing of the axial musculature. Clinical seizures with consistent focal jerking or posturing of one limb are most consistently correctly identified at the bedside and are commonly associated with a focal structural defect, such as a focal perinatal stroke.

- Clinical seizures *sometimes* associated with an EEG seizure pattern:
  - *Myoclonic seizures* consist of single or multiple flexor jerks of the upper or lower limbs. An ictal EEG pattern is not always seen in this group. Fragmentary (multifocal) myoclonus is not always associated with an ictal EEG.
- Clinical seizures *not consistently* associated with an EEG seizure pattern:
  - These include *motor automatisms* characterized by a diversity of signs, including any of the following: wide-eyed staring, rapid blinking, eyelid fluttering, drooling, sucking, repetitive limb movements such as rowing or swimming with the arms or pedaling with the legs, apnea, hyperpnea, tonic eye deviation, and vasomotor skin color changes. This group of **subtle seizures** is generally associated with EEG background abnormalities such as suppression; the seizure itself may not have a consistent EEG correlate. This is reflective of diffuse cerebral dysfunction, such as seen in hypoxic-ischemic encephalopathy or metabolic disorders.
  - Generalized tonic seizures and focal and multifocal myoclonus are also often not associated with neonatal ictal EEG patterns, and when seen in stuporous or comatose children, the jerks may not be epileptic. However, if the EEG is completely normal, it is unlikely that the behaviors of concern represent subtle seizures.

Some simple clinical observations should guide the assessment of neonates with episodic abnormal behaviors. Epileptic behaviors are typically repetitive and stereotyped but are not provoked by stimulation of the child or increased with increasing intensity of a stimulus. Nonepileptic movements may disappear with repositioning of a limb or the child. Gentle restraint of a limb should be able to suppress or abort nonepileptic motor activity, whereas epileptic movements are still palpable. The association of abnormal eye movements with unusual behavior or limb movements suggests a seizure rather than nonepileptic behavior.

The possible etiologic factors are numerous and diverse (Tables 39.15 and 39.16). The most common cause is hypoxic-ischemic encephalopathy (60–65%); it is important to make a positive diagnosis of this historically and to exclude conditions such as perinatal local anesthetic toxicity, pyridoxine-dependent seizures, prenatal injury, and metabolic encephalopathies that may masquerade as perinatal asphyxia.

Diagnostic Investigations

EEG monitoring is useful in the evaluation of suspicious fluctuations in vital signs in neonates who are paralyzed and intubated or comatose, or in neonates with subtle but repetitive episodes of unusual behavior.

Many neonatal intensive care units have the capability to perform amplitude-integrated EEG (aEEG), which is a reduced electrode monitoring method that uses time-compressed baseline trends of two or four channels of EEG to allow the bedside practitioner to look for changes suspicious for seizure. However, both the sensitivity and specificity of aEEG are lower than that of full-montage conventional EEG: <50% if only a single channel of aEEG is available, but up to 76% and 78%, respectively, when two channels of raw EEG are available for comparison and direct review by expert aEEG interpreters. Conventional EEG is recommended over aEEG when both are available; however, the use of aEEG is associated with lower total seizure duration in neonates compared to no monitoring.

Proper treatment must include a thorough search for the cause of the seizures because many conditions necessitate specific treatment.

TABLE 39.15 Causes of Neonatal Seizures

Ages 1–4 Days
Hypoxic-ischemic encephalopathy
Drug withdrawal, maternal drug use of narcotics or barbiturates
Drug toxicity: lidocaine, penicillin
Intraventricular hemorrhage
Acute metabolic disorders
    Hypocalcemia
        Perinatal asphyxia, small for gestational age
        Sepsis
        Maternal diabetes, hyperthyroidism, or hypoparathyroidism
    Hypoglycemia
        Perinatal insults, prematurity, small for gestational age
        Maternal diabetes
        Hyperinsulinemic hypoglycemia
        Sepsis
    Hypomagnesemia
    Hyponatremia or hypernatremia
        Iatrogenic or inappropriate antidiuretic hormone secretion
Inborn errors of metabolism
    Galactosemia
    Glycine encephalopathy
    Urea cycle disorders
    Pyridoxine deficiency (must be considered at any age)

Ages 4–14 Days
Infection
    Meningitis (bacterial), encephalitis (enteroviral, herpes simplex)
Metabolic disorders
    Hypocalcemia
      Diet, milk formula
    Hypoglycemia, persistent
      Inherited disorders of metabolism: galactosemia, fructosemia, leucine sensitivity
      Hyperinsulinemic hypoglycemia
      Anterior pituitary hypoplasia, pancreatic islet cell tumor
      Beckwith syndrome
Drug withdrawal, maternal drug use of narcotics or barbiturates
Benign neonatal convulsions, familial and nonfamilial
Kernicterus, hyperbilirubinemia

Ages 2–8 Wk
Infection
    Herpes simplex or enteroviral encephalitis, bacterial meningitis
Head injury
    Subdural hematoma, child abuse
Inherited disorders of metabolism
    Aminoacidurias, urea cycle defects, organic acidurias
    Neonatal adrenoleukodystrophy
Malformations of cortical development
    Lissencephaly
    Focal cortical dysplasia
Tuberous sclerosis
Sturge-Weber syndrome

Prognosis

The prognosis for normal development after neonatal seizures depends on the cause of the seizures. Approximately 50% of neonates with seizures develop normally, 30% have neurologic sequelae, and 15–20% die. Neonates with seizures caused by CNS infection, hypoglycemia,

TABLE 39.16   Inherited Disorders of Metabolism and Neurodegenerative Diseases Associated with Seizures in Infants

Disorder	Clinical Features and Laboratory Findings	Investigations
Neonates		

These disorders are rare. The clinical features are nonspecific and usually do not distinguish between the inherited disorders of metabolism; however, they may suggest that a search for these conditions is warranted:
Metabolic or degenerative disorder in another sibling
Normal immediately after birth with symptoms and signs developing in the first days to weeks of life
Food intolerance; vomiting, diarrhea, not settling after feedings
Lethargy, may become stuporous after feeding
Hypotonia
Seizures; tonic, clonic, subtle neonatal seizures; myoclonus in some disorders
Late signs: weight loss, failure to thrive, psychomotor retardation
	Initial investigations in neonatal seizures:
	  Glucose, urinalysis, ketones
	  Serum glucose, Na+, K+, Ca2+, Mg2+, blood urea nitrogen, creatinine
	  Serum ammonia, lactate, and pyruvate
	  Liver function tests, complete blood cell count, arterial blood gas measurements
	  Lumbar puncture and CSF analysis
	  EEG
	  CT or MRI scan may be indicated

Maple syrup urine disease	An unusual maple syrup odor of the urine may be detected; severe metabolic acidosis and increased anion gap; urine positive for ketones; boiled urine reacts with 2,4-DNPH to give yellow precipitate	Serum amino acid analysis; elevated serum leucine, isoleucine, and valine

Organic acidurias
  Propionic acid
  Methylmalonic acid
  Isovaleric acid
  Glutaric acid
	Hyperammonemia, metabolic acidosis and increased anion gap, ketosis, low blood urea nitrogen; secondary elevation of lactate and hypoglycemia may be present and secondary carnitine deficiency may occur; glycine level may be elevated in these disorders
	Thrombocytopenia, neutropenia, and anemia
	Characteristic body odor in some of these disorders
		Urine organic acid analysis
		Serum carnitine measurement
		Serum acylcarnitine profile

Urea cycle disorders	Hyperammonemia without hypoglycemia, ketoacidosis or hematologic abnormalities	Serum ammonia. Plasma amino acids and urine orotic acid can help define the specific urea cycle defect
Nonketotic hyperglycinemia D-glyceric acidemia (glycine encephalopathy)	Intractable seizures and severe encephalopathy, often with coma, within the first weeks of life; may have the clinical syndrome of early myoclonic encephalopathy; myoclonic seizures, burst suppression on EEG, severe psychomotor retardation	Elevated urine and plasma glycine levels, normal organic acid pattern and ammonia level. Ratio of CSF:serum glycine necessary to make the diagnosis
Pyridoxine dependency	No specific clinical features; must be suspected in all neonatal seizures without alternative cause and especially in those not responding to simple measures	Therapeutic trial of pyridoxine; high dosage must be given for a period of weeks

Peroxisomal diseases
  Zellweger syndrome
  Adrenoleukodystrophy
  Refsum disease
	Characteristic facies
	Neonatal form
	Infantile form
		Screen with serum very-long-chain fatty acid analysis, specific measurement of phytanic acid, pristanic acid, pipecolic acid, red cell plasmalogens, and bile acids for biochemical diagnosis. Molecular diagnostics using comprehensive gene panels

Infants Pyruvate dehydrogenase deficiency Pyruvate carboxylase deficiency	Metabolic acidosis and increased anion gap, lactic acidosis, with normal lactate-to-pyruvate ratio (10:20); hyperammonemia may be seen; normoglycemic; serum and CSF alanine levels may be elevated Lactate-to-pyruvate ratio is normal or elevated The clinical features are nonspecific: encephalopathy, hypotonia, and seizures; intermittent hyperventilation may be present. Both these disorders can manifest later in childhood with developmental delay and episodic symptoms such as ataxia and vomiting	Serum lactate and pyruvate measurement Serum and CSF amino acids measurement
Biotinidase deficiency	Refractory seizures, rash, alopecia; lactic and organic acidosis	
Phenylketonuria	Onset in infancy with developmental delay and seizures; seizures occur in about 25%, and the infant may have severe epilepsy with West syndrome; deficiency of phenylalanine hydroxylase causes the accumulation of phenylalanine and phenylacetic acid	Nearly 100% identified through newborn screening. Plasma amino acids will identify elevated phenylalanine in affected individuals

TABLE 39.16 Inherited Disorders of Metabolism and Neurodegenerative Diseases Associated with Seizures in Infants—cont'd

Disorder	Clinical Features and Laboratory Findings	Investigations
Infants—cont'd		
Phenylketonuria variant with biopterin deficiency	Hypotonia and seizures develop at or after 6 mo of age; generalized motor seizures, erratic myoclonus, and oculogyric seizures	Nearly 100% identified through newborn screening. Plasma amino acids will identify elevated phenylalanine in affected individuals
Tay-Sachs disease GM$_2$ gangliosidosis	Abnormalities appear in the first weeks to months of life with irritability and acoustic startle or myoclonus, not seizures, in the first months; developmental delay and cherry-red macular spots are present; seizures develop in the second year of life; erratic myoclonus, focal seizures, and slowing of background rhythms on EEG	Blood sample and skin biopsy; hexosaminidase A deficiency detectable in blood lymphocytes and cultured fibroblasts
Sandhoff disease GM$_2$ gangliosidosis type II	Similar in phenotype to Tay-Sachs disease	Hexosaminidase B deficiency detectable in blood lymphocytes and cultured fibroblasts
GM$_1$ gangliosidosis	Dysmorphic features; three clinical subtypes, *infantile* with rapid progression in first 6 mo of life, seizures are frequent without specific characteristics; cherry-red spots on the maculae; *juvenile* or *late-onset* form (6 mo–3 yr); *chronic* form (4–30 yr). Dysmorphic features and skeletal changes similar to Morquio mucopolysaccharide storage disorder	Skin biopsy, blood β-galactosidase deficiency found in blood lymphocytes and cultured fibroblasts
Leigh disease (subacute necrotizing encephalopathy)	A clinical syndrome resulting from various abnormalities of mitochondrial oxidative phosphorylation Usually manifesting in infancy with regression of motor skills, hypotonia, lethargy, respiratory disorders (typically hyperventilation and apnea), and seizures; other features are nuclear and supranuclear oculomotor paralysis, brainstem dysfunction, choreoathetosis, cerebellar ataxia, and pyramidal signs	CSF lactate measurement; MRI of the brain (may show midbrain periaqueductal signal abnormalities) Muscle biopsy for oxidative metabolism analysis and DNA studies
Menkes disease	Sex-linked inheritance on long arm of X chromosome; hypotonia, failure to thrive, abnormal temperature regulation, hypothermia or hyperthermia, fragile wiry hair, poor pigmentation, generalized seizures, often infantile spasms	Deficiency of serum copper and ceruloplasmin
Krabbe disease	Appears before 3–6 mo of age; rigidity develops in an irritable, crying infant; opisthotonic posturing of the neck and trunk; generalized motor seizures may occur, but must be distinguished from tonic spasms; affected children become blind with optic atrophy	Skin biopsy and blood galactocerebrosidase deficiency
Angelman syndrome	Developmental delay from birth, characteristic facies, ataxia with jerky limb movements, inappropriate laughter ("happy puppet"), seizures in 86% of patients	Abnormal methylation of maternally inherited imprinted region of chromosome 15q11.2. Four known genetic mechanisms can cause Angelman syndrome; approximately 70% of cases result from de novo maternal deletions involving chromosome 15q11.2-q13; approximately 2% result from paternal uniparental disomy of 15q11.2-q13; a subset of the remainder result from other imprinting defects and pathogenic variants in the gene encoding the ubiquitin-protein ligase E3A gene (*UBE3A*)
Early infantile type of ceroid-lipofuscinosis Batten disease	Severe myoclonus at 3–18 mo; hypotonia, ataxia, impaired vision, dementia; diffuse cerebellar and cerebral atrophy on EEG; no enzymatic defect identified; diagnosis must be based on clinical features and skin biopsy showing ceroid	Skin biopsy, inclusion bodies on electron microscopy of peripheral lymphocytes (buffy coat EM), rectal biopsy; genetic testing available
Other Rare Metabolic Disorders with Encephalopathy Seizures in Infancy		
Glutaric aciduria type II, multiple acyl-CoA dehydrogenase deficiency Medium-chain acyl–CoA dehydrogenase deficiency Canavan–van Bogaert disease Molybdenum cofactor deficiency		Specific testing based on suspected diagnosis

CoA, coenzyme A; CSF, cerebrospinal fluid; DNPH, dinitrophenylhydrazine; EM, electron microscopy.

TABLE 39.17 Childhood Epileptic Syndromes with Generally Good Prognosis

Syndrome	Comment
Benign neonatal familial convulsions	Dominant, may be severe and resistant during a few days
	Febrile or afebrile seizures (benign) occur later in a minority
Infantile familial convulsions	Dominant, seizures often in clusters (overlap with benign partial complex epilepsy of infancy)
Febrile convulsions plus syndromes	In some families, febrile and afebrile convulsions occur in different members, GEFS+
	The old dichotomy between febrile convulsions or epilepsy does not always hold
Benign myoclonic epilepsy of infancy	Often seizures during sleep, one rare variety with reflex myoclonic seizures (touch, noise)
Partial idiopathic epilepsy with rolandic spikes	Seizures with falling asleep or on awakening; focal sharp waves with centrotemporal location on EEG; genetic
Idiopathic occipital partial epilepsy	Early childhood form with seizures during sleep and ictal vomiting; can occur as status epilepticus
	Later forms with migrainous symptoms; not always benign
Petit mal absence epilepsy	Cases with absences only, some have generalized seizures; 60–80% full remission
	In most cases, absences disappear on therapy but there are resistant cases (unpredictable)
Juvenile myoclonic epilepsy	Adolescence onset, with early morning myoclonic seizures and generalized seizures during sleep; often history of absences in childhood

GEFS+, generalized epilepsy with febrile seizures plus.
Modified from Deonna T. Management of epilepsy. *Arch Dis Child.* 2005;90:5–9; and Seneviratne U. The prognosis of idiopathic generalized epilepsy. *Epilepsia.* 2012;53(12):2079–2090.

structural brain malformations, intraventricular hemorrhage, and hypoxic-ischemic encephalopathy have a higher risk of poor outcome due to the prevalence of global brain injury in these conditions. Fifty percent of neonates with hypoxic-ischemic encephalopathy–related seizures develop normally, but fewer than 10% of neonates with seizures and intraventricular hemorrhage develop normally. In contrast, those infants with seizures caused by hypocalcemia (in the absence of asphyxia), drug withdrawal (from maternal drug use), and focal arterial ischemic stroke usually do well, as these are either caused by reversible, transient, or focal etiologies. The likelihood of recurrent seizures is 15–30% overall.

The EEG may add prognostic information; neonates with a normal background pattern are unlikely to have any neurologic deficits and are less likely to have seizures as a cause for their paroxysmal events, but persistent severe abnormalities of the background rhythms, such as burst-suppression patterns, suppression of background rhythms, and electrocerebral silence, have over 90% chance of a poor outcome, including death. Moderate abnormalities of the EEG in the form of amplitude asymmetries and patterns immature for the patient's conceptional age are associated with intermediate outcomes and are of less value in isolation from other clinical data; these will require long-term neurologic follow-up. Table 39.17 lists neonatal and childhood epileptic disorders with a typically good prognosis.

Treatment

The primary treatment for neonatal seizures is the treatment of the underlying cause. All neonates with seizures should have a trial of pyridoxine and folinic acid treatment if the cause is not identified and seizures persist. Some neonates also require treatment with an AED, traditionally phenobarbital, but levetiracetam and fosphenytoin are also used. Protein binding is lower in neonates than in older children, and the speed of hepatic metabolism changes significantly in the first few days of life, so frequent serum levels of protein-bound, hepatically metabolized AEDs such as phenobarbital or fosphenytoin are necessary for the first several days of treatment, or when making dose adjustments.

At an intravenous loading dose of 18–20 mg/kg, phenobarbital should produce a serum level of approximately 18–20 mg/L. A daily maintenance dose of 3–5 mg/kg, either administered once daily or in two divided doses daily, keeps serum levels in this range. The serum level can be increased to 40–60 mg/L with further loading doses before consideration of a second drug for persistent seizures.

If a self-limited or correctable short-term insult is the cause, the clinician may administer a loading dose with phenobarbital and give no maintenance therapy, simply observing for recurrent seizures. Alternative management would be to administer a loading dose of phenobarbital and give maintenance doses throughout an illness or to treat for a maximum of 3–6 months if the time during which the child is at risk for seizures is uncertain.

Epileptic Syndromes

Benign idiopathic neonatal convulsions, familial and nonfamilial. Some neonatal seizures occur in otherwise healthy neonates without perinatal risk factors or identifiable causes that remit spontaneously and are not followed by developmental delay; these include benign idiopathic neonatal convulsions and benign familial neonatal convulsions. These are diagnoses of exclusion and a complete work-up for other causes of neonatal seizures must be performed before deciding upon these etiologies.

Benign idiopathic neonatal convulsions are common and may account for 2–7% of neonatal seizures. The disorder is sometimes referred to as **fifth-day fits**, although the seizures may begin between 1 and 7 days of age. The seizures are typically focal and multifocal clonic seizures that may, in rare cases, develop into status epilepticus. The seizures remit within hours or days. Although normal at the onset of seizures, affected neonates may become drowsy and hypotonic during the seizures and for a few days after the seizures remit. Long-term follow-up data are not yet complete, but the majority of affected children appear to have normal psychomotor development and no increased risk for the development of epilepsy.

Benign familial neonatal convulsions are less common. There is a distinctive family history of transient neonatal seizures that shows autosomal dominant inheritance. The onset of seizures is usually between 2 and 4 days after birth, but in some cases, onset may occur at 1–3 months of age. The neonates are otherwise healthy without risk factors for seizures. The seizures are usually brief clonic seizures, but some neonates have tonic seizures. This group differs from the nonfamilial cases in that the seizures may persist longer, the interictal EEG is generally nonspecific, and later seizures occur more frequently in approximately 10–15% of children. Abnormalities in two potassium channel genes, *KCNQ2* on chromosome 20 and *KCNQ3* on chromosome 8, have been found in some kindreds (see Table 39.4).

Vitamin-dependent seizures. There are rare metabolic disorders that present in the first few days of life with encephalopathy and refractory seizures; a smaller percentage of these disorders can be treated with early diagnosis and administration of the correct vitamin. Pyridoxine-dependent and folinic acid–dependent seizures are two such disorders; pyridoxine is essential for amino acid metabolism, and folinic acid is necessary for DNA synthesis and repair. Multidisciplinary care with a geneticist and a neurologist is ideal for children with these rare disorders.

Pyridoxine-dependent seizure is a rare autosomal recessive disorder in which seizures usually appear within the first 3 months of life, often within hours of birth, but in rare cases, as late as 2–5 years of age. The EEG may show focal, multifocal, and generalized epileptiform activity, and the child is encephalopathic. The seizures (myoclonic, GTC, and partial) and EEG discharges disappear over hours in response to 100 mg of intravenous pyridoxine (vitamin B_6), which can be repeated 3–5 times as necessary. The children require long-term pyridoxine, 50–100 mg/day.

Folinic acid–responsive seizures present very similarly to pyridoxine-dependent seizures, with medically intractable, relentless seizures of multiple types, often within the first days of life. The seizures respond to 2.5–5 mg of folinic acid twice daily.

These are rare disorders, but as they are neurologically devastating or fatal if untreated, it is reasonable to administer a trial dose of pyridoxine and/or folinic acid to seizing, encephalopathic infants where no other cause has been found for their seizures and encephalopathy. If there is a clinical, and ideally electrographic, response to the vitamin trial, then it is also reasonable to continue the supplement. Nonetheless, even with early diagnosis and treatment, these children may have developmental delays.

Biotin-responsive basal ganglia disease is a subacute encephalopathy syndrome manifest with episodes of dystonia, confusion, seizures, and coma that responds to acute and chronic biotin and thiamine therapy. *SLC19A3* is the responsible gene.

Structural focal epilepsy. **Malformations of cortical development**. Disorders of cell migration within the CNS may result in profound anatomic abnormalities and dysfunction or a spectrum of lesser abnormalities, ranging from focal areas of cortical dysgenesis or dysplasia and clinical deficits to subcortical collections of neurons (heterotopia) seen only under the microscope. Migrational abnormalities are rare but are commonly associated with seizures. Although these abnormalities are present from birth, seizures may develop at any age.

Lissencephaly, or agyria, is a profound abnormality characterized by a smooth brain without development of the normal gyral pattern and sulci; there are often large heterotopias in the white matter, and neuroimaging studies may reveal the appearance of a double cortex.

Hemimegalencephaly is characterized by gross enlargement of one hemisphere with no normal cortical development within that hemisphere. More restricted abnormalities may occur in the form of a limited area of gyral enlargement and distortion called pachygyria.

Schizencephaly refers to unilateral or bilateral clefts in the cerebral hemispheres, usually with abnormal arrangement (polymicrogyria) of the cortical gray matter lining the clefts.

Porencephaly refers to fluid-filled cavities within the brain. Porencephalic cysts communicate with both the subarachnoid space and the ventricular system and are lined not by cortical gray matter but rather by white matter because they result from loss of tissue as a consequence of insults, typically infarction or hemorrhage, during development.

Early-onset generalized epileptic syndromes with encephalopathy. **Early myoclonic encephalopathy** appears in neonates before 2–3 months of age, usually within the first 2 weeks of life. Myoclonus appears at the onset but may be fragmentary. Partial motor seizures, massive myoclonus, or infantile spasms may also occur. The EEG shows a suppression-burst pattern that may later evolve into a hypsarrhythmic pattern. There is a failure or arrest of psychomotor development and a high rate of mortality before 12 months of age. A number of patients have an inborn error of metabolism, including nonketotic hyperglycinemia, D-glyceric acidemia, propionic acidemia, and methylmalonic acidemia; some have a pathologic genetic variant (Table 39.18).

Early epileptic encephalopathy with suppression-burst EEG pattern (Ohtahara syndrome) has an onset during the same period. The affected child experiences intractable tonic seizures or epileptic spasms, and the EEG shows a suppression-burst pattern. Affected children have a severe encephalopathy, and the prognosis for remission from seizures or for normal development is very poor. Many of these patients have pathologic gene variants or malformations of cortical development (see Table 39.18).

There appear to be neonates in whom the EEG features and clinical course of these two syndromes overlap; these syndromes may evolve into West syndrome and Lennox-Gastaut syndrome.

TABLE 39.18 Genetic Variants Associated with Epileptic Encephalopathies

Variant Site	Ohtahara Syndrome	EME	West Syndrome	SMEI	Atypical RTT with Early Epilepsy	EFMR
ARX	Yes		Yes			
CDKL5			Yes		Yes	
ErbB4		Yes				
MAGI2			Yes			
PCDH19				Yes		Yes
PNKP	Yes		Yes			
SCN1A				Yes		
SLC25 A22	Yes					
STXBP1	Yes		Yes			

Only epileptic encephalopathy syndromes presenting during infancy are included. Some variants may also be associated with other conditions; for example, the *SCN1A* variant is associated with generalized epilepsy with febrile seizures.

EFMR, epilepsy and cognitive impairment limited to females; EME, early myoclonic encephalopathy; RTT, Rett syndrome; SMEI, severe myoclonic epilepsy of infancy (also known as Dravet syndrome).

From Beal JC, Cherian K, Moshe SL. Early-onset epileptic encephalopathies: Ohtahara syndrome and early myoclonic encephalopathy. *Pediatr Neurol.* 2012;47:317–323 (Table 2, p. 321).

Infancy

The paroxysmal disorders of infancy (8 weeks to 2 years) are shown in Tables 39.4 and Table 39.19.

Paroxysmal Nonepileptic Disorders

Infantile syncope

Cyanotic infant syncope (breath-holding spells). Cyanotic infant syncope consists of episodes of loss of consciousness followed by tonic stiffening in crying infants. The peak incidence is between 6 and 18

TABLE 39.19 **Paroxysmal Disorders in Infants**

Nonepileptiform Disorders

Infantile syncope*
Cyanotic breath-holding spells
Pallid syncope
Shivering attacks
Paroxysmal torticollis
Extrapyramidal drug reactions, dystonia
Gastroesophageal reflux with dystonia†
Rumination†
Stereotypical movements, autism, Rett syndrome, coexisting deafness and blindness†
Withholding, constipation†
Masturbation
Spasmus nutans
Opsoclonus
Benign paroxysmal vertigo
Myoclonus
Nonepileptic; anxiety, excitement, acute metabolic encephalopathy
Benign myoclonus of early infancy
Hyperexplexia†
Alternating hemiplegia of childhood
Sleep disorders*
Jactatio capitis, head banging

Acute Symptomatic Seizures, Occasional Seizures

Febrile convulsions*
Meningitis, encephalitis*
Head injury, child abuse
Poisoning
Intercurrent medical illness, renal and liver disease, cardiac left-to-right shunt, and embolism
Metabolic disease, rickets

Epileptic Syndromes

Symptomatic focal epilepsy†
West syndrome
Early myoclonic encephalopathy‡
Early infantile encephalopathic epilepsy‡
Malformations of cortical development‡
Neurocutaneous disorders (see Table 39.11)
    Tuberous sclerosis
    Sturge-Weber syndrome
    Incontinentia pigmenti
    Epidermal nevus syndrome
Severe myoclonic epilepsy in infancy (Dravet syndrome and its mimics)

---

*Common.
†See childhood section for discussion.
‡See neonatal section for discussion.

---

months of age, but it may occur in neonates or in children as old as 6 years of age. The typical clinical picture is an infant who is frightened, frustrated, or surprised; begins to cry vigorously; and then becomes apneic and cyanotic before becoming unconscious, stiff, or limp. In rare cases, typical infant syncope may evolve into a brief GTC seizure. The child regains consciousness rapidly after being positioned horizontally or stimulated without a prolonged postictal state, although there may be a tendency to sleep.

These episodes have also been called breath-holding spells, anoxic seizures, and convulsive syncope, but *cyanotic infant syncope* may be a better term because the loss of consciousness appears to be the result of transient impairment of cerebral perfusion. The subsequent tonic posturing in the typical attack is not epileptic but is thought to have the same brainstem origin as decerebrate or decorticate posturing.

Cyanotic infant syncope is common and is seen in 4.6% of a large cohort of children monitored from birth. A thorough history is usually sufficient for diagnosing this condition. The crucial diagnostic point is the history of an external event precipitating the episode. The differential diagnosis is noted in Table 39.20.

Although the spells appear to be unpleasant for the child and can be frightening to the parents, they do not result in neurologic sequelae and do not necessitate intensive investigation. The child should be evaluated for anemia; treatment of iron-deficiency anemia reduces the frequency of syncopal events. Treatment with carbamazepine, phenytoin, or valproate may decrease the frequency or severity of postsyncopal convulsions in the rare child with epileptic seizures triggered by the anoxic event. Children with known brainstem or posterior fossa malformations may also be at higher risk of prolonged syncope and clinically significant anoxia due to their abnormal respiratory drive, and these children may benefit from treatment.

Pallid infant syncope. Pallid infant syncope occurs in response to transient cardiac asystole in children with a hypersensitive cardioinhibitory reflex. This form is much less common than cyanotic syncope but more alarming. There is minimal crying, perhaps only a gasp, and no obvious apnea before the loss of consciousness. Again, there is a precipitating event; the child appears to lose consciousness after minimal injury or fright, collapses limply, and then may have posturing and clonic movements before regaining consciousness (see Table 39.20).

Pallid infant syncope, if frequent and troublesome or if followed by prolonged GTC convulsions, can be treated with atropine, which blocks the vagus nerve–mediated asystole. Most affected children require no medical treatment.

Hyperekplexia. A startle response is normally seen in children and adults in response to sudden, unexpected stimuli. There are two phases to a startle response: the initial startle followed by an orienting response to locate the stimulus. **Hyperekplexia** is characterized by an excessive startle response interfering with daily living, usually causing patients to fall stiffly with preserved consciousness (see Chapter 40). This disorder may present as early as infancy with hypertonia and dramatic startle responses that do not habituate or extinguish with repeated stimuli (meaning they continue to startle, no matter how many times a stimulus is given in a short period of time). The excessive startle and hypertonia (stiffness) can lead to genuinely life-threatening apneas and breath-holding spells when startled or upset. Generalized seizures have been reported in some cases; intellectual disability and delayed motor development occur in patients with complex neurodevelopmental disorders. The background EEG is usually normal. There may be some improvement with benzodiazepines or valproic acid.

Pathogenic variants in glycine receptors and transporter genes have been identified to be causally associated with the phenotype. The specific genes *GLRA1*, *GLRB*, *SLC6A5*, and *ATAD1* have been found in

TABLE 39.20   Differential Diagnosis of Infantile Syncope

Clinical	Cyanotic Infantile Syncope	Pallid Syncope	Tonic-Clonic Seizures	Infantile Spasms
Age range	1–6 yr; peak, 6–18 mo	1–6 yr	All ages	4–12 mo
Precipitating factors	Present (e.g., minor trauma, frustration, fright)	Present (e.g., minor trauma, frustration, fright)	Usually none	None
Occurrence in sleep	Never	Never	Common	At transition from awake to sleep and sleep to awake
Sequence of events	Crying → exhale; apnea → cyanosis, loss of consciousness; opisthotonos → relaxation, resumption of breathing	Upset, usually not crying → sudden pallor → limp fall with fainting → tonic posture, or clonic jerks may occur	Sudden loss of consciousness → increased tone, followed by synchronous jerking of body and limbs → unconsciousness; duration, 1–2 min	Sudden sustained flexion or extension of proximal limbs and trunk; duration, 2–20 sec; seizures usually occur multiple times daily
Postictal symptoms	Usually minimal; infant may be lethargic and irritable	Usually minimal; quick return to normal	Usually marked; unconsciousness initially, then confusion and lethargy	Rapid return to preictal state
Interictal EEG	Normal	Normal	Frequently abnormal with epileptiform discharges	Abnormal background and epileptiform discharges
Ictal EEG	Reflects global cerebral hypoxia, diffuse rhythmic slowing → suppression → slowing with return of consciousness	Reflects global cerebral hypoxia; diffuse, rhythmic slowing → suppression → slowing with return of consciousness	EEG seizure patterns; postictal diffuse suppression, then slowing	High-amplitude slow transient waves → diffuse suppression
Pathophysiology	Respiratory arrest without asystole	Vagal bradycardia or temporary asystole	Primary CNS event	Primary CNS event, age-related epileptic seizure

CNS, central nervous system.

families with an autosomal dominant or recessive inheritance pattern. Glycine is a co-agonist for the *N*-methyl-D-aspartate (NMDA) receptor, which is an excitatory receptor critical for learning and neuronal plasticity. Pontine lesions may be seen in some patients.

Sleep disorders. Also referred to as head banging or rocking, jactatio capitis nocturna consists of rhythmic to-and-fro movements of the head or rocking of the body. It occurs typically at the transition from wakefulness to sleep, early in the evening, or after arousal during the night. This behavior is quite common, occurring in up to 15% of children; it begins in infancy or early childhood but may persist up to 10 years of age. The child is not awake during the episode and does not remember the events, which usually last <15 minutes. In most cases, it is sufficient to ensure that the bed area is padded to prevent injury.

Shivering attacks. Shivering or shuddering attacks are brief episodes characterized by sudden flexion of the head and trunk associated with a rapid tremulous contraction of the musculature. The appearance is similar to that of a sudden brief shudder experienced normally when exposed to cold. In this condition, the shuddering occurs repeatedly. Some infants experience more than 100 brief shudders per day. There may be clustering, with intervals of several weeks free of the episodes. The child may assume a characteristic posture with flexion of the head, trunk, and elbows and adduction of the elbows and knees.

The attacks have been described in children between the ages of 4 months and 10 years, although most often the onset seems to occur in infancy and early childhood. The phenomenon is nonepileptic and benign, eventually disappearing. Some children and their relatives have been reported to have an essential tremor. The shuddering is faster and of lower amplitude than myoclonus and is paroxysmal, not sustained, as occurs with a tremor. An important epileptic disorder that must be ruled out is infantile spasms.

Paroxysmal torticollis. Torticollis is an abnormal posturing of the head and neck, with the head flexed toward the shoulder and the neck rotated with the chin turned toward the opposite shoulder. The posturing is paroxysmal, although variable in duration, lasting minutes or days, and there is no loss of consciousness. Some children have associated pallor, agitation, and vomiting, and the disorder has been suspected to result from labyrinthine dysfunction, like benign paroxysmal vertigo of childhood. The disorder is self-limited and remits in early childhood. There is an association with migraine in patients later in life and among their relatives.

In older children, torticollis may occur as a **focal dystonia** persisting to adulthood. Familial cases have been described, and in some, the torticollis may be the earliest manifestation of a more generalized dystonia (see Chapter 40).

Sustained abnormal posturing should prompt appropriate radiologic investigations to exclude inflammatory or neoplastic disorders of the upper cervical spinal cord, posterior fossa, cervical spine, or soft tissues of the neck (particularly a retropharyngeal abscess). In very rare cases, gastroesophageal reflux manifests with dystonic posturing of the neck and upper trunk. Adverse extrapyramidal reactions to phenothiazines and related drugs may produce dystonic posturing of the neck and trunk.

The pharmacologic treatment for torticollis includes a number of different medication classes, including anticholinergics (trihexyphenidyl), dopamine agonists (pramipexole), nonsteroidal antiinflammatory drugs (NSAIDs), baclofen, benzodiazepines (clonazepam), and β blockers (propranolol). Botox injections may be used for more refractory cases. Physical therapy can also be very helpful. The most severe cases can be evaluated for surgical intervention, such as selective denervation or sternocleidomastoid release.

Infantile masturbation. Episodes of genital self-stimulation may occur in young children. Toddlers may assume stereotyped posturing with tightening of the thighs or applied pressure to the suprapubic or pubic area not associated with manual stimulation of the vulva or rhythmic movements. The episodes vary in duration from minutes to hours and are often accompanied by irregular breathing, facial flushing, and diaphoresis, and the child may be irritated and cry if interrupted. A thorough history or a video of the episodes may be sufficient to make this diagnosis.

Spasmus nutans. Spasmus nutans is a rare disorder usually of unknown origin characterized by nystagmoid eye movements, head nodding, and torticollis. Head nodding may develop before the nystagmus and can be horizontal, vertical, or mixed. Both the head movements and the nystagmus may be paroxysmal, allowing confusion with seizures. There is no loss of consciousness during an episode. Small-amplitude rapid eye movements are typical; they tend to be asymmetric between the eyes and may even be monocular. The eye movements vary in prominence with different directions of gaze.

This is usually a self-limited disorder with onset between 4 and 18 months of age and not persisting after age 3 years, although nystagmus alone may persist in some children. Investigations should include imaging of the brain with special focus on the optic nerves, optic chiasma, and brainstem, because some cases have been associated with CNS tumors.

Benign paroxysmal vertigo. Benign paroxysmal vertigo may be confused with seizures because attacks develop suddenly, are accompanied by ataxia, and may cause the infant or young child to fall. There is pallor, distress, and assumption of a motionless, often supine, position, but no loss of consciousness; older children can recall the event. There may be vomiting with associated nystagmus. Attacks last seconds to minutes and vary in frequency, sometimes occurring daily. Older children can identify symptoms of nausea and vertigo and are less likely to be thought to be experiencing seizures. The children are normal between attacks. The condition is closely related to **migraine**, with many shared symptoms and the later development of more typical migrainous headache (see Chapter 34).

Benign myoclonus of early infancy. This uncommon syndrome may resemble the cryptogenic form of infantile spasms at onset, with bilateral myoclonic jerks developing in a previously normal infant. However, this is a benign, probably nonepileptic condition occurring in infants 3–8 months of age and disappearing after a period of weeks or months. The pattern of myoclonus may differentiate it from infantile spasms, including predominant involvement of the head, neck, and upper limbs with adversive head movements or tremors without involving the lower limbs. The EEG is normal. Myoclonic movements are not accompanied by an EEG seizure pattern. These abnormal movements may necessitate monitoring to establish a nonepileptic diagnosis. There is no arrest of normal development or regression as is seen in West syndrome. Most important, the myoclonus remits, not persisting after 2 years of age, and there is increased risk for other seizure patterns after its cessation.

Alternating hemiplegia of childhood. Alternating hemiplegia of childhood is a rare syndrome of episodic hemiplegia that usually manifests in infancy with the following diagnostic criteria:
1. Onset before age 18 months, often before age 6 months
2. Recurrent episodes of fluctuating hemiparesis or hemiplegia affecting both sides of the body and disappearing during sleep
3. Other paroxysmal phenomena: tonic seizures, dystonic posturing, choreoathetosis, nystagmus, and other paroxysmal oculomotor disturbances; and autonomic dysfunction, occurring during or between hemiplegic episodes
4. Progressive cognitive and neurologic deficits

The pathophysiologic mechanism remains unknown, although there are reports of mitochondrial dysfunction in some cases and an autosomal dominant pattern of inheritance in others (see Chapter 37). The differential diagnosis includes paroxysmal choreoathetosis and dystonia syndromes, familial hemiplegic migraine, transient ischemic attacks associated with cerebral vascular abnormalities such as moyamoya disease or cardiac emboli, mitochondrial disorders, hyperviscosity, sickle cell anemia crises, inherited disorders of metabolism (pyruvate dehydrogenase deficiency and Leigh disease), and epileptic seizures with postictal paralysis. Symptomatic treatment is available with calcium channel blockers; flunarizine is the one commonly cited in the literature but is not available in the United States or Japan. An alternative calcium channel blocker would be nimodipine.

There have been case reports of a similar-appearing disorder with nocturnal paroxysmal events of flaccid hemiplegia lasting up to several hours at a time. The key differentiating factors are that these children are essentially normal prior to diagnosis, the events occur during sleep, and the children appear to outgrow these spells by midchildhood without significant long-term neurologic sequelae. This is known as **benign nocturnal alternating hemiplegia of childhood.** No consistent gene variants have been associated with this disorder, and there is no consistent response to antiepileptics or calcium channel blockers.

Acute Symptomatic Seizures and Occasional Seizures

Febrile convulsions. Febrile convulsions are common and are defined as seizures occurring between the ages of 6 months and 5 years in association with a fever in the absence of intracranial infection. Patients with a history of previous afebrile seizures are not included in the affected population. The temperature elevation is variable. The highest incidence of febrile convulsions occurs between 1 and 2 years of age, and 85% of febrile convulsions occur before the age of 4 years. The incidence is between 2% and 5%; it is slightly more common in males.

The seizures are usually brief with generalized clonic or tonic-clonic motor involvement without any postictal paralysis or a prolonged postictal state of confusion or drowsiness. The seizures generally occur well within the first 24 hours of a febrile illness, not necessarily when the fever is highest; they may be the first indication of illness. **Complex febrile convulsions** are defined as those lasting longer than 15 minutes, recurring during a single febrile illness, having unilateral or focal features, or followed by postictal paralysis. Seizures occurring late in a febrile illness should raise suspicions of encephalitis, brain abscess, or meningitis. Febrile delirium and even rigors may be mistaken for seizure activity.

The initial investigation must include a search for the cause of the febrile illness. For this diagnosis, it is essential that primary CNS infection be ruled out as the cause of both the fever and the seizures. A lumbar puncture is recommended in children younger than 12 months of age if there is any suspicion of intracranial infection, and when features of the seizure or postictal state suggest a focal or lateralized seizure. Herpes simplex encephalitis in particular should be considered in children presenting with evidence of encephalitis and focal seizures. CT, MRI, and EEG may be part of the work-up if an underlying CNS infection is suspected or a neurologic deficit has been revealed by the history or examination.

However, if the history is consistent with a febrile seizure, the child is in the appropriate age range and is developmentally normal, a fever has been documented, and an obvious source of infection has been found, extensive investigations are unnecessary. Many clinicians would not perform a lumbar puncture or obtain an EEG in an otherwise healthy child with an uncomplicated febrile seizure over the age of 2 years who has an obvious source of infection such as otitis media or a urinary tract infection.

Treatment of a child still in convulsion on arrival at the hospital should include prompt attention to protection of the airway and circulation. Giving acetaminophen rectally should lower the fever. Nasal or rectal diazepam or intravenous lorazepam should be administered if the child has been seizing for more than 10 minutes. Some children may require hospital admission. The family should be advised that future fevers with temperatures above 38°C (100.4°F) may be treated with regular acetaminophen or ibuprofen to make the child more comfortable; however, this does not guarantee that future febrile convulsions will be prevented, even if the parents respond to the first elevated temperature.

There is no increased rate of mortality from true febrile convulsions, and the cognitive and neurologic development can be expected to be normal after a simple febrile convulsion. However, approximately 30% of febrile convulsions recur in future febrile illness, and the parents should be warned of this. Recurrence is most likely in the first 6–12 months after the initial febrile convulsion. Other factors that increase the chance of recurrence are onset at a young age, pre-existing neurologic abnormalities, and family history of epilepsy or febrile convulsions.

Most authorities would advise no treatment for almost all children with febrile convulsions. Rare exceptions include children presenting with prolonged (>15 minutes) seizures and children younger than 12 months old with multiple recurrences. For children with recurrent prolonged febrile seizures, rectal diazepam could be considered as an abortive therapy. Children with recurrent episodes of **febrile status epilepticus**, particularly starting under 1 year of age, with focal features, or associated with any insidious neurologic or cognitive decline, should be referred to a neurologist for further evaluation, particularly for sodium channelopathies such as **Dravet syndrome** or **generalized epilepsy with febrile seizures plus (GEFS+)** (Tables 39.4 and 39.21). Informing and reassuring parents of the benign nature and usual course of febrile convulsions are very important and may be of greater value than any medication.

There appears to be an increased risk of epilepsy among children with febrile convulsions. Overall, the risk is approximately 3%. Risk factors increasing the likelihood of future epilepsy include existence of a prior neurologic abnormality, prolonged convulsions (>30 minutes), focal or lateralized features of the seizure, and repeated convulsions within 24 hours. The incidence of epilepsy increases from 3% of those without risk factors to 49% of those with three risk factors. Risk factors for epilepsy with generalized seizures are more than three febrile seizures and epilepsy in a first-degree relative, which suggests that febrile convulsions in these individuals may be a manifestation of an increased predisposition to epilepsy. For epilepsy with focal seizures, the risk factors are prolonged convulsions, focal features of the seizure, and repeated seizures within 24 hours, which suggest either a causative role of febrile convulsions in partial epilepsy or a pre-existing brain lesion. The number of recurrences of febrile seizures has not been shown to be a risk factor for later epilepsy. There is no evidence that AED treatment of febrile seizures affects the risk for later development of afebrile seizures.

Epileptic Syndromes

West syndrome.
- Peak presentation: ages 4–8 months.
- **Red flags**: daily clusters of brief hiccupping or startle-type seizures, particularly upon waking up or falling asleep. Developmental regression.

TABLE 39.21 **Paroxysmal Disorders of Childhood**
Nonepileptiform Disorders
Breath-holding spells*,†
Syncope‡
Migraine and migraine equivalents, recurrent abdominal pain, cyclic vomiting*
Tic*
Spasmodic torticollis†
Drug reactions, dystonia
Paroxysmal choreoathetosis
Gastroesophageal reflux
Benign paroxysmal vertigo†
Myoclonus, nonepileptic; anxiety, excitement, acute metabolic encephalopathy†
Hyperexplexia
Masturbation†
Withholding, constipation*
Daydreaming, staring spells*
Stereotypical movements, autism, coexistent deafness and blindness
Factitious syndrome by proxy (Munchausen syndrome by proxy)
Hyperventilation‡
Psychogenic seizures‡
Transient global amnesia‡
Sleep*
Head banging, jactatio capitis†
Pavor nocturnus
Somnambulism, somniloquy
Acute Symptomatic Seizures, Occasional Seizures
Febrile convulsions*
Brain tumor
Meningitis, encephalitis
Head injury, child abuse
Poisoning
Intercurrent medical illness; renal, liver disease; cardiac right-to-left shunt; and embolism
Metabolic disease, rickets
Epileptic Syndromes
Benign partial epilepsies*
Symptomatic focal epilepsy*
Epilepsia partialis continua
Rasmussen encephalitis
Autosomal dominant nocturnal frontal lobe epilepsy
Epileptic encephalopathy with continuous spike-and-wave pattern during sleep
Benign epilepsy with centrotemporal spikes (benign rolandic epilepsy)
Hemiconvulsion hemiplegia syndrome
Childhood absence epilepsy*
Epilepsy with myoclonic absences
Lennox-Gastaut syndrome
Epilepsy with myoclonic atonia (previously astatic) seizures (Doose syndrome)
Landau-Kleffner syndrome
Febrile seizures plus
Panayiotopoulos syndrome

*Common.
†See infant section for discussion.
‡See adolescent section for discussion.

- Acuity: emergent to urgent; ideally obtain an EEG within a week and call a neurologist if this diagnosis is suspected. Must be managed by a neurologist due to atypical treatment needs (adrenocorticotropic hormone [ACTH]), which may require hospital admission.
- Prognosis: generally poor, particularly if the diagnosis is missed.

West syndrome, or severe encephalopathic epilepsy in infants, is characterized by infantile spasms, the hypsarrhythmic EEG pattern, and developmental delay. It is a severe and devastating form of epilepsy, usually with evidence of diffuse cerebral dysfunction and a poor prognosis in most cases. The incidence is about 1/4,000–6,000 infants with onset between 3 and 12 months of age; peak onset is 4–8 months.

A spasm is a brief bilateral tonic contraction of the muscles of the trunk, neck, and limbs, usually but not always symmetric. These seizures are commonly overlooked by both families and physicians for weeks to months; they can be confused for hiccupping, startling, or the Moro reflex, or be subtle enough to be missed entirely. They classically occur in multiple daily clusters lasting 10–15 minutes, with each cluster containing anywhere from a few spasms to dozens. The clusters occur during the transitions between wakefulness and sleep, so are most common in the early morning and evening, or occasionally around naptimes.

The extent of muscle involvement varies from a powerful contraction that *jackknifes* the body to minimal contraction of truncal muscles that causes only stiffening. Spasms may involve truncal flexion, extension, or both; the child may fling out their arms or elevate them for several seconds. Eye movements are commonly associated with the spasm, either as deviation or as repetitive nystagmoid upward jerks. Apnea is common, but tachypnea is uncommon. Children may cry out or seem to giggle at the end of the spasm.

As the spasms continue, there may be insidious loss of developmental motor milestones such as sitting, rolling, babbling, or head control. Another commonly described regression is a decline in visual attentiveness, meaning that the child no longer easily regards faces, tracks moving objects, or reaches for toys. This is due to the progressive cortical dysfunction caused by the underlying hypsarrhythmic EEG pattern.

The differential diagnosis can include colic, exaggerated Moro reflexes, or normal myoclonic jerks on falling asleep or waking. Multiple myoclonic seizure syndromes, both benign and otherwise, occur in this age group and must be distinguished from infantile spasms by a neurologist.

Evaluation: EEG, MRI. The term **hypsarrhythmia** in an EEG report is specific for a diagnosis of infantile spasms. The hypsarrhythmic EEG pattern is a high-amplitude, chaotic slowing of generalized distribution without interhemispheric synchronization and with multifocal epileptiform discharges throughout. Hypsarrhythmia is more frequent in younger infants and early in the course of the disorder, and it is more common to find some modified variant of it. In a child with a strong clinical suspicion of infantile spasms, sleep must be captured in the EEG, as early in the course, the hypsarrhythmic pattern is only evident during sleep.

Investigation of patients with infantile spasms is directed at determining the cause and then determining whether there is an underlying genetic, structural, or metabolic etiology. Infantile spasms can be caused by a wide variety of neurologic pathology; the most common etiologic factor is perinatal hypoxic-ischemic encephalopathy. Other important associations include intrauterine infection, prematurity, intracranial hemorrhage, malformations of cortical development, tuberous sclerosis, head injury, CNS infection, and inborn errors of metabolism. If infantile spasms are seen in conjunction with agenesis of the corpus callosum and retinal abnormalities on eye examination, this suggests a diagnosis of **Aicardi syndrome**. Genes associated with West syndrome are noted in Table 39.18.

Approximately 95% of children with an identified cause (structural, genetic, or metabolic) have a prognosis of moderate to severe neurologic injury, including refractory epilepsy, cognitive impairment, or permanent developmental sequelae.

Approximately 10–15% of patients have no identifiable underlying cause *and* a history of normal development before the onset of their illness; this subset is referred to as cryptogenic, or idiopathic, West syndrome. This subset of patients is likely to have a much better long-term outcome: 38% of these patients are normal or mildly impaired, in comparison with only 5% of symptomatic patients.

A unique subset of patients who may develop infantile spasms is children with **trisomy 21 (Down syndrome)**. The incidence of infantile spasms in this group is 1–5%. Though they have a genetic disorder and baseline neurologic abnormalities, these children have a particularly high response rate to treatment with ACTH with rapid resolution of the abnormal hypsarrhythmia on EEG.

About 50% of all infants with West syndrome go on to have other seizure types when spasms cease. Persistence of the epilepsy in most of the patients is associated with loss of the spasms and development of other seizure types, such as tonic seizures, focal seizures, and tonic-clonic seizures. Approximately half of children with Lennox-Gastaut syndrome, a combination of cognitive disability, generalized seizures, and a distinctive abnormal EEG pattern, have a history of infantile spasms. Seizures very similar in appearance to infantile spasms (brief myoclonic or tonic seizures occurring in clusters) may recur later in childhood, and these are referred to as epileptic spasms.

Treatment with corticosteroids aborts the spasms in a significant number of infants. There are two approaches: intramuscular injections of synthetic ACTH gel or high-dose oral steroids. Both treatment regimens generally last 8–12 weeks, and both require frequent monitoring for side effects. The spasms should cease, and the EEG patterns improve if the child has responded. The pediatrician may be called upon to monitor electrolytes, blood pressures, or signs of illness while the child is under treatment. Live vaccinations are generally held for 6–12 months after a course of immunomodulatory therapy.

Vigabatrin is another effective AED for infantile spasms, and it has been shown to be particularly effective in the treatment of infantile spasms with tuberous sclerosis or other focal cortical dysplasias. However, this medication is currently strictly regulated in its prescription, and patients on vigabatrin require examinations by an ophthalmologist every 3 months due to the small risk of permanent peripheral vision loss with prolonged use of the medication. Most patients with infantile spasms take vigabatrin for 6 months or less.

Many other antiepileptic medications, including topiramate, lamotrigine, valproic acid, cannabidiols, and benzodiazepines, have had some efficacy in isolated cases, but this response is unpredictable. ACTH, corticosteroids, and vigabatrin are the commonly used medications with the highest efficacy across multiple etiologies.

Severe myoclonic epilepsy in infancy (Dravet syndrome).

- Peak presentation: ages 9–18 months
- **Red flags**: normal development until the onset of multiple episodes of prolonged febrile status epilepticus, often with focal features; seizures provoked by warm ambient temperatures, hot baths, fever, or vaccinations
- Acuity: urgent due to the development of medically refractory epilepsy and potential for multiple episodes of status epilepticus
- Prognosis: poor; identified cause of some cases of so-called vaccine encephalopathy

Severe myoclonic epilepsy in infancy is a rare, generalized epilepsy appearing in the first year of life. The syndrome differs from the myoclonic syndromes already described (early myoclonic encephalopathy and early infantile encephalopathic epilepsy) by its later onset and the EEG findings. Pathogenic variants in the voltage-gated sodium channel gene *SCN1A* and other genes are seen frequently in these cases (see Table 39.4, Fig. 39.7). Although *SCN1A* variants are highly associated with the Dravet phenotype, some patients with these variants do not

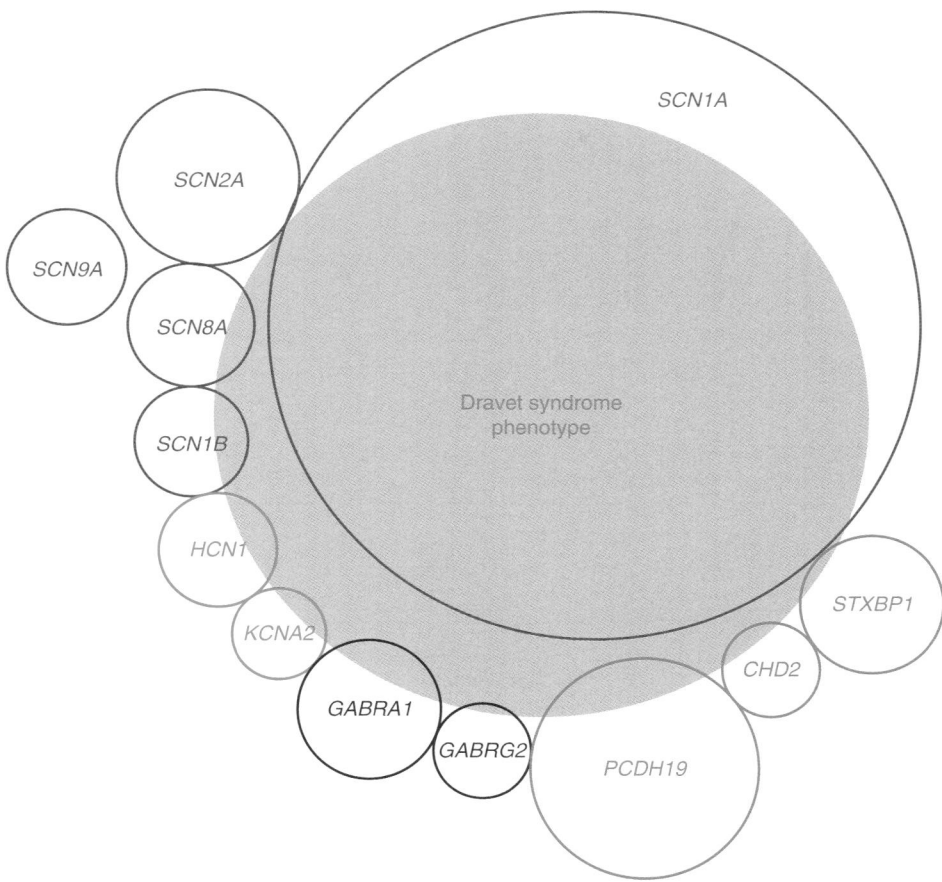

Fig. 39.7 Genes associated with a Dravet syndrome phenotype. *Red*, sodium channels; *green*, potassium channels; *purple*, chloride channels; *blue*, nonchannels. (From Steel D, Symonds JD, Zuberi SM, et al. Dravet syndrome and its mimics: beyond *SCN1A. Epilepsia.* 2017;58[11]:1807–1816 [Fig. 1, p. 1812].)

fit the full diagnostic criteria for Dravet syndrome: some manifest as genetic epilepsy with febrile seizures plus (GEFS+). In addition, multiple other genes overlap with the Dravet phenotype (see Fig. 39.7).

The child may initially present with febrile or afebrile seizures, usually with normal prior psychomotor development preceding the onset of seizures, and often with a family history of epilepsy. The seizures are generalized or unilateral clonic seizures; myoclonic seizures appear later (and may not be a major feature of the disorder, despite the name), between 8 months and 4 years of age; and focal seizures and atypical absences may occur. The interictal EEG may be normal initially and only later show fast, generalized, spike-and-wave epileptiform discharges and focal abnormalities.

The seizures are usually refractory to many commonly used AEDs due to the fact that these AEDs act on sodium channels and this disorder is generally caused by sodium channel mutations. Antiepileptic medications that may worsen seizures or be ineffective in Dravet syndrome include phenytoin, lamotrigine, carbamazepine, oxcarbazepine, and vigabatrin. The natural history, disease progression, and age-related manifestations are noted in Figure 39.8.

Childhood

The paroxysmal disorders of childhood (2–12 years) are given in Table 39.21.

Paroxysmal Nonepileptic Disorders

Migraine and migraine equivalents. Migraine is a common disorder, and some episodes may be confused with seizures because of their paroxysmal nature and association with neurologic deficits or altered consciousness (see Chapter 34). The presentation of migraines in children may also be markedly different than that in adolescents and adults; "migraine equivalents" are paroxysmal disorders that are strongly associated with the later development of migraines and may share similar underlying pathophysiologic mechanisms.

When evaluating paroxysmal events suspected to be migraines or migraine equivalents, the following **red flags** should prompt expedited neuroimaging, specialist evaluation, or emergency room evaluation, depending upon the severity of the symptom and how ill the child appears:
- Sudden severe head pain that awakens the child from sleep
- Positional symptoms, meaning that the child's headache or vomiting dramatically worsens or improves with simple positional changes from lying to sitting
- Abnormal eye movements, such as prominent nystagmus (jerky eye movements) or a forced downward gaze
- Focal neurologic symptoms including focal limb weakness or facial droop
- Altered mental status

In **cyclic vomiting**, recurrent attacks of nausea, vomiting, and abdominal pain occur on a daily or weekly basis without any evidence of intercurrent illness or objective evidence of gastrointestinal pathology. There is no confusion or disorientation associated with these spells. Typically, there are symptom-free intervals lasting weeks to months, and recurrence is unpredictable. There may be a strong family history of migraine, and there appears to be some overlap of the cyclic vomiting with migraine.

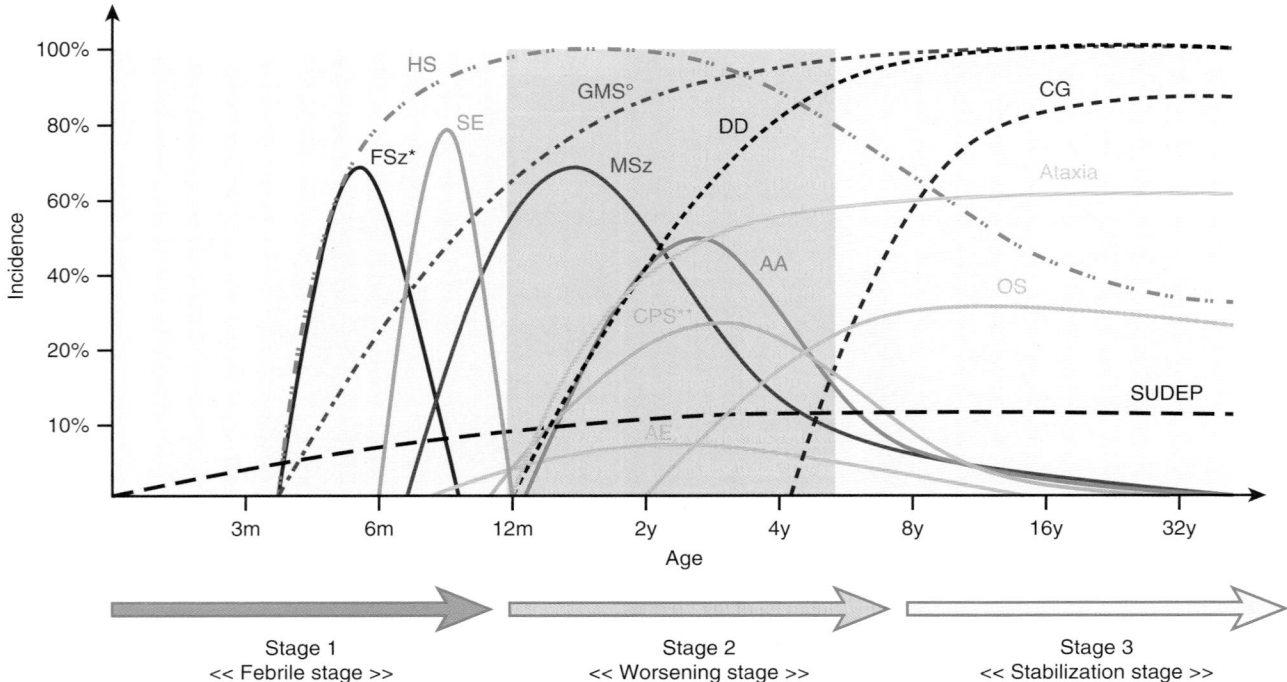

Fig. 39.8 Schematic representation of clinical manifestations of Dravet syndrome and their relative incidence according to age. *Moderate fever for 60%; mostly clonic generalized and unilateral motor seizures. **Difficult distinction between atypical absences and complex partial seizures without ictal EEG recording, so their precise incidence is unknown. °Including generalized tonic-clonic and unilateral seizures. However, unilateral seizures are less frequent after the age of 7 years, whereas sleep seizures increase after 6–7 years and become predominant after the age of 9–10 years. AA, atypical absences; AE, acute encephalopathy; CG, crouching gait; CPS, complex partial seizures; DD, developmental delay; FSz, complex febrile seizures; GMS, generalized motor seizures; HS, hyperthermia sensitivity; MSz, myoclonic seizures; OS, obtundation status; SE, convulsive status epilepticus; SUDEP, sudden unexpected death in epilepsy. (From Gataullina S, Dulac O. From genotype to phenotype in Dravet disease. *Seizure.* 2017;44:58–64 [Fig. 1, p. 59].)

Tic disorders.

- Peak presentation: age 5–7 years
- Classical features: no alteration of awareness, stereotyped behaviors, a sensation of "compulsion" to perform the behavior and "relief" once it is completed
- Acuity: low
- Prognosis: excellent, although disabling tics and psychiatric comorbidities should be addressed, if present

Tics are common and are sudden, brief, purposeless involuntary movements or vocalizations that occur during wakefulness only; children may describe a sense of compulsion and can briefly suppress the behavior but have a sense of relief when performing the suppressed action (Table 39.22) (see Chapter 40). Children may have phonic tics (such as tongue clicking or throat clearing), motor tics (such as blinking, sniffing, or shrugging), or any combination of both. Tics are treated when they become disruptive, socially unacceptable, or physically uncomfortable, but otherwise they are considered benign and normally do not require pharmacologic treatment. Common comorbidities that should be screened for include anxiety, attention-deficit/hyperactivity disorder (ADHD), and obsessive-compulsive disorder.

They often become noticeable in early grade school years, around the time that some children start stimulant medications for ADHD. This temporal association has led to the misconception that the stimulant medications have caused the tics.

α_2-Agonists such as clonidine are common first-line treatments for disruptive or disabling tics; more severe tics can be treated with atypical antipsychotics such as risperidone.

Tourette syndrome is diagnosed when a child has had multiple motor tics and at least one phonic tic present for longer than 1 year. Other tic disorders can be purely motor or purely phonic and are classified according to their symptoms and duration (transient vs chronic).

Table 39.22 outlines some of the clinical features of episodic abnormal movements that may appear in children.

Sleep disorders.

- Peak presentation: age 2–7 years
- Classical features: occurring a few hours after falling asleep ("around midnight"), nonstereotyped behaviors, screaming, agitation, and inconsolability despite being apparently awake, no memory of frightening imagery
- Acuity: low
- Prognosis: excellent, although children with frequent episodes may need to be monitored by their parents to prevent injury during a panicked state

Night terrors and confusional arousals. Night terrors are a common phenomenon in children and are most frequent in boys aged 5–7 years. Up to 15% of children younger than 7 years have experienced some form of these episodes. The attacks are characterized by sudden arousal from sleep, often screaming in terror, and then crying with agitation and tachycardia. There may be vigorous and potentially injurious motor activity in older children, such as running or hitting the bed or wall. The striking feature of these episodes is that the child is inconsolable but seemingly awake. The episodes arise out of slow-wave non–rapid eye movement sleep, usually occurring 1–2 hours after bedtime, and are not responses to dream imagery (i.e., not nightmares). Episodes last several minutes. Prior sleep deprivation, febrile illness, emotional stress, and some medications (sedatives/hypnotics, neuroleptics, stimulants, antihistamines) may be precipitants. In contrast to the experience of nightmares, children are amnestic for the events and their distress in night terrors.

Confusional arousals are less dramatic attacks with similar origin from slow-wave sleep and are more typical in younger children. The affected child stirs and begins crying and whimpering inconsolably. These arousals may be prolonged in infants, lasting up to 30–40 minutes.

There is no specific treatment for these events; parents should be educated about the nature of these arousals and reassured that they are self-limited.

The most important mimic of parasomnias is nocturnal seizures. **Nocturnal frontal lobe seizures** occur during sleep and can have bizarre hypermotor behaviors such as rolling, turning, picking, yelling, and fumbling. In school-aged children, **benign rolandic epilepsy** manifests itself as seizures when coming out of sleep with gurgling, salivation, hemifacial and hemibody twitching, and often partially preserved consciousness of the event. Important distinguishing historical factors between seizures and parasomnias are the time of onset (seizures: shortly after falling asleep or early in the morning), duration (most seizures last 1–2 minutes, and parasomnias can have a significantly longer duration), and any associated tongue bite, urinary incontinence, or insidious behavioral or developmental regression.

Somnambulism. Somnambulism, or sleepwalking, is common in childhood. Approximately 15% of children have walked in their sleep, especially in the 2–3-year-old age group, and 2.5% are habitual sleepwalkers, having episodes at least once a month. The age at onset peaks between 4 and 10 years. There is a family history of sleepwalking and other parasomnias in 60–80% of patients. These episodes of apparent unresponsiveness and "automatisms" could be mistaken for focal dyscognitive seizures or a postictal state.

Self-stimulatory behavior/stereotypies. Repetitive purposeless movements may be performed by children on the autism spectrum or with cognitive disabilities. Combined with unresponsiveness, these behaviors may be mistaken for automatisms in focal dyscognitive seizures. The important features that distinguish such behavior from epileptic activity are the setting in which it occurs, the variable content and duration of the "attacks," and the complete failure of the episodes to interrupt more stimulating activities. However, it may be very difficult to determine the nature of the episodes by interview; video and EEG monitoring may be required. These behaviors are not harmful and may provide soothing sensory input to the child performing them.

Acute Symptomatic Seizures and Occasional Seizures

Febrile convulsions remain one of the most common causes of occasional seizures in early childhood. Head injury is more common in

---

TABLE 39.22 Abnormal Involuntary Movements

Movement	Characteristics	Associations
Tics	Brief involuntary movements (motor tics) or sounds (phonic or vocal tics) occurring against a background of normal motor activity Tics may be simple, sudden brief movements such as shrugging a shoulder, blinking, or grimacing; or complex, more coordinated movements that might appear purposeful, such as hitting or touching Snorting, sniffing, or throat clearing are examples of simple phonic tics, and short utterances, echolalia, or coprolalia are complex phonic tics	Idiopathic tic disorders Tourette syndrome
Tremor	Movements caused by rhythmically alternating contractions of a muscle group and its antagonists The movements may involve proximal and axial muscles Classified as resting, postural, or action tremors according to the response to these maneuvers	Physiologic tremor, essential tremor
Chorea	Random brief limb movements of variable duration; these can be incorporated into voluntary movements by the patient	SLE Wilson disease Rheumatic fever Autoimmune encephalitis Postinfectious
Athetosis	Slow writhing movements of the extremities, often distal extremities The movements are random Often involuntary movements of this type have some features of chorea and are termed *choreoathetoid*	Kernicterus
Dystonia	Sustained muscle co-contraction of agonist and antagonist muscle groups, frequently causing twisting and repetitive movements or abnormal postures The velocity of the movements varies, usually being sustained at the height of the involuntary contraction for 1 sec or longer The duration also varies in different syndromes; in spasmodic torticollis, there may be rhythmic jerks or spasms into the abnormal posture Subclassified by extent (focal, segmental, multifocal, and generalized) and relationship to movement (action and rest)	Idiopathic (inherited) syndromes Postlesional syndromes
Myoclonus	Rapid brief muscle jerks with an irregular or occasionally rhythmic quality Can be epileptic or nonepileptic in origin	Encephalopathies Idiopathic and symptomatic epilepsies
Ballismus	Wild, large-amplitude, irregular limb movements	Postlesional
Asterixis	Repetitive movements caused by sudden, brief, irregular lapses in posture of an extremity	Metabolic encephalopathies
Dyskinesia	Sometimes used as a general term to describe abnormal involuntary movements	

SLE, systemic lupus erythematosus.

childhood than in infancy, but the list of other potential causes of seizures, including brain tumor, intracranial infection, and poisoning, is very similar. In addition, some metabolic and neurodegenerative disorders manifest in childhood, not in infancy (Table 39.23).

Epileptic Syndromes

Benign partial epilepsies of childhood. Focal seizures and focal EEG discharges usually suggest the presence of a localized cerebral lesion. There is a group of idiopathic partial epilepsies beginning in children without abnormalities on neurologic examination or neuroimaging studies, and frequently, with a family history of epilepsy. The benign partial epilepsies of childhood (BPECs) are characterized by focal seizures and focal epileptiform discharges, both with age-dependent spontaneous recovery, in the absence of anatomic lesions.

Clinically, the seizures begin between 18 months and 12 years of age, most often at 8–10 years; there is no neurologic deficit or developmental delay. The seizures are brief and stereotyped in an individual, although they vary among patients. The seizures do not have a prolonged postictal deficit, are usually infrequent, and respond well to AED treatment. The focal epileptiform discharges occur with normal background rhythms. The sharp waves or spikes have a characteristic structure and are often very frequent, increasing during sleep. Rare generalized epileptiform discharges may occur, but if they are prominent, the diagnosis of BPEC should be questioned.

TABLE 39.23 Inherited Disorders of Metabolism and Neurodegenerative Diseases Associated with Seizures in Childhood and Adolescence

Name	Clinical Features and Laboratory Findings	Investigations
Syndrome of Progressive Myoclonus Epilepsy		
Multiple specific disorders cause the clinical syndrome of PME Prominent myoclonus: irregular repetitive, spontaneous or with action, stimulus sensitive Associated seizure types: usually tonic-clonic, but also tonic, absence, and partial seizures Progressive neurologic deterioration, with prominent ataxia and other motor signs developing later Progressive dementia, varying in degree between the specific disorders		
Most Cases Are Caused by the Following Five Disorders:		
Unverricht-Lundborg	Onset, ages 8–15 yr; myoclonus and GTC seizures, cerebellar ataxia, slowly progressive but mild cognitive decline; patients have long survival in comparison to other disorders in this group	Chromosome 21q22; cystatin B variants Clinical diagnosis must exclude other causes of PME syndrome
Myoclonus epilepsy and ragged red fibers (MERRF)	Onset, ages 5–12 yr (range, 3–62 yr); myoclonus, GTC seizures, progressive ataxia, dementia Other features include deafness, optic atrophy, neuropathy, myopathy, pyramidal signs, dysarthria, and nystagmus There may be clinical overlap with other mitochondrial encephalomyopathies: mitochondrial encephalomyopathy with lactic acidosis and strokelike episodes (MELAS) and Kearns-Sayre syndrome	Serum and CSF lactate and pyruvate measurements Muscle biopsy; light microscopy, electron microscopy (EM), biochemical analysis of oxidative metabolism, and DNA studies
Lafora body disease	Onset, ages 10–19 yr; generalized clonic, GTC, and partial seizures with visual auras; myoclonus develops later and becomes very disabling; severe dementia; death within 5 yr of disease onset Lafora bodies (intracellular amyloid inclusions) are found in skin, muscle, neurons, and hepatocytes	Biopsy of skin must include eccrine sweat glands (i.e., axilla) to exclude Lafora bodies Chromosome 6q24; gene *EPM2A* produces laforin
Neuronal ceroid lipofuscinosis		
Late infantile form (Jansky-Bielschowsky)	Onset, ages 2–4 yr; severe epilepsy, myoclonic, GTC, atonic, atypical absence seizures (not tonic, vs Lennox-Gastaut syndrome), progressive severe dementia, ataxia, pyramidal and extrapyramidal signs, visual loss later, usually death in adolescence Ophthalmologic examination necessary; on EEG, marked photic sensitivity to 1-Hz stimulation, electroretinogram (ERG) and visual evoked potential (VEP) abnormalities	Skin, conjunctival, or rectal mucosal biopsy; skin biopsy is the most practical and least morbid. EM of circulating lymphocytes can be used for screening Lipopigment accumulation in lysosomes best seen in eccrine secretory cells; the inclusions have a characteristic structure on EM that differs between the different subtypes of neuronal ceroid lipofuscinosis EEG, ERG, and VEP testing
Juvenile form (Batten-Spielmeyer-Vogt)	Onset, ages 4–10 yr; usually manifests with decreased visual acuity secondary to retinal degeneration, psychomotor delay, cerebellar and extrapyramidal signs, later onset of seizures, and GTC and myoclonus Progressive severe dementia accompanies the other neurologic signs Death in early adulthood ERG and VEP abnormalities	Same as for the late infantile form
Adult onset (Kufs)	Onset, ages 11–50 yr; dementia, psychiatric symptoms, cerebellar signs, and extrapyramidal signs are most prominent; seizures often tonic; visual disturbances are less common; fundi are normal; on EEG, marked photic sensitivity to 1-Hz stimulation	

TABLE 39.23 Inherited Disorders of Metabolism and Neurodegenerative Diseases Associated with Seizures in Childhood and Adolescence—cont'd

Name	Clinical Features and Laboratory Findings	Investigations
Sialidosis		
Type 1	Onset, ages 8–20 yr; decreased visual acuity and macular cherry red spot; action- and stimulus-induced myoclonus; cerebellar ataxia; no dementia or decreased length of survival A peripheral neuropathy may be present	Urine specimen, blood sample for cultured leukocytes, and skin biopsy to obtain cultured fibroblasts for enzyme analysis
Type 2	Onset, ages 10–30 yr; described in Japanese patients Coarse facial features and PME syndrome Elevated excretion of urinary sialylated oligosaccharides, enzyme analysis shows deficiency of α-N-acetylneuraminidase (both type 1 and type 2)	Same as for type 1
Less Common Causes of PME Syndrome in This Age Group:		
Juvenile neuronopathic Gaucher disease; PME, supranuclear palsy, and splenomegaly; no dementia; pancytopenia on CBC, leukocytes show low β-glucocerebrosidase activity		CBC, leukocytes for enzyme analysis
Dentatorubral-pallidoluysian atrophy, seen in Japanese patients; PME is one manifestation		Clinical diagnosis in life
Neuroaxonal dystrophy; may appear as PME; also, chorea, lower motor neuron signs; axon steroids in neurons, may be seen in autonomic nerve endings around eccrine secretory coils		Peripheral nerve biopsy, skin biopsy
Late-onset GM$_2$ gangliosidosis; sensitivity to acoustic stimulus; myoclonus, severe dementia, dystonia, pyramidal signs; cherry red spot may be seen on the macula		Hexosaminidase A activity
Pantothenate kinase associated neurodegeneration (Hallevorden-Spatz disease)		Clinical diagnosis in life
Action myoclonus–renal failure syndrome, described in French-Canadians; tremor, PME, and, later, proteinuria and renal failure; no dementia		Clinical diagnosis, renal function
Other Rare Disorders with Seizures in Childhood and Adolescence		
Juvenile Huntington disease	Onset, age >3 yr; developmental delay; dystonia; parkinsonian features may be present	GTC, atypical absence, myoclonic seizures
Alpers syndrome	Progressive neurologic degeneration of childhood A clinical syndrome; suspected to be a mitochondrial encephalopathy Normal at birth, then failure to thrive with developmental delay, myoclonic jerks, seizures, episodes of status epilepticus, hypotonia, and visual loss followed by spastic quadriparesis Epilepsia partialis continua may be present The spectrum of clinical features includes deafness, ataxia, chorea, and liver disease	Muscle biopsy
Rett syndrome	Onset, ages 1–2 yr; in girls only; delay or regression in motor development, loss of language, ataxia, "hand-ringing" mannerism Seizures occur later; myoclonic, partial, and GTC Episodes of apnea, ataxic breathing, and hyperventilation; pyramidal signs	Muscle biopsy for mitochondrial enzyme analysis and histologic study, although cause is unknown; genetic testing
Maple syrup urine disease	Less severe forms may manifest late, even in adulthood, with episodic symptoms of encephalopathy and ataxia	Serum amino acids and possibly seizures
Porphyria	Onset, late adolescence, after puberty; 15% of affected patients have seizures during an acute attack of porphyria	Urinary and/or stool porphyrins

CSF, cerebrospinal fluid; GTC, generalized tonic-clonic; PME, progressive myoclonus epilepsy.

The most well-defined form of BPEC is **benign epilepsy with centrotemporal spikes and seizures (BECTS)**, often referred to as **benign rolandic epilepsy**. Brief hemifacial motor seizures with anarthria and drooling are typical, frequently when coming out of sleep. Consciousness is typically preserved, although this may not be true with longer seizures. A somatosensory aura involving the tongue, cheek, or gums may precede the motor seizure. Many seizures occur at night as tonic-clonic seizures, presumably secondary generalized with unwitnessed partial onset. Onset is between 3 and 13 years, with a peak onset at 9–10 years; there is a male-to-female predominance of approximately 3:2.

Management depends on seizure frequency; if the typical EEG discharges have been found in a child without seizures or after a first seizure, there is usually no indication to treat with AEDs. If seizures are infrequent and nocturnal, the option of no treatment should be discussed. AED treatment should be considered for patients experiencing more frequent seizures, troublesome seizures during the day, or seizures associated with any morbidity such as postictal headaches or lethargy. The seizures are usually controlled easily with a variety of AEDs, including carbamazepine or levetiracetam.

The seizures of BPEC resolve spontaneously before 16 years of age, and the EEG may be helpful in deciding when to withdraw treatment. Patients older than 14 years who are seizure-free for 1–2 years with normal EEGs should withdraw from treatment; the clinician should strongly consider a trial of withdrawal in patients 10–14 years old who are seizure-free and have a normal EEG. Younger patients with active EEGs are likely to have recurrence of seizures with AED withdrawal;

if seizures and/or abnormal EEGs persist well into the teenage years, syndromic diagnosis should be reconsidered. Subtle neuropsychologic deficits may be present in children with BECTS, suggesting that this disorder may not be entirely as "benign" as once thought.

Benign childhood epilepsy with occipital paroxysms forms a subset of idiopathic partial epilepsies of childhood. There are two types of this subset: one with early onset (peak onset at 3–5 years), nocturnal seizures with tonic eye deviation, and vomiting, and another with later onset (peak onset at 7–9 years) characterized by seizures beginning with visual symptoms, which is consistent with an occipital origin. These are also referred to as **Panayiotopoulos syndrome** and the **benign occipital epilepsy of Gastaut**, respectively. Hemiclonic seizures or the automatisms of temporal lobe complex seizures often follow according to whether the seizure spreads to suprasylvian or infrasylvian regions. A severe headache may follow the visual auras and a diagnosis of childhood migraine is often considered. The EEG typically shows high-amplitude sharp waves or spike-and-wave complexes recurring at 0.5–1 Hz posteriorly, usually maximal in the occipital regions. The discharges are present when the eyes are closed and should disappear with eye opening. There is some controversy about the specificity of the electroclinical features and whether these cases are true variants of benign childhood epilepsy. The conditions are relatively uncommon, and the same EEG pattern may be seen with symptomatic occipital epilepsy.

Acquired epileptic aphasia and continuous spike-and-wave patterns in slow-wave sleep. These two conditions are age-related epileptic encephalopathies with disturbances in language and cognition occurring in association with persistent focal or bilaterally synchronous epileptiform activity and seizures without an underlying structural lesion. In each, the epileptiform activity is thought to disturb synaptogenesis and connectivity in the maturing brain. Although they are rare, some authorities consider them part of the spectrum of benign childhood epilepsy.

Epileptic aphasia, *or* **Landau-Kleffner syndrome,** begins in a previously normal child (peak age at onset, 5–7 years) with the regression of language. There is severe auditory agnosia, speech may disappear, and the child often appears to be deaf due to impairment of cortical processing of sound and language. There is usually a marked deterioration in behavior as well, and social interactions become altered. Childhood psychosis and the autistic spectrum disorders are often considered in the differential diagnosis, although the age of behavioral regression is atypical for those disorders and should be a red flag when this clinical history presents. Seizures occur but are not frequent and cannot explain the language deficits. The EEG in sleep shows almost continuous bilateral epileptiform discharges maximal over the temporal regions. The seizures are partial and easily controlled with medication, but the language regression and the EEG discharges do not remit with conventional AEDs. Treatment with corticosteroids does improve the condition in many children, but more than half have persistent language and learning deficits, despite the eventual disappearance of the EEG abnormalities.

In **continuous spike-and-wave patterns in slow-wave sleep** or **electrical status epilepticus of slow-wave sleep** (CSWS and ESES, respectively), there is a more diffuse cognitive dysfunction, and more than 85% of the sleep EEG record is occupied by epileptiform discharges. The disorder typically manifests at 5–7 years of age, and there is a broader spectrum of seizure types, including absences, atonic seizures, and focal dyscognitive seizures, which may be frequent in some patients. In Landau-Kleffner, the speech and auditory disturbances are the most striking feature, and in CSWS, executive and behavioral dysfunction predominate. Both are caused by heterozygous variants in the ionotropic NMDA glutamate receptor subunit 2A gene *(GRIN2A)* and inherited as autosomal dominant.

Symptomatic focal (localization-related) epilepsy. The most common seizure type in children with focal epilepsy with an identified cause is the **focal dyscognitive seizure**. Focal dyscognitive seizures may arise from temporal, frontal, parietal, or occipital lobes, but most often from the temporal lobe. The causes of focal epilepsy in childhood are diverse and include birth asphyxia, later anoxic episodes, head injury, neoplasms, infection, malformations of cortical development, the cerebral lesions of neurocutaneous syndromes, vascular malformations, and cerebral infarction. MRI is a crucial diagnostic procedure and can reveal a variety of structural abnormalities.

Focal epilepsy commonly evolves as a medically refractory disorder; in some patients, it can be amenable to surgical resection. The investigation of children for epilepsy surgery is a highly specialized process that follows documentation of medical intractability, which is defined as failure of at least two appropriately chosen and optimized antiepileptic medications. Concordant evidence of a single epileptogenic region within the brain must be found with ictal video and EEG monitoring, both structural neuroimaging (MRI) and functional neuroimaging (single-photon emission computed tomography and PET), and neuropsychologic evaluation (see Fig. 39.4). If a focus can be demonstrated, it must be shown that resection of that area will not cause unacceptable loss of sensorimotor or cognitive function.

Childhood absence epilepsy. Childhood absence epilepsy is an idiopathic generalized epilepsy beginning in previously normal children between 4 and 12 years of age, with peak incidence at 6–7 years of age; females are more frequently affected. It accounts for only about 8–10% of school-aged children with epilepsy. There is a family history of epilepsy in approximately 15–25% of patients. The absence seizures are simple, or more often, complicated with mild automatisms or other motor features. Absence seizures are very frequent, occurring daily, but they generally respond well to antiepileptic therapy. The EEG is normal apart from runs of 3-Hz spike-and-wave complexes; clinical seizures are associated with discharges lasting more than 2–3 seconds. The discharges and clinical seizures can be produced by hyperventilation. Prognosis is generally favorable, with remission in approximately 80% of cases by late adolescence. GTC seizures occur in 40–50% of patients with childhood absence epilepsy. They typically develop years after the onset of absences and may appear after remission from the absence seizures. Usually, the tonic-clonic seizures are infrequent and medically controllable.

Treatment with ethosuximide or valproate controls absence seizures in most patients. However, ethosuximide offers no protection against tonic-clonic seizures, whereas valproate is also effective against tonic-clonic seizures. Therefore, valproate is the drug of choice if both seizure types are present. If either ethosuximide or valproate proves ineffective after an adequate trial at maximum tolerated doses, a trial of the other should be commenced. Combination ethosuximide and valproate therapy has been effective in some patients with absence seizures not controlled by either drug alone. Clonazepam may also be effective, but it is associated with sedative and behavioral side effects. Alternatives may include lamotrigine, topiramate, or zonisamide; medications such as carbamazepine or phenytoin that are specific for focal-onset seizures will in fact exacerbate absence seizures.

Epilepsia partialis continua and Rasmussen encephalitis. Epilepsia partialis continua describes continuous focal motor seizures usually manifesting as repetitive clonic jerks of the face, upper limb, lower limb, or larger portion of one half of the body that continue in this localized manner for hours to days or months. These seizures are caused by cortical processes that directly overlie the motor cortex that include vascular lesions, focal cortical dysplasia, neoplasms, and unidentified focal areas of atrophy. More generalized metabolic disorders such as mitochondrial encephalomyopathy with lactic acidosis and strokelike episodes (MELAS) and an inherited disorder of metabolism (nonketotic hyperglycinemia) have also been reported to cause epilepsia partialis continua.

The focal seizures in this condition are generally impossible to control with AEDs, and surgical management with a limited cortical resection may be necessary. The risk of motor and sensory deficits limits possible resections, and careful mapping of the site of seizure onset and its relationship to functional cortex is required.

Rasmussen encephalitis is a clinically defined syndrome of predominantly hemispheric cerebral dysfunction, with onset of seizures between 2 and 10 years of age. A variety of seizure types can occur, including focal motor seizures and focal dyscognitive seizures with secondary generalization, myoclonus, and epilepsia partialis continua; they are refractory to management with AEDs. The disorder is characterized by a progressive hemiparesis, language disturbances if the dominant hemisphere is affected, and intellectual decline. Progressive hemispheric atrophy, maximal in the central, temporal, and frontal regions, can be documented with neuroimaging studies. Pathologic specimens show nonspecific changes suggestive of immune-mediated encephalitis, although no etiologic agent has been identified. Worsening of the neurologic deficits can be expected over time, although the seizures may lessen and even "burn out."

Functional hemispherectomy performed early in the course of the disease before complete hemiparesis should control seizures, arrest the motor deterioration, and, in most cases, lead to stabilization or even improvement in language and intellectual function. However, significant morbidity and mortality rates are associated with the surgery, and the child is left with a paretic upper limb, although he or she can walk unaided.

Lennox-Gastaut syndrome. Lennox-Gastaut syndrome is characterized by generalized seizures and epileptiform discharges with delayed cognitive development and behavioral problems beginning between the ages of 1 and 8 years. The patients have a mixed seizure disorder with multiple seizure types; the typical seizures are tonic seizures, atypical absences, and atonic seizures, although patients may also have tonic-clonic, myoclonic, and focal dyscognitive seizures. The seizures are not easily controlled and are usually frequent, often with several occurring per day. Episodes of status epilepticus are common, and nonconvulsive stupor with continuous spike-and-wave discharges or a stuporous state with repeated tonic seizures is typical. The waking EEG has abnormally slow background activity, and the EEG correlates of sleep may also be poorly organized. The epileptiform abnormalities consist of slow (<3 Hz) spike-and-wave discharges, multifocal spikes, or sharp waves and paroxysmal fast activity (>10 Hz) in sleep.

Treatment is always indicated, but AEDs are rarely able to control seizures completely. More often, some reduction in the frequency and severity of seizures may be obtained. Patients commonly need combinations of AEDs to address their multiple seizure types. Valproate should be used as a first-line agent for patients with atonic, tonic, and myoclonic seizures and may be helpful with tonic-clonic seizures. Patients with refractory tonic-clonic seizures or focal seizures as well as generalized seizures may benefit from the addition of lamotrigine. Combinations of AEDs must be monitored carefully for drug toxicity and unwanted interactions. Carbamazepine has been reported to exacerbate atypical absence seizures in some patients. Phenytoin can be an effective drug in controlling GTC and tonic seizures. Barbiturates may be effective, although they are often poorly tolerated in children with abnormalities of tone, and drug-related drowsiness may exacerbate tonic seizures in some patients. Other alternatives include clonazepam, topiramate, and levetiracetam. Felbamate and cannabidiols have been reported to improve control of the debilitating tonic or atonic "drop attacks" in patients with this syndrome.

A major source of morbidity and an important management issue are repeated falls associated with tonic and atonic seizures. Appropriate restriction in daily activities and the wearing of helmets with face protection are often required. Division of the anterior portion of the corpus callosum (anterior corpus callosotomy) has been successful in controlling the falls associated with tonic or atonic seizures, but it is considered a palliative and not a curative surgical procedure, and the goal is not complete seizure freedom.

Adolescence

The paroxysmal disorders of adolescence (12–18 years) are shown in Table 39.24.

TABLE 39.24 **Paroxysmal Disorders of Adolescence**
Nonepileptiform Disorders
More Common
Syncope
Migraine
Psychogenic nonepileptic behavioral events
Dissociative states, conversion disorders
Panic attacks, hyperventilation
Daydreaming
Sleep
Nocturnal myoclonus, hypnic jerks
Narcolepsy
Somnambulism
Somniloquy
Less Common
Episodic rage
Malingering
Paroxysmal choreoathetosis
Tremor
Tic
Drug reactions, dystonia
Transient global amnesia
Acute Symptomatic Seizures, Occasional Seizures
More Common
Drug abuse
Reflex seizures (see Table 39.1)
Head injury
Meningitis and encephalitis
Less Common
Brain tumor
Intercurrent medical illness, endocrine disorder, systemic neoplasia
Epileptic Syndromes
More Common
Reflex seizures (see Table 39.1)
Symptomatic localization-related epilepsy
Juvenile myoclonic epilepsy
Less Common
Juvenile absence epilepsy
Epilepsy with generalized tonic-clonic seizures on awakening
Epilepsia partialis continua (Kojewnikow syndrome)
Rasmussen encephalitis
Progressive myoclonic epilepsy
Autosomal dominant epilepsy with auditory features (ADEAF)

Paroxysmal Nonepileptiform Disorders

Syncope. Loss of consciousness with falling is the salient feature of syncope (see Chapter 7 and Table 39.25). Children may be able to describe a distinct trigger, such as needles or the sight of blood, and often describe palpitations, tunnel vision, and nausea. There may be a family history of vasovagal syncope. Cardiac arrhythmias should be ruled out; autonomic testing may be beneficial in patients with very frequent syncope.

Paroxysmal psychiatric events. Psychogenic nonepileptic seizures (PNESs) are events where the patient may have dramatic convulsions, stiffening, unresponsiveness, or dissociative symptoms including amnesia of the events. They are common but are frequently misdiagnosed as epileptic seizures, leading to unnecessary interventions including intubation, hospitalization, invasive testing, or simply years of antiepileptic medications that do not help the patient (Table 39.26). Most cases are best thought of as a manifestation of psychiatric illness, such as post-traumatic stress disorder, anxiety, or depression. Nonepileptic behavioral events should be treated compassionately by the physician as a sign of significant psychiatric distress, and not as malingering or a factitious disorder.

TABLE 39.25 Differential Diagnosis of Syncope

Clinical	Syncope	Tonic-Clonic Seizures
Precipitating factors	Almost always patient is standing; environment is warm; fright; pain	Usually none, although sleep deprivation or awakening may be contributory
Prodrome	Lightheaded, dizzy, queasy; vision dims; loss of color, "gray out"; sweating May be averted by head down or recumbency	Aura or sense of déjà vu or jamais vu may be present
Occurrence in sleep	Never	Common
Evolution	Limp faint → fall → motionless unconsciousness, often with pallor, clammy skin; there may be a tonic phase with generalized stiffening	Sudden loss of consciousness → increased tone and massive truncal flexion or extension, followed by synchronous jerking of body and limbs with rubor or cyanosis and sweating → unconsciousness
Skin	Pale and cool	Flushed, cyanosed, warm
Incontinence	Rare	Occasional
Self-injury	Rare	Common (biting tongue)
Degree of postictal confusion	Minimal	Marked
Family history	Often positive for syncope	May be positive for seizures
Interictal EEG	Usually normal	Frequently abnormal, epileptiform discharges

TABLE 39.26 Differential Diagnosis of Psychogenic Nonepileptic Seizures

Clinical Factors	Psychogenic Seizures	Epileptic Seizures
Age at onset	Usually older than 8–10 yr Predominates in girls; 15–30% of patients are boys	Either sex; no sex predominance
Duration of seizures	May be very prolonged	Usually seconds to minutes
Evolution	May have a very gradual onset and ending	Usually more abrupt onset
Quality of convulsive movements	Thrashing, asynchronous limb movements, often with partial responsiveness	Usually rhythmic and synchronous with loss of consciousness
Stereotypical attacks	Typically variable	Typically stereotyped
Examination during the seizure	May resist examination, combative	Usually unresponsive and amnestic for ictal events
Self-injury	Rare	Common in GTC seizures
Incontinence	Rare	Common in GTC seizures
During sleep	No; may occur nocturnally, but while the patient is awake	Common
Changes in seizure frequency with medication	Rare	Usual
Interictal EEG	Repeatedly normal	Often abnormal
Ictal EEG	No EEG seizure patterns; normal rhythms while patient is unresponsive	EEG seizure patterns
Pitfalls in diagnosis	1. Psychologic factors may not be immediately apparent 2. Misleading information may be given by parents (as in factitious [Munchausen] syndrome by proxy)	1. Asynchronous vigorous automatisms are found in frontal lobe seizures 2. Bilateral limb movements and posturing without loss of consciousness occur in supplementary motor seizures 3. EEG seizure patterns may be absent during some seizures (e.g., auras, SMA)

GTC, generalized tonic-clonic; SMA, supplementary motor area.

Among adults, 20% of patients referred with refractory seizures are found to have psychogenic nonepileptic behavioral events; in children, the number is smaller. *Both epileptic seizures and nonepileptic behavioral events can coexist in the same person*, likely due to the high incidence of anxiety and depression in people living with epilepsy, as well as the stress associated with an unpredictable chronic illness. Typically, they are characterized by marked motor activity such as pelvic thrusting, arching of the back, thrashing of the limbs, and even self-injury. The episodes may have a gradual onset with buildup of motor activity, and they usually last longer than epileptic seizures (see Table 39.26). Other forms that the psychogenic nonepileptic behavioral events may take include a gradual slump to a motionless supine position with unresponsiveness and eyes closed, often with some flickering of the eyelids.

Other types of paroxysmal psychiatric events include panic attacks *and* rage attacks. **Panic attacks** may begin without the patient being able to identify an external precipitant, and then the sense of dread or fear may be mistaken for a psychic aura. Many of the symptoms experienced, including palpitations, paresthesia, formication, lightheadedness, and carpopedal spasm, result from hyperventilation and tachycardia. There may be some apparent disturbance of consciousness. Historically, the sequence of events is important, especially the hyperventilation and associated symptoms. The patient may be asked to hyperventilate in the office to see whether symptoms are reproduced; hyperventilation must continue for 3–5 minutes with good effort for a negative result to be useful.

Rage attacks may also be confused with epileptic seizures. Often seen in intellectually impaired patients, they represent intense frustration in the presence of an inability to vent the frustration in other ways or to communicate it. Rage attacks may also occur in children with normal intelligence or in those taking anabolic steroids.

The interictal EEG is repeatedly normal in patients with psychogenic nonepileptic behavioral events but may be abnormal in children with both epileptic and nonepileptic events. For definitive diagnosis, it may be necessary to record a clinical episode with continuous video and EEG monitoring.

Treatment of psychogenic nonepileptic behavioral events must include an identification of underlying psychosocial and psychiatric problems. Major mood disorders and severe environmental stress, especially sexual abuse, are common among children and adolescents with psychogenic seizures and should be considered in every case. This history, though uncomfortable for both parties to discuss, must be specifically asked about and may require multiple visits to develop the necessary rapport to receive a truthful answer.

Presentation of a nonepileptic diagnosis to the patient after monitoring of a typical spell must be positive ("These attacks are not epileptic and will not necessitate chronic medication or further neurologic investigation") and truthful ("We don't know exactly what is causing them, but emotional factors are clearly playing a major role"). This diagnosis can be received with disbelief or hostility by families for multiple reasons. First, the societal stigma against psychiatric illness may make it difficult for parents to accept that a child has a psychiatric disorder; a genuine neurologic disorder is almost preferable to some families and they may visit multiple medical centers searching for a positive organic diagnosis. Second, even if the family accepts the diagnosis, there may be the perception that these events are "all in the child's head" or "attention-seeking," leading to a nontherapeutic familial and medical response to the diagnosis. If the child has been having events for a prolonged period of time, there is immense social pressure to continue having events, as they may feel that their peers, family, and school would react negatively to the psychiatric diagnosis after having been supportive of the presumptive epileptic diagnosis.

Terminology and phrasing are critical when discussing this diagnosis with families. Referring to them as "psychiatric" or "hysteric" or "conversion disorders" may come across as dismissive, particularly given the stigma around mental illness.

The prognosis of nonepileptic behavioral events in the pediatric population is much better than in adults, with 80% of patients seizure-free at the 3-year follow-up. Involvement of psychiatry and counseling is critical; in particular, cognitive-behavioral therapy appears to be specifically helpful in allowing people to achieve some conscious control over the physical symptoms of their psychiatric illness and to modulate their stress responses. However, the practitioner should be familiar with the concept of nonepileptic behavioral events. The degree and duration of pretreatment disability (school withdrawal, etc.) is a prognostic marker of response to treatment.

Acute Symptomatic Seizures and Occasional Seizures

The causes of acute symptomatic seizures in adolescence include those described in the preceding neonatal and childhood sections, except for febrile convulsions. Head injury may be more common among adolescents because participation in contact sports and motor vehicle accidents occur in the middle to late teen years. Recreational drug use can be associated with seizures.

Epileptic Syndromes

Juvenile myoclonic epilepsy. Juvenile myoclonic epilepsy has an onset between 12 and 18 years of age. The hallmark of the disorder is early-morning myoclonus involving axial and upper limb muscles, usually with sparing of the facial muscles. Episodes typically occur on awakening. Tonic-clonic seizures occur in the majority of patients. A history of early-morning myoclonic jerks may not be volunteered and should be asked of all patients presenting with GTC seizures. The patients may not have identified the myoclonus and instead describe nervousness, shakiness, or clumsiness for the first 1–2 hours of a morning, such as dropping their toothbrush or spilling their cereal. Fatigue, sleep deprivation, stress, and alcohol exacerbate the seizures; some patients have their first seizure shortly after starting college due to a combination of the aforementioned risk factors. The tonic-clonic seizures typically begin with a clustering of repeated myoclonic jerks. Absence seizures occur in 15–40% of patients. Neurologic examination findings, brain MRI, and cognition are normal. The interictal EEG shows spike-and-wave complexes at 3.5–6 Hz. Linkage analysis of patients and their family members has suggested that the disorder is linked to chromosome 21.

Valproate is the preferred AED, as it has efficacy on all seizure types in this disorder. Lamotrigine is another effective agent and is preferentially used in adolescent and adult women because of the potential side effect profile of valproate (weight gain, teratogenicity, and potential hormonal disturbances including polycystic ovarian syndrome). Alternatives may include topiramate, zonisamide, and benzodiazepines, although extensive data concerning their efficacy in this setting are not available.

The seizures are well controlled in 80–90% of patients, but lifelong treatment is required. It is estimated that more than 90% of patients suffer relapse within the first 6–12 months after cessation of AEDs, and relapse is still common, even with prolonged periods of seizure freedom. Although many benign childhood-onset epilepsies remit with adolescence, most adolescent-onset epilepsies do not remit.

Juvenile absence epilepsy. In comparison with *childhood* absence epilepsy, juvenile absence epilepsy has a later onset, at about the time of puberty, and the seizures are less frequent (less than daily). Neurologic examination findings and IQ are normal. The EEG shows generalized spike-and-wave discharges, usually at rates faster than 3 Hz. Tonic-clonic seizures may occur, usually on awakening, more frequently than in childhood absence epilepsy.

The treatment is the same as that for childhood absence epilepsy, but the prognosis for complete remission therapy is less favorable.

Epilepsy with generalized tonic-clonic seizures on awakening. This idiopathic generalized epilepsy involves GTC seizures occurring more than 90% of the time within 2 hours of awakening or in an early-evening period of relaxation. Sleep deprivation and disruption are often potent precipitants of seizures. The age at onset of the seizures is usually between 10 and 20 years; a family history of epilepsy occurs in approximately 10–13% of cases. Myoclonic and absence seizures may also be present, and the distinction between juvenile myoclonic epilepsy and juvenile absence epilepsy is not clear. The EEG may show generalized spike-and-wave complexes or polyspikes.

Treatment starts with valproate, although barbiturates may be very effective. Lamotrigine is also used because of concern about the side effects of valproate. Topiramate and zonisamide may also be helpful. The prognosis for complete control of seizures with therapy is very good: 65–79% of patients have experienced remission with therapy. Avoidance of precipitating factors that disrupt sleep patterns is important. The relapse rate if AEDs are stopped is high (83%) (Fig. 39.9 and Table 39.27).

RARE STATUS EPILEPTICUS SYNDROMES

FIRES (febrile infection–related epilepsy syndrome), a subgroup of NORSE (new-onset refractory status epilepticus), is a rare, devastating disorder of presumed immunologic etiology. FIRES occurs in previously healthy children (mean age ~8 years) and manifests with a nonspecific febrile illness 24 hours to 2 weeks before the onset of acute, recurrent, multiple difficult-to-treat seizures (status epilepticus). The interictal periods are characterized by severe depressed levels of consciousness (Fig. 39.9 and Table 39.27). The cerebrospinal fluid may be normal or reveal a mild pleocytosis. MRI may initially be normal or nonspecific. The differential diagnosis must include other causes of severe encephalopathy with status epilepticus (Table 39.28). Patients with FIRES have no evidence of autoimmune encephalitis antibodies or pathogens noted on brain biopsy. In addition, there is no evidence for pathologic variants in fever-sensitive epilepsy genes. In contrast, adult patients with a NORSE-like phenotype may have identifiable etiologies in ~50% of cases (Table 39.29).

The acute phase of FIRES lasts ~3 weeks but then transitions into a chronic phase characterized by drug-resistant epilepsy, severe cognitive impairment, and bilateral mesial temporal atrophy.

PRINCIPLES OF ANTIEPILEPTIC DRUG USE

The goal of AED therapy is to use a single agent in adequate dosages to completely control seizures. If seizures recur, the dosage of an AED should be gradually increased to achieve the maximum tolerated dose for the patient without causing symptoms of drug toxicity. Therapeutic ranges are derived from population studies in which the serum levels of patients with seizures controlled by an AED were compared with those of patients experiencing side effects. The therapeutic levels should be used as a guide and may also be used to assess compliance.

Around 67% of all seizure patients achieve seizure freedom on their first antiepileptic medication; the response rate is strongly tied to underlying etiology. If one agent does not control the seizures, another AED should be substituted and tried as monotherapy with a period of overlap during the transition period from one antiepileptic to another. An adequate trial of therapy entails the maximum tolerated dose of an AED for a period of time in which several of the patient's seizures (or clusters of seizures) would usually occur or for at least 2 months, whichever is longer. This interval may be shortened in infants and children with very frequent seizures. Changes in AED dosages and regimens should be made gradually, and due regard must

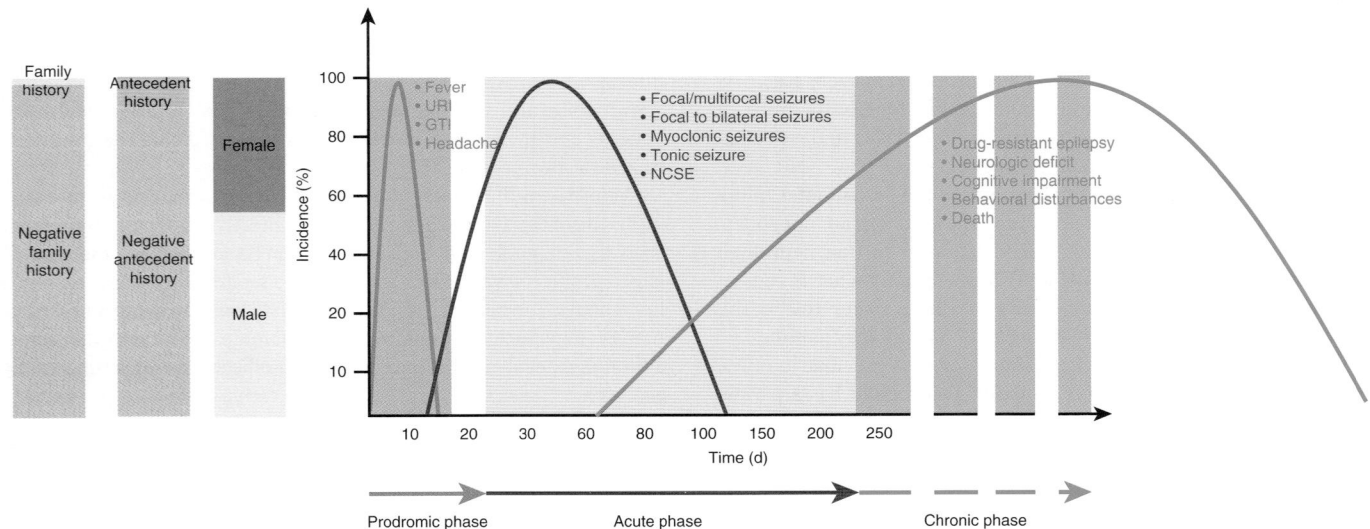

Fig. 39.9 Clinical findings in FIRES (febrile infection–related epilepsy syndrome) and NORSE (new-onset refractory status epilepticus), including family history, antecedents, and sex predominance. The graph shows the symptoms during the prodromic phase, type of seizures in the acute phase, and clinical findings during the chronic phase. GTI, gastrointestinal tract infections; NCSE, nonconvulsive status epilepticus; URI, upper respiratory infection. (From Specchio N, Pietrafusa N. New-onset refractory status epilepticus and febrile infection-related epilepsy syndrome. *Dev Med Child Neurol.* 2020;62:897–905, Fig. 1, p. 899.)

TABLE 39.27 Clinical Features of Febrile Infection–Related Epilepsy Syndrome (FIRES)

Age of onset: 2–17 (median 8) yr

Medical history: febrile seizures in rare cases, no epilepsy or other chronic disease, normal psychomotor development

Family history: uninformative, e.g., no allergies and especially no other family member with FIRES

Prodromal phase:
Different types of febrile infections often flulike
Frequently followed by an afebrile and asymptomatic interval of 1–2 days resulting in a consistent neurologic syndrome

Neurologic syndrome:
Peracute/explosive onset of multifocal or generalized seizures of different types directly evolving into super-refractory status epilepticus
Without other neurologic features (pure seizure phenotype)

EEG: global slowing or multifocal discharges with bilateral frontotemporal predominance, or both

CSF: normal or pleocytosis, normal protein concentration, no oligoclonal bands

MRI (during the acute phase of status epilepticus):
No or nonextensive bitemporal or diffuse abnormalities
Sporadic involvement of the basal ganglia, diffuse cortical edema, and/or hydrocephalus

Cause: extensive infectiologic (e.g., brain biopsies), metabolic (e.g., muscle biopsy), and genetic investigations (e.g., *POLG*, *SCN1A*, *PCDH19* genes, CNVs, exome sequencing) without causative findings

Coexisting autoimmunities: some patients with autoantibodies (e.g., TPO or GluR antibodies)

Treatment: resistance to nearly all drugs and even anesthetics

Outcome:
Almost always chronic epilepsy without silent period
Often global brain atrophy after a few weeks with mild to severe neuropsychologic impairments

CNVs, copy number variants; GluR, glutamate receptor; TPO, thyroid peroxidase.
From van Baalen A, Vezzani A, Hausker M, et al. Febrile infection-related epilepsy syndrome: clinical review and hypotheses of epileptogenesis. *Neuropediatrics.* 2017;48:5–18 (Table 1, p. 6).

TABLE 39.28 Differential Diagnoses of FIRES

Febrile seizure and febrile status epilepticus

Infectious encephalitis: can occur without significant CSF pleocytosis or MRI changes

Limbic encephalitis and other neuronal antibody-associated epileptic encephalitis

Hashimoto encephalopathy/steroid responsive encephalopathy

Posterior reversible encephalopathy syndrome

Alpers disease: hepatic mitochondrial DNA depletion caused by *POLG1* variants affecting the posterior cortex

Acute necrotizing encephalopathy caused by *RANP2* variants

Acute-onset epilepsy triggered by fever in young girls associated with *PCDH19* variants

Dravet syndrome

Primary angiitis of the CNS in childhood

Biotin- (and/or thiamin-) responsive basal ganglia disease with *SLC19A3* variants

Citrullinemia with elevation of the amino acid citrulline in the CSF, mimicking encephalitis

CNS, central nervous system; CSF, cerebrospinal fluid; FIRES, febrile infection–related epilepsy syndrome.
Adapted from van Baalen A, Vezzani A, Hausler M, et al. Febrile infection-related epilepsy syndrome: clinical review and hypotheses of epileptogenesis. *Neuropediatrics.* 2017;48:5–18.

Special considerations for women with epilepsy who take antiepileptic medications and are of childbearing age include the *teratogenicity of several antiepileptic medications*, including valproic acid. Additionally, valproic acid is known to increase the risk of polycystic ovarian syndrome, with its attendant hormonal and metabolic disturbances. Finally, several antiepileptic medications have significant interactions with hormonal contraception, and the provider should familiarize themselves with these interactions to avoid failure of either medication.

Stopping Antiepileptic Drugs

Most children (60–75% of patients) remain seizure-free when AEDs are withdrawn after a seizure-free interval on medication for more than 2 years. If relapse occurs, it is generally in the first few months after cessation of medication, and 60–80% of the relapses occur before 12 months after cessation. Patients with underlying neurologic disorders and deficits and those with multiple seizure types are more likely to suffer relapse. A long duration of epilepsy before remission carries a slightly higher risk of relapse. The EEG is a strong predictor in idiopathic epilepsy; among patients with frequent epileptic discharges that are recorded in generalized epilepsy, the rate of relapse is higher. For most children with epilepsy, it is recommended that children who have been seizure-free for 2 years undergo a trial of AED withdrawal.

LIFESTYLE

Parents should be encouraged to let their children lead a normal lifestyle, although some activities are inherently more dangerous for people with epilepsy. In general, climbing to significant heights, bathing, and swimming alone are not safe for children with active epilepsy. However, the clinician must stress the importance of avoiding overprotection of the child. Participation in sports and other school activities should be encouraged within the limits of avoiding dangerous activities such as rock climbing and scuba diving, in which even a brief loss of

be given to time taken to reach steady-state serum concentrations on the new regimen (see Fig 39.6; Tables 39.30 and 39.31). Drug changes can be made gradually on an outpatient basis, but the physician must warn the parents and child that AED toxicity or an increase in the seizure frequency may occur during the changeover period. More rapid medication changes, especially if barbiturates are to be stopped, often require that the patient be admitted to the hospital during the changeover period.

Only about an additional 10% of patients achieve better control with the addition of a second drug to the first; 20–30% of patients with epilepsy have medically refractory epilepsy. Failure to respond to two AEDs at maximum tolerated doses should prompt a referral for assessment in a specialty epilepsy program. In some patients, resistance to AEDs may be genetically determined by mutations affecting drug transport or in metabolizing proteins such as the multidrug resistance–associated family of drug transporters.

It is important to design dosage schedules that are realistic. Dosing more often than 3 times a day may result in a high incidence of poor compliance. Parents must be advised to be careful with other prescribed and over-the-counter medications. Many medications may interfere with AED metabolism.

TABLE 39.29 NORSE: Prominent Presentation Features of the Most Frequent Etiologies

Categories	*	Most Frequent Findings	Clinical Clues
Unknown	50%		No specific findings
			Prodromal mild febrile illness in 65% of cases
			Typically severe and prolonged SE
Inflammatory and autoimmune encephalitis	40%	Paraneoplastic limbic encephalitis (Anti-Hu, -Ma2/Ta, -CV2/CRMP-5, -amphiphysin, -VGCC, -mGluR5)	Cognitive, especially memory impairment, behavioral changes, temporal lobe seizures, sleep disturbance
			Hu: often more diffuse encephalomyelitis
			Ma2/Ta: hypothalamic dysfunction
			CV2/CRMP5: diffuse encephalomyelitis, chorea
		Surface-binding autoantibodies	
		Anti-NMDAr	Mostly young females
			Prodromal fever, short-term memory loss, psychiatric symptoms, hallucinations, orolingual dyskinesia, autonomic and respiratory failure
			Children: behavioral changes, movement disorders
			EEG: extreme delta brushes (50%)
		Anti-VGKC complex	Mostly elderly males
			LGI-1: limbic encephalitis, faciobrachial dystonic seizures, SIADH
			Caspr2: episodic ataxia
		Anti-GABA(B)r	Limbic encephalitis
		Anti-GABA(A)r	Multifocal neocortical encephalitis
		Anti-AMPAr	Prominent psychiatric symptoms, cerebellar ataxia
		Anti-Glycine-r	No specific features
		Anti-GAD	No specific features
		Steroid-responsive encephalopathy with autoimmune thyroiditis	Rapid-onset dementia, myoclonus, strokelike episodes
			Anti-TPO, anti-TG
Infectious encephalitis	10%	HSV1	Temporal involvement
		Enterovirus	Rash, acute lower motor neuron syndrome
		CMV	Immunodeficiency: gastrointestinal symptoms, retinitis, pneumonitis
		EBV	Adenopathies, ataxia
		VZV	Immunodeficiency: CNS lymphoma
		Mycoplasma pneumoniae	Rash
		Bartonella henselae	Respiratory symptoms, EEG: extreme spindles
		Arboviruses (WNV, tick-borne virus, etc.)	Children: cat-scratch disease with skin lesion and regional adenopathy
			Flulike episode
			WNV: parkinsonism, acute lower motor neuron syndrome, EEG: triphasic waves
Genetic disorders	Rare	SCN1A	Dravet syndrome
		PCDH19	Epilepsy and cognitive impairment limited to female
		CADASIL	Migraine, strokes, visual problems, cognitive deterioration
		Mitochondrial disorders	Elevated CSF lactate and strokelike episodes
		MELAS	Occipital seizures, epilepsia partialis continua, liver failure, nystagmus, ataxia.
		POLG1	

*Proportions mainly reflect adult population. There is a lack of data in pediatric population.
AMPA, α-amino-3-hydroxy-5-méthylisoazol-4-propionate; CADASIL, cerebral autosomal dominant arteriopathy with subcortical infarcts and leukoencephalopathy; CMV, cytomegalovirus; CNS, central nervous system; CSF, cerebrospinal fluid; EBV, Epstein-Barr virus; GABA, γ-aminobutyric acid; GAD, glutamic acid decarboxylase; HSV, herpes simplex virus; LGI1, leucine-rich glioma inactivated 1; MELAS, syndrome of mitochondrial encephalomyopathy, lactic acidosis, and strokelike episodes; NMDA, *N*-methyl-ᴅ-aspartate; PCDH, protocadherin; POLG1, mitochondrial DNA polymerase gamma; SIADH, syndrome of inappropriate antidiuretic hormone secretion; SCN, neuronal voltage-gated sodium channel; SE, status epilepticus; TG, thyroglobulin; TPO, thyroperoxidase; VGKC, voltage-gated potassium channel complex; VZV, varicella-zoster virus; WNV, West Nile virus.
From Sculier C, Gaspard N. New onset refractory status epilepticus (NORSE). *Seizure Eur J Epilepsy.* 2019;68:72–78 (Table 1, p. 74).

TABLE 39.30 Established Efficacy of Antiseizure Medications by Seizure Type (FDA Indications and Class I–III Evidence)

Antiseizure Medication	Monotherapy	Adjunctive	Focal	Generalized Tonic-Clonic	Absence	Myoclonic	LGS	IS	Therapy and Seizure Type
Phenobarbital	X	X	X						
Primidone	X	X	X						
Phenytoin	X	X	X	X					
Methsuximide	X	X			X				Two class IV trials supporting efficacy for focal-onset seizures
Ethosuximide	X	X			X				
Clonazepam	X	X			X	X			
Carbamazepine	X		X	X					
Valproate	X	X	X	X	X	X			Initial monotherapy for generalized tonic-clonic and myoclonic seizures
Felbamate	Conversion to monotherapy	X	X	X			X		
Gabapentin		X	X						Initial monotherapy for focal seizures
Lamotrigine	Conversion to monotherapy	X	X	X			X		Initial monotherapy for absence seizures
Topiramate	X	X	X	X			X		
Tiagabine		X	X						
Levetiracetam		X	X	X		X			Initial monotherapy for focal seizures
Oxcarbazepine	X	X	X						
Zonisamide		X	X						Initial monotherapy for focal seizures
Pregabalin		X	X						
Lacosamide	X	X	X						
Rufinamide		X					X		
Vigabatrin	X	X	X					X	
Ezogabine/retigabine		X	X						
Clobazam		X					X		
Perampanel	X	X	X	X					Efficacy against myoclonic seizures
Eslicarbazepine	X	X	X						
Brivaracetam	X	X	X						
Cannabidiol		X					X (also DS)		
Cenobamate	X	X	X						

DS, Dravet syndrome; FDA, US Food and Drug Administration; IS, infantile spasms; LGS, Lennox-Gastaut syndrome.
From Jankovic J, Mazziotta JC, Pomeroy SL, et al., eds. *Bradley's Neurology in Clinical Practice.* 8th ed. Philadelphia: Elsevier; 2022:1651, Table 100.3.

TABLE 39.31 Management of Seizures Refractory to Medical Therapy

Incorrect Diagnosis

Review seizure type

Focal dyscognitive seizures may be mistaken for absence seizures

Reflex epilepsy with uncontrolled precipitating factors, photosensitivity, reading epilepsy

Repeat EEG with hyperventilation, photic stimulation, and sleep recording
If results are negative, consider nonepileptic paroxysmal disorders

Psychogenic nonepileptic behavioral events (see Table 39.26)

Migraine

Porphyria, hypoglycemia, hypocalcemia

Continuing seizures: admit for video/EEG monitoring to record the event

Inappropriate Medication

Review anticonvulsant levels

A second AED may have caused a drop in the serum level of a first-line drug

Review seizure type

Phenobarbital and carbamazepine may exacerbate atypical absence seizures

Drowsiness caused by phenobarbital and benzodiazepines may exacerbate tonic seizures

Phenytoin often worsens the function of patients with progressive myoclonus epilepsy syndromes

Noncompliance with Medication or Medical Advice

Check AED levels; ask patient to record medication doses taken

Check sleep habits, drug use; arrange review by social worker, psychiatrist

Inability to cope with epilepsy and avoidance of precipitating factors (adolescence, low intelligence, dysfunctional home situation)

Review all patient's prescribed and over-the-counter medications; urine drug screen for drug abuse

Exacerbation by other medication or toxins

Intercurrent Illness or Metabolic Complication from Another Medication

Serum Na^+, K^+, glucose, Ca^{2+}, Mg^{2+}, creatinine, liver function studies, complete blood cell count, pregnancy test

Intractable Epilepsies

Up to one third of cases of symptomatic focal epilepsy are refractory to current medical therapy

After an adequate attempt with two first-line medications and available new AEDs, refer for epilepsy surgery assessment

Symptomatic generalized epilepsies such as West syndrome and Lennox-Gastaut syndrome are often refractory

Need to reassess goals of therapy

Refer for surgical assessment if there are recurrent falls caused by tonic or atonic seizures in an older child

Epilepsy with progressive neurologic deterioration: e.g., brain tumor, inherited disorders of metabolism, degenerative neurologic disease, progressive myoclonus epilepsy, phakomatosis, systemic or cerebral vasculitis

Review history, family history, and physical examination; repeat neuroimaging; repeat EEG studies

AED, antiepileptic drug.

awareness could result in serious injury or death. If seizures are well controlled, minimal restrictions apply. In children with active seizures characterized by loss of consciousness, the physician makes judgments on the basis of an individual assessment considering the nature of the seizures, their frequency, and the degree of supervision during the activity in question. Driving restrictions vary from state to state; it is advisable that an adolescent be seizure-free for at least 2 years before applying for a driver's permit. In general, heavy-impact contact sports such as football are best avoided by children with active epilepsy but are not contraindicated for children in remission. In adolescents, some advice regarding birth control may be necessary because many adolescents are unaware of the interaction of AEDs and oral contraceptives.

BIBLIOGRAPHY

A bibliography is available at ExpertConsult.com.

40

Movement Disorders in Childhood

S. Anne Joseph

The clinical evaluation of childhood movement disorders depends on the crucial step of phenomenology that precedes and guides evaluation and management. Historically, many of the chronic movement disorders were identified as phenotypic syndromes based on clinical presentation, associated symptoms, and disease course. With the growing availability of genetic testing, more of the underlying metabolic and heredodegenerative disorders causing chronic movement disorders are being identified, producing a clearer understanding of the full clinical spectrum of these disorders (Fig. 40.1).

MOVEMENT DISORDERS

Movement disorders are a group of disorders where there is excessive movement or a paucity of voluntary movement (Table 40.1). The problem is not primarily due to weakness or abnormality of tone (spasticity). This group of disorders is characterized by difficulty initiating movement, abnormal control of voluntary movement, abnormalities of posture, or the presence of unwanted involuntary movements. Primary movement disorders imply a dysfunction in the basal ganglia and its connections or dysfunction of the cerebellum and its connections.

Movements disorders in general can be divided into two main categories. There may be a paucity of normal voluntary movements (**hypokinetic**) or the presence of abnormal involuntary movements (**hyperkinetic**). The hyperkinetic movement disorders include dystonia, ataxia, tremor, chorea, athetosis, ballismus, tics, and myoclonus. In the hypokinetic disorders there is a paucity or decreased amplitude of normal voluntary movements (hypokinesia), slow voluntary movements or difficulty initiating voluntary movement (bradykinesia), or loss of movement (akinesia). One example of a hypokinetic movement disorder is parkinsonism (resting tremor, slow voluntary movements, rigidity).

CHIEF COMPLAINT

The presenting symptom or chief complaint in a child with a movement disorder may be any of the following:
- Inability to sit still
- Gait abnormality
- Twitching
- "Weakness" or dropping things
- Shaking/trembling of the hands
- Unsteadiness
- Abnormal movements

The goal of the history and examination is to confirm the presence of the abnormal movement and correctly characterize it. Phenomenology is the study or observation of the abnormality. The clinical evaluation of movement disorders emphasizes the question "What type of abnormal movement is present?" or "What is the phenomenology?" rather than "Where is the lesion in the neurologic axis?" Phenomenology is determined by clinical examination, observation, and, when necessary, videotape review. Videotape review is especially useful when a paroxysmal movement is not witnessed during the clinic visit. Phenomenology links directly to potential differential diagnosis as well as choice of symptomatic therapy.

HISTORY

The clinical history in the child with a suspected movement disorder should include the course of the problem, whether acute or chronic. Specific information on whether the movements are paroxysmal (episodic) should be obtained. If the abnormal movements are paroxysmal, the history should indicate whether the abnormal movements are task specific (e.g., writer's cramp, which is a task-specific focal dystonia) and whether there are specific triggers that provoke the abnormal movements. Initiation of sudden movement that triggers dystonia is the hallmark of paroxysmal kinesigenic dystonia or dyskinesia (Table 40.2). Anticipation, emotional change, and stress can increase the frequency of tics. Excitement and emotional distress tend to bring out stereotypies. In general, abnormal movements do not awaken a child from sleep. Most movement disorders disappear in deep sleep except for ballismus and severe torsion dystonia. An abnormal movement that awakens a child from sleep should raise the suspicion for seizures.

The history should clarify the areas of the body affected, severity, and degree of functional impairment. Associated neurologic symptoms such as weakness, visual disturbance, seizures, and mental status changes imply a more widespread neurologic process than that primarily affecting the basal ganglia. Symptoms such as fever, rash, and pharyngitis suggest the presence of systemic illness.

The impact of the abnormal movement on the child's day-to-day function as well as limitations of function should be documented.

A detailed academic, behavioral, and psychiatric history should be obtained as movement disorders are often accompanied by behavioral, emotional, cognitive, and psychiatric comorbidities.

The history should include medications that have been recently started or stopped as well as chronic medications.

The child's birth and developmental history clarify whether the movement disorder occurred in a child who had no preceding neurologic conditions or in a child who had prior neurologic/developmental difficulty. The age of onset may provide a clue to the diagnosis (Fig. 40.2 and Table 40.3).

Family history of similar symptoms or a variation of the same type of problem suggests a genetically inherited disorder.

PHYSICAL EXAMINATION

The general physical examination should determine the presence of systemic signs.

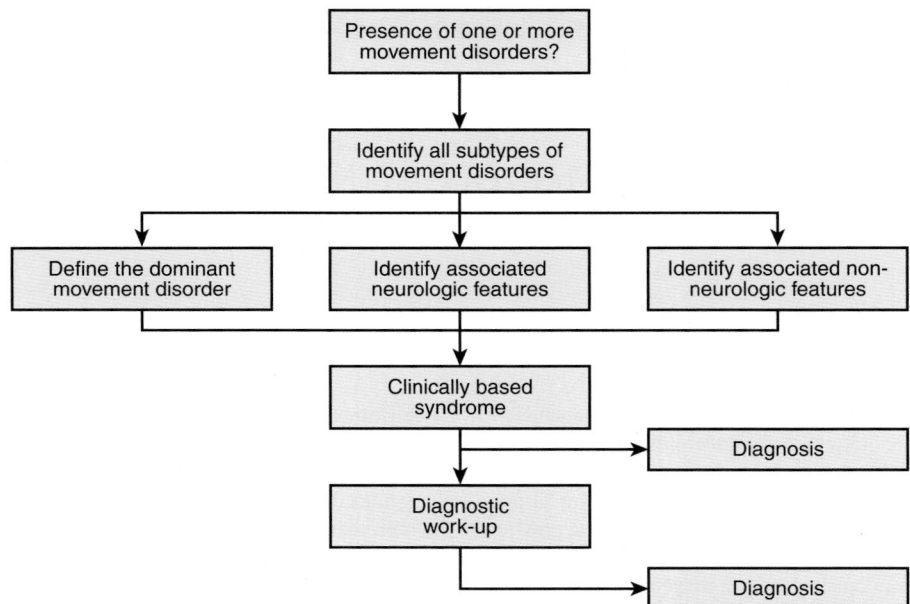

Fig. 40.1 A systematic approach to diagnosis in patients presenting with movement disorders. (From Abdo WF, van de Warrenburg BPC, Burn DJ, et al. The clinical approach to movement disorders. *Nat Rev.* 2010;6:29–37 [Fig. 1, p. 34].)

TABLE 40.1	Types of Childhood Movement Disorders
Dystonia	
Chorea, athetosis, ballismus	
Myoclonus	
Tremor	
Ataxia	
Stereotypies	
Tics	

The comprehensive neurologic examination determines whether there are other neurologic abnormalities besides involuntary movements. The mental status examination should include observations about alertness, attention, behavior, mood, and emotions. Cranial nerve examination should specifically determine whether there is nystagmus, limitation of eye movements, or weakness of the face, tongue, and jaw muscles. In general, the motor exam portion of the neurologic examination tends to emphasize muscle tone, strength, and the muscle stretch reflexes (deep tendon reflexes). This portion of the motor exam is effective in identifying the presence of weakness, spasticity, or hypotonia. Some features of involuntary movements such as the inability to maintain a voluntary contraction may be detected during the general motor examination. The template of the motor examination that starts with muscle tone, then goes on to testing of strength, and ends with reflex testing is useful for localization but insufficient for characterization of abnormal movements. Although it is assumed that general observation of the patient occurs throughout the visit, this alone is often insufficient for accurate characterization of the movement disorder. Therefore, once the motor exam that assesses tone, strength, and reflexes is completed, an additional portion of time should be allocated specifically for the observation of the involuntary movements to categorize them (phenomenology).

Posture and abnormal movements should be observed while the patient is in the recumbent position, in the seated position, standing upright with arms by the side, and then standing with arms and fingers outstretched. The child's ability to maintain a voluntary posture or voluntary muscle contraction should be assessed. This includes the ability to maintain grip while holding the examiner's hands and the ability to maintain tongue protrusion. Observation of tasks such as picking up, grasping, playing with small toys, pouring water from glass to glass, and writing is useful in the characterization of involuntary movements affecting the upper extremities, trunk, and neck. Stance, gait, swivel, running, stooping, and recovering should be assessed. Observation of speech is important as abnormal movements of the tongue, palate, lower face, and jaw affect the quality of speech. Abnormal movements of the laryngeal muscles affect voice production and quality. Motor impersistence and parakinesia (described in the section on chorea) should be recognized and identified when present. Paroxysmal movements such as tics may be briefly suppressible during a voluntary motor task, only to emerge once the task is accomplished. Tics when mild may not be witnessed in the clinic. Paroxysmal kinesigenic dystonia is often provoked by getting up from the seated position or at the beginning of a short sprint (see Table 40.2). Paroxysmal movements that occur between periods of normalcy may not be witnessed during the examination. When a paroxysmal movement is not witnessed in the clinic, videotape review is often helpful.

The gait examination is an essential component of the neurologic examination in a child with a movement disorder. The various gait abnormalities linked to the different movement disorders are listed in Table 40.4.

DYSTONIA

Dystonia is defined as a movement disorder in which involuntary sustained or intermittent muscle contractions cause twisting and repetitive movements, abnormal postures, or both. Dystonia is often initiated or worsened by voluntary action and associated with overflow muscle activation.

Dystonia can affect any part of the body. Terms used to describe the distribution of dystonia include focal, segmental, multifocal, and

TABLE 40.2 Classification of Primary and Epilepsy Paroxysmal Dyskinesias

	PKD	PNKD	PED	PHD*
Inheritance	AD	AD	AD	Usually sporadic
Gender M:F	4:1	2:1	2:3	7:3
Age at onset, yr	<1–20	<1–20s	2–30	4–20s
Phenomenology of abnormal movements	Dystonia with or without chorea/ballism, uni- or bilateral	Dystonia with or without choreoathetosis, uni- or bilateral, rarely spasticity	Dystonia, sometimes in combination with choreoathetosis, uni- or bilateral	Dystonia, chorea, ballism
Triggers	Sudden movement, change in direction, acceleration, startle	Alcohol, caffeine, emotions, fatigue	Prolonged exercise, muscle vibration	Sleep
Duration of paroxysms	Seconds up to 5 min	2 min–4 hr	5 min–2 hr	30 min up to 50 min
Frequency of paroxysms	1 per month to 100 per day	Few per week to few in a lifetime	Few per month	Few per year to few per night
Genetics	1. EKD1: 16p11.2-q12.1 (DYT10) with *PRRT2* gene within this region 2. EKD2: 16q13-q22.1 (DYT19) 3. EKD3: no variant on chromosome 16	1. *PNKD*: 2q35 (DYT8) 2. *SCL2A1*: chromosome 1 (DYT9) 3. *KCNMA1*: 10q22 4. Locus on 2q31 (DYT20)	1. *SCL2A1*: 1p35-p31.3 (DYT18)	1. *CHRNA4*: 20q13.2-q13.3 2. *CHRNB2*: chromosome 1q21 3. Locus on chromosome 15q24 4. Locus on chromosome 8p21
Treatment	Anticonvulsants (carbamazepine, phenytoin, others)	Avoiding triggers, benzodiazepines (clonazepam)	Avoiding triggers, ketogenic diet (in GLUT-1 deficiency)	Anticonvulsants

*Also known as autosomal dominant nocturnal frontal lobe epilepsy.
AD, autosomal dominant; AR, autosomal recessive; PED, paroxysmal exercise-induced dyskinesia; PHD, paroxysmal hypogenic dyskinesia (a seizure disorder); PKD, paroxysmal kinesigenic dyskinesia; PNKD, paroxysmal nonkinesigenic dyskinesia.

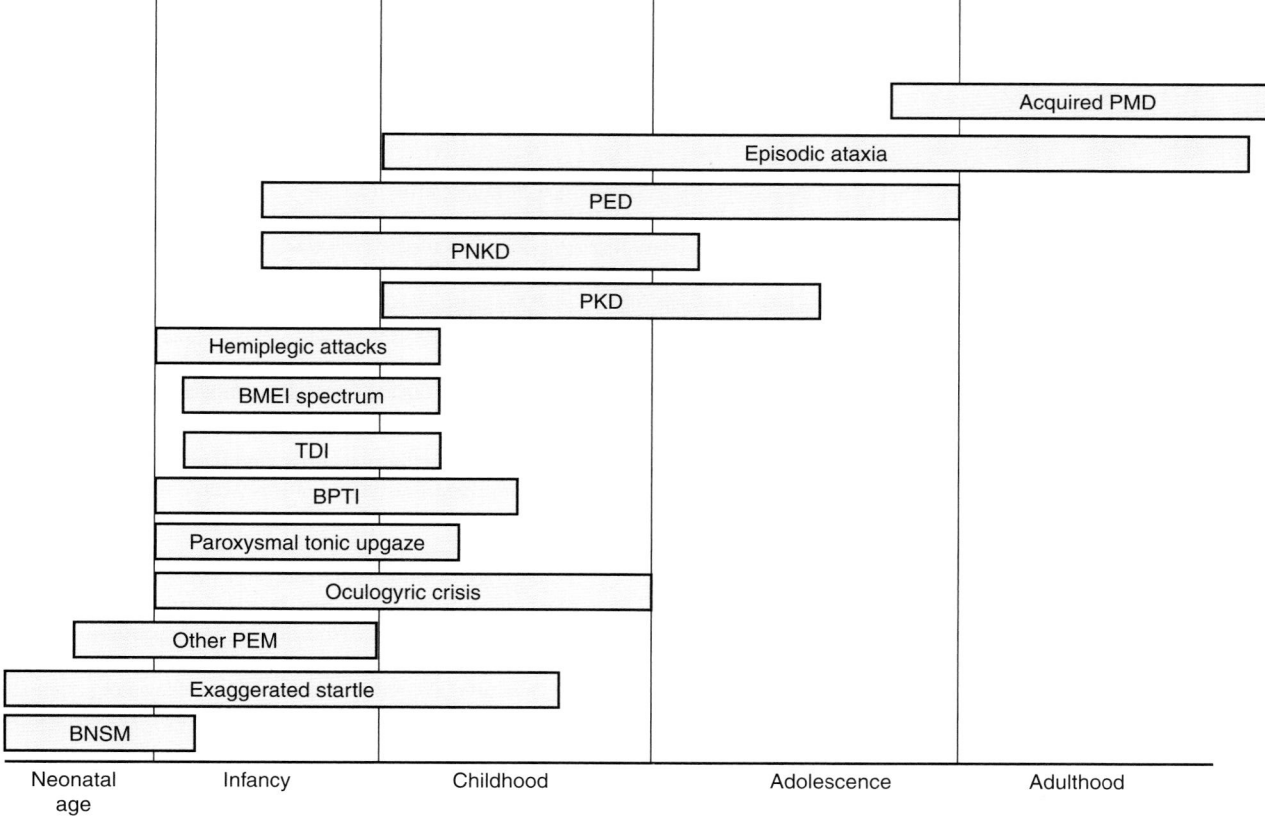

Fig. 40.2 Onset of different paroxysmal movement disorders (PMDs) according to age. BNSM, benign neonatal sleep myoclonus; BMEI, benign myoclonus of early infancy; BPTI, benign paroxysmal torticollis of infancy; PEM, paroxysmal eye movements; PED, paroxysmal exercise-induced dyskinesia; PKD, paroxysmal kinesigenic dyskinesia; PNKD: paroxysmal nonkinesigenic dyskinesia. (From Garone G, Capuano A, Travaglini L, et al. Clinical and genetic overview of paroxysmal movement disorders and episodic ataxias. *Intern J Mol Sci.* 2020;21:3630, Fig. 1.)

TABLE 40.3   IEMs Associated with Movement Disorder by Age at Onset

Prenatal	Neonatal	Infancy and Childhood	Adolescence and Adulthood
• Atypical Gaucher disease due to saposin C deficiency • Glycine encephalopathy	• Hyperekplexia or hyperexcitability: SUOX—isolated sulfite oxidase deficiency • Absence of voluntary movements or HRS: CLPB 3-methylglutaconic aciduria disorder, ADSL adenylosuccinate lyase deficiency, and PC pyruvate carboxylase deficiency • Myoclonic jerks: GLDC and ATM-glycine encephalopathy • Tremor, jitteriness, dystonia: HTRA2 3-methylglutaconic aciduria type 8	• Most of the IEMs presenting with MD begin in this age group • Onset before 2 yr of age: disorders of purine and creatine metabolism, neurotransmitter disorders, propionic and methylmalonic acidemia, glutaric aciduria type 1, disorders of cobalamin metabolism, biotinidase deficiency, manganese disorders (SLC39A8), GLUT-1 deficiency, mitochondrial disorders (including Leigh syndrome), SNX14 deficiency, CLN14 disease, Niemann-Pick type C, sialidosis, PMM2-CDG and other congenital disorders of glycosylation	• Adult-onset ataxia: 3-methylglutaconyl-CoA hydratase deficiency, 3-phosphoglycerate dehydrogenase deficiency, g-glutamylcysteine synthetase deficiency, OPA1 deficiency, very long-chain fatty acid elongase 4 deficiency, very long-chain fatty acid elongase 5 deficiency, abetalipoproteinemia, hereditary coproporphyria, complex MD (tremor, ataxia, myoclonus, perioral dyskinesias), cathepsin F deficiency (myoclonus, cerebellar ataxia, parkinsonism), neuronal ceroid lipofuscinosis type 4 (Parry type)

Many IEMs presenting with MD do not have a specific age of onset, and hence this parameter may not be extremely valuable in evaluating a particular case.

IEMs, inborn errors of metabolism; MD, movement disorder.

From Ortigoza-Escobar JD. A proposed diagnostic algorithm for inborn errors of metabolism presenting with movements disorders. *Front Neurol.* 2020;11:582160, Table 2.

TABLE 40.4   Gait Abnormalities in Movement Disorders

Ataxia	Wide-based stance. Extra steps to the side or backward to maintain balance while standing still. Extra steps to the side and a "drunken"-type gait with trunk sway when walking. Veering to the side and falls especially when turning or changing direction. Hurls self forward while running with a tendency to fall at the end of the run. In general, the mildly ataxic child tends to have a harder time standing still or walking slowly compared to running. When severe, standing, walking, and running are all significantly impaired.
Choreoathetosis	Lurching-type gait. Difficulty standing still or motionless with intermittent, random jerky movements of arms, neck, trunk, legs, and face giving rise to a "fidgety" appearance.
Tics	Normal gait and coordination.
Stereotypies	Normal gait.
Dystonia	If dystonia is focal and does not involve the legs or trunk, gait may be normal. In generalized dystonia, look for twisting and/or prominent lordosis of the trunk or twisting inward or medially of the legs. The feet may be inverted and plantarflexed. The abnormality tends to become more noticeable the longer the patient walks or runs. When dystonia is severe, the affected limbs tend to move "en bloc" with little apparent flexibility at the joints.
Tremor	Gait can be normal. In the parkinsonian patient there is difficulty initiating movement and the gait is often slow and "stiff." In the patient with orthostatic tremor, standing brings out the tremor in the legs. The tremor disappears or improves when seated or walking.
Myoclonus	Gait is usually normal. If myoclonus affects the trunk or legs, lightning-like jerks depending on the amplitude can result in falls.

generalized. Focal dystonia affects a single body part. Examples of focal dystonia include blepharospasm (involuntary spasms of the eyelids), torticollis (dystonia of the neck muscles), and writer's cramp (dystonia of the hand). Dystonia that affects two contiguous body parts is referred to as segmental dystonia (e.g., neck and arm or face and arm). Dystonia of two noncontiguous body parts is referred to as multifocal dystonia. Dystonia on one side of the body (e.g., left leg and left arm) is described as hemidystonia. Dystonia of more than one limb with involvement of the trunk is termed generalized dystonia. Dystonia may affect the larynx in isolation as a focal dystonia or as part of a more generalized dystonia giving rise to a "strangled," "whispery," or "breathy" quality of voice production. The distribution of dystonia may be sometimes helpful in localization. For example, acute hemidystonia may be due to pathology in the contralateral basal ganglia. The documentation of the distribution of dystonia also helps in the clinical detection of progression of disease over time.

The clinical evaluation of a patient with dystonia should delineate the time course of symptoms (acute, subacute, or chronic), distribution, whether it is present all the time or paroxysmal (if paroxysmal, whether it is provoked by initiation of movement), whether there is a diurnal variation (worse toward the end of the day), presence of other symptoms, and family history of similar conditions.

The etiology or underlying causes of pediatric dystonia are quite heterogenous. It is helpful in the clinical setting to differentiate acute dystonia from subacute or chronic dystonia. Acute dystonia in general suggests that the dysfunction in the brain is acute and therefore should be evaluated urgently. Associated symptoms of fever or systemic symptoms suggest a primary central nervous system (CNS) infection or inflammation that requires urgent evaluation.

Subacute and chronic dystonia are usually due to more slowly progressive acquired conditions, genetic disorders, or heredodegenerative conditions.

Acute Dystonia

When faced with a child presenting with acute dystonia, the evaluation should be conducted rapidly considering drugs/toxins, infection, inflammation, and acute ischemia as possible causes (Table 40.5).

TABLE 40.5   Differential Diagnosis of Acute Dystonia

Drugs: L-dopa, dopamine antagonists, fenfluramine, antipsychotics, antiemetics, anticonvulsants, flecainide, ergots, some calcium channel blocking agents

Toxins: carbon monoxide, magnesium, carbon disulfide, cyanide, methanol, disulfiram, wasp sting

Structural: stroke or lesion involving the basal ganglia

Infection: viral or bacterial encephalitis; other infections with focal brain lesions: tuberculosis, neurocysticercosis

Inflammation: involving the basal ganglia: acute disseminated encephalomyelitis (ADEM), *N*-methyl-D-aspartate receptor (NMDAR) encephalitis, rarely antiphospholipid antibody syndrome

TABLE 40.6   Differential Diagnosis of Paroxysmal Dystonia

Paroxysmal kinesigenic dystonia

Paroxysmal nonkinesigenic dystonia

Sandifer syndrome

Benign paroxysmal dystonia

Seizures

Alternating hemiplegia of childhood

In these situations, dystonia is often not isolated and is often accompanied by systemic symptoms and signs or other abnormalities in the neurologic system such as mental status changes, seizures, or acute psychiatric symptoms.

Infections

Viral or bacterial encephalitis may affect the basal ganglia, giving rise to an acute movement disorder with dystonia, usually in the setting of systemic symptoms and symptoms arising from multifocal involvement of the brain.

Inflammation

Postinfectious syndromes such as acute disseminated encephalomyelitis (ADEM) may present with a mixed movement disorder with dystonia.

N-methyl-D-aspartate receptor (NMDAR antibody) encephalitis is one of the more well-defined autoimmune disorders presenting with both movement disorders (chorea, dystonia) and neuropsychiatric symptoms. The symptoms usually evolve in a subacute to chronic fashion occasionally with acute worsening. A clinical suspicion of the condition, often with MRI signal changes in the hippocampi, mesial temporal lobes, thalamus, and brainstem (not all cases have MRI changes), with NMDAR antibody positivity in serum and cerebrospinal fluid (CSF) help clinch the diagnosis. Screening for an underlying tumor should be undertaken. Cases in children and adolescents have been linked to ovarian or testicular teratoma, seminoma, and small-cell lung cancer. The incidence of tumors in children with this condition is lower than that of adults. Management is with immune therapy following tumor resection (in the cases linked to tumors).

Acute Dystonic Reactions from Medications

Areas affected include the jaw muscles (trismus), neck (torticollis), back (opisthotonus), and extraocular muscles (oculogyric deviation of eyes). The patient may also have trouble chewing or swallowing. Although these sudden movements can mimic seizures, the patient remains fully aware of their surroundings and the dystonia resolves almost immediately with intravenous Benadryl. Commonly used medications such as antiemetics, anticonvulsants, and neuroleptics with dopamine-blocking properties can give rise to acute or delayed dystonic reactions.

Paroxysmal Dystonia

Paroxysmal dystonia in sleep should raise the suspicion of seizures and appropriate neurophysiologic evaluation may be needed to differentiate seizures from a movement disorder. Paroxysmal dystonic movements with alteration of consciousness should also raise the suspicion of seizures (Table 40.6).

Paroxysmal Kinesigenic Dyskinesia

Paroxysmal dystonia or choreoathetosis triggered by the initiation of movement suggests the diagnosis of paroxysmal kinesigenic dyskinesia (PKD) (see Table 40.2). PKD appears to be a heterogenous disorder in which initiation of movement triggers episodes of dystonia or choreoathetoid movements. The symptoms are often unilateral. Onset of symptoms is between ages 1 and 20 years. The episodes of dystonia are clinically distinct from seizures because consciousness is fully preserved, and the episodes are triggered by the initiation of movement. There is no associated pain with these episodes. The episodes last seconds to less than a minute. Some patients have additional neurologic disorders such as benign infantile epilepsy. Infantile convulsions followed by PKD in late childhood or adolescence is thought to be a variant form of PKD.

The diagnosis of PKD is confirmed by the absence of organic disease or structural abnormality on neuroimaging and the response to anticonvulsant medications such as carbamazepine, usually in low doses. This condition may be sporadic or familial. Familial PKD can be caused by variants in the proline-rich transmembrane protein 2 (*PRRT2*). However, this gene is found in only a portion of individuals with PKD. Variants in *KCNA1* are identified in some families with PKD. A diagnostic approach to paroxysmal dyskinesias is noted in Fig. 40.3.

Sandifer Syndrome

Episodic arching or dystonic posture of the neck and back in an infant or child can be seen in the setting of reflux. These episodes are usually related to feeds.

Benign Paroxysmal Torticollis

This is thought to be a migraine variant. In this condition children have paroxysmal episodes of head and/or trunk tilt that can last for hours or days, usually without other symptoms. Onset can be as early as the first year of life. Usually these episodes gradually decrease with age and resolve or evolve into episodes of migraine as the child grows older. At initial presentation, a detailed clinical evaluation should be undertaken, with appropriate testing to rule out organic causes. Careful monitoring should occur to determine whether these symptoms evolve into those of migraine or change to suggest a chronic neurogenetic dystonia that would warrant further evaluation.

Alternating Hemiplegia of Childhood

Alternating hemiplegia of childhood (AHC) is a rare condition presenting in childhood with episodes of temporary paralysis, often affecting one side of the body (hemiplegia). The episodes usually occur before age 18 months and last from minutes to days. Although not primarily a movement disorder, individuals can also have episodic choreoathetosis or dystonia in addition to episodes of hemiplegia. The episodes of abnormal movements can occur during or separate from the episodes of paralysis. These episodes can occur with triggers of stress, cold, or extreme tiredness. Sometimes there is no recognizable trigger. Other potential symptoms include

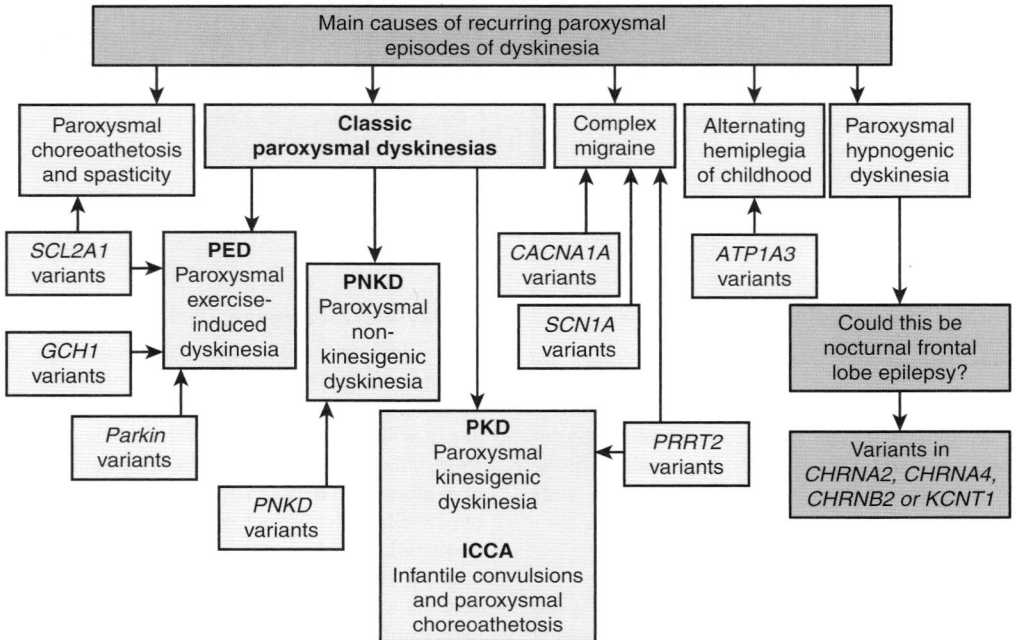

Fig. 40.3 Main genetic causes of recurring paroxysmal episodes of dyskinesia. (From Swaiman KF, Ashwal A, Ferriero DM, et al., eds. *Swaiman's Pediatric Neurology.* 6th ed. Philadelphia: Elsevier; 2018:722, Fig. 94-1.)

developmental delay, abnormal eye movements, and seizures. Most individuals have pathogenic variants in *ATP1A3*, and a smaller number have variants in *ATP1A2*. There is a high rate of de novo (sporadic) events, so many patients do not have a family history of similar symptoms. When there is a family history, it tends to follow an autosomal dominant pattern. Several treatments have been used including flunarizine, benzodiazepines, topiramate, oral adenosine triphosphate (ATP), coenzyme Q, acetazolamide, aripiprazole, and dextromethorphan, with various rates of success in aborting attacks or decreasing their frequency.

Chronic Dystonia

Classification of chronic dystonia is linked to etiology (Tables 40.7 and 40.8).

Primary pure dystonia: Dystonia is the only clinical symptom and there is no identifiable exogenous cause or other inherited degenerative disease.

Primary dystonia plus syndromes: Dystonia may be a prominent or early sign but there are other abnormal movements such as myoclonus, ataxia, or parkinsonism, and there is no evidence of neurodegeneration.

Primary paroxysmal dystonia: Dystonia occurs in brief episodes with normalcy in between. These disorders can be familial or sporadic.

Secondary dystonia: Dystonia is a symptom of an identified neurologic condition such as brain tumor, stroke, infection, inflammation, drugs, or toxins.

Heredodegenerative: Dystonia is one of many other neurologic signs or symptoms of a heredodegenerative or metabolic disorder (see Table 40.8).

Primary Dystonia

Early-Onset Dystonia

Early-onset idiopathic torsion dystonia caused by variants in *DYTI* (*TOR1A*/torsin A) represents the most common and most severe form of pure primary chronic dystonia in childhood. Previously referred to as dystonia musculorum deformans, it accounts for 16–53% of pediatric-onset dystonia in the non-Jewish population and for 80–90% of cases in the Ashkenazi Jewish population. The dystonia usually

TABLE 40.7   Types of Chronic Dystonia

PRIMARY (PURE) DYSTONIA

Autosomal Dominant
Idiopathic torsion dystonia: DYTI *(TOR1A)*
Idiopathic torsion dystonia/whispering dysphonia: DYT4 *(TUBB4A)*
Adolescent/early adulthood onset: DYT6 *(THAP1)*
DYT13

Autosomal Recessive
DYT17

PRIMARY DYSTONIA PLUS SYNDROMES

Autosomal Dominant
Guanosine triphosphate (GTP) cyclohydrolase-1: DYT5 (dopa-responsive dystonia)
Dystonia myoclonus: DYT11: epsilon sarcoglycan gene variant
Rapid-onset dystonia parkinsonism: DYT12
Alcohol-responsive dystonia myoclonic dystonia: DYT15

Autosomal Recessive
Young-onset dystonia parkinsonism: DYT16

PRIMARY PAROXYSMAL DYSTONIA
Paroxysmal kinesigenic dyskinesia (PKD): DYT10 *(PxMD-PRRT2)*
Paroxysmal nonkinesigenic dyskinesia (PNKD1): DYT8 *(PxMD-PNKD)*
Paroxysmal exercise-induced dyskinesia (PED): DYT18 *(PxMD-SLC2A1)* gene variants

SECONDARY DYSTONIA
Structural defects: stroke, tumor
Infection/inflammation
Drugs, toxins
Hypoxic-ischemic encephalopathy
Rasmussen syndrome

DYT, prefix nomenclature for numbering monogenic dystonias.

TABLE 40.8 Diseases with Complex Symptoms and Dystonia: Inherited Neurodegenerative/Metabolic Disorders

Disorder	MOI	Gene(s)	Clues to the Diagnosis
Neurodegenerative Diseases			
DRPLA (dentatorubral-pallidoluysian atrophy)	AD	*ATN1*	Huntington disease–like; prominent myoclonus
Huntington disease (Westphal variant juvenile- or childhood-onset HD)	AD	*HTT*	Family history; caudate atrophy on MRI
Huntington disease–like 2	AD	*JPH3*	African ancestry
Rett or Rett-like syndrome	XL, AD	*MECP2, FOXG1, GNB1*	Unusual stereotypies; autism
Parkin type of early-onset Parkinson disease	AR	*PARK2*	Abnormal DaTscan
Chorea-acanthocytosis	AR (and possible AD)	*VPS13A*	Acanthocytes in blood smear
McLeod neuroacanthocytosis syndrome	XL	*XK*	Weak expression of Kell antigens; acanthocytes in blood smear
Neuronal intranuclear inclusion disease	AD or sporadic	Unknown	MRI: high-intensity signal in cortico-medullary junction on DWI images; intranuclear inclusions on skin biopsies
Disorders Leading to Brain Calcification			
Primary familial brain calcification	AD	*PDGFB, PDGFRB, SLC20A2, XPR1*	MRI/CT: calcifications in basal ganglia, white matter, and cerebellum
Disorders of Heavy Metal Metabolism			
Wilson disease	AR	*ATP7B*	↓ Plasma ceruloplasmin; Kaiser-Fleischer corneal ring; face of the giant panda sign on MRI
Hypermanganesemia with dystonia, polycythemia, and cirrhosis	AR	*SLC30A10*	T1-weighted hyperintensities in basal ganglia and cerebellum on MRI
	AR	*SLC39A14*	
Neurodegeneration with Brain Iron Accumulation (NBIA)			
Mitochondrial membrane protein-associated neurodegeneration	AR	*C19orf12*	T2-weighted hypointensities in substantia nigra and globus pallidus on MRI; T2-weighted hyperintense streaking between hypointense internal globus pallidus and external globus pallidus
Aceruloplasminemia	AR	*CP*	MRI: hypointensity of basal ganglia, thalamus, red nucleus, occipital cortex, and cerebellar dentate nuclei on T2-weighted images
Woodhouse-Sakati syndrome	AR	*DCAF17*	Dystonia deafness syndrome; hypogonadism; alopecia
Fatty acid hydroxylase–associated neurodegeneration	AR	*FA2H*	MRI: hypointensity of the globus pallidus, confluent hyperintensities of white matter on T2-weighted images, pontocerebellar atrophy, thin corpus callosum
Neuroferritinopathy	AD	*FTL*	MRI: cystic lesions in the basal ganglia, bilateral pallidal necrosis; hypointensity of caudate, globus pallidus, putamen, substantia nigra, and red nuclei on T2-weighted images
Pantothenate kinase–associated neurodegeneration	AR	*PANK2*	Eye-of-the-tiger sign on MRI
PLA2G6-associated neurodegeneration	AR	*PLA2G6*	Cerebellar hypoplasia and T2-weighted high signal in the cerebellum on MRI
β-Propeller protein–associated neurodegeneration	XL	*WDR45*	MRI: hypointense globus pallidus and substantia nigra on T2-weighted images
Lipid Storage Disorders			
Neuronal ceroid-lipofuscinoses	AR; adult-onset AD or AR	*ATP13A2, CLN3, CLN5, CLN6, CLN8, CTSD, CTSF, DNAJC5, GRN, KCTD7, MFSD8, PPT1, TPP1*	Dementia; epilepsy; visual loss in children
Fucosidosis	AR	*FUCA1*	MRI: hypointensity of globus pallidus and substantia nigra on T2-weighted images; dysostosis multiplex
Niemann-Pick disease type C	AR	*NPC1, NPC2*	Supranuclear gaze palsy, splenomegaly, ↑ oxysterol blood levels
Sphingolipidosis			
Arylsulfatase A deficiency	AR	*ARSA*	Progressive demyelination

Continued

TABLE 40.8 Diseases with Complex Symptoms and Dystonia: Inherited Neurodegenerative/Metabolic Disorders—cont'd

Disorder	MOI	Gene(s)	Clues to the Diagnosis
Lysosomal Storage Diseases			
Krabbe disease	AR	GALC	Progressive demyelination, enlargement of optic nerve and chiasm
GM1-gangliosidosis	AR	GLB1	MRI: hyperintensity of caudate nucleus and putamen with signs of diffuse hypomyelination on T2-weighted images
GM2-gangliosidosis, AB variant	AR	GM2A	Indistinguishable from GM1-gangliosidosis
Leukodystrophies			
Creatine deficiency syndromes		GAMT, GATM, SLC6A8	MR spectroscopy: no creatine peak
Pelizaeus-Merzbacher disease	XL	PLP1	Hypomyelination on MRI
Disorders of Purine Metabolism			
Lesch-Nyhan syndrome	XL	HPRT1	Self-mutilation; ↑ uric acid in plasma and urine
Mitochondrial Disorders			
Leigh syndrome	AR, mt	Pathogenic variants in the mtDNA; nuclear genes*	Bilateral basal ganglia lesions on MRI; ↑ lactate levels on magnetic resonance spectroscopy
Leber hereditary optic neuropathy	Mt	Pathogenic variants in the mtDNA	Optic nerve changes on fundoscopy
MELAS (mitochondrial encephalomyopathy, lactic acidosis, and strokelike episodes)	Mt	Pathogenic variants in the mtDNA	Deep white matter changes and strokelike lesions on MRI
MERRF (myoclonus epilepsy associated with ragged-red fibers)	Mt	Pathogenic variants in the mtDNA	Progressive myoclonus, epilepsy, and ataxia; muscle biopsy showing ragged-red fibers; ↑ lactate in serum and CSF
POLG-related disorders	AR, AD	POLG	Progressive external ophthalmoplegia, ataxia
Deafness-dystonia-optic neuronopathy syndrome (Mohr-Tranebjaerg syndrome)	XL	TIMM8A	Dystonia (particularly oromandibular) and deafness
Other dystonia-deafness syndromes	AD	SERAC1, SUCLA2	Dystonia and deafness
	XL	DDP	Dystonia and deafness
Organic Acidurias			
D-2-hydroxyglutaric aciduria	AR	D2HGDH	Newborn screening
Glutaric aciduria type 1	AR	GCDH	Newborn screening
Methylmalonic acidemia	AR	MCEE, MMAA, MMAB, MMADHC, MMUT	Newborn screening
Aminoacidurias			
Homocystinuria caused by cystathionine β-synthase deficiency	AR	CBS	Homocysteine levels ↑ in blood
Phenylketonuria	AR	PAH	Newborn screening
Hartnup disorder	AR	SLC6A19	Levels of neutral amino acids ↑ in urine
Disorders of Biotin Metabolism			
Biotinidase deficiency	AR	BTD	Newborn screening
Disorders of Thiamine Metabolism			
Biotin-thiamine-responsive basal ganglia disease	AR	SLC19A3	Recurrent subacute encephalopathy; symmetric and bilateral edematous lesions in caudate nucleus, putamen, and cortex on MRI
Disorders of Galactose Metabolism			
Classic galactosemia and clinical variant galactosemia	AR	GALT	Newborn screening
Encephalopathy with Uncertain Pathogenesis			
Aicardi-Goutières syndrome	AD, AR	ADAR, RNASEH2A, RNASEH2B, RNASEH2C, SAMHD1, TREX1	Early-onset encephalopathy; chilblain lesions

Disorders with ataxia as a predominant feature, particularly AD SCA (e.g., SCA3) and AR early-onset ataxias (e.g., ataxia-telangiectasia)

*Genes associated with mitochondrial DNA-associated Leigh syndrome and NARP: *BCS1L, C20ORF7, C8ORF38, COX10, COX15, FOXRED1, MTFMT, NDUFA2, NDUFA9, NDUFA10, NDUFA12, NDUFAF2, NDUFAF6, NDUFS1, NDUFS3, NDUFS4, NDUFS7, NDUFS8, SDHA, SURF1.*
AD, autosomal dominant; AR, autosomal recessive; CSF, cerebrospinal fluid; DWI, diffusion-weighted imaging; MOI, mode of inheritance; mt, mitochondrial; SCA, spinocerebellar ataxia; XL, X-linked.

Klein C, Lohmann K, Marras C, et al. Hereditary dystonia overview. In: *GeneReviews* [Internet]. Seattle: University of Washington, 1993–2021. 2003 Oct 28 [updated 2017 Jun 22], Table 4.

begins in childhood or early adolescence as a focal dystonia either in the hand or foot and gradually progresses. Rarely the neck or facial muscles may be involved first. Treatment is symptomatic.

Dopa-Responsive Dystonia

This group of disorders with onset in childhood, adolescence, or early adulthood presents with dystonia with dramatic and sustained response to levodopa. This condition was initially referred to as dopa-responsive dystonia (DRD) with marked diurnal fluctuation or Segawa syndrome. Symptoms have marked diurnal fluctuation, with mild or minimal dystonia in the morning (after overnight sleep), progressively worsening toward the end of the day. Several clinically similar conditions with dystonia have been described, all with the common features of diurnal variation and responsiveness to levodopa. The collective group of DRD appears to be a fairly heterogenous group with either a dominant or recessive pattern of inheritance. Although most cases of DRD in childhood are due to pathogenic variants in guanosine triphosphate (GTP) cyclohydrolase 1 (*GCH1*), other abnormalities such as compound heterozygous variants in *GCH1*, tyrosine hydroxylase (*TH*), sepiapterin reductase (*SPR*), or 6-pyruvoyltetrahydropterin synthase (*6-PTS*) genes have been found. Older adolescents with symptoms of DRD have been linked to juvenile parkinsonism and *Parkin* gene variants. Not all clinical forms have an identified genotype. CSF neurotransmitter metabolites show abnormalities in the dopamine metabolites neopterin and biopterin.

The age of onset is around 6 years, often with dystonia of the foot as the first presenting symptom. This gradually progresses to generalized dystonia. However, onset can be as young as infancy with dystonia and rigidity. *It is not uncommon for such young children to be misdiagnosed as having cerebral palsy.* Treatment with levodopa results in a dramatic improvement. In a child with chronic dystonia without an identified etiology, a trial of levodopa should be considered.

Symptomatic Dystonia

Acute or subacute hemidystonia should alert the clinician of the possibility of a space-occupying lesion in the contralateral basal ganglia such as a tumor or a stroke.

Hemidystonia has been reported as a symptom of Rasmussen syndrome.

Dystonia has also been reported as an early symptom of ataxia-telangiectasia occurring prior to the onset of ataxia.

Wilson Disease

Wilson disease is an autosomal recessive disorder of copper metabolism that manifests with damage to hepatic cells and the basal ganglia. The disorder in childhood usually presents with hepatic symptoms (see Chapter 18). Adolescent patients present with psychiatric and behavioral manifestations, while in young adults, dystonia, parkinsonism, tremor, and abnormal gait can be seen. Although rare, movement disorders have been reported in younger children with Wilson disease. Children with Wilson disease and movement disorder present with dystonia, tremor, ataxia, or gait abnormality with rigidity. The initial presentation may be any one of these in isolation or in combination, remaining stable for years before progression occurs. The presence of Kayser-Fleischer (K-F) rings in the eyes (due to copper deposition in the Descemet membrane of the cornea) is a helpful sign but not pathognomonic when present (Fig. 40.4). This can sometimes be seen with bedside ophthalmoscopy but often requires a slit-lamp examination to be visualized. The diagnosis of Wilson disease is made with a low serum copper and ceruloplasmin, increased 24-hour urinary copper excretion, and the presence of K-F corneal rings or detection of biallelic *ATP7B* pathogenic variants on molecular genetic testing.

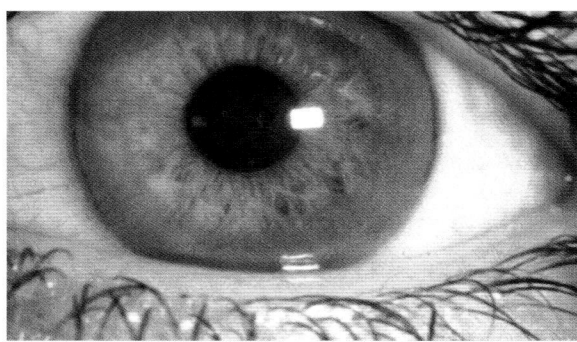

Fig. 40.4 Kayser-Fleischer ring. There is a brown discoloration at the outer margin of the cornea because of the deposition of copper in the Descemet membrane. Here it is clearly seen against the light green iris. Slit-lamp examination is required for secure detection. (From Ala A, Walker AP, Ashkan K, et al. Wilson's disease. *Lancet*. 2007;369:397–408.)

When a diagnosis remains unclear, the definitive test is a liver biopsy for measurement of copper concentration in liver tissue. Treatment is lifelong with copper chelating agents.

Lesch-Nyhan Syndrome

This X-linked condition is characterized by severe, impulsive self-mutilatory behaviors. It results from a deficiency of the enzyme hypoxanthine-guanine-phosphoribosyltransferase (HGPRT), which is associated with hyperuricemia, developmental delays, and severe intellectual disability. Symptoms of motor dysfunction and dystonia or choreoathetosis often precede the self-mutilatory behavior, with children mistakenly given a diagnosis of cerebral palsy. Serum uric acid levels are elevated, and diagnosis is confirmed with enzyme testing or gene sequencing.

Rasmussen Syndrome

This immune-based disorder usually affects one side of the brain causing refractory focal seizures and progressive unilateral loss of motor function (hemiparesis) and intellectual disability. The progressive loss of function occurs because of chronic inflammation and atrophy of one hemisphere of the brain.

Although primarily linked to focal seizures and epilepsia partialis continua, basal ganglia involvement resulting in unilateral dystonia or chorea has been reported.

Niemann-Pick Type C

Niemann-Pick type C is a lysosomal storage disorder caused by defects in intracellular cholesterol and lipid transport. The clinical manifestations typically begin in childhood or early adulthood and include slowly progressive dementia, often with seizures. Most patients also have progressive ataxia with a *supranuclear vertical gaze palsy*, although other phenotypes with dystonia, spasticity, myoclonus, or parkinsonism may also occur.

Management of Dystonia

Management in primary dystonia is symptomatic. Anticholinergic medications, dopamine-blocking and -depleting agents, baclofen, and benzodiazepines have been utilized, often with incomplete benefit and with side effects limiting dose escalation. Botulinum toxin can be effective in focal dystonia. In generalized dystonia, botulinum toxin injections can be helpful when administered to the most disabling sites. Levodopa is the mainstay of treatment for DRD. Other forms of dystonia may respond partially to levodopa. Since complete response to levodopa can be clinically diagnostic for DRD, a trial of levodopa should be considered in every child who presents with a primary dystonia.

Deep brain stimulation has been utilized with some success in cases refractory to medication.

Management for secondary dystonia targets the underlying etiology as well as symptom treatment.

CHOREA/ATHETOSIS/BALLISMUS

Chorea is defined as an ongoing random-appearing sequence of one or more discrete involuntary movements or movement fragments.

Ballismus is defined as chorea that affects proximal joints such as the shoulder or hip. This leads to more dramatic, large-amplitude movements with a "flinging" or "flailing" quality.

Athetosis is defined as a slow, continuous, writhing movement that prevents maintenance of a stable posture.

Chorea and athetosis often coexist and are referred to as choreoathetosis.

Choreic movements appear random due to their timing, duration, and anatomic location. These movements are usually rapid and tend to have a jerky quality. Chorea is present during voluntary movements as well as at rest. Children with chorea tend to appear "fidgety." Chorea is distinguished from tremor by its randomness and lack of rhythmicity.

Choreoathetosis is usually accompanied by two clinical phenomena. Motor impersistence observed in choreoathetosis is the inability to sustain voluntary contraction of muscles. The individual often drops objects in their grasp. During the examination when asked to grasp the examiner's hand and sustain a grip, repetitive intermittent involuntary relaxation and voluntary contraction trying to maintain this muscle contraction give rise to the **milkmaid grip**. The combination of random, jerky movements of chorea and motor impersistence gives rise to the **piano playing movements** of fingers while trying to hold arms and fingers outstretched. If chorea is generalized or affects the buccolingual muscles, there is inability to keep the tongue protruded (**darting tongue**).

The second phenomenon seen in chorea is **parakinesia**. These are voluntary movements made to mask or camouflage the involuntary movements.

Chorea can be acquired or occur in the setting of an underlying chronic disorder.

Acute Chorea

Acute chorea tends to be acquired (Table 40.9) and should be evaluated urgently. In a child with acute chorea the following questions should be answered at the initial evaluation:

1. Is there evidence for a primary CNS infection or a postinfectious condition such as ADEM or Sydenham chorea?
2. If the chorea is unilateral, is there evidence of a focal lesion such as an acute stroke or lesion in the basal ganglia?
3. Is there evidence of systemic involvement?
4. Is there evidence for cardiac involvement?
5. Are any of the following tests needed:
   a. ECG/echocardiogram
   b. Neuroimaging: MRI of the brain with magnetic resonance angiography
   c. ASO titers and anti-DNase B titers
   d. Antinuclear antibody (ANA), antiphospholipid antibody panel
   e. Throat swab for culture
   f. CSF analysis for infection or inflammation

Sydenham Chorea

This is one of the most common causes of acquired chorea affecting children between the ages of 5 and 15 years. The onset is often insidious

---

TABLE 40.9 **Causes of Acute Choreoathetosis**

Acute infection/encephalitis

Autoimmune: Sydenham chorea, lupus, antiphospholipid antibody syndrome, acute disseminated encephalomyelitis (ADEM), *N*-methyl-D-aspartate receptor (NMDAR) encephalitis, system lupus erythematosus (SLE)

Drug induced: withdrawal emergent syndrome (abrupt discontinuation of a dopamine receptor antagonist), anticonvulsants (phenytoin, carbamazepine), tardive dyskinesia (long-term side effects of dopamine receptor antagonists and neuroleptics), amphetamines, cocaine, tricyclic antidepressants

Toxins: alcohol, anoxia, carbon monoxide, toluene, thallium, mercury, manganese

Systemic disease: hyperthyroidism, hypoparathyroidism, hypoglycemia, hyperglycemia

Vascular: bilateral chorea has been linked to cardiopulmonary bypass surgery: Stroke from ischemia, embolus, hemorrhage, moyamoya disease, midsize vessel cerebral vasculopathy usually unilateral at onset

---

and occurs after a streptococcal infection. The chorea is usually generalized but can affect one side more than the other at onset. Sydenham chorea is considered a major clinical criterion of acute rheumatic fever. The onset of chorea and emotional lability in an otherwise healthy child should raise the suspicion of this condition. The diagnosis is based on finding a link to a previous streptococcal infection with a throat swab (culture) and high blood titers of streptococcal antibodies (ASO, anti-DNase B), or the presence of arthritis, carditis, or cardiac valvular disease. This condition occurs anywhere from a few weeks to 8 months after the acute streptococcal infection or exposure to streptococcus. Therefore, at the onset of choreoathetosis, the characteristic signs of an acute streptococcal pharyngitis are no longer present. About 25% of individuals with rheumatic fever develop Sydenham chorea, and in one series, up to 50% of individuals who presented with Sydenham chorea had cardiac involvement. Differential diagnosis in the absence of laboratory tests that support previous streptococcal exposure includes other inflammatory conditions such as antiphospholipid antibody syndrome or lupus. In most cases, the chorea in Sydenham chorea gradually resolves but can take anywhere from weeks to a year to disappear. In some cases, chorea persists chronically. *Sydenham chorea can recur with reinfection.* Antiepileptic agents such as levetiracetam, carbamazepine, benzodiazepines, valproate, and low-dose dopamine-depleting agents have been utilized for symptomatic treatment to decrease the chorea in Sydenham chorea. There has been some support for using a short course of oral steroids or intravenous immunoglobulin based on the idea that ongoing inflammation is contributing to the symptoms. In every child suspected of Sydenham chorea a cardiology evaluation is recommended, and once the diagnosis is confirmed, management is similar to that of rheumatic fever, with long-term antibiotic prophylaxis against streptococcal infection. Neuroimaging of the brain with MRI is done to rule out alternative causes.

Acute Disseminated Encephalomyelitis

ADEM is thought to be an immune-based disorder of the brain and spinal cord, triggered by a preceding environmental stimulus such as a viral/bacterial infection or immunization.

The diagnosis is made based on the acute presentation of a child with neurologic signs and symptoms pointing to multifocal brain disease, diffuse/scattered fairly discrete signal changes on the MRI of the brain and/or spinal cord, occasional involvement of the optic nerves (optic neuritis), the absence of a primary CNS infection (bacterial or viral), and either normal CSF or mild CSF pleocytosis with elevated protein. The patient often looks ill and may have a fever. Although this condition is thought to predominantly affect white matter, signal changes are often seen in the basal ganglia and abnormal movements such as choreoathetosis can be part of the presenting symptoms. At presentation acute encephalitis and ADEM can be difficult to differentiate. When suspected, the evaluation, which includes neuroimaging and CSF evaluation, should be performed urgently. The treatment of ADEM targets suppressing inflammation with intravenous corticosteroids. Intravenous immunoglobulins or plasmapheresis may benefit children who fail to respond to corticosteroids.

Drug-Induced Chorea

Chorea can be seen when dopamine receptor blocking drugs are abruptly withdrawn. This is referred to as **withdrawal emergent syndrome**. The chorea gradually resolves within weeks to months. Slow tapering of the medication when possible instead of abrupt withdrawal decreases the risk of this syndrome. **Tardive syndromes** or tardive dyskinesia can be seen with the chronic use of neuroleptic agents for psychiatric disorders, as well as some neurologic and gastrointestinal disorders. Neuroleptics such as phenothiazines, haloperidol, risperidone, quetiapine, and olanzapine, and antiemetics such as

metoclopramide and prochlorperazine, have been linked to the occurrence of chorea late in the course of treatment. The risk of tardive dyskinesia in children appears lower than adults but has been reported as high as 9.8% after long-term exposure.

Chronic Chorea

Chronic choreoathetosis in childhood is due to disorders that may be static (perinatal hypoxic ischemic encephalopathy or malformations of brain development) or progressive (genetic, metabolic, or heredodegenerative diseases).

Disorders that present with chronic chorea are broadly considered as isolated (Table 40.10), in which chorea may be the only symptom, or a part of more complex disorders (Table 40.11), with other neurologic symptoms as well as chorea.

TABLE 40.10 Genetic Disorders with Chorea as the Primary Symptom

Benign hereditary chorea
Paroxysmal kinesigenic dyskinesia
Paroxysmal nonkinesigenic dyskinesia

TABLE 40.11 List of Monogenic Causes of Chorea

Gene	Main Associated Phenotype	Gene Product	Inheritance	Age of Onset	Diagnostic Clues
HTT	Huntington disease	Huntingtin	AD (CAG expansion)	Childhood to late adulthood	Cognitive decline, psychiatric disturbances Progressive course MRI: caudate nucleus head atrophy
PRNP	HDL1	Prion protein	AD (octapeptide coding repeat expansion)	Adulthood	Dementia and psychiatric features Possible parkinsonism at onset and longer survival than HD
JPH3	HDL2	Junctophilin 3	AD (CAG/CTG expansion)	Adulthood	Parkinsonism may be first manifestation High frequency in people with Black African ancestry
TBP	HDL4 Spinocerebellar ataxia type 17	TATA box-binding protein	AD (CAG expansion)	Childhood to adulthood	Ataxia and cognitive decline Frequent parkinsonism MRI: cerebellar atrophy
ATN1	Dentatorubral-pallidoluysian atrophy	Atrophin-1	AD (CAG expansion)	Childhood to adulthood	Seizures, myoclonus, and cognitive decline MRI: cerebellar and brainstem atrophy (especially pons) High frequency in Japan
C9orf72	FTD/MND	Chromosome 9 Open reading frame 72	AD (GGGGCC expansion)	Childhood to adulthood	Prominent cognitive and psychiatric features Pyramidal signs MRI: diffuse cerebral atrophy
FTL	Neuroferritinopathy	Ferritin light chain	AD	Teenage to late adulthood	Action-specific facial dystonia Reduced ferritin plasma levels MRI: iron deposition in basal ganglia and cortical pencil lining
SLC20A2	Idiopathic basal ganglia calcification (IBGC)	Na-dependent phosphate transporter type 2	AD	Symptoms: early to late adulthood	CT scan: basal ganglia, cerebellar dentate nuclei, and subcortical white matter calcification
PDGFB		Platelet-derived growth factor β polypeptide		Calcium deposition: childhood to adolescence	
PDGFRB		Platelet-derived growth factor receptor β			
XPR1		Xenotropic and polytropic retroviruses receptor			

Continued

TABLE 40.11   List of Monogenic Causes of Chorea—cont'd

Gene	Main Associated Phenotype	Gene Product	Inheritance	Age of Onset	Diagnostic Clues
VPS13A	Chorea-acanthocytosis	Chorein	AR	Early adulthood	Severe oromandibular dystonia with lip and tongue biting Head drops Peripheral axonal neuropathy Elevated serum CK MRI: caudate nucleus head atrophy
XK	McLeod syndrome	Kell blood group protein	X-linked recessive	Adulthood	Peripheral sensorimotor neuropathy Cardiomyopathy Elevated serum CK
ATM	Ataxia-telangiectasia	Ataxia-telangiectasia mutated gene	AR	Childhood to adulthood	Oculocutaneous telangiectases Sensorimotor neuropathy Elevated serum α-fetoprotein Predisposition to malignancy MRI: cerebellar atrophy
APTX SETX PNKP	Ataxia with oculomotor apraxia (AOA) types 1, 2, and 4	Aprataxin Senataxin Polynucleotide kinase 3′-phosphatase	AR	Childhood to adulthood	Sensorimotor neuropathy Hypoalbuminemia in AOA1 Hypercholesterolemia in AOA1 and AOA4 Elevated α-fetoprotein in AOA2 and AOA4 MRI: cerebellar atrophy
RNF216	Gordon-Holmes syndrome	Ring finger protein 216	AR	Adulthood	Hypogonadism MRI: cerebellar atrophy
NKX2-1	NKX2-1-related chorea	Thyroid transcription factor 1	AD/de novo	Infancy	Nonprogressive course Hypotonia and early falls Learning difficulties Frequent pulmonary and thyroid dysfunction
ADCY5	ADCY5-related chorea	Adenylate cyclase 5	AD/de novo	Infancy to childhood	Normal cognition Dystonia and myoclonus may become prominent with age Severe diurnal and nocturnal exacerbations Axial hypotonia and delayed milestones in most severe cases
PDE10A	PDE10A-related chorea	Phosphodiesterase 10A	De novo/AR	Infancy to childhood	Delayed milestones and language development and dysarthria in cases with recessive variants MRI: symmetric T2-hyperintense bilateral striatal lesions in cases with dominant de novo variants
GPR88	GPR88-related chorea	G protein–coupled receptor 88	AR	Childhood	Language delay and learning disabilities
GNAO1	Early infantile epileptic encephalopathy type 17 (Ohtahara syndrome)	Gαo	De novo	Infancy to childhood	Progressive and severe movement disorder associated with developmental delay, with or without seizures
FOXG1	Congenital Rett disease	Forkhead box G1	De novo	Infancy to early childhood	Severe intellectual disability, absent language, acquired microcephaly MRI: corpus callosum abnormalities, frontal or frontotemporal underdevelopment, mild cerebellar hypoplasia, and delayed myelination
SYT1	Severe motor delay and intellectual disability	Synaptotagmin-1	De novo	Infancy	Severe delayed motor development without seizures
SCN8A	Early infantile epileptic encephalopathy type 13 BFIS	NaV1.6α-subunit of voltage-gated Na channels	AD/de novo	Infancy to childhood	Paroxysmal dystonia/chorea triggered by sudden movements or emotional stress Focal EEG abnormalities during attacks

AD, autosomal dominant; AR, autosomal recessive; BFIS, benign familial infantile seizures; CK, creatine kinase; HD, Huntington disease; HDL, Huntington disease–like.

From Menacci NE, Carecchio M. Recent advances in genetics of chorea. *Curr Opin Neurol.* 2016;29(4):486–495.

Benign Hereditary Chorea

Benign hereditary chorea (BHC) was initially described clinically as a rare autosomal dominant disorder presenting with chorea in early childhood and a family history of the same. Although it was recognized that some children with this condition also had associated hypotonia, mildly delayed motor development, and tremor, there was usually no progression of symptoms and apart from chorea children usually remained well. The family history often helped confirm this clinical diagnosis. The disorder is caused by a pathogenic variant in the *NKX2.1* (*TITF1*) gene. Since the identification of the genetic etiology, there has been a phenotypic expansion leading to the consideration of *NKX2-1*-related disorders that range from BHC to choreoathetosis, congenital hypothyroidism, and neonatal respiratory distress (known as **brain-lung-thyroid syndrome**). Interestingly, some of the original families described as having BHC did not harbor identifiable variants in this gene, suggesting that this disorder may be genetically heterogeneous.

Classical BHC presents with hypotonia in infancy and delayed motor milestones, with the onset of chorea around age 2 years or earlier. The chorea is generalized, increasing with excitement or stress. Usually the chorea remains stable with some improvement in adolescence and young adulthood. Other types of movements seen in individuals who have pathogenic variants in *NKX2.1* include dystonia, ataxia, tremor, sudden falls (nonepileptic drops), and tics. These symptoms may occur with or without chorea. Speech difficulty consisting of dysarthria or stuttering have been reported in BHC. Cognitive skills were previously thought to be normal in BHC; however, recent studies show conflicting results, with some individuals having higher cognitive skills than expected for age, and some lower. Depression, psychosis, attention-deficit/hyperactivity disorder (ADHD), and obsessive-compulsive disorder (OCD) have all been reported with *NKX2.1* gene variants. *NKX2.1* testing should be considered in individuals with neonatal hypotonia, motor developmental delay, and early-onset chorea and/or dystonia. The presence of lung or thyroid symptoms should further increase the suspicion of this disorder.

Treatment

Treatment of chorea should target the underlying cause. Symptom treatment can be with dopamine receptor blocking agents (neuroleptics and tetrabenazine), although potential side effects of these medications should be taken into consideration. Other medications that have been used for symptomatic treatment of chorea include anticonvulsants, specifically sodium valproate, levetiracetam, and the benzodiazepines.

ATAXIA

Ataxia is unsteadiness out of proportion to the degree of weakness and involuntary movements. True ataxia implies a disorder of the cerebellum and its connections.

Many of the ataxic disorders have myoclonus, chorea, and dystonia as part of the phenotype. These abnormal movements when present do not directly cause the unsteadiness. The presence of other abnormal movements and symptoms in an ataxic child may be helpful in identification of the underlying cause.

The clinical exam in a child suspected of having ataxia should focus on the presence of cerebellar tremor (intention tremor), nystagmus, dysarthria, and truncal titubation. Stance, gait, and coordination are important parts of the examination of the ataxic child. The clinical exam should also determine whether other abnormal movements such as choreoathetosis, myoclonus, or dystonia are present. In every child with ataxia, careful observation of eye movements should occur specifically looking for the presence of opsoclonus. This sign may be subtle and difficult to detect, especially if the child is irritable. Signs that point

TABLE 40.12 Causes of Ataxia
Acute Ataxia
Cerebellar stroke: embolic/dissection/thrombosis of the vertebral arteries, hemorrhage
Acute hydrocephalus
Acute decompensation from a posterior fossa tumor (astrocytoma, ependymoma, medulloblastoma), primitive neurectodermal tumor (PNET), cerebellar hemangioblastoma (von Hippel–Lindau syndrome)
Postinfectious: postinfectious cerebellar ataxia, acute disseminated encephalomyelitis (ADEM), Miller Fisher variant of Guillain-Barré syndrome (acute inflammatory demyelinating polyradiculoneuropathy [AIDP])
Drug ingestion/toxins
Subacute Ataxia
Paraneoplastic: opsoclonus-myoclonus ataxic encephalopathy
Brain tumor: posterior fossa/cerebellar/brainstem tumors
Hydrocephalus
Celiac disease

to the underlying etiology include cutaneous/conjunctival telangiectasia (ataxia telangiectasia) and opsoclonus (opsoclonus-myoclonus ataxic encephalopathy) (Tables 40.12, 40.13, and 40.14).

Opsoclonus-Myoclonus Ataxic Encephalopathy/Opsoclonus Myoclonus Syndrome

The diagnosis of this syndrome is entirely clinical. In this condition, otherwise healthy children between the ages of 1 and 4 years (mean age of onset about 18 months) develop ataxia over days to weeks. At onset the condition may mimic acute cerebellar ataxia, which tends to be a self-limiting postinfectious disorder, resolving within a few weeks. However, in opsoclonus myoclonus syndrome (OMS) the ataxia does not resolve within a few weeks but tends to gradually worsen, or remain the same, with gradual increase in irritability and the occurrence of myoclonus and opsoclonus. Myoclonus and opsoclonus may be present at onset but may occur after the onset of ataxia. When opsoclonus and myoclonus are mild, they can be missed during the examination of an irritable ataxic child. The clinical diagnosis is much easier to arrive at when the triad of symptoms—myoclonus, opsoclonus, and ataxia—are present from onset or when opsoclonus is severe. However, the diagnosis may be missed for months when opsoclonus is mild and starts indolently a few weeks after the onset of ataxia.

Opsoclonus is defined as chaotic, multidirectional, rapid, conjugate eye movements. There is often a subtle eyelid flutter accompanying the darting eye movements. When opsoclonus is mild, the child has difficulty maintaining eye contact or maintaining gaze on a toy. Quick darting movements of the eyes when the child is asked to visually focus on an object may initially appear to suggest that the child is volitionally looking away. However, with careful observation of eye movements, it gradually becomes apparent that the multidirectional jerky, involuntary eye movements interfere with visual focus. When severe or dramatic, parents usually notice the movement and bring it to the clinician's attention, often using descriptive terms that illustrate why the disorder was historically referred to as "dancing eyes–dancing feet syndrome."

Myoclonus is easily recognizable when large in amplitude. When subtle, the isolated, lightning-like jerks may be easier to feel rather than detect visually.

Encephalopathy in OMS is usually profound and consists of irritability, sleep disturbance, and rage attacks. With time, encephalopathy worsens and is accompanied by potentially irreversible neurologic regression.

TABLE 40.13 Ataxias in Which Specific Abnormalities May Confirm or Point to the Diagnosis*

Disorder	Diagnosis
Abetalipoproteinemia	Low vitamin E levels, abnormal lipoprotein electrophoresis
Aceruloplasminemia	Cognitive changes, craniofacial dyskinesia, ataxia, retinal degeneration, low serum copper, absent ceruloplasmin, abnormal MRI brain; variants in the ceruloplasmin gene
Adrenomyeloneuropathy	Ataxia, neuropsychiatric changes, abnormal MRI, elevated serum long-chain fatty acids; variants in the *ABCD2* gene
Ataxia with coenzyme Q10 (CoQ10) deficiency	Low CoQ10 in muscle biopsy
AOA1	High serum cholesterol, low albumin
AOA2	High α-fetoprotein
AT	High α-fetoprotein, low immunoglobulin (Ig)
Celiac disease	Antitissue transglutaminase antibody
Cerebrotendinous xanthomatosis	Intestinal symptoms, spastic ataxia, cognitive impairment, tendon xanthoma, high serum cholestanol; variants in the *CYP27A1* gene
Late-onset Tay-Sachs (LOTS)	Ataxia, neurogenic weakness, cognitive changes; hexosaminidase levels, hex-A variant analysis
Niemann-Pick type C (NPC) disease	Vertical gaze palsy, hepatosplenomegaly, fibroblast and *NPC* variants
Pyruvate dehydrogenase complex (PDHC) deficiency	Plasma and CSF lactate; PDHC in fibroblasts; variants in *PDHC* complex genes
Refsum disease	Ataxia, neural deafness, retinitis pigmentosa, ichthyosis, elevated plasma phytanic acid; variants in *PHYH* and *PEX 7* genes
Syndromes of myoclonic epilepsy	Many associated with ataxia
Vanishing white matter disease	MRI and MRS
Wilson disease	Serum copper, ceruloplasmin

AOA, ataxia with oculomotor apraxia; AT, ataxia-telangiectasia; CNS, central nervous system; CSF, cerebrospinal fluid; MRS, magnetic resonance spectroscopy.
*Some also appear in Table 40.14, and many have additional CNS features. Clinical features summarized only for those not described in main text.
From Daroff RB, Jankovic J, Mazziotta JC, et al., eds. *Bradley's Neurology in Clinical Practice.* 7th ed. Philadelphia: Elsevier; 2016:1470, Table 97.3.

The condition is thought to be a neuroinflammatory, often paraneoplastic disorder. Once the diagnosis is made, a careful search for a neuroblastoma (in the chest/abdomen/pelvis) should be undertaken. In about 50% of children, a remote neuroblastoma is found. However, resection of tumor alone is insufficient to reverse or stop the progression of OMS. Long-term immune therapy with continued surveillance for tumor recurrence or detection is the mainstay of management. The challenge is to consider this condition early in the differential diagnosis of acute or subacute ataxia, exclude other conditions that cause acute ataxia in children, and shorten the time to treatment.

TABLE 40.14 Phenotypic Clues to Specific Gene Variants in the Dominant Ataxias

Clue	Related Dominant Ataxia
Age at onset	Young adult: SCA1, 2, 3, 7; childhood onset: DRPLA, SCA7, SCA13 Older adult: SCA6
Degree of anticipation in age at onset	Often large in SCA7, DRPLA Often seen in all CAG repeat–related SCAs
Benign course	SCA6
Upper motor neuron signs	SCA1, 5, 7, 8; MJD Rare in SCA2
Akinetic-rigid syndrome	MJD, SCA2
Chorea	Prominent in DRPLA; may occur late in other SCAs
Action tremor	SCA12, SCA15/16
Very slow saccades	SCA2, 7; may occur late in SCA1, 3; uncommon in SCA6
Downbeat nystagmus	SCA6, EA2
Generalized areflexia	SCA2, 4 SCA3 with older-adult onset
Visual loss	SCA7
Seizures	SCA10; early-onset cases of DRPLA and SCA7
Dementia/psychiatric features	SCA12, 17, 27; DRPLA
Myoclonus	DRPLA, SCA14
Intellectual disability	SCA13
Episodic symptoms	EA1 and EA2

DRPLA, dentatorubral-pallidoluysian ataxia; EA, episodic ataxia; MJD, Machado-Joseph disease; SCA, spinocerebellar ataxia.
From Daroff RB, Jankovic J, Mazziotta JC, et al., eds. *Bradley's Neurology in Clinical Practice.* 7th ed. Philadelphia: Elsevier; 2016:1471, Table 97.4.

Clinical Observations in Children with Ataxia

When ataxia is mild, young children tend to have an easier time running compared to standing still. Running may be easier as children tend to launch themselves forward to compensate for their difficulty with balance. Standing still, with feet together, is often accompanied by steps backward or to the side to maintain balance. Changing direction while walking or turning around is often accompanied by a step to the side to maintain balance. Stooping and recovering may be difficult. When the ataxia is mild, children can stoop and recover but tend to do so with feet placed wide apart. When ataxia is severe, standing, walking, running, and even sitting become difficult and require support.

The muscle stretch reflexes (deep tendon reflexes) should be evaluated in all children as part of the neurologic examination. In cerebellar disorders the reflexes may be blunted. However, if there is peripheral nerve involvement (e.g., in the Miller Fisher variant of Guillain-Barré), reflexes are lost.

Acute Cerebellar Ataxia

This condition is usually seen in children between ages 2 and 7 years (see Table 40.12). The onset is usually explosive with ataxia that is maximal on the day of onset. Often the symptom of ataxia is preceded by a febrile illness. The condition is thought to be postinfectious in nature. Infectious agents that have been linked to acute cerebellar ataxia include coxsackievirus, echoviruses, Epstein-Barr virus, hepatitis A, measles, mumps, parvovirus B19, *Borrelia burgdorferi,* and *Mycoplasma pneumoniae.* Acute cerebellar ataxia is usually self-limited, with recovery occurring within a few days and resolution of symptoms within weeks to months. The diagnosis in the acute phase is one of exclusion, with exclusion of other postinfectious conditions (ADEM, Miller Fisher variant of Guillain-Barré syndrome) and posterior fossa structural abnormalities. The diagnosis is fully confirmed retrospectively once the course of recovery has taken place. Most children get neuroimaging at the onset to evaluate for other conditions such as posterior fossa abnormalities and ADEM. CSF analysis is indicated after neuroimaging if encephalitis is suspected. Children with acute cerebellar ataxia should be monitored closely to make sure that they are following the expected course of recovery. If recovery does not continue as expected, alternative diagnoses such as OMS should be considered.

Causes of Chronic Ataxia

Chronic ataxia is often due to a structural abnormality of brain development such as Dandy-Walker syndrome or due to a progressive hereditary or neurodegenerative disorder (Tables 40.15, 40.16, and 40.17).

TABLE 40.15 Autosomal Recessive Ataxias

Entity	Gene Locus/Gene/Protein	Variant
Friedreich ataxia	9q/*FRDA*/frataxin	Homozygous GAA expansion; rarely heterozygous expansion and point mutation in second allele
MIRAS	15q/*POLG 1*/polymerase γ	Point mutations
IOSCA	6p/*C10orf2*/Twinkle	Point mutations
Abetalipoproteinemia	8q/αTTP/αTTP	Frameshift or missense variants
Cayman ataxia	19q/*ATCAY*/caytaxin	Missense variants
Ataxia-telangiectasia	11q/*ATM*/ATM	Deletions, missense variants, insertions
AOA1	9p/*APTX*/aprataxin	Point mutations
AOA2	9q/*SETX*/senataxin	Point mutations
ATLD	11q/*mRE11*/mRE11	Missense, nonsense variants
SCAN1	14q/*TDP1*	Missense, nonsense variants
ARSACS	13q11/*SACS*/sacsin	Missense, nonsense variants
MSS	5q/*SIL1*/BiP-associated protein	Point mutations
ARCA1	6q/*SYNE1*/SYNE 1	Point mutations
ARCA 2	Several genes in CoQ 10 pathway	

AOA1, ataxia with oculomotor apraxia type 1; AOA2, ataxia with oculomotor apraxia type 2; ARCA1, 2, autosomal recessive cerebellar ataxia type 1 and 2; ARSACS, autosomal recessive ataxia of Charlevoix-Saguenay; ATLD, ataxia-telangiectasia–like disorder; IOSCA, infantile-onset spinocerebellar ataxia; MIRAS, mitochondrial recessive ataxia syndrome; MSS, Marinesco-Sjögren syndrome; SCAN1, spinocerebellar ataxia with axonal neuropathy.
From Daroff RB, Jankovic J, Mazziotta JC, et al., eds. *Bradley's Neurology in Clinical Practice.* 7th ed. Philadelphia: Elsevier; 2016:1465, Table 97.2.

The progressive hereditary ataxias are often accompanied by additional neurologic signs and symptoms. Clinical features that may be seen in the progressive genetic ataxias include other abnormal movements, encephalopathy, peripheral nerve involvement, and spasticity. Hyperkinetic movements such as dystonia, myoclonus, chorea, and tremor have been reported to occur in about one third of patients with progressive autosomal recessive ataxia. The presence of ataxia, with involuntary movements with progressive loss of reflexes, should raise suspicion for Friedreich ataxia.

Glucose Transporter-1 Deficiency Syndrome

The glucose transporter-1 (GLUT-1) deficiency syndrome is caused by variants in the *SLC2A1* gene, which encodes for the glucose transporter protein type 1. GLUT-1 deficiency was previously recognized as a cause

TABLE 40.16 Autosomal Dominant Ataxias Related to Nucleotide Expansions

Disease	Gene/Protein	Repeat	Locus
SCA1	*ATXN1*/ataxin-1	CAG	6p
SCA2	*ATXN2*/ataxin-2	CAG	12q
SCA3 (MJD)	*ATXN3*/ataxin-3	CAG	14q
SCA6	*CACNA1A*/calcium channel	CAG	19p
SCA7	*ATXN7*/ataxin-7	CAG	3p
SCA8	*ATXN8*/untranslated	CTG-CAG	13q
SCA10	*ATXN10*/untranslated	ATTCT	22q
SCA12	*PP2R2B*/phosphatase	CAG	5q
SCA17	*TBP*/TATA binding protein	CAG	6q
SCA 31	Unknown	TGGAA insertion	
SCA 36	*NOP56*	GGCCTG untranslated	
DRPLA	ATN	CAG	12p

ATN, atrophin; ATXN, ataxin; MJD, Machado-Joseph disease; SCA, spinocerebellar ataxia; TBP, TATA binding protein.
From Daroff RB, Jankovic J, Mazziotta JC, et al., eds. *Bradley's Neurology in Clinical Practice.* 7th ed. Philadelphia: Elsevier; 2016:1474, Table 97.5.

TABLE 40.17 Autosomal Dominant Ataxias with Defined Variants Unrelated to Nucleotide Expansions

Disease	Gene	Locus	Mutation
SCA5	*SPTBN2*	11p	Deletions, point mutation
SCA11	*TTBK2*	15q	Insertion/deletion
SCA13	*KCNC3*	19q	Point mutations
SCA14	*PRKCG*	19q	Deletions, point mutations
SCA15/16	*ITPR1*	3p	Deletions, point mutations
SCA20*	Unknown	11q	Duplication
SCA27	*FGF14*	13q	Point mutations
SCA28	*AFG3L2*	18p	Point mutations

*In SCA20, the region duplicated has multiple genes.
SCA, spinocerebellar ataxia.
From Daroff RB, Jankovic J, Mazziotta JC, et al., eds. *Bradley's Neurology in Clinical Practice.* 7th ed. Philadelphia: Elsevier; 2016:1474, Table 97.6.

of infantile epilepsy, developmental delay, cognitive impairment, spasticity, and ataxia. The GLUT-1 protein is involved in moving glucose across the blood-brain barrier. The diagnosis is suspected when the CSF glucose is lower than expected when compared with serum glucose and confirmed by erythrocyte glucose uptake studies and by *GLUT-1* gene sequencing. With the availability of genetic testing, the spectrum of symptoms from this disorder has expanded. This disorder can present not only with seizures and movement disorders but also exclusively with movement disorders. The most common movement disorder in GLUT-1 deficiency is ataxia and dystonia often combined with spasticity. Gene variants in the *GLUT-1* gene have also been described as a cause of dominant and sporadic paroxysmal exertion-induced dyskinesia (PED/DYT18) and slowly progressive spastic paraparesis combined with PED (DYT19). The spectrum of movement disorders that can be seen in GLUT-1 deficiency includes gait disturbance, dystonia, chorea, cerebellar action tremor, myoclonus, dyspraxia, episodic ataxia, weakness, parkinsonism, exercise-induced dyskinesias, and nonkinesigenic dyskinesia. Treatment with the ketogenic diet may lead to symptomatic improvement. With the availability of a potential treatment linked to symptomatic improvement, it becomes important to consider this condition in children who present with chronic and paroxysmal movement disorders.

Ataxia-Telangiectasia

Ataxia-telangiectasia (AT) is an autosomal recessive disorder characterized by ataxia, cutaneous telangiectasia, immune dysfunction, cancer susceptibility, and radiation sensitivity (Fig. 40.5). Although there is a wide variability in severity of symptoms between affected individuals, in general, motor dysfunction starts in infancy. Ataxia may be subtle and noticed when the child starts to ambulate. Dystonia or chorea may be present prior to the onset of frank ataxia. Immune dysfunction with frequent sinopulmonary infections may be noted in early childhood. Cutaneous telangiectasias tend to develop after age 2 years, sometimes much later. Usually they first appear on the conjunctiva. Other areas where they may be seen include the ears, flexor surfaces of the limbs, and face.

AT has been clinically referred to as a chromosomal instability syndrome, a neurocutaneous syndrome, and a DNA repair disorder. Most but not all patients with AT have high serum α-fetoprotein levels. About 80% have decreased levels of immunoglobulin A (IgA), immunoglobulin E (IgE), and immunoglobulin G (IgG) (selective deficiency of IgG-2 subclass).

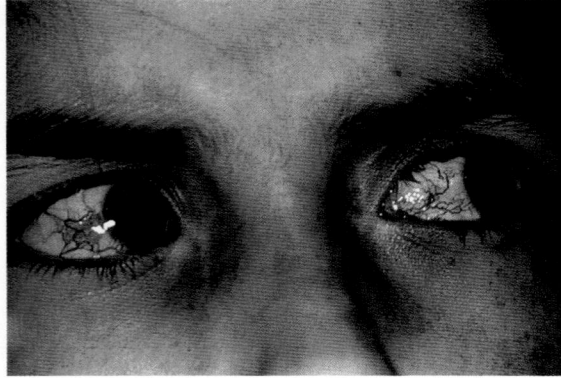

Fig. 40.5 Conjunctival telangiectasia in a patient with ataxia-telangiectasia. (From Daroff RB, Jankovic J, Mazziotta JC, et al., eds. *Bradley's Neurology in Clinical Practice*. 7th ed. Philadelphia: Elsevier; 2016:1468, Fig. 97.6.)

Individuals with AT have an increased risk of malignancies, especially lymphoma and leukemia. They are also highly sensitive to radiation, which produces cellular and chromosomal damage and may be a precipitant in the development of neoplasia.

The diagnosis should be suspected in a child with chronic ataxia. Serum α-fetoprotein is utilized as a screening tool but may be normal in a minority of patients. MRI of the brain may be normal initially with cerebellar degeneration becoming apparent later. The diagnosis of AT can be confirmed by the absence or deficiency of ataxia-telangiectasia mutated (ATM) protein and/or ATM kinase activity in cell lines established from lymphocytes or skin biopsies, or the identification of pathologic variants in the *ATM* gene. With the availability of whole exome sequencing (WES) and its use in children with undiagnosed neurologic or motor symptoms, milder and atypical forms of AT are being identified.

Management is supportive, targeting motor dysfunction, infections, immune function, and pulmonary function. Exposure to radiation should be minimized.

Evaluation and Testing in a Child with Ataxia

Overall, the evaluation of a child with acute or subacute ataxia is different from that of a child with chronic ataxia. In a child with acute ataxia an acquired etiology requiring rapid diagnosis and treatment is assumed. Chronic ataxia is often due to a heredodegenerative disorder or chronic structural brain abnormality.

Consideration for testing in a child with acute ataxia should include neuroimaging with MRI. Consider both brain and spine if a postinfectious cause such as ADEM is suspected with assessment of cerebral vasculature if ischemia/stroke is suspected. Contrast with neuroimaging is indicated if infection or inflammation is suspected. Evaluation of CSF for infectious agents, pleocytosis, autoimmune markers, glucose (with simultaneous serum glucose), protein, and lactate should be performed if a primary CNS infection or inflammation is suspected. If acute ataxia continues to evolve and takes on a subacute course, celiac disease and OMS should be considered. OMS tends to be overlooked if not considered, leading to irreversible neurologic regression.

In chronic ataxia treatable causes should be screened for. Screening should include serum α-fetoprotein, vitamin E levels, antitissue transglutaminase antibody (for celiac disease), and lipoprotein profile. Serum α-fetoprotein may be elevated in AT. Although AT is not treatable, it would be important to identify individuals with this condition to avoid unnecessary radiation, which could predispose them to future tumors. In all children with chronic ataxia with or without seizures, testing for GLUT-1 deficiency should be strongly considered. Further tiered testing should proceed for children with chronic ataxia who remain undiagnosed, eventually proceeding to WES or targeted next-generation sequencing panels.

TREMOR

Tremor is an involuntary, rhythmic oscillatory movement of a body part. In general, the limbs and head when unsupported exhibit a slight tremor. This is referred to as a physiologic tremor. Physiologic tremor is usually not visible, unless it is enhanced by fatigue, anxiety, or medication. A pathologic tremor is usually visible under normal circumstances.

Tremor is classified by its frequency, amplitude, distribution (what parts of the body are affected), whether it is present at rest, whether it is induced by trying to sustain posture (sustension) or by motion (action or kinesis), and whether it increases at the end point of motion.

The clinical examination should note which parts of the body are involved and activation conditions (what conditions bring out the tremor). Activation conditions consist of either rest or action. Action implies voluntary muscle contraction either while maintaining posture (postural) or during voluntary movement of the affected area (kinesis).

Resting tremor is a tremor in a body part in conditions where that body part is at rest and not voluntarily activated. This is examined with the specific body part relaxed and completely supported.

Action tremor occurs while voluntarily maintaining a position against gravity (postural and orthostatic tremor) or during voluntary movement of that body part (kinetic tremor). Kinetic tremor is further subdivided into simple kinetic tremor (tremor is roughly the same throughout the movement) and intention tremor (tremor that is present during movement of that body part and increases as the body part approaches its target).

Once the tremor is confirmed and classified, the next clinical determination is whether it is isolated or associated with other symptoms or signs (e.g., seizures, other movement disorders, or systemic signs such as hepatomegaly, K-F ring, or exophthalmos).

The aforementioned describes phenomenology and not etiology. However, once the tremor is classified, the search for an underlying cause is undertaken based on the diseases linked to the tremor syndrome (Table 40.18). A tremor syndrome may have multiple etiologies. Intention tremor implies a lesion or dysfunction in the cerebellum or its connections. Combined tremor syndromes usually have an underlying structural, metabolic, or heredodegenerative basis.

Unless the child or adolescent presents with an isolated tremor that has the clinical features of an isolated essential tremor combined with a strong family history of the same, further evaluation to determine the cause should be undertaken.

Essential Tremor

This condition causes an isolated tremor syndrome. The tremor is a postural, mid-amplitude, mid-frequency tremor usually starting in the adolescent age group without any other associated neurologic/movement disorder symptoms. A family history is helpful, but usually diagnosis is made in the absence of other etiologies and with normal neuroimaging. Longitudinal follow-up is necessary to make sure no other symptoms emerge with time indicating an alternative underlying disorder. Treatment is usually not needed. However, if tremor impairs fine motor skills, symptomatic treatment with propranolol or primidone can be attempted.

TABLE 40.18 Causes of Tremor

Metabolic/electrolyte derangement: abnormality of glucose, calcium, magnesium

Endocrine: thyroid, parathyroid dysfunction

Drugs/medication: antiepileptic agents (lamotrigine, valproate), β2-adrenergic agonists, nicotine, caffeine stimulants, antihistamines, tricyclic antidepressants, theophylline, neuroleptics

Heredodegenerative disorders: Wilson disease

Screening Tests to Consider for the Child Who Presents with Tremor

Thyroid function
Serum copper and ceruloplasmin
Glucose and electrolytes
MRI of the brain
Eye exam

Shudder Attacks

These are discrete episodes of a rapid tremor of the head, shoulder, and arms, often accompanied by facial grimacing. The episodes last several seconds and can occur multiple times a day. There is no alteration of consciousness with these episodes. Onset is usually in infancy or early childhood. They typically abate as the child grows older. There has been some suggestion that shudder attacks may be the earliest manifestation of essential tremor, but this link has not been proven. Seizures with shuddering semiology have been described; therefore, an EEG to capture and characterize the movements may be warranted. The EEG should remain normal during a shudder if indeed the shudder is a movement and not a seizure.

TICS

Tics are repeated, intermittent movements or movement fragments that are almost always briefly suppressible and are usually associated with awareness of an urge to perform the movement. Tics can be motor (movement) or vocal.

Simple motor tics consist of repetitive movements in one small muscle group, for example, blinking or eyebrow elevation. Complex motor tics consist of a sequence of stereotyped movements involving multiple muscle groups, for example, flailing of arms with a simultaneous facial grimace and neck thrust.

Simple vocal tics consist of rudimentary sounds such as sniffing or throat clearing or a repetitive simple sound such as "uh" or "ah." Complex vocal tics consist of repetitive words or phrases, for example, "gotta go." Tics have two additional phenomena. They are often preceded by an unpleasant sensory feeling or "premonitory urge," and they can be voluntarily suppressed for brief periods. Tics are most often seen in the setting of a tic disorder or Tourette disorder.

Tourette Disorder

Both multiple motor and one or more vocal tics have been present at some time during the illness, waxing and waning for more than a year since first tic onset before age 18 years, not due to the direct physiologic effects of a substance (e.g., cocaine) or a general medical condition (e.g., Huntington disease, encephalitis).

Chronic Motor Tic or Vocal Tic Disorder

Single or multiple motor or vocal tics, but not both, have been present at some time during the illness, waxing and waning for more than a year since tic onset, starting prior to age 18 years, not due to a substance such as cocaine or a general medical condition such as encephalitis.

Provisional Tic Disorder

Single or multiple motor and/or vocal tics have been present for less than a year with onset prior to age 18 years, not due to the direct effect of a substance (such as stimulants) or a general medical condition (e.g., postviral encephalitis).

Comorbidities that can be seen in individuals with a tic disorder include ADHD, learning difficulties, obsessive compulsions/OCD, anxiety, depression, behavior difficulty (oppositional defiance, disruptive behavior, explosive outbursts), and sleep difficulty. Comorbidities, when present, tend to manifest earlier than tics. Tics in childhood tend to start around the early school years. A positive family history is present in about one half of patients. Reports indicate that tic severity in general may decline during adolescence. By early adulthood tic symptoms in the greater proportion of patients with Tourette syndrome may be greatly diminished.

Treatment is aimed at the comorbidities that interfere with academic and social function. Treatment of tics is purely symptomatic, and the goal is not for complete tic suppression but rather a reduction in tics to decrease the secondary psychosocial impairment. Most children have mild tics that do not interfere with activity and do not require treatment. However, tics can be disabling and cause social embarrassment. Treatments that have been used to suppress tics include non-neuroleptic medications (guanfacine, clonidine, topiramate), neuroleptics (pimozide, haloperidol, aripiprazole), and behavior therapy. Although tic-suppressing typical and atypical neuroleptics are often effective, their side effects often limit their usefulness. Comprehensive behavior interventions for tics (CBIT) can improve symptoms of Tourette syndrome.

STEREOTYPIES

Stereotypies are repetitive, simple movements that can be voluntarily suppressed. These are involuntary, patterned, purposeless movements such as body rocking; head nodding; head shaking; head banging; hand flapping; repetitive, sequential finger movements; fluttering fingers in front of face; and head nodding. These primary movements may be accompanied by stereotypic jumping or jaw opening. Stereotypies tend to occur when the child is excited, stressed, distracted, or engrossed. Stereotypies can be stopped by distraction. They can continue for many minutes if the child is not distracted by another activity. Stereotypies can be seen in typically developing children as well as in children with autism spectrum disorder, developmental disorders, sensory deprivation, and adaptive and language difficulty. They can be seen in individuals with tic disorders but are distinct from tics and do not respond to the usual medications used to suppress tics. Stereotypies typically begin before age 3 years.

MYOCLONUS

Myoclonus is a sequence of repeated, often nonrhythmic, brief, shock-like jerks due to sudden involuntary contraction or relaxation of one or more muscles.

Myoclonus can either be a movement disorder (Table 40.19) or epileptic. The EEG is a useful tool in differentiating the two, as myoclonic seizures are associated with epileptiform discharges on the EEG. Although sometimes difficult to clinically differentiate, myoclonic seizures are distinct from myoclonus (movement disorder) in their mechanism. However, myoclonic seizures and myoclonus can both be present together in certain specific progressive neurologic diseases.

Neonatal Sleep Myoclonus

This is a self-limiting disorder seen in otherwise normal neonates during sleep. The myoclonic jerks can affect the arms, legs, or face; are often fragmented, typically occurring in clusters of jerks over a few seconds; only occur in sleep; and disappear as soon as arousal occurs. Waking the baby while the movement is occurring causes the movements to cease. Benign sleep myoclonus begins in the first month of life, gradually diminishing and resolving by age 6 months. Due to the possibility of myoclonic seizures in this age group, an EEG is usually done. In benign neonatal sleep myoclonus, the EEG remains normal during the myoclonic jerk. Inadvertent treatment with benzodiazepines or sedating medications can exacerbate the myoclonus in benign neonatal sleep myoclonus.

Hereditary Hyperekplexia

Hyperekplexias are a group of nonepileptic, exaggerated stimulus-induced startle disorders (see Chapter 38). Tactile, auditory, or emotional stimuli provoke an excessive myoclonic or startle response. The phenomenology involves myoclonic-type jerks that simultaneously involve the neck, trunk, and arms. When the onset occurs in infancy, there is often "stiffness" or persistent hypertonia with superimposed repetitive startles, thus leading to the descriptive term **stiff baby syndrome**. There are several genetically distinct hyperekplexias, some associated with epileptic seizures and others remaining a pure movement disorder. The pure movement disorder forms tend to gradually improve with age and respond well to benzodiazepines such as valium or clonazepam.

Essential Myoclonus

Onset of myoclonus is in the first 2 decades of life. There should be no associated epilepsy, cognitive impairment, ataxia, or other movement disorders. Differential diagnosis in adolescence includes juvenile myoclonic epilepsy (JME) and in a younger child, Jeavons syndrome. In JME, epileptic myoclonic and absence seizures in the first few hours after waking up in the morning often remain unrecognized as seizures until the onset of a generalized tonic-clonic seizure several years later. **Jeavons syndrome** is a type of generalized epilepsy characterized by childhood-onset eyelid myoclonia, with or without absence seizures, photosensitivity, and, in some patients, generalized tonic-clonic seizures. Differentiating the epilepsy syndromes with myoclonic seizures from a movement disorder is fairly straightforward in the presence of generalized tonic-clonic seizures or absence seizures. When the diagnosis is in doubt, an EEG capturing the myoclonus is helpful. In essential myoclonus, the EEG remains normal during the myoclonic jerk, differentiating it from myoclonic epilepsy.

DYSKINETIC CEREBRAL PALSY

Cerebral palsy is a descriptive term used for a motor disorder appearing early in life, caused by a nonprogressive injury or lesion in the developing brain. The most common form of cerebral palsy affects tone (spastic hemiparesis, spastic quadriparesis, spastic diplegia). The second most common is dyskinetic (involuntary movements) cerebral palsy caused by nonprogressive abnormality or damage in the basal ganglia or thalamus. Often a child with cerebral palsy will have both spasticity and dyskinesias (mixed-type cerebral palsy). Mixed-type cerebral palsy and dyskinetic cerebral palsy together account for a large portion of childhood movement disorders. The involuntary movements in dyskinetic cerebral palsy are commonly dystonia, chorea, or both. Pure dyskinetic cerebral palsy appears to be the dominant type of cerebral palsy found in term babies with perinatal hypoxic-ischemic encephalopathy.

The diagnosis of dyskinetic cerebral palsy is clinical and illustrates the contrast between adults and children with neurologic problems. In contrast to adults, the clinical picture in an infant or young child with motor dysfunction can evolve or change over time with brain maturation. However, when there is an evolution of clinical symptoms over time, the concern for a progressive neurologic disorder or alternative diagnosis arises. The presence of an identifiable injury such as perinatal hypoxic ischemia, kernicterus, or MRI changes indicating old ischemia or a recognized malformation of the brain assists in confirming a nonprogressive insult. However, in the absence of an identifiable injury, diseases that "mimic" dyskinetic cerebral palsy including metabolic and other neurologic disorders should be considered. These disorders would include those listed under heredodegenerative causes of secondary dystonia as well as the disorders causing chronic chorea and chronic ataxia (see Tables 40.7, 40.11, and 40.15). In addition to these, Table 40.20 lists some of the conditions that mimic dyskinetic cerebral palsy.

TABLE 40.19 Etiologic Classification of Myoclonus

Physiologic Myoclonus (Normal Subjects)

Sleep jerks (hypnagogic jerks)

Anxiety-induced

Exercise-induced

Hiccup (singultus)

Benign infantile myoclonus with feeding

Essential Myoclonus (No Known Cause and No Other Gross Neurologic Deficit)

Hereditary (phenotype may be pure myoclonus or myoclonus-dystonia)

Sporadic

Epileptic Myoclonus (No Known Cause and No Other Gross Neurologic Deficit)

Fragments of epilepsy

Isolated epileptic myoclonic jerks

Epilepsia partialis continua

Idiopathic stimulus-sensitive myoclonus

Photosensitive myoclonus

Myoclonic absences in petit mal

Childhood myoclonic epilepsies

Infantile spasms

Myoclonic astatic epilepsy (Lennox-Gastaut syndrome)

Cryptogenic myoclonus epilepsy

Myoclonic epilepsy of Janz

Benign familial myoclonic epilepsy (Rabot syndrome)

Progressive myoclonic epilepsy: Baltic myoclonus (Unverricht-Lundborg syndrome)

Symptomatic Myoclonus (Progressive or Static Encephalopathy Dominates)

Storage diseases

Lafora body disease

Lipidoses, such as GM2 gangliosidosis, Tay-Sachs disease, Krabbe disease

Ceroid lipofuscinosis (Batten disease, Kufs disease)

Sialidosis (cherry red spot)

Spinocerebellar degeneration

Ramsay Hunt syndrome (many causes)

Friedreich ataxia

Ataxia-telangiectasia

Basal ganglia degenerations

Wilson disease

Torsion dystonia

Hallervorden-Spatz disease

Progressive supranuclear palsy

Huntington disease

Parkinson disease

Corticobasal degeneration

Pallidal degenerations

Multiple system atrophy

Mitochondrial encephalopathies, including myoclonic epilepsy and ragged-red fibers

Dementias

Creutzfeldt-Jakob disease

Alzheimer disease

Viral encephalopathies

Subacute sclerosing panencephalitis

Encephalitis lethargica

Arbovirus encephalitis

Herpes simplex encephalitis

Postinfectious encephalitis

Metabolic

Hepatic failure

Renal failure

Dialysis syndrome

Hyponatremia

Hypoglycemia

Infantile myoclonic encephalopathy (polymyoclonus, with or without neuroblastoma)

Nonketotic hyperglycemia

Multiple carboxylase deficiency

Toxic encephalopathies

Bismuth

Heavy metal poisons

Methyl bromide, dichlorodiphenyltrichloroethane

Drugs, including L-dopa, tricyclic antidepressants

Physical encephalopathies

Posthypoxia (Lance-Adams syndrome)

Post-traumatic

Heat stroke

Electric shock

Decompression injury

Focal central nervous system damage

Poststroke

Post-thalamotomy

Tumor

Trauma

Olivo-dentate lesions (palatal myoclonus)

Spinal cord lesions (segmental or spinal myoclonus) disease

From Daroff RB, Jankovic J, Mazziotta JC, et al., eds. *Bradley's Neurology in Clinical Practice*. 7th ed. Philadelphia: Elsevier; 2016:243, Box 23-10.

TABLE 40.20   Diseases That Mimic Dyskinetic Cerebral Palsy

Lesch-Nyhan syndrome
Glutaric aciduria type 1
Ataxia-telangiectasia
Rett syndrome
Angelman syndrome
Dopa-responsive dystonia
Glucose transporter deficiency
Pyruvate dehydrogenase complex deficiency
Creatine transporter deficiency
Mitochondrial disorders
Familial idiopathic basal ganglia calcification
Neuroacanthocytosis
Early-onset Parkinson disease
Wilson disease

From Debopam S. Management of alternating hemiplegia of childhood: a review. *Pediatr Neurol.* 2020;103:12–20.

CONDITIONS THAT MIMIC MOVEMENT DISORDERS

Epilepsia Partialis Continua

Epilepsia partialis continua (EPC) is a condition in which focal non-rhythmic jerking usually in one limb occurs for hours or weeks without alteration of consciousness. The phenomenology is that of myoclonus. Sometimes the movements can mimic chorea. However, the persistent, focal nature of the fragmented jerks affecting a single limb should raise the possibility of EPC. A high index of clinical suspicion followed by EEG helps confirm the diagnosis of EPC. Underlying conditions causing EPC include focal structural abnormalities of the cerebral cortex, focal infection (cerebritis), cerebral ischemia, and Rasmussen syndrome.

Psychogenic Movement Disorders

Tremor, dystonia, myoclonus, and gait difficulty have all been reported. The mean age at symptom onset is ~14 years, with no patient younger than 7 years. Psychogenic movement disorders (PMDs) tend to be paroxysmal, abrupt in onset, with selective disability. Organic movement disorders that are often mistakenly diagnosed as PMDs include paroxysmal dystonia or paroxysmal dyskinesias, episodic ataxia, task-specific dystonia, and drug-induced dystonia. Little is known about the long-term prognosis of childhood-onset PMDs.

Chronic movement disorders not only affect motor function but also are often accompanied by behavioral, social, cognitive, academic, and psychiatric difficulties. Symptom treatment is aimed at the symptoms that impair daily function. Management in the chronic movement disorders is usually multidisciplinary, with the management team consisting of pediatricians, physical medicine and rehabilitation specialists, physical and occupational therapists, geneticists and metabolic specialists, neurologists, orthopedics, developmental specialists, school counselors, and teachers.

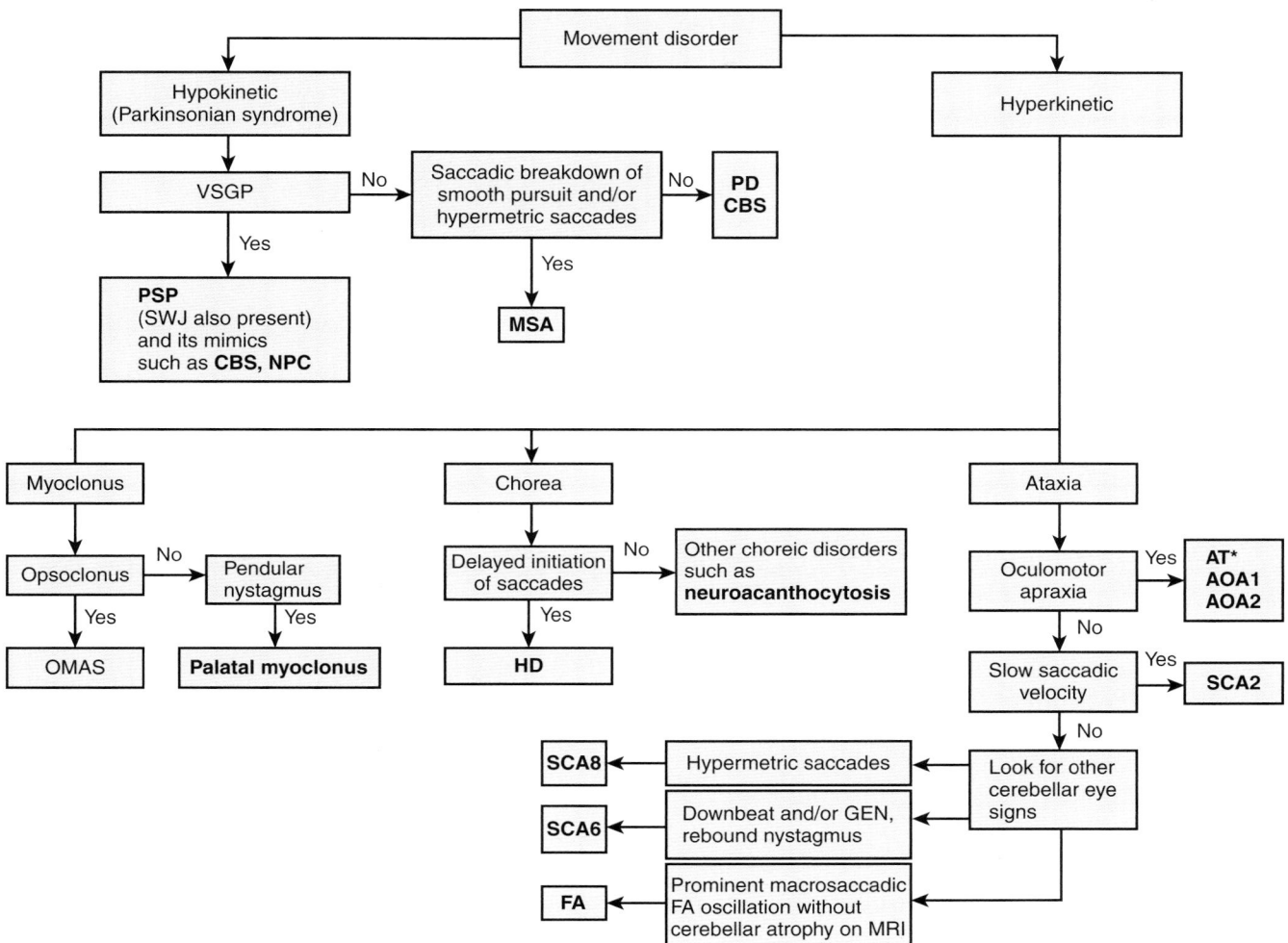

Fig. 40.6 An algorithmic approach to movement disorders utilizing phenomenology and saccades. The approach starts with classifying the patient as hypokinetic or hyperkinetic. Various saccadic abnormalities can help lead to the final diagnosis in each phenomenology. *Cerebellar eye movement abnormalities including downbeat, upbeat, position, gaze-evoked nystagmus, and saccadic dysmetria are also common in ataxia-telangiectasia. AOA1, ataxia with oculomotor apraxia type 1; AOA2, ataxia with oculomotor apraxia type 2; AT, ataxia-telangiectasia; CBS, corticobasal syndrome; FA, Friedreich ataxia; GEN, gaze-evoked nystagmus; HD, Huntington disease; MSA, multiple system atrophy; NPC, Niemann-Pick type C; OMAS, opsoclonus-myoclonus ataxia syndrome; PD, Parkinson disease; SCA2, spinocerebellar ataxia type 2; SCA6, spinocerebellar ataxia type 6; SCA8, spinocerebellar ataxia type 8; SWJ, square wave jerks; VSGP, vertical supranuclear gaze palsy. Y = Yes; N = No. (From Termsarasab P, Thammongkolchai T, Rucker JC, et al., The diagnostic value of saccades in movement disorder patients: a practical guide and review. *J Clin Move Disord.* 2015;2:14, Fig. 4.)

TABLE 40.21 Commonly Seen Movement Disorder Mimics

Mimics of Parkinsonism
- Depression
- Obsessive slowness
- Hypothyroidism
- Spasticity
- Dystonic tremor
- Frozen shoulder
- Slowing due to normal aging
- Catatonia

Mimics of Craniocervical Dystonia (Torticollis)
- Retropharyngeal abscess
- Atlantoaxial subluxation
- Congenital muscular torticollis
- Correcting head tilt in cranial nerve palsy ("ocular torticollis")
- Space-occupying lesion in posterior fossa
- Sandifer syndrome with head tilt
- Dropped head syndrome in neuromuscular disease

Mimics of Limb Dystonia
- Contracture
- Spasticity
- Abnormal posture due to paresis or atrophy
- Myotonia or neuromyotonia
- Sensory ataxia and/or pseudoathetosis
- Stiff-person syndrome
- Tonic spasms
- Seizures or epilepsia partialis continua

Mimics of Facial Dystonia
- Ptosis or pseudoptosis
- Trismus
- Hemimasticatory spasm
- Hemifacial spasm (tonic component)
- Myotonia
- Tetanic spasms
- Apraxia of eyelid opening (levator inhibition)

Mimics of Myoclonus
- Tics
- Tremor
- Fasciculations (spontaneous contractions of muscle fibers supplied by a single motor unit that are too small to cause movement across a joint)
- Myokymia (involuntary, subtle, continuous, rippling quivering of muscles, which does not produce movement across a joint)
- Chorea

From Abdo WF, van de Warrenburg BPC, Burn DJ, et al. The clinical approach to movement disorders. *Nature Rev Neurol.* 2010;6:29–37 (Box 2, p. 35).

TABLE 40.22 Commonly Seen "Mixed" Movement Disorders

Combinations	Possible Etiology
Tremor and akinesia	Parkinson disease or atypical parkinsonism
Parkinsonism, ataxia, autonomic dysfunction, spasticity, myoclonus	Multiple system atrophy
Vertical supranuclear gaze palsy and falls, symmetric parkinsonism	Progressive supranuclear palsy
Akinesia, rigidity, myoclonus, dystonia and apraxia, asymmetric clinical phenotype	Corticobasal degeneration
Chorea, dystonia, and bradykinesia	Huntington disease
Dystonia plus tremor	Primary dystonia
Tremor (rest and postural), dystonia, akinetic–rigid syndrome	Wilson disease
Ataxia and myoclonus (Ramsay-Hunt syndrome, "progressive myoclonic ataxia")	Mitochondrial disease; celiac disease; Unverricht-Lundborg disease

From Abdo WF, van de Warrenburg BPC, Burn DJ, et al. The clinical approach to movement disorders. *Nature Rev Neurol.* 2010;6:29–37 (Table 2, p. 36).

TABLE 40.23 Medications with Movement Disorder as Side Effects

Medication	Parkinsonism	Myoclonus	Dystonia	Ataxia	Tremor	Chorea
Anticonvulsants	✓	✓	✓	✓	✓	✓
Antipsychotics	✓	✓	✓		✓	
Antidepressants		✓	✓	✓	✓	
Antihypertensives		✓				
Antiparkinson drugs		✓	✓			
Antibiotics		✓			✓	
Antineoplastic		✓		✓	✓	
Opiates		✓				
Anxiolytics		✓		✓		
Anaesthetics		✓				
Oral contraceptives						✓
Antiemetics			✓		✓	
Immunosuppressants				✓	✓	
Corticosteroids			✓		✓	

From Brandsma R, Vanegmond ME, Tijssen MA, et al. Diagnostic approach to paediatric movement disorders: a clinical practice guideline. *Dev Med Child Neurol.* 2020. doi:10.1111/dmcn.14721.

TABLE 40.24 Inborn Errors of Metabolism Presenting with Paroxysmal Movement Disorders

Ataxia	Dystonia	Chorea	Dyskinesia
• Pyruvate dehydrogenase complex deficiency • *BTD*-biotinidase deficiency • Hartnup disease • *GLDC* and *AMT*-glycine encephalopathy • *HTD*-tyrosinemia type III • *SLC2A1*-GLUT1 deficiency	• *SLC2A1*-GLUT1 deficiency • *ECHS1*-mitochondrial short-chain enoyl-CoA hydratase 1 deficiency • *HIBCH*-3-hydroxyisobutyryl-CoA hydrolase deficiency • Pyruvate dehydrogenase complex deficiency	• OTC-ornithine transcarbamylase deficiency	• *ABAT*-GABA transaminase deficiency • *ALDH5A1*-succinic semialdehyde dehydrogenase deficiency • *PARK2*-Parkin deficiency

From Ortigoza-Escobar JD. A proposed diagnostic algorithm for inborn errors of metabolism presenting with movements disorders. *Front Neurol.* 2020;11:582160, Table 3.

SUMMARY AND RED FLAGS

A stepwise approach to the evaluation of a child with a movement disorder should be undertaken (see Fig. 40.1).

1. Delineate the phenomenology.
2. Determine whether symptoms are acute or chronic.
3. Formulate differential diagnoses.
4. Decide on urgency of evaluation and treatment based on differential diagnoses.
5. Perform tiered testing in the child with a chronic movement disorder, with emphasis on the treatable conditions.

A diagnostic approach is noted in Fig. 40.6. Mimics and mixed movement disorders are noted in Tables 40.21 and 40.22, respectively.

In addition, drugs may produce more than one pattern of movement disorder (Table 40.23). Furthermore, inborn errors of metabolism must be considered in the differential diagnosis (Table 40.24). Management includes treatment of the underlying condition (when treatable), symptom treatment of the movement when necessary, and treatment of comorbid conditions.

Red flags include chronicity, developmental regression, intellectual disability, seizures, syndromic phenotype, and systemic organ involvement.

BIBLIOGRAPHY

A bibliography is available at ExpertConsult.com.

41

Altered Mental Status

Tracey H. Liljestrom

ALTERED MENTAL STATUS

Altered mental status (AMS) refers to a broad range of nonspecific symptoms indicating a change in brain function from a patient's baseline and can include confusion, alteration in consciousness, disorientation, decreased awareness, amnesia, and change in behavior. Accurate diagnosis and management rely on rapidly characterizing the change in mental status and prioritizing the identification of life-threatening causes. AMS can be divided into *hyperactive states* (increased psychomotor activity, labile mood, behavioral disturbances) and *hypoactive states* (decreased psychomotor activity, alteration in consciousness). Hypoactive states often correspond to a decrease in level of consciousness, which must be managed as a life-threatening emergency until proven otherwise.

Altered level of consciousness refers to decreases in arousal and responsiveness to the environment. Intact consciousness requires two components: wakefulness and awareness both of self and of the environment. Abnormal states of consciousness present along a spectrum and range from lethargy to obtundation to stupor and finally coma (Table 41.1). **Coma** is the lack of any awareness of self and environment despite painful or other external stimulation. **Delirium**, in contrast, follows a fluctuating course of alertness and attention; waxing and waning periods of irritability, agitation, lack of contact with the environment, disorientation, and confusion may be observed. Periods of lucidity may alternate with the delirious state, and patients may proceed rapidly from delirium to lethargy or coma. Both delirium and coma represent final common pathways of multiple processes that lead to global central nervous system (CNS) failure. *Any alteration in the level of consciousness, whether delirium, lethargy, obtundation, stupor, or coma, must be managed as a life-threatening emergency until proven otherwise.*

ALTERED STATES OF CONSCIOUSNESS

Arousal and awareness form the foundation for normal cognitive function and consciousness. **Arousal** is determined in the brainstem's ascending reticular activating system (ARAS), which is also known as the "sleep center" of the brain. **Awareness** and behavior are generated in the cortex of the bilateral cerebral hemispheres. The cortex is the central processing center that interprets neuronal input and generates awareness. Diffuse injury to the cerebral hemispheres, injury to the ARAS, or both create an alteration in consciousness. Because the ARAS is located near several brainstem reflexes, injury to the ARAS is often accompanied by dysfunction of these reflexes including altered pupillary light reflex (controlled by cranial nerves II and III) and altered eye movement reflexes (oculocephalic and oculovestibular reflexes, which are controlled by cranial nerves III, VI, and VIII and the medial longitudinal fasciculus). Conversely, intact pupillary light, oculocephalic, and oculovestibular reflexes suggest dysfunction of both cerebral hemispheres. ARAS dysfunction is usually a result of structural causes, while diffuse cerebral dysfunction is usually caused by medical causes such as toxic or metabolic encephalopathies.

Classification Systems

Standardized language is necessary to properly diagnose and treat alterations in consciousness because terms such as lethargy, obtundation, stupor, *and* coma *are qualitative descriptions.* Rating scales permit different observers to follow the progression of the patient's mental status over time and facilitate effective communication of clinical information. The most widely used grading system is the **Glasgow Coma Scale (GCS)** (Table 41.2), which has been modified for children younger than 5 years of age based on their age-appropriate developmental abilities (Table 41.3). This 15-point scale evaluates three areas of CNS function: eye opening, verbal response, and motor response. A score of 15 indicates full function, whereas a score of 3 indicates no function. The first area of assessment is eye opening, in which the arousability and alertness of the patient are evaluated. Spontaneous eye opening indicates intact arousal mechanisms but does not imply awareness. The second area, verbal response, requires a high degree of integration within the CNS. Oriented responses indicate awareness of person, place, and time. The third area, motor functioning, reflects mentation as well as the integrity of the major CNS pathways. For purposes of gauging global brain function, the best motor response from any limb is taken as the score. Variation in response from one side of the body to the other is indicative of an asymmetric brain lesion. Spinal cord lesions resulting in paralysis or significant orthopedic injuries to the extremities prevent evaluation of the motor portion of the GCS.

The GCS can provide a general assessment of consciousness but is not intended to take the place of a complete neurologic evaluation (Table 41.4). The GCS is an objective measure of the patient's level of consciousness and should be used serially over time to monitor improvement or worsening of consciousness. Interventions are often based on the score; for example, most patients with a score of 8 or less should undergo endotracheal intubation. Deterioration of a patient's score by 2 or more points indicates a need for urgent re-evaluation of the patient and the possible need for further interventions such as endotracheal intubation and diagnostic studies such as a brain CT scan.

The GCS has also been shown to correlate with prognosis in patients presenting with decreased levels of consciousness. In traumatic brain injury, it may take days to weeks for patients with initial scores of 3–5 to become conscious as opposed to a few days in patients with scores of ≥6. Children presenting after near-drowning with an initial score of ≥6 have good outcomes. Patients presenting with a score of ≤5 have a high probability of mortality or profound neurologic sequelae. A score of 3 on transfer to an intensive care unit after near-drowning has been associated with a nearly 100% rate of poor outcome.

Although the GCS is a widely applied tool for assessment, it does not assess *brainstem function* and fails to discriminate between low

TABLE 41.1 States of Altered Consciousness or Unresponsiveness

Coma: a state of unarousable unresponsiveness; even strong exteroceptive stimuli fail to elicit recognizable psychologic responses; unresponsive to pain

Stupor: spontaneous unarousability interruptible only by vigorous, direct external stimulation; responsive only to pain

Hypersomnia, pathologic drowsiness, obtundation: terms applied to an increase above the patient's normal sleep/wake ratio, often accompanied during wakefulness by reduced attention and interest in the environment; responsive to pain and other stimuli

Delirium: an acute or subacute reduction in awareness, attention, orientation, and perception ("clouding of consciousness"), fluctuating and accompanied by abnormal sleep/wake patterns and often psychomotor disturbances, which can be hypo- or hyperactive

Syncope: brief loss of consciousness caused by global failure of cerebrovascular perfusion

Dementia: a sustained or permanent multidimensional or global decline in cognitive functions

Vegetative state: a sustained, complete loss of cognition, with sleep/wake cycles and other autonomic functions remaining relatively intact; can either follow acute, severe bilateral cerebral damage or develop gradually as the end stage of a progressive dementia

Locked-in state: preservation of intellectual activity accompanied by severe or total incapacity to express voluntary responses as a result of damage to or dysfunction of descending motor pathways in the brain or peripheral motor nerves; most, but not all, such patients can use vertical eye movements to signal by code

Modified from Plum F. Neurology/disturbances of consciousness and arousal. In: Wyngaarden JB, Smith LH, Bennett JC, eds. *Cecil Textbook of Medicine*. 19th ed. Philadelphia: WB Saunders; 1992:2049.

scores in intubated patients. The **Full Outline of Unresponsiveness (FOUR) Scale** is another tool to assess consciousness and evaluates eye response, motor response, brainstem reflexes, and respiratory effort on a 4-point scale. The FOUR score eye and motor responses are defined similarly to the GCS (see Table 41.2). The assessment of brainstem response focuses on the pupillary and corneal reflexes. The respiratory assessment includes ways to score for an intubated patient along with respiratory effort. Because the FOUR score includes brainstem responses and differentiates between intubated and nonintubated patients, this scale is better able to discriminate between patients with a GCS score of 3. Regardless of the scoring system used, reporting the score for each element can improve the precision of the assessment of the level of consciousness to guide management decisions.

Other scales have been developed to measure the level of consciousness in specific disease states, such as poisonings and hepatic failure. The **Reed classification** of coma has been used in the setting of poisoning or intoxication (Table 41.5) and is used to evaluate increasing depths of coma encountered with CNS-depressant drugs. The cardiovascular system is included in this classification because toxic ingestions may depress myocardial contractility or cause vasodilation. Neurologic function in a patient with **hepatic encephalopathy** is staged according to the scoring system of symptoms, signs, and EEG (Table 41.6).

Differential Diagnosis

The differential diagnosis in AMS is extensive. When AMS is associated with decreased level of consciousness, the differential can be broadly categorized as structural brain disease, nonstructural or medical disease, and psychogenic causes. Structural etiologies can result in either focal or nonfocal neurologic signs and include traumatic head injuries, hydrocephalus, tumors, intracranial hemorrhages, and cerebral vascular accidents. Nonstructural etiologies usually are associated

with nonfocal neurologic exams and result in a decreased level of consciousness through diffuse neuronal injury. Nonstructural etiologies include infections, metabolic encephalopathies, toxic ingestion, hypoxic-ischemic events, inflammatory brain diseases, and seizures (Table 41.7). The age of the patient can help the clinician differentiate the likely causes of coma, although there is considerable overlap (Table 41.8). Patients with delirium must be differentiated from an acute psychotic event (Table 41.9) (see Chapter 31). In addition, in patients who are awake but presenting with AMS, performing an appropriate mental status exam may help evaluate the degree of impairment and potential etiology (Table 41.10). The mental status exam is most abnormal with medical (encephalopathy, encephalitis) causes of altered behavior and mental status. *In primary psychiatric disorders, the neurologic exam is nonfocal and level of wakefulness often remains intact despite changes in behavior, orientation, and/or responses.*

Simultaneous Diagnosis and Management Approach

Many causes of AMS are life-threatening medical emergencies. Rapid assessment and diagnosis are therefore crucial and must happen simultaneously alongside management of identified life-threatening etiologies. The approach to the child with AMS can be divided into four parts: (1) stabilization, (2) rapid clinical assessment, (3) reversal of immediately treatable toxic or metabolic causes, and (4) detailed investigation including determination of the level of CNS function and of the cause of the coma (Fig. 41.1).

Stabilization

Initial stabilization for all patients includes assessment of the patient's airway, breathing, and circulation (ABCs). The first step in management is evaluating the patient's airway and responding appropriately to ensure patency. This may involve positioning, suctioning, or intubating. This is closely tied to the assessment of breathing and the respiratory drive via auscultation, observation, respiratory rate, and pulse oximeter. Obtunded, stuporous, or comatose patients usually require intubation unless their mental status is improving or can be readily reversed. Intubation in these patients allows the airway to be secured, treatment of hypoventilation or hypoxia (which may be contributing to the patient's AMS), and protection of the airway if a gag reflex is not present. Manipulation of the neck, particularly extension, should be avoided when an airway is being stabilized or secured, unless the cervical spine has already been cleared via history or imaging.

After a patient's airway and breathing are stabilized, the next step in management is assessment and stabilization of circulation. Initial assessment includes heart rate, blood pressure, presence and volume of peripheral pulses, capillary refill time, and adequacy of end-organ perfusion. **Shock** is defined as inadequate supply of oxygen to meet metabolic needs in the body's tissues. If shock leads to hypoperfusion of the brain, AMS and decreased levels of consciousness result (see Chapter 10). Assessment of vital signs may also suggest the presence of increased intracranial pressure (bradycardia, hypertension, irregular respirations) or a toxidrome.

Rapid Clinical Assessment

After initial stabilization of the airway, breathing, and circulation, attention should turn to rapid clinical assessment with the goal of quickly identifying life-threatening and reversible causes of AMS. The rapid clinical assessment should include a focused history from available friends, family, witnesses, first responders, and the medical record as applicable, and a focused physical exam with a targeted neurologic examination.

Rapid History

Initially, history gathering should focus on rapid detection of possible life-threatening causes of AMS. Pertinent questions include recent

TABLE 41.2 Glasgow Coma Scale Versus Full Outline of Unresponsiveness Score

Glasgow Coma Scale (GCS)		Full Outline of Unresponsiveness (FOUR)	
Eye Opening:		**Eye Response:**	
1	Does not open eyes	4	Eyelids open and comply with verbal stimuli
2	Opens eyes in response to noxious stimuli	3	Eyelids open but not tracking
3	Opens eyes in response to voice	2	Eyelids closed but open to loud noise
4	Opens eyes spontaneously	1	Eyelids closed but open to noxious stimuli
		0	Eyelids remain closed
Verbal Response:		**Motor Response:**	
1	No verbal response	4	Thumbs up, fist or peace sign
2	Incomprehensible sounds	3	Localize to pain
3	Inappropriate words	2	Flexion to pain
4	Confused and disoriented fluid speech	1	Extension to pain
5	Oriented with normal speech	0	No response to pain or myoclonus
Motor Response:		**Brainstem Reflexes:**	
1	No movements	4	Pupil and corneal reflexes present
2	Extension to noxious stimuli	3	One pupil wide and fixed
3	Flexion to noxious stimuli	2	Pupil or corneal reflex absent
4	Withdrawal to pain	1	Pupil and corneal reflexes absent
5	Localizes to pain	0	Absent pupil, corneal, and cough reflex
6	Obeys commands		
		Respirations:	
		4	Regular breathing pattern
		3	Cheyne-Stokes respirations
		2	Irregular breathing
		1	Intubated but breathing above the vent
		0	Breathing at vent rate or apnea
TOTAL SCORE 3–15		TOTAL SCORE 0–16	

TABLE 41.3 Pediatric Glasgow Coma Scale

Activity	Best Response	Score
Eye opening	Spontaneously	4
	To speech	3
	To pain	2
	None	1
Verbal	Oriented	5
	Words	4
	Vocal sounds	3
	Cries	2
	None	1
Motor	Obeys commands	5
	Localizes pain	4
	Flexion to pain	3
	Extension to pain	2
	None	1
Normal Total Score Based on Age		
Birth–6 mo		9
7–12 mo		11
1–2 yr		12
2–5 yr		13
>5 yr		14

Modified from Simpson D, Reilly P. Pediatric coma scale. *Lancet.* 1982;2:450.

TABLE 41.4 The Neurologic Examination in Coma

1. Guarantee vital functions.
2. Feel the scalp for hematomas (overlying fracture lines); be sure the neck is not fractured; test gently for stiff neck.
3. Test language. Test arousability by words, loud sounds, noxious stimuli. If vocalizations occur, check quickly for appropriate phrases, actual words, and presence or absence of aphasia.
4. Perform a neuro-ophthalmologic examination.
   Funduscopy (if difficult, can be deferred until patient is stabilized)
   Papilledema (increased intracranial or venous sinus pressure)
   Hemorrhages (subarachnoid hemorrhage; hypertensive encephalopathy; hypoxic-hypercarbic encephalopathy)
   Pupils
   Light reaction: Use bright flashlight and, if necessary, a magnifying glass to be certain of findings. Absence means potentially fatal deep sedative poisoning or acute or chronic structural brainstem damage.
   Equality: 15% of normal patients have mild anisocoria, but new or >2 mm dilatation means parasympathetic (third nerve) palsy.
   Extraocular movements: Absence acutely means deep drug poisoning, severe brainstem damage, polyneuropathy, or botulism.
   Dysconjugate deviation: At rest, this means an acute third, fourth, or sixth nerve palsy or internuclear ophthalmoplegia. Tonic conjugate deviation toward a paralytic arm and leg means forebrain seizures or a contralateral pontine destructive lesion; such deviation away from the paralytic arm and leg means forebrain gaze paralysis.
   Spontaneous eye movements: In comatose patients, nystagmus, bobbing, and independently moving eyes all mean brainstem damage.
   Oculocephalic (away from direction of head turning) or oculovestibular (toward cold caloric irrigation) responses: Absence of responses means drug overdose or severe brainstem disease; dysconjugate responses with equal pupils mean internuclear ophthalmoplegia; responses with unequal pupils mean third nerve disease.
5. Examine the motor systems.
   Strength
   Unilateral weakness or motionlessness of arm and leg means contralateral supraspinal upper motor neuron lesion, most often cerebral; if of arm, leg, and face, contralateral cerebral lesion. Occasionally, arm and leg weakness reflects contralateral brainstem lesion.
   Weakness or motionlessness of all four extremities implies metabolic disease; less likely is brainstem disease (tone and reflexes increased) or peripheral disease (tone and reflexes decreased).
   Attempt to Elicit Reflex Posturing
   Arm flexed, leg extended: contralateral deep cerebral-thalamic lesion
   Arm and leg extended: thalamic or mesencephalic lesion
   Arms extended and legs flexed or flaccid: pontine lesion
   Legs flexed, arms flaccid: pontomedullary or spinal lesion
   Compare side-to-side reflexes and examine plantar responses.
6. Seek seizure activity or abnormal movements: (1) generalized, (2) focal, (3) multifocal, and (4) myoclonic.
   Control (1) immediately, (2) and (3) deliberately; if (4) is present, treat underlying disease.
   Acute tremor, asterixis, multifocal myoclonus: Seek metabolic cause.
7. Inspect breathing.
   Regular hyperpnea: metabolic acidosis; pulmonary infarction; congestive failure or alveolar infiltration; sepsis; salicylism; hepatic coma
   Cyclically irregular (Cheyne-Stokes): low cardiac output plus bilateral cerebral or upper brainstem dysfunction
   Irregular gasping, slow or weak: lower, brainstem dysfunction (including hypoglycemia, drug effects); less often, peripheral ventilatory paralysis
8. Proceed with laboratory tests and emergency management as described in text.

Modified from Plum F. Neurology/sustained impairments of consciousness. In: Wyngaarden JB, Smith LH, Bennett JC, eds. *Cecil Textbook of Medicine*. 19th ed. Philadelphia: WB Saunders; 1992:2057.

history preceding the change in mental status, timing of onset and progression of AMS, and the patient's medical history such as diabetes, seizures, substance abuse, or immunocompromise. Questions regarding any traumatic injuries over the previous few days should be asked, and even if trauma is denied, concern for nonaccidental trauma should be raised if the story is inconsistent or nonspecific for the presenting clinical scenario. History should also include fevers or other signs or symptoms of infection as well as signs of increased intracranial pressure such as vomiting, ptosis, and headaches. Infants with rising increased intracranial pressure may present with irritability, lethargy, increasing head circumference, and poor feeding. A dietary history in infants presenting with a depressed level of consciousness is paramount and may raise suspicion of hypoglycemia (from fasting or emesis) or hyponatremia (from ingestion of free water). Exposure to drugs or toxins should be suspected in any patient with a sudden onset of unexplained symptoms (coma, seizures) or a gradual onset of symptoms preceded by a period of confusion or delirium. The caregivers should be asked directly about possible access to medications, recreational drugs, and environmental toxins.

Rapid Physical Exam

After quickly collecting the available historical information, the next phase in management is completing a focused physical exam including a rapid neurologic assessment, which should take no more than a few minutes.

General Physical Exam

The general physical exam should include assessment of vital signs with emphasis on the cardiovascular, respiratory, and head and neck exams as well as a general assessment. Special attention should be paid to identify any physical exam findings that may suggest a specific toxidrome. The absence of a history of trauma or physical findings suggestive of a rapidly progressive intracranial process does not preclude a traumatic or an anatomic cause of coma. Traumatic injuries can result in life-threatening illnesses at any age, including in newborns. The head and neck should be carefully inspected, and the skull palpated for evidence of trauma (Table 41.11). In infants, a bulging fontanel suggests raised intracranial pressure, which may have various causes. A bulging fontanel in the absence of a febrile illness should raise the suspicion of trauma, including abusive head trauma. Retinal hemorrhages are often present on funduscopic examination in children with abusive head trauma. In addition to abusive head trauma, a child may have a subarachnoid hemorrhage (ruptured aneurysm, arteriovenous malformation) or hydrocephalus without any of the aforementioned signs or symptoms of raised intracranial pressure. An ear exam should be performed to evaluate hemotympanum. Hemotympanum, clear drainage from the nose or ear, Battle sign (bruising behind the ear), and raccoon eyes may indicate a basilar skull fracture (see Table 41.11).

Hyperventilation can be observed in midbrain structural lesions but also in toxic-metabolic encephalopathies as a primary response to stimulation of the respiratory center (salicylates, theophylline, hyperammonemia, hepatic coma) or as a compensatory response to a metabolic acidosis. This pattern is also seen with raised intracranial hypertension. **Hypoventilation** with a normal rhythm, particularly if associated with a symmetrically depressed motor examination, usually implies global CNS depression secondary to drug ingestion such as opioids or benzodiazepines (Fig. 41.2).

Neurologic Exam

After completing a brief general physical exam and noting impaired consciousness, a rapid neurologic assessment is required. Level of consciousness should be assessed using a validated scoring system such at the GCS or FOUR scores. In children with altered level of consciousness, the neurologic assessment should focus on identifying lateralizing or focal findings, assessing for signs of increased intracranial pressure, and recognizing brainstem dysfunction. Intrinsic to this assessment is differentiating between bilateral cerebral hemisphere dysfunction, ARAS dysfunction, or both. Bilateral cerebral hemisphere involvement may be further divided into unilateral lesions with mass effect versus diffuse bilateral injury. If the ARAS is affected, additional evidence of brainstem dysfunction is usually present.

Motor System and Focal Findings

The presence of focal findings can be determined by comparison of either side of the child's body. Careful attention should be paid to asymmetry of tone and movement between extremities, asymmetry of the face either at rest or with movement, and asymmetry of reflexes, such as the pupillary and deep tendon reflexes. Examination of the motor system includes observation first of body position, then spontaneous movements, and finally response to noxious stimuli (Fig. 41.3). Throughout the exam, the examiner should note asymmetry between sides and muscle tone.

A normal body position usually denotes an intact brainstem, as do spontaneous, nonposturing movements. **Hemiparesis** or **hemiplegia** implies a structural lesion in the contralateral hemisphere or subcortical region or an ipsilateral spinal cord injury. The presence of **hypertonia** or **hyperreflexia** suggests previous corticospinal tract disease or an acute brainstem injury at the midbrain-pontine level. It can also be observed in patients with severe metabolic derangements, such as hepatic coma, hypoglycemia, anoxia, and uremia. **Hypotonia** implies bilateral hemispheric dysfunction or a medullary or spinal cord lesion. In patients with severe depression of brain function, motor function can be assessed only after the application of a noxious stimulus, such as a sternal rub or increasing subungual pressure to the fingernails or toenails. If the response to a noxious stimulus includes verbalization, eye opening, or a normal motor response (e.g., localization of the stimulus, withdrawal of the limb, or movement away from the stimulus), this indicates that the ascending sensory pathways to the cerebral hemispheres are intact, and descending motor pathways are functioning.

Signs of Increased Intracranial Pressure

Indications of clinically significant intracranial hypertension can be assessed through the pupillary responses (Fig. 41.4), vital signs, and motor responses (Tables 41.12 and 41.13). The cranial vault contains brain, blood, and cerebrospinal fluid (CSF), and an increase in volume in one area necessitates a decrease in volume in another area. This increase in volume may occur secondary to space-occupying lesions, edema, intracranial hemorrhage, or hydrocephalus. The volume compensation mechanisms within the cranial vault are limited, and if volume cannot

TABLE 41.5	Reed Classification of Coma
Grade 0*	Asleep Can be aroused Will answer questions
Grade 1*	Comatose Withdraws from painful stimuli Intact reflexes
Grade 2*	Comatose Does not withdraw from painful stimuli No respiratory, circulatory depression Intact reflexes
Grade 3†	Comatose Reflexes absent No respiratory, circulatory depression
Grade 4†	Comatose Reflexes absent Respiratory or circulatory problems

*Good prognosis.
†Very serious, may need measures to enhance elimination.
Modified from Ellenhorn MJ, Barceloux DE. *Medical Toxicology: Diagnosis and Treatment of Human Poisoning.* New York: Elsevier Science; 1988:17.

TABLE 41.6	Stages of Hepatic Encephalopathy			
	I	**II**	**III**	**IV**
Symptoms	Periods of lethargy, euphoria; reversal of day-night sleeping; may be alert	Drowsiness, inappropriate behavior, agitation, wide mood swings, disorientation	Stupor but arousable; confused, incoherent speech	Coma: IVa responds to noxious stimuli; IVb no response
Signs	Trouble drawing figures, performing mental tasks	Asterixis, fetor hepaticus, incontinence	Asterixis, hyperreflexia, extensor reflexes, rigidity	Areflexia, no asterixis, flaccidity
EEG	Normal	Generalized slowing, Q waves	Markedly abnormal triphasic waves	Markedly abnormal bilateral slowing, delta waves, electrocortical silence

From Kliegman RM, St. Geme JW III, Blum NJ, et al., eds. *Nelson Textbook of Pediatrics.* 21st ed. Philadelphia: Elsevier; 2020:2135, Table 391.1.

TABLE 41.7 Etiologic Classification of Altered Mental Status in Children

Infectious	Metabolic/Systemic	Toxic*	Traumatic*	Anatomic	Hypoxic-Ischemic	Epileptic	Vascular	Inflammatory	Psychologic
Viral	Hypoglycemia*	Sympathomimetics	Concussion*	Tumor	Cardiac arrest	Postictal state*	Embolism	Autoimmune encephalitis	Conversion disorders*
Aseptic meningitis*	Inborn errors of metabolism*	Anticholinergics	Cerebral contusion	Hydrocephalus	Cardiac arrhythmia	Status epilepticus*	Spontaneous intraparenchymal hemorrhage	ADEM	Catatonia
Encephalitis*	Hyperammonemia	Phenothiazines	Epidural hematoma	Hydrocephalus with shunt malfunction	Severe shock	Absence status	Subarachnoid hemorrhage	NMO	Intensive care unit delirium
? Reye syndrome	Hepatic failure	PCP	Subdural hematoma	Subdural hematoma	Near-drowning	Complex partial seizure	Venous sinus thrombosis	Multiple sclerosis	Psychogenic nonepileptic seizures
? Hemorrhagic shock and encephalopathy syndrome	Renal diseases	LSD	Brainstem	Epidural hematoma	Neonatal asphyxia*	Epilepsy-encephalopathy syndromes	Vasculitis	Rasmussen encephalitis	
Postinfectious encephalomyelitis	Uremic encephalopathy	Marijuana	Epidural contusion	Brain abscess	Hypoxemic respiratory failure		Lupus erythematosus	Neurosarcoidosis	
Systemic infection with shock	Hypertensive encephalopathy	Cocaine	Diffuse axonal shear injury	Subdural empyema	Carbon monoxide poisoning		Hypertensive encephalopathy	Hashimoto encephalopathy	
Bacterial	Dialysis encephalopathy (dysequilibrium syndrome)	Heavy metals (lead, arsenic, mercury)	Cerebral edema*	Epidural empyema	Cyanide toxicity		Acute confusional migraine*	HLH	
Brain abscess	Hyperosmolar states	Salicylates	Intraparenchymal hemorrhage	Cerebral edema	Anaphylaxis				
Epidural empyema	Hypernatremia	Organophosphates and carbamates	Intraventricular hemorrhage (neonate)*	Intracranial hemorrhage	Asthma				
Subdural empyema	Hyperglycemia–diabetes mellitus*	Antihistamines	Obstructive hydrocephalus	Cerebrovascular accident/stroke					
Systemic infection with shock	Hypo-osmolar states	Industrial solvents (inhaled)	Post-traumatic seizure						
Toxic shock syndrome	Hyponatremia*	Alcohols	Fat embolism						
Rickettsial infection	Rapid decrease in osmolality in hyperosmolar states	Opioids							
Fungal	Adrenal insufficiency	Sedative-hypnotics							
Fungal meningitis	Hyperthyroidism and hypothyroidism	Barbiturates							
Fungal brain abscess	Hyperparathyroidism	Carbon monoxide							
Protozoan	Hypercalcemia	Tricyclic antidepressants							
Meningitis	Hypocalcemia	Carbamazepine							
Abscess	Hypermagnesemia	Cyanide							
Postimmunization encephalopathy	Hypomagnesemia	Methaqualone							
	Hypophosphatemia	Burn encephalopathy							
	Hypercapnia	Selective serotonin reuptake inhibitors							
	Hypoxia*	Serotonin-norepinephrine reuptake inhibitor							
	Shock*	Monoamine oxidase inhibitors							
	Vitamin deficiency and toxicity states	Penicillins							
	Nicotinic acid	Carbapenems							
	Pantothenic acid	Methotrexate							
	Pyridoxine	Valproate							
	Thiamine	Vigabatrin							
	Vitamin B_{12}	Levetiracetam							
		Cyclosporine							
		Tacrolimus							

Continued

TABLE 41.7	Etiologic Classification of Altered Mental Status in Children—cont'd								
Infectious	Metabolic/ Systemic	Toxic*	Traumatic*	Anatomic	Hypoxic-Ischemic	Epileptic	Vascular	Inflammatory	Psychologic
	Intussusception encephalopathy Methemoglobinemia Acidosis Alkalosis Porphyria Reye syndrome Mitochondrial encephalopathies								

*Common.
ADEM, acute disseminated encephalomyelitis; HLH, hemophagocytic lymphohistiocytosis; LSD, lysergic acid diethylamide; NMO, neuromyelitis optica; PCP, phenylcyclohexyl piperidine (phencyclidine HCl).

TABLE 41.8 Common Causes of Altered Mental Status by Age

Neonate	Infant	Child	Adolescent
Hypoglycemia	Meningitis	Meningitis	Meningitis
Birth asphyxia	Bacterial	Bacterial	Bacterial
Congenital anomalies of the central nervous system	Viral	Viral	Viral
Systemic infection with shock	Trauma	Encephalitis	Encephalitis
Cardiogenic shock	Abuse/shaken baby syndrome	Trauma	Intentional ingestion
Congenital infection	Asphyxia	Ingestion	Recreational drug/alcohol use
Bacterial meningitis	Brief resolved unexplained event	Reye syndrome	Suicide gesture or attempt
Inborn errors of metabolism	Intentional suffocation	Systemic infection with shock	Often involves multiple agents
Hypocalcemia	Systemic infection with shock	Seizure	Trauma
Intraventricular hemorrhage	Ingestion	Near-drowning	Seizures
Seizures	Inborn errors of metabolism	Hypoglycemia	Diabetic ketoacidosis
Birth trauma	Hypoglycemia	Intussusception	Systemic infection with shock
	Hyponatremia	Acute demyelinating encephalomyelitis	Toxic shock syndrome
	Hypocalcemia	Diabetic ketoacidosis	Reye syndrome
	Encephalitis		Spontaneous intracranial hemorrhage
	Postimmunization encephalopathy		Psychologic
	Hemorrhagic shock and encephalopathy syndrome		Lupus
	Intussusception encephalopathy		
	Seizures		

TABLE 41.9 Special Problems in the Differential Diagnosis of Delirium*

Clinical Feature	Delirium	Dementias	Schizophrenia	Depression
Course	Acute onset; hours, days, or more	Insidious onset[†]; months or years; progressive	Insidious onset, 6 mo or more; acute psychotic phases	Insidious onset, at least 2 wk, often months
Attention	Markedly impaired attention and arousal	Normal early; impairment later	Normal to mild impairment	Mild impairment
Fluctuation	Prominent in attention arousal; disturbed day/night cycle	Prominent fluctuations absent; lesser disturbances in day/night cycle	Absent	Absent
Perception	Misperceptions; hallucinations, usually visual, fleeting; paramnesia	Perceptual abnormalities much less prominent[‡]; paramnesia	Hallucinations, auditory with personal reference	May have mood-congruent hallucinations
Speech and language	Abnormal clarity, speed, and coherence; disjointed and dysarthric; misnaming; characteristic dysgraphia	Early anomia; empty speech; abnormal comprehension	Disorganized, with a bizarre theme	Decreased amount of speech
Other cognition	Disorientation to time, place; recent memory and visuospatial abnormalities	Disorientation to time, place; multiple other higher cognitive deficits	Disorientation to person; concrete interpretations	Mental slowing; indecisiveness; memory retrieval difficulty
Behavior	Lethargy or delirium; nonsystematized delusions; emotional lability	Disinterested; disengaged; disinhibited; delusions and other psychiatric symptoms	Systematized delusions; paranoia; bizarre behavior	Depressed mood; anhedonia; lack of energy; sleep and appetite disturbances
EEG	Diffuse slowing; low-voltage fast activity; specific patterns	Normal early; mild slowing later	Normal	Normal

*The characteristics listed are the usual ones and are not exclusive.
†Patients with vascular dementia may have an abrupt decline in cognition.
‡Patients with dementia with diffuse cortical Lewy bodies often have a fluctuating mental status and hallucinations.
From Mendez MF, Padilla CR. Delirium. In: Daroff RB, Jankovic J, Mazziotta JC, et al., eds. *Bradley's Neurology in Clinical Practice.* 7th ed. Philadelphia: Elsevier; 2016:32, Table 4.2.

TABLE 41.10   MMC (Mini-Mental State Examination for Children)

Function	Tests	Score
Orientation	Name, surname, age, sex	0-1-2-3-4
	Name of parents, state, city, place	0-1-2-3-4
	Age, month, day of month, day of week	0-1-2-3-4
Object naming	Pen, watch, glasses	0-1-2-3
Digit span—forward	5-3	0-1-2-3-4
	4-7-2	
	5-9-3-1	
	2-7-5-9-4	
Digit span—backward	3-6	0-1-2-3
	2-9-5	
	4-1-9-7	
Recall	Pen, watch, glasses	0-1-2-3
Naming body parts	Naming body part indicated by the examiner: hand, foot, knee, nose, ear	0-1-2-3-4-5
Command	"Take the paper in your right hand, fold it in half, and put it on the floor" ("Pegue o papel com a mão, dobre-o ao meio e coloque-o no chão")	0-1-2-3
Verbal string repetition	"No ifs, ands, or buts" ("Nem aquí, nem lá, nem acolá")	0-1
Reading	"Read this and do what it says" ("Close your eyes")	0-1
Writing	"Write your name"	0-1
Constructional praxis	"Copy the drawings. Do it as best you can" (vertical line at age 3 yr, cross at age 4 yr, circle at age 5 yr, square at age 6 yr, and diamond at age 7 yr)	0-1
Maximum total score		**37**

Adapted version of the MMSE (Mini-Mental State Examination). From Moura R, Andrade PMO, Fontes PLB, et al. Mini-Mental State Exam for Children (MMC) in children with hemiplegic cerebral palsy. *Dement Neuropsychol.* 2017;11(3):287–296. https://www.ncbi.nlm.nih.gov/pmc/articles/PMC5674673/table/t5/?report=objectonly

be decreased in another area, intracranial pressure increases. The first signs of increasing intracranial pressure are often headache and vomiting followed by decreased consciousness, which is then followed by posturing, and finally vital sign changes followed by death. Sixth cranial nerve palsy or inability to abduct the eye can be an early sign of increased intracranial pressure caused by stretching of the sixth cranial nerve. Papilledema is also associated with increased intracranial pressure but takes ≥12 hours to develop and therefore may be absent in acute increased intracranial pressure. As intracranial pressure continues to increase, it eventually leads to brain herniation and the vital sign changes of **Cushing triad**: hypertension, bradycardia, and irregularities of respiration.

Brain herniation can occur at several different locations. The most common type of herniation is transtentorial herniation, which can be divided into uncal and central herniation. **Uncal herniation** occurs when the uncus (the inner part of the temporal lobe) herniates over the tentorium. This puts pressure on the midbrain, which contains the third cranial nerve. Pressure on the third cranial nerve impairs its parasympathetic fibers, leading to ipsilateral pupillary dilatation. Therefore, a unilaterally fixed and dilated pupil in a patient who is not awake represents uncal herniation. **Central herniation** occurs when central brain structures (diencephalon and temporal lobes) herniate through the tentorium cerebelli. Pressure on the hypothalamus at first causes small reactive pupils, which then progress to pupils that are fixed at midposition. Other types of herniation include **subfalcine herniation,** in which the cingulate gyrus herniates under the falx cerebri and presents with unilateral or bilateral weakness and can progress to central herniation. **Tonsillar herniation** or foramen magnum herniation results from the cerebellar tonsils being forced through the foramen magnum causing compression on the medulla oblongata and the cervical spinal cord leading to downbeat nystagmus, bradycardia, bradypnea, and hypertension. These signs can sometimes be worsened with neck flexion and improved with neck extension.

Brainstem Functioning

Brainstem function is evaluated by observing the child's respiratory pattern, pupillary reflexes, corneal reflexes, and eye movement reflexes. Dysfunction of brainstem reflexes implies disruption of the ARAS and is a red flag indicating a serious and life-threatening disease process.

Breathing Patterns

Significant brainstem dysfunction is usually associated with an abnormal breathing pattern (see Fig. 41.2). **Cheyne-Stokes respiration** is a pattern of breathing in which periods of hyperpnea alternate with shorter apneic phases, observed in the presence of bilateral hemispheric or diencephalic dysfunction. It may also precede transtentorial herniation. The hyperpneic periods have a characteristic smooth, crescendo-decrescendo pattern. **Central neurogenic hyperventilation** is encountered with midbrain dysfunction; patients with this problem are tachypneic and hyperpneic. **Apneustic breathing** is associated with damage in the middle to lower pontine region. This pattern is characterized by a prolonged pause at full inspiration. Clusters of breaths separated by periods of apnea may be observed in patients with low pontine to upper medullary lesions, whereas medullary lesions result in ataxic or irregular breathing, slow regular breathing, or agonal respiration.

Pupillary Light Reflexes

Pupillary light reflexes are generally preserved in metabolic encephalopathy, whereas their absence strongly suggests a structural lesion. The only exception to the latter is certain drug effects, particularly with potent anticholinergic compounds, such as glutethimide, atropine, or scopolamine, which produce fixed and dilated pupils. The balance between sympathetic and parasympathetic stimulation, which results in pupillary dilatation and constriction, normally determines pupillary size and reactivity. A **unilaterally dilated and fixed pupil** is a sign of uncal herniation with entrapment of the oculomotor nerve. Parasympathetic fibers innervating the eye accompany the oculomotor nerve. Sympathetic fibers originate from at least four hypothalamic nuclei so that diencephalic dysfunction results in small, reactive pupils. Hypothalamic damage often results in ipsilateral miosis associated with **Horner syndrome** (miosis, ptosis, and anhidrosis).

Injury to nuclei located in the midbrain disrupts both sympathetic and parasympathetic pathways, resulting in midsized, fixed pupils. Damage to the midbrain tectal regions also produces midposition or slightly large, fixed pupils. In contrast to nuclear damage, however, accommodation may be intact, so that pupillary size fluctuates spontaneously. Pontine lesions, principally hemorrhage, interfere with descending sympathetic fibers, causing symmetrically small pupils for which a magnifying glass may be needed to detect a light reflex. Lateral medullary lesions may also produce Horner syndrome, whereas central herniation results in fixed, dilated pupils. Figure 41.4 summarizes pupillary findings in comatose patients.

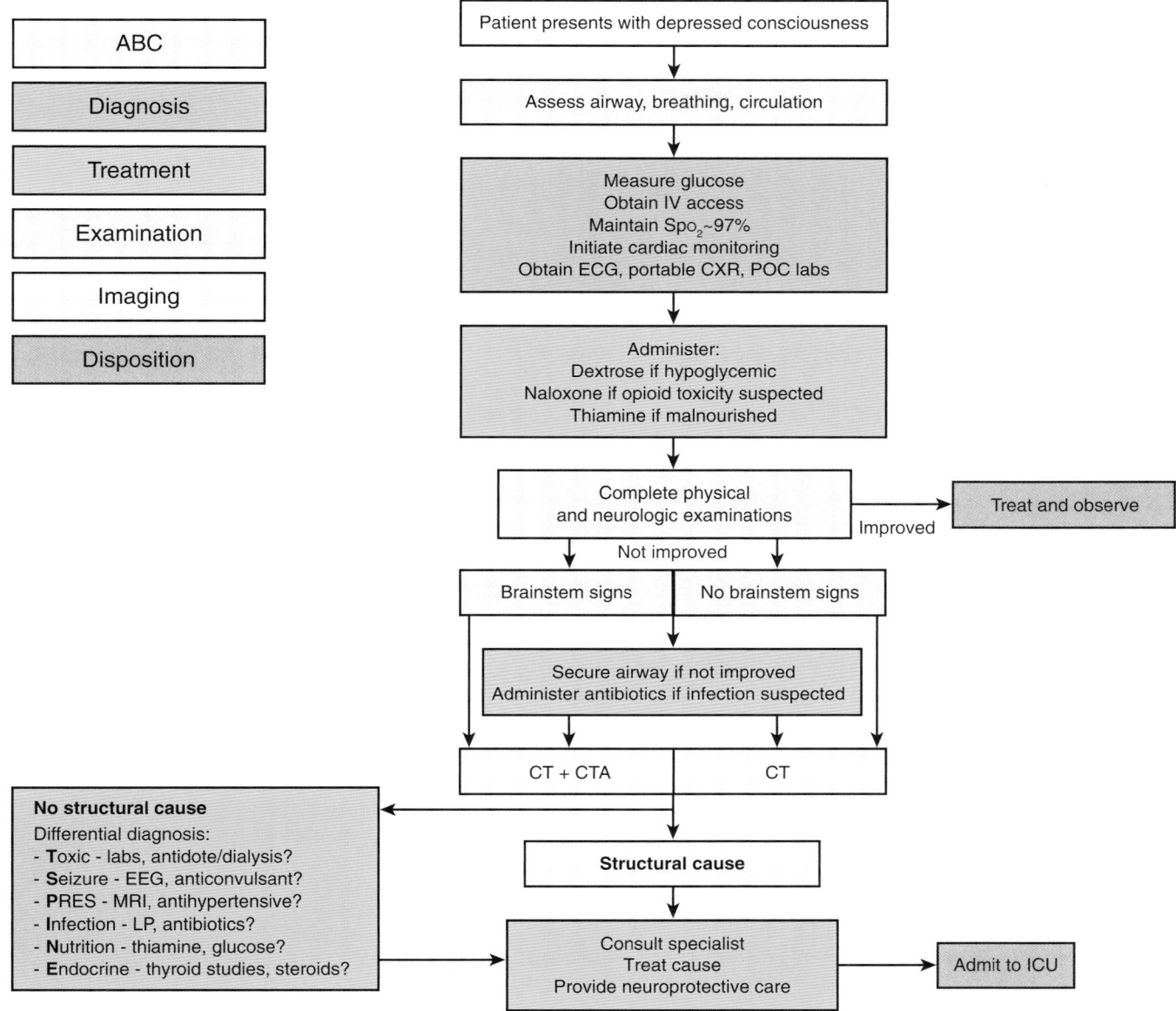

Fig. 41.1 Algorithm for diagnostic and management approach to depressed consciousness and coma. ABC, airway, breathing, circulation; CTA, computed tomography angiography; CXR, chest x-ray; ICU, intensive care unit; IV, intravenous; LP, lumbar puncture; POC, point of care; PRES, posterior reversible encephalopathy syndrome; Spo$_2$, oxygen saturation. (From Walls RM, Hockberger RS, Gausche-Hill M, eds. *Rosen's Emergency Medicine Concepts and Clinical Practice.* 9th ed. Philadelphia: Elsevier; 2018:130, Fig. 13.2.)

TABLE 41.11	Signs of Head Trauma Possibly Associated with Intracranial Disease
General	**Signs of Basilar Skull Fracture**
Lacerations	Hemotympanum
Hematomas	CSF rhinorrhea
Ecchymosis	CSF otorrhea
Swelling	"Raccoon eyes"
Palpable crepitations	Battle sign
Step-off of skull	

CSF, cerebrospinal fluid.

Eye Movement Reflexes

Evaluation of eye movements is helpful in differentiating hemispheric from brainstem causes of coma. Frontal regions of the cerebral hemispheres are responsible for voluntary eye movements, the quick phase of nystagmus, and control over brainstem reflexes that determine eye movements. Bilateral hemispheric depression may result in roving eye movements if brainstem function is intact. Because stimulation of a frontal gaze center causes conjugate deviation of the eyes to the opposite side, tonic lateral deviation of the eyes implies a seizure emanating from the contralateral hemisphere. Eye deviation may also result from an ipsilateral hemispheric injury with unopposed stimulation from the undamaged hemisphere or from a contralateral pontine lesion. The degree of eye deviation is usually more dramatic with hemispheric damage than with brainstem damage.

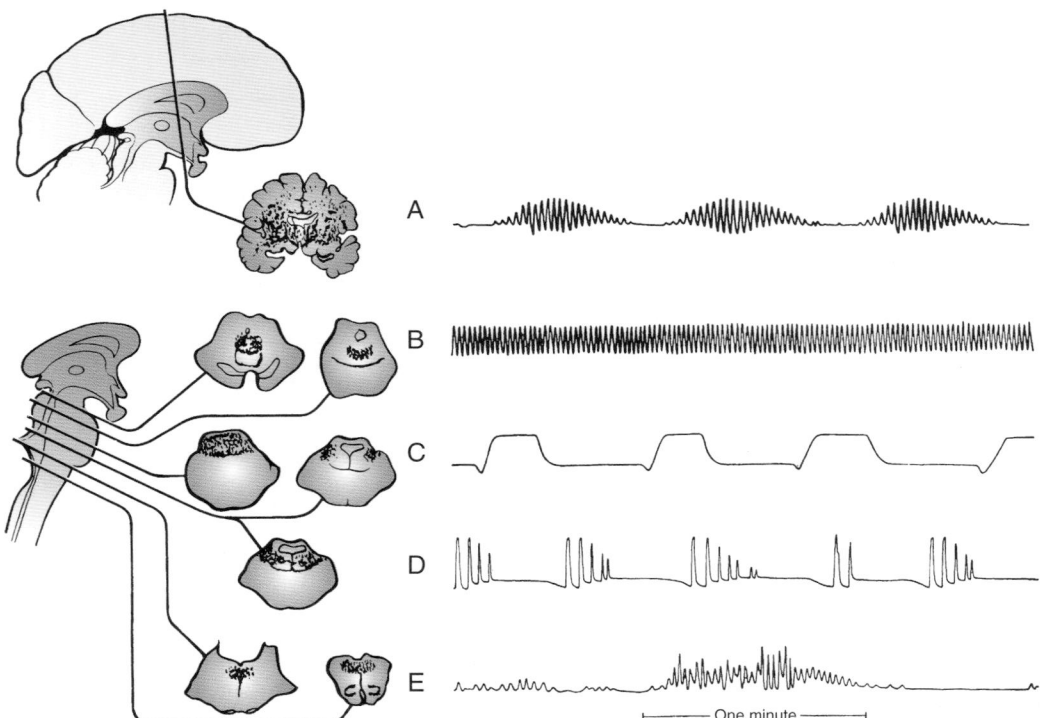

Fig. 41.2 Abnormal respiratory patterns. *A,* Cheyne-Stokes respiration. *B,* Central neurogenic hyperventilation. *C,* Apneusis. *D,* Cluster breathing. *E,* Ataxic breathing. *Shaded areas* show location of brain pathology associated with abnormal respiratory pattern.

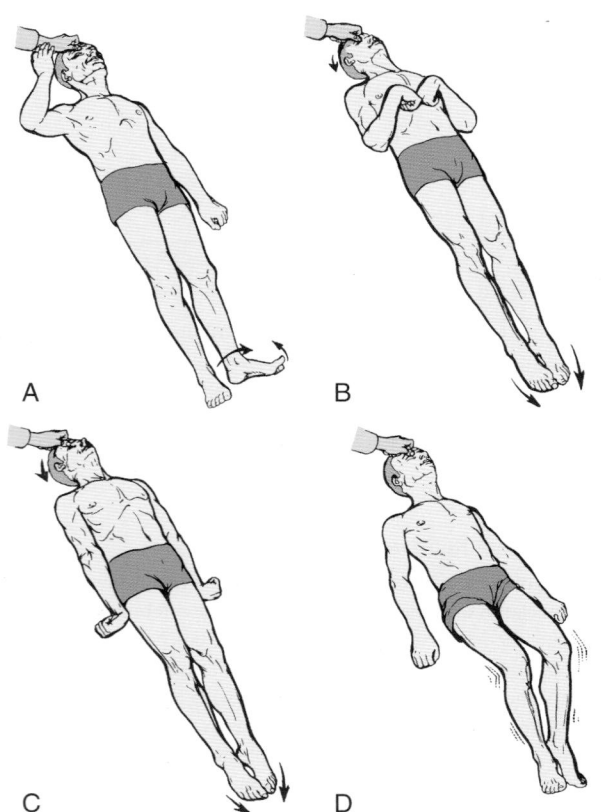

Fig. 41.3 Motor response to noxious stimuli. *A,* Localization. *B,* Decorticate posturing. *C,* Decerebrate posturing. *D,* Opisthotonos posturing.

If the patient's eyes are not moving, then reflex eye movements are tested by the oculocephalic and oculovestibular responses (Fig. 41.5). These maneuvers involve the same major neuronal pathways. Afferent fibers from the labyrinth, cerebellum, and cervical muscles reach the vestibular nuclei (cranial nerve VIII) in the medulla. Fibers from the vestibular nuclei then course to the ipsilateral abducens nuclei (cranial nerve VI). Fibers from the abducens nuclei then decussate in the midpons and ascend in the medial longitudinal fasciculus to reach the contralateral oculomotor nuclei (cranial nerve III). Intact reflexes indicate the absence of cortical input on an intact brainstem.

The oculocephalic reflex is elicited by rotating the child's head from side to side and observing the eye movements. *This reflex should not be checked unless a cervical spine injury has been ruled out.* If brainstem function is intact, the eyes deviate in a direction opposite to the head movement. Both left and right lateral rotation should be tested. This reflex is then tested in a vertical plane by rapidly flexing and extending the neck. A positive response is upward gaze when the neck is flexed and downward deviation when the head is extended.

The oculovestibular reflex is tested by instilling ice water into the ear canal. The ear canal must be visualized to ensure that there is no obstruction and that the tympanic membrane is intact. The head is then placed at a 30-degree angle from the horizontal so that the semicircular canal is vertical, and up to 120 mL of ice water is then injected slowly into the external ear canal over a few minutes through an angiocatheter. After a minimum of 5 minutes, the other ear may be tested; this interval allows time for the oculovestibular system to re-equilibrate. A positive response in an awake patient is nystagmus with the slow component toward the irrigated ear and the fast component away from the stimulus. With bilateral hemispheric depression, the fast phase of nystagmus dissipates, and the eyes are tonically deviated toward the irrigated ear.

Both the oculocephalic and oculovestibular reflexes are absent in patients with low brainstem lesions because neurotransmission between

METABLIC

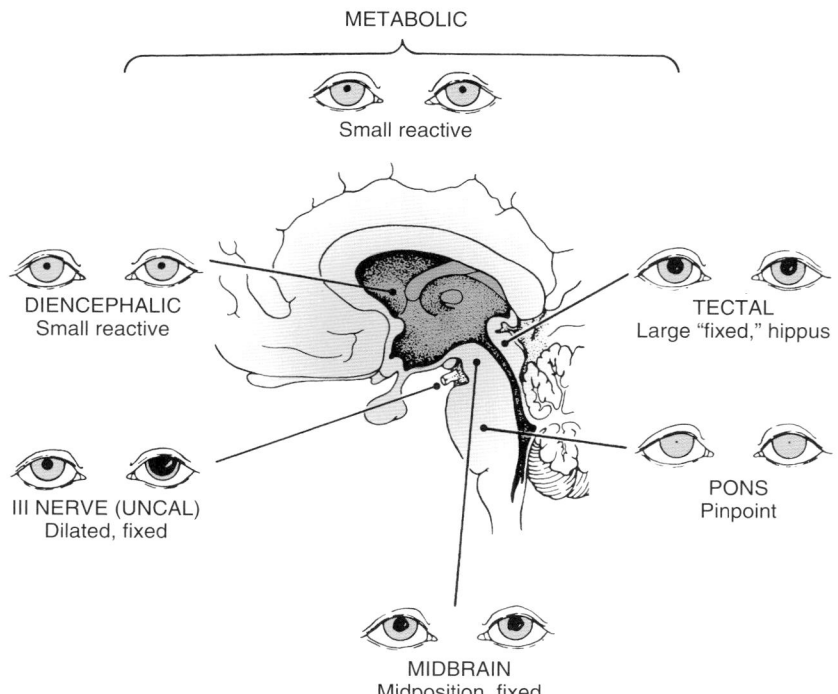

METABOLIC
Small reactive

DIENCEPHALIC
Small reactive

TECTAL
Large "fixed," hippus

III NERVE (UNCAL)
Dilated, fixed

PONS
Pinpoint

MIDBRAIN
Midposition, fixed

Fig. 41.4 Pupils in comatose patients.

TABLE 41.12 Signs of Incipient Downward Herniation

	Central	Uncal
Arousal	Impaired early, before other signs	Impaired late, usually with other signs
Breathing	Sighs, yawns, sometimes Cheyne-Stokes respiration	No early change
Pupils	First, small reactive (hypo-thalamus); then one or both approach midposition	Ipsilateral pupil dilates, followed by somatic third nerve paralysis
Oculocephalic responses	Initially sluggish, later tonic conjugate	Unilateral third nerve paralysis
Motor signs	Early hemiparesis opposite to hemispheric lesion followed late by ipsilateral motor paresis and extensor plantar response	Motor signs late, sometimes ipsilateral to lesion

From Plum F. Neurology/sustained impairments of consciousness. In: Wyngaarden JB, Smith LH, Bennett JC, eds. *Cecil Textbook of Medicine*. 19th ed. Philadelphia: WB Saunders; 1992:2050.

TABLE 41.13 Characteristics of Supratentorial Lesions Leading to Coma

Initiating symptoms usually cerebral-focal: aphasia; focal seizures; contra-lateral hemiparesis, sensory change, or neglect; frontal lobe behavioral changes; headache

Dysfunction moves rostral to caudal: e.g., focal motor → bilateral motor → altered level of arousal

Abnormal signs usually confined to a single or an adjacent anatomic level (not diffuse)

Brainstem functions spared unless herniation develops

From Plum F. Neurology/sustained impairments of consciousness. In: Wyngaarden JB, Smith LH, Bennett JC, eds. *Cecil Textbook of Medicine*. 19th ed. Philadelphia: WB Saunders; 1992:2050.

of a blink in response to a loud noise or bright light implies dysfunction of the pontine reticular formation secondary to either metabolic or structural causes. Unilateral absence of a blink implies a facial nerve lesion. The afferent limb of the corneal reflex is carried by the trigeminal nerve (cranial nerve V). The normal effector response involves both upward deviation of the eye (oculomotor nerve) and closure of the eyelid (facial nerve). A normal reflex suggests that the integrity of pathways between the midbrain and the pons has not been violated.

Body Position

In patients with decreased level of consciousness, the body's position in response to noxious stimuli can indicate hemispheric verses brainstem dysfunction. **Decorticate posturing** occurs when the upper extremities are held flexed at the elbow, wrist, and fingers and implies hemispheric dysfunction with an intact brainstem. **Decerebrate posturing** occurs when arms are internally rotated and adducted at the shoulder, extended at the elbow, pronated at the forearm, and flexed at the fingers (see Fig. 41.3). Opisthotonos with clenched teeth is a severe form of decerebration. Decerebrate posturing usually suggests brainstem compression or a severe structural injury to the midbrain-pontine region. It can also occur in association with severe metabolic diseases, such as hepatic coma, anoxia, and hypoglycemia. Less commonly, decerebrate

the vestibular and abducens nuclei is interrupted. In patients with damage to the medial longitudinal fasciculus, the ipsilateral eye fails to adduct on irrigation of the contralateral ear canal. However, the opposite eye abducts normally. With a lesion in the left medial longitudinal fasciculus, the right eye abducts, but the left eye does not, in response to irrigating the right ear canal. This reaction is caused by disruption of fibers between the abducens and the contralateral oculomotor nuclei (see Fig. 41.5).

Corneal Reflex

In addition to assessing ocular motility, the examiner should test the corneal reflex and determine the presence or absence of a blink. The absence

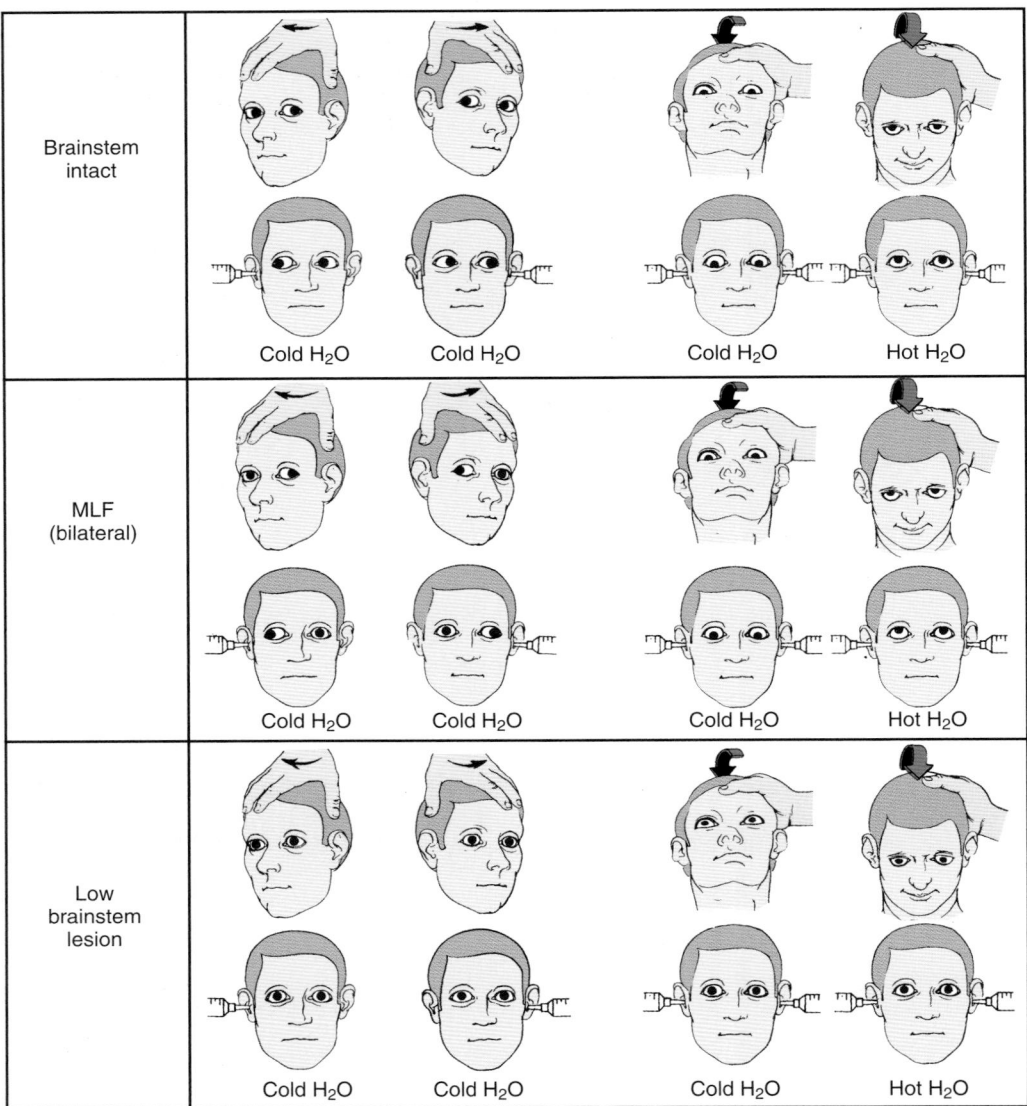

Fig. 41.5 Ocular reflexes. MLF, medial longitudinal fasciculus.

posture may represent delayed cortical demyelination after a hypoxic-ischemic injury. Pontomedullary or spinal cord damage is associated with a flaccid response to noxious stimulation.

Determining the Level of CNS Dysfunction

The origin of coma (hemispheric vs brainstem) and its cause (metabolic vs structural) can be elucidated by synthesizing the findings from examining pupillary size and reactivity, eye movements, motor responses, and respiratory pattern. Putting together the elements of the neurologic exam can help distinguish between global bilateral hemispheric dysfunction more likely to be caused by toxic-metabolic insults versus structural insults as well as suggest the level of CNS dysfunction (Table 41.14). Focality or asymmetry in the neurologic exam, signs of increased intracranial pressure, and signs of brainstem involvement all suggest a structural cause to the AMS.

Absent or asymmetric corneal reflexes or abnormal oculocephalic or oculovestibular reflexes suggest serious brainstem involvement. Normal brainstem responses combined with withdrawal to pain suggest a supratentorial abnormality. Roving but conjugate eye movements suggest an intact brainstem, whereas vertical malalignment suggests the

brainstem is affected. Asymmetric pupils in an altered patient indicate herniation from increased intracranial pressure.

Reversal of Immediately Treatable Toxic or Metabolic Causes

If the etiology for altered consciousness is not immediately apparent from the rapid clinical assessment, emphasis should shift to a systematic review of the reversible causes. A blood glucose level should be obtained as soon as possible on all children presenting with AMS. Hypoglycemia is a medical emergency that must be treated immediately because sustained hypoglycemia may result in permanent neurologic damage. Hypoglycemia in an altered child can be treated with intravenous dextrose, glucagon injection, or glucose gel applied to the oral mucosa. If obtaining a blood glucose level is delayed for any reason, empiric treatment for hypoglycemia should be given. In the absence of a central line, the percent dextrose solution used may vary; however, the absolute dose of glucose remains the same. Depending on the underlying etiology of the hypoglycemia, some patients will require a continuous infusion of glucose and electrolytes to prevent rebound hypoglycemia after the dextrose bolus. Regardless, any child found to

TABLE 41.14 Neurologic Findings That Help to Localize Site of Structural Brain Disease by Location of Lesion

Bilateral hemispheric	Spontaneous eye movements (roving, dipping,* ping-pong, nystagmoid jerks)
	Upward or downward eye deviation
	Intact oculovestibular reflexes
	Intact pupillary and corneal reflexes
	Variable motor responses
	Adventitious limb movements (subtle manifestations of seizures, myoclonus, asterixis)
Brainstem displacement from a hemispheric mass	Anisocoria or unilateral fixed and dilated pupil (predominant lateral displacement)
	Midposition fixed pupils (predominant downward displacement)
	Extensor or flexor posturing
	Central hyperventilation (diencephalic)
Brainstem displacement from a cerebellar mass	Direction-changing or vertical nystagmus from the cerebellar lesion
	Ocular bobbing†
	Absent corneal reflexes with intact pupillary reflexes
	Extensor or flexor posturing
	Facial or abducens nerve palsy
	Skew deviation (vertical misalignment of eyes)
	Internuclear ophthalmoplegia
Intrinsic brainstem lesion	Vertical nystagmus or bobbing
	Miosis (with pontine lesions)
	Internuclear ophthalmoplegia
	Variable pupillary and corneal reflexes (can both be absent)
	Absent oculocephalic and oculovestibular responses
	Extensor or flexor posturing
	Ataxic breathing (pontomedullary damage)

*Slow eye movement down followed by rapid return up to the midplane.

†Rapid eye movement up followed by slow return down to the midplane.

From Edlow JA, Rabinstein A, Traub SJ, et al. Diagnosis of reversible causes of coma. *Lancet.* 2014;382:2064–2076.

TABLE 41.15 Contraindications to Lumbar Puncture

Clinically important cardiorespiratory compromise in a neonate or young infant

Signs of raised intracranial pressure (pupillary changes, ptosis, hypertension, bradycardia, posturing, cranial nerve VI palsy, retinal changes)

Skin or soft tissue infection overlying area where lumbar puncture is to be performed

Focal neurologic findings

Suspected brain abscess (illness duration longer than expected for meningitis; focality)

chronic benzodiazepine use or who has ingested multiple agents such as tricyclic antidepressants, which may precipitate seizures.

When there are clinical signs or symptoms of infection present, the patient should be evaluated for signs of sepsis as well as CNS infection such as meningitis, encephalitis, or a parameningeal infection. Sepsis is a medical emergency; blood cultures should be obtained, and antibiotics started within an hour of recognition. If meningitis or encephalitis is suspected, a lumbar puncture should be performed, an opening pressure obtained, and CSF sent for Gram stain, culture, protein, glucose, and rapid identification of pathogens by polymerase chain reaction (PCR). Contraindications to a lumbar puncture are listed in Table 41.15. Antibiotics should not be delayed in order to perform a lumbar puncture. Suspicion for meningitis or encephalitis increases with the presence of a fever, bulging fontanel, nuchal rigidity, and Kernig or Brudzinski signs. Prior administration of antibiotics does not affect meningeal irritation. Most (85%) children with meningitis have AMS (53% lethargic, 22% stuporous, 10% comatose). If a contraindication to a lumbar puncture exists or if CSF is unable to be obtained, the child should be stabilized, receive empirical antimicrobial therapy, and undergo head CT imaging. The patient should undergo lumbar puncture as soon as it is no longer contraindicated. If a patient presents with sudden nuchal rigidity not preceded by a prodromal illness, a subarachnoid hemorrhage should be suspected, and a CT scan performed before the lumbar puncture.

If history is concerning for seizures and the physical exam reveals concern for ongoing seizure, such as continued rhythmic jerking of extremities or tonic deviation of the eyes, then a benzodiazepine such as intravenous lorazepam or intranasal midazolam should be given empirically and the patient monitored for effects.

If signs of increased intracranial pressure are present, treatment should be initiated with raising the head of the bed 30 degrees and hypertonic saline or mannitol should be given. If signs of imminent herniation are present, hyperventilation either manually through a bag-mask or with a ventilator in intubated patients can be initiated as a temporizing intervention until more definitive treatment is available. Emergent head CT and neurosurgical consultation should be obtained. In addition to an elevated head position, other neuroprotective principles include avoiding constrictive items around the neck; avoiding hypoxia or hyperoxia; avoiding hypotension, hypoglycemia, hyperglycemia, and hyperthermia; and preventing and treating seizures.

Reasons to obtain an emergent head CT include focal neurologic findings, concern for trauma, or other signs or symptoms consistent with a structural cause of AMS. If the cause of AMS continues to remain unknown and particularly if the exam is consistent with nonstructural causes, initial laboratory investigation should be obtained including CBC, electrolytes, magnesium, calcium, and phosphorus, BUN, creatinine, liver function tests including serum bilirubin and ammonia, lactic acid, arterial or venous blood gas, urine and serum toxicology screens, urine analysis with urine ketones and urine reducing substances, and appropriate cultures (blood, urine, CSF).

have hypoglycemia will need close monitoring of their blood glucose levels until stabilized (see Chapter 57).

Reversible ingestions should be considered next. Naloxone should be administered to children who have marked depression of consciousness without an obvious cause, particularly if hypoventilation is observed and opioid ingestion is suspected. Miosis is not a necessary finding because ingestion of multiple agents, including narcotics, may not result in small, constricted pupils. Organophosphates, clonidine, Lomotil, cholinesterase inhibitors (for myasthenia gravis), and valproate may cause miosis. Meperidine does not produce miosis. Diseases producing miosis include cluster headaches, Horner syndrome, Lyme disease, and uveitis. Large ingestions of narcotics may necessitate larger single doses of naloxone because of the competitive nature of its antagonistic effect. Even if initial improvement is noted, patients may require multiple doses or even a continuous infusion of naloxone because its half-life is shorter than that of many opioids. Benzodiazepine ingestion can also cause depressed levels of consciousness and can be reversed with flumazenil. Flumazenil, a specific competitive antagonist of benzodiazepines, should only be given if acute benzodiazepine overdose is suspected as administration of flumazenil to a patient with

DETAILED INVESTIGATION

Once the patient has been stabilized and life-threatening causes of AMS have been excluded, the coma can be considered stable if (1) focal neurologic findings are not present, (2) there is no evidence of significant brainstem dysfunction, (3) intracranial pressure is not raised, (4) there is no evidence of head trauma or CNS infection, and (5) the child does not have a rapidly reversible toxic or metabolic cause. At this point a detailed physical examination and expanded laboratory evaluation can be undertaken to confirm the level of CNS function and the cause of the coma.

Further history should be reviewed that was not able to be obtained earlier including detailed family history, social history, and further exposures including sources of carbon monoxide, animal exposures or bites, travel history, toxins or medications in the house, and pill counts if applicable. Collateral information should be reviewed if not available earlier. A detailed physical examination may provide further clues to the cause of the coma (Table 41.16), and careful attention should be paid to ensure full exposure and a thorough physical exam. If not already performed, attention should be paid to the skin, thyroid, and abdominal exam. In addition to the neurologic exam described previously focused on emergent findings, further detailed neurologic examination should also be performed.

Once further history is gathered and a detailed physical exam is performed, further laboratory and electrophysiology studies and imaging may be warranted based on the clinical scenario (Tables 41.17 and 41.18). In addition to the labs mentioned previously, second-line studies may include thyroid function tests; cortisol; carboxyhemoglobin; coagulation studies; ammonia; lactic acid; inflammatory markers; and antibody testing. An osmolal gap, as well as an anion gap, should be calculated. The osmolal gap is the difference between the measured and calculated serum osmolality (normal is <5–10 mOsm/kg H_2O) (Table 41.19). Both serum and urine toxicology screens should be sent when suspecting ingestions; however, the results must be interpreted cautiously. Because toxicology screens are not standardized, a "negative" result does not rule out an undetermined ingestion and clinicians should be familiar with what is tested on their local toxicology screens. Screening for certain agents, such as methanol and ethylene glycol, needs to be requested specifically. Depending on the compound, both false negatives and false positives may be a concern. ECG should be considered particularly if concerned for electrolyte derangement or intoxication in order to assess for cardiac conduction abnormalities. Other laboratory testing may include heavy metal levels, porphyria testing, and testing for inborn errors of metabolism (plasma amino acids, plasma carnitine, plasma pyruvate, urinary amino acids, and urinary organic acids and acylcarnitine profile). In infants and young children, a positive stool guaiac may suggest **intussusception,** which can occasionally present with decreased level of consciousness (encephalopathy), and further work-up with abdominal ultrasound for confirmation should be pursued.

Further infectious work-up may include fungal and mycobacterial cultures and antigen or serologic studies for specific infectious etiologies such as enterovirus, herpes simplex virus, Epstein-Barr virus (EBV), cytomegalovirus (CMV), HIV, *Borrelia burgdorferi, Bartonella henselae, Rickettsia,* arboviral encephalitides, rabies, cryptosporidium, mycobacterium tuberculous, syphilis, histoplasmosis, and mycoplasma. In the appropriate endemic areas or in returning travelers, the clinician should also consider testing for dengue, malaria, Japanese encephalitis, viral hemorrhagic fevers, and parasitic meningitis, particularly if eosinophils are present in the CSF (≥10 eosinophils/mL[3] or pleocytosis with ≥10% eosinophils).

For patients who remain altered without a clear etiology, lumbar puncture should be performed if not done already. CSF should be sent for cell count and differential, glucose, protein, Gram stain, bacterial culture, and herpes simplex virus PCR. Other CSF testing should be obtained based on risk factors and clinical scenario. In immunocompromised patients, fungal and mycobacterial cultures should be sent as well as additional testing for cryptococcal antigen, histoplasma antigen, human herpes virus 6, and CMV. Multiplex or individual PCR and antibody testing of the CSF for bacterial and viral pathogens should be considered.

If concerned for an **autoimmune** process, the appropriate antibodies such as antinuclear antibody (ANA) and antineutrophil cytoplasmic antibodies (ANCAs) should be obtained, and complement levels and autoimmune antibody testing of the CSF should be performed.

If not already performed, brain imaging should be considered. Head imaging should only be obtained after the patient has been stabilized and the risks of transporting an acutely ill child for the study have been weighed against the diagnostic benefit. CT scan offers the quickest modality for head imaging and the modality of choice when concerned for a structural cause of coma. Head CT will reveal intracranial bleeding, hydrocephalus, cerebral edema, herniation, and abnormal fluid collections. Limitations of head CT scan include exposure to radiation, limited evaluation of the posterior fossa, and decreased sensitivity to changes in the brain parenchyma. If the etiology of the altered level of consciousness is not found on head CT, an MRI of the brain should be obtained, which is more sensitive for acute stroke, demyelination, lesions in the posterior fossa, epileptic foci, and changes associated with infectious or autoimmune encephalitis. Limits of an MRI include longer imaging time, which often necessitates sedation of infants and young children. If there is concern for stroke, sinus venous thrombosis, or other vascular abnormality, appropriate vascular imaging should be obtained such as CT or magnetic resonance angiography and/or venography (MRA and MRV, respectively). For otherwise stable neonates and young infants, head ultrasound can be obtained as an *initial* head imaging modality and can be used to identify intracranial hemorrhage, subdural collections, edema, and signs of increased intracranial pressure.

Other important investigations include EEG monitoring over time to detect **nonconvulsive status epilepticus** in patients with decreased level of consciousness. EEG is indicated if there is concern for secondary seizures due to trauma, structural lesions, encephalitis, or encephalopathy. If there is concern for **catatonia,** consultation with psychiatry should be obtained and a trial of lorazepam with monitoring for improvement in mental status can be considered (see Chapter 31).

TRAUMA

Traumatic brain injury (TBI) accounts for approximately half of the incidence of childhood coma and is the leading cause of pediatric trauma death. Falls and motor vehicle crashes account for the most common mechanisms of injury, and the risk of TBI tends to increase throughout childhood. Severe TBI can lead to AMS through a variety of mechanisms including diffuse axonal injury, brain contusion, intraparenchymal brain hemorrhage, subdural hemorrhage, epidural hemorrhage, and subarachnoid hemorrhage. The mechanism of brain injury is caused both by the primary injury and by secondary injury caused by edema, hypoxia, hypoperfusion, increased intracranial pressure, and metabolic derangements such as acidosis and hypoglycemia. After initial stabilization, a patient presenting with any known trauma and AMS should have a head CT and the appropriate neurosurgical consultation and intervention. Even without a clear history of trauma, TBI should be suspected in patients presenting with AMS and other signs of trauma including bruising, lacerations, fractures, raccoon eyes, Battle sign (bruising posterior to the ear), and hemotympanum.

TABLE 41.16 Physical Examination and Diagnosis of Coma

System	Sign	Disorder
Skin	Dry	Dehydration, myxedema, adrenal insufficiency, anticholinergic poisoning
	Moist, sweating	Syncope, hypoglycemia, hyperthyroidism
	Pigment	Addison disease, porphyria
	Nevi	Tuberous sclerosis with seizures
	Petechiae	Bacteremia, bacterial endocarditis, idiopathic thrombocytopenia purpura
	Ecchymosis	Coagulopathy, intracranial hemorrhage
	Cyanosis	Hypoxia, congenital heart disease with cerebral embolism, methemoglobinemia
	Pallor	Shock, hemorrhage, severe anemia
	Erythema	Carbon monoxide, atropine, or mercury intoxication: toxic shock syndrome, heat stroke
	Butterfly rash	Lupus erythematosus, tuberous sclerosis, dermatomyositis
	Desquamation	Vitamin A intoxication, scarlatina, Kawasaki disease
	Jaundice	Hepatic disease, hemolytic anemia
	Nail changes	Splinter hemorrhage–endocarditis
		Candida infection, hypoparathyroidism, Addison disease
		Periungual fibroma (tuberous sclerosis)
Breath odor	Fruity	Diabetic ketoacidosis; amyl nitrate, alcohol, isopropyl alcohol poisoning
	Feculent	Hepatic encephalopathy
	Garlic	Selenium toxicity, arsenic poisoning, organophosphate poisoning
	Almonds	Cyanide poisoning
	Wintergreen	Methyl salicylate poisoning
	Ammoniacal	Uremia
	Acrid (pearl-like)	Paraldehyde, chloral hydrate poisoning
Scalp	Contusions	Trauma
	Vasodilation	Sagittal sinus thrombosis
Eyes	Chemosis	Cavernous sinus thrombosis
	Periorbital ecchymosis	Blow-out orbital fracture
	Subhyaloid hemorrhage	Subarachnoid hemorrhage
	Vasospasm (retina)	Hypertensive encephalopathy
	Miosis	Opioids, organophosphates, clonidine, Horner syndrome
	Mydriasis	Anticholinergic agents, antihistamines
	Retinal hemorrhages	Trauma, child abuse
Ears	Hemorrhage	Basilar skull fracture
	Purulent otitis media	Brain abscess, lateral sinus thrombosis
Nose	Cerebrospinal fluid rhinorrhea	Basilar skull fracture
Mouth	Bitten tongue and buccal mucosa	Seizure disorder
	Pigmentation	Addison disease
	Lead lines	Plumbism (lead intoxication)
Neck	Rigid	Meningitis, pneumonia, subarachnoid hemorrhage, encephalitis
Thyroid	Enlarged	Myxedema, thyrotoxicosis, Hashimoto encephalopathy
Heart	Murmur	Subacute endocarditis, brain abscess
Abdomen	Hepatomegaly	Leukemia, hepatic failure, heart failure
	Splenomegaly	Leukemia, lymphoma, hepatic failure
Extremities	Fracture	Trauma, fat embolism
	Ecchymosis	Trauma, hemorrhagic diathesis, shock, vasculitis
	Osler nodes	Endocarditis
	Muscle rigidity	Neuroleptic malignant syndrome, serotonin syndrome

Modified from Tait VF, Dean JM, Hanley DF. Evaluation of the comatose child. In: Rogers MC, ed. *Textbook of Pediatric Intensive Care.* 2nd ed. Baltimore: Williams & Wilkins; 1992:741.

TABLE 41.17　Laboratory Evaluation of Metabolic Brain Disease

Test	Reason for Test
Immediate	
Glucose	Hypoglycemia, DKA, hyperosmolar coma
Na⁺	Sodium dysregulation, osmolar abnormalities
Electrolytes	Electrolyte imbalances, including Mg^{2+}
Ca^{2+}	Hypercalcemia or hypocalcemia
BUN	Uremia
Arterial blood pH, Pco_2, Po_2, oxygen saturation	Acidosis, alkalosis, hypoxia, CO, or methemoglobin
Lumbar puncture	Infection, hemorrhage, meningeal carcinomatosis
CBC with differential	Infection, anemia
Later	
Liver function tests, ammonia level	Hepatic encephalopathy, Reye syndrome, urea cycle defect
Lactic acid	Sepsis, inborn errors of metabolism
Drug levels	Overdose
Blood and CSF culture	Sepsis, encephalitis, meningitis
Hormone levels including TFTs and cortisol	Myxedema coma, thyroid storm, adrenal crisis
Coagulation profile	Intravascular coagulation, coagulation disorders
EEG	Seizure disorder

CO, carbon monoxide; CSF, cerebrospinal fluid; DKA, diabetic ketoacidosis; Pco_2, partial pressure of carbon dioxide; Po_2, partial pressure of oxygen; TFTs, thyroid function tests.
Modified from Plum F. Neurology/sustained impairments of consciousness. In: Wyngaarden JB, Smith LH, Bennett JC, eds. *Cecil Textbook of Medicine.* 19th ed. Philadelphia: WB Saunders; 1992:2053.

Most pediatric patients presenting with head injury will have minor injuries. Patients with AMS or loss of consciousness do not fall within the low-risk category and require further observation and head imaging. In addition to the more severe forms of TBI, mild TBI can also lead to AMS in the form of confusion, disorientation, or lethargy. In mild injury (GCS score 13–15), the neurologic exam is nonfocal, and there are no physical exam findings concerning for skull fracture. The definition of mild TBI includes one or more of the following: confusion or disorientation; post-traumatic amnesia for <24 hours; loss of consciousness for <30 minutes; transient seizure or focal neurologic signs or symptoms; and GCS score 13–15 at 30 minutes or longer after the injury. Concussion is defined as trauma-induced brain dysfunction without structural injury on neuroimaging and symptoms include headache, dizziness, confusion, drowsiness, nausea, amnesia, irritability, and transient loss of consciousness.

Infants with head trauma may have evidence of intracranial hypertension: bulging fontanel, decerebrate posturing, and tachypnea. The clinical picture in a young infant may be confused with meningitis. In the absence of a febrile illness, trauma should be suspected, and the patient should be treated as if there is a rapidly progressive intracranial process. Infants are at increased risk for abusive head trauma, formerly referred to as shaken baby syndrome or nonaccidental trauma. The first 2 years of life present a high-risk period with an estimated incidence of 16–33 cases/100,000 children affected. Injury occurs by many

different mechanisms including blunt force, acceleration/deceleration, penetrating trauma, or asphyxiation. Infants with abusive head trauma often present with nonspecific concerns and without clear history of trauma. Presenting symptoms can include lethargy (77%), respiratory depression or seizure (43–50%), developmental delay (12%), or nonspecific findings such as irritability, decreased oral intake, and vomiting (15%). The key to diagnosis is to maintain a high index of suspicion (see Chapter 30).

PRIMARY BRAIN DISEASES

Diseases that primarily affect the brain leading to AMS can be divided into those causing structural lesions and those causing diffuse injury to the brain. Overlap does occur: A CNS infection may cause both diffuse disease and structural damage such as encephalitis or meningitis complicated by a brain abscess.

Structural Brain Disease

Various forms of primary structural brain diseases can lead to AMS. Symptoms associated with structural brain disease vary depending on the location of the lesion. If level of consciousness is affected, then either the bilateral cerebral hemisphere or ARAS is involved as discussed earlier. In space-occupying structural lesions, this most commonly occurs through increased intracranial pressure. Such lesions include intracranial hemorrhages, tumors, hydrocephalus, and vascular abnormalities. Structural brain lesions can also cause more subtle changes in mental status such as behavior changes depending on their location within the brain.

Intracranial Hemorrhage and Thrombosis

The vast majority of intracranial hemorrhages in children result from TBI, but more rare causes include hemorrhagic conversion of ischemic stroke, ruptured aneurysms, vascular malformations, brain tumors, CNS infections, vasculitis, vasculopathies, and moyamoya disease. The risk of intracranial hemorrhage is increased in the context of bleeding disorders and evaluation for a congenital or acquired bleeding disorder should be undertaken in patients with otherwise unexplained intracranial bleeding.

Arteriovenous malformations (AVMs) are the most dangerous vascular malformation with approximately 50% of children having hemorrhage as their initial presentation. Other symptoms can include seizure or focal neurologic deficit. Brain AVMs most often present with intraparenchymal bleeding but can also cause intraventricular or subarachnoid bleeding depending on the location of the AVM. **Cavernous malformations** (cavernous angiomas or cavernomas) can also present with hemorrhage, seizures, and progressive neurologic deficits and can be sporadic or familial. Diagnosis is usually made on neuroimaging including angiography.

Ischemic stroke is rare in children and is most often related to an underlying pathology that increases the risk of stroke. Such pathologies include congenital heart disease, prothrombotic clotting disorders, sickle cell disease, leukemias and lymphomas, infection, trauma, and certain genetic predispositions. Ischemic stroke most often presents with focal neurologic findings and is much less likely to present with decreased level of consciousness than hemorrhagic strokes. In the minority of ischemic strokes, decreased level of consciousness may be seen as an effect of the predisposing condition, location within the brainstem, or secondary effects of large strokes such as edema (see Chapter 37).

In addition to arterial thrombosis **cerebral sinus venous thrombosis** (CSVT) can also cause AMS. Risk factors include genetic conditions predisposing to thrombophilia, oral contraceptives, malignancy, infection, and head injury. In childhood, CSVT has its highest incidence

TABLE 41.18 Neuroimaging and Electrophysiologic Techniques and Findings in Disorders of Consciousness

Technique	Measurement	Strengths	Limitations	Vegetative State	Minimally Conscious State	Comatose
FDG-PET	Metabolic	Relatively direct measure of neuronal energy use (glucose uptake)	Ionizing (limited repeated measures)	Voxel-based: hypometabolism in lateral and medial frontoparietal cortices	Metabolic dysfunction in left hemisphere	
fMRI	CBF	High-resolution structural imaging of gray-white matter (DTI) and functional imaging (spectroscopy, resting, passive, and active CBF paradigms)	Sensitive to movement artifacts requiring sedation/anesthesia. Incompatible with ferromagnetic material (deprivation, pumps, electrodes)	Activation fMRI: low-level cortical activation DMN—partially preserved	Activation fMRI: near-normal high-level cortical activation	
EEG/ERPs	Electrical	Repeatable, portable, and inexpensive	Muscle, eye, and dysautonomia artifacts. Challenging source reconstruction		EEG: slow-wave activity through night and periods of REM sleep	ERP-poor outcome with absence of a cortical response to electrical stimulation of median nerves
EEG-TMS	Electrical	Stereotaxic stimulation connectivity studies	Stimulation areas are limited by muscle artifacts	TMS triggers a simple, local EEG response similar to deep sleep/anesthesia	Complex activations in distant cortical areas	

CBF, cerebral blood flow; DMN, default model network; DTI, diffuse tensor imaging; ERPs, event-related potentials; FDG, ^{18}F-fluorodeoxyghicose; fMRI, functional magnetic resonance imaging; REM, rapid eye movement; TMS, transcranial magnetic stimulation.
From Parrillo JE, Dellinger RP. *Critical Care Medicine: Principles of Diagnosis and Management in the Adult.* 5th ed. Philadelphia: Elsevier; 2019.

TABLE 41.19 Toxins and Disease States Causing Elevated Anion and/or Osmolal Gaps

Anion Gap	Osmolal Gap
Ethanol	Ethanol
Ethylene glycol	Ethylene glycol
Methanol	Methanol
Toluene	Acetone
Iron	Propylene glycol
Isoniazid	Ethyl ether
Salicylates	Isopropyl alcohol
Paraldehyde	Mannitol
Strychnine	Trichloromethane
Renal failure	Renal failure
Diabetic ketoacidosis	Diabetic ketoacidosis
Lactic acidosis	

in the neonatal period, presenting with diffuse brain injury leading to decreased level of consciousness and seizures. Neonatal risk factors include perinatal complications including birth hypoxia and maternal infection, dehydration, and head and neck disorders. Older children may have a wider variability in presentation with headache being the most common symptom. More severe presentations can lead to venous infarction and hemorrhage, which can result in seizures, focal deficits, and encephalopathy leading to confusion and decreased level of consciousness.

INTRACRANIAL TUMOR

Intracranial tumors, including both malignant and nonmalignant tumors, can present with subacute changes in mental status both from increased intracranial pressure and from effects at the location of the tumor itself. Mechanisms for acute AMS in the context of a CNS tumor include intracranial bleeding and seizures. Primary malignant CNS tumors are the second most common type of childhood malignancies and the leading cause of cancer mortality in children. The most common symptoms of CNS tumors are consistent with increased intracranial pressure and focal findings that are dependent on the location of the tumor. In infants and young children this includes macrocephaly, irritability, bulging fontanel, splayed sutures, and developmental delay. For older children, headache, ataxia, behavioral changes, and decreased school performance can be seen. Nausea and vomiting occur at all ages. Neuroimaging is required for diagnosis and is indicated in any patient presenting with decreased level of consciousness with signs or symptoms of increased intracranial pressure or focal neurologic signs.

Hydrocephalus

Hydrocephalus can also lead to AMS, both acutely and more slowly depending on the timing of onset of the hydrocephalus. **Obstructive hydrocephalus** refers to accumulation of CSF secondary to blockage within the ventricular system and is the most common form of hydrocephalus seen in children. **Communicating hydrocephalus** refers to decreased absorption of CSF in the subarachnoid space. Both forms of hydrocephalus most commonly present with signs of increased intracranial pressure. Changes in mental status may include behavioral changes such as irritability, aggressive behavior, indifference, and, in young children, developmental delay. As the hydrocephalus progresses, lethargy and drowsiness may be seen as pressure is placed on the midbrain and brainstem. Physical exam in infants may reveal macrocephaly, frontal bossing, and prominent scalp veins. Neurologic exam may reveal spasticity secondary to stretching of the fibers from the motor cortex, extraocular muscle paresis secondary to compression of the third or sixth cranial nerves, and in severe cases inability to gaze upward leading to the sclera being visible caudal to the iris ("setting-sun" sign). Diagnosis is made with neuroimaging revealing ventriculomegaly in the context of increased intracranial pressure. Ventriculomegaly without increased intracranial pressure is more likely to represent reduced brain volume in the proper clinical setting. Etiologies of hydrocephalus are diverse and include both congenital and acquired causes. **Shunt malfunction** remains high on the differential for children with a history of hydrocephalus and shunt placement who present with signs of increased intracranial pressure, particularly AMS.

Nonstructural or Medical Primary Brain Disease

Seizures

In generalized and focal seizures with altered awareness (previously complex partial seizures), the seizure itself presents with altered awareness and decreased responsiveness. This is followed by a postictal period characterized by decreased level of consciousness. In Todd paralysis, the postictal period is associated with focal neurologic deficits that resolve spontaneously with recovery from the postictal period. While seizures are most often short-lived, status epilepticus (ongoing or frequent seizure activity) can cause prolonged altered level of consciousness. Particularly in the setting of *nonconvulsive status epilepticus*, diagnosis may be delayed. Children younger than 2 years of age are very unlikely to present with tonic-clonic and absence seizures and more likely to present with sudden loss of muscle tone (focal or generalized), posturing, abrupt change in behavior, and clonic jerking of extremities or eyelids. Seizures in neonates can be subtle and a high index of suspicion must be maintained for infants with abnormal movements. Mimics of seizures vary depending on the age of the patient. In neonates, jitteriness (whether benign or associated with drug withdrawal, hypoglycemia, hypocalcemia, or hypoxic-ischemic encephalopathy), benign neonatal sleep myoclonus, and apnea may all be mistaken for seizure and often require EEG to differentiate. The differential in older infants includes breath-holding spells, Sandifer syndrome, dystonia, and sleep-related rhythmic movement disorders. With the exception of hypoglycemia, hypocalcemia, and hypoxic-ischemic encephalopathy, these mimics are not associated with prolonged periods of AMS. AMS in infants with concern for seizure indicates a serious underlying pathology. The differential in older children includes migraine syndromes, psychogenic nonepileptic seizures, syncope, movement disorders, and sleep disorders. EEG monitoring can help distinguish epileptic seizures from other events in difficult-to-distinguish cases. Prolonged altered level of consciousness in these patients is a red flag for more severe underlying pathology and should prompt a thorough work-up as indicated earlier (see Chapter 39).

Central Nervous System Infections

CNS infection represents the most common cause of nontraumatic decreased level of consciousness, accounting for approximately a third of nontraumatic cases. Children presenting with decreased level of consciousness without a clear etiology should undergo lumbar puncture with CSF studies to evaluate for infection unless a contraindication to a lumbar puncture exists. CNS infections range from meningitis, encephalitis, and brain abscesses to empyema of the epidural or subdural spaces. In some patients, a combination of these may be present.

CSF studies may be falsely reassuring in infections that do not communicate with the CSF such as in an intraparenchymal brain abscess or epidural abscess or in encephalitis. Intracranial abscesses often require neuroimaging with contrast for diagnosis. Causative pathogens of CNS infections are broad and include numerous viruses, bacteria, fungus, and protozoa (see Chapter 42). While CNS infection should remain at the top of the differential for patients presenting with fever and AMS, the less common causes include drug ingestions that cause hyperthermia (amphetamines, cocaine, salicylates, selective serotonin reuptake inhibitors, anticholinergics), heat stroke, and autoimmune-mediated disorders.

Inflammatory Diseases of the Central Nervous System

A variety of immune-mediated and inflammatory disorders can affect the CNS and cause AMS. These include autoimmune encephalitis, demyelinating disease, and CNS vasculitis. All of these disorders are rare but important to recognize as early detection and treatment in many can reduce morbidity and mortality.

Autoimmune encephalitis is a common cause of encephalitis and AMS characterized by brain inflammation mediated by autoantibodies most commonly against cell-surface antigens of neurons or intracellular proteins. Common presenting symptoms include new-onset subacute behavioral changes, psychiatric disturbances, cognitive decline, seizures, abnormal movements, and, as the disease progresses, decreased level of consciousness and coma. Some autoimmune encephalitis syndromes are associated with specific triggers including tumors (paraneoplastic) or preceding infections, although childhood-onset autoimmune encephalitis is less likely than adult onset to be associated with an underlying tumor.

Anti-NMDA (N-methyl-D-aspartate) receptor encephalitis is the most common autoimmune encephalitis in children and adolescents. A prodrome of headache, fever, and viral-like symptoms progress over a few days to psychiatric symptoms (anxiety, bizarre behavior, hallucinations, delusions, disorganized thinking), insomnia, memory deficits, seizures, dyskinesias, and language dysfunction, which can progress to decreased level of consciousness and coma sometimes associated with catatonic features and autonomic instability. Although anti-NMDA receptor encephalitis has been described in children as young as 8 months of age, the incidence is higher in adolescence and has been associated with underlying teratomas as well as preceding herpes simplex virus (HSV) encephalitis. While half of patients will have a normal MRI, the other half will have a transient nonspecific T2 or fluid-attenuated inversion recovery (FLAIR) signal hyperintensities in multiple cortical and subcortical areas. EEG most commonly shows focal and diffuse slowing with variable epileptiform activity. Diagnosis is confirmed with detection of anti-NMDA receptor antibodies in the CSF. Anti-NMDA receptor antibodies can also be detected in serum with lower sensitivity.

Many other autoantibodies have been described in children with autoimmune encephalitis with variable clinical presentations (Table 41.20). The differential for autoimmune encephalitis includes infection encephalitis, acute disseminated encephalomyelitis (ADEM), angiitis of the CNS, toxic-metabolic disturbances, CNS tumors, primary psychiatric disease, seizure disorders, inborn errors of metabolism, and mitochondrial cytopathies. Neurologic findings, even if subtle, in patients presenting with psychiatric symptoms should be considered a red flag and prompt further investigation, including for autoimmune encephalitis (see Chapter 31). Autoimmune encephalitis should be considered in patients with a history of a viral encephalitis who present with a recurrence of encephalitis because viral encephalitis has been associated with later development of autoantibodies and autoimmune encephalitis.

Certain demyelinating disorders can also lead to encephalopathy and AMS. **ADEM** is an autoimmune disorder mediated through auto-antibodies to myelin as well as T-cell-mediated damage. Immune dysfunction is often triggered by an antecedent infection, most often viral, with many pathogens being implicated as possible triggers including coronavirus, coxsackievirus, CMV, EBV, HSV, HIV, influenza, measles, rubella, varicella zoster, West Nile virus, *B. burgdorferi*, chlamydia, mycoplasma, rickettsia, and β-hemolytic *Streptococcus*. ADEM predominantly affects children ages 5–8 years and has a male predominance. Neurologic symptoms typically present 4–13 days after the initial triggering infection and include irritability, confusion, decreased level of consciousness, hemiparesis, cerebellar ataxia, optic neuritis, myelopathy, and seizures. At presentation, patients often have fever, headache, vomiting, and meningismus followed by the progression of neurologic findings. In severe cases, encephalopathy, difficult-to-control seizures, and/or respiratory failure from paralysis of the diaphragm may necessitate intensive care admission and mechanical ventilation. ADEM is a self-limited disorder with resolution of symptoms in 2–4 weeks. Diagnosis is aided with neuroimaging with MRI showing large (>1–2 cm) tumefactive T2 lesions of similar age with variable enhancement in either the brain or spine. CSF may be normal or may show signs of inflammation with CSF pleocytosis usually <100 cells/mL or increased protein. The criteria for diagnosis include the first multifocal episode of CNS demyelinating disease with encephalopathy that cannot be explained by other etiologies with absence of new clinical or MRI findings 3 months or more after onset.

The differential for demyelinating encephalopathies includes **neuromyelitis optica** (NMO) and pediatric multiple sclerosis. NMO can occasionally present with encephalopathy similar to that seen in ADEM, although it more commonly presents with optic neuritis, transverse myelitis, or focal brainstem findings. Diagnosis requires signs of optic neuritis, longitudinal lesions of the spinal cord involving at least three vertebral segments, brain imaging not meeting criteria for multiple sclerosis, and the detection of aquaporin-4 (AQP4)-immunoglobulin G (IgG) serum antibodies. Brain imaging in a patient with NMO will typically have less defined hemispheric lesions.

Pediatric multiple sclerosis (MS) is defined as onset of MS prior to age 18 years with demyelinating lesions separated over time and space.

	Disorder	Associated Antibody	Signs and Symptoms	Key Findings
Antibody-mediated autoimmune encephalitis	Anti-NMDA receptor encephalitis	Anti-NMDAR	Psychiatric disturbance Movement disorders Cognitive decline Speech dysfunction Seizures Movement disorders	Anti-NMDAR antibodies Associated with teratomas and preceding HSV encephalitis
	Anti-GABA$_A$R encephalitis	Anti-GABA$_A$R	Refractory seizures Confusion Behavioral changes Movement disorders	MRI with multifocal, extensive cortical and subcortical T2 hyperintensities
	Anti-GABA$_B$R encephalitis	Anti-GABA$_B$R	Seizures Memory loss Confusion Limbic encephalitis	MRI normal or with increased signal in medial temporal lobes
	Anti-GlyR encephalitis	Anti-Gly receptor	Stiff-person syndrome Limbic encephalitis Seizures Movement disorders Brainstem involvement	MRI is normal or with nonspecific findings
	Anti-mGlu R5 receptor encephalitis	Anti-mGlu R5	Confusion Psychiatric disturbance Encephalopathy	Associated with Hodgkin lymphoma
	Anti-dopamine D2 receptor encephalitis	Anti-D2 receptor antibodies	Lethargy Dystonia Parkinsonism Psychiatric disturbance	MRI with increased signal in basal ganglion
Demyelinating disorders	ADEM	Anti-MOG	Polyfocal neurologic deficits Encephalopathy	MRI with large white matter lesions No new clinical symptoms or MRI changes for 3 mo
	NMO	Anti-AQP4 Anti-MOG	Optic neuritis Myelitis Less likely to cause encephalopathy	Spinal cord lesions involving at least three vertebral segments
	Multiple sclerosis	n/a	At least two monofocal or polyfocal neurologic deficits separated in time and space Less likely to cause encephalopathy	Oligoclonal bands in the CSF

TABLE 41.20 Summary of Inflammatory Brain Disorders

Continued

TABLE 41.20 Summary of Inflammatory Brain Disorders—cont'd

	Disorder	Associated Antibody	Signs and Symptoms	Key Findings
Other inflammatory brain conditions	Rasmussen encephalitis	n/a	Refractory seizures Unilateral cortical deficits Cognitive decline	Progressive unilateral hemispheric and brainstem atrophy with contralateral cerebellar atrophy

	Hemophagocytic lymphohistiocytosis	n/a	Seizures
			Decreased consciousness
			Focal motor deficits
			Systemic symptoms:
			  Fever
			  Hepatomegaly
			  Splenomegaly
			  Lymphedema
				Associated with systemic inflammation
				Pancytopenia
				Low fibrinogen
				High ferrin
				High triglycerides

	Hashimoto encephalopathy	Antithyroid antibodies	Decreased consciousness Seizures Myoclonus Tremor Hyperreflexia	May be euthyroid, hypothyroid, or hyperthyroid
	Granulomatous inflammatory brain disease	n/a	Facial nerve palsy Seizures Cognitive dysfunction Encephalopathy Hydrocephalus Myelopathy	May be associated with symptoms of sarcoidosis elsewhere (uveitis, cough, renal disease, polyarthritis) MRI may have meningeal enhancement or white matter lesions

	cPACNS	n/a	Large vessel:
			  Unilateral, focal neurologic deficits
			  Ischemic stroke
			Small vessel:
			  Encephalopathy
			  Seizures
			  Fever
			  Fatigue
				MRA in large vessel reveals stenosis/dilatation of large vasculature
				Imaging is normal in small vessel and diagnosis often requires biopsy

ADEM, acute disseminated encephalomyelitis; AQP4, aquaporin-4; cPACNS, childhood primary angiitis of the central nervous system; $GABA_AR$, gamma-aminobutyric acid A receptor; $GABA_BR$, gamma-aminobutyric acid B receptor; GlyR, glycine receptor; mGlu R5, metabotropic glutamate receptor 5; MOG, myelin oligodendrocyte glycoprotein; NMDA, *N*-methyl-D-aspartate; HSV, herpes simplex virus; NMO, neuromyelitis optica.

In children, MS is most likely to follow a relapsing-remitting course. Although much less likely than ADEM, episodes of MS may present with encephalopathy, but MS requires additional episodes of demyelination separated in time that are not associated with encephalopathy and with new lesions on MRI for diagnosis. Pediatric MS typically presents in adolescence with monofocal neurologic deficits. However, cases in those younger than 10 years have also been described and are more likely to have initial episodes with polyfocal dysfunction and encephalopathy, making distinction from ADEM challenging. Lumbar puncture is performed to evaluate for other diseases and is more likely to reveal oligoclonal bands in MS than ADEM or other monophasic demyelinating diseases. Detection of anti–myelin oligodendrocyte glycoprotein (anti-MOG) antibody may suggest an alternative diagnosis of ADEM or NMO, and detection of AQP4-IgG is most consistent with NMO.

CNS vasculitis can be both primary (independent) or secondary to a systemic disease; presentation depends on the size of the blood vessels affected. *Large-vessel* vasculitis is more likely to present with sudden-onset focal neurologic deficits and ischemic stroke, although occasionally patients can present with more diffuse neurologic complaints such as decreased cognition and change in behavior. *Small-vessel* vasculitis is more likely to present with encephalopathy, extensive focal deficits, and status epilepticus and can be difficult to distinguish from other inflammatory brain conditions such as autoimmune encephalitis (see Table 41.20). **Childhood primary angiitis of the central nervous system** (cPACNS) is divided into three subtypes: angiography-positive, nonprogressive cPACNS; angiography-positive, progressive cPACNS; and angiography-negative, brain biopsy–positive, small-vessel cPACNS. Diagnosis of large-vessel vasculitis is made on imaging with MRI that reveals ischemic lesions in large-vessel distributions in combination with MRA demonstrating irregular unilateral stenosis or dilatation in the distal internal carotid artery and proximal segments of the anterior cerebral artery and/or middle cerebral artery. Nonprogressive cPACNS usually shows unilateral distribution of lesions, while progressive cPACNS is more likely to show bilateral lesions in multiple vascular territories. For small-vessel cPACNS, MRI reveals gadolinium enhancement of lesions and meninges or inflammatory lesions in the subcortical or cortical areas usually without ischemic lesions, but it can also be normal. MRA is normal. Many patients require angiography or brain biopsy to confirm the diagnosis.

Secondary causes of vasculitis in children include infections (both active and postinfectious), systemic rheumatic disease (systemic lupus erythematous, ANCA-associated vasculitis, scleroderma, dermatomyositis, Behçet disease), inflammatory diseases (inflammatory bowel disease, hemophagocytic lymphohistiocytosis, Kawasaki disease), malignancy (especially CNS lymphoma), and drugs (cocaine,

TABLE 41.21 Changes in Level of Consciousness Observed with Specific Drug Intoxications

Coma	Agitation	Confusions and/or Hallucinations	Seizures
Anticholinergics	Sympathomimetics	Anticholinergics	Cocaine
Antihistamines	Methylxanthines	Psychotropics	Amphetamines
Cholinergic agents	Phencyclidine	Lysergic acid diethylamide	Methylxanthines
Sedative-hypnotics	Salicylates	Mescaline	Tricyclic antidepressants
Alcohols	Alcohol	Marijuana	Cholinergic agents
Opiates		Antihistamines	Neuroleptics
Neuroleptics			Salicylates
Tricyclic antidepressants			Camphor
Phencyclidine			Isoniazid
Salicylates			Phenytoin
Heavy metals			Antihistamines
Hypoxia			
Carbon monoxide			
Cyanide			

amphetamine). These secondary causes of CNS vasculitis are associated with systemic signs and symptoms. Work-up typically includes inflammatory markers, CBC with differential, ANA, ANCA, extractable nuclear antigens (ENAs), anti–double-stranded deoxyribonucleic acid (anti-dsDNA), complement components 3 and 4, von Willebrand factor (vWF) antigen, lumbar puncture with oligoclonal bands, neuronal antibodies, tests for infection, and cytology.

TOXIC ENCEPHALOPATHY

Toxic compounds are common causes of altered consciousness in children. More than 90% of poisonings in young children are unintentional and involve a single substance, many of which are prescription medications. Children in certain age groups are at greater risk of being poisoned; 44% and 59% of all cases of poisonings reported to poison control centers occur in children younger than 3 and 6 years of age, respectively. Of these ingestions, opioid, sedative-hypnotic, and cardiovascular medication ingestions are the most common. Intentional ingestions are far more common in adolescents. In addition, some medications, even when taken as prescribed, can have adverse reactions that cause AMS and encephalopathy including valproate, vigabatrin, levetiracetam, methotrexate, corticosteroids, cyclosporine, tacrolimus, penicillins, cephalosporins, quinolones, macrolides, and metronidazole. The clinician's index of suspicion should be dependent not only on the age of the patient but also on the history of the present illness; a poisoning should be suspected in a previously healthy child who presents with a sudden onset of unexplained symptoms (seizures, mental status changes, vomiting, hematemesis) or a gradual onset of symptoms preceded by a period of confusion or delirium. *Medications and toxins within the house as well as recent medication changes should be reviewed.* A correct diagnosis is usually established by integrating information from the history, physical examination, and ancillary tests and then identifying a **toxidrome**, a symptom complex associated with a given class of ingested drug. The most important aspects of the physical examination to identify a toxidrome are the level of consciousness, the pupillary examination, and the vital signs.

Level of Consciousness

Table 41.21 lists common agents responsible for different changes in mental status. Toxic exposures may also occur via routes other than the oral route; organophosphates may be absorbed through the skin, whereas other compounds, such as carbon monoxide, are inhaled.

TABLE 41.22 Effect of Drugs on Pupillary Findings

Dilated	Constricted	Nystagmus
Sympathomimetics	Opiates	Barbiturates
Anticholinergics	Phenothiazines	Alcohol
Cocaine	Cholinergic agents	Phenytoin
Tricyclic antidepressants	Benzodiazepines	Carbamazepine
Glutethimide	PCP	PCP
LSD	Clonidine	Glutethimide

LSD, lysergic acid diethylamide; PCP, phenylcyclohexyl piperidine (phencyclidine HCl).

Pupillary Examination

When the pupils are evaluated for size and reactivity, the presence of nystagmus should also be noted (Table 41.22). Most drugs cause horizontal nystagmus; however, phenytoin may produce upbeat nystagmus, whereas phencyclidine (PCP) may cause rotary nystagmus.

Vital Signs

Although fever is typically indicative of infection or a metabolic disturbance, such as the hemorrhagic shock and encephalopathy syndrome, many toxic compounds may induce **hyperthermia** (Table 41.23). The most common causes of fever in intoxicated children include anticholinergic compounds, antihistamines, salicylates, and sympathomimetic agents. Less common causes of fever include agents producing the serotonin syndrome and neuroleptic malignant syndromes. **Hypothermia** may also be a sign of drug exposure (Table 41.24). Sedative-hypnotic agents, including ethanol, are common causes of hypothermia.

Bradycardia or **tachycardia** may result directly from the autonomic effect of a drug or may be a reflex response to a change in blood pressure. Intoxication with a β blocker, calcium channel blocker, α_2-adrenergic agonist (clonidine), or cholinergic agonist (organophosphate) characteristically manifests with bradycardia with or without hypertension. In mild clonidine ingestions or in the early stage of clonidine intoxication, the patient may be hypertensive as a result of the partial α_1-agonist effect of the drug. Bradycardia may be a reflex response to the precipitation of hypertension by a vasoconstrictor agent, such as an ergotamine, or an α-adrenergic agonist, such as phenylpropanolamine. A β-adrenergic agonist or anticholinergic agent intoxication usually manifests with tachycardia as part of the symptom complex. Intoxication with drugs

TABLE 41.23   Compounds and Conditions Inducing Hyperthermia

Muscular Hyperactivity or Rigidity
Agents producing serotonin syndrome
Agents producing neuroleptic malignant syndrome
Amoxapine
Amphetamines
Cocaine
Ethanol or sedative-hypnotic withdrawal
Lithium
LSD
MAO inhibitors
Phencyclidine
Tricyclic antidepressants

Increased Metabolic Rate
Dinitrophenol
Pentachlorophenol
Salicylates
Thyroid hormone

Impaired Heat Dissipation or Thermoregulation
Anticholinergic agents
Antihistamines
Antipsychotic agents
Tricyclic antidepressants

Other/Unknown Mechanisms
Metal fume fever

LSD, lysergic acid diethylamide; MAO, monoamine oxidase.
Modified from Olson KR, Pentel PR, Kelley MT. Physical assessment and differential diagnosis of the poisoned patient. *Med Toxicol.* 1987;2:40. Permission granted by AIDS International, Inc.

TABLE 41.24   Compounds and Conditions Inducing Hypothermia

Ethanol
Sedative-hypnotic agents (e.g., barbiturates, benzodiazepines)
Hypoglycemia
Isopropyl alcohol
Opiates
Phenothiazines
Tricyclic antidepressants

Adapted from Olson KR, Pentel PR, Kelley MT. Physical assessment and differential diagnosis of the poisoned patient. *Med Toxicol.* 1987;2:41. Permission granted by AIDS International, Inc.

that possess both α- and β-adrenergic agonist properties may manifest with both tachycardia and hypertension, whereas several classes of compounds may cause hypotension with a reflex tachycardia. Examples of the latter include direct vasodilators or α-adrenergic blockers (hydralazine, phenothiazines, tricyclic antidepressants) and compounds that cause third-space fluid losses (acute iron intoxication). The anticholinergic properties of the phenothiazines and tricyclic antidepressants contribute to the tachycardia seen with these agents. Cholinergic compounds, such as organophosphates and carbamates, may cause tachycardia instead of bradycardia because acetylcholine is the neurotransmitter found at nicotinic receptors in the sympathetic chain ganglion.

Tachypnea or hyperpnea may result from a central effect of a drug (salicylates, methylxanthines) or from a metabolic acidosis (salicylates,

alcohols, lactic acid) in addition to structural CNS lesions or cardiopulmonary compromise. Slow or shallow breathing should always raise the suspicion of drug ingestion, particularly with CNS depressants, such as narcotics and sedative-hypnotics. Hypoventilation may also be a presenting symptom of a clonidine overdose as a result of its opiate-like effects. In addition, organophosphate or carbamate intoxications may manifest with hypoventilation secondary to weakness of the respiratory muscles.

Odors emanating from the breath or clothing may offer invaluable clues as to the diagnosis. Not only do certain metabolic diseases, such as diabetic ketoacidosis and hepatic failure, produce characteristic breath odors but also so do a number of chemical compounds, including cyanide (bitter almonds); isopropyl alcohol, methanol, and salicylate (acetone); methyl salicylate (wintergreen); arsenic, thallium, and organophosphates (garlic); and turpentine (violets). Inspection of the skin and mucous membranes may also be helpful (Table 41.25).

Although a single sign or symptom may be attributable to many classes of drugs, combinations of symptoms (toxidrome) enable the clinician to narrow down the number of possible agents. Sympathomimetic agents, anticholinergics, and tricyclic antidepressants all cause mydriasis and tachycardia. If these symptoms occur in a patient with a prolonged QRS interval on an ECG, the most likely cause is a tricyclic compound, whereas if the former symptoms occur in a diaphoretic, tremulous patient, a sympathomimetic agent would be suspected. Table 41.26 outlines toxidromes of common classes of compounds ingested by children.

Management of most ingestions includes prevention of further absorption and supportive therapy. Activated charcoal is one method for decreasing absorption of stomach contents. Gastric decontamination should be withheld if a nontoxic substance is ingested, if a nontoxic quantity of a toxic compound is ingested, if absorption is likely to be complete, or if a caustic agent is ingested. Under these circumstances, gastric decontamination carries risks but no benefits. Induction of emesis is contraindicated in patients with a depressed mental status or who are at risk for a sudden deterioration of their mental status.

Very few specific antidotes exist for substances that are ingested. If an antidote exists, its use depends on the patient's prognosis if it were not administered. Not all children require treatment with *N*-acetylcysteine after acetaminophen poisoning. If the patient is asymptomatic and has a serum acetaminophen concentration in a nontoxic range when plotted on the Rumack-Matthew nomogram, *N*-acetylcysteine therapy is not indicated. Table 41.27 is a partial list of available antidotes. Although not a true antidote, sodium bicarbonate is included as an antidote for salicylate and tricyclic antidepressant ingestions because its use can reduce symptoms by reducing tissue distribution of these compounds.

Some drugs lend themselves to procedures aimed at enhancing drug elimination from the body. These procedures include changing urinary pH (alkalinization to enhance salicylate excretion), using multiple doses of charcoal (theophylline, phenobarbital, carbamazepine), and performing extracorporeal drug removal (peritoneal or hemodialysis, charcoal hemoperfusion, exchange transfusion). Either patient-related or drug-related criteria should be met before the institution of extracorporeal drug removal (Table 41.28). When the management approach is not known, a resource such as a poison control center or a clinical pharmacologist should be consulted.

METABOLIC ENCEPHALOPATHIES

Metabolic derangements cause AMS through global cerebral dysfunction in the absence of primary brain disease, either structural or nonstructural. These disorders are important to quickly recognize as many are reversible if treated early but may lead to permanent effects or death if treatment is delayed. Derangement of this neuronal homeostasis results in neuronal dysfunction, which first affects complex brain functions such as consciousness. If untreated, progression of neuroinflammation through cytokine release can lead to neuronal cell death, prompting further inflammation and compromise to the blood-brain barrier leading to brain edema, herniation, and death. Metabolic encephalopathy is often characterized by lack of focal neurologic deficits and preserved pupillary reactions (Table 41.29).

Hypoxia causes AMS in the immediate short term as well as causing hypoxic-ischemic encephalopathy (HIE) if a hypoxic insult is not immediately reversed. Treatment of hypoxia should happen immediately during the initial stabilization of the patient to prevent further injury. The hypoxic insult is often obvious from the prior history. Perinatal insults are a common cause of neonatal HIE, while drowning and airway obstruction may precipitate HIE in older children. Other inciting events include cardiopulmonary arrest, severe hypotension from any etiology, or severe disruption of hemoglobin's oxygen-carrying capacity such as in carbon monoxide poisoning.

Sepsis from any source can also cause an encephalopathy likely through multiple mechanisms including hypotension, hypoperfusion, and direct effects of the immune response on the blood-brain barrier and brain parenchyma. When sepsis causes encephalopathy in the absence of CNS infection or direct effects from other end-organ failure, the term *sepsis-associated encephalopathy* (SAE) is used. SAE can range from delirium and agitation to lethargy and coma. EEG can be normal, but as level of consciousness decreases, theta waves appear followed by the delta waves, generalization of triphasic waves, and burst-suppression patterns. Treatment is geared toward treating the underlying infection and metabolic derangements caused by sepsis.

TABLE 41.25 Skin Manifestations of Intoxication

Manifestation	Toxin/Condition
Bullous lesions	Barbiturates, carbon monoxide, sedative-hypnotics, opioids
Diaphoresis	Cholinergic agents (organophosphates), sympathomimetics, mercury, arsenic, salicylates
Dry skin (and mucous membranes)	Anticholinergics, antihistamines, narcotics
Diffuse erythema	Anticholinergics, carbon monoxide, cyanide, boric acid, mercury
Cyanosis	Hypoxia, methemoglobinemia, ergotamines
Needle tracks	Opiates, phencyclidine, amphetamine
Jaundice	Acetaminophen

TABLE 41.26 Toxidromes of Common Classes of Drugs

Drug Class	Level of Consciousness	Pupils	Vital Signs	Other
Sympathomimetics (amphetamines, cocaine, ephedrine, methylphenidate [Ritalin])	Agitation; psychosis	Dilated	↑ HR; ↑ BP; ↑ T	Tremors, sweating, arrhythmias; seizures
Anticholinergics (antihistamines, scopolamine, atropine, jimson weed, nightshade, phenothiazines, tricyclics)	Confusion; hallucinations	Dilated	↑ HR; ↑ T; ±↑ BP	Flushed; dry skin and mucous membranes; urinary retention; decreased bowel sounds
Opiates	Euphoria; coma	Pinpoint	↓ RR; ±↓ HR; ±↓ BP	Shallow respirations; dry mucous membranes
Cholinergic syndrome (organophosphates; carbamates, bethanechol, *Amanita* mushrooms)	Coma	Miosis	↓ or ↑ HR; ↓ or ↑ BP	Salivation, lacrimation, urination, defecation, bronchorrhea; muscle twitching before flaccidity; seizures
Sedative-hypnotics (alcohol, barbiturates, benzodiazepines)	Coma	± Miosis	↓ RR (shallow); hypothermia; ↓ BP	Ataxia; nystagmus; slurred speech
Neuroleptics (phenothiazines, butyrophenones)	Coma	Miosis (except thioridazine [Mellaril])	↑ HR; ↓ BP; ↓ or ↑ T	Dystonic reactions; ataxia; neuroleptic malignant syndrome; prolonged Q-T interval
Tricyclic antidepressants	Confusion; agitation; coma	Dilated	↑ HR; ↓ or ↓ BP; ↑ T; ↓ RR	Quinidine-like effect: prolonged QRS or Q-T interval and ventricular arrhythmias; seizures; anticholinergic effects (see above)
Salicylates	Disorientation; hyperexcitability; coma (severe)	—	↑ T; ↓ or ↑ RR + depth	Vomiting; tinnitus; metabolic acidosis; hypokalemia
Carbon monoxide	Lethargy; coma	—	—	Headache, nausea, flulike syndrome, dizziness, blurred vision
Theophylline	Agitation	—	↑ HR; ↓ BP; ±↑ RR; ± ↑ T	Protracted vomiting; tremors, seizures, arrhythmias
Phencyclidine	Delirium; combativeness; catatonia; coma	Miosis	—	Rotary nystagmus; seizures
SSRIs	Drowsiness; agitation; delirium; coma	Dilated or unreactive	↑ HR; ↑ T; ↓ BP	Nausea, vomiting, tremor, rigidity, myoclonus, hyperreflexia, diaphoresis

BP, blood pressure; HR, heart rate; RR, respiratory rate; SSRI, selective serotonin reuptake inhibitor; T, temperature.

TABLE 41.27   Specific Toxins and Their Antidotes

Toxin	Antidote	Toxin	Antidote
Acetaminophen	N-Acetylcysteine	Iron	Deferoxamine
Anticholinergics	Physostigmine	Lead	EDTA; dimercaprol; dimercaptosuc-cinic acid; penicillamine
Arsenic	Dimercaprol		
Benzodiazepines	Flumazenil	Mercury	Dimercaprol
β Blockers	Glucagon*	Methanol	Ethanol or fomepizole
Calcium channel blockers†	Calcium	Opiates	Naloxone
Carbamate insecticides	Atropine	Nitrites	Methylene blue
Carbon monoxide	Oxygen	Organophosphates	Atropine; pralidoxime
Cyanide	Amyl nitrite or sodium nitrate plus sodium thiosulfate	Phenothiazines‡	Diphenhydramine or benztropine
		Salicylates	Sodium bicarbonate
Digitalis	Digoxin-specific antibody fragments	Tricyclic antidepressants	Sodium bicarbonate
Ethylene glycol	Ethanol or fomepizole	Warfarin	Vitamin K
Heparin	Protamine		

*May reverse cardiac toxicity.
†Usually requires saline infusion as well for bradyarrhythmias or conduction abnormalities.
‡Dystonic reactions only.
EDTA, ethylenediaminetetraacetic acid.

TABLE 41.28   Indications for Extracorporeal Drug Removal*

Patient Related

Severe intoxication refractory to medical management (e.g., refractory seizures)

Impairment of normal excretion routes that may lead to prolonged intoxication

Drug Related

Ingestion and probable absorption of a potentially lethal dose determined after gut decontamination

Documentation of a potentially lethal drug level

Presence of a significant quantity of a compound that is metabolized to a toxic metabolite (e.g., methanol)

*Patient- and drug-related criteria for extracorporeal drug removal. Only one criterion needs to be met.

TABLE 41.29   Characteristics of Metabolic Encephalopathy

Confusion, lethargy, delirium often precede or replace coma

Motor signs, if present, usually symmetric

Bilateral asterixis, myoclonus appear

Pupillary reactions usually preserved; tonic caloric reflex often present

Sensory abnormalities usually absent; hypothermia common

Abnormal signs reflect incomplete brain dysfunction at multiple anatomic levels

From Plum F. Neurology/sustained impairments of consciousness. In: Wyngaarden JB, Smith LH, Bennet JC, eds. *Cecil Textbook of Medicine.* 19th ed. Philadelphia: WB Saunders; 1992:2052.

Hypoglycemia is a common cause of metabolic encephalopathy in children; evaluation and treatment should happen concurrently with rapid stabilization and assessment of the child presenting with AMS. Children with AMS secondary to hypoglycemia may present with confusion, delirium, or coma. Occasionally, focal neurologic deficits may be present that resolve with treatment of the hypoglycemia. The most common cause of hypoglycemia is **ketotic hypoglycemia** in the setting of ill or fasting infants and young children with decreased oral intake and glycogen stores (see Chapter 57).

Electrolyte derangements of various kinds can present with AMS and include both elevated and decreased serum levels of sodium, calcium, and magnesium (see Chapter 59).

A variety of endocrinopathies can also present with AMS. The most common of these is **diabetic ketoacidosis** (DKA), which occurs in children with underlying diabetes mellitus (DM), most commonly type 1, but occasionally in type 2. Symptoms include nausea, vomiting, abdominal pain, Kussmaul breathing, and decreased level of consciousness. Even without a history of DM, a child's initial presentation of DM may be in DKA, which also increases the risk of cerebral edema, an uncommon but dangerous complication of DKA. Children with DM type 2 may present with **hyperosmolar hyperglycemic state** (HHS) indicated by severe hyperglycemia without ketoacidosis. The hyperosmolarity of HHS leads to a decreased level of consciousness and coma and carries a higher risk of mortality than DKA. Other rare endocrine disorders that present with AMS include **myxedema coma** in the setting of severe hypothyroidism. Clinical signs include hypothermia, bradycardia, hypoventilation, and hypoxia, and it is often triggered by infection, burns, or medications in untreated or undertreated hypothyroidism. **Thyroid storm** or severe hyperthyroidism can lead to agitation, irritability, psychosis, seizures, and, in rare cases, coma. Other symptoms consistent with hyperthyroidism are usually present and include tremor, tachycardia, hypertension, hyperthermia, and cardiac arrhythmias. **Adrenal crisis** can also lead to confusion, behavioral changes, psychosis, and decreased level of consciousness progressing to coma. Associated systemic signs include hypotension, nausea, vomiting, abdominal pain, fever, hyponatremia, and hyperkalemia. Adrenal crisis is often triggered by stress-including dehydration, trauma, surgery, infection, or sudden cessation of exogenous steroid treatment in the setting of Addison disease, congenital adrenal hypoplasia, or chronic exogenous steroid use.

End-organ failure, particularly of the liver or kidneys, can also lead to AMS and decreased level of consciousness. **Hepatic encephalopathy** occurs in the setting of both acute and chronic hepatic failure (see Chapter 18). In the setting of chronic liver failure, hepatic encephalopathy can be triggered by infection, excessive protein intake,

TABLE 41.30   Select Inborn Errors of Metabolism Associated with Neurologic and Laboratory Manifestations in Neonates

DETERIORATION IN CONSCIOUSNESS	SEIZURES AND HYPOTONIA
Metabolic Acidosis Organic acidemias Disorders of pyruvate metabolism Fatty acid oxidation defects Fructose-1,6-bisphosphatase deficiency Glycogen storage diseases Mitochondrial respiratory chain defects Disorders of ketone metabolism **Hypoglycemia** Fatty acid oxidation defects Disorders of gluconeogenesis Disorders of fructose and galactose metabolism Glycogen storage diseases Disorders of ketogenesis Organic acidemias Hyperinsulinemic hypoglycemias Mitochondrial respiratory chain defects Neonatal intrahepatic cholestasis caused by citrin deficiency Pyruvate carboxylase deficiency Carbonic anhydrase VA deficiency **Hyperammonemia** Urea cycle disorders Organic acidemias Fatty acid oxidation disorders Disorders of pyruvate metabolism *GLUD1*-related hyperinsulinemic hypoglycemia Carbonic anhydrase VA deficiency	Antiquitin deficiency (pyridoxine-dependent epilepsy) Pyridoxamine 5'-phosphate oxidase (PNPO) deficiency (pyridoxal phosphate-responsive epilepsy) Folate metabolism disorders Multiple carboxylase deficiency (holocarboxylase synthetase deficiency and biotinidase deficiency) Urea cycle disorders Organic acidemias Fatty acid oxidation disorders Disorders of creatine biosynthesis and transport Disorders of neurotransmitter metabolism Molybdenum cofactor deficiency and sulfite oxidase deficiency Serine deficiency disorders Glycine encephalopathy Asparagine synthetase deficiency Mitochondrial respiratory chain defects Zellweger spectrum disorders Congenital disorders of glycosylation Purine and pyrimidine metabolism defects **NEONATAL APNEA** Glycine encephalopathy Asparagine synthetase deficiency Urea cycle disorders Organic acidemias Disorders of pyruvate metabolism Fatty acid oxidation defects Mitochondrial respiratory chain defects

From Kliegman RM, St. Geme JW III, Blum NJ, et al., eds. *Nelson Textbook of Pediatrics*. 21st ed. Philadelphia: Elsevier; 2020:690, Table 102.3.

gastrointestinal bleeding, or nonadherence to medications. Initial signs include sleep disturbance, confusion, and asterixis, which can progress to lethargy, seizures, coma, and posturing. Hepatic encephalopathy in acute liver failure is a poor prognostic sign without transplant. Advanced kidney failure, whether acute or chronic, can lead to **uremic encephalopathy,** which presents with lethargy, confusion, hallucinations, and occasionally coma. Other symptoms include tremor, myoclonus, asterixis, seizures, and tetany. Treatment with hemodialysis usually resolves symptoms. Encephalopathy that occurs during or immediately after dialysis may represent **dialysis disequilibrium syndrome** and is thought to be related to rapid removal of urea leading to cerebral edema.

Hypertensive encephalopathy occurs in the setting of severe hypertension and causes headache, nausea, vomiting, seizures, and AMS, which improve with treatment of the hypertension. Hypertension may also be associated with **reversible posterior leukoencephalopathy syndrome** (RPLS) (also known as posterior reversible encephalopathy syndrome [PRES] or hypertensive encephalopathy), which is also an acute encephalopathy characterized by cortical and white matter changes on T2 and FLAIR MRI that usually improves with treatment of hypertension. Predisposing factors include renal disease, uremia, and preeclampsia/eclampsia. Other causes of RPLS have been described including autoimmune disorders, chemotherapy, immunosuppressive therapy, and infection.

Inborn Errors of Metabolism

Inborn errors of metabolism are complex and encompass many conditions. Table 41.30 provides a partial list of inborn errors of metabolism that may manifest in the neonate with deterioration in consciousness, seizures, hypotonia, and/or apnea. Many of these conditions relate to defective enzymes that lead to accumulation of a toxic product. Newborn screening has increased the number of infants diagnosed and effectively treated during the asymptomatic phase of a disease. The clinical manifestations of metabolic disease in the neonate can be nonspecific (Table 41.31). The infants are often thought to have sepsis and are evaluated and treated for presumptive infection. The presence of a documented infection does not preclude metabolic disease because some of these infants are prone to infection (e.g., galactosemia and *Escherichia coli* sepsis). A family history of a previous infant dying from an unexplained illness or other children in the family with neurologic disorders may provide clues to a metabolic cause. Laboratory abnormalities that may be seen in metabolic disease are listed in Table 41.32.

Infants with urea cycle defects often manifest AMS, coma (recurrent), and emesis. They cannot metabolize waste nitrogen to urea; this leads to accumulation of ammonia in the blood. These disorders are inherited as autosomal recessive traits, except for ornithine transcarbamylase deficiency, which is X-linked. The keys to the diagnosis of inborn errors of metabolism in the neonate are a high degree of suspicion, the appropriate screening studies (see Table 41.32), and, if the results are positive, a more detailed laboratory evaluation under the guidance of a specialist in metabolic diseases (Table 41.33).

Metabolic encephalopathy resulting from inborn errors of metabolism may also manifest in older children or adolescents. The onset of symptoms may be triggered by changes in dietary intake, fasting, dehydration, illness, medications, childbirth, trauma, or surgery.

TABLE 41.31   Clinical Manifestations of Inborn Errors of Metabolism in the Neonatal Period

Lethargy
Coma
Seizures
Increased or decreased muscle tone
Poor suck and feeding
Vomiting
Diarrhea
Apnea
Tachypnea and/or hyperpnea
Respiratory failure
Jaundice
Unusual odors
Cardiomegaly
Hepatomegaly

TABLE 41.32   Laboratory Evidence of Metabolic Disease

Acidosis,* alkalosis
Hypoglycemia
Hyperammonemia
Elevated lactate levels
Elevated liver enzyme levels
Direct hyperbilirubinemia
Urine-reducing substance
Urine ketones present in excess or absent when expected to be present

*High anion gap if increased organic acids (ketoacids, lactic acid) are produced. Normal anion gap if associated renal tubular acidosis (type I glycogen storage disease, galactosemia) is present.

TABLE 41.33   Laboratory Evaluation of Suspected Inborn Errors of Metabolism

Plasma ammonia
Arterial blood gas
Plasma amino acids
Plasma carnitine
Plasma pyruvate and lactate
Urinary amino acids
Urinary organic acids and acylcarnitine profile

TABLE 41.34   Characteristics and Categories of Coma

Supratentorial Mass Lesion Affecting Diencephalon/Brainstem
- Initial focal cerebral dysfunction
- Dysfunction progresses rostral to caudal
- Signs reflect dysfunction at one level
- Signs often asymmetric

Subtentorial Structural Lesion
- Symptoms of brainstem dysfunction or sudden-onset coma
- Brainstem signs precede or accompany the coma
- Cranial nerve and oculovestibular dysfunction
- Early onset of abnormal respiratory patterns

Metabolic-Toxic Coma
- Confusion or stupor precede motor signs
- Motor signs usually symmetric
- Pupil responses generally preserved
- Myoclonus, asterixis, tremulousness, and generalized seizures common
- Acid-base imbalance common, with compensatory ventilatory changes

Psychogenic Coma
- Eyelids squeezed shut
- Pupils reactive or dilated, unreactive (cycloplegics)
- Oculocephalic reflex unpredictable, nystagmus on caloric tests
- Motor tone normal or inconsistent
- No pathologic reflexes
- Awake-pattern EEG

From Vincent JL, Abraham E, Moore FA, et al., eds. *Textbook of Critical Care.* 7th ed. Philadelphia: Elsevier; 2017:241, Box 48-3.

Additionally, less severe forms of disorders that classically present in infancy such as urea cycle disorders or organic acidemias may also present in older children with episodes of vomiting, lethargy, seizures, or psychomotor abnormalities. Recurrent hypoglycemia, frequent hospitalizations for dehydration, metabolic decompensation out of proportion to the severity of acute illness, recurrent vomiting, developmental delay, poor growth or failure to thrive, cramping after exercise, and protein or carbohydrate (fructose) aversions may all signal concern for inborn errors of metabolism. Like in infants, work-up is influenced by the presenting signs and symptoms and often requires consultation with a specialist in inborn errors of metabolism.

SUMMARY AND RED FLAGS

AMS is a common symptom related to a wide variety of underlying pathologies and particularly when associated with a decreased level of consciousness indicates a serious manifestation of potentially life-threatening but at times reversible disorders. Initial diagnosis and management are focused on stabilization, rapid clinical assessment, and treatment of immediately reversible causes such as hypoglycemia. Red flags indicating structural causes include signs of increased intracranial pressure, focal neurologic deficits, and signs of brainstem dysfunction. Red flags indicating life-threatening toxic-metabolic causes include signs of intracranial infections, sepsis, and hemodynamic instability. Common causes vary by age, but toxic ingestion, trauma, seizures, infections, and metabolic disturbances, including inborn errors of metabolism, must be considered. Finding one etiology of AMS does not preclude other contributing comorbid conditions as many initial causes of AMS may progress to others. For example, severe head trauma may lead to seizures and dysregulation of sodium and increase the risk for subsequent infection. The location and etiology of AMS may have characteristic patterns or manifestations (Table 41.34).

BIBLIOGRAPHY

A bibliography is available at ExpertConsult.com.

42

Encephalitis

Robert M. Kliegman

Encephalitis, or inflammation of the brain, and **myelitis**, or inflammation of the spinal cord, cause myriad symptoms and signs because of the subtle behavioral phenotypes and varying locations of the inflammation. The lesions are hard to categorize or quantify and are not generally accessible to biopsy. The challenge in relatively nonverbal children compounds the problem. **Encephalopathy**, or dysfunction of alertness, attention, cognition, and speech, has a much broader differential diagnosis (see Chapter 31). For this reason, the diagnosis of encephalomyelitis (EM) usually requires fevers or an objective neurologic sign to open the investigation (Table 42.1).

Encephalitis is uncommon (0.3–0.5/100,000 population) and is only one of many etiologies of altered mental status including the broad category of noninfectious noninflammatory encephalopathies (see Chapter 41). Indeed, encephalitis may be due to infections of the central nervous system, as well as immune-mediated processes (active, postinfectious), autoimmune (N-methyl-D-aspartate receptor [NMDAR] antibody, others), or overlapping (HSV with NMDAR encephalitis, COVID-19 with acute disseminated encephalomyelitis [ADEM]).

ETIOLOGY

Encephalitis may be infectious, postinfectious, autoinflammatory, or autoimmune (Table 42.2). The approach to the epidemiology of encephalitis must take age (see Table 42.2) and exposure (Table 42.3) into consideration. Exposures include other affected people in addition to insects (mosquitoes, ticks, others), animals (bats, dogs, cats, raccoons, sheep, goats), ingestion or inhalation (water, soil, foods), the season, and travel to endemic areas. Although many cases of encephalitis have no identifiable exposures, particularly autoimmune encephalitis, a careful history may improve the ability to make a diagnosis and provide specific therapy (brucellosis, *Baylisascaris procyonis*, *Naegleria fowleri*).

In addition to infectious etiologies, autoimmune encephalitis must always be considered in the differential diagnosis (Tables 42.4, 42.5, 42.6, and 42.7). Subacute or chronic encephalitis, particularly in immunosuppressed patients, has a different epidemiology (Table 42.8). In addition, many systemic disorders mimic encephalitis (Table 42.9) (see Chapter 31).

Herpes simplex is the most important treatable infectious endemic cause of encephalitis in the United States. Seasonal fluctuations of aseptic meningitis and/or encephalitis are often due to enteroviruses/parechoviruses and arboviruses (arthropod-borne virus) such as West Nile, Powassan, St. Louis, California, Eastern and Western equine, and La Crosse viruses. Zika, dengue, and Chikungunya are also arboviruses. In endemic areas and during the appropriate season, tick-borne diseases (Lyme disease) should be considered.

Autoimmune encephalitis, ADEM, and neuromyelitis optica spectrum disorder (NMOSD) are important, recognizable, noninfectious-inflammatory treatable disorders that commonly present with an encephalitis-like picture.

Autoimmune Encephalitis

Autoimmune encephalitis is often associated with behavioral or psychiatric changes and seizures; the MRI may be normal, but the EEG will universally be abnormal. The presence of restricted diffusion or contrast enhancement is unusual in autoimmune encephalitis. The most common form of autoimmune encephalitis is caused by antibodies to the NMDA receptor (NMDAR), which in children is often associated with agitation, hallucination, sleep disorder, movement disorders (or catatonia), ataxia, mutism, and seizures. Inflammatory markers are often normal. NMDAR encephalitis is uncommonly paraneoplastic in children (more so in adolescents) and usually of ovarian origin. NMDAR encephalitis can be triggered by HSV encephalitis and Japanese encephalitis virus, which confounds the primary diagnosis. Other relatively antibody-mediated syndromes include myelin oligodendrocyte glycoprotein (MOG) and GAD65.

The most common, *cell-mediated autoimmune encephalitis* is **acute disseminated encephalomyelitis (ADEM)**, a bilateral, asymmetric demyelinating syndrome presenting 2–4 weeks after a minor respiratory or gastrointestinal infection; it has also been reported after measles, historical smallpox and neural tissue–derived rabies vaccines, trauma, or surgery. Encephalopathy is present in >90% of patients; fever is not. Often there is paresis of the cranial nerves or extremities. Imaging is usually abnormal in most cases (Fig. 42.1). ADEM is cell mediated, but a subset of patients, usually with more severe disease, show peripheral antibodies to MOG; some with MOG antibodies have a course distinct from ADEM. Epidemiologic (Fig. 42.2) and MRI findings (Table 42.10) may help differentiate ADEM from MS. Corticosteroids are often used despite inconclusive evidence; rapid withdrawal of corticosteroids may result in relapse.

Acute transverse myelitis (TM) clinically mimics cord transection (sensory, motor, and sphincter impairment) at a precise spinal level, but MRI usually demonstrates cord inflammation extending more than three vertebral bodies. It is essential to emergently exclude spinal cord compression by epidural abscess, hematoma, or tumor. Sparing of proprioception and vibration suggests possible anterior spinal artery disease (vasculitis, infarction, syphilis, schistosomiasis). Therapy is not established, and outcomes vary. **Acute flaccid myelitis** (AFM) (or acute flaccid paralysis) is a syndrome associated with TM with anterior horn cell involvement, typically in younger children, occurring seasonally. Recovery is variable. There has been irregular geographic coincidence with outbreaks of enterovirus (EV) D-68 and coxsackievirus A-16, but virus is usually not detected in CSF. Outbreaks of AFM have occurred in other regions without detection of these viruses despite aggressive diagnostic surveillance.

The most common treatable cause of sporadic encephalitis at all ages is caused by **herpes simplex virus**. Apart from the neonatal period, when the virus spreads hematogenously, encephalitis is mediated by reactivation of the virus in the trigeminal nerve and spread to the innervated base of the brain (frontal and temporal lobes). The

TABLE 42.1   Comparison of Encephalitis and Encephalopathy

	Encephalitis	Encephalopathy
Clinical Features		
Fever >38°C	Common	Uncommon
Headache	Common	Uncommon†
Depressed mental status >24 hr*	May fluctuate	Steady decline in mental status
Focal neurologic signs	Common	Uncommon
Seizures	Occasional	Uncommon
Types of seizures	Generalized or focal	Generalized
Laboratory Results		
CBC	Leukocytosis occasional	Leukocytosis uncommon
Cerebrospinal fluid	Pleocytosis common	Pleocytosis uncommon
EEG	Diffuse slowing and occasional focal abnormalities or periodic patterns	Diffuse slowing
MRI	May have focal abnormalities	No focal abnormalities

*Lethargy, irritability, coma, change in behavior or personality.
†Unless increased intracranial pressure.
Modified from Bennett JE, Dolin R, Blaser MJ. *Mandell, Douglas, and Bennett's Principles and Practice of Infectious Diseases*. 9th ed. Vol 1. Philadelphia: Elsevier; 2020:1227, Table 89.1.

TABLE 42.2   Causes of Encephalitis at Different Ages

Age Group	Inflammation	Autoimmune	Infectious	Mimics
0–24 mo	Cryopyrin disorders Interferonopathies Complement disorders (HUS/TTP) Aicardi-Goutieres syndrome	Paraneoplastic Rare under 12 mo	Congenital infections Enteroviruses Arboviruses (including WNV) HSV HIV-1	Urea cycle disorders, maple syrup urine disease, Reye (MCAD deficiency), CPT2, mitochondrial disorders (Leigh) Bacterial meningitis Brain malformations Intoxication Epilepsy Dravet (SCNA1) and other epilepsy encephalopathy syndromes Acute adrenal crisis Hydrocephalus HLH Glioma AFP: SMA, botulism, pseudoparesis
2–5 yr	Complement disorders (HUS/TTP)	ADEM NMOSD VZV AFP: TM, AFM, NMOSD	HSV Enteroviruses Influenza Arboviruses EBV Adenovirus Mycoplasma Bartonella Rabies	Bacterial meningitis Intoxication Reye (MCAD deficiency) Epilepsy Dravet (SCNA1) and other epilepsy encephalopathy syndromes HUS, infectious HLH Mitochondrial disorders (MELAS) Glioma; CNS lymphoma
School age		ADEM NMDAR NMOSD VZV AFP: TM, AFM, NMOSD	HSV Enteroviruses Influenza EBV Adenovirus Mycoplasma Bartonella Lyme Rabies	Epilepsy Dravet (SCNA1) and other epilepsy encephalopathy syndromes CNS lymphoma HLH Mitochondrial disorders (MELAS) Vasculitis (primary, rickettsia, VZV) Glioma; CNS lymphoma AFP: AFM

TABLE 42.2 Causes of Encephalitis at Different Ages—cont'd

Age Group	Inflammation	Autoimmune	Infectious	Mimics
Pubertal		ADEM NMDAR NMOSD VZV SLE AFP: TM, NMOSD	HSV Enteroviruses Influenza EBV Mycoplasma HIV-1 Lyme Rabies	Intoxication Psychosis Wilson disease HLH Pseudotumor cerebri Multiple sclerosis Mitochondrial disorders (MELAS) Vasculitis (primary, rickettsia, VZV) Tumor metastases AFP: Guillain-Barré
Young adult		ADEM NMDAR NMOSD SLE Paraneoplastic AFP: TM, NMOSD	HSV Enteroviruses Influenza EBV Mycoplasma HIV-1 Lyme Rabies	Intoxication Psychosis Wilson disease HLH Periarteritis nodosa, Takayasu, giant cell, ANCA+ arteritis Acute intermittent porphyria Multiple sclerosis Mitochondrial disorders (MELAS) Vasculitis (primary, rickettsia, VZV) Tumor metastases AFP: Guillain-Barré
Adult		Limbic encephalitis SLE AFP: NMOSD NMDAR	HSV Enteroviruses Influenza HIV-1 Lyme WNV Rabies	Intoxication Glioma; CNS lymphoma TTP Neurodegeneration Tumor metastases HLH Periarteritis nodosa, Takayasu, giant cell, ANCA+ arteritis Multiple sclerosis Mitochondrial disorders (MELAS) Vasculitis (primary, rickettsia, VZV) Glioma; CNS lymphoma; tumor metastases AFP: Guillain-Barre

ADEM, acute disseminated encephalomyelitis; AFM, acute flaccid myelitis; AFP, acute flaccid paralysis; ANCA, antineutrophil cytoplasmic antibody; CNS, central nervous system; CPT2, carnitine palmitoyltransferase-2; EBV, Epstein-Barr virus; HLH, hemophagocytic lymphohistiocytosis; HSV, herpes simplex virus; HUS, hemolytic uremic syndrome; MCAD, medium-chain acylcarnitine deficiency; MELAS, mitochondrial encephalopathy lactic acidosis syndrome; NMDAR, N-methyl-D-aspartate receptor; NMOSD, neuromyelitis optica spectrum disorders; SCNA1, sodium voltage-gated channel alpha subunit 1; SLE, systemic lupus erythematosus; SMA, spinal muscular atrophy; TM, transverse myelitis; TTP, thrombotic thrombocytopenia purpura; VZV, varicella-zoster virus; WNV, West Nile virus.

proximity of the innervated dura to CSF explains the remarkably high sensitivity of polymerase chain reaction (PCR) tests for HSV encephalitis (93%) relative to those for hematogenous neonatal HSV encephalitis (70%). The virus is highly cytolytic, causing tissue necrosis. Early CSF findings do not distinguish HSV from other encephalitides; hemorrhagic CSF with a high protein level signifies necrotic brain lesions. Acyclovir requires a virally expressed thymidine kinase for activity, which directly matches potential cellular toxicity with antiviral effect. Acyclovir will crystalize in the kidneys unless hydration is aggressive.

The most common cause of **epidemic infectious encephalitis** is the enteroviruses. Enteroviruses cause summer outbreaks of aseptic meningitis without measurable neurologic deficits. Why they should on occasion mimic necrotizing HSV encephalitis in unclear; the rarity of the event raises consideration for a second-hit hypothesis. Enteroviruses include poliomyelitis viruses, the historical cause of epidemic acute flaccid paralysis worldwide. Nonpolio enteroviruses have been associated temporally with biannual outbreaks of AFM, with different clinical, radiologic, and virologic patterns than polio. Acute

poliomyelitis is restricted to anterior motor neurons in the spine, causing *asymmetric* flaccid paralysis with leg pain but without sensory or autonomic disturbances. Detection of virus in the CSF is common. Enteroviruses are naturally cleared by immunoglobulins, so patients with hypogammaglobulinemia are at high risk of a slow, chronic encephalitis due to enteroviruses.

Influenza viruses cause yearly outbreaks of severe respiratory illness and may be the most common precipitant of acute metabolic diseases causing *encephalopathy*, including Reye syndrome (medium-chain acylcarnitine deficiency [MCAD] deficiency), acute hemorrhagic shock and encephalopathy, acute necrotizing (thalamic, RANBP2) encephalopathy, acute encephalopathy with biphasic seizures and restricted diffusion, hemiconvulsion/hemiplegia syndrome, and mild encephalopathy with reversible splenial lesions. These syndromes are characterized by acute febrile illness, brain edema, hepatitis and disseminated intravascular coagulation (DIC) in some, and seizures. Syndromes vary by ethnicity and geography. All respiratory viruses associated with these syndromes are common and several are restricted

TABLE 42.3   Exposures Associated with Agents Causing Encephalitis and Encephalitis-Like Syndrome

Exposure and/or Reservoir	Agent	Risk Factors and Epidemiology
Arthropods		
Mosquitoes	**Alphaviruses**	
	Chikungunya virus	Tropical Africa and Southeast Asia, Indian Ocean and parts of Europe, Caribbean countries, South and Central America
	Western equine encephalitis (WEE) virus	Summer and early fall onset; western USA and Canada, Central and South America; rare cause of encephalitis, with 640 cases reported in the USA from 1964 to 1999. There have been only 4 cases of neuroinvasive disease due to WEE since 1989, with no cases reported in the last 10 yr (through 2009)
	Eastern equine encephalitis virus	Eastern and southern coastal states; children and elderly disproportionately affected; rare cause of encephalitis, with 260 cases reported in the USA from 1964 to 1999
	Venezuelan equine encephalitis virus	Mexico, Central and South America; rarely in border states of USA (Texas, Arizona)
	Semliki Forest virus	Africa
	Flaviviruses	
	West Nile virus	Epidemic encephalitis throughout USA, Europe; endemic in Middle East; cases also found in Africa, Caribbean, India, Australia, Russia, and Southeast Asia; peak incidence adults >50 yr
	Japanese encephalitis virus	Most common worldwide cause of encephalitis, endemic throughout Asia; vaccine preventable
	St. Louis encephalitis virus	Endemic to western USA; with periodic outbreaks in central/eastern USA, peak incidence in adults >50 yr
	Murray Valley encephalitis virus	Australia and New Guinea
	Bunyaviruses	
	California/La Crosse virus	USA with most cases in upper midwestern states (MN, WI, IA, IL, IN, OH) and more recently in mid-Atlantic and southeastern states (WV, VA, KY, NC, and TN); peak incidence in school-aged children
	Phleboviruses	
	Rift Valley fever virus	Africa and Arabia
Ticks	Powassan virus	In the USA, endemic in the Upper Midwest, Great Lakes, New England, and New York; endemic in eastern Canada
	Anaplasma phagocytophilum	Endemic to New England and north central and western USA
	Ehrlichia ewingii	Endemic to southeastern and central USA
	Ehrlichia chaffeensis	Endemic to northeastern USA and Midwest
	Rickettsia rickettsii	Rocky Mountain spotted fever has been reported throughout the USA with the exceptions of Hawaii and Vermont; states with highest incidence are Oklahoma, North Carolina, Arkansas, Tennessee, and Missouri
	Tickborne encephalitis virus	Endemic to Eastern and Central Europe, East and Southeast Asia
	Borrelia burgdorferi	Encephalitis in early disseminated Lyme disease; encephalopathy in late disease
	Kyasanur Forest disease virus	India
Sandflies	*Bartonella bacilliformis*	Colombia, Ecuador, and Peru
	Toscana virus	Italy, Mediterranean
	Chandipura virus	India
Tsetse flies	*Trypanosoma brucei gambiense*	West Africa and India; central nervous system (CNS) illness can occur years after infection
	Trypanosoma brucei rhodesiense	East Africa; CNS illness can occur years after infection

TABLE 42.3   **Exposures Associated with Agents Causing Encephalitis and Encephalitis-Like Syndrome—cont'd**

Exposure and/or Reservoir	Agent	Risk Factors and Epidemiology
Wild or Domestic Animals		
Bats	Rabies virus	Vaccine preventable. Between 1995 and 2009, 43 rabies cases were recognized in the USA; 10 of these cases were imported (usually from a canine strain), and the remaining cases were acquired in the USA mostly related to bat exposures and often with an unknown bite exposure
	Nipah virus	Epidemics in Southeast Asia; also found in Bangladesh and India. Reservoir host is fruit bat, but humans generally acquire disease through direct contact with infected swine
	Histoplasma capsulatum	Eastern and central USA; occupational or recreational activities where there is exposure to disturbed soil, such as gardening; playing in barns, hollow trees, bird roosts, or caves; and examination, demolition, or renovation of contaminated buildings
Deer	Borrelia burgdorferi	Deer is reservoir host, but infection usually is transmitted to humans via tick vector
Elk	Anaplasma phagocytophilum	Deer is reservoir host, but infection usually is transmitted to humans via tick vector
	Brucella abortus	Almost total eradication in cattle in the USA, but the disease still occurs in some elk herds and wild bison in the western USA
Dogs	Rabies virus	Vaccine preventable; dogs important in developing countries; worldwide distribution
	Toxocara canis	Dogs, especially puppies, shed eggs in feces, and organism survives in soil for prolonged period
Cats	Bartonella henselae	Typically follows scratch or bite from cat or kitten; highest incidence in children
	Toxoplasma gondii	Cats and other felines are reservoir hosts; they shed oocytes in feces, and the soil becomes contaminated. Sheep, goats, swine, cattle serve as intermediate hosts
	Rabies virus	Vaccine preventable; most common vector in the USA is bat, and bites often unrecognized; cats are second to dogs in importance in developing countries; worldwide distribution
	Toxocara cati	Cats, especially kittens, shed eggs in feces, and organism survives in soil for prolonged period
Rodents	Lymphocytic choriomeningitis virus	Peak incidence in fall and winter; chronic infection in laboratory or house mice, hamsters, and guinea pigs; humans infected by inhalation or ingestion of dust or food contaminated by urine, feces, blood, nasopharyngeal secretions of infected rodents
	Leptospira spp.	Rodents (and other animals) excrete organism in urine, and the organism remains viable in soil or water for weeks to months
Raccoons	Baylisascaris procyonis	Pica, particularly near raccoon latrine
	Rabies virus	"Raccoon strain" extends along eastern seaboard of the USA and has reached as far north as Ontario and New Brunswick in Canada
Sheep, goats	Brucella melitensis	Direct contact with infected animals or their secretions (note that B. melitensis has been eradicated in the USA since early 1970s)
	Coxiella burnetii	Inhalation; either direct exposure to animal or exposure to contaminated materials (e.g., wool, straw)
Birds	Cryptococcus neoformans	Inhalation of soil contaminated with bird feces
	Chlamydophila psittaci	Healthy and sick birds can harbor and transmit organism to humans; usually acquired via inhalation of fecal dust/sections of birds
	West Nile virus	Birds are reservoir hosts, but infection usually is transmitted to humans via mosquito vector
Old World monkeys	Herpes B virus	Bite of Old World monkey (e.g., macaque)
Horses	Hendra virus	Endemic in Australia; associated with excretions/tissues from horses
Swine	Nipah virus	Epidemics in Southeast Asia; close contact with pigs
	Brucella suis	No longer found in domestic swine but present in some wild hog populations

Continued

TABLE 42.3   Exposures Associated with Agents Causing Encephalitis and Encephalitis-Like Syndrome—cont'd

Exposure and/or Reservoir	Agent	Risk Factors and Epidemiology
Skunks	Rabies virus	Skunk populations are widely distributed in the USA; cases found in California, Arizona, north central USA, eastern coast of the USA
Squirrels	Bornavirus	Only three human cases described to date, exposure to squirrels in Germany
Parturient animals (especially farm animals)	*Coxiella burnetii*	Humans generally acquire via inhalation; either direct exposure to animal or exposure to contaminated materials (e.g., wool, straw)
Ingestion or Inhalation		
Fresh water	*Naegleria fowleri*	Swimming or diving in warm, natural bodies of water (rarely poorly chlorinated pools reported)
	Leptospira spp.	Organisms excreted in animal urine or placental tissue and can remain viable for weeks to months in soil or water; recreational exposure associated with wading or swimming in contaminated water (particularly after floods)
Soil	*Balamuthia mandrillaris*	Contact with soil seems to be important risk factor, presumably through inhalation or inoculation
	Acanthamoeba spp.	Contact with soil seems to be important risk factor, presumably through inhalation or inoculation
	Baylisascaris procyonis	Pica, particularly near raccoon latrine; raccoons infected with *B. procyonis* appear to be common in many parts of the USA; human cases reported in California, Oregon, New York, Pennsylvania, Illinois, Michigan, Georgia, Minnesota, and Missouri
	Coccidioides spp.	Also known as *valley fever*. Infection is seasonal and is acquired by inhalation of soil or dust or laboratory acquired; endemic in certain areas of Arizona, California, Nevada, New Mexico, Texas, Utah, and northwestern Mexico. Also found in northern Argentina, northwest Brazil, Colombia, Paraguay, Venezuela, and Central America
	Histoplasma capsulatum	Inhalation of airborne spores from soil. Outbreaks have occurred in endemic areas with exposure to bird, chicken, or bat droppings or recently contaminated soil. Globally distributed, with the Ohio and Mississippi River basin, Mexico, and Central and South America being endemic areas in which as many as 80% of children have been infected. Also found in Africa, East Asia, Australia, and rarely Europe
	Blastomyces dermatitidis	Endemic areas include the midwestern, southwestern, and south central USA and the Canadian provinces near the Great Lakes and the St. Lawrence Seaway
	Toxocara canis/Toxocara cati	Eggs in sandboxes and playgrounds; organisms survive long periods in soil
Undercooked pork or beef (rarely chicken)	*Toxoplasma gondii*	Consuming raw or undercooked infected meat; worldwide
Undercooked freshwater fish, chicken, or pork	*Gnathostoma* spp.	Southeast Asia and Mexico
Freshwater crayfish or crabs	*Paragonimus westermani*	Mostly in Asia but some reports from Africa and South America
Raw or undercooked meat	*Trichinella* spp.	Mostly associated with pigs but has been found in other mammals (e.g., horses, bears, foxes)
Frogs, snakes	*Gnathostoma spinigerum*	Southeast Asia and some areas in South and Central America
Raw or undercooked freshwater prawns, crabs, or frogs, or unwashed produce (with snails or slugs)	*Angiostrongylus cantonensis*	Reported in Louisiana, Hawaii, the South Pacific, Pacific Islands, Southeast Asia, Asia, Australia, and the Caribbean
Raw vegetables	*Toxoplasma gondii*	Consumption of raw, unwashed vegetables
Unpasteurized milk	*Coxiella burnetii*	Animal exposures (particularly placenta and amniotic fluid)
	Tickborne encephalitis virus	Tick bite or ingestion of unpasteurized milk; endemic to Eastern and Central Europe, East and Southeast Asia
	Listeria monocytogenes	Can be found in about 5% of unpasteurized milk samples and products
	Toxoplasma gondii	Consumption of raw goat milk

TABLE 42.3 **Exposures Associated with Agents Causing Encephalitis and Encephalitis-Like Syndrome—cont'd**

Exposure and/or Reservoir	Agent	Risk Factors and Epidemiology
Season		
Fall	Enteroviruses	Peak incidence in late summer and early fall; enterovirus 71 a cause of large outbreaks in Asia, with children primarily affected
	Arthropod-borne pathogens	Geographically specific agents/risks
Winter	Influenza virus, other respiratory viruses	Sporadic cases in children, with most reports from Japan and Southeast Asia
Spring	Enteroviruses	Peak incidence in late summer and early fall; enterovirus 71 a cause of large outbreaks in Asia, with children primarily affected
	Arthropod-borne pathogens	
Summer	Enteroviruses	Peak incidence in late summer and early fall; enterovirus 71 a cause of large outbreaks in Asia, with children primarily affected
	Naegleria fowleri	Swimming or diving in brackish freshwater lakes or ponds
	Arthropod-borne pathogens	Geographically specific agents/risks
Recreation		
Camping or hunting	Arthropod-borne pathogens	Geographically specific agents/risks
Spelunking	Rabies virus	Airborne transmission has been reported rarely in caves inhabited by millions of bats
	Histoplasma capsulatum	Inhalation of spores from soil contaminated with bat guano
Sexual activity	HIV	Global risk
	Treponema pallidum	Global risk
	Herpes simplex virus 2 (HSV-2)	HSV-1 also can be transmitted by sexual activity
Water sports	*Naegleria fowleri*	Swimming or diving in brackish freshwater lakes or ponds
	Leptospira spp.	Exposure to water contaminated with urine of infected animals via swallowing water or skin contact
Blood Transfusion or Organ Transplantation		
	Toxoplasma gondii	Infection can occur through blood transfusion or organ transplantation
	Rabies virus	Rare case reports of transmission via organ transplantation
	Balamuthia mandrillaris	Rare case reports of transmission via organ transplantation
	Lymphocytic choriomeningitis virus	Rare case reports of transmission via organ transplantation
Foreign Travel		
Global	West Nile virus	Geographically specific risks
	Rabies virus	Dog bites are the most common mode of acquisition in developing countries
	HSV-1 and HSV-2	Sporadic
	Influenza	Seasonal by region
	Measles	Measles subacute sclerosing panencephalitis can occur despite history of immunization (child generally had unrecognized infection before measles vaccine)
	Enteroviruses	Seasonal by region
	HIV	Sexual activity and bloodborne
	Plasmodium spp.	Tropical and subtropical areas
Africa	Chikungunya virus	Particularly Tanzania
	Poliovirus	Wild poliovirus transmission occurs in Nigeria
	Histoplasma capsulatum	Microfoci throughout Africa
	Taenia spp.	East Africa, particularly in underdeveloped communities with poor sanitation and where people eat raw or undercooked pork

Continued

TABLE 42.3 **Exposures Associated with Agents Causing Encephalitis and Encephalitis-Like Syndrome—cont'd**

Exposure and/or Reservoir	Agent	Risk Factors and Epidemiology
Asia	Chikungunya virus	Particularly India, Indonesia, Thailand, and Indian Ocean islands
	Japanese encephalitis virus	Including Southeast Asia
	Tickborne encephalitis virus	Central Europe to Japan
	Borrelia burgdorferi	Temperate forested regions throughout northern Asia
	Histoplasma capsulatum	Microfoci throughout eastern Asia
	Gnathostoma spinigerum	Southeast Asia, particularly Thailand, and Japan
	Nipah virus	Southeast Asia, particularly Malaysia
	Taenia spp.	Southeast Asia, particularly in underdeveloped communities with poor sanitation and where people eat raw or undercooked pork
	Poliovirus	Wild type present in India, Pakistan, Afghanistan
Australia	Murray Valley encephalitis virus	Also in New Guinea
	Japanese encephalitis virus	Northern Australia
	Histoplasma capsulatum	Microfoci throughout Australia
	Hendra virus	Exposure to body fluids and excretions of infected horses is important
Caribbean	Venezuelan equine encephalitis virus	Trinidad
Europe	Tickborne encephalitis virus	Central Europe to Japan
	Chikungunya virus	Italy (northeastern), France (southern)
	Anaplasma phagocytophila	Temperate zones, particularly Germany, Portugal, and Denmark
	Toscana virus	Italy, Mediterranean
	Borrelia burgdorferi	Temperate forested regions throughout Europe, particularly eastern and central Europe
	Taenia spp.	Eastern Europe, particularly in underdeveloped communities with poor sanitation and where people eat raw or undercooked pork
Mediterranean	Toscana virus	Central Italy, France, Spain, Portugal, Greece, Cyprus
North America	Powassan virus	Northeastern and central USA, Canada
	California/La Crosse virus	Midwestern and eastern USA
	St. Louis encephalitis virus	Geographic range extends from Canada to Argentina, but most human cases in the western USA, with periodic outbreaks in central and eastern USA
	Ehrlichia chaffeensis	Southern and central USA, and mid-Atlantic and coastal states
	Anaplasma phagocytophila	Wooded areas of the north and northeastern USA, mid-Atlantic, Midwest, West Coast
	Rickettsia rickettsii	Throughout southern Canada and North America, with peak incidence in southeast and south central USA, northern and southwestern Mexico, Costa Rica, and Panama
	Eastern equine encephalitis	Highest incidence in Atlantic and Gulf states
	Venezuelan equine encephalitis virus	Florida and southwestern USA, rarely in border states (Texas, Arizona); tropical latitudes of Mexico and Central America
	Western equine encephalitis virus	Most cases occur in western USA and prairie provinces in Canada, but WEE also occurs in Mexico and Central America; infection associated with residence in rural areas and with agricultural occupations and other outdoor activities that lead to contact with the vector mosquito
	Borrelia burgdorferi	Eastern USA, Upper Midwest, and Pacific Northwest; epidemics in summer months when ticks actively seek hosts and human outdoor activity is greatest
	Coccidioides spp.	Semiarid regions of southwestern USA and Mexico
	Blastomyces dermatitidis	Southeastern and central states, midwestern states bordering the Great Lakes; thrives in decaying vegetation or wet soil
	Histoplasma capsulatum	Endemic in Mississippi, Ohio, and Missouri River valleys in the USA and other microfoci throughout the USA, Mexico, and Central America
	Balamuthia mandrillaris	Highest number of cases reported from Arizona, California, and Texas in the USA; also occurs in Mexico and Central America
	Taenia spp.	Mexico and Central America, especially in underdeveloped communities with poor sanitation and where people eat raw or undercooked pork
	Gnathostoma spinigerum	Mexico and Central America; humans become infected by eating undercooked fish or poultry containing third-stage larvae, or reportedly by drinking water containing infective second-stage larvae

TABLE 42.3 Exposures Associated with Agents Causing Encephalitis and Encephalitis-Like Syndrome—cont'd

Exposure and/or Reservoir	Agent	Risk Factors and Epidemiology
Russia	Taenia spp.	More prevalent in underdeveloped communities with poor sanitation and where people eat raw or undercooked pork
	Tickborne encephalitis virus	Eastern Russia
South America	Venezuelan equine encephalitis virus	Tropical latitudes, particularly Colombia, Venezuela, Peru, and Ecuador
	St. Louis encephalitis virus	From Canada to Argentina, but most human cases occur in the USA
	Western equine encephalitis virus	Associated with residence in rural areas and with agricultural occupations and other outdoor activities that lead to contact with the vector mosquito
	Rickettsia rickettsii	Brazil and Argentina
	Coccidioides spp.	Semiarid regions
	Histoplasma capsulatum	Microfoci throughout South America
	Gnathostoma spinigerum	Consuming undercooked fish or poultry containing third-stage larvae, or reportedly by drinking water containing infective second-stage larvae
	Bartonella bacilliformis	Middle altitudes of Andes Mountains
	Taenia spp.	More prevalent in underdeveloped communities with poor sanitation and where people eat raw or undercooked pork

From Long SS, Prober CG, Fischer M. *Principles and Practice of Pediatric Infectious Diseases*. 5th ed. Philadelphia: Elsevier; 2018:306–310, Table 44-1.

TABLE 42.4 Diagnostic Criteria for Definite Autoimmune Limbic Encephalitis

Diagnosis can be made when all four* of the following criteria have been met:
1. Subacute onset (rapid progression of <3 mo) of working memory deficits, seizures, or psychiatric symptoms suggesting involvement of the limbic system
2. Bilateral brain abnormalities on T2-weighted fluid-attenuated inversion recovery MRI highly restricted to the medial temporal lobes[†]
3. At least one of the following:
   - CSF pleocytosis (white blood cell count of >5 cells/mm^3)
   - EEG with epileptic or slow-wave activity involving the temporal lobes
4. Reasonable exclusion of alternative causes

CSF, cerebrospinal fluid.
*If one of the first three criteria is not met, a diagnosis of definite limbic encephalitis can be made only with the detection of antibodies against cell-surface, synaptic, or onconeural proteins.
[†]18-Fluorodeoxyglucose (18F-FDG) PET can be used to fulfill this criterion. Results from studies from the past 5 yr suggest that 18F-FDG-PET imaging might be more sensitive than MRI to show an increase in FDG uptake in normal-appearing medial temporal lobes.
From Graus F, Titulaer MJ, Balu R, et al. A clinical approach to diagnosis of autoimmune encephalitis. *Lancet Neurol*. 2016;15:391–404 (Panel 2, p. 395).

TABLE 42.5 Diagnostic Criteria for Definite Acute Disseminated Encephalomyelitis

Diagnosis can be made when all five of the following criteria have been met:
1. A first multifocal, clinical CNS event of presumed inflammatory demyelinating cause
2. Encephalopathy that cannot be explained by fever
3. Abnormal brain MRI:
   - Diffuse, poorly demarcated, large (>1–2 cm) lesions predominantly involving the cerebral white matter
   - T1-hypointense lesions in the white matter in rare cases
   - Deep gray matter abnormalities (e.g., thalamus or basal ganglia) can be present
4. No new clinical or MRI findings after 3 mo of symptom onset
5. Reasonable exclusion of alternative causes

CNS, central nervous system.
From Graus F, Titulaer MJ, Balu R, et al. A clinical approach to diagnosis of autoimmune encephalitis. *Lancet Neurol*. 2016;15:391–404 (Panel 3, p. 396).

TABLE 42.6   Diagnostic Criteria for Anti-NMDA Receptor Encephalitis

Probable Anti-NMDA Receptor Encephalitis*

Diagnosis can be made when all three of the following criteria have been met:

1. Rapid onset (<3 mo) of at least four of the six following major groups of symptoms:
   - Abnormal (psychiatric) behavior or cognitive dysfunction
   - Speech dysfunction (pressured speech, verbal reduction, mutism)
   - Seizures
   - Movement disorder, dyskinesias, or rigidity/abnormal postures
   - Decreased level of consciousness
   - Autonomic dysfunction or central hypoventilation
2. At least one of the following laboratory study results:
   - Abnormal EEG (focal or diffuse slow or disorganized activity, epileptic activity, or extreme delta brush)
   - CSF with pleocytosis or oligoclonal bands
3. Reasonable exclusion of other disorders

Diagnosis can also be made in the presence of three of the above groups of symptoms accompanied by a systemic teratoma

Definite Anti-NMDA Receptor Encephalitis*

Diagnosis can be made in the presence of one or more of the six major groups of symptoms and IgG anti-GluN1 antibodies,[†] after reasonable exclusion of other disorders (appendix)

CSF, cerebrospinal fluid; IgG, immunoglobulin G; NMDA, *N*-methyl-D-aspartate.

*Patients with a history of herpes simplex virus encephalitis in the previous weeks might have relapsing immune-mediated neurologic symptoms (post–herpes simplex virus encephalitis).

[†]Antibody testing should include testing of CSF. If only serum is available, confirmatory tests should be included (e.g., live neurons or tissue immunohistochemistry, in addition to cell-based assay).

From Graus F, Titulaer MJ, Balu R, et al. A clinical approach to diagnosis of autoimmune encephalitis. *Lancet Neurol.* 2016;15:391–404 (Panel 4, p. 397).

TABLE 42.7   Diagnostic Criteria for Bickerstaff Brainstem Encephalitis

Probable Bickerstaff Brainstem Encephalitis

Diagnosis can be made when both of the following criteria have been met:

1. Subacute onset (rapid progression of <4 wk) of all the following symptoms:
   - Decreased level of consciousness
   - Bilateral external ophthalmoplegia
   - Ataxia
2. Reasonable exclusion of alternative causes

Definite Bickerstaff Brainstem Encephalitis

Diagnosis can be made in the presence of positive IgG anti-GQ1b antibodies even if bilateral external ophthalmoplegia is not complete or ataxia cannot be assessed, or if recovery has occurred within 12 wk after onset

IgG, immunoglobulin G.

From Graus F, Titulaer MJ, Balu R, et al. A clinical approach to diagnosis of autoimmune encephalitis. *Lancet Neurol.* 2016;15:391–404 (Panel 5, p. 398).

TABLE 42.8   Subacute and Chronic Central Nervous System Presentations: Microbiologic Causes

Viruses

Measles virus (inclusion body encephalitis)
Varicella-zoster virus (causes a multifocal leukoencephalopathy)
Cytomegalovirus
Herpes simplex virus (especially HSV-2)
Human herpes virus 6
Enteroviruses
HIV (dementia)
Measles virus (subacute sclerosing panencephalitis)
JC/BK* virus (progressive multifocal leukoencephalopathy)

Bacteria

Mycobacterium tuberculosis
Treponema pallidum (syphilis)
Borrelia burgdorferi (Lyme neuroborreliosis)
Tropheryma whipplei (Whipple disease)

Fungi

Cryptococcus neoformans

Parasites

Trypanosoma brucei spp. (African trypanosomiasis)
Toxoplasma gondii (toxoplasmosis)

Prions

Creutzfeldt-Jakob disease

*JC and BK viruses are named after the initials of the patients from whom they were first isolated.

Viral agents often seen in immunocompromised or immunocompetent patients; other pathogens in all patients.

Modified from Solomon T, Hart I, Beeching NJ. Viral encephalitis: a clinician's guide. *Pract Neurol.* 2007;7:288–305; and Solomon T. Arboviruses. In: Gill GV, Beeching NJ, eds. *Lecture Notes: Tropical Medicine.* 6th ed. Oxford: Wiley-Blackwell; 2009:287–288.

to mucosal surfaces (e.g., influenza, respiratory syncytial virus [RSV], rotavirus). Half of patients (other than those with splenial lesions) have neurologic sequelae. MRI findings confirm the anatomic diagnosis. The presence of cardiomyopathy or liver failure with encephalopathy may also suggest a mitochondrial disorder. The empirical use of nucleoside analogs as antivirals in patients with possible mitochondrial disorders risks unbalancing nucleoside pools to cause further mitochondrial DNA loss.

CNS vasculitis and **vasculopathies** are mostly secondary to other inflammatory processes (see Chapter 37). The distinction of encephalitis and CNS vasculitis is partly semantic because encephalitis involves the neurovascular unit and perivenular inflammation is a regular pathologic finding in encephalitis. Systemic infections (rickettsia), virus reactivations (varicella-zoster virus [VSV]), and toxins (Shiga toxin, hemolytic uremia syndrome [HUS]/thrombotic

TABLE 42.9   Conditions Mimicking Infectious Encephalitis

Immune Mediated
- Anti-*N*-methyl-ᴅ-aspartate receptor-associated (NMDAR) and other autoimmune encephalitides*
- Rheumatologic causes (systemic lupus erythematosus, Sjögren syndrome, Behçet disease, sarcoidosis)
- Small-vessel vasculitis
- Corticosteroid-responsive encephalopathy associated with Hashimoto thyroiditis
- Acute disseminated encephalomyelitis (ADEM)

Toxic Encephalopathy
- Bacterial toxins (*Shigella* spp., *Campylobacter jejuni*, *Salmonella* spp.)
- Reye syndrome
- Acute toxic ingestion
- Lead intoxication
- Hyperpyrexic encephalopathy and shock syndrome

Inborn Error of Metabolism
- Ornithine transcarbamylase deficiency, heterozygote
- Glutaric acidemia type 1
- Medium-chain acyl coenzyme A dehydrogenase deficiency
- Mitochondrial encephalopathy with lactic acidosis and stroke syndrome
- Acute intermittent porphyria

Acquired Metabolic
- Hypoglycemia
- Electrolyte disturbances
- Uremia
- Hepatic encephalopathy
- Endocrine disorder
- Vitamin deficiency (thiamine, B_{12})

Tumor
Brainstem glioma
Other neoplasms (primary or metastatic; paraneoplastic disease)

Other Central Nervous System Conditions
- Stroke
- Pseudotumor cerebri
- Acute confusional migraine
- Brain malformations
- Psychosis
- Epilepsy encephalopathy syndromes (genetic)
- Bacterial meningitis
- Brain or parameningeal abscess
- Endocarditis complicated by brain embolism
- Venous sinus thrombosis
- Subdural or epidural hematoma
- Head injury
- Connective tissue disorder
- FIRES
- Hypertensive encephalopathy (PRES)

*Two broad categories of antigens: (1) intracellular paraneoplastic antigens, including Hu, Ma2, CV2, and CRMP5, and (2) cell surface antigens, such as voltage-gated potassium channels and others.
FIRES, febrile infection related epilepsy syndrome; PRES, posterior reversible encephalopathy syndrome.
From Long SS, Prober CG, Fischer M. *Principles and Practice of Pediatric Infectious Diseases*. 5th ed. Philadelphia: Elsevier; 2018:310, Box 44-1.

thrombocytopenic purpura [TTP]) cause secondary vasculitis and encephalopathy. Autoimmune forms of vasculitis include innate inflammopathies (pyrin, interferon, and complement disorders) as well as antibody-mediated (system lupus erythematosus [SLE]) and cell-mediated (Rasmussen) processes. Primary small-vessel vasculitis has a long prodrome and often presents subtly, including encephalopathies, developmental regression, and behavioral and psychiatric symptoms. Inflammatory markers are elevated and oligoclonal bands are present in one third of cases. MRI may be normal or demonstrate demyelination (but with meningeal enhancement) or cord lesions. Contrast enhancement is variable; there is no restricted diffusion. Diagnosis may require brain biopsy but does not require targeting of a radiologic lesion. Granulomatous inflammation is more common in adults than children.

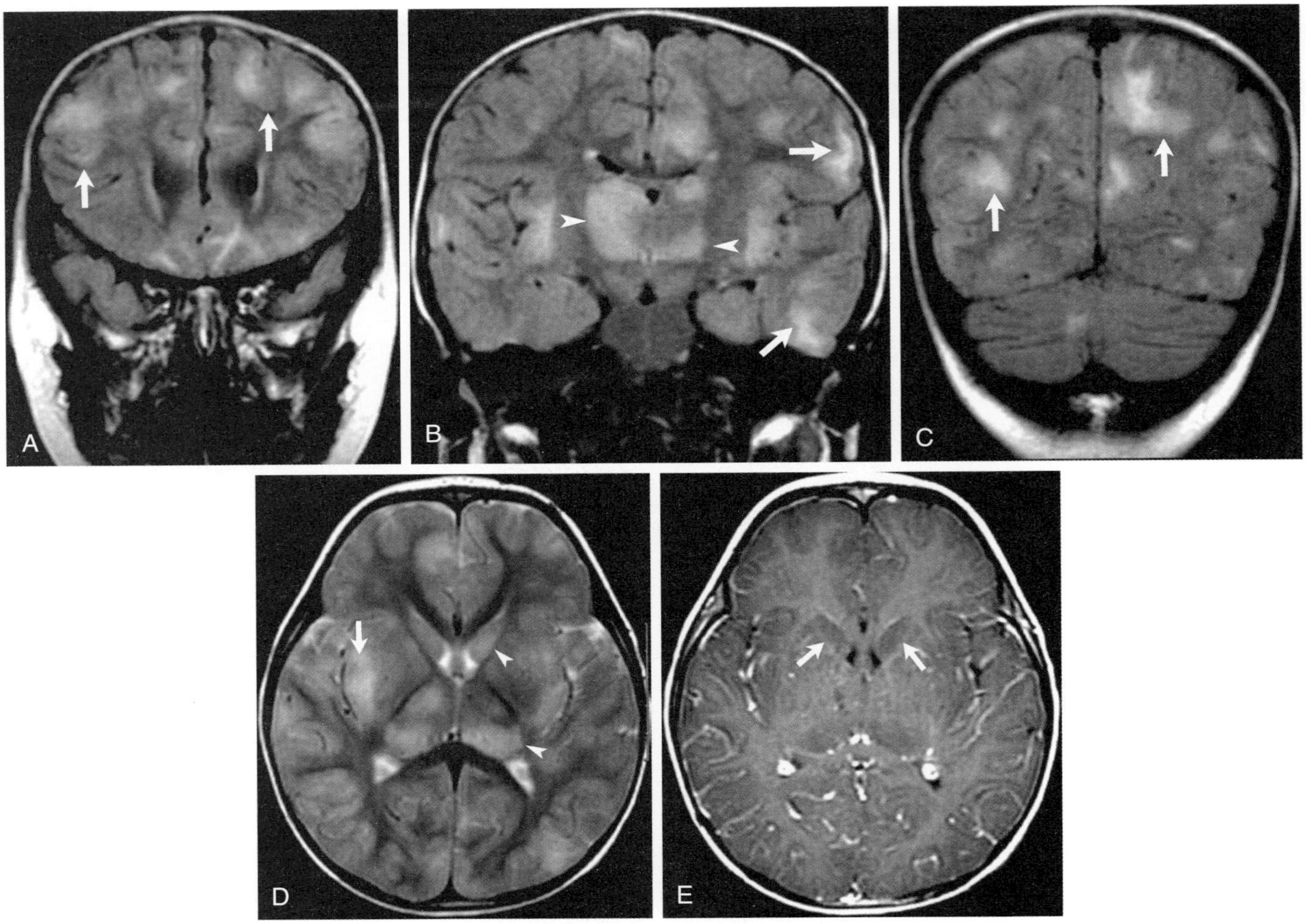

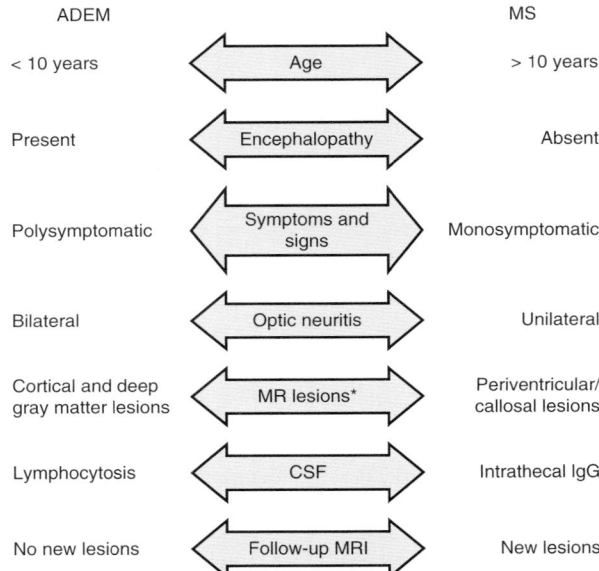

Fig. 42.1 Acute disseminated encephalomyelopathy (ADEM). Twenty-two-month-old male with lethargy, hypotonia, ataxia, and decreased righting reflexes preceded by an antecedent upper respiratory illness. Sequential coronal fluid-attenuated inversion recovery images from anterior to posterior *(A–C)*, axial T2-weighted *(D)*, and axial postcontrast T1-weighted *(E)* MRI. There are patchy areas of bilateral subcortical white matter T2 prolongation *(arrows* in *A–D)*, as well as abnormal T2 prolongation within the central gray structures *(arrowheads* in *B* and *D)*. There is no significant contrast enhancement noted; however, the central gray structures appear to stand out in relief on the postcontrast images *(arrows* in *E)* likely secondary to abnormal T1 prolongation. (From Rothenberg Maddocks AB, Pollock AN. Infection and inflammation. In: Coley BD, ed. *Caffey's Pediatric Diagnostic Imaging.* 13th ed. Philadelphia: Elsevier; 2019:339–340, Fig. 34.26.)

ADEM		MS
< 10 years	Age	> 10 years
Present	Encephalopathy	Absent
Polysymptomatic	Symptoms and signs	Monosymptomatic
Bilateral	Optic neuritis	Unilateral
Cortical and deep gray matter lesions	MR lesions*	Periventricular/callosal lesions
Lymphocytosis	CSF	Intrathecal IgG
No new lesions	Follow-up MRI	New lesions

Fig. 42.2 Clinical and investigation differences between ADEM and MS (trends only). *MR lesions other than white matter. ADEM, acute disseminated encephalomyelitis; CSF, cerebrospinal fluid; IgG, immunoglobulin G; MS, multiple sclerosis. (From Dale RC, Branson JA. Acute disseminated encephalomyelitis or multiple sclerosis: can the initial presentation help in establishing a correct diagnosis? *Arch Dis Child.* 2005;90:636–639 [Fig. 3, p. 638].)

TABLE 42.10 MRI Characteristics in ADEM vs MS

MRI Characteristics	ADEM: Typical	MS: Typical
Deep gray matter and cortical involvement	Yes	No
Bilateral diffuse lesions	Yes	No
Poorly marginated lesions	Yes	No
Large globular lesions	Yes	No
Periventricular pattern of lesions	No	Yes
Lesions perpendicular to long axis of corpus callosum	No	Yes
Ovoid lesions	No	Yes
Lesions confined to corpus callosum	No	Yes
Sole presence of well-defined lesions	No	Yes
Black holes (on T1 sequence)	No	Yes

ADEM, acute disseminated encephalomyelitis; MS, multiple sclerosis.
From Pohl D, Alper G, Van Haren K, et al. Acute disseminated encephalomyelitis. *Neurology.* 2016;87(Suppl 2):S38–S45 (Table 2, p. S40).

TABLE 42.11 Examination Findings of Importance in Assessing a Patient with Suspected Encephalitis

- Airway, breathing, circulation
- Mini-mental state, cognitive function, behavior (when possible)
- Evidence of prior seizures (tongue biting, injury)
- Subtle motor seizures (mouth, digit, eyelid twitching)
- Meningism
- Focal neurologic signs
- Papilledema
- Flaccid paralysis (anterior horn cell involvement)
- Rash (purpuric—meningococcus; vesicular—hand, foot, and mouth disease; varicella-zoster; rickettsial disease)
- Injection sites of drug abuse
- Bites from animals (rabies) or insects (arboviruses)
- Movement disorders, including parkinsonism

From Kneen R, Michael BD, Menson E, et al. Management of suspected viral encephalitis in children—Association of British Neurologists and British Paediatric Allergy, Immunology, and Infection Group National Guidelines. *J Infect.* 2010;64:499–477 (Table 7, p. 456).

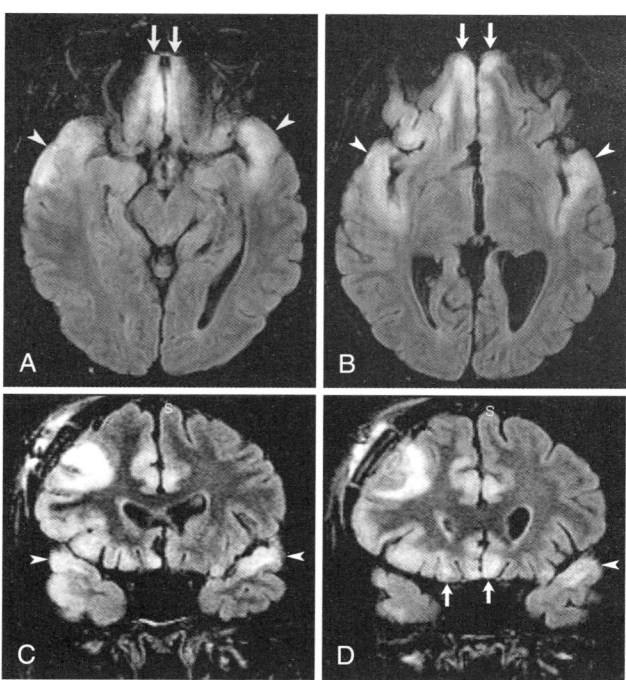

Fig. 42.3 Herpes simplex virus (HSV). Patient with seizures and decreased level of consciousness. Axial fluid-attenuated inversion recovery (FLAIR) *(A and B)* and coronal FLAIR *(C and D)* MRIs were obtained. There is abnormal signal intensity within both frontal lobes *(arrows)* and temporal lobes *(arrowheads)* indicative of HSV encephalitis. The bilateral temporal lobe involvement is a clue to the underlying causative agent of HSV. (From Rothenberg Maddocks AB, Pollock AN. Infection and inflammation. In: Coley BD, ed. *Caffey's Pediatric Diagnostic Imaging.* 13th ed. Philadelphia: Elsevier; 2019:344, Fig. 34.34.)

Evaluation

Evaluation is considered in cases of encephalitis or encephalopathy in association with fevers or focal neurologic signs. Symptoms are difficult to elicit in preverbal children, but speech, behavior, and sleep are often affected. Important findings on physical exam are noted in Table 42.11. Objective motor signs include myoclonus, myoclonic seizures, tremors, dyskinesias, abnormalities of tone, and ataxia. Dysautonomia is often present. CT of the head is rarely useful other than to detect gross edema, midline shifts, obstructive hydrocephalus, intracranial hemorrhage, or calcifications. MRI provides exquisite detail and can differentiate strokes, gray matter involvement, demyelination, and large-vessel vasculitis (see Chapter 37) (Fig. 42.3). MRI should include T2, fluid-attenuated inversion recovery (FLAIR), diffusion-weighted imaging (DWI), and intravenous contrast to differentiate disorders. Magnetic resonance angiography or magnetic resonance spectroscopy may be indicated. EEG is generally not specific but universally has an abnormal background with or without seizures; EEG is normal in pediatric autoimmune neuropsychiatric disorders associated with streptococcal infections (PANDAS)/pediatric acute-onset neuropsychiatric syndrome (PANS) and psychiatric disorders.

There are myriad causes of autoimmune and infectious encephalitis (Tables 42.12, 4.13, and 4.14).

TABLE 42.12 Diagnostic Algorithm for Initial Evaluation of Encephalitis in Children*

Routine Studies

CSF[†]

Collect at least 5 mL fluid, if possible; freeze unused fluid for additional testing

Opening pressure, WBC count with differential, RBC count, protein, glucose

Gram stain and bacterial culture

HSV-1/2 PCR

Enterovirus PCR

Serum

Routine blood cultures

EBV serology (VCA IgG and IgM and EBNA IgG)

Mycoplasma pneumoniae IgM and IgG

Hold acute serum and collect convalescent serum 10–14 days later for paired antibody testing

Imaging

Neuroimaging (MRI preferred to CT, if available)

Neurophysiology

EEG

Other Tissues/Fluids

Mycoplasma pneumoniae PCR from throat sample

Enterovirus PCR and/or culture of throat and stool

When clinical features of extra-CNS involvement are present, we recommend additional testing (e.g., biopsy of skin lesions; bronchoalveolar lavage and/or endobronchial biopsy in those with pneumonia/pulmonary lesions; throat swab PCR/culture in those with upper respiratory illness; stool culture in those with diarrhea); also see below

Conditional Studies

Host Factors

Age <3 yr—parechovirus PCR (CSF)

Immunocompromised—CMV PCR, HHV 6/7 PCR, HIV PCR (CSF); cryptococcal antigen; *Toxoplasma gondii* serology and/or PCR; MTB testing[‡]; fungal testing[§]; WNV testing[‖]

Geographic Factors

Africa—malaria (blood smear); trypanosomiasis (blood/CSF smear, serology from serum and CSF); dengue testing[‖]

Asia—Japanese encephalitis virus testing[‖]; dengue testing[‖]; malaria (blood smear); Nipah virus testing (serology from serum and CSF; PCR, immunohistochemistry, and virus isolation in a BSL4 lab can also be used to substantiate diagnosis)

Australia—Murray Valley encephalitis virus testing[‖]; Kunjin virus testing[‖]; ABLV testing[¶]

Europe—tickborne encephalitis virus (serology); if Southern Europe, consider WNV testing,[‖] Toscana virus testing[‖]

Central and South America—dengue testing[‖]; malaria (blood smear)

North America—geographically—appropriate arboviral testing (e.g., WNV, Powassan, La Crosse, Eastern equine encephalitis viruses,[‖] Lyme [serum ELISA and Western blot])

Season and Exposure

Summer/fall—arbovirus[‖] and tickborne disease** testing

Cat (particularly if with seizures, paucicellular CSF)—*Bartonella* antibody (serum), ophthalmologic evaluation

Tick exposure—tickborne disease testing**

Animal bite/bat exposure—rabies testing[¶]

Swimming or diving in warm fresh water or nasal/sinus irrigation—*Naegleria fowleri* (CSF wet mount and PCR[††])

Specific Signs and Symptoms

Abnormal behavior (e.g., new-onset temper tantrums, agitation, aggression), psychotic features, seizures or movement disorder—NMDAR antibody (serum, CSF), oligoclonal bands, IgG index, rabies testing[¶]

Behavior changes followed by myoclonic spasms/jerks: measles IgG (CSF and serum)

Vesicular rash—VZV PCR from CSF (sensitivity may be low; if test available, consider CSF IgG and IgM); VZV IgG and IgM from serum

Rapid decompensation (particularly with animal bite history or prior travel to rabies-endemic areas)—rabies testing[¶]

Respiratory symptoms—chest imaging (chest x-ray and/or CT scan); respiratory virus testing[‡‡]; *Mycoplasma pneumoniae* PCR (CSF)

Acute flaccid paralysis—arbovirus testing[‖]; rabies testing[¶]

Parkinsonism—arbovirus testing[‖]; toxoplasma serology

Nonhealing skin lesions—*Balamuthia, Acanthamoeba* testing[††]

Prominent limbic symptoms—autoimmune limbic encephalitis testing,[§§] HHV-6/7 PCR (CSF)

TABLE 42.12   Diagnostic Algorithm for Initial Evaluation of Encephalitis in Children*—cont'd

Laboratory Features

If EBV serology is suggestive of acute infection, perform EBV PCR (CSF)

Elevated transaminases—rickettsia serology, tickborne disease testing**

CSF protein >100 mg/dL, or CSF glucose <2/3 peripheral glucose, or lymphocytic pleocytosis with subacute symptom onset—MTB testing[‡]; fungal testing[§];
  Balamuthia mandrillaris testing[††]

CSF protein >100 mg/dL or CSF glucose <2/3 peripheral glucose and neutrophilic predominance with acute symptom onset and recent antibiotic use—CSF PCR for
  Streptococcus pneumoniae and *Neisseria meningitidis*

CSF eosinophilia—MTB testing[‡]; fungal testing[§]; *Baylisascaris procyonis* antibody (serum and CSF); *Angiostrongylus cantonensis, Gnathostoma* sp. testing[||||]

Hyponatremia—MTB testing[‡]

M. pneumoniae serology or throat PCR positive—*M. pneumoniae* PCR (CSF)

Neuroimaging Features

Frontal lobe—*N. fowleri* (CSF wet mount and PCR[††])

Temporal lobe—HSV, HHV-6/7 PCR (CSF)

Basal ganglia and/or thalamus—respiratory virus testing[‡‡]; arbovirus testing[||]; MTB testing[‡]

Brainstem—respiratory virus testing[‡‡]; arbovirus testing[||]; *Listeria* PCR (if available); *Brucella* antibody (serum); MTB testing[‡]

Cerebellum—VZV PCR from CSF (sensitivity may be low; if test available, consider CSF IgG and IgM); VZV IgG and IgM from serum; EBV PCR (CSF)

Diffuse cerebral edema—respiratory virus testing[‡‡]

Space-occupying and/or ring-enhancing lesions—MTB testing[‡]; fungal testing[§]; *B. mandrillaris* and *Acanthamoeba* testing[††]; *Toxoplasma gondii* serology

Hydrocephalus and/or basilar meningeal enhancement—MTB testing[‡]; fungal testing[§]; *B. mandrillaris* testing[††]

Infarction or hemorrhage—MTB testing[‡]; fungal testing[§]; respiratory virus testing[‡‡]

White matter lesions—oligoclonal bands, IgG index, Lyme (serum ELISA and Western blot); *Brucella* (serology or CSF culture)

Measles virus testing for SSPE; *Baylisascaris procyonis* antibody (serum and CSF); *B. mandrillaris* testing[††]

ABLV, Australian bat lyssavirus; BSL4, biosafety level 4; CMV, cytomegalovirus; CNS, central nervous system; CSF, cerebral spinal fluid; EBNA, Epstein-Barr virus nuclear antigen; EBV, Epstein-Barr virus; ELISA, enzyme-linked immunosorbent assay; HHV, human herpesvirus; HSV, herpes simplex virus; IgG, immunoglobulin G; IgM, immunoglobulin M; MTB, *Mycobacterium tuberculosis*; NMDAR, N-methyl-D-aspartate receptor; PCR, polymerase chain reaction; RBC, red blood cell; RT, reverse transcriptase; SSPE, subacute sclerosing panencephalitis; VCA, viral capsid antigen; VGKC, voltage-gated potassium channel; VZV, varicella-zoster virus; WBC, white blood cell; WNV, West Nile virus.

*This table is not intended to encompass all causes of encephalitis, nor all epidemiologic or laboratory-based risk factors. We recommend utilizing this table as a guideline for initial management of acute encephalitis in children beyond the neonatal period. For additional information, we recommend consulting Tunkel et al. 2008, Steiner et al. 2010, Kneen et al. 2012 (see Bibliography). Consultation with local health authorities is also recommended.

[†]Although some members of the consortium recommended *M. pneumoniae* CSF PCR as routine testing for all children, a consensus was not reached given the challenges of establishing a diagnosis of encephalitis due to *M. pneumoniae* (see text).

[‡]MTB testing includes CSF smear for acid-fast bacilli and CSF mycobacterial culture along with one or more of the number of MTB PCR tests for CSF now commercially available. Sensitivity of smear and culture increases with the volume of CSF analyzed; we recommend consulting with the laboratory regarding optimal volumes of CSF to be analyzed. Given the varying sensitivity of these tests, systemic MTB testing including tuberculin skin test (may be negative) or interferon-γ release assay, stains and cultures from sputum, and tissue from biopsies from any potential systemic sites of infection.

[§]Fungal testing should be tailored to specific geographic region and prior travel history/place of residence, and typically consists of serology, antibody testing from urine and/or CSF, and cultures from blood and CSF.

[||]Arbovirus testing should be tailored to specific geographic region and typically consists of IgG and IgM from serum and CSF; PCR (serum, CSF) can be performed for select arboviruses (i.e., WNV, California serogroup viruses), and is particularly useful in immunocompromised patients.

[¶]Rabies/ABLV testing includes serologic analysis of serum and CSF; virus isolation or RT-PCR from saliva; and tests for viral antigen or histopathology on either a brain biopsy or full-thickness biopsy of the nape of the neck. Testing should be conducted in concert with a local or regional public health department.

**Tickborne disease testing should be tailored to specific geographic region and typically consists of serology (i.e., *Borrelia, Ehrlichia, Rickettsia* sp., *Anaplasma phagocytophilum*, tickborne encephalitis virus) and blood PCR (*Ehrlichia, Anaplasma*).

[††]*N. fowleri, B. mandrillaris,* and *Acanthamoeba* spp. testing is only available at specialized laboratories (e.g., Centers for Disease Control and Prevention) and includes serum immunofluorescence assay, immunohistochemistry on brain or other tissue, and PCR testing on brain or other tissue and CSF. In addition, CSF wet mount is recommended for *N. fowleri* testing. Brain tissue from affected region offers optimal sensitivity and specificity but other specimens can be tested.

[‡‡]Respiratory virus testing includes either culture or respiratory PCR panel from respiratory specimens (e.g., nasopharyngeal swab, nasal wash). Respiratory virus testing should include influenza A and B (during influenza season). Testing for other respiratory viruses including parainfluenza 1–4, adenovirus, and human metapneumovirus should be considered, although their role in causing CNS illness is controversial.

[§§]Autoimmune limbic encephalitis evaluation includes testing for antibodies to VGKC, GAD, AMPA receptor, GABA_b receptor, mgluR5, Hu, CV2, Ma2, and amphiphysin.

[||||]Limited testing may be available through research laboratories and includes examination of CSF or other affected tissues (i.e., eye, muscle) for presence of parasite or detection of antibody in serum or CSF.

From Venkatesan A, Tunkel AR, Bloch KC, et al. Case definitions, diagnostic algorithms, and priorities in encephalitis: consensus statement of the International Encephalitis Consortium. *CID.* 2013;57:1114–1128 (Table 3, pp. 1119–1120).

TABLE 42.13   Initial CSF Testing for Encephalomyelitis at Children's Wisconsin: Consensus Recommendations of Infectious Disease and Neurology Services

Test
Opening pressure
CSF complete (cells, glucose, protein)
Meningoencephalitis NAAT CSF panel (BioFire panel includes *Escherichia coli* K1, *Haemophilus influenzae, Listeria monocytogenes, Neisseria meningitidis, Streptococcus agalactiae, Streptococcus pneumoniae,* cytomegalovirus, enterovirus/parechovirus, herpes simplex virus 1 and 2, human herpesvirus-6, varicella-zoster virus, *Cryptococcus neoformans/gattii*)
Bacterial culture and Gram stain
Cytology
Encephalopathy, autoimmune panel (Mayo panel includes antibodies to GAD65, VGKC, ANNA-1, ANNA-2, ANNA-3, PCA-1, PCA-2, PCA-Tr, amphiphysin, CRM-5 Ig, AGNA-1, NMDA receptor, AMPA receptor, GABA-B receptor)
CSF oligoclonal bands (CSF + serum)
Additional CSF
In summer (May–October) add:
Arbovirus Ab panel CSF (includes Eastern equine encephalitis IgG+IgM, St. Louis encephalitis IgG+IgM, California/La Crosse encephalitis IgG+IgM, Western equine encephalitis IgG+IgM)
West Nile virus Ab IgM CSF

Ab, antibody; *CSF,* cerebral spinal fluid; *IgG,* immunoglobulin G; *IgM,* immunoglobulin M; *NAAT,* nucleic acid amplification test.

TABLE 42.14   Initial Blood Testing for Encephalomyelitis at Children's Wisconsin: Consensus Recommendations of Infectious Disease and Neurology Services

Test
ESR
CRP
Ferritin
CPK
Aldolase
EV/PeV PCR
Blood cultures
HIV-1 rapid test
RPR
ANA evaluation with reflex ENA and dsDNA
Antithyroid antibody panel
Brucella panel (obtain CSF panel if positive)
Bartonella Ab IgG IgM with reflex
Lyme Ab with reflex Western blot (obtain CSF Ab if positive)
EBV Ab panel (obtain CSF PCR if positive)
HIV-1 RNA PCR
HTLV1/HTLV2 screen blood
NMO antibody
Vitamin B$_{12}$
Anticardiolipin antibody panel
CSF oligoclonal bands (blood)
Serum special collection (hold)
In summer (May–October) add:
Tickborne panel NAAT anaplasma/ehrlichia/babesia

Ab, antibody; *AFP,* α-fetoprotein; *ANA,* antinuclear antibody; *CPK,* creatine phosphokinase; *CSF,* cerebral spinal fluid; *ENA,* extractable nuclear antigen; *EV,* enterovirus; *HTLV,* human T-lymphotropic virus; *IgG,* immunoglobulin G; *IgM,* immunoglobulin M; *NAAT,* nucleic acid amplification test; *NMO,* neuromyelitis optica; *PeV,* parechovirus; *RPR,* rapid plasma reagin.
*Shaded items were adapted for acute flaccid myelitis (AFM) outbreaks.

DIAGNOSTIC EMERGENCIES: OTHER DISEASES TO EXCLUDE

Encephalomyelitis

- **Bacterial meningitis.** Highly damaging; screening by blood culture, CSF, Gram stain, and CSF cytochemical profile; easily diagnosed by culture and with highly effective antibacterial therapies. Most common bacteria are detected by CSF nucleic acid amplification test (NAAT) panels. Lumbar puncture should be performed immediately if no localizing signs are present by exam (see Chapter 52). Ultrasonography for optic nerve sheath diameter (ONSD) at bedside accurately estimates intracranial pressure to enable prompt lumbar puncture. Increased ONSD can also be detected by MRI in coronal and axial views. Practitioners must consider obtaining enough CSF to avoid delays in other time-sensitive diseases, such as herpes simplex encephalitis.
- **Herpes simplex encephalitis.** The most common cause of sporadic encephalitis (HSV-1), and causal of an aseptic meningitis syndrome (HSV type 2) during genital flares. Highly necrotizing but can be diagnosed with high sensitivity (93%) by NAAT testing in CSF when symptoms present for more than 4 days (otherwise requiring a later sample) and with safe, effective antiviral therapies. Screening for HSV is included in most clinical CSF NAAT panels.
- **Fever-associated epileptic encephalopathies.** Various genetic or idiopathic disorders characterized by preceding or concurrent fever may manifest with seizures (often refractory status epilepticus) *and* encephalopathy. **Dravet syndrome** (*SCN1A*, unknown), **Alpers syndrome** (*POLG1*), and early epileptic encephalopathy type 9 (*PCDH19*) are examples of genetic epilepsy encephalopathies precipitated by fever. **Febrile infection–related epilepsy syndrome (FIRES) and new-onset refractory status epilepticus (NORSE)** are catastrophic idiopathic disorders preceded by a febrile illness 24 hours to 2 weeks prior to the onset of the epileptic encephalopathy.

Acute Flaccid Paresis/Paralysis (Without Encephalopathy)

- Bacterial epidural abscess, hematoma, and tumor must be excluded. Screening requires exam of the spine and bedside ultrasonography and MRI before lumbar puncture.

ADEM

- **CNS lymphoma.** Rare but empirical corticosteroid therapy for ADEM may compromise later diagnostic profiling and chemotherapeutic response. Diagnostics and therapeutics are well based on evidence. Screening requires cytology of CSF cells.
- **Hemophagocytic lymphohistiocytosis (HLH).** Rare, genetic or secondary to another disease. Often requires chemotherapy and stem cell transplantation. Diagnostics and therapeutics are well based on evidence. Screening is aided by cytology of CSF cells (hemophagocytosis) and high serum ferritin. May *initially* present with only CNS symptoms.

COVID-19 ASSOCIATED CNS MANIFESTATIONS

Severe neurologic manifestations of SARS-CoV-2 infections are noted in ~5% of hospitalized patients with respiratory failure and those with multisystem inflammatory syndrome in children (MIS-C). Potential etiologies of neurologic disorders in patients with COVID-19 include cytokine hyperinflammation and neuroimmune (antibody or T-cell) induced direct CNS injury. The spectrum of manifestations is broad and includes encephalopathy, seizures, delirium, ADEM, psychosis, Guillain-Barré syndrome, and MERS (mild encephalopathy with reversible splenial lesions). In addition to neuroimmune-mediated inflammations, patients are also at risk for cerebrovascular disease (ischemic or hemorrhagic stroke).

■ SUMMARY AND RED FLAGS

Depending on the epidemiology, the etiology of infectious encephalitis becomes readily apparent with MRI and examining the CSF or other fluids. Presumptive diagnosis of autoimmune encephalitis or ADEM may initially be facilitated by diagnostic criteria including MRI and EEG; therapy should not be delayed while waiting for results on autoimmune antibody panels (see Tables 42.4 to 42.7).

Red flags include coma, papilledema or signs of impending brain herniation, hemiplegia, autonomic dysfunction, a distinct cord level, exposure to high-risk vectors (rabies, etc.), being immunosuppressed, and travel to endemic areas.

BIBLIOGRAPHY

A bibliography is available at ExpertConsult.com.

43

Eye Disorders

Deborah M. Costakos

EYE AND VISUAL SYSTEM ANATOMY

The anatomies of the eye and visual system are shown in Figs. 43.1 and 43.2. The optic nerves, made up of the converging nerve fiber layer of the retina, have intraocular, intraorbital, intracanalicular, and intracranial portions. Partial decussation of the optic nerve fibers occurs in the chiasm, which gives binocular visual input to each side of the brain. The visual cortex is where the conscious process of seeing occurs.

DEVELOPMENT OF THE EYE AND VISUAL SYSTEM

The eyes and vision of a newborn are immature and require several years to reach adult proportions and functional status. By the ninth month of gestation, the retinal vessels have reached the periphery of the retina (an important factor in the pathogenesis of retinopathy of prematurity [ROP]), the optic nerve has completed myelination, and the pupillary membrane has disappeared. Postnatal reorganization of neuron-to-neuron connections in the visual cortex improves the poor visual acuity and other visual processes, which are not fully developed at birth. The visual acuity of the newborn has been estimated to be 20/400–20/600 and may reach the normal 20/20 level as early as 6–12 months of age as tested with visual evoked cortical responses. Acuity of 20/20 is not reached with other types of testing such as preferential looking with Teller acuity cards until ages 3–5 years. Visual acuity measured with conventional letter or symbol recognition methods does not reach 20/20 until 6 years of age because of cognitive factors. Binocular vision, including establishment of normal ocular alignment and depth perception, and improved facility of accommodation, the ability to focus on images at different distances, develop rapidly in the first year of life. The rapid maturation of visual function in the first year of life accounts for the critical period of visual development and the extreme sensitivity of the visual system to abnormal visual input from strabismus or cataracts. Children deprived of vision in this critical period will have limited visual potential and may develop nystagmus (abnormal eye movements).

The majority of newborns are moderately hyperopic. Heredity contributes to the refractive status of the eyes and the environment and visual experience also plays a role.

AMBLYOPIA AND VISION SCREENING

Amblyopia is defined as a unilateral or, less commonly, bilateral reduction in visual acuity that cannot be immediately corrected with glasses or surgery. In children whose visual acuity can be accurately measured, a practical definition of amblyopia is a two-line or greater difference between the best-corrected visual acuity of the eyes. For preverbal children, differences between the eyes in fixation and following behavior or fixation preference are used to diagnose amblyopia. Automated photoscreeners can aid in the diagnosis of risk factors for amblyopia and strabismus, particularly in preverbal children who perform poorly on subjective testing. Amblyopia results from abnormal visual experience early in life during the critical period for visual development. The sensitive period for amblyopia starts in early infancy and continues to at least the age of 6 years and sometimes beyond the age of 8 years. There is a suggestion of cortical plasticity in adults that may allow for some vision improvement into adulthood. The prevalence of amblyopia in the North American population is 2–4%.

Unilateral amblyopia results from three types of abnormal visual experience: strabismus, anisometropia (unequal refractive errors), and monocular visual deprivation (e.g., cataract, corneal opacity, hemangioma [severe ptosis]). **Bilateral amblyopia** results from bilateral media opacities or significant bilateral refractive errors (ametropia). Nearly all amblyopia is reversible if discovered at an early age and treated appropriately. Treatment effectiveness declines after the age of 5 years.

Detection strategies for amblyopia can involve early recognition of factors that give rise to amblyopia or actual measurement of reduced visual acuity that may be caused by amblyopia. Most amblyopia risk factors can be detected through routine pediatric screening such as ocular history, red reflex evaluation, ocular motility, and vision assessment. Recommended screening and referral guidelines are shown in Table 43.1. Whenever possible, a line of symbols or isolated symbols with surrounding crowding bars is recommended for screening (Fig. 43.3). Isolated symbols can lead to overestimates of the visual acuity of an eye with amblyopia due to a crowding phenomenon or contour interaction in which symbols of a given size are more difficult to recognize if they are surrounded by similar symbols. Hence, visual acuity obtained with single optotypes without crowding bars can result in failure to detect amblyopia.

The treatment of amblyopia involves eliminating amblyopia risk factors, providing a focused retinal image with appropriate optical correction, and forcing use of the amblyopic eye through occlusion of the sound eye or blurring the image the sound eye receives. For patients with visual deprivation amblyopia, the depriving factor must be addressed medically or surgically. Optical correction including a bifocal is required for patients who have had cataract surgery. Intraocular implants are not generally placed in children under 1 year of age due to the high postoperative complication rates. For patients with anisometropic amblyopia, optical correction usually involves spectacles or, less commonly, contact lenses.

An adhesive patch worn over the sound eye most commonly achieves forced use of the amblyopic eye. Occlusive devices can be attached to glasses but may be less reliable since the child can peek over the glasses or around the occlusive device. The use of the potent cycloplegic agent atropine sulfate may also be used to encourage use of the amblyopic eye. A drop of atropine is applied to the sound eye each day; this temporarily impairs its accommodative ability and, in the presence of sufficient hyperopia, prevents that eye from obtaining

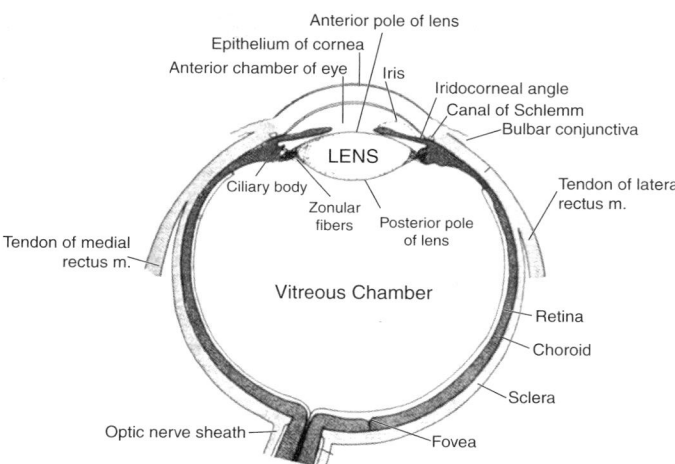

Fig. 43.1 Anatomy of the right eye as seen in cross section. (Modified from Reilly BM. *Practical Strategies in Outpatient Medicine.* 2nd ed. Philadelphia: WB Saunders; 1991:36.)

a clear retinal image. Atropine "penalization" for amblyopia works best in hyperopic patients with mild to moderate amblyopia (visual acuity of 20/100 or better). Close follow-up of patients being treated for amblyopia is important for monitoring compliance with treatment and for preventing the development of iatrogenic reverse amblyopia in the sound eye from excessive occlusion or penalization.

VISUAL FIELDS

Quantitative testing of the visual field of most children is difficult before the age of 10 years (see Fig. 43.2). Confrontation field tests can be performed to detect gross abnormalities of the visual field (hemianopsias), but even these are not reliable and need to be confirmed at an older age. Visual field defects in children are uncommon despite parental concerns about a child who seems to bump into objects frequently. Unilateral retinal or optic nerve disease can produce unilateral visual field defects, but these are almost always associated with reduced visual acuity in the involved eye. Bilateral visual field defects, particularly if symmetric (homonymous), indicate disease of the optic radiations or visual cortex. Visual acuity may be entirely normal. Causes of bilateral visual field defects in children include cerebrovascular accidents, pituitary or hypothalamic tumors, or congenital central nervous system (CNS) abnormalities.

STRABISMUS

Strabismus is derived from the Greek word *strabismos*, "to squint to look obliquely or askance." It implies misalignment of the eyes in such a way that they are not simultaneously viewing the same object. Terms to describe eye alignment and movement are noted in Table 43.2. Strabismus can be constant or intermittent and can be the same in all directions of gaze (comitant) or greater in one direction of gaze than in others (incomitant). Furthermore, it can be categorized as congenital or acquired, monocular or alternating. The direction of misalignment can be vertical or horizontal. Vertical strabismus is referred to as a hypertropia of the higher eye. Horizontal strabismus can be convergent (esotropia) or divergent (exotropia). *The importance of strabismus detection derives primarily from the fact that it is the leading cause of amblyopia.* Other reasons for detecting strabismus are the possibility of being able to restore normal binocular use of the eyes, improving depth perception, and minimizing the social and economic drawbacks to strabismus in society.

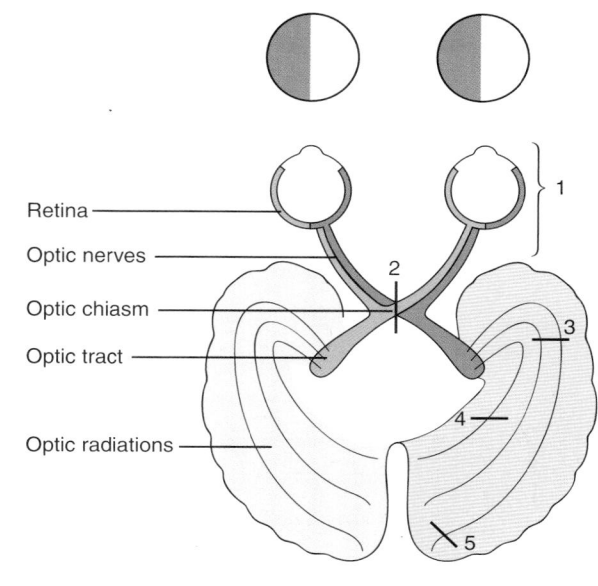

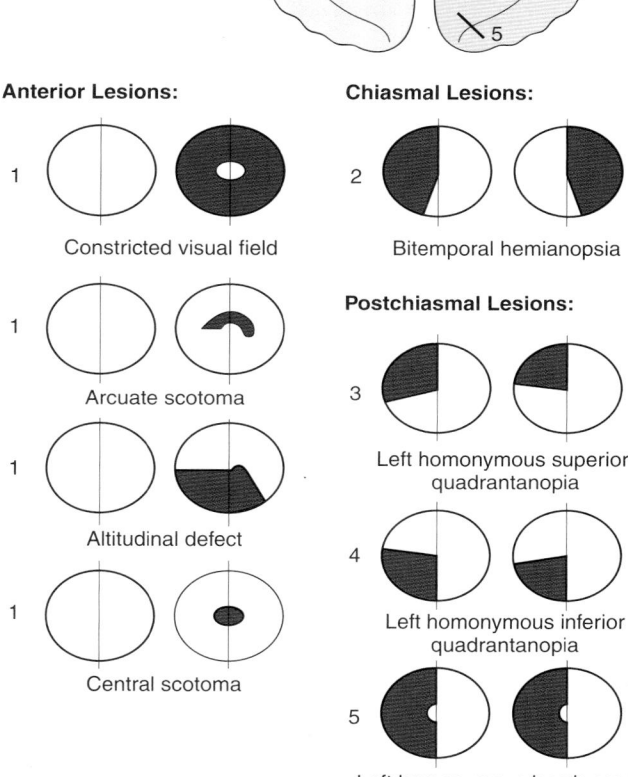

Anterior Lesions:

1 Constricted visual field

1 Arcuate scotoma

1 Altitudinal defect

1 Central scotoma

Chiasmal Lesions:

2 Bitemporal hemianopsia

Postchiasmal Lesions:

3 Left homonymous superior quadrantanopia

4 Left homonymous inferior quadrantanopia

5 Left homonymous hemianopsia with macular sparing

Retina
Optic nerves
Optic chiasm
Optic tract
Optic radiations

Fig. 43.2 Anatomy of the visual pathways. The anatomy of the visual pathways appears at the top of the figure, the *pink shading* indicating how visual information from the left visual space eventually courses to the right brain. Visual field defects are at the bottom of the figure. Anterior defects (labeled *1* from disease of the optic nerve or retina) characteristically affect one eye and cause defects *(red shading)* that may cross the vertical meridian (i.e., the vertical meridian is the vertical line bisecting each visual field). Chiasmal defects (labeled *2*) and postchiasmal defects (labeled *3* for a lesion in the anterior temporal lobe, *4* for the parietal lobe, and *5* for the occipital cortex) characteristically affect both eyes and respect the vertical meridian. (Modified from McGee S. *Evidence-Based Physical Diagnosis.* 3rd ed. Philadelphia: Elsevier; 2012:514.)

TABLE 43.1   Vision Screening Recommendations

Age	Tests	Referral Criteria Comments
Newborn to 12 mo	• Ocular history • Vision assessment • External inspection of the eyes and lids • Ocular motility assessment • Pupil examination • Red reflex examination	• Poor tracking after 3 mo of age • Abnormal red reflex • Ptosis • Positive ocular history of retinoblastoma in a parent or sibling • Positive history of metabolic disease with risk of cataract • Abnormal ocular alignment (strabismus) in infant older than 3 mo of age • Pupil asymmetry of >1 mm
12–36 mo	• Ocular history • Vision assessment • External inspection of the eyes and lids • Ocular motility assessment • Pupil examination • Red reflex examination • Visual acuity testing • Objective screening device "photoscreening" • Ophthalmoscopy	• Fail photoscreening • Visual acuity worse than 20/50 in one or both eyes • Visual acuity difference of two or more lines • Strabismus • Abnormal head position • Chronic tearing or discharge • Abnormal exam

36 mo–5 yr	• Ocular history
	• Vision assessment
	• External inspection of the eyes and lids
	• Ocular motility assessment
	• Pupil examination
	• Red reflex examination
	• Visual acuity testing (preferred) or photoscreening
	• Ophthalmoscopy
		• Visual acuity thresholds below
		  • Ages 36–47 mo: must correctly identify the majority of the optotypes on the 20/50 line to pass
		  • Ages 48–59 mo: must correctly identify the majority of the optotypes on the 20/40 line to pass
		• Fail photoscreening
		• Visual acuity difference of two or more lines
		• Strabismus
		• Abnormal exam

5 yr and older*	• Ocular history • Vision assessment • External inspection of the eyes and lids • Ocular motility assessment • Pupil examination • Red reflex examination • Visual acuity testing • Ophthalmoscopy	• Children who cannot read at least 20/30 with either eye. Must be able to identify the majority of the optotypes on the 20/30 line • Visual acuity difference of two or more lines • Strabismus • Abnormal exam

*Repeat screening every 1–2 yr after the age of 5 yr.
From American Academy of Pediatric Ophthalmology and Strabismus Techniques for Pediatric Vision Screening, May 2014.

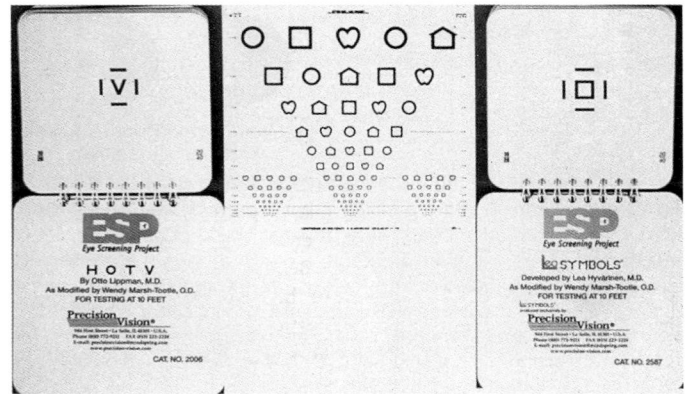

Fig. 43.3 The Lea symbols in chart format *(middle)* and the Lea symbols and HOTV tests with crowding bars *(right and left)*. All tests should be administered at a distance of 10 feet.

Strabismus detection can be simple, as in patients with a large angle of deviation (Fig. 43.4), or difficult, as in patients with more subtle deviations or no deviation at all (pseudostrabismus) (Fig. 43.5). Evaluation of the symmetry of the corneal light reflexes from a penlight directed at the eyes can reliably detect many cases (see Fig. 43.4). With smaller angles of strabismus or when the results of the corneal light reflex are in doubt, the cover test should be performed (Fig. 43.6). It is important to provide attractive fixation targets for the child to view during the test.

Infantile esotropia is defined as convergent strabismus with onset within the first 6 months of life (see Fig. 43.4). Transient crossing or divergence of the eyes is common in newborns and is probably not significant unless it persists beyond 3 months of age. In the classic form of infantile esotropia, there is a large-angle, constant deviation. The child may alternate fixation (cross-fixate), in which case the visual acuity is usually good in both eyes. Cross-fixation may mimic bilateral sixth nerve palsy. If the crossing is present in only one eye, amblyopia occurs in the nonfixating eye. Binocular vision is disrupted in infantile esotropia. The cause of infantile esotropia is not known, but hereditary factors play a definite role. The incidence of infantile esotropia is <1% among neurologically normal infants.

Early surgical correction of infantile esotropia may result in full or nearly full restoration of normal binocular function, a result not believed to be obtainable with correction of misalignment at older ages. The ideal timing of surgery for infantile esotropia is not known, but children operated on before 2 years of age are more likely to obtain

TABLE 43.2 Description of Alignment and Movement

Normal Ocular Alignment: Orthophoria

Latency

-phoria: development of abnormality only during certain conditions (fatigue, illness, cover test)

-tropia: abnormality present during normal conditions; deviation may be constant or intermittent

Direction of Deviation

Eso-: inward, horizontal deviation ("crossing")

Exo-: outward, horizontal deviation ("wall eye")

Hyper-: upward, vertical deviation

Hypo-: downward, vertical deviation

Incyclo-: nasal torsional deviation of the superior pole of the cornea

Excyclo-: temporal torsional deviation of the superior pole of the cornea

Equality of Deviation

Concomitant: misalignment is equal in all positions of gaze

Noncomitant: misalignment varies significantly in different positions of gaze

Neuromuscular Dysfunction

Paralytic: misalignment secondary to a cranial nerve palsy, muscle weakness, or mechanical restriction (usually noncomitant)

Nonparalytic: no underlying neuromuscular dysfunction; usually concomitant but can be noncomitant

Tandem Movements of Both Eyes

-version: both eyes move in same direction (conjugate); direction of movement: levo- (left), dextro- (right), supra- (up), infra- (down)

-vergence: eyes move in opposite directions (disconjugate); convergence (inward movement), divergence (outward movement)

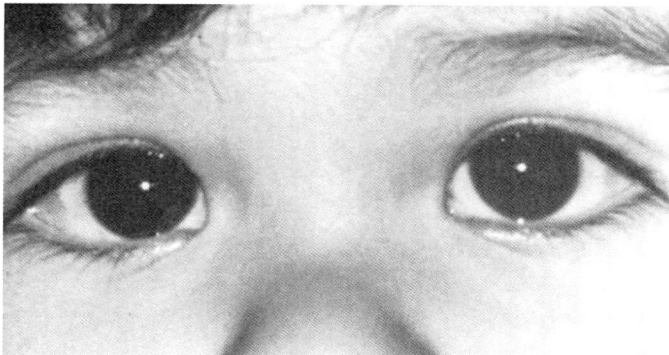

Fig. 43.5 A child with pseudoesotropia. Note that the wide nasal bridge and prominent epicanthal folds create the illusion of an esotropia. The corneal light reflexes are centered in each eye; therefore, the eyes are straight. (From Lavrich JB, Nelson LB. Diagnosis and treatment of strabismus disorders. *Pediatr Clin North Am.* 1993;40:741.)

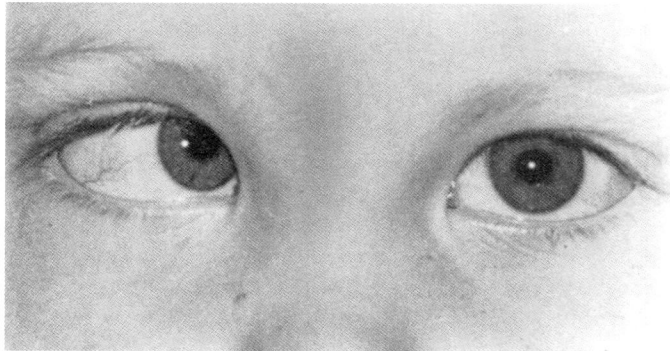

Fig. 43.4 Corneal light reflex test reveals an asymmetrically placed reflex that is laterally displaced in the right eye. This indicates an inward deviation of the eye (esotropia). (From Lavrich JB, Nelson LB. Diagnosis and treatment of strabismus disorders. *Pediatr Clin North Am.* 1993;40:739.)

binocular single vision. Early detection and prompt referral of infants with suspected esotropia are indicated.

A second category of esotropia occurs in children whose eyes are initially straight but start to cross, usually intermittently at first, at 1–3 years of age. These children have excessive hyperopia and an abnormal relationship between accommodation and convergence. This type of esotropia is called **accommodative esotropia.** Amblyopia frequently develops. Treatment consists of correcting amblyopia and providing spectacles to correct hyperopia, thereby modulating the amount of accommodation required by the child (Fig. 43.7). Bifocal spectacles may also be necessary for some forms of accommodative esotropia.

Esotropia caused by paralysis of a lateral rectus muscle, a sixth cranial nerve palsy, occurs much more frequently in children than in infancy (Fig. 43.8). Approximately 30% of children will have an intracranial tumor (brainstem glioma, medulloblastoma, ependymoma, craniopharyngioma). Other causes include head trauma or a recent benign viral illness. The sixth nerve palsy may resolve spontaneously if the cause is benign. Other acquired etiologies include acute demyelinating encephalomyelitis (ADEM) or multiple sclerosis (MS), Lyme disease, pontine vascular malformations, raised intracranial pressure (nonlocalizing), and middle ear infection complicated by petrous apicitis (Gradenigo syndrome). An older child may present with complaints of diplopia or a face turn or closure of one eye to avoid diplopia, whereas a younger child may present with only the esotropia because of rapid development of suppression to eliminate diplopia. Neurologic investigation is indicated if the history does not support a benign etiology or the paralysis does not spontaneously abate in a few weeks (a so-called benign sixth nerve palsy believed to be postviral in origin) or if the child demonstrates other neurologic impairment or has papilledema.

Infantile exotropia is much less common than infantile esotropia. Infantile exotropia presents as a large deviation of the eyes prior to 6 months of age. Infantile exotropia is uncommon in otherwise healthy infants. It is, however, commonly associated with craniofacial disorders or neurologic impairment. Surgery may be done early in life, but these patients are less likely to obtain good binocular vision than infantile esotropia.

Intermittent exotropia is the most common type of exotropia. This usually manifests by 5 years of age. Parents will notice that the eyes deviate out at times and yet not at others. The deviation is most likely to occur when the child is tired or ill. Because the child maintains the ability to keep the eyes aligned part of the time, amblyopia is uncommon. Diplopia is prevented by active cortical suppression of input from the portion of the retina of the deviated eye that overlaps the central view of the fixating eye. When the eyes are straight, the child generally maintains normal binocular function, including stereopsis. The clinical management of intermittent exotropia is not clear. Treatment is not necessarily indicated as observation of children 3–11 years old shows that <15% of children are unlikely to develop a constant exotropia or amblyopia or lose stereopsis. Part-time patching, additional minus power spectacles in patients with myopia, and orthoptic exercises are treatment options, but there is insufficient evidence that these

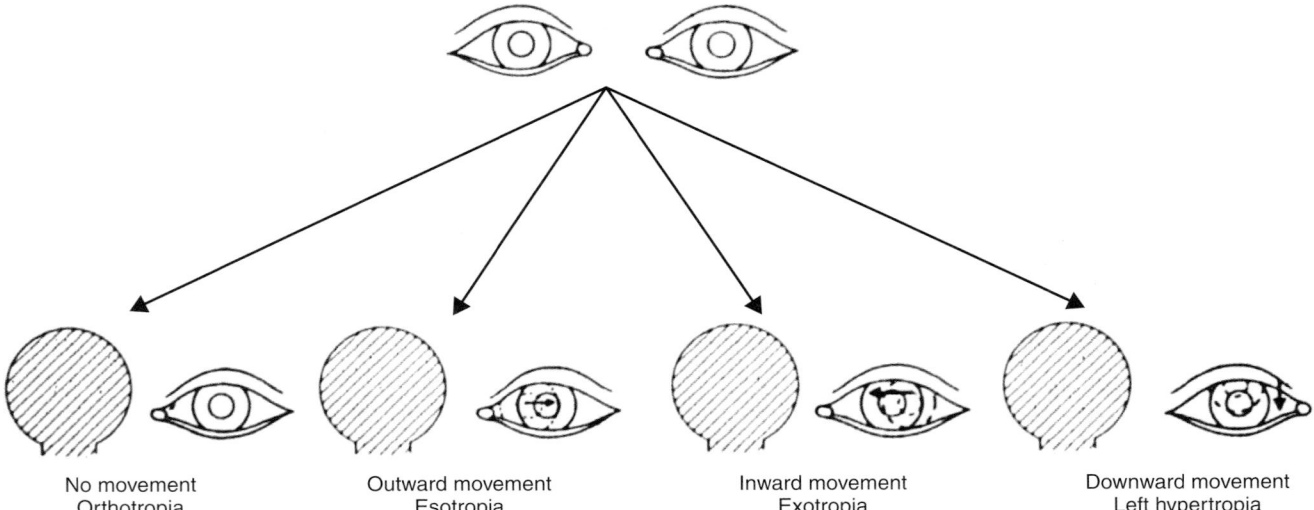

No movement
Orthotropia

Outward movement
Esotropia

Inward movement
Exotropia

Downward movement
Left hypertropia

Fig. 43.6 The cover test. In each instance, the occluder is placed over the right eye while the patient is viewing a fixation target and the examiner is watching for movement of the patient's left eye. If the left eye is not aligned, it will need to move to look at the fixation target. If there is no movement of the left eye, the test needs to be repeated by occluding the left eye and watching for movement of the right eye.

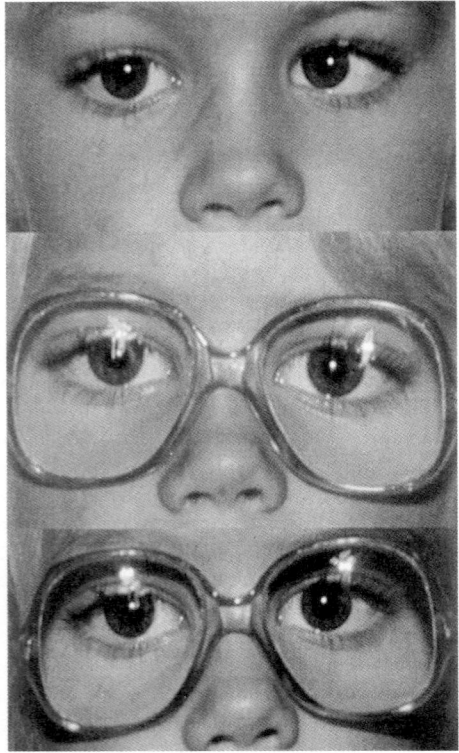

Fig. 43.7 Accommodative esotropia *(top)*. The deviation is completely controlled with glasses at both distant *(middle)* and near *(bottom)* fixation distances.

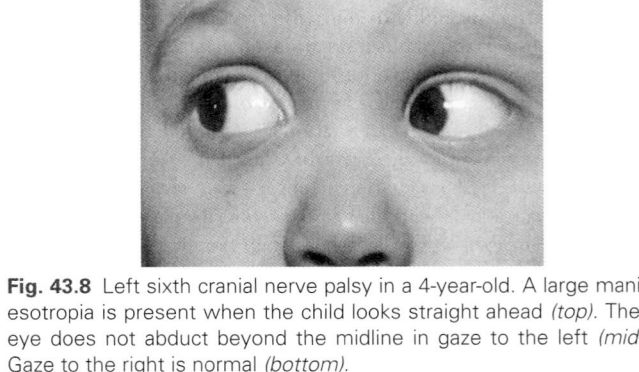

Fig. 43.8 Left sixth cranial nerve palsy in a 4-year-old. A large manifest esotropia is present when the child looks straight ahead *(top)*. The left eye does not abduct beyond the midline in gaze to the left *(middle)*. Gaze to the right is normal *(bottom)*.

treatments are more effective than observation. For those patients whose control over an intermittent exotropia deteriorates, surgery can be offered.

Primary vertical strabismus is far less common than horizontal strabismus. A small vertical deviation (hypertropia or hypotropia) in association with a larger amount of horizontal strabismus, however, is common, and is managed in conjunction with the horizontal deviation. A common cause of hypertropia in children is congenital paralysis of the superior oblique muscle, a fourth cranial nerve paralysis. In some children, the "paralysis" is actually caused by an anatomic abnormality

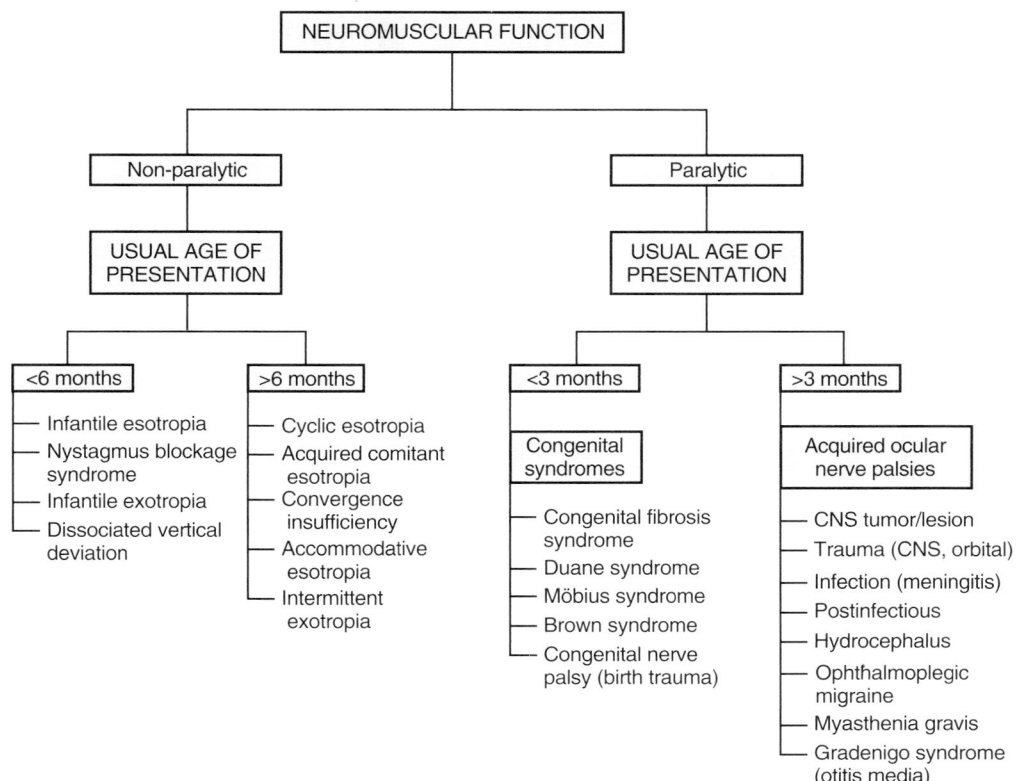

Fig. 43.9 Evaluation of strabismus. CNS, central nervous system.

of the superior oblique tendon. Acquired causes of a superior oblique palsy include trauma, CNS abnormalities, or brain tumors. Children with a superior oblique paralysis of any cause frequently present with a head tilt and face turn toward the side opposite the paralyzed superior oblique muscle. If there is a question as to the timing of the onset of the superior oblique palsy, a review of pictures at a younger age may be helpful in determining chronicity. Superior oblique paralysis is one of the more common causes of **ocular torticollis**. An eye muscle disorder needs to be ruled out in any child with a chronic abnormality of head position. The anomalous head position and hypertropia caused by a superior oblique paralysis can be improved by eye muscle surgery in most instances. An approach to the evaluation of strabismus is noted in Fig. 43.9, and less common forms of strabismus are listed in Table 43.3.

REFRACTIVE ERRORS

Refractive errors include myopia (nearsightedness), hyperopia (farsightedness), and astigmatism. Refractive errors may be similar (isometropia) or different (anisometropia) between the two eyes. Bilateral amblyopia may result from a high refractive error that is isometropic. Full-time spectacle correction will often correct bilateral amblyopia. Unilateral amblyopia may result from anisometropia. Patching or atropine penalization may be necessary in these children.

Myopia

In patients with myopia (nearsightedness), the parallel rays of light in the resting (nonaccommodating) eye are focused in front of the retina. The symptoms of myopia are squinting, holding or viewing an object more closely than normal, and complaining of blurred far vision.

The incidence and degree of myopia increase with age, especially during growth spurts, as in adolescence. There is a complex interaction between genetic and environmental factors in the development of myopia. The incidence of myopia varies with ethnicity and geographic regions and has been increasing in prevalence over the past 50 years. There have been several genetic markers linked to myopia, but the increasing frequency among younger generations suggests environment plays an important role. The increase in prevalence from 10% to 90% in some populations is a public health concern, particularly with high myopia. Myopia can be associated with increased risk of retinal detachment, early cataract, and glaucoma. In very high myopia there can be thinning of the retina and retinal degeneration. This can result in decreased vision even with spectacle or contact lens correction. A promising strategy to slow the progression of myopia is application of a dilute formulation of atropine. Increasing the time spent outdoors appears to slow progression.

Myopia may be associated with other ocular abnormalities, such as keratoconus (central conical protrusion of the cornea), cataracts, ectopia lentis (dislocated lens), spherophakia (overly spherical lens), glaucoma, and medullated (myelinated) nerve fibers. There is an increased prevalence of myopia in premature infants, especially with ROP (retinopathy of prematurity). Children with high degrees of myopia may have an underlying systemic association, such as Marfan, Stickler, Noonan, or Down syndrome. If myopia is sufficient to produce visual symptoms, spherical concave (minus) lenses in the form of spectacles or contact lenses are prescribed to correct the refractive error. Prescription changes may be needed every 1–2 years and more often during growth spurts.

Hyperopia

In patients with hyperopia (farsightedness), parallel rays of light in the nonaccommodating eye would be focused behind the retina. The process of accommodation (focusing), which alters the shape of the lens, can compensate for some degrees of hyperopia. Because most children have a tremendous range of accommodation, mildly hyperopic children can see clearly without any visual symptoms. Moderate to severely

TABLE 43.3   Less Common Forms of Strabismus

Type of Strabismus	Presenting Symptoms and Signs	Cause	Treatment
Duane syndrome	Esotropia with deficient abduction or exotropia with deficient adduction of one eye; head turn	Absence of sixth nerve nucleus and aberrant innervation of lateral rectus muscle from third cranial nerve	Strabismus surgery for correction of large deviations or abnormal head position
Dissociated vertical deviation	One eye turns up intermittently, especially with fatigue	Eye movement abnormality related most commonly to congenital esotropia	Eye muscle surgery on superior rectus and inferior oblique muscles
Brown syndrome	Head tilt; inability to elevate eye in adduction	Restriction of free passage of superior oblique tendon through trochlea	Observation if not severe; superior oblique tendon surgery if severe
Möbius syndrome	Masklike facies; inability to abduct both eyes; difficulty closing eyes	Bilateral sixth and seventh nerve palsies	Protect corneas from exposure; strabismus surgery
Congenital fibrosis syndrome	Chin-up head position; inability to elevate eyes; ptosis	Autosomal dominant gene on chromosome 16 in some patients; superior division of third nerve in others	Surgical release of tight extraocular muscles
Third nerve palsy	Exotropia and hypertropia; ptosis; dilated, nonreactive pupil	Congenital absence of third nerve; trauma; tumor	Ptosis and strabismus surgery
Double elevator palsy	Chin-up head posture; inability to elevate one eye	Paresis of superior rectus muscle	Transposition strabismus surgery
Orbital floor fracture	Vertical diplopia; chin-up head position	Entrapment of orbital tissues in fracture	Repair of floor fracture; release of inferior rectus muscle restriction
Myasthenia: congenital or acquired	Variable ptosis and eye movement abnormalities	Blockage of acetylcholine receptor sites by immune complexes	Treatment of systematic myasthenia; strabismus surgery if patient is stable
Mitochondrial disorders	Ptosis, progressive external ophthalmoplegia, optic neuropathy, cardiomyopathy, peripheral myopathy	Various mitochondrial variants	Supportive

hyperopic children may be unable to fully compensate through accommodation. The greater accommodative effort may lead to symptoms of "eyestrain," which consist of headaches, fatigue, or eye rubbing. These symptoms may lead to a lack of interest in reading or in prolonged close work. Some children may also develop accommodative esotropia. Some children have a decreased ability to accommodate, or accommodative insufficiency, and are symptomatic even with low degrees of hyperopia. If hyperopia produces symptoms, decreases vision, or causes esotropia, spherical convex (plus) lenses usually in the form of glasses are prescribed to correct the refractive error.

Astigmatism

In astigmatism, the refractive power differs in various meridians of the eye. In most cases, astigmatism is caused by abnormal curvature of the cornea; although rare, lens abnormalities or dislocation may cause astigmatism. Infants and children with corneal distortion secondary to scarring (trauma or infection) or to external compression (neurofibroma or hemangioma of eyelid) are at an increased risk for astigmatism. Moderate levels of astigmatism may produce blurring of vision (far and near), leading to squinting, fatigue, headaches, and lack of interest in close-up work in older children and amblyopia in younger children. Cylindric or spherocylindric lenses (usually glasses) are used to improve vision and comfort.

Anisometropia

In patients with anisometropia, the refractive error of one eye differs significantly from that of the other eye. The difference in refraction can be spherical (hyperopia or myopia) or cylindric (unequal amounts of astigmatism). Mild degrees of anisometropia usually cause no visual symptoms and do not lead to amblyopia. Amblyopia develops with higher degrees of anisometropia because the child uses the less ametropic eye and suppresses vision in the other. Strabismus frequently coexists with anisometropia, and both conditions may be involved in the pathophysiologic mechanisms of amblyopia. Anisometropia may initially be detected by comparison of the red reflex between the two eyes (Brückner test). The affected eye has the duller red reflex. Early detection and treatment of anisometropia are essential for the development of optimal visual function.

VISION IMPAIRMENT IN CHILDREN

Vision impairment is formally defined as best-corrected visual acuity of 20/70 or worse in both eyes. Impairment of vision exists as a continuum from 20/70 to no light perception. Unrestricted, noncommercial driver's license has a requirement of best-corrected vision of 20/40 or better in most states. Legal blindness is said to be present when best-corrected visual acuity is 20/200 or less in each eye. Constricted visual fields may also play a role in the diagnosis of vision impairment or legal blindness. An infant or child whose visual acuity and visual field cannot be quantitated may be judged visually impaired on the basis of inability to fixate on and follow movement of the examiner's face or other objects or, in severe instances, inability to perceive light. Milder vision impairment may be suspected on the basis of associated eye signs but can be difficult to confirm in a preverbal child because of compensatory behavior (holding objects close, a face turn) that allows the child to have relatively normal overall function and development. Observation of the child's behavior in the examination room, examination of the eyes (Table 43.4), and a detailed history (Table 43.5) taken from the parents about the child's visual behavior at home can be important in establishing the degree of impairment. Many visually impaired infants and children have objective signs such as nystagmus, sluggish pupillary light reflexes, or anatomic abnormalities such as optic nerve hypoplasia or chorioretinal scarring. Visual evoked potential (VEP) and electroretinogram (ERG) can help delineate optic nerve or retina pathology, respectively.

TABLE 43.4   Red Flags in Inspection and Direct Ophthalmoscopy in Evaluating Visual Impairment

Physical Findings	Possible Pathologic Process
Inspection	
Globe	
Small	High hyperopia, persistent hyperplastic primary vitreous, phthisis bulbi (shrinkage related to deteriorating eye disease)
Large	Glaucoma, high myopia
Red eye	Inflammatory disease (infection, uveitis), trauma, tumor, glaucoma
Protrusion	Retrobulbar or orbital infection/tumor, hyperthyroidism, nonspecific orbital inflammation (orbital pseudotumor), sarcoidosis
Sunken	Orbital fracture, Horner syndrome, atrophy, microphthalmia
Misalignment	Impairment of extraocular muscles: congenital weakness, muscle entrapment (tumor/trauma), cranial nerve palsy (infection, tumor, stroke, congenital)
Ophthalmoscopy	
Cloudy cornea	Anterior segment dysgenesis (Peter anomaly), glaucoma, trauma, infection, metabolic storage diseases (mucopolysaccharidoses)
Lens	
Cloudy	Cataracts (congenital vs systemic diseases)
Dislocated	Homocystinuria, Marfan syndrome
Cloudy vitreous	Retinoblastoma, detached retina, endophthalmitis, uveitis, hemorrhage
Optic disk	
Pale	Optic atrophy (congenital, trauma, tumor, hydrocephalus, degenerative neurologic disease)
Swollen	Increased intracranial pressure, optic neuritis
Hemorrhage	Optic neuritis, increased intracranial pressure
Retina/choroid	
Abnormal color	Retinitis pigmentosa (spicule pattern), chorioretinitis (atrophy with hyperpigmentation), Tay-Sachs disease (cherry-red macula), albinism
Exudates	Diabetes mellitus, Coats disease, increased intracranial pressure, sickle cell, arteriovenous malformations
Hemorrhage	Hypertension, diabetes mellitus, increased intracranial pressure, trauma, blood disorders
Phakomatoses	Tuberous sclerosis (yellow plaques, nodules), von Hippel–Lindau disease (reddish globular mass), Sturge-Weber syndrome (choroidal hemangioma), neurofibromatosis (yellow plaques)
Blood vessels	
Constricted	Hypertension
Microaneurysm	Diabetes mellitus
Perivascular sheathing, cuffing, leakage, occlusion	Retinal vasculitis

TABLE 43.5   Red Flags in History for Visual Impairment

Manifestation	Possible Pathologic Process
Child's Complaint	
Generalized blurred vision	
Far vision only	Myopia
Near vision only	Hyperopia, disorder of accommodation
Both far and near	Astigmatism or defect of visual pathways
Focal blurred vision (veil, shadow)	
Unilateral	Ipsilateral retinal or optic nerve
Bilateral	Chiasmal, postchiasmal, or bilateral prechiasmal lesion
Ghost/double vision	
With binocular vision	Cranial nerve or extraocular muscle
With monocular vision	Ocular media or macular disease
Changes in special visions	
Poorer color vision	Retinal or optic nerve disease
Poorer night vision	Retinal disease (retinitis pigmentosa), congenital stationary night blindness, vitamin A deficiency
Visual sensations	
Floaters, spots	Uveitis, retinal detachment, or hemorrhage
Shimmering lines or scotoma	Migraines
Visual hallucinations	Cerebral lesion, psychogenic, autoimmune encephalitis
Parents' Observations	
Age-appropriate infant does not track	Severe ocular (myopia, cataracts) or systemic (meningitis) pathologic process
Objects viewed too closely	Decreased visual acuity related to refractive error; ocular or neurologic disorder
Squinting	Decreased visual acuity related to refractive error; ocular or neurologic disorder
Roving or wandering eyes	Nystagmus or strabismus; rule out ocular or neurologic disorder
Head tilting	Compensatory posturing for nystagmus, strabismus, astigmatism, or visual field defect
Bumping into objects	Visual field defect, decreased visual acuity
Reading problems	Visual impairment, visual processing disorder

Visual inattentiveness in an infant deserves special attention because of the possibility that the child has a treatable but not obvious form of vision impairment such as bilateral congenital cataracts. Even if the cause of impairment is not remediable, early diagnosis is important for referral of the infant for physical and occupational therapy for visual impairment since these children have very specific needs. Vision impairment (monocular or binocular) acquired after infancy obligates the physician to search for a cause such as a retinal degeneration because some causes are treatable (Tables 43.6, 43.7, and 43.8).

Optic neuropathies may be isolated or part of a broader multisystem disease. Leber hereditary optic neuropathy, a mitochondrial disorder, presents with subacute and severe vision loss (Table 43.9). Other mitochondrial disorders with optic atrophy include Leigh syndrome

TABLE 43.6 Childhood Amaurosis (Blindness): Principal Neurologic Considerations

Congenital Malformations
Optic nerve hypoplasia
Congenital hydrocephalus
Hydranencephaly
Porencephaly
Microencephaly
Encephalocele, particularly occipital type

Phakomatoses
Tuberous sclerosis
Neurofibromatosis (special association with optic glioma)
Sturge-Weber syndrome
von Hippel–Lindau disease

Tumors
Retinoblastoma
Optic glioma
Perioptic meningioma
Craniopharyngioma
Cerebral glioma
Posterior and intraventricular tumors when complicated by hydrocephalus

Neurodegenerative Diseases
Cerebral storage disease
Gangliosidoses, particularly Tay-Sachs disease Sandhoff variant, generalized gangliosidosis
Other lipidoses and ceroid lipofuscinoses, particularly the late-onset such as Jansky-Bielschowsky and Batten-Mayou-Spielmeyer-Vogt
Mucopolysaccharidoses, particularly Hurler syndrome and Hunter syndrome
Leukodystrophies (dysmyelination disorders), particularly metachromatic leukodystrophy and Canavan disease
Demyelinating sclerosis (myelinoclastic diseases), especially Schilder disease and Devic neuromyelitis optica
Special types: Dawson disease, Leigh disease, Bassen-Kornzweig syndrome, Refsum disease
Retinal degenerations: "retinitis pigmentosa" and its variants, Leber congenital type
Optic atrophies: congenital autosomal recessive type, infantile and congenital autosomal dominant types
Leber disease, and atrophies associated with hereditary ataxias: Behr, Marie, and Sanger-Brown
Usher syndrome

Infectious Processes
Encephalitis, especially in the prenatal infection syndromes due to *Toxoplasma gondii*, cytomegalovirus, rubella virus, *Treponema pallidum*
Meningitis; arachnoiditis
Optic neuritis
Chorioretinitis

Hematologic Disorders
Leukemia with central nervous system involvement

Vascular and Circulatory Disorders
Inflammatory vascular diseases (lupus, sarcoidosis, granulomatosis with polyangiitis, vasculitis)
Coats disease*
Arteriovenous malformations: intracerebral hemorrhage, subarachnoid hemorrhage
Susac syndrome[†]

Trauma
Contusion or avulsion of optic nerves or chiasm
Cerebral contusion or laceration
Intracerebral, subarachnoid, or subdural hemorrhage

Drugs and Toxins

*Coats disease: poor vision, leukocoria, retinal telangiectasia, and exudation.
[†]Susac syndrome: branch retinal artery occlusions, hearing deficits, central nervous system dysfunction.

and myoclonus epilepsy with ragged-red fibers (MERRF) syndrome. Hereditary neuropathies (Charcot-Marie-Tooth, familial dysautonomia, spinocerebellar ataxia, Friedreich ataxia), some leukodystrophies, and lipidosis are also associated with optic neuropathy.

RETINOPATHY OF PREMATURITY

Premature infants are at risk for the development of ROP because the retinal vessels have not yet grown out to the periphery of the retina and are susceptible to a variety of postnatal influences, including oxygen that can adversely affect retinal vessel maturation. In advanced stages of ROP, retinal neovascularization and fibrosis may lead to traction on the retina and result in a retinal detachment, the most common cause of blindness in premature infants. In most cases, fortunately, ROP spontaneously resolves.

The international classification system for the acute stages of ROP describes the location, extent, and stage of the disease according to the position of the advancing wave of retinal vessels (Fig. 43.10). The retina is divided into zones I, II, and III. Zone I is centered on the optic nerve, from which the retinal arterioles emerge, and zone III exists as a crescent of retina on the temporal side; zone II occupies the midportion of the retina in all four quadrants. The severity is indicated by stages 1–5, with stage 1 representing mild ROP and stage 5 representing a total retinal detachment.

The management of ROP begins with a systematic program of eye examinations at well-defined times in infants judged to be at risk for developing ROP. The frequency of examinations is dependent on the findings and progression of the disease. Infants with a birthweight of <1,500 g are first examined 4–6 weeks after birth. Follow-up examinations are performed at regular intervals until the retina is fully

TABLE 43.7 Causes of Monocular Visual Loss

Disorder	Timing	Pattern of Loss	Other Clues	Fundus Appearance	Pupil
Refractive error	Gradual*	Varies	Improves with pinhole	Normal	Normal
Cataract	Very gradual	Tunnel?	Opacity visible	Normal	Normal, but red reflex decreased
Corneal disease	Acute or chronic	Murky	Opacity visible or positive fluorescein	Normal	Normal, but red reflex decreased
Iritis	Acute or chronic	Murky	Pain Ciliary flush	Normal	Small Disfigured?
Open-angle glaucoma	Gradual	Varies	Elevated pressures	Normal	Normal
Angle-closure glaucoma	Acute	Varies	Pain Steamy cornea Patient ill	Normal	Dilated Fixed
Central retinal occlusion	Acute	Varies	Painless Abrupt	Pale with cherry-red macula	Normal
Retinal detachment	Acute	Varies	Painless Floaters	Unremarkable or diagnostic	Afferent pupillary defect if extensive
Vitreous hemorrhage	Acute	"Dark"	Cannot see in the eye	Obscured	Normal, but red reflex decreased
Amaurosis fugax	Acute Transient	5–10 min	Carotid or heart disease, migraine	Normal	Normal
Migraine	Acute Transient	5–30 min	Headache History Scintillations	Normal	Normal
Optic neuropathy, neuritis	Gradual or acute	Central scotoma	Decreased visual acuity, loss of color vision, pain on eye movement, may also have spinal cord lesion	Normal Pale optic disk?	Afferent defect
Diffuse retinopathy	Gradual	Varies	Genetic AIDS	Retinal lesions	Afferent defect?
Papilledema (chronic)	Late	Varies	CNS tumor Pseudotumor cerebri Hypertensive crisis	Diagnostic; optic atrophy	Normal
Endophthalmitis	Varies	Varies	Corneal, systemic infection Penetrating injury Systemic inflammation or injury Hypopyon	Varies Often obscured	Varies

*Refractive error may be more acute when caused by diabetes mellitus.
CNS, central nervous system.
Modified from Reilly BM. *Practical Strategies in Outpatient Medicine*. 2nd ed. Philadelphia: WB Saunders; 1991:60.

TABLE 43.8 Organic Causes of Vision Loss in Neonates

Condition	Physical Findings	Comments
Corneal Disease		
Corneal forceps injury	Cloudy cornea	May lead to astigmatism and amblyopia; associated with intraocular hemorrhage, retinal detachment
Sclerocornea	Opaque cornea	Scleralization of cornea; familial or sporadic; keratoplasty possibly needed to provide vision
Anterior microphthalmia	Small cornea	Familial inheritance; associated with congenital cataracts, glaucoma, and/or coloboma
Anterior Chamber Diseases		
Peter anomaly	Corneal opacity with iridocorneal/lenticulocorneal adhesions	Maldevelopment of anterior segment of eye; associated with glaucoma and lens abnormalities
Persistent pupillary membrane	Bands or membranes obscuring pupil	Rupture of vessels in membranes may lead to hyphema; membrane may need to be removed to restore vision

Continued

TABLE 43.8 Organic Causes of Vision Loss in Neonates—cont'd

Condition	Physical Findings	Comments
Anterior Chamber Diseases—cont'd		
Glaucoma	Tearing, enlarged eye, photophobia, cloudy cornea, pale optic disk	Increased intraocular pressure leading to blindness (optic nerve damage) Causes: anomalies of anterior segment, intraocular hemorrhage, ocular inflammatory disease, intraocular tumors Treatment: surgery
Iris and Lens Disorders		
Aniridia	Large, irregular, unreactive pupil	Hypoplasia of iris—may be heritable or sporadic, which is associated with a deletion of chromosome 11 and Wilms tumor or WAGR syndrome
Cataracts	Lens opacity	Multiple causes, ranging from familial inheritance to drugs
Anterior PHPV	Leukocoria (white pupillary reflex), lens opacity, cloudy cornea, small lens and eye	Persistence of fetal hyaloid vascular system, resulting in fibrovascular plaque on back of lens; as plaque contracts, ciliary process and lens become distorted Complications: glaucoma, cataract, intraocular hemorrhage, rupture of posterior capsule Treatment: removal of membrane, lens aspiration Prognosis: poor visual outcome
Retinal and Optic Nerve Disorders		
Posterior PHPV	Fibroglial veils around disk/macula, vitreous opacities (membrane, vessels)	Persistence of posterior fetal hyaloid vascular system; remnants of vascular system may cause traction detachment of retina
Chorioretinitis	Diffuse or local retinal atrophy demarcated by hyperpigmentation	Inflammation of posterior uvea with retinal involvement Causes: toxoplasmosis, histoplasmosis, herpes simplex, cytomegalic inclusion virus, syphilis, tuberculosis, and toxocariasis Other complications: glaucoma, detached retina
Retinoblastoma	Leukocoria	Neoplastic tumor with locus on chromosome 13; high incidence of secondary malignancy; poor prognosis with extraorbital metastasis
Retinopathy of prematurity	Leukocoria, cloudy vitreous; retinal white lines and ridges	Abnormal vascularization of retina; associated with retinal traction and detachment
Leber congenital retinal amaurosis	Normal findings to degeneration of retina	Failure of both rods and cones in retina; reduced or absent response to electroretinography; autosomal recessive
Achromatopsia	Color cannot be detected, photophobia	Failure of cone system in retina; autosomal recessive, or X-linked; diagnosed with ERG
Congenital stationary night blindness	Disk anomalies, poor night vision	Defect in rod system of retina; autosomal recessive, dominant, or X-linked recessive
Optic nerve hypoplasia	Pale, small optic disk; peripapillary halo of pigmentation	Secondary to failure in differentiation or degeneration of retinal ganglion cell axons Some causes: septo-optic dysplasia (hypopituitary, midline CNS defects), chromosomal defects (trisomy 13), albinism, fetal drug exposure (phenytoin, ethanol), infant of diabetic mother, CNS defects (hydrocephalus, anencephaly, encephalocele)
Optic nerve aplasia	Absence of retinal vessels and optic disk	Maldevelopment of optic nerve; associated with severe eye and CNS anomalies
Morning glory disk anomaly	Enlarged, funnel-shaped disk	Associated with retinal detachments and midline defects (cleft palate, encephalocele, agenesis of corpus callosum)
Coloboma	White, wedge-shaped retinal defect; visual field loss	Malclosure of embryonic fissure that leaves a gap in the retina, hence exposing sclera; defect may extend to lens; associated with many congenital syndromes
Aicardi syndrome	Retinal lacunae, coloboma of optic disk	Occurs mostly in females; associated with agenesis of corpus callosum, seizures, intellectual disability, vertebral anomalies
Albinism	Photophobia; blue-gray to yellow-brown iris; macular hypoplasia	Defect in formation of melanin, resulting in lack of pigment in eyes and sometimes skin; increases risk of skin cancer with hypopigmented skin

CNS, central nervous system; ERG, electroretinogram; PHPV, persistent hyperplastic primary vitreous; WAGR, Wilms tumor, sporadic aniridia, genitourinary malformations, and mental retardation.

vascularized. If treatment is required, laser ablation of immature retina or intravitreal injections of anti–vascular endothelial growth factor (VEGF) medication such as bevacizumab are options. The choice of treatment depends on the zone and the rate of progression of disease. Insulin-like growth factor (IGF)-1 supplementation or alterations may be a means to prevent ROP in the future.

LEUKOCORIA AND RETINOBLASTOMA

Leukocoria or "white pupil" is a sign, not a specific disease (Table 43.10). True leukocoria mandates prompt referral to an ophthalmologist as the causes may threaten either vision and/or life. Retinoblastoma is the most feared cause of leukocoria because of its potential to

TABLE 43.9 Genetic and Clinical Features of Primary Hereditary Optic Atrophies and Their Respective Genes

	OPA1	LHON	OPA3	TMEM126A	WFS1
Inheritance	Autosomal dominant	Maternal	Autosomal dominant	Autosomal recessive	Autosomal dominant
Age of onset	Childhood	Young adult, male >> female	Late childhood	Childhood	Childhood to adult
Ophthalmologic features	Slowly progressive, tritanomaly	Sudden visual loss Frequently beginning unilateral	Often additional cataract	Early manifestation and progression	Highly variable
Loss of visual acuity	Moderate-severe	Pronounced visual impairment	Moderate	Severe visual loss	Variable
Possible extraocular signs	~20% of patients have neurologic symptoms (e.g., ataxia, neuropathy)	Mild neurologic symptoms possible; multiple sclerosis–like symptoms	Late in life; mild neurologic signs possible late in life	Subclinical hearing impairment	Hearing impairment, disturbed glucose tolerance, behavioral abnormalities

LHON, Leber hereditary optic neuropathy; OPA1, optic atrophy type 1; OPA3, optic atrophy type 3; TMEM126A, optic atrophy type 7; WFS1, Wolfgram syndrome.
From Neuhann T, Rautenstrauss B. Genetic and phenotypic variability of optic neuropathies. *Expert Rev Neurother.* 2013;13(4):357–367.

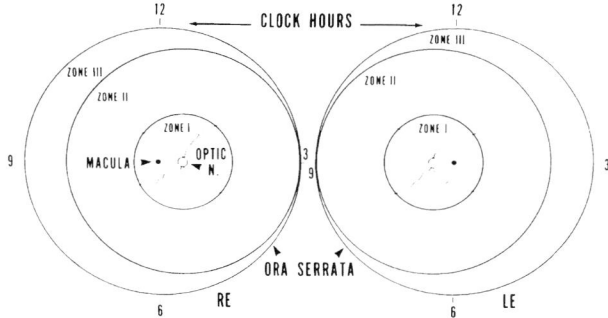

Fig. 43.10 The international classification of retinopathy of prematurity (ROP). The stage of ROP is determined by the location, extent, and stage of disease according to the position of the advancing waves of retinal vessels. LE, left eye; RE, right eye.

metastasize and cause death. It is the most common malignant ocular tumor of childhood, with an incidence of about 1/15,000. Leukocoria, the most common presenting sign, is caused by light reflection from the tumor's white surface (Fig. 43.11) as opposed to the usual red reflex from the retina. Approximately 25% present with strabismus. Less common presentations include periocular inflammation, glaucoma, and proptosis. Imaging is helpful to evaluate for calcifications that occur in retinoblastoma and to help confirm the diagnosis as well as to evaluate for pinealoblastoma and extension of the tumor into the orbit. MRI should be done because CT scan poses concern for radiation exposure and the development of secondary cancers, for which patients with retinoblastoma are at increased risk. Referral of a patient with suspected retinoblastoma to an ophthalmologist experienced in its diagnosis and management is critical. Genetic counseling is indicated, as is examination of parents and siblings. In about 1% of cases a parent will have a regressed retinoblastoma or retinocytoma. Treatment options are focused on vision-sparing therapies including ophthalmic artery chemosurgery, laser photocoagulation, cryotherapy, intravitreal chemotherapy, systemic chemotherapy, and enucleation depending on laterality, location, extent of tumor, and vision potential. There is concerted effort to save the globes through advances in therapies, and in most cases, this can be achieved.

CHILDHOOD CATARACTS

Congenital cataracts are a common cause of unilateral or bilateral vision loss in children, usually resulting from irreversible amblyopia

TABLE 43.10 Differential Diagnosis of Leukocoria (White Pupillary Reflex)

Common Causes
Cataracts
Cicatricial retinopathy of prematurity
Coloboma
Exudative retinopathy
Fundus coloboma
Larval granulomatosis (toxocariasis)
Persistent hyperplastic primary vitreous
Retinoblastoma

Other Causes
Atrophic chorioretinal scars
Coats disease
Congenital retinal fold
Endophthalmitis
Glioneuroma
Hemangioma
Hamartoma
Leukemic ophthalmopathy
Incontinentia pigmenti
Medullated nerve fibers
Medulloepithelioma
Morning glory disk anomaly
Norrie disease
Organized vitreous hemorrhage
Phakomatoses
Retinal gliosis
Retinal dysplasia
Retinoschisis
Toxoplasmosis
Vitreoretinopathy (exudative)

in one or both eyes and occasionally from other accompanying structural ocular abnormalities (Table 43.11). Many infants with cataracts have leukocoria, but all visually significant cataracts can be detected by careful evaluation of the red reflex (Figs. 43.12 and 43.13). Infants with bilateral, visually significant cataracts may present with visual inattentiveness or nystagmus, signs that significant impairment of vision has already occurred.

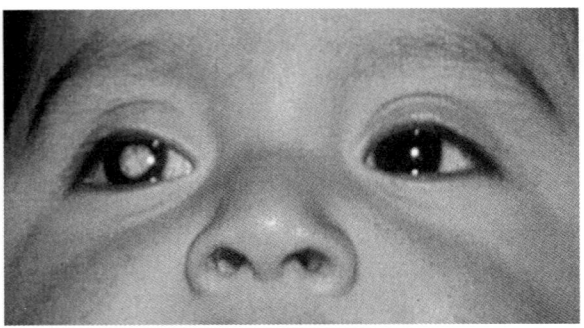

Fig. 43.11 Infant with leukocoria of right eye caused by retinoblastoma.

Most cases of unilateral cataract are idiopathic in origin or associated with other ocular anomalies (persistent hyperplastic primary vitreous, anterior segment dysgenesis). Bilateral cataracts have a known genetic basis in about 60–70% of the cases, but this is increasing as novel pathologic genetic variants continue to be described. Cataracts are commonly inherited in an autosomal dominant manner but may be inherited in an autosomal recessive or X-linked pattern. They can be associated with metabolic disease such as galactosemia or Fabry syndrome. Cataracts found to be a result of a metabolic disease may be reversible by removal of the offending agent; galactosemic cataracts are potentially reversible if lactose is eliminated from the diet promptly. Intrauterine TORCH(S) infections (*t*oxoplasmosis, *r*ubella,

---

TABLE 43.11   Differential Diagnosis of Cataracts

Developmental Variants
Prematurity ("γ" suture vacuoles) with or without retinopathy of prematurity

Genetic Disorders

Simple Mendelian Inheritance
Autosomal dominant (most common)
Autosomal recessive
X-linked

Major Chromosomal Defects
Trisomy disorders (13, 18, 21)
Turner syndrome (45X)
Deletion syndromes (11p13, 18p, 18q)
Duplication syndromes (3q, 20q, 10q)

Multisystem Genetic Disorders
Alport syndrome (hearing loss, renal disease)
Alström disease (nerve deafness, diabetes mellitus)
Apert syndrome (craniosynostosis, syndactyly)
Bardet-Biedl syndrome
Cockayne syndrome (premature senility, skin photosensitivity)
Conradi syndrome (chondrodysplasia punctata)
Crouzon syndrome (dysostosis craniofacialis)
Hallermann-Streiff syndrome (microphthalmia; small, pinched nose; skin atrophy; and hypotrichosis)
Hypohidrotic ectodermal dysplasia (anomalous dentition, hypohidrosis, hypotrichosis)
Ichthyosis (keratinizing disorder with thick, scaly skin)
Incontinentia pigmenti (dental anomalies, intellectual disability, cutaneous lesions)
Lowe syndrome (oculocerebrorenal syndrome: hypotonia, renal disease)
Marfan syndrome
Meckel-Gruber syndrome (renal dysplasia, encephalocele)
Myotonic dystrophy
Nail-patella syndrome (renal dysfunction, dysplastic nails, hypoplastic patella)
Marinesco-Sjögren syndrome (cerebellar ataxia, hypotonia)
Nevoid basal cell carcinoma syndrome (autosomal dominant, basal cell carcinoma erupts in childhood)
Peter anomaly (corneal opacifications with iris-corneal dysgenesis)
Reiger syndrome (iris dysplasia, myotonic dystrophy)
Rothmund-Thomson (poikiloderma: skin atrophy)
Rubinstein-Taybi syndrome (broad great toe, intellectual disability)
Smith-Lemli-Opitz syndrome (toe syndactyly, hypospadias, intellectual disability)
Sotos syndrome (cerebral gigantism)
Spondyloepiphyseal dysplasia (dwarfism, short trunk)
Stickler syndrome
Werner syndrome (premature aging in second decade of life)

Inborn Errors of Metabolism
Abetalipoproteinemia (absent chylomicrons, retinal degeneration)
Cerebrotendinous xanthomatosis (CTX)
Fabry disease (α-galactosidase A deficiency)
Galactokinase deficiency
Galactosemia (galactose-1-phosphate uridyltransferase deficiency)
Homocystinemia (subluxation of lens, intellectual disability)
Hyperferritinemia
Infantile ceroid-lipofuscinosis
Mannosidosis (acid α-mannosidase deficiency)
Niemann-Pick disease (sphingomyelinase deficiency)
Refsum syndrome (phytanic acid α-hydrolase deficiency)
Wilson disease (accumulation of copper leads to cirrhosis and neurologic symptoms)
Zellweger syndrome

Endocrinopathies
Hypocalcemia (hypoparathyroidism)
Hypoglycemia
Diabetes mellitus

Congenital Infections
Toxoplasmosis
Cytomegalovirus infection
Syphilis
Rubella
Perinatal herpes simplex infection
Measles (rubeola)
Poliomyelitis
Influenza
Varicella-zoster

Ocular Anomalies
Microphthalmia
Coloboma
Aniridia
Mesodermal dysgenesis
Persistent pupillary membrane
Posterior lenticonus
Persistent hyperplastic primary vitreous
Primitive hyaloid vascular system
Retinitis pigmentosa

Miscellaneous Disorders
Atopic dermatitis
Drugs (corticosteroids)
Radiation
Trauma

Idiopathic

cytomegalovirus, *h*erpes simplex, and *s*yphilis) can also cause cataracts. Usually these are bilateral but in the case of congenital rubella infection unilateral cataract may occur. Evaluation for a systemic cause should include a pediatric physical examination, ophthalmologic examination of the infant and family members, urine for reducing substances after lactose-containing milk feeding, and labs for TORCH infections, calcium, phosphorus, and glucose. Other metabolic studies, chromosomal evaluation, and genetic consultation may be indicated.

Cataracts in older children may be newly acquired due to a metabolic disease, drug exposure such as steroids, or a manifestation of progressive congenital cataracts. Cataract may rarely be the initial manifestation of diabetes type 1 but can occur as a complication particularly in patients with poor glycemic control. Bilateral cataracts are often the presenting sign in patients with unrecognized cerebrotendinous xanthomatosis (CTX). These patients usually have had chronic diarrhea without a known cause. Unfortunately, CTX is often diagnosed late after mental and neurodegeneration has started to occur. Since chenodeoxycholic acid can be used to prevent mental and neurologic deterioration, CTX should be considered in the presence of a juvenile-onset cataract and chronic diarrhea. Occasionally cataracts, unilateral or bilateral, are caused by an underlying congenital lens defect, which develops into a visually significant cataract at a later age. Trauma is a common cause of an acquired unilateral cataract.

Ideally, unilateral cataracts must be removed, and amblyopia treatment begun in the first or second month of life. Bilateral cataracts judged to be visually significant must be treated in the first 3 months of life to facilitate an optimal outcome. After this critical period maximum visual potential is decreased. Aphakic correction in infants younger than 6–12 months with bilateral cataracts is generally provided with extended-wear contact lenses or spectacles. Unilateral aphakia in this age group is best managed with a contact lens. A posterior chamber intraocular lens may be placed in children over the age of 1 year unless the child has an underlying inflammatory condition such as juvenile idiopathic arthritis (JIA). An intraocular lens may be placed in a child with a traumatic cataract if the intraocular structures that support the lens are intact. The management of a cataract goes well beyond cataract surgery. Amblyopia must be treated with occlusion of the sound eye, often for several years, until stable visual acuity can be demonstrated. Most children (80%) will develop strabismus by age 5 years. Those who have had cataract surgery must be monitored indefinitely to evaluate for delayed complications such as glaucoma and retinal detachment.

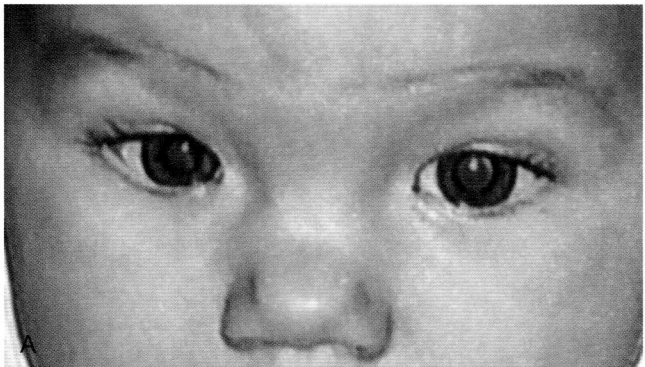

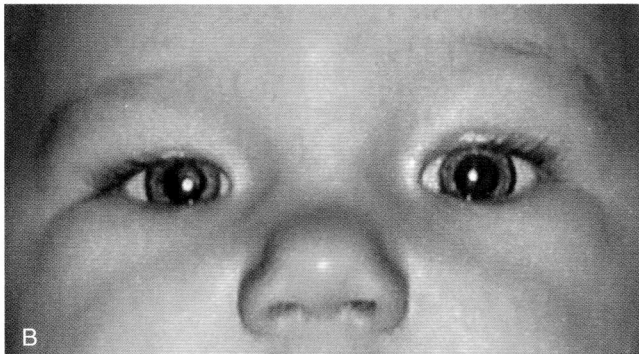

Fig. 43.12 *A,* Photograph of an infant taken when 4 months of age showing normal red reflexes in both eyes. *B,* Photograph of the same infant 2 months later showing loss of the red reflex in the right eye. At the time of cataract surgery, the right eye was found to have a dense central cataract and persistent fetal vasculature. (From Lambert SR, Lyons CJ, eds. *Taylor & Hoyt's Pediatric Ophthalmology and Strabismus.* 5th ed. Philadelphia: Elsevier; 2017:353, Fig. 37-22.)

GLAUCOMA IN CHILDHOOD

Pediatric glaucomas result from abnormalities of the aqueous outflow pathways (primary congenital glaucoma) or abnormalities that affect other parts of the eye (secondary glaucoma) (Table 43.12). Several genes causing primary congenital glaucoma, usually autosomal recessive, have been identified. Primary congenital glaucoma is bilateral in about 65% of patients. This presents as a classic triad consisting of blepharospasm, photophobia, and epiphora (Fig. 43.14). The cornea may be cloudy due to edema resulting from elevated intraocular pressure. The cornea also enlarges and the axial length of the eye may increase with elevated intraocular pressure. Onset usually occurs in the first year of life, but only 25% are present at birth. If glaucoma presents

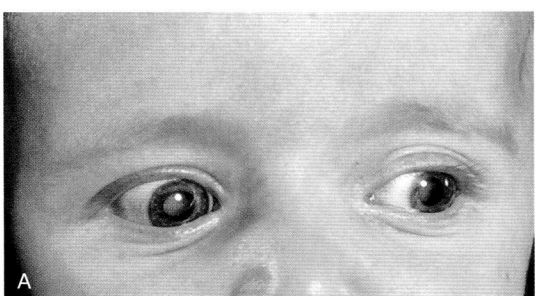

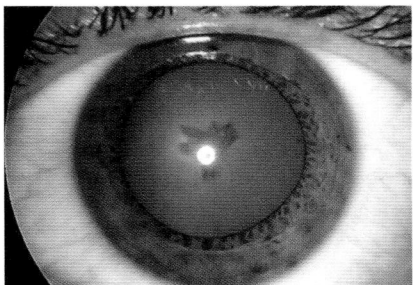

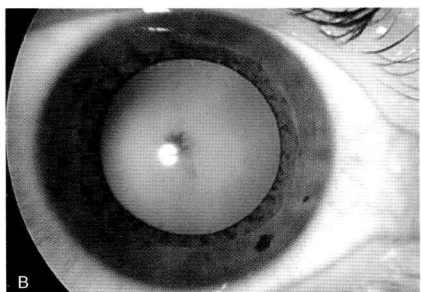

Fig. 43.13 Autosomal dominant cataracts. *A,* A 3-month-old infant with bilateral dense cataracts. *B,* His mother has mild cataracts. (From Lambert SR, Lyons CJ, eds. *Taylor & Hoyt's Pediatric Ophthalmology and Strabismus.* 5th ed. Philadelphia: Elsevier; 2017:354, Fig. 37-23.)

TABLE 43.12 Classifications of Childhood Glaucomas

PRIMARY CHILDHOOD GLAUCOMA

Primary congenital glaucoma (isolated trabeculodysgenesis)

    Neonatal or newborn onset (0–1 mo)

    Infantile onset (>1 mo–2 yr)

    Late onset or late recognized (>2 yr)

    Spontaneously arrested (nonprogressive buphthalmos, Haab striae, normal intraocular pressure [IOP] and optic nerves)

    Juvenile open-angle glaucoma

SECONDARY CHILDHOOD GLAUCOMA

Glaucoma Associated with Nonacquired Ocular Anomalies

Conditions with predominantly ocular anomalies *present at birth* that may or may not be associated with systemic signs:

    Axenfeld-Rieger anomaly ("syndrome" if systemic associations)

    Peters anomaly ("syndrome" if systemic associations)

    Congenital ectropion uveae

    Congenital iris hypoplasia

    Aniridia

    Persistent fetal vasculature (PFV) (if glaucoma present before cataract surgery)

    Oculodermal melanocytosis (nevus of Ota)

    Microphthalmos/microcornea

    Ectopia lentis

    Simple ectopia lentis (no systemic associations)

    Ectopia lentis et pupillae

Glaucoma Associated with Nonacquired Systemic Disease or Syndrome

Conditions predominantly with known syndromes, systemic anomalies, or systemic disease *present at birth* that may be associated with ocular signs:

    Phakomatoses

        Sturge-Weber syndrome

        Neurofibromatosis (NF-1)

        Klippel-Trenaunay-Weber syndrome

SECONDARY CHILDHOOD GLAUCOMA—CONT'D

Chromosomal disorders such as trisomy 21 (Down syndrome)

    Connective tissue disorders

        Marfan syndrome

        Weill-Marchesani syndrome

        Stickler syndrome

    Metabolic disorders

        Homocystinuria

        Lowe syndrome

        Mucopolysaccharidoses

    Rubinstein-Taybi

    Congenital rubella

Glaucoma Associated with Acquired Condition

Conditions that are not inherited or present at birth but that *develop after birth:*

    Uveitis

    Trauma (hyphema, angle recession, ectopia lentis)

    Steroid induced

    Tumors (benign/malignant, ocular/orbital)

    Retinopathy of prematurity (ROP)

    Postsurgery other than cataract surgery

Glaucoma Following Cataract Surgery

Subdivided into three categories based upon cataract type and there being *no glaucoma prior to cataract surgery:*

    Congenital idiopathic cataract

    Congenital cataract associated with ocular anomalies/systemic disease or syndrome

    Acquired cataract

Adapted from Beck A, Chang TCP, Freedman S. Definition, classification and differential diagnosis. In: Welnreb RN, Grajewskl A, Papadopoulos M, et al., eds. *Childhood Glaucoma, WGA Consensus Series - 9.* Amsterdam: Kugler Publications; 2013:3–10.

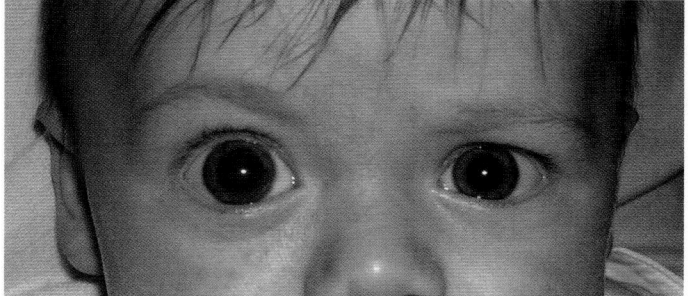

Fig. 43.14 Infant with right buphthalmos. (From Lambert SR, Lyons CJ, eds. *Taylor & Hoyt's Pediatric Ophthalmology and Strabismus.* 5th ed. Philadelphia: Elsevier; 2017:363, Fig. 38-1.)

after the age of 5 years, it is known as primary juvenile open-angle glaucoma. The natural history of untreated primary congenital glaucoma is blindness resulting from progressive corneal opacification and optic nerve damage. Treatment is surgical, although eye pressure–lowering medications such as topical β blockers and topical or oral carbonic anhydrase inhibitors may be used as temporizing measures. Even with treatment, final visual acuity is worse than 20/50 in more than 50% of the patients.

Secondary glaucoma may present similarly to primary glaucoma but is associated with other factors such as ocular trauma, inflammation, prolonged steroid use, or cataract. Some systemic conditions such as neurofibromatosis and Sturge-Weber syndrome are also associated with secondary glaucoma. The differential diagnosis of congenital glaucoma includes anterior segment dysgenesis and conditions that demonstrate corneal opacities (Table 43.13) or an enlarged cornea (Table 43.14). Epiphora also occurs with

TABLE 43.13 STUMPED: Differential Diagnosis of Neonatal Corneal Opacities

Diagnosis	Laterality	Opacity	Ocular Pressure	Other Ocular Abnormalities	Natural History	Inheritance
S – Sclerocornea	Unilateral or bilateral	Vascularized, blends with sclera, clearer centrally	Normal (or elevated)	Cornea plana	Nonprogressive	Sporadic
T – Tears in endothelium and Descemet membrane						
Birth trauma	Unilateral	Diffuse edema	Normal	Possible hyphema, periorbital ecchymoses	Spontaneous improvement in 1 mo	Sporadic
Infantile glaucoma	Bilateral	Diffuse edema	Elevated	Megalocornea, photophobia and tearing, abnormal angle	Progressive unless treated	Autosomal recessive
U – Ulcers						
Herpes simplex keratitis	Unilateral	Diffuse with geographic epithelial defect	Normal	None	Progressive	Sporadic
Congenital rubella	Bilateral	Disciform or diffuse edema, no frank ulceration	Normal or elevated	Microphthalmos, cataract, pigment epithelial mottling	Stable, may clear	Sporadic
Neurotrophic – exposure	Unilateral or bilateral	Central ulcer	Normal	Lid anomalies, congenital sensory neuropathy	Progressive	Sporadic
M – Metabolic (rarely present at birth) (mucopolysaccharidoses IH, IS; mucolipidoses type IV)*	Bilateral	Diffuse haze, denser peripherally	Normal	Few	Progressive	Autosomal recessive
P – Posterior corneal defect	Unilateral or bilateral	Central, diffuse haze or vascularized leukoma	Normal or elevated	Anterior chamber cleavage syndrome	Stable; sometimes early clearing or vascularization	Sporadic, autosomal recessive
E – Endothelial dystrophy						
Congenital hereditary endothelial dystrophy	Bilateral	Diffuse corneal edema, marked corneal thickening	Normal	None	Stable	Autosomal dominant or recessive
Posterior polymorphous dystrophy	Bilateral	Diffuse haze, normal corneal thickness	Normal	Occasional peripheral anterior synechiae	Slowly progressive	Autosomal dominant
Congenital hereditary stromal dystrophy	Bilateral	Flaky, feathery stromal opacities; normal corneal thickness	Normal	None	Stable	Autosomal dominant
D – Dermoid	Unilateral or bilateral	White vascularized mass, hair, lipid arc	Normal	None	Stable	Sporadic

*Mucopolysaccharidosis IH, Hurler syndrome; mucopolysaccharidosis IS, Scheie syndrome.
From Nelson LB, Calhoun JH, Harley RD. *Pediatric Ophthalmology.* 3rd ed. Philadelphia: WB Saunders; 1991:210.

conjunctivitis, corneal trauma, and nasolacrimal duct obstruction (NLDO). Photophobia is observed in infants with corneal trauma, corneal deposits, cystinosis, and inflammation (uveitis). Corneal opacification can also be found in infants with corneal dystrophies, metabolic storage diseases such as mucopolysaccharidoses, and forceps-related obstetric trauma.

The diagnosis of primary congenital glaucoma or secondary glaucoma is generally confirmed by performing an examination with the patient under anesthesia. The child needs to be quiet and very cooperative in order to get an accurate intraocular pressure reading and a careful examination of the cornea and anterior segment structures. The diagnosis rests on a constellation of abnormal ocular findings, including elevated intraocular pressure, corneal enlargement, increased axial length, anomalies of the drainage angle, and signs of damage to the optic nerve in conjunction with medical history.

TABLE 43.14   Differential Diagnosis of Enlarged Cornea

Anterior	Primary Infantile Simple Megalocornea	Megalophthalmos	Glaucoma with Buphthalmos
Inheritance	Autosomal dominant (?)	X-linked recessive (male preponderance)	Sporadic
Time of appearance	Congenital	Congenital	First year of life
Bilaterality	Bilateral	Bilateral	Unilateral or bilateral
	Symmetric	Symmetric	Asymmetric
Natural history	Nonprogressive	Nonprogressive	Progressive
Symptoms	None	None	Photophobia, epiphora
Corneal clarity	Clear	Clear or mosaic dystrophy	Diffuse edema, tears in Descemet membrane
Intraocular pressure	Normal	Elevated in some adults	Elevated
Corneal diameter	13–18 mm	13–18 mm	13–18 mm
Corneal thickness	Normal	Normal	Thick
Keratometry	Normal	Normal; astigmatism	Flat
Gonioscopy	Normal	Excessive mesenchymal tissue	Excessive mesenchymal tissue
Globe diameter (A scan)	23–26 mm	23–26 mm	27–30 mm
Major ocular complications	None	Lens dislocation; cataract, <40 yr; secondary glaucoma	Optic disk damage, late corneal edema
Associated systemic disorders	None	Occasionally Marfan and other skeletal abnormalities	None consistent

From Nelson LB, Calhoun JH, Harley RD. *Pediatric Ophthalmology*. 3rd ed. Philadelphia: WB Saunders; 1991:201.

CHILDHOOD UVEITIS

Uveitis is defined as inflammation of the uveal tissue of the eye, which includes the iris, ciliary body, and choroid. Inflammation can involve any or all of these structures, and terms such as iritis (Fig. 43.15), iridocyclitis, choroiditis, and chorioretinitis are used to designate which portion of the uveal tissue is involved. Anatomic location such as anterior, posterior, intermediate, or panuveitis or associated with meningitis is useful in determining etiology (Table 43.15). Masquerade syndromes such as lymphoma or leukemia can mimic uveitis since they can have a leukocyte response that can be mistaken for inflammation.

JIA (juvenile idiopathic arthritis) is the most common cause of childhood anterior uveitis. JIA uveitis is most common in the pauciarticular form, when the onset occurs before the age of 7 years, and when the antinuclear antibody blood test is positive. Females are at higher risk than males; 10–15% of children with JIA develop uveitis and 10% of those who develop uveitis do so prior to the diagnosis of JIA. It is common for children with JIA to have no symptoms of inflammation in the eye. Despite the lack of symptoms, uveitis can cause severe vision loss due to the development of edema or deposition of calcium (band keratopathy) in the cornea or retinal edema (Fig. 43.15). A cataract and/or glaucoma may result from inflammation in the eye or chronic use of steroids used to quiet the inflammation. The pupil may have an irregular shape as a result of adhesions to the underlying lens (posterior synechiae). Visual impairment occurs in up to 40% of children with JIA uveitis and blindness occurs in 10% of affected eyes. For this reason there are screening guidelines for the recommended frequency of eye exams based on the risk factors that predispose patients with JIA to uveitis including category of arthritis (oligoarthritis vs polyarthritis), age of onset of arthritis, presence of antinuclear antibody positivity, and duration of disease (Fig. 43.16).

The diagnosis of uveitis can be made from an eye examination. Because uveitis can be caused by infections, trauma, or autoimmune disorders and often is idiopathic, evaluation of the cause of the uveitis requires a thorough pediatric physical examination as well as supplementary radiologic and laboratory testing. A chest radiograph may demonstrate tuberculosis and sarcoidosis. Serologic evaluation may include tests for syphilis, sarcoidosis, JIA, Lyme disease, herpes, measles, and toxoplasmosis. In males, haplotype testing for human leukocyte antigen B27 may be indicated because of the association between iritis and pauciarticular arthritis that may later evolve into ankylosing spondylitis.

The management of iritis in children is the elimination of intraocular inflammation. In some cases of noninfectious uveitis, local treatment with topical corticosteroid drops or periocular corticosteroid injections may control the inflammation. In many cases, local corticosteroids are not sufficient to control chronic uveitis. Immunomodulatory agents such as oral corticosteroids and corticosteroid-sparing agents, including nonsteroidal antiinflammatory drugs (NSAIDs), antimetabolites, T-cell inhibitors, alkylating agents, and antitumor necrosis factor biologic agents, are options. Short courses of corticosteroids may be used, but corticosteroid-sparing drugs are the first-line therapy for long-term use due to the many side effects of corticosteroids. Biologic agents are commonly used in severe disease or when the child has not responded to NSAIDs. Mydriatic drops are used to prevent the formation of posterior synechiae.

Toxoplasmosis caused by the intracellular parasite *Toxoplasma gondii* is the most common cause of posterior uveitis in children. Most ocular toxoplasmosis in the pediatric age group is probably acquired from the mother during pregnancy. In some instances, the infection is inactive at birth and goes unrecognized until inflammation occurs. Toxoplasmosis that is active at birth may result in widespread fetal tissue damage or may be associated with chorioretinitis, encephalomyelitis, and visceral disease. The diagnosis of toxoplasmosis is based on clinical findings, intracranial calcification in some children, and laboratory tests for specific immunoglobulin G (IgG) and immunoglobulin M antibodies. Isolated ocular toxoplasmosis does not require

TABLE 43.15 Differential Diagnosis and Etiology of Uveitis

Anterior Uveitis
Juvenile idiopathic arthritis
Trauma
Herpes
Syphilis
Lyme disease
Fuchs heterochromic iridocyclitis
Kawasaki syndrome
Tubulointerstitial nephritis and uveitis syndrome
Enthesitis related arthritis
Orbital pseudotumor
Ulcerative colitis
Idiopathic

Intermediate Uveitis
Pars planitis
Sarcoidosis
Tuberculosis
Juvenile xanthogranuloma
Lyme disease
Idiopathic

Posterior Uveitis and Panuveitis
Toxoplasmosis
Toxocariasis
Herpes, rubella, rubeola, measles
Histoplasmosis
Syphilis
Sympathetic ophthalmia
Sarcoidosis
Bartonella
Candida albicans
Lyme disease
Familial juvenile systemic granulomatosis (Blau syndrome)
Diffuse unilateral subacute neuroretinitis (DUSN)
Tuberous sclerosis
Vogt-Koyanagi-Harada syndrome
Behçet disease
Idiopathic

Uveo-Meningeal Syndromes
Vogt-Koyanagi-Harada disease
Behçet
Sarcoidosis
Granulomatosis with polyangiitis
Cat-scratch disease
Whipple disease
Syphilis
Lyme disease
Acute posterior multifocal placoid pigment epitheliopathy
Lymphoma
Herpes simplex
Cytomegalovirus

From Basic and Clinical Science Course, Section 6. *Ophthalmology and Strabismus*. San Francisco: American Academy of Ophthalmology; 2013–2014:268, Table 22-1.

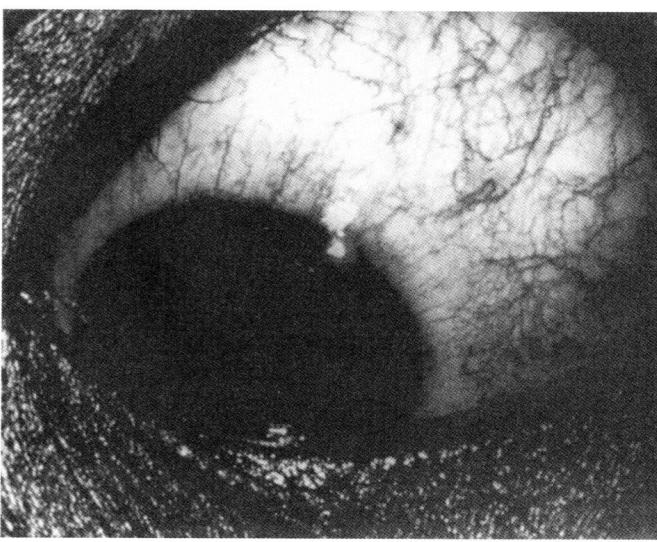

Fig. 43.15 Ciliary flush associated with iritis. Note the straight, radially oriented vessels extending out from the iris. (From Reilly BM. *Practical Strategies in Outpatient Medicine*. 2nd ed. Philadelphia: WB Saunders; 1991:41.)

treatment unless it threatens vision. When treatment is indicated, it involves the use of one or more antimicrobial drugs. The most common therapy consists of combination therapy with pyrimethamine and sulfadiazine. Steroids may be given in combination with antibiotics. Intravitreal clindamycin with dexamethasone may be as effective as systemic therapies. Several other entities can simulate uveitis in children and must be considered. These entities include retinoblastoma, leukemia, lymphoma, juvenile xanthogranuloma, and an intraocular foreign body.

NASOLACRIMAL PROBLEMS IN CHILDHOOD

The nasolacrimal system consists of tear-secreting glands and a drainage system. The lacrimal gland, located in the superotemporal orbit, is the primary producer of tears; accessory lacrimal glands in the upper eyelid supplement its output. The lacrimal drainage apparatus begins with puncta on the nasal aspect of the upper and lower eyelid margins. The puncta continue as canaliculi that course nasally to empty into the lacrimal sac. The lacrimal sac in turn drains inferiorly through the nasolacrimal duct just under the inferior turbinate in the nose (Fig. 43.17).

The most common developmental anomaly of the nasolacrimal drainage system is **nasolacrimal duct obstruction (NLDO)**, which occurs in up to 20% of infants. A thin mucosal membrane at the distal end of the duct, the valve of Hasner, is the most common cause of obstruction. Typically, the infant has epiphora and a mucopurulent discharge that causes matting of the eyelids beginning at about 1 month of age. Pressure applied to the lacrimal sac with a finger or cotton swab often results in reflux of cloudy fluid from the puncta. If infected, the source is usually polymicrobial, but a bacteriologic diagnosis is not necessary for clinical management. Eyelash washes with dilute baby shampoo can decrease the frequency of infections. Topical antibiotics can be used to decrease purulence, but this likely leads to resistant organisms. Recurrent infections may be considered an indication for early probing. Lacrimal sac massage may push fluid through the mucosal membrane and thereby open the duct, but the pressure applied to the lacrimal sac needs to be forceful. Most NLDOs will spontaneously resolve. If resolution does not occur within the first year of life, probing of the duct can be done and is effective in 90% of cases. Effectiveness of

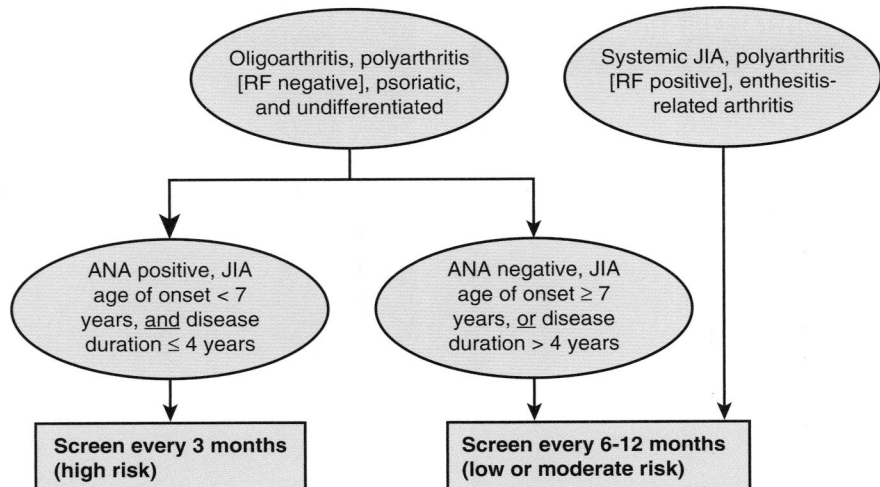

Fig. 43.16 Ophthalmology screening recommendations. ANA, antinuclear antibody; JIA, juvenile idiopathic arthritis; RF, rheumatoid factor. (From Angeles-Han ST, Ringold S, Beukelman T, et al. 2019 American College of Rheumatology/Arthritis Foundation Guideline for the Screening, Monitoring, and Treatment of Juvenile Idiopathic Arthritis-Associated Uveitis. *Arthritis Care Res (Hoboken)*. 2019;71(6):703–716.)

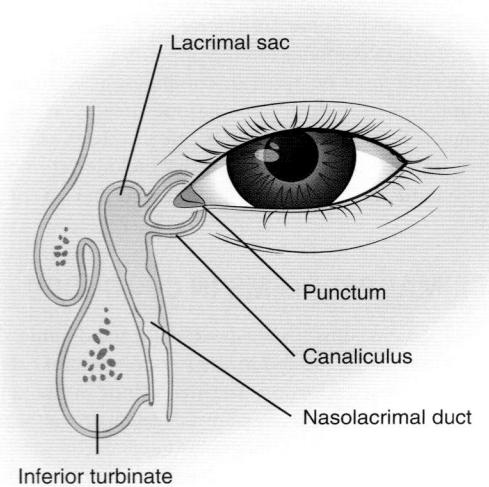

Fig. 43.17 Anatomy of the nasolacrimal drainage system. (Modified from *Rev Ophthalmol.* 2001;8:122. Reprinted with permission from Jobson Publishing: New York.)

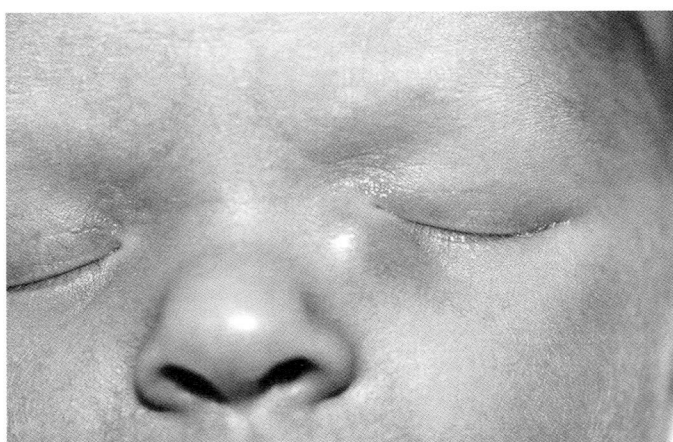

Fig. 43.18 Dacryocystocele of the left lacrimal sac in a 2-week-old infant. The dacryocystocele resolved with a probing of the left tear duct.

nasolacrimal duct probing decreases after the age of 18 months. A silicon stent can be placed temporarily to maintain an open duct, which increases the success of long-term patency.

NLDO must be differentiated from atresia of the puncta or canaliculi causing tearing but not infection and lacrimal-cutaneous fistula causing tears to drain to the skin surface. These conditions require surgery to re-form the canalicular system and puncta and repair the fistula if present. NLDO should be differentiated from infectious conjunctivitis, especially gonococcal, chlamydial, and herpetic infections. Chronic tearing also occurs in congenital glaucoma in addition to blepharospasm and photophobia.

A **dacryocystocele** is a variation of congenital NLDO that occurs in newborns. These infants present with a bluish mass in the naso-orbital region below the medial canthal tendon. This mass is a dilated lacrimal sac that has both distal obstruction from a membrane and proximal obstruction from a one-way valve effect from an incompetent valve of Rosenmüller (Fig. 43.18). A hemangioma or dermoid cyst may have a bluish hue, but hemangiomas typically do not present at birth. An encephalocele or dermoid cyst may also appear to be a bluish mass but will lie above the medial canthus. On occasion, the dilated sac is accompanied by bulging of the nasal mucosa at the distal end of the nasolacrimal duct. The nasal mucocele can compromise the infant's breathing. Imaging may help determine the location of the medial canthus in the presence of swelling, confirm the suspected diagnosis, and evaluate for the presence of a nasal mucocele, which is important for surgical planning. If the dacryocystocele fails to resolve with topical antibiotics and massage, or if cellulitis develops, systemic antibiotics and surgical decompression must be considered. Decompression is accomplished by relieving the distal obstruction by probing the nasolacrimal duct, removing any nasal cyst, and possibly placing a stent.

RED EYE

The term *red eye* usually refers to inflammation of the conjunctiva that causes the eye to appear red. Much less commonly (and much more seriously), the sclera is injected. Causes of red eye include infection of the ocular surface (cornea, conjunctiva, and sclera), allergy, intraocular inflammation, glaucoma, foreign body, and trauma. Evaluation must be directed toward discerning whether a child's red eye is caused by a benign condition that will spontaneously resolve (viral conjunctivitis)

or easily be treated with topical medication (bacterial conjunctivitis) or whether the cause is potentially vision threatening (iritis, corneal ulceration, glaucoma) and requires urgent ophthalmologic evaluation (Table 43.16). Signs that should raise concerns for a serious etiology of red eye are in an immunocompromised host, severe pain,

TABLE 43.16   The Red Eye

Condition	Cause	Signs/Symptoms	Treatment
Bacterial conjunctivitis	*Haemophilus influenzae, H. influenzae aegyptius, Streptococcus pneumoniae, Neisseria gonorrhoeae, Staphylococcus aureus, Yersinia* species, cat-scratch bacillus less common	Mucopurulent unilateral or bilateral discharge, normal vision, photophobia usually absent Conjunctival injection and edema (chemosis); gritty sensation	Topical antibiotics: systemic ceftriaxone for gonococcus, *H. influenzae*
Viral conjunctivitis	Adenovirus, ECHO virus, coxsackievirus, herpes simplex virus, coronavirus	As above; may be hemorrhagic, unilateral enlarged preauricular lymph nodes	Self-limited
Neonatal conjunctivitis	*Chlamydia trachomatis*, gonococcus, chemical (silver nitrate), *S. aureus*	Palpebral conjunctival follicle or papillae; as above	Ceftriaxone for gonococcus and oral erythromycin for *C. trachomatis*
Allergic conjunctivitis	Seasonal pollens or allergen exposure	Itching, incidence of bilateral chemosis (edema) greater than that of erythema, tarsal papillae	Antihistamines, steroids, cromolyn
Keratitis	Herpes simplex, adenovirus, *S. pneumoniae, S. aureus, Pseudomonas* species, *Acanthamoeba* species, chemicals	Severe pain, corneal swelling, clouding, limbus erythema, hypopyon, cataracts; contact lens history with amebic infection	Specific antibiotics for bacterial/ fungal infections; keratoplasty, acyclovir for herpes
Endophthalmitis	*S. aureus, S. pneumoniae, Candida albicans*, associated surgery or trauma	Acute onset, pain, loss of vision, swelling, chemosis, redness; hypopyon and vitreous haze	Antibiotics
Anterior uveitis (iridocyclitis)	JIA, reactive arthritis, sarcoidosis, Behçet disease, Kawasaki disease, inflammatory bowel disease	Unilateral/bilateral; erythema, ciliary flush (in circumcorneal area), irregular pupil, iris adhesions; pain, marked photophobia, small pupil, poor vision, no discharge	Topical steroids, plus therapy for primary disease
Posterior uveitis (choroiditis)	Toxoplasmosis, histoplasmosis, *Toxocara canis*	No sign of erythema, decreased vision, no discharge	Specific therapy for pathogen
Episcleritis/scleritis	Idiopathic autoimmune disease (e.g., SLE, Henoch-Schönlein purpura)	Localized pain, intense erythema, unilateral; blood vessels bigger than in conjunctivitis; scleritis may cause globe perforation, no discharge	Episcleritis is self-limiting; topical steroids for fast relief
Foreign body	Occupational exposure	Unilateral, red, gritty feeling; visible or microscopic size	Irrigation, removal; check for ulceration
Blepharitis	*S. aureus, S. epidermidis*, seborrheic, blocked lacrimal duct: rarely, molluscum contagiosum, *Pthirus pubis, Pediculosis capitis*	Bilateral, irritation, itching, hyperemia, crusting, affecting lid margins	Topical antibiotics, warm compresses
Dacryocystitis	Obstructed lacrimal sac: *S. aureus, H. influenzae*, pneumococcus	Pain, tenderness, erythema and exudate in area of lacrimal sac (inferomedial to inner canthus); tearing (epiphora); possible orbital cellulitis	Systemic, topical antibiotics; surgical drainage
Dacryoadenitis	*S. aureus, Streptococcus* species, CMV, measles, EBV, enteroviruses, trauma, sarcoidosis, leukemia	Pain, tenderness, edema, erythema over gland area (upper temporal lid); fever, leukocytosis	Systemic antibiotics; drainage of orbital abscesses
Orbital cellulitis	Paranasal sinusitis: *H. influenzae, S. aureus, S. pneumoniae*, other *Streptococcus* species Trauma: *S. aureus* Fungi: *Aspergillus, Mucor* species if immunodeficient	Rhinorrhea, chemosis, vision loss, painful extraocular motion, proptosis, ophthalmoplegia, fever, lid edema, leukocytosis *S. aureus*	Systemic antibiotics (postseptal cellulitis), drainage of orbital abscesses
Periorbital cellulitis	Trauma: *S. aureus, Streptococcus* species Bacteremia: *H. influenzae*, pneumococci, *S. pyogenes, S. aureus*	Cutaneous erythema, warmth, normal vision, minimal involvement of orbit, fever, leukocytosis, toxic appearance	Systemic antibiotics (preseptal cellulitis)

CMV, cytomegalovirus; *EBV*, Epstein-Barr virus; *ECHO*, enteric cytopathogenic human orphan; *JIA*, juvenile idiopathic arthritis; *SLE*, systemic lupus erythematosus.
Modified from Behrman RE, Kliegman RM. *Nelson Essentials of Pediatrics*. 3rd ed. Philadelphia: WB Saunders; 1998; with data from Rosenbaum JT, Nozik RA. Uveitis: many diseases, one diagnosis. *Am J Med*. 1985;79:545–547; Elkington AR, Khaw PT. The red eye. *BMJ*. 1988;296:1720–1724; Wilhemus KR. The red eye. Infectious conjunctivitis, keratitis, endophthalmitis, and periocular cellulitis. *Infect Dis Clin North Am*. 1988;2:99–116; Forrester JV. Uveitis: pathogenesis. *Lancet*. 1991;338:1498–1501; Gioliotti F. Acute conjunctivitis of childhood. *Pediatr Ann*. 1993;22:353–356.

proptosis, limitation of eye movements, opacified cornea, abnormal pupil response, or lack of response to therapy.

In taking the history, the examiner should inquire about laterality, onset, associated illnesses, contact with others with "pink eye," the presence of pain or itching, the characteristics of any discharge (watery, mucoid, purulent), and blurring of vision. The examination of the child should start with as precise a measurement of visual acuity as possible. The presence and type of discharge should be noted. Inspection of the surface of the eye with a penlight should determine whether the cornea is clear. Fluorescein staining of the cornea to assess for a corneal abrasion should be done. The red reflex should be checked. The presence of foreign bodies should be considered.

The most common cause of a red eye in a child is infectious conjunctivitis (Table 43.17). *Streptococcus pneumoniae* is the most frequent bacterial pathogen, followed by some *Haemophilus* species and *Moraxella*. However, infections from *Haemophilus* species have decreased because of immunization. In hospitalized patients, staphylococcal infections (including methicillin-resistant *Staphylococcus aureus*) are more common. A bacterial culture is not necessary in mild cases of suspected bacterial conjunctivitis because the infection tends to be self-limiting but may last up to 2 weeks. Treatment with a broad-spectrum *topical* antibiotic may relieve symptoms and shorten the course of infection, allowing the child to return to school or daycare. Topical antibiotic options include trimethoprim–polymyxin B, erythromycin, gentamicin or tobramycin, ciprofloxacin, moxifloxacin, gatifloxacin, azithromycin, and sulfacetamide. Sulfacetamide preparations are inexpensive but have a narrower range of effectiveness and cause a great deal of stinging. Sulfa drugs also have an association with Stevens-Johnson syndrome. Gentamicin can cause redness, which can cause difficulty in determining whether or not the conjunctivitis is treated. The aminoglycosides are less effective with gram-positive

organisms, particularly streptococcal species. Trimethoprim sulfate/ polymyxin B is bacteriostatic and a 7–10-day course of therapy is recommended. The fluoroquinolones are rapidly effective but have different dosing recommendations. Azithromycin has a very short course. Steroid-antibiotic combinations should be avoided because of the risk of worsening a bacterial corneal ulcer or an unsuspected herpes simplex infection.

Viral conjunctivitis tends to be associated with a watery or mucoid discharge. Follicles may be visible with low magnification on the palpebral conjunctiva, and a preauricular lymph node can often be palpated. Adenovirus is a common pathogen; epidemic outbreaks are frequent. In children as old as 2 years, adenovirus can manifest with severe periorbital edema and erythema that mimics bacterial preseptal or orbital cellulitis; a conjunctival pseudomembrane is common in this setting. Adenovirus types 8, 19, and 35; enterovirus 70; and coxsackie 24 are associated with subconjunctival hemorrhages or hemorrhagic conjunctivitis. Pharyngoconjunctival fever, conjunctivitis accompanied by a sore throat and fever, is associated with adenovirus types 3 and 7. Cultures are not usually necessary but can be performed if there is a question of etiology. Antibiotics are ineffective in adenovirus infections. Treatment is largely supportive, with cool compresses and artificial tears providing symptomatic relief. Adenovirus is highly contagious so careful attention to hygiene should be taken among family members, caregivers, and contacts to prevent the spread of infection.

Less frequent causes of viral conjunctivitis are herpes simplex and varicella. These may be associated with vesicular involvement of the eyelid and face. Treatment with oral antiviral medications can be used if lesions are very near the cornea or there is corneal involvement. Oral antivirals are also considered in individuals who are immunocompromised. Topical antivirals are also used in patients with corneal involvement. Topical corticosteroid medications are contraindicated in

TABLE 43.17   Conjunctivitis: Differential Diagnosis

Cause	Unilateral or Bilateral	Discharge	Lids	Onset/Course	Treatment
			CLINICAL FINDINGS		
Viral* (usually adenovirus)	Bilateral	Thin, mucoid	Follicular	Gradual Upper respiratory tract infection? Preauricular adenopathy	Compresses
Herpes simplex	Unilateral	Thin, mucoid	Follicular	Gradual Keratitis Dendritic ulcer	Acyclovir
Bacterial	Unilateral or bilateral	Purulent	Papillary, purulent	Gradual	Topical antibiotics
Gonococcal	Unilateral	Purulent	Edema, inflamed	Hyperacute	Systemic antibiotics
Chlamydial	Unilateral or bilateral	Thin, mucoid	Follicular	Indolent Persistent Neonatal period Sexually active	Oral erythromycin any age or tetracycline (>10 yr of age)
Allergic	Bilateral	Watery	Papillary	Gradual Seasonal Pruritic	Topical vasoconstrictors Systemic antihistamine Topical steroids
Vernal	Bilateral	Watery	Giant papillary	Adolescence Seasonal	Cromolyn?
Contact lens irritation	Bilateral	Watery	Giant papillary	Lenses	Adjust lens Change solution
Chemical	Unilateral or bilateral	Watery	Variable	Acute	Irrigate Remove irritant

*Undifferentiated viral conjunctivitis, not caused by herpes virus infection.
Modified from Reilly BM. *Practical Strategies in Outpatient Medicine*. 2nd ed. Philadelphia: WB Saunders; 1991:46.

herpetic infections because of the potential for worsening the infection. However, the ophthalmologist often uses topical steroids to control inflammation after the viral infection has been treated.

The DNA poxvirus *Molluscum contagiosum* can cause a chronic conjunctivitis when lesions are located on the eyelid margin (Fig. 43.19). The conjunctivitis is caused by release of poxvirus particles into the tear film. Additional waxy, umbilicated lesions are oftentimes found elsewhere on the face. The infection may be self-limited, but treatment of more severe cases requires incision and debridement of the central core from each lesion.

Allergic conjunctivitis manifests with a bilateral watery or mucoid discharge and must always be considered in the differential diagnosis of bilateral red eyes. The child may rub the eyes because of pruritus; nasal allergic symptoms may also be present. About 80% of individuals with allergies have ocular symptoms and these may occur in isolation. A more severe form of allergic conjunctivitis, **vernal keratoconjunctivitis (VKC)**, tends to occur in males in the first 2 decades of life and is seasonal, occurring in the spring and fall. Ulceration of the cornea can occur. Usually the ulceration is sterile but it can impair vision. Treatment of allergic conjunctivitis includes topical antihistamines, mast cell stabilizers, or a combination of the two. Systemic treatment of allergies often improves the ocular symptoms. In severe cases of allergic conjunctivitis or VKC, steroids or cyclosporines can be used.

Systemic syndromes must also be considered in a child with a red eye. In Stevens-Johnson syndrome, conjunctival inflammation is associated with other mucous membrane or cutaneous involvement. This disease can have severe ophthalmic consequences as a result of conjunctival scarring, changes of the eyelid position, and dry eye syndrome. Kawasaki syndrome is a febrile illness of young children who frequently manifest bilateral nonpurulent conjunctival injection and, in rare cases, iritis. Similarly, self-limited conjunctivitis can also be seen in COVID-19–associated multisystem inflammatory syndrome in children (MIS-C) and COVID-19 infections. Ophthalmic consultation may be indicated to assist in the diagnosis and management of children with Stevens-Johnson syndrome.

EYELID ABNORMALITIES

Congenital abnormalities of the eyelids can be severe as in the case of cryptophthalmos, in which there is a failure of differentiation of eyelid structures and the skin passes uninterrupted from the forehead to the cheek. This is often associated with corneal abnormalities and systemic abnormalities. Colobomas of the eyelid can occur and are usually on the upper lid and can range in severity from a notch to the entire length of the eyelid. Eyelid colobomas are often associated with Goldenhar and CHARGE (*c*oloboma, *h*eart defects, choanal *a*tresia, *r*etardation,

and *e*ar abnormalities) syndromes. Surgery can be done to reconstruct the eyelids. More common eyelid abnormalities include entropion (inward turning of the eyelid margin), ectropion (eversion of the eyelid margin), epiblepharon (in which a horizontal fold of skin in the lower eyelid causes the lashes to rub against the cornea), and distichiasis (in which an accessory row of eyelashes is more posterior than the normal ones and can rub against the cornea). All these may resolve spontaneously or, if necessary, can be corrected with eyelid surgery. Epiblepharon tends to be well tolerated by patients. Epicanthus, a crescent-shaped fold of skin, is usually most prominent in the upper eyelid that can make the child appear esotropic by obscuring the underlying nasal sclera.

Congenital ptosis (Fig. 43.20*A*), droopiness of the upper eyelid, is usually caused by abnormal development of the levator muscle. Other causes in children are trauma, congenital third nerve palsy, and congenital Horner syndrome. Acute onset of ptosis in the absence of trauma requires evaluation for new-onset Horner syndrome, which may be associated with neuroblastoma, and evaluation for a third nerve palsy, which may be associated with an intracranial mass. A child with congenital ptosis needs to be monitored for deprivational amblyopia due to the eyelid occluding their visual axis. Also, these children are at risk of refractive amblyopia since they commonly have refractive errors. Treatment of ptosis is delayed until the child is several years old unless it is causing amblyopia due to occlusion of the visual axis or astigmatism that is difficult to treat with glasses, or when severe chin-up head posture is necessary to allow the child to see (Fig. 43.20*B*). Surgical correction consists of resection of the levator muscle or suspension of the upper eyelid to the frontalis muscle with a silicon sling or autogenous or cadaveric fascia lata.

A diagnostic approach to congenital and acquired ptosis is noted in Figs. 43.22 and 43.23, respectively.

ORBITAL TUMORS

Orbital tumors, either benign or malignant, may occur in children. The space-occupying lesions can present with proptosis, swelling or

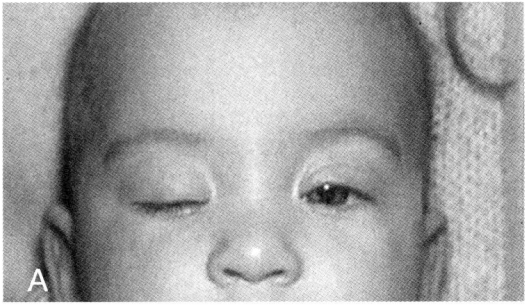
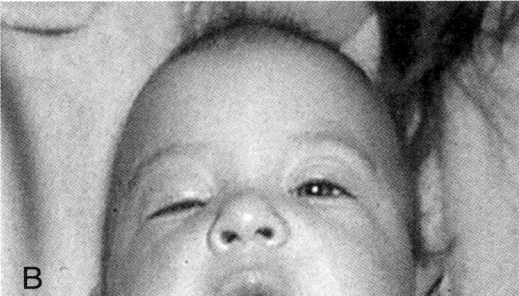

Fig. 43.20 *A,* Congenital ptosis of the right upper eyelid. *B,* The child adopted a compensatory chin-up head posture to allow use of both eyes together and did not have amblyopia.

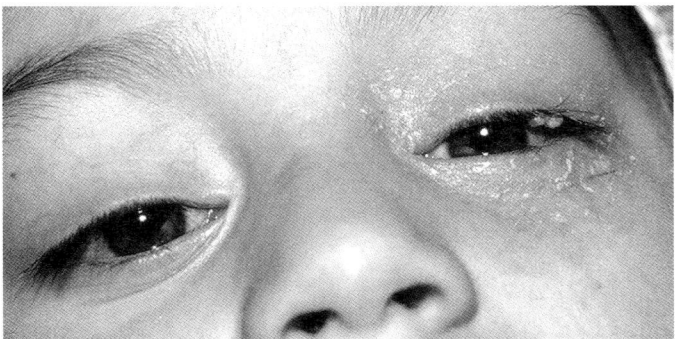

Fig. 43.19 Chronic eczematoid and follicular conjunctivitis in only the left eye, caused by *Molluscum contagiosum,* in a 5-year-old. Note the elevated lesions on the lateral aspect of the left upper eyelid.

discoloration of the eyelids, ptosis, or strabismus. Some of the most common benign tumors are vascular lesions. **Hemangiomas** occur in 1–3% of term newborns and are more common in premature infants. Hemangiomas are classified by depth of skin involvement and type of orbital involvement. The natural history involves rapid proliferation over the first several months of life. Ulceration, hemorrhage, and occlusion or induced astigmatism of the eye causing amblyopia (Fig. 43.21) can occur. After the first year of life, the lesion begins to regress. Systemic diseases such as PHACE syndrome (*p*osterior fossa malformations, *h*emangiomas, *a*rterial anomalies, *c*oarctation of the aorta and cardiac defects, *e*ye abnormalities) and multiple cutaneous hemangiomas with hepatic hemangiomas may have an orbital or eyelid hemangioma as the presenting finding. First-line treatment consists of oral propranolol 1–3 mg/kg/day divided into three oral doses. Side

effects include bradycardia, hypoglycemia, hypotension, somnolence, bronchospasm, and cough. Treatment initiation is done under medical supervision and care is taken to administer the medicine with feeds to limit the side effects. Topical timolol maleate may be used with minimal side effects for superficial skin lesions but is not effective in deeper or orbital lesions. A pulsed dye laser can also be used to treat the superficial lesions.

Lymphangiomas may cause proptosis. Most commonly these present in the second or third decade but may present in infancy. The size may increase with the onset of an upper respiratory infection. Lymphangiomas are usually managed conservatively but short courses of steroids can be used. Rapid expansion may occur if bleeding into the lesion occurs. This may require surgical intervention if the pressure in the orbit is threatening damage to the optic nerve.

Dermoid cysts are benign choristomas that arise from primitive dermal elements that develop in fetal suture lines. This tissue forms a keratinized epithelium cyst and includes hair follicles, sweat glands, and sebaceous glands. It most commonly occurs superotemporally in the zygomatic frontal suture but may be superonasal in the frontal-nasal suture. Imaging can be valuable in confirming the diagnosis and determining if the dermoid extends into the orbit. If the cyst ruptures, a marked inflammatory reaction ensues, so removal is recommended prior to the child becoming very active, which increases the chances of the child rupturing the cyst traumatically.

Malignant tumors of the orbit can rapidly enlarge, which makes them difficult to differentiate from inflammatory and infectious causes. **Rhabdomyosarcomas** are the most common primary pediatric orbital tumor. Average age of onset is 5–7 years. Usually the tumor arises in the orbit but it can arise in the conjunctiva, eyelid, or uveal tissue. Patients present with rapidly progressing proptosis. Tumors need to be removed completely and chemotherapy or radiation may also be needed.

Neuroblastoma is the most common metastatic orbital tumor of childhood. It usually arises from the adrenal gland or sympathetic ganglion chain, hence the association with acquired Horner syndrome. Unilateral or bilateral proptosis and eyelid ecchymosis are the classic

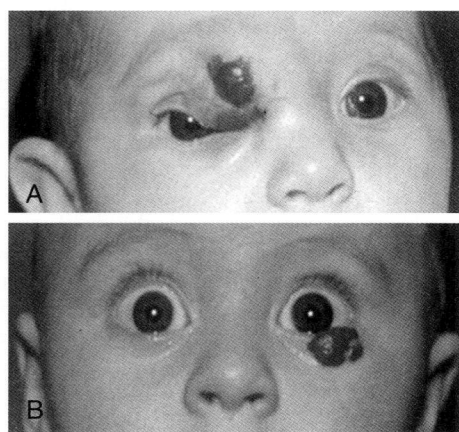

Fig. 43.21 *A,* A capillary hemangioma of the right upper eyelid and anterior orbit. This lesion necessitated treatment because it was causing amblyopia from astigmatism as a result of pressure against the globe and by occlusion of the visual axis. *B,* This capillary hemangioma of the left lower eyelid is not causing amblyopia and does not necessitate treatment unless it grows substantially.

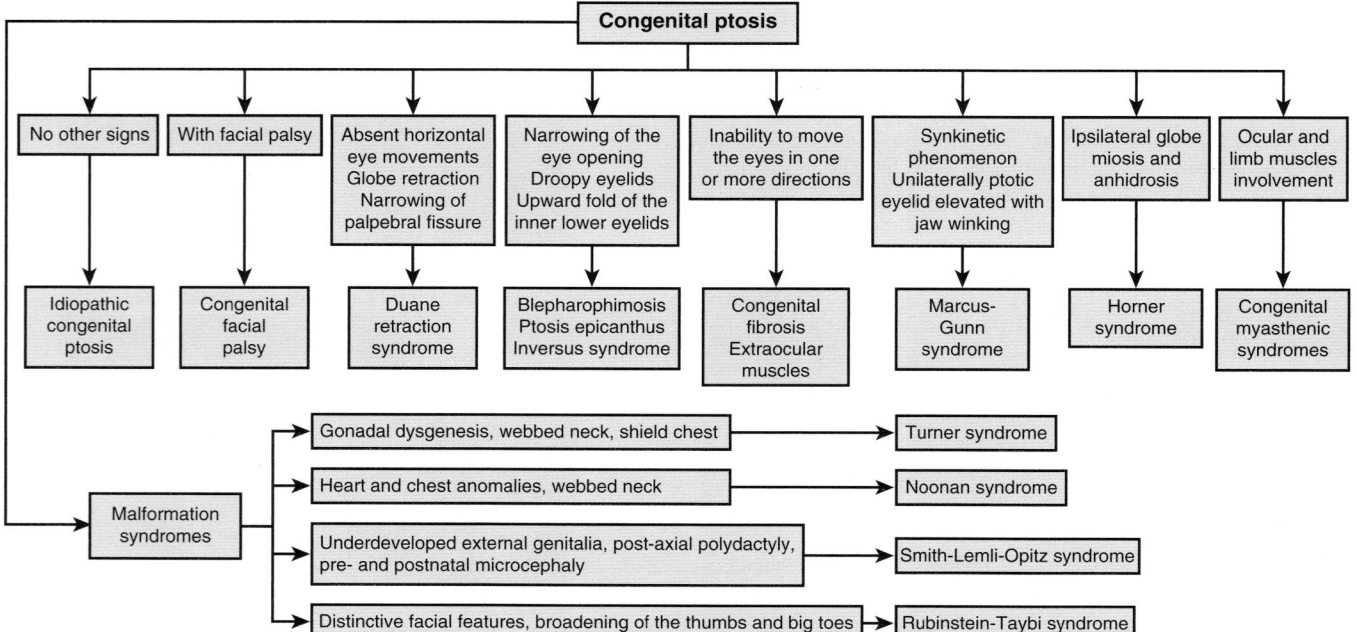

Fig. 43.22 Flow chart outlining congenital types of ptosis. (From Pavone P, Cho YC, Pratico AD, et al. Ptosis in childhood: a clinical sign of several disorders. *Medicine.* 2018 Sep;97[36]:e12124, Fig. 8A.)

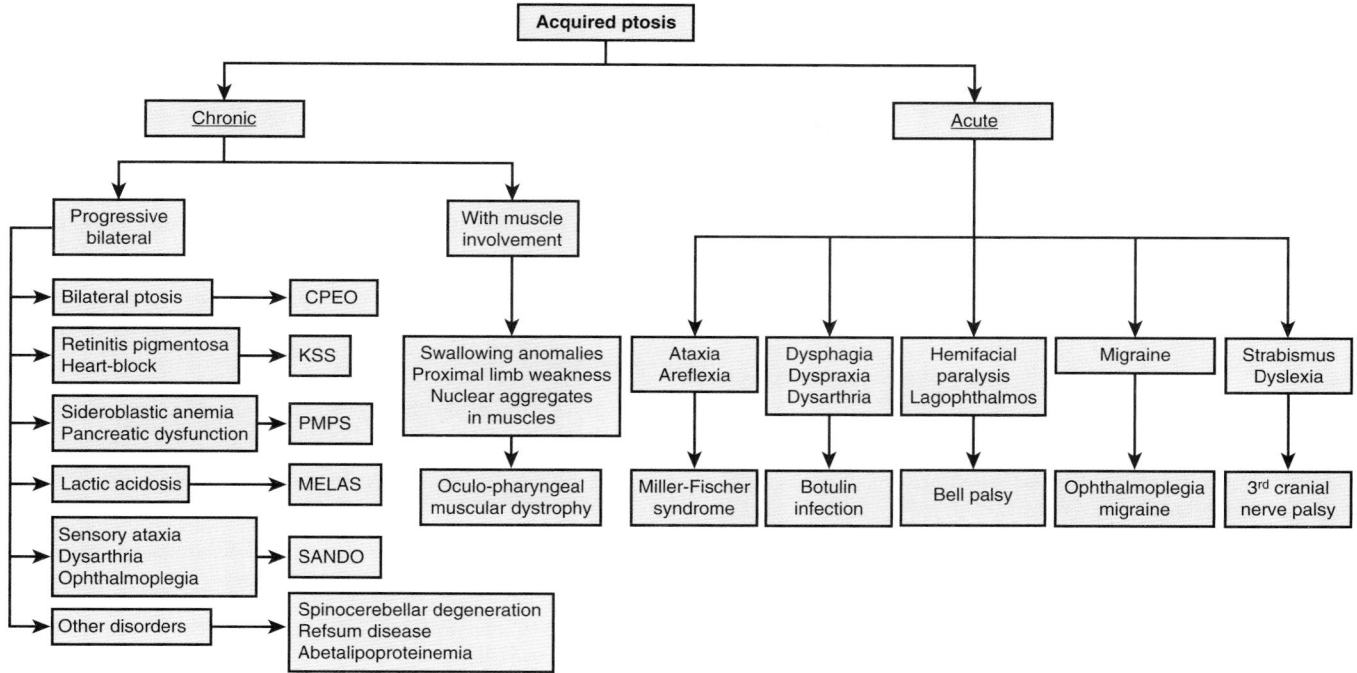

Fig. 43.23 Flow chart outlining acquired types of ptosis. CPEO, chronic progressive external ophthalmoplegia; KSS, Kearns-Sayre syndrome; MELAS, mitochondrial encephalopathy, lactic acidosis, and strokelike episodes; PMPS, Pearson marrow pancreas syndrome; SANDO, sensory ataxic neuropathy, dysarthria, and ophthalmoparesis. (From Pavone P, Cho YC, Pratico AD, et al. Ptosis in childhood: a clinical sign of several disorders. *Medicine.* 2018 Sep;97[36]:e12124, Fig. 8B.)

presentations. **Opsoclonus** (rapid, multidirectional eye movements) is a paraneoplastic syndrome associated with neuroblastoma and is not related to orbital involvement. The mean age of diagnosis of orbital metastasis of neuroblastoma is 2 years.

Other, less common orbital tumors in childhood are Ewing sarcoma, Burkitt lymphoma, leukemia, and Langerhans cell histiocytosis. Ewing sarcoma is the second most common solid tumor metastatic to the orbit (after neuroblastoma). Orbital involvement occurs in 1–2% of children with leukemia and this must be differentiated from orbital infections.

Nonspecific Orbital Inflammation/Idiopathic Orbital Inflammation/Orbital Pseudotumor

Nonspecific orbital inflammation (NSOI) is an acute or subacute benign idiopathic inflammatory process associated with multiple orbital structures. After thyroid-associated disease and lymphoproliferative disorders, it is the third most common noninfectious masslike inflammatory lesion of the orbit. It is unilateral in ~75% of patients who often present with periorbital edema, blepharoptosis, limited extraocular motion, pain, proptosis, conjunctival injection, or decreased visual acuity. There are five subtypes involving specific orbit tissues: dacryoadenitis (Fig. 43.24), myositis (Fig. 43.25), anterior orbit (Fig. 43.26), orbit apex (optic nerve) (Fig. 43.27), and diffuse. There is an association with IgG4-related disease, which may also manifest with inflammation and fibrosis in extraorbital tissue (pancreas, retroperitoneal); systemic IgG4-related disease is more common in patients with bilateral lacrimal gland involvement.

The differential diagnosis of NSOI includes sarcoidosis, granulomatosis with polyangiitis, lymphoma, and thyroid orbitopathy. Biopsy is not initially needed for patients with a typical presentation (usually myositis) or a higher risk (orbital apex-optic nerve). Therapy is usually initiated with systemic corticosteroids.

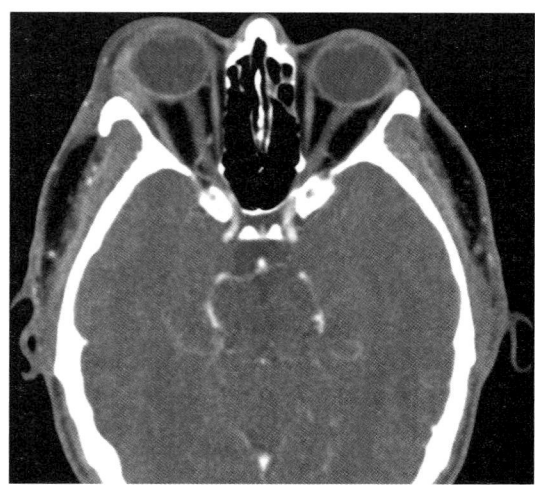

Fig. 43.24 Noncontrast axial CT study exhibiting right acute dacryoadenitis with inflammation adjacent to the lateral orbital wall and lateral rectus muscle. (From Maamari RN, Couch SM. Nonspecific orbital inflammation. *Adv Ophthalmol Optom.* 2018;3[1]:315–335, Fig. 3.)

OCULAR MANIFESTATIONS OF SYSTEMIC DISEASE

Neurologic Disease

Ocular abnormalities frequently accompany neurologic disease, and their detection can help in the localization and diagnosis of a specific condition. Abnormal findings of pupillary reaction, decreased visual acuity, or decreased color vision can indicate abnormities of the optic nerve, which can be associated with other neurologic conditions. An afferent pupillary defect is an important finding that may signify unilateral optic nerve disease. The condition may be intrinsic to the optic

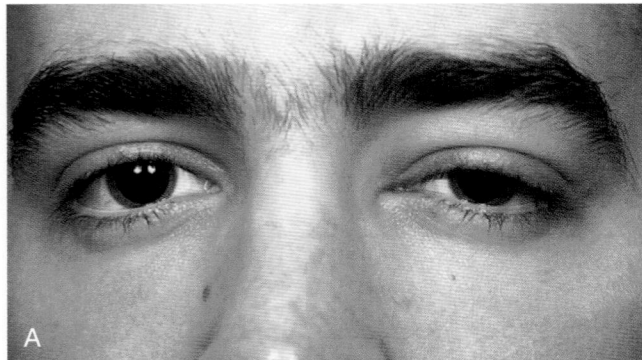

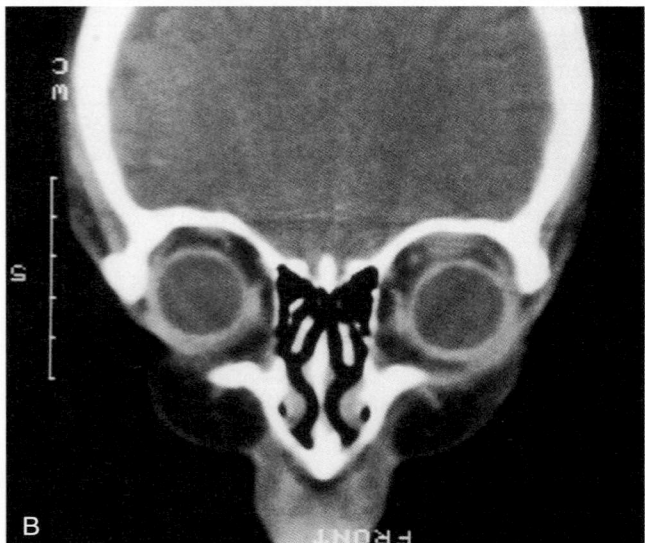

Fig. 43.25 Left superior rectus myositis in a 16-year-old boy. Ptosis *(A)* and pain limitation of upgaze with diplopia were the presenting signs; this was due to left superior rectus myositis shown as a thickened muscle complex on CT scan *(B)*. (Patient from the University of British Columbia.) (From Lambert SR, Lyons CJ, eds. *Taylor & Hoyt's Pediatric Ophthalmology and Strabismus.* 5th ed. Philadelphia: Elsevier; 2017:277, Fig. 30-8.)

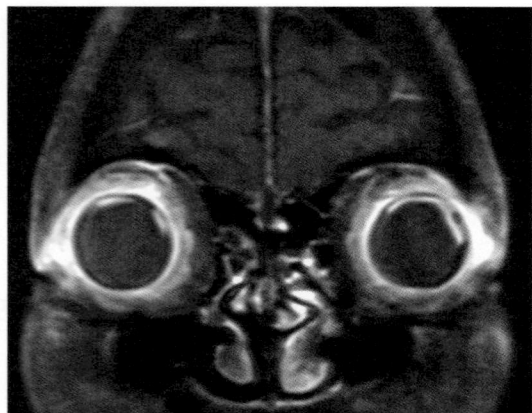

Fig. 43.26 Bilateral anterior orbital nonspecific orbital inflammation. Contrast-enhanced, T1-weighted, coronal MRI with fat suppression demonstrating bilateral scleritis and enhancement of the Tenon space. Dilated fundus examination also revealed bilateral choroidal effusions. (From Maamari RN, Couch SM. Nonspecific orbital inflammation. *Adv Ophthalmol Optom.* 2018;3[1]:315–335, Fig. 6.)

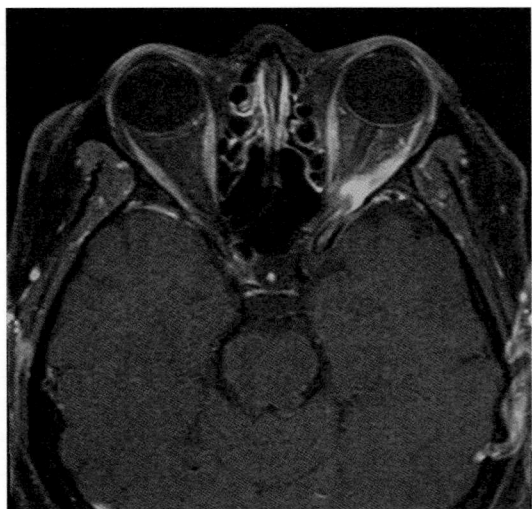

Fig. 43.27 Nonspecific orbital inflammation involving the orbital apex. Contrast-enhanced, T1-weighted, axial MRI with fat suppression showing inflammatory tissue at the left orbital apex resulting in compression and obliteration of the optic nerve. (From Maamari RN, Couch SM. Nonspecific orbital inflammation. *Adv Ophthalmol Optom.* 2018;3[1]:315–335 [Fig. 7, p. 322].)

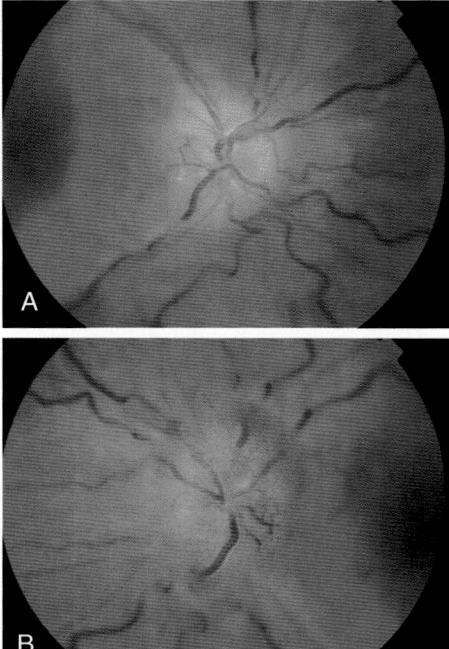

Fig. 43.28 Right *(A)* and left *(B)* fundi showing acute papilledema. (From Lambert SR, Lyons CJ, eds. *Hoyt and Taylor Pediatric Ophthalmology and Strabismus.* 4th ed. Philadelphia: Elsevier; 2013:593, Fig. 55.1.)

nerve such as a glioma in neurofibromatosis type 1, extrinsic such as an orbital tumor, applying pressure on the nerve, or inflammation of the optic nerve as seen with **optic neuritis** in MS, neuromyelitis optica, and ADEM. Color perception and the visual acuity of the affected eye are usually reduced in comparison with that of the normal eye. The presence of an afferent pupillary defect necessitates a comprehensive eye examination and imaging studies of the orbit and brain.

Optic nerve edema (Fig. 43.28) is a worrisome sign because of its association with conditions that cause increased intracranial pressure.

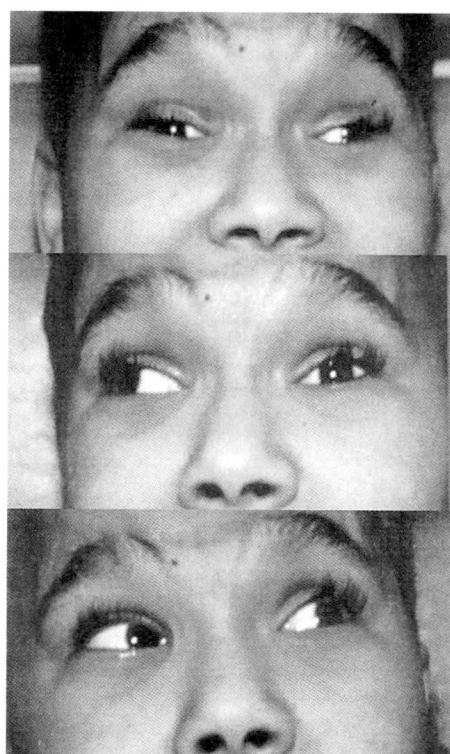

Fig. 43.29 Left third cranial nerve palsy. The boy has exotropia *(top)*, limitation of adduction of his left eye *(middle)*, and normal gaze to his left *(bottom)*.

The elevation of the optic nerve and blurring of the disk margins must be differentiated from optic nerve drusen, which can have similar clinical appearances. Autofluorescent photography and ultrasound (B-scan) of the optic nerves can help differentiate optic nerve edema and optic nerve drusen. Papilledema, swelling of the optic nerve as a result of increased intracranial pressure, is almost always bilateral. Visual acuity may be normal initially but decreases with chronic or severe optic nerve swelling. Color vision may be decreased prior to a decrease in visual acuity.

Strabismus of truly acute onset is most often incomitant and caused by paralysis of extraocular muscles innervated by the third or sixth cranial nerves. Cranial trauma, brain tumors, and viral infections are the most common causes of acute, incomitant strabismus in children. A sixth nerve palsy is of less localizing value than a third nerve palsy because of the more tortuous intracranial course of the sixth nerve. This nerve can be affected by direct pressure from a mass and indirectly by conditions that cause diffuse increased intracranial pressure. A patient with an acute sixth nerve paralysis typically has esotropia that increases when they gaze toward the affected side (see Fig. 43.8). The patient may have a compensatory face turn toward the side of the lesion to allow fusion and prevent diplopia. A third nerve paralysis usually causes exotropia and hypotropia of the involved eye (Fig. 43.29). There may also be ipsilateral ptosis and a dilated, nonreactive pupil. *A verbal child will typically complain of diplopia at the onset.* A general approach to an acquired diplopia is noted in Fig. 43.30.

The **neurocutaneous syndromes** are a group of inherited disorders featuring multiple, discrete lesions of two or more organ systems, most commonly the skin and brain. These include neurofibromatosis, tuberous sclerosis, angiomatosis of the retina and cerebellum (von Hippel–Lindau disease), and encephalofacial or encephalotrigeminal angiomatosis (Sturge-Weber syndrome).

Sometimes ataxia-telangiectasia, incontinentia pigmenti, and racemose angioma are included in neurocutaneous syndromes. Ocular involvement is common and may be a site of comorbidity or may serve as a marker for the overall condition. Lisch nodules are benign tan, smooth-surfaced lesions on the iris surface that look somewhat gelatinous and are seen in **neurofibromatosis** type 1 (NF-1). They are usually not present until 3 years and thereafter about 10% of patients develop Lisch nodules per year. They do not have malignant potential. Other ocular features of NF-1 are plexiform neurofibromas of the eyelid that give the eyelid margin a sigmoid shape and cause a variable amount of ptosis, astigmatism, and possibly amblyopia. Glaucoma is a significant problem in patients with NF-1. It is usually unilateral and associated with an ipsilateral plexiform neurofibroma of the upper eyelid. This is generally managed surgically. Visual prognosis in patients who develop glaucoma is poor.

Optic gliomas, such as low-grade pilocytic astrocytomas, have the potential to cause severe vision loss in patients with NF-1. The gliomas can involve one or both optic nerves as well as the optic chiasm. They are found prospectively in 15% of patients with NF-1 but cause visual symptoms such as vision loss or proptosis in only 1–5% of patients. Treatment of optic gliomas is reserved for lesions that are documented to be growing and causing visual morbidity, although it is difficult to determine which patients require treatment before vision loss occurs. NF-2 is much less common than NF-1 and involves primarily the acoustic nerves. Ocular involvement can consist of posterior lens opacities and hamartomas of the retina.

Tuberous sclerosis is an autosomal dominant disorder localized to chromosome 9. In children with tuberous sclerosis, angiofibromas of the eyelids and retinal lesions known as astrocytic hamartomas can occur but rarely cause significant problems with vision. The retinal lesions are not pathognomonic of tuberous sclerosis, inasmuch as similar lesions have been reported in NF-1 and in unaffected individuals.

Von Hippel–Lindau disease is autosomal dominant. Both benign and malignant tumors can occur in affected individuals as a result of a variant in a tumor suppressor gene. Hemangioblastomas of the retina can produce a lipid exudate in the retina as a result of leakage from the thin vessel walls. This can lead to vision loss and ultimately a retinal detachment. Symptoms of vision loss do not occur until extensive leakage or retinal detachment occurs. More than 65% of lesions can be treated effectively with laser photocoagulation. Because lesions are most effectively treated prior to the development of symptoms, children known to have von Hippel–Lindau disease should have regular eye examinations beginning at the age of 5 years.

Sturge-Weber syndrome results from a somatic pathologic genetic variant in *GNAQ*. Ocular involvement is common. Abnormalities of the ocular circulation can occur when the eyelids are affected. These abnormalities range from increased conjunctival vascularity to angiomas of the choroid. Choroidal angiomas usually remain asymptomatic in childhood but can thicken in adolescence and cause degeneration of the overlying retina. Glaucoma is the most serious ocular complication and occurs in 70% of affected patients. Regular eye examinations in infancy are necessary to rule out glaucoma. Treatment of glaucoma associated with Sturge-Weber syndrome may be difficult. Topical drops may be effective in initially lowering eye pressure, but the patient may eventually require surgical intervention.

Ataxia-telangiectasia syndrome is an autosomal recessive disorder. Oculomotor abnormalities may be early manifestations of this syndrome. In 90% of patients, telangiectasia develops in the conjunctiva in children between the ages of 3 and 5 years.

Incontinentia pigmenti syndrome is an X-linked dominant condition in which proliferative retinal vasculopathy develops in about 30% of affected patients. The retinal changes can mimic ROP with

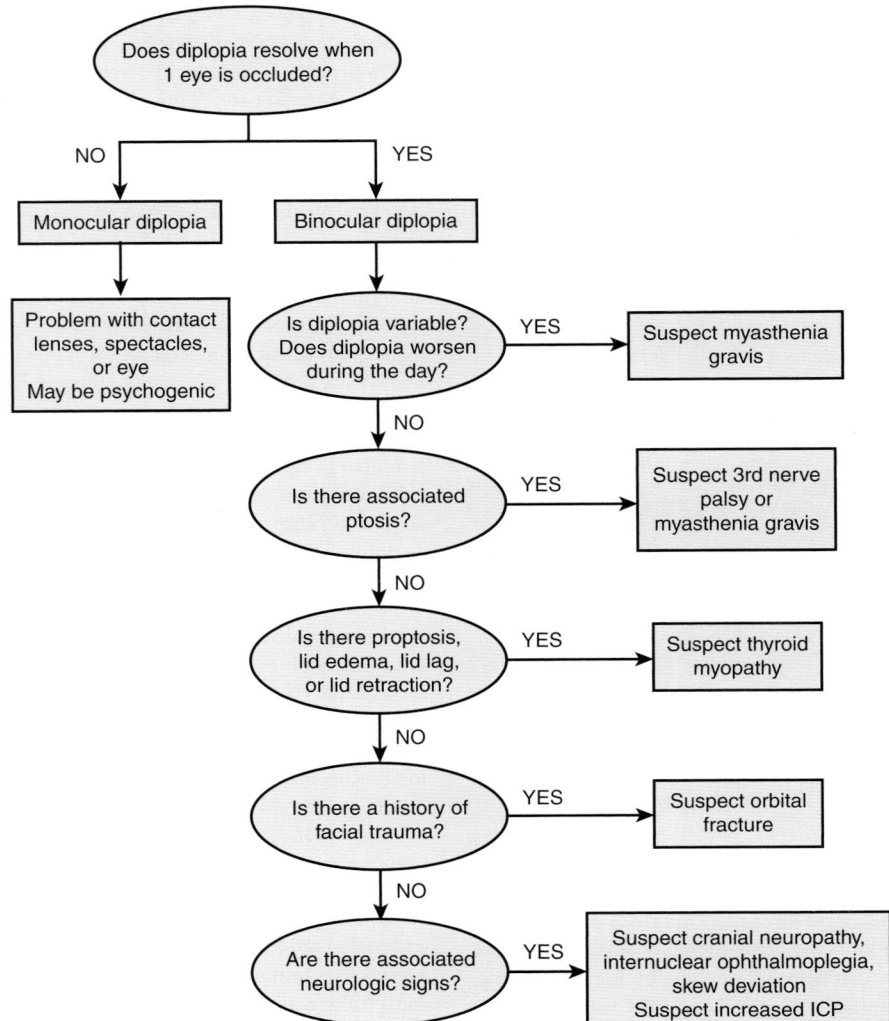

Fig. 43.30 General approach to diplopia. The clinician should first distinguish monocular from binocular diplopia and, in patients with binocular diplopia, address the five questions on the right side of the figure. Only then should the clinician identify which muscle is weak, although this is unnecessary if the clinician already suspects myasthenia (from fatigability) or full third nerve palsy (from weakness of the medial rectus, superior rectus, inferior rectus, and inferior oblique muscles, with or without a dilated pupil). Uncommon causes of diplopia and associated ptosis, not presented in the figure, are botulism, the Miller-Fisher variant of Guillain-Barré syndrome, and aberrant regeneration of the third nerve. Uncommon causes of diplopia and associated orbital findings (e.g., proptosis) are carotid-cavernous fistula (which causes an orbital bruit), orbital tumor, and pseudotumor. ICP, intracranial pressure. (From McGee S. *Evidence-Based Physical Diagnosis*. 3rd ed. Philadelphia: Elsevier; 2012:522, Fig. 57-1.)

incomplete peripheral retinal vascularization. Retinal detachment can occur. Treatment includes laser photocoagulation or cryotherapy, but these treatments have varying degrees of success.

In **Wyburn-Mason syndrome,** an arteriovenous malformation syndrome can affect the retina with shunting of blood directly from arteries to veins. Vision can be normal or markedly reduced, depending on the location of the lesion.

Dermatologic Disease

Albinism is a heterogeneous group of genetic disorders resulting from absence of melanin in the eye, skin, or both. Clinically, albinism is divided into ocular and oculocutaneous forms. Oculocutaneous albinism (OCA) results from variants in the tyrosinase gene (*TYR*) or *OCA1* gene. There are two subtypes and hair color can range from

blond to light brown as the most prevalent type of albinism worldwide. Ocular albinism is autosomal recessive or an X-linked gene variant in the *OCA1* gene. Ocular albinism mainly affects pigmentation in the visual system and the most common ocular finding is iris transillumination, which may be observable in a darkened room by placing a penlight against the lower eyelid and noting the red reflex and passage of light from both the pupil and the iris. Other frequent ocular findings are nystagmus, light fundus pigmentation (blonde fundus), foveal hypoplasia, and high refractive errors. Visual acuity usually ranges from 20/40 to 20/400. The **Chédiak-Higashi** and **Hermansky-Pudlak** syndromes can manifest features of albinism. If either of these conditions is suspected, hematologic consultation is recommended because of the lethal nature of these forms of albinism. All patients with OCA are at an increased risk of skin cancer and should be counseled as such.

Stevens-Johnson syndrome is an acute inflammatory condition affecting skin and mucous membranes. Drugs, particularly sulfonamide medications, are common precipitating factors. Microbial agents, especially *Mycoplasma pneumoniae*, have also been implicated in this condition. Ocular involvement, which occurs in half of the patients, consists of eyelid edema and ulceration, conjunctival injection with vesicle formation, and, in severe cases, conjunctival scar formation that may result in adhesions between the palpebral and bulbar conjunctiva (symblepharon). The severity of late ocular complications depends primarily on the extent of conjunctival involvement. Malposition of the eyelids with corneal irritation from inward-turned eyelashes (trichiasis) can occur from severe conjunctival scarring. The most serious complication is dry eye syndrome, caused by damage to the ducts of the lacrimal glands and obliteration of conjunctival mucus-forming cells (goblet cells). Eyelid surgery may be required, and the child with a dry eye may face a lifetime of needing ocular lubrication from artificial tears and ointments. Aggressive lubrication during the acute phase of the disease is recommended to keep tissues moist and prevent conjunctival adhesions. Treatments may include regular debridement of the fornices of the eye or placement of symblepharon rings or amniotic membranes in severe cases.

Hyperkeratotic disorders such as lamellar ichthyosis can cause scaling of the eyelids, ectropion, lagophthalmos, and exposure keratopathy. Although eyelid surgery may be required, the mainstay of treatment is ocular lubrication with artificial tears and ointments. **Connective tissue disorders** such as Marfan syndrome, Stickler syndrome, Ehlers-Danlos syndrome, and pseudoxanthoma elasticum (PXE) are associated with particular ocular abnormalities. Patients with Stickler syndrome, Marfan syndrome, and Ehlers-Danlos syndrome have myopic retinal degeneration and can develop retinal detachment. Lens subluxation is common in Marfan syndrome. Cracks in the Bruch membrane of the retina, known as angioid streaks, occur in 85% of patients with PXE, and 70% of these patients experience vision loss from hemorrhage, extension into the macula, choroidal sclerosis, and atrophy of the retinal pigment epithelium. Angioid streaks rarely occur before the second decade of life.

Skin disorders causing neoplasia such as juvenile xanthogranuloma can affect the eye, sometimes even in the absence of typical skin lesions. Ocular complications from juvenile xanthogranuloma occur most commonly in infants and consist of nodular tumors of the iris and ciliary body. The iris lesions have thin-walled vessels that are prone to bleeding and to causing a hyphema. Glaucoma and iridocyclitis can also occur. The iris lesions may respond to topical corticosteroids.

Hematologic Disorders

The **hemoglobinopathies** can have direct ocular consequences. Patients with hemoglobin SC or S thalassemia are more prone to retinal vascular occlusive disease because of a higher hematocrit and greater blood viscosity than are patients with hemoglobin SS, but retinal complications are frequently not seen until adolescence or early adulthood. Patients develop hemorrhages, angioid streaks, and arterial occlusions. Patients with sickle cell disease or sickle cell trait are at higher risk of complications of trauma, particularly hyphema. These patients may develop glaucoma, optic nerve damage, and artery occlusion in this setting and require close monitoring.

Leukemia in children is usually acute. All ocular structures may be affected by direct infiltration of leukemic cells, hemorrhage, or infection. Conjunctival thickening, hypopyon, corneal ulcers, iris infiltrates, retinal hemorrhages, and neovascularization may occur. Infiltration of the optic nerve can be difficult to distinguish from papilledema secondary to CNS relapse. Infectious processes may present with similar findings as leukemia and can be difficult to discern from leukemic infiltrates. Papilledema and intraocular infection are true emergencies as the findings not only threaten vision but also are highly correlated with CNS involvement. Prompt diagnosis and treatment are necessary.

Congenital Heart Disease

Eye disease can be related to congenital heart disease by association, which is not surprising because there is a temporal relationship between the embryogenesis of the heart and that of the eyes; an embryopathic insult may result in malformations of both systems. CHARGE syndrome is a result of a pathologic genetic variant in the CHD7 transcription regulator of tissue-specific genes. The effects are tissue and developmental stage dependent. Colobomas of the eyelid, iris, retina, choroid, and optic nerve occur. They are usually bilateral and the effects on vision are determined by the extent of the coloboma. If the macula is involved, the visual prognosis is poor. Congenital heart disease can be a cause of eye disease as a direct effect of complications such as cyanosis or systemic hypertension. Severe hypoxia can cause cortical visual impairment or damage to the optic nerve resulting in optic atrophy.

Gastrointestinal Disorders

Ocular manifestations of inherited metabolic abnormalities of the gastrointestinal system occur primarily in the cornea and retina. **Wilson disease** is an autosomal recessive disorder of copper metabolism. The excess copper is deposited in the liver, basal ganglia, cornea, and kidney. Liver damage and neurologic and psychiatric disorders result at a young age. The deposition of copper in the Descemet membrane of the cornea creates the Kayser-Fleischer ring, which is pathognomonic of the disease. Copper may also be deposited in the lens. The corneal deposition of copper is not generally symptomatic, but lens deposition may adversely affect vision.

Alagille syndrome, an autosomal dominant condition with intrahepatic bile duct hypoplasia, is associated with a peripheral corneal finding known as posterior embryotoxon. This finding consists of thickening and anterior displacement of the Schwalbe line, which is the peripheral extent of the Descemet membrane of the cornea. It can best be seen with a slit-lamp biomicroscope. Posterior embryotoxon occurs in more than 90% of patients with Alagille syndrome, but because it also occurs in up to 15% of normal individuals, it is not pathognomonic for this syndrome.

Inflammatory bowel disease also can be associated with ocular disease. Anterior uveitis occurs in both Crohn disease and ulcerative colitis. Uveitis is diagnosed in almost half of cases of Crohn disease and fewer in ulcerative colitis. In turn, untreated chronic uveitis can lead to cataracts, glaucoma, and retinal edema. Conjunctivitis, keratitis, and retinal vasculitis are less frequent complications of these diseases.

Genitourinary Disease

Oculorenal syndromes may result from chromosomal abnormality syndromes or from inherited metabolic or developmental defects. The **Wilms tumor** gene *WT1* lies near the *PAX6* gene locus on 11p13. A chromosomal deletion of both results in Wilms tumor and aniridia. A larger deletion may result in WAGR syndrome (*W*ilms tumor, sporadic *a*niridia, *g*enitourinary malformations, and mental *r*etardation). Any child with nonfamilial aniridia is at risk for Wilms tumor and needs appropriate genetic evaluation.

The **Bardet-Biedl syndrome** is an autosomal recessive disorder combining retinal dystrophy, polydactyly, obesity, renal abnormalities, and hypogenitalism. An ERG may be the earliest means of detecting the cone-rod dystrophy in suspected cases. Visual acuity and the funduscopic appearance may be normal in early childhood. Vision may then decrease and pigmentary retinopathy, which appears around the age of 8 years, becomes more prominent with age.

Cystinosis is also an autosomal recessive disorder of cystine transport from lysosomes that leads to intracellular accumulation of cystine in many tissues, including the eyes and kidneys. Cystine crystals accumulate in the anterior layer of the cornea beginning in the first year of life. This can cause photophobia, which can be severe. Retinal deposits of cystine can lead to focal degeneration of the retinal pigment epithelium. Frequent topical administration of cysteamine drops (6–12 times per day) can clear the cornea of cystine crystals and relieve ocular discomfort.

Alport syndrome is an X-linked syndrome characterized by nephritis, hearing loss, and ocular signs, particularly of the lens. An "oil droplet" appearance can be seen in the pupil with an ophthalmoscope. This represents an abnormality in the anterior capsule of the lens, anterior lenticonus, which can sometimes be associated with a cataract. Perimacular flecks are frequently present in the retina but do not tend to reduce visual acuity.

The **Lowe oculocerebrorenal syndrome** is also an X-linked disorder comprising congenital cataracts, intellectual disability, and renal tubular dysfunction. Glaucoma develops in a high proportion of affected boys and men. The carrier state can frequently be detected in girls and women by the appearance of numerous punctate opacities of the lens.

Endocrine Disease

Optic nerve hypoplasia is the most common congenital optic nerve anomaly. It can involve only a segment of the optic nerve. A superior segmental hypoplasia sometimes occurs in children of diabetic mothers. Optic nerve hypoplasia can occur with other CNS abnormalities. Patients with optic nerve hypoplasia may have **septo-optic dysplasia,** which denotes the absence of the septum pellucidum and agenesis of the corpus callosum or additional findings including pituitary abnormalities and cerebral hemisphere abnormalities. Evaluation of hypothalamic and pituitary functions is indicated in patients found to have pituitary abnormalities on imaging or if there is clinical suspicion of endocrine abnormalities such as neonatal jaundice, hypoglycemia, or difficulty with temperature control.

Diabetes mellitus (DM) results in retinopathy at some point in nearly all persons with insulin-dependent type 1 diabetes. The prevalence of retinopathy is directly proportional to the duration of disease after puberty. It rarely occurs within 5 years of diagnosis, occurs in about 50% of patients at 7 years after diagnosis, and is seen in 90% at 15 years after diagnosis. Funduscopic signs of diabetic retinopathy are microaneurysms, retinal hemorrhages, cotton wool spots, and hard exudates. Proliferative diabetic retinopathy with neovascularization is uncommon in children. Intensive glucose control as monitored by hemoglobin A_{1c} decreases the incidence and progression of diabetic retinopathy. Type 2 DM patients are more likely to develop diabetic retinopathy at a younger age. Screening for diabetic retinopathy can be done by dilated eye exam or retinal photography. In type 1 DM, screening should start by age 11 or at the onset of puberty, younger when the patient has had DM for a minimum of 3 years. Children with type 2 DM should undergo a dilated eye exam at the time of diagnosis.

Diabetic cataracts caused by sorbitol accumulation in the lens are also complications of DM in children. Refractive changes such as myopia can occur with rapid rises in blood sugar because of osmotic changes in the lens.

Thyroid ophthalmopathy related to **Graves disease** occurs in children much less frequently than in adults. It can be a cause of proptosis, lid edema, eyelid retraction, or restrictive strabismus due to lymphocytic infiltration of the muscles.

Infectious Diseases

Intrauterine or maternally transmitted infections can cause tissue damage or malformation. The common types of congenital infections are the **TORCH**. The infectious agent, *T. gondii*, is acquired transplacentally or postnatally and has particular affinity for the CNS, including the retina. Chorioretinitis and uveitis may occur and resolution leaves scarring. Reactivation can occur and thus serial eye examinations are necessary. The macula is commonly involved, and vision can be quite poor. Intrauterine rubella infection has become a rarity in the United States because of immunization with the measles-mumps-rubella vaccine. A fetus infected transplacentally in the first trimester of pregnancy is prone to multiple congenital defects, including heart disease, microcephaly with intellectual disability, and deafness. Ocular sequelae include cataracts, glaucoma, and chorioretinitis. Cataracts may be unilateral. Permanent visual impairment despite cataract surgery is common in these children. **Cytomegalovirus (CMV)** is the most common congenital infection in humans occurring in 1% of infants, although over 90% are asymptomatic and may not require treatment. Ophthalmic manifestations include retinochoroiditis, optic nerve anomalies, microphthalmos, cataract, and uveitis. CMV retinitis can be acquired in children who are immunocompromised.

Herpes simplex virus (HSV) may be acquired during passage through the birth canal or by close contact. Skin lesions on the eyelids (Fig. 43.31), keratoconjunctivitis, uveitis, or retinitis may occur. Acute retinal necrosis may occur in conjunction with CNS involvement. Keratitis is treated with topical antivirals, while systemic disease or retinitis is treated with oral or intravenous antiviral therapy. **Congenital syphilis** may occur following maternal infection. Early eye involvement is rare and symptoms may occur as late as adolescence. Chorioretinitis appears as a salt-and-pepper granularity. Uveitis, glaucoma, or interstitial keratitis may occur. Affected children are treated with intravenous penicillin G and monitored until serologic tests become nonreactive or the titer has decreased fourfold.

Ophthalmia neonatorum is defined as conjunctival infection or inflammation occurring in the first month of life. Almost any bacterial pathogen can cause conjunctivitis in a newborn, but infection with *Neisseria gonorrhoeae* is of particular concern because it produces a hyperacute, profusely purulent conjunctivitis that can lead to corneal perforation and blindness. The U.S. Preventive Services Task Force recommends prophylactic topical 1% tetracycline or 0.5% erythromycin ointment administered within 24 hours after birth for prevention of gonococcal neonatorum. A 2.5% solution of povidone-iodine is used effectively and inexpensively in other countries but has not been approved for this use in the United States at this

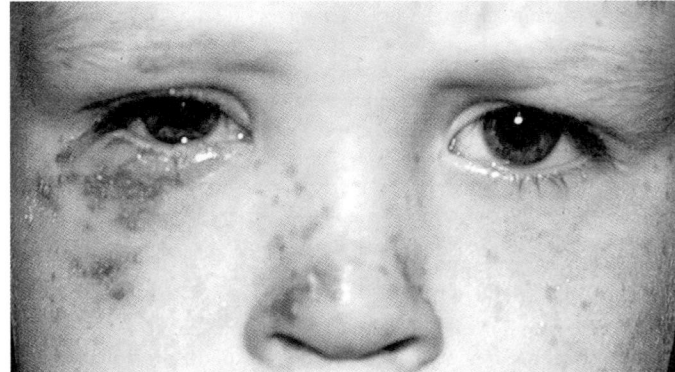

Fig. 43.31 Vesicular eruptions of the right lower eyelid and the right side of the nose, caused by primary herpes simplex infection. The cornea was not involved.

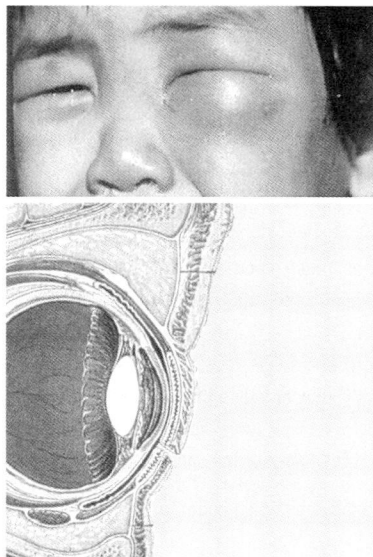

Fig. 43.32 Preseptal cellulitis in a young girl. The infection is confined to the space anterior to the superior and inferior orbital septa and does not involve the orbit.

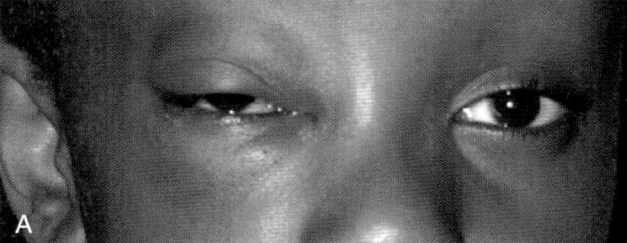

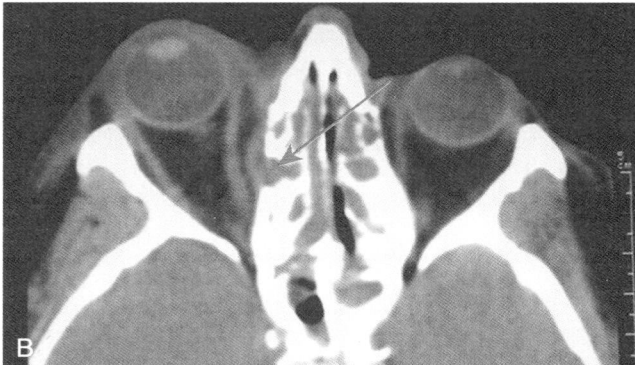

Fig. 43.33 *A,* A 7-year-old child with right orbital cellulitis, proptosis, white eye, limitation of eye movements, but no optic nerve compromise. *B,* CT scan shows ethmoid sinusitis, significant proptosis, and a small medial subperiosteal abscess *(arrow)*. He was successfully treated with antibiotics alone and did not need surgical intervention. (From Lambert SR, Lyons CJ, eds. *Taylor & Hoyt's Pediatric Ophthalmology and Strabismus.* 5th ed. Philadelphia: Elsevier; 2017:95, Fig. 14.11.)

time. *Chlamydia trachomatis* (also known as trachoma–inclusion conjunctivitis or TRIC) is a common cause of neonatal conjunctivitis and is acquired from an infected cervix during delivery. Because this organism can also cause pneumonia, systemic treatment with oral erythromycin is indicated for treatment. In a child presenting with ophthalmia neonatorum it is important to obtain the history of whether prophylaxis has been given, particularly in cases of home births, where this is unlikely. Evaluation with Gram and Giemsa stains and bacterial cultures are indicated. Polymerase chain reaction (PCR) testing can be done for suspicion of HSV infection. *Chlamydia* can be diagnosed by culture, fluorescent antibody-staining techniques, or enzyme immunoassays.

Preseptal cellulitis, defined as infection confined to the eyelid tissues anterior to the orbital septum, is a common infection in children and needs to be distinguished from infection involving the orbit (Fig. 43.32). Preseptal infections may result from trauma and insect bites involving the eyelids, severe conjunctivitis, primary bacteremia, or upper respiratory infection, or they may spread to the eyelids from the paranasal sinuses. The affected eyelids are swollen and red, and the infection can spread further into the eyebrow, forehead, and cheek. Proptosis and limitation or pain of eye movements do not occur in preseptal cellulitis, but confirmation of this can be problematic because of the difficulty of opening the eye. *S. aureus,* group A streptococcus, and *S. pneumoniae* are the most common pathogens. Patients with signs and symptoms of systemic toxicity should be hospitalized for intravenous antibiotics; milder cases of preseptal cellulitis may be managed with oral antibiotics as long as appropriate follow-up is ensured.

Orbital cellulitis is an infection of the orbit that involves the tissues posterior to the orbital septum. Most frequently, this is a result of spread of infection from the ethmoid or frontal sinuses. Ocular signs include eyelid edema and erythema, proptosis, and inferior and lateral displacement of the globe with limited eye movements. Ocular movement is painful; visual activity may be reduced. If orbital cellulitis is suspected, CT of the orbit and sinuses is indicated. Children younger than 9 years are more likely to have an infection caused by a single aerobic pathogen, whereas children older than 9 years may have complex infections with multiple pathogens. Often, orbital cellulitis begins as

a subperiosteal abscess that forms in the potential space between the periorbital (analogous to the periosteum of long bones) and the orbital bones (Fig. 43.33). Left untreated, this space-occupying mass can apply pressure to the optic nerve and cause permanent damage to vision. It can also spread into the intracranial space and result in a cavernous sinus thrombosis, a subdural empyema, or cerebral abscess. Systemic toxicity is quite common and severe with orbital cellulitis. Most children younger than 9 years who have small- to medium-sized subperiosteal abscesses can be treated successfully with broad-spectrum intravenous antibiotics (ceftriaxone and vancomycin, ampicillin/sulbactam, or piperacillin/tazobactam). Close observation with periodic checks of vision and pupillary function is important in the first 24–48 hours of treatment. Older children, those with large subperiosteal abscesses, and children who fail to respond to intravenous antibiotics within 48 hours require surgical drainage of the abscess. Emergency drainage is indicated in a patient of any age where there is compromise of the optic nerve.

NYSTAGMUS

Nystagmus is defined as an involuntary rhythmic, to-and-fro movement of the eyes. Horizontal nystagmus is the most common form of nystagmus, but vertical nystagmus and torsional nystagmus also occur (Table 43.18). Nystagmus may be congenital or acquired. Gaze positions can affect the eye movement. Congenital nystagmus is somewhat of a misnomer because the abnormal eye movements are generally not noted until an infant is 1 or 2 months of age, when the fixation reflex becomes established. The etiologies of nystagmus are varied. A child presenting with infantile nystagmus without neurologic symptoms is more likely to have an ocular etiology than neurologic. Non-nystagmus eye movements are noted in Table 43.19.

TABLE 43.18   Specific Patterns of Nystagmus

Pattern	Description	Associated Conditions
Latent nystagmus	Conjugate jerk nystagmus toward viewing eye	Congenital vision defects, occurs with occlusion of eye
Manifest latent nystagmus	Fast jerk to viewing eye	Strabismus, congenital idiopathic nystagmus
Periodic alternating	Cycles of horizontal and horizontal-rotary movements that change direction	Caused by both visual and neurologic conditions
Seesaw nystagmus	One eye rises and intorts as other eye falls and extorts	Usually associated with optic chiasm defects
Retraction nystagmus	Eyes jerk back into orbit or toward each other	Caused by pressure on mesencephalic tegmentum (Parinaud syndrome)
Gaze-evoked nystagmus	Jerk nystagmus in direction of gaze	Caused by medications, brainstem lesion, or labyrinthine dysfunction
Gaze-paretic nystagmus	Eyes jerk back to maintain eccentric gaze	Cerebellar disease
Downbeat nystagmus	Fast-phase beating downward	Posterior fossa disease, drugs
Upbeat nystagmus	Fast-phase beating upward	Brainstem and cerebellar disease, and some visual conditions
Vestibular nystagmus	Horizontal-torsional or horizontal jerks	Vestibular system dysfunction
Asymmetric or monocular nystagmus	Pendular vertical nystagmus	Disease of retina and visual pathways
Spasmus nutans	Fine, rapid, pendular nystagmus	Torticollis, head nodding; idiopathic or gliomas of visual pathways

TABLE 43.19   Specific Patterns of Non-Nystagmus Eye Movements

Pattern	Description	Associated Conditions
Opsoclonus	Multidirectional conjugate movements of varying rate and amplitude	Hydrocephalus, diseases of brainstem and cerebellum, neuroblastoma
Ocular dysmetria	Overshoot of eyes on rapid fixation	Cerebellar dysfunction
Ocular flutter	Horizontal oscillations with forward gaze and sometimes with blinking	Cerebellar disease, hydrocephalus, or central nervous system neoplasm
Ocular bobbing	Downward jerk of eyes from primary gaze; eyes remain for a few seconds, then drift back	Pontine disease
Ocular myoclonus	Rhythmic to-and-fro pendular oscillations of the eyes, with synchronous nonocular muscle movement	Damage to red nucleus, inferior olivary nucleus and ipsilateral dentate nucleus

Idiopathic infantile motor nystagmus syndrome (INS) in some patients is associated with variants in the *GPR143* gene, which is an X-linked recessive disorder that also produces isolated ocular albinism. Patients with idiopathic infantile nystagmus with this variant do not have decreased ocular pigmentation. In these patients, visual acuity is only moderately impaired, and the fundus examination findings and the ERG are normal. Usually an affected individual will have a null point or a preferred position in which the eye movements are minimized. This may affect the head position as the patient tries to keep the eyes in the null point. In patients with INS there is often dampening or quieting of the nystagmus with convergence. Vision may be quite good (20/40 or better) in the patient's preferred gaze and head position. Sometimes surgery is done on the eye muscles to move them into a position such that the head is straighter. A family history of nystagmus can frequently be ascertained.

Congenital sensory nystagmus occurs with disorders that impair normal image formation (bilateral congenital cataracts) or image processing in both eyes (a retinal dystrophy or bilateral optic nerve atrophy or hypoplasia). Eye movements may be searching and there is no null point. Visual acuity is more severely impaired than in idiopathic congenital nystagmus (20/200 or less), and visual loss may be progressive in some instances. The evaluation of a child with congenital nystagmus entails a thorough health and family history, a general physical examination, and an eye examination by an ophthalmologist with expertise in pediatric eye disorders. Electroretinography, VEPs, or optical coherence tomography (OCT) may be useful in establishing a specific diagnosis.

A cranial MRI scan is indicated when the optic nerves are anomalous, the child is delayed or has neurologic abnormalities, or the nystagmus is acquired. Early determination of the etiology of nystagmus is important with the availability of gene therapy treatments for specific retinal dystrophies. Gene therapy for Leber congenital amaurosis is U.S. Food and Drug Administration approved for children as young as 1 year old, and multiple clinical trials for other retinal dystrophy therapies are ongoing. **Acquired nystagmus** is less common than congenital nystagmus. Nystagmus that is truly acquired beyond the first few months of life is of concern and may represent a significant neurologic abnormality. It may be caused by CNS disorders, particularly of the cerebellum, brainstem, or suprasellar region. In children, the most common tumor causing acquired nystagmus is a craniopharyngioma. Vertically oriented nystagmus is also of concern; it may be associated with the Arnold-Chiari malformation or with pharmacologic agents such as lithium, tranquilizers, or anticonvulsants.

Spasmus nutans is a special form of acquired nystagmus with onset in the first 2 years of life. The usual triad of findings consists of nystagmus (often a shimmering type of nystagmus that is frequently asymmetric or even monocular), head nodding, and torticollis. This form of nystagmus is generally benign and disappears by the age of 3–4 years. In some cases, spasmus nutans can be associated with chiasmal or suprachiasmal lesions or retinal dystrophies. Neuroradiologic investigation is indicated.

Opsoclonus is a special form of eye movement abnormality that is not truly nystagmus in that the bizarre, seemingly random oscillations of the eyes are not rhythmic and are frequently multivectorial. The most common cause of opsoclonus in children is acute cerebellar ataxia. The child presents with "dancing eyes and dancing feet." Opsoclonus can occur also with occult neuroblastoma, as a paraneoplastic phenomenon, with viral encephalitis, and with hydrocephalus.

OCULAR TRAUMA

Trauma is a major cause of acquired visual loss in children. Ninety percent of trauma cases are preventable and 50% occur in the home. The nature of the traumatic injury varies by age but there is a persistent male preponderance. In school-aged children, sports-related injuries are the most common cause of ocular injury, accounting for 25% of hospitalizations. There is some effort to reduce injuries by legislation. The incidence of eye injuries from ice hockey are almost zero since the institution of mandatory face masks in children playing organized hockey. Projectile injuries from firearms, air guns, and fireworks are relatively frequent in the United States; however, these injuries are very rare in countries without easy access to guns or fireworks.

The extent of the eye examination is determined by the child's level of cooperation. If the circumstances of the injury suggest a high likelihood of a perforating injury (from a sharp object that could go through the cornea or sclera), the eye should not be forced open but rather should be covered with a protective shield to prevent further injury until the child can be seen by an ophthalmologist and an exam under anesthesia can be done if necessary. If a perforating injury is considered unlikely (a blunt or scratching type of injury), a sterile, topical ophthalmic anesthetic agent can be applied to the eye to reduce surface pain, which is a major cause of the child's reluctance to open the eye. The eye can then be inspected for foreign bodies or corneal abrasion. Fluorescein dye may be of help in diagnosing a corneal abrasion. The fluorescein may have a linear pattern of staining that suggests a foreign body may be on the tarsal conjunctiva under the upper eyelid and during an eye blink the cornea is being abraded. Lid eversion is needed to investigate this possibility. The inferior fornix should also be inspected for foreign bodies.

Corneal or conjunctival foreign bodies can sometimes be irrigated out of the eye. Otherwise, the foreign body may be removed at a slit-lamp using topical anesthesia if the patient is cooperative. If not, the patient will require anesthesia. Management of a corneal abrasion entails relief of pain, prevention of infection, and promotion of healing of the corneal epithelium. Ibuprofen or similar analgesics are usually sufficient for pain relief. Topical anesthesia, while used in the office, should not be used at home as it prevents epithelial healing and can be toxic to the cornea with longer-term use. A drop of a cycloplegic agent (cyclopentolate) may provide comfort by relieving ciliary spasm. Application of a topical antibiotic ointment such as erythromycin helps prevent infection and provides lubrication to the ocular surface to allow the new epithelium to form and adhere to the basement membrane of the cornea. Patching the eye has not been shown to be of any additional benefit. Close follow-up is indicated to make sure that the cornea is healing and has not developed an infection that could lead to a corneal ulcer. Most abrasions heal completely within 24–48 hours.

Hyphema

Any child with blunt trauma to the eye should be evaluated for blood in the anterior chamber of the eye, known as a hyphema (Fig. 43.34). The visual acuity of the injured eye should be measured if possible. The anterior segment and pupillary function should be assessed if

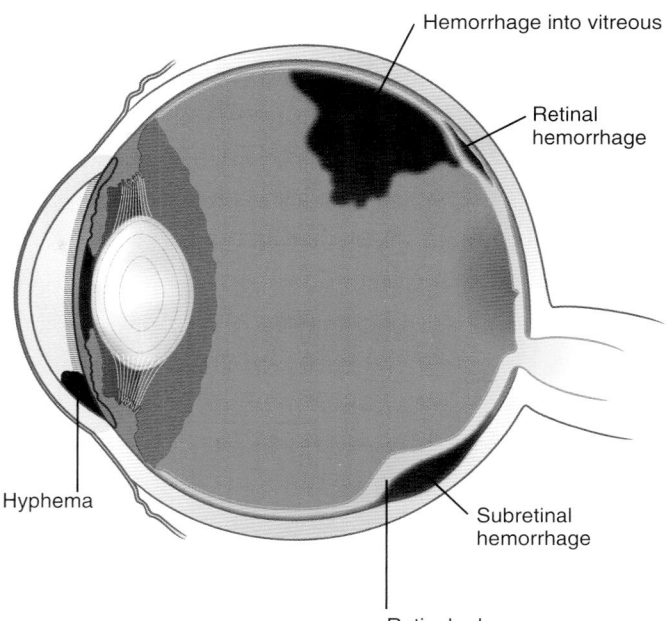

Fig. 43.34 Various types of ocular hemorrhage after blunt trauma to the globe. (From Reilly BM. *Practical Strategies in Outpatient Medicine*. 2nd ed. Philadelphia: WB Saunders; 1991:68.)

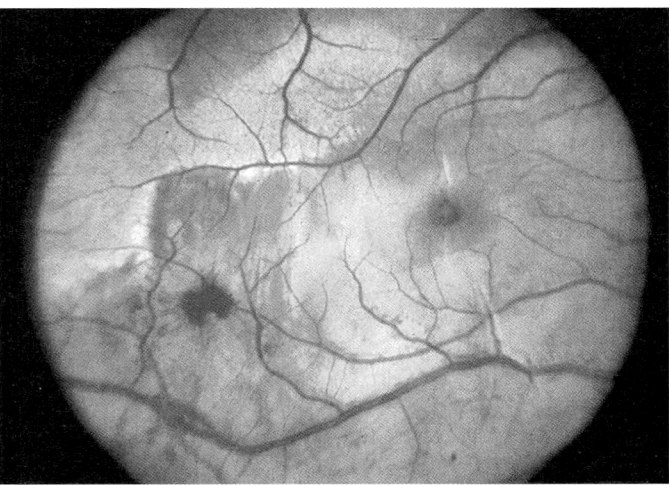

Fig. 43.35 Hemorrhage and edema of the retina from blunt ocular trauma (commotio retinae).

the hyphema only partially fills the anterior chamber. Fundoscopy should be attempted to look for associated retinal hemorrhage, edema (Fig. 43.35; also see Fig. 43.34), or detachment. The view of the retina may be obscured by blood. If necessary, ultrasound can be used to determine if the retina is attached. Usually the blood will resolve if the patient can limit their activity. *NSAIDs should be avoided.* The complications of hyphema include glaucoma, corneal blood staining, and rebleeding. The glaucoma may be managed initially with topical medications but the blood may need to be washed out of the anterior chamber surgically if the intraocular pressure cannot be controlled, blood is not resolving, or corneal blood staining is severe and threatening vision.

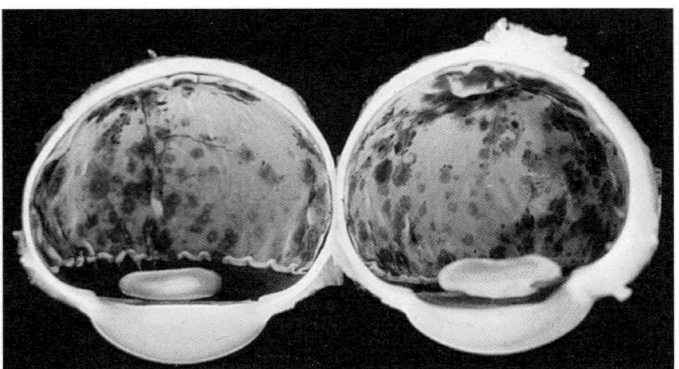

Fig. 43.36 Gross pathologic specimen from an infant who died of shaken baby syndrome. Note the diffuse retinal hemorrhages.

Eye Injuries in Child Abuse

In cases of child abuse, the presenting sign may involve the eye. Ocular injuries are also detected in the course of examining many other child abuse injuries. Blunt injuries to the eyelids and anterior segment of the eye from fingers, fists, or belts may cause eyelid ecchymosis, subconjunctival hemorrhage, hyphema, cataract, and lens dislocation. The finding of such an injury should alert the physician to the possibility of child abuse. Abusive head trauma is caused by forceful acceleration and deceleration motion such as shaking, which results in subdural hemorrhage and retinal or vitreous hemorrhages (Fig. 43.36). The vitreous is adherent to the retina and the traction of the moving vitreous results in multiple retinal hemorrhages, often in all layers of the retina. In severe cases, the optic nerve may be avulsed. Vitreous or retinal hemorrhage may take a long time to resolve and the child is at risk for amblyopia during the time the vision is obscured by blood. In cases of persistent hemorrhage, a vitrectomy may need to be done to clear the blood in the visual axis. Cortical brain damage also has a role in limiting visual function. Fewer than half of the patients diagnosed with abusive head trauma with retinal or vitreous hemorrhage see better than 20/40 after recovery.

FUNCTIONAL VISION LOSS

Some patients complain of vision loss or blurring or other visual disturbances (seeing spots, colors, or patterns) while the eye exam is normal. Functional visual disturbances occur most commonly in girls of ages 8–15 years. The key to confirming functional vision loss is to demonstrate objective findings that indicate better vision than the subjective responses. The patient's responses to visual acuity testing are frequently inconsistent. Stereoacuity testing may demonstrate better visual acuity than the patient is reporting. There are several examining techniques that the ophthalmologist can employ to get this information. There are also objective tests available to further delineate etiologies of possible vision loss; however, these are rarely needed. These include imaging tests such as OCT, fluorescein angiogram, ERG, or VEPs. The relationship of functional vision loss to true psychologic disease is unclear but it is worth keeping in mind that there is a higher incidence of functional vision loss in children who are experiencing psychologic stressors. Some children willfully complain of vision loss because they want glasses. The treatment should consist of reassurance. It may be of benefit to refer the patient to a psychiatrist if the symptoms do not subside.

VISUAL COMPLAINTS OF CHILDREN

Frequently, a child is brought to the pediatrician because of a subjective visual complaint from the child rather than because of an abnormality observed by a parent. Symptoms associated with reading are common and include seeing blurred print, words "swimming" together, and skipping words or lines. Other children complain primarily of blurred distance vision. Uncommon visual phenomena may include seeing colored lights, objects appearing larger or smaller, seeing spots, and double vision. Eye pain localized to one or both eyes is also common. There may be physiologic explanations for each of the complaints, and the child is usually interested in an explanation of the reason proposed for their complaint. A careful history of the exact nature of the complaint and any associated concerns should be sought and a screening eye examination performed. Specifically, distance and near visual acuity should be measured in each eye. A cover test or stereopsis test rules out manifest strabismus. An external eye examination may reveal a reason for eye pain (conjunctival injection, tearing, corneal abrasion, foreign body). Pupillary reactions should be assessed. Fundoscopy should be done to evaluate optic nerve and retinal status. A color vision test may be helpful. Having the child read an age-appropriate passage may reveal information about the child's reading ability and the severity of the reading complaint. If the examination is normal, simple reassurance may ease the concerns of the child and parent, particularly if combined with an offer to follow up on the complaint if it persists or if the parent notes objective changes in the child's eyes. If difficulty reading persists despite correction of any refractive error and an otherwise normal eye exam, the child may have learning disabilities that warrant further evaluation. Behavioral vision therapy has not been proven to improve reading skills, learning disabilities, or dyslexia and is not recommended.

▌ SUMMARY AND RED FLAGS

Ocular manifestations of vision loss, strabismus, and nystagmus may be caused by isolated ocular pathologic processes or by significant systemic disease. Vision screening and basic evaluations done in the pediatrician's office are important for detection of vision loss. Impaired visual function resulting from strabismus, cataracts, or other conditions may produce amblyopia and blindness. It is important to detect amblyopia because in most cases, amblyopia is reversible if discovered early and treated appropriately. Symptoms and signs that suggest potentially life- or vision-threatening diseases are listed in Table 43.20.

TABLE 43.20 Concerning Symptoms and Signs That Should Raise Red Flags

Symptom or Sign	Most Worrisome or Urgent Cause
Leukocoria	Retinoblastoma
Acute onset of strabismus	Cranial nerve palsy from brain tumor, ↑ICP
Acute vision loss	Compression or infiltration of optic nerve by an orbital or intracranial lesion
Proptosis	Rhabdomyosarcoma
Sudden onset of ptosis	Third nerve palsy from tumor, ↑ICP
Severe progressive headaches	↑ICP
Black eye	Trauma with associated hyphema
Light sensitivity	Uveitis
Head tilt or turn	Cranial nerve palsy causing strabismus, ↑ICP
Loss of corneal luster	Corneal edema from glaucoma or uveitis
Purulent conjunctivitis in a newborn	Gonococcal infection
Acquired anisocoria	Horner syndrome caused by cervical neuroblastoma, ↑ICP
Bilateral cataracts in a newborn	Galactosemia
Retinal hemorrhage in an infant or toddler	Child abuse
Onset of nystagmus after early infancy	Brainstem or posterior fossa tumor

↑ ICP, increased intracranial pressure.

BIBLIOGRAPHY

A bibliography is available at ExpertConsult.com.

44

Arthritis

James J. Nocton

Musculoskeletal complaints are among the most frequent reasons for children to present to a primary care office, walk-in clinic, or emergency room. While the child and parents may be focusing on what they perceive to be a localized problem, complaints involving the musculoskeletal system (e.g., arthralgia, myalgia, joint swelling, poorly localized extremity pain, limping, or refusal to walk) may be associated with a long list of potential systemic illnesses. Children or their parents rarely arrive in the clinic expressing a concern for "arthritis" or "patellofemoral syndrome." Instead, they typically describe symptoms such as pain, swelling, limping, or other limitations of activity and function. These children might have complaints as a result of chronic inflammatory arthritis or an associated systemic rheumatic disease, a traumatic or overuse condition, a mechanical or anatomic problem, or a pain syndrome, among other possible explanations.

The differential diagnosis of extremity pain is extensive (Table 44.1). For many of these diagnoses, the history and physical examination are sufficient to confirm a diagnosis; for others, specific laboratory tests, imaging studies, or rarely tissue biopsy will additionally be required to confirm a suspected diagnosis. Musculoskeletal symptoms may indicate pathologic processes isolated to a single extremity or joint, disease restricted to the musculoskeletal system, or a systemic illness of which the joint symptoms may be just one feature.

Arthritis is a specific sign indicating objective inflammation of the joint and can be defined as (1) swelling of the joint or (2) limitation of motion combined with one of the following: tenderness, warmth, or pain on motion. Arthritis should be distinguished from arthralgia (Table 44.2), myalgia, neuralgia, bone pain, cutaneous pain, and allodynia, because if arthritis is present, the diagnostic possibilities are limited to more specific categories of disease (Fig. 44.1). Arthritis is not a specific disease; there are infectious, postinfectious/reactive, hematologic, metabolic, oncologic, and rheumatic causes of arthritis. The cause of the arthritis is determined by establishing the characteristics of the arthritis, including the number and location of the joints affected; the severity, degree of disability, and chronicity of the arthritis; and the pattern of any associated systemic signs and symptoms.

HISTORY

Although the parents and child are usually the principal historians, it is helpful to determine whether other adults have seen signs or have been aware of the child's symptoms. Have daycare providers reported problems to the parents? Has the school staff, coach, or physical education teacher noticed any problems similar to those seen at home?

Obtaining consistent information from several observers in different settings determines the frequency and consistency of the symptoms, as well as how disabling the symptoms have been, and may often help to confirm the reliability of the history. If there are inconsistencies, it becomes increasingly difficult to formulate a diagnosis, and information from the physical examination, along with potential laboratory and imaging studies, may be needed to resolve these inconsistencies.

Pain Location

Pain directly over a joint or joints may indicate synovial inflammation (arthritis), arthralgia secondary to viral infection, or mechanical joint problems such as joint laxity or ligament trauma. Pain near a joint may represent disease in the muscle, bone, tendon, enthesis (tendon insertion sites), or bursa, or may be referred from a nearby joint. There are several possible sites of extremity pain (Fig. 44.2). Pain may involve a whole limb or limbs, or isolated regions of a limb, in which case it may be secondary to neuropathy, myalgia, or a regional pain syndrome. Complaints of pain "all over" may suggest diffuse pain related to a systemic illness or, if chronic, an amplified or myofascial pain syndrome. Intense pain localized to a single small area is seen with infection, trauma, fracture, or tumor. Migrating arthritis or arthralgia is more suggestive of diagnoses such as acute rheumatic fever or immune complex–mediated disease (e.g., from infection or drug reaction) and is less consistent with trauma, tumors, osteomyelitis, or septic arthritis, except for the migratory polyarthritis-tenosynovitis-dermatitis seen in certain instances of disseminated *Neisseria gonorrhoeae* infection or endocarditis.

Pain Character

Arthritis is an aching discomfort that is usually not severe; some children with arthritis may not complain of pain at all. Complete disability secondary to arthritis is rare and should prompt a search for an alternative explanation. Severe pain should increase the suspicion of a pain syndrome or bone disease such as osteomyelitis, leukemia, metastatic neuroblastoma, fracture, or bone tumors. Sporadic episodes of extreme pain interspersed with pain-free intervals are seen with pain syndromes such as growing pains, myofascial pain, and complex regional pain syndrome, or in situations in which psychologic and behavioral factors, such as stress, anxiety, or depression, contribute to the pain. Sharp, radiating, or throbbing pain is unusual for arthritis and suggests an alternative explanation such as neuropathic pain, trauma, or psychogenic pain.

TABLE 44.1 Conditions Causing Arthritis or Extremity Pain

Rheumatic and Inflammatory Diseases
Juvenile idiopathic arthritis
Systemic lupus erythematosus
Juvenile dermatomyositis
Polymyositis
Polyarteritis nodosa
Scleroderma
Sjögren syndrome
Behçet disease
Mixed connective tissue disease
Granulomatosis with polyangiitis
Microscopic polyangiitis
Eosinophilic granulomatosis with polyangiitis
Sarcoidosis
Kawasaki disease
Henoch-Schönlein purpura (immunoglobulin A vasculitis)
Hypersensitivity vasculitis
Chronic recurrent multifocal osteomyelitis (chronic nonbacterial osteomyelitis)
Autoinflammatory syndromes including familial Mediterranean fever
Juvenile ankylosing spondylitis
Inflammatory bowel disease
Psoriasis
Relapsing polychondritis

Infectious Illnesses
Septic arthritis (e.g., *Staphylococcus aureus*, *Streptococcus pneumoniae*, *Kingella kingae*, *Neisseria gonorrhoeae*, *Haemophilus influenzae*)
Osteomyelitis
Lyme disease (*Borrelia burgdorferi*)
Viral illness (e.g., parvovirus, rubella, mumps, Epstein-Barr virus, hepatitis B and C, Chikungunya fever, HIV, human T-lymphotropic virus-1 [HTLV-1], Zika)
Pyomyositis
Fungal arthritis
Mycobacterial infection
Endocarditis

Hematologic Disorders
Hemophilia
Hemoglobinopathies (including sickle cell disease)
Thalassemia

Immunodeficiencies
Hypogammaglobulinemia
Immunoglobulin A deficiency
HIV
Common variable immunodeficiency
Complement deficiency
DiGeorge syndrome
Ataxia-telangiectasia
Wiskott-Aldrich syndrome

Congenital and Metabolic Disorders
Gout
Pseudogout (calcium pyrophosphate dihydrate crystal deposition disease)
Mucopolysaccharidoses
Fucosidoses
Glycogen storage diseases
Thyroid disease (hypothyroidism, hyperthyroidism)
Hyperparathyroidism
Vitamin C deficiency (scurvy)
Vitamin D deficiency (rickets)
Hereditary connective tissue disease (Marfan syndrome, Ehlers-Danlos syndrome)
Fabry disease
Farber disease

Orthopedic Disorders
Trauma
Tendonitis
Patellofemoral syndrome
Hypermobility syndrome
Overuse syndrome
Osteochondritis dissecans
Avascular necrosis (including Legg-Calvé-Perthes disease)
Pigmented villonodular synovitis
Hypertrophic osteoarthropathy
Slipped capital femoral epiphysis
Osteolysis
Benign bone tumors (including osteoid osteoma)
Synovial chondromatosis
Idiopathic multicentric osteolysis

Neuropathic Disorders
Peripheral neuropathies
Carpal tunnel syndrome
Charcot joints (neuropathic osteoarthropathy)

Neoplastic Disorders
Leukemia
Neuroblastoma
Lymphoma
Bone tumors (osteosarcoma, Ewing sarcoma)
Benign cartilage tumor (e.g., chondroma)
Chondrosarcoma
Histiocytic syndromes
Synovial tumors

Reactive Arthritis
Acute rheumatic fever
Postinfectious arthritis (meningococcus, *H. influenzae b*, postenteritis, posturethritis)
Serum sickness
Transient synovitis of the hip
Postimmunization

Pain Syndromes
Fibromyalgia
"Growing" pains
Depression (with somatization)
Anxiety
Stress
Complex regional pain syndrome
Myofascial pain syndromes

Miscellaneous Disorders
Plant-thorn synovitis (*Pantoea agglomerans*, *Nocardia* sp.)
Myositis ossificans
Eosinophilic fasciitis
PAPA (pyogenic arthritis, pyoderma gangrenosum, acne)
SAPHO (synovitis, acne, hyperostosis, osteitis)
Raynaud phenomenon
Erythromelalgia
Sweet syndrome

TABLE 44.2   **Distinguishing Characteristics of Arthritis and Arthralgia**

Arthritis	Arthralgia
Prominent swelling	Minimal or no swelling
Morning stiffness	No morning stiffness
Symptoms improve with activity	Symptoms are exacerbated by activity
Stiffness follows rest	Pain constant or improves with rest
Limited range of motion	Normal or excessive range of motion
Warmth of joint	No warmth
Symptoms usually daily, consistent with minor variation	Symptoms variable, constant, or intermittent

HISTORY AND PHYSICAL EXAMINATION

ARTHRITIS

Common
  Septic arthritis
  Reactive arthritis
  Rheumatic disease

Uncommon
  Malignancy
  Metabolic disease
  Hemophilia

NO ARTHRITIS

Common
  Orthopedic or
    traumatic disorder
  Viral illness
  Pain syndrome

Uncommon
  Malignancy
  Benign bone lesion
  Metabolic disease

Fig. 44.1 Algorithm for determining the cause of extremity pain based on the presence or absence of arthritis.

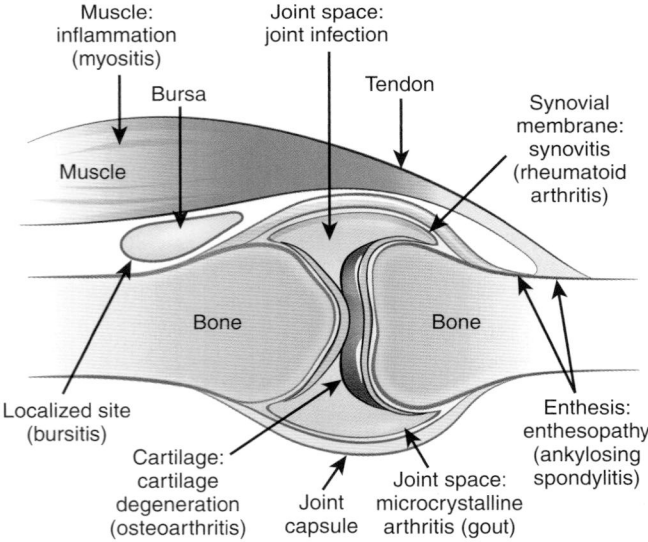

Fig. 44.2 Location of musculoskeletal disease processes by site, pathophysiologic process, and typical disease *(parentheses).* (From Fries JF. Approach to the patient with musculoskeletal disease. In: Wyngaarden JB, Smith LH, Bennett JC, eds. *Cecil Textbook of Medicine.* 19th ed. Philadelphia: WB Saunders; 1992:1488.)

Pain Timing

Arthritis usually causes consistent patterns of daily discomfort with minor variability from day to day. Stiffness or pain-related discomfort occurs on awakening in the morning or after other periods of inactivity, such as prolonged sitting in class or taking a long car ride. The stiffness may last for hours but generally improves with activity during the day. Some forms of arthritis, such as Lyme arthritis or enthesitis-related arthritis, a subtype of juvenile idiopathic arthritis (JIA), may be more episodic. Lyme arthritis classically causes symptoms for days to weeks, usually in a single knee, interspersed with periods of improvement. Enthesitis-related arthritis can cause sudden swelling and discomfort in one or more joints for several weeks to months at a time, followed by gradual spontaneous improvement.

Discomfort that occurs with activities and improves with rest is more suggestive of mechanical pain associated with patellofemoral syndrome, hypermobility, tendonitis, overuse, or muscle strain. Affected children do not have significant symptoms in the morning or after naps, and these conditions are generally not associated with signs of significant inflammation such as warmth, prominent or chronic swelling, or limited range of motion.

Nocturnal pain that wakes children from sleep may be seen in conditions such as leukemia, bone tumors, or infections, but may also occur with less critical conditions such as growing pains, muscle cramps, or psychogenic pain. Children with benign causes of nocturnal pain will lack systemic symptoms, are well during the day, and have normal physical examination findings, whereas those with inflammatory illnesses typically have additional signs and symptoms.

Pain Acuity

Most chronic arthritis is insidious in onset and affected children often have symptoms for weeks to months before they seek medical attention. If the onset is sudden and severe, the evaluation should focus on excluding diagnoses that require urgent treatment, such as trauma, fracture, atraumatic hemarthrosis, septic arthritis, or osteomyelitis. Acute rheumatic fever, reactive arthritis, and viral-associated arthritis or myositis may also manifest suddenly.

Children who describe having extremity pains for many months or years often have mechanical causes of their discomfort such as hypermobility syndrome or patellofemoral syndrome, psychogenic pain, or other relatively benign conditions such as growing pains.

Signs of Inflammation

The swelling and warmth of arthritis are often apparent to the child and parents. Exceptions may include the shoulder and hip, in which the joints are too deep for these signs to be visible, and the spinal, temporomandibular, and sacroiliac joints, in which the articular surfaces are small in relation to the surrounding soft tissues. In these areas, physical examination may reveal tenderness or limitation of motion in the absence of signs of inflammation.

Disability

The chief complaint associated with arthritis may often be a disability such as limping, trouble running or climbing stairs, or difficulty dressing. Some children have associated pain and signs of inflammation, whereas others have little or no discomfort, instead presenting with an isolated decrease in functional ability.

If the chief complaint is the disability, it is helpful to localize the source of the disability to the joint, the bones, the muscles, or the nerves. Muscle or nerve disease manifests primarily as weakness, although some children with sensory neuropathies or myositis, particularly acute viral or bacterial myositis, will also have pain. Dermatomyositis and polymyositis cause symmetric proximal weakness in the upper and lower extremities. The characteristic symptoms are difficulties climbing stairs, rising from the floor, taking the big step onto a bus or into the family minivan, and washing or combing the hair, as well as fatigue and poor endurance. Isolated lower extremity or asymmetric weakness should increase suspicion of neurologic disease.

Disabilities from arthritis are caused by limited range of motion or discomfort in the joint rather than weakness. Limping, particularly in the mornings; unilateral toe-walking because of inability to extend the knee; and difficulty running and jumping are seen with lower extremity arthritis. The child with hand or wrist arthritis has difficulty opening bottles, turning doorknobs, manipulating buttons or snaps on clothing, and gripping pencils or utensils.

Medical History

Numerous genetic syndromes and metabolic diseases are associated with arthritis and arthropathy (see Table 44.1). Endocrine disorders such as diabetes, hyperparathyroidism, and hypothyroidism may be associated with arthropathy, periosteal inflammation, and muscle weakness, respectively. Arthritis is more frequent in patients with psoriasis and inflammatory bowel disease. Bone pain is common in hemoglobinopathies such as sickle cell disease. Cystic fibrosis and other chronic pulmonary diseases increase the likelihood of painful **hypertrophic osteoarthropathy:** the clinical triad of arthritis, digital clubbing, and ossifying periostitis of the long bones. Arthritis or arthralgia may occur after viral diseases or immunization, particularly with immunization against rubella and hepatitis B, presumably secondary to immune complex deposition in the joint.

Medications

Medications may directly cause joint or periarticular symptoms, either via serum sickness–like reactions associated with immune complex arthritis or swelling related to anaphylaxis. Response to medications may also provide further insight into the etiology of arthritis. In most children, an adequate dose of nonsteroidal antiinflammatory drugs (NSAIDs) improves the discomfort of arthritis to some degree. In rheumatic fever, NSAIDs often result in dramatic improvement in symptoms. Conversely, the patient who continues to have severe pain despite adequate doses of antiinflammatory and analgesic medication is more likely to have an infection, a fracture, a tumor, or psychogenic pain.

Family History

For some diseases, a positive family history increases the likelihood that other individuals in the family have that disease, but the genetics of the rheumatic diseases are complex, and none of the genetic associations are strong enough to confirm or eliminate a diagnosis based solely on family history. Within the rheumatic diseases, the family history is most helpful when diagnostic possibilities include enthesitis-related arthritis, psoriatic arthritis, or lupus. Ankylosing spondylitis, reactive arthritis, or inflammatory bowel disease in the family increases the likelihood that the child's arthritis is caused by one of these entities. The presence of the human leukocyte antigen (HLA)-B27 in these family members may increase the likelihood of enthesitis-related arthritis in the child. Approximately 30% of patients with lupus will have a first-degree relative affected by lupus. Less common familial illnesses that may cause rheumatic complaints include familial Mediterranean fever and other autoinflammatory syndromes that cause periodic fevers, mucopolysaccharidoses, fucosidoses, hemophilia, and muscular dystrophies. A family history of adults with osteoarthritis or other forms of degenerative arthritis is generally not helpful, since these entities are relatively common in adults and rarely relevant to a child's joint symptoms.

Social History

Determining the extent to which the problem has limited usual activities helps to gauge the severity of the problem. Has the child missed school because of their symptoms? Has the child been able to participate in physical education, organized sports, and other physical activities? Is the child participating in social activities with friends? In some instances, the limitations are directly related to discomfort or disability from arthritis, but school absences and the discontinuation of sports and social activities may also be secondary to depression or psychogenic pain. It is helpful to ask the parents whether the child's mood or personality has changed recently and whether there have been any recent known psychosocial stressors such as problems at school or with friends or discord within the family. Chronic amplified pain syndromes in children are frequently associated with a history of psychosocial stress, anxiety, or depression.

Travel history is important in considering certain infectious arthritides. The spirochete *Borrelia burgdorferi*, the causative agent of **Lyme disease**, is transmitted by the bite of a deer tick that has a specific geographic distribution. Lyme arthritis characteristically causes episodic joint effusions in one or several large joints, most commonly the knee. A small percentage of patients develop chronic arthritis. In the United States, endemic regions include the Northeast (Connecticut, Rhode Island, and Massachusetts), mid-Atlantic (Long Island, New York City suburbs, New Jersey, southeastern Pennsylvania, Delaware, and Maryland), and the upper Midwest (parts of Minnesota, Illinois, and Wisconsin). Although these endemic areas have been gradually expanding, a child who does not live in or has not traveled to these areas is unlikely to have Lyme disease. Arthritis may be the only symptom of Lyme disease and may not appear until up to 2 years after the tick bite; a history of the classic rash (**erythema migrans**) is helpful but not necessary for a diagnosis of Lyme disease. **Rickettsiosis** and **ehrlichiosis** tend to produce arthralgia but occasionally result in frank arthritis; residing in or traveling to endemic regions should increase suspicion of these vector-borne infections. The geographic distribution of **Chikungunya virus** has been widening; in addition to established endemicity in Africa, Asia, regions of Europe, and areas within the Indian and Pacific Oceans, transmission has been documented throughout North and South America and the Caribbean. Acute infection is often accompanied by rash and, when present in combination with fever, small and large joint polyarthritis, arthralgia, and myalgia, may mimic systemic JIA. Some patients may go on to develop chronic joint symptoms; inquiring about travel to endemic regions may hint at the diagnosis in both the acute and chronic stages of infection. Other viruses confined to a specific geographic area include Zika (South America, Africa, Asia), Ross River (South Pacific), o'nyong-nyong (Africa), and Sindbis (Africa, Middle East, Philippines).

REVIEW OF SYSTEMS

Constitutional Symptoms

Some rheumatic diseases, including several forms of childhood arthritis, are generalized systemic illnesses and cause fevers, poor appetite, weight loss, and fatigue. The absence of these symptoms helps eliminate specific illnesses as diagnostic possibilities. When fevers are present, establishing the pattern of fever is important. Systemic JIA typically produces one or two high temperature spikes each day, with many afebrile hours in between (Fig. 44.3). More persistent fevers tend to be seen with infections or Kawasaki disease. A periodic fever pattern, in which fevers occur for several days, followed by weeks without fever, is seen in familial Mediterranean fever, cyclic neutropenia; the syndrome of periodic fever, aphthous stomatitis, pharyngitis, and adenopathy (PFAPA); and other autoinflammatory syndromes. Systemic lupus erythematosus (SLE), vasculitis, rheumatic fever, serum sickness, inflammatory bowel disease, sarcoidosis, leukemia, and neuroblastoma may cause fevers associated with arthritis or extremity pains. These illnesses do not cause specific patterns of fever.

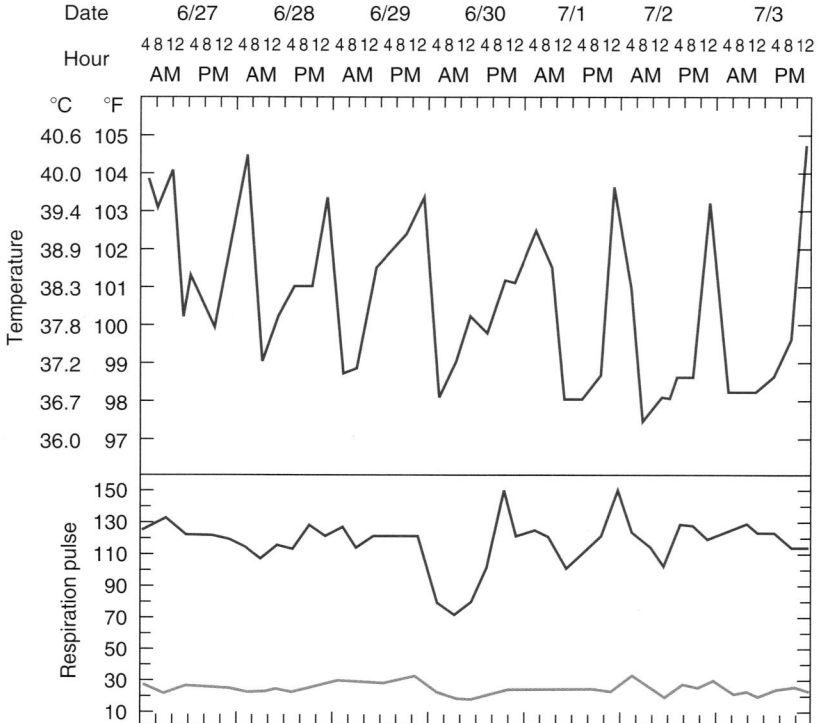

Fig. 44.3 Intermittent fever of systemic-onset juvenile idiopathic arthritis in a 3-year-old girl. (From Petty RE, Laxer RM, Lindsley CB, et al., eds. *Textbook of Pediatric Rheumatology.* 7th ed. Philadelphia: Elsevier; 2016:206.)

Decreased appetite is common in many arthritides, but when associated with documented weight loss, may indicate more severe or systemic illness. Although most children with JIA do not have significant appetite changes, those with systemic JIA may have substantial appetite and growth disturbances. Severe polyarticular JIA may cause some appetite changes and mild weight loss. Children with Crohn disease or ulcerative colitis, both of which are often accompanied by abdominal pain and diarrhea, may demonstrate poor appetite and failure to thrive. Vasculitis, SLE, scleroderma, malignancies, and chronic infections such as tuberculosis are additional causes of significant weight loss. An increase in weight should raise the suspicion of hypothyroidism or fluid retention.

Fatigue is common with any systemic illness, and it may be present in systemic or polyarticular JIA, SLE, hypothyroidism, polymyositis, dermatomyositis, rheumatic fever, and chronic pain syndromes. The clinician should attempt to distinguish between generalized fatigue and specific muscle weakness. The presence of proximal muscle weakness, often associated with fatigue and poor endurance, is characteristic of polymyositis and dermatomyositis.

Skin Changes

Systemic JIA is nearly always accompanied by evanescent pink or salmon-colored macules, often a few centimeters in diameter or smaller but sometimes coalescing to form larger patches (Fig. 44.4). These may be generalized or localized to the trunk or extremities. The macules usually appear with the fever spikes, are not pruritic, and may resolve completely when the fever is absent. Sometimes parents do not notice the rash because of its fleeting nature. Acute rheumatic fever is associated with a specific rash, **erythema marginatum**, though only in approximately 5% of cases. Erythema marginatum is also a fleeting rash, changing in distribution over time, and consists of erythematous patches with serpiginous borders that tend to migrate, usually

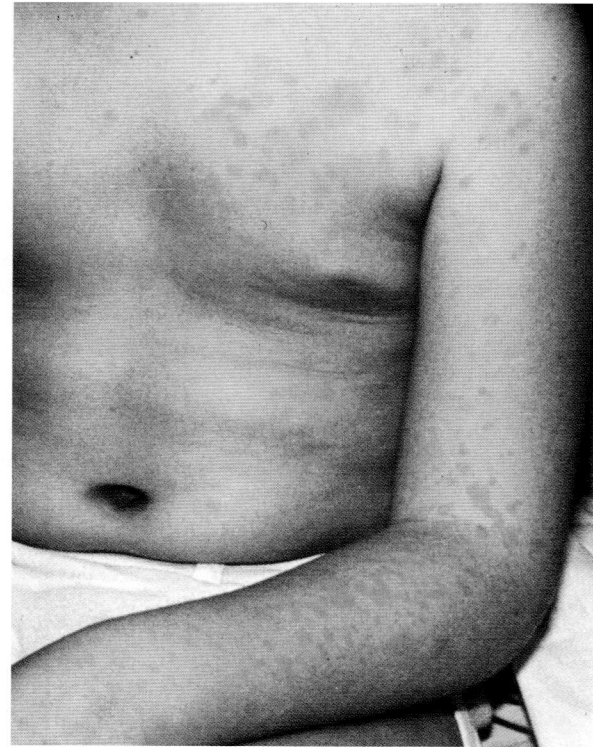

Fig. 44.4 Systemic juvenile idiopathic arthritis rash, a salmon-colored, macular rash that is nonpruritic. The individual lesions are transient, appear in crops, and may be in a linear distribution after minor trauma such as scratching the surface of the skin (Koebner phenomenon). (From Petty RE, Laxer RM, Lindsley CB, et al., eds. *Textbook of Pediatric Rheumatology.* 7th ed. Philadelphia: Elsevier; 2016:206.)

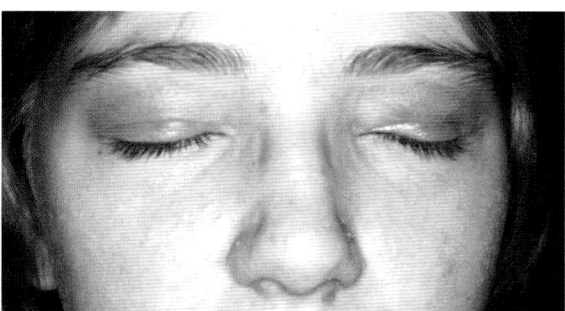

Fig. 44.5 Heliotrope rash with edema of the eyelids in juvenile dermatomyositis. (From Petty RE, Laxer RM, Lindsley CB, et al., eds. *Textbook of Pediatric Rheumatology.* 7th ed. Philadelphia: Elsevier; 2016:359.)

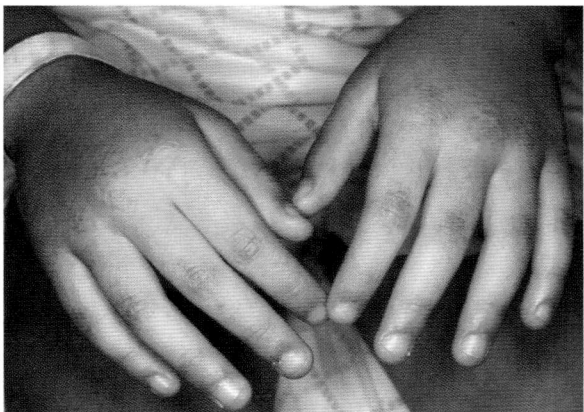

Fig. 44.6 Symmetric, scaly, erythematous plaques and papules over the metacarpopharyngeal and proximal interphalangeal joints of the hands in juvenile dermatomyositis. *C,* Atrophic, pale lesions may also occur. (From Petty RE, Laxer RM, Lindsley CB, et al., eds. *Textbook of Pediatric Rheumatology.* 7th ed. Philadelphia: Elsevier; 2016:359.)

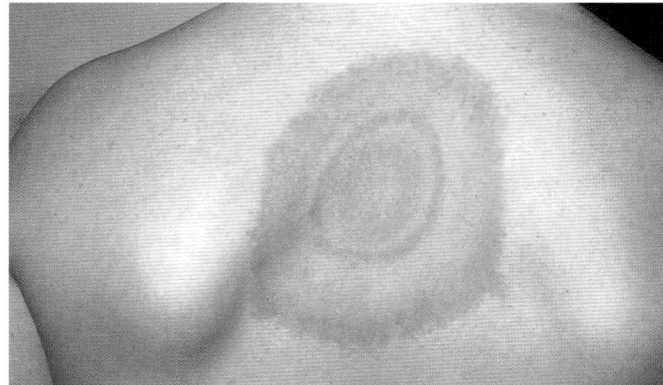

Fig. 44.7 Erythema migrans. Lesions begin as red macules that expand to form large rings that often have a typical "bull's-eye" appearance. (From Petty RE, Laxer RM, Lindsley CB, et al., eds. *Textbook of Pediatric Rheumatology.* 7th ed. Philadelphia: Elsevier; 2016:554.)

over the trunk and proximal extremities. Because of these changes in distribution, families often confuse both of these rashes with urticaria. The **malar rash** of SLE is a fixed, erythematous, nonblanching patch over the cheeks and nasal bridge that tends to spare the nasolabial folds; SLE may also cause vasculitic rashes, as well as nonspecific erythematous macular or papular lesions. Vasculitic rashes consist of palpable purpura and can sometimes be ulcerative. The characteristic skin lesions in dermatomyositis are pathognomonic: **heliotrope rash** is a violaceous discoloration of the upper eyelid, often accompanied by edema. The heliotrope may sometimes be accompanied by more widespread facial erythema (Fig. 44.5). **Gottron papules** are erythematous plaques or papules that appear on the extensor surface of the metacarpophalangeal and proximal interphalangeal joints of the hands (Fig. 44.6) in individuals with dermatomyositis. These are sometimes scaly, are sometimes pale or atrophic, and can be confused with psoriasis or eczema if not for the distribution. Lesions similar to the Gottron papules occasionally appear on the extensor surfaces of the elbows and knees and over the medial malleoli. In addition, erythematous patches may appear on the shoulders, chest, or face (see Fig. 44.5C), where the appearance can cause confusion with the malar rash of SLE.

Erythema migrans occurs in up to 80% of cases of Lyme disease in children and appears days to weeks after the tick bite. The lesion expands, beginning as a small papule and then forming a large erythematous, circular patch, usually at least 5 cm in diameter and often

with some clearing in the center to produce a target-like appearance (Fig. 44.7). If Lyme disease is left untreated, the lesion usually lasts for several weeks and then gradually resolves. If dissemination occurs, some individuals develop multiple secondary lesions that appear similar to the primary lesion.

Various mucocutaneous findings are present in up to half of patients with acute Chikungunya virus infection. Rash tends to be a generalized morbilliform maculopapular eruption that spares the face and appears within several days of the onset of fever, before subsiding within a week. Patients may also experience areas of hyperpigmentation, often in the centrofacial region and restricted to the nose, a finding termed the **Chick sign**. Up to a third of patients with acute Chikungunya will develop a chronic arthritis that may mimic JIA; therefore, inquiring about a remote history of characteristic skin findings, as well as constitutional symptoms such as a brief febrile illness temporally correlated with travel to regions where Chikungunya is endemic, may prompt testing for prior exposure to Chikungunya.

The history of other types of rashes or skin lesions may suggest other diagnoses. Measles and parvovirus infections, for example, have characteristic rashes. A history of photosensitivity is suggestive of SLE. Petechiae may be seen with SLE, vasculitis, immune thrombocytopenia, or leukemia. Pallor or cyanosis of the digits, hands, and feet upon exposure to cold temperatures suggests **Raynaud phenomenon**, which is most often seen in those with no underlying systemic illness but may be associated with several rheumatic diseases, most commonly SLE, mixed connective tissue disease (MCTD), and scleroderma. **Scleroderma** causes tightening, thickening, and the development of a waxy texture to the skin, and it frequently begins on the hands, feet, and face.

Additional Symptoms

Questioning the parents about cognitive difficulties, including declining school performance or memory loss, helps screen for the possibility of subtle central nervous system involvement that may be associated with SLE or central nervous system vasculitis. Seizures or frank psychosis may also occur in these illnesses. Alopecia is frequently seen with SLE and may also occur with hypothyroidism. Ocular symptoms, such as pain or redness of the eye, may occur with uveitis or with nonspecific orbital inflammation (also known as orbital pseudotumor) potentially associated with a number of rheumatic diseases. Acute anterior uveitis (involving the iris and/or ciliary body) can be seen with reactive arthritis and enthesitis-related arthritis. Chronic anterior uveitis is most common in younger children with oligoarticular or polyarticular JIA and is usually asymptomatic. Sarcoidosis in children may be associated with both anterior and posterior uveitis. Ulcerations of the nose or hard palate may be present in SLE. Both uveitis and oral aphthous ulcerations can be seen with inflammatory bowel disease and also with Behçet disease, which can also include genital aphthous ulceration. Frequent sinusitis is often an early manifestation of granulomatosis with polyangiitis (GPA).

Chest pain that is worse when the patient lies supine and improves with sitting up and leaning forward may represent pericarditis, which is most commonly associated with SLE and systemic-onset JIA but may occur in rheumatic fever. Dysphagia suggests esophageal dysmotility, which may occur with inflammatory myopathies and scleroderma. Asking whether the child needs to cut food into small pieces, needs to drink an unusual amount of fluid with meals, or takes a long time to complete a meal are helpful ways of assessing dysphagia. Abdominal pain, vomiting, and diarrhea are nonspecific but if severe or associated with melena or hematochezia, might suggest Henoch-Schönlein purpura (HSP), also known as immunoglobulin A (IgA) vasculitis, as well as inflammatory bowel disease, polyarteritis nodosa with vasculitis of the intestine, or the rare intestinal vasculitis associated with SLE or dermatomyositis. Testicular pain is seen with some forms of vasculitis, particularly IgA vasculitis (HSP) and polyarteritis nodosa. Peripheral edema, sacral edema, or periorbital edema may be present with illnesses causing glomerulonephritis, such as SLE and the antineutrophil cytoplasmic antibody (ANCA)-associated vasculitides.

PHYSICAL EXAMINATION

Observing the child ambulate or explore the examination room provides a sense of the severity of the illness and the degree of disability. Particularly with young children, this period of observation may give a better sense of the range of motion or the degree of discomfort in the joints than the formal examination, when the child may be uncooperative.

The examination begins by reviewing the vital signs. Fever, especially in the child with arthritis or localized extremity pain, may suggest an infectious process. Systemic-onset JIA is the only subtype of JIA associated with fever. Abnormalities in other vital signs are not expected with isolated arthritis and suggest that a systemic disease may be present. Tachycardia may be caused by fever, anxiety, pericarditis, or myocarditis. Tachypnea suggests the presence of cardiac or pulmonary disease, and hypertension increases the suspicion of renal involvement.

In any child with joint complaints, it is critical to examine all the joints, even those that are asymptomatic. Children or their parents may focus on the joint that is most painful or causes the most disability and are often unaware of the presence of arthritis in other joints. The neck and the joints of the upper extremities are best examined with the child in a sitting position. Children with inflammation in the joints of the cervical spine usually have limitations in extension, lateral flexion, and rotation. This is tested by asking the child to look up at the ceiling, touch each ear to the ipsilateral shoulder, and touch the chin to each shoulder.

Arthritis of the temporomandibular joint is common with polyarticular JIA and might easily be overlooked. Children with chronic arthritis of these joints develop micrognathia and often retrognathia as a result of delayed mandibular growth. The oral opening is often decreased in size, and there may be pain with opening and closing of the jaw or tenderness to palpation directly over the joint.

Shoulder arthritis is identified by detecting limited range of motion and pain with motion. With the upper arm abducted to 90 degrees and the elbow flexed to 90 degrees, the clinician can then rotate the upper arm superiorly and inferiorly (external and internal rotation of the humerus, respectively), noting any limitation or pain. Alternatively, the patient can be asked to abduct and internally rotate the arm, reaching

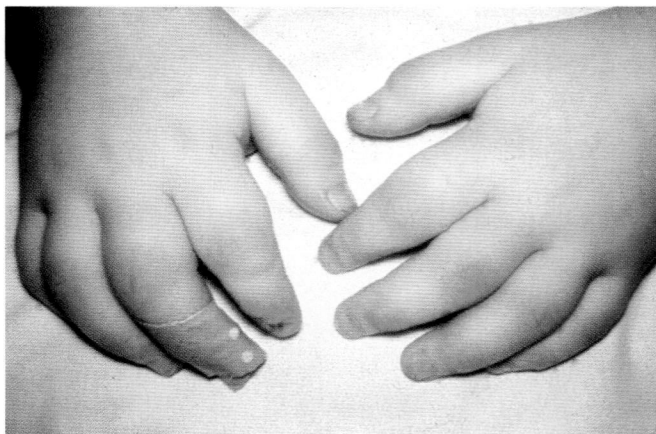

Fig. 44.8 The joints of the wrists and hands of a 2-year-old male are swollen, warm, and painful with limited extension of the fingers. (From Petty RE, Laxer RM, Lindsley CB, et al., eds. *Textbook of Pediatric Rheumatology.* 7th ed. Philadelphia: Elsevier; 2016:194.)

behind the head to touch the contralateral scapula, and then to adduct and internally rotate the arm, reaching behind the back and upward, again touching the contralateral scapula. The acromioclavicular joints and the sternoclavicular joints are occasionally affected by arthritis and should be palpated, noting any swelling or tenderness.

In the elbow, arthritis often produces detectable swelling and warmth, usually identified posteriorly, proximal to the olecranon. Elbow extension and flexion should also be tested, along with supination of the forearm and hand. Many children can normally hyperextend their elbows, and the degree of extension is variable; therefore, it is helpful to compare the range of motion of each elbow to the contralateral side.

The wrists are inspected for swelling and palpated for warmth and tenderness. Many children with wrist arthritis develop swelling on the dorsal aspect of the wrist that is usually nontender. Extension tends to be more limited than flexion in wrist arthritis, and radial deviation tends to be more limited than ulnar deviation. Children with wrist arthritis frequently complain of pain or withdraw their arm with maneuvers to test flexion and extension of the wrist.

The metacarpophalangeal (MCP) joint and the proximal interphalangeal (PIP) and distal interphalangeal (DIP) joints should be individually palpated, and any swelling, tenderness, or warmth should be noted (Fig. 44.8). The examiner should flex and extend the MCP joints, looking for limitations. To test the range of motion of the PIP and DIP joints, the child should try to supinate the hand and flex all the digits, attempting to touch the fingertips to the palm. To examine the first MCP and thumb interphalangeal joint, the child should try to touch the tip of the thumb to the base of the fifth finger. Grip strength is determined by having the child tightly squeeze two of the clinician's fingers. Arthritis of the wrist or any of the small joints of the hand decreases grip strength.

The child should next lie in a supine position, either in the parent's lap or on the examination table so that the lower extremities can be examined. Each hip is taken through its range of motion, beginning with flexion by trying to bring the knee as close to the chest as possible. Any pain or limitation is noted. With the hip and knee each flexed to 90 degrees, internal and external rotation are tested by keeping the knee in a fixed position and turning the lower leg laterally and medially, thereby rotating the femur. The hip and knee are then extended back to a neutral supine position and abduction is tested. With the child in the prone position, the examiner evaluates hip extension by placing a hand on the child's ipsilateral iliac crest and lifting the child's thigh posteriorly with the knee extended. Hip arthritis most often causes limitations with internal rotation and extension, usually in association with pain in the inguinal area.

The knee is inspected for effusions and other obvious deformities. Palpation of the knee assesses for warmth, a common finding in knee arthritis; synovial swelling (producing a "spongy" feel); or an effusion (often feels like a "water balloon"). Applying pressure in the suprapatellar area with one hand while palpating on either side of the patella with the other allows for the detection of effusions more readily because this forces excessive joint fluid that has accumulated in the suprapatellar area into the synovial space lateral and medial to the patella. Small effusions may be detected by eliciting a **bulge sign**. This is done by milking the medial and lateral depressions around the patella superiorly to push the fluid into the suprapatellar space and then gently pushing either medially or laterally just superior to the patella. This releases the fluid inferiorly, causing the area medial to the patella to bulge out. The popliteal fossa should be palpated, because fluid within the knee joint may track posteriorly as it accumulates, producing fullness in the popliteal fossa and sometimes a frank cyst.

Palpating around the edges of the patella causes pain in many adolescents with **patellofemoral syndrome** (also known as chondromalacia patellae), a common cause of knee pain in active adolescents. In another maneuver that elicits pain in this syndrome, the patient relaxes the quadriceps muscles while the examiner displaces the patella inferiorly by pushing on the superior pole of the patella. While the examiner maintains pressure on the patella, the patient contracts the quadriceps. In patients with patellofemoral syndrome, pain elicited by this maneuver is referred to as a positive **patellar apprehension test**, while a grinding sensation felt by the examiner constitutes a positive **patellar grind sign**. The tibial tubercle and patellar tendon should be inspected and palpated for swelling and tenderness associated with **Osgood-Schlatter disease** and **patellar tendonitis**, respectively.

Flexing and extending the knee tests range of motion. Most young children can normally touch their heel to their buttocks and can hyperextend the knee slightly. The examiner can detect subtle limitations in extension by standing at the foot of the table and lifting the heels of the child off the table as the child relaxes their legs in a fully extended position. If one knee is limited with extension, the patella on that side may appear slightly more elevated.

Swelling in the ankles is often best seen when inspecting and palpating the posterior aspect of the ankle, where fullness on either side of the ankle may be appreciated between the Achilles tendon and the malleoli. Warmth is common with ankle arthritis. Testing range of motion in the ankle should include both the tibiotalar ankle joint and the subtalar talocalcaneal joint. Cupping the heel with one hand and using the other hand to grasp the forefoot allows the examiner to move the forefoot superiorly (dorsiflexion) and inferiorly (plantar flexion) to evaluate the tibiotalar joint. The hand cupping the heel is then rocked laterally and medially to check inversion and eversion associated with motion at the subtalar joint. Holding the heel firmly with a cupped hand and gently rotating the forefoot with the other hand tests the joints of the midfoot. Each of the metatarsophalangeal (MTP) joints is palpated along with each of the toes. The MTP joints are flexed and extended noting any limitations or pain, and as with other joints, also noting any asymmetry with the contralateral MTP joints. The toes are inspected for the presence of swelling. The plantar fascia and the Achilles tendon are palpated, and any tenderness or swelling is noted.

The child should stand so that the examiner can evaluate the back. The sacroiliac joints are palpated, any tenderness is noted, and the child is asked to keep the knees extended and bend forward, touching the hands to the ground if possible. The lumbar spine should curve forward normally without flattening. The **modified Schober measurement**, which reveals whether the lumbar spine flexes normally, is done by marking the lumbar spine at a point where a horizontal line connecting the lateral lumbar indentations intersects the spine. Then the examiner measures 10 cm above and 5 cm below that spot while the child is standing. When the child bends forward, the distance between the top and bottom marks should increase to at least 21 cm as the vertebral bodies separate during flexion. A shorter distance suggests limitation in mobility of the spine and potential spondylitis. Scoliosis is detected by noting any asymmetric elevation of the shoulder and upper back while the child bends forward.

Hypermobility is a very common cause of pain associated with sports and other activities; it tends to improve with rest. Hypermobility, patellofemoral syndrome, frequent ankle sprains, and pes planus are frequently seen together. The hypermobile child or adolescent can hyperextend the knees and elbows, appose the thumb to the forearm while flexing the wrist, hyperextend the MCP joints so that the digits are parallel to the forearm when the wrist is extended, and easily put the palms flat on the floor while bending forward from a standing position with the knees locked. Extreme hypermobility is seen in some individuals with Ehlers-Danlos syndrome or Marfan syndrome. Obtaining a Beighton score may help the examiner more objectively assess the degree of hypermobility (see Chapter 47).

Myofascial pain syndromes are often associated with the presence of specific **trigger points**, exquisitely tender, well-localized points often detected in the following locations: the occiput, trapezius muscles, medial borders of the scapula, upper outer quadrant of the buttocks, the second cervical space anteriorly, the second costochondral space just distal to the lateral epicondyle on the forearm, the greater trochanter in the proximal leg, and the medial aspects of the knees. Their presence in the older child with diffuse pain, fatigue, and difficulty sleeping is highly suggestive of a myofascial pain syndrome.

Proximal muscle strength testing and an evaluation of muscle bulk should be performed in any patient complaining of weakness or fatigue. The deltoids, biceps, triceps, psoas, quadriceps, and hamstrings are tested. Neck flexor weakness is common in dermatomyositis and polymyositis and is tested by having the child lie supine and lift only their head. Most children can lift and keep the head elevated, even if asked to resist pressure from the examiner's hand against the forehead. To test proximal leg strength, the child rises from a sitting position on the floor. Chronic knee arthritis or hip disease leads to atrophy of the ipsilateral quadriceps. Similarly, ankle arthritis causes the gastrocnemius to atrophy; wrist arthritis leads to wasting of the forearm muscles; and elbow contractures cause atrophy of the triceps muscle. Atrophy is easily overlooked, and it is sometimes helpful to measure the circumference of the thigh, calf, or upper arm to detect asymmetry.

The skin and mucous membranes should be examined carefully, as there may be clues to the presence of systemic disease (Table 44.3). Systemic JIA, SLE, acute rheumatic fever, and dermatomyositis are associated with characteristic rashes. Petechiae or palpable purpura suggests vasculitis. Nodules are seen with acute rheumatic fever and polyarticular rheumatoid factor–positive JIA. Thickening and tightening of the skin, particularly over the distal extremities and face, are suggestive of scleroderma. Nasal or palatal ulcers suggest SLE, whereas aphthous ulceration may be seen with inflammatory bowel disease or Behçet disease, the latter particularly if on the genitals in the absence of sexually transmitted infection. Alopecia, either localized or diffuse, may be apparent to the examiner without being recognized by the patient. The presence of peripheral or periorbital edema increases the suspicion of glomerulonephritis.

The remainder of the physical examination including head, eyes, ears, chest, heart, and abdomen should also be performed carefully,

TABLE 44.3 Skin Manifestations of Rheumatic Disease

Physical Finding	Possible Disease
Petechiae, purpura	Vasculitis (may be palpable) Leukemia Meningococcemia Other infections SLE
Erythema nodosum	Inflammatory bowel disease Streptococcal infection Sarcoidosis Drug reaction Tuberculosis Fungal infection
Gottron papules	Dermatomyositis
Alopecia	SLE, hypothyroidism
Calcification	Dermatomyositis, scleroderma
Subcutaneous nodules	Polyarticular JIA, rheumatic fever
Oral ulcers	SLE, Behçet disease, inflammatory bowel disease, reactive arthritis
Genital ulcers	Behçet disease
Digital ulcers	Vasculitis, SLE, scleroderma
Tight, thickened skin	Scleroderma
Livedo reticularis	Antiphospholipid syndrome, SLE, cutaneous polyarteritis nodosa
Nail dystrophy or pits	Psoriasis
Edema	SLE, vasculitis, scleroderma, eosinophilic fasciitis, serum sickness, Henoch-Schönlein purpura
Desquamation	Kawasaki disease, scarlet fever
Cyanosis	Raynaud phenomenon, hypertrophic osteoarthropathy

JIA, juvenile idiopathic arthritis; SLE, systemic lupus erythematosus.

with attention to potential signs that might indicate systemic and/or organ-specific disease.

LABORATORY STUDIES

Laboratory testing should be considered when the diagnosis is unclear and systemic disease is a concern. It is important to recognize that laboratory tests are not diagnostic of JIA. Tests frequently seen in "arthritis panels" such as those for antinuclear antibody (ANA), rheumatoid factor (RF), ESR, and CRP are not specific for arthritis and may be abnormal in healthy children or in those with infections and other coincidental diseases.

A CBC with manual differential is useful in decreasing the suspicion of an acute infection or leukemia as the etiology of bone pain, joint pain, or even frank arthritis. A normal CBC is reassuring, but it is also helpful to compare the platelet count to the ESR when concerned about leukemia. Because platelets are an acute-phase reactant, they should increase as the ESR increases. A normal or low platelet count in a child with markedly elevated ESR increases the suspicion of leukemia or another cause for platelet destruction or decreased bone marrow platelet production.

An elevated peripheral white blood cell (WBC) count is often present in septic arthritis or osteomyelitis but is neither sensitive nor specific for these infections. In systemic-onset JIA, the WBC count may be markedly elevated to 20,000 WBCs/mm³ or greater

and the hemoglobin may be as low as 6 or 7 g/dL; the platelet count is typically significantly elevated. For many of the other inflammatory diseases that are associated with arthritis or extremity pain, a mild to moderate normocytic anemia and a mild thrombocytosis are common. SLE may be associated with anemia, leukopenia, and thrombocytopenia.

The ESR is helpful when physical examination is inconclusive for signs of inflammation. In children who are uncooperative or whose body habitus precludes adequate assessment, it may be difficult to detect small effusions or subtle limitations in the range of motion. In these instances, an elevated ESR increases the suspicion of arthritis, although a normal ESR does not exclude it. In children who clearly have rheumatic disease or infection, the ESR is not useful diagnostically, but it may be useful as a means of monitoring disease activity over time. CRP is often elevated in systemic-onset JIA, polyarticular JIA, and infectious arthritis but is often normal in oligoarticular arthritis. Procalcitonin is typically normal in JIA and elevated in bacterial osteoarticular infections.

Vasculitis or SLE may result in glomerulonephritis; proteinuria or red blood cell casts can be detected on urinalysis, and the serum creatinine level will be elevated if glomerulonephritis has resulted in renal insufficiency. Severe proteinuria will also lead to hypoalbuminemia. Kawasaki disease is associated with sterile pyuria.

Serum aminotransferases are elevated in patients with hepatitis and occasionally in patients with SLE. In those with myositis, elevations in aminotransferases often occur concomitantly with increased creatine kinase, lactate dehydrogenase, and aldolase levels.

Antinuclear Antibody

The ANA test is a sensitive screen for SLE or overlap syndromes that include features of SLE, being positive in approximately 99% of these patients. **The ANA is not a useful screen for any other rheumatic disease, including JIA, because it is neither sensitive nor specific enough for these other conditions;** furthermore, the ANA is positive in many healthy children and adults, and it may be positive in infections and other autoimmune and systemic illnesses (Table 44.4). Therefore, it does not necessarily indicate the presence of disease and should only be ordered as a diagnostic screening test when there is a strong suspicion of SLE or an overlap syndrome.

Those with SLE and overlap syndromes usually have high ANA titers, typically with values of 1:640 or higher, although there is no level of titer elevation that is sufficiently specific or sensitive enough to either diagnose or exclude the possibility of SLE, and further testing will be necessary in children with features of SLE and an elevated ANA. The pattern of the ANA is rarely helpful. Homogeneous and speckled patterns are the most common and are not specific. A peripheral or "rim" pattern is usually associated with anti–double-stranded DNA (anti-dsDNA) antibodies and is more specific for SLE. A nucleolar pattern suggests the presence of anti–Scl-70 antibodies, which may be seen in patients with scleroderma.

Rheumatoid Factor

The RF test is not sensitive or specific for JIA. Only approximately 5% of children with JIA have a positive RF result, usually in teenagers with polyarticular arthritis. RF is an immunoglobulin M antibody directed against immunoglobulin G. In children with polyarthritis, the presence of RF is a poor prognostic factor; these children have a high likelihood of developing chronic, erosive arthritis. A positive test result for RF can be seen with other illnesses associated with the formation of immune complexes, including rheumatic diseases such as SLE or vasculitis, and with infectious diseases such as bacterial endocarditis, infectious mononucleosis, and hepatitis B or C. RF should not be ordered, and

TABLE 44.4 Autoantibodies in Children

Test	Characteristics
Antinuclear antibody (ANA)	99% sensitive in SLE; very nonspecific; present in healthy children, endocarditis, autoimmune hepatitis, JIA, Hashimoto thyroiditis, lymphoma, psoriatic arthritis, dermatomyositis, scleroderma, mononucleosis
Anti–double-stranded DNA (dsDNA)	Up to 80% sensitive for SLE; highly specific (nearly 100%)
Anti-Smith (Sm)	Up to 50% sensitive in SLE; nearly 100% specific
Anti-SSA (Anti-Ro)	Up to 50% sensitive in SLE; seen in asymptomatic children; present in Sjögren syndrome and scleroderma; can be associated with neonatal lupus
Anti-SSB (Anti-La)	Up to 15% sensitive in SLE; seen in similar conditions as anti-SSA; can be associated with neonatal lupus
Antiribonucleoprotein (RNP)	Up to 40% sensitive in SLE; also seen in mixed connective tissue disease
Antihistone	Drug-induced SLE-like syndromes
Rheumatoid factor (RF)	30% of SLE patients; 5% of JIA; also seen in infections
Antiproteinase 3 (c-ANCA)	90–95% sensitive and specific for granulomatosis with polyangiitis
Antimyeloperoxidase (p-ANCA)	75% sensitive for microscopic polyangiitis; seen in other vasculitides, inflammatory bowel disease, other inflammatory diseases
Anti-RBC membrane (Coombs positive)	Up to 50% sensitive in SLE; nonspecific, seen also in Evans syndrome, isolated hemolytic anemia
Anticardiolipin	Seen in SLE; nonspecific, seen in asymptomatic children and in those with antiphospholipid syndrome

ANCA, antineutrophil cytoplasmic antibody; JIA, juvenile idiopathic arthritis; RBC, red blood cell; SLE, systemic lupus erythematosus; SSA and SSB, Sjögren syndrome type A and type B.

will not be helpful diagnostically, in individuals who do not have polyarthritis on physical examination.

Additional Antibody Testing

If the history and physical examination findings suggest SLE and an individual has an elevated ANA, additional autoantibody testing is helpful (see Table 44.4). Anti-dsDNA antibodies and anti-Smith antibodies are highly specific for SLE. Antiribonucleoprotein (anti-RNP) antibodies may be seen in patients with SLE; anti-RNP antibodies along with an elevated ANA and without anti-dsDNA or anti-Smith antibodies suggest the specific overlap syndrome **mixed connective tissue disease**, which has a combination of clinical features seen with SLE, dermatomyositis, and scleroderma. Anti–Sjögren syndrome type A (anti-SSA; also known as anti-Ro) and anti–Sjögren syndrome type B (anti-SSB; also known as anti-La) antibodies are occasionally seen in patients with SLE but are not specific. They are seen in Sjögren syndrome, an illness producing chronic inflammation of the salivary and lacrimal glands and resulting in xerostomia and xerophthalmia. These antibodies may also be seen in asymptomatic, healthy individuals.

Anticardiolipin antibodies, one of several antiphospholipid antibodies, may be present in SLE, but they are also seen in asymptomatic

TABLE 44.5 Criteria for Diagnosing Lyme Disease

Characteristic clinical presentation
- Early localized disease: erythema migrans at the site of a recent tick bite, possible constitutional symptoms (malaise, headache, mild neck stiffness, myalgia, arthralgia), possible fever
- Early disseminated disease: multiple erythema migrans lesions at sites distinct from initial lesion, cranial nerve palsies (particularly cranial nerve VII), lymphocytic meningitis, polyradiculitis, constitutional symptoms, carditis
- Late disease: arthritis, polyneuropathy, encephalomyelitis

Exposure in an endemic area*

Positive Lyme EIA, confirmed by positive Western blot

Western blots are considered positive if the following are present:
For IgM, two of the following three bands must be present:
23, 39, 41 kD
For IgG, 5 of the following 10 bands must be present:
18, 21, 28, 30, 39, 41, 45, 58, 66, 93 kD

*Mid-Atlantic and southern New England coastal regions, northwestern Wisconsin, and eastern Minnesota are considered the most endemic regions in North America. Even within these regions, the incidence of infection can vary widely.
EIA, enzyme immunoassay; Ig, immunoglobulin; kD, kilodaltons.

individuals and in those with the antiphospholipid antibody syndrome, in which clinical manifestations are a result of the hypercoagulable state associated with these antibodies. These manifestations include venous and arterial thromboses and recurrent spontaneous abortions. Many patients with SLE have a false-positive Venereal Disease Research Laboratory (VDRL) test result because this test also detects antiphospholipid antibodies. A positive direct Coombs test result, indicative of an autoimmune hemolytic anemia, is common in patients with SLE, although rarely is the hemolysis clinically significant.

GPA and the other ANCA-associated vasculitides are the only types of vasculitis that can be diagnosed on the basis of serologic testing. Antiproteinase 3 antibodies, identified on immunofluorescence testing as cytoplasmic-staining or c-ANCA, are 95% sensitive and specific for GPA. The antimyeloperoxidase antibody (corresponding to peripheral-staining or p-ANCA on immunofluorescence testing) is much less specific; it may be present in those with other vasculitides and also in those with a variety of infectious and inflammatory illnesses.

Viral infections such as human parvovirus B19, Epstein-Barr virus, Chikungunya, and rubella may be associated with arthralgia or arthritis, and testing for antibodies to these viruses may be helpful in some situations. For diagnosing Lyme disease, the enzyme-linked immunosorbent assay (ELISA) is a very sensitive, but not specific, screening test. A positive ELISA should therefore be confirmed by Western blot (Table 44.5).

Complement

The complement proteins C3 and C4 are often depressed in patients with active SLE, which indicates consumption secondary to the formation of immune complexes. Low levels of complement can be seen occasionally with some vasculitides and in other illnesses in which immune complexes form, such as bacterial endocarditis. The CH_{50} is a functional assay that measures the activity of the entire classical pathway of complement. If any single complement protein is sufficiently depressed, this may cause a decrease in the CH_{50}. The CH_{50} is less sensitive and less specific than testing for the individual complement components.

DIAGNOSTIC IMAGING

Radiographs

Plain radiographs of bones and joints may be useful to evaluate for potential infections, trauma, leukemia, or solid bone tumors. Acute osteomyelitis usually causes periosteal elevation, which may be seen on radiographs after approximately 1 week of illness. Chronic osteomyelitis causes abscesses of the bone that are often evident on plain radiographs. Fractures, including stress fractures and small avulsion fractures, are occasionally detected even when the clinical information is not strongly suggestive. Leukemia can cause lucency within the metaphyses of the long bones. Solid tumors, including osteosarcoma, Ewing sarcoma, and the benign osteoid osteoma, may all be identified on plain radiographs. Because knee pain may reflect referred pain from the hip, any child with unexplained knee or thigh pain should also have pelvis and hip radiographs performed, including a "frog-leg" view. The young, limping child may have Legg-Calvé-Perthes disease as a result of avascular necrosis of the femoral head. A slipped capital femoral epiphysis is classically seen in overweight patients in their early teens (see Chapter 45).

In the child with arthritis, soft tissue swelling or effusions within the joint may be identified on plain radiographs; however, normal radiographs do not exclude the possibility of joint inflammation. Chronic arthritis may demonstrate bone erosions and juxta-articular osteopenia. Radiographs can be useful in monitoring the course of the disease and can sometimes help guide management.

In children with suspected SLE, a chest radiograph may reveal an enlarged cardiac silhouette, suggestive of a pericardial effusion or the presence of pleural effusions. If GPA is a consideration, a chest radiograph may reveal bilateral cavitating pulmonary nodules. Pulmonary hemorrhage, with bilateral alveolar infiltrates, can be seen with GPA, SLE, microscopic polyangiitis (MPA), and rarely IgA vasculitis.

Ultrasound

Ultrasonography is a portable, convenient, noninvasive, and efficient tool for imaging joints, tendons, and soft tissues. It may be useful in identifying synovitis, tenosynovitis, and joint effusions when the physical examination is difficult or inconclusive. When used with Doppler, ultrasonography can also identify sites of increased blood flow, which might be an indication of active inflammation.

Magnetic Resonance Imaging

MRI is useful when plain radiographs either are unrevealing or have poorly defined abnormalities. MRI, a sensitive test for septic arthritis, osteomyelitis, suppurative myositis, and avascular necrosis, can also reveal small joint effusions that are not apparent on physical examination. MRI helps distinguish hemarthrosis from other forms of joint swelling and detects ligamentous and meniscal tears. MRI provides better visualization and characterization of tumors than plain radiographs. If myositis is suspected, MRI may reveal increased signal within the muscle as a result of inflammation and can help determine a potential biopsy site. MRI is relatively sensitive for arthritis, allowing very good visualization of synovial tissue.

Bone Scan

A bone scan is useful when plain radiographs are unremarkable and when the source of pain cannot be adequately localized. It is a sensitive test for inflammation in the bones and joints, and it can often help distinguish arthritis from osteomyelitis, fractures, and tumors. Bone scans, like plain radiographs, are not as sensitive for osteomyelitis if obtained very early in the disease process, and a second scan should be considered if the initial study is negative. A bone scan may detect osteoid osteomas that are not apparent on plain radiographs. Complex regional pain syndrome (CRPS) may be associated with an abnormal bone scan, often demonstrating asymmetric increased uptake on the affected side.

Additional Imaging Studies

Echocardiography is useful when acute rheumatic fever is a consideration. Clinically silent valvulitis with resulting insufficiency, as seen in the context of rheumatic fever, may be detected only by echocardiography. The echocardiogram may also detect pericardial effusions in patients with SLE and coronary artery aneurysms in patients with Kawasaki disease.

Conventional angiography, CT with angiography, and magnetic resonance angiography are useful for the diagnosis of medium- or large-vessel vasculitis such as polyarteritis nodosa or Takayasu arteritis. High-resolution CT of the chest without contrast is helpful in visualizing pulmonary nodules in patients with GPA and in detecting basilar lung fibrosis in those with scleroderma.

Joint Fluid Aspiration

Synovial fluid analysis in childhood is most helpful for confirming or excluding three possible problems: (1) infectious arthritis, (2) hemarthrosis (either secondary to trauma or a bleeding diathesis), and very rarely (3) crystal diseases such as gout or pseudogout. A fourth condition, the rare entity of **pigmented villonodular synovitis,** is suggested by the aspiration of a "chocolate brown" synovial fluid from the knee.

Among these possibilities, only infection is a common consideration in childhood and is typically suspected based on the history and physical examination findings. The child with septic arthritis is often febrile and has acute joint pain, swelling, warmth, and occasionally erythema, most commonly in a single joint (Table 44.6), over a period of hours to days. When septic arthritis is suspected, arthrocentesis is necessary, and the joint fluid is sent for cell count, protein quantification, glucose measurement, Gram stain, and microbiologic studies, including bacterial culture and polymerase chain reaction (PCR) testing for *Kingella kingae* (Table 44.7). Additional microbiologic assays might include fungal culture and mycobacterial testing if suspected. Some infectious arthritides develop more indolently, such as gonococcal arthritis, tuberculous arthritis, and opportunistic infections in immunocompromised hosts. Adolescents with monoarticular arthritis (Table 44.8) or with acute polyarthritis should undergo joint aspiration if they have risk factors for gonococcal disease. Likewise, if there has been exposure to tuberculosis or if a child is immunocompromised, joint fluid aspiration should be considered.

If the child has sustained trauma and it is unclear from the history and physical examination whether a joint effusion is inflammatory or hemorrhagic, joint fluid analysis may be helpful. Similarly, if there is history of a bleeding disorder in the family or in the child, joint aspiration should be considered (see Table 44.7), as should assessment of coagulation parameters if the child does not have an established history of a bleeding disorder but one is suspected based on presentation or family history.

Gout and pseudogout are unusual in childhood. Conditions that result in elevated serum uric acid levels predispose a child to gout, and if children with these conditions develop arthritis, the joint fluid should be analyzed for crystals. These conditions include leukemia, tumor lysis syndrome, renal failure, Down syndrome, Lesch-Nyhan syndrome, and type I glycogen storage disease (von Gierke disease).

TABLE 44.6 Frequency of Infected Joints in Children with Septic Arthritis (%)

Joint	Fink and Nelson (N = 591)	Welkon et al. (N = 95)	Speiser et al. (N = 86)	Wilson and Di Paola (N = 61)	Overall
Knee	40	46	30	29	39
Hip	23	25	29	40	25
Ankle	13	15	17	21	14
Elbow	14	5	11	3	12
Shoulder	4	4	2	3	4
Wrist	4	—	1	1	3
PIP, MCP, MTP	1	—	10	—	2
Other	1	5	—	1	1

MCP, metacarpophalangeal; MTP, metatarsophalangeal; PIP, proximal interphalangeal.
Data from Petty RE, Laxer RM, Lindsley CB, et al., eds. *Textbook of Pediatric Rheumatology.* 7th ed. Philadelphia: Elsevier; 2016:534; Fink CW, Nelson JD. Septic arthritis and osteomyelitis in children. *Clin Rheum Dis.* 1986;12(2):423–435; Speiser JC, Moore TL, Osborn TG, et al. Changing trends in pediatric septic arthritis. *Semin Arthritis Rheum.* 1985;15(2):132–138; Wilson NI, Di Paola M. Acute septic arthritis in infancy and childhood. 10 years' experience. *J Bone Joint Surg.* 1986;68(4):584–587; Welkon CJ, Long SS, Fisher MC, et al. Pyogenic arthritis in infants and children: a review of 95 cases. *Pediatr Infect Dis.* 1986;5(6):669–676.

TABLE 44.7 Characteristics of Synovial Fluid

	Appearance	Viscosity	Cells per mm³	% PMNs	Crystals	Microbiology
Normal	Transparent	High	<200	<10%	Negative	Negative
JIA	Translucent	Low	2,000–50,000	Variable	Negative	Negative
Reactive arthritis	Translucent	Low	2,000–50,000	Variable	Negative	Negative
Gout	Translucent to cloudy	Low	200 to >50,000	>90%	Needle-shaped, negatively birefringent monosodium urate monohydrate crystals	Negative
Bacterial arthritis*	Cloudy	Variable	50,000 to >100,000	>90%	Negative	Usually positive
PVNS	Hemorrhagic or "chocolate brown"	Low	Variable	Variable	Negative	Negative
Hemarthrosis	Hemorrhagic	Low	Variable	Variable	Negative	Negative
Lyme disease	Xanthochromic or cloudy	Variable	500 to >100,000 (average 25,000)	Predominantly PMNs	None	Negative

*Includes spirochetal, gonococcal, and mycobacterial infections.
JIA, juvenile idiopathic arthritis; PMNs, polymorphonuclear neutrophils; PVNS, pigmented villonodular synovitis.
Modified from El-Gabalawy HS. Synovial fluid analyses, synovial biopsy, and synovial pathology. In: *Kelley's Textbook of Rheumatology.* 9th ed. Philadelphia: Saunders; 2013:755, Table 53-1.

Invasive Testing

If weakness is present, an electromyogram (EMG) and a nerve conduction study may distinguish myopathies and myositis from neuropathies. Children with inflammatory myositis have a characteristic, albeit nondiagnostic, abnormal EMG. Peripheral neuropathies confirmed by nerve conduction studies may suggest the presence of a vasculitis or SLE.

Biopsies are most helpful in confirming the presence of vasculitis (Table 44.9) and to determine the extent of renal disease in a child with SLE. Kawasaki disease, GPA, MPA, eosinophilic granulomatosis with polyangiitis (EGPA), Takayasu arteritis, polyarteritis, and IgA vasculitis are vasculitides that may be diagnosed on the basis of either clinical criteria alone (Kawasaki disease, IgA vasculitis), a combination of clinical criteria and arteriography (Takayasu arteritis, polyarteritis), or clinical criteria and serologic profiles (antiproteinase 3 and antimyeloperoxidase antibodies in GPA, MPA, and EGPA). Biopsies of affected tissue are often necessary to confirm a diagnosis for many of the vasculitides. The most accessible affected tissue is acquired for biopsy first. If there are no cutaneous lesions easily accessible for biopsy, muscle and nerve samples may be taken for biopsy when EMG and nerve conduction studies reveal the presence of myositis or neuropathy. If neither of these sites is affected, then the risks and benefits of biopsy of affected organs should be evaluated.

Synovial biopsy is rarely useful in the evaluation of arthritis. Biopsy may help to distinguish sarcoid arthropathy from JIA; sarcoid arthropathy is suspected when the young child has erythema nodosum, uveitis, and arthritis, as well as particularly "boggy" synovial effusions. In rare cases, synovial tumors, chronic indolent infections, or foreign bodies may be detected by biopsy.

JUVENILE IDIOPATHIC ARTHRITIS

JIA is not a single disease, but rather a group of chronic diseases that share arthritis as a primary manifestation. JIA is categorized into several different subtypes, each with characteristic clinical and laboratory

TABLE 44.8 Differential Diagnosis of Monoarticular vs Polyarticular Arthritis and Arthralgia

Usually Monoarticular	Often Polyarticular
Common	
Infectious arthritis	Polyarticular JIA
• Bacterial	Psoriatic arthritis
• Mycobacterial	Reactive arthritis
• Fungal	Enthesitis-related arthritis
Avascular necrosis	• Ulcerative colitis
Hemarthrosis	• Crohn disease
Coagulopathy	Serum sickness
Trauma/overuse	Henoch-Schönlein purpura
Oligoarticular JIA	Systemic lupus erythematosus
Congenital hip dysplasia	Viral arthritis
Osteochondritis dissecans	Immune complex–mediated post-
Complex regional pain syndrome	bacteremia (*Neisseria meningitidis,*
Stress fracture	*Haemophilus influenzae*)
Osteomyelitis	Hypermobility
Metastatic tumor (neuroblastoma, leukemia)	Hemoglobinopathies
Rare	
Pigmented villonodular synovitis	Undifferentiated connective tissue
Plant thorn synovitis	disease
Familial Mediterranean fever	Relapsing polychondritis
Synovioma	Whipple disease
Synovial metastasis	Sarcoidosis
Intermittent hydrarthrosis	Systemic JIA
Pancreatic fat necrosis	Pulmonary hypertrophic
Gaucher disease	osteoarthropathy
Behçet disease	Chondrocalcinosis-like syndromes
Regional migratory osteoporosis	caused by ochronosis,
Amyloidosis	hemochromatosis, Wilson disease
Synovial osteochondromatosis	Acute rheumatic fever
	Dialysis arthropathy
	Crystal-induced arthropathies

JIA, juvenile idiopathic arthritis.
Modified from McCune WJ. Monoarticular arthritis. In: Kelley WN, Harris ED, Ruddy S, et al., eds. *Textbook of Rheumatology.* 4th ed. Vol 1. Philadelphia: WB Saunders; 1993:369.

TABLE 44.9 Classification of Childhood Vasculitis

- Predominantly large-vessel vasculitis
  - Takayasu arteritis
- Predominantly medium-vessel vasculitis
  - Childhood polyarteritis nodosa
  - Cutaneous polyarteritis
  - Kawasaki disease
- Predominantly small-vessel vasculitis
  - Granulomatous
    - Granulomatosis with polyangiitis
    - Eosinophilic granulomatosis with polyangiitis
  - Nongranulomatous
    - Microscopic polyangiitis
    - IgA vasculitis (Henoch-Schönlein purpura)
    - Isolated cutaneous leukocytoclastic vasculitis
    - Hypocomplementemic urticarial vasculitis
- Other vasculitides
  - Behçet disease
  - Vasculitis secondary to infection (including hepatitis B–associated polyarteritis nodosa), malignancy, and medication (including hypersensitivity vasculitis)
  - Isolated vasculitis of the central nervous system
  - Cogan syndrome
  - Unclassified

IgA, immunoglobulin A.
Modified from Ozen S, Ruperto N, Dillon MJ, et al. EULAR/PReS endorsed consensus criteria for the classification of childhood vasculitis. *Ann Rheum Dis.* 2006;65:936–941.

arthritis of the knee. This subtype affects primarily young children with an average age of onset of 2 years. Affected children have morning stiffness, mild discomfort, swelling, and warmth of the affected joint or joints but usually remain functional and are systemically well. The arthritis has a good prognosis and in some cases may eventually remit. Most children with this subtype of JIA have a positive ANA test result and are at high risk for associated chronic anterior uveitis.

Polyarticular Juvenile Idiopathic Arthritis

There are two subtypes of polyarticular JIA: RF positive and RF negative. RF-positive disease is most likely the same disease as adult-onset rheumatoid arthritis and tends to affect older children and adolescents. RF-negative polyarticular JIA is much more common and affects all ages. The arthritis in these subtypes is symmetric and affects both small and large joints. Involvement of the small joints of the hands and feet, as well as the wrists, is very common. Chronic anterior uveitis may occur; it is more common in younger patients, especially if ANA test results are positive. The prognosis for those with polyarticular JIA is less favorable, with many children continuing to have some signs and symptoms of arthritis into adulthood.

Enthesitis-Related Arthritis

The term *spondyloarthropathy* encompasses a group of diseases that potentially affect the spine and includes ankylosing spondylitis, psoriatic arthritis, inflammatory bowel disease–associated arthritis, and reactive arthritis. These diseases are grouped together because they share common clinical features such as male predominance, enthesitis, dactylitis, peripheral oligoarticular disease, axial arthritis, acute symptomatic anterior uveitis, and an association with HLA-B27. Within the current JIA classification criteria, psoriatic arthritis is

findings. The diagnosis of JIA is based on history and physical examination. The classification criteria define JIA and the subtypes, but it is important to note that these criteria are intended to be useful for research purposes and are less useful diagnostically (Table 44.10). According to these criteria, JIA is defined as inflammatory arthritis of unknown etiology beginning before age 16 years and persisting for at least 6 weeks. These criteria also specify that the determination of the subtype of JIA should be made based on the findings present 6 months after the onset of disease. Several noninflammatory conditions can closely mimic JIA and are listed in Table 44.11.

Oligoarticular Juvenile Idiopathic Arthritis

This is the most common form of JIA, affecting approximately half of all children with JIA. Oligoarticular JIA can be further classified depending on whether fewer than four joints are affected for the entire course of the disease ("persistent") or if more than four joints are affected after the first 6 months of disease ("extended"). Persistent oligoarticular JIA is the most common form and most often manifests as monoarticular

TABLE 44.10 Classification Criteria for Juvenile Idiopathic Arthritis

General Definition of Juvenile Idiopathic Arthritis
- Arthritis that begins before the 16th birthday and persists for at least 6 wk
- Other known causes of arthritis are excluded

Categories

Systemic Arthritis
- Arthritis in one or more joints with or preceded by fever of at least 2-wk duration that is documented to be daily ("quotidian") for at least 3 days, and accompanied by one or more of the following:
  - Evanescent (nonfixed) erythematous rash
  - Generalized lymph node enlargement
  - Hepatomegaly and/or splenomegaly
  - Serositis

Oligoarthritis
- Arthritis affecting one to four joints during the first 6 mo of disease
- Subcategories:
  - Persistent oligoarthritis: affecting not more than four joints throughout the disease course
  - Extended oligoarthritis: affecting a total of more than four joints after the first 6 mo of disease

Polyarthritis (RF Negative)
- Arthritis affecting five or more joints during the first 6 mo of disease
- Negative test for RF

Polyarthritis (RF Positive)
- Arthritis affecting five or more joints during the first 6 mo of disease
- Two or more positive tests for RF, separated by at least 3 mo during the first 6 mo of disease

Psoriatic Arthritis
- Arthritis and psoriasis or suspicion of underlying psoriasis as evidenced by:
  - Formal diagnosis of psoriasis, or
  - At least two of the following:
    - Dactylitis
    - Nail pitting or onycholysis
    - Psoriasis in a first-degree relative

Enthesitis-Related Arthritis
- Arthritis and enthesitis, or
- Arthritis or enthesitis with at least two of the following:
  - History of sacroiliac joint tenderness and/or inflammatory lumbosacral pain
  - Positive HLA-B27 antigen
  - Onset of arthritis in a male over 6 yr of age
  - Acute (symptomatic) anterior uveitis
  - History of ankylosing spondylitis, enthesitis-related arthritis, sacroiliitis with inflammatory bowel disease, reactive arthritis, or acute anterior uveitis in a first-degree relative

Undifferentiated Arthritis
- Arthritis that fulfills criteria in no category or in two or more of the above categories

HLA, human leukocyte antigen; RF, rheumatoid factor.
Criteria from Petty RE, Southwood TR, Manners P, et al. International League of Associations for Rheumatology classification of juvenile idiopathic arthritis: second revision, Edmonton, 2001. *J Rheumatol.* 2004;31:391–392.

TABLE 44.11 Noninflammatory Mimics of Juvenile Idiopathic Arthritis

Disease	Distinguishing Features
Idiopathic multicentric osteolysis	Usually young children; restricted movement in wrists and ankles followed by rapid progressive resorption of carpal and tarsal bones; plain radiography with early extensive osteolytic changes
Mucopolysaccharidosis	Joint stiffness and contractures in the absence of systemic inflammation; characteristic facial features; multiorgan involvement
Fucosidosis	Polyarticular arthritis; developmental delay; joint findings may precede systemic features, such as visceromegaly, angiokeratomata, growth delay, recurrent infections
Camptodactyly–arthropathy–coxa vara–pericarditis syndrome	Camptodactyly of the fifth fingers; swelling of interphalangeal joints, wrists, and knees without associated inflammation; lack of joint pain and morning stiffness; lack of systemic inflammation; progressive coxa vara; occasionally pericarditis
Progressive pseudorheumatoid dysplasia	Presentation in early childhood with progressive flexion contractures and stiffness of the interphalangeal joints, metaphyseal bony overgrowth of the metacarpals and phalanges, gradual but progressive involvement of remainder of axial skeleton and disproportionate short stature
Pachydermodactyly	Asymptomatic thickening and swelling of the skin and soft tissues around the proximal interphalangeal joints of the hands

classified separately, and the other spondyloarthropathies are designated as enthesitis-related arthritis (ERA) because of the recognition that these forms of arthritis do not always affect the spine, especially during childhood. In addition to chronic arthritis, the JIA classification criteria designate a patient as having ERA if they have two of the following criteria: persistent sacroiliac joint tenderness and/or inflammatory lumbosacral pain, positive HLA-B27 antigen, acute symptomatic anterior uveitis, presence of symptoms in a male over 6 years of age, and, finally, a first-degree relative with a history of ankylosing spondylitis, ERA, sacroiliitis with inflammatory bowel disease, reactive arthritis, or acute anterior uveitis. This subtype of JIA affects older children and has a variable prognosis, with an increased risk of spondylitis over time.

Psoriatic Arthritis

The JIA criteria designate a patient with psoriatic arthritis if they have chronic arthritis accompanied either by a personal diagnosis of psoriasis or by a combination of two other clinical criteria (dactylitis, nail pitting/onycholysis, or psoriasis in a first-degree relative). Psoriatic arthritis in children may occur at any age and has an initial peak incidence between ages 2 and 3 years that appears clinically similar to oligoarticular JIA and a later peak incidence between ages 10 and 12 years that appears clinically similar to ERA. The early-onset form of psoriatic arthritis is more likely to affect females than boys, more often has associated dactylitis and a positive ANA, and is less often associated with a positive HLA-B27. In contrast, the later-onset form is more likely to occur in boys, is more often associated with

TABLE 44.12   European League Against Rheumatism/American College of Rheumatology Classification Criteria for Macrophage Activation Syndrome Complicating Systemic Juvenile Idiopathic Arthritis (2016)

A febrile patient with known or suspected juvenile idiopathic arthritis is classified as having macrophage activation syndrome if the following criteria are met:

Ferritin >684 ng/mL *and* any two of the following:

- Platelet count <181 × 10⁹/L
- Aspartate aminotransferase >48 units/L
- Triglycerides >156 mg/dL
- Fibrinogen <360 mg/dL

Laboratory abnormalities should not be otherwise explained by the patient's condition, such as concomitant immune-mediated thrombocytopenia, infectious hepatitis, visceral leishmaniasis, or familial hyperlipidemia.

a negative ANA and positive HLA-B27, and is more likely to manifest with enthesitis and axial arthritis. Psoriasis usually precedes the development of arthritis, but in some, arthritis can precede the skin disease, sometimes by many years. Up to 30% of patients with psoriasis will have associated arthritis, and patients with nail involvement are more likely to develop arthritis. The severity of the arthritis does not typically correlate with the severity of the skin disease, and the prognosis is variable, with some having only occasional episodic arthritis in a few joints and others having severe, chronic arthritis in multiple joints.

Systemic Juvenile Idiopathic Arthritis

Systemic JIA (SJIA) affects children of all ages but is most commonly seen between the ages of 1 and 5 years. In SJIA, any number of joints may be affected, but most patients eventually develop polyarticular involvement. Children with SJIA initially have a characteristic quotidian fever pattern, consisting of one or two high fever spikes each day with rapid return to normal or lower-than-normal temperature. An evanescent pink macular rash appears with the fever and may resolve completely as the child's fever abates (see Figs. 44.3 and 44.4). Constitutional symptoms such as fatigue, poor appetite, and weight loss are common. Generalized lymphadenopathy and hepatosplenomegaly are also common; pericarditis or pleural effusions may occur. These children feel and appear ill during the fever spikes but may appear much improved once the fever abates. Peripheral leukocytosis of 20,000 WBCs/mm³ or greater, anemia, and thrombocytosis are characteristic laboratory findings. Tests of ANA and RF are usually negative, and uveitis is very rare. In most patients, the fevers and rashes eventually subside and chronic arthritis persists as an isolated manifestation.

Patients with SJIA are at risk for **macrophage activation syndrome**, a life-threatening complication of uncontrolled immune activation resulting in persistent, unremitting fever; petechial/purpuric rashes in some; hepatosplenomegaly; and potentially multiorgan dysfunction. Laboratory examination demonstrates elevated CRP and markedly elevated ferritin with a paradoxically falling ESR due to consumption of fibrinogen. Cytopenias, particularly thrombocytopenia, are observed, as are hypertriglyceridemia and hypoalbuminemia. Hemophagocytosis is observed in various tissues, most commonly in the bone marrow and cerebrospinal fluid. Diagnostic criteria for macrophage activation syndrome are presented in Table 44.12. If clinical suspicion for macrophage activation syndrome remains high despite serum laboratory markers failing to satisfy diagnostic criteria, cerebrospinal fluid or bone marrow investigation for hemophagocytosis should strongly be considered.

Diagnosis

The diagnosis of JIA and the determination of the subtype of JIA is based on clinical features (see Table 44.10). The differential diagnosis is broad (Tables 44.13 and 44.14; see Table 44.1). When there is isolated monoarthritis of the knee and a child has been in an endemic area, Lyme disease should be considered (Table 44.15). Residing in or traveling to endemic areas, particularly if associated with a suggestive prodromal illness, should prompt investigation for other infectious arthritides (Table 44.16). Laboratory tests and imaging studies are used when necessary to exclude other illnesses. The RF and ANA tests are used to classify the subtype of JIA and to determine the risk of uveitis, but **these tests are not sensitive or specific enough to be helpful as either screening tests or diagnostic tests for JIA**. Ophthalmologic slit-lamp evaluations are necessary at specific intervals to screen for anterior uveitis, because usually the uveitis is asymptomatic and can progress to affect visual acuity before it causes other signs and symptoms.

SYSTEMIC LUPUS ERYTHEMATOSUS

In SLE, clinical manifestations are the result of increased production of both specific and nonspecific autoantibodies, with subsequent immune complex formation and deposition throughout the body. The cause of SLE is unknown; it is more common in females, Black individuals, and persons with a first-degree relative with SLE. In childhood, the peak onset is during the early teen years and rarely occurs in children younger than 5 years. The potential clinical manifestations of SLE are numerous, and the illness demonstrates significant interindividual variability. Children with SLE have more severe disease than adults, with a greater incidence of renal involvement.

Diagnosis

SLE is suggested by the common manifestations of fever, malar rash (Fig. 44.9), photosensitivity, and arthritis. The arthritis is most often symmetric and polyarticular and frequently involves the small joints of the hands and feet. In contrast to JIA, the arthritis is typically nondeforming and does not result in erosions. The European League Against Rheumatism (EULAR) and the American College of Rheumatology (ACR) classification criteria for SLE can be a guide to diagnosis (Fig. 44.10). Other clinical manifestations of SLE are listed in Table 44.17.

The ANA test is extremely sensitive, positive in more than 95% of children with SLE, and usually in a high titer; however, it is not specific. Testing for anti-dsDNA antibodies, anti-Smith antibodies, anti-RNP antibodies, and anti-SSA and anti-SSB antibodies should be performed in all children suspected of having SLE (see Table 44.4). Anti-dsDNA antibodies and anti-Smith antibodies are highly specific for SLE. Leukopenia, lymphopenia, thrombocytopenia, and autoimmune hemolytic anemia, frequently with a positive direct Coombs test, are common. Urinalysis is mandatory to screen for nephritis, and proteinuria should increase the suspicion of associated glomerulonephritis. The complement proteins C3 and C4 are low in children with active SLE. Monitoring C3 and C4 levels helps guide therapy; the levels should increase to normal as the illness is better controlled.

Monogenic causes of SLE should be suspected in young children (younger than 5 years), in families with a history of SLE, and in patients with difficult-to-treat SLE. The most common genes associated with SLE are part of the **type 1 interferonopathy group** (Table 44.18). Mimics of SLE are noted in Table 44.19.

TABLE 44.13 Differential Diagnosis of Juvenile Idiopathic Arthritis: Rheumatic Disease

	Rheumatic Fever	Juvenile Idiopathic Arthritis	Systemic Lupus Erythematosus	Kawasaki Disease	Dermatomyositis
Sex predilection	None	Dependent on subgroup	Females > males	None	Girls 3:2
Age at onset	3 yr or older	1 yr or older	Usually >8 yr	4 yr or younger	2 yr or older
Joint manifestations	Transient migratory arthritis of primarily large joints	Oligoarticular or polyarticular; chronic (≥6 wk)	Arthralgia; transient arthritis; chronic arthritis	Pain and swelling of hands and feet; arthritis occasionally	Joint contractures; arthritis occasionally
Extra-articular manifestations	Fever Cardiac disease Chorea Rash Nodules	Dependent on subgroup: Systemic JIA: fever, rash, lymphadenopathy Oligoarticular, polyarticular, psoriatic JIA: chronic iridocyclitis	Often multisystem disease, including nephritis	Fever Conjunctivitis Oral changes Polymorphous rash Lymphadenopathy Coronary vasculitis	Rash Muscle weakness Myalgia Gut vasculitis Respiratory muscle weakness
Diagnostic studies	Prior streptococcal infection Evidence of carditis on echocardiogram or ECG	May have ANA, RF	ANA Autoantibodies Low complement Anti-dsDNA antibody	Coronary dilatation or aneurysm on echocardiogram	Elevated muscle enzymes Myopathic electromyography Abnormal muscle biopsy
Pathogenesis	Poststreptococcal	Unknown	Immune complexes	Unknown	Unknown
Diagnosis	Clinical (Jones criteria)	Clinical (JIA criteria)	Clinical plus laboratory (EULAR/ACR criteria)	Clinical (Kawasaki criteria)	Clinical: rash plus myositis Muscle biopsy
Natural history	Arthritis—transient Carditis may cause permanent damage	Chronic: arthritis may be destructive	Chronic or recurrent May be fatal	Self-limited Coronary vasculitis May be fatal	Chronic May be fatal

ANA, antinuclear antibody; anti-dsDNA, anti–double-stranded DNA; JIA, juvenile idiopathic arthritis; RF, rheumatoid factor; EULAR/ACR, European League Against Rheumatism/American College of Rheumatology.
Modified from Behrman RE, ed. *Nelson Textbook of Pediatrics.* 14th ed. Philadelphia: WB Saunders; 1992:620.

TABLE 44.14 Differential Diagnosis of Juvenile Idiopathic Arthritis: Nonrheumatic Disease

	Septic Arthritis	Lyme Disease	Osteomyelitis	Viral Arthritis	Childhood Malignancy	Structural, Genetic	Growing Pains, Psychogenic
Sex predilection	None	None	None	Females > males	None	Dependent on condition	Growing pains: boys > girls Psychogenic: girls > boys
Age at onset	Any	>2 yr	Any	More common in older children and adults	Any	Any	Growing pains: 2–8 yr Psychogenic: ≥6 yr
Joint manifestations	85% monoarticular; joints swollen, red, hot, painful	Oligoarticular; episodic, recurrent	Sterile joint effusion adjacent to infected bone	Transient arthritis; often polyarticular	Severe bone/joint pain, night pains	Local bone/ joint pain or dysfunction	None or features of complex regional pain syndrome
Extra-articular manifestations	Fever SIRS Other signs dependent on causative organism	Flulike illness Erythema migrans Meningitis Cranial nerve palsies Heart block	Fever SIRS Bone pain	Dependent on causative organism	Signs of underlying malignancy; no high fever, rash, or morning stiffness	Dependent on underlying condition Dysmorphism Structural abnormalities	Growing pains: none Psychogenic: atypical
Diagnostic studies	Cultures: synovial fluid, blood, genital if *Neisseria gonorrhoeae* suspected	Serologic: antibody to *Borrelia burgdorferi*	Blood and bone culture Bone scan	Viral culture/ PCR Rise in antibody titers	Hematologic abnormalities Abnormal radiograph or scan	Demonstration of abnormal structure or metabolic abnormality	Normal

Continued

TABLE 44.14   Differential Diagnosis of Juvenile Idiopathic Arthritis: Nonrheumatic Disease—cont'd

	Septic Arthritis	Lyme Disease	Osteomyelitis	Viral Arthritis	Childhood Malignancy	Structural, Genetic	Growing Pains, Psychogenic
Pathogenesis	Direct synovial infection; immune complex deposition in gonococcal and meningococcal arthritis	Synovial and systemic infection with *B. burgdorferi*	Hematogenous infection of bone	Viral infection of synovium; immune complex deposition in some	Primary bone or periarticular tumor; bony metastasis	Idiopathic or genetic	No organic disease
Diagnosis	Demonstration of organisms in joint fluid	Clinical and serologic	Demonstration of organisms in blood/bone; MRI of bone scan (early); plain radiographs (late)	Clinical; serologic; positive viral culture or PCR from synovial fluid	Bone marrow; tissue biopsy	Recognition of condition or syndrome; positive genetic or biochemical assay	Clinical
Natural history	Joint destruction	Self-resolving	Bone/joint destruction	Self-resolving	Joint manifestations may wax/wane	Chronic	Growing pains: benign Psychogenic: may become chronic and disabling

PCR, polymerase chain reaction; SIRS, systemic inflammatory response syndrome.
Modified from Behrman RE, ed. *Nelson Textbook of Pediatrics*. 14th ed. Philadelphia: WB Saunders; 1992:619.

TABLE 44.15   Manifestations of Lyme Disease by Stage

Early Localized Infection (occurs 3–30 days after tick bite)
Erythema migrans (EM) in 80–90% of patients; single lesion, occasionally associated with fever, malaise, neck pain or stiffness, arthralgia, and myalgia
Systemic symptoms noted above in the absence of EM during summer months
Borrelial lymphocytoma (rare, seen primarily in Europe)

Early Disseminated Infection (occurs weeks to months after tick bite)
Profound malaise and fatigue common
Multiple EM lesions with systemic symptoms similar to early localized infection
Migratory polyarthralgia and myalgia
Carditis (<3% of untreated patients)
    Varying degrees of atrioventricular nodal block
    Mild myopericarditis
Neurologic (<10% of untreated patients)
    Cranial neuropathies (especially facial nerve palsy)
    Lymphocytic meningitis
    Radiculoneuropathies
    Encephalomyelitis

Late Disease (occurs months to years after tick bite)
Arthritis (<10% of patients)
    Acute monoarticular or migratory oligoarticular inflammatory arthritis, usually involving the knee
    Chronic postinfectious arthritis (<10% of patients with arthritis)
Neurologic (very rare)
    Peripheral neuropathies
    Encephalomyelitis (primarily seen in Europe)
Acrodermatitis chronica atrophicans (primarily seen in Europe)

Modified from Bockenstedt LK. Lyme disease. In: Firestein GS, Budd RC, Gabriel SE, et al., eds. *Kelley's Textbook of Rheumatology*. 9th ed. Philadelphia: Saunders; 2013, Chapter 110, Table 110-1.

TABLE 44.16   Infectious Mimics of Systemic Juvenile Idiopathic Arthritis

Nocardia
Brucella canis
Coxiella burnetii
Scrub typhus
Rickettsial diseases
Ehrlichiosis
Chikungunya virus
Zika virus
Dengue virus

DERMATOMYOSITIS

Dermatomyositis is characterized by perivascular inflammation in muscles and skin. Dermatomyositis is more common in females and can occur at any age, with an average age at onset of 8 years. The main manifestations include characteristic skin findings and proximal muscle weakness, specifically involving the neck flexors, deltoids, biceps, triceps, quadriceps, psoas, and hamstrings. These symptoms are occasionally accompanied by mild muscle pain, fatigue, or poor endurance. Early symptoms may include difficulties rising from the floor, climbing stairs, climbing in and out of a motor vehicle, and combing the hair; however, these symptoms are often subtle and not recognized early in the course of the disease. Some children with dermatomyositis may have arthralgia or arthritis that is usually mild and transient.

Skin manifestations include Gottron papules, which are scaly, erythematous plaques or papules that appear over the MCP and PIP joints on the hands (see Fig. 44.6). Similar lesions are seen on the extensor surfaces of the elbows and knees and over the medial malleoli. The distribution of the rash is an early clue to the diagnosis. The periungual capillaries may become grossly dilated and may develop

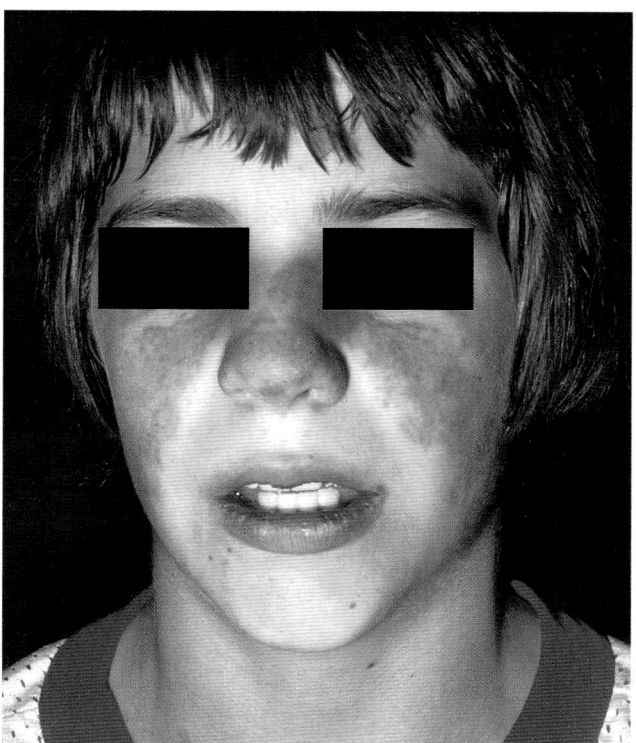

Fig. 44.9 The malar rash of systemic lupus erythematosus crosses the nasal bridge and spares the nasolabial folds, a distribution that is referred to as a "butterfly rash." (From Petty RE, Laxer RM, Lindsley CB, et al., eds. *Textbook of Pediatric Rheumatology.* 7th ed. Philadelphia: Elsevier; 2016:299.)

thromboses that can be visualized either with the naked eye or with mild magnification. Heliotrope rash is a violaceous discoloration of the upper eyelids that is often accompanied by mild edema (see Fig. 44.5) and is pathognomonic for dermatomyositis. Some children develop more extensive erythroderma that may appear over the shoulders, termed the shawl sign, or in a V-neck distribution on the anterior upper chest. With severe disease, some patients also develop skin ulcerations.

Diagnosis

The diagnosis is suggested by the rash and proximal muscle weakness detected on physical examination. Muscle enzymes are elevated in most, but not all, children with dermatomyositis. There may be elevations in only one or a few enzymes and therefore testing for aspartate aminotransferase, alanine aminotransferase, lactate dehydrogenase, creatine kinase, and aldolase should be performed. The child with a characteristic rash, definite proximal muscle weakness, and elevated muscle enzyme levels does not require additional testing for diagnosis. If weakness is questionable, or if the rash is not characteristic, an EMG can confirm the presence of muscle inflammation. MRI is a sensitive test for muscle inflammation and may be a less invasive method of evaluation. If there is any doubt regarding the diagnosis, a muscle biopsy is performed. The site for biopsy is determined by weakness on physical examination or localization by EMG or MRI. The quadriceps or the deltoids are the most commonly accessed biopsy sites. Involvement of the muscle may be spotty, and a normal finding on muscle biopsy does not exclude dermatomyositis. Typical findings on biopsy include perivascular inflammation and perifascicular atrophy. Biopsy can help exclude other muscle diseases such as muscular dystrophies and metabolic myopathies.

SCLERODERMA

Scleroderma is classified into systemic sclerosis and localized scleroderma (Table 44.20). Localized scleroderma, which includes morphea and linear scleroderma, is limited to the skin and subcutaneous tissues, is much more common in childhood, and rarely progresses to involve internal organs. Systemic sclerosis can be life threatening, as it has the potential to involve internal organs and cause severe and widespread skin disease. Arthralgia is relatively common with scleroderma, but significant synovitis is unusual.

Morphea

Morphea is a patch of hardened skin that appears spontaneously on any part of the body. The skin becomes firm, stiff, atrophic, and discolored. Hair is absent. Initially, the lesion appears violaceous, but then it fades to a yellowish-brown or dusky appearance in most individuals. The patches are nontender, and children are otherwise asymptomatic. The natural history of morphea lesions is to gradually fade and soften after an initial period of expansion. Biopsy reveals excessive amounts of collagen in the dermis with absent hair follicles and diminished vascular structures.

Linear Scleroderma

Linear scleroderma is histologically similar to morphea, though lesions consist not of isolated patches, but rather of bands that may extend through an entire limb, through part of the limb, or across the scalp and face, a finding termed a *coup de sabre* lesion. Cosmetically and functionally, linear scleroderma is much more severe than morphea, as the impacted areas may involve the face or limit limb use. Growth of the limb may be affected, and involvement of the digits can cause significant functional difficulty. *Coup de sabre* lesions may be associated with neurologic abnormalities such as seizures; children with these lesions should have a careful neurologic examination and brain MRI as part of their evaluation.

Systemic Sclerosis

Systemic sclerosis typically begins with severe Raynaud phenomenon, followed by thickening and tightening of the skin over the digits and hands and then the face, and then by varying degrees of progressive skin changes over the extremities and trunk. Difficulty opening the mouth and decreased facial expression are signs of facial involvement. As the skin over the hands tightens and hardens, pigment changes may occur, and flexion contractures of the small joints may develop. Renal disease, pulmonary fibrosis, pulmonary hypertension, esophageal and gut dysmotility, and cardiac disease may all occur. Anti–Scl-70 antibodies (antitopoisomerase I) are present in approximately 30–40% of patients with systemic sclerosis and are very specific. There are no other helpful serologic tests. High-resolution CT of the chest, esophagography, and echocardiography should be performed to screen for organ involvement and repeated at periodic intervals. The course of systemic sclerosis is variable; patients with rapid progression tend to have a less favorable outcome. The CREST syndrome (calcinosis, Raynaud phenomenon, esophageal dysmotility, sclerodactyly, and telangiectasias) has less severe cutaneous involvement than systemic sclerosis; however, these patients can develop life-threatening pulmonary hypertension. CREST syndrome is associated with anticentromere antibodies.

RHEUMATIC FEVER

Acute rheumatic fever is a poststreptococcal illness, resulting from a cross-reactive immune response to group A streptococcal

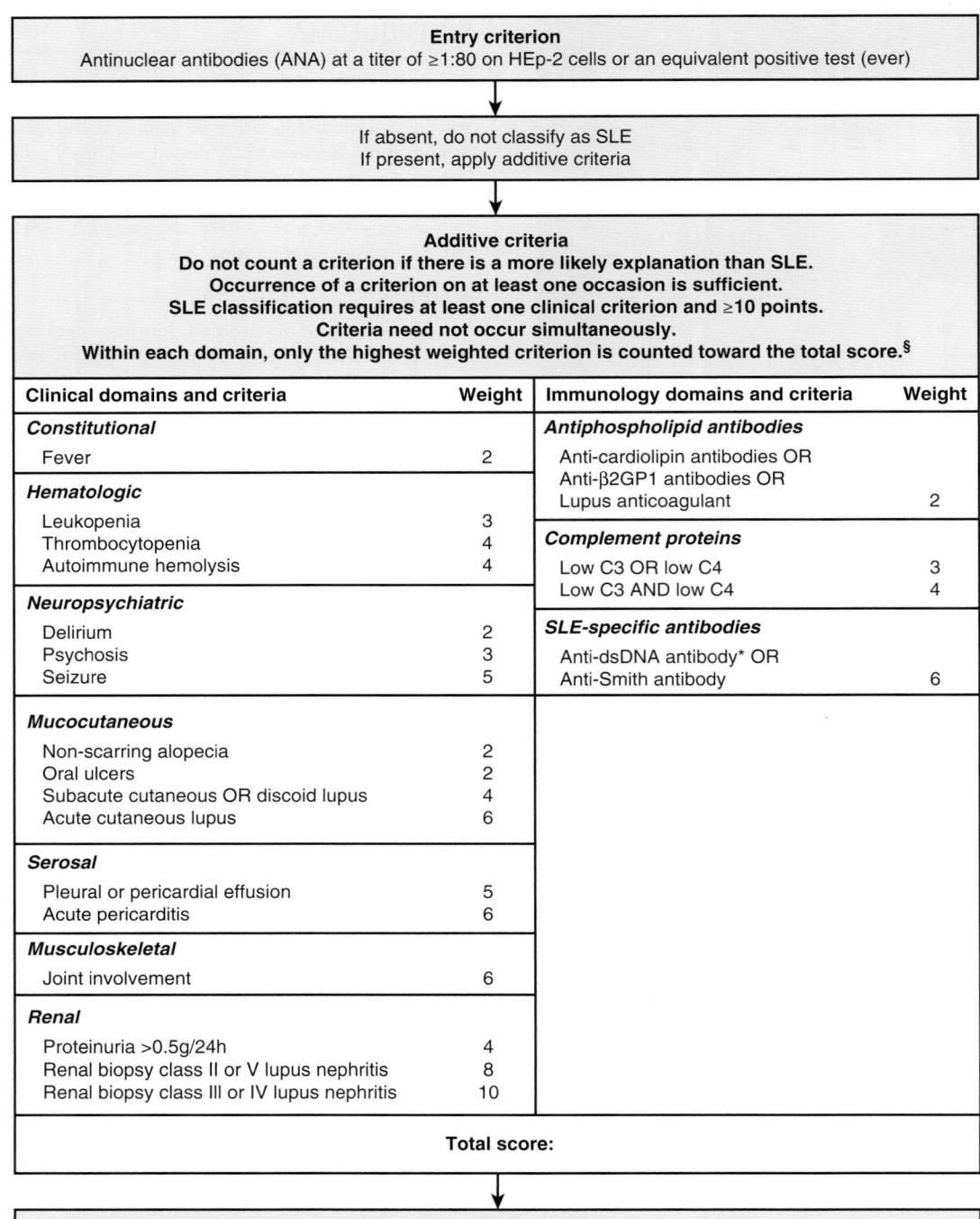

Entry criterion
Antinuclear antibodies (ANA) at a titer of ≥1:80 on HEp-2 cells or an equivalent positive test (ever)

↓

If absent, do not classify as SLE
If present, apply additive criteria

↓

Additive criteria
Do not count a criterion if there is a more likely explanation than SLE.
Occurrence of a criterion on at least one occasion is sufficient.
SLE classification requires at least one clinical criterion and ≥10 points.
Criteria need not occur simultaneously.
Within each domain, only the highest weighted criterion is counted toward the total score.[§]

Clinical domains and criteria	Weight	Immunology domains and criteria	Weight
Constitutional		***Antiphospholipid antibodies***	
Fever	2	Anti-cardiolipin antibodies OR Anti-β2GP1 antibodies OR Lupus anticoagulant	2
Hematologic		***Complement proteins***	
Leukopenia	3	Low C3 OR low C4	3
Thrombocytopenia	4	Low C3 AND low C4	4
Autoimmune hemolysis	4		
Neuropsychiatric		***SLE-specific antibodies***	
Delirium	2	Anti-dsDNA antibody* OR Anti-Smith antibody	6
Psychosis	3		
Seizure	5		
Mucocutaneous			
Non-scarring alopecia	2		
Oral ulcers	2		
Subacute cutaneous OR discoid lupus	4		
Acute cutaneous lupus	6		
Serosal			
Pleural or pericardial effusion	5		
Acute pericarditis	6		
Musculoskeletal			
Joint involvement	6		
Renal			
Proteinuria >0.5g/24h	4		
Renal biopsy class II or V lupus nephritis	8		
Renal biopsy class III or IV lupus nephritis	10		
Total score:			

↓

Classify as systemic lupus erythematosus with a score of 10 or more if entry criterion fulfilled.

Fig. 44.10 Classification criteria for systemic lupus erythematosus (SLE). *In an assay with ≥90% specificity against relevant disease controls. [§]Additional criteria items within the same domain will not be counted. (From Aringer M, Costenbader K, Daikh D, et al. 2019 European League Against Rheumatism/American College of Rheumatology classification criteria for systemic lupus erythematosus. *Arthritis Rheum.* 2019;71[9]:1400–1412.)

pharyngitis (see Chapters 2 and 9). It is most common in children older than 5 years and occurs more often after infection with certain serotypes of group A streptococci. There may also be genetic reasons that predispose some children and adults to the illness. Signs and symptoms of rheumatic fever typically develop 1–3 weeks after streptococcal pharyngitis. Clinical manifestations have been

grouped according to the Jones criteria, which separate major from minor criteria (Table 44.21).

The arthritis of rheumatic fever is usually very painful and is disproportionate to the degree of swelling on physical examination. It is usually a migratory arthritis of the large joints, rarely affecting the fingers, spine, or toes, tending to last in one joint for several days and then

TABLE 44.17 Additional Manifestations of Systemic Lupus Erythematosus

Target Organ	Potential Clinical Manifestations
Constitutional	Fatigue, anorexia, weight loss, fever, lymphadenopathy
Musculoskeletal	Arthritis, myositis, tendonitis, arthralgia, myalgia, avascular necrosis, osteoporosis
Skin	Malar rash, discoid (annular) rash, photosensitive rash, cutaneous vasculitis (petechiae, palpable purpura, digit ulcers, gangrene, urticaria), livedo reticularis, periungual capillary abnormalities, Raynaud phenomenon, alopecia, oral and nasal ulcers, panniculitis, chilblains, alopecia
Renal	Hypertension, proteinuria, hematuria, edema, nephrotic syndrome, renal failure
Cardiovascular	Pericarditis, myocarditis, conduction system abnormalities, Libman-Sacks endocarditis
Neurologic	Seizures, psychosis, cerebritis, stroke, transverse myelitis, depression, cognitive impairment, headaches, migraines, pseudotumor, peripheral neuropathy (mononeuritis multiplex), chorea, optic neuritis, cranial nerve palsies, acute confusional states, dural sinus thrombosis, aseptic meningitis, anxiety disorder
Pulmonary	Pleuritis, interstitial lung disease, pulmonary hemorrhage, pulmonary hypertension, pulmonary embolism
Hematologic	Immune-mediated cytopenias (hemolytic anemia, thrombocytopenia, or leukopenia), anemia of chronic inflammation, hypercoagulability, thrombotic thrombocytopenic microangiopathy
Gastroenterology	Hepatosplenomegaly, pancreatitis, vasculitis affecting the bowel, protein-losing enteropathy, peritonitis
Ocular	Retinal vasculitis, scleritis, episcleritis, papilledema, dry eyes, optic neuritis

Modified from Sadun RE, Ardoin SP, Schanberg LE. Systemic lupus erythematosus. In: Kliegman RM, St. Geme JW, Blum NJ, et al., eds. *Nelson Textbook of Pediatrics*. 21st ed. Philadelphia: Elsevier; 2020:1275, Table 183.1.

migrating to a different joint. The duration of joint symptoms is rarely longer than 3–4 weeks in untreated patients. If patients are treated with NSAIDs, the arthritis usually responds dramatically within 1–2 days. When rheumatic fever is a consideration and the diagnosis is unclear, it may be helpful to avoid NSAID use early in the course to avoid diagnostic confusion.

In the absence of carditis, rheumatic fever may be difficult to distinguish from early SJIA, Kawasaki disease, and viral-induced fever, rash, and joint pain. The diagnosis is clinical. The Jones criteria were developed as a diagnostic aid and include echocardiographic evidence of valvulitis and, in populations with a higher risk of rheumatic fever, monoarthritis or polyarthralgia as less stringent major criteria (see Table 44.21). The presence of two of the major criteria or of one major and two minor criteria plus evidence of recent streptococcal infection is consistent with acute rheumatic fever. Either a positive throat culture or elevations of the antistreptococcal antibodies (i.e., anti–streptolysin O, anti–DNase B) are the standard indicators of potential recent streptococcal infection. Fulfilling these criteria is not specific for rheumatic fever, especially when the evidence of recent streptococcal infection is based on mildly elevated serologic test results. Conversely, there are children with isolated chorea or classic rheumatic carditis who have rheumatic fever without necessarily fulfilling the Jones criteria. When a diagnosis of rheumatic fever is considered in a child with joint symptoms, it is important to distinguish arthritis from arthralgia and to evaluate the nature of the arthritis when present. If the arthritis is nonmigratory and is not exquisitely tender, or if it involves unusual joints such as those in the hands, feet, or spine or lasts longer than 1 week in a single joint, then alternative diagnoses are more likely.

Careful consideration of the diagnosis is especially important because of future implications regarding prognosis and treatment. Children with rheumatic fever may develop carditis with future episodes of streptococcal pharyngitis; each episode of carditis can produce additional heart valve damage. Therefore, prophylactic antibiotic treatment is recommended to minimize streptococcal infections, even for patients who do not have carditis with the initial attack.

IGA VASCULITIS/HENOCH-SCHÖNLEIN PURPURA

IgA vasculitis is an acute self-limited systemic vasculitis of children characterized by palpable purpura and often arthritis, gastrointestinal symptoms, and nephritis. It occurs most commonly between the ages of 3 and 15 years. The presence of palpable purpura is essential for the diagnosis of HSP. Typically, the rash presents as petechiae that coalesce into larger purpura on dependent areas such as the buttocks and legs. The rash is often edematous and on occasion can become ulcerative. Arthritis occurs in up to 80% of children with HSP, is typically acute with significant pain and limitation of range of motion, and usually resolves within days to a week. Large joints tend to be affected and the arthritis is nonmigratory. In most cases, the rash of HSP precedes the development of arthritis, but occasionally, the arthritis may occur a few days before the rash. Other features that might suggest a diagnosis of HSP are gastrointestinal symptoms, nephritis, or angioedema. Gastrointestinal symptoms result from gut vasculitis causing intestinal edema and potentially ischemia and infarction of the gut. Gastrointestinal disease often presents as episodic abdominal pain from intussusception or with abdominal angina (postprandial abdominal pain related to intestinal ischemia). Rarely, hematochezia or currant jelly–like stools can result from intestinal necrosis. In up to a third of cases, abdominal pain will precede the rash. Nephritis may occur at any time up to 6 months after the initial presentation and may manifest with hypertension or with proteinuria, hematuria, or casts on urinalysis. As such, serial urinalysis is recommended until 6 months after the initial presentation to screen for the development of nephritis. Angioedema can occur on the dorsum of the hands or feet, scalp, forehead, eyelids, and scrotum. The acute manifestations of HSP usually resolve in 1–2 weeks and may recur episodically for several weeks after. Nephritis is potentially the most concerning complication that requires longer monitoring and prompt referral to a pediatric nephrologist if urinary abnormalities persist.

MYALGIA

In the child with extremity pain, muscle pain needs to be distinguished from joint pain, bone pain, and the less common neuropathic pain. If the complaint is localized to the muscles, the differential diagnosis is narrowed considerably. Intermittent benign bilateral myalgia of the calves or thighs is one of the more common muscle pain presentations encountered in young children. These pains occur in an active child who has normal physical examination findings without evidence of weakness or systemic illness. Symptoms typically occur in the evening and resolve with massage or mild analgesics such as acetaminophen or ibuprofen, usually within an hour. The frequency of pain can vary and in some children may escalate periodically. Additional evaluation or treatment is unnecessary in most children, and eventually the pains resolve completely.

TABLE 44.18   Reviewed Proteins and Genes Associated with Monogenic Forms of Systemic Lupus Erythematosus

Protein	Gene	Inheritance	Mechanism	Female-to-Male Patient Ratio	Associated Symptoms
C1q	C1QA, C1QB, C1QC	Autosomal recessive	Complement deficiency	1:1	SLE (cutaneous, renal, CNS, arthritis, ANA), young age onset, recurrent bacterial infections
C1r/s	C1R, C1S	Autosomal recessive	Complement deficiency	1:1	SLE (fever, cutaneous, arthritis, renal, ANA, ENA), recurrent infections, encapsulated bacteria, Hashimoto thyroiditis
C2	C2	Autosomal recessive	Complement deficiency	7:1	SLE (cutaneous, arthritis), young age onset, type 1 diabetes
C4	C4A, C4B	Autosomal recessive	Complement deficiency	1:1	SLE (severe photosensitive rash, renal, ANA, Ro), young age onset
TREX1	TREX1	Autosomal dominant (FCL), autosomal recessive and dominant (AGS)	Abnormal DNA clearance leading to IFN activation	Likely 1:1	FCL, AGS, SLE
MDA5	IFIH1	Autosomal dominant	Activation of IFN production	Likely 1:1	AGS, SLE, FCL, IgA deficiency
SAMHD1	SAMHD1	Autosomal recessive and dominant	Abnormal DNA or RNA clearance leading to IFN production	Likely 1:1	AGS, SLE, FCL, photosensitivity
RNaseH2	RNASH2	Autosomal dominant and recessive	Abnormal RNA clearance leading to IFN production	Likely 1:1	AGS, SLE
ADAR1	ADAR1	Mainly autosomal dominant	Abnormal RNA clearance leading to IFN production	Likely 1:1	AGS, SLE
STING	TMEM173	Autosomal dominant	Activation of IFN production	1:1	SAVI, FCL, SLE
DNase I	DNASE1	Autosomal dominant	Abnormal DNA clearance-break intolerance	Female	SLE (dsDNA), adolescent onset, Sjögren syndrome
DNase 1-like-3	DNASE1L3	Autosomal recessive	Abnormal DNA clearance-break intolerance	1:2	SLE (hypocomplementemia, dsDNA, cANCA, renal), HUVS

AGS, Aicardi-Goutières syndrome; ANA, antinuclear antibody; ANCA, antineutrophil cytoplasmic antibody; CNS, central nervous system; dsDNA, double-stranded DNA; ENA, extractable nuclear antigen antibody; FCL, familial chilblain lupus; HUVS, hypocomplementemic urticarial vasculitis syndrome; IFN, interferon; IgA, immunoglobulin A; SAVI, STING-associated vasculopathy with onset in infancy; SLE, systemic lupus erythematosus. From Hiraki LT, Silverman ED. Genomics of systemic lupus erythematosus: insights gained by studying monogenic young-onset systemic lupus erythematosus. *Rheum Dis Clin N Am.* 2017;43:415–434 (Table 1, p. 417).

TABLE 44.19   Mimics of Systemic Lupus Erythematosus

Drug induced (medication or biologic agents)
Kikuchi disease (histiocytic necrotizing lymphadenopathy)
Evans syndrome (autoimmune hemolytic anemia and thrombocytopenia)
Castleman disease (multicentric)
Lymphoma
Type 1 interferonopathy
Autoimmune lymphoproliferative syndrome (ALPS)
Prolidase deficiency
Graft versus host disease
Parvovirus B19
Endocarditis

TABLE 44.20   Classification of Scleroderma

Systemic Sclerosis

- Diffuse cutaneous: systemic fibrosis, including widespread skin involvement (face, trunk, and both proximal and distal extremities) and internal organ involvement (lungs, kidneys, gastrointestinal tract, heart)
- Limited cutaneous (includes CREST syndrome): skin fibrosis limited to the distal extremities, face, and neck; internal organ involvement occurs late, if at all, with pulmonary hypertension often being the most significant development
- Overlap: features of a second rheumatic disease

Localized Scleroderma

- Morphea: a single, discrete patch of fibrotic skin; no organ involvement
- Generalized morphea: multiple discrete patches of fibrotic skin; no organ involvement
- Linear scleroderma: band of fibrosis on the face *(coup de sabre)* or along an extremity, sometimes extending the entire length; no organ involvement
- Mixed
- Pansclerotic: severe joint contractures

CREST, calcinosis, Raynaud phenomenon, esophageal dysmotility, sclerodactyly, and telangiectasias.

TABLE 44.21 Jones Criteria for Diagnosis of Rheumatic Fever

All patient populations must demonstrate evidence of a preceding GAS infection

Initial ARF: two major manifestations OR one major plus two minor manifestations

Recurrent ARF: two major OR one major and two minor OR three minor manifestations

Major Criteria

Carditis: clinical (audible murmur) or subclinical (echocardiographic evidence of valvulitis)

Subcutaneous nodules

Erythema marginatum

Chorea

Low-risk populations*: polyarthritis

Moderate- and high-risk populations: polyarthritis, monoarthritis, or polyarthralgia†

Minor Criteria

Fever (≥38.5°C)

Peak ESR ≥30 mm/hr and/or CRP ≥3.0 mg/dL‡

Prolonged P-R interval, after accounting for age variability (unless carditis is a major criterion)

Low-risk populations: polyarthralgia

Moderate- and high-risk populations: monoarthralgia

*Low-risk populations are those with an ARF incidence ≤2/100,000 school-aged children or an all-age rheumatic heart disease prevalence of ≤1/1000 population per year.
†Polyarthralgia should only be considered as a major manifestation in moderate- to high-risk populations after exclusion of other causes. As in past versions of the criteria, erythema marginatum and subcutaneous nodules are rarely "stand-alone" major criteria. Additionally, joint manifestations can only be considered in either the major or minor categories, but not both in the same patient.
‡The CRP value must be greater than the upper limit of normal for the laboratory. Because ESR may evolve during the course of ARF, peak ESR values should be used.
ARF, acute rheumatic fever; GAS, group A streptococcal.
Modified from Gewitz MH, Baltimore RS, Tani LY, et al. Revision of the Jones criteria for the diagnosis of acute rheumatic fever in the era of Doppler echocardiography. *Circulation.* 2015;131:1806–1818.

As myalgia may accompany polymyositis and dermatomyositis, every child complaining of muscle pain should undergo careful muscle strength testing. Myalgia may also be seen with vasculitis and SJIA. Many children with acute-onset diffuse myalgia have a transient viral illness, and pain usually resolves within several days; however, infection with influenza can cause an exquisitely painful myositis of the gastrocnemius muscles with difficulty ambulating. This condition is

TABLE 44.22 Potential Pitfalls in Diagnosis

Do

1. Examine **all** joints.
2. Order radiographs of both affected and contralateral joints.
3. Ask parents to photograph swelling and rashes.
4. Explore the complete history including the psychosocial history in all patients.
5. Perform a **thorough** physical examination.
6. Consider the presence of MAS in patients with JIA or SLE.

Do Not

1. Indiscriminately order ANA tests, RF tests, or Lyme antibody tests in patients who do not have clinical features consistent with SLE, polyarthritis, or Lyme disease, respectively.
2. Confuse arthralgia (joint pain) with arthritis (inflammation).
3. Treat with prednisone before a diagnosis is clear, or before malignancy has been excluded.
4. Assume laboratory test results are accurate; repeat tests if necessary.
5. Be impatient; many illnesses associated with arthritis take time to either resolve or evolve; patience is often required to make an accurate diagnosis.

ANA, antinuclear antibody; JIA, juvenile idiopathic arthritis; MAS, macrophage activating syndrome; RF, rheumatoid factor; SLE, systemic lupus erythematosus.

usually distinguished easily from a chronic inflammatory muscle disease by the sudden onset and localization to these specific muscles. The creatine kinase level may be very elevated. Myoglobinuria may ensue and potentially affect renal function; therefore, affected children should undergo urinalysis to determine if myoglobinuria is present. Myoglobin in the urine will yield positive results for heme in the absence of erythrocytes on microscopic examination. The myositis associated with influenza and other viruses typically resolves within 1 week and treatment is symptomatic.

COMPLEX REGIONAL PAIN SYNDROME

Complex regional pain syndrome is rare in childhood and poorly understood (see Chapter 33). After a seemingly minor injury, affected children develop intense pain in an extremity or part of an extremity. Additional symptoms include intermittent autonomic changes such as discoloration, coolness, and localized excessive sweating. The pain leads to progressive disability of the extremity, occasionally resulting in fixed posturing of a hand, foot, or limb. Severely affected children become disabled, are unable to ambulate at times, and are often unable to attend school. Psychosocial comorbidity is common. The treatment is analgesia, intense physical and occupational therapy, education, and psychologic counseling. Some children improve dramatically within a few days of instituting therapy, whereas in others, the pain and disability persist, and the process lasts indefinitely. In some instances, sympathetic nerve blockade is helpful.

▮ SUMMARY AND RED FLAGS

The differential diagnosis of arthritis is extensive. Thorough history and physical examination, especially repeated over time, are essential in establishing a diagnosis and initiating a treatment plan. Potential diagnostic pitfalls are noted in Table 44.22. Red flags include manifestations suggestive of septic arthritis (fever, single joint involvement, erythema, extreme tenderness, leukocytosis), malignancy (severe polyarthralgia, night pain, nonarticular bone pain, absence

of obvious swelling or stiffness, positive radiographic changes, and cytopenias), and Lyme disease. The presence of associated systemic signs and symptoms are an indication that the joint complaints are potentially part of a systemic rheumatic disease such as SLE, JIA, MAS, or rheumatic fever.

A variety of noninflammatory conditions may mimic JIA; furthermore, several infectious entities may produce arthritis and systemic symptoms that mimic SJIA. The child with a history of injury and the acute onset of extremity pain may have a fracture or traumatic hemarthrosis, which requires prompt evaluation and management. Any child with extremity pain, including children with arthritis, may have leukemia or neuroblastoma. Systemic symptoms, such as fatigue and poor appetite with weight loss, may accompany the pain and increase suspicion of malignancy. Deep bone pain caused by marrow invasion may not be accompanied by any obvious physical findings.

A normal or slightly low platelet count with an elevated ESR increases the suspicion of malignancy. If leukemia is suspected, a CBC should be obtained, a peripheral smear reviewed, and a bone marrow aspiration performed. This is particularly important if treatment with steroids or other immunosuppressive medications is being considered. Steroids may alleviate inflammation and discomfort but may also place a child with leukemia at risk for relapse with steroid-resistant disease.

BIBLIOGRAPHY

A bibliography is available at ExpertConsult.com.

45

Gait Disturbances

Alicia C. Zolkoske and Shayne D. Fehr

Most gait disturbances are benign and resolve with normal growth and development. Others are pathologic in origin and necessitate treatment (Table 45.1).

GAIT CYCLE

The normal gait cycle is described by foot placement. The gait cycle begins with right heel strike; is followed by left toe-off, left heel strike, and right toe-off; and ends with right heel strike. These five events describe one gait cycle and include two phases: stance and swing. The **stance phase** is the period of time during which one of the two feet is on the ground. The **swing phase** is the period during which a limb is being advanced forward without ground contact.

Measuring the duration of the gait cycle makes it possible to calculate the time required for each of the five phases. During normal gait, the duration of each phase is as follows: for weight acceptance, 11%; for single limb stance, 39%; for weight release, 11%; and for swing phase, 39%. Velocity, cadence, step length, stride length, and step width may be calculated from the timed and measured gait cycle.

DEVELOPMENT OF GAIT

Central nervous system maturation is necessary for the development of normal gait and accounts for the normal progression of developmental milestones. The typical milestones for locomotion include independent sitting at 6 months of age, crawling at about 9 months, walking without assistance at 12–15 months, and running at 18 months. A normal 1-year-old child has a wide-based stance and a rapid cadence with short steps; the elbows are flexed and reciprocal arm motion is not present. Foot strike occurs without an initial heel strike. A 2-year-old child shows increased velocity, step length, and diminished cadence in comparison with a 1-year-old child. Most of the adult gait patterns are present in children by 3 years, with changes in velocity, stride, and cadence continuing to 7 years of age. The gait characteristics of a 7-year-old child are similar to those of an adult.

CLINICAL EVALUATION OF GAIT DISTURBANCES

History

The clinician should inquire about the pregnancy and delivery, the age at which developmental milestones occurred, the presence of any systemic illnesses (including chronicity, fever, rash, weight loss, and other organ system involvement), and whether there is a family history of any congenital musculoskeletal abnormalities or syndromes. With regard to the gait disturbance, it is important to inquire when it was first observed, whether it is unilateral or bilateral, whether it is associated with any injuries or intercurrent systemic illnesses, if there is

associated pain or weakness, and whether there has been a history of improvement or worsening with time.

Physical Examination

General Musculoskeletal Examination

Although most of the findings in gait disturbances are confined to the lower extremities, the upper extremities and spine may be involved as part of an underlying disease process. A general assessment of all extremities and the spine should be performed to identify any abnormal motion, tenderness, swelling, deformity, or increased warmth.

The lower extremity musculoskeletal examination should begin with the child ambulating in the examination room or adjacent hallway. The child must be adequately undressed and be observed from a distance while walking so that the trunk and lower extremities can be clearly visualized. The positions of the thighs, knees, lower legs, and feet should be observed during ambulation. Combining gait observation with the history typically allows for diagnosing most of the common gait disturbances such as torsional variations (in-toeing and out-toeing), equinus gait (toe-walking), and limping.

Examination of the lower extremities should include measurement of lower extremity lengths and assessment of the hip, knee, ankle, and subtalar joints. The thighs, lower legs, and feet are inspected for evidence of asymmetry, soft tissue swelling, or injury. Palpation for tenderness or areas of increased warmth is performed. The shape of the foot is assessed for possible intrinsic deformity.

Lower extremity length measurements. The most accurate method of measuring lower extremity length is with radiographs; however, if radiographs are not readily available, this assessment is best performed by having the child stand on a firm, level surface with the examiner standing behind the child and placing index fingers over the lateral aspect of each of the child's iliac crests. The presence or absence of pelvic obliquity is observed, and blocks of various heights are placed beneath the child's foot on the short side until the pelvis is level. The height of the blocks indicates the amount of lower extremity length discrepancy. Measurements obtained by use of a tape measure can also be performed but are less accurate. The most common measurements using this method are from the anterior-superior iliac spine to the distal aspect of the medial malleolus. These landmarks are sometimes difficult to palpate accurately, and there can be considerable error using this method. The Galeazzi test can assess for femoral or tibial length discrepancy or hip dislocation leading to a perceived limb length disturbance (Fig. 45.1). Tibial length can also be assessed by having the patient in a prone position and knees flexed to 90 degrees and then observing the relative height of the feet.

Joint assessment. The ranges of motion of the hips, knees, ankles, and subtalar joints must be assessed. Hip flexion is measured, as are any flexion contractures. With the hip in extension, the degrees of abduction, adduction, internal rotation, and external rotation are

TABLE 45.1	Causes of Gait Disturbances

Mechanical
Acute injuries (accidental or nonaccidental)
Overuse conditions (mainly sports-related)
Dysplastic lesions
Limb length discrepancy

Osseous
Legg-Calvé-Perthes disease
Osteochondritis dissecans of knee and talus
Slipped capital femoral epiphysis
Osteomyelitis
Diskitis
Osteoid osteoma or other primary bone tumor

Articular
Developmental hip dysplasia
Septic arthritis
Transient synovitis
Rheumatic disease (JIA, SLE)
Hemophilia-related hemorrhage
Ankylosis of a joint

Neurologic
Guillain-Barré syndrome and other peripheral neuropathies
Intoxication
Cerebellar ataxia
Brain tumor
Lesion occupying spinal cord space
Posterior column spinal cord disorders
Myopathy
Hemiplegia
Complex regional pain syndrome
Cerebral palsy
Acute flaccid myelitis

Hematologic/Oncologic
Sickle cell pain crisis
Leukemia, lymphoma
Metastatic tumor
Langerhans cell histiocytosis

Other
Soft tissue infection
Myositis
Fasciitis
Bursitis
Kawasaki disease
Conversion disorder/functional disorder
Gaucher disease
Phlebitis
Scurvy
Rickets
Peritonitis

JIA, juvenile idiopathic arthritis; SLE, systemic lupus erythematosus.

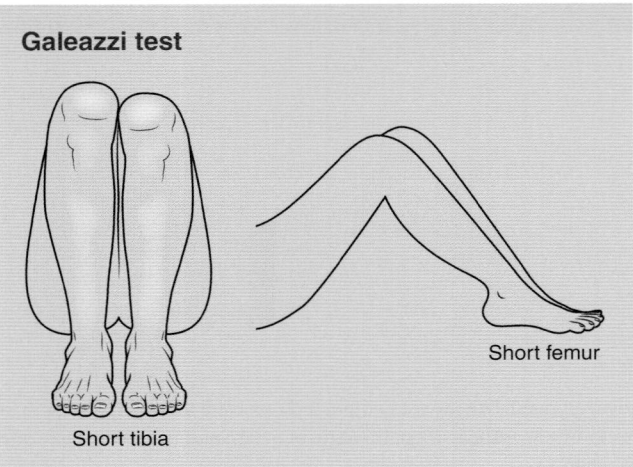

Fig. 45.1 The Galeazzi test assesses for developmental dysplasia of the hip in infants and can be used to screen for femoral or tibial length discrepancy in older children and adults. With the patient in a supine position, the hips are flexed to 45 degrees and the knees to 90 degrees with the feet flat on the examining table. Inequality in the height of the knees is considered a positive Galeazzi sign and in infants is often related to developmental dysplasia of the hip. The test may produce a false negative if there is bilateral developmental dysplasia of the hip. For leg length discrepancy, in instances of tibial shortening, the knee on the affected side will be shifted inferiorly or caudally relative to the unaffected side (left-hand side of figure). In instances of femoral shortening, the knee on the affected side is shifted cephalad (right-hand side of figure). (From Tillotson L, Fieraru G, Briant-Evans T. Examination of the hip for MRCS OSCE. *Surgery [Oxford].* 2020;38:65–69, Fig. 3.)

measured, preferably with a goniometer, and are recorded. Hip rotation is most accurately measured with the child in the prone position with the knees flexed. Older children and adolescents are typically more comfortable when measured in the supine position with hips and knees flexed to 90 degrees. Knee flexion and extension, ankle dorsiflexion, and plantar flexion, as well as subtalar motion, must be assessed and recorded.

Spinal evaluation. Spinal mobility should be assessed because abnormalities such as spondylolysis, nerve root impingement, diskitis, and tumors may manifest as a gait disturbance. The child's ability to flex forward and to reverse lumbar lordosis is a sign of normal mobility (see Chapter 46). Areas of vertebral bone tenderness and muscle spasm are determined by direct palpation.

Neurologic Evaluation

Many gait disturbances have a neurologic cause or association. The neurologic examination should include assessment of unilateral or bilateral involvement, the presence of paresthesia, and muscle strength testing, sensory assessment (particularly to establish the specific level or distribution of any potential sensory deficits), deep tendon reflexes, and pathologic reflexes, such as the Babinski sign. Abnormal rectal tone or bladder distention is concerning for a spinal lesion.

Radiographic Assessment

The need for radiographic evaluation is based on the differential diagnosis. For many gait disturbances, radiographic assessment is not required. When necessary, plain radiographs of the lower extremities, pelvis, or spine are obtained first, followed by special diagnostic studies, such as anteroposterior (AP) leg length radiographs to assess for discrepancy, technetium bone scan to localize occult lesions such as avascular necrosis or stress fracture, and CT to characterize specific lesions. MRI is helpful in the diagnosis of occult or soft tissue lesions, such as infection, tumors, or metabolic bone disease, as well as other pathologic structural processes of the spine, such as syrinx, tethered cord, or disk anomaly.

TABLE 45.2 Common Causes of In-Toeing and Out-Toeing

In-Toeing	Out-Toeing
Medial (internal) femoral torsion	Lateral (external) femoral torsion
Medial (internal) tibial torsion	Lateral (external) tibial torsion
Metatarsus adductus	Calcaneovalgus feet
Talipes equinovarus (clubfoot)	Hypermobile pes planus

Laboratory Tests

Tests such as CBC with differential, ESR, and CRP level are indicated if an infectious, rheumatic, or otherwise inflammatory condition is suspected. Rheumatoid factor and antinuclear antibody determinations are less helpful in the diagnosis of rheumatic causes of gait disturbances (see Chapter 44). Other tests may be indicated for the diagnosis of specific disorders. Electromyography, nerve conduction studies, muscle biopsies, and nerve biopsies are frequently necessary in the diagnosis of myopathic or neuropathic disorders (see Chapter 35). Determinations of creatine phosphokinase, aldolase, and aspartate aminotransferase levels are important in the evaluation of striated muscle function and should be ordered if an underlying myopathy or myositis is suspected.

GAIT DISTURBANCES

The three most common categories of gait disturbances of childhood are torsional variations (in-toeing and out-toeing), toe-walking (equinus gait), and limping.

Torsional Variations

The presence of in-toeing or out-toeing does not necessarily imply an abnormality of the foot; rather, it indicates only the direction in which the foot is pointing during ambulation. Torsional variations can be located from the proximal (i.e., the hip) to the distal (i.e., the foot) region in the involved extremity. Some causes, such as clubfeet, are obvious, whereas others are subtle. Most torsional variations resolve with normal growth and development. The common causes of in-toeing and out-toeing are listed in Table 45.2.

Normal Developmental Alignment

In utero positioning affects the alignment of the lower extremities of infants. In the typical in utero position, the hips are flexed, abducted, and externally rotated; the knees are flexed; and the lower legs are internally rotated. The feet are in a supinated position against the posterolateral aspect of the opposite thigh. The musculoskeletal examination of an infant characteristically shows 20- to 30-degree hip flexion contractures, 50–60 degrees of abduction, 80–90 degrees of external rotation in extension, and minimal or no internal rotation. The knees have 20- to 30-degree flexion contractures, and internal tibial torsion is present. These are normal findings. The increased external rotation of the hip is caused not by femoral retroversion but rather by a posterior hip capsule contracture, which begins to resolve at the time of independent ambulation.

The combination of external rotation at the hip and internal rotation of the lower leg results in **physiologic genu varum**, a bowed appearance of the lower extremities, particularly when in the weight-bearing position, that reflects this physiologic torsional combination. After the child attains independent ambulation, this bowed appearance improves over a 6- to 12-month period with expected resolution by 2 years of age in over 95% of children. Exaggerated bowing under

the age of 2 years, failure to progress through the anticipated developmental stages of limb alignment, asymmetry, pain, or deformity isolated to the tibia may be signs of pathologic genu varum warranting further evaluation; the primary differential diagnosis of pathologic genu varum consists of tibia vara (**Blount disease**), rickets and other metabolic bone diseases, and asymmetric growth following infection or trauma or in the setting of benign or malignant neoplasms. Initial evaluation typically consists of anteroposterior radiographs of the bilateral lower extremities with the knees moved into a forward-facing position so as to minimize confounding from external rotation at the knees. **Tibia vara** is characterized by pathologic disruption of growth at the medial aspect of the proximal tibial physis and may be described as infantile (presentation prior to age 4 years) or adolescent (presentation in later childhood or adolescence); infantile tibia vara is more often bilateral, whereas adolescent disease may be either unilateral or bilateral. In addition to bowing, gait observation may reveal *varus thrust*, which consists of sudden lateral movement of the knee during the stance phase. In tibia vara, the anteroposterior radiographs of the bilateral lower extremities with the knees in a forward-facing position reveal medial beaking and downward sloping of the proximal tibia metaphysis. Patients with **rickets** often have short stature and may additionally present with pathologic fractures. Bone density may be decreased on radiography, though bone mineralization may appear normal as well; patients with severe rickets may have widened and cupped physes and flared metaphyses. Initial serum evaluation of rickets consists of determining levels of parathyroid hormone, calcium, and inorganic phosphorus concentrations; investigations for underlying liver or kidney disease should be undertaken as well. **Congenital pseudoarthrosis of the tibia** and **congenital pseudoarthrosis of the fibula** are very rare forms of angular deformity of the lower extremity that result in bowing; pathogenesis is believed to be related to abnormalities of the periosteum. Both are associated with neurofibromatosis type 1. Affected patients typically present not with a pseudoarthrosis, but with anterolateral bowing of the lower leg that is noted at birth. Rather, pseudoarthroses typically arise following pathologic fracture and subsequent nonunion of the affected bone, usually after the patient begins ambulating. Despite aggressive surgical management, nonunion and progressive deformity may persist.

Physiologic or **developmental genu valgum** ("knock knees") is seen between 3 and 4 years of age. This is true genu valgum, an angular phenomenon, and is not the result of torsional variations. This condition resolves with growth and normal adult knee alignment is obtained between 5 and 8 years of age. Newborns have a mean varus alignment of 15 degrees that corrects to neutral alignment between 18 and 20 months of age. The maximum valgus of 12 degrees occurs by 3–4 years of age. By 7 years of age, the valgus alignment corrects to that of a normal adult (8 degrees in females, 7 degrees in males). Overall, 95% of cases of developmental genu valgum resolve with growth, even in children with more pronounced findings. In some children, the condition may not completely correct until adolescence or may resolve incompletely; in the absence of known trauma or underlying metabolic disease, short stature, or infection, persistent bilaterally symmetric genu valgum is considered idiopathic. The differential diagnosis of nonidiopathic, bilaterally symmetric genu valgum includes rickets, other metabolic diseases such as mucopolysaccharidosis, and skeletal dysplasias. Pathologic genu valgum may also be unilateral; unilateral valgus deformity is often secondary to previous trauma, such as a nondisplaced tibial metaphyseal fracture. Other etiologies include post-traumatic or postinfectious partial physeal arrest; conditions associated with benign neoplasms, such as Ollier disease (multiple enchondromas) or multiple hereditary exostosis; or asymmetric manifestations of metabolic disease or skeletal dysplasia.

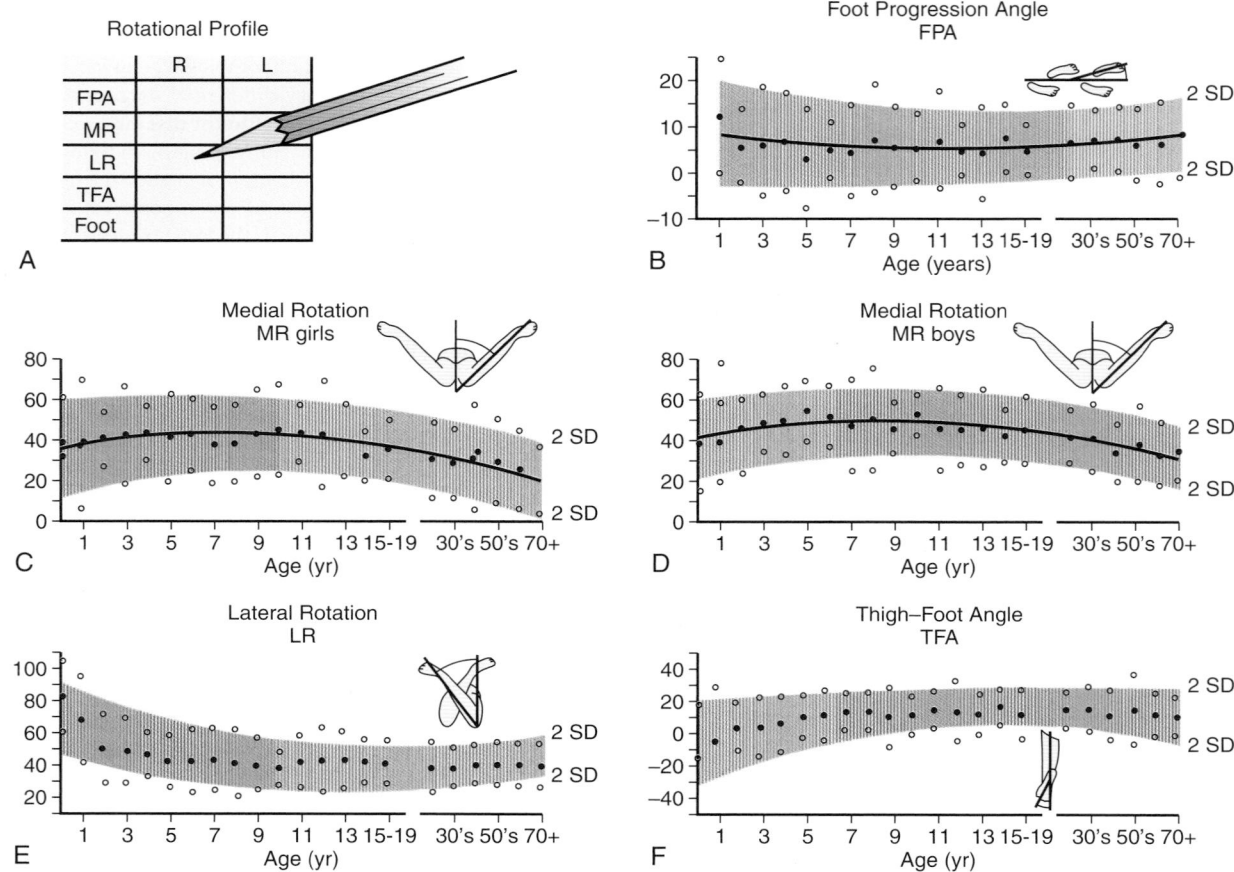

Fig. 45.2 The torsional or rotational profile from birth to maturity. *A,* The rotational profile is assessed and tracked at each visit. *B,* Mean foot progression angle (FPA) by age. *C,* Mean femoral medial rotation in girls by age. *D,* Mean femoral medial rotation in boys by age. *E,* Mean lateral rotation by age. *F,* Mean thigh-foot angle. All graphs include 2 standard deviations from the mean. (From Morrissey RT, Weinstein SL, eds. *Lovell and Winter's Pediatric Orthopaedics.* 3rd ed. Philadelphia: Lippincott Williams & Wilkins; 1990.)

Torsional Profile

The torsional or rotational profile aids in the diagnosis and sequential follow-up of children with torsional variations (Fig. 45.2).

Foot progression angle. The foot progression angle, which is the direction of the long axis of the foot with regard to the direction in which the child is walking (Fig. 45.3), should be measured. Inward rotation is given a negative value and outward rotation a positive value. A normal foot progression angle in children and adolescents is 10 degrees (range, −3 to +20 degrees). The foot progression angle defines whether the gait is normal or if there is an in-toeing or out-toeing gait. Recording the angle allows for comparison during follow-up evaluations.

Hip rotation. Measuring hip rotation allows for indirect assessment of femoral version. Typically, the femoral neck creates an anteriorly directed angle with the transcondylar axis of the distal femur (Fig. 45.4). This anterior angulation is known as femoral anteversion and decreases from approximately 40 degrees at birth to 15 degrees by maturity. Increased internal rotation at the hip indicates excessive anteversion; increased external rotation at the hip indicates retroversion. Hip rotation is assessed with the child in the prone position with the knees together and flexed 90 degrees (Fig. 45.5). In this position, the hip is in neutral alignment. Rotating the lower leg outwardly produces internal rotation of the hip; rotating the lower leg inwardly produces external rotation of the hip. A newborn hip in extension typically rotates externally 80–90 degrees and has a limited internal rotation of 0–10 degrees. By 1

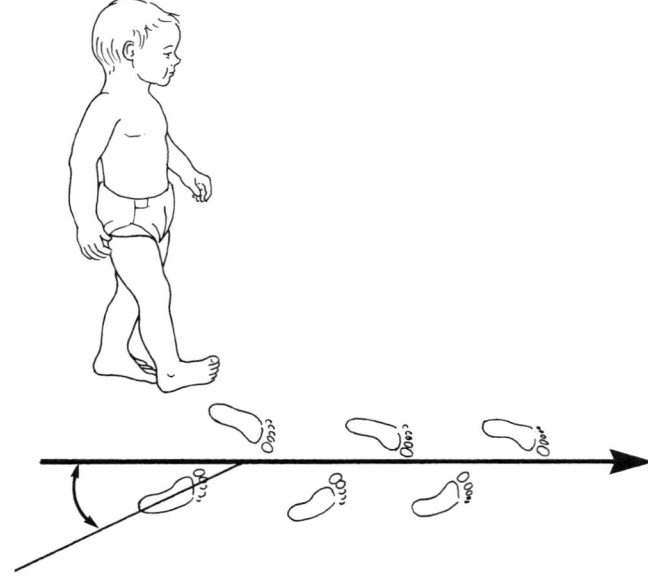

Fig. 45.3 Foot progression angle. The long axis of the foot is compared with the direction in which the child is walking. If the foot points outward, the angle is positive. If the foot points inward, the angle is negative.

year of age, there is approximately 30–40 degrees of internal rotation. Hip rotation should be bilaterally symmetric. Asymmetric rotation is often indicative of a hip disorder and necessitates radiographs of the pelvis. The mean hip internal rotation in extension in older males is 50 degrees (range, 25–65 degrees), and that in females is 40 degrees (range, 15–60 degrees).

Thigh-foot angle. With the child in the prone position and the knees approximated and flexed 90 degrees, the long axis of the foot in the neutral or simulated weight-bearing position can be compared with the long axis of the thigh (Fig. 45.6). Inward rotation is given

a negative value, whereas outward rotation is given a positive value. Inward rotation is indicative of internal tibial torsion, and outward rotation represents external tibial torsion. This angle must be accurately measured and recorded. The mean thigh-foot angle is 10 degrees (range, −5 to +30 degrees) from middle childhood through adult life. Infants have a mean thigh-foot angle of −5 degrees (range, −35 to +40 degrees) as a consequence of the normal in utero position.

Foot shape. With the child again in the prone position, the shape of the foot is easily appreciated, allowing for assessment of children with metatarsus adductus or a calcaneovalgus foot. The mobility of the ankle and subtalar joint can also be evaluated with the child in this position.

In-Toed Gait

Internal femoral torsion. Increased femoral anteversion, also referred to as internal femoral torsion, is the most common cause of in-toeing in children 3 years of age or older and occurs twice as often in girls as in boys. Many affected children have generalized **ligamentous laxity**. Increased femoral anteversion is secondary to excessive or persistent infantile femoral anteversion and is almost always a benign condition that typically improves by 8–9 years of age. Severe anteversion or lack of progressive improvement by late childhood warrants referral to an orthopedic surgeon.

Children with increased anteversion often run with a circumduction gait secondary to internal rotation at the hip, and the parents may

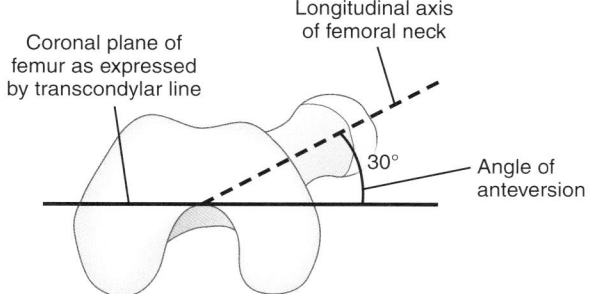

Fig. 45.4 Femoral version. Typically, the femoral neck creates an anteriorly directed angle with the transcondylar axis of the distal femur.

Coronal plane of femur as expressed by transcondylar line

Longitudinal axis of femoral neck

30°

Angle of anteversion

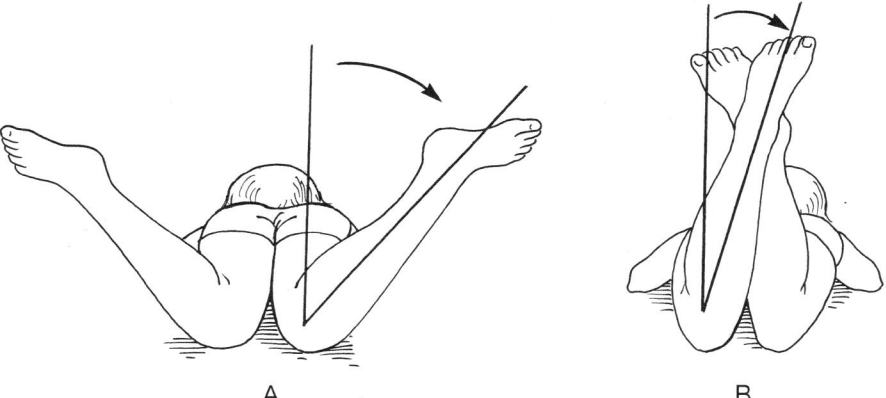

A
B

Fig. 45.5 Hip rotation in extension. The child is in the prone position, with the knees flexed 90 degrees. The lower leg is vertically oriented. This is considered the neutral position. Outward rotation *(A)* of the leg produces internal hip rotation; inward rotation *(B)* produces external hip rotation.

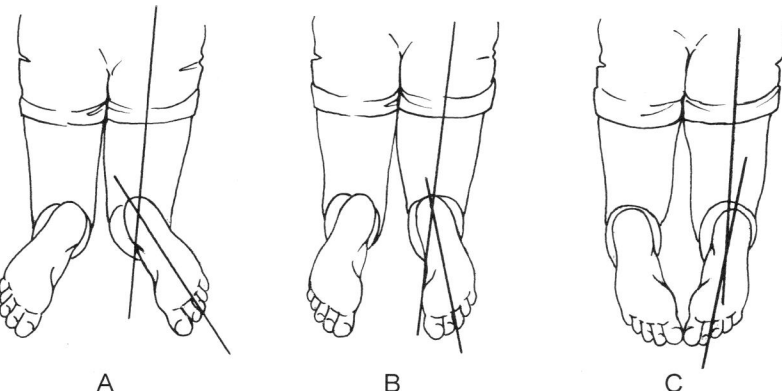

A
B
C

Fig. 45.6 Thigh-foot angle. With the child in the prone position and the knees flexed and approximated, the long axis of the foot can be compared with the long axis of the thigh. The long axis of the foot bisects the heel and the third or middle toe. *A,* External tibial torsion produces excessive outward rotation. *B,* Normal alignment is characterized by slight external rotation. *C,* Internal tibial torsion produces inward rotation.

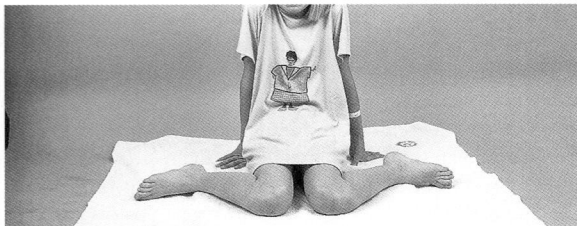

Fig. 45.7 W-sitting is the position of comfort for children with increased femoral anteversion.

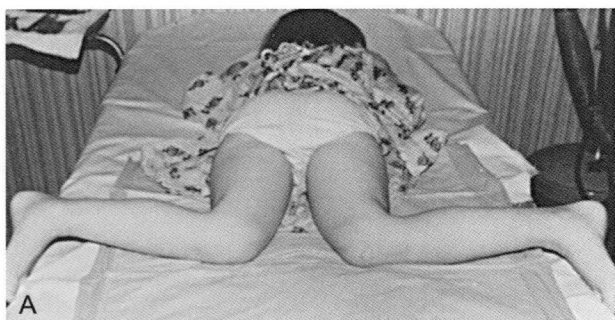

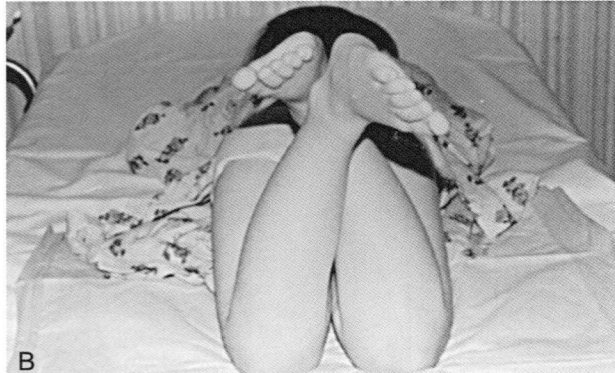

Fig. 45.8 *A,* Clinical photograph of a 5-year-old girl demonstrating internal femoral torsion. She has approximately 80 degrees of internal rotation bilaterally. *B,* External rotation is limited to approximately 15 degrees, for a total arc of rotation of 90–95 degrees.

note that the child W-sits rather than sitting cross-legged (Fig. 45.7). W-sitting is of no concern developmentally, is the position of comfort for the child, and does not cause or worsen in-toeing in children. Children will typically stop sitting in this position after sufficient improvement in the internal torsion allows them to sit cross-legged more comfortably. Common femoral anteversion should not be viewed as a reason for decreased athletic ability or as a risk factor for arthritis, bunions, or back pain. A relationship with patellofemoral pain has been reported in some populations.

Physical examination. Gait assessment reveals that the entire lower extremity is inwardly rotated during ambulation. Foot progression angle is typically negative and a circumduction-type gait may be noted. Hip rotation assessment characteristically reveals 80–90 degrees of internal rotation in the prone, extended position (Fig. 45.8). External rotation, as a consequence, is limited to 0–10 degrees. Features of generalized ligamentous laxity are often present, including elbow, wrist, and finger hyperextension; thumb hyperabduction; knee hyperextension; and hypermobile pes planus.

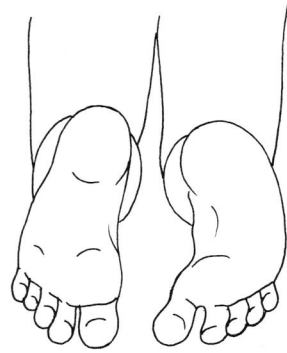

Fig. 45.9 Foot shape. In the same position as for measurement of the thigh-foot angle, the shape of the foot can also be evaluated. In this illustration, the left foot has normal alignment and the right foot demonstrates metatarsus adductus.

Radiographic evaluation. Radiographic evaluation of internal femoral torsion is not necessary. Anteroposterior radiographs of the pelvis are typically normal, but there may be the appearance of a relatively vertical femoral neck angle, or coxa valga. If coxa valga is noted, repeating the radiograph with the hips in 15 degrees of abduction and 30–40 degrees internal rotation will typically reveal a normal femoral neck angle. In more severe cases, MRI, CT, or ultrasonography of the proximal and distal femur can be used to accurately measure the degree of torsion.

Internal tibial torsion. Internal tibial torsion is the most common cause of in-toeing in children younger than 2 years and is secondary to normal in utero positioning. This condition is commonly seen during the second year of life and may be associated with metatarsus adductus. Significant improvement usually does not occur until the child begins to pull up to standing and walk independently. Spontaneous resolution with normal growth and development can be anticipated typically by 4–5 years of age. Rarely, persistent or severe internal tibial torsion in an older child or adolescent may necessitate surgical derotation.

Physical examination. The degree of tibial torsion can be assessed by measuring the thigh-foot angle (see Fig. 45.6). The measurements should be recorded on each visit to the physician to document improvement.

Radiographic evaluation. Radiographic evaluation of internal tibial torsion is not necessary. MRI and CT can assess the degree of tibial torsion, but these are rarely required.

Metatarsus adductus. Metatarsus adductus is the most common congenital foot deformity, occurs equally in boys and girls, and is bilateral in approximately 50% of cases. Metatarsus adductus has hereditary tendencies and is more common in first-born children, most likely as a result of increased molding from the more rigid primigravida uterus and abdominal wall. Up to 10% of children with metatarsus adductus have **developmental dysplasia of the hip**. Significant metatarsus adductus persisting or manifesting after 4 years of age may require surgical correction.

Physical examination. In metatarsus adductus, the forefoot is adducted and occasionally supinated, while the hindfoot and midfoot are normal. A visual line bisecting the heel should normally pass through the second toe or second web space; in metatarsus adductus this line intersects the forefoot more laterally. The lateral border of the foot is convex, the base of the fifth metatarsal is prominent, and the medial border of the foot is concave. There is usually an increased interval between the first and second toes, with the great toe being held in an inwardly rotated or varus position (Fig. 45.9). Ankle range of motion is normal. Forefoot mobility, assessed by stabilizing the hindfoot and midfoot in a neutral position and applying pressure over the first metatarsal head with the opposite hand, can vary from flexible to rigid. Most cases of flexible metatarsus adductus resolve by several months of age; rigid deformities may require casting or surgical correction. In the walking child with an uncorrected or partially corrected metatarsus adductus, there is an in-toed gait, abnormal shoe wear, and possible discomfort from shoe pressure.

Radiographic evaluation. Radiographs of the foot are not necessary for routine, flexible metatarsus adductus. When obtained, anteroposterior and lateral weight-bearing radiographs demonstrate adduction of the metatarsals at the tarsometatarsal joint and an increased intermetatarsal angle between the first and second metatarsals. The midfoot and hindfoot are usually normal. Radiographs should be obtained if the deformity is rigid or if there are any suspected abnormalities of the midfoot or hindfoot.

Talipes equinovarus (clubfoot). Talipes equinovarus is classified as either positional or congenital. **Positional clubfoot** is a normal foot that has been held in the deformed position in utero, and which is flexible on examination in the newborn nursery. **Congenital clubfoot** represents a deformity not only of the foot but also of the entire lower leg and is categorized as either idiopathic or syndromic. There is a spectrum of severity, but clubfoot associated with neuromuscular diagnoses or syndromes is typically rigid and more difficult to treat. Clubfoot is also extremely common in patients with spinal dysraphism, arthrogryposis, and chromosomal syndromes such as trisomy 18 and chromosome 22q11.2 deletion syndrome.

Congenital clubfoot, when diagnosed and treated in infancy with serial casting, typically does not produce a gait disturbance. However, foot contact pressures may remain high, indicating that gait is not entirely normal following correction. In-toeing secondary to persistent internal tibial torsion is common after appropriate treatment. A mild lower extremity length discrepancy of up to 2 cm may be seen in adolescence but usually does not produce a limp or necessitate treatment. On occasion, residual muscle imbalance may cause the child to walk on the lateral border of the foot, leading to discomfort and an antalgic gait that may require further surgical correction.

Out-Toed Gait

External femoral torsion. Femoral retroversion, also referred to as external femoral torsion, is a rare disorder that usually causes no significant functional impairment unless it is associated with a **slipped capital femoral epiphysis (SCFE)**. If the femoral retroversion is caused by SCFE, the slip is treated surgically. On occasion, persistent femoral retroversion following surgical treatment of SCFE can lead to ongoing functional impairment, such as a severe out-toed gait and difficulty in approximating the knees in the sitting position, and may require further surgical correction.

Physical examination. Children with external femoral torsion demonstrate limited internal rotation and excessive external rotation when the hip is examined in the extended position. The hip externally rotates 70–90 degrees, whereas internal rotation is only 0–20 degrees. Idiopathic external femoral torsion is usually bilateral. If the deformity is unilateral, especially in an obese older child or a young adolescent, SCFE must be considered and evaluated.

Radiographic evaluation. Anteroposterior and frog-leg lateral radiographs of the pelvis are necessary for any child or adolescent presenting with external femoral torsion, especially one who is obese, has atraumatic or referred anterior thigh or knee pain, or has unilateral deformity. Approximately 20% of children with SCFE have simultaneous bilateral involvement. The typical changes of SCFE include widening of the physis and an abnormal relationship between the capital femoral epiphysis (CFE) and the femoral neck. The femoral

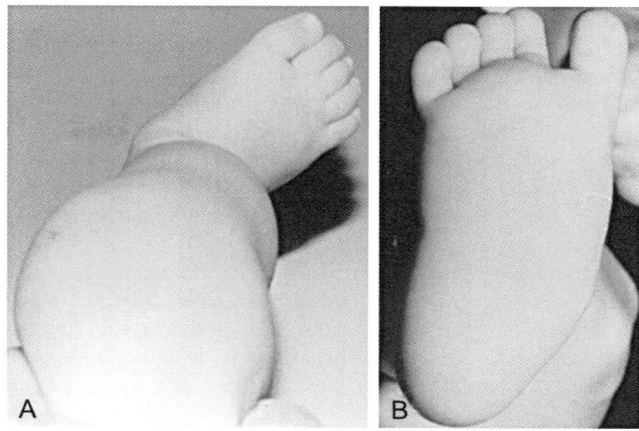

Fig. 45.10 *A,* A clinical photograph of a 2-month-old girl demonstrating excessive external tibial torsion. This reverse or anterior thigh-foot angle shows approximately 50 degrees of external tibial torsion. *B,* A calcaneovalgus foot with forefoot abduction and increased hindfoot valgus in the same infant. There is also hyperdorsiflexibility of the foot in the ankle.

head appears to be slipped inferiorly and posteriorly, but in actuality, the femoral neck is displaced anteriorly and superiorly.

External tibial torsion. External tibial torsion is common and is secondary to a normal variation of in utero positioning in which the plantar surface of the foot is against the wall of the uterus, forcing it into a hyperdorsiflexed, everted position. This rotated alignment produces external tibial torsion and typically an associated calcaneovalgus foot (Fig. 45.10). When this alignment of the lower leg and foot is combined with the exaggerated external rotation of the normal newborn hip, the lower extremity appears to have severe out-toeing and external rotation. This condition follows the same clinical course as internal tibial torsion in that significant improvement does not occur during the first year of life. With the onset of independent ambulation, spontaneous improvement begins and is typically complete by 2–3 years of age.

Physical examination. External tibial torsion results in a positive thigh-foot angle of 30–50 degrees.

Radiographic evaluation. Radiographic assessment for external tibial torsion is not necessary.

Calcaneovalgus foot. The calcaneovalgus foot is common in newborns and is secondary to in utero positioning (see Fig. 45.10). The foot is hyperdorsiflexed with varying degrees of eversion and forefoot abduction. External tibial torsion is usually present. Calcaneovalgus foot is typically unilateral but may occasionally be bilateral. The hyperdorsiflexion of the foot usually resolves during the first 3–6 months of life. On occasion, resistant feet may require passive stretching, taping, or casting into a plantarflexed position. Usually, by the time the child begins to pull to standing and walk independently, the calcaneovalgus condition has resolved. The external tibial torsion, however, persists and follows the same natural history as internal tibial torsion.

Physical examination. The involved extremity demonstrates out-toeing, the dorsum of the foot can easily be brought into contact with the anterior aspect of the lower leg, and the forefoot has an abducted appearance. The increased dorsiflexion should not be confused with the increased joint mobility of premature infants. The deformity is flexible, and plantarflexion of the ankle is normal or almost normal. External tibial torsion of 30–50 degrees is a common associated finding.

Calcaneovalgus foot must be distinguished from the following three conditions: (1) congenital vertical talus, (2) posteromedial bowing of the tibia, and (3) neuromuscular abnormalities, such as paralysis of the gastrocnemius muscle. Differentiation is typically based on physical examination findings, though radiographs may be required. **Congenital vertical talus** results in a rocker-bottom appearance to the foot. The deformity in congenital vertical talus is rigid with inability to achieve passive ankle plantarflexion, as opposed to the flexible deformity seen with a calcaneovalgus foot. In posteromedial bowing of the tibia, the apex of the deformity is in the distal tibia, whereas the apex of the deformity in a calcaneovalgus foot is located at the ankle.

Radiographic evaluation. Simulated weight-bearing anteroposterior and lateral radiographs with forced plantarflexion of the foot may be necessary to differentiate between the calcaneovalgus foot and a congenital vertical talus. In a calcaneovalgus foot, the radiographs either are normal or reveal an increase in hindfoot valgus. In the congenital vertical talus, the hindfoot is in equinus, whereas the midfoot and the forefoot are dorsally displaced, producing a rocker-bottom appearance. The talus is also noted to be out of plane with the metatarsals. Anteroposterior and lateral radiographs of the tibia and fibula are necessary if there is bowing of the lower leg.

Hypermobile pes planus. Hypermobile, flexible, or pronated feet are **flatfeet**, a common cause of concern to parents. Children with this deformity are usually asymptomatic and have no limitation of activities. An individual may present for concerns of out-toeing because of the overpronation of the midfoot and hindfoot, which may allow the forefoot to become abducted. Flexible flatfeet are also common in neonates and toddlers as a result of the associated laxity in the bone-ligament complexes of the feet and the abundant fat in the area of the medial longitudinal arch. Most children with flatfeet improve by 6 years of age. In the older child, flexible flatfeet are usually secondary to generalized ligamentous laxity. Most older children and adolescents with flexible flatfeet or hypermobile pes planus are asymptomatic, though feet that are symptomatic with vigorous physical activity usually respond readily to the use of commercially available medial longitudinal arch supports. When the child has excessive heel valgus, pronation, or abnormal shoe wear that is unresponsive to a commercially or custom-made arch support, the use of a custom orthosis may be beneficial. Surgery is rarely indicated.

Physical examination. In the non–weight-bearing position in the older child with a flexible flatfoot, the normal medial longitudinal arch is visible, but in the weight-bearing position, the foot becomes pronated with varying degrees of pes planus and hindfoot valgus. Instead of bearing weight over the lateral column of the foot, the weight is shifted medially, producing pronation. Subtalar motion is examined with the ankle in the neutral position and should be normal or slightly increased. Loss of subtalar motion may indicate a rigid flatfoot. Common causes of rigid flatfeet include neuromuscular disorders, tarsal coalition, and Achilles tendon contracture, which may present with external foot progression due to associated limited subtalar motion. Rigid flatfeet may also be a familial trait. Other joints, especially the elbows, hands, and knees, usually demonstrate generalized ligamentous laxity in patients with flexible flatfeet. Children with flexible flatfeet should be evaluated for external tibial torsion.

Radiographic evaluation. Radiographs of asymptomatic flexible flatfeet are usually not indicated. Standing anteroposterior oblique and lateral weight-bearing radiographs are obtained, if necessary. The most common indication is the presence of pain (Table 45.3). Anteroposterior radiographs reveal an increase in the talocalcaneal angle (>25 degrees) caused by the excessive hindfoot valgus. The lateral view shows distortion of the normal straight-line relationship between the long axis of the talus and the first metatarsal and flattening of the normal medial longitudinal arch.

TABLE 45.3 Differential Diagnosis of Foot Pain According to Age

Age Group	Diagnostic Considerations
0–6 yr	Poorly fitting shoes Fracture Puncture wound Foreign body Osteomyelitis Cellulitis Juvenile idiopathic arthritis Hair tourniquet Dactylitis Leukemia
6–12 yr	Poorly fitting shoes Trauma (fracture, sprain) Juvenile idiopathic arthritis (enthesopathy) Puncture wound Sever disease (calcaneal apophysitis) Accessory tarsal navicular bone Hypermobile flatfoot Tarsal coalition Oncologic (Ewing sarcoma, leukemia)
12–18 yr	Poorly fitting shoes Stress fracture Trauma (fracture, sprain) Foreign body Ingrown toenail Metatarsalgia Plantar fasciitis Achilles tendinopathy Accessory ossicles (navicular, os trigonum) Tarsal coalition Avascular necrosis of metatarsal (Freiberg infarction) or navicular (Kohler disease) bones Plantar warts

From Marcdante K, Kliegman R, eds. *Nelson Essentials of Pediatrics.* 7th ed. Philadelphia: Saunders; 2015.

Equinus Gait (Toe-Walking)

Toe-walking can be a normal finding in children up to 3 years of age. Persistent toe-walking thereafter or acquired toe-walking at a later age is considered abnormal and necessitates careful evaluation. The differential diagnosis for persistent or acquired toe-walking includes the following:

1. Neuromuscular disorders, such as cerebral palsy, Duchenne muscular dystrophy, or spinal cord abnormality resulting from a tethered spinal cord or diastematomyelia
2. Congenital Achilles tendon contracture (idiopathic toe-walking)
3. Habitual toe-walking
4. Lower extremity length discrepancy

The differentiation of toe-walking can usually be determined from the history and the physical examination. The examiner should establish the time at onset, the amount of time a child spends walking on his or her toes, whether it can be voluntarily corrected, and whether there has been improvement or worsening over time.

Neuromuscular Disorders

The neuromuscular disorder most likely to produce an equinus gait, either unilateral or bilateral, is **cerebral palsy**. The most common type of cerebral palsy is spastic diplegia, a disorder in which the lower extremities are more involved than the upper extremities. Prematurity is a common risk factor for spastic diplegia. It can be symmetric or asymmetric, with one side being slightly more involved than the other. Spastic diplegia tends to produce a bilateral equinus gait. Spastic hemiplegia, in which only one side is involved, is usually caused by birth trauma (asphyxia), perinatal stroke, or underlying congenital malformation and results in unilateral toe-walking.

Acquired or late-onset toe-walking is usually a result of a developing neuromuscular disorder, including hereditary and acquired peripheral neuropathies. Weakness and sensory changes in peripheral neuropathies tend to progress in a distal-to-proximal fashion (see Chapter 35). Dystrophinopathies, such as Duchenne muscular dystrophy, tend to produce proximal weakness first, though can also result in toe-walking (see Chapter 35). As fat and fibrous tissues replace muscle, equinus and other contractures occur. There is usually a history of progressive clumsiness and frequent episodes of falling. The diagnosis of muscular dystrophy is usually made when the child is between 3 and 5 years of age. The diagnosis is suggested by markedly elevated creatine kinase (CK) levels and is confirmed by muscle biopsy or genetic testing. In a spastic equinus gait without contracture, physical therapy and orthoses (daytime, nighttime, or both) may be beneficial. If a contracture has developed, serial casting may be performed in young children, whereas surgical lengthening of the Achilles is usually necessary in older children.

Physical examination. The examination of a child with toe-walking secondary to cerebral palsy reveals either an Achilles contracture or a spastic equinus gait without contracture, as well as abnormal neurologic findings. These findings include increased muscle tone, spasticity, hyperactive deep tendon reflexes, and pathologic reflexes, such as a positive Babinski sign. Hamstring tightness, in addition to ankle equinus, may be a subtle sign of underlying mild cerebral palsy.

Children with peripheral neuropathy tend to have mixed motor and sensory findings that develop in a distal-to-proximal fashion. Children with Duchenne muscular dystrophy typically demonstrate **pseudohypertrophy** of the calves in addition to equinus contracture. They have proximal muscle weakness first, and then generalized weakness, and perhaps decreased or absent upper extremity and patellar tendon reflexes, depending on the stage of progression. Ankle reflexes are usually preserved.

Radiographic evaluation. Radiographic evaluation of a child with toe-walking is rarely necessary. MRI of the brain and spine is occasionally required during the evaluation of a possible neuromuscular disorder.

Other testing. Dynamic electromyography, nerve conduction studies, and gait analysis studies can be helpful in distinguishing among toe-walking caused by mild cerebral palsy, neuropathy, myopathy, or a congenital Achilles contracture. Serum muscle enzyme (CK, aspartate aminotransferase, and aldolase) levels and muscle biopsies are required for children with suspected Duchenne muscular dystrophy or other myopathies. Targeted gene panels or genomic sequencing, as well as functional and genetic mitochondrial studies, can assist in establishing the etiology of neuromuscular disorders.

Lower Extremity Length Discrepancy

Lower extremity length discrepancy is a common cause for a unilateral equinus gait in older children and adolescents. Usually, mild discrepancies of less than 2 cm can be adequately compensated for during normal gait with minimal, if any, limping or toe-walking. Greater discrepancies may result in toe-walking and may require surgical correction. The differential diagnosis of a lower extremity length discrepancy is extensive (Table 45.4).

TABLE 45.4 Causes of Lower Extremity Length Discrepancy

Shortening	Lengthening
Congenital	**Congenital**
Hemiatrophy*	Hemihypertrophy*
Skeletal dysplasias	Local vascular malformation
Short femur	
Proximal focal femoral deficiency*	
Fibular, tibial hemimelia	
Developmental dysplasia of the hip*	
Tumor: Developmental	**Tumor: Developmental**
Neurofibromatosis	Neurofibromatosis
Multiple exostosis	Soft tissue hemangioma
Enchondromatosis (Ollier disease)	Arteriovenous malformation
Osteochondromatosis	Hemihypertrophy with Wilms
Fibrous dysplasia (Albright syndrome)	tumor
Punctate epiphyseal dysplasia	Aneurysm
Dysplasia epiphysealis hemimelica (Trevor disease)	
Radiation therapy before skeletal maturity (physeal arrest)*	
Resection of benign or malignant neoplasm	
Infection	**Infection: Inflammation**
Osteomyelitis*	Metaphyseal osteomyelitis
Septic arthritis	Rheumatoid arthritis
Tuberculosis	Hemarthrosis (hemophilia)
Trauma	**Trauma**
Physeal injury*	Metaphyseal, diaphyseal fracture
Failed joint replacement	Diaphyseal operations (bone
Osteotomy, atrophic nonunion	grafts, osteosynthesis,
Overlapping, malposition of fracture fragments*	periosteal stripping)
Burns	
Neuromuscular Disease	
Poliomyelitis	
Cerebral palsy*	
Myelomeningocele	
Peripheral neuropathy	
Focal cerebral lesions (hemiplegia)	
Other	
Legg-Calvé-Perthes disease*	
Slipped capital femoral epiphysis	
Russell Silver syndrome	
Klippel-Trenaunay-Weber syndrome	

*Common.
Modified from Moseley C. Leg-length discrepancy. *Pediatr Clin North Am.* 1986;33(6):1385; Tachdjian M. *Pediatric Orthopedics.* 2nd ed. Philadelphia: WB Saunders; 1990; reprinted and modified from Behrman RE, ed. *Nelson Textbook of Pediatrics.* 14th ed. Philadelphia: WB Saunders; 1992:1702.

Physical examination. Examination of a child with a lower extremity length discrepancy shows shortness of the involved extremity; this can be measured by placing blocks of various heights beneath the foot until the pelvis is level. The range of motion of the joints of the involved extremity, especially of the hips, must be assessed. The neurologic examination is also important. Children with subtle neurologic disorders, such as cerebral palsy, may also have a very mild lower extremity length discrepancy that contributes to an equinus gait.

Radiographic evaluation. Children with a lower extremity length discrepancy require radiographic assessment. Lower extremity lengths are typically measured radiographically by one of several methods, including the teleoroentgenogram, orthoroentgenogram, scanogram, and low-dose biplanar radiography. Digital teleoroentgenograms and orthoroentgenograms are currently preferred, but low-dose biplanar radiography is becoming more commonplace. The teleoroentgenogram is a single radiographic exposure of both lower extremities in the standing position. Limb length can be measured using tools within the digital radiography software. Advantages include single exposure and detection of angular deformities. The orthoroentgenogram consists of overlapping exposures centered on the hips, knees, and ankles on a long cassette. Like the teleoroentgenogram, an advantage of this type of radiograph is that it shows associated angular deformities. A scanogram consists of three strip exposures of the hips, knees, and ankles on a standard-sized cassette with a radiographic ruler adjacent to the extremity. This is an accurate method of assessing limb length but does not demonstrate angular deformities. Low-dose biplanar radiography is a three-dimensional imaging method with superior accuracy and decreased radiation exposure but requires skilled interpretation to correctly align the limbs for computer-assisted measurement. CT-based measurement is accurate but is not commonly used secondary to the amount of radiation exposure required. Radiographs of the left hand and wrist for bone age are also obtained to assess when skeletal maturity will occur.

Habitual Toe-Walking

Habitual toe-walking occurs in a child who is walking on their toes voluntarily. Toe-walking occurs relatively commonly in young walkers. History and physical examination findings are entirely normal; this is a diagnosis of exclusion. The treatment of habitual toe-walking is observation. As the child becomes heavier and the central nervous system matures, the toe-walking should resolve.

Physical examination. The findings in the examination of the child with habitual toe-walking are normal. The ankle has a full range of motion, and there is no evidence of an underlying neuromuscular disorder.

Radiographic evaluation. Radiographic evaluation is not indicated.

Idiopathic Toe-Walking

Idiopathic toe-walking is defined as the presence of an equinus gait in a child over 2 years of age with or without Achilles tendon contracture in the absence of other etiologies, including habitual toe-walking. The birth and developmental history and the neurologic findings are usually normal. However, mild developmental delays, especially in speech and in fine and gross motor skills, are seen in some children, as are possible deficits in sensory processing. A family history of Achilles contracture, male predominance, and learning disabilities are common findings. Muscle biopsy samples have shown an increase in type I fibers, suggesting a neuropathic process. Serial casting typically leads to resolution, though, in some children, surgical lengthening of the Achilles tendon may be required.

Physical examination. If present, Achilles tendon contracture leads to an inability to dorsiflex the foot to the neutral or plantigrade position. Examination of the ankle shows a 10- to 15-degree fixed equinus contracture. The assessment of an Achilles contracture should be performed with the hindfoot held in a slightly supinated position to bring the calcaneus beneath the talus. If this position is not used, dorsiflexion of the foot produces hindfoot valgus with the appearance of more dorsiflexion than is actually present. Dorsiflexion should

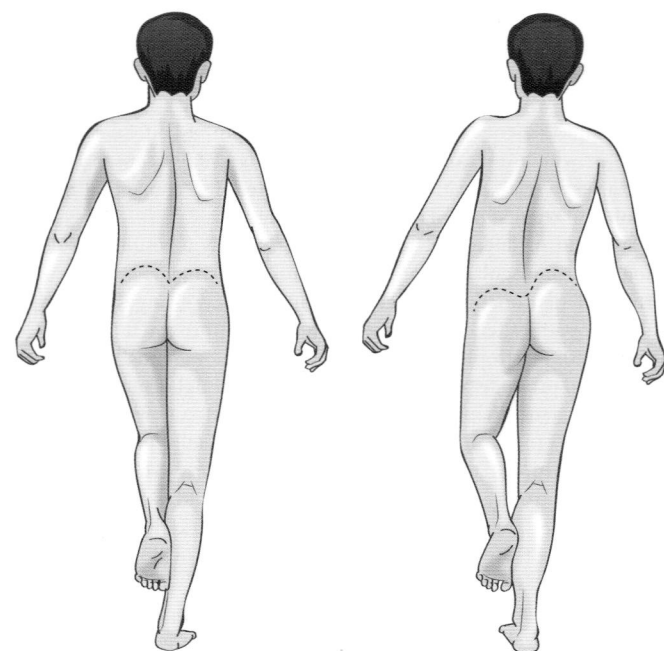

Fig. 45.11 Trendelenburg gait. With functional weakness of the hip abductor muscles, it is difficult to support the body's weight on the affected side; the pelvis tilts down and away from the weak side, and the patient leans toward the affected side.

be assessed with knee in flexion and extension to evaluate tension in the gastrocnemius. In congenital Achilles contractures, no other musculoskeletal or neurologic abnormalities are present.

Radiographic evaluation. Radiographs are not necessary unless an associated abnormality within the foot is thought to be present. Should this occur, anteroposterior and lateral weight-bearing radiographs of the foot should be obtained.

Limping

Limping is categorized as either painful (antalgic gait) or nonpainful (Trendelenburg gait), depending on the length of the stance phase. With an **antalgic gait**, the stance phase is shortened because the child decreases the time spent on the painful extremity. In a **Trendelenburg gait** (Fig. 45.11), which indicates underlying proximal muscle weakness (e.g., muscular dystrophy) or hip instability (e.g., developmental hip dysplasia), the stance phase is the same for the involved and uninvolved sides, but the child leans over the involved side to shift the center of gravity for balance. If the disorder is bilateral, it produces a **waddling gait**. The differential diagnosis is extensive (Table 45.5). Most causes involve the lower extremity, but spinal disorders can also produce limping or difficulty walking, especially if there is spinal cord, nerve root, or peripheral nerve involvement, as can intraabdominal pathology, such as appendicitis or torsion of the testes or ovaries. Painful (antalgic) gaits are predominantly caused by trauma, infection, neoplasia, and rheumatic disorders. Trendelenburg gaits are generally caused by congenital, developmental, or neuromuscular disorders. Thus, antalgic gaits typically result from *acute* disorders, whereas Trendelenburg gaits usually result from *chronic* disorders. The type of gait, the presence or absence of systemic symptoms, and the anatomic location of the symptoms can usually be determined from the history and physical examination findings.

Antalgic Gait

Congenital origin: Tarsal coalition. Tarsal coalition, also called **peroneal spastic flatfoot**, is characterized by a painful, rigid valgus

TABLE 45.5   Differential Diagnosis of Limping in Children

Age Group	Diagnostic Considerations	Age Group	Diagnostic Considerations
Early walker: 1–3 yr of age	**Painful Limp** Septic arthritis and osteomyelitis Iliopsoas abscess Testicular torsion Ovarian torsion Transient synovitis Occult trauma ("toddler's fracture") Nonaccidental trauma Intervertebral diskitis Malignancy	Child: 3–10 yr of age—cont'd	**Painless Limp** Developmental dysplasia of the hip Legg-Calvé-Perthes disease Lower extremity length inequality Neuromuscular disorder Polio Cerebral palsy Stroke Muscular dystrophy (Duchenne)
	Painless Limp Developmental dysplasia of the hip Neuromuscular disorder Cerebral palsy Stroke Lower extremity length inequality	Adolescent: 11 yr of age to maturity	**Painful Limp** Septic arthritis, osteomyelitis, myositis Iliopsoas abscess Testicular torsion Ovarian torsion Trauma Discoid meniscus Rheumatic disorder Slipped capital femoral epiphysis: acute; unstable Osgood-Schlatter disease Chondrolysis Malignancy Nerve entrapment syndromes
Child: 3–10 yr of age	**Painful Limp** Septic arthritis, osteomyelitis, myositis Iliopsoas abscess Testicular torsion Ovarian torsion Transient synovitis Trauma Discoid meniscus Rheumatic disorders Juvenile idiopathic arthritis Intervertebral diskitis Malignancy		**Painless Limp** Slipped capital femoral epiphysis: chronic; stable Developmental dysplasia of the hip: acetabular dysplasia Lower extremity length inequality Neuromuscular disorder Nerve entrapment syndrome Hereditary neuropathy with liability to pressure palsies Stroke

From Marcdante K, Kliegman R, eds. *Nelson Essentials of Pediatrics*. 7th ed. Philadelphia: Saunders; 2015.

or pronation deformity of the midfoot and hindfoot, in association with peroneal muscle spasm but without true spasticity. This condition represents a congenital fusion or failure of segmentation between two or more tarsal bones. However, any condition that alters the normal motion of the subtalar joint may produce the clinical appearance of a tarsal coalition. Thus, congenital malformation, inflammatory disorders, infection, neoplasms, and trauma involving the subtalar joint can manifest with pain, limping, or other symptoms similar to those of a tarsal coalition.

The most common coalitions occur between the calcaneus and navicular (calcaneonavicular) and the middle or medial facet between the talus and calcaneus (talocalcaneal). Coalitions can be fibrous, cartilaginous, or osseous. The incidence of tarsal coalition is approximately 1%, and it appears to be inherited as an autosomal dominant trait. Approximately 60% of calcaneonavicular and 50% of talocalcaneal coalitions are bilateral. Casting and orthotics may provide some relief of symptoms, though surgical repair is typically required.

Physical examination. The onset of symptoms is insidious and usually occurs during late childhood or early adolescence. Although mild limitation of subtalar motion and a valgus or pronated hindfoot may have been present since early childhood, the onset of symptoms varies with the age at which the fibrous or cartilaginous coalition begins to ossify and further decrease motion. The talonavicular coalition ossifies between the ages of 3 and 5 years, the calcaneonavicular coalition between 8 and 12 years, and the middle facet talocalcaneal

coalition between 12 and 16 years of age. The pain is typically felt laterally in the hindfoot and radiates proximally along the lateral malleolus and distal fibula into the peroneal muscle region. Symptoms are usually aggravated by sports or other vigorous activities and are relieved by rest. The foot is pronated in both the weight-bearing and the non–weight-bearing positions. Subtalar joint motion is diminished or absent, and attempts at motion produce pain.

Radiographic evaluation. The diagnosis of tarsal coalition is made radiographically. The initial radiographs should include anteroposterior, oblique, and lateral weight-bearing radiographs of the foot. The oblique view is helpful for identifying changes at the calcaneonavicular joint. Beaking of the anterior aspect of the talus in the lateral view suggests a talocalcaneal coalition. Axial views of the hindfoot can be useful in the diagnosis of a middle facet talocalcaneal coalition. CT has traditionally been the diagnostic procedure of choice for coalition, but MRI is useful for detecting fibrous coalitions. Either CT or MRI should be performed on all coalitions for surgical planning because more than one coalition can be present.

Developmental origin

Legg-Calvé-Perthes disease. Legg-Calvé-Perthes disease (LCPD) is idiopathic avascular necrosis of the CFE and its associated complications in an immature, growing child. This disorder is caused by an interruption of the blood supply to the CFE, occurs predominantly in males (up to 5:1), and is bilateral in approximately 20% of affected children. Children with LCPD have delayed skeletal or bone age, disproportionate growth, and

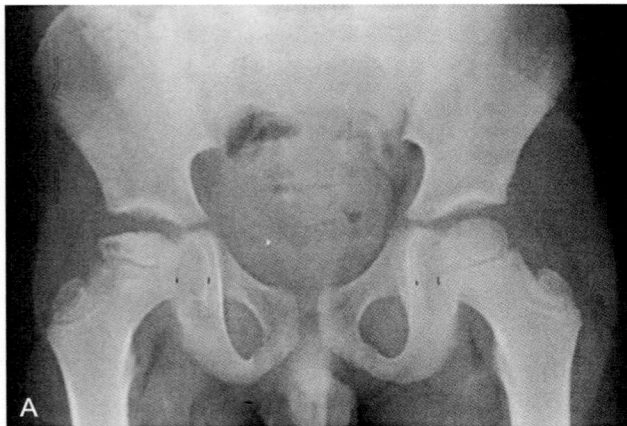

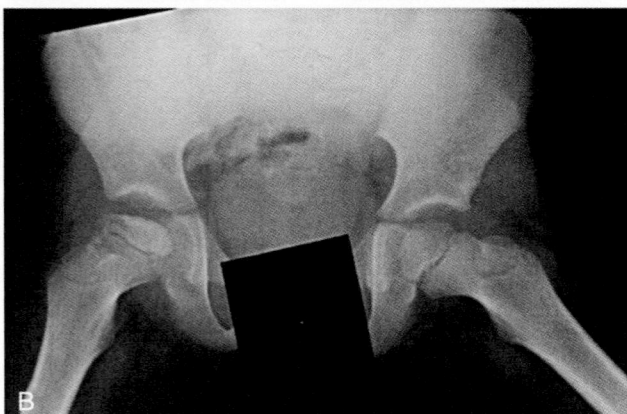

Fig. 45.12 *A,* An anteroposterior radiograph of the pelvis demonstrating Legg-Calvé-Perthes disease (LCPD) of the right hip. The capital femoral epiphysis (CFE) is collapsing, and there is mild widening of the medial joint space. The left CFE is normal. *B,* A frog-leg lateral radiograph of the pelvis demonstrating limited hip abduction caused by LCPD.

mildly short stature. Secondary osteonecrosis is seen in patients with sickle cell anemia. LCPD is a local, self-healing disorder. Prevention of femoral head deformity and secondary degenerative osteoarthritis in adulthood is the only indication for treatment.

Physical examination. The symptomatic onset of LCPD typically occurs between 2 and 12 years of age, at a mean age of 7 years. Younger age at presentation is a positive prognostic indicator. Most of these children present to care with a limp and mild or intermittent pain in the anterior thigh or knee, such that this condition is often referred to as a "painless limp." Pertinent early physical findings include antalgic gait; muscle spasm with mild restriction of hip motion, especially abduction and internal rotation; proximal thigh atrophy; and mild short stature.

Radiographic evaluation. The diagnosis is typically made from anteroposterior and frog-leg lateral radiographs of the pelvis (Fig. 45.12). The radiographic characteristics can be divided into five distinct stages, depending on the interval from the onset of symptoms: (1) cessation of CFE growth, (2) subchondral fracture, (3) resorption or fragmentation, (4) reossification, and (5) healed, or residual. The symptoms are usually most pronounced during the phase of the subchondral fracture and fragmentation. A child with LCPD has the potential for collapse and extrusion of the femoral head, which results in a permanent deformity. If plain radiographs do not demonstrate LCPD in suspected cases, a bone scan or MRI is helpful.

Slipped capital femoral epiphysis. SCFE is the most common adolescent hip disorder. It generally occurs in obese adolescents with

delayed skeletal maturation, or in tall and thin adolescents who have had a recent growth spurt. SCFE can also occur as a complication of an underlying endocrine disorder, such as hypothyroidism and pituitary disorders. When SCFE occurs before puberty, a hormonal abnormality or systemic disorder should be suspected. The histopathologic features of SCFE indicate that mechanical factors are the ultimate cause of slippage. The initial abnormality is most likely secondary to endocrine changes during early adolescence. Obesity produces high shear forces across a weakened and obliquely oriented CFE, resulting in slippage. Surgical stabilization is required.

Physical examination. The physical findings depend on the degree of slippage and the classification. The disorder is classified as either stable or unstable. In an unstable or acute SCFE, the CFE is separated from the femoral neck. This is extremely painful, and the adolescent is unable to stand or bear weight. In a stable or chronic SCFE, the most common type, the CFE and femoral neck are in continuity, and the slippage is occurring slowly by plastic deformation. The adolescent has an antalgic, out-toed gait. The hip range of motion demonstrates a lack of internal rotation and an increase in external rotation; as the hip is flexed, it becomes progressively more externally rotated. Limitation of flexion and abduction in extension may also be present as a result of the deformity of the proximal femur.

Radiographic evaluation. The diagnosis of SCFE is confirmed radiographically. Anteroposterior and frog-leg lateral radiographs of the pelvis must be obtained (Fig. 45.13). Both hips should be visualized on each radiograph for simultaneous comparison. The earliest sign of SCFE is widening of the physeal plate without slippage, which is considered a pre-slip condition. If slippage occurs, the CFE remains in the acetabulum, whereas the femoral neck rotates anteriorly and superiorly, resulting in varus orientation and retroversion of the femoral head and neck. The severity of slippage can be classified by the degree of displacement of the CFE on the femoral neck. Hip pain and limping following surgical correction of SCFE can be related to **chondrolysis,** rapidly progressive destruction of the articular cartilage of the hip. Chondrolysis can also occur following infection of the hip or may be idiopathic.

Trauma

Sprains, strains, and contusions. Sprains are ligamentous injuries, whereas **strains** are musculotendinous injuries. **Contusions** are the result of a direct injury and involve the skin and the subcutaneous tissues as well as underlying muscle.

Sprains are divided into three grades:

Grade I: mild with only slight stretching of the ligament

Grade II: a moderate injury with partial tearing of the ligament but normal stability

Grade III: a severe injury with ligamentous disruption and instability

Sprains, strains, and contusions of the lower extremities are among the most common injuries that produce limping. There is usually a history of trauma, and the location is readily apparent because of soft tissue swelling, ecchymosis, and pain. Most of these injuries occur during athletic activities, but they can also be the result of falls or other minor injuries. In the absence of an associated physeal injury or other fracture, treatment is typically bracing and/or brief immobilization with a gradual return to activity.

Physical examination. In sprains, the physical examination typically reveals that the involved ligament is tender to direct palpation. There may be soft tissue swelling as well as ecchymoses. The range of motion of the involved joint is typically decreased because of pain. On occasion, a mild joint effusion or hemarthrosis may be present.

Strains involve the muscles, and there is usually tenderness to palpation, soft tissue swelling, and pain with joint motion as a result of stretching of the involved muscle. A palpable defect within the muscle

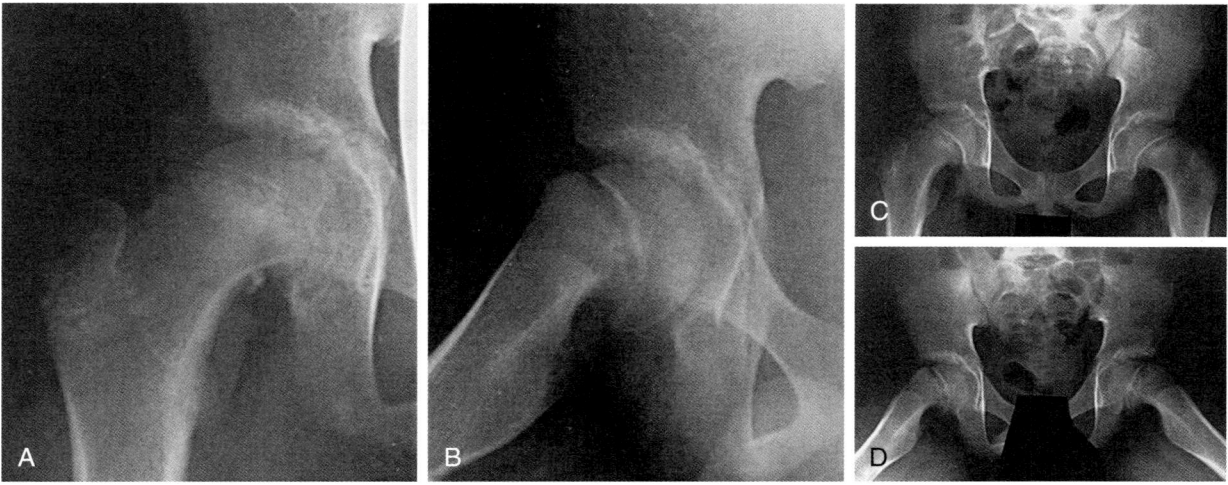

Fig. 45.13 *A,* An anteroposterior radiograph of the right hip in a 13-year-old obese boy who had been limping and complaining of anterior thigh and knee pain for approximately 2 months. There is a mild stable or chronic slipped capital femoral epiphysis (SCFE). Klein line, a line drawn along the superior aspect of the femoral neck, does not intersect the lateral portion of the capital femoral epiphysis (CFE) and thereby indicates slippage. Also, the physis is wide and irregular. *B,* A frog-leg lateral radiograph clearly demonstrates the slippage of the CFE with respect to the femoral neck. *C,* An anteroposterior radiograph of the pelvis demonstrates an asymptomatic mild stable or chronic left SCFE. It is always important to order radiographs of the pelvis rather than individual views of the right or left hip. *D,* A frog-leg lateral radiograph confirms bilateral SCFE.

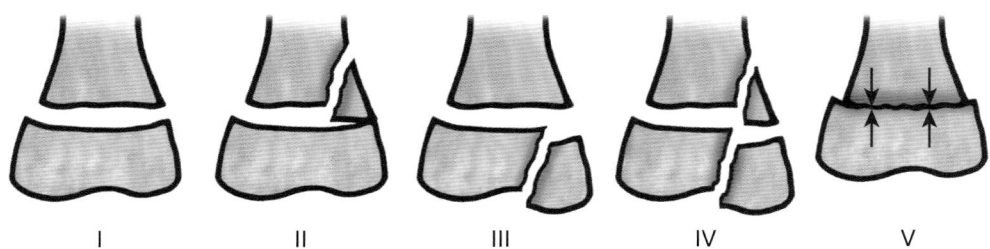

Fig. 45.14 Salter-Harris classification of physeal fractures, types I–V.

is uncommon except in the most severe injuries. These injuries usually limit the excursion of the muscle and its associated joints.

Radiographic evaluation. In children who sustain severe sprains, strains, or contusions evidenced by limping, swelling, or deformity, anteroposterior and lateral radiographs should at least be obtained. A word of caution regarding sprains is necessary: In children, ligaments are usually stronger than the adjacent physes. Therefore, a physeal injury known as a **Salter-Harris fracture** may be present and may have nearly the same clinical features as a sprain (Fig. 45.14 and Table 45.6). Even with negative radiographs a subtle physeal injury may be present. Bony tenderness over the physis is a distinguishing physical exam finding of a Salter-Harris fracture.

Occult fractures. Occult fractures of the tibia are a relatively common cause of limping or refusal to bear weight in very young children. They can also occur in the femur and fibula. These fractures can be the result of very innocuous trauma, such as tripping while walking, stepping on a toy, or falling from a height. Frequently, the injury may not have been observed, and the child cannot convey to the parents what happened, confounding diagnosis.

The most common occult fracture in early childhood is the **"toddler's fracture"** of the tibia. This is a spiral fracture of the distal third of the tibia without an associated fibula fracture. It most commonly occurs in children younger than 4 years of age. Occult tibia fractures can also occur in

TABLE 45.6	**Salter-Harris Classification**
Salter-Harris Type	**Characteristics**
I	Separation through the physis, usually through the zones of hypertrophic and degenerating cartilage cell columns
II	Fracture through a portion of the physis but extending through the metaphysis
III	Fracture through a portion of the physis extending through the epiphysis and into the joint
IV	Fracture across the metaphysis, physis, and epiphysis
V	Crush injury to the physis

From Baldwin KD, Shah AS, Wells L, et al. Common fractures. In: Kliegman RM, St. Geme JW III, Blum NJ, et al., eds. *Nelson Textbook of Pediatrics.* 21st ed. Philadelphia: Elsevier; 2020, Table 703-1.

the metaphyseal regions, usually distally, but only rarely in the diaphysis. Diaphyseal fractures are more commonly the result of child abuse.

Physical examination. Physical findings in a child with an occult fracture can be subtle. There is usually minimal, if any, soft tissue swelling. There is mild tenderness and perhaps increased warmth on palpation over the fracture. On occasion, the increased warmth may be indicative of osteomyelitis. Stress examination of the involved bone increases discomfort.

Radiographic evaluation. Anteroposterior and lateral radiographs should be obtained (Fig. 45.15). The characteristic finding of a toddler's fracture is a faint oblique fracture line crossing the distal third of the tibia. More proximal fractures, or tibial spiral fractures in nonambulatory children, are concerning for nonaccidental trauma and require further directed evaluation or consultation. On occasion, oblique radiographs may be helpful in revealing the fracture. Frequently, initial radiographs reveal no abnormality. If these initial plain radiographs are normal, the child has no systemic symptoms, and an occult fracture of the tibia is suspected, simple immobilization in a long-leg cast is indicated. Another set of radiographs in 1–2 weeks usually reveals the fracture and evidence of healing. If, however, the child has systemic symptoms, such as low-grade fever, and if osteomyelitis is thought to be present, evaluation including a CBC with differential, blood culture, CRP level, ESR, and an MRI should be obtained.

Neoplasia. Benign and malignant neoplastic lesions that involve bone, cartilage, or soft tissue of the spine, pelvis, and lower extremities can manifest as a mass, can cause pain, and can produce an antalgic gait. Leukemia or metastatic neuroblastoma of the bone marrow may produce deep bone pain and limp without objective findings of swelling or tenderness on physical examination. Night pain is a common characteristic of both benign and malignant primary or metastatic tumors. Osseous lesions can usually be diagnosed on plain radiographs, whereas for those of cartilage or soft tissue, MRI or other special imaging studies may be required for diagnosis.

Benign neoplasms. The most common benign lesions that produce limping include a unicameral (simple) bone cyst and osteoid osteoma (Table 45.7). Other less common benign lesions that can produce pain and limping include eosinophilic granuloma of the bone, osteochondroma, and chondroblastoma. Chondroblastoma typically involves the epiphysis.

In **unicameral bone cysts**, the symptoms are usually caused by a nondisplaced pathologic fracture. On occasion, a displaced fracture may occur. The most common location for a unicameral bone cyst is the proximal humerus, followed by the proximal femur. These can occur in any of the bones of the lower extremities, including the foot.

Osteoid osteomas have a highly vascularized nidus, which incites an intense, painful, inflammatory reaction that produces sclerosis of the surrounding bone. The pain is typically worse at night and is characteristically relieved by nonsteroidal antiinflammatory drugs (NSAIDs) and aspirin, though this medication is not recommended in children due to risk of Reye syndrome.

Radiographic evaluation. Most benign neoplasms are visible on anteroposterior and lateral radiographs of the symptomatic area. Characteristics of benign lesions include well-circumscribed lesions without periosteal new bone formation or soft tissue mass. If a lesion is suspected but not visible on plain radiographs, such as may occur in an osteoid osteoma, a technetium bone scan may be helpful. Further evaluation can be achieved with CT or MRI. Diagnosis is further aided by surgical biopsy, which may also allow for surgical treatment.

Malignant neoplasms. Leukemia is the most common childhood malignancy and is frequently accompanied by musculoskeletal complaints, such as limping, fever, bone pain, pallor, bruising, and weight loss (Fig. 45.16). Common malignancies involving the musculoskeletal system include osteogenic sarcoma, Ewing sarcoma, and intraspinal tumors, such as astrocytomas (Table 45.8). Intraspinal tumors tend to produce neurologic symptoms, such as muscle

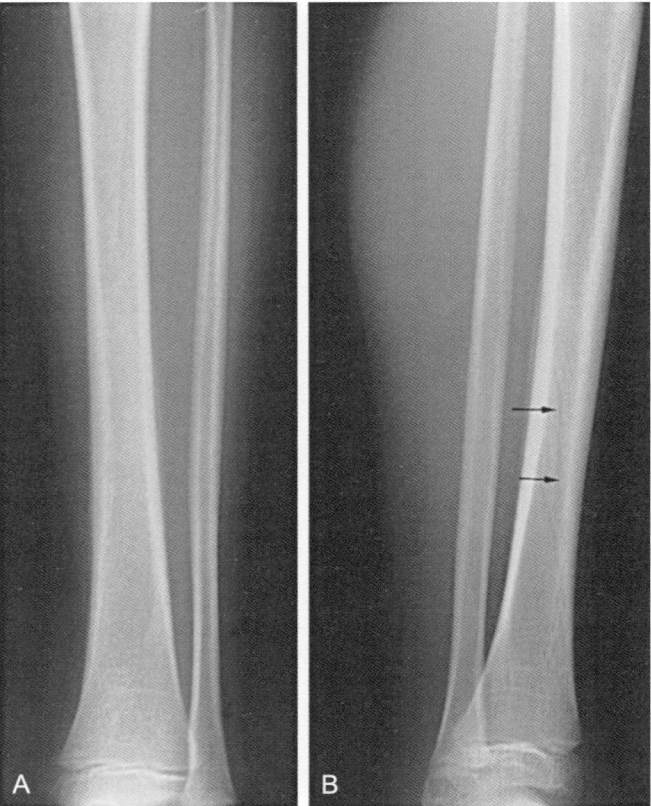

Fig. 45.15 *A,* An anteroposterior radiograph of the lower leg of a 2-year-old girl who had been limping on the left lower leg for approximately 1 week. There was no history of trauma. No obvious abnormality is visible in this view. *B,* A lateral radiograph showing a faint oblique fracture line *(arrows).* This is characteristic of the "toddler's fracture." There is already early subperiosteal new bone or callus formation posteriorly.

weakness, as the cause of limping. The other lesions may produce a mass, bone weakness, and possible pathologic fractures. Weight loss, fever, and pain are common associated complaints.

Physical examination. A careful musculoskeletal and neurologic examination is necessary for any child with a suspected neoplasm. In many cases, a mass, either in the involved bone or in adjacent soft tissues, may be palpable. These are typically tender and warm. These lesions are frequently adjacent to joints and may result in decreased range of motion. Neurologic evaluation may show evidence of muscle weakness or abnormal reflexes, suggestive of spinal cord or peripheral nerve involvement.

Radiographic evaluation. Anteroposterior and lateral radiographs of the involved area usually reveal the presence of a neoplasm. Characteristics of a malignant osseous lesion include bone destruction, permeative or infiltrative appearance, periosteal new bone formation (Codman triangle), and an associated soft tissue mass (see Table 45.8). Radiographic abnormalities associated with acute leukemia include diffuse osteopenia, metaphyseal bands, periosteal new bone formation, geographic lytic lesions, sclerosis, and permeative distraction. Additional studies, such as a bone scan or MRI, may be helpful in localizing the lesion.

Infection and inflammation

Septic arthritis and osteomyelitis. Bone and joint infections are common causes of limping in toddlers and children. When the infection is confined to the synovium of a joint, the condition is

TABLE 45.7 Benign Bone Tumors and Cysts

Disease	Characteristics	Radiographic Findings	Treatment	Prognosis
Osteochondroma (osteocartilaginous exostosis)	Common; distal metaphysis of the femur, proximal humerus, proximal tibia; painless, hard, nontender mass	Bony outgrowth; sessile or pedunculated	Excision, if symptomatic	Excellent; malignant transformation rare
Multiple hereditary osteochondromas	Osteochondroma of long bones; bone growth disturbances	As above	As above	Multiple lesions develop until skeletal maturity, after which no new lesions develop; malignant transformation rare
Osteoid osteoma	Pain relieved by aspirin; femur and tibia; found predominantly in boys	Dense sclerosis surrounds small radiolucent nidus <1 cm	As above	Excellent
Osteoblastoma (giant osteoid osteoma)	As above, but more destructive	Osteolytic component; size >1 cm	As above	Excellent
Enchondroma	Tubular bones of hands and feet; pathologic fractures, swollen bone; Ollier disease if multiple lesions are present	Radiolucent diaphyseal or metaphyseal lesion; may calcify	Excision or curettage	Excellent; malignant transformation rare
Nonossifying fibroma	Silent; rare pathologic fracture; late childhood, adolescence	Incidental radiographic finding; thin sclerotic border, radiolucent lesion	None or curettage with fractures	Excellent; heals spontaneously
Eosinophilic granuloma	Age 5–10 yr; skull, jaw, long bones; pathologic fracture; pain	Small, radiolucent without reactive bone; punched-out lytic lesion	Biopsy, excision rare; irradiation	Excellent; may heal spontaneously
Brodie abscess	Insidious local pain; limp; suspected as malignancy	Circumscribed metaphyseal osteomyelitis; lytic lesions with sclerotic rim	Biopsy; antibiotics	Excellent
Unicameral bone cyst (simple bone cyst)	Metaphysis of a long bone (femur, humerus); pain, pathologic fracture	Cyst in medullary canal, expands cortex; fluid-filled unilocular or multilocular cavity	Curettage; steroid injection into lesion	Excellent; some heal spontaneously
Aneurysmal bone cyst	As above; contains blood, fibrous tissue	Expands beyond metaphyseal cartilage	Curettage, bone graft	Excellent

Modified from Marcdante K, Kliegman R, eds. *Nelson Essentials of Pediatrics.* 7th ed. Philadelphia: Saunders; 2015.

termed septic arthritis. If the primary focus of the infection is within bone, even if the joint is secondarily involved, the condition is termed osteomyelitis. Bacterial pathogens are the most frequent cause of osteoarticular infections in children, with *Staphylococcus aureus* being the most frequent etiology. In neonates, group B streptococcus and gram-negative bacteria are common. Beyond the neonatal period, *Kingella kingae* is the second most frequent cause in children under 5 years of age. In older children and adolescents with puncture wounds of the foot, *Pseudomonas aeruginosa, S. aureus,* and streptococci are commonly implicated. Lyme arthritis should be considered in endemic areas. Sexually active adolescents may develop septic arthritis as a result of gonococcal infections. Patients with sickle cell anemia may develop osteomyelitis as a result of *Salmonella* species or pneumococcal infection.

Acute hematogenous osteomyelitis most commonly involves the femoral neck, the distal femoral metaphysis, and the proximal tibial metaphysis. Acute septic arthritis usually involves the hip, knee, or ankle. Children with these infections may be acutely ill; many may just have fever, limp, and localized pain. Treatment is with surgical drainage as needed and with prolonged antibacterials.

Subacute osteomyelitis, which has very distinct manifestations, occurs most commonly in the knee (Fig. 45.17). These children are usually afebrile and have night pain; hematologic studies yield normal findings. Radiographs show sclerotic metaphyseal lesions that occasionally cross the growth plate into the epiphysis. Culture specimens are positive only occasionally and typically show *S. aureus.*

Recurrent episodes of noninfectious, multifocal bone inflammation are the hallmark of **chronic nonbacterial osteomyelitis**, sometimes referred to as chronic recurrent multifocal osteomyelitis, which can produce a painful limp with involvement of the hip or lower extremities. The disorder is autoinflammatory in nature, begins in late childhood or early adolescence, and affects females more frequently than males. Chronic nonbacterial osteomyelitis may mimic acute hematogenous osteomyelitis at onset, particularly if there is initially one focus of bone inflammation. Inflammatory markers and imaging findings are similar to those in acute hematogenous osteomyelitis, although microbiologic studies are universally negative. The diagnosis becomes more apparent as multiple episodes of bone inflammation, affecting distinct anatomic sites, develop over time.

Recurrent episodes of nonbacterial osteomyelitis are also a feature of **SAPHO syndrome** (synovitis, acne, pustulosis, hyperostosis, osteitis), a rare disorder of immune disregulation, and **Majeed syndrome**, an autosomal recessive disorder (*LPIN2* gene) characterized by recurrent episodes of nonbacterial osteomyelitis, congenital dyserythropoietic

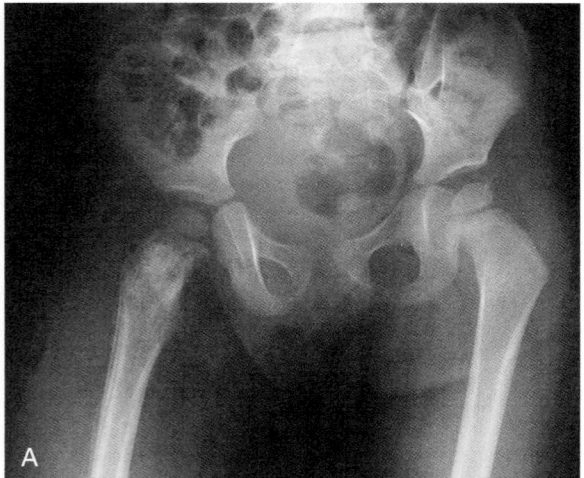

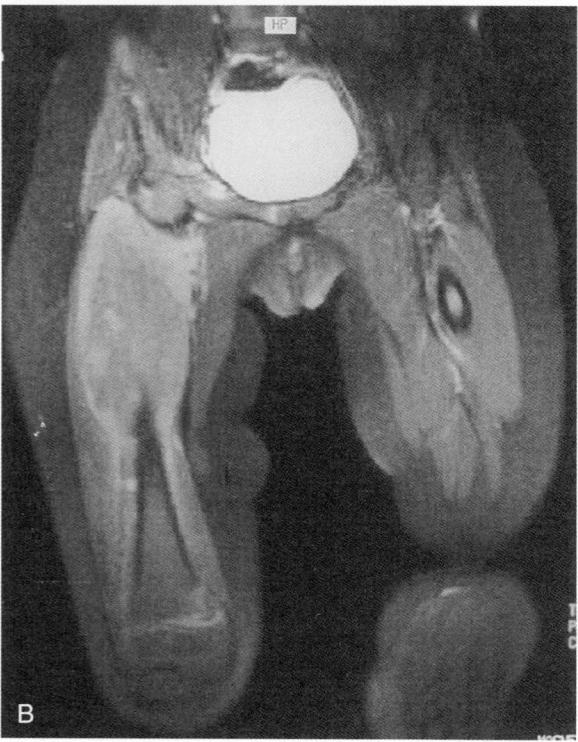

Fig. 45.16 *A,* Anteroposterior pelvic radiograph of a 2-year-old girl who had been limping for 4 months. There is an extensive destructive lesion on the right proximal femur. *B,* A large soft tissue mass is demonstrated on MRI scan. The preoperative diagnosis was Ewing sarcoma, but at biopsy the diagnosis was acute lymphoblastic leukemia.

anemia, joint inflammation, and neutrophilic dermatosis, as well as systemic inflammatory conditions such as inflammatory bowel disease or psoriasis. **Deficiency of interleukin-1 receptor antagonist (DIRA)** presents in infancy with sterile osteitis and periostitis plus a pustular rash, often without fever. Multifocal osteolytic lesions are present in long bones, the clavicle, and ribs. This is an autosomal recessive disorder (*IL1RN* gene).

Physical examination. Children with acute bone and joint infections may exhibit bacteremia and signs of infection, including elevations in temperature, white blood cell count, ESR, and CRP level. Some infants present only with **pseudoparalysis** of the affected limb. When the hip joint is involved, the child holds the hip in a position of flexion, abduction, and external rotation. This position unwinds the

hip capsule and allows it to hold the greatest volume of intracapsular fluid. This initially decreases pressure, but as the pus continues to accumulate, even this position fails to relieve symptoms. A hip joint effusion is usually not palpable, but there may be overlying soft tissue swelling and tenderness.

Infections of peripheral joints, such as the knee, are more easily diagnosed. There is typically a joint effusion and perhaps soft tissue swelling, erythema, and increased warmth over the metaphysis if osteomyelitis is present. Osteomyelitis typically manifests with point tenderness over the involved site; with continued bone destruction and rupture of pus into the periosteum, tenderness becomes more diffuse. Infections can also occur about the ankle and foot. Infection of the foot is less common except as a sequela to puncture wounds through a tennis shoe, producing the classic *P. aeruginosa* or staphylococcal osteomyelitis-osteochondritis.

Radiographic evaluation. Plain radiographs are not helpful in the first 7–10 days of acute hematogenous osteomyelitis, inasmuch as they are usually normal, but must be obtained in the assessment of the child. After 10–14 days of active infection, bone destruction or periosteal bone elevation is seen. MRI, or alternately bone scan, is both sensitive and specific for osteomyelitis and septic arthritis, even early in the course of the disease (Figs. 45.18 and 45.19).

If a septic process about the hip is suspected, an ultrasound study may be beneficial in demonstrating an effusion. If this is present, arthrocentesis or hip aspiration is necessary. The synovial fluid analysis should include a cell count, measurement of protein and glucose levels, Gram stain, cultures, and sensitivity studies. *K. kingae* polymerase chain reaction (PCR) testing should be performed, particularly in younger children. Infections of peripheral joints, such as the knee, are more readily diagnosed by arthrocentesis.

If an osteomyelitis of a metaphyseal region is suspected based on imaging studies, the subperiosteal space and bone may be directly aspirated with a large-bore needle. The material should be sent for bacterial culture, as well as for *K. kingae* nucleic acid amplification testing in younger children, and Lyme testing in endemic areas. Any positive bacterial culture results should have antibacterial susceptibility testing performed so as to guide therapy. Despite these interventions, microbiologic studies may frequently fail to yield results.

Spondylodiskitis. Diskitis, inflammation of the vertebral disk that is often related to infection, may produce refusal to walk and/or limping via disk or bone inflammation, referred pain, or intraspinal extension (see Chapter 46) (Fig. 45.20).

Rheumatic causes. Juvenile inflammatory arthritides affecting the hip, knee, or ankle joints can result in an antalgic gait (see Chapter 44). Immunoglobulin A vasculitis (Henoch-Schönlein purpura) can also produce arthritis or enthesitis that can result in a painful limp (see Chapter 44). Autoimmune and autoinflammatory disorders characterized by bone inflammation were discussed previously.

Transient synovitis. Transient synovitis of the hip (also known as toxic synovitis) is the most common cause of limping in children. It can occur in all age groups, but the mean age at onset is 6 years; most patients are between 3 and 8 years of age. Hip transient synovitis is characterized by acute onset of monoarthritic hip pain, an associated limp, and mild restriction of hip motion, especially abduction and internal rotation. The pain is felt in the groin, anterior thigh, or knee. Any child with atraumatic anterior thigh or knee pain must be carefully evaluated for hip disease because these are the sites of referred pain. Septic arthritis and osteomyelitis must be excluded.

The cause of this disorder remains uncertain. Suspected causes include active or recent systemic viral infection, trauma, and allergic hypersensitivity. Approximately 70% of affected children have had a nonspecific viral upper respiratory infection 7–14 days before the onset of symptoms.

TABLE 45.8 Comparison of Osteogenic and Ewing Sarcoma

	Osteogenic Sarcoma	Ewing Sarcoma
Age	Adolescence	Childhood and adolescence
Ancestry	All	Predominantly non-Hispanic White
Sex (M:F ratio)	1.5:1	1.5:1
Cell	Spindle cell, osteoid	Nonosseous, small round cell
Predisposing risk factors	Retinoblastoma Radiotherapy Alkylating agents	None
Site	Metaphysis, epiphysis; distal femur > proximal tibia > proximal humerus	Diaphysis, medullary cavity, cortical bone, soft tissue; femur > pelvis > tibia > humerus
Presentation	Local pain	Pain, fever, increased ESR, FUO, weight loss
Roentgenogram	Lytic, sclerotic Sunburst pattern	Mottled, lytic Onion-skin pattern
Differential diagnosis	Ewing sarcoma, osteomyelitis	Osteomyelitis, eosinophilic granuloma, lymphoma, neuroblastoma, rhabdomyosarcoma
Metastasis	Lung, bones Skip lesions in the same bone	Lung, bones
Treatment	Surgery, chemotherapy Limb salvage if tumor is resectable and the patient is near adult height	Surgery, radiotherapy Chemotherapy
Outcome	50–60% survival	60% survival without metastasis; 5–15% with metastasis, primary site dependent
Poor prognosis	Onset at age <10 yr, large tumor size (>15 cm), symptoms <2 mo, metastasis	Pelvis, soft tissue tumor, increased LDH, metastasis, increased circulating PMNs, decreased circulating lymphocytes

F, female; FUO, fever of unknown origin; LDH, lactate dehydrogenase; M, male; PMN, polymorphonuclear neutrophil.
Modified from Behrman RE, ed. *Nelson Textbook of Pediatrics*. 14th ed. Philadelphia: WB Saunders; 1992:1312.

Physical examination. The patient is usually ambulatory, and the hip is not held in a position of flexion, abduction, or external rotation unless a significant effusion has developed. The child walks with an antalgic gait on the involved side and is usually afebrile. Laboratory findings are usually within normal limits, but occasionally a minimal elevation of the white blood cell count or ESR may be seen.

Radiographic evaluation. Anteroposterior and frog-leg lateral radiographs of the pelvis are obtained to rule out the presence of other lesions. The radiographs in transient synovitis are normal. On occasion, ultrasonography of the hip may be useful in demonstrating a small joint effusion. MRI is helpful in identifying septic joints or other causes of pain when there is doubt regarding the diagnosis. Bone scans as well may be helpful in difficult or unusual cases; in synovitis, these results are always normal. When the diagnosis of transient synovitis is in doubt, hip arthrocentesis may be necessary. The fluid that is aspirated shows a low white blood cell count (typically well under 25,000 cells/μL), and the cultures are negative.

Trendelenburg Gait

Developmental anomalies

Developmental dysplasia of the hip. Developmental dysplasia of the hip (DDH) refers to the condition of increased laxity of the hip joint and encompasses the following classifications: (1) acetabular dysplasia, (2) hip subluxation, and (3) hip dislocation. Developmental dysplasia of the hip is considered either typical, in which no underlying genetic or syndromic association is identified, or teratologic. Early identification and management improve the functional outcome of surgical repairs. If not identified and appropriately treated, DDH

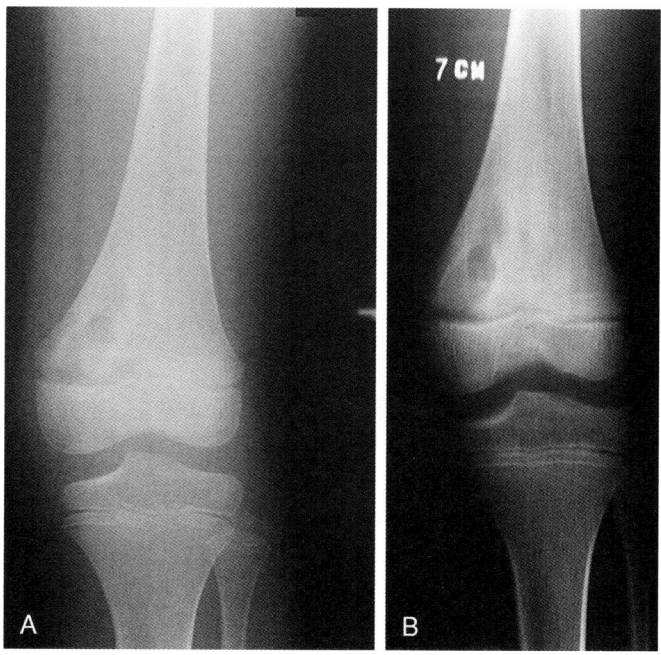

Fig. 45.17 *A,* Anteroposterior radiograph of the distal femur in a 12-year-old girl with limping and nighttime knee pain for 6 months. There is a lucent lesion with surrounding sclerosis in the metaphysis. The lesion crosses the epiphysis; this is characteristic of a subacute osteomyelitis. *B,* Anteroposterior tomography clearly demonstrates the lucent nature of the lesion and its surrounding sclerosis.

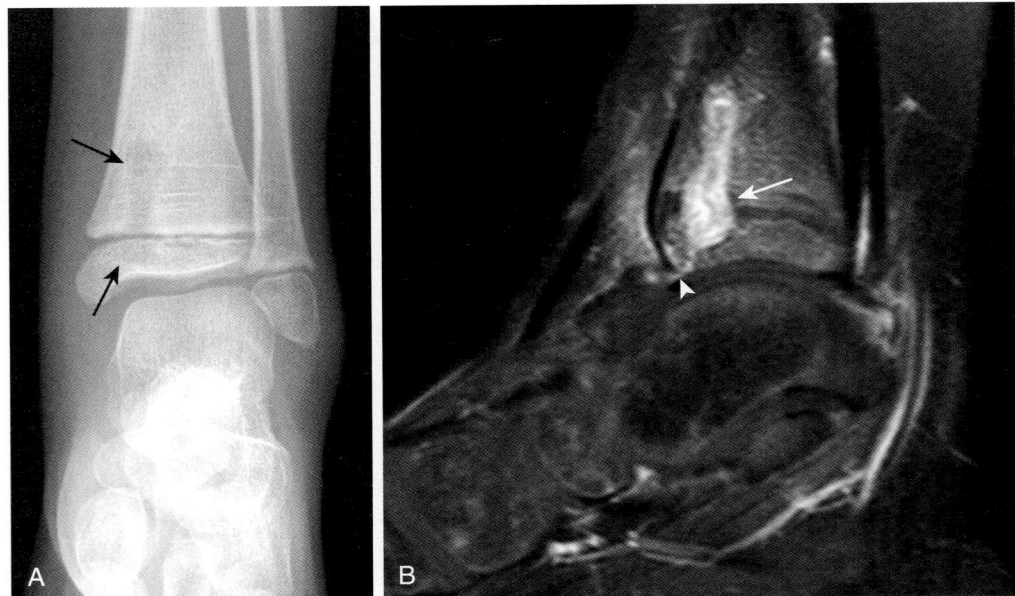

Fig. 45.18 *A,* A frontal radiograph demonstrates a lytic lesion in the distal tibial metaphysis extending into the epiphysis *(arrows).* *B,* A T1-weighted fat-saturated postgadolinium sagittal view demonstrates a thick, rim-enhancing lesion with a small amount of nonenhancing fluid consistent with early abscess formation with epiphyseal extension *(arrow)* and a small cloaca *(arrowhead)* extending to the tibiotalar joint. (From Kan JH, Azouz EM. Musculoskeletal infections. In: Coley BD, ed. *Caffey's Pediatric Diagnostic Imaging.* 12th ed. Vol II. Philadelphia: Elsevier; 2013:1472.)

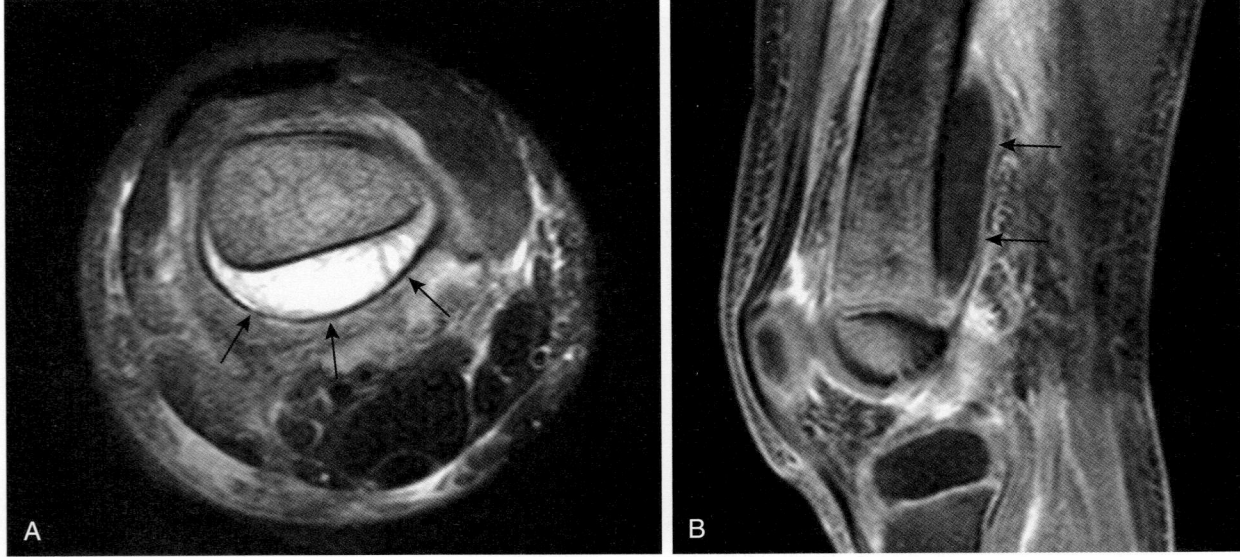

Fig. 45.19 Acute osteomyelitis of the distal femur in a 5-year-old boy. *A,* T2-weighted fat-saturated axial MRI shows a large subperiosteal abscess *(arrows)* at the posterior aspect of the femur. Increased signal is seen within the bone, and there is adjacent soft tissue edema. *B,* T1-weighted fat-saturated postgadolinium sagittal MRI shows the longitudinal extent of the subperiosteal abscess with an enhancing wall *(arrows).* (From Kan JH, Azouz EM. Musculoskeletal infections. In: Coley BD, ed. *Caffey's Pediatric Diagnostic Imaging.* 12th ed. Vol II. Philadelphia: Elsevier; 2013:1476.)

will present with limping, toe-walking, or both. When the problem occurs unilaterally, the child walks with a mild Trendelenburg gait or demonstrates toe-walking. With bilateral involvement, the child stands with an increased lumbar lordosis and has a waddling gait. There is functional impairment resulting from a lack of stability and associated muscle weakness, particularly in the hip abductors.

Physical examination. The most common physical finding in the older child with a developmentally dysplastic hip is limited hip abduction on the involved side. There may be a mild hip flexion contracture and apparent shortening of the extremity. The greater trochanter lies above a line between the anterior superior iliac spine and the ischial tuberosity (Nélaton line). In bilateral dislocations, the

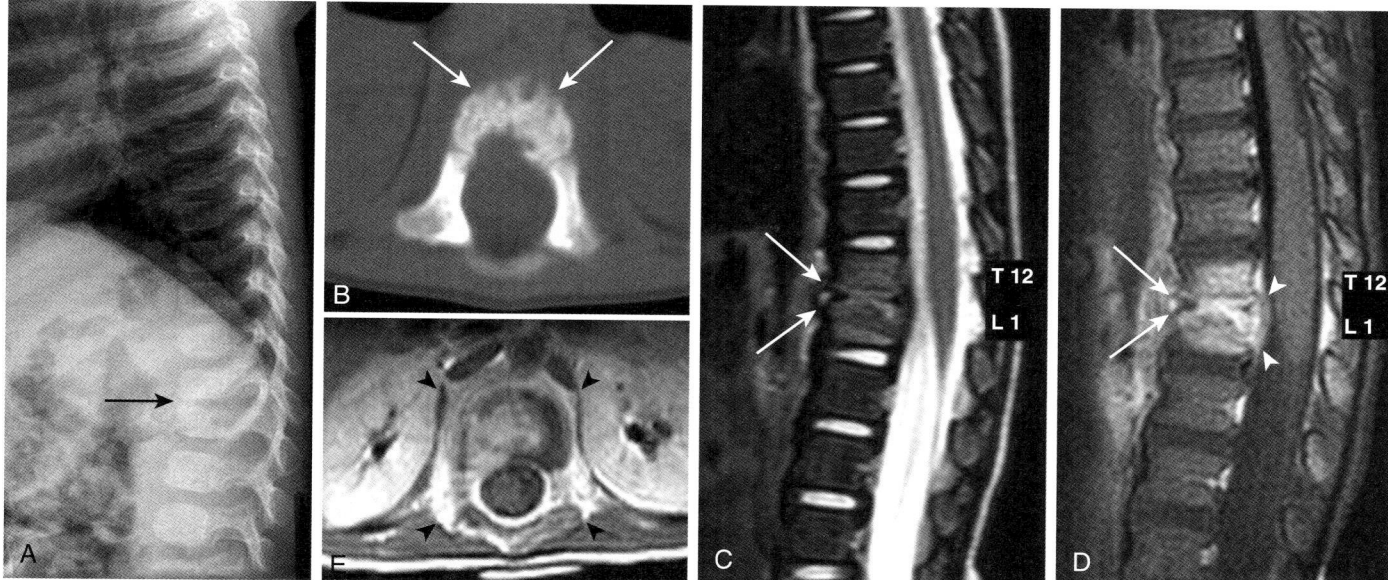

Fig. 45.20 A 15-month-old girl with an abnormal gait and concern for an intraspinal mass had diskitis/osteomyelitis. Lateral spine radiographs demonstrate narrowing of the T12-L1 intervertebral disk space *(arrow in A)*. An axial bone window from a noncontrast CT scan of the spine demonstrates irregularity to the vertebral end plates *(arrows in B)*. A sagittal T2-weighted image *(C)*, a sagittal fat-saturated T1-weighted postcontrast image *(D)*, and an axial T1-weighted postcontrast image *(E)* of the thoracolumbar junction demonstrate loss of height of the T12-L1 intervertebral disk space with adjacent T2 prolongation of the adjacent end plates *(arrows in C)*, with corresponding abnormal enhancement in the same regions *(arrows in D)*, and surrounding masslike soft tissue enhancement *(arrowheads in E)*. Note the thickening/elevation and enhancement of the posterior longitudinal ligament *(arrowheads in D)*. (From Pollock AN, Henesch SM. Infections of the spine and spinal cord. In: Coley BD, ed. *Caffey's Pediatric Diagnostic Imaging.* 12th ed. Vol I. Philadelphia: Elsevier; 2013:465.)

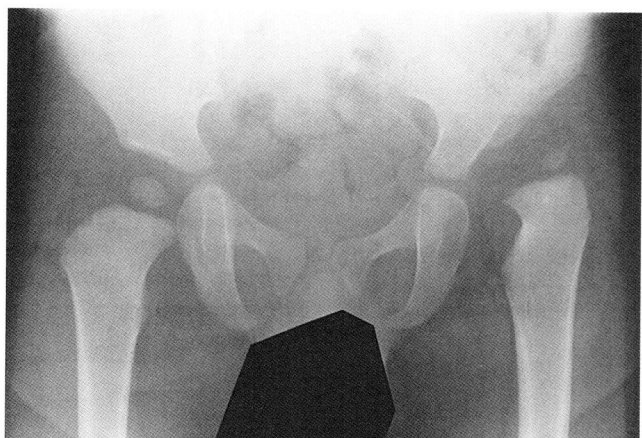

Fig. 45.21 An anteroposterior radiograph of the pelvis of an 18-month-old girl demonstrating a developmental dislocation of the left hip. The acetabulum is severely dysplastic, there is delayed ossification in the capital femoral epiphysis compared to the normal right hip, and the femoral head is displaced laterally and superiorly.

physical findings are more symmetric but there is still limitation of hip abduction. Positive Trendelenburg signs are present on the involved sides. The normal response to a Trendelenburg test occurs when the patient stands on the uninvolved leg and the abductor muscles are able to maintain balance by elevating the contralateral pelvis. A positive Trendelenburg sign, resulting from weakness, is demonstrated when the abductor muscles are unable to maintain pelvic balance and the patient compensates by leaning to the affected side (see Fig. 45.11).

Radiographic evaluation. The diagnosis can be made from routine anteroposterior and frog-leg lateral radiographs of the pelvis (Fig. 45.21). Specialized studies, such as MRI and CT, are usually not necessary. Ultrasound study is not usually necessary in an ambulatory child older than 6 months of age because the CFE is ossified.

Lower extremity length discrepancy. Lower extremity length discrepancy in older children and adolescents has been discussed earlier in this chapter.

Neuromuscular Origin

Cerebral palsy (see Chapter 38). Children with spastic hemiplegia or diplegia may have an associated painless limp caused by muscle spasticity and concomitant weakness of the antagonist muscles. The history should focus on risk factors for cerebral palsy, prematurity, and other congenital anomalies external to the central nervous system, followed by a physical examination, with particular attention to the neurologic system. The neurologic examination reveals evidence of increased muscle tone, spasticity, hyperactive deep tendon reflexes, and pathologic reflexes, such as Babinski signs.

Nerve entrapment syndromes (mononeuropathies). Nerve entrapment lower extremity mononeuropathies may produce a limp or abnormal gait secondary to pain or muscle weakness (Table 45.9). Peroneal nerve entrapment at the level of the head of the fibula is the most common entrapment mononeuropathy. The common fibular (peroneal) nerve wraps around the head of the fibular bone and connects to the periosteum, making it susceptible to trauma or external compression (Fig. 45.22). Workers who squat (farmers, carpet layers), habitual leg crossing, neuromas, Baker cysts, and ankle sprains (traction injury) are risk factors. Pain, foot drop, and paresthesia are common manifestations.

TABLE 45.9 Lower Limb Mononeuropathies

Condition	Etiology	Symptoms	Testing	Results
Femoral neuropathy	Trauma, retroperitoneal hematoma caused by anticoagulation, cardiac catheterizations	Weak quadriceps muscle, weakness of knee extension, absent knee jerk, groin pain, and decreased sensation over medial and anterior thigh and lower leg in the saphenous nerve distribution	Motor nerve conduction to quadriceps Saphenous sensory study EMG of quadriceps as well as other L3 and L4 muscles (e.g., the adductor muscles); consider an EMG screen for radiculopathy	Reduced amplitude or absent saphenous nerve response Reduced CMAP over rectus femoris On EMG, fibrillations in the femoral nerve–innervated muscles
Lateral femoral cutaneous nerve entrapment at thigh (meralgia paresthetica)	Repeated low-grade trauma, obesity, pregnancy, tight clothing most commonly under the lateral end of the ilioinguinal ligament	Pure sensory syndrome at the lateral thigh including unpleasant paresthesias, burning, or a dull ache; no motor symptoms Can be aggravated by prolonged standing or walking	Lateral femoral cutaneous study Femoral evaluation as above should be considered	Reduced amplitude in lateral femoral cutaneous nerve This nerve is technically challenging to study and side-to-side comparisons are useful
Peroneal nerve entrapment at the head of the fibula	Fractures, plaster casts, tight stockings, improper positioning, excessive weight loss, farm work, tumors, crossing legs for a long time	Foot drop, weakness of eversion, numbness on the dorsum of the foot, and pain	SPS testing Motor nerve conduction below and across the fibular head recorded from EDB or tibialis anterior if EDB is atrophied Exclude L5 radiculopathy by EMG Test an additional motor and sensory nerve in the same leg	Reduced or absent SPS response Conduction block across the fibular head Conduction velocity reduced in fibular head segment by >10 m/sec compared with leg segment Fibrillations in muscles innervated by fibular (peroneal) nerve
Tibial nerve entrapment at tarsal tunnel under flexor retinaculum of medial malleolus	Compression from shoes, casting, post-traumatic fibrosis, overuse, ganglion cysts	Pain in foot and ankle, wasting and weakness in feet, sensory impairment at toes and sole of the foot	Plantar sensory (mixed) nerve conductions Tibial motor to AH muscle Another motor and sensory nerve to exclude polyneuropathy EMG of intrinsic foot muscles Consider EMG screen for radiculopathy or sciatic neuropathy	Prolonged or absent latencies or low amplitudes in plantar nerves Prolonged, absent, or small distal responses across tarsal tunnel Fibrillations in the AH or other intrinsic foot muscle innervated by the tibial nerve Normal EDB EMG and sural sensory nerve

AH, abductor hallucis; CMAP, compound muscle action potential; EDB, extensor digitorum brevis; EMG, electromyography; SPS, superficial fibular (peroneal) sensory nerve
Modified from Cifu DX, ed. *Braddom's Physical Medicine and Rehabilitation*. 6th ed. Philadelphia: Elsevier; 2021, Table 8-19.

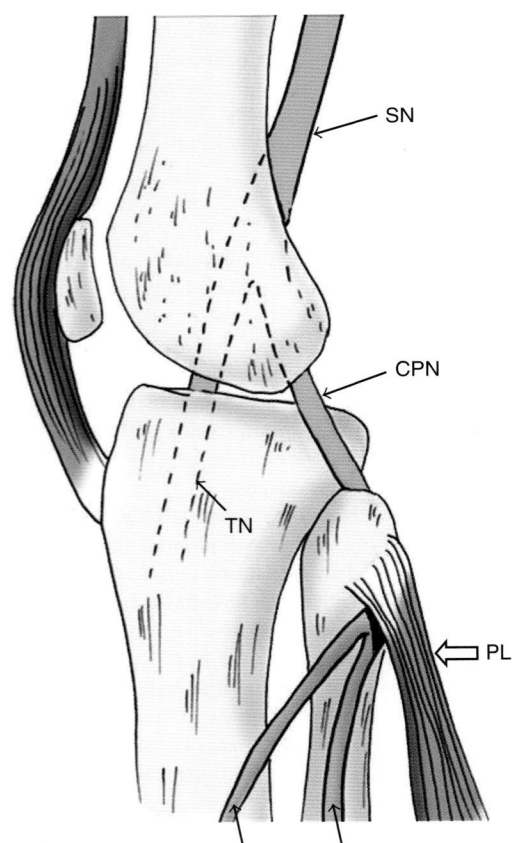

Fig. 45.22 The intimate relationship of the peroneal nerve to the fibular head is demonstrated. CPN, common peroneal (fibular) nerve; PL, peroneus longus; SN, sciatic nerve; TN, tibial nerve. (From Dong Q, Jacobson JA, Jamadar DA, et al. Entrapment neuropathies in the upper and lower limbs: anatomy and MRI features. *Radiol Res Pract*. 2012;2012:230679, Fig. 17.)

Hereditary neuropathy with liability to pressure palsies is another potential mononeuropathy; when the lower extremity is involved, unilateral paresthesias and motor weakness may be present. This is an autosomal dominant disorder due to a deletion or pathologic variant in the *PMP22* gene.

SUMMARY AND RED FLAGS

Conditions associated with limp must be divided into acute, painful lesions and chronic, painless lesions; on occasion, presentations may be mixed. Infection and trauma must be considered emergencies, as should conditions that are joint or limb threatening, such as septic arthritis and osteomyelitis of the hip, avascular necrosis, or SCFE. In addition, signs of spinal cord involvement (see Chapter 46) suggest acute processes that warrant immediate attention to prevent permanent paralysis.

Red flags include acute hip pain, fever with limp, neurologic manifestations (including bowel and bladder dysfunction or paresthesias), point tenderness, the presence of a mass, night awakening pain, and signs of weight loss or hematologic abnormalities such as pallor or bruising.

BIBLIOGRAPHY

A bibliography is available at ExpertConsult.com.

46

Back Pain

Kevin D. Walter

The incidence of pediatric back pain increases with age and has a prevalence of nearly 40% by 18 years of age. While back pain is often related to overuse in sports, work, or a specific traumatic event, it may also be idiopathic, infectious, inflammatory, neoplastic, or secondary to anatomic lesions. While back pain may be mild and resolve spontaneously in athletically active adolescents, back pain in younger children is more unusual and may suggest significant disease (tumor, infection). Persistent back pain in children necessitates a thorough evaluation to rule out disorders that can result in significant morbidity, such as infection or tumor. Back pain is not a disease but a symptom and is often associated in adolescents with headaches, emotional problems, daytime tiredness, and behavioral disorders. Activity modification and rehabilitation or exercises for the spine may help reduce risk for recurrent episodes. *Severe or persistent back pain necessitates a thorough history, physical examination, and appropriate imaging studies to evaluate the child for potentially serious pathologic processes.*

NORMAL ANATOMY, GROWTH, AND DEVELOPMENT OF THE SPINE

The back is often defined as the area from the first thoracic vertebra to the top of the sacrum. The spinal column is composed of vertebral bodies that articulate with each other through intervertebral disks. Each vertebral body has a posterior arch, which includes the spinal and transverse processes, as well as the articulation of the superior and inferior facets.

Vertebral growth occurs in an orderly manner throughout childhood and adolescence. About 50% of vertebral column height is present by the age of 2 years. Each vertebral body contains superior and inferior growth plates, which typically ossify at approximately 4 years of age and close in late adolescence. Acceleration of vertebral growth occurs during the adolescent growth spurt but contributes less to total height than does lower limb growth; the sitting heights of siblings in early and late adolescence are often remarkably similar. Spinal growth slows at menarche in girls and at the time of voice change in boys and is usually complete 2–3 years later. Developmental abnormalities of the column, such as idiopathic scoliosis, most commonly first appear just before the growth spurt. Alterations in spinal configuration caused by congenital deformities of vertebral segments change most rapidly during periods of rapid spinal growth: before the age of 2 years and at the time of the adolescent growth spurt.

There is a strong association of genitourinary, neurologic, gastrointestinal, and dermatologic system abnormalities in patients with congenital abnormalities of the spine. Warning signs of more systemic pathology in patients with congenital spine deformities include leg length inequality, foot size asymmetry, high foot arches, hairy patches or hemangiomas or a mass over the spine, sacral dimpling, enuresis, toe-walking, asymmetry or abnormality in the lower extremity deep tendon reflexes, and lower extremity weakness.

NORMAL SPINAL ALIGNMENT

The normal trunk is symmetric when viewed from the front or the back (Fig. 46.1). The shoulders and pelvis are parallel to each other and to the ground. The distance between the right and left elbows and the sides of the trunk is equal. When the trunk is viewed from the side, a series of curves is present (see Fig. 46.1). A convex anterior lordotic curve is present in the cervical region. The thoracic spine is concave anteriorly in a kyphotic pattern. The normal lumbar spine is lordotic, and the sacrum and coccygeal regions are kyphotic. Normal adult sagittal alignment develops gradually; children younger than 10 years typically have less cervical lordosis and more lumbar lordosis than adults. Injuries, infections, tumors, inflammation, and developmental abnormalities of the spine often produce alterations in these expected contours. Range of motion is demonstrated in Fig. 46.2.

EVALUATION OF THE PEDIATRIC SPINE

Examination of the spine should be part of the routine physical examination in the healthy child and adolescent. Patients presenting with a chief complaint of back pain require a detailed history and thorough physical examination (Table 46.1).

When findings on screening examinations are abnormal or when a patient presents with complaints of back pain, a more detailed examination is required. The spinal vertebral column, spinal cord, and spinal nerves are intimately related, and disorders affecting any of these elements may produce symptoms and signs in the others. Detailed examination of strength in the muscles of the spine and lower extremities (Fig. 46.3), sensation (Fig. 46.4), abdominal and lower extremity reflexes, anal sphincter tone, and perianal sensation should be performed when the primary examination suggests involvement of the neural structures that pass through the spinal column.

BACK PAIN OF BRIEF DURATION

In children younger than 10 years of age, extremity injuries are more common than back pain related to routine play and organized sports activities. When the trunk is involved, contusions and abrasions are much more common than ligament sprains and muscle strains.

When a child presents with back pain of brief duration after a play- or sports-related injury, a careful examination should be performed. If there are no other associated injuries and the screening examination shows no alterations in trunk configuration or lower extremity strength or sensation (see Figs. 46.3 and 46.4), no further work-up is necessary. A brief period of rest for 1–2 days, followed by gradual resumption of activities, is appropriate treatment. Imaging studies are not necessary when the duration of symptoms is short and the physical examination findings are normal. Signs of systemic illness (fever, weight loss) or neurologic deficits warrant an immediate, more in-depth evaluation.

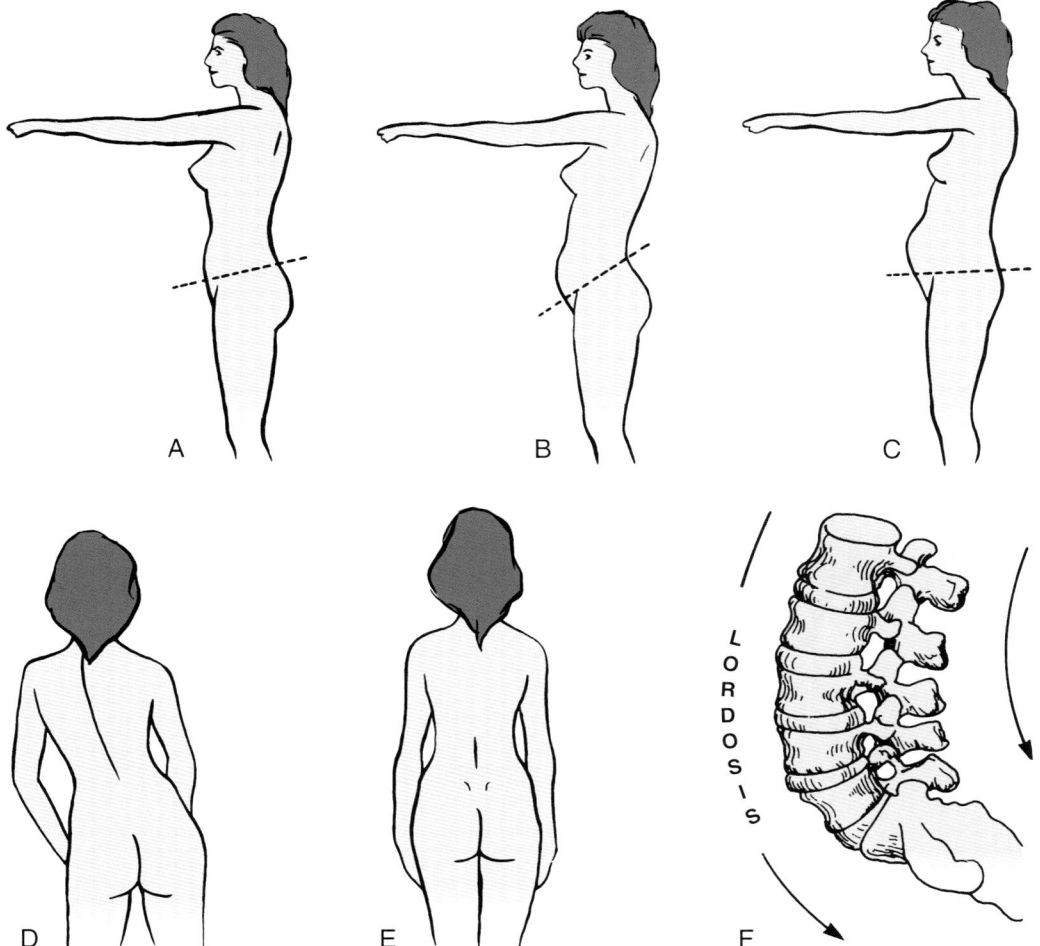

Fig. 46.1 *A,* Normal posture with normal lumbar lordosis. *B,* Exaggerated lumbar lordosis caused by pelvic tilting. *C,* "Paunchy" posture. *D,* Spastic scoliosis caused by muscle spasm. *E,* Normal posture without scoliosis. *F,* The normal orientation of the lumbar spine is that of mild lordosis. Exaggerated lordosis may predispose the patient to mechanical back pain. (From Reilly BM. *Practical Strategies in Outpatient Medicine.* 2nd ed. Philadelphia: WB Saunders; 1991:908.)

Acute back injuries occur more frequently in adolescence, as the sizes of participants and potential forces generated in recreational activities increase. If there are no other associated injuries and the screening examination findings are normal, no further imaging work-up is necessary. A brief period of rest followed by gradual resumption of activities remains appropriate treatment. The importance of a comprehensive and balanced conditioning exercise program should be stressed to young athletes. Sport-related injuries can be reduced by preparticipation conditioning, appropriate warm-up, careful supervision, and resting when fatigued.

Trauma sufficient to cause acute spine fractures may occur because of motor vehicle or bicycle crashes, falls, and diving and gymnastic injuries. The frequency and severity of spine trauma rises in later adolescence as exposure to these events increases. In such cases, there is a clear relationship between the trauma and the onset of symptoms. Injury to the spinal column should be suspected in all individuals whose level of consciousness is impaired after a crash or sports injury, regardless of the presence or absence of symptoms.

Children with suspected acute spinal injury should be immobilized on backboards designed for children until definitive imaging studies can be performed and interpreted. Immobilization of the child's cervical spine on a solid backboard should be avoided. The child's occiput projects farther posteriorly than an adult's, causing cervical flexion if the child's neck is immobilized on a standard backboard. Spinal immobilization boards for children are readily available and have a cut-out section to accommodate the occiput. When such boards are not available, a blanket or firm mattress should be interposed between the trunk and the backboard to prevent neck flexion.

PERSISTENT BACK PAIN

Persistent or severe back pain is uncommon in young children but is more common in athletically active adolescents. Mechanical low back pain is said to be present in the patient with no definable pathology on physical exam or imaging studies, but frequent exam findings include tight hamstrings, poor posture, weak core musculature, and discomfort with paraspinal muscle palpation. This is the situation in over 50% of patients presenting with low back pain. The implications of severe or persistent back pain are more serious in younger patients than in adolescents. Persistent back pain in young children is usually not the result of a congenital spinal deformity or developmental disorders of the spine but may be due to infection or tumor. As a child enters and passes through the adolescent growth spurt, back pain may arise from a small number of congenital and developmental disorders of the spinal column. Degenerative disorders of the spine such as intervertebral disk herniation are uncommon causes of back pain

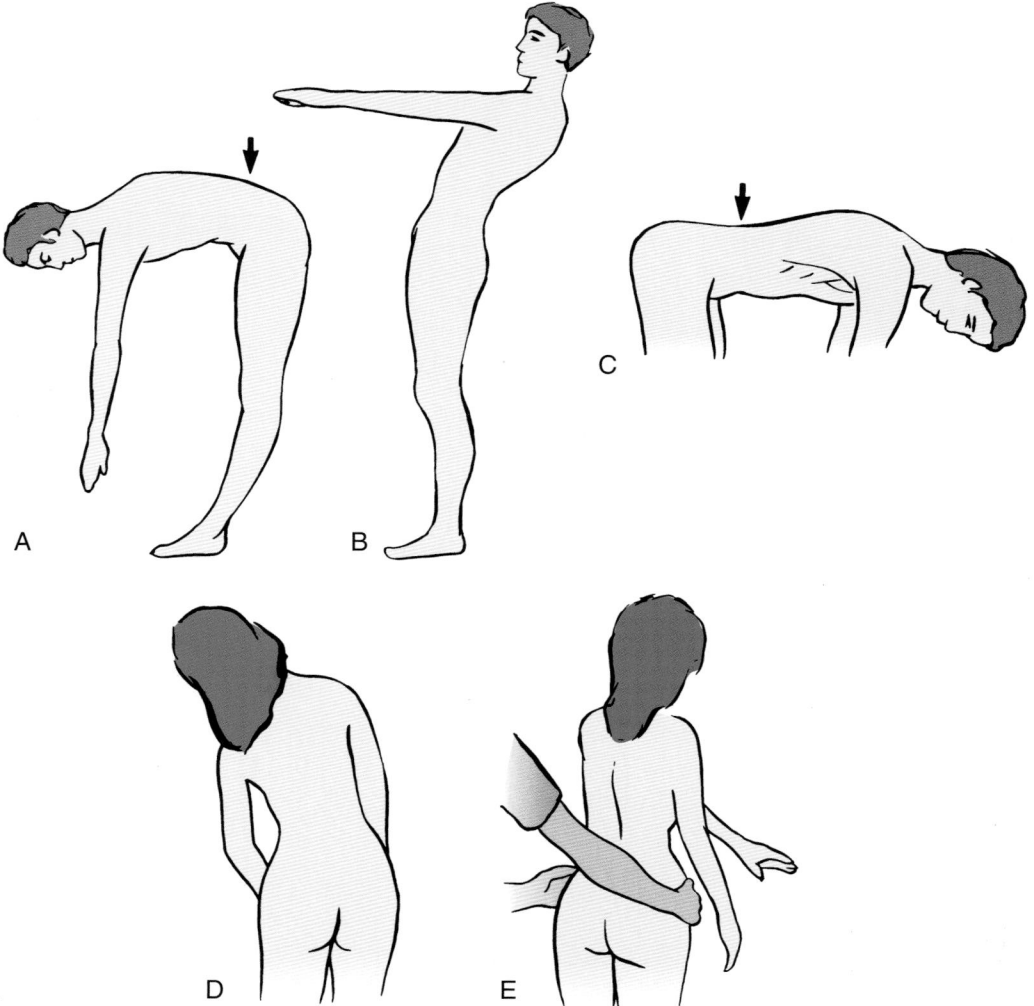

Fig. 46.2 Back range of motion. *A*, Flexion. Note the normal reversal of lumbar lordosis during flexion *(arrow)*. *B*, Extension. *C*, Persistent lordosis during back flexion as a result of muscle spasm *(arrow)*. *D*, Lateral flexion. *E*, Lateral torsion *(rotation)*. (From Reilly BM. *Practical Strategies in Outpatient Medicine*. 2nd ed. Philadelphia: WB Saunders; 1991:909.)

TABLE 46.1	Guidelines for Primary Examination of the Back

History

Is there a history of back pain? If so, what is the:
   Frequency?
   Duration?
   Relationship to activity?
Antecedent trauma?
Is there associated pain in the legs?
Is there incontinence or enuresis?
Is walking painful?
Have there been systemic signs of chronic illness?
Is there a family history of deformity?
Is there a family history of disc disease?

Physical Examination
General Appearance and Palpation
Are the right and left sides of the trunk symmetric?
Are there hairy patches, nevi, sinuses, or dimpling over the midline of the spine?
Are the pelvis and shoulders level?
Is there normal kyphosis and lordosis?
On forward bending, is a rib hump present?
Is there muscle atrophy?
Is there localized tenderness?

Motion
Can the patient easily bend forward and touch their toes?
Is there pain with range of motion?
Is normal hamstring flexibility present?
Is the gait normal?

Lower Extremities
Are leg lengths equal?
Is strength normal in the major motor groups of the lower limbs?
Is sensation normal in the lower limbs?
Are reflexes normal at the knees and ankles?
Are pathologic reflexes present?
What is the response to straight leg *and* cross straight leg raising maneuvers?

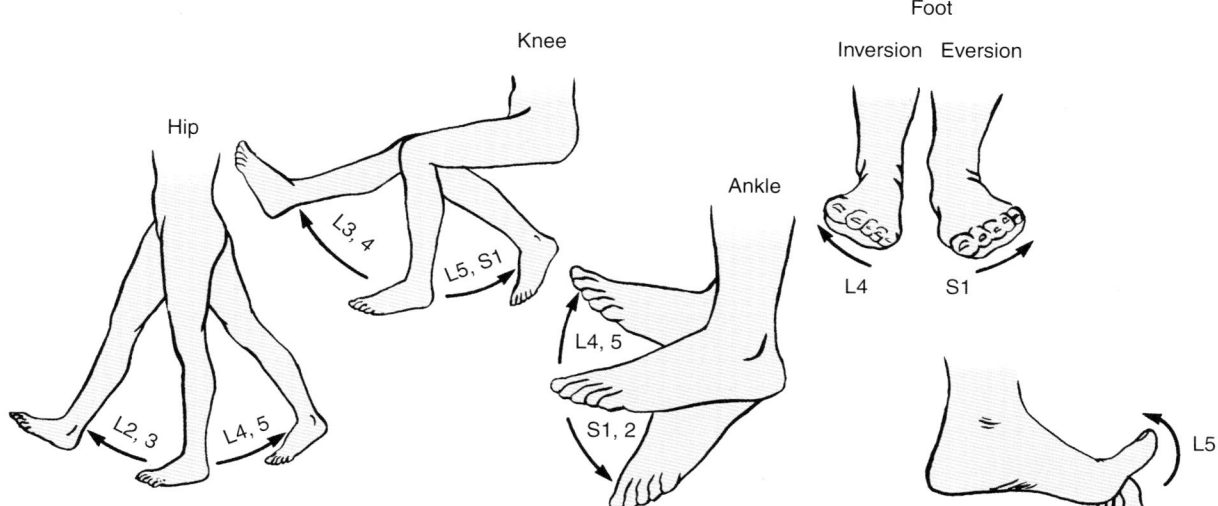

Fig. 46.3 Motor control of the lower extremity. (From Reilly BM. *Practical Strategies in Outpatient Medicine.* 2nd ed. Philadelphia: WB Saunders; 1991:926.)

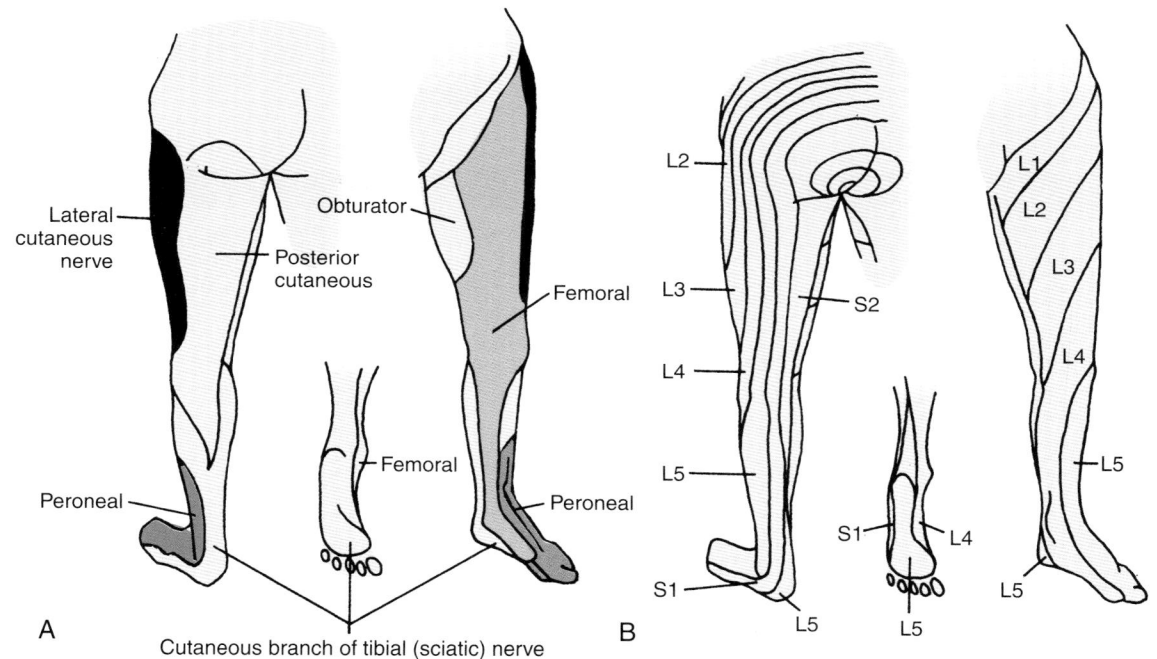

Fig. 46.4 Sensory innervation of the lower extremity. *A,* Peripheral nerve innervation. *B,* Dermatomal (root) innervation. (From Reilly BM. *Practical Strategies in Outpatient Medicine.* 2nd ed. Philadelphia: WB Saunders; 1991:927.)

in childhood. In evaluating a patient, it is important to try to distinguish musculoskeletal-mechanical disorders from those with more generalized systemic signs or those suggestive of a neoplasia (Fig. 46.5). Concerns for neoplastic or infectious etiologies herald the need for advanced imaging; if the MRI shows no definitive pathology, then patients are considered to have mechanical low back pain. Pediatric multidisciplinary pain clinics also help those who have persistent pain that is not responding to usual treatment.

Differential Diagnosis (Table 46.2)

The differential diagnosis for pediatric back pain varies with age. In neonates and infants, infection, neoplasm, and nonaccidental trauma should be considered. As patients age, it becomes easier to obtain a history and physical exam. In children younger than 10 years, there is still heightened concern for both bone and hematologic neoplasm (osteoblastoma, leukemia, lymphoma). Infectious disorders like spondylodiskitis (diskitis and osteomyelitis) tend to be more localized. At this time, rheumatologic disorders may begin to appear. In older children and adolescents, infectious, neoplastic, and rheumatologic disorders should remain in the differential diagnosis list. Congenital and developmental variations in the formation of the spine may cause back pain. Most commonly, the period of rapid growth and increase in physical activity and athletics results in a greater frequency of musculoskeletal injuries (strains, stress fractures, disk pathology).

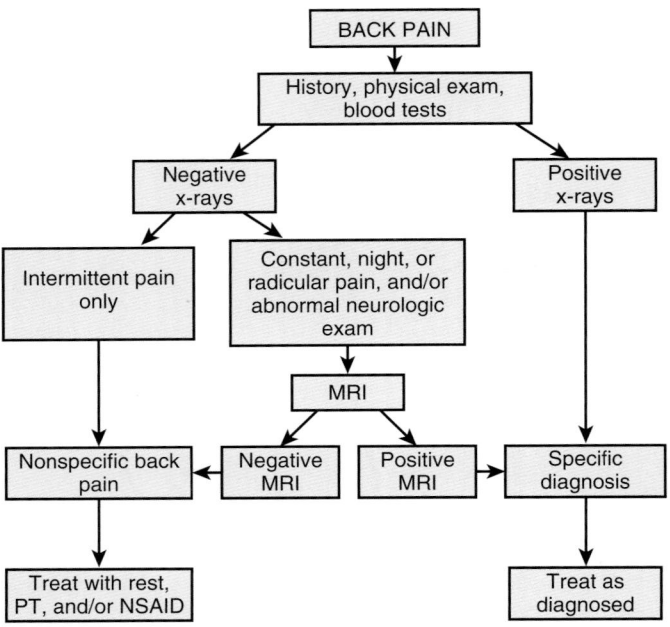

Fig. 46.5 Pediatric back pain algorithm for children 4 years of age and older. NSAID, nonsteroidal antiinflammatory drug; PT, physical therapy. (From Feldman D, Straight J, Badra M, et al. Evaluation of an algorithmic approach to pediatric back pain. *J Pediatr Orthop.* 2006;26: 353–357.)

SPECIFIC DIAGNOSES

Spondylodiskitis

Diskitis and vertebral osteomyelitis represent a single bacterial infectious process involving both the disk space and the adjacent vertebral bodies (Fig. 46.6). Spondylodiskitis is most common in toddlers and in early adolescence. Diskitis may begin as a microabscess within the vertebral body adjacent to the vertebral end plate. The disk becomes infected from perforating vascular channels across the end plate. Vascular channels may also perforate the end plate on the opposite side of the disk, leading to involvement of the opposite vertebral body.

Most commonly, diskitis is a bacterial infection, usually caused by *Staphylococcus aureus*. Other pathogens include *Kingella* and *Brucella* organisms. *Mycobacterium tuberculosis* should be considered in patients who have spent significant time outside the United States, in patients who have recently immigrated, or in high-risk, immunocompromised patients (Fig. 46.7).

Clinical Findings

Three age-dependent patterns of presentation have been noted for spondylodiskitis. Children younger than 3 years (the most common age) often present with irritability and refusal to walk *and* sit, and may have apparent dysfunction (limp, antalgic gait) of the lower extremities. Patients may have loss of lumbar lordosis (the lumbar spine is the most common site) and refusal to allow passive motion of the lumbar spine. Patients between the ages of 3 and 8 years often have pain

TABLE 46.2 Differential Diagnosis of Back Pain

Inflammatory and Infectious Diseases	Mechanical Trauma and Abnormalities
Spondylodiskitis: diskitis* and vertebral osteomyelitis (pyogenic, tuberculosis)	Muscle strain/sprain*
Spinal epidural abscess	Overuse syndromes (common with athletic training and in gymnasts and dancers)*
Transverse myelitis	Hip/pelvic anomalies
Pyelonephritis*	Herniated disk
Perinephric abscess	Juvenile osteoporosis (rare)
Pancreatitis	Vertebral stress fractures
Paravertebral muscle abscess, myositis	Apophyseal ring fracture
Psoas abscess	Lumbosacral sprain*
Endocarditis	Seatbelt injury
Pelvic osteomyelitis or myositis	Trauma (direct injury; e.g., motor vehicle crash)*
Pelvic inflammatory disease	Strain from heavy backpacks
Rheumatologic Diseases	**Neoplastic Diseases**
Pauciarticular juvenile idiopathic arthritis*	Primary vertebral tumors (osteogenic sarcoma, Ewing sarcoma)
Reactive arthritis	Metastatic tumor (neuroblastoma, rhabdomyosarcoma)
Ankylosing spondylitis	Primary spinal tumor (astrocytoma, ependymoma, lipoma, cysts)
Psoriatic arthritis	Malignancy of bone marrow (ALL, lymphoma)
Ulcerative colitis, Crohn disease	Benign tumors (eosinophilic granuloma, osteoid osteoma, osteoblastoma,
Fibromyalgia, fibrositis	aneurysmal bone cyst)
Developmental Diseases	**Other**
Spondylolysis (in adolescence)*	Disk space calcification (idiopathic, S/P diskitis)
Spondylolisthesis (in adolescence)*	Conversion reaction
Scheuermann syndrome (in adolescence)*	Sickle cell anemia*
Lumbar Scheuermann syndrome	Nephrolithiasis
Scoliosis	Hemolysis (acute)
Chiari malformation type 1 with or without syringomyelia	Hematocolpos
Spinal dysraphism	S/P lumbar puncture

*Common.
ALL, acute lymphocytic leukemia; S/P, status post.
Modified from Behrman R, Kliegman R, eds. *Nelson Essentials of Pediatrics.* 2nd ed. Philadelphia: WB Saunders; 1994:711.

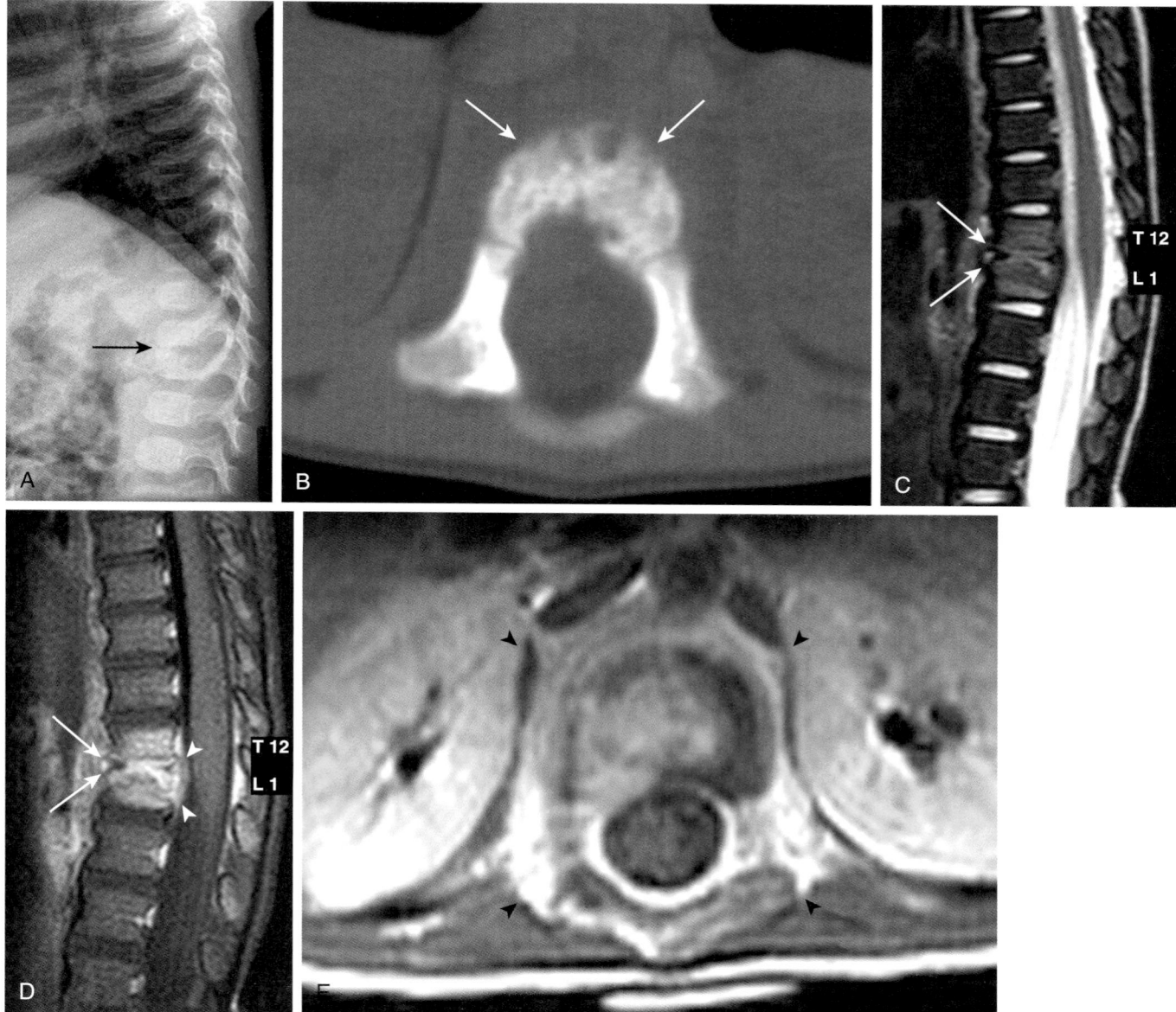

Fig. 46.6 Diskitis/osteomyelitis in a 15-month-old female with abnormal gait and concern for intraspinal mass. *A,* Lateral spine radiographs demonstrate narrowing of the T12–L1 intervertebral disk space *(arrow).* *B,* Axial noncontrast CT of the spine demonstrates irregularity to the vertebral end plates *(arrows).* Sagittal T2-weighted *(C)* and sagittal fat-saturated postcontrast T1-weighted *(D)* images and axial postcontrast T1-weighted MRI *(E)* of the thoracolumbar junction demonstrate loss of height of the T12–L1 intervertebral disk space with T2 prolongation of the adjacent end plates *(arrows in C),* with corresponding abnormal enhancement in the same regions *(arrows in D)* and surrounding masslike soft tissue enhancement *(arrowheads in E).* (From Rothenberg Maddocks AB, Pollock AN. Infections of the spine and spinal cord. In: Coley BD, ed. *Caffery's Pediatric Diagnostic Imaging.* 13th ed. Philadelphia: Elsevier; 2019:421, Fig. 44.7.)

referred to the abdomen, particularly when the disk involves the lower thoracic spine. Preteens and adolescents (next most common age) with diskitis often have back pain; the discomfort often radiates into both legs. Additional features at all ages include fever in ~50%; refusal to bear weight (sitting or standing); refusal to bend forward; and, if intraspinal inflammation is present, decreased lower extremity muscle tone and strength, and alterations of deep tendon reflexes. Both *S. aureus* and tuberculosis may also involve adjacent paravertebral soft tissue abscesses (psoas, iliopsoas muscles).

Radiographs of the spine in nontuberculosis disease may be normal early in the disease. Over about 3 to 4 weeks, radiographs may reveal disk space narrowing with subsequent erosion and sclerosis of the vertebral end plates. Radiographic findings often lag behind clinical presentation with diskitis. MRI is the definitive imaging study (see Figs. 46.6 and 46.7). The MRI reveals the extent of the inflammatory process better and can delineate the degree of bone destruction (if any), the presence of paravertebral or epidural abscess formation, or intraspinal inflammation. Tuberculous spondylodiskitis (**Pott disease**) often has multiple levels of vertebral involvement as well as noncontiguous lesions, while bacterial spondylodiskitis usually involves one disk space and the adjacent vertebral bodies. CBC is normal in ~50%; however, the ESR is elevated in >90%. Blood culture should be obtained as well, but this is also usually negative. If positive, a blood culture can help identify appropriate antibiotic treatment.

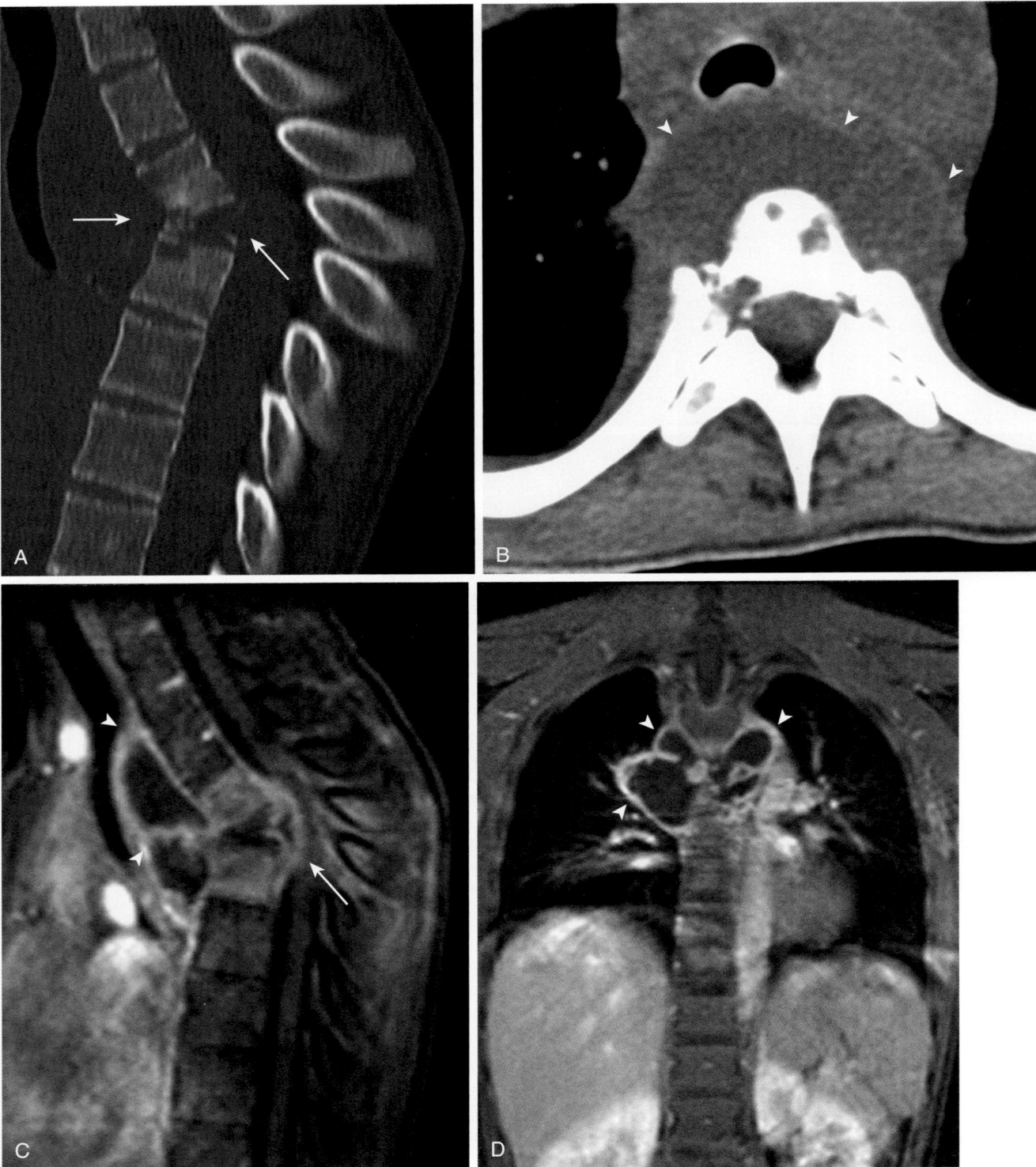

Fig. 46.7 Tuberculous osteomyelitis in a 13-year-old female with progressive loss of strength and coordination in legs. Sagittal reformatted *(A)* and axial soft tissue window *(B)* images from a CT of the spine, and sagittal *(C)* and coronal *(D)* fat-saturated postcontrast T1-weighted MRI of the thoracic spine demonstrate marked kyphosis at site of bony collapse at the level of the midthoracic spine *(arrows in A and C)*, as well as surrounding soft tissue abscess *(arrowheads in B–D)*, predominately anteriorly, at the same level. (From Rothenberg Maddocks AB, Pollock AN. Infections of the spine and spinal cord. In: Coley BD, ed. *Caffery's Pediatric Diagnostic Imaging*. 13th ed. Philadelphia: Elsevier; 2019:422, Fig. 44.8.)

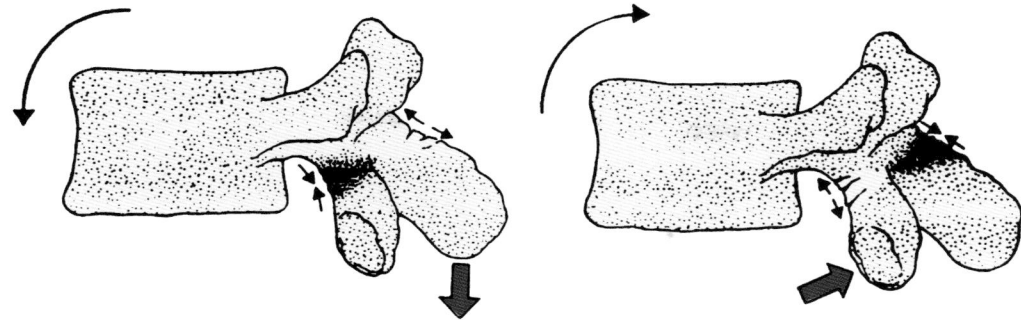

Fig. 46.8 Stress leading to fracture of the pars interarticularis.

Treatment

The diagnosis of bacterial spondylodiskitis should be suspected in patients with fever and unexplained back or leg pain and in previously healthy toddlers who become irritable and refuse to walk. Spinal cord and vertebral tumors are major considerations in the differential diagnosis, which can usually be diagnosed with MRI. After appropriate laboratory studies, including blood cultures, have been performed, treatment should be started. In patients with a positive blood culture, targeted antibiotic therapy should be started. Patients with negative blood cultures should begin broad-spectrum antibiotics, ensuring coverage of *S. aureus*. Consultation with pediatric infectious disease specialists may be helpful. Initial therapy should be intravenous; oral antibiotics can be considered as pain decreases and laboratory studies return to normal. A total of 4–6 weeks of therapy is recommended for patients with bacterial spondylodiskitis. Pain control and immobilization of the spine may be helpful in reducing symptoms.

Patients who remain ill or worsen (or those with epidural or paraspinal abscesses) after the initiation of antibiotic treatment should undergo surgical biopsy and drainage. Biopsy should also be performed in patients in whom tuberculous intervertebral disk space infection is suspected (positive exposure history, positive purified protein derivative, pulmonary lesions, or positive QuantiFERON results).

Radiographic changes continue long after the inflammatory process has resolved. Progressive disk space narrowing, intervertebral disk space calcification, and spontaneous intervertebral arthrodesis are potential late findings.

Spondylolysis and Spondylolisthesis

The most common cause of low back pain in the adolescent (particularly those active in athletic activity) is spondylolysis. This is a fracture at the pars interarticularis, or the junction between the superior and inferior facet in the posterior arch of the vertebral body. The prevalence of spondylolysis has been reported in up to 8% of the population and nearly 50% of adolescent athletes with low back pain. The frequency is increasing in younger children due to the dramatic rise in year-round training for youth sports. In 80% the spondylolysis is bilateral; some develop spondylolisthesis, a deformity where the superior vertebral body translates or slips anteriorly on the vertebral body beneath it (Figs. 46.8, 46.9, and 46.10).

Spondylolysis and spondylolisthesis in children and adolescents usually involve the fifth lumbar and first sacral units. Less commonly, spondylolysis and spondylolisthesis can occur at L4, L3, and L2. Spondylolysis appears to be less common in Black persons and much more common in some North American Eskimo groups; the lowest incidence has been reported in Black females, and the highest in White males. The male-to-female ratio is 2:1. The disorder appears to be multifactorial; both hereditary and mechanical factors have been implicated.

Spondylolysis can be secondary to underlying dysplasia of the posterior spine. It is not present at birth, but with growth and activity, it is

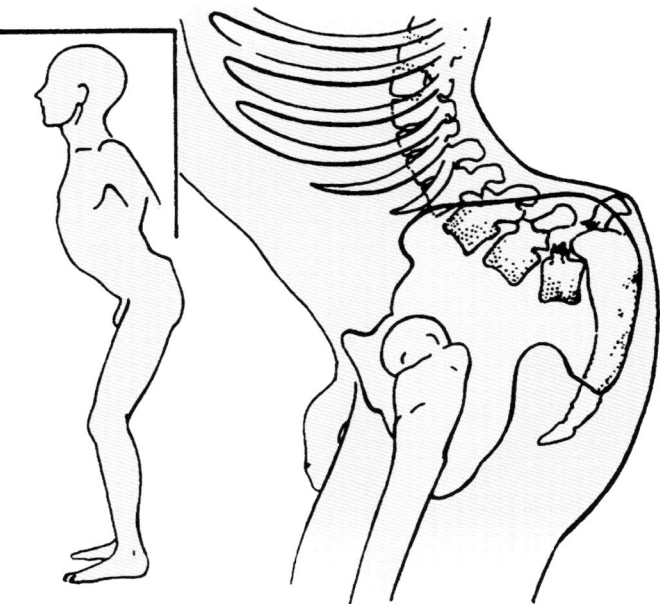

Fig. 46.9 Clinical picture of severe spondylolisthesis.

seen by age 6 years in about 4% of children and 6% of adults. A high rate of spondylolysis has been reported in Scheuermann disease (thoracic kyphosis), which may be related to compensatory excessive lumbar lordosis. In addition, an increased incidence of spondylolisthesis has been noted among both patients with neural tube defects and those with cerebral palsy. It can also result from acute trauma, although fracture/dislocation of the spine from violent trauma are other causes.

Most commonly, spondylolysis is secondary to repeated stress from activity and sport, especially sports that require repetitive trunk flexion and extension like gymnastics, dance, and football linemen, but can occur in any sport. These forces cause stress or fatigue fracture of the posterior elements of L5 and may be responsible for acutely painful spondylolysis in some preadolescent and adolescent athletes.

Clinical Findings

Symptoms in patients with spondylolysis and spondylolisthesis are quite variable; many patients are asymptomatic. Some patients with minimal slips have extreme pain, while others with moderate to severe slips have little or no discomfort. Most patients will complain of aching low back pain that is exacerbated by activity and somewhat reduced by rest. Pain is often reported with prolonged sitting or standing as well. Activity that involves back extension tends to be particularly painful. Buttock and

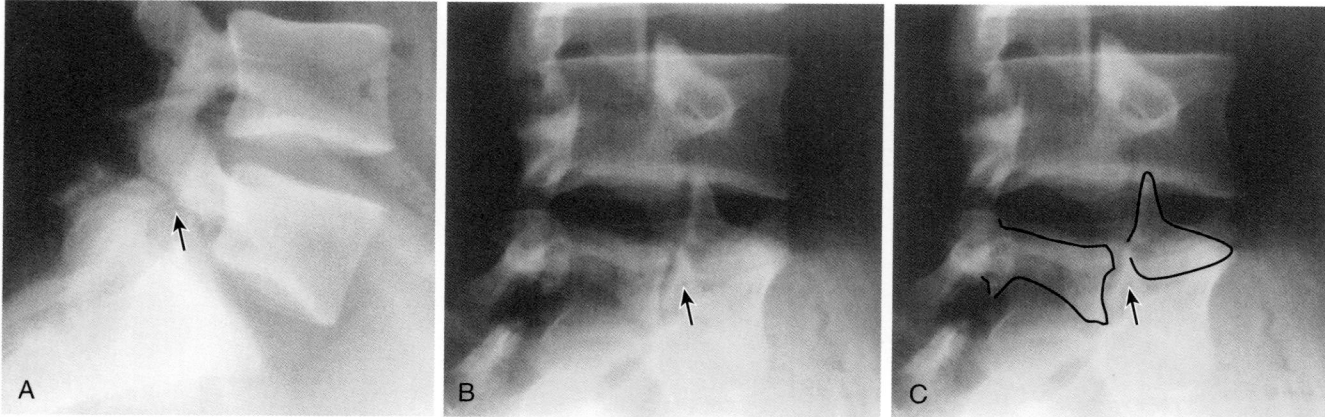

Fig. 46.10 *A,* Radiograph features of spondylolysis showing lytic defect *(arrow)* in the pars interarticularis. *B,* In isthmic defects, this appears as the collar *(arrow)* of the "Scotty dog" sign. *C,* Collar of the Scotty dog sign outlined on film. (From Rathjen KE. Back pain. In: Herring JA, ed. *Tachdjian's Pediatric Orthopaedics.* 5th ed. Philadelphia: Elsevier; 2014:95.)

posterior thigh pain may be present, but radicular symptoms of nerve root compression are usually absent; however, severe spondylolisthesis may cause radicular symptoms and bowel and bladder dysfunction.

On physical examination, patients will have increased pain with back extension, as this movement loads the posterior elements of the spine. A positive "stork test," or back extension while balancing on a single leg, has been associated with spondylolysis, but the test does not have a high level of specificity or sensitivity. Patients often have discomfort to palpation near the midline of the spine near the injury and also the paraspinal musculature. Patients with spondylolisthesis may have a palpable "step-off" or loss of prominence to palpation of the spinous process. Hamstring and hip flexor tightness are frequently observed, as is core weakness on manual muscle testing. Patients often have increased lumbar lordosis. Neurologic evaluation of the lower extremities is usually normal, although severe spondylolisthesis may have nerve involvement.

If spondylolysis or spondylolisthesis is suspected, standing anteroposterior and lateral radiographs of the lumbar spine should be obtained. Unilateral spondylolysis may appear on radiographs as a lucency or defect near the pars interarticularis or hypertrophy of the contralateral side. Previous recommendations included oblique radiographs to assess for the "Scotty dog" sign, but current research has shown no increased sensitivity in diagnosis from oblique views (see Fig. 46.10). Given the added radiation exposure and cost, oblique radiographs have fallen out of favor. The lateral radiograph will allow for spondylolisthesis grading using the Meyerding classification based on the severity of anterior translation (Fig. 46.11). Grade 1 spondylolisthesis is 0–25%, grade 2 is 25–50%, grade 3 is 50–75%, and grade 4 is 75–100%, and spondyloptosis is complete anterior displacement.

While radiographs show spondylolisthesis, they are commonly normal with spondylolysis. If there is a high clinical suspicion for spondylolysis with normal radiographs, providers should proceed to advanced imaging. MRI is the procedure of choice in assessing spondylolysis. Not only does MRI eliminate radiation exposure, but also it has the added benefit of showing stress reactions prior to complete fracture and is better at assessing other pathologies, like disk herniation or infection.

Treatment

In asymptomatic patients with a low-grade spondylolisthesis, serial evaluations until linear growth is finished and encouraging lower body flexibility and core strength are recommended, as the likelihood of progression is low. However, if significant progression occurs (even if a

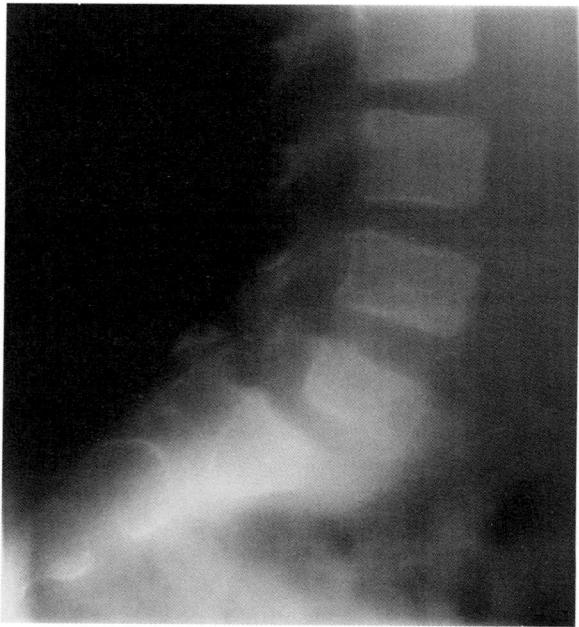

Fig. 46.11 Spondylolisthesis. Slippage of L5 on the underlying body of S1 has occurred as a consequence of the defective formation of the posterior elements of L5. In this case, slippage is moderate, measuring slightly more than 25% of the width of the S1 vertebral segment.

patient is asymptomatic) or if the slip exceeds 50%, the likelihood of continued progression and neurologic impairment is high, so surgical intervention (spinal fusion) is recommended.

Initial treatment of patients with symptomatic spondylolysis and grade 1 or 2 spondylolisthesis without neurologic impairment is nonoperative. Treatment strategies focus on rest or activity reduction, pain control with nonsteroidal antiinflammatory drugs (NSAIDs), and physical therapy to improve flexibility and core strengthening. Bracing with a lumbosacral orthotic to improve posture and prevent extension can be used but is controversial. Athletes should be told to expect at least 6 weeks away from sport before gradually returning to activity if pain-free and progressing in physical therapy. Most patients with symptomatic spondylolysis or mild spondylolisthesis respond to conservative therapy and are able to return to sports; however, a small percentage of patients do not respond to nonoperative therapy and surgical intervention may be necessary.

Intervertebral Disk Herniation

Intervertebral disk herniation is much less common in children than in adults. Estimates show that <10% of adolescents with low back pain have a lumbar disk herniation. Most patients have a significant history of trauma, as opposed to degenerative change common in adults. There may be an association with congenital anomalies of the lumbar spine, such as transitional vertebra or spina bifida occulta. There may be a family history of low back pain or herniated disk, as an autosomal dominant trait has been linked to the *COL9A2* collagen IX gene.

Clinical Findings

The symptoms of a herniated lumbar disk in adolescents differ somewhat from those in adults. The initial complaint in adolescents is significant low back discomfort. While adults more commonly have lower extremity radicular symptoms early on, it is only months later that the symptoms of leg discomfort become more noticeable or prominent in the pediatric population. Pain is typically aggravated by activity, forward flexion, and Valsalva maneuver, and relieved with rest. Paraspinal muscular spasm and loss of lumbar lordosis is common. Hamstring tightness, positive straight leg raise, and slump test are often present. A thorough neurologic evaluation should be performed, but abnormal findings are less likely in the adolescent with herniated disc than in the affected adult. Clues to suggest a lumbosacral radiculopathy include abnormal straight leg or cross straight leg raising responses, weak ankle dorsiflexion, calf wasting, diminished ankle reflex, and decreased sensation.

Plain radiographs are needed as an initial study, but these are usually normal except for loss of lumbar lordosis. MRI is the procedure of choice for diagnosing a disk herniation (Fig. 46.12). In rare cases,

adolescents (often weightlifters) may develop a *vertebral apophyseal ring fracture*, where the bone displaces posteriorly into the spinal canal and acts like a herniated disk. This is an avulsion fracture that is identified with either a CT scan or MRI. Presentation and treatment for apophyseal ring fracture are similar to disk herniation.

Treatment

Most adolescents will benefit from nonoperative treatment. The cornerstones are rest from activity, pain control, and physical therapy focusing on core strength and extension-based exercises. Bracing or a lumbar corset may be helpful in reducing pain for some patients. Patients should expect a slow recovery with a gradual return to activity.

Patients who do not respond to conservative therapy or patients who present with progressive neurologic deficits may benefit from surgical intervention. Surgical correction has been successful at providing symptom relief to the young patient.

Idiopathic Kyphosis

Abnormal increases in expected thoracic kyphosis in children and adolescents produce round back deformities (Fig. 46.13). These may be congenital, neuromuscular, or idiopathic in origin. Mild to moderate

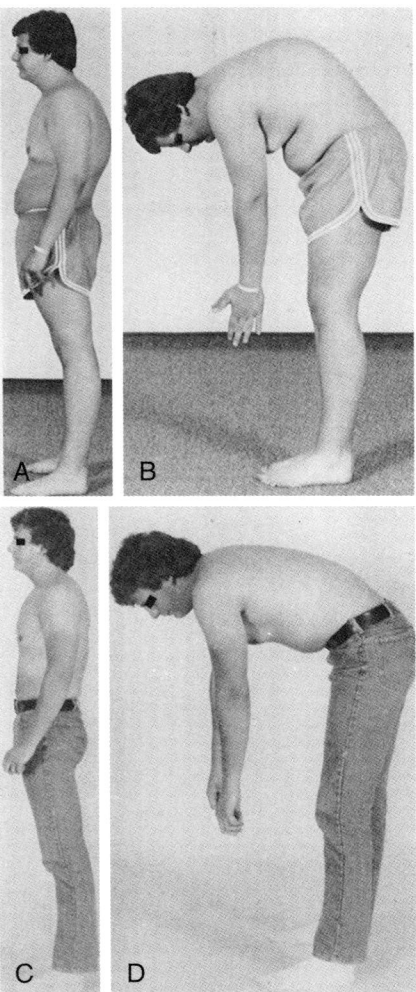

Fig. 46.13 Preoperative *(A, B)* and postoperative *(C, D)* views of an adolescent boy with severe kyphosis secondary to Scheuermann disease. He required both anterior and posterior spinal fusion. He now has a markedly improved appearance and no further progression of the kyphosis. (From Renshaw TS. *Pediatric Orthopedics*. Philadelphia: WB Saunders; 1986:53.)

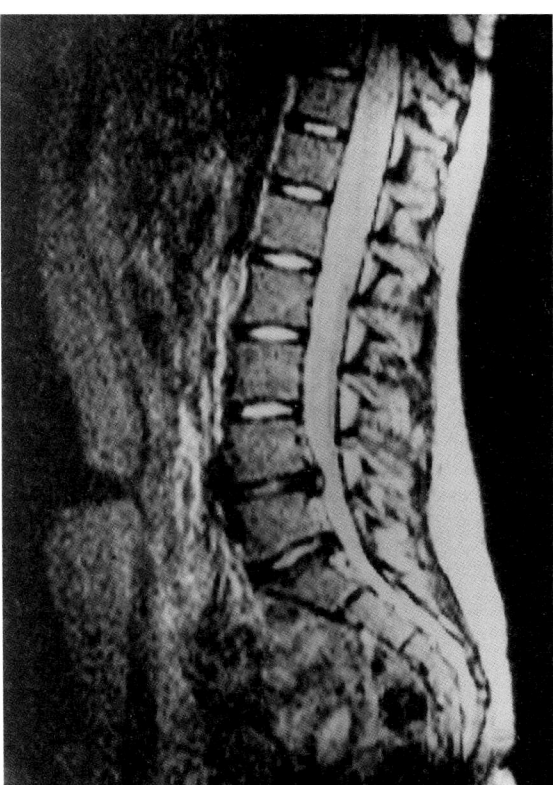

Fig. 46.12 MRI of herniated disk at L4–5. (From Rathjen KE. Back pain. In: Herring JA, ed. *Tachdjian's Pediatric Orthopaedics*. 5th ed. Philadelphia: Elsevier; 2014:94, Fig. 7-3.)

increases in kyphosis cause little deformity and few symptoms. Severe kyphosis is disfiguring, often causes midscapular back pain, and may lead to spinal cord compromise.

Round back posture is often encountered in otherwise healthy adolescents during screening examinations. Although their parents often report poor posture, affected patients are usually asymptomatic. A history should be obtained and physical examination performed. Complaints of severe back pain or leg pain, enuresis, and findings of lower extremity weakness or increased reflex tone in patients with round back are ominous findings and warrant further evaluation and referral.

When accentuated kyphosis is present, radiographs are indicated. Patients with 20- to 45-degree thoracic kyphotic curves on the lateral radiograph and no underlying structural vertebral changes are less concerning. Usually such curves correct easily on passive or active hyperextension. For such children, no treatment except for a thoracic hyperextension exercise program to improve posture and periodic follow-up examination is necessary.

Scheuermann kyphosis is a progressive (usually thoracic) kyphosis, which occurs in approximately 5–8% of the population. This is typically found in adolescents and affects males 5 to 10 times more often than females. The etiology remains unknown. Patients will have a kyphotic curve over 45 degrees with anterior vertebral body wedging in three consecutive vertebrae on lateral radiographs. In addition, disk herniation into the vertebral body may be present (**Schmorl nodules**). Scheuermann kyphosis is treated with antiinflammatory medications and physical therapy exercises focused on back extension. Patients with more severe kyphosis often have kyphotic curves >60 degrees and show little correction with hyperextension. Radiographs show vertebral wedging, end plate irregularity, and kyphosis (Fig. 46.14). Cardiopulmonary complications can result from very significant curves (>100

degrees). **Lumbar Scheuermann** kyphosis is less common and associated with overuse injury producing microfractures.

Treatment depends on the degree of deformity and the age of the patient. Skeletally immature individuals with significant deformity may improve with a program of exercise and use of a Milwaukee or modified Boston brace. Bracing does not reverse a deformity, but it may prevent progression. Skeletally mature patients will not respond to bracing but may improve with a back-strengthening exercise program. Patients with unacceptable deformity who are too old for brace treatment require surgical correction.

Congenital vertebral malformations that produce kyphotic deformities develop during the first trimester of gestation and, like other congenital abnormalities of the spine, are often associated with abnormalities of the genitourinary tract or the spinal cord. Kyphosis that results from congenital vertebral deformities is often obvious early in life and may be rapidly progressive (Fig. 46.15). The spinal cord may become tented over the apex of the deformity, producing symptoms and signs of spasticity in the lower extremity and bladder. Progression of deformity is dangerous; congenital kyphosis is the spinal deformity most often associated with paraplegia. Patients should be promptly referred for orthopedic evaluation.

Scoliosis

Idiopathic scoliosis is a combination of lateral deviation and rotation of vertebral bodies that may produce back pain in ~30% of patients. When painful scoliosis is present, a careful search for the cause of the symptoms must be undertaken. Infection, tumor, a spinal cord syringomyelia or diastematomyelia *(more common with left thoracic curves)*, and occult fractures may produce clinical findings that resemble idiopathic scoliosis but, in contrast to idiopathic scoliosis, cause significant chronic pain as well. Any patient with painful scoliosis should have a careful evaluation for other spinal anomalies causing the pain.

Etiology

Idiopathic scoliosis begins in the immature spine, although progression of pre-existing curvatures may occur in adult life. The cause of

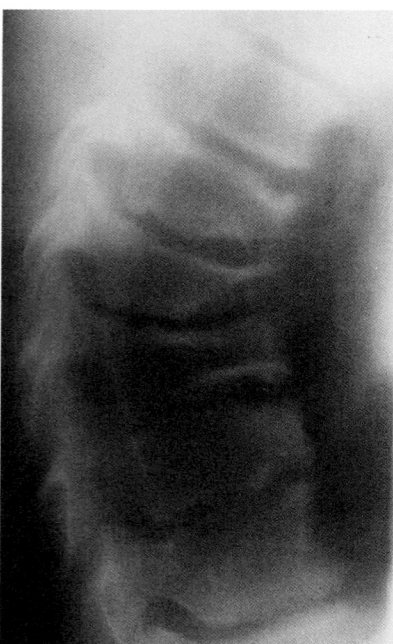

Fig. 46.14 Scheuermann kyphosis. Lateral radiographs of the midthoracic spine in an asymptomatic 16-year-old male with moderately severe kyphosis. There is severe wedging, loss of vertebral height, and end plate irregularity present on these films. His radiographic findings appear far worse than his symptoms and signs. If further collapse were to develop and the kyphosis became more severe, surgical intervention would be necessary.

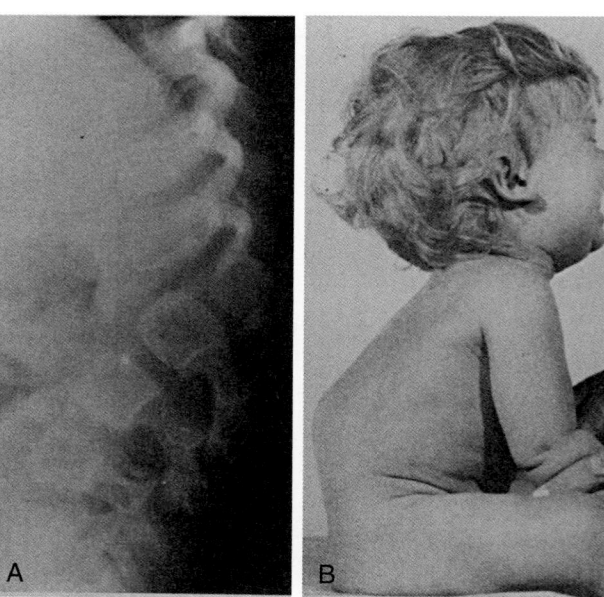

Fig. 46.15 *A,* Congenital kyphosis secondary to failure of vertebral bodies to form at T12 and L1. *B,* The clinical appearance of the child. Thoracolumbar kyphosis is obvious. (From Renshaw TS. *Pediatric Orthopedics.* Philadelphia: WB Saunders; 1986:44.)

idiopathic scoliosis remains unclear. Hormonal factors appear to play a role in curve progression, inasmuch as severe curves occur much more often in girls. Some studies have demonstrated abnormalities of proprioception and vibratory sensation in affected patients, suggesting that abnormalities of posterior column function may contribute to the development of curvature. Other investigators have implicated cerebellar or muscular (myopathy) dysfunction as a possible cause of spinal imbalance.

No clear genetic pattern has been established. Curves occur more frequently in individuals with affected first-degree relatives, but transmission is not Mendelian. Although curvature is more likely to develop in the daughters of affected mothers than in other children, the magnitude of curvature in an affected individual is not related to the magnitude of curvature in relatives. It appears likely that a combination of genetic predisposition and other undefined factors is responsible for development and progression of idiopathic scoliosis.

Classification

Idiopathic curves are grouped into infantile (birth–3 years), juvenile (4–10 years), and adolescent categories on the basis of age at onset of curvature. The infantile form is considered a distinct entity, while the difference between juvenile and adolescent scoliosis is not as sharp.

Infantile idiopathic scoliosis. Infantile idiopathic scoliosis is rare in the United States, accounting for <1% of new cases of idiopathic scoliosis. It is more common in Europe. The majority of patients are males, and most curves are convex toward the left rather than the right, as in the other varieties of idiopathic scoliosis. Some infants suspected of having idiopathic deformity actually have subtle congenital vertebral abnormalities. The diagnosis of idiopathic deformity is appropriate only when radiographic studies show no evidence of congenital vertebral anomalies (e.g., hemivertebra) and there are no signs of spinal dysraphism or of neuropathic or myopathic disorders.

Although many infantile curves resolve spontaneously, others progress relentlessly and are very difficult to effectively treat. Observation is appropriate until 6 months of age in infants with mild idiopathic scoliosis, but prompt referral should be made if curves persist or increase during the period of observation.

Juvenile idiopathic scoliosis. Juvenile idiopathic scoliosis begins before the adolescent growth spurt. Some curves are probably undetected cases of infantile scoliosis. Others, particularly those that occur in older children, may be early manifestations of adolescent idiopathic scoliosis. Some curves remain small and, in fact, may resolve spontaneously. Others remain stable until the onset of the growth spurt and then progress unless treated. Still others progress steadily throughout childhood and adolescence. Some are associated with intraspinal anomalies (**syrinx**). There is no reliable method of predicting the behavior of juvenile curves at the time of diagnosis, but, in general, high-magnitude curves in young patients are more likely to increase with growth than smaller curves in older children.

The majority of patients with juvenile curves >25 degrees at the time of diagnosis require some form of active treatment. Treatment must begin at the time progression is first documented to reduce risk for development of severe deformity.

Adolescent idiopathic scoliosis. Most cases of idiopathic scoliosis in North America develop around the time of the adolescent growth spurt (Figs. 46.16 and 46.17). Often parents and children are unaware of the presence of curvature at the outset. Nerve root impingement, intervertebral disk disease, and spinal cord compression are uncommon in young patients with idiopathic scoliosis. Large curves are seven times more common in females than in males. Pain is so rare that children and adolescents with painful curves must be carefully evaluated to exclude neoplastic and inflammatory processes of the

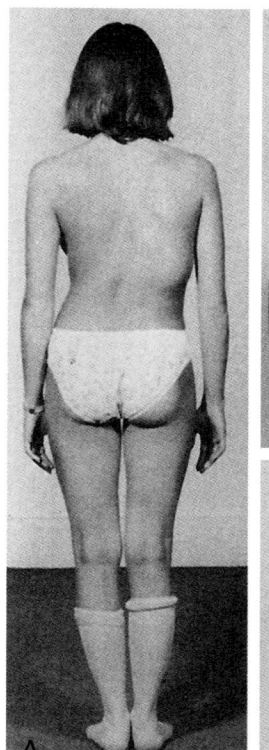
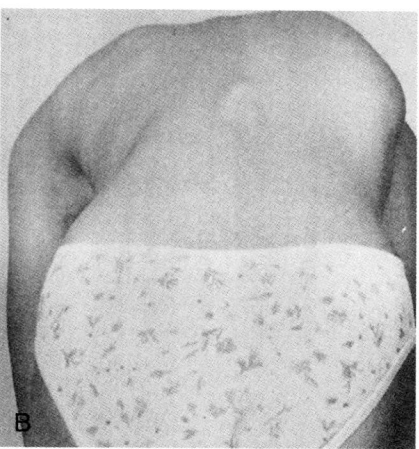
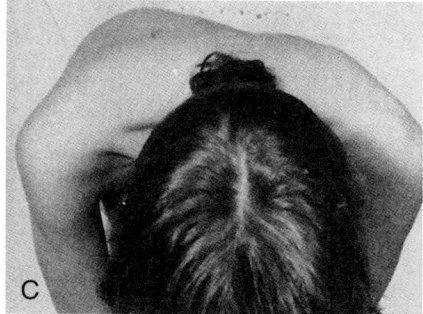

Fig. 46.16 *A,* Adolescent idiopathic scoliosis, viewed from the back. Note the right-sided thoracic prominence. When the patient bends forward *(B),* the rib prominence is even more apparent. This is secondary to rotation of the ribs and spine. The rib prominence is also quite evident when viewed from the front *(C).* (From Renshaw TS. *Pediatric Orthopedics.* Philadelphia: WB Saunders; 1986:47.)

spinal column or neural canal. Idiopathic scoliosis is usually a painless disorder during childhood and adolescence. Severe structural curves may cause no pain until degenerative changes develop in adulthood.

School Screening Programs

School screening programs for spinal deformity concentrate on children in the late juvenile and early adolescent periods. The most common screening method employed is the forward-bend test, based anatomically on the vertebral rotation that accompanies lateral spinal deviation (see Fig. 46.16). Associated clinical findings include shoulder asymmetry, unequal distances between the medial borders of the elbows and the flanks, and apparent leg length inequality or pelvic tilt. Breast asymmetry, caused by forward rotation of the chest wall on the side of the curve concavity and backward displacement of the chest wall on the convex side of the curve, is often present in affected girls.

The threshold for "identification" on screening examination is subjective, and the incidence of spine asymmetry detected by school screening programs varies with the method of screening and the experience of the examiner. A range of 3–20% has been reported. Follow-up radiographic studies of children thought to have abnormal curvatures on school screening examinations indicate an incidence of scoliosis in screened children of <15% (range, 0.4–14%). The incidence of curves >20 degrees at the time of primary screening is probably <0.5%. Simple devices such as the scoliometer determine spine asymmetry by measuring the angle of trunk rotation at the apex of the rib hump. An angle of >7 degrees is an appropriate criterion for referral.

The initial response to a positive school screening examination is a repeat physical evaluation in clinic. If asymmetry is confirmed, a single standing posteroanterior spine film, including vertebral levels T1 to S1, should be obtained. Lateral films, bending films, and oblique views are not necessary. Referral is appropriate for skeletally immature children or adolescents with curves >20 degrees.

Natural History

The natural history of curvature in patients with spine asymmetry is highly variable. Factors that appear to be associated with risk of progression include the magnitude of curvature at the time of detection, the chronological and skeletal age of the patient, the pattern of curvature, and the menarchal status. Immature patients with large-magnitude curves are far more likely to experience progression than are more mature patients with smaller curves. Progression of idiopathic thoracic curves of <30 degrees after skeletal growth has finished is uncommon; however, progression is likely to occur in patients with curves >50 degrees at skeletal maturity.

Uncontrolled curve progression causes significant problems in adult life. Unacceptable deformity, back pain, chronic fatigue, and decreased work capacity are common. Premature degenerative arthritis and nerve root impingement caused by deformity and osteophytic spurring occur in patients with lumbar curves or double thoracic-lumbar curves. Asymptomatic decreased vital capacity is common in patients with thoracic curves; symptomatic cardiopulmonary compromise (cor pulmonale) may develop in patients with curves >80 degrees.

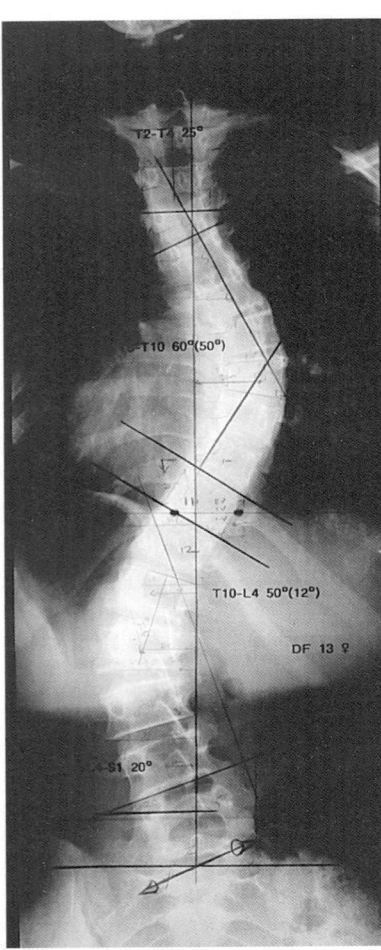

Fig. 46.17 Adolescent idiopathic scoliosis. The patient, a 13-year-old girl, had a severe double-curve pattern with significant accompanying deformity but no pain. Surgical treatment was warranted to halt progression and restore spinal alignment.

Treatment

The goal of treatment in idiopathic scoliosis is to bring a patient to skeletal maturity with a cosmetically acceptable, balanced, and stable curve that is unlikely to progress in adult life. Mature adolescents with curves <30 degrees need no treatment beyond initial evaluation. Further progression of curvature is unlikely to occur in these individuals. Patients with juvenile scoliosis and less mature adolescents with curves between 10 and 20 degrees should be monitored at 6-month intervals with single standing posteroanterior spine radiographs. If progression occurs, they should be referred for orthopedic care.

Active treatment is indicated for growing patients with curves >30 degrees. Brace treatment remains the standard method of nonoperative treatment of idiopathic curvature. Surgical treatment is appropriate for patients with curves too severe for brace treatment. Documented progression in spite of nonoperative treatment is another indication for surgical intervention.

Improved instrumentation and internal fixation devices, intraoperative monitoring of spinal cord function, and autologous transfusion have improved the safety and efficacy of surgical correction. In most cases, patients can be out of bed the day after surgery and are discharged within 5 days of surgery. Return to school is usually possible within 3 weeks; most activities of normal life, including sports, can be resumed within 6 months. In many instances, no postoperative immobilization is required; in other cases, a removable lightweight plastic orthosis can be employed. Prolonged periods of immobilization in a plaster cast are uncommon.

Syringomyelia

Syringomyelia (syrinx) is a fluid-filled cavitation of the spinal cord that may be congenital or acquired. Predisposing conditions include Chiari malformation, trauma, intraspinal tumor, scoliosis, and arachnoiditis. Most patients have headaches and back (constant, gradual) pain that may be aggravated by Valsalva maneuvers (coughing, sneezing). If the cavity enlarges, long tract signs may develop including sensory loss, dysesthesias, weakness, muscle atrophy, and abnormal deep tendon reflexes. MRI is the diagnostic study of choice (Figs. 46.18 and 46.19).

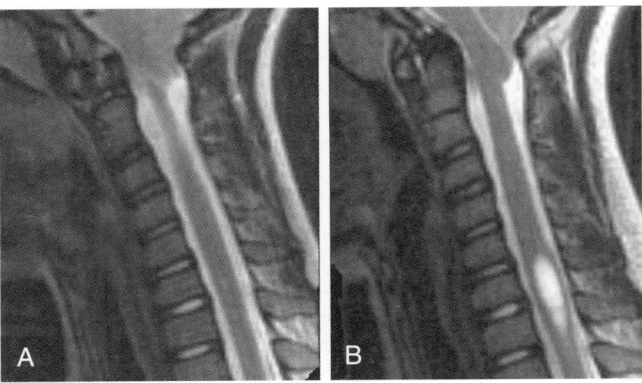

Fig. 46.18 Sagittal T2-weighted images of the cervical spine in an 8-year-old male. *A,* Image was obtained after a brain magnetic resonance examination identified a Chiari 1 malformation. *B,* Image was obtained 10 months later, after the child developed numbness and tingling in the left arm and leg. In most cases of syrinx-complicating Chiari 1 malformation, the spinal cord lesion is apparent at the time of diagnosis, but there is a risk of syringomyelia developing over time in this patient population. (From Jones BV. Cord cystic cavities: syringomyelia and prominent central canal. *Semin Ultrasound CT MRI.* 2017;38:98–104 [Fig. 3, p. 100].)

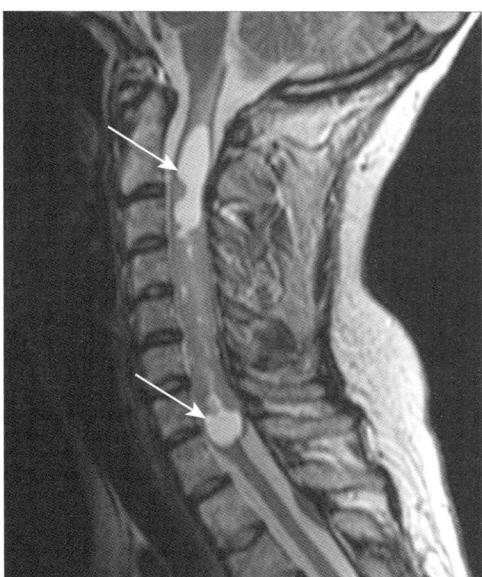

Fig. 46.19 Sagittal T2-weighted image of the cervical spine in a 24-year-old patient with neurofibromatosis type 2 and a cervical cord ependymoma shows syrinx cavities cephalad and caudad to the tumor *(arrows)*. (From Jones BV. Cord cystic cavities: syringomyelia and prominent central canal. *Semin Ultrasound CT MRI.* 2017;38:98–104 [Fig. 4, p. 101].)

Tumors of the Spinal Column

Persistent and progressive back pain, muscle spasm, and abnormal trunk posture and signs of spinal cord compression are ominous findings in children. Neoplastic disease must be considered in patients with no other obvious source of pain (see Table 46.2). Prompt referral is essential when spinal neoplasia is suspected. The success of treatment depends in large part on early discovery and intervention.

Primary Lesions of Bone

The most common primary bone tumors affecting the spinal column in children are osteoid osteomas and osteoblastomas, with eosinophilic granuloma and aneurysmal bone cyst also in the differential. Although benign, these lesions may cause considerable back pain and local bone destruction. **Osteoid osteoma** pain usually increases throughout the day and may awaken the child at night. It is classically relieved with NSAID use. Osteoid osteoma lesions are small and often difficult to see on plain radiographs, but if seen will have slight sclerosis. Therefore, advanced imaging with MRI or CT scan is helpful (Fig. 46.20). Osteoid osteoma does not undergo malignant transformation and can be treated with radiofrequency ablation or surgical excision. **Osteoblastomas** are often larger and do not respond to medication like osteoid osteomas. Radiographs often show cystic lesions with local destruction of bone (Fig. 46.21). Osteoblastoma can undergo malignant transformation and is usually treated with surgical excision.

Malignant bone lesions, such as osteosarcoma and Ewing sarcoma, can occur in the spine but are more common in long bones. These lesions usually occur in the vertebral body and can cause spinal cord compression. Unexplained pain is the hallmark of spinal neoplasia and is usually the presenting complaint. Malignancies often have associated systemic signs, such as fever, night sweats, and unexplained weight loss. These lesions are frequently seen on radiographs due to their destructive nature, but advanced imaging is routinely obtained to assist with treatment and surgical planning.

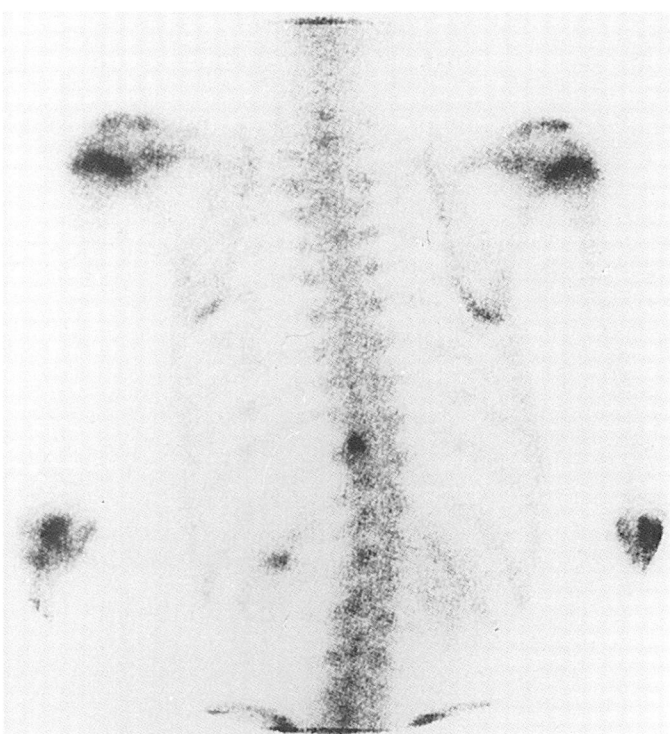

Fig. 46.20 Osteoid osteoma of the spine. Technetium bone scanning shows increased uptake in the T10 vertebral body in a 15-year-old boy. Note the scoliosis that accompanies this painful lesion. The condition did not respond to antiinflammatory medications, and surgical excision was necessary.

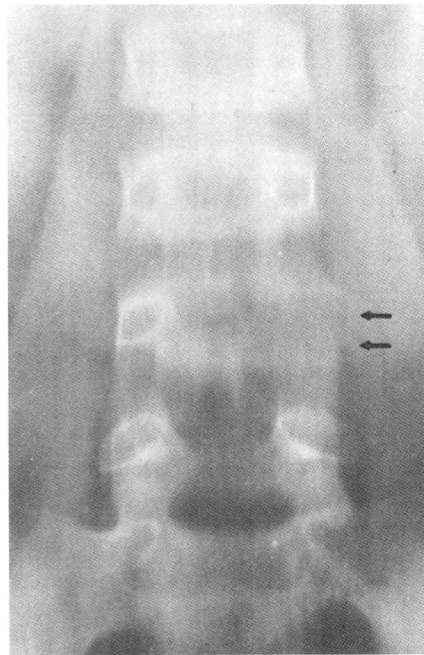

Fig. 46.21 The patient presented with left-sided lumbar back pain. Note the destruction of the vertebral pedicle at L4 *(arrows)*. This proved to be an osteoblastoma. Children with back pain should be suspected of having a tumor of the spine or spinal cord until it is proven otherwise. (From Renshaw TS. *Pediatric Orthopedics.* Philadelphia: WB Saunders; 1986:57.)

TABLE 46.3 Red Flags: Most Common Indications from History and Examination for Pathologic Findings Needing Special Attention and Sometimes Immediate Action

- Children younger than 18 yr old with considerable pain
- History of violent trauma
- Nonmechanical nature of pain (i.e., constant pain not affected by movement; pain at night)
- History of cancer
- Systemic steroid use
- Drug use
- HIV infection or other immunocompromised patients
- Unintentional weight loss
- Systemically ill, particularly signs of infections such as fever or night sweats
- Persisting severe restriction of motion or intense pain with minimal motion
- Structural deformity including scoliosis, Chiari malformation, tethered cord
- Difficulty with micturition
- Loss of anal sphincter tone or fecal incontinence, saddle anesthesia
- Progressive motor weakness or gait disturbance, paresthesias, pes cavus, foot drop
- Marked morning stiffness
- Peripheral joint involvement
- Iritis, skin rashes, colitis, urethral discharge, or other symptoms of rheumatologic disease
- Inflammatory disorder such as ankylosing spondylitis suspected
- Family history of rheumatologic disease or structural abnormality

Modified from Nachemson A, Vingard E. Assessment of patients with neck and back pain: a best-evidence synthesis. In: Nachemson AL, Johnsson B, eds. *Neck and Back Pain: The Scientific Evidence of Causes, Diagnosis, and Treatment.* Philadelphia: Lippincott Williams & Wilkins; 2001.

Tumors of Neural Elements

Back pain, lower extremity weakness, and sphincter disturbances are common manifestations of neoplasms of the spinal cord. Although such lesions are rare, they must be suspected in children with unexplained back or leg pain, weakness, sensory or reflex abnormalities, bowel or bladder incontinence, or unexplained gait abnormalities. Neuroblastoma is the most common lesion, but sarcomas (including Ewing sarcoma, rhabdomyosarcoma, and hemangiosarcoma) and astrocytomas or ependymomas also occur in the neural contents of the spinal canal.

In such patients, standard radiography often shows only loss of lordosis or scoliosis secondary to muscle spasm. MRI demonstrates the abnormality, but definitive diagnosis usually requires biopsy.

Leukemia and Lymphoma

Skeletal involvement is common in patients with leukemia and lymphoma. Back pain or limb pain may be the presenting symptom in some children. Proliferation of abnormal hematopoietic tissue in the marrow of long bones or vertebral bodies causes pain and weakens their structure.

Clinical symptoms and signs in children with leukemic skeletal involvement may be confusing. The history should include questions on fever, localized pain and swelling, and history of unusual bruising and bleeding. Elevations of the white blood cell count and ESR may be mistaken as signs of septic arthritis, osteomyelitis, or intervertebral disk space infection. The presence of abnormal white blood cells on the peripheral blood cell count or of thrombocytopenia increases the likelihood of bone marrow tumor rather than infection.

Leukemia and lymphoma can show osteopenia, periosteal elevation, and metaphyseal lucencies on radiographs of long bones, but these findings are difficult to detect with spine radiographs. Vertebral compression and wedging are sometimes present and may mimic acute fracture or, on occasion, osteomyelitis. The absence of a history of trauma should alert the examiner to search for other causes of the radiographic abnormality. Preservation of intervertebral disk space height with collapse of adjacent vertebral segments is an indication that the vertebral bodies rather than the intervertebral disk are the sites of the abnormality. MRI can identify areas of involvement and extent of intraspinal infiltration.

The diagnosis of leukemia can be established by bone marrow aspiration. Biopsy of involved vertebral segments is rarely necessary. Support of the spine in a custom-fabricated orthosis is useful for relieving pain and preventing further vertebral collapse during the initial phases of treatment. Prolonged brace treatment may be necessary to prevent vertebral compression fractures that may accompany the osteopenia resulting from steroid therapy. Surgical decompression and fusion may be required in rare cases of acute vertebral compression and spinal cord compromise.

Mechanical Back Pain

Many pediatric patients have no identifiable cause for their back pain. These patients are thought to have mechanical or myofascial back pain. It is felt that tight hamstrings, poor posture, and weak core musculature are major contributing factors. It is critical to ensure that all other causes of back pain have been ruled out before making a diagnosis of mechanical back pain. Treatment for these patients is avoiding activities that increase pain, pain control, and physical therapy to improve the aforementioned concerns. If the pain is persistent, then involvement of a multidisciplinary pain program with behavioral health can be helpful.

■ SUMMARY AND RED FLAGS

Back pain in children may be referred pain from intraabdominal or retroperitoneal disease (see Table 46.2) or may represent direct involvement of the spinal cord, vertebral bodies, or paraspinal musculature. The prevalence of back pain in the pediatric population is greater than previously estimated; the prevalence increases with both sedentary lifestyle and increased physical activity/athletic participation. Acute back pain associated with physical activity should respond to reduced activity levels, NSAIDs, and exercises fairly quickly.

Chronic persistent back pain, pain with associated neurologic deficits (lower extremity or bowel and bladder), cutaneous lesions over the lumbar spine, systemic signs (fever, night waking, weight loss), and tenderness with neurologic dysfunction after trauma are red flags (Table 46.3).

Spinal cord involvement above T10 produces symmetric weakness, increased deep tendon reflexes, up-going toes, and an appropriate sensory loss; conus medullaris involvement (T10 to L2) produces symmetric weakness, increased knee and decreased ankle deep tendon reflexes, a saddle-type anesthesia, and up- or down-going toes on Babinski testing; and cauda equina involvement (below L2) produces asymmetric weakness, loss of deep tendon reflexes, and down-going toes. Signs of cord involvement are particularly ominous and are medical emergencies.

BIBLIOGRAPHY

A bibliography is available at ExpertConsult.com.

47

Hypermobility

Donald Basel

It is estimated that up to 25% of the population reports the presence of joint hypermobility, but a quarter of the population does not have an associated connective tissue disorder, nor is the increased mobility deemed a health concern; nonetheless, hypermobility may be associated with a connective tissue disorder. In addition, there is a vast spectrum of comorbidities attributed to the presence of hypermobility (Fig. 47.1 and Table 47.1).

EVALUATING HYPERMOBILITY

There have been several methodologies used to accurately define the presence of joint hypermobility; the most universally accepted method is the Beighton score (Fig. 47.2 and Tables 47.2 and 47.3). Possible reasons for the estimated high incidence of hypermobility in the general population is the incorrect application of the criteria listed in the Beighton score or not applying the relevant age-appropriate adjustment to the score (see Table 47.3). It is important to strictly adhere to the guide in Fig. 47.2 and to use a goniometer to ensure accurate measurement of joint angles. Patients tend to overestimate their own hypermobility; one should avoid unnecessary diagnostic evaluations that might not add value to the purpose of assessing the underlying etiology of the presenting symptoms. The Beighton score has typically been reserved for children older than 6 years of age because it may be unreliable in younger children who have a propensity for natural joint hypermobility. One revision of the Beighton score that includes ankle dorsiflexion has been reported as a reliable indicator for children up to the age of 5 years.

CONNECTIVE TISSUE AND ITS ROLE IN THESE DISORDERS

The structural integrity of connective tissues ensures normal articular surfaces, normal bone structure and strength, normal tendon insertion, and both macroscopic and microscopic support for muscles. The range of disorders involving primary connective tissue integrity extends from bone dysplasia, muscle dystrophy, and myopathy to the more well-recognized hereditary disorders of connective tissue such as Ehlers-Danlos syndrome (Table 47.4). Hypermobility is also a common feature seen in chromosomal aneuploidies and neurodevelopmental syndromes such as Down syndrome. A review of a commonly used database for matching phenotypes with syndromic traits identified >500 entries spanning these broad groups within the differential diagnostic consideration for hypermobility (Table 47.5).

The *functional impact* of disregulating connective tissues is neither well characterized nor well understood. There is recognition that *functional disorders* co-segregate with disorders that impact connective tissues. Functional gastrointestinal disorders (constipation, gastroparesis, bloating, and pain) as well as dysautonomia in the cardiovascular system (orthostatic intolerance, tachy-/bradycardias) are frequently documented complaints and their presence often triggers the evaluation for hypermobility or a more diffuse underlying connective tissue disorder. The range of common symptoms frequently associated with hypermobility is detailed in Table 47.1 and Figs. 47.3, 47.4, 47.5, and 47.6.

Hypermobility Spectrum Disorders

The classification of hypermobility as a disease has undergone numerous changes, with the emphasis being discerning "benign familial hypermobility" from more serious connective tissue disorders. The most recent of these classifications is derived from the International Consortium on the Ehlers-Danlos Syndromes meeting in 2017 (Table 47.6).

This classification for hypermobile Ehlers-Danlos syndrome (hEDS) has been criticized for being too restrictive because several individuals who previously met clinical diagnosis based on the Villefranche classification no longer meet these criteria despite a family history supporting the diagnosis. There are good reasons for this more restrictive diagnosis given the clinical pleiotropy of associated symptoms (see Table 47.1) and lack of a defining molecular diagnosis. It is widely believed that hEDS is not a single disorder but represents the involvement of several gene pathways. This does not help the clinician because there are more individuals who are diagnosed with hypermobility spectrum disorder (HSD) who share complex medical histories. Utilization of the 5-point hypermobility questionnaire can be helpful in identifying affected patients with a history of hypermobility (Table 47.7).

The age and gender at diagnosis vary and tend to favor females through puberty and young adulthood. There is often a preceding significant life event such as a motor vehicle crash or injury, hospitalization for an infection, or some other significant medical issue. It is not clear how this relates to the clinical manifestation, either as a trigger for closer medical inspection or a true epigenetic phenomenon that initiates a cascade with an evolving phenotype.

DIAGNOSTIC CHARACTERIZATION OF HYPERMOBILITY

The evaluation of hypermobility extends beyond the joints. A detailed head-to-toe evaluation is necessary to assess for possible syndromic disorders (see Chapter 29), primary neuromuscular disorders, and other chameleons or mimics that overlap with the primary hypermobility

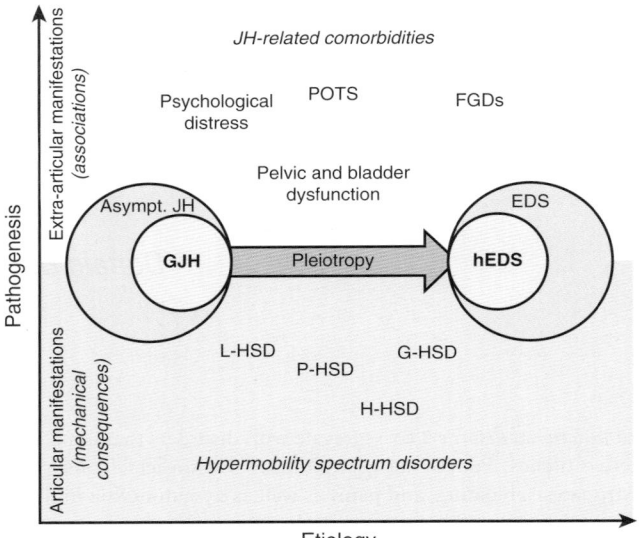

Fig. 47.1 Schematization of the novel terminology introduced by the new nosology of Ehlers-Danlos syndrome and joint hypermobility. The two-dimensional variability is represented by the vertical (pathogenesis) and horizontal (etiology) lines. In the middle are the relationships between the domains of asymptomatic joint hypermobilities and Ehlers-Danlos syndrome. Generalized joint hypermobility and hypermobile Ehlers-Danlos syndrome are highlighted as the closest phenotypes within the corresponding domains. Pleiotropy is the concept bridging the two domains. Below them is the "realm" of the hypermobility spectrum disorders. Hypermobility spectrum disorders group together all those phenotypes presenting joint hypermobility plus one or more of its secondary manifestations but not satisfying the criteria for any Ehlers-Danlos syndrome variant, also comprising the hypermobile type. Above the two domains is the wide spectrum of joint hypermobility–related comorbidities that may occur in all the phenotypes lying beneath. Joint hypermobility–related comorbidities comprise an expanding group of common disorders (i.e., psychological distress, functional gastrointestinal disorders, cardiovascular dysautonomia, and pelvic prolapses—not otherwise defined) that show a statistical association with joint hypermobility, but their etiopathogenesis is complicated by a variety of acquired factors.
EDS, Ehlers-Danlos syndrome (various types); FGDs, functional gastrointestinal disorders; G-HSD, generalized hypermobility spectrum disorder; GJH, generalized joint hypermobility; hEDS, hypermobile Ehlers-Danlos syndrome; JH, joint hypermobility (various types); H-HSD, historical hypermobility spectrum disorder; L-HSD, localized hypermobility spectrum disorder; P-HSD, peripheral hypermobility spectrum disorder; POTS, postural orthostatic tachycardia syndrome. (From Castori M, Tinkle B, Levy H, et al. A framework for the classification of joint hypermobility and related conditions. *Am J Med Genet C [Semin Med Genet]*. 2017;175C:148–157 [Fig. 2, p. 150].)

TABLE 47.1	Clues Suggestive of a Hereditary Connective Tissue Disorder
System	**Symptom/Sign**
Integument	Striae (see Fig. 47.4)
	Easy and frequent bruising
	Skin hyperextensibility (see Fig. 47.5)
	Poor wound healing, easy scarring (see Fig. 47.6)
Cardiovascular	Dizzy spells
	Postural orthostatic tachycardia or orthostatic intolerance
	Palpitations
Musculoskeletal	Joint instability/frequent ankle sprains/subluxations (knee, shoulder)/congenital hip dislocation
	Temporomandibular joint pain
	Scoliosis
	Chronic fatigue; exercise intolerance
	Pes planus
	Genu recurvatum
	Chronic musculoskeletal pain syndromes (focal or generalized)
Neurologic	Headache (orthostatic; intracranial hypotension)
	Anxiety
	Sleep disturbance
	Fibromyalgia
	Restless leg syndrome
	Chiari type I
	Delayed locomotor development
	Poor handwriting
	Cerebrospinal fluid leaks
Gastrointestinal	Irritable bowel syndrome (bloating, pain)
	Constipation/gastroparesis
	Abdominal migraine
	Nausea/cyclic vomiting
	Rectal prolapse
	Hernias
	Absent lingual frenulum
Urogenital	Uterine prolapse
	Cervical incompetence
	Frequency; stress incontinence
	Vulvodynia

spectrum disorders. The algorithm illustrated in Fig. 47.7 provides a framework for approaching the diagnostic evaluation for a patient with generalized joint hypermobility.

The primary differential diagnoses for hypermobility are other forms of hereditary connective tissue disorders. These are detailed in Tables 47.5 and 47.8 (see also Table 29.10 for Marfan syndrome) in addition to the individual syndrome-defining characteristics.

There is a broad range of disorders to consider in the differential when assessing hypermobility (Table 47.9). In the context of syndromic hypermobility (i.e., in association with learning difficulties, dysmorphisms, or major malformations), it is important to refer to a genetics specialty service so that additional evaluation and testing can be considered. Similarly, if muscle weakness or suspicion for a bone dysplasia is suspected, those patients should be further evaluated by a specialist with expertise in the field.

CLOSING CONSIDERATIONS

The presentation of a young adolescent with chronic fatigue, dysautonomia, or diffuse or regional pain syndromes in the presence of hypermobility requires careful consideration. These nonspecific symptom complexes can overlap with hEDS, syndromic disorders such as

1. Passive dorsiflexion of the fifth metacarpophalangeal joint. Score is positive if ≥ 90°

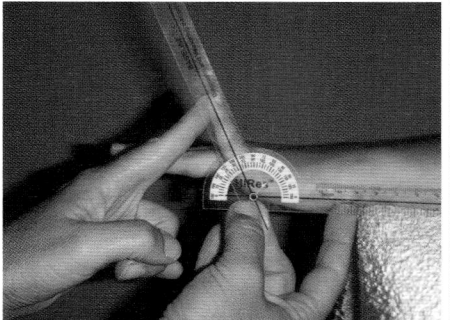

4. Passive apposition of the thumb to the flexor side of the forearm, while shoulder is 90° flexed, elbow extended and hand pronated. Score is positive if the whole thumb touches the flexor side of the forearm.

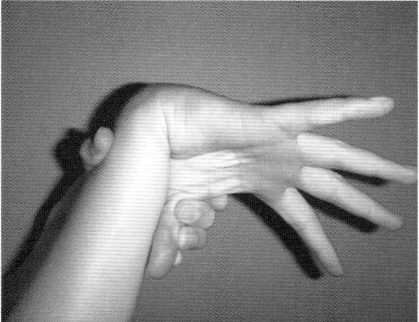 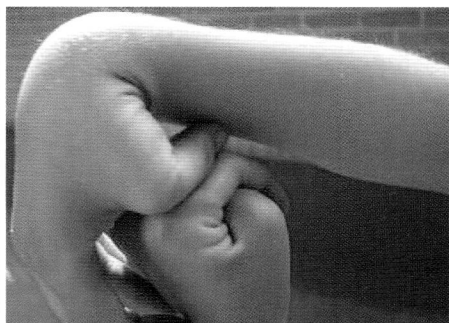

Score: Positive   Score: Negative

2. Passive hyperextension of the elbow. Score is positive if ≥ 10°

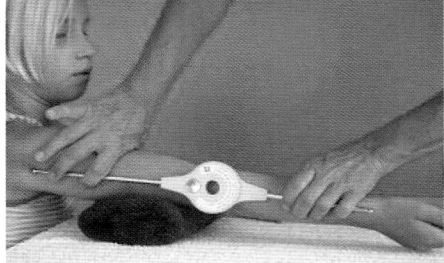

5. Forward flexion of the trunk, with the knees straight. Score is positive if the hand palms rest easily on the floor.

3. Passive hyperextension of the knee. Score is positive if ≥ 10°

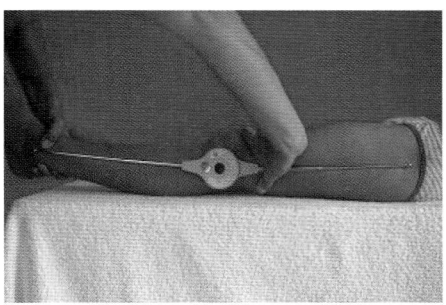

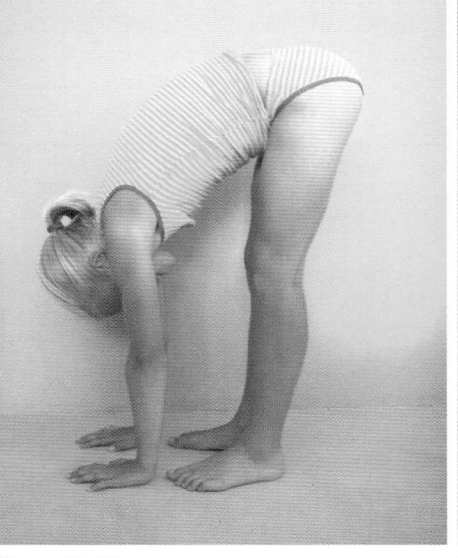 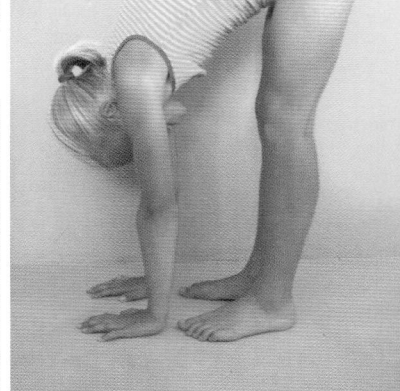

*Males positive if > 180° for measure 2 and 3.   Score: Positive   Score: Negative

Fig. 47.2 Beighton score. The range of motion of several key small and large joints is measured to provide an overview of joint hypermobility. Instability is not assessed. Scoring: 2 points for each bilateral measure in nos. *1* to *4* and 1 point for no. *5,* equaling a total possible score of 9. Hypermobility is considered significant with a score of ≥6 between the ages of 6 and 35. (Modified from Smits-Engelsman B, Klerks M, Kirby A. Beighton score: a valid measure for generalized hypermobility in children. *J Peds.* 2011;158[1]:119–123.e4.)

TABLE 47.2 9-Point Beighton Score of Hypermobility

Description	Bilateral Testing	Scoring (Max. Points)
Passive dorsiflexion of the fifth metacarpophalangeal joint to ≥90 degrees	Yes	2
Passive hyperextension of the elbow >190 degrees in females and >180 degrees in males	Yes	2
Passive hyperextension of the knee >190 degrees in females and >180 degrees in males	Yes	2
Passive apposition of the thumb to the flexor side of the forearm while the shoulder is flexed 90 degrees, elbow is extended, and hand is pronated	Yes	2
Forward flexion of the trunk, with the knees straight, so that the hand palms rest easily on the floor	No	1
Total		**9**

TABLE 47.3 Age-Associated Beighton Scores for Significant Joint Hypermobility

Age range	< Puberty	Puberty–50 yr	>50 yr	Any age with joint injury
Positive Beighton Score	≥6	≥5	≥4	Age score − 1

TABLE 47.4 Classification of Ehlers-Danlos Syndrome

Type	Gene	Skin Findings	Joint Changes	Inheritance	Other Comments
Classic	COL5A1, COL5A2 (usually haploinsufficiency)	Hyperextensibility, bruising, velvety skin, widened atrophic scars, molluscoid pseudotumors, spheroids	Hypermobility and its complications, joint dislocations	AD	Mitral valve prolapse, hernias
	COL1A1-specific pathogenic variant c934C>T			AD	Blue sclerae, short stature, osteopenia/fractures; may have late arterial rupture
Classic Variants					
Cardiac valvular	Biallelic loss of function for COL1A2	Classic EDS features		AR	Severe cardiac valve issues as adult
Periodontal	C1R C1S	Can have classic EDS features	Can have hypermobility	AD	Periodontitis, marfanoid habitus, prominent eyes, short philtrum
Classic-like	TNXB	Hyperextensibility, marked hypermobility, severe bruising, velvety skin, no scarring tendency	Hypermobility	AR	Parents (especially mothers) with one TNXB gene variant; can have joint hypermobility
Hypermobility	Unknown	Mild hyperextensibility, scarring textural change	Hyperextensibility, chronic joint pain, recurrent dislocations	AD	Sometimes confused with joint hypermobility syndrome
Vascular	COL3A1 Rare variants in COL1A1	Thin, translucent skin, bruising, early varicosities, acrogeria	Small joint hypermobility	AD	Abnormal type III collagen secretion; rupture of bowel, uterus, arteries; typical facies; pneumothorax
Kyphoscoliosis	PLOD (deficient lysyl hydroxylase) FKBP14	Soft, hyperextensible skin; bruising; atrophic scars	Hypermobility	AR	Severe congenital muscle hypotonia that improves a little in childhood, congenital kyphoscolioses, scleral fragility and rupture, marfanoid habitus, osteopenia, sensorineural hearing loss
Variants with Kyphoscoliosis					
Spondylocheirodysplastic form	SLC39A13, which encodes the ZIP 13 zinc transporter β4GALT7 or β3GalT6, encoding galactosyltransferase I or II, key enzymes in GAG synthesis	Similar to kyphoscoliotic form		AR	Spondyloepimetaphyseal dysplasia; can have bone fragility and severe progressive kyphoscoliosis without congenital hypotonia, moderate short stature, loose facial skin, wrinkled palms with thenar and hypothenar atrophy, blue sclerae, curly hair, alopecia
Brittle cornea syndrome	ZNF469 or PRDM5	Skin hyperextensibility	Joint hypermobility	AR	Kyphoscoliosis; characteristic thin, brittle cornea; ocular fragility; blue sclera; keratoconus
Musculocontractural	CHST14 (encoding dermatan 4-O-sulfotransferase) DSE (encoding dermatan sulfate epimerase)	Fragile, hyperextensible skin with atrophic scars and delayed wound healing	Hypermobility	AR	Progressive kyphoscoliosis, adducted thumbs in infancy, clubfoot, arachnodactyly, contractures, characteristic facial features, hemorrhagic diathesis

TABLE 47.4 Classification of Ehlers-Danlos Syndrome—cont'd

Type	Gene	Skin Findings	Joint Changes	Inheritance	Other Comments
Variants with Kyphoscoliosis—cont'd					
Myopathic	COL12A1	Soft, hyperextensible	Hypermobile small joints, large joint contractures (hip, knees, elbows)	AD or AR	Characterized by muscle hypotonia and weakness
Arthrochalasis	Exon 6 deletion of COL1A1 or COL1A2	Hyperextensible, soft skin with or without abnormal scarring	Marked hypermobility with recurrent subluxations	AD	Congenital hip dislocation, arthrochalasis, multiplex congenita, short stature
Dermatosparaxis	Type I collagen N-peptidase ADAMTS2	Severe fragility; sagging, redundant skin		AR	Also occurs in cattle

AD, autosomal dominant; AR, autosomal recessive; EDS, Ehlers-Danlos syndrome; GAG, glycosaminoglycan.
From Malfait F, Francomano C, Byers P, et al. The 2017 international classification of the Ehlers-Danlos syndromes. *Am J Med Genet C [Semin Med Genet.]* 2017;175(1)8–26; and Kliegman RM, St. Geme JW III, Blum NJ, et al., eds. *Nelson Textbook of Pediatrics.* 21st ed. Philadelphia: Elsevier; 2020:3526–3527, Table 679-1.

TABLE 47.5 Selected Conditions Associated with Hypermobility

Marfan Syndrome
- Tall and thin
- Arm span greater than height
- Lower ratio of upper body segment to lower body segment (long legs); normal ratio is 0.85 in Whites and 0.92 in Blacks
- Arachnodactyly
- Pectus excavatum or carinatum
- Kyphoscoliosis
- Dislocation of the lens of the eye
- Aortic root dilatation
- Heart murmurs, midsystolic click
- Hernias
- Autosomal dominant disorder due to pathogenic variants of fibrillin gene on chromosome 15

Homocystinuria
- Marfanoid habitus
- Major risk of thrombotic events
- Autosomal recessive disorder usually associated with cystathionine β-synthase deficiency

Stickler Syndrome
- Typical facial appearance: malar hypoplasia, depressed nasal bridge, epicanthal folds, micrognathia
- Cleft palate (Pierre Robin sequence)
- Severe myopia (may lead to retinal detachment)
- Sensorineural hearing loss
- Mitral valve prolapse
- Genetically heterogenous, autosomal dominant inheritance associated with pathogenic variants in collagen type II and type XI and rare recessive subtype associated with pathogenic variants in collagen type IX

Ehlers-Danlos Syndromes
- Skin abnormalities: thin, hyperelastic, cigarette paper scars, easy bruising
- Dislocation of joints
- Rarely, artery aneurysms; hollow organ rupture
- Heterogeneous conditions; at least nine types with different inheritance patterns

Osteogenesis Imperfecta
- Blue sclerae
- Fragile bones with multiple fractures and deformities
- Short stature
- Spinal deformity
- Different types; usually autosomal dominant inheritance
- Genetically heterogenous with end effect impacting collagen 1 function or structure

Williams Syndrome
- Short stature
- Characteristic elfin facial appearance
- Hoarse voice
- Friendly and loquacious
- Developmental delay
- Supravalvular stenosis
- Occasionally hypercalcemia
- Initially hypermobile but later become hypomobile without pain
- Sporadic and inherited cases due to deletion of elastin allele on chromosome 7

Down Syndrome (Trisomy 21)
- Hypotonia
- Developmental delay
- Characteristic facial appearance; epicanthal folds
- Short stature
- Endocardial cushion defects
- Broad hands with simian creases
- Brushfield (depigmented) spots of the iris
- Usually occurs in a sporadic fashion

For further details about these conditions, the reader is referred to Jones KL. *Smith's Recognizable Patterns of Human Malformation.* 5th ed. Philadelphia: Saunders; 1997; and Beighton P. *McKusick's Heritable Disorders of Connective Tissue.* 5th ed. St. Louis: Mosby; 1993.
From LeBlanc C, Houghton K. Noninflammatory musculoskeletal pain. In: *Textbook of Pediatric Rheumatology.* 7th ed. Elsevier; 2016:665, Box 51-3.

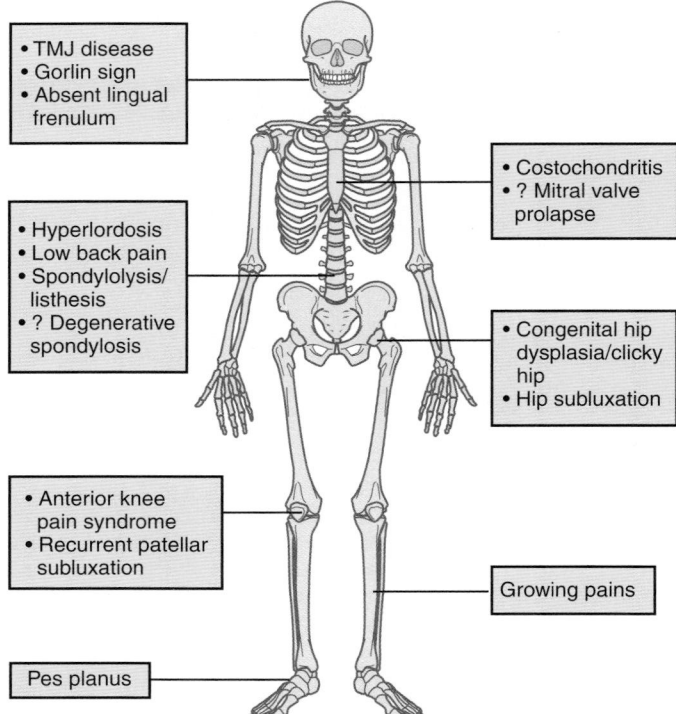

Fig. 47.3 Clinical features and symptom complexes seen in children and adolescents with joint hypermobility syndrome. TMJ, temporomandibular joint. (From Murray KJ. Hypermobility disorders in children and adolescents. *Best Prac Res Clin Rheumatol.* 2006;20[2]:329–351 [Fig. 1, p. 333].)

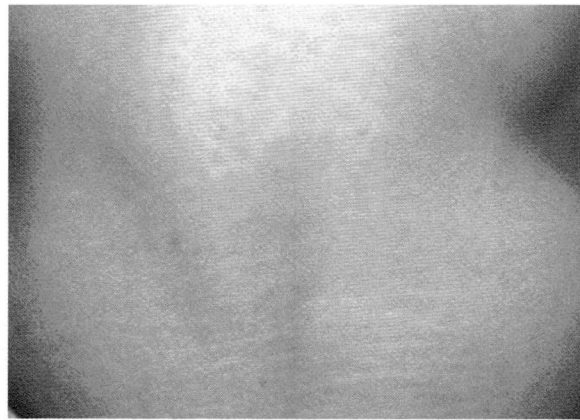

Fig. 47.4 Abnormal striae. (From Hakim AJ, Sahota A. Joint hypermobility and skin elasticity: the hereditary disorders of connective tissue. *Clin Dermatol.* 2006;24:521–533 [Fig. 1A, p. 538].)

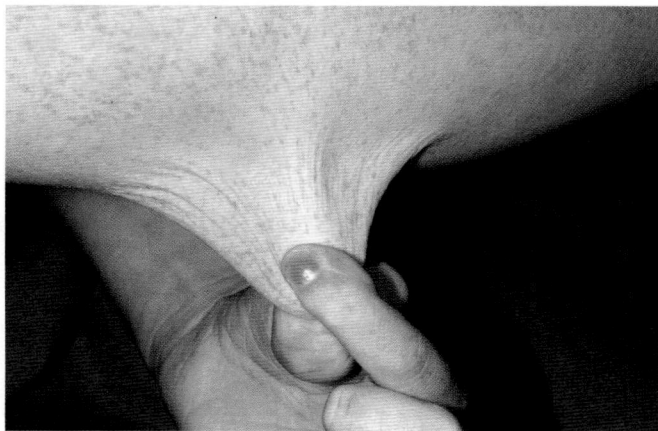

Fig. 47.5 Ehlers-Danlos syndrome. Skin hyperextensibility on the arm. This sign does not demonstrate laxity because on release the skin quickly returns to normal. (From Paller AS, Mancini AJ, eds. *Hurwitz Clinical Pediatric Dermatology.* 5th ed. Elsevier; 2016:121, Fig. 6-1.)

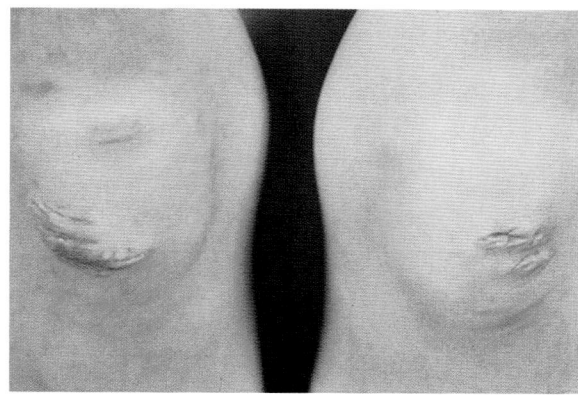

Fig. 47.6 Large "cigarette paper" scars on the knees of a child with Ehlers-Danlos type 1. (From Weston WL, Lane AT, Morelli JG, eds. *Color Textbook of Pediatric Dermatology*. 3rd ed. Mosby; 2002:268, Fig. 18-10.)

TABLE 47.6 Diagnostic Criteria for the Diagnosis of Hypermobile Ehlers-Danlos Syndrome

CRITERION 1: GJH
Must meet Beighton Score for age

CRITERION 2: At least two features must be present

Age	Beighton Score	Feature A: Systemic manifestations of CTD (need ≥5)	Feature B: Family history (one or more first-degree relatives must meet criteria)
Prepubescent or adolescent	≥6	1. Unusually soft/velvety skin 2. Mild skin hyperextensibility 3. Unexplained striae distensae/rubrae 4. Bilateral piezogenic papules of heel 5. Recurrent/multiple abdominal hernia	Feature C: MSK complications (need ≥1) 1. MSK pain in ≥2 limbs, recurring daily for ≥3 mo 2. Chronic widespread pain for ≥3 mo 3. Recurrent joint dislocations or frank joint instability, in the absence of trauma (a or b)
Pubescent up until age 50	≥5	6. Atrophic scarring in ≥2 sites 7. Pelvic floor, rectal, and/or uterine prolapse in children, men, or nulliparous women	a. ≥3 atraumatic dislocations in same joint or ≥2 more atraumatic dislocations in 2 different joints occurring at different times
Over age 50	≥4	8. Dental crowding and high or narrow palate 9. Arachnodactyly	b. Medical confirmation of joint instability at two or more sites not related to trauma
Patients with AJLs	BS 1 point under age requirements AND a positive 5PQ	10. Arm span-to-height ≥1.05 11. Mitral valve prolapse 12. Aortic root dilatation with z score > +2	

CRITERION 3: All three prerequisites must be met

1. Absence of unusual skin fragility
2. Exclusion of other heritable and acquired connective tissue disorders. In patients with an acquired connective tissue disorder, additional diagnosis of hEDS requires meeting both features A and B of Criterion 2. Feature C of Criterion 2 cannot be counted in this situation
3. Exclusion of alternative diagnoses that may also include joint hypermobility by means of hypotonia and/or connective tissue laxity

5PQ, 5-Point Questionnaire; AJLs, acquired joint limitations; BS, Beighton score; CTD, connective tissue disorder; GJH, generalized joint hypermobility; hEDS, hypermobile Ehlers-Danlos syndrome; MSK, musculoskeletal.
From Kohn A, Chang C. The Relationship Between Hypermobile Ehlers-Danlos Syndrome (hEDS), Postural Orthostatic Tachycardia Syndrome (POTS), and Mast Cell Activation Syndrome (MCAS). *Clin Rev Allergy Immunol*. 2020;58(3):273–297; and Malfait F, Francomano C, Byers P, et al. The 2017 International Classification of the Ehlers-Danlos syndromes. *Am J Med Genet C Semin Med Genet*. 2017;175(1)8–26.

TABLE 47.7 Hypermobility 5-Point Questionnaire

1. Can you now (or could you ever) place your hands flat on the floor without bending your knees?
2. Can you now (or could you ever) bend your thumb to touch your forearm?
3. As a child, did you amuse your friends by contorting your body into strange shapes or could you do splits?
4. As a child or teenager, did your shoulder or kneecap dislocate on more than one occasion?
5. Do you consider yourself double-jointed?

A yes answer to two or more questions suggests joint hypermobility with 80–85% sensitivity and 80–90% specificity.

Adapted from Colombi M, Dordoni C, Chiarelli N, et al. Differential diagnosis and diagnostic flow chart of joint hypermobility syndrome/Ehlers-Danlos syndrome hypermobility type compared to other heritable connective tissue disorders. *Am J Med Genet C Semin Med Genet*. 2015;169C(1):6–22.

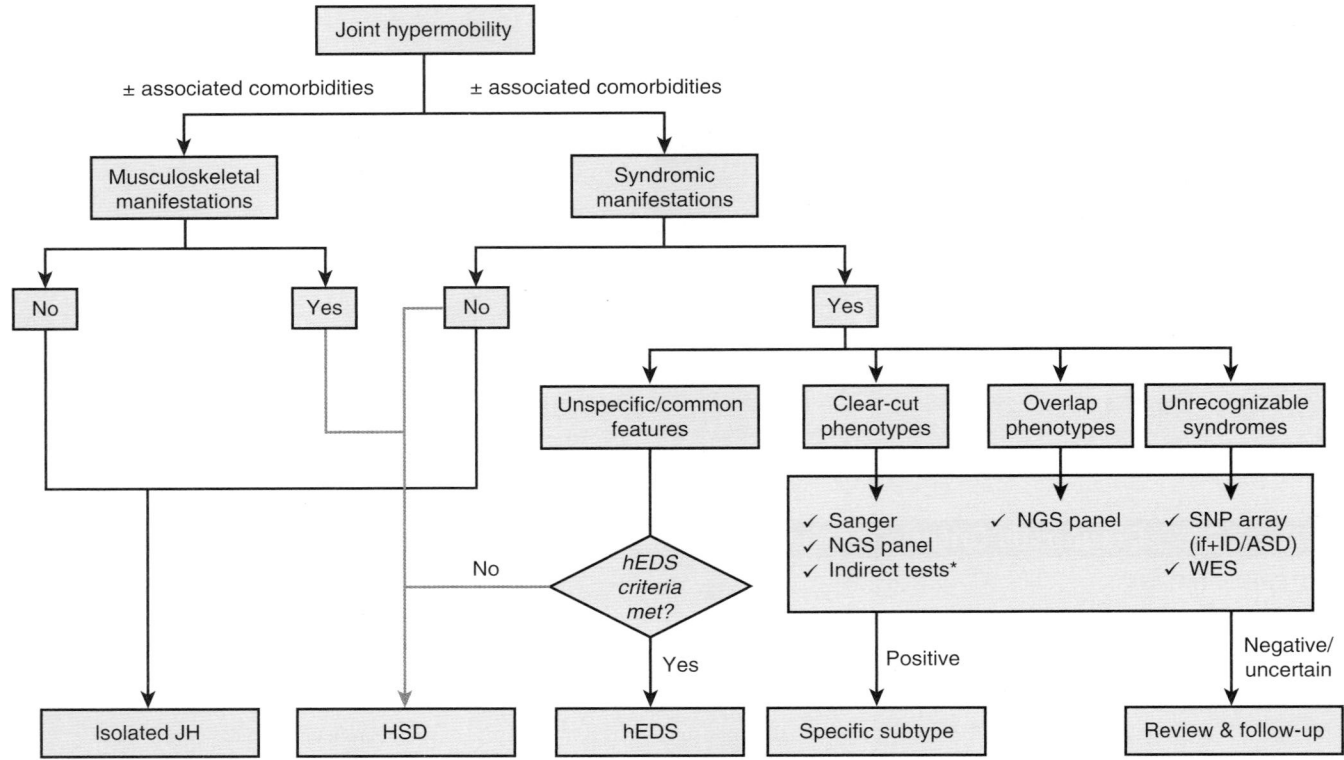

Fig. 47.7 Diagnostic approach for a patient with generalized joint hypermobility (JH). JH without associated musculoskeletal and syndromic manifestation should be considered a benign and common trait. In the presence of systemic involvement, possible scenarios include specific/common phenotypes (see Table 47.9). Once all other partially overlapping conditions have been excluded, the presence of musculoskeletal manifestations in the absence of appreciable systemic involvement prompts a diagnosis of HSD. If the conditions for hEDS are met (see Table 47.7), then a clinical diagnosis of hEDS is made; no molecular testing required. When a well-defined HCT is suspected, additional testing in the form of CVS imaging and molecular testing can formalize the diagnosis. The final scenario refers to JH phenotypes with overt syndromic association in the absence of a clearly identifiable Mendelian disorder. In these cases, additional testing is directed by the presence of dysmorphic features, ASD, or ID. ASD, autism spectrum disorder; HCT, hereditary disorders of connective tissue; hEDS, hypermobile Ehlers-Danlos syndrome; HSD, hypermobility spectrum disorder; ID, intellectual disability; NGS, next-generation sequencing; SNP, single nucleotide polymorphism; WES, whole exome sequencing. (From Guarnieri V, Castori M. Clinical relevance of joint hypermobility and its impact on musculoskeletal pain and bone mass. *Curr Osteoporos Rep.* 2018;16:333–343 [Fig. 2, p. 337].)

TABLE 47.8   Hereditary Disorders of the Connective Tissues Featuring Joint Hypermobility

Ehlers-Danlos Syndromes	Gene	Inheritance	Distinguishing Features
Classic	*COL5A1, COL5A2, COL1A1*	AD	Papyraceous and hemosiderotic scars; velvety, hyperextensible skin
Classic-like	*TNXB*	AR	Velvety, hyperextensible skin; absence of papyraceous scars
Hypermobile	Unknown	AD	Hypermobility; meets 2017 criteria; comorbid extramusculoskeletal manifestations
Vascular	*COL3A1*	AD	Extensive easy bruising; vascular aneurysms and ruptures; sudden death
Kyphoscoliotic	*PLOD1, FKBP14*	AR	Congenital, progressive scoliosis; congenital hypotonia
Dermatosparaxis	*ADAMTS2*	AR	Extreme skin fragility; velvety, hyperextensible skin; acquired cutis laxa
Cardiac-valvular	*COL1A2*	AR	Severe cardiac valvular involvement; velvety, hyperextensible skin
Arthrochalasia	*COL1A1,COL1A2*	AD	Congenital hip dysplasia/subluxation
Musculocontractural	*CHST14, DSE*	AR	Contractures; velvety, hyperextensible skin
Periodontal	*C1R, C1S*	AD	Severe and early-onset periodontitis; tibial plaques
Brittle cornea syndrome	*ZNF469, PRDM5*	AR	Keratoconus; thin cornea
Spondylodysplastic	*B4GALT7, B3GALT6, SLC39A13*	AR	Congenital hypotonia; short stature; bowed limbs
Myopathic	*COL12A1*	AD, AR	Congenital hypotonia; proximal contractures
Hypermobility Spectrum Disorder	Unknown		Exclusion of other clear causes of hypermobility and does not meet 2017 criteria

TABLE 47.8 Hereditary Disorders of the Connective Tissues Featuring Joint Hypermobility—cont'd

Ehlers-Danlos Syndromes	Gene	Inheritance	Distinguishing Features
Disorders of the *TGFB* Pathway			
Marfan syndrome	*FBN1*	AD	Lens dislocation; thoracic aorta dilatation/dissection
Loeys-Dietz syndrome	*TGFBR1, TGFBR2, TGFB2, TGFB3, SMAD2, SMAD3*	AD	Dysmorphic; thoracic aorta dilatation/dissection; middle arteriopathy
Shprintzen-Goldberg syndrome	*SKI*	AD	Craniosynostosis; dysmorphic; thoracic aorta dilatation/dissection
Meester-Loeys syndrome	*BGN*	X-linked	Mild skeletal dysplasia; dysmorphic; thoracic aorta dilatation/dissection
Lateral meningocele syndrome	*NOTCH3*	AD	Multiple Tarlov cysts and spinal meningoceles; dysmorphic
Arterial tortuosity syndrome	*SLC2A10*	AR	Arterial tortuosity; middle arteriopathy; thoracic aorta dilatation/dissection; acquired cutis laxa
Cutis Laxa Syndromes			
ALDH18AI-related cutis laxa	*ALDH18A1*	AR	Intellectual disability; cataracts; poor growth
De Barsy syndrome	*PYRC1*	AR	Intellectual disability; pseudo-athetoid movements; eye anomalies; poor growth
EFEMP2-related cutis laxa	*EFEMP2*		Emphysema; middle arteriopathy; diaphragmatic hernia
ELN-related cutis laxa	*ELN*	AD	Thoracic aorta dilatation/dissection
FBLN5-related cutis laxa	*FBLN5*	AD, AR	Emphysema; peripheral pulmonary stenosis
Geroderma osteodysplasticum	*GORAB*	AR	Osteopenia; fractures; poor growth
LTBP4-related cutis laxa	*LTBP4*	AR	Peripheral pulmonary stenosis; congenital heart defect; diaphragmatic hernia
PYCR1-related cutis laxa	*PYCR1*	AR	Intellectual disability; hypoplasia of the corpus callosum

Adapted from Baban A, Castori M. Pharmacological resources, diagnostic approach, and coordination of care in joint hypermobility-related disorders. *Exp Rev Clin Pharmacol.* 2018;11(7):689–703, Table 1. doi:10.1080/17512433.2018.1497973.

TABLE 47.9 Disorders Featuring Joint Hypermobility

OMIM	Syndromic Disorders	OMIM	Chromosomal Aneuploidies	OMIM	Skeletal Dysplasias
100050	Aarskog syndrome		Chromosome instability disorder, Wegner type	100800	Achondroplasia
103285	ADULT syndrome		Chromosome 1, del 1p(p21-p32)	102500	Hajdu-Cheney syndrome
112240	Cole-Carpenter syndrome		Chromosome 1, del 1q(q21-q25)	105835	Angel-shaped phalangoepiphyseal dysplasia
113310	Fibular aplasia		Chromosome 1, dup 1p(p21.2-p13.2)	108300	Stickler syndrome
115150	Cardiofaciocutaneous syndrome		Chromosome 2, interstitial del 2q(q13q22)	113500	Dominant brachyolmia
117550	Sotos syndrome		Chromosome 2, microdeletion 2q33.1	119600	Cleidocranial dysplasia
129490	Ectodermal dysplasia, hypohidrotic hair/tooth type		Chromosome 2, partial trisomy 2p	146000	Hypochondroplasia
130070	Larsen syndrome		Chromosome 2, terminal del 2q/2q37 deletion	150230	Langer-Giedion syndrome
130650	Beckwith-Wiedemann syndrome		Chromosome 3, interstitial del 3q	151050	Lenz-Majewski hyperostotic dwarfism
135500	Zimmermann-Laband syndrome		Chromosome 3, microduplication 3q13.31	156400	Metaphyseal chondrodysplasia, Jansen type
135900	Coffin-Siris syndrome		Chromosome 4, microdeletion 4p16.3	156530	Metatropic dysplasia
136140	Floating-Harbor syndrome		Chromosome 4, interstitial del 4q	166200	Osteogenesis imperfecta, type 1
146510	Pallister-Hall syndrome		Chromosome 4, microdeletion 4q25	177170	Pseudoachondroplasia
147920	Kabuki syndrome		Chromosome 6, del 6q27	184260	Odontochondrodysplasia
158350	Cowden syndrome		Chromosome 6, interstitial del 6q	184840	Weissenbacher-Zweymuller syndrome
161200	Nail-patella syndrome		Chromosome 6, microdeletion 6q14	201250	Acromesomelic dysplasia, Hunter-Thompson
162200	Neurofibromatosis 1		Chromosome 7, partial dup 7p	210600	Seckel syndrome
163950	Noonan syndrome		Chromosome 7, partial dup 7q	216550	Cohen syndrome
162400	Hereditary sensory neuropathy type IA; HSAN1A		Chromosome 8, interstitial dup 8p	217980	Toriello-Carey syndrome
175050	Juvenile polyposis, hereditary hemorrhagic telangiectasia syndrome		Chromosome 8, mosaic tetrasomy 8p	218040	Costello syndrome

Continued

TABLE 47.9   Disorders Featuring Joint Hypermobility—cont'd

OMIM	Syndromic Disorders	OMIM	Chromosomal Aneuploidies	OMIM	Skeletal Dysplasias
175100	Familial adenomatous syndrome, Gardner syndrome	608156	Chromosome 8, microdeletion 8q22.1	223800	Dyggve-Melchior-Clausen syndrome
176270	Prader-Willi syndrome		Chromosome 9, dup 9q	239850	Cantu syndrome
180849	Rubinstein-Taybi syndrome		Chromosome 9, microdeletion 9q22.3	248010	Magaepiphyseal dysplasia, McAlister-Coe type
192430	Velocardiofacial syndrome		Chromosome 9, partial dup 9p	250215	Metaphyseal acroscyphodysplasia
201200	Acrogeria, Gottron type	158170	Chromosome 9, partial del 9p	250230	Metaphyseal chondrodysplasia, Kaitila type
190350	Trichorhinophalangeal syndrome, type 1		Chromosome 9, trisomy 9	250250	Cartilage-hair hypoplasia
218600	Baller-Gerold syndrome		Chromosome 10, duplication 10q	250420	Metaphyseal dysplasia, deafness, intellectual disability
223370	Dubowitz syndrome		Chromosome 10, mosaic trisomy 10	251450	Desbuquois dysplasia 1
230740	GAPO syndrome			263520	Short rib-polydactyly syndrome, Majewski type
241519	Cerebral calcification, opalescent teeth, phosphaturia		Chromosome 11, microdeletion 11q13.2q13.4	264180	Pseudodiastrophic dysplasia
243800	Johanson-Blizzard syndrome		Chromosome 11, partial dup lip	271510	Sponastrime dysplasia
248800	Marinesco-Sjögren syndrome		Chromosome 12, del 12p	271640	Spondyloepimetaphyseal dysplasia, joint laxity, type 1
249310	Megalocornea-intellectual disability, type 1		Chromosome 12, duplication 12q23q24	2736S0	Thanatophoric dysplasia
249620	Blepharophimosis-intellectual disability syndrome, Ohdo type		Chromosome 12, microdeletion 12ql3.13	273740	Thoraco-limb dysplasia
256690	Neurofaciodigitorenal syndrome		Chromosome 12, microdeletion 12ql4	309350	Melnick-Needles syndrome
257910	Oculo-palato-cerebral syndrome		Chromosome 12, mosaic partial dup 12q	313420	Spondylometaphyseal dysplasia, X-linked
257970	Oculo-renal-cerebellar syndrome		Chromosome 12, partial dup 12q	600373	CODAS syndrome
258360	Onychotrichodysplasia, neutropenia, intellectual disability		Chromosome 13, dup 13q11-q13.2	607095	Anauxetic dysplasia
261540	Peters-plus syndrome		Chromosome 13, partial dup 13q		
264800	Pseudoxanthoma elasticum		Chromosome 14, deletion 14q23		**Myopathies and Muscular Dystrophies**
265050	3MC syndrome		Chromosome 14, microdeletion 14q24	254000	Congenital muscular dystrophy, gonadal dysgenesis
267750	Knobloch syndrome		Chromosome 14, partial dup 14q	254090	Ullrich congenital muscular dystrophy
268050	Mirhosseini-Holmes-Walton syndrome		Chromosome 15, interstitial del 15q(q21q25)	256030	Nemaline myopathy
268400	Rothmund-Thomson syndrome		Chromosome 15, inv dup(15)	618323	Myasthenic syndrome, congenital
269880	SHORT syndrome		Chromosome 15, trisomy 15		
271270	Spinocerebellar ataxia, dysmorphic facies	613406	Chromosome 15, microdeletion 15q24		**Metabolic Disorders/Inborn Errors of Metabolism**
273750	3M syndrome		Chromosome 16, partial dup 16p	210200	3-Methylcrotonylglycinuria
275900	Spastic paraplegia 20 (SPG20)	136570	Chromosome 16, microdeletion 16p12.1	208400	Aspartylglucosaminuria
300000	Opitz G syndrome		Chromosome 17, mosaic trisomy 17	236200	Homocystinuria
300194	Alport syndrome, intellectual disability, elliptocytosis		Chromosome 17, partial dup 17p	252500	Mucolipidosis 2
300049	Periventricular heterotopia disorder		Chromosome 17, partial dup 17q	253000	Morquio syndrome
300422	FG syndrome	610443	Chromosome 17, microdeletion 17q21.31	277400	Methylmalonic aciduria/ homocystinuria, cblC (MAHCC)
300624	Fragile X syndrome (FXS)	601808	Chromosome 18, partial del 18q	277900	Wilson disease
303600	Coffin-Lowry syndrome		Chromosome 19, deletion 19p13.3	300352	Creatine deficiency syndrome, X-linked
305000	Dyskeratosis congenita syndrome	613026	Chromosome 19, microdeletion 19q13.11	304150	Occipital horn syndrome
305600	Focal dermal hypoplasia		Chromosome 20, partial dup 20p	600721	D-2-hydroxyglutaric aciduria
309520	Lujan-Fryns syndrome	190685	Chromosome 21, trisomy 21/Down syndrome		
601803	Pallister-Killian syndrome	611867	Chromosome 22, proximal 22q11 deletion		

TABLE 47.9 Disorders Featuring Joint Hypermobility—cont'd

OMIM	Syndromic Disorders	OMIM	Chromosomal Aneuploidies	OMIM	Skeletal Dysplasias
602342	Pierpont syndrome		Chromosome X, duplication Xq		
602535	Marshall-Smith syndrome		Chromosome X, dup Xp11.22-21.1		
602501	Megalencephaly, capillary malformation, polymicrogyria				
606170	Genitopatellar syndrome				
609442	Fetal valproate syndrome				
613805	Meier-Gorlin syndrome				
615879	Tatton-Brown-Rahman syndrome				
616580	Au-Kline syndrome				
616721	Congenital disorders of glycosylation				
617140	ZTTK syndrome				
618332	Menke-Hennekam syndrome 1 (MKHK1)				
618371	Turnpenny-Fry syndrome (TPFS)				

ADULT, acro-dermato-ungual-lacrimal-tooth; CODAS, cerebral, ocular, dental, auricular, skeletal anomalies; GAPO, growth retardation, alopecia, pseudoanodontia, and optic atrophy; ZTTK, Zhu-Tokita-Takenouchi-Kim.

Noonan syndrome, myopathies, metabolic disorders including disorders of energy (mitochondrial) metabolism, or creatine uptake disorders. A detailed history of exacerbating circumstances can help define some of these disease mimics along with appropriate serum and biochemical testing or consideration for gene sequencing. Specialist referral is often necessary to help guide the evaluation, but it is the primary care physician who recognizes and initiates many of these investigations.

BIBLIOGRAPHY

A bibliography is available at ExpertConsult.com.

48

Lymphadenopathy and Neck Masses

Brett J. Bordini

Given the role of the lymphatic system in developing adaptive responses to numerous antigenic challenges and the rate at which the immune system is exposed to novel antigens early in life, enlarged lymph nodes are regularly encountered both incidentally and within the context of many childhood illnesses. The challenge for the clinician is determining when a change in the size or quality of a lymph node is physiologic or when such a change represents pathology. A thorough history, physical examination, and recognition of the anatomic drainage patterns of the lymphatic system will oftentimes sufficiently narrow the differential diagnosis of lymphadenopathy such that complicated or invasive diagnostic evaluations are unnecessary. It is equally important to consider other non–lymph node disorders in the differential diagnosis (parotids, brachial cleft cysts, primary tumors).

MECHANISM OF LYMPHADENOPATHY

The lymphatic system is a network of vessels and tissues that collects excess fluid from the cellular interstitium and returns it to the peripheral circulation. This interstitial fluid is similar in composition to plasma, though it may contain additional proteins, pathogens, other antigens, and antigen-presenting cells. The collected fluid, termed **lymph**, enters the lymphatic system via specialized lymphatic capillaries and passes into nearby lymph nodes via afferent lymphatic vessels. The lymph nodes contain both B and T lymphocytes lying in a supportive framework within a connective tissue capsule (Fig. 48.1). Additional lymphocytes may enter lymph nodes from the peripheral venous circulation via postcapillary high endothelial venules. Antigens, antigen-presenting cells, and pathogens within the lymph interact with the lymphocytes, allowing for the production of B- and/or T-cell immune responses in an effort to clear the antigen or pathogen. Efferent lymphatic vessels then carry lymph and antigen-sensitized lymphocytes from the nodes back to the peripheral circulation via the thoracic duct.

Enlargement of lymph nodes can come about via a variety of mechanisms. First, **physiologic hyperplasia** can occur as nodal and circulating lymphocytes proliferate within nodes in response to antigenic stimulation. Second, bacteria that have been transported to the nodes may stimulate the recruitment of polymorphonuclear cells and the elaboration of inflammatory mediators that can lead to the edema, erythema, and tenderness characteristic of **bacterial lymphadenitis** or to suppuration and abscess formation. Third, **malignant cells** may arise within the node itself and proliferate, causing enlargement, or arrive from distant cancerous sites and infiltrate the nodal tissue. Fourth,

certain **immune disorders** (hemophagocytic lymphohistiocytosis) or immune reactions to medications can cause lymphadenopathy either directly or as part of a serum sickness–like reaction. Finally, in rare **genetic storage diseases** (e.g., Niemann-Pick, Gaucher diseases), macrophages laden with abnormally metabolized lipids may lodge within lymph nodes, causing enlargement.

The regional drainage pattern of each lymph node group is important in determining the cause of lymphadenopathy, particularly when localized to an individual node or contiguous group of nodes (Fig. 48.2 and Tables 48.1 and 48.2). The cervical lymph nodes drain lymph from distinct areas of the head, neck, and throat and may enlarge if a local infection is present. Consequently, because otitis media and pharyngitis are common infections in children, head and neck lymphadenopathy is one of the more frequently encountered regional lymphadenopathy patterns in small children. The axillary nodes drain lymph from the arms, lateral breasts, and superficial chest and upper abdomen, and isolated enlargement of these nodes may suggest pathology in these areas. The inguinal nodes drain the lower extremities, genitourinary system, and perineum, which may indicate lower extremity pathology or the presence of a sexually transmitted infection in patients with an exposure history. Supraclavicular lymphadenopathy is a concerning finding and should prompt investigation for an underlying neoplasm, fungal infection, tuberculosis, or sarcoidosis. **Generalized lymphadenopathy**, defined as the presence of enlarged or abnormal lymph nodes in two or more noncontiguous lymph node groups (with or without hepatosplenomegaly), is often indicative of a systemic response to an infectious or otherwise inflammatory process but may also indicate malignant proliferation of lymphocytes (Table 48.3).

History

History should be aimed at establishing the time course of the development of lymphadenopathy, whether the lymphadenopathy is restricted to a particular anatomic region or is generalized, and if there are any associated signs, symptoms, or exposures that may suggest an etiology.

Lymphadenopathy that develops rapidly over several days is more suggestive of an acutely inflammatory, often infectious process, whereas more indolently developing lymphadenopathy may suggest malignancy, chronic disease, or an atypical infection. The sudden onset of unilateral inguinal adenopathy shortly following lower extremity trauma suggests an infection in the traumatized extremity. In contrast, progressive enlargement of multiple noncontiguous nodal groups over the course of weeks or months that is accompanied by weight loss, fevers, or night sweats suggests a systemic illness such as lymphoma or tuberculosis. When establishing the time period over which the lymphadenopathy developed, clarifying both when the node was first noted to be abnormal and the last time the node was felt to be normal is essential, particularly if associated symptoms, overlying skin changes, and tenderness are absent, since more slowly developing lymphadenopathy may not be noticed until the node or nodes are quite enlarged, or if lymphadenopathy was noted only incidentally when dressing, grooming, or bathing.

The age of the child with lymphadenopathy is similarly important in the consideration of the cause (see Table 48.3). Neonatal lymphadenopathy is typically indicative of exposure to an infectious agent in utero, such as cytomegalovirus (CMV), syphilis, HIV, rubella, or toxoplasmosis, though may less frequently be associated with congenital malignancy, immune disorders, or storage diseases. In contrast, toddlers and children with adenopathy tend to have either focal infections that drain into the affected nodal chain, or systemic viral infections, resulting in diffusely enlarged nodes. Adolescents may acquire exposures that place them at risk for sexually transmitted infections and inguinal adenopathy. Just as exposure to certain infectious agents may vary with age, the risk of hematologic malignancy varies as well: Acute leukemias are more common in toddlers and young children, non-Hodgkin lymphoma is more common in school-aged children, and Hodgkin lymphoma is more common in adolescents.

The past medical history and review of systems should be explored for conditions that may either cause lymphadenopathy directly or place the patient at increased risk for opportunistic infections, such as congenital or acquired immunodeficiency. The clinician should inquire about any signs or symptoms that would suggest an acute infectious process or more slowly progressive constitutional symptoms that may suggest malignancy or indolent infection. The quality of oral hygiene practices and dentition should be assessed as **odontogenic infections** may not readily be appreciated as a source of cervical lymphadenopathy. The use of any prescription medications, over-the-counter medicines, or traditional remedies should be ascertained: In addition to identifying medications that may directly cause lymphadenopathy, this information may identify medications that may cause a serum sickness–like reaction with resultant lymphadenopathy or that may be used to treat autoimmune or rheumatologic conditions that are associated with generalized lymphadenopathy (see Table 48.3).

After determining the timing and distribution of the lymphadenopathy and placing these findings within the context of the child's age and past medical history, the clinician should inquire about any exposures that may have led to the development of lymphadenopathy, focusing in particular on diet, travel history, and contact with individuals, animals,

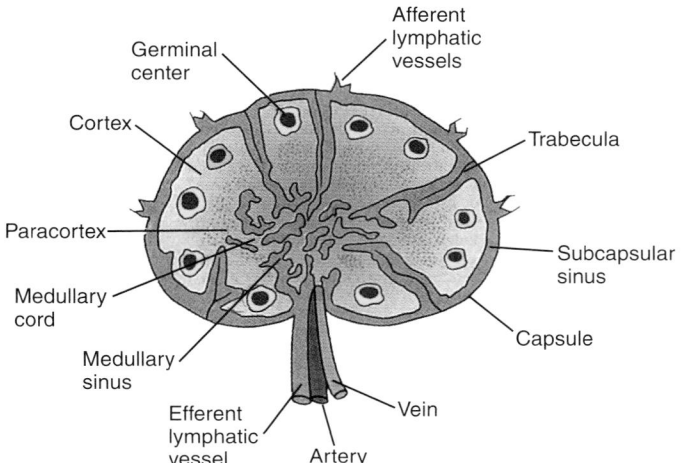

Fig. 48.1 Diagrammatic representation of the structure of a lymph node. (From Faller DV. Diseases of the lymph nodes and spleen. In: Wyngaarden JB, Smith LH, Bennett JC, eds. *Cecil Textbook of Medicine.* 19th ed. Philadelphia: WB Saunders; 1992:979.)

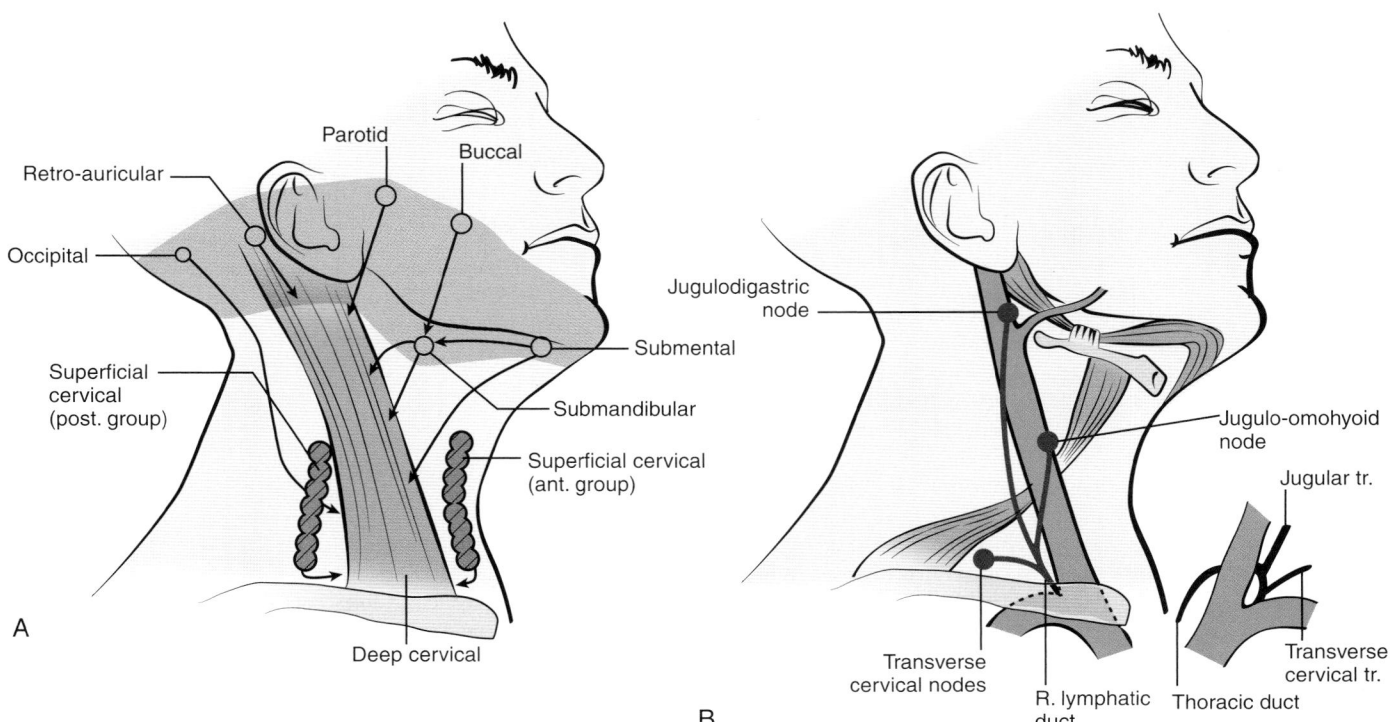

Fig. 48.2 The superficial *(A)* and deep cervical *(B)* lymph nodes that drain the head and neck. Ant., anterior; post., posterior; R, right; superfic., superficial; tr., tributary. (From O'Rahilly RO. *Gardner-Gray-O'Rahilly Anatomy: A Regional Study of Human Structure.* 5th ed. Philadelphia: WB Saunders; 1986:719.)

TABLE 48.1   Drainage Areas of Regional Nodes

Abdominal and Pelvic
Abdomen, lower extremity, pelvic organs

Axillary
Arm, breast, chest wall, hand, upper and lateral abdominal wall

Cervical
External ear; larynx; parotid; superficial tissues of the scalp, head, and neck; thyroid; tongue; trachea

Epitrochlear
Forearm, hand

Iliac
Bladder, lower abdomen, part of the genitalia, urethra

Inguinal
Gluteal region, lower anal canal, lower extremity, perineum, vulva and vagina in females, scrotum and penis in males, skin of the lower abdomen

Mediastinal
Thoracic viscera

Occipital
Posterior scalp

Popliteal
Knee joint, skin of the lateral lower leg and foot

Preauricular
Cheek, conjunctivae, eyelid, temporal scalp

Submaxillary/Submental
Buccal mucosa, gums, teeth, tongue

Supraclavicular
Abdomen, arms, head, lungs, mediastinum, neck, superficial thorax
Left supraclavicular adenopathy is usually due to an intraabdominal problem
Right supraclavicular adenopathy is usually due to an intrathoracic problem

TABLE 48.2   Sites of Regional Lymphadenopathy and Associated Diseases

Cervical
Oropharyngeal infection (viral, group A streptococcal, or staphylococcal)
Scalp infection (tinea)
Mycobacterial lymphadenitis (tuberculous and nontuberculous mycobacteria)
Viral infection (EBV, CMV, HHV-6, measles)
Cat-scratch disease
Kawasaki disease
Multisystem inflammatory syndrome in children (MIS-C) associated with COVID-19
Thyroid disease
Kimura disease
Rosai-Dorfman (sinus histiocytosis)
Periodic fever, aphthous stomatitis, pharyngitis, cervical adenopathy (PFAPA) syndrome
Kikuchi-Fujimoto disease
Unicentric Castleman disease

Anterior Auricular
Conjunctivitis or other eye infections
Oculoglandular tularemia, cat-scratch disease, EBV, adenovirus

Posterior Auricular
Otitis media
Viral infection (especially rubella, parvovirus)

Supraclavicular
Malignancy or infection in the mediastinum (right)
Metastatic malignancy from abdomen (left)
Lymphoma
Tuberculosis

Epitrochlear
Hand infection, arm infection*
Lymphoma†
Sarcoidosis
Syphilis
EBV
HIV

Inguinal
Urinary tract infection
Sexually transmitted infection (especially syphilis or lymphogranuloma venereum)
Lower extremity suppurative infection
Plague

Hilar (Not Palpable, Found on Chest Radiograph or CT) (see Table 48.4)
Tuberculosis†
Histoplasmosis†
Blastomycosis†
Coccidioidomycosis†
Leukemia/lymphoma†
Hodgkin disease†
Metastatic malignancy*
Sarcoidosis†
Castleman disease

Axillary
Cat-scratch disease
Arm infection
Malignancy of chest wall
Leukemia/lymphoma
Brucellosis

CMV, cytomegalovirus; EBV, Epstein-Barr virus; HHV-6, human herpesvirus 6.
*Unilateral.
†Bilateral.

or environments that may pose a risk for disease transmission. Contact with or consumption of raw or undercooked meats, particularly pork, lamb, and venison, may transmit *Toxoplasma gondii*, leading to toxoplasmosis. Similarly, contact with agricultural animals or ingestion of unpasteurized dairy products may place patients at risk for acquiring certain pathogens, such as *Brucella* species or *Mycobacterium bovis*; infection with either may lead to generalized lymphadenopathy. Potential exposures in the home environment should be assessed, including the risk of contaminated drinking water and whether there are concerns for mold exposure, particularly in immunocompromised patients. The presence of pets, either within the home or in the area, should be determined. Cats or kittens that may scratch the child and transmit *Bartonella henselae*, the etiologic agent of **cat-scratch disease**, are often omitted from the history unless such questions are specifically asked. Furthermore, some families may deny the presence of household pets but forget to mention that the child plays with a pet present in a barn or around the neighborhood. Travel history should determine whether the child is from or has been exposed to geographic areas associated with a higher risk for acquiring certain infections, such as tuberculosis in endemically affected nations or histoplasmosis in the Ohio River valley. The clinician should inquire whether any family members or

close contacts are ill or taking medications, whether any have recently traveled to or immigrated from other countries, and whether any have recently been incarcerated. Adolescents should be questioned about risk factors for HIV and sexually transmitted infections, such as syphilis or lymphogranuloma venereum, which may cause generalized or inguinal lymphadenopathy, respectively.

The family history should also focus on potentially heritable conditions, such as autoimmune or rheumatologic disorders, certain hematologic and soft tissue malignancies, and storage diseases that may be associated with noninfectious forms of lymphadenopathy.

TABLE 48.3 Differential Diagnosis of Generalized Lymphadenopathy

Neonate	Child	Adolescent
Common Causes		
CMV	Nonspecific viral infections	Viral infections
HIV	EBV	EBV
Syphilis	CMV	CMV
Toxoplasmosis	HIV	HIV
	Toxoplasmosis	Measles
	Measles	Toxoplasmosis
		Syphilis
Rare Causes		
Chagas disease (congenital)	Serum sickness	Serum sickness
Congenital leukemia	SLE, JIA	SLE, JIA
Congenital tuberculosis	Leukemia/lymphoma	Leukemia/lymphoma
Reticuloendotheliosis	Tuberculosis (miliary)	Tuberculosis
Metabolic storage disease	Sarcoidosis	Sarcoidosis
Histiocytic disorders	DRESS	DRESS
Listeria sepsis	Fungal infections	Fungal infections
	Plague	Plague
	Leptospirosis	Leptospirosis
	Brucellosis	Brucellosis
	Langerhans cell histiocytosis	Drug reaction (immune)
	Macrophage activation syndrome	Castleman disease
	Hemophagocytic lymphohistiocytosis	Rickettsial infection
	Castleman disease (very rare in this age group)	
	Chronic granulomatous disease	
	Sinus histiocytosis (Rosai-Dorfman disease)	
	Kikuchi Fujimoto disease	
	Autoimmune lymphoproliferative disease (ALP)	
	Rickettsial infection	

CMV, cytomegalovirus; DRESS, drug reaction, eosinophilia, systemic symptoms; EBV, Epstein-Barr virus; JIA, juvenile idiopathic arthritis (as Still disease); SLE, systemic lupus erythematosus.

Physical Examination

Physical examination should assess general appearance and look for findings that may reveal the underlying cause of lymphadenopathy. Examination of the lymphatic system should establish the size, quality, and distribution of any abnormal lymph nodes and should assess for the presence of tenderness or changes in the overlying skin or surrounding tissues.

Size

The threshold beyond which a particular node is considered enlarged varies by nodal group. In general, nodes over 1 cm in diameter are considered enlarged; exceptions include epitrochlear nodes >0.5 cm in diameter and inguinal nodes >1.5 cm in diameter.

Quality

The quality of the nodes often yields some clues as to the cause of the adenopathy. The clinician should assess consistency, mobility, shape, tenderness, and whether any changes to the overlying skin or soft tissues are present. The following general patterns are worth noting:

- Erythematous, tender, and warm: acute bacterial infection with suppurative adenitis
- Tender, nonerythematous, and soft: viral infection or other systemic infection
- Firm, hard, rubbery, and nontender: lymphoma or other infiltrating tumor
- Hard, matted, immobile, and nontender: primary or metastatic tumor; fibrotic changes following acute infection

Distribution

All areas in which lymphadenopathy is commonly present should be palpated, including the cervical, auricular, axillary, epitrochlear, inguinal, and supraclavicular areas. If more than two noncontiguous nodal groups are abnormal, without evidence of distinct focal infections inciting the lymphadenopathy within each group, the lymphadenopathy is generalized.

Regional lymphadenopathy usually reflects pathologic processes within the lymphatic drainage distribution of that particular nodal chain (see Table 48.2). Several patterns of regional lymphadenopathy should prompt further evaluation. The presence of palpable supraclavicular nodes is often a red flag for a serious illness such as malignancy. **Supraclavicular nodes** that are palpated on the right side often reflect a mediastinal tumor or invasive mediastinal infection, such as histoplasmosis. Supraclavicular nodes on the left side are often the result of metastatic spread of an abdominal tumor. The presence of either type of node mandates an urgent evaluation, including a CBC with differential; imaging with chest radiography, CT, MRI, or PET scan; and consideration of biopsy. **Epitrochlear nodes**, if unilateral, commonly indicate the hand or arm as a source of distal infection; however, palpable bilateral epitrochlear lymph nodes usually reflect systemic illness, such as syphilis, sarcoidosis, or lymphoma. **Inguinal** node enlargement is common and is usually caused by the frequent occurrence of minor trauma and infections in the lower extremities of children. Significantly enlarged inguinal nodes may also be present with sexually transmitted infections, such as syphilis, chlamydial urethritis, or lymphogranuloma venereum, or with urinary tract infection, lymphoma, or abdominal tumors.

Mediastinal adenopathy (or mass) may be detected incidentally, secondary to chest symptoms, or during the evaluation of peripheral but generalized lymphadenopathy. The differential diagnosis is noted in Table 48.4.

Evaluation and Management Strategies

Many previously healthy children with acute lymphadenopathy require few, if any, laboratory or imaging studies. No laboratory testing may be required for well-appearing children whose acute, localized adenopathy can be attributed to an infection in the vicinity of the node; similarly, generalized lymphadenopathy clearly associated with a systemic viral infection may not require further evaluation. The differential diagnosis of lymphadenopathy is developed in a stepwise fashion, first by determining whether the lymphadenopathy is regional or generalized. Next, the time course of the lymphadenopathy should be defined as acute or chronic, the latter defined as being present for a period of more than 4 weeks. Finally, the quality of the nodes and the presence of any associated signs or symptoms should be ascertained, as the extent of evaluation is dictated by both the characteristics of the lymphadenopathy and the presence of

TABLE 48.4 Differential Diagnosis of Mediastinal Masses

Anterior Mediastinum

Lymphoma
Thymic cyst
Thymic hyperplasia
Benign teratoma
Malignant germ-cell tumor
Thymoma
Langerhans cell histiocytosis (from bone)

Middle Mediastinum

Lymphoma
Tuberculosis
Histoplasmosis
Sarcoidosis

Posterior Mediastinum

Neuroblastoma
Ganglioneuroma
Neurofibroma
Sarcoma
Duplication cyst

From Alexander S, Ferrando AA. Pediatric lymphoma. In: Orkin SH, et al., eds. *Nathan and Oski's Hematology and Oncology of Infancy and Childhood.* 8th ed. Philadelphia: Elsevier; 2015;2:1627, Box 53-2.

associated signs and symptoms. Using this approach, a comprehensive differential diagnosis and evaluation plan can then be developed (Figs. 48.3 and 48.4).

Regional Lymphadenopathy: General Evaluation Principles

The typical child with acute regional lymphadenopathy presents with enlarged nodes, commonly in the cervical region. A thorough history and careful physical examination should reveal whether nodes are definitely involved, as opposed to other non-nodal structures, such as salivary glands. In many cases, no other abnormalities are found on examination, systemic signs are minimal, and no further evaluation is required. **Acute cervical lymphadenopathy** in the presence of upper respiratory infectious symptoms often requires only observation. In the child whose presenting features are only fever and an acutely inflamed unilateral cervical lymph node, bacterial lymphadenitis should be considered. Laboratory tests should include a CBC and differential as well as measurement of inflammatory markers such as the ESR, CRP, or procalcitonin level. A trial of oral antibiotics (with activity against mouth flora, streptococci, and staphylococci) may be considered; if the lymphadenopathy persists or worsens, intravenous antibiotics may be indicated, as should be consideration of diagnoses other than acute unilateral bacterial lymphadenitis, such as lymphadenitis from tuberculosis or atypical mycobacteria. In those instances, if clinical signs or exposure history are suggestive, a purified protein derivative (PPD) or interferon gamma release assay should be undertaken, and if the results are negative and symptoms improve on the intravenous antibiotics, it is reasonable to complete the antimicrobial course orally.

In contrast, if the lymphadenopathy continues or becomes frank lymphadenitis with erythema and tenderness despite antimicrobial therapy, further work-up is indicated. Imaging the involved area is helpful but not always necessary. Although ultrasonography can reveal enlarged nodes or a fluid-filled abscess or cyst, contrast-enhanced CT of the area is the best method for defining the extent of inflamed nodes

and whether an abscess is present (Fig. 48.5). If an abscess is found, incision and drainage, followed by appropriate bacterial and mycobacterial cultures and stains, are appropriate. If atypical mycobacteria are suspected on the basis of a borderline positive PPD or cross-reacting gamma interferon release array result or clinical presentation, fine-needle aspiration or excisional biopsy is preferred because incision and drainage often lead to draining sinus tracts that are difficult to heal (Fig. 48.6). Enlarged nodes that do not recede in several weeks with appropriate antimicrobial therapy and without explanation (such as acute Epstein-Barr virus [EBV] infection) should also raise the suspicion of malignancy.

The presence of additional signs or symptoms should prompt consideration of alternate diagnoses. Acute cervical lymphadenopathy accompanying pharyngitis in children older than 18 months may necessitate testing for group A streptococci. The additional presence of hepatomegaly or splenomegaly should raise suspicion of EBV-related infectious mononucleosis, in which case a CBC with white blood cell differential (to identify lymphocytosis and atypical lymphocytes) (Table 48.5) and EBV titers (or a monospot heterophile antibody test in older children) may be helpful.

Supraclavicular adenopathy, acute cervical adenopathy accompanied by respiratory distress, or prolonged cervical adenopathy warrants anteroposterior and lateral radiographs of the neck and/or chest, a CBC with white blood cell differential, and interferon gamma release assay or placement of PPD tuberculin skin test. CT with contrast is necessary in certain situations to fully delineate cervical adenopathy that is excessively large or that impinges on the airway, or to determine whether mediastinal adenopathy is also present. Empiric glucocorticoid therapy, often considered in an attempt to reduce discomfort associated with inflamed nodes, usually in the head and neck area, *should not* be administered without definitively establishing the etiology of lymphadenopathy, as such treatment can delay or obscure the diagnosis of hematologic malignancy, and prior glucocorticoid therapy in the setting of hematologic malignancy can portend a higher risk classification and ineligibility for certain oncology treatment protocols. Exceptions may be considered in instances of impending critical airway obstruction secondary to severely enlarged cervical lymph nodes.

Generalized Lymphadenopathy: General Evaluation Principles

In the child with generalized lymphadenopathy, the cause may be infectious, immunologic, or malignant. Infectious causes, such as HIV, EBV, CMV, toxoplasmosis, and secondary syphilis, can generally be determined relatively quickly through serologic or nucleic acid–based testing. Noninfectious causes, such as systemic lupus erythematosus, macrophage activation syndrome, hemophagocytic lymphohistiocytosis, and serum sickness, can also generally be excluded by a thorough history and specific laboratory studies. Drugs may cause serum sickness or produce hypersensitivity reactions, either of which may result in generalized lymphadenopathy. Medications associated with drug-induced lymphadenopathy include allopurinol, atenolol, captopril, carbamazepine, gold, hydralazine, penicillins, phenytoin, primidone, procainamide, pyrimethamine, quinidine, sulfonamides, sulindac, and tetracyclines. If the generalized lymphadenopathy cannot be attributed to a definite cause, if the nodes fail to recede within several weeks, and especially if there are systemic symptoms, malignancy must be considered. An abnormal CBC demonstrating anemia, leukopenia, or thrombocytopenia, or radiologic evidence of mediastinal adenopathy or pleural disease is highly suggestive of malignancy. HIV, EBV, and CMV studies (culture, polymerase chain reaction [PCR], and serologic profiles) may be obtained

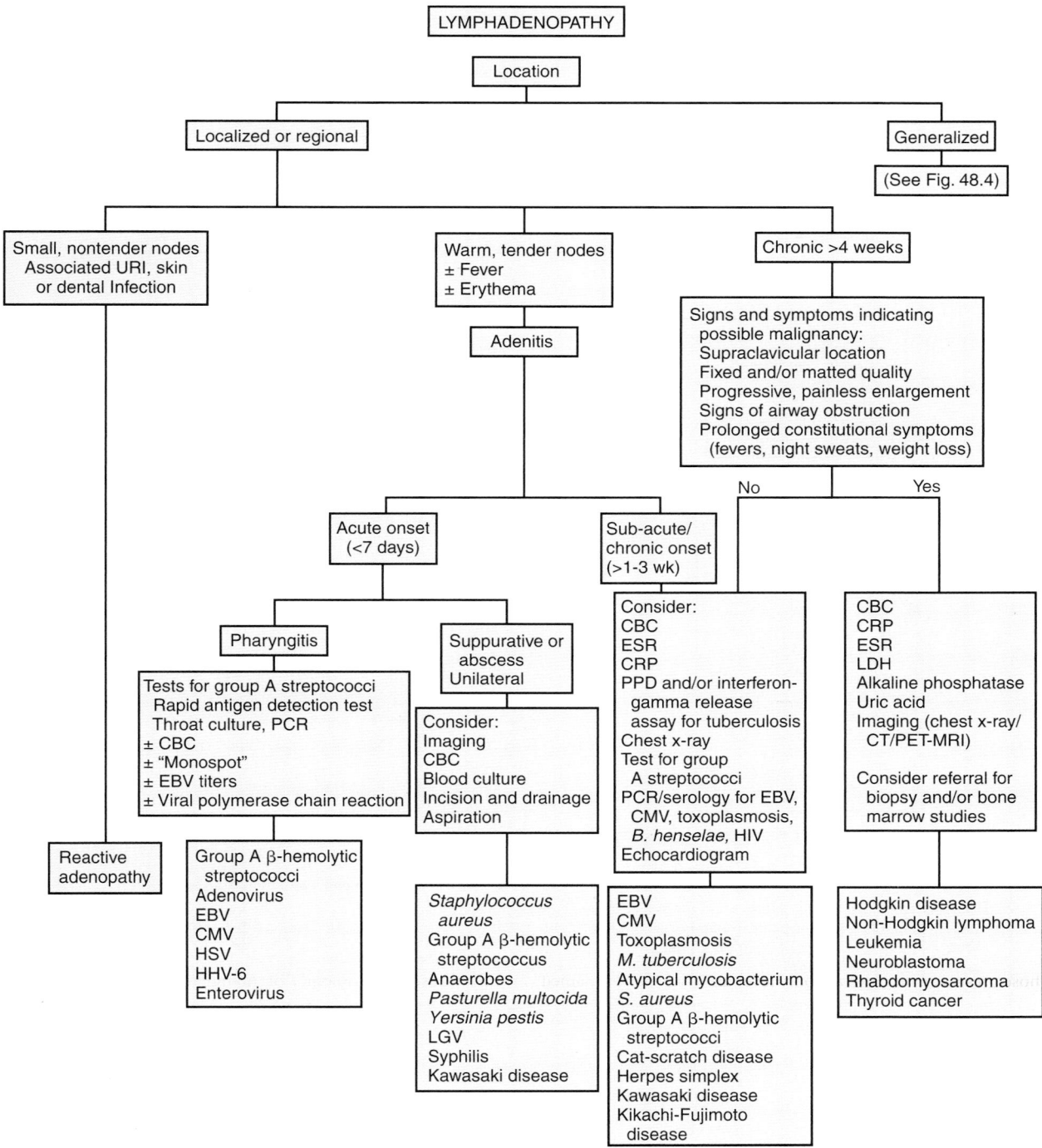

Fig. 48.3 Diagnostic algorithm for the evaluation of regional lymphadenopathy. *CMV,* cytomegalovirus; *EBV,* Epstein-Barr virus; *HHV,* human herpesvirus; *HSV,* herpes simplex virus; *LDH,* lactate dehydrogenase; *LGV,* lymphogranuloma venereum; *PCR,* polymerase chain reaction; *PET,* position emission tomography; *PPD,* purified protein derivative (tuberculosis skin test); *RPR,* rapid plasma reagin; *URI,* upper respiratory infection; *VDRL,* Venereal Disease Research Laboratory. (Modified from Pomeranz AJ, Sabnis S, Busey SL, et al. *Pediatric Decision-Making Strategies.* 2nd ed. Philadelphia: Elsevier; 2016:229.)

for some children. Because the diagnoses of leukemia (through bone marrow aspiration, biopsy), lymphoma (through bone marrow aspiration, biopsy), systemic lupus erythematosus (through antinuclear antibody, double-stranded DNA antibodies), and cat-scratch disease (through biopsy and/or *B. henselae* serologic profile) require more invasive and expensive tests, the physician should first consider all

aspects of the history and physical examination before ordering laboratory studies. Because serious disseminated infections, such as tuberculosis and histoplasmosis, can manifest in a similar manner, fine-needle aspiration or biopsy of an involved node or bone marrow aspiration is crucial. Excision of a node is preferred in some cases to obtain adequate tissue for pathologic study, stains, or cultures.

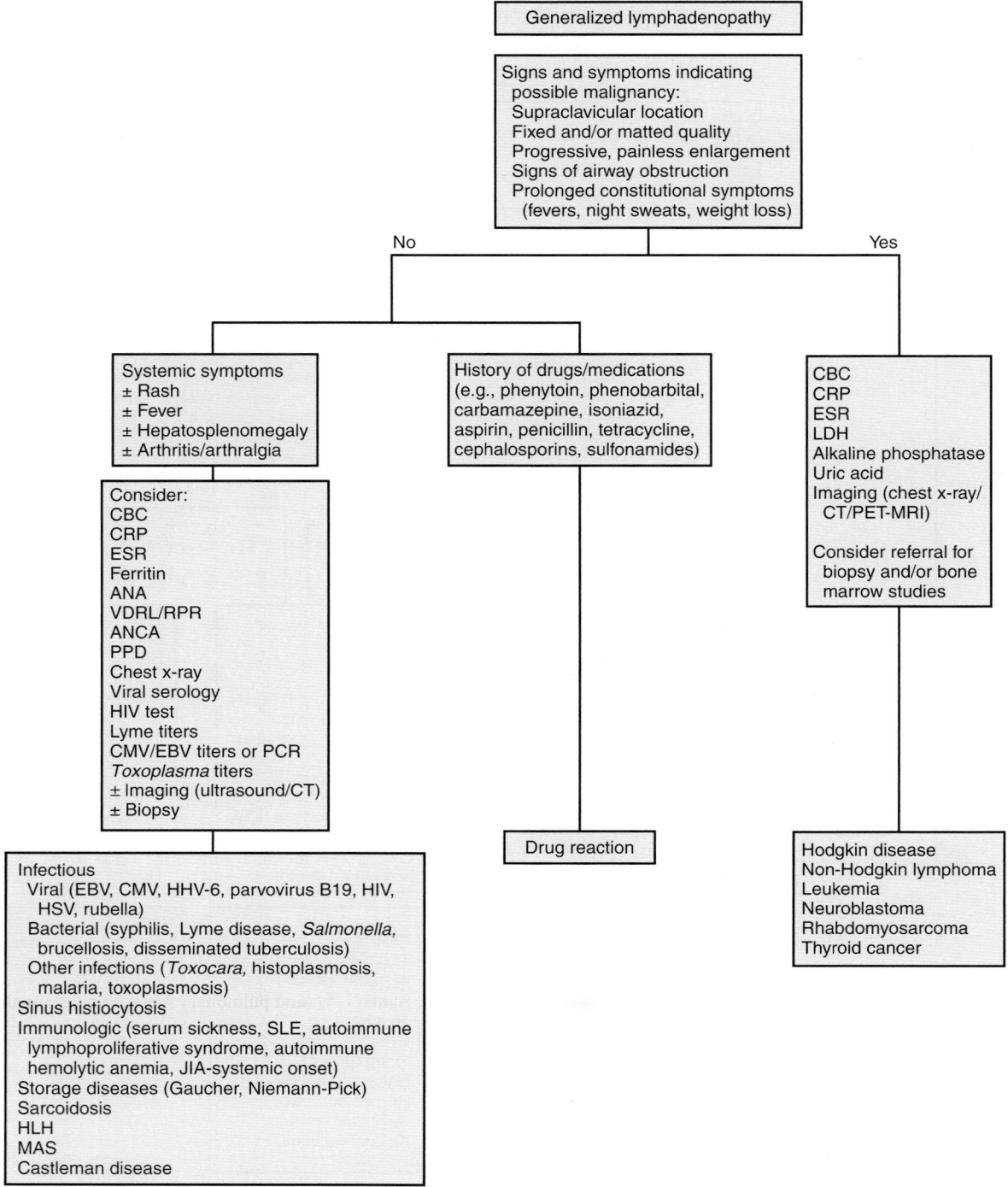

Fig. 48.4 Diagnostic algorithm for generalized lymphadenopathy. ANA, antinuclear antibody; ANCA, antineutrophil cytoplasmic antibody; CMV, cytomegalovirus; EBV, Epstein-Barr virus; HHV-6, human herpesvirus 6; HLH, hemophagocytic lymphohistiocytosis; HSV, herpes simplex virus; JIA, juvenile rheumatoid arthritis; LDH, lactate dehydrogenase; MAS, macrophage activation syndrome; PCR, polymerase chain reaction; PET, position emission tomography; PPD, purified protein derivative (tuberculosis skin test); RPR, rapid plasma reagin; SLE, systemic lupus erythematosus; VDRL, Venereal Disease Research Laboratory. (Modified from Pomeranz AJ, Sabnis S, Busey SL, et al. *Pediatric Decision-Making Strategies.* 2nd ed. Philadelphia: Elsevier; 2016:231.)

Lymphadenopathy Patterns

Several patterns of lymphadenopathy and their underlying causes deserve special mention, due either to the frequency with which they are encountered in pediatric practice or to the potential severity of the underlying cause.

Infections of the oropharynx. Pharyngeal infection is the most common cause of regional lymphadenopathy in children (see Chapter 2). Many of these pharyngeal infections are associated with cervical lymphadenopathy and are viral in origin. Frequent viral causes include adenovirus, parainfluenza, influenza, rhinovirus, coronaviruses

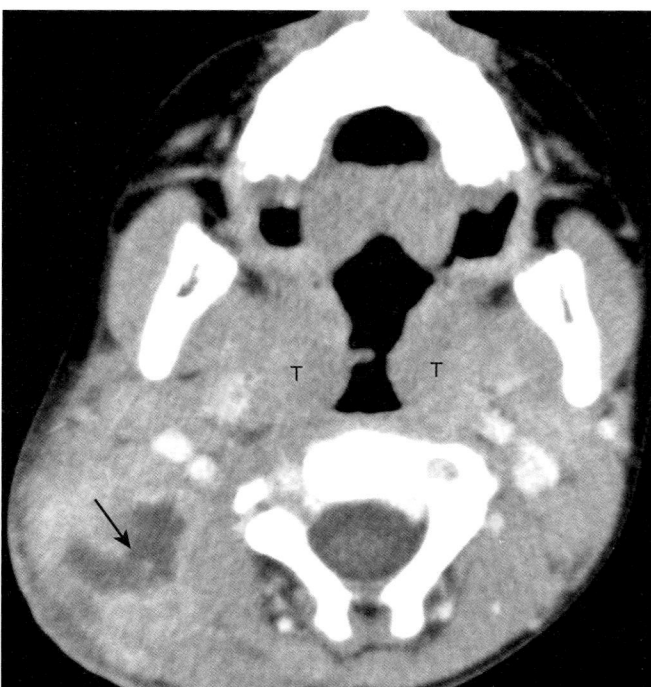

Fig. 48.5 Suppurative lymphadenitis in a 5-year-old female with neck swelling and redness. Contrast-enhanced CT image reveals a group of enlarged nodes in the right posterior triangle with central hypoattenuating necrosis *(arrow)*. Also, note the enlarged tonsils (T) in this child with recurrent tonsillitis. (From Lowe LH, Smith CJ. Infection and inflammation. In: Coley BD, ed. *Caffey's Pediatric Diagnostic Imaging*. 12th ed. Philadelphia: Elsevier; 2013;1:139.)

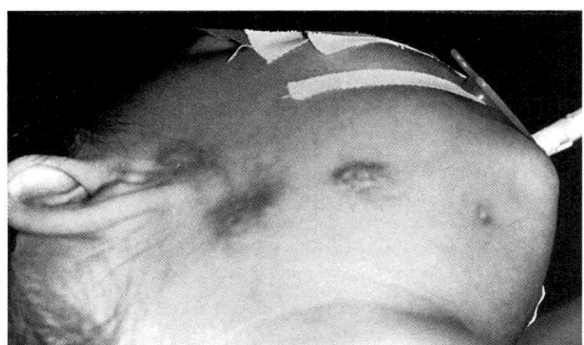

Fig. 48.6 Atypical mycobacterial infection frequently involves the submandibular triangle and preauricular regions. (From Rizzi MD, Wetmore RF, Potsic WP. Differential diagnosis of neck masses. In: Lesperance MM, ed. *Cummings Pediatric Otolaryngology*. Philadelphia: Elsevier; 2015:252, Fig. 19.14.)

(including severe acute respiratory syndrome-coronavirus 2 [SARS-CoV-2]), and enterovirus. EBV and CMV also commonly cause exudative pharyngitis and cervical lymphadenopathy. The chief complaint usually includes pain with swallowing and with talking, as well as tender, enlarged lymph nodes in the neck. Systemic manifestations, such as fever, myalgia, chills, and rhinorrhea, may also be present. An examination of the throat typically reveals a symmetrically erythematous posterior oropharynx with enlarged tonsils that often contain exudates. Exudates can be seen with both viral and bacterial causes of pharyngitis and adenopathy, and thus do not reliably discriminate between the two causes. Herpes stomatitis with mucocutaneous involvement and

TABLE 48.5 Differential Diagnosis of Atypical Lymphocytosis

Epstein-Barr virus primary infection (infectious mononucleosis)
Cytomegalovirus primary infection (heterophile-negative mononucleosis)*
Human herpesvirus 6 primary infection (roseola)
Primary HIV infection
Toxoplasmosis
Acute viral hepatitis
Rubella, mumps
Drug hypersensitivity reaction (e.g., phenytoin, sulfa) (DRESS)

*Cytomegalovirus is the most common cause of heterophile-negative mononucleosis.
DRESS, drug reaction, eosinophilia, systemic symptoms.
From Bennett JE, Dolin R, Blaser MJ. *Mandell, Douglas, and Bennett's Principles and Practice of Infectious Diseases*. 9th ed. Vol. 2. Philadelphia: Elsevier; 2020:1884, Table 138.8.

herpes pharyngitis with oropharyngeal vesicles are also associated with bilaterally enlarged, tender, nonerythematous cervical nodes.

Bacterial infection of the pharynx is also commonly associated with enlarged, tender cervical lymph nodes. Strains of group A β-hemolytic streptococci are the most common causes of such infections and are difficult to differentiate clinically from viral causes of pharyngitis and lymphadenopathy; thus, throat culture, PCR, or rapid antigen detection is necessary. An associated sandpapery rash and beefy-red tonsils with palatal petechiae are not usually seen with viral pathogens and should make the examiner consider group A streptococci and toxin-mediated scarlet fever as a likely cause. Other bacteria can cause pharyngitis and cervical adenopathy, including non–group A streptococci and anaerobic organisms, such as *Fusobacterium* species. Anaerobic organisms can lead to painful oral gingivitis or stomatitis and pharyngitis (**Vincent angina**) that may progress to peritonsillar abscess. Asymmetry in the tonsils and surrounding tissues, as well as deviation of the uvula away from the affected side, may be seen with peritonsillar abscesses, along with unilateral tender, enlarged cervical lymph nodes ipsilateral to the abscess. Complications of acute bacterial pharyngitis may also include **Lemierre syndrome**, the findings of which include high fever and unilateral lateral neck swelling that may be confused with adenopathy. Lemierre syndrome is due to septic thrombosis of the internal jugular vein (and pulmonary septic emboli), usually caused by invasion of the bloodstream by *Fusobacterium* organisms, and should lead to prompt hospitalization, blood cultures, treatment with intravenous antibiotics, and imaging of the internal jugular vein via Doppler flow ultrasonography or contrast-enhanced CT.

Acute cervical lymphadenitis—inflammation of the cervical lymph nodes with tender enlargement—is most likely to occur with group A streptococcal or *Staphylococcus aureus* infection. There may or may not be a history of sore throat or pharyngeal inflammation on examination. Infection with other oral bacteria, including non–group A streptococci and anaerobes such as *Fusobacterium* or *Arcanobacterium* species, may also occur, presumably with the pharynx as the portal of entry. Other common sites for acute lymphadenitis are the submandibular nodes. Usually, these nodes quickly diminish in size after institution of appropriate antibiotic therapy, providing some degree of retrospective diagnosis while simultaneously being therapeutic.

Suppuration and spontaneous drainage of the nodes are less common than adenitis and are not typically seen in the setting of viral infections. Acute suppurative cervical adenitis can be seen in infections of the face and scalp and is usually caused by infection with group A streptococci or *S. aureus*. Management of suppuration includes incision and drainage or excision of the suppurative node. Gram stain and bacterial, fungal, and mycobacterial cultures of the drainage should be obtained. If there is concern for mycobacterial disease, a tuberculin skin test should be placed and/or interferon-γ release assay should be performed. Total excision should be performed if atypical mycobacterial infection is suspected, because draining fistulas may form if a needle biopsy or partial resection is performed. Fine-needle aspiration may reduce the risk of sinus formation.

Infections of the extremities. Bacterial infections of the skin and soft tissues are common causes of localized lymphadenopathy and adenitis and can lead to axillary or inguinal adenopathy if these infections originate in the extremities. Primarily caused by group A β-hemolytic streptococci or *S. aureus*, these infections may drain into and inflame single or multiple regional lymph nodes. Any laceration or insect bite that becomes infected may yield adenopathy upstream in the nodal drainage basin of the infected site. Occasionally, penetrating injuries to the feet occurring through damp shoes or in wet areas may yield infections with other bacteria, such as *Pseudomonas aeruginosa*. These penetrating infections usually manifest with cellulitis or osteomyelitis; lymphadenopathy is noted during the physical examination. The most common sites of infection include the foot or leg, leading to unilateral inguinal lymphadenitis, and the hand or arm, causing axillary lymphadenitis or unilateral inflammation of the epitrochlear nodes. *Sporothrix schenckii*, a fungus found in soil and on plant surfaces, can also produce regional lymphadenopathy after a minor penetrating injury, such as pricking a finger or toe on a rose thorn. **Sporotrichosis** presents as a small nontender nodule at the site of entry that over days to weeks spreads via lymphatic channels, producing ulcerating nodules along the lymphatic drainage pathway and either axillary or inguinal adenopathy, depending on the site of inoculation.

Epstein-Barr virus infection. Infection with EBV is a common cause of both regional (bilateral cervical) and diffuse lymphadenopathy (see Chapter 2). This virus classically causes a mononucleosis syndrome in adolescents (Fig. 48.7), consisting of acute pharyngitis that may have a prolonged course, with tender and firm cervical adenopathy, malaise, fever, weight loss, and anorexia. Nearly half of patients will have generalized lymphadenopathy as well. More than 80% of patients have mild hepatitis (transaminitis) that is clinically silent but can be documented with liver enzyme studies; approximately 10% become jaundiced. Splenomegaly is present in more than 50% of patients and, in rare cases, progresses to splenic rupture. A small number of patients also have parapharyngeal and tonsillar lymphoid hyperplasia, which causes difficulty swallowing or breathing and can produce significant problems, leading to dehydration or airway obstruction. Small children with EBV infection often present with atypical symptoms or may be completely asymptomatic. In these children, fever and mild cervical adenopathy may be the major symptoms on presentation, or the child may be significantly ill with high fever and pharyngitis. In some, a nonspecific rash, appearing often after beginning empiric antibiotic therapy with penicillins, will suggest the diagnosis. Young children with acute EBV infection are more likely to have hepatosplenomegaly, rash, and eyelid edema than are young adults.

The diagnosis of EBV infection in older children focuses on the characteristic clinical syndrome and a relative lymphocytosis of 40–50% seen in the differential white blood cell count, with up to 20% atypical lymphocytes. Heterophile immunoglobulin M (IgM) antibodies, which are non-EBV directed and agglutinate sheep and horse red blood cells, are found in more than 80% of young adults with EBV and are at maximal titer 3–4 weeks after infection. Heterophile antibodies are rarely found in children younger than 5 years with EBV infections. In young children, antibody titers directed to specific EBV antigens are necessary to confirm the diagnosis

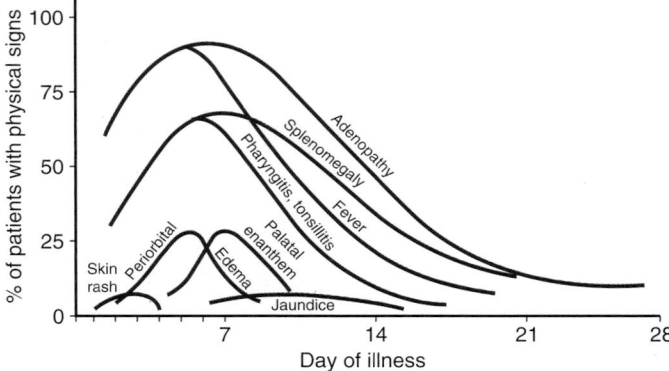

Fig. 48.7 The clinical course of acute Epstein-Barr mononucleosis. Adenopathy occurs early in the infection and can persist for weeks. (Modified from Rapp CE, Hewston JF. Infectious mononucleosis and the Epstein-Barr virus. *Am J Dis Child*. 1978;132:78.)

(Table 48.6). Temporally, IgM and immunoglobulin G (IgG) antibodies develop against the viral capsid antigen (VCA) first, followed by antibodies directed against early antigen (EA). Antibodies to nuclear antigens develop weeks later and, if present with EA IgG, are indicative of infection in the recent past. Approximately 20% of children present after the VCA IgM has already declined. In these children, VCA and EA IgG are present.

Organ transplant and other immunosuppressed patients may develop a **lymphoproliferative syndrome** due to EBV that presents with generalized lymphadenopathy, hepatosplenomegaly, and fever. Diagnosis is based on the EBV viral load determined by PCR on blood.

Because group A streptococcal infection can present in a similar manner, or be present simultaneously with EBV infection, and because other viruses can cause pharyngitis and tender, enlarged cervical lymph nodes, differentiating these various causes of pharyngitis and lymphadenopathy is important. Acute streptococcal pharyngitis can be identified on throat culture, PCR, or antigen testing and improves after institution of penicillin therapy; EBV infections do not improve with antibiotics, tend to result in a diffuse rash if treated with penicillins, and have a more prolonged clinical course. In addition, severe malaise and splenomegaly do not occur with most bacterial or viral causes of pharyngitis and cervical lymphadenopathy, and these findings should prompt the clinician to consider EBV infection. Similarly, most viral causes of cervical adenopathy and pharyngitis, with the exception of CMV, are not associated with the brisk atypical lymphocytosis commonly seen with EBV infections, and they are not usually associated with abnormal liver function results.

Cytomegalovirus infection. Infection with CMV in immunocompetent children can result in a mononucleosis syndrome with atypical leukocytosis and lymphadenopathy. CMV mononucleosis is associated with fever and malaise similar to that seen in EBV; in contrast to EBV, CMV mononucleosis does not usually cause severe, exudative tonsillopharyngitis or the production of heterophile-specific or EBV-specific antibodies. Women who are pregnant when they have primary CMV infections are at risk of delivering a child with **congenital CMV infection** through transplacental infection; approximately 10% of these neonates will have severe systemic findings. Lymphadenopathy may be present in congenital CMV but is not a common finding. Intrapartum transmission via cervical secretions or postpartum transmission via breast milk typically does not result in clinically apparent infection. Identifying CMV in the urine of the neonate in the first week of life confirms congenital infection.

TABLE 48.6   Antibodies to Epstein-Barr Virus

Antibody Specificity	Time of Appearance in Infectious Mononucleosis	Percentage of EBV-Induced Mononucleosis Cases with Antibody	Persistence	Comments
Viral Capsid Antigens				
IgM VCA	At clinical presentation	100	4–8 wk	Highly sensitive and specific major diagnostic utility
IgG VCA	At clinical presentation	100	Lifelong	High titer at presentation and lifelong persistence make IgG VCA more useful as epidemiologic tool than as diagnostic tool in individual cases
Early Antigens				
Anti-EA-D	Peaks at 3–4 wk after onset	70	3–6 mo	Correlated with severe disease; also seen in nasopharyngeal carcinoma
Anti-EA-R	2 wk to several months after onset	Low	2 mo to >3 yr	Occasionally seen with unusually severe or protracted illness, also seen in African Burkitt lymphoma
Latent Antigen				
EBV nuclear antigen	3–4 wk after onset	100	Lifelong	Late appearance helpful in diagnosis of heterophile-negative cases

EA, early antigen; EBV, Epstein-Barr virus; IgG, immunoglobulin G; IgM immunoglobulin M; VCA, viral capsid antigen.
From Bennett JE, Dolin R, Blaser MJ. *Mandell, Douglas, and Bennett's Principles and Practice of Infectious Diseases.* 9th ed. Vol. 2. Philadelphia: Elsevier; 2020:1884, Table 138.9.

The diagnosis in older children is usually made serologically, in tests measuring both IgM and IgG antibodies directed to CMV. Simultaneous testing for EBV may reveal cross-reactivity, with some patients with positive CMV titers also demonstrating low-level positivity for EBV; a similar phenomenon may be seen in patients with EBV who demonstrate low-level cross-reactivity with CMV. Viral culture and nucleic acid amplification assays can also identify CMV from blood, throat swab, and urine specimens. Although CMV culture (especially from the urine) is frequently positive in children with CMV infection, many children, especially those in daycare, are silently infected and excrete CMV in the absence of clinical signs and symptoms. Therefore, CMV culture is less useful in the toddler age group.

Cat-scratch disease. Cat-scratch disease is caused by a small gram-negative bacillus, *B. henselae*, which can also cause bacillary angiomatosis in patients with HIV infection. Cat-scratch disease occurs several days after the scratch or bite of an infected cat or kitten. A papule at the site of the trauma usually develops, followed 1–3 weeks later by regional lymphadenopathy; there is no lymphangitis. Most patients with cat-scratch disease have a single enlarged, usually nonsuppurative lymph node. Nodes may be tender, particularly in the up to 30% of patients whose nodes suppurate. Axillary nodes are the most common to be enlarged, likely secondary to the upper extremities being the part of the body most frequently scratched or bitten. The next most common sites for adenopathy are the neck and jaw, followed by the inguinal region. Although single nodes are most commonly affected, regional adenopathy may also occur. Generalized lymphadenopathy is unusual in the immunocompetent host.

Approximately half the patients have low-grade fever and malaise, but a small number have high fevers (>39.5°C) and more severe systemic symptoms. In most patients, the swollen, inflamed nodes regress spontaneously within several weeks, though almost one-third of patients progress to have purulent drainage that is culture negative by standard techniques. Uncommon complications include a spontaneously resolving encephalopathy, erythema nodosum, oculoglandular syndrome of Parinaud (in which *B. henselae* is inoculated into the eye and causes conjunctivitis and preauricular adenopathy), thrombocytopenia, hepatitis or splenitis with granulomas, transverse myelitis, and

in rare cases osteolytic bone lesions. Other causes of **oculoglandular syndrome** include tularemia, adenoviruses, and enteroviruses.

The diagnosis is based on the history of contact with kittens or cats and the classic clinical manifestations; evaluation should include a careful search for an entrance site papule. Confirmatory testing is difficult, as *B. henselae* is a fastidious organism and is difficult to isolate via conventional culture techniques. Acute and convalescent antibody titers are typically employed, though the clinician should exercise caution in interpretation given the high rate of seroprevalence in the general population and the potential for cross-reactivity with other infections. Pathologic samples of tissue from the involved node may provide further evidence if they demonstrate granulomas, central necrosis, and organisms on Warthin-Starry silver stain. The decision to perform a biopsy is usually predicated on there being no clear history of a preceding contact with a cat or kitten or when the presentation is atypical and cannot be differentiated from other, more serious illnesses, such as mycobacterial adenitis.

Chronic granulomatous disease. Chronic granulomatous disease (see Chapter 54) comprises a group of rare inherited disorders of neutrophil function, characterized by recurrent pyogenic infections that are often accompanied by lymphadenopathy and/or abscess formation. Most cases are inherited in an X-linked manner; the remining one-third are autosomal recessive. Chronic granulomatous disease should be considered in a young child (often a male) who presents with recurrent fevers and infection, pneumonia, adenopathy, and abdominal pain. Family history often reveals another relative with the disease or includes a death from an infection in a young child. Common pathogens contain catalase and include *S. aureus* and *Aspergillus* species.

The diagnosis is established via neutrophil function tests, such as nitroblue tetrazolium testing, which demonstrate the defective neutrophil oxidation. Positive findings on neutrophil function tests are confirmed via molecular genetic analysis that demonstrates pathogenic variants in genes that encode subunits of phagocyte nicotinamide adenine dinucleotide phosphate (NADPH) oxidase: X-linked disease is caused by pathogenic variants in *CYBB*; autosomal recessive disease is caused by pathogenic variants in *CYBA*, *NCF1*, *NCF2*, and *NCF4*.

Human immunodeficiency virus. Initial infection with HIV may manifest as a heterophile-negative mononucleosis-like acute retroviral syndrome consisting of diffuse lymphadenopathy, fever, sore throat, rash, myalgia, diarrhea, leukopenia, thrombocytopenia, and general malaise. Patients with HIV infection who are not diagnosed and treated go on to have weight loss or poor weight gain and acquire thrush and other opportunistic infections, such as pneumonia caused by *Pneumocystis jirovecii*; the presence of such infections should prompt consideration of congenital or acquired immunodeficiency (see Chapter 54). HIV-infected children are also more likely than immunocompetent hosts to have other infectious causes of lymphadenopathy, such as tuberculosis, atypical mycobacterium, CMV, or fungi, or noninfectious causes, such as lymphoma or Kaposi sarcoma (human herpesvirus type 8 [HHV-8]). *Regional* lymphadenopathy is not a common manifestation of HIV infection unless the regional adenopathy represents a distinct focal infection. The diagnosis of HIV infection is typically established via a rapid combined antibody/antigen immunoassay that detects antibodies to HIV-1 and HIV-2, as well as the p24 antigen present in early stages of HIV-1 infection. Patients for whom this combined immunoassay is negative should not require further testing unless there is concern for very early infection or recent significant exposure, in which case HIV-1 nucleic acid testing should be performed immediately and the immunoassay repeated after a short interval. Patients for whom the initial immunoassay is positive require further testing to determine whether infection is due to HIV-1 or HIV-2. Negative or indeterminate results on this further testing should be followed by nucleic acid amplification testing for HIV-1 or by repeating the testing algorithm if HIV-2 is suspected.

Mycobacterial infections. Tubercular cervical adenitis is not common in the United States, though can be associated with ingestion of raw, contaminated milk and infection with *M. bovis.* Regional or diffuse lymphadenopathy caused by infection with *Mycobacterium tuberculosis* is also unusual in nonendemic nations; it is increasing in frequency in children in the United States as a result of an increase in the number of adults actively infected with tuberculosis. This increase is attributable to several issues, including immigration from endemic areas, reduction in tuberculosis control programs, the likelihood of HIV-infected individuals to have a high mycobacterial burden, noncompliance by infected individuals with multidrug treatment regimens, and drug resistance by the organism. Most adenitis caused by mycobacteria in the United States is caused by atypical strains that are not serious pathogens in the immunocompetent host.

Several historical and clinical criteria can be used to differentiate tuberculous adenitis from atypical mycobacterial infections. Most children with tuberculosis have a history of exposure to an adult with active tuberculosis. Infection with atypical mycobacteria is more common in the southern parts of the United States. Children with tuberculous adenitis may have hilar lymphadenopathy because the lungs are usually the source of primary infection. Evidence of extralymphatic disease is also common in children with tuberculosis; such disease includes pneumonia, pleural effusions, bone marrow suppression, liver function abnormalities, and disseminated (miliary) disease. Miliary tuberculosis may manifest with diffuse lymphadenopathy and should be considered if pulmonary infiltrates and systemic symptoms are present. Such extralymphatic disease and diffuse lymphadenopathy are rare in immunocompetent children with adenitis caused by atypical mycobacteria but may occur in the setting of HIV infection.

The most common mycobacterial infection in children in the United States is the infection of the lymph nodes with the **atypical mycobacteria**, primarily *Mycobacterium avium-intracellulare* complex, *Mycobacterium kansasii*, *Mycobacterium scrofulaceum*, and *Mycobacterium marinum.* The involved lymph nodes are usually tender, unilateral, and

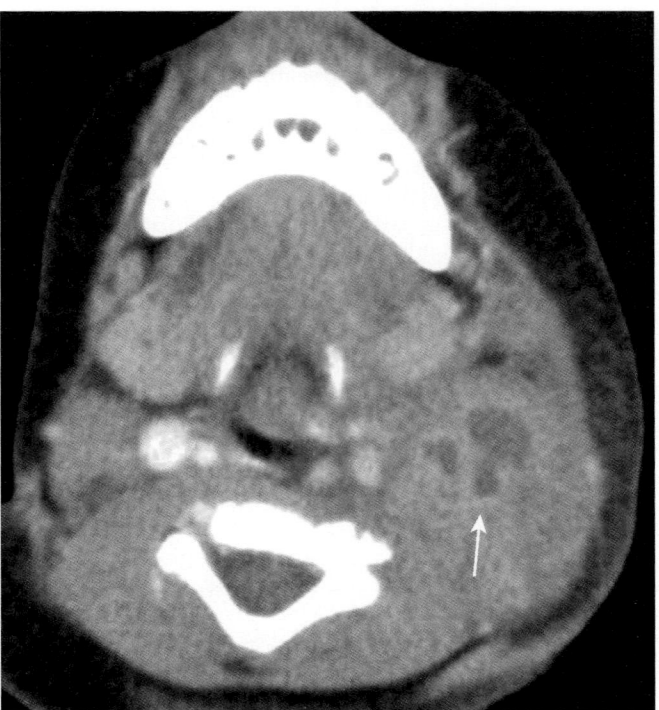

Fig. 48.8 Nontuberculous mycobacterial infection in a 10-year-old male with left neck swelling. Axial contrast-enhanced CT image shows a cluster of enlarged nodes in the left neck containing low-attenuation necrotic centers *(arrow).* (From Lowe LH, Smith CJ. Infection and inflammation. In: Coley BD, ed. *Caffey's Pediatric Diagnostic Imaging.* 12th ed. Philadelphia: Elsevier; 2013;1:139.)

cervical in most infections, presumably because the organism enters via the oropharynx. Most frequently, a previously healthy child presents with a mass that is really unilateral lymphadenitis or adenopathy in the cervical, submandibular, or submaxillary region (Figs. 48.6 and 48.8). Although fever may be present, other significant systemic symptoms are usually not present. In a small number of patients, the affected node spontaneously ruptures and drains before the visit to the physician. The drainage is not usually grossly purulent and may be a clue that atypical mycobacteria are the cause of the infected node. Regional adenopathy may also be seen after immunization with bacille Calmette-Guérin (BCG) vaccine.

The gold standard for diagnosis of lymphadenitis caused by atypical mycobacteria is acid-fast staining and culture of the excised node. Incision and drainage of these nodes may lead to chronically draining sinus tracts, which may leave scars; thus, this method is contraindicated. The usual scenario involves a young, preschool-aged child with an enlarged cervical node (or nodes) that responds poorly to antibiotics. The child has no history of contact with cats and is otherwise well. A tuberculin skin test often yields 5–9 mm of induration because atypical mycobacteria have antigens cross-reactive to those of tuberculosis. This amount of induration is considered indeterminate for tuberculosis in low-risk patients and suggests that the adenopathy is caused by an atypical mycobacterium. **Interferon-γ release assays** will be positive for *M. tuberculosis, M. bovis,* and some atypical mycobacterium (*M. marinum, M. kansasii*) but will be negative for BCG and infection with *M. avium-intracellulare* complex. Gradual resolution of lymphadenitis sometimes occurs in children with atypical mycobacterial infections. Excisional biopsy is not necessary if the diagnosis is made presumptively from skin test results of <10 mm induration, if other infections are ruled out, if resolution occurs, and if the child is at low risk for infection with *M. tuberculosis* (see Chapter 3). If the node does not improve, continues to enlarge, or spontaneously drains, excision is recommended and is usually curative. Fine-needle aspiration (for culture and acid-fast staining) may also be used if the node is in an area where excision is impractical.

Toxoplasmosis. *Toxoplasma gondii* is a protozoan organism that is a parasite of cats. Many other animals, including humans, can be incidentally and chronically infected hosts in which the parasite cannot complete its life cycle. Human acquisition of toxoplasmosis can result from contact with cat feces or soil that contains oocysts, which infect the host upon ingestion. Alternatively, the ingestion of tissue cyst-containing raw or undercooked meat, particularly lamb or pork, may lead to infection. Adults in the United States are more likely to be infected from ingestion of raw meat than from contact with oocysts in cat feces or soil. Finally, infection can be transmitted to the fetus, especially when a pregnant woman is acutely infected with toxoplasmosis. Although many fetal infections are asymptomatic, transplacental infection with toxoplasmosis can result in severe neurologic damage, chorioretinitis, aseptic meningitis, and significant systemic illness manifesting with the classic triad of hepatosplenomegaly, intracranial calcifications, and hydrocephalus. Although lymphadenopathy can occur in the newborn with congenital toxoplasmosis, it is a more common symptom of acute toxoplasmosis in older children and young adults.

The most common symptoms in children who acquire toxoplasmosis are lymphadenopathy, fever, malaise, myalgia, and pharyngitis. Most commonly affected are the anterior and posterior cervical and axillary nodes, which may be tender; involvement is usually bilateral. The lymph node enlargement seen in toxoplasmosis is caused by reticular hyperplasia and inflammation. Most laboratory results are normal, but the white blood cell count may show an absolute lymphocytosis with atypical lymphocytes, which can cause confusion with EBV, HIV, or CMV mononucleosis.

The diagnosis is made primarily with serologic studies. Various diagnostic techniques can be used on the patient's serum, including indirect immunofluorescence, complement fixation, and enzyme-linked immunosorbent assay. A fourfold rise in IgG titer or the presence of IgM antibodies is diagnostic. In neonatal infections, tests measuring IgM have become more sensitive and specific. If biopsy is performed, actual parasite forms can sometimes be demonstrated. Antigen tests and cultures that grow the parasite are also available but primarily on an investigational level.

Syphilis. Syphilis, caused by the spirochete *Treponema pallidum*, is common in the United States (see Chapter 21). The natural course of noncongenital syphilis includes three major clinical manifestations:
- Primary syphilis, in which the individual develops a painless chancre at the site of inoculation
- Secondary syphilis, in which the organism disseminates hematogenously to many organs
- Tertiary syphilis, in which gummatous lesions develop in end organs, such as the brain, heart, and bones

Lymphadenopathy can be seen as one of the manifestations of syphilis in several situations. In primary syphilis, in which the inoculation site is usually the genital area, regional lymphadenopathy with painless, firm nodes occurs at the time that a chancre is observed. Inguinal adenopathy in an adolescent who is sexually active mandates further examination and work-up for sexually transmitted infections such as syphilis. In secondary syphilis, the organism has disseminated, with multiple organs involved. The classic manifestations are protean and usually include nonvesicular rashes and systemic symptoms that may include fever, malaise, anorexia, and weight loss. Lymphadenopathy, regional or generalized, is common and often includes epitrochlear nodes.

Pregnant women with syphilis who are untreated readily transmit the disease to the fetus, causing congenital syphilis, often with significant sequelae. Infants with congenital syphilis may also have generalized lymphadenopathy, although this finding is less common than other systemic symptoms, such as hepatosplenomegaly, snuffles, and periosteal reactive disease.

The diagnosis has been complicated by the inability to grow the organism in vitro. Dark-field examination of exudate from a chancre or other superficial lesion, nasal discharge, or placental tissue shows numerous spirochetes, but dark-field methods are often unavailable to routine laboratories. The organism can be detected via nucleic acid–based testing, though such assays have not been approved for clinical use; serologic assays continue to be the primary mode of diagnosis. Nontreponemal serologic studies rely on host production of antibodies to nonspecific lipoidal host tissue antigens that arise as a result of infection with the spirochete. These tests include the Venereal Disease Research Laboratory (VDRL) test, the serologic test for syphilis, and the rapid plasma reagin (RPR) test. Levels of these antibodies decline after adequate treatment and are useful in confirming eradication of the infection. False-positive reactions can occur, particularly in individuals with connective tissue disorders or mononucleosis. False-negative results can be seen in early primary syphilis, in latent infection, late in congenital syphilis, or in the presence of high antibody concentrations, in which case retesting a diluted specimen can produce a true-positive result. In contrast to nontreponemal assays, the fluorescent treponemal antibody absorption test (FTA-ABS) measures antibodies directed specifically to *T. pallidum* and can be used as a confirmatory test in individuals with positive results on nontreponemal tests. These antibodies usually remain present for the life of the infected individual, even if the patient receives adequate therapy. Thus, in contrast to nontreponemal tests, the FTA-ABS has little use in monitoring the efficacy of treatment.

Acute leukemia, lymphoma, and other malignancies. Lymphadenopathy is frequently among the presenting findings in patients with leukemia or lymphoma. Enlarged lymph nodes may be noted in an isolated, regional, or generalized distribution, with or without classic systemic symptoms, such as fever, malaise, night sweats, weight loss, and anorexia. Malignant nodes are usually firm, rubbery, fixed, and nontender, and may be matted. Unlike many of the acute lymphadenopathies caused by infectious agents, most lymph nodes that are malignant increase in size gradually. Additional findings suggestive of malignancy include age older than 10 years, size >2.5 cm, duration >6 weeks (and increasing in size), and supraclavicular location.

Approximately 50% of children with **acute lymphoblastic leukemia** have adenopathy at the time of diagnosis. Nodal disease may be either generalized or localized to regional nodal groups, often the cervical chains. Nodal disease is frequently accompanied by other signs and symptoms, including fevers, malaise, weight loss, pallor, bone pain, petechiae and bruising, splenomegaly, or hepatomegaly. The CBC usually demonstrates anemia, thrombocytopenia, leukocytosis or leukopenia, circulating blasts, or some combination thereof. Some patients may have normal peripheral blood laboratory results on initial evaluation. Acute myelogenous leukemia is less common in children but may manifest in a similar manner. Bone marrow biopsy and aspiration must be performed, and the findings are diagnostic.

Non-Hodgkin lymphoma is a relatively common childhood malignancy and often manifests with mediastinal or pleural disease. Adenopathy in the supraclavicular, cervical, or axillary regions is usually present and may occur in the absence of chest involvement. Systemic symptoms are variable at the time of diagnosis. Lymph nodes, as in other malignancies, tend to be firm, nontender, and rubbery, and their size may increase relatively rapidly over several weeks. Because lymphoblastic lymphoma may represent a variant of acute lymphoblastic leukemia, the signs and symptoms of leukemia and lymphoma may merge. Non-Hodgkin lymphoma of B-cell origin (Burkitt and

TABLE 48.7	Ulceroglandular Disorders
Anthrax	
Tularemia	
Herpes simplex	
Pasteurella multocida (dog or cat bite)	
Rickettsialpox	
Tick-borne lymphadenopathy syndrome	
Mediterranean spotted fever	
African tick bite fever	
Typhus	
Cat-scratch disease	
BCG immunization	
Spirillary rat-bite fever	
Plague	
Nocardiosis	
Actinomycosis	
Cutaneous diphtheria	
Cutaneous coccidioidomycosis	
Cutaneous histoplasmosis	
Cutaneous leishmaniasis	
Cutaneous tetanus	
Monkeypox	

BCG, bacille Calmette-Guérin.

non-Burkitt lymphoma) in children in the United States usually originates in an intraabdominal site, and regional adenopathy, if present, is then in the inguinal or iliac regions. The African variety of Burkitt lymphoma often manifests as an expanding jaw mass.

Hodgkin disease often presents with painless cervical or supraclavicular lymphadenopathy in older school-aged children and adolescents. Nodes are firmer than those seen in patients whose nodes are enlarged in reaction to infections. In a small number of children with Hodgkin disease, the size of the nodes may wax and wane for several months before a definitive diagnosis is made. Supraclavicular nodes usually indicate intrathoracic disease, which is present in 60–70% of patients at the time of diagnosis. Axillary or inguinal nodes may also be the sites of presenting lymphadenopathy. Approximately 30% of patients with Hodgkin disease have systemic symptoms at presentation, including fatigue, weight loss, fevers, night sweats, and poor appetite. Some patients with Hodgkin disease also have unusual symptoms, such as pruritus, hemolytic anemia, and chest pain after alcohol ingestion. Such systemic symptoms with lymphadenopathy are red flags for immediate work-up for malignancy. Diagnosis is confirmed by biopsy of involved nodes and/or bone marrow aspiration, if the tumor has spread to the bone marrow.

Disseminated neuroblastoma may manifest as diffuse adenopathy in younger children. Such children often have primary adrenal or paraspinal masses with bone metastasis and have nonspecific systemic symptoms, abdominal mass, bone pain, and, sometimes, symptoms of spinal cord compression. Other tumors, such as rhabdomyosarcoma and thyroid cancer, manifest in rare cases with lymphadenopathy caused by local or disseminated metastasis.

Ulceroglandular disorders. Ulceroglandular (lymphocutaneous) disorders usually involve an initial injury or bite to an extremity with a resulting cutaneous lesion (ulcer, eschar, or papule) and enlarged regional nodes, with or without lymphangitis (Table 48.7). In some, the cutaneous lesion is secondary to hematogenous spread; in these circumstances the lymph node enlargement may then be generalized (e.g., monkeypox).

Kimura disease. Kimura disease is characterized by the development of benign, nontender subcutaneous nodules in the head and neck with associated regional lymphadenopathy, blood and tissue eosinophilia, and elevations in serum immunoglobulin E. Lesions typically appear in adolescence or early adulthood; the condition is more common in

biological males of Asian descent. Biopsies should be performed to rule out malignancy. Histologic specimens show massive eosinophilic infiltration of the nodules and affected lymph nodes. Up to 60% of affected patients may develop kidney disease, oftentimes nephrotic syndrome. Treatment modalities include surgery, radiation therapy, and glucocorticoids, though are typically reserved for patients with functional or aesthetic impairments secondary to the lesions.

Kikuchi-Fujimoto disease (histiocytic necrotizing lymphadenitis). Kikuchi disease is a rare, usually self-limiting disease with onset in late childhood through early adolescence, usually presenting as firm unilateral posterior cervical adenitis, fever, malaise, elevated ESR, atypical lymphocytosis, and leukopenia. Nodes are often as large as 3 cm, though some can be larger. Nodes are painful or tender in approximately 50% of cases, may be multiple in number, and must be differentiated from lymphoma. Node involvement may occasionally be bilateral or present in locations other than the cervical region, such as in the axillary or supraclavicular regions.

The etiology is presumed to be secondary to an abnormal immune response; diagnosis is established via lymph node biopsy. Histologic features include necrosis with karyorrhexis (i.e., fragmentation of the nucleus with breakup of chromatin), a histiocytic infiltrate, crescentic plasmacytoid monocytes, and an absence of neutrophils. The disease is self-limiting and usually spontaneously resolves within 6 months, although relapses may occur. Therapy with systemic steroids is reserved for cases with severe symptoms. Autoimmune diseases have been associated with Kikuchi disease, most commonly systemic lupus erythematosus.

Sinus histiocytosis with massive lymphadenopathy (Rosai-Dorfman disease). This rare non-Langerhans histiocytosis typically presents with massive, bilateral, painless, and mobile cervical lymphadenopathy with associated fever, leukocytosis, and elevated ESR; polyclonal elevation of IgG may be present. Night sweats and weight loss are common; autoimmune hemolytic anemia is a less common associated finding.

Other nodal chains may be involved. Extranodal disease occurs in 40% of cases; the most common sites are the skin, followed by the nasal cavity and sinuses, palate, orbit, bone (lytic lesions), and central nervous system. Patients presenting with features suggestive of Rosai-Dorfman disease (RDD) should undergo a comprehensive evaluation aimed at identifying conditions that may predispose to RDD and excluding alternate diagnoses such as malignancy or hemophagocytic lymphohistiocytosis (see Chapter 54), as well as establishing the extent of any extranodal involvement. Predisposing conditions include a family history (pathogenic variants in *SLC29A3* and *TNFRSF* have been associated with RDD), concurrent lymphoma, autoimmune disease (in particular, systemic lupus erythematosus and juvenile idiopathic arthritis), and elevated IgG4 levels. Diagnosis requires biopsy: histology demonstrates pale S100[+], CD68[+], and CD1a[−] histiocytes containing engulfed lymphocytes. These histologic findings, in conjunction with expected clinical features, are diagnostic. Spontaneous remission may occur after a prolonged course, though most patients benefit from treatment, which may include glucocorticoids, surgical resection, immunomodulators such as sirolimus, chemotherapy, or radiation therapy.

Castleman disease (angiofollicular lymph node hyperplasia). Castleman disease is an uncommon lymphoproliferative disease usually seen in adolescents or young adults. Enlargement of a single node, most often in the mediastinum or abdomen, is the most common localized presentation. Some patients may have fever, night sweats, weight loss, and fatigue. Management includes surgery and/or radiation therapy.

Multicentric Castleman disease is a systemic lymphoproliferative disorder that causes lymphadenopathy, hepatosplenomegaly, fever, anemia, overexpression of interleukin-6 (IL-6), and polyclonal hypergammaglobulinemia. Multicentric Castleman disease is classified as being associated with human herpesvirus-8 infection or as being idiopathic;

rarely, some patients with idiopathic multicentric Castleman disease develop a potentially life-threatening variant characterized by *t*hrombocytopenia, *a*nasarca, *f*evers, *r*eticulin myelofibrosis, and *o*rganomegaly (**TAFRO syndrome**). Treatment options include glucocorticoids, chemotherapy, and immunomodulating therapy directed against CD20 or the IL-6 pathway.

Kawasaki disease. Kawasaki disease (see Chapter 53) is a medium-vessel vasculitis of childhood of uncertain etiology. The hallmark of Kawasaki disease is a high, unremitting, and prolonged fever of 5 or more days' duration in the presence of specific associated symptoms; diagnostic criteria for classic Kawasaki disease include four or more of the following: cervical lymphadenopathy that is typically >1.5 cm in diameter and unilateral; a polymorphous rash; bilateral nonexudative bulbar conjunctivitis; extremity changes (acutely, palmar erythema or swelling of the hands and feet; subacutely, periungual peeling of the fingers and toes), and changes in the lips or oral cavity (e.g., redness, lip cracking, strawberry tongue, mucosal injection).

Mimics of Kawasaki disease include certain viral infections such as adenovirus, though the identification of a specific viral pathogen in the setting of findings strongly consistent with Kawasaki disease does not preclude the possibility that the virus induced an aberrant host response resulting in Kawasaki disease. Features of Kawasaki disease are also shared with **multisystem inflammatory syndrome in children (MIS-C) associated with COVID-19 infection.** Estimated to affect <1% of children infected with SARS-CoV-2, MIS-C typically presents with prolonged fevers of approximately 5 days' duration,

prominent gastrointestinal symptoms (e.g., abdominal pain, vomiting, or diarrhea), rash, altered sensorium, mucous membrane changes, and conjunctivitis. Lymphadenopathy is a less frequent presenting symptom and is found in approximately 15% of cases. Some patients with MIS-C present critically ill, with findings suggestive of toxic shock syndrome, and have hypotension, myocardial dysfunction, serositis, and multisystem organ involvement; coagulation abnormalities may also present (see Chapter 53).

MIMICS OF HEAD AND NECK LYMPHADENOPATHY: HEAD AND NECK MASSES

Given the density of anatomic structures within the head and neck and the frequency with which these structures may be confused for enlarged lymph nodes, congenital and acquired lesions of these head and neck structures, many of which are benign, may mimic lymphadenopathy and deserve consideration. Primary among these structures and lesions are the salivary glands, including the parotid gland, as well the thyroid gland, branchial cleft cysts, hemangiomas, cystic hygromas, and non-nodal soft tissue malignancy. History and physical examination should provide sufficient information to arrive at an appropriate differential diagnosis and evaluation strategy of these mimics. Important factors in distinguishing lymphadenopathy from non-nodal congenital or acquired lesions of the head and neck include the age of the child, anatomic position, presence of signs of inflammation, associated symptoms, and the time course of the development of symptoms (Figs. 48.9 and 48.10).

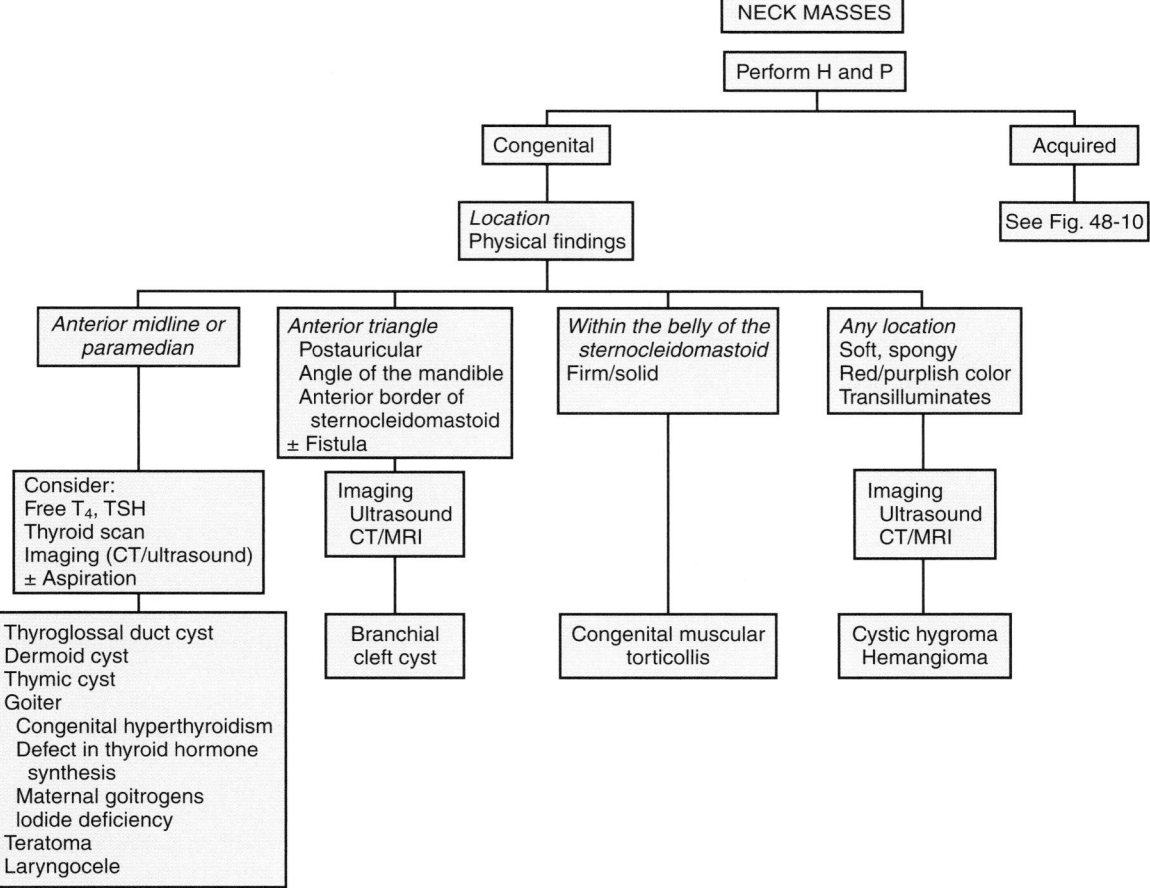

Fig. 48.9 Diagnostic algorithm for congenital neck masses. H and P, history and physical examination; T$_4$, thyroxine; TSH, thyroid-stimulating hormone. (Modified from Pomeranz AJ, Sabnis S, Busey SL, et al. *Pediatric Decision-Making Strategies.* 2nd ed. Philadelphia: Elsevier; 2016:9.)

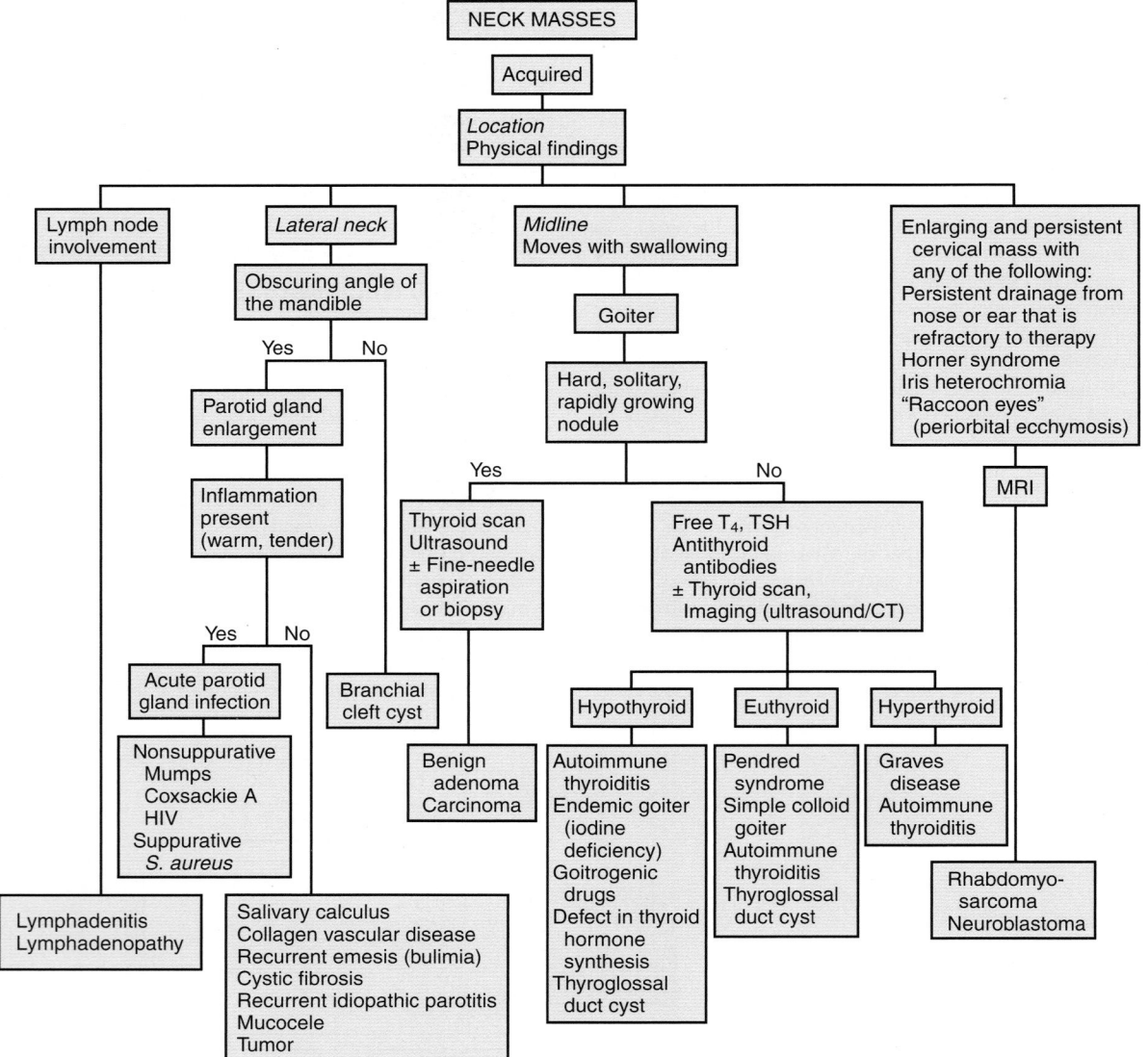

Fig. 48.10 Diagnostic algorithm for acquired neck masses. T₄, thyroxine; TSH, thyroid-stimulating hormone. (Modified from Pomeranz AJ, Sabnis S, Busey SL, et al. *Pediatric Decision-Making Strategies.* 2nd ed. Philadelphia: Elsevier; 2016:11.)

Salivary Gland Lesions

Enlargement and inflammation of the salivary glands may be mistaken for lymphadenopathy and most frequently affect the parotid glands in children. Infectious etiologies include acute suppurative sialadenitis, which is typically caused by *S. aureus*, as well as viral mumps or HIV-related parotitis. Noninfectious inflammatory conditions may be primary, part of a systemic inflammatory disorder, or related to obstruction (i.e., sialolithiasis). Diagnosis involves distinguishing the involved salivary gland from adjacent structures such as submandibular lymph nodes, identifying findings on physical examination that suggest salivary gland involvement (such as the expression of pus into the oral cavity from the salivary duct upon massaging an acutely suppurative gland or the inability to express normal saliva from the duct when obstructed), and obtaining imaging (CT, MRI, or ultrasound) and fine-needle aspiration as needed, particularly if there is concern for solid malignancy.

Thyroid Lesions

Diffuse enlargement of the thyroid gland, or **goiter**, may present at any age, including in neonates. Goiter is typically readily distinguished from cervical lymphadenopathy by virtue of its midline location and, in older children able to follow commands, its mobility upon mimicking a swallow during physical examination. Congenital goiter may be due to inborn defects in thyroid hormone biosynthesis, developmental anomaly, or exposure to maternal antithyroid antibodies or antithyroid medications given for maternal hyperthyroidism. In older children and adolescents in areas of the world with adequate iodine supplementation, goiter is typically due to autoimmune thyroiditis; however, iodine-deficiency goiter is the most common cause worldwide. Acquired goiter is associated with hypothyroidism, hyperthyroidism, or a euthyroid state. A diffusely enlarged thyroid gland without nodules should be investigated with determination of the free thyroxine and thyroid-stimulating hormone levels, assessment for the presence of

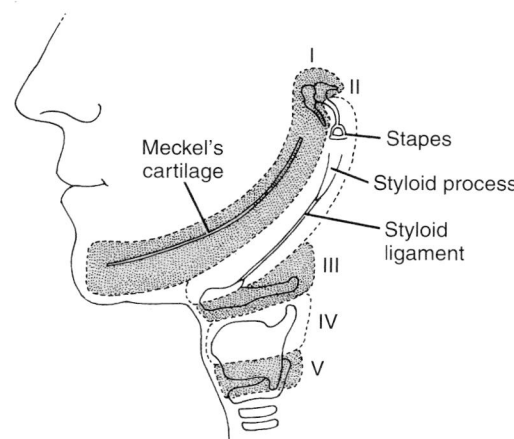

Fig. 48.11 Skeletal derivatives of the branchial arches. (From Flint PW, Haughey BH, Lund VJ, et al., eds. *Cummings Otolaryngology Head & Neck Surgery.* 5th ed. Philadelphia: Elsevier; 2010:2583, Fig. 181.10.)

antithyroid antibodies, and consideration of ultrasound imaging (see Fig. 48.10). Isolated thyroid nodules may be more difficult to distinguish from lymphadenopathy, suggest benign adenoma or carcinoma, and should be investigated with a thyroid scan, ultrasound, and either fine-needle aspiration or biopsy to obtain histologic diagnosis.

Developmental Anomalies and Soft Tissue Tumors

Infantile hemangioma (lymphangioma) is a venous malformation that typically enlarges to the point of being noticed within the first year of life. Superficial lesions are often readily distinguished by their red, blue, or violaceous appearance and by being blanchable. Deeper lesions may be mistaken for an enlarged lymph node if overlying skin changes are not overt, requiring ultrasonography to establish the diagnosis. Isolated lesions tend to spontaneously regress in early childhood, though lesions that are large or that have negative functional or aesthetic sequelae may be treated, oftentimes with enteral propranolol. Multiple head and neck hemangiomas may be associated with PHACE (*p*osterior fossa anomalies, *h*emangioma, *a*rterial anomalies, *c*ardiac anomalies, and *e*ye anomalies) syndrome (see Chapter 37).

Cystic hygroma typically presents as a large translucent soft tissue mass in the lateral neck, axilla, or chest wall that is often detected on prenatal ultrasound or noted at the time of or shortly after birth. Though a malformation of lymphatic vessels, the lesion is rarely confused for lymphadenopathy unless small. Cystic hygroma is associated with chromosomal abnormalities such as trisomy 21, Turner syndrome, and Noonan syndrome in approximately 50% of cases.

Branchial cleft cysts make up approximately 20% of congenital neck masses and often remain asymptomatic until late childhood, when they become infected, typically by oropharyngeal flora or sinopulmonary pathogens. Given that the majority are located anterior to the sternocleidomastoid muscle, an acutely inflamed cyst may be confused with a suppurative lymph node and the two can be distinguished via CT, MRI, or fluoroscopic studies (Figs. 48.11 and 48.12).

Thyroglossal duct cysts are distinguished by their midline position in the anterior neck and are rarely confused with lymphadenopathy (Fig. 48.13). Most remain asymptomatic though may be diagnosed after developing secondary bacterial infection in the context of an upper respiratory tract infection. Thyroid studies and imaging should be obtained; surgical resection is typically advised.

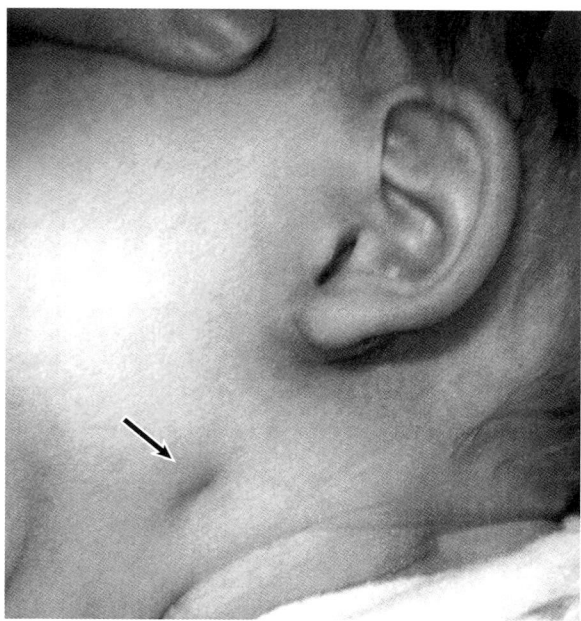

Fig. 48.12 First branchial derivatives present as a pit or a mass near the angle of the mandible *(arrow)*. They frequently originate in or near the external canal and, during their course, involve the facial nerve. (From Rizzi MD, Wetmore RF, Potsic WP. Differential diagnosis of neck masses. In: Lesperance MM, ed. *Cummings Pediatric Otolaryngology.* Philadelphia: Elsevier; 2015:248, Fig. 19.3.)

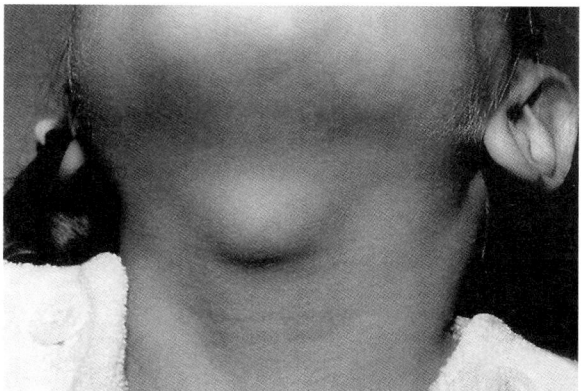

Fig. 48.13 Thyroglossal duct cysts are often found in the midline of the neck at or near the hyoid bone. (From Rizzi MD, Wetmore RF, Potsic WP. Differential diagnosis of neck masses. In: Lesperance MM, ed. *Cummings Pediatric Otolaryngology.* Philadelphia: Elsevier; 2015:248, Fig. 19.5.)

Rare soft tissue masses of the head and neck include congenital cervicofacial teratoma and rhabdomyosarcoma. The former may involve the orbit, nasopharynx, oropharynx, tongue, palate, or anterior neck, and, if interfering with in utero swallowing, may be associated with pulmonary hypoplasia and fetal hydrops and require fetal surgery to correct. The latter may be confused with congenital muscular torticollis and may be difficult to distinguish on ultrasonography or even MRI. Gadolinium administration with MRI will reveal heterogeneous enhancement, allowing for presumptive diagnosis as well as surgical planning.

■ SUMMARY AND RED FLAGS

Lymphadenopathy is a common manifestation of many childhood illnesses. Most often, regional adenopathy is associated with a bacterial infection in the vicinity of the node or with viral pharyngitis. Generalized adenopathy does not always indicate a serious underlying disease. Adenopathy usually resolves either spontaneously or after appropriate antibiotic therapy. When adenopathy is accompanied by weight loss, recurrent fevers, night sweats, or other systemic signs or symptoms, a more serious cause must be vigorously sought. The presence of supraclavicular nodes is usually a red flag for serious illness such as malignancy. Adenopathy associated with hepatomegaly, splenomegaly, or an abdominal mass must be quickly investigated. Furthermore, if the adenopathy does not diminish or resolve after antibiotic therapy or after 3 weeks, a more thorough evaluation is necessary. A chest x-ray must be performed for children with peripheral lymphadenopathy who are suspected of having a malignancy to look for mediastinal nodes. In children with known immunodeficiency, the cause of the adenopathy may be far more serious. These children are more prone to opportunistic infections; malignancies also occur at a higher frequency in immunosuppressed children than in the general population. Several conditions may mimic head and neck lymphadenopathy, including salivary gland and thyroid disorders, as well as developmental anomalies such as branchial cleft cysts, hemangiomas, or cystic hygromas.

BIBLIOGRAPHY

A bibliography is available at ExpertConsult.com.

49

Pallor and Anemia

Jacquelyn M. Powers and Amanda M. Brandow

Pallor, a perceptible reduction in the usual color and tone of the skin and/or mucosa, is a highly nonspecific finding that may be a manifestation of a diversity of diseases or may be normal for a given individual. It may result from alterations of cutaneous blood flow, anemia, or unknown mechanisms. Under normal circumstances the pink appearance of the lips, mucosa, and skin is influenced by the nature and character of these tissues, the adequacy of vascular perfusion, and the level of hemoglobin. Because pallor is most often associated with anemia, parental perception of it frequently generates considerable anxiety. However, a broad diagnostic approach is most appropriate (Table 49.1).

Anemia is the condition in which hemoglobin level (or hematocrit) is more than 2 standard deviations below the mean for age. Anemia is clinically relevant only when the low hemoglobin level results in decreased oxygen-carrying capacity of the blood. By definition, 2.5% of the general population has a hemoglobin or hematocrit level below the defined limits of normal. This fact must be kept in mind when evaluating children with mild anemia for which no explanation can be identified. Hemoglobin level varies considerably with age and sex (Table 49.2). Newborns have relatively high levels of circulating hemoglobin due to intrauterine adaptation to a relatively hypoxic environment. The postnatal oxygen rich environment results in decreased erythropoietin production, and hemoglobin production markedly diminishes for the first 2 months of life until a physiologic nadir occurs. The mean hemoglobin level rises gradually during childhood equally for both males and females until puberty when boys achieve a level approximately 20% higher than that of females.

Under normal conditions, the body's red blood cell (RBC) mass is maintained at a level appropriate to support tissue oxygen needs through the oxygen-sensing regulatory feedback stimulus of the hormone erythropoietin. Produced in the kidney, erythropoietin stimulates the production of mature RBCs within the bone marrow. Over a 3- to 5-day period, RBC precursors mature into reticulocytes that are released into the peripheral blood. In 24–48 hours, reticulocytes become mature RBCs that circulate in the peripheral blood for approximately 120 days. Senescent RBCs are removed from the circulation by reticuloendothelial cells within the spleen, liver, and bone marrow. A metabolic by-product of hemoglobin catabolism is bilirubin. The iron from senescent RBCs is efficiently recycled for the production of new erythrocytes. Anemia occurs as the result of one or a combination of three pathophysiologic mechanisms:

- Acute blood loss
- Impaired bone marrow production of RBCs
- Increased peripheral destruction of RBCs (hemolysis)

HISTORY

There are several important aspects of the history that can assist in the evaluation of a patient with pallor and suspected anemia.

Assessment of sun exposure and familial patterns of complexion are crucial because many patients are intrinsically pale, and a child with pallor is not necessarily anemic. A careful evaluation of the medical history is fundamental in the assessment of a patient with suspected pallor (Table 49.3).

A neonatal history of hyperbilirubinemia supports a possible diagnosis of congenital hemolytic anemia such as hereditary spherocytosis. This can be further supported by a family history of anemia, blood transfusions, splenectomy, and/or cholecystectomy.

Obtaining a dietary history is very important when evaluating a patient for anemia. Infants delivered prematurely or exclusively breast-fed infants without adequate iron supplementation from infant foods in the second half of their first year of life are at risk for iron-deficiency anemia. Toddlers who consume large amounts of cow's milk and children and adolescents who consume little meat are also at risk for iron-deficiency anemia. In addition, patients and breast-fed infants of mothers who follow a strict vegan diet may become deficient in vitamin B_{12}.

Clinical history should also include assessment for blood loss. In adolescent females, menstrual history suggestive of abnormal uterine bleeding and/or heavy menstrual bleeding increases risk for iron deficiency. All children should be assessed for gastrointestinal (GI) symptoms that would be suggestive of occult or gross GI blood loss as well. Pulmonary hemorrhage is a rare source of blood loss in children but should be considered in a child with iron-deficiency anemia and recurrent pulmonary issues including pneumonia or wheezing.

Medication history is pertinent because certain drugs, including antimalarial agents and sulfonamide antibiotics, can induce oxidant-associated hemolysis in the patient deficient in glucose-6-phosphate dehydrogenase (G6PD), whereas other medications may cause immune hemolysis (penicillin) or decreased RBC production (chloramphenicol). Travel history may suggest exposure to infections such as malaria.

PHYSICAL EXAMINATION

The general appearance of the child can provide clues to the severity and chronicity of the problem. Severe anemia that develops slowly over weeks or months is often well tolerated. Vital signs (including orthostatic blood pressure), height, weight, and growth offer further insight into the severity and chronicity of the problem. Isolated pallor in a well-appearing child who does not have evidence of systemic disease is less ominous than pallor noted in a child who is ill appearing or who has bruising, petechiae, lymphadenopathy, hepatosplenomegaly, or abdominal mass. Pallor at any site increases the likelihood of anemia; pallor of the face, nail beds, tongue, palms, and palmar creases and conjunctival pallor enhance the likelihood of anemia. Conjunctival rim pallor when compared to the usually more fleshlike pallor of the deeper posterior region of the palpebral conjunctiva is highly specific in adult

TABLE 49.1 Causes of Pallor in Children Based on Etiologic Mechanism

I. Anemia
II. Decreased Tendency of the Skin to Pigment
   A. Physiologic (fair-skinned individuals)
   B. Limited sun exposure
III. Alteration of the Consistency of the Subcutaneous Tissue
   A. Edematous states, increased intravascular hydrostatic pressure (e.g., congestive heart failure), decreased intravascular oncotic pressure (hypoproteinemia), increased vascular permeability (e.g., vasculitis)
   B. Hypothyroidism
IV. Decreased Perfusion of the Cutaneous/Mucosal Vasculature
   A. Hypotension, cardiogenic shock (pump failure or rhythm disturbance), hypovolemia (blood loss, dehydration), anaphylaxis, sepsis, acute adrenal insufficiency, vasovagal syncope
   B. Vasoconstriction, increased sympathetic activity (hypoglycemia, pheochromocytoma), neurologic complications (head trauma, seizures, migraine)
   C. Frostbite
V. Chronic Conditions
   A. Malignant disease
   B. Atopy
   C. Chronic inflammatory disease, juvenile idiopathic arthritis, inflammatory bowel disease
   D. Cardiopulmonary disease (including cystic fibrosis)
   E. Diabetes mellitus
   F. Congenital and acquired immunodeficiencies
   G. Ocular cutaneous albinism
   H. Panic attack
   I. Presyncope
   J. Food protein–induced enterocolitis syndrome

From Reece RM. *Manual of Emergency Pediatrics*. 4th ed. Philadelphia: WB Saunders; 1992.

patients with anemia. Table 49.4 outlines physical examination findings that may provide clues to the underlying cause of anemia.

Prominent cheekbones, dental malocclusion, and frontal bossing may occur in patients with chronic hemolytic anemias (i.e., thalassemia major) because of the expansion of bone marrow space. Tortuosity of conjunctival vessels occurs in sickle cell disease. Splenomegaly is often present in children with congenital hemolytic anemia. Lymphadenopathy and hepatosplenomegaly may indicate the presence of infiltrative disease of the bone marrow and visceral organs such as leukemia. Purpura in the anemic child is suggestive of associated thrombocytopenia that may accompany aplastic anemia or leukemia.

Many congenital anomalies and/or dysmorphic features have been associated with hematologic conditions, particularly bone marrow failure syndromes. Patients with Fanconi anemia are often short and have hyperpigmentation, hypoplastic "finger-like" thumbs, radial bone anomalies, and structural renal abnormalities. Patients with Diamond-Blackfan anemia are often short and have a "curious, intellectual" facial expression.

When pallor and anemia are seen in the context of other signs that suggest chronic inflammation, infection, or systemic disease, a diligent general physical examination may yield substantive information. Hypertension and short stature may suggest chronic renal disease. Joint swelling and/or pain may suggest rheumatologic disorders. Digital clubbing may suggest advanced cyanotic cardiopulmonary diseases. Abdominal pain, diarrhea, and poor growth may suggest an underlying GI disorder such as inflammatory bowel disease. Recurrent pneumonia or wheezing may suggest pulmonary hemorrhage.

New onset of pallor is suggestive of anemia. The child who has always appeared pale but is otherwise well with normal growth and development likely has an intrinsic constitutional characteristic. In such instances, the child and other family members often have light hair and skin complexion. An unremarkable general medical history and physical examination support a physiologic explanation for pallor. Some children may appear pale because of limited sun exposure as might occur during the winter in cooler climates.

TABLE 49.2 Values (Normal Mean and Lower Limits of Normal) for Hemoglobin, Hematocrit, and MCV Determination

Age (yr)	HEMOGLOBIN (G/DL)		HEMATOCRIT (%)		MCV (FL)	
	Mean	Lower Limit	Mean	Lower Limit	Mean	Lower Limit
0.5–1.9	12.5	11.0	37	33	77	70
2–4	12.5	11.0	38	34	79	73
5–7	13.0	11.5	39	35	81	75
8–11	13.5	12.0	40	36	83	76
12–14						
Female	13.5	12.0	41	36	85	78
Male	14.0	12.5	43	37	84	77
15–17						
Female	14.0	12.0	41	36	87	79
Male	15.0	13.0	46	38	86	78
18–49						
Female	14.0	12.0	42	37	90	80
Male	16.0	14.0	47	40	90	89

MCV, mean corpuscular volume.
From Nathan DC, Oski F. *Hematology of Infancy and Childhood*. 4th ed. Philadelphia: WB Saunders; 1993.

TABLE 49.3 Historical Clues in Evaluation of Anemia

Variable	Comments
Age	Iron deficiency rare in the absence of blood loss before 6 mo in term or before doubling birthweight in preterm infants
	Neonatal anemia with reticulocytosis suggests hemolysis or blood loss; with reticulocytopenia it suggests bone marrow failure or rarely severe autosomal recessive hereditary spherocytosis
	Sickle cell anemia and β-thalassemia appear as fetal hemoglobin disappears (4–8 mo of age)
	Nutritional iron deficiency in young children up to 4 yr of age
	Iron deficiency due to menstrual blood loss in adolescent females 12 to 18 yr of age
Family history and genetic considerations	X-linked: G6PD deficiency
	Autosomal dominant: spherocytosis, elliptocytosis, stomatocytosis, ovalocytosis
	Autosomal recessive: sickle cell, Fanconi anemia (most cases)
	Family member with early age of cholecystectomy (bilirubin stones) or splenectomy: hemolysis
	Ethnicity: thalassemia with Mediterranean origin; G6PD deficiency in blacks, Greeks, and Sephardic Jews
	Race: β-thalassemia in Whites; α-thalassemia in Blacks and Asians; SC and SS in Blacks
Nutrition	Cow's milk diet and iron deficiency (young children)
	Strict unsupplemented vegetarian and vitamin B_{12} or iron deficiency
	Goat's milk and folate deficiency
	Pica: plumbism (lead poisoning) and iron deficiency
	Cholestasis: malabsorption and vitamin E deficiency
Drugs	G6PD-susceptible agents
	Immune-mediated hemolysis (e.g., penicillin)
	Bone marrow suppression
	Phenytoin: increases folate requirements
Diarrhea	Malabsorption of vitamins B_{12} and E and iron
	Inflammatory bowel disease and anemia of chronic disease or blood loss with concomitant iron deficiency
	Milk protein allergy colitis–induced blood loss
	Intestinal resection and vitamin B_{12} deficiency
Infection	*Giardia* and iron malabsorption
	Intestinal bacterial overgrowth (blind loop) and vitamin B_{12} deficiency
	Fish tapeworm and vitamin B_{12} deficiency
	Epstein-Barr virus, cytomegalovirus, and bone marrow suppression
	Mycoplasma and hemolysis
	Parvovirus and bone marrow suppression
	Chronic infection
	Endocarditis
	Malaria and hemolysis
	Hepatitis and aplastic anemia

G6PD, glucose-6-phosphate dehydrogenase; SC, sickle cell C disease; SS, sickle cell S disease.

Children with malignant disease or chronic illness (e.g., rheumatologic disorders, inflammatory bowel disease, chronic cardiopulmonary disorders, diabetes) may have a pale appearance that is unrelated or out of proportion to the degree of associated anemia. Atopic children often have distinctly pale mucosa related to local edema. Children with generalized edema caused by hypoproteinemia, congestive heart failure, or vasculitis often appear pale because of excess interstitial fluid within the mucosal or cutaneous tissues. Patients with hypothyroidism are pale because of myxedematous changes in the skin, subcutaneous tissue, and mucosa.

LABORATORY EVALUATION

The initial laboratory test in a child with pallor should be a CBC including a manual white blood cell (WBC) differential and reticulocyte count. Significant pallor from anemia usually does not occur until the hemoglobin level falls below 8 g/dL. Appropriate sample collection is important. "False anemia" (resulting from laboratory error or sampling difficulty) should be considered when laboratory findings are not consistent with clinical impressions. Capillary blood sampling can be associated with substantial error, depending on the difficulty in performing the procedure and the use of mechanical force necessary to promote blood flow. When laboratory or sampling errors are suspected, a venipuncture sample should be obtained for confirmation. By definition, 2.5% of the general population has hemoglobin levels below the lower limit of normal, which is termed "statistical anemia." This phenomenon should be considered when mild, unexplained normocytic anemia is identified in a healthy child. Statistical anemia is a diagnosis of exclusion and therefore requires that other etiologies of normocytic anemia such as undiagnosed kidney disease, hypothyroidism, or underlying inflammation be ruled out.

Most laboratories perform CBCs with automated technology systems. Hemoglobin concentration (grams per deciliter), RBC count (cells per cubic millimeter), and mean corpuscular volume (MCV) (expressed in femtoliters [fL]) are directly measured. Hematocrit value, mean corpuscular hemoglobin (MCH), and MCH concentration (MCHC) are derived values and therefore are less accurate. Other important information reported includes RBC distribution width (RDW), WBC count (cells per cubic millimeter), and platelet count. In addition to the hemoglobin values, careful attention should be given to the MCV, RDW, RBC morphology, platelet count, WBC count, and reticulocyte count.

CLASSIFICATION OF ANEMIA

Reticulocyte Count

The reticulocyte count, reported as a percentage of total RBCs, is essential in categorizing anemia. An elevated reticulocyte count implies a bone marrow response to either increased RBC destruction (hemolysis) or acute or chronic blood loss. In cases of acute blood loss, bone marrow response demonstrated by reticulocytosis occurs at an average of 3–4 days. Thus, in the setting of acute blood loss, the reticulocyte count is most helpful when the bleeding and subsequent anemia have been present for more than a few days. Likewise, in patients with nutritional anemias, a reticulocyte count should be checked several days after the initiation of therapy (e.g., iron supplementation) to assess appropriate response.

Anemias are categorized on the basis of the adequacy of the reticulocyte response. The reticulocyte count is expressed as a percentage of the total number of RBCs. In the setting of a normal hemoglobin, the reticulocyte count is about 1–2%. In patients with moderate or severe anemia, the reticulocyte count may appear elevated, but in absolute terms, it may be insufficient for the degree of anemia. Therefore, the reticulocyte count must be corrected using the following formula:

$$\text{Corrected reticulocyte count} = \frac{\text{reticulocyte count} \times \text{hemoglobin}}{(\text{normal hemoglobin for age})}$$

TABLE 49.4 Physical Findings in the Evaluation of Anemia

System	Observation	Significance
Skin	Hyperpigmentation	Fanconi anemia, dyskeratosis congenita
	Café-au-lait spots	Fanconi anemia
	Vitiligo	Vitamin B_{12} deficiency
	Partial oculocutaneous albinism	Chediak-Higashi syndrome
	Jaundice	Hemolysis, hepatitis
	Petechiae, purpura	Bone marrow infiltration, autoimmune hemolysis with autoimmune thrombocytopenia, hemolytic uremic syndrome
	Erythematous rash	Parvovirus, Epstein-Barr virus
	Butterfly rash	SLE
Head	Frontal bossing	Thalassemia major, chronic subdural hematoma
	Microcephaly	Fanconi anemia
Eyes	Microphthalmia	Fanconi anemia
	Retinopathy	Hemoglobin SS, SC disease
	Optic atrophy, blindness	Osteopetrosis
	Blocked lacrimal gland	Dyskeratosis congenita
	Kayser-Fleischer ring	Wilson disease
	Blue sclera	Iron deficiency
Ears	Deafness	Osteopetrosis
Mouth	Glossitis	Vitamin B_{12} deficiency; iron deficiency
	Angular stomatitis	Iron deficiency
	Cleft lip	Diamond-Blackfan syndrome
	Pigmentation	Peutz-Jeghers syndrome (intestinal blood loss)
	Telangiectasia	Osler-Weber-Rendu syndrome (blood loss)
	Leukoplakia	Dyskeratosis congenita
Chest	Shield chest or widespread nipples	Diamond-Blackfan syndrome
	Murmur	Endocarditis; prosthetic valve hemolysis
Abdomen	Hepatomegaly	Hemolysis, infiltrative tumor, chronic disease, hemangioma, cholecystitis
	Splenomegaly	Hemolysis, sickle cell disease (early), thalassemia, malaria, lymphoma Epstein-Barr virus, portal hypertension, hemophagocytic syndromes
	Nephromegaly or absent kidney	Fanconi anemia
Extremities	Absent thumbs	Fanconi anemia
	Thenar eminence hypoplasia; triphalangeal thumb	Diamond-Blackfan syndrome
	Spoon nails	Iron deficiency
	Beau line (nails)	Heavy metal intoxication, severe illness
	Mees line (nails)	Heavy metals, severe illness, sickle cell anemia
	Dystrophic nails	Dyskeratosis congenita
	Edema	Milk-induced protein-losing enteropathy with iron deficiency, renal failure
Rectal	Hemorrhoids	Portal hypertension
	Heme-positive stool	Intestinal hemorrhage
Nerves	Irritable, apathy	Iron deficiency
	Peripheral neuropathy	Deficiency of vitamins B_1 and B_{12} and lead poisoning
	Dementia	Deficiency of vitamins B_{12} and E
	Ataxia, posterior column signs	Deficiency of vitamins B_{12} and E
	Stroke	Sickle cell anemia, paroxysmal nocturnal hemoglobinuria, severe iron-deficiency anemia

SC, sickle cell C disease; SLE, systemic lupus erythematosus; SS, sickle cell S disease.
Modified from Scott JP. Hematology. In: Behrman RE, Kliegman RM, eds. *Nelson Essentials of Pediatrics*. 2nd ed. Philadelphia: WB Saunders; 1994:520.

If the corrected reticulocyte count is >2%, then the bone marrow is producing RBCs at an accelerated pace (Fig. 49.1).

Red Blood Cell Size

The MCV is vital to the classification of anemia. High MCV is termed *macrocytosis*, and low MCV is termed *microcytosis*. MCV in the normal range is termed *normocytic*. Normal standards for MCV are age related; a simple guideline is that the lower normal limit of MCV for children older than 6 months is 70 fL plus the patient's age in years

until the adult standard of 80–100 fL is reached (see Table 49.2). The MCV must always be interpreted in conjunction with a review of the peripheral blood smear, RDW, and reticulocyte count. A varied population of both smaller and larger RBCs (e.g., reticulocytes) may yield a falsely normal MCV and be diagnostically misleading. A high RDW in the setting of a normal MCV is a clue that two populations of RBCs exist. Microcytosis (low MCV) is associated with iron deficiency, thalassemia, and long-standing anemia of inflammation (Table 49.5). Macrocytosis (high MCV), an unusual finding in children, is associated

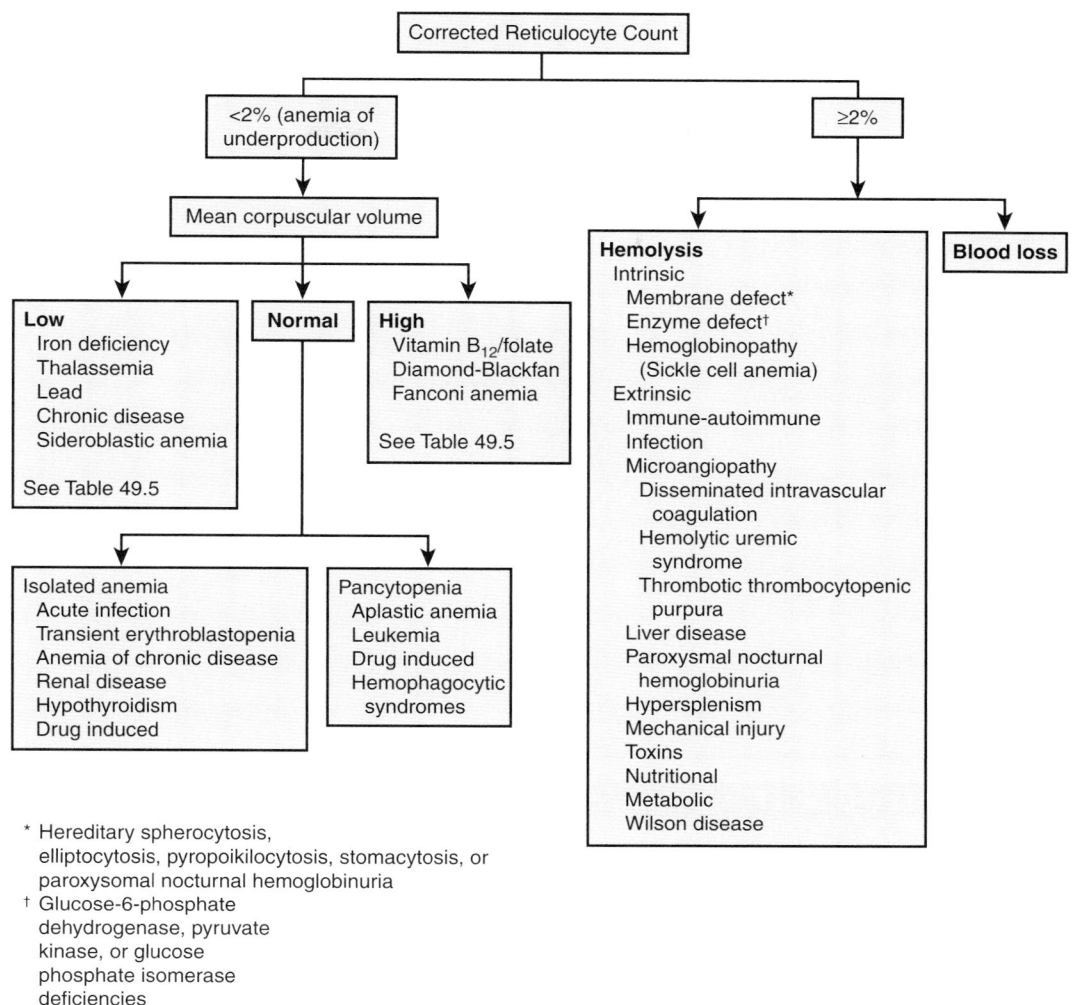

Fig. 49.1 Diagnostic approach to anemia.

with vitamin B_{12} or folate deficiency, bone marrow failure syndromes (e.g., Fanconi anemia, Diamond-Blackfan anemia), and some cases of hypothyroidism (see Table 49.5).

An individual with small RBCs may have a normal or near-normal hemoglobin level if the RBC count is increased as occurs in patients with thalassemia minor who often have RBC counts of more than 5 × 10^6. The MCHC reflects the level of hemoglobin per cell and would be expected to be low in patients with anemias in which RBCs are "under-hemoglobinized," such as the hypochromic anemia of iron deficiency.

The RDW is derived from the histogram of RBC volumes. A normal RDW (11.5–14.5%) implies a uniform population of RBCs that are similar in size. In α-thalassemia trait or β-thalassemia trait, a uniform population of small cells exists; hence, the MCV is low and the RDW is normal or minimally elevated. An elevated RDW is seen in iron deficiency where the population of small cells is variably sized; hence, the MCV is low and the RDW is elevated. The RDW is often the last hematologic parameter to normalize after successful therapy for iron deficiency. In some hemolytic anemias the RDW is elevated because of the presence of large reticulocytes (Table 49.6). An elevated RDW in the setting of a normocytic anemia suggests two populations of RBCs, namely large cells (elevated MCV) and small cells (low MCV), and is concerning for a combined anemia (e.g., concomitant iron deficiency and vitamin B_{12} or folate deficiency).

Red Blood Cell Morphology

Abnormalities of RBC structure may be readily apparent on inspection of the peripheral blood smear and provide helpful diagnostic hints (Table 49.7 and Fig. 49.2).

Other Laboratory Abnormalities Associated with Anemia

Evaluation of the WBC count, differential, and platelet count is imperative in the setting of anemia. Leukopenia, neutropenia, and/or thrombocytopenia occurring in a patient with anemia of underproduction are suggestive of aplastic anemia or infiltrative bone marrow disease such as leukemia (see Chapter 50). The presence of immature leukocytes on a smear associated with either a high or a low WBC count is suggestive of leukemia. Mild neutropenia may be seen in patients with transient erythroblastopenia of childhood but children are otherwise well appearing, in contrast to children with underlying malignancy. Thrombocytosis may be present in patients with iron deficiency, blood loss, inflammatory disease, infection, malignancy, or asplenia.

Elevated serum indirect bilirubin, lactate dehydrogenase, and urinary urobilinogen levels occur in patients with increased rates of RBC destruction (hemolysis). Immune-mediated hemolytic anemia should be suspected when anemia, jaundice, reticulocytosis, splenomegaly, and microspherocytes are noted. To investigate the underlying cause

TABLE 49.5 Causes of High or Low Mean Corpuscular Volume

Low Mean Corpuscular Volume

Iron deficiency
Thalassemias
Lead toxicity
Anemia of chronic disease
Copper deficiency
Sideroblastic anemia
Hemoglobin E
Hereditary pyropoikilocytosis

High Mean Corpuscular Volume

Normal newborn
Elevated reticulocyte count
Vitamin B_{12} or folate deficiency
Diamond-Blackfan anemia (congenital hypoplastic anemia)
Fanconi anemia
Aplastic anemia
Down syndrome
Hypothyroidism (occasionally)
Orotic aciduria
Lesch-Nyhan syndrome
Drugs (zidovudine, chemotherapy)
Chronic liver disease
Paroxysmal nocturnal hemoglobinuria
Thiamine-responsive megaloblastic anemia
Myelodysplasias
Dyserythropoietic anemias

TABLE 49.6 Red Blood Cell Distribution Width (RDW) in Common Anemias of Childhood

Anemia	MCV
Elevated RDW (Nonuniform Population of RBCs)	
Hemolytic anemia with elevated reticulocyte count	High
Iron-deficiency anemia	Low
Anemias due to red blood cell fragmentation: DIC, HUS, TTP	Low
Megaloblastic anemias: vitamin B_{12} or folate deficiency	High
Normal RDW (Uniform Population of RBCs)	
Thalassemias	Low
Acute hemorrhage	Normal
Fanconi anemia	High
Aplastic anemia	High

DIC, disseminated intravascular coagulation; HUS, hemolytic uremic syndrome; MCV, mean corpuscular volume; RBC, red blood cell; TTP, thrombotic thrombocytopenic purpura.

TABLE 49.7 Peripheral Blood Morphologic Findings in Various Anemias

Microcytes

Iron deficiency
Thalassemias
Lead toxicity
Anemia of chronic disease

Macrocytes

Newborns
Vitamin B_{12} or folate deficiency
Diamond-Blackfan anemia
Fanconi anemia
Aplastic anemia
Liver disease
Down syndrome
Hypothyroidism

Spherocytes

Hereditary spherocytosis
Immune hemolytic anemia (newborn or acquired)
Hypersplenism

Sickled Cells

Sickle cell anemias (SS disease, SC disease, $S\beta^+$thalassemia, $S\beta^0$thalassemia)

Elliptocytes

Hereditary elliptocytosis
Iron deficiency
Megaloblastic anemia

Target Cells

Hemoglobinopathies (especially hemoglobin C and SC and thalassemia)
Liver disease
Xerocytosis

Basophil Stippling

Thalassemia
Lead intoxication
Myelodysplasia

Red Blood Cell Fragments, Helmet Cells, Burr Cells

Disseminated intravascular coagulation
Hemolytic uremic syndrome
Thrombotic thrombocytopenic purpura
Kasabach-Merritt syndrome
Waring blender syndrome (artificial heart valve)
Uremia
Liver disease

Hypersegmented Neutrophils

Vitamin B_{12} or folate deficiency

Blasts

Leukemia (ALL or AML)
Severe infection (rarely)

Leukopenia/Thrombocytopenia

Fanconi anemia
Aplastic anemia
Leukemia
Hemophagocytic histiocytosis

Howell-Jolly Bodies

Asplenia, hyposplenia
Severe iron deficiency

Dacrocytes (teardrop cells)

Myelodysplasia
Leukemia
Neuroblastoma

ALL, acute lymphocytic leukemia; AML, acute myeloid leukemia; SC, sickle cell C disease; SS, sickle cell S disease.

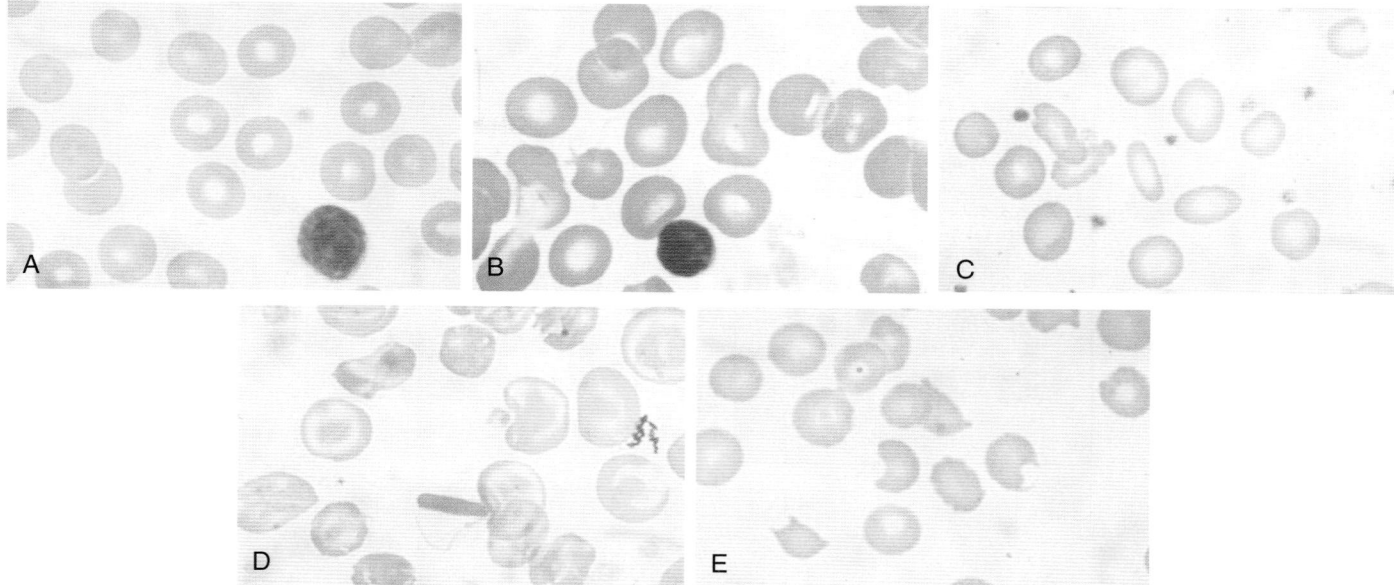

Fig. 49.2 Morphologic abnormalities of the red blood cell. *A,* Normal. *B,* Macrocytes. *C,* Hypochromic microcytes. *D,* Target cells. *E,* Schizocytes. (Courtesy of Dr. E. Schwartz.)

of the hemolysis, a direct Coombs test should be performed to detect the presence of an autoantibody on the RBC surface. An iron panel, ideally drawn when fasting, that demonstrates a low serum iron level, elevated total iron-binding capacity, and a low percentage of iron saturation (% saturation = serum iron/total iron-binding capacity × 100) and/or decreased serum ferritin level is helpful in establishing a diagnosis of iron deficiency. Hemoglobin identification via electrophoresis or high-performance liquid chromatography is necessary to identify hemoglobinopathies such as sickle cell disease or thalassemia. Assessment of RBC enzyme levels (e.g., G6PD) may be necessary when infection- or medication-related hemolytic anemia is suspected in a male of Mediterranean or African descent. True macrocytic anemia with megaloblastic neutrophils should prompt assessment for vitamin B_{12} or folate deficiency. Bone marrow aspirate and biopsy should strongly be considered when other cytopenias exist such as thrombocytopenia or neutropenia.

DIAGNOSTIC WORK-UP

From a clinical perspective, it is best to consider the differential diagnosis of pallor in the context of the acuity and severity of the clinical findings (Fig. 49.3). The well-appearing child may only need a CBC to confirm normal counts and provide reassurance. The pale child who appears mildly or moderately ill requires a CBC and other potential studies to detect any suspected underlying disease. The pale child who appears seriously ill requires urgent evaluation and appropriate therapeutic intervention. A CBC should be obtained for all children with other laboratory assessments dictated based on the suspected diagnosis. If hemorrhage or severe anemia is suspected, a type and cross-match must be sent to the blood bank, intravenous access should be secured, and frequent serial evaluations of hemoglobin, blood pressure, pulse, perfusion, and end-organ function must be performed.

DIFFERENTIAL DIAGNOSIS OF ANEMIA

The differential diagnosis of anemia is presented in Figs. 49.1 and 49.4.

Anemia Secondary to Acute Blood Loss

Significant blood loss on an acute or subacute basis results in anemia. In subacute bleeding, the fall in hemoglobin occurs gradually and a period of about 24 hours may be required for full intravascular equilibration after acute blood loss. When severe acute blood loss occurs, intravascular volume depletion is the primary concern, which cannot be assessed by hemoglobin level. Therefore, in the setting of severe blood loss, blood pressure, heart rate, adequacy of peripheral perfusion, and mental status are the best ways to assess patients. In most instances, an obvious history of blood loss is apparent (e.g., epistaxis, heavy menstrual bleeding, hematemesis, lower GI bleeding, trauma). In some cases, intraabdominal bleeding can occur that is not clinically apparent. Large amounts of blood may accumulate in the GI tract before the development of hematemesis, hematochezia, or melena. Intraabdominal bleeding may occur after trauma or may result from an ulcer (see Chapter 16) and may be associated with progressive anemia in the absence of an obvious source of bleeding. The clinical history coupled with the physical examination (including rectal examination) and tests for occult blood in the stool generally define the source of blood loss. Pulmonary hemorrhage may not be readily apparent, especially if chronic; thus, evaluation with pulse oximetry and chest X-ray or chest CT scan may be indicated in a child with concerns for blood loss without an obvious source.

In anemia associated with blood loss, the RBC size and morphology are normal and appropriate reticulocytosis should occur within 3–5 days from the start of the blood loss. If hemorrhage has ceased, the hemoglobin level should gradually increase unless supervening factors such as iron deficiency exist.

Severe hemorrhage associated with intravascular volume depletion warrants immediate intervention to avoid shock. RBC transfusions are necessary until hemorrhage has ceased. Less severe hemorrhage that is not associated with intravascular volume depletion will likely manifest with moderate to severe anemia. Transfusions may be necessary when the oxygen-carrying capacity of the blood is diminished to the point of impending tissue hypoxia. In these cases, the need for transfusion therapy is based on clinical symptoms including tachycardia, dyspnea,

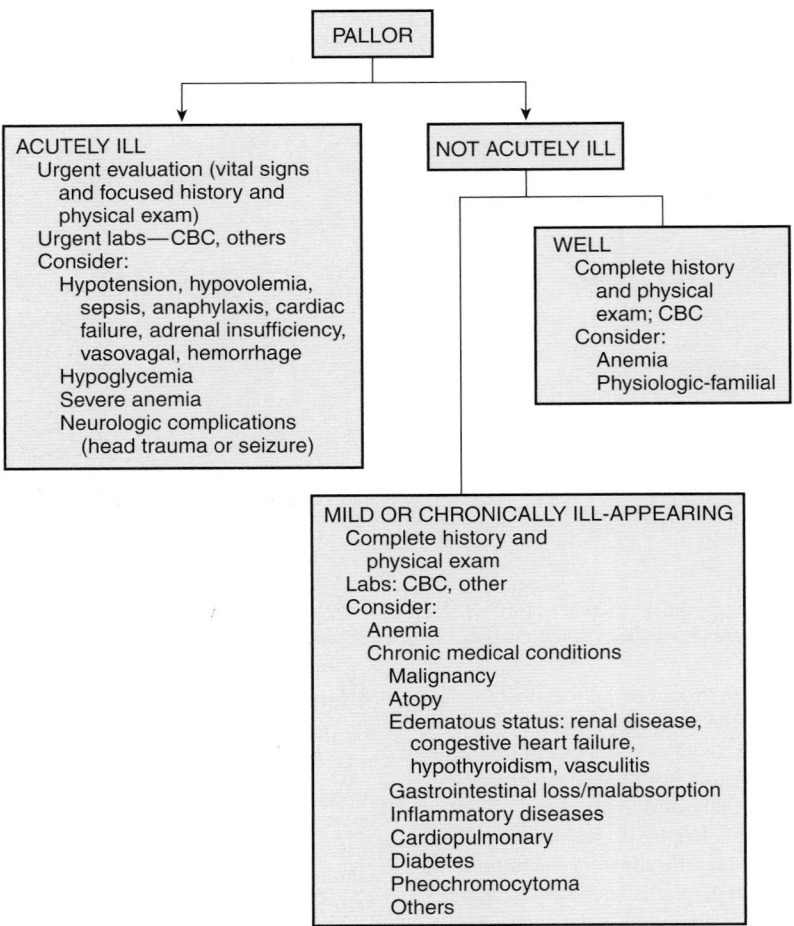

Fig. 49.3 Approach to the pale child.

heart failure, fatigue, or lightheadedness. If hemorrhage has ceased, intravascular volume is replete, and if the patient is not manifesting signs of cardiorespiratory compromise, transfusion therapy may be avoided. In such instances, it is appropriate to supply therapeutic doses of iron with close follow-up to ensure adequacy of the reticulocyte response (Table 49.8).

Anemia Secondary to Underproduction

Anemia caused by the underproduction of RBCs (see Figs. 49.1 and 49.4) is characterized by a suboptimal bone marrow response to the anemia reflected by a corrected reticulocyte count of <2%. Associated clinical symptoms can provide clues to the etiology of underproduction, especially for nonhematologic causes of anemia. Common nonhematologic causes of underproduction include chronic renal disease, chronic inflammation, or infection. Hematologic causes of underproduction are outlined in subsequent text. Anemia due to underproduction of RBCs should be evaluated in the context of RBC size: microcytic, normocytic, or macrocytic.

Microcytic Anemias

Hemoglobin, the chief intracellular component of the RBC, is composed of heme (iron and protoporphyrin IX) and globin chains (α and β). Any factor that diminishes the availability or utilization of these components results in microcytic anemia. The automated MCV represents the mean RBC volume and does not address variations in cell size. The RDW, however, describes variation in RBC size and if normal defines a relatively uniform population of cells. Review of the peripheral blood smear also

provides additional evidence regarding variability in cell size and shape. It is important to note that MCV is age related (see Table 49.2). When the diagnosis is not immediately apparent, it is helpful to carefully select from a variety of available laboratory studies to further differentiate the cause of the microcytic anemia (Table 49.9). Hepcidin levels (low in iron deficiency; high in anemia of chronic disease) may also be helpful.

Iron-Deficiency Anemia. Iron deficiency is the most common nutritional deficiency that causes anemia. Iron deficiency occurs due to either insufficient nutritional intake to meet demands associated with growth or excessive blood loss. Iron is a key component of the hemoglobin molecule; its deficiency leads to anemia associated with reduced hemoglobin production (hypochromia) and small RBCs (microcytosis). Infants are at particular risk for the development of iron deficiency since their rapid growth and expanding blood volume impose considerable iron demands. Premature infants are at the highest risk because most in utero iron is transferred from the mother to the fetus during the last trimester of pregnancy and postnatal growth rate is rapid. In addition, exclusively breast-fed infants are also susceptible to iron deficiency in the second half of their first year of life if adequate supplemental iron via solid food intake is not provided. Toddlers are at high risk for the development of iron deficiency due to excessive cow's milk intake leading to decreased intake of dietary sources of iron, and GI blood loss from milk protein sensitivity. Thus, appropriate counseling should be provided to the family to ensure that cow's milk is limited to no more than 24 oz/day. Unsupplemented vegans are also at risk for iron deficiency. Adolescent females are at very high risk due to menstrual blood loss and poor nutrition. Risk for iron deficiency is high in adolescent females especially during the first year

I. Acute blood loss with hemodilution

II. Anemia of RBC underproduction (i.e., inadequate reticulocyte count)

Microcytic
1. Iron deficiency
2. Lead intoxication
3. Thalassemia syndromes
4. Anemia of chronic diseases

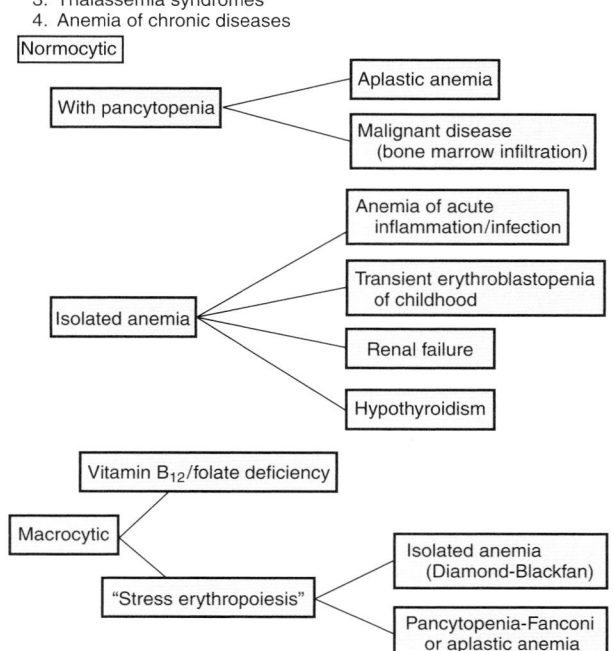

III. Anemia due to increased destruction = hemolysis (i.e., adequate reticulocyte count)

Intrinsic RBC defect
1. Hemoglobinopathies (sickle cell anemia, unstable hemoglobins)
2. Membrane defects (hereditary spherocytosis, elliptocytosis)
3. Enzymopathies (G6PD, pyruvate kinase deficiency)

Extrinsic defects
1. Immune hemolysis
2. Infection (bacterial, viral, other)
3. Microangiopathy (disseminated intravascular coagulation, hemolytic uremic syndrome, thrombotic thrombocytopenic purpura)
4. Liver disease
5. Paroxysmal nocturnal hemoglobinuria
6. Hypersplenism
7. Mechanical injury (e.g., burns)
8. Toxins
9. Nutritional (vitamin E deficiency)
10. Metabolic (galactosemia)
11. Wilson disease

Fig. 49.4 Differential diagnosis of anemia. G6PD, glucose-6-phosphate dehydrogenase; RBC, red blood cell.

TABLE 49.8   Therapy for Iron Deficiency

Infants and Children

3 mg/kg of elemental iron given as a single daily dose (ideally before breakfast)

Adolescents

65–130 mg of elemental iron given in a single daily dose

Duration of Prescription

Continue *therapeutic dose* of iron for 2–3 mo after hemoglobin level has been corrected (to replete stores), after which both maintenance nutritional needs and underlying etiology (i.e., control of blood loss, if present) must be met

---

TABLE 49.9   Laboratory Findings in Microcytic Anemia

	Fe	TIBC	Pb	HbA$_2$	Ferritin	sTfR	RDW
Iron deficiency	↓	↑	nl	nl	↓	↑↑	↑
α-Thalassemia (Bart hemoglobin)	nl	nl	nl	nl	nl	↑	↓
β-Thalassemia (homozygous)	nl	nl	nl	↑	nl	↑	↑
Lead poisoning	nl	nl	↑	nl	nl	nl*	nl*
Anemia of chronic disease	↓	↓	nl	nl	nl or ↑	nl*	nl*

*Unless iron deficient.
Fe, iron; HbA$_2$, hemoglobin A$_2$; nl, normal; Pb, lead; RDW, red blood cell distribution width; sTfR, serum transferrin free receptor; TIBC, total iron-binding capacity.

TABLE 49.10   Nonhematologic Consequences of Iron Deficiency

Impairment of cognitive development
Pica
Epithelial abnormalities (gastrointestinal mucosal lesions, glossitis; spoon-shaped nails)
Exercise intolerance (muscle weakness)
Behavioral manifestations
Poor growth
Impaired collagen synthesis (blue sclera)

---

after menarche. *When iron deficiency occurs outside of the setting of infancy, toddlers, or adolescent females (i.e., school-age children or adolescent males), a pathologic source of blood loss must be strongly considered and occult GI bleeding is an important source to consider as iron-deficiency anemia can be the first clue to the presence of inflammatory bowel disease or other GI disease.*

Nutritional sources of iron include iron-fortified infant formula (12 mg/L), iron-fortified infant cereal, beef, fish, and fowl. Ascorbic acid (vitamin C) may enhance the absorption of iron. The American Academy of Pediatrics recommends iron-fortified infant formula or breast milk until the age of 1 year and the introduction of iron-rich foods after 6 months of age. Cow's milk is a very poor source of nutritional iron and should not be given to infants younger than 1 year of age. After 1 year of age, infants should consume no more than 24 oz/day. Iron supplementation is necessary for preterm infants, many adolescent females, vegans, and pregnant women and should be strongly considered for all exclusively breast-fed infants regardless of diet. Iron deficiency must be viewed as a systemic deficiency disorder, only one manifestation of which is anemia (Table 49.10).

Iron-deficiency anemia may be detected by routine hemoglobin screening. This should be performed initially in children between 9 and 12 months of age. It is recommended again between 18 and 24 months of age as toddlers become especially vulnerable to iron deficiency after transition from formula to cow's milk at 12 months of age. Adolescent females should be screened 1–2 years after menarche. Laboratory confirmatory studies are necessary when iron-deficiency anemia is suspected in patients who are not at high risk for nutritional deficiency or in those in whom anemia is moderately severe (see Table 49.9). A serum ferritin level of <15 ng/dL or an iron saturation of <15% confirms the diagnosis.

Symptomatic iron deficiency in young children is infrequent, but when it occurs, it is generally noted in infants who consume large amounts of cow's milk and have intestinal blood loss as a result of asymptomatic milk protein–induced enterocolitis. Such children may have pallor, irritability, fatigue, glossitis, blue sclera, and in extreme cases signs and symptoms of high-output cardiac failure (i.e., dyspnea, diaphoresis, pallor, tachycardia, gallop rhythm, and hepatomegaly), protein-losing enteropathy, or stroke. Blood loss may be intermittent; a negative stool test for blood does not rule out the diagnosis. Mild anemia in otherwise well infants between 6 and 24 months of age, particularly in association with ingestion of large amounts of cow's milk, is most likely caused by iron deficiency.

When mild anemia is detected in the healthy, menstruating adolescent female, chronic blood loss is usually the etiology. Empirical iron therapy is often prescribed in such circumstances (see Table 49.8). If the hemoglobin level has normalized after 1 month of therapy, a presumptive diagnosis has been established and the patient should receive an additional 2–3 months of therapeutic doses of iron to replete stores. An appropriate response to iron therapy is the diagnostic "gold standard." If unrecognized, iron-deficiency anemia in adolescent females can progress to severe anemia resulting in headache, dizziness, restless legs, and syncope. Hemostatic evaluation should be performed and hormonal therapy strongly considered to minimize ongoing blood loss to prevent persistent or recurrent iron-deficiency anemia.

Recurrent iron-deficiency anemia in infants and children, despite limitation of cow's milk intake and compliance with supplemental iron, should raise the suspicion for blood loss, particularly GI blood loss. Rarely, *pulmonary hemorrhage* can be a source of chronic blood loss. This condition is called **Heiner syndrome** and is due to severe cow's milk protein hypersensitivity. Heiner syndrome should be considered when chronic iron-deficiency anemia exists with associated cough, wheeze, or diagnosis of "asthma." Chest radiograph reveals pulmonary infiltrates consistent with hemorrhage. Pulmonary vascular anomalies and systemic vasculitis are other causes of pulmonary hemorrhage.

Iron-refractory iron-deficiency anemia. Iron deficiency that begins early in infancy that is unresponsive to therapeutic doses of oral iron may be due to iron-refractory iron-deficiency anemia (IRIDA), an autosomal recessive disorder due to pathologic variants in *TMPRSS6*, which is involved in iron homeostasis. There is a microcytic hypochromic anemia, low iron levels, and transferrin saturations but normal to high ferritin or hepcidin levels. Because of iron malabsorption, oral iron is usually ineffective and intravenous iron is indicated. The differential diagnosis includes celiac disease and *Helicobacter pylori* or autoimmune atrophic gastritis.

Standard-of-care treatment of iron-deficiency anemia with oral iron is outlined in Table 49.8. Intravenous iron therapy is often useful upfront in certain situations (poor compliance, iron malabsorption in patients with celiac disease, intestinal bacterial overgrowth syndrome, inflammatory bowel disease, and genetic causes affecting iron absorption; children receiving hemodialysis). It may also be considered in iron-deficiency anemia patients with long-standing anemia or who have failed oral iron therapy for any reason, including nonadherence. The optimal approach to iron-deficiency anemia in infants and children is prevention.

Thalassemia syndromes. The thalassemia syndromes represent a heterogeneous group of inherited disorders of decreased globin production that lead to microcytic anemia, which can be mistaken for iron deficiency. The child with microcytic anemia, without evidence of iron deficiency, should be evaluated for thalassemia (Fig. 49.5).

Two genes, one inherited from each parent, code for the production of the β-globin chains of hemoglobin. When one gene is affected by the β-thalassemia gene variant, a moderate diminution in the production of the β-globin chain occurs, resulting in mild microcytic anemia of underproduction. β-Thalassemia occurs most commonly in individuals of Mediterranean, Asian, or African descent. Patients with **β-thalassemia trait** are asymptomatic and the diagnosis is frequently made when anemia and microcytosis are noted at the time of routine screening for iron deficiency or incidentally when a CBC is obtained for the assessment of acute or chronic symptoms. Typically patients have mild anemia and a low MCV. For an equivalent degree of anemia, the MCV is substantially lower than that seen in iron deficiency.

This phenomenon is reflected in the Mentzer index calculated by dividing the MCV by the RBC count (in millions). The RBC count is usually elevated in thalassemia. Thus, an index of <13 is suggestive of thalassemia trait, whereas an index of >13 is generally suggestive of iron-deficiency anemia. A normal MCV virtually excludes a diagnosis of β-thalassemia. A normal or mildly elevated RDW is usually seen in thalassemia and reflects a relatively uniform population of microcytic RBCs. This is in contrast to iron deficiency wherein the RDW is uniformly elevated reflecting variation in cell size.

The peripheral blood smear demonstrates microcytosis, hypochromia, and target cells. Occasional fragments and basophilic stippling may be seen. Newborn hemoglobinopathy screening will be normal in patients with β-thalassemia trait. Hemoglobin analysis performed at 6 months of age or older will demonstrate an elevation of hemoglobin A2. The significance of diagnosing β-thalassemia trait is twofold: (1) its confusion with iron deficiency (hence, patients may be treated unnecessarily with repeated courses of iron and undergo repeated unnecessary blood studies) and (2) its genetic implications. A child from two individuals with β-thalassemia trait carries a 25% risk per pregnancy of being affected with homozygous β-thalassemia (thalassemia major), a severe hematologic disorder. Parents and siblings of a child with a diagnosis of β-thalassemia trait should be appropriately screened and counseled. For purposes of screening, a normal, age-adjusted MCV essentially excludes a diagnosis of β-thalassemia trait.

Homozygous β-thalassemia, also known as β-thalassemia major or Cooley anemia, results from the inheritance of the β-thalassemia trait variant from each parent. This results in a severe deficiency of β-globin chain production with an excess of α-globin chains. These α-globin chains precipitate within developing erythroid elements in the marrow and lead to brisk intramarrow destruction of developing erythroid elements (ineffective erythropoiesis). As a result, patients with β-thalassemia major present during infancy at 6–12 months of age with severe anemia and an inadequate reticulocyte count during the time when transition from fetal hemoglobin to adult hemoglobin occurs. Children with β-thalassemia major typically present with fatigue, irritability, pallor, jaundice, and marked hepatosplenomegaly that is caused by extramedullary hematopoiesis. Frontal bossing and prominent cheek bones (maxillary hyperplasia) may be noted and result from expansion of the marrow space to compensate for the severe anemia. Most patients are of Mediterranean or Asian descent.

Laboratory findings include severe anemia and a decreased age-adjusted MCV. The peripheral blood smear is markedly abnormal, demonstrating severely under-hemoglobinized (hypochromic) RBCs and target cells and wide variability in cell shape and size (increased RDW). Chronic transfusion therapy sufficient to suppress ineffective erythropoiesis (maintaining hemoglobin level >10 g/dL) may be associated with relatively normal growth, development, and functional capabilities. Long-term iron chelation for management of iron overload allows for prolonged survival and decreases complications of transfusional hemosiderosis (hepatic, endocrine, and cardiac dysfunction). Bone marrow transplantation is curative and a potential treatment option for younger patients who have a human leukocyte antigen–identical healthy sibling or matched unrelated donor.

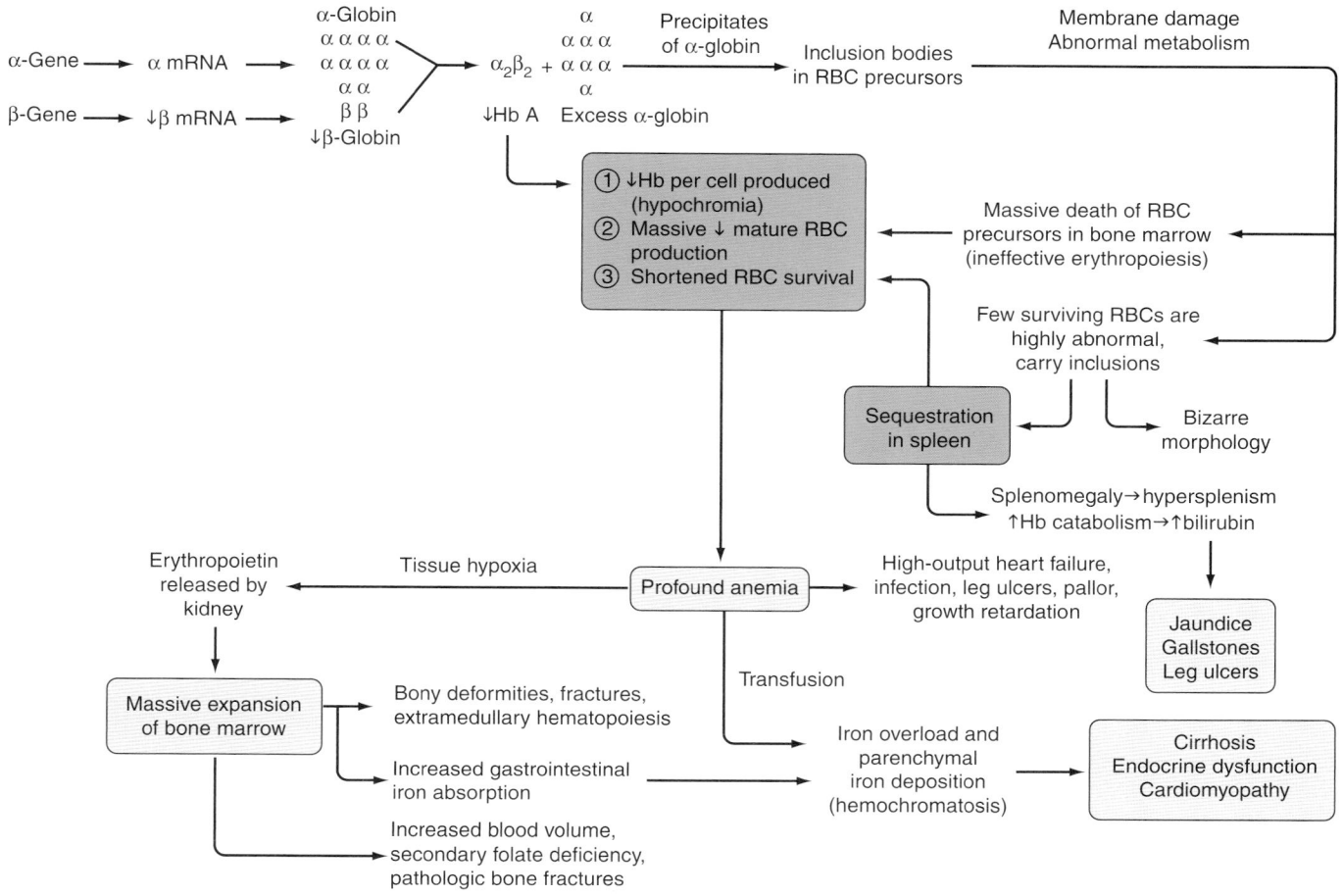

Fig. 49.5 Pathophysiology of severe forms of β-thalassemia. The diagram outlines the pathogenesis of clinical abnormalities resulting from the primary defect in β-globin chain synthesis. Hb, hemoglobin; RBC, red blood cell. (From Chapin J, Giardina PJ. Thalassemia syndromes. In: Hoffman R, Benz EJ Jr, Silberstein LE, et al., eds. *Hematology: Basic Principles and Practices.* 7th ed. Philadelphia: Elsevier; 2018:550, Fig. 40-4.)

Four genes code for the α-globin chains of hemoglobin: two genes on each chromosome 16. Deletions of one, two, three, or four of these genes account for the variable laboratory and clinical findings associated with the **α-thalassemia syndromes**. Decreased α-globin chain production leads to an excess of β-globin chains, which then precipitate within developing RBCs in the bone marrow, leading to destruction. Mature RBCs are mildly hypochromic and microcytic and may appear to be targeted.

Deletion of one α-thalassemia gene is known as the "silent carrier" state because it is not associated with anemia or microcytosis. This occurs in about 30% of individuals of African or Asian descent.

Deletion of two genes represents **α-thalassemia trait**. Similar to β-thalassemia trait, such patients manifest mild anemia and microcytosis with MCVs generally in the mildly decreased range (less microcytosis than is generally seen in β-thalassemia trait). The presence of Hb Barts on newborn screen confirms the diagnosis. Hemoglobin analysis beyond the newborn period cannot diagnose α-thalassemia trait.

A three-gene deletion leads to **hemoglobin H disease**, which is associated with moderate hemolytic anemia, microcytosis, reticulocytosis, and splenomegaly.

A four-gene deletion represents **α-thalassemia major** or hemoglobin Bart disease, in which the fetus is unable to produce any α-chains. Hence, nearly all in utero hemoglobin is Bart type (composed of four β-chains). Hemoglobin Bart disease has an extremely high oxygen affinity and leads to severe tissue hypoxemia and resultant fetal hydrops and death. On occasion, babies with hemoglobin Bart disease have been saved by extraordinary measures (intrauterine transfusion and early delivery), but they are then committed to lifelong transfusion support and/or bone marrow transplantation.

Hemoglobin H disease and α-thalassemia major occur almost exclusively in individuals of Asian descent. This is because Asians and Africans have different chromosomal arrangements of the abnormal genes. When α-thalassemia minor (two-gene deletion) occurs in the Asian population, deletions may be *cis* (both genes deleted from the same chromosome) or *trans* (each chromosome missing one gene). In individuals of African descent, α-thalassemia minor (two-gene deletion) occurs only on the basis of a *trans* distribution; hence, a child from two individuals with the African variety of α-thalassemia trait is affected with only two α genes deleted (α-thalassemia minor). A child from two individuals of Asian descent who have α-thalassemia minor may be affected with all four genes deleted (α-thalassemia major). The implication of a diagnosis of α-thalassemia trait in individuals of African descent usually relates primarily to its confusion with iron deficiency. Individuals of Asian descent must be appropriately counseled regarding the potential for transmission of serious hematologic disease if two individuals with α-thalassemia trait have a child.

Lead poisoning. The occurrence of elevated serum and total body burdens of lead is a major public health problem. This is of particular importance for infants and young children from families living in old housing with lead-based paint. Elevated lead levels may decrease erythropoiesis because lead inhibits several enzymes along the path of protoporphyrin synthesis. Lead may also produce hemolysis.

Anemia is usually seen in association with lead levels of 60–70 µg/dL or higher. Anemia is mild, variably microcytic, and associated with prominent basophilic stippling of RBCs. Coexistent iron deficiency is common because iron deficiency promotes increased lead absorption. The presence of mild microcytic anemia in children with mild to moderate lead burdens is usually due to concomitant iron deficiency. Lead chelation therapy is appropriate when lead levels are higher than 40–45 µg/dL. Additional features of marked lead toxicity include intestinal colic, lead lines in long bone radiographs, behavioral changes, renal tubular defects, and lead encephalopathy associated with increased intracranial pressure.

Anemia of inflammation. In a wide variety of chronic inflammatory or infectious disorders, mild to moderate anemia, termed **anemia of inflammation** (previously known as anemia of chronic disease), may be present. The MCV is usually normal to mildly decreased. Chronic inflammation or infection impairs the transfer of iron from reticuloendothelial cells within the marrow to developing erythroid elements. This results in some degree of iron-restricted erythropoiesis despite adequate marrow stores of iron. This impaired transfer of iron is due in part to the iron regulatory hormone hepcidin, which is elevated during times of inflammation. Often the history and physical examination findings point to acute inflammation or chronic illness, but occasionally patients have no obvious manifestations of systemic disease. The presence of unexplained normocytic or mild microcytic anemia should alert the clinician to the possibility of occult systemic disease. An elevated ESR or CRP is usually noted in patients with chronic inflammatory or infectious states. Anemia of inflammation is characterized by no specific abnormalities on peripheral smear other than mild hypochromia and microcytosis. Serum ferritin levels are elevated in inflammatory states and are thus a poor reflection of iron status. Serum iron level and total iron-binding capacity are generally decreased, but the percentage of iron saturation is often within the low to normal range, distinguishing it from iron-deficiency anemia.

Rare causes of microcytic anemia. **Sideroblastic anemias** are a group of very rare congenital (often X-linked) inherited diseases associated with impairment of protoporphyrin synthesis and variable microcytic anemia. The bone marrow examination demonstrates evidence of developing erythroid cells with excess iron deposited in mitochondria that tend to form a circular appearance around the nucleus, hence the term *ringed sideroblast* (Table 49.11). **Copper deficiency** is another rare cause of microcytic anemia. Associated features include neutropenia and scurvy-like bone changes (periosteal elevation). Only under unusual circumstances, when prominent microcytic anemia is otherwise unexplained, should these rare disorders be considered.

Normocytic Anemia Secondary to Underproduction

When normocytic anemia secondary to underproduction is identified in a patient, the key issue is whether anemia is occurring in isolation or is associated with other cytopenias (see Chapter 50 and Fig. 49.6; also see Fig. 49.4). Normocytic anemia with an inadequate reticulocyte response and pancytopenia raises the possibility of serious primary or secondary bone marrow failure syndromes (see Chapter 50) or malignancy. The history and physical examination findings are often predictive of the presence of thrombocytopenia (easy bruising, petechiae, ecchymosis) and/or neutropenia (fever, signs of infection). Adenopathy and hepatosplenomegaly are suggestive of bone marrow infiltration caused by malignancy.

TABLE 49.11	**Classification of Sideroblastic Anemia**
Hereditary (Nonsyndromic)	
X-linked	
Autosomal dominant or recessive	
Acquired	
Idiopathic acquired* (refractory anemia with ring sideroblasts)	
Associated with previous chemotherapy, irradiation, or in transition myelodysplasia or myeloproliferative diseases	
Drugs	
Alcohol	
Isoniazid	
Chloramphenicol	
Other drugs	
Rare Causes	
Erythropoietic protoporphyria	
Copper deficiency or zinc overload	
Hypothermia	
Hereditary (Syndromic)	
X-linked sideroblastic anemia with ring sideroblasts and cerebellar ataxia	
Myopathy, lactic acidosis, and sideroblastic anemia	
Pearson syndrome	
Thiamine-responsive megaloblastic anemia	
Sideroblastic anemia with immunodeficiency, fevers, and developmental delay	

*Trial of pyridoxine indicated.
From Hoffman R, Benz EJ Jr, Silberstein LE, et al., eds. *Hematology: Basic Principles and Practices.* 7th ed. Philadelphia: Elsevier; 2018:507, Table 38-5.

Acquired aplastic anemia is a rare disorder of childhood characterized by pancytopenia (neutropenia, anemia, thrombocytopenia) and a markedly hypoplastic bone marrow (see Chapter 50). Clinical manifestations may include pallor, fatigue, purpura, bleeding (cutaneous petechiae and ecchymosis, epistaxis, gingival oozing), and/or recurrent infection. Adenopathy and hepatosplenomegaly are not features of this condition. The cause is often idiopathic but may be related to prior infection (hepatitis, Epstein-Barr virus), toxin exposure (benzene, other volatile compounds), or medications (chloramphenicol, anticonvulsants). The peripheral blood smear demonstrates normal-appearing RBCs, an absence of polychromasia, and few leukocytes and platelets. The MCV may be elevated. A bone marrow biopsy demonstrates hypoplasia involving all cell lines.

Disorders associated with bone marrow infiltration including **leukemia** and **metastatic malignancy** often manifest with normocytic anemia secondary to RBC underproduction, thrombocytopenia, and either neutropenia or leukocytosis. Teardrop erythrocytes (dacrocytes) may be present in the peripheral smear (see Table 49.7). The MCV may be elevated. Many children with leukemia come to medical attention because of pallor, fatigue, and purpura. Limping and skeletal pain are also common with childhood leukemia. Pallor, purpura, adenopathy, and hepatosplenomegaly are often seen on physical examination. Peripheral blood smear usually but not always has leukemic blasts. Bone marrow examination findings are diagnostic.

When normocytic anemia secondary to underproduction is isolated *without* associated thrombocytopenia or neutropenia, several diagnostic entities must be considered. Mild anemia commonly accompanies acute infections and inflammatory illness. Children are

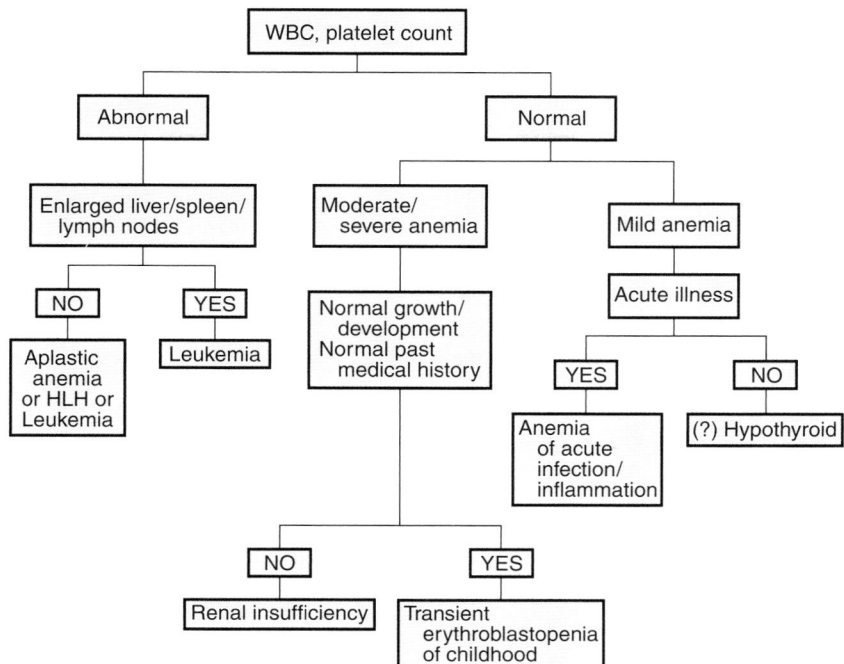

Fig. 49.6 Diagnostic scheme of normochromocytic anemia of underproduction. HLH, hemophagocytic lymphohistiocytosis; WBC, white blood cell.

often incidentally found to be anemic several days to a few weeks after having childhood infectious illnesses including viral upper respiratory tract infections, gastroenteritis, or undifferentiated febrile illnesses. Anemia reflects impaired erythrocyte production because of bone marrow–suppressive mediators of the immune/inflammatory response including interleukins, interferons, and tumor necrosis factor. Cessation of RBC production leads to a fall in hemoglobin level of about 1 g/dL/wk. Mild anemia discovered during or shortly after acute illness does not necessitate an extensive evaluation; rather, a follow-up hemoglobin determination should be obtained several weeks later. Persistent anemia necessitates further evaluation.

Transient erythroblastopenia of childhood (TEC), occurring predominantly in infants and toddlers (85% between 1 and 4 years), represents a temporary arrest of erythropoiesis. The underlying mechanism is hypothesized to be secondary to immunoglobulin G (IgG) antibodies that cross-react with early erythroid precursor cells. Infection is thought to be one impetus for the development of this condition. Patients may present with pallor and fatigue that occurs gradually over several weeks to months. Because of the very gradual fall in hemoglobin, most affected children are remarkably well compensated. Physical examination usually shows only marked pallor and mild tachycardia. Adenopathy and hepatosplenomegaly are not present. Congestive heart failure occurs only if anemia is very severe. The CBC demonstrates a normocytic anemia and profound reticulocytopenia. The WBC and platelet counts are normal in most patients; however, 25% of patients have mild neutropenia at the time of presentation. The peripheral blood smear is unremarkable. Recovery is spontaneous, and treatment is supportive. Blood transfusion is indicated only for patients with severe, symptomatic anemia. TEC may be difficult to differentiate from congenital hypoplastic anemia (Diamond-Blackfan anemia), particularly in children younger than 1 year (Table 49.12). In Diamond-Blackfan anemia, a constitutional RBC aplasia syndrome, MCV and fetal hemoglobin levels are usually elevated for the patient's age, providing clues to the diagnosis (see Chapter 50). Patients with

TABLE 49.12 Distinguishing Features Between Diamond-Blackfan Anemia (DBA) and Transient Erythroblastopenia of Childhood (TEC)

	DBA	TEC
Etiology	Genetic	Acquired
Immune mediated	None	Common
Family history	≈10%	Occasional siblings with concurrent TEC
Antecedent history	None	Viral infection
Age at diagnosis	90% by 1 yr	6 mo–4 yr
Physical anomalies	≈50%	None
Neurologic findings	None	Occasional
Transfusion dependence	Yes, if steroid refractory	None
Course	Chronic	Full recovery
Risk of cancer	Increased	Not increased
Risk of MDS or leukemia	Increased	Not increased
Laboratory findings at diagnosis:		
RBC size	Macrocytic	Normocytic
HbF	Increased	Normal*
i Antigen	Increased	Normal*
RBC enzyme activities	Fetal levels	Adult levels
RBC adenosine deaminase	Increased in 40–90%	Normal

*During spontaneous recovery, values may be increased.
HbF, fetal hemoglobin; MDS, myelodysplasia syndrome; RBC, red bood cell.
From Hoffman R, Benz EJ Jr, Silberstein LE, et al., eds. *Hematology: Basic Principles and Practices.* 7th ed. Philadelphia: Elsevier; 2018:377, Table 29-7.

TEC are otherwise healthy with no abnormal physical exam findings aside from those associated with anemia. Nonetheless, transient neurologic findings may be seen in TEC; these include papilledema, ataxia, hemiparesis, and seizures.

A patient with previously undiagnosed chronic hemolytic anemia (sickle cell anemia, hereditary spherocytosis) may present with normocytic anemia and severe reticulocytopenia if transient RBC hypoplasia occurs based on a viral infection such as commonly seen with parvovirus B19. Because of a shortened RBC life span in patients with chronic hemolysis, a transient arrest of RBC production can cause severe anemia that evolves over several days. Patients may have a history of neonatal jaundice and/or intermittent icterus, and they often have splenomegaly and an abnormal peripheral smear related to the underlying hemolytic disease.

Isolated anemia secondary to underproduction occurs in children with **chronic renal disease** because of erythropoietin deficiency. Clinical and laboratory findings often suggest a diagnosis of renal insufficiency such as poor growth, hypertension, edema, abnormal urinalysis, and elevated serum urea nitrogen and creatinine levels. The anemia of chronic renal disease can be successfully treated by recombinant human erythropoietin in conjunction with intravenous iron therapy.

Macrocytic Anemia (see Figs. 49.1 and 49.4)

Anemia due to bone marrow failure syndromes. **Diamond-Blackfan anemia** is a constitutional pure RBC aplasia syndrome that manifests during the first year of life with isolated severe anemia and reticulocytopenia (see Chapter 50). The remainder of the CBC is unremarkable. Because synthesis of RBCs containing adult hemoglobin is markedly impaired, RBCs generally manifest fetal characteristics, including elevated MCV, increased levels of fetal hemoglobin, and the "i" surface antigen. Bone marrow aspirate demonstrates pure RBC aplasia.

Fanconi anemia usually manifests with macrocytic anemia secondary to underproduction and pancytopenia. It is a constitutional disorder frequently associated with physical stigmata in ~50% of patients (see Chapter 50). Most patients do not present with overt hematologic manifestations until 4 or 5 years of age. Thumb and radial anomalies should alert the clinician to possible Fanconi anemia even in the absence of cytopenias. RBCs tend to have fetal characteristics including increased MCV and elevated fetal hemoglobin level. There are at least 15 genes responsible for Fanconi anemia; sequencing may confirm the diagnosis.

Megaloblastic anemia (vitamin B_{12} deficiency or folate deficiency). Megaloblastic anemia, characterized by macrocytic RBCs with variable abnormalities of WBCs and platelets, is usually caused by vitamin B_{12} deficiency or folate deficiency. Albeit rare in children, it can occur secondary to nutritional or congenital etiologies. If severe, associated pancytopenia can occur (see Chapter 50). In addition to large ovoid RBCs, hypersegmented neutrophils (more than 5 lobes/cell) are often seen on the peripheral smear (Fig. 49.7); large platelets can be present. It is appropriate to suspect vitamin B_{12} deficiency or folate deficiency in patients with otherwise unexplained macrocytic anemia. Documenting the presence of vitamin B_{12} deficiency or folate deficiency requires an assessment of nutrition and GI absorption. Prompt diagnosis of vitamin B_{12} deficiency is imperative due to the associated neurologic manifestations that can occur. Importantly, the degree of anemia can be inversely proportional to the neurologic symptoms. The diagnosis of vitamin B_{12} deficiency and folate deficiency cannot be made solely on the levels of vitamin B_{12} deficiency or folate. The precursors of methylmalonic acid (MMA) and homocysteine must also be evaluated since normal vitamin B_{12} levels can still be associated with vitamin B_{12} deficiency. Elevated MMA despite normal B_{12} levels is diagnostic of

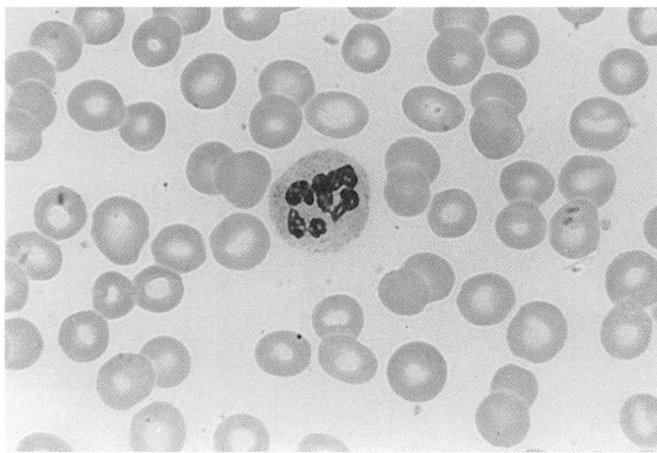

Fig. 49.7 Hypersegmented polymorphonuclear leukocyte as seen in vitamin B_{12} deficiency or folate deficiency.

B_{12} deficiency. RBC folate and not serum folate should be evaluated to accurately assess folate levels.

Nutritional vitamin B_{12} deficiency may occur in breast-feeding infants of mothers on strict vegetarian diets that exclude milk and egg products. **Congenital pernicious anemia** is a rare syndrome associated with vitamin B_{12} malabsorption that is caused by gastric intrinsic factor deficiency. Children who have had resection of the terminal ileum, the site of absorption of vitamin B_{12}, may develop megaloblastic anemia. Vitamin B_{12} malabsorption may occur in patients affected with autoimmune gastritis or with inflammatory disease involving the terminal ileum such as Crohn disease or ulcerative colitis. Rare congenital disorders that affect vitamin B_{12} transport, absorption (i.e., Imerslund-Grasbeck syndrome), or metabolism can also occur.

Unlike body stores of vitamin B_{12}, which may provide several years' reserve, folate stores are limited to several weeks' supply. Folate is ubiquitous in food sources; hence, nutritional deficiency is unusual. Infants fed unsupplemented goat's milk may develop profound folate deficiency. Malabsorption of folate can occur in children who have limited small bowel absorptive capacity because of surgical resection or inflammatory disease.

Anemia Caused by Increased Red Blood Cell Destruction

The hemolytic disorders (see Figs. 49.1 and 49.4) are characterized by shortened RBC survival and compensatory reticulocytosis. Normal RBCs survive approximately 120 days in the circulation. New RBCs are manufactured at a rate equivalent to the destruction of senescent RBCs so that under normal circumstances an appropriate hemoglobin level is maintained. Intrinsic or extrinsic RBC factors can lead to accelerated RBC destruction. Several clinical and laboratory hallmarks are associated with hemolysis (Table 49.13). It is imperative that a technically adequate peripheral blood smear be examined whenever hemolysis is suspected. Although normal RBC structure does not exclude a diagnosis of hemolytic anemia, most hemolytic diseases are associated with morphologic abnormalities (Table 49.14). Depending on the cause of the hemolysis, RBCs may be removed from the circulation by reticuloendothelial cells (*extravascular* hemolysis) or may lyse within the circulation (*intravascular* hemolysis). With intravascular hemolysis, hemoglobin is released into the plasma and bound by the serum protein haptoglobin. In states of brisk intravascular hemolysis, haptoglobin may be depleted and free hemoglobin may be filtered by the kidney, resulting in a pink appearance of the urine. A urinary dipstick test result is positive for blood, but the microscopic examination of the urinary sediment does not demonstrate intact RBCs.

TABLE 49.13 Clinical and Laboratory Features Suggestive of Hemolytic Anemia

Pallor
Icterus
Dark or tea-colored urine
Splenomegaly
Gallstones
History of neonatal jaundice
Positive family history of anemia, splenectomy, cholecystectomy
↑ Reticulocyte count
↑ RDW (due to ↑ reticulocyte count)
Abnormal RBC morphology
↑ Indirect bilirubin (normal direct bilirubin)
↓ Serum haptoglobin level
↑ Urinary urobilinogen level
Hemoglobinuria (+ dipstick test result for blood; no RBCs in urine)
↑ LDH level

LDH, lactate dehydrogenase; RBC, red blood cell; RDW, red blood cell distribution width.

TABLE 49.14 Hemolytic Anemia: Diagnostic Clues Based on Red Blood Cell Structure

Sickle cells: sickle cell disease
Target cells: hemoglobinopathies (HbC, HbS, thalassemia), liver disease
Schistocytes/burr cells/helmet cells/RBC fragments: microangiopathic hemolytic anemia—DIC, HUS, TTP
Spherocytes: hereditary spherocytosis, autoimmune hemolytic anemia
Cigar-shaped cells: hereditary elliptocytosis
"Bite" cells: G6PD deficiency
Poikilocytosis, microcytosis, fragmented erythrocytes, elliptocytes: hereditary pyropoikilocytosis

DIC, disseminated intravascular coagulation; G6PD, glucose-6-phosphate dehydrogenase; Hb, hemoglobin; HUS, hemolytic uremic syndrome; RBC, red blood cell; TTP, thrombotic thrombocytopenic purpura.

Disturbances of any of the three key components of the RBC—the membrane, enzymes, and hemoglobin—may lead to ongoing or intermittent hemolysis.

Membrane Defects

The prototypic intrinsic red cell membrane defect is **hereditary spherocytosis**, which is an inherited disorder that can be inherited as autosomal dominant or autosomal recessive or be a new variant. This disorder occurs in approximately 1/5,000 live births. It is seen most typically in individuals of Northern European descent but may be identified in any population. The basic defect is an abnormality of a membrane protein (spectrin, protein 3, or ankyrin) that allows the RBC membrane to lose its redundancy and the usual biconcave disk shape resulting in a small, dense cell of spheroid configuration (see Fig. 49.2). Hemolysis occurs because the spheroid RBCs are far less distensible and are unable to successfully traverse the microcirculation of the spleen. Characteristic clinical findings include anemia, reticulocytosis, and the presence of abundant microspherocytes on peripheral smear. Associated nonspecific findings of chronic hemolysis are often present including pallor, icterus, and splenomegaly. In autosomal dominant forms the family history is often positive for anemia, splenectomy, or cholecystectomy.

Newborns with hereditary spherocytosis frequently develop jaundice within the first 24 hours after birth, necessitating phototherapy and occasionally exchange transfusion. Diagnosis may be confirmed by an osmotic fragility test reflecting the limited capacity of the RBC to expand when incubated in a hypotonic solution. The clinical spectrum of disease is broad. Some patients have mild, well-compensated hemolysis and the condition is detected during their adult years after a diagnosis in one of their children. Other patients may have brisk hemolysis during infancy necessitating intermittent transfusion support. Most patients have a disease course characterized by mild to moderate anemia, reticulocytosis, and splenomegaly. Patients are susceptible to exacerbations of anemia because of virus-induced hyperhemolysis or transient RBC hypoplasia. Parvovirus B19 may cause superimposed transient RBC hypoplasia of about 1 week's duration, resulting in moderate to severe anemia that requires transfusion.

A severe form of autosomal recessive hereditary spherocytosis due to *SPTA1* variants can present with fetal anemia and often require intrauterine transfusion support to prevent progression to hydrops. At birth, infants have severe anemia with reticulocytopenia that can be difficult to distinguish from Diamond-Blackfan anemia. These patients are often transfusion dependent and share many clinical characteristics to patients with ineffective erythropoiesis such as thalassemia.

Hereditary elliptocytosis represents a heterogeneous group of inherited disorders characterized by variable chronic hemolysis and abundant elliptical RBCs on peripheral smear. The clinical and laboratory findings are similar to those seen in hereditary spherocytosis. Splenectomy is appropriate in patients with moderate to severe hemolytic disease.

Hereditary pyropoikilocytosis is an autosomal recessive membrane disorder that manifests in the newborn period and is characterized by marked jaundice and anemia, reticulocytosis, and striking aberrations of RBC structure (see Table 49.14). Hemolysis lessens with advancing age.

Enzyme Defects

The most common RBC enzyme defect is G6PD deficiency. An X-linked disorder, G6PD deficiency occurs most commonly in individuals of African and Mediterranean descent and should always be considered in the differential diagnosis of acute hemolytic anemia in males (though rarely females can be affected). Deficiency of G6PD activity renders hemoglobin susceptible to oxidant insult, leading to precipitation of hemoglobin, membrane damage, and ultimately RBC destruction. Oxidant injury may occur because of intercurrent infection or ingestion of various substances, including medications (i.e., classically sulfa drugs), toxins, and foods such as fava beans (Table 49.15).

The common African variant of G6PD, termed *G6PD deficient variant A–*, is not necessarily associated with chronic hemolysis but usually manifests as mild acute hemolytic anemia related to specific precipitating factors. Rarely is hemolysis sufficiently severe to warrant transfusion therapy. Patients are often incidentally found to be anemic with evidence of an appropriate reticulocyte response. A peripheral blood smear may demonstrate "bite" cells as portions of the RBC (precipitates of hemoglobin) are removed by reticuloendothelial cells (Fig. 49.8). G6PD enzyme assay is necessary for the establishment of a diagnosis, but the test must be performed on a sample that has been depleted of reticulocytes because newly released RBCs have greater amounts of G6PD. The Mediterranean variety of G6PD deficiency tends to be more severe and may be associated with chronic hemolysis as well as hemolysis with superimposed acute events caused by infection or medication leading to symptomatic anemia and the occasional need for transfusion therapy.

Although rare, **pyruvate kinase deficiency (PKD)** is the second most common enzyme deficiency after G6PD deficiency. Inheritance of PKD is autosomal recessive. PKD is characterized by absence of or

TABLE 49.15 Factors Known to Promote Hemolysis in Patients with G6PD Deficiency

Viral or bacterial infection
Fava beans
Vitamin C (large doses)
Mothballs (naphthalene)
Benzene and other volatiles
Medications
    Sulfonamides*
    Antimalarial drugs†
    Nitrofurantoin
    Nalidixic acid
    Chloramphenicol
    Vitamin K analogs
    Methylene blue
    High-dose aspirin
    Stibophen
    Niridazole
    Probenecid
    Dimercaprol (BAL)
    Toluidine blue
    Phenylhydrazine
    Local anesthetics such as lidocaine, benzocaine

*Sulfanilamide, sulfapyridine, sulfadimidine, sulfacetamide, sulfafurazole, salicylazosulfapyridine (Azulfidine), dapsone, sulfoxone, co-trimoxazole (Septrin).
†Primaquine, pamaquine, chloroquine (use with caution).
G6PD, glucose-6-phosphate dehydrogenase.

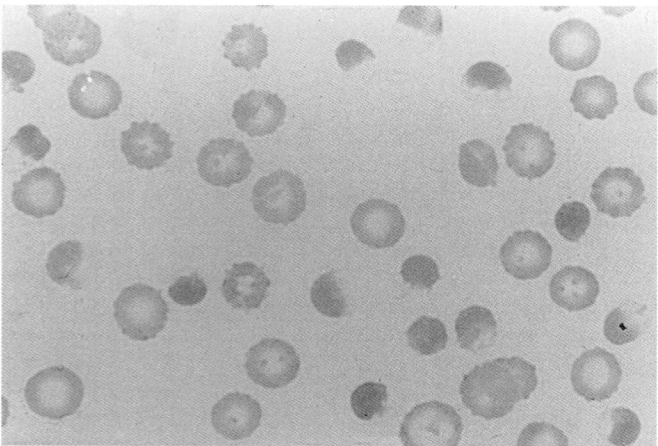

Fig. 49.8 "Bite" cells and burr cells as seen in glucose-6-phosphate dehydrogenase deficiency hemolysis.

significantly reduced levels of the intracellular RBC enzyme pyruvate kinase. Lack of this enzyme leads to decreased levels of ATP and subsequent brisk hemolysis. The clinical spectrum of PKD is variable but can result in severe chronic hemolytic anemia that is present in utero and postnatally. In its most severe form, hemolysis is extremely brisk, and it is not uncommon for patients with PKD to maintain reticulocyte counts of 40% or higher. Peripheral blood smear appears relatively unremarkable but may demonstrate spiculated RBCs. Specific enzyme assay can be performed by specialized laboratories to aid in the diagnosis. Patients with PKD usually require lifelong RBC transfusions that often result in transfusional iron overload. Splenomegaly is often present. Splenectomy is not curative but can ameliorate the condition by resulting in an increment in hemoglobin by 1–2 g/dL, thereby reducing

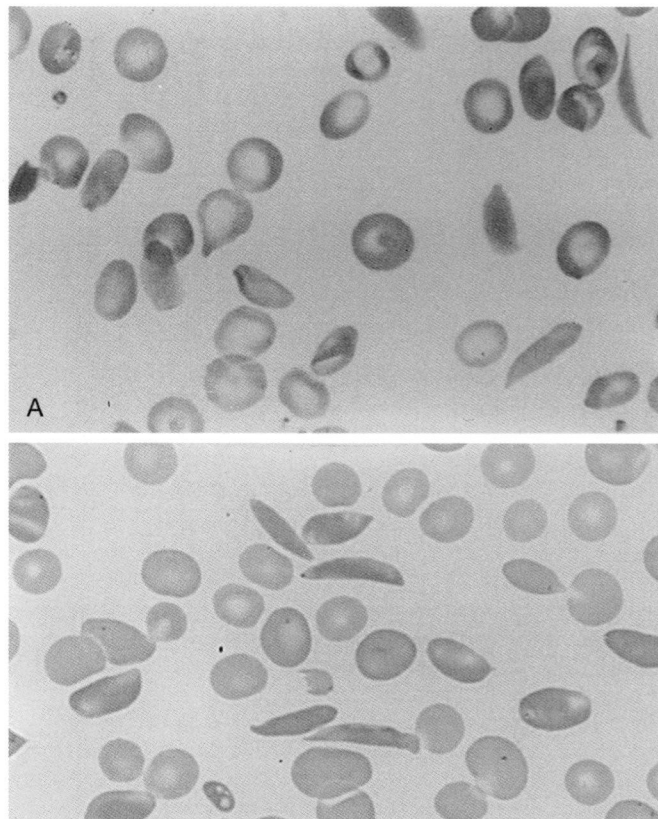

Fig. 49.9 Sickle cell anemia. *A, B,* Sickled erythrocytes and target cells.

the number of required transfusions. Following splenectomy, the reticulocyte count increases further. Patients with PKD are also extremely susceptible to transient RBC hypoplasia caused by parvovirus B19 infection.

Hemoglobinopathies

Hemoglobinopathies usually occur because of a single amino acid substitution in α- or β-globin chains. Hemoglobinopathies are among the most common causes of chronic hemolytic disease. α- and β-Thalassemia syndromes were previously discussed. Sickle cell syndromes are the most frequently encountered hemoglobinopathies.

The sickle hemoglobinopathy syndromes are a group of genetically inherited disorders encountered most frequently in individuals of African descent. Thus, a form of **sickle cell disease** should be considered in the differential diagnosis of anemia in any Black child. These disorders occur less frequently in individuals of Mediterranean or Arabic background.

Sickle hemoglobin is characterized by a single amino acid substitution of valine for glutamic acid in the number 6 position of the β-globin chain. Sickle hemoglobin tends to form insoluble fibers and polymerization within the RBC when deoxygenated. This ultimately leads to the formation of the characteristic crescent-shaped sickled erythrocytes (Fig. 49.9). When sickle hemoglobin trait is inherited from both parents in an autosomal recessive fashion, the child has homozygous hemoglobin SS disease. This is the most severe form of sickle cell disease. Sickle hemoglobin may also be co-inherited with other β-globin gene defects such as hemoglobin C or β-thalassemia and give rise to other heterozygous forms of sickle cell disease that can be less severe than hemoglobin SS disease. Approximately 1 in 400 African Americans has sickle cell disease.

TABLE 49.16 Hemoglobin Electrophoresis Diagnosis of Sickle Hemoglobinopathy

Disease	Hemoglobin Type
Normal	A
SS, Sβ⁰ disease	S (no hemoglobin A)
S trait	A > S
SC disease	S + C (about equal proportions)
S-β-thalassemia	S > A (S predominant hemoglobin)

TABLE 49.17 Clinical Manifestations of Sickle Cell Anemia*

Manifestation	Comments
Anemia	Chronic onset, 3–4 mo of age; hematocrit usually 18–26%
Aplastic crisis	Parvovirus infection, reticulocytopenia, acute and reversible
Sequestration crisis	Massive splenomegaly, shock; treat with transfusion
Hemolytic crisis	May be associated with G6PD deficiency
Dactylitis	Hand-foot swelling in early infancy
Painful crisis	Microvascular painful vasoocclusive infarctions of muscle, bone, bone marrow, lung intestines; other etiologies likely contribute that are under investigation
Cerebral vascular accidents (overt and silent)	Large- and small-vessel sickling and thrombosis (stroke); necessitates chronic transfusion
Acute chest syndrome	Infection, infarction, hypoventilation, bone marrow emboli, severe hypoxemia, infiltrate, dyspnea, rales
Chronic lung disease	Pulmonary fibrosis, restrictive lung disease, cor pulmonale, pulmonary artery hypertension
Priapism	Causes eventual impotence; treat with transfusion, oxygen, or corpora cavernosa to spongiosa shunt, local injection of α-adrenergic agents
Ocular	Retinopathy
Gallbladder disease	Bilirubin stones; cholecystitis
Renal	Hematuria, papillary necrosis, renal-concentrating deficit; nephropathy; chronic renal failure
Cardiomyopathy	Heart failure (fibrosis)
Leg ulceration	Seen in older patients
Infections	Functional asplenia, defects in properdin system; pneumococcal bacteremia, meningitis, and arthritis; deafness from meningitis, *Haemophilus influenzae* sepsis, *Salmonella* and *Staphylococcus aureus* osteomyelitis; severe *Mycoplasma* pneumonia; *Escherichia coli*; urinary tract infection
Growth failure, delayed puberty	May respond to nutritional supplements
Neurocognitive deficits	Poorer school performance
Psychosocial issues	Depression, anxiety, attention-deficit/hyperactivity disorder (ADHD)

*Clinical manifestations with sickle cell trait are unusual but include renal papillary necrosis (hematuria), sudden death on exertion, intraocular hyphema extension, and sickling in unpressurized airplanes.

G6PD, glucose-6-phosphate dehydrogenase.

Modified from Scott JP. Hematology. In: Behrman RE, Kliegman RM, eds. *Nelson Essentials of Pediatrics*. 2nd ed. Philadelphia: WB Saunders; 1994:530.

Approximately 8% of African Americans are carriers of the hemoglobin S gene, which is also termed **sickle cell trait** and results in approximately 30–40% of hemoglobin S. Sickle cell trait is rarely associated with clinical disease except under states of unusually severe arterial hypoxemia. Spontaneous hematuria may occasionally occur in sickle trait as a result of the induction of sickling in the extremely hypertonic environment of the renal medulla. Patients with sickle cell trait are distinctly not anemic and have a normal peripheral blood smear.

The diagnosis of sickle cell disease is usually straightforward. Children are variably anemic with reticulocytosis. The peripheral blood smear demonstrates characteristic sickled erythrocytes (see Fig. 49.9). The definitive diagnosis must be established by hemoglobin identification methods (Table 49.16). The hemoglobin solubility test (sickle preparation, Sickledex) should not be used to make the diagnosis as false-negative tests can occur. Diagnosis in newborns is routinely and accurately performed in most locations within the United States as a component of state-mandated universal neonatal screening programs.

Sickle cell disease is a multiorgan system disease. The clinical manifestations are extremely broad but generally include (1) chronic hemolytic anemia, (2) vasoocclusion resulting in ischemic injury to tissue, (3) susceptibility to infection, (4) acute and chronic pain, (5) cerebrovascular complications (e.g., stroke), (6) cardiopulmonary complications, and (7) renal disease (Table 49.17). Infants younger than 4–6 months usually show no clinical manifestations because of naturally high levels of fetal hemoglobin. By 1–2 years of age, most affected patients have had a specific sickle cell–related manifestation.

Patients may appear variably pale and icteric depending on the degree of hemolysis. Splenomegaly can be seen in children between 6 and 36 months of age in patients with hemoglobin SS disease and may persist into adolescence in some patients with milder variants (SC disease, S-β⁺-thalassemia). Autoinfarction from microvascular occlusion ultimately leads to fibrosis of splenic tissue by age 3–4 years in most patients with hemoglobin SS disease. Gallstones occur regularly and may lead to symptoms of cholelithiasis, acute cholecystitis, biliary tract obstruction, and/or pancreatitis. Many patients have delayed growth and pubertal development but ultimately achieve normal adult height. Exacerbation of anemia can occur as a result of infection-induced hyperhemolysis or transient RBC aplasia commonly associated with parvovirus B19 infection. Hyperhemolytic episodes may also occur in male patients with concomitant G6PD deficiency. RBC transfusions are necessary when progressive anemia occurs in the context of splenic sequestration or aplastic crises or due to other clinical complications such as acute chest syndrome.

Hemoglobin E is seen with considerable frequency among individuals of Asian descent. Hemoglobin E trait is characterized by mild anemia and mild microcytosis. There are no significant clinical implications. The diagnosis is confirmed by hemoglobin electrophoresis. When hemoglobin E occurs in the double heterozygous state with β-thalassemia, patients often have a moderately severe thalassemic syndrome; hence, genetic counseling is advisable.

Acquired Autoimmune Hemolytic Anemia

This condition may occur as a transient, postviral process or in conjunction with underlying immunologic dysfunction (immunodeficiency, autoimmune disease, HIV infection, lymphoid malignancy).

TABLE 49.18   Characteristics of Antibodies in Immune Hemolytic Anemia

	Warm-Antibody	Cold Agglutinin Disease	Paroxysmal Cold Hemoglobinuria	Drug-Related Immune, Type 1	Drug-Related Immune, Type II
Antibody isotype	IgG (rarely IgA)	IgM	IgG	IgG	IgM, IgG
Optimum temperature of reaction	37°C	0°C	0°C	37°C	37°C
Direct Coombs test	IgG ± C3	C3 only	C3 only	IgG only	C3 only
Agglutination in saline	None (rarely +)	++++	+	0 to +	0 to ++ (with drug)
Lysis by complement in vitro	Rare	Poor	Well	None	Sometimes well
Clinical severity	Mild to very severe	Mild to moderate	Moderate to severe	Mild to moderate	Mild to severe
Response to prednisone	Often	None	Often	If needed	Not needed
Response to splenectomy	Often	Rare	None	Not needed	Not needed

IgA, IgG, and IgM, immunoglobulins A, G, and M; +, strength of agglutination response.
From Rose MG, Berliner N. Disorders of red blood cells. In: Andreoli TE, Carpenter CJ, Bennett JC, et al., eds. *Cecil Essentials of Medicine.* 4th ed. Philadelphia: WB Saunders; 1997:389.

Hemolysis is usually brisk; thus, most patients are symptomatic and present with pallor, jaundice, tea-colored urine, fatigue, and tachycardia. Splenomegaly is variably present. The degree of anemia is highly variable, and the reticulocyte count is elevated in most patients; however, a minority of patients present with a low reticulocyte count because of immune destruction of reticulocytes. The peripheral smear demonstrates microspherocytes. The direct Coombs test is positive, confirming the diagnosis. Consideration should be given to evaluating immunologic dysfunction, infection, and malignancy (immunoglobulin levels, T and B lymphocyte counts, HIV and Epstein-Barr virus studies, chest radiography). The characteristics of the antibody types are noted in Table 49.18. Warm antibodies (usually IgG) may be idiopathic or associated with lymphoma, HIV or Epstein-Barr virus infections, rheumatologic disorders (lupus), primary immunodeficiency diseases, or most likely a nonspecific infectious phenomenon. Cold antibodies (usually immunoglobulin M [IgM]) may also be seen in response to viral infections and *Mycoplasma pneumoniae* and syphilis infections, or in the context of autoimmune disorders.

Aggressive therapy is recommended because life-threatening anemia is known to occur. Corticosteroids (prednisone) should be administered in most patients found to have warm autoimmune hemolytic anemia. An exception is patients with EBV-related autoimmune hemolytic anemia in whom the hemoglobin has stabilized. RBC transfusion should be considered based on the degree of the anemia; however, cross-matching blood is likely to be difficult due to the autoantibody. Intravenous immunoglobulin and high-dose steroids (methylprednisolone) should be considered in severe cases. Close hemoglobin monitoring and reticulocyte counts should be done to follow the rate of hemolysis. The role of steroids in the treatment of cold autoimmune hemolytic anemia is less clear and is classically reserved for prolonged cases requiring frequent RBC transfusions. Recombinant antibodies directed to B lymphocytes such as rituximab have been effective in refractory cases.

ANEMIA IN THE NEONATE

Neonatal anemia should be viewed in the context of three possible pathophysiologic pathways (Table 49.19): (1) acute blood loss, (2) anemia of underproduction, and (3) anemia associated with increased destruction. Familial genetic disorders may manifest in the neonatal period or any time during infancy (Table 49.20).

TABLE 49.19   Anemia in the Neonate

Blood Loss (Common)

Placenta previa
Abruptio placentae
Twin-twin transfusion
Fetal–maternal hemorrhage (acute vs chronic)
Neonatal hemorrhage

Decreased RBC Production (Unusual)

Diamond-Blackfan anemia
Autosomal recessive hereditary spherocytosis
Congenital leukemia
Transient myeloproliferative syndrome in Down syndrome
Osteopetrosis

Hemolysis

Intrinsic RBC defect (uncommon)
    Membrane (hereditary spherocytosis or elliptocytosis)
    Enzyme (G6PD, PK)
    Hemoglobin (α or γ chain abnormality)
Extrinsic RBC defect
    Immune (ABO, Rh, minor group incompatibilities) (common)
    Infection (intrauterine infection, bacterial, viral, protozoal)
    DIC
    Kasabach-Merritt syndrome
    Galactosemia
    TTP *(ADAMTS13)*

DIC, disseminated intravascular coagulation; G6PD, glucose-6-phosphate dehydrogenase; PK, pyruvate kinase; RBC, red blood cell; TTP, thrombotic thrombocytopenic purpura.

The full-term infant has a normal hemoglobin value (hemoglobin, 15–21 g/dL; hematocrit, 45–65%) that is substantially higher than that in older infants and young children. This finding represents a functional adaptation to the relatively hypoxic in utero environment. The reticulocyte count is elevated to about 7–8% during the first 3 days of life, after which there is an abrupt cessation of erythropoiesis until 2 months of age, when a physiologic hemoglobin nadir of about 9.5–10 g/dL is reached. This physiologic anemia of infancy is exaggerated in preterm infants whose hemoglobin levels may fall to approximately 7 g/dL at about 1–1.5 months of age. This fall in hemoglobin value

TABLE 49.20 Genetic Disorders Associated with Anemia in the Neonate

Syndrome	Genetic Characteristics	Hematologic Phenotype
Diamond-Blackfan syndrome	Autosomal recessive (AR); sporadic variants and autosomal dominant (AD) inheritance have been described	Steroid-responsive hypoplastic anemia after 5 mo of age
Fanconi anemia	AR, probably abnormalities in multiple genes (at least five genetic subtypes have been identified)	Steroid-responsive hypoplastic, macrocytic anemia DNA is hypersensitive to injury
Hereditary spherocytosis	AR (*SPTA1* variant)	Present with fetal anemia and reticulocytopenia, often requiring intrauterine transfusion
Aase syndrome	AR, possible AD	Steroid-responsive hypoplastic anemia; macrocytic; improves with age
Pearson syndrome	Mitochondrial DNA abnormalities, X-linked or AR	Hypoplastic sideroblastic anemia unresponsive to pyridoxine
Lethal osteopetrosis	AR, caused by defective resorption of immature bone	Hypoplastic anemia due to marrow encroachment
Congenital dyserythropoietic anemia (CDA)	AR	Type I: megaloblastoid erythroid and nuclear chromatin bridges between cells
		Type II: hereditary erythroblastic multinuclearity and positive acidified serum test results (HEMPAS)
		Type III: erythroblastic multinuclearity and macrocytosis
Peutz-Jeghers syndrome	AD	Iron deficiency, anemia from chronic blood loss
Dyskeratosis congenita	X-linked recessive, locus on Xq28; some cases with AD inheritance	Hypoplastic anemia; usually present between 5 and 15 yr of age
X-linked α-thalassemia/intellectual disability (ATR-X and ATR-16) syndromes	ATR-X: X-linked recessive, mapped to Xq13.3; ATR-16: mapped to 16p13.3; deletions of α-globin locus	ATR-X: hypochromic, microcytic anemia, mild form of hemoglobin H disease; ATR-16: more significant hemoglobin H disease and anemia are present
Thrombocytopenia with absent radius (TAR) syndrome	AR	Hemorrhagic anemia, possibly hypoplastic anemia as well
Osler hemorrhagic telangiectasia syndrome	AD, mapped to 9q33-34	Hemorrhagic anemia

From Ohls RK. Evaluation and treatment of anemia in the neonate. In: Christensen RD, ed. *Hematologic Problems of the Neonate*. Philadelphia: Saunders; 2000:153.

represents a physiologic response to the oxygen-rich extrauterine environment, which decreases erythropoietin production.

Neonatal Anemia Caused by Blood Loss

Anemia caused by blood loss is often obvious. It occurs in placenta previa, abruptio placentae, or a large cephalohematoma. Other etiologies of hemorrhage may be occult and include intracranial and intrahepatic hematomas. Internal hemorrhage is much more likely to occur in difficult deliveries. If twin-twin transfusion occurs, one infant will develop anemia while the other develops polycythemia. Fetal–maternal hemorrhage is sufficiently severe to cause anemia in only a small percentage of neonates. The Kleihauer-Betke test may detect the presence of fetal RBCs in the maternal circulation but may yield false-negative results, particularly in mothers with type O blood who have antibodies against infant A, B, or AB blood cells. Fetal–maternal hemorrhage must always be suspected when otherwise unexplained anemia occurs in a newborn.

The time course and extent of blood loss determine the clinical presentation. If blood loss is mild or chronic, infants may appear normal or have mild pallor and tachycardia. In the event of severe acute blood loss, the newborn may present with signs of acute illness including lethargy, tachycardia, hypotension, and respiratory distress. The hemoglobin value is a poor index of the severity of acute blood

loss because equilibration of fluid compartments may take 24–36 hours. Blood loss as a cause of anemia should always be suspected in cases of obstetric complications, multiple births, or difficult and traumatic deliveries. In cases of severe blood loss, emergency transfusion therapy is appropriate. In the neonate who is hemodynamically stable but has experienced significant blood loss, a more conservative approach is recommended.

Neonatal Anemia Caused by Decreased Red Blood Cell Production

Anemia caused by decreased RBC production in the newborn is unusual. Infants with congenital hypoplastic anemia (Diamond-Blackfan anemia) are usually only mildly anemic during the newborn period. Congenital leukemia is a rare disorder characterized by infiltration of the bone marrow leading to anemia, thrombocytopenia, and leukocytosis in association with hepatosplenomegaly and occasionally cutaneous leukemic infiltrates manifesting as blue papular lesions ("blueberry muffin" spots). Infants with Down syndrome may present with a clinical and hematologic picture identical to that of congenital leukemia, which is a transient myeloproliferative process that spontaneously remits over several months. Infantile osteopetrosis (marble bone disease), a disorder characterized by a limited ability to degrade bone, usually does not cause pancytopenia until a few months after birth.

Neonatal Anemia Caused by Increased Red Blood Cell Destruction

Anemia caused by increased RBC destruction (hemolytic anemia) places the neonate at risk for indirect hyperbilirubinemia because of the limited hepatic bilirubin-conjugating ability during the first weeks of life. Even relatively small increases in the rate of RBC destruction can lead to marked increases in serum bilirubin level. All infants who have elevations of indirect bilirubin levels above the normal range during the first 3 days of life should be evaluated for possible hemolysis, with a CBC, reticulocyte count, peripheral blood smear, maternal and infant blood type assessments, and direct Coombs test.

Intrinsic disorders of the erythrocyte may manifest in the neonate. Infants with hereditary spherocytosis, pyropoikilocytosis, or elliptocytosis may develop anemia and extreme hyperbilirubinemia that necessitate phototherapy and, rarely, exchange transfusion. A peripheral blood smear and family history may be helpful in identifying an intrinsic RBC membrane defect. A severe form of autosomal recessive hereditary spherocytosis may present with fetal anemia requiring intrauterine transfusion support. At the time of birth infants will have severe anemia with reticulocytopenia with or without indirect hyperbilirubinemia.

G6PD deficiency can occur in newborn males (rarely females) of African or Mediterranean descent. Because of the increased susceptibility of neonatal RBCs to oxidant injury, anemia, reticulocytosis, and hyperbilirubinemia may occur without an obvious precipitating oxidant insult. Hemoglobinopathies rarely manifest during the neonatal period. β-Globin chain defects such as sickle cell disease and thalassemia are not clinically apparent until about 4–6 months of age because of the predominance of fetal hemoglobin in the perinatal period.

Severe α-thalassemia, including α-thalassemia major or hemoglobin Bart disease, can affect the fetus. Such infants develop severe in utero anemia with resultant hydrops fetalis because of the limited ability of hemoglobin Bart disease to release oxygen to tissues.

Isoimmune hemolytic anemia is the most common cause of hemolytic anemia in the newborn. It is caused by incompatibility between maternal and fetal blood groups, including Rh, ABO, or minor blood group antigens. In **Rh incompatibility**, the mother is Rh negative, and the infant is Rh positive (inherited from the father). If the mother has been exposed to Rh-positive blood cells through prior pregnancy, miscarriage, therapeutic abortion, or mismatched blood transfusion, IgG antibodies may develop that traverse the placenta and cause immune destruction of fetal Rh-positive cells. In such instances hemolysis occurs in utero and in the neonatal period. In severe circumstances the fetus may be extremely anemic, which results in heart failure, hydrops fetalis, and death. In less serious instances infants may be born quite anemic and develop brisk hyperbilirubinemia, which can lead to kernicterus. The severity of Rh immune hemolytic disease increases with successive pregnancies. This disorder is uncommon because of the routine practice of administering Rh immunoglobulin to Rh-negative mothers who are 28–30 weeks pregnant and within 72 hours of delivery or after spontaneous or therapeutic abortion. Prenatal management of the affected fetus may include ultrasonographic assessment of fetal well-being (vascular resistance, hydrops) and in high-risk situations serial fetal hemoglobin levels obtained by ultrasonographically guided aspiration of umbilical cord blood (cordocentesis). When the fetus demonstrates progressive in utero severe anemia, intrauterine intravascular blood transfusion therapy has been shown to decrease the risk for fetal

demise. Management of the neonate relates largely to the severity of the hemolysis. Hyperbilirubinemia must be treated aggressively with phototherapy and, if severe, exchange transfusion. RBC transfusions are appropriate for symptomatic anemia. On occasion, anemia is detected several weeks after Rh hemolysis and may be associated with a profoundly depressed reticulocyte count. This late anemia is of uncertain origin, but inappropriately low erythropoietin levels have been noted. Symptomatic infants may require transfusion therapy. Affected infants have been successfully treated with human recombinant erythropoietin.

Immune incompatibility in the **ABO system** is common and usually occurs when mothers with type O blood have newborns whose blood type is A or B. The degree of hemolysis is usually much less severe than in Rh disease. Fetal hydrops is extremely rare. Most babies with ABO incompatibility manifest jaundice from indirect hyperbilirubinemia during the first 1–2 days after birth. Hemoglobin levels are often within the normal to mildly anemic range, but moderate anemia occasionally occurs. The reticulocyte count is usually mildly elevated, and the peripheral blood smear may show microspherocytes. Results of the Coombs test are usually weakly or moderately positive, but false-negative results do occur. Treatment is generally directed toward hyperbilirubinemia and may require phototherapy. Intravenous immunoglobulin therapy has been helpful in some patients. Exchange transfusion is rarely necessary. Anemia occasionally necessitates blood transfusion. Immune incompatibility may also occur on the basis of minor blood group antigens such as the Duffy or Kell antigen systems. Clinical and laboratory findings are similar to those in ABO hemolytic disease except that the direct Coombs test result is usually strongly positive.

Other causes of hemolytic anemia in the newborn include bacterial sepsis and intrauterine infection (cytomegalovirus, toxoplasmosis, herpes, rubella, and syphilis). Intrauterine infectious syndromes can cause mild to moderate hemolytic anemia of several months' duration. Such infants may demonstrate physical stigmata including small size for gestational age, microcephaly, chorioretinitis, hepatosplenomegaly, intracranial calcifications, and "celery stalking" of the long bones on radiographic study.

Microangiopathic hemolytic anemia can occur in the newborn as a result of disseminated intravascular coagulation (DIC). In the neonate, DIC is usually caused by serious infection, hypoxemia resulting from respiratory distress syndrome in the preterm infant, or ischemic tissue injury related to birth asphyxia. Newborns with hemolysis resulting from infection or DIC are often extremely ill and require RBC transfusion support.

Microangiopathic hemolytic anemia and consumptive thrombocytopenia can occur in Kasabach-Merritt syndrome, which is associated with cavernous hemangiomas and localized intravascular coagulation. Some infants have obvious expansive cutaneous and subcutaneous lesions, but occult visceral hemangiomas, particularly in the liver, can occur. The peripheral blood smear demonstrates evidence of RBC fragments and burr cells. Kasabach-Merritt syndrome may necessitate treatment with plasma and platelet transfusions if consumptive coagulopathy is severe. Corticosteroids and interferon therapy have been helpful in some affected infants.

The diagnostic approach to anemia in the neonate requires a careful assessment of maternal, prenatal, and perinatal history as well as the clinical status of the neonate (Fig. 49.10). CBC, reticulocyte count, peripheral blood smear, maternal and infant blood types, and direct Coombs tests are virtually always necessary laboratory studies. Other studies must be dictated by the clinical and initial laboratory findings.

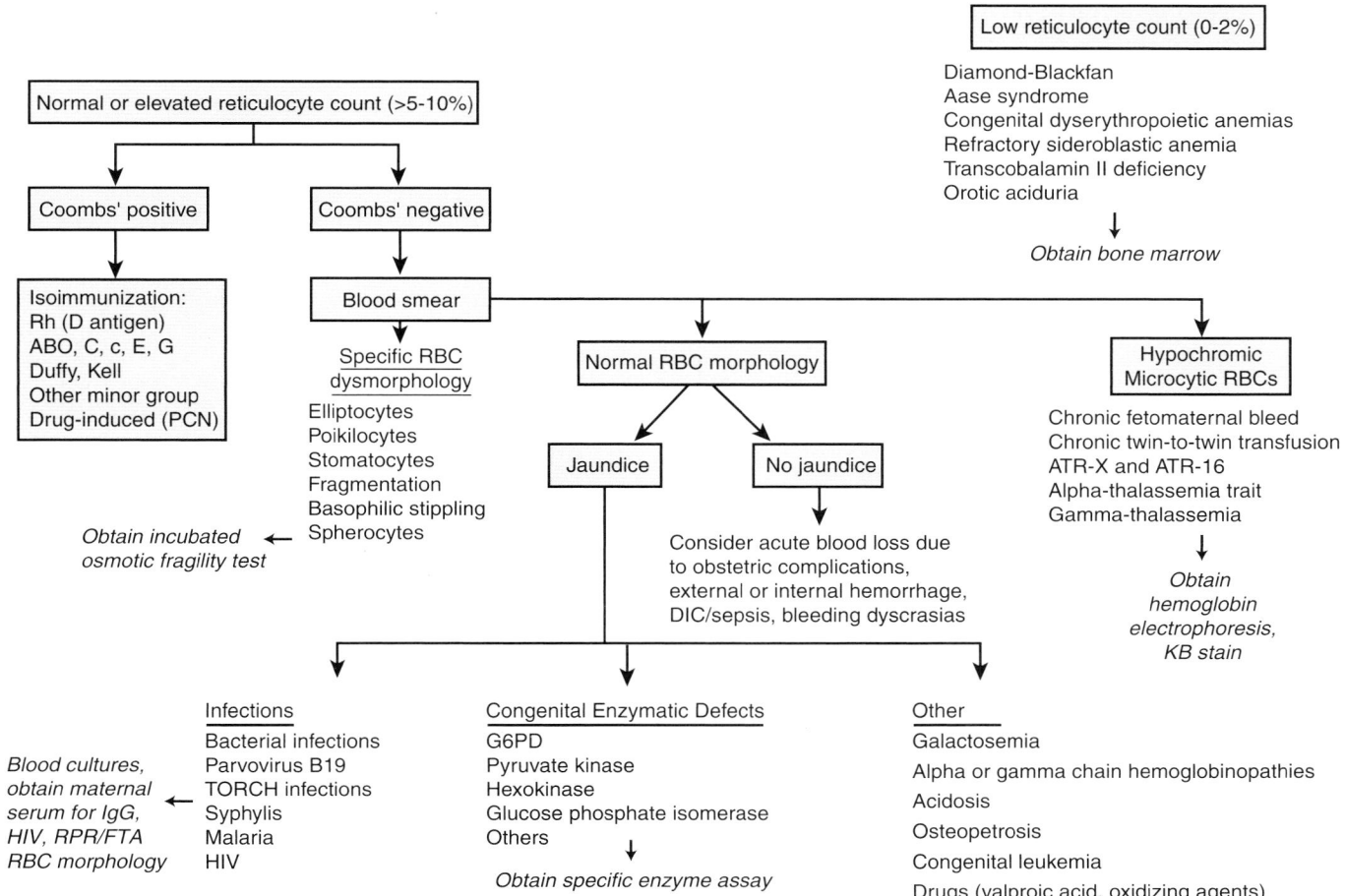

Fig. 49.10 Differential diagnosis of neonatal anemia. The physician first seeks information from the family, maternal, and labor and delivery histories and then obtains initial laboratory tests: hemoglobin, reticulocyte count, blood type, direct Coombs test, peripheral smear, red blood cell (RBC) indices, and bilirubin concentration. Results are used to navigate the diagnostic flow chart. ATR-16, α-thalassemia retardation syndrome, chromosome 16–linked; ATR-X, α-thalassemia retardation syndrome, X-linked; DIC, disseminated intravascular coagulation; FTA, fluorescent treponemal antibody test; G6PD, glucose-6-phosphate dehydrogenase; KB, Kleihauer-Betke; PCN, penicillin; RPR, rapid plasma reagin test; TORCH, toxoplasmosis, other infections, rubella, cytomegalovirus, and herpes simplex. (From Ohls RK. Evaluation and treatment of anemia in the neonate. In: Christensen RD, ed. *Hematologic Problems of the Neonate*. Philadelphia: Saunders; 2000:162.)

■ SUMMARY AND RED FLAGS

Anemia is a relatively common finding in children. A complete and thorough evaluation of clinical findings by a detailed history and physical examination is the most important element in the establishment of a diagnosis and in defining appropriate therapy.

Anemia may be a primary event reflecting intrinsic hematologic disease or it may be a manifestation of a wide variety of systemic disorders involving any organ system. Anemia must always be fully evaluated in view of the potential diagnostic and therapeutic implications. Patients who appear acutely ill should have a more thorough and prompt evaluation because acute blood loss must be treated quickly. If acute blood loss is not suspected, acute hemolysis or splenic sequestration of RBCs must be considered.

Anemia is often a sign of underlying acute or chronic disease. In such cases, anemia is not usually an isolated finding. Therefore, symptoms such as shortness of breath, extreme pallor, weight loss, fevers, lethargy, and fatigue should prompt a thorough evaluation of the patient.

On physical examination, the findings of abnormal vital signs, failure to thrive, bleeding or bruising, adenopathy, or organomegaly should lead the examiner to suspect that a potentially serious underlying disorder is present (Table 49.21). When a CBC is obtained, a low hemoglobin value accompanied by any abnormality of MCV, WBC, or platelet count should be taken seriously and should be more thoroughly investigated. The diagnostic evaluation should be directed accordingly based on these abnormal findings.

TABLE 49.21   Red Flags

Anemia Accompanied by:

Abnormal vital signs (tachycardia, hypotension, hypertension)
Congenital anomalies
Neutropenia and/or thrombocytopenia
High MCV with normal RDW
Blasts on the peripheral smear
Lymphadenopathy (generalized)
Bruising or bleeding
Weight loss, failure to thrive
Shortness of breath, fatigue
Fever
Hypoxia
Hepatosplenomegaly
Edema
Oliguria-anuria
Bloody diarrhea
Red urine (hemoglobinuria)
Family history of anemia, splenectomy, cholecystectomy, transfusions

MCV, mean corpuscular volume; RDW, red blood cell distribution width.

BIBLIOGRAPHY

A bibliography is available at ExpertConsult.com.

50

Pancytopenia/Aplastic Anemia/Bone Marrow Failure

Amy Moskop and Julie Talano

Pancytopenia is defined by a decrease in all peripheral blood cell lines, including leukocytes, red blood cells (RBCs), and platelets. All of these cells are produced by the bone marrow, and therefore an evaluation of the bone marrow is often required (Table 50.1). Aplastic anemia is a serious cause of pancytopenia with multiple etiologies (Tables 50.2 and 50.3).

Patients often present with fevers and infections related to leukocytopenia and/or neutropenia, anemia (pallor, tachycardia), and thrombocytopenia (bleeding, bruising, petechiae). In pediatrics, one must consider the age of the patient for normal ranges of cell lines, as these change with age (Table 50.4).

HISTORY

The predisposing risk factors for pancytopenia may help guide the diagnostic approach (Tables 50.5 and 50.6).

In addition to a thorough *personal* history review, a *family* history should also include questions related to congenital anomalies, syndromes associated with leukemias, thalassemias, sickle cell disease, and early or unusual childhood illnesses or death in relatives.

Physical Findings

Patients with isolated pancytopenia might present with evidence of anemia and thrombocytopenia including pallor, petechiae, and purpura or with more severe hemorrhages. Additionally, if leukopenia or neutropenia is present, they might present with mild or severe infections. Symptoms such as fever, rhinorrhea, cough, congestion, conjunctivitis, lymphadenopathy, hepatosplenomegaly, and rash can be seen in common viral illnesses, cytomegalovirus (CMV) or Epstein-Barr virus (EBV) infections, and acute leukemia. One should also look for signs of jaundice or scleral icterus. Hepatomegaly and splenomegaly might be present and can be found in liver disease or in malignant causes, such as acute leukemias.

Because there are several syndromes associated with pancytopenia, a careful review for congenital anomalies is important (Tables 50.7 and 50.8 and Figs. 50.1 and 50.2).

Laboratory Evaluation

(Tables 50.3, 50.8, 50.9, and 50.10 and Fig. 50.3)

HYPOCELLULAR MARROW

Inherited

Fanconi Anemia

Fanconi anemia (FA) is an autosomal recessive genetic disorder associated with congenital anomalies, cancer predisposition, and pancytopenia due to bone marrow failure (see Fig. 50.1). The classic physical exam findings include short stature, skin hyperpigmentation, and upper limb anomalies (such as absent, hypoplasia, or bifid thumb). Because ~50% of patients with FA have normal physical findings, they are often undiagnosed until they present with hematologic abnormalities. This is typically in the first decade of life.

The test of choice for FA detects chromosomal breakage in cells exposed to diepoxybutane (DEB) and mitomycin C (MMC), cross-linking agents. There are multiple genes in the FA pathway and their protein products are involved in the DNA damage recognition and repair pathways; these lead to the chromosome fragility seen in FA (see Tables 50.3 and 50.10).

Marrow failure classically begins with thrombocytopenia followed by granulocytopenia, macrocytosis, and then macrocytic anemia. The marrow will often show decreased or absent megakaryocytes, hypocellularity, and fatty replacement. About 10% of patients will present with acute myeloid leukemia (AML). Because of the fragility to alkylating agents, these patients cannot be treated with the typical intensive therapy used in AML.

The curative therapy for FA is hematopoietic stem cell transplantation (HSCT). The HSCT therapy must avoid the associated chromosome fragility seen in FA, and the timing of transplant is often delayed as long as safely possible. Long-term survival outcomes following a matched sibling transplant is ~80%.

Dyskeratosis Congenita

Dyskeratosis congenita (DC) is an inherited (X-linked, autosomal recessive or dominant) bone marrow failure syndrome (see Tables 50.3 and 50.10). Patients first present with lacy skin pigmentation on the face, neck, chest, and arms and nail dystrophy followed by oral mucosal leukoplakia (see Fig. 50.2). Marrow failure will become apparent by their teen years.

Telomeres protect the ends of chromosomes; their length decreases with each cell cycle. Stem cells are able to activate telomerase, which allows for self-renewal. Gene variants seen in DC lead to inheritance of short telomeres and defects in the maintenance of telomeres, leading to stem cell exhaustion and eventually producing pancytopenia.

Patients will initially present with isolated thrombocytopenia, which will then evolve into pancytopenia. There is also macrocytosis and elevated fetal hemoglobin levels. In addition to hypocellularity of marrow, there can be signs of myelodysplasia or leukemia.

The anabolic steroid oxymetholone can improve marrow function. About 60% of patients will respond to this therapy, which can have a long-lasting effect. HSCT can be used in DC; however, the survival rate remains poor at 50%. There is significant morbidity and mortality following HSCT specific to DC including pulmonary fibrosis and gastrointestinal (GI) bleeding secondary to vascular anomalies.

TABLE 50.1   Differential Diagnosis of Pancytopenia

Pancytopenia with Hypocellular Bone Marrow

Acquired aplastic anemia
Inherited aplastic anemia (Fanconi anemia and others)
Some myelodysplasia syndromes
Rare aleukemic leukemia (acute myelogenous leukemia)
Some acute lymphoblastic leukemias
Some lymphomas of bone marrow

Pancytopenia with Cellular Bone Marrow

Primary bone marrow diseases
Myelodysplasia syndromes
Paroxysmal nocturnal hemoglobinuria
Myelofibrosis
Some aleukemic leukemias
Myelophthisis
Bone marrow lymphoma
Secondary to systemic diseases
Systemic lupus erythematosus, Sjögren syndrome
Primary immunodeficiency diseases
Hypersplenism
Vitamin B_{12}, folate deficiency (familial defect)
Overwhelming infection
Alcohol
Brucellosis
Ehrlichiosis
Sarcoidosis
Tuberculosis and atypical mycobacteria

Hypocellular Bone Marrow ± Cytopenia

Q fever
Legionnaires disease
Mycobacteria
Tuberculosis*
Anorexia nervosa, starvation
Hypothyroidism

*Pancytopenia in tuberculosis only rarely is associated with a hypocellular bone marrow at biopsy or autopsy. Marrow failure in the setting of tuberculosis is almost always fatal; exceptional patients probably had underlying myelodysplasia or acute leukemia.
From Hoffman R, Benz EJ Jr, Silberstein LE, et al., eds. *Hematology: Basic Principles and Practice.* 7th ed. Philadelphia: Elsevier; 2018:395, Table 30.1.

TABLE 50.2   Etiology of Aplastic Anemia

Irradiation
Drugs and Chemicals
Cytotoxic agents
Benzene
Idiosyncratic reactions
Chloramphenicol
Nonsteroidal antiinflammatory drugs
Antiepileptics
Gold
Other drugs and chemicals

Viruses
Epstein-Barr virus (infectious mononucleosis)
Hepatitis virus (non-A, non-B, non-C, non-G hepatitis)
Parvovirus (transient aplastic crisis, some pure red cell aplasia)
HIV (AIDS)

Immune Diseases
Immune mediated (idiopathic)
Eosinophilic fasciitis
Hyperimmunoglobulinemia
Thymoma and thymic carcinoma
Graft versus host disease in immunodeficiency
Paroxysmal nocturnal hemoglobinuria

Other
Pregnancy

Modified from Hoffman R, Benz EJ Jr, Silberstein LE, et al., eds. *Hematology: Basic Principles and Practice.* 7th ed. Philadelphia: Elsevier; 2018:395, Table 30.2.

The most common hematologic finding in SDS is neutropenia, which predisposes to bacterial and fungal infections. About 10–65% of patients will present with pancytopenia; the majority of patients will have elevated fetal hemoglobin levels. Marrow cellularity can be variable; there is also a risk for myelodysplastic syndrome (MDS) and AML.

Management of SDS includes granulocyte colony-stimulating factor (G-CSF) for patients with severe neutropenia as well as transfusions for anemia and thrombocytopenia. The management of exocrine pancreatic insufficiency involves oral pancreatic enzyme replacement and fat-soluble vitamin supplements. HSCT is used in SDS with improved outcomes if performed prior to the development of leukemia, but data are limited and outcomes remain poor.

Congenital Amegakaryocytic Thrombocytopenia

Congenital amegakaryocytic thrombocytopenia (CAMT) is an autosomal recessive disorder that begins in infancy with isolated thrombocytopenia. Patients with CAMT present with signs of thrombocytopenia, cerebellar and cerebral atrophy, developmental delay, and various congenital heart defects. *MPL* is a gene for the receptor of thrombopoietin that impacts megakaryocytic proliferation as well as apoptotic regulation and survival of stem cells. Pathologic gene variants of *MPL* have different effects on thrombopoietin receptor function, which produces a wide spectrum of severity.

The marrow findings will initially demonstrate amegakaryocytosis with normal cellularity. Among patients who progress to pancytopenia, the marrow cellularity decreases, and fatty infiltration is noted. These patients are also at risk for development of MDS and AML. Androgens

Shwachman-Diamond Syndrome

Shwachman-Diamond syndrome (SDS) is an autosomal recessive inherited disorder. The typical clinical characteristics include exocrine pancreas insufficiency, which presents as fat malabsorption; skeletal changes including delayed bone maturation, metaphyseal dysostosis, short or flared ribs, and bifid thumbs; and bone marrow failure (Table 50.11).

The pathologic gene *SBDS* seen in SDS is involved in ribosomal biogenesis, which is associated with pancytopenia, although the exact mechanism is not completely understood. Failure of pancreatic acinar development leads to fatty infiltration of the pancreas and associated exocrine dysfunction. Marrow failure is a result of dysfunctional stem cells, apoptosis of progenitor cells, and inability of the microenvironment to support hematopoiesis. Diagnosis is made based on clinical findings and genetic variant analysis for *SBDS*.

TABLE 50.3 Genetic Conditions Commonly Associated with Bone Marrow Failure

Gene	Inheritance	Condition	Gene	Inheritance	Condition
ABCB7	X-linked	Sideroblastic anemia with ataxia	JAGN1	AR	SCN6
ACD	AR and AD	Dyskeratosis congenita	LAMTOR2 (ROBLD3)	AR	p14 deficiency
ADA2 (CECR1)	AR	Vasculitis, autoinflammation, immunodeficiency, and hematologic defects syndrome	LIG4	AR	LIG4 syndrome
			LYST	AR	Chediak-Higashi syndrome
AK2	AR	Reticular dysgenesis	MPL	AR	Congenital amegakaryocytic thrombocytopenia
AP3B1	AR	Hermansky-Pudlak type 2	MRTFA (MKL1)	AR	Neutropenia with combined immune deficiency
ATM	AR	Ataxia-telangiectasia			
ATR	AR	Seckel syndrome	MYSM1	AR	Familial bone marrow failure syndrome type 4
BLM	AR	Bloom syndrome			
BRCA1, BRCA2 (FANCD1), BRIP1 (FANCJ), ERCC4 (FANCQ), FANCA, FANCB, FANCC, FANCD2, FANCE, FANCF, FANCG, FANCI, FANCL, FANCM, MAD2L2, PALB2 (FANCN), RAD51, RAD51C (FANCO), RFWD3, SLX4 (FANCP), UBE2T, XRCC2	AR; except: FANCB — X-linked RAD51 — AD	Fanconi anemia	NAF1	AD	Pulmonary fibrosis and emphysema
			NBN	AR	Nijmegen breakage syndrome
			NHEJ1	AR	Severe combined immunodeficiency with microcephaly, growth retardation, and sensitivity to ionizing radiation
			NHP2 (NOLA2)	AR	Dyskeratosis congenita
			NOPIO (NOLA3)	AR	Dyskeratosis congenita
CD40LG	X-linked	X-linked hyper-IgM syndrome	NSMCE3	AR	Lung disease, immunodeficiency, and chromosome breakage syndrome
CLPB	AR	3-methylglutaconic aciduria type VII, with cataracts, neurologic involvement, and neutropenia			
			PARN	AD and AR	Dyskeratosis congenita; pulmonary fibrosis and/or bone marrow failure
CSF3R	AD, AR, and somatic	Severe congenital neutropenia 7 (SCN7) (germline); predisposition to myelodysplastic syndrome (somatic)			
			POT1	AD	Familial chronic lymphocytic leukemia
CTC1	AR	Coats plus syndrome	RAB27A	AR	Griscelli syndrome type 2
CXCR2	AR	Myelokathexis	RAC2	AR	Neutrophil immunodeficiency syndrome
CXCR4	AD	WHIM syndrome			
DKC1	XR	Dyskeratosis congenita or Hoyeraal-Hreidarsson syndrome	RBM8A	AR	Thrombocytopenia-absent radius syndrome
DNAJC21	AR	Familial bone marrow failure syndrome type 3	RMRP	AR	Cartilage-hair hypoplasia
			RNF168	AR	RIDDLE syndrome
EFL1	AR	Shwachman-Diamond syndrome	RPL5, RPL9, RPL11, RPL15, RPL18, RPL26, RPL27, RPL31, RPL35, RPL35A, RPS7, RPS10, RPS15, RPS15A, RPS17, RPS19, RPS24, RPS26, RPS27, RPS27A, RPS28, RPS29, TSR2	AD; except: TSR2 — X-linked	Diamond-Blackfan anemia
EIF2AK3	AR	Wolcott-Rallison syndrome			
ELANE (ELA2)	AD	SCN1			
EPO	AR, AD	Diamond-Blackfan anemia; erythrocytosis			
ERCC6L2	AR	Familial bone marrow failure syndrome type 2			
G6PC3	AR	SCN4, nonsyndromic SCN, Dursun syndrome	RTEL1	AD and AR	Dyskeratosis congenita
			RUNX1	AD and somatic	Familial platelet disorders (germline); acute myeloid leukemia (germline); predisposition to myelodysplastic syndrome/acute myeloid leukemia (somatic)
GATA1	X-linked	GATA1-related X-linked cytopenia			
GATA2	AD	GATA2 deficiency			
GFI1	AD	SCN2			
HAX1	AR	SCN3, Kostmann syndrome			
HYOU1	AR	Immunodeficiency and hypoglycemia	SAMD9	AD	MIRAGE syndrome
			SAMD9L	AD	Ataxia-pancytopenia syndrome

Continued

TABLE 50.3   Genetic Conditions Commonly Associated with Bone Marrow Failure—cont'd

Gene	Inheritance	Condition	Gene	Inheritance	Condition
SBDS	AR	Shwachman-Diamond syndrome (SDS)	TP53	AD and somatic	Familial bone marrow failure syndrome 5 (germline); transformation to myelodysplastic syndrome/acute myeloid leukemia in patients with Shwachman-Diamond syndrome (somatic)
SLC37A4	AR	Glycogen storage disease type IB			
SMARCD2	AR	Specific granule deficiency 2			
SRP54	AD	Congenital neutropenia			
SRP72	AD	Familial bone marrow failure syndrome type 1			
STK4	AR	STK4 deficiency	USB1	AR	Clericuzio-type poikiloderma with neutropenia
STN1	AR	Coats plus syndrome with telomere defects			
			VPS13B	AR	Cohen syndrome; congenital neutropenia with retinopathy
TAZ	X-linked	Barth syndrome			
TCIRG1	AR, AD	Osteopetrosis (AR), congenital neutropenia (AD)	VPS45	AR	SCN5
			WAS	X-linked	Wiskott-Aldrich syndrome, X-linked
TCN2	AR	Transcobalamin II deficiency			
TERC (hTR)	AD	Dyskeratosis congenita	WDR1	AR	WDR1 deficiency
TERF2IP	AD	Familial melanoma	WIPF1	AR	Wiskott-Aldrich syndrome
TERT	AD and AR	Dyskeratosis congenita	WRAP53 (TCAB1, WDR79)	AR	Dyskeratosis congenita, Revesz syndrome, Hoyeraal-Hreidarrson syndrome
TINF2	AD	Classic or severe DC, Revesz syndrome, Hoyeraal-Hreidarrson syndrome; AD 3			

AD, autosomal dominant; AR, autosomal recessive; RIDDLE, radiosensitivity, immunodeficiency, dysmorphic features, and learning difficulties; WHIM, warts, hypogammaglobulinemia, immunodeficiency, myelokathexis.
Courtesy of the Laboratory of Genetics and Genomics, Cincinnati Children's Hospital Medical Center, University of Cincinnati, https://www.cincinnatichildrens.org/service/b/bone-marrow/therapies/bone-marrow-failure-syndromes.

TABLE 50.4   Age-Specific Blood Cell Indices

Age	Hb (g/dL)*	HCT (%)*	MCV (fL)*	MCHC (g/dL RBC)*	Reticulocytes	WBCs (×10³/mL)[†]	Platelets (10³/mL)[†]
26–30 wk gestation[‡]	13.4 (11)	41.5 (34.9)	118.2 (106.7)	37.9 (30.6)	—	4.4 (2.7)	254 (180–327)
28 wk	14.5	45	120	31.0	(5–10)	—	275
32 wk	15.0	47	118	32.0	(3–10)	—	290
Term[§] (cord)	16.5 (13.5)	51 (42)	108 (98)	33.0 (30.0)	(3–7)	18.1 (9–30)[‖]	290
1–3 days	18.5 (14.5)	56 (45)	108 (95)	33.0 (29.0)	(1.8–4.6)	18.9 (9.4–34)	192
2 wk	16.6 (13.4)	53 (41)	105 (88)	31.4 (28.1)	—	11.4 (5–20)	252
1 mo	13.9 (10.7)	44 (33)	101 (91)	31.8 (28.1)	(0.1–1.7)	10.8 (4–19.5)	—
2 mo	11.2 (9.4)	35 (28)	95 (84)	31.8 (28.3)	—	—	—
6 mo	12.6 (11.1)	36 (31)	76 (68)	35.0 (32.7)	(0.7–2.3)	11.9 (6–17.5)	—
6 mo–2 yr	12.0 (10.5)	36 (33)	78 (70)	33.0 (30.0)	—	10.6 (6–17)	(150–350)
2–6 yr	12.5 (11.5)	37 (34)	81 (75)	34.0 (31.0)	(0.5–1.0)	8.5 (5–15.5)	(150–350)
6–12 yr	13.5 (11.5)	40 (35)	86 (77)	34.0 (31.0)	(0.5–1.0)	8.1 (4.5–13.5)	(150–350)
12–18 yr							
Male	14.5 (13)	43 (36)	88 (78)	34.0 (31.0)	(0.5–1.0)	7.8 (4.5–13.5)	(150–350)
Female	14.0 (12)	41 (37)	90 (78)	34.0 (31.0)	(0.5–1.0)	7.8 (4.5–13.5)	(150–350)
Adult							
Male	15.5 (13.5)	47 (41)	90 (80)	34.0 (31.0)	(0.8–2.5)	7.4 (4.5–11)	(150–350)
Female	14.0 (12)	41 (36)	90 (80)	34.0 (31.0)	(0.8–4.1)	7.4 (4.5–11)	(150–350)

*Data are mean (− 2 SD).
[†]Data are mean (± 2 SD).
[‡]Values are from fetal samplings.
[§]1 mo, capillary hemoglobin exceeds venous: 1 hr: 3.6-g difference; 5 day: 2.2-g difference; 3 wk: 1.1-g difference.
[‖]Mean (95% confidence limits).
Hb, hemoglobin; HCT, hematocrit; MCHC, mean cell hemoglobin concentration; MCV, mean corpuscular volume; RBC, red blood cell; WBC, white blood cell.
From Gajjar R, Jalazo E. Hematology, Table 14-1 Age-Specific Blood Cell Indices. In: *Harriet Lane Handbook: A Manual for Pediatric Housestaff.* 20th ed. Philadelphia: Saunders; 2014:305–306.

TABLE 50.5 History Clues for the Etiology of Pancytopenia

General Cause	History Clues to Review
Viral	Fever, viral symptoms, sick contacts, rashes, conjunctivitis, jaundice
Malignant	Fevers, bony pain, weight loss, lymphadenopathy, hepatosplenomegaly, night sweats
Liver failure	Jaundice, abdominal pain, encephalopathy
Environmental	History of radiation or chemotherapy, environmental toxins
Medication	See Table 50.6
Immunodeficiency	Recurrent or opportunistic infections, skin infections, mouth sores, eczema, failure to thrive, positive newborn screen
Dietary	Vegan diet, goat milk ingestion, short bowel syndrome
Genetic	Bone marrow failure syndromes; see Table 50.3

TABLE 50.6 Classification of Drugs and Chemicals Associated with Aplastic Anemia

I. Agents That Regularly Produce Marrow Depression as a Major Toxic Effect When Used in Commonly Used Doses or Normal Exposures

- Cytotoxic drugs used in cancer chemotherapy
- Alkylating agents (busulfan, melphalan, cyclophosphamide)
- Antimetabolites (antifolic compounds, nucleotide analogs), antimitotics (vincristine, vinblastine, colchicine)
- Some antibiotics (daunorubicin, doxorubicin [Adriamycin])
- Benzene (and less often benzene-containing chemicals: kerosene, carbon tetrachloride, Stoddard solvent, chlorophenols)

II. Agents Probably Associated with Aplastic Anemia but with a Relatively Low Probability Relative to Their Use

- Chloramphenicol
- Insecticides
- Antiprotozoals (quinacrine and chloroquine)
- Nonsteroidal antiinflammatory drugs (including phenylbutazone, indomethacin, ibuprofen, sulindac, diclofenac, naproxen, piroxicam, fenoprofen, fenbufen, aspirin)
- Anticonvulsants (hydantoins, carbamazepine, phenacemide, ethosuximide)
- Gold, arsenic, and other heavy metals such as bismuth and mercury
- Sulfonamides as a class
- Antithyroid medications (methimazole, methylthiouracil, propylthiouracil)
- Antidiabetes drugs (tolbutamide, carbutamide, chlorpropamide)
- Carbonic anhydrase inhibitors (acetazolamide, methazolamide, mesalazine)
- D-Penicillamine
- 2-Chlorodeoxyadenosine

III. Agents More Rarely Associated with Aplastic Anemia

- Antibiotics (streptomycin, tetracycline, methicillin, ampicillin, mebendazole and albendazole, sulfonamides, flucytosine, mefloquine, dapsone)
- Antihistamines (cimetidine, ranitidine, chlorpheniramine)
- Sedatives and tranquilizers (chlorpromazine, prochlorperazine, piperacetazine, chlordiazepoxide, meprobamate, methyprylon, remoxipride)
- Antiarrhythmics (tocainide, amiodarone)
- Allopurinol (can potentiate marrow suppression by cytotoxic drugs)
- Ticlopidine
- Methyldopa
- Quinidine
- Lithium
- Guanidine
- Canthaxanthin
- Thiocyanate
- Carbimazole
- Cyanamide
- Deferoxamine
- Amphetamines

From Hoffman R, Benz EJ Jr, Silberstein LE, et al., eds. *Hematology: Basic Principles and Practice*. 7th ed. Philadelphia: Elsevier; 2018:399, Table 30.3.

and corticosteroids have been used to treat pancytopenia with some improvement, but HSCT remains the only curative option.

Other Genetic Syndromes

There are several other genetic syndromes that can develop pancytopenia. These include Down syndrome, Noonan syndrome, Dubowitz syndrome, Seckel syndrome, reticular dysgenesis, Schimke immunoosseous dysplasia, cartilage-hair hypoplasia, and familial aplastic anemia (Table 50.12). In addition, cytopenias including pancytopenia may occur in primary immunodeficiency diseases (Fig. 50.4). These include common variable immunodeficiency (CVID), autoimmune lymphoproliferative syndrome (ALPS), and immune disregulation polyendocrinopathy enteropathy X-linked (IPEX) and IPEX-like syndromes.

ACQUIRED

Acquired aplastic anemia, a rare but severe hematologic disorder, is different from inherited bone marrow failure syndromes and can be a result of drugs, chemicals, radiation, infections, or immune disorders (see Tables 50.1 and 50.2). A bone marrow evaluation reveals hypocellularity; severity is graded based on the Camitta criteria (Table 50.13).

There must be a thorough review of drug and chemical exposures (see Table 50.6). Medications can result in pancytopenia either by direct toxicity, metabolite-driven toxicity, or antibody-mediated destruction. Chemotherapeutic agents, radiation, benzene, chloramphenicol, antiepileptics, gold, nonsteroidal antiinflammatory drugs (NSAIDs), and several antibiotics are notable exposures.

Infections

Several viruses may result in acquired aplastic anemia. These include parvovirus B19, EBV, CMV, hepatitis viruses, herpesviruses, and HIV. Other infections such as mycobacterial infections can also lead to pancytopenia.

Immune Diseases

It is thought that immune-mediated, previously identified as idiopathic aplastic, anemia is a result of immune-mediated destruction of bone marrow stem cells. This is often a diagnosis of exclusion following a broad work-up for other acquired causes and must be distinguished from inherited bone marrow failure syndromes before treatment can begin. Autoimmune disorders, such as systemic lupus erythematosus or rheumatoid arthritis, can have hematologic abnormalities including pancytopenia.

Pregnancy

Aplastic anemia is a rare complication of pregnancy; the cause remains unknown. Management must be weighed with the risk to the fetus and

TABLE 50.7 Specific Types of Anomalies in Fanconi Anemia*

Skin (40%)
Generalized hyperpigmentation on the trunk, neck, and intertriginous areas; café-au-lait spots; hypopigmented areas

Body (40%)
Short stature, delicate features, small size, underweight

Upper Limbs (35%)
Thumbs (35%): absent or hypoplastic; supernumerary, bifid, or duplicated; rudimentary; short, low set, attached by a thread; triphalangeal, tubular, stiff, hyperextensible
Radii (7%): absent or hypoplastic (only with abnormal thumbs); absent or weak pulse
Hands (5%): clinodactyly; hypoplastic thenar eminence; six fingers; absent first metacarpal; enlarged, abnormal fingers; short fingers; transverse crease ulnae (1%): dysplastic or absent

Lower Limbs (5%)
Feet: toe syndactyly, abnormal toes, flat feet, short toes, clubfeet, six toes, supernumerary toe
Legs: congenital hip dislocation, Perthes disease, coxa vara, abnormal femur, thigh osteoma, abnormal legs

Gonads
Males (25%): hypogenitalia, undescended testes, hypospadias, abnormal genitalia, absent testis, atrophic testes, azoospermia, phimosis, abnormal urethra, micropenis, delayed development
Females (2%): hypogenitalia; bicornuate uterus; abnormal genitalia; aplasia of uterus and vagina; atresia of uterus, vagina, and ovary

Other Skeletal Anomalies
Head (20%) and face (2%): microcephaly, hydrocephalus, micrognathia, peculiar face, birdlike face, flat head, frontal bossing, scaphocephaly, sloped forehead, choanal atresia, dental abnormalities
Neck (1%): Sprengel deformity; short, low hairline; webbed spine (2%): spina bifida (thoracic, lumbar, cervical, occult sacral)
Spine (2%): spina bifida (thoracic, lumbar, cervical, occult sacral), scoliosis, abnormal ribs, sacral agenesis, sacrococcygeal sinus, Klippel-Feil syndrome, vertebral anomalies, extra vertebrae

Eyes (20%)
Small eyes, strabismus, epicanthal folds, short or almond-shaped palpebral fissures, hypertelorism, ptosis, slanting, cataracts, astigmatism, blindness, epiphora, nystagmus, proptosis, small iris

Ears (10%)
Deafness (usually conductive); abnormal shape; atresia; dysplasia; low set, large, or small; infections; abnormal middle ear; absent eardrum; dimples; rotated; canal stenosis

Kidney (20%)
Ectopic or pelvic; abnormal, horseshoe, hypoplastic, or dysplastic; absent; hydronephrosis or hydroureter; infections; duplicated; rotated; reflux; hyperplasia; no function; abnormal artery

Gastrointestinal System (5%)
High-arched palate, atresia (esophagus, duodenum, jejunum), imperforate anus, tracheoesophageal fistula, Meckel diverticulum, umbilical hernia, hypoplastic uvula, abnormal biliary ducts. megacolon, abdominal diastasis, Budd-Chiari syndrome

Urogenital
Males (25%): micropenis, penile-scrotal fusion, undescended or atrophic or absent testes, hypospadias, chordae, phimosis, azoospermia
Females (2%): bicornuate uterus, aplasia or hypoplasia of vagina and uterus, atresia of vagina, hypoplastic uterus, hypoplastic or absent ovary, hypoplastic fused labia

Cardiopulmonary System (6%)
Patent ductus arteriosus, ventricular septal defect, abnormal heart, peripheral pulmonic stenosis, aortic stenosis, coarctation, absent lung lobes, vascular malformation, aortic atheromas, atrial septal defect, tetralogy of Fallot, pseudotruncus, hypoplastic aorta, abnormal pulmonary drainage, double aortic arch, cardiac myopathy

Central Nervous System (3%)
Hyperreflexia, Bell palsy, CNS arterial malformation, moyamoya syndrome, Arnold-Chiari malformation, stenosis of internal carotid artery, small pituitary gland, absent corpus callosum, slow development (10%)

*Abnormalities are listed in the approximate order of frequency within each category.
Adapted from Shimamura A, Aher BP. Pathophysiology and management of inherited bone marrow failure syndromes. *Blood Rev.* 2010;24:101–122.
From *Nelson Textbook of Pediatrics.* 21st ed. Philadelphia: Elsevier; 2020:2571, Table 495.2.

TABLE 50.8 Inherited Causes of Bone Marrow Failure

Disease	Supportive Clinical Findings	Supportive Laboratory Findings	Inheritance Pattern
Fanconi anemia	Skeletal abnormalities (radius, thumb); small stature; urogenital abnormalities; 40% with no physical findings	Increased chromosomal breakage in response to mitomycin C or diepoxybutane	AR (most) or XLR
Dyskeratosis congenita	Leukoplakia; nail dystrophy; lacy skin pigmentation; pulmonary fibrosis	Genetic testing (a negative result does not rule out disease)	AR, XLR, or AD
Shwachman-Diamond syndrome	Exocrine pancreatic insufficiency	Genetic testing (a negative result does not rule out disease); normal sweat chloride	AR
Congenital amegakaryocytic thrombocytopenia	Sequelae of severe thrombocytopenia	Genetic testing (a negative result does not rule out disease); elevated thrombopoietin levels	AR
Hemophagocytic lymphohistiocytosis	Fever; splenomegaly; hepatitis; neurologic symptoms; rash	Hemophagocytosis; hypertriglyceridemia; hypofibrinogenemia; low/absent NK-cell activity; elevated serum ferritin; soluble CD25 >2,400 U/mL	AR or XLR

AD, autosomal dominant; AR, autosomal recessive; NK, natural killer; XLR, X-linked recessive.
Modified from Weinzierl EP, Arber DA. The differential diagnosis and bone marrow evaluation of new-onset pancytopenia. *Am J Clin Pathol.* 2013;139:9–29 (Table 1, p. 10).

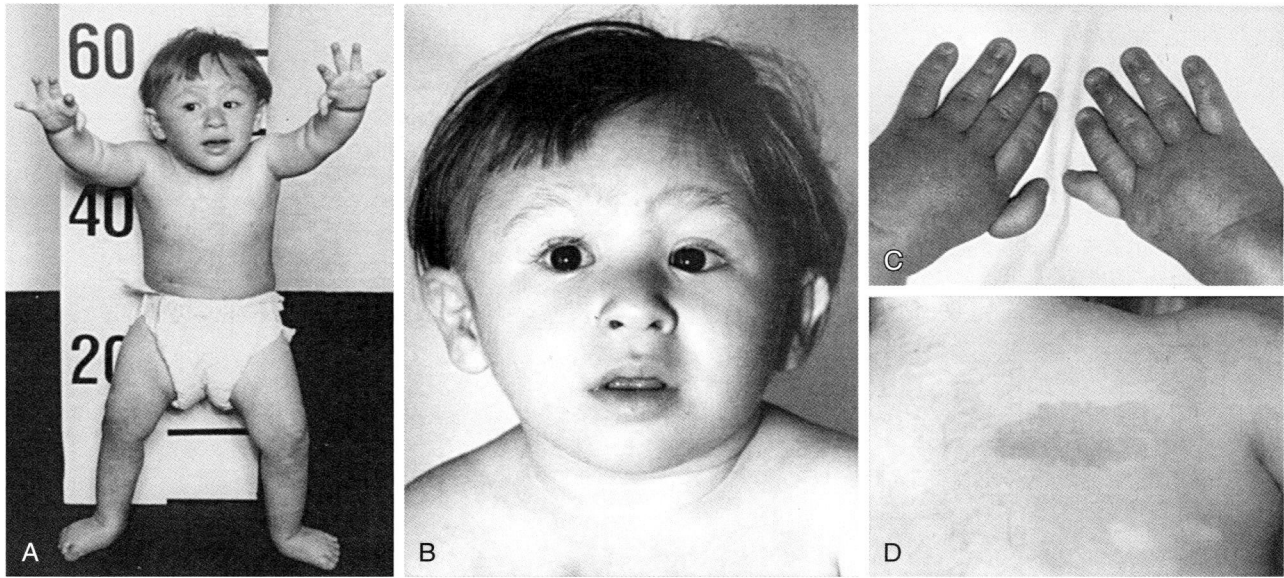

Fig. 50.1 A 3-year-old boy with Fanconi anemia who exhibits several classic phenotypic features. *A,* Front view. *B,* Face. *C,* Hands. *D,* Back right shoulder. The features to be noted include short stature, dislocated hips, microcephaly, a broad nasal base, epicanthal folds, micrognathia, thumbs attached by a thread, and café-au-lait spots with hypopigmented areas beneath. (From Nathan DC, Orkin SH, Ginsburg D, et al., eds. *Nathan and Oski's Hematology of Infancy and Childhood.* 6th ed. Vol. I. Philadelphia: Saunders; 2003:285.)

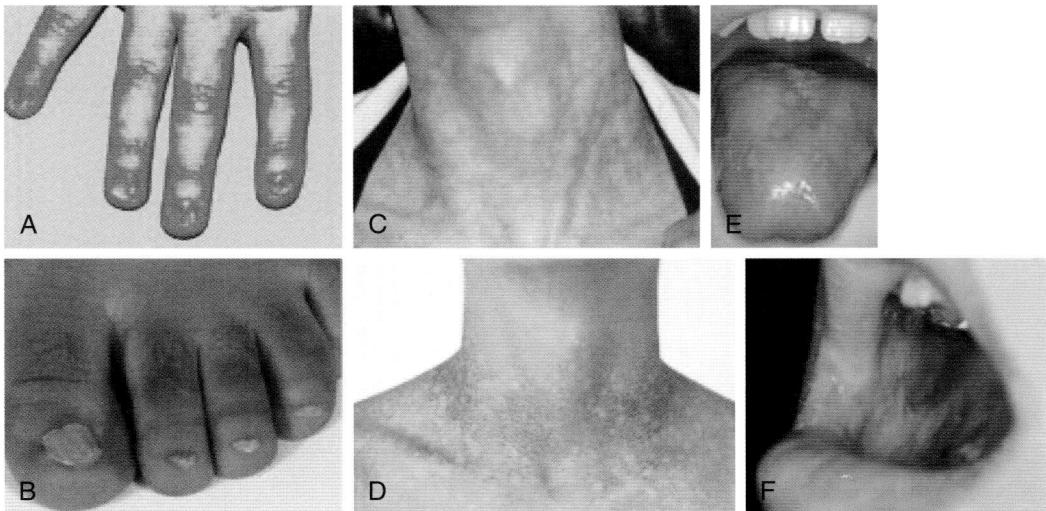

Fig. 50.2 Features of the diagnostic triad in dyskeratosis congenita. *A, B,* Dystrophic nails on hands and feet. *C, D,* Lacy reticular pigmentation on neck and upper thorax. *E, F,* Oral leukoplakia on tongue and buccal mucosa. (*A–C* and *E,* From Shimamura A, Alter BP. Pathophysiology and management of inherited bone marrow failure syndromes. *Blood Rev.* 2010;24:101–122, Fig. 8; *D* and *F,* from Savage SA, Alter BP. Dyskeratosis congenita. *Hematol Oncol Clin North Am.* 2009;23:215–231.)

mother and often requires transfusion support to minimize the risk of hemorrhage.

Paroxysmal Nocturnal Hemoglobinuria

Paroxysmal nocturnal hemoglobinuria (PNH) is another cause of acquired aplastic anemia. A pathologic gene variant leads to a clonal population of stem cells that are more susceptible to complement-mediated destruction. The majority of pediatric patients with PNH will have marrow failure. Associated symptoms include thrombosis (classically abdominal venous thrombosis), nocturnal hemoglobinuria, chronic hemolysis, and cytopenias. The diagnostic method includes flow cytometry looking for decreased expression of both CD55 and CD59 markers.

Marrow Replacement

A marrow evaluation for pancytopenia may reveal abnormal development of stem cells *or* replacement of normal marrow elements. This requires a careful morphologic review of the bone marrow aspirate and biopsy as well as cytogenetic studies.

TABLE 50.9 Laboratory Evaluation for Pancytopenia

CBC, differential, peripheral blood smear review Reticulocyte count	
Cell destruction	Direct Coombs test, haptoglobin, LDH, hemoglobinuria, total bilirubin
Cell consumption	PT, PTT, fibrinogen, creatinine
Viral marrow suppression	CMV, EBV, HIV, coronavirus disease 2019 (COVID-19), brucellosis, TB, Q fever, Legionnaires disease, hepatitis, parvovirus, dengue, measles, mumps, rubella, varicella, influenza A
Bone marrow evaluation Stains, chromosomal and flow cytometry Cellularity, myelofibrosis, infiltrative process, storage diseases	

CMV, cytomegalovirus; EBV, Epstein-Barr virus; LDH, lactate dehydrogenase; PT, prothrombin time; PTT, partial thromboplastin time; TB, tuberculosis.

TABLE 50.10 Inherited Bone Marrow Failure Syndromes and Associated Genes

Syndrome	Genes
FA	FANC: A, B, C, D1/BRCA2, D2, E, F, G, I, J, L, M, N, O
DC	X-linked: DKC1 AD: TINF2, TERC, TERT AD: NOP10, NHP2
SDS	SBDS
CAMT	MPL

CAMT, congenital amegakaryocytic thrombocytopenia; DC, dyskeratosis congenita; FA, Fanconi anemia; SDS, Shwachman-Diamond syndrome.

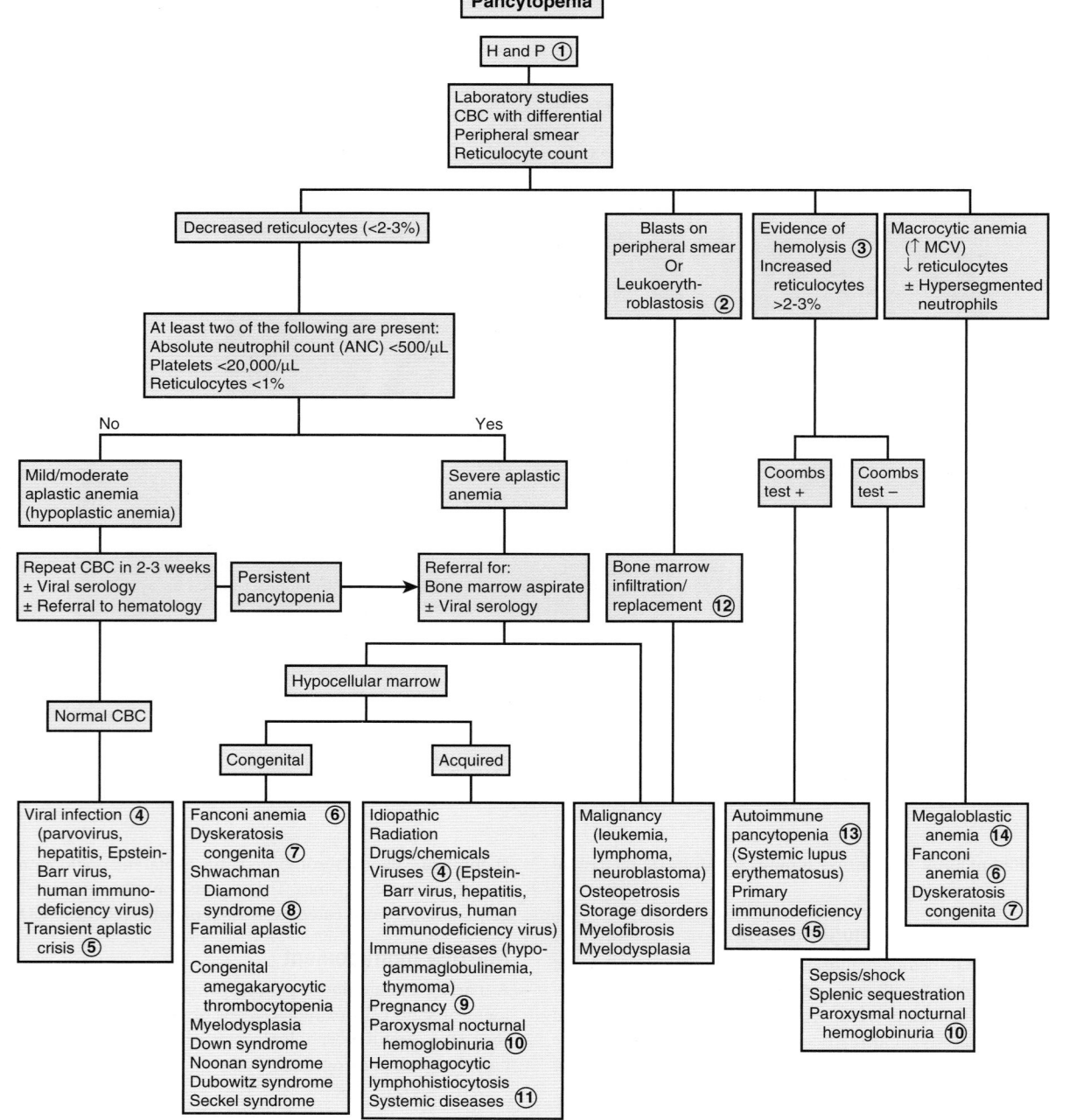

Fig. 50.3 Pancytopenia diagnostic algorithm. *1,* History should include exposure to agents that are potentially myelosuppressive. These include radiation and chemotherapy (e.g., 6-mercaptopurine, methotrexate, nitrogen mustard). Other drugs include chloramphenicol, sulfonamides, phenylbutazone, and anticonvulsants. Chemicals and toxins include benzene and other aromatic hydrocarbons present in insecticides and herbicides. A history and physical examination compatible with certain viral infections should be sought. An increased susceptibility to infection may suggest an immunodeficiency syndrome. A family history of congenital anomalies, aplastic syndromes, and leukemias may indicate syndromes associated with constitutional aplastic pancytopenias. Physical examination may reveal the effects of the cytopenias, including anemia, which results in tachycardia and pallor; thrombocytopenia, which may cause bleeding, bruising, epistaxis, petechiae, or ecchymoses; and neutropenia, which may be associated with oral ulcerations and fevers. Examination should include identification of congenital anomalies associated with Fanconi and other syndromes (e.g., Down syndrome). *2,* When blasts are seen on peripheral smear, it indicates leukemia requiring referral for bone marrow examination. Leukoerythroblastosis (myelophthisic anemia) is usually due to invasion of the bone marrow and resulting release of immature cells including erythroblasts (nucleated erythrocytes), immature neutrophils, and giant platelets. *3,* Laboratory findings suggesting hemolysis include abnormal cell morphology, increased reticulocyte count, increased red blood cell distribution width, indirect bilirubin, urine urobilinogen, lactate dehydrogenase, decreased serum haptoglobin, and hemoglobinuria. *4,* The most common cause of mild or moderate pancytopenias in healthy patients is suppression due to infectious agents. Specific viruses include human parvovirus B19, hepatitis viruses (B, C, non-A, non-B, and non-C), dengue virus, cytomegalovirus, human herpesvirus 6, and Epstein-Barr virus. Patients with HIV may have pancytopenia for a number of reasons, including opportunistic infections, drugs used in treatment, and neoplasms associated with the disease. Other viruses that may cause cytopenias include measles, mumps, rubella, varicella, and influenza A. If a viral etiology is suggested, it is reasonable to recheck the CBC in a few weeks. If the pancytopenia persists or becomes more severe, referral to a hematologist for further evaluation is recommended. *5,* Patients with hemolytic anemia who have shortened red blood cell survival time are at risk of transient aplastic crisis. This is most commonly associated with parvovirus and may occur in children with sickle cell disease, thalassemia, hereditary spherocytosis, and other types of erythroid stress. *6,* Fanconi anemia is an autosomal recessive condition. Two-thirds of affected children have congenital anomalies. These include microcephaly, microphthalmia, absent radii and thumbs, and heart and kidney abnormalities. There may be hypopigmentation of the skin and short stature. *7,* Dyskeratosis congenita is a rare form of ectodermal dysplasia associated with pancytopenia. Dermatologic manifestations include hyperpigmented skin, dystrophic nails, and mucous membrane leukoplakia. *8,* Shwachman-Diamond syndrome is characterized by neutropenia with exocrine pancreatic insufficiency (e.g., malabsorption, steatorrhea, failure to thrive). About 50% develop aplastic anemia. *9,* Pregnancy may be associated with aplastic anemia; estrogens may play a role. *10,* Paroxysmal nocturnal hemoglobinuria is characterized by intravascular hemolysis and hemoglobinuria as well as venous thrombosis. There is a strong association with aplastic anemia. *11,* Systemic diseases may be associated with pancytopenias. These may include systemic lupus erythematosus, metabolic diseases, brucellosis, sarcoidosis, and tuberculosis. *12,* Replacement of the marrow by malignant or nonhematopoietic cells may cause pancytopenias. Conditions include leukemia, lymphomas, and neuroblastoma metastases to the bone marrow. Osteopetrosis may cause obliteration of the marrow. Myelofibrosis may also be a cause. Myelodysplastic syndrome is rare in children; there is an increased risk of development with Down syndrome, Kostmann syndrome, Noonan syndrome, Fanconi anemia, trisomy 8 mosaicism, neurofibromatosis, and Shwachman syndrome. *13,* In autoimmune pancytopenia the Coombs (direct antiglobulin) test is usually positive. There is evidence of hemolysis with autoimmune hemolytic anemia. It is known as Evans syndrome when the patient has autoimmune hemolytic anemia and immune thrombocytopenic purpura (ITP). There may also be an associated autoimmune neutropenia. It may be associated with disorders such as systemic lupus erythematosus (SLE). *14,* Megaloblastic anemia (large RBCs with abnormal hypersegmented neutrophils due to vitamin B_{12} or folate deficiency) is rare in children. Neutropenia and thrombocytopenia may be present, particularly in patients with long-standing and severe deficiencies. *15,* Including autoimmune lymphoproliferative syndrome (ALPS), common variable immune deficiency (CVID), and immune disregulation, polyendocrinopathy, endocrinopathy, X-linked (IPEX). MCV, mean corpuscular volume. (From Pomeranz A, Busey S, Sabnis S, et al. *Pediatric Decision-Making Strategies.* Philadelphia: Saunders; 2002:361. Data from Sills R. *Practical Algorithms in Pediatric Hematology and Oncology.* Basel, Switzerland: Karger; 2003:114.)

Malignant Infiltration

Acute leukemias are the most common cause of marrow replacement secondary to malignancies in children. Acute lymphoblastic and myeloid leukemias often present with pancytopenia with peripheral lymphoblasts or myeloblasts as well as a marrow filled with blasts leading to pancytopenia. Some patients have no blasts in their peripheral blood smears. The diagnosis can be confirmed with morphologic review of the marrow, flow cytometry, and cytogenetics to confirm the cells of origin. There are other malignancies that can infiltrate the marrow including lymphomas, neuroblastoma, and Langerhans cell histiocytosis, as well as other solid tumors.

Myelodysplasia

MDS typically presents with isolated cytopenias but also pancytopenia. MDS is a disorder of ineffective hematopoiesis. There is also a risk for MDS to develop into AML. Pediatric MDS classification is described in Table 50.14. Patients with inherited bone marrow syndromes or other genetic predisposition syndromes are at high risk for developing MDS. *Treatment-related* MDS can also be seen after exposure to alkylating agents and topoisomerase II inhibitors during treatment for other malignancies. Because of the aggressive nature of MDS in children, most patients require HSCT shortly after diagnosis. Options that have been used for patients without a matched donor include

TABLE 50.11 Major Clinical Features of Shwachman-Diamond Syndrome

Clinical Feature	% Present
Hematologic*	
Neutropenia	90%
Severe (≤500/μL)	46%
Anemia	46%
Thrombocytopenia	42%
Pancytopenia	21%
Gastrointestinal	
Exocrine pancreatic insufficiency*	98%
Liver (elevated transaminases)	61%
Skeletal abnormalities	70%
Metaphyseal dysostosis	53%
Rib cage abnormalities	35%
Short stature (<3rd percentile)	66%

*Hematologic abnormalities and exocrine pancreatic insufficiency are defining features of SDS, thus the near-100% incidence of these findings. Data from Ginzberg H, Shin J, Ellis L, et al. Shwachman syndrome: phenotypic manifestations of sibling sets and isolated cases in a large patient cohort are similar. *J Pediatr.* 1999;135:81–88; Cipolli M, D'Orazio C, Delmarco A, et al. Shwachman's syndrome: pathomorphosis and long-term outcome. *J Pediatr Gastroenterol Nutr.* 1999;29:265–272; and Kuijpers TW, Alders M, Tool AT, et al. Hematologic abnormalities in Shwachman-Diamond syndrome: lack of genotype-phenotype relationship. *Blood.* 2005;106:356–361. From *Nelson Textbook of Pediatrics.* 21st ed. Philadelphia: Elsevier; 2020:2573, Table 495.3.

immunosuppressive therapy, tyrosine kinase inhibitors (TKIs), and DNA hypomethylating agents.

Syndromes associated with increased risk of developing MDS include:

- CAMT
- Diamond-Blackfan anemia
- Dyskeratosis congenita
- Fanconi anemia
- Severe congenital neutropenia
- Shwachman-Diamond syndrome
- Bloom syndrome
- Li-Fraumeni syndrome
- Neurofibromatosis type 1
- Noonan syndrome
- Wiskott-Aldrich syndrome

GATA2 deficiency is another genetic cause of MDS. Half of the patients with *GATA2* deficiency have de novo gene variants that effect proliferation of hematopoietic stem cells. It is associated with immunodeficiencies, aplastic anemia, MDS, and progression to AML. A history of warts, lymphedema, hearing loss, or thrombosis might be clues to this underlying diagnosis. The natural history is variable but typically begins with cytopenias, including aplastic anemia and immune dysregulation in the first decade of life followed by increased infections and transformation to MDS in the second decade of life. Infectious complications include nontuberculosis mycobacterial, bacterial, fungal (aspergillosis), and viral infections, including human papillomavirus (HPV) and EBV. A bone marrow evaluation will initially show hypocellularity but then progress to hypercellular marrow, which is

TABLE 50.12 Additional Genetic Syndromes Associated with Pancytopenia

Syndrome	Classic Clinical Features	Possible Bone Marrow Findings
Down syndrome	Up-slanted palpebral fissures, flattened nasal bridge, nuchal folds, single palmar flexion crease, clinodactyly of the fifth finger, hypotonia	Aplastic anemia MDS Acute leukemias
Noonan syndrome	Hypertelorism, ptosis, short neck, low-set ears, short stature, congenital heart disease, and multiple skeletal and hematologic abnormalities	JMML Amegakaryocytic thrombocytopenia Pancytopenia
Dubowitz syndrome	Eczema, small stature, mild microcephaly, micrognathia	Pancytopenia Hypoplastic anemia Bone marrow hypoplasia Aplastic anemia
Seckel syndrome	Growth failure, developmental delay, microcephaly, hypoplastic face with prominent nose	Aplastic anemia Malignancies
Reticular dysgenesis	Severe combined immunodeficiency with congenital agranulocytosis	Lymphopenia and neutropenia Variable anemia and thrombocytopenia Aplastic anemia
Schimke immunoosseous dysplasia	Pigmentary skin changes, discolored and configured teeth, renal dysfunction, nephrotic syndrome	Pancytopenia
Cartilage-hair hypoplasia	Metaphyseal dysostosis and other skeletal findings; short-limbed dwarfism; fine, sparse hair; GI abnormalities	Macrocytic anemia Neutropenia, lymphopenia, lymphoma

GI, gastrointestinal; JMML, juvenile myelomonocytic leukemia; MDS, myelodysplastic syndrome.

typically associated with MDS. Nearly 75% of patients will develop a myeloid neoplasm by age 40 years. The curative therapy is HSCT, but it is unknown when best to proceed with transplant. It is thought that undergoing HSCT prior to developing the severe complications seen later in life will improve outcomes.

Nonmalignant Causes of Infiltration That Lead to Pancytopenia

Hemophagocytic lymphohistiocytosis (HLH) is a group of life-threatening syndromes that results from an overactivation of the immune system (Table 50.15). HLH is characterized by proliferation of macrophages that produce excessive cytokines leading to widespread organ dysfunction. HLH is manifest with fever, hepatosplenomegaly, rash, high ferritin levels, pancytopenia, liver dysfunction, and hypofibrinogenemia. The diagnostic criteria can be seen in Table 50.16. HLH can be familial or acquired, with the latter being more common.

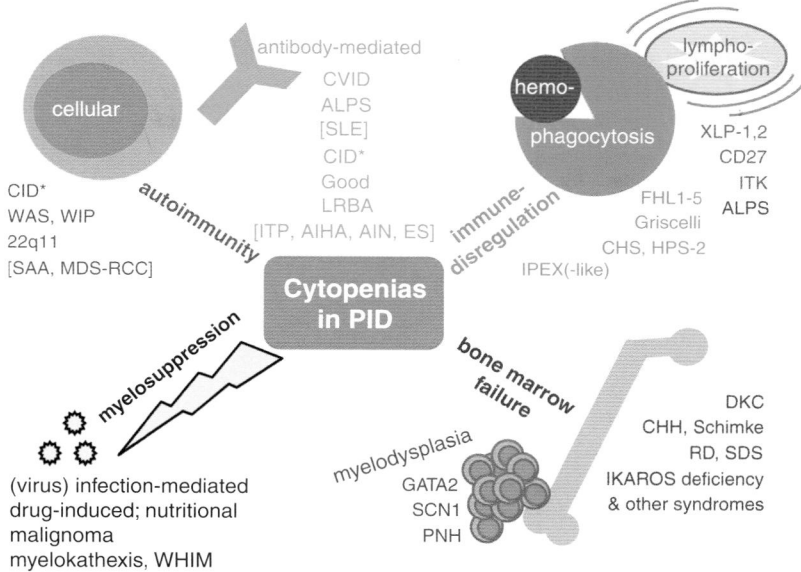

Fig. 50.4 Synopsis of cytopenias in primary immunodeficiency (PID). Conceptual overview, excluding primary defects of phagocyte number or function, inherited non-PID bone marrow failure syndromes, and disorders of isolated lymphopenia (without other cytopenia). *Includes hypomorphic gene variants in SCID genes, CD40, CD40L, and other combined immunodeficiencies such as radiosensitive disorders, defects in the Ca^{2+} channel, and activating PI3K syndrome. AIHA, autoimmune hemolytic anemia; AIN, autoimmune neutropenia; ALPS, autoimmune lymphoproliferative syndrome; CHH, cartilage hair hypoplasia; CHS, Chediak-Higashi syndrome; CID, combined immunodeficiency; CVID, common variable immunodeficiency; DKC, dyskeratosis congenita; ES, Evans syndrome; FHL1-5, familial hemophagocytic lymphohistiocytosis 1-5; HPS-2, Hermansky-Pudlak syndrome 2; IPEX, immune dysregulation, polyendocrinopathy, and enteropathy X-linked syndrome; ITK, IL-2–inducible T-cell kinase deficiency; ITP, immune thrombocytopenia; LRBA, lipopolysaccharide-responsive beigelike anchor deficiency; MDS, myelodysplastic syndrome; PNH, paroxysmal nocturnal hemoglobinuria; RCC, refractory cytopenia of childhood; RD, reticular dysgenesis; SAA, severe aplastic anemia; SCN1, severe congenital neutropenia 1; SDS, Shwachman-Diamond syndrome; SLE, systemic lupus erythematosus; WHIM, warts, hypogammaglobulinemia, immunodeficiency, myelokathexis; WIP, WAS protein–interacting protein; XLP-1,2, X-linked lymphoproliferative disease 1,2. (From Seidel MG. Autoimmune and other cytopenias in primary immunodeficiencies: pathomechanisms, novel differential diagnoses, and treatment. *Blood.* 2014;124(15):2337–2344 [Fig. 1, p. 2338].)

TABLE 50.13 Camitta Criteria for Severity of Aplastic Anemia	
Moderate or Nonsevere	**Decreased Bone Marrow Cellularity and Cytopenias but not Fulfilling Severe Criteria**
Severe	Bone marrow cellularity <25% AND at least two of the following: • ANC <500 • Platelet count <20,000 • Reticulocyte count <60,000
Very severe	Severe criteria AND • ANC <200

ANC, absolute neutrophil count.
Adapted from Hartung H, Olson, T, Bessler M. Acquired aplastic anemia in children. *Pediatr Clin North Am.* 2013;60(6):1311–1336, Box 1, p. 2.

Familial HLH is a result of genetic defects and secondary HLH can be a result of underlying malignancy or infection.

Leukoerythroblastosis is the presence of leukocytosis and erythroid and myeloid blasts in the peripheral blood. This is typically indicative of marrow stress leading to immature cells being pushed out to peripheral blood. It can be seen with underlying malignancies, infections, storage diseases, medications, myelofibrosis, and osteopetrosis.

The bone marrow can be replaced with underlying pathology leading to pancytopenia, but often many of the cell lines are preserved.

There are reports of leukoerythroblastosis in infants with underlying intrauterine parvovirus B19 infection. It has also been reported in a patient with a severe malaria episode with bacterial superinfection as well as a child with a bacterial abscess. Infections can lead to diffuse infiltrates or granulomata (necrotizing or non-necrotizing).

Glycogen storage and **lysosomal storage** disorders are inherited metabolic disorders caused by specific enzyme deficiencies. Glycogen storage disorders lack the enzyme responsible for glycogen metabolism and lead to accumulation of glycogen within liver or muscle. Type 1a glycogen storage disease, a deficiency in glucose-6-phophatase, leads to hepatosplenomegaly and hypoglycemia in infancy and can develop hypertension, renal insufficiency, and hepatic adenomas. Type 1b is associated with neutropenia and inflammatory bowel disease later in life. Patients can also have severe anemia, often related to underlying adenoma (type 1a) or inflammatory bowel disease (type 1b); type 1b can have neutropenia, increased risk of bacterial infection, and the risk of developing AML.

Lysosomal storage disorders, due to the inability to degrade macromolecules, lead to the accumulation of these macromolecules within multiple organs including the bone marrow. Mucopolysaccharidoses, Tay-Sachs disease, Fabry disease, Gaucher disease, Krabbe disease, and Pompe disease are all examples of these disorders. The associated symptoms vary, but in general there is accumulation of macromolecules in the liver, spleen, brain, and bones leading to physical features

TABLE 50.14   World Health Organization Classification of Pediatric Myelodysplastic Syndrome (MDS)

	Peripheral	Marrow
MDS with single-lineage dysplasia	<1% blasts	<5% blasts ≥10% unilineage dysplasia <15% ringed sideroblasts
MDS with ring sideroblasts	No blasts	<5% blasts ≥15% ring sideroblasts
MDS with multilineage dysplasia	<1% blasts No Auer rods $<1 \times 10^9$ monocytes	<5% blasts ≥10% dysplasia in two or more myeloid lineages ±15% sideroblasts No Auer rods
MDS with excess blasts-1	<5% blasts No Auer rods $<1 \times 10^9$ monocytes	5–9% blasts Single or multilineage dysplasia No Auer rods
MDS with excess blasts-2	5–19% blasts Auer rods $<1 \times 10^9$ monocytes	10–19% blasts Single or multilineage dysplasia Auer rods
MDS with isolated del(5q)	Anemia <1% blasts Normal to increased platelet count	<5% blasts No Auer rods Normal to increased megakaryocytes (hypolobulated nuclei) Isolated del(5q)
MDS-unclassifiable	Cytopenias ≤1% blasts	<5% blasts <10% dysplasia in one or more myeloid lineages Cytogenetic abnormality associated with MDS (i.e., unbalanced: +8, –7 or del(7q), –5 or del(5q), del(20q), –Y, i(17q) or t(17p), –13 or del(13q), del(11q), del(12p) or t(12p), del(9q), idic(X)(q13); balanced: t(11;16)(q23;p13.3), t(3;21)(q26.2;q22.1), t(1;3)(p36.3;q21.2), t(2;11)(p21;q23), inv(3)(q21q26.2), t(6;9)(p23;q34))

Adapted from Arber et al. The 2016 revision to the World Health Organization classification of myeloid neoplasms and acute leukemia. *Blood.* 2016;127(2):2391–2405, Table 1, p. 2392; National Cancer Institute. Childhood acute myeloid leukemia/other myeloid malignancies treatment, Table 3, "World Health Organization (WHO) Classification of Bone Marrow and Peripheral Blood Findings for Myelodysplastic Syndromes (MDS)," https://www.cancer.gov/types/leukemia/hp/child-aml-treatment-pdq#link/_74; and Arceci R, Meshinchi S. Acute myeloid leukemia and myelodysplastic syndromes. In: Pizzo P, Poplack D, Adamson P, et al., eds. *Principles and Practice of Pediatric Oncology.* 7th ed. Philadelphia: Wolters Kluwer; 2016:498–505.

characteristic of each. There can also be accumulation within the bone marrow leading to replacement of normal hematopoietic stem cells and cytopenias as well as leukoerythroblastosis; Gaucher disease is the prototype of these disorders affecting the marrow.

Medications have been reported to cause leukoerythroblastosis, also known as leukemoid reaction. These include G-CSF, corticosteroids, tetracycline, streptokinase, and antiepileptic drugs.

Myelofibrosis is a clonal disorder of stem cells that can lead to cytopenias, hepatosplenomegaly, and bone marrow fibrosis. Primary myelofibrosis is rare in pediatrics but can be aggressive and often requires HSCT.

Osteopetrosis is characterized by arrest or dysfunction of osteoclast formation, which leads to increased bone mass. Patients are also prone to fractures. The classic radiographic finding is a "bone-in-bone" appearance (Fig. 50.5). The increased bone mass prevents normal development of bone marrow leading to extramedullary hematopoiesis. Patients can present with anemia, thrombocytopenia, or even pancytopenia. Bone growth around cranial nerve foramina may produce vision and hearing impairment.

Megaloblastic Anemia

Megaloblastic anemia is characterized by macrocytic anemia but can often present with pancytopenia. Peripheral blood smear may show hypersegmented neutrophils; marrow evaluation reveals megaloblastic morphology affecting erythroid, myeloid, and platelet precursors. This is often a result of nutritional deficiencies, such as vitamin B_{12} or folate.

Vitamin B_{12}

Vitamin B_{12}, or cobalamin, must be obtained through dietary intake; deficiency often occurs in patients with unsupplemented vegan diets or minimal meat intake. Cobalamin is absorbed in the ileum so patients with poor absorption, such as celiac disease, inflammatory bowel disease, or diseases requiring bowel resection, are also at risk. Intrinsic factor is responsible for the absorption of cobalamin. Pernicious anemia, an acquired deficiency of intrinsic factor, is the most common cause of severe cobalamin in adults. Rarely, infants can have a congenital **intrinsic factor deficiency**; there are several rare inborn errors of cobalamin uptake and transport. In addition to the hematologic manifestations of cobalamin deficiency, patients can also present with neurologic (central or peripheral) symptoms; heart failure may develop when there is severe anemia. Neurologic symptoms can be irreversible without treatment and include developmental delay; posterior column deficits, such as loss of vibration and proprioception; paresthesia; peripheral neuropathy; weakness; ataxia; and seizures. Significant cobalamin deficiency can occur *without* hematologic changes; the neurologic findings can precede the megaloblastic anemia. Diagnostic testing includes low serum cobalamin as well the cobalamin precursors because some patients can have vitamin B_{12} levels in the normal range,

TABLE 50.15 Hemophagocytic Lymphohistiocytosis (HLH)

Disease	Gene	Protein	Percentage of fHLH	Immune Impairment	Unique Clinical Characteristics
fHLH-1	Unknown 9q21.3–22		Rare		
fHLH-2	*PRF1*	Perforin	~20–37,789 50delT mainly in African American/African descent	Cytotoxicity; forms pores in APCs	
fHLH-3	*UNC13D*	Munc13–4	20–33	Cytotoxicity; vesicle priming	Increased incidence of CNS HLH
fHLH-4	*STX11*	Syntaxin 11	<5	Cytotoxicity; vesicle fusion	Mild, recurrent HLH and colitis
fHLH-5	*STXBP2*	Syntaxin binding protein 2	5–20	Cytotoxicity; vesicle fusion	Colitis and hypogammaglobulinemia
Syndromes with Partial Oculocutaneous Albinism					
Griscelli syndrome	*RAB27A*	Rab27A	~5	Cytotoxicity; vesicle docking	Partial albinism and silver-gray hair
Chediak-Higashi syndrome	*LYST*	Lyst	~2	Cytotoxicity; heterogeneous defects in NK cells	Partial albinism, bleeding tendency, and recurrent infections
Hermansky-Pudlak syndrome type II	*AP3B1*	AP-3 complex subunit β1	Rare	Cytotoxicity; vesicle trafficking	Partial albinism and bleeding tendency
EBV-Driven and Rare Causes					
XLP1	*SH2D1A*	SAP	~7	Signaling in cytotoxic NK and T cells	Hypogammaglobulinemia and lymphoma
XLP2	*BIRC4*	XIAP	~2	NK T-cell survival and NF-κB signaling	Mild, recurrent HLH and colitis
ITK deficiency	*ITK*	ITK	Rare	IL-2 signaling in T cells	Hypogammaglobulinemia, autoimmunity, and Hodgkin lymphoma
CD27 deficiency	*CD27*	CD27	Rare	Signal transduction in lymphocytes	Combined immunodeficiency and lymphoma
XMEN syndrome	*MAGT1*	MAGT1	Rare	Magnesium transporter, induced by TCR stimulation	Lymphoma, recurrent infections, and CD4 T-cell lymphopenia

EBV, Epstein-Barr virus; ITK, interleukin-2–inducible T-cell kinase; NF-κB, nuclear factor kappa-B; TCR, T-cell receptor.
Data from Bondarenko EI. Experiences in the medical service for miners [article in Russian]. *Med Sestra.* 1978 Nov;37(11):47–49; and Kliegman RM, Bordini BJ, eds. Undiagnosed and rare diseases in children. *Pediatr Clin North Am.* 2017;64(1):91–109 (Table 1, p. 95).

TABLE 50.16 Hemophagocytic Lymphohistiocytosis (HLH) Diagnostic Criteria

HLH Can Be Established if Either A or B Is Fulfilled			
A	A molecular diagnosis is consistent with HLH (see Table 50.15)		
B	Diagnostic criteria (five out of the eight criteria below)		Cause
	1	Fever	Increased IL-1 and IL-6 levels
	2	Splenomegaly	Organ infiltration by lymphocytes and histiocytes
	3	• Cytopenias (affecting two of three lineages on peripheral blood) • Hemoglobin <9 g/dL (or infants <4 wk old, use <10 g/dL) • Platelets <100 × 10⁹/L • Neutrophils <1 × 10⁹/L	Increased TNF-α and IFN-γ
	4	• Hypertriglyceridemia and/or hypofibrinogenemia • Fasting triglycerides ≥265 mg/dL • Fibrinogen ≤1.5 g/L	Increased TNF-α inhibits lipoprotein lipase Activated macrophages secrete plasminogen activator, which results in high plasmin levels and hyperfibrinolysis
	5	Hemophagocytosis in bone marrow or spleen or lymph nodes	Activated macrophages
	6	Low or absent NK-cell activity (using local laboratory reference)	
	7	Ferritin ≥500 mg/L*ᵃ	Activated macrophages secrete ferritin
	8	Soluble CD25 (i.e., soluble IL-2 receptor) ≥2,400 U/mL	From activated lymphocytes (sIL-2R)

*A ferritin level of >500 ng/mL is nonspecific and can be seen in a variety of diseases, including shock, chronic transfusions, immunodeficiency, liver disease, cystic fibrosis, malignancy, after transplant, and autoimmune diseases. Experts often use a ferritin level of >2,000 ng/mL as concerning and >10,000 ng/mL as highly suspicious for HLH. The sensitivity and specificity for HLH with a ferritin level >10,000 ng/mL are ~90% and >95%, respectively.
IFN, interferon; IL, interleukin; TNF, tumor necrosis factor.
Data from Allen CE, McClain KL. Pathophysiology and epidemiology of hemophagocytic lymphohistiocytosis. *Hematology Am Soc Hematol Educ Program.* 2015;2015:177–182; Janka GE. Hemophagocytic syndromes. *Blood Rev.* 2007;21:245–253. Henter J, Horne A, Aricó M, et al. HLH-2004: diagnostic and therapeutic guidelines for hemophagocytic lymphohistiocytosis. *Pediatr Blood Cancer.* 2007;48:124–131.

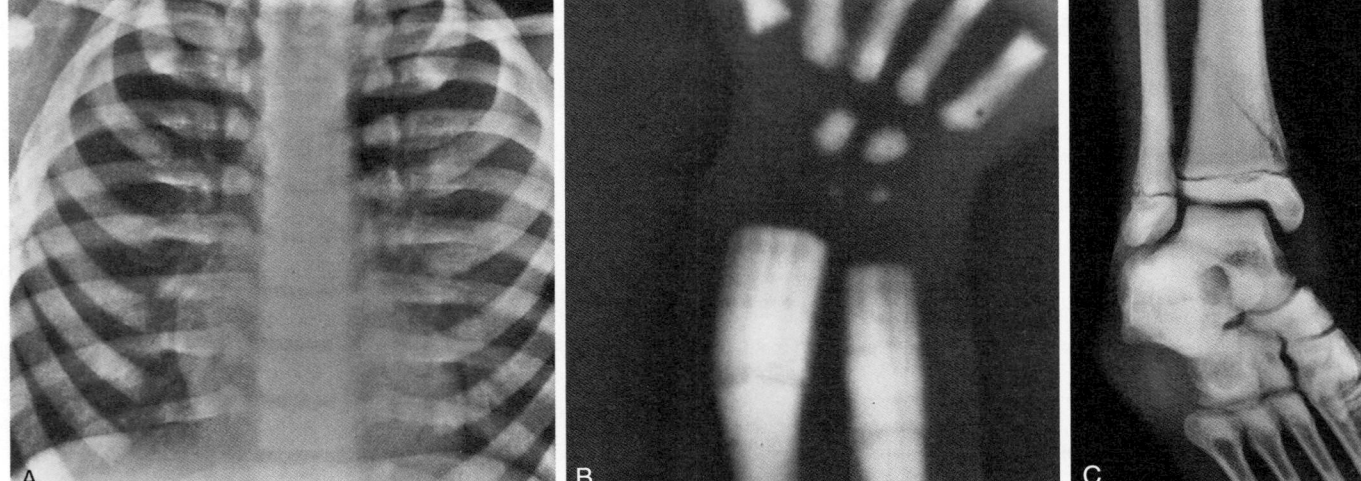

Fig. 50.5 Osteopetrosis. Frontal radiograph of the chest *(A)* and posteroanterior image of the right wrist *(B)* demonstrate diffusely dense bones in a young child with osteopetrosis. *C,* Mortise view of the right ankle in an older child shows a pathologic fracture through the distal tibia in the setting of diffusely increased bone density. The "bone within bone" or "picture frame" appearance is noted, most pronounced in the metatarsals. (From Walters MM, Robertson RL. *Pediatric Radiology: The Requisites.* 4th ed. Philadelphia: Elsevier; 2017:211, Fig. 7.43.)

but because methylmalonic acid and homocysteine accumulate in cobalamin deficiency, these levels are helpful in making this diagnosis. Patients are treated with supplemental cobalamin often in intramuscular replacements until response with simultaneous dietary changes or indefinitely for patients with absorption etiologies.

Folate Deficiency

Folate is widely available in many foods, and since folate fortification of foods in the United States, this nutritional deficiency remains rare. It is seen in severe malnutrition and alcohol use. Patients with poor folate absorption due to inflammatory bowel disease, intestinal resection, or certain medications (antiepileptic drugs, methotrexate, trimethoprim) are also at risk of folate deficiency. Goat's milk is low in folate, so a careful review of infants' and young children's milk intake is necessary. Patients present similarly to those with cobalamin deficiency and have the same hematologic and bone marrow findings. Serum folate levels are low within 2 weeks of deficiency and the RBC folate level decreases slowly over 3–4 months. Homocysteine will also be increased, but unlike cobalamin deficiency, there is no accumulation of methylmalonic acid. Supplemental folic acid and improvement in dietary intake are essential to treating this deficiency.

Myelodysplasia often presents similarly to other causes of megaloblastic anemia with macrocytosis, megaloblastic changes, and pancytopenia. Bone marrow evaluation and cytogenetics will help differentiate the underlying etiology, which can guide appropriate therapy. Drugs that cause megaloblastic anemia include antineoplastic agents, immunomodulators, antibiotics, antimalarial medications, and antiepileptic medications.

Dyserythropoietic anemia is characterized by abnormal erythropoiesis leading to defective RBC production. This can be inherited, such as congenital dyserythropoietic anemias, or acquired. In addition to defective production of RBCs and reticulocytopenia, hemolysis can also be seen in these conditions. Patients present with anemia, jaundice, and splenomegaly. In addition to the anemia and hemolysis, marrow findings reveal dyserythropoietic changes and megaloblastic changes. Management includes supportive blood transfusions, and there are reports of successful bone marrow transplantation for some of these patients.

Increased Reticulocytes/Evidence of Hemolysis
Coombs Positive

A patient presenting with pancytopenia but with increased reticulocyte count indicates a possible cellular destructive etiology. Other evidence of hemolysis might be present, such as jaundice, hemoglobinuria, and elevated indirect bilirubin. The direct Coombs test, or direct antiglobulin test (DAT), can further narrow the differential diagnosis. The DAT can identify antibodies and complement components on the surface of circulating erythrocytes. When the DAT is positive, this is indicative of an antibody-mediated destruction of RBCs. Destruction of other cell lines can also be seen with concomitant immune destruction of RBCs leading to autoimmune pancytopenia.

Autoimmune

Autoimmune hemolytic anemia (AIHA) is antibody-mediated destruction of RBCs and can be classified into primary or secondary. *Warm-reactive* AIHA is the most common form and involves immunoglobulin G autoantibodies that lead to hemolysis. Other less common forms include paroxysmal cold hemoglobinuria and cold-agglutinin disease. Secondary AIHA is a result of another underlying diagnosis including autoimmune disorders, malignancies, medications, primary immunodeficiency diseases, and infections. These secondary causes often result in antibody-mediated destruction of other cell lines, which can result in pancytopenia. **Evans syndrome** classically is associated with AIHA and immune-mediated thrombocytopenia but can have autoimmune neutropenia. Evans syndrome may be idiopathic or due to systemic lupus erythematosus, CVID, ALPS, or IPEX syndromes.

Coombs Negative
Sepsis/Shock

DAT-negative hemolysis and pancytopenia can be a result of diminished cell production or increased cell destruction.

Disseminated intravascular consumption (DIC) is an acquired disorder of hemostasis that is characterized by increased thrombin formation, decreased anticoagulation, activation and impairment of fibrinolysis, and activation of inflammatory pathways. This is often associated with thrombocytopenia, but pancytopenia can be seen. Patients can have both bleeding and thrombosis as a result of the consumption of both procoagulant and anticoagulant factors. In addition to cytopenias, there are prolonged prothrombin time (PT) and partial thromboplastin time (PTT) and low fibrinogen all consistent with this consumption. Peripheral blood smear may reveal schistocytes. The most common cause of DIC in children is shock. Management of DIC is supportive but focused on identifying and treating the underlying cause.

Splenic Sequestration and Hypersplenism

The spleen filters all RBCs daily and removes any abnormal cells. In the setting of AIHA, sickle cell anemia, portal hypertension, and various erythrocyte membrane disorders, the erythrocytes can be trapped within the spleen. Splenic sequestration, or enlargement of the spleen when blood cannot exit the spleen during filtration, leads to pooling of blood and expansion of the spleen. **Hypersplenism** starts as expansion of the spleen due to RBC pooling and then becomes a reservoir for all blood cells, which can lead to other cytopenias. Splenomegaly can also occur in the setting of liver disease due to portal hypertension. This can result in hypersplenism leading to cytopenias over time.

RED FLAGS

Pancytopenia often becomes evident by bleeding (purpura, petechiae) or pallor. A CBC confirms the presence of anemia, neutropenia, and thrombocytopenia. Persistent, congenital, familial, and severe pancytopenia are potentially life-threatening conditions. Red flags include fevers, lymphadenopathy, hepatosplenomegaly, bone pain, blasts noted on the peripheral smear, hemophagocytosis, and congenital anomalies. Disorders not to miss include leukemia, lymphoma, HLH, and genetic causes of bone marrow failure.

BIBLIOGRAPHY

A bibliography is available at ExpertConsult.com.

51

Bleeding and Thrombosis

Brian R. Branchford and Veronica H. Flood

Hemostasis is a process that maintains normal blood flow through healthy vessels but, when a vessel is damaged, rapidly generates a platelet plug (primary hemostasis) and subsequent thrombin clot (secondary hemostasis) at the site of vascular injury. The major components of the hemostatic mechanism are the platelets, the anticoagulant proteins, the procoagulant proteins, and the various components of the vascular wall. Normal hemostasis is an interactive process in which each element cooperates closely to generate a rapid, cohesive, focused reaction. An abnormality of one element destabilizes the system, but significant clinical symptoms often manifest only when two components are affected. Typical examples include the patient with hemophilia who bleeds after sustaining trauma and the antithrombin (AT)-deficient woman in whom thrombosis develops during pregnancy. The astute clinician is aware of situations that may exacerbate preexisting conditions. Pretreatment of known predisposing conditions can prevent complications, as exemplified by infusion of factor VIII (factor 8*) concentrate before and after surgery to a patient with hemophilia A to prevent excessive bleeding. Table 51.1 shows common bleeding symptoms and the most common disorders that trigger these symptoms.

COAGULATION CASCADE

Two opposing systems generate local clots but limit the clot to the area of vascular damage. Fig. 51.1 shows the sequence of activation of coagulation. The cascade is capable of rapid response because generation of a small number of activated factors at the "top" of the cascade leads to thousands of molecules of thrombin (factor 2). Deficiencies of proteins at or below factors 11 or 7 in the coagulation cascade sequence result in clinical bleeding symptoms, whereas deficiencies of factor 12, prekallikrein, and high-molecular-weight kininogen do not. The coagulation mechanism is continuously generating a small amount of thrombin. If there is trauma, tissue factor (TF) and factor 7 combine to activate factor 10 to factor 10a both directly and indirectly via factor 9. Factor 10a then forms a complex on a membrane surface (provided by the activated platelet) with factor 5 and calcium, resulting in even more thrombin generation. Platelets adhere to exposed subendothelial material in areas of vessel injury, thus generally restricting thrombin generation and clot formation to the area of damage.

Thrombin exerts positive feedback on the system by acting on factor 11 to trigger the intrinsic system, cleaving factors 5 and 8 to activate

---

*Established international nomenclature refers to the clotting factors by their respective Roman numerals. However, for this general pediatrics textbook, we have chosen here to use Arabic numerals to avoid confusion that results on occasion from use of Roman numerals.

them, further accelerating thrombin generation, aggregating platelets, and activating factor 13. Clotting proteins, along with enzymes and zymogens, circulate in concert and a rapid activation cascade ensues with the exposure to damaged endothelium. This dynamic system concept allows for expeditious cessation of bleeding but underscores the impact of deficiencies in anticoagulant protein when thrombin is being continuously generated. A deficiency of an inhibitory enzyme or a cofactor removes part of the "brakes" on the system and causes increased thrombin generation.

COAGULATION INHIBITORS

Four key systems interact to inhibit the coagulation mechanism:
- AT
- Protein C/S system
- Fibrinolytic system
- Tissue factor pathway inhibitor (TFPI)

Antithrombin

AT is a member of the serine protease inhibitor family (serpins) that inhibits thrombin, factor 10a, and, less efficiently, factors 9a and 11a. When AT is bound to heparin, this reaction is accelerated 1,000-fold. AT is the active anticoagulant operative during heparin therapy; if AT is deficient, the activity of heparin is compromised. Heparin-like molecules are synthesized by endothelial cells and interact with AT on the vessel wall to inhibit coagulation. Both congenital and acquired AT deficiencies are associated with a predisposition toward thrombosis. AT is consumed during clotting.

Protein C/Protein S System

The protein C (PC)/protein S (PS) system is complex and limits clot extension by inactivating the rate-limiting coenzymes of the coagulation cascade, factors 5 and 8. To prevent extension of the clot, the anticoagulant mechanism must limit thrombin formation to areas of vascular damage. First, thrombin binds to the protein thrombomodulin on intact endothelial cells. Thrombomodulin-bound thrombin then converts protein C into its activated form, activated protein C (APC). APC then combines with protein S to inactivate factors 5 and 8. In addition, APC may promote fibrinolysis. Thrombin itself is inactivated when bound to thrombomodulin and simultaneously augments the anticoagulant response by generating APC. APC limits the amount of thrombin that can be generated subsequently.

AT, PC, and PS are important inhibitors of clotting because deficiencies of each of these proteins, either inherited or acquired, are associated with an increased risk for thrombosis. A gene variant in factor 5 (factor 5 Leiden) that makes it less susceptible to proteolysis by APC (resistance to APC) is the most common hereditary predisposition to

TABLE 51.1 Common Causes of Clinical Bleeding Symptoms

Mucocutaneous Bleeding

Immune thrombocytopenic purpura

Child abuse

Trauma

Poisoning with anticoagulants (rat poison)

von Willebrand disease

Platelet function defect or deficiency: acquired or genetic

Marrow infiltration: malignancy

Marrow failure/aplasia

Collagen vascular defect

Deep/Surgical Bleeding

Hemophilia

Vitamin K deficiency

von Willebrand disease

Trauma

Generalized Bleeding

Disseminated intravascular coagulation

Vitamin K deficiency

Liver disease

Uremia

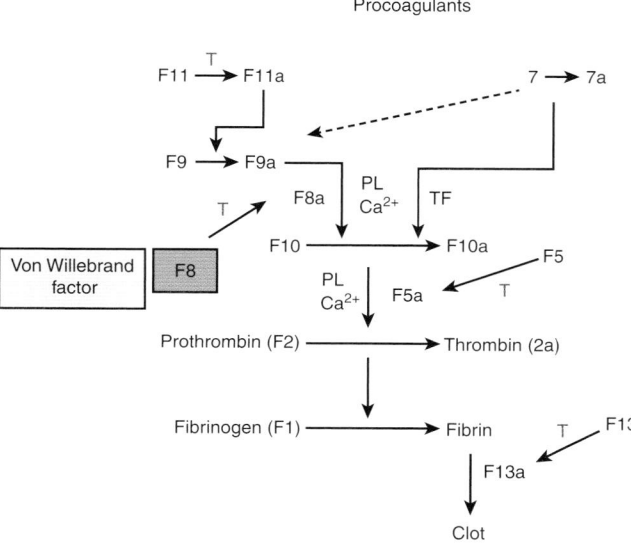

Fig. 51.1 The coagulation cascade and the critical positive feedback role of factor 2a (thrombin) (T) on multiple aspects of the coagulation cascade. In addition, thrombin aggregates platelets and thereby contributes to platelet plug formation. The *dotted line* connecting factor 7a with factor 9 depicts the physiologic pathway of factor 9 activation in vivo. Factor 8 circulates bound to von Willebrand factor. After activation by thrombin, factor 8a can participate with factor 9a in the activation of factor 10. Factor 13a cross-links fibrin and stabilizes the fibrin clot. Ca²⁺, calcium; PL, platelet phospholipid surface; TF, tissue factor. (Modified from Montgomery RR, Scott JP. Hemorrhage and thrombotic diseases. In: Behrman RE, Kliegman RM, Jenson HB, eds. *Nelson Textbook of Pediatrics.* 16th ed. Philadelphia: WB Saunders; 1999:1505.)

thrombosis, although it imparts only a modest increase in absolute risk. TFPI is an inhibitor of factor 7a (Fig. 51.2).

Fibrinolytic System

The fibrinolytic system dissolves and removes clots from the vascular system so that normal flow through vessels can be restored. Endothelial cells synthesize two activators of plasminogen: tissue-type plasminogen activator (tPA) and urokinase, both of which convert plasminogen to plasmin, the enzyme that degrades fibrin. Normally, plasminogen activator and its inhibitor, plasminogen activator inhibitor (PAI-I), are synthesized in equimolar amounts and are released from endothelial cells in parallel, leading to minimal amounts of active fibrinolysis. Increased activation or damage to the vascular system can alter this balance, however, and result in increased tPA release, thus generating plasmin and lysing local clots. Plasminogen activator has been synthesized in a recombinant form (rtPA) and is an effective pharmacologic fibrinolytic agent in vivo.

PLATELET-ENDOTHELIAL CELLS AXIS

Clotting is initiated when platelets adhere to damaged endothelium (Fig. 51.3). In areas of vascular damage, the adhesive protein, von Willebrand factor (VWF), binds to the exposed subendothelial collagen matrix and undergoes a conformational change. VWF then binds to its platelet receptor, glycoprotein Ib, and activates platelets. Activated platelets secrete adenosine diphosphate (ADP), which induces nearby circulating platelets to aggregate. Platelet-to-platelet cohesion is mediated by the binding of fibrinogen (clotting factor 1) to its platelet receptor, glycoprotein IIb/IIIa ($\alpha_{iib}\beta_3$). Therefore, both VWF and fibrinogen play essential roles in normal platelet function in vivo. Simultaneously with the platelet adhesion-aggregation response, coagulation is being activated. The phospholipid-rich platelet membrane brings the reactants of the cascade into close proximity, promoting rapid, effective factor catalysis and accelerating the reactions 1,000-fold faster than would occur in the absence of the appropriate surface.

Normally, endothelial cells provide an antithrombotic surface through which blood flows without interruption. The endothelial cell is capable of a rapid change in function and character so that it can augment coagulation after stimulation with a variety of modulating agents, including lymphokines and cytokines, as well as noxious agents such as endotoxin and infectious viruses (Fig. 51.4). Widespread alteration of endothelial cell function can shift and disregulate the hemostatic response and promote activation of clotting, which is the probable mechanism by which sepsis induces the clinical syndrome of disseminated intravascular coagulation (DIC).

DEVELOPMENTAL HEMOSTASIS

Hemostatic disorders in newborns are more common than at any other pediatric age. The neonate is relatively deficient in most procoagulant and anticoagulant proteins. Platelet function may also be impaired. Blood flow characteristics in the newborn are unique because of the high hematocrit, small-caliber vessels, low blood pressure, and special areas of vascular fragility. Table 51.2 presents the normal values for coagulation screening tests and procoagulant proteins in preterm and full-term infants, as well as in older children. Table 51.3 presents age-specific values for the anticoagulant and fibrinolytic proteins.

Levels of factors 5 and 8, fibrinogen, VWF, and platelets become normal by 28 weeks of gestation. PS levels are also close to normal at birth, but levels of other anticoagulant proteins, especially PC, AT, and plasminogen, are low in full-term infants and are even lower in

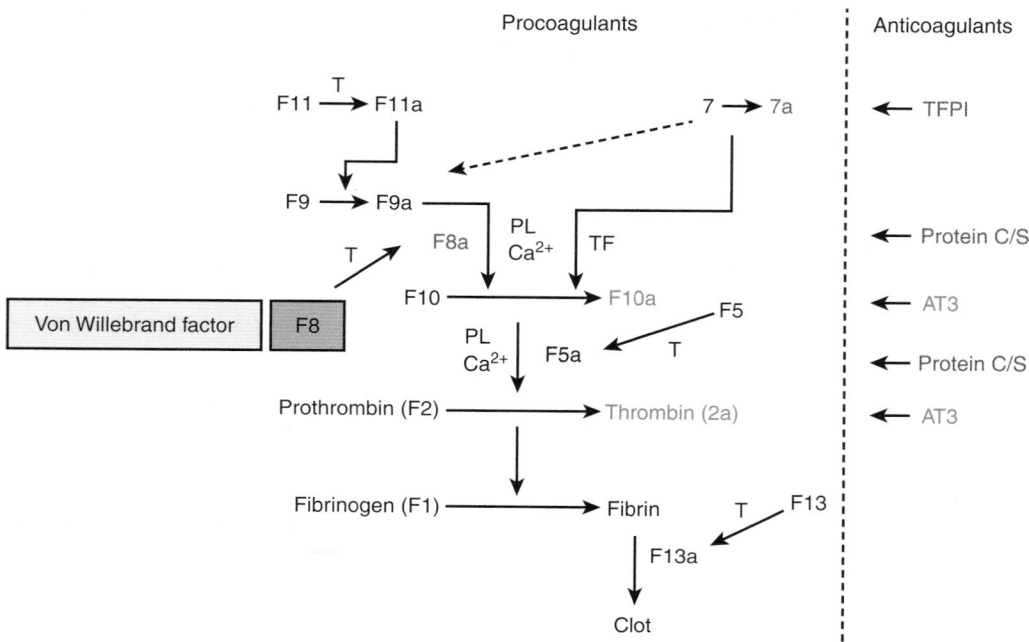

Fig. 51.2 The major sites of action of the physiologic anticoagulants. Antithrombin (AT) irreversibly binds and inactivates factor 10a and thrombin. Thrombin binds to endothelial thrombomodulin and activates protein C. The activated protein C/protein S complex (protein-C/S) proteolyses and inactivates factors 5a and 8a. The tissue factor pathway inhibitor (TFPI) binds to the complexes of factor 7a–tissue factor–factor 10a and inactivates factor 7a. Ca^{2+}, calcium; PL, platelet phospholipid surface; TF, tissue factor. (Modified from Montgomery RR, Scott JP. Hemorrhage and thrombotic diseases. In: Behrman RE, Kliegman RM, Jenson HB, eds. *Nelson Textbook of Pediatrics.* 16th ed. Philadelphia: WB Saunders; 1999:1505.)

Blood vessel

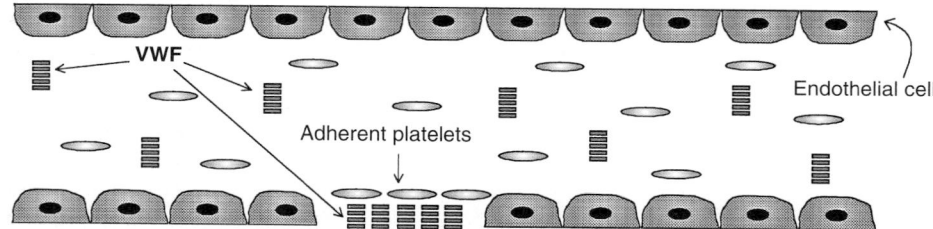

Adherence of platelets to damaged endothelium is VWF-dependent

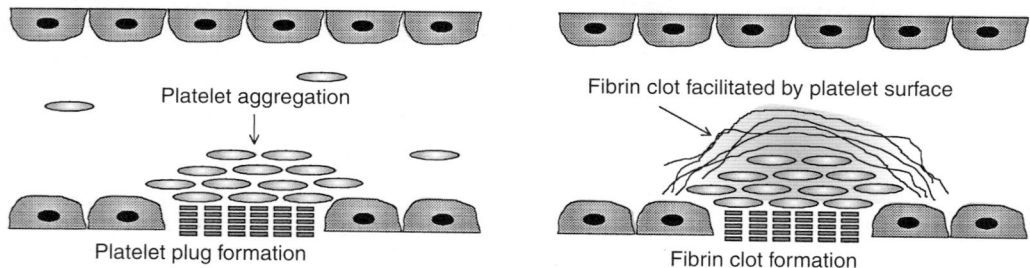

Fig. 51.3 The endothelial cell–platelet–von Willebrand factor (VWF) interaction that results in initiation of the normal platelet plug by the adhesion of platelets to damaged endothelium, mediated by VWF with subsequent formation of the platelet plug and fibrin clot. (Courtesy R.R. Montgomery.)

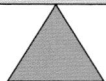

Antithrombotic   **Prothrombotic**

(endotoxin)
(cytokines)
(viral agents)

Thrombomodulin
Heparin
Surface charge   Tissue factor generation
ADPase   Synthesis of clotting factors
Tissue plasminogen activator   and von Willebrand factor
Prostacyclin generation   Reaction surface
Nitric oxide   Plasminogen activator inhibitor
                              Platelet activating factor

Fig. 51.4 Endothelial balance. The pivotal role of the endothelium in maintaining a balance between antithrombotic and prothrombotic activities, as influenced by endotoxins, viruses, and immunomodulatory cytokines. ADPase, adenosine diphosphatase.

premature neonates. The levels of most procoagulant and anticoagulant proteins increase throughout gestation; therefore, the most immature infant has the lowest levels of these proteins and is at the highest risk for either bleeding or thrombotic complications.

Vitamin K deficiency is a particular problem of the newborn. Vitamin K is a fat-soluble vitamin that induces the post-translational γ-carboxylation of the vitamin K–dependent substances (factors 2, 7, 9, and 10; PC; and PS). This carboxylation step occurs after the protein is synthesized in the liver and must occur for a vitamin K–dependent coagulation factor to bind calcium, the bridge to the membrane surface on which these proteins form complexes with other members of the clotting cascade and catalyze subsequent reactions. Vitamin K deficiency effectively renders these proteins unable to bind to a surface. Most of the vitamin K in adults originates from the diet and from bacterial production in the intestine. The breast-fed neonate is at high risk for vitamin K deficiency because human milk is relatively deficient in vitamin K, the neonatal liver itself is immature with reduced carboxylation function, and the newborn's gut requires several days to develop normal bacterial flora.

Severe vitamin K deficiency in neonates, vitamin K–dependent bleeding (VKDB), occurs in breast-fed infants who have not received intramuscular vitamin K prophylaxis. VKDB can be classified by age of onset into early (<24 hours), classical (days 1–7), and late (>1 week to <6 months), and by etiology into idiopathic and secondary. In secondary VKDB, in addition to breast-feeding, other predisposing factors are apparent, such as poor intake or malabsorption of vitamin K (hepatobiliary disease). Such infants may experience diffuse bleeding and even central nervous system hemorrhage. VKDB is an extraordinarily rare event in the United States, occurring in <2% of live births, because of nearly universal neonatal administration of vitamin K. In the evaluation of bleeding in a newborn, the clinician should confirm that vitamin K has been administered. Patients with disorders of the gastrointestinal tract, those taking broad-spectrum antibiotics, those born of mothers who received phenobarbital or phenytoin during pregnancy (very–early-onset VKDB), and those with cholestasis and malabsorption (late-onset VKDB) are at higher risk for vitamin K deficiency.

CLUES FROM HISTORY AND PHYSICAL EXAMINATION

History

Table 51.4 is an outline of historical questions that are important for the diagnosis of bleeding disorders as it is critical to obtain quantifiable, precise information. Easy bruising and nosebleeds are common in children, although the presence of large (>2 inches in diameter) bruises at multiple sites, prolonged nosebleeds (>15–30 minutes), and hematoma formation are seen in up to 20–40% of children with a bleeding disorder. Bleeding postcircumcision should raise the suspicion of hemophilia, while bleeding from the umbilical cord stump is associated with factor 13 deficiency. Some helpful questions include "What was the biggest bruise you ever had, and what caused it?" and "Have you ever noted little red dots (petechiae) on your skin?"

A personal or family history of gynecologic bleeding is often valuable. Menorrhagia causing iron-deficiency anemia, bleeding after childbirth, or need for red blood cell transfusion or early hysterectomy because of bleeding is often inappropriately assumed to have anatomic causes ("dysfunctional uterine bleeding"). The clinician must ascertain the number of pads used per day, in addition to the length and frequency of each menstrual cycle. If the majority of females in a family have an underlying bleeding disorder, then that family's "normal menstrual periods" may be quite abnormal. Many adolescent females with menorrhagia caused by an underlying bleeding disorder respond to oral contraceptive agents; *therefore, improvement in bleeding symptoms after starting oral contraceptive agents does not rule out a bleeding disorder.*

Historical information is equally important in deciding who requires evaluation for a predisposition to thrombosis. Virtually all pediatric patients in whom a blood clot develops in the absence of major vascular instrumentation, catheter placement, underlying infection, or other inflammatory state merit careful laboratory screening for a prothrombotic state (a hereditary or acquired disorder that predisposes to clotting). Even in the situation of a provoked thrombosis, a detailed family history should be documented for early-onset stroke; early myocardial infarction; and blood clots in the veins, arteries, or lungs.

Physical Examination

The most important determination is whether the patient appears acutely or chronically ill, including vital signs and growth parameters. The nose should be examined for ulcers or anatomic bleeding sites, and the heart should be examined for the presence of murmurs (as occur in anemia and endocarditis). Joints should be examined for chronic arthropathy (as occurs in hemophilia) or joint laxity (as occurs in Ehlers-Danlos syndrome), and the extremities are examined for thumb or radial anomalies (thrombocytopenia–absent radius syndrome, or Fanconi anemia). The abdomen and lymph nodes should be examined for the presence of hepatosplenomegaly and adenopathy.

The examination of the skin should include a search for pallor, hematomas, petechiae, ecchymoses, telangiectasias, poor wound healing (large or abnormal scars), lax (loose) skin, and varicose veins (possible deep venous thrombosis). Petechiae are pinpoint, flat, dark red lesions caused by capillary bleeding into the skin. Ecchymoses are larger lesions (bruises) that are flat and usually not palpable. Hematomas are accumulations of blood in the skin or deeper tissues; in the skin, hematomas are raised and palpable. Bruises should be described in detail, including whether hematomas are associated with bruises and whether petechiae are present. Petechiae and ecchymoses are usually painless. Purpura refers to any group of disorders characterized by the presence of dark-red, purplish, or brown lesions of the skin and mucous membranes. The discoloration is caused by the leakage of red blood cells from affected vessels. Purpuric lesions can be caused by abnormalities of the platelets, of coagulation proteins, or of vessel walls. Since all these lesions result from visualization of extravascular blood under the skin, blanching will not occur with manual pressure.

TABLE 51.2   Reference Values for Coagulation Tests in Healthy Children*

Test	19–27 Wk Gestation†	28–31 Wk Gestation†	30–36 Wk Gestation	Full Term	1–5 Yr	6–10 Yr	11–18 Yr	Adult
PT (sec)	—	15.4 (14.6–16.9)	13.0 (10.6–16.2)	13.0 (10.1–15.9)	11 (10.6–11.4)	11.1 (10.1–11.4)	11.2 (10.2–12.0)	12 (11.0–14.0)
INR	—	—	1.0 (0.61–1.7)	1.00 (0.53–1.62)‡	1.0 (0.96–1.04)	1.01 (0.91–1.11)	1.02 (0.93–1.10)	1.10 (1.0–1.3)
aPTT (sec)	—	108 (80–168)	53.6 (27.5–79.4)‡§	42.9 (31.3–54.3)‡	30 (24–36)	31 (26–36)	32 (26–37)	33 (27–40)
Fibrinogen (factor 1)	1.00 (±0.43)	2.56 (1.60–5.50)	2.43 (1.50–3.73)‡§	2.83 (1.67–3.99)	2.76 (1.70–4.05)	2.79 (1.57–4.0)	3.0 (1.54–4.48)	2.78 (1.56–4.0)
Bleeding time (min)	—	—	—	—	6 (2.5–10)‡	7 (2.5–13)‡	5 (3.8)‡	4 (1–7)
Prothrombin (factor 2)	0.12 (±0.02)	0.31 (0.19–0.54)	0.45 (0.20–0.77)‡	0.48 (0.26–0.70)‡	0.94 (0.71–1.16)‡	0.88 (0.67–1.07)‡	0.83 (0.61–1.04)‡	1.08 (0.70–1.46)
Factor 5	0.41 (±0.10)	0.65 (0.43–0.80)	0.88 (0.41–1.44)§	0.72 (0.34–1.08)‡	1.03 (0.79–1.27)	0.90 (0.63–1.16)‡	0.77 (0.55–0.99)‡	1.06 (0.62–1.50)
Factor 7	0.28 (±0.04)	0.37 (0.24–0.76)	0.67 (0.21–1.13)‡	0.66 (0.28–1.04)‡	0.82 (0.55–1.16)‡	0.86 (0.52–1.20)‡	0.83 (0.58–1.15)‡	1.05 (0.67–1.43)
Factor 8 procoagulant	0.39 (±0.14)	0.79 (0.37–1.26)	1.11 (0.5–2.13)	1.00 (0.50–1.78)	0.90 (0.59–1.42)	0.95 (0.58–1.32)	0.92 (0.53–1.31)	0.99 (0.50–1.49)
VWF	0.64 (±0.13)	1.41 (0.83–2.23)	1.36 (0.78–2.10)	1.53 (0.50–2.87)	0.82 (0.60–1.20)	0.95 (0.44–1.44)	1.00 (0.46–1.53)	0.92 (0.50–1.58)
Factor 9	0.10 (±0.01)	0.18 (0.17–0.20)	0.35 (0.19–0.65)†§	0.53 (0.15–0.91)†‡	0.73 (0.47–1.04)‡	0.75 (0.63–0.89)‡	0.82 (0.59–1.22)‡	1.09 (0.55–1.63)
Factor 10	0.21 (±0.03)	0.36 (0.25–0.64)	0.41 (0.11–0.71)‡	0.40 (0.12–0.68)‡	0.88 (0.58–1.16)‡	0.75 (0.55–1.01)‡	0.79 (0.50–1.17)	1.06 (0.70–1.52)
Factor 11	—	0.23 (0.11–0.33)	0.30 (0.08–5.2)‡§	0.38 (0.40–0.66)‡	0.97 (0.52–1.50)‡§	0.86 (0.52–1.20)	0.74 (0.50–0.97)‡	0.97 (0.67–1.27)
Factor 12	0.22 (±0.03)	0.25 (0.05–0.35)	0.38 (0.10–0.66)†§	0.53 (0.13–0.93)‡	0.93 (0.64–1.29)	0.92 (0.60–1.40)	0.81 (0.34–1.37)‡	1.08 (0.52–1.64)
PK		0.26 (0.15–0.32)	0.33 (0.09–0.89)‡	0.37 (0.18–0.69)‡	0.95 (0.65–1.30)	0.99 (0.66–1.31)	0.99 (0.53–1.45)	1.12 (0.62–1.62)
HMWK		0.32 (0.19–0.52)	0.49 (0.09–0.89)‡	0.54 (0.06–1.02)‡	0.98 (0.64–1.32)	0.93 (0.60–1.30)	0.91 (0.63–1.19)	0.92 (0.50–1.36)
Factor 13a			0.70 (0.32–1.08)‡	0.79 (0.27–1.31)‡	1.08 (0.72–1.43)	1.09 (0.65–1.51)	0.99 (0.57–1.40)	1.05 (0.55–1.55)
Factor 13b			0.81 (0.35–1.27)‡	0.76 (0.30–1.22)‡	1.13 (0.69–1.56)‡	1.16 (0.77–1.54)‡	1.02 (0.60–1.43)	0.98 (0.57–1.37)

*All factors except fibrinogen (mg/mL) are presented as U/mL, where pooled normal plasma contains 1 U/mL. All data are expressed as the mean followed by the upper and lower boundaries encompassing 95% of the normal population.

†Levels for 19–27 wk and 28–31 wk are from multiple sources and cannot be analyzed statistically.

‡Values are significantly different from those of adults.

§Values are significantly different from those of full-term infants.

aPTT, activated partial thromboplastin time; HMWK, high-molecular-weight kininogen; INR, international normalized ratio; PK, prekallikrein; PT, prothrombin time; VWF, von Willebrand factor.

Data from Andrew M, Paes B, Johnston M. Development of the hemostatic system in the neonate and young infant. *Am J Pediatr Hematol Oncol.* 1990;12:95–104; and Andrew M, Vegh P, Johnston M, et al. Maturation of the hemostatic system during childhood. *Blood.* 1992;80:1998–2005.

TABLE 51.3 Reference Values for the Inhibitors of Coagulation in Healthy Children in Comparison with Adults*

Inhibitor	19–27 Wk Gestation[†]	28–31 Wk Gestation[†]	30–36 Wk Gestation	Full Term	1–5 Yr	6–10 Yr	11–18 Yr	Adult
AT3	0.24 (±0.03)[‡]	0.28 (0.20–0.38)[‡]	0.38 (0.14–0.62)[‡,§]	0.63 (0.39–0.87)[‡]	1.11 (0.82–1.39)	1.11 (0.90–1.31)	1.06 (0.77–1.32)	1.0 (0.74–1.26)
Protein C	0.11 (±0.03)[‡]	—	0.28 (0.12–0.44)[‡,§]	0.35 (0.17–0.53)[‡]	0.66 (0.40–0.92)[‡]	0.69 (0.45–0.93)[‡]	0.83 (0.55–1.11)[‡]	0.96 (0.64–1.28)
Protein S	—	—	—	—	—	—	—	—
Total (U/mL)	—	—	0.26 (0.14–0.38)[‡,§]	0.36 (0.12–0.60)[‡]	0.86 (0.54–1.18)	0.78 (0.41–1.14)	0.72 (0.52–0.92)	0.81 (0.61–1.13)
Free (U/mL)	—	—	—	—	0.45 (0.21–0.69)	0.42 (0.22–0.62)	0.38 (0.26–0.55)	0.45 (0.27–0.61)
Plasminogen (U/mL)	—	—	1.70 (1.12–2.48)[‡]	1.95 (1.25–2.65)[‡]	0.98 (0.78–1.18)	0.92 (0.75–1.08)	0.86 (0.68–1.03)	0.99 (0.77–1.22)
TPA (ng/mL)	—	—	8.48 (3.00–16.70)	9.6 (5.0–18.9)	2.15 (1.0–4.5)[‡]	2.42 (1.0–5.0)[‡]	2.16 (1.0–4.0)[‡]	1.02 (0.68–1.36)
α2AP (U/mL)	—	—	0.78 (0.40–1.16)	0.85 (0.55–1.15)	1.05 (0.93–1.17)	0.99 (0.89–1.10)	0.98 (0.78–1.18)	1.02 (0.68–1.36)
PAI–1	—	—	5.4 (0.0–12.2)[‡]	5.42 (1.0–10.0)	5.42 (1.0–10.0)	6.79 (2.0–12.0)[‡]	6.07 (2.0–10.0)[‡]	3.60 (0–11.0)

α2AP, α2-antiplasmin; AT3, antithrombin 3; PAI-1, plasminogen activator inhibitor type 1; TPA, tissue plasminogen activator.
*All values are expressed in U/mL, where pooled plasma contains 1 U/mL, with the exception of free protein S, which contains a mean of 0.4 U/mL. All values presented as the mean by the upper and lower boundaries encompassing 95% of the population.
[†]Levels for 19–27 wk and 28–31 wk are from multiple sources and cannot be analyzed statistically.
[‡]Values are significantly different from those of adults.
[§]Values are significantly different from those of full-term infants.
Data from Andrew M, Paes B, Johnston M. Development of the hemostatic system in the neonate and young infant. *Am J Pediatr Hematol Oncol.* 1990;12:95–104; and Andrew M, Vegh P, Johnston M, et al. Maturation of the hemostatic system during childhood. *Blood.* 1992;80:1998–2005.

Coagulation Screening Tests

After obtaining a history and performing a physical examination, the clinician must determine the need for a hemostatic evaluation (Fig. 51.5). The history is likely to be the most sensitive screening tool for a significant bleeding disorder, although its use in a very young child, especially before toddler age, is limited and attention must shift to the perinatal and family history. For patients with clinical clues of a coagulation disorder, the initial screening studies should assess the clotting factors and platelet function. No set of screening tests is complete and capable of detecting the panorama of hemorrhagic disorders, but the screen should include:

- CBC to evaluate hemoglobin and platelet count
- Prothrombin time (PT)
- Partial thromboplastin time (PTT)
- Functional fibrinogen level or thrombin time (TT)
- VWF testing

If there is high suspicion for an underlying bleeding disorder, specific screening for von Willebrand disease (VWD) and platelet function defects should be considered even if the PT and PTT are normal. There are no simple tests to screen for a thrombotic tendency.

Prothrombin Time and Partial Thromboplastin Time

The PT and PTT (Fig. 51.6) are measures of all the coagulation factors except factor 13. Fibrinogen function should be measured as fibrinogen activity or TT. The PTT is the screening test that checks for deficiency of all clotting factors except factors 7 and 13. The PTT can be prolonged either by a deficiency of a clotting factor or by the presence of an agent in the plasma that delays the clotting time (an inhibitor). The PT is especially sensitive to deficiencies of factor 7.

To test for an inhibitor, one part of the patient's plasma is mixed with one part of pooled normal plasma obtained from 20–50 healthy adults. Pooled normal plasma provides a 100% level of each clotting

factor. If mixed 1:1 with plasma that is deficient in one or several factors, the mixture should possess at least a 50% level of each factor and the PTT should correct to the normal range. If an inhibitor is present, the PTT usually does not correct to normal. The most common types of inhibitors include anticoagulants, such as heparin, and autoantibodies directed against either specific clotting factors (factor 8 inhibitors) or the phospholipid substances used in the PTT (lupus-type anticoagulants).

The PTT is especially sensitive to deficiencies of factors 8, 9, and 11 (hemophilia A, B, and C, respectively), as well as 12. A prolonged PTT in an asymptomatic child is most commonly caused by factor 12 deficiency or by a lupus-type anticoagulant, neither of which cause clinically significant coagulopathy. The PTT can also yield a false result if preanalytic variables are not adequately controlled:

1. When poor venipuncture technique, by adding TF to the blood, activates clotting and artifactually shortens the PTT
2. When insensitive laboratory reagents fail to detect clinically significant deficiencies (most common in mild factor 9 deficiency)
3. When the citrate concentration is not corrected for blood with a high hematocrit (in neonates and in patients with cyanotic congenital heart disease), leading to a prolonged PTT

Bleeding Time

The bleeding time is an indirect measure of platelet number and a more direct measure of platelet function, vascular integrity, and platelet interaction with the vascular subendothelium. As such, the bleeding time is usually abnormal in patients with thrombocytopenia, platelet function abnormalities, abnormal collagen (Ehlers-Danlos syndrome), and VWD. Unfortunately, because of its insensitivity and high level of variability, the bleeding time is a relatively poor tool for detecting the milder forms of these hemostatic disorders and cannot be used to rule out VWD and mild or moderate platelet function deficits. It is rarely used in the United States.

TABLE 51.4 History of a Bleeding Disorder

I. HISTORY OF DISORDER
  A. Onset of symptoms
    1. Age
    2. Acute vs lifelong
    3. Triggering event
    4. Timing of bleeding after injury: immediate vs delayed
  B. Sites of bleeding
    Clarify single site (potential anatomic issue) vs multiple sites (more likely presentation of systemic bleeding disorder).
    1. Mucocutaneous*
      a. Epistaxis
        (1) Duration, frequency, seasonal tendency
        (2) Associated trauma (nose picking, allergy, infection)
        (3) Resultant anemia, emergency department evaluation, cautery
      b. Oral (gingiva, frenulum, tongue lacerations, bleeding after tooth brushing, after dental extractions requiring sutures/packing)
      c. Bruising (number, sites, size, raised [other than extremities], spontaneous vs trauma, knots within center, skin scarring)
      d. Gastrointestinal bleeding
    2. Deep
      a. Musculoskeletal
        (1) Hemarthroses, unexplained arthropathy
        (2) Intramuscular hematomas
      b. Central nervous system hemorrhage
      c. Genitourinary tract
    3. Surgical
      a. Minor (sutures, lacerations, poor or delayed wound healing)
      b. Major
        (1) Tonsillectomy and adenoidectomy
        (2) Abdominal surgery
  C. Perinatal history
    1. Superficial (bruising, petechiae)
    2. Deep
      a. Circumcision
      b. Central nervous system bleeding
      c. Gastrointestinal bleeding
      d. Cephalohematoma
      e. Unexplained anemia or hyperbilirubinemia
      f. Delayed cord separation, bleeding after cord separation
    3. Vitamin K administration
    4. Maternal drugs
  D. Obstetric/gynecologic bleeding
    1. Menorrhagia
      a. Onset, duration, amount (number of pads), frequency, persistence after childbirth
      b. Resultant anemia, iron deficiency
    2. Bleeding at childbirth (onset, duration, transfusion requirement, history of traumatic delivery, recurrences with subsequent pregnancies, spontaneous abortions)
  E. Medications
    1. Aspirin and nonsteroidal antiinflammatory drugs
    2. Anticoagulants
    3. Antibiotics
    4. Anticonvulsants
  F. Diet
    1. Vitamin K
    2. Vitamin C

II. FAMILY HISTORY
  Draw family tree. The items just listed should be applied to immediate family members, especially a history of easy bruising, epistaxis, excessive bleeding after surgery, menorrhagia, excessive bleeding after childbirth, or a family history of others with diagnosed or suspected bleeding disorders. Attempt to deduce inheritance pattern.

*Significant historical information is presented in boldface type.

Platelet Function Analysis

The sensitivity and specificity of platelet function analysis are insufficient for diagnosis, but it may have utility as a screen for severe platelet function defects in very small infants where rapid results are needed and size prohibits collection of large volumes of blood needed for platelet aggregation testing.

Figs. 51.7 and 51.8 provide an approach to evaluate the patient with an isolated prolongation of the PT or PTT.

Thrombin Time and Reptilase Time

The TT and reptilase time are tests that measure the conversion of fibrinogen to fibrin. The thrombin time is sensitive to heparin effect, whereas the snake venom reptilase time remains normal in the presence of heparin. Both the thrombin time and the reptilase time are prolonged by uremia, by dysfibrinogenemia, and by low fibrinogen levels (<75 mg/dL).

MUCOCUTANEOUS BLEEDING

Mucocutaneous bleeding occurs within the skin or mucous membranes. Common complaints include prolonged, frequent nosebleeds; gum bleeding; prolonged bleeding after tooth extraction; menorrhagia; and easy bruising with or without petechiae formation. Mucocutaneous bleeding is usually associated with abnormalities of platelet number or function, of platelet cofactors such as VWF, or of the vessel wall. The well-appearing child who presents with the acute onset of petechiae and purpura, often in association with nosebleeds or bleeding gums, and otherwise normal examination findings typically has **acute immune thrombocytopenic purpura (ITP)**. The majority of affected children have an antecedent viral illness. After exposure to the viral infection, an antibody that binds to the platelet membrane develops, leading to the premature destruction of the antibody-coated platelets in the spleen.

The peak ages for the presentation of ITP are 1–4 years of age and adolescence, but ITP occurs throughout childhood and adolescence. Females are more commonly affected in adolescence but not in childhood, likely due to menarche occurring in the interim. The work-up of a child with thrombocytopenia should include a careful history aimed at detecting symptoms (e.g., weight loss, fever, bone pain, anorexia) of other pre-existing illnesses (e.g., leukemia, systemic lupus erythematosus [SLE], endocarditis, HIV), exposures to drugs or toxins, and a personal or family history of thrombocytopenia. The physical examination must be detailed and include a search for signs of malignancy (e.g., lymphadenopathy, hepatosplenomegaly), chronic illness, and congenital malformations. When evaluating the CBC, the clinician should ensure that the hemoglobin, white blood cell count, differential, indices, and peripheral smear are normal, which would make the diagnosis of a hematologic malignancy or other marrow failure syndrome unlikely. The presence of large platelets on the smear or measured as a high mean platelet volume suggests accelerated thrombopoiesis and increased platelet destruction, consistent with ITP. The differential diagnosis of thrombocytopenia is noted in Table 51.5; genetic disorders are noted in Table 51.6.

After the presumptive diagnosis of ITP, a Coombs test may be considered to rule out a simultaneous autoimmune hemolytic anemia. The role of studies for platelet antibodies is unclear; there are no data indicating that these studies are either diagnostic or prognostic in children. If the child is male, is young, and has a history of eczema or recurrent infection, immunoglobulin levels to rule out **Wiskott-Aldrich syndrome** are indicated. Platelets are also often below average size in this disorder. Similarly, in older children, especially girls as they approach adolescence, an antinuclear antibody (ANA) test to rule out **SLE** manifesting as thrombocytopenia may be considered, although it

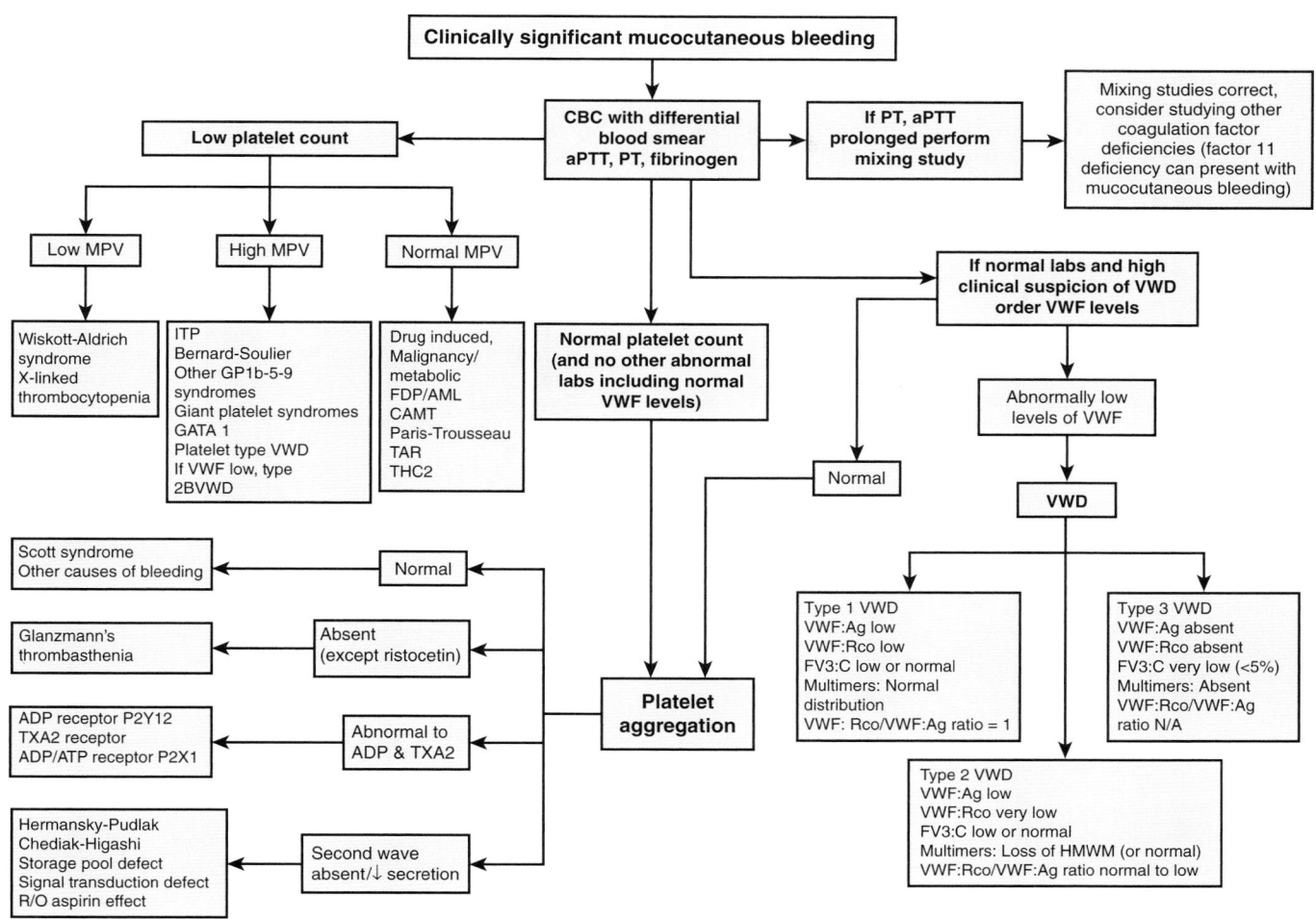

Fig. 51.5 Guide to the staged work-up of clinically significant mucocutaneous bleeding. ADP, adenosine diphosphate; Ag, antigen; aPTT, activated partial thromboplastin time; ATP, adenosine triphosphate; CAMT, congenital amegakaryocytic thrombocytopenia; FDP/AML, familial platelet disorder with predisposition to acute myelogenous leukemia; GP, glycoprotein; HMWM, high-molecular-weight multimer; ITP, immune thrombocytopenia; MPV, mean platelet volume; PT, prothrombin time; Rco, ristocetin cofactor test; R/O, rule out; TAR, thrombocytopenia with absent radii syndrome; THC2, thrombocytopenia 2; TXA2, thromboxane A2; VWD, von Willebrand disease; VWF, von Willebrand factor. (From Orkin SH, Fisher DE, Ginsburg D, et al., eds. *Nathan and Oski's Hematology and Oncology of Infancy and Childhood.* 8th ed. Philadelphia: Elsevier; 2015:1005, Fig. 29.1.)

is more likely to yield positive results in children with chronic ITP. **HIV** infection occasionally manifests as ITP. The diagnostic yield of bone marrow examination in a child with normal findings on a careful physical examination (no lymphadenopathy or hepatosplenomegaly) and a completely normal CBC including a manual white blood cell differential, other than isolated thrombocytopenia, is negligible and therefore not recommended.

Once a diagnosis of ITP is made, several therapeutic options are available, including close observation and education. The family should be advised that the child must avoid activities that increase the risk of head injury. Treatment should be reserved for children at high risk for clinical bleeding (platelet count <20,000/mm³ and children with petechiae and mucosal hemorrhages). Some clinicians believe that patients with mucous membrane purpura are at higher risk and definitely require treatment. Treatment is not recommended for patients without bleeding symptoms. The major cause of mortality in ITP is related to intracranial hemorrhage, which has been observed in fewer than 0.5–1% of patients. Table 51.7 provides a perspective on treatment alternatives for ITP. Options for initial therapy

for patients in need of treatment include intravenous immunoglobulin (IVIG) and prednisone, and some clinicians may consider anti-D immune globulin in patients with Rh-positive blood type. Transfusion of platelets should be reserved for life-threatening bleeding because transfused platelets are rapidly destroyed. Thrombopoietin receptor agonists have been approved for use in adults and children with chronic ITP with bleeding symptoms not responsive to IVIG, steroids, or splenectomy.

Ten to 20% of children with ITP have persistence of thrombocytopenia for more than 6 months (**chronic ITP**). These patients are more likely to be older (adolescent) girls or to have had an insidious onset of symptoms. The clinician must look carefully for predisposing causes, including SLE; HIV infection; autoimmune lymphoproliferative syndrome (ALPS); common variable immune deficiency (CVID); immune disregulation polyendocrinopathy enteropathy, X-linked (IPEX); or medications. The treatment of chronic ITP is evolving and includes repeated doses of IVIG, prolonged steroid use, and consideration of rituximab, thrombopoietin receptor agonists, and/or splenectomy. Because of improved medical therapy weighted against infectious and

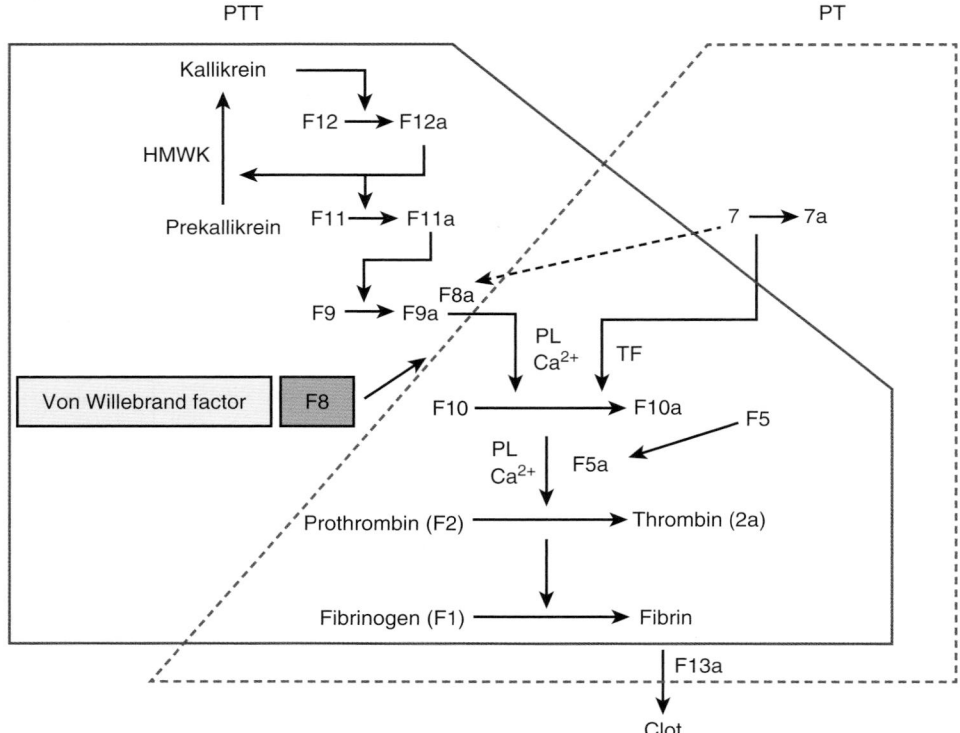

Fig. 51.6 Elements of the coagulation cascade measured by the prothrombin time (PT) and the partial thromboplastin time (PTT). Note that prekallikrein (PK), high-molecular-weight kininogen (HMWK), and factor 12 are shown in this figure and not in the depiction of the coagulation cascade in Fig. 51.1, because a deficiency of PK, HMWK, or factor 12 can cause a prolongation of the PTT. However, a deficiency of any of these proteins alone is not associated with a clinical bleeding disorder. Ca^{2+}, calcium; PL, platelet phospholipid surface; TF, tissue factor. (Modified from Montgomery RR, Scott JP. Hemorrhage and thrombotic diseases. In: Behrman RE, Kliegman RM, Jenson HB, eds. *Nelson Textbook of Pediatrics*. 16th ed. Philadelphia: WB Saunders; 1999:1505.)

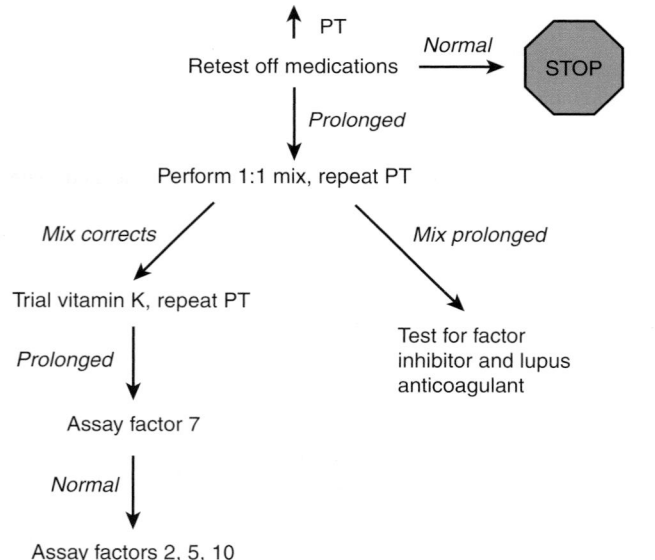

Fig. 51.7 Flow diagram for the evaluation of a patient with an isolated prolongation of the prothrombin time (PT).

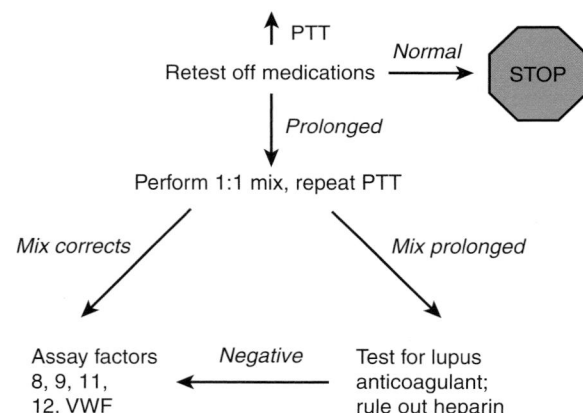

Fig. 51.8 Flow diagram for the evaluation of a patient with an isolated prolongation of the partial thromboplastin time (PTT). To rule out heparin effect, the thrombin time is compared with the reptilase time. If the thrombin time is significantly longer than the reptilase time, heparin is present in the sample. VWF, von Willebrand factor.

TABLE 51.5 Differential Diagnosis of Thrombocytopenia in Children

I. Destructive Thrombocytopenias		II. Impaired or Ineffective Production	
Primary platelet consumption syndromes	Immune thrombocytopenic purpura Drug-induced thrombocytopenia Infection-induced thrombocytopenia (HIV)	Congenital and hereditary disorders	TAR syndrome Other congenital thrombocytopenias with megakaryocytic hypoplasia Fanconi aplastic anemia Bernard-Soulier syndrome*
Immunologic	Post-transfusion purpura Autoimmune or lymphoproliferative disorders Neonatal immune thrombocytopenias Allergy and anaphylaxis Post-transplantation thrombocytopenia Chronic microangiopathic hemolytic anemia and thrombocytopenia Heparin or vaccine associated	Primary hematologic processes	May-Hegglin anomaly* Wiskott-Aldrich syndrome* Miscellaneous hereditary thrombocytopenias (X-linked or autosomal)* Mediterranean thrombocytopenia Associated with trisomy 13 or 18
Nonimmunologic	Hemolytic uremic syndrome Thrombotic thrombocytopenic purpura Catheters, prostheses, or cardiopulmonary bypass (mechanical destruction) Congenital or acquired heart disease	Metabolic inborn errors	Holocarboxylase synthetase deficiency Isovaleric acidemia Some mitochondrial disorders Methylmalonic acidemia Ketotic glycinemia
Combined platelet and fibrinogen consumption syndromes	Disseminated intravascular coagulation Kasabach-Merritt syndrome Other causes of local consumption coagulopathy	Acquired disorders	Aplastic anemia Marrow infiltrative processes Drug or radiation induced Nutritional deficiency states (iron, folate, or vitamin B_{12})
Miscellaneous causes	Phototherapy Perinatal aspiration syndromes Persistent pulmonary hypertension Rhesus alloimmunization	**III. Sequestration**	Hypersplenism Hypothermia
Specific to the neonate	Status post–exchange transfusion Polycythemia Metabolic inborn errors of metabolism Maternal HELLP syndrome Glomerular disease Preeclampsia		

*These hereditary thrombocytopenias can be associated with normal or increased bone marrow megakaryocytes.
HELLP, hypertension, elevated liver enzymes, low platelets; TAR, thrombocytopenia–absent radius. Modified from Schultz Beardsley D. Platelet abnormalities in infancy and childhood. In: Nathan DG, Oski FA, eds. *Hematology of Infancy and Childhood*. 4th ed. Philadelphia: WB Saunders; 1993;2:1566.

thrombotic risk, splenectomy is limited to patients with severe, refractory chronic ITP.

Neonatal Thrombocytopenia

Thrombocytopenia is common, especially in sick newborns. The differential diagnosis of neonatal thrombocytopenia includes most of the causes seen in older children and a few additional specific to the newborn (Fig. 51.9, in the shaded areas; see also Table 51.5). When evaluating the thrombocytopenic newborn, the physician must know the perinatal history including the mother's health during this and prior pregnancies, history of current or previous low platelets, or children dying of hemorrhage. A maternal history of fever, viral infection (cytomegalovirus, rubella), sexually transmitted infections (syphilis, HIV), medications, toxemia, or collagen vascular disease (SLE) is informative. The family history should be evaluated for bleeding disorders, recurrent infections, or malignancies, especially in siblings, both as neonates and at any age.

During examination of the newborn, the most important element to determine is the child's general well-being. The examiner should look especially for signs of systemic illness, as well as lymphadenopathy, hepatosplenomegaly, mass lesions, hemangiomas, bruits, and congenital anomalies, especially of the radial bones. The examiner should carefully evaluate the hemoglobin, the white blood cell count, and the

differential for the presence of abnormal immature cells (blasts). Red blood cell structure should be examined for signs of microangiopathy. Small platelets (low mean platelet volume) suggest abnormal thrombopoiesis, whereas large platelets are found with accelerated platelet destruction (see Fig. 51.5). *Thrombocytopenia can be caused by synthetic failure, sequestration, or destructive processes.* The destructive processes are most common and are either immune or nonimmune in origin. Nonimmune causes of platelet consumption—for example, DIC, sepsis, congenital infections, or thrombotic events—are usually associated with obvious clinical findings. When evaluating the ill-appearing neonate or child for thrombocytopenia, the examiner should perform coagulation studies to detect fibrinogen consumption (fibrinogen level, D-dimer). Neonates with immune-mediated platelet destruction usually appear healthy.

After the clinician obtains a thorough history, performs a careful physical examination, and evaluates the CBC, the initial step in management of the child with thrombocytopenia depends on the cause and severity of the thrombocytopenia. In the neonate with severe thrombocytopenia (platelet count <40,000/mm³) delivered vaginally, an ultrasound study of the head should be done to rule out intracranial bleeding. Platelet transfusion for thrombocytopenia can serve both as a therapeutic tool for stopping the bleeding and as a diagnostic maneuver. In patients with decreased platelet synthesis, survival of transfused

TABLE 51.6 Inherited Platelet Disorders

Platelet Defect	Gene Defect (Chromosomal Location)	Pathophysiology	Clinical and Laboratory Characteristics	Bleeding Treatment
Defects in Platelet Adhesion				
Bernard-Soulier syndrome (BSS)	Autosomal recessive: GP1BA (17p13) GP1BB (22q11) GP9 (3q21) Autosomal dominant: Ala156Val, GP1BA—Bolzano variant	Defective GPIb-IX-V receptor, impaired adhesion to VWF	Often severe bleeding phenotype Thrombocytopenia Large platelets Platelet aggregation: absent ristocetin-induced response Flow cytometry: reduced or absent CD42a (GPIX)/CD42b (GP1bα) GP1BA and GP1BB gene sequencing	Supportive care Platelet transfusion (risk of alloantibodies) Antifibrinolytics rF7a
Velocardiofacial/ DiGeorge syndrome (VCFS)	22q11.2 deletion including GP1BB	Defective GPIb-IX-V receptor	Thrombocytopenia Large platelets and α-granules Cardiac, thymus, parathyroid, facial, and cognitive abnormalities	Supportive care
Platelet-type von Willebrand disease (PT-VWD)	Autosomal dominant: gain-of-function variants in GP1BA	Defective GPIb-IX-V, gain-of-function interaction between VWF-GP1bα	Thrombocytopenia Large platelets Platelet clumping Decreased VWF:Ag, VWF multimers Platelet aggregation: low-dose ristocetin-induced platelet agglutination GP1BA gene sequencing	Supportive care Platelet transfusion Antifibrinolytics rF7a
Defects of Platelet Aggregation				
Glanzmann thrombasthenia (GT)	Autosomal recessive: ITGA2B (17Q21.32) ITGB3 (17q21.32)	Defective integrin αIIbβ3 (GPIIb/IIIa, CD41/CD61) Impaired fibrinogen-mediated platelet aggregation	Often severe bleeding phenotype Normal platelet count and morphology Platelet aggregation: absent response to all agonists except ristocetin Flow cytometry: absent or reduced CD41 and CD61	Supportive care rF7a (considered the first line) Platelet transfusion (risk of HPA alloantibodies) Antifibrinolytics
Defects in Agonist Receptors				
Thromboxane-prostanoid (TP) receptor defects	Autosomal recessive: TBXA2R (19p13.3)	Defective TP receptor, abnormal response to TXA2	Mild bleeding phenotype Platelet aggregation: abnormal response to arachidonic acid and U46619 TBXA2R gene sequencing	Supportive care
ADP receptor defects P2Y12	Autosomal recessive: P2RY12 (3q23–25)	Defective ADP receptor, abnormal response to ADP, de-aggregation with high-dose ADP	Mild bleeding phenotype Platelet aggregation: abnormal response to ADP P2RY12 gene sequencing	Supportive care
Collagen receptor defects GPVI	Autosomal recessive: GP6 (19q13.4)	Defective GPVI receptor, impaired response to collagen	Mild bleeding phenotype Platelet aggregation: abnormal response to collagen GP6 gene sequencing	Supportive care
Platelet Granule Defects (α-Granules)				
Gray platelet syndrome (GPS)	Autosomal recessive: NBEAL2 (3p21)	Defective development of α-granules, loss of α-granule cargo proteins into bone marrow and spleen	Progressive myelofibrosis Thrombocytopenia Large pale platelets on blood smears Absent α-granules on TEM NBEAL2 gene sequencing	Supportive care Antifibrinolytics DDAVP Platelet transfusion Splenectomy
Arthrogryposis, renal dysfunction, and cholestasis syndrome (ARC syndrome)	Autosomal dominant: VPS33B (15q26) VIPAS39 (14q24)	Abnormal intracellular vesicle trafficking and membrane fusion	Thrombocytopenia Large pale platelets on blood smears Absent α-granules on TEM Lethal early in life VPS33B and VIPAS39 sequencing	Supportive care Platelet transfusion Antifibrinolytics

TABLE 51.6 Inherited Platelet Disorders—cont'd

Platelet Defect	Gene Defect (Chromosomal Location)	Pathophysiology	Clinical and Laboratory Characteristics	Bleeding Treatment
Quebec platelet disorder (QPD)	Autosomal recessive: Tandem duplication of *PLAU* (10q22.2)	Increased expression and storage of releasable urokinase plasminogen activator due to a gain-of-function defect	Delayed-onset bleeding not responding to platelet transfusion Variable thrombocytopenia Abnormal urokinase in platelets detected with immunoblot or ELISA *PLAU* duplication testing	Supportive care Antifibrinolytics
Paris-Trousseau/Jacobsen syndrome (PTS)	Autosomal dominant: Deletion of chromosome 11q23–24 Hemizygous deletion of *FLI1* (11q24.1–q24.3)	Unknown	Thrombocytopenia Large platelets Giant α-granules on TEM Immature megakaryocytes in the bone marrow Cognitive, cardiac, and facial abnormalities	Supportive care Antifibrinolytics Platelet transfusion
Platelet Granule Defects (δ-Granules)				
Hermansky-Pudlak syndrome (HPS)	Autosomal recessive HPS1–10 (*HPS1, AP3B1, HPS3, HPS4, HPS5, HPS6, DTNBP1, BLOC1S3, BLOC1S6,* and *AP3D1*)	Defective intracellular biogenesis and trafficking of lysosome-related organelle δ-granules (DG) and melanosomes	Decreased to absent δ-granules Lumiaggregometry: decreased/absent ATP release Whole-mount EM Gene sequencing of 10 candidate genes Oculocutaneous albinism	Supportive care Antifibrinolytics Platelet transfusion DDAVP
Chédiak-Higashi syndrome (CHS)	Autosomal recessive: *LYST* (1q42–1q42.2)	Defective vesicular protein and membrane trafficking resulting in giant granules	Giant eosinophilic inclusions in neutrophils Decreased to absent δ-granules Lumiaggregometry: decreased/absent ATP release Hypopigmentation and immunodeficiency	Supportive care
Platelet Cytoskeletal Defects				
Wiskott-Aldrich syndrome (WAS)/X-linked thrombocytopenia	X-linked *WAS* (Xp11.23–p11.22) encoding WAS protein	Loss/defective WAS protein (WASp) leading to defective actin remodeling by actin-related protein 2/3 (Arp2/3) complex	Thrombocytopenia Small platelets Recurrent infections and eczema Decreased/absent intracellular WASp per immunoblot/ELISA *WAS* gene sequencing	Supportive care Platelet transfusion Antifibrinolytics Splenectomy (not recommended)
ARPC1B deficiency	Autosomal recessive: *ARPC1B* (7q22.1)	Loss of ARPC1B in hematopoietic cell Arp2/3 complex	Small platelets Inflammatory disease, recurrent infections, small vessel vasculitis, abnormal platelet function Decreased/absent intracellular ARPC1B per immunoblot *ARPC1B* gene sequencing	Supportive care Antifibrinolytics Platelet transfusion
MYH9-related disease (MYH9-RD)	Autosomal dominant: *MYH9* (22q12–13) encoding nonmuscle myosin heavy chain IIA	Defective nonmuscle myosin IIA motor protein	Thrombocytopenia Large platelets Döhle-like inclusions in neutrophils Myosin IIA aggregates in neutrophils—immunofluorescence microscopy Variable degree of renal disease, sensorineural hearing loss, presenile cataract	Supportive care Platelet transfusion Antifibrinolytics THPO receptor agonists

ADP, adenosine diphosphate; DDAVP, desmopressin; ELISA, enzyme-linked immunosorbent assay; EM, electron microscopy; HPA, human platelet antigen; r7a, recombinant activated factor 7; TEM, transmission electron microscopy; THPO, thrombopoietin; TXA2, thromboxane A2; VWF, von Willebrand factor.

From Al-Huniti A, Kahr WH. Inherited platelet disorders: diagnosis and management. *Transfus Med Rev.* 2020;34(4):277–285, Table 1.

TABLE 51.7 **Common Treatment Alternatives for Childhood Acute Immune Thrombocytopenic Purpura (ITP)**

Drug	Route of Administration	Pros	Cons	Cost in USD (Assuming Typical 15 kg Toddler)
IVIG	IV	Rapid onset of action Does not rely on patient/family giving medication at home Effective in 75–80% of patients	IV required Either inpatient or prolonged (4–6 hr) visit to clinic Does not alter long-term outcome	$3,000 for 1-mg/kg dose
Prednisone	Oral (can also be given IV)	Outpatient administration Rapid onset of action Effective in 75–80% of patients Does not require placement of an IV Short course likely minimal side effects	Steroid side effects (GI, mood swings, growth issues with long-term use) May need multiple courses No effect on long-term outcome	2-wk course of 2 mg/kg/day: $15
Rituximab	IV	Durable remission in 40–60%	IV administration May cause reactivation of hepatitis	Four doses of 375 mg/m², approximately $5,000–$15,000
Splenectomy	Surgery	Curative in 80% of patients	Expensive Invasive Impairs host defense against encapsulated organisms Reserved for chronic ITP and/or serious bleeding complications	$10,000–$20,000
Thrombopoietin agonists	Oral (options also come as IV, SQ)	Noninvasive Outpatient treatment	Associated with elevation in liver enzymes Require frequent monitoring Not curative, most patients require ongoing administration	1-mo course of 25 mg/day, $3,000

GI, gastrointestinal; IV, intravenous; IVIG, intravenous immunoglobulin; SQ, subcutaneous; USD, US dollars.

platelets should be normal (multiple days), whereas in thrombocytopenic states caused by platelet destruction, transfused platelets should be cleared rapidly (detected with a 1-hour post-transfusion platelet count). For this reason, platelet transfusions are usually contraindicated in thrombocytopenic states caused by accelerated platelet destruction, as in ITP and hemolytic uremic syndrome (except in the event of life-threatening bleeding such as intracranial hemorrhage). The yield and survival of the transfused platelets should be monitored with serial platelet counts after transfusion.

Antibody-mediated thrombocytopenia in the neonate is caused by transfer of maternal immunoglobulin G (IgG) antibodies that react with the neonate's platelets. A mother with active ITP or a history of previous ITP is at risk for delivering a thrombocytopenic baby. There is no definitive, noninvasive method to determine the newborn's risk of thrombocytopenia, although the actual risk for severe bleeding during delivery appears low. In contrast, children born to mothers who are sensitized to paternal alloantigens present on the fetal platelets have a higher risk for perinatal hemorrhage and symptomatic thrombocytopenia. This disorder, **neonatal alloimmune thrombocytopenia (NAIT)**, is the platelet equivalent of maternal Rh isoimmunization and differs from Rh disease in that first-born children are commonly affected. The importance of this diagnosis is that it is commonly associated with prenatal intracranial hemorrhage with a resultant high rate of morbidity and mortality (15%). Therefore, recognition of the diagnosis in the first pregnancy can have a major impact on the management of subsequent pregnancies. Transfusion of washed maternal platelets that lack the paternal alloantigen toward which the maternal antibody is directed will correct the platelet count and prevent further bleeding. Random donor platelets are rapidly destroyed. Newborns with NAIT can be easily differentiated from thrombocytopenic newborns of mothers with ITP on the basis of the mother's platelet count. Mothers

with ITP are thrombocytopenic unless they have had a splenectomy. Mothers of infants with NAIT have normal platelet counts.

Although the initial diagnosis of NAIT is usually made by studying the reaction of maternal serum against paternal platelets, prenatal diagnosis is performed with molecular biologic techniques to detect the allelic differences between the mother and the fetus by analysis of various fetal DNA sources. After prenatal diagnosis, treatment of the mother with IVIG has been shown to raise the fetal platelet count and prevent fetal bleeding. In addition, postnatal treatment of the neonate with IVIG and corticosteroids may be helpful after restoration of a normal platelet count by transfusion of washed maternal platelets. *All blood products administered to the neonate with thrombocytopenia should be irradiated to prevent graft versus host disease mediated by the recipient's reaction to potential rare donor lymphocytes that persist in the platelet product despite leukofiltration, because some patients may have a congenital immunodeficiency syndrome manifested by thrombocytopenia.*

Child Abuse

The most common cause of remarkable bruising and bleeding with normal hemostatic screening studies in infancy is child abuse. Child abuse may mimic a bleeding disorder and it is important to obtain screening studies in the evaluation of potential child maltreatment.

Chronic/Insidious Onset of Mucocutaneous Bleeding

When symptoms of skin and mucous membrane bleeding are lifelong, the most common cause is VWD. Congenital platelet function defects are almost as common, while congenital thrombocytopenic syndromes and abnormalities of the vessel wall are less common. VWD, the deficiency of VWF, is the most common hereditary bleeding disorder, with a prevalence of approximately 1/1,000 in the milder forms. The inheritance of VWD is usually autosomal dominant. VWF is a large,

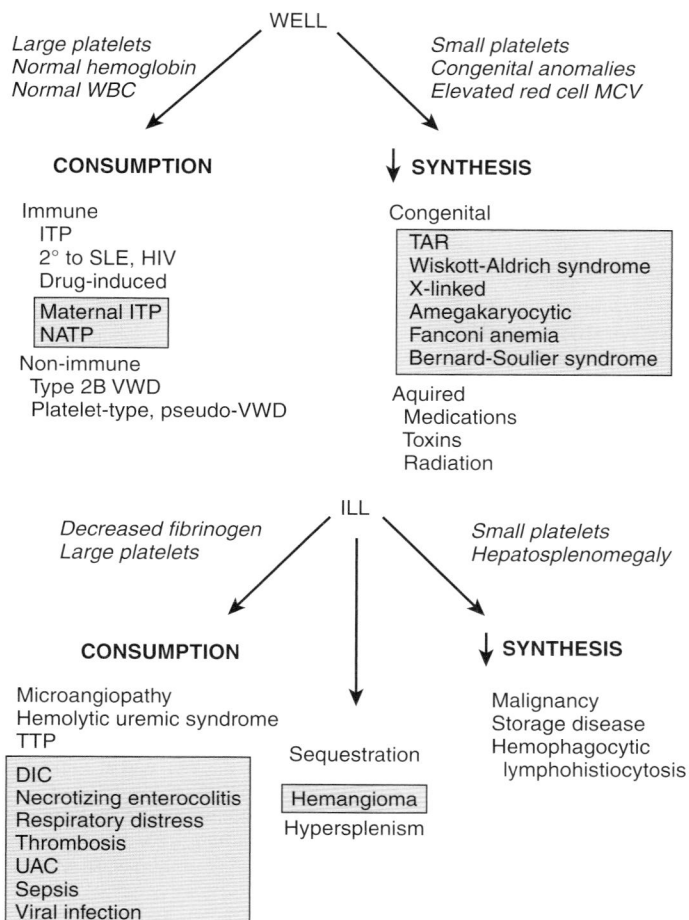

Fig. 51.9 Differential diagnosis of childhood thrombocytopenic syndromes. The syndromes are initially separated by their clinical appearance. Clues leading to the diagnosis are presented in italics. The mechanisms and common disorders leading to these findings are shown in the lower part of the figure. Disorders that commonly affect neonates are listed in the shaded boxes. DIC, disseminated intravascular coagulation; ITP, idiopathic immune thrombocytopenic purpura; MCV, mean corpuscular volume; NATP, neonatal alloimmune thrombocytopenic purpura; SLE, systemic lupus erythematosus; TAR, thrombocytopenia–absent radius (syndrome); TTP, thrombotic thrombocytopenic purpura; UAC, umbilical artery catheter; VWD, von Willebrand disease; WBC, white blood cell; 2°, secondary.

multimeric protein that functions as the bridge between platelets and damaged vessel walls; therefore, deficient or dysfunctional VWF causes delayed formation of the platelet plug (see Fig. 51.3). In addition, VWF serves as a carrier protein for factor 8. A profound deficiency of VWF is associated with low levels of factor 8, so that the patient with severe VWD has the clinical manifestations of both VWD and hemophilia.

The presentation of VWD is highly variable. Mucocutaneous bleeding or no symptoms are the most common findings. Because neonatal VWF levels are often elevated after vaginal delivery, the onset of clinical symptoms for mild and moderate VWD is usually during the toddler stage or later. The only presenting complaint may be abnormal preoperative screening coagulation studies. The laboratory diagnosis of the disease is particularly challenging because there is no single test that optimally measures VWF function.

The PTT and bleeding time are only abnormal in about half of patients VWD. A von Willebrand screen, including VWF antigen (to measure total protein) and activity (to measure protein function) is recommended to fully assess for VWD. The need for additional work-up is defined by the clinical clues, including the patient's personal history of bleeding, the family history, and the potential for surgery (Fig. 51.10).

The diagnosis of VWD is further complicated by the observation that VWF is a labile protein and levels can be increased by stress, medication, trauma, pregnancy, and difficult venipuncture. VWF levels are also elevated following vaginal delivery in some infants with VWD. This can be helpful in terms of ability to perform circumcision in some males with potential VWD, but problematic in terms of making an immediate diagnosis. It remains unclear whether there is a physiologically different hemostatic level of VWF for different blood groups. Age has been shown to influence VWF levels in adults, but this has not been adequately investigated in children. Furthermore, there are multiple variants of VWD; the clinician should perform repeated studies if there is a high index of suspicion or abnormal positive screening tests.

VWD can be classified as **type 1** (classic disease with mild or moderate quantitative deficiency), **type 2** (a dysproteinemia or qualitative deficiency), or **type 3** (severe disease: virtual absence of VWF [near-complete quantitative deficiency] as well as low levels of factor 8). The treatment of the disease is dependent on the type and the response to 1-deamino(8-D-arginine) vasopressin (DDAVP). DDAVP is a synthetic vasopressin analog that induces the release of VWF and factor 8. Levels of these factors rise three- to fivefold after a dose of 0.3

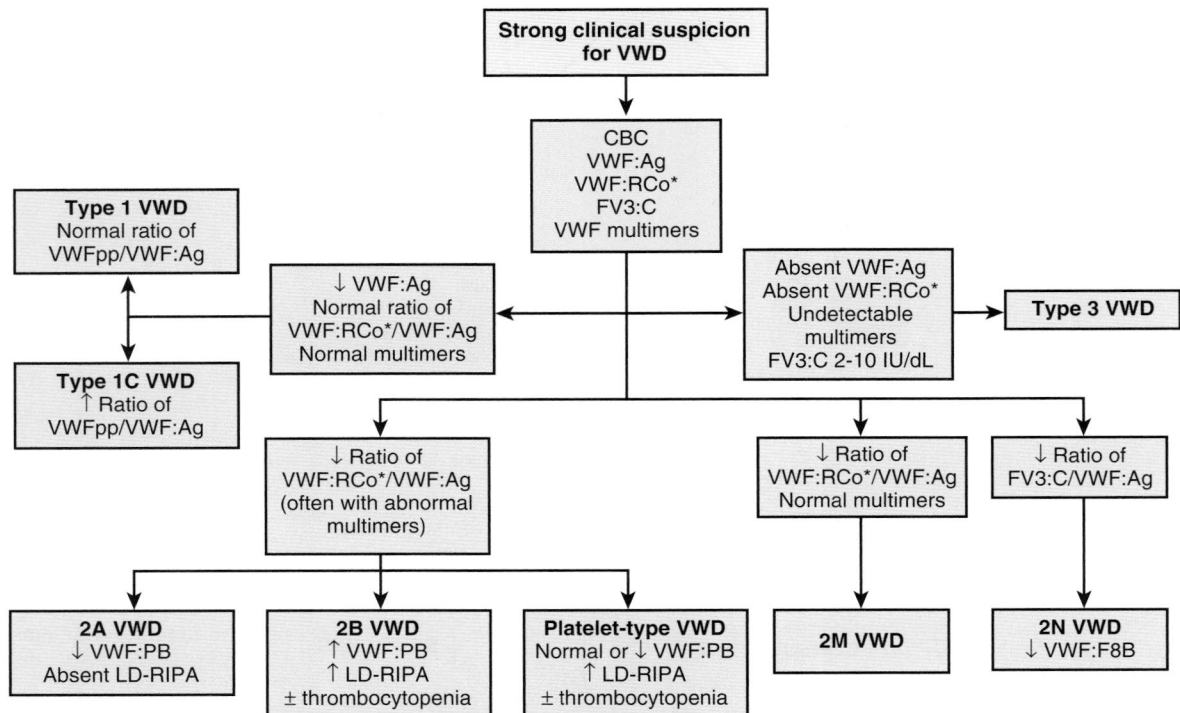

Fig. 51.10 Desmopressin (DDAVP, 0.3 µg/kg intravenously) was administered to 40 patients with type 1 von Willebrand disease (VWD). Plasma samples were obtained before infusion and at 1 and 4 hours after infusion. The *left-hand* panel illustrates the mean and 1–standard deviation range for these 40 individuals. The *right-hand* panels illustrate the consistency of the response in these 40 individuals for both von Willebrand factor antigen (VWF:Ag) and ristocetin cofactor (VWF:RCo) activity. LD-RIPA, low-dose ristocetin-induced platelet aggregation; PB, platelet binding. *Or VWF:GPIbM. (Courtesy J. P. Scott and R. R. Montgomery.)

µg/kg. For most cases of VWD, DDAVP is the treatment of choice. A therapeutic trial with measurements of VWF before and both 1 hour and 4 hours after DDAVP administration should be performed to document the efficacy of DDAVP before surgery. The late time-point is useful to identify clearance defects, such as type 1C, which may demonstrate an initial response but lack the sustained response critical for clinical use of DDAVP. Patients with rare variant forms of VWD (type 2A, type 2B, and platelet type) may have no response or an adverse response to DDAVP; therefore, while some screening evaluations such as an activity-to-antigen ratio <0.6, for example, can raise suspicion for type 2 disease, full studies to identify the subtype are needed before a trial of DDAVP. These studies correlate functional levels of VWF with the amount of protein measured antigenically (VWF antigen), the multimeric size of the protein (VWF multimers), and the aggregation response of the patient's platelet-rich plasma to high and low concentrations of ristocetin or VWF binding to platelet GPIb (VWF activity).

Most patients with mild and moderate type 1 VWD have a satisfactory response to intranasal or intravenous DDAVP; hemostasis for most surgical procedures can be provided with daily doses of DDAVP on consecutive days, but use beyond 3 days is not recommended due to limited effect after this time as endothelial stores of VWF and factor 8 will have been exhausted. For severely affected patients or those with variant forms of the disease noted previously (type 2A, type 2B, platelet type), treatment should be individualized. Some patients with type 2A respond to DDAVP. Severely affected patients with VWD and those with the 2B variant should receive a clotting factor concentrate containing a full complement of normal VWF multimers (Humate-P and Wilate are the currently approved products for children, and Vonvendi

[recombinant VWF concentrate] is approved for use in adults) in doses similar to those outlined for factor 8 in Table 51.8.

Platelet Function Defects

For patients with mucocutaneous bleeding but a normal platelet count and normal VWF studies, platelet aggregation studies should be performed to evaluate for a primary or secondary platelet function defect, especially if abnormality is detected on a screening platelet function assay (PFA). Many medications may induce an acquired abnormality of platelet number and/or function. A careful history to elicit exposure to medications and to determine whether clinical symptoms correlate with exposure to specific drugs is critical. Common medications that alter platelet number or function are aspirin, nonsteroidal antiinflammatory drugs, alcohol, penicillin in high doses, and valproic acid.

Most primary platelet function defects cause relatively mild mucocutaneous bleeding symptoms (see Table 51.6). In these disorders, there is most commonly an abnormality of the storage granules or release mechanism within the platelet, causing delayed or diminished response to agonists that induce platelet aggregation, such as collagen. Platelet function defects, like most other hemostatic defects, are accentuated by medications that impair platelet function. In rare instances, a patient demonstrates impressive petechiae and hematomas at birth because of an absence of one of the essential platelet membrane receptors for the adhesive proteins VWF or fibrinogen. These disorders, **Glanzmann thrombasthenia** (deficiency of glycoprotein αIIbβ3, the fibrinogen receptor) and **Bernard-Soulier syndrome** (deficiency of glycoprotein Ib, the von Willebrand receptor), represent the most severe types of platelet function defects. The platelet count is normal

TABLE 51.8 Characteristics of Factors 8 and 9 and Respective Modes of Treatment for Bleeding Episodes Caused by Hemophilia A or B

	Factor 8	Factor 9
Yield	1.5–2%/U/kg infused	0.7–1%/U/kg infused
Half-life	8–12 hr	18–24 hr
Goal therapeutic level:		
Life and limb-threatening, acute hemarthrosis treatment	80–100%	80–100%
Minor bleeds (gingival bleeding, epistaxis)	40–50%	30–50%
Dose computation*	[(Level desired— baseline level) × weight (kg)] × 0.5	[(Level desired— baseline level) × weight (kg)] × 1.3
Therapeutic alternatives	Desmopressin[†] Plasma-derived factor 8 concentrate	Plasma-derived factor 9 concentrate Prothrombin complex concentrate[‡]

*Assumes use of a standard half-life recombinant factor replacement product.
[†]After adequate response has been demonstrated.
[‡]Repeat doses have been associated with increased risk for thrombosis.

in Glanzmann thrombasthenia thrombocytopenia, but patients with Bernard-Soulier syndrome usually have thrombocytopenia with remarkably large platelets.

Milder thrombocytopenia syndromes have been well characterized due to advances in genetics; a defect in the myosin heavy chain 9 gene (*MYH9*) causes **congenital macrothrombocytopenia**, associated in some cases with deafness, ocular abnormalities, or nephritis. **Congenital amegakaryocytic thrombocytopenia** is caused by a defect in the thrombopoietin receptor c-Mpl, while **X-linked thrombocytopenia** is caused by a defect in *GATA-1*. Patients with mild or moderate platelet function defects often respond to DDAVP (though the exact mechanism of this response remains unknown), but more severe bleeding may necessitate platelet transfusions.

Chronic Thrombocytopenic Syndromes

Patients with long-standing thrombocytopenia usually present with mucocutaneous bleeding. Mechanisms of the thrombocytopenia include impaired marrow synthesis, sequestration, and increased destruction (see Fig. 51.9). These can be acquired or congenital. The **congenital thrombocytopenic syndromes** usually manifest at the time of birth or early in infancy. These syndromes may be associated with congenital anomalies (thrombocytopenia–absent radius syndrome and Fanconi anemia) or be part of a complex hereditary syndrome (Wiskott-Aldrich syndrome with small platelets, eczema, and immunodeficiency) in addition to thrombocytopenia. Small platelets are a frequent finding in many of the syndromes associated with decreased platelet production. During the physical examination of patients with suspected congenital thrombocytopenia, the clinician must search not only for the signs of bleeding but also for subtle congenital anomalies, including abnormal growth parameters, the presence of skin hyperpigmentation or café-au-lait spots, and anomalies of the limbs, axial skeleton, and urinary tract.

The **acquired causes of thrombocytopenia** resulting from decreased production usually have an insidious onset of symptoms and are often associated with other abnormalities in the blood count. The **aplastic syndromes** (congenital aplastic anemia and acquired aplastic anemia) are associated with the gradual onset of thrombocytopenia, usually in association with a falling granulocyte count and anemia. Platelets are small, and the mean corpuscular volume is usually elevated.

Infiltration of the marrow by malignant cells or storage cells interferes with normal thrombopoiesis and commonly results in thrombocytopenia. Common malignancies associated with thrombocytopenia include acute lymphoblastic leukemia, lymphomas, Langerhans cell histiocytosis, and metastatic solid tumors (neuroblastoma). Abnormalities of other blood elements, as well as findings of adenopathy, hepatosplenomegaly, or masses, are clues to the presence of an infiltrative disorder.

Disorders of the vessel walls may present either acutely or chronically. Vasculitic disorders often manifest with lesions of the skin and mucous membranes that appear hemorrhagic and are associated with clinical symptoms related to involvement of other organ systems (gastrointestinal, renal, central nervous system). Paradoxically, patients with these disorders usually have normal coagulation studies and normal platelet counts. Henoch-Schönlein purpura is an example; it manifests with a purpuric rash, including both petechiae and larger palpable purpuric lesions of the lower extremities and buttocks, often found in association with arthritis, cramping abdominal pain, and focal glomerulonephritis.

Petechiae and ecchymoses are also common symptoms of disorders of the collagen matrix. Patients with Ehlers-Danlos syndrome have lax joints, hyperelastic skin, and abnormal wound healing. These patients frequently present with ecchymoses and rarely with petechiae. Bleeding time is usually prolonged, but other ex vivo hemostatic assays are usually normal, and so the diagnosis is made on the basis of clinical findings and, in some cases, genetic evaluation.

DEEP BLEEDING

Bleeding into the tissues of the muscles or joints is characteristic of hemophilia. The presentation of the patient with hemophilia varies with severity, age, and exposure to trauma. Only 30% of boys with hemophilia bleed excessively at circumcision, and neonatal intracranial bleeding is rare despite the trauma of a vaginal delivery. After the neonatal period, children with hemophilia usually present as toddlers with either intramuscular hematomas or hemarthroses. In the toddler stage, the most commonly affected joints are the ankles and elbows; the knees, hips, and shoulders are affected later. The affected children, who are usually boys due to the X-linked genetic nature of this disease, bruise easily and hematomas frequently develop over areas of common trauma (the forehead, arms, and legs, especially pretibial). Other common bleeding sites include the frenulum and sites of venipuncture. Sites of life-threatening bleeding include the central nervous system (the most common cause of death from hemorrhage); the mouth and throat, resulting in airway obstruction; and the retroperitoneal area or gastrointestinal tract, leading to exsanguination.

Red flags for the diagnosis of hemophilia are:
- Persistent bleeding after circumcision
- Hemarthrosis/intramuscular hematoma
- Bleeding frenulum

The deficiency of factor 8 (hemophilia A) or factor 9 (hemophilia B) causes bleeding because delayed thrombin formation results in a large, friable clot. Often there is an initial hemostatic plug that breaks down hours after the injury (secondary bleeding). Because factors 8 and 9 are necessary for normal wound healing, patients with inadequate replacement or untreated hemophilia frequently have poorly healed wounds.

Hemophilia A occurs in 1/10,000 live births and hemophilia B in about 1/40,000. The PTT is prolonged and should correct on 1:1 mix with normal plasma. Specific assays for factors 8 and 9 should be performed to identify the deficient factor. Severity is determined by the level of the deficient clotting factor. Severe hemophilia is defined by the World Health Organization as <1% factor activity, moderate as 1–5% activity, and mild as >5% activity. These factor levels correlate approximately with clinical symptoms: Patients with severe deficiency bleed spontaneously; patients with moderate deficiency bleed with minor trauma; and patients with mild deficiency bleed only after significant trauma, and their condition may go undiagnosed for many years. Because hemophilia A and B are transmitted as X-linked traits, the family history may be informative if there is a history of male maternal relatives with a bleeding disorder. Approximately 33% of affected patients have new gene variants and therefore have a negative family history. Bleeding complications have occurred in female carriers, especially at surgery; thus, all obligate carriers should have factor levels measured to determine if perioperative hemostasis management is indicated.

Treatment of hemophilia requires prompt replacement or correction of the deficient factor with the safest available material. Table 51.8 provides dosing information and therapeutic alternatives for factors 8 and 9 deficiency. Treatment of bleeding episodes is first aimed at stopping the hemorrhage, and then should be continued until the wound has healed. Recombinant factor 8 or 9 concentrate is a commonly used treatment product, with purified plasma-derived factor as an alternative choice with some evidence that suggests a lower risk for inhibitor formation in previously untreated patients with this latter approach. Extended half-life factor products have been developed and may improve quality of life by reducing the frequency of infusions but still allow for peak levels that may be protective against bleeding during sports or other activities. A shift was seen with the approval of emicizumab, a subcutaneously administered bispecific antibody therapy that can be administered as rarely as monthly and has been recently approved for use in children and adults with hemophilia A with and without inhibitors. This product provides a steady-state level of a factor 8 mimetic that binds factors 9a and 10 similarly to the tenase complex in the intrinsic system. For patients with mild hemophilia A who respond to DDAVP with adequate levels, DDAVP is the treatment of choice. Prophylaxis with factor concentrates has revolutionized the care of children with hemophilia by preventing chronic arthropathy and muscular atrophy. Patients with hemophilia should be monitored at comprehensive treatment centers that are experienced in the medical, social, physical, and financial impact of hemophilia care.

The common complications of hemophilia treatment can be divided into those of immunologic origin and those caused by infectious organisms. In 15–25% of patients with hemophilia A and a smaller percentage of patients with hemophilia B, **inhibitors to clotting factor** replacement material develop. These inhibitors, usually IgG antibodies, lead to rapid inactivation and clearance of infused replacement material. The presence of an inhibitor should be suspected and tested for in any patient with hemophilia who does not respond appropriately to factor replacement. The treatment of patients with inhibitors is problematic and should be relegated to experts in hemophilia care. The management of acute bleeding episodes may require administration of an activated clotting factor concentrate to "bypass" the inhibitor.

Infectious complications of hemophilia therapy have been curtailed by donor screening, sophisticated viral inactivation processes, and chemical purification techniques used in the preparation of plasma-derived replacement material. Recombinant factor concentrates represent the culmination of these efforts. Older patients treated before 1983 with concentrates were exposed to HIV, hepatitis C, and sometimes hepatitis B. Most patients exposed to HIV became infected and manifested the spectrum of signs and symptoms of HIV infection. Viral inactivation techniques in conjunction with intense donor screening for hepatitis C antibody have greatly decreased the risk for hepatitis C exposure. Nevertheless, chronic non-A, non-B hepatitis is a common finding in older patients with hemophilia who were treated with plasma-derived factor concentrates.

The need for intravenous access to provide factor infusions creates another complication with the use of indwelling central venous catheters to facilitate factor delivery to young children with poor venous access. While some patients can be treated with less frequent dosing through peripheral veins, some patients undergo surgery for placement of a central venous catheter (CVC). Although these catheters undoubtedly increase adherence to prophylactic treatment, they can serve as a nidus for infection or thrombosis or lead to complications due to surgery required for insertion or removal. The complicated decision-making around CVC use is one factor driving the consideration of emicizumab, which does not require IV access.

A new frontier in hemophilia therapy is on the horizon with the development of gene therapy and gene-editing techniques, of which several are currently in phase II and III clinical trials. Long-term real-world safety and efficacy have yet to be shown definitively, primarily due to the relatively short duration of the trials to date, but there is real potential for a possible "cure" for hemophilia with this approach.

Surgical Bleeding

Aside from technical causes, most surgical bleeding results from a failure to recognize a pre-existing coagulopathy. VWD and primary or secondary platelet dysfunction are the most common causes of bleeding after ear, nose, and throat surgery. Significant hemorrhaging after general surgery is often a manifestation of previously undiagnosed mild or moderate hemophilia or vitamin K deficiency.

When elective surgery is planned, the decision to perform preoperative hemostatic screening is influenced by the patient's age (and therefore previous exposure to trauma), personal and family histories of bleeding, and type of surgery. Certain surgeries, such as tonsillectomy, scoliosis repair, and central nervous system surgery, provide major challenges to hemostasis, having a high frequency of bleeding complications. In contrast, most general surgical procedures, such as hernia repair, rarely involve clinical bleeding. The diagnostic yield of preoperative studies before tonsillectomy and adenoidectomy remains controversial.

GENERALIZED BLEEDING

Generalized bleeding is a manifestation of a major disorder of hemostasis, usually caused by a deficiency of multiple factors in association with deficient or dysfunctional platelets. Generalized bleeding occurs most commonly in the context of DIC in seriously ill patients.

DIC is a generalized consumption of clotting factors, anticoagulant proteins, and platelets triggered by a life-threatening illness and usually accompanied by ischemia, hypoxia, and shock (Table 51.9). DIC may be either a hemorrhagic or a thrombotic disorder, or both, as the clinical manifestations of this generalized coagulopathy are highly variable. Laboratory studies usually demonstrate a prolonged PT, decreased fibrinogen level, and decreased platelet level (these are the most reliable indicators of DIC), in addition to elevated D-dimer levels and a prolonged PTT.

Several mechanisms can trigger acute DIC, including widespread endothelial damage induced directly or indirectly by infectious organisms and release of procoagulant material after trauma. Virtually any life-threatening illness or injury can trigger DIC. In acute DIC, activation of the clotting mechanism leads to consumption of clotting factors (1, 2, 5, 8), anticoagulant proteins (PC, PS, AT, plasminogen), and platelets. In the syndrome known as purpura fulminans, microvascular thromboses develop in the skin, causing painful purpuric lesions that

TABLE 51.9 Causes of Disseminated Intravascular Coagulation

Infection

Meningococcemia (purpura fulminans)

Other gram-negative bacteria (*Haemophilus* species, *Salmonella* species, *Escherichia coli*)

Gram-positive bacteria (group B streptococci, staphylococci)

Rickettsiae (Rocky Mountain spotted fever)

Virus (SARS-CoV-2, cytomegalovirus, herpes, hemorrhagic fevers)

Malaria

Fungus

Tissue Injury

Central nervous system trauma (massive head injury)

Multiple fractures with fat emboli

Crush injury

Profound shock or asphyxia

Hypothermia or hyperthermia

Massive burns

Malignancy

Acute promyelocytic leukemia

Acute monoblastic or myelocytic leukemia

Widespread malignancies (neuroblastoma)

Venom or Toxin

Snake bites

Spider bites, bee stings

Scorpion

Microangiopathic Disorders

"Severe" thrombotic thrombocytopenic purpura or hemolytic uremic syndrome

Giant hemangioma (Kasabach-Merritt syndrome)

Gastrointestinal Disorders

Fulminant hepatitis

Severe inflammatory bowel disease

Hereditary Thrombotic Disorders

Antithrombin deficiency

Homozygous protein C deficiency

Neonatal Disorders

Maternal toxemia

Group B streptococcal infections

Abruptio placentae

Severe respiratory distress syndrome

Necrotizing enterocolitis

Congenital viral disease (cytomegalovirus, herpes)

Erythroblastosis fetalis

Miscellaneous Disorders

Severe acute graft rejection

Acute hemolytic transfusion reaction

Severe collagen vascular disease

Kawasaki disease

Heparin-induced thrombosis

Infusion of "activated" prothrombin complex concentrates

Hyperpyrexia/encephalopathy, hemorrhagic shock syndrome

SARS-CoV-2, several acute respiratory syndrome–coronavirus-19.

Modified from Montgomery RR, Scott JP. Hemostasis: disease of the fluid phase. In: Nathan DG, Oski FA, eds. *Hematology of Infancy and Childhood*. 4th ed. Philadelphia: WB Saunders; 1993;2:1639.

TABLE 51.10 Differential Diagnosis of Coagulopathies That Can Be Confused with Disseminated Intravascular Coagulation

	Prothrombin Time	Partial Thromboplastin Time	Fibrinogen	Platelets	Clinical Keys
DIC	Increased	Increased	Decreased	Decreased	Shock
Liver failure	Increased	Increased	Decreased	Normal or decreased	Jaundice
Vitamin K deficiency	Increased	Increased	Normal	Normal	Malabsorption, GI or liver disease
Sepsis without shock	Increased	Increased	Normal	Normal	Fever

DIC, disseminated intravascular coagulation; GI, gastrointestinal.

progress to localized necrotic lesions. Table 51.10 presents laboratory findings in DIC in comparison with those in other acquired coagulopathies that potentially could be confused with DIC. Because DIC is virtually always seen in a child with a life-threatening illness, the clinical diagnosis is usually made on the basis of the child's clinical appearance in association with laboratory abnormalities. Clotting factor and anticoagulant protein levels are confirmatory but seldom necessary to reach a diagnosis of DIC. The only diagnosis difficult to differentiate from DIC in the laboratory is that of severe hepatic disease with impending liver failure. The patient with severe liver disease is markedly jaundiced and the thrombocytopenia is relatively mild.

The treatment of DIC focuses on the underlying cause of the DIC, on the altered homeostasis that sustains the coagulopathy, and on the bleeding or thrombotic complications that ensue. Shock itself plays a critical role in DIC because shock reduces the reticuloendothelial clearance of activated clotting factors and complexes. Reduced hepatic blood flow causes decreased synthesis of depleted clotting and anticoagulant proteins.

To summarize the treatment of DIC:

1. Treat the initiating and propagating events.
2. Optimize cardiorespiratory status by improving perfusion and correcting acidosis.

TABLE 51.11   **Commonly Used Hemostatic Agents***

Component	Contents	Usual Dose	Comments/Disadvantages
FFP (unit)	1 U/mL of each clotting factor	10–15 mL/kg	Large volume Infectious risk
Cryoprecipitate (1 bag)	100 units factor 8/bag 150 mg fibrinogen/bag Factor 13, fibronectin	0.2 bag/kg	Infectious risk
Platelets (unit)	5.0–7.0×10^{10} platelets in 30–60 mL of plasma	½–1 single donor apheresis unit	Infectious risk
Factor concentrates (unit)	Units as labeled	Factor 8, 20–50 U/kg Factor 9, 30–130 U/kg	Recombinant
Desmopressin	4 µg/mL	0.3 µg/kg/dose	Increases factor 8 and VWF Improves platelet function Also used in uremia, liver disease Risk for hyponatremia (rare if fluid restriction observed)
AT concentrate	Units as labeled	(Desired AT – baseline AT) × weight (kg)/1.4	Plasma derived or recombinant available

*Key points to transfusion: (1) Determine deficiency state. (2) Use appropriate dose and material. (3) Measure response 1–2 hr and 24 hr after transfusion.
AT, antithrombin; DDAVP, 1-deamino(8-D-arginine) desmopressin; FFP, fresh frozen plasma; VWF, von Willebrand factor.

3. Replace deficient platelets, clotting factors, and anticoagulant proteins (Table 51.11) if needed. Specific indications for replacement are variable and depend on the patient's clinical condition and severity of bleeding.

The following are rough guidelines for treatment:
- Fresh-frozen plasma, 10–15 mL/kg every 6–12 hours, to provide clotting factors in physiologic balance with anticoagulant proteins
- Platelets, ½–1 single donor apheresis unit for platelet count <50,000/mm³
- Cryoprecipitate, 1 bag/5 kg for fibrinogen level <100 mg/dL
- Prothrombin complex concentrate (indicated for urgent reversal of acquired coagulation factor defect from vitamin K antagonist therapy in adults), dosing based on pretreatment international normalized ratio (INR)
- Anticoagulant therapy for major vessel thrombosis

The efficacy of anticoagulant therapy in DIC has not been proved in controlled prospective studies. Heparin has been used for the treatment of purpura fulminans, acute promyelocytic leukemia, and thromboses that develop in conjunction with DIC. Most patients with DIC have a coagulopathy that consumes procoagulant proteins and causes clinical oozing or bleeding; in a small percentage of patients, however, thrombosis develops. In these patients, anticoagulant therapy may decrease morbidity and should be considered for administration in a manner similar to that for those patients who have major vascular thrombosis (Table 51.12), though the risk assessment evaluations as well as type and dose of anticoagulant for thromboprophylaxis in children is currently an area of intense study. Deficient clotting factors and platelets should be transfused to prevent further development of thrombosis or bleeding during anticoagulation.

Neonatal Purpura Fulminans

The differential diagnosis of a neonate who presents with multiple purpuric lesions over the buttocks, trunk, extremities, and face (nose, ears) that change from dark red to purple and black over a few minutes in association with abnormal neurologic findings or an abdominal mass includes sepsis with DIC and a generalized viral infection. A key finding in such a neonate for a homozygous PC deficiency is the presence of painful petechiae and purpura (purpura fulminans). After viral and bacterial cultures, diagnostic studies should include a CBC and coagulation screening for DIC, as well as measurements of PC, PS, AT, and plasminogen.

To confirm this diagnosis, the clinician must differentiate DIC from congenital PC deficiency. DIC is characterized by the consumption of clotting factors, anticoagulant proteins, and platelets. Although PC levels fall in DIC, patients with congenital PC deficiency have strikingly low levels of PC. Anticoagulant proteins are routinely consumed in situations of widespread activation of the clotting mechanism. Therefore, mildly depressed levels of PS, AT, and plasminogen would be expected when there is generalized intravascular coagulation. In congenital PC deficiency, the PC level is strikingly lower than that of the other anticoagulant proteins, which increases the likelihood that the deficiency of PC represents the primary cause of the coagulopathy. To determine whether the deficiency is hereditary, the next step is to obtain blood samples from the parents to measure levels of the deficient protein or proteins. In homozygous deficiencies, the levels of both parents should be reduced. Deficiency of PC, PS, or AT usually manifests as venous thromboembolic disease in adulthood and is inherited as a codominant trait. Congenital severe, symptomatic PC deficiency is usually inherited in an autosomal recessive manner from asymptomatic parents.

Therapy must be instituted promptly to replace the deficient anticoagulant protein with fresh frozen plasma. Fresh frozen plasma contains all of the clotting factors and anticoagulant proteins in an unconcentrated form. PC has a short half-life and may need to be infused every 6–12 hours to maintain measurable levels. This, unfortunately, may lead to problems with fluid and protein overload if repeated doses of plasma are necessary. *PC concentrate* is now available as specific therapy for patients with PC deficiency. The patient should also undergo anticoagulation with heparin to limit further thromboses. A striking improvement after administration of PC, either as plasma or as concentrate, is strong evidence of the diagnosis. Warfarin therapy has been effective in managing such patients on a chronic basis.

Other Causes of Generalized Bleeding

A coagulopathy is a common complication of severe liver disease with synthetic dysfunction, resulting from deficient production of multiple clotting factors and anticoagulant proteins in association with increased D-dimer formed as a result of hyperfibrinolysis. This may contribute to inhibition of platelet function.

TABLE 51.12 Comparison of Antithrombotic Agents

	Fibrinolytic Therapy	Standard Heparin	Low-Molecular-Weight Heparin	Warfarin	Direct Oral Anticoagulants (DOACs)
Indication	Recent onset of life- or limb-threatening thrombus	Thrombus of indeterminate age	Thrombus of indeterminate age	Long-term oral anticoagulation	Long-term oral anticoagulation
Dose	rTPA, 0.1–0.2 mg/kg/hr IV	50–75 U/kg bolus, then 20–25 U/kg/hr continuous IV infusion	1–1.25 mg/kg SQ every 12 hr (1.5 mg/kg if <2 mo of age)	0.1–0.2 mg/kg/day PO	Varies depending on medication
Adjustment	Increase dose for lack of clinical effect	Adjust dose by 5–10% every 6 hr until desired level or PTT achieved	Check level after second or third dose No further monitoring required once in goal range	Daily until stable INR	None indicated
Course	1–72 hr	5–14 days	5 days–mo	Weeks to months to years	Weeks to months to years
Monitor by:	"Lytic state" with D-dimer	PTT, 2–2.5× control value	Low-molecular-weight heparin level, 0.5–1.0	INR, 2.0–3.0	
Mechanism	Activation of plasminogen to plasmin	Accelerates AT-dependent inactivation of factors 2a (thrombin) and 10	Accelerates AT-dependent inactivation of factor 10	Impairs vitamin K–dependent carboxylation of factors 2, 7, 9, 10	
Risk for bleeding	Medium/high	Low	Low	Low	

AT, antithrombin; INR, international normalized ratio; IV, intravenously; PO, per os (orally); PTT, partial thromboplastin time; rTPA, recombinant tissue-type plasminogen activator; SQ, subcutaneous.

Uremia results in a diffuse bleeding diathesis, with mucosal bleeding (epistaxis, gastrointestinal bleeding) as a major manifestation. The major underlying mechanism in uremic bleeding appears to be increased nitric oxide generation, leading to decreased platelet function. Many patients with bleeding caused by uremia or liver disease respond to DDAVP.

Vitamin K deficiency manifests as generalized bleeding into the skin, gastrointestinal tract, and central nervous system. Children at highest risk are breast-fed neonates, malnourished individuals, those receiving broad-spectrum antibiotics, those with cholestatic liver disease and subsequent vitamin K malabsorption, and those who have ingested rat poison (warfarin). The treatment of patients with vitamin K deficiency is parenteral vitamin K. The response is usually rapid, but in emergency situations, transfusion of fresh frozen plasma corrects the coagulopathy faster. Differentiation of some of these syndromes from DIC is presented in Table 51.10.

THROMBOSIS

Thromboembolic disease in pediatrics has a bimodal age distribution. Venous and arterial thrombi are common in newborns, especially in premature neonates, because of the combination of low levels of anticoagulant proteins, decreased blood flow, elevated blood viscosity because of high hematocrit, and, in particular, the placement of intravascular catheters for monitoring and nutrition. The second peak of thromboembolic disease, usually venous in character, is in adolescence, when patients with primary deficiencies of anticoagulant proteins typically present and when secondary disorders (e.g., vasculitis, pregnancy, malignancy, surgery, major trauma, inflammatory bowel disease, and infection) induce a higher frequency of venous thrombosis.

Venous Thromboembolic Disease

Diagnostic Approach

Venous thromboembolic disease classically manifests with a warm, swollen, tender extremity or affected organ. The differential diagnosis

in such cases includes trauma, infection, stasis without thrombosis, lymphedema, edema, and neoplasm. In children and adolescents, thrombi may develop within major internal organs with distinctive clinical manifestations, including sagittal sinus thrombosis with resultant increased intracranial pressure; hepatic vein thrombosis with the **Budd-Chiari syndrome**; portal vein thrombosis associated with splenomegaly and varices; and **renal vein thrombosis** with a resultant abdominal mass, hematuria, and proteinuria. Long-term central venous access is associated with a significant risk for asymptomatic venous thrombosis. **Pulmonary emboli** may manifest as "atypical" pneumonia resulting in chest pain, tachycardia, tachypnea, shortness of breath, and/or hypoxemia in the absence of fever. The hypoxemia may occur in the presence of minimal findings on routine chest radiographs.

The clinician should obtain a careful history for antecedent trauma, infection, or other predisposing causes of thromboembolic disease (Table 51.13). The abdomen and extremities should be carefully examined for mass lesions leading to venous stasis. The presence of a bruit or hemihypertrophy of the affected limb is a clue to an arteriovenous malformation. In addition, masses within the bone, abdominal tumors, and lymphatic obstruction should be considered. Initial laboratory studies should include a CBC, platelet count, and evaluation for DIC, as well as cultures of the blood if the patient is febrile. During the process of a localized thrombosis, there may be consumption of clotting factors, but rarely is the consumption significant enough in older children and adults to induce abnormal results on routine coagulation screening tests (platelets, PT, PTT, fibrinogen). Tests for fibrin breakdown (D-dimer) may be positive. Unfortunately, these tests are nonspecific and not necessarily diagnostic of vascular thrombosis. Studies in adults have indicated that lack of elevated D-dimer has a strong negative predictive value for pulmonary embolus, especially when combined with a clinical algorithm for risk assignment such as the Wells criteria (Table 51.14). The diagnostic approach to a patient with suspected venous thrombosis is presented in Fig. 51.11.

TABLE 51.13 Hypercoagulable States/Risk Factors for Thrombosis

Primary Disorders (Congenital)

Factor 5 Leiden (activated protein C resistance)

Prothrombin 20210 variant

Protein C deficiency

Protein S deficiency

Antithrombin deficiency

Plasminogen deficiencies

Homocystinuria

Dysfibrinogenemia

Elevated plasminogen activator inhibitor (PAI-1)

Elevated factor 8

Absence of inferior vena cava

Secondary Disorders (Acquired)
Coagulopathies

Lupus anticoagulant (antiphospholipid syndrome)

Nephrotic syndrome

Estrogen-containing contraceptives

Malignancy

Therapy with activated prothrombin complex concentrates

Pregnancy

Autoimmune disorders

Other medications such as tamoxifen, thalidomide, asparaginase, corticosteroids

HIV/AIDS

Platelet Disorders

Diabetes mellitus

Myeloproliferative disorders

Thrombocythemia

Paroxysmal nocturnal hemoglobinuria

Heparin or vaccine-induced thrombocytopenia

Flow and Vessel Disorders

Polycythemia-hyperviscosity

Marfan syndrome

Vasculitis

COVID-19 including MIS-C

Vessel grafts/prosthetic valves

Vascular stasis

Trauma

Indwelling catheters

Surgery

Immobilization

Iliac vein compression syndrome (May-Thurner syndrome)

Thoracic outlet obstruction (Paget-Schroetter syndrome)

MIS-C, multisystem inflammatory syndrome in children.
Modified from Schafer A. The hypercoagulable states. *Ann Intern Med.* 1985;102:814; and from Scott JP, Flood V, Raffini L. Hemorrhagic and thrombotic diseases. In: Kliegman RM, St. Geme JW III, Blum NJ, et al., eds. *Nelson Textbook of Pediatrics.* 21st ed. Philadelphia: Elsevier; 2020:2604.

TABLE 51.14 Diagnosis of Pulmonary Embolism: The Wells Criteria

Wells Criteria	Score
Clinical signs and symptoms of deep vein thrombosis (DVT)	3
Alternative diagnosis less likely	3
Heart rate >100	1.5
Immobilization for 3 or more consecutive days in the previous week	1.5
Definite history of pulmonary embolism or DVT	1.5
Hemoptysis	1
Recent history of malignancy	1

A Wells score of 0–1, low risk; 2–6, moderate risk; >6, high risk.
From Meaney JFM, Doran SP. Current status of imaging for interventional procedures. In: Adam A, Dixon AK, Gillard JH, et al., eds. *Grainger and Allison's Diagnostic Radiology.* 7th ed. Philadelphia: Elsevier; 2056: 2021.

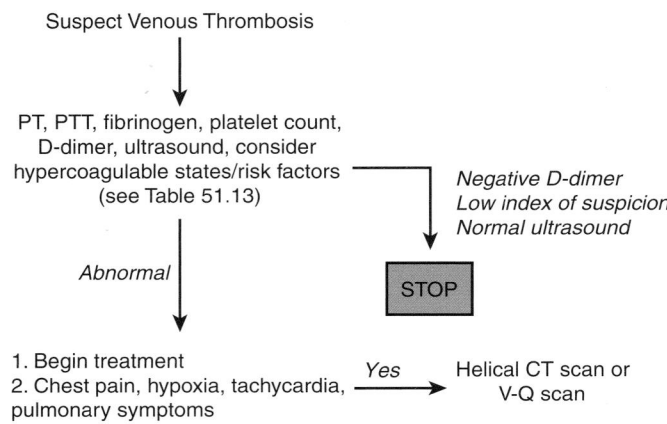

Fig. 51.11 Flow diagram for the approach to a patient with venous thromboembolic disease. The international normalized ratio (INR) corrects the PT for institutional differences in reagents and instruments. When a patient is taking a stable warfarin dosage, the INR is calculated by a ratio of the patient's PT to the control PT raised to a correction factor (the International Sensitivity Index) that allows for comparison of different PT reagents and machines in different laboratories. For all patients receiving chronic warfarin therapy, their anticoagulant therapy should be measured as the INR. The INR level should be maintained between 2.0 and 3.0 for effective, safe anticoagulant therapy. An INR exceeding 3.0 has been associated with increased risk for bleeding without improved therapeutic effects for patients with venous thromboembolic disease. PT, prothrombin time; PTT, partial thromboplastin time; V-Q, ventilation-perfusion.

Specific Diagnostic Studies

Compression ultrasonography is generally used to assess for the presence of a lower extremity thrombosis and many episodes of upper extremity thrombosis. While ultrasound with Doppler flow studies to look at flow of red blood cells through arteries or veins may be sufficient for diagnosis of renal or hepatic thrombosis as well, consideration should be given to other modalities, including CT scan, echocardiogram, and venography. MRI and magnetic resonance venography can be useful in diagnosis of venous dural sinus thrombosis or evaluation of proximal extent of a lower extremity into the large vessels of the pelvis and/or abdomen.

If pulmonary embolism is suspected, a spiral CT scan is the diagnostic study of choice. CT scan is indicated in any patient with a venous thrombosis and cardiac and/or respiratory symptoms, including tachycardia, tachypnea, and hypoxia. Pulmonary embolism may be present without significant respiratory distress and should be considered in patients with chest pain or hemoptysis, particularly following surgery and immobilization.

Thrombophilia Testing

In children, the diagnosis of venous thrombosis in the setting of risk factors, such as surgery, immobilization, or catheter placement, does not generally warrant any additional work-up. Adult guidelines specifically recommend against thrombophilia testing in thrombosis in the setting of major transient risk factors. *An unprovoked, or recurrent, thrombosis merits work-up for a congenital or acquired thrombophilic condition.* Some clinicians may also pursue this work-up for thrombi in unusual anatomic sites, with extremely large thrombus burden, or in patients with family history of thrombosis.

The most severe inherited thrombophilias are deficiencies of anticoagulants PC, PS, and AT. Although rare, these are associated with a higher relative risk for thrombosis than the more common thrombophilias. Levels of PC, AT, and plasminogen may be depleted/consumed after development of deep vein thrombosis, pulmonary emboli, or both; low levels at the time of thrombosis do not necessarily imply a congenital deficiency. If low levels are found, consideration should be given to performing studies on the parents to establish the inheritance of the deficiency because all these are inherited as autosomal codominant traits. Alternatively, or in addition, the patient's levels should be re-evaluated several months after the acute event; the clinician should remember that warfarin reduces functional levels of all the vitamin K–dependent proteins, including PC and PS.

Less severe, but more common, inherited thrombophilias include **factor 5 Leiden and the prothrombin gene variant.** These occur in up to 5% of the U.S. population and have a lower relative risk for thrombosis. Testing of asymptomatic family members is not generally required, although affected females should probably be counseled to avoid estrogen-containing oral contraceptives due to a higher risk for thrombosis.

The **lupus anticoagulant** (LA) is one of several antiphospholipid antibodies (others including anticardiolipin and β-2-glycoprotein-Ib antibodies) that acts as an acquired thrombophilia. This causes a prolonged PTT that fails to correct on mixing with normal plasma because of the presence of an antibody that reacts with the phospholipid reagent in the PTT. The lupus anticoagulant does not bind in vivo to the platelet membrane; thus, the whole blood clotting time is normal. Paradoxically (considering the name), the LA is associated with venous and arterial thromboembolic disease and spontaneous abortions but is usually not a cause of clinical bleeding. If these study findings are negative, the thrombin time should be measured or a comparison of functional and antigenic levels of fibrinogen should be done to detect a dysfibrinogenemia. The presence of an LA occurs frequently in patients with SLE, but it is by no means exclusive to this disease. Indeed, approximately 5% of healthy children may develop transient, self-resolving LA after infection, trauma, or surgery.

Arterial Thrombosis

Arterial thrombi are rare in older children and adolescents and are frequently a manifestation of a systemic disorder resulting in vascular damage or embolic disease such as sickle cell anemia, Kawasaki disease, bacterial endocarditis, vasculitis syndromes, homocystinuria, or cocaine use. The presence of an intraarterial catheter is an obvious nidus for thrombosis. Neck trauma that is often mild can cause carotid or vertebral artery dissection or aneurysms. These dissections or aneurysms can result in emboli to the brain. A history of neck trauma should be sought in older children who present with arterial stroke.

ANTICOAGULANT THERAPY

Parenteral Therapy
Unfractionated Heparin

Unfractionated heparin (UFH) is the most commonly used agent for the initial treatment of venous or arterial thrombosis and is administered either intravenously (IV) or subcutaneously. Heparin functions as an anticoagulant by binding to AT and accelerating the AT-dependent inactivation of thrombin and factor 10a, as well as of factors 9a and 11a. Although most studies of heparin pharmacokinetics have been performed in adults, there are important differences in the pharmacologic features of heparin in children and especially neonates. Thirty-nine percent of children achieve a prolongation of the PTT within the target range after a bolus dose of 50 U/kg. Children younger than 1 year require an average of 28 U/kg/hr to maintain a therapeutic level of the PTT. In contrast, most children older than 1 year are satisfactorily maintained on 20 U/kg/hr of heparin. A representative treatment protocol may begin with an initial IV bolus of 50–75 U/kg of heparin, with 20–25 U/kg/hr for a minimum of 5 days to maintain a PTT of approximately 2–2.5 times the control value. Reports in adults suggest that the heparin level (UFH-calibrated anti-Xa assay) is superior for monitoring heparin therapy compared to the PTT. The heparin level or PTT should be checked every 4–6 hours after a dose change until a satisfactory level is attained, and then at least every 6 hours after that. Studies have documented an increased risk for progressive or recurrent thrombi in patients who fail to achieve adequate anticoagulant levels promptly. Sometimes this delay can be seen in patients with concomitant bleeding concerns that preclude the use of an up-front bolus, or those with significant clinical inflammation that may increase levels of circulating heparin-binding proteins. Anti-Xa levels are especially useful in premature and full-term newborns who may have a "normal" prolonged PTT. A therapeutic range of 0.3–0.7 U/dL has been demonstrated to be safe and effective.

Low-molecular-weight heparin (LMWH) provides an alternative to standard UFH therapy. Pediatric experience with LMWH given subcutaneously is similar to that in adults. LMWH given to infants and children with thromboses appears to be as effective as standard heparin, with a similar or reduced risk for bleeding. LMWH requires much less laboratory monitoring. Reasonable age-based starting doses of the LMWH enoxaparin in pediatrics are approximately 1.75 mg/kg (for patients younger than 1 month), 1.64 mg/kg (1 month to 1 year), 1.5 mg/kg (1 to 6 years), and 1.0 mg/kg (older than 6 years of age). Similar to UFH, a LMWH-calibrated anti-Xa assay can be used to adjust dosing as needed to achieve a level between 0.5 and 1.0 U/dL. Dalteparin, another LMWH, is the only other anticoagulant approved by the U.S. Food and Drug Administration as of this writing.

Total length of therapy for provoked clots typically extends for 3 months, while therapy for unprovoked clots may extend to 6–12 months or even indefinitely, depending on the presence of other prothrombotic conditions and personal/family thrombotic history.

Heparin and LMWH may induce thrombocytopenia (heparin-induced thrombocytopenia [HIT]). **Type I HIT** is a nonimmunologic heparin-induced platelet sequestration, while **type II HIT** is immune mediated (heparin platelet factor antibody) and associated with thrombosis (deep venous, pulmonary embolism, necrotizing cutaneous lesions).

TABLE 51.15	**Direct Oral Anticoagulants (DOACs)**				
	Dabigatran	**Rivaroxaban**	**Apixaban**	**Edoxaban**	**Betrixaban**
Factor target	2a	10a	10a	10a	10a
Half-life (hr)	12–17	5–13	8–14	10–14	20–30
Renal clearance (%)	80	33	25	35–50	5–7
Drug metabolism	P-glycoprotein	P-glycoprotein and *CYP34A*	P-glycoprotein and *CYP34A*	P-glycoprotein	P-glycoprotein
Drug reversal	Idarucizumab	Andexanet alfa	Andexanet alfa	Andexanet alfa	Andexanet alfa

From Kliegman RM, St. Geme JW III, Blum NJ, et al., eds. *Nelson Textbook of Pediatrics.* 21st ed. Philadelphia: Elsevier; 2020:2606, Table 506.3.

Fibrinolytic Therapy

Fibrinolytic therapy is indicated for serious and potentially life-threatening thrombosis because it provides a more rapid lysis of clots than standard anticoagulant treatment with heparin and is clinically effective in both arterial and venous clots. Because bleeding complications are many times higher than those with heparin in older individuals, the clinical severity of the clot must justify the use of lytic therapy, such as a life- or limb-threatening extremity clot or a pulmonary embolus resulting in cardiac compromise. For smaller thrombi or those in nonvital locations, heparin is safe and effective. Lytic therapy is best used early in the evolution of the thrombus. If the clot has been long-standing, it is unlikely that fibrinolytic therapy will be efficacious.

The presence of any intracranial process, recent major surgery, or recent significant bleeding is an absolute contraindication to fibrinolytic therapy and a relative contraindication to heparin treatment. In patients with a normal cranial sonogram (or CT) and complete occlusion of the aorta or evidence of compromise of major organ function, fibrinolytic therapy has been safely and successfully administered with very careful monitoring. Table 51.12 outlines dose and monitoring studies for two commonly used fibrinolytic agents: recombinant TPA and urokinase. Fibrinolytic therapy appears to result in a more rapid return of pulmonary artery flow after pulmonary emboli and may decrease the likelihood and/or severity of postphlebitic syndrome after deep vein thrombosis, though this is a starkly understudied area in pediatrics.

Input from an interventional radiologist may be useful to discuss various options, such as systemic vs local (catheter-directed) thrombolysis and any potential role for mechanical lysis.

Warfarin

Warfarin has long been the anticoagulant of choice for long-term oral therapy, though direct oral anticoagulants (DOACs) are becoming more well studied in children. Warfarin acts by blocking the vitamin K–dependent post-translational modification of factors 2, 7, 9, and 10

and of PC and PS. The usual warfarin starting dose is 0.1–0.2 mg/kg/day. Younger children appear to require higher doses to achieve a therapeutic level of the INR. Due to the changes in warfarin metabolism that may occur because of concomitant medications or varying amounts of vitamin K in a diet, frequent blood testing may be needed to maintain an adequate INR. If warfarin therapy is started early in the course of heparin therapy for thrombotic disease, effective oral anticoagulant effect is often achieved by day 5, at which time levels of all the vitamin K–dependent factors should be depressed by warfarin. Early in the course of treatment with warfarin, the PT is affected first because factor 7 has the shortest half-life of the vitamin K–dependent procoagulants and factor 7 levels fall briskly after warfarin treatment. The next levels that fall are PC and PS, followed by the other clotting factors. Therefore, in the first several days warfarin must be coadministered with UFH or LMWH so as to avoid a temporary hypercoagulable state. The aim of warfarin therapy for venous thromboembolic disease is to achieve a stable INR of approximately 2.0–3.0, though specific range may vary based on clinical indication. For example, for prevention of embolization from prosthetic valves, a higher INR may be preferable. Patients with PC or PS deficiency are at risk for warfarin-induced skin necrosis when warfarin therapy is initiated, particularly if high doses are used. These individuals should be given heparin before warfarin is started, and they should not receive a loading/high dose of warfarin.

Warfarin may be reversed by administration of either IV or oral vitamin K. Although IV vitamin K may work slightly faster, response rates at 24 hours are identical and IV vitamin K carries the associated risk for overcorrection and prolonged subtherapeutic INRs. Therefore, oral administration is preferable for non–life-threatening bleeding.

Direct Oral Anticoagulant Therapy

DOACs appear to be at least as effective as warfarin and possibly safer (Table 51.15). It should be noted that some specific diagnoses may still require warfarin, including patients with antiphospholipid antibody syndrome and some patients with cardiac issues.

■ SUMMARY AND RED FLAGS

Bleeding and thrombotic problems are often familial but may also be acquired. A family history and personal history that quantitate bleeding episodes are of utmost help in planning an evaluation. Red flags include anemia; signs of end-organ bleeding or vascular occlusion, particularly the central nervous system; signs of a systemic disorder (pancytopenia, hypotension, rash, weight loss, chronic fever, liver–renal–pulmonary system involvement); and signs of hemorrhagic shock.

BIBLIOGRAPHY

A bibliography is available at ExpertConsult.com.

Fever

Anna R. Huppler

Fever is a common symptom associated with a range of infectious and noninfectious etiologies. Two-thirds of all children visit a physician for fever before they reach the age of 2 years. The appropriate evaluation for fever depends on age, duration of illness, comorbidities, and associated signs and symptoms. The etiology of fever is often revealed with careful history and physical examination, though the precise microbiologic or genetic etiology for fever may need to be elucidated with further diagnostic testing in appropriate situations.

DEFINITIONS

- **Fever without source (FWS):** A child with fever of recent onset with no obvious historical or physical explanation for the fever is said to have FWS. Most patients with FWS, regardless of age, have a self-limited viral illness. Bacterial pathogens account for a small but clinically significant number of cases. The challenge is to identify which children have fever caused by bacteria or other pathogens that would require treatment. Evaluation decisions must balance the risk of morbidity and mortality associated with delayed treatment with the risks of testing or treatment when neither is needed. The risk of bacterial infection decreases with increasing age and is highest for infants younger than 3 months of age, compared to infants and toddlers 3–36 months of age, and even lower for children over the age of 36 months. High suspicion for serious infection should also be considered in immunocompromised patients or those with indwelling hardware such as central venous access lines or ventriculoperitoneal shunts.
- **Fever with localizing signs:** Fever in children most commonly presents with signs or symptoms that indicate a likely diagnosis. Examples include fever accompanied with vomiting and diarrhea (gastroenteritis: see Chapter 14), sore throat (pharyngitis: see Chapter 2), or dysuria and flank pain (pyelonephritis: see Chapter 21).
- **Fever of unknown origin (FUO):** The term *FUO* broadly refers to prolonged fevers with no etiology found after an initial evaluation. Varying specific definitions are found in the literature. In adults, classic FUO is defined as an illness lasting more than 3 weeks with fever higher than 38.3°C (101°F) on several occasions and uncertainty of diagnosis after a 1-week study in the hospital. Shorter duration of fever (as little as 3 days) may prompt evaluation in cases of health care–associated fever or underlying immunodeficiency. In pediatrics, the defined duration of FUO is variable, from 8 days to 3 weeks (average, 2 weeks), and may depend on the age of the patient, with shorter periods of fever tolerated in young infants and

more traditional adult standards tolerated in adolescent patients. A practical diagnosis of FUO in pediatrics is the presence of daily temperatures higher than 38°C (100.4°F) for at least 8–14 days and no diagnosis after an initial evaluation including history, physical examination, and basic laboratory and radiologic tests.

PATHOPHYSIOLOGY OF FEVER

Temperature is controlled by the thermoregulatory center, located in the preoptic area of the anterior hypothalamus. The thermoregulatory center receives input from peripheral receptors and the temperature of the blood bathing the hypothalamus and acts on autonomic, endocrine, and behavioral mechanisms to maintain the body temperature at a particular set point. The hypothalamic set point normally maintains body temperature around 37°C, but there can be significant variation among individuals. Normal temperatures range from 36°C to 37.8°C, depending on the time of day, with the peak in the afternoon (5–7 P.M.) and the trough in the early morning (2–6 A.M.). Although the circadian rhythm is not well established in infancy, it becomes more reliable by the second year of life.

The febrile response not only produces an elevation in body temperature but also causes physiologic changes that enhance the individual's ability to eliminate infection, including the production of acute-phase reactants and alterations in metabolism and endocrine function. **Acute-phase reactants**—proteins that are produced in response to infection or injury—include ceruloplasmin, CRP, haptoglobin, amyloid A, complement, ferritin, and fibrinogen. Hormones and cytokines, some of which are endogenous pyrogens, regulate the production of acute-phase proteins. Exogenous pyrogens, such as bacteria or endotoxins, generate the production of endogenous pyrogens, which play a vital role in prostaglandin-related set point elevation and regulation of acute-phase responses.

Fever results when the thermoregulatory set point is elevated above the normal set point; the hypothalamus then generates physiologic changes involving endocrine, metabolic, autonomic, and behavioral processes. Diversion of blood from peripheral vessels to central vessels causes coolness of the extremities but helps increase core temperature. Shivering increases metabolic activity and heat production. The affected patient may feel cold and seek a warmer environment or add clothing to feel warmer and prevent heat loss. Once these processes have resulted in increasing the core temperature to match the elevated set point, the thermoregulatory center works to maintain the temperature at that point, as it does during normothermia. The thermoregulatory point returns to normal once the infection is resolved. The hypothalamus then produces physiologic changes to decrease the core temperature; these changes include sweating, dilatation of cutaneous blood vessels, and the sensation of feeling hot, which may lead to behaviors such as removing clothing or seeking a cooler environment.

Fever has both positive and negative effects. High body temperatures may impair the reproduction and survival of some invading microorganisms by decreasing required nutrients, such as free iron, or by optimizing immunologic responses, such as phagocytosis. However, at extremely high temperatures, immunologic responses may be impaired. Fever increases the basal metabolic rate by 10–12% for each degree Celsius elevation in temperature. This change in metabolic rate increases oxygen consumption, carbon dioxide production, and fluid and caloric needs. Fluid requirements increase 100 mL/m^2/day for each 1°C rise in temperature above 37.8°C.

Elevated body temperature occurring in the absence of infectious or inflammatory stimuli is termed **hyperthermia**. Hyperthermia can result from excessive heat production, inadequate heat dissipation, or hypothalamic dysfunction (Table 52.1). **Heat stroke** is a form of heat illness in which excessive heat production and inadequate heat dissipation can result in extreme elevations in temperature despite a

normal hypothalamic set point. Prompt restoration of normal body temperature is mandatory to prevent multiorgan dysfunction and death.

FEVER WITHOUT SOURCE

The evaluation of FWS aims to identify the etiology of the fever and determine the severity of illness. All patients should undergo a thorough history and physical examination. The scope of laboratory and radiographic evaluation depend on the patient age and severity of illness. FWS of long duration may meet criteria for FUO.

History

A detailed history may reveal a potential source for infection. A complete history addresses several important issues: (1) duration and pattern of fever; (2) height of fever; (3) mode of temperature measurement; (4) administration and response to medications, including antipyretics, antibiotics, or home remedies; (5) associated symptoms; (6) environmental exposures; (7) ill contacts; (8) immunization history including recent administrations, and (9) recent travel. In addition, inquiry into the child's past medical history may reveal important historical information such as recurrent febrile illnesses, primary or acquired immunodeficiency, or underlying diseases that predispose to infection or fevers. A personal history of or exposure to COVID-19 suggests the possibility of multisystem inflammatory syndrome in children (MIS-C).

Temperature Measurement

Rectal temperature measurement is the gold standard for children 3 years of age or younger. The most widely accepted definition of fever is rectal temperature of 38°C (100.4°F) or higher. It is important to consider that infants, especially those younger than 2 months of age, may have a blunted febrile response or develop hypothermia with infection. Hence, lack of fever should not be used as a criterion for ruling out infection in infants. Rectal temperature measurement should be avoided in neutropenic immunocompromised patients, in whom rectal manipulation may result in translocation of bacteria to the bloodstream.

Oral temperature measurement is reliable for cooperative patients who are older than 4–5 years of age. **Axillary temperature** measure is commonly performed but is less precise than rectal temperatures. There is a general correlation between axillary and rectal temperature measurements; the axillary temperature is usually 0.5–0.85°C *lower*. **Tympanic membrane thermometers** are often inaccurate in children. **Temporal artery temperature** measurement correlates well with rectal temperature in some studies, but it has been shown to be inferior when patients are febrile. It can be considered in settings when children are not likely to be febrile and are over 3 months of age. When detection of fever is critical for diagnosis and management, rectal temperatures should be used in the child 3 years of age and younger.

Physical Examination

The physical examination is vitally important to classify the febrile child as ill- or well-appearing. This classification informs the requirement for and urgency of laboratory and radiographic evaluation, as well as the subsequent management. Ill-appearing children are typically lethargic or irritable. They may show signs of shock, including weak peripheral pulses, tachycardia, poor perfusion, respiratory distress, mottling, cyanosis, or decreased mental status (Table 52.2). Additional worrisome signs include petechiae or purpura and signs of meningitis. After thorough clinical and laboratory evaluation, ill-appearing children should

---

TABLE 52.1 Causes of Hyperthermia

Excessive Heat Production

Exertion

Heat stroke (exertion)

Malignant hyperthermia (anesthesia induced)

Neuroleptic malignant syndrome

Catatonia

Tetanus

Status epilepticus

Delirium

Endocrine disorders (hyperthyroidism, pheochromocytoma)

Drugs (cocaine, amphetamines, ephedrine, phencyclidine, tricyclic antidepressants, lysergic acid diethylamide [LSD], lithium, thyroid hormone, salicylates)

Diminished Heat Dissipation

Heat stroke

Occlusive dressings

Dehydration

Extensive burns (including severe sunburn)

Anhidrotic ectodermal dysplasia

Anticholinergic-like drugs (atropine, antihistamines, phenothiazines, tricyclic antidepressants)

Autonomic neuropathy

Spinal cord level paralysis (spinal crisis)

Possible overbundling (especially in a warm environment)

Overheating in automobile exposed to sun or heat

Therapeutic hyperthermia

Hypothalamic Dysfunction*

Stroke

Encephalitis

Granulomatous processes (sarcoid, tuberculosis, eosinophilic)

Trauma

Central: idiopathic

Phenothiazines

Hemorrhage

*Usually associated with hypothermia.

TABLE 52.2 International Consensus Definitions for Pediatric Sepsis

Infection	Suspected or proven infection or a clinical syndrome associated with high probability of infection

SIRS	Two of four criteria, one of which must be abnormal temperature or abnormal leukocyte count:
	1. Core temperature >38.5°C (101.3°F) or <36°C (96.8°F) (rectal, bladder, oral, or central catheter)
	2. Tachycardia:
	   Mean heart rate >2 SD above normal for age in absence of external stimuli, chronic drugs, or painful stimuli
	   or
	   Unexplained persistent elevation over 0.5–4 hr
	   or
	   In children <1 yr old, persistent bradycardia over 0.5 hr (mean heart rate <10th percentile for age in absence of vagal stimuli, β-blocker drugs, or congenital heart disease)
	3. Respiratory rate >2 SD above normal for age or acute need for mechanical ventilation not related to neuromuscular disease or general anesthesia
	4. Leukocyte count elevated or depressed for age (not secondary to chemotherapy) or >10% immature neutrophils

Sepsis	SIRS plus a suspected or proven infection

Severe sepsis	Sepsis plus one of the following:
	1. Cardiovascular organ dysfunction, defined as:
	   Despite >40 mL/kg of isotonic intravenous fluid in 1 hr:
	   • Hypotension <5th percentile for age or systolic blood pressure <2 SD below normal for age
	   or
	   • Need for vasoactive drug to maintain blood pressure
	   or
	   • Two of the following:
	     • Unexplained metabolic acidosis: base deficit >5 mEq/L
	     • Increased arterial lactate: >2 times upper limit of normal
	     • Oliguria: urine output <0.5 mL/kg/hr
	     • Prolonged capillary refill: >5 sec
	     • Core-to-peripheral temperature gap >3°C (5.4°F)
	2. ARDS as defined by the presence of a Pao_2/Fio_2 ratio ≤300 mm Hg, bilateral infiltrates on chest radiograph, and no evidence of left heart failure
	   or
	Sepsis plus two or more organ dysfunctions (respiratory, renal, neurologic, hematologic, or hepatic)

Septic shock	Sepsis plus cardiovascular organ dysfunction as defined above
MODS	Presence of altered organ function such that homeostasis cannot be maintained without medical intervention

ARDS, acute respiratory distress syndrome; Fio_2, fraction of inspired oxygen; MODS, multiple organ dysfunction syndrome; Pao_2, partial pressure arterial oxygen; SIRS, systemic inflammatory response syndrome.

From Turner DA, Cheifetz IM. Shock. In: Kliegman RM, St. Geme JW III, Blum NJ, et al., eds. *Nelson Textbook of Pediatrics.* 21st ed. Philadelphia: Elsevier; 2020:578, Table 88.7.

be admitted to the hospital and likely require empiric antibiotic treatment while microbiologic and other diagnostic assays are pending.

Observational Scales

It is challenging to determine the subsequent evaluation and management of infants and children with FWS who do not appear ill. The physician's ability to make a hypothesis about the child's degree of illness, on the basis of observation, may simultaneously allow for identification of serious infection as well as eliminate administration of unnecessary testing or treatment. An objective scoring measure may be used to assess serious illness in young febrile children. The Acute Illness Observation Scale (AIOS) (Table 52.3), also known as the Yale Observation Score, is a 6-item predictive model graded on a scale of 1–5. Use of the AIOS in conjunction with the history and physical examination has a higher sensitivity for identifying serious illness than history and physical examination alone. While helpful in determining the severity of illness, the AIOS cannot be used to confirm or exclude serious bacterial infection.

Differential Diagnosis

Most children who present with FWS are subsequently determined to have a self-limited benign viral infection. In a study of children with FWS aged 2–36 months, 76% had one or more known pathogenic viruses found, most commonly adenovirus, human herpesvirus 6 (HHV-6: roseola), enterovirus, or parechovirus. Other identifiable viruses include respiratory syncytial virus, parainfluenza viruses, influenza viruses, varicella (chickenpox), human metapneumovirus, and parvovirus (fifth disease/erythema infectiosum). Measles, mumps, and rubella are uncommon in countries with sufficiently high rates of immunization but have been reported in epidemics following imported cases or in underimmunized communities. Although rapid testing for viral pathogens is often readily available, a detailed and costly investigation to identify a viral pathogen is not necessary unless the confirmation of a viral infection will change the acute diagnostic plan, there is potential for antiviral therapy (e.g., herpes simplex virus [HSV], influenza), fever is prolonged (FUO), or end-organ involvement is identified (e.g., hepatitis, myocarditis, encephalitis, or meningitis).

Although less common than viral infections, bacterial infections are notable causes of FWS, especially in younger children. Bacterial infections most likely to manifest in the absence of localizing symptoms include urinary tract infections, bacteremia, and meningitis. Bacterial superinfection concurrent with or after viral infection may also occur. Well-documented examples include croup due to parainfluenza virus predisposing to bacterial tracheitis, influenza accompanied by bacterial pneumonia, and varicella complicated by invasive group A streptococcal (GAS) infection. In many cases, there is a clear biphasic pattern to the symptoms with improvement in the initial viral symptoms followed by recurrent fever or worsening symptoms. These bacterial superinfections are unusual causes of FWS since localizing signs and symptoms in the respiratory tract or skin are usually present.

Noninfectious conditions manifesting as FWS are rare. Historical clues (recurrences, chronicity) or systemic signs usually indicate malignancy or rheumatic disorders. Similarly, history should suggest conditions associated with hyperthermia, such as heat-related illness or drug ingestion. Recent receipt of immunizations may cause fever at a characteristic interval. The 1–2-week delay between measles, mumps, and rubella (MMR) or varicella vaccine and fever onset may result in decreased recognition of this fever source. Many noninfectious inflammatory conditions are elusive to diagnosis in the early days of fever. However, some inflammatory conditions in children, such as

TABLE 52.3 Acute Illness Observation Scale

Observation Item	1 Normal	3 Moderate Impairment	5 Severe Impairment
Quality of cry	Strong with normal tone or Content and not crying	Whimpering or Sobbing	Weak or Moaning or High-pitched
Reaction to parent stimulation	Cries briefly, then stops or Content and not crying	Cries off and on	Continual cry or Hardly responds
State variation	If awake → stays awake or If asleep and stimulated → wakes up quickly	Eyes close briefly → awakens or Awakes with prolonged stimulation	Falls asleep or Will not rouse
Color	Pink	Pale extremities or Acrocyanosis	Pale or Cyanotic or Mottled or Ashen
Hydration	Skin normal, eyes normal and Mucous membranes moist	Skin, eyes normal and Mouth slightly dry	Skin doughy or Skin tented and Dry mucous membranes and/or Sunken eyes
Response (talk, smile) to social overtures	Smiles or Alert (≤2 mo)	Brief smile or Alert briefly (≤2 mo)	No smile; face anxious, dull, expressionless or No alertness (≤2 mo)

From McCarthy PL, Sharpe MR, Spiesel SZ, et al. Observation scales to identify serious illness in febrile children. *Pediatrics.* 1982;70:802.

Kawasaki disease and MIS-C, require early intervention to prevent severe sequelae or severe illness.

Urinary Tract Infections

Urinary tract infections (UTIs) are the most common serious bacterial infection in children younger than 36 months of age who present with FWS. UTIs are often occult in children younger than 24 months because the symptoms, except for fever, are nonspecific or nonexistent. UTI occurs in 7% of febrile children younger than 2 years. The prevalence of UTI varies by height of the fever, duration of the fever, age, gender, race, and circumcision status. Children with FWS >39°C are at a higher risk of UTIs. Males with fever for more than 2 days and females with fever for more than 1 day are more likely to have a UTI. Higher rates of UTIs are found in females, especially those younger than 12 months of age. For febrile males younger than 3 months of age, 20.1% of those who are uncircumcised have a UTI; for circumcised males, the rate is 2.4%. UTI rates are higher among children with abnormal genitourinary tract anatomy or neurogenic bladder.

Urine specimens should be obtained from the following children with FWS: those with a history of UTI, those with a history of urinary tract anomalies or vesicoureteral reflux, females younger than 12–24 months, uncircumcised males younger than 12 months, and circumcised males younger than 6 months. Prompt evaluation of the urine in all febrile infants younger than 2 months is mandatory. There is an age-associated risk of bacteremia with UTIs, particularly in infants. The incidence of bacteremia in patients with UTI who are younger than 2 months ranges from 4% to 15% depending on the setting. Opinions regarding when to obtain blood cultures in infants with UTI differ, but a reasonable approach would be to obtain blood cultures in children younger than 2–6 months with suspected UTI and in older infants with UTI if they are ill-appearing.

Bacteremia

Occult bacteremia is defined by the presence of a positive blood culture for pathogenic bacteria in a febrile patient who does not appear extremely ill and who has no focus of infection, excluding otitis media. Prior to the introduction of conjugate pneumococcal vaccines, *Streptococcus pneumoniae* was a common cause of occult bacteremia in young children. With the introduction of the 7-valent conjugate pneumococcal vaccine in 2000, rates of pneumococcal bacteremia decreased from 74.5 to 10 cases per 100,000 per year. The expansion to 13-valent conjugate pneumococcal vaccine (PCV-13) in 2010 correlated with a further threefold decline in pneumococcal bacteremia. In immunized febrile children 3–36 months of age, the likelihood of detecting a contaminant on blood culture may be double the incidence of true occult bacteremia in the post–PCV-13 era. Risk factors for recurrent occult bacteremia include functional or anatomic asplenia (including sickle cell anemia) as well as defects in the innate immune system, including abnormalities in the toll-like receptor signaling pathway, which may also result in a blunted host immune response and decrease the likelihood of associated signs or symptoms when bacteremic.

Overall, *most cases of bacteremia in children are not occult.* Children with bacteremia are likely to either be ill-appearing or have a focus of infection, such as a UTI. *Escherichia coli* is the most common cause of bacteremia in children aged younger than 12 months, all associated with UTI. Other less common causes of bacteremia in young children beyond the neonatal period are *Neisseria meningitidis*, nontyphoidal *Salmonella*, *Staphylococcus aureus*, and GAS. *N. meningitidis* bacteremia is frequently associated with serious sequelae, including shock and meningitis. Nontyphoidal *Salmonella* bacteremia is often accompanied or preceded by enteritis. In some instances, particularly in young infants, the diarrhea is mild or even absent. The prevalence of *Salmonella* bacteremia among patients with *Salmonella* enteritis has been reported to be between 2% and 45%; fever is not always present. *Salmonella* infection seldom causes serious complications in patients with normal host defenses and resolves spontaneously. Infants younger than 3 months, malnourished children, and immunocompromised individuals are at high risk for serious and disseminated *Salmonella* infection.

Meningitis

Bacterial and viral meningitis/meningoencephalitis are important causes of FWS in young infants. The most common etiologic agents in neonates are *E. coli*, group B *Streptococcus* (GBS), *Listeria monocytogenes*, HSV, and enterovirus. Pneumococcus and meningococcus become more common after 1 month of age.

Role of Diagnostic Testing in Patients with Fever Without Source

Evaluation is usually divided into four different age ranges: younger than 1 month, 1–3 months, 3–36 months, and older than 36 months. Testing for each individual age group is based on risks for diseases and prevalence of pathogens.

Complete Blood Count and Other Markers of Inflammation

The white blood cell (WBC) count is the most commonly used test in young children with FWS. CBC is less useful as a marker for invasive disease caused by *E. coli* than by *S. pneumoniae*; thus, its utility has declined with the reduced incidence of invasive pneumococcal disease. Similarly, band counts are less informative except in the 29–60-day-old infant as part of identifying a low-risk cohort. A WBC count of 5,000–15,000 is generally considered normal for children over 1 month of age. A WBC count of <15,000/mm^3 or even leukopenia may be found in children with *N. meningitidis* bacteremia. A minority of children with occult nontyphoidal *Salmonella* bacteremia have been found to have a WBC count exceeding 15,000/mm^3. CRP and procalcitonin combined with a UA can be used to screen for bacterial infection. This combination of tests has been validated for children 7 days to 36 months of age.

Molecular Testing

Polymerase chain reaction (PCR, also known as nucleic acid amplification tests or NAAT) is useful in identifying the cause of acute fever from common viruses such as respiratory syncytial virus, influenza viruses, parainfluenza viruses, enteroviruses, parechovirus, adenoviruses, coronaviruses including severe acute respiratory syndrome–coronavirus 2

(SARS-CoV-2), rhinoviruses, and HSV. Appropriate specimens include nasopharyngeal (respiratory viruses and enterovirus), stool (adenovirus and enterovirus), cerebrospinal fluid (CSF) (enterovirus and HSV most commonly), skin (HSV), and blood (enterovirus, adenovirus, and HSV). Typically, PCR testing is reserved for patients with serious illness or pathogens that are amenable to treatment, such as HSV, or in circumstances when the identification of a specific viral etiology would allow for the discontinuation of empiric antibacterial therapy. PCR testing is also available for some bacterial pathogens from select body fluids (CSF, pleural fluid).

Additional methods are available in select laboratories to identify serious bacterial infections. **Gene expression profiles** of peripheral blood leukocytes demonstrate different biosignatures of RNA production associated with bacterial or viral infections, though this method does not identify the specific pathogen. **Rapid multiplex PCR** combined with standard blood culture methods may identify a specific pathogen much sooner (~20 hours) than standard blood culture techniques. Specific bacteria may be identified using **16S ribosomal RNA** bacterial gene detection in tissue biopsies or blood. This method does not require bacterial growth but may lack sensitivity with low inoculum.

Blood Cultures

Blood cultures are the gold standard for identification of bacteremia. Blood culture methodology allows for continuous and automated detection of bacterial growth. Blood cultures are easy to perform and provide essential information in the diagnosis and management of patients with possible bacteremia. Pathogen growth is usually detected within 24–48 hours of collection, with positive identification of most organisms within 2–24 hours of growth. Rapid diagnostic techniques such as multiplex PCR on positive blood culture bottles and matrix-assisted laser desorption/ionization time-of-flight mass spectrometry (MALDI-TOF MS) on growing bacteria have further shortened the interval to pathogen identification.

False-negative blood culture results may be due to prior treatment with antibiotics, presence of intermittent bacteremia, or sampling error due to small specimen volume. Alternatively, too much blood inoculated into the blood culture bottle may yield a false-negative result because of ongoing killing of bacteria by neutrophils. Reference ranges for the appropriate volumes of blood are available based on the patient size and type of blood culture bottle. False-positive results are most commonly due to inadequate skin preparation, leading to contamination with skin flora.

Urinalysis and Urine Culture

Recommendations for the diagnosis of UTI include a UA that has pyuria (defined as >5 WBCs/high-power field [hpf] on the microscopic examination or a positive leukocyte esterase on dipstick) and a positive urine culture for a uropathogen in an appropriately collected specimen; 50,000 to 100,000 colonies of a single organism is considered positive (see Chapter 21). Children should have a catheterized urine specimen obtained, unless they are toilet-trained and can supply a clean voided specimen. Suprapubic aspiration allows for noncontaminated urine collection but requires technical expertise, and parents often perceive it as unsuitably invasive; it may be the only alternative for males with severe phimosis. The use of plastic receptacles attached to the perineum should be discouraged because contamination from skin and fecal flora commonly occurs.

Lumbar Puncture

Lumbar puncture (LP) to obtain CSF is indicated if the patient is younger than 28 days or if a diagnosis of sepsis, meningitis, or encephalitis is considered, regardless of the child's age. Normal CSF findings, including chemistry, cell count with differential, Gram stain, PCR, and culture, help exclude the diagnosis of meningitis. Less than 1% of children with normal preliminary CSF results have a positive culture; in most of these, the pathogen is *N. meningitidis*. Thus, even in the presence of normal preliminary CSF results, close follow-up is essential.

Chest Radiographs

Chest radiographs are usually normal in children who have FWS. Respiratory signs or symptoms, such as tachypnea, retractions, crackles, wheezing, rhonchi, nasal flaring, grunting, cough, or hypoxia, may predict chest radiograph findings consistent with pneumonia. In practice, pneumonia can often be diagnosed solely based on the clinical findings of fever, tachypnea, and crackles; chest radiographs are not always necessary. However, chest radiographs may be useful in evaluating for the presence of pleural effusion or other complications of pneumonia, or in instances where lower-lobe or lingular pneumonia produces vague referred abdominal pain that is more pronounced than respiratory signs or symptoms.

Stool Cultures

Most acute febrile diarrhea episodes in developed countries are caused by viral pathogens. Stool testing for bacterial pathogens by culture or enteric pathogen PCR is indicated if there are risk factors in the history, such as blood in the stool or certain exposures (petting zoos, ingestion of potentially contaminated food) (see Chapter 14).

Evaluation and Management

Children Younger Than 3 Months

Febrile infants younger than 3 months have a higher incidence of serious bacterial infections than older infants and therefore deserve special consideration. The relatively high incidence of bacterial disease probably results from a combination of factors unique to this age group: decreased opsonin activity, decreased macrophage function, decreased neutrophil function, poor immunoglobulin G (IgG) antibody response to encapsulated bacteria, and susceptibility to bacterial pathogens such as GBS, gram-negative enteric organisms such as *E. coli*, and *L. monocytogenes*. The incidence of early-onset GBS infections has decreased with routine screening and the intrapartum treatment of GBS-positive pregnant women; the incidence of late-onset GBS (>1 week) has not decreased. In contemporary studies, *E. coli* is the most common organism causing bacterial infections in neonates and young infants.

In very young infants, clinical evaluation alone is insufficiently sensitive to exclude bacterial infections such as UTI, bacteremia, or meningitis. In addition, abnormal initial laboratory results are often insufficiently specific to definitively diagnose these infections. Various investigators developed clinical prediction models to identify febrile infants at low risk for serious bacterial infection (Table 52.4). Application of these criteria allowed for decreased laboratory testing and/or hospitalization in select infants who were unlikely to have bacterial meningitis, bacteremia, or UTI. In 2021, the American Academy of Pediatrics (AAP) with the assistance of the Agency for Healthcare Research and Quality published new guidelines for the evaluation and management of well-appearing febrile infants 8 to 60 days old. Notable changes from those earlier clinical prediction models included changes in tests used to guide decision making, with increased emphasis on CRP and procalcitonin, and new age-based risk stratification.

Management of well-appearing febrile infants **younger than 21 days** includes evaluation of the blood, urine, and CSF for bacterial infection, as well as any other sites based on presenting findings (e.g., chest radiograph in neonates with respiratory distress or cough) and hospitalization for parenteral antimicrobial therapy pending culture results. The reasoning for this conservative approach lies in the difficulty in

TABLE 52.4 Low-Risk Criteria in a Child 0–3 Months Old with Fever

Boston Criteria

Infants are at low risk if they appear well, have a normal physical examination, received no antimicrobials or DTaP vaccine in the previous 48 hr, have a caretaker reachable by telephone, and if laboratory tests are as follows:

- CBC: <20,000 WBC/mm³
- Urine: negative leukocyte esterase or <10 WBC/hpf
- CSF: leukocyte count <10 cells/mm³
- Chest radiograph: no infiltrate (if respiratory symptoms)

Philadelphia Protocol

Infants are at low risk if they appear well and have a normal physical examination, caregiver available to be contacted, and if laboratory tests are as follows:

- CBC: <15,000 WBC/mm³; immature: total neutrophil ratio <0.2
- Urine: <10 WBC/hpf; no bacteria on Gram stain
- CSF: <8 WBC/mm³; no bacteria on Gram stain; nonbloody specimen
- Chest radiograph: no infiltrate
- Stool: no RBC; few to no WBCs (if abnormal stools)

Pittsburgh Guidelines

Infants are at low risk if they appear well and have a normal physical examination; no history of prematurity, illness, hospitalization, antibiotics, or siblings with GBS disease; and if laboratory tests are as follows:

- CBC: 5,000–15,000 WBC/mm³; peripheral absolute band count ≤1,500/mm³
- Urine (enhanced urinalysis): ≤9 WBC/mm³ and no bacteria on Gram stain
- CSF: ≤5 WBC/mm³ and negative Gram stain; if bloody tap, then WBC:RBC ≤1:500
- Chest radiograph: no infiltrate (if respiratory symptoms)
- Stool: <5 WBC/hpf (if diarrhea)

Rochester Criteria

Infants are at low risk if they appear well and have a normal physical examination; previous healthy, full-term gestation, no recent antibiotics, and no unexplained hyperbilirubinemia; and if laboratory findings are as follows:

- CBC: 5,000–15,000 WBC/mm³; absolute band count ≤1,500/mm³
- Urine: <10 WBC/hpf, no bacteria on Gram stain
- Chest radiograph: no infiltrate (if respiratory symptoms)
- Stool: <5 WBC/hpf (if abnormal stools)

CSF, cerebrospinal fluid; hpf, high-powered field; RBC, red blood cell; WBC, white blood cell.

evaluating the behavioral state of neonates, the rapid clinical deterioration of infants with bacterial infections, the immature neonatal immune system, and the possibility of life-threatening viral infections caused by HSV and enteroviruses. Evaluation should include bacterial cultures of the CSF, blood, and urine; a CBC with differential; examination of the CSF for cell count and differential, protein, and glucose; and UA. Inflammatory markers such as procalcitonin and CRP may also be obtained. Testing for HSV (surface swabs, blood, and CSF PCR) and empiric treatment for possible HSV infection should be considered in patients at increased HSV risk. While the risk of vertical transmission of HSV is highest during a primary maternal infection of genital herpes at or near the time of delivery, the presence of maternal HSV infection is often unknown. Additional risk factors for neonatal HSV include a known maternal history of genital HSV lesions or peripartum fevers, as well as neonatal seizures, hypothermia, vesicles, mucous membrane ulcers, leukopenia, thrombocytopenia, elevated alanine aminotransferase levels, or CSF pleocytosis with a Gram stain that is negative for organisms.

A combination of age, clinical evaluation, and laboratory studies is used to define a specific population of **well-appearing febrile infants** who are at low risk for bacterial infections. With the 2021 AAP guidelines, the relevant age range is **22–60 days old**, with additional evaluation steps recommended for the infants **aged 22–28 days.** Infants at low risk for bacterial infections are those who are well-appearing with no evident focus of bacterial infection on physical examination and who have negative laboratory screening results. Historically, **low-risk screening criteria** included normal total WBC, band count, immature-to-total

neutrophil ratio, UA WBC, CSF WBC, and lack of organisms observed in fluid stains (see Table 52.4). Based on existing evidence, the updated 2021 AAP guidelines focus instead primarily on UA results and inflammatory markers for risk stratification. Abnormal inflammatory markers are defined as temperature >38.5°C, procalcitonin >0.5 ng/mL, CRP >20 mg/L, and absolute neutrophil count (ANC) >4000–5200 cells/mm³. A positive UA result should be followed with bladder catheterization or suprapubic aspiration for urine culture. Decision on the performance of an LP depends on the age group of the child (22–28 days versus 29–60 days old) and the result of the inflammatory marker testing (Table 52.5). In most circumstances, patients with increased inflammatory

TABLE 52.5 Management of Fever Without Source

Group	Management
Any toxic-appearing child 0–36 mo and temperature ≥38°C (100.4°F)	Hospitalize, broad cultures plus other tests,* parenteral antibiotics
Child <22 days and temperature ≥38°C (100.4°F)	Hospitalize, broad cultures plus other tests,* parenteral antibiotics
Child 22–60 days and temperature ≥38°C (100.4°F)	**Three-Step Process** 1. Determine risk based on history, physical examination, and laboratory studies. Low risk: • Uncomplicated medical history • Well-appearing physical examination • Normal laboratory studies • Urine: negative leukocyte esterase, nitrite ≤5 WBC centrifuged, and <10 WBC/hpf uncentrifuged • Inflammatory markers: temperature ≤38.5°C, procalcitonin ≤0.5 ng/mL, CRP ≤20 mg/L, absolute neutrophil count ≤4000–5200/mm³ • Stool studies if diarrhea (no RBC and <5 WBC/hpf) 2. If child fulfills all low-risk criteria, use age to determine need for LP, parenteral antimicrobials, and hospital observation. • Age 22–28 days: May perform LP. May administer parenteral antimicrobials. Observe in hospital. • Age 29–60 days old: Need not perform LP. Need not administer antimicrobials. Observe closely at home with follow-up within 24–36 h. 3. If child does not fulfill all low-risk criteria, use age and lab results to determine need for LP, antimicrobials, and hospital observation. • Age 22–28 days with abnormal UA and normal inflammatory markers: May perform LP. Administer parenteral antimicrobials. Observe in hospital. • Age 22–28 days with abnormal inflammatory markers: Perform LP. If CSF pleocytosis, CSF uninterpretable, or abnormal UA, administer parenteral antimicrobials and observe in hospital. If CSF and UA are normal, may observe at home after parenteral antimicrobials or observe in the hospital with or without parenteral antimicrobials. • Age 29–60 days with abnormal UA and normal inflammatory markers: Administer oral antimicrobials. May observe closely at home with follow-up in 12–24 h. • Age 29–60 days with abnormal inflammatory markers: May perform LP. If CSF pleocytosis, administer parenteral antimicrobials and observe in hospital. If CSF is normal, may administer parenteral or oral antimicrobials and may observe closely in hospital or at home. If CSF is not available or uninterpretable, administer parenteral antimicrobials and may observe closely in hospital or at home.
Child 2–36 mo and temperature 38–39°C (100.4–102.2°F)	Reassurance that diagnosis is likely self-limited viral infection, but advise return with persistence of fever, temperatures >39°C (102.2°F), and/or new signs and symptoms.
Child 2–36 mo and temperature >39°C (102.2°F)	**Two-Step Process** 1. Determine immunization status. 2. If received conjugate pneumococcal and *Haemophilus influenzae* type b vaccines, obtain urine studies (urine WBC, leukocyte esterase, nitrite, and culture) for all girls, all boys <6 mo old, all uncircumcised boys <2 yr, and all children with recurrent urinary tract infections. If did not receive conjugate pneumococcal and *H. influenzae* type b vaccines, manage according to the 1993 Guidelines (see Baraff et al. *Ann Emerg Med.* 1993;22:1198–1210).

*Other tests may include chest radiograph, stool studies, herpes simplex virus polymerase chain reaction.

hpf, high-powered field; LP, lumbar puncture; RBC, red blood cell; WBC, white blood cell.

Adapted from Nield LS, Kamat D. Fever without a focus. In: Kliegman RM, Stanton BF, St Geme JW III, et al, eds. *Nelson Textbook of Pediatrics.* 20th ed. Philadelphia: Elsevier; 2016: Table 177.3; with data from Pantell RH, Roberts KB, Adams WG, et al. Evaluation and Management of Well-Appearing Febrile Infants 8 to 60 Days Old. *Pediatrics.* 2021;148(2).

markers or positive UA results should be administered parenteral antibiotics. Select patients can be treated with oral antimicrobials or be observed without antimicrobial therapy in hospital or at home. Regardless of whether the clinician chooses to treat the patient with empiric antibiotics, all low-risk infants should be re-evaluated within 24 hours. Those who appear ill or who have positive culture results should be hospitalized for parenteral antibiotics. If a child appears well and all culture results are negative, close follow-up should be continued and a second return visit made in 24 hours.

Although most of the original studies on management of well-appearing febrile infants included infants up to 3 months of age, most infants aged 2–3 months can be managed safely according to the guidelines for infants and children aged 3–36 months (see Table 52.5). Special consideration should also be given to febrile infants with recent receipt of vaccinations. Fever within the first 48 hours after immunization occurs in greater than 40% of young infants.

All ill-appearing febrile infants regardless of age must be evaluated for bacteremia, meningitis, or pyelonephritis and treated immediately after cultures are obtained.

Children Aged 3–36 Months

The risk of bacteremia for children with FWS in this age group has decreased with the routine use of pneumococcal vaccines. The most common occult bacterial infection in this age group is UTI. However, children in this age group who appear ill should undergo a full sepsis evaluation (see Table 52.5).

Screening UA for UTI should be considered in children with a history of UTI; children with a history of urinary tract anomalies or vesicoureteral reflux; females younger than 12–24 months, especially when the temperature is >39.0°C; uncircumcised males younger than 12 months; and circumcised males younger than 6 months. Blood cultures are recommended for children with probable UTIs who are younger than 6 months of age. A febrile child with moderate leukocyte esterase on macroscopic UA or pyuria on an appropriately collected specimen should be treated presumptively for a UTI. Urine cultures should be obtained for any patient with a suspected UTI. The choice of antibiotics should be guided by knowledge of the common pathogens that cause UTIs and by patterns of antibiotic sensitivity in the community. Hospitalization should be considered for the child who is vomiting, dehydrated, or ill-appearing; for those in whom compliance is likely to be poor; and for any patient with underlying renal or urologic anomalies.

Evaluation for meningitis with an LP is necessary in any child with unexplained sepsis, signs or symptoms of central nervous system (CNS) infection, or blood culture positive for *N. meningitidis* or *H. influenzae* type B. Admission to the hospital for parenteral antibiotics is necessary while awaiting the results of CSF studies.

Outpatient management of children with FWS is acceptable for those with a low probability of meningitis, good follow-up, and reliable caregivers. The clinical evolution and results of cultures dictate the next stage of management. The child with occult pneumococcal bacteremia who appears well and is afebrile when returning for a follow-up may be managed as an outpatient with parenteral ceftriaxone followed by oral antibiotics according to the sensitivity of the organism. If blood culture is positive for nontyphoidal *Salmonella* organisms and the child is younger than 3 months, full sepsis evaluation and intravenous antibiotics are recommended. Oral antibiotics and close follow-up are recommended for older children with *Salmonella* bacteremia. Children with continued FWS should be re-evaluated every 48 hours until fever resolution to assess for the emergence of new signs and symptoms, as well as changes in the severity of illness. Laboratory work-up such as CBC with differential, comprehensive metabolic profiles, and inflammatory markers may be indicated, such as when evaluating for incomplete Kawasaki disease.

Children Older Than 36 Months

Evaluation and management of ill-appearing children older than 36 months with FWS are similar to those of younger children. History to evaluate for potential sources is more reliable in this age group, thus decreasing the incidence of FWS. Close attention should be paid to environmental exposures and ill contacts because of the high likelihood of increased contacts in this school-aged cohort. For children in this age group with true FWS who do not appear ill, no screening diagnostic tests are indicated. For children in the 3–36-month age range, repeat evaluation every 48 hours may be necessary until fever resolves or a diagnosis is reached.

Fever with Localizing Signs: Focus on Central Nervous System Infections

Bacterial Meningitis

Bacterial meningitis is usually a disease of infants and young children. It is seen during all seasons; however, there may be a seasonal correlation between the presence of preceding respiratory pathogens in the upper respiratory tract and the subsequent development of bacterial meningitis. Bacterial meningitis usually occurs sporadically, although clusters of cases have been noted in daycare centers, colleges, and other closed communities. The incidence of meningitis is increased in children with traumatic fractures of the cribriform plate or paranasal sinuses or with a cochlear implant (pneumococci); children who have undergone neurosurgical procedures such as ventricular shunts (*S. aureus, Staphylococcus epidermidis, Cutibacterium acnes*); children with congenital or acquired immunodeficiencies (pneumococci, *L. monocytogenes*, meningococci); children with anatomic or functional asplenia (pneumococci, meningococci); and children with sickle hemoglobinopathies (pneumococci).

Bacterial meningitis manifests in two patterns. In the first, the symptoms develop slowly over several days, the initial symptoms being those of a nonspecific illness. The signs and symptoms of meningitis develop subsequently. In the second pattern, the disease develops suddenly and quickly with signs and symptoms of meningitis and/or sepsis.

The manifestations of meningitis depend on the child's age. In infants, the findings are usually nonspecific and may be subtle; they include vomiting, diarrhea, irritability, lethargy, poor feeding, respiratory distress, seizures, hypothermia, and jaundice. Only 50% of affected infants have fever, but fever may also be the only presenting symptom. It is uncommon for affected young infants to have a stiff neck, and only 30% have a bulging fontanel.

Older children present with more specific meningeal signs. The classic presenting symptoms are headache that is described as severe, generalized, and constant, and stiff neck, caused by inflammation of the cervical dura and reflex spasm of the extensor muscles of the neck. Pain and limitation of motion occur with flexion of the neck, but lateral movement of the neck may be normal and pain-free. Other symptoms may include nausea, vomiting, anorexia, and photophobia.

On examination, patients with meningitis demonstrate irritability, mental confusion or altered consciousness, nuchal rigidity, and, occasionally, hyperesthesia and ataxia. The clinician demonstrates nuchal rigidity by feeling resistance and observing a painful response while flexing the patient's neck. The stiffness may not be recognized until the end of flexion. The neck usually can be rotated without symptoms. In the child who is crying and tensing the muscles, nuchal

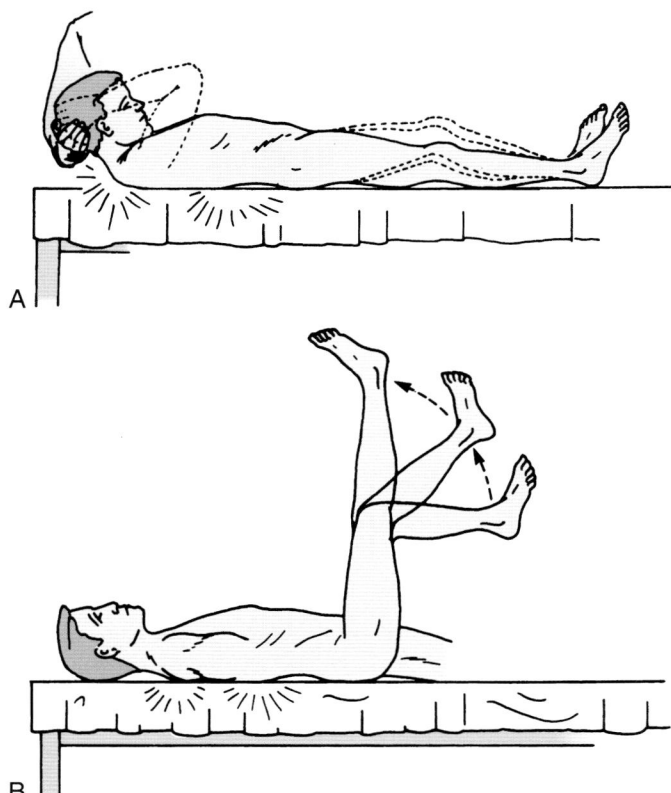

Fig. 52.1 *A,* Brudzinski sign. The patient lies supine, and the head is passively elevated from the table by the examiner. The patient complains of neck and low back discomfort and attempts to relieve the meningeal irritation by involuntary flexion of the knees and hips. *B,* Kernig sign. The patient lies supine, with the hips and knees flexed. The knees are then gradually extended. Complaints of pain in the lower back, neck, and/or head are suggestive of meningeal irritation. (From Reilly BM. *Practical Strategies in Outpatient Medicine.* 2nd ed. Philadelphia: WB Saunders; 1991:95.)

rigidity may be demonstrated if the examiner places one hand under the occiput of the supine patient and lifts the child. If the neck does not flex, it is stiff. Alternatively, a sitting child may be observed following an object as it falls to the floor. The child who flexes the neck to look at the object does not have nuchal rigidity. In the presence of meningitis, flexion of the neck causes spontaneous flexion of the legs at the hips and knees, known as the **Brudzinski sign** (Fig. 52.1). The **Kernig sign** is elicited when the patient lies supine and, with the knee flexed, the leg is flexed at the hip. The knee is then extended. A positive sign is present if this movement is limited by contraction of the hamstrings and causes pain. Nuchal rigidity is absent in 1.5% of older children with meningitis; it may be absent in children who have overwhelming infections, who are deeply comatose, or who have focal or global neurologic impairment.

As many as 15% of children with bacterial meningitis initially present in a **comatose** or semi-comatose state (see Chapter 41). Because of the short duration and inconsistent development of increased intracranial pressure, **papilledema** is usually not seen at presentation. When it is present, venous sinus thrombosis, subdural effusion, or an intracranial abscess must be considered. **Seizures** occur before hospital admission in up to 20% of affected patients.

Children with meningitis may also present with cutaneous findings. Although commonly associated with meningococcal disease, purpura, petechiae, or a diffuse nonspecific maculopapular rash may be present

in meningitis caused by any of the common bacterial pathogens (see Chapter 53).

Septic arthritis may be seen simultaneously with bacterial meningitis. This has been assumed to be caused by simultaneous localizing infection after a primary bacteremia. Reactive arthritis caused by immune complex deposition is also seen with bacterial meningitis. This arthritis affects a single large joint and appears 5–7 days after initiation of treatment for meningitis. In general, arthritis occurring acutely with meningitis should be assumed to be infectious (see Chapter 44).

Various eye disorders have also been described with acute bacterial meningitis, including photophobia, transient cataracts, paralysis of the extraocular muscles, pupillary dysfunction, dendritic ulcers, endophthalmitis, cortical blindness, and conjunctivitis.

Recurrent episodes of bacterial meningitis occur rarely. Potential etiologies include congenital CSF fistulas (inner ear, dermal sinus, neuroenteric cysts, lumbosacral sinus tracts), traumatic or surgical CSF fistula (skull fracture, postoperative nasal surgery, cochlear implant), immunodeficiency states, and parameningeal infections (mastoiditis, sinusitis, craniofacial osteomyelitis). Recurrent nonbacterial lymphocytic meningitis (**Mollaret meningitis**) may be due to HSV-1, HSV-2, or Epstein-Barr virus (EBV); HaNDL (headache and neurologic deficits with CSF lymphocytes) is another recurrent syndrome that mimics meningitis.

Diagnostic studies

Lumbar puncture and cerebrospinal fluid analysis. The definitive diagnosis of meningitis is based on examination of the CSF. The CSF is usually obtained via an LP (or spinal tap). The LP is performed by introducing a small-bore, short-beveled spinal needle with a stylet into the subarachnoid space at the L3–L4 or L4–L5 level. Approximately 3 mL of fluid is removed for analysis.

There are a few contraindications for the performance of an LP. The first is cardiorespiratory compromise. Performance of the LP requires that the child be held in flexion to open the intervertebral spaces. In seriously ill children or children with significant cardiac or pulmonary compromise, this positioning may be enough to cause respiratory arrest. The LP may need to be postponed, be performed cautiously with continuous cardiorespiratory monitoring, or be performed with the patient in the sitting position.

Second, children with **increased intracranial pressure** from a focal CNS lesion, such as brain abscess or tumor or from illnesses associated with cerebral edema, have a risk of cerebral herniation after an LP. If signs or symptoms of increased intracranial pressure are present, the LP should be postponed until the increased pressure is lowered with appropriate treatment. *If an LP is delayed, appropriate antibiotic therapy should be initiated without further delay.* Third, the LP should not be done if the spinal needle must pass through an area of infection on its way to the subarachnoid space. To do so might introduce pathogens into the CNS that could cause meningitis.

Complications of LP are uncommon. In children with underlying or temporary bleeding disorders, epidural hematomas causing lower limb paralysis may occur. In children with hemophilia, disseminated intravascular coagulopathy, or thrombocytopenia, LP should be postponed until the bleeding disorder is corrected. Extra care should be taken to avoid a traumatic LP, and patients should be monitored for postprocedure neurologic deficits. *Empirical therapy may be started while the coagulopathy is corrected.* Other, rarer complications of LP include cortical blindness from compression of the posterior cerebral artery against the tentorium cerebelli and cervical spinal cord infarction from herniation of the cerebellar tonsils through the foramen magnum. Post-LP headache may occur in up to 10% of older children and adults; it is presumably caused by persistent CSF leakage at the puncture site.

Opening pressure measurements are obtained with the head of the bed flat and with the child relaxed and in the lateral decubitus position with the back no longer tightly flexed. The upper limit of normal opening pressure depends on age (5 cm H_2O in premature infants, 10 cm H_2O in infants, and 25–28 cm H_2O in children 1–18 years of age). Opening pressure measurements are elevated if the LP is performed with the patient in the sitting position and if the patient is combative or performing the Valsalva maneuver. Obstructive hydrocephalus, hyperventilation, or removal of fluid can all lead to lowering of the measurement. Children with bacterial meningitis have a mean opening pressure of 18 ± 7 cm H_2O.

The CSF is examined for red blood cell (RBC) number, WBC number and differential, glucose, protein, and the presence of pathogenic organisms by stain, rapid testing (antigen and PCR), or culture.

Normal CSF is clear and colorless (Table 52.6). Blood in the CSF indicates a traumatic LP (also known as a "traumatic tap") or a CNS hemorrhage. A traumatic tap occurs when the spinal needle is advanced through the subarachnoid space and penetrates the richly vascularized ventral epidural space. Blood is thereby introduced into the subarachnoid space, and the CSF appears bloody. Obtaining an RBC count on tubes 1 and 3 may be informative because the count is unchanged in CNS hemorrhage but may decline in traumatic taps. Centrifugation of

TABLE 52.6 Cerebrospinal Fluid Findings in Central Nervous System Disorders

Condition	Pressure (cm H_2O)	Leukocytes (cells/mm³)	Protein (mg/dL)	Glucose (mg/dL)	Comments
Normal	<28	<5, ≥75% Lymphocytes In neonates: <20	20–45	>50 (or 66–75% serum glucose)	
Common Forms of Meningitis					
Acute bacterial meningitis	Usually elevated	100–10,000 or more; usually 300–2,000; PMNs predominate	Usually 100–500	Decreased, usually <40 (or <50% serum glucose)	Organisms usually seen on Gram stain and isolated by culture
Partially treated bacterial meningitis	Normal or elevated	5–10,000; PMNs usual but mononuclear cells may predominate if pretreated for extended period	Usually 100–500	Normal or decreased	Organisms may be seen on Gram stain. Pretreatment may render CSF sterile. PCR-based assays may detect bacterial DNA
Viral meningitis or meningoencephalitis	Normal or slightly elevated	Rarely >1,000 cells. Eastern equine encephalitis and lymphocytic choriomeningitis may have cell counts of several thousand. PMNs early but mononuclear cells predominate through most of the course	Usually 50–200	Generally normal; may be decreased to <40 in some viral diseases, particularly mumps (15–20% of cases)	HSV encephalitis is suggested by focal seizures or by focal findings on MRI or CT scans or EEG. Most arboviruses detected by serology. Most other viruses detected by PCR of CSF
Uncommon Forms of Meningitis					
Tuberculous meningitis	Usually elevated	10–500; PMNs early, but lymphocytes predominate through most of the course	100–3,000; may be higher in presence of block	<50 in most cases; decreases with time if treatment is not provided	Acid-fast organisms rarely seen on smear. Large volumes of CSF required for recovery of organisms. *Mycobacterium tuberculosis* may be detected by PCR of CSF
Fungal meningitis	Usually elevated	5–500; PMNs early but mononuclear cells predominate through most of the course. Cryptococcal meningitis may lack pleocytosis. Coccidioidal meningitis may have eosinophilia	25–500	<50; decreases with time if treatment is not provided	Budding yeast may be seen. Organisms may be recovered in culture. Cryptococcal antigen (CSF and serum) may be positive in cryptococcal infection
Syphilis (acute) and leptospirosis	Usually elevated	50–500; lymphocytes predominate	50–200	Usually normal	Positive CSF serology. Spirochetes not demonstrable by usual techniques of smear or culture; dark-field examination may be positive
Amebic (*Naegleria*) meningoencephalitis	Elevated	1,000–10,000 or more; PMNs predominate	50–500	Normal or slightly decreased	Mobile amoebae may be seen by wet-mount microscopy of CSF

TABLE 52.6 Cerebrospinal Fluid Findings in Central Nervous System Disorders—cont'd

Condition	Pressure (cm H₂O)	Leukocytes (cells/mm³)	Protein (mg/dL)	Glucose (mg/dL)	Comments
Brain Abscesses and Parameningeal Focus					
Brain abscess	Usually elevated	5–200; CSF rarely acellular; lymphocytes predominate; if abscess ruptures into ventricle, PMNs predominate and cell count may reach >100,000	75–500	Normal unless abscess ruptures into ventricular system	CSF cultures are only positive in 24% of cases unless abscess ruptures into ventricular system
Subdural empyema	Usually elevated	100–5,000; PMNs predominate	100–500	Normal	No organisms on smear or culture of CSF unless meningitis also present; organisms found on tap of subdural fluid
Cerebral epidural abscess	Normal to slightly elevated	10–500; lymphocytes predominate	50–200	Normal	No organisms on smear or culture of CSF
Spinal epidural abscess	Usually low, with spinal block	10–100; lymphocytes predominate	50–400	Normal	No organisms on smear or culture of CSF
Chemical (drugs, dermoid cysts, myelography dye)	Usually elevated	100–1,000 or more; PMNs predominate	50–100	Normal or slightly decreased	Epithelial cells may be seen within CSF by use of polarized light in some children with ruptured dermoids
Noninfectious Causes					
Sarcoidosis	Normal or elevated slightly	0–100; mononuclear	40–100	Normal	No specific findings
Systemic lupus erythematosus with CNS involvement	Slightly elevated	0–500; PMNs usually predominate; lymphocytes may be present	100	Normal or slightly decreased	No organisms on smear or culture. Positive neuronal and ribosomal P protein antibodies in CSF
Tumor, leukemia	Slightly elevated to very high	0–100 or more; mononuclear or blast cells	50–1,000	Normal to decreased (20–40)	Cytology may be positive
Acute disseminated encephalomyelitis	Normal or elevated	~100 lymphocytes	Normal to elevated	Normal	MRI adds to diagnosis
Autoimmune encephalitis	Normal	~100 lymphocytes	Normal to elevated	Normal	Anti-NMDAR antibody positive (CSF is more sensitive than serum)

CSF, cerebrospinal fluid; HSV, herpes simplex virus; NMDAR, N-methyl-ᴅ-aspartate receptor; PCR, polymerase chain reaction; PMN, polymorphonuclear neutrophils.

From Janowski AB and Hunstad DA. Central nervous system infections. In: Kliegman RM, St. Geme JW III, Blum NJ, et al., eds. *Nelson Textbook of Pediatrics*, 21st ed. Philadelphia: Elsevier; 2020:322–323, Table 621.1.

the CSF sample may also help differentiate between a traumatic tap and a CNS hemorrhage. When blood has been present in the CSF for several hours, the CSF is xanthochromic after centrifugation. However, if the blood was recently mixed with CSF, as in the case of a traumatic tap, the supernatant is clear. Xanthochromic CSF can also be caused by icterus or an elevated CSF protein concentration.

The normal values for CSF WBC are shown in Table 52.6. Most children with bacterial meningitis have a WBC count of at least 100/mm³ in their CSF, but in general, more than 5 cells/mm³ in children after the neonatal period is considered abnormal. Normal CSF WBC values for neonates are higher than for older children, but reference ranges have been revised to lower numbers with the availability of high-quality data on noninfected neonates. Mean CSF WBC in the absence of viral or bacterial meningitis is 8.6 cells/mm³ and 3.6 cells/mm³ in the first week of life and weeks 1–8, respectively. A CSF absolute neutrophil count exceeding 3 neutrophils/mm³ is also considered abnormal and evidence of a bacterial infection. Although rapidly fulminant meningitis may not be accompanied by CSF pleocytosis on initial examination, the CSF of 98% of children with bacterial meningitis has pleocytosis with a differential of more than 50% neutrophils. CSF with at least 200–400 WBCs/mm³ will appear visually turbid.

It is sometimes difficult to know whether the WBCs seen on examination of the CSF are caused by CSF pleocytosis or are peripheral blood WBCs contaminating the CSF. To aid in this determination, the ratio of WBCs to RBCs in the CSF is compared with the ratio of WBCs to RBCs in the patient's peripheral blood collected around the same time. A higher ratio in the CSF can indicate the presence of CSF pleocytosis. When the CSF ratio is at least 10 times higher than the blood ratio, bacterial meningitis is favored, with a sensitivity of 88% and a specificity of 90%. Conversely, the negative predictive value for the presence of bacterial meningitis of a <10-fold difference between the ratios is 99%. Traumatic taps usually do not alter the CSF glucose,

Gram stain, or culture findings, which are often abnormal with bacterial meningitis. When there is doubt about the validity of the cell count after a potentially traumatic tap, the LP should be repeated after several hours by introducing the spinal needle one intervertebral space above the original tap site.

In normal CSF, the glucose concentration is two-thirds that of serum glucose concentration. The CSF glucose concentration is low in most infants and younger children with bacterial meningitis and in 45% of school-aged children with bacterial meningitis. In children older than 2 months of age, a CSF/serum glucose ratio of <0.4 is 80% sensitive and 98% specific for the presence of bacterial meningitis. The presence of RBCs in a CSF sample that is promptly analyzed does not affect the glucose concentration.

The normal CSF protein concentration is <45 mg/dL in children older than 2 months. The mean CSF protein concentration is 90 (range, 20–170) in full-term infants and 115 (range, 65–150) in preterm infants. The CSF protein concentration is elevated in more than 90% of younger children with bacterial meningitis but in only 60% of infected school-aged children. Every 1,000 RBCs in the CSF (from a traumatic tap) increases the protein concentration by approximately 1 mg/dL.

Microscopic examination of a CSF Gram stain for bacteria should be performed routinely, with results used to expand the differential diagnosis. Due to inherent inaccuracies in the technique, antibiotics should never be narrowed based on Gram stain results alone. The sensitivity of this test is directly related to the number of organisms in the CSF and is inversely related to the age of the patient. Additional stains (fungal, mycobacterial) may be indicated depending on the clinical circumstances. Rapid pathogen identification can be accomplished with antigen testing (such as for *Cryptococcus* species) and PCR. Targeted PCR, most commonly for enterovirus and HSV, and multiplex PCR panels have proven to be sensitive diagnostic tools in the evaluation of CNS infections. Indiscriminate use of multiplex PCR panels may increase costs and identify the presence of organisms that are not contributing to the current illness (such as chromosomally integrated HHV-6). PCR for bacterial organisms may increase the diagnostic yield in patients treated with antibiotics before CSF is obtained. Culture remains the gold standard for the identification of bacterial pathogens and permits the assessment of antibiotic susceptibility. In circumstances in which the causative pathogen remains elusive, unbiased next-generation sequencing (NGS) of CSF may be used.

In patients who have been treated with antibiotics before the LP is performed, bacterial meningitis cannot be ruled out based on Gram stain or culture alone. The presence of abnormalities of CSF cell count (including elevated leukocytes), protein concentration, and glucose concentration is compatible with the diagnosis of bacterial meningitis and will likely result in presumptive treatment for bacterial meningitis based on age and comorbidities. If an organism is identified by culture or PCR, definitive antibiotic treatment is administered. If no organism is identified, the decision to continue treatment depends on the clinical suspicion of bacterial meningitis and the exclusion of other causes of aseptic meningitis (Tables 52.7 and 52.8).

TABLE 52.7 **Clinical Conditions and Infectious Agents Associated with Aseptic Meningitis**

Viruses	Bacteria
Arboviruses: La Crosse, eastern equine, western equine, Venezuelan equine, St. Louis encephalitis, Powassan and California encephalitis, chikungunya, Colorado tick fever, dengue, Jamestown Canyon, Japanese encephalitis, Rift Valley fever, tick-borne encephalitis, West Nile virus, Zika	Mycobacterium tuberculosis (early and late)
	Leptospira species (leptospirosis)
	Treponema pallidum (syphilis)
	Borrelia species (tick-borne relapsing fever or hard tick relapsing fever)
Enteroviruses (coxsackievirus, echovirus, enterovirus, poliovirus)	*Borrelia burgdorferi* (Lyme disease)
Parechovirus	*Nocardia* species
Herpes simplex (types 1 and 2)	*Brucella* species
Varicella-zoster virus	*Bartonella* species (cat-scratch disease)
Epstein-Barr virus	*Rickettsia rickettsiae* (Rocky Mountain spotted fever)
Cytomegalovirus	*Rickettsia prowazekii* (typhus)
Human herpesvirus (types 6 and 7)	*Ehrlichia* species
Parvovirus B19	*Anaplasma* species
Adenovirus	*Coxiella burnetii*
Variola (smallpox)	*Mycoplasma pneumoniae*
Measles	*Mycoplasma hominis*
Mumps	*Chlamydia trachomatis*
Rubella	*Chlamydia psittaci*
Influenza A and B	*Chlamydia pneumoniae*
Parainfluenza	*Ureaplasma* species
Rhinovirus	Partially treated bacterial meningitis
Rabies virus	
Lymphocytic choriomeningitis	**Bacterial Parameningeal Focus**
Rotaviruses	Sinusitis
Cardiovirus A	Mastoiditis
Hendra and Nipah viruses	Brain abscess
Astroviruses	Subdural-epidural empyema
Coronaviruses	Cranial osteomyelitis
Human T-cell lymphotropic virus (HTLV-1)	
HIV	

TABLE 52.7 Clinical Conditions and Infectious Agents Associated with Aseptic Meningitis—cont'd

Fungi

Coccidioides immitis (coccidioidomycosis)

Blastomyces dermatitidis (blastomycosis)

Cryptococcus neoformans (cryptococcosis)

Histoplasma capsulatum (histoplasmosis)

Candida species

Other fungi (*Alternaria, Aspergillus, Cephalosporium, Cladosporium, Bipolaris hawaiiensis, Paracoccidioides brasiliensis, Pseudallescheria boydii, Sporothrix schenckii, Ustilago* species, zygomycetes)

Parasites (Eosinophilic)

Angiostrongylus cantonensis

Gnathostoma spinigerum

Baylisascaris procyonis (raccoon roundworm)

Strongyloides stercoralis

Trichinella spiralis

Toxocara canis

Taenia solium (cysticercosis)

Paragonimus westermani

Schistosoma species

Fasciola species

Parasites (Noneosinophilic)

Toxoplasma gondii (toxoplasmosis)

Acanthamoeba species

Naegleria fowleri

Balamuthia mandrillaris

Malaria

Postinfectious

Vaccines: rabies, influenza, measles, poliovirus

Demyelinating or allergic encephalitis

Systemic or Immunologically Mediated

Acute disseminated encephalomyelitis (ADEM)

Autoimmune encephalitis

Bacterial endocarditis

Kawasaki disease

Systemic lupus erythematosus

Vasculitis, including polyarteritis nodosa

Sjögren syndrome

Mixed connective tissue disease

Rheumatoid arthritis

Behçet syndrome

Granulomatosis with polyangiitis

Lymphomatoid granulomatosis

Granulomatous arteritis

Sarcoidosis

Familial Mediterranean fever

Vogt-Koyanagi-Harada syndrome

Neonatal onset multisystem inflammatory disease (NOMID)

Sweet syndrome (acute febrile neutrophilic dermatosis)

Aicardi-Goutières syndrome

Malignancy

Leukemia

Lymphoma

Metastatic carcinoma

Central nervous system tumor (e.g., craniopharyngioma, glioma, ependymoma, astrocytoma, medulloblastoma, teratoma)

Drugs

Intrathecal injections (contrast media, serum, antibiotics, antineoplastic agents)

Nonsteroidal antiinflammatory agents

OKT3 monoclonal antibodies

Carbamazepine

Azathioprine

Intravenous immunoglobulin

Antibiotics (trimethoprim-sulfamethoxazole, sulfasalazine, ciprofloxacin, isoniazid)

Miscellaneous

Heavy metal poisoning (lead, arsenic)

Foreign bodies (shunt, reservoir)

Subarachnoid hemorrhage

Postictal state

Postmigraine state

Mollaret syndrome (recurrent)

Intraventricular hemorrhage (neonate)

Familial hemophagocytic syndrome

Postneurosurgical procedure

Dermoid-epidermoid cyst

Syndrome of transient headache and neurologic deficits with cerebrospinal fluid lymphocytosis (HaNDL)

Data from Bronstein DE, Glaser CA. Aseptic meningitis and viral meningitis. In: Cherry J, Demmler-Harrison GJ, Kaplan SL, et al., eds. *Feigin and Cherry's Textbook of Pediatric Infectious Diseases*. 7th ed. Philadelphia: WB Saunders; 2014:484–492; and from Romero JR. Aseptic and viral meningitis. In: Long SS, Pickering LK, Prober CG, eds. *Principles and Practice of Pediatric Infectious Disease*. 4th ed. Philadelphia: Saunders; 2012:292–297.

Computed tomography. Routine CT of the head is not indicated in children with suspected meningitis. Nonfocal increases in intracranial pressure typical of bacterial meningitis do not result in cerebral herniation with LP and may appear normal on CT. CT should be reserved for children who show clinical signs of herniation or cerebral edema and for those with focal symptoms concerning for an intracranial mass.

Other laboratory tests. Bacterial meningitis is usually accompanied by elevated peripheral blood WBC and platelet counts, but leukopenia and thrombocytopenia may also be seen in the case of overwhelming infection. The sensitivity (70%), specificity (54%), and

negative predictive value (81%) of the differential WBC count are too low to render the differential WBC examination useful in making the diagnosis of bacterial meningitis.

Blood cultures may be useful in identifying the bacterial pathogen of meningitis. However, blood culture is negative in up to 33% of children with meningococcal, 20% with pneumococcal, and 10% with *H. influenzae* type b meningitis. Sensitivity of blood culture further decreases with prior antibiotic exposure. In addition, there is a negative correlation between the length of illness before diagnosis and the rate of positive blood cultures. A bacterial meningitis score has been developed to attempt to distinguish between bacterial and aseptic (i.e.,

TABLE 52.8   Characteristics of the Most Common Causes of Aseptic Meningitis

Organism	Age Group	Season	Prodrome	Clinical Characteristics	Epidemiologic Characteristics	Agent Identification	Serologic Diagnosis
Common							
Enteroviruses	Infants, young children	Summer, fall	None, or mild GI or pharyngitis syndrome for 1–3 days	Exanthem, myopericarditis, conjunctivitis, pleurodynia, hand-foot-mouth disease, herpangina, myositis, hepatitis	Epidemic	PCR of CSF, blood, throat, stool	Paired IgG (rarely used)
Arboviruses	Children, elderly	Summer, early fall	Fever, rash, malaise for 1–5 days	Encephalitis or aseptic meningitis	Geographic area, contact with insect vector, encephalitis in community or animals	PCR of CSF for some	IgM, paired IgG (serum or CSF)
Herpes simplex type 2	Neonates, young adults	Year round	Fever (neonate), genital vesicles for 1–7 days	Associated primary herpes lesions	Perinatal or sexual exposure	PCR or culture of genital/skin lesions; PCR (CSF)	IgM, paired IgG
Borrelia burgdorferi (Lyme disease)	Children, adults	Spring–late fall	Erythema migrans; secondary symptoms weeks to months later	Facial palsy or other cranial nerve palsy; radiculitis; heart block	Endemic area, deer tick exposure (often unrecognized)	PCR (CSF) (low sensitivity)	EIA screen with Western blot confirmation
Less Common							
Mumps	5–9 yr olds	Late winter–spring	Parotitis, orchitis: 2–10 days	Parotitis, orchitis, oophoritis, pancreatitis	Exposure to mumps or vaccination	PCR (CSF or throat)	IgM, paired IgG
HIV	Young adults	Year round	Fever, arthralgias, maculopapular rash, pharyngitis, adenopathy	Same as prodrome; meningitis may occur 1–5 days into the illness	2–6 wk after sexual or blood exposure	PCR (RNA, blood)	Fourth-generation Ag/Ab test (may be negative at this stage)
Lymphocytic choriomeningitis virus	Older children, young adults	Fall, early winter	Fever and flulike syndrome, 5–21 days	Orchitis, alopecia	Exposure to mice, hamsters	PCR (CSF or blood)	IgG
Mycobacterium tuberculosis	Infants (primary infection), young adults (reactivation)	Year round	Fever	Pneumonia, basilar inflammation with cranial nerve palsy and intracranial hypertension	History of tuberculosis or exposure, HIV risk factors	Culture, PCR (CSF)	None
Leptospira	Young adults	Late summer, early fall	Hepatitis and hematuria, 1–7 days	Conjunctivitis, splenomegaly, jaundice, nephritis, rash	Exposure to animals, water contaminated with animal urine	Culture (blood, CSF, or urine)	Paired IgG
Fungal	Premature infant, young adult	Year round	Fever	Basilar inflammation on CT or MRI, cranial nerve findings	Endemic area (blastomycosis, histoplasmosis) Immunodeficiency (cryptococcosis) Prematurity (candidiasis)	Culture (CSF), antigen (select species), meningeal biopsy	Specific IgG
Mycoplasma organisms	Children, young adults	Fall, winter	Fever, malaise, sore throat, cough	Cough, rash, hemolytic anemia	Family or community epidemic	PCR (CSF or nasopharyngeal)	IgM (false positive common)

CSF, cerebral spinal fluid; EIA, enzyme immunoassay; GI, gastrointestinal; IgG and IgM, immunoglobulins G and M; PCR, polymerase chain reaction.

Modified from Connolly KJ, Hammer SM. The acute aseptic meningitis syndrome. *Infect Dis Clin North Am.* 1990;4:599–622; and from Davis LE. Aseptic and viral meningitis. In: Long SS, Pickering LK, Prober CG, eds. *Principles and Practice of Pediatric Infectious Disease.* New York: Churchill Livingstone; 1997:331.

nonbacterial) meningitis in patients with CSF pleocytosis. The risk of bacterial meningitis is low if *none* of the following criteria are present: history of a seizure with the illness, blood neutrophil count ≥10 × 10⁹ cells/L, positive CSF Gram stain, CSF protein ≥80 mg/dL, or CSF neutrophil count ≥1 × 10⁹ cells/L. This diagnostic tool is 99% sensitive and 62% specific for bacterial meningitis. It should only be applied to non–ill-appearing children older than 2 months without petechiae, purpura, or other concerning findings on examination who have not been pretreated with antibiotics.

Aseptic Meningitis

Aseptic meningitis is an inflammatory process of the meninges, most often characterized by acute signs and symptoms of meningeal irritation; mononuclear CSF pleocytosis (predominance of monocytes, macrophages, and/or lymphocytes); a normal or, less frequently, elevated CSF protein concentration; normal or, less often, low CSF glucose concentration; and no organisms demonstrable by Gram stain or bacterial cultures. There are many causes of aseptic meningitis (see Table 52.7). The most common cause is viral infection; up to 90% of cases are caused by enteroviruses and arboviruses (see Chapter 42). The definitive diagnosis is made by identifying the organism in the CSF. However, this is not always possible, and other causes must be excluded by history, presence or absence of associated symptoms, and appropriate laboratory tests (see Tables 52.7 and 52.8).

Viral meningitis. The most common pathogens to cause viral meningitis are enteroviruses. Enteroviral meningitis occurs most often during the summer and early fall months. Transmission is via the fecal-oral route, and young children exhibit increased transmission of the viruses and more severe disease in comparison with other age groups. Initially, patients may have a respiratory tract infection, a nonspecific febrile illness, or vomiting and diarrhea. Viral infection of the meninges occurs 7–10 days after initial exposure. The clinical course may be biphasic. Virus from the oropharynx can be cultured only during the first 5–7 days of the illness but may be excreted in stool for 6–8 weeks.

Children with viral meningitis present with fever, nuchal rigidity, irritability, headache, and vomiting. Less common symptoms are anorexia, drowsiness, photophobia, myalgia, and malaise. Affected young infants often lack meningeal signs. In addition, children may have an altered sensorium, but focal neurologic signs are rare. Seizures are more common in infants.

The number of WBCs in the CSF varies from zero to several thousand (see Table 52.6). Up to 75% of *initial (early in the illness)* CSF specimens contain a predominance of polymorphonuclear cells. Mononuclear cells predominate by 2 days after the onset of symptoms. Of children with enteroviral meningitis, 18% may have decreased CSF glucose concentrations, whereas 12% may have elevated CSF protein. Aseptic meningitis secondary to parechovirus may have no CSF pleocytosis. *Meningitis due to Lyme disease may mimic viral meningitis in both clinical presentation and CSF findings.* It is important to differentiate viral meningitis from Lyme meningitis (which is treatable) in endemic areas.

Treatment of enteroviral meningitis is supportive. Admission to the hospital may be required while bacterial meningitis is being ruled out and for intravenous hydration. Analgesics and antipyretics may also be indicated. The LP performed to diagnose viral meningitis is often helpful in ameliorating the acute symptoms. The mechanism for this is not clear.

The outcome is quite good for children in whom common viral pathogens cause aseptic meningitis. Multisystem organ involvement may occur in neonates with enterovirus infections, including septic shock, hepatitis, myocarditis, and respiratory failure. Long-term adverse outcomes are more common (but unusual) in children who have viral

meningitis during the first year of life. Speech and language development may be affected. Treatment and outcome for the other types of aseptic meningitis depend on the underlying cause.

Tuberculous meningitis. Tuberculous meningitis is an important treatable cause of aseptic meningitis. During the primary pulmonary tuberculous infection and subsequent lymphohematogenous spread to extrapulmonary sites, tubercle bacilli produce local microscopic granulomas in the CNS and meninges. If this primary CNS infection is not contained by host defense mechanisms (T lymphocytes, monocytes), or if host defense mechanisms fail at a later period, tuberculous meningitis may result. Meningitis occurs weeks to months after the primary pulmonary process. Miliary tuberculosis is a risk factor for TB meningitis.

The symptoms of tuberculous meningitis are insidious and subacute (weeks to months). Stage 1 is a prodrome with nonspecific manifestations (apathy, poor school function, irritability, weight loss, fever, night sweats, nausea); stage 2 is heralded by the onset of neurologic signs (headache, cranial neuropathy, nuchal rigidity, signs of increased intracranial pressure); and stage 3 manifests with altered levels of consciousness (lethargy, stupor, coma). Meningismus may be absent.

The diagnosis is supported by a history of contact with adults with known active tuberculosis, a chronic cough, or HIV disease, or by a history of immigration, poverty, or homelessness. In addition, the patient's chest radiograph is consistent with active or, often, quiescent tuberculosis (parenchymal-hilar node calcifications, infiltrates, hilar adenopathy, and, in rare cases, endobronchial or cavitary lesions), and the patient's tuberculin skin test or interferon-γ release assay may yield a positive result (see Chapter 3). Cranial CT or MRI may show the intense meningeal inflammation around the base of the brain or inflammatory mass lesions (tuberculomas). The CSF results (see Table 52.6) include profound hypoglycorrhachia, a high CSF protein, lymphocyte- or monocyte-predominant cells (usually 500 cells/mm³), increased opening pressure, and, on occasion, organisms on acid-fast staining. PCR amplification of *Mycobacterium tuberculosis* DNA aids in making a more rapid diagnosis than does culture of CSF, sputum, or gastric aspirates, which traditionally requires 2–6 weeks. The differential diagnosis depends on the stage of the illness.

Encephalitis and Meningoencephalitis

Encephalitis is inflammation of the brain parenchyma, whereas **meningoencephalitis** is inflammation of the brain accompanied by inflammation of the meninges (see Chapter 42). Meningoencephalitis is distinguished from aseptic meningitis by evidence of brain parenchymal involvement, including behavior or personality changes; altered level of consciousness (including agitation or coma); generalized seizures; focal neurologic signs, including focal seizures and focal motor defects (hemiparesis or ataxia); or movement disorders. The differential diagnosis is broad, inclusive of both infectious and noninfectious etiologies. Despite broad diagnostic testing, an etiologic agent is identified in less than half of cases.

Enteroviruses and arboviruses are the most commonly identified causes of infectious encephalitis in children. Enterovirus encephalitis, uncommon without meningeal involvement, is suggested by epidemic occurrence and presence of typical prodrome or associated findings (see Table 52.8); diagnosis is by PCR for enterovirus in CSF, blood, throat, or stool specimens. A CSF or blood specimen is preferred because enterovirus persists in the throat and especially stool for weeks after the primary infection has resolved and its presence in stool is nonspecific. Arbovirus encephalitis is suggested by mosquito or tick exposure and epidemic occurrence and is diagnosed by findings of arbovirus immunoglobulin M (IgM) in CSF or blood or by paired serologic findings (acute and convalescent serology) for IgG.

HSV is a treatable cause of encephalitis. In neonates, HSV encephalitis usually occurs between 7 and 21 days of age; may produce focal or generalized CNS disease; and may occur with or without conjunctivitis, oral mucosal involvement, vesicles on skin, or disseminated disease (hepatitis, pneumonia, septic appearance). After the neonatal period, HSV encephalitis is usually isolated to the CNS and classically produces necrotizing encephalitis with a focus in the temporal lobe. Symptoms in persons with HSV encephalitis range broadly from those suggesting mild aseptic meningitis to the presence of status epilepticus and coma and then death. In addition to elevated WBC, CSF examination later in infection may show increased numbers of erythrocytes and elevated protein due to parenchymal brain involvement. CT, MRI, and EEG may suggest a temporal lobe focus. Specific diagnosis is by PCR of CSF for HSV DNA. In the appropriate clinical setting, presumptive therapy with high-dose intravenous acyclovir is indicated while awaiting the results of PCR of CSF for HSV.

Autoimmune encephalitis, such as anti-N-methyl-D-aspartate receptor (anti-NMDAR) encephalitis, is a relatively common form of noninfectious encephalitis. Data from the California Encephalitis Project showed that anti-NMDAR encephalitis was the most common *identifiable* cause of encephalitis in their cohort, which included patients from 6 months to 30 years. Most of the cases occurred in children and adolescents. Patients present with features similar to viral encephalitis, but seizures, language dysfunction, psychosis, autonomic dysfunction, movement disorders, and EEG abnormalities are more common in these patients.

FEVER OF UNKNOWN ORIGIN

Daily fevers lasting more than a week with no diagnosis apparent after initial history and physical examination are termed FUO. The differential diagnosis for FUO in children is broad (Table 52.9). The most commonly identified etiology for FUO in children is infection, with rates as high as 51% depending on the practice setting and availability of diagnostic testing. Infections identified included UTI and tuberculosis in all children; osteomyelitis and bartonellosis in countries with higher baseline socioeconomic status; and brucellosis and typhoid in countries with lower baseline socioeconomic status. Other significant causes of FUO are collagen vascular disease, malignancy, Kawasaki disease, and inflammatory bowel disease. Often patients with FUO have atypical manifestations of common childhood bacterial or viral diseases rather than unusual or uncommon disorders. Approximately one quarter of FUO resolves without diagnosis.

The evaluation of a child with FUO centers on serial histories and physical examinations. Repeated history taking is useful because parents often remember important details after the initial interview. The physical examination findings may also change during the course of the investigation, revealing important clues (Fig. 52.2 and Table 52.10). Clues to the diagnosis are noted in Tables 52.11 and 52.12.

History

The detailed history should include the time of day of the fever, who measured the temperature, and the instrument that was used to measure the temperature. Increased temperatures after exercise and in the

---

TABLE 52.9   Etiology of Fever of Unknown Origin (FUO) in Children

Abscesses
Brain
Hepatic
Intraabdominal*
Odontogenic (dental)
Pelvic*
Perinephric and renal
Psoas
Rectal
Subphrenic

Bacterial Diseases
Actinomycosis
Bartonella henselae (cat-scratch disease)*
Brucellosis
Campylobacter
Chlamydia
Francisella tularensis (tularemia)
Fusobacterium (Lemierre syndrome)
Leptospirosis
Listeria monocytogenes (listeriosis)
Lymphogranuloma venereum
Meningococcemia (chronic)
Mycoplasma pneumoniae
Psittacosis
Rat-bite fever (*Streptobacillus moniliformis*; streptobacillary form of rat-bite fever)
Salmonella
Tuberculosis*
Whipple disease
Yersiniosis

Localized Infections
Bacterial endocarditis*
Cholangitis
Ludwig angina
Mastoiditis
Osteomyelitis*
Pericarditis
Pneumonia
Pyelonephritis*
Sinusitis
Spondylodiskitis

Spirochetes
Borrelia burgdorferi (Lyme disease)
Leptospirosis
Rat-bite fever (*Spirillum minus*; spirillary form of rat-bite fever)
Relapsing fever (*Borrelia recurrentis, Borrelia miyamotoi*)
Syphilis

Fungal Diseases
Blastomycosis (extrapulmonary)
Coccidioidomycosis (disseminated)
Cryptococcosis
Histoplasmosis (disseminated)

Rickettsiae-like Organisms
Anaplasmosis
Ehrlichiosis
Q fever
Rocky Mountain spotted fever
Tick-borne typhus

TABLE 52.9 Etiology of Fever of Unknown Origin (FUO) in Children—cont'd

Viruses
Arboviruses
Cytomegalovirus*
Epstein-Barr virus*
Hantavirus
Hepatitis viruses
HIV
Human herpesviruses (HHV-6 and HHV-7)
Lymphocytic choriomeningitis
Respiratory viruses (especially, adenovirus and enteroviruses)*

Parasitic Diseases
Amebiasis
Babesiosis
Baylisascaris
Malaria
Naegleria
Toxoplasmosis
Trichinosis
Trypanosomiasis
Visceral larva migrans (Toxocara)

Rheumatologic Diseases
Autoimmune hepatitis
Behçet syndrome
Chronic noninfectious osteomyelitis (CNO)
Juvenile dermatomyositis
Juvenile idiopathic arthritis* ± macrophage activation syndrome
Rheumatic fever
Systemic lupus erythematosus*
Vasculitis syndromes (granulomatous, nongranulomatous)

Hypersensitivity Diseases
Drug fever
Hypersensitivity pneumonitis
Hypersensitivity vasculitis/reactive arthritis*
Serum sickness
Weber-Christian disease

Neoplasms
Atrial myxoma
Cholesterol granuloma
Hodgkin lymphoma
Inflammatory pseudotumor
Langerhans cell histiocytosis
Leukemia
Lymphoma*
Pheochromocytoma
Neuroblastoma
Wilms tumor

Granulomatous Diseases
Crohn disease
Granulomatous hepatitis
Polyangiitis with granulomatosis
Sarcoidosis

Familial and Hereditary Diseases
Anhidrotic ectodermal dysplasia
Autoimmune lymphoproliferative syndrome (ALPS)
Autonomic neuropathies
Fabry disease
Familial dysautonomia
Familial Hibernian fever
Familial Mediterranean fever and the many other autoinflammatory (periodic fever) diseases (see Chapter 54)
Hypertriglyceridemia
Ichthyosis
Sickle cell crisis
Spinal cord/brain injury

Miscellaneous
Addison disease
Allergic alveolitis
Castleman disease (see Chapter 48)
Cyclic neutropenia
Diabetes insipidus (non-nephrogenic and nephrogenic)
Factitious fever
Hemophagocytic syndromes
Hypereosinophilia syndromes
Hypothalamic-central fever
Infantile cortical hyperostosis
Inflammatory bowel disease*
Kawasaki disease*
Kikuchi-Fujimoto disease
Metal fume fever
Multisystem inflammatory syndrome in children (MIS-C)
Pancreatitis
Poisoning
Pulmonary embolism
Thrombophlebitis
Thyrotoxicosis, thyroiditis

*Most common identified causes of FUO in children.

afternoon often represent normal variations. The appearance of the child while febrile is also important. Increased temperature without sweating might be seen in a child with ectodermal dysplasia or factitious fever. Increased temperature without signs of fatigue or malaise is less likely to be true fever.

The pattern of fever should be noted (Fig. 52.3). Sustained fever, intermittent fever, and relapsing fever are associated with different disease states. Sustained or remittent fever remains elevated with little variation during the day and is associated with enteric (typhoid) fever, tularemia, and rickettsial diseases such as typhus and Rocky Mountain spotted fever. Intermittent fever normalizes at least once a day and is associated with tuberculosis, abscesses, lymphomas, juvenile idiopathic arthritis (JIA), and some forms of malaria. Children with relapsing fever have afebrile days between febrile episodes. Relapsing fever is associated with rat-bite fever, Borrelia species (tick-borne and hard tick relapsing fever), malaria, brucellosis, subacute bacterial endocarditis,

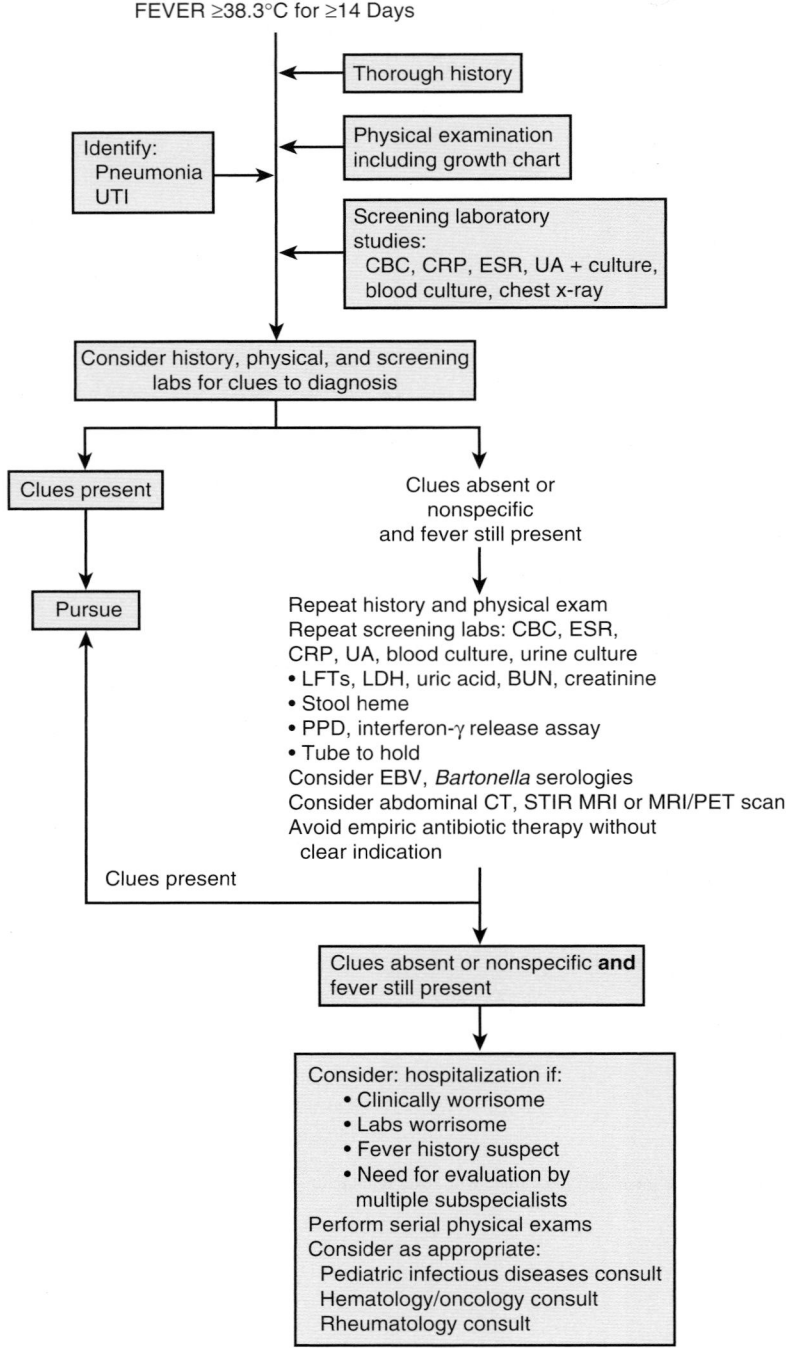

Fig. 52.2 Approach to the evaluation of fever of unknown origin (FUO). EBV, Epstein-Barr virus; LDH, lactate dehydrogenase; LFT, liver function test; PPD, purified protein derivative; STIR, short tau inversion recovery rapid MRI; UTI, urinary tract infection.

African trypanosomiasis, lymphoma, and Lyme disease. Saddle-back or double-hump fever lasts a few days, is followed by an afebrile day or two, and then returns. This pattern is associated with viruses such as enterovirus and dengue fever. Double quotidian fever (two fever spikes each day) occurs in visceral leishmaniasis, malaria, and gonococcal endocarditis. Unfortunately, neither the fever pattern nor the duration is sufficient to determine a cause.

Other patterns of fever are rarely due to infection. This includes periodic fevers and prolonged fevers lasting more than 1 year. Periodic fevers occur as acute stereotypical febrile episodes separated by prolonged afebrile, healthy periods. Diseases to consider include cyclic neutropenia, familial Mediterranean fever, and the syndrome of periodic fever, aphthous stomatitis, pharyngitis, and adenitis (PFAPA). Periodic fever syndromes have different prevalence patterns in different ethnic groups and different inheritance patterns. A detailed family history is particularly important when these diagnoses are considered (see Chapter 54). Fevers lasting for more than 1 year are not usually infectious; factitious fever, rheumatic or granulomatous disorders, familial diseases, or malignancies need to be considered in these patients.

TABLE 52.10 Examples of Subtle Physical Findings Having Special Significance in Patients with Fever of Unknown Origin

Body Site	Physical Finding	Diagnosis
Head	Sinus tenderness	Sinusitis
	Scalp redness or tenderness	Infantile cortical hyperostosis (Caffey disease)
Oropharynx	Ulceration	Disseminated histoplasmosis, SLE, Behçet syndrome, IBD
	Tender tooth	Periapical abscess
Fundi or conjunctivae	Choroid tubercle	Disseminated granulomatosis*
	Petechiae, Roth spot	Endocarditis
Thyroid	Enlargement, tenderness	Thyroiditis
Heart	Murmur	Endocarditis, rheumatic fever
Abdomen	Enlarged iliac crest lymph nodes, splenomegaly	Lymphoma, endocarditis, disseminated granulomatosis*
Rectum	Perirectal fluctuance, tenderness	Abscess
	Perianal skin tags, fistula	IBD
Genitalia	Testicular nodule	Periarteritis nodosa, tumor
	Epididymal nodule	Disseminated granulomatosis*
Lower extremities	Deep venous tenderness	Thrombosis or thrombophlebitis; malignancy, autoimmune disease
Skin and nails	Petechiae, splinter hemorrhages, subcutaneous nodules, clubbing	Vasculitis, endocarditis, chronic pulmonary disease
Muscles	Weakness, tenderness	Myositis
Joints	Swelling, stiffness, erythema	SLE, JIA, IBD

*Includes tuberculosis, histoplasmosis, coccidioidomycosis, sarcoidosis, and syphilis.
IBD, inflammatory bowel disease; JIA, juvenile idiopathic arthritis; SLE, systemic lupus erythematosus.
Modified from Wright WF. Fever of unknown origin. In: Bennett JE, Dolin R, Blaser MJ, eds. *Mandell, Douglas, and Bennett's Principles and Practices of Infectious Diseases*. 9th ed. Philadelphia: Elsevier; 2020:790–800, Table 56.7.

TABLE 52.11 Examples of Potential Diagnostic Clues to Infections Presenting as Fever of Unknown Origin

Etiology	Historical Clues	Physical Clues
Anaplasmosis	Transmitted by the bite of an *Ixodes* tick in association with outdoor activity in north central and eastern USA	Fever, headache, arthralgia, myalgia, pneumonitis, thrombocytopenia, lymphopenia, and elevated liver enzymes
Babesiosis	Transmitted by the bite of an *Ixodes* tick in association with outdoor activity in the northeastern USA	Arthralgia, myalgia, relative bradycardia, hepatosplenomegaly, anemia, thrombocytopenia, and elevated liver enzymes
Bartonellosis	Recent travel to the Andes mountains with fever and bacteremia (Oroya fever, *Bartonella bacilliformis*), association with homelessness in urban settings *(Bartonella quintana)* or contact with either fleas or the scratch of an infected kitten or feral cat *(Bartonella henselae)*	Conjunctivitis, retroorbital pain, anterior tibial bone pain, macular rash, nodular plaque lesions, and/or regional lymphadenopathy
Blastomycosis	Contact with soil adjacent to the Mississippi and Ohio River valleys, Saint Lawrence River in New York and Canada, and North American Great Lakes, or exposure to infected dogs	Arthritis, atypical pneumonia, pulmonary nodules, and/or fulminant adult respiratory distress syndrome; verrucous, nodular, or ulcerative skin lesions; and prostatitis
Brucellosis	Associated with contact with or consumption of products from infected goats, pigs, camels, yaks, buffalo, or cows and with abattoir work	Arthralgia, hepatosplenomegaly, suppurative musculoskeletal lesions, sacroiliitis, spondylitis, uveitis, hepatitis, and pancytopenia
Coccidioidomycosis	Exposure to soil or dust in the southwestern USA	Arthralgia, pneumonia, pulmonary cavities, pulmonary nodules, erythema multiforme, and erythema nodosum
Ehrlichiosis	Transmitted by the bite of an *Amblyomma, Dermacentor,* or *Ixodes* tick in association with outdoor activity in midwestern and southeastern USA	Pneumonitis, hepatitis, thrombocytopenia, and lymphopenia
Enteric fever (*Salmonella enterica* serovar typhi)	Recent travel to a third world country with consumption of potentially contaminated food or water	Headache, arthritis, abdominal pain, relative bradycardia, hepatosplenomegaly, and leukopenia

Continued

TABLE 52.11 Examples of Potential Diagnostic Clues to Infections Presenting as Fever of Unknown Origin—cont'd

Etiology	Historical Clues	Physical Clues
Histoplasmosis	Exposure to bat or black bird excreta in roosts, chicken houses, or caves in the region surrounding the Ohio and Mississippi River valleys of the USA or regions of Central and South America, Africa, Asia, and Australia	Headache, pneumonia, pulmonary cavities, mucosal ulcers, adenopathy, erythema nodosum, erythema multiforme, hepatitis, anemia, leukopenia, and thrombocytopenia
Leishmaniasis (visceral disease)	Associated with recent travel to areas endemic for sand flies	Hepatosplenomegaly, lymphadenopathy, and hyperpigmentation of the face, hand, foot, and/or abdominal skin (kala azar)
Leptospirosis	Occupational exposure among workers in sewers, rice and sugar cane fields, and abattoirs; recreational water sports and exposure to contaminated waters or infected dogs	Bitemporal and frontal headache, calf and lumbar muscle tenderness, conjunctival suffusion, hepatic and renal failure, and hemorrhagic pneumonitis
Malaria	Recent travel to endemic areas in Asia, Africa, and Central and South America	Fever, headaches, nausea, emesis, diarrhea, hepatomegaly, splenomegaly, and anemia
Psittacosis *(Chlamydia psittaci)*	Associated with contact with birds, especially psittacine birds	Fever, pharyngitis, hepatosplenomegaly, pneumonia, blanching maculopapular eruptions, erythema multiforme, erythema marginatum, and erythema nodosum
Q fever *(Coxiella burnetii)*	Associated with farm, veterinary, or abattoir work; consumption of unpasteurized milk; and contact with infected sheep, goats, or cattle	Atypical pneumonia, hepatitis, hepatomegaly, relative bradycardia, and/or splenomegaly
Rat-bite fever *(Streptobacillus moniliformis)*	Recent bite or scratch by a rat, mouse, or squirrel and/or ingestion of food or water contaminated by rat excrement	Headaches, myalgia, polyarthritis, and maculopapular, morbilliform, petechial, vesicular, or pustular rash over the palms, soles, and extremities
Relapsing fever *(Borrelia recurrentis)*	Associated with poverty, crowding, and poor sanitation (louse borne); or with camping (tick borne), particularly in the Grand Canyon	High fever with rigors, headache, delirium, arthralgia, myalgia, and hepatosplenomegaly
Rocky Mountain spotted fever	Associated with outdoor activity in the South Atlantic or southeastern USA and exposure to *Dermacentor* tick bites	Headache, petechial rash involving the extremities, hand palms, and feet soles
Tuberculosis	Recent contact with tuberculosis, recent immigration from an endemic country, and work or residence in homeless shelters, correctional facilities, or health care facilities	Night sweats, weight loss, atypical pneumonia, cavitary pulmonary lesions
Tularemia	Associated with bites by *Amblyomma* or *Dermacentor* ticks, deer flies, and mosquitoes or direct contact with the tissues of infected animals such as rabbits, squirrels, deer, raccoons, cattle, sheep, and swine	Ulcerated skin lesions at a bite site, pneumonia, relative bradycardia, lymphadenopathy, and conjunctivitis
Whipple disease *(Tropheryma whipplei)*	Potential association with exposure to sewage	Chronic diarrhea, arthralgia, weight loss, malabsorption, and malnutrition

From Bennett JE, Dolin R, Blaser MJ. *Mandell, Douglas, and Bennett's Principles and Practices of Infectious Diseases*. 9th ed. Vol. 1. Philadelphia: Elsevier; 2020:798, Table 56.8.

TABLE 52.12 Discriminating Features of Noninfectious Causes of Fever of Unknown Origin

Causes of Fever	Exposure or Condition	Features	Diagnostic Method
Infectious Causes			
Kikuchi-Fujimoto disease		Regional or generalized lymphadenopathy; elevated inflammatory markers	Biopsy or histology
Inflammatory pseudotumor	History of nonspecific illness (presumed host-controlled infection)	Insidious; malaise, weight loss, vague abdominal pain or tenderness; anemia; elevated inflammatory markers	Abdominal CT; biopsy or histology
Kawasaki disease (incomplete)		Asynchronous or incomplete features of Kawasaki disease; elevated inflammatory markers; thrombocytosis	Clinical constellation; echocardiogram
Juvenile idiopathic arthritis	Familial, sporadic	Hepatosplenomegaly, lymphadenopathy, exanthem; anemia, elevated inflammatory markers	Clinical constellation
Systemic lupus erythematosus	Familial, sporadic	Malaise, weight loss; then multisystem involvement (kidneys, joints, skin)	Serum antinuclear antibody, anti–double-stranded DNA, anti–smooth muscle antibody

TABLE 52.12   Discriminating Features of Noninfectious Causes of Fever of Unknown Origin—cont'd

Causes of Fever	Exposure or Condition	Features	Diagnostic Method
Hemophagocytic lymphohistiocytosis	Virus associated; familial rheumatic disorder	Severe, rapidly progressive illness; hepatomegaly, lymphadenopathy, exanthem; cytopenias; extreme elevations of inflammatory markers	Ferritin, triglyceride levels, other diagnostic criteria; erythrophagocytosis by macrophages; natural killer cell, CD8⁺ T lymphocyte dysfunction
Vasculitis syndromes	Familial, sporadic	Specific hallmarks (renal, neurologic, stomatitis or perianal ulcers, uveitis, pulmonary)	Clinical constellation; specific autoantibodies; biopsy or histology
Sarcoidosis	Geography; race	Fatigue, weight loss, leg pain; anemia; elevated inflammatory markers; mediastinal lymphadenopathy; uveitis	Clinical constellation; biopsy or histology; soluble interleukin-2 receptor level
Inflammatory bowel disease	Familial; sporadic	Linear growth failure, subtle gastrointestinal symptoms or abdominal tenderness; perirectal skin tag; iron-deficiency anemia; elevated inflammatory markers	Abdominal CT; barium study
Lymphoreticular malignancy		Weight loss, fatigue; nonarticular bone pain; lymphadenopathy; cytopenias	Bone marrow or tissue biopsy
Drug hypersensitivity	Prescription or nonprescription drug exposure	Preserved sense of well-being; exanthems; eosinophilia; organ dysfunction (renal, cardiac, pulmonary)	Clinical constellation; withdrawal of drug
Factitious fever or Munchausen syndrome by proxy	Predisposing parent-patient dynamic	Discordant temperature and vital signs; discordant parent-measured temperature and urine temperature; normal inflammatory markers	Clinical constellation; verification of temperature in medical setting
Hypothalamic dysfunction, diabetes insipidus, dysautonomia, or absent corpus callosum	Underlying condition; genetic syndrome; anatomic abnormality	Normal inflammatory markers; hypernatremia; no response to nonsteroidal antiinflammatory drugs	Clinical constellation; laboratory tests and imaging

Modified from Long SS, Prober CG, Fischer M, eds. *Principles and Practice of Pediatric Infectious Diseases.* 5th ed. Philadelphia: Elsevier; 2018:121, Table 15.2.

A complete review of systems is essential in the evaluation of FUO. Subtle respiratory or gastrointestinal symptoms may suggest back-to-back viral illnesses, commonly occurring during the first year in school or daycare. A history of rash is important for diagnosing Lyme disease, JIA, and acute rheumatic fever (see Chapter 53). The review of systems may reveal heat intolerance, palpitations, tremors, and declining quality of schoolwork in a child with hyperthyroidism. The overall state of health, including growth, energy, and appetite, can classify the severity of the illness and urgency of diagnostic testing.

Exposure history can be informative for uncommon causes of fever (see Table 52.12). A history of pica with fevers is associated with visceral larva migrans and toxoplasmosis. Exposure to domesticated and wild animals should be identified to exclude zoonoses (see Chapter 53). The food history should be detailed and should include water sources (particularly inquiring about well water), use of game meats, and consumption of undercooked meats or unpasteurized dairy products (e.g., milk or cheese). Travel history is critically important in the establishment of a differential diagnosis. Areas visited, accommodations, activities, prophylactic treatments, animal and insect exposures, and water and food sources should be reviewed. Coccidioidomycosis, histoplasmosis, malaria, Lyme disease, and Rocky Mountain spotted fever have regional distributions in the United States; travel to and within countries where other diseases are endemic should be ascertained as well (Table 52.13).

Previous medical records should be reviewed. Weight loss is important for diagnosing many chronic diseases such as lymphoma, tuberculosis, and inflammatory bowel disease. Poor weight gain and growth, with or without gastrointestinal symptoms, may be the only historical clue to inflammatory bowel disease (see Chapter 14). HIV risk factors in the parents and child should be reviewed. The types and frequency of prior infections may suggest an immunodeficiency. Past and current medications may reveal additional medical history. A history of severe head trauma may be associated with hypothalamic dysfunction and central fevers.

Physical Examination

Whenever possible, the patient should be examined during a febrile episode. Accompanying tachycardia and tachypnea can differentiate true fever from normal diurnal variation or factitious fever. Certain signs, such as rash, may only be present during the fever.

Eyes

The ophthalmologic examination should include assessment of visual acuity, extraocular motion, visual field integrity, and gaze, as well as inspection of external structures and ophthalmoscopic examination (see Chapter 43). Conjunctivitis, iritis-uveitis-scleritis, or both may be seen in a variety of infectious conditions, including EBV infection, leptospirosis, rickettsial infection, and cat-scratch disease. Conjunctivitis, uveitis, or both occur with Kawasaki disease, systemic lupus erythematosus (SLE), polyarteritis nodosa, and JIA. Sarcoidosis may be associated with conjunctival and uveal tract nodules. A thorough ophthalmoscopic evaluation (and, if needed, slit-lamp examination) should be performed. Sarcoidosis may be accompanied by vascular occlusions, hemorrhages, vascular sheathing, and preretinal inflammatory exudates. Cytomegalovirus (CMV) produces chorioretinitis associated with white infiltrates near vessels and confluent depigmented

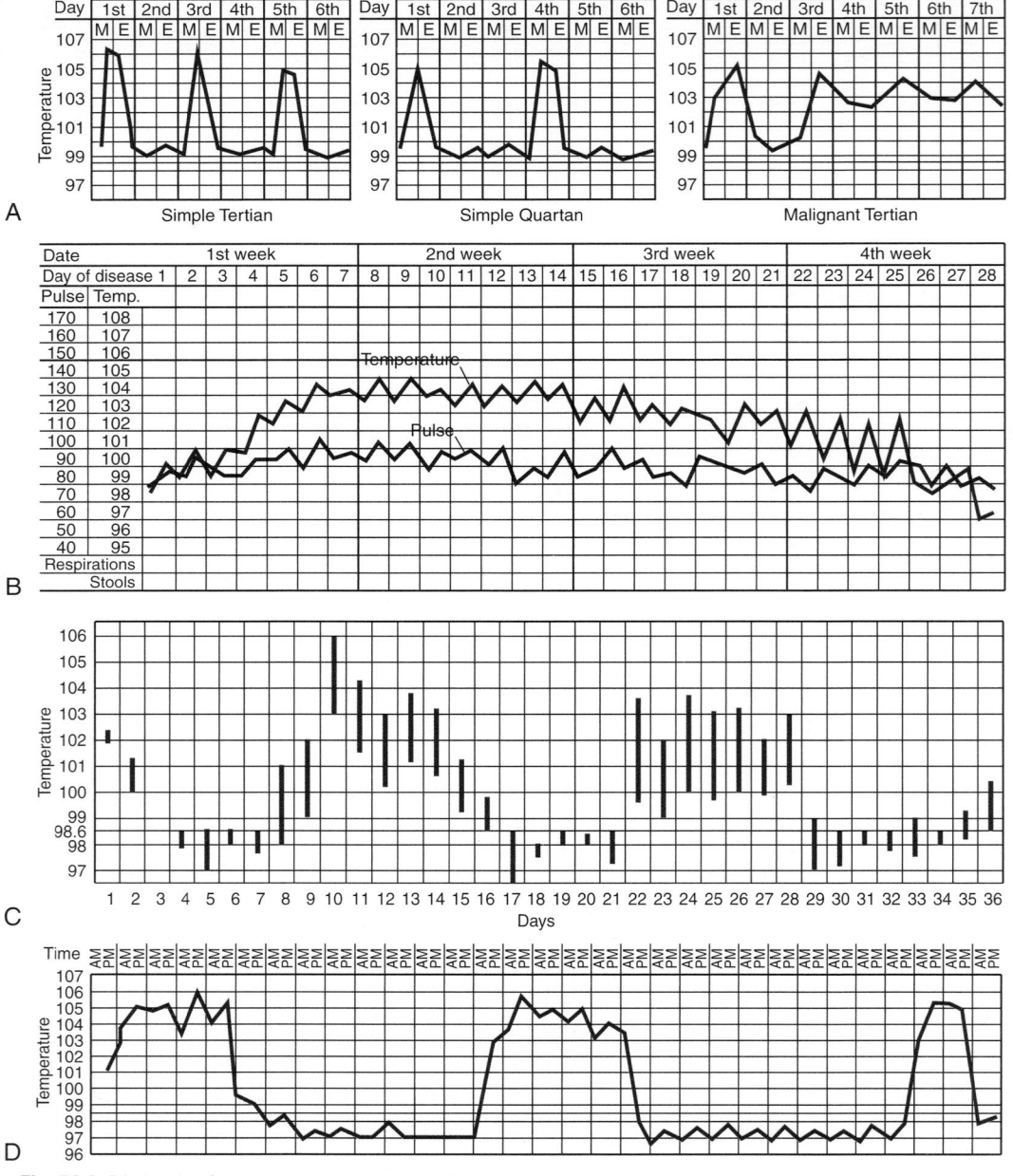

Fig. 52.3 Distinctive fever patterns. *A*, Malaria. *B*, Typhoid fever (demonstrating relative bradycardia). *C*, Hodgkin disease (Pel-Ebstein pattern). *D*, Borreliosis (relapsing fever pattern). (Data from Woodward TE. The fever pattern as a clinical diagnostic aid. In: Mackowiak PA, ed. *Fever: Basic Mechanisms and Management.* 2nd ed. Philadelphia: Lippincott-Raven; 1997:215–236.)

areas. Histoplasmosis causes small atrophic spots and, in rare cases, focal granulomas of the retina and choroid. *Toxoplasma gondii* is a common cause of recurrent retinochoroiditis. Retinal changes also occur with bacterial endocarditis. Tuberculosis can cause formation of choroidal tubercles and ulcerative palpebral conjunctival lesions. Slit-lamp examination may also reveal iridocyclitis in JIA, Behçet syndrome, and inflammatory bowel disease.

Ears, Nose, and Throat

The frontal and maxillary sinuses should be palpated for tenderness. The nares should be inspected for inflamed mucosa, aphthae, and purulent discharge. Tympanic membranes should be viewed and insufflated (see Chapter 5). The mouth should be checked for lesions, inflammation, and tooth tenderness. Behçet syndrome may manifest with oral aphthous lesions. Inspection of teeth and gums may reveal a dental abscess; percussing each tooth with a wooden tongue blade may produce pain in the abscessed tooth that may not otherwise be appreciated on visual inspection. Pharyngitis with and without exudate is associated with EBV infection, tularemia, leptospirosis, and CMV. PFAPA syndrome is characterized by periodic fever, aphthous stomatitis, pharyngitis, and cervical adenopathy. *Candida* infection in the mouths of children older than 6 months may result from immunodeficiency such as HIV, from stasis of oral secretions in children who are not orally fed, or from improper technique with inhaled steroids.

TABLE 52.13　Causes of Fever in the Returned Traveler

Diagnosis	%
Malaria	30–40
Hepatitis	3–6
Respiratory infection*	2–11
Urinary tract infection/pyelonephritis	2–4
Dysentery	4–5
Dengue fever	2–6
Enteric (typhoid) fever	1–2
Tuberculosis	1–2
Rickettsial infection	~1
Acute HIV infection	<1
Amebic liver abscess	<1
Other miscellaneous infections	4–9
Miscellaneous noninfectious causes	1–6
Undiagnosed	~25

*Includes upper respiratory tract infection, pneumonia, and bronchitis.
Modified from Suh KN, Kozavsky PE, Keystone JS. Evaluation of fever in the returned traveler. *Travel Med.* 1999;83:997–1017.

Neck

The neck should be examined for adenopathy or thyroid enlargement (see Chapter 48). The rest of the lymphatic system should be carefully examined. A single tender node may be seen with cat-scratch disease or nontender node with lymphoma. Generalized adenopathy can be seen in CMV, EBV, HIV, and systemic JIA (see Chapter 44).

Heart, Lungs, and Abdomen

Careful auscultation of the heart and lungs is essential. A mitral or aortic regurgitant murmur may be the initial finding of infectious endocarditis or of carditis in children with acute rheumatic fever. A pericardial friction rub may also suggest JIA, SLE, rheumatic fever, malignancy, or viral pericarditis. The abdomen must be carefully palpated for evidence of masses or hepatosplenomegaly (see Chapters 17 and 20). Abdominal tenderness may be present with abdominal abscesses, hepatosplenomegaly, and inflammatory bowel disease. A rectal examination should be performed, and stool should be tested for occult blood. Sexually active girls should have a pelvic examination. Pain on movement of the uterus during the pelvic examination may indicate pelvic inflammatory disease.

Musculoskeletal Evaluation

The musculoskeletal examination should include assessments of strength and of active and passive range of motion and evaluation for warmth, tenderness, or swelling of joints. Irritability and pain on palpation over a bone or pseudoparalysis may be the first clue to osteomyelitis. Bone pain may also result from neoplastic infiltration of the bone marrow or sickle cell anemia. Unexplained fever, arthralgia, and arthritis may be present with acute rheumatic fever, JIA, Lyme disease, Kawasaki disease, SLE, polyarteritis nodosa, and Behçet syndrome (see Chapter 44). Myalgia occurs commonly with viral diseases such as influenza, and may be present with rickettsial diseases, polyarteritis nodosa, Takayasu arteritis, and dermatomyositis.

Skin

The skin must be inspected for evidence of rashes and other lesions (see Chapter 53). JIA may manifest with an evanescent, salmon-colored macular rash over the trunk and joints that may appear and disappear rapidly and be evident only during febrile periods. Dermatomyositis is characterized by a heliotropic rash of the upper eyelids and an erythematous eruption (vasculitis) over the extensor surfaces (Gottron sign). SLE may manifest with a butterfly rash over the nose and malar regions, signs of photosensitivity in sun-exposed areas, or vasculitis. The rash of Kawasaki disease is erythematous and may manifest in many forms; it is most commonly a diffuse maculopapular rash. In Rocky Mountain spotted fever, there are erythematous macules on the wrists, ankles, or forearms that may become maculopapular and expand centripetally to the proximal extremities and torso; palms and soles may be involved and petechiae may develop later in the course of the illness. Endocarditis may be associated with splinter hemorrhages, Janeway lesions (painless, small, erythematous, or hemorrhagic lesions on the palms and soles), or Osler nodes (small, tender nodules on the palms). Lyme disease usually manifests with erythema migrans. This nontender, erythematous rash expands over hours and may have a pale center ("bull's eye rash," occurring in ~50% of erythema migrans). The rash begins at the site of the tick bite during early localized Lyme disease; secondary lesions may appear at other sites during early disseminated Lyme disease. Tularemia, salmonellosis, listeriosis, and EBV infections may feature generalized maculopapular rashes.

Diagnostic Studies

Laboratory evaluation should proceed in a stepwise, focused manner with emphasis on identifying serious illnesses with defined interventions (see Fig. 52.2). Initial studies should include a CBC with differential, ESR, CRP, blood cultures, UA, urine culture, and chest radiograph.

The CBC with differential is neither specific nor diagnostic, except in rare circumstances, such as seeing lymphoblasts on the blood smear. Approximately 30% of patients have abnormal WBC counts; 46% may have a left shift (i.e., increased band neutrophil percentage), lymphocytosis, atypical lymphocytes, or blasts. An elevated ESR or CRP indicates inflammation. The ESR is usually high in children with FUO caused by infectious pathogens, malignancies, and rheumatic diseases. Of patients with an ESR <10 mm/hr, 90% have a self-limited viral disease.

UA and urine culture identify occult infections, particularly in young girls. The UA may also be abnormal in patients with endocarditis and rheumatic and other inflammatory disorders.

Chest radiographs should be examined for unexpected consolidations, calcifications, interstitial changes, perihilar adenopathy, mediastinal masses, or cardiomegaly (heart failure, pericarditis). Chest films are abnormal in up to 15% of patients with FUO.

Further studies should be directed by information obtained from detailed histories and physical examinations, as well as the initial laboratory studies. Leukopenia, thrombocytopenia, and hyponatremia may be a sign of certain tick-borne infections. Abnormalities in the physical exam or laboratory values may suggest diagnostic yield for biopsy of lymph nodes, skin, liver, or bone marrow.

In many cases, the etiology is still unknown after the initial evaluation and fever persists, necessitating performance of a second tier of testing. The initial laboratory studies may be repeated, especially to assess for trends in inflammatory markers. Additional studies may include a complete metabolic panel (CMP, to include assessments of kidneys and liver), lactate dehydrogenase (LDH), uric acid, fibrinogen, ferritin, immunoglobulins, and fecal occult blood. The presence of transaminitis suggests the need to evaluate for associated viral infections, such as hepatitis A, CMV, EBV, adenovirus, and enterovirus. Elevation in LDH and uric acid suggests increased cell turnover due to an occult malignancy. Marked abnormalities in fibrinogen, ferritin, or immunoglobulins may suggest a more serious cause of FUO such as immune disregulation. The presence of fecal occult blood can point toward inflammatory bowel disease; if symptoms or the presence of fecal occult blood suggest inflammatory bowel disease, fecal calprotectin can assess for bowel inflammation and suggest the need for endoscopic studies and biopsy. All children with FUO should be assessed for tuberculosis (tuberculin skin tests or interferon-γ release assay) and HIV (fourth-generation antibody/antigen screen; see Chapter 48). After 10–14 days of fever have elapsed, additional infections may be identified by serologies. Organism-specific IgG and IgM can be used to diagnose CMV, EBV (with the addition of EBV nuclear antigen antibody [EBNA] to aid with timing of the infection), and *Bartonella* infection. PCR-based bacteria detection from whole blood may also detect nonculturable organisms. Depending on travel and exposure history, additional serologic testing for toxoplasmosis, brucellosis, tularemia, and leptospirosis may be indicated. Expanded radiologic studies should include abdominal imaging. In well-appearing children, abdominal ultrasound may be performed first. With ill appearance or continued elusive diagnosis, abdominal CT is appropriate. Additional imaging that may be of benefit include sinus CT, whole-body MRI (to evaluate for occult osteomyelitis, malignancy, or histiocytic disorders), and PET/CT or MRI. Specialized radiologic studies performed without specific diagnostic clues from the history, physical examination findings, or initial laboratory evaluation results have a low yield.

Finally, hospitalization may be considered at any time if the clinical assessment or laboratory values are worrisome for a serious cause of fever (see Table 52.13). In some cases, hospitalization is used to verify the presence of fever or facilitate evaluation by multiple subspecialists, such as infectious diseases, hematology/oncology, or rheumatology. In most well-appearing children, serial physical examinations and diagnostic evaluation can be performed safely in an outpatient setting.

Cause

Most of the causes of FUO eventually develop localizing signs, symptoms, or abnormal laboratory studies. The following list of etiologies may either initially present with isolated fever or atypically present with fever.

Infectious Syndromes Causing Fever of Unknown Origin

A wide variety of infectious syndromes have been identified in children with FUO including subacute bacterial endocarditis, UTI, sinusitis, abscesses, osteomyelitis, and rheumatic fever.

Bacterial endocarditis. Bacterial endocarditis is rare in children; incidence increases with advancing age and history of pre-existing heart disease (see Chapter 9). A new murmur or a change in the characteristic of an existing murmur may not be initially evident. Vegetations also may not be visible initially by transthoracic echocardiography; repeat transthoracic echocardiography or a transesophageal approach for patients with larger body habitus may be more sensitive. Large-volume blood cultures separated in space and time are necessary for definitive diagnosis. PCR-based blood assays may help diagnose culture negative endocarditis.

Urinary tract infection. Both upper and lower UTIs may present without localized pain or dysuria. Leukocytes may be absent in urine early in infection (see Chapter 21). Sterile pyuria may be present with tuberculosis, nongonococcal urethritis, viral cystitis, Kawasaki disease, reactive arthritis, interstitial nephritis, well-circumscribed renal abscess, and certain rheumatic diseases. Renal ultrasonography may show areas of decreased echogenicity, enlarged echogenic kidneys, and renal or perinephric abscesses. A CT scan with contrast may reveal infected parenchyma as a nonenhancing lucency. Nuclear medicine renal scans can be used to identify active areas of infection and old scars.

Sinusitis. Factors that decrease the size and patency of the ostium or impair the mucociliary transport system predispose a child to sinusitis. Ethmoid and maxillary sinuses are present at birth. The frontal sinuses usually appear near 5 or 6 years of age but may be asymmetric or absent. Sphenoid sinuses may be seen radiographically by 9 years of age. Prolonged nasal congestion, headache, purulent nasal discharge, sore throat, daytime cough, tender teeth, and halitosis may be present in children with sinusitis. CT will demonstrate opacification of the sinuses but may not differentiate viral and bacterial infections. Rhinoscopy may show purulent material at the ostium of an infected sinus. Three distinct clinical presentations can identify high probability of bacterial sinusitis: (1) acute onset of high fever with severe purulent nasal discharge, (2) recurrent fever with onset of purulent nasal discharge during a period of apparent recovery from a viral URI, and (3) prolonged (>10–14 days) fever and nasal drainage. Infectious complications of sinusitis include dural space empyema or brain abscess.

Abscesses. Focal abscess not apparent on physical examination may present with FUO. Liver abscess may manifest with right upper quadrant tenderness and hepatomegaly. Blood cultures and laboratory assessments of the liver are often normal. Pelvic abscesses should be suspected in children with FUO who have abdominal, rectal, or pelvic tenderness even in the absence of a mass. Congenital anomalies, such as a patent urachus, may become superinfected and present with fever. The diagnosis of deep-seeded abscesses is usually made with MRI, CT with contrast, or ultrasonography. CT or ultrasound guidance may be used to direct percutaneous drainage of many abscesses for diagnostic and therapeutic purposes.

Osteomyelitis. Bacterial osteomyelitis in childhood is usually seeded from a hematogenous source, but it sometimes follows penetrating injury. Refusal to use the affected limb or tenderness to palpation over the infected site is common; localizing symptoms may be initially absent in infants. Abnormalities in plain radiographs appear late, typically 2 weeks or more after onset. MRI is the imaging modality of choice. The blood or bone culture is often positive and markers of inflammation (CRP, procalcitonin, and ESR) are elevated. Suppurative myositis may mimic osteomyelitis and manifest as an FUO. Chronic noninfectious osteomyelitis (CNO), including chronic recurrent multifocal osteomyelitis (CRMO), may present with fever and pain at one or more sites of sterile inflammation. The presence of recurrent sterile bone and joint inflammation accompanied by acne and pustulosis is highly suggestive of SAPHO syndrome (*s*ynovitis, *a*cne, *p*ustulosis, *h*yperostosis, and *o*steitis), a rare multisystem inflammatory disorder.

Rheumatic fever. Acute rheumatic fever may initially present as FUO, but diagnosis requires the development of a localizing sign or symptom. Early acute rheumatic fever may only manifest as polyarthralgia and elevation of inflammatory markers. Elbows, wrists, knees, and ankles are frequently involved. The diagnosis is made by fulfillment of the Jones criteria, which requires at least one objective major criterion (see Chapter 9).

Bacterial Pathogen Causes of Fever of Unknown Origin

Bacterial syndromes that cause FUO in children include Lyme disease, cat-scratch disease, Q fever, rat-bite fever, tularemia, brucellosis, leptospirosis, chlamydial infections, and rickettsial infections.

Lyme disease. Lyme disease is caused by the spirochete *Borrelia burgdorferi* and is transmitted by the *Ixodes scapularis* and *Ixodes pacificus* ticks. Although fever may be the only presenting symptom, careful history and examination invariably reveals one of the specific manifestations of Lyme disease. The usual manifestation of early Lyme disease is with a single (early localized) or multiple (early disseminated) erythema migrans lesions—an erythematous, annular, nontender, expanding rash with or without central clearing (see Chapter 53). The rash is self-limited and resolves in 1–30 days (usually 2 weeks). Other manifestations of early disseminated Lyme disease include facial nerve palsy, peripheral neuropathy, cardiac conduction defects, myocarditis, and aseptic meningitis. Patients with early localized or disseminated Lyme may also exhibit fever, chills, fatigue, headaches, malaise, myalgia, and arthralgia. Late disseminated Lyme disease presents as monoarticular arthritis, typically with marked swelling but preservation of some range of motion. Although a history of exposure to outdoor activities or ticks is common in patients with Lyme disease at any stage, recognition of the specific tick bite resulting in disease transmission is unusual. Diagnosis in early localized Lyme disease should be made clinically on the basis of an erythema migrans lesion. Serology in early infection lacks sensitivity and specificity. Diagnosis of early disseminated and late disseminated Lyme disease requires a typical clinical illness and serologic evidence of infection with a two-tier testing strategy. The initial test is an enzyme-linked immunosorbent assay (ELISA) or immunofluorescence assay (IFA) screen. If this result is equivocal or positive, a Western immunoblot is performed to confirm the presence of at least five IgG antibodies ("bands") specific to *B. burgdorferi* infection. Western blot should not be performed if the ELISA is negative or has not been performed because it lacks specificity in this setting.

Cat-scratch disease. Cat-scratch disease is a febrile illness associated with cats (usually kittens or cats in the first 2 years of life) and, more rarely, dogs. *Bartonella henselae*, which may be transmitted by the cat flea and cat saliva, is the etiologic agent. After a scratch or bite, a papule forms and may persist from days to months. Regional lymphadenopathy with one or more nodes occurs proximal to the skin site 1–9 weeks after inoculation. The node or nodes become enlarged and tender and may have overlying erythema. The lymphadenopathy usually resolves after 2–4 months but may last up to 3 years. Affected children may have adenopathy with fever, headache, malaise, anorexia, sore throat, and conjunctivitis (see Chapter 48). Atypically, cat-scratch disease can present with isolated fever (FUO) or disseminated disease (culture-negative endocarditis, encephalopathy, bone lesions, or liver or spleen granulomas). Diagnosis is established with serology.

Q fever. Q fever occurs as an acute or chronic infection caused by *Coxiella burnetii*. It manifests with headache, fever, chills, malaise, and, on occasion, respiratory symptoms. Gastrointestinal tract symptoms are also common in children. Severe disease with hepatic, cardiac, or CNS involvement is rare. Domesticated farm animals including cattle, sheep, and goats are the primary reservoirs for human infection. Humans acquire the organism through inhalation of infected aerosols, particularly after livestock birthing, or ingestion of unpasteurized dairy products. Diagnosis is made by serologic testing.

Rat-bite fever. Rat-bite fever is a relapsing fever caused by *Streptobacillus moniliformis* or *Spirillum minus*. Both organisms live in the upper respiratory tract of rodents and can be transmitted to humans through rodent bites, exposure to rodent oral secretions, or ingestion of contaminated food or water. Initial symptoms include relapsing fever, chills, malaise, and muscle aches. Rash, including palm and sole involvement, and migratory polyarthritis or arthralgia are common. Complications include abscesses, pneumonia, endocarditis, myocarditis, and meningitis. Diagnosis is made by blood culture or culture of other infected fluid, such as abscess aspiration.

Tularemia. *Francisella tularensis* is the causative agent of tularemia. The disease is spread by contact with wild animals, such as rabbits and prairie dogs; insects that bite these animals, such as ticks and deer flies; or contaminated water or aerosols. A maculopapular nodule forms at the portal of entry and later becomes ulcerated with associated regional lymphadenopathy, a phenomenon termed ulceroglandular disease. Children may also present with fever and other disease variants based on the site of inoculation. Pharyngitis, conjunctivitis, hepatosplenomegaly, and pneumonia may occur. Diagnosis is made by serologic study.

Brucellosis. Brucellosis is caused by several bacterial species including *Brucella abortus*, *Brucella melitensis*, *Brucella suis*, and *Brucella canis*. The microorganisms are found in wild and domesticated animals. Infection may occur by airborne spread or by ingestion of meat or milk, with most childhood cases in the United States resulting from ingestion of unpasteurized milk or cheese. The infected child may present with fever, chills, malaise, headache, arthralgia, or myalgia. Pneumonia, cardiac involvement, and CNS involvement occur in rare cases. Diagnosis is made by special culture techniques and serologic study.

Leptospirosis. Leptospirosis is caused by members of the spirochete genus *Leptospira*. Infection is spread by contact with the urine of wild or domestic animals. In 1–2 weeks after exposure, patients experience the abrupt onset of fever, chills, nausea, vomiting, headache, and occasionally conjunctival suffusion and rash. The initial acute septicemia phase may be followed by a second immune-mediated phase with fever, aseptic meningitis, and uveitis. Severe illness with renal failure, jaundice, myocarditis, shock, and pulmonary hemorrhage may occur. Diagnosis is made by special culture techniques and serologic testing.

Chlamydial infection. Psittacosis and lymphogranuloma venereum are chlamydial causes of FUO. *Chlamydia psittaci* may be transmitted by infected birds and produces respiratory illness with fever. Cardiac, liver, CNS, and thyroid involvement are possible though are rare. Diagnosis is made serologically. *Chlamydia trachomatis* is a sexually transmitted organism that causes urogenital infections, perihepatitis, invasive lymphadenopathy (lymphogranuloma venereum), neonatal conjunctivitis, and neonatal pneumonia. Diagnosis is by PCR of infected body fluids.

Rickettsial infections. Transmission of the causative agent for Rocky Mountain spotted fever, *Rickettsia rickettsii*, occurs by tick bite. This disease is a small-vessel vasculitis that manifests with fever, headache, intense myalgia, and abdominal symptoms. A characteristic rash is usually present by the sixth day of illness, includes palms and soles, and progresses from macular to petechial. Characteristic laboratory findings include leukopenia, thrombocytopenia, and hyponatremia. Mortality rates are high, necessitating prompt therapy when the diagnosis is suspected. Diagnosis is confirmed by PCR testing of blood or serology.

Anaplasmosis and ehrlichiosis are caused by *Anaplasma phagocytophila* and multiple *Ehrlichia* species. Organisms are transmitted by *I. scapularis* or the Lone Star tick (*Amblyomma americanum*). These illnesses are usually seen in the southeastern and upper midwestern United States and present with fever, severe headache, gastrointestinal symptoms, and myalgia. Rash is inconsistent but more common in children than in adults. Symptoms and general laboratory perturbations are similar to Rocky Mountain spotted fever. Diagnosis is confirmed by PCR or serology.

Fungal Pathogen Causes of Fever of Unknown Origin
Fungal causes of FUO include blastomycosis, histoplasmosis, coccidioidomycosis, and cryptococcoses.

Blastomyces dermatitidis is a saprophytic fungus with both yeast and mycelial forms; it is found in the soil all over the world but is common in the Americas. It is endemic in the Southeast and Midwest regions of North America (Great Lakes). Infections with this fungus may localize to the lungs or disseminate to the brain, bone, or skin. The diagnosis is made by antigen testing on urine, fungal culture from respiratory or tissue samples, or visualization of broad-based budding yeast on fungal stains.

Histoplasma capsulatum is a yeast found in soil in the Ohio and Mississippi River valleys and other locations in the United States and causes pulmonary and disseminated disease. Its many disease presentations make it one of the "great mimics" in medicine. Diagnosis is made by the demonstration of the microorganism in biopsy or respiratory specimens, antigen testing on urine, or serology.

Coccidioides immitis is found in soil in the southwestern United States. Infections in humans are associated with a febrile pulmonary disease characterized by cough, rash, and chest pain. Diagnosis is usually made serologically.

Cryptococcus neoformans is often found in pigeon droppings and can cause pulmonary or CNS infection in immunocompromised patients. The diagnosis is made by culture, antigen in blood or CSF, or identification of encapsulated yeast in collected specimens.

Viral Pathogen Causes of Fever of Unknown Origin

Fever associated with most viral infections resolves within 7–10 days. For this reason, laboratory work-up of FUO is usually deferred until after this interval in the well-appearing child. Although certain respiratory viruses such as adenovirus can cause prolonged fevers, the classic viral infections associated with FUO are CMV, EBV, and HIV.

Cytomegalovirus. CMV may cause a mononucleosis-like syndrome (heterophile-negative mononucleosis) in children. Generalized or cervical adenopathy may be seen along with fatigue, malaise, fever, hepatosplenomegaly, and abdominal pain (see Chapter 48). A morbilliform rash may occur. CMV retinitis, hepatitis, colitis, and pneumonitis are usually limited to children with impaired immune systems. The virus is transmitted by contact with infected secretions. Infection is diagnosed by PCR (blood, urine) or by serology, although care must be taken to differentiate acute infection from reactivation.

Epstein-Barr virus. Infectious mononucleosis is typically caused by EBV and may manifest with fever, exudative pharyngitis, malaise, and fatigue (see Chapter 48). The appearance of rash is sometimes preceded by amoxicillin therapy, but rash may occur without antibiotic administration. Tender lymphadenopathy and hepatosplenomegaly may occur. The diagnosis may be made by nonspecific tests (heterophile antibody or monospot) in older patients, but these studies are unreliable for young children. Specific antibody tests against viral capsid antigen, early antigen, and nuclear antigen are recommended in younger children.

Human immunodeficiency virus. Infection with HIV may cause FUO in children. The fever is typically due to associated opportunistic infections or malignancies that occur as a result of chronic immunodeficiency. Diagnosis is made with fourth-generation antigen/antibody tests or PCR if acute infection is suspected (see Chapter 48).

Parasitic Pathogen Causes of Fever of Unknown Origin

FUO in children may be caused by parasitic infections, including babesiosis, toxoplasmosis, and toxocariasis.

Babesiosis is caused by *Babesia microti* and is a parasite of rodents transmitted to humans by tick bite. Infection may result in fever, chills, nausea, vomiting, night sweats, myalgia, and arthralgia. Identification of the organism in a thick smear of RBCs, blood PCR, or serology is diagnostic.

Toxoplasma gondii is a protozoan parasite. Children become infected from eating contaminated, undercooked meat or from exposure to the feces of domestic cats. Most infections acquired postnatally are asymptomatic, but children may develop a mononucleosis-like illness (see Chapter 48). Diagnosis is by serology.

Toxocariasis (visceral larva migrans or ocular toxocariasis) results from ingestion of larvae of *Toxocara canis* or from *Toxocara cati* shed in dog and cat feces, respectively. Heavy or repeated infection results in fever, intense eosinophilia, hepatomegaly, and hypergammaglobulinemia. Lung, heart, and CNS involvement is rare. In ocular toxocariasis, the eye is infected, resulting in inflammation and scarring. Diagnosis is based on serology, but care must be taken to differentiate prior or asymptomatic infection from active infection.

Infections in Children with Fever of Unknown Origin Who Live in or Have Traveled to Countries with Certain Endemic Infections or Lower Baseline Socioeconomic Status

In a child who has traveled to or lives in a country with lower baseline socioeconomic status, consideration must be given to the location, water sources, and activities. Some causes of FUO to consider include malaria, viral hepatitis, typhoid fever, tuberculosis, and amebic liver abscess (see Table 52.13).

Malaria

Malaria is transmitted by the bite of an infected mosquito carrying one of the five species of the *Plasmodium* genus that cause disease in humans. The patient experiences chills, rigors, high fever, diaphoresis, and headaches. The incubation period varies among species, from 1 week to several months. Demonstration of the parasite on thick peripheral blood smear is diagnostic. The endemicity of malaria in various countries can be checked at http://www.cdc.gov/malaria.

Viral Hepatitis

Hepatitis A may be contracted by ingestion of contaminated food or water. Hepatitis B and C viruses are transmitted through blood products or sexual contact. Symptoms can include fever, malaise, jaundice, hepatomegaly, nausea, and anorexia. Hepatitis B and C can become chronic (see Chapter 18). Initial diagnosis is by serologic testing, with PCR testing for active disease in hepatitis B and C.

Typhoid Fever (Enteric Fever)

Enteric fever is caused by infection with *Salmonella enterica* serovars typhi, paratyphi A, paratyphi B, and paratyphi C. After ingestion of contaminated water or food, the incubation period is usually 1–2 weeks, but may be as long as 8 weeks. Persistent fever, headache, malaise, anorexia, splenomegaly, and rose spots are clinical hallmarks of enteric fever. Diagnosis is by blood culture.

Tuberculosis

Tuberculosis may manifest as FUO in children (see Chapters 3 and 48). Affected children may have pulmonary or extrapulmonary disease. The signs and symptoms of pulmonary disease may vary greatly from weight loss, tuberculin skin test conversion, and low-grade fever to mass effect from mediastinal lymphadenopathy and fulminant disseminated pulmonary involvement with miliary infiltrates or, in rare cases, cavitation. Pulmonary tuberculous presents as an FUO less commonly than nonpulmonary tuberculosis. Hematogenous spread may cause CNS, liver, heart, or renal involvement. Ingested bacilli may result in gastrointestinal tuberculosis. The diagnosis requires demonstration of acid-fast bacilli or positive PCR from sputum, gastric aspirate, or the affected organ. Skin testing or interferon-γ release assays may yield negative results in the case of active tuberculosis.

Amebiasis

Intestinal infection with *Entamoeba histolytica* may produce invasion of the mucosal lining and spread to other organs such as the liver. Amebic liver abscess may manifest with fever, weight loss, right upper quadrant pain, and anorexia. The patient may have painful hepatomegaly without splenomegaly. The abscess may be localized with abdominal ultrasonography or CT. Diagnosis is by ova and parasite examination of the stool and serology.

Rheumatic Causes of Fever of Unknown Origin

Rheumatic diseases are the second most common identified cause of FUO after infections. In a systematic review, the most common causes were JIA and SLE (see Chapter 44).

Juvenile Idiopathic Arthritis

JIA is a diagnosis that requires time to identify all manifestations and to exclude other entities. JIA is defined by arthritis of unknown origin that begins in a child younger than 16 years and persists for a minimum of 6 weeks. JIA is divided into three subtypes: systemic, polyarticular, and oligoarticular. The systemic form often manifests with prolonged high fever. Affected children often have a daily fever and may have a fine macular rash, arthralgias, arthritis, hepatosplenomegaly, or pericardial involvement. Characteristic laboratory findings include leukocytosis, thrombocytosis, and elevated ESR. Polyarticular JIA may manifest with arthritis, low-grade fever, morning stiffness, anorexia, and weight loss. There is no diagnostic laboratory test for JIA.

Polyarteritis

Polyarteritis is a necrotizing vasculitis that may manifest with myalgia, arthralgia, fever, vasculitic skin lesions, and abdominal pain. Cardiac, CNS, and renal involvement may also occur. The ESR is usually markedly elevated. Biopsy and the presence of antibodies to proteinase 3 and myeloperoxidase (antineutrophil cytoplasmic antibodies) aid with diagnosis.

Systemic Lupus Erythematosus

SLE may manifest with fever, photosensitivity, mouth sores, weight loss, rash, myalgias, malaise, fatigue, and hepatosplenomegaly. Patients may also have serositis and renal involvement. Cytopenias are typical. The presence of autoantibodies is common, including antinuclear antibody (ANA), double-stranded DNA (dsDNA), antibodies to extractable nuclear antigens (ENAs, such as anti-Smith antibody, anti-ribonuclear protein antibody, anti-Ro antibody, and anti-La antibody), and antiphospholipid antibodies.

Behçet Syndrome

Behçet syndrome is very rare in children but may manifest with FUO. Patients may have aphthous stomatitis, arthritis, genital ulcers, uveitis, and erythema nodosum.

Neoplasms

Hodgkin lymphoma, lymphoma, neuroblastoma, and leukemia may all manifest as FUO. In young children, leukemia, neuroblastoma, and lymphoma should be suspected, whereas in adolescents, Hodgkin lymphoma and Ewing sarcoma are more common as causes of FUO.

Hodgkin Lymphoma

Hodgkin lymphoma may manifest with firm, nontender adenopathy; fever; night sweats; and weight loss. Some patients present with a mediastinal mass with or without respiratory symptoms. Diagnosis is made through biopsy.

Lymphoma

Non-Hodgkin lymphoma may manifest as painless adenopathy, cough or dyspnea from a mediastinal mass, abdominal mass, nerve compression, bone pain, fever, and weight loss. Adenopathy and masses may be inapparent on physical examination but found on chest or abdominal imaging. Diagnosis is by biopsy.

Neuroblastoma

Neuroblastoma may manifest as abdominal, thoracic, or pelvic masses; spinal cord compression; bone pain; hypertension; hepatomegaly; diarrhea; and fever (see Chapter 20). Diagnosis is aided by radiologic studies and urinary catecholamine measurements and is confirmed by biopsy.

Leukemia

Both acute lymphocytic leukemia and acute nonlymphocytic leukemia may manifest with lethargy, pallor, bleeding, fever, bone pain, lymphadenopathy, and arthralgia. Diagnosis is made by blood smear and bone marrow biopsy.

Pheochromocytoma

Pheochromocytomas are rare catecholamine-secreting tumors; 10% occur in children. These tumors manifest with paroxysmal or sustained hypertension, headache, excessive sweating, fever, hyperglycemia, and palpitations. The tumors are usually in the adrenal medulla, but 35% of those occurring in children are multiple or extra-adrenal. Diagnosis is made by measuring urinary or plasma metanephrine or catecholamine levels. Localization of tumor is by CT, MRI, or iodine 131-metaiodobenzylguanidine scanning.

Miscellaneous Causes of Fever of Unknown Origin

Genetic Diseases (See Chapter 54)

Familial Mediterranean fever is an autosomal recessive trait seen in people of Sephardic Jewish descent and people of Middle Eastern descent. The fever may be accompanied by joint, abdominal, and chest pain. Anhidrotic ectodermal dysplasia is an X-linked recessive disorder associated with decreased ability to sweat, dental abnormalities, and sparse hair. Eyebrows and eyelashes may be absent. Fever may result from the inability of the body to cool itself. Diagnosis is made by skin biopsy that shows an absence of eccrine glands.

Drug Fever

Drug fever is a diagnosis of exclusion. Some drugs are more likely than others to cause drug fever (α-methyldopa, phenytoin, penicillins). There is no characteristic fever pattern. The lag time between the initiation of the drug and onset of fever is highly variable. There is an infrequent association with rash or eosinophilia. Some drugs may cause fever by virtue of physiologic side effects. Anticholinergic drugs may decrease sweating and diminish the body's ability to cool itself. Chronic salicylate intoxication can cause increased heat production by uncoupling oxidative phosphorylation.

Kawasaki Disease

Kawasaki disease may manifest with a variety of signs, including rash; lymphadenopathy; conjunctival hyperemia; strawberry tongue; erythematous lips; swelling of hands and feet; arthralgia; arthritis; myocarditis; late desquamation of hands, feet, and perineal area; and sterile pyuria. Fever may be high and spiking. Diagnosis is by fulfillment of clinical criteria (see Chapter 53). A subset of patients with MIS-C will present with features of Kawasaki disease with additional findings, such as coagulopathy, cardiac dysfunction, or shock. A known prior history of infection with the SARS-CoV-2 virus or demonstration of prior infection via positive IgG in an unvaccinated individual in the setting of a hyperinflammatory illness suggests MIS-C rather than Kawasaki disease.

Inflammatory Bowel Disease

Inflammatory bowel disease (ulcerative colitis, Crohn disease) may manifest with FUO. Ulcerative colitis may manifest with bloody diarrhea, fever, fecal urgency, and straining (see Chapter 14). Pyoderma gangrenosum, arthritis, and erythema nodosum can also be seen. Crohn disease (regional enteritis) may manifest with abdominal pain, fever, anorexia, and growth failure. Diarrhea may develop later. Arthritis, erythema nodosum, and finger clubbing may also occur. Diagnosis of inflammatory bowel disease is by endoscopy and histology.

Thyrotoxicosis

Hyperthyroid states may manifest with FUO. Physical examination may reveal tremor, tachycardia, palpitations, exophthalmos, lid lag, eyelid retraction, and smooth, flushed skin with diaphoresis. Diagnosis is made from thyroid function studies.

Factitious Disorders

Factitious fever may be a form of factitious disorder imposed on self (formerly Munchausen syndrome) or medical child abuse (formerly

TABLE 52.14	**Red Flags for Potentially Serious Febrile Conditions**
History	**Screening Laboratory Tests**
Poor appetite	Anemia
Weight loss (unintentional)	Hypoalbuminemia
Sleep perturbation	Lactate dehydrogenase or uric acid elevation
Focal complaints	Immunoglobulin elevation
High fever longer than 5 days	
Oliguria	**Elevated Inflammatory Markers**
	Marked leukocytosis or neutropenia
Physical Examination	Bandemia
Hepatomegaly	Pronounced thrombocytosis or thrombocytopenia
Splenomegaly	
Lymphadenopathy	**Markedly Elevated**
Rash (especially petechiae or purpura)	ESR
Wasting	CRP
Clubbing	Procalcitonin
Altered mental status	Ferritin
Focal findings	Fibrinogen (elevated or low)
Shock (tachycardia hypotension)	

From Chusid MJ. Fever of unknown origin in childhood. *Pediatr Clin North Am.* 2017;64(1):205–230, Box 1.

Munchausen syndrome by proxy) (see Chapter 30). A variety of techniques have been used to falsely elevate a recorded temperature. A mercury thermometer may be rubbed between hands or placed near a light bulb. Hot liquids may be placed in the mouth before an oral temperature is taken. Hot rectal douches have also been reported to raise a rectally taken temperature. Even with pathologic fevers, there is some circadian rhythm to the temperature curve; with factitious fever there is no rhythm. In addition, there is usually no vasoconstriction, sweating, tachypnea, or tachycardia. If factitious fever is suspected, the temperature should be obtained while the patient is observed. The temperature of freshly voided urine can also be recorded.

Other patients may produce actual diseases that cause true fevers, such as by injecting infected pyogenic material subcutaneously or intravenously or by taking toxic levels of thyroid hormone. Once the diagnosis is documented and the safety and security of the child ensured, psychiatric care is indicated.

Patients with Fever of Unknown Origin in Whom No Diagnosis Is Made

If no diagnosis is made, most patients are clinically well and asymptomatic on follow-up. Some may be determined to be healthy from the start; most are in good health at follow-up, whereas few have symptoms at the end of evaluation. Some may have relapses of fever for a few months. Diseases such as JIA, inflammatory bowel disease, and PFAPA syndrome may not be immediately diagnosed but usually manifest typical symptoms and signs within 2 years of the onset of the FUO.

SUMMARY AND RED FLAGS

Many children with fever will have a source identified on their initial history and physical examination. Red flags include patients with symptoms or signs of sepsis (tachycardia, hypotension) or meningitis or encephalitis (fever, headache, irritability, altered mental status, and, for the older child, meningismus). Affected infants with meningitis are more likely than older children to have subtle and nonspecific symptoms.

A child with fever of recent onset with no adequate historical or physical explanation for the fever is said to have FWS. Because of the high volume of children with FWS, it is important to have a reliable system for individual patient evaluation and management. Although most patients with FWS have a self-limited viral illness, up to 10% have an invasive bacterial infection, with young infants at highest risk. Because of the potential for morbidity and mortality from the organisms that cause invasive disease, identification of patients at high risk is essential. Although there is no single, timely series of tests that correctly categorizes all patients, the combination of careful clinical evaluation and appropriate laboratory screening criteria can help identify a level of risk in children of different ages. The reduction of bacteremia due to vaccine-serotype pneumococcus has led to a careful reduction in diagnostic testing, especially in the 3–36-month-old child with FWS. Red flags include a history of immunodeficiency or other chronic medical illness, prior episodes of bacteremia, anatomic or functional asplenia, no prior immunizations, toxic appearance, signs of shock, petechiae or purpura, poor responsiveness, and other signs of altered mental status.

Some children who are initially thought to have FWS develop into patients with FUO. A practical definition of FUO is a temperature higher than 38°C (100.4°F) daily for at least 8–14 days and no diagnosis after an initial evaluation. Work-up of the patient with FUO should proceed in a stepwise manner. It should be kept in mind that many patients with FUO have unusual, atypical, or complicated manifestations of common childhood illness, mainly infections. Red flags include weight loss, night sweats, signs of organ system dysfunction or failure, or unstable vital signs suggestive of sepsis (Table 52.14). Only this last category requires empiric antibiotics or deviation for the usual stepwise evaluation of FUO.

BIBLIOGRAPHY

A bibliography is available at ExpertConsult.com.

53

Fever and Rash

Michelle L. Mitchell

The coexistence of fever and rash suggests a relatively wide spectrum of pathologic entities for diagnostic consideration. This spectrum includes local or systemic infection with a wide range of microbial pathogens; toxin-mediated disorders, including those associated with bacterial superantigen production; inflammatory conditions including vasculitides and rheumatologic diseases; and hypersensitivity disorders. While most conditions causing fever and rash are benign and self-limited, a thorough clinical evaluation is crucial to identify those caused by life-threatening diseases or those requiring specific treatment. The essential elements for accurate diagnosis include a detailed history and a thorough physical examination including a careful systematic observation of the patient for evidence of toxicity. Because this approach lacks perfect sensitivity, the laboratory may play an important role in the diagnostic process.

FEVER AND RASH

History

Information about the features of the rash includes when it occurred in relation to the fever, its evolution or progression, its anatomic distribution, and whether it is pruritic or painful (Table 53.1). Degree of illness should be evaluated, especially in the infant and toddler, by assessing oral intake, activity level, and urine output. A description of the fever pattern can be useful (see Chapter 52) and immunization status will help prioritize the differential diagnosis. Essential information from the epidemiologic and social history should include season of the year; geographic location of the patient's residence; exposure to known ill contacts; recent travel or exposure to individuals from different geographic areas; exposure to pets, wildlife, or insects; recent immunizations; ingestion of raw meat or fish, unpasteurized dairy, and/or potentially contaminated meat or produce; a detailed list of medications; previous blood transfusion; and, for the adolescent patient, intravenous drug use and sexual activity.

The medical and family history should be used to assess the overall health of the patient over time, as well as that of family members, to determine the possibility of underlying primary or acquired immunodeficiency or diseases associated with autoimmunity or chronic inflammation. A history of increased susceptibility to infection, as manifested by chronic or recurrent infections after infancy such as pneumonia, sinusitis, bronchitis, otitis media, diarrhea, and bacteremia, is an important indicator of underlying immunodeficiency disease (see Chapter 54). In addition, the occurrence of an unusually severe infection or an infection with a pathogen of low virulence (e.g., *Pneumocystis jiroveci*) should raise suspicion for an immunodeficiency state. A history of hemolytic anemia, leukopenia, thrombocytopenia, or arthritis suggests an autoimmune disorder or malignancy, which may also be associated with impairment in immune function (see Chapter 44).

In a thorough systems review, the clinician should assess the probability of a subacute or chronic underlying infectious, inflammatory, or malignant disease by inquiring about anorexia, nausea, vomiting, weight loss or failure to thrive, night sweats, fatigue, cough, and exercise intolerance. The clinician should seek symptoms suggesting multisystem disease, such as myalgias, arthralgias, headache, precordial pain or pain with inspiration, abdominal pain, jaundice, skin photosensitivity, peripheral edema, alopecia, Raynaud phenomenon, and hematuria. In patients with symptoms that indicate the presence of multisystem disease, a thorough survey of the functional status of the central, peripheral, and autonomic nervous systems is clinically relevant. Specific inquiries into visual disturbances, photophobia, disordered mentation, neck stiffness, paresthesia, weakness, or seizure activity are essential and may reveal potentially life-threatening infection within the central nervous system or a systemic vasculitis involving the nervous system, such as systemic lupus erythematosus (SLE) or polyarteritis nodosa.

Examination

The physical examination is used to refine the probability of underlying serious illness, to identify rashes typical of a specific diagnosis, to look for noncutaneous disease manifestations, and to identify if further testing or treatment is indicated (Tables 53.2 and 53.3; also see Chapters 52 and 61).

A critical first step is an assessment of the patient's vital signs and degree of toxicity. Lethargy, irritability, altered mental status, decreased activity, poor perfusion, pallor, mottled skin, decreased pulses, or cyanosis indicates serious illness; resuscitation and treatment directed at the most likely diagnoses should be initiated without delay. The importance of the height of fever in predicting the risk of serious illness is unclear. Underlying chronic illness and degree of toxicity are more useful for risk assessment than fever height. The presence of tachycardia and tachypnea in any patient with fever and rash suggests the possibility of sepsis. Tachycardia may also be seen in endocarditis or in myocarditis secondary to certain viruses, Kawasaki disease (KD), multisystem inflammatory syndrome children (MIS-C), or acute rheumatic fever. Evidence of alteration in mental status suggests either sepsis associated with decreased organ perfusion or primary meningoencephalitis. The presence of hypotension usually indicates septic shock, but other disorders such as toxic shock syndrome (TSS), dengue hemorrhagic shock syndrome, KD shock syndrome, MIS-C, hemorrhagic fever with renal syndrome caused by hantavirus, and lupus myocarditis must also be considered in this context. Hypertension may be noted in association with vasculitic disorders involving small- to medium-sized arteries, such as polyarteritis and SLE.

The clinical characteristics of the rash are often helpful in establishing an etiologic diagnosis. A morphologic nomenclature of cutaneous manifestations helps the clinician with differential diagnosis,

TABLE 53.1   Essential Elements of the History in the Clinical Assessment of Fever and Rash

Demographic Data

Age

Sex

Ethnicity

Season

Geographic area; resident or travel to endemic areas

Diet history (raw meats, shellfish; unpasteurized dairy, etc.)

Ill contacts (home, daycare, school, workplace)

Sexual contacts

Pets (dogs, cats, reptiles, turtles, rodents, birds), wildlife, insects (especially ticks)

Medications and drugs

Transfusions

Immunizations

Occupational

Features of Rash

Temporal associations (onset relative to fever)

Progression and evolution

Location and distribution

Pain or pruritus

Timing and pattern of desquamation

Associated Symptoms

Focal (suggesting organ-specific illness)

Systemic (suggesting generalized or multisystem illness)

Prior Health Status

Medical and surgical history

Growth and development

Recurrent infectious illnesses

Family History

TABLE 53.2   Essential Elements of the Physical Examination in the Clinical Assessment of Fever and Rash

Degree of Toxicity

Vital Signs

Fever pattern

Tachycardia or bradycardia

Tachypnea

Hypotension or hypertension

Characteristics of Rash

Macular

Papular

Maculopapular

Petechiae or purpura

Diffuse erythroderma

Accentuation in flexural creases

Desquamation with stroking (Nikolsky sign) or spontaneous

Localized erythroderma

Expansile

Painful

Urticaria

Vesicles, pustules, bullae

Nodules

Ulcers

Distribution and Localization of Rash

Generalized or localized

Symmetric or asymmetric

Centripetal or centrifugal

Associated Enanthem

Buccal mucosa

Palate

Pharynx and tonsils

Genitals

Associated Findings (Isolated or in Clusters)

Ocular

Cardiac

Pulmonary

Gastrointestinal

Musculoskeletal; myalgia

Neurologic

Lymphadenopathy

Hepatosplenomegaly

Arthritis/arthralgia

documentation, and communication (see Chapter 61). An **exanthem** is defined as a skin eruption occurring as a sign of a generalized disease. An **enanthem** is an eruption on the mucous membranes that occurs in the context of generalized disease. Exanthems and enanthems may be macular, maculopapular, vesicular, urticarial, petechial, or diffusely erythematous. Rashes are usually classified according to their most typical lesion morphology. However, morphology may vary as rashes evolve; the rash of Rocky Mountain spotted fever is classically described as petechial, but it may initially be maculopapular. In addition, the rash of chickenpox begins as a papule that progresses to vesicular that then forms crusted lesions; all stages are present at the same time. Because a wide variety of infectious agents, including viruses and a broad range of bacteria (including rickettsiae), as well as drugs and inflammatory conditions can cause exanthems and enanthems, few of these eruptions are pathognomonic (Tables 53.4, 53.5, and 53.6).

Specific Skin Lesions

Maculopapular Eruptions

Macules are flat, nonpalpable circumscribed lesions, while **papules** are <1 cm, circumscribed palpable lesions. Maculopapular lesions

may coalesce into a more confluent morbilliform (measles-like) eruption. A rash with multiple small papules that feels like sandpaper is described as **scarlatiniform**. Maculopapular rashes are usually seen in viral illnesses, drug eruptions, and immune complex–mediated disorders. The classic childhood exanthems such as measles, rubella, erythema infectiosum (fifth disease, caused by parvovirus B19), and roseola (exanthem subitum, caused by human herpesvirus types 6 and 7) produce a maculopapular rash and are usually clinically

TABLE 53.3 Rashes Involving Palms and Soles

Bacterial
Meningococcemia
Disseminated gonococcemia
Endocarditis
Rocky Mountain spotted fever
Rat-bite fever
Secondary and congenital syphilis
Murine typhus
Pseudomonas folliculitis

Viral
Hand-foot-mouth disease
Chickenpox
Measles
Chikungunya
Parvovirus B19 (papular-purpuric gloves and socks syndrome)
Monkeypox

Infestation
Scabies

Immunologic
Palmoplantar pustulosis (SAPHO syndrome)
Keratoderma blennorrhagica (reactive arthritis)
Vasculitis
Kawasaki disease
MIS-C
SLE
Stevens-Johnson syndrome
Erythema multiforme
Graft versus host disease
Id reaction to fungi
Guttate psoriasis

Other
Langerhans cell histiocytosis

MIS-C, multisystem inflammatory syndrome in children; SAPHO, synovitis, acne, plantar pustulosis, hyperostosis, osteitis; SLE, systemic lupus erythematosus.

hypersensitivity syndrome, formerly anticonvulsant hypersensitivity syndrome).

Inflammatory diseases can also present with fever and maculopapular rash. Systemic juvenile idiopathic arthritis (SJIA, Still disease) classically presents with an evanescent, salmon-colored macular rash on the trunk and proximal extremities that coincide with fever spikes (see Chapter 44). Many of the hereditary periodic fever syndromes manifest with macular, maculopapular, or urticarial rashes associated with fever (see Chapter 54).

Petechiae and Purpura

Extravasation of red blood cells from the vasculature into the skin produces petechiae and purpura. These lesions do not blanch with applied pressure. **Petechiae** are pinpoint lesions (<3 mm). **Purpura** are larger lesions and can be either palpable or nonpalpable. While the majority of patients with fever and petechiae have a benign illness, their presence, especially in a child younger than 24 months, is of particular concern. Between 2% and 20% of affected patients have an underlying bacterial infection, and depending on the clinical setting, 0.5–10% have sepsis caused by *Neisseria meningitidis*. Other potentially serious infections signaled by a petechial rash and fever include bacterial endocarditis and Rocky Mountain spotted fever. Group A streptococcal (GAS) pharyngitis is the most common bacterial cause of fever and petechiae, with up to 20% of patients with fever and petechiae being diagnosed with GAS pharyngitis in some studies. Common viral causes include enterovirus and adenovirus. Febrile children may develop petechiae after coughing or vomiting; petechiae in this setting are almost always located in the superior vena cava distribution above the nipple line. Further, petechiae confined solely to the area above the nipple line is rarely associated with invasive bacterial disease. Noninfectious causes of fever and petechiae include drug eruptions and acute leukemia. Not all children with fever and petechiae have thrombocytopenia.

Diffuse purpuric lesions may be noted in a wide variety of disorders. These include infectious diseases associated with organisms with a predilection for vascular endothelium, such as *N. meningitidis* (Fig. 53.6) and rickettsiae (Fig. 53.7), uncommon bacterial diseases such as rat-bite fever (Fig. 53.8) and *Vibrio vulnificus* or Brazilian purpuric fever caused by *Haemophilus aegyptius*, and a number of viral hemorrhagic fever diseases. Purpura is also associated with disseminated intravascular coagulation (DIC) and profound thrombocytopenia, such as in idiopathic thrombocytopenic purpura (see Chapter 51). Purpura followed by subsequent necrosis of skin is referred to as **purpura fulminans**, a severe, life-threatening condition that has been reported after relatively benign infections such as varicella or with more serious disorders (meningococcemia) (Fig. 53.9). Purpura can also occur in the noninfectious vasculitides, such as Henoch-Schönlein purpura (HSP) and granulomatosis with polyangiitis. Discrete, raised purpuric lesions (palpable purpura) distributed predominantly over the buttocks and lower extremities are typical for this disorder. While bacteremia must be considered for all febrile patients presenting with diffuse or discrete purpuric lesions (see Figs. 53.6, 53.7, 53.8, and 53.9), patients with HSP are generally well-appearing but may have significant discomfort from arthritis or abdominal pain.

Vesiculobullous Eruptions

Vesicular rashes (sharply demarcated, raised lesions containing clear fluid), **bullae** (vesicles exceeding 1 cm in diameter), or **pustules** (raised lesions containing cloudy fluid composed of serum and inflammatory cells) may be suggestive of focal or disseminated infection with various pathogens or signal a serious drug reaction. **Localized vesicles** may suggest infection with herpes simplex virus (HSV) type 1 or 2 (especially if the vesicles are grouped on an erythematous base),

recognizable (Figs. 53.1 and 53.2; see Table 53.6). Other organisms that commonly cause a maculopapular rash include enteroviruses, Epstein-Barr virus (EBV), cytomegalovirus, adenovirus, acute HIV, and hepatitis B virus. **Erythema migrans,** the distinctive rash of Lyme disease (caused by the tick-borne spirochete *Borrelia burgdorferi*), begins as a papule at the site of a recent tick bite and slowly expands over days to weeks to form an erythematous, annular lesion, sometimes with partial central clearing (Fig. 53.3). The rash of southern tick-associated rash illness (STARI) appears similarly. **Erythema marginatum,** a rare but major manifestation of acute rheumatic fever, is also distinctive (Fig. 53.4).

Morbilliform drug eruptions are often indistinguishable from viral exanthems and typically present 7–14 days after exposure to a drug (Fig. 53.5). As with most viral exanthems, the rash starts on the trunk and spreads to the extremities. Examples of causative agents include aminopenicillins, cephalosporins, antiepileptics, and sulfonamides. Morbilliform drug eruptions usually resolve spontaneously after discontinuation of the culprit drug, but sometimes they are the first sign of the potentially life-threatening syndrome drug rash with eosinophilia and systemic symptoms (**DRESS**, also known as drug-induced

TABLE 53.4 Differential Diagnosis of Fever and Rash

Lesion	Pathogen or Associated Factor
Maculopapular or Macular Rash	**Viruses** Measles (confluent), rubella (discrete), roseola (human herpesvirus 6),* fifth disease (parvovirus),* EBV,* enteroviruses,* hepatitis B virus (papular acrodermatitis or Gianotti-Crosti syndrome), HIV, dengue virus, adenovirus, chikungunya virus
	Bacteria Rheumatic fever (group A streptococcus), scarlet fever, erysipelas, *Arcanobacterium haemolyticum*, secondary syphilis, leptospirosis, *Pseudomonas*, meningococcal infection (early), *Salmonella* (typhoid rose spots), Lyme disease, STARI, *Mycoplasma pneumoniae*,* *Listeria monocytogenes*, *Brucella melitensis*, *Coxiella burnetii* (Q fever), rat-bite fever
	Rickettsiae Early Rocky Mountain spotted fever, typhus (scrub, murine, endemic), ehrlichiosis (monocytic)
	Other Kawasaki disease,* *Coccidioides immitis*, drug reactions, SJIA, hereditary fever syndromes, HLH, toxoplasmosis, MIS-C
Diffuse Erythroderma	**Bacteria** Scarlet fever (group A streptococcus),* other streptococci, toxic shock syndrome (*Staphylococcus aureus* and group A streptococcus),* staphylococcal scarlet fever, ehrlichiosis *(Ehrlichia chaffeensis)*, MIS-C
	Fungi *Candida albicans*
Urticarial Rash	**Viruses** EBV, hepatitis B and C, HIV, enteroviruses
	Bacteria *M. pneumoniae*, group A streptococci, *Shigella*, meningococcus, *Yersinia*, *Borrelia burgdorferi*
	Other Various parasites, insect bites, food-drug allergens (usually afebrile)
Vesicular, Bullous, Pustular	**Viruses** Herpes simplex,* varicella-zoster,* coxsackieviruses,* echoviruses, vaccinia, variola, monkeypox, chikungunya
	Bacteria Staphylococcal scalded skin syndrome, staphylococcal bullous impetigo, group A streptococcal crusted impetigo, gonococcemia,* *Vibrio vulnificus*, rat-bite fever, anthrax
	Other Toxic epidermal necrolysis, Stevens-Johnson syndrome,* rickettsialpox

Lesion	Pathogen or Associated Factor
Petechial-Purpuric	**Viruses** Atypical measles, congenital rubella, cytomegalovirus, enterovirus, HIV, hemorrhagic fever viruses, hemorrhagic varicella, EBV, hepatitis B, adenovirus, yellow fever, parvovirus, chikungunya
	Bacteria Sepsis (meningococcal,* gonococcal, pneumococcal,* *S. aureus**), endocarditis, rat-bite fever (*Spirillum minus* or *Streptobacillus moniliformis*), *Pseudomonas aeruginosa*, group A streptococcus, *Capnocytophaga canimorsus*, *Yersinia pestis*
	Rickettsiae Rocky Mountain spotted fever,* epidemic and murine typhus, ehrlichiosis
	Other Vasculitis, thrombocytopenia, Henoch-Schönlein purpura,* malaria
Erythema Nodosum	**Viruses** EBV, hepatitis B and C, HSV, HIV
	Bacteria Group A streptococcus, tuberculosis, *Yersinia*, *Bartonella henselae* (cat-scratch disease), brucellosis, Q fever, *M. pneumoniae*, tularemia, syphilis, mycobacteria, *Chlamydia* spp., meningococcus, *Campylobacter* spp.
	Fungi Coccidioidomycosis, histoplasmosis, blastomycosis, sporotrichosis, cryptococcosis
	Other Sarcoidosis, inflammatory bowel disease, estrogen-containing oral contraceptives, systemic lupus erythematosus, Behçet disease, lymphoma, ascaris, filariasis

Distinctive Rashes	
Ecthyma gangrenosum	*P. aeruginosa* (main cause), *Vibrio vulnificus*, and various other gram-negative bacteria; *Staphylococcus aureus*; *Streptococcus pyogenes*; various molds
Erythema migrans	Lyme disease, STARI
Necrotic eschar	Scrub typhus, aspergillosis, mucormycosis, cutaneous anthrax, rickettsialpox and other rickettsiae (early)
Erysipelas	Group A streptococcus (main cause), *Capnocytophaga canimorsus*
Koplik spots	Measles
Erythema marginatum	Acute rheumatic fever (group A streptococcus)
Erythema multiforme	Herpes simplex virus or *M. pneumoniae*
Rose spots	Salmonella

*Common.

EBV, Epstein-Barr virus; HLH, hemophagocytic lymphohistiocytosis; HSV, herpes simplex virus; MIS-C, multisystem inflammatory syndrome in children; SJIA, systemic juvenile idiopathic arthritis; STARI, southern tick-associated rash illness.

Modified from Prince A. Infectious diseases. In: Behrman RE, Kliegman RM, eds. *Nelson Essentials of Pediatrics.* 2nd ed. Philadelphia: WB Saunders; 1994:299.

varicella-zoster virus (especially if grouped vesicles are distributed in a dermatomal pattern) (Fig. 53.10), or infection with nonviral pathogens, such as *Rickettsia akari* (the cause of **rickettsialpox**, a mouse mite–borne rickettsiosis found worldwide but common in New York City). Localized pustules and bullae are usually suggestive of pyodermas caused by *Staphylococcus aureus*, but pustular lesions distributed on the palms and soles in the context of fever may represent infective emboli with microabscess formation (Janeway lesions), which are often caused by *S. aureus* endocarditis.

Vesicles distributed in a more **generalized pattern**, especially with a concentration of lesions over the head and trunk in various stages of evolution, are suggestive of primary varicella-zoster virus infection (**chickenpox**). A more generalized pattern with a concentration over the extremities is suggestive of enteroviral infection, especially with coxsackievirus A16 (**hand-foot-and-mouth disease**), or A6 in even more severe presentations. Orthopoxviruses such as monkeypox, like smallpox, cause a systemic febrile rash illness with lesions that progress from papules to vesicles to pustules concentrated on the face and extremities. **Acute generalized exanthematous pustulosis (AGEP)** is a rare cutaneous hypersensitivity reaction characterized by numerous sterile pustules beginning on the face and spreading to the trunk and limbs. It typically presents within 24 hours after exposure to an offending drug, usually a β-lactam or macrolide antibiotic. The clinician evaluating the sexually active patient presenting with asymmetric generalized pustules or vesicopustular lesions should also consider disseminated infection with *Neisseria gonorrhoeae*. Diffuse vesiculobullae may be noted in Stevens-Johnson syndrome (SJS) or in toxic epidermal necrolysis (TEN), life-threatening mucocutaneous hypersensitivity diseases usually related to drugs.

Nodules

Nodules (discrete, raised, firm, well-demarcated lesions without fixation to the overlying skin) may be associated with a number of underlying infectious or inflammatory disorders, such as polyarteritis nodosa and Sweet syndrome (acute febrile neutrophilic dermatosis). Red, pink, or plum-colored nodules distributed in a seemingly random manner over the skin surface may represent leukemic infiltrates. The subcutaneous nodules of acute rheumatic fever are usually located over bony extensor surfaces near tendons and are found in <5% of patients with acute rheumatic fever. They may also be found in patients with polyarticular JIA and dermatomyositis.

Erythema nodosum (erythematous and painful nodules usually distributed over the extremities) may be associated with viral infections including hepatitis B and C; bacterial infectious agents including group A β-hemolytic streptococcus (most common), chlamydia, *Brucella* species, and *Yersinia* species; mycobacterial infections; fungal infections, particularly *Coccidioides immitis* and less often *Histoplasma capsulatum*, *Blastomyces dermatitidis*, or *Cryptococcus neoformans*; or drug reactions, especially in response to oral contraceptives and sulfonamides. Other noninfectious causes include SLE, sarcoidosis, and inflammatory bowel disease.

Ulcers

Ulcers are depressed lesions in which the epidermis and some or all of the dermis has been destroyed. In immunocompromised hosts, infection with HSV may manifest with shallow erosive or ulcerative lesions. In immunocompetent hosts, cutaneous ulcerations may be noted in noninfectious disorders associated with vasculitis, such as SLE, polyarteritis nodosa, and HSP.

Pyoderma gangrenosum and **ecthyma gangrenosum** are painful cutaneous ulcerative lesions with an erythematous, raised edge. The lesions usually begin as a papule and break down rapidly with central necrosis. It may be seen in immunocompromised patients, typically in

the setting of neutropenia, often with systemic infections with bacterial pathogens (typically gram-negative), such as *Pseudomonas aeruginosa* or *Stenotrophomonas maltophilia* (ecthyma). In immunocompetent patients, the lesion may manifest in the context of inflammatory bowel disease (pyoderma gangrenosum), PAPA (pyogenic arthritis, pyoderma gangrenosum, acne), or rheumatoid arthritis. Digital ulcerations may be noted in patients with small-vessel vasculitis, such as SLE. Oral ulcerations may be noted in those with herpes simplex or coxsackievirus (hand-foot-and-mouth disease) or as a manifestation of Behçet disease, SLE, PFAPA (periodic fever, aphthous stomatitis, pharyngitis, adenitis), cyclic neutropenia, or inflammatory bowel disease.

Erythema

Diffuse erythema (**erythroderma**) is associated with toxin-mediated disorders characterized by superantigen production. Bacterial superantigens cause nonspecific T-cell stimulation resulting in several acute rash-fever disorders, such as staphylococcal scalded skin syndrome (SSSS; Fig. 53.11), streptococcal scarlet fever, staphylococcal or streptococcal TSS, and possibly KD.

Localized erythema in the context of acute fever is strongly suggestive of cellulitis, erysipelas, or abscess. The presence of warmth, tenderness, and associated lymphangitis is highly indicative. Organisms causing cellulitis or abscess formation are usually inoculated directly into the skin as a result of trauma. However, bacteremic localization is well described among young children with preseptal or facial cellulitis associated with *Haemophilus influenzae* type b (pre–*H. influenzae* type b vaccine) or *Streptococcus pneumoniae*.

Patients with SLE or dermatomyositis may present with an isolated erythematous malar rash (butterfly rash), which is exacerbated by exposure to sunlight. The acute onset of intense "slapped-cheek" erythema of the face suggests erythema infectiosum, a recognizable exanthem caused by parvovirus B19, and should be differentiated easily from the malar rash of SLE, which usually manifests other characteristics, such as chronicity as well as hyperkeratosis and follicular plugging. In addition, patients with erythema infectiosum tend to have a maculopapular, lacelike rash over the arms, which may spread to the buttocks and thighs (Fig. 53.12; see Table 53.6).

Patients with **dermatomyositis** may have localized lilac-colored lesions over the eyelids (heliotrope rash), which may be associated with periorbital edema. Such patients characteristically, but not invariably, have an erythematous, scaly eruption on the face, neck, knees, elbows, and phalanges. When the rash is localized over the knuckles, it resembles dripped wax and has been referred to as Gottron papules. Patients with autoinflammatory disorders (periodic fever syndromes) may present with localized erythema or fasciitis (see Chapter 54).

Other Physical Examination Findings

Joint Manifestations

Pain, swelling, tenderness, and limited range of motion involving one joint or multiple joints, or that migrate from joint to joint, or discrete pain at the insertion of tendons, ligaments, or fascia (enthesopathy) may indicate a primary infectious illness, a "reactive" (immunologically mediated) disorder, or a systemic inflammatory condition. Primary infectious illnesses associated with this finding include *N. gonorrhoeae*, *B. burgdorferi* (Lyme disease), parvovirus, and rubella, including vaccine-associated strains. Reactive disorders, such as reactive arthritis (arthritis/enthesitis, conjunctivitis, urethritis), may be associated with infection caused by enteric pathogens, such as *Salmonella* and *Shigella* organisms, or genital pathogens, such as *N. gonorrhoeae* or *Chlamydia* species, but may also include diseases of unknown origin, such as inflammatory bowel disease, in which the rash is usually erythema nodosum. A **serum sickness–like reaction** can be seen after treatment

TABLE 53.5　Common Bacterial Exanthems

Disease	Cause	Age	Season	Transmission	Incubation (Days)	Prodrome
Scarlet fever	Group A streptococcus	School age	Fall, winter, spring	Direct contact, droplets	1–4	Sore throat, headache, abdominal pain, cervical lymphadenopathy, fever, 0–2 days, acute onset
Staphylococcal scalded skin syndrome (SSSS)	*S. aureus*–producing exfoliative toxin	Neonates, infants, young children	Any	Colonization, contact	Unknown	None
Toxic shock syndrome (TSS)	*S. aureus*–producing toxic shock syndrome toxin-1 (TSST-1) and staphylococcal enterotoxins (SEs) Group A streptococcus–producing *Streptococcus pyogenes* exotoxins (SPEs)	Adolescent females if menstrual; others variable	Any	Colonization, contact	Variable, often 1–5	Myalgias, fevers, and gastrointestinal symptoms May be secondary to wound infection, trivial mucosal or respiratory infection, or necrotizing fasciitis or myositis
Meningococcemia	*Neisseria meningitidis*	Any (<5 yr and adolescents)	Winter, spring, follows influenza epidemics	Close, prolonged contact	5–15	Fever, malaise, myalgia, 1–10 days
Rocky Mountain spotted fever (RMSF)	*Rickettsia rickettsii*	Any (>5 yr), male > female	Summer	Carrier ticks	3–12	Fever, myalgia, headache, malaise, ill appearance, 2–4 days
Rickettsialpox	*Rickettsia akari*	Any	Any	Mouse mite	7–14	Fever, chills, headache, malaise, 4–7 days

TABLE 53.5 Common Bacterial Exanthems—cont'd

Features and Rash Structure	Enanthem	Complications	Prevention/Treatment	Comments
Diffuse erythema with "sandpaper" feel; accentuation of erythema in flexural creases (Pastia lines); circumoral pallor, lasts 2–7 days; may exfoliate	Palatal petechiae, strawberry tongue	Peritonsillar abscess, rheumatic fever, glomerulonephritis	Prevent rheumatic fever with penicillin within 10 days of onset of pharyngitis, treat with penicillin	Similar syndrome may be noted with *Arcanobacterium haemolyticum* in adolescents; group A streptococci may also produce toxic shock or true bacteremic shock syndromes in addition to cellulitis, lymphangitis, and erysipelas; *Staphylococcus aureus* may produce a scarlatiniform rash
Sudden onset, tender erythroderma progressing to diffuse flaccid bullae; significant perioral, perinasal peeling; eventual diffuse exfoliation (positive Nikolsky sign), possibly conjunctivitis, purulent rhinorrhea	Unusual	Shock	Treat with intravenous antibacterial active against *S. aureus*	—
Diffuse sunburn-like erythroderma; hypotension, diarrhea, emesis, mental status changes; late desquamation	Conjunctivitis	Shock, multisystem organ dysfunction/failure	Treat with intravenous antibacterial active against *S. aureus*; penicillin if group A streptococcus suspected; clindamycin; possible intravenous immune globulin; prevent menstrual-associated TSS by frequent changes of tampon	—
Erythematous, nonconfluent, discrete papules (early); petechiae, purpura present on trunk, extremities, palms, soles	Petechiae	Shock, meningitis, pericarditis, arthritis, endophthalmitis, gangrene, disseminated intravascular coagulation	Contacts: rifampin; general: vaccine; treat with ceftriaxone, penicillin (if sensitive)	*Neisseria gonorrhoeae*, pneumococcus, *Haemophilus influenza* type b, group A streptococcus may produce similar clinical manifestations
Early maculopapular, then petechial or, rarely, purpuric; present on extremities, then trunk, palms, and soles	Petechiae variable	Shock, myocarditis, encephalitis, pneumonia	Remove ticks as soon as possible; use tick repellants; treat with doxycycline	*Ehrlichia chaffeensis* and other rickettsiae may produce similar illnesses with or without a rash
At primary bite site, eschar; secondary papulovesicles in same stage throughout illness; fewer vesicles than in chickenpox (5–30); present on trunk and proximal extremities	Occasional, transient lesions in the oral cavity similar to that seen on the body	Usually none	Treat with doxycycline	Often confused with chickenpox; may be more common than expected, especially in crowded urban settings with poor housing

TABLE 53.6   Common Viral Exanthems

Disease	Cause	Age	Season	Transmission	Incubation (Days)	Prodrome
Measles (rubeola)	Measles virus	Any	Winter, spring	Respiratory droplet	10–12	High fever, cough, coryza, conjunctivitis, 2–4 days
Rubella (German measles)	Rubella virus	Infants, young adults	Winter, spring	Respiratory droplet	14–21	Malaise, fever <101°F, posterior auricular, cervical, occipital adenopathy, 0–4 days
Roseola (exanthem subitum)	Human herpesvirus type 6 (HHV-6), human herpesvirus type 7 (HHV-7)	Infants/toddlers (6 mo–2 yr) for HHV-6, can be older children for HHV-7	Any	Secretions of asymptomatic close contacts	9–10 (HHV-6); unknown (HHV-7)	Irritability, high fever 3–7 days, cervical, occipital adenopathy
Fifth disease (erythema infectiosum)	Parvovirus B19	Prepubertal children, schoolteachers	Winter, spring	Respiratory droplets; blood transfusion, placenta	5–15	Headache, malaise, myalgia; often afebrile
Chickenpox (varicella)	Varicella-zoster virus	1–14 yr (most) but can vary	Late fall, winter, early spring	Respiratory droplet	10–21	Fever
Enteroviruses	Coxsackievirus, echovirus, and others	Often infants and young children but varies	Summer, fall	Fecal-oral, respiratory, vertical, and possibly fomites	4–6	Variable: irritable, fever, sore throat, myalgias, headache
Mononucleosis	Epstein-Barr virus	Children, adolescents	Any	Close contact, saliva, blood transfusion	28–49	Fever, adenopathy, eyelid edema, sore throat, hepatosplenomegaly, malaise; atypical lymphocytosis
Gianotti-Crosti syndrome (papular acrodermatitis of childhood)	EBV, hepatitis B virus (uncommon where vaccination rates are high), coxsackieviruses, others	1–6 yr (primarily)	Any	Variable; fecal, sexual, blood products for hepatitis B	Unknown; 50–180 days for hepatitis B	Usually none except for specific viral disease; arthritis-arthralgia for hepatitis B

CNS, central nervous system; EBV, Epstein-Barr virus; HBIG, hepatitis B virus immune globulin; VZIG, varicella-zoster immune globulin.

TABLE 53.6   Common Viral Exanthems—cont'd

Features and Rash Structure	Enanthem	Complications	Prevention/Treatment	Comments
Maculopapular (confluent), begins on face, spreads to trunk; lasts 3–6 days Brown color develops; fine desquamation; toxic, uncomfortable appearance, photophobia; rash may be absent in HIV infection	Koplik spots on buccal mucosa before rash	Febrile seizures, otitis, pneumonia, encephalitis, laryngotracheitis, thrombocytopenia; delayed subacute sclerosing panencephalitis	General: measles vaccine at 12–15 mo and again at 4–6 yr Exposure: measles vaccine if within 72 hr; immune globulin if within 6 days of exposure (must then wait 6–8 mo to vaccinate) World Health Organization recommends treatment with vitamin A in all patients with measles	Reportable to public health department; epidemics reported, contagious 3 days before symptoms until 4 days after rash Increasing incidence as vaccination rates are decreasing
Discrete, nonconfluent, rose-colored macules and papules, begins on face and spreads downward; lasts 1–3 days	Variable erythematous macules on soft palate	Arthritis, thrombocytopenia, encephalopathy; fetal embryopathy	General: rubella vaccine at 12–15 mo and again at 4–6 yr; exposure: possibly immune serum globulin	Reportable to public health department; epidemics reported, contagious 2 days before symptoms and 5–7 days after rash
Discrete macules on trunk, neck; sudden-onset rash with defervescence; lasts 0.5–2 days; some patients have no rash	Variable erythematous macules on soft palate	Single or recurrent febrile seizures; encephalopathy; dissemination (e.g., liver, CNS, lung) in immunosuppressed patients	None	No epidemics
Local erythema of cheeks (slapped cheek appearance); lacy pink-red erythema of trunk and extremities, ± pruritus; rash may lag prodrome by 3–7 days; lasts 2–4 days, may recur 2–3 wk later	Rare, ill-described, on buccal mucosa	Arthritis, aplastic crisis in patients with chronic hemolytic anemia (e.g., sickle cell), fetal anemic hydrops, vasculitis, Wegner granulomatosis	Isolation of patients with aplastic crisis but not normal host with fifth disease	Epidemics reported; once rash is present, the normal host is not contagious; patients with aplastic crisis often have no rash
Pruritic papules, vesicles in various stages, 2–4 crops and then crusts; distributed on trunk and then face, extremities; lasts 7–10 days; recurs years later in dermatomal distribution (zoster, shingles)	Oral mucosa, tongue	Staphylococcal or streptococcal skin infection, arthritis, cerebellar ataxia, encephalitis, thrombocytopenia, Reye syndrome (with aspirin), myocarditis, nephritis, hepatitis, pneumonia; dissemination in immunocompromised	VZIG for exposed immunosuppressed patients, susceptible pregnant women, preterm neonates, and infants at birth whose mother developed varicella 5 days before and 2 days after birth; active immunization with live attenuated vaccine at 12 mo	Acyclovir therapy for immunosuppressed and possibly normal patients (controversial); contagious 1–2 days before rash until all lesions are crusted
Hand-foot-and-mouth: vesicles in those locations; others: nonspecific, usually fine nonconfluent, macular or maculopapular rash, rarely petechial, urticarial, or vesicular; lasts 3–7 days	Yes	Aseptic meningitis, hepatitis, myocarditis, paralysis: usually in younger patients	None	Rash may appear with fever or after defervescence; rash may be present in <50% of enteroviral illnesses; epidemics possible, contagious up to 2 wks
Maculopapular or morbilliform on trunk, extremities; may be confluent; often elicited by simultaneous administration of ampicillin or allopurinol; rash in 15% and in 50% with drug-induced form, lasts 2–7 days	Variable	Anemia, thrombocytopenia, aplastic anemia, hepatitis, encephalitis; rarely hemophagocytic lymphohistiocytosis, lymphoproliferative syndrome	None	Cytomegalovirus and toxoplasmosis also produce mononucleosis-like illness; monospot or heterophile tests negative
Papules, papulovesicles, discrete or confluent; face, arms, extremities, often spares trunk; lasts 4–10 days	Variable	As per specific disease	Hepatitis B: HBIG plus vaccine	—

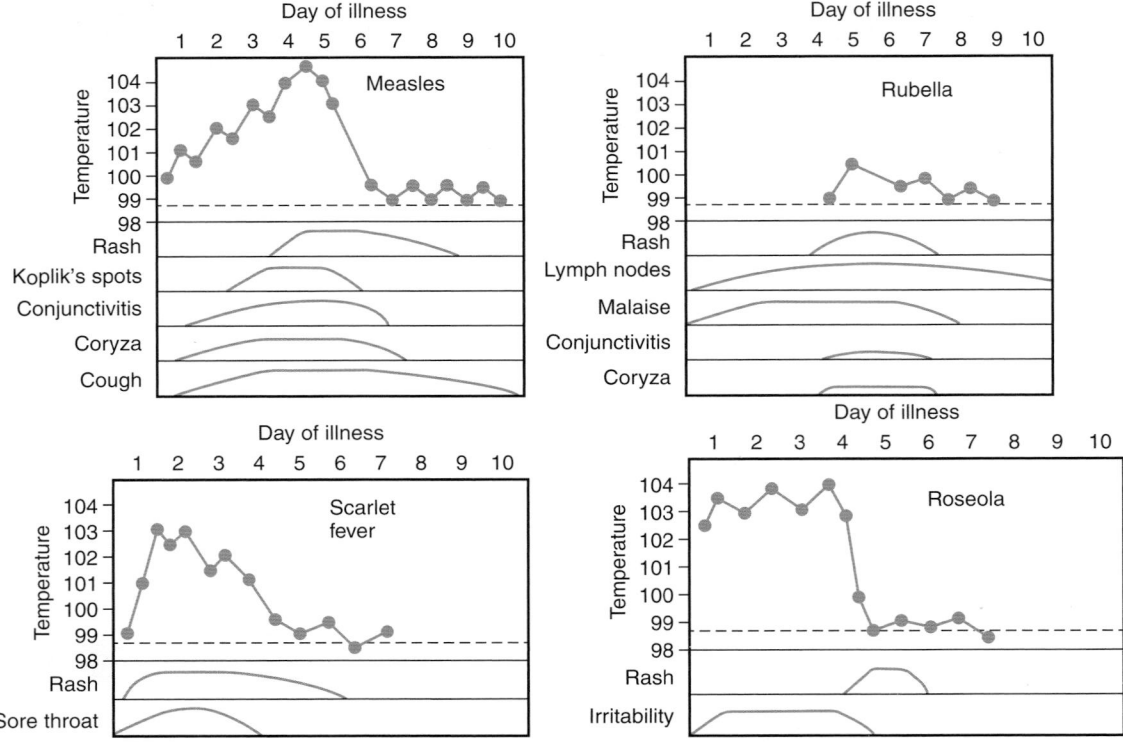

Fig. 53.1 Schematic diagrams illustrating differences among four acute exanthems characterized by maculopapular eruptions. (Modified from Gershon AA, Hotez PJ, Katz SL, eds. *Krugman's Infectious Diseases of Children.* 11th ed. Philadelphia: Mosby; 2004:927, Fig. 45.1.)

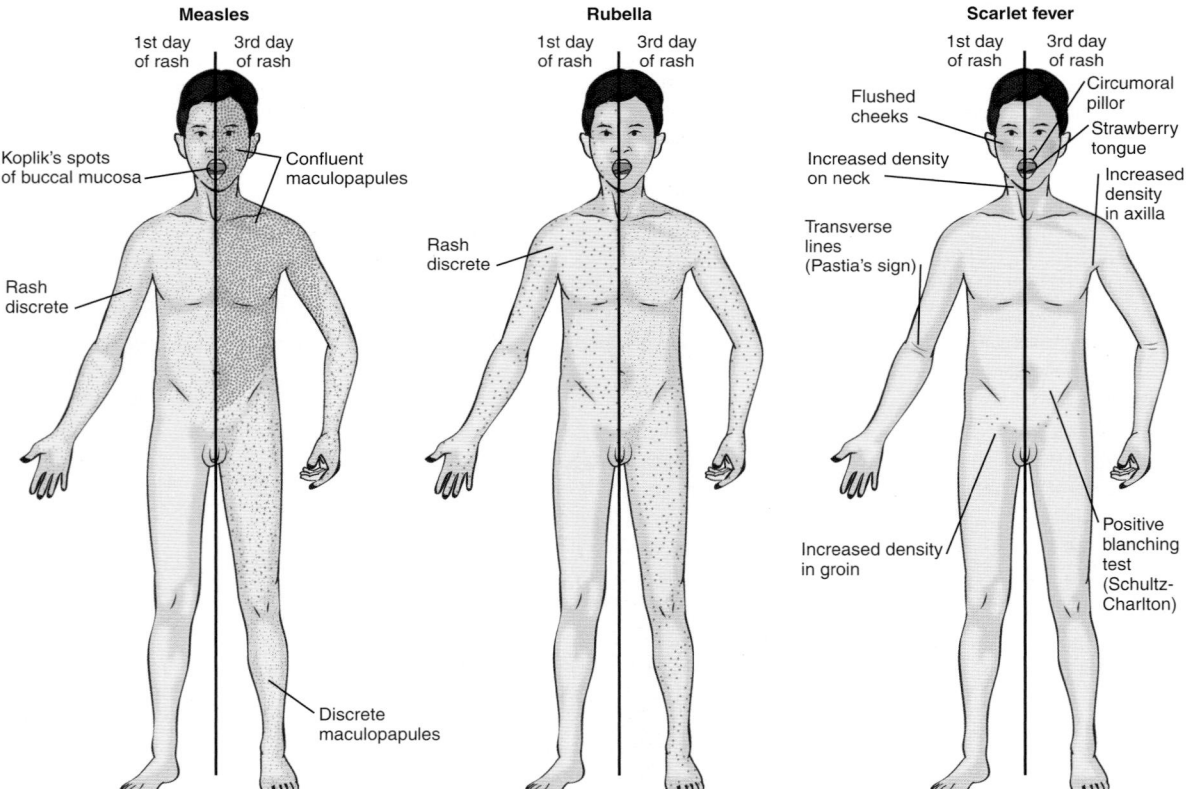

Fig. 53.2 Schematic drawings illustrating difference in appearance, distribution, and progression of rashes of measles, rubella, and scarlet fever. (From Gershon AA, Hotez PJ, Katz SL, eds. *Krugman's Infectious Diseases of Children.* 11th ed. Philadelphia: Mosby; 2004:928.)

with antibiotics. Children with systemic inflammatory conditions including KD, HSP, polyarteritis, SLE, SJIA, acute rheumatic fever, and some of the hereditary periodic fever syndromes may also have joint manifestations (see Chapters 44 and 54).

Cardiac Manifestations

Cardiac manifestations may accompany acute rheumatic fever, bacterial endocarditis, KD, MIS-C, or SJIA (see Chapter 44). The presence of

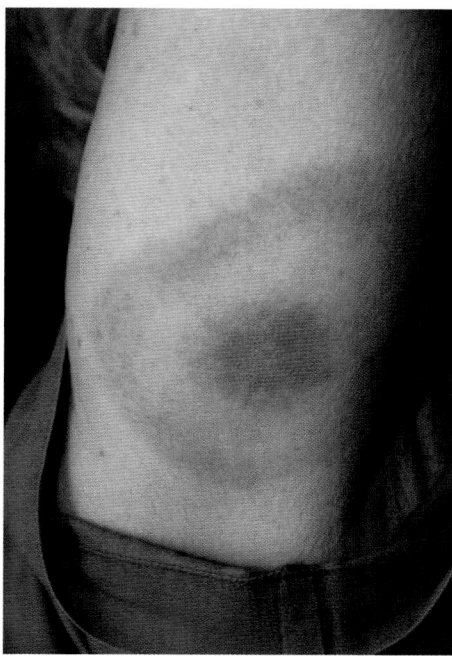

Fig. 53.3 Erythema migrans—erythematous target-like plaque of Lyme disease. The primary skin lesion of *Borrelia burgdorferi* infection is noted for centrifugal expansion, sometimes leaving a central clearing. The rash of southern tick–associated rash illness (STARI) is also similar to the rash of early Lyme disease. (Courtesy James Gathany; Content Providers CDC/James Gathany—this media comes from the Centers for Disease Control and Prevention's Public Health Image Library [PHIL], with identification number #9875. From Borchers AT, Keen CL, Huntley AC, et al. Lyme disease: a rigorous review of diagnostic criteria and treatment. *J Autoimmun.* 2015;57:82–115.)

tachycardia out of proportion to the severity of the fever may be indicative of sepsis or the carditis accompanying acute rheumatic fever, KD, MIS-C, viral myocarditis, or DRESS. A precordial friction rub is suggestive of pericarditis, which is noted frequently in patients with SJIA. The presence of a new murmur or a changing murmur on auscultation can be suggestive of bacterial endocarditis, whereas the detection of the apical systolic murmur of mitral regurgitation or the diastolic murmur of aortic insufficiency can be suggestive of acute rheumatic fever (see Chapter 9). A gallop rhythm on auscultation indicates underlying myocarditis, which may accompany coxsackievirus or other viral infection, rheumatic disease, KD, or MIS-C.

Ocular Manifestations

Isolated ocular manifestations in the setting of fever, such as conjunctival injection and frank conjunctivitis, may be suggestive of infection with measles or adenovirus, leptospirosis, KD, or onset of SJS, TEN, or reactive arthritis. The skin, eye, mouth form of neonatal HSV can infect the eyes, causing conjunctivitis and keratitis. **Anterior uveitis** (redness with accompanying photophobia or pain or change in vision) may indicate KD, SJIA, sarcoidosis, ulcerative colitis, Behçet syndrome, or, uncommonly, an infection such as leptospirosis (see Chapter 43). Retinal hemorrhages seen on funduscopy may indicate bacterial endocarditis.

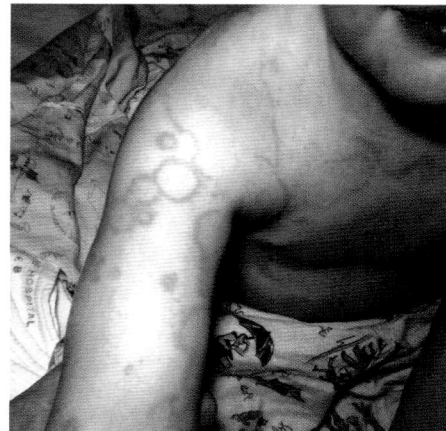

Fig. 53.4 Polycyclic red borders of erythema marginatum in a febrile child with acute rheumatic fever. (From Schachner LA, Hansen RC, eds. *Pediatric Dermatology.* 3rd ed. Philadelphia: Mosby; 2003:808.)

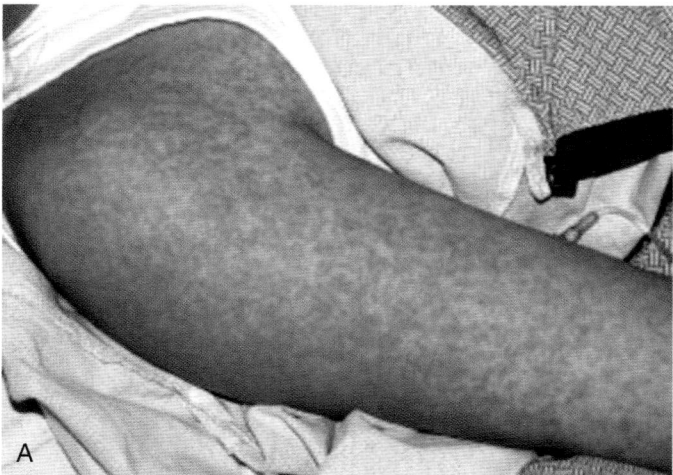

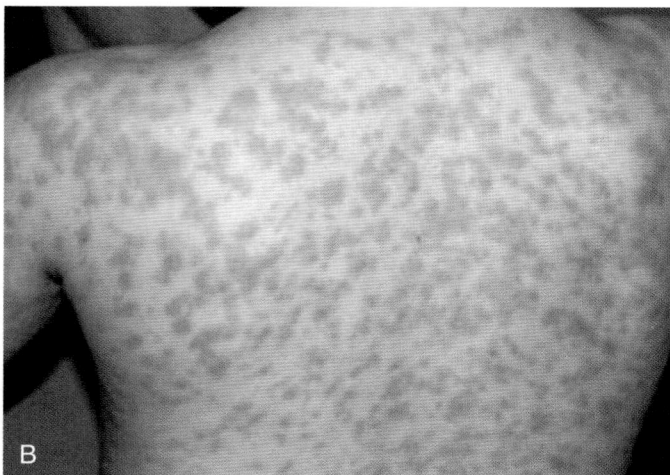

Fig. 53.5 Morbilliform drug eruptions. *A,* Fine, pink macules and thin papules becoming confluent on the posterior upper arm, which is a dependent area in this hospitalized patient. *B,* More edematous ("urticarial") pink papules; unlike true urticaria, these lesions are not transient. (From Julie V. Schaffer, MD. Fever and rash. In: Bolognia JL, ed. *Dermatology Essentials.* Philadelphia: Elsevier; 2014;3:28–38.)

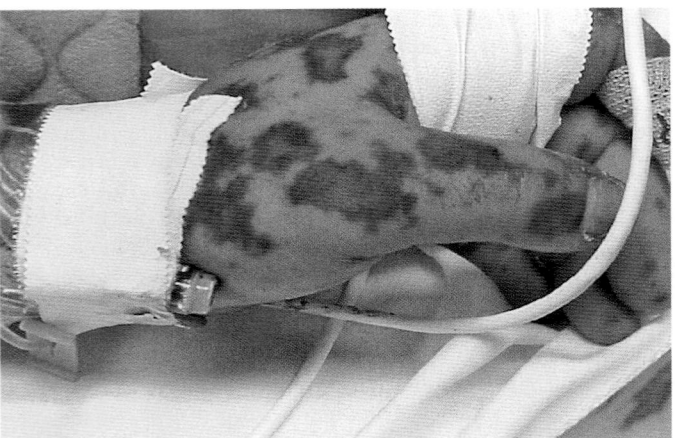

Fig. 53.6 Widespread purpura of meningococcemia. (From Callen JP, ed. *Dermatological Signs of Internal Disease*. 4th ed. Philadelphia: Elsevier; 2009:256, Fig. 28-14.)

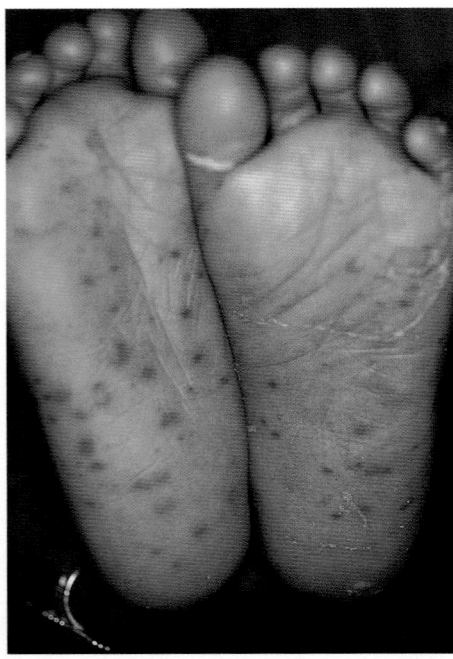

Fig. 53.7 Purpuric lesions in a patient with Rocky Mountain spotted fever. (From Callen JP, ed. *Dermatological Signs of Internal Disease*. 4th ed. Philadelphia: Elsevier; 2009:258, Fig. 28-16.)

Neurologic Manifestations

Neurologic findings accompanying fever and rash may be indicative of specific infectious or immunologically mediated disorders. Mental status findings suggestive of recent-onset psychosis may indicate cerebritis, which can accompany SLE. Significant alteration in mental status accompanied by seizure or focal motor impairment or cerebellar dysfunction may be suggestive of primary infectious encephalitis associated with arbovirus, herpes simplex, measles, varicella-zoster virus, rickettsia, West Nile virus, or *Mycoplasma pneumoniae* infection. Nuchal rigidity, the Kernig sign, or the Brudzinski sign indicates meningeal irritation, which may accompany infection caused by the enteroviruses; bacteria such as *S. pneumoniae*, *N. meningitidis*, or spirochetes such as *B. burgdorferi*; fungi such as *H. capsulatum*; or inflammation caused by underlying SLE, sarcoidosis, or KD. Cranial nerve palsies, ataxia, or peripheral neuropathy may accompany infection with *B. burgdorferi* early in the course of **Lyme disease** (especially Bell palsy), or it may indicate an underlying vasculitis, such as SLE. Movement abnormalities, particularly chorea, may be suggestive of either SLE or acute rheumatic fever. **Hemophagocytic lymphohistiocytosis (HLH)** is a life-threatening syndrome of excessive immune activation that can have varied neurologic manifestations including seizure, mental status changes, and ataxia. The rash associated with HLH is also variable and can be maculopapular, erythrodermic, petechial, or purpuric. When seen in a patient with SJIA, the syndrome is called macrophage activation syndrome.

Pulmonary Manifestations

The presence of isolated lower respiratory tract findings (decreased breath sounds, rales, expiratory wheezing, respiratory distress, and cyanosis) indicates underlying pulmonary infection with an organism such as measles, adenovirus, *M. pneumoniae*, or *Legionella pneumophila*. Although sarcoidosis, collagen vascular disease, and systemic vasculitis (granulomatosis with polyangiitis, eosinophilic granulomatosis

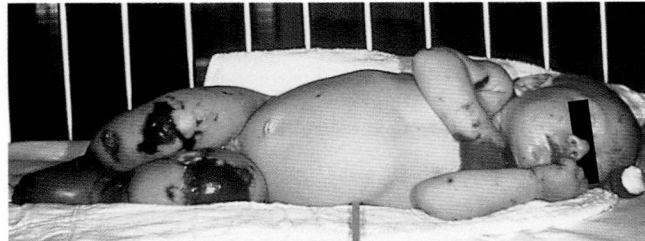

Fig. 53.9 Purpura fulminans. Bacterial septicemia results in necrosis, small-vessel thrombosis, and disseminated intravascular coagulation and is often associated with multiorgan failure. Several amputations may be required. (From Dinulos GHJ. *Habif's Clinical Dermatology*. 7th ed. Philadelphia: Elsevier; 2021:371, Fig. 9.65.)

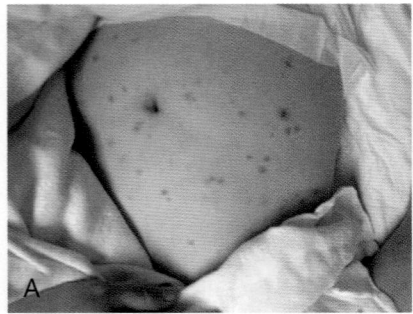
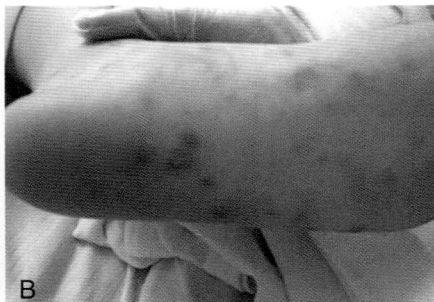
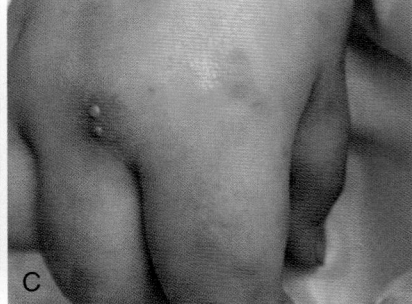

Fig. 53.8 Rat-bite fever. *A*, Erythematous papules on the abdomen. *B*, Purpuric pustules on the sole of the left foot. *C*, Pustules on erythematous bases on the right dorsal hand. (From Miraflor AP, Ghajar LD, Subramaniam S, et al. Rat-bite fever: an uncommon cause of fever and rash in a 9-year-old patient. *JAAD Case Rep.* 2015;1[16]:371–374 [Fig. 1, p. 372].)

with polyangiitis, HSP) may involve the lower respiratory tract, isolated pulmonary findings are infrequently indicative of these disorders. The acute respiratory distress syndrome can develop in any patient with a serious systemic inflammatory condition such as sepsis, SJS, TEN, HLH, and DRESS.

Clusters of Findings

Clusters of findings on examination that are of diagnostic importance include the following.

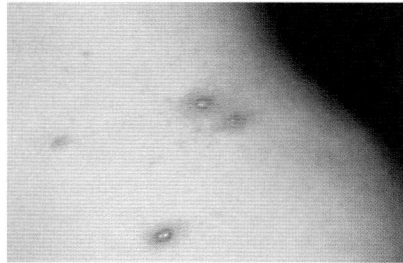

Fig. 53.10 Skin lesions of chickenpox. Note the varying stages of development (macules, papules, and vesicles) present at the same time. (From Paller AS, Mancini AJ. *Hurwitz Clinical Pediatric Dermatology.* 5th ed. Philadelphia: Elsevier; 2016.)

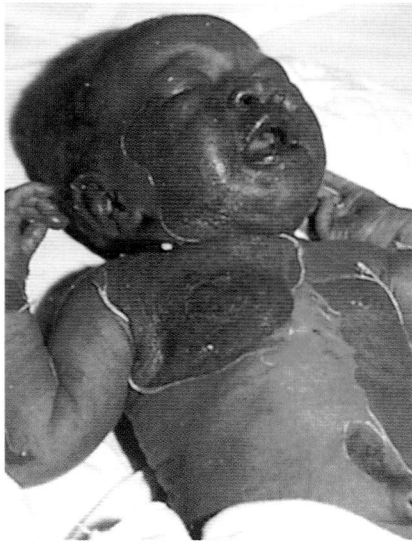

Fig. 53.11 An infant with staphylococcal scalded skin syndrome. (From Kliegman RM, Stanton BF, St Geme JW III, et al., eds. *Nelson Textbook of Pediatrics.* 20th ed. Philadelphia: Elsevier; 2016.)

The **mucocutaneous–lymph node** cluster (bilateral conjunctival injection, palmar-plantar erythema/indurative edema of the hands and feet, erythema of the oropharyngeal mucosa/"strawberry" tongue, cervical lymphadenopathy) is suggestive of KD, TSS, SJS, streptococcal scarlet fever, Rocky Mountain spotted fever, dengue, leptospirosis, or MIS-C.

The **reticuloendothelial cell hyperplasia cluster** (hepatosplenomegaly with or without generalized adenopathy) is suggestive of (1) disseminated infectious disease caused by bacteria (*Salmonella typhi* or other enteric fever pathogens), virus (cytomegalovirus, HIV-1, EBV), rickettsia (*Orientia tsutsugamushi* in "scrub typhus"), protozoa (malaria), or fungus (*H. capsulatum, C. immitis*); (2) disseminated malignancy including Langerhans cell histiocytosis, leukemia, and lymphoma; (3) sarcoidosis; (4) HLH; or (5) rheumatologic disease.

The **mononucleosis-like syndrome cluster** (exudative pharyngitis and regional adenopathy with or without splenomegaly) is suggestive of infection with group A streptococcus, *Arcanobacterium haemolyticum*, *Francisella tularensis*, EBV, HIV, toxoplasmosis, cytomegalovirus, coxsackievirus, or DRESS.

Diagnostic Studies

The history and physical examination together determine the prior probability of a specific disease. In the context of a very high or very low prior probability of a specific disease, laboratory testing adds very little useful information. Thus, ancillary testing is most useful when the prior probability of specific disease is equivocal.

Laboratory Tests

In an ill-appearing child, basic laboratory testing including CBC with smear, CRP, ESR, procalcitonin, chemistries, blood cultures, and possibly cerebral spinal fluid culture should be obtained. Coagulation studies should be completed in patients with petechiae, purpura, bleeding, or concern for DIC.

A Gram stain of any ulcerative, pustular, petechial, or purpuric lesion can be useful. The identification of bacteria suggests pyogenic infection, which may be localized or disseminated. The presence of only polymorphonuclear white blood cells in the fluid of pustular lesions does not exclude bacterial infection from consideration, especially disseminated infection with *N. gonorrhoeae.* Specimens of these lesions or any fluid from a pustule should also be obtained for bacterial culture and possibly fungal or mycobacterial culture depending on the level of suspicion for these types of pathogens.

Vesicular and bullous lesions in a febrile child with an uncertain diagnosis can be unroofed, scraped at the base, and submitted for microscopic examination after Tzanck preparation. The presence of multinucleated giant cells or eosinophilic intranuclear inclusions indicates infection with herpesvirus or varicella-zoster virus. The sensitivity of the Tzanck preparation for cutaneous herpes simplex infection is 64% and

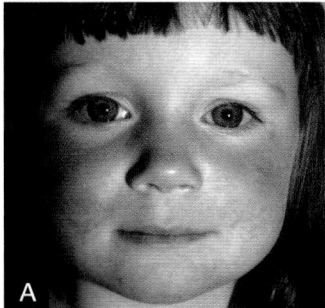
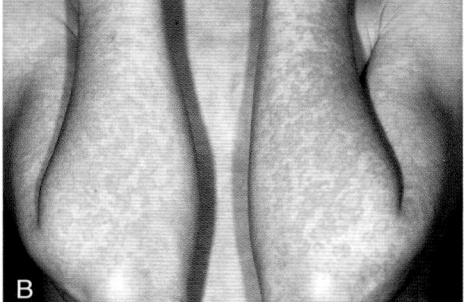
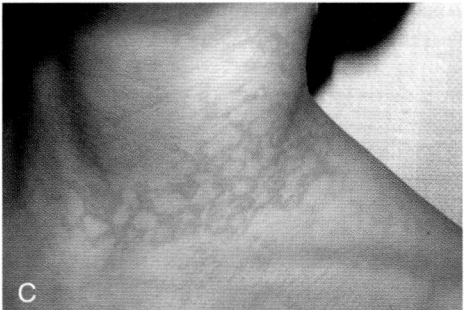

Fig. 53.12 *A,* Erythema infectiosum. Facial erythema ("slapped cheek"). The red plaque covers the cheek and spares the nasolabial fold and the circumoral region. *B,* A macular eruption appears on the extensor extremities. *C,* The eruption fades into a lacy netlike pattern. (From Dinulos GHJ. *Habif's Clinical Dermatology.* 7th ed. Philadelphia: Elsevier; 2021:536, Figs. 14.19, 14.20.)

the specificity is 86%. Because the sensitivity of the procedure is low, a negative result does not exclude the diagnosis of herpes simplex infection. Thus, to identify the virus, a specimen of the lesion should also be obtained for polymerase chain reaction (PCR), which is more sensitive than culture.

Diagnosing a systemic infectious illness may necessitate the use of specific bacterial, viral, or fungal culture techniques; paired acute- and convalescent-phase serologic study; antigen detection systems; or molecular techniques such as PCR or 16S (bacterial) and 28S (fungal) ribosomal DNA. Culture techniques are most specific when normally sterile tissue or body fluids are sampled and inoculated directly into liquid or solid media. Interpretation of bacterial cultures obtained from nonsterile sites, such as the tonsils and nasopharynx, is subject to increased rates of false-positive results because of recovery of organisms that colonize these areas.

Serologic techniques are potentially useful in establishing a diagnosis of a specific infection. Confirmation of infection with the rickettsiae and several other atypical bacteria and viruses is probably best accomplished through serologic techniques demonstrating a fourfold increase in titer, but also highly suggestive with a high immunoglobulin G (IgG) at least 2 weeks from illness onset if a first sample is negative or not obtained. Similarly, detection of a recent infection with group A streptococci may be accomplished by demonstrating very elevated or rising antibody titers to streptolysin O (ASO titer) or to deoxyribonuclease B (anti–DNase B).

Antigen detection systems are useful for rapid diagnosis. A solid-phase detection system, such as enzyme-linked immunosorbent assay (ELISA), has the advantage of being independent of the need for intact cellular material but is affected by antigen or antibody cross-reactivity in the sample (which limits specificity) and by poor antigen-antibody affinity (which limits sensitivity). Nonetheless, ELISA is the preferred technique for the serologic diagnosis of a wide spectrum of infectious agents, including *B. burgdorferi* (Lyme disease pathogen) (as the first part in a two-tier serologic assay, the second being a Western immunoblot; see Chapter 52) and hepatitis B virus.

Latex particle agglutination is an alternative solid-phase antigen detection system that does not require intact cellular material and whose advantages include rapidity of use and ease of interpretation. Latex particle agglutination is used for the rapid identification of patients with GAS pharyngitis or with invasive disease caused by encapsulated bacteria, such as *S. pneumoniae*, *H. influenzae* type b, *N. meningitidis*, group B streptococci, and *Escherichia coli* BK1. Latex particle agglutination is limited by factors similar to those affecting ELISA. Latex agglutination tests for group A streptococci have specificities of more than 90%, which facilitates their use for clinical confirmation of infection, but their sensitivities are only 60–90%, which limits their use in excluding infection.

PCR has replaced many of the previously commonly used latex agglutination assays. PCR testing is available for diagnosis of GAS pharyngitis and may preclude the need for culture confirmation. Multiplex PCRs of respiratory and diarrhea specimens provide higher sensitivity and specificity compared to antigen tests, as well as offering the potential benefit of testing for multiple potential pathogens with one test. Multiplex PCR testing of cerebrospinal fluid (CSF) for common bacterial and viral pathogens is also available. CSF PCR testing should be in addition to CSF culture given current limited experience, unclear sensitivity, and specificity issues.

PCR from blood is available for certain bacteria and viruses. For DNA viruses that establish latency (e.g., cytomegalovirus and EBV), serologic testing is still utilized to help diagnose primary versus past infection that PCR cannot reliably differentiate between. However, PCR for these viruses also offers quantitation of viral load, which is useful in the care of immunocompromised hosts. Blood PCR is also used in the diagnostic work-up of rickettsiae, but due to limited sensitivity, serologic testing is often needed. Neither PCR nor serology is useful in early management of rickettsial infections due to the typical turnaround time, so treatment

needs to be determined based on clinical presentation. The identification of patients with noninfectious systemic illness caused by underlying rheumatologic disease, immune complex disease, or vasculitis is best accomplished through serologic techniques combined with other indirect laboratory evidence of active inflammation or tissue injury (see Chapter 44). Diagnoses of autoinflammatory diseases are based on clinical criteria and can be confirmed with genetic testing (see Chapter 54).

Histopathology

Punch biopsy for light and electron microscopy and immunohistologic studies should be considered for diagnostic purposes for patients presenting with fever and bullous lesions that are clearly not typical pyodermas; fever and nodular lesions; or lesions suggestive of vasculitis (palpable purpura, livedo reticularis). A punch biopsy with indirect immunofluorescent antibody staining may also be useful for patients with petechial lesions, especially in an acral distribution, for the early diagnosis (within 48 hours of antibiotic initiation) of infection with *R. rickettsii*. This procedure has a sensitivity of 70% and a specificity of 100%. The low sensitivity and restricted availability (Centers for Disease Control and Prevention [CDC] and some academic centers) of the test limits its use in decision making in the acute care setting.

Other Diagnostic Studies

Echocardiography and ECG are part of the diagnosis of some fever and rash syndromes. The 2015 revision of the Jones criteria for diagnosis of acute rheumatic fever adds echocardiography to diagnose cardiac involvement even when it is not clinically evident. Prolonged P-R interval on ECG remains one of the minor Jones criteria. In incomplete KD and presumed MIS-C, echocardiography is used to help guide diagnosis when patients do not meet all classic criteria.

Diagnosis and Decision Making

Accurate diagnosis depends on careful synthesis of selected data obtained from the clinical assessment. Because most children with acute episodes of fever and rash have a common, self-limited infectious disease, a specific diagnosis can often be established simply by pattern recognition alone (e.g., visual recognition of the common exanthems of childhood or a specific lesion such as erythema migrans) or with minimal use of adjunctive testing (a rash consistent with scarlet fever accompanied by a positive PCR or latex agglutination test for group A streptococcus). In some cases the spectrum of possible infectious pathogens may be broad, the presenting complaints or features of the rash may be atypical, or the diagnosis may not yield easily to simple pattern recognition. In these situations, empirical use of the laboratory may prove useful to the clinician. It may also be preferable to "watchful waiting" and serial clinical follow-up when the patient is judged to be at risk for a treatable illness associated with significant subsequent morbidity (e.g., streptococcal infection leading to acute rheumatic fever) or when specific information is necessary to advise parents of the risk of contagion to other children, to immunocompromised contacts, or to pregnant women.

Well-appearing immune-competent patients with fever and petechial rash present a challenge to the clinician. Such patients with cough or emesis *and* petechiae only above the nipple line, and a positive streptococcal antigen or PCR test, or patients with normal leukocyte, absolute neutrophil, and platelet counts and a normal prothrombin time are exceedingly unlikely to have an invasive bacterial illness such as meningococcemia.

The subset of patients with fever and rash who have shock or appear toxic, have unstable vital signs, or have altered mental status must have a comprehensive evaluation and a diagnosis confirmed as quickly as possible to detect potentially life-threatening underlying infection. Patients with thrombocytopenia and an abnormal coagulation profile should be admitted for further evaluation and treatment of DIC, which may have an underlying infectious or inflammatory cause. Patients with thrombocytopenia and a normal coagulation profile may have infection with tick-borne rickettsial pathogens, *Ehrlichia chaffeensis*, EBV, an autoimmune disease such as SLE, or a primary hematologic-oncologic disorder, such as idiopathic thrombocytopenic purpura or leukemia, associated with an intercurrent infection; such patients should be evaluated for these disorders. Patients with eosinophilia and elevated transaminases may have DRESS.

Several serious diseases present with features that resemble benign processes; it is crucial to distinguish these as early in the clinical course as possible so definitive treatment can be given (Table 53.7).

Clinical Syndromes

In certain instances, the diagnostic approach to disorders manifesting with fever and rash is wholly dependent on an aggregation of signs, symptoms, and laboratory results. These disorders either have many underlying causes manifesting with overlapping features or have unknown causes for which no confirmatory tests have yet been devised. These diseases are diagnosed by recognizing patterns and sometimes by excluding other diagnoses; some are based on formalized aggregation, termed *syndromic diagnosis*. Although syndromic diagnosis is based on explicit clinical criteria, some of the clusters of

TABLE 53.7   Potentially Life-Threatening Conditions with Initial Skin Findings That Can Mimic a More Common Benign Disorder

Potentially Life-Threatening Condition	Benign Disorder That Is Mimicked Early in the Course	Clues to the Diagnosis as the Condition Evolves
DRESS/DIHS*	Morbilliform/urticarial drug eruption > viral exanthem	• Facial swelling • High fever • Prominent lymphadenopathy • Marked peripheral blood eosinophilia, atypical lymphocytes • Elevated transaminases, other signs of internal organ involvement
Stevens-Johnson syndrome/ toxic epidermal necrolysis	Morbilliform/urticarial drug eruption > viral exanthem	• Early involvement of palms and soles • Duskiness of blistering (often initially in the center of lesions) • Painful/tender skin • Mucosal erosions (oral, nasal, ocular, genital)
RMSF/other rickettsial spotted fevers	Viral exanthem	• Potential exposure to ticks (e.g., season [spring to late summer for RMSF], geographic location) • High fever, myalgias, headache (often for 2–5 days prior to rash) • Rash begins on wrists/ankles, spreads centripetally (± palms/soles) • Petechiae within erythematous macules/papules
Meningococcemia	Viral exanthem	• Petechiae → retiform purpura • Fever with chills, myalgias • Headache, stiff neck • Leg pain, cold hands/feet, abnormal skin color
Kawasaki disease	Viral exanthem, morbilliform/urticarial drug eruption, erythema multiforme, "diaper dermatitis" (for early perineal eruption)	• Early perineal erythema → desquamation • Conjunctival injection • "Chapped" lips, "strawberry" tongue • Acral erythema and edema • Continued high-spiking fever >5 days • Prominent unilateral lymphadenopathy
Staphylococcal scalded skin syndrome	Seborrheic dermatitis, viral exanthem	• Painful/tender skin • Periorificial (around mouth and eyes) edema and (later) radial scale-crusts • Confluent erythema → superficial erosions/peeling, especially in intertriginous sites
Toxic shock syndrome	Scarlatiniform exanthem	• Strawberry tongue • Mucositis • Rapid evolution • Hypotension
Necrotizing fasciitis	Cellulitis	• Tense, "woody" induration • Extreme pain or (later) anesthesia • Rapid evolution • Erythema → dusky gray color • Watery, malodorous discharge
MIS-C	Viral exanthem, scarlatiniform exanthem	• Fever • Multisystem involvement • Recent SARS-CoV-2 infection or exposure to COVID-19 • Lab studies with multiorgan involvement and elevated inflammatory markers

*In general, begins ≥2 wk after the drug is initiated and has a relatively limited set of culprit medications.
DIHS, drug-induced hypersensitivity syndrome; DRESS, drug reaction with eosinophilia and systemic symptoms; RMSF, Rocky Mountain spotted fever; MIS-C, multisystem inflammatory syndrome in children; SARS-CoV-2, severe acute respiratory syndrome–coronavirus 2.
Modified from Bolognia J, Schaffer JV, Duncan KO, et al. Fever and rash. In: Bolognia J, Schaffer JV, Duncan KO, et al., eds. *Dermatology Essentials*. Oxford: Saunders; 2014:35, Table 3.1.

signs, symptoms, and laboratory findings were established originally for epidemiologic purposes (case definition) to facilitate exploration of an underlying cause. As such, although they are usually quite specific, these criteria may be less sensitive when they are applied in the acute care setting for the purposes of clinical diagnosis.

Kawasaki Disease

KD is a medium-vessel vasculitis of childhood with a predilection for the coronary arteries. It is the second most common vasculitis of childhood after HSP, and it is the most common cause of acquired heart disease in children in the United States. Etiology is unknown, but epidemiologic studies support an infectious trigger. A genetic role is suspected given the 10- to 20-fold increased incidence in Japan as compared to the United States and United Kingdom. The majority (75–85%) of affected children are younger than 5 years old. Infants aged younger than 6 months and children over 5 years old are at the highest risk for coronary artery aneurysms.

The fever of KD is usually high and unremitting; patients are often irritable and ill-appearing. Rash is seen in more than 80% of patients with KD and is polymorphic. It is often morbilliform but may also be erythema multiforme–like (fixed erythematous target lesions; Fig. 53.13), urticarial, scarlatiniform, or pustular. Erythema and early

desquamation (within 48 hours) of the perineum is common. Vesiculobullous lesions and petechiae are unexpected.

Diagnosis is made on clinical grounds (Table 53.8 and Figs. 53.14, 53.15, 53.16, 53.17, and 53.18). Fewer than 75% of patients meet the

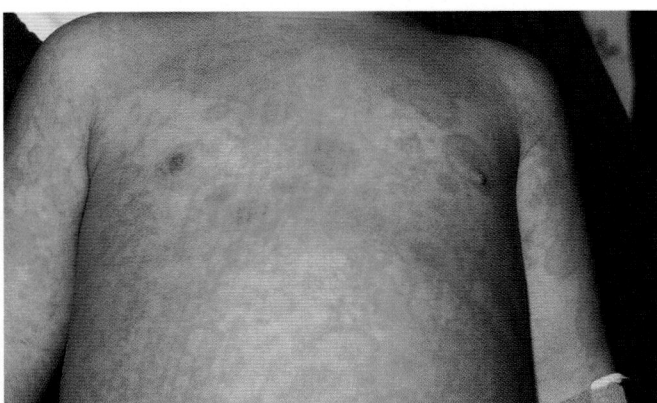

Fig. 53.13 Erythema multiforme in a child with Kawasaki disease. (From Paller AS, Mancini AJ. *Hurwitz Clinical Pediatric Dermatology.* 5th ed. Philadelphia: Elsevier; 2016.)

TABLE 53.8   Diagnosis of Classic Kawasaki Disease (KD)

Classic KD is diagnosed in the presence of fever for at least 5 days (the day of fever onset is taken to be the first day of fever) together with at least four of the five following principal clinical features. In the presence of four or more principal clinical features, particularly when redness and swelling of the hands and feet are present, the diagnosis of KD can be made with 4 days of fever, although experienced clinicians who have treated many patients with KD may establish the diagnosis with 3 days of fever in rare cases:

1. Erythema and cracking of lips, strawberry tongue, and/or erythema of oral and pharyngeal mucosa
2. Bilateral bulbar conjunctival injection without exudate
3. Rash: maculopapular, diffuse erythroderma, or erythema multiforme–like
4. Erythema and edema of the hands and feet in acute phase and/or periungual desquamation in subacute phase
5. Cervical lymphadenopathy (≥1.5 cm diameter), usually unilateral

A careful history may reveal that one or more principal clinical features were present during the illness but resolved by the time of presentation.

Patients who lack full clinical features of classic KD are often evaluated for incomplete KD. If coronary artery abnormalities are detected, the diagnosis of KD is considered confirmed in most cases.

Laboratory tests typically reveal normal or elevated white blood cell count with neutrophil predominance and elevated acute-phase reactants such as CRP and ESR during the acute phase. Low serum sodium and albumin levels, elevated serum liver enzymes, and sterile pyuria can be present. In the second week after fever onset, thrombocytosis is common.

Other clinical findings may include the following:

Cardiovascular
  Myocarditis, pericarditis, valvular regurgitation, shock
  Coronary artery abnormalities
  Aneurysms of medium-sized noncoronary arteries
  Peripheral gangrene
  Aortic root enlargement

Respiratory
  Peribronchial and interstitial infiltrates on CXR
  Pulmonary nodules

Musculoskeletal
  Arthritis, arthralgia (pleocytosis of synovial fluid)

Gastrointestinal
  Diarrhea, vomiting, abdominal pain
  Hepatitis, jaundice
  Gallbladder hydrops
  Pancreatitis

Nervous system
  Extreme irritability
  Aseptic meningitis (pleocytosis of cerebrospinal fluid)
  Facial nerve palsy
  Sensorineural hearing loss

Genitourinary
  Urethritis/meatitis, hydrocele

Other
  Desquamating rash in groin
  Retropharyngeal phlegmon
  Anterior uveitis by slit-lamp examination
  Erythema and induration at BCG inoculation site

The differential diagnosis includes other infectious and noninfectious conditions, including the following:

  Measles
  Other viral infections (e.g., adenovirus, enterovirus)
  Staphylococcal and streptococcal toxin-mediated diseases (e.g., scarlet fever and toxic shock syndrome)
  Drug hypersensitivity reactions, including Stevens-Johnson syndrome
  Systemic onset juvenile idiopathic arthritis

With epidemiologic risk factors:
  Rocky Mountain spotted fever or other rickettsial infections
  Leptospirosis

BCG, bacillus Calmette-Guerin; CXR, chest radiography.
From Dinulos GHJ. *Habif's Clinical Dermatology.* 7th ed. Philadelphia: Elsevier; 2021:544, Table 14.3.

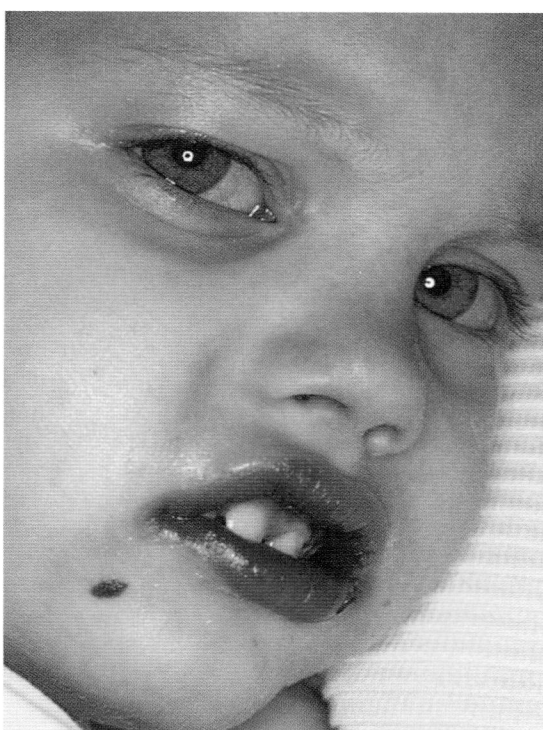

Fig. 53.14 Kawasaki disease. Nonpurulent conjunctival injection and "cherry red" lips with fissuring and crusting are early signs of the disease. (Courtesy Anne W. Luckey, MD.)

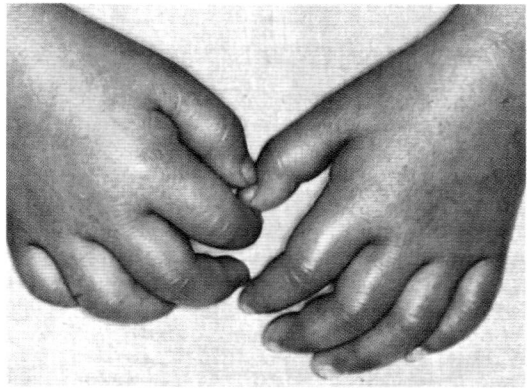

Fig. 53.15 Indurative edema of the hands in Kawasaki disease. (From Kliegman RM, Stanton BF, St. Geme JW III, et al., eds. *Nelson Textbook of Pediatrics.* 20th ed. Philadelphia: Elsevier; 2016.)

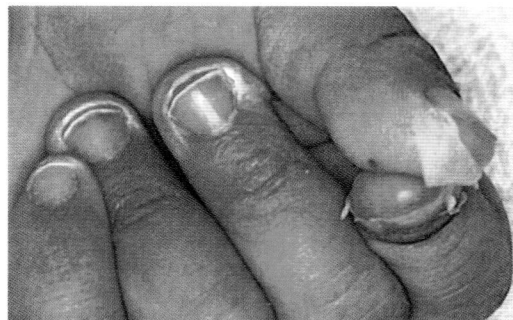

Fig. 53.16 Desquamation of the fingers in a patient with Kawasaki disease, convalescent stage. (From Kliegman RM, Stanton BF, St. Geme JW III, et al., eds. *Nelson Textbook of Pediatrics.* 20th ed. Philadelphia: Elsevier; 2016.)

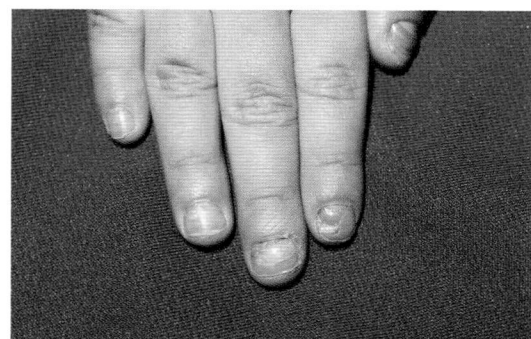

Fig. 53.17 Beau lines, a horizontal groove on the nails of a patient with Kawasaki disease, convalescent stage. (From Paller AS, Mancini AJ. *Hurwitz Clinical Pediatric Dermatology.* 5th ed. Philadelphia: Elsevier; 2016.)

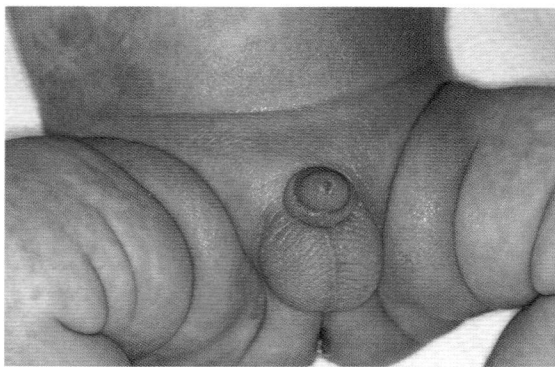

Fig. 53.18 A scarlet fever–like rash that desquamates in a child with Kawasaki disease. (From Habif TP. *Clinical Dermatology.* 6th ed. Philadelphia: Elsevier; 2016.)

classic complete criteria at presentation; diagnosis of incomplete KD may be made with less than four criteria with the addition of laboratory and echocardiographic criteria (Fig. 53.19). Application of this algorithm increases sensitivity for KD to 97%. Early diagnosis is crucial to decrease the risk of coronary artery aneurysms, which decreases to <5% in promptly treated patients at 7-week follow-up.

The differential diagnosis of KD includes scarlet fever, TSS, Rocky mountain spotted fever, Stevens-Johnson syndrome, measles, and MIS-C (Tables 53.9 and 53.10 and Fig. 53.20). **MIS-C** is a potentially life-threatening illness that has been epidemiologically linked to severe acute respiratory syndrome–coronavirus 2 (SARS-CoV-2) infection. Patients present with multiple systemic symptoms including fever, rash, mucocutaneous changes, conjunctivitis, gastrointestinal symptoms, and/or altered mental status. Signs include multiorgan involvement, often with elevated troponin, B-type natriuretic peptide (BNP), or proBNP. There may also be acute kidney injury, elevated liver enzymes, and, in severe cases, hemodynamic instability or frank shock. Significant elevation of CRP has been almost uniformly present. The features may overlap with TSS and KD for which some patients may meet full or partial diagnostic criteria (see Table 53.9). Patients with MIS-C may have a negative nasopharyngeal test for SARS-CoV-2 but a positive antibody titer.

Toxic Shock Syndrome

TSS is a life-threatening illness caused by superantigen-producing strains of group A streptococcus and *S. aureus.* The syndrome is defined by fever, diffuse macular erythroderma with convalescent desquamation, hypotension, mucositis, strawberry tongue, and

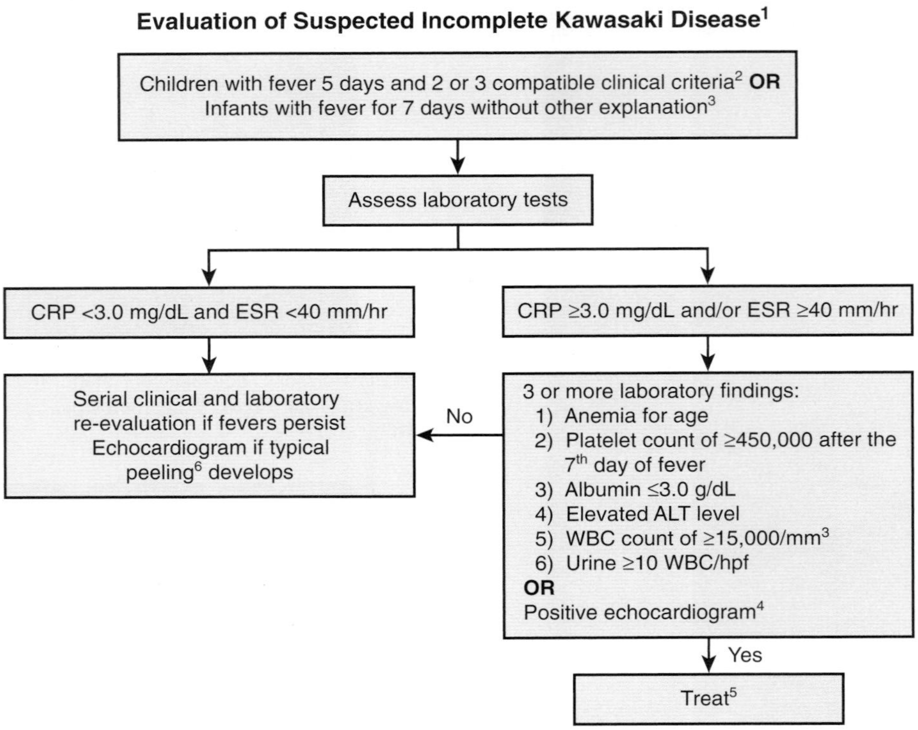

Evaluation of Suspected Incomplete Kawasaki Disease[1]

Fig. 53.19 Evaluation of suspected incomplete Kawasaki disease. [1]In the absence of a "gold standard" for diagnosis, this algorithm cannot be evidence based but rather represents the informed opinion of the expert committee. Consultation with an expert should be sought any time assistance is needed. [2]Characteristics suggesting that another diagnosis should be considered include exudative conjunctivitis, exudative pharyngitis, ulcerative intraoral lesions, bullous or vesicular rash, generalized adenopathy, or splenomegaly. [3]Infants 6 months of age or younger are the most likely to develop prolonged fever without other clinical criteria for Kawasaki disease; these infants are at particularly high risk of developing coronary artery abnormalities. [4]Echocardiography is considered positive for purposes of this algorithm if any of three conditions are met: z score of left anterior descending coronary artery or right coronary artery ≥2.5; coronary artery aneurysm is observed; or three or more other suggestive features exist, including decreased left ventricular function, mitral regurgitation, pericardial effusion, or z scores in left anterior descending coronary artery or right coronary artery of 2–2.5. [5]If the echocardiogram is positive, treatment should be given within 10 days of fever onset or after the 10th day of fever in the presence of clinical and laboratory signs (CRP, ESR) of ongoing inflammation. [6]Typical peeling begins under the nail beds of fingers and toes. ALT, alanine transaminase; hpf, high-powered field; WBC, white blood cell. (Reprinted with permission from McCrindle BW, Rowley AH, Newburger JW, et al. Diagnosis, treatment, and long-term management of Kawasaki disease: a scientific statement for health professionals from the American Heart Association. *Circulation.* 2017;135[17]:e927–e999.)

multiorgan dysfunction. Menstrual staphylococcal TSS classically affects menstruating teenage females secondary to vaginal colonization with toxic shock syndrome toxin 1 (TSST-1)-producing strains of *S. aureus*. TSST-1 and other staphylococcal exotoxins also cause TSS in the setting of abscess, wound infections or burns, nasal packing, or other infections. Streptococcal TSS is often associated with severe cutaneous infections but has no identified source of entry in ~50% of patients. Diagnostic criteria are slightly different for each syndrome.

Staphylococcal Toxic Shock Syndrome

Laboratory criteria for diagnosis include negative results on the following tests, if obtained: blood or CSF cultures (blood culture may be positive for *S. aureus*) and serologies for Rocky Mountain spotted fever, leptospirosis, or measles. A probable case meets the laboratory criteria and four of five clinical criteria and a confirmed case meets the laboratory and all five clinical criteria:

Fever: temperature ≥102°F (≥38.9°C)

Rash: diffuse macular erythroderma

Desquamation: 1–2 weeks after onset of rash

Hypotension: systolic blood pressure ≤90 mm Hg for adults or <5th percentile by age for children aged younger than 16 years

Multisystem involvement (three or more of the following organ systems):

1. Gastrointestinal: vomiting or diarrhea at the onset of illness
2. Muscular: severe myalgia or creatine phosphokinase level at least twice the upper limit of normal
3. Mucous membrane: vaginal, oropharyngeal, or conjunctival hyperemia
4. Renal: blood urea nitrogen or creatinine at least twice the upper limit of normal for laboratory or urinary sediment with pyuria (≥5 leukocytes/high-power field) in the absence of urinary tract infection
5. Hepatic: total bilirubin, alanine aminotransferase enzyme, or aspartate aminotransferase enzyme levels at least twice the upper limit of normal for laboratory
6. Hematologic: platelets <100,000/mm³
7. Central nervous system: disorientation or alterations in consciousness without focal neurologic signs when fever and hypotension are absent

TABLE 53.9   CDC Case Definition for MIS-C

All **four** diagnostic criteria must be met:
1. Age <21 yr
2. Clinical presentation should include **all** of the following:
   a. Fever ≥38.0°C for ≥24 hr or report of subjective fever lasting ≥24 hr
   b. Laboratory evidence of inflammation, including, but not limited to, **one or more** of the following:
      - Elevated CRP
      - Elevated ESR
      - Elevated fibrinogen
      - Elevated procalcitonin
      - Elevated D-dimer
      - Elevated ferritin
      - Elevated lactic acid dehydrogenase (LDH)
      - Elevated interleukin-6 (IL-6)
      - Elevated neutrophils
      - Reduced lymphocytes
      - Low albumin
   c. Evidence of clinically severe illness requiring hospitalization
   d. Multisystem (**≥2**) organ involvement (cardiac, renal, respiratory, hematologic, gastrointestinal, dermatologic, or neurologic)
3. No alternative plausible diagnoses
4. Positive for current or recent SARS-CoV-2 infection by RT-PCR, serology, or antigen test; or COVID-19 exposure within the 4 wk prior to the onset of symptoms

CDC, Centers for Disease Control and Prevention; MIS-C, multisystem inflammatory syndrome in children; RT-PCR, reverse transcriptase polymerase chain reaction; SARS-CoV-2, severe acute respiratory syndrome–coronavirus 2.
Source: United States Centers for Disease Control and Prevention. Multisystem inflammatory syndrome in children (MIS-C) associated with coronavirus disease 2019 (COVID-19). 2020. Available at https://emergency.cdc.gov/han/2020/han00432.asp.

TABLE 53.10   Comparing and Contrasting Multisystem Inflammatory Syndrome in Children (MIS-C) with Kawasaki Disease

MIS-C	Kawasaki Disease
Mean age 8–12 yr	Mean age <5 yr
Non-Hispanic Blacks at higher risk	Asians at higher risk
Fever >24 hr	Fever >5 days
GI symptoms common (severe abdominal pain)	GI complaints not common
Myocarditis/myocardial dysfunction (left ventricular dysfunction)	Myocardial function normal/mildly reduced*
Coronary artery dilation or aneurysms (25–50%)	Coronary artery abnormalities such as aneurysms common if untreated
Renal involvement more common	Renal involvement rare
Proinflammatory state common	Proinflammatory state common
Lymphopenia common	Lymphopenia not common
Thrombocytopenia	Thrombocytosis

GI, gastrointestinal.
*Except in Kawasaki shock syndrome.
From Naka F, Melnick L, Gorelik M, et al. A dermatologic perspective on multisystem inflammatory syndrome in children. *Clin Dermatol.* [published online ahead of print, 2020 Sep. 23], Table 5.

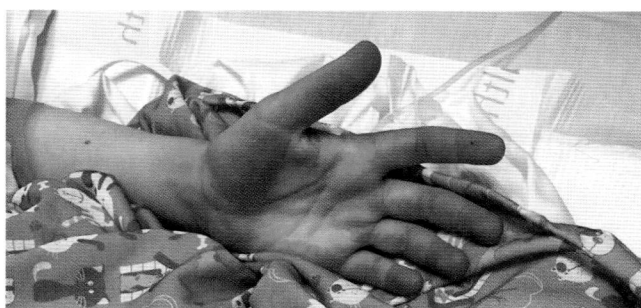

Fig. 53.20 Multisystem inflammatory syndrome in children. (From Naka F, Melnick L, Gorelik M, et al. A dermatologic perspective on multisystem inflammatory syndrome in children. *Clin Dermatol.* [published online ahead of print, 2020 Sep. 23].)

Streptococcal Toxic Shock Syndrome

Confirmed case: isolation of group A streptococci from a normally sterile site (blood; cerebrospinal, pleural, or peritoneal fluid; tissue biopsy; surgical wound; etc.); or
Probable case: isolation of group A streptococci from a nonsterile site (throat, sputum, vagina, superficial skin lesion), and
Clinical signs of severity:
1. Hypotension: systolic blood pressure ≤90 mm Hg in adults or below 5th percentile for age in children, and
2. Two or more of the following signs:
   - Renal impairment: creatinine ≥177 μmol/L (≥2 mg/dL) for adults or ≥2 times the upper limit of normal for age; in patients with pre-existing renal disease, a twofold or greater elevation over the baseline level
   - Coagulopathy: platelets ≤100 × 10⁹/L (≤100,000/mm³) or DIC defined by prolonged clotting times, low fibrinogen level, and the presence of fibrin degradation products
   - Liver involvement: serum aspartate aminotransferase, alanine aminotransferase, or total bilirubin levels ≥2 times the upper limit of normal for age; in patients with pre-existing liver disease, a twofold or greater elevation over the baseline level
   - Acute respiratory distress syndrome defined by acute onset of diffuse pulmonary infiltrates and hypoxemia in the absence of cardiac failure, or evidence of diffuse capillary leak manifested by acute onset of generalized edema, or pleural or peritoneal effusions with hypoalbuminemia
   - A generalized erythematous macular rash that may desquamate
   - Soft tissue necrosis, including necrotizing fasciitis or myositis, or gangrene

Erythema Multiforme

Erythema multiforme (EM) is a self-limited immune reaction that predominantly occurs in the setting of infection, most often HSV. *M. pneumoniae* and rarely drugs or systemic disease are causes of EM. It is characterized by the abrupt onset of fixed erythematous papules that evolve into target lesions (see Fig. 53.13). The basic lesions are round macular targets symmetrically distributed especially over the palms, soles, and extensor surfaces of the extremities. Severe mucosal lesions can also develop (EM major). Though it has potentially overlapping features with SJS (Stevens-Johnson syndrome), it is a distinct disease.

Stevens-Johnson Syndrome, Toxic Epidermal Necrolysis, and Staphylococcal Scalded Skin Syndrome

SJS and TEN are rare, life-threatening mucocutaneous exfoliative dermatoses that are usually drug related (Table 53.11). They are thought to be associated with an immune response to an antigenic complex

TABLE 53.11 **Classification of Stevens-Johnson Syndrome (SJS), Toxic Epidermal Necrolysis (TEN), and Stevens-Johnson Syndrome–Toxic Epidermal Necrolysis (SJS-TEN) Overlap**

	SJS	SJS-TEN	TEN
Lesional morphology	Targetoid lesions, dusky red macules, bullae	Targetoid lesions, dusky red macules, bullae	Targetoid lesions, dusky erythematous macules and plaques, detachment of epidermis
Localization of skin lesions	May be scattered and isolated; may be confluent, especially on the trunk and face	May be scattered and isolated; often confluent	Usually extensive involvement with widespread confluence
Involved skin	<10%	10–30%	>30%
Biopsy features	More interface dermatitis	Significant interface dermatitis + necrolysis	Predominantly necrolysis
Mucosal changes	Prominent	Prominent	May be less than in SJS
Systemic involvement	Often present	Always present	Always present

From Paller AS, Mancini AJ, eds. *Hurwitz Clinical Pediatric Dermatology.* 5th ed. Philadelphia: Elsevier; 2016:478, Table 20.3.

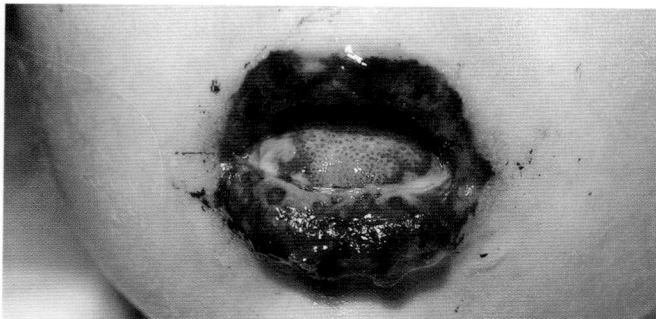

Fig. 53.21 Stevens-Johnson syndrome. Mucous membrane involvement with severe swelling and hemorrhagic crusting of the lips. (From Paller AS, Mancini AJ. *Hurwitz Clinical Pediatric Dermatology.* 5th ed. Philadelphia: Elsevier; 2016.)

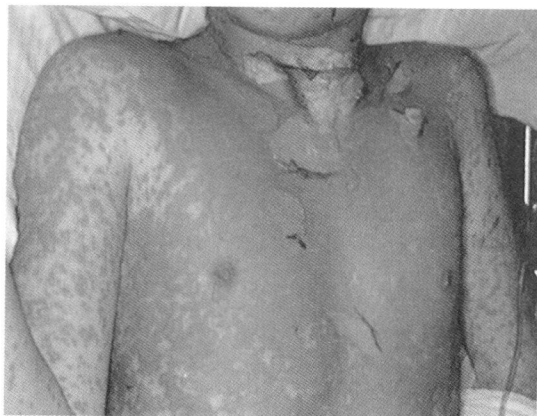

Fig. 53.22 Stevens-Johnson syndrome. Confluent erythema, blisters, and exfoliation of the epidermis are present. (From Hurwitz S. *Clinical Pediatric Dermatology: A Textbook of Skin Disorders of Childhood and Adolescence.* 2nd ed. Philadelphia: WB Saunders; 1993:528.)

formed by the reaction of intermediate drug metabolites with host tissues. SJS and TEN are characterized by diffuse cutaneous erythema and full-thickness necrosis of the epidermis with detachment of the skin at the dermal-epidermal junction. They differ in the percentage of involved total body surface area (BSA); SJS involves ≤10% BSA, SJS/TEN overlap involves between 10% and 30% BSA, and TEN involves ≥30% BSA. They differ histopathologically from SSSS, which also manifests clinically with diffuse erythema and blistering in its cleavage plane. In SSSS, blistering is produced more superficially by disruption of the epidermal granular cell layer in response to one of two staphylococcal exfoliative toxins (ET-A or ET-B). This results in easy disruption of skin with firm rubbing (Nikolsky sign). SSSS is usually seen in infants and young children, whereas SJS and TEN are seen in older children. The key feature that distinguishes SJS and TEN from SSSS is the presence of blistering lesions, which may involve the lips, eyes, nasal mucosa, genitalia, or rectum (Figs. 53.21 and 53.22). Extensive ocular involvement, including corneal ulceration, uveitis, and panophthalmitis, may develop. Pulmonary and renal involvement have also been reported. Representative medications frequently associated with SJS and TEN include aminopenicillins, carbamazepine, phenytoin, trimethoprim-sulfamethoxazole, and nonsteroidal antiinflammatory medications. Prognosis is related to the speed with which the responsible medication is withdrawn, so a timely diagnosis is critical.

Serum Sickness and Serum Sickness–Like Reaction

Serum sickness is a systemic hypersensitivity condition resulting from immune complex deposition in tissue and blood vessels that causes tissue damage through complement activation. It is classically associated with the administration of animal serum proteins, but the availability

of alternative therapies, including monoclonal antibodies of human origin, has decreased the incidence of true serum sickness. A serum sickness–like reaction can be triggered by antibiotics or other drugs (particularly cefaclor, penicillins, sulfonamides, phenytoin, carbamazepine) and presents 1–2 weeks after exposure. Symptoms include fever, rash, arthralgia or arthritis, and lymphadenopathy. The rash of serum sickness–like reaction is morbilliform or large fixed serpiginous and cyclic urticarial plaques; it can be confused with other circular rashes such as giant urticaria and EM (Fig. 53.23). Serum sickness–like reactions do not exhibit the hypocomplementemia, vasculitis, circulating immune complexes, and renal lesions that are seen in serum sickness. Critical to making the diagnosis is identification of exposure to a drug in the preceding 1–2 weeks. A watchful waiting approach may support the diagnosis, inasmuch as the syndrome should resolve within approximately 4 weeks if exposure to the purported offending agent has been curtailed. Persistence of findings beyond this period indicates another disorder associated with immune complex–mediated vasculitis.

Henoch-Schönlein Purpura (IgA Vasculitis)

HSP is usually a self-limited immunoglobulin A (IgA)-mediated vasculitis representing the most common vasculitis of childhood. It affects vessels in the skin, joints, gastrointestinal tract, and kidneys. The clinical manifestations include a rash, which initially is urticarial and then frequently evolves into a maculopapular eruption; after this eruption, petechiae and then purpuric plaques distributed predominantly on the buttocks and over the lower extremities develop (Fig. 53.24). These

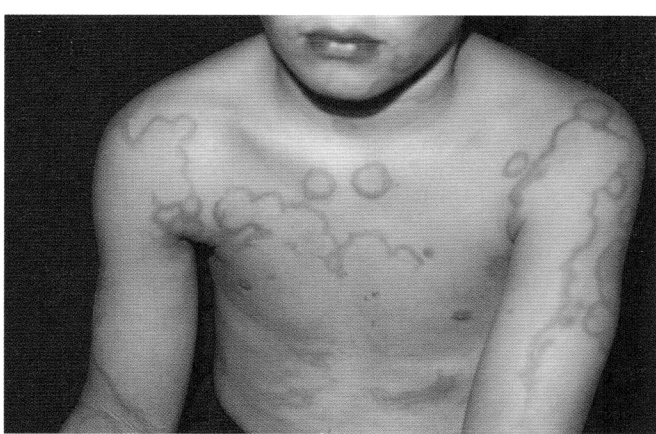

Fig. 53.23 Serum sickness–like reaction. Urticarial wheals occurred 2 weeks after exposure to cefaclor. (From Paller AS, Mancini AJ, eds. *Hurwitz Clinical Pediatric Dermatology.* 5th ed. Philadelphia: Elsevier; 2016:475, Fig. 20.13.)

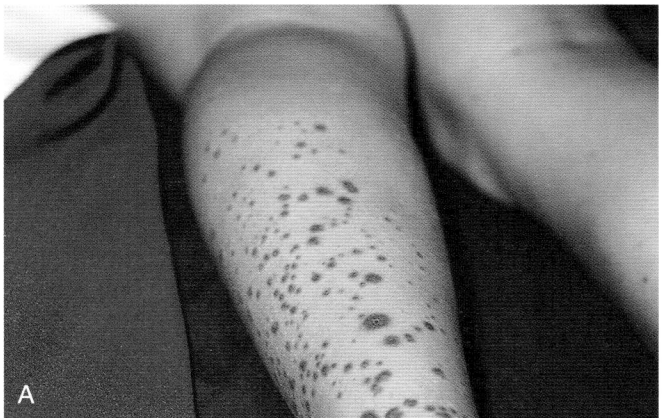

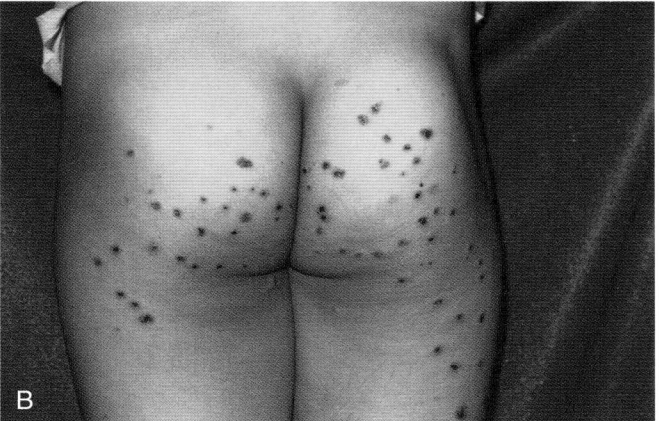

Fig. 53.24 *A,* Henoch-Schönlein purpura. Palpable purpuric papules and plaques. *B,* Palpable purpura of the buttocks, a classic site of involvement in Henoch-Schönlein purpura. (From Paller AS, Mancini AJ, eds. *Hurwitz Clinical Pediatric Dermatology.* 5th ed. Philadelphia: Elsevier; 2016:497, Figs. 21.3, 21.5.)

plaques usually are raised from the skin surface, which gives the rash its characteristic feature of "palpable purpura." Associated findings that are variably present include arthralgias and arthritis; edema of the feet, hands, face, scrotum, and scalp; melena, which may accompany intussusception; and an abnormal UA that demonstrates hematuria and

proteinuria. Fever, if present, is low grade and not a dominant feature of HSP. Laboratory testing is not necessary but can be of use to the clinician in excluding the infectious or hematologic causes of purpura if the patient does not present with classic features. Specifically, the results of both the platelet count and the coagulation profile are normal, and blood cultures are sterile. A Gram stain of the lesion is not usually needed, but the results are negative. Skin biopsy demonstrates the characteristic leukocytoclastic vasculitis involving the vessels in the dermis with IgA deposition.

Other Disorders

The diagnosis of other disorders manifesting with fever and rash is also based on formal syndromic criteria. SJIA (see Chapter 44), acute rheumatic fever (see Chapter 9), HLH (see Chapter 54), and SLE are examples. Representative diagnoses usually necessitating tissue confirmation are sarcoidosis and other vasculitides, such as polyarteritis nodosa or Wegener granulomatosis.

Management of Fever and Rash

Treatment of patients with fever and rash includes both anticipatory guidance and specific interventions. Anticipatory guidance alone usually suffices for patients who have a clearly identifiable, acute, self-limited, and noninvasive infectious or hypersensitivity disorder. Parents should be informed of the probable duration of illness, the expected evolution of clinical manifestations, potential complications and how to recognize them, and when to recontact the physician (see Tables 53.5 and 53.6).

The use of antipyretics as supportive therapy for patients with fever remains controversial. Arguments in favor of such therapy include decreasing symptomatic discomfort associated with the febrile state and reducing the undesirable metabolic and cardiopulmonary effects. Inadvertent overdose or unwanted side effects of over-the-counter antipyretics argue against their routine use.

Empirical therapy with antibiotics is an appropriate strategy for patients with focal cutaneous infection, such as cellulitis and erythema migrans; for patients with petechial or purpuric rash who are thought to have invasive infectious disorders; or for patients who appear toxic or manifest signs of cardiovascular instability. If epidemiologic evidence or clinical features are suggestive of rickettsial infection, the antimicrobial regimen should include doxycycline, even for children younger than 8 years. Suspected neonatal HSV infection should be treated with parenteral acyclovir.

Patients for whom a diagnosis is established by pattern recognition, case finding, syndromic aggregation, biopsy, or exclusion of other disorders may receive definitive interventions, as available, if the treatment benefits outweigh the risks. SSSS should be treated with an intravenous antistaphylococcal antibiotic. Staphylococcal TSS should be treated by removing vaginal foreign material if present, or otherwise effectively draining the source of the infection, and administering intravenous vancomycin; toxin and cytokine production should be curtailed with a bacterial protein synthesis inhibitor such as clindamycin. If methicillin-sensitive *S. aureus* is confirmed by vaginal or other culture, an antistaphylococcal penicillin plus clindamycin is appropriate. Streptococcal TSS should be treated with surgical debridement if indicated, and parenteral penicillin and clindamycin. Intravenous immune globulin (IVIG) may be used as adjunctive therapy for streptococcal TSS to neutralize bacterial exotoxins. Treatment of acute rheumatic fever is directed at group A streptococcus with treatment-dose penicillin followed by prophylactic doses of penicillin to decrease the risk of recurrent rheumatic fever. Diseases caused by drug toxicity are treated by discontinuing the offending medication. SJS and TEN are treated with supportive care, often in a burn center; meticulous skin and ophthalmologic care; and IVIG.

Infections with HSV or varicella-zoster virus may be treated with oral or intravenous acyclovir. Intravenous therapy is particularly appropriate for immunocompromised patients. The benefits of acyclovir therapy for HSV or varicella-zoster virus in immunocompetent hosts are less clear but traditionally utilized as it appears to shorten the duration of symptoms, particularly if given early in the course of infection.

Pharmacologic interventions in the systemic inflammatory disorders include antiinflammatory agents such as the nonsteroidal agents, corticosteroids, and immunosuppressant or modulating agents. Administration of IVIG is a definitive intervention in all patients with KD to reduce coronary aneurysm formation. The most effective treatment regimen for patients with KD of <10 days' duration is one dose of IVIG (2 g/kg) given over 12 hours with adjunctive aspirin therapy for at least 6–8 weeks to prevent thrombotic complications. Because 10% of patients may have persistent fever (>48 hours) or recrudescence of fever after the one-dose IVIG regimen, repeated treatment with IVIG is often necessary. Treatment of IVIG nonresponders is more controversial and may consist of corticosteroids, infliximab, or other immunosuppressant agents.

Patients with MIS-C often require admission to an intensive care unit and require organ-specific support for heart, kidney, or lung dysfunction in addition to IVIG, methylprednisolone, and anticoagulant therapy.

SUMMARY AND RED FLAGS

Most childhood episodes of fever and rash represent benign, self-limited viral illnesses with little or no sequelae. Diseases with potentially significant sequelae, such as meningococcemia, Rocky Mountain spotted fever, acute rheumatic fever, KD, SJS, DRESS, MIS-C, TSS, and SSSS, require efficient evaluation and timely treatment. Red flags include toxic appearance, unstable vital signs, meningismus, or fever with petechiae or purpura.

BIBLIOGRAPHY

A bibliography is available at ExpertConsult.com.

54

Recurrent Fever, Immune Deficiency, and Autoinflammatory Disorders

James W. Verbsky and John M. Routes

The immune system functions to prevent and impede the local establishment or systemic dissemination of bacteria, viruses, fungi, and protozoa. This highly complex system has to recognize the pathogen, initiate inflammation, and generate antibodies and T-cell responses with the goal of clearing the pathogen while retaining immunologic memory toward the pathogen. Furthermore, it must accomplish this task without excessive inflammation or the development of autoimmunity, both of which can lead to tissue damage. A common symptom of the immune response to infection is fever.

The differential diagnosis for patients with recurrent fevers is formidable in view of the complexity of the immune system, as well as the multitude of causes of fever. Fever can occur with any inflammatory stimulus, whether that be infections, autoimmune disorders, malignancy, or due to rare genetic variants that lead to spontaneous inflammation or autoimmunity, known as **autoinflammatory disorders** or **immune disregulation disorders,** respectively. Fever is a challenging issue for providers and causes considerable angst in families. It is helpful to have a consistent stepwise approach to a patient with recurrent fevers, keeping the differential diagnosis of fevers in mind.

Evaluation of fever should always start with a history and physical exam to look for an infectious source. Fevers without a clear infectious source should raise the possibility of an autoimmune disorder or malignancy as fevers in these disorders can be episodic; however, other symptoms are usually present that persist following resolution of the fever. Recurrent or persistent rashes, arthritis, weight loss, or abdominal pain may initiate a work-up for autoimmune diseases such as inflammatory bowel disease or juvenile arthritis or could represent an immune disregulation disorder. Basic lab testing to look for progressive hematologic abnormalities may lead to a work-up for malignancy. Inflammatory markers, including ESR or CRP, can be useful between febrile episodes, as normalization of inflammatory markers between fever episodes is unusual in ongoing autoimmune diseases or malignancies.

Recurrent infections need to be assessed by their severity and location, the responsible organisms, and the age of the patient. A young child with intermittent viral upper respiratory or gastrointestinal infections or recurrent ear infections is the norm, and reassurance and follow-up are all that is necessary with the expectation that these episodes will improve and eventually resolve over time. Recurrent bacterial infections may initiate a more in-depth immune work-up to evaluate for a primary immune deficiency, particularly if these are persistent or occur in unusual sites or with unusual organisms. Although there are no established rules regarding immunologic work-up of a patient with infections, an evaluation should be considered for at least one of the following: (1) more than two systemic bacterial infections (sepsis, meningitis, osteomyelitis); (2) two or more serious respiratory infections (pneumonia) or bacterial infections (cellulitis, draining otitis media, lymphadenitis) per year; (3) the presence of an infection at an unusual site (hepatic or brain abscess); (4) infections with unusual pathogens (*Aspergillus* pneumonia, disseminated candidiasis, or infection with *Serratia marcescens*, *Nocardia* species, or *Burkholderia cepacia*); (5) infections of unusual severity (pneumonias complicated by empyema or abscesses); and (6) recurrent mycobacterial infections or invasive infections with atypical mycobacteria. Persistent and recurrent fever episodes without infectious sources that don't resolve over time could represent an autoinflammatory disorder, and genetic testing could be pursued.

HISTORY AND PHYSICAL EXAMINATION

History

The history must determine the frequency of fevers, associated symptoms, presence of an infection, and whether the patient returns to a normal state of health in between these episodes. Resolution of fever but persistence of other symptoms or lab abnormalities (e.g., anemia, ESR, CRP) should raise the possibility of autoimmune disease or malignancy. Regarding recurrent fevers with infections, the clinician must determine (1) the frequency, location, severity, and complications of the infections; (2) the accuracy of how infections were documented; (3) the presence or absence of a symptom-free interval; (4) the microbiologic features of any isolate; and (5) the response to antibiotic therapy. A single chronic infection may wax and wane with intermittent, inadequate treatment and may manifest as a series of infections. Furthermore, a detailed history can elucidate other risk factors for recurrent infections. Many nonimmune disorders are characterized by an increased susceptibility to infection that must also be considered (Table 54.1). Approximately 30% of children with recurrent sinopulmonary symptoms can be categorized as **atopic** (genetic predisposition to develop allergic diseases). These subjects have normal growth and development, and episodes of recurrent illness may be afebrile, respond poorly to antibiotics, and be accompanied by upper respiratory symptoms such as coughing, sneezing, or wheezing. There may be a family history of atopic disease, and the patient's past medical history may include episodic wheezing, protracted cough after upper respiratory tract infection (URI), hay fever, allergies to foods, or eczema. The physical examination of allergic school-aged children may reveal typical characteristics including the following: dark circles under the eyes; open mouth with dry lips; coated tongue; evidence of nasal obstruction; transverse nasal crease; boggy, pale nasal mucosa; mucus in the pharynx; posterior pharyngeal "cobblestoning"; and postnasal drip.

Malnutrition and specific vitamin deficiencies may alter immune cell function. Protein-losing states due to gastrointestinal (e.g., inflammatory bowel disease, protein-losing enteropathy) or renal disease (e.g., nephrotic syndrome) may lead to hypocomplementemia, hypogammaglobulinemia, and recurrent infections. Chronic treatment with corticosteroids and other immunosuppressants can result in acquired

TABLE 54.1   Secondary Causes of Recurrent Infections

Predisposing Causes	Organism and Type of Infection
Alteration of Mucocutaneous Barriers	
Indwelling Catheter	
Central venous catheter (Broviac, Hickman)	*Staphylococcus aureus, Staphylococcus epidermidis,* and *Bacteroides, Candida, Pseudomonas* species: bacteremia, fungemia
Urinary catheter	*Escherichia coli, Enterococcus* species, *Staphylococcus saprophyticus:* pyelonephritis
Tenckhoff catheter (continuous ambulatory peritoneal dialysis)	*S. epidermidis, S. aureus, Escherichia coli, Pseudomonas aeruginosa, Candida* species: peritonitis
Cerebrospinal fluid shunts	*S. epidermidis, S. aureus,* diphtheroid, *Bacillus* species: meningitis
Aspirated pulmonary foreign body	*S. aureus,* anaerobes: pneumonia, pulmonary abscess, empyema
Burns	*P. aeruginosa, S. epidermidis, Candida* species: cutaneous lesions, sepsis
Inhalation Therapy: Contaminated Solutions	*P. aeruginosa, Serratia marcescens, Legionella* species: pneumonia
Surgical Wounds	
Abdominal	Gram-negative bacteria, *S. aureus, S. epidermidis, Candida* species: peritonitis
Nongastrointestinal	*S. aureus, S. epidermidis,* streptococci, gram-negative bacteria: wound abscess, sepsis
Fistula-Sinus Communications	
Neurocutaneous fistula	*S. aureus, S. epidermidis, E. coli:* meningitis
Neuroenteric fistula	Gram-negative bacteria: meningitis
Otic, facial sinus–meningeal sinus tract	Pneumococcus: meningitis
Facial sinus fracture (CSF rhinorrhea)	Pneumococcus: meningitis
Intravenous Drug Abuse	*S. aureus, P. aeruginosa,* streptococci: endocarditis, osteomyelitis: hepatitis B, C, D viruses: AIDS
Prosthetic Devices	
Cardiac valves	*S. epidermidis,* streptococci, *S. aureus,* diphtheroid, *Candida* species: endocarditis
Pacemaker	*S. epidermidis, S. aureus, Candida* species: subcutaneous pocket or endocardial infection
Chronic Disease	
Malnutrition	Measles; tuberculosis; herpes simplex virus; bacterial, parasitic, and viral diarrhea; gram-negative bacteria: sepsis, pneumonia
Cystic fibrosis	*S. aureus, H. influenzae,* mucoid *P. aeruginosa, Burkholderia cepacia;* pneumonia
Diabetes mellitus	Urinary tract infections, *Mucor,* and other fungi: sinus-orbital infection
Nephrotic syndrome	*Pneumococcus, E. coli:* peritonitis
Uremia	*S. aureus,* gram-negative bacteria, fungi: sepsis, soft tissue infection
Cirrhosis, ascites	*Pneumococcus, E. coli:* peritonitis
Prolonged broad-spectrum antibiotic therapy	*Candida* species, *Enterococcus* species, multidrug-resistant gram-negative or gram-positive bacteria: sepsis
Spinal cord injury	Gram-negative or gram-positive bacteria: pneumonia, pyelonephritis, pressure sores, abscesses, osteomyelitis
Sickle cell anemia	*Pneumococcus:* sepsis, meningitis, osteoarticular infection
	Salmonella species, *S. aureus:* osteomyelitis
Congenital heart disease	*S. aureus, Streptococcus viridans* group: endocarditis
Urinary tract anomaly	*E. coli, S. saprophyticus, Enterococcus* species: pyelonephritis
Kartagener syndrome (dysmotile cilia)	*H. influenzae, Moraxella catarrhalis, Pneumococcus:* pneumonia, sinusitis
Eczema/atopic disease	*S. aureus, Streptococcus* species, varicella, herpes simplex, molluscum: cutaneous infection, cellulitis
Protein-losing enteropathy (lymphangiectasia)	Pneumococcus: sepsis, peritonitis
	Giardia species: diarrhea
Periodontitis	*Fusobacterium* species: cellulitis, facial space infection
Splenic Dysfunction (e.g., Sickle Cell Anemia/Asplenia)	*S. pneumoniae:* sepsis, meningitis
	H. influenzae type b: sepsis, meningitis
	N. meningitidis: sepsis, meningitis
	Capnocytophaga canimorsus
	Babesiosis
	Malaria
	Group B *Streptococcus*
	Enterococcus
	Bacteroides
	Salmonella

CSF, cerebrospinal fluid.

immunodeficiency with hypogammaglobulinemia, lymphopenia, and recurrent infections.

Perinatal History

The clinician should determine if there was exposure to maternal viral infection during gestation (HIV, cytomegalovirus [CMV], herpes simplex virus, rubella) or a history of prematurity, blood transfusions, respiratory distress syndrome, or other pertinent neonatal illnesses. Infants previously placed on ventilators may develop chronic obstructive lung disease (bronchopulmonary dysplasia), predisposing them to recurrent pulmonary infections. Most perinatal HIV infections are seen in children whose mother or mother's partner has engaged in high-risk behavior (i.e., multiple sex partners or use of intravenous drugs). Attention should be paid to the time of umbilical cord separation since infants with a history of delayed umbilical cord separation and recurrent episodes of sepsis or pneumonia should be evaluated for **leukocyte adhesion deficiency**.

Anatomic Abnormalities

Recurrent infections in primary immune deficiencies typically affect different anatomic locations. Structural or anatomic defects often result in recurrent infections that are generally localized to the affected organ system. Approximately 10% of children with recurrent infections have an underlying chronic disease or a structural defect that predisposes them to recurrent infections (see Table 54.1).

Eustachian tube abnormalities or cleft palate results in recurrent or chronic otitis media; congenital heart disease results in an increased risk of endocarditis; and posterior urethral valves, vesicoureteral reflux, or ureteral pelvic junction obstruction results in recurrent urinary tract infections. Recurrent pneumonia may result from congenital malformations (trachea-esophageal fistulas, cystic adenomatoid malformation, or sequestration), from aspiration of a foreign body (peanut, small toys) or chronic aspiration (gastroesophageal reflux, swallowing disorders, neurologic diseases), and from bronchopulmonary dysplasia. Repeated pneumonias in dependent lobes warrant evaluation for recurrent aspiration. Chronic illnesses that result in recurrent pulmonary infections include cystic fibrosis, primary ciliary dyskinesia, or α_1-antitrypsin deficiency. Recurrent sinus infections can occur due to anatomic defects of the sinuses (polyps, stenotic os). Endotracheal intubation predisposes the patient to recurrent pulmonary infections with nosocomial organisms. Right middle lobe syndrome and sequestered lung can appear as recurrent pneumonia in the same anatomic location.

Any direct communication to the cerebrospinal fluid that bypasses the blood-brain barrier predisposes patients to a central nervous system infection. Basilar skull fractures and dermal sinus tracts or fistulas may communicate with the subarachnoid space or neural tissue. Other conditions predisposing patients to opportunistic infections of the central nervous system include penetrating foreign body, cerebrospinal fluid shunts, myelomeningocele, and encephalocele. Local infections of the sinuses or of the middle ear may spread to contiguous structures to form cerebral abscesses or subdural-epidural empyema. Intravenous drug use, bacterial endocarditis, and heart disease with right-to-left shunt are associated with an increased risk of central nervous system infections.

ASPLENIA

The spleen plays a particularly important role in preventing invasive infections, especially during the first year of life before specific immunity to certain bacteria has developed. The spleen is able to bind and phagocytose encapsulated bacteria and produces natural antibodies against polysaccharides that cross react with the cell walls of bacterial pathogens, thereby providing a critical role in preventing sepsis in immunologically immature subjects from encapsulated bacteria. The spleen is also an important location for the phagocytosis of complement and antibody opsonized bacteria, and a key location for the production of antibodies.

Functional asplenia occurs in children with sickle cell disease, initially as a result of vascular occlusion by the sickle cells in the splenic circulation. Congenital absence of the spleen may occur alone or as part of an asplenia syndrome with congenital heart disease. Heterotaxy and disorders of left-right patterning can result in polysplenia in which the spleens are not functional. Genetic variants in NKX2 and ribosomal protein SA have been found in a small number of patients with congenital asplenia. Trauma and surgical splenectomy are also important causes of asplenia.

Individuals without spleens (anatomic or functional) are subject to a severe form of sepsis that is rapid in onset and can lead to sudden death if it is not recognized and treated promptly. Pneumococci are responsible for more than 50% of such infections; infections with *Haemophilus influenzae*, *Staphylococcus aureus*, group A streptococci, gram-negative enteric bacilli, and meningococci also occur (see Table 54.1).

The diagnosis of anatomic or functional asplenia is suggested by the presence of red blood cell inclusions, particularly Howell-Jolly bodies on peripheral blood smear. Failure of uptake of technetium 99–sulfur colloid, which is normally taken up by the entire reticuloendothelial system, and lack of erythrocyte pitting are also noted in asplenic patients. Lack of a spleen by ultrasonography of the abdomen is suggestive of asplenia, but accessory splenic tissue may still be present. Functional tests of splenic tissue are a better indicator of asplenia.

The risk of fulminant infection in patients who have undergone splenectomy (from surgery or trauma) or in those with functional asplenia or congenital asplenia is highest in the first few years. The risk is lower in older children and in adults, probably because they have developed opsonizing antibodies through previous exposure. The management of functional or anatomic asplenia lies mainly in prevention. When splenectomy becomes necessary, partial protection against life-threatening infections can be obtained by immunizing patients with conjugated and polyvalent pneumococcal, *H. influenzae* type b, and meningococcal vaccines. Booster immunization may be needed because of waning immunity with time. Prophylactic antibiotics may be given continuously in a single daily dose for 1–3 years or up to the age of 16 years (some authorities suggest longer periods or even for life) after splenectomy. Parents of older asplenic children are advised to have their children seen by a physician or to administer the antibiotics at the first sign of a febrile illness.

Family History

Specific patterns of inheritance have been determined for a variety of immunologic defects resulting in immune deficiency or autoinflammatory disorder. Genetic defects of immunity can be inherited as X-linked, autosomal recessive, or autosomal dominant disorders. Monogenic primary immunodeficiencies and autoinflammatory disorders may exhibit reduced penetrance (some people with the genetic abnormality do not exhibit a clinical phenotype) and variable expressivity (different signs and symptoms with the same genetic defect). A family history of unexplained infant deaths or serious infection should be sought, particularly in male infants since a number of important immune deficiencies are X-linked. Evidence of consanguinity should also be established as many serious primary immune deficiencies are autosomal recessive. Since allergic diseases can appear as recurrent infections, a family history of atopy is important. A child who has one allergic parent or two allergic parents will develop an atopic disease in 25% and 50% of cases, respectively. Some autoinflammatory disorders are more prevalent in subjects from certain geographic regions (e.g., familial Mediterranean fever), and many have an autosomal dominant inheritance pattern, and therefore a family history of fevers should be sought.

Environmental History

Respiratory and dermatologic findings are a result of exposure to environmental allergens and toxins. Specific bacteriologic and parasitic exposures are associated with certain pets (i.e., *Salmonella* organisms and iguanas or turtles; psittacosis and birds; *Bartonella* organisms in kittens). A travel history may suggest exposure to unusual organisms that are regionally endemic, such as certain parasites and specific insect or animal bites, or to contaminated water. A move to a new house or to a new nursery school or exposure to a new babysitter, pet, or housekeeper may suggest possible allergic and infectious risks.

Physical Examination

The physical examination may provide important clues to the diagnosis of a primary immune deficiency or autoinflammatory disorder. Longitudinal evaluation of height and weight is crucial in identifying infants with failure to thrive or acute weight loss. Some immune deficiencies are associated with skeletal dysplasia or growth deficiency in addition to failure to thrive. Chronic upper respiratory infections are suggested by scarred tympanic membranes, postnasal drip, and cervical adenopathy. Transverse nasal creases, circles under the eyes, and posterior pharyngeal "cobblestoning" suggest respiratory allergy. Recurrent cough, wheezing, digital clubbing, and chest deformity are suggestive of pulmonary disease. Recurrent aphthous stomatitis can be a sign of a serious systemic disorder such as immune deficiency, an autoinflammatory disorder, autoimmunity, or inflammatory bowel disease. Auscultation of the apex of the heart in the right side of the thorax (dextrocardia) may be accompanied by ciliary motility abnormalities or asplenia. Lymphadenopathy, hepatosplenomegaly, pallor, wasting, and recent weight loss are suggestive of systemic disease. Absence of lymph tissue (tonsils and lymph nodes) is suggestive of a B-cell deficiency, while absence of thymic tissue on chest radiograph in an infant is suggestive of T-cell deficiency. Parotid enlargement with lymphadenopathy and hepatosplenomegaly is suggestive of HIV infection. Skin abnormalities including alopecia, eczema, pyoderma, pustules, livedo, and telangiectasia can be important clues to immunodeficiency or autoinflammatory disorders. Evidence of hematologic disease, such as pallor, petechiae, and jaundice, can be associated with immunodeficiencies. Generalized lymphadenopathy and splenomegaly may be suggestive of HIV disease, a phagocyte disorder with recurrent infections, or a lymphoproliferative disorder.

Diagnostic Categories

The information obtained from the history and physical examination is usually sufficient to make a tentative classification:

The patient who is probably healthy
The atopic or allergic patient
The patient with a nonimmunologic defect in host defense
The patient with hereditary autoinflammatory or fever syndrome
The patient with a primary immunodeficiency
The patient with an immune disregulation disorder

The Patient Who Is Probably Healthy

Many healthy children have repeated minor infections or have a relatively brief history of repeated infections or a single prolonged illness from which recovery has been delayed. Most URIs last <7 days, and duration of >14 days is unusual. Most children younger than 1 year who have a large family or who attend daycare develop respiratory or gastrointestinal infections about 6 times during the first year of life. The onset of the recurrent infection may coincide with entry into daycare,

preschool, or kindergarten. The healthy child has normal growth and development before the illness and usually a normal physical examination finding. When a discrepancy exists between the severity of an illness as reported by the parent and the child's physical appearance, it is often prudent to delay a detailed evaluation until more objective findings are documented by repeat examinations during acute episodes. Laboratory testing might include a CBC, inflammatory markers (i.e., ESR, CRP) to exclude rheumatic disorders or occult infections, and measurement of serum immunoglobulin levels (IgG, IgA, IgM, IgE) and vaccine-specific titers as a screen. Cultures and imaging of the affected area may provide additional data. With reassurance of the parents, these children recover spontaneously. Simple measures, rather than a complex set of laboratory studies, are often the only treatment required.

THE PATIENT WITH HEREDITARY INFLAMMATORY DISORDERS

Autoinflammatory syndromes, formerly known as **periodic fever syndromes**, are a heterogeneous and ever-increasing group of rare inflammatory disorders that manifest with recurrent fevers and/or inflammatory episodes (Table 54.2). Recurrent fevers or inflammation can often be mistaken for recurrent infections. Patients exhibit characteristic physical findings during these episodes, such as fever, various rashes, lymphadenopathy, aphthous stomatitis, arthritis, and serositis with abdominal, chest, or testicular pain. Not all of the features of a particular autoinflammatory syndrome may be present in young children, and these features may develop over time. These episodes can be periodic or sporadic, but the characteristic features occur with each episode (Table 54.3). Laboratory evaluation may show elevated white blood cell (WBC) counts and elevated inflammatory markers during the episode that typically resolve between episodes. Importantly, infectious evaluations are often repeatedly negative, and the patient is typically well between febrile episodes. Diagnosis of these disorders requires genetic testing; there are large panels of immunologically relevant genes that can be ordered to test for these disorders.

Familial Mediterranean Fever

Familial Mediterranean fever (FMF) is caused by variants in the *MEFV* gene that encodes the protein pyrin (see Table 54.2). Although FMF is considered an autosomal recessive disorder, a substantial percentage of patients with clinical FMF have only one demonstrable variant in *MEFV*. FMF is characterized by short episodes of fever (i.e., 1–3 days), serositis/peritonitis, prominent arthritis, and erythematous rash (Fig. 54.1). Early in life fever may be the only symptom. More classic features typically appear within 3 years. The arthritis is typically monoarticular, and aspirates of affected joints are sterile with a predominance of neutrophils. In some cases, splenomegaly and systemic vasculitis can ensue. The most serious long-term comorbidity with FMF is amyloidosis, which occurs frequently in patients who are not compliant with colchicine prophylaxis. Pyrin interacts with the inflammasome, a macromolecular complex involved in the processing of interleukin-1β (IL-1β), and variants that result in FMF result in greater IL-1 production. Daily colchicine prophylaxis prevents many of the long-term complications of this disorder.

Pyogenic Arthritis, Pyoderma Gangrenosum, and Acne Syndrome

Pyogenic arthritis, pyoderma gangrenosum, and acne (PAPA) is an autosomal dominant inherited syndrome caused by variants in *PST-PIP1* (see Table 54.2), which leads to hyperphosphorylation of PST-PIP1 and increased interaction with pyrin, leading to increased IL-1β production. PAPA begins in childhood with episodes of sterile monoarticular arthritis, and later in life pyoderma gangrenosum–like

TABLE 54.2 Autoinflammatory Disorders

Disease	Genetic Defect/ Presumed Pathogenesis	Inheritance	Functional Defects	Associated Features
Familial Mediterranean fever	*MEFV* (leads to gain of pyrin function, resulting in inappropriate IL-1β release)	AR, rarely AD	Reduced phosphorylation of mutated pyrin by protein kinases, resulting in activation of pyrin, inflammasome activation, and ASC-induced IL-1 processing and inflammation	Recurrent fever, serositis, and inflammation responsive to colchicine. Predisposes to vasculitis and inflammatory bowel disease
Mevalonate kinase deficiency (hyper-IgD syndrome)	*MVK*	AR	Affecting cholesterol synthesis and defective prenylation of proteins such as RhoA, which inhibits pyrin activation	Periodic fever and leukocytosis with high IgA and IgD levels, lymphadenopathy
Familial cold autoinflammatory syndrome	*NLRP3; NLRP12*	AD	Same as above	Nonpruritic urticaria, arthritis, chills, fever, and leukocytosis after cold exposure
Muckle-Wells syndrome	*NLRP3* (leads to constitutive activation of the NLRP3 inflammasome)	AD	Defect in cryopyrin, increased IL-1 processing by inflammasome	Urticarial-like rash from birth, aseptic meningitis with hearing loss or eye involvement, joint abnormalities, amyloidosis
Neonatal-onset multisystem inflammatory disease (NOMID) or chronic infantile neurologic cutaneous and articular syndrome (CINCA)	*NLRP3* (see above)	AD	Same as above	Similar to above but severe and early onset
Deficiency of IL-1 receptor antagonist (DIRA)	LOF variants in *IL1RN*	AR	Loss of IL-1 receptor antagonist	Pustular rash, osteopenia, lytic bone lesions, and prominent systemic inflammation
TNF receptor–associated periodic syndrome (TRAPS)	*TNFRSF1A*	AD	Variants of 55-kDa TNF receptor leading to intracellular receptor retention or diminished soluble cytokine receptor available to bind TNF	Recurrent fever, serositis, rash, and ocular or joint inflammation
Pyogenic sterile arthritis, pyoderma gangrenosum, and acne (PAPA) syndrome	*PSTPIP1*, binds pyrin and activates inflammasome	AD	Disordered actin reorganization leading to compromised physiologic signaling during inflammatory response	Destructive arthritis, inflammatory skin rash, myositis
Blau syndrome	GOF variants in *NOD2* (also called CARD15) lead to NF-κB activation	AD	Variants in nucleotide binding site of CARD15, possibly disrupting interactions with lipopolysaccharides and NF-κB signaling	Uveitis, granulomatous synovitis, camptodactyly, rash, and cranial neuropathies, 30% develop Crohn disease
Majeed syndrome (chronic recurrent multifocal osteomyelitis and congenital dyserythropoietic anemia)	*LPIN2* (increased expression of the proinflammatory genes)	AR	Undefined	Chronic recurrent multifocal osteomyelitis, transfusion-dependent anemia, cutaneous inflammatory disorders
Deficiency of adenosine deaminase 2 (DADA2)	LOF variants in *CECR1* (ADA2)	AR	Unclear mechanism of action	Fevers, CNS strokes, vasculitis, rash, cytopenias, hypogammaglobulinemia
AFEC (autoinflammation with infantile enterocolitis)	GOF variants in *NLRC4*	AD	Spontaneous activation of the inflammasome with IL-1 and IL-18 production	Fevers, vomiting, secretory diarrhea, duodenitis, splenomegaly, and rash
Acardia Goutières syndrome	LOF variant in *TREX1*, a 3′ repair exonuclease	AR or AD	Defects lead to accumulation of intracellular nucleic acids and an interferon response	Leukoencephalopathy with calcifications, cerebral atrophy, hepatosplenomegaly, anemia
STING-associated vasculopathy of infancy (SAVI)	GOF variants in *TMEM173* (STING)	AD	Spontaneous activation of STING induces interferon production	Fever; vasculitic rash with infarction on fingers, face, ears, nose; pulmonary disease
Chronic atypical neutrophilic dermatosis with lipodystrophy and elevated temperature (CANDLE)	LOF variants of *PSMB8*, others	AR	Defective proteasome function leads to interferon production	Fevers, purpuric skin rash, neutrophilic dermatosis, lipodystrophy, developmental delay, basal ganglion calcification
A20	LOF variants in *TNFAIP3*	AD	Haploinsufficiency results in enhanced NF-κB activation	Oral and genital ulcerations, uveitis, fevers; mimics familial Behçet disease

Continued

TABLE 54.2 Autoinflammatory Disorders—cont'd

Disease	Genetic Defect/ Presumed Pathogenesis	Inheritance	Functional Defects	Associated Features
Otulipenia	LOF variants in *FAM105B* (otulin)	AR	Enhanced NF-κB activation	Recurrent fevers, joint swelling, painful nodular red rash, GI inflammation/ diarrhea, failure to thrive
Autoinflammation with episodic fever and lymphadenopathy (AIEFL)	LOF variants of *RIPK1*	AD	Activation of proinflammatory cytokines and chemokines such as IL-6, TNF, and IFNγ	Recurrent fever beginning in early infancy, lymphadenopathy and occasional hepatosplenomegaly, no rash or ulcers

AD, autosomal dominant; *AR*, autosomal recessive; *GOF*, gain of function; *IFN*, interferon; *Ig*, immunoglobulin; *IL*, interleukin; *LOF*, loss of function; *NF-κB*, nuclear factor-κB; *TNF*, tumor necrosis factor.

TABLE 54.3 Features of Autoinflammatory Syndromes That May Narrow Diagnosis

Clinical Features	Autoinflammatory Syndrome
Age of Onset	
Birth	NOMID, DIRA, FCAS
Infancy	HIDS, FCAS
Toddler/late childhood	PFAPA syndrome
Onset in adulthood	TRAPS, DITRA
Ethnicity and Geography	
Armenians, Turks, Italians, Sephardic Jews	FMF
Arabs	FMF, DITRA
Dutch, French, German	HIDS, MWS
United States	FCAS
Triggers	
Vaccines	HIDS
Cold exposure	FCAS
Stress, menses	FMF, TRAPS, MWS, DITRA
Minor trauma	MWS, TRAPS, HIDS
Exercise	FMF, TRAPS
Pregnancy	DITRA
Duration of Episode	
<24 hr	FCAS, FMF
1–3 days	FMF, MWS, DITRA
3–7 days	HIDS, PFAPA syndrome
>7 days	TRAPS
Constant episode	NOMID, DIRA
Interval Between Episodes	
3–6 wk	PFAPA syndrome, HIDS
>6 wk	TRAPS
Unpredictable	All others

DIRA, deficiency of the IL-1 receptor antagonist; *DITRA*, deficiency of the IL-36 receptor antagonist; *FCAS*, familial cold autoinflammatory syndrome; *FMF*, familial Mediterranean fever; *HIDS*, hyperimmunoglobulin D syndrome; *MWS*, Muckle-Wells syndrome; *NOMID*, neonatal-onset multisystem inflammatory disease; *PFAPA*, periodic fever, aphthous stomatitis, pharyngitis, and cervical adenitis; *TRAPS*, tumor necrosis factor receptor–associated periodic syndrome.
Adapted from Hashkes PJ, Toker O. Autoinflammatory syndromes. *Pediatr Clin N Am.* 2012;59:447–470.
From *Zitelli and Davis' Atlas of Pediatric Physical Diagnosis*. 7th ed. Philadelphia: Elsevier; 2018:273, Table 7.11.

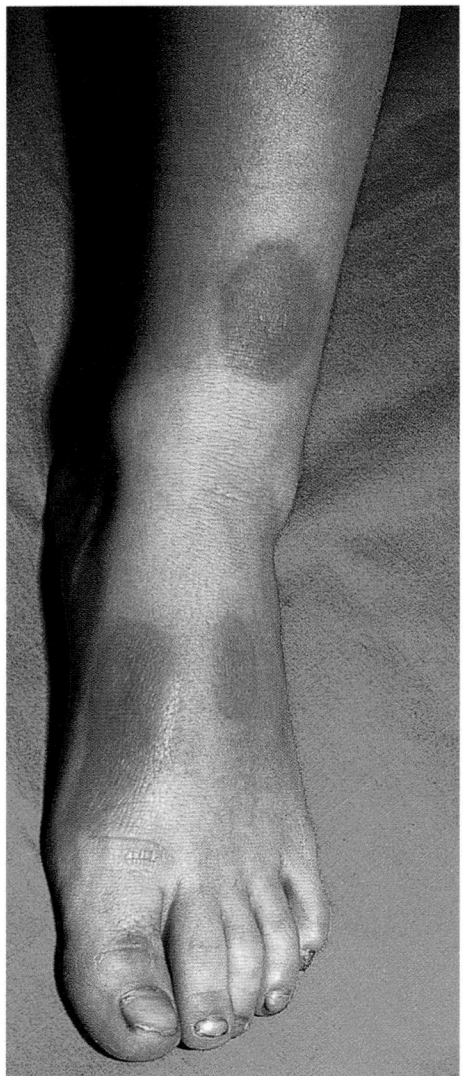

Fig. 54.1 Familial Mediterranean fever. Erythematous rash on the dorsal aspect of the foot and pretibial area of an affected child. (From Paller AS, Mancini AJ, eds. *Hurwitz Clinical Pediatric Dermatology.* 5th ed. Philadelphia: Elsevier; 2016:584, Fig. 25-24.)

ulcerative skin lesions and cystic acne (Fig. 54.2). The episodes of arthritis are the most common presentation, start in early childhood, and typically affect one to three joints at a time. The joint effusions are typically neutrophil-rich and sterile. Treatment of the arthritis with surgical drainage or treatment with intraarticular or systemic steroids has shown benefit in resolving arthritis. Several reports demonstrated

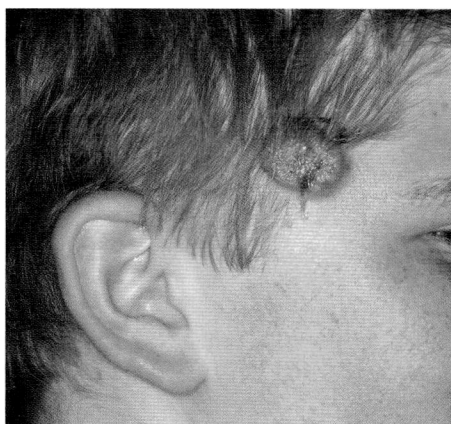

Fig. 54.2 Pyogenic sterile arthritis, pyoderma gangrenosum, and acne (PAPA) syndrome. This 11-year-old boy had small inflammatory papules of acne, which rapidly became purulent plaques (as shown) and then ulcerated to form pyoderma gangrenosum, leaving residual scars. He also had arthritis. His disease was brought under control with golimumab (tumor necrosis factor inhibitor) and isotretinoin. (From Paller AS, Mancini AJ, eds. *Hurwitz Clinical Pediatric Dermatology.* 5th ed. Philadelphia: Elsevier; 2016:589, Fig. 25-29.)

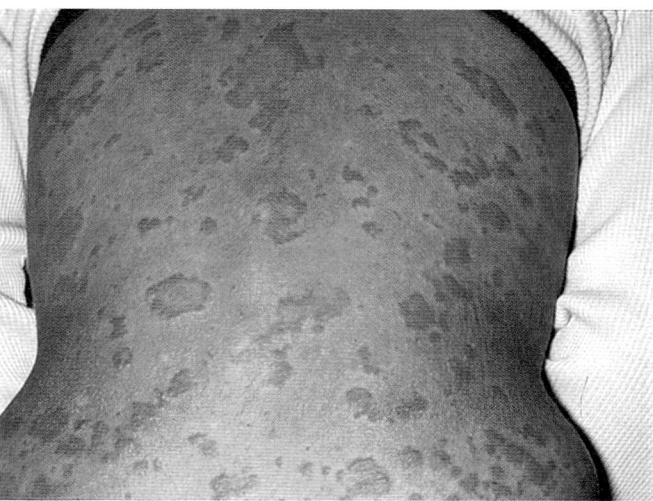

Fig. 54.3 Urticarial rash is the most common skin manifestation seen in Muckle-Wells syndrome. (From Barron K, Kastner DL. Periodic fever syndromes and other inherited autoinflammatory diseases. In: Petty RE, Laxer RM, Lindsley CB, et al, eds. *Textbook of Pediatric Rheumatology.* 8th ed. Philadelphia: Elsevier; 2020, Fig. 39.4.)

successful treatment with an IL-1 receptor antagonist (anakinra) or other IL-1 blockers (rilonacept, canakinumab).

Cryopyrin-Associated Periodic Syndromes

Cryopyrin-associated periodic syndromes (CAPSs) are a spectrum of autoinflammatory disorders that are inherited in an autosomal dominant manner due to variants in the *NLRP3* gene (see Table 54.2). *NLRP3* encodes cryopyrin, a protein that is part of the inflammasome. Variants that cause CAPS prevent autoinhibition of the cryopyrin protein, resulting in spontaneous activation of the inflammasome and excessive production of IL-1β.

CAPS consists of three diseases: familial cold autoinflammatory syndrome (FCAS), Muckle-Wells syndrome (MWS), and neonatal-onset multisystem inflammatory disorder (NOMID), which represent a spectrum of disorders that present with recurrent or continual systemic inflammation, rash, fevers, arthritis, neurologic deficits, and amyloidosis. **FCAS** is the mildest form of this disorder that presents with fevers, an evanescent rash, headache, conjunctivitis, and joint pain after generalized cold exposure. Although the rash can have some visual features of urticaria, it is macular without signs of mast cell degranulation, and is histologically characterized by a neutrophilic infiltrate. **MWS** presents similarly to FCAS, but cold exposure is not necessary for symptoms to occur (Fig. 54.3). Unlike FCAS, chronic meningitis occurs with papilledema and sensorineural hearing loss, joint pain and swelling is more severe, and untreated, amyloidosis develops over time. **NOMID** is the most severe variant of CAPS. Like MWS, all patients with NOMID exhibit a rash at or shortly after birth (Fig. 54.4). Neurologic symptoms, such as aseptic meningitis, headache, cerebral atrophy, uveitis, hearing loss, and intellectual disability, are common and severe. In NOMID and MWS, chronic inflammation of the joints leads to a chronic arthropathy with epiphyseal and patellar overgrowth. FCAS, MWS, and NOMID exhibit laboratory evidence of an acute-phase response with leukocytosis, neutrophilia, anemia, thrombocytosis, and elevated ESR and CRP levels.

IL-1 inhibitors (anakinra, rilonacept, canakinumab) are now the treatment of choice for these disorders based on their ability to induce rapid and sustained clinical response. Laboratory abnormalities typically normalize in days, and the rash responds rapidly. Importantly, IL-1 blockade improves long-term morbidity such as hearing loss, joint deformity, and amyloidosis.

Hyperimmunoglobulin D Syndrome

Hyperimmunoglobulin D syndrome (HIDS) is an autoinflammatory disorder caused by variants in the mevalonate kinase *(MVK)* gene (see Table 54.2). MVK is an enzyme involved in the biosynthesis of cholesterol and isoprenoids. Patients with HIDS have low but detectable MVK enzyme activity resulting in elevated levels of mevalonic acid in the urine, particularly during attacks. Complete absence of MVK results in mevalonic aciduria, an inborn error of metabolism, which is also associated with fevers. It is unclear how variants in MVK lead to an autoinflammatory disease.

The clinical manifestations of HIDS occur at an early age with recurrent fevers with lymphadenopathy, abdominal pain, arthralgia and arthritis, and painful migratory erythematous macules. These episodes may last 4–7 days and are often triggered by stress, trauma, or vaccination. Serum IgD and IgA levels are usually elevated but may be normal. Acute-phase reactants are elevated during attacks. Although high-dose corticosteroids and tumor necrosis factor-α (TNF-α) antagonists have been used with variable success, IL-1β inhibitors appear more effective at preventing the inflammatory episodes. Amyloidosis may occur but is relatively rare.

Deficiency of the Interleukin-1 Receptor Antagonist

Deficiency of the IL-1 receptor antagonist (DIRA) is an autosomal recessive disorder due to variants in the IL-1 receptor antagonist gene *(IL-1RN)* (see Table 54.2). IL-1 receptor antagonist (IL-1RA) is a decoy protein that binds to the IL-1 receptor but does not result in signaling, and the absence of IL-1RA in patients with DIRA leads to cellular hyperresponsiveness to IL-1β.

The clinical manifestations of DIRA occur within the first 2 weeks of life and include pustular rash, osteopenia, lytic bone lesions, and prominent systemic inflammation. All patients develop cutaneous pustulosis, and biopsies of the skin lesions revealed a neutrophilic predominance (Fig. 54.5). Respiratory distress, aphthous ulcers, hepatomegaly, and failure to thrive occur, with approximately one-third of infants expiring prior to diagnosis and effective treatment. Bone is prominently involved, with osteopenia, multiple osteolytic lesions, and rib widening. Laboratory abnormalities reflect an acute-phase response with elevated ESR and CRP, leukocytosis, anemia, and thrombocytosis.

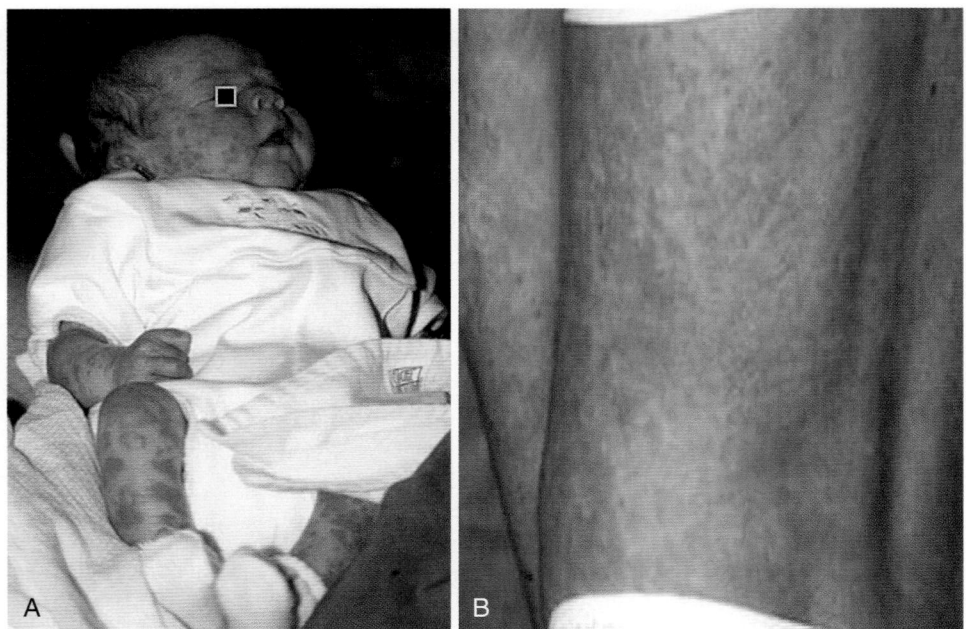

Fig. 54.4 Neonatal-onset multisystem inflammatory disorder. *A,* An urticaria-like rash is usually present at birth or during the first months of life. *B,* The rash is nonpruritic and papular. (Courtesy Dr. Raphaela Goldbach-Mansky, NIAID, NIH.)

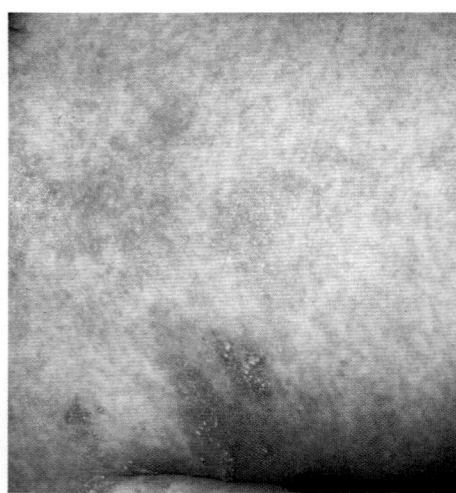

Fig. 54.5 Deficiency of interleukin-1 receptor antagonist. This young male with failure to thrive and multifocal lytic lesions of bone showed numerous plaques of erythematous pustules. (From Paller AS, Mancini AJ, eds. *Hurwitz Clinical Pediatric Dermatology.* 5th ed. Philadelphia: Elsevier; 2016:587, Fig. 25-25.)

Anakinra, a recombinant IL-1RA, is highly effective in the treatment of DIRA. Anakinra essentially replaces the IL-1RA that patients with DIRA cannot synthesize. The longer-acting anti–IL-1 agents canakinumab and rilonacept also work with the advantage of less frequent dosing compared to anakinra but are considerably more expensive.

TNF Receptor–Associated Periodic Syndrome

TNF receptor–associated periodic syndrome (TRAPS) is an autosomal dominant disease associated with missense variants in the extracellular domain of the TNF receptor 1 (TNFR1) gene *(TNFRSF1A)* (see Table 54.2). The clinical manifestations of TRAPS include recurrent and often prolonged fevers, abdominal pain, and arthralgias. A migratory rash with underlying fascial inflammation and myalgia can be seen, as well as conjunctivitis and periorbital edema (Fig. 54.6). Increased serum levels of CRP, ESR, leukocytosis, and thrombocytosis are evident during and in between attacks. Initial insights into the pathophysiology of this disorder came when patients with TRAPS exhibited low serum levels of soluble TNFR1, suggesting that shedding of TNF receptors acts as a natural antagonist to TNF-α. In support of this, the TNF-α antagonist etanercept has been shown to reduce the severity of symptoms in some cases of TRAPS. However, not all patients with TRAPS have low serum TNFR1 levels, and TNF-α inhibition is not completely effective. Reports have also shown the beneficial effects of IL-1 inhibition and the anti–IL-6 receptor antibody tocilizumab.

Deficiency of Adenosine Deaminase 2

Deficiency of adenosine deaminase 2 (DADA2) is an autosomal recessive disorder due to loss of function of *CECR1*, which encodes adenosine deaminase 2 (ADA2) (see Table 54.2). The clinical manifestations of DADA2 begin in childhood with intermittent fevers, recurrent lacunar strokes, organomegaly, hypogammaglobulinemia, and systemic vasculitides. Pure red cell aplasia, immune thrombocytopenia, neutropenia, and bone marrow failure have been observed. The lacunar strokes begin before the age of 5 years and typically occur during inflammatory episodes. A livedo-like rash is a prominent feature with biopsies showing a predominance of neutrophils and macrophages as well as vasculitis in medium-sized vessels. Some of these patients are diagnosed with early-onset polyarteritis nodosa. Treatment with glucocorticoids, TNF-α inhibitors, and IL-1 blockers has been utilized with some benefit. Hematopoietic stem cell transplantation is increasingly the treatment of choice for this disorder.

Interferonopathies

Another group of disorders that result in spontaneous inflammation are known as **interferonopathies** (Fig. 54.7 and Table 54.4). Interferonopathies are genetic defects that result in the spontaneous

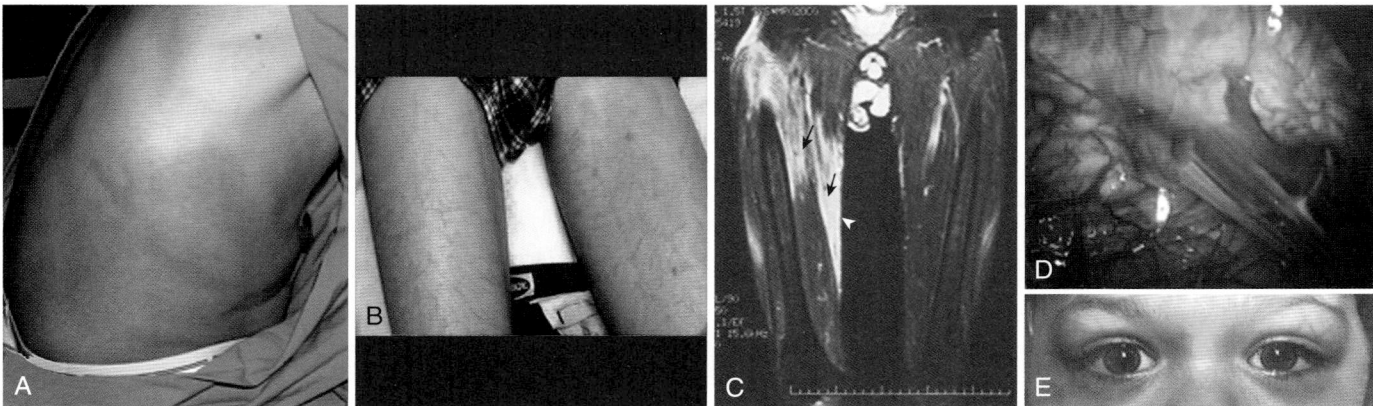

Fig. 54.6 Cutaneous findings associated with tumor necrosis factor receptor–associated periodic syndrome (TRAPS) may consist of macular areas of erythema on the torso *(A)* or on an extremity *(B)*. *C,* Sagittal views of the proximal thighs of a TRAPS patient demonstrating edematous changes within muscle compartments *(black arrows)*, here and extending to the skin *(white arrows)*. *D,* Peritoneal inflammation can lead to adhesions. *E,* Periorbital edema is commonly observed in TRAPS patients during a flare. (From Barron K, Kastner DL. Periodic fever syndromes and other inherited autoinflammatory diseases. In: Petty RE, Laxer RM, Lindsley CB, et al, eds. *Textbook of Pediatric Rheumatology*. 8th ed. Philadelphia: Elsevier; 2020, Fig. 39.2.)

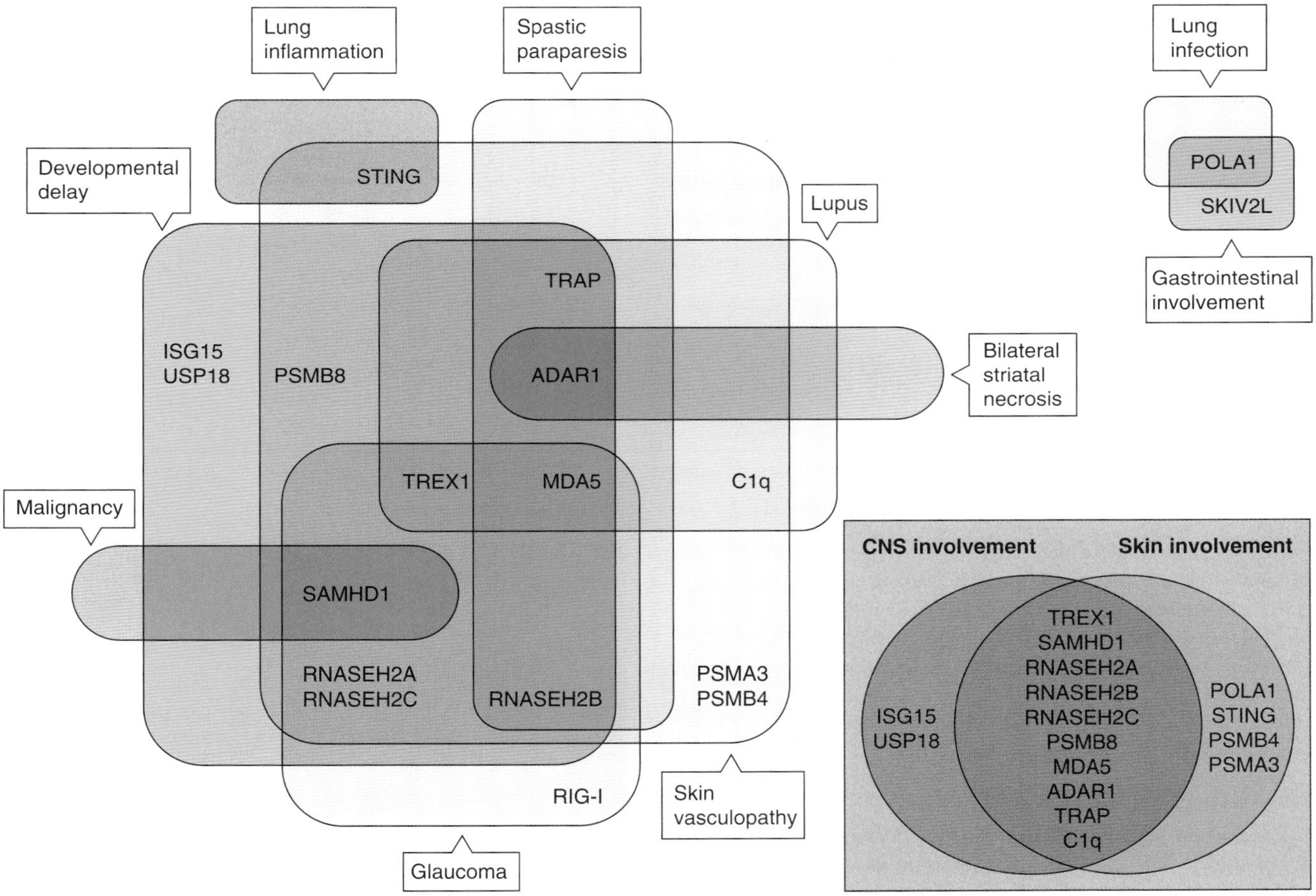

Fig. 54.7 Specific and overlapping features of monogenic type 1 interferonopathies. In the broadest sense, central nervous system (CNS) and skin disease are the most common features of the type 1 interferonopathies. Discrete neurologic phenotypes associated with variants in AGS-associated genes include "nonsyndromic" spastic paraparesis (RNASEH2B, ADAR1, and IFIH1) and bilateral striatal necrosis (ADAR1). Glaucoma is a common feature of AGS and is also seen in the Singleton-Merten syndrome phenotype associated with gain-of-function variants in IFIH1 and DDX58 (RIG-I). Systemic lupus erythematosus (lupus) is most frequently associated with variants in ACP5 and C1q. Malignancy has only been reported in the context of SAMHD1. Lung inflammation is so far restricted to patients with variants in TMEM173 (STING). The phenotypes associated with variants in POLA1 and SKIV2L appear distinct. (From Rodero MP, Crow YJ. Type 1 interferon-mediated monogenic autoinflammation: the type I interferonopathies, a conceptual overview. *J Exp Med*. 2016;21:2527–2538 [Fig. 2, p. 2531].)

TABLE 54.4   Mutated Gene, Protein Function, Pattern of Inheritance, and Main Symptoms of Known Type 1 Interferonopathies

Disease	Gene	Protein Function	Inheritance	Symptoms
Aicardi-Goutières syndrome (AGS) type 1	TREX-1	3'-5' DNA exonuclease	AR and AD	Classical AGS
AGS2	RNASEH2B	Components of RNase H2 complex. Removes ribonucleotides from RNA-DNA hybrids	AR	Classical AGS
AGS3	RNASEH2C			Classical AGS
AGS4	RNASEH2A			Classical AGS with dysmorphic features
AGS5	SAMHD1	Restricts the availability of cytosolic deoxynucleotides	AR	Mild AGS, mouth ulcer, deforming arthropathy, cerebral vasculopathy with early-onset stroke
AGS6	ADAR	Deaminates adenosine to inosine in endogenous dsRNA, preventing recognition by MDA5 receptor	AR and AD	Classical AGS, bilateral striatal necrosis
AGS7	IFIH1	Cytosolic receptor for dsRNA	AD	Classic or mild AGS, asymptomatic
Retinal vasculopathy with cerebral leukodystrophy (RVCL)	TREX-1	3'-5' DNA exonuclease	AD	Adult-onset loss of vision, stroke, motor impairment, cognitive decline, Raynaud, and liver involvement
Spondyloenchondrodysplasia (SPENCD)	ACP5	Lysosomal phosphatase activity	AR	Spondyloenchondrodysplasia, immune disregulation, and in some cases combined immunodeficiency
STING-associated vasculopathy with onset in infancy (SAVI)	TMEM173	Transduction of cytoplasmic DNA-induced signal	AD	Systemic inflammation, cutaneous vasculopathy, pulmonary inflammation
Proteasome-associated autoinflammatory syndrome (PRAAS)	PSMB8	Part of the proteasome complex	AR	Autoinflammation, lipodystrophy, dermatosis, hyperimmunoglobulinemia, joint contractures, short stature
ISG15 deficiency	ISG15	Stabilizes USP18, a negative regulator of type 1 interferon	AR	Brain calcifications, seizures, mycobacterial susceptibility
Singleton-Merten syndrome (SMS)	IFIH1	Cytosolic receptor for dsRNA	AD	Dental dysplasia, aortic calcifications, skeletal abnormalities, glaucoma, psoriasis
Atypical SMS	DDX58	Cytosolic receptor for dsRNA	AD	Aortic calcifications, skeletal abnormalities, glaucoma, psoriasis
Trichohepatoenteric syndrome (THES)	SKIV2L	RNA helicase	AR	Severe intractable diarrhea, hair abnormalities (trichorrhexis nodosa), facial dysmorphism, immunodeficiency in most cases

From Volpi S, Picco P, Caorsi R, et al. Type 1 interferonopathies in pediatric rheumatology. *Pediatr Rheumatol*. 2016;14:35: https://doi.org/10.1186/s12969-016-0094-4

production of type 1 interferons, which leads to inflammation and characteristic features. The genetic defects occur in genes that process or detect intracellular nucleic acids, a sign of viral infections, resulting in the production of type 1 interferon and subsequent systemic inflammation. Since interferons signal through Janus kinases, which results in inflammation, targeted therapies with Janus kinase inhibitors have shown promise.

STING-Associated Vasculopathy

STING-associated vasculopathy of infancy (SAVI) is an autoinflammatory disorder that presents with intermittent low-grade fevers; rashes on the cheeks, nose, or digits; myositis; arthritis; and evidence of interstitial lung disease (see Table 54.2). The vascular involvement can be significant resulting in ulceration of the distal extremities with tissue infarcts (Fig. 54.8). Autosomal dominantly inherited variants in the signaling molecule STING, which senses altered intracytoplasmic double-stranded DNA levels, lead to its spontaneous activation and the production of type 1 interferon. Currently there is no treatment, although Janus kinase inhibitors are available based on in vitro studies and case reports.

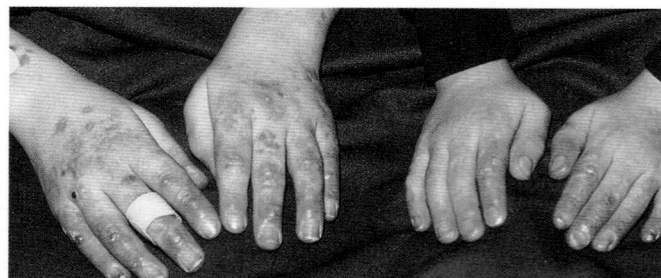

Fig. 54.8 Stimulator of interferon genes (STING)-associated vasculopathy with onset in infancy (SAVI) syndrome. These two unrelated boys both show the acral telangiectatic vasculopathy of SAVI syndrome. One of these boys died at 14 years of age because of his pulmonary disease. (From Paller AS, Mancini AJ, eds. *Hurwitz Clinical Pediatric Dermatology*. 5th ed. Philadelphia: Elsevier; 2016:587, Fig. 25-26.)

Chronic Atypical Neutrophilic Dermatosis with Lipodystrophy and Elevated Temperature

Misfolded or damaged proteins are degraded by the proteasome, and defects in the proteasome lead to buildup of dysfunctional or misfolded proteins. This buildup occurs during viral infections and is sensed by the cell with resultant interferon production. Chronic atypical neutrophilic dermatosis with lipodystrophy and elevated temperature (CANDLE) occurs due to genetic defects in the proteasome with resultant type 1 interferon production (see Table 54.2). Mild infections, cold, or stress affects metabolic demands, which can precipitate episodes of inflammation in this disorder. Features include early-onset recurrent fevers; rashes on the fingers, toes, face, and ears; and erythematous or violaceous periorbital and perioral edema. Erythematous nodules, plaques, and purpuric lesions can occur, and biopsies demonstrate leukocytoclastic vasculitis with fibrinoid necrosis and panniculitis. Labs are significant for elevated inflammatory markers, chronic anemia, thrombocytosis, and hypergammaglobulinemia. Over time lipodystrophy, aseptic meningitis, and synovitis develop. Autosomal recessive loss-of-function variants in the *PSMB8* gene, which codes for the proteasome subunit β5i, is the classic defect, but genetic variants in the other subunits of the proteasome may also result in CANDLE syndrome.

NF-κB Related Disorders

Nuclear factor-κB (NF-κB) family members are sequestered in the cytoplasm bound to inhibitory proteins, and when activated these proteins are degraded via the ubiquitin pathway, allowing for the nuclear translocation of NF-κB and the transcription of many inflammatory proteins. De-ubiquitinating enzymes inhibit this process, and genetic variants in two of these proteins, otulin and A20, lead to autoinflammatory disorders. **Otulipenia**, due to homozygous loss-of-function variants in the *FAM105B* gene that encode otulin, may present with episodes of recurrent fevers, joint swelling, painful nodular red rash, gastrointestinal inflammation with diarrhea, and failure to thrive. Biopsies of the rash will show a neutrophilic dermatosis and small/medium-vessel vasculitis. **A20 haploinsufficiency** is an autosomal dominantly inherited autoinflammatory disorder caused by genetic variants in the *TNFAIP3* gene (see Table 54.2). Patients present with systemic inflammation, oral and genital ulcers, uveitis, and fevers similar to familial Behçet disease. Other autoinflammatory disorders, such as Blau syndrome, have also been postulated to lead to NF-κB activation. **Blau syndrome** is an autosomal dominant disease caused by variants in NOD2 that result in spontaneous activation of the NOD2 protein, activation of NF-κB, and production of proinflammatory cytokines. Blau syndrome was originally described as a granulomatous disease affecting the skin, joints, and uveal tract and should be considered in any individual presenting with early-onset sarcoidosis. Blau syndrome presents with a boggy synovitis of large joints, particularly the wrists and ankles, and an erythematous papular rash similar to erythema nodosum. Biopsy of these lesions demonstrates noncaseating granulomas. Unlike sarcoidosis, respiratory involvement and hilar adenopathy are rare, although granulomatous liver disease, cranial neuropathies, and large-vessel vasculitis can occur. Laboratory studies in Blau syndrome are typically normal, although elevated ESR and angiotensin-converting enzyme levels can be seen, and hypergammaglobulinemia can occur. Most patients with Blau syndrome have been treated with corticosteroids, although limited reports have shown effectiveness of infliximab, thalidomide, and possibly anakinra.

THE IMMUNODEFICIENT PATIENT

Approximately 5–10% of children with recurrent infections have an underlying primary immunodeficiency. Frequently, the onset of infections occurs between the ages of 6 and 12 months, but delays in diagnosis are not uncommon. In addition, certain immune deficiencies such as common variable immunodeficiency disease (CVID) can present in adolescence or young adulthood; thus, it is critical to consider immune defects in children of any age. Infections in patients with primary immune deficiencies often vary in type, location, and severity, although sinopulmonary infections are common. Failure to thrive may occur and can be a sign of a serious immune defect. Patients with primary immune defects often require repeated courses of antibiotics or intravenous antibiotics or may have infections with unusual organisms or exhibit unexpected complications. Such children may respond to antibiotics but become ill when the medications are discontinued.

In a patient with recurrent infections and recurrent fevers, it can be difficult to pinpoint the cause of the infections. The immune system has four primary components:

1. **Antibody-mediated immunity (humoral or B-cell immunity)** is mediated by bone marrow–derived B lymphocytes and plasma cells (differentiated antibody-producing cells), which release antibodies (immunoglobulins) into secretions, plasma, and interstitial spaces. Antibodies work to opsonize and promote phagocytosis of organisms, prevent infection by pathogens, neutralize toxins, and lyse pathogens (with the aid of complements).
2. **Cell-mediated immunity (T-cell immunity)** is mediated by thymus-derived T lymphocytes (i.e., CD4 and CD8 T cells) that are activated by antigen-presenting cells (e.g., dendritic cells, macrophages) and antigens. Although T cells do not produce immunoglobulin, CD4 T cells are necessary for optimal B-cell function. CD4 T cells also express cytokines that activate phagocytes to efficiently clear intracellular pathogens. CD8 T cells lyse virally infected cells.
3. The **phagocytic system** consists of tissue macrophages and dendritic cells, as well as blood-borne monocytes and neutrophils. In response to specific signals, phagocytes ingest and kill invading microorganisms. Dendritic cells also serve as antigen-presenting cells for T cells.
4. The **complement system** acts synergistically with antibodies and the remainder of the immune system to help clear microbial infections both directly (complement-mediated cytolysis) and indirectly (recruitment of phagocytic cells, opsonization of microbes).

The different arms of the immune system are interconnected, and thus similar infections may occur as a manifestation of phagocyte, humoral, cell-mediated, or complement disorders that can be inherited or acquired (Table 54.5). Alternatively, highly characteristic infections can point to a defect in a particular arm of the immune system (Tables 54.6, 54.7, and 54.8). Most patients with recurrent infections do not have an underlying identifiable primary immunodeficiency, but they frequently have allergic rhinitis, asthma, or other risks for recurrent infections (see Table 54.1). Because of the low probability of identifying a discrete immune defect, the primary physician faces the difficult decision about the extent of the evaluation and which patients merit a complete evaluation.

Diagnostic Approach to the Patient with Recurrent Infections

Patients with recurrent, severe, or unusual infections involving multiple sites or organ systems should be investigated for an immunodeficiency (Fig. 54.9). Initial tests are recommended for patients suspected of a primary immune deficiency, although a variety of immune defects can occur despite normal screening tests. *Thus, it is recommended that advanced testing be performed in consultation with a clinical immunologist.*

A CBC with *manual* differential should always be obtained in the evaluation of any child suspected of immunodeficiency. A neutrophil count below 500/mm³ might indicate an associated immune defect, severe congenital neutropenia, cyclic neutropenia, idiopathic neutropenia, marrow failure, or replacement of marrow by leukemia or a

TABLE 54.5 Cause and Mechanism of Recurrent Infection in Immunodeficiency States

Disorder	Pathogen	Deficiency
Primary Immunodeficiencies		
Humoral immunodeficiency syndromes (predominantly B-cell defects)	Bacterial pathogens, enteroviruses, *Giardia lamblia*	Reduced phagocytic efficiency, failure of lysis and agglutination of bacteria, inadequate neutralization of virus and bacterial toxins
Cellular immunodeficiency syndromes (predominantly T-cell defects)	CMV, VZV, warts, *Strongyloides stercoralis; Mycobacterium, Listeria, Nocardia; Cryptococcus, Candida* species; *Pneumocystis carinii*	Absence of or impaired delayed hypersensitivity response; absence of T-cell cooperation for B-cell synthesis of antibodies to T-cell–specific antigens; absence of T-cell cytokines that activate mononuclear phagocytes, failure of T-cell clearance of viruses
Complement Deficiencies		
C1, C2, C3, C4, and factor B	*Streptococcus pyogenes, Streptococcus pneumoniae, Staphylococcus aureus, Haemophilus influenzae, Klebsiella* species	Defective chemotaxis and opsonization of microbes
C5–C8 and properdin deficiencies	*Neisseria meningitidis, Neisseria gonorrhoeae*	Defective membrane attack mechanism
Phagocyte Defects		
Neutropenia (ANC < 500/mm³)	Pyogenic bacteria or fungi, *Pseudomonas* species, *Staphylococcus aureus*	Decreased neutrophil numbers
Chronic granulomatous disease	Catalase-positive organisms, e.g., *S. aureus, Serratia* species, *Burkholderia cepacia, Nocardia* species, *Candida* species, *Aspergillus* species	Impaired neutrophil bactericidal activity secondary to impaired production of hydrogen peroxide
Secondary Immunodeficiencies		
AIDS	CMV, VZV, adenovirus, HBV, *Giardia lamblia, Entamoeba histolytica, Mycobacterium avium–intracellulare, Toxoplasma gondii, Mycobacterium tuberculosis, Cryptococcus neoformans, Pneumocystis jirovecii; Campylobacter, Candida, Isospora, Aspergillus, Nocardia, Strongyloides,* and *Cryptosporidium* species	CD4 lymphopenia with reduced TH1 response
Cancer	VZV, HSV, *Escherichia coli; Pseudomonas, Klebsiella, Listeria, Cryptococcus, Pneumocystis,* and *Mycobacterium* species	Neutropenia, lymphopenia, impaired cellular immunity
Immunosuppression	HSV, VZV, CMV, EBV, hepatitis virus, *Pseudomonas* species, *E. coli; Klebsiella, Acinetobacter, Serratia, Candida, Aspergillus, Mucor,* and *Cryptococcus* species	Dependent on agent used, leads often to impaired cellular immunity and neutropenia, lymphopenia
Transplantation	CMV, HSV, VZV, hepatitis virus, *S. aureus; Pseudomonas, Klebsiella, Candida, Aspergillus, Nocardia,* and *Pneumocystis* species; EBV	Related to use of immunosuppressive agents
Malnutrition	Measles, HSV, VZV, *Mycobacterium* species	Impaired T-cell function, reduction in complement activity

ANC, absolute neutrophil count; CMV, cytomegalovirus; EBV, Epstein-Barr virus; HBV, hepatitis B virus; HSV, herpes simplex virus; VZV, varicella-zoster virus.

tumor if other hematopoietic cell lines are affected (Table 54.9). Analysis of the peripheral blood smear is important as this can detect neutrophil abnormalities (e.g., abnormal granules in Chédiak-Higashi) or evidence of asplenia (i.e., Howell-Jolly bodies).

Serum immunoglobulin levels (IgG, IgA, IgM, IgE) are essential to the work-up of suspected primary immunodeficiency. Antibody levels vary with age, with normal adult values of IgG at birth from transplacental transfer of maternal IgG, a physiologic nadir occurring between 3 and 6 months of age, and a gradual increase to adult values over several years. IgA and IgM are low at birth and levels increase gradually over several years, with IgA taking the longest to reach normal adult values. When IgG levels are low, albumin levels should be measured because increased loss of proteins, as in protein-losing enteropathy or nephrotic syndrome, can result in hypogammaglobulinemia. High immunoglobulin levels suggest intact B-cell immunity and can be found in diseases with recurrent infections, such as chronic granulomatous disease (CGD), immotile cilia syndrome, cystic fibrosis, HIV

infection, autoimmune diseases (lupus), and other disorders leading to chronic inflammation. Elevated IgE levels can be found in a number of immune deficiencies such as hyper-IgE syndrome but more likely represent atopic disease. Undiagnosed asthma is frequently a cause of prolonged or frequent URIs, which masquerades as a primary immunodeficiency.

Specific antibody titers after childhood vaccination (tetanus, diphtheria, *H. influenzae* type b, or *Streptococcus pneumoniae*) reflect the capacity of the immune system to synthesize specific antibodies and to develop memory B cells. If titers are low, immunization with a specific vaccine and obtaining titers 4–6 weeks later should be performed to confirm a response to the immunization. Poor response to bacterial polysaccharide antigens is often found before 24 months of age; even in older individuals the antibody response to polysaccharide vaccines is typically less robust and less long-lived than protein antigens. The development of protein-conjugate polysaccharide vaccines to *S. pneumoniae* and *H. influenzae* has dramatically reduced invasive

TABLE 54.6 Characteristic Pathogens Affecting Immunocompromised Patients

I. Humoral Defects

A. Antibody Deficiency (B-Cell Defects)
1. Bacteria
Staphylococcus aureus (sepsis, sinopulmonary infection)
Haemophilus influenzae (sepsis, meningitis, arthritis, sinopulmonary infection)
Streptococcus pneumoniae (sepsis, meningitis, arthritis)
Pseudomonas aeruginosa (sepsis, pneumonia)
Mycoplasma species (arthritis, pneumonia)
Salmonella species (enteritis)
Campylobacter species (enteritis)
2. Viruses
Enterovirus, including polio vaccine (encephalitis, paralysis, myositis, arthritis)
Rotavirus (enteritis)
3. Protozoa
Giardia lamblia (enteritis)
B. Complement Deficiencies
1. C1, C2, C3, C4, factor B
Streptococcus pyogenes
S. pneumoniae, S. aureus, H. influenzae, Neisseria meningitidis, Klebsiella species (sepsis, meningitis, arthritis)
2. C5–C8, properdin deficiency
N. meningitidis, Neisseria gonorrhoeae (meningitis, sepsis, arthritis)

II. Combined B- and T-Cell Defects (Congenital, AIDS, Immunosuppression Malignancies)

A. Bacteria
Listeria monocytogenes (sepsis, meningitis)
Salmonella (sepsis)
Mycobacterium tuberculosis (pneumonia, disseminated disease)
Atypical mycobacteria (*Mycobacterium avium, Mycobacterium intracellulare*) (sepsis, pneumonia, disseminated disease)
Nocardia species (pneumonia, CNS infection)
Legionella species (pneumonia)
B. Fungi
Cryptococcus neoformans (sepsis, meningitis)
Histoplasma capsulatum (pneumonia, disseminated disease)
Coccidioides immitis (pneumonia, meningitis)
C. Viruses
Varicella-zoster (cutaneous and CNS infection, pneumonia, hepatitis)
Cytomegalovirus (bone marrow infection, pneumonia, retinitis, esophagitis, colitis, CNS infection)
Herpes simplex (CNS infection, pneumonia, esophagitis, hepatitis, disseminated disease)
Epstein-Barr virus (lymphoma)
Measles (pneumonia, encephalitis)
Polyomavirus BK (hemorrhagic cystitis, ureteric stenosis, renal insufficiency)
Polyomavirus JC (progressive multifocal leukoencephalopathy)
Papilloma viruses
D. Protozoa
Pneumocystis carinii (pneumonia, rare extrapulmonary spread)
Toxoplasma gondii (CNS infection, myocarditis)
Cryptosporidium species (enteritis)
E. Helminths
Strongyloides stercoralis (enteritis, pneumonia, sepsis, meningitis)

III. Neutropenia (Severe Chronic Neutropenia, Aplastic Anemia, Myelosuppression, Myelophthisis Myelosuppressive Agents, Bone Marrow Transplantation)

A. Bacteria
Escherichia coli (sepsis, pneumonia, pyelonephritis)
Klebsiella pneumoniae (sepsis, pneumonia)
P. aeruginosa (sepsis, pneumonia, cutaneous lesions)
Mixed anaerobic and aerobic enteric bacteria (typhlitis, perianal abscess)
S. aureus (sepsis, cellulitis, soft tissue infection)
Staphylococcus epidermidis (line infection)
Corynebacterium JK strain (sepsis)
α-Hemolytic streptococci (sepsis)
B. Fungi
Candida species (sepsis, pneumonia, ophthalmitis, liver and spleen abscesses)
Aspergillus species (sepsis, pneumonia, sinusitis, CNS infection, cutaneous lesions)
Mucor (pneumonia, sinusitis, CNS infection)
Fusarium species (sepsis, cutaneous lesions, pneumonia)
Alternaria species (sepsis, cutaneous lesions)

IV. Phagocytic Dysfunction

A. Chronic Granulomatous Disease
Bacteria (soft tissue, lymphadenitis, pneumonia, osteomyelitis)
Catalase-positive organisms (e.g., *S. aureus, Serratia marcescens, Burkholderia cepacia, Nocardia* species)
Fungi (pneumonia, liver infection, soft tissue), *Candida* species, *Aspergillus* species
B. Other Phagocyte Defects (Leukocyte Adhesion Deficiency Hyperimmunoglobulin E, Chédiak-Higashi syndrome, Specific Granule Deficiency, Rac-2 Deficiency)
Bacteria (soft tissue, pneumonia, lymphadenitis)
Pseudomonas species, *S. aureus, E. coli, Klebsiella, Enterobacter* species
Fungus (pneumonia)
Candida infection if diabetic

CNS, central nervous system.

TABLE 54.7 Clinical Aids to the Diagnosis of Immunodeficiency

Suggestive of B-Cell Defect (Humoral Immunodeficiency)

Recurrent bacterial infections of the upper and lower respiratory tracts

Recurrent skin infections, meningitis, osteomyelitis secondary to encapsulated bacteria *(Streptococcus pneumoniae, Haemophilus influenzae, Staphylococcus aureus, Neisseria meningitidis)*

Severe *Giardia lamblia* infections

Paralysis after vaccination with live attenuated poliovirus

Reduced levels of immunoglobulins

Suggestive of T-Cell Defect (Combined Immunodeficiency)

Systemic illness after vaccination with any live virus or bacille Calmette-Guérin (BCG)

Unusual life-threatening complication after infection with benign viruses (giant cell pneumonia with measles; varicella pneumonia)

Chronic oral candidiasis after 6 mo of age

Chronic mucocutaneous candidiasis

Graft versus host disease after blood transfusion

Reduced lymphocyte counts for age

Low level of immunoglobulins

Absence of lymph nodes and tonsils

Small thymus

Chronic diarrhea

Failure to thrive

Recurrent infections with opportunistic organisms

Generalized, recurrent, recalcitrant warts

Suggestive of Macrophage Dysfunction

Disseminated atypical mycobacterial infection, recurrent *Salmonella* infection

Fatal infection after BCG vaccination

Congenital Syndromes with Immunodeficiency

Ataxia-telangiectasia: ataxia, telangiectasia

Autoimmune polyglandular syndrome: hypofunction of one or more endocrine organs, chronic mucocutaneous candidiasis

Cartilage-hair hypoplasia: short-limbed dwarfism, sparse hair, neutropenia

Wiskott-Aldrich syndrome: thrombocytopenia, male gender, eczema

Chédiak-Higashi syndrome: oculocutaneous albinism, nystagmus, recurrent bacterial infections, peripheral neuropathies

DiGeorge syndrome (22q deletion syndrome): unusual facies, heart defect, hypocalcemia

CHARGE syndrome: coloboma, heart defects, atresia choanae, retarded growth, genital hypoplasia, ear anomalies/deafness

Short-limb skeletal dysplasia with combined immune deficiency: metaphyseal dysplasia, ADA deficiency, or Omenn syndrome

X-linked agammaglobulinemia with growth hormone deficiency: hypogammaglobulinemia, growth hormone deficiency

Kabuki syndrome: long palpebral fissures, prominent eyelashes, congenital heart disease

Timothy syndrome: prolonged QT, congenital heart disease, developmental delay

PTEN tumor hamartoma syndrome: multiple hamartomas, cancer

Suggestive of Asplenia

Heterotaxia, complex congenital heart disease, Howell-Jolly bodies on blood smear, sickle cell anemia

ADA, adenosine deaminase.

TABLE 54.8 Sentinel Infections and Related Genes

Infections	Recognized Gene Defects and Well-Characterized Syndromes
Viruses	
Herpes simplex encephalitis	*TBK1, TLR3, TRAF3, TRIF, UNC93B*
Cutaneous herpes simplex	Severe T-cell defects, *DOCK8, GATA2, WAS*
EBV—chronic	*CD21, CD27, CORO1A, ITK, MAGT1, PRKCD, CXCR4*
EBV—HLH	*AP3B1, LYST1, PRF1, RAB27A, SH2D1A, STX11, UNC13D, XIAP*
CMV	Severe T-cell defects, Good syndrome, *DOCK8, GATA2, STIM1, WAS*
Papilloma virus	Idiopathic CD4 lymphopenia, *ATM, CD40L, EVER1, EVER2, DOCK8, GATA2, IKBKG, MST1, RORH, STK4, CXCR4*
Fungi	
Candida	*AIRE, CARD9, IL17F, IL17RA, STAT1*
Aspergillus	Idiopathic CD4 lymphopenia, *CYBA, CYBB, DOCK8, GATA2, ITGB2, NCF1, NCF2, NCF4, STAT3*
Bacteria	
Pseudomonas	Congenital neutropenia, *IRAK4, ITGB2, MYD88, BTK* (neutropenia), *CD40LG* (neutropenia)
Salmonella	*CYBB, IFNGR1, IFNGR2, IL12B, IL12RB1*
Serratia	*CYBA, CYBB, NCF1, NCF2, NCF4*
Neisseria	*C5, C6, C7, C8A, C8B, C8G, C9, CFD, CFH, CFI, CFP*
Streptococcus pneumoniae	*C1QA, C1QB, C1QC, C4A+C4B, C2, C3, IRAK4, MYD88*
Mycobacteria	
Mycobacteria	*CYBA, CYBB, GATA2, IFNGR1, IFNGR2, IKBKG, IL12, IL12RB1, IRF8, NCF1, NCF2, NCF4, STAT1, TYK2*

HLH, hemophagocytic lymphohistiocytosis.

From Sullivan KE, Stiehm ER, eds. *Stiehm's Immune Deficiencies.* 2nd ed. London: Elsevier; 2020, Table 1.2.

infections with these organisms in early childhood by improving the response to vaccination. Antibody responses to the *S. pneumoniae* serotypes found in the 23-valent polysaccharide vaccine, but not in the conjugate vaccine, can be used to test antibody responses to polysaccharide antigens.

Complement assays include the CH50 test, which measures the presence of proteins in the classical pathway of complement (C1, C2, C3, C4), and the AH50 test, which tests the proteins of the alternative pathway of complement (C3, factor B, properdin). In patients with deficiencies in complement protein, the CH50 levels or AH50 levels are generally zero, whereas they are low but not absent in disorders leading to complement consumption (e.g., systemic lupus erythematosus). If both the CH50 and AH50 levels are abnormal, a defect in the common

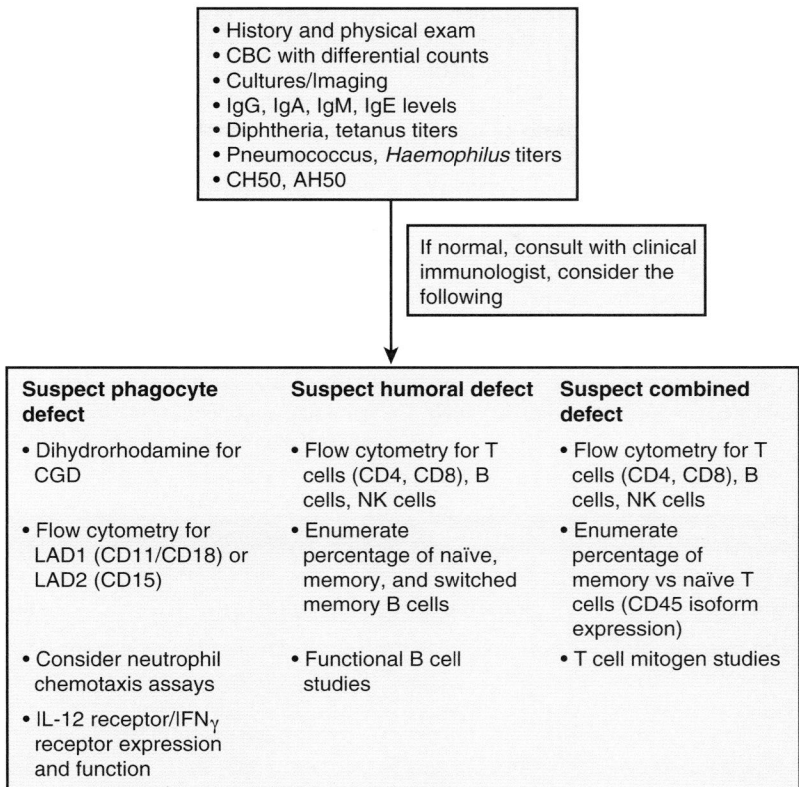

Fig. 54.9 Initial work-up and follow-up studies of patients with suspected immune deficiency. Consultation with a clinical immunologist is recommended to guide advanced testing and interpret results. CGD, chronic granulomatous disease; Ig, immunoglobulin; LAD, leukocyte adhesion defect; NK, natural killer; IL, interleukin; IFN, interferon.

TABLE 54.9 Neutropenia-Associated Immune Deficiencies

Phenotype	Gene Defect
Severe congenital neutropenia	HAX1
	ELANE
	G6PC3
	WAS
	VPS45
Moderate neutropenia	GSPT1
	PNP
	CXCR4
	Dyskeratosis congenital genes
	VPS13B
	SBDS
	TAZ
	RMRP
	LAMTOR2
Intermittent neutropenia	BTK
	CD40L
Hemophagocytic disorders	LYST
	RAB27A
	AP3B1
	SH2D1A
	XIAP

From Sullivan KE, Stiehm ER, eds. *Stiehm's Immune Deficiencies*. 2nd ed. London: Elsevier; 2020, Table 1.7.

pathway is likely (C5–C9). Specialized laboratories can measure the presence or function of specific complement proteins.

If the aforementioned studies are normal but a primary immune deficiency is still suspected, advanced studies can be performed. One such advanced study is **flow cytometry** to enumerate the percentage and absolute numbers of T cells, B cells and markers of B-cell maturation, and natural killer (NK)-cell subsets. Flow cytometry can also test for the presence of surface proteins that are necessary for normal immunity, such as major histocompatibility complex molecules or adhesion molecules. Functional T-cell tests include T-cell proliferation assays in response to mitogens (phytohemagglutinin or concanavalin A) or antigens (tetanus toxoid or *Candida*). These in vitro assays assess the capacity of T cells to proliferate in response to a nonspecific stimulus (mitogens) or antigen-specific memory T cells (antigens). T-cell proliferation in response to specific antigens requires a prior exposure to that unique antigen. Delayed-type hypersensitivity skin tests to protein antigens such as tetanus, diphtheria, *Candida,* or mumps demonstrate the presence and function of both antigen-specific T cells and antigen-presenting cells. If delayed-type hypersensitivity skin test results are negative, one may consider a booster vaccination and retesting 4 weeks later.

Tests for **neutrophil function** include the dihydrorhodamine 123 (DHR) or nitroblue tetrazolium (NBT) test. The DHR assay is the most commonly used and preferred test for the diagnosis of CGD. In the DHR test, oxygen radicals generated by the enzyme nicotinamide adenine dinucleotide phosphate (NADPH) oxidase in activated neutrophils generate H_2O_2, which oxidizes DHR, resulting in the emission of light that is detected by flow cytometry. In all forms of CGD, NADPH oxidase in neutrophils is either poorly functional or nonfunctional. Therefore, neutrophils that are activated in patients with CGD cannot generate oxygen radicals and therefore they have an abnormal DHR test (no increase in light emitted from activated neutrophils).

Genetic testing to ascertain or confirm the diagnosis of a primary immunodeficiency is often essential to make the diagnosis of a primary immunodeficiency. Defining a genetic cause of a primary immunodeficiency is important in deciding on the optimal course of treatment, determining the natural history and prognosis of the disease, genetic counseling, and prenatal diagnosis. Genetic panels, which include genes known to be implicated in specific types of immunodeficiencies such as phagocytic defects, humoral deficiencies, or severe combined immunodeficiency, are frequently performed. More extensive genetic testing, such as exome sequencing, may be used in particularly complicated cases or when genetic panels fail to yield a diagnosis.

HUMORAL IMMUNE DISORDERS

Immune disorders that result in impaired immunoglobulin production can result in recurrent infections, typically of the sinopulmonary tract (pneumonia, sinusitis, otitis media), although more disseminated infections can occur (meningitis, sepsis, cellulitis) (Table 54.10). These individuals do not typically have infections with opportunistic pathogens such as *Cryptosporidium, Pneumocystis,* or fungi that are characteristic of combined immune deficiencies (T-cell- or cell-mediated defects).

X-Linked Agammaglobulinemia

X-linked agammaglobulinemia (XLA; Bruton agammaglobulinemia) is caused by variants in the gene that encodes Bruton tyrosine kinase (BTK) and accounts for approximately 85% of all inherited forms of agammaglobulinemias (see Table 54.10). BTK is a cytoplasmic tyrosine kinase that is essential for pre–B-cell differentiation into mature B cells.

TABLE 54.10 Humoral Immune Deficiencies

Disease	Genetic Defect/Presumed Pathogenesis	Inheritance	Serum IgG	Associated Features
Severe Reduction in All Serum Immunoglobulin Isotypes with Profoundly Decreased or Absent B Cells				
BTK deficiency	*BTK,* a cytoplasmic tyrosine kinase activated by cross-linking of the BCR	XL	All isotypes decreased in majority of patients; some patients have detectable immunoglobulins	Severe bacterial and enteroviral infections
μ Heavy chain deficiency	*IGHM;* essential component of the pre-BCR	AR	All isotypes decreased	Severe bacterial and enteroviral infections
λ5 Deficiency	*IGLL1;* part of the surrogate light chain in the pre-BCR	AR	All isotypes decreased	Severe bacterial and enteroviral infections
Igα deficiency	*CD79A;* part of the pre-BCR and BCR	AR	All isotypes decreased	Severe bacterial and enteroviral infections
Igβ deficiency	*CD79B;* part of the pre-BCR and BCR	AR	All isotypes decreased	Severe bacterial and enteroviral infections
BLNK deficiency	*BLNK;* a scaffold protein that binds to BTK	AR	All isotypes decreased	Severe bacterial and enteroviral infections
PI3 kinase deficiency	*PIK3R1;* a kinase involved in signal transduction in multiple cell types	AR	All isotypes low	Severe bacterial infections
Severe Reduction in at Least Two Serum Immunoglobulin Isotypes with Normal or Low Number of B Cells				
Common variable immunodeficiency disorders	Unknown	Variable	Low IgG and IgA and/or IgM	Clinical phenotypes vary: Most have recurrent infections, some have polyclonal lymphoproliferation, autoimmune cytopenias, and/or multisystemic granulomatous disease
ICOS deficiency	*ICOS;* a costimulatory molecule expressed on T cells	AR	Low IgG and IgA and/or IgM	Recurrent infections; autoimmunity, gastroenteritis, granuloma in some
CD19 deficiency	*CD19;* transmembrane protein that amplifies signal through BCR	AR	Low IgG and IgA and/or IgM	Recurrent infections; may have glomerulonephritis
CD81 deficiency	*CD81;* transmembrane protein that amplifies signal through BCR	AR	Low IgG, low or normal IgA and IgM	Recurrent infections; may have glomerulonephritis
CD20 deficiency	*CD20;* a B-cell surface receptor involved in B-cell development and plasma cell differentiation	AR	Low IgG, normal or elevated IgM and IgA	Recurrent infections
CD21 deficiency	*CD21;* also known as complement receptor 2 and forms part of the CD19 complex	AR	Low IgG; impaired antipneumococcal response	Recurrent infections

TABLE 54.10 Humoral Immune Deficiencies—cont'd

Disease	Genetic Defect/Presumed Pathogenesis	Inheritance	Serum IgG	Associated Features
Severe Reduction in at Least Two Serum Immunoglobulin Isotypes with Normal or Low Number of B Cells—cont'd				
TACI deficiency	*TNFRSF13B* (TACI); a TNF receptor family member found on B cells and is a receptor for BAFF and APRIL	AD or AR or complex	Low IgG and IgA and/or IgM	Variable clinical expression
BAFF receptor deficiency	*TNFRSF13C* (BAFF-R); a TNF receptor family member found on B cells and is a receptor for BAFF	AR	Low IgG and IgM	Variable clinical expression
AID deficiency	*AICDA* gene	AR	IgG and IgA decreased; IgM normal or increased	Bacterial infections, enlarged lymph nodes, and germinal centers
UNG deficiency	*UNG*	AR	IgG and IgA decreased; IgM normal or increased	Bacterial infections, enlarged lymph nodes, and germinal centers
Selective IgA deficiency	Unknown	Variable	IgA decreased/absent	Usually asymptomatic; may have recurrent infections with poor antibody responses to carbohydrate antigens; may have allergies or autoimmune disease; a very few cases progress to CVID, and others coexist with CVID in the family

AD, autosomal dominant; AR, autosomal recessive; BCR, B-cell receptor; CVID, common variable immunodeficiency disease; Ig, immunoglobulin; TNF, tumor necrosis factor; XL, X-linked.

Affected children exhibit severe reductions in serum immunoglobulins and a serious risk for recurrent and sometimes life-threatening infections. Expression of the BTK gene also occurs in myeloid cells and appears to be essential in preventing apoptosis in neutrophils due to cellular stress early in life. This biological function of BTK may account for the **neutropenia** associated with this condition, which typically occurs with serious infection at the time of initial presentation.

Although some affected children are asymptomatic until the age of 2 years, most show symptoms between 6 and 9 months of age when maternal transplacental acquired antibodies disappear. Affected individuals develop recurrent infections (recurrent otitis media, sinusitis, pneumonia, meningitis) with pyogenic bacteria, such as pneumococci, staphylococci, streptococci, and *Haemophilus* species. They also have an unusual susceptibility to infection by enteroviruses, which can lead to chronic diarrhea, hepatitis, pneumonitis, and persistent meningo-encephalitis. Most live attenuated viral or bacterial vaccines are contraindicated in patients with XLA. The live attenuated polio vaccine is particularly problematic and has caused paralysis in some XLA patients. XLA patients have marked hypoplasia of lymphoid tissue (adenoids, tonsils, lymph nodes) with absence of germinal centers and rare plasma cells. The diagnosis should be considered if the serum IgG, IgM, and IgA levels are <5% of age-adjusted control values in a patient with normal T-cell function. In most patients, the number of B cells in the peripheral blood is severely reduced or absent. Treatment includes aggressive antibiotic management of infections and replacement immunoglobulin therapy, although chronic pulmonary and gastrointestinal diseases may still occur.

A variety of genetic defects involved in B-cell development also lead to agammaglobulinemia, including μ heavy chain, λ5, Igα, Igβ, *PI3KR1*, and *BLNK* (see Table 54.10). These are inherited in an autosomal recessive manner and exhibit similar clinical and laboratory phenotype.

Common Variable Immunodeficiency

CVID is a heterogeneous immunodeficiency characterized by hypogammaglobulinemia developing after an initial period of normal immune function, most commonly in the second and third decades of life (see Table 54.10). The etiology of CVID in the majority of cases is unknown, although a minority of patients have variants in the genes encoding for ICOS ("inducible costimulator" on activated T cells), TACI (transmembrane activator and calcium-modulating cyclophilin ligand interactor), CD19, CD21, CD81, or BAFF-R (see Table 54.10).

Patients with CVID are susceptible to frequent respiratory tract infections due to *pneumoniae, H. influenzae* type b, and *Mycoplasma*. Bronchiectasis due to recurrent pyogenic lung infections is a frequent complication. Gastrointestinal infections with *Giardia, Campylobacter, Salmonella, Helicobacter,* and enteroviruses are common. Bacterial overgrowth in the gut may lead to diarrhea, steatorrhea, malabsorption, and protein-losing enteropathy. Patients exhibit normal-sized or enlarged tonsils and lymph nodes and frequently have splenomegaly.

In addition to the infectious complications of CVID, noninfectious complications of CVID are common and the most common cause of death. Autoimmune hemolytic anemia and autoimmune thrombocytopenia occur frequently. Multisystemic granulomatous disease occurs in approximately 20–30% of patients, with noncaseating granulomas occurring most frequently in the lung, liver, spleen, and skin. When the granulomatous inflammation affects the lungs, it causes an interstitial lung disease known as **granulomatous and lymphocytic interstitial lung disease (GLILD)**. GLILD is frequently misdiagnosed as sarcoidosis and may lead to significant pulmonary fibrosis causing respiratory failure. Enteropathy is another serious complication of CVID and can be confused with celiac disease and lead to chronic diarrhea, protein loss, and poor nutrition. Patients with CVID are also at increased risk for inflammatory bowel disease. Nodular regenerative hyperplasia of the liver is the most common liver disease in CVID, is characterized initially by an increased alkaline phosphatase and relatively normal alanine transaminase (ALT) and aspartate transaminase (AST), and is frequently complicated by clinically significant portal hypertension early in the course of the disease. Patients with CVID are at high risk to develop B-cell lymphomas, which are Epstein-Barr virus (EBV) negative. The etiology of these noninfectious complications of CVID is unknown. GLILD, gastrointestinal tract disease, in particular enteropathy, liver disease, and B-cell lymphomas are independent risk factors for early mortality in CVID.

The diagnosis of CVID requires that age-adjusted serum IgG levels be <2 standard deviations (SD) below normal values together with low serum IgA levels (mg/dL) and/or low serum IgM levels. Specific antibody production following immunization with polysaccharide antigens (e.g., unconjugated pneumococcal vaccine) is low or absent, and responses to protein antigens (e.g., tetanus and diphtheria) may be impaired. T-cell numbers and function are highly variable, and B-cell numbers are usually normal but may be low. It is important to exclude XLA, X-linked lymphoproliferative disease, or hyper-IgM syndrome as well as other causes of hypogammaglobulinemia, such as hypogammaglobulinemia associated with thymoma, hypogammaglobulinemia secondary to protein-losing enteropathy or other protein-losing states, or hypogammaglobulinemia secondary to medications (rituximab, systemic corticosteroids), before making the diagnosis of CVID.

Transient Hypogammaglobulinemia of Infancy

The fetus is capable of producing IgM or IgG by the 20th week of gestation when adequately stimulated (intrauterine infection), but under normal conditions neonatal levels of IgG are a reflection of prior maternal immunity via transplacental passage of maternal IgG. Significant antibody production does not normally begin until the second or third month of life; elevated IgA and IgM in a newborn can be a sign of an intrauterine or perinatal infection. Because maternal antibodies have a half-life of approximately 30 days, the term infant may develop a variable *physiologic* hypogammaglobulinemia between the ages of 4 and 9 months. In *transient* hypogammaglobulinemia of infancy, the immunoglobulin nadir at 6 months of age is accentuated, with immunoglobulin levels <200 mg/dL. Immunoglobulin levels remain diminished throughout the first year of life and usually increase to normal, age-appropriate levels, generally by 2–4 years of age. If the hypogammaglobulinemia is profound in extent or duration, recurrent viral and pyogenic infections can occur. The diagnosis is supported by normal levels of both B and T cells and normal antibody responses to protein antigens such as diphtheria and tetanus toxoids. The transient nature of this disorder cannot be confirmed, however, until immunoglobulin levels return to normal ranges. Most patients do not require immune globulin replacement therapy.

Immunoglobulin A Deficiency

Selective IgA deficiency is defined as serum IgA levels <10 mg/dL with normal levels of other immunoglobulins. The diagnosis cannot be confirmed until the patient is at least 4 years of age when IgA levels should reach adult levels. Selective IgA deficiency is the most common immune disorder, occurring in approximately 1 in 500 individuals. Most patients with selective IgA deficiency are asymptomatic. In others, it is associated with recurrent sinopulmonary infections, food allergy, autoimmune disease, or celiac disease. IgA deficiency rarely occurs in families and can exhibit either autosomal recessive or autosomal dominant inheritance with variable penetrance. Antibody replacement therapy is not indicated for IgA deficiency. In patients with IgA deficiency and increased infections, other reasons for recurrent infection should be sought (atopic disease). Blood products often contain IgA, and IgA-deficient patients may develop antibodies against IgA. Therefore, IgA-deficient patients may be prone to anaphylactic reactions upon administration of blood products containing IgA; this is a relatively rare complication of IgA deficiency.

Specific Antibody Deficiency

Specific antibody deficiency syndrome is characterized by recurrent sinopulmonary infections with normal immunoglobulin levels and normal lymphocyte numbers and subsets, but a decreased ability to make specific antibodies in response to polysaccharide vaccines, such as to the 23-valent pneumococcal vaccine. Children younger than 2 years of age may not respond well to polysaccharide vaccines, so interpreting these results must include consideration of the age of the child. The pathogenesis of this disorder is unknown. Lack of specific antibody titers to polysaccharide vaccines and recurrent sinopulmonary infections with encapsulated bacteria may necessitate the use of prophylactic antibiotics or uncommonly replacement antibody therapy. Specific antibody deficiency many times resolves as the child becomes older.

Hyperimmunoglobulin M Syndrome

Hyperimmunoglobulin M (hyper-IgM) syndrome results from a failure of B cells to undergo class switching from IgM to IgA, IgG, or IgE. The failure to efficiently class switch can result in recurrent infections. Hyper-IgM syndrome was first described as a result of defects in CD40 ligand or CD40, although these disorders are actually combined immunodeficiency disorders and are discussed later. Deficiencies in activation-induced cytidine deaminase (AID) and uracil DNA-glycosylase (UNG), two enzymes involved in class switch recombination, can result in hyper-IgM syndrome without cell-mediated defects (see Table 54.10). Quantitative immunoglobulins in AID and UNG deficiency demonstrate a low IgG and IgA and a normal or elevated IgM. The clinical manifestations are similar to other significant antibody deficiencies.

COMBINED IMMUNODEFICIENCY DISORDERS

T cells are required to activate macrophages and to optimally activate B lymphocytes, and thus disorders of T lymphocytes result in defects in both cell-mediated and humoral immunity and are termed combined immune deficiencies. Patients with combined defects in T- and B-cell function have infections with the usual community-acquired pathogens as well as opportunistic or unusual pathogens, and infections may be more severe or in unusual anatomic sites compared to normal individuals (see Tables 54.5, 54.6, and 54.7). In many cases they may have other associated problems such as autoimmune problems, malignancies, or failure to thrive.

Severe Combined Immunodeficiency

Severe combined immunodeficiency (SCID) is a primary immunodeficiency caused by variants in one of several genes whose function is essential for the normal development of T cells (Table 54.11). In all forms of SCID there are profound abnormalities in T cells and subsequently B-cell function is abnormal. Clinical manifestations of SCID generally begin within the first 4 months of life with the waning of maternal antibody and include failure to thrive; severe bacterial, viral, or fungal infections; and intractable diarrhea. Infections with opportunistic pathogens such as *Pneumocystis jiroveci* and *Cryptosporidium* are common. Infections with *Candida* frequently involve the mucous membranes (mouth, esophagus, vagina), face, and diaper area, which are difficult to treat. Chronic viral infections including pneumonitis caused by adenovirus or CMV, disseminated varicella, and measles infections occur. Chronic infection following immunization with live viral vaccines (measles, mumps, rubella, varicella, rotavirus) are frequent. Fatal, disseminated mycobacterial infection following bacille Calmette-Guérin (BCG) vaccination is frequently seen in parts of the world that use the BCG vaccine.

Patients with SCID may have skin disease similar to eczema due to graft versus host disease (GVHD) from engraftment of maternal lymphocytes or Omenn syndrome. **Omenn syndrome**, a variant form of

TABLE 54.11 Severe Combined Immunodeficiency (SCID)

Disease	Genetic Defect/ Pathogenesis	Inheritance	Circulating T Cells	Circulating B Cells	Serum Ig	Associated Features
γc Deficiency	*IL-2RG*: defect in γ chain of receptors for IL-2, -4, -7, -9, -15, -21	XL	Markedly decreased	Normal or increased	Decreased	Markedly decreased NK cells
JAK3 deficiency	*JAK3*: defect in Janus-activating kinase 3	AR	Markedly decreased	Normal or increased	Decreased	Markedly decreased NK cells
IL7Rα deficiency	*IL7RA*: defect in IL-7 receptor α chain	AR	Markedly decreased	Normal or increased	Decreased	Normal NK cells
CD45 deficiency	*PTPRC*: defect in CD45	AR	Markedly decreased	Normal	Decreased	Normal γ/δ T cells
CD3δ deficiency	*CD3D*: defect in CD3δ chain of T-cell antigen receptor complex	AR	Markedly decreased	Normal	Decreased	Normal NK cells, no γ/δ T cells
CD3ε deficiency	*CD3E*: defect in CD3ε chain of T-cell antigen receptor complex	AR	Markedly decreased	Normal	Decreased	Normal NK cells, no γ/δ T cells
CD3ζ deficiency	*CD3Z*: defect in CD3ζ chain of T-cell antigen receptor complex	AR	Markedly decreased	Normal	Decreased	Normal NK cells, no γ/δ T cells
SCID Characterized by Lack of T and B Cells (DNA Recombination Defects)						
RAG 1 deficiency	*RAG1*: defective VDJ recombination; defect of recombinase-activating gene (RAG) 1	AR	Markedly decreased	Markedly decreased	Decreased	
RAG 2 deficiency	*RAG2*: defective VDJ recombination; defect of recombinase-activating gene (RAG) 2	AR	Markedly decreased	Markedly decreased	Decreased	
DCLRE1C (Artemis) deficiency	*ARTEMIS*: defective VDJ recombination; defect in Artemis DNA recombinase repair protein	AR	Markedly decreased	Markedly decreased	Decreased	Radiation sensitivity
DNA PKcs deficiency	*PKRDC*: defective VDJ recombination; defect in DNA PKcs recombinase repair protein	AR	Markedly decreased	Markedly decreased	Decreased	Radiation sensitivity, microcephaly, and developmental defects
Reticular dysgenesis, AK2 deficiency	*AK2*: defective maturation of lymphoid and myeloid cells (stem cell defect)	AR	Markedly decreased	Decreased or normal	Decreased	Granulocytopenia and deafness
Adenosine deaminase (ADA1) deficiency	*ADA1*: defective ADA activity	AR	Absent from birth or progressive	Decreased or normal	Decreased	Decreased NK cells, often with costochondral junction defects, neurologic features; partial ADA activity may result in delayed or milder presentation

AR, autosomal recessive; Ig, immunoglobulin; NK, natural killer cell; XL, X-linked.

SCID, is characterized by erythroderma and desquamation, lymphadenopathy, hepatosplenomegaly, marked eosinophilia, elevated serum IgE, and impaired T-cell function. Omenn syndrome is caused by hypomorphic variants that preserve limited function in SCID-causing genes, usually *RAG1, RAG2,* or Artemis *(DCLRE1C).* Patients with Omenn syndrome have T cells in the periphery, but these T cells are typically expanded oligoclonal Th2 cells that secrete high levels of IL-4 and IL-5, which lead to the clinical phenotype. Omenn syndrome is fatal unless corrected by bone marrow transplantation. Patients with SCID are extremely susceptible to fatal GVHD from T lymphocytes in blood transfusions, and these patients should always receive irradiated blood products. Fatal CMV infections may also develop in patients with SCID receiving blood products from CMV-positive donors. Therefore, all blood products in these patients should be from CMV-negative donors.

Patients with SCID exhibit severe deficits in immunoglobulin synthesis and the responses to specific antigens are impaired. B cells may be absent or increased, but a profound decrease in naive T cells is always present. The number of T cells in the peripheral blood is generally fewer than 10% of normal (<200 cells/mm³), and T cells show decreased proliferative responses to mitogens, decreased cytotoxicity, and decreased immunoregulatory activity. SCID is uniformly fatal without definitive treatment, which is hematopoietic stem cell transplantation (HSCT) or in some cases gene therapy. **Newborn screening for SCID** using the T-cell receptor excision circle (**TREC**) assay occurs in all of the United States and in an increasing number of countries. TRECs are formed during DNA recombination of the T-cell receptor, are biomarkers of naive T cells, and can be enumerated on the dried blood spots obtained for routine newborn screening tests. The TREC assay is highly sensitive at detecting SCID in newborns before life-threatening infectious complications occur. Early detection and treatment of newborns with SCID using the TREC assay improves long-term survival to >90%.

X-linked recessive SCID, which is caused by variants in the common gamma chain of the IL-2 receptor gene *(IL2RG)*, is the most common form of SCID (see Table 54.11). The IL2RG protein is shared by several interleukin receptors (IL-2, IL-4, IL-7, IL-9, IL-15, and IL-21). The lack of T and NK cells is due to defective signaling through the IL-7 and IL-15 receptors, respectively. IL-21 is required for efficient B-cell function. Female carriers can be identified because lymphocytes and NK cells exhibit nonrandom inactivation of the X chromosome.

Autosomal recessive SCID is less common than X-linked SCID and is caused by many different genetic defects that can be broken down based on the cell types that are lacking. A lack of T cells but not B cells is seen in genetic defects in T-cell signaling proteins including *JAK3*, *IL7R*, and *CD3* subunits (see Table 54.11). A lack of T and B cells is seen in defects in genes that affect DNA recombination, which is required to generate T- and B-cell receptors, including *RAG1*, *RAG2*, and *DCLRE1C*

(artemis) (see Table 54.11). **Adenosine deaminase (ADA) deficiency**, an autosomal recessive trait, results in an inability to catalyze the conversion of adenosine and deoxyadenosine to inosine and deoxyinosine, respectively. Deficiency of ADA results in the accumulation of deoxyadenosine and deoxyadenosine triphosphate, which is toxic to lymphocytes, resulting in loss of T, B, and NK cells. Regardless of the genetic cause of SCID, all patients have extremely low numbers of naive T cells and all exhibit the typical clinical features in terms of susceptibility to infection, failure to thrive, and 100% mortality without definitive treatment.

COMBINED IMMUNE DEFICIENCIES

Combined immunodeficiencies are genetic defects that result in defective T-cell function with or without intrinsic B-cell abnormalities (Table 54.12). Because T-cell function is abnormal, B-cell function is also compromised leading to a combined immunodeficiency, albeit less severe than SCID.

TABLE 54.12 Combined Immune Deficiencies

Disease	Genetic Defect/ Presumed Pathogenesis	Inheritance	Circulating T Cells	Circulating B Cells	Serum Ig	Associated Features
CD40L deficiency	*CD40LG* (also called TNFSF5 or CD154)	XL	Normal	B-cell numbers may be normal or increased	IgG and IgA decreased; IgM normal or increased	Bacterial and opportunistic infections, neutropenia, autoimmune disease
CD40 deficiency	*CD40* (also called TNFRSF5)	AR	Normal	B-cell numbers may be normal or increased	IgG and IgA decreased; IgM normal or increased	Bacterial and opportunistic infections, neutropenia, autoimmune disease
Purine nucleoside phosphorylase (PNP) deficiency	*PNP*, absent PNP, and T-cell and neurologic defects from elevated toxic metabolites, especially dGTP	AR	Progressive decrease	Normal	Normal or decreased	Autoimmune hemolytic anemia, neurologic impairment
ZAP70 deficiency	*ZAP70* intracellular signaling kinase, acts downstream of TCR	AR	Decreased CD8, normal CD4 cells	Normal	Normal	Autoimmunity in some cases
MHC class I deficiency	*TAP1, TAP2,* or *TAPBP* (tapasin) genes giving MHC class I deficiency	AR	Decreased CD8, normal CD4	Normal	Normal	Vasculitis; pyoderma gangrenosum
MHC class II deficiency	MHC class II proteins (*CIITA, RFX5, RFXAP, RFXANK* genes)	AR	Normal number, decreased CD4 cells	Normal	Normal or decreased	Failure to thrive, diarrhea, respiratory tract infections, liver/biliary tract disease
AD hyperimmunoglobulin E syndrome (HIES) (Job syndrome)	Dominant negative heterozygous variants in STAT3	AD; often de novo defect	Normal Th-17 and T follicular helper cells decreased	Normal; switched and nonswitched memory B cells are reduced; BAFF level increased	Elevated IgE; specific antibody production decreased	Distinctive facial features (broad nasal bridge), eczema, osteoporosis, and fractures; scoliosis, delay of shedding primary teeth, hyperextensible joints, bacterial infections (skin and pulmonary abscesses, pneumatoceles) due to *Staphylococcus aureus*, candidiasis, aneurysm formation

TABLE 54.12	Combined Immune Deficiencies—cont'd					
Disease	Genetic Defect/ Presumed Pathogenesis	Inheritance	Circulating T Cells	Circulating B Cells	Serum Ig	Associated Features
DOCK8 deficiency	*DOCK8*—regulator of intracellular actin reorganization	AR	Decreased impaired T-lymphocyte proliferation	Decreased, low CD27+ memory B cells	Low IgM, increased IgE	Low NK cells with impaired function, hypereosinophilia, recurrent infections; severe atopy, extensive cutaneous viral and bacterial *(Staphylococcus)* infections, susceptibility to cancer
Omenn syndrome	*RAG1, RAG2, artemis, IL7RA, RMRP, ADA, LIG4, IL2RG, AK2,* or associated with DiGeorge syndrome; some cases have no defined gene variant	Variable	Present; restricted T-cell repertoire, and impaired function	Normal or decreased	Decreased, except increased IgE	Erythroderma, eosinophilia, adenopathies, hepatosplenomegaly
ITK deficiency	ITK encoding IL-2-inducible T-cell kinase required for TCR-mediated activation	AR	Progressive decrease	Normal	Normal or decreased	EBV-associated B-cell lymphoproliferation, lymphoma, normal or decreased IgG
Activated PI3K-δ	*PIK3CD*	AD; gain of function			High IgM, low IgA or IgG. Reduced IgG2 and impaired antibody to pneumococci and *Haemophilus*	Respiratory infections, bronchiectasis; autoimmunity; chronic EBV and EBV-induced lymphoproliferative disease and CMV infection

AD, autosomal dominant; AR, autosomal recessive; CMV, cytomegalovirus; dGTP, deoxyguanosine triphosphate; EBV, Epstein-Barr virus; Ig, immunoglobulin; IL, interleukin; MHC, major histocompatibility complex; NK, natural killer; TCR, T-cell receptor; XL, X-linked.

Hyper-IgM syndrome is characterized by normal or increased concentrations of IgM and IgD but decreased levels or absence of IgG, IgA, and IgE (see Table 54.12). The most common form of these disorders is X-linked hyper-IgM syndrome, which is due to a variant in the gene encoding the T-cell surface protein CD40 ligand *(CD40L)*. A rarer, autosomal recessive form of this disorder is caused by variants in the *CD40* gene, which is expressed on the surface of B cells and antigen-presenting cells (see Table 54.12). The CD40/CD40L pathway is essential for B-cell isotype switching, which allows a B cell to maintain antigen specificity while altering immunoglobulin function. Isotype class switching requires specific cytokines and the interaction between CD40 ligand on CD4 T cells and CD40 on B cells. All patients with hyper-IgM syndrome due to genetic defects in CD40L or CD40 have increased susceptibility to sinopulmonary infections with pyogenic bacteria. These individuals are also susceptible to opportunistic infections including *P. jiroveci (carinii)* and *Cryptosporidium parvum*. Signaling via CD40 on B cells accounts for the defects in antibody production and class switching, while defective CD40 signaling in phagocytes and antigen-presenting cells accounts for the susceptibility to opportunistic pathogens. In addition, as many as 50% of patients with CD40L deficiency will exhibit neutropenia.

Signal transduction via CD40 activates several signaling molecules and transcription factors, including NF-κB, and two enzymes, AID and UNG, which are also required for class switching. Damaging variants in AID or UNG cause a failure of immunoglobulin isotype switching without opportunistic infections since these proteins function only in isotype class switching and not cell-mediated immunity.

The hyper-IgM phenotype is seen in a number of primary immune deficiencies including an X-linked immunodeficiency associated with ectodermal dysplasia resulting from defects in the gene encoding the **NF-κB essential modulator (NEMO)**. NF-κB signaling is important for function of both innate and adaptive immune systems. Therefore, patients with defects in NEMO have a combined immunodeficiency and are susceptible to a wide spectrum of viruses and bacteria, in particular pyogenic bacteria (e.g., *S. pneumoniae, H. influenzae*) and atypical mycobacteria.

Gain-of-function variants in the catalytic domain of PI3 kinase *(PIK3CD)* can also lead to elevated IgM levels, and initial patients with this disease were misdiagnosed as having hyper-IgM syndrome. PIK3CD is expressed in B cells and T cells, and therefore gain-of-function variants in PIK3CD lead to the constitutive activation of PI3 kinase, resulting in impaired T-cell and B-cell function. These patients present with recurrent sinopulmonary infections and have an increased susceptibility to infection with herpes viruses. Autoimmunity, lymphoproliferation (including an increased incidence of EBV-induced lymphoproliferative disease and B-cell lymphomas), and structural lung disease (bronchiectasis) commonly occur.

Purine Nucleoside Phosphorylase Deficiency

Purine nucleoside phosphorylase (PNP) is an enzyme that follows adenosine deaminase in the purine salvage pathway and catalyzes the conversion of inosine and guanosine to hypoxanthine and guanine, respectively (see Table 54.12). PNP deficiency, which is inherited as an autosomal recessive disorder, leads to the intracellular buildup of deoxyguanosine triphosphate (deoxy-GTP), which is toxic to rapidly dividing cells. Although PNP is ubiquitously expressed, PNP deficiency affects T cells and not B cells and leads to T-cell lymphopenia with preserved numbers of B cells. Although serum immunoglobulins are usually normal, specific antibody production is impaired. A low serum uric acid level is suggestive of PNP deficiency. Patients with PNP deficiency are predisposed to infection with common and opportunistic pathogens. Autoimmunity and neurologic manifestations are also common. The only curative treatment for PNP deficiency is HSCT.

Hyperimmunoglobulin E Syndrome

Classic hyperimmunoglobulin E syndrome (HIES), also known as **Job syndrome,** is an autosomal dominant disorder caused by variants in signal transducer and activator of transcription 3 (STAT3), an important signaling molecule required for the signaling of several cytokines such as IL-6 and IL-10 (see Table 54.12). Classic HIES is characterized by markedly elevated levels of serum IgE, early-onset severe eczematous dermatitis, recurrent bacterial infections (skin, respiratory tract, bone), and chronic candidiasis (thrush, onychomycosis). Other associated features include coarse facial features, manifested by a broad nasal bridge, prominent nose, dental abnormalities, and irregular proportional cheeks and jaw. The eczematous rash is typically papular and pruritic, involving the face and extensor surfaces of arms and legs, and may start at birth or soon thereafter. The skin abscesses typically due to *S. aureus* are remarkable for their absence of surrounding erythema or warmth, leading to the term *cold abscesses.* By 5 years of age, all patients have had a history of recurrent skin abscesses and recurrent pneumonias with pneumatoceles, along with chronic otitis media and sinusitis. Patients may also develop septic arthritis, cellulitis, or osteomyelitis. Fungal infections with *Candida albicans* and *Aspergillus* species occur. Serum IgE levels typically exceed 2,500 IU/mL. Usually, patients with HIES have normal concentrations of IgG, IgA, and IgM, and frequently have eosinophilia. The clinical manifestations of **DOCK8 deficiency** display considerable overlap with classic HIES, with high IgE levels, eczema, and recurrent infections (see Table 54.12). However, patients with DOCK8 deficiency typically lack pneumatoceles and bone and tooth abnormalities. The optimal treatment of classic HIES is largely supportive and includes antimicrobial therapy and, in selected patients, replacement antibody. In contrast, HSCT is curative for DOCK8 deficiency.

IMMUNODEFICIENCIES WITH SYNDROMIC FEATURES

Several genetic defects that affect the immune system also affect other organ systems and thus represent a clinical syndrome (Tables 54.7 and 54.13). A careful history and exam can lead a clinician to the diagnosis. Most of these conditions present with combined T- and B-cell defects.

Wiskott-Aldrich Syndrome

Wiskott-Aldrich syndrome (WAS) is an X-linked recessive disorder caused by variant in the gene that encodes the WAS protein, or WASP. WASP controls the assembly of actin filaments and intracellular vesicle transport in lymphocytes and megakaryocytes. WAS is characterized by abnormalities in lymphocyte, platelet, and phagocyte function (see Table 54.13). Classic WAS is characterized by the triad of recurrent infections involving encapsulated bacteria and opportunistic pathogens, hemorrhage secondary to thrombocytopenia and platelet dysfunction, and atopic dermatitis. Variants in the WAS gene can also cause X-linked neutropenia and X-linked thrombocytopenia. The clinical manifestations of WAS begin in early infancy with pneumonia, otitis media, meningitis, and bleeding. Patients are susceptible to recurrent and severe infections with encapsulated bacteria and viruses (herpes simplex virus, varicella, EBV, CMV). Fungal and pneumocystis infections may occur as well. Autoimmunity is common and includes cytopenias, vasculitis, arthritis, and inflammatory bowel disease. Patients are also susceptible to malignancy, in particular lymphoreticular malignancies. In classic WAS there is thrombocytopenia with abnormally small platelets. Deficiency of this protein results in elevated levels of IgE and IgA, decreased IgG and/or IgM, poor responses to polysaccharide antigens, and waning T-cell function. One-third of patients with WAS die as a result of hemorrhage, and two-thirds die as a result of recurrent infection caused by bacteria, CMV, *P. jiroveci,* or herpes simplex virus. In classic WAS, HSCT is the treatment of choice and long-term survival is excellent in patients with appropriately human leukocyte antigen (HLA)-matched donors.

Ataxia-Telangiectasia

Ataxia-telangiectasia (AT) is an autosomal recessive disorder characterized by neurologic dysfunction, endocrine abnormalities, oculocutaneous telangiectasia, immunodeficiency, and radiation sensitivity with a high rate of malignancy (see Table 54.13). The defective gene is the AT mutated gene *(ATM)* that encodes for a phosphatidylinositol 3-kinase involved in sensing DNA damage and DNA repair. Cerebellar ataxia is usually the first clinical manifestation, occurring when the child begins to walk. The patient's neurologic status often worsens, and choreoathetosis and oculomotor abnormalities develop. Telangiectasias first appear in the bulbar conjunctivae between 2 and 5 years of age and later spread to areas of trauma. Endocrine abnormalities, such as insulin-resistant diabetes mellitus and hypogonadism, are common. There is a 15% risk of malignancy, with non-Hodgkin lymphoma being the most common. Patients with AT are extremely sensitive to ionizing radiation, and radiographic studies should be avoided if possible. Radiation sensitivity accounts for the high incidence of chromosomal translocations involving chromosomes 7 and 14 at the site of T-cell receptor genes and immunoglobulin heavy-chain genes.

The degree of immunodeficiency in AT is quite variable and may include abnormalities in T cells and B cells. Respiratory tract disease is an important cause of morbidity and mortality and includes sinopulmonary infection with encapsulated organisms, interstitial lung disease, and lung disease associated with neuromuscular deficits including recurrent aspiration. Opportunistic respiratory tract infections are uncommon. There is no curative therapy for AT, although antimicrobial prophylaxis and intravenous immunoglobulin (IVIG) replacement are used to prevent infections.

DiGeorge Syndrome (22q Deletion Syndrome) and Other Thymic Defects

22q Deletion syndrome is a disorder caused in the majority of cases by microdeletion at chromosome 22q11.2, although a deletion at a second locus at chromosome 10p13 results in a similar clinical picture. 22q Deletion syndrome, also known as velocardiofacial syndrome, is characterized by a constellation of clinical features that include dysmorphic facies, hypoparathyroidism, congenital heart defects, and T-cell lymphopenia (see Table 54.13). The clinical anomalies are caused by maldevelopment of structures derived from the first through the sixth branchial pouches during embryogenesis, resulting in variable hypoplasia of the thymus, parathyroid glands, face, ears, aortic arch, and heart. Congenital heart defects include truncus arteriosus, ventricular septal defect, interrupted aortic arch, and tetralogy of Fallot. Hypocalcemia with tetany is often the initial problem in the first and second

TABLE 54.13 Combined Immune Deficiencies with Syndromic Features

Disease	Genetic Defect/ Presumed Pathogenesis	Inheritance	Circulating T Cells	Circulating B Cells	Serum Ig	Associated Features
Wiskott-Aldrich Syndrome (WAS)	*WAS*; cytoskeletal and immunologic synapse defect affecting hematopoietic stem cell derivatives	XL	Progressive decrease, abnormal lymphocyte responses to anti-CD3	Normal	Decreased IgM: antibody to polysaccharides particularly decreased; often increased IgA and IgE	Thrombocytopenia with small platelets; eczema; lymphoma; autoimmune disease; IgA nephropathy; bacterial and viral infections. XL thrombocytopenia is a mild form of WAS, and XL neutropenia is caused by missense variants in the GTPase binding domain of WAS protein
Ataxia-telangiectasia	*ATM*; disorder of cell cycle checkpoint; and DNA double-stranded break repair	AR	Progressive decrease	Normal	Often decreased IgA, IgE, and IgG subclasses; increased IgM monomers; antibodies variably decreased	Ataxia; telangiectasia; pulmonary infections; lymphoreticular and other malignancies; increased α-fetoprotein and increased radiosensitivity
Cartilage-hair hypoplasia	*RMRP* (RNase MRP RNA) involved in processing of mitochondrial RNA and cell cycle control	AR	Varies from severely decreased (SCID) to normal; impaired lymphocyte proliferation	Normal	Normal or reduced; antibodies variably decreased	Short-limbed dwarfism with metaphyseal dysostosis, sparse hair, bone marrow failure, autoimmunity, susceptibility to lymphoma and other cancers, impaired spermatogenesis, neuronal dysplasia of the intestine
CHARGE syndrome	Variable defects of the thymus and associated T-cell abnormalities often due to deletions or variants in *CHD7*, *SEMA3E*, or as-yet-unknown genes	De novo defect (majority) or AD	Decreased or normal; some have <1,500 CD3 T cells/μL	Normal	Normal or decreased	Coloboma, heart anomaly, choanal atresia, retardation, genital and ear anomalies
22q Deletion syndrome (includes DiGeorge anomaly)	Contiguous gene defect in 90% affecting thymic development; may also be due to heterozygous variant in *TBX1* (chromosome 22q11.2 deletion or TBX1 haploinsufficient syndrome)	AD; often de novo	Decreased or normal; 5% have <1,500 CD3 T cells/μL	Normal	Normal or decreased	Hypoparathyroidism, conotruncal malformation; abnormal facies; large deletion (3 Mb) in 22q11.2 (or rarely a deletion in 10p)

AD, autosomal dominant; AR, autosomal recessive; Ig, immunoglobulin; XL, X-linked.

months after birth. Facial abnormalities include microstomia, hypertelorism, and low-set ears.

The degree of immunodeficiency is highly variable and related to the extent of residual thymic function. In *complete* DiGeorge syndrome, which occurs in <1% of patients, severe T-cell deficiency leads to a disorder resembling SCID with failure to thrive, and recurrent infections with opportunistic organisms (*P. jiroveci*, viruses, and fungi). In contrast, many other patients with 22q deletion syndrome exhibit relatively normal immune function or relatively minor immunodeficiency. Autoimmunity, including autoimmune cytopenias, is common. The total T-cell count may vary from severely depressed to normal. No correlation has been shown between the severity of congenital defects and the severity of immunodeficiency, and immune function often improves with age.

The diagnosis is established by chromosomal microarray or fluorescent in situ hybridization to detect the usual deleted region in chromosome 22q11.2. Approximately 10% of patients have hypogammaglobulinemia with a minority requiring antibody replacement therapy. Importantly, due to intrinsic defects in the thymus, patients with 22q deletion syndrome cannot be treated with HSCT, although transfer of mature T cells during transplant may confer some immune function.

CHARGE syndrome (coloboma, heart anomaly, choanal atresia, retardation of growth, genital and ear anomalies) can be rarely seen with features of DiGeorge syndrome when thymic aplasia is present. Variants in *CHD7* are the most common known cause of CHARGE syndrome, although variants in *SEMA3E* are found in a minority of patients (see Table 54.13). The degree of immunodeficiency is related to the extent of thymic hypoplasia and T-cell numbers and can be highly variable. Similar to DiGeorge syndrome, some variants of CHD7 are a cause of SCID with a profound T-cell lymphopenia.

Cartilage-Hair Hypoplasia

Cartilage-hair hypoplasia (CHH) is an autosomal recessive disease caused by variants in the ribonuclease mitochondrial RNA-processing (RMRP) gene. CHH is characterized by metaphyseal dysostosis, sparse and thin hair, and variable immunodeficiency (see Table 54.13). Lymphocyte counts over time become low in all patients due to low numbers of T cells. Proliferative responses to mitogens are generally depressed, and immune function may deteriorate with time. The immunodeficiency can range from mild to severe, but in many affected patients it is relatively mild. Patients benefit most from replacement immunoglobulin. Patients may have moderate to severe neutropenia, making them susceptible to both viral and bacterial infections.

COMPLEMENT SYSTEM DEFICIENCIES

The complement system consists of plasma and membrane proteins that function in the innate immune response as well as facilitating adaptive immunity. Complement proteins can kill pathogens with or without antibodies, opsonize pathogens to facilitate their uptake by phagocytes, or mediate inflammation. The complement system can be activated through three pathways—the classical, alternative, or lectin pathways—that involve the sequential activation of complement factors resulting in an amplified response. Disorders of the complement system predispose to recurrent infection, autoimmunity, and angioedema (Table 54.14 and Fig. 54.10).

TABLE 54.14 Complement Defects

Disease	Genetic Defect/Presumed Pathogenesis	Inheritance	Functional Defect	Associated Features
C1q deficiency	*C1QA, C1QB, C1QC:* classical complement pathway components	AR	Absent CH50 hemolytic activity; defective activation of the classical pathway, diminished clearance of apoptotic cells	SLE, infections with encapsulated organisms
C1r deficiency	*C1R:* classical complement pathway component	AR	Absent CH50 hemolytic activity; defective activation of the classical pathway	SLE, infections with encapsulated organisms
C1s deficiency	*C1S:* classical complement pathway component	AR	Absent CH50 hemolytic activity; defective activation of the classical pathway	SLE, infections with encapsulated organisms
C4 deficiency	*C4A, C4B:* classical complement pathway components	AR	Absent CH50 hemolytic activity; defective activation of the classical pathway, defective humoral immune response to carbohydrate antigens in some patients	SLE, infections with encapsulated organisms
C2 deficiency	*C2:* classical complement pathway component	AR	Absent CH50 hemolytic activity; defective activation of the classical pathway	SLE, infections with encapsulated organisms, atherosclerosis
C3 deficiency	*C3:* central complement component	AR, gain-of-function AD	Absent CH50 and AH50 hemolytic activity; defective opsonization, defective humoral immune response	Infections; glomerulonephritis, aHUS with gain-of-function variants
C5 deficiency	*C5:* terminal complement component	AR	Absent CH50 and AH50 hemolytic activity; defective bactericidal activity	Neisserial infections
C6 deficiency	*C6:* terminal complement component	AR	Absent CH50 and AH50 hemolytic activity; defective bactericidal activity	Neisserial infections
C7 deficiency	*C7:* terminal complement component	AR	Absent CH50 and AH50 hemolytic activity; defective bactericidal activity	Neisserial infections
C8 α–γ deficiency	*C8A, C8G:* terminal complement components	AR	Absent CH50 and AH50 hemolytic activity; defective bactericidal activity	Neisserial infections
C8b deficiency	*C8B:* terminal complement component	AR	Absent CH50 and AH50 hemolytic activity; defective bactericidal activity	Neisserial infections
C9 deficiency	*C9:* terminal complement component	AR	Reduced CH50 and AH50 hemolytic activity; deficient bactericidal activity	Mild susceptibility to neisserial infections
C1 inhibitor deficiency	*C1NH:* regulation of kinins and complement activation	AD	Spontaneous activation of the complement pathway with consumption of C4/C2; spontaneous activation of the contact system with generation of bradykinin from high-molecular-weight kininogen	Hereditary angioedema
Factor B	*CFB:* activation of the alternative pathway	AD	Gain-of-function variant with increased spontaneous AH50	aHUS
Factor D deficiency	*CFD:* regulation of the alternative complement pathway	AR	Absent AH50 hemolytic activity	Neisserial infections
Properdin deficiency	*CFP:* regulation of the alternative complement pathway	XL	Absent AH50 hemolytic activity	Neisserial infections

Disease	Genetic Defect/Presumed Pathogenesis	Inheritance	Functional Defect	Associated Features
Factor I deficiency	*CFI*: regulation of the alternative complement pathway	AR	Spontaneous activation of the alternative complement pathway with consumption of C3	Infections, neisserial infections, aHUS, preeclampsia, membranoproliferative glomerulonephritis
Factor H deficiency	*CFH*: regulation of the alternative complement pathway	AR	Spontaneous activation of the alternative complement pathway with consumption of C3	Infections, neisserial infections, aHUS, preeclampsia, membranoproliferative glomerulonephritis
MASP1 deficiency	*MASP1*: cleaves C2 and activates MASP2	AR	Deficient activation of the lectin activation pathway, cell migration	Infections, candida infections

TABLE 54.14 Complement Defects—cont'd

AD, autosomal dominant; aHUS, atypical hemolytic uremic syndrome; AR, autosomal recessive; SLE, systemic lupus erythematosus; XL, X-linked.

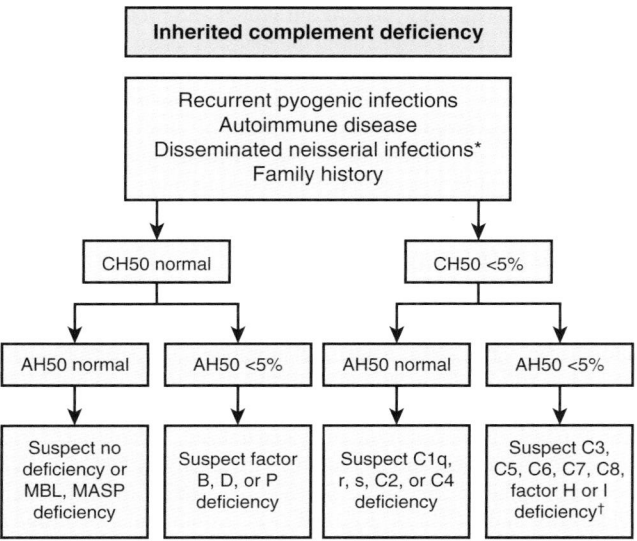

Fig. 54.10 Flow chart for the evaluation of inherited complement deficiencies using hemolytic screening assays for the classical (CH50) and alternative (AH50) pathways. For each assay, the entire activation pathway, including the membrane attack complex, is required for lysis. MASP, MBL-associated serine protease; MBL, mannose-binding lectin. *Gonococcal and meningococcal. † C9 deficiency may have up to 30% normal CH50 with low AH50. (From Kliegman RM, St. Geme JW III, Blum NJ, et al., eds. *Nelson Textbook of Pediatrics.* 21st ed. Philadelphia: Elsevier; 2020:1152, Fig. 160.1.)

The three pathways for complement activation are initiated by different mechanisms. The classical pathway is activated by antigen-antibody complexes. The alternative pathway may be activated by C3b generated through the classical pathway or by spontaneous hydrolysis of C3 on microbial surfaces. The lectin pathway is initiated by the interaction of mannose-binding lectin with microbial carbohydrate. Activation of the classical pathway by an antigen-antibody complex is initiated by the binding of C1q to the Fc portion of an antibody molecule in the immune complex. C1r autoactivates and cleaves C1s, which cleaves C4 and then C2, forming the C3 convertase C4b2b. C4b2b is activated by the lectin pathway when mannose-binding protein binds to sugar residues on the surface of pathogens, and mannose-binding protein–associated proteases (MASPs) cleave C4 and C2. The alternative pathway is always active at a low level and is amplified when active C3 binds to a surface that lacks regulatory proteins. C3b generated from C3 binds to factor B, which is cleaved by factor D to form the alternative pathway C3 convertase C3bBb. Properdin binds to and stabilizes the C3 convertase. The C3 convertase can cleave C3, resulting in further C3b deposition and activation of the alternative pathway, which acts as an amplification loop by generating more C3b, or it can form the C5 convertase, which initiates the formation of a membrane attack complex (MAC). The MAC is a complex of C5b, C6, C7, C8, and several C9 molecules that is common to all three pathways. The MAC generates pores in the cell membrane, leading to lysis of the cells.

C3a and C5a, produced by cleavage of C3 and C5, respectively, release histamine from mast cells and basophils, leading to increased vascular permeability and smooth muscle contraction. In addition, C5a has chemotactic activity, attracting phagocytes to the site of complement activation, and it can cause degranulation of phagocytic cells. C3b acts as an opsonin when attached to the surface of a pathogen by binding to phagocytes.

The complement system is under tight regulation because it has potent inflammatory activity and the potential to cause significant damage to host cells, and therefore there are a number of complement regulatory proteins. C1 inhibitor regulates the cascade by blocking active sites on C1r, C1s, and the MASP. Factor I destabilizes C3 convertase complexes and degrades the active fragments. Other inhibitors include membrane proteins, such as decay accelerating factor (DAF), CR1, membrane cofactor protein (MCP), and plasma proteins such as C4 binding protein. Formation of the MAC can be blocked by cell surface CD59. Deficiency of any of these regulatory proteins can result in an inflammatory response, tissue damage, or excessive complement consumption. Deficiency in the expression of CD59 results in paroxysmal hemoglobinuria. Deficiencies in the complement regulatory proteins (factor H, factor I, and MCP) result in atypical hemolytic uremic syndrome and membranoproliferative glomerulonephritis type II, and have been linked to age-related macular degeneration (see Table 54.14).

Although protein deficiencies or abnormalities have been identified for components in the classical complement pathway, the severity and the type of infection vary because of the considerable overlap between the two pathways (see Table 54.14). Disorders of complement proteins can result from inherited deficiency or can be secondary to increased consumption. Deficiencies of early components of the classical pathway (C1, C2, or C4) are not usually associated with severe infections, although patients with C2 deficiency may present with recurrent respiratory tract infections with encapsulated bacteria. Patients with C1, C2, or C4 deficiency are susceptible to autoimmune diseases, especially systemic lupus erythematosus. The exact mechanism of this susceptibility is not known but is thought to arise from the role of these early components of complement in clearing immune complexes. Deficiency of C3, the major opsonin, due to a genetic defect or secondary to excessive consumption or protein loss (e.g., nephrotic syndrome, systemic lupus erythematosus) predisposes patients to infections, especially with encapsulated organisms. Deficiency of one of the terminal components that compose the MAC or properdin predisposes patients to invasive infections (e.g., meningitis, septicemia) with *Neisseria meningitidis* and *Neisseria gonorrhoeae*. Complement deficiency may be found in 40% of patients presenting with recurrent neisserial infections, particularly with meningococcal disease caused by uncommon serogroups (see Table 54.14).

C1 inhibitor deficiency causes **hereditary angioedema**, an autosomal dominant disorder that results in disregulation of the classical complement pathway. After minor trauma, affected patients develop local angioedema without urticaria, pain, or erythema. The angioedema may be severe and untreated leads to significant morbidity and mortality. Angioedema involving the larynx or upper airways can be life-threatening, and involvement of the bowel leads to abdominal pain, vomiting, and diarrhea. Lack of inhibition of plasma kallikrein by C1 inhibitor and disregulated production of bradykinin is the cause of the angioedema. Treatment of hereditary angioedema includes administration of C1 inhibitor, administration of a pharmacologic inhibitor of plasma kallikrein (ecallantide), or administration of a bradykinin β_2-antagonist (icatibant).

Diagnosis of Complement Deficiencies

The CH50 test is a widely available test of classical complement pathway function based on an antibody-dependent hemolytic assay. The CH50 test depends on the function of all nine complement proteins, C1 through C9. The AH50 test, which activates the alternative pathway, depends on the alternative pathway components and C5–C9. An abnormal CH50 but not AH50 is consistent with defects in C1, C2, or C4. Alternatively, an abnormal AH50 but normal CH50 indicates a defect in properdin or factor B. Abnormal results of both tests indicate a deficiency in a terminal component common to both pathways (C3, C5–C9). If the CH50 or AH50 levels are abnormal, individual components can be analyzed in specialized laboratories. In hereditary angioedema, C4 levels are generally low, but C3 levels are normal. Determination of C1 inhibitor levels and/or function is needed to definitively diagnose hereditary angioedema. Low C3 and C4 levels are seen when the classical pathway is activated (e.g., systemic lupus erythematosus), whereas activation of the alternative pathway characteristically results in low C3 levels and normal C4 levels.

Specific treatment of complement deficiencies with component replacement is not available. Frequent courses of antibiotics or prophylactic antibiotics have been utilized. Immunization of patients and close contacts with pneumococcal and meningococcal vaccines may be useful, but infections may still occur in immunized complement-deficient patients. Replacement of complement proteins by plasma transfusion has been used in some patients with C2 deficiency, factor H deficiency, or factor I deficiency. MCP deficiency presenting with atypical hemolytic uremic syndrome is treated with renal transplantation since it is a membrane protein.

PHAGOCYTIC DISORDERS

Neutrophils are important in protecting the skin, mucous membranes, and the lining of the respiratory and gastrointestinal tracts. They form the first line of defense against microbial invasion. During the critical first 2–4 hours after tissue invasion by pathogenic organisms, the arrival of phagocytic cells at the site of infection is crucial for the containment of the infection, limiting the size of the local lesion, and preventing

dissemination. Monocytes/macrophages are also important in cell-mediated immunity, and in response to T-cell cytokines (interferon-γ [IFNγ]), these cells become effective killers of intracellular pathogens.

Neutrophils develop in the bone marrow from hematopoietic stem cells, and upon leaving the bone marrow mature neutrophils are found in the circulation or roll along the endothelium (known as the marginating pool). Adhesion molecules are necessary for neutrophils to roll and adhere to vascular endothelium and extravasate from the blood into sites of infection, where they phagocytose and kill pathogens, especially those coated by complement or antibodies. Chemotactic factors, including the complement fragment C5a, IL-8, leukotriene B$_4$, and bacterial formylated peptides (fMLP), mobilize neutrophils to enter tissues and sites of infections. Once in tissues these cells ingest the offending organisms (phagocytosis) and activate biochemical pathways important in intracellular microbial killing (degranulation and oxidative metabolism). The respiratory burst consists of the de novo synthesis of highly toxic and often unstable derivatives of molecular oxygen. Degranulation is the process by which lysosomal granules, containing preformed polypeptide antibiotics and proteases, fuse with the phagocytic vacuoles containing the ingested microbes.

Patients with neutrophil disorders are susceptible to a variety of bacterial infections and certain fungi. Infections associated with neutrophil disorders include infections of mucosal surfaces (e.g., respiratory tract infections, rectal and vaginal infections, gingivostomatitis), abscesses in the skin and viscera, lymphadenitis, poor wound healing, delayed umbilical cord separation, or absence of pus.

Disorders of Neutrophil Numbers

Neutropenia is defined as an absolute neutrophil count (ANC) <1,500/mm^3 for children 1 year of age or older, although African American children can have lower neutrophil numbers. The susceptibility to infection is minimally increased until the ANC is <1,000/mm^3. Most patients do well with an ANC >500/mm^3. At these levels, localized infections are more common than generalized bacteremia. Serious bacterial infections are more common with an ANC <200/mm^3. Neutropenia may be congenital and caused by variants in several genes (Tables 54.9 and 54.15) or acquired (e.g., autoimmune neutropenia, drug reactions, marrow replacement with cancer cells).

Inherited Forms of Neutropenia

Severe congenital neutropenia (Kostmann syndrome) is an autosomal recessive disorder caused by variants in the HCLS-associated protein X-1 *(HAX1)* gene and is characterized by severe persistent neutropenia (ANC <500 cells/mm^3) and recurrent bacterial infections (see Table 54.15). Affected patients often have increased plasma concentrations of granulocyte colony-stimulating factor (G-CSF) as well as circulating eosinophils and monocytes. In severe congenital neutropenia, the neutrophil counts increase in response to exogenous G-CSF despite the elevated level of G-CSF at baseline.

Autosomal dominant inherited variants in the elastase 2 gene *(ELA2)* are the most common cause of **cyclic neutropenia,** although the disorder may present as persistent neutropenia as well. In the cyclic form of neutropenia, there are periodic episodes of profound neutropenia (ANCs <200 cells/mm^3), generally lasting 3–6 days and occurring in 21-day cycles (see Table 54.15). During the episodes of neutropenia, individuals develop aphthous ulcers, gingivitis, stomatitis, and cellulitis. Death from overwhelming infection with *Clostridium perfringens* occurs in about 10% of patients.

Severe congenital neutropenia, which may be either persistent or cyclic, is also seen in **Shwachman-Diamond syndrome**, an autosomal recessive syndrome of pancreatic insufficiency accompanying bone marrow dysfunction. Metaphyseal dysostosis and dwarfism may occur.

TABLE 54.15 Phagocyte Disorders

Disease	Genetic Defect/ Presumed Pathogenesis	Inheritance	Affected Cells	Affected Function	Associated Features
Severe congenital neutropenia 1 (ELANE deficiency)	*ELANE:* misfolded protein response, increased apoptosis	AD	N	Myeloid differentiation	Susceptibility to MDS/leukemia
SCN2a (GFI1 deficiency)	*GFI1:* loss of repression of ELANE	AD	N	Myeloid differentiation	B/T lymphopenia
SCN3 (Kostmann disease)	*HAX1:* control of apoptosis	AR	N	Myeloid differentiation	Cognitive and neurologic defects in patients with defects in both HAX1 isoforms, susceptibility to MDS/leukemia
SCN4 (G6PC3 deficiency)	*G6PC3:* abolished enzymatic activity of glucose-6-phosphatase, aberrant glycosylation, and enhanced apoptosis of N and F	AR	N + F	Myeloid differentiation, chemotaxis, O⁻ production	Structural heart defects, urogenital abnormalities, inner ear deafness, and venous angiectasias of trunks and limbs
SCN5	*VPS45:* controls vesicular trafficking	AR	N + FM	Myeloid differentiation, migration	Extramedullary hematopoiesis, bone marrow fibrosis, nephromegaly
Cyclic neutropenia	*ELANE:* misfolded protein response	AD	N	Differentiation	Oscillations of other leukocytes and platelets
X-linked neutropenia/ myelodysplasia	*WAS:* regulator of actin cytoskeleton (loss of autoinhibition)	XL, gain of function	N + M	Mitosis	Monocytopenia
Leukocyte adhesion deficiency type 1 (LAD1)	*ITGB2:* adhesion protein (CD18)	AR	N + M + L + NK	Adherence, chemotaxis, endocytosis, T/NK cytotoxicity	Delayed cord separation, skin ulcers, periodontitis, leukocytosis
Leukocyte adhesion deficiency type 2 (LAD2)	*SLC35C1* GDP-fucose transporter	AR	N + M	Rolling, chemotaxis	Mild LAD type 1 features plus hh-blood group plus mental and growth retardation
Leukocyte adhesion deficiency type 3 (LAD3)	*KINDLIN3:* Rap1-activation of β1–3 integrins	AR	N + M + L + NK	Adherence, chemotaxis	LAD type 1 plus bleeding tendency
Rac 2 deficiency	*RAC2:* regulation of actin cytoskeleton	AD	N	Adherence, chemotaxis, O⁻ production	Poor wound healing, leukocytosis
X-linked chronic granulomatous disease (CGD)	*CYBB:* electron transport protein (gp91phox)	XL	N + M	Severe NADPH oxidase activity with decreased superoxide production, impaired pathogen killing by phagocytic cells.	Recurrent bacterial infection, susceptibility to fungal infection, inflammatory gut manifestations; McLeod phenotype in patients with deletions extending into the contiguous Kell locus
Autosomal recessive CGD – p22 phox deficiency	*CYBA:* electron transport protein (p22phox)	AR	N + M	Same as X-CGD	Recurrent bacterial infection, susceptibility to fungal infection, and inflammatory gut manifestations
Autosomal recessive CGD – p47 phox deficiency	*NCF1:* adapter protein (p47phox)	AR	N + M	Same as X-CGD	Recurrent bacterial infection, susceptibility to fungal infection, and inflammatory gut manifestations
Autosomal recessive CGD – p67 phox deficiency	*NCF2:* activating protein (p67phox)	AR	N + M	Same as X-CGD	Recurrent bacterial infection, susceptibility to fungal infection, and inflammatory gut manifestations
Autosomal recessive CGD – p40 phox deficiency	*NCF4:* activating protein (p40phox)	AR	N + M	Killing (faulty O⁻ production)	Inflammatory gut manifestations only
IL-12 and IL-23 receptor β1 chain deficiency	*IL-12RB1:* IL-12 and IL-23 receptor β1 chain	AR	L + NK	IFN-γ secretion	Susceptibility to *Mycobacteria* and *Salmonella*

Continued

TABLE 54.15   Phagocyte Disorders—cont'd

Disease	Genetic Defect/ Presumed Pathogenesis	Inheritance	Affected Cells	Affected Function	Associated Features
IL-12p40 deficiency	*IL-12B:* subunit p40 of IL-12/IL-23	AR	M	IFNγ secretion	Susceptibility to *Mycobacteria* and *Salmonella*
IFNγ receptor 1 deficiency	*IFNGR1:* IFNγR ligand binding chain	AR, AD	M + L	IFNγ binding and signaling	Susceptibility to *Mycobacteria* and *Salmonella*
IFNγ receptor 2 deficiency	*IFNGR2:* IFNγR accessory chain	AR	M + L	IFNγ signaling	Susceptibility to *Mycobacteria* and *Salmonella*
STAT1 deficiency (AD form)	*STAT1* (loss of function)	AD	M + L	IFNγ signaling	Susceptibility to *Mycobacteria*

AD, autosomal dominant; AR, autosomal recessive; B/T, B and T cells; IFN, interferon; IL, interleukin; L, lymphocyte; M, monocyte/macrophage; MDS, myelodysplasia syndrome; N, neutrophil; NK, natural killer cell; XL, X-linked.

A gain-of-function variant in the WAS protein has also been associated with an X-linked form of severe congenital neutropenia. Severe congenital neutropenia may be associated with SCID in reticular dysgenesis, a disorder of hematopoietic stem cells affecting all bone marrow lineages due to variants in the *AK2* gene.

The mainstay of treatment of all congenital neutropenias is recombinant human granulocyte colony-stimulating factor (rhG-CSF). Approximately 10% of patients with the diagnosis of severe congenital neutropenia and Shwachman-Diamond syndrome develop myelodysplasia/acute myelogenous leukemia. No cases of malignant transformations have been observed in patients with either cyclic or idiopathic neutropenia.

Acquired Neutropenia

Isoimmune neutropenia occurs in neonates as the result of transplacental transfer of maternal antibodies to fetal neutrophil antigens. The mother produces antibodies to specific neutrophil antigens on the surface of fetal leukocytes that are inherited from the father and are not present on maternal cells. Isoimmune neonatal neutropenia, similar to isoimmune anemia and thrombocytopenia, is a transient process that resolves as maternal antibodies wane. Cutaneous infections are common, and sepsis is rare. Early treatment of infection while the infant is neutropenic is the major goal of therapy. Intravenous immune globulin may decrease the duration of neutropenia. *Autoimmune neutropenia* usually develops in children 5–24 months of age. Neutrophil autoantibodies may be IgG, IgM, IgA, or a combination of these. Usually, the condition spontaneously resolves in 6 months to 4 years. Although intravenous immune globulin and corticosteroids have been used, most patients respond to G-CSF.

Disorders of Neutrophil Adhesion and Chemotaxis

Leukocyte adhesion deficiency type 1 (LAD-1) is an autosomal recessive inherited disorder resulting from variants in the gene encoding the β₂ integrin CD18. CD18 is the common β-subunit of lymphocyte function-associated antigen-1 (LFA-1) (CD11a/CD18), Mac-1 (CD11b/CD18), and P150,95 (CD11c/CD18), proteins that are expressed on lymphocytes, monocytes/macrophages, and neutrophils, respectively. Diminished or absent surface expression of these proteins accounts for a profound impairment of neutrophil and monocyte cell migration and phagocytosis. The severity of the immunodeficiency is dependent on the level of expression of CD18. Infants affected with this disorder may present in early infancy with failure of separation of the umbilical cord (often 2 months after birth) with attendant omphalitis and sepsis (see Table 54.11). Cutaneous, respiratory, gingival, and mucosal infections are common, and sepsis may lead to death in early childhood. Due to a failure of neutrophils to adhere normally to vascular endothelium (marginate), ANCs are usually >20,000/mm³ even when patients are not infected. The diagnosis of LAD-1 can be made measuring the amount of LFA-1 on the surface of lymphocytes by flow cytometry. Hematopoietic stem cell transplantation is curative.

Leukocyte adhesion deficiency type 2 (LAD-2) is an autosomal recessive congenital disorder of glycosylation (type iic) caused by variants in the *SLC35C1* gene. The *SLC35C1* gene encodes a GDP-fucose transporter, and variant in this gene results in the absence of sialylated Lewis X blood group on the surface of neutrophils and other leukocytes, resulting in failure to roll and subsequently adhere to vascular endothelium. Patients with LAD-2 manifest with growth retardation, dysmorphic features, and neurologic deficits in addition to the increased susceptibility to infection. LAD-3 is a rare disorder caused by defects in the KINDLIN-3 protein resulting in defective neutrophil adhesion as well as platelet defects. Patients with LAD-3 present similarly to those with LAD-1 with recurrent severe infections as well as a bleeding disorder.

Depressed neutrophil chemotaxis has been observed in a wide variety of clinical conditions (see Table 54.15). In addition to LAD-1 and LAD-2, defective migration of neutrophils has been described in hyper-IgE syndrome due to STAT3 variants and with variants in the *RAC2* gene (see Table 54.15). RAC2 is the predominant GTPase in human neutrophils, and it is integral to the function of the actin cytoskeleton. Deficiency in RAC2 is associated with decreased neutrophil chemotaxis, superoxide generation, and decreased degranulation in response to formylated peptides.

Disorders of Neutrophil Function

Chronic granulomatous disease (CGD) is a disorder of phagocytes due to variants in any one of the subunits of the enzyme NADPH oxidase (see Table 54.15). NADPH oxidase consists of five subunits (gp91ᵖʰᵒˣ, p22ᵖʰᵒˣ, p47ᵖʰᵒˣ, p67ᵖʰᵒˣ, and cytochrome B-245/Eros) and is responsible for the generation of the respiratory burst, which involves the catalytic conversion of molecular oxygen to superoxide (O_2^-) that is essential for the killing of a variety of bacterial and fungal pathogens by neutrophils and macrophages. Variants in the gene encoding the gp91ᵖʰᵒˣ protein are inherited in an X-linked manner and account for approximately 65% of CGD. All other forms of CGD are inherited in an autosomal recessive manner.

Although the clinical manifestations are variable, several clinical features suggest the diagnosis of CGD. The onset of clinical signs and symptoms may occur from early infancy to young adulthood, and the attack rate and severity of infections are dependent on the amount of residual oxidase activity generated by NADPH oxidase in affected individuals. Affected patients may have recurrent lymphadenitis, bacterial hepatic abscesses, or osteomyelitis. Infections also occur in the lungs, middle ear, gastrointestinal tract, skin, and urinary tract. Patients characteristically exhibit lymphadenopathy, hypergammaglobulinemia, hepatosplenomegaly, dermatitis, failure to thrive, anemia, chronic diarrhea, and abscesses. Granulomas are prominent and may obstruct the pylorus or ureters or lead to inflammatory bowel disease. The most common pathogen is *S. aureus*, and infection with *S. marcescens*, *B. cepacia*, *Aspergillus* sp., *C. albicans*, or *Salmonella* sp. can occur. The diagnosis of CGD is made by either the DHR test or the NBT dye test.

The treatment of CGD is rapidly evolving. CGD is traditionally treated with prophylactic trimethoprim-sulfamethoxazole, itraconazole, long-term continuous IFNγ therapy, and prompt treatment of acute infections. Steroids and antibiotics are used to treat granulomatous complications of the gastrointestinal, urinary, and respiratory tracts. Definitive treatment of CGD by HSCT in properly HLA-matched patients has achieved excellent outcomes (>90% survival) even for patients at high risk for transplant-associated morbidity and mortality.

DISORDERS OF MACROPHAGE FUNCTION

The IFNγ/IL-12 axis is crucial to host defense against intracellular pathogens, including mycobacteria, *Listeria*, and *Salmonella* species. Dendritic cells and macrophages produce IL-12 in response to bacterial pathogens that in turn stimulate the secretion of IFNγ by T cells and NK cells. IFNγ binds to receptors on macrophages, stimulating the production of TNF-α and inducible nitric oxide synthetase, promoting antigen presentation, and augmenting the respiratory burst and bactericidal activities of macrophages.

The classic members of this group of disorders involve variants in the IFNγ receptor, the IL-12 receptor, or IL-12. The IFNγ receptor contains two chains: IFNγ receptor 1 (IFNγ-R1), which binds ligand, and IFNγ receptor 2 (IFNγ-R2), which is necessary for ligand-induced signaling. Complete absence of IFNγ-R1 or IFNγ-R2 is inherited in an autosomal recessive manner and causes the most severe disease, manifesting early in infancy often with disseminated atypical mycobacterial infection, recurrent *Salmonella* infection, or fatal infection after BCG vaccination. Partial IFNγ-R1 or IFNγ-R2 defects typically have milder disease and present often in early childhood, but nonetheless with increased susceptibility to nontuberculous mycobacterial disease. Patients with partial IFNγ-R1 deficiency are especially prone to osteomyelitis due to atypical mycobacteria. Variants leading to a deficiency in the production of the p40 subunit of IL-12 or in the expression of the IL-12Rβ1 receptor are inherited in an autosomal recessive manner. These patients have an increased susceptibility to serious infection with environmental mycobacteria, BCG, and *Salmonella* sp. Unexpectedly, these patients are also susceptible to skin and, rarely, invasive infections with *C. albicans*. Variants in STAT1, which mediates the signal transduction following the binding of IFNγ with the IFNγ receptor, also causes susceptibility to mycobacterial infections and is inherited in an autosomal recessive pattern. In addition, these patients are susceptible to a variety of viral pathogens since STAT1 is required for signal transduction of IFNα/β in addition to IFNγ.

IMMUNE DISREGULATION SYNDROMES

Immune disregulation disorders are genetic defects in the regulation of the adaptive immune system (T and B cells) resulting in early-onset inflammatory bowel disease, eczema, autoimmune cytopenias, and other autoimmune or inflammatory complications. Abnormalities of immune regulation are frequently important components of the clinical manifestations in patients with primary immune deficiencies, which have been described previously in this chapter. Unlike autoinflammatory disorders, these disorders are not episodic and are associated with autoimmune manifestations. Additionally, the clinical phenotype includes varying degrees of susceptibility to infection.

Hemophagocytic Lymphohistiocytosis

Hemophagocytic lymphohistiocytosis (HLH) is caused by variants in the gene encoding perforin or genes encoding other proteins involved in the cytotoxic function of NK cells and CD8 cells, such as Munc13-4, syntaxin11, and syntaxin11 binding protein (Table 54.16).

TABLE 54.16 Disorders of Immune Regulation

Disease	Genetic Defect	Inheritance	Affected cells	Functional Defect	Associated Features
Perforin deficiency (FHL2)	*PRF1*; perforin induces pores in target cell membrane	AR	CTL and NK cells	Decreased to absent NK and CTL cytotoxicity, normal degranulation	Fever, hepatosplenomegaly (HSMG), hemophagocytic lymphohistiocytosis (HLH), cytopenias
UNC13D/Munc13-4 deficiency (FHL3)	*UNC13D*; required to prime vesicles for fusion	AR	CTL and NK cells	Decreased to absent NK and CTL cytotoxicity, abnormal degranulation	Fever, HSMG, HLH, cytopenias
Syntaxin 11 deficiency (FHL4)	*STX11*, required for secretory vesicle fusion with the cell membrane	AR	CTL and NK cells	Decreased to absent NK and CTL cytotoxicity, abnormal degranulation	Fever, HSMG, HLH, cytopenias
STXBP2/Munc18-2 deficiency (FHL5)	*STXBP2*, required for secretory vesicle fusion with the cell membrane	AR	CTL and NK cells	Decreased to absent NK and CTL cytotoxicity, abnormal degranulation	Fever, HSMG, HLH, cytopenias
Chédiak-Higashi syndrome	*LYST*, impaired lysosomal trafficking	AR	CTL and NK cells, others	Decreased to absent NK and CTL cytotoxicity, abnormal degranulation	Partial albinism, recurrent infections, fever, HSMG, HLH, giant lysosomes, neutropenia, cytopenias, bleeding tendency, progressive neurologic dysfunction

Continued

TABLE 54.16 Disorders of Immune Regulation—cont'd

Disease	Genetic Defect	Inheritance	Affected cells	Functional Defect	Associated Features
Griscelli syndrome, type 2	RAB27A encoding a GTPase that promotes docking of secretory vesicles to the cell membrane	AR	CTL and NK cells, others	Decreased to absent NK and CTL cytotoxicity, abnormal degranulation	Partial albinism, fever, HSMG, HLH, cytopenias
SH2D1A deficiency (XLP1)	SH2D1A encoding an adaptor protein regulating intracellular signaling	XL	CTL and NK cells, others	Partially defective NK-cell and CTL cytotoxic activity	Clinical and immunologic features triggered by EBV infection: HLH, lymphoproliferation, aplastic anemia, lymphoma, hypogammaglobulinemia, absent iNK T cells
XIAP deficiency (XLP2)	XIAP encoding an inhibitor of apoptosis	XL	Many	Increased T-cell susceptibility to apoptosis to CD95 and enhanced activation-induced cell death (AICD)	EBV infection, splenomegaly, lymphoproliferation, HLH, colitis, IBD, hepatitis, low iNK T cells
IPEX, immune disregulation, polyendocrinopathy, enteropathy, X-linked	FOXP3, encoding a T-cell transcription factor	XL	T-regulatory cells	Lack of (and/or impaired function of) CD4+ CD25+ FOXP3+ regulatory T cells (Tregs)	Autoimmune enteropathy, early-onset diabetes, thyroiditis, hemolytic anemia, thrombocytopenia, eczema, elevated IgE, IgA
CD25 deficiency	IL2RA, encoding IL-2Rα chain	AR	T cells, T-regulatory cells	No CD4+ C25+ cells with impaired function of Tregs, absent in vitro proliferative responses	Lymphoproliferation, autoimmunity; impaired T-cell proliferation
STAT5b deficiency	STAT5B, signal transducer, and transcription factor, essential for normal signaling from IL-2 and IL-15, key growth factors for T and NK cells	AR	Many	Impaired development and function of γδ T cells, Tregs, and NK cells, low T-cell proliferation	Growth hormone–insensitive dwarfism, dysmorphic features, eczema, lymphocytic interstitial pneumonitis, autoimmunity
LRBA deficiency	LRBA (lipopolysaccharide-responsive beigelike anchor protein)	AR	T cells, T-regulatory cells	Decreased CTLA4 cell surface expression	Recurrent infections, hypogammaglobulinemia, inflammatory bowel disease, autoimmunity; EBV infections
CTLA4	Variants or deletions in CLTA4	AD	T cells, T-regulatory cells	Decreased CTLA4 cell surface expression	Recurrent infections, autoimmune cytopenias, hypogammaglobulinemia, lung disease, brain inflammation
APECED (APS-1), autoimmune polyendocrinopathy with candidiasis and ectodermal dystrophy	AIRE, encoding a transcription regulator needed to establish thymic self-tolerance	AR	T cells, T-regulatory cells	AIRE/1 serves as checkpoint in the thymus for negative selection of autoreactive T cells and for generation of Tregs	Autoimmunity: hypoparathyroidism, hypothyroidism, adrenal insufficiency, diabetes, gonadal dysfunction, and other endocrine abnormalities; chronic mucocutaneous candidiasis, dental enamel hypoplasia, alopecia areata, enteropathy, pernicious anemia
ALPS-FAS	TNFRSF6, encoding CD95/Fas cell surface apoptosis receptor	AR		Apoptosis defect FAS mediated, increased CD4− CD8− TCRα/β double-negative (DN) T cells	Splenomegaly, adenopathies, autoimmune cytopenias, increased lymphoma risk, IgG and IgA normal or increased, elevated FasL and IL-10, vitamin B$_{12}$
ALPS-FASLG	TNFSF6, Fas ligand for CD95 apoptosis	AR	Lymphocytes	Apoptosis defect FAS mediated, increased DN T cells	Splenomegaly, adenopathies, autoimmune cytopenias, SLE; soluble FasL is not elevated
ALPS–caspase 10	CASP10, intracellular apoptosis pathway	AD	Lymphocytes	Defective lymphocyte apoptosis, increased DN T cells	Adenopathies, splenomegaly, autoimmunity

TABLE 54.16 Disorders of Immune Regulation—cont'd

Disease	Genetic Defect	Inheritance	Affected cells	Functional Defect	Associated Features
ALPS–caspase 8	*CASP8*, intracellular apoptosis, and activation pathways	AR	Lymphocytes	Defective lymphocyte apoptosis and activation, increased DN T cells	Adenopathies, splenomegaly, bacterial and viral infections, hypogammaglobulinemia
FADD deficiency	*FADD* encoding an adaptor molecule interacting with FAS, and promoting apoptosis	AR	Lymphocytes	Defective lymphocyte apoptosis, increased DN T cells	Functional hyposplenism, bacterial and viral infections, recurrent episodes of encephalopathy and liver dysfunction
Early-onset inflammatory bowel disease	Variants in *IL-10* (results in increase of many proinflammatory cytokines)	AR	Monocyte/ macrophage, activated T cells	IL-10 deficiency leads to increase of TNFγ and other proinflammatory cytokines	Enterocolitis, enteric fistulas, perianal abscesses, chronic folliculitis
Early-onset inflammatory bowel disease	*IL-10RA* (see above)	AR	Monocyte/ macrophage, activated T cells	Variants in IL-10 receptor alpha leads to increase of TNFγ and other proinflammatory cytokines	Enterocolitis, enteric fistulas, perianal abscesses, chronic folliculitis
Early-onset inflammatory bowel disease	*IL-10RB* (see above)	AR	Monocyte/ macrophage, activated T cells	Variants in IL-10 receptor beta leads to increase of TNFα and other proinflammatory cytokines	Enterocolitis, enteric fistulas, perianal abscesses, chronic folliculitis

AD, autosomal dominant; AR, autosomal recessive; CTL, cytotoxic T lymphocyte; EBV, Epstein-Barr virus; IBD, inflammatory bowel disease; Ig, immunoglobulin; IL, interleukin; iNK, invariant natural killer; NK, natural killer cell; SLE, systemic lupus erythematosus; TCR, T-cell receptor; TNF, tumor necrosis factor; XL, X-linked.

HLH is a life-threatening disorder of infants and is characterized by high fever, rash, hyperferritinemia, coagulopathy, and hematologic cytopenias. HLH is typically triggered in response to viral infections, in particular EBV and CMV. The various molecular defects that underlie HLH all result in ineffective clearance of viral infections by NK cells and CD8 T cells, resulting in prolonged antigen exposure and protracted activation of CD8 T cells and NK cells. CD8 T cells and NK cells produce large amounts of IFNγ that activate macrophages, resulting in phagocytosis of bone marrow elements and end-organ damage. This disorder is fatal if not treated aggressively with combined immunosuppressive medications and chemotherapy. HSCT is the only curative treatment.

Chédiak-Higashi syndrome (CHS), an abnormality of secondary granules, is an autosomal recessive disorder caused by a variant in the *LYST* gene, which encodes a cytoplasmic protein thought to be involved in organellar protein trafficking resulting in fusion of the primary and secondary granules in neutrophils. Despite normal ingestion of particles and normal production of superoxide, neutrophils and macrophages in patients with CHS have delayed killing of microorganisms. Large azurophilic lysosomal granules are present in all granule-bearing cells including neutrophils and melanocytes. A smear of peripheral blood can demonstrate these giant granules in neutrophils, which are virtually pathognomonic of CHS when other features are present.

Recurrent infections affect the skin, respiratory tract, and mucous membranes and are caused by both gram-positive and gram-negative bacteria as well as by fungi. *S. aureus* is the most common organism. Despite normal platelet counts, patients with CHS have prolonged bleeding times due to a platelet storage pool abnormality. Patients usually have partial oculocutaneous albinism. Most patients progress to an accelerated phase associated with EBV infection and characterized by a lymphoproliferative syndrome with generalized lymphohistiocytic infiltrates, fever, jaundice, hepatomegaly, lymphadenopathy, and pancytopenia (see Table 54.16). Neuropathy, which can be sensory or motor, and ataxia may be present.

X-Linked Lymphoproliferative Disease Type 1 and Type 2

X-linked lymphoproliferative disease type 1 (XLP-1) is caused by a variant in the gene called *SH2D1A*, which encodes for an adapter protein involved in signal transduction of T cells and NK cells. XLP-2 is a similar disorder caused by variants in *XIAP*. XLP-1 is characterized by fulminant infection with EBV with immunodisregulation and/or lymphoma. Boys with this disease may be relatively normal until infected with EBV, which is acutely fatal in 80% of patients and due to the development of HLH. Boys who survive the initial EBV infection develop hypogammaglobulinemia and are at high risk for developing aplastic anemia and B-cell lymphomas. XLP-2 presents similarly with HLH following EBV infection but can also present with early-onset colitis. Definitive therapy of both forms of XLP is HSCT.

Immune Disregulation, Polyendocrinopathy, Enteropathy, X-Linked and Related Disorders

The maintenance of peripheral tolerance is critically dependent on T-regulatory cells, CD4+ T cells that prevent autoimmunity and excessive immune responses. These cells are generated in the thymus to self-antigens, express the transcription factor Foxp3, and constitutively express high levels of the IL-2 receptor (CD25). T-regulatory cells express numerous immunosuppressive molecules including cytotoxic T-lymphocyte antigen 4 (CTLA4), which inhibits T-cell activation, and IL-10 and transforming growth factor-β (TGF-β).

Immune disregulation, polyendocrinopathy, enteropathy, X-linked (IPEX) is caused by variants in the *FOXP3* gene, an X-linked transcription factor essential for the production and function of T-regulatory cells (see Table 54.16). In males with a null variant in FOXP3, the clinical manifestations begin at birth or soon thereafter, and consist of inflammatory gastrointestinal tract disease, failure to thrive, autoimmune diabetes mellitus, thyroiditis, Addison disease, severe food allergies, eczema, and autoimmune cytopenias. Hypomorphic variants in Foxp3 that encode a protein with residual functional activity lead to a later onset and milder clinical phenotype, but allergic disease and failure to thrive are common.

Patients with this disorder are aggressively immunosuppressed to be stabilized, but bone marrow transplantation is the only curative therapy.

CD25 Deficiency

CD25 (α chain of the high-affinity IL-2 receptor) deficiency is an autosomal recessive disorder due to variants in the *IL2RA* gene (see Table 54.16). T-regulatory cells constitutively express CD25 and respond to IL-2 generated by T cells during an immune response for their immunoregulatory functions. CD25 deficiency results in a syndrome similar to IPEX with severe enteropathy, diabetes mellitus, autoimmune hemolytic anemia, eczema, and lymphoproliferation. Importantly, patients with CD25 deficiency exhibit several unique features not seen in IPEX, namely chronic herpetic viral infections (e.g., CMV, EBV) and an increased susceptibility to infections.

Signal Transducer and Activator of Transcription Protein 5B Deficiency

STAT5b deficiency is an autosomal recessive disorder due to variants in the STAT5b gene, one of two STAT5 proteins involved in IL-2 signaling (see Table 54.16). Similar to CD25 deficiency, STAT5b deficiency results in T-regulatory cell dysfunction leading to a syndrome of immune deficiency with autoimmunity. These infants also suffer from autoimmune diseases such as autoimmune thrombocytopenia and hemolytic anemia, eczema, and arthritis. Unlike IPEX or CD25 deficiency, growth failure occurs in STAT5b since this signaling protein is required for growth hormone signaling. Additionally, patients with STAT5b deficiency also develop pulmonary disease that pathologically resembles interstitial lymphocytic pneumonia, although whether this represents an autoimmune phenomenon or a response to infectious episodes is unclear.

Cytotoxic T-Lymphocyte Antigen 4 Deficiency

CTLA4 deficiency is an autosomal dominant inherited disorder due to variants of the gene encoding for the CTLA4 protein (see Table 54.16). Not all patients who have damaging variants in CTLA4 develop a clinical phenotype (i.e., reduced penetrance), and the onset of the disease and clinical manifestations are variable (variable expressivity). The clinical manifestations of CTLA4 deficiency may occur in early childhood or adulthood. The most common clinical manifestations include enteropathy; granulomatous and lymphocytic lung infiltration; lymphocytic infiltration of the bone marrow, brain, kidney, or liver; respiratory tract infections; splenomegaly; lymphadenopathy; and immune cytopenias. Patients frequently have hypogammaglobulinemia, which explains their propensity to infection, and may appear to have CVID at presentation. Autoimmune thyroiditis and psoriasis also

occur. Treatment of CTLA4 deficiency includes the use of replacement immunoglobulin therapy for patients with hypogammaglobulinemia and recombinant CTLA4 for the autoimmune manifestations.

A phenotypically similar disorder is caused by variants in the lipopolysaccharide-responsive vesicle trafficking, beach and anchor containing *(LRBA)* gene, which regulates the expression of CTLA4 on the surface of T cells. CTLA4 is essential for the function of T-regulatory cells, which explains the common autoimmune and autoinflammatory features of both LRBA deficiency and CTLA4 deficiency. HSCT is increasingly being performed with good outcomes if performed early, prior to end-organ damage.

Autoimmune Polyendocrinopathy–Candidiasis–Ectodermal Dystrophy

Autoimmune polyendocrinopathy–candidiasis–ectodermal dystrophy (APECED) is an autosomal recessive disorder caused by variants in the gene encoding the autoimmune regulator *(AIRE)* gene (see Table 54.16). *AIRE* is a transcription factor that is essential for expression of peripheral tissue antigens in the thymus, allowing for deletion of self-reactive T cells in the thymus (i.e., negative selection) and for the production of T-regulatory cells with the correct antigen specificity. The clinical manifestation of APECED includes chronic or recurrent *Candida* infections of the mucous membranes, skin, and nails; autoimmune hypoparathyroidism; and Addison disease. Other autoimmune disorders, such as vitiligo, thyroiditis, and pernicious anemia, may occur. The insidious and variable onset of the endocrinopathies requires the need for frequent evaluation for autoimmune endocrine disorders. The propensity to develop fungal infections is explained by autoantibodies to certain immune cytokines, such as IL-17, that are critical to the defense of fungal infections.

Autoimmune Lymphoproliferation Syndrome

Autoimmune lymphoproliferation syndrome (ALPS) is a group of disorders most commonly caused by variants in the *FAS* gene or less commonly the FAS ligand *(FASL)* gene (see Table 54.16). Other genetic causes of ALPS have been described. FAS is a protein that is involved in the normal apoptotic pathway of lymphocytes, and defective apoptosis due to defects in FAS or FASL underlies the autoimmune manifestations of this disorder. The clinical manifestations of ALPS include lymphoproliferation (i.e., splenomegaly and lymphadenopathy) and autoimmune manifestations, particularly autoimmune thrombocytopenia and autoimmune hemolytic anemia, and an increased susceptibility to lymphoma. Autoimmune manifestations are usually responsive to immunosuppressive medication.

▉ SUMMARY AND RED FLAGS

Fevers and recurrent *benign* infections are common, especially in large families or in daycare settings, in which children may manifest 6–10 URIs or gastroenteritis episodes a year. These infections usually last <1 week. The child continues to grow and develop normally and their activities are not restricted. Screening tests to evaluate immune function are typically normal. Red flags to consider disorders of the immune system include absent lymphoid tissue, failure to thrive,

digital clubbing, chronic diarrhea, prolonged infections, infections with unusual organisms, repeated serious infections, bronchiectasis, eczematous dermatitis, a family history of early childhood deaths (presumably from infection), and other diseases associated with increased risks for infection (sickle cell anemia, malignancy, asplenia). In these cases, immunologic work-up, genetic testing, and consultation with a clinical immunologist can lead to a diagnosis and definitive treatment.

BIBLIOGRAPHY

A bibliography is available at ExpertConsult.com.

Disorders of Puberty

Peter M. Wolfgram and Bethany Auble

Puberty is defined by both biologic and social standards. Puberty is the time when there is an increase in sex steroid production, resulting in physical changes such as breast development in females and testicular enlargement in males, as well as maturation of processes required for future fertility. Puberty, also known as adolescence, is the time when children make the transition to adult patterns of behavior, which involve maturity, responsibility, and sexuality.

NORMAL PUBERTAL DEVELOPMENT

Terminology

Various terms are used to discuss puberty (Table 55.1). **Bone age** refers to the degree of epiphyseal calcification, width, and proximity to adjacent metaphyses and is a marker of physical maturity that normally corresponds to chronologic age. **Dental age** generally correlates with bone age. Bone age is derived by comparing a radiograph of the left hand and wrist to gender-appropriate standards in Greulich and Pyle's bone age atlas. In infants and toddlers, a more accurate assessment of bone age can be determined from a radiograph of the hemi-skeleton, with primary attention to epiphyses of the long bones. Delayed or advanced bone age occurs in many conditions; bone age is strongly influenced by sex steroid production. The timing of the onset of puberty is usually more closely linked to the bone age than to the chronologic age when the two are significantly discordant. Regardless of chronologic age, linear growth ceases when the bone age reaches 15 years in females and 18 years in males.

Anatomy

Puberty is controlled by the production of gonadotropin-releasing hormone (GnRH) in the anterior hypothalamus. GnRH-containing cell bodies project axons to the median eminence, where they terminate on the hypothalamic portal vessels. This system is referred to as the **GnRH pulse generator**. After GnRH reaches the anterior pituitary gland via the portal vasculature, it stimulates the production of both follicle-stimulating hormone (FSH) and luteinizing hormone (LH) by the gonadotroph cells. In females, both FSH and LH are required for estrogen production by ovarian granulosa cells. The regulated secretion of FSH and LH is also required for follicle growth, ovulation, and maintenance of the corpus luteum. In males, FSH regulates spermatogenesis by Sertoli cells within the seminiferous tubules, and LH activates Leydig cells to produce testosterone (Fig. 55.1). Androgens cause development of male internal and external reproductive organs and secondary sexual characteristics in both sexes by binding to receptor

proteins in the cells of target tissues. Sex steroids also exert a negative feedback effect on the pituitary gland and hypothalamus.

Physiology

Perinatal Period and Infancy

Maternal estrogens stimulate breast development in both male and female fetuses. Maternal estrogens also stimulate uterine developmental and endometrial growth; at birth, withdrawal of the high levels of maternal estrogen and placental progesterone causes the infant endometrium to regress or even slough and manifests as vaginal bleeding.

At birth, levels of LH and FSH in both sexes rise markedly and remain elevated for several months. In the female, FSH stimulates ovarian granulosa cells to produce 17β-estradiol sufficient to maintain prenatal breast development for up to 8 months of life. Estrogen-induced vaginal cornification is generally evident as abundant vaginal discharge at birth and is maintained as long as estrogens are produced. Ovarian size from birth to 3 months ranges from 0.7 to 3.6 cm^3, decreasing to 2.7 cm^3 by 12 months and to 1.7 cm^3 by 24 months; this size persists until the onset of puberty. Ultrasound studies of the ovaries in normal infants show many microcysts.

Male breast development regresses rather quickly after birth. Elevated LH levels after birth stimulate Leydig cell production of testosterone for 6–12 months, leading to further genital development. Penis length increases from 3–5 cm in the full-term newborn to 4.5–6 cm by 2–3 years.

Childhood

By 2 years of age, serum gonadotropin levels decrease, and thus serum sex steroid levels also decrease, frequently to levels undetectable by conventional assays.

Beginning approximately at ages 6–7 years in females and 7–8 years in males, adrenal androgen production begins to increase and can be detected by the presence of increasing concentrations of the weak adrenal androgen dehydroepiandrosterone (DHEA) and its sulfated derivative, DHEA sulfate (DHEAS). Despite these serum levels, there is initially no secondary sexual (pubic or axillary) hair development.

Adolescence

Beginning on average at about 10.5 years in females and 11.5 years in males, there is the return of activity of the hypothalamic GnRH pulse generator, leading to increased serum levels of FSH and LH. The kiss-peptin (*KISS1* gene)/G-protein-coupled receptor (GPR54) (also called KISS1 receptor) system stimulates the GnRH neurons and is involved in the feedback regulation of the hypothalamic-pituitary-gonadal axis by gonadal steroids. The trigger mechanism for this resurgence is unknown, but it may be linked to attainment of a critical body mass or fat mass. Leptin, a hormone produced by fat cells, may be the connection between weight (fat mass) and pubertal events. In early puberty, the activity of the hypothalamic GnRH pulse generator is mostly

TABLE 55.1   Puberty Terminology

Gonadarche: maturation of the gonads under the control of the hypothalamus (GnRH) and pituitary gland (FSH and LH)

Thelarche: presence of breast development in girls

Gynecomastia: presence of breast development in boys

Adrenarche or development of androgen-regulated pubarche: secondary sexual characteristics, including pubic hair, axillary hair, apocrine (underarm) odor, and acne, in both sexes

Menarche: time of the first menstrual period

Spermarche: time when a boy is first able to produce sperm

FSH, follicle-stimulating hormone; GnRH, gonadotropin-releasing hormone; LH, luteinizing hormone.

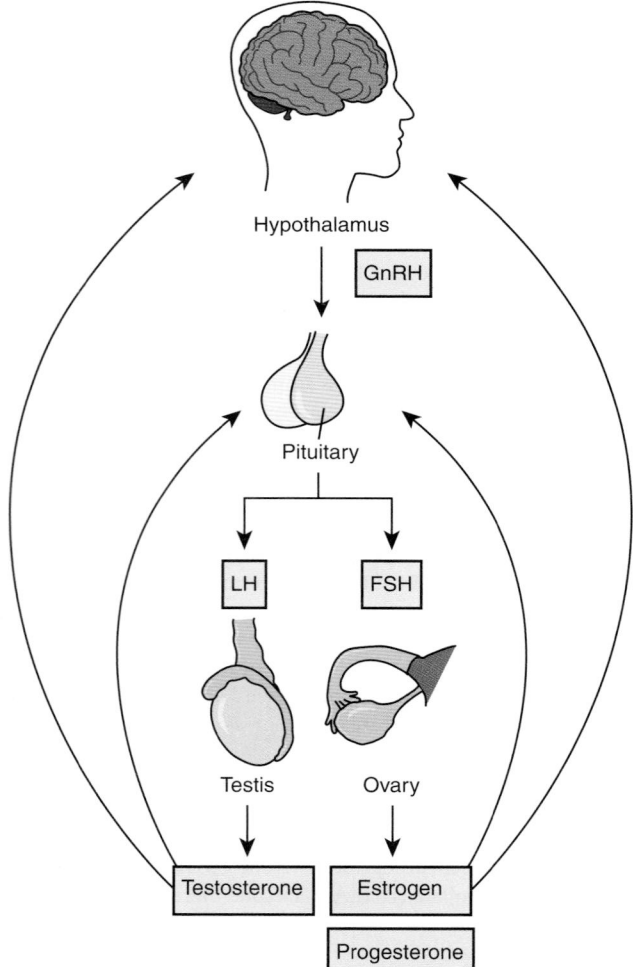

Fig. 55.1 Normal hypothalamic-pituitary-gonadal axis. FSH, follicle-stimulating hormone; GnRH, gonadotropin-releasing hormone; LH, luteinizing hormone. (Courtesy of Sex Development: Genetics and Biology: An initiative of the Research Program in Disorders of Sex Development, funded by the NHMRC Australia. http://www.dsdgenetics.org/index.php?id=48.)

evident overnight (sleep-entrained), with pulses increasing in number and amplitude and eventually occurring every 60–90 minutes. Over time, this process begins to occur during the daytime; there is always greater gonadotropin secretion at night. Because of the longer half-life of sex steroids, serum levels of estradiol and testosterone show little, if any, diurnal variation. Testosterone levels may be slightly higher in the morning with advancing puberty. There is central sensitivity to the negative feedback effects of sex steroids, leading to significant elevations of gonadotropins when sex steroid production is impaired. The function of the hypothalamic GnRH pulse generator can be accelerated in the setting of obesity, and LH and FSH secretion can revert to the prepubertal pattern in the setting of significant weight loss, as occurs in females with anorexia nervosa.

Usually within 6 months of the onset of this heightened GnRH pulse generator activity in females, there is also increasing production of androgens by the adrenal glands, the major source of androgens in females. In males, the testes are the main source of androgens, although male adrenarche also begins about 6 months after gonadarche.

Sex Steroid Effects

In response to FSH, both testes and ovaries enlarge, starting gonadarche. Ovarian granulosa cells produce 17β-estradiol, which causes estrogen effects that generally occur in a fixed order (Table 55.2). Growth increase is one of the early effects of estrogen. Growth is stimulated by estrogen-stimulated increased production of growth hormone and insulin-like growth factor 1. Estrogens along with growth hormone and thyroid hormones increase bone mineralization and growth.

In response to LH, testicular Leydig cells produce testosterone, which is converted to dihydrotestosterone (DHT), leading to androgen effects that generally occur in the same order (Table 55.3).

Note that growth is not stimulated early in puberty by rising testosterone; in fact, during the phase when testosterone levels are beginning to rise, growth is usually slowed perceptibly from a prepubertal height velocity of perhaps 5 cm/yr to a velocity as slow as 4 cm/yr for 12–18 months. As levels of testosterone increase closer to 400 ng/dL and testis volume increases to between 10 and 12 mL, males make the transition to rapid growth. Rapid growth for males thus occurs for about 2 years in middle puberty, and slower growth continues for 2–3 more years.

TABLE 55.2   Estrogen Effects

Vaginal and urethral cornification

Breast development, often asymmetric

Linear growth

Fat development

Uterine development

Menarche: 2–2.5 yr after breast buds

TABLE 55.3   Androgen Effects

Psychologic changes

Skin and hair oils, sweat odors

Areolar growth and pigment

Sexual skin pigment and folding

Phallic growth

Voice change

Sexual hair growth

Hairline recession

Statural growth

Muscle mass/strength

Benign adolescent gynecomastia occurs in as many as 40–60% of normal males; enough estrogen relative to the amount of testosterone is produced so that breast development occurs. Gynecomastia usually starts in early to middle puberty (peak age, 13 years), before adult male concentrations of testosterone are achieved. It typically starts on one side and resolves within 2 years. Gynecomastia is more common in obese males, although true breast tissue in this setting is often difficult to distinguish from fat tissue (lipomastia).

Chronology of Puberty

Females

Females begin puberty at an average age of 10.5 years (range, 8–13 years; mean ± 2.5 standard deviations [SD]). There are data suggesting that female puberty begins at an earlier age and that African-American females begin puberty about 1 year earlier than White females, but this is not universally accepted. In 85% of females, the first clinically detectable sign of puberty is breast development (**thelarche**), although ovarian enlargement, which is not clinically detectable in a strict sense, occurs first. Breast buds appear as small nodules either directly underneath the nipples or slightly off center, causing the areolae and nipples to be pushed out and sometimes cause minor, transient discomfort or itching as the skin around the nipple is stretched. Breast development may be unilateral and asymmetric in its earliest stages. Pubic hair usually begins to develop within the next 6 months; in approximately 15% of females, pubic hair precedes breast development. Such discordance has no clinical significance. The female adolescent growth spurt commences near the onset of thelarche, generally spanning a 2-year period between the ages of 11 and 13 years. Axillary hair generally begins, on average, between 12 and 13 years. Menarche, a rather late event in female puberty, occurs on average between 12.2 and 12.8 years, typically 2–2.5 years following thelarche. Menarche is often preceded by a whitish, non–foul-smelling vaginal discharge (physiologic leukorrhea) for up to 6 months. At the time of menarche, an adolescent female has reached 96.5% of her adult height potential. However, more linear growth may remain in clinical situations in which menarche occurs at a younger bone age than is typical for the average adolescent female. Menstrual cycles for the first 2 years after menarche are often anovulatory and irregular in frequency.

Males

Males begin puberty at an average age of 11.5 years (range, 9–14 years; mean ± 2.5 SD). The first clinically detectable sign of puberty is testicular enlargement, a fact generally unknown to patients and their parents. From birth to the start of puberty, male testicular volumes range between 1 and 2 mL as determined by using an orchidometer, a series of ellipsoid models of varying volumes (Fig. 55.2). Stretched penile length (measured with a rigid tape measure on the dorsum of the penis from the pubic symphysis to the tip of the nonerect penis without considering any foreskin tissue) averages about 3.5 cm (range, 2.8–4.2 cm) at birth and grows by an average of 2.5 cm until the start of puberty. The onset of male puberty is considered to have begun when at least one of the two testicles reaches 4 mL in volume. It takes approximately 5–6 years for the testicles to reach the average adult volume of 18 mL. Approximately 75–80% of the adult testicle consists of seminiferous tubules; testosterone-producing Leydig cells make up the remainder.

Within 6 months after the start of testicular enlargement, pubic hair can be found; pubic hair precedes testicular enlargement in approximately 15%. The presence of pubic hair is incorrectly considered the first evidence of puberty in males by both patients and parents. Pubic hair is followed by the development of axillary hair at approximately 14 years of age. During this time, penile enlargement also occurs, reaching a mean adult length of 12.4 ± 1.6 cm at 20 years of age. The male adolescent growth spurt typically occurs between the ages of 13 and 15 years, commencing when the testicular volumes reach 12 mL. By age 15 years, a male has attained 98% of his final adult height. The ability of adolescent males to produce sperm, as evidenced by detection of spermatozoa in urine samples, begins between 13.5 and 15 years.

Clinical Staging of Puberty

Standardized staging of pubertal development in both sexes allows for comparison between children, as well as longitudinal monitoring of individual children (Fig. 55.3).

Breast development in females, genitalia in males, and pubic hair in both sexes are scored according to five-stage systems referred to as Tanner stages 1–5. Axillary hair in both sexes is rated by a three-stage system referred to as stages 1–3. Puberty itself is not staged because different components of puberty may occur at different stages.

Females

For breast development, Tanner stage 1 refers to no breast development; Tanner stage 2, to the presence of just breast buds (one or two); Tanner stage 3, to the beginning of formation of the peripheral mound with elevation of the breast; Tanner stage 4, to a further increase in breast size, with the formation of the so-called "double contour," in which the areola and papilla are both raised off the surface of the whole breast; and Tanner stage 5, to adult size, with a return to the single contour in which the surface of the areola is again flush with that of the breast. It may be difficult to differentiate between Tanner stages 3 and 5 because the only difference between these two stages is breast size (determined mostly by fat content). Thus, small breasts, especially in an older adolescent female, should not necessarily be construed as Tanner stage 3, especially if she has already menstruated, which typically occurs when the breasts have reached Tanner stage 4 and/or if women in the family typically have small breasts.

Males

For external genitalia, Tanner stage 1 refers to the prepubertal state (testes <4 mL in volume); Tanner stage 2, to slight enlargement of the testes and scrotum; Tanner stage 3, to lengthening of the penis and further

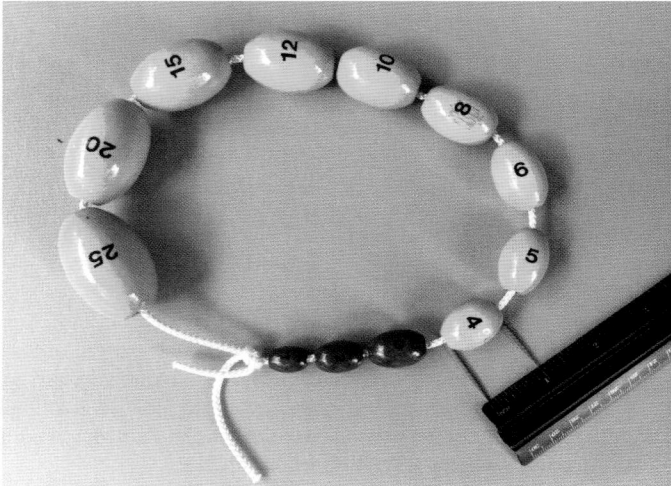

Fig. 55.2 Prader orchidometer is a series of plastic or wooden ovoid-shaped pieces attached by a string representing different testicular volumes (1 mL, 2 mL, 3 mL, 4 mL, 5 mL, 6 mL, 8 mL, 10 mL, 12 mL, 15 mL, 20 mL, and 25 mL). (From Zitelli BJ, McIntire, SC, Nowalk AJ, eds. *Zitelli and Davis' Atlas of Pediatric Physical Diagnosis.* 7th ed. Philadelphia: Elsevier; 2018:348, Fig. 9.5.)

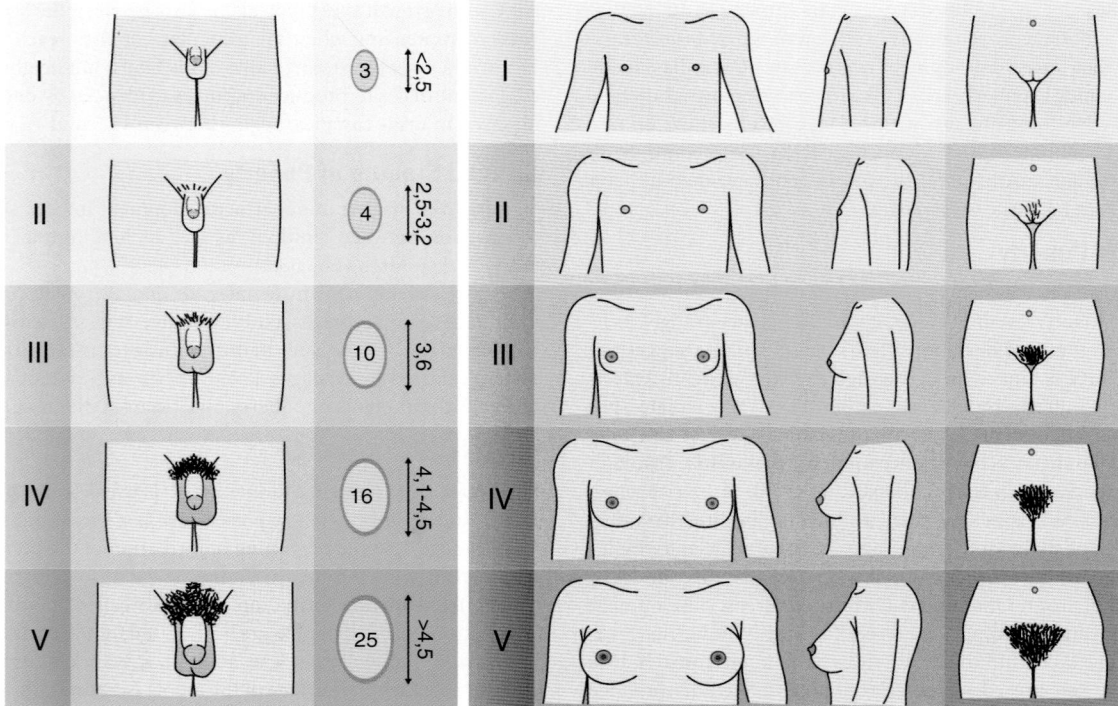

Fig. 55.3 Tanner stages. (Illustrations by Michał Komorniczak.)

enlargement of the testes and scrotum; Tanner stage 4, to continued penile growth in both length and width with development of the glans; and Tanner stage 5, to adult appearance. An alternative, simplified, and equally accurate approach involves only sizing of the testicles, whereby 4 mL represents the start of puberty, 12 mL correlates with the start of the growth spurt, and 18 mL is the average adult size. In some cases, the appearance of pubic hair does not occur until the testicular volumes reach 12–15 mL. Testicular volumes may differ at all stages between sides but not usually by more than one size on a standard orchidometer. It is important not to confuse a hydrocele with an enlarged testis.

Females and Males

Tanner staging of pubic hair is similar in both sexes. Tanner stage 1 is defined by having no pubic hair. Tanner stage 2 is characterized by the presence of a few, countable strands of curly, coarse, pigmented hair along the labia minora in females or at the base of the penis and/or on the scrotum in males. Lighter and softer hair (lanugo) in the pubic region is not pubic hair. On occasion, especially in individuals from ethnic populations from Mediterranean countries or Northern India, there may be an extension of coarse body hair (hypertrichosis) to the pubic region that can be difficult to discern from pubic hair. Tanner stage 3 refers to the presence of coarser, darker, and curlier hairs, the number of which is no longer countable, which have spread more laterally. Tanner stage 4 refers to a thick, fully triangular pattern of hair growth, without spread to the thighs. Finally, Tanner stage 5 refers to the adult pattern in which there is spread of hair to the medial thighs. The designation Tanner stage 6 is used to describe hair growing up the linea alba, referring to the so-called male escutcheon.

Axillary hair is the simplest component of puberty to quantify. Stage 1 refers to the absence of any hair. Stage 2 refers to a countable number of curly, coarse, pigmented strands in at least one armpit. Stage 3 refers to the adult complement, which is merely more hair than is present in stage 2. For the individual with shaved axillae, it is safe to assume either stage 2 or stage 3 hair is present.

Family Patterns

The timing of puberty is affected by familial patterns; both parents' histories are important in assessing the child with early or late puberty. The following information is useful for establishing the parental effect:

- Age of their mother's menarche
- Age their father began shaving on a daily basis
- Age when their parents stopped growing

PRECOCIOUS PUBERTY

Definition

The onset of puberty, at least in females, may be occurring earlier than in the past; therefore, the definition of precocious puberty has been modified to refer to the appearance of any feature of puberty before 8 years of age in females and before 9 years of age in males. Some experts would argue that the definition of precocious puberty in African-American and Hispanic females would be younger than 7 years, but the strict definition remains younger than 8 years. The family pattern must also be considered; an early onset of puberty is frequently familial.

Normal Variants

Idiopathic Isolated Premature Thelarche

This common condition is the development of breast tissue in females before 8 years of age in White children and 7 years of age in African-American children, with no other manifestations of puberty (Fig. 55.4). Elevated serum estrogen levels for age have been difficult to demonstrate, although higher levels than in age-matched normal females have been measured by an ultrasensitive estradiol assay. Development of breast tissue commonly begins between 2 and 3 years of age; it may be present from birth. The observed tissue may be asymmetric, unilateral, or bilateral. When asymmetric or unilateral, parents are typically concerned about the possibility of malignancy, an extremely rare occurrence in childhood. The early breast tissue frequently regresses without intervention, but it may persist. If it persists, the degree of development

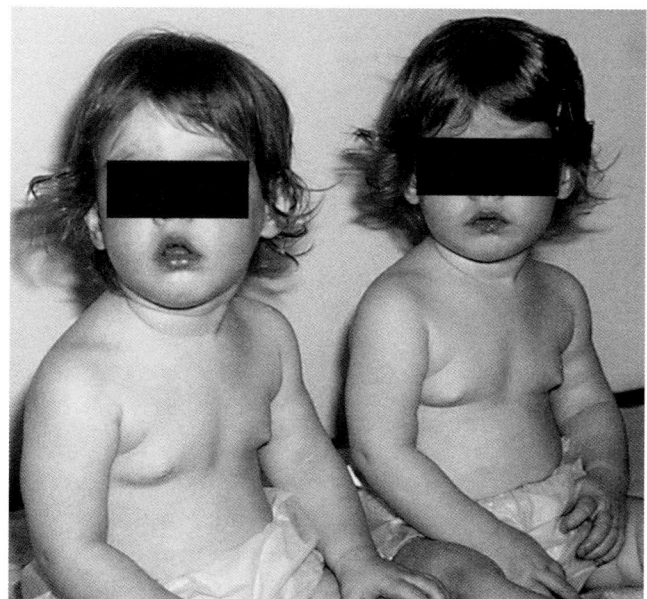

Fig. 55.4 Two-year-old twin sisters with idiopathic isolated premature thelarche manifested by isolated breast development to Tanner stage 3.

does not usually exceed Tanner stage 3. The bone age, if determined, is not frequently advanced, and there is no associated growth spurt. If these simple clinical criteria are met, no hormonal studies or additional radiologic procedures are necessary.

Physiologic breast enlargement also occurs in neonates from placental transfer of estrogens. Most marked in the first weeks of life, it usually regresses by 1–2 months.

Idiopathic Isolated Precocious Adrenarche

This common, normal variant is characterized by the development of pubic hair, axillary hair and odor, and/or a small amount of acne in White females before the age of 8 years, in African-American females before the age of 7 years, and in males before the age of 9 years. It appears to result from early production of adrenal androgens. Precocious adrenarche occurs much more commonly in females than in males and develops most often in obese and/or African-American females and in brain-injured children. There is no associated evidence of virilization (no growth spurt, no significant advancement of bone age, no increase in muscle bulk, no voice deepening, and no temporal hair recession). In females, there is no associated clitoromegaly and no evidence of estrogen-mediated components of puberty; in males, there is no phallic or testicular enlargement. If a child presents at a very young age, it is generally presumed that an organic cause (such as congenital adrenal hyperplasia) will be found. However, in infant males with isolated scrotal hair, typically no cause is found, and the hair subsequently falls out. In most cases of idiopathic precocious adrenarche (benign premature adrenarche), serum levels of DHEA and/or DHEAS are consistent with the reference range of Tanner staging of the hair growth, and the 8:00 a.m. 17-hydroxyprogesterone level is normal. If these criteria are met, no additional laboratory studies are indicated. This pubertal variant was considered benign and self-limited, but data suggest that at least in females with associated low birthweight, it may suggest an increased risk for **polycystic ovary disease**.

Isosexual Central Precocious Puberty

Central sexual precocity results from activation of the hypothalamic-pituitary-gonadal axis at an earlier-than-normal age (Figs. 55.1 and

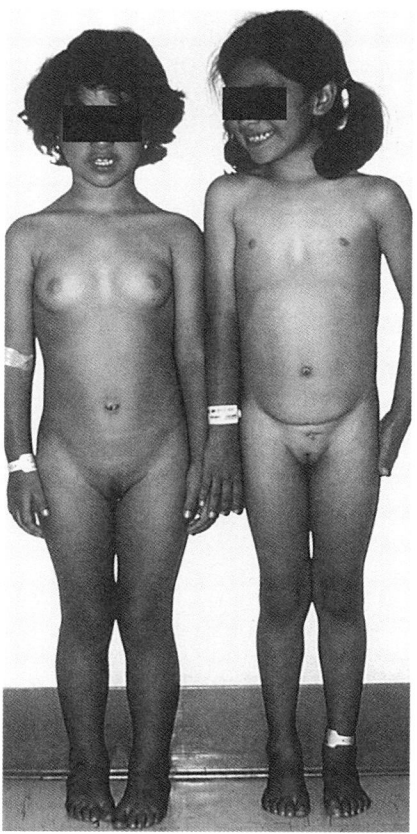

Fig. 55.5 A 3-year-old girl *(left)* with isosexual central precocious puberty characterized by both breast and pubic hair development, and tall stature, contrasted to a normal 5-year-old prepubertal girl *(right)*.

55.5). *Isosexual* development refers to pubertal changes appropriate for the sex of the child, such as breast budding in females and testicular enlargement in males. This is to be distinguished from *contrasexual* development, in which the pubertal features in females are mediated by male hormones (clitoromegaly) and those in males are mediated by female hormones (breast development).

Causes of isosexual precocious puberty are listed in Tables 55.4 and 55.5 and Figs. 55.5 and 55.6. The majority of cases in females, who are at least 10-fold more likely to be affected than males, are idiopathic, whereas only a small percentage of affected males have no definable cause. Ovarian size, as seen on an ultrasound, is generally a reflection of ovarian estrogen production. In true central puberty, pituitary gonadotropins cause both ovaries to increase in size.

In true male central puberty, testes enlarge and androgen production increases. The size of testis enlargement sufficient to determine puberty is debatable. In general, prepubertal testes are <4 mL in volume and 2 cm in length. If on examination both testes are enlarged and androgen signs are present, it is likely puberty is underway and testis-derived testosterone levels are increasing. If basal pituitary gonadotropins are increasing, or if LH levels increase markedly after GnRH stimulation, the diagnosis is central precocious puberty.

Hypothalamic hamartomas, which may be associated with ectopic secretion of GnRH or transforming growth factor-α, are common causes of precocious puberty. Approximately 3% of children with neurofibromatosis type 1 develop central precocity, usually caused by a hypothalamic optic glioma.

Central precocious puberty in the setting of untreated or undertreated peripheral causes of puberty, such as **virilizing congenital**

TABLE 55.4   Classification of Sexual Precocity

TRUE PRECOCIOUS PUBERTY OR COMPLETE ISOSEXUAL PRECOCITY (GnRH-DEPENDENT SEXUAL PRECOCITY OR PREMATURE ACTIVATION OF THE HYPOTHALAMIC GnRH PULSE GENERATOR)

Idiopathic true precocious puberty
CNS tumors
Optic glioma associated with neurofibromatosis type 1
Hypothalamic astrocytoma
Other CNS disorders
Developmental abnormalities including hypothalamic hamartoma of the tuber cinereum
Encephalitis
Static encephalopathy
Brain abscess
Sarcoid or tubercular granuloma
Head trauma
Hydrocephalus
Arachnoid cyst
Myelomeningocele
Vascular lesion
Cranial irradiation
True precocious puberty after late treatment of congenital virilizing adrenal hyperplasia or other previous chronic exposure to sex steroids
True precocious puberty due to gain-of-function pathologic variants in *KISS1R/KISS1* genes
Central precocious puberty due to loss of function in *MKRN3* or *DLK1* genes (Figs. 55.6 and 55.7)

INCOMPLETE ISOSEXUAL PRECOCITY (HYPOTHALAMIC GnRH INDEPENDENT)
Males
Gonadotropin-secreting tumors
hCG-secreting CNS tumors (e.g., chorioepitheliomas, germinoma, teratoma)
hCG-secreting tumors located outside the CNS (hepatoma, teratoma, choriocarcinoma)
Increased androgen secretion by adrenal gland or testis
Congenital adrenal hyperplasia (CYP21 and CYP11B1 deficiencies)
Virilizing adrenal neoplasm
Leydig cell adenoma
Familial testotoxicosis (sex-limited autosomal dominant pituitary gonadotropin-independent precocious Leydig cell and germ cell maturation)
Cortisol resistance syndrome

Females
Ovarian cyst
Estrogen-secreting ovarian or adrenal neoplasm
Peutz-Jeghers syndrome

Both Sexes
McCune-Albright syndrome
Hypothyroidism
Iatrogenic or exogenous sexual precocity (including inadvertent exposure to estrogens in food, drugs, or cosmetics)

VARIATIONS OF PUBERTAL DEVELOPMENT
Premature thelarche
Premature isolated menarche
Premature adrenarche
Adolescent gynecomastia in boys
Macro-orchidism

CONTRASEXUAL PRECOCITY
Feminization in Males
Adrenal neoplasm
Chorioepithelioma
CYP11B1 deficiency
Late-onset adrenal hyperplasia
Testicular neoplasm (Peutz-Jeghers syndrome)
Increased extraglandular conversion of circulating adrenal androgens to estrogen
Iatrogenic (exposure to estrogens)

Virilization in Females
Congenital adrenal hyperplasia
CYP21 deficiency
CYP11B1 deficiency
3β-HSD deficiency
Virilizing adrenal neoplasm (Cushing syndrome)
Virilizing ovarian neoplasm (e.g., arrhenoblastoma)
Iatrogenic (exposure to androgens)
Cortisol resistance syndrome
Aromatase deficiency

CNS, central nervous system; CYP11B1, 11-hydroxylase; CYP21, 21-hydroxylase; GnRH, gonadotropin-releasing hormone; hCG, human chorionic gonadotropin; 3β-HSD, 3β-hydroxysteroid dehydrogenase 4,5-isomerase.
Modified from Grumbach MM. True or central precocious puberty. In: Kreiger DT, Bardin CW, eds. *Current Therapy in Endocrinology and Metabolism, 1985–1986*. Toronto, Canada: BC Decker; 1985:4–8.

---

adrenal hyperplasia, is caused by premature activation of the GnRH pulse generator, presumably as a result of continuous central nervous system exposure to high levels of androgens (or androgens aromatized to estrogens). Precocious puberty with thelarche and menarche in the setting of long-standing severe untreated **primary hypothyroidism** (Van Wyk–Grumbach syndrome) can occur, although the mechanism is not clear. It is clinically distinguished by the usual manifestations of hypothyroidism, including delayed growth and bone age, rather than the advanced bone age present with other causes of precocious puberty.

Incomplete Isosexual Precocity (Precocious Pseudopuberty)

Precocious pseudopuberty refers to gonadal or adrenal sex steroid secretion *not* resulting from activation of the hypothalamic-pituitary-gonadal axis (pituitary independent). It is caused by excessive production of or exposure to either androgens or estrogens (see Table 55.4).

Androgen Exposure or Overproduction

Anabolic steroids have been taken by males and females to improve muscle development and athletic performance. In males, if anabolic steroids are taken at the age of puberty, secondary sexual development will progress, but the testes will remain small. In females, anabolic steroids can produce clitoral enlargement (particularly in diameter), acne, and hirsutism, as well as emotional lability.

Females. **Ovarian tumors** producing androgens (thecoma) and sometimes also estrogen may be palpable on physical examination and are usually easily seen on a pelvic ultrasound. Arrhenoblastoma, a virilizing ovarian tumor, is rare in children. Gonadoblastomas, which

TABLE 55.5   Differential Diagnosis of Sexual Precocity

Disorder	Plasma Gonadotropins	LH Response to GnRH	Serum Sex Steroid Concentration	Gonadal Size	Miscellaneous
Gonadotropin Dependent					
True precocious puberty	Prominent LH pulses (premature reactivation of GnRH pulse generator)	Pubertal LH response initially during sleep	Pubertal values of testosterone or estradiol	Normal pubertal testicular enlargement or ovarian and uterine enlargement	MRI of brain to rule out CNS tumor or other abnormality; skeletal survey for McCune-Albright syndrome (by US)
Incomplete Sexual Precocity (Pituitary Gonadotropin Independent)					
Males					
Chorionic gonadotropin-secreting tumor in males	High hCG, low LH	Prepubertal LH response	Pubertal value of testosterone	Slight to moderate uniform enlargement of testes	Hepatomegaly suggests hepatoblastoma; CT scan of brain if chorionic gonadotropin-secreting CNS tumor suspected
Leydig cell tumor in males	Suppressed	No LH response	Very high testosterone	Irregular, asymmetric enlargement of testes	
Familial testotoxicosis	Suppressed	No LH response	Pubertal values of testosterone	Testes symmetric and >2.5 cm but smaller than expected for pubertal development; spermatogenesis occurs	Familial; probably sex-limited, autosomal dominant trait
Virilizing congenital adrenal hyperplasia	Prepubertal	Prepubertal LH response	Elevated 17-OHP in CYP21 deficiency or elevated 11-deoxycortisol in CYP11B1 deficiency	Testes prepubertal	Autosomal recessive; may be congenital or late-onset form, may have salt loss in CYP21 deficiency or hypertension in CYP11B1 deficiency
Virilizing adrenal tumor	Prepubertal	Prepubertal LH response	High DHEAS and androstenedione values	Testes prepubertal	CT, MRI, or US of abdomen
Premature adrenarche	Prepubertal	Prepubertal LH response	Prepubertal testosterone, DHEAS, or urinary 17-ketosteroid values appropriate for pubic hair stage 2	Testes prepubertal	Onset usually after 6 yr of age; more frequent in CNS-injured children
Females					
Granulosa cell tumor (follicular cysts may present similarly)	Suppressed	Prepubertal LH response	Very high estradiol	Ovarian enlargement on physical examination, CT, or US	Tumor often palpable on physical examination
Follicular cyst	Suppressed	Prepubertal LH response	Prepubertal to very high estradiol	Ovarian enlargement on physical examination, CT, or US	Single or recurrent episodes of menses and/or breast development; exclude McCune-Albright syndrome
Feminizing adrenal tumor	Suppressed	Prepubertal LH response	High estradiol and DHEAS values	Ovaries prepubertal	Unilateral adrenal mass
Premature thelarche	Prepubertal	Prepubertal LH, pubertal	Prepubertal or early estradiol response	Ovaries prepubertal	Onset usually before 3 yr of age
Premature adrenarche	Prepubertal	Prepubertal LH response	Prepubertal estradiol; DHEAS or urinary 17-ketosteroid values appropriate for pubic hair stage 2	Ovaries prepubertal	Onset usually after 6 yr of age; more frequent in brain-injured children
Late-onset virilizing congenital adrenal hyperplasia	Prepubertal	Prepubertal LH response	Elevated 17-OHP in basal or corticotrophin-stimulated state	Ovaries prepubertal	Autosomal recessive

Continued

TABLE 55.5   Differential Diagnosis of Sexual Precocity—cont'd

Disorder	Plasma Gonadotropins	LH Response to GnRH	Serum Sex Steroid Concentration	Gonadal Size	Miscellaneous
In Both Sexes					
McCune-Albright syndrome	Suppressed	Suppressed	Sex steroid pubertal or higher	Ovarian enlargement (visible on US); slight testicular enlargement	Skeletal survey for polyostotic fibrous dysplasia and skin examination for café-au-lait spots
Primary hypothyroidism	LH prepubertal; FSH may be slightly elevated	Prepubertal FSH may be increased	Estradiol may be pubertal	Testicular enlargement; ovaries cystic	TSH and prolactin elevated; T₄ low

CNS, central nervous system; CYP, P450 cytochrome isoenzyme; DHEAS, dehydroepiandrosterone sulfate; FSH, follicle-stimulating hormone; GnRH, gonadotropin-releasing hormone; hCG, human chorionic gonadotropin; LH, luteinizing hormone; 17-OHP, 17-hydroxyprogesterone; T_4, thyroxine; TSH, thyroid-stimulating hormone; US, ultrasonography.

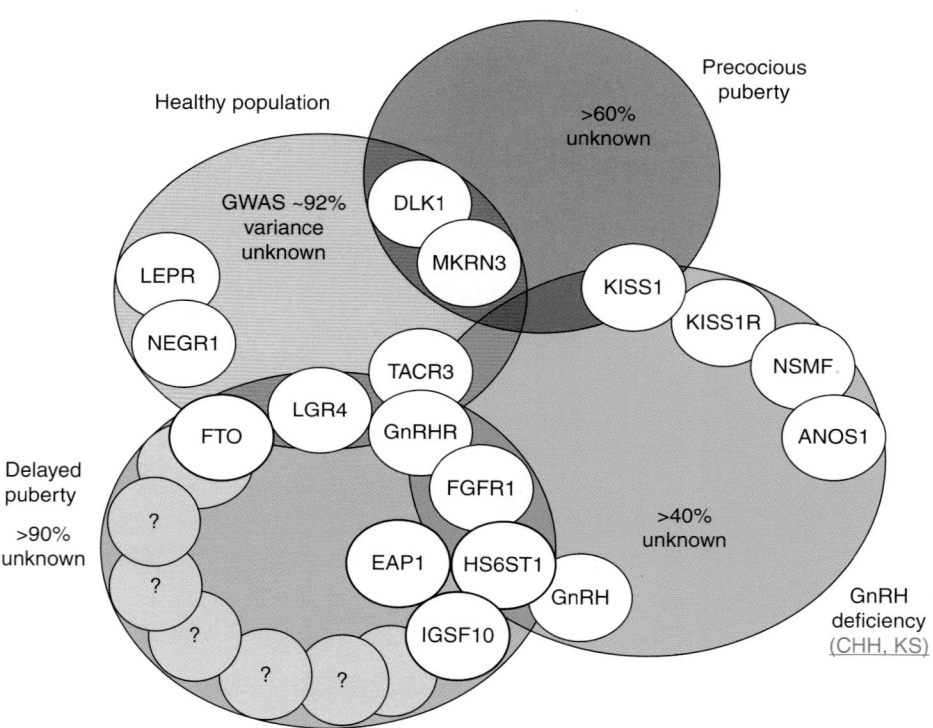

Fig. 55.6 Established genetic basis of common genetic variants of pubertal timing from genome-wide association studies (GWAS), conditions of GnRH deficiency (CHH and KS), precocious puberty, and delayed puberty and their overlap. Activating and inactivating pathologic variants in KISS1 and KISS1R cause the opposite phenotypes, precocious puberty and CHH, respectively. Bold circles highlight those genes whose pathologic gene variants have been identified in familial delayed puberty. CHH, congenital hypogonadotropic hypogonadism; KS, Kallmann syndrome. (From Howard SR. The genetic basis of delayed puberty. *Front Endocrinol (Lausanne)*. 2019;10:423 [published 2019 Jun 26], Fig. 5.)

are not always virilizing, typically occur in phenotypic females who have Y chromosome material. Granulosa cell tumors usually cause estrogen overproduction but occasionally cause virilization due to excessive androgen production.

Adrenal tumors can be detected with ultrasonography, CT, or MRI. Androgens produced by adrenal tumors are not suppressed by dexamethasone. Excessive adrenal androgens may also be produced as a result of late-onset or nonclassical **congenital adrenal hyperplasia**, but the androgen production can be suppressed by dexamethasone. The enzymatic deficiency in late-onset congenital adrenal

hyperplasia is mild, inasmuch as it does not cause ambiguity of genitalia at birth; however, it is associated with an accelerated growth rate and advanced bone age and may be clinically recognized any time after birth.

Males. If both testes are slightly increased in volume and testosterone levels are increased but LH and FSH levels are low, there are two possibilities: either the testes are being stimulated by human chorionic gonadotropin (hCG), which acts like LH and does not increase testicular volume, as with FSH, or the testes are functioning autonomously. hCG levels must be determined, and if they are

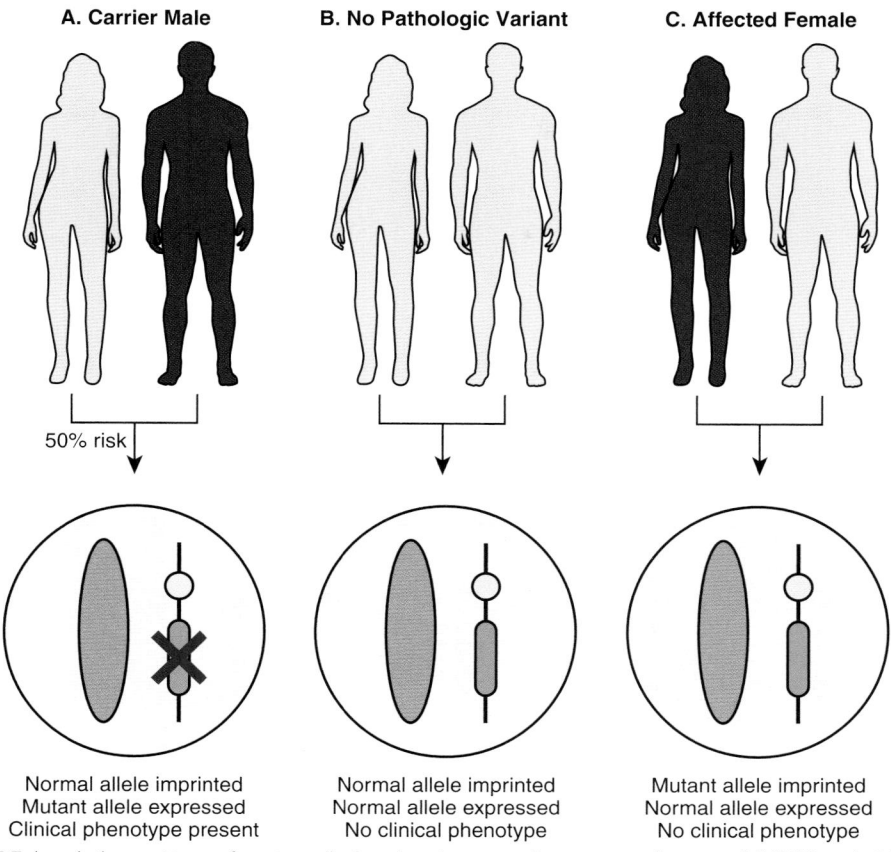

A. Carrier Male

B. No Pathologic Variant

C. Affected Female

50% risk

Normal allele imprinted
Mutant allele expressed
Clinical phenotype present

Normal allele imprinted
Normal allele expressed
No clinical phenotype

Mutant allele imprinted
Normal allele expressed
No clinical phenotype

Fig. 55.7 Imprinting pattern of maternally imprinted, paternally expressed genes *MKRN3* and *DLK1*. *A,* Maternal allele is imprinted or silenced; mutant paternal allele is expressed, resulting in phenotype of central precocious puberty. *B,* Maternal allele is normally imprinted and normal paternal allele is expressed, resulting in normal puberty. *C,* Maternal allele containing pathologic variant is imprinted; normal paternal allele is expressed, resulting in no pathologic phenotype (i.e., normal puberty). (Modified figure courtesy Ross McGowan, Department of Zoology, University of Manitoba.)

increased, tumors producing hCG must be identified and removed; such tumors may include hepatoma, germinoma, hepatoblastoma, teratoma, and chorioepithelioma.

If both testes are producing testosterone autonomously without gonadotropin stimulus, the condition of **testotoxicosis** is probable. Children with this autosomal dominant disorder have signs of puberty by 4 years of age (Fig. 55.8). Testosterone production and Leydig cell hyperplasia occur in the setting of prepubertal serum LH levels, because of a gain-of-function pathologic variant in the gene for the LH receptor, resulting in its constitutive activation. Affected males are fertile. Females who carry this pathologic variant do not develop precocious puberty.

If one testis is enlarged, a Leydig cell adenoma in that testicle is probably producing excess testosterone; the tumor must be removed. The high levels of testosterone suppress LH and FSH secretion, so the other testicle remains small. Depending on age, a testicular prosthesis may be inserted to replace the removed testicle.

If androgen signs are developing steadily but neither testis has enlarged, the androgen is presumed to be either from the adrenal glands or from an exogenous source. Inappropriate adrenal production of androgens results from tumors or abnormalities in steroid synthesis enzymatic activity. An adrenal tumor would have affected growth whenever the gland started to function, but not necessarily beginning at birth. A defect in steroid synthesis caused by an enzymatic deficiency (usually 21-hydroxylase) may be congenital, as in congenital adrenal hyperplasia, and the excess androgen production resulting from the enzymatic deficiency would have been produced from the time of birth,

leading to increased growth velocity from early life. *Children with congenital adrenal hyperplasia may have severe adrenal crises during an illness or surgery.* A late-onset or nonclassical form of adrenal hyperplasia may also occur. A tumor can be identified by CT, ultrasonography, or MRI and must be removed.

Estrogen Overproduction

The most common cause of premature progressive breast development is simple premature thelarche. In this case, a pelvic ultrasound study may show prepubertal ovaries varying from 1 to 3 mL in volume with many small estrogen-producing follicular cysts. Some cysts may be larger (persistent follicular cysts). Estradiol is produced by the granulosa cells lining the follicles and causes vaginal discharge and breast development. Estradiol may cause uterine development as well but generally does not cause increased growth velocity. LH and FSH levels are low, and if estradiol is measured, it might be elevated but minimally so. The follicular cysts regress spontaneously (90% of the time) within a few weeks to months, and the vaginal cornification is lost within 1 week of cyst regression. The breast tissue then softens but can remain for months and may never completely regress. Typically, premature thelarche due to persistent follicular cysts is usually benign and self-limited. However, 10% of the cysts may persist and enlarge, with some follicular cysts becoming large enough to threaten ovarian torsion and to necessitate surgical treatment.

Granulosa cell tumors are usually isolated occurrences but may occur as part of **Peutz-Jeghers syndrome** (oral melanosis and intestinal

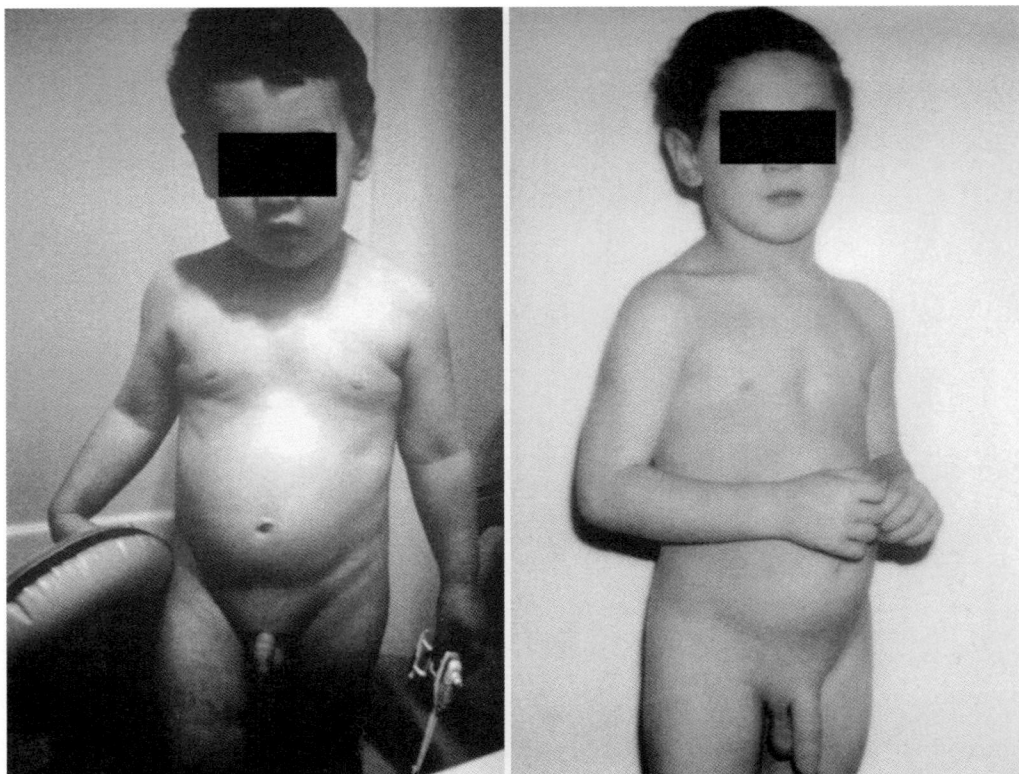

Fig. 55.8 A boy with familial testotoxicosis associated with significant penile enlargement, moderate pubic hair growth, and mild to moderate testicular enlargement over a 1.75-year period. *Left,* At 2 years of age. *Right,* At 3.75 years of age.

polyps). Aromatase is the enzyme that is responsible for conversion of androgen to estrogen; aromatase excess is an autosomal dominant disorder that can lead to increased estradiol levels.

McCune-Albright syndrome. This disorder (Fig. 55.9) consists of the clinical triad of polyostotic fibrous dysplasia, hyperpigmented macules (café-au-lait spots) with irregular borders ("coast of Maine"), and multiple autonomous endocrinopathies (most commonly gonadotropin-independent precocious puberty, but also hyperthyroidism, acromegaly, and hypercortisolemia) (Table 55.6). Precocious puberty occurs much more commonly in females than in males. Patients have a somatic mutation in their *GNAS1* gene that occurs early in embryogenesis and results in somatic mosaic constitutive activation of adenylyl cyclase in affected tissues. This activation leads to the autonomous function of involved tissues, resulting, in the case of affected endocrine glands, in unregulated production of hormone. Precocity in females, often heralded by menstrual bleeding, frequently occurs before 2 years of age. The ovaries are enlarged and have many follicular cysts; the patient has elevated levels of estradiol. Later, when the GnRH pulse generator is activated subsequent to unabated sex steroid exposure, the patient may transition from gonadotropin-independent to central precocious puberty.

Neurofibromatosis type 1. Neurofibromatosis type 1 can present with precocious puberty secondary to a hypothalamic tumor. Pseudothelarche/gynecomastia can present due to a plexiform neurofibroma deep to the areola with either asymmetric (more common) or bilateral apparent breast tissue growth. Management is dependent on the rate of growth and degree of tissue involvement. Surgery is typically delayed until normal breast tissue has matured, but with the introduction of MEK inhibitor therapy, consideration for reducing a large tumor burden prior to surgery could be considered.

Vaginal Bleeding

The usual progression of puberty in females dictates that breast and uterine development begin about 2 years before the menses. When the rate of pubertal progression is accelerated, menses may start as early as 1–1.5 years after thelarche; if the rate is slow, menses may start perhaps 3–4 years after thelarche. In any case, vaginal bleeding is always a much later sign than breast development, and whenever vaginal bleeding occurs too early—especially if it ever occurs before breast development starts—it must be investigated thoroughly.

Gynecomastia

Breast tissue frequently develops in males during mid-puberty, when the production of estrogen from testosterone in the testes temporarily overbalances the testosterone effects. Only rarely does breast tissue develop in prepubertal males, inasmuch as young males do not respond to transient gonadotropin stimulation with estrogen production. Differential diagnosis includes estrogen-producing tumors (gonadal or adrenal), exogenous estrogen, hCG-producing tumors, aromatase excess, certain types of male pseudohermaphroditism, and Klinefelter syndrome. Certain medications and illicit drugs are associated with gynecomastia. A **prolactinoma** should be considered, especially in the setting of **galactorrhea**.

Evaluation of gynecomastia in prepubertal males may include karyotyping and measurement of gonadotropins, estradiol, testosterone, hCG, TSH, and prolactin level. Imaging is dictated by the results.

Diagnostic Approach to Precocious Puberty

In the initial evaluation of the child with precocious puberty, the clinician attempts to determine:

- Whether the process is a normal variant or pathologic
- The rate of progression of the pubertal changes

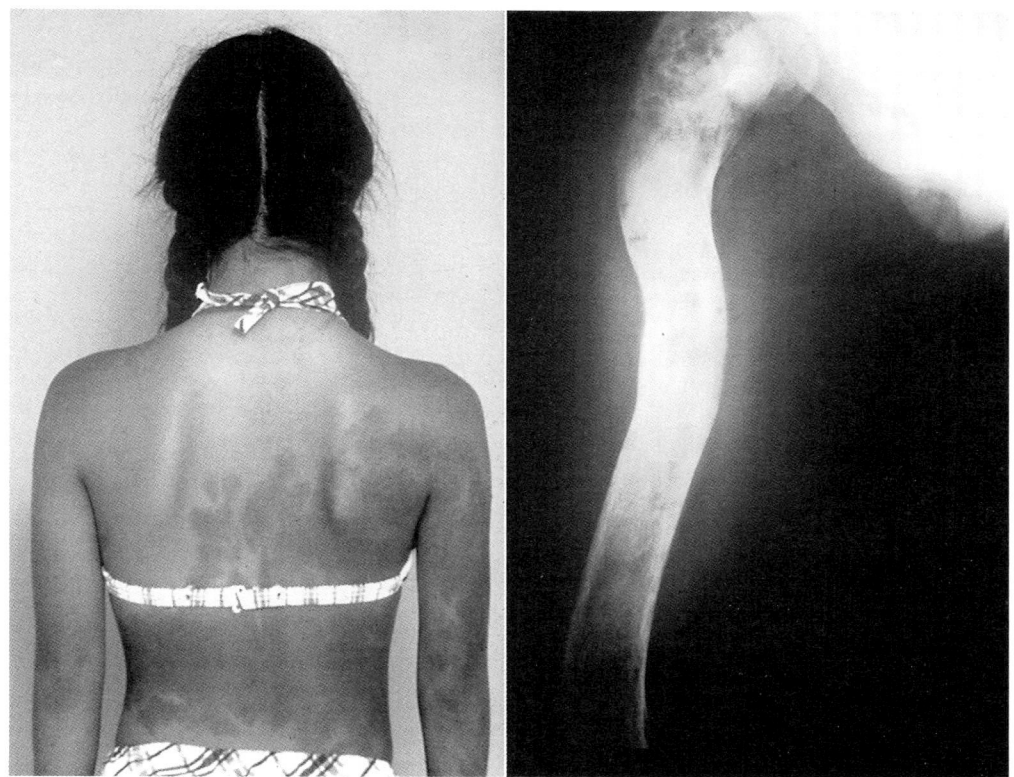

Fig. 55.9 A 12-year-old girl with McCune-Albright syndrome with a café-au-lait spot with an irregular border ("coast of Maine") on the back *(left)* and representative lesion of fibrous dysplasia involving the left humerus *(right)*.

TABLE 55.6 Clinical Manifestations of McCune-Albright Syndrome in 158 Reported Patients*

Manifestation	Total (n = 158)	Male (n = 53)	Female (n = 105)	Mean Age at Diagnosis (yr) and Range	Comments
Fibrous dysplasia	97	51	103	7.7 (0–52)	Polyostotic more common than monostotic
Café-au-lait lesion	85	49	86	7.7 (0–52)	Variable size and number of lesions, irregular border (coast of Maine)
Sexual precocity	52	8	74	4.9 (0.3–9)	Common initial manifestation
Acromegaly/gigantism	27	20	22	14.8 (0.2–42)	17/26 of patients with adenoma on MRI/CT
Hyperprolactinemia	15	9	14	16.0 (0.2–42)	23/42 of acromegalic patients with PRL
Hyperthyroidism	19	7	23	14.4 (0.5–37)	Euthyroid goiter is common
Hypercortisolism	5	4	5	4.4 (0.2–17)	All primary adrenal
Myxomas	5	3	5	34 (17–50)	Extremity myxomas
Osteosarcoma	2	1	2	36 (34–37)	At site of fibrous dysplasia, not related to prior radiation therapy
Rickets/osteomalacia	3	1	3	27.3 (8–52)	Responsive to phosphorus plus calcitriol
Cardiac abnormalities	11	8	9	(0.1–66)	Arrhythmias and CHF reported
Hepatic abnormalities	10	6	10	1.9 (0.3–4)	Neonatal icterus is most common

% OF PATIENTS (header above Total, Male, Female columns)

*Evaluations include clinical and biochemical data; other rarely described manifestations include metabolic acidosis, nephrocalcinosis, developmental delay, thymic and splenic hyperplasia, and colonic polyps.
CHF, congestive heart failure; PRL, prolactin.
Modified from Ringel MD, Schwindinger WF, Levine MA. Clinical implications of genetic defects in G proteins: the molecular basis of McCune-Albright syndrome and Albright hereditary osteodystrophy. *Medicine (Baltimore).* 1996;75:171–184.

- Whether the process originates centrally or peripherally

Initial evaluation should include:

- Medical history: prenatal and birth history, growth patterns; excessive responses to illness (adrenal crisis); exposure to exogenous sex steroids; history of intracranial insults (hydrocephalus, meningitis, or encephalitis)
- Review of symptoms: growth records, head size since birth, vision problems, headache, age at onset of androgen signs (behavior changes, need for increased hair washing because of oiliness, need for deodorant), age at onset of estrogen signs (vaginal discharge or breast budding), café-au-lait spots ("coast of Maine" in McCune-Albright syndrome or "coast of California" in neurofibromatosis)
- Family history: timing of maternal and paternal growth and pubertal development; siblings and cousins with early development; neurofibromatosis
- Physical examination: vital signs, height, weight, head circumference, tooth age, café-au-lait spots, neurofibromata, pubic and axillary hair, body odor, skin and hair oils, visual fields, optic discs, breast development, vaginal cornification/discharge, penis/clitoris size, scrotal/labial development, testicular volume, pubic hair stages, facial asymmetry or bone abnormalities (fibrous dysplasia of McCune-Albright syndrome), neurologic status, affect or mood, intellectual ability

The first test is usually a determination of bone age; if the bone age is not significantly advanced (within 1 year or 2 SD) and not associated with an increase in height velocity, the results suggest a normal variant, a slowly progressive process, or a process of relatively short duration. If the bone age is significantly advanced, an evaluation is mandatory (Table 55.7). Clinical and laboratory findings in sexual precocity are listed in Table 55.5.

For females with breast development, pelvic ultrasonography and determination of central precocity are the initial diagnostic tests. Because of the pulsatile secretion of serum gonadotropins, random measurements of LH and FSH even by ultrasensitive immunochemiluminescent assay (ICMA) are occasionally low and appear prepubertal even in the setting of central activation. If this occurs and there is clinical suspicion nonetheless of maturation of the GnRH pulse generator, a GnRH stimulation test should be performed. With central precocity, as with normal puberty, endogenous GnRH that "primes" the pituitary gonadotrophs is being produced, so that after administration of a single pharmacologic dose of GnRH (Leuprolide), there is copious release of LH. If, on the other hand, the precocity has a peripheral basis, the high levels of circulating estradiol, through central negative feedback, prevent the gonadotrophs from releasing LH in response to the exogenous GnRH bolus.

If a female with advanced bone age presents only with contrasexual androgenic effects (specifically, evidence of virilization), measurement of gonadotropins and estradiol is not indicated as an adrenal cause should be considered. Measurement of serum 17-hydroxyprogesterone is the diagnostic test for 21-hydroxylase deficiency, the most common enzyme abnormality associated with nonclassical or late-onset adrenal hyperplasia. On occasion, an adrenocorticotropic hormone (ACTH) stimulation test may need to be performed to determine the specific enzymatic deficiency. Screening for Cushing syndrome with a 24-hour urine collection with measurement of free cortisol (and creatinine to document completeness of the collection) or midnight salivary cortisol may also be indicated if the appropriate "cushingoid" body habitus is present. Linear growth is *attenuated* with Cushing syndrome, which is in contrast to most other causes of precocious puberty. Given the typical lack of ovarian involvement in the pathology of virilization in girls, MRI of the head is not usually indicated.

For males, the testicular examination guides the evaluation by suggesting whether there is a testicular or adrenal source of the androgens.

TABLE 55.7 Diagnostic Approach to Precocious Puberty

Females with Breast Development, with or Without Androgen Effects

Random serum FSH and LH measurement by ICMA; estradiol measurement

GnRH stimulation test (if random FSH and LH levels are uninformative)

Pelvic ultrasonography

Prepubertal ovaries: ultrasonography (or other radiologic imaging) to image adrenal glands and question about exogenous sources

One enlarged ovary: either functioning ovarian cyst or solid granulosa cell tumor

Bilaterally enlarged ovaries for age: GnRH test to distinguish between central precocity (usual) or McCune-Albright syndrome (rare)

Head MRI with contrast medium (if central precocity is confirmed biochemically and is progressive)

Females with Contrasexual Androgen Effects (Virilization)

Serum total testosterone (provides an index of the severity of the process)

17-Hydroxyprogesterone (for CAH)

ACTH stimulation test (for CAH) (optional)

Midnight salivary cortisol or 24-hr urine free cortisol and creatinine (for Cushing syndrome)

Abdominal/pelvic MRI (if testing suggests either an adrenal or ovarian tumor)

Males with Isosexual Precocity

Prepubertal testes: ultrasonography (or other radiologic imaging) of the adrenal glands; question about exogenous sources

One enlarged testis: ultrasonography (or other radiologic imaging) of this testis for an androgen-producing tumor

Bilaterally enlarged testes for age: GnRH test to distinguish between central precocity and other causes (familial testotoxicosis, hCG-producing tumor, CAH with adrenal rests, or hypothyroidism)

If central precocity is confirmed biochemically, head MRI with contrast

Tests to Consider, in Either Sex, Depending on Clinical Presentation

Serum hCG

Prolactin

T_4 and TSH

ACTH, adrenocorticotropic hormone; CAH, congenital adrenal hyperplasia; FSH, follicle-stimulating hormone; GnRH, gonadotropin-releasing hormone; hCG, human chorionic gonadotropin; ICMA, immunochemiluminescent assay; LH, luteinizing hormone; T_4, thyroxine; TSH, thyroid-stimulating hormone.

Testotoxicosis and hCG-producing tumors cause some testicular enlargement but less than expected for the degree of virilization.

Treatment of Precocious Puberty

General Issues

Not all cases of precocious puberty necessitate treatment. Cases of idiopathic precocious thelarche and adrenarche should be monitored, because their manifestations are not typically progressive and there is no significant early onset of the other components of puberty or short stature. In addition, not all children with central precocious puberty require treatment, inasmuch as a significant number of cases are either slowly progressive and/or transient. Unless there is rapid progression and/or significant psychosocial difficulties, most children with central precocity should be observed for a 3- to 6-month period before therapy is initiated. The reasons that favor treatment include preservation of acceptable final height, prevention of psychologic trauma

TABLE 55.8 Objectives for the Management and Treatment of True Precocious Puberty

Detection and treatment of an expanding intracranial lesion

Arrest of premature sexual maturation until the normal age at onset of puberty

Regression of secondary sexual characteristics already present

Attainment of normal mature height; suppression of the rapid rate of skeletal maturation

Prevention of emotional disorders and handicaps and alleviation of parental anxiety; promotion of understanding by counseling, early sex education, and acceleration of social age

Reduction of risk of sexual abuse and early sexual debut

Prevention of pregnancy in girls

Preservation of future fertility

Diminishment of the increased risk of breast cancer associated with early menarche

From Grumbach MM. True or central precocious puberty. In: Krieger DT, Bardin CW, eds. *Current Therapy in Endocrinology and Metabolism, 1985–1986.* Toronto, Canada: BC Decker; 1989:4–8.

TABLE 55.9 GnRH Analogs Used to Treat Precocious Puberty

Leuprolide acetate (Lupron Depot) given as an intramuscular injection every 1–3 mo*

Leuprolide acetate (Lupron) given as a daily subcutaneous injection

Nafarelin acetate (Synarel) given b.i.d. by an intranasal route

*Preferred because of infrequent dosing.
b.i.d., twice a day; GnRH, gonadotropin-releasing hormone.

(menstruation at an early age), reversal of mature physical appearance to decrease the risk of pregnancy in females (because other people assume that affected children are older than they appear), and reduction of aggressiveness and preoccupation with sexuality. Serious psychologic effects of early puberty are not usually encountered. If a decision is made to initiate treatment, the goal of therapy is to inhibit secretion and/or effects of estrogens in females and androgens in males (Table 55.8).

Central Precocious Puberty

The goal of therapy is to inhibit secretion of gonadotropins and reduce production of sex steroids by the administration of GnRH agonist analogs with a prolonged duration of action (Table 55.9). This causes downregulation of pituitary GnRH receptors, preventing the response to endogenous GnRH and thus decreasing LH and FSH secretion. Several doses of GnRH are necessary to produce the antagonistic response because the treatment initially stimulates the axis and only later results in downregulation of pituitary GnRH receptors. Accurate verification of adequate suppression of the axis typically requires repeat GnRH testing, although random LH-ICMA levels may be sufficient.

Therapy is stopped around 11 years in females and 12 years in males so that puberty can resume and be concordant with peers. Successful GnRH agonist treatment is associated with a stabilization of androgen effects in males and estrogen effects in females; there is no effect on androgen-mediated events in females as androgens are predominately produced by the adrenal glands. Complete reversal of physical changes to the prepubertal state is unusual. Height velocity and the rate of bone age maturation should slow; on some occasions, height velocity becomes subnormal. This is not necessarily problematic as long as bone age maturation slows commensurately. Final height is optimized with earlier initiation of therapy. Once GnRH analog therapy

TABLE 55.10 Treatment of Precocious Pseudopuberty (Incomplete Isosexual Precocity)

Tumors
    Surgical removal
    Chemotherapy and/or radiation as indicated

Illicit or unintentional administration of exogenous estrogens or androgens should be uncovered and eliminated

Familial testotoxicosis: ketoconazole or spironolactone and testolactone

Adrenal hyperplasia: exogenous glucocorticoid

Hypothyroidism: levothyroxine

McCune-Albright syndrome: testolactone or anastrozole

GnRH agonist therapy may need to be added to any of the above medical therapies if central puberty becomes superimposed at an early age

GnRH, gonadotropin-releasing hormone.

is discontinued, reactivation of the hypothalamic-pituitary-gonadal axis occurs within 12 months. Long-term fertility data in individuals treated with GnRH analogs as children continue to grow, but studies suggest successful childbearing in women and normal testicular function in young adult men following GnRH therapy.

Large tumors in the hypothalamic-pituitary region are surgically removed, and both the tumor and the surgery can precipitate central precocious puberty. However, hypothalamic hamartomas are benign and tend to grow very slowly; therefore, surgery is usually not recommended.

Precocious Pseudopuberty (Incomplete Isosexual Precocity)

Treatment is directed at the underlying cause (Table 55.10). The precocious puberty of McCune-Albright syndrome is treated with inhibitors (testolactone or anastrozole) of aromatase, the enzyme that converts androgen to estrogen. The results of this approach are variable, and sometimes a GnRH agonist must be added if central puberty is also present. Ketoconazole is an effective therapy for familial testotoxicosis (due to a constitutively active LH receptor) because it has the desirable and reversible side effect of interfering with sex steroid synthesis; spironolactone is an androgen receptor blocker.

DELAYED OR ABSENT PUBERTY

Delayed puberty is the failure of development of any pubertal feature by 13 years of age in females or by 14 years of age in males. A lower cutoff may be appropriate in a child with a strong familial pattern of early puberty.

Differential Diagnosis

Delay or absence of puberty is caused by:
- Constitutional (self-limited) delay: a variant of normal
- Hypogonadotropic hypogonadism: low gonadotropin levels as a result of a defect of the hypothalamus and/or pituitary gland (Tables 55.11 and 55.12 and Fig. 55.10)
- Hypergonadotropic hypogonadism: high gonadotropin levels as a result of a lack of negative feedback because of a primary gonadal problem (see Tables 55.11 and 55.12). Girls may have isolated absence of adrenarche with normal breast development (see later discussion).

Constitutional (Self-Limited) Delay of Growth and Puberty

This is the most common cause of delayed puberty and is thought to be a normal variant. It is usually diagnosed in males, probably as a result

TABLE 55.11 Classification of Delayed Puberty and Sexual Infantilism

Idiopathic (Constitutional or Self-Limited) Delay in Growth and Puberty (Delayed Activation of Hypothalamic LRF Pulse Generator)	***Miscellaneous Disorders—cont'd***
	Chronic gastroenteric disease
Hypogonadotropic Hypogonadism: Sexual Infantilism Related to Gonadotropin Deficiency	Börjeson-Forssman-Lehmann syndrome
	Chronic renal disease
CNS Disorders	Malnutrition
	Anorexia nervosa
Tumors	Bulimia
Craniopharyngiomas	Psychogenic amenorrhea
Germinomas	Impaired puberty and delayed menarche in female athletes and ballet dancers
Other germ cell tumors	(exercise amenorrhea)
Hypothalamic and optic gliomas	Hypothyroidism
Astrocytomas	Diabetes mellitus
Pituitary tumors (including MEN-1, prolactinoma)	Cushing disease
	Hyperprolactinemia
Other Causes	Marijuana use
Langerhans histiocytosis	Gaucher disease
Postinfectious lesions of the CNS	
Vascular abnormalities of the CNS	***Hypergonadotropic Hypogonadism***
Radiation therapy	*Males*
Congenital malformations, especially associated with craniofacial anomalies	The syndrome of seminiferous tubular dysgenesis and its variants (Klinefelter
Head trauma	syndrome)
Lymphocytic hypophysitis	Other forms of primary testicular failure
	Chemotherapy
Isolated Gonadotropin Deficiency	Radiation therapy
Kallmann syndrome	Testicular steroid biosynthetic defects
With hyposmia or anosmia	Sertoli cell–only syndrome
Without anosmia	LH receptor pathologic variant
LHRH receptor pathologic variant	Anorchia and cryptorchidism
Congenital adrenal hypoplasia (*DAX1* pathologic variant)	Trauma/surgery
Isolated LH deficiency	
Isolated FSH deficiency	*Females*
Prohormone convertase 1 deficiency (PCI)	The syndrome of gonadal dysgenesis (Turner syndrome) and its variants
	XX and XY gonadal dysgenesis
Idiopathic and Genetic Forms of Multiple Pituitary Hormone Deficiencies Including *PROP1* Pathologic Variant (see Table 55.12 and Figs. 55.6 and 55.10)	Familial and sporadic XX gonadal dysgenesis and its variants
	Familial and sporadic XY gonadal dysgenesis and its variants
	Aromatase deficiency
Miscellaneous Disorders	Other forms of primary ovarian failure
Prader-Willi syndrome	Premature menopause
Bardet-Biedl syndrome	Radiation therapy
CHARGE syndrome	Chemotherapy
Functional gonadotropin deficiency	Autoimmune oophoritis
Adrenal hypoplasia congenita	Galactosemia
Chronic systemic disease and malnutrition	Glycoprotein syndrome type 1
Septo-optic dysplasia	Resistant ovary
Sickle cell disease	FSH receptor pathologic variant
Hartsfield syndrome	LH/hCG resistance
Cystic fibrosis	Polycystic ovarian disease
Gordon Holmes syndrome	Trauma/surgery
AIDS	Noonan or pseudo-Turner syndrome
Solitary median maxillary incisor syndrome	Ovarian steroid biosynthetic defects

CNS, central nervous system; CHARGE, coloboma, heart malformations, choanal atresia, growth retardation, genital anomalies, ear anomalies; FSH, follicle-stimulating hormone; hCG, human chorionic gonadotropin; LH, luteinizing hormone; LHRH, luteinizing hormone–releasing hormone; LRF, luteinizing hormone–releasing factor; MEN, multiple endocrine neoplasia.

of ascertainment bias of referral patterns. The cause is unknown, but approximately 50% of affected patients have a first-degree relative with delayed puberty and/or late growth. This tendency can occur in a child of the same gender as the affected parent or in a child of the opposite gender. An affected child typically presents in early adolescence when peers are beginning to develop and having growth spurts, but the patient is not. The patient's height is usually at or below the 3rd percentile (see Chapter 56). In the classic case, the affected child had a normal

TABLE 55.12 Molecular Basis for Developmental Disorders Associated with Hypogonadotropic Hypogonadism

Gene	Phenotype	Complex Phenotype
Isolated Hypogonadotropic Hypogonadism		
Kallmann Syndrome or Normosmic Idiopathic Hypogonadotropic Hypogonadism (with the Same Variant Gene) (See Table 55.13)		
KAL1 (Xp22.3)	X-linked Kallmann syndrome	Anosmia/hyposmia, renal agenesis, dyskinesia
FGFR1 (8p11.2)	Autosomal dominant Kallmann syndrome (± recessive)	Anosmia/hyposmia, cleft lip/palate
FGF8 (ligand for FGFR1) (10q25)		
NSMF (9p34.3)	Autosomal dominant/oligogenetic Kallmann syndrome	
PROK2 (3p21.1)	Autosomal recessive Kallmann syndrome	
PROKR2* (20p12.3)		
CHD7 (8p12.1)	Autosomal dominant (some)	CHARGE syndrome; includes hyposmia
Normosmic Isolated Hypogonadotropic Hypogonadism		
GNRH1 (8p21-11.2)	Autosomal recessive	
GNRHR* (4q13.2-3)	Autosomal recessive (± dominant)	
GPR54* (19p13.3)	Autosomal recessive	
SNRPN		Prader-Willi syndrome, obesity
Lack of function of paternal 15q11-q13 region or maternal uniparental disomy		
LEP (7q31.3)	Autosomal recessive	Obesity
LEPR (1p31)	Autosomal recessive	Obesity
NROB1 (X21.3-21.2)	X-linked recessive	Adrenal hypoplasia
TAC3 (12q13-12)	Autosomal recessive	
TACR3 (4q25)	Autosomal recessive	
Multiple Pituitary Hormone Deficiencies		
PROP1 POU1F1	Autosomal recessive GH, PRL, TSH, and LH/FSH (less commonly, later-onset ACTH deficiency)	
HESX1	Autosomal recessive and heterozygous pathologic variants	Septo-optic dysplasia
	Multiple pituitary deficiencies including diabetes insipidus, but LH/FSH uncommon	
LHX3	Autosomal recessive GH, PRL, TSH, FSH/LH	Rigid cervical spine
PHF6	X-linked; GH, TSH, ACTH, LH/FSH	Börjeson-Forssman-Lehmann: intellectual disability; coarse facies

*A G protein–coupled receptor.
ACTH, corticotrophin; FGF, fibroblast growth factor; FSH, follicle-stimulating hormone; GH, growth hormone; GnRH, gonadotropin-releasing hormone; LH, luteinizing hormone; PRL, prolactin; TSH, thyroid-stimulating hormone.

length at birth, a slowdown in height velocity between 6 months and 2 years of age that resulted in short stature, and a normal or near-normal height velocity thereafter along the child's current height percentile. The physical examination findings are unremarkable, and, depending on the age, the child may have delayed puberty. The cardinal diagnostic result is a bone age that is moderately delayed in comparison with chronologic age. There may also be a history of delayed dentition. Without intervention, final adult height usually reaches or approximates the target height range. However, children with constitutional delay may have a blunted pubertal growth spurt in relation to their peers, and therefore may not reach their genetic target height range.

Hypogonadotropic Hypogonadism

A variety of central nervous system insults may disrupt production of gonadotropins. The GnRH pulse generator may be disrupted by an interfering substance, such as excess prolactin (with or without hypothyroidism), or by stress, chronic illness, malnutrition, or excessive physical activity. The hypothalamic arcuate nucleus may be damaged by trauma, radiation, infection, infiltration, increased intracranial pressure, or surgery. The most common mass lesions are craniopharyngiomas, gliomas, and cysts. Congenital conditions or malformations may have allowed enough GnRH for infantile development but not enough for pubertal needs.

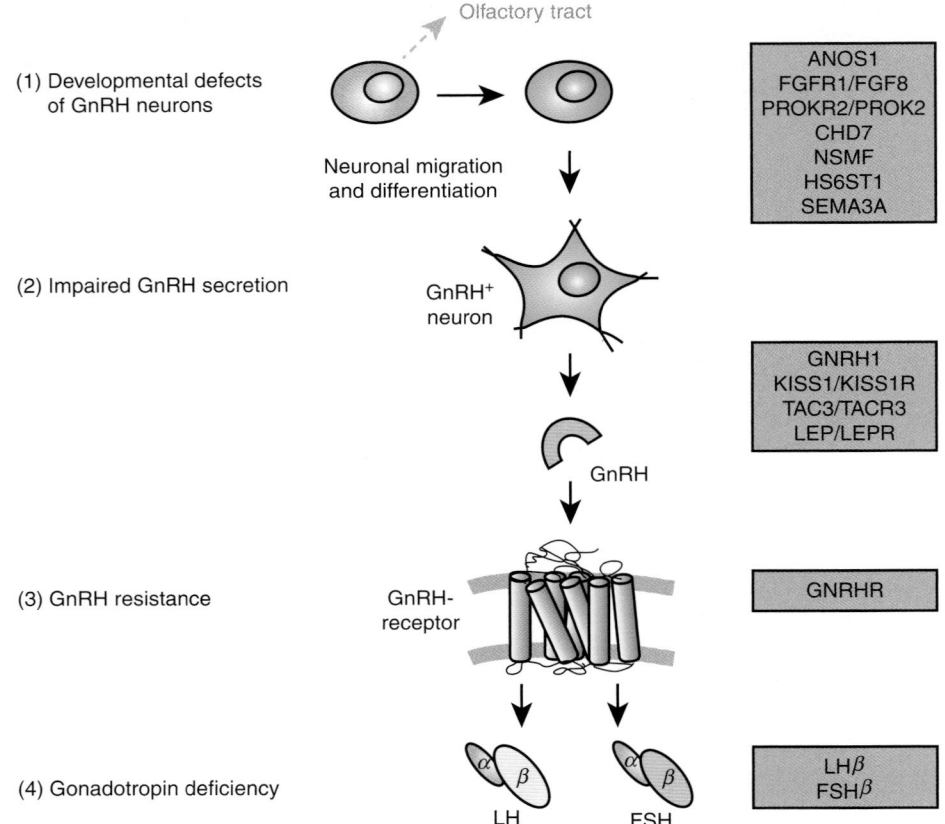

(1) Developmental defects
of GnRH neurons

Olfactory tract

Neuronal migration
and differentiation

ANOS1
FGFR1/FGF8
PROKR2/PROK2
CHD7
NSMF
HS6ST1
SEMA3A

(2) Impaired GnRH secretion

GnRH⁺
neuron

GNRH1
KISS1/KISS1R
TAC3/TACR3
LEP/LEPR

GnRH

(3) GnRH resistance

GnRH-
receptor

GNRHR

(4) Gonadotropin deficiency

LHβ
FSHβ

LH   FSH

Fig. 55.10 Pathologic variants in single genes at many levels of the hypothalamic-pituitary-gonadal axis can cause hypogonadotropic hypogonadism. FSH, follicle-stimulating hormone; GnRH, gonadotropin-releasing hormone; LH, luteinizing hormone. (Modified from Beate K, Joseph N, de Roux N, Wolfram K. Genetics of isolated hypogonadotropic hypogonadism: role of GnRH receptor and other genes. *Int J Endocrinol.* 2012;2012:147893, Fig. 1.)

Kallmann syndrome. This is the combination of an impaired or absent sense of smell and gonadotropin deficiency. Other features include color blindness, atrial septal defects, and renal structural anomalies (unilateral renal agenesis). The X-linked form is caused by a mutation of the *KAL* gene; there are autosomal recessive and autosomal dominant forms (Table 55.13).

LH and FSH deficiencies may also be isolated or caused by multiple pituitary hormone deficiencies. The latter condition may be a result of pituitary damage from trauma, radiation, infection, sickle cell disease, compression by infiltrate or tumor, or autoimmune processes. In differentiating primary pituitary deficiency from that secondary to hypothalamic deficiency, the clinician should remember that all pituitary hormones except prolactin are stimulated by hypothalamic releasing hormones; prolactin is inhibited by hypothalamic prolactin inhibitory factor. Therefore, if all pituitary hormones, including prolactin, are deficient, the problem is in the pituitary gland. If prolactin levels are present or even elevated but the other pituitary hormones are deficient, the problem is above the pituitary gland in the stalk or hypothalamus. In the case of isolated LH and FSH deficiencies, the primary abnormality may lie within the pituitary or hypothalamic neurons producing GnRH; however, increasingly there is evidence of primary abnormalities being further upstream. In particular, defects in molecules required for proper migration of GnRH neurons (including the *KAL* gene) or lack of necessary signaling to GnRH-producing neurons (e.g., defects in kisspeptin or neurokinin B and their receptors) can result in LH and FSH deficiency through inappropriate GnRH secretion.

Hypergonadotropic Hypogonadism: Males

If the testes are small, they may have been damaged by torsion, sickle cell disease, infection, autoimmune disease, chemotherapy, or radiation and may not be able to respond to LH and FSH stimulation. If the bone age is >10 years and the hypothalamus has probably matured, the serum LH and FSH may then be high.

When the testis size is prepubertal and LH is present but testosterone is not increasing, there may be a problem with the LH receptor.

Klinefelter syndrome. This occurs in 1:500 males and is often associated with a 47,XXY karyotype; common features include cognitive delays, adolescent gynecomastia (often pronounced), and small, firm testes. The testes rarely exceed 5 mL in volume (approximately 25% of the average adult volume). Patients, often tall and thin with an eunuchoid habitus, may have delayed puberty. Virilization may be incomplete, the phallus is often smaller than average, and infertility nears 100%. These children will need testosterone treatment to fully attain secondary sexual characteristics.

Hypergonadotropic Hypogonadism: Females

In this condition, the ovary may be unable to synthesize estrogen (an inherited metabolic defect, possibly associated with excess adrenal mineralocorticoid and hypertension), the ovary may not be formed normally (dysgenesis), or the ovary may have been damaged by any of the factors listed for testicular damage and by galactosemia.

The ovary may be intact but may not be stimulated by gonadotropins. Gonadotropins are present but not effective if there is an FSH receptor problem.

TABLE 55.13 Genetic Heterogeneity of Kallmann Syndrome

Location	Phenotype	Inheritance	OMIM	Gene
1q32.1	Hypogonadotropic hypogonadism 13 with or without anosmia	AR	614842	KISS1
2q14.3	Hypogonadotropic hypogonadism 15 with or without anosmia	AD	614880	HS6ST1
3p14.3	Hypogonadotropic hypogonadism 18 with or without anosmia	AR/AD/Digenic	615267	IL17RD
3p13	Hypogonadotropic hypogonadism 4 with or without anosmia	AD	610628	PROK2
4q13.2	Hypogonadotropic hypogonadism 7 with or without anosmia	AR	146110	GNRHR
4q24	Hypogonadotropic hypogonadism 11 with or without anosmia	AR	614840	TACR3
4q27	Hypogonadotropic hypogonadism 25 with or without anosmia	AD	618841	NDNF
5q31.3	Hypogonadotropic hypogonadism 17 with or without anosmia	AD	615266	SPRY4
7q21.11	Hypogonadotropic hypogonadism 16 with or without anosmia	AD	614897	SEMA3A
7q31.32	Hypogonadotropic hypogonadism 22 with or without anosmia	AR	616030	FEZF1
8p21.3	Hypogonadotropic hypogonadism 20 with or without anosmia	AD	615270	FGF17
8p21.2	Hypogonadotropic hypogonadism 12 with or without anosmia	AR	614841	GNRH1
8p11.23	Hypogonadotropic hypogonadism 2 with or without anosmia	AD	147950	FGFR1
8q12.2	Hypogonadotropic hypogonadism 5 with or without anosmia	AD	612370	CHD7
9q34.3	Hypogonadotropic hypogonadism 9 with or without anosmia	AD	614838	NSMF
10q24.32	Hypogonadotropic hypogonadism 6 with or without anosmia	AD	612702	FGF8
10q26.12	Hypogonadotropic hypogonadism 14 with or without anosmia	AD	614858	WDR11
11p14.1	Hypogonadotropic hypogonadism 24 with or without anosmia	AR	229070	FSHB
12q13.3	Hypogonadotropic hypogonadism 10 with or without anosmia	AR	614839	TAC3
12q21.33	Hypogonadotropic hypogonadism 19 with or without anosmia	AD	615269	DUSP6
19p13.3	Hypogonadotropic hypogonadism 8 with or without anosmia	AR	614837	KISS1R
19q13.33	Hypogonadotropic hypogonadism 23 with or without anosmia	AR	228300	LHB
20p12.3	Hypogonadotropic hypogonadism 3 with or without anosmia	AD	244200	PROKR2
20p12.1	Hypogonadotropic hypogonadism 21 with or without anosmia	AD	615271	FLRT3
Xp22.31	Hypogonadotropic hypogonadism 1 with or without anosmia	XLR	308700	ANOS1

AD, autosomal dominant; AR, autosomal recessive; OMIM, Online Mendelian Inheritance in Man (www.OMIM.org); XLR, X-linked recessive.

Turner syndrome. The two most common features of Turner syndrome are short stature (involving the limbs to a greater degree than the trunk) and ovarian insufficiency (Fig. 55.11). Lymphedema and a webbed neck are diagnostic features present in a neonate. Additional features include a shield chest, increased carrying angle (cubitus valgus), short fourth metacarpal, hypoplastic nails, renal anomalies, and left-sided heart defects (coarctation of the aorta, bicuspid aortic or mitral valves, etc.). Approximately 50% of affected females have no stigmata except short stature and thus are typically identified later. About 20% may have spontaneous puberty with functioning ovaries for at least a short period of time, which is in large part dependent on the child's karyotype, but the infertility rate is >99%.

Females with Delayed or Absent Adrenarche

If a female has advanced breast development but no androgen signs, she may have a deficiency of androgen receptors, as occurs in **androgen insensitivity syndrome** (testicular feminization). In females, the androgens come predominantly from the adrenal glands (adrenarche). If the bone age has not passed 8 years, when DHEAS generally increases, adrenarche may simply be delayed (delayed adrenarche). If bone age is advanced, however, there is a deficiency in androgen production. In addition, there may be an inherited problem in androgen synthesis from an enzyme deficiency or the adrenal glands may be damaged secondary to autoimmune, infectious, or hypoxic injury. In these latter conditions, other signs of adrenal insufficiency would be evident.

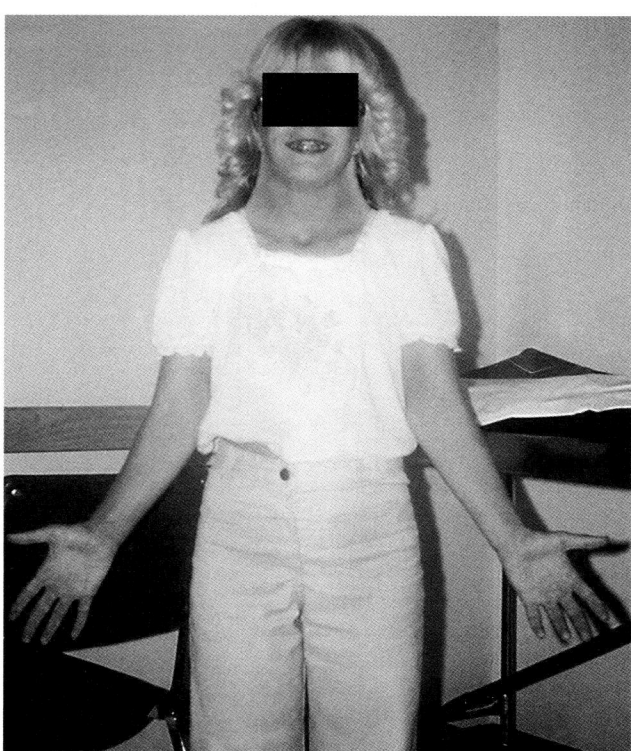

Fig. 55.11 A 16-year-old girl with Turner syndrome (45,XO), characterized by short stature, absence of thelarche, webbed neck, and increased carrying angles.

Diagnostic Approach to Delayed Puberty

A normal growth rate with delayed, but not absent, puberty and a family history of "late blooming" suggests the diagnosis of constitutional delay of growth and puberty, which is the most commonly encountered cause (see Tables 55.11 and 55.12). A bone age that correlates with the patient's pubertal status confirms the clinical impression; no other testing is necessary.

Initial evaluation should include:

- Medical history: trauma, illness, medications (e.g., stimulants, chemotherapy), radiation, infection, malnutrition, autoimmune problems, sickle status, stresses, growth records, galactosemia
- Review of symptoms: vision problems, headache, vomiting, inability to detect odors (hyposmia or anosmia), age at onset of androgen signs, age at onset of estrogen signs, small genitalia at birth, signs of primary adrenal insufficiency such as hyperpigmentation, need for deodorant, need to wash hair more frequently
- Family history: timing of maternal and paternal growth and pubertal development; siblings and cousins with delayed development

- Physical examination: signs of chronic disease, temperature, blood pressure, height, weight, head circumference, dental age, tanning (hyperpigmentation), pubic and axillary hair, adult body odor, skin and hair oils, visual fields, optic discs, ability to detect odors, breast development, vaginal cornification/discharge, penis size, scrotal development, testicular volume, pubic hair stages, neurologic status, affect or mood, intellectual ability, dysmorphic features

Initial laboratory evaluation screens for chronic disease include CBC, chemistry profile, and sedimentation rate, as well as free thyroxine and thyroid-stimulating hormone (hypothyroidism) and prolactin level (hyperprolactinemia). If growth is slow, the clinician should measure insulin-like growth factor-1 level (a marker of basal growth hormone activity) and consider growth hormone testing. The clinician should measure testosterone levels in males and estradiol levels in females.

Measurements of random FSH and LH and results of a GnRH stimulation test may differentiate between hypogonadotropic hypogonadism and primary gonadal failure (Figs. 55.12 and 55.13). Elevated

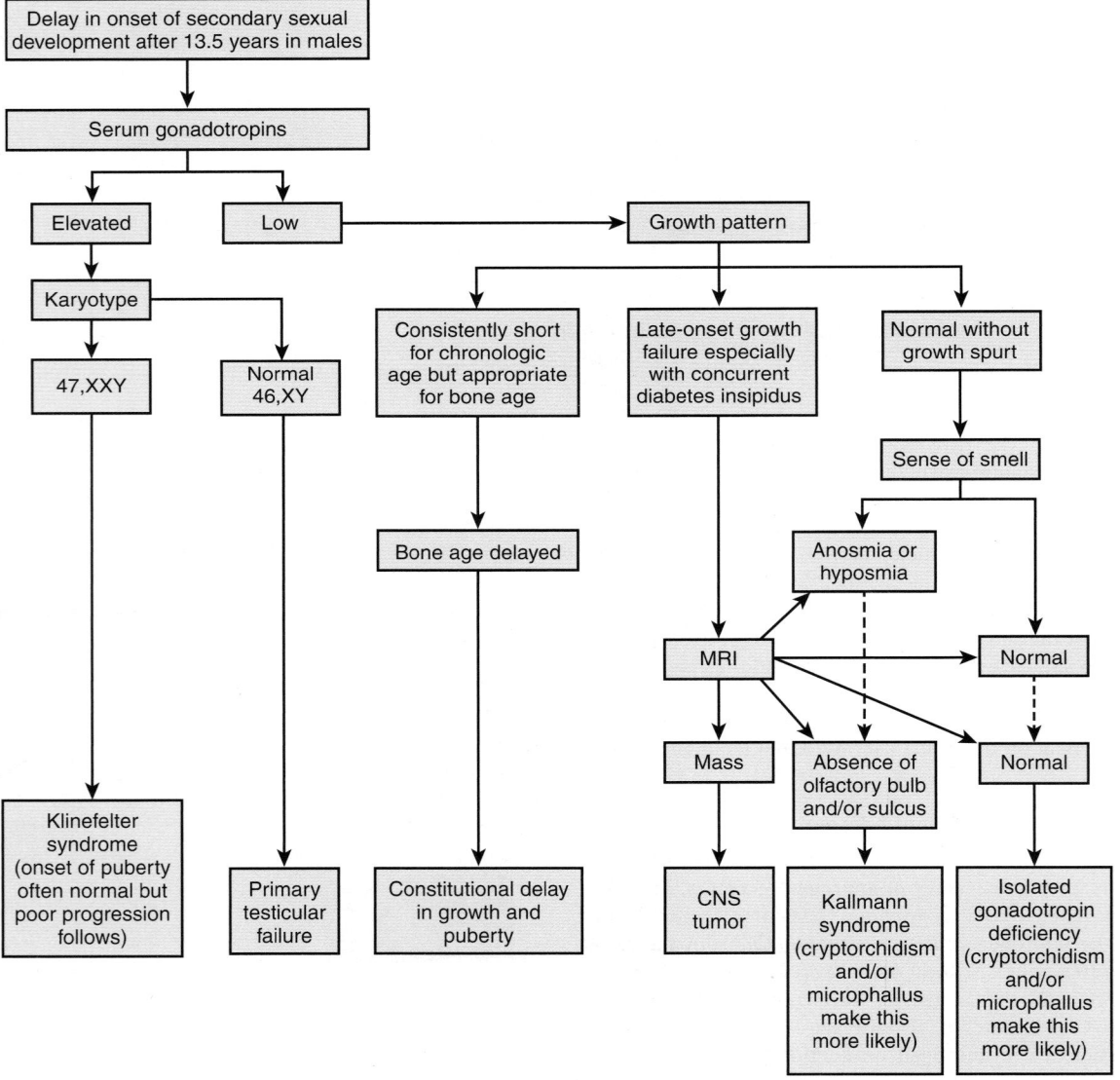

Fig. 55.12 Flow chart for the evaluation of delayed puberty in males. A brain MRI with absent olfactory bulb and/or sulcus is consistent with Kallmann syndrome, while a normal MRI suggests isolated gonadotropin deficiency. CNS, central nervous system. (From Melmed S, Polonsky KS, Larsen PR, et al., eds. *Williams Textbook of Endocrinology*. 13th ed. Philadelphia: Elsevier; 2016:1156.)

gonadotropin levels support a diagnosis of primary gonadal failure. Chromosomal karyotyping is then performed (Klinefelter syndrome in males and Turner syndrome in females). GnRH stimulation testing, with measurement of serum LH levels over 3–4 hours, is often employed. Its rationale is based on the fact that a child in puberty has a significant rise in serum LH over baseline. Unfortunately, the GnRH test is not helpful in distinguishing between constitutional delay and hypogonadotropic hypogonadism because in both cases, the LH response is blunted secondary to lack of endogenous GnRH priming of the gonadotrophs. However, the child with constitutional delay eventually develops an appropriate pubertal response to GnRH stimulation testing.

If **Kallmann syndrome** is being considered, an MRI scan may show abnormalities in the olfactory region. If a 46,XX female has unexplained ovarian failure, ovarian antibodies (21-hydroxylase antibodies) are obtained and müllerian-inhibiting substance or anti-müllerian hormone (AMH) can also be utilized in females to assess ovarian follicle reserve and potential fertility. An hCG stimulation test to evaluate ability to produce testosterone and a serum level of müllerian-inhibiting substance (secreted by Sertoli cells) are useful for determining whether functional testicular tissue is present.

Treatment of Delayed Puberty

If delayed puberty is **physiologic**, there is no medical necessity for initiating sex steroid replacement. "Watchful waiting" is usually the appropriate course of action. Adolescent males with constitutional delay of growth and puberty who are short, underdeveloped, and

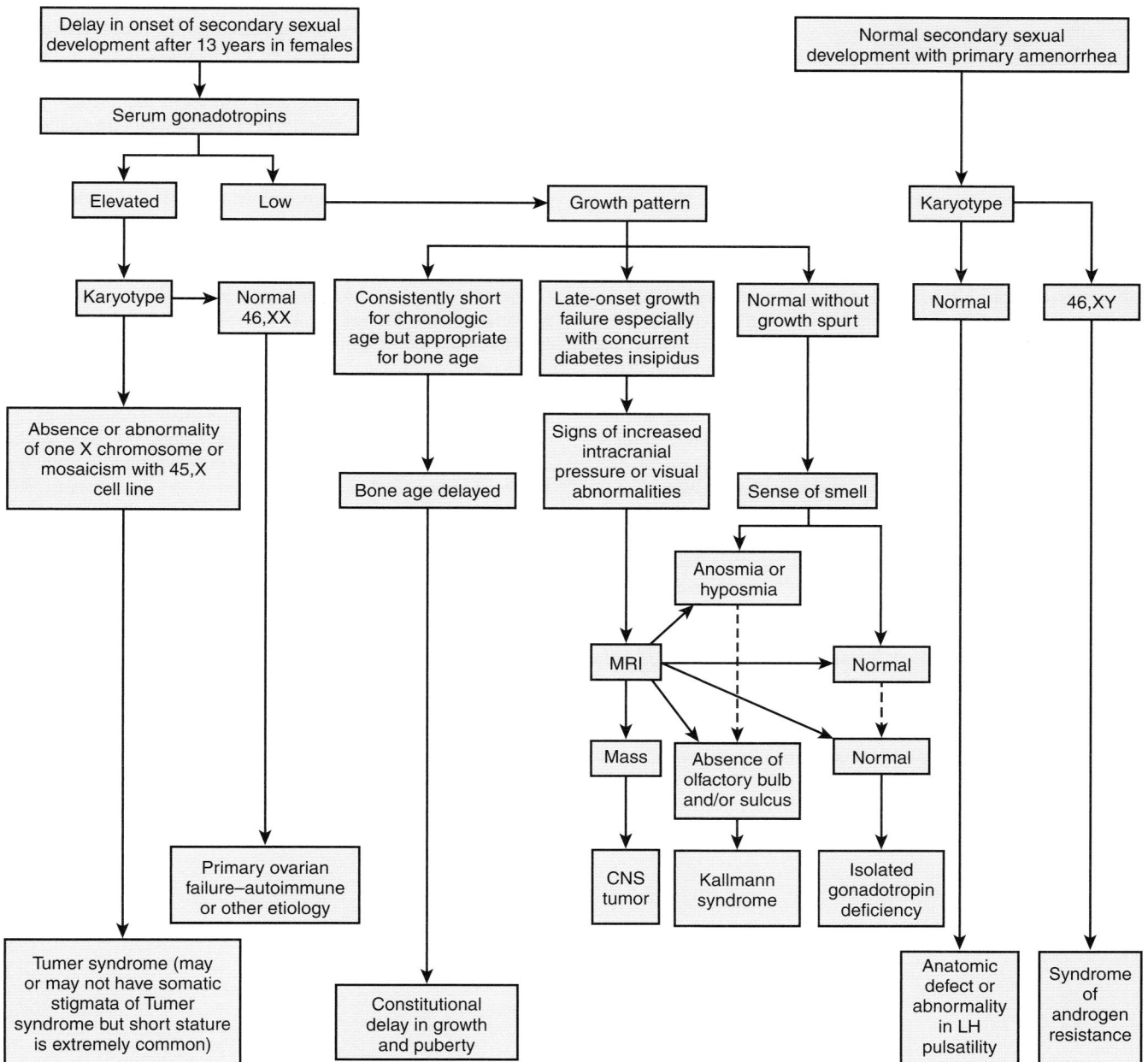

Fig. 55.13 Flow chart for the evaluation of delayed puberty in females. A brain MRI with absent olfactory bulb and/or sulcus is consistent with Kallmann syndrome, while a normal MRI suggests isolated gonadotropin deficiency. CNS, central nervous system; LH, luteinizing hormone. (From Melmed S, Polonsky KS, Larsen PR, et al., eds. *Williams Textbook of Endocrinology*. 13th ed. Philadelphia: Elsevier; 2016:1157.)

TABLE 55.14	Red Flags Related to Puberty
Pubertal changes in African-American females beginning before age 6 yr (excluding isolated thelarche from birth to 2 yr of age)
Pubertal changes in White females beginning before age 7 yr (excluding isolated thelarche from birth to 2 yr of age)
Pubertal changes in all males beginning before 9 yr of age
Absence of pubertal changes in females by 13 yr of age
Absence of pubertal changes in males by 14 yr of age
Neurologic signs and symptoms (headaches, visual disturbances)
Vaginal bleeding before breast development
Significantly asymmetric gonadal size in either sex (males, by clinical examination; females, by pelvic ultrasonography)
Testicular underdevelopment
Females with advancing breast development but no androgen signs
Galactorrhea
Pelvic mass

TABLE 55.15	Things Not to Miss with Regard to Puberty
Dysmorphic features
Unusual thinness or obesity
Cutaneous findings
Penis or clitoris diameter and length
Size of testes in patients with gynecomastia
Associated endocrine deficiencies or excesses

psychologically affected frequently benefit from a short course of testosterone therapy. This is usually given as long-acting intramuscular testosterone at a dosage of 50–100 mg every 4 weeks for typically 6 months. Treatment is generally begun at about 13 years of age and, if possible, when the testes are about 6–8 mL in volume. These doses stimulate height and weight gain, allow adequate virilization (increased pubic and axillary hair growth and penile enlargement), and do not typically suppress pituitary FSH and LH secretion, thereby allowing simultaneous endogenous pubertal progression (testicular enlargement). This narrows the physical gap between the patient and peers without causing undue advancement of bone age. Acne is the principal side effect, and the final adult height is not altered. It is the hope that at the conclusion of treatment, the male will continue to grow and develop rapidly with the testosterone treatment perceived as a "jump starter" of endogenous puberty. A short course of low-dose anabolic steroids, such as oxandrolone or fluoxymesterone, can also be employed in prepubertal and pubertal males, and low-dose estradiol has been used in prepubertal and pubertal females with constitutional delay.

Treatment of **hypogonadism** is aimed at mimicking normal physiology with stepwise replacement of testosterone in males and estrogen and progesterone in females. For males with hypogonadism, low-dose parenteral testosterone is initiated at 50 mg every 4 weeks, with increases in 50-mg increments made over a 2- to 3-year period. Most adult men receive 200 mg every 2 weeks, which is based on the daily adult male testosterone production rate of 6 mg. Some adult men are treated with 300 mg every 2 weeks. Adult men can use testosterone by patch, which is often associated with local irritation, or by alcohol-based gel, but typically in growing adolescents, intramuscular testosterone is prescribed.

For females, daily estrogen therapy is given for 1 year. This can be either in the form of conjugated estrogens (Premarin) at 0.3 mg daily for the first 6 months and 0.625 mg daily for the second 6 months, or with an analogous schedule of ethinyl estradiol replacement or through a weekly applied 17β-estradiol patch. This duration does not place the uterus at undue risk for hyperplasia and malignancy, but after 2 years of therapy (or if spotting occurs prior), progesterone should be added. Options to consider when adding progesterone include continuing the purely estrogen-containing pills (conjugated estrogens or ethinyl estradiol) or the 17β-estradiol patches in conjunction with oral medroxyprogesterone acetate (Provera) or switching the patient over to conventional oral contraceptives. If the patient is not put on a conventional oral contraceptive, the estrogen (pill or patch) is prescribed on days 1–23 of the calendar month with addition of medroxyprogesterone acetate on days 10–23. With this approach, withdrawal bleeding generally occurs between day 23 and the end of the month, although there can be some variability in the timing between patients.

Patients of either sex with hypogonadotropic hypogonadism are potentially fertile, but sex steroid therapy alone is ordinarily not sufficient to initiate gametogenesis, although there are rare cases in males in which testosterone replacement alone has stimulated spermatogenesis. The general approach to fertility induction in either sex involves the addition of either cyclic gonadotropin therapy or pump-driven GnRH therapy at the age of desired conception. *Finally, if hypogonadotropic hypogonadism is present as one component of hypopituitarism, it is critical to adequately replace all deficient hormones.* In contrast, patients with primary hypogonadism have intrinsic gonadal damage and are normally infertile.

SUMMARY AND RED FLAGS

Early, late, or asynchronous puberty can indicate underlying pathology. Red flags related to puberty are listed in Table 55.14. Important findings not to miss are listed in Table 55.15.

BIBLIOGRAPHY

A bibliography is available at ExpertConsult.com.

56

Short Stature

Omar Ali

Short stature (usually defined as height >2 standard deviations [SD] below the mean for age) and **growth failure** (a subnormal height velocity that leads to decline in growth percentiles, usually height velocity >1.5 SD below the mean for age) are *symptoms, not diseases*. Of the two, short stature is more likely to be noticed, *but growth failure is more likely to be pathologic.*

Short stature may represent a normal variant or it may be a signal of serious physical or emotional illness. Because linear growth is a crucial component of childhood, growth is in many ways an index of childhood well-being. Illnesses, even those not involving aberrations of growth-regulating hormones, often interfere with growth. Therefore, the measurement and charting of heights sequentially on standardized growth charts constitute a central part of a child's medical evaluation, and the finding of short stature, particularly if associated with a subnormal height velocity, deserves close attention and appropriate evaluation.

DEFINITION

Short stature is defined as height more than 2 SD below the mean for age, which is at the 2.3 percentile (Fig. 56.1*A*, *B*). On growth charts (and in clinical practice) it is more common to define short stature as height below the 3rd percentile for age, which is −1.88 SD. Implicit in this definition is the understanding that height is a normally distributed characteristic; therefore, a proportion of normal individuals have heights more than 2 SD above or below the mean. Since height is strongly heritable (i.e., a large proportion of the observed variation between individuals is hereditary), stature that is inappropriately low for the child's genetic endowment may also be a cause for concern.

Growth failure is defined as a subnormal rate of growth, a height velocity that is below the norm for that age. Since sustained height velocity below the 25th percentile is insufficient to maintain a child's position on the growth chart, growth failure is sometimes defined as height velocity below the 25th percentile for age. Other authorities prefer to use >1.5 SD below the average height velocity for that age as the cut-off (see Chapter 12).

Short stature should be distinguished from "failure to thrive." The latter term refers primarily to *poor weight gain* in infants and young children (although linear growth may be secondarily affected), whereas short stature refers primarily to subnormal linear growth in childhood and adolescence (see Chapter 12).

Normal Growth

Height is highly heritable, but the genetic program underlying this regulation is not fully understood. The growth of individual organs as well as the growth of the skeleton as a whole is regulated by negative feedback mechanisms that slow and eventually stop growth as organs and the organism reach their final size. This gradual deceleration of growth with age does not appear to be driven primarily by changes in the endocrine system, since levels of growth hormone (GH) and the insulin-like growth factors remain elevated even as growth slows in the latter part of puberty. The final height and growth pattern of any given individual are affected by subtle variations in many genes, while more significant variants in *individual-specific* genes cause the various genetic forms of short stature and skeletal dysplasias (Fig. 56.2).

FETAL GROWTH AND BIRTH SIZE

A human being experiences the most rapid linear growth in the *prenatal* period (growing from near-zero to about 50 cm in length in just 9 months). While genetic factors play a major role in postnatal growth, *fetal* growth and birth size mainly reflect maternal and placental factors, including maternal or uterine size, parity, multiparity, nutrition, and placental function. Many congenital disorders such as Turner syndrome and congenital GH deficiency that markedly stunt postnatal growth have only minimal effects on prenatal growth and birth size. Birth size is generally a poor predictor of the eventual growth pattern in most children. An exception is the neonate who is small for gestational age as a result of **intrauterine growth restriction (IUGR)** (Table 56.1). While most infants with IUGR (caused by nutritional problems or poor placental function) show catch-up growth (a period of rapid growth that occurs spontaneously after relief from the adverse intrauterine condition that had suppressed the rate of growth), 10–20% remain shorter than expected beyond infancy and early childhood, making IUGR one of the causes of childhood short stature.

Postnatal Growth Patterns

Infancy is also a period of relatively rapid growth (faster than at any other time in postnatal life). Growth then gradually slows as the infant gets older, declining to its lowest point just before puberty, before accelerating again during the pubertal growth spurt and finally ending with the completion of linear growth about 5 years after the onset of puberty (Table 56.2 and Fig. 56.3).

Since birth length is mostly determined by maternal and placental factors, size at birth may not reflect the infant's genetic growth potential. *It is during the first 2 years of life that infants gradually transition from their birth size to their own genetically determined height potential.* Therefore, it is normal for infants to shift linear growth percentiles during this period; 65% of infants will exhibit such shifts, moving up or down on the growth chart. By 24 months, these shifts are complete, and most children have entered a specific "growth channel" or linear growth percentile in relation to peers and any significant deviation from this channel should evince concern.

After a period of slow but steady growth during childhood, many children experience a further "prepubertal dip" in height velocity, reaching a nadir just before onset of puberty. Height velocity then

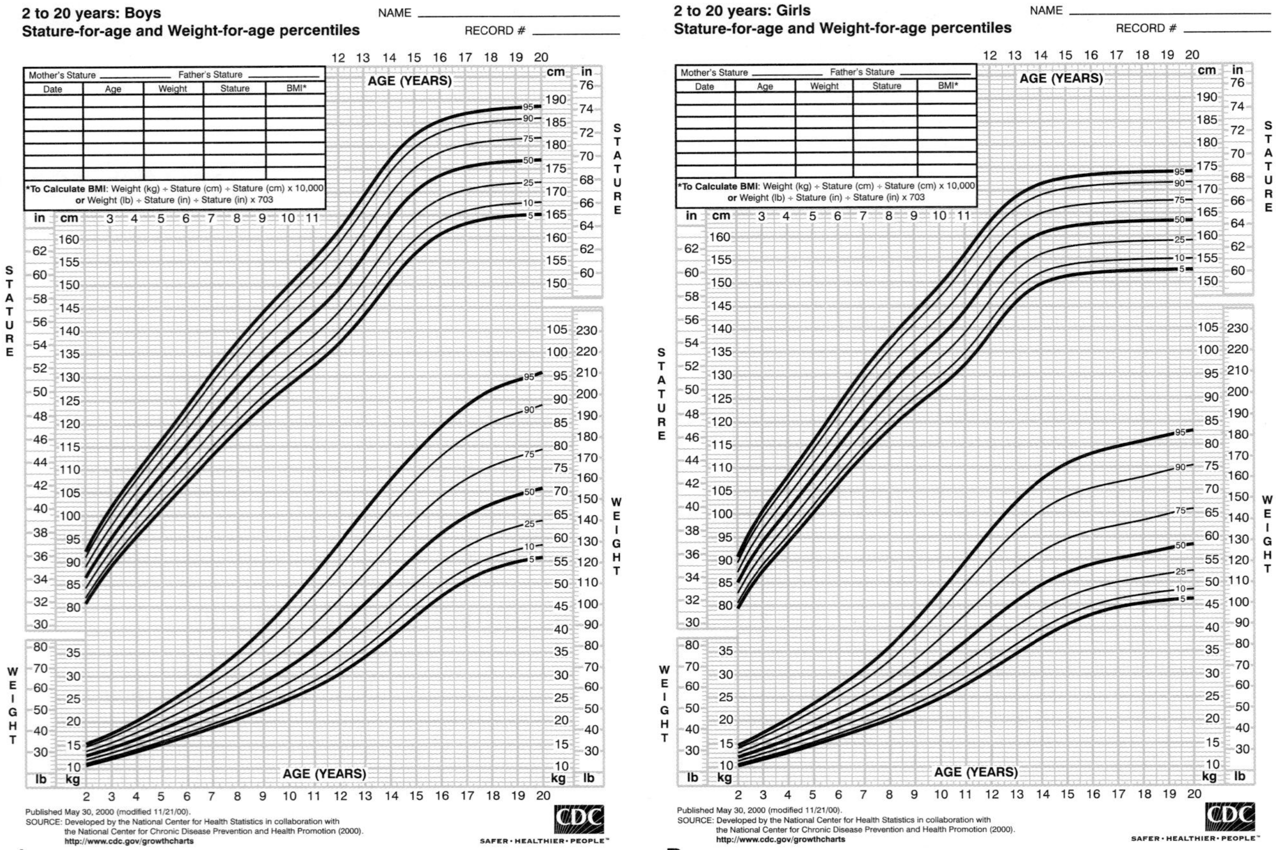

2 to 20 years: Boys
Stature-for-age and Weight-for-age percentiles

A

Fig. 56.1 Centers for Disease Control and Prevention (CDC) growth charts for ages 2–20. *A,* Males, stature for age. *B,* Females, stature for age.

2 to 20 years: Girls
Stature-for-age and Weight-for-age percentiles

B

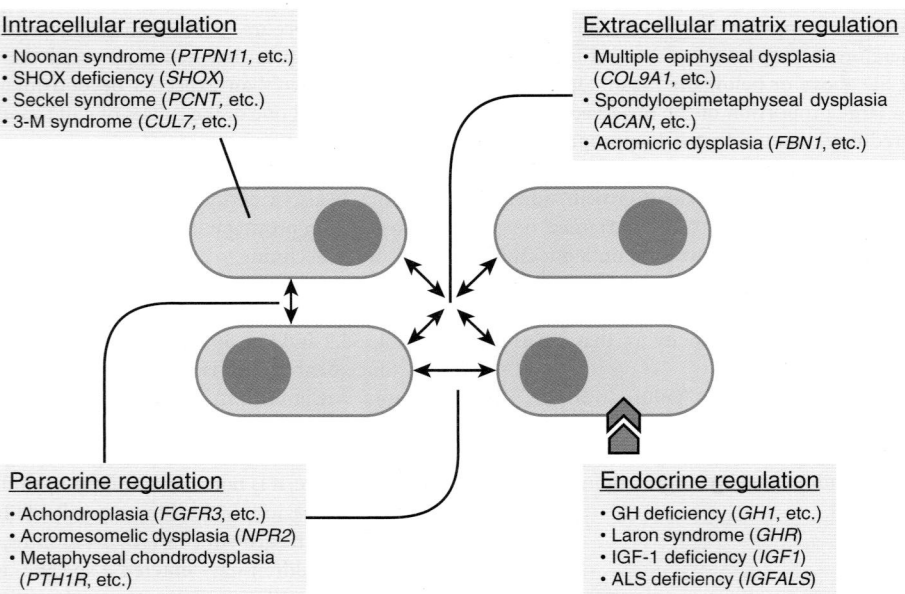

Intracellular regulation
- Noonan syndrome (*PTPN11*, etc.)
- SHOX deficiency (*SHOX*)
- Seckel syndrome (*PCNT*, etc.)
- 3-M syndrome (*CUL7*, etc.)

Extracellular matrix regulation
- Multiple epiphyseal dysplasia (*COL9A1*, etc.)
- Spondyloepimetaphyseal dysplasia (*ACAN*, etc.)
- Acromicric dysplasia (*FBN1*, etc.)

Paracrine regulation
- Achondroplasia (*FGFR3*, etc.)
- Acromesomelic dysplasia (*NPR2*)
- Metaphyseal chondrodysplasia (*PTH1R*, etc.)

Endocrine regulation
- GH deficiency (*GH1*, etc.)
- Laron syndrome (*GHR*)
- IGF-1 deficiency (*IGF1*)
- ALS deficiency (*IGFALS*)

Fig. 56.2 Molecular mechanisms of short stature. Short stature is caused by multiple molecular defects, including intracellular signaling, extracellular matrix, and paracrine and endocrine regulation. *Ovoid shapes* represent growth plate chondrocytes. *Arrows* indicate mechanisms regulating chondrocytes. Examples of clinical syndrome and the genetic cause under different molecular mechanisms are shown in each box. GH, growth hormone; IGF, insulin-like growth factor. (From Jee YH, Andrade AC, Baron J, et al., Genetics of short stature. *Endocrinol Metab Clin N Am.* 2017;46[2]:259–281, Fig. 1.)

TABLE 56.1 Factors Often Associated with Intrauterine Growth Restriction

FETAL

Chromosomal and genetic disorders

Chronic fetal infections (cytomegalic inclusion disease, congenital rubella, syphilis)

Congenital anomalies—syndrome complexes

Irradiation

Multiple gestation

Pancreatic hypoplasia

Insulin deficiency (production or action of insulin)

Insulin-like growth factor type 1 deficiency

PLACENTAL

Decreased placental weight, cellularity, or both

Decrease in surface area

Villous placentitis (bacterial, viral, parasitic)

Infarction

Tumor (chorioangioma, hydatidiform mole)

Placental separation

Twin transfusion syndrome

MATERNAL/PATERNAL

Toxemia

Hypertension or renal disease, or both

Hypoxemia (high altitude, cyanotic cardiac or pulmonary disease)

Malnutrition (micronutrient or macronutrient deficiencies)

Chronic illness

Sickle cell anemia

Drugs (narcotics, alcohol, cigarettes, cocaine, antimetabolites)

IGF2 gene variant (paternal)

From Kliegman RM, St. Geme JW III, Blum NJ, et al., eds. *Nelson Textbook of Pediatrics.* 21st ed. Philadelphia: Elsevier; 2020, Table 117.4.

TABLE 56.2 Growth Velocity at Various Ages

Age Interval	Average Height Velocity
Prenatal	66 cm/yr
0–1 yr	25 cm/yr
1–2 yr	12 cm/yr
2–3 yr	8 cm/yr
3–5 yr	7 cm/yr
5 yr–onset of puberty	5–6 cm/yr
Pubertal growth spurt	Girls 8–12 cm
	Boys 10–14 cm

accelerates once again as puberty advances. This acceleration of growth during puberty reaches a peak known as the "pubertal growth spurt." The timing of the pubertal growth spurt differs between females and males. Females generally begin pubertal development at 10 to 11 years of age and their pubertal growth spurt starts coincidentally with breast development and peaks before menarche. For females with an average tempo of puberty, peak growth velocity (8–9 cm per year) is reached at 11–12 years of age. After menarche (which generally occurs 2–2.5 years after onset of puberty), the growth rate declines and growth finally stops about 2 years after menarche, with girls gaining an average of 7 cm in height after menarche.

In males, testicular enlargement is generally the first sign of puberty and occurs at approximately 11.5 years on average (range, 9–14.3 years). In males with an average tempo of pubertal development, peak growth velocity occurs about 2 years after onset of puberty (so it is later than girls in absolute terms, as well as in terms of stage of puberty) at approximately 13–14 years, with an average rate of 10.3 cm (4 inches) per year. *It is worth noting that prepubertal males and females grow at very similar rates; the ultimate taller stature of males relative to females is mostly the result of a longer period of growth and a higher peak growth velocity during puberty.*

These are the *average* timings of puberty and pubertal growth, but it should be kept in mind that there are large variations in the timing of puberty—and therefore in growth rates—among individuals of the same age during the period of adolescence.

Because of these characteristic patterns of growth during childhood and adolescence, the rate of growth (centimeters per year or inches per year) is a key variable in evaluating a short child. Growth rates may vary somewhat with season and can be affected by transient illness, but a child should maintain a relatively set growth channel on the linear growth percentile charts after 2–3 years of age. A persistently slow rate of growth in relation to age-appropriate norms is alarming and is likely to reflect an underlying medical disorder.

MEASURING A CHILD

Stature is evaluated as supine length until 2 years of age and as standing height thereafter (Fig. 56.4). For measurement of supine length, an infant lies on an inflexible ruled horizontal surface, at one end of which one person holds the infant's head in contact with a fixed board; a second person extends the infant's leg as much as possible and brings a movable plate in contact with the infant's heel. *Recumbent measurements average 1 cm (0.4 inch) more than standing height.*

After 2 years of age, children are measured standing and barefoot with a device such as a Harpenden stadiometer; a vertical metal bar is affixed to an upright board or wall, and height is measured at the top of the head by a sliding perpendicular plate or block. *Measurements of length using pen marks on the examining table at the head and foot of infants are often grossly inaccurate, as are height measurements using a flexible metal rod atop a standard weight scale.*

With the use of optimal techniques, the variation in measurement among observers is <0.3 cm (0.1 inch). It is then possible to determine changes in height over 3- to 4-month intervals to estimate the annualized growth rate. However, because of normal seasonal variations in growth rates, a longer interval between measurements (6–12 months) is more reliable in the calculation of height velocity.

Measurements are then plotted on standard growth charts; it is recommended that World Health Organization (WHO) growth charts be used for infants from birth to 2 years of age and Centers for Disease Control and Prevention (CDC) growth charts for children from ages 2 to 18 years (see Fig. 56.1). These CDC and WHO growth charts are available at http://www.cdc.gov/growthcharts/ and https://www.who.int/childgrowth/standards/en/.

For children with specific disorders, such as Turner syndrome, there are disorder-specific standardized growth curves for many of these disorders. Children with known disorders should be plotted on these curves to avoid unintentional evaluation for growth failure, as they may appear to be abnormally short on the standard growth charts. Calculated growth rates (centimeters per year or inches per year) should be evaluated in relation to age-related norms with growth velocity charts for North American children for children over 2 years of age (see Fig. 56.3).

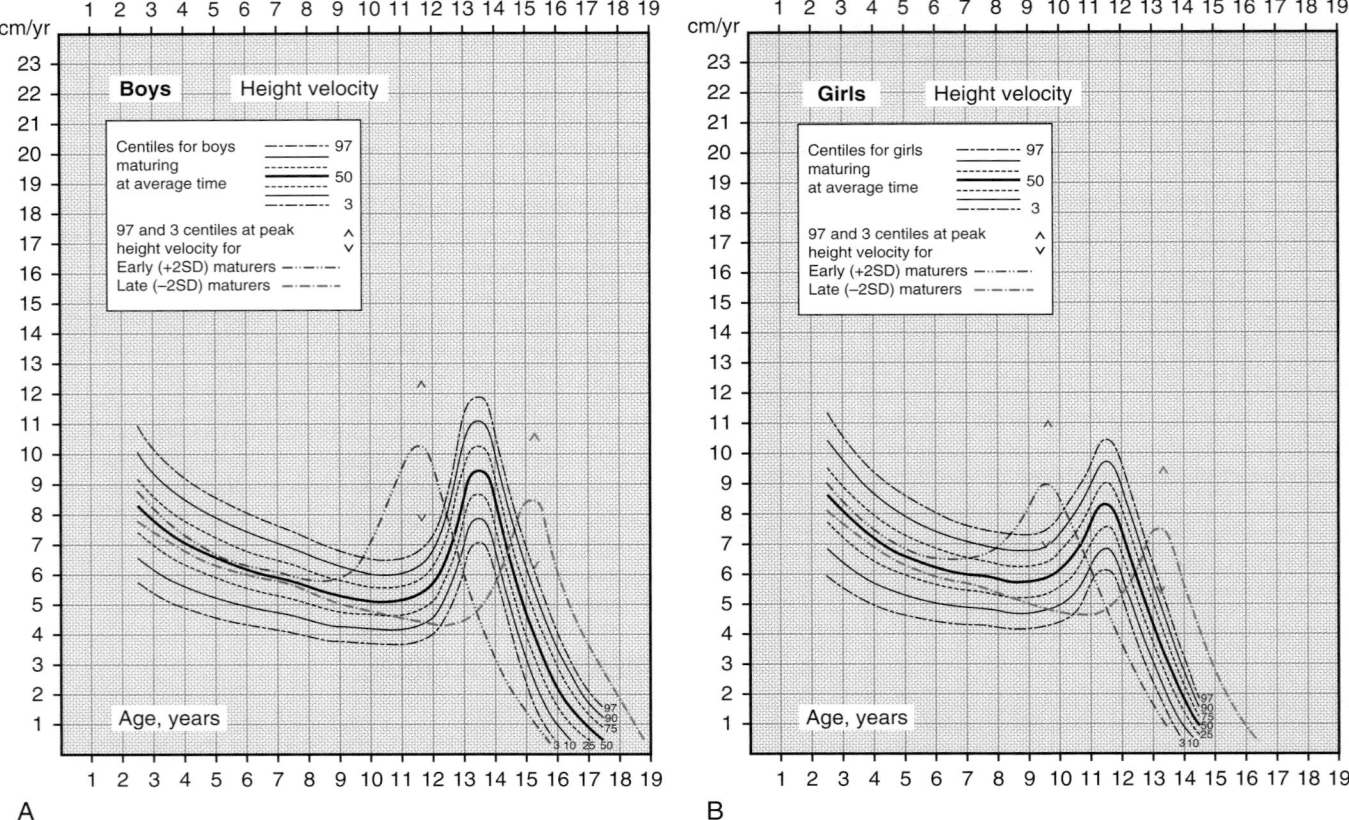

Fig. 56.3 *A,* Height velocity for American males. Lines with early velocity refer to the 50th centile for boys 2 standard deviations (SD) early in growth tempo; lines with late or gradual velocity refer to the 50th centile for boys 2 SD late in growth tempo. ^ and v, 97th and 3rd centiles for peak velocities of early and late maturers, respectively. *B,* Height velocity for American females. Lines with early velocity refer to the 50th centile for girls 2 SD early in growth tempo; lines with late or gradual velocity refer to the 50th centile for girls 2 SD late in growth tempo. ^ and v, 97th and 3rd centiles for peak velocities of early and late maturers, respectively. (Redrawn from Tanner J, Davies P. Clinical longitudinal standards for height and height velocity in North American children. *J Pediatr.* 1985;107:317–329.)

BODY PROPORTIONS

The cephalo-caudal ratios change with age until adult height is attained (Fig. 56.5). Thus, apart from linear height, it is also useful to assess the upper-to-lower segment ratio (U/L) (Fig. 56.6) and the arm span. The U/L is determined by measuring the lower segment (vertical distance between the top of the symphysis pubis and the floor, with the child standing) and the upper segment (height minus lower segment). Arm span is the distance between the outstretched middle fingertips with the child standing against a flat board or wall. The U/L and arm span are used to determine whether the child is normally proportioned or not (in Europe it is more common to assess sitting height vs standing height for the same purpose).

The U/L gradually declines with age throughout childhood (see Fig. 56.6). Since infants have relatively short legs, the U/L is high (an average of 1.7) at birth. It then declines throughout childhood as the legs increase in length relative to the upper body, decreasing to a mean of 0.9 by late puberty (in males; in females the ratio may be closer to 0.95). The arm span as compared to the height is another measure of body proportions and is normally shorter than the height in younger children and increases to become slightly longer than the height by late puberty (about 5 cm more than height in boys, 1.2 cm more than height in girls). Deviations from the norm in the U/L and the arm span may point to syndromic conditions such as skeletal dysplasias,

Turner syndrome, or longstanding hypothyroidism (increased U/L, i.e., relatively short extremities) and radiation-induced spinal damage or genetic disorders like Klinefelter or Marfan syndrome and homocystinuria (low U/L, due to a relatively short trunk or unusually long extremities).

Weight should also be considered in relation to a child's stature. Undernutrition is generally caused by nonendocrine factors (poor nutritional intake, malabsorption, systemic illness) and typically leads to a decrease in weight before a decrease in linear growth. Obesity in childhood is usually exogenous; exogenous obesity is generally associated with an accelerated growth rate. In contrast, endocrine disorders that cause poor growth and short stature are often associated with weight gain and obesity (Cushing syndrome, hypothyroidism, and, in some instances, GH deficiency). Therefore, the obese child who has a slow growth velocity is more likely to have an endocrine cause of short stature, while the undernourished child with short stature likely has short stature secondary to poor weight gain and is unlikely to have an endocrine disorder.

Familial and Genetic Factors

Both parental height and parental pattern of growth are key determinants of a child's growth pattern. This strong familial influence on height is not detectable at birth but is manifested by 2–3 years of age. Final adult height is strongly heritable with heritability estimates ranging

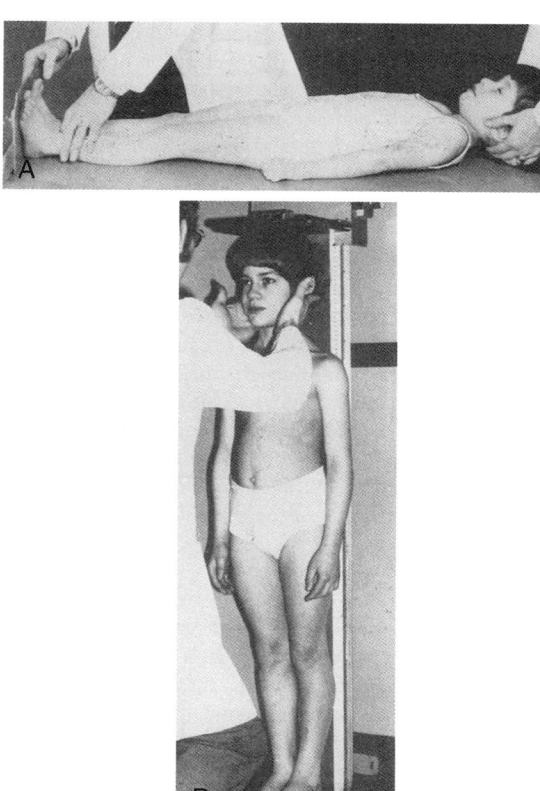

Fig. 56.4 *A,* Technique for measuring length. *B,* Technique for measuring erect height. (From Wilson JD, Foster DW, eds. *Williams Textbook of Endocrinology.* 8th ed. Philadelphia: WB Saunders; 1992:1106–1107.)

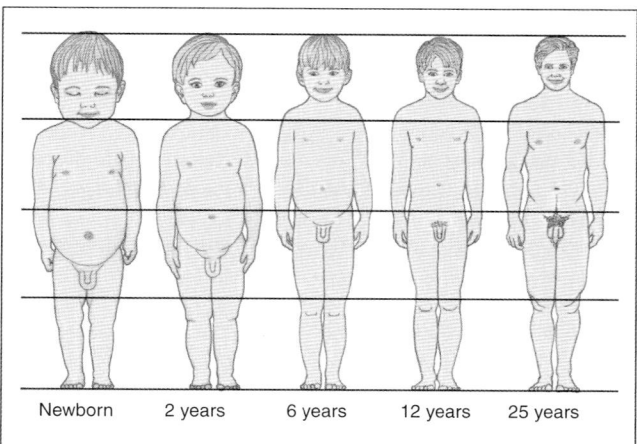

Fig. 56.5 Approximate changes in body proportions from birth through adulthood. (Modified from Leifer G. *Introduction to Maternity & Pediatric Nursing.* Philadelphia: Saunders; 2011:347–385, Fig. 15-2.)

from 0.8 to 0.95 (i.e., 80–95% of the observed variation is explained by hereditary rather than environmental factors). The midparental height (MPH) is used as a measure of the child's genetic growth potential and is an average of the height of both parents *after correcting for gender.* Because the average adult male is taller than the average adult female by 13 cm (5 inches), 13 cm is added to the mother's height in the case of a male child, while 13 cm is subtracted from the father's height in the case of a female child; the parental heights, after correction for gender, are then averaged to obtain the MPH.

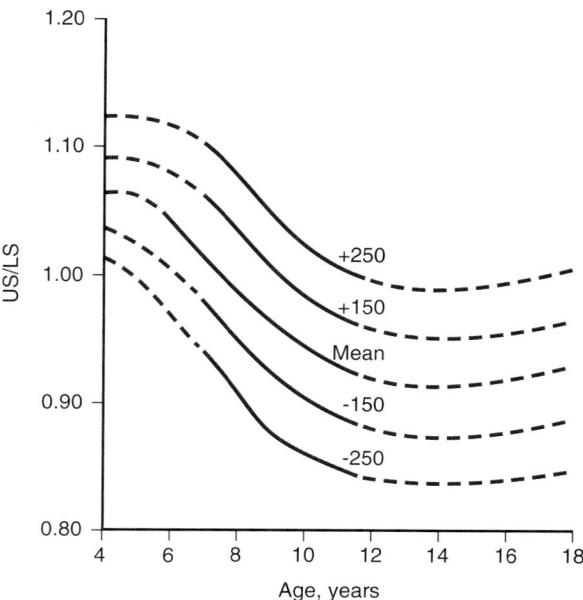

Fig. 56.6 Normal upper-to-lower segment ratios (US/LS) for White children. (From McKusick V. *Hereditable Disorders of Connective Tissue.* 4th ed. St. Louis: CV Mosby; 1972.)

MPH is determined in the following manner:

Males: [father's height in cm + (mother's height in cm + 13 cm)]/2

Females: [(father's height in cm − 13 cm) + mother's height in cm] /2

The MPH is a good index of the child's genetic height potential but tends to become less accurate if one parent is unusually tall or short; that is, the offspring of an exceptionally tall parent or exceptionally short parent will be closer to the average height than is predicted by the MPH because of the phenomenon of *regression to the mean.*

In addition to the influence on final adult height, parents' *patterns* of growth are also often repeated in their children. In particular, many males who were "late bloomers" with delayed onset of puberty and delayed but normal growth spurts have sons with a similar growth pattern.

Ethnic Factors and Secular Trend

The average height of various populations across the globe is not the same; Northern European populations are taller than many (but not all) other ethnic groups and it therefore seems to make sense to use population-specific standards of growth because a child from a generally short ethnic group may be labeled as "short stature" by Northern European standards, but may be normal for their own ethnic group. Two additional observations need to be kept in mind though:

1. Migrants from countries where the average height is lower tend to have children who are taller than their parents when they move to a country with a higher standard of living. This indicates that at least some of the observed height difference may be environmental (most likely related to nutrition and childhood disease burden) and that this height difference may shrink or disappear in subsequent generations.
2. The Northern European populations were themselves much shorter in the 18th and 19th centuries and average heights have steadily increased as living standards improved (reflecting improvements in nutrition and other public health measures). This "secular trend"

in height slows down and plateaus over time (most likely because a "genetic ceiling" is reached) but is much more marked in populations that have recently seen an improvement in living standards.

Practitioners should make allowances for ethnic differences in height when evaluating children from different ethnic backgrounds but should not automatically assume such differences as the sole explanation for short stature in children from historically shorter populations. *Growth velocity in particular should not be abnormal even in historically shorter populations, and a subnormal growth velocity should trigger an evaluation in the same way as it would in children from a Northern European background.*

GENERAL WELL-BEING

Because growth is a barometer of a child's health and general well-being, freedom from serious illness is necessary for a child to achieve their genetic growth potential. Chronic illnesses that are not primarily problems of stature often interfere with growth secondarily, and short stature may be the presenting feature of such conditions as inflammatory bowel disease, celiac disease, and renal disease.

Psychological Factors

Under normal circumstances, emotional and psychological factors do not have a great effect on growth. However, in certain cases, *emotional deprivation* can lead to very significant growth failure (sometimes labeled "deprivation dwarfism" or "psychosocial dwarfism") via mechanisms that are still poorly understood.

Endocrine Regulation of Growth

Growth hormone (GH) is produced by the anterior pituitary under the control of growth hormone–releasing hormone (GHRH) from the hypothalamus and is essential for normal growth in childhood and adolescence (though it appears to play a relatively small role in prenatal growth). GH is secreted in brief pulses and peak secretion occurs during sleep, so random serum levels have little utility in the evaluation of GH deficiency except in the immediate newborn period (when random GH levels are usually elevated and a level below 7 ng/mL is very likely to reflect GH deficiency).

GH exerts its growth-promoting effect mainly through stimulating the production of **insulin-like growth factor 1 (IGF-1)** (primarily in the liver, but also in some target tissues), though there is also some direct actions of GH on bone. Most circulating IGF-1 is bound to IGF-binding proteins, with the largest proportion being bound in a ternary complex with **IGF-binding protein-3 (IGFBP3)** and a protein named the acid-labile-subunit (ALS). Because IGF-1 levels in the blood are stable through the day and reflect the integrated effect of GH secretion, measurement of IGF-1 is often used as a surrogate measure of GH secretion.

Thyroid hormone also has a relatively limited role in prenatal growth but is essential for normal postnatal linear growth, both via direct actions on the epiphyseal growth plate and via a permissive effect on GH secretion. **Hypothyroidism** can therefore lead to very profound growth failure and an evaluation of thyroid hormone status is essential in the investigation of growth failure.

Glucocorticoids do not play any significant role in normal growth but are powerful inhibitors of growth when present in excess. Persistent exposure to excess corticosteroids (whether endogenous or exogenous) can lead to very severe growth failure (along with significant weight gain). Deficiency of glucocorticoids generally does not adversely affect growth if the child is otherwise healthy.

Sex steroids mediate the pubertal growth spurt (see Chapter 55). This involves direct effects of sex steroids on bone growth as well as steroid-induced amplification of GH secretion. Most of the bone-maturing action of sex steroids is mediated by estrogen in *both* sexes; while testosterone has some direct effect on bone strength and thickness, most of the effects of testosterone on linear growth and the maturation of growth plates in males also occur via the action of estrogen produced by the peripheral conversion of testosterone. Consequently, even in males, bone maturation can be affected by genetic defects in the production or action of estrogen, as well as by pharmacologic inhibition of this pathway (e.g., by using aromatase inhibitors that block the conversion of testosterone to estrogen). **Sexual precocity** (true precocious puberty, exogenous exposure, or congenital adrenal hyperplasia) tends to accelerate linear growth transiently as a result of premature or excessive production of sex steroids (see Chapter 55). But, if left untreated, these conditions eventually advance osseous maturation, leading to premature epiphyseal fusion and short final adult height. Absence of sex steroids (**hypogonadism**), in the absence of other abnormalities, blunts the pubertal growth spurt but tends not to limit final height as bone maturation and epiphyseal fusion are also delayed by the lack of estrogen in these patients.

BONE AGE

Osseous maturation follows a very predictable pattern during the growth and development of the child and an X-ray of the *nondominant hand* can be used to assess bone age (i.e., the degree of maturation of the bones compared to age-matched standards). Bone age is usually estimated by comparing the child's radiologic findings with a standard set of radiologic images, or by using various scoring algorithms. These readings are subject to observer bias and error (other methods that use artificial intelligence to automatically assess bone age may bypass this issue) but are still useful as long as this inherent subjectivity is kept in mind. Bone age is very closely correlated with pubertal maturation, and an assessment of bone age can be especially useful in cases of precocious puberty, delayed puberty, and constitutional growth delay. Except in cases of precocious puberty, bone age is rarely useful in the evaluation of short stature in a child younger than 5 years of age.

Causes of Short Stature

Understanding the factors that influence childhood growth leads directly to an understanding of the causes of short stature and to the differential diagnosis of short stature for an individual child (Tables 56.3, 56.4, 56.5, 56.6, and 56.7). While a very large number of conditions can potentially lead to short stature and growth failure, the vast majority of children with short stature either are normal variants (familial short stature, constitutional delay of growth and puberty) or have no discernible cause (idiopathic short stature). It is also important to remember that the child with *growth failure* is far more likely to have an underlying pathology than a child who happens to be short but has a normal growth velocity.

Normal Variants

The two most frequent causes of short stature in children are **familial short stature** and **constitutional delay of growth and puberty**. These are considered normal variants and their recognition can help avoid expensive and unnecessary testing and interventions.

Familial Short Stature

The term *familial short stature* is usually reserved for familial forms of mild to moderate short stature that do not have a specific identifiable genetic defect; since hundreds of genes play a role in growth, this height potential reflects the influence of multiple loci of small effect or a few loci of relatively moderate effect. Genetic disorders that result in severe short stature, or that are associated with other abnormal physical

TABLE 56.3 Classification of Growth Disorders

I. PROPORTIONAL SHORT STATURE
  A. GENETIC CAUSES
    Single-gene disorders (GHRH-receptor, GH gene, SHOX, etc.)
    Syndromic short stature (Prader-Willi syndrome, Russell-Silver syndrome, etc.)
    Polygenic (familial) short stature
    Chromosomal abnormalities
      Turner syndrome
      Down syndrome
  B. SECONDARY GROWTH DISORDERS
    A. Malnutrition
    B. Chronic disease
      Cardiac disorders
        Left-to-right shunts
        Congestive heart failure
      Pulmonary disorders
        Cystic fibrosis
      Gastrointestinal disorders
        Inflammatory bowel disease
        Celiac disease
        Malabsorption
        Chronic diarrhea
      Hematologic disorders
        Chronic anemia (including sickle cell disease, thalassemias)
      Renal disorders
        Chronic renal failure
        Renal tubular acidosis
      Immunologic disorders
        Congenital immunodeficiency
        HIV
    C. Intrauterine growth restriction
    D. Endocrine disorders
      Hypothyroidism
      Growth hormone deficiency
      IGF-1 deficiency or resistance
      Cushing syndrome
      Pseudohypoparathyroidism
      Vitamin D–deficient or –resistant rickets
  C. IDIOPATHIC SHORT STATURE (ISS)
  D. CONSTITUTIONAL DELAY OF GROWTH AND PUBERTY
II. DISPROPORTIONATE SHORT STATURE (skeletal dysplasias) (see Table 56.4)

GH, growth hormone; GHRH, growth hormone–releasing hormone; IGF-1, insulin-like growth factor 1.

TABLE 56.4 Nosology and Classification of Genetic Skeletal Disorders: 2019 Revision

1. FGFR3 chondrodysplasia group
2. Type 2 collagen group
3. Type 11 collagen group
4. Sulphation disorders group
5. Perlecan group
6. Aggrecan group
7. Filamin group and related disorders
8. TRPV4 group
9. Ciliopathies with major skeletal involvement
10. Multiple epiphyseal dysplasia and pseudoachondroplasia group
11. Metaphyseal dysplasias
12. Spondylometaphyseal dysplasias (SMDs)
13. Spondylo-epi-(meta)-physeal dysplasias (SEMDs)
14. Severe spondylodysplastic dysplasias
15. Acromelic dysplasias
16. Acromesomelic dysplasias
17. Mesomelic and rhizo-mesomelic dysplasias
18. Bent bone dysplasia group
19. Primordial dwarfism and slender bones group
20. Dysplasias with multiple joint dislocations
21. Chondrodysplasia punctata (CDP) group
22. Neonatal osteosclerotic dysplasias
23. Osteopetrosis and related disorders
24. Other sclerosing bone disorders
25. Osteogenesis imperfecta and decreased bone density group
26. Abnormal mineralization group
27. Lysosomal storage diseases with skeletal involvement (dysostosis multiplex group)
28. Osteolysis group
29. Disorganized development of skeletal components group
30. Overgrowth (tall stature) syndromes with skeletal involvement
31. Genetic inflammatory/rheumatoid-like osteoarthropathies
32. Cleidocranial dysplasia and related disorders
33. Craniosynostosis syndromes
34. Dysostoses with predominant craniofacial involvement
35. Dysostoses with predominant vertebral with and without costal involvement
36. Patellar dysostoses
37. Brachydactylies (without extraskeletal manifestations)
38. Brachydactylies (with extraskeletal manifestations)
39. Limb hypoplasia–reduction defects group
40. Ectrodactyly with and without other manifestations
41. Polydactyly-syndactyly-triphalangism group
42. Defects in joint formation and synostoses

From Mortier GR, et al. Nosology and classification of genetic skeletal disorders: 2019 revision. *Am J Med Genet.* 2019;179A:2393–2419.

findings (syndromes), or that are caused by known genetic defects (see Table 56.7), are conventionally treated separately from familial short stature. In familial short stature the child's height is in keeping with their genetic endowment, and the child is otherwise healthy. Typically, one or both parents (and often other family members) are about 1.5 to 2 SD below the mean in height. This relatively short genetic potential is reflected in short MPH, and if the child continues to grow along the current percentile, the child would fall within 9 cm of this MPH (this is approximately 2 SD of the MPH); by age 2 the child is usually noted to be small in relation to peers. Although the growth channel is low, it should *parallel the normal growth curve* from that point onward. Continued deviation away from the normal growth curve (indicating a subnormal growth velocity) is *not* typical and should raise concerns about a disorder other than familial short stature. Stature that is extremely low

(2.5–3 or more SD below the mean) raises concerns even if the parents are short, since this degree of short stature may reflect a specific genetic cause of short stature (e.g., a mild defect in GH secretion or action, or a form of hypochondroplasia) in the parents as well as the child.

The review of systems is generally negative in the otherwise healthy child, as are the physical examination findings (aside from short stature). The height-to-weight ratio, body proportions, muscularity, and pubertal development are normal for age. Abnormalities found on review of systems or physical examination should prompt consideration of other diagnoses.

Laboratory studies are not mandatory but if done are all normal. The bone age is also normal. Prediction of adult height can be made on the basis of bone age but the accuracy is variable; the predicted height is within 9 cm of the MPH.

TABLE 56.5 Genetic Defects of the GH-IGF Axis Resulting in Somatotroph Dysfunction and GH Deficiency

Factor	Gene Function	Affected Cell Types	Clinical Phenotype	Mode of Inheritance
Gene Variants in Factors Resulting in Growth Hormone and Associated Hormone Deficiencies				
Hesx1	• Paired-like homeobox gene • Early marker for pituitary primordium and Rathke pouch • Requires Lhx3 for maintenance and PROP1 for repression	Somatotrophs, thyrotrophs, gonadotrophs (posterior pituitary may also be affected)	• Isolated GH deficiency or multiple hormone deficiency (including diabetes insipidus) • Puberty may be delayed • Associated with septo-optic dysplasia • Abnormal MRI findings: pituitary hypoplasia, ectopic posterior pituitary, midline forebrain abnormalities	AD, AR
Lhx3 (Lim 3, P-LIM)	• Member of LIM-homeodomain family of gene regulatory proteins • Required for survival and proliferation of Rathke pouch • Activates α-GSU promoter • Acts with Pit1 to activate TSH-β gene promoter	Somatotrophs, lactotrophs, thyrotrophs, gonadotrophs, possibly corticotrophs	• Patients may present with rigid cervical spine causing limited neck rotation • Hypoplastic anterior/intermediate pituitary lobe	AR
Lhx4	• A LIM protein with close resemblance to Lhx3 • Important for proliferation and differentiation of cell lineages • May have overlapping function with PROP1 and POU1F1	Somatotrophs, lactotrophs, thyrotrophs, gonadotrophs, corticotrophs	• Combined pituitary hormone deficiencies with predominant GH deficiency • Severe anterior pituitary hypoplasia, ectopic neurohypophysis	AD
SIX6	• Member of the *SIX/sine oculis* family of homeobox genes • Expressed early in hypothalamus, later in Rathke pouch, neural retina, and optic chiasma	Somatotrophs, gonadotrophs	• Bilateral anophthalmia • Pituitary hypoplasia • Associated with deletion at chromosome 14q22-23	Unknown
FGF8, FGFR1, PROKR2	• Ventral diencephalon	Somatotrophs, gonadotrophs	• Septo-optic dysplasia	AD

PITX2 (RIEG1)	• Bicoid-related homeobox gene expressed early in Rathke pouch
	• Important in maintaining expression of *Hesx1* and *PROP1*
		Somatotrophs, lactotrophs, thyrotrophs, reduced expression of gonadotrophs	• Associated with Rieger syndrome:
			  • Anterior-chamber eye anomalies
			  • Dental hypoplasia
			  • Protuberant umbilicus
			  • Intellectual disability
			  • Pituitary dysfunction
				AD

PROP1 (Prophet of Pit1)	• Paired-like homeodomain transcription factor required for *PIT1* expression • Coexpressed with *Hesx1*	Somatotrophs, lactotrophs, thyrotrophs, gonadotrophs, corticotrophs (delayed)	• Combined pituitary deficiencies (GH, TSH, PRL, and late-onset ACTH reported) • Gonadotropin insufficiency or normal puberty with later onset of deficiency • Several gene variants noted in nonconsanguineous families	AR
POU1F1 (PIT1)	• Member of the POU transcription factor family • Important for activation of *GH1, PRL,* and *TSH-β* genes	Somatotrophs, lactotrophs, thyrotrophs	• Combined pituitary deficiencies (GH, TSH, PRL, and late-onset ACTH reported); TSH secretion may initially be normal • Pituitary hypoplasia	AD, AR
Otx2	• Bicoid-type homeodomain gene required for forebrain and eye development • Antagonizes *FGF8* and *SHH* expression • May have importance in activation of *Hesx1*	Somatotrophs, thyrotrophs, corticotrophs, and probably gonadotrophs	• Severe ocular malformation including anophthalmia • Combined pituitary hormone deficiencies with LH/FSH deficiency • Anterior pituitary hypoplasia with ectopic posterior pituitary	Unknown

TABLE 56.5 Genetic Defects of the GH-IGF Axis Resulting in Somatotroph Dysfunction and GH Deficiency—cont'd

Factor	Gene Function	Affected Cell Types	Clinical Phenotype	Mode of Inheritance
SOX2	• Member of SOXB1 subfamily as *SOX1* and *SOX3* expressed early in development	Somatotrophs, gonadotrophs (and, in animal models, thyrotrophs)	• Hypogonadotropic hypogonadism • Anterior pituitary hypoplasia • Bilateral anophthalmia/microphthalmia • Midbrain defects, including corpus callosum and hippocampus • Sensorineural defects • Esophageal atresia and learning difficulty	De novo
SOX3	• Member of SOX (SRY-related HMG box) • Developmental factor expressed in developing infundibulum and hypothalamus	Somatotrophs, additional anterior pituitary cell types	• Duplications of Xq26-27 in affected males (female carriers unaffected) • Variable intellectual disability • Hypopituitarism with abnormal MRI • Anterior pituitary hypoplasia • Infundibular hypoplasia • Ectopic/undescended posterior pituitary • Abnormal corpus callosum • Murine studies suggest SOX3 dosage critical for normal pituitary development	X-linked
Isolated Growth Hormone Deficiency				
GLI2	• Member of the *GLI* gene family; transcription factors that mediate SHH signaling	Somatotrophs	• Heterozygous loss-of-function gene variants in patients with holoprosencephaly • Penetrance variable • Pituitary dysfunction accompanied by variable craniofacial abnormalities	Unknown
GHRHr	• Encodes GHRH receptor	Somatotrophs	• Short stature • Anterior pituitary hypoplasia	AR
GH1	• Encodes GH peptide • Several gene variants shown to affect GH secretion or function	Somatotrophs	• Short stature • Abnormal facies • Presentation includes bioactive GH	AR, AD, or X-linked

ACTH, adrenocorticotropic hormone; AD, autosomal dominant; AR, autosomal recessive; FSH, follicle-stimulating hormone; GH, growth hormone; GHRH, growth hormone–releasing hormone; α-GSU, glycoprotein α subunit; HMG, high-mobility group; IGF, insulin-like growth factor; LH, luteinizing hormone; PRL, prolactin; SHH, Sonic hedgehog; TSH, thyroid-stimulating hormone (thyrotropin).
From Melmed S, Auchus RJ, Goldfine AB, et al., eds. *Williams Textbook of Endocrinology.* 14th ed. Philadelphia: Elsevier; 2020:962–963, Table 25.2.

Constitutional Delay of Growth and Puberty

Constitutional delay of growth and puberty is a growth pattern that is also considered a variant of normal. These children appear to have a slowed maturational pattern and their bone age is delayed relative to their peers. As part of this slowed maturation, they also enter puberty later than their peers. This variant occurs in both sexes but is more common in males and is recognized predominantly in them for this reason, as well as for cultural reasons (greater attention being paid to short stature in adolescent males than females).

These children often begin to show moderate short stature (height −1.5 to −2.5 SD) during early to middle childhood but are otherwise healthy. They have delayed onset of puberty and therefore a delayed growth spurt. One or both parents (or other family members) may have a history of delayed puberty and a late adolescent growth spurt, with eventual cessation of growth during late adolescence or even into the third decade of life. The affected parent usually is of normal adult stature. Otherwise, the history and review of systems are negative. The physical examination findings are normal except for delayed onset of puberty in children of an appropriate age.

Laboratory tests are not mandatory but are normal if performed, with the important exception of a delayed bone age (bone age <

chronologic age). It is important to note that IGF-1 levels normally increase with onset of puberty and should be compared with standards for the child's pubertal stage and bone age rather than the chronologic age. The delayed bone age suggests that the child has more "room to grow" than the average age-matched child and that the child is likely to reach an adult height taller than that suggested by the current height percentile. Some children have *mixed* familial short stature and constitutional delay in growth and development; they tend to have both delayed puberty and a short-predicted adult height.

Chronic illness may mimic constitutional delay in growth and development and should be considered in the differential diagnosis. It is sometimes difficult to distinguish children with constitutional delay in growth and development from the more unusual condition of central (hypothalamic/pituitary) hypogonadism; a positive family history of delayed but normal puberty and growth, a normal sense of smell (to exclude Kallmann syndrome), and normal neurologic findings favor constitutional delay. Evaluation for permanent **central hypogonadism** is indicated if puberty fails to begin by age 13 in females or 14 in males, particularly if there is no family history of constitutional growth delay.

Females with delayed puberty are more likely to have an underlying pathologic cause, so the threshold for investigation is lower in

TABLE 56.6 Clinical Features of Growth Hormone Insensitivity

Parameter	Clinical Finding
Growth and Development	
Birthweight	Near normal
Birth length	May be slightly decreased
Postnatal growth	Severe growth failure
Bone age	Delayed, but may be advanced relative to height age
Genitalia	Micropenis in childhood; normal for body size in adults
Puberty	Delayed 3–7 yr
Sexual function and fertility	Normal
Craniofacies	
Hair	Sparse before age 7 yr
Forehead	Prominent; frontal bossing
Skull	Normal head circumference; craniofacial disproportion due to small facies
Facies	Small
Nasal bridge	Hypoplastic
Orbits	Shallow
Definition	Delayed eruption
Sclerae	Blue
Voice	High pitched
Musculoskeletal/Metabolic/Miscellaneous	
Blood glucose	Hypoglycemia in infants and children; fasting symptoms in some adults
Waking and motor milestones	Delayed
Hips	Dysplasia; avascular necrosis of femoral head
Elbow	Limited extensibility
Skin	Thin, prematurely aged
Bone mineral density	Osteopenia

From Melmed S, Auchus RJ, Goldfine AB, et al., eds. *Williams Textbook of Endocrinology*. 14th ed. Philadelphia: Elsevier; 2020:973, Table 25.4.

females. On the other hand, benign constitutional delay is common in males and in the presence of a positive family history further evaluation may be delayed even beyond the age of 14. The possibility of **central hypogonadism** becomes stronger the longer the onset of puberty is delayed, but it should be noted that cases of spontaneous development of normal puberty can occur up to and even beyond the age of 18.

In most cases only reassurance and an explanation of the growth pattern is required, but if the parents *and* the child are eager to hasten pubertal development (usually because of involvement in sports or because of bullying and other psychosocial considerations), then a short course of low-dose sex steroids can accelerate the onset of puberty. Such intervention does not change the final height but hastens the child's progression to that height. Treatment options are discussed in detail later in this chapter.

Idiopathic Short Stature

Idiopathic short stature (ISS) is a clinical description rather than a disease. ISS is generally considered a normal variant of growth (since pathologic causes are excluded, by definition). The exact definition varies from country to country; in the United States, the Food and Drug Administration (FDA) used a definition of height >2.25 SD below the age mean (which is the 1st percentile for height) in children in whom no specific cause of short stature has been identified after a thorough evaluation. This corresponds to an adult height <160 cm (5 feet 3 inches) for males and <150 cm (4 feet 11 inches) for females.

In many cases these children have familial short stature and their height is not inappropriate for parental height. But in most definitions they are included in the category of ISS because the purpose of the definition was to identify children who may not have any pathology, but whose short stature per se constitutes a possible reason to treat them with GH. This notion remains controversial because there is no universal agreement about the psychosocial or economic impact of ISS. Those who support treatment of these children argue that such a degree of short stature may have adverse psychological, social, and economic consequences and deserves to be treated even if no underlying pathology is identified. Opponents argue that there is no convincing evidence that short stature of this degree itself leads to any significant handicaps that would justify prolonged invasive therapy with an extremely expensive medication that may itself have future adverse health consequences. Third-party payers often regard such treatment as cosmetic

TABLE 56.7 Genetics of Syndromic Short Stature

Genes	Function	Disorder	Key Clinical Features
FGD1	Guanine nucleotide exchange factor	Aarskog-Scott (faciogenital dysplasia)	IUGR, hypertelorism, ptosis, everted lower lip vermilion, joint hyperextension, finger abnormalities, shawl scrotum
PRKAR1A	cAMP-dependent regulatory subunit of protein kinase A	Acrodysostosis, type 1	IUGR, skeletal dysplasia, severe brachydactyly, facial dysostosis, nasal hypoplasia, advanced bone age, obesity, hormone resistance
PDE4D	cAMP-specific 3′,5′-cyclic phosphodiesterase 4D	Acrodysostosis, type 2	IUGR (variable), skeletal dysplasia, accelerated bone age progression, variable hormone resistance
GNAS	G-protein α subunit	Albright hereditary osteodystrophy	IUGR, obesity, round-shaped face, subcutaneous ossifications, brachymetacarpal bone (fourth and fifth)
RPS6KA3	Serine/threonine kinase in RAS-MAPK pathway	Coffin-Lowry syndrome	No IUGR, microcephaly, facial dysmorphism, skeletal abnormalities, intellectual disability, hypotonia, X-linked disorder
HRAS	Signal transduction with GTPase activity in RAS-MAPK pathway	Costello (faciocutaneoskeletal syndrome)	No IUGR, delayed development, intellectual disability, distinctive facial features, loose folds of extra skin (especially, hands and feet), flexible joints

TABLE 56.7   Genetics of Syndromic Short Stature—cont'd

Genes	Function	Disorder	Key Clinical Features
PTPN11, RAF1, BRAF	Protein-tyrosine phosphatase/RAS-MAPK regulation	Multiple lentigines syndrome (LEOPARD syndrome)	No IUGR, lentigines, hypertrophic myopathy, electrocardiographic conduction abnormalities, ocular hypertelorism, pulmonic stenosis, abnormalities of genitalia, sensorineural deafness
NF1	RAS signal transduction	Neurofibromatosis type 1	No IUGR, café-au-lait spot, malignancy (pheochromocytoma and gastrointestinal stromal tumor), Lisch nodules, osteoporosis
PTPN11, BRAF, SOS1, KRAS, RAF1, NRAS, RASA2, SHOC2, CBL, RIT1 (activating)	Protein-tyrosine phosphatase/RAS-MAPK regulation	Noonan syndrome or Noonan-like syndrome	No IUGR, distinctive facial appearance, a broad or webbed neck, congenital heart defects, coagulopathy, skeletal malformations, developmental delay
ROR2, WNT5A, DVL1	Cell surface receptor, secreted signaling protein	Robinow syndrome (acral dysostosis with facial and genital abnormalities)	IUGR (variable); short-limb dwarfism; costovertebral segmentation defects; abnormalities of head, face, and external genitalia; chest deformities; rib fusions; scoliosis; brachydactyly; aplasia/hypoplasia of the phalanges and metacarpal/metatarsal bones
LARP7	Transcriptional regulator of polymerase II genes	Alazami syndrome	IUGR (variable), facial dysmorphism (triangular face), intellectual disability, tendon or skeletal abnormalities
SOX9	Chondrocyte differentiation factor	Campomelic dysplasia	IUGR, born with bowing of the long bones, short legs, dislocated hips, ambiguous genitalia, distinctive facial features
BRF1	RNA polymerase III transcription initiation factor	Cerebello-facio-dental syndrome	IUGR, facial dysmorphism, hypoplastic cerebellum, markedly delayed bone age
SOX11	Transcriptional regulation of GDF5	Coffin-Siris syndrome	IUGR (variable), intellectual disability, facial dysmorphism, hearing or vision impairment, severe scoliosis
MLL2 (KMT2D), KDM6A	Histone methyltransferase/histone demethylase	Kabuki syndrome	IUGR (variable), facial features that resemble the make-up worn by actors of Kabuki (long eye openings slanting upward, arched eyebrows, prominent ears, and corners of the mouth turning downward), mild to moderate intellectual disability; problems involving heart, skeleton, teeth, and immune system
ANKRD11	Transcription regulator	KBG syndrome	IUGR (variable), facial dysmorphism, hearing loss, congenital heart defect, skeletal anomalies, global developmental delay, seizures, intellectual disability
SHOX	Transcription factor	Leri-Weill dyschondrosteosis, mesomelic dysplasia (Langer type)	No IUGR, skeletal dysplasia, Madelung deformity
CREBBP, EP300	Transcriptional coactivator	Rubinstein-Taybi syndrome	IUGR (variable), facial dysmorphism, moderate to severe intellectual disability, broad thumbs and first toes
BLM	DNA repair enzyme	Bloom syndrome	IUGR (as case report); increased risk of cancer; sun-sensitive skin changes on face, hands, and/or arms; a high-pitched voice; distinctive facial features, including a long, narrow face, small lower jaw, large nose, and prominent ears
ERCC6, ERCC8	DNA repair	Cockayne syndrome	IUGR (variable), microcephaly, photosensitivity progeroid appearance, progressive pigmentary retinopathy, sensorineural deafness
FANCA, FANCC, FANCG	DNA repair	Fanconi anemia	IUGR, absence of thumb, hyperpigmentation, early-onset bone marrow failure, predisposition to cancers
LIG4	DNA repair	LIG 4 syndrome	No IUGR, distinctive facial features, microcephaly, pancytopenia, various skin abnormalities, immune deficiency
NSMCE2	DNA repair	Microcephalic primordial dwarfism–insulin resistance syndrome	No IUGR reported, microcephaly, insulin resistance
NBN (NBS1)	DNA repair	Nijmegen breakage syndrome	No IUGR, microcephaly, distinctive facial features, immunodeficiency, and cancer predisposition
SMARCAL1	DNA repair	Schimke immunoosseous dysplasia	IUGR, kidney disease, immune deficiency, stroke, bone marrow failure, kidney failure
ATR, ATRIP, CENPJ, CEP152, CEP63, DNA2, PCNT, PLK4, RBBP8, XRCC4	DNA repair, centrosome maintenance, DNA stability	Seckel syndrome	IUGR, microcephaly, beaklike protrusion of nose, facial dysmorphism

Continued

TABLE 56.7	**Genetics of Syndromic Short Stature—cont'd**		
Genes	**Function**	**Disorder**	**Key Clinical Features**
CUL7, OBSL1, CCDC8	Microtubule stabilization and genome stability	3-M syndrome	IUGR, facial dysmorphism (triangular face), relatively large head circumference, prominent fleshy heels
ALMS1	Microtubule organization	Alström syndrome	No IUGR, vision and hearing abnormalities, childhood obesity, diabetes mellitus, heart disease, and slowly progressive kidney dysfunction
SMARCB1, SMARCE1, SMARCA4, ARID1A, ARID1B	Chromatin remodeling	Coffin-Siris syndrome	IUGR (variable), intellectual disability, facial dysmorphism, hearing or vision impairment, severe scoliosis
NIPBL (50%), SMC1A, HDAC8, RAD21, SMC3	Cohesin pathway (sister chromatid cohesion)	Cornelia de Lange syndrome	IUGR, dysmorphic facial features (facial hirsutism), microcephaly, limb reduction defects, cardiac defect, and intellectual disability
SRCAP	Chromatin remodeling	Floating-Harbor syndrome	IUGR (variable), facial dysmorphism, abnormal thumb, delayed bone age, early puberty, delay in expressive language
LMNA	Nuclear stability	Hutchinson-Gilford progeria	No IUGR, failure to thrive, distinctive facial features (aged-looking skin), alopecia, loss of subcutaneous fat, joint abnormalities
RNU4ATAC	Minor intron splicing	MOPD I	IUGR, microcephaly, dysmorphic face, skin and skeletal abnormalities, developmental delay
PCNT	Mitotic spindle/chromosome segregation	MOPD II	IUGR, facial dysmorphism, microcephaly, near-normal intelligence, cancer susceptibility
TRIM37	Peroxisomal protein, possibly ubiquitin-dependent degradation	Mulibrey nanism	IUGR, dysmorphic craniofacial features, heart disease (constrictive pericardium), hepatomegaly, Wilms tumor
CRIPT	Interaction with cytoskeleton	Primordial dwarfism	IUGR (not established), facial dysmorphism, microcephaly, ophthalmologic abnormalities, intellectual disabilities, skeletal abnormalities, pigmentation abnormalities
POC1A	Centriole assembly/ciliogenesis	SOFT syndrome	IUGR, disproportionate short stature, onychodysplasia, facial dysmorphism, hypotrichosis
DHCR7	Steroid biosynthesis	Smith-Lemli-Opitz syndrome	IUGR; distinctive facial features; microcephaly; intellectual disability or learning problems; behavioral problems; malformations of heart, lungs, kidneys, gastrointestinal tract, and genitalia
COL2A1	Extracellular matrix, collagen	Achondrogenesis (type II), hypochondrogenesis, Kniest dysplasia, spondyloepiphyseal dysplasia congenita, Stickler syndrome type 1	IUGR, skeletal abnormalities, problems with vision and hearing
FBN1	Extracellular matrix, fibrillin 1	Acromicric dysplasia, geleophysic dysplasia 2	No IUGR; short hands and feet; thickened skin and joint contractures; limited range of motion in fingers, toes, wrists, and elbows; cardiac issue
COL11A1	Extracellular matrix, collagen 11	Fibrochondrogenesis	IUGR (variable), skeletal dysplasia, broad long bone metaphyses, pear-shaped vertebral bodies, flat midface with a small nose and anteverted nares, significant shortening of all limb segments
COL10A1	Extracellular matrix, collagen 10	Metaphyseal dysplasia, Schmid type	No IUGR, coxa vara, relatively short limbs, bow legs, waddling gait
MATN3, COL9A1, COL9A2, COL9A3	Extracellular matrix, cartilage oligomeric matrix protein, collagen, matrilin-3	Multiple epiphyseal dysplasia	No IUGR, skeletal dysplasia, joint pain, joint deformity, waddling gait
COMP	Extracellular matrix, cartilage oligomeric matrix protein	Multiple epiphyseal dysplasia, pseudoachondroplasia	No IUGR, short arms and legs, a waddling walk, early-onset joint pain (osteoarthritis), limited range of motion at elbows and hips
HSPG2	Extracellular matrix, perlecan	Schwartz-Jampel syndrome	IUGR (not established), permanent myotonia (prolonged failure of muscle relaxation), skeletal dysplasia, kyphoscoliosis, bowing of diaphyses and irregular epiphyses
ACAN	Extracellular matrix, aggrecan	Spondyloepimetaphyseal dysplasia, aggrecan/Kimberly type	IUGR, macrocephaly, severe midface hypoplasia, short neck, barrel chest, brachydactyly, advanced bone age
FGFR3 (activating)	Fibroblast growth factor receptor	Achondroplasia, hypochondroplasia	IUGR, short upper arms and thighs, limited range of motion at elbows, relative macrocephaly with a prominent forehead, trident hand

TABLE 56.7   Genetics of Syndromic Short Stature—cont'd

Genes	Function	Disorder	Key Clinical Features
IHH	Secreted signaling molecule, Indian hedgehog	Acrocapitofemoral dysplasia, brachydactyly, type A1	No IUGR, brachydactyly
NPR2 (inactivating)	CNP receptor	Acromesomelic dysplasia, Maroteaux type	IUGR (variable), short limbs and hand/foot malformations
BMPR1B, GDF5	BMP receptor/interacting protein (ligand)	Brachydactyly, type A1 and A2	No IUGR, brachydactyly
PTHLH	Secreted signaling molecules (PTH-related protein)	Brachydactyly, type E2	No IUGR, shortening of fingers mainly in metacarpals and metatarsals
IGF2	Secreted signaling molecule (insulin-like growth factor 2)	IGF-2 deficiency	IUGR, Silver-Russell–like facies
PTH1R	PTH and PTHrP receptor	Metaphyseal chondrodysplasia (Jansen type), Eiken dysplasia, chondrodysplasia (Blomstrand type)	No IUGR, skeletal dysplasia, micrognathia, failure of tooth eruption, low-set/posteriorly rotated ears, proptosis
IGFALS	Acid-labile subunit	ALS deficiency	IUGR (variable), low IGF-1 and IGF-BP3
GH1, GHRHR, SOX3, BTK	GH production	GH deficiency	No IUGR, GH deficiency
IGF1	IGF-1	IGF-1 deficiency	IUGR, microcephaly, intellectual disability, low IGF-1 level
IGF1R	Insulin-like growth factor receptor	IGF-1 insensitivity	IUGR, normal to high IGF-1 level
STAT5B	Growth hormone signaling	Immune deficiency and GH resistance	No IUGR, elevated random GH but low IGF-1 or IGFBP3, immunodeficiency
GHR	Growth hormone receptor	Laron syndrome	IUGR, elevated GH and low IGF-1

ALS, acid labile subunit; BMP, bone morphogenetic protein; cAMP, cyclic adenosine monophosphate; CNP, C-type natriuretic peptide; GH, growth hormone; GTP, guanosine triphosphate; GWA, genome-wide association; IGF-1, insulin-like growth factor 1; IUGR, intrauterine growth restriction; MAPK, mitogen-activated protein kinase; MOPD, microcephalic osteodysplastic primordial dwarfism; PTH, parathyroid hormone; PTHrP, PTH-related protein; RAF, rapidly accelerated fibrosarcoma; RAS, rat sarcoma.
Modified from Jee YH, Andrade AC, Baron J, et al. Genetics of short stature. *Endocrinol Metab Clin N Am* 2017;46(2):259–281 (Table 1, pp. 262–269).

and may not approve requests for therapy. It should be noted that in most cases there are no consistent adverse effects of short stature on quality of life in children at or just below the 1st percentile; however, some studies do indicate that practical and psychosocial difficulties increase in those with extreme degrees of short stature.

ISS is a diagnosis of exclusion; history, physical examination, laboratory studies, and imaging studies do not reveal any specific cause of short stature in an otherwise normal child. How much investigation is needed before a child can be labeled as having ISS remains a matter of controversy and clinical practice can vary significantly within and between different countries. Treatment with GH was approved by the FDA in 2003 but remains controversial and may not be approved by third-party payers. Treatment is more likely to be beneficial in those with more extreme degrees of short stature. A predicted adult height <136 cm (about 4 feet 6 inches) in females and less than 149 cm (about 4 feet 11 inches) in males is *very* likely to be associated with quality-of-life issues and deserves treatment even in the absence of any underlying cause.

Small for Gestational Age

Children who are born small for gestational age (SGA) usually catch up with their peers by 2–3 years of age, but 10–20% of children born SGA will fail to catch up and will continue to be below the 3rd percentile.

This is more likely in children who are born premature as well as SGA and in those most severely affected at birth. The mechanism underlying this failure of catch-up growth is not well understood. Children with IUGR also have an increased future risk of metabolic disorders like type 2 diabetes. Children who were SGA typically have normal proportions and no other physical findings; in some cases, the IUGR is just one component of a genetic syndrome (see Tables 56.3, 56.6, and 56.7) and other features of the syndrome are present.

Children who were born SGA with poor postnatal growth typically have normal or even elevated GH levels but lower average values of IGF-1 and IGFBP3 (though most are still in the normal range), indicating some degree of GH resistance in at least some of these children. GH treatment increases final height by about 1 SD on average (about 6 cm) if started early in life and continued for at least 7 years. In the United States, treatment is approved by the FDA for children who were born SGA and whose height remains >2 SD below the mean at age 2. In Europe, treatment is approved for children whose height is >2.5 SD below the mean by age 4. These children can be mildly GH resistant and may therefore require GH doses at the higher end of the dose range. Since individual response varies, GH treatment can be started at the usual dose (30–50 μg/kg/day) and then increased if needed based on growth response and IGF-1 levels.

ENDOCRINE DISORDERS

Growth Hormone Deficiency

GH is essential for postnatal growth, and children who lack it are extremely stunted. GH deficiency may be congenital or acquired. The **congenital** form may be associated with other pituitary hormone deficiencies (multiple pituitary hormone deficiency, MPHD) and may be associated with **midline craniofacial defects** (absence of the septum pellucidum and optic nerve hypoplasia [septo-optic dysplasia], cleft palate, holoprosencephaly, single central incisor). Genetic testing has revealed underlying genetic variants in transcription factors involved in the development of the anterior pituitary in many (but not all) of these cases (see Table 56.5). Isolated congenital GH deficiency is relatively rare (i.e., it is more common to see congenital GH deficiency as a component of multiple pituitary hormone deficiencies). Some of these isolated cases are related to genetic abnormalities in the growth hormone–releasing hormone receptor (GHRHR variants) and others to variants in the GH gene itself. Variants in the GH receptor or in downstream signaling molecules lead to various rare forms of GH resistance. Variants in the IGF-1 gene, in the ALS protein (a component of the IGF-IGFBP3-ALS ternary complex), and in the IGF-1 receptor can also lead to growth failure on rare occasions. But most cases of GH deficiency discovered during the evaluation of short stature are not due to known genetic variants in the GH-IGF axis and are regarded as **idiopathic.**

GH deficiency may also be **acquired** secondary to birth injury, head trauma, midline tumors (most commonly craniopharyngioma), histiocytic infiltrative disorders, and cranial irradiation. Most such cases are associated with deficiencies of other pituitary hormones, but isolated GH deficiency may also occur after such insults. Injury to the anterior pituitary during childhood most often affects GH secretion, followed by gonadotropins, thyroid-stimulating hormone (TSH), and adrenocorticotropic hormone (ACTH) in that order (in adults, gonadotropins may be affected more than GH). It is therefore possible to see isolated GH deficiency after a cranial injury, while it is very unusual to see central hypothyroidism or adrenal insufficiency in the absence of GH deficiency.

Growth Hormone Deficiency Presenting in the Neonatal Period

Isolated congenital GH deficiency that *presents* in the newborn period is uncommon. If GH deficiency presents in the newborn period, it usually does so in the setting of MPHD. It may be associated with midline defects (central incisor, septo-optic dysplasia, holoprosencephaly, cleft palate). Affected infants are often normal in birth size, although statistical analysis suggests that, as a group, they are somewhat small. These newborns have an increased incidence of hypoglycemia and may also have jaundice with a hepatitis-type picture and conjugated hyperbilirubinemia (there are cases that have been mistaken for biliary atresia). Males frequently have micropenis; cryptorchidism may be seen in cases with concomitant gonadotropin deficiency. Hypoglycemia may be worsened by associated ACTH deficiency, which may also lead to hypotension and hypothermia. Associated central hypothyroidism may also cause hypothermia, poor growth, poor feeding, and prolonged jaundice.

Laboratory testing reveals a low random GH level (this is the only stage in life at which a random GH level is useful; levels <7 ng/mL in the first week of life are considered abnormal), as well as low levels of IGF-1 (not very useful because the normal range overlaps with the deficient range) and low IGFBP3. Associated central hypothyroidism, if present, is suggested by a low thyroxine (T_4) and an *inappropriately*

normal (or even slightly elevated) TSH level; one would have expected the TSH level to be markedly elevated in a baby with low T_4, but instead it is either normal or just minimally elevated. A low cortisol level (especially in the face of hypoglycemia or other stressful situations) and low or low-normal ACTH level may hint at central ACTH deficiency; an ACTH stimulation test may be required to confirm the diagnosis. Gonadotropin levels may be affected and, if so, will remain low instead of rising in the first 2–3 months of life as they normally do in infants. GH stimulation testing is *not* required for the diagnosis of GH deficiency in the newborn period. Genetic testing may show pathogenic variation in one of several genes involved in the normal development of the pituitary and the GH-producing cells of the pituitary (*POUF1, PROP1, HESX1, LXH3, LHX4,* and *SOX3*) (see Table 56.5). Treatment with GH (*and* with other pituitary hormones that are frequently deficient in these neonates) will permit normal growth and development and prevents hypoglycemia and other complications.

Growth Hormone Deficiency in Childhood

Most children who are diagnosed with GH deficiency in childhood demonstrate no manifestations in the neonatal period. A very small proportion has specific genetic defects in GH secretion or action that did not present (or were not obvious) in the newborn period; these children will usually exhibit very profound growth failure by the second or third year of life. They typically look younger than their actual age and are classically described as chubby or cherubic; their heights are depressed more than their weights. They may have high-pitched voices, delayed dentition, and poor musculature. On testing, they are found to have very low IGF-1 and IGFBP3 levels; GH stimulation testing reveals peak GH levels that are almost always lower than 5 ng/mL. Bone age is typically delayed and an MRI of the brain may show a hypoplastic pituitary gland, an empty sella, or an abnormal pituitary bright spot. Genetic testing may show defects in the GHRHR gene or the GH gene (see Table 56.5). Defects in other genes involved in regulating GH secretion may be seen, but all are extremely rare. These children typically respond very dramatically to GH replacement therapy and will grow very poorly in the absence of such therapy

Much more common is the phenomenon of the child who presents with short stature in childhood but does not have any known genetic or acquired cause of GH deficiency. These children are diagnosed as GH deficient based on a combination of auxologic and laboratory criteria and are candidates for GH therapy. But unlike children with neonatally apparent GH deficiency or children with obvious causes of acquired GH deficiency (tumors, trauma, radiation), these children are frequently not GH deficient when retested after puberty. This **idiopathic growth hormone deficiency** may be due to multiple genetic loci of small effect or a few loci of moderate effect, but the exact cause usually remains unknown. Poor linear growth usually becomes evident by age 3 years, but many cases are not brought to the attention of physicians until later in childhood. Diagnosis and treatment of children with idiopathic GH deficiency is based on consensus guidelines and expert opinion and may vary from country to country. In most cases, children are investigated for idiopathic GH deficiency if they are below the normal range for height (>2 SD below the mean, or <3rd percentile) or are extremely short for their genetic target height (projected adult height more than 9 cm below the MPH). A subnormal growth velocity (growth velocity <25th percentile or >1.5 SD below the mean) is seen and no other obvious cause of short stature can be found.

No single test can be regarded as the gold standard for making this diagnosis. Most children will have an IGF-1 level that is low for age (and in older children, for pubertal stage and bone age), but occasionally a child who meets all other criteria for GH deficiency will have a normal IGF-1 level, while in other cases the IGF-1 level may be low because of malnutrition or chronic disease in a child who is not GH deficient. IGFBP3 level is also frequently used as a measure of GH secretion but is less sensitive than the IGF-1 level and may not be helpful in most cases. Bone age is almost always delayed. If the diagnosis is suspected as a result of auxologic findings (short stature, subnormal growth velocity), a delayed bone age, and low IGF-1 and/or IGFBP3 levels, then most authorities recommend performing two GH stimulation tests. In these tests, GH secretion is provoked by one of several pharmacologic agents and multiple GH levels are drawn over the next 2–3 hours. Glucagon, arginine, L-dopa, and clonidine are the most commonly used agents in children; insulin-induced hypoglycemia is considered by many to be the gold standard test in adults *but is associated with the risk of life-threatening hypoglycemia and is not recommended in children*. If all levels remain below an arbitrary cut-off (10 ng/mL in the United States), then the child is considered GH deficient. It should be noted that provocative testing is known to have both false-positive and false-negative results and should only be interpreted in the context of all available auxologic, laboratory, and imaging information. Because of these issues, some authorities recommend using auxologic criteria and growth factor levels to make the diagnosis of GH deficiency without performing any provocative tests of GH secretion.

Any child diagnosed as having GH deficiency should have cranial imaging performed to rule out intracranial pathology before treatment is started. Once imaging (usually an MRI of the brain with fine cuts through the pituitary region) has been performed, treatment can be started with GH. The usual starting dose ranges from 30 to 50 μg/kg/day and this can then be increased in case of poor response. Doses of 70 μg/kg/day or higher may be needed in some cases. IGF-1 levels can be used to assess biochemical response and to see if there is room to increase GH dose any further. Some authorities have recommended IGF-based dosing (adjusting the GH dose to keep the IGF-1 level in the high-normal range), but very high doses of GH may be required in some children to achieve such levels and because of safety concerns this method has not been widely adopted.

Acquired Growth Hormone Deficiency

In acquired forms of GH deficiency, there may be a history of a precipitating event (cranial irradiation, head trauma) or a history suggestive of an intracranial lesion (headaches, vomiting, visual disturbances). Affected children often have normal growth until the onset of the disorder; thereafter, their growth is attenuated.

On physical examination, there may be evidence of the underlying disturbance (bitemporal hemianopsia, optic atrophy, or papilledema in midline tumors such as craniopharyngioma; dermatitis, scalp lesions, or hepatosplenomegaly in Langerhans cell histiocytosis). The typical case will either be a child with a known history of conditions that can affect the anterior pituitary (head injury, irradiation, tumor) who shows deceleration of growth or a child who was growing normally and then has an obvious growth failure. Lab tests will show decreased IGF-1 levels (and in some cases, abnormal levels of other pituitary hormones); cranial imaging (usually an MRI with and without contrast) should then be done in all such cases. Bone age may not be delayed if the onset of GH deficiency was relatively recent. The diagnosis of GH deficiency is usually confirmed by provocative testing and patients can then be treated with the usual doses of GH. In patients with brain tumors, treatment is usually delayed for at least 1 year after completion of therapy because of the theoretical risk that GH therapy may increase the size of any tumor that is present.

Traditionally, GH therapy for GH deficiency was continued until linear growth was completed (i.e., until the closure of epiphyses), though it could be stopped at any point before that if the child is satisfied with their attained height. Because of the extremely high cost of GH therapy ($50,000–$100,000 per year in the United States), many third-party payers require cessation of therapy once a reasonable adult height has been reached (exact targets vary depending on the plan).

Growth Hormone Insensitivity

GH action may be impaired due to variants of the GH receptor (**Laron syndrome**), defects in postreceptor signaling, variants in the IGF-1 gene, deficiency of the ALS protein, and defects in IGF-1 action (see Tables 56.3, 56.5, 56.6, and 56.7). All of these conditions are very rare and constitute only a tiny fraction of the cases of short stature and growth failure seen in clinical practice.

The GH receptor consists of an extracellular ligand-binding domain, a single membrane-spanning domain, and a cytoplasmic signaling component. Circulating GH-binding protein (GHBP) is just the extracellular domain of the GH receptor protein. Pathologic variants in this receptor lead to various forms of **Laron syndrome**, characterized by GH resistance (hence elevated GH levels), low IGF-1 and IGFBP3, and extreme degrees of growth failure. In some (but not all) cases, the extracellular domain of the receptor is involved, so GHBP level is also low.

Other clinical features of Laron syndrome include small head circumference, characteristic facies with saddle nose and prominent forehead, delayed skeletal maturation, small genitalia and testes, short limb length compared to trunk length, and abnormal body composition, with osteopenia and obesity. Intellectual development is normal or only modestly impaired. Prenatal growth is near normal, but postnatal growth is profoundly affected, with heights as low as −10 SD.

It is worth noting that *untreated* children do not have a shortened lifespan and have a *lower*-than-average risk for cancer.

Defects in the post-GH receptor signaling pathway can also cause short stature. Several patients have been described with GH insensitive caused by a homozygous missense variant in the gene encoding STAT5B protein, which is an essential component of the JAK-STAT signaling pathway that is activated by the GH receptor. These patients have severe postnatal growth failure as well as immune disregulation related to the role of STAT5B in the immune system.

Variants in the gene encoding IGF-1 cause profound prenatal as well as postnatal growth failure. Complete absence of IGF-1 is probably lethal in humans, but individuals have been described with deletions in the IGF-1 gene causing partial loss of function. These patients also have microcephaly, significant developmental delay, and hearing loss.

IGF-1 is carried in the bloodstream primarily as part of a ternary complex with IGFBP3 and ALS. **ALS deficiency** leads to low circulating IGF-1 levels (probably via accelerated IGF-1 metabolism) and leads to mild short stature and pubertal delay.

IGF-1 receptor variants are extremely rare in liveborn babies and present with profound prenatal and postnatal growth failure. These children may have normal or only mildly abnormal cognitive development. Unlike the other GH insensitivity syndromes, circulating levels of IGF-1 are normal or elevated in these patients.

All forms of GH insensitivity (except rare IGF-1 receptor defects) lead to IGF-1 deficiency. The FDA has approved treatment of these disorders with recombinant IGF-1 in cases where height *and* IGF-1 levels are more than 3 SD below the mean, with elevated or normal GH levels, and no response to GH therapy. Commercial availability of this product has varied and obtaining supplies for therapy may sometimes be a problem.

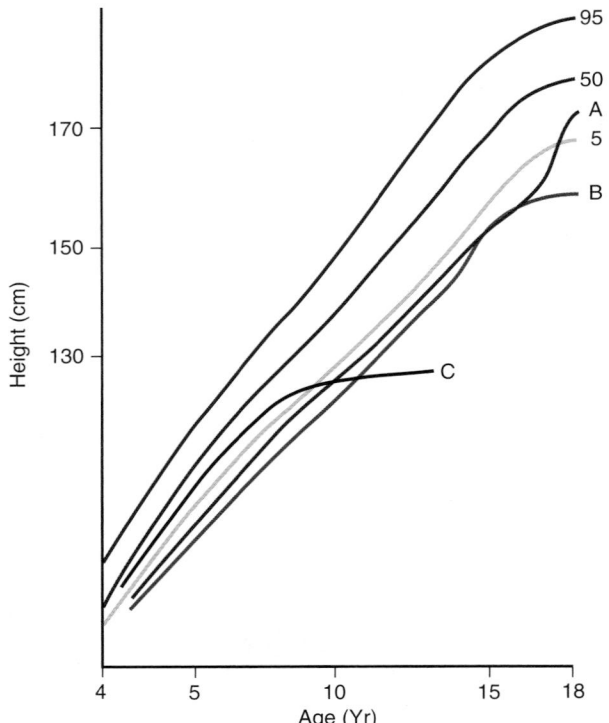

Fig. 56.7 Patterns of linear growth. Normal growth percentiles (5th, 50th, 95th) are shown along with typical growth curves for constitutional delay of growth and adolescence *(A)*, familial short stature *(B)*, and acquired pathologic growth failure *(C)* (e.g., acquired primary hypothyroidism). (From Styne DM. Endocrine disorders. In: Behrman RE, Kliegman RM, eds. *Nelson Essentials of Pediatrics.* 2nd ed. Philadelphia: WB Saunders; 1994:616.)

HYPOTHYROIDISM

Hypothyroidism impairs linear growth (Fig. 56.7). Thyroid deficiency may be congenital or acquired (Fig. 56.8). In view of the usefulness of neonatal thyroid screening programs, it is very uncommon for congenital hypothyroidism to go untreated and cause short stature.

Acquired hypothyroidism in children usually results from **autoimmune thyroiditis**. Children with Turner syndrome, Down syndrome, Klinefelter syndrome, celiac disease, or diabetes mellitus are at increased risk for autoimmune hypothyroidism, as are children with a family history of autoimmune disease. Acquired hypothyroidism tends to manifest most commonly in older children and teenagers. Often there are few complaints except for slow growth (after previously normal growth), weight gain, a goiter, or a combination of these. Other symptoms (dry hair or skin, constipation, cold intolerance) are less common. Postmenarchal females may have menorrhagia, amenorrhea, or, in rare cases, galactorrhea. School performance is generally not impaired. On physical examination, the major features are a height suggestive of deceleration from the previous growth curve, a goiter, and relative obesity (weight age > height age). The physical examination may also reveal bradycardia, dry hair or skin, and delayed reflexes.

In acquired hypothyroidism, the laboratory test results include a high level of TSH and a low or low-normal T_4 level or free thyroxine level (FT_4). The presence of positive thyroid antibodies (antithyroperoxidase and antithyroglobulin antibodies) is consistent with autoimmune thyroiditis. The bone age is often significantly delayed in hypothyroidism.

Central hypothyroidism is uncommon. In the newborn period it usually (but not always) presents as a component of MPHD with TSH levels that are normal or even mildly elevated but that are inappropriately low for the decreased T_4 level. Acquired central hypothyroidism is usually due to known injury to the anterior pituitary (e.g., central nervous system [CNS] tumors, granulomas, irradiation, head trauma) and is associated with other pituitary hormone deficiencies. In practice, it is much more common to see low T_4 and normal or mildly elevated TSH levels in children who have another illness and have the syndrome of **nonthyroidal illness (NTI)** (previously known as euthyroid sick syndrome) leading to temporarily abnormal thyroid function tests.

The treatment of hypothyroidism is thyroid replacement therapy (L-thyroxine).

Glucocorticoid Excess (Cushing Syndrome)

Cushing syndrome results from excessive levels of glucocorticoids. Whether endogenous or exogenous, glucocorticoids markedly stunt growth. In general, because such conditions are acquired, the history reveals a child previously growing well whose growth velocity slows. The child typically continues to gain weight at a rapid rate, even though linear growth is attenuated. This is in contrast to exogenous obesity, in which affected children tend to grow at normal or rapid rates. The history may indicate that the child was treated with oral, topical (especially with occlusive dressings), or intradermal glucocorticoids at high doses or for long durations. Alternate-day oral glucocorticoids are much less likely to attenuate growth than are daily doses. Cushing syndrome is very unlikely with inhaled corticosteroids (ICSs), but a small effect on linear growth may be seen with the use of high-potency ICSs.

Physical findings in endogenous Cushing syndrome may include acne, virilization, and increased appetite. Hyperpigmentation may occur when Cushing syndrome is secondary to excessive ACTH levels. This may be caused by ACTH from a pituitary tumor (Cushing disease) or (less commonly) from a nonpituitary source (ectopic ACTH syndrome).

The physical examination usually reveals short stature with relative obesity. Many affected children have the moon face and plethora characteristic of Cushing syndrome. A buffalo hump, large purple striae, acne, and hypertension may also be present. Marked virilization is worrisome because it may indicate an adrenal tumor.

The diagnosis of endogenous Cushing syndrome is based on demonstrating abnormally high glucocorticoid production (on 24-hour urine sample for free cortisol, normalized to creatinine) and failure to suppress cortisol production adequately in response to exogenous glucocorticoid. A screening test for capacity to suppress cortisol secretion in response to exogenous glucocorticoid is the overnight dexamethasone suppression test. This involves the child taking 0.3 mg/m^2 of dexamethasone at 11:00 P.M. (the standard dose of dexamethasone in adults is 1 mg), followed by a measurement of circulating cortisol the following morning; a normal cortisol level after dexamethasone suppression is <2 mcg/dL (<55 nmol/L). False-positive results may occur in the setting of obesity, chronic illness, or stress. If the child shows biochemical evidence of Cushing syndrome, further investigations, including CT, MRI, and measurement of ACTH levels, are needed to determine whether a pituitary tumor (commonest cause), an adrenal tumor, or ectopic ACTH production is present. Exogenous Cushing syndrome is usually evident from the history and physical examination results.

Treatment involves the removal of excess glucocorticoids by either reducing or discontinuing exogenous steroids if medically feasible or, in the case of endogenous hypercortisolism caused by a pituitary or adrenal tumor, by surgery.

Genetic Causes of Short Stature

A large number of single gene defects and copy number variants are known to be associated with short stature (see Table 56.7). Some of

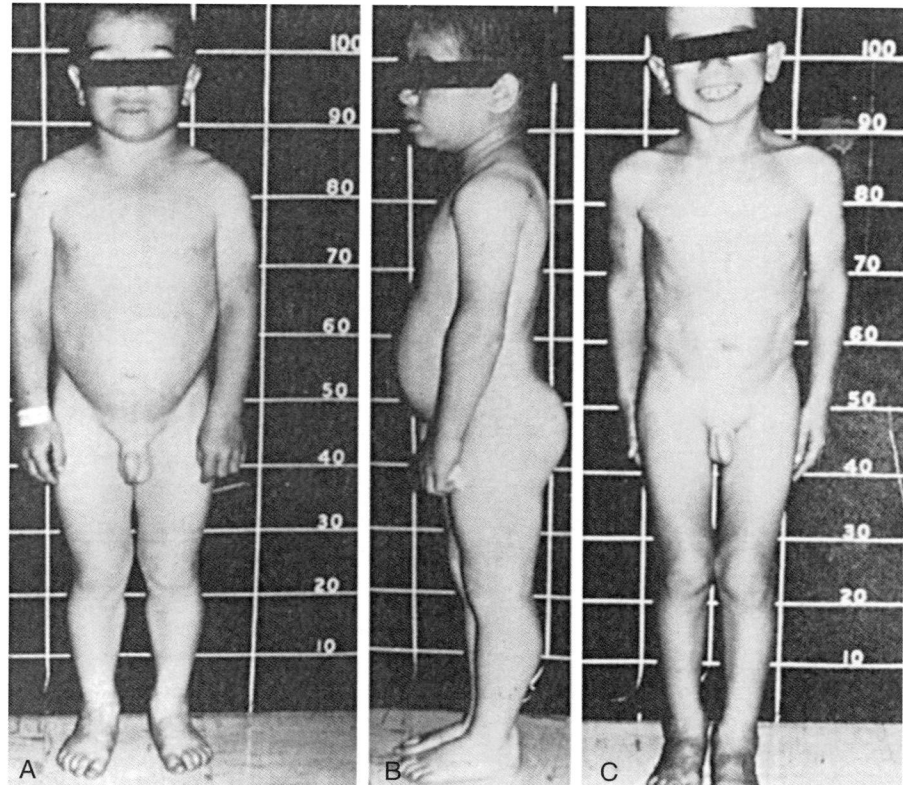

Fig. 56.8 *A, B,* A 10-year-old boy with acquired hypothyroidism, before treatment. Note short stature, immature body proportions, sleepy expression, generalized myxedema, and protuberant abdomen. *C,* After 4 months of thyroid hormone therapy, the child has grown, has lost myxedema, and has a bright facial expression. (From Kaplan SA, ed. *Clinical Pediatric and Adolescent Endocrinology.* Philadelphia: WB Saunders; 1982:93.)

them cause other abnormal physical findings (syndromic), but genetic causes of short stature are also found in children who do not have any other physical finding. Genes that have been found to be associated with short stature include variants in PAPPA2, ACAN (aggrecan), NPPC (C-natriuretic peptide, CNP), NPR2 (CNP receptor), PTPN11 (and other RASopathies), FBN1, IHH, and BMP2. It is not routine practice to obtain genetic tests in otherwise normal children with short stature, but as technology progresses this may become standard of care in the future. Several chromosomal aneuploidies are associated with significant short stature, but apart from Turner syndrome and Down syndrome, these are relatively uncommon causes of short stature. Because of the relatively high prevalence of Turner syndrome, a karyotype is indicated in the evaluation of all prepubertal females with significant short stature.

Turner Syndrome

Turner syndrome is relatively common, with an incidence of 1 per 2,500 liveborn females, and is caused by the absence or abnormality of an X chromosome. Short stature is the *single most common physical finding* in Turner syndrome and may occur in the absence of any other physical finding (Fig. 56.9). The mechanism by which short stature occurs in Turner syndrome is multifactorial, but haplo-insufficiency (absence of one copy) of the **S**hort **S**tature **H**omeobo**X** gene (SHOX) is believed to play a major role. This gene is located within the pseudo-autosomal region of the X chromosome, which escapes X-inactivation and is therefore normally expressed from both copies of the X chromosome. It is highly active in skeletal tissues and its absence in Turner syndrome (where only one X chromosome is present, or if present, the

second X chromosome is abnormal) leads to haplo-insufficiency and causes severe short stature.

Linear growth is only mildly affected in utero and birth size is normal or near normal. By early childhood, marked short stature is usually noted and there is progressive deviation of height away from the normal growth curve. Linear growth is further attenuated during the teenage years and mean adult height ranges from 142 cm to 146 cm in various populations. Even in females with Turner syndrome, adult height is influenced by the height of the parents, and females with Turner syndrome who are born to tall parents tend to be taller. Breast enlargement and menses generally fail to occur as a result of ovarian failure. However, the presence of pubertal development should not deter consideration of the diagnosis because approximately 10% of patients have some residual ovarian tissue rather than streak gonads. In a few cases, even fertility has been reported.

In addition to short stature and ovarian failure, there may be various dysmorphic features, including webbed neck, low posterior hairline, lymphedema beginning in the neonatal period (manifesting mainly as puffy hands and feet), increased carrying angle of the arm, pigmented nevi, short fourth metacarpals, nail abnormalities, and renal and cardiac anomalies (coarctation of the aorta). But any or all of these may be absent and short stature may be the only abnormality in some females with Turner syndrome (particularly in those with chromosomal mosaicism, which can occur in up to a third of cases). *Therefore, the absence of dysmorphic features should not preclude consideration of Turner syndrome in short females.*

A karyotype analysis is necessary to confirm or rule out the diagnosis of Turner syndrome in any female with short stature of unknown

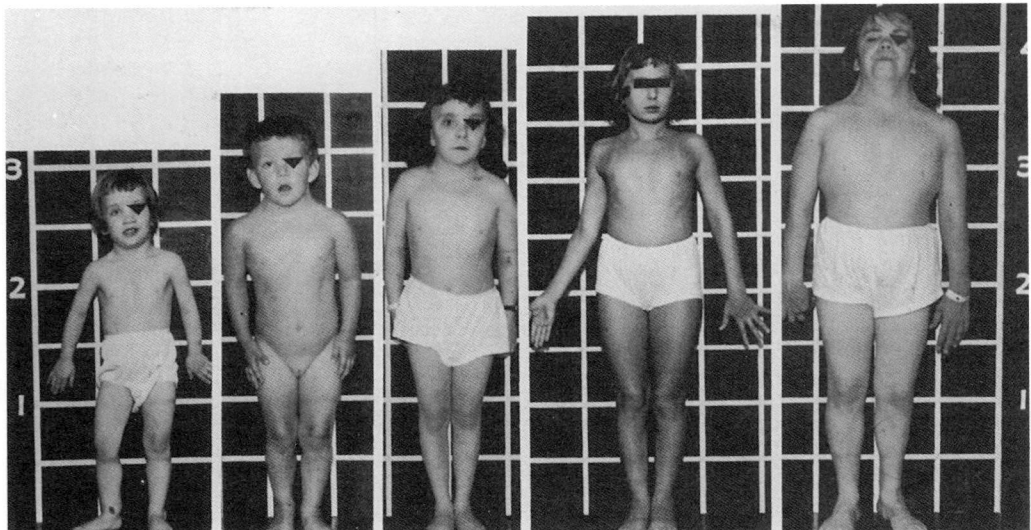

Fig. 56.9 Five different females with 45,XO syndrome illustrating the variability of features such as webbed neck and broad chest. (From Lemli L, Smith D. The XO syndrome. A study of the differentiated phenotype in 25 patients. *J Pediatr.* 1963;63:577–588.)

origin. This should initially be performed on a blood sample, but if there is a high index of suspicion, other tissues (such as a skin biopsy for fibroblast analysis) should be screened due to the high prevalence of mosaicism. Additional laboratory features may include abnormally high levels of the gonadotropins, luteinizing hormone, and follicle-stimulating hormone (FSH), which are indicative of ovarian failure; however, levels may be normal in middle childhood because of normal CNS suppression of gonadotropin secretion at that time.

Although short stature in Turner syndrome is not believed to result from GH deficiency, treatment of Turner syndrome with GH therapy (typically in higher doses than those required for classical GH deficiency) increases final height and is recommended. Addition of low-dose oxandrolone may further increase the growth of females with Turner syndrome and is a useful adjunct in females who are diagnosed relatively late and who may not reach a normal height with GH therapy alone.

Down Syndrome

Short stature is a prominent feature in Down syndrome, but the mechanism by which trisomy 21 causes impaired growth is not known. It is independent of the hypothyroidism that may also occur in this condition. Specific treatment for short stature is typically not recommended in this condition.

Prader-Willi Syndrome

Prader-Willi syndrome (PWS) is characterized by hypotonia, failure to thrive with poor suck during infancy, hypogonadism (manifested as cryptorchidism in males), short stature with small hands and feet, hyperphagia leading to morbid obesity beginning in early childhood, developmental delay/intellectual disability, and behavioral issues, including obsessive-compulsive disorder. Average adult height is 147 cm (4 feet, 9 inches) in females and 155 cm (5 feet, 1 inch) in males. PWS is caused by the absence or inactivity of a segment of the paternally inherited chromosome 15 (15q11.2-13), whereas deletion of the same chromosomal segment in the maternally inherited chromosome causes **Angelman syndrome**. It is thus a classic example of genomic imprinting, a phenomenon in which the expression of a gene or genomic region differs depending on the chromosome's parent of origin.

PWS may be due to a deletion of the PWS region of the paternal chromosome (about 65% of cases) or the inheritance of two complete copies of the maternal chromosome 15 and the absence of the paternal chromosome (a condition labeled maternal uniparental disomy, responsible for 30–35% of the cases). In about 2% of the cases it appears to be due to a defect in the imprinting center rather than the absence of the paternal genes. DNA methylation probes will detect almost all cases by revealing whether the patient has maternal and paternal methylation patterns (normal), absence of the paternal pattern (causing PWS), or absence of the maternal pattern (causing Angelman syndrome). Further genetic testing is then needed to determine whether the cause is a deletion, a disomy, or an imprinting center defect.

Early treatment with GH increases final height, and it also improves body composition and the achievement of developmental milestones. It may also decrease the incidence of morbid obesity. *For these reasons, most authorities consider early treatment with GH (starting between 4 months and 2 years of age) to be standard of care in PWS.* Because of some reports of possible increase in the rate of sudden death from upper airway obstruction in the first months of treatment, a sleep study and/or an ear, nose, and throat (ENT) consult may be recommended before initiating treatment, with the sleep study repeated 6–12 weeks after starting treatment and annually thereafter.

Russell-Silver Syndrome/Silver-Russell Syndrome

Russell-Silver syndrome is characterized by severe IUGR that persists in postnatal life. These children have proportionate short stature, a normal head circumference, triangular facies, downturned corners of the mouth, and a prominent forehead. A clinical diagnosis is made when the presence of four or more of the Netchine-Harbison criterion are present (Table 56.8). Molecular testing only identifies a causal variation in 60% of cases. Other features may include fifth finger clinodactyly, multiple café-au-lait macules, fasting hypoglycemia, and excessive sweating. These children usually have feeding difficulties and may exhibit mild developmental delay.

Russell-Silver syndrome is associated with methylation abnormalities in an imprinting control region on the paternal chromosome 11p15.5 in ~60% of subjects. In another 10% it is caused by maternal uniparental disomy of chromosome 7 (absence of the paternal chromosome 7). Rare sequence variants can be seen involving the genes

TABLE 56.8 Netchine-Harbison Clinical Scoring System (NH-CSS) for Silver-Russell Syndrome

Small for gestational age (birthweight and/or length ≥2 standard deviations (SD) below the mean for gestational age)

Postnatal growth failure (length/height ≥ SD below the mean at 24 mo)

Relative macrocephaly at birth (head circumference >1.5 SD above birthweight and/or length)

Frontal bossing or prominent forehead (forehead projecting beyond the facial plane on a side view as a toddler [1–3 yr])

Body asymmetry (limb length discrepancy ≥0.5 cm, or <0.5 cm with two or more other asymmetric body parts)

Feeding difficulties or body mass index ≤2 SD at 24 mo or current use of a feeding tube or cyproheptadine for appetite stimulation

A score of 4 or more indicates a high likelihood for clinical diagnosis and molecular testing is warranted. Adapted from Aziz S, et al. A prospective study validating a clinical scoring system and demonstrating phenotypical-genotypical correlations in Silver-Russell syndrome. *J Med Genet*. 2015;52(7):446–453.

IGF2, CDKN1C, PLAG1, and *HMGA2.* No genetic cause is identified in up to 40% of remaining children and the diagnosis is based on clinical criteria. Treatment with GH increases height, but the doses required may be higher than average because of some element of GH resistance.

Short Stature HomeoboX *(SHOX)* Gene Variants

The short stature homeobox *(SHOX)* gene is located within the pseudoautosomal region of the X and Y chromosomes. This region escapes X-inactivation and so it is normally expressed from both X chromosomes in females. In males the gene is expressed from the X as well as the Y chromosomes. Haplo-insufficiency of the *SHOX* gene (variants affecting one copy of the gene) leads to short stature that may be associated with other skeletal findings such as the Madelung deformity (a dinner fork deformity of the distal forearm and wrist), mesomelia (shortening of the forearm and leg), cubitus valgus, and dislocation of the ulna. The combination of short stature and several of the aforementioned significant skeletal abnormalities is labeled **Leri-Weill dyschondrosteosis** and is more common in females (ratio 4:1). In other cases, the skeletal abnormalities may be relatively subtle and isolated short stature may be the only notable finding.

Screening for *SHOX* gene variants is reserved for children with any combination of the following physical findings: increased U/L, reduced arm span/height ratio, increased sitting height/height ratio, above-average body mass index, Madelung deformity, cubitus valgus, short or bowed forearm, dislocation of the ulna at the elbow, or the appearance of muscular hypertrophy. In otherwise short children who do not have any of these associated findings, the yield from testing for *SHOX* variants is very low. Treatment with GH can increase final height, though higher-than-average doses may be required.

Noonan Syndrome

Noonan syndrome has an incidence of 1 in 1,000–2,500 live births. Molecular testing of the 13 genes known to be causally associated with Noonan syndrome identifies a pathogenic variant in *PTPN11* in 50% of affected individuals; SOS1 is the next most frequent seen in approximately 13%, while *RAF1, RIT1,* and *KRAS* are seen in approximately 5% each, respectively. The remaining genes are noted in fewer than 1% of cases. They include *BRAF, LZTR1, NRAS, PPP1CB, MRAS, SHOC2, RRAS2,* and *SOS2.* In about 20% of the patients, no causally

associated pathogenic variant is detected. One of the reasons for this is that RAS-related disorders are known to have a relatively high degree of somatic mosaicism. The syndrome is characterized by minor facial dysmorphism (hypertelorism, downward eye slant, and low-set ears), proportionate short stature, and right-sided heart disease, most often pulmonic stenosis and hypertrophic cardiomyopathy. Other common findings include a short, webbed neck; chest deformity (pectus excavatum); cryptorchidism; intellectual disability; bleeding diathesis; and lymphedema. GH therapy is recommended to treat short stature associated with Noonan syndrome and is an FDA-approved indication for the use of GH.

Malnutrition

Worldwide, malnutrition resulting from poverty is still the commonest cause of short stature. In North America, malnutrition may arise from inadequate intake secondary to poverty or deprivation, poor intake secondary to overt or occult chronic illness (e.g., inflammatory bowel disease, renal failure), or inability to utilize food intake (malabsorption). In all these conditions, weight tends to be depressed to a greater degree than height. The history should include review of the child's food intake (often best obtained by a 3-day diet record), appetite, and detailed review of systems. Specific nutritional disorders, such as rickets, may also lead to short stature. Appropriate treatment leads to acceleration of linear growth, typically lagging a few weeks or months behind weight gain. Catch-up growth occurs but may not compensate for all of the lost height potential in longstanding cases, leading to a permanent height deficit.

Chronic Illness

Chronic illnesses, such as inflammatory bowel disease, celiac disease, renal dysfunction, and chronic inflammation, can lead to short stature. The mechanisms of impaired growth include poor appetite or poor intake (inflammatory bowel disease, renal dysfunction), malabsorption (celiac disease), medications (chronic glucocorticoids for severe asthma), chronic acidosis (renal tubular acidosis), and secondary endocrine dysfunction (GH resistance associated with systemic inflammation). Although the primary disorder is evident in many cases, short stature is sometimes the presenting feature of the chronic disease. This occurs notably in inflammatory bowel disease, celiac disease, and renal dysfunction.

Gastrointestinal Disease: Children usually have a greater deficit in weight than height. Gastrointestinal symptoms are frequently present, but short stature alone may be the initial presentation of celiac disease and inflammatory bowel syndrome. The growth failure in inflammatory bowel disease is due to a combination of decreased food intake, malabsorption, and the inflammatory process (mediated by proinflammatory cytokines). This may be further aggravated by the use of high-dose glucocorticoids for treatment. GH therapy has been shown to increase height velocity in some small trials in inflammatory bowel disease, but no consensus exists yet about its role in these children. Celiac disease responds to a gluten-free diet and height velocity normalizes with adequate treatment.

Renal Disease: Children with chronic kidney disease may develop growth failure due to chronic metabolic acidosis, uremia, poor nutrition, anorexia, anemia, calcium and phosphorus imbalance, renal osteodystrophy, and impairment of GH action. It may also be aggravated by the use of high-dose glucocorticoids. GH therapy is recommended for children with profound growth failure and is typically continued until renal transplantation.

Pulmonary Disease: Growth failure in cystic fibrosis is secondary to both its pulmonary and gastrointestinal manifestations. Chronic infection and systemic inflammation contribute to short stature.

Severe asthma may interfere with growth directly as well as via the effect of glucocorticoid therapy. Daily use of systemic glucocorticoids for any significant length of time will lead to growth suppression, but potent ICSs may also have noticeable systemic effects in some cases (probably due to individual differences in technique and sensitivity). Alternate-day dosing and drug holidays can reduce this risk of growth suppression from oral corticosteroids. In the case of ICSs, the use of the minimum effective potency and dose may help ameliorate systemic effects in children who exhibit signs of growth failure.

Immunodeficiencies: Both congenital and acquired immunodeficiencies (HIV infection) are associated with growth failure. Mechanisms include anorexia, malabsorption, diarrhea, chronic infection, and systemic inflammation. Diagnosis is usually evident but an occasional child with common variable immune deficiency may present with growth failure before clues in the history and physical examination lead to an evaluation of immune status. Successful treatment of the underlying disease will usually lead to an improvement in growth.

In most of these systemic illnesses, the history typically reveals that the child had been growing normally until some point. Then the growth rate slowed, which is suggestive of onset of an illness. The history may reveal a clear earlier diagnosis of chronic illness or may include symptoms suggestive of the underlying disorder (e.g., loss of appetite, diarrhea, mouth sores, and fever). The physical examination typically shows that the weight is more depressed than the height, but typically head circumference is preserved. If there is microcephaly, a primary genetic etiology should be considered. There may also be features indicative of the underlying disorder (e.g., pallor in anemia, perianal findings in Crohn disease).

Laboratory studies that screen for chronic illness (CBC, ESR, chemistry profile, UA) may at times provide clues to the diagnosis. Screening for celiac disease with tissue transglutaminase immunoglobulin A (IgA) antibody testing may be indicated, especially if failure to thrive appears after a period of normal growth or if weight is affected more than height. If indicated by the clinical features and/or screening laboratory studies, definitive diagnosis requires directed tests (e.g., endoscopy and biopsy for inflammatory bowel disease or celiac disease, sweat chloride test for cystic fibrosis).

The management of these conditions rests on specific therapy directed at the underlying condition (e.g., gluten-free diet for celiac disease). When the disease is adequately treated, the growth rate often improves but catch-up growth may not compensate for all of the lost height potential in long-standing cases, leading to a permanent height deficit. GH therapy may be indicated if the height deficit is severe and is unlikely to correct with treatment of the underlying disease alone. GH is specifically approved for the treatment of short stature in children with renal insufficiency.

Emotional Deprivation

Deprivation can stunt growth in two ways. First, a child may be deprived of food (an example of malnutrition); in this case, the child's weight is generally depressed more than the height. Second (and more rarely), a child who is emotionally deprived (and emotional deprivation, rather than actual physical abuse, seems to be key) may have profound short stature without apparent malnutrition (**psychosocial dwarfism**). In this case, the height is depressed more than the weight (Fig. 56.10). Such a child may (in some but not all cases) have the clinical features of GH deficiency and may in fact show laboratory evidence of hypopituitarism. But when placed in a more nurturing environment, the child grows markedly, and the GH levels revert to normal. This disorder may be difficult to diagnose, and the social history is critical. The diagnosis ultimately rests on significant improvement of growth once the environment improves.

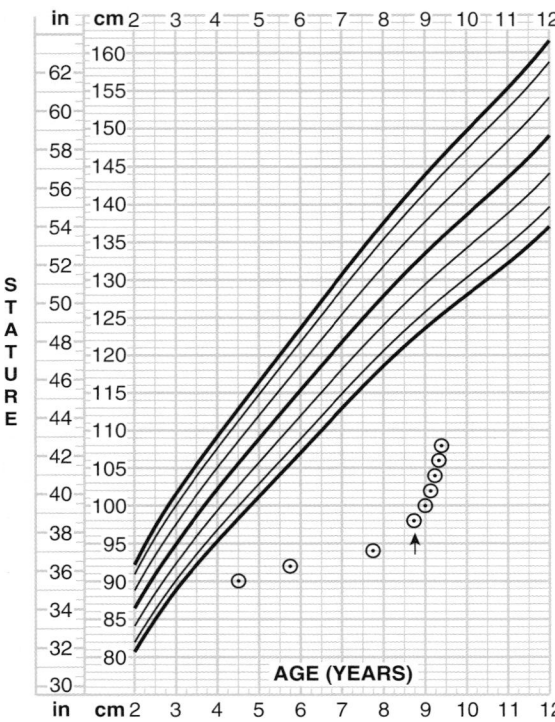

Fig. 56.10 Growth chart of a boy with deprivation dwarfism (psychosocial dwarfism). Between ages 6 and 8⁷/₁₂ years, he had chemical evidence of growth hormone (GH) deficiency. After placement in a chronic care facility *(arrow)*, his growth rate improved markedly, and his GH levels reverted to normal. NCHS, National Center for Health Statistics. (From Styne DM. Growth. In: Greenspan FS, Forsham PH, eds. *Basic and Clinical Endocrinology.* 3rd ed. Los Altos, CA: Appleton & Lange; 1991.)

Iatrogenic Causes

Treatments for medical conditions may secondarily impair growth. The classic example is glucocorticoids. This is obviously a risk with prolonged systemic steroid use but even inhaled or topical steroids (especially if used over a wide area or under occlusive cover) may suppress growth. A significant proportion of the dose of ICSs is deposited in the oral cavity and oropharynx and after being swallowed is absorbed via the gastrointestinal tract. Much of this is metabolized to inactive metabolites in the liver (first-pass metabolism), but some still escapes inactivation and may have systemic effects. Systemic effects are generally mild, but long-term studies show that high-potency ICSs (budesonide, fluticasone) do have a small but measurable impact on linear growth. The final adult height may be decreased by 1–2 cm in long-term users of ICSs. Since poorly controlled asthma is a serious condition and may have an even bigger impact on growth, this relatively small effect should not prevent the use of ICSs in asthmatics who need it. But an occasional child may have more significant slowing of growth based on individual differences in sensitivity, metabolism, and technique, and this possibility should be kept in mind as a possible cause of slow growth.

Spinal irradiation for treatment of malignancies may stunt growth by limiting further spinal growth; this is associated with a high U/L. Treatments for hyperactivity (sympathomimetic agents suppress appetite) may interfere with growth and cause a small but measurable decrease in final height in some children.

BONE DYSPLASIAS

Skeletal dysplasias constitute a broad group of genetic disorders in which there is innate failure of normal bone or cartilage development.

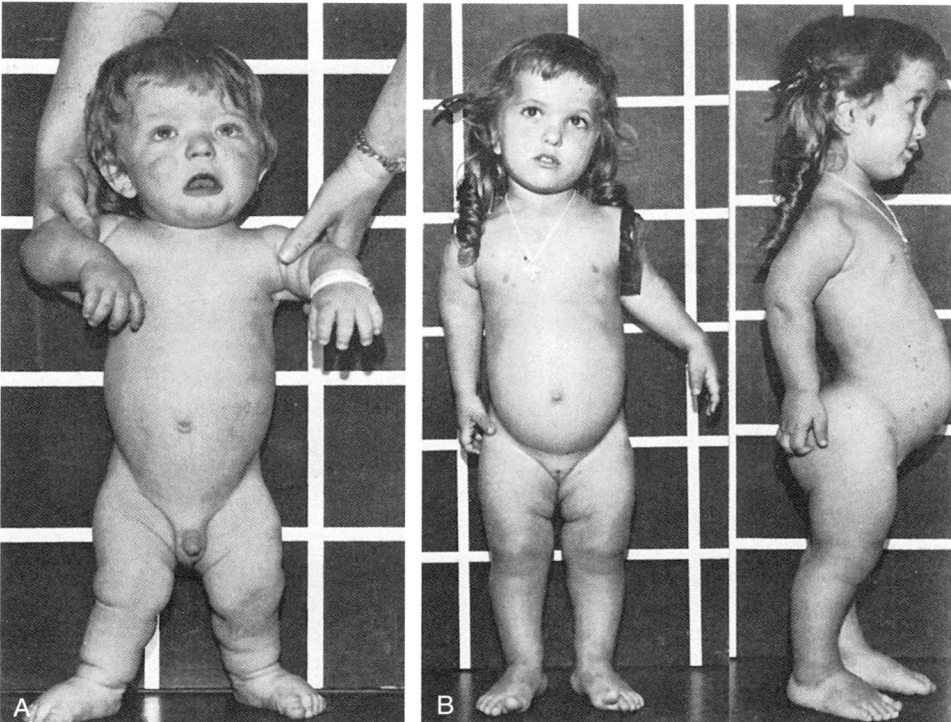

Fig. 56.11 Achondroplasia. *A,* One-year-old boy with height age of 4 months. *B,* Four-year-old girl with height age of 20 months. (*A,* From Smith DW. Compendium on shortness of stature. *J Pediatr.* 1967;70:504; *B,* from Jones KL, ed. *Smith's Recognizable Patterns of Human Malformation.* 4th ed. Philadelphia: WB Saunders; 1988.)

There are 461 unique skeletal disorders classified into 42 groups (see Table 56.4).

Abnormal body proportions are characteristic of these conditions (disproportionate short stature), although there are some exceptions. Bone ages are not reliable indicators of osseous maturity in these conditions.

Achondroplasia

Achondroplasia is the classic example of an osteochondrodystrophy (Fig. 56.11). The incidence is 1 per 20,000. This condition is caused by the autosomal dominant pathogenic variant p.Gly380Arg in the fibroblast growth factor receptor 3 (FGFR3) in 98% of cases; approximately 80% are due to de novo variation (i.e., spontaneous new pathogenic variant in offspring). Short stature, body disproportion with short limbs, hypotonia, and a relatively large head with midface hypoplasia are often noted at birth. Progressive deceleration of growth rate begins in infancy, and the humerus and femur are particularly shortened (rhizomelia, i.e., proximal shortening of the limbs). The hands may show a three-pronged configuration (trident hand). In addition, there may be hydrocephalus as a result of narrowing of the foramen magnum, kyphosis, stenosis of the spinal canal, and vertebral disk lesions. The diagnosis is clinical and is supported by characteristic radiologic features that include small cuboid vertebral bodies and anterior beaking of the first or second lumbar vertebra. The average adult height is 125 cm (4 feet, 1 inch) in girls and 131 cm (4 feet, 3 inches) in boys. Treatment with an agent that antagonizes the gain-of-function effect on chondrocyte maturation results in an increased annualized growth velocity. Longitudinal studies are ongoing to determine the impact on the foramen magnum and risk for spinal stenosis.

Hypochondroplasia

Hypochondroplasia is an allelic variant of achondroplasia and manifests with short stature and dysmorphic features that are often milder than in achondroplasia. In particular there are few craniofacial abnormalities, and body disproportion may be subtle. Newborns may be slightly small, but short stature generally becomes apparent by age 3 years. The short stature is minimally disproportionate with relatively short limbs. The hands and feet are usually stubby. Genu varum may occur. Radiologic hallmarks include metaphyseal indentation and flaring as well as hypoplasia of the ilia with small greater sciatic notches. Some reports suggested a beneficial effect of GH but this remains a nonstandard indication for GH treatment.

Spondyloepiphysial dysplasias are a heterogeneous group of dysplasias that primarily affect the epiphyses and the vertebral bodies. Most forms are characterized by short-trunk dwarfism (preferential shortening of the trunk as compared with the extremities) and vertebral anomalies. These conditions may lead to spinal cord compression due to subluxation of the cervical spine. GH therapy is not recommended.

Osteogenesis Imperfecta

Moderate and severe forms of osteogenesis imperfecta are associated with proportional short stature. The diagnosis is typically made on the basis of bone fragility and fractures; short stature is not a presenting feature.

EVALUATING THE CHILD WITH SHORT STATURE

Statistically, most children with short stature will turn out to have one of the normal variant causes of short stature (familial short stature or constitutional delay) or will have ISS. An extensive evaluation will *not* reveal a specific cause in most patients. On the other hand, short stature in general and growth failure in particular may be the first sign of serious systemic disease or endocrine disorder and appropriate evaluation is essential to make the correct diagnosis. It is best to start the evaluation with a thorough history (including a family history and direct measurement of the heights of both parents if possible) and physical examination (including careful measurement and plotting of height on appropriate growth charts) and then order laboratory tests and imaging studies based on this evaluation and specifically tailored to the particular child instead of simply ordering a certain panel of tests on every child with short stature.

At the first contact with a short child, the physician usually does not know if the height velocity is also abnormal. If the initial history and examination do not indicate that a specific cause may be present, it is best to schedule a second visit in 4–6 months to reassess the height and to accurately measure the height velocity. But if the initial history and examination indicate possible pathology, or if the short stature is unusually severe (more than 2.5 SD below the mean is a good cut-off), then some immediate lab tests and a bone-age X-ray may be performed at the first visit.

At any stage, the finding of a subnormal growth velocity is more concerning than the finding of short stature. Normal growth variants are not characterized by a subnormal growth velocity, and (barring mismeasurement) a growth rate below the normal range is a cause of concern and should trigger an evaluation. A figure of 5 cm per year is frequently used as a rough measure of the minimum height velocity in childhood (after age 3), though strictly speaking, normal height velocity may be as low as 4 cm per year for boys and 4.5 cm per year for girls in children between age 6 and puberty.

Initial screening labs should include an IGF-1 level (to assess GH secretion), a TSH (to evaluate the thyroid gland), and a bone-age X-ray to assess bone maturation and obtain an estimate of the final adult height. A CBC (to rule out anemia) and a creatinine level (to assess renal function) as well as an ESR or CRP to identify systemic inflammation may be indicated as well. *A karyotype is mandatory in any female with significant short stature* because of the possibility of Turner syndrome. Beyond that, the testing will be guided by the history, the physical examination, and the results of initial screening labs.

IMPORTANT CONSIDERATIONS IN THE HISTORY

Pregnancy and Birth History

Did the mother have illnesses or take medication during the pregnancy? Maternal illness or use of certain drugs can cause poor fetal growth.

What was the birthweight and length? IUGR may lead to continuing small stature.

Did the baby have perinatal problems such as unexplained hypoglycemia, prolonged jaundice, or, in males, a small phallus? These are all suggestive of congenital GH deficiency.

Did the neonate have other perinatal problems (birth asphyxia, puffy extremities)? These may provide clues to the underlying cause of short stature (significant hypoxia may lead to hypopituitarism; puffy extremities in a female are suggestive of Turner syndrome).

Infancy and Childhood

What was the child's growth pattern? The child who is short but growing at a normal rate and paralleling the 3rd percentile is more likely to have familial or constitutional short stature. The child whose height deviates progressively away from the normal curve (especially after 24 months of age) is much more likely to have an underlying medical disorder. When this progressive deviation occurs from early childhood and continues, it often represents a congenital disorder (e.g., Turner syndrome, congenital GH deficiency). However, growth attenuation that occurs after a sustained period of normal growth suggests that a disorder has been acquired (e.g., acquired GH deficiency, inflammatory bowel disease).

What were the child's developmental milestones? How is the school performance? Slow development or poor school performance may indicate a central disorder or may represent part of a syndrome (e.g., PWS). Hypothyroidism acquired after age 3 years usually does not interfere with school performance, although inadequately treated congenital hypothyroidism often leads to intellectual impairment. This question may also elicit a history of emotional problems.

Has the child had any serious illnesses or been on medication? Chronic illness often impedes growth, as do certain medications (glucocorticoids). A history of nonendocrine medical problems may also provide clues to the underlying disorder (e.g., the presence of aortic coarctation may be suggestive of Turner syndrome).

Review of Systems

How is the child's appetite? What does the child eat in a typical 3-day period (often best described by a formal diet record)? Adequate caloric intake is needed for growth. Inadequate intake may be a symptom of underlying chronic disease.

Does the child have abdominal pain, diarrhea, unexplained fevers, mouth or anal sores, or joint pain? These symptoms suggest occult inflammatory bowel disease.

Does the child have neck swelling, lethargy, constipation, cold intolerance, or weight gain without much increase in height? These are among the symptoms of acquired hypothyroidism.

Does the child have headaches, vomiting, or visual disturbances? Symptoms of CNS dysfunction, raised intracranial pressure, or both suggest the possibility of acquired hypopituitarism in association with a central lesion such as a tumor or hydrocephalus.

Has the child begun pubertal development? Puberty influences growth. Children with constitutional delay in growth and development have delayed puberty and often have an exaggerated nadir of growth velocity before puberty begins. However, the more puberty is delayed, the greater the likelihood of a medical disorder such as hypogonadism. Delayed puberty may also be a manifestation of hypogonadism (Turner syndrome), or it may be secondary to a growth-impeding disorder (hypothyroidism, malnutrition, chronic illness). *Precocious puberty is not a cause of growth failure (it should accelerate growth), but it may lead to short final adult height because of premature fusion of the epiphyses.*

Family History

What were the heights of parents and other family members at the child's age, and when did they undergo puberty? What are the current heights of parents and family members? The most frequent causes of short stature are familial short stature and constitutional delay in growth and development. In the former, a family history of short stature is elicited. In the latter, a family history of delayed puberty is elicited.

Physical Examination

Height and weight should each be plotted carefully on growth charts. The degree of short stature in relation to peers is ascertained. Previous height measurements provide an index of the child's pattern of growth. Weight that is depressed more than height in a short child is suggestive of chronic illness or malnutrition. In contrast, a child who is short but chubby is more likely to have an endocrine disorder or syndrome (e.g., GH deficiency, hypothyroidism, Cushing syndrome, PWS).

Exogenous obesity is usually associated with relatively tall stature. Disproportionate short stature is characteristic of skeletal dysplasias (short limbs in the case of achondroplasia and hypochondroplasia, short trunk in some rare forms of skeletal dysplasia) and may also be seen in long-standing hypothyroidism.

The presence of dysmorphic features is often suggestive of a syndrome or genetic disorder (e.g., Turner syndrome, Noonan syndrome). Midline craniofacial defects are suggestive of hypopituitarism.

Goiter, delayed dentition, bradycardia, dry hair or skin, or delayed reflexes may be suggestive of hypothyroidism.

Cherubic or doll-like appearance, high-pitched voice, delayed dentition, poor musculature, or relative adiposity may be suggestive of GH deficiency.

Bitemporal hemianopsia, papilledema, optic atrophy, or accelerating head circumference in a young child is suggestive of a CNS abnormality (craniopharyngioma) causing hypopituitarism.

The stage of puberty is noted. Delayed puberty is compatible with constitutional delay in growth and development, hypogonadism, panhypopituitarism, severe hypothyroidism, or chronic illness.

THERAPEUTIC OPTIONS

Specific Treatment of the Primary Disorder

If a child is found to have a clear medical condition causing short stature and for which treatment is available (e.g., hypothyroidism, GH deficiency), the appropriate treatment (thyroid replacement therapy or GH therapy, respectively) improves growth markedly as long as the epiphyses remain open. Often, such children experience accelerated (catch-up) growth for some time after appropriate treatment is instituted. Complete compensation for growth failure is unlikely to occur if the disorder was many years in duration or occurred very close to the onset of normal puberty.

Sex Steroids

Sex steroid treatments may be administered to adolescents with constitutional delay of growth and development. Males with delayed puberty may be treated with testosterone enanthate or cypionate (50–100 mg/mo intramuscularly or subcutaneously for 3–6 months; smaller doses given more frequently may be more physiologic and are preferred by some practitioners) to gradually bring about secondary sexual characteristics and accelerated linear growth. This is often gratifying for males and is usually followed by spontaneous pubertal development. The low dose of testosterone is designed to avoid undue advancement of bone age and loss of growth potential. Oxandrolone is a testosterone derivative with less androgenic effects than testosterone, and does not aromatize to estrogen, so theoretically it may be preferable to depot-testosterone injections. Several small studies report beneficial effects of oxandrolone in males with constitutional delay of growth and puberty. The usual dose is 2.5 mg daily for anywhere from 3 to 12 months. Giving oxandrolone (in addition to GH therapy) to females with Turner syndrome leads to better height outcomes than GH alone, so this is frequently done at around age 8–10 years in females who are still well short of a normal height. Females with Turner syndrome who started GH relatively early in life are less likely to require the addition of oxandrolone. The usual dose is 0.03–0.05 mg/kg/day. Side effects at this dose are rare, but signs of virilization should prompt a reduction in dose.

Estrogen

Just as males with constitutional delay are treated with androgens, females with pubertal delay and mild short stature may be treated with a short course of estrogen therapy. However, benign constitutional delay is less likely in females (who are more likely to have an underlying pathologic cause such as Turner syndrome) and such treatment is relatively rare. If it is contemplated, care should be taken to exclude other causes of pubertal delay and to use low doses of estrogens because estrogens promote epiphyseal closure.

Counseling

Reassurance and counseling should be available for all patients. For many children with familial short stature or constitutional delay in growth and development, it is reassuring to be told that they are normal and are likely to reach a normal adult height or one in keeping with the family heights. This is particularly true for children with delayed puberty, in whom the discrepancy in height in comparison with peers (who have gone through their pubertal growth spurts) is disconcerting. It is helpful if parents do not dwell on the child's height but focus on the child's strengths. Gymnastics, wrestling, soccer, and swimming are often activities at which short children are not at a disadvantage and in which they may excel.

Growth Hormone Therapy

There is a broad consensus for the use of GH therapy in children with short stature caused by classical GH deficiency, Turner syndrome, Noonan syndrome, SHOX haplo-insufficiency, PWS, Russell-Silver syndrome, and chronic renal failure. Children who were born SGA and fail to catch up to the normal range of height by age 2 (by age 4 in Europe) are also candidates for GH therapy. The FDA has approved GH for children with ISS, but this treatment remains controversial and the cost-benefit ratio remains uncertain.

Side effects of GH therapy include fluid retention that is usually mild and tends to resolve with continued treatment. Mild headaches are also common and are usually benign. Increased intracranial pressure (**pseudotumor cerebri**) is a rare but serious dose-related side effect. It usually resolves if treatment is stopped, and after resolution, treatment can frequently be restarted at a lower dose. The incidence of **slipped capital femoral epiphyses** is increased and **scoliosis** may be worsened during GH therapy, likely secondary to accelerated growth. GH-neutralizing antibodies may appear but are rarely of clinical significance. GH can accelerate the growth of existing nevi and can induce insulin resistance, but this does not appear to be clinically significant.

Because of its growth-promoting effects, there has long been concern about a possible increase in the incidence of cancer. No significant increase in common childhood cancers has been noted yet in surveillance studies, but (somewhat unexpectedly) in one French study (the Safety and Appropriateness of Growth hormone treatments in Europe [SAGhE] study) the group treated with GH had a standardized mortality ratio (SMR) of 1.33 (95% confidence interval [CI], 1.08–1.64) compared to controls. Cardiovascular disease was responsible for most of the excess mortality. Although all-type cancer-related mortality was not increased in the French cohort, bone tumor–related mortality was increased. There were weaknesses in the design of this study and a smaller study from Belgium, the Netherlands, and Sweden did not show the same results, but the study did raise concerns about long-term safety. More long-term follow-up data is being collected to determine the true long-term safety profile of GH. Until more information becomes available, most authorities do not recommend any changes in current practice, but this may change if new studies reveal new hazards. It should be kept in mind that GH therapy on a large scale did not begin until 1985, so even the earliest treated subjects are not very old at this time; impact on the risk of cancer or heart disease in the elderly (if any) may not be detectable in various study cohorts at this time.

OTHER TREATMENTS

Recombinant human IGF-1 is indicated for the treatment of extremely short children with primary IGF-1 deficiency (both height *and* IGF-1 >3 SD below the mean for age) caused by severe GH insensitivity (e.g., Laron syndrome and IGF-1 gene defects). Availability may be an issue. Possible side effects include hypoglycemia, increased intracranial pressure, and adenotonsillar hypertrophy.

TABLE 56.9   Red Flags in the Evaluation of Short Stature

Height >2–2.5 standard deviations below the mean for age
Subnormal growth velocity
Abnormal body proportions
Abnormal height:weight ratio
Dysmorphic features including midline facial defects
Goiter
Abnormal central nervous system (headache, cranial neuropathies) and ophthalmologic (visual field defects, papilledema) examinations
Acquired growth failure in a previously growing child

TABLE 56.10   Conditions Not to Miss

Hypoglycemia in a child with no risk factors for hypoglycemia	Consider hypopituitarism in the differential
Hypoglycemia, jaundice, and microphallus in a newborn boy	Rule out growth hormone deficiency
Obesity in a child who is short	Rule out hypothyroidism, growth hormone deficiency, Cushing syndrome, Prader-Willi syndrome, Laurence-Moon-Biedl syndrome
Shortness in a child with a goiter	Rule out hypothyroidism
Shortness in a child with headache, vomiting, or visual disturbance	Rule out hypopituitarism secondary to central nervous system lesion, including craniopharyngioma or hydrocephalus

SUMMARY AND RED FLAGS (TABLES 56.9 AND 56.10)

Short stature may be a variant of normal development or may indicate a serious underlying problem (see Tables 56.3, 56.5, 56.7, and 56.9). When short stature is associated with a slow growth velocity, progressive deviation from the child's previous growth channel, obesity, headache, vomiting, dysmorphic features, or a goiter, or if short height is inconsistent with the family history, a search for an underlying medical disorder should be undertaken. Understanding how to measure a child accurately, performing simple proportion measurements, and calculating growth velocity are skills that all pediatricians must have to diagnose short stature and identify associated disease states and syndromes.

BIBLIOGRAPHY

A bibliography is available at ExpertConsult.com.

57

Hypoglycemia

Alvina R. Kansra

Hypoglycemia, although rare in children beyond the newborn period, is an acute, life-threatening medical emergency that may result in seizures, permanent brain injury, or even sudden death. Hypoglycemia may represent a serious underlying disorder due to hormonal deficiencies, metabolic defects, genetic disorders, drugs, or toxins. Therefore, to evaluate hypoglycemia either in a child or newborn, a comprehensive strategy for diagnosis and treatment is crucial. Hypoglycemia occurs when there is a disruption in the normal response of the metabolic and endocrine systems during the transition from fed to fasted state resulting in an imbalance in glucose homeostasis, either excessive glucose removal from the circulation or deficient glucose delivery into the circulation, or both. To make the accurate diagnosis, it is essential to obtain labs at the time of hypoglycemia that includes plasma and urine specimens for critical hormones, as well as metabolic products before initiating treatment. However, treatment should never be delayed if there is uncertainty as to what critical labs are required. Obtaining a "red top" and "green top" blood collection tube will allow for most all studies to be run.

DEFINITION OF HYPOGLYCEMIA

The precise definition of hypoglycemia, one applicable to all age groups, is controversial. Historically, a working definition for significant hypoglycemia was initially developed based on the clinical manifestations of low blood sugars in neonates.

Attempts have been made to define hypoglycemia by using operational thresholds or a clinical approach. An operational threshold is based on the glucose in plasma or whole blood that prompts the intervention and is defined as blood glucose <40 mg/dL (plasma glucose levels <45 mg/dL); the clinical approach defines the blood glucose concentration threshold at which clinical signs and symptoms appear (and disappear by correcting the low glucose concentration). The wide range of blood glucose concentrations at which clinically overt signs may appear has led to uncertainty in definition.

Regardless of the wide fluctuations in glucose levels (between fed and fasting states), plasma blood glucose is normally maintained within a very narrow range of 70–100 mg/dL. A plasma glucose value below 40 mg/dL is commonly taken as the clinical definition of hypoglycemia. However, subtle signs and symptoms of neuroglycopenia can be documented at plasma glucose levels below 70 mg/dL and are more apparent at glucose levels below 60 or 50 mg/dL. For provocative tests, such as fasting studies, a glucose level of 50 mg/dL can be taken as sufficiently low for judging fuel and hormonal responsiveness. The response to a given level of plasma glucose can vary, depending on the underlying disorder. Patients with glucose-6-phosphatase deficiency (type 1 glycogen storage disease) may appear asymptomatic at glucose levels below 40 mg/dL because they have concomitant elevations of plasma lactate and ketones, which can partially spare the glucose

utilization by the brain. On the other hand, children with defects in fatty acid oxidation can become very ill at plasma glucose levels as high as 60 mg/dL because they have no alternative fuels (ketones) to glucose as a substrate for the brain, heart, and skeletal muscle.

When comparing reported glucose values, the clinician must recognize some technical factors. Unless a free-flow blood sample is obtained from the infant with minimal pain, the glucose values are likely to be unreliable. Second, whole blood glucose values are slightly lower than those of plasma because of the dilution by the fluid in the red blood cells. Finally, hematocrit also influences the blood glucose concentration. This is particularly important in newborns whose hematocrit values are higher than older infants and children. A high hematocrit level results in lower blood glucose concentration; the opposite is true for low hematocrit values.

It was once common practice to accept lower standards for glucose levels in newborns because of the high frequency of low plasma glucose levels on the day of birth. It should be stressed that these lower values represent a purely "statistical" definition of normal; there is no evidence that the neonatal brain has less need for glucose than do the brains of older children or adults. Specific maturational delays in several of the fasting systems (metabolic, endocrine) adequately explain why neonates have such a high risk of hypoglycemia during the first 12–24 hours after delivery. The use of different glucose standards for newborns should be discouraged, and the same treatment goals for hypoglycemia should be applied to newborns and older children: that is, to maintain plasma glucose levels above 60 mg/dL.

REGULATION OF BLOOD GLUCOSE CONCENTRATION

The brain is solely dependent upon glucose as a *primary* source of energy. However, during the period of starvation, it can also use ketones as an alternative *(but not sole)* source for energy production. Glucose is derived from either the intestinal absorption of dietary carbohydrates (exogenous source) or endogenous production (glycogenolysis or gluconeogenesis). Within 2–3 hours after a meal, glucose absorption from the intestine ceases, and the liver becomes the major source of glucose for the brain and other tissues. The liver produces glucose through a combination of glycogenolysis and gluconeogenesis (Fig. 57.1). Gluconeogenesis provides approximately 25% of hepatic glucose production in the early phases of fasting; the rate of gluconeogenesis is determined largely by rates of proteolysis and remains constant throughout fasting. Hepatic glycogenolysis provides most of the glucose production early in a fast, but by 12 hours, liver glycogen stores become depleted. The body must then begin to depend on release of fatty acids by lipolysis from stores of fat in adipose tissue. Most tissues can oxidize free fatty acids (FFAs) directly and thus minimize their use of glucose. The major exception is the brain, which is unable to directly oxidize FFAs because

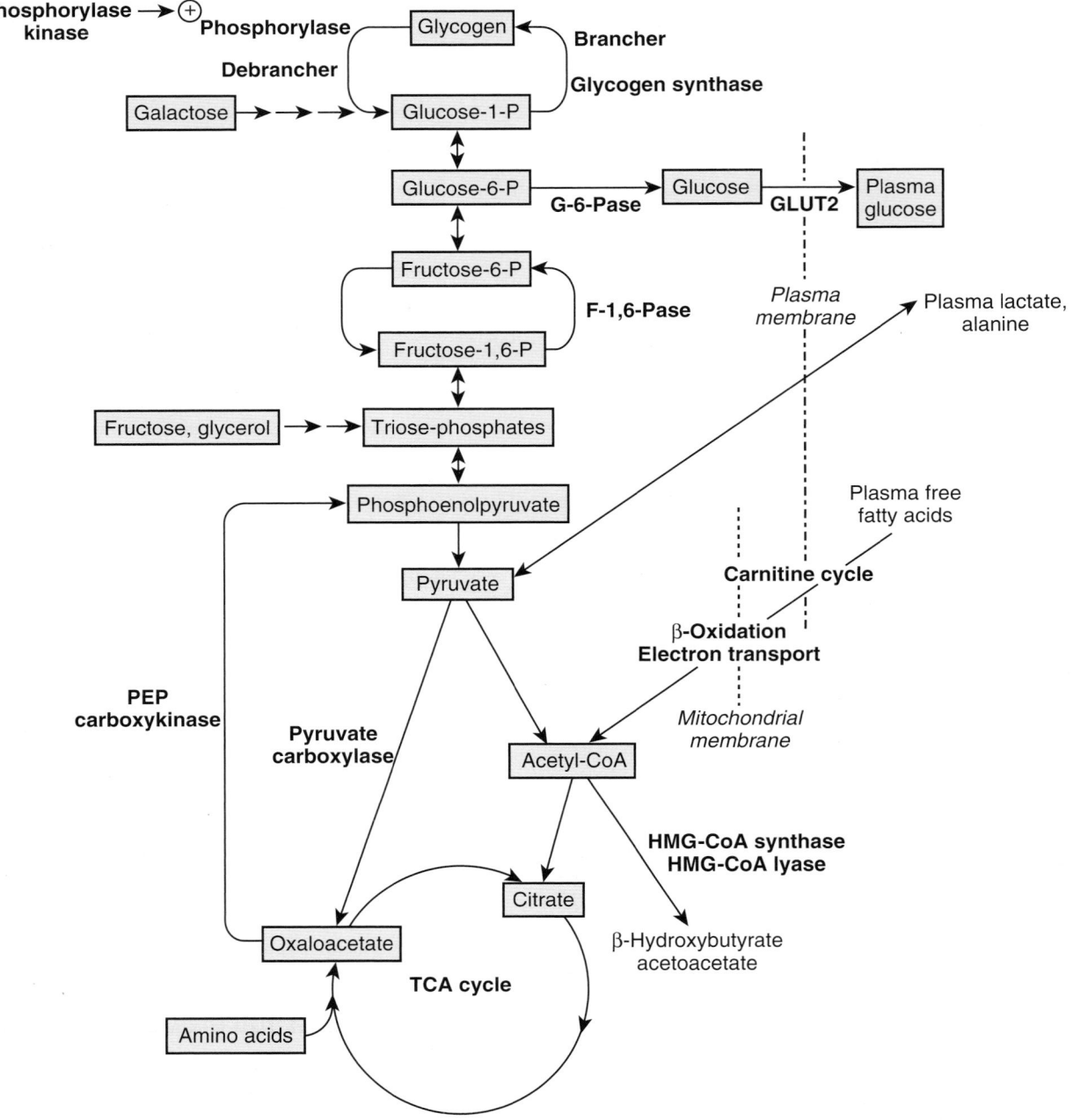

Fig. 57.1 Metabolic systems of fasting adaptation. Shown are the pathways of hepatic gluconeogenesis, glycogenolysis, and ketogenesis. Key enzyme steps are in boldface. Enzyme steps in gluconeogenesis: pyruvate carboxylase, phosphoenolpyruvate (PEP) carboxykinase, fructose-1,6-bisphosphatase (F-1,6-Pase), glucose-6-phosphatase (G-6-Pase), and the plasma membrane glucose transporter 2 (GLUT2). Enzyme steps in glycogenolysis: glycogen synthase, glycogen brancher enzyme, glycogen phosphorylase kinase, glycogen phosphorylase, and glycogen debrancher enzyme. Steps in ketogenesis include a series of enzyme steps in the carnitine cycle for transporting fatty acids across the mitochondrial membrane, enzymes of the β-oxidation cycle, enzymes of electron transport, and enzymes of ketone synthesis (3-hydroxy-3-methylglutaryl-coenzyme A [HMG-CoA] synthase and HMG-CoA lyase). P, phosphate; TCA, tricarboxylic acid.

FFAs cannot cross the blood-brain barrier. Partial oxidation of FFAs in the liver produces ketones (β-hydroxybutyrate and acetoacetate), which are readily oxidized by the brain, thus sparing cerebral glucose consumption.

Metabolic systems and hormones normally prevent hypoglycemia during fasting (Tables 57.1 and 57.2). The integration of these systems is demonstrated by the changes in plasma concentrations of the major fuels and hormones during fasting (Fig. 57.2). Plasma glucose concentrations gradually decline over the course of the fast as liver glycogen reserves are depleted. In infants and young children, with their larger ratio of brain to body mass, glucose levels fall faster than in older children and adults and may reach 50 mg/dL by 24–30 hours of fasting. Plasma levels of lactate, a representative gluconeogenic precursor, decline while fasting as hepatic gluconeogenesis is stimulated and protein turnover slows. Plasma FFA levels begin to rise quickly after 12–20 hours of fasting in response to the fall in insulin concentrations as glucose levels decline. The increased availability of FFAs is accompanied by a 10- to 20-fold rise in plasma ketone levels as hepatic oxidation of FFAs is activated. Determining the circulating levels of these fuels and hormones at the point of hypoglycemia provides the most critical information for diagnosing the cause of hypoglycemia.

CLINICAL MANIFESTATIONS

A variety of signs and symptoms may occur in patients with hypoglycemia (Table 57.3). They can be divided into two categories. Those in the first category result from activation of the autonomic nervous system and release of the counter-regulatory hormone epinephrine (neurogenic). Those in the second category are secondary to inadequate delivery of glucose to the brain (neuroglycopenia).

CAUSES OF TRANSIENT NEONATAL HYPOGLYCEMIA

Hypoglycemia is a common problem in newborns. Most cases are transient, although the neonatal period is also the time when inherited disorders are most likely to manifest. The differential diagnosis of hypoglycemia is extensive (Tables 57.4 and 57.5).

Normal Newborns

As many as 30% of normal, full-term newborns and those appropriate for gestational age may be unable to maintain plasma glucose levels above 50 mg/dL if they fast during the first 6 hours after delivery. By the second day of life, the frequency of plasma glucose concentrations below 50 mg/dL decreases to <1%, which indicates a rapid maturation of fasting metabolic adaptation. The poor fasting tolerance on the day

of birth can be explained by lack of development of key enzymes in the pathways of both hepatic gluconeogenesis and ketogenesis. Transcription of these genes is delayed until after delivery but becomes well activated by the end of the first 24 hours. Glucagon and cortisol may be important for activation of enzymes involved in gluconeogenesis. Ingestion of long-chain fats (e.g., in colostrum) may be important for triggering transcription of the two enzymes of ketogenesis. Thus, on the day of birth, all newborns can be viewed as having impaired fasting adaptation. In the absence of other risk factors, hypoglycemia in the first day may necessitate only feeding and follow-up blood glucose determination to ensure that further work-up is not necessary. Breast-fed babies are at special risk for hypoglycemia when there are problems initiating milk production.

Newborns Small for Gestational Age and Premature Infants

Hypoglycemia is significantly more common in premature infants and those small for gestational age because of decreased stores of glycogen, fat, and protein. In addition, the enzymes necessary for gluconeogenesis may be less developed than in normal full-term infants.

Infants of Diabetic Mothers

Infants born to mothers with any type of diabetes, including gestational diabetes, are at risk for hypoglycemia due to increased insulin secretion before birth that persists for the first few days after delivery. This transient neonatal hyperinsulinemia occurs because maternal hyperglycemia stimulates fetal insulin secretion and, after delivery, affected infants have difficulty in downregulating insulin secretion to adapt to the withdrawal of the hyperglycemia. Because of the growth-stimulating effects of insulin on the fetus, infants of diabetic mothers are often large for gestational age. Blood glucose levels should be monitored after birth until they stabilize in the normal range. Enteral feedings should be initiated as soon as possible to prevent fasting hypoglycemia. Hypoglycemia should be treated with intravenous glucose; the problem should resolve promptly, within 1–2 days. Prolonged hyperinsulinism (HI) in infants of diabetic mothers should raise the suspicion of either a genetic form of HI or perinatal stress-induced HI.

Perinatal Stress-Induced Hyperinsulinism

Some infants with birth asphyxia or intrauterine growth restriction may have severe problems with hypoglycemia for prolonged periods, ranging from a few days to a few months after birth. This form of transient HI has not been well characterized, but it is probably not rare. The mechanism appears to be HI; oral diazoxide, which decreases insulin secretion, provides good control of hypoglycemia in these infants.

Erythroblastosis Fetalis

An association between hypoglycemia and erythroblastosis fetalis caused by Rh incompatibility occurs in infants who are anemic at birth (cord hemoglobin <10 g/dL). The low blood glucose levels in these

---

TABLE 57.1 Metabolic Systems and Hormones Regulating Blood Glucose

Metabolic Systems
Hepatic gluconeogenesis
Hepatic glycogenolysis
Adipose tissue lipolysis
Fatty acid oxidation (liver and peripheral organs) and hepatic ketogenesis

Hormonal Systems
Insulin
Counter-regulatory hormones
    Glucagon
    Cortisol
    Growth hormone
    Epinephrine

TABLE 57.2 Hormonal Regulation of Fasting Metabolic Systems

Hormone	Hepatic Glycogenesis	Hepatic Glucogenesis	Adipose Tissue Lipolysis	Hepatic Ketogenesis
Insulin	Inhibits	Inhibits	Inhibits	Inhibits
Glucagon	Stimulates	—	—	—
Cortisol	—	Stimulates	—	—
Growth hormone	—	—	Stimulates	—
Epinephrine	Stimulates	Stimulates	Stimulates	Stimulates

From Sperling MA, ed. *Pediatric Endocrinology*. 2nd ed. Philadelphia: Elsevier; 2002.

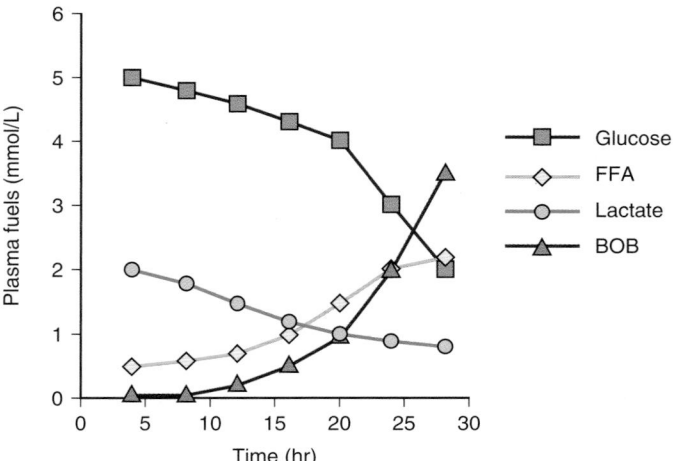

Fig. 57.2 Changes in plasma levels of key fuels during fasting in a normal child. Note that plasma glucose declines toward hypoglycemic values by 24 hours as hepatic glycogen reserves become depleted. Plasma levels of lactate, a representative gluconeogenic substrate, decline gradually during the fast as hepatic gluconeogenesis is activated. Late in fasting, levels of plasma free fatty acids (FFAs) increase as lipolysis is stimulated, followed by a dramatic rise in β-hydroxybutyrate that reflects the increase in the rates of hepatic fatty acid oxidation and ketone synthesis. BOB, β-hydroxybutyrate.

infants have been attributed to high plasma insulin concentration. The cause of these high insulin levels remains undefined. The current prevention and management of Rh sensitization have markedly reduced the incidence of erythroblastosis and of fetal and neonatal anemia. Nonetheless, such infants require careful monitoring of plasma glucose concentration soon after birth.

Intrapartum Maternal Glucose Administration

Administration of excessive glucose quantities to the mother during labor results in maternal as well as fetal hyperglycemia. Increased fetal glucose concentration causes increased fetal insulin secretion and fetal HI. If the glucose has been administered to the mother immediately before the infant's birth, the infant is born with high insulin levels. An acute administration of large amounts of glucose-containing fluids to prevent hypotension in women receiving conduction anesthesia could result in acute fetal hyperglycemia, HI, and metabolic acidosis due to increased lactate concentration, resulting in transient HI that leads to hypoglycemia in a fetus. This effect is more pronounced if the mother has received glucose infusion for a prolonged period of time.

Maternal Drug Therapy

The various pharmacologic agents administered to the mother for the treatment of medical problems that can influence blood glucose levels in the newborn can be divided into two broad categories:

1. Some drugs, including oral hypoglycemic agents, can directly affect blood glucose. Oral hypoglycemic agents, such as chlorpropamide, metformin, and sulfonylureas, are administered by some physicians for the treatment of gestational diabetes. These drugs are easily transported across the placenta, and the infant is born with a certain amount of drug present in the circulation. These drugs, particularly those with prolonged effects, may result in profound hypoglycemia that tends to persist until the drug is removed, either by its own clearance or by exchange transfusion.

2. Some drugs are administered to the mother with indirect effects (the more common contributor to neonatal hypoglycemia). β-Sympathomimetic agents commonly used for the prevention and

TABLE 57.3	**Symptoms of Hypoglycemia**
Neurogenic Symptoms Due to Activation of Autonomic Nervous System*	
Sweating	
Shakiness, trembling	
Tachycardia	
Anxiety, nervousness	
Weakness	
Hunger	
Nausea, vomiting	
Pallor	
Hypothermia	
Neuroglycopenic Symptoms Due to Decreased Cerebral Glucose Use	
Headache	
Visual disturbances	
Lethargy, lassitude	
Restlessness, irritability	
Difficulty with speech and thinking, inability to concentrate	
Mental confusion	
Somnolence, stupor, prolonged sleep	
Loss of consciousness, coma	
Hypothermia	
Twitching, convulsions, "epilepsy"	
Bizarre neurologic signs	
Motor disturbances	
Sensory disturbances	
Loss of intellectual ability	
Personality changes	
Bizarre behavior	
Outburst of temper	
Psychologic disintegration	
Manic behavior	
Depression	
Psychoses	
Permanent mental or neurologic damage	

*Some features may be attenuated by β-adrenergic blocking agents. From Langdon DR, Stanley CA, Sperling, MA. Hypoglycemia in the toddler and child. In: Sperling MA, ed. *Pediatric Endocrinology*. 4th ed. Philadelphia: Elsevier; 2014:922.

treatment of premature labor can result in maternal hyperglycemia by increasing hepatic glucose production and decreasing glucose utilization. Maternal hyperglycemia, in turn, can initiate fetal hyperglycemia and HI, which can cause hypoglycemia in the newborn.

Beckwith-Wiedemann Syndrome

Beckwith-Wiedemann syndrome (BWS) is an overgrowth and cancer predisposition disorder with macrosomia, macroglossia, abdominal wall defects, hemihypertrophy, and hypoglycemia in the neonatal period. Most cases of BWS are sporadic, although approximately 15% have autosomal dominant inheritance. BWS appears to be caused by abnormal genomic imprinting involving multiple genes at chromosome 11p15.

Approximately 50% of newborns with BWS have hypoglycemia; 80% of cases are mild and transient. The remaining 20% of cases are more prolonged and difficult to control. Early recognition of hypoglycemia is extremely important for appropriate clinical management because there is an association in BWS between hypoglycemia and intellectual impairment. Any infant born with an omphalocele should be monitored for potential hypoglycemia. HI is the principal mechanism of the hypoglycemia in BWS

TABLE 57.4 Classification of Hypoglycemia in Infants and Children

NEONATAL TRANSITIONAL (ADAPTIVE) HYPOGLYCEMIA

Associated with Inadequate Substrate or Immature Enzyme Function in Otherwise Normal Neonates
Prematurity

Small for gestational age

Normal newborn

Transient Neonatal Hyperinsulinism
Infant of diabetic mother

Small for gestational age

Discordant twin

Birth asphyxia

Rhesus hemolytic disease

Infant of toxemic mother

HNF4A/HNF1A

NEONATAL, INFANTILE, OR CHILDHOOD HYPERINSULINEMIC HYPOGLYCEMIAS
Recessive K_{ATP} channel HI

Recessive *HADH* (hydroxyl acyl-CoA dehydrogenase) variant HI

Recessive *UCP2* (mitochondrial uncoupling protein 2) variant HI

Focal K_{ATP} channel HI

Dominant K_{ATP} channel HI

Atypical congenital hyperinsulinemia (no variants in *ABCC8* or *KCNJ11* genes)

Dominant glucokinase HI

Dominant glutamate dehydrogenase HI (hyperinsulinism/hyperammonemia syndrome)

Dominant variants in *HNF-4A* and *HNF-1A* (hepatic nuclear factors 4α and 1α) HI with monogenic diabetes of youth later in life

Dominant variant in *SLC16A1* (the pyruvate transporter)—exercise-induced hypoglycemia

Acquired islet cell adenoma

Beckwith-Wiedemann syndrome

Factitious disorder: insulin administration (Munchausen syndrome by proxy)

Oral sulfonylurea drugs

Congenital disorders of glycosylation

Exercise-induced hyperinsulinemic hypoglycemia

Counter-Regulatory Hormone Deficiency
Panhypopituitarism

Isolated growth hormone deficiency

Adrenocorticotropic hormone deficiency

Addison disease

Epinephrine deficiency

Glycogenolysis and Gluconeogenesis Disorders
Glucose-6-phosphatase deficiency (GSD 1a)

Glucose-6-phosphate translocase deficiency (GSD 1b)

Amylo-1,6-glucosidase (debranching enzyme) deficiency (GSD 3)

Liver phosphorylase deficiency (GSD 6)

Phosphorylase kinase deficiency (GSD 9)

Glycogen synthetase deficiency (GSD 0)

Fructose-1,6-diphosphatase deficiency

Pyruvate carboxylase deficiency

Galactosemia

Hereditary fructose intolerance

GLUT 1-2-3 transporter defects

Lipolysis Disorders

Fatty Acid Oxidation Disorders
Carnitine transporter deficiency (primary carnitine deficiency)

Carnitine palmitoyltransferase-1 deficiency

Carnitine translocase deficiency

Carnitine palmitoyltransferase-2 deficiency

Secondary carnitine deficiencies

Long-, medium-, short-chain acyl-CoA dehydrogenase deficiencies

Disorders of ketone synthesis/utilization

OTHER ETIOLOGIES

Substrate-Limited
Ketotic hypoglycemia

Poisoning—drugs

Salicylates

Alcohol

Oral hypoglycemic agents

Insulin

Propranolol

Pentamidine

Quinine

Disopyramide

Ackee fruit (unripe)—hypoglycin

Vacor (rat poison)

Trimethoprim-sulfamethoxazole (with renal failure)

Liver Disease
Reye syndrome

Hepatitis

Cirrhosis

Hepatoma

AMINO ACID AND ORGANIC ACID DISORDERS
Maple syrup urine disease

Propionic acidemia

Methylmalonic acidemia

Tyrosinemia

Glutaric aciduria type 2

3-Hydroxy-3-methylglutaric aciduria

Adenosine kinase deficiency

Mitochondrial disorders

SYSTEMIC DISORDERS
Sepsis

Carcinoma/sarcoma (secreting insulin-like growth factor 2)

Heart failure

Malnutrition

Malabsorption

Anti-insulin receptor antibodies

Anti-insulin antibodies

Neonatal hyperviscosity

Renal failure

Diarrhea

Burns

Shock

Postsurgical

Pseudohypoglycemia (leukocytosis, polycythemia)

Excessive insulin therapy of insulin-dependent diabetes mellitus

Factitious

Nissen fundoplication (dumping syndrome)

Falciparum malaria

GSD, glycogen storage disease; HI, hyperinsulinemia; K_{ATP}, regulated potassium channel.

From Sperling MA. Hypoglycemia. In: Kliegman RM, Stanton BF, St. Geme JW III, et al., eds. *Nelson Textbook of Pediatrics*. 20th ed. Philadelphia: Elsevier; 2016:776.

TABLE 57.5   Syndromic Forms of Hyperinsulinemic Hypoglycemia*

Syndrome Name	Gene (Location) Genetic Etiology	Clinical Characteristics
Pre- and Postnatal Overgrowth (Macrosomia)		
Beckwith-Wiedemann	(11p15)	Macroglossia, abdominal wall defects, ear lobe pits/creases, hemihypertrophy, tumor risk
Sotos	NSD1(5q35)	Macrocephaly, frontal bossing, pointed chin, developmental delay, tumor risk
Simpson-Golabi-Behmel	GPC3(Xq26), GPC4(Xp22)	Coarse facial features, broad feet, polydactyly, cryptorchidism, hepatomegaly, tumor risk
Perlman	DIS3L2(2q37)	Inverted V-shaped upper lip, prominent forehead, developmental delay, hypotonia, tumor risk
Postnatal Growth Failure (Short Stature)		
Kabuki	KMT2D(12q13), KDM6A(Xp11.3)	Arched eyebrows, long eyelashes, developmental delay, fetal finger pads, scoliosis, heart defects, hypotonia
Costello	HRAS (11p15)	Deep palmar/plantar creases, developmental delay, coarse facial features, heart abnormalities, papillomas, tumor risk
Chromosomal Abnormality		
Mosaic Turner	(Loss of X in some cells)	Milder Turner syndrome phenotype (short stature, coarctation of aorta, gonadal dysgenesis)
Patau	Trisomy 13	Developmental delay, microphthalmia, heart and neural defects
Congenital Disorders of Glycosylation		
Types 1a, 1b, and 1d	PMM2(16p13.2), MPI(15q24.1), ALG3(3q27.1)	Developmental delay, hypotonia, growth failure
Contiguous Gene Deletion Affecting the ABCC8 Gene		
Usher	11 genes	Hearing loss, visual impairment
Abnormalities in Calcium Homoeostasis		
Timothy	CACNA1C(12p13.33)	Long QT syndrome, syndactyly, developmental delay, immune deficiency
Insulin Receptor Variant		
Insulin resistance syndrome (leprechaunism)	INS(19p13)	Hypo- and hyperglycemia, pre- and postnatal growth restriction, elfin-like features, hirsutism
Other Syndromes		
Congenital central hypoventilation syndrome	PHOX2B(4p13)	Central hypoventilation, "box-shaped" face, neurocristopathies (Hirschsprung disease, tumor risk)

*Various developmental syndromes have been described with the gene/s linked to the condition and the common clinical features.
From Guemes M, Rahman SA, Kapoor RR, et al. Hyperinsulinemic hypoglycemia in children and adolescents: recent advances in understanding of pathophysiology and management. *Rev Endocrine Metabol Dis.* 2020;21:577–597 (Table 2, p. 583).

and occurs in 30–60% of children. Hypertrophy and hyperplasia of the islet of Langerhans have been observed. Hypoglycemia in children with BWS is usually transient, lasting for a few days. In some patients, HI hypoglycemia may persist longer and will require continuous feeding, medical therapy, or, in rare cases, partial pancreatectomy. Medical treatment generally includes diazoxide and octreotide, and if managed medically, the hypoglycemia eventually resolves over weeks to months of care.

CAUSES OF PERSISTENT HYPOGLYCEMIA IN INFANTS AND CHILDREN

Hyperinsulinism

Congenital HI is the most common cause of persistent hypoglycemia in infants and children. It was previously referred to as nesidioblastosis, leucine-sensitive hypoglycemia, or idiopathic hypoglycemia of infancy. Most affected patients present during infancy; macrosomia may be present at birth because of high fetal insulin levels, which act as a growth factor in utero. Excessive insulin secretion during fasting suppresses all the fasting systems, including hepatic glucose production, lipolysis, and ketogenesis. Hypoglycemia is a consequence of increased utilization and underproduction of glucose. Because lipolysis and ketosis are inhibited, alternative fuel levels remain low, which increases the risk of seizures and permanent brain injury. There are several genetic defects of pancreatic β-cell insulin secretion in children with HI (Fig. 57.3 and Table 57.6; see also Table 57.4). In the presence of severe hypoglycemia, there is often an inappropriately normal plasma insulin level but low FFA and ketone levels. The response to glucagon demonstrates an increase in blood glucose levels of >30 mg/dl; the glucose infusion rate is often very high (>8 mg/kg/min) (Table 57.7).

TABLE 57.6 Correlation of Clinical Features with Molecular Defects in Persistent Hyperinsulinemic Hypoglycemia in Infancy

Type	Macrosomia	Hypoglycemia/ Hyperinsulinemia	Family History	Molecular Defects	Associated Clinical, Biochemical, or Molecular Features	Response to Medical Management	Recommended Surgical Approach	Prognosis
Sporadic	Present at birth	Moderate/severe in first days to weeks of life	Negative	*ABCC8/KCNJ11A* gene variants not always identified in diffuse hyperplasia	Loss of heterozygosity in microadenomatous tissue	Generally poor; may respond better to somatostatin than to diazoxide	Partial pancreatectomy if frozen section shows β-cell crowding with small nuclei—suggests microadenoma Subtotal >95% pancreatectomy if frozen section shows giant nuclei in β cells—suggests diffuse hyperplasia	Excellent if focal adenoma is removed, thereby curing hypoglycemia and retaining sufficient pancreas to avoid diabetes Guarded if subtotal pancreatectomy (>95%) is performed; diabetes mellitus develops in 50% of patients; hypoglycemia persists in 33%
Autosomal recessive	Present at birth	Severe in first days to weeks of life	Positive	*ABCC8/KCNJ11A*	Consanguinity a feature in some populations	Poor	Subtotal pancreatectomy	Guarded
Autosomal dominant	Unusual	Moderate onset usually post–6 mo of age	Positive	Glucokinase (activating) Some cases gene unknown	None	Very good to excellent	Surgery usually not required Partial pancreatectomy only if medical management fails	Excellent
Autosomal dominant	Unusual	Moderate onset usually post–6 mo of age	Positive	Glutamate dehydrogenase (activating)	Modest hyperammonemia	Very good to excellent	Surgery usually not required	Excellent
Beckwith-Wiedemann syndrome	Present at birth	Moderate, spontaneously resolves post–6 mo of age	Negative	Duplicating/ imprinting in chromosome 11p15.1	Macroglossia, omphalocele, hemihypertrophy	Good	Not recommended	Excellent for hypoglycemia; guarded for possible development of embryonal tumors (Wilms hepatoblastoma)
Congenital disorders of glycosylation	Not usual	Moderate/onset post–3 mo of age	Negative	Phosphomannose isomerase deficiency	Hepatomegaly, vomiting, intractable diarrhea	Good with mannose supplement	Not recommended	Fair

From Sperling MA. Hypoglycemia. In: Kliegman RM, Stanton BF, St. Geme JW III, et al., eds. *Nelson Textbook of Pediatrics.* 20th ed. Philadelphia: Elsevier; 2016:778.

TABLE 57.7 Diagnostic Criteria for HH: Cutoff Values for Each Analyte to Aid in Diagnosis of HH

Serum Analyte	Result in Patients with HH
Blood Glucose <3.0 mmol/L (54 mg/dL) and	
Insulin	Detectable
C-peptide	Detectable (≥0.5 ng/mL)
Free fatty acids	Low or suppressed (<1.5 mmol/l* or <1.7 mmol/l†)
Ketone bodies	Low or suppressed (3-β-hydroxybutyrate <2 mmol/l* or <1.8 mmol/l†)
IGFBP-1	Low (≤110 ng/mL†) as insulin negatively regulates IGFBP-1 expression
Ammonia	Normal; can be raised in HI/HA syndrome
Hydroxybutyrylcarnitine	Normal; raised in HH due to *HADH* variant
Cortisol, growth hormone	Raised; generally cortisol >20 μg/dL (500 nmol/L); growth hormone >7 ng/mL—younger children might have poor counter-regulatory response
Amino acids and urine organic acids	Normal; leucine, isoleucine, and valine may be suppressed in HH
Proinsulin	>20 pmol/L
Additional Information When Diagnosis of HH Uncertain	
Glucose infusion rate	>8 mg/kg/min to achieve euglycemia
IM or IV glucagon administration or SC octreotide administration	30 mg/dL (positive glycemic response)

HI/HA, hyperinsulinemic hypoglycemia/hyperammonemia syndrome; HADH: short-chain L-3-hydroxyacil-CoA dehydrogenase; IGFBP-1, insulin growth factor–binding protein-1; IM: intramuscular; IV, intravenous; SC, subcutaneous.

*Low.

†Suppressed.

From Guemes M, Rahman SA, Kapoor RR, et al. Hyperinsulinemic hypoglycemia in children and adolescents: recent advances in understanding of pathophysiology and management. *Rev Endocrine Metabol Dis.* 2020;21:577–597 (Table 3, p. 585).

Recessive KATP Channel Hyperinsulinism

This is the most severe form of congenital HI. Affected infants are usually large for gestational age and present with symptoms of hypoglycemia in the first days after birth. The hypoglycemia is often incredibly severe, and treatment may require intravenous glucose infusions at 20–30 mg/kg/min (4–6 times normal) to maintain plasma glucose in the normal range of 70–100 mg/dL. This disorder is caused by genetic defects of the β-cell plasma membrane adenosine triphosphate–dependent potassium (KATP) channel (Fig. 57.4). The channel is encoded by two adjacent genes located on chromosome 11p: *ABCC8*, which encodes the sulfonylurea receptor type 1 (SUR1) protein subunit, and *KCNJ11A*, which encodes the potassium channel, inwardly rectifying, Kir6.2 subunit. Common founder variants of *ABCC8* have been identified in Ashkenazi Jews and in Finland, but most affected patients have one of many "private" (rare and unique) variants. Medical management with diazoxide or octreotide (which acts like somatostatin) may be tried (see Figs. 57.3 and 57.4) but is rarely effective. Most infants require surgical near-total (98%) pancreatectomy to achieve control of hypoglycemia. Approximately 50% of infants with severe HI who require surgery have diffuse disease caused by these recessive KATP channel variants; the remainder have focal lesions that are potentially curable by partial surgical resection.

Focal KATP Channel Hyperinsulinism

Approximately half the infants with severe neonatal-onset HI have focal lesions of the pancreas that are potentially curable by surgical resection. The molecular defect in these infants involves the same KATP channel genes as in recessive KATP channel HI through a two-hit mechanism: loss of heterozygosity for the maternal chromosome 11p and expression of a paternally derived *ABCC8* or *KCNJ11A* variants. Histologically, the focal lesions usually appear as adenomatosis. The clinical features are identical to those of infants with recessive KATP channel HI, including diazoxide unresponsiveness and hypoglycemia that is extremely difficult to control. Methods to diagnose and localize focal pancreatic adenomatosis preoperatively include acute insulin response tests to secretagogues such as calcium and tolbutamide, selective pancreatic arterial calcium stimulation of insulin release with pancreatic venous sampling, and PET.

Dominant KATP Channel Hyperinsulinism

HI caused by a dominantly expressed variant of the *ABCC8* gene, rather than the usual recessive disease inheritance, is reported in one family previously.

Dominant Glutamate Dehydrogenase Hyperinsulinism

Dominantly expressed gain-of-function variants of glutamate dehydrogenase have been identified in children with the unusual combination of HI plus asymptomatic hyperammonemia (HI/HA). Most cases arise from de novo variants, and only 20% are familial. Hypoglycemic symptoms often do not manifest in the neonatal period, and the disorder may not be recognized until the affected patient is an adult. Birthweights of affected infants are normal.

In addition to hypoglycemia, affected individuals have persistent but asymptomatic HA in the range of 70–150 μmol/L (see Fig. 57.3). The variants affect the pathway of leucine-stimulated insulin secretion, and patients can have protein-sensitive hypoglycemia, as well as fasting hypoglycemia. Diazoxide is effective in controlling hypoglycemia.

Dominant Glucokinase Hyperinsulinism

This rare disorder causes mild fasting hypoglycemia as a result of a dominant gain-of-function variant of islet glucokinase (see Fig. 57.3). Birthweights of affected infants are normal, and the age at onset of hypoglycemic symptoms ranges from infancy to adulthood. Diazoxide therapy has been effective in controlling plasma glucose levels.

Insulinoma

Acquired **insulinomas** are the most common form of HI in adults but are rare in childhood, especially in early infancy. These are usually isolated, benign tumors, but multiple adenomas may be associated with familial multiple endocrine neoplasia (MEN) syndromes. In contrast to focal congenital HI, insulinomas may be detectable by imaging procedures such as CT, MRI, PET scans, or transduodenal ultrasonography. Surgical resection is the treatment of choice.

Insulin Reaction, Oral Hypoglycemic Agents, and Surreptitious Insulin Administration

Insulin-induced hypoglycemia is a common occurrence in insulin-treated diabetic patients and may also occur in patients with type 2 diabetes who are taking oral hypoglycemic agents, such as glyburide, that stimulate insulin secretion. Surreptitious insulin administration should always be included in the differential diagnosis of unexplained hypoglycemia and, in young children, may occur as part of factitious disorder by proxy (Munchausen syndrome by proxy). Exogenous human or animal insulin use can be demonstrated by assays showing elevated plasma insulin values with simultaneous suppression of

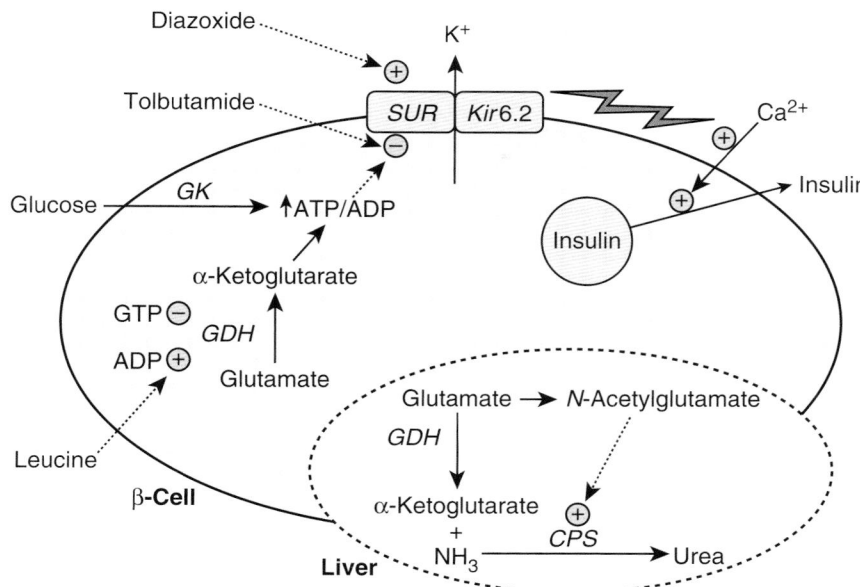

Fig. 57.3 Pathways of pancreatic β-cell insulin secretion. Increases in plasma concentrations of glucose lead to increased pancreatic β-cell glucose oxidation rates and elevations of intracellular adenosine triphosphate (ATP). The increase in the ratio of ATP to adenosine diphosphate subsequently acts via the sulfonylurea receptor type 1 (SUR1) component of the ATP-sensitive potassium (KATP) channel to inhibit potassium efflux, resulting in membrane depolarization and activation of a voltage-gated calcium ion channel. The rise in intracellular calcium triggers the release of insulin from secretory granules into the plasma. Genes involved in congenital hyperinsulinism include glucokinase; glutamate dehydrogenase (GDH); SUR1; and the ion pore component of the KATP channel, Kir6.2. Note that leucine triggers β-cell insulin secretion by allosterically activating GDH to increase oxidation of glutamate, which subsequently leads to inhibition of the KATP channel. As shown in the *inset* of liver pathways of glutamate metabolism, in the hyperinsulinism/hyperammonemia syndrome, overactivity of GDH leads to excessive ammonia production from glutamate and also decreases the availability of glutamate for synthesis of *N*-acetylglutamate, a required allosteric activator of the first step in ureagenesis. Note that SUR1 mediates both tolbutamide activation of insulin release and diazoxide inhibition of insulin release. Somatostatin inhibits insulin release at a more distal site in the pathway. ADP, adenosine diphosphate; CPS, carbamoyl phosphate synthetase; GK, glucokinase; GTP, guanosine triphosphate; SUR, sulfonylurea receptor.

plasma C peptide (use of insulin lispro may not be detectable with some insulin immunoassays).

Counter-Regulatory Hormone Deficiencies

Hypopituitarism

Isolated deficiency of growth hormone, or both growth hormone and adrenocorticotropin hormone deficiency, predisposes to fasting hypoglycemia. In affected older infants, hypoglycemia may occur after 10–14 hours of fasting. Newborns with hypopituitarism sometimes present with much more severe hypoglycemia, which can closely mimic the KATP channel form of congenital HI, including increased glucose requirements of 10–20 mg/kg/min and an inappropriate glycemic response to glucagon when patients are hypoglycemic. A liver disease resembling progressive cholestatic jaundice may occur in these newborns and does not resolve until replacement therapy is begun for the deficient hormones. Hypotonia and, in affected boys, a small phallus may also be present.

Several syndromes, such as midline craniofacial defects, septo-optic dysplasia, and Russell-Silver dwarfism, may be associated with hypopituitarism. Infant boys characteristically have microphallus, which is a useful diagnostic sign.

Isolated Cortisol Deficiency

Fasting hypoglycemia may occur in infants and children with adrenal insufficiency of various causes, including adrenocorticotropin hormone deficiency and primary adrenal insufficiency (Addison disease), or because of adrenal suppression resulting from exogenous glucocorticoid administration. Hypoglycemia is uncommon in the presentation of newborns with congenital adrenal hyperplasia, but once glucocorticoid replacement treatment is begun, these children are also at risk for adrenal crises and hypoglycemia if not given supplemental doses during intercurrent illness.

Epinephrine Deficiency

Catecholamine deficiency is extremely rare and has been described as secondary to adrenal hemorrhage in infants small for gestational age. These patients may present for the first time during childhood with hypoglycemia during fasting. The diagnosis is confirmed by measurement of plasma or urinary catecholamine levels. Some affected children may show evidence, on abdominal films, of previous adrenal hemorrhage in the form of adrenal calcification.

Fasting hypoglycemia has been observed occasionally in children treated with **β-blocking agents**, such as propranolol. The mechanism appears to be suppression of lipolysis because of the interference with epinephrine stimulation of adipose tissue; this suppression impairs the third stage of fasting adaptation. Hypoglycemia may occur after 12 or more hours of fasting. Hypoglycemic attacks may be associated with acute hypertension because of the unopposed α-adrenergic effects of epinephrine.

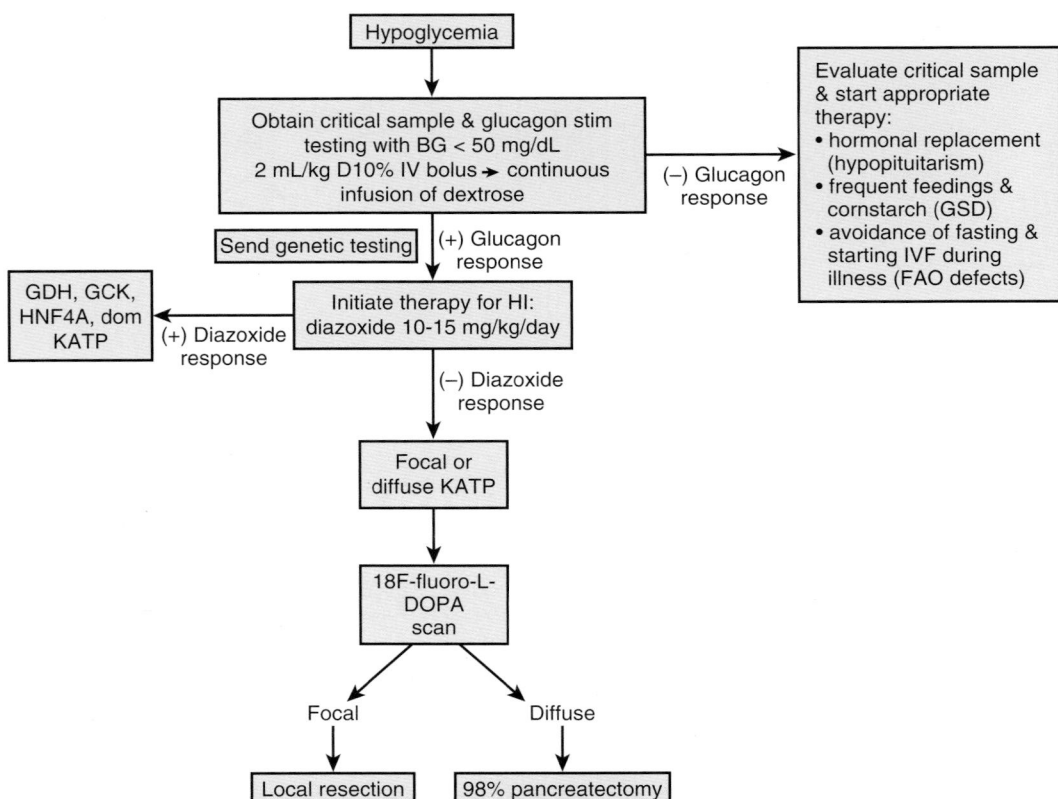

Fig. 57.4 Diagnostic and treatment approach in cases of hyperinsulinism. BG, blood glucose; D, dextrose; dom, dominant; FAO, fatty acid oxidation; GCK, glucokinase; GDH, glutamate dehydrogenase; GSD, glycogen storage disease; HNF4A, hepatic nuclear factor 4-alpha; IV, intravenous; IVF, intravenous fluids; KATP, adenosine triphosphate–dependent potassium channel. (From De León DD, Thornton PS, Stanley CA, et al. Hypoglycemia in the newborn infant. In: Sperling MA, ed. *Pediatric Endocrinology*. 4th ed. Philadelphia: Elsevier; 2014:171, Fig. 6.8.)

Metabolic Enzyme Defects

Hepatic Gluconeogenesis

The genetic metabolic defects in hepatic gluconeogenesis lead to fasting hypoglycemia associated with increased plasma concentrations of gluconeogenic precursors, such as lactate and alanine.

Glucose-6-phosphatase deficiency (glycogen storage disease type 1a and type 1b). This is the most common form of the glycogen storage disorders, although (see Fig. 57.1) deficiency of glucose-6-phosphatase is a gluconeogenic defect because it blocks the release of glucose from *both* gluconeogenesis and glycogenolysis. Hypoglycemia occurs within 2–3 hours after a meal, once intestinal carbohydrate absorption is complete. Affected infants usually do not present with symptomatic hypoglycemia, because the associated elevations of lactate provide an alternative fuel for the brain when the glucose level is low. Instead, the manifestation is usually growth failure late in the first year. The liver is massively enlarged because of fat and glycogen deposition and extends into the left upper quadrant and down into the pelvis. Associated abnormalities include elevations of plasma triglyceride (up to 2,000–4,000 mg/dL) and hyperuricemia due to shunting of the excessive glucose-6-phosphate via other pathways, causing excessive production of lactic acid, lipid synthesis, and hyperuricemia. Treatment is aimed at avoiding fasting hypoglycemia by using a combination of high-carbohydrate meals and uncooked cornstarch or continuous intragastric dextrose infusions to prevent growth failure. Carbohydrates that cannot be converted to glucose, such as galactose in milk, fructose in fruits, and sucrose, should be limited. The type 1b variant is caused by deficiency of the microsomal glucose-6-phosphate translocase and is associated with the additional problem of neutropenia, leading to mouth ulcers and skin infections. Treatment with granulocyte colony-stimulating factor has been beneficial in these patients.

Glucose transporter 2 deficiency (Fanconi-Bickel syndrome). A small number of infants have been described with a combination of hepatomegaly, increased liver glycogen store, renal Fanconi syndrome, and galactose intolerance. Pathogenic variants that cause this recessive inherited disorder are in the gene *SLC2A2*, which encodes glucose transporter 2 (GLUT2), a plasma membrane glucose transporter expressed in liver, kidney, and pancreatic β cells. GLUT2 is necessary to export free glucose from the cytosol into the plasma (see Fig. 57.1). The deficiency of GLUT2 interferes with glucose release from the liver not only from glycogenolysis but also from gluconeogenesis and from other sugars, such as galactose and fructose.

Fructose-1,6-diphosphatase deficiency. This defect blocks gluconeogenesis immediately above the triose-phosphates (see Fig. 57.1). Affected children present in the first year or the neonatal period with life-threatening attacks of hypoglycemia and lactic acidemia provoked by fasting stress. Moderate fatty hepatomegaly is commonly seen together with hyperuricemia. Fructose ingestion can precipitate hypoglycemia and lactic acidemia. During controlled fasting, plasma glucose can be maintained in the normal range until 8–12 hours, because glycogenolysis remains normal. Treatment with avoidance of prolonged fasting and restriction of fructose-containing foods and glycerol is effective in avoiding hypoglycemia.

Pyruvate carboxylase deficiency. Pyruvate carboxylase is one of the four key gluconeogenic enzymes (see Fig. 57.1). It also plays an important role in pyruvate oxidation because it generates oxaloacetate needed to maintain tricarboxylic acid (TCA) cycle activity. The clinical features are often dominated by the defect in pyruvate oxidation and include those of **Leigh syndrome** and **congenital lactic acidemia**. However, affected infants are also susceptible to the development of symptomatic hypoglycemia after 8–10 hours of fasting.

Hepatic Glycogenolysis

Defects in hepatic glycogenolysis are associated with abbreviated fasting tolerance, leading to hypoglycemia and hyperketonemia. Defects can occur in either the synthesis or breakdown of hepatic glycogen (see Fig. 57.1). Debrancher enzyme deficiency is the most severe of these defects.

Debrancher enzyme deficiency (type 3 glycogen storage disease). Children with this disorder usually present in the first year of life with growth delay and massive hepatomegaly. Symptomatic hypoglycemia is not common, because plasma ketone levels are usually elevated and provide the brain with alternative substrate when the glucose level is low. Hypoglycemia develops quickly, often within 3–6 hours after a meal. Treatment with uncooked cornstarch to prolong glucose absorption is useful in preventing hypoglycemia and improving growth. Problems caused by hypoglycemia are ameliorated later in childhood as body mass increases. However, half or more of patients with debrancher enzyme deficiency are at risk for developing progressive muscle weakness and/or cardiomyopathy by the second and third decades of life.

Phosphorylase/phosphorylase kinase deficiency. The manifestations of either of these two enzyme defects clinically resemble a very mild form of debrancher enzyme deficiency. Affected infants present with enlarged livers, often in association with impaired growth. Symptomatic hypoglycemia is unusual. Fasting tests show a pattern of accelerated starvation with early onset of hyperketonemia. Treatment to reduce fasting intervals to less than 4–6 hours (e.g., with uncooked cornstarch) is helpful in correcting the failure to thrive. As in debrancher enzyme deficiency, the fasting disturbance becomes less apparent as body mass increases, and the hepatomegaly and growth delay may totally resolve by the end of the first decade. Liver phosphorylase deficiency is recessively inherited; both recessive inheritance and X-linked inheritance have been reported for phosphorylase kinase deficiency.

Glycogen synthase deficiency. A small number of patients with deficiency of glycogen synthase have been reported. They have presented with episodes of symptomatic, hyperketotic hypoglycemia after fasts of 10–12 hours. Mild hepatomegaly may be present because of the increased deposition of triglycerides that is common in all of the glycogenoses. Treatment with uncooked cornstarch at bedtime may be helpful in avoiding symptomatic episodes of early-morning hypoglycemia.

Fatty Acid Oxidation Disorders

Genetic defects in fatty acid oxidation interfere with the ketotic phase of fasting adaptation. The most common of the disorders is medium-chain acyl-coenzyme A (CoA) dehydrogenase (MCAD) deficiency. Children with MCAD deficiency present with acute attacks of life-threatening coma and **hypoketotic hypoglycemia** that are usually precipitated by fasting stresses of 12 hours or longer. Attacks are triggered by intercurrent illnesses that impair feeding, especially gastroenteritis. The clinical features mimic Reye syndrome, with coma, elevated liver transaminase levels, and mild hepatomegaly with steatosis. More severe forms of fatty acid oxidation disorders

also involve skeletal and cardiac muscle and may manifest with cardiomyopathy and chronic muscle weakness or acute episodes of rhabdomyolysis. More than 12 different defects in the pathway of fatty acid oxidation have been identified; all are recessively inherited. Many states have neonatal screening programs in which dual tandem mass spectrometry of blood spot acyl-carnitine profiles are used to detect MCAD deficiency and several of the other fatty acid oxidation disorders. This is important for presymptomatic detection and treatment because the mortality rate at the first presentation may be higher than 25%.

Other Metabolic Causes of Hypoglycemia

Glucose transporter 1 deficiency. Isolated hypoglycorrhachia (low cerebrospinal fluid glucose level) in association with normal concentrations of plasma glucose has been demonstrated in several infants with intractable seizures in early infancy caused by a deficiency of glucose transporter 1 (GLUT1). GLUT1 is the plasma membrane carrier protein responsible for glucose transport across the blood-brain barrier, as well as into red blood cells. Affected patients are heterozygous for a GLUT1 variant and have persistently low levels of spinal fluid glucose, ranging from 20 to 30 mg/dL. Seizures may begin in the neonatal period and respond poorly to treatment with antiseizure drugs. Progressive brain damage, microcephaly, and developmental delay occur in untreated patients. Several patients have been reported to respond very well to treatment with a ketogenic diet, which restricts carbohydrates and keeps plasma levels of ketones elevated to 3–6 mEq/L.

Hereditary fructose intolerance. Hereditary fructose intolerance is caused by a recessively inherited deficiency of hepatic fructose-aldolase, which transforms fructose-1-phosphate to the triose-phosphates. Affected patients cannot metabolize dietary fructose or sucrose (table sugar) in the liver or intestinal mucosa for conversion to glucose. Chronic fructose intake in young infants may cause liver dysfunction, acidemia, failure to thrive, hyperuricemia, and, ultimately, liver failure. In affected older children, ingestion of fructose causes severe abdominal pain, and these children may learn by experience to avoid fructose and thus escape identification. Fasting tolerance is normal, but ingestion of large amounts of fructose may provoke postprandial hypoglycemia by tying up intracellular phosphate and thus blocking glycogenolysis. Treatment is avoidance of dietary sources of fructose.

Galactosemia (galactose-1-phosphate uridyl transferase deficiency). This is a serious inborn error of metabolism wherein many of the long-term consequences of the metabolic defect can potentially be prevented by early intervention. For this reason, all infants born in the United States are screened for galactosemia in the neonatal period. Absence of galactose-1-phosphate uridyl transferase prevents the conversion of galactose to glucose and results in accumulation of galactose-1-phosphate in the liver and other tissues. It has been suggested that accumulation of this metabolite inhibits the enzyme involved in the conversion of glucose-1-phosphate to glucose-6-phosphate and thus decreases the production of glucose from glycogen, thereby producing hypoglycemia. Depending on the magnitude of the defect, affected infants may present in the immediate neonatal period or later in infancy. The patients do not tolerate galactose or lactose. Intolerance to lactose in milk, the major nutrient containing galactose, is evident soon after birth when feedings are initiated. The infant may present with vomiting, failure to thrive, hepatomegaly, and indirect or direct hyperbilirubinemia. In severe or untreated cases, lenticular opacities, aminoaciduria, and intellectual disability may occur. In untreated patients, progressive hepatomegaly, cirrhosis, and hepatic failure may develop. Affected infants are at increased risk for *Escherichia coli* sepsis.

Any infant with persistent jaundice, hepatomegaly, and failure to thrive should be tested for galactosemia. A presumptive diagnosis can be made by the presence of reducing sugar (Clinitest positive) that is not glucose (i.e., the glucose enzyme test result is negative) in the urine. This test should be performed while the infant is being fed a galactose-containing formula. The diagnosis should be confirmed by measuring the enzyme activity in the red blood cells.

Treatment consists of elimination of galactose from the diet. Despite treatment, which results in prevention of hepatic disease and of intellectual disability, many affected older children demonstrate learning and behavior problems.

Reactive Hypoglycemia

Reactive or postprandial hypoglycemia is extremely rare in the pediatric age range and, even in adults, may be overdiagnosed. Three situations in infants and children present with reactive hypoglycemia:

Glutamate dehydrogenase-hyperinsulinism, hyperinsulinism/hyperammonemia syndrome. Affected children have fasting hypoglycemia but, because of their leucine sensitivity, may also develop symptomatic hypoglycemia within 30–90 minutes of eating a high-protein meal.

Post–Nissen fundoplication hypoglycemia (late dumping syndrome). Like patients who have had gastric surgery, infants who have undergone Nissen fundoplication procedures for gastroesophageal reflux can develop recurrent attacks of postprandial hypoglycemia. The hypoglycemia may be severe enough to produce seizures and permanent brain damage. The mechanism is thought to involve rapid gastric emptying that leads to a rapid rise in plasma glucose accompanied by a delayed but excessive insulin response, which is followed by a precipitous fall in plasma glucose to hypoglycemic levels 30–90 minutes after a meal.

Hereditary fructose intolerance. Patients with this disorder develop acute abdominal discomfort and hypoglycemia within a short period of time after an oral load of fructose (e.g., fruit, fruit juice, or sucrose).

Ketotic Hypoglycemia

Idiopathic ketotic hypoglycemia (IKH) is the most frequent cause of hypoglycemia in children between 1 and 5 years of age and typically occurs after a period of poor food intake. Due to the overlap with signs of other common diseases like psychiatric disorders, migraine, gastric disorders, or visual disturbances, diagnosis of IKH is often delayed. If a child with normal growth and psychomotor development presents with a first episode of symptomatic hypoglycemia that improves quickly with glucose administration, IKH should be considered. Obtaining urinary ketones to assess for ketonuria at the time of hypoglycemia is helpful to make the diagnosis and other hormonal and metabolic work-up can safely be deferred. However, if the child presents with frequent recurrences, extensive work-up to assess for adrenal insufficiency or growth hormone deficiency or metabolic pathway defects (glycogen storage disease) should be considered. Hypoglycemic attacks secondary to IKH can be prevented by supplying frequent snacks containing complex carbohydrates, so-called "slow sugars," particularly at bedtime.

DIAGNOSIS OF HYPOGLYCEMIA

Critical Samples

Tests on the specimens of blood and urine obtained at the time of hypoglycemia provide the key information for diagnosis (Tables 57.7 and 57.8 and Fig. 57.5). Ideally, these specimens are collected during hypoglycemia, immediately before treatment is begun. It is best to collect some extra tubes of plasma and urine just before giving intravenous dextrose, to set aside for later decisions about which other tests

to order. Tests should include plasma glucose measurement and various metabolic precursors and hormones involved in glucose counter-regulation, including glucose, bicarbonate, insulin, growth hormone, cortisol, lactate, pyruvate, ammonia, β-hydroxybutyrate, FFA, carnitine, acyl-carnitine profile, and a urine sample for organic acid analysis and ketones. Additional tests to consider include transaminases, uric acid, triglycerides, and creatinine kinase levels. Fig. 57.5 shows a paradigm for diagnosis of different hypoglycemic disorders that is based on analysis of the critical samples.

Fasting Study

In some cases, a formal fasting test is advised to establish the etiology of hypoglycemia. This should only be done in a well-controlled setting with adequate monitoring by experienced medical and nursing staff. Fasting is usually begun at 8 P.M. after bedtime snack or sometimes in the morning, especially in younger patients, to make sure that there is enough supervision and staff available during the time hypoglycemia occurs.

Useful "Casual Specimen" Tests

Only a few tests are informative except at times of hypoglycemia. These include plasma acyl-carnitine profiles and plasma total and free carnitine levels (for suspected fatty acid oxidation defects) and plasma ammonia (for the HI/HA syndrome).

Glucagon Stimulation

If HI is suspected, a glucagon stimulation test at the onset of hypoglycemia (50 mg/dL) may be confirmatory. A glycemic response exceeding 30 mg/dL is consistent with HI, because the normal response would be to have depleted liver glycogen reserves well before reaching hypoglycemia.

Acute Insulin Response Tests for Hyperinsulinism

β-Cell responsiveness to different secretagogues (calcium, leucine, glucose, tolbutamide) can be used to define specific genetic forms of HI and to distinguish focal from diffuse pancreatic disease preoperatively.

Plasma Acyl-Carnitine Profile

Dual tandem mass spectrometry methods have been developed for analyzing plasma acyl-carnitine profiles and other metabolites in small samples, such as filter paper blood spots. These assays are useful for screening for most of the genetic fatty acid oxidation disorders (e.g., MCAD deficiency) and should be performed before patients suspected to have such a defect begin a formal fasting test. Many states incorporate these methods for neonatal screening of up to 30 different inborn errors of metabolism. Some fatty acid oxidation defects do not cause abnormal acyl-carnitine profiles; examples include carnitine palmityl-transferase 1 deficiency, carnitine transporter deficiency, and β-hydroxy-β-methylglutaryl-CoA dehydrogenase deficiency. These disorders must be investigated with additional in vivo and in vitro tests.

Urinary Organic Acid Quantitation

Assays of urinary metabolites by gas chromatography–mass spectrometry are also useful in identifying specific defects in fatty acid oxidation. Abnormalities are most pronounced during activation of lipolysis, such as at the end of a diagnostic fasting test or in the "critical sample" urine collected at the time of an acute illness.

Cultured Cells

For in vitro diagnosis of fatty acid oxidation defects, cultured cells from patients, such as skin fibroblasts or lymphoblasts, may be useful for testing overall pathway activity, for assaying activities of candidate enzymes,

TABLE 57.8 Clinical Manifestations and Differential Diagnosis in Childhood Hypoglycemia

Condition	Hypoglycemia	Urinary Ketones or Reducing Sugars	Hepatomegaly	SERUM		EFFECT OF 24–36-HR FAST ON PLASMA				GLYCEMIC RESPONSE TO GLUCAGON		GLYCEMIC RESPONSE TO INFUSION OF	
				Lipids	Uric Acid	Glucose Insulin	Ketones	Alanine	Lactate	Fed	Fasted	Alanine	Glycerol
Normal	0	0	0	Normal	Normal	↓	↑	↓	Normal	↑	↓		Not indicated
Hyperinsulinemia	Recurrent severe	0	0	Normal or ↑	Normal	↑↑	↓↓	Normal	Normal	↑	↑		Not indicated
Ketotic hypoglycemia	Severe with missed meals	Ketonuria +++	0	Normal	Normal	↓	↑↑	↓↓	Normal	↑	↓↓		Not indicated
Fatty acid oxidation disorder	Severe with missed meals	Absent	0 to + Abnormal liver function test results	Abnormal ↑		Contraindicated				↑	↓		Not indicated
Hypopituitarism	Moderate with missed meals	Ketonuria ++	0	Normal	Normal	↓	↑↑	↓↓	Normal	↑	↓↓	↑	↑
Adrenal insufficiency	Severe with missed meals	Ketonuria ++	0	Normal	Normal	↓	↑↑	↓↓	Normal	↑	↓↓	↑	↑
Enzyme deficiencies	Severe-constant	Ketonuria +++	+++	↑↑	↑↑	↓	↑↑	↑↑	↑↑	0	0-↓↓	0	0
Glucose-6-phosphatase debrancher	Moderate with fasting	++	++	Normal	Normal	↓	↑↑	↓↓	Normal	↑	0-↓↓	↑	↑
Phosphorylase	Mild-moderate	Ketonuria ++	+	Normal	Normal	↓	↑↑	↓↓	Normal	0-↑	0-↑	↑	↑
Fructose-1, 6-diphosphatase	Severe with fasting	Ketonuria +++	+++	↑↑	↑↑	↓	↑↑	↑↑	↑↑	↑	0-↓↓	↓	↓
Galactosemia	After milk or milk products	0 Ketones; (s) +	+++	Normal	Normal	↓	↑	↓	Normal	↑	0-↓↓	↑	↑
Fructose intolerance	After fructose	0 Ketones; (s) +	+++	Normal	Normal	↓	↓	↓	Normal	↑	0-↓↓	↑	↑

Details of each condition are discussed in the text.

0, absence; ↑ or ↓, small increase or decrease, respectively; ↑↑ or ↓↓, large increase or decrease, respectively; +, less likely; ++, likely; +++, definitively.

From Sperling MA. Hypoglycemia. In: Kliegman RM, Stanton BF, St. Geme JW III, et al., eds. *Nelson Textbook of Pediatrics.* 20th ed. Philadelphia: Elsevier; 2016:780.

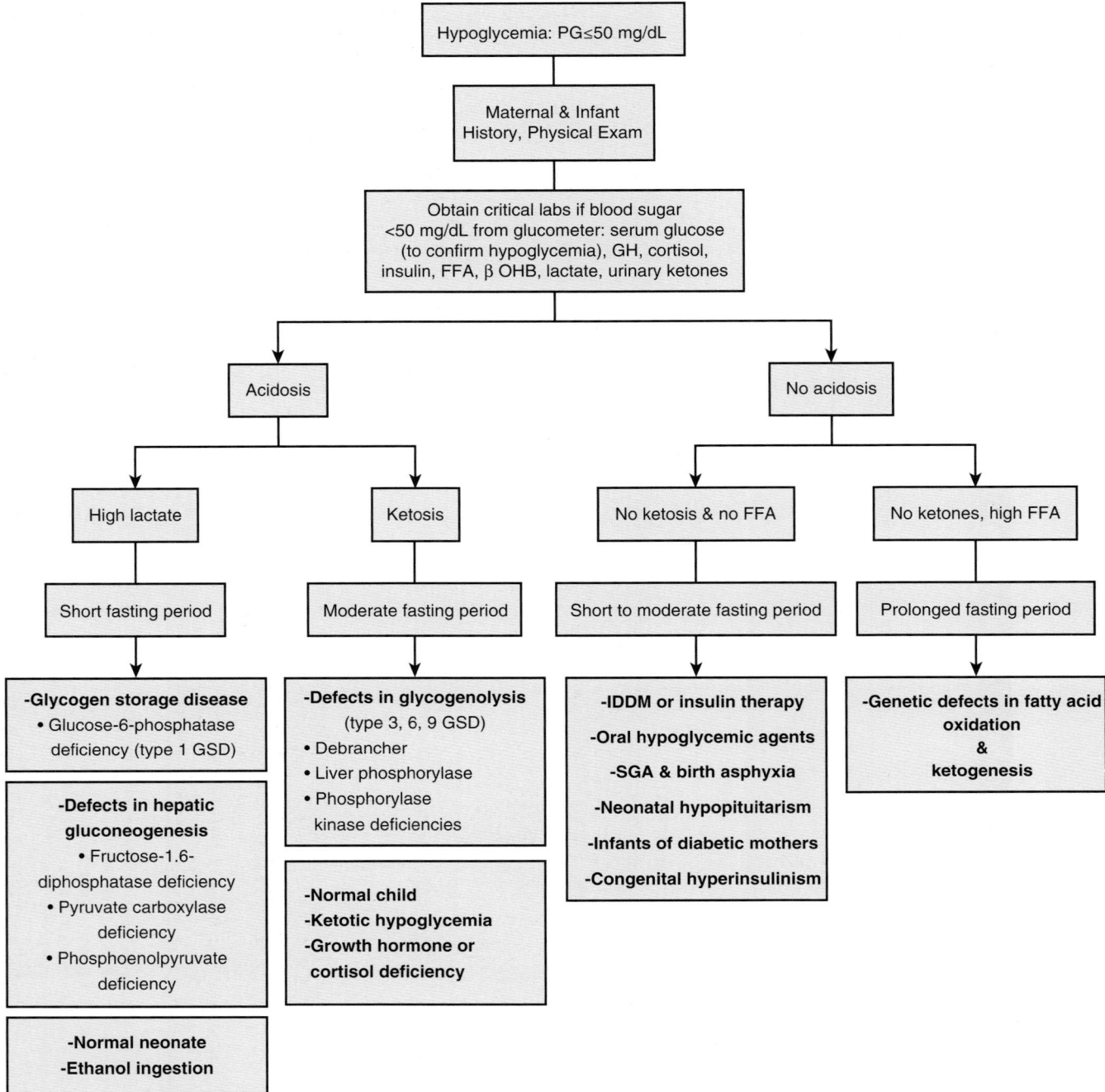

Fig. 57.5 Diagnostic algorithm for determining the etiology of hypoglycemia in children. OHB, hydroxybutyrate; FFA, free fatty acid; GH, growth hormone, GSD, glycogen storage disease; PG, plasma glucose. (Modified from Melmed S, Auchus RJ, Goldfine AB, Koenig RJ, Rosen CJ. *Williams Textbook of Endocrinology.* 14th ed. Elsevier; 2020:1547, Fig. 38.14.)

or as a source of DNA for variant analysis. Most enzymes in the pathway are expressed in cultured cells, except for 3-hydroxy-3-methylglutaryl–CoA synthase, which is restricted to liver, intestine, and kidney.

Genetic Analysis

Genetic variant identification is useful for confirmation of diagnosis and genetic counseling. In a limited number of disorders, common variants that can be easily screened for as a primary diagnostic test have been identified. These include MCAD deficiency, glucose-6-phosphatase deficiency, and hyperinsulinemia due to ATP-binding cassette transporter 8 *(ABCC8)*, ATP sensitive inward rectifier potassium channel

11 *(KCNJ11A)*, mitochondrial glutamate dehydrogenase 1 *(GLUD1)*, hepatic nuclear factor 4-alpha *(HNF4A)*, glucokinase *(GCK)*, mitochondrial hydroxyacyl-coenzyme A *(HADH)*, and mitochondrial uncoupling protein 2 *(UCP2)*. Easy access to information about disease-associated variants is available through the Online Mendelian Inheritance in Man (OMIM) website (http://www.ncbi.nlm.nih.gov/Omim/).

TREATMENT OF HYPOGLYCEMIA

The initial treatment of hypoglycemia is to promptly raise the plasma glucose level to normal and maintain it in the range of 80–100 mg/dL.

For long-term management, the minimum goal of therapy is always to keep the plasma glucose level above 60 mg/dL.

Whenever treatment begins in a patient with new-onset hypoglycemia, every effort should be made to collect the critical samples for diagnosis. One extra tube of 5 mL of plasma or serum (green-top or red-top tube) is sufficient to measure key chemistry levels, fuels, and hormones. An extra tube of 10 mL or more of urine should also be collected for urinary organic acid quantitation.

For emergency treatment of hypoglycemia, an intravenous bolus of dextrose, 200 mg/kg, is given rapidly, and then a continuous intravenous infusion is begun to run at a rate equal to at least normal hepatic glucose output (about 4–6 mg/kg/min). With 10% dextrose solutions, this means a bolus of 2 mL/kg followed by continuous infusion at maintenance rates. Infants with HI may require considerably higher rates of dextrose infusion, up to 20–30 mg/kg/min. Infants with fatty acid oxidation disorders should receive sufficient dextrose to ensure that insulin secretion is stimulated enough to suppress lipolysis—that is, 10% dextrose at 8–10 mg/kg/min—and to maintain all plasma glucose levels slightly above 100 mg/dL. Glucagon may be used to treat hypoglycemia on an emergency basis, but only if the hypoglycemia is known to be caused by HI; a dose of 1 mg should be used at all ages to avoid undertreatment.

SUMMARY AND RED FLAGS

Hypoglycemia has many manifestations and must be thought of as a cause of nonspecific signs in newborns. It is a readily treatable cause of lethargy, coma, and seizures. Other affected children have signs of catecholamine excess. Untreated symptomatic hypoglycemia is life-threatening and can produce significant, irreversible central nervous system injury.

Red flags include metabolic acidosis (inborn errors of metabolism, sepsis); a positive family history (inborn errors of metabolism, hyperinsulinism, hypoglycemic agents); hypoketonuria (hyperinsulinemia, fatty acid oxidation defects) and high glucose infusion rates (hyperinsulinism); onset during adolescence (drugs or alcohol); hepatomegaly (glycogen storage disease, other inborn errors of metabolism); feeding intolerance (galactosemia); or recurrent or a family history of emesis, lethargy, coma, or sudden infant death syndrome (medium-chain acyl dehydrogenase deficiency).

BIBLIOGRAPHY

A bibliography is available at ExpertConsult.com.

58

Polyuria and Urinary Incontinence

Cynthia G. Pan

POLYURIA AND URINARY INCONTINENCE

Urinary incontinence is a normal developmental stage. When present beyond a certain age defined by parental and societal expectations, it can cause concern and anxiety in the patient and family. Urinary incontinence can also be a symptom of significant pathologic processes. The challenge to the clinician is identifying the child with an organic disorder among the many who are proceeding along a normal developmental track.

VOIDING PHYSIOLOGY

Urinary continence is dependent on normal bladder function and normal urine production. Normal development of bladder function results in the storage and release of urine in a socially and physically acceptable way. During storage, the detrusor muscle is relaxed, and the capacity of the bladder allows urine to be held for several hours. Micturition is then voluntary, with coordinated detrusor contraction and sphincter relaxation, resulting in complete bladder emptying. The bladder capacity in children learning to be toilet trained is variable, being dependent on their own sensation of bladder fullness. The maximum functional bladder capacity may differ greatly among children when measured by home diaries. Cystometry, a method of measuring bladder volume, can be estimated by the following formula:

Cystometric bladder capacity (ounces) = $(2 \times$ age [years]$) + 2$

In children 2 years of age or older:

Cystometric bladder capacity (ounces) = $\dfrac{\text{age (years)}}{2} + 6$

Although the innervation of the bladder is predominantly autonomic, bladder function is under control of cortical function. Thus, a complex integration of visceral and somatic innervation is necessary for normal voiding, which perhaps explains the wide spectrum in the ages for urinary continence. Parasympathetic neural activity provides the primary input during micturition, leading to relaxation of the urethral smooth muscle and initiating detrusor contractions. Pelvic nerves conducting parasympathetic activity form a reflex arc with the centrally located pontine micturition center. The thoracolumbar sympathetic branch, via hypogastric and pelvic sympathetic nerves, innervates the detrusor to relax and the urinary sphincter to contract during urine storage.

Urinary continence thus relies on the abilities to (1) store urine without leakage, (2) release urine voluntarily and completely, and (3) interrupt micturition voluntarily. The third ability is indicative of fully coordinated cortical-autonomic function.

TOILET TRAINING

The age at which toilet training is achieved is influenced by cultural factors as well as psychosocial factors. The achievement of daytime urinary continence follows the attainment of bowel control. There is evidence that the age of daytime and nighttime continence has increased worldwide in the past century. Data suggest a change in parental attitudes toward the toilet training process and their expectations. Among social factors reported, children of single parents are successfully toilet trained at an earlier age, whereas enrollment in daycare does not have a significant influence. There is no consensus on age of readiness for toilet training in Western society. Nearly two dozen signs of readiness have been reported, but no evidence-based studies are available to indicate which readiness signs and how many are needed for a child to successfully toilet train. Consistent predictive factors include that females are toilet trained earlier than males and Black children are trained earlier than White children. Techniques for toilet training are varied and range from the child-oriented approach to single-day training intensive methods to the use of daytime wet alarms.

URINE VOLUME AND SOLUTE DIURESIS

Polyuria is the overproduction of urine. Polyuria is a symptom that is fixed and therefore occurs during both the daytime and the nighttime. "Nocturnal polyuria," a symptom proposed in a subset of patients with primary nocturnal enuresis, is discussed separately. Overproduction of urine indicates a defect in one of several mechanisms regulating water and solute homeostasis. Identification of children with incontinence caused by polyuria is essential for diagnosing a variety of disorders (Table 58.1).

Urine production varies depending on the intake of fluids and solute, activity, caloric expenditure, and the environment. The volume reflects the maintenance of normal fluid and electrolyte balance (1) through the regulation of plasma osmolality by vasopressin and through the thirst mechanism and (2) by the regulation of extracellular volume and solute (mainly sodium) homeostasis by the kidney. The sensation of thirst occurs when plasma osmolality rises above a threshold of 280–290 mOsm/L. Release of vasopressin, a peptide produced by the hypothalamus, parallels the sensation of thirst and then acts on receptors in the collecting ducts of the kidney to diminish water excretion and to concentrate the urine. Hypovolemia is also a stimulant for vasopressin. Once serum osmolality is restored to normal, vasopressin release is inhibited, and renal water excretion increases. Maintenance of extracellular fluid volume depends on sodium homeostasis and directly affects urine volume. It involves the interaction of several systems, including (1) the renin-angiotensin system, (2) the atrial natriuretic peptide, and (3) the sympathetic nervous system.

TABLE 58.1 Causes of Urinary Incontinence
With Polyuria
Diabetes mellitus
Primary polydipsia (psychogenic, behavioral)
Central diabetes insipidus
Nephrogenic diabetes insipidus
Primary
Genetic
Secondary
Obstructive uropathy: concurrent (anatomic, neurogenic) or postobstructive
Polyuric phase of acute kidney injury
Chronic renal failure
Juvenile nephronophthisis
Fanconi syndrome (e.g., cystinosis)
Hypokalemia
Hypercalcemia
Bartter syndrome
Gitelman syndrome
Sickle cell disease
Renal tubular acidosis
Medications (e.g., lithium)
Interstitial nephritis
Without Polyuria
Primary nocturnal enuresis*
Dysfunctional voiding syndromes
Neuropathic bladder
Anatomic defects of the urinary tract

*Some cases may be characterized by nocturnal polyuria.

TABLE 58.2 Secondary and Acquired Forms of Nephrogenic Diabetes Insipidus–Like Disorders
Acquired
Chronic pyelonephritis
Tubulointerstitial nephritis
Chronic renal failure secondary to obstructive uropathy
Drug-induced tubulopathy
Hypokalemia
Hypercalcemia
Congenital
Renal tubular acidosis
Nephrocalcinosis
Cystinosis
Sickle cell nephropathy
Juvenile nephronophthisis
Renal dysplasia
Cystic kidney disease
Bartter syndrome
Storage, metabolic diseases (tyrosinemia, Fabry disease)

Among patients with primary nocturnal enuresis, there is a subset of patients with "nocturnal polyuria," in which larger volumes of more dilute urine are produced than in patients who remain dry. Responsiveness to the administration of vasopressin analogs, such as desmopressin acetate (1-deamino[8-D-arginine] vasopressin [DDAVP]), differentiates such patients into responders and nonresponders.

History

The history should begin with determining if urinary incontinence is limited to primary nocturnal enuresis versus daytime urinary incontinence (DUI). The next step is to inquire whether it is primary or secondary. Primary nocturnal enuresis is considered a separate disorder and unlikely to have organic etiology, whereas the determination of secondary nocturnal enuresis or secondary DUI should call for careful evaluation. Questions to determine whether the patient has polyuria are important as the presence of polyuria suggests a variety of metabolic, systemic, and kidney diseases. The absence of polyuria directs more focus on the lower urinary tract (Table 58.2; see also Table 58.1).

Polyuria

Polyuria, the excessive production of urine, can result from the absence of release of antidiuretic hormone (ADH), failure of the kidney to respond to ADH, or an osmotic diuresis. This can lead to urinary incontinence, especially in young children. Polyuria always results in polydipsia. It is often easier to query parents as to whether the volume of fluid intake by the child is excessive rather than to obtain an estimate of the volume of urine output. The first clue to polydipsia in infants is irritability and "hunger" after a successful feeding of formula or breast milk. In young children, favoring water over solids or milk, as well as seeking water in unusual places (e.g., toilets), can be a sign of

polydipsia. Waking to seek fluids at night in a consistent pattern is also a sign of polydipsia. Parental stories of bed linens being soaked despite a "double diaper" or training pull-on diaper are remarkable, especially when recounted by experienced parents.

An osmotic diuresis leading to polyuria may be an early sign of diabetes mellitus. The previously dry child may develop secondary nocturnal or even daytime enuresis. Associated symptoms include polydipsia and polyphagia with poor weight gain and fatigue. Children with central diabetes insipidus (CDI) and the genetic forms of nephrogenic diabetes insipidus (NDI) produce very large amounts of hypotonic urine. Along with polyuria and enuresis, these children may have a history of frequent hospitalizations for dehydration, often provoked by relatively minor illnesses. The dehydration is often associated with moderate or severe hypernatremia. Failure to thrive may develop because of a preference for low-calorie-containing fluids over solid foods. The secondary causes of NDI may include a partial defect in the mechanism for renal concentrating, and urinary incontinence may be the only symptom (see Table 58.2). Conversely, other children may also have growth retardation because of associated chronic renal failure or the associated metabolic abnormalities (e.g., metabolic acidosis in renal tubular acidosis [RTA] or rickets in Fanconi syndrome, metabolic alkalosis in Bartter syndrome). Polydipsia can also result from a behavioral problem and result in polyuria, but patients will demonstrate normal urinary concentrating ability using appropriate testing.

Voiding History

In the presence of enuresis but the absence of polyuria, a voiding history helps to determine whether additional evaluation is warranted. Is the urinary incontinence nocturnal only, or is daytime incontinence also present? Does the patient have stool incontinence? Voiding frequency is sometimes difficult to ascertain in a school-age child, and an assignment to keep a diary of voiding can be given on the first visit. This should include information on both bladder and bowel habits, specifically urine volumes and when urinary incontinence occurs. Voiding postponement, or urine holding patterns, with overflow incontinence is most easily identifiable with a diary. Incontinence can be a symptom of a urinary tract infection (UTI) (see Chapter 21). Associated symptoms may include dysuria, frequency, and urgency. Other urinary symptoms such as dysuria, urgency, dampness in the underwear, or other signs of UTI can all be signs of voiding dysfunction. Asking parents for specific observations—such as (1) the sudden urge to void followed by incontinence or (2) maneuvers to prevent urine leakage, such as squatting and pressing the heel of the foot into the perineum—elicits clues to a hyperactive detrusor muscle. Incontinence may occur with giggling, with physical stress while jumping, or with activities that require Valsalva maneuvers.

Secondary enuresis is defined as enuresis occurring after a dry period of at least 6 consecutive months and can be the first sign of an acquired renal or metabolic disease. Fecal soiling or constipation may be an accompanying sign of voiding dysfunction, but it should first raise suspicion for an occult spinal lesion such as spina bifida or a tethered cord. In addition, continuous dribbling, a poor urinary stream, or recurrent infections may be a sign of anatomic or neuropathic lesions (see Table 58.1).

Primary Nocturnal Enuresis

The patient with nocturnal enuresis (bedwetting) is typically without any major daytime symptoms. Enuresis is considered primary when the patient has not had any dry periods for >6 months. Toilet training for daytime control is often achieved easily. The frequency of wet nights should be ascertained to gauge the magnitude of the problem. Approximately 5–10% of 7-year-old children are affected and for some the problem persists into adolescence and even adulthood. A family history of nocturnal enuresis increases a patient's risk for nocturnal enuresis. If both parents have a history of enuresis, the rate of occurrence in offspring may be as high as 70–80%. If the father had primary nocturnal enuresis, the child has a fivefold to sevenfold increase in risk. The pathophysiologic mechanism is multifactorial; explanations include defects in osmoregulation (nocturnal polyuria), nocturnal detrusor over-reactivity, and disorders of sleep or arousal states.

Behavioral Issues

Social stressors should be ascertained because psychologic factors are important in the occurrence of secondary enuresis. There are reports of other psychiatric issues, such as attention-deficit/hyperactivity disorder, autism, and conduct disorders, associated with a higher incidence of daytime and nighttime incontinence. It has been widely accepted, however, that many affected children are often emotionally well adjusted. Nonetheless, care should be taken not to underestimate the sequelae of both enuresis and DUI in the older school-age child, who may feel "abnormal" among peers. Evaluation of the patient should always include inquiring how the patient and other family members are reacting to the problem and whether it may be interfering socially, with school issues, and with quality of life.

Finally, primary nocturnal enuresis may be a sleep disorder or a disorder of arousal. Patients with severe nocturnal enuresis may have defects in arousal to auditory stimuli. Inquiry into symptoms of sleep apnea should also be made, such as snoring or restless sleep, as it may lead to altered arousal states, leading to nocturnal enuresis in patients with sleep apnea (see Chapter 6).

Physical Examination

In all affected patients, their growth should be evaluated, because failure to thrive can be seen in many of the metabolic disorders that produce polyuria. The presence of hypertension suggests underlying renal or urologic abnormalities. Careful evaluation of the lower back may reveal cutaneous abnormalities such as hair tufts, pits, dimpling, or vascular malformations, which are possible signs of spina bifida occulta or tethered cord. A significant deviation of the gluteal cleft may also suggest the possibility of spinal dysraphism. The abdominal examination is important for detecting a distended bladder, suprapubic tenderness, or significant stool retention. A neurologic examination should include

assessment of lower extremity deep tendon reflexes, observation of the gait, and evaluation of perineal sensation and anal sphincter tone, again screening for the possibility of a neuropathic bladder. Anatomic abnormalities leading to incontinence should be sought by inspection of the genitalia. In females, the examination includes a search for fused labial folds and dribbling urine from an ectopic ureter. In males, the phallus should be inspected for the presence of epispadias or undescended testicles.

Diagnosis

The presence or absence of polyuria helps guide the necessary laboratory and radiologic testing (Figs. 58.1 and 58.2). An immediate UA is critical for differentiating the glycosuria of diabetes mellitus from the low specific gravity (osmolality) of diabetes insipidus or the proteinuria and/or hematuria of chronic renal disease.

A water deprivation test to examine urine concentrating capacity of patients when diabetes insipidus is suspected should be done in a hospital setting, with close observation of and attention to urine and serum osmolarity, urine output, and weight loss. In patients with significant polyuria, dehydration and hyperosmolarity are easily precipitated with several hours of water deprivation. For patients with a less suspect history of polyuria, a first morning void after an overnight fast should be sufficient for checking urine osmolarity or specific gravity.

In some patients, the problem can be better defined with a home voiding diary, which outlines how often and how much they are voiding and when urinary incontinence, constipation, or encopresis occurs.

Laboratory Assessment

Routine laboratory examination in patients with monosymptomatic nocturnal enuresis includes a UA and then is diagnosed by taking a good history and performing a complete physical examination. In patients with DUI or secondary nocturnal enuresis, or when polyuria or polydipsia is present, a screening UA, followed by appropriate blood chemistry studies, is important for evaluating for diabetes mellitus or electrolyte disorders such as metabolic acidosis (RTA), metabolic alkalosis (Bartter syndrome), hypercalcemia, and hypokalemia. Hypernatremia can be seen in the severe forms of diabetes insipidus. UTI should be sought in most patients with incontinence by obtaining a UA and urine culture. A UA also helps screen for occult, chronic glomerular or tubular renal disease. Hematuria or proteinuria can be a sign of renal disease, although its absence does not exclude this possibility. Glycosuria, when associated with normal serum glucose, can indicate tubulointerstitial disease, where proximal tubular injury results in a lowered threshold for glucose reabsorption.

Imaging and Cystometry

Radiologic imaging is not necessary in most patients with primary nocturnal enuresis. In select patients with secondary enuresis, daytime symptoms, or a suspect history or UA, renal ultrasonography may provide information regarding acquired or congenital renal diseases. Images of the bladder can reveal urologic abnormalities, including poor bladder emptying or thickened bladder wall. A voiding cystourethrogram is indicated only in patients with a questionable urinary stream, continuous dribbling (aberrant ectopic ureter), or suspected spinal cord lesions with lower extremity neurologic signs. MRI of the lower spine should be reserved for patients with cutaneous signs, neurologic or orthopedic symptoms of the lumbar-sacral spine, or complex spinal bone deformities seen on plain radiographs (Table 58.3 and Figs. 58.3 and 58.4). All patients with CDI must undergo cerebral MRI with specific focus on the hypothalamic-pituitary region.

Cystometry examination is useful for a select group of patients with a history of dysfunctional voiding symptoms whose response to

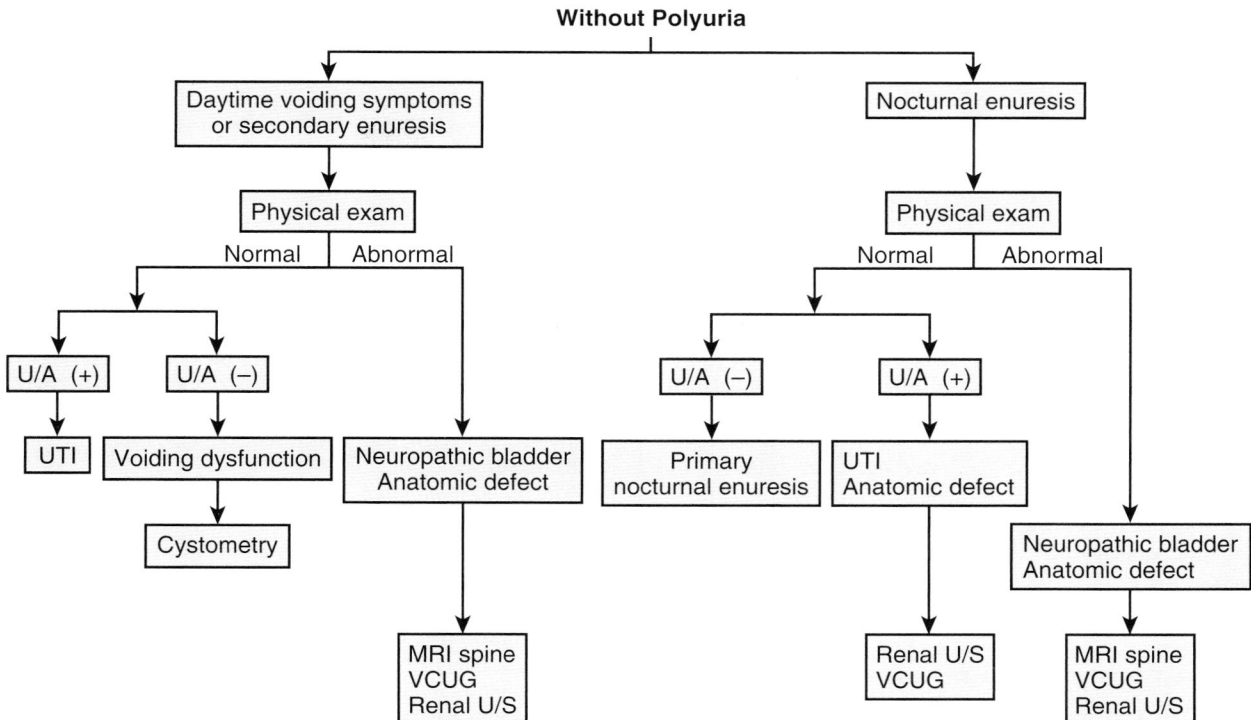

Fig. 58.1 Diagnosis of enuresis without polyuria. U/S, ultrasonography; UTI, urinary tract infection; VCUG, voiding cystourethrogram; +, positive; –, negative.

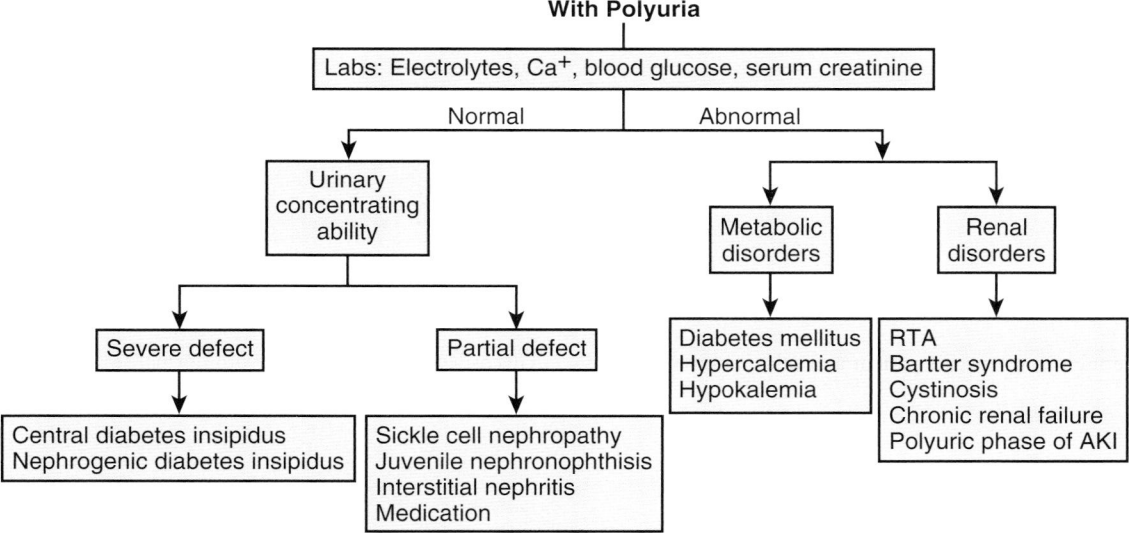

Fig. 58.2 Diagnosis of enuresis with polyuria. AKI, acute kidney injury; RTA, renal tubular acidosis.

therapy is poor. Bladder instability is characterized by involuntary contractions at more than 15 cm of water pressure during filling. Small bladder capacity is almost always a functional problem, not anatomic.

Differential Diagnosis

Primary Nocturnal Enuresis

Primary nocturnal enuresis (bedwetting) is considered abnormal in most social contexts after the age of 5 years. In the *Diagnostic and Statistical Manual of Mental Disorders*, fifth edition (DSM-5), primary enuresis is defined as wetting clothes or the bed at least twice a week for more than 3 consecutive months. Most affected patients have no daytime symptoms. It is a common problem, but only a small proportion of patients seek medical advice. The incidence of pure primary nocturnal enuresis without other symptoms is twice as common among males as among females.

Daytime Urinary Incontinence

DUI is defined as involuntary, intermittent leakage during the day in children older than 5 years of age with a frequency of once a month and persisting for >3 months. This occurs when there is an imbalance or lack of coordination of activity between the detrusor muscle activity (bladder contracture) and the bladder neck or external sphincter activity (bladder outlet control). This poor coordination can, over time, cause a wide spectrum of disorders, including incontinence. The severity depends on the balance of forces among the detrusor activity, bladder neck, and external sphincter. In the extreme case, high bladder pressures produce acquired urologic abnormalities, including hydronephrosis, vesicoureteral reflux (VUR), and renal damage. Dysfunctional voiding can be classified as mild, moderate, or severe. Early recognition can lead to proper management and avoidance of long-term sequelae.

Mild voiding dysfunction. Daytime urinary frequency is characterized by frequency and urgency as often as every 15–20 minutes. This is usually associated with incontinence or mild pain and occurs in children aged 3–8 years. The condition is also usually self-limiting. A thorough history should be documented, a careful physical examination conducted, and UA performed to rule out other pathologic processes.

Moderate voiding dysfunction. There are two extremes in the spectrum of moderate dysfunctional voiding. Over time, *voiding postponement*, or *urine holding*, as infrequent as once every 8–12 hours, results in incontinence and recurrent UTIs. This can be a consequence of behaviors developed when the young child is learning voluntary contraction of the external sphincter muscle while toilet training. It

may also develop when a child goes to school or camp and does not want to use an unfamiliar toilet or be in an embarrassing situation. The child learns additional maneuvers to void infrequently, such as squatting and pressing the heel of the foot in the perineum. This turns into dysfunctional voiding when over time the child is unable to relax the external sphincter in coordination with detrusor activity during voiding. This results in incomplete and inefficient bladder emptying.

The *overactive bladder*, or *urge syndrome*, is also a common abnormality in DUI. Low-quantity, frequent voiding leading to incontinence is secondary to delayed resolution of uninhibited bladder contractions that normally resolve as the child matures. This asynchronous activity between detrusor muscle and sphincter contraction leads to higher intravesical pressures. Urgency and urge incontinence are the most common symptoms, but recurrent UTIs and VUR may result as well. Complications may include thickening, trabeculations, or diverticula of the bladder. High bladder pressure can also cause hydroureter and hydronephrosis.

Severe dysfunctional voiding. This is often referred to as the *non-neurogenic neurogenic bladder* (Hinman syndrome), a syndrome representing the extreme end of the spectrum of dysfunctional voiding. Inappropriate voluntary contraction of the external sphincter during voiding produces high intravesical pressure and a functional outlet obstruction, leading to abnormal bladder function, hydronephrosis, and possibly renal failure. With time, the voiding pattern becomes habitual, and the anatomic changes in the bladder impede the ability to void normally. Biofeedback and clean intermittent straight catheterization may restore bladder emptying and function and prevent renal failure.

Special considerations. **Giggle incontinence** is most often seen in females and is characterized by incontinence after laughter. It too is usually self-limiting. **Stress incontinence** follows athletic activities such as running or jumping and landing; it is common with activities such as gymnastics and cheerleading. Timely bladder emptying before exercise is effective in preventing this problem. **Urethrovaginal reflux** can lead to postvoid dribbling and can occur in young females who develop habits of incomplete voiding or can result from urine that is collected in the vagina during voiding. Sitting with the knees slightly apart or sitting on the toilet facing backward eliminates this problem. Anatomic issues such as meatal anomalies and labial adhesion can also be a cause of this form of incontinence.

Neuropathic Bladder

The neuropathic bladder most often occurs in patients with spina bifida, an open or closed congenital spinal cord fusion defect. This results in distortion of normal neural tissues in the spinal cord or nerve

---

TABLE 58.3 Cutaneous Lesions Associated with Occult Spinal Dysraphism

Imaging Indicated
Subcutaneous mass or lipoma
Hairy patch
Dermal sinus or cyst
Atypical dimples (deep, >5 mm, >25 mm from anal verge)
Vascular lesion, e.g., hemangioma or telangiectasia
Skin appendages or polypoid lesions, e.g., skin tags, tail-like appendages
Scarlike lesions (aplasia cutis)

Imaging Uncertain
Hyperpigmented patches
Deviation of the gluteal fold

Imaging Not Required
Simple dimples (<5 mm, <25 mm from anal verge)
Coccygeal pits

From Williams H. Spinal sinuses, dimples, pits and patches: what lies beneath? *Arch Dis Child Educ Pract Ed.* 2006;91:ep75–ep80.

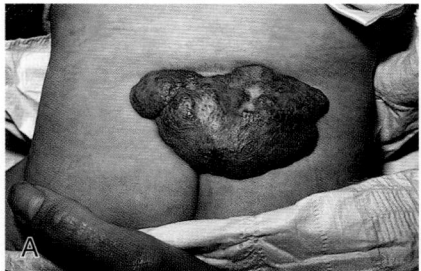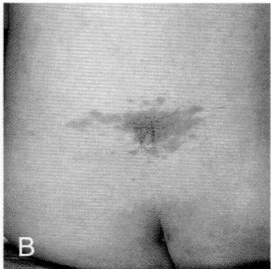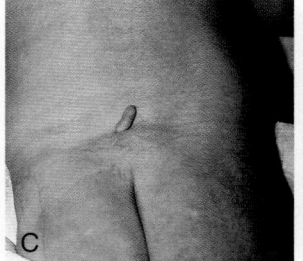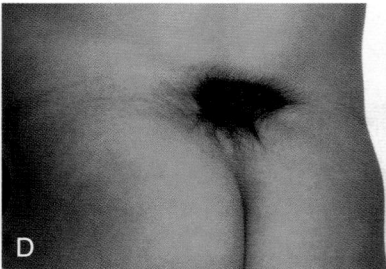

Fig. 58.3 Clinical aspects of congenital median lumbosacral cutaneous lesions. *A,* Midline sacral hemangioma in a patient with an occult lipomyelomeningocele. *B,* Capillary malformation with a subtle patch of hypertrichosis in a patient with a dermal sinus. *C,* Human tail with underlying lipoma in an infant with lipomyelomeningocele. *D,* Midline area of hypertrichosis (faun tail) overlying a patch of hyperpigmentation. (*A–C,* From Kos L, Drolet BA. Developmental abnormalities. In: Eichenfield LF, Frieden IJ, Esterly NB, eds. *Neonatal Dermatology.* 2nd ed. Philadelphia: WB Saunders; 2008; *D,* from Spine and spinal cord: developmental disorders. In Schapira A, ed. *Neurology and Clinical Neuroscience.* Philadelphia: Mosby; 2007.)

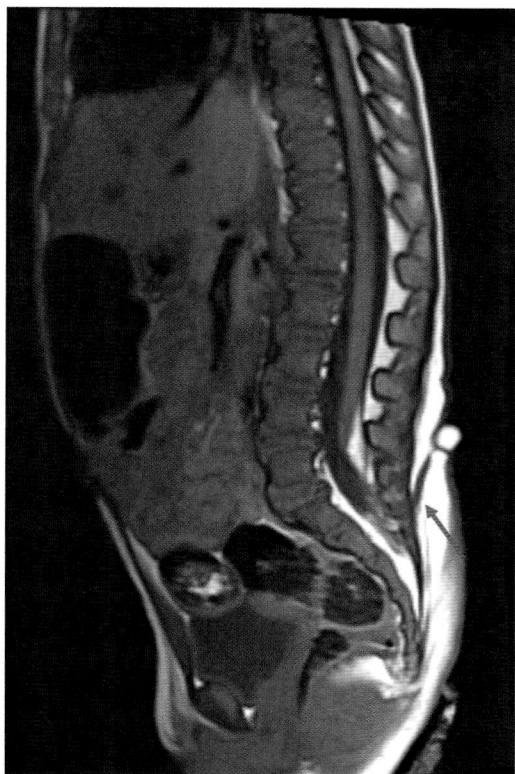

Fig. 58.4 Dermal sinus tract—similar to a lipomyelomeningocele but with an additional fibrous tract *(red arrow)* extending from a superficial skin dimple to the placode. (From Martin RJ, Fanaroff AA, Walsh MC, eds. *Fanaroff' & Martins's Neonatal-Perinatal Medicine.* 11th ed. Philadelphia: Elsevier; 2020:1075, Fig. 58.4.)

roots. The range of anomalies includes meningocele, lipomeningocele, primary tethered cord, dermoid cyst, syrinx, and sacral agenesis (see Fig. 58.4). Closed defects can be initially asymptomatic and manifest during toilet training years with incontinence, recurrent UTIs, or orthopedic problems in later childhood. Many children who present with symptoms have a cutaneous finding over the lumbosacral spine noted since birth. The severity of the symptoms does not seem to predict the severity of the bladder dysfunction or renal damage. Despite lesser neurologic deficits in closed spina bifida, affected patients have demonstrated bladder dysfunction as severe as that observed in open spina bifida. Acute spinal injury (trauma), compression (tumor), or infection (transverse myelitis) may produce similar bladder conditions such as acute urinary retention.

Anatomic Defects

Posterior urethral valves and urethral obstruction. This is the most common form of urinary obstruction leading to kidney failure in male infants and children. It is a result of persistence of fetal folds in the posterior urethra, which act as a valve to create urinary obstruction. Poor urinary stream and bladder distention are the most common urinary complaints, but dribbling and incontinence are also observed. UTI can be the presenting problem, and when it is diagnosed in young males, especially infants, posterior urethral valves should always be sought.

Eagle-Barrett, or prune-belly, syndrome is another important cause of urethral obstruction. Early obstruction during embryogenesis leads to hydronephrosis, hydroureter, abdominal distention, abdominal musculature deficiency, and excessive skin folds, thus giving the wrinkly "prune" appearance of the abdomen in severe cases. A spectrum of renal dysplasia and chronic kidney disease can result in both conditions.

Renal duplication. This is a result of duplication of the ureteric bud during embryogenesis, causing a double collecting system, or two ureters. Duplicated ureters can open separately inside the bladder, but in rare cases, an ectopic ureter can end in the vagina, urethra, or vestibule, leading to dribbling and incontinence.

Vesicoureteral reflux. VUR is the retrograde flow of urine from the bladder into the ureters and kidney. Normal insertion of the ureter into the bladder submucosal wall forms a flap-valve mechanism that prevents urine backup during filling and contraction. Congenital VUR is secondary to shorter ureteric segments in the bladder wall. Urine flow mechanics are disrupted by the constant filling of the bladder with urine that has flowed backward and then returns to the emptied bladder. The inability to completely empty the bladder eliminates an important defense against UTIs. Secondary VUR can be associated with dysfunctional voiding. Dyssynergia between detrusor contraction and sphincter relaxation may result in VUR and recurrent UTIs. Urethral obstruction leading to high intravesical pressure also leads to VUR, poor bladder emptying, and thus UTIs and incontinence.

Metabolic Disorders

Hypercalcemia. This is an uncommon electrolyte disorder in children but can be observed in primary hyperparathyroidism, vitamin D intoxication, immobilization, Williams syndrome, malignancy, and idiopathic hypercalcemia of infancy. Polyuria is a symptom of hypercalcemia and is a result of its inhibitory effect on Na$^+$, K$^+$-ATPase function in renal tubules. This leads to renal sodium and water losses and thus to polyuria and volume contraction. In chronic hypercalcemia, increased calcium excretion over time can lead to nephrocalcinosis, tubular damage, and poor urinary concentrating ability, thus enhancing polyuria.

Hypokalemia. This is another electrolyte disorder that induces polyuria. In children, it occurs as a result of diuretic use, aldosterone excess states, Cushing syndrome, and intrinsic renal disorders that affect potassium handling. The latter includes disorders such as RTA, Bartter syndrome, or renal injury from nephrotoxic medications. Hypokalemia interferes with water reabsorption in the collecting duct of the kidneys.

Diabetes mellitus. Polyuria and urinary incontinence can be the first symptoms of diabetes mellitus and are secondary to hyperglycemia and the osmotic diuresis resulting from chronic glycosuria. The renal threshold for reabsorption of glucose is exceeded when the blood glucose level is higher than approximately 180 mg/dL. If oral intake of fluid decreases, as occurs when diabetic ketoacidosis causes anorexia and emesis, significant dehydration and shock frequently develop.

Central Diabetes Insipidus

In CDI, the lack of circulating ADH prevents concentration of the urine, leading to high quantities of dilute urine. The defect can be complete or partial, and thus the degree of polyuria is variable. In complete CDI, the massive polyuria can lead to severe dehydration and hypernatremia. CDI can be secondary to congenital malformations of the pituitary gland, intracranial surgery, head trauma, or tumor involving the nuclei of the hypothalamus (where ADH is produced) or the neurohypophysial axis itself. There is also an idiopathic form and familial forms of CDI. Abnormalities in the *AVP* gene are the most common familial form inherited in most patients as an autosomal dominant trait; X-linked or autosomal recessive inheritance has also been reported. In the idiopathic form, infiltrative diseases such as Langerhans cell histiocytosis (Letterer-Siwe syndrome) should be sought. A significant proportion of young children initially diagnosed with idiopathic CDI have been found to have histiocytosis in subsequent years. Treatment is with ADH or its analogs.

Renal Concentrating Defects

Renal tubular acidosis. In distal **(type 1) RTA**, the most common form of RTA, there is a defect in the tubular secretion of hydrogen ions and decreased formation of NH_4^+ cations in the urine. In children, the presentation includes failure to thrive, polyuria, and polydipsia. Hypokalemia is a common finding and can be profound, leading to weakness. Hypercalciuria and low urine citrate excretion combine to produce nephrocalcinosis. The autosomal recessive form of the disease is frequently associated with hearing loss. There are also autosomal dominant forms of the disease. Distal RTA may be secondary to medications (e.g., amphotericin) or a variety of conditions, including interstitial nephritis, obstructive uropathy, nephrocalcinosis, renal transplantation, sickle cell disease, and systemic lupus erythematosus (see Chapter 59).

Proximal RTA is less common and is a primary defect in bicarbonate reabsorption in the proximal tubule. When associated with other proximal tubular defects, such as salt wasting, phosphate wasting, glycosuria, and aminoaciduria, it is referred to as Fanconi syndrome. Manifesting in infancy to early adulthood, cystinosis is the most common cause of proximal RTA in children. This autosomal recessive disorder results from a defect in cystine transport and results in the lysosomal accumulation of cystine throughout the body. The infantile form usually manifests in the first year of life. Without intervention, this form results in end-stage renal failure. Acidosis, rickets, polyuria, and severe failure to thrive are hallmarks of the disease. Early intervention with oral cysteamine to bind cysteine has dramatically improved the outcome in affected patients. Proximal RTA is a feature of several other genetic disorders manifesting in childhood (such as galactosemia, tyrosinemia, hereditary fructose intolerance, glycogen storage disease type I, Lowe syndrome, Wilson disease, osteopetrosis) or ingestion of toxins (e.g., heavy metals) (see Chapter 59).

Sickle cell disease. Hemoglobin S is a genetic defect in hemoglobin A that results in red blood cells that deform under low oxygen tension (see Chapter 49). The renal medulla is a site with high osmolality, low oxygen tension, and relative acidosis, all conditions that promote sickling. This results in occlusion of blood vessels and damage to the renal medulla, the primary site where the urine is concentrated. The resultant decreased ability to concentrate leads to a higher incidence of nocturnal enuresis in affected patients.

Nephronophthisis. Juvenile nephronophthisis is an autosomal recessive disorder that leads to end-stage renal failure between preadolescence and early adulthood. Patients have high urine output because of poor renal concentrating ability and renal salt wasting. Patients may have primary or secondary nocturnal enuresis. The salt wasting causes salt craving, and patients prefer salty foods or even eat salt directly from the saltshaker. A small percentage of these patients have retinitis pigmentosa, which may cause blindness at birth or later in life. Patients may present with symptoms of chronic renal failure.

Nephrogenic diabetes insipidus. The congenital form of NDI is often diagnosed before toilet training, but it can lead to urinary incontinence in later childhood. Infants may present with poor growth, severe dehydration, seizures, and central nervous system injury or death. In families in which the diagnosis has already been made, early intervention in infants can prevent these symptoms and lead to an excellent outcome. Ninety percent of patients have the X-linked form of the disease, which is caused by a gene variant ADH receptor. Female carriers may be mildly affected. The autosomal recessive and autosomal dominant forms of NDI are caused by variants in aquaporin, the water channel that allows uptake of water in the collecting duct. Treatment is with indomethacin, sodium restriction, and thiazide diuretics.

Treatment
Primary Nocturnal Enuresis

Establishing whether the primary nocturnal enuresis is the only symptom (monosymptomatic) or whether there are associated symptoms such as DUI, constipation, sleep disorders, or behavioral issues is necessary before a treatment strategy is developed.

Many families whose child has monosymptomatic nocturnal enuresis simply want reassurance that there is not an organic explanation. It is also helpful to let the family and child know that almost all patients "outgrow" primary nocturnal enuresis. Positive reinforcement for dry nights, dispelling any negative attitudes, and avoiding blame enhance the child's self-esteem. If treatment is sought, the enuresis alarm has a high success rate, but patient selection is important. These devices are designed to awaken patients when micturition begins and result in the development of increased bladder capacity. Its effect may not be seen for up to 12 weeks, and therefore the family and patient must be highly motivated. Older patients who are ready to take charge of the problem and who do not have difficulty waking are the best candidates.

Pharmacologic therapy for primary nocturnal enuresis includes the use of DDAVP, an ADH analog. There is probably a subpopulation of patients with enuresis who have "nocturnal polyuria," which led to the drug's popularity, but there is evidence that this is independent of vasopressin secretion. DDAVP is most effective in children with a positive family history of primary nocturnal enuresis, with normal bladder capacity, and who are older than 7 years. Its safety profile has been excellent, but patients should be given careful instruction on restricting fluid intake after the bedtime dose. There are occasional reports of hyponatremic seizures in children who drink excessively while taking DDAVP.

Patients with small bladder capacity and diurnal symptoms tend not to respond to DDAVP; these patients may benefit from anticholinergic therapy, such as oxybutynin. Combination therapy involving a bed alarm plus DDAVP or DDAVP plus anticholinergic therapy may be helpful in select patients.

Imipramine, a tricyclic antidepressant, has been shown to be effective, but its side effects and toxicity have limited its use for this benign condition. Patients with enuresis and other behavioral problems who take selective serotonin reuptake inhibitors have reported improvement in the enuresis. This may be an appropriate option in this population.

Daytime Urinary Incontinence

Treatment of mild functional forms of DUI should begin with nonpharmacologic management, or urotherapy, that is individualized to patient symptoms. Patients should receive education on bowel and bladder function, and also be instructed to void on a regular schedule, even if they do not feel the urge to void. This encourages voiding when the patient is relaxed and will lead to fewer contractions of the external sphincter during micturition. They may also benefit from counseling on posture, fluid intake, and diet. Keeping a diary of the voiding schedule involves the child in management and makes them more aware of bladder and bowel habits. Aggressive management of constipation (see Chapter 19) improves good bladder emptying and decreases bladder instability. These nonpharmacologic approaches to urotherapy are often enough to treat the majority of neurologically and anatomically intact children.

When DUI continues despite nonpharmacologic methods, pharmacologic therapy is used as an adjunct. Anticholinergic therapy is the mainstay of drug treatment, especially in the child with an overactive bladder or urge syndrome, blocking receptors in the bladder and suppressing bladder contractility. Oxybutynin should be started at a low dosage and titrated to its maximum dosage if necessary. The minimum effective dosage should be used to minimize side effects (dry mouth, flushing, constipation, concentration problems, and blurred vision). Use of the extended-release form of oxybutynin bypasses the first-pass metabolism and is reported to result in better tolerance. The use of α-adrenergic antagonists (e.g., doxazosin, tamsulosin, terazosin) is currently reserved for off-label use in the treatment of non-neurogenic bladder dysfunction, reducing bladder outlet resistance.

Patients with recurrent UTIs who develop urine-holding patterns that lead to overflow incontinence may benefit from a trial of antibiotic prophylaxis. This may keep the child free of infection and may prevent the painful urination that reinforces exaggerated external sphincter contraction and urine holding. Botulinum toxin is a neurotoxin that inhibits acetylcholine release at the presynaptic junction and is approved for sphincteric injections. It is not approved for voiding dysfunction in children. The off-label use in children with neuropathic bladders and treatment-resistant non-neurogenic bladders has shown reports of favorable outcomes.

Biofeedback is reserved for patients with moderate to severe dysfunctional voiding. Patients can learn to increase bladder capacity and inhibit detrusor contractions through this method. Neuromodulation using transcutaneous electrical nerve stimulation (TENS) has shown promise in reducing incontinence episodes and urgency in randomized controlled trials. More evidence is needed, but it remains an adjunct therapy in children.

Polyuria

The treatment of polyuria depends on the cause. In certain disorders, such as diabetes mellitus, hypokalemia, or hypercalcemia, the underlying disorder can be corrected. The high urine output in CDI decreases markedly with the use of DDAVP. In contrast, there is no effective therapy for reducing urine output in patients with disorders such as juvenile nephronophthisis or obstructive uropathy.

The hereditary forms of NDI cause massive polyuria. A combination of sodium restriction and a thiazide diuretic can decrease this high urine output by producing a subtle volume depletion that results in less water being delivered to the collecting duct. The addition of

TABLE 58.4	Red Flags
Polyuria	
Polydipsia	
Failure to thrive	
Poor urinary stream	
Encopresis	
Secondary enuresis	
Abnormal gait, including toe walking	
Recurrent urinary tract infections	
Cutaneous lesions over lumbosacral spine	
Diminished lower extremity reflexes	
Abnormal genitalia	
Palpable bladder	
Hypertension	
Headache	
Visual disturbances	
Obstructive sleep apneas	
Recurrent fevers	

indomethacin or other nonsteroidal antiinflammatory drugs can, by reducing renal blood flow, further decrease urine output in patients with NDI. The use of indomethacin also reduces the high urine output in Bartter syndrome. Despite therapy, patients with Bartter syndrome and NDI continue to have high urine output, and the family should be counseled that a delay in achieving nighttime continence is expected.

Neuropathic Bladder and Anatomic Disorders

The treatment of these disorders depends on the specific defect. In patients with neuropathic bladders resulting from spina bifida, chronic intermittent catheterization of the bladder may be the only way to achieve continence. Uninhibited bladder contractions may necessitate anticholinergic therapy as an adjunct.

Anatomic disorders such as posterior urethral valves or VUR may still necessitate medical therapy or biofeedback after corrective surgery. Urodynamic testing can be very helpful in this population to define the problem leading to incontinence.

SUMMARY AND RED FLAGS

Most children with urinary incontinence do not have an organic problem. The work-up consists of a thorough history and physical examination with laboratory analysis when indicated. Red flags that indicate the need for diagnostic tests are shown in Table 58.4.

BIBLIOGRAPHY

A bibliography is available at ExpertConsult.com.

59

Acid–Base and Electrolyte Disturbances

Sarah Vepraskas, Heather Toth, and Michael Weisgerber

The presence of an acid–base or an electrolyte disorder may explain a patient's symptoms or may lead to a specific diagnosis.

ACID–BASE BALANCE

Normal acid–base balance is maintained by the lungs and kidneys. Carbon dioxide, a by-product of normal metabolism, is a weak acid. The lungs are able to prevent an increase in the partial pressure of carbon dioxide (Pco_2) in the blood by excreting the carbon dioxide (CO_2) produced by the body. The pulmonary response to changes in the CO_2 concentration is fast, as it occurs via central sensing of the Pco_2, and there is a subsequent increase or decrease in ventilation to maintain a normal Pco_2 (35–45 mm Hg). There is an inverse relationship between Pco_2 and ventilation because an increase in ventilation decreases the Pco_2, and a decrease in ventilation increases the Pco_2.

The kidneys are responsible for excreting acid produced by the body. Sources of hydrogen ions include protein metabolism and incomplete metabolism of carbohydrates and fat; urine or stool losses of bicarbonate may contribute to acidemia. The hydrogen ions formed from endogenous acid production are neutralized by bicarbonate from the bicarbonate buffer system. The bicarbonate buffer system, based on the relationship between carbon dioxide and bicarbonate (HCO_3^-), is displayed by the following equation:

$$CO_2 + H_2O \leftrightarrow H^+ + HCO_3^-$$

This equation can help us understand how changes in CO_2 or HCO_3^- affect the acid–base balance.

ACID–BASE DISORDERS

A pH <7.35 is defined as acidosis, and a pH >7.45 is defined as alkalosis. An acid–base disorder is **respiratory** in etiology when it is caused by a primary abnormality in respiratory function (a change in $Paco_2$) and is **metabolic** when the primary change is due to a variation in bicarbonate concentration. Acid–base disorders may also be mixed, which occurs when two or even three primary events act to alter the acid–base state at the same time.

In metabolic disorders, extracellular buffers (bicarbonate) rapidly titrate the presence of strong acids or bases. Intracellular buffers chiefly accomplish the buffering of respiratory disorders. Secondary respiratory compensation for metabolic acid–base disorders begins within minutes by changes in ventilation and is usually complete in 12–24 hours. In contrast, secondary metabolic compensation for respiratory disorders occurs more slowly, beginning within hours but requiring 2–5 days for completion. The kidneys increase net acid excretion in response to a primary respiratory acidosis; renal net acid excretion also increases during a metabolic acidosis if the kidneys themselves are not the cause of the metabolic acidosis. The expected compensation for

primary acid–base disorders is shown in Table 59.1. *These compensatory mechanisms never return the pH back to normal until the underlying disease process has subsided or has been effectively treated.*

When only one primary acid–base abnormality occurs and its compensatory mechanisms are activated, the disorder is classified as a simple acid–base disorder. When a combination of acid–base disturbances occurs, the disorder is classified as a mixed acid–base disorder. The latter should be suspected if the compensation in a given patient differs from the predicted values (see Table 59.1). Interpretation of data in infants and young children requires caution. Crying results in hyperventilation and can quickly change Pco_2 and consequently the pH.

SYMPTOMS OF ACID–BASE DISORDERS

History and clinical evaluation are the first steps in assessing a patient with an acid–base disorder. Although the signs and symptoms associated with an acid–base abnormality can be nonspecific, there are certain clues that one can obtain from manifestations that can assist in the diagnosis of the acid–base disorder. **Metabolic acidosis** results in increased minute ventilation (manifesting as increased respiratory rate and/or effort) because of respiratory compensation. A patient may have tachypnea with a metabolic acidosis from a diarrheal illness, dehydration, poisoning, diabetic ketoacidosis, inborn errors of metabolism, or infection. In more severe acidosis (pH <7.20), the respiratory pattern is characterized by deep and rapid breaths (Kussmaul respiration). Severe acidosis may also lead to hypotension, pulmonary edema, and asystole; its harmful effects are accentuated in the presence of hypoxia. Chronic metabolic acidosis leads to poor growth and hypercalciuria with subsequent bone disease because bone buffering of acid produces marked mineral losses.

A child with **metabolic alkalosis** may be asymptomatic. In some cases, careful examination of the child may detect hypoventilation. One should consider metabolic alkalosis in a child who has been vomiting or in a child who has had chronic diuretic use. Severe alkalosis (pH >7.55) can lead to tissue hypoxia, mental confusion, obtundation, muscular irritability, tetany, and an increased risk of seizures and cardiac arrhythmias. Some of these signs and symptoms are related to decreased concentration of serum ionized calcium as a result of its increased binding to protein in the presence of alkalosis. Acid–base disturbances can be assessed through laboratory analysis by obtaining a basic chemistry panel and/or a blood gas analysis.

RENAL REGULATION OF ACID–BASE BALANCE

The kidneys are the principal regulator of bicarbonate homeostasis. The renal regulation of HCO_3^- can be divided into two processes: reabsorption of HCO_3^- and excretion of H^+. The first role of the kidneys is to reabsorb the filtered HCO_3^- so that this important extracellular buffer

TABLE 59.1 Changes in P_{CO_2}, HCO_3^-, and pH in Primary Acid–Base Disorders*

Disorder	Primary Event	Degree of Initial Disturbance	Compensation	Degree of Compensation
Metabolic acidosis	↓ $[HCO_3^-]$	For every 10 mEq/L ↓ in HCO_3^-, pH ↓ by 0.15	↓ P_{CO_2}	For 1 mEq/L ↓ $[HCO_3^-]$, P_{CO_2} ↓ 1–1.5 mm Hg
Metabolic alkalosis	↑ $[HCO_3^-]$	For every 10 mEq/L ↑ in HCO_3^-, pH ↑ by 0.15	↑ P_{CO_2}	For 1 mEq/L ↑ $[HCO_3^-]$, P_{CO_2} ↑ 0.5–1 mm Hg
Respiratory acidosis		For every 10 mm Hg ↑ in P_{CO_2}, pH ↓ by 0.08		
Acute (<12–24 hr)	↑ P_{CO_2}		↑ $[HCO_3^-]$	For 10 mm Hg ↑ P_{CO_2}, $[HCO_3^-]$ ↑ 1 mEq/L
Chronic (3–5 days)	↑ P_{CO_2}		↑↑ $[HCO_3^-]$	For 10 mm Hg ↑ P_{CO_2}, $[HCO_3^-]$ ↑ 4 mEq/L
Respiratory alkalosis		For every 10 mm Hg ↓ in P_{CO_2}, pH ↑ by 0.08		
Acute (<12 hr)	↓ P_{CO_2}		↓ $[HCO_3^-]$	For 10 mm Hg ↓ P_{CO_2}, $[HCO_3^-]$ ↓ 1–3 mEq/L
Chronic (1–2 days)	↓ P_{CO_2}		↓↓ $[HCO_3^-]$	For 10 mm Hg ↓ P_{CO_2}, $[HCO_3^-]$ ↓ 1–3 mEq/L

*Normal serum $[HCO_3^-]$ is 24 mEq/L, and normal arterial partial pressure of carbon dioxide (P_{CO_2}) is 40 mm Hg.
↓, decrease; ↓↓, greater decrease; ↑, increase; ↑↑, greater increase.
Modified from Brewer ED. Disorders of acid-base balance. *Pediatr Clin North Am.* 1990;37:429–447.

is not excreted in the urine. The second role of the kidneys is to excrete H^+ that is produced from protein and phospholipid catabolism.

Most (80–90%) of the filtered HCO_3^- is reabsorbed in the proximal tubule. Bicarbonate reabsorption at this site is increased by the contraction of the extracellular fluid (ECF) volume, activation of the renin-angiotensin system (mainly through the effect of angiotensin II), elevated P_{CO_2}, and hypokalemia. Conversely, HCO_3^- reabsorption is decreased when there is expansion of the ECF volume, inhibition of angiotensin II, a fall in P_{CO_2}, and an elevation of the parathyroid hormone level.

The distal tubule and collecting duct regenerate bicarbonate via H^+ ion secretion into the tubular lumen by an H^+-adenosine triphosphatase (H^+-ATPase) pump in the luminal membrane. This active secretion can generate an H^+ ion gradient of 1,000:1 between tubular fluid and cells, permitting the urine pH to fall to as low as 4.5. The active H^+ secretion is significantly influenced by the luminal electronegativity caused by active Na^+ reabsorption in the cortical collecting duct. Thus, in the cortical collecting duct, H^+ excretion is influenced by distal Na^+ delivery and reabsorption. In contrast, in the outer medullary portion of the collecting duct, aldosterone stimulates the H^+ excretion independently of Na^+ delivery or reabsorption. Some of the H^+ secreted is consumed in reclaiming the small amount of HCO_3^- that escaped reabsorption at proximal sites; the rest of the H^+ is excreted in the urine. The ability to excrete a large amount of H^+ ions is dependent on the presence of buffers. The H^+ ions are buffered by phosphates and, to a lesser extent, by other non-reabsorbable anions. The other very important urinary buffer is ammonia (NH_3), which combines with a secreted H^+ to generate an ammonium ion (NH_4^+). The proximal tubular cells generate ammonia through the metabolism of the amino acid glutamine. For every H^+ that is finally excreted, an HCO_3^- is added to the ECF compartment. Metabolic acidosis by itself enhances NH_4^+ production and excretion. Ammonia genesis by proximal tubular cells is also stimulated by hypokalemia, whereas hyperkalemia inhibits ammonia genesis. The ability of the kidney to produce ammonia is markedly decreased in conditions such as chronic renal failure as a result of reduced renal mass and in some types of renal tubular acidosis (RTA). The ability to lower urine pH and increase net acid excretion may not be achieved until 4–6 weeks of age.

METABOLIC ACIDOSIS

A metabolic acidosis can result from addition of H^+ to the body, failure to excrete H^+, or loss of HCO_3^-. The differential diagnosis of metabolic acidosis is simplified by classifying the causes into those associated with a normal anion gap (also known as a hyperchloremic metabolic acidosis) and those associated with an increased anion gap (Table 59.2).

The anion gap is easily calculated: $Na^+ − (Cl^- + HCO_3^-)$. The anion gap is normally 8–16 mEq/L. When a strong acid (e.g., lactic acid) is added to or produced in the body, hydrogen ions are neutralized by bicarbonate, HCO_3^- is consumed by the H^+, and the bicarbonate concentration falls. The accompanying anion, such as lactate, is a new unmeasured anion, which increases the anion gap. The increase in the anion gap is usually proportional to the fall in serum (HCO_3^-). In contrast, when HCO_3^- is lost from the body, no new anion is generated. In this situation, there is a reciprocal increase in the serum Cl^- to maintain electroneutrality. The anion gap does not change; the rise in (Cl^-) is proportional to the fall in (HCO_3^-).

Normal Anion Gap (Hyperchloremic) Metabolic Acidosis
Renal Tubular Acidosis
RTA is a group of disorders characterized by impairment of renal HCO_3^- reabsorption and/or H^+ excretion in the presence of a relatively normal glomerular filtration rate (GFR). On the basis of the distinctive pathophysiologic features, three types of RTA—type I (distal or classic), type II (proximal or bicarbonate wasting), and type IV (hyperkalemic)—are recognized (Table 59.3).

Type I RTA is caused by the inability to secrete H^+ in the **distal tubule**, resulting in hypokalemic hyperchloremic metabolic acidosis. These patients have a tendency to develop nephrocalcinosis and nephrolithiasis, which results from the excretion of large quantities of calcium, combined with an alkaline urine pH and hypocitraturia. In addition to the deficient H^+ secretion, these patients are unable to increase ammonia genesis. The patient's urine pH remains alkaline (>5.5) despite extreme systemic metabolic acidosis. Type I RTA may occur as an isolated condition or may develop secondary to several diseases, medications, or toxins (Table 59.4). Type I RTA due to variants in the *ATP6V1B1* gene is associated with early severe deafness, while variants in *SLC4A1* may be associated with congenital hemolytic anemia.

Type II RTA is caused by an impairment of HCO_3^- reabsorption in the **proximal tubule**, resulting in hypokalemic hyperchloremic metabolic acidosis. Because the distal acidification mechanisms are intact, these patients can lower the urine pH to <5.5 and can excrete adequate amounts of NH_4^+ when the serum HCO_3^- is below the filtration threshold. As a result, their acidosis is usually less profound than that which occurs in distal RTA. In some patients, there may be

TABLE 59.2   Causes of Metabolic Acidosis

NORMAL ANION GAP

Diarrhea

Renal tubular acidosis (RTA):

    Distal (type I) RTA (OMIM 79800/602722/267300)*

    Proximal (type II) RTA (OMIM 604278)†

    Hyperkalemic (type IV) RTA (OMIM 201910/264350/177735/145260)‡

Urinary tract diversions

Post-hypocapnia

Ammonium chloride intake

INCREASED ANION GAP

Lactic Acidosis

Tissue hypoxia

    Shock

    Hypoxemia

    Severe anemia

    Cyanide poisoning

    Carbon monoxide poisoning

    Methemoglobinemia

Liver failure

Lymphoma, leukemia, solid tumors

Intestinal bacterial overgrowth

Inborn errors of metabolism

Thiamine deficiency

Medications

    Nucleoside reverse transcriptase inhibitors

    Metformin

    Propofol

Other Causes

Ketoacidosis

    Diabetic ketoacidosis

    Starvation ketoacidosis

    Alcoholic ketoacidosis

Kidney failure/uremia

D-Lactic acidosis

Poisoning

    Ethylene glycol

    Methanol

    Salicylate

    Toluene

    Paraldehyde

    Cocaine

*Along with these genetic disorders, distal RTA may be secondary to renal disease or medications.

†Most cases of proximal RTA are not caused by this primary genetic disorder. Proximal RTA is usually part of Fanconi syndrome, which has multiple etiologies.

‡Hyperkalemic RTA can be secondary to a genetic disorder (some of the more common are listed) or other etiologies.

OMIM, database number from the Online Mendelian Inheritance in Man (http://www.ncbi.nlm.nih.gov/omim).

From Greenbaum LA. Electrolyte and acid-base disorders. In Kliegman RM, St. Geme JW III, Blum NJ, et al., eds. *Nelson Textbook of Pediatrics.* 21st ed. Philadelphia: Elsevier; 2020:416.

TABLE 59.3   Differentiation of RTA Types

Factor	Type I	Type II	Type IV
Serum K⁺	Low or normal	Low	High, salt wasting
Renal function	Normal or near normal	Normal or near normal	Stage 3, 4, or 5 chronic kidney disease
Urine pH during acidosis	High >5.5	Low <5.5 or normal	Low or high
Serum HCO₃⁻ (mmol/L)	10–20	16–18	16–22
Urine P_{CO_2} (mm Hg)	<40	<40	>70
Urine citrate	Low	High	Low
Fanconi syndrome	No	May be present	No

Type III RTA combines features of type I and II RTA in patients with osteopetrosis.

From Palmer BF. Metabolic acidosis. In: Johnson RJ, Feehally J, Floege J, eds. *Comprehensive Clinical Nephrology.* 5th ed. Philadelphia: Saunders; 2015:153.

of multiple defects in proximal tubule reabsorption and, in addition to type II RTA, includes excessive urinary losses of glucose, amino acids, phosphate, and uric acid. The excessive losses of phosphate often cause hypophosphatemic rickets. There are many causes of type II RTA (see Table 59.4).

Type IV RTA results from low circulating aldosterone concentrations, partial or complete end-organ resistance to aldosterone, or aldosterone antagonism. Because of the lack of aldosterone effect, there is decreased distal acidification and decreased distal sodium reabsorption with hyperkalemic hyperchloremic acidosis. The hyperkalemia seen in type IV RTA is the most characteristic feature and differentiates it from the other two types.

The examination of a child with RTA may be normal. Poor skin turgor may be present from dehydration. Muscle weakness and muscle aches from hypokalemia may occur. Low back pain and bone pain may be present in patients with abnormalities of calcium metabolism (type II). All forms of RTA are associated with growth failure. Patients with Fanconi syndrome have severe rickets/osteomalacia and malnutrition.

Laboratory evaluation in all patients with RTA shows metabolic acidosis with hyperchloremia and a normal anion gap. The urine pH always exceeds 5.5 in type I RTA but can be <5.5 in type II and type IV RTA.

Type I and II RTA are treated with oral sodium bicarbonate titrated to correct the acidosis. Potassium supplementation is needed in hypokalemic patients. Type IV RTA can be treated with furosemide to lower elevated potassium levels, along with sodium bicarbonate to correct significant acidosis. Fludrocortisone can be used to correct mineralocorticoid deficiency. In patients with secondary proximal RTA, treatment should be aimed at the primary disorder.

There needs to be frequent monitoring of potassium levels in type IV RTA. Because of the common occurrence of nephrocalcinosis and nephrolithiasis in type I RTA, renal ultrasound can be used to monitor these patients. A skeletal survey to look for bone disease should also be done, especially in cases of type II RTA. Patients with Fanconi syndrome should be evaluated for cystinosis, the most common cause of Fanconi syndrome in children. Some patients with inherited distal RTA have sensorineural deafness; therefore, infants and children with established distal RTA need routine audiograms.

an increase in urinary calcium excretion, but because citrate excretion is normal, nephrocalcinosis is uncommon. Type II RTA may rarely occur as an isolated defect, but it usually coexists with other defects in proximal tubule function. **Fanconi syndrome** is the combination

TABLE 59.4   Common Causes of Renal Tubular Acidosis (RTA)

PROXIMAL RTA/TYPE II RTA

Primary

Sporadic (common)

Inherited

- Inherited renal disease (idiopathic Fanconi)
- Autosomal dominant
- Autosomal recessive
- X-linked (Dent disease)
- Inherited syndromes
- Cystinosis
- Tyrosinemia type 1
- Galactosemia
- Oculocerebral dystrophy (Lowe syndrome)
- Wilson disease
- Hereditary fructose intolerance
- Glycogen storage disease type 1

Secondary

Intrinsic renal disease

- Autoimmune diseases (Sjögren syndrome)
- Hypokalemic nephropathy
- Renal transplant rejection

Hematologic disease

- Myeloma

Drugs

- Gentamicin
- Cisplatin
- Ifosfamide
- Sodium valproate

Heavy metals

- Lead
- Cadmium
- Mercury

Organic compounds

- Toluene

Nutritional

- Kwashiorkor

Hormonal

- Primary hyperparathyroidism

DISTAL RTA/TYPE I RTA

Primary

Sporadic

Inherited

- Inherited renal diseases
- Autosomal dominant
- Autosomal recessive
- Autosomal recessive with early-onset hearing loss
- Autosomal recessive with later-onset hearing loss
- Inherited syndromes associated with type I RTA
- Marfan syndrome
- Wilson syndrome
- Ehlers-Danlos syndrome
- Familial hypercalciuria

DISTAL RTA/TYPE I RTA—cont'd

Secondary

Intrinsic renal

- Interstitial nephritis
- Pyelonephritis
- Transplant rejection
- Sickle cell nephropathy
- Lupus nephritis
- Nephrocalcinosis
- Medullary sponge kidney

Urologic

- Obstructive uropathy
- Vesicoureteral reflux
- Hepatic
- Cirrhosis

Toxins or medications

- Amphotericin B
- Lithium
- Toluene
- Cisplatin

HYPERKALEMIC RTA/TYPE IV RTA

Primary

Sporadic

Genetic

- Hypoaldosteronism
- Addison disease
- Congenital adrenal hyperplasia
- Pseudohypoaldosteronism (type I or II)

Secondary

Urologic

- Obstructive uropathy

Intrinsic renal

- Pyelonephritis
- Interstitial nephritis

Systemic

- Diabetes mellitus
- Sickle cell nephropathy

Drugs

- Trimethoprim/sulfamethoxazole
- Angiotensin-converting enzyme inhibitors
- Cyclosporine
- Prolonged heparinization

Addison disease

From Sreedharan S, Avner ED. Renal tubular acidosis. In: Kliegman RM, Stanton BF, St Geme JW, et al., eds. *Nelson Textbook of Pediatrics*. 20th ed. Philadelphia: Elsevier; 2016:2530.

Additional Causes of Renal Loss of Bicarbonate

Carbonic anhydrase inhibitors such as acetazolamide inhibit the carbonic anhydrase present in the proximal tubule, thus preventing the reabsorption of HCO_3^-. The net effect is similar to that of proximal RTA.

Potassium-sparing diuretics such as spironolactone or amiloride can impair H^+ secretion by the distal nephron by blocking Na^+ absorption in this segment.

Gastrointestinal Loss of Bicarbonate

Diarrhea is the most common cause of non–anion gap hyperchloremic metabolic acidosis in children. The acidosis is secondary to loss of stool bicarbonate. The degree of dehydration should be assessed, and appropriate fluid resuscitation should be given, which should help correct the acidosis. If there is persistent acidosis, one should consider additional etiologies such as worsening infection/sepsis, an inborn error of metabolism, adrenal insufficiency, or bacteria-associated production of methemoglobinemia or D-lactate.

Miscellaneous Causes of Hyperchloremic Acidosis

Recovery from ketoacidosis. During recovery from diabetic ketoacidosis (DKA), many patients may eliminate the organic anions (through increased renal clearance and utilization) faster than their acidosis resolves. The clinical picture can resemble normal anion gap acidosis. Excessive fluids with isotonic chloride levels may contribute to this acidemia.

Dilutional acidosis. The rapid expansion of ECF volume with fluids that do not contain HCO_3^- leads to a dilution of HCO_3^- and mild metabolic acidosis. In addition, the expansion of ECF volume by itself promotes urinary HCO_3^- loss, possibly contributing to the dilutional acidosis.

Parenteral alimentation. Amino acid infusions without concomitant administration of alkali (or alkali-generating precursors) may produce a normal anion gap acidosis in a manner similar to that of addition of HCl.

Increased Anion Gap Acidosis

Increased Acid Production

Diabetic ketoacidosis. In DKA, the lack of insulin and excess of glucagon shunt free fatty acids into ketone body formation. The rate of formation of ketone bodies, principally β-hydroxybutyrate and acetoacetate, exceeds the capacity for their peripheral utilization and renal excretion. Accumulation of ketoacids (both of which are relatively strong acids and dissociate rapidly into H^+ and the ketoacid anions) results in metabolic acidosis. Acetone is formed by nonenzymatic conversion of acetoacetate and is responsible for the fruity odor of the patient's breath (see Chapter 58).

Patients with DKA typically present with polyuria and polydipsia in addition to altered mental status (ranging from confusion and drowsiness, which can progress to obtundation and loss of consciousness) and deep, sighing respirations (Kussmaul respirations). Additional clinical manifestations of DKA can be dehydration, nausea, vomiting, abdominal pain, and tachypnea. Laboratory analysis of a patient with DKA is significant for a severely increased anion gap metabolic acidosis with pH values that may be lower than 7.0. Initially, the increase in the anion gap is in proportion to the decrease in HCO_3^-, but once the patients start recovering with successful management, the kidneys clear the ketoacid anions, and the increase in the anion gap becomes less than the fall in HCO_3^-. The loss of ketoacid anions in urine increases the urinary losses of Na^+ and K^+ as the accompanying cations.

The diagnosis of DKA is made by the combination of increased anion gap metabolic acidosis, hyperglycemia, and demonstration of serum (or urine) ketoacid anions. The therapy for DKA includes careful volume repletion, insulin, and correction of electrolyte disturbances.

Severe acidosis is reversible by fluid and insulin replacement. Insulin inhibits ketosis and allows ketoacids to be metabolized, which generates bicarbonate. Treatment of hypovolemia improves tissue perfusion and renal function, thereby increasing the excretion of organic acids. Most patients with DKA present with considerable total body deficits of potassium, magnesium, and phosphorus, even though serum levels, particularly of potassium, may actually be high on presentation.

Lactic acidosis. Under normal conditions, lactate is formed in relatively small amounts and is further metabolized by the liver. Pathologic conditions associated with either local or systemic hypoxia or ischemia, hypotension (shock), impaired oxidative metabolism, or impaired hepatic clearance can cause significant lactic acidosis.

The diagnosis of lactic acidosis must be considered in all forms of increased anion gap metabolic acidosis. The diagnosis can be confirmed by measuring the serum lactate level, and treatment must be directed at the underlying pathophysiologic process (see Table 59.2).

GRACILE syndrome (growth retardation, amino aciduria, cholestasis, iron overload, lactic acidosis, and early death) is a rare lethal autosomal recessive disease caused by a point variant in the *BCS1L* gene encoding a mitochondrial protein. In a Finnish study describing 17 newborn infants with this disorder, the infants presented with aminoaciduria and failure to thrive, with 9 of them dying by 12 days of life and the 8 other infants dying by age 1–4 months. The autosomal recessive mode of inheritance makes GRACILE syndrome different from neonatal hemochromatosis and hepatitis and should be considered in a neonate presenting with significant fetal growth disturbance and severe lactic acidosis.

Inborn errors of metabolism. Most patients with inborn errors of metabolism that cause a metabolic acidosis present in the neonatal period or shortly thereafter. Organic acidemias, aminoacidopathies, disorders of fatty acid oxidation, mitochondrial disorders, and defects in carbohydrate metabolism are associated with acidosis. Associated presenting signs and symptoms may include vomiting, failure to thrive, lethargy, seizures, developmental abnormalities, hepatomegaly, and elevated blood or urine levels of a particular metabolite. Some of these disorders will be detected by the state newborn screening protocols. In contrast, urea cycle disorders during the first few days of life manifest with respiratory alkalosis because of stimulation of the respiratory center by increased ammonia levels. Congenital lactic acidosis may be due to mitochondrial gene variants or enzymes involved in glucose metabolism (pyruvate dehydrogenase complex); the latter presents with severe lactic acidosis after birth, while the presentation of mitochondrial gene variants can be variable.

Poisonings. A variety of toxic agents may be associated with increased anion gap metabolic acidosis; these include salicylate intoxication, ethylene glycol (a component of antifreeze), and methanol. Carbon monoxide, cyanide poisoning, or methemoglobinemia induces hypoxic acidosis.

Classically, **salicylate intoxication** is described as causing respiratory alkalosis (stimulation of the respiratory center), followed by increased anion gap metabolic acidosis (accumulation of salicylic acid itself and lactic acidosis as a result of uncoupling of mitochondrial oxidative phosphorylation). However, children may present with simple increased anion gap metabolic acidosis. Nausea, tinnitus, noncardiogenic pulmonary edema, and prolonged prothrombin time are other associated features. Alkalization of the blood and urine with sodium bicarbonate is beneficial despite the potential problems associated with its use in acute metabolic acidosis. Alkalization of the plasma decreases the diffusion of salicylate into the central nervous system, and alkaline urine improves renal excretion. In severe poisoning, hemodialysis is quite effective at removing salicylate from the body. In cases of poisonings, dialysis serves the dual purposes of removing the poison (if dialyzable) and correcting the acid–base and electrolyte abnormalities.

Propofol-related infusion syndrome (PRIS) usually results with prolonged (>48 hour) high-dose (>4 mg/kg/hr) infusions and manifests with lactic acidosis, rhabdomyolysis, cardiac failure, and shock. PRIS may result from propofol-induced mitochondrial impairment.

Failure of Acid Excretion

In both acute and chronic renal failure, the kidneys fail to excrete the acid produced from normal daily metabolism. Both H^+ and anions accumulate in the body, resulting in slow consumption of bicarbonate stores. However, the acidosis is generally not severe unless a markedly catabolic state occurs or other associated conditions coexist. In acute renal failure, there is abrupt and complete inhibition of acid excretion, whereas in chronic renal failure, there initially is enhanced ammonia genesis by the remaining nephrons. As renal failure progresses, excretion of both NH_4^+ and phosphate declines. In addition, the secondary hyperparathyroidism seen with chronic renal failure decreases proximal tubular HCO_3^- reabsorption and adds a component of hyperchloremic acidosis to the increased anion gap acidosis.

Treatment of Metabolic Acidosis

The morbidity and mortality caused by metabolic acidosis are determined not only by the severity of acidosis but also by the amenability of the underlying disorder to medical management. During treatment of metabolic acidosis, the primary effort should focus on the management of the underlying condition. The recommendations and goals of buffer therapy differ for acute acidotic disorders such as DKA and for chronic acidotic states such as RTA.

During the correction of acute metabolic acidosis, particular attention should be paid to ensure an appropriate potassium balance. During an episode of metabolic acidosis, potassium shifts from the intracellular space to the extracellular space in exchange for H^+, and thus the presence of a total body potassium deficit may not be appreciated. Hypokalemia may become evident only as the pH increases and potassium returns to the intracellular space. Chronic metabolic acidosis slows linear growth and interferes with bone mineralization. In chronic metabolic acidosis, there is a need for alkali therapy.

METABOLIC ALKALOSIS

Metabolic alkalosis (pH >7.45) occurs as a result of a primary increase in the serum HCO_3^-, which may occur as a result of (1) net loss of H^+, (2) net gain of HCO_3^- (or its precursors), or (3) loss of fluid with more Cl^- than HCO_3^-. Normally functioning kidneys can excrete large amounts of HCO_3^- and should offset any increase in serum HCO_3^- resulting from these causes. Therefore, factors that prevent the kidneys from excreting HCO_3^- also must be present to maintain the metabolic alkalosis.

Factors Initiating Metabolic Alkalosis

The H^+ can be lost externally, either through the gastrointestinal tract or through the kidneys. For every H^+ lost at these sites, the body gains one HCO_3^- ion. This is because H^+ production at both these sites (gastric parietal cell and renal tubular cells) is associated with generation of an equivalent number of HCO_3^- molecules. H^+ can also be "lost" internally, by shifting into the intracellular compartment. This occurs in states of severe potassium depletion (H^+ moves in, whereas K^+ exits the cell, to maintain electroneutrality).

The administration of HCO_3^- or its precursors (such as lactate, citrate, and acetate) at a rate greater than normal metabolic production of acid can lead to net gain of HCO_3^- by the body.

External loss of fluid (gastric fluid) containing more Cl^- than HCO_3^- raises the concentration of HCO_3^- in the body. One of the factors responsible for this type of alkalosis is the associated volume contraction, which leads to increased bicarbonate reabsorption by the proximal tubule of the kidney.

Factors Responsible for Sustaining Alkalosis

Decrease in effective blood volume and kidney perfusion causes increased Na^+ reabsorption in both the proximal tubule (angiotensin II effect) and the distal renal tubule (mineralocorticoid effect), thereby increasing H^+ excretion.

Increased mineralocorticoid levels directly increase H^+ secretion in the outer medullary collecting duct.

Chloride depletion increases HCO_3^- reabsorption in the proximal tubule. This effect is independent of ECF volume status.

Hypokalemia sustains metabolic alkalosis by decreasing bicarbonate loss. Hypokalemia promotes hydrogen ion secretion in the distal nephron and stimulates ammonia genesis in the proximal tubular cells. When produced, ammonia enhances renal excretion of hydrogen ions.

Hypercapnia induces a state of intracellular acidosis, which increases H^+ secretion. Although Pco_2 increases as a normal compensatory response to metabolic alkalosis, the elevated Pco_2 prevents the renal correction of alkalosis.

Differential Diagnosis of Metabolic Alkalosis

The causes of metabolic alkalosis can be divided into two categories on the basis of the urinary chloride level. The alkalosis in patients with low urinary chloride is maintained by volume depletion; volume repletion is needed to correct the alkalosis. In the process of volume depletion, there are losses of sodium, potassium, and chloride, but the loss of chloride is usually greater than the losses of sodium and potassium combined. Since chloride losses are the main cause of the volume depletion, these patients require chloride to correct the volume deficit and metabolic alkalosis; these patients have chloride-responsive metabolic alkalosis. Conversely, patients with alkalosis and an elevated urinary chloride concentration do not respond to volume repletion and have chloride-resistant metabolic alkalosis. Blood pressure can also be useful when considering the etiology of a patient's chloride-resistant metabolic alkalosis (Table 59.5).

Urinary Chloride Level Lower Than 15 mEq/L

Chloride-deficient diet. Although uncommon in developed countries, the ingestion of milk formula with low chloride content has been shown to result in hypochloremic metabolic alkalosis and failure to thrive in infants and to result in later neurodevelopmental abnormalities in childhood.

Upper gastrointestinal losses. The gastric fluid has a high H^+ concentration; loss of gastric fluid by vomiting or by nasogastric drainage leads to a net gain of HCO_3^- in the body. Although this is the initiating factor, the alkalosis is sustained by concomitant Cl^- and K^+ losses. Secondary hyperaldosteronism, resulting from volume contraction, promotes further urinary potassium and H^+ excretion, worsening the hypokalemia and alkalosis; urine is the source of most of the potassium losses caused by emesis. The degree of metabolic alkalosis associated with vomiting is generally mild except in conditions in which gastric secretions are greatly stimulated (e.g., Zollinger-Ellison syndrome) or there is protracted vomiting (e.g., pyloric stenosis).

Metabolic alkalosis can also be seen in newborns of mothers with eating disorders (bulimia). The baby reflects the electrolyte changes of the mother and sustains alkalosis because of the Cl^- deficiency.

TABLE 59.5   Causes of Metabolic Alkalosis

Chloride Responsive (Urinary Chloride <15 mEq/L)

Gastric losses
    Emesis
    Nasogastric suction
Diuretics (loop or thiazide)
Chloride-losing diarrhea (OMIM 214700)
Chloride-deficient formula
Cystic fibrosis (OMIM 219700) (pseudo-Bartter syndrome)
Seasonal (extreme heat)
Post-hypercapnia

Chloride Resistant (Urinary Chloride >20 mEq/L)

High blood pressure
    Adrenal adenoma or hyperplasia
    Glucocorticoid-remediable aldosteronism (OMIM 103900)
    Renovascular disease
    Renin-secreting tumor
    17-β-Hydroxylase deficiency (OMIM 202110)
    11-β-Hydroxylase deficiency (OMIM 202010)
    Cushing syndrome
    11-β-Hydroxysteroid dehydrogenase deficiency (OMIM 218030)
    Licorice ingestion
    Liddle syndrome (OMIM 177200)
Normal blood pressure
    Gitelman syndrome (OMIM 263800)
    Bartter syndrome (OMIM 607364/602522/241200/601678)
    Autosomal dominant hypoparathyroidism (OMIM 146200)
    EAST/SeSAME syndrome (OMIM 612780)
    Base administration

EAST, epilepsy, ataxia, sensorineural hearing loss, and tubulopathy; OMIM, database number from the Online Mendelian Inheritance in Man (http://www.ncbi.nlm.nih.gov/omim); SeSAME, seizures, sensorineural deafness, ataxia, mental retardation, and electrolyte imbalances.
Modified from Greenbaum LA. Electrolyte and acid-base disorders. In Kliegman RM, St. Geme JW III, Blum NJ, et al., eds. *Nelson Textbook of Pediatrics.* 21st ed. Philadelphia: Elsevier; 2020:419.

Chloride-secreting diarrhea. This is a rare congenital syndrome characterized by a defect in small- and large-bowel chloride absorption that leads to a chronic diarrhea with high chloride losses in the stool. The ongoing chloride depletion leads to a sustained metabolic alkalosis.

Diuretic therapy. Chronic use of loop and thiazide diuretics may cause a metabolic alkalosis. The alkalosis is sustained because of hypochloremia, hypokalemia, and volume contraction with resultant secondary hyperaldosteronism. The urinary Cl⁻ may be high if the diuretics have been ingested recently. The metabolic derangements caused by loop diuretics are identical to those seen in Bartter syndrome.

Hypercapnia. Chronic hypercapnia, as seen in bronchopulmonary dysplasia or cystic fibrosis, leads to an elevated serum bicarbonate concentration from metabolic compensation. The increase in serum bicarbonate is balanced by a decrease in serum chloride. Affected patients have chloride depletion, which may be worsened by concomitant diuretic use. With resolution of the hypercapnia, the bicarbonate concentration remains high until the chloride depletion is corrected.

Seasonal hypokalemic metabolic alkalosis. Occasionally reported in infants with cystic fibrosis during excessive heat waves, chloride loss in sweat together with dehydration produces this syndrome. It may rarely be seen in children without cystic fibrosis.

Urinary Chloride Level Higher Than 20 mEq/L with Hypertension

Pediatric patients with hypertension either have increased levels of aldosterone or act as if they do. Increased aldosterone "effects" cause renal retention of sodium, which results in elevated blood pressure. The disorders of mineralocorticoid excess are characterized by volume expansion and hypertension (see Table 59.5). The mineralocorticoid excess stimulates the renal excretion of H⁺ and K⁺, resulting in metabolic alkalosis and hypokalemia. The various causes can be differentiated by evaluating the renin-aldosterone axis. Treatment is aimed at removing or correcting the source of the mineralocorticoid excess.

Urinary Chloride Level Higher Than 20 mEq/L with Normal Blood Pressure

Bartter syndrome and Gitelman syndrome. These uncommon disorders result from defects in various ion transporters within the nephron. Bartter syndrome is a severe disorder that is characterized by urinary chloride wasting, hypokalemia, metabolic alkalosis, and increased serum levels of aldosterone and renin. Hypercalciuria is also common and leads to nephrocalcinosis in some patients. Affected patients present with a history of failure to thrive, polyuria, polydipsia, and a tendency for dehydration. In neonatal Bartter syndrome, there is usually a history of polyhydramnios and premature delivery. Gitelman syndrome, in contrast, is a milder disorder characterized by hypokalemia, metabolic alkalosis, and hypomagnesemia caused by urinary magnesium wasting; calcium excretion is normal. The growth retardation is not as severe. Children with Gitelman syndrome, however, are more prone to febrile seizures and tetanic episodes.

The genetics of additional variants of Bartter and Gitelman syndromes have been identified, most of which have autosomal recessive inheritance, although there are some exceptions (Table 59.6). See Table 59.7 for the distinguishing features of Bartter and Gitelman syndrome variants.

Treatment of Metabolic Alkalosis

Treatment focuses on correcting the underlying disorder and depends on the pathophysiologic mechanisms of the alkalosis. Patients with a chloride-responsive metabolic alkalosis (urine Cl⁻ <15 mEq/L) respond to volume repletion; both sodium and potassium chloride are necessary. In rare cases, if alkalosis persists despite chloride supplementation, the carbonic anhydrase inhibitor acetazolamide can be used to increase urinary bicarbonate losses. In patients undergoing persistent gastric drainage, administration of either an H₂ blocker or H⁺ pump inhibitor can be beneficial by decreasing the gastric H⁺ secretion.

Treatment of chloride-resistant metabolic alkalosis with hypertension (urinary Cl⁻ >20 mEq/L) mandates interference with the mineralocorticoid (or mineralocorticoid-like substance) that is maintaining renal H⁺ losses. This can sometimes be accomplished pharmacologically (e.g., with spironolactone or with other distal potassium-sparing diuretics such as amiloride).

RESPIRATORY ACIDOSIS

Respiratory acidosis results when there is an inappropriate increase in blood P_{CO_2} that is secondary to impaired pulmonary ventilation. Respiratory acidosis can result from either pulmonary disease, such as in severe bronchiolitis, or nonpulmonary disease, such as a narcotic overdose. In acute compensation, plasma bicarbonate increases by 1 for each 10 mm Hg increase in the P_{CO_2}. In chronic respiratory acidosis, the kidneys increase acid secretion. Renal compensation starts in 12–24 hours and reaches maximum in 3–5 days. In chronic compensation, plasma bicarbonate increases by 3–5 for each 10 mm Hg increase in the P_{CO_2}.

TABLE 59.6 Types of Bartter Syndrome, Gitelman Syndrome, and Related Conditions

Disorder	OMIM, Gene	Gene Product	Inheritance	Features
BS Variants				
BS I (ABS, HPES)	601678, *SLC12A1*	NKCC2	AR	Polyhydramnios, prematurity, hypokalemic hypochloremic alkalosis, nephrocalcinosis, with or without concentrating defect
BS II (ABS with transient hyperkalemia and acidosis, HPES)	241200, *KCNJ1*	ROMK1	AR	Polyhydramnios, prematurity, transient hyperkalemia and acidosis, then hypokalemic hypochloremic alkalosis, nephrocalcinosis, with or without concentrating defect
BS III (CBS)	607364, *CLCNKB*	ClC-Kb	AR; many sporadic	Variable age at presentation with severity corresponding to type of gene variant; hypokalemic hypochloremic alkalosis
BS IVa and BS IVb (ABS or HPES with sensorineural deafness)	602522, *BSND, CLCNKA, CLCNKB*	Bartter ClC-Ka and ClC-Kb	AR	Polyhydramnios, prematurity, hypokalemic hypochloremic alkalosis, sensorineural deafness, with or without concentrating defect
BS V (transient ABS)	300971, M*AGED2*	MAGED2	XR	Severe polyhydramnios, hypokalemic hypochloremic alkalosis with symptoms resolving within the first few months of life
AD hypocalcemic hypercalciuria	601199, *L12SP*	CaSR	AD	Hypocalcemic hypocalciuria, hypokalemic hypochloremic alkalosis, suppressed PTH
GS Variants				
GS	263800, *SLC12A3*	NCC	AR	Present in later childhood or adulthood with weakness, lethargy, carpopedal spasm, hypokalemic alkalosis, hypomagnesemia, hypermagnesuria, and hypocalciuria
EAST syndrome (SeSAME)	612780, *Kir4.1*	KCNJ10	AR	Epilepsy, ataxia, sensorineural deafness, hypokalemic hypochloremic alkalosis
Other Variants				
CLDN10 variants	617579, *CLDN10*	Claudin-10	AR	Hypokalemic metabolic alkalosis with hypocalciuria but normal to elevated magnesium

AD, autosomal dominant; AR, autosomal recessive; BS, Bartter syndrome; CaSR, calcium-sensing receptor; ClC-Ka, chloride channel-Ka; ClC-Kb, chloride channel-Kb; GS, Gitelman syndrome; MAGED, melanoma-associated antigen-D2; NCC, thiazide-sensitive NaCl co-transporter; NKCC2, furosemide-sensitive Na-K-2Cl co-transporter; OMIM, Online Mendelian Inheritance in Man; PTH, parathyroid hormone, ROMK, renal outer medullary K channel; SeSAME, seizures, sensorineural deafness, ataxia, mental retardation, and electrolyte unbalances; XR, X-linked recessive.
From Fulchiero R, Seo-Mayer P. Bartter syndrome and Gitelman syndrome. *Pediatr Clin North Am.* 2019;66:121–134, Box 1.

TABLE 59.7 Features That Distinguish Bartter and Gitelman Syndrome Variants

Variant	Age of Onset	Serum K	Serum Cl	Serum Mg	Serum Renin, Aldosterone	Urine Ca/Cr	Other Distinct Features
BS I	AN	Low	Low	Normal	High, high	High	—
BS II	AN	High, then low	Low	Normal	High, high	High	Transient hyperkalemia
BS III	N, C, A	Low	Very low	Normal	High, high	Low, normal, or high	—
BS IVa, IVb	AN	Low	Low	Normal	High, high	Normal or high	Sensorineural deafness
BS V	AN	Low	Low	Normal	High, high	—	Transient features
Hypocalcemic hypercalciuria	—	Low	Low	Normal	High, high	High	Family history, hypocalcemia, suppressed PTH
GS	C, A	Low	Low	Low	High, high	Low	—
EAST syndrome	—	Low	Low	Low	High, high	Low	Epilepsy, ataxia, sensorineural deafness

A, adult; AN, antenatal; BS, Bartter syndrome; C, child; Ca/Cr, spot calcium-to-creatinine ratio; GS, Gitelman syndrome; Mg, magnesium; N, neonate.
From Fulchiero R, Seo-Mayer P. Bartter syndrome and Gitelman syndrome. *Pediatr Clin North Am.* 2019;66:121–134, Box 3.

Patients with a respiratory acidosis are often tachypneic as they are trying to correct the inadequate ventilation. The degree of hypercarbia drives the symptoms in a patient with respiratory acidosis. Patients with acute respiratory acidosis have more symptoms than patients with chronic respiratory acidosis. Hypoxia is usually seen in a patient with acute respiratory acidosis who is breathing room air. There may also be central nervous system manifestations of respiratory acidosis, which can include, but are not limited to, anxiety, dizziness, headache, confusion, hallucinations, myoclonic jerks, seizures, psychosis, and coma.

The management of respiratory acidosis is directed toward improving alveolar ventilation and treating the underlying disorder.

RESPIRATORY ALKALOSIS

Respiratory alkalosis occurs when there is an inappropriate decrease in Pco_2 as a result of pulmonary hyperventilation. In a spontaneously breathing child, this can result from fever, sepsis, mild asthma, panic attack, or central nervous system disorders. In the intensive care unit, the most common cause is mechanical overventilation of an intubated child. A metabolic response to an acute respiratory alkalosis is mediated by hydrogen ion release from nonbicarbonate buffers and occurs within minutes. In this acute compensation, plasma bicarbonate falls by 2 for each 10 mm Hg decrease in Pco_2. In chronic respiratory alkalosis, the kidneys decrease H^+ secretion, which produces a decrease in the serum HCO_3^- concentration. Metabolic compensation for a respiratory alkalosis develops gradually and takes 2–3 days. In chronic compensation, plasma bicarbonate falls by 4 for each 10 mm Hg decrease in the Pco_2. Chronic respiratory alkalosis is the only acid–base disorder in which the pH may be completely normalized by the compensatory mechanisms.

Symptoms of acute respiratory alkalosis may be chest tightness, palpitations, lightheadedness, circumoral numbness, or extremity paresthesias. Less commonly, tetany, seizures, muscle cramps, or syncope can be seen. The lightheadedness and syncope are felt to be a result of the decrease in cerebral blood flow that is caused by hypocapnia. The paresthesias, tetany, and seizures are thought to be related to the decrease in ionized calcium that occurs because alkalemia causes more calcium to bind to albumin. The treatment is management of the underlying process.

MIXED ACID–BASE DISORDERS

Mixed acid–base disorders occur when two or three primary events act to alter the acid–base state at the same time. The deviations in pH are more marked when two primary events block the compensation of each other, such as the combination of a metabolic acidosis and a respiratory acidosis seen in a patient with shock and respiratory failure. In contrast, in the presence of two opposing primary events, the pH may be normal or only minimally abnormal, as can be seen with combined vomiting and diarrhea. A mixed acid–base disorder is commonly seen when neonates with respiratory acidosis caused by chronic lung disease also receive diuretics, which can cause a metabolic alkalosis.

The diagnosis of mixed acid–base disorder should be suspected in the following situations:

If the compensation for the primary event is absent or is out of the expected range.

If the deviation in anion gap and/or serum Cl^- is out of proportion to the change in HCO_3^-.

If the anion gap is significantly increased in the presence of a near-normal pH.

POTASSIUM DISORDERS

Potassium is the major intracellular cation with a normal serum concentration of 3.5–5.5 mEq/L. The differential distribution of potassium between the intracellular (150 mEq/L) and extracellular compartments, sustained by the action of the Na^+,K^+-ATPase pump, is the chief determinant of the resting membrane potential. Not surprisingly, both hyperkalemia (serum K^+ >5.5 mEq/L) and hypokalemia (serum K^+ <3.5 mEq/L) have a profound effect on the excitability of the neuromuscular tissue, especially the cardiac tissue. As a result, fatal cardiac arrhythmias are possible sequelae of hypokalemia or hyperkalemia.

Almost all dietary potassium is absorbed. The kidney is the major organ responsible for K^+ excretion, eliminating more than 90% of the daily K^+ intake. However, after an acute ingestion of K^+, the kidneys excrete only half of it over the first 4–6 hours; the remainder is transiently redistributed intracellularly before the kidneys eventually excrete it. This intracellular redistribution has a very important role in offsetting acute changes in serum K^+, but it has a limited capacity to do so. Redistribution of a very small fraction (1–2%) of intracellular K^+ into the ECF can easily increase serum K^+ to a dangerous level. A number of factors affect the distribution of K^+ between the intracellular

TABLE 59.8 Factors Affecting Potassium Distribution Between Extracellular Fluid and Intracellular Fluid

Insulin	Excess causes hypokalemia
	Deficiency causes hyperkalemia
Catecholamines	β-agonists cause hypokalemia
	β-antagonists cause hyperkalemia
Acid–base status	Metabolic alkalosis causes hypokalemia
	Metabolic acidosis (especially inorganic) causes hyperkalemia
Tissue injury	Causes hyperkalemia

From Chadha V, Alon US. Acid-base and electrolyte disturbances. In: Kliegman RM, Greenbaum LA, Lye PS, eds. *Practical Strategies in Pediatric Diagnosis and Therapy.* 2nd ed. Philadelphia: Elsevier; 2004:455.

space and the ECF (Table 59.8). The colonic excretion of K^+ is of no significance under normal conditions, but in patients with chronic renal failure, it becomes an important route of K^+ elimination, when colonic excretion increases substantially.

Because the kidney is the major route of potassium elimination from the body, a disturbance in renal potassium handling can be the cause of excessive loss or retention.

In clinical practice, spironolactone, amiloride, and triamterene decrease urinary K^+ excretion. Whereas spironolactone is an aldosterone antagonist, amiloride and triamterene block the Na^+ conductance channels present in the principal cell luminal membrane. The antimicrobial trimethoprim prevents K^+ secretion by the same mechanism as amiloride.

HYPOKALEMIA

Hypokalemia (Table 59.9 and Fig. 59.1) may result from (1) increased renal losses, (2) increased extrarenal losses, (3) redistribution, or (4) prolonged decreased intake of potassium. When interpreting cases of hypokalemia, the clinician should pay careful attention to blood pressure and obtain laboratory data concerning acid–base status, electrolytes, osmolality of blood and urine, and the renin-aldosterone axis.

Increased Renal Losses with Hypertension

Mineralocorticoid Excess

The presence of excess mineralocorticoid hormone, regardless of its source, results in stimulation of potassium secretion by the distal tubular cells of the nephron. Mineralocorticoid excess can result from primary hyperaldosteronism, rare forms of congenital adrenal hyperplasia (17α-hydroxylase or 11β-hydroxylase deficiency), syndrome of apparent mineralocorticoid excess, glucocorticoid remediable aldosteronism, and Cushing syndrome. The hypokalemia in these conditions is associated with increased sodium chloride retention, causing hypertension. The expansion of the extracellular volume eventually leads to the suppression of Na^+-retaining mechanisms, but the K^+ losses continue unabated. Metabolic alkalosis develops as a result of enhanced proximal ammonium production secondary to potassium depletion.

Liddle Syndrome

Liddle syndrome is characterized by a primary increase in sodium reabsorption in the collecting tubule and associated with increased potassium secretion. The sodium reabsorption is increased through activation of the amiloride-sensitive renal sodium channel. Because serum aldosterone levels are low, spironolactone is ineffective, but amiloride and triamterene, which block the sodium channel, decrease potassium losses and help ameliorate the hypokalemia and the hypertension.

TABLE 59.9 Differential Diagnosis of Hypokalemia

INCREASED RENAL LOSSES (TTKG >6)

With Hypertension

Mineralocorticoid excess
    Primary aldosteronism
    Congenital adrenal hyperplasia
        17-α-Hydroxylase deficiency
        11-β-Hydroxylase deficiency
    Hyperreninemic hyperaldosteronism
    Glucocorticoid-suppressible hyperaldosteronism
    Exogenous mineralocorticoid
    Cushing syndrome
    Liddle syndrome

With Normal Blood Pressure

With Acidosis

Renal tubular acidosis
Diabetic ketoacidosis

With Alkalosis

Vomiting
Diuretics
Congenital chloride diarrhea
Bartter syndrome
Gitelman syndrome
Magnesium depletion
Normotensive hyperaldosteronism

With Normal Acid–Base

Recovery from acute tubular necrosis
Postobstructive diuresis
Drugs (penicillins, amphotericin B)

EXTRARENAL LOSSES (TTKG <2)

Diarrhea/GI fistulas
Laxative abuse
Profuse sweating

REDISTRIBUTION

Alkalosis
β-Adrenergic agonists
Barium intoxication
Familial hypokalemic periodic paralysis

TTKG, transtubular potassium gradient.
From Chadha V, Alon US. Acid-base and electrolyte disturbances. In: Kliegman RM, Greenbaum LA, Lye PS, eds. *Practical Strategies in Pediatric Diagnosis and Therapy.* 2nd ed. Philadelphia: Elsevier; 2004:456.

Increased Renal Losses with Normal Blood Pressure

The hypokalemia associated with Bartter syndrome, Gitelman syndrome, RTA, DKA, and vomiting are discussed in the section on acid–base disorders.

Hypomagnesemia of any cause can lead to K+ depletion, and correction of hypokalemia is not possible until magnesium balance is restored. These effects are believed to be secondary to magnesium's effect on aldosterone secretion and K+ channels. Magnesium replacement in this situation should be done with magnesium oxide, because the sulfate ion of magnesium sulfate can increase the urinary K+ losses.

The polyuric recovery phase of acute tubular necrosis and the postobstructive diuresis after relief of urinary tract obstruction are commonly encountered clinical conditions that may be associated with excess urine potassium losses. Penicillins can increase urinary K+ losses by increased delivery of sodium and nonabsorbable anions to the distal nephron. Amphotericin B enhances urinary K+ loss by increasing the tubular K+ permeability and also by causing type I RTA.

Increased Extrarenal Losses

Diarrhea is a very common cause of hypokalemia in pediatric practice. Profuse sweating is a much less frequent cause of hypokalemia (seasonal pseudohypokalemia).

Redistribution

Alkalosis causes potassium to enter cells in exchange for H+. β-Adrenergic agonists increase intracellular movement of potassium. **Familial hypokalemic periodic paralysis** is a rare disorder characterized by recurring transient episodes of net K+ transfer from ECF to intracellular fluid (ICF). The autosomal dominant form manifests between the ages of 10 and 19 years. The dominant finding is muscle weakness, which may advance to paralysis. Episodes typically occur after large carbohydrate-rich meals, strenuous exercise, or insulin administration. Hyperthyroid states may also produce hypokalemic paralysis. Therapy is largely symptomatic; empirical treatment with acetazolamide has yielded some results.

EAST (epilepsy, ataxia, sensorineural deafness, and tubulopathy) syndrome, also known as SeSAME syndrome (seizures, sensorineural deafness, ataxia, mental retardation, and electrolyte imbalances), is a rare disorder caused by a variant in the K(+) channel KCNJ10 (Kir4.1), found in the basolateral membrane of the renal distal convoluted tubule. Inheritance is autosomal recessive and the loss-of-function variant seen in EAST/SeSAME syndrome gives patients a similar clinical picture as Gitelman syndrome, with hypokalemic alkalosis, hypomagnesemia, and hypocalciuria. Urinary studies have demonstrated potassium, magnesium, and sodium wasting, and salt craving, enuresis, and polydipsia/polyuria have been reported in patients with EAST syndrome, consistent with renal salt wasting.

Consequences of Hypokalemia

Hypokalemia produces functional alterations in skeletal muscle, smooth muscle, and the heart. The cardiac conduction effects are the most serious consequence of hypokalemia. The characteristic ECG changes include flattening of the T wave with appearance of the U wave (Fig. 59.2). Skeletal muscle weakness usually starts in the limbs before involving the trunk and respiratory muscles. Paralytic ileus and gastric dilatation reflect smooth muscle dysfunction. Rhabdomyolysis is a dramatic and serious complication of hypokalemia. Hypokalemia is particularly dangerous in patients taking digoxin.

In the kidney, potassium deficiency may result in vacuolar changes in the tubular epithelium. The renal concentrating capacity is decreased, causing polyuria. Prolonged and sustained hypokalemia leads to systemic alkalosis.

Treatment of Hypokalemia

The immediate objective of potassium replacement is to prevent life-threatening cardiac conduction and muscle complications. The ultimate goal is to replenish total body potassium stores. There is no method of determining the potassium deficit, because there is no definite correlation between the plasma potassium concentration and body potassium stores. A decrease of 1 mEq/L in serum potassium concentration secondary to potassium loss generally corresponds to a loss of approximately 10–30% of body potassium. In conditions

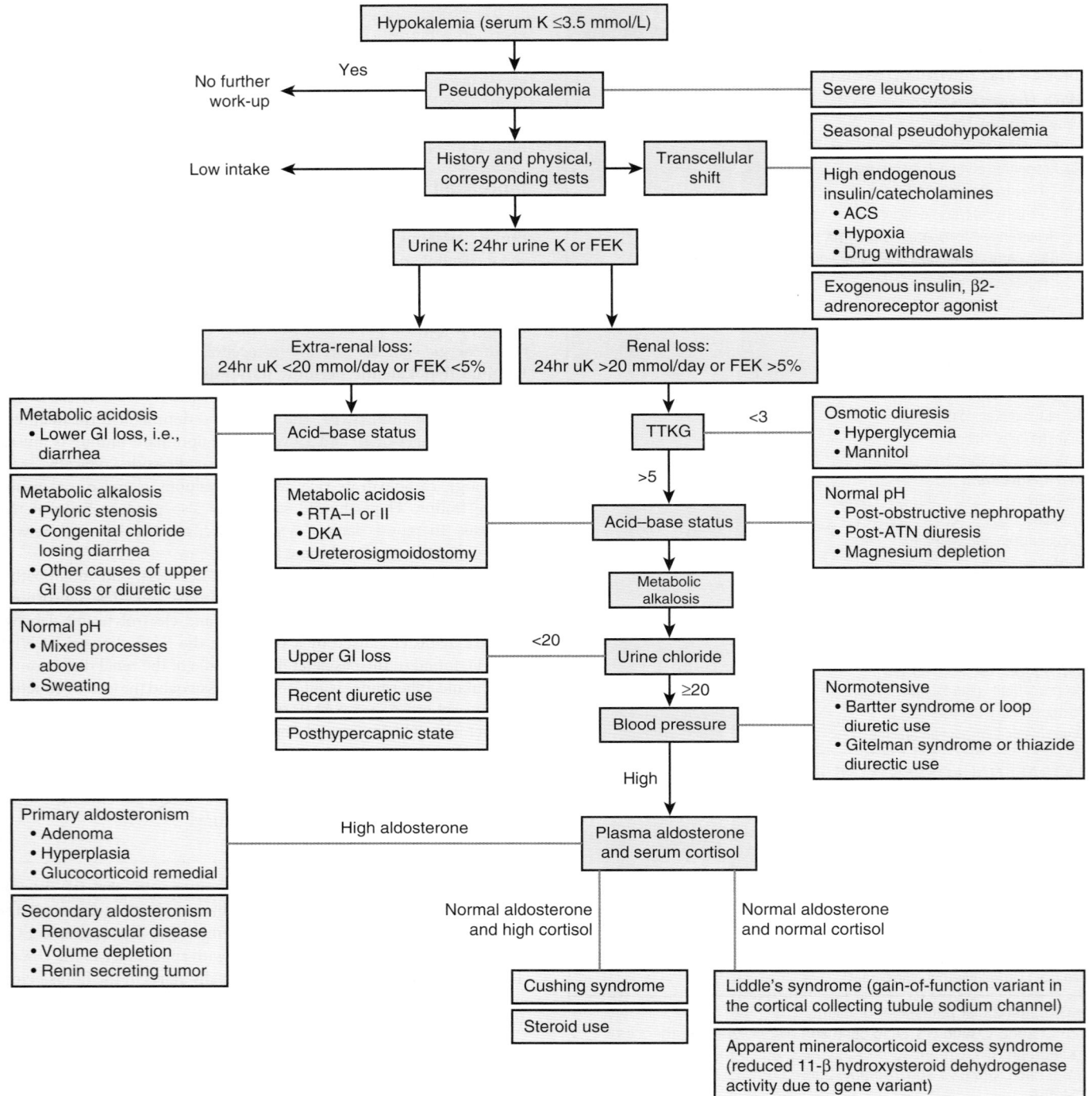

Fig. 59.1 The diagnostic approach to hypokalemia. ACS, acute coronary syndrome; ATN, acute tubular necrosis; DKA, diabetic ketoacidosis; FEK, fractional excretion of K; GI, gastrointestinal; RTA, renal tubular acidosis; TTKG, transtubular potassium gradient; uK, urine K. (Modified from Kellerman RD, Rakel DP, eds. *Conn's Current Therapy.* Philadelphia: Elsevier; 2020:340, Fig. 1.)

with associated acidosis and/or hyperosmolality (e.g., RTA, DKA), the plasma potassium concentration may underestimate potassium stores, and correction of acidosis with bicarbonate in these conditions may rapidly lower the serum potassium concentration.

The safest route to administer potassium is by mouth, but in states of severe symptomatic hypokalemia or when there are gastrointestinal problems, potassium must be given intravenously. The usual concentration of potassium in intravenous fluid solutions is up to 40 mEq/L.

Higher concentrations of up to 60–80 mEq/L can be given in a central vein under continuous ECG monitoring. Dextrose should be avoided in the initial fluids because its administration with secondary increased insulin secretion may result in further lowering of the plasma potassium concentration. The choice of potassium salt depends on the clinical situation. Under most circumstances, when hypovolemia coexists, potassium chloride is appropriate. Potassium bicarbonate (or, more often, other salts such as citrate or acetate, which generate bicarbonate)

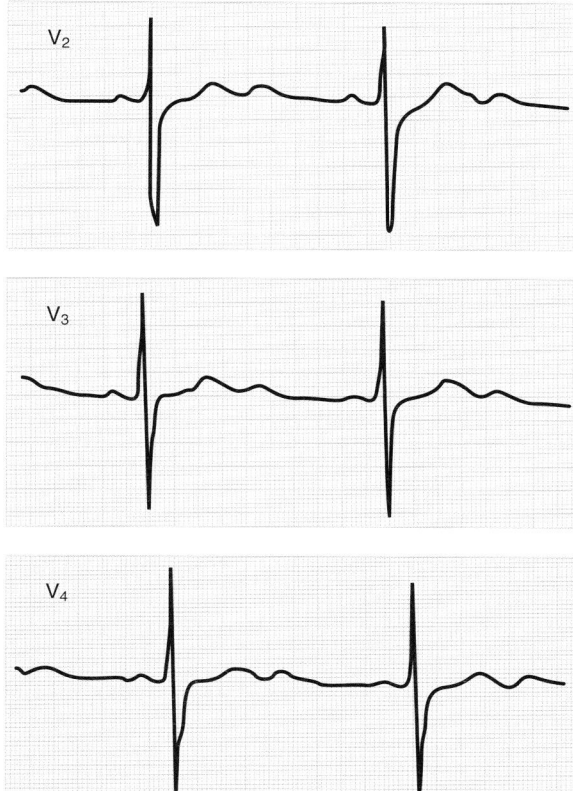

Fig. 59.2 The ECG manifestations of hypokalemia. The serum potassium concentration was 2.2 mEq/L. The ST segment is prolonged, primarily because of a U wave following the T wave, and the T wave is flattened. (From Goldman L, Schafer AI, eds. *Goldman-Cecil Medicine.* 26th ed. Philadelphia: Elsevier; 2020:727, Fig. 109.1.)

can be given in the presence of coexistent *metabolic acidosis.* If there is an associated phosphate deficiency (as in DKA), potassium phosphate can be used. It is important to remember that correction of total body potassium deficits can take days to weeks.

HYPERKALEMIA

Moderate (6.1–7.0 mEq/L) to severe (>7.0 mEq/L) hyperkalemia, especially if it develops acutely, can lead to grave consequences and requires prompt treatment. **Pseudohyperkalemia** can occur as a result of the release of intracellular potassium (e.g., hemolysis caused by mechanical trauma during venipuncture), and it can also be seen in conditions with marked leukocytosis and thrombocytosis. It can be avoided by minimizing trauma and hand clenching during venipuncture, by rapidly separating red blood cells, and by using plasma rather than serum for potassium measurements. *An unexpected elevated potassium level should be immediately repeated.*

Hyperkalemia can be caused by (1) reduced urinary potassium excretion, (2) increased potassium intake, (3) release of intracellular potassium, and/or (4) impaired cellular potassium uptake (Table 59.10 and Fig. 59.3).

Reduced Urinary Potassium Excretion

Renal potassium excretion decreases when the GFR is decreased or when there is a defect in tubular potassium excretion resulting from lack of aldosterone, medications, or a primary defect in tubular potassium excretion.

TABLE 59.10 Differential Diagnosis of Hyperkalemia
PSEUDOHYPERKALEMIA
Hemolysis
Thrombocytosis
Leukocytosis
REDUCED URINARY POTASSIUM EXCRETION (TTKG <5)
Renal Failure
Acute
Chronic
Hypoaldosteronism
Addison disease
Hereditary adrenal enzyme defects
21-Hydroxylase deficiency
Hyporeninemic hypoaldosteronism
Pseudohypoaldosteronism (Gordon syndrome)
Drugs
ACE inhibitors
Potassium-sparing diuretics
Spironolactone
Amiloride
Triamterene
Cyclosporine
Trimethoprim
Heparin
Nonsteroidal antiinflammatory agents
Primary Tubular Defects
Post–renal transplantation
Lupus nephritis
AIDS
RTA type IV (chloride shunt)
INCREASED INTAKE/TISSUE RELEASE (TTKG >10)
Intravenous/oral administration
Hemolysis (endogenous or transfused blood)
Rhabdomyolysis
Tumor lysis
REDISTRIBUTION
Acidosis
Insulin deficiency (diabetes)
Familial hyperkalemic periodic paralysis
Digitalis toxicity
β-Adrenergic blockade
Succinylcholine

ACE, angiotensin-converting enzyme; RTA, renal tubular acidosis; TTKG, transtubular potassium gradient.
From Chadha V, Alon US. Acid-base and electrolyte disturbances. In: Kliegman RM, Greenbaum LA, Lye PS, eds. *Practical Strategies in Pediatric Diagnosis and Therapy.* 2nd ed. Philadelphia: Elsevier; 2004:457.

Renal Failure

Potassium excretion is decreased in both acute and chronic renal failure. Severe hyperkalemia occurs more commonly in acute renal failure. In contrast, in patients with chronic renal failure, hyperkalemia does not occur unless the GFR is lower than 10 mL/min or some other factor

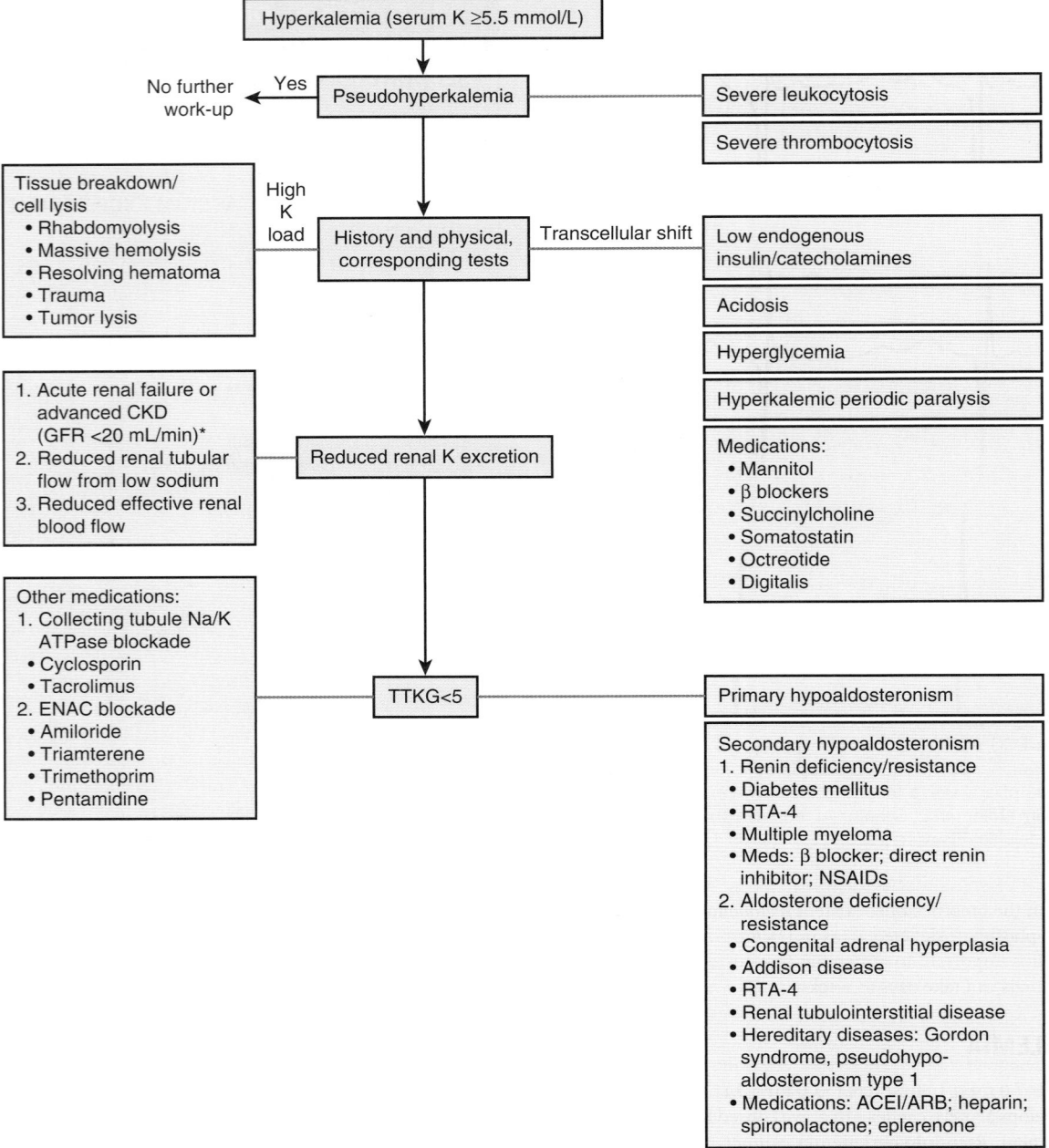

Fig. 59.3 The diagnostic approach to hyperkalemia. *Hyperkalemia may occur with higher GFR if K load is excessive. ACEI, angiotensin-converting enzyme inhibitor; ARB, angiotensin receptor blocker; CKD, chronic kidney disease; ENAC, epithelial sodium channel; GFR, glomerular filtration rate; NSAIDs, nonsteroidal antiin-flammatory drugs; RTA, renal tubular acidosis; TTKG, transtubular potassium gradient. (Modified from Kellerman RD, Rakel DP, eds. *Conn's Current Therapy*. Philadelphia: Elsevier; 2020:341, Fig. 2.)

predisposing to hyperkalemia is present. In patients with chronic renal failure, potassium balance is maintained by increased K⁺ secretion per functioning nephron and also by enhanced excretion of K⁺ through the gastrointestinal tract.

Hypoaldosteronism

Low levels or absence of aldosterone (or aldosterone receptor defects) may result from a variety of conditions (Addison disease, congenital adrenal hyperplasia [deficiency of 21-hydroxylase], and hyporenine-mic hypoaldosteronism). In addition to hyperkalemia, hyponatremia

and hyperchloremic metabolic acidosis are the associated features in these disorders. The diagnosis can be confirmed by measurement of renin activity and aldosterone levels.

Drugs

Several drugs are known to be associated with hyperkalemia; they can either impair renin-aldosterone secretion or action (angiotensin-converting enzyme inhibitors, spironolactone, cyclosporine, or heparin) or impair renal tubular potassium secretion (amiloride, tri-amterene, trimethoprim, or cyclosporine).

Primary Tubular Defects

In some patients, hyperkalemia occurs because of low urinary K^+ excretion despite normal renin and aldosterone levels. The presence of a selective defect in K^+ secretion has been described in subjects with renal transplant rejection and lupus nephritis.

Increased Potassium Intake/Tissue Release

Acute increases in potassium intake, usually through parenteral administration, may result in hyperkalemia. The hyperkalemia is typically transient because normal kidneys have a large capacity for excreting potassium. Sustained hyperkalemia is seen only when renal excretory mechanisms are impaired.

In **tumor lysis syndrome** and rhabdomyolysis, massive amounts of K^+ are released from the intracellular compartment, but hyperkalemia does not usually occur unless acute renal failure supervenes. Similarly, trauma, intravascular hemolysis, transfusion of stored blood, and catabolic states such as infection or high fever are associated with release of K^+ from the cells; however, hyperkalemia is uncommon as long as renal function is normal and normal to high urine output is maintained with fluid therapy.

Redistribution

Acidosis and insulin deficiency result in egress of intracellular potassium. β_2-Receptor blockers, digitalis (by inhibiting the Na^+,K^+-ATPase pump), and succinylcholine (by inhibiting cellular repolarization) cause hyperkalemia by impairing cellular potassium uptake.

Consequences of Hyperkalemia

Overt clinical manifestations are uncommon with hyperkalemia, but cardiac arrhythmias are potentially life-threatening. Generalized muscular weakness and paralysis can occur. The characteristic ECG findings seen with increasing $[K^+]$ are tall, peaked T waves; widening of the QRS complex; decreased amplitude of the P wave; and fusion of the QRS complex with the T wave, forming a sine wave (Fig. 59.4). This can be rapidly followed by atrioventricular dissociation and ventricular tachycardia or fibrillation. Cardiac arrest is more common with hyperkalemia than with hypokalemia.

Treatment of Hyperkalemia

The treatment of hyperkalemia depends on the magnitude of the hyperkalemia, the severity of ECG changes, and the anticipated future rise in $[K^+]$. The specific therapy should always focus on the underlying cause. However, a plasma potassium concentration higher than 7.0 mEq/L or marked ECG changes are potentially life-threatening and necessitate immediate treatment. A normal ECG result should not lead to a more casual approach, because significant ECG changes can appear over a short period of time. All potassium intake (parenteral nutrition, medications with potassium salt) and medications that cause hyperkalemia, such as potassium-sparing diuretics, angiotensin-converting enzyme inhibitors, and trimethoprim, should be discontinued. The treatment modalities usually belong to the following three categories: (1) antagonism of membrane excitability, (2) shifting of potassium into the intracellular compartment, and (3) elimination of excess potassium (Table 59.11).

Calcium protects the heart from fatal arrhythmias caused by hyperkalemia by normalizing the difference between the resting and threshold potentials. This protective effect is quite rapid but relatively short-lived; therefore, other measures to reduce the concentration of serum potassium are necessary.

Potassium can be shifted from the extracellular to the intracellular compartment by administration of glucose and insulin, or β_2-adrenergic agonists, as detailed in Table 59.11. Although the intracellular shift of

Lead V_3

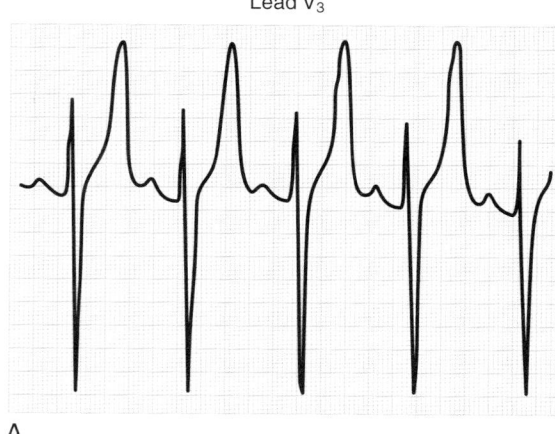

A

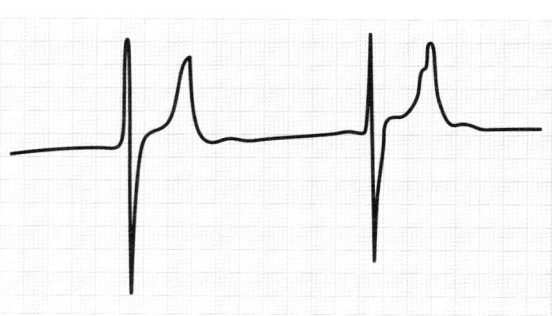

B

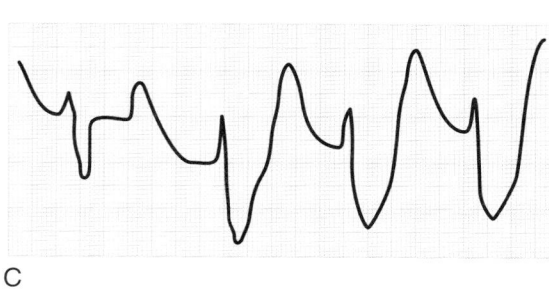

C

Fig. 59.4 The effects of progressive hyperkalemia on the electrocardiogram. All of the illustrations are from lead V_3. *A,* Serum potassium concentration $([K^+]) = 6.8$ mEq/L; note the peaked T waves together with normal sinus rhythm. *B,* Serum $[K^+] = 8.9$ mEq/L; note the peaked T waves and absent P waves. *C,* Serum $[K^+] > 8.9$ mEq/L; note the classic sine wave with absent P waves, marked prolongation of the QRS complex, and peaked T waves. (From Goldman L, Schafer AI, eds. *Goldman-Cecil Medicine.* 26th ed. Philadelphia: Elsevier; 2020:727, Fig. 109.2.)

potassium can be accomplished rather quickly, this is only a temporary measure, and further steps should be taken to establish a negative potassium balance.

Loop or thiazide diuretics increase renal potassium excretion. In patients with aldosterone deficiency, fludrocortisone increases renal potassium excretion. Alkalinizing the urine through systemic base administration can further enhance urinary potassium losses.

Cation exchange resins (enteric) remove potassium from the body and are effective in acute situations, particularly when poor renal function is present. Dialysis is needed in patients with severe hyperkalemia, especially in the presence of advanced renal failure or when accompanied by a hypercatabolic state or severe tissue necrosis. For urgent potassium removal, hemodialysis is more effective than continuous hemodiafiltration or peritoneal dialysis.

TABLE 59.11   **Treatment of Hyperkalemia**
Antagonism of Membrane Excitability
Calcium gluconate 10% (elemental calcium, 0.45 mEq/mL), 0.5–1.0 mL/kg body weight (maximum = 10 mL), injected intravenously and slowly over 5–10 min, with continuous monitoring of heart rate)
Shift of Potassium into the Intracellular Compartment
• Sodium bicarbonate, 1–2 mEq/kg body weight intravenously over 10–20 min; usefulness is limited in patients with volume expansion
• Glucose, 1 g/kg body weight, and insulin, 1 unit per every 4 g of glucose, intravenously over 20–30 min
• β₂-Adrenergic agonists, such as albuterol, intravenously or by nebulizer or aerosol
Elimination of Excess Potassium
• Loop/thiazide diuretics
• Fludrocortisone (0.05–0.1 mg/day); should be avoided or given with great caution to hypertensive patients
• Cation exchange resin, sodium polystyrene sulfonate, 1 g/kg body weight (maximum, 15 g/dose), administered orally or rectally in 20–30% sorbitol or 10% glucose, 1 g resin/4 mL (additional 70% sorbitol syrup may be given if constipation occurs)
• Peritoneal dialysis, hemodialysis, or hemodiafiltration

Modified from Hellerstein S, Alon US, Warady BA. Renal impairment. In: Ashcraft KW, Murphy JP, Sharp RJ, et al., eds. *Pediatric Surgery.* 3rd ed. Philadelphia: Saunders; 2000:47–57.

SODIUM DISORDERS

Sodium is the principal cation of the ECF compartment, and total body sodium content is the major determinant of ECF volume. A normal ECF volume is essential for maintaining an adequate circulating blood volume. The sodium concentration determines cell volume by directing water movement between the ECF compartment and the intracellular compartment. An increase in ECF osmolality causes water to move out of cells, and a decrease in ECF osmolality causes water to move into cells. Sodium homeostasis is coupled with water homeostasis; therefore, disorders of sodium homeostasis usually occur as a result of imbalances of both sodium and water rather than an isolated imbalance of either sodium or water.

The kidneys are pivotal regulators of sodium and water balance. Sodium excretion, which is regulated by the renin-angiotensin-aldosterone system and atrial natriuretic peptide, increases in response to an expanded intravascular volume, as may occur with a high sodium intake. In response to a decreased intravascular volume, the urine can be made virtually sodium free.

A detailed history of the underlying disease, food and fluid intake, and fluid losses in the form of stool, emesis, and urine should be obtained. The physical examination focuses on an evaluation of the patient's volume status, including the nature and rate of peripheral pulses, blood pressure, fullness of the fontanel, level of consciousness, dryness of mucous membranes, coolness of extremities, and capillary refill time. Urinary sodium concentration can provide valuable information regarding the child's effective blood volume, but it can be misleading if the patient is receiving diuretics or has abnormal renal sodium handling. The clinical features associated with alterations in plasma osmolality are nonspecific. Osmolality is regulated by thirst and vasopressin production, which determines renal water excretion. A low serum osmolality may produce lethargy and confusion, whereas a high serum osmolality may lead to irritability, a high-pitched cry, and a doughy skin texture. The determination of plasma osmolality requires

a direct laboratory measurement or can be estimated from the following formula:

$$\text{Serum osmolality}_{(mOsm)} = 2 \times [Na^+]_{mEq/L} + [glucose]_{mg/dL}/18 + [urea]_{mg/dL}/2.8$$

HYPONATREMIA

Hyponatremia is defined as a plasma sodium <135 mEq/L and is generally characterized as a disproportionate concentration of water to sodium. This may arise from either water retention or sodium losses. Hyponatremia should be differentiated from pseudohyponatremia and factitious hyponatremia. **Pseudohyponatremia** occurs in the presence of excessive amounts of plasma proteins and lipids, which decrease the percentage of plasma water and thus artificially lower the plasma sodium concentration. The measured plasma osmolality of these patients is normal, inasmuch as lipids and proteins do not contribute significantly to osmolality because of their large size. Therefore, a gap between measured and calculated osmolalities can indicate pseudohyponatremia.

Factitious hyponatremia results from high plasma concentrations of impermeable solutes such as glucose or mannitol that cause movement of water from the intracellular to the extracellular space. In contrast to pseudohyponatremia, the low plasma sodium concentration in these situations is a true value, and plasma osmolality is increased as a result of the presence of the extra solutes. The decrease in plasma sodium is approximately 1.6 mEq/L for every 100 mg/dL increase in the plasma glucose concentration.

In true hyponatremia, the plasma osmolality is low (<280 mOsm/kg), and the pathophysiologic processes are caused by (1) loss of both plasma sodium and water (sodium losses exceeding water losses), (2) increase in plasma water (without edema), or (3) increase in both total body water and sodium (increase in water exceeding that of sodium; usually with edema). Estimating the status of the ECF volume (hypovolemia, euvolemia, or hypervolemia) is therefore useful in narrowing the differential diagnosis (see Figs. 59.1, 59.5, 59.6).

Hypovolemic Hyponatremia

Hypovolemia hyponatremia occurs when urinary and/or gastrointestinal sodium losses exceed those of water; fluids are sequestered into third spaces such as the peritoneal cavity, subcutaneous tissue, or bowel lumen; or, uncommonly, sodium is lost in sweat for patients with cystic fibrosis or in excessively hot climatic zones. The most common cause of hypovolemic hyponatremia in children is gastroenteritis. Fistulas and various types of gastrointestinal drainage tubes can also lead to a similar clinical picture. The normally functioning kidneys respond by conserving sodium, and the urine sodium concentration is usually <20 mEq/L.

The kidneys can be the source of excessive sodium loss in premature infants (tubular immaturity), in patients receiving diuretics, and in those having an osmotic diuresis (DKA). The presence of increased urinary bicarbonate, as seen in certain patients with metabolic alkalosis and RTA, leads to obligatory losses of sodium in the urine. The urinary sodium losses are increased during the recovery phase of acute tubular necrosis, after relief of urinary tract obstruction, and in certain renal diseases (salt-wasting nephropathies) such as medullary cystic disease, polycystic kidney disease, and tubulointerstitial diseases. All of these disorders are usually accompanied by hypokalemia. The presence of hyperkalemia and normal renal function in patients with hypovolemic hyponatremia suggests mineralocorticoid deficiency or type IV RTA.

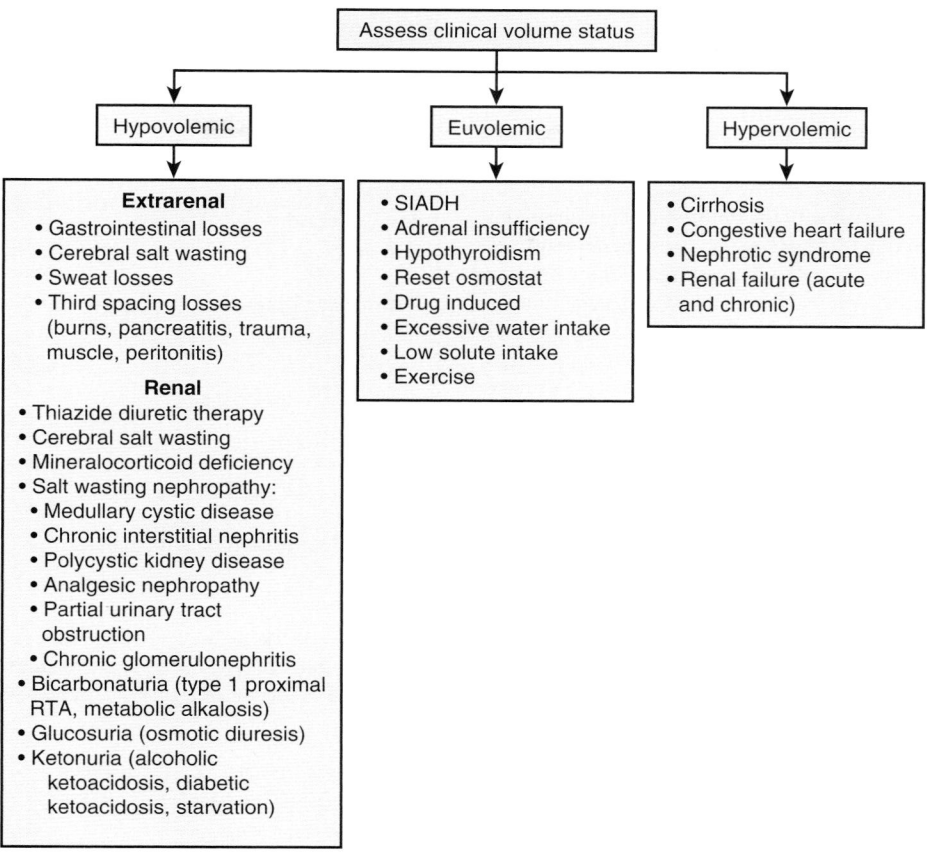

Fig. 59.5 The differential diagnosis of hypo-osmolar hyponatremia. RTA, renal tubular acidosis; SIADH, syndrome of inappropriate antidiuretic hormone. (From Kellerman RD, Rakel DP, eds. *Conn's Current Therapy.* Philadelphia: Elsevier; 2020:343, Fig. 1.)

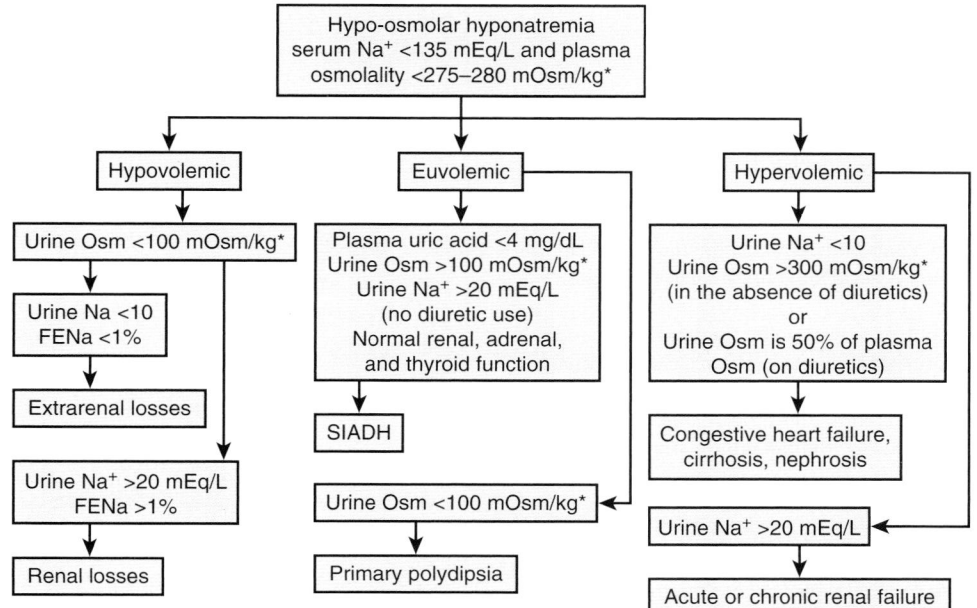

Fig. 59.6 Laboratory findings in hypo-osmolar hyponatremia. FENa, fractional excretion of sodium; Osm, osmoles; SIADH, syndrome of inappropriate antidiuretic hormone. *Per kg water. (From Kellerman RD, Rakel DP, eds. *Conn's Current Therapy.* Philadelphia: Elsevier; 2020:344, Fig. 2.)

Some children with acute or chronic central nervous system injury (closed-head trauma, neurosurgery, tumors, subarachnoid hemorrhage, or meningitis) present with excessive renal sodium losses and develop hypovolemic hyponatremia. The condition known as **cerebral (renal) salt-wasting** syndrome is controversial and may possibly occur because of secretion of atrial natriuretic hormone or other undetermined factors. Cerebral salt wasting is usually associated with hypovolemia but may be confused with the syndrome of inappropriate antidiuretic hormone secretion (SIADH), which does not demonstrate volume depletion. In cerebral (renal) salt wasting, sodium balance (intake-excretion) is negative. Adrenal insufficiency and renal tubular injury are important disorders in the differential diagnosis of cerebral salt wasting. Apart from managing the underlying condition, patients with cerebral salt-wasting syndrome require replacement of urinary sodium and water losses.

In all patients with renal losses of sodium as a cause of hypovolemic hyponatremia, the urinary sodium concentration is usually >20 mEq/L, despite the presence of hypovolemia.

Euvolemic Hyponatremia

The ECF volume status of patients in this group is usually normal; some persons have a slightly increased ECF volume, but they are not edematous. Owing to slight ECF volume expansion, urinary sodium concentration is usually >20 mEq/L.

The **syndrome of inappropriate antidiuretic hormone secretion (SIADH)** is a common cause of euvolemic hyponatremia. Exogenous administration of DDAVP (synthetic analog of vasopressin) can produce a similar clinical picture. SIADH, which has multiple causes (e.g., central nervous system infections, trauma, hypoxia, and various malignancies), results from antidiuretic hormone (ADH) secretion despite the absence of increased plasma osmolality or volume depletion, the normal stimuli for ADH secretion. Rarely is SIADH due to a vasopressin-independent mechanism such as vasopressin-receptor sensitivity to vasopressin (Table 59.12). The diagnostic criteria are as follows:

1. Hypo-osmolar hyponatremia
2. Urine osmolality higher than serum osmolality
3. Normal renal function
4. Normal adrenal and thyroid function
5. High urinary sodium concentration (this is not an absolute criterion, inasmuch as urinary sodium concentrations may be low in patients who are severely sodium depleted)
6. Absence of hypovolemia or edema
7. Hypouricemia

In the absence of any obvious clinical signs, the incidental laboratory finding of hyponatremia is usually the first clue to the presence of SIADH.

Because SIADH is a problem of water retention and not of sodium depletion, the most appropriate treatment is water restriction. Attempts to correct the hyponatremia with sodium administration cause an increase in urinary sodium excretion and little change in the plasma sodium concentration. Nonetheless, sodium administration is needed if severe hyponatremia leads to neurologic symptoms.

Glucocorticoid and thyroid hormone deficiency can cause hyponatremia similar to that of SIADH. Adrenal insufficiency may also produce volume depletion and an Addisonian crisis. The hyponatremia resolves with appropriate hormonal replacement therapy.

Acute water intoxication is an uncommon cause of euvolemic hyponatremia in children receiving hypotonic intravenous fluids; it is likely to happen only if there is an associated impairment of free water excretion capability. Postoperative patients are at particularly increased risk because of high ADH secretion secondary to pain and emotional stress. As the free water excretion ability of infants is limited

in comparison with that in older children, they are at increased risk of developing hyponatremia from excessive oral water intake. Infants younger than 6 months fed water without electrolytes may develop hyponatremia and associated symptoms such as lethargy, seizures, and hypothermia. Symptoms correct rapidly with water restriction.

TABLE 59.12 Causes of the Syndrome of Inappropriate ADH Secretion

Ectopic ADH Production from Tumors
Bronchogenic carcinoma
Bronchial carcinoid
Non-Hodgkin lymphoma
Hodgkin disease
Thymoma

Pulmonary Disease
Tuberculosis
Pneumonia
Aspergillosis with cavitation
Lung abscess
Chronic chest infections
Positive pressure mechanical ventilation

Central Nervous System Disease
Brain tumor
Encephalitis
Meningitis
Brain abscess
Head injury
Subarachnoid hemorrhage
Guillain-Barré syndrome
Systemic lupus erythematosus
Acute intermittent porphyria
Stress
Hydrocephalus

Drug Induced
Carbamazepine
Desmopressin
Oxytocin
Vincristine
Interferons
Nicotine
Cyclophosphamide
Morphine
Amitriptyline
Selective serotonin reuptake inhibitors
3,4-Methylenedioxymethamphetamine (Ecstasy)
Phenothiazines
Barbiturates
ACE inhibitors
Omeprazole
Tricyclic antidepressants

ACE, angiotensin-converting enzyme; ADH, antidiuretic hormone. Modified from Goldman L, Schafer AI, eds. *Goldman-Cecil Medicine.* 26th ed. Philadelphia: Elsevier; 2020:717, Table 108-3.

Medications may also cause hyponatremia, through a variety of mechanisms, such as impairing urinary diluting capacity (i.e., thiazide and loop diuretics) or renal salt wasting (Bactrim). Other medications that can induce hyponatremia are angiotensin-converting enzyme inhibitors, mannitol, and nonsteroidal antiinflammatory medications (see Table 59.12).

Intoxication of traditional amphetamines and synthetic cathinones (β-ketone amphetamine analogs) such as "bath salts" can result in hyponatremia, which may cause profound central nervous system disturbances. Other electrolyte abnormalities may also be seen with amphetamine intoxication including hypokalemia, hyponatremia, hypermagnesemia, and elevated anion gap metabolic acidosis.

Hypervolemic Hyponatremia

In the absence of renal disease, patients with hypervolemic hyponatremia have decreased effective circulating blood volume but with resulting sodium and water retention. Urine sodium concentration is low. The edema-forming states such as heart failure, cirrhosis, and nephrosis are characterized by decreased effective blood volume (despite an increased ECF) that leads to stimulation of the renin-angiotensin-aldosterone axis as well as ADH secretion. Although both sodium and water are retained, hyponatremia develops because of proportionately greater water retention. The urinary sodium is usually <10 mEq/L because of avid sodium reabsorption due to decreased effective blood volume and decreased renal perfusion.

Clinical Signs and Symptoms of Hyponatremia

Most patients with mild degrees of hyponatremia (plasma sodium levels, 125–135 mEq/L) are asymptomatic. Once the serum sodium concentration falls below 120 mEq/L, serious sequelae, especially involving the central nervous system, may follow. Cerebral edema develops because the decrease in plasma osmolality causes water to move into the cells. Cerebral overhydration can manifest with varied symptoms, such as headache, vomiting, altered consciousness, seizures, and coma. The severity of symptoms is dependent on both the magnitude and rapidity of the fall in the plasma sodium concentration. Although seizures are common with acute hyponatremia, patients with chronic hyponatremia may manifest focal neurologic deficits and ataxia. The brain is protected during chronic hyponatremia by adaptive changes involving loss of intracellular osmolytes. However, the same protective changes can be responsible for the harmful effects seen when chronic hyponatremia is corrected too rapidly (see later discussion).

Patients with hypovolemic hyponatremia can develop shock at lesser degrees of body water depletion in comparison with patients with normal or increased serum sodium concentration, because of the associated fluid shift from the ECF to the ICF compartment. The decrease in the intravascular volume is a stimulus for ADH secretion, which serves to perpetuate the hyponatremia by limiting renal water excretion.

Treatment of Hyponatremia

The treatment of hyponatremia depends on its severity, its duration, and the ECF volume status. The primary goal should be to treat the underlying condition giving rise to hyponatremia (e.g., management of diarrhea, mineralocorticoid deficiency, nephrosis, or heart failure). However, management of hypovolemia often requires initiation of corrective therapy before the underlying disease is controlled.

Patients with severe hypovolemia should promptly receive parenteral fluids to restore the circulating blood volume and normalize tissue perfusion. Blood and urine specimens should ideally be obtained as soon as possible to assess serum electrolytes, BUN level, creatinine level, and urinary sodium excretion. *Because correction of severe hypovolemia takes precedence over normalization of osmolality, isotonic solutions can be safely administered before the blood chemistry results are available.* Crystalloids are the preferred replacement fluids except if blood transfusion is required in cases of hemorrhagic shock. Isotonic crystalloids such as 0.9% saline (sodium level, 154 mEq/L) or lactated Ringer solution (sodium level, 130 mEq/L) are administered at a rate of 10–20 mL/kg over a short period of time. Fluid boluses can be repeated as needed until clinical improvement has occurred. The correction of hypovolemia helps in reversing the pathophysiologic factors causing water retention, thus ameliorating the hyponatremia. In patients with known cardiac, renal, or pulmonary diseases, fluid should be administered with caution, and concomitant measurement of central venous pressure and respiratory function is desirable.

After correction of acute hypovolemia, the remaining fluid deficit should be corrected slowly over 24–48 hours; additional fluid should be given to accommodate ongoing losses.

Patients with significant symptoms attributable to severe hyponatremia should receive hypertonic (3%) saline. Central nervous system symptoms almost always lessen when the serum sodium concentration is increased by 10 mEq/L. It is recommended that the initial serum sodium correction not exceed 125 mEq/L with this treatment.

Patients with SIADH require water restriction. In this group of patients, it is difficult to raise the plasma sodium concentration even with hypertonic saline, unless the ECF volume is simultaneously reduced. Whereas water restriction is enough for patients with mild hyponatremia, patients with symptoms should receive intravenous furosemide followed by intravenous hypertonic saline. In chronic SIADH, demeclocycline and vaptans (vasopressin-receptor antagonist) are effective because they diminish the renal response to ADH.

Patients with hypervolemic hyponatremia require salt and water restriction. Any effort to increase the serum sodium concentration by saline administration causes further ECF volume expansion and may worsen the patient's condition. In cases of severe salt and water overload associated with renal failure, dialysis is the most effective therapy.

The management of patients with chronic hyponatremia is controversial. These patients usually have very subtle symptoms because the brain has time to adapt to the disturbance with a decrease in the intracellular osmolytes. Rapid correction of hyponatremia can lead to cellular shrinkage and can cause an **osmotic demyelination syndrome**, particularly in the pons; patients with extensive lesions can have flaccid quadriplegia, dysphagia, and dysarthria.

HYPERNATREMIA

Hypernatremia is a plasma sodium level >145 mEq/L and usually occurs as a result of (1) loss of both body sodium and water (water losses exceeding those of sodium), (2) isolated loss of water, and rarely (3) increase in body sodium. The development of hypernatremia is often prevented by thirst and renal concentrating mechanisms. Thirst is so effective that even patients with complete diabetes insipidus (DI) avoid hypernatremia by spontaneously increasing fluid intake. Hypernatremia develops only when hypotonic fluid losses occur in combination with a disturbance in water intake, as a result of inadequate access (as in comatose, developmentally delayed, or very young patients), or as a result of a primary abnormality of the thirst mechanism (e.g., hypothalamic adipsic syndrome). Establishing the differential diagnosis of hypernatremia is aided by determining the patient's ECF volume status (hypovolemia, euvolemia, or hypervolemia) (Fig. 59.7).

Hypovolemic Hypernatremia

Disorders associated with losses of both sodium and water but with a relatively greater loss of water lead to hypovolemic hypernatremia. Many of the common causes (e.g., diarrhea, diuretic use) are similar to those that cause hypovolemic hyponatremia. Hypernatremia in these situations develops because of failure to ingest hypotonic fluids. Hypernatremic dehydration and failure to thrive often develop in neonates who nurse poorly, especially if the mother's breast milk has not come in. If the losses are extrarenal (e.g., through diarrhea, vomiting, profuse sweating), the urinary sodium concentration is <10 mEq/L. The renal causes are usually associated with a urine sodium concentration >20 mEq/L.

Euvolemic Hypernatremia

Pure water losses do not lead to volume contraction unless the water losses are large; these patients therefore *appear* euvolemic. In addition, hypernatremia develops only when the hypotonic losses are not accompanied by appropriate water intake. Although water loss can occur through the skin or the respiratory tract, the most important disorder in this group is DI.

Patients with DI have a very low urine osmolality. Central DI is caused by a failure to secrete ADH; nephrogenic DI is secondary to a renal resistance to ADH. Acquired forms of central and nephrogenic DI are more common than the hereditary forms.

Hereditary central DI can be either autosomal dominant or, less commonly, autosomal recessive. The autosomal recessive form occurs in association with diabetes mellitus, optic atrophy, and deafness (**Wolfram syndrome**). The acquired causes of central DI include central nervous system trauma, infections, tumors, granulomatous infiltration, and vascular malformations.

Congenital nephrogenic DI is a rare X-linked disorder affecting mainly males, with variable penetrance in females. The **acquired form of nephrogenic DI** can be seen in association with chronic renal diseases (e.g., polycystic disease, medullary cystic disease, ureteral obstruction), electrolyte disorders (e.g., hypokalemia, hypercalcemia), drugs (e.g., lithium, demeclocycline, amphotericin, foscarnet), and sickle cell disease/trait.

Older children with DI have polyuria, polydipsia, and nocturia. The urine is hypo-osmolar and remains so even when these children develop dehydration and consequently increased serum osmolality. During infancy, DI can manifest with recurrent episodes of unexplained dehydration and fever of unknown origin (FUO). Repeated episodes of hypernatremic dehydration can lead to permanent neurologic sequelae.

Performing a fluid deprivation test and then determining the response to injectable vasopressin can help diagnose DI and differentiate between the central and nephrogenic forms. Primary treatment should focus on the underlying cause. Central DI is managed with hormonal replacement therapy with desmopressin (DDAVP). There is considerable individual variation in the required dosage, and it is important to allow patients to revert to mild polyuria before the next dose is given, to prevent excessive water accumulation. An intravenous form of ADH can be used in sick and comatose patients.

Therapy for nephrogenic DI should ensure a sufficient intake of water to replace the large urinary losses. Because obligatory urinary

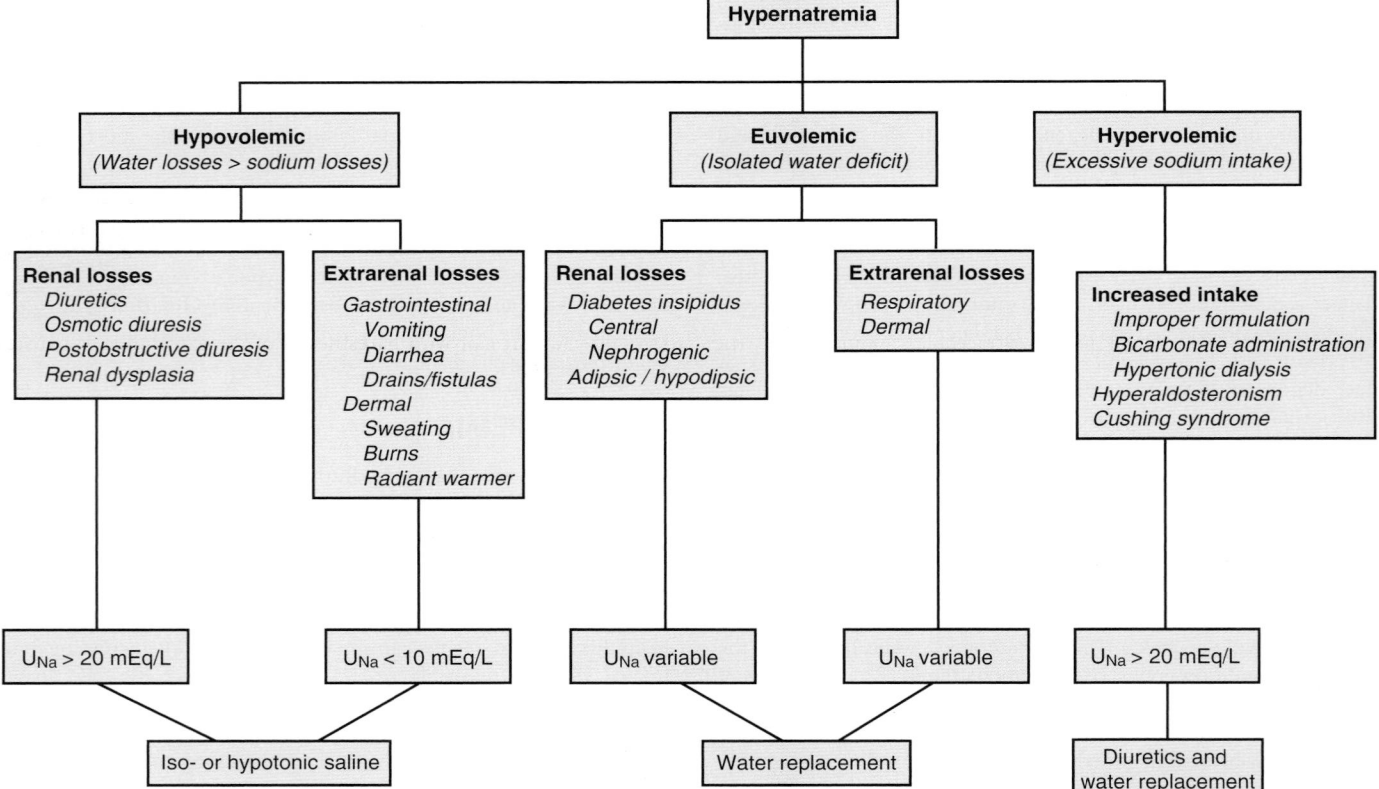

Fig. 59.7 Classification, diagnosis, and treatment of hypernatremic states. (Modified from Beri T, Schrier RW. Disorders of water metabolism. In: Schrier RW, ed. *Renal and Electrolyte Disorders*. Philadelphia: Lippincott-Raven; 1997.)

water losses increase with increasing solute load, restriction of sodium intake reduces the urine output. Administration of diuretics, such as thiazides and amiloride, keeps these patients in a mildly dehydrated state, which leads to increased water reabsorption in the more proximal segments of the nephron, thereby decreasing urine output. Nonsteroidal antiinflammatory drugs such as indomethacin also reduce polyuria and may be used in combination with diuretics. Careful attention should be paid to the fluid balance in these patients when they are sick and have poor oral fluid intake because they require large quantities of water replacement. Frequent monitoring of serum electrolytes is mandatory during these periods.

Medications such as amphotericin B, dexamethasone, lithium, ofloxacin, and foscarnet can result in hypernatremia by causing a nephrogenic DI, and electrolytes should be monitored in patients on these medications for prolonged time periods.

Adipsic/hypodipsic hypernatremia (essential/neurogenic hypernatremia, osmoreceptor dysfunction) characterizes a group of patients who have persistent hypernatremia, absence or attenuation of thirst, and in some partial DI. Adipsic hypernatremia may be idiopathic or associated with hypothalamic sarcoidosis, histiocytosis, tumors, hemorrhage, anterior communicating artery aneurysm, hydrocephalus, trauma, or congenital malformations (holoprosencephaly). These patients require regimental intake of fluids; they may need supplementation with DDAVP.

Hypervolemic Hypernatremia

This is the least common type of hypernatremia. Most of the causes are iatrogenic (administration of improperly formulated oral rehydration solution, administration of intravenous fluids, excessive bicarbonate administration during resuscitative efforts, inadvertent dialysis against a high sodium concentration dialysate, salt poisoning, and seawater drowning).

Salt poisoning is often evident without signs of dehydration or weight loss (weight gain may occur); the fractional excretion of sodium is elevated, urine output is sustained, and an elevated sodium level in the gastric aspirate may be noted.

Other less common causes of hypernatremia include primary hyperaldosteronism and Cushing syndrome.

Clinical Signs and Symptoms of Hypernatremia

Hypernatremia causes intracellular dehydration by movement of water from the intracellular to the extracellular compartment. The consequences of intracellular dehydration are particularly marked in the brain and manifest with irritability, altered sensorium, lethargy, and hyperreflexia and eventually seizures, coma, and death. Brain hemorrhages can result from tearing of small blood vessels when the brain contracts as a result of intracellular dehydration. **Hypernatremia and dehydration may predispose to dural sinus thrombosis**. During chronic hypernatremia, the brain cells adapt to the increased ECF osmolality by accumulating idiogenic osmoles (which are mostly amino acids, particularly taurine). They increase intracellular osmolality, consequently restoring intracellular volume. This protective response has significant implications for therapy and the speed with which hypernatremia should be corrected.

Treatment of Hypernatremia

The treatment of hypernatremia is guided by its severity, its chronicity, and the ECF volume status of the patient.

It is important to realize that patients with hyperosmolality maintain the ECF space at the expense of the ICF compartment, and, therefore, the degree of sodium and fluid losses may be profound before clinical signs of hypovolemia develop. Large volumes of isotonic crystalloid may be necessary to replace the fluid deficit.

Once initial fluid resuscitation has been performed, the serum sodium concentration should be restored slowly over a minimum period of 48 hours. The total water deficit can be estimated as follows (FW, free water; NA, sodium):

$$FW \ deficit \ (child) = 0.6 \times weight \ (kg) \times ((current \ NA \ / \ 140) - 1)$$

Hypernatremia is corrected especially slowly when it is more severe and chronic. The rate of fall in plasma sodium concentration should be <1 mEq/L/hr. During the correction of hypernatremia, the idiogenic osmoles that brain cells produce to prevent cellular dehydration dissipate slowly. If hypernatremia is corrected too rapidly, the increased intracellular osmolality from the idiogenic osmoles can lead to cerebral edema. In patients with salt poisoning, the first line of therapy is restriction of salt intake, followed by administration of hypotonic fluid; acute salt ingestion does not generate idiogenic osmols, permitting a more rapid treatment.

CALCIUM DISORDERS

Serum calcium concentration in the ECF is regulated by parathyroid hormone (PTH), which acts on the kidney and bones, and by 1,25-dihydroxyvitamin D, which acts on the intestines and bones. About 50% of the calcium is in the ionized form, 40% is protein bound (mainly to albumin), and 10% is associated with anions, such as bicarbonate, citrate, sulfate, phosphate, and lactate. It is important to remember that serum albumin levels and pH affect calcium levels. There is a direct relationship between serum albumin concentration and total serum calcium. An alkaline pH will increase protein binding, leading to decreased ionized calcium levels. It is important to obtain an ionized calcium level when evaluating calcium derangements.

Hypocalcemia

There are many causes of hypocalcemia, and measurements of PTH can help classify the etiology of hypocalcemia (Fig. 59.8). Hypocalcemia is defined as a total serum calcium level below 8.5 mg/dL and an ionized serum calcium level below 4.65 mg/dL. Patients with mild hypocalcemia are usually asymptomatic. With severe hypocalcemia, patients may present with paresthesias of the extremities, Chvostek sign, Trousseau sign, muscle cramps or spasm, laryngospasm, tetany, and seizures. Cardiac manifestations of hypocalcemia include a prolonged QT interval, which can progress to heart block. In a child presenting with severe hypocalcemia, especially one with a past medical history significant for constipation, clinicians should be sure to take a thorough medication history, including whether they have received sodium phosphate enemas, as there are reports of patients presenting with marked hypocalcemia after receiving phosphate-containing enemas.

Hypercalcemia

Similar to hypocalcemia, there are also many causes of hypercalcemia (Fig. 59.9). Hypercalcemia usually occurs through one of three mechanisms: increased bone resorption, increased gastrointestinal absorption of calcium, and decreased renal excretion. Hypercalcemia is defined as total serum calcium above 10.5 mg/dL and an ionized serum calcium above 5.25 mg/dL. Patients with mild hypercalcemia usually do not have symptoms. Patients with severe hypercalcemia may have neurologic manifestations ranging from drowsiness to coma.

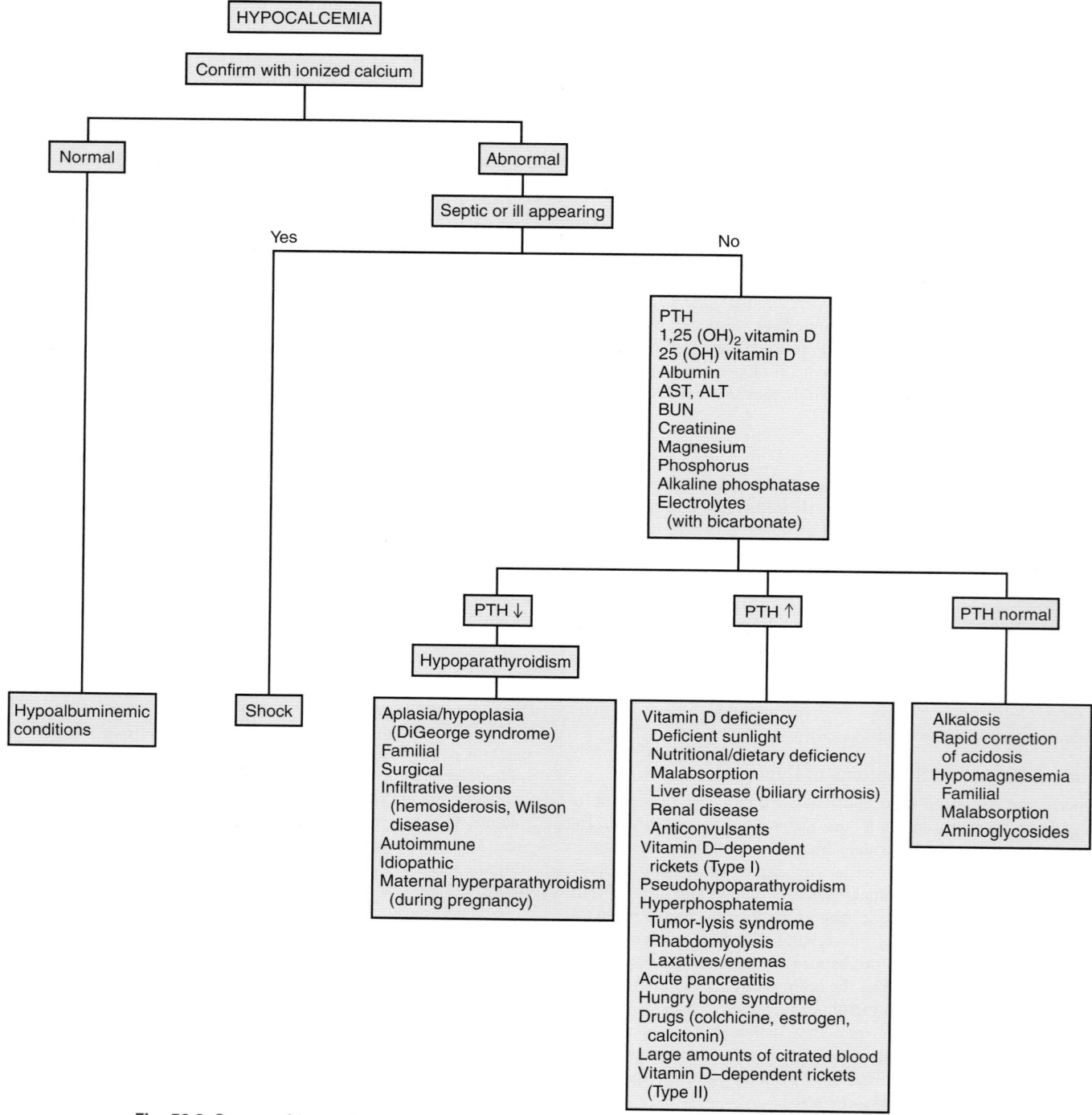

Fig. 59.8 Causes of hypocalcemia. ALT, alanine aminotransferase; AST, aspartate aminotransferase; PTH, parathyroid hormone. (From Pomeranz AJ, Sabnis S, Busey SL, et al. Hypocalcemia. In: Pomeranz AJ, Sabnis S, Busey SL, et al., eds. *Pediatric Decision-Making Strategies*. 2nd ed. Philadelphia: Elsevier; 2016:335.)

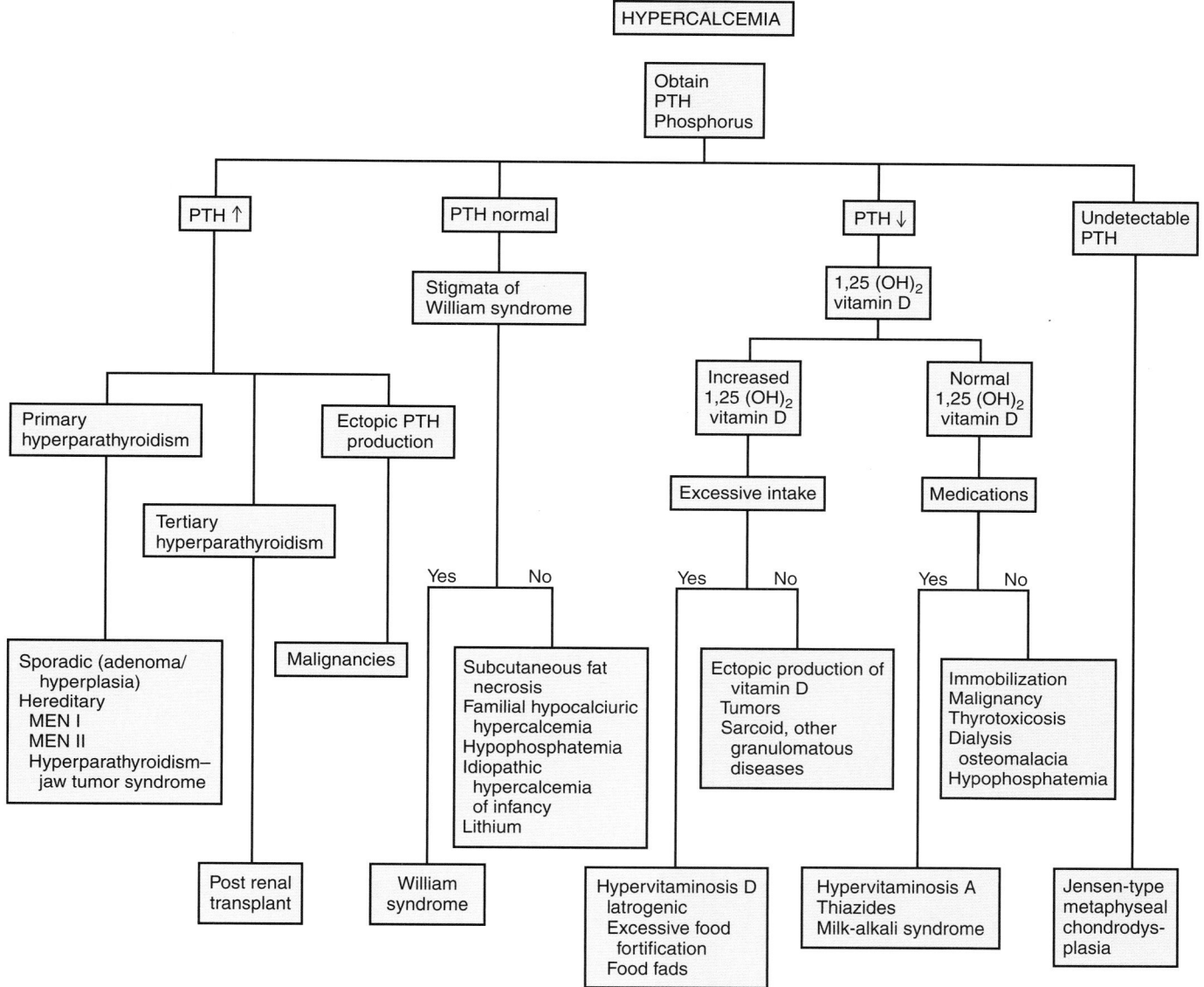

Fig. 59.9 Causes of hypercalcemia. MEN, multiple endocrine neoplasia; PTH, parathyroid hormone. (From Pomeranz AJ, Sabnis S, Busey SL, et al. Hypocalcemia. In: Pomeranz AJ, Sabnis S, Busey SL, et al., eds. *Pediatric Decision-Making Strategies*. 2nd ed. Philadelphia: Elsevier; 2016:337.)

RICKETS

Rickets is a disease caused by deficient mineralization of the osteoid matrix before closure of the epiphyseal plate that results in softening and weakening of bones in infants and children. In patients with rickets, the growth plate cartilage and osteoid continues to expand but mineralization is inadequate, and as a result, the growth plate thickens. The circumference of the growth plate and the metaphysis also increases, which expands bone width at the location of the growth plates and causes some of the classic clinical manifestations, such as widening of the wrists and ankles. There is also softening of the bones that can lead to bone deformities and causes them to bend easily, especially when subject to certain forces.

Rickets is usually caused by nutritional and less often malabsorptive vitamin D deficiency. Risk factors include limited sun exposure, ages 6–24 months, prematurity, solely breast-fed infants, use of anticonvulsants, and darker skin pigmentation. Rickets is still a significant problem in developing countries, likely due to nutritional vitamin D deficiency and inadequate calcium intake.

Clinical Manifestations

Most clinical features of rickets are due to skeletal changes (Figs. 59.10 and 59.11). Craniotabes is a softening of the cranial bones, which can be appreciated by applying pressure at the occiput or over the parietal bones. Widening of the costochondral junctions produces a rachitic rosary, which can be detected on exam by moving one's fingers along the costochondral junctions from rib to rib, named because it feels like the beads of a rosary. Increased circumference of the wrists and ankles is a result of growth plate widening. Patients with rickets may have an indentation of the lower ribs, known as a Harrison groove, which occurs from the pulling of the softened ribs by the diaphragm during inspiration. Softening of the ribs can impair

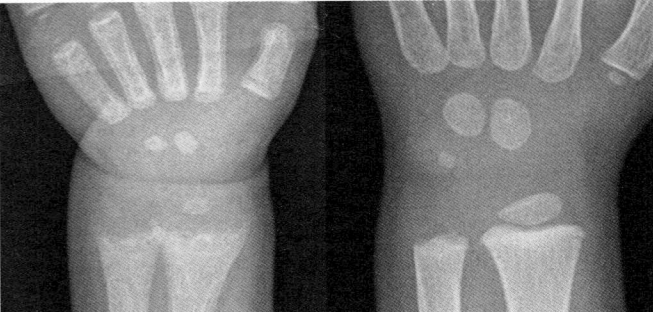

Fig. 59.10 Vitamin D deficiency rickets. A 14-month-old child with growth failure and severe rickets who responded well to vitamin D therapy. The initial image *(left)* shows loss of definition of the zones of provisional calcification for the distal radial and ulnar metaphyses along with metaphyseal fraying and concavity ("cupping") and physeal widening with an increased distance between the epiphysis and visualized portion of the metaphysis. Periosteal new bone also is present that is seen best along the metacarpals but also is present along the distal radius. With healing *(right)*, the zone of provisional calcification is well mineralized and the other findings have resolved. (From Coley BD, ed. *Caffey's Pediatric Diagnostic Imaging.* 13th ed. Philadelphia: Elsevier; 2019:1397, Fig. 139.1.)

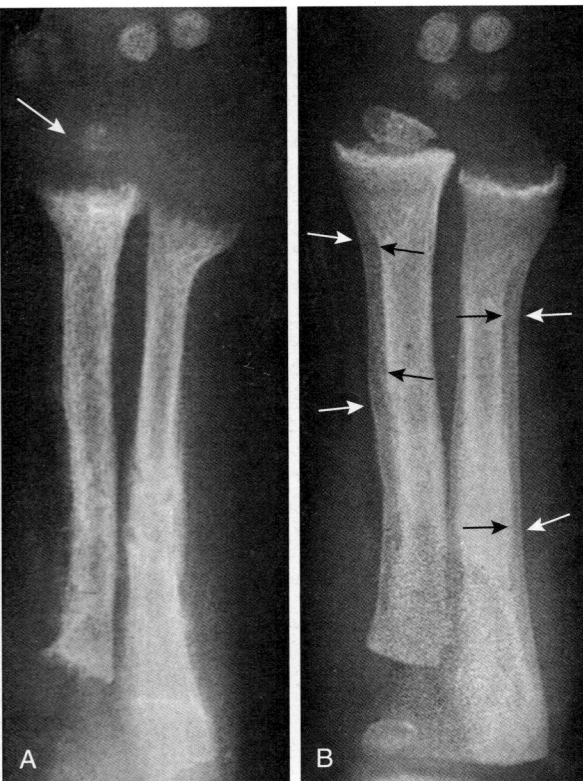

Fig. 59.11 Diaphyseal findings in a patient with severe vitamin D deficiency rickets. Radiographs of the forearm during the active phase *(A)* show coarse demineralization and subperiosteal bone resorption, which are indicative of hyperparathyroidism as a result of rickets. Also note the severe rachitic findings in the metaphysis and poor mineralization of the distal radial epiphysis *(arrow)* with loss of the zones of provisional calcification. With healing 3 months later *(B)*, extensive periosteal new bone is seen *(white arrows)* with calcification of previously nonmineralized osteoid *(black arrows)* produced by periosteal osteoblasts. (From Coley BD, ed. *Caffey's Pediatric Diagnostic Imaging.* 13th ed. Philadelphia: Elsevier; 2019:1398, Fig. 139.4)

TABLE 59.13 Clinical Features of Rickets

General

Failure to thrive (malnutrition)

Listlessness

Protruding abdomen

Muscle weakness (especially proximal)

Hypocalcemic dilated cardiomyopathy

Fractures (pathologic, minimal trauma)

Increased intracranial pressure

Head

Craniotabes

Frontal bossing

Delayed fontanel closure (usually closed by 2 yr)

Delayed dentition

    No incisors by age 10 mo

    No molars by age 18 mo

Caries

Craniosynostosis

Chest

Rachitic rosary

Harrison groove

Respiratory infections and atelectasis*

Back

Scoliosis

Kyphosis

Lordosis

Extremities

Enlargement of wrists and anides

Valgus or varus deformities

Windswept deformity (valgus deformity of one leg with varus deformity of other leg)

Anterior bowing of tibia and femur

Coxa vara

Leg pain

Hypocalcemic Symptoms†

Tetany

Seizures

Stridor caused by laryngeal spasm

*These features are most frequently associated with the vitamin D deficiency disorders.

†These symptoms develop only in children with disorders that produce hypocalcemia.

From Greenbaum LA. Vitamin D deficiency (rickets) and excess. In: Kliegman RM, St. Geme JW III, Blum NJ, et al., eds. *Nelson Textbook of Pediatrics.* 21st ed. Philadelphia: Elsevier; 2020:375, Table 64.3.

air movement and predisposes patients to atelectasis and pneumonia. In addition to the skeletal manifestations, rickets can present with hypocalcemia, hypophosphatemia, and tetany (Table 59.13). It is important to note that most children are asymptomatic, and rickets is diagnosed through an incidental finding on physical or radiologic examination.

There is some variation in the clinical presentation of rickets based on the etiology. Changes in the lower extremities tend to be the

TABLE 59.14   Causes of Rickets

Vitamin D Disorders	Phosphorus Deficiency
Nutritional vitamin D deficiency	Inadequate intake
Congenital vitamin D deficiency	Premature infants (rickets of prematurity)
Secondary vitamin D deficiency	Aluminum-containing antacids
Malabsorption	
Increased degradation	**Renal Losses**
Decreased liver 25-hydroxylase	X-linked hypophosphatemic rickets*
Vitamin D–dependent rickets types 1A and 1B	Autosomal dominant hypophosphatemic rickets*
Vitamin D–dependent rickets types 2A and 2B	Autosomal recessive hypophosphatemic rickets types 1 and 2*
Chronic kidney disease	Hereditary hypophosphatemic rickets with hypercalciuria
	Overproduction of fibroblast growth factor-23
Calcium Deficiency	Tumor-induced rickets*
Low intake	McCune-Albright syndrome*
Diet	Epidermal nevus syndrome*
Premature infants (rickets of prematurity)	Neurofibromatosis*
Malabsorption	
Primary disease	
Dietary inhibitors of calcium absorption	

*Disorders secondary to fibroblast growth factor-23.
From Greenbaum LA. Vitamin D deficiency (rickets) and excess. In: Kliegman RM, St. Geme JW III, Blum NJ, et al., eds. *Nelson Textbook of Pediatrics.* 21st ed. Philadelphia: Elsevier; 2020:376, Table 64.2.

TABLE 59.15   Laboratory Findings in Various Disorders Causing Rickets

Disorder	Ca	Pi	PTH	25-(OH)D	1,25-(OH)₂D	ALP	Urine Ca	Urine Pi
Vitamin D deficiency	N, ↓	↓	↑	↓	↓, N, ↑	↑	↓	↑
VDDR type 1A	N, ↓	↓	↑	N	↓	↑	↓	↑
VDDR type 1B	N, ↓	↓	↑	↓	N	↑	↓	↑
VDDR type 2A	N, ↓	↓	↑	N	↑↑	↑	↓	↑
VDDR type 2B	N, ↓	↓	↑	N	↑↑	↑	↓	↑
Chronic kidney disease	N, ↓	↑	↑	N	↓	↑	N, ↓	↓
Dietary Pi deficiency	N	↓	N, ↓	N	↑	↑	↑	↓
XLH*	N	↓	N, ↑	N	RD	↑	↓	↑
ADHR*	N	↓	N	N	RD	↑	↓	↑
HHRH	N	↓	N, ↓	N	↑	↑	↑	↑
ARHR type 1 or type 2*	N	↓	N	N	RD	↑	↓	↑
Tumor-induced rickets†	N	↓	N	N	RD	↑	↓	↑
Fanconi syndrome	N	↓	N	N	RD or ↑	↑	↓ or ↑	↑
Dent disease	N	↓	N	N	N	↑	↑	↑
Dietary Ca deficiency	N, ↓	↓	↑	N	↑	↑	↓	↑

1,25-(OH)₂D, 1,25-dihydroxyvitamin D; 25-(OH)D, 25-hydroxyvitamin D; ADHR, autosomal dominant hypophosphatemic rickets; ALP, alkaline phosphatase; Ca, calcium; HHRH, hereditary hypophosphatemic rickets with hypercalciuria; N, normal; Pi, inorganic phosphorus; PTH, parathyroid hormone; RD, relatively decreased (because it should be increased given the concurrent hypophosphatemia); VDDR, vitamin D–dependent rickets; XLH, X-linked hypophosphatemic rickets; ↓, decreased; ↑, increased; ↑↑, extremely increased.
*Elevated fibroblast growth factor-23 (FGF-23).
†FGF-23 elevated in some patients.
From Greenbaum LA. Vitamin D deficiency (rickets) and excess. In: Kliegman RM, St. Geme JW III, Blum NJ, et al., eds. *Nelson Textbook of Pediatrics.* 21st ed. Philadelphia: Elsevier; 2020:375, Table 64.4.

dominant feature in X-linked hypophosphatemic rickets. Symptoms secondary to hypocalcemia occur only in those forms of rickets associated with decreased serum calcium (Table 59.14).

Diagnosis of rickets is usually made by radiographic examination of the long bones. Laboratory values can support the diagnosis. Laboratory values may show decreased calcium and phosphorus, increased alkaline phosphatase, decreased 25-(OH) vitamin D_3 levels, increased 1,25-(OH)₂ vitamin D levels, and increased PTH levels. The increased PTH is indicative of the hormonal response that tries to maintain normal calcium (Table 59.15). The appropriate treatment depends on the underlying etiology.

SUMMARY AND RED FLAGS

Acid–base and electrolyte disturbances have many causes that reflect abnormalities of regulation or compensation of these systems. For many acid–base or electrolyte disturbances, the underlying condition needs to be treated before consideration of the electrolyte or acid–base disturbance. This is true in all causes of shock, such as dehydration, adrenal crisis, severe trauma, or systemic hemorrhage. The circulating blood volume must be quickly reestablished; this is usually performed as part of the resuscitation phase of treating dehydration or shock. Thereafter, specific acid–base or, more often, electrolyte abnormalities can be attended to during the replacement phase to correct electrolyte deficits. In general, electrolyte disturbances must be corrected slowly.

This is particularly true for sodium abnormalities. The major exceptions are hyperkalemia and acute hypercarbic respiratory acidosis, which must be treated immediately.

Each of the discussed acid–base and electrolyte disturbances is important, and hyperkalemia remains the one of most concern and the most dangerous.

Anuria or polyuria, hypotension or hypertension, weight loss, seizures, coma, hypoglycemia, muscle cramps, tetany, hyperglycemia, apnea, and arrhythmias are additional concerning signs and symptoms. Moreover, the clinician must remain vigilant in identifying the primary reason or reasons for any of these acid–base or electrolyte disturbances.

BIBLIOGRAPHY

A bibliography is available at ExpertConsult.com.

Congenital Cutaneous Lesions and Infantile Rashes

Stephen R. Humphrey

RASHES (TABLE 60.1)

Papules and Pustules—Diffuse or Scattered

Erythema toxicum is a benign condition that occurs in 30–70% of White full-term infants. Erythema toxicum occurs less frequently in premature infants. The eruption is characterized by blotchy, erythematous macules or patches with central papules, pustules, or vesicles that give the infant a "flea-bitten" appearance (Fig. 60.1). The lesions develop most commonly between the second and fourth days after birth; however, they may appear during the first 2–3 weeks. They are self-limiting and usually resolve within several days. Typical sites of involvement include the face, trunk, and proximal extremities. There may be very few to hundreds of lesions.

A Giemsa or Wright stain of the intralesional contents reveals sheets of *eosinophils* with a relative absence of neutrophils. Peripheral eosinophilia may be present in up to 20% of affected infants. Erythema toxicum is occasionally confused with transient neonatal pustular melanosis, congenital cutaneous candidiasis, impetigo neonatorum, milia, herpes simplex, or miliaria rubra (prickly heat).

Transient neonatal pustular melanosis, seen in up to 4% of neonates, occurs more often in Black infants. Typically present at birth, the initial lesions are 2- to 5-mm pustules distributed over the face, neck, and upper chest and, less often, on the sacrum, trunk, thighs, palms, and soles (Fig. 60.2). In contrast to the lesions of erythema toxicum, there is no erythema surrounding each pustule, and a Wright stain of pustular contents reveals many neutrophils. In both disorders, the pustules are sterile and should be distinguished from those seen in potentially serious infections caused by herpes simplex virus (HSV), *Staphylococcus aureus*, or *Candida* species.

The superficial pustules of transient neonatal pustular melanosis rupture spontaneously within the first few days after birth, leaving hyperpigmented macules that have collarettes of fine scale. It is common to see only the hyperpigmented macules at birth. These brown spots slowly fade over several weeks to months.

Miliaria results from sweat retention and is exacerbated by heat and humidity. Affected newborns are frequently in incubators or receiving phototherapy. Keratinous plugging of the eccrine ducts and subsequent release of eccrine sweat into the surrounding skin produces two distinct clinical manifestations with different sites of eccrine duct obstruction. In miliaria crystallina, obstruction occurs just below the stratum corneum, resulting in superficial, noninflammatory 1- to 2-mm vesicles. In miliaria rubra, or "prickly heat," obstruction occurs in the mid-epidermis. This is associated with an inflammatory response

exhibited by vesicles, papules, or papulovesicles surrounded by a rim of erythema. The lesions occur in clusters on the trunk, face, scalp, and intertriginous regions. Neither type of miliaria warrants therapy, but improvement occurs with cooling of the skin and avoidance of excessive warmth and moisture.

Eosinophilic pustular folliculitis is another disorder of infancy characterized by recurrent crops of vesicles and pustules, beginning in the first year of life. Lesions are often present on the forehead and scalp. The condition tends to occur in a cyclic pattern and is very pruritic. Scraped material from the pustules subjected to Wright stain demonstrates a large number of eosinophils but no evidence of infectious organisms. A CBC may show peripheral eosinophilia. In rare cases, skin biopsy may be necessary. Histopathologic study demonstrates a perifollicular and dermal infiltrate of eosinophils, as well as lymphocytes and histiocytes. Because the clinical condition is very similar to infantile acropustulosis, some authors contend that eosinophilic pustular folliculitis may be part of the same clinical spectrum. This condition is not associated with systemic disease, and the first-line treatment is symptomatic with topical corticosteroids and antihistamines. Oral and topical indomethacin has been effective in recalcitrant cases. Eosinophilic pustular folliculitis usually resolves spontaneously by 2–3 years of age.

Acropustulosis of infancy is a condition that may present at birth or during the first few weeks or months afterward. The disorder is characterized by recurrent eruptions of pruritic pustules or vesicles involving the hands and feet (Fig. 60.3). On occasion, involvement includes other sites such as the trunk or abdomen. The lesions frequently begin in crops, which typically last approximately 1 week, and resolve with desquamation, followed by postinflammatory hyperpigmentation.

Acropustulosis is often confused with infantile scabies. Family history and examination of scrapings of the involved area may help differentiate between these two diagnoses. However, there is some thought that it may occur after a previous scabies infection. Scrapings of lesions in acropustulosis often demonstrate neutrophils. Bacterial infection should also be ruled out by wound cultures. Treatment is symptomatic and consists of control of pruritus with low- to mid-potency topical corticosteroids and antihistamines. Parents should be advised that lesions tend to occur episodically until approximately 2–3 years of age.

Neonatal cephalic pustulosis (neonatal acne) develops in approximately 20% of newborns. Typically, it is not present at birth but appears during the first few weeks after birth. Characterized by papules and pustules located on the face or trunk, this condition usually resolves within the first several months of life (Fig. 60.4). Neonatal acne is a

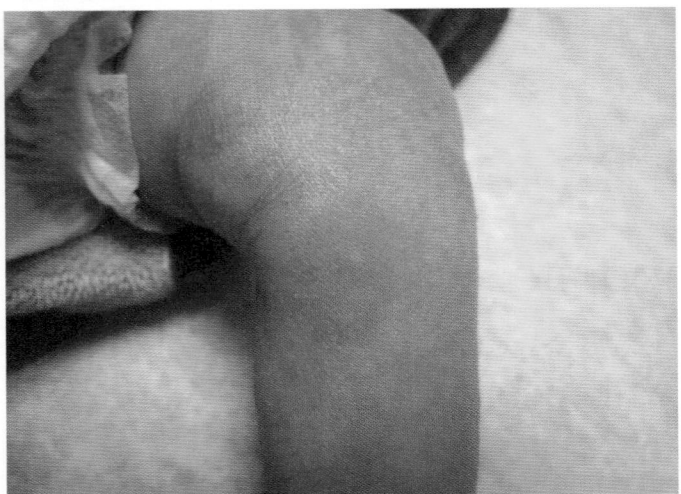

Fig. 60.1 Papules surrounded by erythema are characteristic of erythema toxicum. Typically it is located on the trunk but can be on the extremities as well.

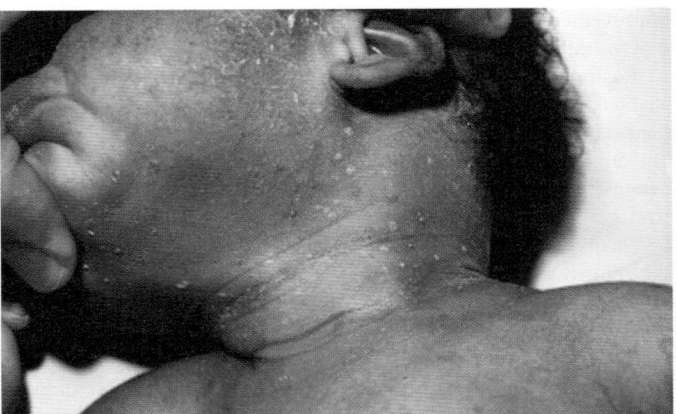

Fig. 60.2 Transient neonatal pustular melanosis. Papules and papulopustules rupture to leave a collarette of fine scales and eventual hyperpigmentation. (From Paller AS, Mancini AJ. Cutaneous disorders of the newborn. In: Paller AS, Mancini AJ, eds. *Hurwitz Clinical Pediatric Dermatology*. 4th ed. Philadelphia: Elsevier; 2011:18.)

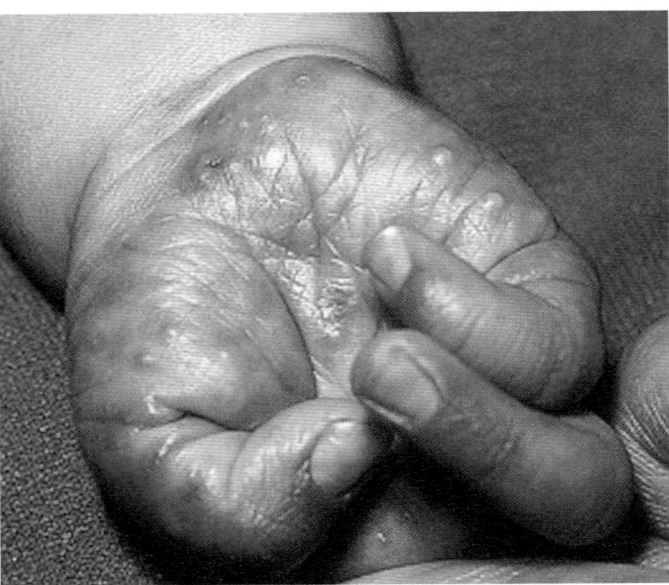

Fig. 60.3 Acropustulosis of infancy. Multiple tense erythematous papules and pustules on the palm of this 4-month-old girl. (From Paller AS, Mancini AJ. Cutaneous disorders of the newborn. In: Paller AS, Mancini AJ, eds. *Hurwitz Clinical Pediatric Dermatology*. 4th ed. Philadelphia: Elsevier; 2011:19.)

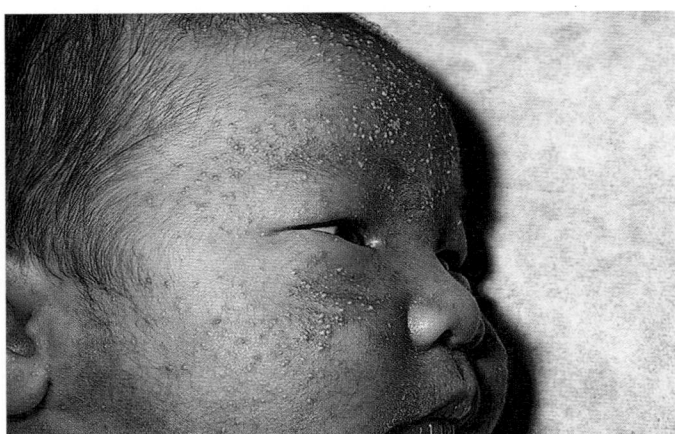

Fig. 60.4 Neonatal acne (cephalic pustulosis) is usually found on the cheeks and scalp in the first 2–4 weeks of life; small red papules and pustules without comedones are evident. (Modified from Eichenfield LF, Frieden IJ, Esterly NB. *Textbook of Neonatal Dermatology*. Philadelphia: Saunders; 2001:94.)

misnomer as neonatal cephalic pustulosis is likely caused by *Malassezia* yeast species. Therapeutic intervention is rarely required, but ketoconazole 2% cream may be of some use.

Langerhans cell histiocytosis (LCH) is a rare disorder, affecting about 5 per 1 million children, which is characterized by a proliferation of clonal dendritic cells, called Langerhans cells. There are four main types, two of which are most frequently seen in neonates and infants, though there is substantial overlap among the types.

Congenital self-healing reticulohistiocytosis (**Hashimoto-Pritzker disease**) typically presents at birth or within the first few days of life and is limited to the skin. There is a diffuse eruption of red to purple-brown papules and nodules that will crust and remit after several weeks. While it is considered a benign, self-limited condition, it can rarely progress to other, more aggressive forms of LCH.

Letterer-Siwe disease is the more acute, diffuse form of LCH that has multisystem involvement. It commonly presents before 1 year of age with the majority of patients having skin findings of small 1- to 2-mm papules, pustules, and vesicles, typically on the scalp, intertriginous areas, and trunk (Fig. 60.5). The lesions are often crusted and may

have secondary bacterial infections. Fissures and confluence of papules can be seen. It can be confused with seborrheic dermatitis and other forms of diaper dermatitis (Table 60.2).

Patches and Plaques

Patches are confluent, flat lesions over 1 cm in size, while plaques are slightly raised lesions over 1 cm in size. Many of these conditions have overlapping features but can often be distinguished by their location, distribution, and response to certain treatments (see Table 60.1).

Neonatal lupus erythematosus is a unique annular erythematous eruption during the neonatal period. It affects 1 in 12,000–20,000 live births. Congenital cases are even more uncommon. Lesions of neonatal lupus are often scaly, annular plaques that usually occur on the face and scalp and may affect the periorbital and malar areas, creating

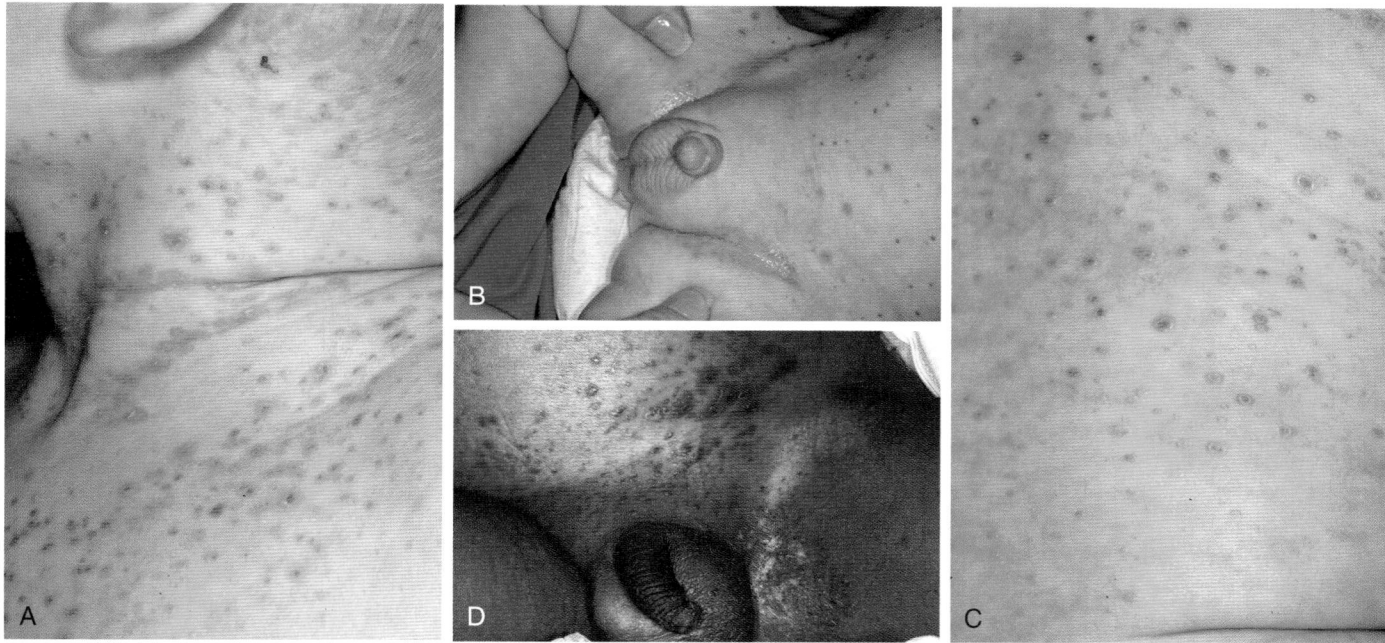

Fig. 60.5 Langerhans cell histiocytosis (LCH). *A–C,* Erythematous and eroded papules in the neck fold and inguinal creases and over the trunk. Note the associated crusting, purpura, and umbilicated nature of some of the papules. *D,* Eroded, erythematous, and hemorrhagic papules in the groin of this infant with disseminated LCH. Note the associated jaundiced appearance, a result of massive liver involvement. (From Paller AS, Mancini AJ, eds. *Hurwitz Clinical Pediatric Dermatology.* 5th ed. Philadelphia: Elsevier; 2016:232, Fig. 10-2.)

TABLE 60.1 Neonatal and Infantile Cutaneous Lesions

RASHES

Papules and Pustules

Erythema toxicum	Occurs first few days of life
	Blotchy red macules with central papule, pustule, or vesicle
Transient neonatal pustular melanosis	Present at birth
	More common in African-American infants
	Pustules resolve with hyperpigmented macules
Miliaria	Associated with overheating
	Vesicles and pustules in occluded areas
Eosinophilic pustular folliculitis	Onset during infancy
	Pruritic pustules on the head and neck
Acropustulosis of infancy	Onset during infancy
	Pruritic pustules on the hands and feet
Neonatal cephalic pustulosis (neonatal acne)	Pink papules, predominately on face
Langerhans cell histiocytosis	Crusted papules, predominately on the scalp and intertriginous areas
Herpes simplex virus	Onset from birth to 2 wk
	Grouped vesicles and papulopustules favor scalp and trunk
Varicella	Diffuse vesicles and papules
	Associated with sepsis, fever/hypothermia
Scabies	Pruritic papules, vesicles, and pustules
	Can be widespread in infants, but concentrated in intertriginous areas
Syphilis	Widely scattered scaly red-brown papules and plaques

Patches and Plaques

Neonatal lupus	Bright red annular patches and plaques distributed on cheeks and periorbital skin
	Heart block is most common extracutaneous finding
Seborrheic dermatitis	Pink patches on the scalp, face, ears, and intertriginous areas
	May have yellow, greasy scale
	Erosions and fissures can be seen
Diaper dermatitis	Pink patches with erosions in the groin and buttocks
	Can be multifactorial

FIXED LESIONS

Macules, Papules, and Pustules

Milia	Pinpoint white-yellow papules without erythema
	Typically on face, gingiva, or palate
	Resolves with time
Sebaceous gland hyperplasia	Skin-colored to yellow tiny papules on cheeks and nose
	Secondary to maternal androgens
	Resolve in first few months
Subcutaneous fat necrosis	Firm, indurated, tender plaques on back, arms, shoulders of newborns
	Due to perinatal trauma, hypothermia, or hypoxemia
	Monitor for hypercalcemia

Continued

TABLE 60.1   Neonatal and Infantile Cutaneous Lesions—cont'd

Macules, Papules, and Pustules—cont'd

Juvenile xanthogranuloma	Solitary yellow-pink plaques on the face and scalp May ulcerate and usually resolve spontaneously
Mastocytoma	Yellow to pink solitary plaques Can urticate or swell with friction or rubbing Composed of mast cells Can be seen in infants but typically more common with toddlers
Urticaria pigmentosa	Condition with several mastocytomas Rare in infants Typically presents with lesions that will urticate Over time, they become hyperpigmented Rarely associated with systemic symptoms
Spider angioma	Rare in infants Small blanching capillaries with "feeder vessel" on the trunk and face
Pyogenic granuloma	Solitary, small vascular papules that develop rapidly and bleed profusely Typically seen in toddlers and occasionally infants

Patches and Plaques

Pink (Vascular or Other)

Hemangioma	Benign vascular tumors, typically present in first month of life Grow rapidly for first several months and then involute slowly over a couple of years
PHACE/PELVIS	Syndromes associated with hemangiomas in particular locations on the face or back
Capillary malformation	Stable, pink, vascular patches; typically unilateral In V1 distribution, can be associated with Sturge-Weber syndrome
Nevus simplex	Pink patches on glabella, eyelids, nape of neck, typically Usually fade over first couple of years
Cutis marmorata telangiectasia congenita	Lacy, reticulated vascular patches Do not resolve with rewarming of infant May have atrophic changes or ulcerate
Kaposiform hemangioendothelioma	Rare vascular tumor Firm, violaceous, and tends to proliferate Can lead to consumptive coagulopathy (Kasabach-Merritt syndrome)
Venous/lymphatic malformation	Slow-flow vascular malformations Typically present at birth May be associated with atrophy or overgrowth

Hyperpigmented or Darker Pigment

Congenital melanocytic nevus	Pigmented macules, papules, patches, and plaques Present in 2–3% of population
Neurocutaneous melanosis	Defined by a giant melanocytic nevus or greater than two CMNs Associated with melanocytic infiltration of leptomeninges Clinically symptomatic lesions have worse prognosis

Café-au-lait macules	Well-demarcated tan maculesor patches Seen in 10–20% of population Multiple lesions can be associated with neurofibromatosis
Dermal melanocytosis	Large, poorly demarcated, slate-gray to blue patches on buttocks and lumbosacral region Occurs normally in darker skin tones Typically fades over time

Hypopigmented or Depigmented

Nevus depigmentosus	Hypopigmented patch that persists through life
Ash leaf spots	Hypopigmented macules that present in first few months to years of life Typically seen with tuberous sclerosis
Piebaldism	Well-circumscribed areas of depigmentation on the skin Tends to be symmetric and stable in size
Waardenburg syndrome	White forelock, white patches on skin Can have heterochromia of irides and hearing loss
Albinism	Diffuse congenital hypopigmentation of skin Usually involves eyes and hair Should be monitored closely by ophthalmologists Evaluate for hearing loss Patients need lifelong photoprotection

Other

Nevus sebaceus	Sebaceous gland hamartoma, usually present at birth Yellow-orange and smooth plaque Thickens during puberty
Dermoid cyst	Typically found in head/neck region Potential for intracranial connection
Aplasia cutis	Congenital absence of skin, typically on scalp Can resemble scars when child is older
Hair collar sign	Ring of dense, darker hair encircling a scalp lesion Can be a sign of spinal dysraphism
Hypertrichosis of lumbar area	Normal variant in certain ethnicities Can be indicator of spinal dysraphism
Sacral dimples	Commonly seen Large dimples along gluteal crease need to be evaluated for spinal dysraphism Can be associated with hypertrichosis

TRANSIENT/CHANGING LESIONS

Patches

Segmental

Cutis marmorata	Lacy, reticulated vascular patches, often bilateral Resolve with warming of infant and disappear over time

Diffuse

Harlequin color change	Marked erythema on dependent side Simultaneous blanching on nondependent side Transient

Distal Extremities

Acrocyanosis	Bluish-purple discoloration of hands, feet, and lips Occurs with crying and cold stress

CMN, congenital melanocytic nevi; PELVIS, perineal hemangioma, external genitalia malformations, lipomyelomeningocele, vesicorenal abnormalities, imperforate anus, and skin tag; PHACE, posterior fossa malformations, hemangiomas, arterial anomalies, cardiac defects, and eye abnormalities.

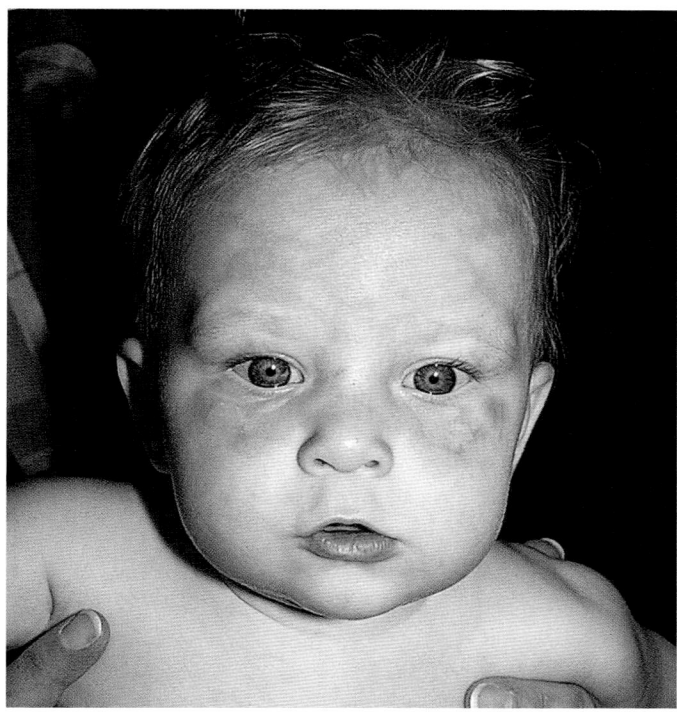

Fig. 60.6 "Raccoon eyes" eruption of neonatal lupus erythematosus. (From Eichenfield LF, Frieden IJ, Esterly NB. *Textbook of Neonatal Dermatology*. Philadelphia: Saunders; 2001:297.)

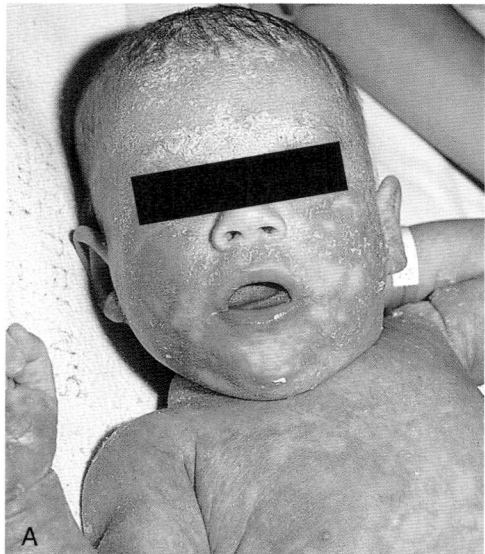

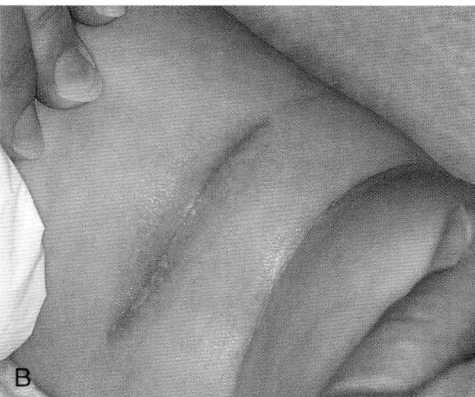

Fig. 60.7 *A*, Seborrheic dermatitis may occasionally be widespread. *B*, The body folds are often involved in seborrheic dermatitis. (From Eichenfield LF, Frieden IJ, Mathes EF, et al., eds. *Neonatal and Infant Dermatology*. 3rd ed. Philadelphia: Elsevier; 2015:225, Figs. 15.11 and 15.12.)

a "raccoon eyes" appearance (Fig. 60.6). Other manifestations may include transient hypopigmentation with epidermal atrophy or telangiectasia. Cutaneous lesions may be present at birth but often appear within the first 2–4 months of life. The lesions are usually exacerbated by sun exposure and are typically photodistributed. The majority of skin findings are transient, lasting up to 6–9 months.

Cutaneous findings and congenital heart block are each present individually in approximately 50% of affected infants; some studies have shown congenital heart block to be much less common. An overlap of both is present in approximately 10% of affected infants. The major morbidity and mortality of neonatal lupus result from congenital heart block.

The diagnosis of neonatal lupus includes examination of anti-Ro, anti-La, and anti-U1RNP autoantibodies in both the infant and mother. Ninety-five percent of mothers of infants with neonatal lupus have anti-Ro antibodies. Skin biopsy is usually not necessary. Work-up should include an ECG, platelet count, and liver function tests because approximately 35% of affected infants have liver disease or thrombocytopenia. Rare reports of multisystem involvement, including neurologic and respiratory findings, have been reported.

Mothers with high titers of anti-Ro antibodies or with systemic lupus erythematosus have a higher risk of delivering an infant with neonatal lupus and should be counseled appropriately. Mothers with positive anti-Ro or anti-La antibodies will have an approximately 2% risk of their baby having neonatal lupus. Despite high antibody titers, fewer than half of mothers of affected infants are symptomatic at the time of delivery. In most of these mothers, evidence of connective tissue disease, usually Sjögren syndrome or subacute cutaneous lupus, develops over time.

Differential diagnosis should include annular erythema of infancy, tinea corporis, and cutis marmorata telangiectatica congenita (CMTC). Treatment consists of photoprotection and topical steroids. Most

cutaneous changes resolve spontaneously by 6–9 months of age as a result of a gradual decrease in maternal antibodies.

Seborrheic dermatitis, common during infancy, typically manifests within the first several weeks after birth. Characterized by erythema and a yellow, greasy scale, it usually resolves spontaneously within several months. The eruption occurs at sites where sebaceous glands are concentrated, such as the face, chest, posterior auricular scalp, and intertriginous areas (Fig. 60.7). *Malassezia* colonization plays a part in the development of seborrheic dermatitis. "Cradle cap" is seborrhea that is confined to the scalp. Involvement of the diaper area is characterized by salmon-colored patches that arise in skinfolds and spread to the genitalia, suprapubic area, and upper medial thighs. Scale may not be as apparent in intertriginous areas. Unlike atopic dermatitis, this eruption is not very pruritic. Secondary candidal or bacterial infection is common, particularly if erosions or fissures are seen.

The diagnosis is established clinically. The presence of greasy yellow scales and salmon-colored patches, involvement of the scalp and intertriginous areas, early onset, and lack of pruritus or atopic history help distinguish seborrheic from atopic dermatitis. However, some infants have an overlap of seborrheic dermatitis and atopic dermatitis. Seborrheic dermatitis should also be differentiated from LCH, in which the

TABLE 60.2   **Diaper Dermatitis**

Disease	Clinical Manifestation	Other Features	Treatment
Friction	Inner surface of thighs, genitalia, buttocks, abdomen	Course waxes and wanes Aggravated by talc	Responds well to diaper changes Avoidance of diapers
Irritant	Mild erythema with shiny surface and occasional papules Confined to convex surfaces Spares intertriginous areas	Exacerbated by heat, moisture, and sweat retention	Gentle cleansing Regular diaper changes Barrier creams (zinc oxide, Vaseline) Low-potency topical steroids can help
Allergic contact	Typically confined to convex surfaces Skin involved is in direct contact with offending agent Mild cases: diffuse erythema, papules, vesicles, scaling Severe cases: papules, plaques, psoriasiform lesions, ulcerations, infiltrative nodules	Often related to topical antibiotics (neomycin, bacitracin) Certain emulsifiers in topical products Preservatives in wet wipes can be an offender	Remove offending agent Judicious use of low-potency topical steroids Barrier creams/ointments
Seborrheic dermatitis	Salmon-colored patches Often have yellow, greasy scale Fissures, erosions, maceration, and weeping can be seen	Axillae, ear creases, and neck are often involved "Cradle cap" on scalp Hypopigmentation often seen in patients with darker skin tones	Low-potency topical steroids If coexistent infection—antifungal or antibacterial agents
Candidiasis	Usually involves intertriginous areas and convex surfaces Bright-red papules and plaques Satellite lesions on abdomen and thighs	Oral thrush may be present Often occurs after treatment with systemic antibiotics or local topical steroid use	Topical anticandidal agent, including nystatin
Intertrigo	Well-demarcated, macerated plaques with weeping Gluteal cleft and fleshy folds of thighs	May be associated with miliaria	Avoiding excessive heat Cool clothing
Psoriasis	Bright red, scaly, well-demarcated plaques Can persist for months Less responsive to topical treatment	Red, sometimes scaly Can be present on extremities or trunk Nail changes seen Family history	Low-potency topical steroids Moisturizers
Staphylococcal infection	Many thin-walled pustules with pink-red base Collarette of scale after rupturing		Antistaphylococcal therapy
Acrodermatitis enteropathica (zinc deficiency)	Early lesions are vesicular and pustular Become confluent, pink, dry, scaly, crusty plaques	Perioral skin typically also involved Irritability or listlessness Failure to thrive, alopecia, diarrhea	Secondary to zinc deficiency or inborn error of zinc transporter Treat with zinc replacement
Langerhans cell histiocytosis	May mimic candidiasis or seborrheic dermatitis Persistent, does not improve with standard treatments Clusters of infiltrative, crusted, hemorrhagic papules Ulceration can be seen	Involvement of groin, axillae, periauricular skin, hairline, and scalp Anemia, thrombocytopenia, hepatosplenomegaly, and osseous lesions	Chemotherapy

lesions are typically purpuric, erosive, or crusted, and from psoriasis (see Chapter 61). Skin biopsy findings, as well as hepatosplenomegaly, purpura, lymphadenopathy, anemia, thrombocytopenia, external otitis, interstitial pneumonia, and osseous lesions, further distinguish LCH from seborrheic dermatitis.

Treatment of the scalp consists of mild keratolytic shampoos, such as those containing selenium sulfide or zinc pyrithione. Ketoconazole 2% shampoo can be efficacious, particularly with controlling overgrowth of the yeast. Mineral oil may be helpful in removing thick, adherent scales. The scalp and diaper dermatitis may be treated with low-potency topical corticosteroids and barrier ointments. Topical antifungal or antibacterial agents should be used for coexisting candidiasis or impetigo.

Diaper dermatitis is one of the most common dermatologic disorders of infants and toddlers (see Table 60.2). It comprises a group of inflammatory conditions that involve the lower abdomen, genitalia, upper thighs, and buttocks. Clinical manifestations include erythema, edema, erosions, vesicles, and pustules. Secondary changes of postinflammatory hyperpigmentation or hypopigmentation are common.

Diaper dermatitis is often multifactorial, including irritation from feces/urine, skin breakdown from maceration, and bacterial or fungal components. Although urinary ammonia was thought to be the primary factor in the development of diaper dermatitis, feces now appear to play a more important role. Fecal ureases, by converting urea to ammonia, cause the elevation of skin pH, which in turn increases fecal protease and lipase activity. These proteases and lipases cause the disruption of the epidermal barrier. Skin wetness, friction, maceration, and contact with feces, urine, and microbes further compromise epidermal integrity. This results in increased permeability of the skin to irritants such as soaps, powders, and detergents. Diaper dermatitis may begin as early as 1–2 months of age and may become a chronic or recurrent problem in older infants as well.

Allergic contact dermatitis is another component to consider, although it is more common in toddlers and children than neonates.

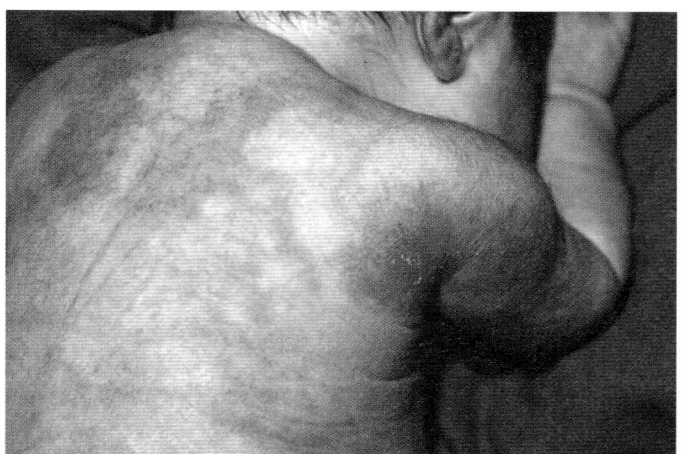

Fig. 60.8 Subcutaneous fat necrosis. Indurated, erythematous plaques on the shoulders and back of this 1-week-old boy. (From Paller AS, Mancini AJ. Cutaneous disorders of the newborn. In: Paller AS, Mancini AJ, eds. *Hurwitz Clinical Pediatric Dermatology.* 4th ed. Philadelphia: Elsevier; 2011:14.)

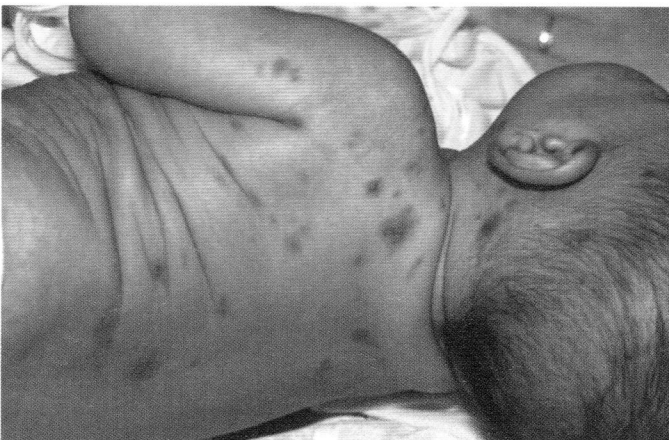

Fig. 60.9 Urticaria pigmentosa.

Offenders can be dispersed dyes from disposable diapers and methylisothiazolinone in wet wipes. The differential diagnosis may also include seborrheic dermatitis, skin or perianal infections (particularly due to group A streptococcus), and psoriasis (see Chapter 61).

FIXED LESIONS

Macules, Papules, and Pustules

Milia are pinpoint white or yellow papules that are commonly present in 40–50% of neonates. Located predominantly on the face, they may also be seen in the oral cavity, where they are referred to as Epstein pearls (palate) or Bohn nodules (gingiva). The lesions represent keratin-filled epidermal inclusion cysts, which usually resolve spontaneously during the first few weeks of life. Unusually widespread or persistent lesions may be associated with defects such as hereditary trichodysplasia, oral-facial-digital syndrome, or particular subtypes of epidermolysis bullosa (EB). Milia may be present in several genodermatoses, including Bazex-Dupré-Christol, Rombo, and Brook-Spiegler syndromes; atrichia with papular lesions; and pachyonychia congenita type 2. Treatment is typically not needed, though topical retinoids have been used.

Sebaceous gland hyperplasia is characterized by the presence of multiple flesh- to yellow-colored tiny papules primarily on the nose and cheeks of full-term infants. The increased sebaceous cell size and number as well as sebaceous gland volume may result from maternal androgen stimulation. Spontaneous resolution occurs within the first 4–6 months of life.

Subcutaneous fat necrosis is a condition of otherwise healthy infants that is associated with preceding trauma, cesarean section, cold injury (including therapeutic hypothermia), or hypoxia. Over half of patients will develop lesions within the first week of life. This disorder occurs primarily in healthy full-term and postmature infants. It is thought to be due to the higher ratio of saturated to unsaturated fat in neonates, thereby predisposing the fat to crystallization with colder temperatures. Single or multiple erythematous to violaceous, indurated, tender nodules or plaques arise on the buttocks, thighs, back, cheeks, and arms. In rare cases, lesions liquefy, ulcerate, and drain an oily substance (Fig. 60.8). The diagnosis can be confirmed by the histopathologic findings of fat lobules containing pathognomonic needle-shaped clefts surrounded

by a mixed inflammatory infiltrate of lymphocytes, histiocytes, and foreign body giant cells. Intact lesions heal spontaneously within several months, whereas ulcerated lesions may heal more slowly and result in scarring. All patients should be screened for hypercalcemia, which may be present in nearly 70% of patients. Fortunately, hypercalcemia tends to be asymptomatic, without evidence of irritability, hypotonia, or weight loss, though life-threatening hypercalcemia may occur. The hypercalcemia may be delayed, with normal serum calcium early in the course of this disorder but elevated levels arising several weeks later. In most patients, the hypercalcemia resolves within 4 weeks of initial detection. Some recommend screening at 30, 45, and 60 days following resolution of skin lesions. The differential diagnosis includes cold panniculitis, cellulitis, and sclerema neonatorum.

Juvenile xanthogranulomas (JXGs) are rare, benign, solitary collections of non–Langerhans cell histiocytes, thought to be reactive in nature. They typically present during the neonatal and infantile period and usually resolve over subsequent months or years. Multiple lesions may exist and should raise suspicion for extracutaneous disease. The incidence of extracutaneous JXG is rare, and the eye is thought to be the most common site, occurring in 0.24% of patients. Multiple JXGs should trigger a thorough review of symptoms, as neurofibromatosis (NF)-1 is associated with multiple JXGs. Recommendations for ophthalmology examinations are somewhat controversial and are likely low yield, unless there are ocular or visual symptoms. A skin biopsy is diagnostic and shows collections of histiocytes and multinucleated giant cells called Touton giant cells.

A **mastocytoma** is a solitary skin-colored to light red or tan papule or plaque that is often located on the trunk, extremities, or neck. Some lesions may have a yellow or pink hue. The lesion may appear at birth or within the first few months of life. Histopathologic study reveals the dermis densely infiltrated with mast cells. The characteristic finding on physical examination is that stroking the lesion causes histamine release that results in tense edema within the lesion and an erythematous flare, known as the Darier sign. A skin biopsy and special stains for mast cells may confirm the clinical diagnosis. Symptoms such as pruritus or flushing, when present, are usually mild. Treatment is not usually necessary unless the patient has symptoms of excessive histamine release. The condition is self-limited and resolves spontaneously over several years. The lesions do not need to be excised.

Urticaria pigmentosa is characterized by the development of multiple mastocytomas, usually within the first 8–12 months of life (Fig. 60.9). The lesions may vary in size from a few millimeters to several centimeters. Some lesions may not become pigmented until the child is approximately 6 months of age or older. Therefore, early lesions of

TABLE 60.3 Types of Vascular Tumors and Vascular Malformations

Vascular Tumors	Vascular Malformations
Hemangioma	Capillary malformation
Kaposiform hemangioendothelioma	Venous malformation
Tufted hemangioma	Lymphatic malformation
Noninvoluting congenital hemangioma (NICH)	Arteriovenous malformation (AVM)
Rapidly involuting congenital hemangioma (RICH)	Mixed

TABLE 60.4 Differentiation of Infantile Hemangiomas vs Vascular Malformations

Infantile Hemangioma	Vascular Malformations
Up to 55% present at birth	90% recognized at birth
Rapid postnatal growth and slow involution	Static malformation of dysplastic vessels that grows proportionally with child
Rapid endothelial cell turnover	Normal endothelial cell turnover and proliferation
Increased incidence in female-to-male ratio (3:1–5:1)	Female-to-male incidence ratio 1:1

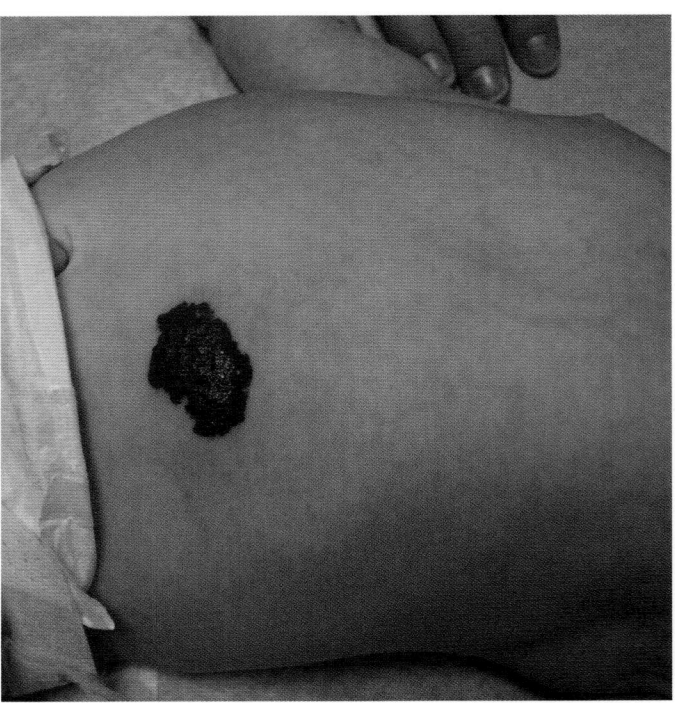

Fig. 60.10 A superficial hemangioma on the abdomen.

urticaria pigmentosa may resemble recurrent urticaria until pigmentation is noted. The Darier sign, or urtication of the lesions upon rubbing, is seen in urticaria pigmentosa as well. Rarely, these lesions may produce enough histamine release to cause flushing, diarrhea, vomiting, tachycardia, and hypotension. Parents should be counseled about the avoidance of mast cell–degranulating agents.

Antihistamines should be used in any patient who experiences prominent histamine effects. Patients should be monitored closely for any symptoms that suggest systemic mastocytosis. In rare cases, other organs may be involved, including the intestines, bone, liver, spleen, and bone marrow. Intestinal involvement may be manifested by chronic diarrhea. The liver and spleen should be palpated for hepatosplenomegaly, and the patient should be monitored for any symptoms of bone involvement. Routine bone marrow and hematologic examinations are not required. Systemic manifestations are more common in adults; infants or children with significant systemic symptoms may require further evaluation. In most infants and young children, urticaria pigmentosa remits spontaneously by adulthood. Children who present at an older age tend to have a more persistent condition that is less likely to resolve.

Plaques and Patches

Pink (Vascular or Other)

Vascular birthmarks can be classified into two groups: tumors and malformations (Table 60.3). Infantile hemangiomas are the most common of the vascular tumors, and their behavior is characterized by a growth phase (endothelial proliferation), followed by a plateau or stabilization phase and then an involutional phase. Vascular malformations are usually apparent at birth and tend to be relatively stable developmental abnormalities of vessels, including any combination of capillaries, veins, arteries, and lymphatic vessels (Table 60.4).

Infantile hemangiomas are the most common benign tumors occurring in children. These lesions develop in approximately 4% of

White infants by 1 year of age. Females are affected approximately 3 times as often as males. The incidence is higher in premature infants. Other risk factors for hemangiomas include low birthweight and multiple gestations. The natural course of infantile hemangiomas includes proliferative and involutional phases that end in complete, spontaneous regression in most cases. There is some thought that infantile hemangiomas may be triggered by hypoxia, either through maternal events or the infant factors.

There are three types of infantile hemangiomas:

1. Superficial hemangiomas, once referred to as strawberry marks, are the most common type (60%). They are bright red with well-demarcated borders (Fig. 60.10). Often, a pale pink stain or bruise-like patch is noted at birth before taking its more characteristic form.
2. Deep hemangiomas, previously known as cavernous hemangiomas, are the least common of the three types (15%). They typically have a blue-violaceous to skin-colored surface. These lesions involve the deep reticular dermis and subcutaneous tissue. These may not be noted until the infant is a few months old.
3. Mixed hemangiomas (25%) possess both superficial and deep components (Fig. 60.11).

Most infantile hemangiomas occur on the head and neck, but any area of the body may be involved. Infantile hemangiomas may be indistinguishable from port-wine stains in the early weeks of life. Lesions must be followed closely during the first few weeks after birth to determine whether a proliferative phase is present. Although the cause of infantile hemangiomas is not clear, their natural course has been well documented. The initial lesion may be a white macule with central threadlike telangiectases or a red macule resembling a port-wine stain. A peripheral zone of pallor representing vasoconstriction may be noted at this stage. Within the first few months of life, the macule becomes raised and enlarges. During the first 6 months of life, infantile hemangiomas proliferate at a rapid rate, and after 6 months, the lesions grow at a slower rate. Deep hemangiomas (and to a lesser extent mixed hemangiomas) have a slightly delayed onset of growth but also have sustained growth when compared to superficial hemangiomas. Involution may begin as early as the first year of life and is heralded by a color change from bright cherry red to dull red violet. Deep hemangiomas start to lose their blue-violet hue. In time, the central portion of the superficial hemangioma develops a grayish-white color that eventually extends to the periphery of the lesion. Lesions on the lips and nose and deep hemangiomas usually involute more slowly. It is not possible to predict precisely how long an infantile hemangioma will take to involute. Statistically, 50% of lesions are gone by 5 years of age, 70% by 7 years, and more than 90% by 9 years. Once resolved, residual skin

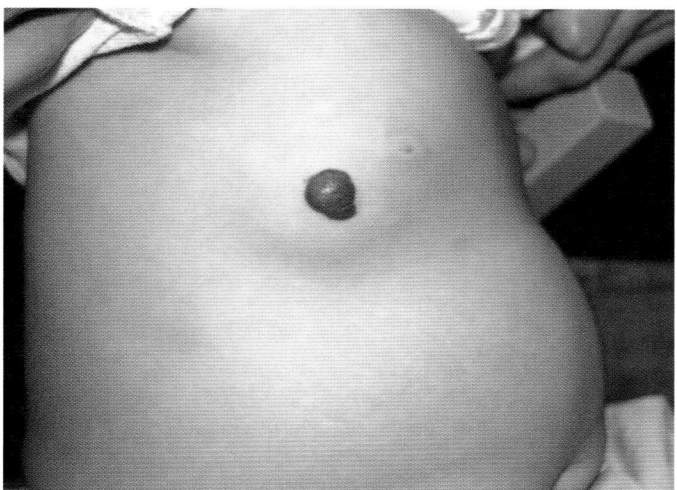

Fig. 60.11 A mixed hemangioma with prominent deep component on the trunk.

changes such as hypopigmentation, atrophy, and telangiectases may be present in up to 10–20% of affected patients. If infantile hemangiomas have grown rapidly during their proliferative phase or were very exophytic, residual fibrofatty tissue may also be seen.

Infantile hemangiomas have many potential complications and associations (Table 60.5). For most, no treatment is needed. Management of infantile hemangiomas is based on a variety of factors. These include the size of the lesion, location of the lesion, age of the patient, rate of growth/involution at the time of presentation, and risk or presence of complications. β Blockers, such as oral propranolol or topical timolol 0.5% solution, are the initial treatment of choice. The most common adverse events are sleep changes and cool extremities, but more serious concerns are hypotension, bradycardia, and hypoglycemia, though these are rare. A pretreatment screening should include clinical examination to identify patients who are at risk for cardiac or pulmonary abnormalities.

Lesions that may need to be treated include those on the midface, labial, periorbital, genital, or diaper area. These lesions warrant close clinical observation during the rapid growth phase of early infancy. Additional therapeutic modalities that are more rarely used include intralesional steroids, pulsed dye laser therapy, surgery, embolization, and sclerosing agents.

Location of infantile hemangiomas (segmental on face or beard distribution) as well as on the spine and lower back should raise concern for PHACE syndrome or PELVIS/SACRAL syndrome, respectively.

Posterior fossa malformations, hemangiomas, arterial anomalies, cardiac defects, and eye abnormalities (PHACE) syndrome is a rare syndrome that affects a subgroup of infants with infantile hemangiomas. It is likely the most common vascular neurocutaneous disorder. The cutaneous findings tend to be larger hemangiomas (>5 cm) and also tend to be segmental, rather than arising from one point. These hemangiomas can be more confluent, have a telangiectatic appearance,

TABLE 60.5	Complications and Syndromes of Infantile Hemangiomas
Location	**Complication**
Lips/perineal/lumbosacral area	Seen in rapidly growing lesions, especially of oral mucosa and genital area
	Risk for infection, scarring, hemorrhage; can be very painful
High output, extensive lesions	Congestive heart failure; hypothyroidism
	Extensive lesions with a large vascular supply may compromise cardiac function
"Beard" distribution	Symptomatic subglottic hemangiomas may occur in 50–60% of patients with extensive "beard" involvement
	Refer for laryngoscopy to evaluate risk for respiratory or airway compromise
	Often manifests within first 2–3 mo of life
Periorbital distribution	Associated ocular complications in up to 80% of patients
	Screening by an ophthalmologist to rule out astigmatism or amblyopia
Ear lesions	Location can cause the obstruction of auditory canal or decreased auditory conduction
	Monitor for otitis media or speech delay
Lumbosacral hemangiomas	High risk for spinal dysraphism; imaging of all midline lumbosacral hemangiomas should be considered
	Increased risk with other lumbosacral abnormalities (e.g., hypertrichosis, dimple, tags)
	Associated urogenital/anogenital anomalies may be present
Large, extensive cervicofacial hemangiomas	PHACE syndrome
Benign neonatal hemangiomatosis	Multiple cutaneous hemangiomas without evidence of visceral hemangiomatosis
	History taking/physical examination should be performed thoroughly to rule out systemic involvement
	Consider liver ultrasound for infants with five or more cutaneous hemangiomas
	Benign clinical course with involution of hemangiomas within first year
Disseminated neonatal hemangiomatosis	Multiple cutaneous hemangiomas with evidence of visceral hemangiomatosis
	Liver most commonly affected; can affect lungs, gastrointestinal tract, eyes, mouth, and tongue
	Work-up necessary to determine the extent of systemic involvement; aggressive treatment usually needed

PHACE, posterior fossa malformations, hemangiomas, arterial anomalies, cardiac defects, and eye abnormalities.

or be composed of grouped papules. They are nearly always located on the head or face. It is important to distinguish them from capillary malformations. Approximately 20% of all infants with segmental facial hemangiomas have extracutaneous anomalies.

Criteria for PHACE syndrome include one segmental hemangioma of the head (>5 cm in diameter) *plus* one major criterion or two minor criteria. Major and minor criteria involve a group of cerebrovascular, structural brain, cardiovascular, ocular, and ventral/midline defects.

Cerebral vascular anomalies are the most common extracutaneous manifestation. The changes tend to be arterial, unlike Sturge-Weber syndrome, which involves capillaries. Imaging (MRI/magnetic resonance angiography [MRA] of the head and neck) greatly aids in the work-up of a patient with a segmental hemangioma on the face/head, looking for arterial changes, as a subset of patients are at increased risk for vasculopathy and ischemic stroke, though this remains a poorly understood complication.

Many congenital brain abnormalities have been noted in patients with PHACE syndrome: The most common ones are malformations of the posterior fossa and cerebellum. Most patients with congenital lesions will have normal neurologic examinations during infancy, and, thus, screening should not be based on abnormalities with the neurologic examination.

Cardiovascular anomalies may be seen on echocardiogram in up to 40% of patients and include coarctation of the aorta (most common), aberrant subclavian aneurysm, ventricular septal defect, and arterial aneurysms. Ocular abnormalities are somewhat rare in PHACE syndrome but include microphthalmia, optic nerve hypoplasia, persistent fetal vasculature, and morning glory disk anomalies. Midline defects including sternal cleft, supraumbilical abdominal raphe, and subtle changes such as sternal pits, dimples, or papules can be seen. A screening echocardiogram should be done for children who are at risk for PHACE syndrome.

Treatment typically is propranolol, and for patients with life-threatening hemangiomas, it can be initiated prior to obtaining imaging results. Propranolol is typically well tolerated in patients with PHACE syndrome, though it is recommended that they undergo a physical exam and echocardiogram prior to initiation, to make sure there is not coarctation of the aortic arch.

PELVIS, LUMBAR, and SACRAL syndromes are all different acronyms to describe disorders that include a segmental hemangioma of the perineal area or midline lower back with underlying abnormalities. The acronyms PELVIS (perineal hemangioma, external genitalia malformations, lipomyelomeningocele, vesicorenal abnormalities, imperforate anus, and skin tag) and SACRAL (spinal dysraphism, anogenital anomalies, cutaneous anomalies, renal and urologic anomalies, associated with angioma of lumbosacral localization) have been used to describe associations with occult spinal dysraphism. The risk of a spinal anomaly is ~35% with a solitary lumbosacral hemangioma. MRI is more sensitive than ultrasound in evaluating for underlying spinal abnormalities in lumbosacral lesions, such as tethered cord.

Capillary malformations (also known as port-wine stains or nevus flammeus) occur in 0.3% of all newborns. They are present at birth and represent progressive ectasia of the superficial vascular plexus. These lesions do not undergo spontaneous resolution. They are usually unilateral and segmental but can be bilateral (Fig. 60.12). The face and neck are the most commonly affected sites. Capillary malformations are typically pink to red during infancy and darken to reddish-purple hues with advancing age. Affected adults frequently have thickened, nodular port-wine stains that may be associated with soft tissue hypertrophy. Capillary malformations occur as isolated cutaneous lesions or in conjunction with other abnormalities.

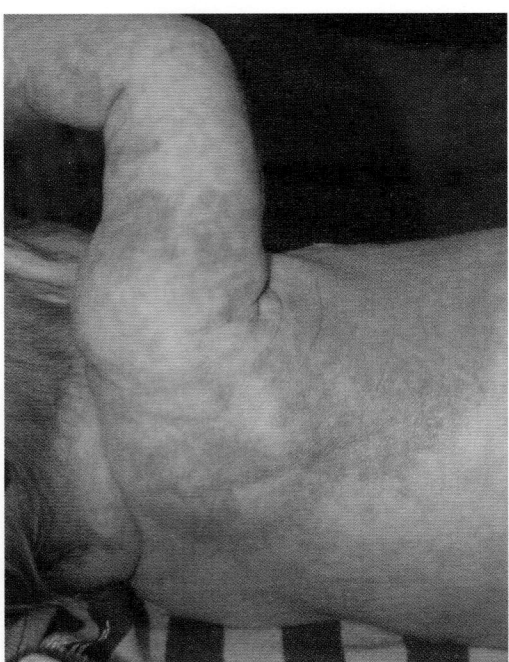

Fig. 60.12 Capillary malformation of the back and flank, extending down the right arm.

Sturge-Weber syndrome includes ipsilateral association of a facial capillary malformation, almost always involving the V1 distribution of the trigeminal nerve, eye abnormalities (primarily glaucoma), and vascular malformations of the ipsilateral leptomeninges and brain. The incidence of Sturge-Weber syndrome is approximately 5–10% in infants with a capillary malformation of the V1 distribution of the trigeminal nerve. Consequences of Sturge-Weber syndrome may include seizures, developmental delay, hemiplegia, and glaucoma. Neuroimaging may be helpful in demonstrating the characteristic calcifications of the leptomeninges and the abnormal cerebral cortex, although these changes may be quite subtle with early studies. Having MRI findings to diagnose Sturge-Weber syndrome prior to developing symptoms does not necessarily result in better outcomes. Newborns at risk for Sturge-Weber syndrome should have careful clinical follow-ups, including monitoring eye pressure for glaucoma. Early referral to a pediatric neurologist for education of parents to help monitor for neurologic symptoms is also recommended.

Other syndromes associated with capillary malformations include Klippel-Trenaunay syndrome and Parkes-Weber syndrome. **Klippel-Trenaunay syndrome** is characterized by a capillary malformation, venous and/or lymphatic malformation, and soft tissue and/or bone overgrowth of the affected limb. **Parkes-Weber syndrome** is the association of arteriovenous malformations, limb overgrowth, and the variable presence of lymphedema and multiple arteriovenous shunts. Klippel-Trenaunay syndrome is a slow-flow capillary-venous malformation, whereas Parkes-Weber syndrome is a fast-flow arterial-venous malformation. Both entities can result in overgrowth and hypertrophy of the affected limb; however, Parkes-Weber syndrome usually results in increased morbidity and clinical consequences.

Treatment of a capillary malformation is best accomplished with the pulsed dye laser. Several treatments are generally required over months to years to achieve desired fading. Depending on the location of the capillary malformation, the response to the pulsed dye laser may be limited. Many experts believe that early initiation of pulsed dye laser therapy results in superior cosmetic results.

Nevus simplex (salmon patch) is the most common vascular lesion in infancy. These lesions consist of ectatic capillaries and are present at birth in about 40% of infants. These pink to red macules can be located on the nape of the neck, glabella, forehead, upper eyelids, and nasolabial regions. More atypical locations include the lateral forehead, nose, upper and lower lip, and back. Unusually persistent or prominent nevus simplex can be associated with Beckwith-Wiedemann syndrome, Nova syndrome, nevus simplex with odontodysplasia, macrocephaly-capillary malformation syndrome, and Roberts-SC syndrome.

No treatment is necessary because most of these fade by 1–2 years of age. Persistent lesions can be treated successfully with the pulsed dye laser if cosmetically disturbing.

Cutis marmorata telangiectatica congenita (CMTC) manifests as an erythematous to dark, bluish-purple, reticulated vascular patch that does not resolve with physiologic warming. This disorder is characteristically more segmental and asymmetric than physiologic cutis marmorata. The clinical findings are most often noted within the first few days of life. Associated features may include cutaneous atrophy and ulcerations of the skin. CMTC has also been reported to be associated with additional abnormalities, including body asymmetry (hypotrophy or hypertrophy of affected limb), other vascular malformations, developmental delay, and glaucoma (with lesions in the V1/V2 trigeminal nerve distribution). CMTC may be difficult to differentiate from a reticulated capillary malformation. The clinical course of CMTC is characterized by gradual fading within the first 1–2 years of life, and treatment is generally not required.

Kasabach-Merritt phenomenon is the presence of thrombocytopenia, hemolytic anemia, hypofibrinogenemia, and consumptive coagulopathy in association with a vascular tumor. Kasabach-Merritt phenomenon is associated with distinct vascular lesions: namely, kaposiform hemangioendothelioma (KHE) or tufted angioma, but not infantile hemangiomas. KHE and tufted angiomas are rare vascular tumors thought to exist on a spectrum. They can be locally destructive, infiltrating underlying soft tissue. Clinical examination findings, histologic findings, and the behavior of associated vascular tumors differ from those of conventional infantile hemangiomas. These lesions are often firm and violaceous with a shiny texture and may proliferate for several years. This condition can be life-threatening and may warrant aggressive multimodal therapeutic modalities. Treatment of choice is complete excision, if possible, but may not be feasible given location, size, or tissue infiltration. Other treatments include sirolimus, high-dose systemic corticosteroids, compression therapy, embolization, irradiation, low-molecular-weight heparin, and interferon alfa. Sirolimus has been used with promising results.

Venous and lymphatic malformations are slow-flow vascular malformations that are often present at birth. **Venous malformations** are bluish, poorly demarcated, compressible masses. The characteristic bluish hue is caused by the presence of ectatic venous channels in the dermis. Often there may be associated swelling with changes in position or activity. Venous malformations can be segmental or more generalized, and radiologic imaging may assist in determining the extent of the lesion. Evaluation for central nervous system abnormalities with cranial imaging is recommended for patients with venous malformations of the face, to rule out developmental intracranial venous abnormalities that usually are asymptomatic. Many lesions manifest with pain caused by muscle involvement or with episodes of thrombosis or hematoma. Other associated risks include bone abnormalities (thinning, demineralization, or hypoplasia) and chronic localized intravascular coagulation. Treatment is aimed at correcting disfigurement and functional impairments. Therapy can include sclerotherapy, deep laser surgery, compression, and surgical excision. In many cases, it may be best to not intervene and to treat symptomatically.

Lymphatic malformations, previously referred to as lymphangiomas, are usually skin-colored masses that may have superficial clear or hemorrhagic vesicles that occasionally leak lymphatic fluid. These lesions can be classified as macrocystic, microcystic, or mixed. Macrocystic malformations often occur on the head and neck and are frequently diagnosed by prenatal ultrasonography. When such a large lymphatic malformation occurs on the head and neck region, it is often referred to as cystic hygroma. Microcystic malformations are usually more superficial lesions with a "frog spawn" appearance (hemorrhagic and clear vesicles) that intermittently leak lymphatic fluid. This characteristic lesion was previously referred to as lymphangioma circumscriptum. These lesions usually become more evident in childhood rather than infancy. Large lymphatic malformations may impinge on vital structures and cause severe compromise in the neonatal period. Cellulitis is a potential complication of lymphatic malformations and may require prophylactic antibiotics if recurrent. Treatment includes sclerotherapy, sirolimus, and surgery in select lesions; surgical therapy of these lesions is often difficult and may result in recurrences and complications.

Hyperpigmented or Darker Pigmented Lesions

Several hyperpigmented or darker pigmented lesions can be seen during the neonatal period and infancy, while others can present later in childhood (Table 60.6).

Congenital melanocytic nevi (CMN) are pigmented macules, papules, patches, or plaques that are present at birth or early infancy in approximately 2–3% of children. The lesions are often tan at birth and become darker and hairier during infancy and childhood. Congenital nevi can be divided into small (<1.5 cm), medium (1.5–20 cm), large (20–40 cm), and giant (>40 cm) lesions on the basis of their projected adult size. In neonates and infants, lesions larger than 9 cm on the head and larger than 6 cm on the body constitute giant CMN (Fig. 60.13). Most CMN are small to medium in size. The incidence of giant melanocytic nevi is approximately 1/20,000 live births. The majority of CMN have a variant in *NRAS*.

The malignant potential of CMN remains an area of great controversy. The risk for malignant transformation in the general population for small and medium congenital nevi is thought to be <1%, and there are no universal guidelines for their management. For comparison, the overall risk for melanoma in the general population in the United States is 2%. Removal of these nevi can wait until later childhood, when local anesthesia and outpatient surgery are feasible.

The risk for malignant transformation of *giant* CMN is another controversial issue. Interestingly, long-term prospective studies have shown melanoma of the central nervous system to be more common than melanoma of the skin. The incidence of melanoma is approximately 8% in those with CMN >60 cm with projected adult size. These large lesions warrant close observation and serial photography. Careful annual or semiannual examinations with palpation of the nevi are essential, as melanoma can arise from deep portions of the nevi with little or no apparent surface alterations. Removal of giant congenital nevi is also controversial from a future-melanoma-risk standpoint. Removal may require extensive grafting as well as soft tissue expansion procedures.

Neurocutaneous melanosis is defined as the presence of giant (>40 cm) and/or multiple CMN, in association with benign or malignant melanocytic infiltration of the leptomeninges. Clinically symptomatic neurocutaneous melanosis substantially worsens the prognosis of large or giant CMN and usually presents around or before 2 years of age, but some may not show symptoms until the second or third decade of life. Most symptomatic patients die within 3 years of the onset of initial neurologic symptoms, typically from central nervous system

TABLE 60.6   Congenital and Acquired Disorders of Hyperpigmentation

Disorder	Congenital or Acquired	Clinical Features
Freckles (ephelides)	Acquired	Small tan to brown, 1- to 5-mm macules Increase in number and pigmentation in summer and spring due to sunlight Seen in fair-skinned individuals in sun-exposed areas
Lentigines	Acquired	Uniform, dark, brown/black 2- to 5-mm macules No seasonal variation or change with sun exposure Can be anywhere on the body, including mucous membranes
Café-au-lait spots	Congenital or acquired	May be seen at birth or later in life Tan to brown discrete macules or patches Round or oval Six or more lesions >5 mm in prepubertal persons meets diagnostic criteria for neurofibromatosis (NF) NF lesions are smooth and well demarcated McCune-Albright syndrome spots are larger and more jagged
Dermal melanocytosis (mongolian spots)	Congenital	Brown, blue-gray patches often seen on lower trunk Seen usually in African-Americans, Asians, or Native Americans Usually fades over time
Nevus of Ota	Congenital or acquired	50% present at birth; 50% develop in second decade Unilateral, blue-gray pigmentation in trigeminal nerve distribution Commonly involves ipsilateral sclera May darken or enlarge over time
Nevus of Ito	Congenital or acquired	Patchy blue-gray pigmentation of shoulder, supraclavicular area May increase in size and color over time
Congenital melanocytic nevus	Congenital	Tan, brown, dark brown macules, patches, plaques, seen at birth or early infancy Variable color and texture Large, giant, or multiple nevi increase risk for neurocutaneous melanosis
Nevus spilus (speckled lentiginous nevus)	Congenital or acquired	Well-demarcated, hyperpigmented patch with smaller, darker macules and papules within larger patch May be extensive and segmental in distribution Small risk for malignant transformation
Acquired melanocytic nevi	Acquired	May start as hyperpigmented macules (junctional melanocytic nevi) Over time, can become elevated papules (compound melanocytic nevi) Peaks in number during second and third decade of life Abnormalities in color, borders, size, symmetry may suggest malignancy
Melanoma	Acquired	Variegation in color, texture, or border of congenital or acquired melanocytic nevi Rare in childhood or infancy Risk correlated with family history and sun exposure in childhood

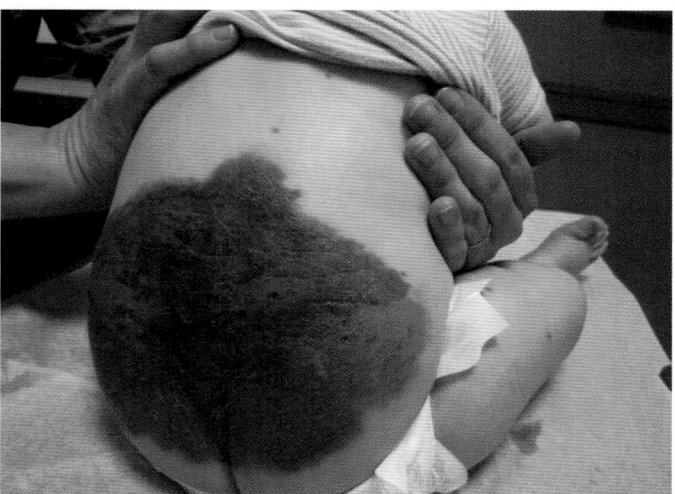

Fig. 60.13 Giant congenital melanocytic nevus of the lower back. Imaging should be considered to evaluate for tethered cord or spinal dysraphism, as well as melanosis of the spine or brain.

melanoma or mechanical obstruction. The most frequent clinical manifestations include hydrocephalus, seizures, papilledema, headaches, increase in head circumference, paresis, and developmental delay. Location overlying the axial skeleton and many satellite lesions are predictors of neurocutaneous melanosis.

Screening MRI of the central nervous system is currently the best predictor of all adverse outcomes. MRI with contrast of the head *and* spine within the first 6 months of life is suggested in newborns with giant CMN, particularly in the posterior axial distribution and especially if satellite nevi are present. An MRI is also recommended for any infant with two or more CMN, regardless of size. MRI abnormalities of the brain have been identified in asymptomatic patients with giant or multiple CMN. The most common imaging abnormalities in asymptomatic patients seen were T1 shortening in the cerebellum, temporal lobes, pons, and medulla. Radiologic findings can be very subtle and may be missed by radiologists unfamiliar with this entity. The risk of melanoma is higher in those with multiple CMN, particularly if neurologic abnormalities are noted on screening MRI.

Café-au-lait macules are well-circumscribed tan macules that usually measure <0.5 cm but may be as large as 15–20 cm in diameter. The

TABLE 60.7	Congenital and Acquired Disorders of Hypopigmentation and Depigmentation	
Disorder	**Congenital or Acquired**	**Clinical Features**
Piebaldism	Congenital	Autosomal dominant inheritance Leukoderma of frontal scalp White forelock Usually involves face, neck, trunk, flank, and extremities Waardenburg syndrome is a variant, with sensorineural deafness, limb defects, and Hirschsprung disease
Nevus depigmentosus	Congenital	Well-circumscribed hypopigmented patch (not typically depigmented) May be isolated or segmental Usually present at birth or infancy Wood lamp may aid in diagnosis Often found on trunk or extremities
Hypomelanosis of Ito	Congenital	Whorls or streaks of hypopigmentation that follow lines of Blaschko Usually present at birth, but may present in first few years of life Can be associated with central nervous system, eye, or musculoskeletal abnormalities
Nevus anemicus	Congenital	Rubbing or temperature change causes erythema of surrounding skin Often unilateral and on trunk Not accentuated by Wood lamp Asymptomatic
Ash leaf spot	Congenital	Hypopigmented macules/patches often present at birth Wood lamp may aid in diagnosis Solitary lesion often of no significance Multiple lesions are associated with tuberous sclerosis
Vitiligo	Acquired	Complete loss of pigment in involved areas May be segmental in distribution Hyperpigmentation can be seen at the edges of lesions Infrequently seen with autoimmune disorders, such as hypothyroidism
Albinism	Congenital	Complete depigmentation or hypopigmentation in skin Affects eyes and hair Increased risk for skin cancer

lesions are found on any cutaneous site and may be present at birth or appear during early childhood. Although café-au-lait spots are seen in 10–20% of normal individuals, the presence of many macules should raise the clinical suspicion of NF or other genetic disorders (see Table 60.6). The presence of six or more café-au-lait spots (>0.5 cm in prepubertal children; >1.5 cm in postpubertal children) fulfills one of the diagnostic criteria for NF-1. Although the lesions are not pathognomonic, they are present in most patients with NF and tend to be larger and more numerous. Café-au-lait spots have also been associated with tuberous sclerosis, McCune-Albright syndrome, Turner syndrome, Bloom syndrome, ataxia-telangiectasia, Russell-Silver syndrome, Fanconi anemia, epidermal nevus syndrome, Gaucher disease, and Chédiak-Higashi syndrome.

Dermal melanocytosis (mongolian spots) are large, poorly demarcated, slate-gray to blue-black patches usually located over the buttocks or lumbosacral region of normal infants. The condition occurs in approximately 80–90% of Black infants, 75% of Asian infants, and 10% of White infants. Dermal melanocytosis may be single or multiple and frequently measure up to 10–20 cm in diameter. This benign disorder is present at birth, usually fades during early childhood, and necessitates no therapeutic intervention. In rare cases, the lesions may persist into adulthood and may benefit from therapy with lasers that treat dermal pigmentation. These lesions should not be confused with bruises. Dermal melanocytosis is also seen in Hurler, Hunter, GM1 gangliosidosis, Niemann-Pick, mucolipidosis, and mannosidosis syndromes.

The nevus of Ota and nevus of Ito are special variants of dermal melanocytosis commonly seen in Asian and Black individuals. In contrast to mongolian spots, these conditions tend to persist throughout adulthood. The **nevus of Ota** is a slate-gray to blue-black patch located in the distribution of the trigeminal nerve. The condition is usually unilateral and involves the forehead, temple, periorbital region, nose, and cheek. Pigmentation of the sclera, iris, and choroid occurs in about 50% of affected individuals. The disorder may be cosmetically disfiguring, and laser treatment may be promising in some cases. The **nevus of Ito** is a similar lesion occurring in the distribution of the lateral supraclavicular and brachial nerves. The condition is usually unilateral and involves the shoulder, neck, upper arm, scapular, and/or deltoid regions. It may be seen alone or in conjunction with the nevus of Ota.

Hypopigmented and Depigmented Lesions

These conditions are often cosmetically disfiguring and persistent. They can be markers of serious systemic diseases. Pigmentary disorders may be localized or generalized; congenital or acquired; and transient, stable, or progressive (Table 60.7).

Nevus depigmentosus is a benign, solitary, hypopigmented macule or patch that is noted at birth. It is not depigmented as the name suggests. It typically remains stable in size and may grow in proportion to the patient as they grow. It should be differentiated from vitiligo.

Ash leaf spots are hypopigmented macules, sometimes present at birth or within the first few months or years of life, that allow early identification of individuals with tuberous sclerosis (Fig. 60.14). Although occasionally observed in normal infants, the characteristic lesions are present in up to 90% of patients with tuberous sclerosis. They are

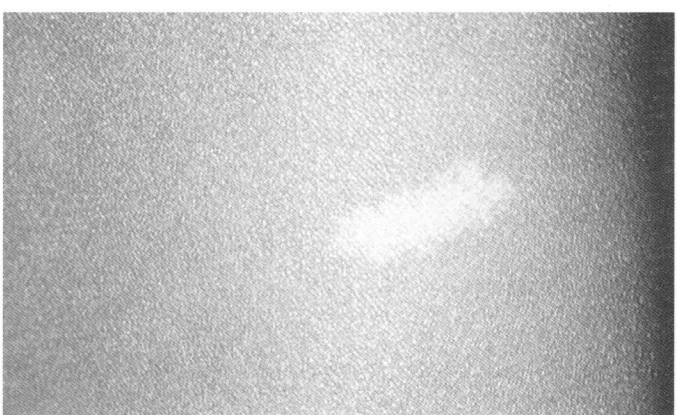

Fig. 60.14 Ash leaf macule of tuberous sclerosis.

usually 2–3 cm in size and are located on the trunk and extremities. The macules may be lancet shaped or may have a confetti-like or irregularly shaped appearance. *Wood lamp examination may facilitate identification.* Although tuberous sclerosis is an autosomal dominant disorder, spontaneous gene variants are responsible for up to 50% of new cases. Other cutaneous findings include facial angiofibromas (adenoma sebaceum), periungual or subungual fibromas, gingival fibromas, shagreen patches (connective tissue hamartomas), and fibrous plaques (typically on the forehead). Systemic manifestations include seizures, intellectual disability, cardiac rhabdomyomas, renal angiomyolipomas and cysts, retinal nodular hamartomas, and pulmonary cysts. Imaging studies of the brain may demonstrate cortical tubers or subependymal nodules, which are pathognomonic for tuberous sclerosis.

Piebaldism is characterized by circumscribed areas of depigmentation in the newborn. The leukoderma is usually located on the frontal scalp and is associated with a white forelock; however, the depigmented patches characteristically involve the trunk, upper arms, and legs. Hyperpigmented or normally pigmented macules or patches may occur within the depigmented patches. This rare condition is transmitted in an autosomal dominant pattern. The disorder is usually present at birth but may not be recognized until later because of the light color of neonatal skin. A Wood lamp may enhance the contrast between depigmented and normal skin.

Piebaldism is a stable condition throughout life, and most affected individuals are otherwise normal. Sun protection and cosmetic camouflage of the depigmented skin are the mainstays of therapy.

Waardenburg syndrome is a rare genetic disorder characterized by a white forelock, areas of leukoderma, congenital sensorineural deafness, heterochromia of the irides, and lateral displacement of the medial canthi. Other features may include a flattened nasal bridge, confluent eyebrows, hypoplasia of the nasal alae, speech impairment that may or may not be related to presence of a cleft lip or palate, and various skeletal abnormalities. It is most commonly inherited in an autosomal dominant fashion, though autosomal recessive inheritance patterns are sometimes seen.

Albinism is manifested by diffuse congenital hypopigmentation or depigmentation of the skin, hair, and eyes. This heterogeneous group of disorders is composed of approximately 10 types of oculocutaneous albinism and 5 forms of ocular albinism. Most types of oculocutaneous albinism are inherited in an autosomal recessive pattern. The variants of ocular albinism are transmitted in an X-linked or autosomal recessive mode of inheritance.

The various forms of albinism can usually be diagnosed by findings on physical examination. These features include absent or reduced pigmentation of skin and hair and ophthalmologic findings such as foveal hypoplasia, nystagmus, photophobia, transillumination of the irides, fundal depigmentation, and decreased visual acuity. Patients should be monitored closely by ophthalmologists and evaluated for hearing loss. In White persons, the skin is usually milk white and the hair is white, blond, or light brown. The pupils are usually pink, and the irides are blue or gray. In African-Americans, the skin may appear tan or white and is frequently freckled. The hair is usually blond or red, and the eyes are blue or hazel.

Treatment of albinism includes photoprotection and sun avoidance. Individuals are predisposed to severe actinic damage and should be monitored closely for the development of actinic keratoses, basal cell carcinomas, squamous cell carcinomas, and melanomas.

Other

Nevus sebaceus of Jadassohn is a hamartoma of sebaceous gland derivation. Typically present at birth, these lesions are variable in size, usually solitary, and located on the scalp, face, and neck. During infancy, they are well-circumscribed, hairless, yellowish-orange, smooth, velvety, or waxy plaques. These nevi tend to thicken and become verrucous during puberty.

Because up to 15% of these lesions develop secondary benign or malignant neoplasms during adolescence or adulthood, prophylactic surgical excision is recommended before puberty.

Dermoid cysts are nontender, noncompressible, firm, congenital subcutaneous nodules found along sites of closure of embryonic clefts. Dermoids are lined by stratified squamous epithelium that contains mature adnexal structures. Although these lesions can be noted in newborns, they may not be detected until later in infancy or in childhood after the lesion enlarges or becomes inflamed. Lesions are often described as rubbery and may be blue to skin-colored in appearance. A tuft of hair may be seen protruding from an orifice in the dermoid. Dermoid cysts are often found in the head and neck region, often the lateral portion of an eyebrow.

The most important concern with dermoid cysts is the potential for an intracranial connection. Up to 25% of midline or nasal dermoid cysts may have an intracranial connection; all midline head and spinal lesions should be imaged. If a connection is present, the patient is at risk for infection because the dermoid cyst and sinus can serve as a portal of entry for bacteria. These patients should be referred to neurosurgery for removal and repair. Dermoid cysts that are not midline, including those commonly seen at the lateral brow area, should also be excised because of the potential risk for infection and bony erosion. After surgical excision, lesions do not usually recur.

Aplasia cutis congenita is a heterogeneous group of disorders in which there is a congenital absence of skin (Fig. 60.15). This disorder may involve the epidermis, dermis, and subcutaneous tissues. The most common type of aplasia cutis is membranous aplasia cutis. These lesions are well-demarcated, small, oval, 1- to 5-cm defects on the vertex of the scalp. They are easily identified by their classic "punched-out" appearance and may have an atrophic surface with a glistening, membrane-like surface at birth. In older children, these lesions resemble scars. If the lesion is associated with a hair collar or midline in location, the clinician should evaluate for the potential of cranial dysraphism.

The defect is usually solitary; however, in a minority of patients, multiple sites may be affected. Aplasia cutis can also occur on the trunk and limbs, where the defects are often bilateral and symmetric; extremity lesions must be distinguished from EB. Aplasia cutis in the midline lumbosacral area is of particular importance because it may be associated with spinal dysraphism.

Lesions of membranous aplasia cutis usually necessitate no further investigation, and gradual epithelialization typically occurs spontaneously. However, large, deep, or widespread lesions with underlying bone defects may necessitate surgical intervention to facilitate healing.

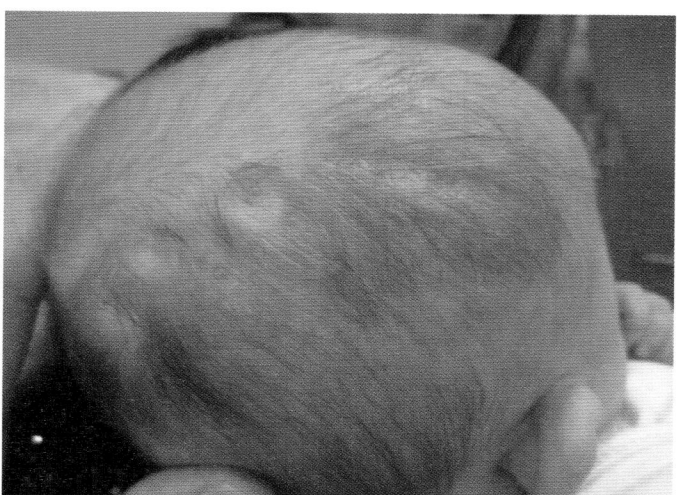

Fig. 60.15 Congenital absence of skin (aplasia cutis congenita) on the scalp of a neonate; multiple lesions can be seen.

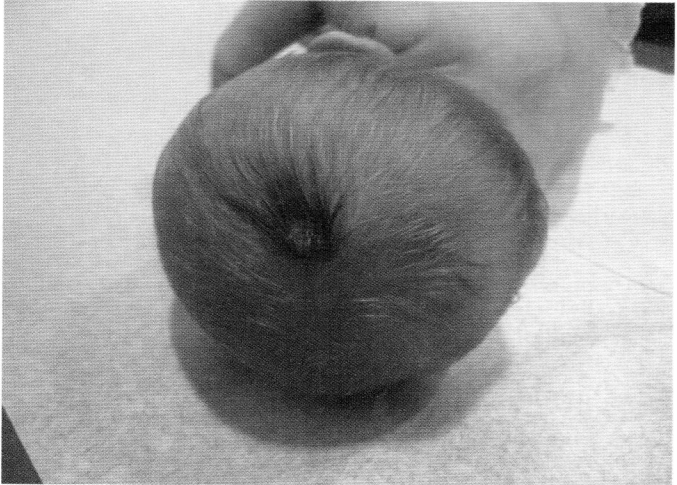

Fig. 60.16 A classic hair collar sign (from aplasia cutis).

The term **hair collar sign** is a designation for hypertrichosis that usually either partly or completely encircles a congenital scalp lesion (Fig. 60.16). Usually the ring of hair is denser, darker, and coarser in texture than the normal scalp hair. A hair collar sign surrounding a congenital scalp nodule is a marker for cranial dysraphism, including encephaloceles and meningoceles. If a hair collar sign is seen in combination with a capillary malformation or aplasia cutis, the risk for cranial dysraphism is increased substantially. Therefore, all congenital midline lesions with a hair collar sign should be imaged to evaluate for an intracranial connection. MRI is the gold standard, but it occasionally misses a small intracranial connection. Lack of a hair collar sign in aplasia cutis correlates with a negative predictive value of abnormal imaging findings. Therefore, MRI is likely not needed in patients with aplasia cutis who do not have a hair collar sign.

Aplasia cutis typically is an isolated finding, but it can be associated with some syndromes, including Adams-Oliver syndrome. This rare condition also includes CMTC and limb defects. In the setting of aplasia cutis, a good physical and evaluation for limb abnormalities is recommended.

Lumbosacral hypertrichosis may be a normal variant, especially in certain ethnic groups. However, hypertrichosis in this area in association

with other stigmata indicative of a neurologic defect is highly suggestive of spinal dysraphism. The area may be poorly circumscribed, and the hair can be light or dark. The hypertrichosis is often present at birth. Complete neurologic examination should be performed. There are no defined parameters to determine further evaluation of isolated hypertrichosis, though suspicion for spinal dysraphism is higher if additional cutaneous markers, such as a vascular stain or a mass, are also present. If a spinal defect is suspected, further evaluation by MRI of the spine is necessary.

Lumbosacral dimples are common findings in neonates. Large, deep dimples that are located in the superior portion of the gluteal crease should be radiologically imaged to rule out dermal sinuses communicating directly with the spinal canal. These dimples should not be probed because of the potential communication with the spinal canal. Sacral dimples seen in association with other cutaneous findings such as hypertrichosis, vascular birthmarks, a mass, or a deviated gluteal cleft carry particularly high risk for spinal dysraphism. Imaging should be performed with MRI of the spine as ultrasound has low sensitivity for subtle findings.

Infantile hemangiomas that overlie the midline of the back are strong markers for spinal dysraphism, most often lipomyelomeningocele, intraspinal lipoma, or a tethered cord. Infantile hemangiomas that are larger than 4 cm and overlap the midline appear to carry greater risk for spinal dysraphism, and MRI should be performed. The risk for spinal dysraphism is increased when hemangioma is seen in association with other cutaneous findings such as sacral dimples, hypertrichosis, or a deviated gluteal cleft.

A solitary midline capillary malformation of the back without additional clinical findings may be a marker for spinal dysraphism, but this association is less clear. All affected infants should be evaluated for additional neurocutaneous stigmata. If a lumbosacral capillary malformation is detected with other cutaneous markers of spinal dysraphism, imaging is warranted.

TRANSIENT AND PHYSIOLOGIC CHANGES TO THE SKIN

Many entities unique to newborns are caused by physiologic phenomena in response to the infant's transition to the new environment. Most such entities are benign and self-limited.

Cutis Marmorata

Cutis marmorata is characterized by symmetric reticulated cyanosis involving the trunk and extremities. This marbled appearance usually appears when the skin is cool and resolves upon rewarming of the infant. This benign condition typically improves with age. When this vascular pattern is seen in older infants or children, it may be associated with Down syndrome, Cornelia de Lange syndrome, or hypothyroidism.

Cutis marmorata should be differentiated from CMTC. The persistent cutis marmorata of CMTC is characteristically asymmetric; often segmental, mottled, or marble-like; and more localized than physiologic cutis marmorata. In addition, the reticulated mottling of CMTC is darker in color and does not resolve with rewarming. Although CMTC improves with age, the abnormal vascular pattern is more persistent than that seen in physiologic cutis marmorata. It may be an isolated entity or may have distinct associations, including atrophy or hypertrophy of the affected extremity, ulcerations, or coexistent vascular malformations and tumors, and other extracutaneous anomalies. If CMTC is generalized or involves the face, patients should be evaluated for glaucoma as well.

Harlequin Color Change

The harlequin color change is a distinctive condition observed in infants lying on their sides. It is characterized by marked erythema on the dependent side of the infant's body with simultaneous blanching

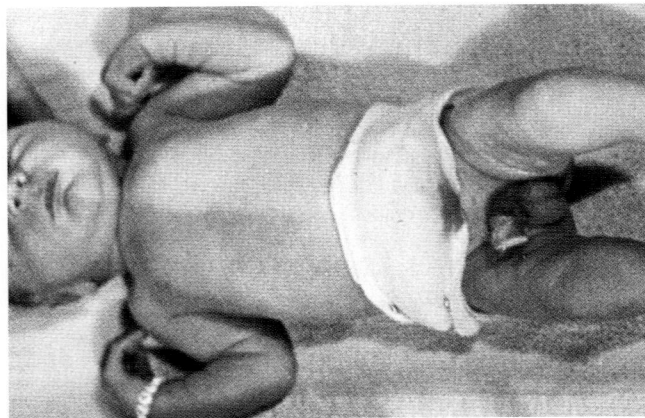

Fig. 60.17 The dependent side is bright red in this infant with the harlequin color change. (From Cohen BA, ed. *Pediatric Dermatology*. 4th ed. Philadelphia: Elsevier; 2013:19, Fig. 2.10.)

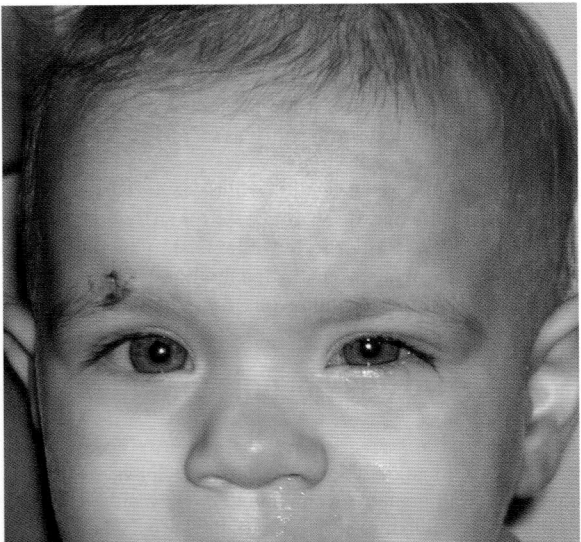

Fig. 60.18 Harlequin syndrome. Transient unilateral flushing associated with hyperhidrosis, tearing, and rhinorrhea. (From Eichenfield LF, Frieden IJ, Mathes EF, et al., eds. *Neonatal and Infant Dermatology*. 3rd ed. Philadelphia: Elsevier; 2015:420, Fig. 25.17.)

of the nondependent side (Fig. 60.17). This phenomenon occurs more often in premature infants but may be observed in full-term newborns. The change may be caused by autonomic immaturity, which results in altered peripheral vascular tone.

Although it typically occurs within the first 3 weeks of life, harlequin color change is most often noted at 2–5 days of age. The changes develop abruptly and usually resolve within 20 minutes.

The **harlequin syndrome** is characterized by hemifacial flushing, tearing, and rhinorrhea with contralateral hypohidrosis (Fig. 60.18). **Frey syndrome** (auriculotemporal nerve syndrome) is characterized by unilateral (occasionally bilateral) facial flushing and sweating, triggered by the introduction of solid foods.

Acrocyanosis

The normal newborn usually displays a bluish-purple discoloration of the hands, feet, and lips. Referred to as acrocyanosis, this typically occurs in association with crying or cold stress and can be seen in >30% of infants. It results from increased peripheral arteriolar tone, which leads to vasospasm and subsequent venous pooling.

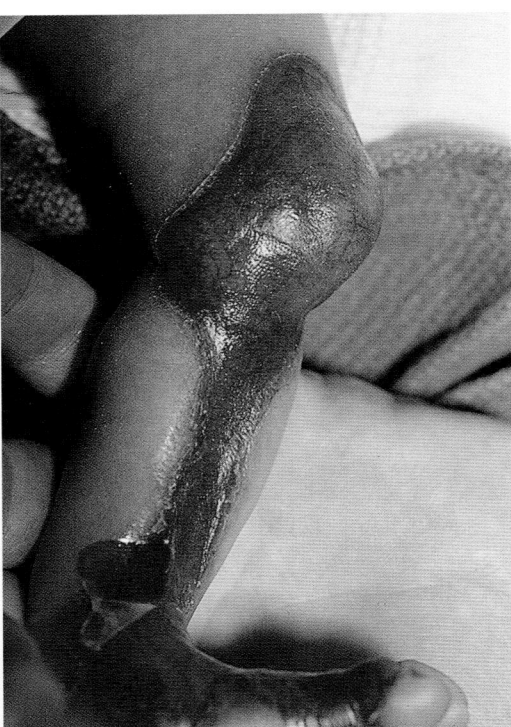

Fig. 60.19 Congenital localized absence of skin can be seen in all types of epidermolysis bullosa. (From Eichenfield LF, Frieden IJ, Mathes EF, et al., eds. *Neonatal and Infant Dermatology*. 3rd ed. Philadelphia: Elsevier; 2015:143, Fig. 11.2.)

Acrocyanosis should be differentiated from central cyanosis, which is noted on mucosal surfaces. Physiologic acrocyanosis gradually resolves spontaneously during the neonatal period.

RARE AND GENETIC DISORDERS

Epidermolysis Bullosa

EB represents a group of diseases manifested by spontaneous or friction (trauma)-related skin and oral mucosa–related fragility and bulla formation, inherited as autosomal or dominant disorders. Subgroups include:

EB simplex (suprabasal, basal) (Figs. 60.19 and 60.20 and Table 60.8)
EB junctional (Herlitz, other) (Table 60.9)
EB dystrophic (dominant, recessive) (Table 60.10) and Kindler syndrome

Neonates may present at birth with lower extremity ulcerations (congenital localized absence of skin: Bart syndrome) that may resemble cutis aplasia (see Fig. 60.19). Blisters, bulla, and erosions also develop after birth secondary to minor trauma (see Fig. 60.20).

More severe subtypes may heal with scarring; infection is a risk in all subtypes. EB is also associated with congenital pyloric outlet obstruction; airway (laryngeal involvement) obstruction is a less common complication.

Ichthyosis

These heterogeneous disorders are characterized by cutaneous scaling in a syndromic or nonsyndromic pattern, presenting in the newborn as lamellar ichthyosis, congenital ichthyosiform erythroderma, or collodium baby (Figs. 60.21, 60.22, and 60.23 and Table 60.11).

Neutrophilic Dermatosis

Sweet syndrome is an acute febrile neutrophilic dermatosis that is often associated with another primary disorder including congenital

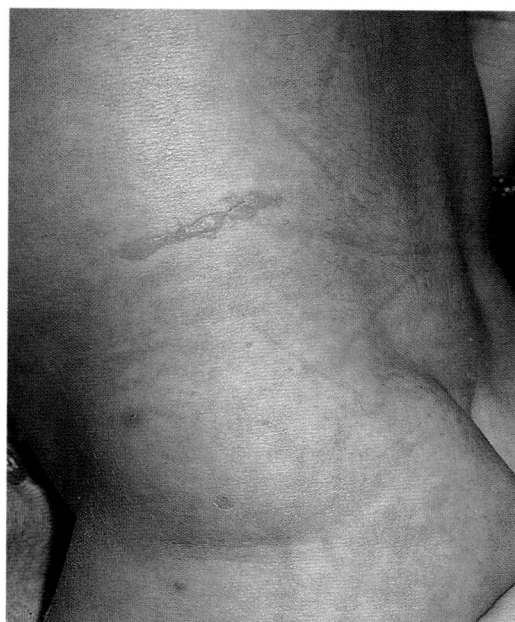

Fig. 60.20 Blistering caused by the edge of a diaper in an infant with a milder form of epidermolysis bullosa. (From Eichenfield LF, Frieden IJ, Mathes EF, et al., eds. *Neonatal and Infant Dermatology*. 3rd ed. Philadelphia: Elsevier; 2015:143, Fig. 11.3.)

TABLE 60.8 Characteristics of Major Forms of Epidermolysis Bullosa Simplex (EBS), Basal

Type	Clinical Manifestations
EBS, localized (formerly Weber-Cockayne)	Easy blistering on palms and soles
	May be focal keratoderma of palms and soles in adults
	~25% show oral mucosal erosions
	Rarely show reticulated pigmentation, especially on arms and trunk, and punctate keratoderma (EBS with mottled pigmentation)
EBS, generalized, intermediate (formerly Koebner)	Generalized blistering
	Variable mucosal involvement
	Focal keratoderma of palms and soles
	Nail involvement in 20%
	Improves with advancing age
EBS, generalized, severe (formerly Dowling-Meara)	Most severe in neonate, infant; improves beyond childhood
	Large, generalized blisters; later, smaller (herpetiform) blisters
	Mucosal blistering, including esophageal
	Nails thickened, shed but regrow
	May have natal teeth
EBS with mottled pigmentation	Reticulated hyperpigmentation, especially on arms and trunk
	Punctate keratoses and keratoderma

From *Hurwitz Clinical Pediatric Dermatology*. 5th ed. Philadelphia: Elsevier; 2016:319, Table 13-2.

TABLE 60.9 Characteristics of Major Forms of Junctional Epidermolysis Bullosa (JEB)

Type	Clinical Manifestations
JEB, generalized severe (formerly Herlitz)	50% of patients die by 2 yr old
	Blisters heal with atrophic scarring but no milia
	Periungual and fingerpad blistering, erythema
	Blistering of oral and esophageal mucosae
	Laryngeal and airway involvement with early hoarseness
	Later, perioral granulation tissue with sparing of lips
	Anonychia
	Dental enamel hypoplasia, excessive caries
	Growth retardation
	Anemia
JEB, generalized intermediate (formerly non-Herlitz)	Less severe, but similar manifestations to Herlitz type, including dental, nail, and laryngeal involvement
	Granulation tissue is rare
	Perinasal cicatrization
	Less mucosal involvement
	Alopecia
	Anemia but not as severe as JEB, generalized severe
JEB, localized	Localized blisters without residual scarring or granulation tissue
	Minimal mucosal involvement
	Dental and nail abnormalities as in JEB, generalized severe
JEB, generalized with pyloric atresia	Usually lethal in neonatal period
	Generalized blistering, leading to atrophic scarring
	May be born with large areas of cutis aplasia
	No granulation tissue
	Nail dystrophy or anonychia
	Pyloric atresia, genitourinary malformations
	Rudimentary ears
	Dental enamel hypoplasia (survivors)
	Variable anemia, growth retardation, mucosal blistering

From *Hurwitz Clinical Pediatric Dermatology*. 5th ed. Philadelphia: Elsevier; 2016:321, Table 13-4.

usually on the face and upper extremities (Fig. 60.24). Pathologic variants in *POMP* are associated with immune deficiency, autoimmunity, and neonatal-onset Sweet syndrome.

CANDLE (early-onset chronic atypical neutrophilic dermatitis with lipodystrophy and elevated temperature) presents in the newborn with recurrent lesions and fevers similar to Sweet syndrome. CANDLE is due to pathologic variants in *PSMB8*, which is a component of immunoproteasome. The rash precedes the lipodystrophy (Fig. 60.25) and is seen on the trunk, limbs, fingers, and face. The rash is annular and produces hyperpigmentation after an acute episode.

Immune Disregulation

Neonatal-onset multisystem inflammatory disease (NOMID), also known as chronic infantile neurologic cutaneous and articular syndrome (CINCA), may manifest at birth or infancy with intermittent fevers and a papular urticaria-like nonpruritic rash (Fig. 60.26). During episodes there may be arthralgias and arthritis leading in

infection (HIV), immune deficiency (common variable immune deficiency, chronic granulomatous disease), neoplasia, inflammatory bowel disease, lupus, and autoinflammatory disorders. It is characterized by high fevers with erythematous, painful raised papular nodules

TABLE 60.10 Characteristics of Major Forms of Dystrophic Epidermolysis Bullosa

Type	Clinical Manifestations
Dominant dystrophic	Onset at birth to early infancy
	Blistering predominates on dorsum of hands, elbows, knees, and lower legs
	Milia associated with scarring
	Some patients develop scarlike lesions, especially on the trunk
	80% have nail dystrophy
Recessive dystrophic, severe generalized	Present at birth
	Widespread blistering, scarring, milia
	Deformities: pseudosyndactyly, joint contractures
	Severe involvement of mucous membranes, nails; alopecia
	Growth retardation, poor nutrition
	Anemia
	Mottled, carious teeth
	Osteoporosis, delayed puberty, cardiomyopathy, glomerulonephritis, renal amyloidosis, IgA nephropathy
	Predisposition to squamous cell carcinoma in heavily scarred areas
Recessive dystrophic, generalized intermediate	Generalized blisters from birth with milia, scarring
	Less anemia, growth retardation, mucosal but more esophageal issues with advancing age

IgA, immunoglobulin A.
From *Hurwitz Clinical Pediatric Dermatology*. 5th ed. Philadelphia: Elsevier; 2016:323, Table 13-6.

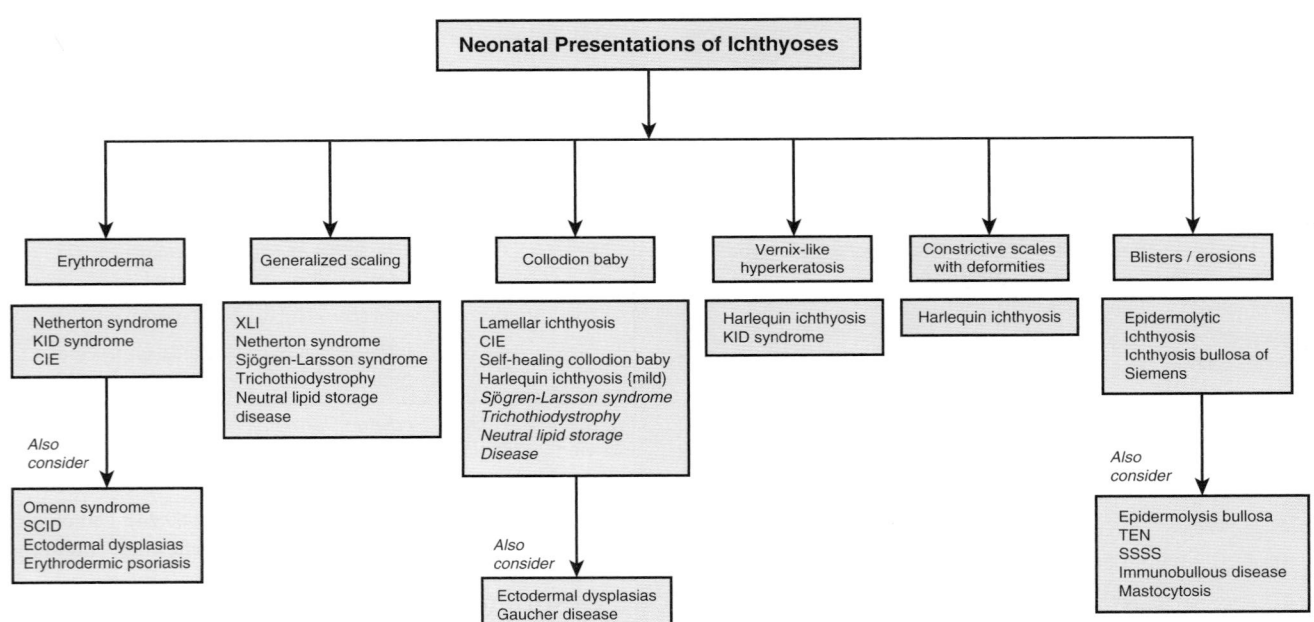

Fig. 60.21 Neonatal presentations of ichthyoses. The spectrum of possible presentations of ichthyosis in the neonate and the possible underlying forms of ichthyosis. In some cases, disorders beyond ichthyosis must be considered ("*also consider*"). Sjögren-Larsson syndrome, trichothiodystrophy, and neutral lipid storage disease are italicized, as they rarely present as collodion babies. CIE, congenital ichthyosiform erythroderma; KID syndrome, keratitis-ichthyosis-deafness syndrome; SCID, severe combined immunodeficiency; SSSS, staphylococcal scalded skin syndrome; TEN, toxic epidermal necrolysis; XLI, X-linked ichthyosis. (From Craiglow BG. Ichthyosis in the newborn. *Semin Perinatol.* 2013;37:26–31 [Fig. 2, p. 28].)

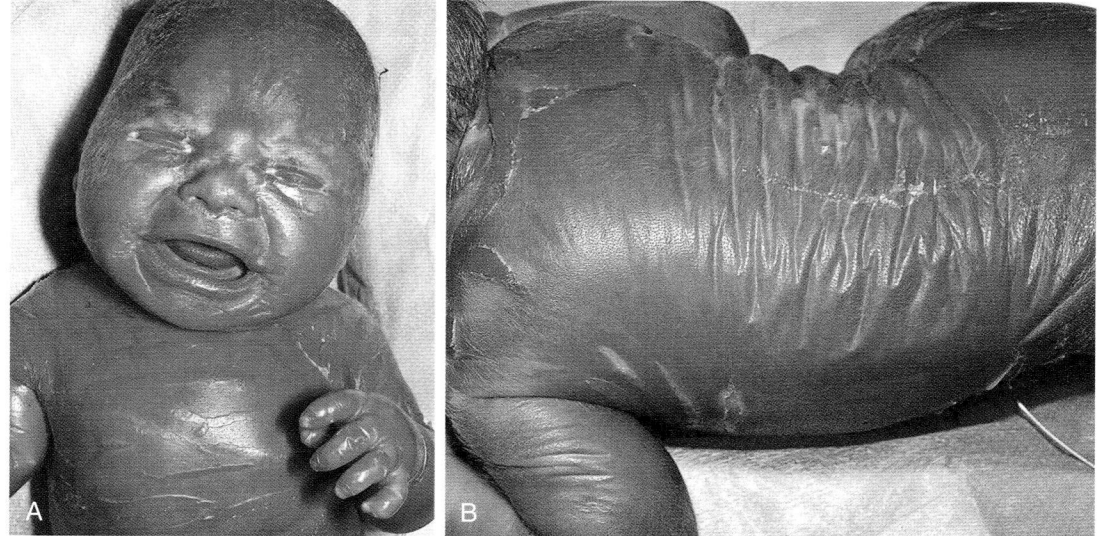

Fig. 60.22 Collodion baby. *A,* A shiny transparent membrane covered this baby at birth. *B,* She later developed lamellar ichthyosis. (From Cohen BA, ed. *Pediatric Dermatology.* 4th ed. Philadelphia: Elsevier; 2013:26, Fig. 2.29.)

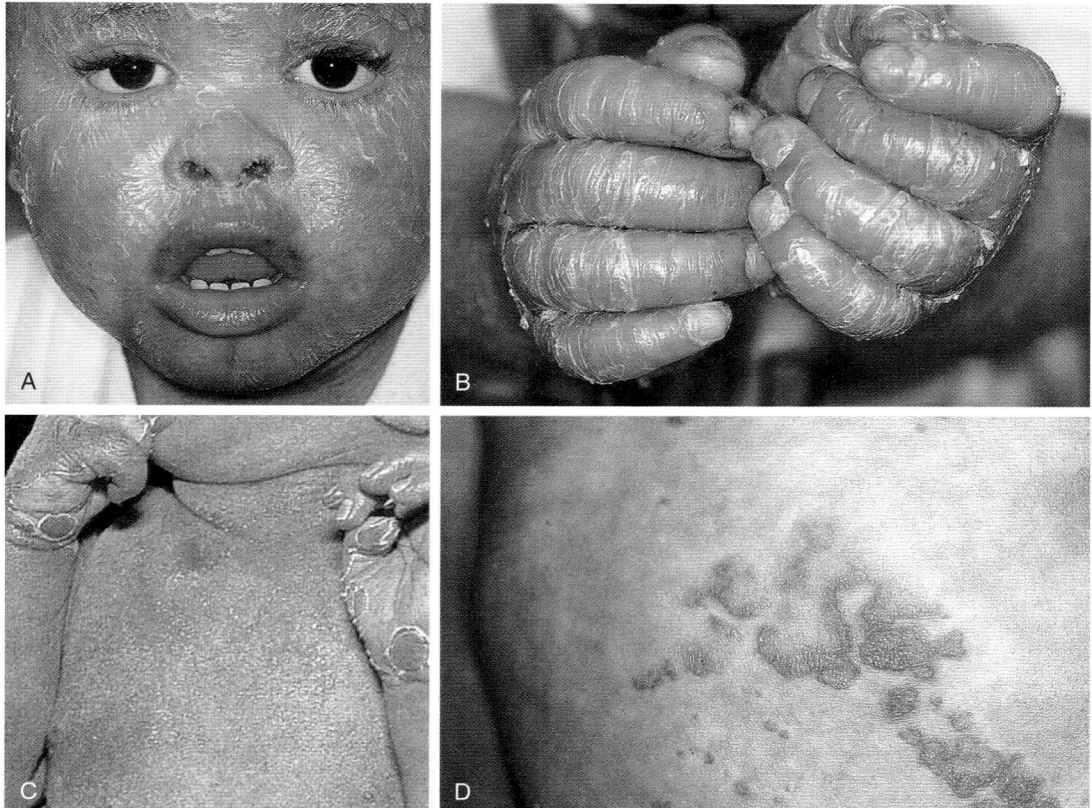

Fig. 60.23 Congenital ichthyosiform erythroderma in two children. *A,* Congenital erythroderma persisted in this child. *B,* Note the marked scaling on her hands. *C,* Generalized erythema with fine scaling was noted on the first day of life. *D,* Shortly after his first birthday, he developed a new pattern of migrating, scaly, erythematous plaques typical of Netherton syndrome. Microscopic examination of his hair revealed trichorrhexis invaginata (bamboo hair). (From Cohen BA, ed. *Pediatric Dermatology.* 4th ed. Philadelphia: Elsevier; 2013:28, Fig. 2.31.)

TABLE 60.11   Ichthyoses and Ichthyosis Syndromes

VARIANT	Genetics	Incidence	Clinical Features	Onset
Congenital ichthyosiform erythroderma OMIM #242100	Autosomal recessive *TGM-1, ABCA12, NIPAL4 (ICHTHYIN) ALOX12B, ALOXE3*	1/50,000–1/100,000	Collodion baby Fine white scale on trunk, face, and scalp Large scale on legs Variable erythroderma	Birth
Lamellar ichthyosis OMIM #242300	Autosomal recessive *TGM-1, ABCA12, NIPAL4 (ICHTHYIN), CYP4F22, LIPN*	1/100,000	Collodion baby Generalized large, dark, platelike scale Ectropion, eclabium Mild palmoplantar keratoderma	Birth
Epidermolytic hyperkeratosis OMIM #113800	Autosomal dominant (most common) Autosomal recessive, sporadic *KRT1, KRT10*	Rare	Widespread blisters at birth Increased erythema, scale with age Marked scale in intertriginous areas, palms, soles Malodor from bacterial overgrowth	Birth
Ichthyosis vulgaris OMIM #146700	Autosomal dominant *FILAGGRIN*	1/250 (may be higher)	Generalized mild scale sparing flexures Improves with age	After 3 mo
X-linked ichthyosis OMIM #308100	X-linked recessive Steroid sulfatase gene	1/2,000–1/6,000 males	Large "dirty" scales on trunk, extremities sparing flexures Variable in female carriers Corneal opacities in Descemet membrane Cryptorchidism Placental sulfatase deficiency with prolonged maternal labor	Within first 3 mo
Harlequin ichthyosis OMIM #242500	Autosomal recessive *ABCA12*	Very rare	Thick plates of "armor"-like scale in neonate Overall survival just over 50% Death in first 3 mo of life most common	Birth

SYNDROMIC

Syndrome/Disease	Genetics	Clinical Features
Netherton syndrome OMIM #256500	Autosomal recessive *SPINK5*	Hair shaft anomaly (trichorrhexis invaginata most common), ichthyosis linearis circumflexa, severe atopic dermatitis, failure to thrive
Refsum disease, infantile OMIM #266510	Autosomal recessive *PEX1, PXMP3, PEX26*	Retinitis pigmentosa, cerebellar ataxia, chronic polyneuritis with deafness, skin resembles ichthyosis vulgaris
Sjögren-Larsson syndrome OMIM #270200	Autosomal recessive *ALDH3A2* (fatty aldehyde dehydrogenase gene)	Spastic paralysis, intellectual disability, seizures, glistening dots on retina, dental bone dysplasia, similar skin findings to congenital ichthyosiform erythroderma
Conradi-Hunermann syndrome (chondrodysplasia punctata type 2) OMIM #302900	X-linked dominant *EBP* gene	Chondrodysplasia punctata, alopecia, skeletal anomalies, cataracts, dysmorphic facies, ichthyosiform erythroderma
KID (keratitis-ichthyosis-deafness) syndrome OMIM #148210	Autosomal dominant (sporadic) *GJB2* encoding connexin 26	Fixed keratotic plaques, keratoderma, atypical ichthyosis with prominent keratoses on extremities and head, neurosensory deafness, keratoconjunctivitis
CHILD syndrome OMIM #308050	X-linked recessive *NSDHL*	Congenital hemidysplasia, unilateral ichthyosiform nevus (epidermal nevus), limb defects, cardiovascular and renal anomalies

From Cohen BA. *Pediatric Dermatology.* 4th ed. Philadelphia: Saunders/Elsevier; 2013:27–28, Tables 2.2 and 2.4.

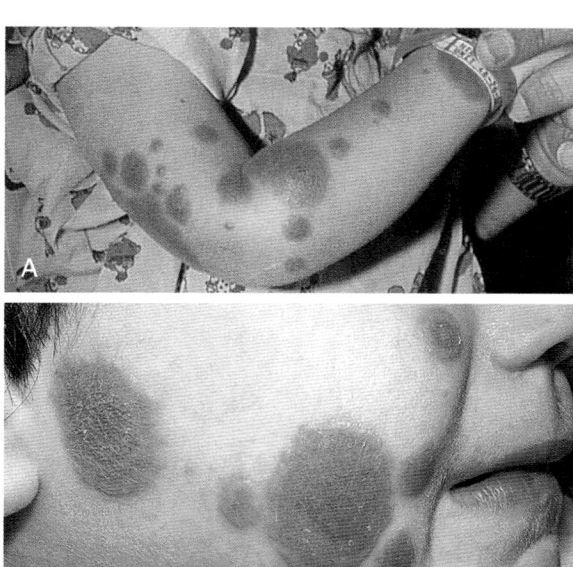

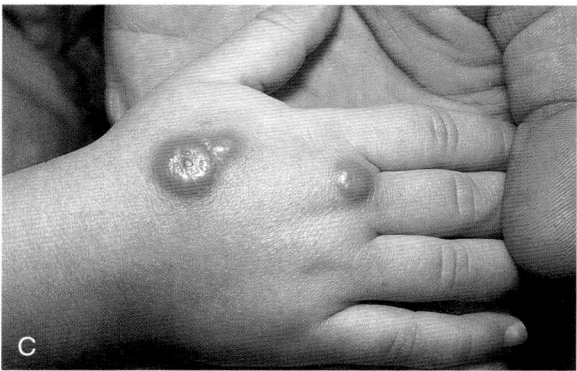

Fig. 60.24 *A–C,* Sweet syndrome. A 2-year-old girl developed fever, arthritis, leukocytosis, and widely disseminated, red-to-violaceous plaques and nodules, which demonstrated intense neutrophilic inflammation on skin biopsy. An extensive evaluation failed to reveal any underlying disease. Although she responded quickly to systemic corticosteroids, it took nearly a year to wean her because of frequent recurrences. (From Cohen BA, ed. *Pediatric Dermatology.* 4th ed. Philadelphia: Elsevier; 2013:189, Fig. 7.32.)

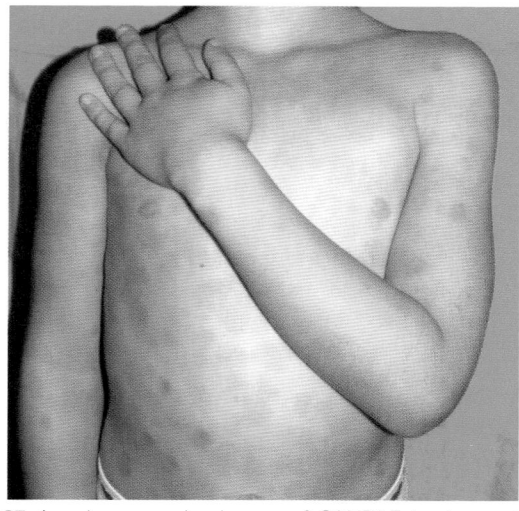

Fig. 60.25 Annular, purpuric plaques of CANDLE (early-onset chronic atypical neutrophilic dermatitis with lipodystrophy and elevated temperature) syndrome. (From Torrelo A. CANDLE syndrome as a paradigm of proteasome-related autoinflammation. *Frontiers Immunol.* 2017;8:927, Fig. 5.)

some to permanent joint deformity. Neurologic manifestations include chronic aseptic meningitis, cerebral atrophy, cognitive decline, optic nerve edema, and hearing loss. Leukocytosis and elevations of CRP and ESR indicate the inflammatory state. This cryopyrin-associated autoinflammatory disease is due to pathologic variants in *NLRP3* (see Chapter 54).

STING-associated vasculopathy with onset in infancy (SAVI) is due to a gain-of-function pathologic variant in *TMEM173* (*STING1*) and presents as an autoinflammatory disease with neonatal or infancy onset. Manifestations include failure to thrive, recurrent fevers, spontaneous or cold-induced (malar or digits) rash (Fig. 60.27), gingivostomatitis, interstitial lung disease, polyarthritis, and increased inflammatory markers including CRP, ESR, and antinuclear antibody (ANA). Heterozygous variants in *STING1* are also associated with familial chilblain lupus (see Chapter 44).

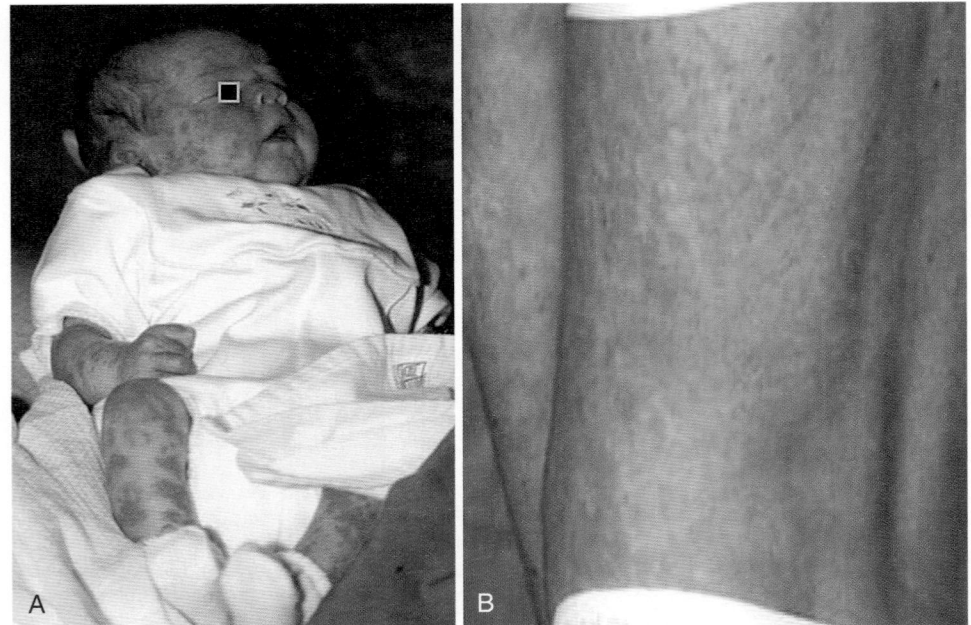

Fig. 60.26 Neonatal-onset multisystem inflammatory disease (NOMID). *A,* An urticaria-like rash is usually present at birth or during the first months of life. *B,* The rash is nonpruritic and papular. (Courtesy Dr. Raphaela Goldbach-Mansky.)

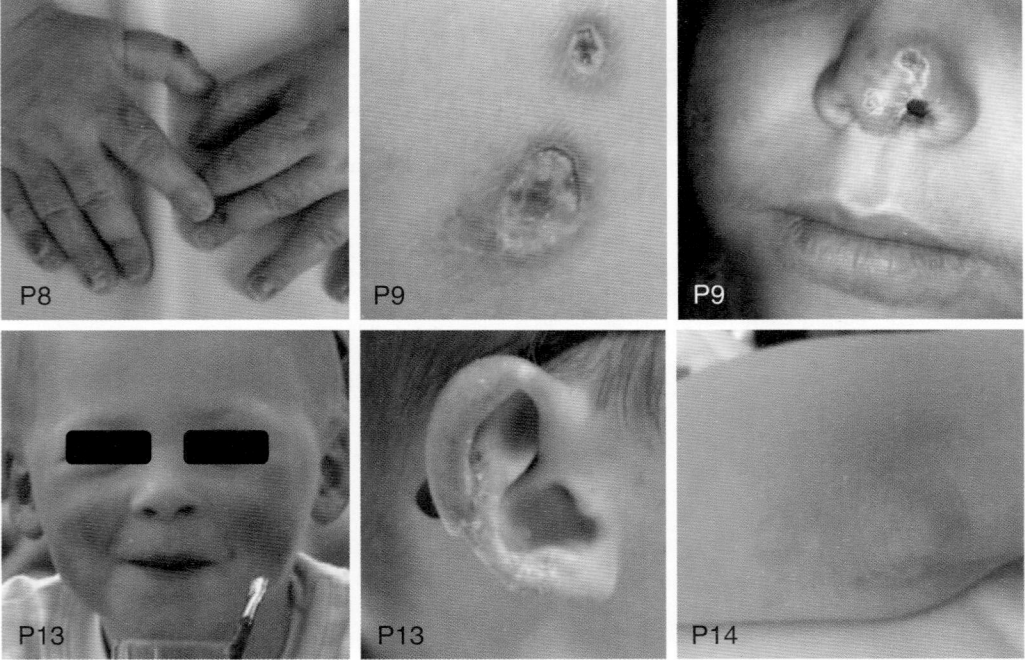

Fig. 60.27 STING-associated vasculopathy with onset in infancy (SAVI). Cutaneous involvement observed in patients. Representative cutaneous involvement observed in four patients of the cohort, demonstrating erythematous infiltrated plaques with ulcerations on the dorsal side of the fingers and mild nail dystrophy *(P8)*, roundlike ulcerations on the dorsal side of the right leg and ulceration of the nose and the right cheek *(P9)*, facial erythema and telangiectatic lesions of the cheeks and erythema and ulceration of the outer helix of the right ear *(P13)*, and urticarial-like lesions of the right elbow *(P14)*. (From Fremond ML, Hadchouel A, Berteloot L, et al. Overview of STING-associated vasculopathy with onset in infancy (SAV1) among 21 patients. *J Allergy Clin Immunol: In Practice.* 2021;9[2]:803–818 [Fig. 2A, p. 808].)

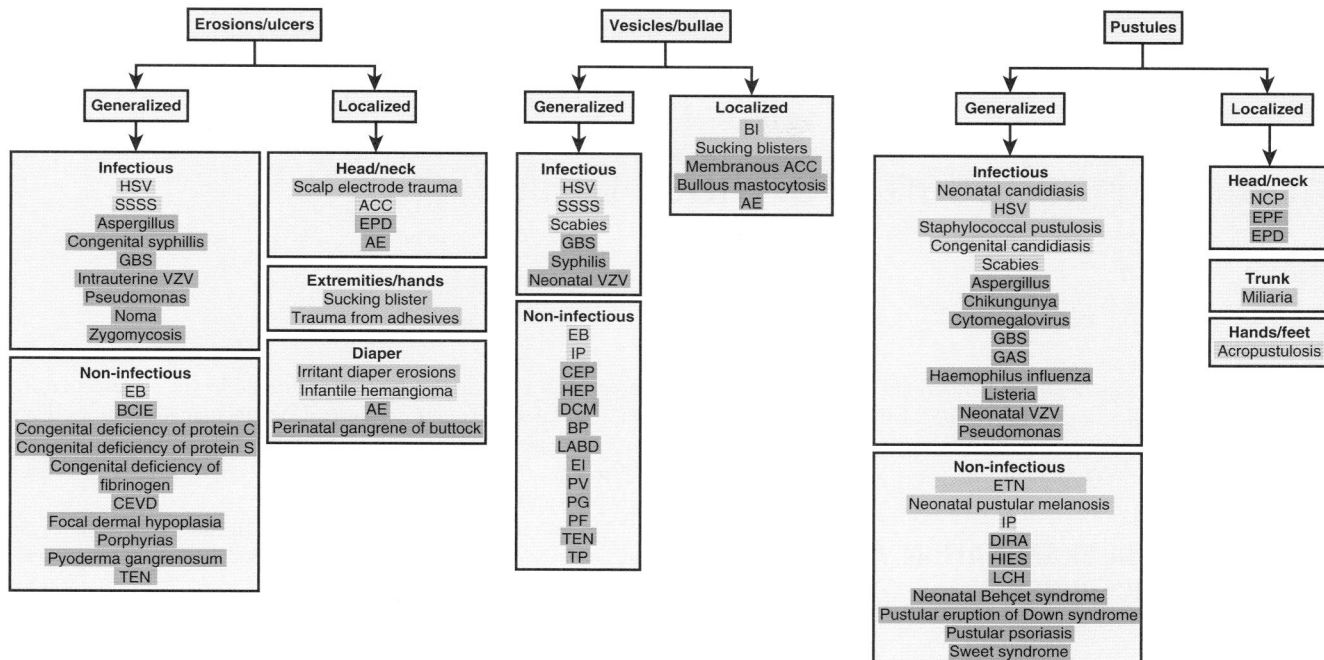

Fig. 60.28 Diagnostic algorithm for vesiculopustular eruptions in neonates based on primary lesion morphology and distribution. Conditions highlighted in green are common, yellow are uncommon, and red are rare. ACC, aplasia cutis congenita; AE, acrodermatitis enteropathica; BCIE, bullous congenital ichthyosiform erythroderma; BI, bullous impetigo; BP, bullous pemphigoid; CEP, congenital erythropoietic porphyria; CEVD, congenital erosive and vesicular dermatosis; DCM, diffuse cutaneous mastocytosis; DIRA, deficiency of interleukin-1 receptor antagonist; EB, epidermolysis bullosa; EI, epidermolytic ichthyosis; EPD, erosive pustular dermatosis of the scalp; EPF, eosinophilic pustular folliculitis; ETN, erythema toxicum neonatorum; GAS, group A streptococcus; GBS, group B streptococcus; HEP, hepatoerythropoietic porphyria; HIES, hyperimmunoglobulin E syndrome; HSV, herpes simplex virus; IP, incontinentia pigmenti; LABD, linear immunoglobulin A bullous dermatosis; LCH, Langerhans cell histiocytosis; NCP, neonatal cephalic pustulosis; PF, pemphigus foliaceus; PG, pemphigoid gestationis; PV, pemphigus vulgaris; SSSS, staphylococcal scalded skin syndrome; TEN, toxic epidermal necrolysis; TP, transient porphyrinemia; VZV, varicella zoster virus. (From Lalor LE, Chiu YE. Rare vesiculopustular eruptions of the neonatal period. *Clin Perinatol.* 2020;47[1]:53–75 [Fig. 1, p. 54].)

SUMMARY AND RED FLAGS

Neonates and infants can have a variety of congenital birthmarks and transient rashes. It is necessary to identify the primary skin lesion, any secondary skin lesions or changes, and the size, color, distribution, and configurations of the lesions to develop an appropriate differential diagnosis. Many entities unique to neonates are benign and self-limited and often require only reassurance to the parents.

Red flags are lesions consistent with HSV, *Staphylococcus aureus*, or LCH (see Table 60.2); those consistent with neurocutaneous diseases, such as ash leaf spots; or a capillary malformation in V1 distribution (see Table 60.1). The location of infantile hemangiomas in a beard distribution or on the spine and lower back should raise concern for PHACE or PELVIS/SACRAL syndrome (see Table 60.5). Lesions found on the midline of the back or head such as hemangiomas or hair collar sign can be associated with spinal dysraphism (see Table 60.1 and Fig. 60.12).

An approach to the diagnosis of erosive, vesicular, bullous, and pustular lesions is noted in Fig. 60.28.

BIBLIOGRAPHY

A bibliography is available at ExpertConsult.com.

Acquired Rashes in the Older Child

Kristen E. Holland

Many skin findings in childhood are benign and self-limited conditions. Other dermatologic complaints may be the first manifestation of a systemic disease or associated condition, recognition of which facilitates appropriate evaluation and treatment.

HISTORY, PHYSICAL EXAMINATION, AND DIAGNOSTIC PROCEDURES

History

A careful and focused history is necessary to diagnose pediatric skin disorders. It may be helpful to examine the patient first and then proceed with a relevant line of questioning. Important questions to ask include the following:
1. When did the eruption begin?
2. How did the eruption evolve (distribution, spread, change in the structure of individual lesions)?
3. Are the lesions pruritic or painful?
4. Have there been previous similar episodes?
5. Are there associated systemic symptoms?
6. Are there exacerbating or alleviating factors?
7. Has treatment been rendered? If so, what effect has it had?
8. Are there affected family members or close contacts?
9. Is there a family history of skin disease?

Physical Examination

Precise morphologic descriptions are critical for establishing a differential diagnosis (Figs. 61.1 and 61.2). For every eruption, the primary and secondary skin lesions are identified, and then the size, color, distribution, and configuration of the lesions are described. Palpation of cutaneous lesions provides additional information, such as firmness, tenderness, mobility, temperature, and ability to blanch with pressure. Examination of the hair, nails, and mucosal surfaces should be included. Certain diseases have pathognomonic findings.

Primary Lesions

Macules and Patches. Macules are flat, circumscribed lesions that are detected because of a change in color. Pink or red macules may be caused by inflammation or vasodilation. Brown, black, or white lesions may be caused by alterations in melanin synthesis. Purple hues may represent extravasation of blood into the skin. Macules >1 cm in diameter are usually described as patches.

Papules, Nodules, Plaques, and Tumors. Papules are circumscribed, palpable, elevated solid lesions. Typically <0.5–1 cm in diameter, these lesions may be epidermal or dermal in origin and may be flat-topped or dome shaped. Plaques are elevated flat-topped lesions, larger than 1 cm in diameter, often formed by the coalescence of papules. Nodules are epidermal, dermal, or subcutaneous lesions that may, in some cases, evolve from pre-existing papules; size may range from 0.5 to 2 cm. Tumors are larger nodules >2 cm in diameter that are usually solid and well circumscribed.

Vesicles and Bullae. Vesicles are small fluid-filled lesions. Bullae are large vesicles, usually >1 cm in diameter. The tenseness or flaccidity of the blister indicates whether the level of separation is intraepidermal or subepidermal (Fig. 61.3 and Table 61.1).

Pustules. Pustules are white or yellow well-circumscribed lesions that contain purulent material. Pustules do not always signify an infectious cause.

Wheals. Wheals are edematous, elevated lesions that are transient in nature and variable in shape and size. They may be white or erythematous and often have central pallor.

Telangiectases. Telangiectases are ectatic, dilated superficial blood vessels of the skin that typically blanch when pressure is applied.

Secondary Lesions

Secondary lesions may represent the natural evolution of primary lesions or changes that result from external manipulation, such as scratching.

Crusts. Crusts represent serum, pus, blood, or exudate that has dried on the skin surface.

Scales. Scales appear as yellow, white, or brownish flakes on the skin surface that represent desquamation of stratum corneum.

Erosions. Erosions are moist, erythematous, circumscribed lesions that result from partial or complete loss of the epidermis. They often result from rupture of a vesicle or bulla. Erosions do not involve the dermis or subcutaneous tissue; therefore, they heal without scarring.

Ulcers. Ulcers are deeper than erosions and result from full-thickness loss of the epidermis. As they penetrate the dermis or fat, they usually heal with scarring.

Lichenification. Lichenification, or thickening of the skin, usually results from chronic scratching or rubbing. Accentuation of skin markings or hyperpigmentation is observed.

Fissures. A fissure is a linear crack in the epidermis extending to the dermis.

Atrophy. Atrophy represents loss of substance of the skin. Epidermal atrophy is characterized by loss of skin markings, increased wrinkling, and transparency with visibility of underlying vasculature. Dermal or subcutaneous atrophy results in depression of the skin with minimal, if any, epidermal changes.

Excoriations. Excoriations are linear erosions on the skin caused by scratching.

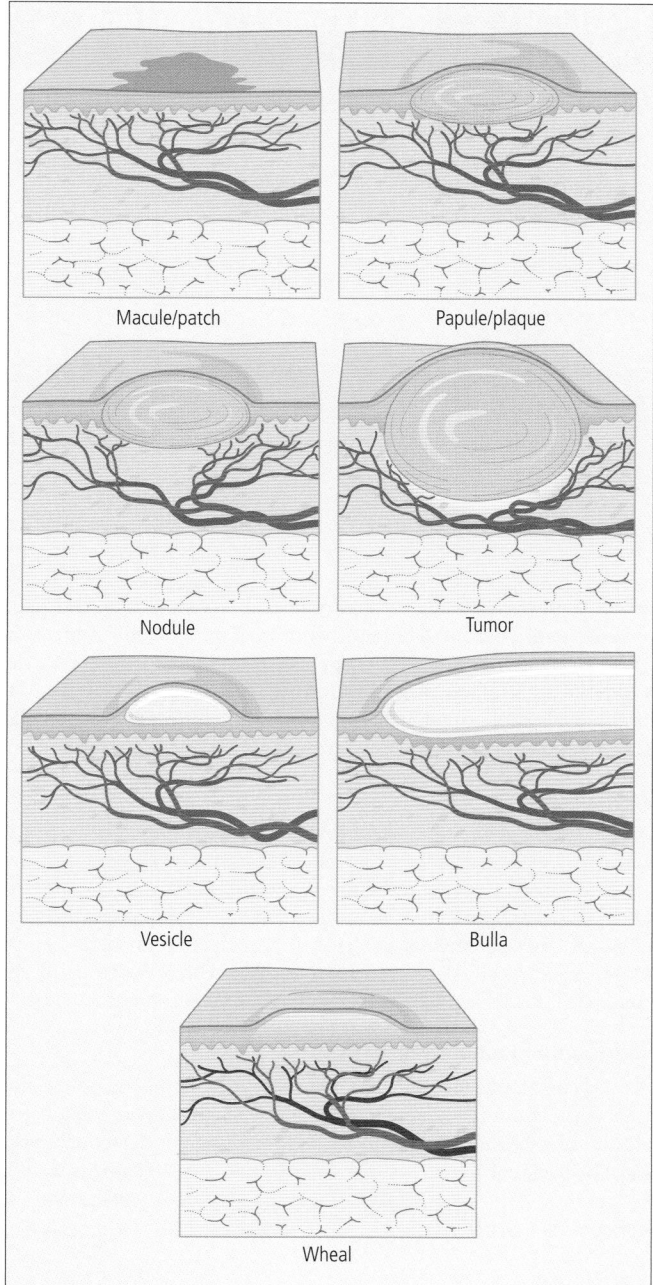

Fig. 61.1 Primary skin lesions. (From Cohen BA. Introduction to pediatric dermatology. In: Cohen BA, ed. *Pediatric Dermatology*. Philadelphia: Saunders; 2013.)

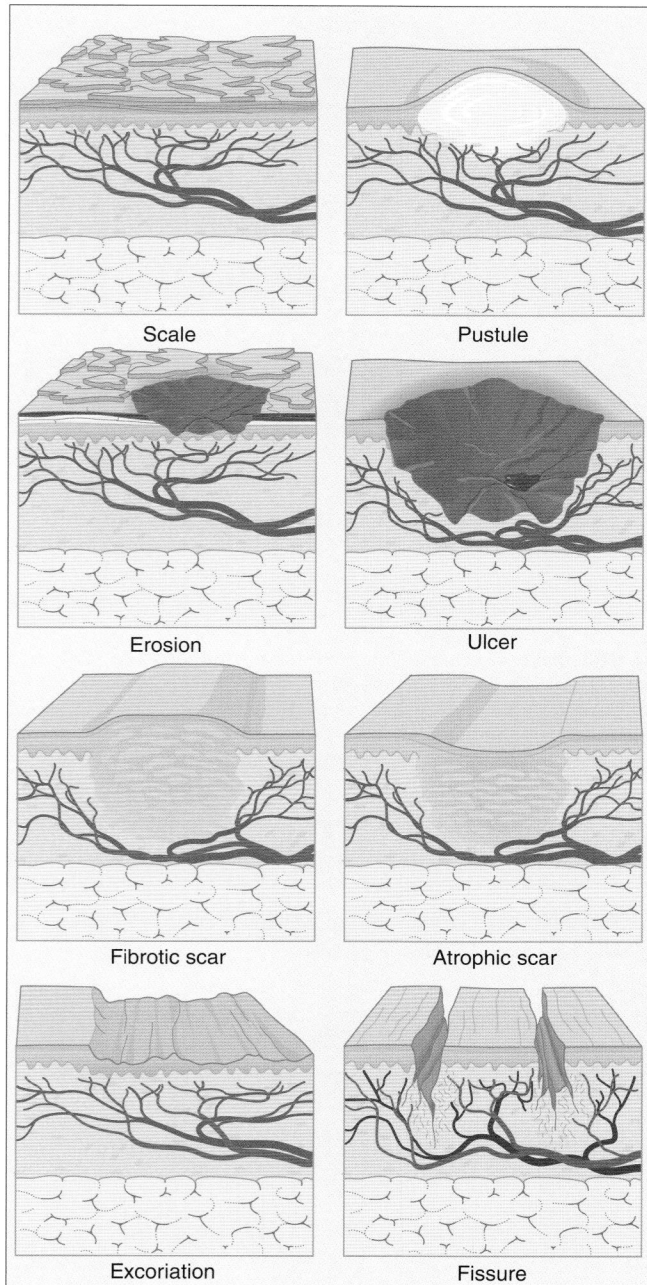

Fig. 61.2 Secondary skin lesions. (From Cohen BA. Introduction to pediatric dermatology. In: Cohen BA, ed. *Pediatric Dermatology*. Philadelphia: Saunders; 2013:1–13.)

Diagnostic Techniques

Potassium Hydroxide Test

This simple and rapid test can confirm the diagnosis of dermatophyte or candidal infections. Scale is scraped with a curved blade onto a microscope slide. Hair or nail fragments can also be examined. A glass coverslip is then placed on the slide after 1–2 drops of 10–20% potassium hydroxide (KOH) are added. The slide is heated gently but not boiled, which can result in KOH crystallization and subsequent difficulty in interpretation. Dermatophyte infections are confirmed by identifying **fungal hyphae**, which appear as long, branching septate filaments. **Pseudohyphae** or **budding spores** are characteristic of candidiasis. Short, broad hyphae and clusters of budding cells resembling "spaghetti and meatballs" are diagnostic of tinea versicolor.

Tzanck Smear

A Tzanck smear can be useful in the diagnosis of varicella-zoster virus and herpes simplex virus (HSV) infections. The smear is prepared by unroofing a blister with a curved blade and gently scraping the blister base and underside of the roof. The material is spread in a thin layer onto a glass slide. The slide is air-dried and stained with Giemsa or Wright stain. Identification of **multinucleated giant cells**, a syncytium of epidermal cells with multiple overlapping nuclei, establishes the diagnosis. These cells may have 2–15 nuclei and are much larger than other inflammatory cells. Although a positive result of Tzanck preparation is confirmatory, a negative test result does not rule out herpes viral infection. Viral specimens should be obtained for culture or polymerase chain reaction (PCR) to differentiate HSV from varicella-zoster virus infections.

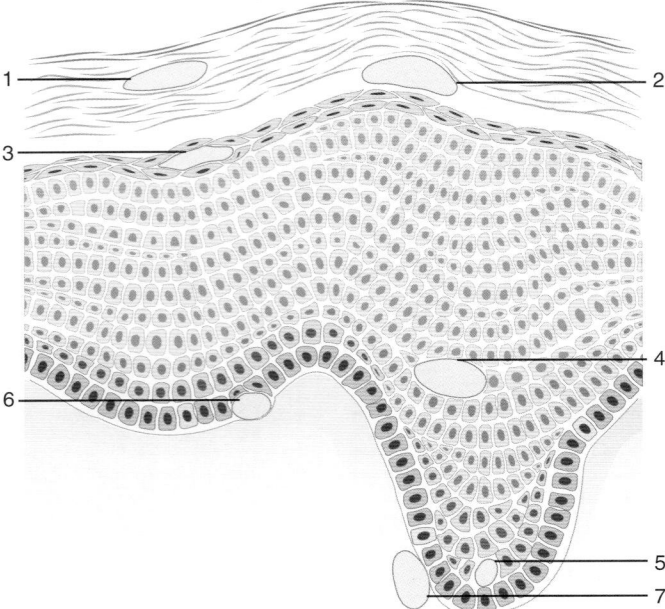

Fig. 61.3 Blister cleavage sites in the skin. *1,* Intracorneal. *2,* Subcorneal. *3,* Granular layer. *4,* Intraepidermal. *5,* Suprabasal. *6,* Junctional (between the basal cell membrane and basement membrane). *7,* Subepidermal. (From Esterly NB. The skin. In: Behrman RE, ed. *Nelson Textbook of Pediatrics.* 14th ed. Philadelphia: WB Saunders; 1992:1640.)

TABLE 61.1 Sites of Blister Formation in Selected Vesiculobullous Diseases

Site of Cleavage	Clinical Examples
Intracorneal	Miliaria crystallina
Granular layer	Bullous impetigo Staphylococcal scalded skin syndrome Pemphigus foliaceus
Intraepidermal	Dermatophytosis Insect bites Incontinentia pigmenti Scabies Viral blisters
Suprabasal	Pemphigus vulgaris
Basal cell layer	Epidermolysis simplex
Junctional	Junctional epidermolysis bullosa
Subepidermal	Toxic epidermal necrolysis Dermatitis herpetiformis Recessive dystrophic epidermolysis bullosa Dominant dystrophic epidermolysis bullosa Linear IgA disease of childhood

IgA, immunoglobulin A.

Scabies Test

A scabies preparation exhibiting the mite, egg, or feces (scybala) confirms the diagnosis of scabies infestation with *Sarcoptes scabiei.* The mite is most often found within burrows (serpiginous or elongated papules), which may have a vesicle or pustule at one end. A drop of mineral oil should be applied to the lesion so that the scraped material adheres to the blade. The site is then scraped firmly with a curved

TABLE 61.2 Wood Lamp Examination Findings

Clinical Appearance	Fluorescence	Organisms/Disease
Brown or red thin plaques on the groin, axillae, or toe webs	Coral, red, pink	Erythrasma (*Corynebacterium minutissimum*)
Hypopigmented or hyperpigmented macules and plaques on the trunk	Pale green or yellow	Tinea versicolor (*Malassezia* spp.)
Infection of the toe web space; often in burn patients	Bright yellow-green	*Pseudomonas aeruginosa*
Scaling of the scalp with patchy hair loss	Yellow-green	Tinea capitis (*Microsporum canis, Microsporum audouinii*) Not *Trichophyton tonsurans*

blade, which occasionally induces minimal bleeding. The material is applied to a microscope slide, another drop of mineral oil is added, and a glass coverslip is placed. Mites are eight-legged arachnids that are easily identified under low magnification. Eggs are frequently observed as smooth ovals approximately half the size of the mite. Feces are smaller than ova and appear as red-brown round pellets, often in clusters.

Gram Stain

A Gram stain can be useful in the diagnosis and treatment of suspected bacterial infections. After the site is disinfected, the pustule or blister roof is carefully removed with a needle or straight blade. The contents of the pustule are removed in a sterile manner and spread thinly onto a glass slide. The specimen is air-dried or heat-fixed, stained, and examined microscopically. Results help determine which antibiotic, if any, is indicated. Bacterial cultures are typically obtained simultaneously.

Wood Lamp Examination

A Wood lamp emits low-intensity ultraviolet light at 365 nm and is useful for accentuating pigmentary alterations such as those of vitiligo, piebaldism, or ash leaf macules in the newborn, and for detecting several fungal or bacterial infections. The examination is performed in a darkened room, and the lamp is held 4–6 inches from the patient's skin. Characteristic color changes of infectious etiologies are outlined in Table 61.2.

Skin Biopsy

A skin biopsy can be performed when a clinical diagnosis is unclear. Histologic evaluation of a small skin specimen may reveal changes in the epidermis, dermis, or subcutaneous tissue that confirm or rule out specific disorders. Direct immunofluorescence testing can be extremely helpful in the diagnosis of collagen vascular and autoimmune bullous diseases (Table 61.3).

DERMATOLOGIC DISORDERS IN OLDER INFANTS AND CHILDREN

Many skin lesions are acquired during childhood and adolescence, ranging from benign self-limited asymptomatic dermatoses to chronic skin disorders. Establishing the symptomatology and time course and evaluating the morphology of the lesions can help distinguish among childhood dermatoses.

TABLE 61.3   Immunofluorescent Findings in Immune-Mediated Cutaneous Diseases

Disease	Involved Skin	Uninvolved Skin	Direct IF Findings	Indirect IF Findings	Circulating Antibodies
Dermatitis herpetiformis	Negative	Positive	Granular IgA ± C3 in papillary dermis	None	IgA antiendomysial and transglutaminase antibodies
Bullous pemphigoid	Positive	Positive	Linear IgG and C3 band in BMZ, occasionally IgM, IgA, IgE	IgG to BMZ	IgG anti-BP180 and anti-BP230
Pemphigus (all variants)	Positive	Positive	IgG in intercellular spaces of the epidermis between keratinocytes	IgG in intercellular spaces of the epidermis between keratinocytes	IgG antidesmoglein 1 and 3 (pemphigus vulgaris and foliaceus) IgA antidesmocollin 1 (IgA pemphigus)
Linear IgA bullous dermatosis (chronic bullous dermatosis of childhood)	Positive	Positive	Linear IgA at BMZ, occasionally C3	Low titer, rare IgA, anti-BP180	None
Discoid lupus erythematosus	Positive	Negative	Linear IgG, IgM, IgA, and C3 at BMZ (lupus band)	None	Usually ANA negative
Systemic lupus erythematosus	Positive	Variable; exposed to sun, 30–50%; nonexposed, 10–30%	Linear IgG, IgM, IgA, and C3 at BMZ (lupus band)	None	ANA Anti-Ro (SSA), anti-La (SSB) Anti-RNP Anti-dsDNA Anti-Sm
Henoch-Schönlein purpura	Positive	Positive	IgA around vessel walls	None	None

ANA, antinuclear antibody; BMZ, basement membrane zone at the dermal-epidermal junction; BP, bullous pemphigoid; C, complement; dsDNA, double-stranded DNA; IF, immunofluorescence; Ig, immunoglobulin; Sm, Smith; SSA/SSB, Sjögren syndrome A/B; RNP, ribonucleoprotein.

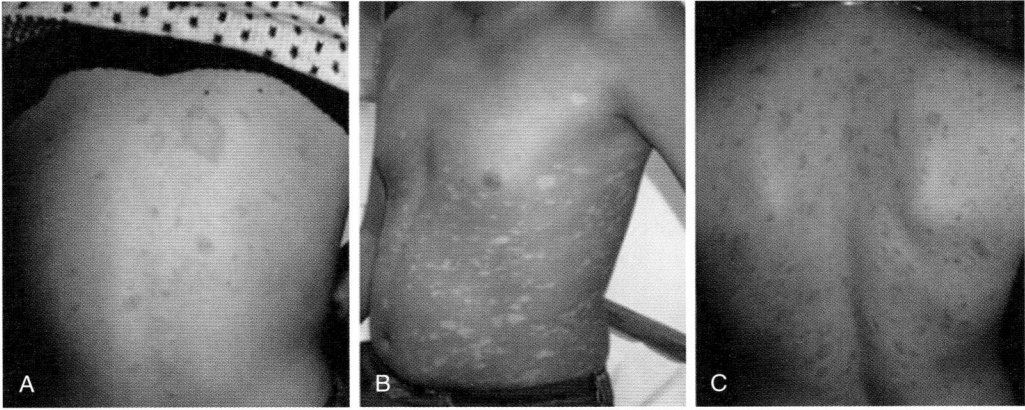

Fig. 61.4 Pityriasis rosea. *A,* The herald patch. *B,* Oval lesions oriented along the lines of skin cleavage on the trunk. *C,* Christmas tree distribution on the back. (From Cohen BA, Davis HW, Gehris RP. Dermatology. In: Zitelli BJ, et al., eds. *Atlas of Pediatric Physical Diagnosis.* Philadelphia: Saunders; 2012:299–368.)

Scaling Disorders

The term *papulosquamous* refers to conditions in which the primary lesions are papules or plaques associated with scale. These disorders are typically benign but can be chronic and therapeutically challenging.

Pityriasis Rosea

Pityriasis rosea is an acute, common, self-limited eruption that has no gender predilection. Although the precise cause is unknown, a viral origin is suspected because there have been reports of epidemics, clusters of cases among closely related individuals, and low recurrence rates. Furthermore, a prodrome of malaise, headache, and respiratory symptoms is occasionally observed. Pityriasis rosea has been associated with systemic reactivation of human herpesvirus (HHV)-6 and HHV-7.

The eruption usually begins with a solitary oval, pink, scaly plaque approximately 3–5 cm in diameter, typically located on the trunk or proximal extremities (Fig. 61.4). Referred to as the **herald patch**, this finding is observed in up to 70% of cases. When the herald patch has an elevated red border and central clearing, it resembles tinea corporis. Performing a KOH preparation can differentiate these two conditions. Within 1–2 weeks after appearance of the herald patch, numerous small, pink, scaly papules or plaques arise over the trunk and proximal extremities, sparing the face and distal extremities. The lesions

TABLE 61.4	Differential Diagnosis of Papulosquamous Disorders (Primary Skin Lesions Are Papules or Plaques Associated with Scale)
Lichen planus
Lupus erythematosus
Lichen striatus
Lichen nitidus
Psoriasis
Guttate psoriasis
Pityriasis rosea
Pityriasis lichenoides (parapsoriasis)
Pityriasis rubra
Dermatophyte infections
Dermatomyositis
Drug eruption
Nummular eczema
Atopic dermatitis
Seborrheic dermatitis
Secondary syphilis
Cutaneous T-cell lymphoma

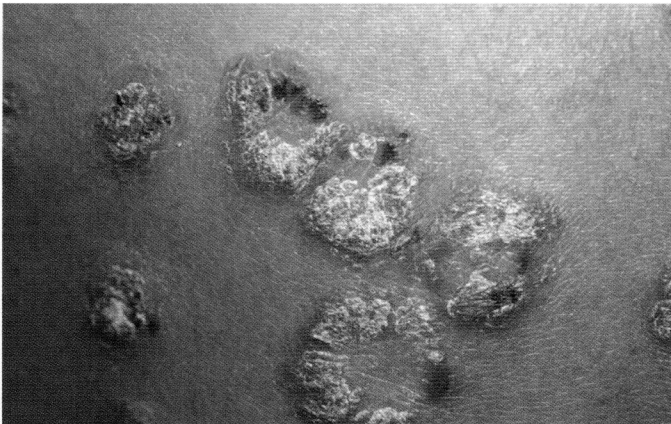

Fig. 61.5 Well-demarcated erythematous, scaly plaques of psoriasis. (From Kliegman RM, et al. Diseases of the epidermis. In: Kliegman RM, et al., eds. *Nelson Textbook of Pediatrics*. 20th ed. Philadelphia: Elsevier; 2015:3160–3162.)

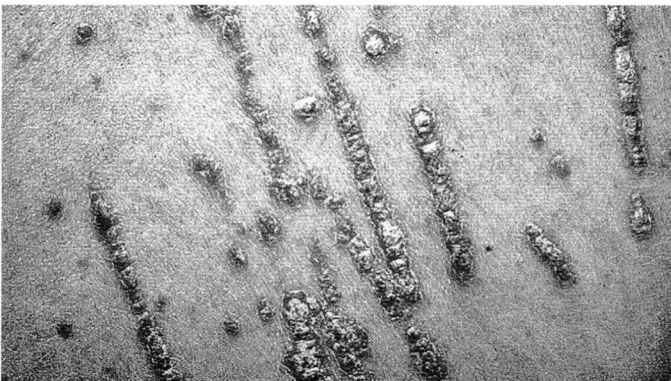

Fig. 61.6 Koebner phenomenon in psoriasis with linear plaques formed in the pattern of excoriations. (From Papulosquamous eruptions. In: Cohen BA, ed. *Pediatric Dermatology*. Philadelphia: Saunders; 2013:68–103.)

classically have a fine cigarette paper–like peripheral collarette of scale. These oval 0.5- to 2-cm lesions have their long axis oriented along skin lines and, when present on the trunk, result in a "Christmas tree" pattern on the back (see Fig. 61.4). Young children, particularly those with darker skin pigmentation, may have an "inverse" type of pityriasis rosea, with most lesions distributed on the distal extremities, face, neck, and intertriginous regions. Other variants seen in children may have lesions that are papular, vesicular, pustular, purpuric, or lichenoid.

The duration of the eruption varies from 2 to 12 weeks. Pityriasis rosea is self-limited and does not necessarily require therapy, though it improves significantly with exposure to ultraviolet light. Emollients, topical corticosteroids, or oral antihistamines help relieve pruritus. Postinflammatory hypopigmentation or hyperpigmentation may persist for weeks to months, especially in dark-skinned patients. Many other dermatoses can resemble pityriasis rosea (Table 61.4). In sexually active adolescents, a rapid plasma reagin (RPR) test should be obtained to rule out the possibility of secondary syphilis, especially if the palms and soles are involved. Persistence of the eruption after 3–4 months necessitates an evaluation for another diagnosis.

Psoriasis

Psoriasis is an immune-mediated inflammatory skin condition characterized by well-demarcated, erythematous scaly papules and plaques located most often on the scalp, elbows, knees, genitalia, and lumbosacral regions. The course is more chronic and unpredictable than that of pityriasis rosea. Psoriasis occurs in up to 3% of the population, with approximately 30% of affected individuals manifesting symptoms before the age of 20 years. Both genders are equally affected in adulthood, but childhood psoriasis has a slight female predominance. The cause is multifactorial, though a familial predisposition is present in many affected individuals, including up to 50% of patients with childhood onset. The association between psoriasis, obesity, and metabolic syndrome has been described in both adult and pediatric patients with psoriasis; metabolic screening for individuals with moderate to severe involvement should be considered.

Psoriasis encompasses a broad spectrum of clinical manifestations, ranging from mild, asymptomatic, virtually undetectable disease to extensive, chronic, debilitating disease. The course is usually marked by recurrent flares and remissions and is often exacerbated by stress, trauma, infection, climate, hormonal factors, and particular medications.

Although morphologic variations exist, the classic lesions of **plaque psoriasis** are well-demarcated erythematous papules or plaques with a silvery-white scale (Fig. 61.5). The lesions usually begin as small erythematous papules that gradually enlarge and coalesce to form plaques up to several centimeters in diameter. The micaceous (mica-like) scale of the psoriatic plaque is more adherent centrally than peripherally. Removal of this scale results in multiple small bleeding points, a finding referred to as the *Auspitz sign* that is secondary to disruption of the dilated blood vessels that are located high in the papillary dermis. Although this finding is seen in psoriasis, it is not pathognomonic. The **Koebner phenomenon**, another characteristic feature of psoriasis that is also observed in a number of dermatologic conditions, is an isomorphic response (i.e., development of new or larger lesions) occurring at sites of injury or trauma such as scratching, sunburn, or surgery (Fig. 61.6).

Psoriatic lesions tend to be distributed symmetrically. Although extensor surfaces are typically involved, a variant of psoriasis known as **inverse psoriasis** affects flexural surfaces, such as the axillae and groin. Facial involvement is more common in children than in adults. Scalp lesions are present in most children with psoriasis, wherein a diffuse, thick white scale may be accompanied by erythema. In contrast

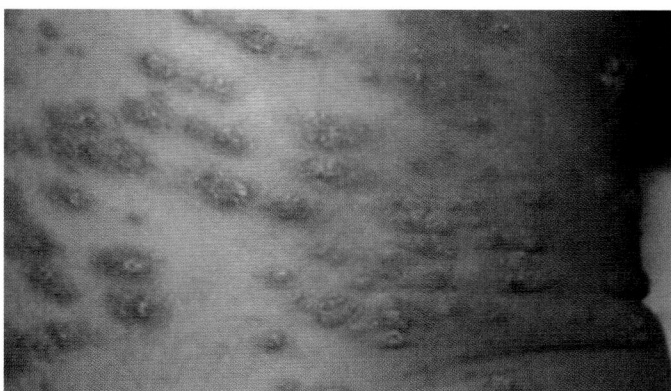

Fig. 61.7 Small droplike plaques of guttate psoriasis. (From Cohen BA, Davis HW, Gehris RP. Dermatology. In: Zitelli BJ, et al., eds. *Atlas of Pediatric Physical Diagnosis*. Philadelphia: Saunders; 2012:299–368.)

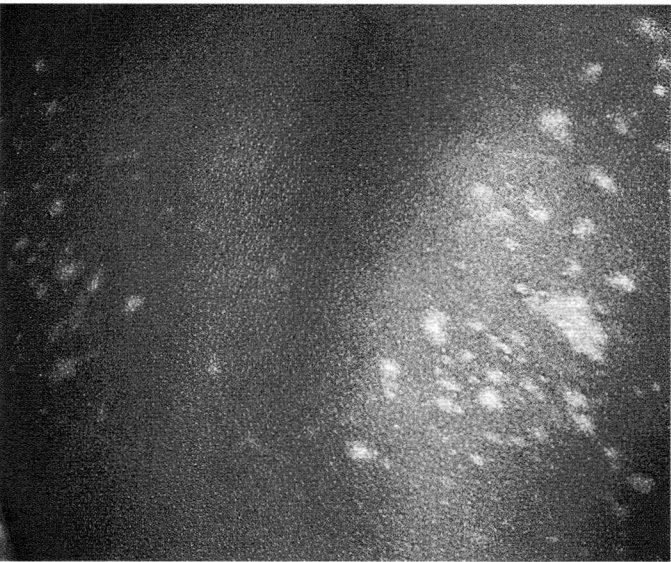

Fig. 61.8 Asymptomatic, hypopigmented, minimally scaly patches on the trunk of a child, which were present for several years and found to be cutaneous T-cell lymphoma. (From Papulosquamous eruptions. In: Cohen BA, ed. *Pediatric Dermatology*. Philadelphia: Saunders; 2013:68–103.)

to seborrhea, psoriasis often extends beyond the hairline, affecting the forehead, ears, and neck. The lesions are variably pruritic and are generally not associated with hair loss. Scalp psoriasis tends to be more resistant to therapy than seborrheic dermatitis.

Nail abnormalities are seen in up to 50% of patients with psoriasis. Nail pits are the most common finding, identified by multiple pinpoint depressions that are irregularly distributed over the nail plate. Although nail pitting is characteristic of psoriasis, it is not pathognomonic, also being found in atopic dermatitis, alopecia areata, and trauma. Other nail changes include separation of the nail plate from the nail bed (onycholysis), subungual hyperkeratosis, discoloration, crumbling, and yellowish-brown "oil spots" on the nail plate.

Guttate psoriasis, characterized by numerous droplike lesions, is a variant commonly seen in children and young adults (Fig. 61.7). The round-to-oval, pinkish red, somewhat scaly papules arise in crops and are widely distributed, particularly on the trunk. Two thirds of affected patients have a history of an upper respiratory tract infection or pharyngitis, usually streptococcal in origin, in the 1–3 weeks preceding the onset of lesions. Lesions often improve following appropriate antibiotic therapy; however, the course may range from spontaneous resolution to chronic disease.

Psoriasis is usually diagnosed from the appearance of skin lesions. However, when the diagnosis is unclear, a skin biopsy may be helpful. Differential diagnosis of psoriasis includes seborrheic dermatitis, dermatophytosis, pityriasis rosea, lichen planus, atopic dermatitis, and subacute cutaneous lupus erythematosus (see Table 61.4).

The course of psoriasis is marked by recurrent flares and remissions, often in an unpredictable fashion. A subset of individuals gradually improves over time. Management of psoriasis varies and depends on age of the child, extent of involvement, functional limitations, and psychosocial impact. For limited disease, topical therapy (e.g., emollients, corticosteroids, vitamin D derivatives, retinoids, tar, keratolytics) alone may afford control. For more extensive or debilitating disease, the addition of phototherapy or a systemic agent (e.g., immunosuppressants, retinoids, or biologic therapy) may be necessary.

Pityriasis Lichenoides

Pityriasis lichenoides can manifest in two forms: pityriasis lichenoides et varioliformis acuta (PLEVA) or pityriasis lichenoides chronica. These diseases most commonly affect children between ages 5 and 15 years, and both are believed to be part of the same clinical spectrum. **PLEVA** is characterized by an abrupt eruption of multiple, 2- to 4-mm, nonpruritic, variably scaly erythematous macules and papules that may progress to vesicular, necrotic, or crusted lesions. The lesions often occur in crops and are thus present in different stages. Distribution is most commonly on the trunk, but lesions may spread to the extremities. The condition may resolve spontaneously within several months, or recurrences and relapses may occur episodically for several years.

Pityriasis lichenoides chronica manifests more gradually and is characterized by pink-to-brown 2- to 5-mm papules with central adherent scale, found primarily on the trunk and proximal extremities. The clinical course is variable, and the lesions may last from months to years. After the papules recede, postinflammatory hypopigmentation or hyperpigmentation commonly occurs. Sequelae are uncommon, and the lesions usually heal without a scar. Pityriasis lichenoides chronica may initially resemble pityriasis rosea and other papulosquamous eruptions (see Table 61.4). Reports of cutaneous T-cell lymphoma (**mycosis fungoides**) in the setting of pityriasis lichenoides chronica exist, and the patient with a persistent or atypical eruption should be evaluated with consideration of a skin biopsy (Fig. 61.8).

Treatment may be limited to topical emollients in an asymptomatic patient. If treatment is required, first-line agents include oral antibiotics with antiinflammatory properties (e.g., erythromycin, doxycycline) for several weeks, which have shown benefit in some children.

Lichen Planus

Lichen planus occurs in patients of all ages but is less commonly seen in children than in adults. It is characterized by the "5 Ps": purple, polygonal, planar, pruritic papules. The primary lesion is a shiny, violaceous, flat-topped papule, often with angulated borders, measuring from 2 mm to more than 1 cm in diameter. The lesions are very pruritic and demonstrate the Koebner phenomenon, which results in the development of new lesions (often in a linear configuration) at sites of scratching. The distribution may be localized or generalized, and lesions may number from few to numerous. Sites of predilection include the volar wrists, forearms, legs, genitalia, and mucous membranes. The presence of **Wickham striae**, a reticulated pattern of delicate white lines or streaks seen on the buccal mucosa or skin, aids in confirming the diagnosis.

Nail changes consisting of longitudinal ridging, generalized nail destruction, red or brown discoloration, subungual hyperkeratosis,

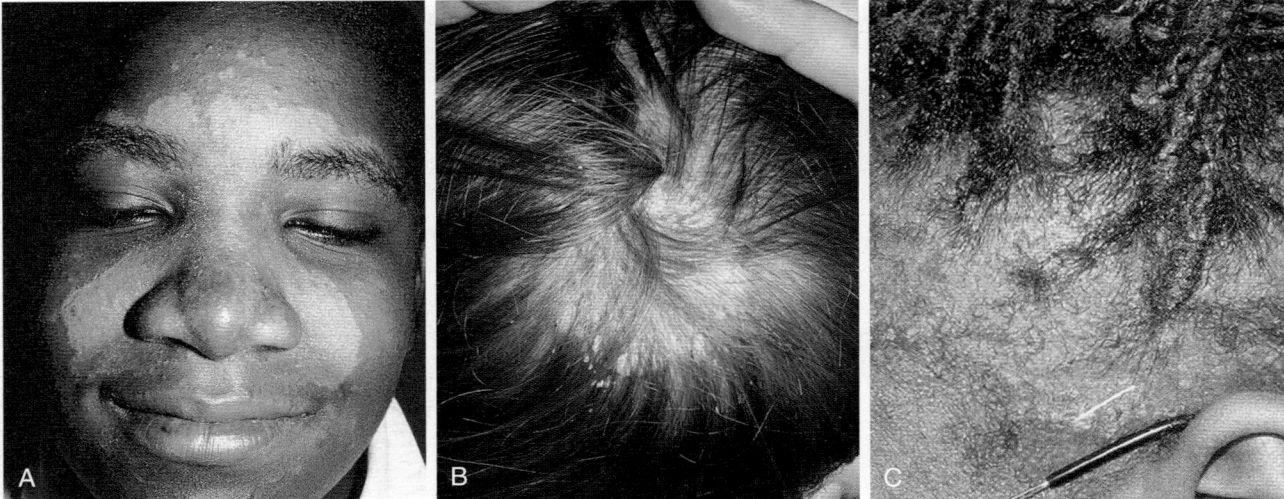

Fig. 61.9 Seborrheic dermatitis in the older child or adolescent. *A,* Scaly, hypopigmented lesions on the face involving eyebrows, nasolabial folds, and nasal bridge. *B,* Thick, yellow, adherent scale in the scalp. *C,* Confluent, scaly patches on the scalp with mild erythema. (From Papulosquamous eruptions. In: Cohen BA, ed. *Pediatric Dermatology.* Philadelphia: Saunders; 2013:68–103.)

and thinning of the nail plate are seen in approximately 10% of patients. Pterygium formation results from the overgrowth of fibrous tissue, which extends from the proximal nail fold to the tip of the nail, obliterating the nail plate.

Drug-induced lichenoid eruptions may mimic lichen planus. Common medications that can produce a lichenoid eruption include antihypertensives (e.g., β blockers, angiotensin-converting enzyme inhibitors), diuretics (e.g., hydrochlorothiazide), antimalarials, penicillamine, and gold salts. Rarely, tetracycline, griseofulvin, nonsteroidal antiinflammatory medications, phenytoin, and carbamazepine can be causes. Unlike other cutaneous medication reactions, the lichenoid reaction may not occur for months or years after medication initiation.

Lichen planus is typically a clinical diagnosis, though if necessary, a skin biopsy specimen can reveal specific findings. The differential diagnosis most often includes psoriasis and drug eruptions (see Table 61.4). If oral lesions are present, possible alternate diagnoses include aphthous stomatitis, erythema multiforme (EM), herpes simplex, or leukoplakia.

Topical corticosteroids are the treatment of choice in most cases. Lichen planus often resolves spontaneously over 1–2 years, but some cases may persist for many years. Generalized eruptions may respond to a short course of systemic corticosteroids. Oral antihistamines provide symptomatic relief.

Seborrheic Dermatitis

Seborrheic dermatitis is characterized by an erythematous, scaly, symmetric eruption that occurs most often in hair-bearing and intertriginous regions. Seborrhea of infancy is discussed in Chapter 60. In adolescents, yellowish, greasy scale of the scalp, eyebrows, nasolabial folds, nasal bridge, posterior auricular regions, and mid-chest may be accompanied by mild erythema (Fig. 61.9). Immunodeficiency and histiocytic disorders may be accompanied by severe, recalcitrant seborrheic dermatitis (Fig. 61.10). Although typical patients usually respond well to therapy, it is a chronic condition characterized by recurrences. It is often responsive to low-potency topical corticosteroids or topical antifungals (e.g., azoles, ciclopirox, selenium sulfide). These preparations may be available in a number of vehicles, including solutions or shampoos for the scalp. Keratolytics may be added when thicker scale is present.

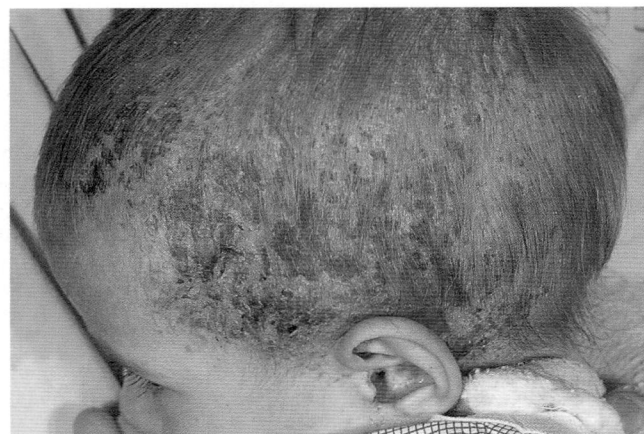

Fig. 61.10 Letterer-Siwe disease. Erythematous, slightly scaly plaques are present on the scalp of this child. (From Piette WW. Cutaneous manifestations of macrophage/dendritic cell proliferative disorders [histiocytosis]. In: Callen JP, Jorizzo JL, Bolognia JL, et al., eds. *Dermatological Signs of Internal Disease.* 4th ed. Philadelphia: Elsevier; 2009:150, Fig. 17-1.)

Atopic Dermatitis

Atopic dermatitis (**eczema**) is a chronic condition characterized by pruritus, a personal or family history of atopy, and an age-dependent distribution. It is common during infancy and childhood. Up to 95% of affected individuals have signs before the age of 5 years.

Typical lesions are pink-to-red crusted or scaly plaques or papules. Some individuals have follicular accentuation, particularly on the trunk, manifested by a goosebump-like texture. **Lichenification** (thickened skin with exaggerated skin markings) is a feature of chronic atopic dermatitis and results from repeated rubbing and scratching. Excoriations are secondary lesions caused by scratching. Postinflammatory pigmentary changes are frequently noted, especially in darker-skinned individuals (Fig. 61.11). Associated findings are noted in Table 61.5.

The distribution of the lesions tends to be age dependent. The cheeks, face, scalp, trunk, and extensor surfaces of the arms and legs are characteristically involved in the infant form. Between the ages of 2 and 10 years (childhood atopic dermatitis), the distribution predominantly

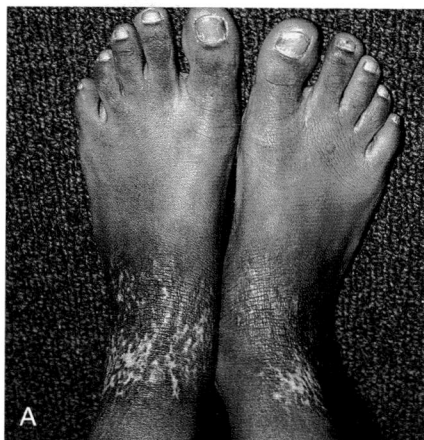

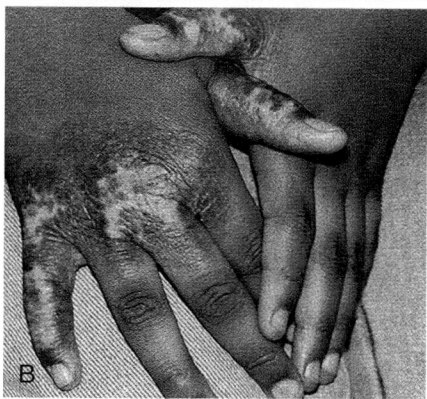

Fig. 61.11 Postinflammatory pigment changes of the ankles *(A)* and hands *(B)*. (From Papulosquamous eruptions. In: Cohen BA, ed. *Pediatric Dermatology*. Philadelphia: Saunders; 2013:68–103.)

TABLE 61.5 Atopic Dermatitis: Associated Findings

Finding	Features
Ichthyosis vulgaris	Affects 20% of patients with atopic dermatitis Primarily involves the legs and trunk
Keratosis pilaris	Asymptomatic hyperkeratotic follicular papules found mainly on the extensor surfaces of the upper arms and anterior thighs, also on the face in children
Pityriasis alba	Hypopigmented patches on the cheeks and occasionally upper body
Hyperlinear palms/soles	Common
Dennie-Morgan fold	A double line found under the lower eyelids Not pathognomonic
Lichen spinulosus	More commonly seen in darker skin Pruritic grouped hyperkeratotic follicular spires
Eye findings	Keratoconjunctivitis, cataracts, keratoconus (abnormally shaped cornea), retinal detachment (rare)
Dyshidrotic eczema	Firm vesicles found on the palms and soles and lateral aspects of digits Frequently associated with hyperhidrosis
Nummular eczema	Well-demarcated, scaly, coin-shaped lesions usually on the lower extremities Associated with xerosis
Juvenile plantar dermatosis	Occasionally exudative lesions Painful erythema, scaling, cracking, and fissuring of weight-bearing surfaces of the feet Often associated with hyperhidrosis Improvement after puberty

involves the neck, wrists, ankles, and flexural surfaces of the extremities (Fig. 61.12). After puberty, atopic dermatitis has a predilection for the face, neck, hands, and feet. The clinical features of the skin lesions are not specific to this condition, as other eczematous eruptions (contact dermatitis, seborrheic dermatitis) have a similar appearance. Laboratory tests are of limited value, and histologic findings reveal nonspecific spongiotic dermatitis. The distribution of lesions, age at onset, and history are most important for establishing the diagnosis. Obtaining a complete personal and family history of atopic diatheses is necessary.

Secondary infections are the most common complication. Individuals with atopic dermatitis have increased colonization with *Staphylococcus aureus*. Most affected children need occasional treatment with antibiotics to eradicate secondary infection, and dilute sodium hypochlorite bleach baths can help reduce infection with *S. aureus*. The presence of pustules, extensive excoriations, or weeping and crusted lesions suggests the need for antibacterial therapy. Topical therapy with mupirocin may be sufficient for limited areas; however, widespread involvement may necessitate the use of oral antimicrobial agents. The increase in methicillin-resistant *S. aureus* (MRSA) infections has limited therapeutic options in some patients. Secondary infection with HSV is referred to as **eczema herpeticum** or **Kaposi varicelliform eruption** (Fig. 61.13). Transmission may occur during routine childcare from a caretaker with a herpetic fever blister, whereby the eczematous skin becomes inoculated with HSV. The hallmark of this condition is the rapid development of numerous umbilicated vesicles and pustules. Later in the course, multiple erosions are seen, and identification of an intact vesicle may be difficult. The infection may be associated with fever and other constitutional symptoms, and expedient treatment with acyclovir is required. Hospitalization may be

necessary in young infants or severely affected individuals. Recurrences of eczema herpeticum can be problematic. Eczema coxsackium is a similar condition due to entroviruses.

Other dermatologic conditions to consider in the differential diagnosis of a rash that looks like atopic dermatitis are presented in Tables 61.6 and 61.7.

An overview of the management of atopic dermatitis is presented in Table 61.8.

Vascular Lesions

Spider Angioma (Nevus Araneus)

Telangiectases are dilated capillaries that appear as red linear stellate or punctate lesions. There are many causes of *primary* telangiectasia (spider angiomas, hereditary hemorrhagic telangiectasia syndrome) and *secondary* telangiectasia, such as collagen vascular disease. Spider angiomas are the most common of the telangiectases. In the pediatric age group, these lesions are typically not associated with systemic disease. Spider angiomas are seen most often on the face and tops of hands. They usually develop after 2 years of age. Small vessels radiate from a central punctum (arteriole), giving the appearance of a "spider." When pressure is applied to the central punctum, the lesion blanches. Treatment, if desired, consists of gentle electrodesiccation or pulsed dye laser therapy. In some cases, spider angiomas clear without treatment.

Pyogenic Granuloma

Pyogenic granulomas are acquired vascular lesions that arise from the connective tissue of the skin or mucous membranes. These vascular

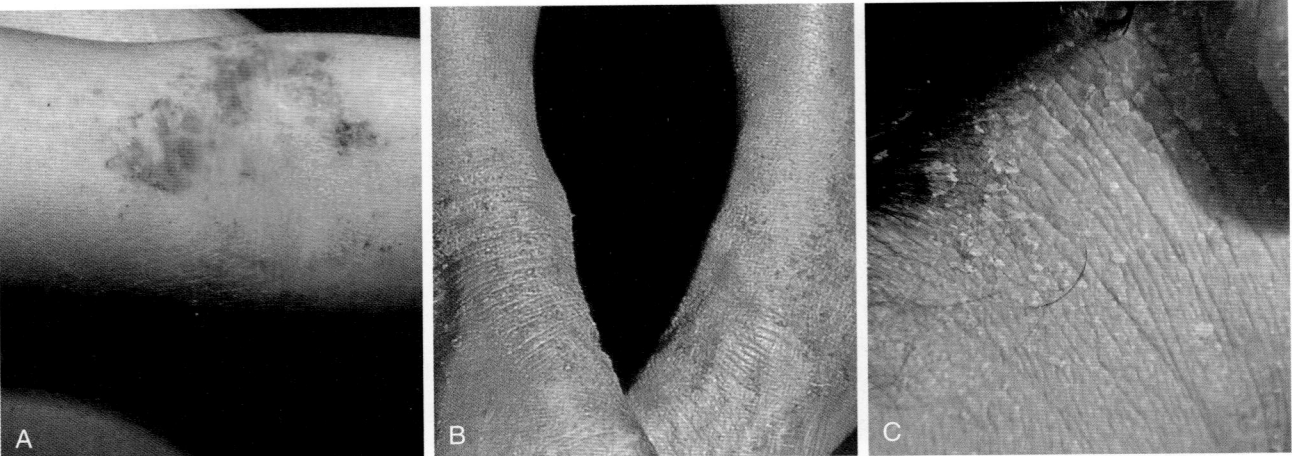

Fig. 61.12 Atopic dermatitis in childhood with lesions of the arm *(A)*, ankles *(B)*, and neck *(C)*. (From Papulosquamous eruptions. In: Cohen BA, ed. *Pediatric Dermatology*. Philadelphia: Saunders; 2013:68–103.)

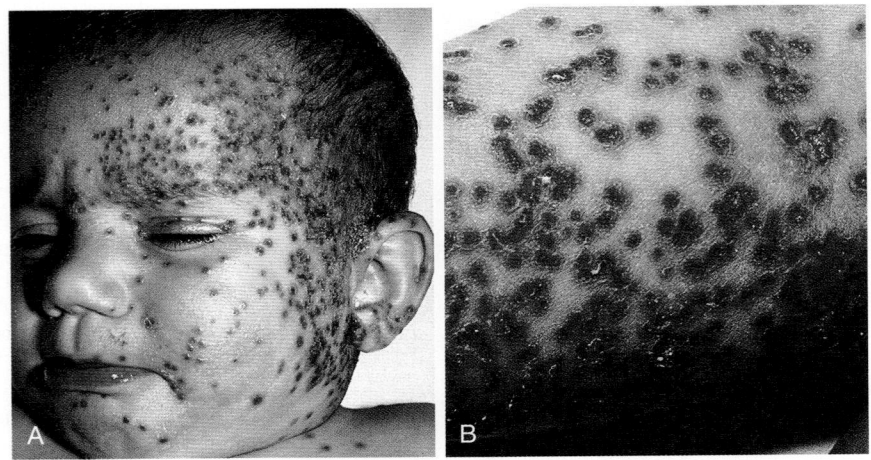

Fig. 61.13 Eczema herpeticum infection in a patient with atopic dermatitis. Numerous punched-out vesicles and erosions involving the face *(A)* and extremities *(B)*. (From Papulosquamous eruptions. In: Cohen BA, ed. *Pediatric Dermatology*. Philadelphia: Saunders; 2013:68–103.)

TABLE 61.6	Differential Diagnosis of Atopic Dermatitis	
Condition	**Similarities**	**Differences**
Seborrheic dermatitis	Scaly plaques	Earlier onset is typical, can be seen in older children
	Erythroderma may be seen when severe	Increased severity associated with immunodeficiency disorders and neurologic dysfunction
		Pruritus minimal or absent
		Well-demarcated lesions
		Characteristic yellowish-salmon greasy lesions with intertriginous distribution
Contact dermatitis		
Primary irritant	Common in infants, young children	Usually less pruritic and less eczematoid
	May have similar distributions depending on the irritant (i.e., cheeks, chin, neck)	Diaper area distribution uncommon in atopic dermatitis
Allergic	Pruritic	Well circumscribed
	Erythematous, papulovesicular eruption	Uncommon in first few months of life
		Involutes spontaneously after the removal of the offending agent

TABLE 61.6   Differential Diagnosis of Atopic Dermatitis—cont'd

Condition	Similarities	Differences
Psoriasis	Scaly, red lesions	Deeper red-violaceous hue Thick micaceous scale Characteristic nail changes Sharply demarcated lesions Distinct distribution Pruritus may be less intense
Scabies	Frequent eczematous changes secondary to scratching, rubbing, or irritating therapy Can be very difficult to distinguish in infancy	Polymorphous with papules, pustules, and hyperpigmented nodules Presence of burrows Isolation of a mite from skin scrapings Acute onset Affected household members
Langerhans cell histiocytosis	Scaly, erythematous eruption Usually begins during first year of life	Primarily children <3 yr of age Presence of purpuric papules Associated hematologic abnormalities, hepatosplenomegaly
Acrodermatitis enteropathica	Vesiculobullous eczematoid lesions Onset during infancy	Acral, periorificial distribution Associated features: failure to thrive, diarrhea, alopecia, nail dystrophy, low serum zinc levels
Phenylketonuria	Eczematous eruption	Hereditary Intellectual disability, seizures Diffuse hypopigmentation, blond hair, photosensitivity Elevated blood phenylalanine levels

TABLE 61.7   Features of Primary Immunodeficiencies Associated with Eczematous Dermatitis

Disease	Gene	Inheritance	Clinical Features	Lab Abnormalities
AD-HIES	*STAT3*	AD, less commonly sporadic	• Cold abscesses • Recurrent sinopulmonary infections • Mucocutaneous candidiasis • Coarse facies • Minimal trauma fractures • Scoliosis • Joint hyperextensibility • Retained primary teeth • Coronary artery tortuosity or dilatation • Lymphoma	• High IgE (>2,000 IU/μL) • Eosinophilia
DOCK8 deficiency	*DOCK8*	AR	• Severe mucocutaneous viral infections • Mucocutaneous candidiasis • Atopic features (asthma, allergies) • Squamous cell carcinoma • Lymphoma	• High IgE • Eosinophilia • With or without decreased IgM
PGM3 deficiency	*PGM3*	AR	• Neurologic abnormalities • Leukocytoclastic vasculitis • Atopic features (asthma, allergies) • Sinopulmonary infections • Mucocutaneous viral infections	• High IgE • Eosinophilia
WAS	*WASP*	XLR	• Hepatosplenomegaly • Lymphadenopathy • Atopic diathesis • Autoimmune conditions (especially hemolytic anemia) • Lymphoreticular malignancies	• Thrombocytopenia (<80,000/μL) • Low mean platelet volume • Eosinophilia is common • Lymphopenia • Low IgM, variable IgG
SCID	Variable, depends on type	XLR and AR most common	• Recurrent, severe infections • Failure to thrive • Persistent diarrhea • Recalcitrant oral candidiasis • Omenn: lymphadenopathy, hepatosplenomegaly, erythroderma	• Lymphopenia common • Variable patterns of reduced lymphocyte subsets (T, B, natural killer cells) • Omenn: high lymphocytes, eosinophilia, high IgE

Continued

TABLE 61.7 Features of Primary Immunodeficiencies Associated with Eczematous Dermatitis—cont'd

Disease	Gene	Inheritance	Clinical Features	Lab Abnormalities
IPEX	FOXP3	XLR	• Severe diarrhea (autoimmune enteropathy) • Various autoimmune endocrinopathies (especially diabetes mellitus, thyroiditis) • Food allergies	• High IgE • Eosinophilia • Various autoantibodies
Netherton syndrome	SPINK5	AR	• Hair shaft abnormalities • Erythroderma • Ichthyosis linearis circumflexa • Food allergies • Recurrent gastroenteritis • Neonatal hypernatremic dehydration • Upper and lower respiratory infections	• High IgE • Eosinophilia

AD, autosomal dominant; AD-HIES, autosomal-dominant hyper-IgE syndrome; AR, autosomal recessive; DOCK8, dedicator of cytokinesis 8 gene; Ig, immunoglobulin; IPEX, immune disregulation, polyendocrinopathy, enteropathy, X-linked syndrome; PGM3, phosphoglucomutase 3; SCID, severe combined immunodeficiency; WAS, Wiskott-Aldrich syndrome.

From Youssef MJ, Chiu YE. Eczema and urticaria as manifestations of undiagnosed and rare diseases. *Pediatr Clin N Am.* 2017;64(1):39–56 (Table 1, pp. 41–42).

TABLE 61.8 Atopic Dermatitis Management

Therapeutic Modality	Indications and Recommendations
Bathing	Recommended daily for 10–15 min with warm, not hot, water. May use fragrance-free bath oils. Hydrates the skin.
Soaps	Mild, fragrance-free cleansers are essential.
Emollients	Best applied immediately after bathing/showering. Should be used as often as possible. Petroleum jelly is an ideal emollient: contains no water, additives, or preservatives and prevents evaporative water loss from the skin. Thick creams are an alternative.
Bleach (sodium hypochlorite)	Depending on the size of the bathtub/amount of water used, 0.25–0.5 U.S. cup (60–120 mL) of common bleach solution (6% sodium hypochlorite) is added to a full bath (40-gallon tub). Performed 2–3 times/wk to reduce *Staphylococcus aureus* colonization.
Compresses	Indicated for acute weeping lesions. Helps cool and dry the skin, reduces inflammation. Use cool tap water or aluminum acetate solutions for 20 min, 2–4 times daily. Follow with topical corticosteroid application.
Topical corticosteroids	Indicated to reduce pruritus and inflammation. The potency of the topical corticosteroid is determined by the age of patient, site of involvement, severity of dermatitis, and duration of therapy. Facial and intertriginous skin should be treated with low-potency preparations. Apply before emollient. Use the lowest potency that is effective. Monitor closely for potential side effects, such as striae and cushingoid features.
Topical immunomodulators	Tacrolimus and pimecrolimus may be effective steroid-sparing agents for mild to moderate focal involvement, particularly on the face or groin.
Antihistamines	Controversial whether effective in this condition. Topical formulations should be avoided. Hydroxyzine may be more effective than diphenhydramine. May induce drowsiness and help some patients sleep. Nonsedating antihistamines include cetirizine, loratadine, and fexofenadine.
Antibiotics	Patients with atopic dermatitis often have increased colonization with *S. aureus*. Use if multiple weeping excoriations, crusts, or pustules suggest secondary infection or if severe or resistant eczema is present. Treat with antistaphylococcal antibiotics; specific antibiotic is based on local susceptibilities.
Ultraviolet light	Useful for severe, uncontrollable atopic dermatitis. May administer narrowband ultraviolet B (NBUVB) light.
Tars	Useful for chronic, dry, lichenified lesions, not for acute dermatitis.
Environmental conditions	Environmental factors may influence the severity of the dermatitis. Some helpful measures: • Avoid fragrances in all topicals and laundry products. • Avoid wool, feathers, dust exposure. • Reduce house dust mites. • Eliminate animal dander. • Use plastic mattress covers. • Reduce stress/anxiety. • Increase environmental humidity to reduce skin evaporative losses. • Avoid smoking.
Systemic immunosuppressants	Oral corticosteroids should be avoided. Dupilumab, an IL-4 receptor α-antagonist, is FDA-approved for the treatment of atopic dermatitis. Cyclosporine, methotrexate, mycophenolate mofetil, and azathioprine have shown some benefit in the management of atopic dermatitis but, given the side effect profile, should be prescribed under the direction of a dermatologist.

FDA, U.S. Food and Drug Administration; IL, interleukin.

nodules may be associated with antecedent trauma and represent a reactive, proliferative process. They are usually solitary, but multiple lesions occur in rare cases (Fig. 61.14). Arising as small red papules, pyogenic granulomas grow rapidly and can ulcerate, leading to profuse bleeding. Histologically, these lesions resemble infantile hemangiomas (IHs). Unlike IHs, onset after the first year of life is typical, bleeding is common, spontaneous regression is rare, and recurrences may be seen. Treatment involves destruction by pulsed dye laser therapy, electrodesiccation, surgical removal, or cryotherapy.

DISORDERS OF PIGMENTATION

These conditions are often cosmetically disfiguring and persistent and can be markers of serious systemic diseases. Pigmentary disorders may be localized or generalized; congenital or acquired; and transient, stable, or progressive (see Chapter 60).

Acquired Disorders of Hypopigmentation or Depigmentation

Postinflammatory Hypopigmentation
Postinflammatory hypopigmentation is a common form of acquired hypopigmentation and may follow any inflammatory skin condition, including bullous disorders, infections, eczema, psoriasis, pityriasis rosea, secondary syphilis, insect bites, acne, pityriasis lichenoides chronica, and burns. More frequently detected in darker-skinned individuals, the clinical findings consist of irregularly shaped hypopigmented patches of variable size, often ill-defined, located at sites of preceding inflammation. Postinflammatory hypopigmentation usually resolves gradually over several months, and no treatment is necessary other than photoprotection.

Pityriasis Alba
Pityriasis alba is characterized by poorly demarcated, slightly scaly, hypopigmented oval macules or patches located on the face (typically the cheeks), upper trunk, or extensor surfaces of the arms (Fig. 61.15). The lesions generally vary from 0.5 to 2 cm in diameter, are often multiple, and are usually asymptomatic. Sun exposure may increase the contrast with normal skin, prompting patients to seek treatment. The condition may at times be associated with atopic dermatitis, and differentiating pityriasis alba from patches of atopic dermatitis–related postinflammatory hypopigmentation may be difficult. In contrast to postinflammatory hypopigmentation, the histology of pityriasis alba demonstrates low-grade inflammation. The hypopigmentation typically persists for several months to years. Although no therapeutic

intervention is required, the use of emollients and low-potency topical corticosteroids may be effective.

Vitiligo
Vitiligo is an acquired disorder characterized by areas of complete loss of skin pigment resulting from the cytotoxic activity of autoreactive T cells against melanocytes. Autoantibodies against melanocyte-specific antigens have also been detected. The condition often manifests during childhood and is believed to be linked to specific pathogenic genetic variants. There is an increased incidence of autoimmune diseases in affected individuals and their families. The incidence of vitiligo (Addison disease, hypothyroidism, pernicious anemia, lupus) in persons with diabetes mellitus is also higher than that in the general population.

The onset of vitiligo may be precipitated by sunburn or other trauma. Physical findings are usually sufficient for establishing the diagnosis. Well-demarcated depigmented macules and patches that are often bilateral and symmetric are distributed over the joints of the extremities, on the periorificial areas, and within skin folds. Segmentally distributed depigmentation is more common in children than in adults. The course is unpredictable. Spontaneous complete repigmentation is unusual; however, partial repigmentation may be seen, especially within lesions of less than 2 years' duration. Repigmentation proceeds gradually and is more likely to occur in children than in adults.

Treatment response often takes months. For limited involvement, topical corticosteroids are most frequently used, and calcineurin inhibitors provide an option in places where it may be preferable to avoid corticosteroids. For more widespread involvement, phototherapy may provide the best chance of repigmentation and may slow progression in rapidly progressive disease. Other interventions may consist of cosmetic camouflage, self-tanners, or photoprotection to reduce the contrast between affected and unaffected sites. Careful photoprotection is also recommended to prevent the development of cutaneous malignancy. Bleaching agents are another option in individuals with depigmentation of >50% of their cutaneous surface.

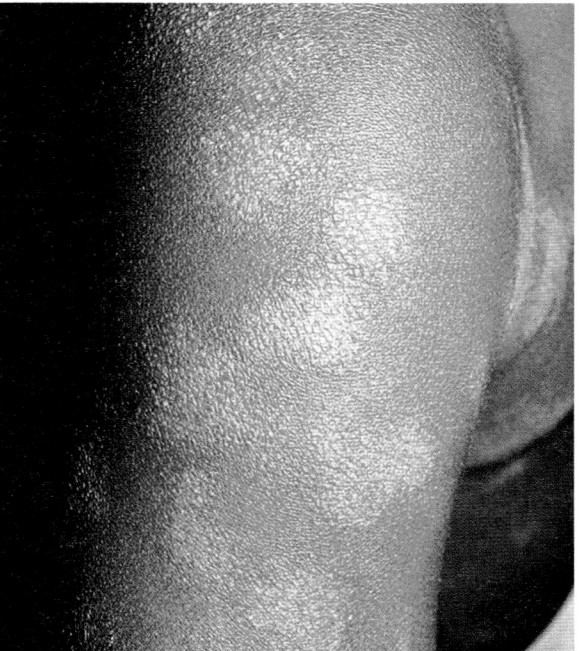

Fig. 61.15 Poorly demarcated areas of hypopigmentation in pityriasis alba. (From Papulosquamous eruptions. In: Cohen BA, ed. *Pediatric Dermatology*. Philadelphia: Saunders; 2013:66–103.)

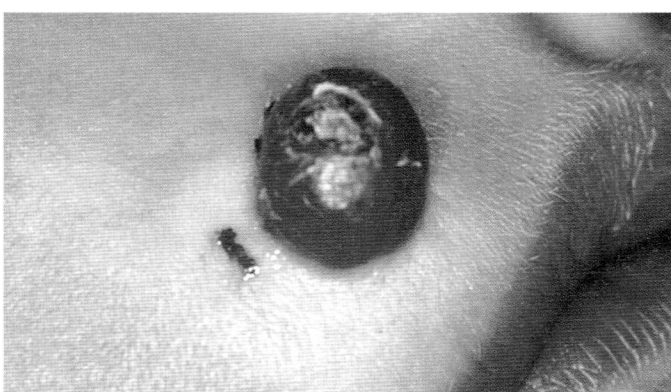

Fig. 61.14 Pyogenic granuloma. Hemorrhagic nodule with a central crust. (From Nodules and tumors. In: Cohen BA, ed. *Pediatric Dermatology*. Philadelphia: Saunders; 2013:126–147.)

Disorders of Hyperpigmentation

Lentigines

Lentigines are 1- to 5-mm macules that are darker than freckles and may occur on any cutaneous site, including the mucous membranes. Lentigines have no seasonal variance, and those that manifest during early childhood often disappear during adulthood. A lentigo may be clinically indistinguishable from a junctional nevus (mole); however, these lesions are histologically distinct.

Several syndromes are associated with multiple lentigines. Patients with multiple lentigines/**LEOPARD syndrome** can present with isolated skin involvement with generalized lentigines or the complete syndrome (multiple lentigines, ECG abnormalities, ocular hypertelorism, pulmonic stenosis, abnormal genitalia, growth retardation, and neural deafness). Lentigines in these patients may not appear until 4–5 years of age and increase rapidly thereafter. Multiple lentigines located on the mucous membranes, especially the vermilion border of the lips and buccal mucosa, should alert the clinician to the possibility of **Peutz-Jeghers syndrome**, which is characteristically associated with intestinal polyposis and subsequent risk of malignant transformation and intussusception. **Laugier-Hunziker syndrome** also presents with lentigines involving the lips and buccal mucosa without the gastrointestinal involvement of Peutz-Jeghers. **Solar lentigines** occur in sun-exposed areas in older children, particularly at sites of prior sunburns.

Café-Au-Lait Macules

Café-au-lait macules are well-circumscribed tan macules that usually measure <0.5 cm and may be as large as 15–20 cm in diameter (Fig. 61.16). The lesions are found on any cutaneous site and may be present

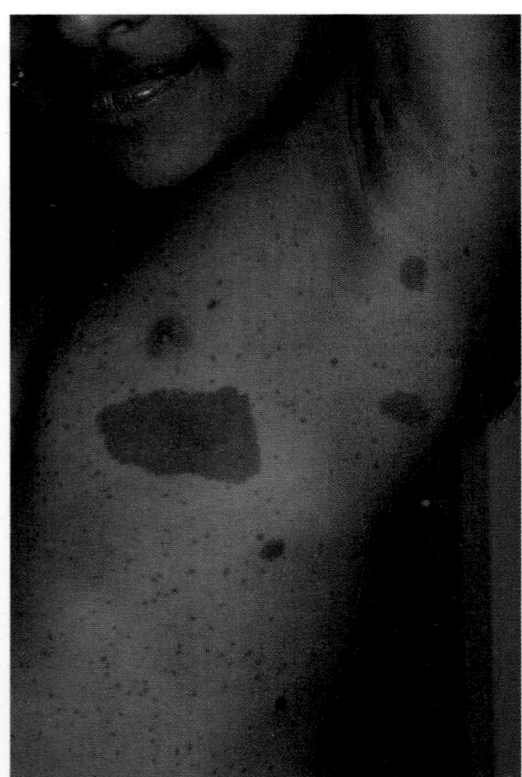

Fig. 61.16 A child with neurofibromatosis 1 and numerous and variously sized café-au-lait macules over the trunk. (From Price HN, Marghoob AA. Disorders of hyperpigmentation and melanocytes. In: Eichenfield LF, Frieden IJ, Mathes EF, et al., eds. *Neonatal and Infant Dermatology.* 3rd ed. Philadelphia: Elsevier; 2015:389, Fig. 24.1.)

at birth or appear during early childhood. Although café-au-lait spots are seen in up to 20% of normal individuals and may be familial, the presence of many macules should raise the clinical suspicion of **neurofibromatosis** (Table 61.9). The presence of six or more café-au-lait spots (>0.5 cm in prepubertal children; >1.5 cm in postpubertal children) fulfills one of the diagnostic criteria for neurofibromatosis type 1. Although the lesions are not pathognomonic, they are present in most patients with neurofibromatosis and tend to be larger and more numerous. Café-au-lait spots have also been associated with Watson syndrome, tuberous sclerosis, McCune-Albright syndrome, Turner syndrome, Bloom syndrome, ataxia-telangiectasia, Russell-Silver syndrome, Fanconi anemia, Gaucher disease, Legius syndrome, ring chromosome syndrome, and Chédiak-Higashi syndrome.

Postinflammatory Hyperpigmentation

Postinflammatory hyperpigmentation is the most common cause of acquired hyperpigmentation in children. This pigmentary alteration can follow any inflammatory insult and is seen commonly after insect bites, acne, drug reactions, or other skin trauma. The clinical features are usually more striking in darkly pigmented individuals and often may be more pronounced than the original inflammatory lesions. The increased pigmentation usually resolves gradually over several months to years.

Acquired Melanocytic Nevi

Acquired melanocytic nevi arise during early childhood as 1- to 2-mm brown macules occurring most often on sun-exposed skin. These early flat nevi usually represent junctional nevi, in which nests of nevus cells are located along the dermo-epidermal junction. Over time, some nevus cells may spread into the dermis, forming compound melanocytic nevi, which appear somewhat larger and more papular than junctional nevi. In some nevi, the nevus cells may become restricted to the dermis. These intradermal nevi are usually fleshy or even pedunculated in appearance. Located usually on the head, neck, or upper trunk, these nevi may clinically resemble skin tags.

There is a gradual increase in the number of nevi during childhood and adolescence. The average individual acquires approximately 20–40 melanocytic nevi. This number peaks at 25 years of age. In general, fair-skinned persons have a greater number of nevi than do darkly pigmented persons.

Melanoma

Although melanomas are very rare in childhood, their incidence is increasing and can present with atypical features compared to the classic criteria of adult cases. The overall lifetime risk of melanoma in White persons in the United States is currently approximately 1 in 50 individuals. Melanoma can arise de novo or from pre-existing congenital or acquired melanocytic nevi. Three subtypes include **spitzoid** (papular, nodular, may be amelanotic, sun and non–sun-exposed distribution), melanoma arising in a **congenital melanotic nevus** (new, rapidly growing nodule in subcutaneous or dermal plane of a nevus), and **conventional melanoma** (sun-exposed skin in adolescents: papule or nodule may be melanotic in children). Nevi should be observed for specific changes that may be indicative of malignancy. These alterations include the following:

1. Rapid growth of the nevi
2. Changes in texture, including nodularity, crusting, ulceration, bleeding, or loss of normal skin lines
3. Changes in pigmentation, especially the development of red, white, or blue hues
4. Border irregularity, especially notched or scalloped edges
5. Symptoms of itching, tenderness, or pain

TABLE 61.9   Neurocutaneous Syndromes

Syndrome	Mode of Inheritance	Cutaneous Findings	Systemic Findings
Tuberous sclerosis	Autosomal dominant	Ash leaf macules Angiofibromas (adenoma sebaceum) Shagreen patches Periungual/subungual fibromas Gingival fibromas	CNS involvement (seizures, intellectual disability, cortical tubers) Cardiac rhabdomyomas Retinal gliomas Renal carcinoma or hamartoma Renal or pulmonary cysts Skeletal abnormalities
Neurofibromatosis (NF) (NF1 >85% of cases)	Autosomal dominant	Café-au-lait macules (more than six measuring ≥1.5 cm in adults and >0.5 cm in children) Axillary, inguinal freckling (Crowe sign) Neurofibromas Blue-red macules and pseudoatrophic macules (involuted neurofibromas) Lisch nodules (melanocytic hamartomas of the iris)	Acoustic neuroma in NF2 Optic glioma may result in exophthalmos, decreased visual acuity Intellectual disability (rarely) Seizure disorders (rarely) Tumors (astrocytomas) Hyperactivity, macrocephaly Learning disabilities, speech delay Osseous defects (up to 50%) Intestinal neurofibromas Endocrine disorders
Incontinentia pigmenti	X-linked dominant	Phase 1: inflammatory vesicles/bullae in crops over trunk and extremities, may persist weeks to months Phase 2: irregular linear verrucous lesions on one or more extremities, resolves spontaneously within several months Phase 3: brown to blue-gray hyperpigmentation, swirl-like formations on extremities and trunk; increases in intensity through second year of life, then remains stable or fades over many years Phase 4: streaked hypopigmented lesions	Eosinophilia CNS involvement (seizures, spasticity, ↓ IQ) in 30% Spasticity Ophthalmic changes (strabismus, cataracts, optic atrophy, retinal damage) Alopecia Skeletal abnormalities Dental abnormalities

CNS, central nervous system; IQ, intelligence quotient.

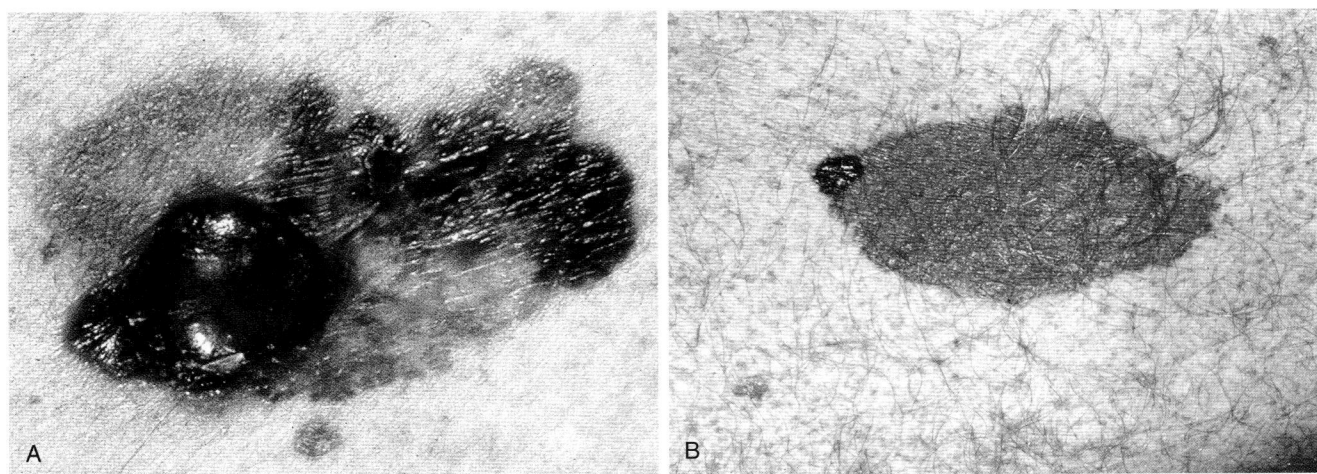

Fig. 61.17 Melanoma. *A,* This lesion shows the irregularity of outline, color, and thickness typical of a melanoma. *B,* A black papule developed in the border of a 3.5 × 1.5–cm congenital pigmented nevus. Biopsy showed a thin melanoma, and the lesion was excised with a 1-cm margin. (From Mavropoulos JC, Cohen BA. Disorders of pigmentation. In: Cohen BA, ed. *Pediatric Dermatology.* 4th ed. Philadelphia: Elsevier; 2013:157, Fig. 6.15.)

Additionally, the **ABCD criteria** include asymmetry, border irregularity, color variegation, and diameter >6 mm.

In general, melanomas occur more frequently in lightly pigmented individuals, in individuals with a high nevus count, and in those with a family history of melanoma. Melanomas usually appear as darkly pigmented nodular masses, often with color variegation, larger than 6 mm

in diameter (Fig. 61.17). They are often asymmetric and tend to have irregular borders and surface characteristics. Melanomas must be differentiated from other benign pigmented lesions, including congenital and acquired melanocytic nevi, blue nevi, Spitz nevi, vascular lesions such as hemangiomas and pyogenic granulomas, and pigmented lesions caused by trauma. Suspect lesions should be referred to a dermatologist.

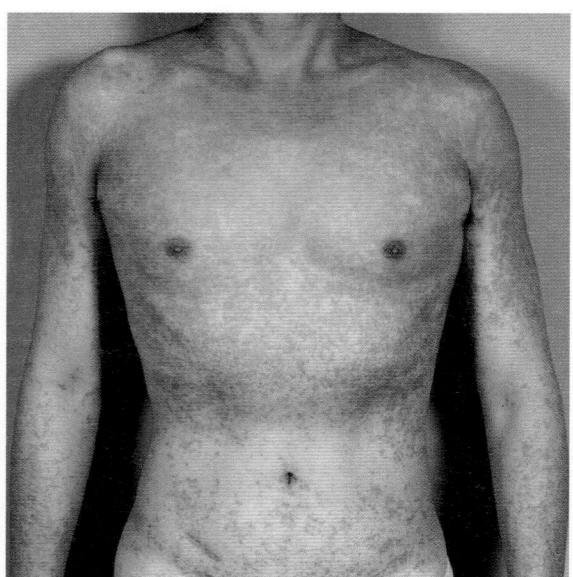

Fig. 61.18 Morbilliform drug eruption due to trimethoprim-sulfamethoxazole (TMP-SMZ). This HIV-positive young man developed a widespread eruption of blanchable erythematous macules and papules 8 days after starting TMP-SMZ. Note the coalescence on the upper trunk. (From Chan RKW, Chio MTW, Koh HY. Cutaneous manifestations of HIV infection. In: Bolognia JL, Schaffer JV, Cerroni L, eds. *Dermatology*. 4th ed. Philadelphia: Elsevier; 2018, Fig 78.18.)

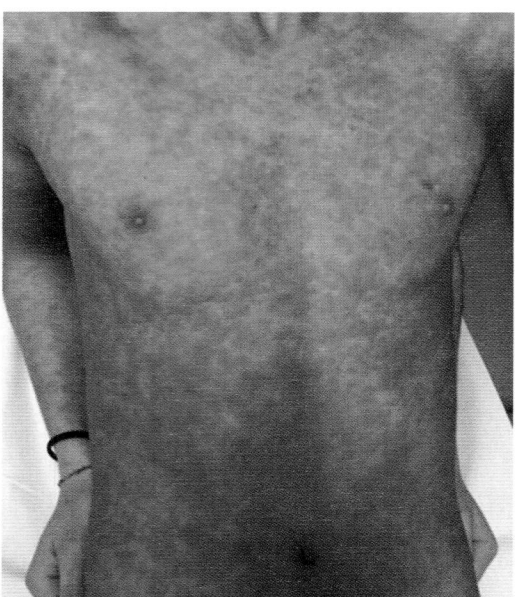

Fig. 61.19 Acute rash in DRESS (drug reaction with eosinophilia and systemic symptoms) syndrome. (Modified from Mori F, Caffarelli C, Caimmi S, et al. Drug reaction with eosinophilia and systemic symptoms [DRESS] in children. *Acta Biomed.* 2019;90[S3]:66–79 [Fig. 1, p. 68].)

The mortality rate of melanoma is estimated to be between 10% and 20%. The prognosis depends on the thickness of the lesion. For lesions <0.75 mm in depth, the prognosis is excellent. Surgical excision is the treatment of choice. Patients should be educated on the importance of photoprotection with broad-spectrum (ultraviolet A and B) sunscreens.

REACTIVE ERYTHEMAS

Morbilliform Drug Eruption

Morbilliform (measles-like) eruptions are the most common cutaneous manifestations of drug-induced eruptions in children. In this eruption, fine erythematous macules and papules are distributed over the trunk (Fig. 61.18). The rash often spreads centripetally from the trunk to the extremities. Lesions may coalesce into large plaques and are usually pruritic. Morbilliform drug eruptions are often difficult to differentiate from viral exanthems. It is believed that concomitant viral infections may predispose susceptible individuals to develop an allergic morbilliform drug eruption.

Many agents, including common antibiotics, can trigger a morbilliform drug eruption. These medications include penicillins, sulfonamides, thiazides, sulfonylureas, nonsteroidal antiinflammatory drugs (NSAIDs), aromatic anticonvulsants, and gold. Treatment includes prompt diagnosis with discontinuation of the offending medication and symptomatic care with antihistamines and emollients. The rash may last an average of 1–2 weeks and sometimes progresses despite discontinuation of the offending medication. In rare cases for which discontinuation of the offending medication is not possible, continuation of the medication with close monitoring for the development of a more severe reaction may be considered as tolerance may develop with subsequent resolution of the eruption.

Severe Cutaneous Adverse Reaction to Drugs

More serious drug reactions include DRESS (drug reaction with eosinophilia and systemic symptoms) (Fig. 61.19), Stevens-Johnson syndrome/toxic epidermal necrolysis (SJS/TEN) (Fig. 61.20), and acute generalized exanthematous pustulosis (AGEP) (Fig. 61.21). Distinguishing features are noted in Table 61.10 and Fig. 61.22. SJS/TEN is also characterized by a positive Nikolsky sign (Fig. 61.23). Responsible drugs are noted for each syndrome in Table 61.11.

Fixed Drug Eruption

A fixed drug eruption is characterized by the sudden development of solitary or multiple well-demarcated, annular, erythematous, or hyperpigmented plaques. One of the distinguishing features is persistent postinflammatory hyperpigmentation, which may last weeks to months after the eruption subsides. The size of the lesion may vary, and the sites of predilection include the lips, trunk, legs, arms, and genitals. In some cases, the lesion may have a central bulla. Systemic symptoms are rare though may consist of local pruritus or a burning sensation.

Discontinuation of the offending medication causes a decrease in the intensity of the erythema and edema; repeated challenge with the same agent causes a reappearance of the lesion in the same location and may produce new lesions. Future outbreaks may be progressively more severe. The most common agents inducing fixed drug eruption include barbiturates, sulfonamides, tetracyclines, phenolphthalein, acetaminophen, salicylates, NSAIDs, and even certain foods that contain the synthetic food coloring yellow 5 (tartrazine). Treatment is aimed at discontinuation and avoidance of the offending agent.

When numerous lesions occur, the condition may resemble erythema multiforme (EM), and the clinical history becomes paramount in establishing the diagnosis, particularly as there is significant histologic overlap.

HYPERSENSITIVITY REACTIONS

Allergic Contact Dermatitis

Allergic contact dermatitis is a type IV delayed hypersensitivity reaction. This T-cell–mediated immune response occurs after the

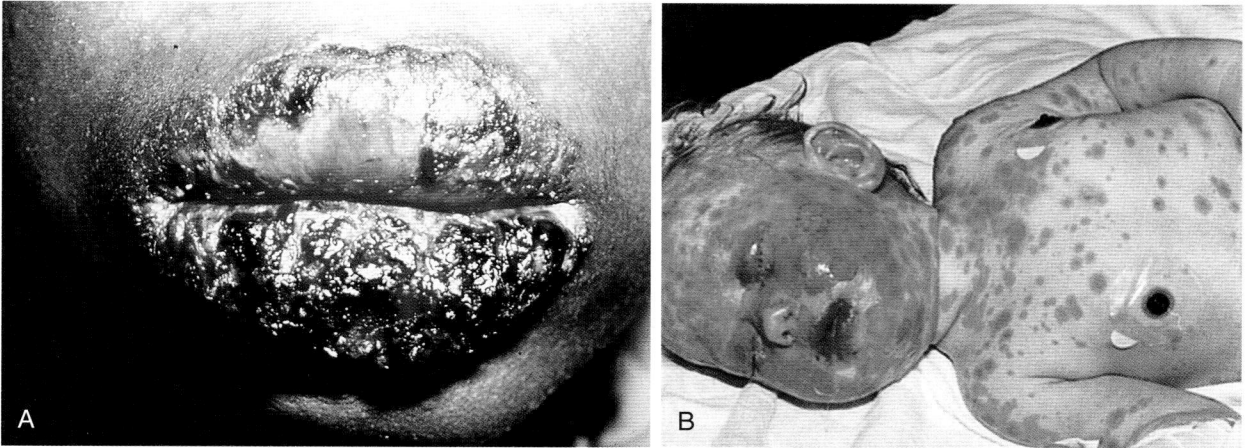

Fig. 61.20 *A,* Erosions and crusting of the lips in Stevens-Johnson syndrome. *B,* Widespread blistering and erosions of the skin and mucous membranes. (From Vesicopustular eruptions. In: Cohen BA, ed. *Pediatric Dermatology.* Philadelphia: Saunders; 2013.)

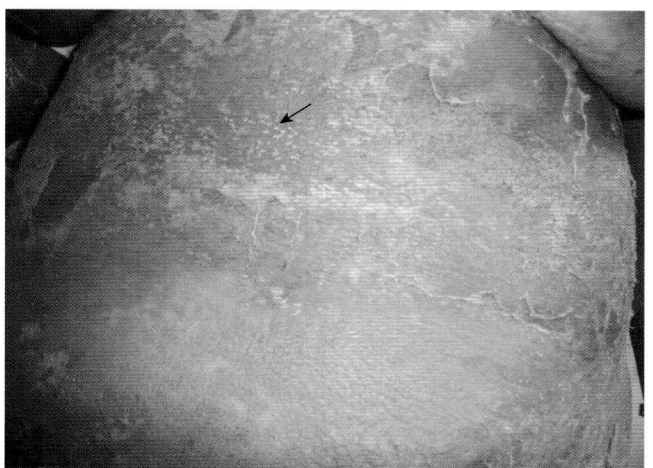

Fig. 61.21 Acute generalized exanthematous pustulosis (AGEP). Nonfollicular pustules *(arrow)* arising on edematous erythema of the trunk. (From Supplement to Duong TA, Valeyrie-Allanore L, Wolkenstein P, et al. Severe cutaneous adverse reactions to drugs. *Lancet.* 2017;390:1996–2011, Fig. S5.)

responsible antigen contacts the skin, resulting in sensitization. Future contact with the same antigen provokes an inflammatory response within hours to several days. Acute contact dermatitis is usually characterized by the sudden onset of erythema, vesiculation, edema, and intense pruritus. Chronic contact dermatitis results in the development of lichenification, scaling, and hyperpigmentation and can be complicated by secondary bacterial infection.

Poison ivy is the most common cause of allergic contact dermatitis (*Rhus* dermatitis) in the United States, in which following sensitization, direct contact of the skin with the sap of poison ivy, oak, or sumac results in an intensely pruritic dermatitis. Contact with clothing or pets that have been exposed to the plant resin and smoke from the fire of such plants being burned are other forms of exposure. Given the relative ease with which the responsible antigens in poison ivy permeate the skin, sensitization can be very rapid. The eruption is usually seen as linear vesicles and papules or plaques. The spread to body sites is caused by exposure to the plant resin, not by the blister fluid. Therefore,

scratching affected skin or contact with affected individuals should not result in spreading of the eruption.

Other common forms of allergic contact dermatitis result from exposure to cosmetics, fragrances, hair dyes, and nickel. **Nickel dermatitis** often results from prolonged contact with the nickel in jewelry or belt buckles (Fig. 61.24). The eczematous changes are usually localized to the sites of contact, including the earlobes, neckline, wrists, and waistline, although generalized lichenoid papular id reactions have been described. The diagnosis of contact dermatitis can usually be determined from history and clinical examination findings. The distribution of linear, geometric, or well-demarcated areas may be helpful in confirming the diagnosis. When allergic contact dermatitis is suspected but the responsible agent is unclear, patch testing with a selected group of antigens may provide useful information. Prevention of future exposure to inciting antigens is necessary.

Usually, treatment with topical corticosteroids, emollients, and antihistamines is sufficient to control the eruption. However, widespread dermatitis or severe involvement of the face may necessitate administration of systemic corticosteroids. Wet compresses with aluminum acetate aid in the drying of weeping, vesicular lesions and provide symptomatic relief.

Urticaria

Urticaria is characterized by transient, edematous, erythematous, often annular wheals (Fig. 61.25). Central clearing may be seen but is not always present. The eruption is often sudden and pruritic, and each lesion rarely lasts longer than a few hours. Although the lesions are transient, they may continue to appear in new locations, and the entire urticarial episode may last hours to years. **Angioedema** is a form of urticaria that manifests with marked swelling of deeper tissue planes that frequently involves the lips, dorsum of the hands or feet, scalp, scrotum, or periorbital tissue.

Giant annular urticaria lesions are usually large, up to 20–30 cm, and polycyclic. A centrally bruised appearance is common within these lesions. Lesions may be of different sizes with bizarre shapes and patterns. Affected patients are often irritable and may have edema of the hands, eyelids, or feet. Giant annular lesions are often confused with the target lesions of EM, although the target lesions of EM are typically smaller (e.g., 1–3 cm). Additional key features differentiate the two disorders. By definition urticarial lesions are transient, with individual

TABLE 61.10 **Main Clinical and Histologic Characteristics of Severe Cutaneous Adverse Reactions (SCARs)**

	Drug-to-SCAR Interval	General Symptoms*	Skin Features	Laboratory Values	Main Organs Involved	Histologic Features
SJS and TEN	4–28 days	Fever ≥38°C, influenza-like syndrome, respiratory tract symptoms	Blisters, large skin detachment, confluent erythema, atypical target lesions, purpura, Nikolsky sign; skin detachment: Stevens-Johnson syndrome <10%, toxic epidermal necrolysis ≥30%, SJS-TEN 10–30%; two or more mucous membranes involved	Lymphopenia, transitory neutropenia, mild cytolysis, renal impairment	Full-thickness epidermal necrosis, focal adnexal necrosis, necrotic keratinocytes, mild mononuclear cell dermal infiltrate, negative direct immunofluorescence test
DRESS syndrome	2–6 wk	Fever ≥38°C, influenza-like syndrome	Maculopapular rash, erythroderma, facial or extremity edema, purpura, pustules, focal monopolar mucous membrane involvement	Eosinophilia >700 cells/μL, atypical lymphocytes, elevated transaminase concentration, impaired renal function, herpesvirus reactivation (HHV-6, HHV-7, EBV, CMV), parvovirus B19 reactivation	Lichenoid infiltrate or eczematous pattern (spongiosis, edema), focal necrotic keratinocytes, mononuclear infiltrate, focal eosinophil and neutrophil infiltrates, mild vasculitis
AGEP	1–11 days	Fever ≥38°C	Intertriginous erythema, edema, widespread nonfollicular sterile pustules, postpustular pinpoint desquamation, Nikolsky sign, rare oral mucous membrane involvement	Hyperleukocytosis, neutrophils ≥7,000 cells/μL, mild eosinophilia	Subcorneal or intraepidermal spongiform or nonspongiform pustules with or without papillary edema, focal necrotic keratinocytes, neutrophilic sometimes with eosinophils, mild vasculitis

*General symptoms can precede or occur at the same time as skin manifestations.
AGEP, acute generalized exanthematous pustulosis; CMV, cytomegalovirus; DRESS, drug reaction with eosinophilia and systemic symptoms; EBV, Epstein-Barr virus; HHV, human herpesvirus; SCAR, severe cutaneous adverse reaction; SJS, Stevens-Johnson syndrome; TEN, toxic epidermal necrolysis.
From Duong TA, Valeyrie-Allanore L, Wolkenstein P, et al. Severe cutaneous adverse reactions to drugs. *Lancet.* 2017;390:1996–2011 (Table 1, p. 1997).

lesions lasting <24 hours, whereas lesions in EM are fixed and usually last 1–2 weeks in the same anatomic location. Outlining the lesions with a marker may help determine whether the lesions are fixed or transient. Another differentiating feature is that the lesions in EM usually have a dusky, necrotic center or blister. A skin biopsy may also aid in differentiating between the two disorders (Table 61.12).

Urticaria may be defined as either acute or chronic. **Acute** urticaria lasts <6 weeks. When hives continue to develop for more than 6 weeks, urticaria is considered **chronic**. Acute urticaria has numerous etiologies but is often caused by medications (particularly antibacterials), foods, infections, or environmental stimuli such as stinging insects (Table 61.13). The cause of **chronic** urticaria is typically difficult to determine, with a broad list of potential etiologies (see Table 61.13). A thorough history and a careful physical examination are the most helpful tools for determining the cause. There are no routine laboratory tests that should be obtained in the evaluation of urticaria; however, if history or physical examination suggests a specific underlying cause, such as infection, then confirmatory testing for that cause should be pursued.

There are physical etiologies of urticaria that tend to recur with exposure to the stimulus (Table 61.14). In addition, urticaria-like lesions have been reported in autoinflammatory diseases (Table 61.15) and other systemic disorders (Table 61.16). An approach to acute and chronic urticaria is noted in Fig. 61.26.

Urticaria is usually self-limited. Treatment consists of eliminating identifiable causes and administering antihistamines. Hydroxyzine and diphenhydramine are often used though often result in drowsiness. Nonsedating antihistamines are preferred, provided there are no potential interactions with concurrent medications. H_1 and H_2 blockers may be combined as needed. Systemic steroids are usually not indicated unless there is airway involvement or anaphylaxis.

Erythema Multiforme

EM is a distinct hypersensitivity eruption associated with numerous etiologies, the most frequent of which is HSV infection, even in the absence of a clinically recognizable herpetic lesion. Additional etiologies include other infections and less commonly medications (Table 61.17). This self-limited condition lacks internal organ involvement and has minimal complications.

Manifestations of EM are variable. The typical lesion in EM is an erythematous papule with a dusky, purpuric, or necrotic center (Fig. 61.27). The lesions are targetoid with concentric zones of color change: a dusky center or blister, a peripheral ring of pale edema, and an erythematous halo; some may not demonstrate the characteristic concentric changes, and the appearance may vary depending on the stage at which the lesion is visualized. Lesions start abruptly and symmetrically as red macules or urticarial papules that expand into a targetoid appearance. They are commonly distributed on the dorsa of the hands,

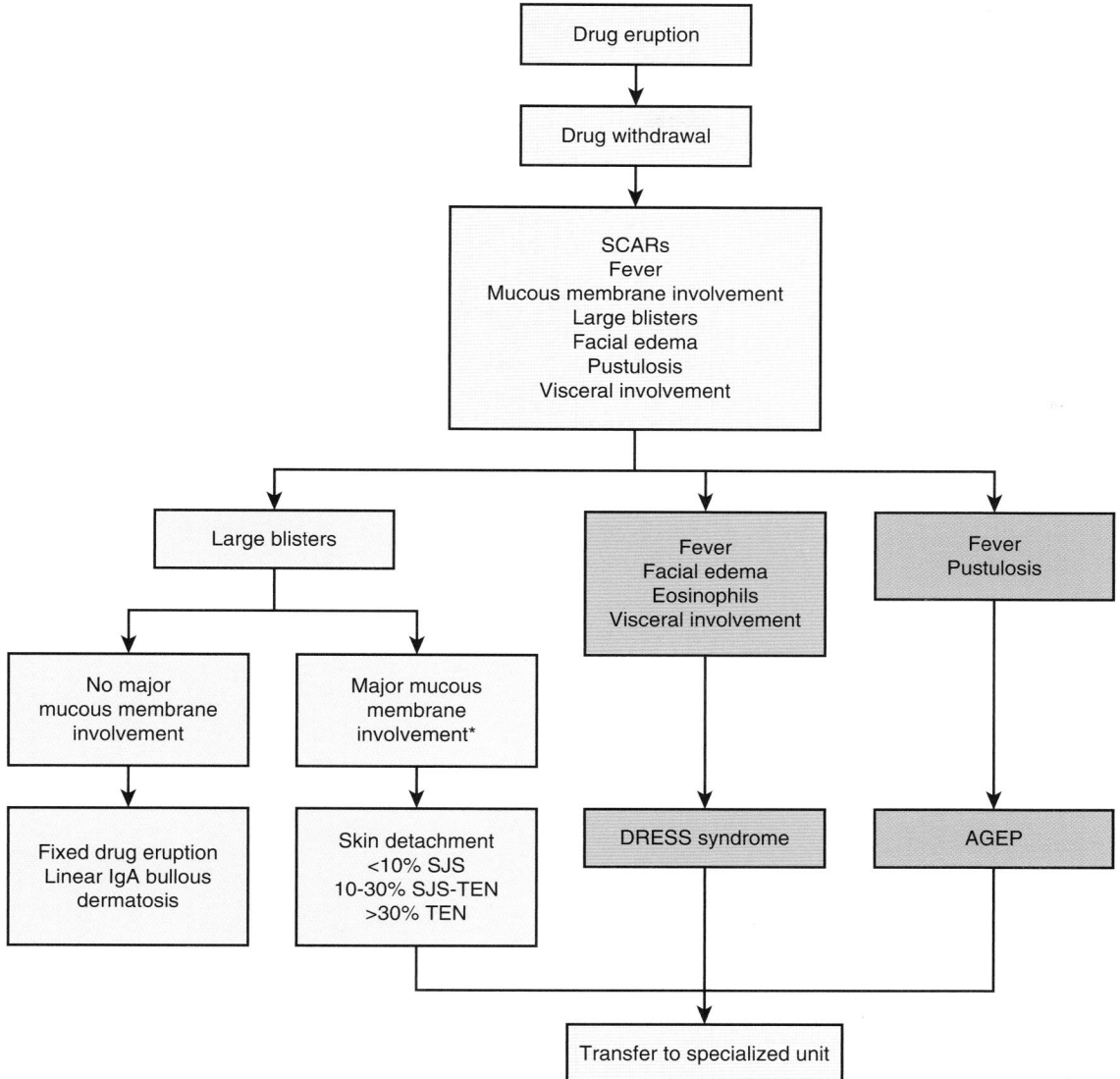

Fig. 61.22 Decisional algorithm for SCARs. Clinical features leading to suspicion of a SCAR and decisional algorithm helping physicians to classify the SCAR at the first visit. *Most patients with SJS or TEN have more than two affected mucous membranes. AGEP, acute generalized exanthematous pustulosis; DRESS, drug reaction with eosinophilia and systemic symptoms; IgA, immunoglobulin A; SCAR, severe cutaneous adverse reaction; SJS, Stevens-Johnson syndrome; TEN, toxic epidermal necrolysis. (From Duong TA, Valeyrie-Allanore L, Wolkenstein P, et al. Severe cutaneous adverse reactions to drugs. *Lancet.* 2017;390:1996–2011 [Fig. 2, p. 2003].)

feet, palms, and soles (see Table 61.12). The Koebner phenomenon may be seen with lesions occurring in areas of injury.

EM minor is often differentiated from *EM major*. EM minor consists of mainly cutaneous lesions with no more than one area of mucosal involvement, typically orolabial. EM major has a similar cutaneous eruption with two or more sites of mucosal involvement with more extensively sized oral lesions. The mucous membranes most commonly involved are the conjunctivae and oral mucosa.

Histopathologic study of the lesions usually demonstrates a perivascular lymphocytic infiltrate with individual keratinocyte necrosis. There may be vacuolar degeneration of the basal layer, spongiosis, papillary dermal edema, and junctional or subepidermal cleft formation. In general, patients with EM major tend to have more extensive inflammation and less extensive epidermal necrosis when compared to patients with SJS.

The disease is usually self-limited and necessitates supportive treatment with analgesics, topical steroids, and antihistamines for symptomatic relief. Systemic steroids may be beneficial in severe cases. Lesions often heal within 1–3 weeks and may leave residual hyperpigmentation. In children with recurrent HSV-associated EM, antivirals may prove helpful.

Stevens-Johnson Syndrome/Toxic Epidermal Necrolysis Complex

SJS and TEN are considered part of a continuum of disease differentiated by body surface area (see Table 61.10). The reaction is often elicited by medications, frequently includes internal organ involvement, and has a high rate of complications and sequelae. In SJS, there is <10% body surface involvement; with 10–30% body surface involvement, the

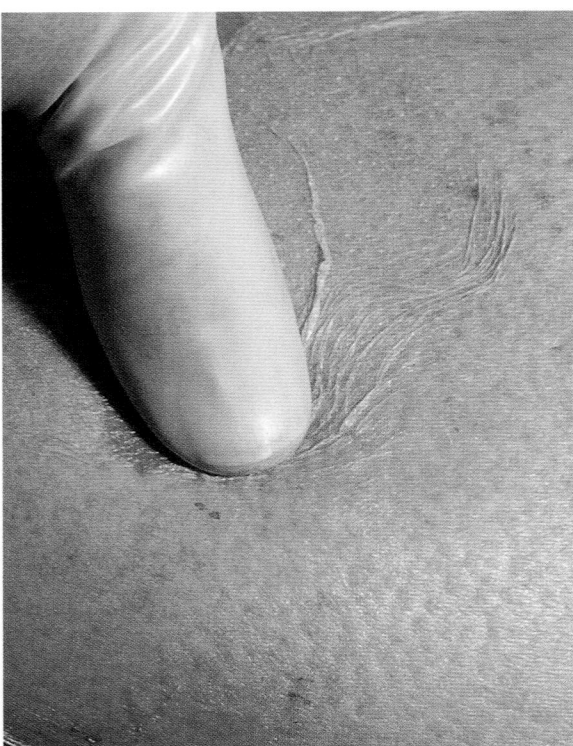

Fig. 61.23 Toxic epidermal necrolysis begins with diffuse, hot erythema. In hours the skin becomes painful, and with slight thumb pressure the skin wrinkles, slides laterally, and separates from the dermis (Nikolsky sign). (From Dinulos GHJ. *Habif's Clinical Dermatology.* 7th ed. Philadelphia: Elsevier; 2021:725, Fig. 18.9B.)

condition is labeled *SJS/TEN overlap*; TEN refers to cases with more than 30% body surface involvement.

SJS is a unique hypersensitivity reaction. Although many factors have been implicated in the origin of SJS/TEN, medications are the most common causes in children. In particular, sulfonamides, anticonvulsants (phenytoin, carbamazepine, lamotrigine, phenobarbital), and NSAIDs are cited as some of the most common triggers. The nature of the reaction is not clearly understood but is believed to be a cytotoxic immune reaction aimed at the destruction of keratinocytes expressing drug-related antigens. In children, infections are also associated with SJS. Classifications such as **Mycoplasma pneumoniae–induced rash and mucositis (MIRM)** and **reactive infectious mucocutaneous eruption (RIME)** have been used when children have documented *M. pneumoniae* or other infection with predominant mucosal involvement and limited cutaneous involvement. Patients with this mucocutaneous hypersensitivity reaction in the setting of infection, referred to as MIRM or RIME, tend to have more limited skin involvement than in traditional SJS.

SJS usually begins with a nonspecific prodrome (often fever, sore throat, and cough) followed by generalized blisters, erosions, erythema, and hemorrhagic crusting of mucous membranes of the mouth, nose, eyes, and/or genitalia as well as the trunk and extremities (see Fig. 61.20). The prodrome associated with SJS can be difficult to distinguish from symptoms of an infection that might precipitate RIME.

To make a diagnosis of SJS, at least two mucous membranes must be involved. The nomenclature surrounding and the distinction between EM major and SJS are controversial as both have skin and mucosal involvement. Lesions in SJS are usually roundish, irregularly shaped, and less targetoid with numerous erythematous to violaceous macules

TABLE 61.11 Delayed Hypersensitivity Drug Rashes by Category

Maculopapular Exanthems—Any Drug Can Produce a Rash 7–10 Days After the First Dose

Allopurinol
Antibiotics: penicillin, ampicillin, sulfonamides
Antiepileptics: phenytoin, phenobarbital
Antihypertensives: captopril, thiazide diuretics
Contrast dye: iodine
Gold salts
Hypoglycemic drugs
Meprobamate
Phenothiazines
Quinine

Drug Rash with Eosinophilia and Systemic Symptoms (DRESS)

Anticonvulsants: phenytoin, phenobarbital, valproate, lamotrigine
Antibiotics: sulfonamides, minocycline, dapsone, ampicillin, ethambutol, isoniazid, linezolid, metronidazole, rifampin, streptomycin, vancomycin
Antihypertensives: amlodipine, captopril
Antidepressants: bupropion, fluoxetine
Allopurinol
Celecoxib
Ibuprofen
Phenothiazines

Erythema Multiforme/Stevens-Johnson Syndrome/Toxic Epidermal Necrolysis

Sulfonamides, phenytoin, barbiturates, carbamazepine, allopurinol, amikacin, phenothiazines
Toxic epidermal necrolysis: same as for erythema multiforme but also acetazolamide, gold, nitrofurantoin, pentazocine, tetracycline, quinidine

Acute Generalized Exanthematous Pustulosis (AGEP)

Antibiotics: penicillins, macrolides, cephalosporins, clindamycin, imipenem, fluoroquinolones, isoniazid, vancomycin, minocycline, doxycycline, linezolid
Antimalarials: chloroquine, hydroxychloroquine
Antifungals: terbinafine, nystatin
Anticonvulsants: carbamazepine
Calcium channel blockers
Furosemide
Systemic corticosteroids
Protease inhibitors

Collagen Vascular or Lupus-Like Reactions

Procainamide, hydralazine, phenytoin, penicillamine, trimethadione, methyldopa, carbamazepine, griseofulvin, nalidixic acid, oral contraceptives, propranolol

Erythema Nodosum

Oral contraceptives, penicillin, sulfonamides, diuretics, gold, clonidine, propranolol, opiates
Fixed drug reactions: phenolphthalein, barbiturates, gold, sulfonamides, meprobamate, penicillin, tetracycline, analgesics

From Duvic M. Urticaria, drug hypersensitivity rashes, nodules and tumors, and atrophic diseases. In: Goldman L, Schafer AI, eds. *Goldman-Cecil Medicine.* 26th ed. Philadelphia: Elsevier; 2020:2635, Table 411-3.

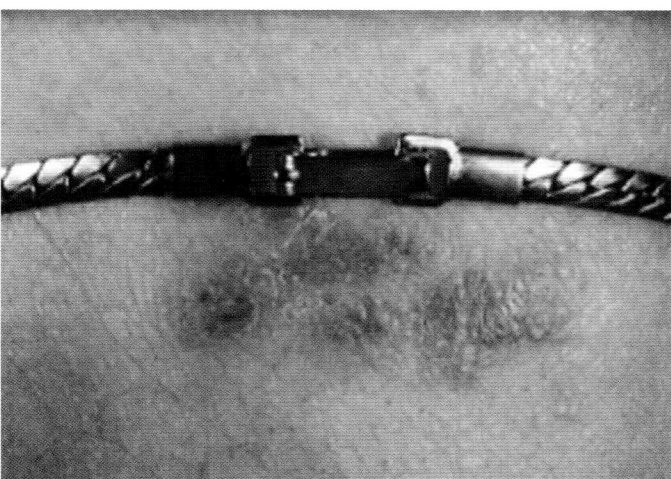

Fig. 61.24 Nickel contact dermatitis. Wrist lesions in the distribution of the nickel bracelet clasp. (From Cohen BA, Davis HW, Gehris RP. Dermatology. In: Zitelli BJ, et al., eds. *Atlas of Pediatric Physical Diagnosis.* Philadelphia: Saunders; 2012:299–368.)

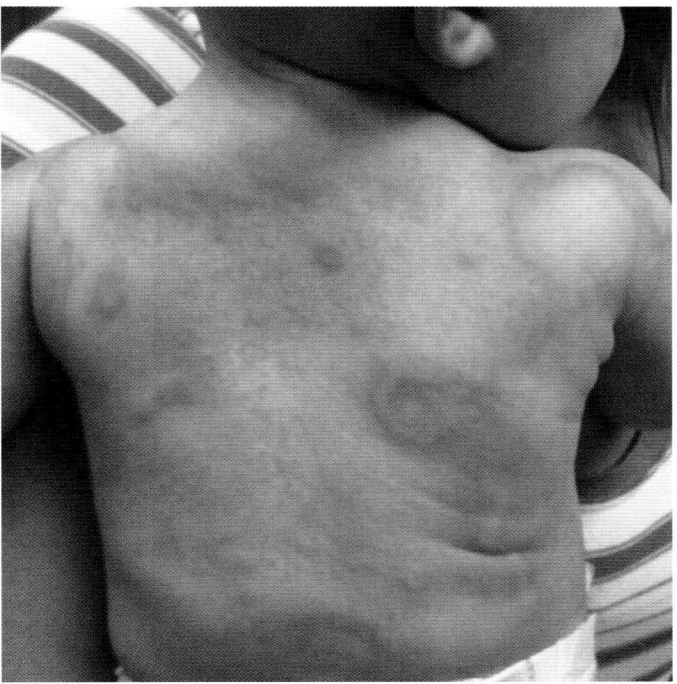

Fig. 61.25 Acute urticaria. Giant annular urticaria with large, bizarre shapes. (From Lee AD, Jorizzo JL. Acute urticaria. In: *Dermatologic Signs of Internal Disease.* 2009:53–62.)

TABLE 61.12 Urticaria vs Erythema Multiforme	
Urticaria	**Erythema Multiforme**
Transient lesions: usually last for hours	Fixed lesions: lasting several days in the same location
Asymmetric, variable, and bizarre shapes	Usually round or oval
Can enlarge to multiple centimeters	Typically less than a few centimeters
No epidermal change: may have central clearing	Epidermal change: usually central necrosis, duskiness, blistering or crusting
Continued appearance of new lesions	All lesions present within first few days
Associated edema of hands/feet, eyelids	No edema
Generalized	Acral distribution

TEN is the most severe hypersensitivity reaction, with an estimated mortality rate as high as 20%. Patients experience tender erythema of the skin that progresses rapidly to blistering and skin fragility with subsequent denudation. Malaise and prolonged fever often accompany these skin changes. Sheets of necrotic epidermis may slough off and leave denuded patches in areas of pressure, such as the back and shoulders (see Fig. 61.23). Mucous membranes are typically involved, and lesions are similar to those seen in SJS with flaccid, hemorrhagic blisters. In severe cases of TEN, sheets of necrotic epidermis may include skin appendages such as fingernails and toenails.

Systemic signs such as fever, weakness, and arthralgia occur commonly. SJS/TEN may be complicated by dehydration, electrolyte imbalance, and bacterial infection that can progress to septic shock. TEN is often accompanied by a systemic toxic state with increased morbidity and mortality. Generalized lymphadenopathy and hepatosplenomegaly may be present. Internal organ involvement, manifesting as tracheal and bronchial symptoms, pneumonitis, hepatitis, acute kidney injury, myocarditis, confusion, and coma, can be prominent in TEN.

Supportive therapy is the mainstay of treatment. Removal of the offending medication or triggering factor is of utmost importance. Careful ophthalmologic monitoring is necessary because corneal scarring may lead to blindness. Affected patients are cared for as if they sustained a severe burn; fluid and electrolyte balance, temperature control, protein loss, and prevention of infection are serious concerns. Affected children usually require initial management in a pediatric intensive care unit or burn center. A number of immunosuppressants or immunomodulators have been used. Systemic corticosteroids remain a topic of controversy with efficacy varying and reports of increased morbidity and mortality. Cyclosporine use has demonstrated decreased morbidity and mortality for SJS/TEN, and tumor necrosis factor-α (TNF-α) inhibitors have shown promise in early studies.

With meticulous supportive care, most children survive; however, there is a high morbidity. Poor prognostic factors include neutropenia, impaired renal function, and extensive skin lesions. Recovery is slow; skin lesions require several weeks to heal, depending on the extent of involvement. Scarring and stricture formation may occur at mucosal sites, as may postinflammatory hypo- or hyperpigmentation.

BULLOUS LESIONS

Staphylococcal Scalded Skin Syndrome

Staphylococcal scalded skin syndrome (SSSS) (Table 61.18) is an exfoliative dermatitis produced by staphylococcal epidermolytic toxins

and papules with dusky centers. The macules may then quickly progress to bullae with skin necrosis. Involvement usually begins more proximally, with a predilection for the face, chest, and neck. There is a striking tendency for coalescence, reminiscent of a diffuse erythema. The eruption in SJS is more generalized and tends to be more truncally distributed than that of EM major.

Histopathologic findings in SJS are characterized by prominent epidermal necrosis with minimal inflammation. Epidermal injury and subepidermal separation may be observed as the result of full-thickness necrosis. Spongiosis and dermal edema are usually absent.

TABLE 61.13   Etiology of Acute and Chronic Urticaria

Etiology of Acute Urticaria

Foods	Eggs, milk, wheat, peanuts, tree nuts, soy, shellfish, fish, strawberries, food additives (direct mast cell degranulation)
Medications	Suspect all medications, even topical, nonprescription, or homeopathic (examples include penicillin, aspirin, sulfonamides, codeine)
Insect stings	Hymenoptera (honeybee, yellow jacket, hornet, wasp, fire ant), biting insects (papular urticaria)
Infections	Bacterial (streptococcal pharyngitis, *Mycoplasma*, sinusitis); viral (hepatitis, mononucleosis [Epstein-Barr virus], coxsackieviruses A and B); fungal (dermatophytes, *Candida*); parasitic (*Ascaris, Ancylostoma, Echinococcus, Fasciola, Filaria, Schistosoma, Strongyloides, Toxocara, Trichinella*)
Contact allergy	Latex, pollen, animal saliva, nettle plants, caterpillars
Transfusion reactions	Blood, blood products, or IVIG administration

Etiology of Chronic Urticaria

Idiopathic/ autoimmune	Approximately 30% of chronic urticaria cases are physical urticaria and 60–70% are idiopathic. Of the idiopathic cases approximately 35–40% have anti-IgE or anti-FcεRI (high-affinity IgE receptor α chain) autoantibodies (autoimmune chronic urticaria)
Physically mediated	Dermatographism Cholinergic urticaria Cold urticaria Delayed pressure urticaria Solar urticaria Vibratory urticaria Aquagenic urticaria
Autoimmune diseases	Systemic lupus erythematosus Juvenile idiopathic arthritis Thyroid (Graves, Hashimoto) Celiac disease Inflammatory bowel disease Leukocytoclastic vasculitis
Autoinflammatory/ periodic fever syndromes	NOMID (neonatal-onset multisystem inflammatory disease) Muckle-Wells syndrome Familial cold autoinflammatory syndrome Cold urticaria, immunodeficiency, autoimmunity as a result of *PLCG2* deficiency
Neoplastic	Lymphoma Mastocytosis Leukemia
Angioedema	Hereditary angioedema (autosomal dominant inherited deficiency of C1-esterase inhibitor) Acquired angioedema Angiotensin-converting enzyme inhibitors

IVIG, intravenous immunoglobulin.
From Lasley MV, Kennedy MS, Altman LC. Urticaria and angioedema. In: Altman LC, Becker JW, Williams PV, eds. *Allergy in Primary Care*. Philadelphia: Saunders; 2000:232–234.

associated with *S. aureus* phage group II. The condition is most common in children younger than 5 years. The condition may be localized, as in the case of bullous impetigo, or become more generalized as the result of hematogenous spread of the epidermolytic toxin from localized sites of infection. The diagnosis of SSSS should be considered in children with generalized tender erythema. The onset of the erythema may be preceded by fever, skin tenderness, malaise, and irritability. The initial sites of involvement are the flexural (neck, groin, and axillae) and periorificial skin. Circumoral erythema with radial crusting and fissuring around the mouth, eyes, and nose is characteristic (Fig. 61.28). A positive **Nikolsky sign**, the ability to laterally spread a blister or slough the skin with the application of light tangential pressure, is seen in most cases. Flaccid bullae, sheets of desquamating skin, or moist red erosions may be present, with the desquamation phase typically beginning 2–5 days after the onset of erythema. As the desquamation is superficial, healing without residual scarring occurs within 1–2 weeks. The diagnosis is usually established from the clinical presentation with the lack of mucosal involvement differentiating between SJS/TEN. *S. aureus* may be isolated from a minority of blood cultures. The organism is more likely to be isolated from distant sites, such as the nares, throat, and conjunctivae, than from the bullae themselves. In some children, the toxin may be produced by an underlying infection, such as pneumonia, osteomyelitis, or septic arthritis.

Localized SSSS or bullous impetigo is typically responsive to oral antibiotics. Children with widespread involvement usually require hospitalization and treatment with intravenous antistaphylococcal antibiotics with antibiotic choice to be based on local resistance patterns to account for the prevalence of methicillin resistance. Clindamycin may be added to inhibit bacterial protein (i.e., toxin) synthesis. Supportive management should be undertaken with close monitoring for fluid and electrolyte imbalances, signs of sepsis, or underlying focal infections. The skin should be handled very carefully, and adhesive bandages should be avoided. Application of an emollient in the desquamation phase may help lubricate the skin and reduce discomfort. Pain control is frequently necessary. The prognosis is good in immunocompetent children.

Epidermolysis Bullosa

Epidermolysis bullosa is a heterogeneous group of inherited blistering disorders characterized by spontaneous and post-traumatic bulla formation (see Chapter 60). It is estimated to occur in approximately 1 in 50,000 births; the severe variants are seen less frequently. There are several distinct variants that are distinguished by the inheritance pattern, cutaneous manifestations, histologic findings, and ultrastructural abnormalities.

In **epidermolysis bullosa simplex (EBS)**, the level of blister cleavage is intraepidermal (see Fig. 61.3). This form results from a defect in the basal cell keratins 5 and 14, which have been localized to chromosomes 12 and 17, respectively, and which are necessary for epidermal integrity. Most of the simplex forms are relatively mild and are autosomal dominant conditions. Bullae formation may be localized or generalized, but it is usually worst in areas of frequent trauma, such as the hands, feet, and joints.

In the **localized form of EBS** (formerly *Weber-Cockayne*), blisters are usually confined to the hands and feet and develop after significant friction or trauma. This form may not become apparent until adolescence or adulthood and may manifest after strenuous activities such as hiking, military training, or golf. There are also generalized forms of EBS in which the bullae are much more extensive and usually apparent at birth and during early infancy. In general, the various EBS subtypes

TABLE 61.14 Comparison of the Physical Urticarias

Urticaria	Relative Frequency	Precipitant	Time of Onset	Duration	Local Symptoms	Systemic Symptoms	Tests	Mechanism	Treatment
Symptomatic dermatographism	Most frequent	Stroking skin	Minutes	2–3 hr	Irregular pruritic attacks	None	Scratch skin	Passive transfer, IgE, histamine, possible role of adenosine triphosphate, substance P, possible direct pharmacologic mechanism	Continual antihistamines
Delayed dermatographism	Rare	Stroking skin	30 min to 8 hr	<48 hr	Burning, deep swelling	None	Scratch skin, observe early and late	Unknown	Avoidance of precipitants
Pressure urticaria	Frequent	Pressure	3–12 hr	8–24 hr	Diffuse, tender swelling	Flulike symptoms	Apply weight	Unknown	Avoidance of precipitants; if severe, low doses of corticosteroids given for systemic effects
Solar urticaria	Frequent	Various wavelengths of light	2–5 min	15 min to 3 hr	Pruritic wheals	Wheezing, dizziness, syncope	Phototest	Passive transfer, reverse passive transfer, IgE, possible histamine	Avoidance of precipitants; antihistamines, sunscreens, antimalarials
Familial cold urticaria	Rare	Change in skin temperature	30 min to 3 hr	<48 hr	Burning wheals	Tremor; headache; arthralgia; fever	Expose skin to cold air	Unknown	Avoidance of precipitants
Essential acquired cold urticaria	Frequent	Cold contact	2–5 min	1–2 hr	Pruritic wheals	Wheezing, syncope, drowning	Apply ice-filled copper beaker to arm, immerse	Passive transfer, reverse passive transfer, IgE (IgM), histamine; vasculitis can be induced	Cyproheptadine hydrochloride, other antihistamines; desensitization; avoidance of precipitants
Heat urticaria	Rare	Heat contact	2–5 min (rarely delayed)	1 hr	Pruritic wheals	None	Apply hot water–filled cylinder to arm	Possibly histamine; possibly complement	Antihistamines; desensitization; avoidance of precipitants
Cholinergic urticaria	Very frequent	General overheating of body	2–20 min	30 min to 1 hr	Papular, pruritic wheals	Syncope; diarrhea; vomiting, salivation; headaches	Bathe in hot water; exercise until perspiring, inject methacholine chloride	Passive transfer; possible immunoglobulin; product of sweat gland stimulation; histamine, reduced protease	Application of cold water or ice to skin; hydroxyzine regimen; refractory period; anticholinergics
Aquagenic urticaria	Rare	Water contact	Several minutes	30–45 min	Papular, pruritic wheals	None reported	Apply water compresses to skin	Unknown	Avoidance of precipitants; antihistamine; application of inert oil
Vibratory angioedema	Very rare	Vibrating against skin	2–5 min	1 hr	Angioedema	None reported	Apply vibration to forearm	Unknown	Avoidance of precipitants

Ig, immunoglobulin.

From Lee AD, Jorizzo JL. Urticaria. In: Callen JP, Jorizzo JL, Bolognia JL, et al., eds. *Dermatological Signs of Internal Disease*. 4th ed. Philadelphia: Elsevier; 2009:59, Table 6-4.

TABLE 61.15   Febrile Autoinflammatory Diseases Causing Urticaria in Children

Disease	Gene (Protein)	Inheritance	Attack Length	Timing of Onset	Cutaneous Features	Extracutaneous Clinical Features
FCAS	*NLRP3* (cryopyrin)	AD	Brief; minutes to 3 days	Neonatal or infantile	Cold-induced urticaria	• Arthralgia • Conjunctivitis • Headache
Muckle-Wells syndrome	*NLRP3* (cryopyrin)	AD	1–3 days	Neonatal, infantile, childhood (can be later)	Widespread urticaria	• Arthralgia/arthritis • Sensorineural hearing loss • Conjunctivitis/episcleritis • Headache • Amyloidosis
Chronic infantile neurologic cutaneous articular syndrome/neonatal-onset multisystem inflammatory disease	*NLRP3* (cryopyrin)	AD	Continuous flares	Neonatal or infantile	Widespread urticaria	• Deforming osteoarthropathy, epiphyseal overgrowth • Sensorineural hearing loss • Dysmorphic facies • Chronic aseptic meningitis, headaches, papilledema, seizures • Conjunctivitis/uveitis, optic atrophy • Growth retardation • Developmental delay • Amyloidosis
HIDS	*MVK* (mevalonate kinase)	AR	3–7 days	Infancy (<2 yr)	• Intermittent morbilliform or urticarial rash • Aphthous mucosal ulcers • Erythema nodosum	• Arthralgia/arthritis • Cervical lymphadenopathy • Severe abdominal pain • Diarrhea/vomiting • Headache • Elevated IgD and IgA antibody levels • Elevated urine mevalonic acid during attacks
Tumor necrosis factor receptor–associated periodic syndrome	*TNFRSF1A* (TNFR1)	AD	>7 days	Childhood	• Intermittent migratory erythematous macules and edematous plaques overlying areas of myalgia, often on limbs • Periorbital edema	• Migratory myalgia • Conjunctivitis • Serositis • Amyloidosis
Systemic-onset juvenile idiopathic arthritis	Polygenic	Varies	Daily (quotidian)	Peak onset at 1–6 yr	• Nonfixed erythematous rash, may be urticarial • With or without dermatographism • With or without periorbital edema	• Polyarthritis • Myalgia • Hepatosplenomegaly • Lymphadenopathy • Serositis
PLAID	*PLCG2*	AD	N/A	Infancy	• Urticaria induced by evaporative cooling • Ulcers in cold-exposed areas	• Allergies • Autoimmune disease • Recurrent sinopulmonary infections • Elevated IgE antibody levels • Decreased IgA and IgM antibody levels • Often elevated antinuclear antibody titers

AD, autosomal dominant; AR, autosomal recessive; FCAS, familial cold autoinflammatory syndrome; HIDS, hyperimmunoglobulin D syndrome; Ig, immunoglobulin; PLAID, PLCγ2-associated antibody deficiency and immune disregulation.

From Youssef MJ, Chiu YE. Eczema and urticaria as manifestations of undiagnosed and rare diseases. *Pediatr Clin N Am.* 2017;64(1):39–56 (Table 2, pp. 49–50).

TABLE 61.16   Diseases Related to Urticaria

Disease	Clinical Features	Histopathology
Urticarial vasculitis	Urticarial lesions >24 hr; residual purpura; more painful than pruritic angioedema in ≤40%; systemic symptoms: fever, arthralgia, arthritis, malaise, lymphadenopathy, and renal and liver involvement	Subtle findings; fibrinoid necrosis of vessel walls, karyorrhexis, extravasation of red blood cells, and endothelial swelling
Serum sickness–like reactions	Urticarial lesions >24 hr; fever, arthralgia, myalgia, arthritis, lymphadenopathy, glomerulonephritis, myocarditis, and neuritis; 1–2 wk after antigen exposure (heterologous serum, or certain infections or drugs)	Leukocytoclastic vasculitis
Mastocytosis	Urticarial lesions; reddish-brown macules and papules; positive Darier sign (urticarial reaction elicited by stroking lesion)	Uniformly spaced mast cells filling papillary dermis with or without reticular dermis; scattered eosinophils
Sweet syndrome (acute febrile neutrophilic dermatosis)	Urticarial plaques >24 hr; fever, leukocytosis; systemic symptoms: arthralgia, malaise, headache, and myalgia	Dense neutrophilic infiltrate in the papillary dermis; pronounced dermal edema
Bullous pemphigoid	Elderly patients; multiple, erythematous, urticarial, pruritic plaques with or without tense blisters	Subepidermal band of inflammatory infiltrate, with an abundance of eosinophils; perilesional DIF: linear complement 3 with or without immunoglobulin G at the BMZ
Insect bites	Long-standing urticarial lesions; central punctum	Variable; intraepidermal and papillary dermal edema; wedge-shaped perivascular and interstitial infiltrate: lymphocytes, eosinophils, and neutrophils

BMZ, basement membrane zone; DIF, direct immunofluorescence.
From Anita C, Baquerizo K, Korman A, et al. Urticaria: a comprehensive review. *J Am Acad Dermatol.* 2018;79:599–614 (Table VIII, p. 609).

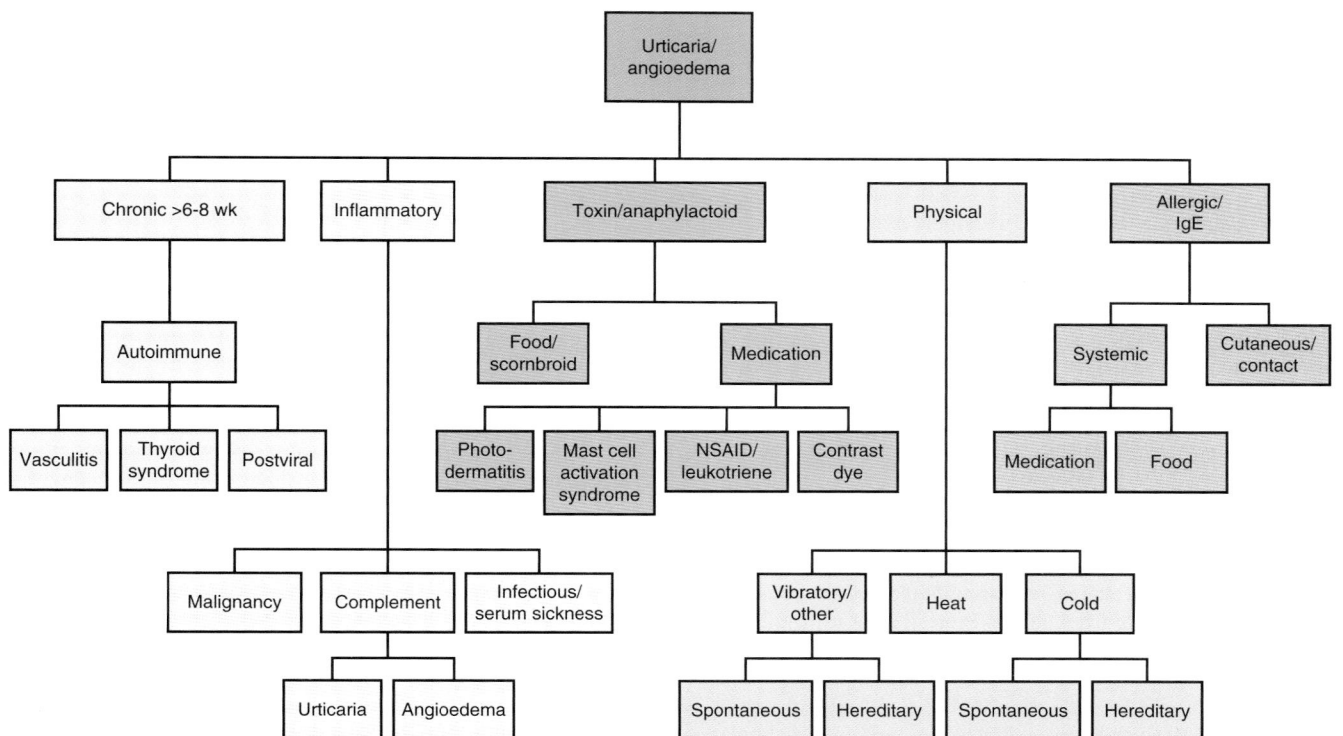

Fig. 61.26 Phenotypic classification of urticaria and angioedema. This figure is intended to provide a framework for clinical use based on the author's and others' experience that most presentations of urticaria and angioedema can be grouped in distinct categories that can predict prognosis and response to therapy. IgE, immunoglobulin E; NSAID, nonsteroidal antiinflammatory drug. (From Dreyfus DH. Differential diagnosis of chronic urticaria and angioedema based on molecular biology, pharmacology, and proteomics. *Immunol Allergy Clin North Am.* 2017;37[1]:201–215.)

TABLE 61.17 Precipitating Factors in Erythema Multiforme–Like Reaction*

Infection (90% of cases)	Viral	Herpes simplex virus (HSV-1, HSV-2)
		Vaccinia (smallpox vaccine)
		Varicella-zoster virus
		Adenovirus
		Epstein-Barr virus
		Cytomegalovirus
		Hepatitis virus
		Coxsackievirus
		Parvovirus B19
		HIV
	Bacterial	*Mycoplasma pneumoniae*
		Chlamydophila (formerly *Chlamydia*) *psittaci*
		Salmonella
		Mycobacterium tuberculosis
	Fungal	*Histoplasma capsulatum*
		Dermatophytes
Medications		Nonsteroidal antiinflammatory drugs
		Sulfonamides
		Anticonvulsants
		Other antibiotics
		Allopurinol
		TNF antibodies
		Taurine-containing energy drinks
		Biologic immune therapies
Exposures (unusual)		Poison ivy
Systemic disease (rare)		Inflammatory bowel disease
		Lupus erythematosus
		Behçet disease

*Most common causes are bolded.
TNF, tumor necrosis factor

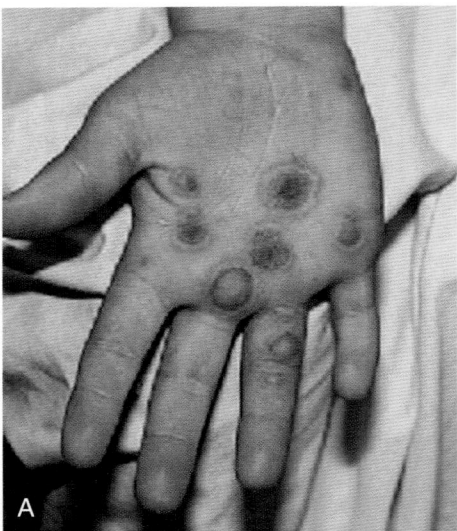

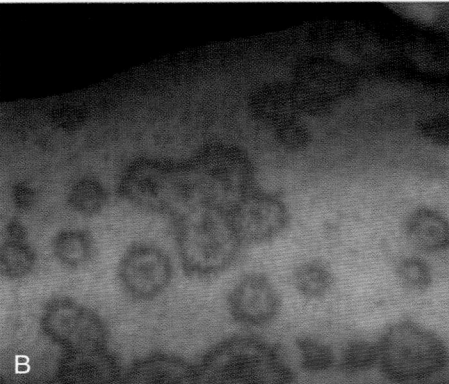

Fig. 61.27 Target lesions of erythema multiforme with characteristic dusky centers on the palms *(A)* and dorsum of the hand *(B)*. (*A*, From Kliegman RM, et al. *Nelson Textbook of Pediatrics*. 20th ed. Philadelphia: Elsevier; 2015:3142; *B*, from Bolognia JL, et al. Erythema multiforme, Stevens-Johnson syndrome, and toxic epidermal necrolysis. In: Bolognia JL, et al. *Dermatology Essentials*. Elsevier; 2014:140–150.)

are characterized by bullae that heal without scarring, mild or no nail changes, and minimal mucosal involvement. There are usually no associated extracutaneous manifestations.

In **junctional epidermolysis bullosa (JEB)**, the cleavage plane is located within the lamina lucida of the dermo-epidermal junction. Most forms are clinically apparent at birth. Inheritance is autosomal recessive. The majority of JEB subtypes result from defects in the laminin 5 protein, which localizes to fibrillar structures within the lamina lucida termed *anchoring filaments*. Other JEB variants are caused by defects in collagen XVII, an important component of the hemidesmosome. There is a wide spectrum of severity across subtypes, ranging from moderate involvement to a more severe, often fatal variant. Some subsets of epidermolysis bullosa are associated with pyloric atresia; the subset resulting from altered expression of plectin is a type of EBS, while the subset resulting from altered expression of $\alpha_6\beta_4$ integrin is a type of JEB. Individuals with these findings may also develop ureterovesical obstruction resulting in recurrent urinary tract infections.

JEB is characterized by widespread bullae that heal with atrophy, not scarring. Dysplastic nails, severe oral lesions, and enamel dysplasia are common. The most severe variant has been referred to as **JEB, generalized severe** (formerly referred to as JEB, Herlitz type). Often fatal by 2 years of age, this variant is characterized by exuberant granulation tissue on the face and around the mouth. Extracutaneous manifestations include pyloric atresia, chronic anemia, and laryngeal involvement that often necessitates tracheostomy.

In **dystrophic epidermolysis bullosa (DEB)**, tissue separation occurs below the dermo-epidermal junction at the level of the lamina densa. The lamina densa is made up of anchoring fibrils composed of type VII collagen. Individuals with the dystrophic form have qualitative or quantitative abnormalities caused by pathogenic variants in the gene for type VII collagen. DEB is further separated into subtypes that may be inherited in either an autosomal dominant or recessive fashion. DEB is usually apparent at birth; there is a wide array of clinical manifestations, but the condition is generally characterized by nail dystrophy and generalized blisters that heal with scarring and milia formation. In the more severe recessive dystrophic form, affected individuals often develop severe interdigital scarring, which results in syndactyly between fingers and eventual encasement of the fingers and thumbs, a finding known as the mitten deformity; similar changes occur in the feet. Severe mucosal involvement is a constant feature of recessive DEB, and esophageal stenosis and obstruction are significant causes of morbidity and mortality. Chronic malnutrition, growth failure, and increased susceptibility to infection may lead to sepsis and death in children with this epidermolysis bullosa subset. Affected patients have multiple extracutaneous manifestations, as well as a very high frequency of aggressive and recurrent squamous cell carcinomas. The

TABLE 61.18   Childhood Vesicular-Bullous Eruptions Categorized by Etiology

Entity	Clinical Clues	Entity	Clinical Clues
I. Hereditary	Bullae at birth in more severe forms	**III. Infectious**	
A. Epidermolysis bullosa (AR, AD)	Localized or widespread	A. Bacterial	
	Dystrophic nails in some forms	1. Staphylococcal scalded skin syndrome (SSSS)	Generalized, tender erythema
	Bullae induced by trauma, friction; may occur spontaneously		Positive Nikolsky sign
			Occasionally associated with underlying infection such as osteomyelitis, septic arthritis, pneumonia
	Mucosal involvement in severe forms		Desquamation, moist erosions observed
B. Incontinentia pigmenti (X-linked recessive)	Crops of blisters at birth or early infancy		More common in children <5 yr of age
	Often linear	2. Bullous impetigo	Localized SSSS
	May have coexistent streaky hyperpigmentation		Transparent flaccid bullae initially, then moist erythematous shallow erosions once bullae disrupted
	Eosinophilia		Covered sites of trunk and perineum likely, can occur on face and extremities
	Associated CNS, dental, ocular, cardiac, skeletal abnormalities	B. Viral	
	Girls affected; boys may have Klinefelter syndrome	1. Herpes simplex virus	Grouped vesicles on erythematous base
C. Porphyria cutanea tarda (AD or acquired)	On dorsal hands, other sun-exposed skin		May be recurrent at the same site: lips, eyes, cheeks, hands
	Heal with milia formation		Reactivated by fever, sunlight, trauma, stress
	Increased fragility of skin		Positive Tzanck smear, herpes PCR
	Hypertrichosis	2. Varicella	Crops of vesicles on erythematous base: "dewdrops on rose petal"
D. Epidermolytic hyperkeratosis (bullous congenital ichthyosiform erythroderma) (AD)	Bullae within the first week after birth		Highly contagious
	Verruciform scales on flexural surfaces		Multiple stages of lesions may be present simultaneously
	Hyperkeratosis after the third month		Associated with fever
	Collodion membrane at birth in some cases		Positive Tzanck smear, varicella-zoster PCR
II. Autoimmune		3. Herpes zoster	Grouped vesicles on erythematous base, limited to one or several adjacent dermatomes
A. Linear IgA disease (chronic bullous disease of childhood)	Onset usually before the age of 6 yr		Usually unilateral
	Sites of predilection: perioral, periocular, lower abdomen, buttocks, anogenital region		Burning, pruritus
	Annular or rosette configuration of tense blisters: "cluster of jewels"		Positive Tzanck smear, varicella-zoster PCR
	Mucous membranes commonly involved		Thoracic dermatomes most commonly involved in children
	Spontaneous remission	4. Hand-foot-and-mouth syndrome (coxsackievirus)	Prodrome of fever, anorexia, sore throat
	DIF shows linear deposits of IgA at DEJ		Oval blisters in acral distribution, usually few in number classically, but more generalized eruptions or concentration in the diaper area may be seen
B. Bullous pemphigoid	Large, tense subepidermal bullae		Shallow oval oral lesions on erythematous base
	Acral involvement common in infants		Highly infectious
	Oral lesions common		Peak incidence: late summer, fall
	DIF shows linear deposits of C3 and IgG at DEJ	C. Fungal	
C. Pemphigus vulgaris	Flaccid bullae, persistent erosions	1. Tinea corporis	Annular scaly plaques, usually with central clearing
	Seborrheic distribution		Pustule formation common
	Mucosal involvement very common, usually the initial manifestation		Positive KOH, fungal culture
	Positive Nikolsky sign	2. Tinea pedis	Vesicles and erosions on instep
	DIF with intercellular (desmosomal) deposits of IgG, C3		Interdigital fissuring
D. Pemphigus foliaceus	Small flaccid bullae or shallow erosions with scaling, crusting		Positive KOH, fungal culture
	Back, scalp, face, upper chest, abdomen; photodistribution	D. Scabies	Interdigital web spaces, genitalia, ankles, lower abdomen, wrist
	Oral lesions uncommon		Intensely pruritic; vesicles on palms and soles
	May resemble a generalized exfoliative dermatitis		Burrow formation
	DIF shows intercellular deposition of IgG, C3 in superficial epidermis		Very contagious
E. Dermatitis herpetiformis	Intensely pruritic		Positive scabies preparation
	Associated with celiac disease		
	Extensor surfaces of elbows, knees, buttocks, shoulders		
	Hemorrhagic lesions on palms and soles		
	DIF shows granular deposition of IgA in dermal papillae		

Continued

TABLE 61.18   Childhood Vesicular-Bullous Eruptions Categorized by Etiology—cont'd

Entity	Clinical Clues	Entity	Clinical Clues
IV. Hypersensitivity		B. Insect bites	Occur occasionally after flea or mosquito bites
A. Erythema multiforme (EM) major	Prodrome of fever, headache, malaise, sore throat, cough, vomiting, diarrhea		May be hemorrhagic bullae
	Involvement of two or more mucosal surfaces; hemorrhagic crusts on lips usually present		Often in linear or irregular clusters
			Very pruritic
	Target lesions progress from central vesiculation to extensive epidermal necrosis; sheets of denuded skin may be present	C. Burns	Irregular shapes and configurations
			May be suggestive of abuse
			Vary from first to third degree; bullae with second and third degree
B. Stevens-Johnson syndrome (SJS)/ toxic epidermal necrolysis (TEN)	SJS has <10% body surface involvement	D. Friction	Usually on acral surfaces
	Associated with infection (e.g., HSV, *Mycoplasma*), medications		May be related to footwear
			Often activity related
	Extension of SJS involving >30% of body surface	**VI. Miscellaneous**	
	Severe exfoliative dermatitis	A. Urticaria pigmentosa	Positive Darier sign (areas where skin is stroked become erythematous, pruritic, and edematous)
	Affects older children, adults		
	Frequently related to medications (e.g., sulfonamides, anticonvulsants)		Coexistent pigmented lesions
			Usually manifests during infancy
	Positive Nikolsky sign		Dermatographism commonly seen
V. Extrinsic		B. Miliaria crystallina	Seen in the setting of fever or overheating
A. Contact dermatitis	Irritant or allergic		Clear, 1–2-mm superficial vesicles occurring in crops, rupturing spontaneously
	Distribution dependent on the irritant/allergen		
	Distribution helpful in establishing diagnosis		Intertriginous areas, especially the neck and axillae

AD, autosomal dominant; AR, autosomal recessive; C, complement; CNS, central nervous system; DEJ, dermo-epidermal junction; DIF, direct immunofluorescence; HSV, herpes simplex virus; IgA and IgG, immunoglobulins A and G; KOH, potassium hydroxide; PCR, polymerase chain reaction.

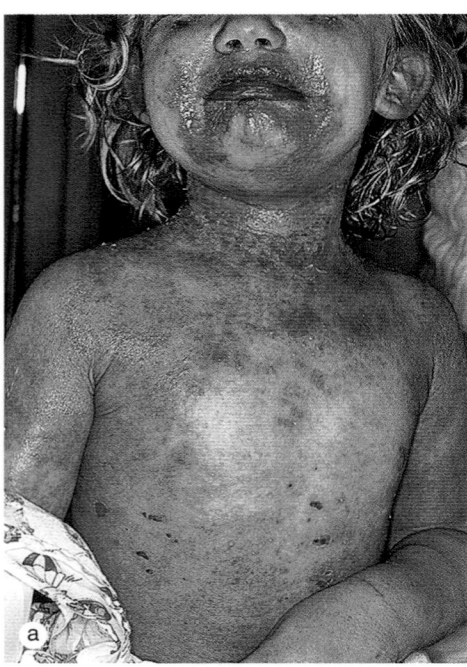

Fig. 61.28 Staphylococcal scalded skin syndrome. Perioral crusting and generalized tender erythematous skin with areas of desquamation. (From Vesicopustular eruptions. In: Cohen BA, ed. *Pediatric Dermatology*. Philadelphia: Saunders; 2013:104–125.)

dominant dystrophic forms are usually more localized and have a better prognosis than recessive DEB.

It is usually impossible to distinguish the variants of epidermolysis bullosa on the basis of clinical manifestations alone; skin biopsies are generally necessary. Immunofluorescence antigen mapping (IFM) and/or transmission electron microscopy on newly induced blisters are used to begin classifying epidermolysis bullosa subtypes. IFM involves use of monoclonal antibodies directed toward the skin basement membrane zone and epidermal antigens to determine the depth of skin cleavage data and presence of proteins. Genetic analysis directed by the results of IFM is recommended for the most precise subclassification.

Treatment modalities depend on the severity of the particular variant. In general, the emphasis is on wound care, infection prevention, and elimination or reduction of mechanical factors likely to induce blister formation. Topical antibiotics and nonadhesive semipermeable dressings may be necessary for recalcitrant wounds. All adhesives should be avoided. In patients with the severe variants of epidermolysis bullosa, a multidisciplinary approach is imperative and should focus on preventive care. All affected patients should undergo genetic counseling.

PURPURA AND PETECHIAE

Purpura refers to the leakage of blood from vessels into the skin or mucous membranes and is associated with diverse causes (Table 61.19). Purpuric lesions do not blanch when pressure is applied. Small lesions that are pinpoint-sized or a few millimeters in diameter are called **petechiae**. Large lesions may be referred to as *ecchymoses*. Raised or palpable purpura is diagnostic of vasculitis and can be seen in conditions such as immunoglobulin A (IgA) vasculitis (formerly referred to as Henoch-Schönlein purpura, HSP), systemic lupus erythematosus, and Rocky Mountain spotted fever. Inflammation and destruction of blood vessel walls are responsible for the raised quality of these lesions. Nonpalpable purpura can be seen with platelet abnormalities, leukemia, and other thrombocytopenic conditions

TABLE 61.19   Causes of Purpura

Infections
Rocky Mountain spotted fever
Sepsis
Bacterial endocarditis
Streptococcal infection
Gonococcemia
Meningococcemia
Hepatitis
Atypical measles
Varicella
COVID-19
Parvovirus 19
Epstein-Barr virus

Collagen Vascular Diseases*
Lupus erythematosus
Dermatomyositis
Rheumatoid arthritis
Ehlers-Danlos syndrome

Hematologic Disorders
Idiopathic thrombocytopenic purpura
Acute lymphocytic leukemia
Aplastic anemia
DIC
Thrombotic thrombocytopenic purpura
Clotting factor deficiencies
Warfarin or heparin use
Malignancy

Medications
Aspirin
Corticosteroids
Penicillins
Sulfonamides
Thiazides
Antiepileptics (phenytoin, valproic acid)

Vasculitis
IgA vasculitis (Henoch-Schönlein purpura)
Polyarteritis nodosa
Polyangiitis with granulomatosis
Cryoglobulinemia

Other
Scurvy
Trauma

*Usually livedo pattern.
DIC, disseminated intravascular coagulation; IgA, immunoglobulin A.

(see Chapter 51); capillaritis (pigmented purpuras); scurvy; viral exanthems; and physical exertion. Petechiae on the upper body (above the nipple line) can result from crying, vomiting, or coughing. Careful clinical examination is important for detecting these lesions and establishing a proper diagnosis.

Immunoglobulin A Vasculitis (Henoch-Schönlein Purpura)

IgA vasculitis, a small-vessel vasculitis that usually occurs in children and young adults, is the most common vasculitis of childhood, with most cases occurring between 3 and 10 years of age (Table 61.20). A leukocytoclastic vasculitis characterized by perivascular IgA deposition in affected tissues can involve the skin, joints, kidneys, and gastrointestinal tract. Given the seasonality and frequency of preceding upper respiratory infections, bacterial (such as streptococcal infections) and viral etiologies are suspected, although the precise nature of the pathogenesis is unclear.

The classic presentation is that of **nonthrombocytopenic palpable purpura** predominantly on the lower extremities and buttocks (Fig. 61.29). However, urticarial and ecchymotic lesions may appear as well. Hemorrhagic bullae and ulcerations can also be present. Edema of the hands, feet, genitalia, and face is common. Systemic involvement is present in approximately two thirds of affected patients, with anginal abdominal pain, arthritis, and arthralgia being the most common extracutaneous symptoms. Arthritis most frequently affects the lower extremities; joint effusions are rare. Gastrointestinal features may include vomiting, colicky abdominal pain, nausea, diarrhea, bleeding, and, in rare cases, intussusception or bowel perforation (see Chapter 13). Renal involvement is the most serious complication and can be manifested by hematuria and/or hypertension (see Chapter 23). Affected patients require close and serial monitoring for nephritis, as renal manifestations can develop several months after diagnosis.

Diagnosis is typically clinical, but a skin biopsy confirms the presence of leukocytoclastic vasculitis in atypical or severe cases. Direct immunofluorescence staining of the skin biopsy specimen reveals IgA deposition around the blood vessels in the superficial dermis (see Table 61.3).

Treatment includes supportive care and analgesics for joint pains. Systemic corticosteroids may be indicated when there is significant gastrointestinal or joint pain as well as renal involvement, but this treatment remains controversial as it does not alter the renal prognosis. Systemic corticosteroids are generally not indicated for skin involvement alone. The clinical course is characterized by acute onset of cutaneous lesions, often associated with fever and malaise. Systemic symptoms usually last for several weeks. Recurrences are common, but spontaneous resolution almost always occurs. The prognosis is excellent, with the primary factor being the extent of renal involvement. Mortality is rare and is usually caused by chronic renal disease.

Livedo Reticularis, Livedo Racemosa (Retiform Purpura)

Livedo reticularis is an ischemic dermopathy characterized by waxing and waning mottling in a reticular violaceous pattern of unbroken rings (branches or nets) with central pallor, most often seen on the lower extremities (Fig. 61.30). It is often primary or idiopathic, but, on occasion, it may be associated with an underlying systemic illness (Table 61.21).

Livedo racemosa (retiform purpura) is associated with an underlying systemic disorder (see Table 61.21) and is characterized by permanent discoloration of large irregular broken rings (nets, branches) with involvement of multiple cutaneous site (trunk, upper and lower extremities) (Figs. 61.30*B* and 61.31).

HAIR LOSS

Alopecia (hair loss) is the most common hair abnormality seen in children. Hair loss can have a number of presentations ranging from focal patches to diffuse thinning. An accurate history alone can often lead to a presumptive diagnosis. Information regarding duration of loss, rate of shedding, medications, trauma, family history of hair disorders, symptoms such as pruritus or burning, breakage, and hair care is particularly important. The scalp should be examined for the pattern and distribution of hair loss, erythema, scaling, scarring, pustules, and

TABLE 61.20 **Types of Vasculitis and Associated Skin Lesions**

Type of Vasculitis	Blood Vessels Involved	Type of Skin Lesion

Small vessel vasculitis:
  Hypersensitivity vasculitis
  IgA vasculitis (Henoch-Schönlein purpura)
  Cryoglobulinemia
  Urticarial vasculitis
  ANCA associated:
    • Microscopic polyangiitis
    • Granulomatosis with polyangiitis (Wegener)
    • Eosinophilic granulomatosis with polyangiitis (Churg-Strauss)
	Dermal capillaries, venules, and occasional small muscular arteries in internal organs
	Dermal small and larger muscular arteries and medium muscular arteries in subcutaneous tissue and other organs
	Small venules, arterioles of dermis, and small muscular arteries
		Purpuric papules and plaques, petechial macules, ecchymotic lesions, hemorrhagic bullae, cutaneous infarctions/necrosis
		Lesions may be urticarial, especially early
		Erythematous, purpuric, and ulcerated nodules, plaques, and purpura
		Ulcerative nodules, peripheral gangrene

Medium-vessel vasculitis:
  Polyarteritis nodosa
  Kawasaki disease
	Small and medium muscular arteries in deep dermis, subcutaneous tissue, and muscle	Deep subcutaneous nodules with ulceration; livedo reticularis; ecchymoses

Large-vessel vasculitis:
  Temporal arteritis
  Polymyalgia rheumatica
  Takayasu disease
	Medium muscular arteries and larger arteries (subclavian, renal, and carotid most common in Takayasu)	Skin necrosis over scalp

Modified from Sunderkotter CH, Zelger B, Chen KR, et al. Nomenclature of cutaneous vasculitis: dermatologic addendum to the 2012 Revised International Chapel Hill Consensus Conference Nomenclature of Vasculitides. *Arthritis Rheumatol.* 2018;70(2):171–184.

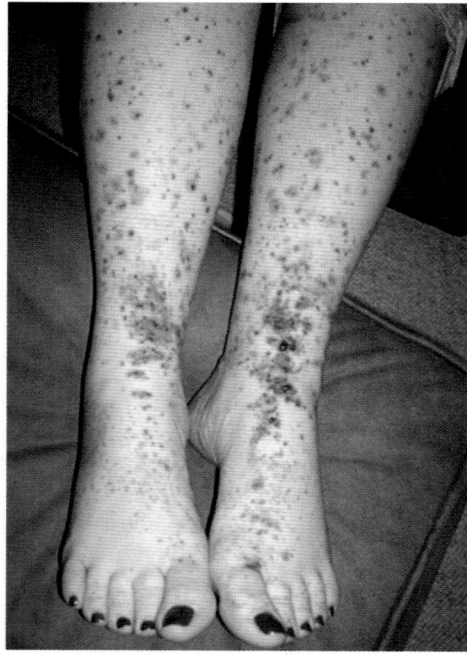

Fig. 61.29 Henoch–Schönlein purpura. Palpable purpura in the lower extremities. (From Kliegman RM, et al. Vasculitis syndromes. In: Kliegman RM, et al., eds. *Nelson Textbook of Pediatrics.* 20th ed. Philadelphia: Elsevier; 2015:1217.)

crusts. Abnormal or broken hairs as well as texture, length, and color should be noted. Associated abnormalities of the teeth, nails, and sweat glands may occur. Hair pulls (gentle pulling on small tufts of hair) and microscopic examination of removed hairs should be performed. Appropriate tests (KOH, fungal culture, scalp biopsy) may be necessary to confirm the clinical suspicions.

It is helpful to determine whether hair loss is acquired or congenital and localized or diffuse. Congenital alopecia usually results from aplasia cutis, intrauterine injury, or nevus sebaceous. Five common

disorders responsible for most cases of childhood hair loss are (1) alopecia areata, (2) tinea capitis, (3) traction alopecia, (4) trichotillomania, and (5) telogen effluvium.

Alopecia Areata

Alopecia areata is a common disorder that affects all ages, particularly children. Although several hypotheses have been proposed, the exact cause is unknown though is generally thought to be an autoimmune condition triggered by genetic and environmental factors. There is a family history of alopecia areata for approximately 20% of affected individuals. Clinically, there is acute onset of hair loss that is occasionally preceded by burning or itching of the scalp. In most cases, well-demarcated, localized areas of alopecia result, and the scalp is usually normal without epidermal changes. **Exclamation point hairs** are pathognomonic and are caused by breakage of abnormally growing hairs. Exclamation point hairs, when pulled out, appear as a tapered or attenuated bulb secondary to atrophy of that portion. When the disease is active, dystrophic anagen hairs can be easily pulled from the periphery of lesions. Nail pitting, often seen in rows, is seen in some cases. Factors that portend a poor prognosis for regrowth include extensive loss, early onset, nail involvement, atopic background, and an ophiasis pattern (involvement of the temporal and occipital hairline).

Treatment consists of topical and intralesional corticosteroids; topical minoxidil; anthralin; and sensitization to contact allergens. Janus kinase inhibitors are currently investigational and may prove beneficial for hair growth. Other supportive measures include camouflage, hairpieces, and support groups. In some cases, hair regrows without medical intervention. Although the course is unpredictable, about half of affected patients have a recurrence.

Tinea Capitis

Tinea capitis (**ringworm**) is a common cause of alopecia in children, although it may not always be associated with hair loss or breakage. The "seborrheic" type of tinea capitis is manifested by diffuse scaling without scalp inflammation. Alopecia is often not noted, but broken hairs are occasionally present. This type of alopecia is frequently misdiagnosed as dandruff. Tinea capitis can also manifest as localized scaly patches, kerions,

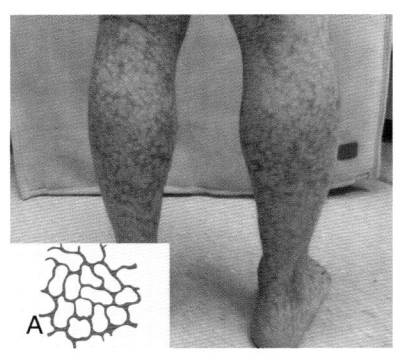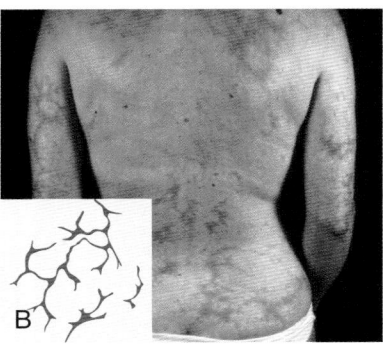

Fig. 61.30 *A,* Livedo reticularis. *B,* Livedo racemosa. (Extracted from Ko CJ. Approach to skin diseases. In: Goldman L, Schafer AI, eds. *Goldman-Cecil Medicine.* 26th ed. Philadelphia: Elsevier; 2020:2602, Table 407-5.)

TABLE 61.21 Pathologic Livedo Reticularis and Livedo Racemosa (Retiform Purpura) with Systemic Associations

Antiphospholipid Antibody Syndrome	**Hematologic/Thrombosis— cont'd**
	Paroxysmal nocturnal hemoglobinuria
Sneddon Syndrome	Disseminated intravascular coagulation
	Livedoid vasculopathy
Autoimmune Disease/Vasculitis	
SLE, rheumatoid arthritis, Sjögren syndrome, dermatomyositis, scleroderma	**Vessel Wall Disorders/Emboli**
Small- and medium-vessel vasculitis (microscopic polyangiitis, SLE/RA-associated vasculitis, systemic and cutaneous PAN, granulomatosis with polyangiitis, eosinophilic granulomatosis with polyangiitis, ADA-2 deficiency)	Calciphylaxis
	Primary hyperoxaluria
	Athero (cholesterol) emboli/septic emboli
	Atrial myxoma
Sarcoidosis	
	Infections
Medications	Various bacteria, spirochetes, rickettsiae, viruses, malaria, *Strongyloides,* COVID-19
Amantadine	
Gemcitabine	**Neurologic Disorders**
Minocycline	Dysautonomias
Pressors (ergotamines, epinephrine/catecholamines, amphetamines, cocaine)	Complex regional pain syndrome
	Paraplegia, stroke, multiple sclerosis
Lopinavir and aripiprazole combination	Divry–van Bogaert syndrome
α and β interferons	Migraine
Quinidine	
Warfarin necrosis	**Neoplasia**
Heparin necrosis	Multiple myeloma, lymphoma, leukemia
	Miscellaneous
Hematologic/Thrombosis	Anorexia nervosa, chronic pancreatitis, homocystinuria, congenital hypogammaglobulinemia, premature PAD, intralymphatic histiocytosis, erythema ab igne, brown recluse spider bite
Cryopathies (cryoglobulinemia, cryofibrinogenemia, cold agglutinins) and paraproteinemias	
Myeloproliferative syndromes	
Pernicious anemia	
Thrombotic thrombocytopenic purpura	

ADA, adenosine deaminase; PAD, peripheral arterial disease; PAN, polyarteritis nodosa; RA, rheumatoid arthritis; SLE, systemic lupus erythematosus.

---

and "black-dot" patches. This latter type features hairs that have broken at the surface of the scalp, resulting in a black-dot appearance. **Kerions** are boggy inflammatory plaques on the scalp that are caused by hypersensitivity to the offending dermatophyte (Fig. 61.32). Pustules and drainage are common, but the purulent material is often sterile. Cervical lymphadenopathy, fever, and elevated white blood cell counts may accompany kerions. The differential diagnosis of tinea capitis includes psoriasis, alopecia areata, trichotillomania, folliculitis, and seborrheic dermatitis.

The most common etiologic agent of tinea capitis is *Trichophyton tonsurans,* a dermatophyte that produces endothrix infections. Because spores are not present on the surfaces of the hair shafts, Wood lamp examination is not useful. If the infection is caused by *Microsporum canis* or another dermatophyte that produces an ectothrix infection, Wood lamp examination results in positive fluorescence (see Table 61.2). Fungal cultures should be performed in all suspected cases of tinea capitis. Fungal culture can be performed with a standard toothbrush and Petri dish. KOH preparations can be useful if positive, but false-negative results are common. Some children may be asymptomatic carriers.

Traditional therapy consists of oral griseofulvin for 6–8 weeks. Selenium sulfide 2.5% shampoo or 2% ketoconazole shampoo should be

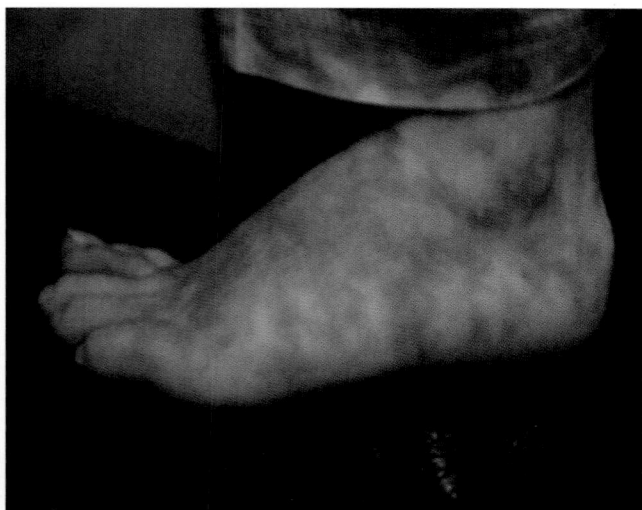

Fig. 61.31 Retiform purpura (livedo racemosa) in a child with deficiency of adenosine deaminase type 2. (From Eleftheriou D, Dusser P, Kone-Paut I. Polyarteritis nodosa. In: Petty RE, Laxer RM, Lindsley CB, et al., eds. *Textbook of Pediatric Rheumatology.* 8th ed. Philadelphia: Elsevier; 2021:469, Fig. 34.3.)

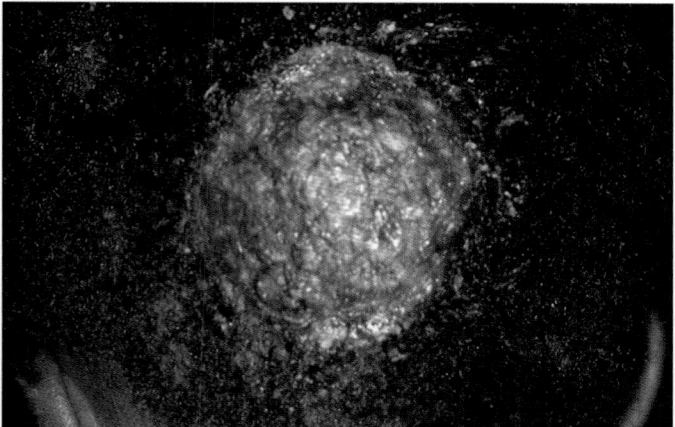

Fig. 61.32 Boggy, purulent mass of the scalp typical of kerions. (From Kliegman RM, et al. Cutaneous fungal infections. In: Kliegman RM, et al., eds. *Nelson Textbook of Pediatrics.* 20th ed. Philadelphia: Elsevier; 2015:3215.)

used to decrease surface spores and reduce spread to other individuals. On occasion, there is a secondary bacterial infection that necessitates antibiotic therapy. Kerions typically respond to griseofulvin, but in severe cases, systemic corticosteroids may be added to decrease inflammation and reduce the risk of scarring. Antifungal agents that may be useful include oral fluconazole, itraconazole, and terbinafine. Incision and drainage are not indicated. A follow-up fungal culture may be obtained to confirm adequacy of treatment.

Traction Alopecia

Traction alopecia is seen in individuals whose hair is tightly braided or pulled into ponytails or cornrows for long periods of time. Chronic tension on the hair shafts leads to breakage and gradual hair loss, often most easily visualized at the frontotemporal hairline. Hairstyle procedures such as straightening or weaving may also result in hair breakage if performed improperly. Physical examination reveals linear areas of hair loss at the part line or throughout the scalp. The alopecia

is reversible in most cases. However, if the traction is maintained for years, the alopecia may become permanent secondary to scarring. Treatment is aimed at avoiding all tension-producing trauma. The patient should be advised to stop all hair chemical procedures, wear loose styles with no braids, avoid wearing heavy objects in the hair or ponytails, and handle hair as gently as possible.

Trichotillomania

In trichotillomania, individuals pull, break, or twist hair from the scalp, eyebrows, eyelashes, and/or pubic hair. In younger children, this form of hair pulling is usually a harmless habit that is outgrown. Trichotillomania in older children and adolescents may represent a more serious psychologic problem with a less favorable prognosis. Psychiatric assistance may be required, and the disorder may be refractory to treatment. On physical examination, there are hairs of varying length in bizarre, often geometric, patterns. The occiput is often spared. Treatment is aimed at identifying underlying psychologic stressors. Supportive therapy and psychologic and/or psychiatric evaluation are usually needed.

Telogen Effluvium

Telogen effluvium is characterized by excessive shedding of telogen (resting) hairs. This may result from medications, febrile illness, crash diets, parturition, surgical procedures or anesthesia, endocrine disorders, or severe emotional stress. A large number of growing hairs enter the resting phase, resulting in a threefold to fivefold increase in the number of resting hairs. Gradually, these numerous telogen hairs are shed over 6–24 weeks. Affected individuals notice increased hair loss and sparser scalp hair 2–4 months after exposure to the inciting factor. The prognosis for this type of diffuse alopecia is excellent. Patient education is important, as is reassurance that regrowth can be expected within approximately 6 months. No treatment is indicated.

INFECTIONS AND INFESTATIONS

Impetigo

Impetigo is the most frequently diagnosed bacterial skin infection. It is a contagious superficial skin infection, occurring most often in infancy and early childhood. The two major pathogens, *S. aureus* and group A β-hemolytic streptococcus *(Streptococcus pyogenes)*, can cause lesions at any body site.

Nonbullous Impetigo

Nonbullous impetigo accounts for the majority of cases and is secondary to infection with either of the aforementioned pathogens. Clinical features do not reliably distinguish staphylococcal from streptococcal impetigo. Lesions typically arise on the face or extremities after trauma such as insect bites, cuts, and abrasions, or after varicella infection. The primary lesion is usually a vesicle or a pustule that develops secondary changes of honey-colored crusting, the clinical hallmark of this condition. In general, the lesions are smaller than 2 cm and may be single or multiple (Fig. 61.33). Although the lesions are generally asymptomatic with little surrounding erythema, regional lymphadenopathy may be present.

The differential diagnosis includes HSV infections, nummular eczema, varicella, kerions, and scabies, which all may become secondarily infected. Nonbullous impetigo usually resolves spontaneously within 2 weeks. It is highly contagious to other parts of the body and to close contacts, however, and should therefore be treated with appropriate antimicrobial agents.

Bullous Impetigo

Bullous impetigo develops on intact skin and is a localized form of SSSS. The initially transparent flaccid bullae are more likely to occur

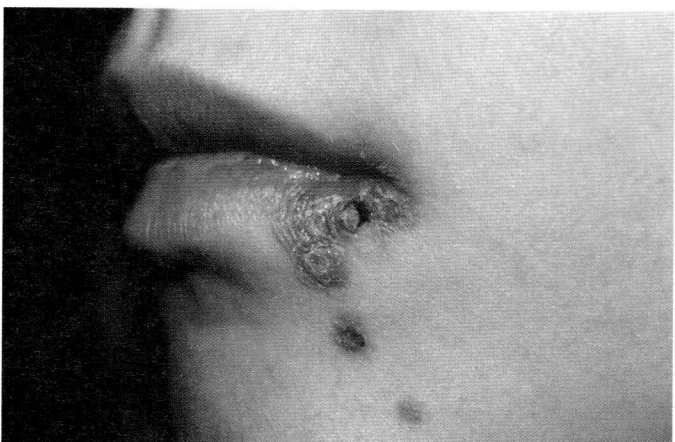

Fig. 61.33 Multiple honey-colored crusted lesions of impetigo. (From Kliegman RM, et al. Cutaneous bacterial infections. In: Kliegman RM, et al., eds. *Nelson Textbook of Pediatrics*. 20th ed. Philadelphia: Elsevier; 2015:3203.)

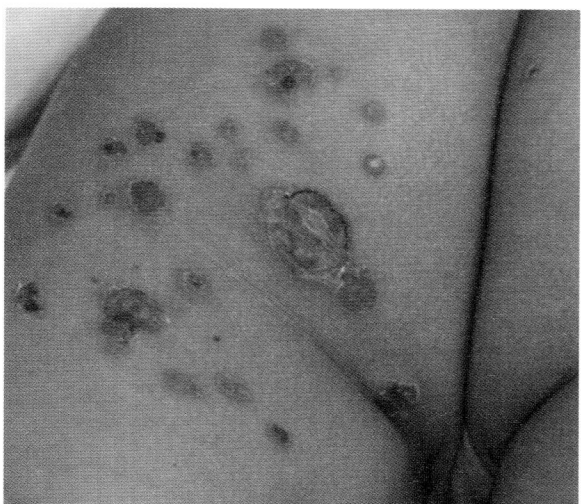

Fig. 61.34 Thin-walled vesicles and shallow erosions with surrounding erythema seen with bullous impetigo. (From Paller AS, Mancini AJ, eds. *Hurwitz Clinical Pediatric Dermatology*. Philadelphia: Elsevier; 2015:334–359.)

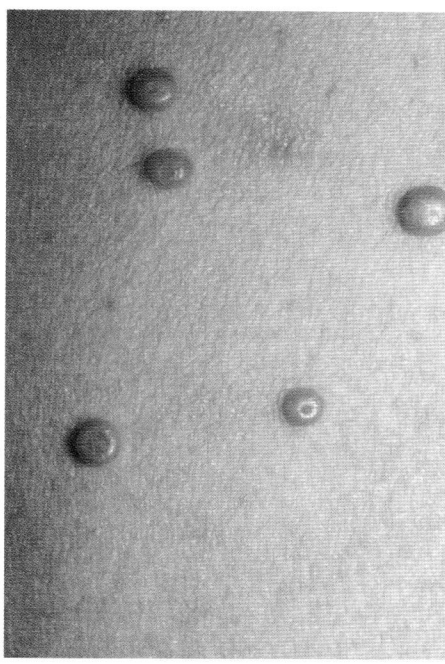

Fig. 61.35 The characteristic umbilicated lesions of molluscum contagiosum. (From Nodules and tumors. In: Cohen BA, ed. *Pediatric Dermatology*. Philadelphia: Saunders; 2013.)

on covered body sites such as the trunk and perineum than are the lesions of nonbullous impetigo. They can, however, occur on the face and extremities as well. Intact vesicles or bullae may be observed, or moist, erythematous shallow erosions may be the sole clinical finding after disruption of the bullae (Fig. 61.34). Bullous impetigo should be differentiated from early SSSS, herpetic infection, allergic contact dermatitis, burns, EM, and inflammatory bullous diseases.

Impetigo may be treated with topical or oral antibiotics depending on the number and locations of the lesions. Topical antibiotics may be acceptable for localized disease.

Systemic therapy is indicated for streptococcal infections or staphylococcal infections with an extensive number of lesions or more severe soft tissue involvement. One of the more cost-effective first-line choices includes cephalexin. However, the incidence of MRSA has increased dramatically, and local resistance patterns should be considered. If MRSA is suspected, initial medication choices include clindamycin, doxycycline (over age 8 years), or sulfamethoxazole-trimethoprim. A culture should be obtained, and antibiotic choice should be based on

susceptibility patterns when available. Recurrent impetigo is often secondary to carriage of *S. aureus*. Although intranasal carriage is common, colonization can also involve the axillae and perineum. Intranasal application of mupirocin may eradicate the organism; however, recolonization occurs over time. Of note, there are reports of increasing resistance with prolonged use of mupirocin. Dilute bleach baths (i.e., sodium hypochlorite) may help reduce recurrent skin infections by decreasing bacterial carriage.

Potential but rare complications of impetigo include pneumonia, cellulitis, osteomyelitis, septic arthritis, and septicemia. Streptococcal infections can also result in scarlet fever, guttate psoriasis, lymphadenitis, and lymphangitis. Furthermore, nephritogenic strains of group A β-hemolytic streptococcus can result in poststreptococcal glomerulonephritis (see Chapter 23). The latency period after impetigo is approximately 3 weeks. Treatment does not prevent poststreptococcal glomerulonephritis but does prevent the spread of the organism to other people.

Molluscum Contagiosum

Molluscum contagiosum, caused by a large DNA poxvirus, is most often seen in children and adolescents. The characteristic well-circumscribed, skin-colored to pearly papules usually arise in crops on the face, trunk, and extremities but have a predilection for the axillary, antecubital, and crural regions (Fig. 61.35). Generally ranging in size from 1 to 5 mm, these asymptomatic papules have a central umbilication, often with a central core. In some individuals, eczematous changes develop at sites of the molluscum lesions, probably representative of a delayed hypersensitivity response. This so-called molluscum dermatitis may be localized or more extensive, is not an uncommon finding, and in fact may be more prominent on examination than the molluscum papules, which are occasionally missed. The associated eczematous dermatitis may resemble nummular eczema or tinea corporis. Molluscum lesions often become inflamed or appear infected shortly before spontaneous involution. Diagnosis is typically clinical; however, skin biopsies or microscopic examination of the cores of the lesions can confirm the diagnosis by revealing molluscum bodies, which are masses of virus-infected epidermal cells. The condition should be differentiated from warts, closed comedones, and milia.

Molluscum contagiosum is both contagious and autoinoculable. The incubation period ranges from 2 weeks to 6 months, and multiple family members are often affected. Immunosuppressed persons are at risk for more aggressive disease, especially patients infected with HIV. Patients with pre-existing atopic dermatitis are also at greater risk for widespread molluscum.

Treatment options include curettage, topical cantharidin, liquid nitrogen, immunotherapy (e.g., with *Candida* antigen), topical retinoids, and imiquimod cream. Most pediatric dermatologists avoid application of cantharidin to facial or genital lesions because of concerns of a possible aberrant reaction. As with other poxvirus infections, these lesions occasionally result in scarring or pits as the lesions resolve.

Warts

Warts are intraepidermal tumors caused by human papillomavirus (HPV), a small DNA virus, and are present in up to 10% of the general population. There are more than 200 types of HPV. The virus produces four major types of warts: common, flat, plantar, and genital (condyloma acuminatum). The incubation period generally varies from 1 to 6 months, depending on HPV type, the size of the inoculum, the site of infection, and the host's immune status. The duration of the wart is variable as well; approximately 65% of the lesions resolve spontaneously within 2 years. Warts can be spread between persons and between body sites by direct or indirect contact. Most warts are located on the fingers, hands, and elbows because trauma to these sites promotes inoculation of the virus. Warts also display the Koebner phenomenon, which results in linear configurations of lesions at sites of trauma (e.g., from shaving or scratching).

Common Warts

Verruca vulgaris, or the common wart, is found commonly on the dorsal surface of the hands or fingers, although it may be located anywhere. The lesions may be solitary or multiple and measure from several millimeters to more than 1 cm. Varying in color from yellowish tan to grayish black, the common wart has a distinct rough, papillated surface. Punctate thrombosed capillaries, clinically manifested as black dots, may be seen on the surface.

Flat Warts

Verrucae plana, or flat warts, are 2- to 5-mm flat-topped papules that are typically skin-colored, tan, or brown. They are distributed on the face, neck, and extremities. They often appear grouped, especially when the Koebner phenomenon has occurred secondary to shaving or other trauma. These lesions are most often confused with lichen planus or lichen nitidus because these disorders also feature flat-topped papules.

Plantar Warts

Verrucae plantaris, or plantar warts, develop on the weight-bearing areas of the toes and heels and the midmetatarsal region. The lesions are pushed into the skin in such a manner that the verrucous surface is even with the surrounding skin. These warts are often very tender and may produce significant discomfort with ambulation. Plantar warts may be difficult to distinguish from corns and calluses.

Genital Warts

Condylomata acuminata, or genital warts, are fleshy papillomatous growths found on the genitalia. In early or mild cases, the only physical finding may be subtle skin-colored, flat-topped papules. Their growth can be exuberant in some patients when untreated, resulting

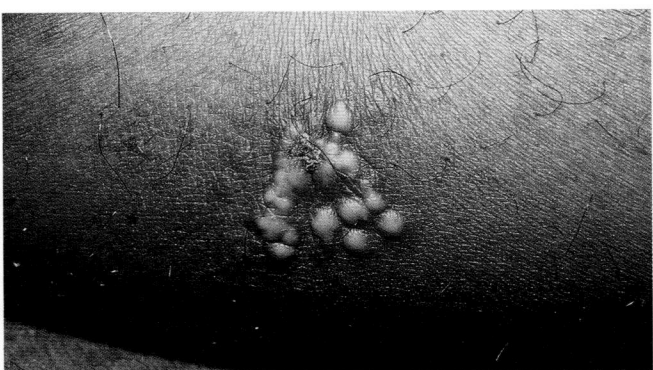

Fig. 61.36 A cluster of vesicopustular lesions on an erythematous base in herpes simplex virus. (From Vesicopustular eruptions. In: Cohen BA, ed. *Pediatric Dermatology*. Philadelphia: Saunders; 2013:104–125.)

in cauliflower-like masses. These genital warts should be differentiated from moist papular or nodular lesions of secondary syphilis (condylomata lata). While consideration for the possibility of sexual abuse should be given when warts are present in the genital area in a child, benign transmission can also occur through vertical transmission at birth, innocent heteroinoculation from a caregiver, and autoinoculation.

Herpes Simplex Virus

HSV is a large DNA virus that is divided into two major antigenic subtypes. Type 1 (HSV-1) has been traditionally associated with oral and nongenital skin herpes infections; type 2 (HSV-2) is generally responsible for genital and neonatal infections. The clinical lesions are indistinguishable but can be differentiated by serologic and molecular tests. HSV infections are categorized as either primary or recurrent. Primary manifestations usually follow an incubation period of approximately 1 week. They range from subclinical infections to localized or generalized vesicular eruptions to life-threatening systemic infections. Primary herpetic infections can involve any cutaneous or mucosal surface.

The classic clinical manifestation consists of grouped thin-walled vesicles on an erythematous base (Fig. 61.36). The lesions usually begin as papules, which evolve into vesicles or, sometimes, pustules within approximately 48 hours. The vesicles rupture and form a crust over the next 5–7 days and generally heal within 2 weeks. The cutaneous eruption is often accompanied by fever, regional lymphadenopathy, or flulike symptoms (see Table 61.18).

After the primary infection, the virus remains dormant until reactivated. Recurrent infections are characterized by localized vesicular eruptions and symptoms such as itching or burning at the same site. Recurrent HSV infections are usually less severe than primary herpes and only occur on keratinized mucosa (vermilion lip, tongue, hard palate, gingiva), sparing the buccal or inner labial mucosa. Location of these can help differentiate from aphthosis, which frequently affects nonkeratinized mucosa. Reactivation of the virus may be triggered by sunburn, cutaneous trauma, febrile illnesses, menstruation, or emotional stress. Oral antivirals, if administered during the prodromal period before the onset of lesions, may abort or shorten recurrent episodes.

Herpetic gingivostomatitis is typically seen in infants and toddlers. Multiple vesicles and subsequent erosions develop on the lips, gingivae, anterior portion of the tongue, or hard palate. The condition is very painful and is often accompanied by inability to eat and drink. Fever, irritability, and cervical lymphadenopathy are frequently observed. The fever typically resolves within 3–5 days, whereas the oral lesions may persist for up to 2 weeks. The lesions may resemble aphthae, which are usually more localized and are not accompanied by systemic symptoms. Enteroviruses may produce similar oral manifestations; however, they tend to spare the gingivae and often affect the posterior pharynx.

The test of choice to confirm the diagnosis of HSV infection is PCR for HSV. Tzanck smear can suggest HSV but is not specific. Treatment is supportive, with an emphasis on pain control and fluid replacement. Systemic antivirals may hasten resolution of the lesions and shorten the course of the illness.

Neonatal herpes is a potentially fatal infection, often with severe central nervous system involvement. Vigilant evaluation to determine extent of infection, intravenous acyclovir, and supportive care are required. Immunocompromised children who develop a herpetic infection should receive intravenous acyclovir and be monitored carefully for evidence of pulmonary, hepatic, and central nervous system involvement.

Another high-risk group consists of children with underlying atopic dermatitis who, if exposed to HSV, are susceptible to rapid spread of herpetic blisters. This condition, referred to as **eczema herpeticum** or **Kaposi varicelliform eruption**, may be accompanied by fever and malaise (see earlier, in Atopic Dermatitis). Oral or intravenous antivirals and supportive care are indicated.

Varicella

Varicella (**chickenpox**) is a very contagious but usually self-limited infection caused by the varicella-zoster virus. Since the introduction of the varicella vaccine, mild and atypical variants of this disease have become more common.

Transmitted by close contact and respiratory droplets, varicella has an incubation period of 10–21 days. The cutaneous manifestation in healthy children is characterized by crops of lesions (usually two or three crops of 50–100 lesions each) that initially appear as 2- to 3-mm red macules and then evolve through papular, vesicular, and finally pustular stages within approximately 24 hours. The vesicular stage has traditionally been described as resembling "dewdrops on a rose petal" (Fig. 61.37). The presence of lesions in various stages is characteristic of varicella. Varicella lesions often appear first on the scalp, face, or trunk and then progress to the extremities. All vesicles become crusted and resolve over several days. Chickenpox usually heals without scarring, except for lesions that have been excoriated or secondarily infected.

The eruption is usually accompanied by fever, intense pruritus, and malaise (see Table 61.18). The exanthem may be more extensive in children with skin disorders.

When the diagnosis is unclear, confirmatory tests include PCR, immunofluorescent staining, and viral culture. A positive Tzanck smear supports the diagnosis but is not specific for varicella. Symptomatic treatment consists of oral antihistamines, aluminum acetate soaks, oatmeal baths, calamine lotion, and cool compresses. Lesions should be observed for signs of secondary bacterial infection. Antiviral therapy is not routinely recommended in otherwise healthy children. Oral antivirals, if given, should be administered within 24 hours of the onset of the eruption. Immunosuppressed individuals usually require intravenous acyclovir.

High-risk individuals (immunosuppressed, immunocompromised, those with malignancies) who have been exposed to varicella should receive gamma globulin prophylaxis as soon as possible. If varicella develops in a pregnant woman within 5 days before delivery or in a mother 48 hours after delivery, the infant should also be treated with gamma globulin prophylaxis. Complications may include visceral organ involvement, coagulopathy, hemorrhage, pneumonia, or encephalitis.

Herpes Zoster

Similar to HSV, the varicella-zoster virus remains dormant in the dorsal root ganglia after initial infection. Reactivation of the virus results in the clinical manifestations of herpes zoster, or shingles. The infection usually manifests as a linear or bandlike papulovesicular eruption affecting one or several dermatomes (Fig. 61.38; see also Table 61.18). Commonly, there is a prodrome of burning, pruritus, or pain of the affected skin that may last several days before the appearance of cutaneous lesions. Vesicles become crusted, and all lesions resolve within a few weeks. The most common dermatomes involved are within the thoracic regions. Up to 10 **satellite lesions** may be encountered outside the primary dermatomes in uncomplicated zoster. An increased number of satellite lesions is observed in **generalized zoster**, which carries a greater risk of systemic involvement. Widespread vesicles should raise the suspicion of an underlying immunodeficiency disorder.

Immunocompromised patients, especially children with lymphoreticular malignancies, are at increased risk for zoster and should be treated with either oral or intravenous acyclovir. As with HSV

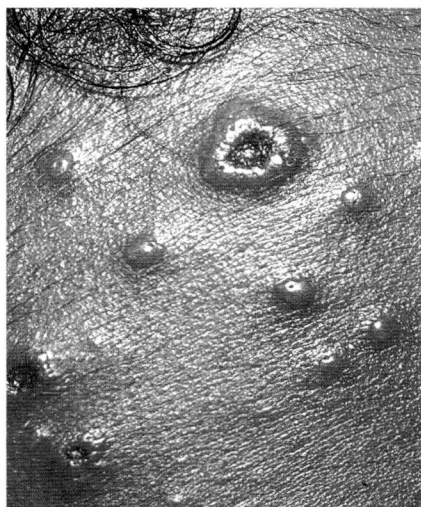

Fig. 61.37 Lesions in various stages of development including the dewdrop on a rose petal appearance characteristic of varicella. (From Vesicopustular eruptions. In: Cohen BA, ed. *Pediatric Dermatology*. Philadelphia: Saunders; 2013:104–125.)

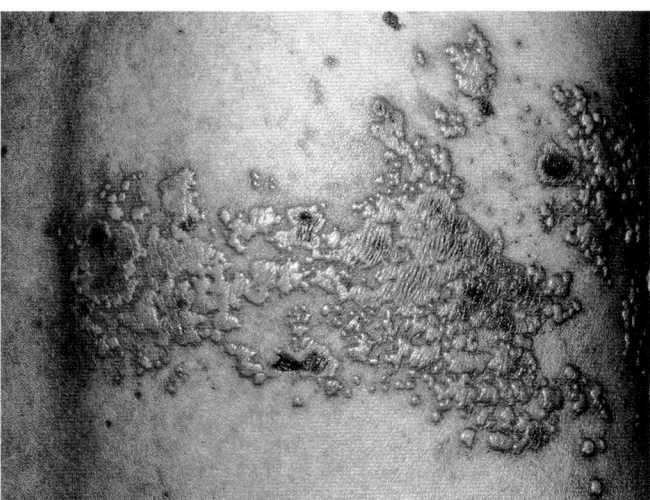

Fig. 61.38 A dermatomal distribution of umbilicated vesicles is characteristic of herpes zoster. (From Vesicopustular eruptions. In: Cohen BA, ed. *Pediatric Dermatology*. Philadelphia: Saunders; 2013:104–125.)

infection, lesions around the eyes, nose, and forehead require careful ophthalmologic examination. Ocular complications occur in approximately 50% of the patients with ophthalmic zoster. The potential for deep keratitis, uveitis, secondary glaucoma, and loss of vision warrants prompt ophthalmologic evaluation. Patients with zoster should avoid contact with high-risk individuals who are susceptible to development of varicella.

Scabies

Scabies is an extremely common eruption. It occurs in persons of all ages and results from infestation of the superficial layers of skin by the human mite *S. scabiei*. The infestation is highly contagious and is therefore seen frequently among individuals living in crowded conditions. Humans are the only source of the mite, which can be passed from one person to another. Fomites can also play an important role in transmission. In previously unexposed individuals, the incubation period varies from 2 to 6 weeks. The incubation period is significantly shortened in individuals who have been previously exposed to the mite.

Although the morphologic appearance of scabies can vary dramatically, the hallmark lesion is the burrow, a serpiginous or linear papule caused by movement of the mite through the epidermis. Although considered to be characteristic of scabies, the burrow is apparent in only a minority of patients. Other typical lesions include papules, vesicles, and pustules, the distribution of which is age dependent. Nodules may appear during active infection and may persist for several weeks to months after treatment; these are common in infantile scabies and on the penis and scrotum of affected males. These persistent nodules are referred to as postscabetic nodules and may be a manifestation of an ongoing hypersensitivity response. In infants, the distribution is generalized and involves the trunk, scalp, face, neck, axillae, palms, and soles. Because the eruption is extremely pruritic, secondary infection and eczematization are common, leading to misdiagnoses of impetigo and atopic dermatitis. In affected older children, adolescents, and adults, the lesions characteristically involve the volar aspects of the wrists, ankles, interdigital web spaces, buttocks, genitalia, groin, abdomen, and axillae (Fig. 61.39). Unlike infantile scabies, the lesions always spare the head.

The diagnosis can be confirmed by scraping the newer lesions, ideally a burrow, with a blade after the application of mineral oil. The scraping may be viewed microscopically, and the presence of mites, ova, or feces is considered diagnostic. Although the yield may be low, suspect lesions should be scraped and an attempt should be made to identify evidence of the mite. In prolonged cases of scabies that have been appropriately treated, the diagnosis of acropustulosis of infancy needs to be considered.

Topical 5% permethrin cream is the treatment of choice for infants over 2 months and children. Permethrin cream is applied to the entire body from the neck down and thoroughly washed off after 8–12 hours. Scalp and neck treatment is often necessary for infants. This treatment should be repeated 1 week later. Lindane is not recommended as first-line treatment for scabies because of its potential for neurotoxicity. Six percent sulfur ointment should be used as an alternative therapy in infants younger than 2 months and in pregnant women. Topical and oral ivermectin are options for resistant infestations. Because scabetic lesions are the result of a hypersensitivity reaction, itching may persist for several weeks despite treatment, which can be relieved with emollients, topical corticosteroids, and antihistamines.

It is critical that all household members as well as close contacts be treated simultaneously to prevent reinfestation. All linens and clothes should be washed and dried in an electric dryer because heat kills the mite. Bulkier linens and stuffed toys can be placed in plastic bags for several days. Mites do not survive without a human host for more than 2–3 days.

Pediculosis

Lice are ectoparasitic insects. *Pediculus humanus capitis*, the head louse, causes the most common form of louse infestation. Because the head louse can survive for more than 2 days off the host's scalp, the condition can be transmitted via shared hats, combs, brushes, towels, or bedding. On physical examination, the nits (ova) can be found close to the scalp on the proximal hair shafts. They appear as small, oval, whitish bodies approximately 0.5 mm in length. They adhere tightly to the hair shaft and are not easily removed. The nits can be more readily identified by their fluorescence under a Wood lamp. Microscopic examination of the proximal hair shaft may further aid in recognition of the nits. The infestation is characterized by intense pruritus, especially at night.

Initial treatment may consist of over-the-counter topical application of 1% permethrin shampoo or pyrethrin combined with piperonyl butoxide products, both of which have good safety profiles. However, resistance to these products has been documented. In treatment failures or known resistance, additional topical agents such as malathion 0.5%, benzyl alcohol, spinosad, and ivermectin lotions are options. Oral ivermectin may be used when lice are resistant to all topical agents. However, each agent's recommended age, weight, and safety profile need to be considered.

It is extremely important to wash and dry all exposed bedding and clothing on a hot cycle. All combs and brushes should be soaked in the pediculicide for 15 minutes, and all items that cannot be machine-washed with hot water or dry-cleaned should be placed in plastic bags for 2 weeks. All household members should be treated at the same time. Nits must be removed with a fine-toothed comb after application of a damp towel to the scalp.

Candidiasis

Candidal species, particularly *Candida albicans*, may be considered part of the normal cutaneous flora in most individuals. However, predisposing factors such as endocrine or genetic disorders, immunosuppressed states, and the administration of systemic corticosteroids or antibiotics may allow for overgrowth of this organism and subsequent infection. Candidiasis refers to an acute or chronic infection of the skin, mucous membranes, or internal organs caused by this pathogenic yeast. Other conditions, such as warmth, moisture, and disruption of

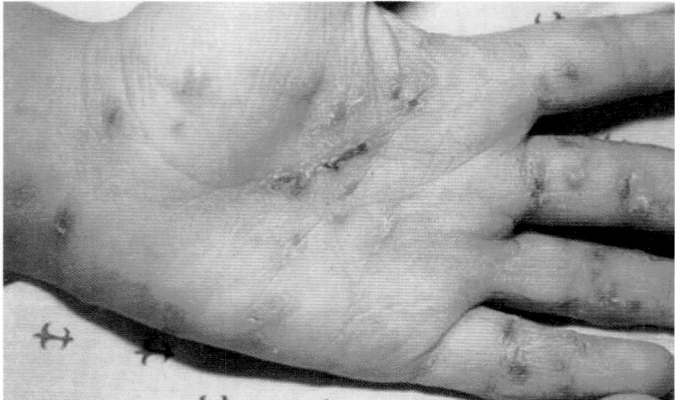

Fig. 61.39 Papulopustular eruption of scabies with burrows visible on the palms and wrist of a child. (From Papulosquamous eruptions. In: Cohen BA, ed. *Pediatric Dermatology*. Philadelphia: Saunders; 2013:68–103.)

the epidermal barrier, further promote invasion and overgrowth. Cutaneous candidiasis can have a variety of clinical manifestations, depending on the site of infection. Some of the most common manifestations include (1) oral candidiasis (thrush), (2) candidal diaper dermatitis, (3) vulvovaginitis, and (4) paronychia.

Oral candidiasis is a common condition of infancy and in immunosuppressed individuals. It is characterized by painful inflammation of the oral cavity with multiple, often confluent, white plaques on an intensely erythematous base. The disorder usually responds to treatment with oral nystatin suspension, which is applied to the oral mucosa 4 times daily until 2 days after the lesions have completely resolved. Oral fluconazole is another therapeutic option for more extensive or resistant cases. Extensive involvement or failure to respond to treatment may suggest an underlying immunodeficiency disease. Cutaneous lesions in the intertriginous and diaper areas are frequently coexistent with thrush.

Candidal paronychia manifests with erythema and edema of the proximal and lateral nail folds, which is usually not associated with tenderness, in contrast to acute bacterial paronychia. The nail is often dystrophic, crumbly, and thick. The condition is seen commonly in thumb suckers. Treatment with topical antifungal creams with yeast coverage, applied nightly under occlusion for several weeks, usually results in clinical resolution.

Dermatophytoses

The dermatophytes are a group of fungi that infect the hair, skin, and nails and result in a collection of clinical syndromes referred to as dermatophytoses. The clinical conditions are referred to as tinea (or ringworm), and the affected body site determines the name of the entity. This group of infections is caused by species of *Trichophyton*, *Microsporum*, and *Epidermophyton*. Dermatophyte infections are usually confined to the epidermis.

Tinea Capitis

Tinea capitis is discussed in the section on alopecia.

Tinea Corporis

Tinea corporis is characterized by one or multiple annular erythematous patches that can occur anywhere on the body. The lesions typically have a papular scaly border and demonstrate central clearing (Fig. 61.40). Vesiculation and pustulation, especially peripherally, are commonly observed. The borders are usually sharply demarcated. Identification of fungal hyphae by KOH examination of scrapings of the lesion's scaly border confirms the diagnosis. Psoriasis, nummular eczema, secondary syphilis, the herald patch of pityriasis rosea, and the annular plaques of granuloma annulare may resemble tinea corporis.

Tinea Pedis

Tinea pedis is diagnosed most often in postpubertal adolescents. The clinical manifestation is variable, but multiple vesicles or erosions on the insteps are characteristic. Other findings include fissures and maceration of the web spaces and a more treatment-resistant variant of tinea pedis, in which there is generalized scaling of one or both soles with extension onto the lateral aspect of the foot. The differential diagnosis includes atopic or contact dermatitis, juvenile plantar dermatosis, psoriasis, and scabies. The clinician should have increased suspicion for tinea pedis if unilateral involvement is present. A positive KOH scraping or fungal culture rules out these other entities.

Tinea Faciei

Tinea faciei, a dermatophyte infection of the face, is commonly seen in children. Erythematous, scaly, and often in a malar distribution, the condition may resemble lupus erythematosus but is less symmetric. Atopic, contact, and seborrheic dermatitis may have similar cutaneous manifestations. The diagnosis can be confirmed by a positive KOH scraping or fungal culture.

Tinea Cruris

Tinea cruris, uncommon before adolescence, is an erythematous scaly eruption involving the inguinal creases and medial thighs. The eruption is usually symmetric, and sometimes the margins are papular. This infection may resemble candidiasis, in which there is also scrotal erythema. *Erythrasma*, an uncommon superficial bacterial infection caused by *Corynebacterium minutissimum*, may also mimic tinea cruris. The coral red fluorescence seen on Wood lamp examination is diagnostic of erythrasma, which can be further differentiated from tinea cruris by a negative KOH preparation and fungal culture.

Dermatophyte infections of the skin can usually be successfully managed with topical antifungal agents such as clotrimazole, econazole, ciclopirox, tolnaftate, or terbinafine creams or lotions. These medications are applied twice daily for approximately 2–4 weeks. They should be continued for several days after clinical resolution is apparent. Widespread eruptions or treatment failures may necessitate systemic antifungal therapy, such as griseofulvin, fluconazole, itraconazole, or terbinafine.

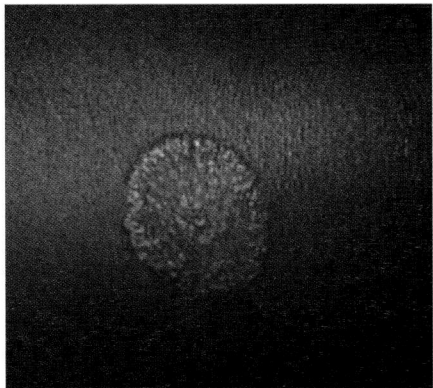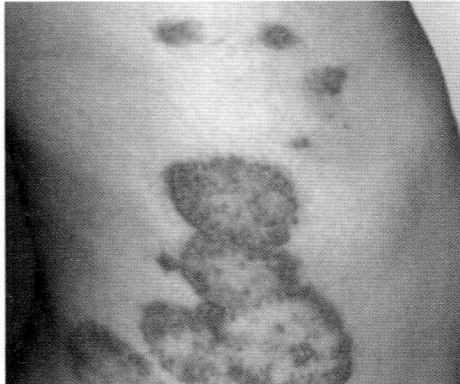

Fig. 61.40 Annular erythematous, scaly plaques with central clearing as seen in tinea corporis. (From Cohen BA, Davis HW, Gehris RP. Dermatology. In: Zitelli BJ, et al., eds. *Atlas of Pediatric Physical Diagnosis*. Philadelphia: Saunders; 2012:299–368.)

Tinea Versicolor

Occurring more frequently in adolescents and adults, tinea versicolor is a superficial fungal infection characterized by multiple slightly scaly macules and patches located on the upper trunk, neck, proximal extremities, and, on occasion, the face. The macular lesions vary in hue (pink, tan, brown, white), hence the name "versicolor." In darkly pigmented or tanned individuals, the macules appear hypopigmented; in fair-skinned persons or during winter months, the lesions usually appear tan-brown. Tinea versicolor is caused by *Malassezia* species, formerly referred to as *Pityrosporum orbiculare* or *Pityrosporum ovale*, a dimorphic fungus that is a skin saprophyte. It is generally present in its yeast form, which does not produce a rash. When proliferation of the filamentous form occurs, the organism produces the characteristic lesions of tinea versicolor. Usually asymptomatic or only slightly pruritic, tinea versicolor is primarily a cosmetic disturbance that occurs most commonly in warm and humid environments.

Although the diagnosis is established by the distinctive clinical presentation, a KOH scraping of the fine scale reveals multiple round spores and short, curved hyphae, giving the characteristic "spaghetti and meatballs" appearance typical of this disorder. Wood lamp examination may demonstrate yellow to yellow-green fluorescence, further supporting the diagnosis (see Table 61.2). The differential diagnosis includes postinflammatory pigment alteration, pityriasis alba, vitiligo, contact dermatitis, seborrheic dermatitis, and pityriasis rosea.

Tinea versicolor is a chronic condition. Although usually responsive to therapy, recurrences are common. Application of 2.5% selenium sulfide shampoo to the affected skin can be very effective used daily and left on for 10 minutes or left on overnight as a single application. Other topical treatments include broad-spectrum antifungal creams or lotions. In extremely widespread or recalcitrant cases, or in immunosuppressed individuals, oral treatment with fluconazole or itraconazole may be indicated. Having patients exercise after medicating may enhance delivery of the medication to the skin, resulting in greater success of treatment. After successful treatment, the lesions remain temporarily hypopigmented or hyperpigmented. Prophylaxis with weekly use of an antiyeast shampoo or soap may help reduce recurrences.

ACNE VULGARIS

Acne is a very common condition in adolescents, but all age groups can be affected. Open and closed comedones, inflammatory papules, pustules, and nodules are characteristic primary lesions. Scarring and sinus tracts are present in moderate to severe forms. Androgens stimulate the hair follicle unit, leading to hyperkeratosis of the follicular epithelium and increased sebum production, resulting in follicular plugging. The microscopically plugged follicle is clinically apparent as a comedo. With further accumulation of keratin and sebum, the follicle wall may rupture and elicit an inflammatory reaction as contents are released into the surrounding dermis. Clinically, this corresponds to inflammatory lesions ranging from inflammatory papules and pustules to nodules or cysts. *Propionibacterium acnes*, an anaerobic follicular diphtheroid, contributes to the inflammatory process.

The diagnosis of acne is a clinical one; skin biopsies and other diagnostic studies are not necessary. In some cases of mid-childhood acne (1–7 years of age) or associated signs or symptoms of androgen excess (e.g., hirsutism, irregular menses), endocrinologic evaluation may be needed to further elucidate the hormonal factors contributing to formation of acne lesions. Medication-induced acne can be seen in all age groups; the offending medications include glucocorticoids, androgens, hydantoin, and isoniazid. The constellation of synovitis, acne, pustulosis, hyperostosis, and osteitis is the hallmark of **SAPHO syndrome**, a rare chronic inflammatory disorder of the bones, joints, and skin.

Other acne-associated autoinflammatory syndromes include **PAPA** (pyogenic sterile arthritis, pyoderma gangrenosum, acne) (Fig. 61.41), **PASH** (pyoderma gangrenosum, acne, suppurative hidradenitis), **PAC** (pyoderma gangrenosum, acne, ulcerative colitis), and **PAPASH** (pyogenic arthritis, pyoderma gangrenosum, acne, suppurative hidradenitis). Hyperandrogen states such as polycystic ovary syndrome, congenital adrenal hyperplasia, **SAHA syndrome** (seborrhea, acne, hirsutism, androgenetic alopecia), and **HAIR-AN syndrome** (hyperandrogenism, insulin resistance, acanthosis nigricans) are also associated with severe acne.

Treatment of acne varies depending on the types of lesions present and individual tolerance to acne medication. Patients should be instructed to use mild cleansers and oil-free, noncomedogenic moisturizers, sunscreen, and makeup. Antibacterial soaps and cleansers may help reduce surface bacteria. Topical medications include

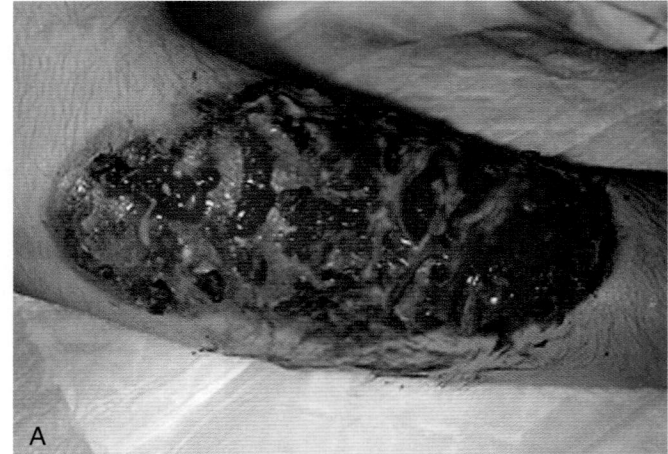

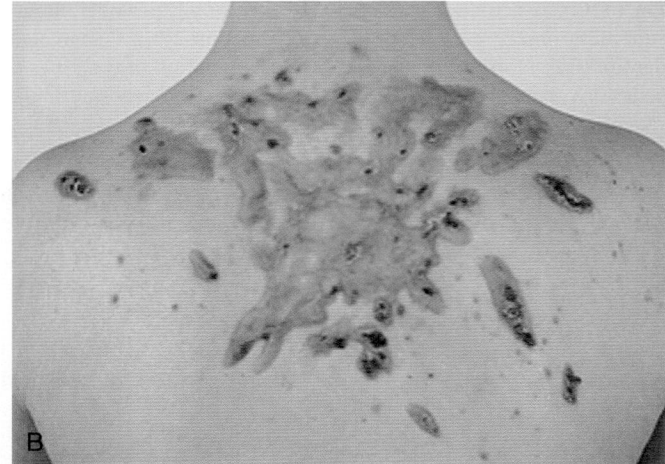

Fig. 61.41 *A*, Aggressive ulcerative skin lesions indistinguishable from pyoderma gangrenosum seen in a patient with pyogenic sterile arthritis, pyoderma gangrenosum, and acne (PAPA). *B*, Cystic acne in PAPA begins in adolescence and persists into adulthood. (From Barron K, Kastner DL. Periodic fever syndromes and other inherited autoinflammatory diseases. In: Petty RE, Laxer RM, Lindsley CB, et al., eds. *Textbook of Pediatric Rheumatology.* 8th ed. Philadelphia: Elsevier; 2021:538, Fig. 39.8.)

TABLE 61.22 Cutaneous Lumps and Bumps: Distinguishing Features

Diagnosed Lesion	Usual Onset	Color	Size	Site	Comments	Therapy
Epidermal cyst	Childhood, adolescence	Skin-colored	1–3 cm	Face, scalp, neck, trunk	Potential for inflammation and infection	Elective excision vs observation
Dermoid cyst	Birth	Skin-colored	1–4 cm	Face, scalp, lateral eyebrow	When midline, may have sinus tract	Elective excision
Pilomatricoma	Any age, 50% before adolescence	Skin-colored, reddish-blue, bluish-gray	0.5–3 cm	Head, neck	Malignant transformation possible but rare	Elective excision vs observation
Dermatofibroma	Adulthood, 20% before age 20 yr	Skin-colored, tan-brown, black	0.3–1 cm	Extremities	May follow trauma	Elective excision vs observation
Neurofibroma	Occasionally at birth Usually childhood or adolescence	Usually skin colored Also pink, blue	2 mm to several centimeters	Any body site	May be associated with neurofibromatosis May see café-au-lait spots	Elective excision vs observation
Juvenile xanthogranuloma	Birth, childhood	Yellow-orange to reddish-brown	0.5–4 cm	Head, neck, trunk, proximal extremities	Extracutaneous lesions involving eye, other organs	Ophthalmology consult; resolves spontaneously
Keloids	Peak between puberty and age 30	Pink to violaceous	Variable	Any site of injury Commonly earlobes after piercing	Often tender or pruritic Familial tendency	Difficult; intralesional steroids, excision
Granuloma annulare	Childhood, adolescence	Skin-colored to red	1–4 cm	Distal extremities	May be generalized in approximately 15% of cases	Observe, self-limited Topical steroids if needed
Lipoma	Puberty, adulthood	Skin-colored	Variable May be >10 cm	Any, but usually neck, shoulders, back, abdomen	Malignant change very rare	Observe, excision
Solitary mastocytoma	Birth, early infancy	Skin-colored to light brown or tan Occasionally pink or yellowish hue	1–5 cm	Any site, but most often on arms, neck, trunk	Positive Darier sign Urticaria with stroking	Usually resolves spontaneously; antihistamines may be helpful

benzoyl peroxide, retinoids, antibiotics, and combination products. Retinoids are most effective in decreasing new comedo formation and promoting expulsion of existing comedones by reducing and preventing abnormal keratinization of the follicular canal. Benzoyl peroxide has mostly antiinflammatory activity as the result of its antibacterial activity with mild comedolytic effects and can be used as an adjunct to retinoid therapy.

Inflammatory acne, particularly with evidence of scarring, often requires the use of antibiotics, either topically or systemically. Oral contraceptives may also provide a significant benefit for the treatment of acne in women, particularly in those with a perimenstrual flare. **Nodulocystic acne** or recalcitrant severe inflammatory acne is best treated with isotretinoin, a synthetic vitamin A derivative. Given the restrictions surrounding its prescription and side effects, referral to a dermatologist is typically needed to pursue this therapy.

LUMPS AND BUMPS

The presence of cutaneous or subcutaneous **nodules** and **tumors** can present a diagnostic challenge. They are also a source of great concern to parents, who fear the possibility of malignancy. Fortunately, most

cutaneous nodules and tumors in children are benign, and cutaneous malignancies are rare (Table 61.22). Nonetheless, certain genodermatoses are associated with cutaneous malignancies (Table 61.23).

Granuloma Annulare

Granuloma annulare is characterized by skin-colored to mildly erythematous dermal papules and nodules that may expand and coalesce into rings. These asymptomatic annular plaques measure 1–4 cm in diameter and appear most commonly on the dorsal hands and feet or extensor surfaces of the extremities (Fig. 61.42). The centers of these lesions usually appear normal but are occasionally hyperpigmented or violaceous in color. The overlying epidermis is unaffected. Multiple lesions are common, particularly in children. Histologically, there is dermal infiltration of lymphocytes and histiocytes surrounding degenerated collagen. The eruption is commonly confused with that of tinea corporis, but tinea has epidermal changes such as scaling, vesiculation, or pustules. Granuloma annulare may be seen in all age groups, but at least 40% of cases occur before 15 years of age. The etiology remains unknown though may result from a cell-mediated immune response. Some cases have been associated with preceding trauma, such as insect bites. In adults, granuloma annulare

TABLE 61.23 Cancer-Associated Genodermatoses

Disease	Associated Cancer	Clinical Manifestations	Genetics
Basal cell nevus syndrome (Gorlin syndrome)	Many basal cell carcinomas (mean age of onset 15 yr) on sun-exposed and non–sun-exposed areas; medulloblastoma; astrocytoma	Many basal cell nevi, palmar and plantar pits, jaw cysts, calcification of the falx cerebri, ovarian fibromas, fused ribs	Autosomal dominant; *PTCH1* gene on chromosome 9q22.32
Hidrotic ectodermal dysplasia (Clouston syndrome)	Squamous cell carcinoma of palms, soles, nail bed	Normal sweating, total alopecia, severe nail dystrophy, palmar and plantar hyperkeratosis	Autosomal dominant *GJB6* gene
Acrokeratosis paraneoplastica (Bazex syndrome)	Basal cell carcinomas of the face (second to third decade)	Follicular atrophoderma, localized anhidrosis and/or generalized hypohidrosis	Autosomal dominant Xq24–q27
Dysplastic nevus syndrome (familial, atypical, multiple-mole syndrome)	Cutaneous and intraocular melanoma, lymphoreticular malignancy, sarcomas	Multiple, large reddish-brown moles with irregular borders and nonuniform colors, usually on trunk and arms; familial occurrence of melanoma	Autosomal dominant genetic heterogeneity
Multiple hamartoma syndrome (Cowden disease)	Carcinoma of the breast, colon, thyroid	Coexistence of multiple ectodermal, mesodermal, and endodermal nevoid neoplasms; punctate keratoderma of the palms; multiple angiomas, lipomas	Autosomal dominant; *PTEN* gene on chromosome 10q23.31
Neurofibromatosis type 1 (von Recklinghausen disease)	Optic pathway gliomas; Malignant peripheral nerve sheath tumors; Fibrosarcomas; Squamous cell carcinomas; Nonlymphocytic leukemia; Pheochromocytoma; Carcinoid meningiomas	Café-au-lait spots; Skeletal anomalies; Neurofibromas; Lisch nodules; Axillary freckling; Xanthogranulomas	Autosomal dominant *NF1* gene; Sporadic variants in 50% of cases
Neurofibromatosis type 2	Acoustic neuromas; Schwannomas; Meningiomas; Astrocytomas	Neurofibromas; ± café-au-lait macules; Cataracts	Autosomal dominant *NF2* gene; *SCH* gene on 22q11–13.1; Sporadic variants in 50% of cases
Multiple mucosal neuroma syndrome (multiple endocrine neoplasia type IIB)	Pheochromocytoma, medullary thyroid carcinoma	Pedunculated nodules on eyelid margins, lips, and tongue with true neuromas	Autosomal dominant; gene locus 10q11.2; sporadic variant in 50% *RET* gene
Intestinal polyposis II (Peutz-Jeghers syndrome)	Adenocarcinoma of the colon, duodenum; granulosa cell ovarian tumors	Pigmented macules on oral mucosa, lips, conjunctivae, digits; intestinal polyps	Autosomal dominant; *STK11/LKB1* gene on chromosome 19p13.3; sporadic variant in 40%
Intestinal polyposis III (Gardner syndrome)	Malignant degeneration of colon, adenomatous polyps; sarcomas, thyroid carcinoma	Polyps of the colon, small intestine; globoid osteoma of mandible with overlying fibromas; epidermoid cysts; desmoids	5q21–q22 *APC* gene
Tuberous sclerosis	Rhabdomyoma of myocardium, gliomas, mixed tumor of kidney	Triad of angiofibromas, epilepsy, intellectual disability; ash leaf macules; shagreen patches; subungual fibromas; intracranial calcification in 50%	Spontaneous in 75%; autosomal dominant in 25%; heterogeneous loci, 9q34 (*TSC1*), 16p13 (*TSC2*)
Epidermolysis bullosa dystrophica dominant	Squamous cell carcinoma in chronic lesions	Lifelong history of bullae; phenotype not as severe as in recessive forms	Autosomal recessive, chromosome 3p21 (collagen type VII gene)
Epidermolysis bullosa dystrophica recessive	Basal, squamous cell carcinoma in skin, mucous membranes (especially esophagus)	Bullae develop at sites of trauma; present at birth or early infancy; may involve mucous membranes, esophagus, conjunctivae, cornea	Autosomal recessive, chromosome 3p (collagen type VII gene)
Albinism	Increased incidence of cutaneous malignancies	Lack skin pigment, incomplete hypopigmentation of ocular fundi, horizontal congenital nystagmus, myopia	Tyrosinase positive: autosomal recessive, gene locus 15q11.2–q12; Tyrosinase negative: autosomal recessive, gene locus 11q14q21

TABLE 61.23   Cancer-Associated Genodermatoses—cont'd

Disease	Associated Cancer	Clinical Manifestations	Genetics
Poikiloderma congenitale (Rothmund-Thomson syndrome)	Cutaneous malignancies Osteosarcoma	Poikiloderma, short stature, cataracts, photosensitivity, nail defects, alopecia, bony defects	Autosomal recessive; gene locus 8q24.3 *RECQL4* gene
Xeroderma pigmentosum	Basal and squamous cell carcinoma of skin, malignant melanoma	Marked photosensitivity, early freckling, telangiectasia, keratoses, papillomas, photophobia, keratitis, corneal opacities	Autosomal recessive; gene loci – complementation group A – 9q22.33 *XPA* gene group B – 2q14.3 *ERCC3* gene group D – 19q13.32 *ERCC2* gene group F – 13p13.12 *ERCC4* gene
Dyskeratosis congenita	Squamous cell carcinoma of oral cavity, esophagus, nasopharynx, skin, anus	Reticulated hypo- and hyperpigmentation of skin, nail dystrophy, leukoplakia of oral mucosa, thrombocytopenia, testicular atrophy	X-linked recessive (most common); gene locus Xq28 *DKC1* gene

Modified from Cohen BA. Nodules and tumors. In: Cohen BA, ed. *Pediatric Dermatology.* 4th ed. Philadelphia: Elsevier; 2013:127–128, Table 5.2.

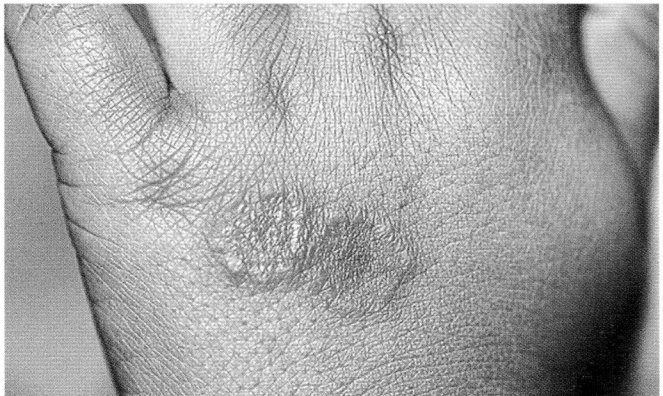

Fig. 61.42 Rings of confluent dermal papules with a depressed center typical of granuloma annulare. (From Cutaneous tumors and tumor syndromes. In: Paller AS, Mancini AJ, eds. *Hurwitz Clinical Pediatric Dermatology.* 5th ed. Philadelphia: Elsevier; 2016, Fig. 9.58.)

is associated with systemic diseases such as diabetes; in children, this association is less robust.

There are several variants of granuloma annulare. Generalized granuloma annulare is characterized by many symmetrically distributed asymptomatic papules. The ringlike lesions may coalesce into reticulated or circinate forms. Subcutaneous granuloma annulare consists of single or multiple deep hard nodules on the extremities, buttocks, and scalp. The lesions of subcutaneous granuloma annulare are most frequently mistaken for rheumatoid nodules; however, the latter are usually larger.

Granuloma annulare resolves spontaneously over several months to years, often with a waxing and waning course. Although more than 50% of cases clear within 2 years, recurrences are common. Treatment is generally unnecessary, but the use of topical or intralesional corticosteroids may hasten resolution.

Juvenile Xanthogranuloma

Juvenile xanthogranulomas (JXGs) are papules, nodules, or plaques within the skin that are distinguished by their characteristic yellow color, though some lesions may be orange, brown, or red. Lesions are solitary or multiple, well demarcated, and rubbery to firm. On examination, an overlying telangiectasia may be visualized. Lesions vary in size, usually from 0.5 to 2 cm, and are commonly located on the head and neck region. The differential diagnosis should include Spitz nevus, solitary mastocytoma, and occasionally nevus sebaceous. Biopsy demonstrates the characteristic histopathologic features of lipid-laden histiocytes and Touton giant cells. Most JXGs are asymptomatic, but occasionally they cause pruritus or pain. The lesions may be noted at birth or present within the first years of life. JXGs are usually benign, and treatment of cutaneous lesions is generally not required. After a brief period of growth, the lesion often stabilizes and involutes spontaneously in months to years.

Multiple lesions should prompt a search for the rare possibility of extracutaneous involvement. The eye is the most common extracutaneous site. Lesions may be found in the iris, and JXG is the most common cause of anterior chamber hemorrhage in children. The incidence of ocular disease in JXGs is approximately 0.4%. Ophthalmologic examination is recommended if a JXG is present near the eye or if there are multiple lesions. Involvement has also been described in other organs including the testes, lungs, liver, spleen, heart, and central nervous system. An increased risk of juvenile myelomonocytic leukemia has been reported in the setting of patients with both neurofibromatosis type 1 and JXGs.

Erythema Nodosum

Erythema nodosum (EN) is an inflammatory, presumed hypersensitivity panniculitis characterized by painful, erythematous subcutaneous nodules classically affecting both shins and less often extensor surfaces of the forearms, thighs, and rarely trunk (Fig. 61.43). Associated features may include a prodrome of malaise, fever, arthralgias, or less often arthritis. The possible predisposing diseases are noted in Table 61.24, although in ~40% no identifiable etiology is detected.

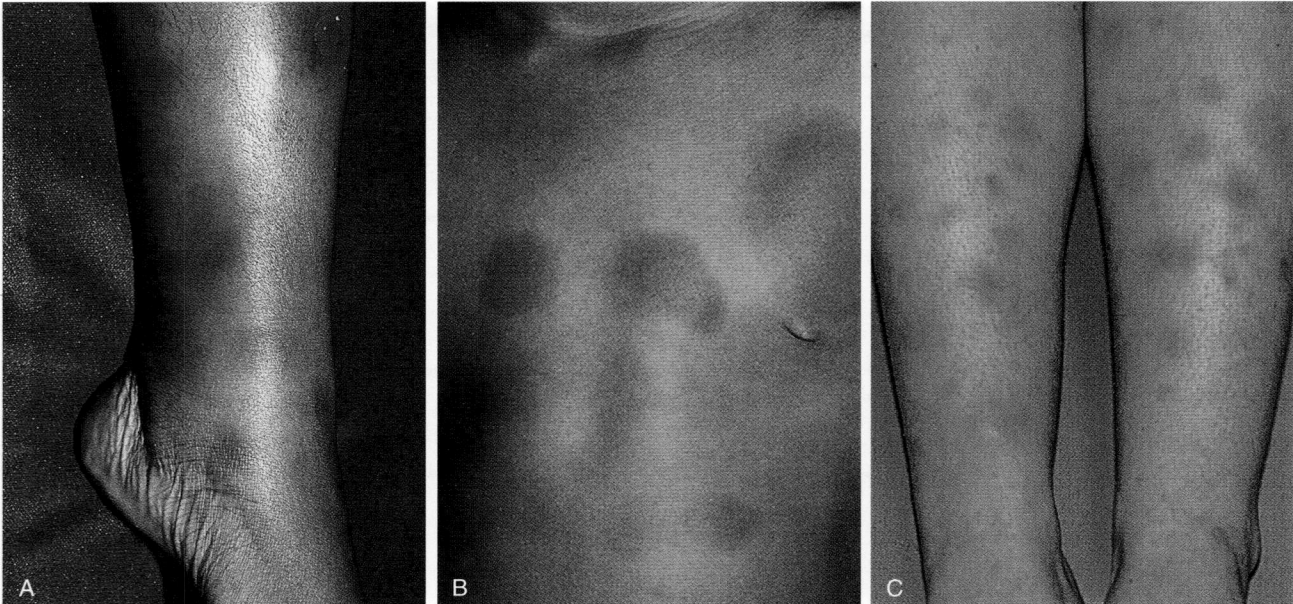

Fig. 61.43 Erythema nodosum. *A,* Tender, deep-seated nodules appeared on the shins of a 16-year-old girl 2 weeks after starting birth control pills. The lesions resolved when the medication was discontinued. *B,* An 18-month-old boy developed (biopsy-proved) erythema nodosum on the chest and abdomen following a cold. The nodules resolved without therapy over several weeks. *C,* This 15-year-old girl developed recurrent biopsy-proven erythema nodosum on her shins with flares of her systemic lupus erythematosus. (From Cohen BA. Reactive erythema. In: Cohen BA, ed. *Pediatric Dermatology.* 4th ed. Philadelphia: Elsevier; 2013:192, Fig. 7.37.)

TABLE 61.24   Erythema Nodosum: Most Common Causes

Bacterial Infections	**Drugs**
Streptococcus	Oral contraceptives
Cat-scratch disease	Sulfonamides
Campylobacter	Sulfonylureas
Lymphogranuloma venereum	Bromides and iodides
Mycobacterium leprae (histologically distinct)	Gold
Mycobacterium tuberculosis	TNF-α inhibitors
Mycoplasma pneumoniae	
Salmonella	**Systemic Illnesses**
Campylobacter	Inflammatory bowel disease
Brucellosis	Acute myelogenous leukemia
Tularemia	Behçet disease
Yersinia enterocolitica	Hodgkin disease
Psittacosis	Löfgren syndrome
	Non-Hodgkin lymphoma
Fungal Infections	Sarcoidosis
Blastomycosis	Internal carcinomas
Coccidioidomycosis	
Histoplasmosis	**Other**
	Pregnancy
Viral Infections	Sweet syndrome
Epstein-Barr virus	Whipple disease
Hepatitis B	Behçet disease

TNF, tumor necrosis factor.
From Dinulos GHJ. *Habif's Clinical Dermatology.* 7th ed. Philadelphia: Elsevier; 2021:727, Box 18.6; and Sunderkotter CH, Zelger B, Chen KR, et al. Nomenclature of cutaneous vasculitis: dermatologic addendum to the 2012 Revised International Chapel Hill Consensus Conference Nomenclature of Vasculitides. *Arthritis Rheumatol.* 2018;70(2):171–184.

SUMMARY AND RED FLAGS

While the time course of dermatosis often is variable, one should be vigilant to re-evaluate skin lesions not following the typical course to identify skin findings that represent manifestations of underlying chronic disorders or life-threatening disease processes. An ill-appearing child with acute skin findings and systemic symptoms should narrow the focus to specific subsets of disease processes. A careful history and physical examination can help differentiate between disease processes of hypersensitivity such as SJS and TEN, DRESS, and infections (SSSS, HSV, meningococcemia) to determine appropriate acute evaluation and management of these life-threatening entities.

BIBLIOGRAPHY

A bibliography is available at ExpertConsult.com.

INDEX

Page numbers followed by "f" indicate figures and "t" indicate tables.